Normal Blood Pressure Ranges of Infants and Children

Age	Systolic (mm Hg)	
Newborn–12 hr (less than 1000 gm)	39–59	16–36
Newborn–12 hr (3000 gm)	50–70	24–45
Newborn–96 hr (3000 gm)	60–90	20–60
Infant	74–100	50–70
Toddler	80–112	50–80
Preschooler	82–110	50–78
School-Age	84–120	54–80
Adolescent	94–140	62–88

Head Circumference Norms for Girls (in cm)

	Percentiles					
Age	3	25	50	75	90	97
Birth	32.5	33.9	34.7	35.4	36	36.6
3 months	37.9	39.2	40	40.8	41.7	42.3
6 months	40.9	42	42.8	43	44.5	45.4
9 months	42.6	43.8	44.6	45.4	46.3	47.2
12 months	43.6	45	45.8	46.7	47.7	48.4
15 months	44.3	45.6	46.5	47.4	48.4	49.1
18 months	44.9	46.2	47.1	48	49	49.8
2 years	45.8	47.2	48.1	49.1	50.1	50.9
3 years	46.8	48.4	49.3	50.3	51.1	52

Head Circumference Norms for Boys (in cm)

	Percentiles					
Age	3	25	50	75	90	97
Birth	33	34.4	35.3	36.2	37	37.5
3 months	38.7	40	40.9	41.5	42.1	43.2
6 months	42.1	43.3	43.9	44.8	45.4	45.9
9 months	43.8	45.1	46	46.5	47.1	47.8
12 months	44.9	46.5	47.3	47.8	48.4	48.9
15 months	45.6	47.1	48	48.5	49.2	49.8
18 months	46.2	47.7	48.7	49.2	49.9	50.6
2 years	47	48.2	49.7	50.2	51	51.7
3 years	47.9	49.6	50.4	51.3	51.9	52.7

Child Health Nursing

*A Comprehensive Approach
to the Care of Children
and Their Families*

Child Health Nursing

A Comprehensive Approach to the Care of Children and Their Families

Debra Broadwell Jackson, PhD, RN

Head and Associate Professor
Department of Health Science
College of Nursing
Clemson University
Clemson, South Carolina

Rebecca B. Saunders, PhD, RNC

Associate Professor
School of Nursing
The University of North Carolina at Greensboro
Greensboro, North Carolina

71 Contributors

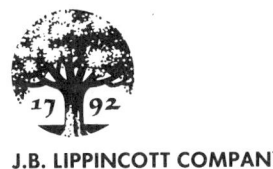

J.B. LIPPINCOTT COMPANY

Philadelphia

Sponsoring Editor: Barbara Nelson Cullen
Senior Developmental Editor: Eleanor Faven
Coordinating Editorial Assistant:
    Jennifer E. Brogan
Project Editor: Dina Kamilatos
Indexer: Ellen Murray
Design Coordinator: Doug Smock
Interior Designer: Susan Blaker

Cover Designer: Susan Blaker
Production Manager: Caren Erlichman
Production Coordinator: Kevin P. Johnson
Compositor: Tapsco, Incorporated
Printer/Binder: R. R. Donnelley & Sons
    Company
Cover Printer: The Lehigh Press, Inc.

We gratefully acknowledge the following sources in providing the assigned photographs:

Kathy Sloan, photographer, courtesy of Children's Hospital, Oakland, California: Units 4, 5, 7, 8, 9, 12, 15

Kathy Sloan, photographer: Units 1, 6, 10, 13, 14, 16, 18; Reviewers photo, Contents photo, Expanded Contents photo, Appendices photo, and Cover photo (extreme right).

Special thanks to Steve Tiger and the nurses at Children's Hospital, Oakland, California, for their time and cooperation in providing a number of photographs in this book.

Peggy Levine, photographer, for the use of photos in Figures 25-2A, C; 25-3A; 25-4A, B; 25-5; 25-6; 25-8; 25-15 A, B; 25-16 A, B, C, D; and 62-14.

6 5 4 3 2 1

Library of Congress Cataloging in Publications Data

Child health nursing: a comprehensive approach to the care of children and their families / [edited by] Debra Broadwell Jackson, Rebecca B. Saunders.
      p.   cm.
    Includes bibliographical references and index.
    ISBN 0-397-54725-0
    1. Pediatric nursing. 2. Teenagers—Diseases—Nursing. 3. Family nursing. I. Jackson, Debra Broadwell, 1949– . II. Saunders, Rebecca B.
    [DNLM: 1. Pediatric Nursing. 2. Professional-Family Relations.
WY 159 C53635]
RJ245.C475 1993
610.73'62—dc20
DNLM/DLC
for Library of Congress   92-49526
                                                              CIP

Any procedure or practice described in this book should be applied by the healthcare practitioner under appropriate supervision in accordance with professional standards of care used with regard to the unique circumstances that apply in each practice situation. Care has been taken to confirm the accuracy of information presented and to describe generally accepted practices. However, the authors, editors, and publisher cannot accept any responsibility for errors or omissions or for any consequences from application of the information in this book and make no warranty express or implied, with respect to the contents of the book.

Every effort has been made to ensure drug selections and dosages are in accordance with current recommendations and practice. Because of ongoing research, changes in government regulations and the constant flow of information on drug therapy, reactions and interactions, the reader is cautioned to check the package insert for each drug for indications, dosages, warnings and precautions, particularly if the drug is new or infrequently used.

To my family: Vince, my husband, for his love and his caring and his support in writing this book; and Katie and Stacey, my daughters, who are so lovingly presented in this book. When this project started I never knew how positively my life would change. Thank you.

D.B.J.

To my husband Dean, for his constancy and sustaining love, and to Reuben, who has been our joy to parent.

R.B.S.

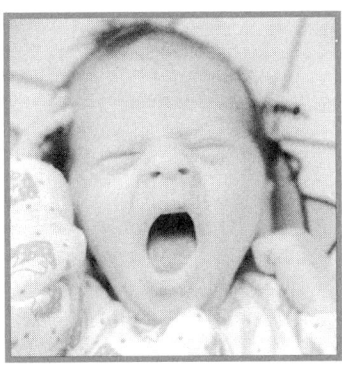

Contributors

Stephanie S. Allen, MS, RN, Lecturer, Baylor University, School of Nursing, Dallas, Texas
Chapter 58: Nursing Assessment and Diagnosis of Gastrointestinal Function

Suzan Banoub-Baddour, DNSc, RN, Associate Professor, Memorial University of Newfoundland, School of Nursing, St. John's, Newfoundland, Canada
Chapter 18: Behavioral and Emotional Responses to Life Stress

Ruth C. Bindler, MS, RNC, Associate Professor, Intercollegiate Center for Nursing Education, Washington State University, Spokane, Washington
Chapter 9: Health Supervision of Children

Marilyn Birchfield, MA, RN, Assistant Professor, Community Health, Loyola University, Marcella Niehoff School of Nursing, Chicago, Illinois
Chapter 11: Health Assessment, Promotion, and Maintenance for the Neonate

Marilyn L. Boos, MS, RN, Clinical Nurse Specialist, Alfred I. DuPont Institute, Wilmington, Delaware
Chapter 62: Nursing Planning, Intervention, and Evaluation for Altered Musculoskeletal Function

Janice Gilyard Brewington, PhD, MSN, RN, Assistant Dean/Associate Professor, North Carolina Agricultural and Technical State University, School of Nursing, Greensboro, North Carolina
Chapter 4: Cultural and Economic Influences on the Family

June S. L. Chan, MSN, RN, Director, Professional Practice and Research, Children's Hospital of The King's Daughters, Norfolk, VA
Chapter 35: Nursing Planning, Intervention, and Evaluation for Altered Head and Neck Function
Chapter 38: Nursing Planning, Intervention, and Evaluation for Altered Respiratory Function

Kathryn Martens Clark, BSN, RN, Clinical Care Coordinator—Pediatrics–Endocrine, University of Michigan, Ann Arbor, Michigan
Chapter 56: Nursing Planning, Intervention, and Evaluation for Altered Endocrine Function

Lucia G. Copeland, MS, RN, Assistant Professor, University of Vermont, School of Nursing, Burlington, Vermont
Chapter 20: The Child With Special Needs

Kay Jackson Cowen, MSN, RN, C, Lecturer, School Nursing, The University of North Carolina at Greensboro, Greensboro, North Carolina
Chapter 23: Hospital Care for Children

Brenda L. Cox, BSN, RN, Clinical Instructor, Dialysis Units, Children's Hospital of Los Angeles, Los Angeles, California
Chapter 47: Nursing Planning, Intervention, and Evaluation for Altered Renal Function

Janet Craig, MS, RN, PNP, CCRN, Pediatric Nurse Educator, University of California, San Francisco, San Francisco, California
Chapter 38: Nursing Planning, Intervention, and Evaluation for Altered Respiratory Function

Joann M. Eland, PhD, RN, NAP, FAAN, Associate Professor of Nursing, The University of Iowa, College of Nursing, Iowa City, Iowa
Chapter 28: Children With Pain

Jane C. Evans, PhD, RN, Director, Center for Nursing Research, Associate Professor, School of Nursing, Medical College of Ohio; Director of Nursing Research, St. Vincent's Medical Center, Toledo, Ohio
Chapter 52: Nursing Assessment and Diagnosis of Neurologic Function
Chapter 53: Nursing Planning, Intervention, and Evaluation for Altered Neurologic Function

Marilyn Lang Evans, PhD, RN, Visiting Associate Professor, School of Nursing, The University of North Carolina at Greensboro, Greensboro, North Carolina
Chapter 7: Health Promotion and Maintenance

Susan A. Fay, MSN, RN, CPNP, Clinical Nurse Specialist, Developmental Pediatrics, James Whitcomb Riley Hospital for Children, Indianapolis, Indiana
Chapter 24: Home Care for Ill Children

Lori St. Dennis Feezle, BSN, RN, CPN, Department of Pediatric Endocrinology, James Whitcomb Riley Hospital for Children, Indianapolis, Indiana
Chapter 56: Nursing Planning, Intervention, and Evaluation for Altered Endocrine Function

Deborah L. Gray, MSN, RN, CPNP, CDE, Clinical Nurse Specialist, Section of Pediatric Diabetes, Adjunct Clinical Instructor, Indiana University School of Nursing; Indiana University Diabetes Research and Training Center, Indianapolis, Indiana
Chapter 56: Nursing Planning, Intervention, and Evaluation for Altered Endocrine Function

Mikel Gray, PhD, NP, CURN, Clinical Urodynamics, Egelston Children's Hospital at Emory, Scottish Rite Children's Medical Center, Shepherd Spinal Center; Clinical Professor, Georgia State University, School of Nursing, Atlanta, Georgia
Chapter 48: Anatomy and Physiology of the Urinary System
Chapter 49: Nursing Assessment and Diagnosis of Urinary Function
Chapter 50: Nursing Planning, Intervention, and Evaluation for Altered Urinary Function

Tina S. Gustin, MSN, RN, Renal Clinical Nurse Specialist, Children's Hospital of The King's Daughters, Norfolk, Virginia
Chapter 46: Nursing Assessment and Diagnosis of Renal Function

Keela A. Herr, PhD, RN, CS, Assistant Professor, The University of Iowa, Iowa City, Iowa
Chapter 28: Children With Pain

Marilyn Hockenberry-Eaton, PhD, RNC, PNP, Associate Professor, Emory School of Nursing, Atlanta, Georgia
Chapter 31: Children With Cancer

Robbie B. Hughes, EdD, RN, Professor, Department of Nursing Science, Clemson University, College of Nursing, Clemson, South Carolina
Chapter 27: Immune Responses

Mary Louise Icenhour, PhD, RN, Assistant Professor, Duke University School of Nursing, Durham, North Carolina
Chapter 5: The High-Risk Family

Debra Broadwell Jackson, PhD, RN, Head and Associate Professor, Department of Health Science, College of Nursing, Clemson University, Clemson, South Carolina
Chapter 6: Child and Family Teaching
Chapter 8: Growth and Development of Children
Chapter 18: Behavioral and Emotional Responses to Life Stress

Kathy Warbritton Janvier, MS, RN, Instructor, Maternal–Child Nursing, Delaware Technical and Community College, Newark, Delaware
Chapter 62: Nursing Planning, Intervention, and Evaluation for Altered Musculoskeletal Function

Cathy Jordan, MN, RN, CPNP, Instructor, Emory School of Nursing, Atlanta, Georgia
Chapter 33: Anatomy and Physiology of the Head and Neck

Jane Hiura Katsura, MS, RN, Clinical Nurse Specialist, Nurse Educator, Children's Hospital, Oakland, Oakland, California
Chapter 39: Anatomy and Physiology of the Cardiovascular System
Chapter 40: Nursing Assessment and Diagnosis of Cardiovascular Function

Virginia McMahon Keatley, PhD, BNC, Lecturer, Widener University, Chester, Pennsylvania; formerly Assistant Professor, Maternal–Child Health Nursing, Loyola University, Marcella Niehoff School of Nursing, Chicago, Illinois
Chapter 10: Health Assessment, Promotion, and Maintenance for the Prenatal Period

Beverly Kopala, PhD, RN, Associate Professor, Loyola University, Marcella Niehoff School of Nursing, Chicago, Illinois
Chapter 51: Anatomy and Physiology of the Nervous System

Kathy S. Lawrence, MN, RN, CS, Pediatric Clinical Nurse Specialist, Children's Hospital of Pittsburgh; Adjunct Assistant Professor, University of Pittsburgh, School of Nursing, Pittsburgh, Pennsylvania
Chapter 41: Nursing Planning, Intervention, and Evaluation for Altered Cardiovascular Function

Jean Libonate, MSN, RN, Associate Director of Nursing, USHAWL, Inc; Cedars–Sinai Artificial Kidney Center, Los Angeles, California
Chapter 45: Anatomy and Physiology of the Renal System

Esma Liss, BSN, RN, CCRN, Clinical Nurse II, Children's Hospital of Pittsburgh, Pittsburgh, Pennsylvania
Chapter 41: Nursing Planning, Intervention, and Evaluation for Altered Cardiovascular Function

Peggy Malague MacKay, MN, RN, Clinical Nurse Specialist in General Pediatrics, Egleston Children's Hospital at Emory University, Atlanta, Georgia
Chapter 34: Nursing Assessment and Diagnosis of Head and Neck Function

Michael J. Mahlmeister, MS, RRT, Education Director, Respiratory Care Services, Assistant Clinical Professor, School of Nursing, Medical Center at the University of California, San Francisco, San Francisco, California
Chapter 38: Nursing Planning, Intervention, and Evaluation for Altered Respiratory Function

Marcia C. Maurer, MS, RN, Assistant Professor Maternal–Child Health Nursing, Coordinator, Graduate Perinatal Program, Loyola University, Marcella Niehoff School of Nursing, Chicago, Illinois
Chapter 36: Anatomy and Physiology of the Respiratory System
Chapter 37: Nursing Assessment and Diagnosis of Respiratory Function

Mary J. McDonald, MS, RN, CEN, Clinical Nurse Specialist, Emergency Center, Children's Medical Center, Dallas, Texas
Chapter 59: Nursing Planning, Intervention, and Evaluation for Altered Gastrointestinal Function

Gail R. McIlvain-Simpson, MSN, RN, C, Clinical Nurse Specialist, Pediatric Rheumatology, Alfred I. duPont Institute, Wilmington, Delaware
Chapter 62: Nursing Planning, Intervention, and Evaluation for Altered Musculoskeletal Function

Janyce H. McLin, BSN, RN, CCTC, Renal Transplant Program Manager, Sentara Norfolk General Hospital, Norfolk, Virginia
Chapter 46: Nursing Assessment and Diagnosis of Renal Function

Kitty Miller, MSN, RN, Manager, Ambulatory Care Services, Children's Hospital of Los Angeles, Los Angeles, California
Chapter 66: Anatomy and Physiology of the Reproductive System
Chapter 67: Nursing Assessment and Diagnosis of Reproductive Function
Chapter 68: Nursing Planning, Intervention, and Evaluation for Altered Reproductive Function

Kathy Stimac O'Brien, MSN, RN, Pediatric Clinical Nurse Specialist, Memorial Miller Children's Hospital, Long Beach, California
Chapter 47: Nursing Planning, Intervention, and Evaluation for Altered Renal Function

Susan Hall Parker, RN, Pediatric Endocrinology and Diabetes Specialist, Charlotte, North Carolina
Chapter 55: Nursing Assessment and Diagnosis of Endocrine Function
Chapter 56: Nursing Planning, Intervention, and Evaluation for Altered Endocrine Function

Lynn C. Parsons, MS, RN, PNP, Nurse Clinician Pediatric Hematology/Oncology, University of Kansas Medical Center, Kansas City, Kansas
Chapter 43: Nursing Assessment and Diagnosis of Hematologic Function

Katherine L. Patterson, MN, RN, Pediatric Hematology/Oncology, Clinical Nurse Specialist, University of Missouri Hospitals and Clinics, Division of Patient Services, Columbia, Missouri
Chapter 43: Nursing Assessment and Diagnosis of Hematologic Function

Kaaren Peterschmidt, RN, MS, Senior Staff Nurse, Pediatric ICU, Lucille Packard Children's Hospital, Palo Alto, California; Pediatric Critical Care Nurse Consultant, Cupertino, California; formerly Nursing Educational Coordinator, Stanford University Medical Center, Pediatric ICU, Palo Alto, California
Chapter 26: Homeostatic Mechanisms and Responses

Janet Pitcher, MSN, RN, Clinical Nursing Specialist, Pediatric Gastroenterology/Nutrition, University of California, Davis Medical Center, Sacramento, California
Chapter 57: Anatomy and Physiology of the Gastrointestinal System

Marcene L. Powell, MN, RN, DSW, Professor of Nursing, Nell Hodgson Woodruff School of Nursing, Emory University, Atlanta, Georgia
Chapter 3: Family-Centered Child Health Care
Chapter 21: Impact of Chronic Illness on Children

Bridget Recker, EdM, RN, Clinical Coordinator, Pediatrics, Maimonides Medical Center, Brooklyn, New York
Chapter 54: Anatomy and Physiology of the Endocrine System

Karen S. Reed, PhD, RN, Associate Professor, University of Akron, Akron, Ohio
Chapter 5: The High-Risk Family
Chapter 19: Mental Health Issues in Childhood and Adolescence

Ellen A. Reynolds, MS, RN, CEN, Clinical Research Nurse Specialist, Ambulatory Care; formerly Trauma Clinical Nurse Specialist, Children's Hospital of Pittsburgh, Pittsburgh, Pennsylvania
Chapter 30: Multiple Traumas in Children

Sherrill Jantzi Rudy, BSN, RN, MSN Student, Parent–Child Health/Nurse Practitioner, University of Pittsburgh, School of Nursing; Chairperson Education Committee, Dermatology Nurses' Association, Pittsburgh, Pennsylvania
Chapter 63: Anatomy and Physiology of the Integumentary System
Chapter 64: Nursing Assessment and Diagnosis of Integumentary Function
Chapter 65: Nursing Planning, Intervention, and Evaluation for Altered Integumentary Function

Deborah DiSchino Ryan, MSN, RN, Assistant Professor of Nursing, Nell Hodgson Woodruff School of Nursing, Emory University, Atlanta, Georgia
Chapter 12: Health Assessment, Promotion, and Maintenance for Infants
Chapter 13: Health Assessment, Promotion, and Maintenance for Toddlers
Chapter 14: Health Assessment, Promotion, and Maintenance for Preschool Children
Chapter 15: Health Assessment, Promotion, and Maintenance for School Age Children
Chapter 16: Health Assessment, Promotion, and Maintenance for Adolescents

Christine Chiarmonte Sanford, MSN, RN, CPN, Faculty, Watts School of Nursing, Durham, North Carolina
Chapter 60: Anatomy and Physiology of the Musculoskeletal System
Chapter 61: Nursing Assessment and Diagnosis of Musculoskeletal Function
Chapter 62: Nursing Planning, Intervention, and Evaluation for Altered Musculoskeletal Function

Rebecca B. Saunders, PhD, RNC, Associate Professor, School of Nursing, The University of North Carolina at Greensboro, Greensboro, North Carolina
Chapter 1: Perspectives on Child Health Nursing
Chapter 2: The Nursing Process
Chapter 8: Growth and Development of Children

Judith Scully, MSN, RN, Instructor, Loyola University, Marcella Niehoff School of Nursing, Chicago, Illinois
Chapter 11: Health Assessment, Promotion, and Maintenance for the Neonate

Margaret C. Slota, MN, RN, Children's Hospital of Pittsburgh, Pittsburgh, Pennsylvania
Chapter 41: Nursing Planning, Intervention, and Evaluation for Altered Cardiovascular Function

Jeff Smith, MS, BSN, RN, College of Nursing and Allied Health, University of Cincinnati, Cincinnati, Ohio
Chapter 53: Nursing Planning, Intervention, and Evaluation for Altered Neurologic Function

Terry Tallman, MSN, RN, Clinical Nurse Specialist, Pediatric Cardiothoracic Surgery, Children's Hospital of Pittsburgh, Pittsburgh, PA
Chapter 41: Nursing Planning, Intervention, and Evaluation for Altered Cardiovascular Function

Donna Ojanen Thomas, MSN, RN, CEN, Director, Emergency Department, Primary Children's Medical Center, Salt Lake City, Utah
Chapter 29: Childhood Emergencies

Mary Ann A. van Dam, MS, RN, PNP, Faculty, Pediatric Nursing Department, San Francisco State University; Clinical Pediatric Nurse, University of California, San Francisco, San Francisco, California
Chapter 38: Nursing Planning, Intervention, and Evaluation for Altered Respiratory Function

Barbara Velsor-Friedrich, PhD, RN, Associate Professor, Maternal–Child Health, Loyola University, Marcella Niehoff School of Nursing, Chicago, Illinois
Chapter 17: Coping With Change

Carolyn Vieweg, MSN, RN, CRNP, Cardiac Clinical Nurse Specialist, Cooper Hospital University Medical Center, Camden, New Jersey; Clinical Instructor, Pediatric Clinical Care, University of Pennsylvania, Philadelphia, Pennsylvania
Chapter 41: Nursing Planning, Intervention, and Evaluation for Altered Cardiovascular Function

Gail Wade, MS, RN, Instructor, University of Delaware, Newark, Delaware
Chapter 62: Nursing Planning, Intervention, and Evaluation for Altered Musculoskeletal Function

Carolyn L. Walker, PhD, RN, Associate Professor, San Diego State University, School of Nursing, San Diego, California
Chapter 32: The Child Who is Dying

Karen Wall, BScN, Red River Community College, Nursing Department, Winnipeg, Manitoba, Canada
Chapter 8: Growth and Development of Children;
Chapter 25: Approaches to Nursing Procedures

Victoria A. Weill, MSN, RNC, CPNP, Pediatric Nurse Practitioner/Clinical Coordinator, Young Family Tract, Primary Care Program, University of Pennsylvania, School of Nursing, Philadelphia, Pennsylvania
Chapter 22: Ambulatory Care for Children

Anita L. Wingate, PhD, BSN, Associate Professor and Academic Coordinator, Division of Nursing Practice, School of Nursing, University of Kansas Medical Center, Kansas City, Kansas
Chapter 42: Anatomy and Physiology of the Hematologic System

Irene Tremaine Winnen, MSN, RN, Pediatric Cardiology Clinical Nurse Specialist, California Pacific Medical Center, San Francisco, California
Chapter 41: Nursing Planning, Intervention, and Evaluation for Altered Cardiovascular Function

Linda G. Wofford, MSN, PNP, Pediatric Nurse Practitioner, Houston, Texas
Chapter 44: Nursing Planning, Intervention, and Evaluation for Altered Hematologic Function

Cynthia J. Wright, MSN, RN, CRRN, Pediatric Rehabilitation Coordinator, Children's National Medical Center, Washington, DC
Chapter 30: Multiple Traumas in Children

Marybeth Young, PhD, RNC, Assistant Professor, Maternal–Child Health Nursing, Loyola University, Marcella Niehoff School of Nursing, Chicago, Illinois
Chapter 10: Health Assessment, Promotion, and Maintenance for the Prenatal Period

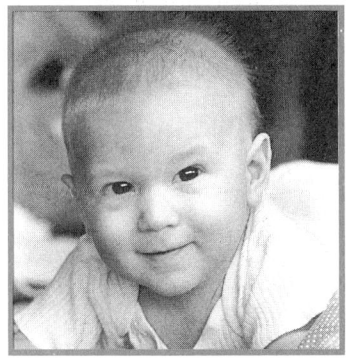

Reviewers

Rose M. Alvin, PhD, CRNP, Assistant Professor, Parent–Child Nursing Graduate Program, School of Nursing, University of Pittsburgh, Pittsburgh, Pennsylvania

Sara Arneson, PhD, RN, Senior Associate Dean and Associate Professor, University of Virginia, School of Nursing, Charlottesville, Virginia

Lois K. Baker, PhD, RN, CPNP, Associate Professor, Nursing, Cedarville College, Cedarville, Ohio

Bonnie L. Barndt-Maglio, RN, MS, formerly Assistant Vice President for Nursing, Critical Care, The Children's Medical Center, Dayton, Ohio

Rosemary A. Bellavance, MS, BSN, RN, Clinical Instructor, Maternal–Child Health, Holy Family Hospital, Methuen, Massachusetts; Clinical Instructor, Pediatrics, Northern Essex Community College, Haverhill, Massachusetts

Patricia Burgess, MS, RNC, Assistant Professor, Orvis School of Nursing, University of Nevada, Reno, Reno, Nevada

Catherine Burns, PhD, RN, PNP, Associate Professor, Oregon Health Sciences University, School of Nursing, Portland, Oregon

Darlene Nebel Cantu, MSN, RNC, Faculty, Baptist Memorial Hospital System, School of Professional Nursing, San Antonio, Texas

Beverly Corbo-Richert, PhD, RN, CCRN, Formerly Assistant Professor, Parent–Child Nursing Graduate Program, University of Pittsburgh, Pittsburgh, Pennsylvania

Nancy Fleming Courts, PhD, RN, NCC, Assistant Professor, School of Nursing, University of North Carolina at Greensboro, Greensboro, North Carolina

Susan B. Crowell, MSN, RN, PNP, Health Education Specialist, School Administration Districts, Maine Public Schools

Susan Fowler-Kerry, MN, BA, BSN, PhD Candidate, Associate Professor, College of Nursing, University of Saskatchewan, Saskatoon, Saskatchewan, Canada

Irene S. DiFlorio, MS, RN, Assistant Professor, Maternal/Child Nursing, Syracuse University, College of Nursing, Syracuse, New York

Beth Donaher-Wagner, MSN, RN, Staff Development Instructor, Pediatrics and Obstetrics, Pocono Medical Center, East Stroudsburg, Pennsylvania

Marilyn S. Hammond, MS, BS, RN, Former Instructor, Brigham Young University, Provo, Utah

Mary R. Hauck, PhD, RN, Clinical Nurse Specialist, Variety Club Children's Hospital, University of Minnesota; Adjunct Clinical Professor, School of Nursing, University of Minnesota, Minneapolis, Minnesota

Patricia Cima Isaacs, EdD, RN, PNP, CNS, Professor of Nursing, Director Graduate Pediatric Nurse Practitioner Program, Brigham Young University, College of Nursing, Provo, Utah

Carole Kenner, DNS, RNC, Professor and Interim Department Chair, Parent–Child Health Nursing, College of Nursing and Health, University of Cincinnati, Cincinnati, Ohio

Eileen Mieras Kohlenberg, PhD, RN, Assistant Professor and Chair, Adult Health Nursing Division, School of Nursing, The University of North Carolina at Greensboro, Greensboro, North Carolina

Sally Lewis, BScn, CDE, Unit Manager, Pediatric Metabolic–Diabetic Clinic, Hôtel Dieu of St. Joseph Hospital, Windsor, Ontario, Canada

Terri H. Lipman, PhD, RN, Lecturer, Nursing of Children Division, University of Pennsylvania, School of Nursing; Clinical Nurse Specialist, Diabetes/Endocrinology, Section of Endocrinology, St. Christopher's Hospital for Children, Philadelphia, Pennsylvania

Cindy K. Lybarger, MSN, RN, CCRN, Clinical Nurse Specialist, Pediatric Critical Care, Vanderbilt University Medical Center, Nashville, Tennessee

Ida M. Martinson, PhD, RN, FAAN, Professor, Department of Family Health Care, School of Nursing, University of California, San Francisco, San Francisco, California

Michelle A. Mendes, MS, RN, Adjunct Instructor, Boston College, Chestnut Hill, Massachusetts

Dianne M. Molsberry, MA, BSN, RNC, Clinical Nurse Specialist, Educational Services—Empire Health Consolidated Services, Spokane, Washington

Eileen O'Brien, PhD, RN, Assistant Professor, Maternal–Child Nursing, University of Maryland, Baltimore, Maryland

Maureen J. Osis, MN, RN, Clinical Nurse Specialist, Health Promotion and Education, Osis Consulting Services, Ltd., Calgary, Alberta, Canada

Judith M. Quinn, MS, Assistant Professor, University of Connecticut, School of Nursing, Storrs, Connecticut

Patricia A. Rieser, BSN, RN, Family Nurse Practitioner–Certified, Pediatric Endocrinology, University of North Carolina at Chapel Hill, Chapel Hill, North Carolina

Edythe M. Tuchfarber, EdD, RN, Assistant Professor, University of New Mexico, College of Nursing, Albuquerque, New Mexico

Carol Jo Wilson, PhD, RN, Associate Professor, Parent–Child Health Nursing, Northern Illinois University, School of Nursing, DeKalb, Illinois

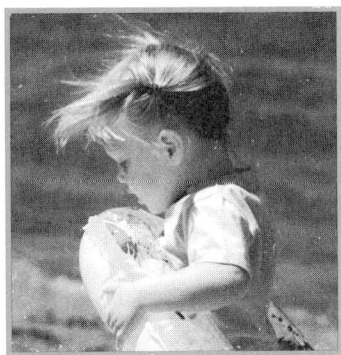

Preface

The population has increased, family structures have changed, and more variety is needed in cultural approaches to health concepts and care. At the same time, health care expenses have escalated, hospital stays are shorter, and more health care is provided in the home. We felt there was a need for a child care textbook with a strong nursing focus to reflect all these changes: a book to address the growing and changing role of nurses in providing care not only for well and sick children but also through anticipatory guidance for their families. With this desire in mind, *Child Health Nursing: A Comprehensive Approach to the Care of Children and Their Families* was developed. Our book is designed and written to prepare nurses in the 1990s to care for children and adolescents in an exciting and ever-changing world.

The text is based on a solid foundation of scientific principles, research findings, and clinical practice. Throughout the text, the family is consistently addressed as the central unit for providing nursing services to children and adolescents. The text's emphasis on health and wellness is underscored by a comprehensive unit covering growth and development from prenatal care through adolescence. The rapidly evolving societal and technological changes have created many new problems and stressors for children and their families, including depression, drug abuse, and suicide. In response, the text emphasizes emotional and psychosocial issues and stressors for children and adolescents. In addition, the many different types of families and the changing family structure are considered for planning appropriate programs and services for children and adolescents.

Features of the Text

We have used a wealth of pedagogical aids to enhance learning and assist the student nurse in preparing for a role in child health nursing. The following are features that appear in many of the chapters:

- **Objectives** provide broad learning goals for each chapter
- **Features of This Chapter** highlight important displays and tables found in the chapter
- **Nursing Care Plans** present specific case studies, NANDA-approved nursing diagnoses, rationales for each intervention, and expected outcomes for a variety of common problems and conditions

- **Child and Family Teaching Plans** give examples of specific situations where the nurse instructs the child and family in discharge planning and well child care
- **Nursing Assessments** aid students in their approaches to planning care for the child and family
- **Nursing Diagnosis** guides the student toward possible diagnoses for children with altered function
- **Nursing Interventions** discuss specific nursing actions for both independent and collaborative interventions
- **Diagnostic Procedures** are outlined in a special in-text display using a consistent format for commonly used procedures
- **Teaching Displays** supply students with important information to share with families
- **Ideas for Nursing Research** help students to begin thinking about the questions and concerns that need to be addressed in the nursing of children
- **Chapter Summaries** provide students with a concise review of the important concepts presented in the chapter
- **Color Plates** illustrate common rashes and lesions associated with infectious diseases and integumentary disorders
- **Photographs, drawings, tables, and displays** clarify text discussion

Organization of the Text

Unit 1 provides an overview of the concepts and theories associated with family-centered child health. Perspectives on child health nursing include historical and future trends that will influence nurses working with families. The presentation of the nursing process describes the method in which we have incorporated the process throughout the text. Gordon's functional health patterns are used for guiding the nursing assessment and diagnosis. Planning, interventions, and evaluation are integral components. The format for the nursing care plan developed in Chapter 2 is used throughout the text to present the nursing process with real-life case studies to help students learn how to develop and implement care plans in actual practice. The family, family-centered care, and cultural and economic influences affecting the family are presented. A special chapter discusses families at high risk for health problems. A foundation of learning and teaching theories and their application for teaching children and adolescents about wellness, health maintenance, and management of disease and treatment round out the unit. The process of developing a family-centered teaching plan is demonstrated in a sequential design. This format for the teaching plan is used in selected situations throughout the text.

Unit 2, which discusses Health Assessment, Promotion, and Maintenance, is a major feature of the text. The unit begins with an overview of well-child supervision, including health assessment strategies and immunization. An exploration of activities needed to promote and maintain health from birth through adolescence is followed by a comprehensive review of physical, psychosocial, moral, and sexual maturation. Health assessment, promotion, and maintenance of well children from prenatal through adolescence using functional health is an organizing framework. The chapters provide suggestions for anticipatory guidance for caregivers and families. The developmental approach helps students understand the importance of the child's age in planning for care. A section on health perception and health maintenance addresses common health concerns with each age. The organization of presenting well children before discussing diseases and disorders helps students understand how normal growth and development may be affected by illness.

Unit 3 presents the emotional and psychosocial considerations of the child and family. The chapters include topics such as the coping process and children's responses to change, behavioral and emotional responses to stress, mental health, special needs, and chronic illness. Emotional and psychosocial issues may relate to healthy children experiencing personal crises or may be associated with particular diseases or treatment, or both. Developmental considerations and parental and sibling coping are discussed.

The advances in health care technology and the ever-increasing cost of medical care has altered the health care delivery system significantly. Unit 4 addresses various delivery systems for children and families, including ambulatory centers, hospital care, and home care. Nursing procedures commonly used with infants, children, and adolescents are reviewed.

Specific responses to physiologic and pathophysiologic changes are common to a variety of diseases and disorders in children and adolescents. Unit 5 examines three processes: homeostatic mechanisms and responses, immune responses, and pain. An overview of pain theories leads to the steps a nurse can take in making a thorough assessment of a child's pain and response to pain medication. Nonpharmacologic management is also outlined.

Childhood emergencies, traumatic injuries, cancer, and dying are topics presented in Unit 6. Throughout these sections the nursing process is presented, incorporating both independent and collaborative interventions. Nurses work with a variety of health professionals when life-threatening events occur.

In the final twelve units, the nursing care of children with altered function of specific body systems are presented. Careful consideration was given to the organization of the text so that the pathophysiology would be presented in a nursing framework and provide the specific disease-related foundation that a nurse needs to care for sick children and adolescents and their families. A sequence of three-chapter units was developed: anatomy and physiology; nursing assessment and diagnosis; and nursing planning, intervention, and evaluation.

The first chapters in units 7 through 18 give an overview of embryonic development, structure and function, and system physiology. These chapters are a review of previous coursework. In the second chapters of these units, the nursing assessment is described and steps in collecting data from the nursing history to a health assessment are included. The assessment is organized by functional health patterns and explores the difference among infants, children, and adolescents, providing the significance of the findings. Prior to formulating a nursing diagnosis, additional data are collected using diagnostic tests. The nurse is responsible for teaching children and families about the tests that will be performed. Assessment data are used in formulating nursing diagnoses based on functional health.

The third chapters in units 7 through 18 present the specific diseases and disorders associated with the system. A common outline has been used for presenting altered function, and includes etiology, pathophysiology, clinical manifestations, significance of findings in diagnostic tests, nursing assessment, nursing diagnosis, goals in planning, interventions, and evaluations. The nursing interventions include independent and collaborative activities. The nurse is in a unique position to observe children's responses to a variety of nursing and medical interventions and then initiate appropriate and timely changes in the care. This text has been developed to assist the nursing student in identifying steps for improving patient care by first understanding the scientific and physiologic implications of symptoms, treatments, and side effects, and then utilizing this data for making appropriate nursing diagnoses and designing effective interventions.

Family-centered nursing care is applied throughout these chapters, as are the developmental considerations of the child as a patient. A nursing care plan and teaching plan using specific examples of children and their families are included. We have identified expert clinicians to develop these chapters. The care of children that contributors recommend has been used in their own practice. They know that nursing interventions make a positive difference in the prognosis and recovery of children and adolescents. They understand what happens within the family when a child is sick. The contributors' experience in working with children and their families is evident throughout the text.

Supplementary Package

The text is complemented by an excellent teaching–learning package. The ancillaries for the book include an Instructor's Manual (available in both U.S. and Canadian versions), a Student Study Guide, a 1000-question Computerized Testbank, and a set of 50 acetate overhead transparencies.

Debra Broadwell Jackson, **PhD, RN**
Rebecca B. Saunders, **PhD, RNC**

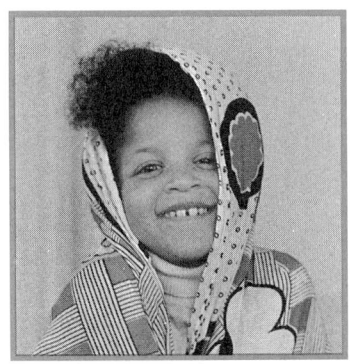

Acknowledgments

We would like to acknowledge several people who have been especially helpful in the development of this text: Eleanor Faven, Senior Developmental Editor, J.B. Lippincott, who started this project with us and has been there every day—through marriage, babies, and hospitalizations; Barbara Nelson Cullen, Acquisitions Editor, J.B. Lippincott, who has had the faith in our abilities to organize the project and to identify the best and brightest contributors in child health nursing; Jeanne Daniels, who provided many photographs of Alexander and Katie for the text; Sue Leopard, Administrative Assistant, Clemson University, for typing and copying and waiting for Federal Express; and Teri Heard, graduate research assistant, Clemson University, who spent many hours in the library researching references. The assistance of Jennifer Brogan, Editorial Assistant, J.B. Lippincott, Dina Kamilatos, Project Editor, J.B. Lippincott, and Susan Blaker, Designer, has been instrumental in the development and production of this text from manuscript to book pages. A special thanks to all of the wonderful parents who allowed us to use photographs of their children.

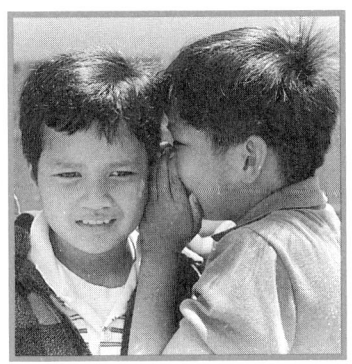

Contents in Brief

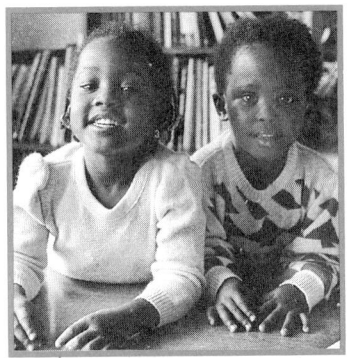

Expanded Contents

Appendices

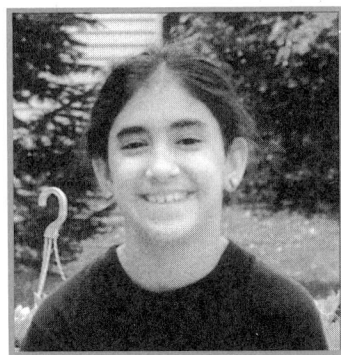

Summary of Special Features

Nursing Assessment Tools

Nursing Interventions Guides

Teaching Displays

Ideas for Nursing Research

Color Plates

Child Health Nursing

*A Comprehensive Approach
to the Care of Children
and Their Families*

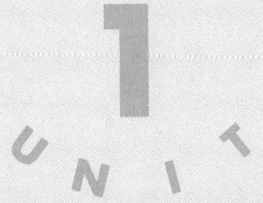
UNIT 1

Family-Centered
Child Health

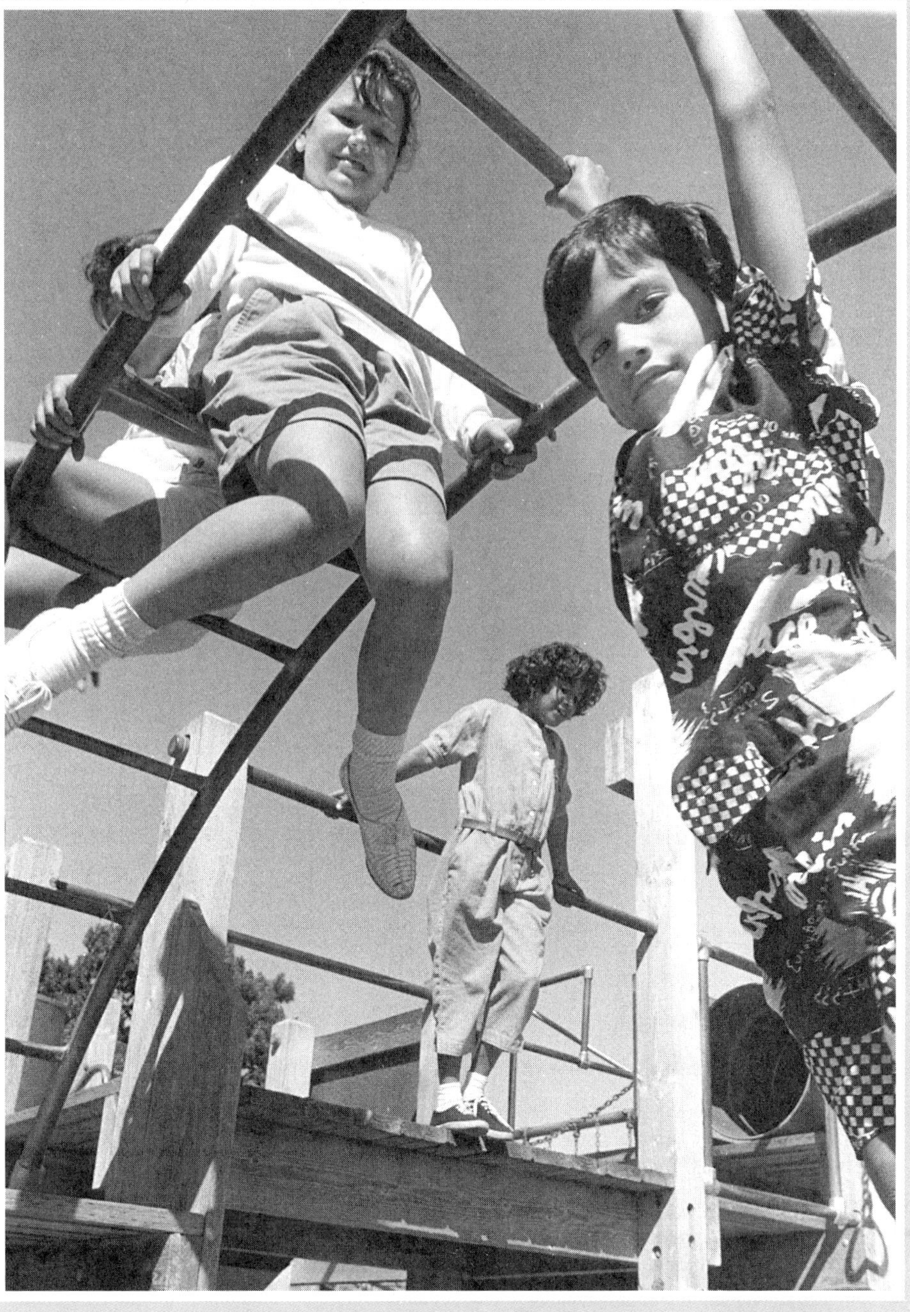

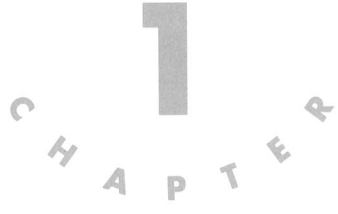

Perspectives on Child Health Nursing

BEHAVIORAL OBJECTIVES

Compare the past status of children in society to their present status.

Discuss the current status of the American child's physical and social health.

Identify elements of family-centered care.

Differentiate between standards of nursing practice and standards of care.

Compare the role of the generalist in child health nursing to the roles of the pediatric nurse practitioner and the clinical nurse specialist.

Describe the impact that ethical and legal concerns have on nursing practice and on nursing research.

Child health nursing is a discipline that requires a broad base of knowledge about the growth and development of children and the host of health and illness issues that affect them. This nursing specialty also requires an understanding of the family's influence on the child and the family's needs related to the health and illness of children. Nurses equipped with this information must also possess a wide range of clinical knowledge and competencies. Therefore, preparation for a role in child health nursing may be considered challenging, yet many nurses choose this specialty because of the scope and diversity of opportunities it offers.

The construction of the essential knowledge base for providing comprehensive nursing care to children and their families may begin with exploration of the context in which that care is delivered. This chapter opens with a historical overview of the phenomenon of childhood, highlighting the vastly different perspective that has evolved over the last 2 centuries. The concept of child health is considered using indicators of physical and social health. The focus of this chapter then turns to nursing for children with a description of family-centered care, nursing roles, and nursing standards (Fig. 1-1). Finally, brief attention is given to some contemporary issues in child health nursing, primarily those related to ethical and legal aspects of care.

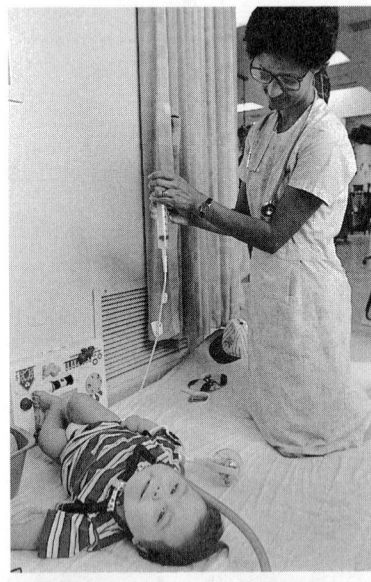
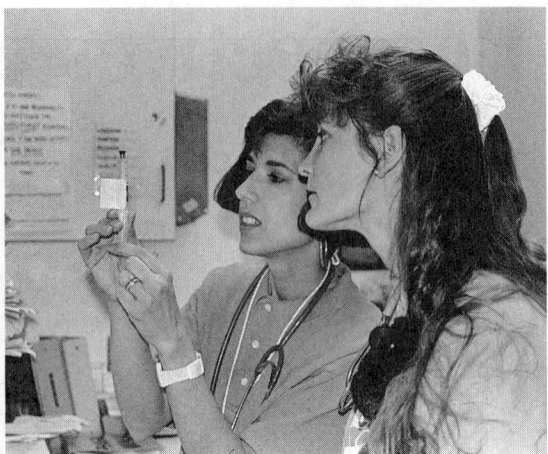
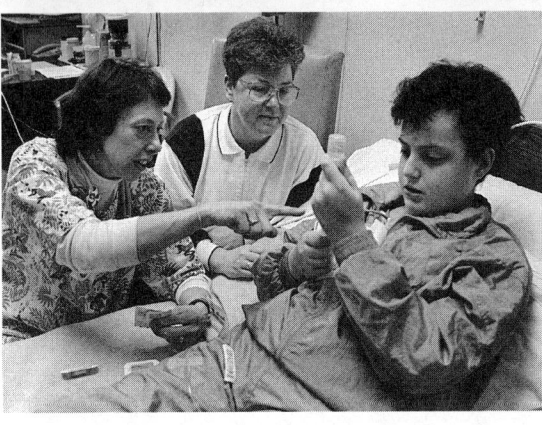

FIGURE 1-1
Nursing practice involves a variety of roles. Pictured here are nurses as care providers, collaborators, and teachers. (Photos by Kathy Sloane. Courtesy of Children's Hospital, Oakland, CA.)

A Perspective on Childhood

Childhood has not always been viewed as a distinct developmental stage, nor have children always enjoyed a central position in family functioning. In fact, the lack of importance attached to children in earlier eras may now seem incredible and disturbing. A historical perspective of childhood is valuable in prompting the nurse's understanding of contemporary attitudes, beliefs, and behaviors toward children.

Children in Antiquity

Archaeological excavations in the Middle East have revealed that children in this region were not valued and were routinely sacrificed in elaborate religious ceremonies. A great number of jars containing the remains of young children have been unearthed in temples built around 1500 B.C.[14] Bones of children also have been found in the walls of many houses, evidence of "foundation sacrifices" offered to invoke the blessing of the gods as construction was begun. In many ancient cultures, children were believed to be born without souls, and their loss was little mourned.

The first historical account of substituting an animal for a child in a sacrificial ceremony is the Biblical story of Abraham and Isaac. Ancient Hebrews valued children highly, and they viewed children as a blessing.[4] The protection and nurturance of children were essential elements of social life, and children were regarded as valuable to the future of their civilization.

These divergent views of the value of children may be recognized later in Greek and Roman cultures. The education and provision for physical needs of children were desirable activities, but sick, disabled, or unwanted children were routinely abandoned or killed. Early Roman law established the father's ownership of his children, who were treated as common property. Fathers could beat, maim, sell, or kill their children under protection of the law.[4] New laws and teachings of the early Christian Church were attempts to curb the inhumane treatment of children, but the practice of infanticide continued into the Middle Ages.[1]

Children in Premodern Eras

During the Middle Ages little distinction was made between the needs and concerns of children and adults. Although cultural information available from this era suggests a growing awareness about differences between adults and children, these ideas were limited and not uniformly applied. Renaissance paintings, for example, failed to show differences in body proportions and clothing between an adult and a child. Children were simply depicted as miniature adults.[7]

During the centuries when diseases and disabilities could not be treated with existing scientific knowledge and technology, the mortality rate among young children was shockingly high. In the absence of effective contraception, parents conceived large numbers of children knowing that only a few were likely to survive. Children who lived long enough to enter childhood were expected to share the responsibility for family survival. At the age of 6 to 8 years, children were often put into apprenticeship systems in which they worked 14-hour days and suffered from deplorable conditions and inhuman treatment. Those who survived to adolescence were quickly entered into marriage contracts that were arranged by their elders to capitalize on their economic value.

Children were considered adults in the legal system. Imprisonment, shipment to a foreign country, and even public execution were acceptable punishments for childhood crimes such as dishonesty, theft, or insubordination. Because children were viewed as innately evil, they needed strict discipline and harsh punishment to ensure that goodness prevailed. The lack of understanding of the childhood developmental process led to unrealistic expectations and inappropriate parenting behaviors.

The view of childhood and the role of children in society subtly began to shift late in the 17th century. Philosophers such as John Locke (1632 to 1704) and Jean-Jacques Rousseau (1712 to 1778) disputed the view that children were innately evil, but recognized the negative influence of many current childrearing practices. These philosophers encouraged parents to engage in activities that positively shaped the personalities of children and to curb their abusive discipline. Although the view of the child's moral depravity and need for punishment remained strong into the 19th century, the alternate view of childhood as a time of physical as well as social and emotional development also grew.

The work of the English biologist Charles Darwin (1809 to 1882) shed new light on growth and behavior in children and stimulated public interest in human origins and development. During the later years of the 19th century eminent American authors wrote passionately about the need to nurture children from infancy onward. Parental authority without violence and the need for moral training in concert with the psychological and neurological development of children were novel ideas that were received sympathetically by many parents and professionals (Fig. 1-2).

Children in the Present Century

As the 20th century dawned, public interest in child development continued to grow. Arnold Gessell (1880 to 1961), founder of the Yale Clinic for Child Development, was the first to use scientific methods to study groups of children over time. His descriptions of age-related development from biological and behavioral perspectives were widely disseminated. Another new idea, that childhood experiences are a precursor to adult behaviors, was advanced by the Austrian physician Sigmund

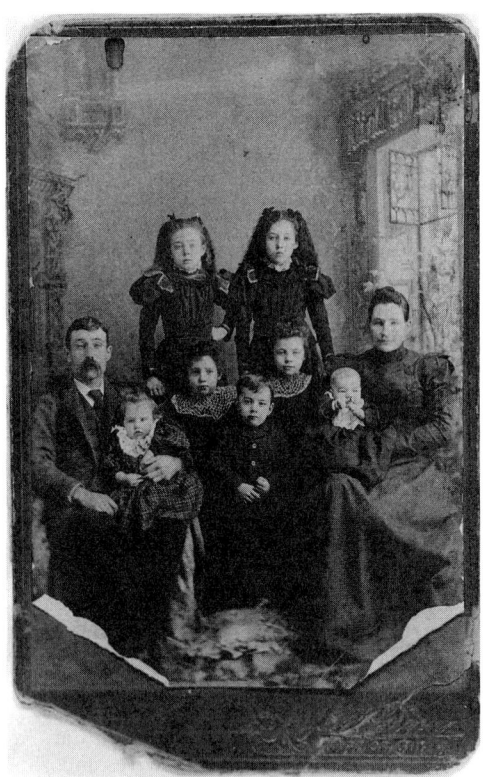

FIGURE 1-2
Children born before the turn of the century dressed like their parents and had important roles in the livelihood of the family. Play was considered frivolous and the privilege of the well-to-do.

Freud (1856 to 1939) and received notable attention. These scientists and other scholars stimulated a desire to understand more about the growth and development of the whole child. Thus, during the first 2 decades of the present century the interest in children was transformed from concern about control and character building to an eagerness to understand development of physical traits, personality, and patterns of behavior throughout childhood.

A spirit of progressivism prevailed during the early years of the 20th century and influenced the enlargement of public and private school systems. Federal labor laws and far-reaching social policies have been enacted as the result of public understanding of the special characteristics and needs of children. National programs have also been established to improve the health of children (see the accompanying display on national efforts to improve child health). Childhood now is viewed as a predictable and formative period; the interaction of heredity and environment in child development is better understood. The value now placed on children in American society stands in stark contrast to the status of children in the past.

A Perspective on Child Health

The general health of a nation may be investigated by studying its vital statistics. These numbers include many aspects of human life, such as birth and death rates, cause of death, and the years of life expectancy. As important

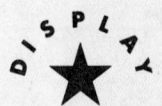

National Efforts to Improve Child Health in the United States

1909—First White House Conference on Dependent Children; organization of prenatal care services; American Association for the Study and Prevention of Infant Mortality founded

1912—Federal Children's Bureau established (continued until 1969 when other agencies took over functions)

1915—National Birth Registry established

1919—White House Conference on Child Welfare Standards

1921—Maternity and Infancy Act (Sheppard-Towner Act) enacted; funding continued until 1929

1928—First National Child Health Day on May 1

1930—White House Conference on Child Health and Protection

1935—Social Security Act; Title V modeled after the Sheppard-Towner Act to provide grants to states to improve maternal and child health and welfare

1940—White House Conference on Children in a Democracy

1943—Emergency Maternity and Infant Care Act made law to provide health care to wives and children of servicemen

1950—Midcentury White House Conference on Children and Youth

1953—U.S. Department of Health, Education, and Welfare formed

1960—White House Conference on Children and Youth

1963—Title V amended to create Maternity and Infant Care programs

1965—Federal Comprehensive Neighborhood Health Centers program established

1966—Special Supplemental Food Program for Women, Infants, and Children (WIC) authorized; implemented in 1972

1967—Medicaid Early and Periodic Screening, Diagnosis, and Treatment program for children enacted

1970—White House Conference on Children; National Health Service Corps established to place health professionals and resources in underserved areas

1979—U.S. Surgeon General's report, *Healthy People,* set national health goals and objectives for maternal and infant health

1981—Title V programs consolidated into the Maternal and Child Health Services Block Grant

1983—The Select Committee on Children, Youth, and Families formed in the U.S. House of Representatives

1985—*Preventing Low Birthweight,* report of the Institute of Medicine

(Adapted from National Commission to Prevent Infant Mortality. [1987]. Inadequate results: National efforts to improve maternal and child health in the United States.)

---

as these indicators of the physical health of children are, they should be studied in comparison with indicators of the social health of children. Together, physical and social health statistics can reveal trends that provide guidance in planning services to improve the well-being of children.

Indicators of Physical Health

A nation's infant mortality rate is often used as an indicator of the adequacy of public health services and medical care made available to women and infants. An infant mortality rate is typically expressed as the number of deaths of infants younger than 1 year per 1000 live births per year. Therefore, an infant mortality rate of 18.1 means that for every 1000 infants born during that year, 18 died before they were 1 year old.

Keeping in mind that reporting procedures are not yet standardized, comparisons can be made among different countries. The United States spends more on child care than any other country (approximately $2.5 billion per year); thus, a very low infant mortality rate would be expected. When compared to the region that was once the Soviet Union, China, Mexico, and India, the infant mortality rate in the United States does compare favorably (Table 1-1). However, the infant mortality rate in the United States is more than twice as high as that in Japan

or Sweden and lags considerably behind other industrialized nations of the world. Approximately 40,000 infants born in the United States die during their first year of life.[2]

The infant mortality rate in the United States, although alarming when compared to other well-developed countries, represents a significant reduction since the turn of the century when the rate was almost 10 times as high (Fig. 1-3). The remarkable progress made in reducing the mortality rate for infants may be attributed to improved nutrition and sanitation, advances in medical treatments and technology, and the American network of public health and social programs for poor mothers and children. The rate has improved very little in recent years, however, especially for minority groups. The mortality rate for African American infants is almost double that for white infants.

The plateau that has been reached in the overall infant mortality rate has been attributed to the fact that medical technology has nearly reached the limits of its ability to save small preterm infants.[2] Two decades ago few infants less than 2 pounds (approximately 900 g) lived more than a short while, but sophisticated technology and medical practice have improved the survival rate of even these small infants. Future advances in this area are unlikely, however, because the viability of an infant is determined by the development and maturation of vital organs and body systems. Only the development of a

TABLE 1-1
Infant Mortality Rates for Selected Nations

Country	Rate
Japan	4.4
Sweden	6.0
Finland	6.3
Switzerland	6.8
The Netherlands	6.8
Canada*	7.2
France*	7.7
United Kingdom*	9.0
Australia*	9.2
United States*	9.9
Soviet Union*	25.1
China†	32.4
Mexico†	47.0
India†	95.0

(Source: United Nations. [1991]. *1989 demographic yearbook.* New York: Department of International Economic and Social Affairs, Statistical Office.)

* Data from 1988.

† Data from 1987.

functioning "artificial womb" is likely to promote future gains in survival rates of very preterm infants.

Low birth weight is one of the major causes of neonatal death. Infants who weigh less than 5.5 pounds at birth are at greatest risk; they are 40 times more likely than infants of normal birth weight to die within the first

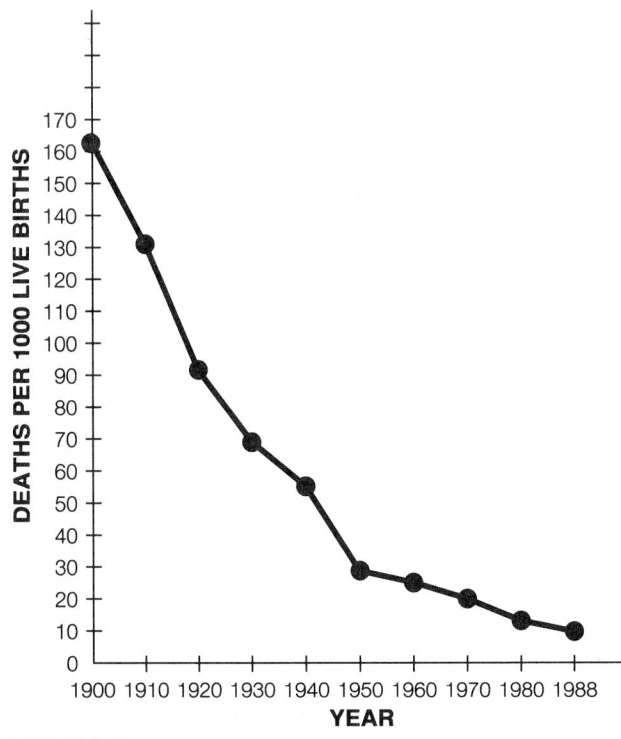

FIGURE 1-3

Infant mortality rate in the United States, 1900 to 1988. (Source: Compiled from several editions of Statistical Abstracts of the United States, U. S. Government Printing Office.)

month of life.[16] Many of these deaths could be avoided if mothers at risk (young and single, undereducated, minority, and poor) had greater access to health care during pregnancy. A national commitment to provide the necessary resources is vital to further reduction of the national infant mortality rate.[2]

Although low birth weight is a major health problem in the United States, it is not the only cause of death in infants younger than 1 year. Congenital anomalies in full-term infants are still common, and sudden infant death syndrome remains an unsolved problem. The mortality rate from these and other causes are listed in Table 1-2. Death for children older than 1 year occurs for a variety of reasons, including disease and injury. When all age groups are considered, accidents are the leading cause of death in children beyond infancy, especially during the teenage years.[24]

Many other statistics related to the physical health of children could be considered. One particularly disturbing finding is that less than half of children younger than age 4 are immunized against communicable diseases.[11] The success that has been achieved in reducing morbidity and mortality from childhood diseases in past years has generated a sense of complacency. Parents may not attend to this important aspect of health maintenance until school entrance requirements are met. Without immunization against measles, mumps, rubella, polio, and other childhood diseases the risk for epidemics and subsequent deleterious effects increases.

Another health problem that has been identified is that approximately one in five children does not have publicly funded or private health insurance.[11] The absence of this coverage may be attributed primarily to economic reasons. Employees who do have coverage are being asked to contribute more to pay for medical insurance that often covers fewer services. Children from middle-income families, particularly those with chronic diseases, are sometimes forced to do without diagnosis or treatment. Children in low-income families are generally covered by Medicaid, but government spending for these programs has declined.

TABLE 1-2
Leading Causes of Death in Infancy, United States, 1989

Cause of Death	Percent Distribution
Congenital anomalies	20.8
Sudden infant death syndrome	14.0
Short gestation and low birth weight	8.4
Respiratory distress syndrome	8.1
Complications of placenta, cord, and membranes	2.3
Infections specific to the perinatal period	2.3
Accidents and adverse effects	2.3
Intrauterine hypoxia and birth asphyxia	2.0
Pneumonia and influenza	1.6
All other causes	34.0

(Source: U.S. Bureau of the Census. [1991]. *Statistical Abstract of the United States: 1991* [111th ed.]. Washington, DC: Author.)

Even if cost were not a factor, the availability of health care services is a problem for many families, especially those in rural areas. Approximately 15% of the population (30 million Americans) has limited or no access to medical care.[19] A single physician or nurse practitioner may be responsible for many people in a widely dispersed geographic region. Children in these areas clearly are at risk for increased morbidity and mortality.

Indicators of Social Health

Until recently no attempt was made to monitor the status of children in terms of their social health, although the federal government has faithfully gathered data on the discrete phenomena that influence the status of social health for infants and children. Agencies such as the Fordham University (New York) Institute for Innovation in Social Policy, however, have begun to systematically investigate the performance of the United States on major social problems. Indicators of the social health of children that are under investigation include child abuse, impoverished children, teen suicide, drug abuse, and dropping out of school. Other problems such as the growth of the homeless population have not been fully addressed.

If these indicators are used to compile an index of social health, it is clear that the well-being of children in America has declined dramatically since 1970 (Fig. 1-4). Particularly devastating to the nation's youth have been sharp increases in the numbers of children and teenagers who are abused, who live in poverty, and who commit suicide.

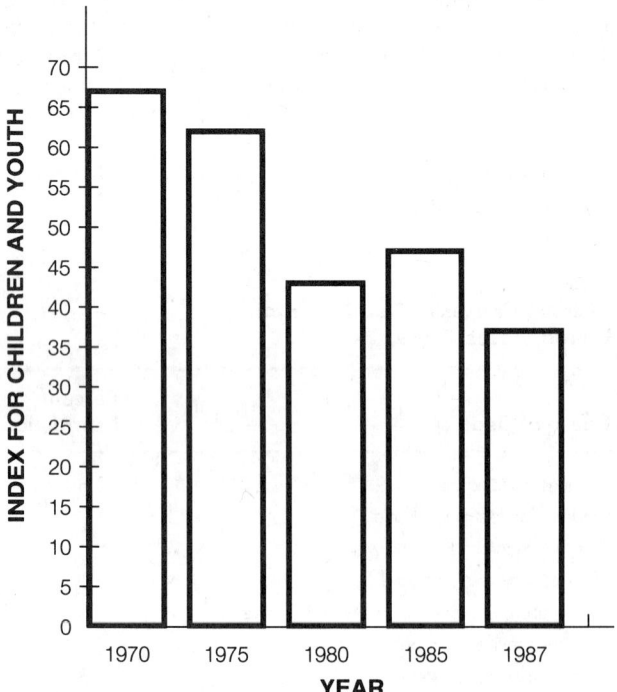

FIGURE 1-4
Index for social health for children and youth, 1970 to 1987. This is a composite measure based on figures from six problem areas (child abuse, children living in poverty, teenage suicide, teenage drug abuse, high school drop-outs, and infant mortality). (Data from Fordham Institute for Innovation in Social Policy, The Index of Social Health: 1989.)

For many years the increase in child abuse rates was partially attributed to improved reporting procedures, yet most of those reporting changes occurred in the early 1980s. The ever-worsening rates suggest that abuse is increasing significantly.

Another key measure of social health is the number of children younger than age 18 who live in poverty; problems such as health, education, and housing are linked to a low income. From 1970 to 1987 the number of children in poverty increased by approximately 25%. As recently as 1987 one of every five children in the United States lived in poverty.[12] Both the physical and social aspects of child and family health are negatively affected by poverty.

The rate of suicide among adolescents has doubled since 1970, but there is speculation that actual numbers of deaths by suicide may be higher than reported figures.[12] When a child dies, suicide may be suspected but not verifiable, and thus it is attributed to natural or accidental causes. This indicator of social health has been the target of increasing investigation and concern.

The remaining indicators of social health are more encouraging.[12] From 1985 to 1987 the rate of drug abuse stabilized, suggesting that recent campaigns waged against this social problem may be influencing American youths. The problem remains, however, one of the most pressing national concerns. Likewise, the problem of high school dropouts has shown gradual improvement throughout the past decade. The slightly worse rate noted in 1987[12] needs to be closely monitored in the future.

A review of these trends indicates that overall the well-being of children in America is declining. The need for public debate and commitment to policies and programs that affect children is vital to retrieving the gains that were attained in the early and middle 1970s. The value placed on the social health of a nation's children is manifested by its domestic social policy. Because children do not vote, they have little political influence. Health care providers who are aware of the facts regarding the social health of children have the opportunity to act as advocates for this population.

Future Health Care Needs of Children

Health care providers who are familiar with the current issues and problems in child health care are concerned about the future. The immense scope and complexity of these problems necessitates that future health needs of children and their families be anticipated now so that priorities can be set and goals clarified. The accompanying display on anticipated health care needs outlines six main categories of need for the year 2000. Nurses with responsibilities in education, administration, practice, and research related to children can use this information to focus their efforts in the years ahead.

Traditional approaches and methods of providing health care for children and families often are inadequate. Innovative thinking and risk taking are necessary for an effective resolution to the problems that have been identified, and professional nurses are in an exciting position

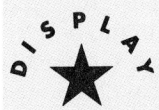

Anticipated Health Care Needs for the Year 2000

Comprehensive health care for children and families to include

- a national health policy with financial support
- goals to support care in the best environment, regardless of ability to pay
- specific programs to provide care in multiple sites with services that are coordinated

Clinical dimensions of care to include

- empowerment of the child and family as active members of the health care team
- atraumatic care in environments where human caring interfaces with technology
- promotion of wellness and early health self-care
- family-focused care

Child health nursing to include

- educational preparation to provide care in multiple sites with advanced knowledge of child development, family systems, and new technology
- care environments that allow more autonomy in decision making
- local health care systems that are nurse based

Nursing research to include

- interdisciplinary investigations to predict positive health outcomes for child and family
- demonstration and evaluation studies to measure outcomes of care
- testing of innovative alternative health care systems

Ethics and ethical decision making to include

- support of the parents, family, and provider
- ethical management of technology

Consumer rights for children to include

- a safe, healthy physical environment, free from abuse and neglect
- families having choices in health care delivery systems
- opportunity to die with dignity

(Adapted from: Feeg, V. D. [1990]. The future of pediatric nursing: Anticipating the health care needs of children. Imprint, 37, p. 75.)

to refocus the care of children. Concepts that are being developed[11] include the following:

- *Case management,* a nursing delivery system in which a nurse views the child and family holistically and coordinates all aspects of care, is gradually replacing other methods of providing care.
- Alternative health and illness care settings are opening to make child health care services more available and accessible.
- Nursing education for child health nurses is expanding to provide a better foundation for the generalist and the specialist.
- Policies related to care of the child and family are being developed or revised to respond to consumer demands within the health care system.
- Ethics committees are increasingly involved in helping to make decisions regarding the health care of children.
- Governments at all levels are responding to public demand for a national children's agenda and health policy legislation.

A Perspective on Nursing of Children

Nurses have a unique opportunity to influence the shaping of new policies and services for children, and professional

nursing organizations are currently involved in these activities. However, nurses who provide direct care for children and their families face a growing challenge to maintain an adequate knowledge base and to improve clinical competencies. Three aspects of nursing care that are emphasized in current practice are the family-centered approach, the development and use of standards, and the expansion of the nurse's role.

Family-Centered Care

The importance of the family to the health and well-being of children has long been recognized. For at least 30 years the term *family-centered care* has permeated nursing literature, and many suggestions for implementing the concept in clinical practice have been offered. However, there is no consensus about the definition of the term, nor is there agreement about how family-centered care is best designed.[29]

One of the most serious problems that health professionals face with families is how to promote more active involvement of children and their families in matters related to child health. The concept of family-centered care calls for family autonomy, self-determination, and control in the care of the child.[25] However, health care providers often inadvertently encourage family dependency, helplessness, and alienation by taking control and doing what is expedient.[27] These actions may be most evident when the child is critically ill. The use of complex technology, the acuity of the child's illness, staff shortages, institutional policies, and economic concerns have been identified as barriers to the delivery of family-centered care.[29]

A comprehensive understanding of the meaning of family-centered care has been facilitated in recent years by the interest of government officials at the national level. For example, a series of seminars began in 1982 with "The Surgeon General's Workshop on Children with Handicaps and their Families."[15] More recently, the Division of Maternal and Child Health of the U.S. Public Health Services has supported the efforts of the Association for the Care of Children's Health (ACCH). One of the goals of the ACCH has been to describe the essential elements of family-centered care, which are listed in the accompanying display. This important work is stimulating health care providers to examine their care practices and question the adequacy of their attempts to promote the concept of family-centered care.

The ability to provide nursing care that is truly family centered demands a recognition of the attitudes and behaviors that limit family involvement. Treating families as partners in the child's care and assisting them to obtain adequate information can result in parent-professional collaboration. The family is thus empowered and can assume responsibility for participating in discussions and making decisions about the child's care.[10]

Nurses have a pivotal role in continuing to clarify how the care of children can become more family centered. They have an opportunity to become involved in testing assumptions and establishing empirical guidelines that can be used by all members of the health team. The significance of the role of nurses in this aspect of patient advocacy cannot be overestimated.

Standards for Child Health Nursing

Professional nurses are accountable for the care they provide to children and families regardless of the setting.

Standards of practice and standards of care are two types of documents used to provide guidance in the delivery and evaluation of the care provided. Standards of practice describe the performance of a professional as determined by an authority in the practice.[5] In contrast, standards of care describe specific patient outcomes and the quality of care that should be provided to children and their families.

General standards for the nursing of children have been developed by the American Nurses Association (ANA) Council on Maternal and Child Nursing. The accompanying display lists maternal and child nursing practice standards. These standards can be used by nurses in all pediatric settings. However, other standards of practice for specific patient populations are available from nursing specialty groups. Specialty practice standards build on the basic standards developed by the ANA, but they are specific to areas of nursing by diagnosis (e.g., renal, cardiovascular, cancer), by age (e.g., neonate, infant, adolescent), or by location (e.g., school, ambulatory clinic, hospital).[3] The accompanying display on outcome standards of pediatric oncology nursing practice is an example of standards of practice developed by a nursing specialty group.

Standards of care are used in quality assurance programs to evaluate the effectiveness of nursing provided for the child or family. Quality assurance is defined as "an estimate of the degree of excellence in the health care provider's performance as reflected by alteration of the patient's health status."[21] The criteria set forth in the standards of care are used to audit child health care services and to implement appropriate changes (see the display on nursing standards for quality assurance). Standards of care are of no value unless they are interpreted and applied to daily nursing practice; if they are, the intent of the standards are realized, and excellence in professional practice is achieved.

In addition to their use in quality assurance programs, professional standards also may be used as a legal yard-

---

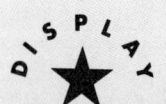

Key Elements of Family-Centered Care

- Recognizing that the family is the constant in a child's life, while the service systems and personnel within those systems fluctuate
- Facilitating parent–professional collaboration at all levels of health care
- Honoring the racial, ethnic, cultural, and socioeconomic diversity of families
- Recognizing family strengths and individuality and respecting different methods of coping
- Sharing with parents, on a continuing basis and in a supportive manner, complete and unbiased information

- Encouraging and facilitating family-to-family support and networking
- Understanding and incorporating the developmental needs of infants, children, and adolescents and their families into health care systems
- Implementing comprehensive policies and programs that provide emotional and financial support to meet the needs of families
- Designing accessible health care systems that are flexible, culturally competent, and responsive to family-identified needs

(Reproduced with permission of the Association for the Care of Children's Health, 7910 Woodmont Ave, Suite 300, Bethesda, MD 20814, from Shelton, T., et al. (1992). Family-centered care for children with special health care needs (2nd ed.). Washington, DC: Association for the Care of Children's Health.)

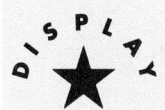

Maternal and Child Nursing Practice Standards

The nurse helps children and parents attain and maintain optimum health.

The nurse assists families to achieve and maintain a balance between the personal growth needs of individual family members and optimum family functioning.

The nurse intervenes with vulnerable clients and families at risk to prevent potential development and health problems.

The nurse promotes an environment free of hazards to reproduction, growth and development, wellness, and recovery from illness.

The nurse detects changes in health status and deviations from optimum development.

The nurse carries out appropriate interventions and treatment to facilitate survival and recovery from illness.

The nurse assists clients and families to understand and cope with developmental and traumatic situations during illness, childbearing, childrearing, and childhood.

The nurse actively pursues strategies to enhance access to and use of adequate health care services.

The nurse improves maternal and child health nursing practice through evaluation of practice, education, and research.

(Adapted from: American Nurses' Association Division on Maternal & Child Health Nursing Practice. [1983]. Standards of Maternal & Child Nursing Practice.)

stick to determine whether care can be considered acceptable nursing practice.[18] Child health nurses, like all professional nurses, are expected to carry out their responsibilities in a reasonably prudent manner. In conjunction with nurse practice acts and other legally binding documents, professional standards clarify what the public and members of the health care system can expect from professional nursing.

Nursing Roles

In providing health care for children, nurses function in many roles, including that of advocate, teacher, care provider, collaborator-coordinator, and researcher. Advocacy for both the child and the family is a major component of nursing care and includes many dimensions from the broad promotion of the rights of the child to

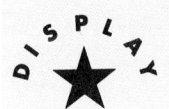

Outcome Standards of Pediatric Oncology Nursing Practice

The child and family possess accurate current information about the disease, options for treatment, consequences or side effects of treatment, potential oncologic emergencies, alternative care settings, and resources to be fully informed partners in the health care team. Information should be specific to the developmental level of the child and family.

The child and family possess adequate information regarding the psychological and physiologic effects of the diagnosis and treatment of cancer on the normal growth and developmental level of the child and family.

The child's physical care is provided by the nurse in collaboration with the child and family. The nurse is responsible for assessing and determining the child's and family's participation in the physical care of the child. The nurse selects interventions that facilitate an appropriate level of self-care.

The child and family maintain psychological, social, and spiritual integrity while living with a diagnosis of cancer.

The child and family possess appropriate knowledge with regard to prevention and early detection of secondary cancer and adult malignancies.

The child and family demonstrate optimal adaptation to long-term survival. This is demonstrated by integration into the family's usual health care practice of current information about possible later psychological or physical consequences from a diagnosis and treatment of cancer in childhood. The child and family also participate in long-term follow-up activities.

The nurse assumes responsibility for improving pediatric oncology nursing practice through evaluation of practice and an ongoing involvement in continuing education, professional development, and research.

(Adapted from: Association of Pediatric Oncology Nurses. [1989]. Outcome Standards of Pediatric Oncology Nursing Practice.)

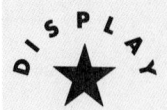

An Example of Nursing Standards Used for Quality Assurance

Topic: ODH-MCH Child Health Standards

Dates of study: 3/24/80–6/9/80

PATIENT Sample 1

Record No.: _____ Page 1 of 4

Name: _____ Date of Audit: _____

B.D. _____ Sex: _____ Clinic: _____

Reviewer: _____

Nursing Standards	Audit Criteria	Exceptions	STD.	EM	ENM	EME	N/A	Notes
Age-appropriate immunization levels: assess current immunization status	Client record shows adequate immunization level according to ODH recommendations and standards	Including but not limited to fever and concurrent acute illness; religious or philosophical reasons; hypersensivitiy	100%					
Inform parent re: possible reaction inherent with the individual immunization	Signed consent forms for immunizations							
Administer immunization according to proper technique	Injection site identified							
Educate parent re: the importance of completing individual's immunization series	Parent teaching completed							
Ascertain that parent received follow-up appointment as indicated	Return appointment							
Ascertain that return appointment kept and above process continuing	Client received subsequent immunization as scheduled							
Initiate appropriate outreach for missed appointments	Outreach effort							

Key: *EM, element met; ENM, element not met; EME, element met by exception; N/A, not appropriate by age/other,* Data sources: *(1) medical summary sheet; (2) case history; (3) attached consent forms; (4) healthy beginning checklist; (5) growth charts.*
(Source: Gurile, P., & Harter, I. C. [1987]. Testing child health standards in a clinical setting. Journal of Pediatric Nursing, 2, *302–307.)*

tapping the resources needed for an individual child or family. As a teacher the nurse explains procedures, protocols, and practices, ensuring that children and families have appropriate information to discuss their options and to enter into the process of making decisions about the child's care. The nurse promotes optimum health through the use of the nursing process: assessment, diagnosis, planning, intervention, and evaluation. Nurses are also expected to collaborate with other professionals on the health care team, and they frequently are given responsibility for coordinating or managing the child's care. Finally, nurses are increasingly responsible for contributing to development of the profession's knowledge base by systematically investigating theoretical or practice issues in child-family nursing.

Not only do nurses function in many roles, but they also practice child-family nursing in a variety of settings. Chapter 22 offers several examples of nurses who provide care to children in ambulatory settings, including physicians' offices, clinics, schools, and camps. Nurses also provide care for children in hospitals (see Chap. 23) and in the home (see Chap. 24). This diversity in care settings has resulted from recent changes within the health care system, chiefly from advances in technology and efforts to contain costs. Other sites for the delivery of health care to children may be expected to emerge in the future.

The growing interest in providing adequate health care for children has also stimulated the development of expanded roles for nurses. The Pediatric Nurse Practitioner (PNP) programs that originated in the 1960s have emphasized health promotion, illness prevention, and wellness maintenance. PNPs possess skill in assessment and treatment of ill children using established protocols. They also provide well-child care and perform developmental screening. In recent years many PNP programs have been incorporated into graduate nursing programs so that a master's degree is obtained in addition to a practitioner's certificate. The additional education provides a broad foundation for advanced nursing practice.

The Clinical Nurse Specialist (CNS) in child health care is another example of an expanded role. Although the CNS role has been poorly defined, recently it has come to indicate graduate education in a specialty area to prepare for practice in that clinical specialty. The CNS in child health care may have wide-ranging responsibilities for all children in a particular health facility, or they may further specialize in an intensive care setting or an oncology unit for children, for example. The multiple roles of the CNS in child and family care provide innumerable opportunities to expand the existing body of knowledge in nursing and to explore methods of improving nursing care practices with children.

A Perspective on Issues Related to Child Health Care

With the expansion of roles and the increasing assumption of responsibilities, child health nurses are faced with numerous issues that affect their practice. Three of these issues are closely tied: ethical decision making, legal obligations, and research on children. Although these issues are discussed separately for clarity in presentation, they are interconnected and difficult to separate in nursing practice.

Ethical Concerns

Ethical dilemmas, situations in which "there is a conflict among duties, loyalties, rights, and/or values,"[22] have become commonplace in the practice of professional nursing. Nurses who work in pediatric settings, particularly those in critical care units, are frequently confronted with difficult decisions about treatment options for children. The question of length of life versus quality of life is one example of ethical dilemmas in which nurses may be involved. Traditional principles of doing good and avoiding harm to patients are no longer an adequate basis for making decisions, because at times there is grave uncertainty about the benefit of a particular course of action.[8]

Parents generally are assumed to know and want what is best for their children.[6] Parental autonomy in making decisions for their children is therefore highly valued and respected. Parental decision making, however, may be difficult when the parents lack the knowledge or skill needed to make decisions or when stress and grief cloud the issues. In these circumstances nurses can facilitate communication between parents and other members of the health care team, but they often "experience conflicting loyalties to themselves, their profession, their colleagues, patients and their families, physicians and health care team members, the institution, and society" about who should make decisions and what the outcome should be.[28]

When disputes arise between parties interested in the child's health, negotiation is needed to resolve the dilemma. The rights and responsibilities of all those involved need to be ensured. Nurses traditionally have been expected to mediate the multiple demands and perspectives in ethical dilemmas of patient care.[6] To prepare themselves for participating in the decision-making process, nurses must learn to clarify values held by themselves and others, know how to use available resources, and understand various ethical theories and principles.[28]

A Code of Ethics has been published by the ANA to guide nursing practice and is shown in the accompanying display. This document focuses on the nurse's accountability to the patient, community, and profession. These guidelines, valuable as general standards, do not constitute a theoretical basis for making ethical decisions. Fry[13] and others have analyzed the basic values of nursing and have proposed the development of a unique theory of nursing ethics. The concept of caring is central to any model that will be developed. Until such a model is refined, nurses will continue to rely on other models derived from biomedical ethics.

Regardless of the theoretical model used, a systematic approach is needed to reduce the stress and anxiety associated with resolving ethical dilemmas. Clough[8] suggests that nurses first clarify their own values about a situation, distinguishing their position from that of others. Second, nurses can prepare others for a crisis before the crisis actually occurs, helping to expose differences of opinion that may exist. Third, nurses need to get as many facts about the situation as possible, exploring what the child and parents feel about the moral issues involved. Fourth, nurses can determine the exact problem, stating the dilemma clearly and concisely for themselves. Fifth, nurses can carefully consider the consequences of each action, knowing that no one action may seem entirely right. Sixth, nurses are ready to take a position regarding the best course of action. This process of decision making increases the probability that nurses will be active participants rather than frustrated bystanders when ethical dilemmas about child health care are being resolved.

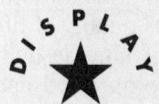

Code of Ethics

1. The nurse provides services with respect for human dignity and the uniqueness of the client unrestricted by considerations of social or economic status, personal attributes, or the nature of health problems.
2. The nurse safeguards the client's right to privacy by judiciously protecting information of a confidential nature.
3. The nurse acts to safeguard the client and the public when health care and safety are affected by the incompetent, unethical, or illegal practice of any person.
4. The nurse assumes responsibility and accountability for individual nursing judgments and actions.
5. The nurse maintains competence in nursing.
6. The nurse exercises informed judgment and uses individual competence and qualifications as criteria in seeking consultation, accepting responsibilities, and delegating nursing activities to others.

7. The nurse participates in the profession's efforts to implement and improve standards of nursing.
8. The nurse participates in the profession's efforts to establish and maintain conditions of employment conducive to high-quality nursing care.
9. The nurse participates in the profession's efforts to protect the public from misinformation and misrepresentation and to maintain the integrity of nursing.
10. The nurse collaborates with members of the health professions and other citizens in promoting community and national efforts to meet the health needs of the public.

(Source: American Nurses' Association. [1985].)

Legal Concerns

Nurses need to know that in addition to basic human rights, children and families possess legal rights. Although declarations of human rights are not legally binding, they may inspire legislative action to ensure that the goals are obtained. For example, the accompanying display on the United Nations' Declaration of the Rights of the Child lists several principles related to the health and well-being of children. The enactment of labor laws, social security programs, and health regulations provides evidence of the government's recognition of those rights and their desire that the rights be observed.

The legal rights of children and families are extensive, and texts on legal issues in nursing can provide a broad range of information (e.g., Creighton[9] and Northrop and Kelly[26]). Of chief concern to child health nurses is the question of consent, because failure to obtain consent leaves nurses and other health care practitioners open to legal charges of battery. A minor cannot give consent for treatment in the health care system; consent must be obtained from the minor's parent or legal guardian.

A child is considered a minor until the age of 18 unless a state has a statute specifying another age.[9] When a minor marries, regardless of age, the parents' control ceases. However, minors may be considered emancipated if parents have relinquished their responsibility to control and care for their child and their rights to a child's services and earnings.[9] Emancipated minors may give consent for their own care.

Three other exceptions to the requirement for parental consent have been identified.[17] First, emergency treatment may be given when the child's life is in danger, when parents are so far away that obtaining consent is not practical, or sometimes if the minor is mature but

unemancipated. Children who can be treated without parental consent can also refuse treatment. Nurses are thus often challenged to provide adequate information so that the decisions are made in the child's best interest.

Research Concerns

In the early years of child development and clinical research, children were studied with little concern about ethical or legal issues, because few regulations or guidelines were available. Some children were subjected to a variety of treatments that today seem unthinkable. Respect for the rights and welfare of children make this type of investigation impossible today. Several agencies concerned with research on children have published ethical guidelines. The major issues concern the right to privacy, informed consent, and truth in experimentation.

A fundamental human right protected by the Constitution gives Americans the *right to privacy*. This right implies that research cannot be conducted when the subjects are unaware that a study is being performed, and the identity of the individuals being studied may not be divulged in reports. Results of the study must be held in strict confidence.

Participants in research also must be informed of the purposes and procedures of the study, and their participation must be voluntary. The application of this principle of *informed consent* to studies of children implies that parents or guardians of those children participating in the study must give their permission based on a clear understanding of the investigation's purpose and the procedures used in the study. Whenever possible, the children should have freedom to choose whether or not to participate in a study and if they do consent, to discon-

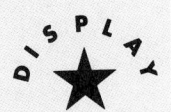

United Nations' Declaration of the Rights of the Child

Preamble

Whereas the peoples of the United Nations have, in the charter, reaffirmed their faith in fundamental human rights, and in the dignity and worth of the human person, and have determined to promote social progress and better standards of life in larger freedom,

Whereas the United Nations has, in the Universal Declaration of Human Rights, proclaimed that everyone is entitled to all the rights and freedoms set forth therein, without distinction of any kind, such as race, color, sex, language, religion, political or other opinion, national or social origin, property, birth or other status,

Whereas the child, by reason of his physical and mental immaturity, needs special safeguards and care, including appropriate legal protection, before as well as after birth,

Whereas the need for such special safeguards has been stated in the Geneva Declaration of the Rights of the Child 1924, and recognized in the Universal Declaration of Human Rights and in the statutes of specialized agencies and international organizations concerned with welfare of children,

Whereas mankind owes to the child the best it has to give

Now Therefore the General Assembly Proclaims

This Declaration of the Rights of the Child to the end that he may have a happy childhood and enjoy for his own good and for the good of society the rights and freedoms herein set forth, and calls upon parents, upon men and women as individuals and upon voluntary organizations, local authorities and national governments to recognize these rights and strive for their observance by legislative and other measures progressively taken in accordance with the following principles:

Principle 1

The child shall enjoy all the rights set forth in this Declaration. All children, without any exception whatsoever, shall be entitled to these rights, without distinction or discrimination on account of race, color, sex, language, religion, political or other opinion, national or social origin, property, birth or other status, whether of himself or of his family.

Principle 2

The child shall enjoy special protection, and shall be given opportunities and facilities, by law and by other means, to enable him to develop physically, mentally, morally, spiritually and socially in a healthy and normal manner and in conditions of freedom and dignity. In the enactment of laws for this purpose the best interests of the child shall be the paramount consideration.

Principle 3

The child shall be entitled from his birth to a name and a nationality.

Principle 4

The child shall enjoy the benefits of social security. He shall be entitled to grow and develop in health; to this end special care and protection shall be provided both to him and to his mother, including adequate pre-natal and post-natal care. The child shall have the right to adequate nutrition, housing, recreation and medical services.

Principle 5

The child who is physically, mentally, or socially handicapped shall be given the special treatment, education and care required by his particular condition.

Principle 6

The child, for the full and harmonious development of his personality, needs love and understanding. He shall, wherever possible, grow up in the care and under the responsibility of his parents, and in any case in an atmosphere of affection and of moral and maternal security; a child of tender years shall not, save in exceptional circumstances, be separated from his mother. Society and the public authorities shall have the duty to extend particular care to

(Continued)

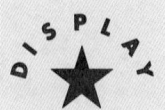

United Nations' Declaration of the Rights of the Child (continued)

children without a family and to those without adequate means of support. Payment of state and other assistance toward the maintenance of children of large families is desirable.

Principle 7

The child is entitled to receive education, which shall be free and compulsory, at least in the elementary stages. He shall be given an education which will promote his general culture, and enable him on a basis of equal opportunity to develop his abilities, his individual judgment, and his sense of moral and social responsibility, and to become a useful member of society.

The best interests of the child shall be the building principle of those responsible for his education and guidance; that responsibility lies in the first place with his parents.

The child shall have full opportunity for play and recreation, which shall be directed to the same purposes as education; society and the public authorities shall endeavor to promote the enjoyment of this right.

Principle 8

The child shall in all circumstances be among the first to receive protection and relief.

Principle 9

The child shall be protected against all forms of neglect, cruelty and exploitation. He shall not be the subject of traffic, in any form.

The child shall not be admitted to employment before an appropriate minimum age; he shall in no case be caused or permitted to engage in any occupation or employment which would prejudice his health or education, or interfere with his physical, mental or moral development.

Principle 10

The child shall be protected from practices which may foster racial, religious and any other form of discrimination. He shall be brought up in a spirit of understanding, tolerance, friendship among peoples, peace and universal brotherhood and in full consciousness that his energy and talents should be devoted to the service of his fellow men.

tinue participation at any time. Informed consent is an attempt to protect the child's best interests and should be obtained in writing.

Another major issue in research involving children is *truth in experimentation*. Deceitful research can have harmful effects on participants, and dishonesty about the purpose of research should be avoided. However, some studies would be impossible to conduct if participants knew all of the specific intents of a study. For example, a researcher who wants to study parent-child interactions for the purpose of predicting child abuse may have difficulty recruiting participants and obtaining unbiased data if purpose was given in detail. Researchers at times must develop descriptions of the study that are honest but may not reveal the entire purpose of the study. A request to participate in research that will "study parent-child relationships," for example, may be sufficient to generate parental approval and consent.

This example shows the overlapping nature of the ethical principles in research of children. It also suggests that gray areas exist to which standards are difficult to apply. Potential benefits of the research must be weighed against the risks to the children involved. Independent

boards of review are thus used to evaluate all aspects of the research proposal and to rule whether or not the research should be conducted. The combined judgment of several researchers serves to keep investigators keenly aware of the ethical issues in their study and promotes more ethical decision making.

Conducting research with children presents special challenges related to data collection.[20] Age and developmental considerations dictate the methodology that may be used to answer the research question. For example, infants and young children without verbal skills may be able to provide other indicators (such as physiological measures or behaviors) that may be used as indicators of the phenomenon being investigated. Innovative solutions often are needed to overcome the problems associated with collection of clinical data.

Because child health nurses view children and families holistically and care for them in numerous and diverse settings, they have endless opportunities to engage in nursing research. These investigations are vital to the continued improvement of care provided to children and their families. Fortunately, nursing administration is increasingly providing support for nursing investigations by approving a variety of research designs, by making resources available, and by integrating research expectations into performance criteria.[23]

Summary

Society's view of childhood has changed through the years, and the care and nurturance of children is considered an important function of the family. The past century has been a time of incredible advances in medical knowledge and technology, enabling health care providers to recognize and treat childhood ailments more effectively. Knowledge of child development processes and norms also has expanded, giving impetus to the notion of health as a multifaceted concept that incorporates social and physical dimensions. The possibility of children living long, productive, and healthy lives has dramatically improved, but much remains to be done to help more children reach their full potential.

Nurses, by virtue of their employment in a wide variety of health care systems and their commitment to providing holistic care, are in an opportune position to advance the cause of child health care. Nursing's interest in developing standards of practice and care speaks to a sense of responsibility for the quality of nursing care provided to children and their families. Furthermore, the sensitivity of nurses to ethical and legal aspects of child and family care helps to ensure that the child's rights and needs will be respected. As nursing knowledge continues to expand through the findings of well-designed research, and as the roles of nurses continue to expand, children and their families will benefit.

References

1. Badinter, E. (1982). *Mother love*. New York: Macmillan.
2. Brecht, M. (1989). The tragedy of infant mortality. *Nursing Outlook, 37*, 18–22.
3. Broadwell, D. (1983). Nursing specialization: The ET nurse. *Journal of Occupational Health Nursing, 31*, 15–19, 45.
4. Brodie, B. (1986). Yesterday, today, and tomorrow's pediatric world. *Children's Health Care, 14*, 168–173.
5. Bru, G. (1990). Using the revised APON standards of practice. *Journal of Pediatric Oncology Nursing, 7*, 17–30.
6. Case, N. K. (1988). Substituted judgment in the pediatric health care setting. *Issues in Comprehensive Pediatric Nursing, 11*, 303–312.
7. Cherry, B., & Carty, R. (1986). Changing concepts of childhood in society. *Pediatric Nursing, 12*(6), 421–424.
8. Clough, J. G. (1988). Making life and death decisions you can live with. *RN, 51*(5), 28–30.
9. Creighton, H. (1986). *Law every nurse should know*. Philadelphia: W.B. Saunders.
10. Dunst, C., et al. (1988). Enabling and empowering families of children with health impairments. *Children's Health Care, 17*, 71–81.
11. Feeg, V. D. (1990). The future of pediatric nursing: Anticipating the health care needs of children. *Imprint, 37*, 70, 72–73, 75, 77.
12. Fordham Institute for Innovation in Social Policy. (1989). *The index of social health*. Tarrytown, NY: Fordham University Graduate Center.
13. Fry, S. T. (1989). Toward a theory of nursing ethics. *Advances in Nursing Science, 11*(4), 9–22.
14. Halley, H. (1965). *Bible handbook*. Grand Rapids, MI: Zondervan.
15. Handmaker, S. D., & Stewart, E. S. (1988). Family-centered care. *Children's Health Care, 17*, 68–70.
16. Institute of Medicine. (1988). *Perinatal care: Reaching mothers, reaching infants*. Washington, DC: National Academy Press.
17. Kelly, M. E. (1987). Maternal and child health nursing. In C. Northrop & M. E. Kelly (Eds.). *Legal issues in nursing* (pp. 157–180). St. Louis: CV Mosby.
18. Kelly, M. E. (1987). Professional negligence overview. In C. Northrop & M. E. Kelly (Eds.). *Legal issues in nursing* (pp. 39–56). St. Louis: CV Mosby.
19. Koop, E. (1989). The health care nun. *Newsweek, CXIV*(9), 10.
20. Kotzer, A. M. (1990). Creative strategies for pediatric nursing research: Data collection. *Journal of Pediatric Nursing, 5*, 50–53.
21. Lane, K., & Peppe, K. (1987). Where are the standards? *Journal of Pediatric Nursing, 2*, 291–294.
22. Levine-Ariff, J., & Groh, D. (1990). *Creating an ethical environment*. Baltimore: Williams & Wilkins.
23. Lynn, M. R. (1990). Research commitment starts at the top. *Journal of Pediatric Nursing, 5*, 136–137.
24. National Safety Council. (1990). *Accident facts 1990 Edition*. Chicago: National Safety Council.
25. Nelkin, V. (1987). Family-centered health care for medically fragile children: Principles and practice. Washington, DC: Georgetown University, National Center for Networking Community Based Services.
26. Northrop, C., & Kelly, M. (1987). *Legal issues in nursing*. St. Louis: CV Mosby.
27. Reid, D. W. (1984). Participatory control and the chronic-illness adjustment process. In H. M. Lefcourd (Ed.). *Research with the locus of control construct: Vol. 2*. Orlando: Academic.
28. Rushton, C. H. (1988). Ethical decision making in critical care. Part 1: The role of the pediatric nurse. *Pediatric Nursing, 14*, 411–412.
29. Rushton, C. H. (1990). Family-centered care in the critical care setting: Myth or reality? *Children's Health Care, 19*, 68–78.

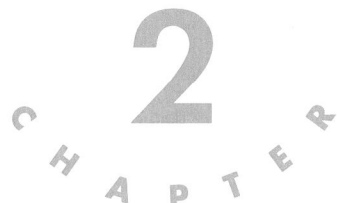

The Nursing Process

BEHAVIORAL OBJECTIVES

Trace the historic origins of the nursing process.

Distinguish between comprehensive and focused nursing assessment.

Explain the value of using functional health as the basis of nursing assessment.

Explain how nursing diagnosis is both an intellectual process and a statement of a health problem.

Differentiate between nursing diagnoses and collaborative problems.

Describe the relationship between client goals and evaluation of nursing care.

The approach to each child who needs nursing care is always unique. Contexts in which the nurse and child meet and individual differences among nurses and children ensure that nursing care for one person is never identical to that for another. This uniqueness does not mean, however, that no patterns exist in the general approach of providing nursing care for children. To the contrary, care is delivered in an organized, systematic manner, and the interactions among nurses and children can be conceptualized in a distinct series of phases known as the nursing process. In this chapter, the components of the nursing process are reviewed, with special attention given to applying the process in the care of children and their families.

Historic Origins of the Nursing Process

Early in the history of nursing, emphasis was placed on performing procedures for the ill to provide a clean environment, comfort, and safety. Florence Nightingale's early efforts to encourage a sound educational basis for the practice of nursing resulted in slow advancement toward a more conceptual approach to the provision of nursing care. After World War II and the tremendous growth in scientific knowledge and technology, nursing underwent rapid change in becoming firmly established as a profession.

One of the most arduous tasks nursing has faced as an emerging profession has been the clarification of what nursing is and does as a practice discipline. Numerous definitions of nursing have been developed, and they continue to be refined. One definition that has gained wide acceptance was presented by the American Nurses' Association in 1980: "Nursing is the diagnosis and treatment of human responses to actual or potential health problems."[2] This definition clearly emphasizes nursing's focus on the phenomena of human responses and not on the illness or health deviation. Some nursing scholars, however, believe that this definition is incomplete without recognition of the role that nurses play in the promotion of wellness.[16] To date, this issue remains unresolved.

As a practice, the delivery of nursing care has been compared to the scientific method because both require that data be collected and analyzed, problems be defined, alternative solutions be considered and tested, and evidence be evaluated. The scientific method, however, is generally considered to be an unbiased, value-free procedure. Human elements in nursing—people working with people—undeniably interject values and bias into nursing practice and require that nursing be considered an art as well as a science.

Although nursing practice can never be reduced to a pure scientific formula, distinct components of care can be identified. The nursing process was so named by Lydia Hall[9] in 1955 and has since been defined as "an organized, systematic method of giving individualized care that focuses on the unique human response of a person or group of people to an actual or potential alteration in health".[2 (p.6)] The nursing process was originally described in a variety of ways by different nurse scholars, but Yura and Walsh's 1967 text[19] portraying the nursing process as a four-step phenomena (assessment, planning, implementation, and evaluation) encouraged consistency in terminology. Today, most nursing leaders believe that nursing diagnosis also should be labeled as a distinct step to emphasize its importance to nursing. The authors of this text adhere to the argument that the nursing process should be discussed as a five-stage process: assessment, nursing diagnosis, planning, intervention, and evaluation.

Conceptual Models for Nursing Care

Although there is general agreement about the basic elements in the process of nursing, there is a diversity of views about the nurse and the nursing role, the person, health, and the environment. Several nurse scholars have developed models of nursing that define these basic concepts and explain interrelationships among them. These models of nursing are important in helping nurses define their roles and guide their collection and understanding of data. Models have been developed, for example, that focus on the life process (Rogers),[17] self-care agency (Orem),[14] adaptation (Roy),[18] behavioral systems (Johnson),[10] and goal attainment (King).[12] This text does not subscribe to a single model of nursing; rather, useful aspects from many different models have been integrated throughout.

Phases of the Nursing Process

A summary of the activities incorporated in each of the phases of the nursing process is presented in Table 2-1. In actual use of the nursing process, the phases are not always well-defined, because they often overlap. Likewise, different aspects of the process may be in place simultaneously as the nurse cares for the child and meets a variety of family needs. The phases of the nursing process are interdependent and interrelated. Therefore, the nursing process may be considered simple in description but complex in application.

Understanding the components of the nursing process encourages the delivery of thoughtful, organized, and effective care to children and their families. The quality of nursing care they receive is thereby improved. Furthermore, communication among members of the health-care team is enhanced when assessments, diagnoses, plans, interventions, and evaluations can be clearly articulated.

Assessment

During the assessment phase, information about the child is collected through a variety of methods to expose actual or potential health problems. On initial encounter with the child and family, the nurse generally does an interview and follows with a physical examination. Information may also be obtained from the records collected in the child's file or chart and from other members of the health-care team who are working with the child and family. Interactions between the child and parents, siblings, or other family members are particularly important and can provide valuable information in the assessment phase of the nursing process. Hence, observation of the child and family behaviors is ongoing as data are collected.

Two types of nursing assessment have been described by Alfaro.[1] The comprehensive assessment done on entry of the child into the health-care system is called "database running assessment" and provides a broad range of information about all aspects of the child's health. This database gives the contextual facts about the child and family that are important in understanding individual differences and needs.

TABLE 2-1
The Nursing Process:
Summary of Activities in Five Phases

Phase	Activity
Assessment	Collection of objective and subjective data about the child's health status from a variety of sources including history, physical examination, and records. Comprehensive and also focused on specific concerns.
Diagnosis	Identification of health problems through analysis of assessment data. Nursing diagnoses are statements of actual, high-risk, or possible health problems that can be treated by nurses independently. Other problems require collaboration with physician.
Planning	Establishment of priorities, setting goals, and writing nursing orders in response to the child's health problems.
Intervention	Use of nursing strategies to help child and family meet goals related to resolving health problems. Nursing orders carried out. Actions may be taken independently or in collaboration with physician's medical plan.
Evaluation	Determination of effectiveness of nursing care plan in assisting the child and family in meeting health goals. Both outcomes and processes are analyzed.

The second type of assessment uses clues from the comprehensive database that actual and potential health problems exist. "Focus assessment" may be started during the initial interview with the child and family to gather more information about a specific concern, but it also is used in subsequent encounters with the child and family to explore further the status of specific problems.

The distinction between comprehensive and focused assessment may be seen in the following example. During the initial interview for comprehensive information, the nurse inquires about the school-age child's patterns of sleep. The child indicates that nighttime sleep is often interrupted several times a week, followed by extreme fatigue the next day. This revelation calls for focused assessment, which may be started at the initial interview and may include how long the problem has existed and how the family manages the episodes. Later, however, as rapport with the child and family builds, the nurse explores the problem in greater depth, seeking clues that assist in making an accurate diagnosis of the child's problem.

Child and Family History Using Functional Health

Although numerous forms and guides have been developed to assist the nurse in collecting data for the comprehensive assessment, the use of functional health patterns has been presented as a standard assessment format that can be used for all clients in all settings.[8] Use of the functional health as a guide for assessment encourages a holistic view of the child and family and permits the identification of both function and dysfunction. This approach to assessment can be used universally, regardless of the nurse's theoretical or philosophic beliefs.[6]

Understanding the use of the functional health typology requires recognition that characteristics of behavior across time are of interest to the interviewer. Although discrete events and responses to health-related issues cannot be overlooked or ignored, the general patterns of behavior that children and families have in responding to those events are of greater significance. Clinical decisions are based on an understanding of how the child and family usually respond to a particular health concern rather than on a single observation or piece of information. The use of functional health as the basis for assessment ensures that data collection is extensive enough to guide accurate evaluation of the child and family's health status.

Gordon's[8] typology of eleven functional health patterns is presented in Table 2-2. Information obtained about these eleven patterns provides an understanding of the complex functioning of the child and family being assessed. Biologic functioning is incorporated, as are aspects of human growth and development, and influences from the environment. The functional health assessment format is easy to learn to use and encourages the movement from the database to nursing diagnosis in the nursing process.

When functional health typology is used for assessment of infants, children, and young adolescents, the questions and observations originally designed for use

TABLE 2-2
Gordon's Functional Health Patterns

Health perception-health management pattern	Describes client's perceived pattern of health and well-being and how health is managed
Nutritional-metabolic pattern	Describes pattern of food and fluid consumption relative to metabolic need and pattern indicators of local nutrient supply
Elimination pattern	Describes pattern of excretory function (bowel, bladder, and skin)
Activity-exercise pattern	Describes pattern of exercise, activity, leisure, and recreation
Cognitive-perceptual pattern	Describes sensory-perceptual and cognitive pattern
Sleep-rest pattern	Describes pattern of sleep, rest, and relaxation
Self perception-self concept pattern	Describes self-concept pattern and perceptions of self (e.g., body comfort, body image, feeling state)
Role-relationship pattern	Describes pattern of role-engagements and relationships
Sexuality-reproductive pattern	Describes client's patterns of satisfaction and dissatisfaction with sexuality pattern; describes reproductive patterns
Coping-stress tolerance pattern	Describes general coping pattern and effectiveness of the pattern in terms of stress tolerance
Value-belief pattern	Describes patterns of values, beliefs (including spiritual), or goals that guide choices or decisions

Gordon, M. (1987). *Nursing diagnosis—Process and application* (2nd ed.), (p. 93). New York: McGraw-Hill.

with adults must be adapted. For example, the nursing interview may be conducted with a parent or guardian if the child is too young to give information. Children's views are elicited as they develop communication skills. Furthermore, assessments are made with acute awareness of developmental norms and environmental influences. Taking the example mentioned above, for example, frequent night waking would not be considered unusual for an infant, but the problem is not considered "normal" in the older school-age child. A guide that may be used to elicit comprehensive information from the parents or guardian and the child about the eleven functional health patterns is outlined in the display.

Physical Examination

The nursing physical examination, another means of expanding the comprehensive database on the child, typically follows the interview in which functional health is assessed. Learning to perform a thorough, systematic examination of the child requires practice under the guidance of an experienced practitioner. The novice examiner develops an organized approach to the physical assessment that is refined as competence in techniques develops. Chapter 9 provides a description of the complete physical examination of the infant and child, and focused examinations for problems within a given system are described in later chapters.

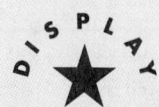

Guidelines for Using Assessment of Functional Health Patterns With Children

A parent report is used until the child can answer the items. The nurse should be familiar with the format and questions so judgment can be rendered in selecting items to be used in the assessment. The age of the child and the reason for seeking entry into the health-care system help determine which questions are appropriate.

I. Health perception-health management pattern
   A. For all children
      1. How is your child's heatlh in general?
      2. How is your child's health today?
      3. What do you do to keep your child well?
         a. Nutrition
         b. Opportunities for exercise and play
         c. Professional health care
         d. Immunization status
         e. Any regular medication? What are they? What is their purpose?
   B. For the hospitalized or ill child
      1. Why was your child admitted to the hospital?
         a. What caused the illness/injury?
         b. When did the illness begin?
      2. What treatment is your child receiving? What is your understanding of the purpose of the treatment? How do you think the treatment is working?
      3. Has your child ever been hospitalized before? For what reason? How did that go for you and the child?
      4. What expectations do you have about this hospitalization?
      5. Do you anticipate any problems in caring for your child at home? What are the anticipated problems?
   C. For both well and ill children: complete for all children under 24 months of age and when appropriate because of related problems (e.g., developmental disabilities, complications of prematurity, and so forth)
      1. Did the mother have prenatal care? How long?
      2. Did the mother take any medications during pregnancy?
      3. Were there any complications during pregnancy?
      4. What were the infant's birth weight and length?
      5. What was the length of gestation?
      6. Were there any complications with the infant during the first month of life?

II. Nutritional-metabolic pattern
   A. How is the child's appetite?
   B. Describe a typical day for your child in terms of what is eaten and drunk at meals and snacks.
      1. Breast-fed
         a. How often?
         b. How long at each feeding?
         c. Any difficulties?
         d. Plans for continuing or weaning
      2. Formula-fed
         a. Name of formula?
         b. Number of feedings in 24 hours?
         c. Amount of formula at each feeding?
         d. Any difficulties perceived?
         e. Plans for continuing or weaning
      3. Solid foods
         a. When begun?
         b. Food groups child eats?
         c. Approximate amounts at each meal?
         d. Describe a typical after-school snack
      4. General
         a. Are there any food restrictions or special diet due to allergies, intolerances, other health problems, or religious practice?
         b. What vitamins and/or supplments does the child take?
         c. How much milk does the child drink in 24 hours?
         d. Does the child use a bottle or cup?
   C. What are the child's special food likes and dislikes?
   D. How often does the child go to "fast-food" restaurants?
   E. How much candy, other sweets, processed snack foods, and soda does your child eat/drink?
   F. What, if any, concerns do you have about your child's appetite, feeding behavior, or diet?

III. Elimination pattern
   A. Bowel
      1. How many stools does your child have daily?
      2. What is the color, amount, and consistency?
      3. Is the child toilet-trained?
      4. Does the child ever need laxatives, enemas, or suppositories? How often? How do you decide that one of the above is necessary?
      5. What is the usual colostomy/ileostomy care (if applicable)?
   B. Bladder
      1. Does your child have any problems with urination?
         a. Bed-wetting (enuresis)
         b. Burning or other dysuria
         c. Dribbling
         d. Oliguria
         e. Polyuria
         f. Urinary retention
      2. Are any assistive devices used?
         a. Intermittent catheterization
         b. Indwelling catheter
         c. Stoma for urinary drinage—describe routine of care

(Continued)

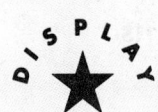

Guidelines for Using Assessment of Functional Health Patterns With Children (continued)

3. Is the child toilet-trained?
   a. Daytime
   b. Nightime
   c. Accidents?
C. Skin—Does your child ever have any trouble with his or her skin (e.g., itching, swelling, rashes, sores, acne, color, or temperature changes)? Describe.

IV. Activity-exercise pattern
A. Gross motor abilities
   1. When did your child roll over? Sit unsupported? Walk alone? Climb stairs? Ride tricycle? and so forth. (Obtain information appropriate to child's age and developmental abilities)
   2. What sports/exercise does your child enjoy and participate in?
   3. What, if any, concerns do you have about your child's abilities in these areas?
B. Fine motor abilities
   1. Does your baby reach for things? Grasp? Transfer objects from one hand to another? Use fingers to pick up objects? Feed self a cracker? Use a spoon?
   2. What hobbies does your child have?
   3. What, if any, concerns do you have about your child's abilities to use his or her hands?
C. Self-care abilities or activities
   1. How independent is your child in self-feeding? Describe the help needed, if any.
   2. How much help does your child need with toileting? If assistive devices are used, is child independent or is help needed? Describe. Does child use diapers, a potty chair, or toilet?
   3. How much help does your child need with dressing (buttons, ties, zippers, and so forth)?
   4. How much help does your child need with hygiene practices (bathing, brushing teeth, and so forth)? Is a shower or tub bath preferred?

V. Sleep-rest pattern
A. How many hours does the child sleep each 24 hours?
   1. At night
   2. Naps
B. What is the child's usual sleep routine?
   1. Bedtime
   2. Naptime
   3. Rituals (stories, drink, and so forth)
   4. Security object(s)
C. Are there any problems related to sleep?
   1. Nightmares, night terrors
   2. Difficulty falling asleep
   3. Refusal at bedtime
   4. Waking up during night

VI. Cognitive-perceptual pattern
A. Does the child have any sensory perception deficits (hearing, smell, sight, touch)? Describe.
B. What grade in school is child?
   1. How does child do in school?
   2. What, if any, problems are perceived by parent, teacher, or child relative to school achievement?

VII. Self-perception pattern
A. How has your child's illness made you feel? What are you most concerned about?
B. For school-age and adolescent child: How does your illness (injury) make you feel? What are you most concerned about?
C. For well older school-age child and adolescent: How do you feel about yourself?

VIII. Role-relationship pattern
A. Communication
   1. Language development
      a. When did child coo? Babble? Say words? Phrases? Sentences? Use pronouns? (Use questions appropriate to child's age and developmental abilities).
      b. Does the child use language appropriate for age?
      c. What, if any, concerns do you have about your child's language development or characteristics of speech?
   2. What language is spoken at home?
B. Relationships
   1. Describe family life
      a. Composition of household (family members, ages)
      b. Cultural background
      c. Roles
      d. Occupations and educational background of adults
      e. Decision-making patterns
      f. Communication patterns
      g. Discipline
      h. Problems (e.g., finances, family violence, problems with parenting, marital problems)
   2. Peer relationships
      a. Does your child play with other children? Describe the quality of the child's play (e.g., solitary, parallel, interactive, cooperative, aggressive).
      b. Does the child have a "best friend" of the same sex? Belong to a "gang"?
      c. Does your child prefer playmates who are older, younger, same age?
      d. Does your child have imaginary playmates?
      e. What concerns, if any, do you have about your child's relationships with others?

(Continued)

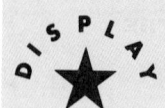

Guidelines for Using Assessment of Functional Health Patterns With Children (continued)

IX. Sexuality-reproductive pattern
   A. What interest does your child show in sexuality/sexual function? How do you feel about this? How do you handle your child's curiosity and behavior?
   B. For adolescent, assess:
      1. Knowledge of sexual functioning
      2. Sexual activity
      3. Use of contraceptives
      4. History of pregnancy
      5. Feelings about opposite sex
X. Coping-stress managment pattern
   A. How do you make decisions? (alone? with whom?)
   B. Have there been any losses or changes in your life in the past year? In your child's (e.g., move,

death of significant other or pet, loss of parental job)?
   C. To whom do you turn for support and help when you are feeling stressed?
   D. How do you manage child care, housework, and other responsibilities? For the teenager: How do you manage schoolwork, sports, and other activities, and work responsibilities?
   E. What can the nurses do to help you during this hospitalization?
XI. Value-belief system
   A. What religious affiliation or preference do you hold?
   B. Is there a religious person or practice (diet, book, ritual) that you desire during your child's hospitalization?

Carpenito, L. J. (1992). Nursing diagnosis: Application to clinical practice *(4th ed.), (pp. 1063–1067). Philadelphia: J. B. Lippincott.*

Record Review

Additional information may be added to the comprehensive database by studying records already compiled for the child. If the child has been incorporated into the health-care system prior to seeing the nurse, the records should be consulted *before* the child and family are approached for an interview or physical examination. A careful review of the records yields valuable information that guides the collection of additional information, and it assists the nurse in avoiding unnecessary repetition of questions answered earlier. The nurse should be thoroughly familiar with all the laboratory studies, x-ray reports, medical history, progress notes, physician's orders, and consultation notes available. Likewise, documentation previously provided by nurses about the child and family should be studied carefully (Fig. 2-1).

Additional Resources

Other resources besides the child, family, and records may be used to develop a more comprehensive database. All providers involved in health care of the child and family may be approached to discuss their observations, findings, and impressions. Social workers, physical therapists, and play therapists, for example, can frequently provide unique information that is essential to delivering holistic nursing care. Finally, written resources in the form of texts, reference books, and professional journals provide valuable information that may be applied to the assessment process. These resources are indispensable to novice nurses as they strive for synthesis and integration of their learning.

The data gathered during initial and ongoing interactions with the child and family may be extensive. Data can be organized by using forms provided by the agency where the child and nurse meet. Agency procedures may require that data be specified as subjective or objective data. Objective data are those that the nurse has observed. For example, information about physical appearance, behavior, vital signs, and laboratory values is concrete and unbiased (objective) data. Subjective data are provided by the child or family and typically refer to their feelings and perceptions. Subjective data may not always be validated by objective data. Quotation marks are used to identify subjective data in written documentation.

Nursing Diagnosis

When the assessment data have been collected and organized, they must be analyzed to identify health problems that can be treated by nursing actions. Theoretical knowledge possessed by the nurse, as well as knowledge acquired through planned clinical activities, is used in thoughtfully studying the database for significant information. Impressions are formed regarding child and family strengths and limitations in patterns of health functioning, and evidence is extracted from the database to support the existence of actual or potential alterations in health. Therefore, nursing diagnosis may be considered both an intellectual process and a statement of a health problem.

Problem Identification: Data Analysis and Conclusions

Analysis is a complex mental process that requires information to be sorted and comparisons to be made between the evidence presented by the child or family and accepted norms. Developing the cognitive skill of

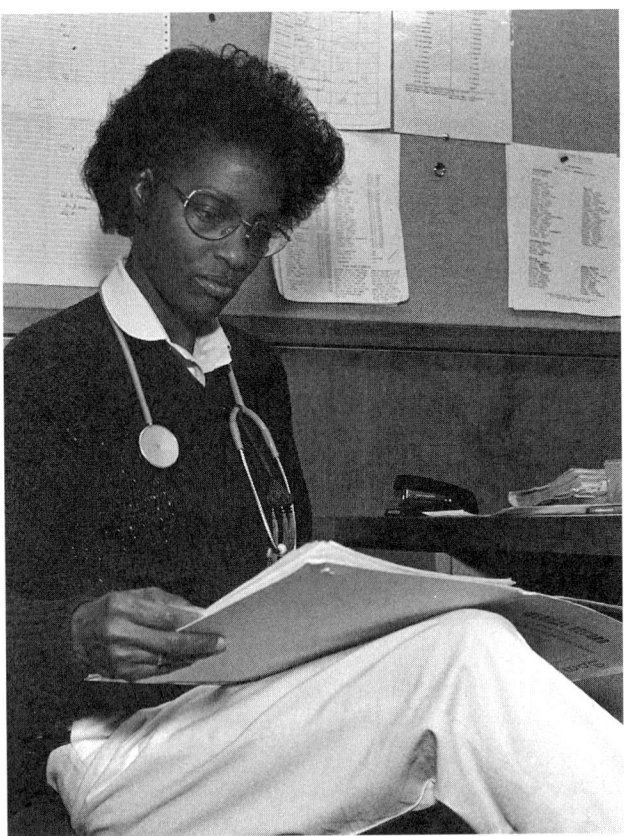

FIGURE 2-1
The nurse reviews records, notes, physician's orders, and other documentation before interviewing or performing a physical examination on the child. (Photo by Kathy Sloane.)

analysis requires patience, practice, and willingness to use the many resources available. Often, written references and other professionals need to be consulted to assist in the data analysis. Above all, a broad view must be taken that gives careful, fair consideration of the data. A hasty leap to conclusive diagnoses jeopardizes the quality of nursing care the child and family receive.

After the data have been analyzed, one of three conclusions may be drawn.[6] First, no health problems may be identified; rather, the child and family may be encouraged to continue using health promotion activities. Nursing's traditional emphasis on wellness and health promotion activities has not been recognized in the classification system for nursing diagnoses.[15] Yet, the North American Nursing Diagnosis Association (NANDA) has encouraged exploration of the issues involved and at their 1988 Conference approved "health-seeking behaviors" as a nursing diagnosis for clinical use and testing.[7] The philosophic debate about wellness-oriented nursing diagnoses has not been resolved, and some believe that health promotion nursing interventions should simply be related to personal outcome goals, not nursing diagnoses.[5]

A second conclusion that may be drawn from analysis of the assessment data is the identification of a problem requiring collaboration with other members of the health-care team (primarily physicians). A collaborative problem is "an actual or potential health problem (complication) that focuses on the physiologic responses of the body (to

trauma, disease, diagnostic studies, or treatment modalities)," that requires both medical and nursing skills to assist in the resolution of the problem.[1] Whenever pathology is present, children may need monitoring to detect onset and changes in the status of complications. These interventions are appropriately included in the domain of nursing, but they are directly linked to the medical diagnosis and treatment plan.

The third conclusion that may be drawn from analysis of the data is that a nursing diagnosis is warranted. The nursing diagnosis describes the "actual or potential health problem that focuses on the human response of a person or group, and that nurses are responsible and accountable for identifying and treating independently."[1 (p.66)] Actual health problems can be validated by the presence of signs and symptoms in the child, and these defining characteristics have been carefully identified by NANDA. The defining characteristics for each nursing diagnosis are published in proceedings of the NANDA conferences (see Carroll-Johnson,[7] for example) and may also be found in texts such as one written by Carpenito.[6]

At times, nurses collect assessment data indicating that the person is more vulnerable to develop a certain health problem than others in similar circumstances. However, defining characteristics of actual problems cannot yet be specified. These potential health problems can be identified with the statement of a "high-risk" nursing diagnosis. This type diagnosis calls for nursing measures that prevent the actual occurrence of health problems.

Sometimes, the nurse suspects that a child has a particular problem; yet, more information is needed to confirm or rule out a nursing diagnosis. Although defining characteristics of the problem are not present, the nurse recognizes certain cues, senses that a problem may exist, and believes that additional exploration of the health pattern should occur. In these instances, a notation regarding a "possible" nursing diagnosis is appropriate.

The discussion of actual, high-risk, and possible nursing diagnoses accurately suggests that developing nursing diagnoses can be a complex process. To further complicate matters, nurses may identify a cluster of actual or high-risk diagnoses that are needed to describe the child's situation. NANDA has used the term "syndrome nursing diagnosis" to describe this phenomenon.[6] The use of this term emphasizes the broad impact of the problem yet avoids the use of many separate nursing diagnoses.

Development of Nursing Diagnoses

Nursing diagnoses of actual problems consists of three parts and may be presented in the "Problem, Etiology, Symptoms" (P E S) format suggested by Gordon.[8] The statement of the diagnostic label, the health problem (P), is followed by etiologic or related factors (E) that have been identified as contributing to the child's health problem. These factors may be related to the child's physiologic functioning, level of maturation, current personal or environmental situation, or to treatments already being given. Finally, the defining characteristics, which are the major criteria for each possible diagnostic judgment, need to be specified. These signs and symptoms

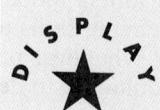

Sample Nursing Diagnosis Written for an Actual Problem in the Problem, Etiology, Symptom (P E S) Format

Actual Nursing Diagnosis

"Impaired skin integrity
    related to
immobility and body cast
    as manifested by
erythema and itching of sacral area."

High-Risk Diagnosis

"High risk for impaired skin integrity
    related to
immobility secondary to body cast."

Three Components

Problem (diagnostic category)
Etiology (contributing
    factors)
Symptom (signs and symptoms)

Two Components

Problem (diagnostic category)
Etiology (contributing
    factors)

(S) have been identified as the essential measure by which the diagnosis may be made, but often additional subjective and objective data can be provided to support the nursing judgment. An example of a nursing diagnosis written in the P E S format is presented in the first part of the display.

Unlike diagnoses for actual health problems, high-risk and possible nursing diagnoses are stated in a two-part statement. The problem at risk is identified (P), followed by etiologic or related factors (E). Instead of signs and symptoms, however, the risk factors are identified as validation of the diagnosis. The second part of the display gives an example of a high-risk nursing diagnosis. The combination of the diagnostic label with contributing factors allows validation of the nursing diagnosis and provides guidance in designing nursing interventions.

Another variation in the development of nursing diagnostic statements is needed when wellness or syndrome nursing diagnoses are justified. In these cases, a one-part statement consisting only of the diagnostic label (P) is used. Phrases concerning etiology and supporting signs and symptoms are omitted. Alfaro,[1] Carpenito,[6] or others may be consulted for more assistance in the development of nursing diagnostic statements.

Nursing diagnoses that lead to independent action should be distinguished from collaborative problems that necessitate the physician's input. Both activities are expected and should be included in the plan for child and family care. Professional nursing legitimately incorporates both types of activities.

The list of health problems diagnosed and treated independently by nurses is not considered complete. New nursing diagnoses are reviewed regularly by NANDA. Acceptance of the diagnoses by the organization simply indicates that the categories are developed enough to be tested clinically. Ongoing refinement of the categories may be expected in the years ahead, especially with consideration of health promotion and illness prevention di-

agnoses. The 1990 list of nursing diagnoses (which include only the "P" statement) have been placed in the functional health patterns categories by Carpenito[6] and are listed in the display on p. 28. Other sources may be consulted for listing of collaborative nursing problems and more discussion regarding nursing diagnoses.

Planning

In the third phase of the nursing process, a plan of care must be devised to address each nursing diagnosis. Likewise, collaborative problems demand attention. The plan for care requires that priorities be set, goals be developed, and nursing orders be written.

Priorities

Learning to assess situations for the purpose of setting priorities in planning care is essential for the contemporary nurse. The nursing shortage and the rising acuity of problems children and their families exhibit in the health-care system demand that nurses become more efficient and effective in their delivery of care. Unfortunately, the setting of priorities often is difficult because of the complex nature of the problems that have been identified.

At times, several health problems need attention simultaneously, and the inexperienced nurse may be unable to determine how to choose among the options. Relationships between one problem and another may also be recognized and make planning for nursing care even more difficult. The hierarchy of human needs described by Maslow[13] or Kalish[11] may help the inexperienced nurse determine which problems need to be addressed first. Certainly, problems that are life-threatening or are contributing to a crisis situation need to be addressed immediately, and less critical problems follow. Novice nurses should not hesitate to ask faculty or other nurses who have advanced experience for assistance in setting priorities.

Client Goals

After priorities for care have been determined, client goals are stated. Ideally, the child and family have been active in providing assessment data and continue providing input in the planning phase of care. Stating desired goals for the client to achieve becomes the joint responsibility of the child–family unit and the nurse. Establishing goals gives clear direction for nursing interactions with children and families, and provides an unmistakable measure of achievement.

Client goals provide a statement of criteria to determine changes that occur in the child's status after nursing care has been provided. The goals are written in measurable terms (i.e., specific behaviors that can be observed are identified). The conditions under which each behavior is expected to occur are stated, and a definite time frame is given. Simply stated, "who, what, how, and when" are written. An example of a client goal is: By the end of the second postoperative day (when), the child (who) is able to walk to the nurses' desk and back to his room (what) without assistance (how).

Stating goals to be achieved when a nursing diagnosis for an actual health problem has been recognized should be a relatively straightforward procedure. Problems arise in stating goals, however, when there are collaborative problems or when the nurse suspects that a health problem exists but needs additional data to rule out or confirm a nursing diagnosis. In these instances, the specific response expected to result from nursing care may be impossible to determine. Therefore, client goals should be stated for only actual or high-risk nursing diagnoses, and they may be omitted for collaborative problems or possible nursing diagnoses.[6]

Determination of appropriate client goals may be facilitated by consulting the available standards of care. Acceptable standards of care are influenced by nurse practice acts, professional nursing organizations, and the institution in which care is to be given. Standards of care available within the institution where the child and family are receiving care give detailed guidelines about interventions typically used in selected patient situations. Although standards of care are not part of the child's permanent record, they encourage efficiency by detailing routine interventions that the nurse is expected to provide.

Nursing Goals

Nurses may be required to distinguish between goals that have been set for the child and family to achieve and goals that the nurse hopes to accomplish in caring for the child and family. Carpenito[6] has clarified that client goals refer to outcomes whereas nursing goals focus on the processes nurses use to achieve those goals. Although the recognition of nursing goals is important, and their identification can promote high-quality nursing care, they generally are not written on the plan of care.

Short-Term and Long-Term Goals

Distinctions are often made between short-term and long-term goals for children and families. Short-term goals can be achieved quickly, perhaps in less than a week. Long-term goals may be difficult to achieve in acute care settings where length of stay has been drastically reduced in recent years. Many long-term goals are achieved in the weeks or months after discharge. Clear communication about goals for the child and family among nurses in the various settings in which the child will be seen enhances verification that goals have been achieved.

Nursing Orders

After client goals and criteria for measuring their achievement have been determined, nursing orders are developed. These specific directions for care refer to the alterations in functional health patterns that were identified earlier in the nursing process. In the P E S format used to develop nursing diagnoses, the "E" (etiologic factors) is the basis for the nursing orders. Nursing orders state the activities required to eliminate or modify factors contributing to the problem. Nursing orders specify the interventions needed to achieve the desired outcomes of care for the child, whether for nursing diagnoses or collaborative problems.

Written Plan

The nursing care plan is designed to accomplish several goals.[3] First, the written care plan facilitates individualized care. Specific health problems can be addressed by nursing orders designed to meet unique needs and circumstances. Second, the care plan gives guidance to members of the nursing team so that consistent, coordinated care is provided for the child and family. Third, the nursing care plan promotes communication among nurses and other members of the health-care team. Finally, the written care plan is useful in guiding the evaluation of the effectiveness of nursing care provided for the child and family.

In the clinical setting, the written plan for care of the child and family takes many forms. *Kardex care plans* typically contain current nursing orders and are altered as the status of the child changes. The Kardex care plan is readily available while the child is hospitalized; however, it is not part of the permanent record. *Standardized care plans* are similar to standards of care, but the standardized care plans are kept as part of the child's permanent chart, and they are designed to allow individualization of goals and interventions.[6]

Computerized care plans use stored memory in generating a care plan for individual children. These automatic systems produce plans similar to standardized care plans. Care plans from the computer also can be individualized by entering data unique to the child. The fact that computerized care plans are easy to update or revise encourages accurate and complete documentation of nursing care.

The individualized written nursing care plan typically required by nursing education programs are rarely required by employing agencies. The time needed to de-

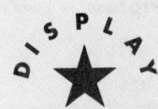

Health Perception—Health Management
  Growth & Development, Altered
  Health Maintenance, Altered
  Health Seeking Behaviors
  Noncompliance
  High Risk for Injury
    High Risk for Suffocation
    High Risk for Poisoning
    High Risk for Trauma
Nutritional—Metabolic
  Body Temperature, High Risk for Altered
    Hypothermia
    Hyperthermia
    Thermoregulation, Ineffective
  Fluid Volume Deficit
  Fluid Volume Excess
  Infection, High Risk for
  ‡Infection Transmission, High Risk for
  Nutrition, Altered: Less than Body Requirements
  Nutrition, Altered: More than Body
    Requirements
  Nutrition, Altered: High Risk for More than Body
    Requirements
    †Breastfeeding, Effective
    Breastfeeding, Ineffective
    Swallowing, Impaired
  †Protection, Altered
    Tissue Integrity, Impaired
      Oral Mucous Membrane, Altered
      Skin Integrity, Impaired
Elimination
  †Bowel Elimination, Altered
    Constipation
    Colonic Constipation
    Perceived Constipation
    Diarrhea
    Bowel Incontinence
  Urinary Elimination, Altered Patterns of
    Urinary Retention
    Total Incontinence
    Funtional Incontinence
    Reflex Incontinence
    Urge Incontinence
    Stress Incontinence
    ‡Maturational Enuresis
Activity—Exercise
  Activity Intolerance
  Cardiac Output, Decreased
  Disuse Syndrome, High Risk for
  Diversional Activity Deficit
  Home Maintenance Management, Impaired
  Mobility, Impaired Physical
  ‡Respiratory Function, Potential Altered
    Ineffective Airway Clearance
    Ineffective Breathing Patterns
    Impaired Gas Exchange
  Self-Care Deficit Syndrome
  (Specify) ‡(Instrumental, Feeding, Bathing/Hy-
    giene, Dressing/Grooming, Toileting)

Tissue Perfusion, Altered (Specify Type) (Cere-
    bral, Cardiopulmonary, Renal, Gastrointes-
    tinal, Peripheral)
Sleep—Rest
  Sleep Pattern Disturbance
Cognitive—Perceptual
  ‡Comfort, Altered
    Pain
    Chronic Pain
  Decisional Conflict
  Dysreflexia
  Knowledge Deficit (specify)
  High Risk for Aspiration
  Sensory–Perceptual Alterations: (Specify) (Vi-
    sual, Auditory, Kinesthetic, Gustatory, Tac-
    tile, Olfactory)
  Thought Processes, Altered
  Unilateral Neglect
Self-Perception
  Anxiety
  Fatigue
  Fear
  Hopelessness
  Powerlessness
  †Self-Concept Disturbance
    Body Image Disturbance
    Personal Identity Disturbance
    Self-Esteem Disturbance
      Chronic Low Self-Esteem
      Situational Low Self-Esteem
Role—Relationship
  ‡Communication, Impaired
    Communication, Impaired Verbal
  Family Processes, Altered
  ‡Grieving
    Grieving, Anticipatory
    Grieving, Dysfunctional
  Parenting, Altered
  Parental Role Conflict
  Role Performance, Altered
  Social Interaction, Impaired
  Social Isolation
Sexuality—Reproductive
  Sexual Dysfunction
  Sexuality Patterns, Altered
Coping—Stress Tolerance
  Adjustment, Impaired
  Coping, Ineffective Individual
    Defensive Coping
    Ineffective Denial
  Coping: Disabling, Ineffective Family
  Coping: Compromised, Ineffective Family
  Coping: Potential for Growth, Family
  Post Trauma Response
    Rape Trauma Syndrome
  ‡Self-Harm, High Risk for
  Violence, High Risk for
Value—Belief
  Spiritual Distress

* The Functional Health Patterns were identified by M. Gordon in Nursing diagnosis: Process and application (New York, McGraw-Hill, 1982) with minor changes by the author.
† These diagnoses were accepted by the North American Nursing Diagnosis Association in 1990.
‡ These diagnoses are not currently on the NANDA list but have been included for clarity and usefulness.
Adapted from Carpenito, L. J. (1992). Nursing diagnosis: Application to clinical practice (4th ed.), (pp. 7–9).

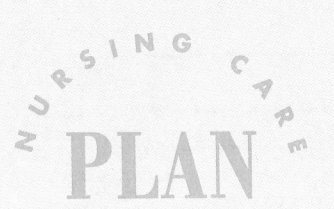

Nursing Care Plan Format and Components Used in This Text

Assessment

Case Study Description   A brief case history of a child and family is related to chapter content.

Assessment Data   Assessment data are presented to permit identification of defining characteristics needed to develop nursing diagnoses.

Nursing Diagnosis	**Intervention**	**Rationale**
The problem statement of the nursing diagnosis is followed by data that support the selection of the nursing diagnosis.	Both independent and collaborative nursing interventions that could be used in managing the health problem are identified.	The choice of nursing intervention is explained.

Evaluation

Measurable behaviors that may validate that the nursing interventions have affected the status of the health problem are listed. A specific time frame is omitted.

---

velop materials that are often repetitive from one child to another is difficult to justify. Writing a plan of care is a valuable experience for the novice nurse, however, because it gives an opportunity to clarify thinking about the nursing process and to demonstrate the application of theory to practice.

Written care plans have been liberally provided in this text to illustrate how nursing care is planned for the children discussed in the case studies. The format used in the written care plans developed for this text appears in this sample Nursing Care Plan. A brief description of content found in each section of the plan is included.

Intervention

After assessments have been made, nursing diagnoses have been established, and the plan for care has been formulated, the implementation phase of the nursing process begins. In this phase, specific nursing interventions are carried out to assist the child and family to achieve the goals they agreed on. Nursing interventions are directed by the nursing orders that were developed for both independent nursing diagnoses and collaborative health problems.

Independent Interventions

Independent nursing interventions are those activities performed by the nurse without a physician's order. Professional nurses provide these interventions by virtue of their education and experience. Identification of all the nurse-initiated, independent functions that nurses perform in providing care to children and their families is the subject of ongoing investigation. Bulechek and McCloskey,[4] however, have identified several independent nursing interventions that can assist the nurse in providing maximum care to children and their families (Table 2-3). More empiric testing is needed to establish guidelines for the use of these interventions.

Collaborative Interventions

Nursing interventions for collaborative problems evolve from the child's pathophysiologic condition and the medical treatment plan. These actions are physician-initiated and include monitoring of the child's status to detect changes and recognize potential complications. Consultation with the physician and other members of the health-care team, such as a physical therapist, dietitian, or respiratory therapist, is often required. The necessity of providing accurate and conscientious nursing interventions for collaborative health problems cannot be overemphasized.

Nursing care for children is implemented in many settings. This text includes chapters on the care of children in ambulatory settings (Chap. 22), in hospitals (Chap. 23), and in the home (Chap. 24). The delivery of nursing interventions is influenced not only by the setting, but also by many other factors including cultural and economic considerations (Chap. 4) and ethical and legal

TABLE 2-3
Examples of Independent Nursing Interventions

Intervention	Description
Active listening	Conscious attending to messages sent by a client to recognize behavior cues that may indicate a health problem
Advocacy	Actions taken on behalf of a client in providing holistic, humanistic nursing care
Assertiveness training	Systematic approach to effective self-expression in a socially appropriate manner
Cognitive reappraisal	Conscious mental processes used to change client perceptions of a situation
Counseling	Interactive helping process characterized by acceptance, empathy, genuineness, and congruency
Culture brokerage	Bridging, negotiating, or linking of orthodox health-care systems with clients of different cultures
Crisis intervention	Systematic problem-solving process to resolve a state of psychologic emergency
Discharge planning	Activities initiated soon after admission to a health-care setting to facilitate continuity of care
Exercise counseling	Therapeutic interactions between the nurse and client to acheive goals related to activity
Group psychotherapy	Interactions among the nurse and several clients to achieve understanding and treatment of interpersonal conflicts
Music therapy	Use of rhythmic, harmonic, and melodic sounds to attain therapeutic goals
Nutritional counseling	Therapeutic interactions between the nurse and client to achieve goals related to foods
Patient contracting	Establishment of mutually acceptable terms for the purpose of changing client behavior
Preoperative teaching	Supportive and educational actions that promote self-health of clients who anticipate an operative procedure
Patient teaching	Use of environmental stimuli to achieve a new thought, skill, attitude, or intention that contributes to change in behavior
Preparatory sensory information	Provision of information about threatening or stressful health-care events before the experience to enhance coping
Presence	Physical and psychologic availability to assist a client in meeting health-care needs
Relaxation training	Internal and external techniques used to produce a health response to stress
Reminiscence therapy	Recall of past experiences to achieve a higher level of wellness
Role supplementation	Therapeutic interactions to improve role transitions and prevent role insufficiency
Self-modification	Application of principles of conditioned learning to help clients make voluntary changes in aspects of their own behavior
Sexual counseling	Use of therapeutic interactions between the nurse and client to achieve goals related to sexuality and body image
Support groups	Provision of social support through the use of a group environment to acheive a mutual goal
Surveillance	Application of behavioral and cognitive processes to collect information systematically for making judgments and predictions about a client's life status
Truth telling	Using honesty in nurse–client interactions to promote client involvement in health care
Values clarification	Techniques used to assist clients to recognize their attitudes, beliefs, and opinions as the basis of making decisions

Adapted from Bulechek, G. M., & McCloskey, J. C. (1985) *Nursing interventions: Treatments for nursing diagnoses.* Philadelphia: W. B. Saunders.

considerations (Chap. 1). The knowledge and skills needed in providing nursing interventions are acquired through the nursing education process in which theoretical content and clinical activities are correlated.

Information about the specific nursing interventions used in the care of the child and family need to be documented as carefully as other aspects of the nursing process. The written care plan, however, may not be used for this purpose. Instead, interventions are often recorded on flowsheets, graphic charts, nurses' progress notes, and other formats designed by the agency. Documenting that nursing orders have been executed accurately is an essential aspect of the nurse's professional responsibilities.

Evaluation

Ongoing appraisal of the progress being made and the care the child and family receive is essential. When nurses provide short-term care for children (less than 2 weeks), evaluation make take the form of status reports on the flowsheet or nursing notes.[6] If, however, the nurse–patient relationship is long-term over weeks or months, the nurse needs to perform a comprehensive evaluation periodically. This last phase of the nursing process requires a careful study of both the outcomes and processes of the nursing care provided.

Evaluation of Outcomes

Evaluation of outcomes is made easier if criteria (the "who, what, how, and when") have been faithfully established when goals were developed with the child and family during the planning phase. Actions or behaviors exhibited by the child and family at the time of evaluation are compared to the written client goals. As in earlier phases of the nursing process, the child and family are also involved in evaluation. They discuss with the nurse whether the goals have been fully achieved and their feelings about the course of care. Variables that have affected success or failure may also be discussed. Thoughtful exploration of the outcome criteria can yield valuable insight into the effectiveness of the plan for nursing. Precise documentation of the evaluation is maintained in the child's permanent record, typically in the nurses' notes, or on the written care plan.

Evaluation of Process

As mentioned earlier, the nurse often mentally recognizes what needs to be done to help children and families achieve their health-related goals. In process evaluation, the nurse considers the appropriateness of assessments, diagnoses, and plans for nursing care. Ability to set priorities, organize responsibilities, and respond to both general and specific changing needs of the child and family is included. Process evaluation requires thoughtful introspection of how the professional nursing role is being managed by the nurse. Linking process evaluation to outcome evaluation has the potential of improving the quality of care provided to children and their families.

Outcome and process evaluation is performed for the purpose of making decisions about the plan of care. Based on evaluation data, decisions may be made to continue with the plan of care that has been designed or to make modifications in the plan. If all goals have been achieved and no new health problems are identified, a decision to terminate nursing care is appropriate. Terminating nursing care, however, requires preparing the child and family to continue the management of the child's health. Discharge planning therefore becomes a vital component of the nursing care plan.

Summary

The nursing process is the sequence of deliberate activities used in providing holistic care for the child and family. Interdependence among the phases of the nursing process (assessment, nursing diagnosis, planning, intervention, and evaluation) is recognized, as is the importance of involving the child and family in each phase and communicating effectively with other members of the health-care team.

Use of the nursing process benefits both the nurse as care provider and the child–family unit as the recipient of that care. For the nurse, efficiency in providing nursing care is improved when an organized, systematic approach is taken. Providing holistic care for children and their

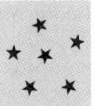

Ideas for Nursing Research

Nursing has made great strides in the past two decades in identifying who we are as nurses and how we function. Research is a vital aspect of this process of clarification. With respect to using the nursing process to provide nursing care to children and their families, the following areas need to be explored through well-designed investigations:

- Refinement of assessment tools and techniques so that accurate information about the child can be obtained, especially when the child cannot communicate verbally.
- Confirmation of the defining characteristics of nursing diagnoses for children, because investigations to date have addressed health problems in adults.
- Development of additional nursing diagnoses that focus on health problems unique to childhood.
- Exploration of nursing interventions for children who are developmentally sensitive.

families demands that creative and innovative approaches be taken in problem solving, thereby enhancing personal satisfaction and professional growth. Children and families who receive care through the nursing process are more likely to have consistent care that is free from duplications, omissions, and errors. They are active participants in the process and are encouraged to assume joint responsibility for meeting their health-related needs. Additionally, continuity of care is promoted for children and families when the plan of nursing care is recorded and clear communications are maintained among members of the health-care team. Conscious use of the nursing process is the keystone to quality nursing care.

References

1. Alfaro, R. (1990). *Applying nursing diagnosis and nursing process: A step-by-step guide* (2nd ed.). Philadelphia: J. B. Lippincott.
2. American Nurses' Association. (1980). *Nursing: A social policy statement.* Kansas City: American Nurses' Association.
3. Bower, F. (1986). *The process of planning nursing care* (3rd ed.). Philadelphia: W. B. Saunders.
4. Bulechek, G. M., & McCloskey, J. C. (1985). *Nursing interventions: Treatments for nursing diagnoses.* Philadelphia: W. B. Saunders.
5. Bulechek, G. M., & McCloskey, J. C. (1989). Nursing interventions: Treatments for potential nursing diagnoses. In R. M. Carroll-Johnson (Ed.), *Classification of nursing diagnoses* (pp. 23–30). Philadelphia: J. B. Lippincott.
6. Carpenito, L. J. (1992). *Nursing diagnosis: Application to nursing practice* (4th ed.). Philadelphia: J. B. Lippincott.
7. Carroll-Johnson, R. M. (Ed.). (1989). *Classification of nursing diagnoses.* Philadelphia: J. B. Lippincott.
8. Gordon, M. (1991). Manual of nursing diagnosis. St. Louis: Mosby.

9. Hall, L. E. (1955). Quality of nursing care. *Public Health News.* Newark, NJ: State Department of Health.

10. Johnson, D. E. (1980). Behavioral system model for nursing. In J. P. Reihl & C. Roy (Eds.), *Conceptual models for nursing practice* (2nd ed.), (pp. 207–216). New York: Appleton-Century-Crofts.

11. Kalish, R. (1983). *The psychology of human behavior* (5th ed.). Monterey, CA: Brooks/Cole.

12. King, I. (1981). *A theory for nursing systems, concepts, process.* New York: Wiley.

13. Maslow, A. (1970). *Motivation in personality.* New York: Harper & Row.

14. Orem, D. (1991). *Nursing: Concepts of practice* (4th ed.). St. Louis: Mosby.

15. Pender, N. (1989). Languaging a health perspective for NANDA taxonomy on research and theory. In R. M. Carroll-Johnson (Ed.), *Classification of nursing diagnoses* (pp. 31–36). Philadelphia: J. B. Lippincott.

16. Popkess-Vawter, S., & Pinnell, N. (1987). Yes: Accentuate the positive. *Am J Nurs, 87,* 1211–1216.

17. Rogers, M. E. (1970). *The theoretical basis of nursing.* New York: Davis.

18. Roy, S. C. (1984). *Introduction to nursing: An adaptation model* (2nd ed.). Englewood Cliffs, NJ: Prentice Hall.

19. Yura, H., & Walsh, M. (1987). *The nursing process: Assessing, planning, implementing, evaluating.* Norwalk: Appleton & Lange.

3
CHAPTER

Family-Centered Child Health Care

BEHAVIORAL OBJECTIVES

Describe family-centered child health care.

Define family.

List current trends in family structure and function.

Discuss family as a system.

Discuss family development and its impact on individual development.

Discuss assessment of the family unit.

Discuss roles and relationships in parenting and among siblings.

The family can be conceptualized as one of the most fundamental and complex of human institutions, with major distinctions that set it apart from other institutions.[8] The family institution is so complex and dynamic that no one theory or discipline defines the family the same.

Family-centered child care can be described as approaches to care that are tailored to meet the special, intricate, and ever-changing needs of all family members, not just the needs of an individual child within the family. A child cannot be provided comprehensive health care in isolation from the family; a family ideally does not receive care without involving all members. Family-centered care and family-centered nursing aim to foster and support the stability of the family. This is in contrast to the past, when the following applied:

- Restricted visiting hours made a young child wait for long periods of time in a hospital bed for contact with a parent.
- Neonates were not allowed with the mother, and mothers were limited in the amount of time they could spend in the simple act of feeding and caring for the newborn.
- Fathers were excluded from the birthing process and were unable to support the mother through labor and birth.
- Hospital or health care agency routines and rituals were given priority over the needs of child patients and their families.
- Families often were kept in the dark, making it difficult for them to make informed decisions about optimal health care interventions.

This chapter begins with concepts of family-centered health care; moves to the uniqueness of the family and its components (structure and function); summarizes theoretical approaches; outlines means of assessing, promoting, and maintaining the family unit; and concludes with a discussion of parenting and

33

sibling relationshipsas part of family-centered care. The dysfunctional family is discussed in Chapter 5.

Concepts of Family-Centered Care

The concept of family-centered nursing care originated with consumerism and research on maternal interactions with infants as well as the unique needs of the family and its members to be active and involved participants in their own health care. It evolved in response to the critical need to re-establish relationships between infants, children, and their family members that earlier had been neglected or disrupted because of forced separation by the health care system. The concept of family care provides the family with autonomy, self-determination, and control.[13] An introduction to family health care was given in Chapter 1, including a display of Elements of Family-Centered Care.

What is especially unique about family-centered care is that it allows the family to participate together in a variety of health care settings, including the home. In essence, the rationale for family-centered care is that agencies must adapt to the needs of the family rather than have the family adapt to the agencies' needs. It established the family's needs as paramount to the health care system's needs (Fig. 3-1). Whether a nurse works with a family in a well-child care setting or in a hospital, the parent may ultimately become the primary care provider. Nursing facilitates the parent's role through caring for the child as a member of the family and teaching the family health care interventions.

Respect for the integrity of the family system is the principle qualification for family-centered care. This qualification demands that nurses know the importance of family theory, apply principles of growth and development in planning care, and assist parents to master their parenting roles. Parents, children, and family members are included as active participants rather than passive recipients. Parents are included in children's care and treated as experts, colleagues, and consultants. Nurses increasingly seek parental input, recommendations, and advice and interact with parents to promote informed decisions and to develop family-centered goals and care plans.

Care in the 1990s

Nurses in the 1990s will be increasingly sensitive to teaching family members to assume greater responsibility for the complex health care needs of children and actively involve the child in his or her own care when the child is cognitively, socially, emotionally, and physically ready to participate in self-care. Increasingly, nurses will make special efforts to assure that all family members are involved in assessment, planning, implementing, and evaluating care for the child and entire family. Concomitant with goals of involving families in more active ways is the objective of encouraging families to promote wellness while preventing or diminishing problems associated with illness. Health promotion and wellness are thus cru-

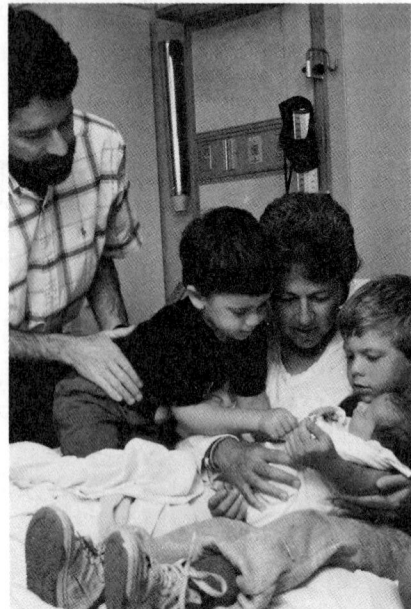

FIGURE 3-1
In family-centered care, the entire family shares in the experience of a new baby.

cial goals of comprehensive family-centered care. These goals are discussed further in Chapter 7.

To achieve aims of excellence in family-centered care, nurses should plan care that reflects scientific knowledge, such as technologic advances and medical breakthroughs. To be successful, a nurse must consider psychosocial information, such as changing family patterns, contemporary health care delivery systems, cost effectiveness, and each family's expectations about their roles and responsibilities. It is essential that nurses assess family members' perceptions of their own roles, responsibilities, and contributions in promoting and maintaining healthy well-being.

An emerging type of nurse-managed care is case management, in which a nurse is responsible for coordinating and managing the care of a child throughout the trajectory of an illness and the treatment. Case management by nurses will ensure better coordination for family-centered care, including coordinating community-based services and referrals. As case managers, nurses will play increasingly pivotal roles in assisting family members to become case managers for their own children.

The Family

Uniqueness of the Family

The family is generally understood to be a simple group of human beings united by certain affiliations, including biologic, emotional, and legal. However, the essential meaning of the word family requires an understanding of the family in a concrete *living* way. To assume that the family is composed of a husband and wife, son, and daughter, and that the husband is the head and the mother the heart of the family is to limit the family and its adaptive principle to a narrow topology, one that is becoming less and less the norm.

Several features of a family make it distinct from any other group. These features are the following:

- Its unbounding *adaptability* and *permeability*, that is, its plasticity
- Its unique *sympathy and mutual feeling* between members
- Its *socioeconomic adaptation* for survival in ingenious ways
- Its enduring *affection* and *emotional ties*

The one integral feature of the family is the power of each of its members to affect the others emotionally. Despite its many diverse forms, the family is a living system, imbued with emotional power that tends to conserve itself and resist outside intrusions. Within its own systems, it can grow purposively but, equally, can become just as unhealthy or dysfunctional. Unconditional affection for one another, sympathy, patience, tolerance, and nurturing—all originate from the emotional wellsprings of the family, but equally does violence, hostility, depression, child abuse, and spouse abuse.

Components of a Family

Several components unique to a family[51] are that the family has a *structure*, carries out *functions* and *assigned roles*, has distinct *modes of interactions*, has available *resources*, progresses through a *life cycle*, has a *history*, and

is made up of *individual members* with special histories. Each of these components is described further in the accompanying display and discussed in the chapter.

Family Structure

American families are not dissolving; they are changing. Family types in North America are more diverse than at any time in history, and nurses should acknowledge the variety within society (Fig. 3-2). Hareven[25] emphasized that variations are not necessarily new. Rather, they reflect a more open society—a society more tolerant of social change, individual preferences and priorities, and alternative opinions.

Extended and Nuclear Families. Historically, the extended family (members of one's family of origin [parents, siblings], family of ascent [grandparents, uncles, aunts, cousins] or families of descent [grandchildren, nephews, nieces]) was antecedent to the nuclear family; its *raison d'etre* being survival. This was primarily because the family was the main unit of economic production. After the Industrial Revolution, members of the family were forced to seek employment in urban centers and the nuclear family became more common.

Nuclear family is defined as a two-generation family of procreation (i.e., parent[s] and child[ren]). The nuclear family form has predominated since the beginning of the nineteenth century. In the recent past the ideal family was viewed as composed of a model two-parent, two-child unit: as such, the children were cared for primarily

---

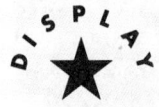

Components of a Family

Structure: organization of members with respect to power or authority and emotional closeness.

Family dynamics: ways in which family members think, feel, and interact with each other and their suprasystems.

Function: tasks that the family carries out for society and its members, such as education, economic structure, socialization, and training.

Assigned roles: prescribed responsibilities, expectations, and rights of each individual member. As a result, one family member may be designated as the breadwinner, another the overseer of discipline, and yet another may assume responsibilities of household operations.

Mode of interaction: style adopted by family members to respond to the environment and with each other as it relates to problem solving and decision making.

Resources: general health of family members, their social support and skills, unique personality characteristics, and financial support.

Family history: myriad of sociocultural factors as well as previous history of illness and strategies of coping with stress or crisis.

Life cycle: developmental stages in a family's life, beginning with marriage and ending with the death of both marital partners. All families move through successive normal transitional steps or stages over time, such as the marriage of a couple, the birth of the first child, children beginning school, children leaving home, and death of a parent or spouse. Each represents a potential crisis point for every family. Each phase of the life cycle is associated with certain developmental tasks in which the successful completion leads to somewhat different levels of family functioning.

Individual member: family member and their unique characteristics, stages of development, contributions they make to the family, their personal concepts and perceptions of themselves and their place in the family, as well as their perception of the family in which they are a part.

Information from Turk, D., & Kerns, R. (1985). The family in health and illness. In Health-illness, and families: A life span perspective (p. 3). New York: John Wiley and Sons.

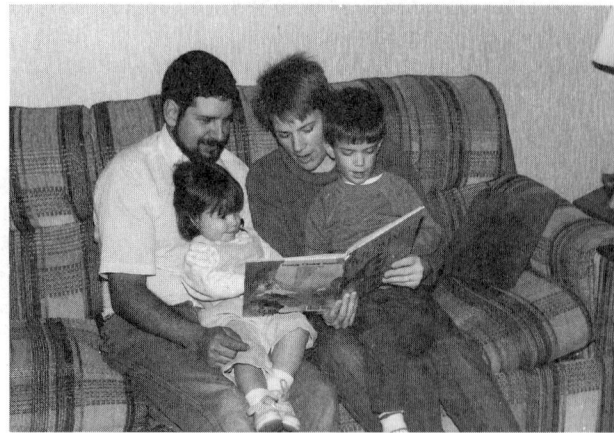
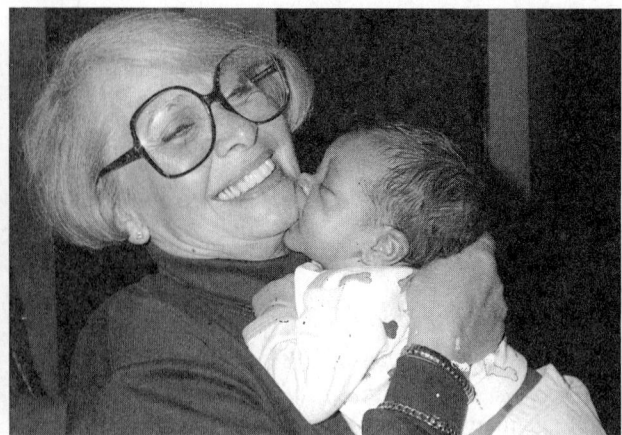
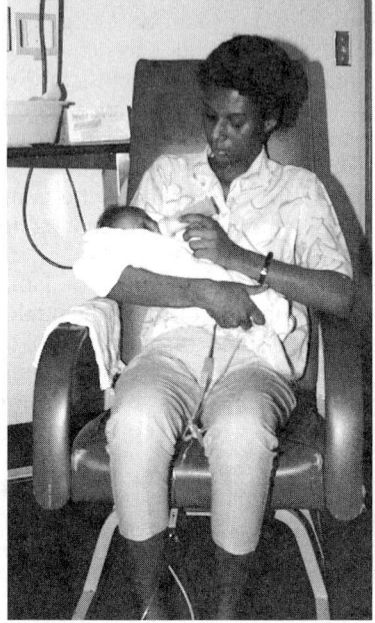
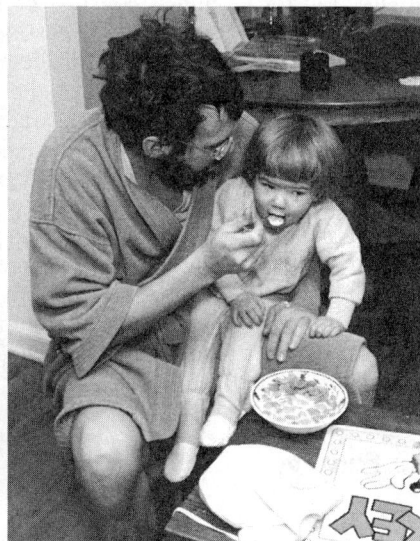
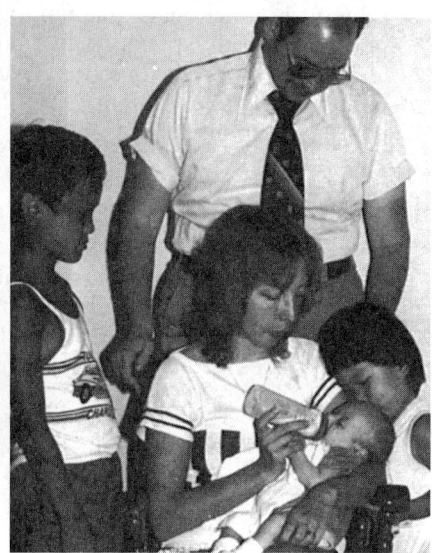

FIGURE 3-2

The changing American family involves a diversity of structures. Shown here are a nuclear family, extended family with grandparents, single-parent family, two-career family where the father shares in childrearing responsibilities, and a family with adopted children.

by the mother, who stayed at home while the father was the exclusive wage earner.[17] There are indications that this unit is showing signs of changes due to economic forces and social dynamics.

Modified Family Structures. Family life continues to be the most significant social unit and organization in all strata of American society,[4] although society continues to experiment with family patterns and nonfamilial living arrangements. Families are modifying traditional roles. For example, both spouses may work, children may go to day care centers, grandparents are raising their grandchildren, the wife may be the primary breadwinner, and the husband may have a lower paying job or may be the sole house manager while the wife works. Characteristics of the following major contemporary family structures are discussed here: single-parent, commuter, empty nest, return to empty nest, and stepfamilies.

Single-Parent Families. More and more children are living in one-parent families for a variety of reasons (Fig. 3-3). For instance, adolescent pregnancies have increased dramatically, and adolescent mothers may choose not to marry. Some professional women are choosing to have children and not marry. In addition, divorce has increased the number of children living in a single-parent home. Men, as well as women, may have primary guardianship of their children.

Two-Career Families. In a two-career family, both the husband and wife work in jobs that are necessary or fulfilling. Economically, it may be necessary for both to work, or neither partner wishes to quit a job to be a housemanager. The numbers of families in which both parents work continues to grow.

Commuter Families. Billingsley[4] used this term to describe the commuter phenomenon that is characteristic of partners who live and work apart for the sake of their

Nuclear Family vs. One-parent Family

□ Two-parent family
▨ One-parent family

**One-parent Family Maintained by Mother vs.
One-parent Family Maintained by Father**

□ Mother
▨ Father

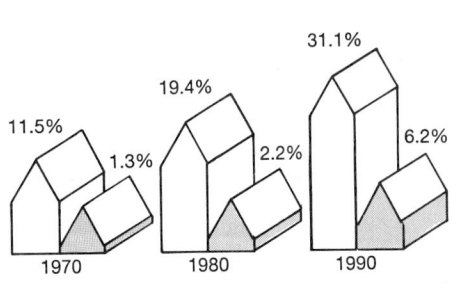

FIGURE 3-3
The changing American family.

commitment to their profession; often one of the partner's occupation is so specialized, it is only found in a certain community. The amount of time the couple spends together varies widely.

Empty-Nest and Return-to-Nest Syndrome. "Empty nest" refers to children who have grown up and left home. They may enter college, get married, or take an apartment with friends. "Return-to-nest" syndrome, or "reverse empty nest" refers to these persons' returning at a later age to take up residence in the parental home again. The cause may be social, economic, or cultural pressures.[4]

Stepfamilies or Blended Families. Stepfamilies are families that have divorced and remarried, bringing with them their children, and forming larger and more complex "blended" family structures. More than 30 million adults constitute stepfamilies, and nearly 20% of all American children live in such families.

Families help members cope with the demands of other organizations in which they must function, to use these organizations for the benefits they provide, and to provide for their member's satisfactions and a mentally and physically healthy environment that is intrinsic to the well-being of the family.

Family Function

The most significant function of the family is reproduction of the individual. The foremost goals of the family are enculturation and socialization to promote the well-being and happiness of its individual members and to set the groundwork for the basis and preparation for children to become citizens in a society.

Duvall[14] identified eight essential tasks for American families: physical maintenance; allocation of resources; division of labor; socialization of members; reproduction, recruitment, and release of family members; maintenance of order; placement of members in the larger society; and maintenance of motivation and morale. These are explained in the accompanying display.

Other functions such as education, religious training, economic production, and protection are now shared by others in communities. Family functions that have emerged include giving affection, providing personal security and acceptance, giving satisfaction and a sense of purpose, assuring continuity of companionship, guaranteeing social placement and socialization, and inculcating controls and a sense of what is right.[15]

Family Theory

Exciting progress has been made in the last three decades in understanding how families function and how and why they become dysfunctional. Several cogent theories have been formulated and subjected to empirical testing. Each develops a different aspect of family organization. Because of the diversity of families, no single theory necessarily applies to all families.

Literature surveys of the late 1960s and early 1970s found the majority of family scholars using symbolic interaction, structural-functional, and developmental frameworks for both theory development and research.[6] The major themes in use today are interactionist, developmental, exchange, and systems theories.[21] These theories are summarized here, although more discussion focuses on family systems and developmental theories. Any of these theories can be used for study of nursing approaches to the family. However, only one framework is recommended initially for any one problem. If frameworks are mixed, the assumptions tend to become confused.[37]

Interactionist Theory

Interactionist theory sees the family as a unit of interacting personalities. The family is studied by analyzing patterns of interactions and communication of the members and their perceived roles. The internal structure of the family is the key focus. Socialization is a key concept,

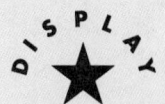

Duvall's Eight Essential Tasks for American Families[15]

Physical maintenance: providing shelter, food, clothing, health care, etc.

Allocation of resources: meeting family needs and costs, apportioning material goods, facilities, space, authority, respect, affection, etc.

Division of labor: deciding who does what, assigning responsibility for procuring income, managing the household, caring for family members, and other specific tasks.

Socialization of members: guiding the internalization of increasingly mature and acceptable patterns of controlling elimination, food intake, sexual drives, aggression, etc.

Reproduction, recruitment, and release of family members: bearing or adopting children and rearing them for release at maturity, incorporating new members by marriage, and establishing policies for inclusion of others: in-laws, relatives, step-parents, guests, family friends, etc.

Maintenance of order: providing means of communication, establishing types and intensity of interaction, patterns of affection, and sexual expression; by administering sanctions, ensuring conformity to group norms.

Placement of members in the larger society: fitting into the community; relating to church, school, organizational life, political, and economic systems; and protecting family members from undesirable outside influences.

Maintenance of motivation and morale: rewarding members for achievements, satisfying individual needs for acceptance, encouragement and affection, meeting personal and family crises, refining a philosophy of life and sense of family loyalty (through rituals, festivals, etc.).

---

because it is the mechanism of transmitting values, goals, sentiments, and meaning to family members.[7]

Exchange Theory

Exchange theory views all human interactions as social exchanges. The rewards and costs of their interactions are weighed. If the exchange is perceived as unequal, one person will be at a disadvantage and the other will control the relationship. The goal of exchange is to minimize costs and maximize rewards.[7]

Family Systems Theory

A general system theory views an individual person as a complex being operating within a system. Therefore, no one member of a family exists in isolation. Focus is on how the parts connect to form a whole, the way the system is organized, and the structure and interaction of the various units.

Epstein and Bishop[18] summarized the major assumptions of family systems theory as follows:

*   The parts of the family are interrelated.
*   One part of the family cannot be understood by simply understanding each of the parts.
*   Family functioning cannot be fully understood by simply understanding each of the parts.
*   A family's structure and organization are important factors determining the behavior of family members.
*   Transactional patterns of the family system shape the behavior of family members.

It is crucial that a family member not lose his or her identity in the system, or forget the power of the family system on an individual person, nor the impact of a person to influence the system. This natural group functions not simply as a collection of individual people but as a unique group with its own rules, roles, structures, and processes.

Family Subsystems: Natural Dyads. The basic unit of family interrelationship is *dyadic*. The term refers to two persons interacting. Dyads and their permutations include, but are not restricted to, the following:

*   Spousal dyad: husband-wife, wife-husband dyad
*   Parental dyad: mother-child, father-child dyad
*   Sibling dyad: brother-sister, sister-sister, brother-brother dyad

It is recognized that, in some families, a spousal dyad may not be present or the dyad may be members of the same sex. The minimal component relationship of the family is the dyad. Because a relationship involves a minimum of two individuals, there is only one individual that remains if the dyad is broken. Any division or loss such as a divorce, separation, death of a member, life-threatening illness, re-marriage, or incarceration leads to destabilization of the family. Thus, interventions that strengthen the dyad relationship, in turn, strengthen the family, conserve equilibrium, and promote stability, integrity, and healthy members.

Developmental Theory: Family Life Cycle

Developmental theory views each family as evolving over time. The family life cycle divides the life history of a family into observable and predictable stages of development.[38] Each stage is characterized by (1) developmental tasks relevant to that stage, and (2) predictable crises associated with the achievement or nonachievement of specific developmental tasks.

The family life cycle can be viewed as an excellent model of evolution of a system, which is changing, yet simultaneously maintaining its integrity.[20] The developmental periods of the children to a large measure define family process. Other life cycle markers include changes in income, family moves, the period when a member seeks health care, or when the mother seeks a job for the first time.

The developmental framework assumes an intact family system as defined by marriage and children. Intact families pass through the same sequences or phases,[22] most of which are marked by a critical transition point such as marriage, birth of the first child, departure from home of the youngest child, empty-nest syndrome, retirement, and death. As Aponte and Van Deusen[2] emphasize, there are potential crisis points that, although challenging, most families succeed in overcoming without overwhelming difficulty.

Duvall[15] pointed out that a longitudinal frame of reference is essential for examining family life. Duvall[15] shows the typical life cycle of an intact family in terms of a circle with eight sectors that include married couples without children, childbearing families, families with preschool children, families with school children, families with adolescents, families as launching centers whereby children leave, middle-aged parents (empty nest, retirement), and aging family members (retirement, death). Although all families will not resemble the model precisely, the circle is useful in plotting the stages through which families typically pass. It is also valuable in predicting the approximate time when each stage will be reached in the family's life cycle.[15]

Carter and McGoldrick[10] viewed life cycle transitions developed within a three-generational family system, as affecting all members simultaneously. The stages of the family life cycle and events are listed in Table 3-1.

Carter and McGoldrick[10] also stressed that "the family is a system passing through time, in a social context which is also changing." Examples of these changes are reflected in the falling birth rate, increasing life expectancy, and rising divorce and remarriage rates.

Characteristics of Functional Families

Several researchers have attempted to distinguish the similarities of families considered healthy and to determine how these families are different from less functional families. Two are presented here. Curran[12] conducted a survey of health care professionals who provided care to families on a regular basis. Curran's research[12] concluded with several characteristics of healthy families. Among the most important findings were that families have the following qualities:

- Communicate effectively
- Respect and support each other
- Respect others outside the family
- Trust each other
- Share time together with play and humor balanced and demonstrated among family members
- Take responsibilities for their actions

- Teach and learn morals that promote the common good and individual welfare
- Enjoy traditions
- Share a religious belief
- Respect each other's privacy

In his own work with families, Framo[20] identified some "ideal" principles of healthy or normal families and marital functioning. These principles include the following:

- Parents are well differentiated, having developed a sense of self before separating from their own families of origin.
- There is a clear separation of generational boundaries within a family. The children should be free of the role of saving a parent or the parental marriage.
- There are realistic perceptions and expectations by parents of each other and their children.
- The loyalty to the family of procreation is greater than to the family of origin.
- The spouses place themselves and each other before anyone else, including the children. The marriage is not a symbiotic one that excludes the children; the children do not feel that to be close to one parent means they are alienating the other.
- Identity development and autonomy are encouraged for all family members.
- Nonpossessive warmth and affection are expressed between parents, between parents and children, and among the siblings.
- There is a capacity to have open, honest, and clear communication as well to respond to issues with each other.
- A realistic, adult-to-adult, caring relationship between each parent and his or her parents and siblings is notable.
- The family is characterized as an open family in the sense of involvement with others outside the family, which includes extended family and friends. In addition, outsiders are permitted inside the family.

Functional families can be beset with internal conflicts and external changes. These families differ from dysfunctional families in that they acknowledge their problems, are able to comment on family rules, and tend to conceptualize their problems, goals, and solutions in nonextremist ways.

Stressors Affecting the Family

Stress, stressors, and coping are discussed further in Chapters 17 and 18. Stress is a normal factor of life, and it can be a positive or negative influence. It is mentioned here because the contemporary family is affected by both visible and hidden stressors. The effects of stress are reflected in increased divorce rates, one-parent families, teenage parents, and step-blended families. The stress can originate from many different sources, most notably illness, economic stress, unemployment, tensions in the workplace that are brought home to the family and, conversely, general boredom owing to lack of immediate and long-term goals and, sometimes, dysfunctional communication. Environmental stressors such as drugs, al-

TABLE 3-1
Stages of the Family Life Cycle

Family Life Cycle Stage	Emotional Process of Transition: Key Principles	Second-Order Changes in Family Status Required to Proceed Developmentally
1. Between families: the unattached young adult	Accepting parent-offspring separation	• Differentiation of self in relation to family of origin • Development of intimate peer relationships • Establishment of self in work
2. The joining of families through marriage: the newly married couple	Commitment to new system	• Formation of marital system • Realignment of relationships with extended family and friends to include spouse
3. The family with young children	Accepting new members into the system	• Adjusting marital system to make space for child(ren) • Taking on parenting roles • Realignment of relationships with extended family to include parenting and grandparenting roles
4. The family with adolescents	Increasing flexibility of family boundaries to include children's independence	• Shifting of parent-child relationship to permit adolescent to move in and out of system • Refocus on mid-life marital and career issues • Beginning shift toward concerns for older generation
5. Launching children and moving on	Accepting a multitude of exits from and entries into the family system	• Renegotiation of marital system as a dyad • Development of adult to adult relationships between grown children and their parents • Realignment of relationships to include in-laws and grandchildren • Dealing with disabilities and death of parents (grandparents)
6. The family in later life	Accepting the shifting of generational roles	• Maintaining own and/or couple functioning and interests in face of physiologic decline; exploration of new familial and social role options • Support for a more central role for middle generation • Making room in the system for the wisdom and experience of the elderly; supporting the older generation without overfunctioning for them • Dealing with loss of spouse, siblings, and other peers and preparation for own death; life review and integration

From Carter, B. & McGoldrick, M. (1988). *The changing family life cycle: A framework for family therapy* (p. 15). New York: Gardner Press.

cohol, population concentration, and violence all converge on the family, affecting the family's equilibrium and adaptive abilities.

Even the developmental crises in the family cycle are stressful. One problem in life-cycle families is the fact that there usually are children of different ages in the family. Thus, the family is addressing several transitions or crises simultaneously. Table 3-2 outlines some of the major issues for children, adults, couples, and parenting at various stages of the life cycle.

The healthy functioning family learns to adapt to these stressors. However, if a family is overly stressed, or is dysfunctional, its problem solving, decision making,

and communication abilities may be seriously impaired. This will affect the members of the family and the overall cohesiveness of the family. High-risk families are discussed in Chapter 5.

Assessing, Promoting, and Maintaining the Family Unit

Americans live in a pluralistic society that has different cultural, racial, ethnic, religious, and sexual values. The nurse should increasingly consider diverse family values

TABLE 3-2
Issues for Children, Adults, Couples, and Parenting Across the Life Cycle

	Transition Into Parenthood	Preschool Children	School-Age Children	Adolescents	Launching Stage
Issues in Child Development	Total dependence Vulnerability Total care, maintenance Attachment	Separation/autonomy Drive for individuation Aggression Gender identity Verbal expression and understanding	Increased impact of other influences Development of moral judgments Achievement (academic, athletic, artistic, etc.) Consolidation of gender identity Development of positive self-concept	Socialization to outside adult world Control of sexual impulses Control of aggressive impulses Maintenance of positive self-concept Independent identity Expression of values	Establishment of independent life style —Financial —Geographic —Emotional —Occupational

Issues in Adult Development	Concerned with making satisfying life investments
	Preoccupied with being productive and performing well
	High financial stress
	High demand on time and energy resources
	Fathers:
	  —Crucial stage of career
	  —May have growing dissatisfaction with "rat race"
	  —May desire to participate in childrearing
	Mothers:
	  —At risk for depression, suicide, marital violence, child abuse
	  —Fulltime homemaker at risk for social isolation, boredom
	  —Employed mothers at risk for overcommitment of resources
				Established economically
				Peak or early decline of earning power
				Generally good health
				Preoccupied with the yield from life investments/taking inventory
				Beginning of biologic decline
				"Middle generation"
				Fathers: slow down of "rat race"
				Mothers: fulltime homemakers—reassessment of future	

Issues for Couples	Adjustment to a triad
	Sharing love with another
	Finding time to be together
	Traditionalization of sex roles
		At risk for end of marital honeymoon
		  —Low ebb of marital satisfaction
		  —Poor communication
		  —Alienation from each other's roles
		  —Disagreements about finances
		  —High demand for decision making
				At risk for reassessment of marriage and marital roles
				  —Disenchantment
				  —"Hollowness" in relationship
				  —Boredom
				  —Further alienation from each other's roles	

Parenting Issues	Attachment
	Type of child care
	Relationship with new grandparents
	Division of parenting responsibilities
	Building of basic trust in child
		Discipline
		Encouragement of positive self-concept in child
		Establishing relationships between
		  —Work and family
		  —Alternative child care and family
		  —School and family
		  —Leisure-recreation and family
		Dealing with childrearing "experts"
				Setting limits
				Allowing participation in adult roles
				Communication
				Programming, i.e., parents vs. adolescent
				Determining activities
				Values (religious, sexual, etc.)
				Distancing, i.e., allowing independence while communicating concern
				Dealing with conflict between parent and adolescent developmental stages	

From McCubbin, H. I., & Figley, C. R. (1983). *Stress and the family* (p. 33). New York: Brunner/Mazel.

and beliefs as well as various modifications of family structures in the care of the child.

Assessment

The research findings from family theorists, clinicians, and practitioners during the last three decades point to the critical necessity for nurses to be objective, systematic, and scientific in their assessment of families.

Child and Family Health History

A functional health approach to taking the family history was discussed in Chapter 2. This section develops the family health history further. It is essential that nurses, at a minimum, assess families to determine the following[26]:

- Structure of the family
- Developmental tasks of each family member
- Phase of family's life cycle
- Developmental stressors present
- Situational stressors present
- Family's perceptions of stress and crisis and meaning assigned to it by the family
- Family's degree of cohesion, flexibility, and adaptability
- Family's resources for responding to change, stress, or crisis
- Family's life context
- Social supports available to family
- Family's problem-solving abilities
- Family's perceptions of own strengths
- Characteristics of healthy family functioning

The nurse can gather data to by observing, interviewing, and interacting with all family members. A series of questions that can be used to initiate the interview assessment is found in Table 3-3.

Developmental Approach

A longitudinal perspective of the family and its life cycle is necessary to determine if its members are accomplishing their respective tasks. By referring to the typical life cycle of an intact family, as outlined in Table 3-1, the nurse can determine if there is a smooth progression, an interruption, obstacles, or complexities in the naturally unfolding family life cycle.

Roberts[38] suggests that it is useful for the nurse to answer the following three questions:

- At what stage of development is this person and his or her family?

TABLE 3-3
Nursing Assessment: Questions for Assessing the Family Unit

Areas of Assessment	Key Questions*
Family size	How many persons are there in your family? Who lives at home?
Expressions of developmental and life cycles	There are several stages to a life cycle. In which stages is your family? Newly married? Family with young children? Family with adolescents? Young adults leaving home?
Knowledge of life cycle crises	What problems does this raise for persons in the family?
Family experience with past life crises	What major problems has your family had to face in the past? Death? Separation? Major physical illness? Major mental illness? Serious financial problems?
Expression of family's coping strategies	Do you think people in the family feel these problems were dealt with satisfactorily?
Expression of chronic problems that may place the family at risk	Does anyone in the family have problems with alcoholism? Drug abuse? Delinquency?
Expression of role assignments	How are major decisions made in the family, and by whom?
	What do you and your partner expect of each of your children on a day-to-day basis? For the future?
	What do you think the children expect of each of you?
	Are all your expectations realistic?
Expression of relationships within the family	What does each person in your family have to do to get attention from others in the family?
Development of self-esteem of family members	How much tolerance of individual differences is there in the family?
Development of values and beliefs in the family	What are the goals, interests, and values (including religious values) of your family?
	Do all the family members work toward these goals?
Determination of socioeconomic level	What is your educational level? In what financial bracket are you?
Relationships with the extended family	Where do your in-laws and other relatives live? Can you count on them for help? Do they create problems for you?
Participation with people outside the family unit	Do you have many friends in the neighborhood? How actively are you involved with them?
	To what groups or clubs do your family members belong?
Development of community support systems	What sorts of community resources has your family used? Describe the experience. Would you use them again?
	Describe any times when you have not used community resources when it would have been appropriate to do so.

* Although these questions are designed to be asked of the parents, most of them may be reworded to be used with other family members.

Adapted from Hennen, B. K. (1980). Family structure and function. In D. B. Shires & B. K. Hennen (Eds.), *Family medicine: A guidebook for practitioners of the art* (p. 19). New York: McGraw-Hill.

- What are the developmental tasks and crises of this unique stage?
- How do the answers and information relate to the person's expressed reason for seeking or obtaining health care?

Answers to these three questions provide the nurse with some essential initial data to identify actual or potential problems in family development. In addition, the nurse also needs to identify family strengths, family resources, and family stressors as well as the family's ability to cope with current health care needs. Being able to differentiate a healthy family from a dysfunctional family is a crucial component of the nursing assessment.

Assessment Tools

In addition, family assessment tools are available to the nurse. These include the Family Functioning Index, Family APGAR, and the Family Adaptability and Cohesion Evaluation Scale (see Appendix). The nurse is encouraged to become informed about these tools, use them with well families first, and administer them to families in different life cycle stages and with different developmental tasks to accomplish. The nurse can practice using these assessment tools, become familiar with their purposes and usefulness, and critique each one, according to its strengths, weaknesses, and value in practice. Not every family requires a comprehensive, complex assessment; however, when the nurse identifies a family at risk for dysfunction or a family confronted with more stress than can be managed effectively, early identification and referral to appropriate family health professionals may prevent long-term dysfunction.

Nursing Diagnoses and Planning

Nursing diagnoses appropriate to family centered nursing care should focus on the needs of the family as well as the needs of the child receiving health care.

Several nursing diagnoses approved by the North American Nursing Diagnosis Association (NANDA) for use with families include Family Coping: Potential for Growth; Altered Family Processes; Ineffective Family Coping: Compromised; and Ineffective Family Coping: Disabling. The first two diagnosis are summarized here because they address the well-functioning family.

Family Coping: Potential for Growth is described by NANDA as "effective managing of adaptive tasks by family members involved with the client's health challenge, who now is exhibiting desire and readiness for enhanced health and growth in regard to self and in relation to the client."[44] This diagnosis is related to a functioning family that is actively seeking to reach its potential.

Altered Family Processes is described by NANDA as "the state in which a family that normally functions effectively experiences a dysfunction."[44] Illness and treatment may be associated with this diagnosis, particularly when the family life is disrupted by the changes resulting from the illness. Frequent trips to the hospital or physician, increased financial burdens, loss of employment, or relocation to be close to medical help may be related.

However, these families are generally able to communicate with one another and are able to adapt.

In addition to developing a plan of care for the child, the nurse should include the family early on in developing a plan of care to promote optimal functioning of all family members.

Interventions

The nurse's roles with families is influenced by the ever increasing dramatic social, economic, and technologic developments that are impacting on changes of the family. The nurse's sensitivity to emerging trends determines his or her ability to respond to the multiple and ever changing needs of the family.

Anticipatory Guidance

Because many of the problems of families are best viewed as difficulties in making a transition from one developmental stage to the next, the nurse considers how the developmental process can be enhanced. The nurse determines whether there are any obstacles in the family's social context or within the family itself that can be eliminated. The nurse observes and determines the cycle that the family is in and whether there is more than one transitional crisis. The nurse also needs to identify the developmental tasks confronting each member, how they have mastered earlier tasks, and the progress each is currently making within the family unit. The nurse offers anticipatory guidance and teaches family members in regard to their developmental tasks, as summarized in Table 3-1, and provides positive comments on the success of the family and its individual members.

Counseling Regarding Hospitalization

In child health nursing, one of the most significant stressors facing a family is hospitalization of the child. Separation, loss of control, fear of the strange new environment, fear of bodily injury and pain, combined with the symptoms and treatments of the illness, create a multitude of family reactions. The nurse's role in educating parents and children about what to expect, what questions to ask, and what they can do are essential in helping families remain intact and supportive.[11] Several chapters in this textbook focus on strategies for managing families stressed by illness or hospitalization.

Evaluation

Evaluation should be based on goals established in planning and determined by interventions based on nursing assessment. Carpenito[11] identified five outcome criteria related to altered family processes: (1) verbalizations of feelings to one another and to others; (2) participation in the care of the sick child or family member; (3) facilitation of the family member from sick to well roles within the family; (4) mutual support for each family member; and (5) use of external support systems.[11]

Roles and Relationships: Parenting

Adequate parenting is the necessary precondition for human development. Gutman[23] emphasizes that "the unique vulnerability of the human child requires a long period of parental service, such that parenthood is generally seen to be coextensive with adulthood."

For the purpose of this section, the following definition of parenting is used. Parenting is "a developmental process carried out by an adult which is aimed at helping a child master successive developmental tasks at different life stages. The process consists of a range and number of learned behaviors that are characterized by interactional styles and change over a period of time".[35]

However, researchers, educators, and clinicians have conceptualized parenting, mothering, and fathering in diverse and inconsistent ways. According to Lidz,[28] the "arrival of the first child transforms spouses into parents and turns marriage into a family." Rossi[39] considered parenthood as a transition point for adults. She was interested in the social aspects of the transition to parenthood and focused on the first pregnancy, rather than marriage, as a major transition point for adults. Her perspectives focused on the woman and were limited in their application because they offered little information about fathers' views of parenting. Much of the early research on parenting studied middle class families with the first child. LeMasters,[27] Dyer,[16] and others found that the first child was associated with being unprepared for bringing the first baby home and assuming total responsibility of the newborn. With appropriate support by nurses and others, families are successful in coping with the demands and changes involved with the responsibilities in caring for a first born.

Realistic Attitudes of Couples

Sometimes partners have unrealistic attitudes about family life. These misconceptions assist in shaping members' interactions, influence the assignment of complementary roles, and partially determine the nature of intrafamilial relationships. The myths outlined in the first column of Table 3-4 feature some common beliefs about successful marriages. If such misconceptions are believed and perpetuated, parenting roles may be hindered. On the other hand, if couples accept the perspectives of the second column of the table, they may have better parental functioning.

Parenting Issues

Parents themselves have identified the following as the greatest parental issues confronting and demanding solutions to avoid the development of a family crisis[45]:

- Discipline
- Illegal drugs and their consequences
- Concern about street crime
- Violence in society
- Violence on television
- The impact of advertising
- Medical care and immunization against disease
- Nutrition and nutrition labeling
- Toy safety
- Education
- Problems associated with working mothers
- Day care
- Problems of communication with their children (drugs, death, sex, drinking, crime and rape, family problems, and money)
- Single parenting

Developmental Tasks

Parents, as adults, face unavoidable developmental tasks throughout their life cycle. While parents are attempting to respond to the changing and complex demands of their own parenting role, they must, according to Boyle,[6] "strive to evolve as individuals in their own rights and to secure a deep and lasting relationship with each other." Boyle formulated a number of propositions that are applicable to most parents, as listed in the display on the developmental tasks of parenthood.

Coping With Stress

Children are born and launched; couples are married and may be divorced and remarried to others; and family members die. All of these transitions require a reclarification of boundaries, cause a major shifting of roles and relationships, and are viewed as potential stressors for parents. McCubbin and Figley[29] propose that "the greater the boundary ambiguity and normative junctures throughout the family life cycle, the higher the marital and individual stress and the greater the risk for marital dysfunction." If the ambiguity is not resolved, the marital couple is at a higher stress level because the regenerative power to reorganize is blocked. When stress and challenges are reconciled, such success contributes to further psychological integration and maturity of both parents and their children.

Parenting Styles

Parenting is different in each family. The four main styles of parenting are authoritative, authoritarian, permissive, and indifferent or uninvolved.[40] Each is discussed here; however, each of these may vary in its degree or scope of application. One parent may use one style whereas the other uses another style, or parents may vary their style depending on the circumstances. Such inconsistency may be difficult for the child. Depending on their age and developmental stage, children may respond differently to different styles.

Authoritative Parenting. Authoritative parents tend to be "child centered." They are accepting of and responsive to the child's needs, desires, and use of persuasive arguments. But they also set clear standards of mature behavior and enforce rules and standards firmly. They encourage open communication, give reasons for their decisions and disciplinary actions, and listen to the

TABLE 3-4
Some Common Myths Concerning Ways to Achieve Marital Happiness

Common Marital Myths	Family Systems Perspective
Marriage and families should be totally happy; each member should expect all or certainly most gratifications to come from the family unit.	A romantic myth; overlooks fact that many of life's satisfactions are commonly found outside family setting.
"Togetherness" through close physical proximity or joint activities leads to satisfactory family life and individual gratification.	Varies greatly from one family to another; cannot be considered ideal pattern for all families under all conditions.
Marital partners should be totally honest with one another at all times.	While openness and frankness are usually desirable, especially in the service of a constructive, problem-solving approach, they may also be damaging if used in the service of hostile, destructive feelings.
In happy marriages, there are no disagreements; when family members fight, it means they hate each other.	Differences between family members are inevitable and often lead to arguments; if these clarify feelings and are not personal attacks, they may be constructive and preferable to covering up differences by always appearing to agree.
Marital partners should see eye to eye on every issue and work toward identical outlook.	Differences in background, experiences, personality make this impossible to achieve; actually different outlooks, if used constructively, may provide family with more options in carrying out developmental tasks.
Marital partners should be unselfish and not think of their individual needs.	Extremes of self-absorption or selflessness are undesirable; satisfactions are needed as an individual, not merely appendage to others (for example, mother lives only to serve family).
Whenever something goes wrong in the family, it is important to determine who is at fault.	Rather than blaming a single individual, dysfunction in the family interactions should be examined so that all members accept responsibilities.
Rehashing the past is helpful when things are not going well at present.	Endless recriminations about past errors usually escalate present problems, not reduce them, because they usually invite retaliation from the partner.
In a marital argument, one partner is right and the other wrong, with the goal of seeing who can score the most "points."	Marriages generally suffer when competition rather than cooperation characterizes marital interactions.
A good sexual relationship inevitably leads to a good marriage.	Good sexual relationship is an important component of a satisfactory marriage, but it does not preclude presence of interpersonal difficulties in other areas
In a satisfactory marriage, the sexual aspect will more or less take care of itself.	Not necessarily; sexual difficulties may be brought into marriage or related to stresses outside of the marriage.
Marital partners understand each other's nonverbal communications and therefore do not need to check things out with one another verbally.	Less likely to be true in dysfunctional families, where misperceptions and misinterpretations of each other's meanings and intent are common.
Positive feedback is not as necessary in marriage as negative feedback.	Positive feedback (attention, compliments) increases the likelihood that desirable behavior will reoccur, rather than taking for granted that it will and focusing on what's wrong with the other's behavior.
Good marriages simply happen spontaneously and require no effort.	Another romantic myth: good marriages require daily input by both partners, with constant negotiation, communication, and mutual problem solving.
Any spouse can (and often should) be reformed and remodeled into the shape desired by the partner.	A poor premise in marriage, and one likely to lead to frustration, anger, and disillusionment. Working on improving the relationship should make partners more compatible and sensitive to each other's needs.
In a stable marriage, things do not change and there are no problems.	All living systems change, grow, and develop over time. Fixed systems sooner or later are out of phase with current needs and developments.
Everyone knows what a husband should be like and what a wife should be like.	Untrue, especially in modern society, where new roles are being explored.
If a marriage is not working properly, having children will rescue it.	On the contrary, children usually become the victims of marital disharmony.
No matter how bad a marriage, it should be kept together for the sake of the children.	Not necessarily true that children thrive better in an unhappy marriage than with a relatively satisfied divorced parent. In marriages where partners stay together as "martyrs" for the children's sake, children usually bear the brunt of resentment partners feel for one another.
If marriage does not work out, an extramarital affair, or divorce and marriage to another spouse, will cure the situation.	Occasionally true, but without gaining insight, similar choices will be made and the same nongratifying patterns repeated.

From Goldenberg, I. & Goldenberg, H. (1985). *Family therapy: An overview* (2nd ed., pp. 82–83). Monterey: Brooks/Cole Publishing.

child's point of view. What are their children like? The children of authoritative parents are generally self-reliant, self-controlled, socially competent, friendly, and have high self-esteem.

Authoritarian Parenting. Authoritarian parents may not balance their demands for mature behavior with an acceptance of the child's needs. They may place strict limits on the child's expression of desires. They characteristically do not discuss their rules and decisions and suppress the child's efforts to challenge their authority. Authoritarian parents exert their greater power through physical punishment and harsh disapproval. Their children tend to fit the image of "speaking when spoken to" — they may lack social competence and spontaneity, are standoffish, and have low self-esteem.

Permissive Parenting. Permissive parents are accepting, responsive, and loving, but they exercise less control over their child's behavior. They characteristically

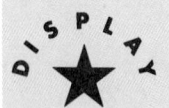

Developmental Tasks of Parenthood

Proposition 1: Parenthood is one of a series of developmental tasks of adult life wherein the parent as well as the child is modified and changed. It is unique in its irrevocability and its power to transform and transcend all other aspects of development.

Proposition 2: The interactional effects between parent and child are stage dependent. Each stage of the child's development present its own goals and challenges, which are faced by parents of widely divergent experiences and developmental stages.

Proposition 3: Parents are frequently caught up in patterns of behavior with their children wherein they re-experience and re-enact an earlier conflict of their own as a child reaches the developmental stage in which the parent's conflict had originated. Such patterns can be, and often are, negative and circular in their functioning.

Proposition 4: Parents bring from their own life experiences expectations and aspirations for themselves and their children of which they are not always aware. Yet these often unconscious motivations significantly influence the childrearing process, with both positive and negative effects.

Proposition 5: A major challenge for parents is to love and bestow affection and caring on significant family members from two distinct generations: their parents and their children. They must also prepare to yield the intensity of their attachments as the parents grow old and the children grow away.

Boyle, M. P. (1983). Evolving parenthood: A developmental perspective. In M. Levine, W. Carey, A. Crocker, & R. Gross (Eds.). Developmental behavioral pediatrics (pp. 50–63). Philadelphia: W. B. Saunders.

avoid, whenever possible, making demands for mature behavior, setting restrictions, and asserting their authority. They allow the child to govern his or her own behavior, often to the point of determining bedtime, mealtime, or television watching. Children of permissive parents tend to be impulsive, aggressive, and lacking the ability to take responsibility.

Indifferent or Uninvolved Parenting. Indifferent or uninvolved parents generally are not highly committed to their role as parents. They try to spend as little time and effort as possible with the child. They tend to be rejecting of and unresponsive to the child's needs, and they provide little guidance and inconsistent discipline. When interacting with the child, their goal often is to increase their own immediate comfort. Children of indifferent or uninvolved parents tend to be hostile, aggressive, disobedient, and disagreeable. They have low self-esteem and may show little regard for other people's rights. Parents who are indifferent and uninvolved can expect problems in response to their uncaring styles and behaviors.

Assessing, Promoting, and Maintaining Parenting Success

Increasingly, nurses are assuming critical roles in planning interventions to strengthen the parent-dyad and, in turn, the parent-child dyad and sibling-dyad. Nye and Berardo[34] indicate that parenting child-care roles include feeding children regularly with adequate diets, providing appropriate clothing, and protecting the child from unintentional physical injury and traumatic experiences.

The nurse needs to be aware of the significance of the parenting role in promoting optimal family and child development. The nurse often has an opportunity to help parents meet their goals in successful childrearing. Also, the nurse must be able to view parents as experiencing clearly identifiable issues of their own. Such observations and insights can be valuable in clarifying concerns and problems and can serve as the springboard for gaining greater parental collaboration in problem solving.

Assessment

Systematic observations and assessments of parenting behaviors are necessary to assist parents in achieving the goals they have established for their children and themselves. The nurse gathers data through observations of parenting styles. Additionally, it is important to obtain parents' perceptions of their own parenting skills, styles, concerns, problems, and priorities. Nurses should be particularly alert for the consistency with which a parent interacts or responds to a child. Nurses can make observations of parents and children in a variety of settings, including the newborn nursery, intensive care unit, hospital unit, child day care center, preschool setting, and school and home settings of children, regardless of whether it be a foster home, natural home, or shelter for homeless children (Fig. 3-4).

The nurse observes how parents identify their children's cues and whether their responses are appropriate. The home may be a more appropriate setting for observing parent-child interactions than a clinic or hospital. The nurse must also include assessments of the home environment (see Appendix) with particular attention to safety for all age groups.

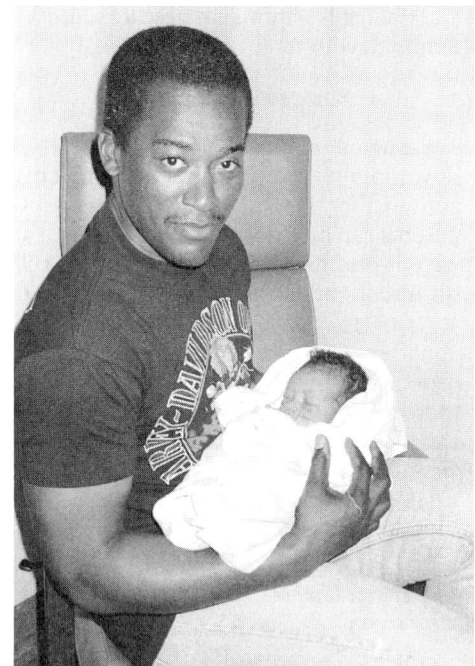

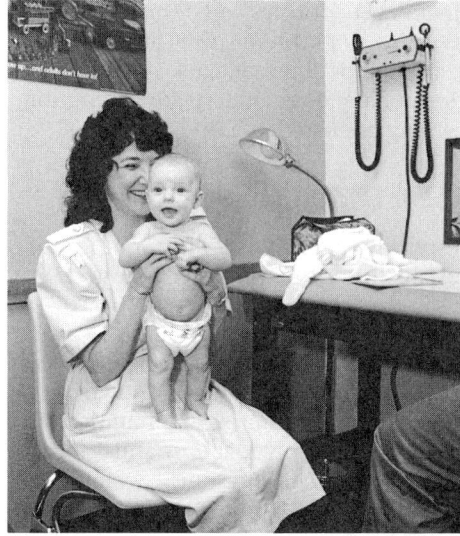

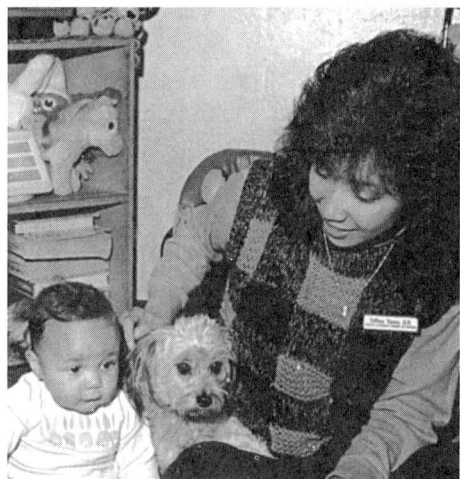

FIGURE 3-4
Parenting can be observed in a variety of settings. Shown here are a father with his newborn in a contemporary maternity center, a mother and daughter in well-child care, and a nursing student visiting in a home. (The last photo is courtesy of Seattle University.)

If parents report concerns regarding crying, sleep, feeding, play, dressing-undressing, language, gross motor skills, or behavioral problems, it is helpful for the nurse to make home visits to gather essential data. Such observations would focus on the parents' perceptions of a concern, the frequency of a concern, its duration, when it most likely occurs, what has been tried to resolve it, the parents' skills in problem-solving, what the parents wish to do next, and what the parents' greatest priority is.

Nursing Diagnoses and Planning

Nursing diagnoses related to family functioning were discussed earlier in this chapter, whereas the dysfunctional family is discussed in Chapter 5. The NANDA diagnoses for altered parenting include Parental Role Conflict, Altered Parenting, and High Risk for Altered Parenting. The first two are discussed here.

Parental Role Conflict is described by NANDA as "the state in which a parent experiences role confusion and conflict in response to crisis."[44] Such a conflict may arise from illness of the care provider or of the child, or a change in the status of care providers. Chronic illnesses and treatment regimens may interfere with the normal parenting functioning.

Altered Parenting is described by NANDA as "the state in which a nurturing figure(s) experiences an inability to create an environment which promotes the optimum growth and development of another human being."[44] Adjusting to parenting is a normal maturational process that requires understanding of development and anticipation of problems. If the parent is unable to provide the necessary environment, parenting effectiveness may become altered.

Together, the parents and nurse establish goals and interventions to address parenting goals.

Interventions

Health care professionals no longer take the child, fix it up, and give it back to the parents. Professionals no longer relegate mothers and fathers to the position of passive recipients of care. Rather, a mutual participation model is used, one in which parents are actively involved in solutions to their children's problems. This model reflects the fact that parents are in charge of their children's welfare. Nurses in a variety of roles can demonstrate respect for parents' ability to problem solve, manage, and respond to their children of different ages.

Approaches for nursing interventions for promotion of functional parenting are listed in Table 3-5.

Reinforcement of Goals

Parents are responsive to encouragement for the realistic goals they establish for their children, the reasonableness of their standards for children, the positive approaches they use, the successes they achieve, the goals they accomplish, and their ability to role model for their children. Parents are receptive to being acknowledged for their ability to reduce stress, improve communication with their children, problem solve, and establish goals with their children, as well as their ability to maintain affectionate and emotional bonds in the midst of stress, struggles, and frustration.

Counseling

To promote positive parenting, nurses have opportunities to base their counseling on parents' realistic expectations of a child, the parents' readiness to change behaviors, and the child's readiness to learn different ways of behaving. Nurses are in strategic positions to also discuss with parents which choices and alternatives they as parents wish to offer to their own children.

Nurses can also be effective in helping parents identify sources of stress and approaches that can reduce or eliminate it. Nurses can serve as exemplary role models for desirable parental behaviors and interactions with children.

Parenting issues are presented in Table 3-2 earlier in the chapter. The nurse provides anticipatory guidance and counsels parents on how to address various stages of family development simultaneously.

Anticipatory Guidance

Nurses' comprehensive knowledge of growth and development can be helpful to parents in the form of anticipatory guidance. Parenting classes for all first-time parents can be extremely helpful when anticipatory guidance is emphasized. Sometimes these classes are carried on in connection with childbirth programs. Telephone services to answer questions give parents more self-confidence in care of the first child. Such services are especially important in clinics or communities where there are adolescent mothers.

Anticipatory guidance is discussed in the health assessment, promotion, and maintenance of well children, Chapters 10 through 16. In many instances, there are Tables addressing anticipatory guidance.

Evaluation

Carpenito[11] identified outcome criteria for parental role conflict and its resolution when related to effects of illness of a child on the family. Such criteria are based on the assumption of knowledgeable parental decision making and active participation in the care of the sick child. Outcome criteria related to altered parenting looks for improved bonding or improved relationship and communication between the parent and child.

Roles and Relationships: Siblings

More than 80% of all children in the United States are siblings; at the turn of the century, there will be at least 62 million children under the age of 18.[31] Although sibling

---

TABLE 3-5
Nursing Intervention: Promoting Positive Parenting Within Families

- Focus on mother's and father's perceptions of child's needs.
- Have continuing dialogue with both parent and child dyads.
- Ask repeatedly about the entire family's perceptions of health or illness to correct misunderstandings.
- Provide verbal and written summaries of child's health care needs and progress.
- Reinforce parents "being in charge" of their child's growth and development and health status.
- Schedule regular follow-up sessions with parents and family members.
- Plan to have both parents present to support each other and reduce stress.
- Encourage parents to ask questions about illness or progress in health.
- Ask family to share their ideas about how to shift priorities and delegate health care tasks to all members of the family.
- Encourage all members of family to change health behaviors to minimize the child's "sick" label.
- Respond to and include parents as consultants to health care team.
- View parents as experts of their own children.
- Provide care based on developmental tasks of children, parents, and family members in the life cycle.
- Focus on long-term and a life course perspective of parents' development tasks within a family system.
- Assist entire family in mobilizing a strong social supportive network; encourage all members to join appropriate groups.
- Provide child with teaching sessions and written instructions that can help increase compliance and reduce feelings of dependence.

- Explain to child's teachers and peers what to expect on child's return to school.
- Focus directly on child to reduce doubts about his or her capabilities and increase strivings for independence and autonomy.
- Provide comprehensive care based on observations of changes and unique needs, and perceived needs of parents and their children.
- Delegate appropriate health-related tasks to mothers, fathers, children, grandparents, and members of extended family.
- Assess parents' mastery of developmental tasks and progress in life cycle.
- Focus on father's needs for anticipatory guidance, principles of growth and development, discipline, ways to promote children's competence, environmental safety, and principles of behavioral management for sleep, feeding, toileting, play, and behavioral problems.
- Teach fathers principles of child care such as diapering, dressing, and health care regimens.
- Support fathers in their home health care responsibilities for children who are ill.
- Encourage fathers to be present for developmental and health assessments of children.
- Support mothers and fathers to address developmental issues beyond infancy, i.e., such topics as temperament, separation, autonomy, independence, industry, identity, and self-esteem, and parental issues such as quality day care, home health care, latch-key children, child neglect and abuse, violence, substance abuse, run-aways, gangs, and teen-age pregnancy.

factors have generally been overlooked in most family research in favor of the parent-parent, mother-child, or father-child dyad,[43] longitudinal studies have found that the sibling bond is generally positive, even when the sibling dyads are of mixed gender.[1]

Characteristics of Relationships

The sibling relationship usually provides the first and most intense peer relationship.[36] (Fig. 3-5). Sibling relationships have distinct characteristics in that they are marked by their intensity, complexity, and longevity.[31,33,43] Whereas most relationships outside the home are essentially brief encounters, a sibling relationship may span six or more decades. Relationships between children and their parents rarely last as long in comparison.

Not only do sibling relationships extend over a long period, but they also are characterized by the intensity of their involvement. Children spend more hours, days, and years with each other in comparison to any other family subsystem.[43]

Siblings may experience ambivalence toward each other. On one hand, they yearn for an equal relationship with someone with whom they can tell secrets, play, and talk about their parents;[43] on the other hand, they compete for parental time and love. These children may vacillate between solidarity and rivalry, loyalty and betrayal, companionship and withdrawal, love and dislike, competition and cooperation, and envy and pride. All of these feelings exert a powerful influence on personality development, relationships, and preparation for later adult roles. (Sibling rivalry is discussed as a preschool problem in Chap. 14.)

Roles

Through forced interactions over the long years of childhood, siblings exert a powerful influence on each other's identity. Even though their actions may be unin-

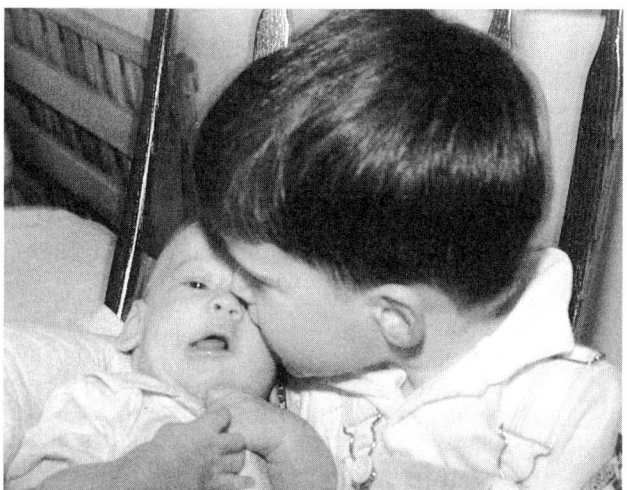

FIGURE 3-5
The sibling relationship is the first and most intense peer relationship. The family setting provides an emotional outlet for children.

tentional, brothers and sisters take on many roles: mentor, supporter, comforter, protector, and socializer. Children who do not have siblings may have to depend on peers, friends, and other family members to interact with them and to fulfill sibling roles.

As *mentors*, siblings serve as teacher and role models for each other. The younger learn from the older. As *supporters*, siblings give affection and help each other during stress and disruptive periods in the family. This may be seen especially in families that are homeless or living in poverty. Minuchin,[32] in direct observation of siblings in underprivileged families, concluded that sibling functions are vital for each other.

As *comforters*, siblings have special methods of sharing problems with each other. Toddlers may become upset at the new baby's crying and suggest ways to comfort the baby. As *protectors*, siblings make an effort to defend each other. This may be seen especially in an older brother's concern for his younger sister. As *socializers*, siblings enrich and expand each other's play and help each other in their psychosocial development and self-definition. Children experience significant social experiences and problems with each other that prepare them for other relationships outside the family.[43] Siblings learn first from their brothers and sisters about competition, domination, conflict, rules, sharing, and taking turns. Through each other they are helped to establish an identity.

Factors Affecting Roles

Despite the fact that most parents make an effort to treat their children equally, each child in the family develops unique interactional patterns. "The truth is that *no two children are ever born into the same family*, even though they share the same parents and the same experiences."[42] The experience of the first child is very different from the experience of the fifth child. The firstborn experience of a new baby is different from the experience of the second born. Among various factors affecting children's development are cultural and ethnic values, gender of children and siblings, family size and spacing, birth position, educational level and ordinal patterns of parents, methods of discipline, socioeconomic level, and location of the household.

Family Size

An only child grows up in an adult world, and a close relationship may develop with the parents. The child may be allowed to participate in adult activities at a young age, for example, be included in family parties or dinners. Parents may be overprotective, and the child may tend to feel he or she is the center of attention for a longer time than normal. These relationships affect the child's behaviors, attitudes, and skills.

A smaller family may have more money and more time for recreational activities. Clothes and toys may be new rather than hand-me-downs for only children. Children may receive a great deal of individual parental attention. Families with fewer children may more easily arrange for their only child to go to college.

However, the larger the family, the more that resources have to be shared. More activities center around the home and family, and the relationship between siblings may be a close one. When there are more children in a family, the parents have to divide their time with more, allowing less time for each individual child. One advantage of a large family is the fact that children may accept more responsibility at an earlier age for both themselves and their siblings.

Altered Function

Roles and relationships change when an altered function occurs in a sibling. Altered function may stimulate or hinder each child's development as well as the interaction between the siblings over the period the illness persists. Featherstone[19] hypothesized that siblings with ill brothers or sisters may long for the "lost relationship that might have been" had an illness not occurred. The way an illness affects the long-term relationship among siblings remains an intriguing but largely unanswered question.[3]

More in-depth discussion of aspects of sibling relationships are discussed in the following chapters: vulnerable child syndrome, Chapter 20; chronic illness, Chapter 21; hospitalization, Chapter 23; and dying and death, Chapter 32. Siblings are also taken into consideration as part of the family throughout the text, including the nursing care plans and teaching plans.

Nurses who provide family-centered child health care must focus on each sibling's developmental tasks. An important question for the nurse to consider is, "Does the altered function affect the ability of siblings to be mentors, supporters, comforters, protectors, and socializers?" Suggestions for nursing interventions in sibling illness are given in Table 3-6. See other chapters for additional interventions.

Summary

Consistent approaches are needed in family-centered care in a diverse and rapidly changing society. Because there is no "typical" American family, nurses should demonstrate greater acceptance of pluralism in family living arrangements, be more flexible in their approaches, and exemplify innovative and creative support for differences exhibited by all family types. Nurses need to develop skills and expertise for a pluralistic society and to respond appropriately to periods of rapid social change affecting family members.

Most families maintain a state of equilibrium during normal transitions and developmental crises; however, keeping a family system in balance requires monitoring of outside forces and consideration of the family values and lifestyles.

As trends in society change and traditional roles in the family are modified, there are more challenges confronting the family. The nurse has vital roles to assume in helping families adapt to transitions and the stressors of change.

Nurses have a wealth of assessment tools and theoretical frameworks to use in assessing and identifying families needing support, especially those at greatest risk for dysfunction. Nurses also have multiple opportunities to enhance healthy child, sibling, parent, and family functioning. By applying theories of child and family development nurses can provide well timed anticipatory guidance, education, referral, and nurturing support to children and families who need it. Most importantly, nurses can apply concepts of family-centered care in practice to enhance optimal functioning in children, parents, and other family members throughout the different stages of the family life cycle. Family-centered care practiced by nurses strengthens and fosters normal family de-

---

TABLE 3-6
Nursing Intervention: Promoting Healthy Function of the Well Sibling

- Concentrate on well child's social needs.
- Assess well sibling for physical symptoms, quality of relationships with family members, social behaviors with peers, communication abilities, and progress in school.
- Assess learning needs of well child and develop appropriate interactional strategies.
- Delegate health care tasks to well sibling commensurate with age, cognitive abilities, and developmental stages.
- Keep well child informed as to sick child's status.
- Thoroughly observe well child for behavior manifestation of bed wetting, thumb sucking, heightened separation anxiety, nightmares, or other clues of regression in development.
- Monitor well child's academic performance and observe for poor grades, underachievement or overachievement, or behavioral problems in school.
- Ask specific questions of well child about where ill child is sick, and how doctors make siblings better.
- Invite well and sick siblings to join support groups (i.e., diabetic or oncology support groups, etc.)
- Meet with well sibling and elicit perceptions of well child's understanding of sick child's illness and the meaning assigned to it by the well child, and answer questions about child's future and responsibilities.
- Encourage well and sick siblings to speak for themselves.

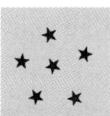

Ideas for Nursing Research

The nurse in well-child settings, school systems, hospitals, clinics, and home settings is in a unique position to explore the relationships between and among family members. The following areas need to be explored:

- Comparison of degree of pain reported by children when parents are present 24 hours a day and when parents' presence is irregular.
- Difference in family interactions when the observations are made in the child's home versus in a clinic setting.
- Single mothers' description of greatest need for their children's health.
- Comparison of feelings of security and self-esteem between children growing up in extended families, nuclear families, and single-parent families.

velopment. By using family-centered care nurses implement important roles to ensure that children will be able to master their unique developmental tasks and fulfill their potential. Parents, too, will be assisted in accomplishing their goals of rearing healthy children and achieving success in their parental roles and responsibilities. The nurse's application of family-centered care approaches fosters each child's and family member's well being and happiness. Through family-centered care nurses can help the family strengthen its bonds, add to its resiliency, and preserve the ideals of family life and its necessary place in today's society.

References

1. Abramovitch, R., Corter, C., Pepler, D. J., & Stanhope, L. (1986). Sibling and peer interaction: A final follow-up and a comparison. *Child Development, 57*(1), 217–229.
2. Aponte, H. J., & Van Deusen, J. M. (1981). Structured family therapy. In A. S. Gurman & D. P. Kniskern (Eds.), *Handbook of family therapy.* New York: Brunner/Muzel.
3. Bank, S., & Kahn, M. D. (1982). *The sibling bond.* New York: Basic Books.
4. Billingsley, A. (1987). Family: Contemporary patterns. In *Encyclopedia of social work.* Silver Springs, MD: National Association of Social Workers.
5. Block, D. A. (1985). The family as a psychosocial system. In S. Henao, & N. P. Grose (Eds.), *Principles of family systems in family medicine.* New York: Brunner/Mazel.
6. Boyle, M. P. (1983). Evolving parenthood: A developmental perspective. In M. Levine, W. Carey, A. Crocker, & R. Gross (Eds.), *Developmental behavioral pediatrics* (pp. 50–63). Philadelphia: W. B. Saunders.
7. Burr W. R., Hill R., Nye F. L., et al (Eds.), (1979). *Contemporary theories about the family,* Vols. 1 and 2. New York: Free Press.
8. Burr, W., & Leigh, K. (1983). Famology: A new discipline. *Journal of Marriage and the Family 45*(3), 467–480.
9. Carter, B., & McGoldrick, M. (1988). *The changing family life cycle: A framework for family therapy.* New York: Gardner Press.
10. Carter, E. A., & McGoldrick, M. (Eds.), (1980). *The family life cycle: A framework for family therapy.* New York: Gardner Press.
11. Carpenito, L. J. (1992). *Nursing diagnosis: Application to clinical practice* (4th ed.). Philadelphia: J. B. Lippincott.
12. Curran, D. D. (1983). *Traits of a healthy family: Fifteen traits commonly found in healthy families by those who work with them.* Minneapolis, MN: Winston Press.
13. Dunst, C., et al. (1988). Enabling and empowering families of children with health impairments. *Children's Health Care 17,* 71–81.
14. Duvall, E. M. (1971). *Family development.* (4th ed.). Philadelphia: J. B. Lippincott.
15. Duvall, E. M. (1977). *Marriage and family development.* Philadelphia: J. B. Lippincott.
16. Dyer, E. D. (1963). Parenthood as crisis: A re-study. *Marriage Family Living, 25,* 196–201.
17. Eidison, B. (1983). Traditional and alternative life styles. In H. Levine, W. Crocher, W. Carey, & R. Crossman (Eds.), *Developmental-behavioral pediatrics.* Philadelphia: W. B. Saunders.
18. Epstein, N., & Bishop, D. (1981). Problem centered systems therapy of the family. In A. Gurman & D. Kniskern (Eds.), *Handbook of family therapy.* New York: Brunner/Mazel.
19. Featherstone, H. (1980). *A difference in the family: Life with a disabled child.* New York: Basic Books.
20. Framo, J. (1981). The integration of marital therapy with sessions with family of origin. In A. S. Gurman & D. P. Kniskern (Eds.), *Handbook of family therapy.* New York: Brunner/Mazel
21. Gillis, C. L., Highley, B. L., Roberts, B. M., & Martinson, I. M.: *Toward a science of family nursing.* New York, Addison-Wesley, 1989
22. Goldenberg, I., & Goldenberg, H. (1985). *Family therapy: An overview* (2nd ed.). Belmont, CA, Wadsworth.
23. Gutman, D. L. (1985). The parental imperative revisited: Towards a developmental psychology of adulthood and later life. *Contemporary Human Development, 14,* 31–60.
24. Handel, G.: *The psychosocial interior of the family.* New York: Aldine Publishing, 1985.
25. Hareven, T. K. (1982). American families in transition: Historical perspectives on change. In F. Walsh (Ed.), *Normal family processes* (p. 13). New York: Guilford Press.
26. Hennen, B. K. (1980). Family structure and function. In D. B. Shires & B. K. Hennen (Eds.), *Family medicine: A guidebook for practitioners of the art* (p. 19). New York: McGraw-Hill.
27. LeMasters, E. E. (1957). Parenthood in crisis. *Marriage Family Living, 9,* 352.
28. Lidz, T. (1986). *The person* (Rev. Ed.). New York: Basic Books.
29. McCubbin, H. I., & Figley, C. R. (1983). *Stress and the family* (p. 33). New York: Brunner/Mazel.
30. McGoldrick, M., & Carter, E. A. (1982). The family life cycle. In F. Walsh (Ed.), *Normal family processes* (p. 175). New York: Guilford.
31. McKeever, P. (1983). Siblings of chronically ill children: A literature review with implications for research and practice. *American Journal of Orthopsychiatry, 53,* 209–218.
32. Minuchin, S. (1974). *Families and family therapy.* Cambridge, MA: Harvard University Press.
33. Moss, C. A. (1987). *Sibling relationships: A study of family adaptation and social support* (Unpublished master's thesis, pp. 19–20). Atlanta: Nell Hodgson Woodruff School of Nursing, Emory University.
34. Nye, F. I., & Berardo, F. M. (1973). *The family: Its structure and interaction* (p. 404). New York: Macmillan.
35. Powell, M. L. (1980). A definition of parenting. Salt Lake City: University of Utah College of Nursing.
36. Powell, T. H., & Ogle, P. A. (1985). *Brothers and sisters—a special part of exceptional families.* Baltimore: Paul H. Brooks.
37. Reeder, S. J., Martin, L. L., & Koniak, D. (1992). *Maternity nursing: Family, newborn, and women's health care* (17th ed.). Philadelphia: J. B. Lippincott.
38. Roberts, L. (1987). The family life cycle in medical practice. In M. Crouch & L. Roberts (Eds.), *The family in medical practice: A family systems primer* (p. 75). New York: Springer-Verlag.
39. Rossi, A. (1980). Transition to parenthood. In J. M. Henslin (Ed.), *Marriage and family in a changing society* (pp. 318–329). New York: Free Press.
40. Sarafino, E. P., & Armstrong, J. W. (1986). Social relations in the family. In *Child and adolescent development* (2nd ed., pp. 330–338). St. Paul: West Publishing.
41. Schulz, D. A., & Rodgers, S. F. (1985). *Marriage, the family and personal fulfillment.* Englewood Cliffs, NJ: Prentice-Hall.
42. Schuster, C. S., & Ashburn, S. S. (1992). *The process of human development: A holistic life-span approach* (3rd ed.). Philadelphia: J. B. Lippincott.
43. Siemon, M. (1984). Siblings of the chronically ill or disabled child: Meeting their needs. *Nursing Clinics of North America, 19*(2), 295–307.
44. Taxonomy I (Revised 1990). St. Louis: North American Nursing Diagnosis Association.
45. *The General Mills American Family Report: 1976–1977: Raising Children in a Changing Society* (pp. 34–37). Minneapolis: General Mills, Inc.
46. Turk, D., & Kerns, R. (1985). The family in health and illness. In *Health-illness and families: A life-span perspective.* New York: John Wiley and Sons.

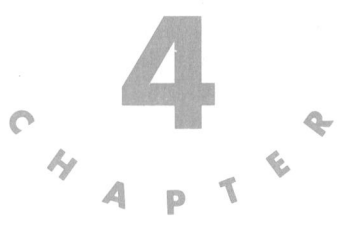

Cultural and Economic Influences on the Family

CHAPTER 4

FEATURES OF THIS CHAPTER

Nursing Assessment: Questions for Assessing Cultural Patterns, Table 4-1

Ideas for Nursing Research

BEHAVIORAL OBJECTIVES

Contrast an ethnocentric perspective to that of cultural pluralism in providing nursing care to children.

Discuss cultural characteristics of selected minority ethnic groups.

Describe the nurse's role in providing culturally relevant health care.

Discuss the impact of cost containment measures on health care for children in minority ethnic groups.

Identify nursing research issues related to cultural and economic influences on the family.

One of the unique characteristics of North America is the variety and number of ethnic groups that comprise its population. Providing optimum health care is an enormous challenge when there are so many cultural variations. Nurses are increasingly aware of the need to understand different cultures and establish patterns of communication with the diversity of children for whom they care.

North American society is also economically diversified. Families living in poverty who are employed or underemployed, families considered as the working poor, and middle income families where one or both parents have become unemployed deserve special attention and consideration. Poverty has no ethnic boundaries, but many ethnic minorities may also be classified as economically poor. Children from these families have numerous health, social, and emotional needs that nurses must be prepared to identify and address.

The focus of this chapter is on cultural and economic influences on children and their families. Cultural aspects such as family structure and kinship bonds, religious beliefs, health beliefs and practices, communication, and interpersonal relations are discussed for the Southeast Asians (Vietnamese), Native Americans (Navajos), Latinos (Mexican Americans), Asian Americans (Chinese), and African Americans. Problems of two other groups, the homeless population and migrant families, are also included. Finally, some of the barriers to health care for children from ethnic minorities and economic aspects of the health care system are reviewed.

Cultural Diversity and Cross-Cultural Nursing

Terminology

Differentiating among terms related to culture, ethnicity, and race is important, but the differences are sometimes complex and confusing. *Culture* is the "central core of each ethnic group; it binds them together with the thread of beliefs, styles of being and adapting."[49] Culture is further described as the behavior patterns of a group or the sum total of a way of life. Culture is the knowledge, beliefs, customs, folkways, mores, religion, and language of a group of people. Culture has long been recognized as a significant determinant of behavior and values within ethnic groups.[25]

When people leave a familiar culture and enter another that is totally unfamiliar, they may experience *culture shock.* Feelings of confusion, anxiety, and fear are common. The process of becoming adapted to new cultural patterns is known as *acculturation.* Newcomers generally try to fit into the mainstream of their new culture. People may become acculturated, but they do not necessarily become assimilated. With *assimilation,* minorities lose their own cultural identity and assume the behaviors of the dominant cultural group.

Race is a biologic label that refers to traits transmitted by birth, such as the clear distinctions between African Americans and whites. Three accepted classifications of racial types are Caucasoid, Mongoloid, and Negroid. These classifications have an impact on how people think and treat each other. The American society tends to use the norms of Anglo-European culture in evaluating the attitudes and behaviors of people from cultural backgrounds different from their own.[25] This biased attitude

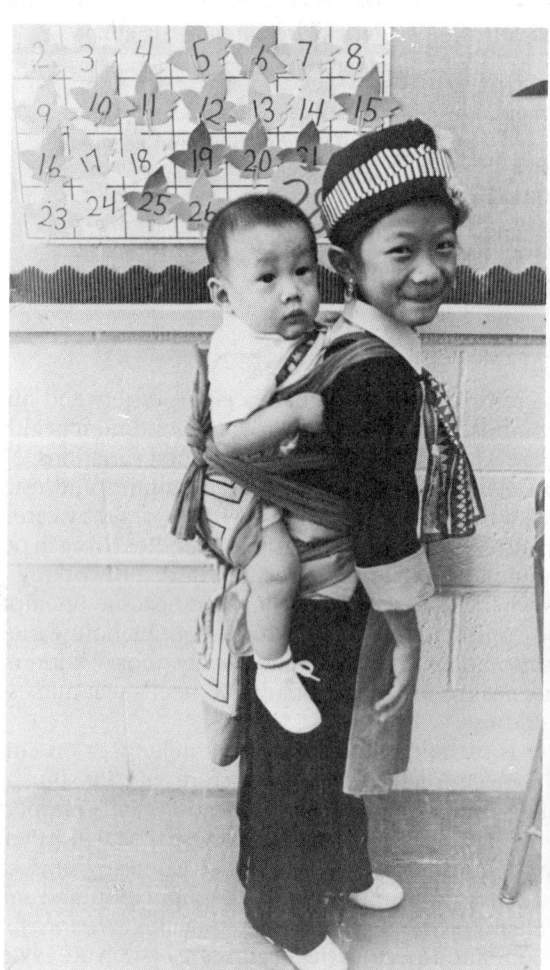
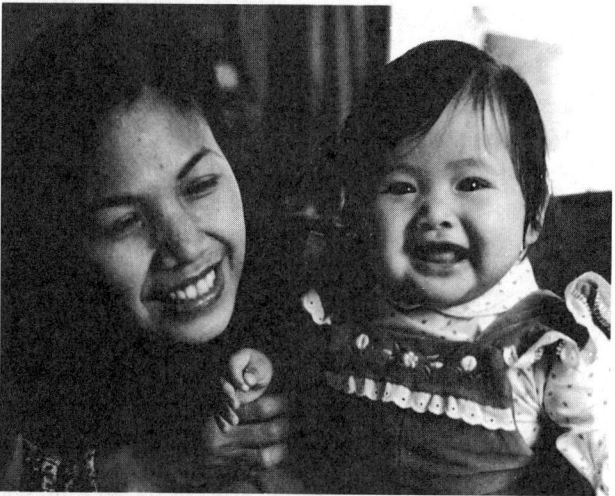
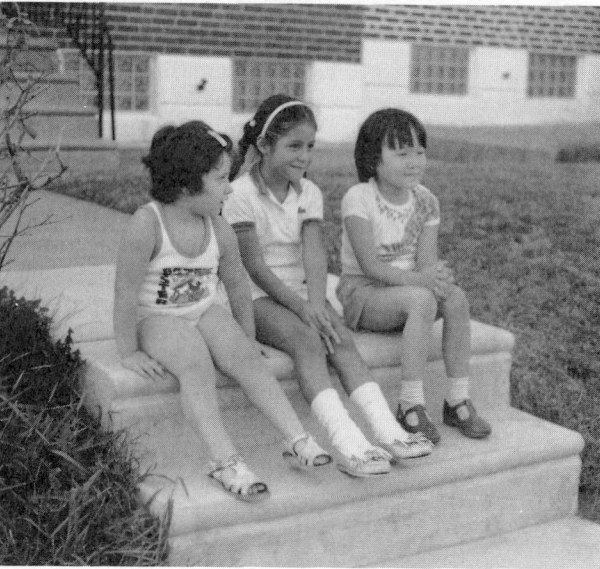

FIGURE 4-1

Perspective of cultural pluralism: cultural heritages should be respected. Pride in one's culture can be fostered by sharing native costumes and customs with teachers and peers. In the second half of the century, Mexican American families have become less isolated and have joined the mainstream. Interactions with peers from other cultures and ethnic groups (Italian, Latino, and Chinese in the lower right) enriches one's values and viewpoints. Children may be acculturated but not assimilated.

is labeled as *ethnocentrism,* the belief that one's own culture is superior to that of any other culture.[25,35] Furthermore, Americans have a tendency to *stereotype* various groups that are culturally different from their own. They apply labels and make generalizations about groups that are often untrue.

One culture cannot be considered inferior or superior to another, and there is no inherent measurement scale to assess the value of a given culture. Many nurses and other health professionals have adopted the perspective of *cultural pluralism,* the understanding that a society is composed of diverse ethnic, racial, religious, and social groups that maintain their traditional cultures and special interests (Fig. 4-1).

Ethnicity can be described as belonging to a particular group in which people share a common sociohistory, have a distinct identity of themselves as a group, and have common geographical, religious, linguistic, racial, and cultural roots. *Ethnic minorities* may be native to the country or immigrant groups. Collectively, ethnic minority groups are rapidly becoming the majority population in the United States; throughout the world, they represent two thirds of the people.[29] Characteristics of several ethnic minority groups are discussed below.

Characteristics of Selected Minorities

The concept of America as a melting pot is a myth suggesting that all differences among groups within the population are blended and lost over time. In contrast, "cultural uniqueness" emphasizes that ethnic minorities have distinct cultures. Although ethnic minority groups do adopt some characteristic behaviors or practices of the dominant culture, many people maintain their own identity and cultural heritage.[19,39]

On the other hand, although similar groups of ethnic minorities share commonalities such a language, color, and historic background, not all members of an ethnic group are alike. There are often subcultures within the dominant culture. For example, Hispanic Americans, Mexican Americans, and Cubans are part of the Latino culture; they have similarities as well as differences.

Southeast Asians (Vietnamese)

Southeast Asians represent a diverse group including Vietnamese, Cambodians, and Laotians (Tai and Hmong). Over the past two decades, the number of Southeast Asians, especially Vietnamese, entering the United States has steadily increased. Many of these newcomers to North America are refugees and not immigrants; that is, they fled their homeland to escape danger or persecution. After coming to the United States, Southeast Asians encountered severe culture shock. Those people with wealth and education have experienced less severe culture shock, but the economically poor Vietnamese people have had more difficulty adjusting to being in North America.[37]

Family Structure and Kinship Bonds. There are strong kinship bonds in the Vietnamese family, and the extended family is the basic unit of the Vietnamese society.[13] Frequently, three or four generations live within one household. The family is traditionally patriarchal; the senior male assumes the position of head of household.[5] As a result of placement in North America, some extended families were separated and family units were disrupted.

Vietnamese do not view themselves independently of family; rather, individuals define themselves as integral parts of the family unit. Decisions are made by the family as a whole, rather than by individual members.[18] Because the family is central to the existence of the Vietnamese, it takes precedence over the individual and country. Thus, the primary goal of the Vietnamese person is to honor, and not to shame or embarrass, the family.

Finally, family lineage is extremely important to the Vietnamese; thus, the order of a person's name is significant. The family name is written first, the middle name second, and the given name last. For example, a female child's name is written as Ngugen Thi Yen, and she should be addressed as Yen.[5] Vietnamese are sensitive about this tradition and are insulted if it is ignored. Nurses who respect this preference when addressing Vietnamese patients can promote effective communication with the child and family.

Religious Beliefs. Vietnamese religious beliefs are derived from a combination of traditions. The dominant religion is Buddhism, but Catholicism and Confucianism are practiced as well as the belief in inanimate and animate good and evil spirits. Religious services are held in the home or in the family temple, and rituals are performed to express thanks or ward off various spirits.[5,13,35] Ancestral altars with incense burners and candlesticks may be found in many homes, and some Catholic homes may have altars with crucifixes and religious pictures.[5]

Religious philosophy is inherent in Vietnamese family health practices. Their holistic approach to health is derived from Buddhist and Chinese philosophy. Following the Buddhist tradition and belief in reincarnation, the Vietnamese believe that illness is the result of bad conduct by an individual or family member in a previous life. Each person is expected to assume responsibility for self cure. Because of this belief, Vietnamese generally do not feel obligated to care for anyone outside their own family.[13]

Health Beliefs and Practices. Vietnamese share the Chinese world view of the concept of harmony which includes the principles of the opposing forces of yin (hot, negative, and female) and yang (cold, positive, and male). Health is the result of the balance between yin and yang; if there is an imbalance, illness occurs. Vietnamese believe that this balance can be disturbed by uncontrolled emotions and improper diet such as an imbalance of yin and yang foods. For example, spicy foods are considered "hot" and bland foods are "cold."[5,13] If a child has a disease considered to be caused by increased yin forces, hot foods are avoided. These beliefs may be assessed by nurses when exploring health maintenance patterns in the process of establishing a comprehensive database.

Home remedies may be used to treat illness, but Vietnamese often use a combination of Western medicine and folk medicine.[5] To maintain equilibrium in the treatment of illness, Western medication and medicinal herbs are categorized according to their properties of hot and cold effects. Western medicines are classified as hot, whereas Oriental medicines are cold.

In addition to herbs, some Vietnamese folk medicinal substances include rice alcohol, deer antlers, dried bumblebees, orange peel, and mint.[5] Treatments practiced by cultural healers include acupuncture, scarification of strategic points on the skin, suction with small tubes or hot cups, and moxibustion (burning a soft substance called moxa on the skin's surface). Moxa is a soft, downy material obtained from a variety of plants including Chinese wormwood. Another folk healing practice called CaoGao ("rubbing out the wind") involves forcefully rubbing certain areas of the body (e.g., neck, head, back of the neck, chest, or back) with the fingers or a coin. Nurses who are unfamiliar with such practices may erroneously diagnose the dark bruises left by such treatment as child abuse.[5,16]

Self-restraint is expected during illness and may be displayed in ways that seem peculiar to Americans. Vietnamese children are taught to avoid open expressions of pain, and they may continue to smile even when intrusive treatments are performed or when they are experiencing extreme discomfort. In caring for the Vietnamese child, the nurse must use astute observational skills to assess accurately the response to pain.

Vietnamese have strong negative perceptions of mental illness and believe it is a stigma, a mark of shame, for the individual and family. Mental illness is thought to be the result of offending a god or demon or committing a sinful act. Because of the traditional belief that physical symptoms are more acceptable, Vietnamese have a tendency to somatize (convert to physical symptoms) any psychological problems. Their traditional views prevent them from readily seeking external help, so they use the family as a support system. When psychological problems are identified in a child, mental health counseling encouraged in a nonthreatening manner is more likely to be accepted.

Communication and Interpersonal Relations. The language barrier between Vietnamese and American health care professionals makes the communication process difficult. A trained interpreter or someone in the family who can speak English well should be present. If possible, the interpreter should be of the same social class, because Vietnamese are class conscious and find talking to anyone outside their social class difficult.[18,37] When discussing a child with Vietnamese parents, the nurse should be formal and polite, treating the family with tact and respect, because being casual is considered offensive. The father or the senior male in the group is addressed as spokesman because of his ascribed position in the family.[18] When questioning Vietnamese parents about their child's illness, it should be done in an indirect manner. Maintaining direct eye contact when conversing is a sign of disrespect. Finally, hand shaking is acceptable only among men.[5,18,37]

Nutritional Patterns. Vietnamese refugees have a daily caloric intake nearly two thirds that of the average American because of Southeast Asians' small stature. This difference is important to remember when assessing nu-

tritional patterns of Vietnamese children. Growth charts used to plot the growth of American children are not appropriate to use in assessing the growth of Vietnamese children because the measurement norms are based on studies of children from predominantly European descent. For example, most American children fall between the 20th and 80th percentiles for height and weight, whereas healthy Southeast Asian children may fall within the 3rd to 10th percentiles. Alarm about the small size of a Vietnamese child is not warranted unless signs of malnutrition are present or if the graphed data fall below the third percentile.[16]

The traditional Vietnamese diet consists of meat (primarily chicken and pork), some fish, fruits, and vegetables such as corn, yams, sweet potatoes, taro root, and green onions. Rice is a dietary staple, and garlic and black pepper are commonly used for seasoning. Tea is the preferred drink. Dairy products are not part of the Vietnamese diet because intolerance of lactose inhibits the absorption and digestion of milk products. Seeking alternate ways for the child to obtain adequate intake of calcium and protein is important in planning nursing care.[12]

Native Americans (Navajos)

There are over 400 different tribes of Native Americans in North America. Half of them live on 40 million acres of reservation in 40 states, and the other half live in urban areas. Several alarming socioeconomic statistics haunt Native Americans.[20] First, the life expectancy is 45 years, far less than any other ethnic group. Second, nearly 60% of the adult population has less than an eighth-grade education. Third, infant mortality is greater than 10% above the national average. Fourth, the majority of Native American families have annual incomes below $4000. Last, the unemployment rate is approximately ten times the national average.

Native Americans dislike the tendency of health care providers and others to classify them broadly as one group. Although they have adopted many of the values and beliefs of the Anglo-Saxon culture, they still value their tribal cultural differences. However, the following general characteristics are recognized across traditional Native American tribes.[21]

- Native Americans are present-oriented and not future oriented. They deal with the here and now.
- Native Americans' emphasis is on completing tasks rather than adhering to rigid schedules and being punctual. Tardiness for an appointment is not an indication of lack of interest, it is secondary to cultural beliefs about time.
- Native Americans place a great value on giving to others and sharing resources. They believe in working together. Competitive behavior is not encouraged.
- Native Americans believe in living in harmony with nature. They take from the environment only what is needed.
- Native Americans have strong kinship bonds, and the extended family is of great importance. Their households consist of relatives along both horizontal and vertical lineage. Grandparents are the official and symbolic leaders.

Navajos represent the largest Indian tribe in North America. There are approximately 150,000 Navajos living on reservations consisting of 24,000 square miles with perhaps another 20,000 to 30,000 living off reservations.[26] Much of the following discussion focuses on their culture.

Family Structure and Kinship Bonds. Family is an integral part of the lives of Navajos. All blood relatives are considered part of the extended family. Cousins are treated as brothers and sisters, and aunts and uncles are treated as grandparents. Even distant relatives are included in the family unit.[23] When children are hospitalized, the expectation of Native American families is that many people will visit.

Family also is an important social network. In many instances, several generations of family members may live in the same household. Family members participate in the care of sick relatives. Nurses can plan to use family members as resources in providing care to Native American children.

Religious Beliefs. Religion is directed toward the maintenance of harmony among nature, humans, and supernatural beings, and illness is a major indication of disharmony. Navajo religious rituals are centered around spirits and are predominantly health oriented.[39] When they are sick or suffer other misfortunes, their religious beliefs and practices help them through the crises. Religion and health are interwoven and not viewed independently of each other.

Health Beliefs and Practices. Navajos believe that disease has four major causes: loss of soul, intrusive objects, spirit possession, and witchcraft. First, it is believed that after birth the soul and wind enter the body and form the person's personality. At death, the wind leaves the body and goes to the afterworld. The first sign of a child's laughter means that the soul has attached itself to the body. Before this event, the Navajos believe that the infant could easily die. During death in old age, the soul becomes detached, but death at this time is considered natural. When a person dies while the wind-soul is well-attached, the person's ghost is thought to be the cause of disease in others.

An alternative view of illness is that an intrusive object enters the body by a special form of witchcraft. Elimination of pain in that part of the body where the object has lodged is accomplished by wizardry.

The third possible cause of illness is spirit intrusion (possession by spirits) in which the wind-soul is displaced by the spirit of a supernatural being. Recorded myths and healing ceremonies describe diseases in terms of spirit possession.[26]

Diseases are also thought to be caused by a form of witchcraft called witchery. Witches are associated with the dead and are considered dangerous.

The medicine man, sometimes called the singer or shaman, is a highly respected tribal leader and the traditional healer for Native Americans. Medicine men are considered diagnosticians, and they perform special ceremonies to determine the cause of disease. Sometimes these ceremonies take days.

Contemporary Navajos tend to use both native and Western medicine for the same illness because of the belief that modern medicine alleviates symptoms whereas Navajo medicine cures.[4,26] Some standard measures used by medicine men to treat disease include sweat baths, bedrest, isolation, diet, and exercise. Many Indians use items such as talismans and herbal medicines that have curative powers. Herbs or mixtures in small cloth bags with strong odors may be brought to the hospital and placed at the bedside. Health professionals should recognize that the two systems (tribal and traditional versus modern American medicine) are not necessarily antagonistic.

Communication and Interpersonal Relations. Some Native Americans are bilingual and others are not; this discrepancy can serve as a barrier to communication.[39] During interviews, notetaking should be avoided because Native American Indians are accustomed to transmitting their history through verbal storytelling. Therefore, they may be offended by a listener's writing during conversation; nurses need to rely on their memory skills when obtaining a health history.

Native Americans have a sensitivity to body language and other nonverbal communication. If health care providers appear rushed or impatient, the family is attuned to this and could become noncommunicative.[39] In many instances, Native Americans are quiet and say little about their condition while being observant of the health care giver's responses. Because direct questioning is considered an invasion of privacy, nurses may use declarative statements to obtain information. For example, if the nurse is examining a child presenting with vomiting, the nurse should respond by saying, "Your child has trouble keeping food on her stomach." Then allow time for the mother to respond. Furthermore, assessment for nonverbal signs of pain is important because Native Americans generally do not outwardly display their discomfort.[39]

Nutritional Patterns. Although some acculturation has occurred, many traditional foods are still eaten routinely by Native Americans. Corn, squash, and beans are a large part of the diet. Corn is also used in some religious rituals because it is thought to have medicinal value. Food restrictions are also observed by some Indians during religious ceremonies, as well as during the prenatal and postpartum period. For example, postpartum food restrictions may include cod, halibut, liver, salt cabbage, and onions.

Malnutrition is a problem experienced by many Indian children. Due to the lack of adequate financial resources, many Native American children suffer from iron deficiency anemia. An accurate nursing assessment of nutritional patterns is essential to identify potential or existing problems and to plan appropriate interventions.[48] Adequacy of iron and calcium intake is especially important.

Latinos (Mexican Americans)

The Latino population is a diverse, heterogeneous group of people from different socioeconomic classes and locations, including South and Central America, Mexico, Spain, and the Caribbean. The three largest and most well-known groups are Mexican Americans, Hispanics, and Puerto Ricans.[30] By the year 2000, it is anticipated that the Latino population will increase to 55.3 million in the United States, thereby becoming the largest minority group. Projected statistics suggest that the median age will be 20.7 in the Latino population, and children under age 5 will outnumber the rest of the Latino population.[49]

The largest of the Latino groups presently living in the United States is Mexican American (also known as the Chicano), and they are emphasized in the folllowing discussion. There is as much variation in the cultures within Latino groups as there is among the Anglo-Saxon group in the United States.[30] Despite their various origins, there are some traditions commonly practiced in all Latino groups.

Family Structure and Kinship Bonds. The membership of Latino households is varied. In some instances, the household may consist of the nuclear family and *abuelitos* (grandparents). Family is important to Latinos, and grandparents are held in high esteem.[28]

The traditional structure of Mexican American families is one of patriarchal-authoritarianism in which a strong sense of masculine pride (machismo) exists. Machismo is related to ''one's manhood, the manly traits of honor and dignity, to the courage to fight, to keeping one's word, and to protecting one's name.''[41,49] In this family pattern, the male is the dominant figure and has responsibility for decision making.

An important implication regarding Latino machismo is that female health professionals, especially whites, should refrain from being too assertive or too forward when providing care to a Mexican American male or members of his family. When administering care to Latino families, the husband and father is consulted when health decisions are being made. The fact that many Latino husbands do not get actively involved with prenatal programs and childrearing should not deter the nurse from including them in prenatal discussions, family planning, and parent education sessions.[28]

In traditional Mexican American families, wives are subservient to their husbands. However, due to the changing roles of women in the American society and acculturation of Latino women, the feminine role of Latino women is changing.[15,49] Many of them are becoming more active in decision making within their families.

Religious Beliefs. Religion is a vital part of Latino culture, and approximately 85% to 90% of Latinos are traditional Catholics. Latinos' attitudes about life, death, wellness, and illness are influenced by their religious beliefs. Many believe that sickness and wellness are related to the will of God. Magico-religious rituals and practices are an integral part of life, and Latinos use their spirituality to assist them to recover from illness.[28] Practices such as visitation of shrines, making promises, offering medals and candles, and praying are used when an illness is severe.[31,39]

Health Beliefs and Practices. Mexican Americans classify diseases, foods, and medicines according to a hot–cold or wet–dry continuum.[9,28] These beliefs are derived from the early Hippocratic theory of disease and the four body humors: (1) blood, hot and wet; (2) yellow bile, hot and dry; (3) phlegm, cold and wet; and (4) black bile, cold and dry. When these humors are balanced, the body is in a state of equilibrium and good health exists. Any imbalance in the relationship of the humors causes diseased states.

This theory of humors provides a mechanism for determining treatment for certain illnesses. For example, if a cold illness occurs, it is treated with a hot remedy. A hot illness is treated with a cold substance. There is no agreement among Latinos as to what constitutes a hot disease and food or a cold disease and food. Careful assessment of these beliefs and practices is important because individual variations do occur.[39,49]

The hot and cold theory is not related to temperature, but it is descriptive of certain substances.[39] The following example provides further explanation of the theory. An expectant mother refrains from eating hot foods after giving birth (a hot experience) or her child will get chincual (diaper rash) after it is born. The mother is given cold foods such as vegetables, fruits, and dairy products to restore balance between hot and cold.[9,39]

Diseases are classified into three categories: dislocation of parts of the body, diseases of emotional origin, and diseases of magical origin. First, dislocation of parts of the body is thought to occur when real or imaginary parts of the body become dislodged from their normal position.

Second, in most parts of Latin America, prolonged emotional states are thought to be the cause of some serious illnesses. Fright (*susto* or *espanto*) and anger (*bilis*) are two of these strong emotional states. *Susto,* which can appear in any person, occurs because the soul is wandering during sleep or a traumatic event.[9] Herbal remedies are used to treat *susto* and *bilis.*

Third, Mexican Americans consider *brujeria* (witchcraft) a cause of disease, accomplished through magical procedures. Spells, prayers, religious objects, (especially pictures of saints), and holy water may be used to rid the body of the evil forces of witchcraft.[9] *Mal ojo,* or evil eye, is a condition found in children that has magical origin. For example, if someone, especially a woman, admires someone else's child and looks at him without touching him, the child may fall ill of *ojo.* Symptoms include headache, fitful sleep, excessive crying without a cause, vomiting, and diarrhea.

Nutritional Patterns. Many Latinos have retained their cultural food practices. Food is a symbol of society, hospitality, and friendship. Diets consist of affordable foods such as corn, beans (especially pinto and kidney beans), potatoes, rice, green bananas, yucca (cassavas), and chili peppers. These foods are high in vegetable protein and carbohydrates but low in calcium, vitamin C, thiamine, niacin, and riboflavin. Latinos often have a low intake of diary products and iron-rich foods.[28]

Nursing assessment of food preparation and dietary habits may reveal deficiencies. A diet that includes foods that are economic and culturally acceptable should be encouraged. To prevent iron deficiency anemia, those foods in the child's diet that are high in iron should be identified and their consumption should be encouraged.

Asian Americans (Chinese Americans)

Members of the Asian American population originate from China, Hawaii, the Philippines, Korea, Indochina, and Japan. Contrary to many Americans' perception of Asian-Americans, they are a heterogeneous group of people with some similarities and many differences. This discussion focuses on the culture of Chinese Americans because they represent the largest ethnic group, and all other Asian groups have some origin from the Chinese.[39]

Family Structure and Kinship Bonds. The Chinese have strong kinship and family bonds. In traditional China, the extended family, including grandparents, parents, siblings, uncles, aunts, and cousins, all lived in the same household. This custom is not prevalent for Chinese Americans in the United States today, but strong emotional bonds still exist among extended family members. In traditional families, there is a distinction between gender roles and obligations. The father is head of the household and, in his absence, the eldest son is in charge. Elderly people are highly respected, and young people do not question their authority.[7] In child rearing, shaming and guilt are used to ensure that the children adhere to the parents wishes. Honor and "face" are of great importance in maintaining the family's and individual's good name.[9]

Religious Beliefs. Three major philosophical and religious roots have influenced Chinese values, health beliefs, attitudes, and behaviors. First, Taoism gives a basic perspective on life. The Taoist view of nature follows cyclic changes: birth and death, the onset of seasons, rhythm of day and night, detachment from the world, and "allowing things to be." Teachings are governed by simplicity and spontaneity. Second, Buddhist teaching focuses on adhering to natural changes by preaching the impermanence of the world. People should be productive and perform good deeds with compassion so high states of being can be reached. Third, Confucian teaching emphasizes rules and regulations for social interaction and the importance of allowing fate to guide one's life. Confucian teaching seems to have more influence on behavior of the Chinese than other religions.[8]

Health Beliefs and Practices. Chinese view health as a state of being in physical and spiritual harmony with nature. Like the Vietnamese, Chinese believe in the duality of yin and yang.

Acupuncture, an ancient Chinese practice, is administered by puncturing the body with various types of needles to alleviate pain and cure illness. The acupuncturist uses approximately nine different needles to diagnose and treat disease.[8]

Moxibustion is another ancient method of treatment. It is performed by burning a soft substance called moxa on the skin over certain meridians.[39] This treatment is used to restore the balance of yin and yang.

Herbal remedies, many of which are available today, are widely used as a treatment for disease. Herbalists prescribe herbs in varying amounts and combinations designated for specific diseases. Criteria for prescribing herbs are the person's age, present health status, and whether the illness is the result of yin and yang imbalance. Herbs are prescribed by trial and error. If symptoms do not subside, clients are told to return the prescription and another herb is prescribed. Because Chinese people have a tendency to shop around and use several different herbalists, a client often obtains several different herbs for treating the same illness.[8] Ginseng is popular and used to treat over two dozen conditions including anemia, colic, depression, indigestion, impotence, and rheumatism.[39,45] When caring for Chinese American children, the nurse should respectfully question Chinese parents about the various kinds of herbs used. Although the value of some herbal treatments cannot be disputed, others may be have an antagonistic or synergistic effect when used in combination with Western medications. The importance of the nurse's obtaining accurate information regarding cultural and individual treatment of illness is evident.

Communication and Interpersonal Relations. Several other cultural values or behaviors influence nursing care of Chinese American children. First, they have a tendency to deny the intensity of pain, and their response to pain may be demonstrated only by covert behavior. Observance of nonverbal responses is necessary to assess accurately the intensity, location, and duration of the pain. The child's lack of verbal complaints and requests for pain medication may be misleading.[8] Second, Chinese Americans are reluctant to be hospitalized. This hesitation is based on several reasons: they think hospitals are unsanitary; surgery, which they view as mutilating, is unnecessary; a client's spirit may get lost and may be unable to find its way home; Chinese food is not served; and there may be no interpreter available.[6,7] Finally, Chinese clients are reluctant to ask for anything because they perceive the health care situation as a dominant-subordinate relationship with the client assuming a subordinate role. When children are hospitalized, nurses may need to explain their professional roles to parents, emphasizing their desire to assist the family. They may also apprise parents of their rights, and explain the need for parent advocacy in making sure their child's needs are met.[7]

African Americans

African American culture has its roots and foundation in the African heritage. Health and health practices were brought to this country by African slaves, some of whom were traditional medicine men. African health beliefs embodied the concept of mind, body, and spirit. In essence, medicine men treated the whole person. The person also was considered part of a larger, external environment.

Family Structure and Kinship Bonds. American society tends to view African American families as matriarchal, but in reality, an African American matriarchy does not exist. Descent and kinship are not traced through the mother. The higher percentage of female-headed households in the African American community, especially in families with low income, reflects the collective misfortunes of divorce, desertion, premature deaths, and illegitimacy.[49] Although sometimes non-traditional in structure, the family is a positive force within the African American culture.[22]

Within the African culture, there were strong kinship bonds, and elderly members of the tribe were highly respected and protected.[2] One general theme that has been threaded throughout African culture is "collective participation." In a majority of healing rituals, for example, participation was required of the client, family, and community under the direction of the medicine man. There is some carry over of this tradition in the health perspective of African Americans today. For example, when an African American child is hospitalized or has surgery, several family members may be present.

The strengths of African American families (especially the significance of the extended family) can be used to plan effective nursing care for African American children. For example, a public health nurse making a home visit may find a multigenerational family living in the same household. The nurse may find that any nursing intervention such as health teaching or nutritional teaching may not be adhered to if the dominant family figure is not included in planning nursing care for the child.[41] Including the grandmother as well as the mother in health teaching would benefit the child.

Religious Beliefs.
Religion has played an integral role in the lives of African Americans, and a majority are Protestants. Historically, the African American church has provided spiritual hope and survival for many African Americans. The African American church has served as the focal point for social movements for African American people. During the 1960s, for example, the church provided impetus and support for the civil rights movement.

The church serves as a haven for African Americans suffering from the despair of poverty and a deprived environment. Furthermore, the church functions to promote a high level of self-esteem and self-respect. Many opportunities exist within the church for children and adults to assume roles of respect and leadership[1] (Fig. 4-2).

Prayer has special meaning in the lives of many African Americans and may be especially important in times of illness. In providing nursing care for the hospitalized

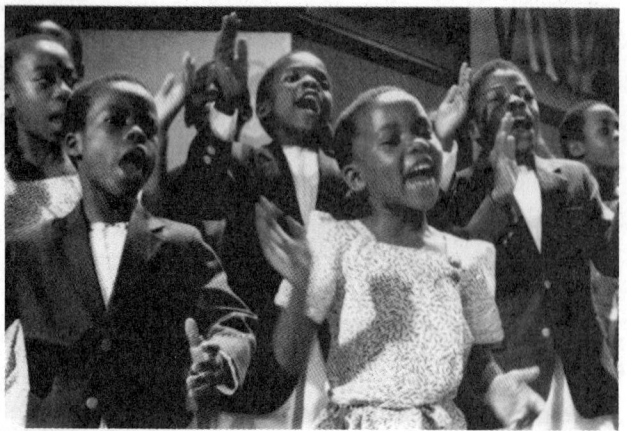

FIGURE 4-2
The church fosters a high level of self-esteem and self-respect. There are opportunities to share in the experiences of the group. (Photograph courtesy of African Children's Choir, sponsored by Friends in the West, Arlington, WA.)

African American child, the family's religious affiliation and beliefs that affect health and healing are assessed. The plan for nursing care includes any religious practices important to the child and family. For example, the family may be asked if they want to pray before taking the child for an operative procedure.

Health Beliefs and Practices.
African Americans' health beliefs and healing practices have evolved from African healing practices and a world view about life and the nature of being: life is a process rather than a state. People have an inherent force of energy that gives them the ability to influence their destiny through the use of knowledge about themselves and the world. For example, a person in a healthy state is in harmony with nature. Disharmony causes illness states within the body.[24,39]

During slavery, African medicine and healing practices were passed on from slaves who were medicine men to women, then from generation to generation. Older men and women with more experience in healing were sought out by others.[2]

Although disease prevention and treatment have origins in African traditions, African Americans have also been influenced by health practices of both Native American Indians and whites. Various methods used to treat illness and have been passed from one family to another. These practices including occult healing, spiritualism, and the use of herbs.

Occult healing occurs through voodoo, witchcraft, hexing, root work, and reading of signs. Voodoo was at one time the most powerful of these cures. It included white magic (harmless) as well as black magic (harmful) rituals. No documentation exists that voodoo is used by African Americans today.[49]

Spiritualism is the belief in the intervention of God. The spiritualist or healer is thought to have received a gift from God to have the power to heal by curing the body of diseases and solving emotional and personal problems.[1,49] Spiritualists are also referred to as faith healers. Many faith healers have a strong following of African Americans today.

Root doctors are people who have a knowledge about the use of herbs, oils, and ointments contrived from secret formulas.[1] Root doctors are also thought to be able to cast a hex or spell on someone. Some African Americans believe that when something evil or bad happens to them, an enemy has had a "root worked on them."

Although some folk remedies used by some African Americans may be harmless, others may be detrimental to their health. Home remedies being used by the family are part of the nursing assessment, as is the determination whether the remedies are harmful. Those practices that are not detrimental to the child's health should be respected. If a harmful practice is identified, the nurse should tactfully explain this to the parents and child.

Not all African Americans share cultural values and practices to the same degree. Factors such as age, social class, financial status, sex roles, regional residence, socialization patterns, individual life styles, and ongoing changes in the environment all account for differences in African American cultural patterns.[1] As in other ethnic groups, upper and middle class African Americans may tend to discard folk medicine. Affluent, educated African

Americans tend to use modern health facilities and adhere to prescribed treatment regimens more readily than African Americans in low socioeconomic conditions.[21]

Communication and Interpersonal Relations. Some African Americans (as well as other ethnic minorities) have a tendency to be especially sensitive to how white health professionals interact with them. When some African Americans enter the health care system, they may exhibit a variety of negative behaviors from submissiveness to aggressiveness. Although this behavior is not unique to one ethnic group, African American clients may exhibit more paranoia about the system than others. This paranoid behavior may be a psychological defense mechanism that African American people use to adapt to their everyday environment.[44] Being aware of the source of this behavior enables nurses to understand that this reaction is not necessarily directed at them as individuals. Addressing African Americans by their surname is one way to demonstrate respect.

Nutritional Patterns. The traditional dietary habits of African Americans are derived from a combination of Southern dietary patterns and dietary habits developed during slavery. "Soul food," a term given to certain foods that have emotional importance, is eaten by many African Americans. Some of these foods include pork products such as pigs' feet, pork ribs, salt pork or "fat back," ham, and chitterlings. Collard greens, mustard, turnip greens, and cornbread are also examples of soul food. This list should not be considered inclusive because what is considered to be soul food varies among African Americans.

Although a detailed diet history is important for all children, it is especially important for African American children with a history of anemia and a family history of hypertension. Dietary plans for children with these diseases should include appropriate allowable ethnic foods. Dietary modifications should also take into account the family's economic status.

Other Groups With Special Needs

Several groups of people are living in poverty with little or no health care. Two of these groups are the homeless and migrant families.

Homeless Families

The homeless population continues to escalate throughout the United States. An estimated 0.5% to 1.0% of the U.S. population is homeless.[33,36] This figure no doubt underestimates the numbers because it is difficult to obtain valid statistics on a mobile group. The homeless population includes the following:[3]

- Patients discharged from mental institutions
- People with alcohol or drug problems
- Women with no financial income
- Jobless youth
- Families who lost former shelter because of unemployment or other financial strains

The homeless are at greater risk than the general population for receiving inadequate health care. Most homeless people seek out medical care only in life-threatening situations. This type of health-seeking behavior exists for several reasons: the negative attitudes of health care providers toward the homeless, the frustration and confusion created by the health care system, and health professionals' lack of understanding of the culture of the homeless. Health care is understandably not a priority for the homeless, because they are fighting for survival on a daily basis. When offered health care services, homeless people are more likely to refuse for the following reasons: they do not perceive a need for the service, referrals are made to agencies that are not part of the person's environment, they lack transportation to designated services, or they lack economic resources needed to maintain their health.

Homeless people are plagued by a number of acute and chronic health problems. Their exposure to environmental conditions makes them vulnerable to problems such as hypothermia, frostbite, heat stroke, heat prostration, and heat cramps, all of which can necessitate hospitalization.[17] Homeless children often contract scabies and lice. They also are susceptible to communicable childhood illnesses such as measles, pertussis, and mumps because of incomplete immunizations. Follow-up care for children with acute and chronic illnesses is a problem because of the transient nature of homeless families.

In providing health care for the homeless family, the nurse assesses the family's ethnic and racial cultural practices and beliefs as well as the culture of the homeless. To preserve the dignity and self-respect of the person, the nurse must provide care in an accepting, nonjudgmental manner. Using effective interpersonal communication skills is necessary to establish a trusting relationship in a short period of time. If homeless clients perceive the environment to be open and trusting, they are more likely to return for follow-up care. Although many programs for the homeless have been established throughout the United States, the numbers are not great enough to solve the problem. The collective involvement of federal, state, and local governments as well as the private sector, and individual citizens is needed to address adequately the concerns of homeless families.

Migrant Families

Migrant workers represent the "true working poor."[38] The migrant worker population is comprised of a diversity of ethnic and racial groups such as African Americans, whites, Jamaicans, Mexican Americans, Hispanics, Native Americans, Southeast Asians, Haitians, and Puerto Ricans. Certain groups are endemic to specific geographic regions. For example, according to the U.S. Department of Agriculture, over one half (53%) of the farm workers in California, Nevada, and Arizona are Hispanic, and about one third (34%) of the workers in eight southern states (Kentucky, Tennessee, North Carolina, South Carolina, Mississippi, Alabama, Georgia, and Florida) are African American.

Identification and tracking of migrant workers is challenging due to factors such as worker mobility, undocumented workers, and rural locations. The Office of Migrant Health, however, reports that nationwide there are approximately 2.7 million migrant and seasonal farm workers and dependents, including 800,000 migrant farm workers and dependents and 1,900,000 seasonal farm workers and dependents.[47]

The only national reporting system currently responsible for tracking migrant workers is the Migrant Student Record Transfer System, which is under the auspices of the Office of Migrant Education in the U.S. Department of Agriculture. This office houses computerized health and academic records of over 700,000 children of migrant workers. Health data include immunization records, results of physical examinations, dental records, abnormal results of health screening, and information on treatment and referrals.[47] These data are readily available to health professionals providing direct care to registered children.

Frequently reported health problems of migrant children fall into four categories: diseases and conditions resulting from poor living conditions and migration, nutritional problems, untreated congenital anomalies, and health problems due to inadequate follow-up and neglect. Some of the conditions related to unsanitary living conditions and migration include viral or bacterial infections, especially upper respiratory infections and gastroenteritis. Crowded living conditions cause these infections to spread rapidly and lead to epidemics. Head lice and scabies are also problems for migrant children. Day care centers and schools should be alerted when these infestations are identified in migrant children who use the facilities.

A second group of health problems is related to nutrition. Anemia is a common problem among migrant children. Families may be referred to the government-sponsored program for food supplements and nutrition counseling for women, infants, and children (WIC). Obesity and hypertension are also prevalent among migrant adults and children.

Untreated congenital anomalies is a third group of problems experienced by migrant children. These children have conditions such as cerebral palsy, deafness, blindness, severe retardation, and hip displacements. When the nurse identifies these problems, the parent's beliefs about the cause of the defects should be discussed and referrals should be made to appropriate agencies.

A fourth category of diseases common to migrant children are those due to inadequate follow-up or neglect. Dental caries, allergies, chronic tonsillitis, visual defects, skin diseases, and parasitic infestations are examples of this category of conditions.[38]

There are many reasons that migrant families receive inadequate or no treatment, and most are related to factors such as lack of money, unfamiliarity with health care services, language barriers, and cultural differences.[34,38] Although the number of health facilities that provide care for migrant families has increased within the past 15 years, most families are ineligible for other services such as Medicaid, because they work and do not meet the requirements. As a result of this constraint and their mobility, migrant workers receive sporadic, episodic illness-related medical care. Migrant workers generally seek care in emergency rooms or clinics for severe illness, complicated pregnancy, and birth.[38]

Because migrant workers represent various ethnic minorities, their primary cultural heritage influences their health care practices. It is important for the nurse to integrate cultural needs with health care.[38] Respect for the migrant worker's religious and healing beliefs can be demonstrated by incorporating family practices or remedies that are not harmful into the child's treatment plan. Bilingual interpreters should be used to enhance communication with the child's family and to explain instructions. Finally, familiarity with the various local, regional, state, and federal programs that provide services for children can help nurses to meet the comprehensive needs of migrant children.

Barriers to Obtaining Access to Health Care

Along with cultural orientations, there are other barriers which prevent ethnic minorities from utilizing health care resources. Language barriers, for example, prevent nurses from making adequate assessments and providing adequate education. Furthermore, some individuals believe that the stereotypical views many health care workers hold for minorities lead to discrimination.

Structure and functional characteristics of the health care system also impede access to health care. These barriers can be described as inadequate health resources such as insufficient funds for special programs, lack of understanding of and general apathy toward problems affecting ethnic minorities, and inaccessible geographic locations of health care facilities.[27,46] Cultural, social, and personal factors can be deterrents to obtaining access to health care. Personal obstacles such as lack of transportation, inadequate financial resources, and lack of health insurance coverage serve as barriers to health care. Psychological barriers include fears, attitudes about receiving free care or "handouts," and cultural beliefs and healing practices. Political barriers include lack of participation of consumers in planning health services. The lack of community agencies and interest groups that can serve as advocates for children and families and have some impact on the establishment of priorities and distribution of services for the poor is also a barrier.[46]

Nursing Implications

Professional nurses need a multicultural perspective in providing care to children from ethnic minorities. This view involves recognition of their own ethnocentrism and how it influences the type of care they provide. The role of the nurse in providing culturally relevant care is to value the uniqueness of a person's cultural heritage, recognize that people are different, and support their right to be different. Nurses must be able to assess individual health beliefs and healing practices and determine which ones can be incorporated into their plan of care without detrimental effects. Table 4-1 provides guidelines for obtaining information related to culture.

In providing cross-cultural nursing care, the nurse should consider the following questions: How does the person view life? What is the person's cultural background, and how does it influence behavior and health

TABLE 4-1
Nursing Assessment: Questions for Assessing Cultural Patterns

Assessment Data	Questions
Ethnic/racial identity	What is the family's ethnic or racial origin? Do both parents belong to the same group?
Birthplace	Where were the parents born? Where were the children born? If parents or any children were born out of the United States, how many years have they lived in the United States?
Geographic location	Does family have easy access to the following places? Shopping center, Place of worship, Grocery store, Health food store, Native food store, School, Community agencies, Health care facilities and physician's office. If they are not accessible, how does family manage?
Mobility	How many places has the family lived? How long did family live in each location? How do the children cope with frequent moving?
Financial status	How does the family meet financial responsibilities? Is there a hardship on the family? Is any contributor unemployed? If yes, what position does this person hold in the family? If there is a financial hardship, is the family interested in obtaining financial assistance?
Utilization of community resources	What community resources does the family use?
Religious beliefs	Are both parents from the same religious background? What types of religious activities does the family participate in? Does any family member have a different religious affiliation?
Health care beliefs and practices	What influence do religious beliefs/practices have on the health beliefs and practices? What types of folk medicine does the family use? Who provides medical care for family members other than a physician? What types of conditions does the family treat at home?
Dietary habits	What specific culture-based foods does the family eat?
Native dress habits	What type of native clothes does the family wear? How often are these worn?
Social networks	What are the family's social support systems? Does the family have access to ethnic activities in the community? Do family members have friends and associations with members of their ethnic group and other ethnic groups? How comfortable are family members interacting with people from other ethnic groups? How important is the extended family? What kind of support does the extended family provide?
Family structure/roles	How are decisions made in the family? Who is the dominant person(s) in the family? Who makes decisions? Who lives in the household?
Childrearing	What type of behavior is expected of the child? How are children disciplined? Who handles the discipline?

Note: These are suggested culturally relevant questions. There are many additional questions that nurses can ask.

care? What is the meaning of health and illness to the person, and what does all of this mean in terms of survival? Answers to these questions, along with general knowledge of the culture, help the nurse to develop the comprehensive database for providing effective nursing care.

General principles for providing care to minorities include the following:

- Treat the person with dignity and respect.
- Address the person by his or her family name or preferred name.
- Be sensitive to the person's cultural heritage.
- Recognize that family participation in care is important for certain groups.
- Use bilingual interpreters when possible.
- Use bilingual educational literature for health teaching or instructions.

Economic Influences on Health Care of Families

Effects of Poverty

Poverty in America has no ethnic boundaries. Millions of Americans—the working poor, African Americans, Hispanics, Native Americans as well as other ethnic groups, migrant farm workers, and scattered rural residents—are living in impoverished environments. Although these groups have better health and easier access to health care than in previous years, their care still lags far behind the standard of care available to the upper and middle classes. The health status of the nation overall has been steadily improving, but the poor are still experiencing an inequitable toll of health problems, as evidenced by high infant mortality, shortened life span, and days of lost work.[16]

The plight of American children living in these impoverished families is symptomatic of national neglect. Statistics for children living in poverty in America are astounding.[16]

- More than one of every four children under the age of 6 years is living in poverty.
- Nearly half of all African American children live in poverty.
- About two of every five Hispanic children are poor.
- Overall infant mortality has been declining about 5% a year since 1965 and is at a low of about 10 infant deaths per thousand live births, but the African American infant mortality rate is almost 100% higher.
- A nonwhite mother is five times more likely than a white mother to die of complications in childbirth.

Children living in poverty are exposed to numerous health and social problems such as malnutrition, iron deficiency anemia, lead poisoning, poor school performance, and high dropout rate.

One of the most distressing facts about the American health care system is that the poorest families experience the most illness. Although there has been a tremendous amount of government-financed medical care coverage for the poor through Medicare and Medicaid, millions of people still receive no benefits. The uninsured poor is a large population of people who cannot pay for medical care because they are unemployed, or because they cannot afford insurance but are not eligible for federal or state medical assistance programs.

Effects of Cost-Containment Measures

Many programs have been established to control and decrease the escalating cost of health care, improve quality care and performance of hospitals and other medical care providers, improve efficiency of medical services, and improve access to medical care. Cost-containment measures such as prospective reimbursement (e.g., diagnosis related groups, known as DRGs) and Medicare or Medicaid reimbursement policies are being used.

The middle or upper class American consumer has a variety of options in the selection of health care facilities as well as providers. Many consumers also have access to alternative modes of health care such as health maintenance organizations (HMOs). However, these same options are not readily available to those living in poverty. The lack of health insurance coverage due to unemployment or inadequate funds to purchase coverage, or being Medicare or Medicaid recipients prevent the poor from having options in selecting their health care provider or facility.

To promote better understanding of the economic aspects of the health care system and their impact on families, some of the alternative modes of health care and health care financing for the indigent are discussed below.

Health Maintenance Organizations

Health maintenance organizations (HMOs) are health care organizations that provide all medical care services needed by families. This form of health delivery allows "corporate practice of medicine to compete with the current fee-for-service delivery."[14] Some of the theoretical advantages of this prepaid health insurance plan are that it: (1) provides incentive for hospital efficiency, (2) ensures less duplication of facilities and services, and (3) minimizes the cost of medical care.

Studies have shown that the total cost of medical care (premium plus out-of-pocket) for HMO enrollees is actually lower than for people with similar coverage using a fee-for-service delivery system and that there are lower hospitalization rates for its members.[14] The majority of these studies, however, were conducted in HMOs in which enrollees were middle class and basically healthy patients with few or no chronic diseases. There were also few elderly patients.

Although many of the accolades given to this method of health care are well-founded, questions must be asked. What does this mean for the nation's poor? Is society, in fact, creating another two-tier system of health care that serves as yet another barrier to health care for the medically indigent?

Even if HMOs made greater efforts to recruit Medicare and Medicaid recipients, and if reimbursement problems under these programs were improved, it is unlikely that these people will opt to receive medical care at these facilities. Low income families are less likely to participate in the mainstream of the health care system.[10] Additionally, low income families are much more likely to receive care from general practitioners rather than specialists, in

a hospital outpatient department rather than in a physician's office, and after traveling for long distances and waiting substantially longer for care.[10] Advocates for health care for the poor must remain informed about legislation and regulations affecting the delivery of health care. Table 4-2 provides a summary of selected programs available to eligible families.

TABLE 4-2
Programs Available to Eligible Families

Type of Program	Description of Program
Aid to Federally Dependent Children (AFDC)	A federally funded program established under the Social Security Act of 1935. Designed to provide financial assistance for needy children who are deprived because of parental death, absence from the home, or physical or mental disability. The program is administered by states.
Medicaid	A federal and state funded program initiated under the Social Security Act in 1965, Title 19. Provides medical assistance to the medically indigent, people receiving public assistance, and people who do not receive public assistance but meet some established eligibility criteria. States are responsible for administering the program.
Food Stamps	Funded and administered by the U.S. Department of Agriculture. Food stamps are coupons that can be used in place of money to pay for food items. The goal of the program is to improve the nutritional status of low socioeconomic families. States are responsible for direct administration of the program.
Supplemental Security Income (SSI)	Federally administered public assistance program that went into effect January 1, 1974, provides income for elderly, blind, or disabled people.
Work Incentive Program (WIN)	A mandatory work requirement program for employable AFDC recipients. Designed to make provisions for job registration, training, and placement services for participants. If people do not register with state employment agencies, their benefits may be terminated. The program has been somewhat controversial.
Early and Periodic Screening, Diagnosis, and Treatment (EPSDT)	Comprehensive program designed to provide health care for Medicaid-eligible children. Legislation was passed in 1971 to implement the program. State Medicaid offices are responsible for making sure all eligible recipients receive these health benefits.
Women, Infants, and Children Food Program (WIC)	A federally funded supplemental food program for low-income pregnant and nursing women, infants, and children (up to 5 years old). The goal of the program is to improve the nutritional status of these people. Vouchers are given to be used for buying essential prescribed high-protein foods and infant formulas. Nutritional counseling and continuous follow-up are maintained.

Wright, R., et al. (1983). *Transcultural perspectives in the human services: Organizational issues and trends.* Springfield, IL: Charles C Thomas; and U.S. Department of Health, Education, and Welfare. EPSDT: Overview. Washington, DC: (HFCA) 77-24534.

Medicaid

Medicaid is a federal–state matching program designed to provide services to the indigent population. The primary responsibility of the federal government is to share program costs with the states, who are responsible for determining clients' eligibility and benefit coverage. Although millions of poor people receive Medicaid, a vast majority of people classified as the "working poor" are not eligible for Medicaid but also cannot afford medical care. Estimates have suggested that approximately one fourth to one third of the population below the poverty level do not receive medical benefits.[10,14]

With the enactment of Medicaid in 1965, states did not foresee the enormous cost of implementing such a program. Inflation and unmanageable program costs have forced many states to make temporary or permanent cutbacks in services. Therefore, more people, especially children, are without medical care. Children from uninsured families are not adequately immunized, do not receive preventive health care services such as physical examinations, and do not receive proper treatment and follow-up for acute and chronic illnesses. The following inequities in the Medicaid program have been cited: (1) wide variation of eligibility standards among states; (2) the discrimination created by diverse eligibility standards and benefit packages; and (3) lack of uniform benefit packages offered by states.[42]

One of the programs sponsored by the Medicaid program is Early and Periodic Screening, Diagnosis, and Treatment (EPSDT). In 1967, Congress passed legislation to create EPSDT, but the program did not get underway until February 1972 because of the complexities in implementing the program. A comprehensive preventive health service for Medicaid-eligible children, EPSDT represents a cooperative effort among physicians, dentists, other health professionals, and the federal government. State agencies are responsible for making sure that these programs are available to eligible children.[43]

EPSDT services include periodic routine physical examination; nutritional, dental, and developmental assessment; blood tests for detection of anemia, abnormal lead levels, and sickle cell anemia; speech, hearing, and vision assessments; and tests for urinary tract infections and tuberculosis. As with any other program for low socioeconomic groups (which includes a large number of ethnic minorities), certain barriers prevent children from receiving the available services. Barriers to use of the services include excessive mobility of families; cultural beliefs or values; low priority given to health care by families struggling for survival; and unwillingness of some physicians to provide care for people who receive Medicaid. To increase the number of eligible children in the program, more outreach services are needed to identify and inform eligible families about EPSDT services. Recruitment of health care professionals is necessary as well.[43]

Diagnostic Related Groups (DRGs)

In 1983, the federal government established a prospective payment system (PPS) for reimbursement to hospitals for inpatient services obtained by Medicare recipients. This method of reimbursement was designed to control escalating medical care costs, specifically inpatient care. The prospective payment system requires that conditions treated within hospitals be grouped into 470 diagnostic related groups (DRGs). The hospital is reimbursed only for the amount of payment allotted under DRG policies. If a patient's condition warrants a longer hospital stay, the additional costs are absorbed by the hospital.[32,40]

DRGs have had detrimental effects on patients, community agencies, hospitals, and families. As a result of DRGs, many patients are discharged from hospitals earlier than usual, thereby placing an additional burden on families. When patients are sent home with subacute problems, home health care agencies may find themselves overloaded. There is also a discriminatory dimension to DRGs in that they are restricted to Medicare patients only and not applicable to patients who have private third party insurance.

Although DRGs have not been enacted for Medicaid recipients, many of whom are children, it is important to mention the potential impact they could have on the health care of children. With more efforts being undertaken by the government to contain health care costs, the potential exists for a similar cost containment measure like DRGs to be expanded to other services that affect children. If such a cost containment measure is instituted for Medicaid patients, children requiring home care would also be affected. Families would need more emotional and financial support. Nurses need to be well informed about governmental regulations and legislation that could affect the health care of children in the future.

Summary

If nurses are to provide quality nursing care for the children of minorities, they must be aware of the impact of cultural and economic factors on the health care of these groups of people. The cultural characteristics of families

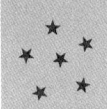

Ideas for Nursing Research

Nursing research related to cultural and economic influences on child health care has received increased attention. The following areas need to be explored:

- The effects of extensive outreach programs on utilization of EPDST services.
- The effects of Maternal Child Health Block Grants on pregnancy outcomes, access to prenatal care, and access to health services for children.
- The effects of the Women, Infants, and Children (WIC) Supplemental Food Program on the nutritional status of infants and children.
- Factors that prevent the homeless from using health care services.
- Types of health facilities the homeless prefer (e.g., mobile clinics, clinics located at shelters for the homeless).

should be an integral part of developing the nursing care plan. To provide culturally relevant nursing care, nurses must become knowledgeable about the various ethnic minorities prevalent in the United States.

Legislation, public policy decisions, and governmental regulations influence the economic and health status of ethnic groups. These factors determine access, availability, and affordability of health care. Nurses must become cognizant of the impact of these dimensions on the plight of children and families within various ethnic groups. Nurses who are well-informed and sensitive to needs of ethnic minority groups may become strong advocates in helping them obtain adequate health care.

References

1. Bloch, B. (1983). Nursing care of black patients. In M. S. Orque, et al. (Eds.), *Ethnic nursing care: A multicultural approach.* St. Louis: Mosby.
2. Branch, M., & Paxton, P. (1976). *Providing safe nursing care for ethnic people of color.* New York: Appleton-Century-Crofts.
3. Brickner, P. W. (1985). Health issues in the care of the homeless. In P. W. Brickner, et al. (Eds.), *Health care of homeless people.* New York: Springer.
4. Bullough, V. L., & Bullough, B. (1982). *Health care for the other Americans.* New York: Appleton-Century-Crofts.
5. Calhoun, M. A. (1985). The Vietnamese women: Health/illness attitudes and behaviors. *Health Care for Women International, 6,* 61.
6. Campbell, T., & Chang, B. (1981). Health care of the Chinese in America. In G. Henderson & M. Primeaux (Eds.), *Transcultural health care.* Menlo Park, CA: Addison-Wesley.
7. Chang, B. (1981). Asian-American patient care. In G. Henderson & M. Primeaux (Eds.), *Transcultural health care.* Menlo Park, CA: Addison-Wesley.
8. Chen-Louie, T. (1983). Nursing care of Chinese Americans. In M. S. Orque, et al. (Eds.), *Ethnic nursing care: A multicultural approach.* St. Louis: Mosby.
9. Clark, M. (1970). *Health in the Mexican American culture: A community study.* Berkeley: University of California Press.
10. Davis, K. (1976). Achievements and problems of Medicaid. *Public Health Reports, 9,* 316.
11. Davis, K. (1984). Health care of low income families. In *The Nation's Health.*
12. Dobbins, E., et al. (1980). Translating the Indochinese diet into English. *RN, 43,* 79.
13. Dobbins, E., et al. (1981). A beginner's guide to Vietnamese culture. *RN, 44,* 44.
14. Feldstein, P. J. (1983). *Health care economics* (2nd ed.). New York: Wiley.
15. Friedman, M. M. (1988). Transcultural family nursing in the United States: Latino and Black families. In J. M. Bell, et al. (Eds.), *Proceedings of the International Family Nursing Conference,* May 24-27, 1988, Calgary, Alberta, Canada.
16. Gallo, R. M., et al. (1980). Little refugees with big needs. *RN, 43,* 45.
17. Goldfrank, L. (1985). Exposure. Thermoregulatory disorders in the homeless patient. In P. W. Brickner, et al. (Eds.), *Health care of homeless people.* New York: Springer.
18. Gordon, V. C., et al. (1980). Southeast Asian refugees. *American Journal of Nursing, 43,* 2031.
19. Henderson, G., & Primeaux, M. (1981). The importance of folk medicine. In G. Henderson & M. Primeaux (Eds.), *Transcultural health care.* Menlo Park, CA: Addison-Wesley.
20. Henderson, G., & Primeaux, M. (1981). Cross-cultural patient care. In G. Henderson & M. Primeaux (Eds.), *Transcultural health care.* Menlo Park, CA: Addison-Wesley.
21. Henderson, G., & Primeaux, M. (1981). American Indian patient care. In G. Henderson & M. Primeaux (Eds.), *Transcultural health care.* Menlo Park, CA: Addison-Wesley.
22. Hill, R. (1971). *The strengths of black families.* New York: Emerson.
23. Hughes, D., et al. (1988). *The health of America's children: Maternal and child health data book.* Washington, DC: Children's Defense Fund.
24. Jacques, G. (1976). Cultural health traditions. In M. Branch & P. Paxton (Eds.), *Providing safe nursing care for ethnic people of color.* New York: Appleton-Century-Crofts.
25. Jones, D. L. (1979). African American clients: Clinical practice issues. *Social Work, 3,* 112.
26. Kunitz, S. J. (1983). *Disease change and the role of medicine: The Navajo experience.* Berkeley: University of California Press.
27. Mechanic, D. (1984). Inequality health status and delivery of health services in the United States. *Journal of Health, Politics, Policy and Law, 9,* 41.
28. Monrroy, L. S. A. (1983). Nursing care of Raza/Latina patients. In M. S. Orque, et al. (Eds.), *Ethnic nursing care: A multicultural approach.* St. Louis: Mosby.
29. Murillo-Rohde, I. (1977). Care for all colors. *Imprint, 24.*
30. Murillo-Rohde, I. (1981). Hispanic American patient care. In G. Henderson & M. Primeaux (Eds.), *Transcultural health care.* Menlo Park, CA: Addison-Wesley.
31. Nall, F. C., & Speilberg, J. (1967). Social cultural factors in the responses of Mexican-Americans to medical treatment. *Journal of Health and Social Behavior, 8,* 302.
32. Newcomer, R., et al. (1985). Medicare prospective payment: Anticipated effect on hospitals, other community agencies, and families. *Journal of Health, Politics, Policy and Law, 10*(2), 275.
33. Nichols, J., et al. (1986). A proposal for tracking health care for the homeless. *Journal of Community Health, 11,* 204.
34. O'Brien, M. E. (1983). Reaching the migrant worker. *American Journal of Nursing, 6,* 895.
35. Orque, M. S., et al. (1983). *Ethnic nursing care: A multicultural approach.* St. Louis: Mosby.
36. Robert Wood Johnson Foundation and Pew Memorial Trust (1984). *Health care for the homeless program.* Application guide.
37. Santopietro, M. C. S., & Lynch, B. A. (1980). What's behind the inscrutable mask? *RN, 43,* 55.
38. Schneider, B. (1986). Providing for the health needs of migrant children. *Nurse Practitioner, 11,* 54.
39. Spector, R. E. L. (1985). *Cultural diversity in health and illness* (2nd ed.). Norwalk, CT: Appleton-Century-Crofts.
40. Spiegel, A. D., & Kavaler, F. (1985). The debate over diagnosis related groups. *Journal of Community Health, 10,* 81.
41. Steiner, S. (1970). *LaRaza.* New York: Harper and Row.
42. Stuart, B., et al. (1985). Medicaid reform: Programming solutions to the equity problem. *Journal of Health Politics, Policy and Law, 10,* 93.
43. U.S. Department of Health, Education, and Welfare. *A guide to administration, diagnosis and treatment: EPSDT.* Washington, DC (HCFA) 77-24534.
44. U.S. Department of Health and Human Services. M. M. Heckler, Secretary. (1985). *Report of the Secretary's task force on black & minority health.* Washington, DC: Government Printing Office.
45. Wallnofer, H., & Von Rottausher, A. (1972). *Chinese folk medicine* (Palmedo, M., Trans.). New York: American Library.
46. Wan, T. T. H. (1977). The differential use of health services: A minority perspective. *Urban Health, 6,* 47.
47. Wilk, V. A. (1986). *The occupational health of migrant and seasonal farmworkers in the United States.* Washington, DC, Farmworkers Justice Fund, Inc..
48. Wilson, U. (1983). Nursing care of American Indian patients. In M. S. Orque, et al. (Eds.), *Ethnic nursing care: A multicultural approach.* St. Louis: Mosby.
49. Wright, R., et al. (1983). *Transcultural perspectives in the human services: Organizational issues and trends.* Springfield, IL: Thomas.

The High-Risk Family

BEHAVIORAL OBJECTIVES

Define the term "high-risk family."

Relate characteristics of high-risk families to potential family dysfunctions.

Discuss the value of multidisciplinary teams in providing health care interventions for high-risk families.

Clarify the nurse's role in planning health care services for the high-risk family.

Explain how either the parental or child subsystems can cause families to be high-risk.

Explain how specific family dysfunctions may influence a child's biopsychosocial health.

The goal of child health nursing is to offer children the best chance for health now and in the future. One of the approaches to this goal is identification of families with potential difficulties that may lead to dysfunctional growth and development. Such families are considered "at risk" or "high risk."

High-risk families are families whose members are not able to function appropriately, or families that, as a unit, are not able to maintain normal function.[8] This group includes families having difficulty managing environmental stressors and those having difficulty with familial interaction. Early interventions can reverse the potential for dysfunction and promote health functioning; therefore, early identification of individual and family needs is essential.[18]

Two main subsystems can be identified in the high-risk family: the parent subsystem and the child subsystem. Parents who are not able to manage stress within themselves or from other sources have difficulty functioning in the parent role. On the other hand, children who have problems also add stress to the family unit and disrupt its functioning. The subsystems are interdependent and should not be viewed in isolation; either may contribute to symptoms of illness within the family unit.

Providing care to families at risk requires the nurse to apply the nursing process not only to individual members but also to the family unit. Increasingly, nursing assessment tools include family assessment data, and consumers of health care are requesting care for family units. This chapter provides guidance in identifying those families at risk and assists the nurse in making appropriate decisions about interventions.

Functional and Dysfunctional Families

Precipitating Factors in High-Risk Families

Although many families with the following characteristics become high risk, not all have an alteration in functioning. Some families have the ability to experience high-risk situations yet are able to maintain equilibrium and cope in a healthy manner. Although more research is needed to explain why not all families react in the same manner to identical situations, some precipitating factors have been identified. One or more of the following may be present, but the more factors involved, the more stress the family will feel.[8]

Family History

Events that have happened in the past may influence the family's ability to adapt to current stressors. Even information about the origins of the family can be important. For example, how did the couple meet? Were the circumstances surrounding the beginning of the family favorable or unfavorable? Were the children planned or unplanned?

Parenting behaviors are learned and passed on to the next generation. Therefore, high-risk parenting behaviors often have been passed down from one generation to the next, creating a long history of unsatisfactory parenting skills. Such behaviors are often difficult to change, but these families may benefit from therapeutic interventions.

Another critical historical factor is the methods the family has used to resolve similar situations in the past. Have they been successful in dealing with previous stressful situations, or is there a pattern of mismanaging stress? These patterns of behavior are also learned from family role models; effective coping strategies may need to be substituted for ineffective actions.

Socioeconomic Factors

The ability to gather resources outside itself is often the deciding factor in whether a family will be able to deal with stressful situations. Inadequate financial resources, for example, is a common problem but may be especially severe in families who have chronically ill children. Health care providers can often help families to identify new resources and to use them effectively.

Present Life Stressors

The identification of current stressors is crucial to understanding the family at risk. If the family is experiencing one stressor, they are often at risk for other stressors. For example, multiple stressors are found in a family where the parents are adolescents with a preterm infant. Also of importance is the strength of magnitude of the stressor. Severe stress can interrupt the ability of even the most healthy family to function effectively.

Family research suggests that single stressors usually do not change the perceived well-being of the family, but an accumulation of stressors has the potential to increase family strain.[7] When new stressors are experienced, prior strains are exaggerated and families become more aware of them as stressors. Yet, the resulting tensions in relationships among family members tend to be more difficult for the family than the new stressor itself.

Family Functioning Continuum

Families can be considered to be on a continuum between functional and dysfunctional, as illustrated in Figure 5-1. *Functional* families are those who are able to deal with situations in a positive manner and possess a high level of well-being. They usually have a history of being able to handle stress in a positive, healthy manner. Functional families use their strengths during crisis or trauma. They are also able to find adequate resources for support.

Potentially dysfunctional families are those who have difficulty handling stressful situations. Carpenito[3] defines high-risk families as those "in which a usually supportive family experiences or is at risk to experience, a stressor that challenges its previously effective functioning." Common contributing factors that are related to decreased functioning include illness, trauma, loss of family members, relocation, or economic crisis. Potentially dysfunctional families do not have the ability to adapt to crisis. Communication among family members becomes strained and difficult. The family often is not able to meet the physical, emotional, social, or spiritual needs of members. Most families are unable to express their feelings and do not seek or accept help appropriately.

Dysfunctional families have clearly identified pathology within the family that disrupts their ability to function.[8] Heiney[9] described the behaviors that are found in dysfunctional families and observed that individual persons within the family have difficulty in conflict resolution and decision making. Three patterns emerge: excessive marital conflict, dysfunction of one of the spouses, and projection of the problems onto a child in the family.

Dysfunctional families are not able to resolve issues or work through problems. Arguments between the marital couple are repetitious, and issues are not resolved. Often, one parent may seem to be extremely competent, whereas the other is unable to function at all. Finally, one or more of the children may begin to "act out" the confusion and fear in the family, and the misbehaving child may thereby give the parents a focus for the problem. A dysfunctional family may be identified when these events are recurrent and effective coping mechanisms are not used.[9]

Each family along the functional-dysfunctional continuum requires a different approach. Functional families may need assistance to maintain their functional status during a specific crisis. In those who are potentially dysfunctional, interventions are aimed at eliminating risk factors to prevent future pathology. In dysfunctional families with identified pathology, interventions are taken to eliminate the factors causing the pathology.[9]

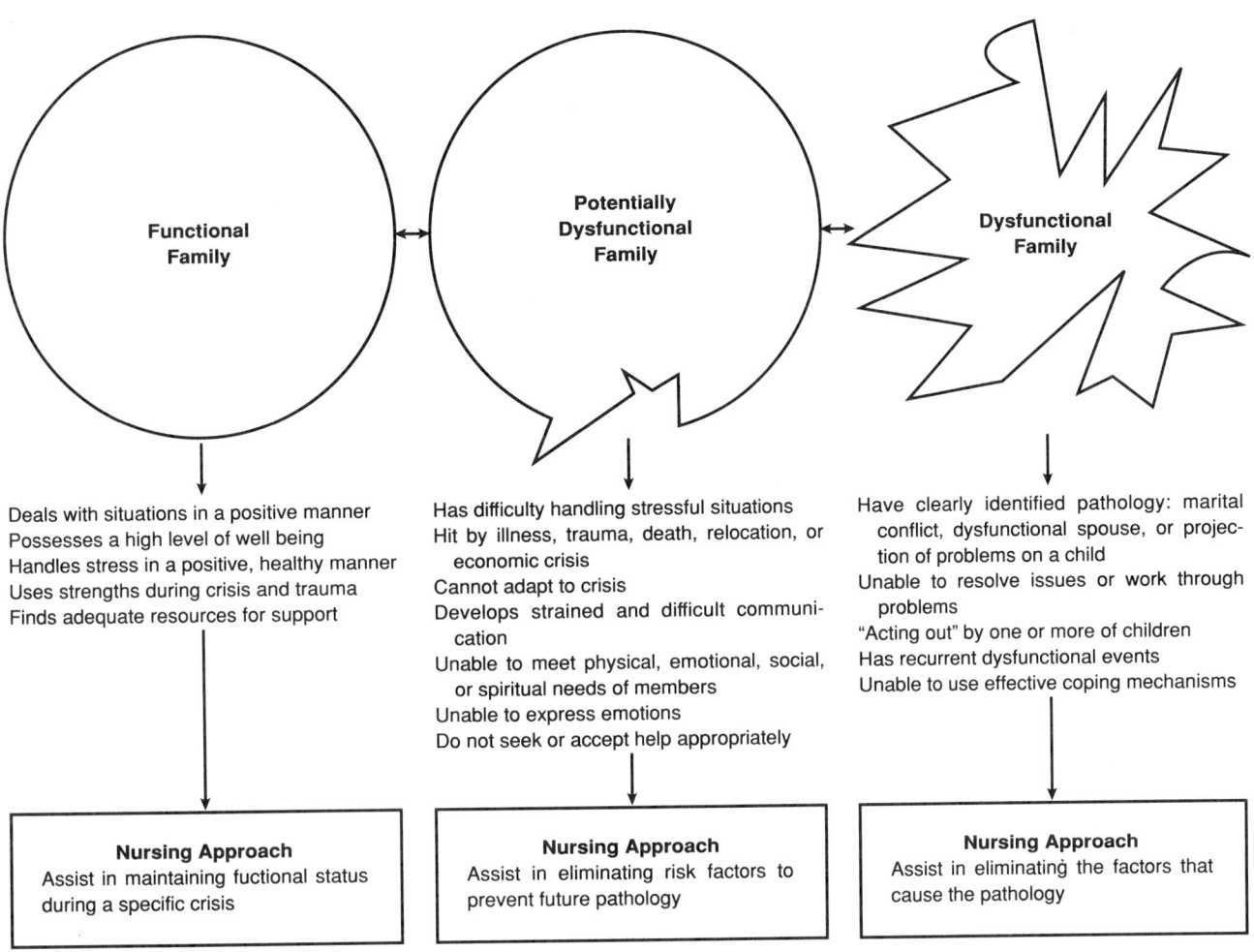

Deals with situations in a positive manner
Possesses a high level of well being
Handles stress in a positive, healthy manner
Uses strengths during crisis and trauma
Finds adequate resources for support

Has difficulty handling stressful situations
Hit by illness, trauma, death, relocation, or economic crisis
Cannot adapt to crisis
Develops strained and difficult communication
Unable to meet physical, emotional, social, or spiritual needs of members
Unable to express emotions
Do not seek or accept help appropriately

Have clearly identified pathology: marital conflict, dysfunctional spouse, or projection of problems on a child
Unable to resolve issues or work through problems
"Acting out" by one or more of children
Has recurrent dysfunctional events
Unable to use effective coping mechanisms

Nursing Approach
Assist in maintaining fuctional status during a specific crisis

Nursing Approach
Assist in eliminating risk factors to prevent future pathology

Nursing Approach
Assist in eliminating the factors that cause the pathology

FIGURE 5-1
Continuum between functional and dysfunctional family. The potentially dysfunctional family can move either way. The nursing approach can assist the family in returning to a functional state.

Interdisciplinary Team Approach

Because clinical nurses with general skills see families in a variety of situations, they are in a unique position to identify high-risk behaviors. Identifying families in possible high-risk situations, however, is only part of the nurse's role. Another is knowing when to relay critical information to other professionals who may be able to provide assistance with the family's care. Family nurse specialists, psychologists, physicians, child development specialists, or social workers, for example, may assist the child care nurse when family problems are identified.

As the health care system becomes increasingly complex, a team approach to human services has become more common. The range of knowledge and skills offered by an interdisciplinary team is much broader than that possessed by a single care provider. A team approach to family care encourages comprehensive assessment of needs and the development of innovative intervention strategies to correct dysfunctional patterns of behavior.[17] The nurse's educational background, experience, system protocols, and available resources will determine the role assumed by that nurse on an interdisciplinary team.

Nursing Implications

Working with families requires the special skills of communication, knowledge of family process, and empathy. The primary objective is to increase the level of family functioning to provide the optimum health state for every family member. As in all clinical situations, the five steps of the nursing process can be applied when caring for families. Assessment skills possessed by professional nurses are essential in diagnosing high-risk families. Then, whether acting alone or as a member of an interdisciplinary team, the nurse may use additional skills in planning and providing interventions, as well as evaluating the outcome of care.

★ **ASSESSMENT**

Family assessment is a process that requires nurses to recognize patterns of behavior rather than just isolated events. For example, a child who occasionally comes into the clinic with a bruise is not considered a victim of child abuse. However, if the child is seen *repeatedly* with bruises, then additional assessment is needed. It is the pattern of behavior over time, not a single event, that generally indicates a family may be at high-risk. Gordon[7] has emphasized that observing the interactions between client and environment is critical to understanding all functional patterns of individual people, families, and communities. For example, levels of communication between and among family members, self-concept and role relationships are influenced by the environment, culture, and the family itself.

Family history has been discussed in Chapters 2 and 3. Assessment tools appear in the Appendix. Assessments in this chapter focus on identifying behavior that place the family at risk.

DETERMINING LEVEL OF RISK

In all family states from functional to dysfunctional, the nurse needs excellent assessment skills to determine the level of family functioning. Gordon[7] suggests that identification of potential problems is as important as diagnosing actual problems. The two critical potential problems are as follows:

- Those persons or families that are at high risk for changing from a potential to an actual problem; for example, risk factors in behavior, situation, or environment.
- Those persons that are at high risk for dysfunctional behavior owing to growth and development issues.

A family determined to be at high risk can include behaviors within each functional pattern grouping as well as growth and development factors. Identification of behaviors indicating high-risk symptoms may occur singularly, in one functional pattern, or in clusters. Gordon[7] observed, "All that is needed for formulating a potential problem are a cluster of risk factors and diagnostic labels to describe them."

During comprehensive assessment of the child, the nurse may recognize cues that suggest further evaluation is warranted. These criteria are in addition to the basic assessment criteria described in Chapters 2 and 3. Additional data are gathered only if the nurse believes that family behavior or interaction indicates a possible cluster of symptoms.

ASSESSMENT USING FUNCTIONAL HEALTH

The assessment criteria presented in Table 5-1 should be used if the nurse has seen a pattern of behaviors that indicate potential dysfunction. Functional health patterns are used to organize the assessment guidelines. The functional patterns of health promotion and health maintenance, activity and exercise, cognition and perception, self-perception and self-concept, role relationships, and coping and stress tolerance have been selected as the most critical factors when assessing the family at risk.

TABLE 5-1
Nursing Assessment: Assessment Criteria for High-Risk Families

Family Cues Indicating Need for Further Assessment	Guidelines to Determine High-Risk Factors
Health Perception and Health Maintenance	
- Alcohol on the breath; especially in the morning - History of chemical dependency in the extended family - Repeated visits to family physician or clinic - Arguments instead of family discussions - Lack of social support systems in the community - Ineffective expression of feelings between and among family members	- Daily use of more than 2 oz of alcohol per day - Use of illegal drugs - Hiding of alcohol or chemicals from any family member - Lack of health maintenance practice, e.g., immunizations, health status examinations - The general mood of the family is depressed and negative - The family appears unkempt, inappropriately dressed - Feelings within the family are not openly expressed - Only certain family members are allowed to express feelings - Negative events are the primary focus of family communication - Children have a subordinate role in family communication - Poor eye contact is used between family members - Infrequent contact with community social systems, e.g., schools, churches, health care delivery facilities - Lack of extended family - Limited willingness or ability to contact community agencies
Nutrition and Metabolism	
- One or more family members are above or below acceptable weight norms - Observation of children eating snacks that are high in sugar or fat - Evidence that the family's daily diet consists mainly of high-carbohydrate foods and lacks proteins, fruits, and vegetables	- The typical family food intake is below acceptable nutritional standards - The family eats irregularly - The family lacks nutritional information - The family has frequent unplanned eating

(Continued)

TABLE 5-1
(Continued)

Family Cues Indicating Need for Further Assessment	Guidelines to Determine High-Risk Factors

Activity and Exercise

- Family identifies few leisure activities outside the home
- Family relies heavily on passive activities, e.g., television with infrequent communication during leisure
- Family has difficulty with budgeting and monthly income to meet financial obligations

- Family has limited exercise
- Family leisure activities involve few community resources
- Family has limited financial resources
- Family lacks knowledge of family budgeting

Cognition and Perception

- Critical family decisions are made by the dominant member; individual family member's concern considered unimportant by the dominant member
- Family decisions are made around present rather than future concerns
- Family language skill suggests lack of understanding of directions for safe compliance with family health care information

- Only one family member makes the decisions
- Family lacks insight into meaning of decisions
- Family lacks understanding of the implications of meeting the health care needs of the children

Self-Perception and Self-Concept

- Family appears downcast; belittles family unit and members within it
- Individual family members dislike time spent within the family unit
- Individual family members are unable or unwilling to speak for themselves; nonassertive behavior demonstrated by one or more family members
- Family admits being overwhelmed by stressors and crises and verbalizes lack of ability to address problems

- Family member affect flat
- Leisure time preferred away from family
- Accepted level of communication is to be negative toward other family members
- Family history of healthy coping during crisis is negative
- External or internal crises lead to dysfunctional behavior
- Family members describe family unit in a negative manner
- Family unable to resolve crises independently

Role Relationships

- Feelings are not freely expressed
- Frequent arguments between the parents
- Inability for the parents to agree on matters involving family functioning
- Parents and children argue openly; lack of emotional warmth in family

- Family members' behavior suggests suppressed anger, e.g., chemical abuse, passive-aggressive verbal responses, manipulation by one or more family members toward the family
- Marital relationship severely impaired due to:
  - Differences in values
  - Lack of communication and caring
  - Maladjusted sexual relationship
  - Individual members unable to meet own interpersonal growth
- Parent-child relationship significantly impaired due to:
  - Inability to bond successfully with the child
  - Behavior control of children harsh and unfeeling
  - Limited open communication between parents and children

Coping and Stress Tolerance

- Presence of chemical or substance abuse, depression, abusive behavior toward family members, unresolved anger within the family
- Presence of the following behaviors in family members:
  - Truancy
  - Neglect
  - Arguments
- Family reacts to normal stressors in an exaggerated manner

- Dysfunctional coping skills demonstrated
- Coping skills used include:
  - Use of illegal substances
  - Unplanned and frequent use of alcohol
  - Overt rage and lack of emotional control in one or more family members

OTHER TOOLS FOR HIGH-RISK FAMILY ASSESSMENT

Other family assessment tools have been developed that emphasize one aspect of the parenting role such as maternal-infant bonding. Some have been developed to detect a special dysfunction in a family, such as child abuse. Family assessment tools used in general assessment situations should detect the family who may have the potential for dysfunction or who is actually dysfunctional. One such tool, the Family APGAR, assesses behaviors that would indicate additional family assessment is needed (see Appendix for the Family APGAR instrument).

SCREEEM Family Assessment Tool. Smilkstein[18] has developed an assessment tool that focuses on the family's ability to respond to stressful events. The acronym SCREEEM is used to guide the evaluation of the family's resources in the area of social, cultural, religious, economic, educational, environmental, and medical. This tool can be used quickly to give an overview of family functioning in selected critical areas. These resources are considered adequate when the following conditions are met:

- Family members are able to communicate and interact openly with one another. Family members also have well-balanced lines of communication to extrafamilial groups such as friends, social groups, and other community organizations.
- Cultural pride or satisfaction can be identified, especially in distinct ethnic groups.
- Religion offers satisfying spiritual experiences as well as contact with a support group.
- The family's economic status allows them to meet the financial demands of everyday life.
- The family's education status allows members to solve or understand most of the problems that arise within their situation.
- Environmental conditions are such that the family is favored by clean air and water and has enough space to satisfy its needs for work, play, and home life.
- Medical resources are available that are satisfactory to meet the family's needs.

This particular assessment tool is not nursing focused; nevertheless, it provides a brief, yet complete, assessment of family functioning.

★ **NURSING DIAGNOSES AND PLANNING**

The development of nursing diagnoses for the family has not progressed as far as those for individuals. Diagnoses approved by the North American Nursing Diagnosis Association (NANDA) for the family and parenting at low risk with normal developmental crises were discussed in Chapter 3. There are few NANDA-approved diagnoses that describe the high-risk family. The diagnosis of Altered Family Processes is related to illness in a family member and concerns a temporary crisis. Other diagnoses have been suggested but have not been approved by NANDA. Some of the nursing diagnoses used in this chapter appear in a list prepared by the University of Toronto Faculty of Nursing. The following diagnoses are used here as examples of what nursing diagnoses for high-risk families might include:

- Family System Disequilibrium: the family group is experiencing distress or disorganization, or both. The family is expected over time to reorganize and stabilize into more satisfying patterns. Contributing factors could be related to changes in composition, roles, relationships, or lifestyle; family strategies for dealing with crisis; insufficient support or role modeling from others; family knowledge deficits; occupational or financial hardships; inadequate stress-relieving strategies; or communication difficulties.
- Family System Dysfunction: Disabling: the family is functioning inadequately in regard to tasks of the nuclear family unit (e.g., provision of basic safety, security, physical survival needs, emotional and social interchange, peaceful coexistence, or sexual differentiation) that lead to the growth of the individual family members. Contributing factors could include the factors mentioned earlier, as well as abusive patterns in families of origin; drug abuse or dependency; long-term avoidance coping; social isolation; absence of bonding; or interpersonal alienation.[25]

Planning care for the high-risk family frequently often is difficult because of family economic factors or the family's reluctance to accept care. However, the professional nurse completes the nursing process with each family whenever possible. If actual interventions cannot be carried out, the nurse may make appropriate referral contacts.

★ **INTERVENTIONS: COLLABORATIVE AND INDEPENDENT**

Interventions focus on interactional family nursing. Such interventions aim at "changing family patterns and the total family system. To accomplish this goal, they predict, at least with some confidence, how changes at the individual and interpersonal systems level and changes in the environment might influence the family systems and its structure."[5] These interventions described by Friedemann can be implemented through three basic supportive functions. Nurses are well within their scope of practice if they intervene in families through support of the child, teaching, and referral.

SUPPORT OF THE CHILD

A critical aspect of intervening in a high-risk family is the recognition of the needs of the child, especially for children who have special health care needs or difficult family circumstances. Because children are vulnerable, the nurse needs to protect them from events that threaten either their physical or psychological safety. This need for protection often requires the help of outside sources such as child protective services. Nurses must know the procedures for referring families to such agencies. Because the legal responsibilities for referral differ from state to state, nurses must learn about the laws governing such actions in the state in which they practice.

TEACHING

Teaching families new ways of managing situations or how to eliminate or decrease high-risk behaviors is important, and content of learning plans can be related to any aspect of functional health. Teaching is also appropriate if there is a learning deficit regarding health maintenance practices or if families want to learn new strategies for coping with stressful situations more effectively. Families also may be taught ways to increase their own social support systems, thereby enhancing their ability to establish useful resources.

Because it is easier to maintain habituated actions than to change, many families continue to use old methods of dealing with stress even though they may not be happy with them. Nurses can intervene by pointing out that the old methods are not working and then help the family explore new ways of managing. Families should be encouraged to discover new ways by themselves. New behaviors are more likely if ideas originate from within the family.

REFERRAL

For a variety of reasons, the nurse often refers the high-risk families to appropriate agencies for needed services. The following circumstances may indicate a need for referral:

- The nurse's role in the practice setting may not permit adequate time or conditions conducive to a positive outcome.
- The complexity of the family dysfunction or potential for dysfunction requires practitioners with more education or expertise.
- Assessment of certain family dysfunctions requires social agencies that specifically address those needs of the family.
- The institutional policy where the nurse is employed restricts certain types of care, such as family therapy.

The nurse's role includes the actual written referral. This can be accomplished only with knowledge of the various local and state agencies and appropriate consultation with the health care team. The process of referral usually is conducted in the following order:

- First, a need for continued intervention is mutually agreed on by the nurse and family.
- Second, the family agrees with the choice of the referral agency by the nurse.
- Third, contact is made with the appropriate agency by telephone or in writing to accomplish the formal referral process. Although contact is usually initiated by the professional, the family also may contact the agency.
- Fourth, a written follow-up report from the referral agency is requested for the family's medical records.

★ EVALUATION

The importance of evaluation of nursing interventions for high-risk family cannot be overstressed. Evaluation assists the nurse in verifying the family's ability to maintain the safety of the child. Evaluation is also a critical tool for monitoring the effectiveness of interventions over time.

Children who grow up in dysfunctional families tend to replicate the same behaviors in their future families. Children who have a range of unmet emotional or educational needs have the potential to experience chronic problems. Using functional health to measure family progress is helpful because of its comprehensive approach to behaviors. Therefore, regardless of the specific nature of the dysfunction, each functional pattern of family behavior needs to be evaluated.

Families at Risk: The Parent Subsystem

Although there are many types of high-risk parenting situations, this section focuses on three frequently seen in today's society: adolescent parents, parents who abuse chemicals, and parents who abuse children. High-risk families rarely have a single explanation of causation, and one area of dysfunction often contributes to another. Attention is given to the effect of dysfunctional parenting on children.

Adolescent Parents

Of the 3.5 million births that occur in the United States, more than 500,000 are termed high risk. These births often occur to adolescent mothers who are poorly prepared to deal with parenthood. The younger the parents, the greater the risks to their children.

Adolescent parenting presents multiple problems for the child, mother, father, extended family, and society. Biologically, the body of an adolescent has not reached full maturity, and adolescent mothers have higher medical risks than their older counterparts. This age group has a high rate of preterm births, pregnancy-induced hypertension, and other perinatal difficulties. In general, adolescents also are deficient in the skills or resources for managing successfully with the problems and frustrations of childbearing and childrearing. Pregnancy interrupts the mother's normal developmental process of resolving issues of self-identity and self-esteem. The normal changes in body image that occur during pregnancy can have ill effects on a teenager who is unsure of her self-image. If the adolescent is unmarried, she must continue to rely on the family of origin for emotional and economic support. This dependency is in direct opposition to the normal adolescent developmental task of breaking away and becoming independent.

The repercussions of childbearing on the life of the adolescent parents are serious and lasting. Mothers under 18 years of age are found less likely to remain with their children or to be interested in their child's progress. They are more likely to have additional children during a 6- to 8-year period following the first-born child. Adolescent parents are also more distractable and dependent.[16]

If marriage is chosen as an option, it too can compound the problems of parenting for the adolescent. The following characteristics have been reported in marriages occurring before the parents are 19 years of age:

- There are fewer life-long assets accumulated. Economic deprivation remains a life-long problem that the parental unit has difficulty reversing.
- There is a likelihood of poor educational achievement. Fewer years of education are the result of the interruption of the normal process of education and training. Once an adolescent becomes pregnant before high school completion, it becomes difficult to return to a formal education program.
- There is more likelihood of divorce or separation. Although many adolescent parents do not marry,

those who do marry tend to have troublesome marriages. There is evidence to suggest that the interruption of normal developmental tasks may explain the higher divorce rate.[23]

Developmental Issues

The very young parent, whether married or single, faces the completion of the normal developmental tasks of adolescence in addition to management of the crisis of parenting. The developmental tasks of identity formation and dealing with intimacy may result in emotional turmoil. Adolescence is also a time of self-discovery and self-concern, but these interests must be put aside while caring for the dependent child. The personal struggle of adolescent parents is to resolve the normal adolescent feelings and responses of dependency-independency and to assume responsibility for their own lives. Because the resolution of personal issues must be accomplished while simultaneously caring for a young infant, the potential for conflict between the role of adolescent and that of a parent is significant (Fig. 5-2).[27]

If an early marriage occurs between adolescents, couples are faced with additional stressors. Not only must they accomplish their individual normal developmental tasks, but they must also meet the needs of the child and their spouse. Adolescent parents often expend so much energy and time on their own developmental issues that they neglect the developmental needs of their children. The implications for the developmental deficits of children born to adolescent parents are extensive. The parents may be immature, thus fostering the possibility of child abuse and poor role modeling for educational advancement and sound decision making in the family.

Economic Issues

One major source of the economic problems of adolescent parents is that the marriage often was precipitated by premarital pregnancy. Quite often, the premarital pregnancy leads to the adolescent's quitting school, a move that essentially ensures a lower socioeconomic status because of the lack of education. Low economic status also lends itself to several health-related problems, including a higher infant mortality rate, higher morbidity rates for all family members, and difficulty in obtaining access to health care. People with low economic status often have difficulty in entering the health care system to obtain services. Therefore, the primary nursing intervention for adolescent parents may be referral to health care agencies that can meet their health care needs.

Health Maintenance Issues

Closely related to the problem of economic deprivation is the practice of health maintenance. Adolescent parents may not possess the knowledge or sensitivity to establish or maintain certain health practices for their children. Indeed, adolescent parents may not have a good health maintenance history themselves. Therefore, the nurse should be aware of the potential for teaching and modeling certain health practices in the family. Teaching needs include every possible aspect of health maintenance, including hygiene, promotion of biologic and psychosocial development, recognizing illness, gaining entry into the health care system, and effectively communicating with health care providers.

Emotional Support Issues

The development of healthy self-concept and positive self-esteem evolves in the family of origin. Children learn from their parents how to feel good about themselves and develop their own positive identity. Healthy self-concept generates the personal belief that the individual possesses positive qualities. Such a self-concept is demonstrated in the confidence to succeed and to meet goals and objectives.

The family unit headed by adolescent parents experiences low self-esteem and negative self-concept for multiple reasons. This problem arises from the adolescent parents' inability to form their own identity due to the pressures of early pregnancy. The resulting poor self-concept may be reinforced by the added pressures of low socioeconomic status and lack of social support systems. It is critical for the nurse to explore this potential dysfunction because of the important influence that low self-esteem has on the children in the family. Children often duplicate their family's self-esteem as they grow older and reinstitute the same level of self-esteem in their future families.

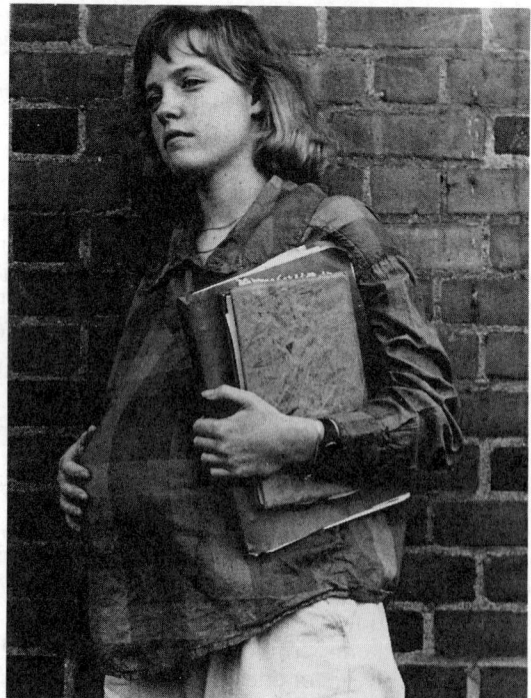

FIGURE 5-2
Adolescent pregnancy presents a major crisis in a young woman's life. Decisions affect the lives of all persons involved (the pregnant mother, the father, the baby, and the baby's biologic grandparents). (From Schuster, C. S. & Ashburn, S. S. [1992]. *The process of human development: A holistic life-span approach* [3rd ed., p. 549]. Philadelphia: J. B. Lippincott)

Nursing Interventions

Nursing interventions for adolescent parents follow the same general guidelines found earlier in the chapter. Supporting the child of adolescent parents is an essential role for the nurse. Teaching adolescents about effective parenting and normal growth and development of children and referring them to agencies where their unique needs and problems can be addressed are also important. Nursing diagnoses and interventions for care of the adolescent parent are given in the accompanying display.

Chemically Dependent Parents

A large number of infants born today have some chemical in their system. National statistics indicate that 8% to 14% of women of childbearing age are addicted to drugs. Estimates are that 2% to 3% are dependent on mood-altering drugs, 2% to 3% are cocaine dependent, 0.5% are opiate dependent, and 5% to 8% are alcohol dependent.[24] A recent study done in California found that 10% of all newborns had a positive urine screen for co-caine, whereas another reported 18% to 21% of the newborns had positive results in a drug screen.[11] The effect of alcohol on newborns has been well documented.[12] Children of alcoholics are at risk for developing intellectual, physical, and psychological problems.[21]

The physical and social impact of any kind of chemical abuse on families is devastating (Fig. 5-3). Parents who are dependent on chemicals are severely limited in their ability to fulfill their parenting roles. The all-consuming need for the chemical takes precedence over all other needs and desires, including the wish to be a good parent. This self-absorption of the parent presents areas of concern for the welfare of the child and the family.

Developmental Issues

The developmental delays of children born to chemically dependent mothers are extensive. It is not clear whether the delays are due to intrauterine exposure to the drugs or from drug withdrawal. Infants who are exposed prenatally to drugs, especially cocaine, are initially unable to respond appropriately to the mother's overtures,

---

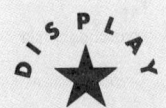

Nursing Diagnoses and Nursing Interventions for Adolescent Parents

Developmental Role Conflicts

Nursing Diagnoses

Personal Identity Disturbance*†
Altered Role Performance*
Role Adaptation Disturbance†
Altered Parenting*
Parenting Difficulty†

Nursing Interventions

- Teach the importance of developmental needs for parents and children.
- Monitor progress in developmental tasks of parents and children.
- Refer to appropriate agencies for help regarding economic issues.

Self-Concept

Nursing Diagnoses

Body Image Disturbance*†
Self-Esteem Disturbance*†

Nursing Interventions

- Assist the family to identify ways to increase their sense of self-worth.
- Assist the family to identify positive qualities.
- Teach assertive behaviors to all family members.

Socioeconomic Issues

Nursing Diagnosis

Impaired Health Care Resources Utilization†

Nursing Interventions

- Refer to appropriate social agency for economic assistance.
- Monitor family's ability to provide for itself economically.

Health Maintenance Issues

Nursing Diagnosis

Impaired Home Maintenance Management*†

Nursing Interventions

- Provide teaching in those areas of identified need.

* Taxonomy I (revised) With Official Nursing Diagnoses. (1991). St. Louis: North American Nursing Diagnosis Association.
† List of Nursing Diagnoses. (1982). Toronto: University of Toronto, Faculty of Nursing.

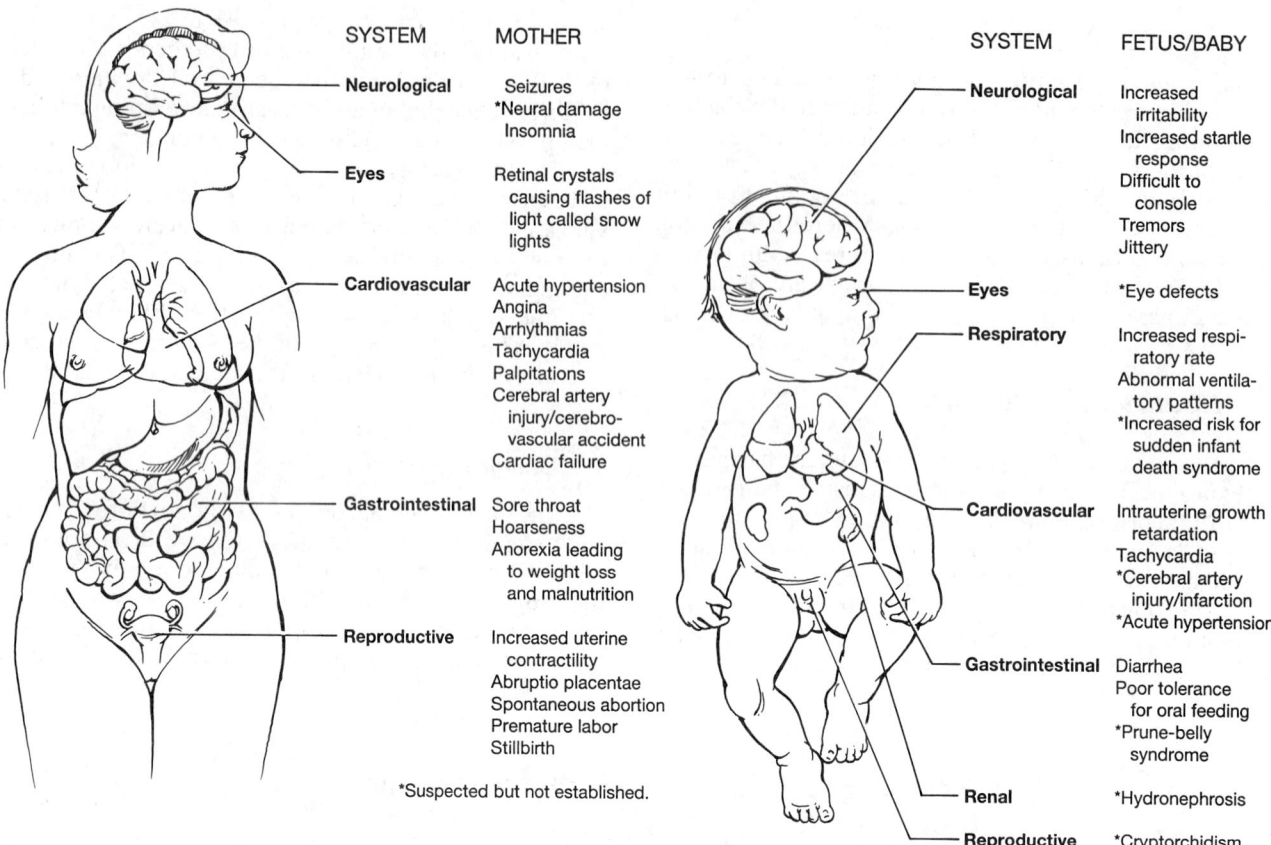

FIGURE 5-3
Substance abuse affects the systems of both the mother and the fetus-neonate.

thus creating difficulty in the attachment process.[1] If the mother and infant are unable to form the initial bond, the chances increase that the parent will not provide an emotional base of security for the child.

Alcoholic parents are unable to provide a consistent environment or role stability, are not dependable, and are not available emotionally for the latency age child. "As a result, when the alcoholic parent is drinking, the children's needs are often ignored. When the alcoholic parent is sober, the lack of emotional availability may continue, or the parent's irritability may alternate with periods of overindulgence in an attempt to alleviate guilt over prior emotional neglect."[13] The impaired parenting patterns are observable in the social and interpersonal responses of the child.

Talashek[21] found that younger adolescents who grow up in a home where one parent was alcoholic had problems with ego development. Because adolescence is a time when children are very sensitive to how they appear to others, they tend to isolate themselves rather than risk the embarrassment of having peers see their parents. The isolation keeps them from social interactions and development of a healthy sense of identity.

Economic Issues

Because the parent's main objective is to obtain and use chemicals, all of the economic resources of the family are typically used to support the habit. The abuse of chemicals not only drains existing economic resources

but future ones as well. As the parents become more and more addicted to the chemical, they are less interested in going to work or engaging in any other productive activity. Thus, the family is deprived of the necessary financial support.

Health Maintenance Issues

Health maintenance is an area of difficulty within the family where the parent abuses chemicals. Health maintenance practices may be altered because of chemical use, lack of motivation, or economic priorities. Frequently chemical use interferes with judgment about the needs of the family concerning health maintenance. For example, parents may value chemical use more than providing adequate food and shelter for their children. This inverted set of priorities has implications for daily caregiving of children and the safety of the home environment.

Emotional Support Issues

Chemical abuse affects many aspects of family functioning, but none so clearly as communication within the family. Use of chemicals alters relationships among family members. If chemicals are repeatedly abused, the content and mode of transmission of communication become impaired. Feelings are expressed in pathologic ways either through overt anger or passive aggressiveness during times of chemical use. Nurses need to be aware of how family members interact with each other and the content of communication.

Families who have members that are chemically dependent usually isolate themselves and avoid social systems within the community. Most families abstain from developing close relationships with others because of their uncertainty of how the dependent family member will behave in a situation. Social isolation increases as the family becomes increasingly dysfunctional. Nurses should be alert for isolative behavior and assist families whenever possible to maintain relationships with community, social, extended family, and religious groups.

Society has often condoned the use of chemicals to facilitate problem solving of everyday difficulties. The popular "martini after work" is an example of socially acceptable chemical use. However, when using chemicals is necessary for making any decision, there is a problem The abuse of substances interferes with healthy decision making and puts parents in a position of becoming a negative role model for the children in the home.

Nursing Interventions

Chemically dependent parents generally need basic education in parenting skills. The central issue in caring for a family in which a parent is chemically dependent, however, is the treatment or the parent with the dependency. Nurses should know the agencies who focus on chemical dependency that are available in their community. Nursing diagnoses and interventions for care of

---

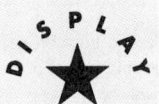

Nursing Diagnoses and Nursing Interventions for the Family That Abuses Chemicals

Addiction and Dependency

Nursing Diagnoses

Drug/Substance Abuse†
Drug Dependence (specify)†

Nursing Interventions

- Monitor extent of chemical use.
- Refer to drug rehabilitation agency for treatment.
- Teach healthy use of chemicals.

Communication Patterns

Nursing Diagnosis

Impaired Communication†

Interventions

- Refer for marriage counseling.
- Teach healthy ways of communicating when emotions and feelings are present.
- Teach about the influence that parents' emotional health has on the psychological health of children.
- Role model healthy communications.

Interactions With Social Systems

Nursing Diagnoses

Impaired Social Interaction*
Inadequate Socialization†
Social Isolation*

Nursing Interventions

- Assist family in maintaining social interaction between themselves and community.
- Teach family ways in which contact with social support groups will enhance family functioning.

Problem-Solving Skills

Nursing Diagnoses

Impaired Problem Solving: Inadequate Insight†
Sensory/Perceptual Alterations (specify)*

Nursing Interventions

- Teach methods of healthy family coping.
- Suggest ways to enhance family problem-solving skills.
- Refer family members who are abusing chemicals to an appropriate community resource to support healthy chemical use.

* Taxonomy I (revised) With Official Nursing Diagnoses. (1991). St. Louis: North American Nursing Diagnosis Association.
† List of Nursing Diagnoses. (1982). Toronto: University of Toronto, Faculty of Nursing.

the family involved with chemicals are listed in the accompanying display.

Abusive Parents

Child abuse frequently evolves from circumstances that already have been identified in this chapter as high-risk factors. Although abuse in the family can be directed at any family member, children are frequently the target because of their vulnerability.

Abuse can take many forms, and often there is a combination of types of abuse. Unfortunately, no consistent or standardized definition of child abuse exists. In the past, the term *abuse* has been primarily a legal concept. The following three characteristics are found in almost all legal definitions:

* The behavior violates a norm of parental conduct.
* The infliction is deliberate and nonaccidental.
* The abuse is severe enough to warrant intervention.[6]

Nine different categories of child have been suggested: physical abuse, sexual abuse, physical neglect, medical neglect, emotional abuse, emotional neglect, educational neglect, abandonment, and multiple maltreatment.[15] It is not the intent of this chapter to describe in detail the different types of abuse that can occur. Rather, it is to give a brief overview of the common characteristics found in abusive families. Sexual abuse is discussed in Chapter 68.

Developmental Issues

One striking characteristic of abusive parents is the generational repetition of abuse; that is, parents who abuse are usually victims of abuse themselves. The pattern of abuse may be seen in three or four generations of one family, although the type of abuse may be different. Experts believe that the reason for the continuous patterns of abuse is a basic inability to provide good parenting. "Parenting is a learned type of behavior, learned through the experience of being a child and of being parented as a baby and small child. The learning is by identification with the caretakers of the earliest months and years. This is true of good parenting as well as inadequate parenting—a perfectly normal process leading to either appropriate or inappropriate parenting behavior depending upon the content of the earliest experience."[20] Children in abusive families do not have the skills of basic trust. Thus, they grow up feeling inferior and worthless (Fig. 5-4). They are more likely to replicate the familiar but destructive environment in their own marriage,[5] thus continuing the patterns of abuse.

Economic Issues

There have been no research findings that directly link socioeconomic status to abuse. The poor, however, are heavily represented in the abusive population. Families in poverty are faced with multiple stressors in their lives. Economic survival is tenuous at best and often un-

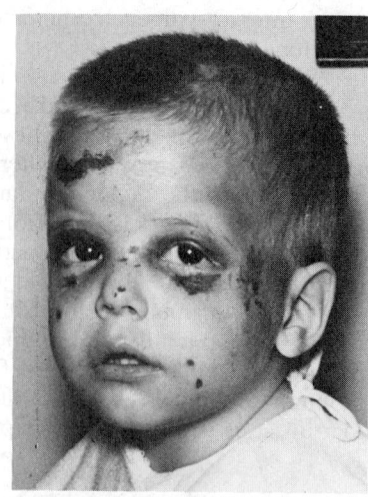

FIGURE 5-4
The child who has been physically abused usually has old *and* fresh bruises about the head, face, and body and may either look sad and forlorn or be actively seeking to please, sometimes even particularly involved with and attentive to the abusing parent.

certain. When parents are dependent on federal or state support to meet basic needs, the families may feel degraded. Low self-esteem and frustration add to the stress already present.[6]

Health Maintenance Issues

Health maintenance issues center around the parents' inability to care for their children without resorting to abusive behaviors. Parents are often unable to nurture their children. They have poor communication skills and are unable to view their children as individuals. Knowledge of normal child development, nutritional needs of children, and safety and discipline guidelines are all issues pertaining to the health of the family.[19]

Emotional Support Issues

The abusive parent displays low self-esteem and problems of identity. Most of these adults have little ability to problem solve and are easily upset when crises occur. Even the normal stress of marriage and day-to-day experiences may be too much for the parent to handle. A lack of problem-solving skills, a history of abuse, and social isolation sets the stage for abuse to occur in the family. Health care workers are often hesitant to provide practical and emotional support for abusive families because they find abusive behavior so repulsive.

Nursing Interventions

Good observational skills and assessment data are of major importance when abuse is suspected. Table 5-2 provides a description of signs of several types of abuse. If the nurse discovers that actual abuse has occurred, the immediate intervention is to relay this finding to the appropriate legal authorities. Every state has individual statutes that protect children and other family members from

TABLE 5-2
Nursing Assessment: Signs of Abuse in Children

Physical Signs	Behavioral Signs
Physical Abuse	
Bruises and welts; may be on multiple body surfaces or soft tissue; may form regular pattern (e.g., belt buckle)	Less compliant than average
	Signs of negativism, unhappiness
Burns: cigar or cigarette, immersion (stocking/glovelike on extremities or doughnut-shaped on buttocks or genitals), or patterned as an electrical appliance (e.g., iron)	Anger, isolation
	Destructive
	Abusive toward others
	Difficulty developing relationships
Fractures: single or multiple; may be in various stages of healing	Either excessive or absent separation anxiety
	Inappropriate caretaking concern for parent
Lacerations or abrasions: rope burns; tears in and around the mouth, eyes, ears, or genitalia	Constantly in search of attention, favors, food, etc.
	Various developmental delays (cognitive, language, motor)
Abdominal injuries: ruptured or injured internal organs	
Central nervous system injuries: subdural hematoma, retinal or subarachnoid hemorrhage	
Physical Neglect	
Malnutrition	Lack of appropriate adult supervision
Repeated episodes of pica	Repeated ingestions of harmful substances
Constant fatigue or listlessness	Poor school attendance
Poor hygiene	Exploitation (forced to beg, steal, etc.; excessive household work)
Inadequate clothing for circumstances	Role reversal with parent
Inadequate medical or dental care	Drug or alcohol use
Sexual Abuse	
Difficulty walking or sitting	Direct or indirect disclosure to relative, friend, or teacher
Thickening and/or hyperpigmentation of labial skin	Withdrawal with excessive dependency
Vaginal opening measures >4 mm horizontally in preadolescence	Poor peer relationships
	Poor self-esteem
Torn, stained, or bloody underclothing	Frightened or phobic of adults
Bruises or bleeding of genitalia or perianal area	Sudden decline in academic performance
Lax rectal tone	Pseudomature personality development
Vaginal discharge	Suicide attempts
Recurrent urinary tract infections	Regressive behavior
Nonspecific vaginitis	Enuresis or encopresis
Venereal disease	Excessive masturbation
Sperm or acid phosphatase on body or clothes	Highly sexualized play
Pregnancy	Sexual promiscuity
Emotional Abuse	
Delays in physical development	Distinct emotional symptoms and/or functional limitations
Failure to thrive	Deteriorating conduct
	Increased anxiety
	Apathy or depression
	Developmental lags

Data from Council on Scientific Affairs (1985). AMA diagnostic and treatment guidelines concerning child abuse and neglect. *Journal of the American Medical Association, 254*(6), 796–800.

abuse. The nurse becomes legally and morally responsible to report such findings if assessments indicate that abuse exists in a family. For those nurses working with children or families, knowledge of the individual state statute regarding neglect or abuse is a critical part of nursing knowledge. Nursing diagnoses and interventions for care of families who abuse children are listed in the accompanying display.

Families at Risk: The Child Subsystem

Families can be at risk owing to stressors that originate from the child rather than the parents. These factors are due to physical illnesses, growth and development issues, or environmental influences. Child factors tend to be

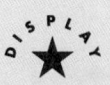

Nursing Diagnoses and Nursing Interventions for Families That Abuse Children

Nursing Diagnoses

Maladaptive Parenting†
High Risk for Violence: Self-Directed or Directed at Others*

Nursing Interventions

- Contact authorities to remove child from environment.
- Refer parents to community or self-help groups.
- Role model parenting behaviors.

* *Taxonomy I (revised) With Official Nursing Diagnoses. (1991). St. Louis: North American Nursing Diagnosis Association.*
† *List of Nursing Diagnoses. (1982). Toronto: University of Toronto, Faculty of Nursing.*

more overt than parental issues and occur either spontaneously (such as prematurity, accidents, and sudden death) or are chronic in nature (as with terminal illness or physical or mental disabilities). The following situations are typical of the child factor of high-risk families.

Preterm Infants

Physical and Developmental Issues

During the last two decades, medical science has made great strides in the ability to save premature neonates. The birth of a preterm infant is a crisis for families. The unexpected birth of a child who may be at physiologic risk can threaten the stability of the family. By the time preterm infants graduate from neonatal intensive care units, the acute care health issues are usually resolved. However, concerns about the long-term physical implications of prematurity are a real source of stress for families.

Preterm birth affects all body organs. The smaller and more immature an infant is at birth, the more likely is multisystem involvement. After the acute situation at birth is resolved, these organs often remain vulnerable to disease. This vulnerability is present over the first 2 years of life but may persist longer.[22] Not only are physical systems as risk, but the children are often developmentally different than full-term infants. Preterm infants tend to be more temperamental, fretful, and distant with their caretakers. These characteristics can negatively affect the parent-child relationship. Given the fact that many of the preterm infants are born to high-risk parents (adolescents or chemically dependent, for example), the stage is set for double vulnerability in the family.

Adding to this potential crisis situation is the fact that health care facilities with the necessary technical equipment are sometimes not available to families in need. Often, the infant must be transported to another hospital

where life support can be given. This situation creates some special issues for the family separated from the infant. Transporting an infant to another facility validates for the family the seriousness of the infant's medical condition. The family sometimes does not visit the infant because of fear of the outcome, but financial issues or lack of transportation also may be a problem.[4]

The differences in the preterm and normal infant are not well known to the general public. Families assume that once the infant has gained weight and is discharged from the hospital, the problems are over. Families presume the infant will follow the normal stages of development. This expectation can be a problem, particularly if the family has experienced a normal birth prior to the preterm one. Discharge planning and follow-up are essential needs that should be provided. Such planning includes educating the family about the differences in preterm versus normal infants, teaching the family how to care for the infant when discharged, and observing interactions between the infant and family members to assess whether the infant will be assimilated into the family. Discharge planning involves assessing the family's needs, their knowledge, and willingness to learn. It also involves planning interventions, instituting the interventions, and evaluating the effectiveness of the entire process.[10]

Economic Issues

The birth of a preterm infant influences every facet of a family's reality, not the least of which is the economic impact. The preterm infant frequently requires weeks or months of expensive hospital care (Fig. 5-5). Payment for such care is often dependent on the parent's economic resources or the availability of public funds such as Medicare or Medicaid. Even though a payment source may be found, parents frequently are liable for uncovered costs, and out-of-pocket payments may cause severe economic hardship. Referrals to social agencies for economic assistance should be made.

Emotional Support Issues

A preterm birth has the potential temporarily or permanently to affect the functioning of the family unit. The abruptness of the preterm birth, the threat to the baby's safety, economic considerations, and projected blame are all possible factors that may alter the parent's marital relationship even after the baby is discharged and healthy.

Parents, especially the mother, are prone to feel guilty about the preterm birth. Parents may speculate about activities that may have initiated labor prematurely. Guilt or blame that develops between the parents may interfere with their ability to support each other during the crisis, thereby placing additional strain on the family. Thus, during such crisis events, it is imperative that the family receive support from outside sources, including nurses and other health care professionals.

Nursing Interventions

Nurses can help parents express their feelings and talk about their fears, anger, and guilt. Health professionals sometimes are uncomfortable listening to such feel-

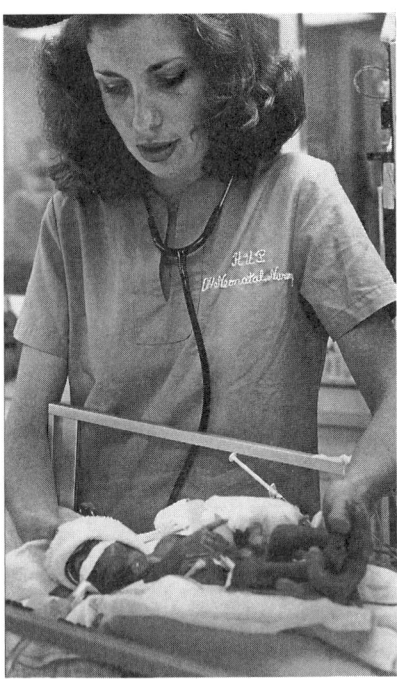

FIGURE 5-5
Hospital care of a preterm infant may require weeks of specialized care with added costs that may not be covered by a financial plan. (Photo courtesty of University of Pennsylvania)

ings and respond by disregarding the importance of such emotions. Many families reach out for spiritual comfort and may benefit from visits by a spiritual counselor, minister, or church member.

If the family is unable successfully to overcome the crisis of preterm birth, they are at risk for continuing dysfunction. Parenting skills are thus inhibited, and the child is affected adversely. Nursing diagnoses and interventions for care of the family with preterm infant are given in the accompanying display.

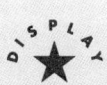

Nursing Diagnoses and Nursing Interventions for Families With a Preterm Infant

Nursing Diagnoses

Ineffective Family Coping: Disabling*
Altered Parenting*
Dysfunctional Grieving*

Nursing Interventions

- Allow parents to verbalize their feelings and concerns.
- Discuss with the parents the emotional impact on the family and marriage that crisis events have precipitated.
- Refer couple to marital counseling.

Taxonomy I (revised) With Official Nursing Diagnoses. (1991). St. Louis: North American Nursing Diagnosis Association.

The Chronically Ill Child

Families who have chronically ill children are similar to families with preterm infants. Consequently, the issues facing the families often follow the same pattern. However, parents of premature infants often have the hope that their child will eventually be normal and healthy, but parents of chronically ill children do not have such assurances. Therefore, the stress and difficulties with the child are of a long-term nature. With continued stress, even families that are relatively stable and healthy have the potential to be at high risk.

Chronic illness can be either of a physical or developmental-emotional nature. Each of the two types have specific problems inherent in the condition. However, there are striking similarities in the effects of either on the family.

Physical and Developmental Issues

As in the case of a preterm infant, the parents' first concern about a child with chronic illness is the child's ability to survive. Children with chronic illness often have physical or mental disabilities that make day-to-day living a struggle. Families must cope with treatment routines that interrupt their normal activities. For example, families with children who have cystic fibrosis must modify the content and methods of preparation of the family diet to incorporate restrictions; recreational activities must be modified so that the child has access to treatment facilities at all times. Arrangements must be made so that the child can have postural drainage at least twice a day. Over the long term, such modifications in family life can be burdensome.[26]

Families with developmentally delayed or emotionally handicapped children face similar frustrations. Although the physical health of the child may not be in question, the ability of the child to function in a normal world certainly is. Children may not be able to dress or feed themselves, placing responsibility for those tasks on other family members. Affected children sometimes have no sense of danger and face safety hazards within the home or in social situations. In addition, parents are often frustrated with the fact that although affected children may look healthy, they are limited in their ability to function independently.

Economic Issues

The economic consequences of chronic illness in a child can be devastating. Although most of the care may be covered by health insurance or other financial support, there are many costs that are not.

Medications, dietary supplements, medical equipment and supplies, transportation to health care facilities, parking fees, and extra expenses for the parents while the child is hospitalized may place a significant financial burden on the family (Fig. 5-6). In addition, the amount of time required to care for the ill child may limit the ability of both parents to work outside the home, thus reducing the family's income. Different employment opportunities may be rejected for fear of losing health in-

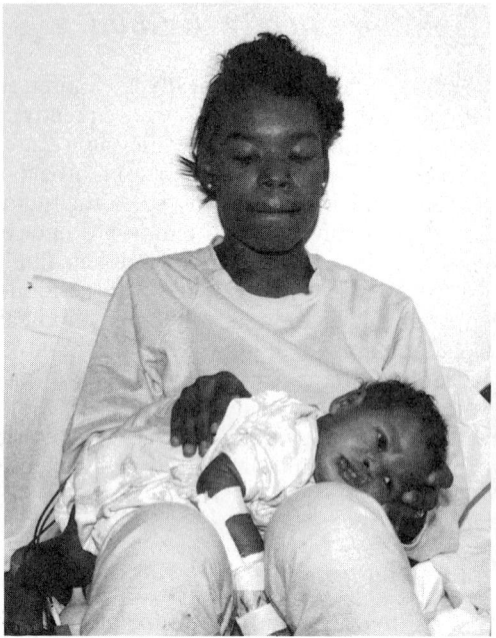
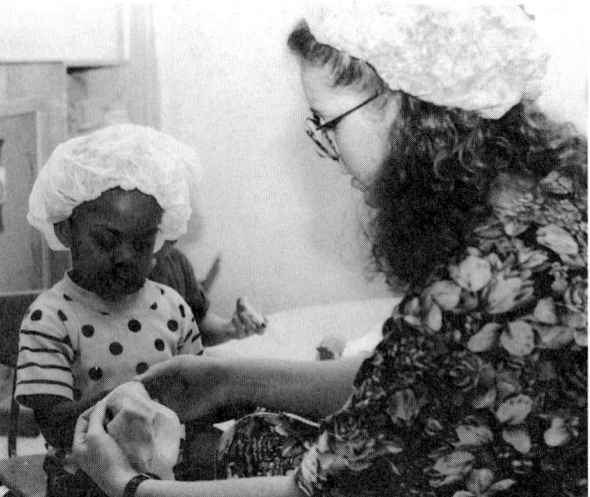

FIGURE 5-6
The family with a chronically ill child may have trouble coping with the investment of time and finances required in providing care and making return visits to the health care facility.

surance coverage or because the job location is too far from a treatment center.[26]

Emotional Support Issues

There are two emotional issues that are universally a part of the family with children who have chronic illness. The first is the guilt associated with somehow failing to produce a perfect child. Whether the chronic illness is a result of genetic or accidental origin, the parents' first reaction is, "What did we do wrong?" "If only" statements are frequently heard from the parents—"if only" they

had done or not done certain things, then the child would not have the illness.

The second emotional issue is one of grieving the loss of the fantasized perfect child. Before birth, all parents expect the child to be a healthy normal child. Each parent envisions how the addition of the child will enhance the quality of the family. Hopes and aspirations for the child's future are a part of the normal process of attaching with the infant. Such dreams are shattered when it becomes clear that the chronically ill child will not be able to fulfill the parents' aspirations. A condition described by Olshansky[14] as "chronic sorrow" is a normal

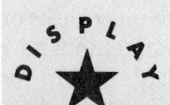

Nursing Diagnoses and Nursing Interventions for Families With a Chronically Ill Child

Grieving and Guilt

Nursing Diagnoses

Anticipatory Grieving*
Dysfunctional Grieving*
Unresolved Guilt†

Nursing Interventions

- Monitor for contributing factors that may delay the grief work.
- Support the family's grief reactions.
- Promote family cohesiveness.
- Identify agencies and support groups that may be helpful.

Altered Roles and Relationships

Nursing Diagnoses

Altered Family Processes*
Powerlessness
Hopelessless

Nursing Interventions

- Facilitate family strengths.
- Intervene when family is unable to carry burden of care.
- Assist family with appraisal of the situation.
- Provide anticipatory guidance.
- Initiate health teaching and referrals as necessary.

* Taxonomy I (revised) With Official Nursing Diagnoses. (1991). St. Louis: North American Nursing Diagnosis Association.
† List of Nursing Diagnoses. (1982). Toronto: University of Toronto, Faculty of Nursing.

parental response in these families. Attempts to deny the problems of the child, or to lead a "normal" life without adjusting to the needs of the child are indications that the family has not been successful in adapting to their life situation. Such a family is at high risk for other types of maladaptive behavior, such as abuse.

Cameron and Orr[2] studied the stress in families of school-age children with delayed mental development. Stress levels were found to be higher in parents who saw their children as less adaptable, less acceptable, more demanding, more moody, more distractable, and less reinforcing to themselves. In addition, parents with high levels of stress were more depressed, less attached to their children, more restricted in their parental roles, and less confident about their competence as parents. Social isolation, less positive relationships with their spouse, and poor health were also evident.

Nursing Interventions

Support is an important element of interventions with the family of a child with a chronic illness—support from the nurse, from outside resources, and from the family to one another. The nurse guides the family through the grieving process, building on existing strengths. Referral may be necessary and can be a positive experience. Health promotion and anticipatory guidance provides the parents with knowledge of care needed by the child. Chapter 21 deals with the child and family with chronic illness. Other chapters in Unit 3 discuss care of the family with various life situations that may be chronic. Nursing diagnoses and interventions for care of the family who has a child with a chronic illness are given in the accompanying display.

Summary

Families that are experiencing various crises or internal pathology must be assessed when the nurse is caring for the child in the family. Using the functional health pattern

format provides an assessment profile in which the nurse can establish the presence of family difficulties. If one or more functional patterns indicate either potential or actual dysfunction, further assessment, planning, and intervention should be undertaken. The nurse in general practice needs to develop assessment skills that assist in case finding high-risk families. Family dysfunction often requires specialized intervention; therefore, referral to other resources within the health care system or community is a common nursing intervention.

References

1. Becker, P., & Burke, S. (1988). Neonatal drug addiction: Analysis from two moral orientations. *Holistic Nursing Practice, 2*(4), 20–27.
2. Cameron, S., & Orr, R. (1989). Stress in families of school-aged children with delayed mental development. *Canadian Journal of Rehabilitation, 2*(3), 137–144.
3. Carpenito, L. (1992). *Nursing diagnosis* (4th ed.). Philadelphia: J. B. Lippincott.
4. Davis, D., & Hawkins, J. (1985). High-risk maternal and neonatal transport: Psychosocial implications for practice. *Dimensions of Critical Care Nursing, 4*(6), 368–379.
5. Friedemann, M. L. (1989). The concept of family nursing. *Journal of Advanced Nursing, 14*(3), 211–216.
6. Getty, C., & Humphreys, W. (1981). *Understanding the family.* New York: Appleton Century Crofts.
7. Gordon, M. (1987). *Nursing diagnosis: Process and application* (2nd ed.). New York: McGraw-Hill.
8. Johnson, S. H. (1986). *Nursing assessment and strategies for the family at risk* (2nd ed.). Philadelphia: J. B. Lippincott.
9. Heiney, S. (1988). Assessing and intervening with dysfunctional families. *Oncology Nursing Forum, 15*(5), 585–589.
10. Julian, K., & Young, C. (1983). Comprehensive health care for the high-risk infant and family: Follow-up of the high risk family. *Neonatal Network, 2*(3), 32–35.
11. Lavee, J. I., McCubbin, H., & Olson, D. H. (1987). Effect of stressful life events and transition on family functioning and well being. *Journal of Marriage and Family, 49*(9), 857–873.
12. Lewis, K., Bennett, B., & Schmeder, N. (1989). The care of infants menaced by cocaine abuse. *American Journal of Maternal Child Nursing, 14*(5), 324–329.
13. Morehouse, E., & Richards, T. (1982). An examination of dysfunctional latency age children of alcoholic parents and problems in intervention. *Journal of Children in Contemporary Society, 15*(1), 21–23.
14. Olshansky, S. (1962). Chronic sorrow: A response to having a mentally defective child. *Social Casework, 43,* 190–193.
15. Pearce, J., & Walsh, K. (1984). Characteristics of abused children: Research findings. *Canada's Mental Health, 32*(2), 2–6.
16. Porter, L. (1984). Parenting enhancement among high-risk adolescents. *Nursing Clinics of North America, 19*(1), 89–102.
17. Saunders, R., Miller, B., & Cates, K. (1989). Pediatric family care: An interdisciplinary team approach. *Children's Health Care, 18*(1), 53–58.
18. Smilkstein, G. (1984). The physician and family function assessment. *Family Systems Review, 2*(3), 263–277.
19. Soditus, C., & Mock, D. (1988). Interrupting the cycle of child abuse. *American Journal of Maternal Child Nursing, 13*(5), 196–199.
20. Steele, B. (1986). Notes on the lasting effects of early child abuse throughout the life cycle. *Child Abuse and Neglect* 10, 283–291.
21. Talashek, M. (1987). Parental alcoholism and adolescent ego identity. *Journal of Community Health Nursing* 4(4), 211–222.

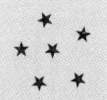

Ideas for Nursing Research

High-risk families present challenging, complex problems for nurses to assess and provide care. The following areas need to be explored:

- Characteristics of families who react quite differently to stressors that appear identical
- Measurement of nursing intervention outcomes for families with adolescent parents
- Needs assessment of families with chemical abuse
- Longitudinal study of nursing needs for families with a chronically ill child
- Interparameter reliability of family-oriented nursing diagnoses

22. Telkoste, K. A., & Bennett, F. C. (1987). The high risk infant: Transitions in health, development, and family during the first years of life. *Journal of Perinatology, 7(4)*, 368–377.

23. Teti, D. M., Lamb, M. E., & Elster, B. B. (1987). Long range socioeconomic and marital consequences of adolescent marriage in three cohort adult males. *Journal of Marriage and Family, 49(3)*, 499–506.

24. US Congress. House Select Committee on Children, Youth and Families. (1986). *Placing infants at risk: Parental addiction and disease.* Washington, D. C.: US Government Printing Office.

25. University of Toronto Faculty of Nursing. (1982). *List of nursing diagnoses and their definitions.* Toronto, University of Toronto.

26. Walker, C. (1988). The clinical challenge of cystic fibrosis. *Journal of Intravenous Nursing 11(6)*, 373–381.

27. Young, M. (1988). Parenting during mid-adolescence: A review of developmental theories and parenting behaviors. *Maternal Child Nursing Journal 17(1)*, 1–12.

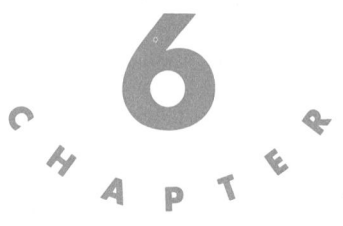

Child and Family Teaching

BEHAVIORAL OBJECTIVES

Describe the role of nurse as an educator of children and their families.

Describe the importance of planning all teaching-learning interactions using a *systems model*.

Identify a variety of opportunities for teaching-learning interactions between nurses and children or families.

Identify the components of a *teaching plan*.

Discuss *learning theory* and the relationship between learning theories and instructional design.

Children and families in contact with health care providers in a variety of settings require facts, new skills, and new perspectives about growing up healthy, managing acute illness, and living with chronic illness.[38] A nurse has the unique opportunity to teach children and families. Every interaction between a nurse and a child and family provides a teaching-learning opportunity.[32] This philosophy of nursing is reflected in the following statement: "Every nurse is a teacher; not to teach is not to nurse."[39]

This chapter focuses on the role of the nurse as a patient educator in formal and informal teaching situations. The realities of acute hospitalization often lead nurses to believe that no time is available for patient education, when in fact every interaction can be used to inform and to teach. More than anyone else in the health care setting, the nurse is able to explain what families can expect when an illness is diagnosed. In well-child settings the nurse can provide hallmarks for normal developmental processes that families can identify as the infants and children grow.[11]

Rationale for Child and Family Educational Programs

The American Hospital Association, the Patient's Bill of Rights, several Nurse Practice Acts, and most Nursing Standards of Practice identify patient teaching as a function of nursing. Nurses report that teaching is a primary role, and nurses are concerned about quality patient education. The nurse has many unique opportunities to assess children and their families for health educational needs and to initiate the teaching process (Fig. 6-1).

Health education is an extremely important concept for nurses working with infants, children, and adolescents and their families. Many studies have documented the cost-effectiveness of preventive health programs, including health education.[8,12,38] Middle-class families are taking more control over their own health care, are better informed, and are asking questions of health care professionals. Mothers and fathers want to know what to expect from their pediatrician, and many are informed during childbirth classes that they should interview prospective pediatricians before selecting one with whom they feel comfortable. Well-baby visits are considered preventive medicine and are not covered by most insurance companies. Many parents cannot afford these services. Public health departments provide clinics for select well-baby services, including immunizations. For some families, this may be the only opportunity to learn about the normal growth and development of their children.[3]

Patient education programs for specific disease treatment and management may be covered by third-party reimbursement. Generally, to be covered the patient teaching must be for diagnosed conditions and be ordered by the physician. The coverage may include inpatient and outpatient education programs. The most commonly covered programs are those for diabetes patient teaching.[12,22,26]

Research has shown that not all patients are comfortable with the quality of information they receive from nurses and physicians.[8] Families have reported that they were never sure what was happening to their children or what to expect. Evidence indicates that nurses and physicians do not view patient education as a priority in hospitals unless specific treatments and self-care skills are needed.[25,31]

When examining factors that facilitate, impede, or act as barriers to patient education, Caffrella[7] found that a lack of staff time to plan, coordinate, and implement patient education; a lack of third party reimbursement; and a lack of physician support inhibited the growth of patient education programs in hospitals. To develop and implement child and family teaching programs nurses should begin to examine more appropriate settings for teaching (homes, outpatient clinics, and hospitals), using multiple settings and times; better use of time, including group and individual teaching sessions; and more family involvement.

Definitions

Patient education is a planned, systematic, and intentional interaction that influences health care behaviors through a variety of strategies, including teaching, counseling, behavior modification, and print and nonprint media and resources.[2,8,33] With patient education the child and family learn new knowledge, skills, or attitudes (Fig. 6-2).

Teaching is defined as activities that assist the learner in knowing factual information, adopting a new attitude, or performing a new skill. The process of teaching implies that there is a relationship between the teacher and the learner.

Learning is defined as "a change in human deposition or capability which can be retained and which is not simply ascribable to the process of growth."[16] When working with children as learners theorists differentiate among learning, maturation, and development. The distinguishing factors between these three concepts often are difficult

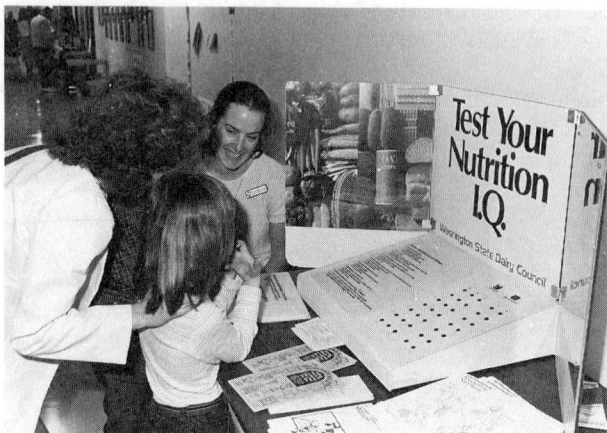

FIGURE 6-1
Nurses can teach by assessing knowledge and initiating interest in a subject. This is an example of preventive health education. (Courtesy of Overlake Hospital Medical Center, Bellevue, WA.)

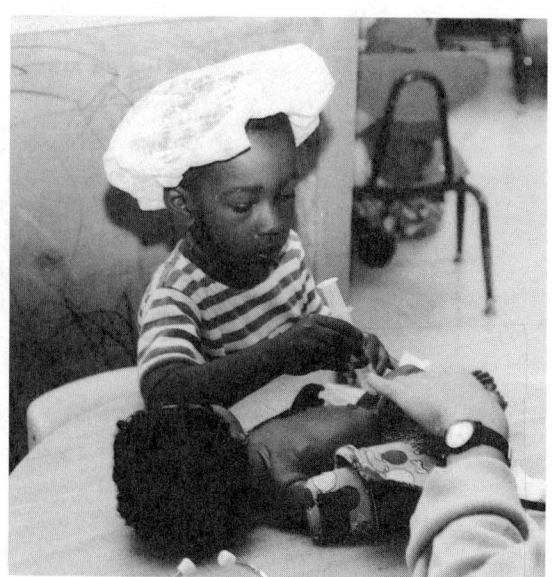

FIGURE 6-2
This child learns about interventions he will undergo by simulating the activity with a doll.

to discern. Bigge[6] defines maturation as a developmental process in which individuals manifest different genetic traits. Developmental changes have been associated with the individual's internal maturation. At various ages children develop the internal skills to be able to do things that they were unable to do before this time. A simplified example is toilet training. The child must have operational neurological pathways, have muscular tone of the bladder, and be able to identify the sensations of a full bladder or a distended rectum and associate these feelings with urination and defecation. Parents teach the child to recognize the feelings and associate them with the need to sit on the toilet. The result is a learned behavior.

The *teaching-learning process* is the interaction between the teacher and the learner, which results in a change in behavior, attitude, or knowledge. The best instruction may not result in learning. Nurses can follow all the guidelines set forth in this chapter and may discover that the patient does not "learn" or comply for a variety of reasons. Ruzicki[35] states that "nurses can assess patient need and readiness, present information in an appropriate manner, provide resources and opportunities for practice, refer and communicate with other care providers. But nurses cannot force patients to learn. Ultimately it is the patient's responsibility for what is done with what was taught."

The teaching-learning process is not checking off information that was provided as the child and family leave the hospital or office. For learning to occur the nurse, the child, and the family must engage in a variety of teaching strategies and interactions. This chapter addresses the various learning theories and teaching strategies that can assist the child and family in learning about well-child development, health promotion, and management of acute and chronic illness.

Learning Theories

The method by which a child or adult learns and remembers information is of interest to nurses involved in patient teaching. Children at various ages are capable of participating in their own care at some level. Nurses, as teachers, have to identify what is possible for each child, what skills can be encouraged, what information can be recalled, and what should not be included. Learning theories provide a base from which a nurse can begin to explore what experts have written about how a person learns; thus, they learn the best way to teach. No one theory explains all aspects of the teaching-learning phenomenon; rather, each provides insight into different aspects of the process.

Three major contemporary models of learning are behavioristic, cognitive, and humanistic perspectives (Table 6-1). The focus of each is centered on how children and adults learn. More recent discussions are focusing on a new arrangement of learning theories into behavioral, cognitive, and interactionist perspectives.[4] Selected theories are discussed in this chapter for application to patient teaching situations.

Behavioral Models of Learning

The two behavioral models that are most often discussed in the educational literature are classical conditioning and operant conditioning.

Pavlov's Classical Conditioning

Every person who participates in an entry-level psychology course is introduced to the concept of Pavlov's classical conditioning. Pavlov is best known for teaching

TABLE 6-1
An Overview of Major Classifications of Learning Theories

Classification and Definition	Major Tenets
Behaviorist: Interprets human behavior as connections between stimuli and responses under the influence of reinforcement.	Respondent behavior results from a specific stimulus (S-R). Operant behavior is emitted as an instrumental act (R-R). Reinforcement increases the probability of operant behavior recurring. Most human behaviors are operant in nature. Punishment decreases the possibility of a response recurring. Continuous reinforcement leads to faster learning. Intermittent reinforcement leads to longer retention of that which is learned.
Cognitivist: Interprets human behavior in terms of cognitive processes such as insight, intelligence, and organizational abilities.	Concerned with the process of decision making, cognitive structure, understanding, perception, and information processing. The emphasis is on the process of learning rather than content.
Humanist: Interprets human behavior as self-centered and directly related to the process of self-actualization.	Learning is an individual internal process. People learn what they perceive to be helpful to maintaining their own structure. Self-actualization is the motivation for learning. Self-actualization and learning involve creative functioning. The organization of the self must not be threatened for new learning to occur.

(Adapted from: Baer, C. L. [1990]. Principles of patient education. In L. E. Lancaster [Ed.]. *Core curriculum for nephrology nurses.* Pitman, NJ: Anthony J. Janetti, with permission.)

dogs to salivate when hearing a tuning fork. This response is called *classical conditioning*. In classical conditioning theory the naturally occurring stimulus-reflex response is unconditioned. A conditioned stimulus (tuning fork) that does not usually evoke a specific behavior is introduced in association with a natural stimulus (food), and it evokes a specific response (salivation). After repeated episodes the behavioral response to a conditioned stimulus has been learned or is a conditioned response; that is, the sound of the turning fork leads to salivation. John B. Watson described the scientific study of behavior based on Pavlov's classical conditioning. Watson believed that human personality developed through the conditioning of various reflexes.[4]

Skinner's Operant Conditioning

B. F. Skinner's *operant conditioning* theory has been the basis of many health-related educational programs, also referred to as behavior modification programs. Skinner defined learning as a change in behavior. Skinner's work is based on the premise that the key to understanding behaviors lies in the understanding of the interrelationships between a stimulus, a response, and the consequences of the response.[4,36,37]

Three important considerations of operant conditioning are Thorndike's law of effect, law of exercise, and law of readiness.[4] The *law of effect* states that the satisfying response to a behavior strengthens the connections between the stimulus and the behavior, and an annoying response weakens the connection. Through trial and error, behaviors are kept or rejected according to the consequences, which can be pleasurable or annoying.[4] Building on the law of effect, Skinner[37] described reinforcement as anything that increases the probability of a behavior occurring more than once. Reinforcements may be positive or negative. Positive reinforcements are straightforward. A behavior is strengthened by the response, stimulus, or event, and the probability that the behavior will occur increases. Negative reinforcement is related to avoidance or escape from the consequences of the stimulus. For example, a child who moves to the door without permission from the teacher is not allowed to go outside with the other children. The probability of the behavioral response occurring (not moving without permission) is increased to avoid the stimulus (remaining in the classroom during recess). In positive and negative reinforcement the probability of the behavior being repeated is increased or strengthened. Punishment is the opposite of reinforcement and decreases the probability that the response will occur. Punishment may be the removal of positive reinforcers or the addition of negative reinforcers. Severe and inescapable punishment can eliminate behavior.

The *law of exercise* implies that the more a child practices a behavior, the greater the probability of a correct response.[37] The *law of readiness* describes the conditions that govern the satisfying or annoying responses that strengthen the connections between the stimulus and the behavioral responses.[36] When a child is not ready to learn a behavior, trying to teach that behavior will increase the chances that learning will be forced and more difficult.

For example, attempting to toilet train a toddler before the child has the ability to remain dry for 2 hours at a time, pull his or her pants up and down, or recognize the need to go to the bathroom will make the teaching more difficult and increase the likelihood of "failure."

In behavior modification programs one behavior is usually replaced by a more "acceptable" or "desired" behavior. For example, if a child has temper tantrums, the behavior modification program may focus on the parent's response to the child's behavior rather than on the child. In this situation children continue temper tantrums regardless of the way in which a parent responds (positive or negative), and the modification is to have parents ignore the child's behavior during the tantrum. Positive parent-child interactions are encouraged related to other behaviors that the parent would like to reinforce.

To effectively use behavioral theories, the nurse and client (child and parents) must be able to identify clearly the behavior that is to be learned. Once the behavior is identified, the nurse can break the behavior into parts or small steps that can be learned and reinforced. The learner can accomplish each component task and thus have success or positive accomplishments toward the goal. The learner should help in identifying the behavior to be learned and the reward systems that will be used to reinforce the behavioral changes.

The concept of behavioral change is easily measured, and the relationship between the stimuli and responses is observable by learner and teacher. Behavioral objectives that are measurable and observable can be developed and used in clinical teaching programs based on the behaviorist models of learning. Short-term and long-term goals can be identified as they relate to the behavioral changes desired.

Cognitive Theories

During the second world war complex skills regarding the operation of sophisticated equipment had to be taught. The behavioral learning principles of reinforcement and practice did not lead to successful instruction.[4] Researchers began to explore methods for designing instruction by topic sequencing and component tasks.[13] Thus, learning theories were shifted to focus on a change in perception or cognitive structure. Learning may or may not result in changes in observable behavior according to cognitive theorists. Learning is a process by which a person gains or changes insights, outlooks, expectations, or thought patterns.[6] Another major change at this time was the focus of educational research. The move from the laboratory and animals to classrooms and student-learners was significant. The results included a move from the "organism" studied by behaviorists to "people," from physical or biological environment to psychological environment, and from action-reaction to interaction.[4,6]

Kurt Lewin, Jean Piaget, and Robert Gagné were influential cognitive theorists. Not only was the question of how people learn being addressed, but the theories also shifted to the question of how instruction could facilitate learning. Each of these theorists are presented briefly.

Lewin

Kurt Lewin's Force Field Theory states that behavior (B) is a function of the person (P) and the psychological environment (E), hence the formula $B = f(P,E)$. Behavior in this theory is assumed to be the outcome of learning and is influenced by the interaction of the person with his or her immediate environment as the person perceives the situation.[4,6,41] The key concepts in Lewin's theory are found in the accompanying display. Behavior depends on the forces in the present field (environment) and includes knowledge gained from experiences and hopes for the future. Lewin described the two types of psychological forces: tendencies to move toward or away from some object or event (driving forces) and obstacles (restraining forces).

Lewin is also credited with identifying the three classical types of conflict situations: approach-approach, approach-avoidance, and avoidance-avoidance,[4] as shown in Figure 6-3. Another important concept identified by Lewin is the difference between cognitive structure and motivational learning. Cognitive structure is learning information, whereas motivational learning is something desirable, such as learning to relax or to like carrots.[4] The two types of learning are different according to Lewin, and therefore the process of learning will be different for cognitive structure and motivational learning.

In addition, Lewin's work on cognitive field theory was expanded to a force field analysis that may be used for behavioral change or planned change. The major categories described in force field analysis are unfreezing, changing, and refreezing. Planned change is used in nursing management strategies and can be applied to changing behaviors.

Piaget

Jean Piaget[28,29] described the developmental process of intellectual life from the activities of the infant to the reasoning processes of the adult. Piaget described the continuous interaction between the individual and the environment as the process of knowledge, that is, the processes of formation from a lesser to a higher degree of knowing. Piaget's conception of cognitive development is derived from his analysis of the biological development of certain organisms.[28,29] His research indicated that biological organisms are not passive; they interact with their environment to adapt to changes. Thus, intelligence is a process of adaptation to the environment.[4] Piaget believed that individuals progress from one level of mental development or knowledge to a higher level through a continual and ever-changing interaction with the environment.[29]

Piaget described three mechanisms of cognitive development and intellectual functioning:

- Fundamental processes involved in interactions with the environment (assimilation, accommodation, and equilibrium)
- Methods of constructing knowledge (physical and logicomathematical experience)
- Qualitative differences in thinking at different stages (sensorimotor, preoperation, concrete operation, and formal operation)[4]

The growth of logical reasoning is a lengthy process that begins at birth.[4] The longitudinal development of logical thinking according to Piaget is influenced by the fundamental processes of assimilation, accommodation, and equilibrium that assist the child in integrating information from the environment within existing cognitive structures and reorganizing structures as understanding increases. The fundamental processes combine in a variety of ways to produce knowledge that is learned from different types of interactions. Empirical abstraction is a process of learning through physical experiences with the environment. The infant hears or touches an object and the physical properties of the object are noted. In reflective abstraction or logicomathematical experience, the infant reflects on his or her actions and reorganizes them. The source of knowing is internal. The four broad stages of cognitive development (sensorimotor, preoperational, concrete operational, and formal operational) are defined in Chapter 8. At each stage of development from sensorimotor to formal operation the cognitive structures change and become more powerful. This is illustrated in Figure 6-4.

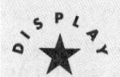

DISPLAY ★ Kurt Lewin's Force Field Theory: Key Concepts

Definition: Force field analysis is a technique used to promote behavioral change by use of a systematic, patient-centered, comprehensive analysis and plan.

Key Concepts

Life space: A personal description of physical, psychosocial, and social factors that relate in a meaningful way.
Force field: The above factors are associated with a force that drives or restrains behavior; the field is described by the person's perceptions of these forces.
   Driving forces: Initiate and maintain change
   Restraining forces: Decrease the effect of driving forces
Time perspective: The force field is dynamic. Behavior depends on forces in the present, which include past experiences and future hopes.

Formula

$$B = f(P,E) \quad B = \text{behavior (learning)}$$

$$P = \text{person} \quad E = \text{environment}$$

Thus, a person's behavior (learning) is determined by the interaction of the person with his or her perceived environment (immediate situation).

(Reference: Vanetzian, E. [1988]. Force field analysis: A person-centered approach to behavior change. Rehabilitation Nursing, 13[1], 23–25.)

I. Approach-approach conflict

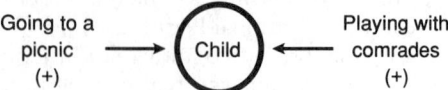

Going to a
picnic ⟶ Child ⟵ Playing with
(+)   comrades
                                 (+)

Child is between two positive valences.

II. Approach-avoidance conflict

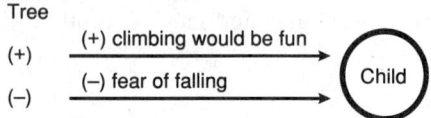

Tree
(+)   (+) climbing would be fun
       (−) fear of falling   Child

(−)

An object or event exerts both positive and
negative forces.

III. Avoidance-avoidance conflict

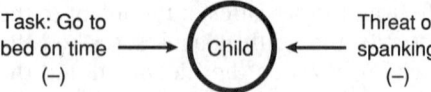

Task: Go to
bed on time ⟶ Child ⟵ Threat of
(−)   spanking
                                 (−)

Child is between two negative valences,
typically, a task he or she does not want
to perform and threat of punishment.

FIGURE 6-3
Examples of Lewin's three types of conflict
situations. (With permission from Bell-Gredler,
M. E. [1986]. Learning and instruction, theory
into practice. New York: Macmillan.)

Piaget's theory has significant implications for teaching and learning interactions with children. Symbolic play and imitation are two ways in which children learn.[28] In symbolic play the young child is developing representational thought and is attempting to place reality into these thoughts. This is learning through assimilation.[4] In imitation the accommodation of behavior to external models is learned. Nurses working with young children can begin to explore ways of teaching that make use of symbolic play and imitation, as well as anticipating the stage of cognitive development at which the child may be functioning. More information on applying Piaget's theory is provided in the next section.

Gagné

Robert Gagné's[13] work on learning theory developed when he was instructing adults on the use of complex military training procedures. The models of learning that focused on reinforcement, distribution of practice, and response familiarity were inadequate for effective learning. Gagné[15] found that effective learning occurred when instruction included a set of component tasks leading to a final task, when each component was mastered, and when sequencing the component tasks allowed for optimal transfer of skills to the final task. Based on this work Gagné developed a theory of instruction, rather than a learning theory, which is a distinction that has significant implications for planning organized programs of instruction. Once discussed as the cumulative learning model, Gagné's work is now referred to as conditions for learning.[4,16,17]

Whereas Piaget's model describes learning as contributing to cognitive development and logical thought, Gagné stated that cumulative learning is primarily responsible for development.[14] Cumulative learning is based on the premise that sequentially ordered skills

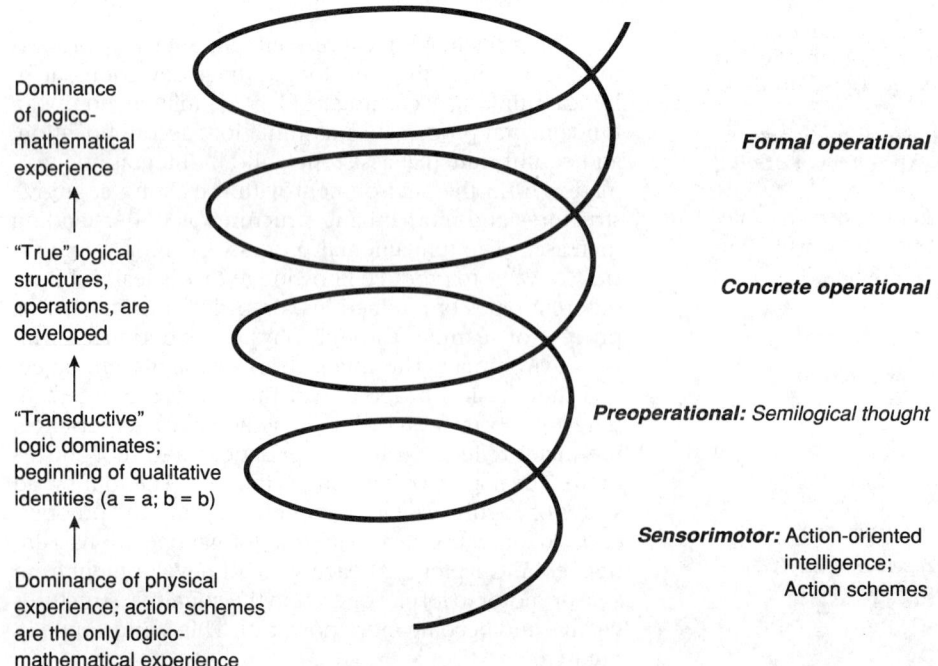

Dominance
of logico-
mathematical
experience

↑

"True" logical
structures,
operations, are
developed

↑

"Transductive"
logic dominates;
beginning of qualitative
identities (a = a; b = b)

↑

Dominance of physical
experience; action schemes
are the only logico-
mathematical experience

Formal operational

Concrete operational

Preoperational: Semilogical thought

Sensorimotor: Action-oriented
intelligence;
Action schemes

FIGURE 6-4
Piaget's cycle of cognitive development.
(With permission from Bell-Gredler,
M. E. [1986]. Learning and instruction,
theory into practice. New York:
Macmillan.)

contribute to the learning of more complex skills. Gagné believes that learning is not a single process and that no one set of characteristics can account for such varied activities, such as learning to define a word or write a paper or lace a shoe.[4,14]

Gagné's theory has been refined and several important concepts are discussed, including components of learning, categories of learning, phases of learning, and the hierarchies of learning.[13,14,16] The components of learning include the internal and external conditions of learning. The internal conditions of learning refer to prerequisite skills and cognitive processing of the individual. These are internal states of the individual. The external or environmental stimuli are the external conditions of learning and include the events of instruction. When the external conditions and internal conditions of learning interact, the outcome is learning (Fig. 6-5).

The five categories of learning include verbal information, intellectual skills, motor skills, attitudes, and cognitive strategies. Each type of learning requires different capabilities and is learned in different ways. This becomes important when outcome objectives and strategies for teaching are developed. For example, if a nurse is teaching a young adolescent to give an insulin injection, one outcome of learning is a *skill*. The nurse would plan the instruction to include the learning of the skills involved (i.e., component tasks), such as calculating the dosage to be given, withdrawing insulin from the bottle, removing air from the syringe, cleansing the skin, injecting the needle, aspirating for blood, and injecting the medication. If the learning was a *change in attitude*, then the instruction would be focused on the steps necessary for a change in attitude, including information about possible actions and their consequences.[4] Learning about diabetes and the role of insulin would result in *verbal information* learning.

Gagné[16] identified nine phases of learning that must occur in sequential order for cognitive processing of concepts to occur. The nine phases in order are attending,

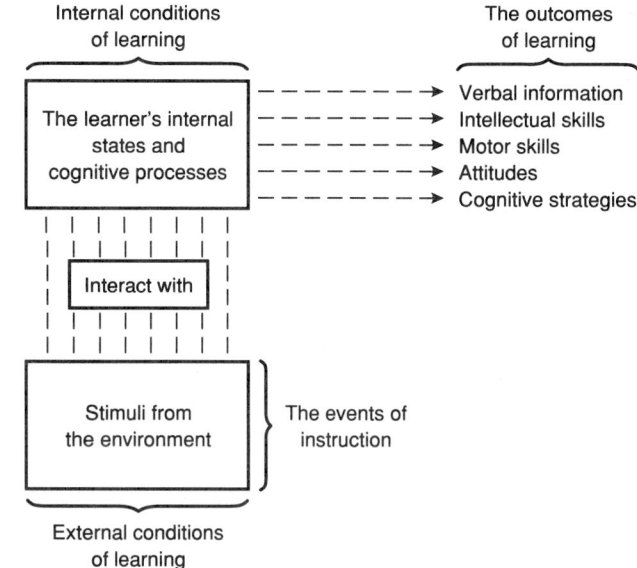

FIGURE 6-5
Gagné's essential components of learning and instruction. (With permission from Bell-Gredler, M. E. [1986]. Learning and instruction, theory into practice. New York: Macmillan.)

expectancy, retrieval, selective perception of stimulus features, semantic encoding, retrieval and responding, reinforcement, cueing retrieval, and generalizability. Bell-Gredler[4] divided the nine phases into three categories of activities: preparation for learning, acquisition and performance, and transfer of learning. Table 6-2 provides the breakdown of the phases into the three categories with a description of the functions that occur during the learning process.

Gagné[13] has described a hierarchy of learning that moves from simple to complex. Each capability is essential to learning the next higher level skill. According to Gagné, the higher skill cannot be learned unless the lower

TABLE 6-2
Summary of the Gagné Nine Phases of Learning

Description	Phases	Function
Preparation for learning	Attending	Alerts the learner to the stimulus
	Expectancy	Orients the learner to the learning goal
	Retrieval (of relevant information or skills) to working memory	Provides recall of prerequisite capabilities
Acquisition and performance	Selective perception of stimulus features	Permits temporary storage of important stimulus features in working memory
	Semantic encoding	Transfers stimulus features and related information to long-term memory
	Retrieval and responding	Returns stored information to the individual's response generator and activates response
	Reinforcement	Confirms learner's expectancy about learning goal
Transfer of learning	Cueing retrieval	Provides additional cues for later recall of the capability
	Generalizability	Enhances transfer of learning to new situations

(From: Bell-Gredler, M. E. [1986]. *Learning and instruction: Theory into practice.* N.Y.: Macmillan.)

TABLE 6-3
Gagné's Hierarchy of Learning

Type of Skill	Description
Discrimination learning	Child responds differentially to characteristics that distinguish objects, such as shape, size, color.
Concept learning	
Concrete concepts	Child identifies object or event as a member of a concept class learned through direct encounters with concrete example, such as triangles.
Defined concepts	Concept cannot be learned through concrete examples; acquired by learning a classifying rule, such as "liberty" or "patriotism."
Rule learning	Child can respond to a class of situations with a class of performances that represents a relationship; for example, a student responds to 5 + 2, 6 + 1, and 9 + 4 by adding each set of integers.
High-order rule learning (problem solving)	Student combines subordinate rules to solve a problem; most effective learning strategy is guided discovery.

(From Bell-Gredler, M. E. [1986]. *Learning and instruction: theory into practice.* N.Y.: Macmillan.)

level is mastered first. The intellectual skills identified are discrimination learning, concept learning, rule learning, and higher-order learning (Table 6-3). At the discrimination level the child begins to distinguish between objects based on shape, size, or color. As children continue to learn about objects they become capable of making different responses to stimuli that are somewhat alike but different. In concept learning the child begins to define objects by applying simple rules. Ultimately, the rules are put together in some fashion (rule learning), and as the child applies a group of rules to solve problems higher-order rule learning has occurred.

Another important point of Gagné's theory is how a person learns to perform procedures. Procedures require motor and intellectual skills.[4] Procedure learning also involves learning step-by-step actions leading to the completed sequence and making decisions about alternative steps at different stages in the procedure. This notion has important implications for teaching children and family health care procedures.

In summary, cognitive learning theorists interpret human behavior in terms of cognitive processes, such as insight, intelligence, and organizational abilities; regard learning as an active process of interaction between the learner and the environment; and view learning as a unique, personal phenomenon. Both Piaget's and Gagné's work may be considered interactionist perspectives rather than purely cognitive theories.[4]

Humanistic Learning Theories

Humanistic learning theorists tend to interpret human behavior as centered on the self with the goal of self-actualization. Learning becomes the process of developing one's full cognitive, affective, and psychomotor potential. The person is viewed as an integrated whole that interacts with the environment. Learning is more subjective than objective, and the affective learning domain is emphasized in humanistic learning. The teacher uses a humanistic approach, including opportunities for active learner participation, self-directed learning experiences, and learning contracts.

Maslow and Rogers are theorists who are considered humanistic in their focus. Maslow's work is presented in Chapter 8 and is not repeated in this chapter. Carl Rogers felt that the purpose of learning was to develop a fully functioning person.[34] Rogers believed that the aim of education was to facilitate learning. He identified three components of positive interpersonal relationships applicable to all human interactions, including teacher-learner interactions. A teacher or facilitator of learning should possess certain attitudinal qualities, including a realness or genuineness; caring, trust, and respect for the learner; and empathic understanding and sensitive listening[34] (Fig. 6-6). These concepts are taught to nursing students as therapeutic communication skills. A trusting relationship between the child, the family, and the nurse educator is also needed. These same qualities are needed when the nurse educator teaches staff or other students.

Additional Theories Applicable to Patient Education

The reader is referred to Chapter 8 for a discussion on information processing theory that addresses how a person's memory, both long and short term, affects learning. The basic assumption of information processing is that human memory is complex and that memory is an active organizer of information.[4] Albert Bandura's social learning theory is also discussed in Chapter 8. Bandura's theory is based on the assumption of a three-way interaction between the person, the environment, and the behavior.

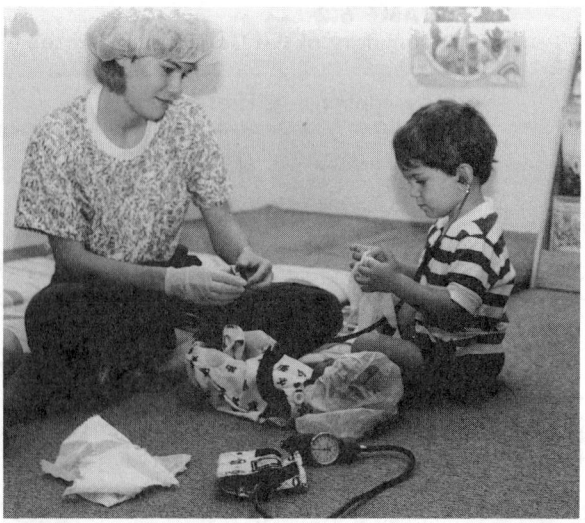

FIGURE 6-6
The teacher's attitudinal qualities are important for developing humanistic teaching environments.

The *health belief model*[30,33] provides another perspective from which to assess and plan educational intervention for children and families (Fig. 6-7). The premise of this model is that certain elements must be in place for people to take health actions. First, people must believe that they can be affected (susceptibility) by a disease or illness; second, the illness would have serious side effects on their lives; third, certain actions can prevent the illness; and fourth, the threat of taking action is not as great as the threat of the illness. While limitations of the model are recognized, research has shown that the model can be used to explain compliance of certain medical regimens.[20] However, the model does make nurse educators think about what influences a person's beliefs about health and their responses to illness and compliance with therapy. Cultural difference as well as socioeconomic factors should be taken into account when planning patient education.

Application of Learning Theories to Child and Family Teaching

Applying learning theories to child and family teaching programs is inherent in the planning process. How the nurse interprets the teaching role in preparing children and families for well-baby visits and immunizations, living with chronic illness, managing acute crises, or preparing for death is based on a personal belief about the importance of the nurse's teaching role and a personal belief about families' and children's abilities to learn.[1] Nurses often teach without considering the process of learning and then wonder why the child and family do not comply with teaching or why they are unable to remember what they have "learned."

Theory is not routinely noted in research studies conducted on the effectiveness of patient education by nurses. Oberst[27] reported that when nurse researchers used theoretical frameworks to guide patient education, the results had more impact on practice and subsequent research. The complex teaching and learning situations that exist in health care should be acknowledged when planning patient education. Children and families must learn about potential life-threatening conditions and their treatments during intense emotional times in unfamiliar settings. Even when nurses discuss normal growth and developmental needs of children, the setting may not be conducive to learning. Multiple theoretical perspectives from nursing, psychology, education, and other fields may provide direction. An eclectic approach to learning and instruction may be more beneficial than a single theoretical approach.[27]

Domains of Learning

Educators routinely discuss domains of learning. The three domains are cognitive (knowledge), psychomotor (skill, behavior), and affective (attitude). The domains are used to provide a guideline for categorizing the outcomes of learning. The approach to teaching will differ depending on the domain. Gagné described five outcomes or categories of learning, including intellectual skills, verbal information, motor skills, attitudes, and cognitive strategies.[15] In planning an instructional sequence, for example, Gagné approached both knowledge and procedural learning as different types. The sequencing of tasks to learn procedures includes knowledge and skills required to accomplish the final task.[4] Another important concept of Gagné's work is that to successfully learn the content or skill, it must be broken into component tasks. Each component task must be learned in sequence, which will lead to successful learning of the final task. For example, if a nurse is teaching a child about leukemia, he or she first explores the parts to be learned, such as the components of blood, the roles of each blood component, the definition of leukemia, the relationship between leukemia and the blood components, the signs and symptoms of leukemia, how these signs and symptoms relate to the components of blood, and so forth. Each phase of instruction would build on the previous learned content until the child and family could explain leukemia to themselves and to others.

Skinner's operant conditioning could be applied to planning for a substitute behavior or new response for a behavior, such as nail biting or temper tantrums. Lewin's field theory also may be applied to behavioral or attitudinal domain outcomes.

Piaget's theoretical framework addresses the way in which children of various ages see the world. This perspective helps teachers to choose their words and examples carefully. Piaget helps teachers to understand the differences between concrete operations and formal operations of cognitive development. During the development of a slide tape program this author was working with a 3-year-old. The child had been promised that nothing would hurt and that only pictures would be taken. When she overheard a discussion with the photographer about the next "shot" she became very upset. Once assured that shot did not refer to injection or needle she was fine. A 6-year-old boy was told in a doctor's office that a benign tumor was going to be "cut" off the side of his neck. He asked his Dad how they were going to put his head on after it was cut off to remove the tumor in his neck. His concern was real and scary for him, and it

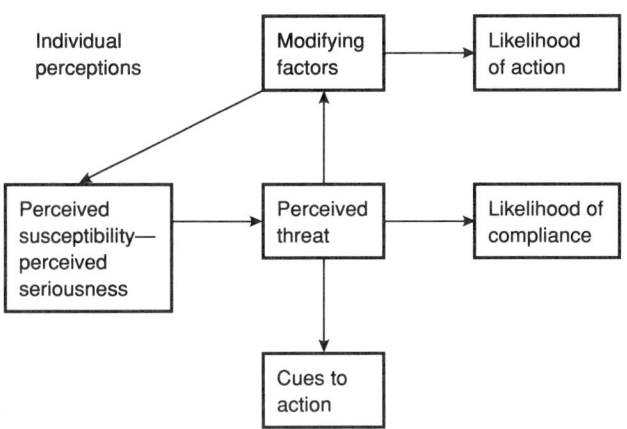

FIGURE 6-7

Health belief model. (Modified from Becker, M. H., Haefner, D. P., Kasl, C. V., et al. [1977]. Selected psychosocial model and correlates of individual health-related behaviors. *Medical Care, 15,* 27–46, with permission.)

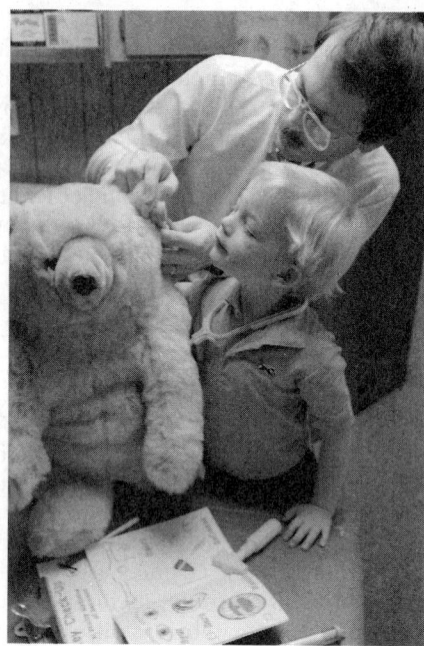

FIGURE 6-8
Teaching should be individualized for the developmental age of the child. Demonstrating on a friendly stuffed animal and using age-appropriate coloring books makes learning fun for this preschooler. (Courtesy of Overlake Hospital Medical Center, Bellevue, WA.)

could have gone unnoticed. The English language is full of words with double meanings that can be confusing for young children who are just learning the language. Parents and caregivers who have English as a second language may find similar problems in understanding commonly used phases that do not translate easily into their native language.

The humanistic theories reinforce the importance of remembering the individual who is being taught (Fig. 6-8). It is essential that in health education nurses listen to the family and child and that they plan goals that reflect the family's and child's needs and plans, not the nurse's. Forming a therapeutic relationship before beginning to develop teaching goals and objectives is essential. Empathy, careful listening, and genuine concern for children and families will help the nurse develop a comprehensive individualized teaching plan. When planning a behavioral change the parent and child, not the nurse or doctor, should identify the behavior to be changed and the appropriate rewards or reinforcement strategies.

Instructional Designs: Models for Developing Patient Teaching

An instructional design is a systematic approach to planning and implementing an educational class or program.[10] A number of different instructional models are available.[1,4,23] Instructional design is a systems approach to educational interventions. In health care settings the instructional design is generally referred to as a teaching plan. Sample teaching plans appear in major chapters of

this book to illustrate important concepts for teaching. Teaching plans ensure that a systematic approach to patient education occurs. A teaching plan allows the primary nurse to outline what is to be taught, when, and in what manner. If the primary nurse is unable to complete the teaching, a teaching plan can be used by other members of the staff to complete the educational program for the child and family. The components of a teaching plan include assessment, planning, implementation, and evaluation. Each of these phases is discussed below.

Assessment

During the assessment phase the nurse educator begins to systematically assess the child and family. Included in the assessment are the following areas: growth and development, environment, physical factors, diagnosis, sociocultural and financial status, emotional and coping skills, personality and learning styles, previous health-related experiences, and beliefs and values regarding health and health care.

The nurse gathers data with the family during this phase. This is the time for discovering what the family and the child need to know. It is easy for health care providers to feel that they know what people need to learn to take care of themselves or their children. The limitation to this perspective is that the child and parent may have questions that the nurse may not address because it is nonessential to the goals identified by the nurse. Occasionally, the family is unable to hear the content because of the fears or anxieties they have about unasked questions or misconceptions. The most effective way to begin is to ask the child and family what questions they have and what they feel they need to know first; then this information can be used to plan their learning goals and objectives.

When working with children and families the nurse often has two clients to teach: the child and the parent-caregiver. This responsibility may require two different teaching plans that have been modified to meet the needs of each. The assessments will reflect that both child and caregiver are being taught. Even young children need to be included in the teaching that is being planned and implemented. A part of the nurse's initial assessment will determine the level and degree to which the child can be involved. Even a 2-year-old needs to be taught in 2-year-old language about the changes he or she will experience. Too often older children are not involved in their care because it is easier and quicker (and sometimes cheaper) for the parents to do the care.

Growth and Development

Assessment of growth and development of a child implies that the nurse is knowledgeable about the normal growth and development of children at various ages. Certain standardized assessment tools can be used, such as the Denver II. Or the nurse may simply observe the child's behaviors in play settings. The nurse can initiate play by providing age-appropriate toys and a setting in which play can occur. If the nurse is teaching specific tasks, a special assessment may be required of the needed skills. Using

Gagné's theory as a framework, nurses should identify what is to be taught and learned first and then break the final task into component parts. The assessment regarding the component parts can then be accomplished.

Home Environment

The home environment should be assessed during this stage of instructional design. Not all parents and children are from middle-class neighborhoods. Not all families consist of a father, mother, and two children. The young, poor, teenage mother may have more limitations when trying to learn to care for her child than an older mother. Family support systems influence the teaching-learning interaction. An assessment of the home will provide the nurse with information about what is available to help the family and what limitations may be present. (Chapter 3 provides an in-depth discussion on family assessment and nontraditional families.) The nurse should determine what facilities are available for the family (i.e., running water, hot water, heat, available space, adaptability). For example, if parents are to give their young child an injection each day, where should the supplies be kept? How many children are in the family? Could other children be hurt if they found the needles? The family can help solve problems and decide on the best location.

Values and Beliefs

Children's and families' attitudes about health and health care also will influence the teaching-learning interaction. For example, the child with a chronic illness may have been in and out of hospitals and clinics. Does the mother feel that no one asks her what she is doing and how it works? Nurses may have limited contact with families and may try to "make the best of the time" without doing a thorough assessment. Listening effectively may eliminate a potential problem. For example, the nurse can ask parents what they are doing at home. "How have you managed Johnny's insulin's injections at home? What is your routine? Can you describe Johnny's diet? How do you feel things are going?" The more open ended the questions, the more information the nurse will obtain.

Readiness to Learn

Readiness to learn implies that a person feels a need to know about something.[33] Physical readiness as well as an intellectual and emotional readiness are part of this desire to learn. In an acute care environment the child and family have a variety of intense stressors that may impede the learning process. Until the family feels a need to know how to manage the care, the teaching may not be successful. If they have indicated a desire for learning, family members may be taught during the early days of hospitalization, and the child may be taught several days later. One of fallacies of the previous statement, however, is the word "days." As hospitalization time is shortened, the time for assessing, planning, and implementing teaching programs is drastically shortened. In outpatient clinics families may be available for teaching sessions on an infrequent basis. Nurses may feel a need to push families toward learning about the care; that is, nurses may want to motivate the family. Mild anxiety may motivate families to learn about their child's illness and care. Severe anxiety, however, may become incapacitating.

Assessment Strategies. Common clues that the nurse can use to assess the overall readiness to learn include whether the child and family are asking questions; whether the family is observing what the nurse is doing (attentive); and whether the family is helping or volunteering to assist the nurse.

A knowledge or skill assessment survey can be developed to evaluate a child or family before continuing to formulate the teaching plan.[26] If the nurse regularly works with a specific illness, it would be helpful to identify a potential resource from the literature or to develop an assessment form for the unit. Table 6-4 provides an example of items in a survey used for assessing adolescents with cancer.

Play therapy and drawing can be used to assess what younger children know about their illness and treatment. An interview of the family also can provide some valuable

---

TABLE 6-4
Nursing Assessment: Knowledge Assessment of Adolescents With Cancer: A Survey Form

1. What causes cancer
2. How long will I be ill
3. How might my illness affect my health later
4. How serious is my illness
5. How can I talk to my friends and relatives about my illness
6. What can I expect if cancer spreads
7. What can I do to aid my future health
8. How will cancer affect my career, social life, and marriage
9. What is the doctor looking for when he or she examines me
10. How can cancer be prevented
11. Why are certain tests done
12. How can I help most with my treatment plan
13. How can the experience of other teenage cancer patients help me solve my problem
14. What are the statistics about the reappearance of cancer
15. What symptoms should I call the doctor about
16. What are the results of the doctor's examinations and tests
17. How will what I eat affect my illness
18. How do my treatments help me
19. What can I expect from each type of treatment
20. What should I do if I forget to take my medicine
21. What are the effects of medicines not prescribed by my doctor on my illness (such as aspirin or cold medicine)
22. What are the effects of cancer and its treatment on my appearance now
23. What are the effects of cancer and its treatment on my appearance in the future
24. How will cancer affect my role in my family in the future (such as my ability to become more independent)
25. What are the effects of alcohol, smoking, or drugs on my illness
26. Will I require physical therapy, use of artificial limbs, and so forth
27. What are the kinds of physical activity I can do
28. How will my illness affect other family members
29. Are there any new facts about cancer research
30. How can I help pay medical bills

(From Levenson, P. M., Pfefferbaum, B., & Overall, J. E. [1983]. A factor analysis of the informational concerns of adolescent cancer patients. *Child Health Care, 11*, 148–153.)

information about their beliefs and expectations and goals. Experiences can provide invaluable data about the family, including what they know, what misconceptions they may have, and what they have previously experienced in the health care system. The more time a nurse spends in the assessment phase, the more likely the teaching plan will reflect the individualized needs of the child and family. Much of the information is gathered when the history and physical are performed at the time of admission. The primary nurse or physician may be another valuable source of assessment data if the patient educator is not the primary nurse.

Motivation

Motivation may be internally or externally perceived. The concepts of positive and negative reinforcement and reward and punishment are basic to the concept of motivation. Self-directed or internal motivation is longer lasting.[33] External motivation requires continuous reinforcement or rewards. Skinner[37] states that certain behaviors, such as interest, enthusiasm, appreciation, and dedication, illustrate motivation. According to Skinner motivation is a result of reinforcements, and eventually the activity is the source of its own reinforcement.[4,37] This phenomenon is easy to identify in classroom situations in which students become excited about learning about a topic and continue to study the areas because of their own interest and enthusiasm. An example of this in health care may be the person who begins exercising to lose weight and subsequently becomes excited about the activity.

Another motivating factor is that people like to learn things that are meaningful to them. If the knowledge or skill is related to their child, the motivation to learn is strong. However, the information needs to be organized in a way that makes sense to them and can be directly related to the care of their child.

Learning Styles

Another important area for assessment is the learning style of the child and family. Research has shown that people learn in different ways.[18,24] The ways in which people perceive and interact with their environment influence how they learn and remember. Kolb[24] describes four ways people learn: active experimentation, reflective observation, concrete experience, and abstract conceptualization. Basically, people learn by doing, watching and listening, feeling, or thinking. The implications for patient education are to identify how people learn and to plan strategies that enhance their learning. Most people use a combination of learning styles. Although formal learning style inventories are available, most are used for research. Children and parents can usually describe how they learn best. For example, if asked, parents may explain that they learn best when they can first observe a procedure (watching and listening) and then try do the task (doing). Other parents may prefer to read about the procedure (thinking) and then observe the process before attempting it. Still other parents may ask to do the procedure with help (active experimentation). Garity[18] rec-

ommends that when patient compliance is essential, patient education programs should be developed from a learning style base. Table 6-5 provides examples of how teaching plans can incorporate learning styles into the methods used for teaching.

Nursing Diagnosis

The use of nursing diagnoses is discussed in Chapter 2. A commonly used nursing diagnosis is "Knowledge Deficit." Dennison and Keeling[9] investigated the appropriateness of Knowledge Deficit as a nursing diagnosis. Content analysis of nursing notes using the label Knowledge Deficit revealed that nurses focused their attention on promoting knowledge as an "entity in itself rather than addressing a specific behavior related to the patient's lack of information." Dennison and Keeling[9] report that nursing diagnoses should reflect observed behaviors related to the defining characteristics of the diagnosis. One intervention is teaching. Jenny[21] also states that Knowledge Deficit does not meet the criteria for legitimacy as a nursing diagnosis. The notion is that information sharing is not the sole role of the nurse. Benner[5] recommends that the function of teaching by the nurse is more "teaching-coaching," which goes beyond the process of information sharing alone. The authors are not recommending that nurses should not teach but that the focus should be on the total plan of patient care with teaching as an intervention related to the underlying problem. For example, a child or family may be anxious about a procedure. The diagnosis may be Anxiety related to the bone marrow aspiration. A form of intervention is teaching the child and family about the procedure.

Planning

After completing the assessment, the planning phase is initiated. During this stage the short- and long-term goals and objectives of the teaching program are developed. The goals should reflect the assessment of the child and family. If the nurse has a goal, it should be added after discussion with and acceptance by the family. The goals and objectives should be clear and attainable. If component parts of the task that lead to the final goal have been outlined, the child and family can achieve success as they master each component task.

TABLE 6-5
Applying Learning Styles to Patient Teaching Strategies

Learning Style	Format	Examples
Thinking	Printed materials	Flyers, booklets, books, handouts
Seeing	Pictorials, visuals	Films, videotapes, slides, pictures
Listening	Auditory stimuli	Lectures, discussions
Doing	Manipulation, tactile stimuli	Models, games, practice sessions

Most hospitals and clinics have learning objectives for clients developed by illness or by diagnosis. Some outpatient settings have learning objectives related to well-child visits. These objectives can be modified after assessing the child and family. Some objectives may be deleted and others added. The nursing care plan and nursing notes can document what changes are made and the rationale based on the assessment.

Behavioral Objectives

Behavioral objectives or performance objectives provide a guide in the development of the content and teaching strategies for patient education plans and evaluation strategies. The objectives are only tools of the planning phase of the instructional design system.

The development of behavioral objectives will vary according to the recommended design of an institution. Gronlund[19] presented a model for developing objectives for teaching that provide for two levels. The first level is an instructional objective, and it guides the teacher in identifying the overall outcome of the teaching-learning interaction. Each instructional objective has specific learning outcomes. These learning outcomes are what nurses commonly refer to as behavioral objectives. In a similar format outcome standards are developed for a classification of disorders or an area of nursing practice. The outcome standards are further broken down into criteria. The criteria for evaluation are the behavioral objectives. The accompanying display on nursing diagnosis provides a sample of outcome standards with criteria for evaluation. The difference between the instructional level (or standard) and specific learning outcomes (or criteria) are the verbs. Behavioral objectives, whether called specific learning outcomes or criteria for evaluation, are always represented by an action-oriented measurable verb. The key to the behavioral objective is being able to observe in some format that a child or parent has performed the stated objective (see the accompanying display on verbs used for developing behavioral objectives).

The unmeasurable verbs, such as know, understand, appreciate, value, and believe, are difficult to measure. Gronlund[19] uses these verbs in his instructional objectives to guide the teacher. For example, the nurse educator wants the child and family to understand the implication of being diagnosed with acute lymphocytic leukemia. This is the goal of the nurse in planning the teaching. However, the nurse must then identify the behavioral objectives or specific learning outcomes that can be used to guide the instruction and evaluation of the outcome of learning. Examples of behavioral objectives include to following:

- Identifies the normal components of blood
- Describes the functions of red blood cells, white blood cells, and platelets
- Lists the symptoms of leukemia
- Describes the relationship between the functions of the blood and the symptoms

Each of these behavioral objectives can be evaluated after the teaching session.

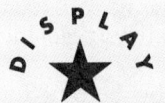

Nursing Diagnosis: Altered Self-Concept Related to Pressure Sores

Outcome Standard

Patient demonstrates positive self-concept as evidenced by

- Active participation and compliance with treatment plans if possible
- Resumption of role-related responsibilities and relationships if possible

Process Standards: Assessment

Nursing assessment includes

- Value attached to the altered body
- Coping styles and strategies (e.g., sharing concerns, informtion gathering, denial, exercise, relaxation, ability to problem solve)
- Lifestyle and social activities
- Personal support systems
- Evidence of negative self-concept (e.g., poor self-care, negative attitude and remarks, social isolation).

Process Standards: Intervention

- Encourage patient to articulate thoughts and feelings regarding pressure sores and the altered body.
- Provide realistic, honest feedback.
- Reinforce or teach appropriate coping strategies to the patient and family.
- Provide support, counseling, and appropriate information to the patient and family.
- Provide information regarding pressure sore prevention and treatment.
- Help patient establish achievable goals and identify progress.
- Refer for professional counseling (e.g., psychiatric nurse, psychologist, psychiatric social worker) when indicated.
- Documentation reflects the nursing process. Evaluation and revision is a continuous process reflecting the patient's response to the plan of care and changing needs.

(With permission, IAET Standards of Care: Dermal Wounds. [1987]. Costa Mesa, CA: International Association for Enterostomal Therapy.)

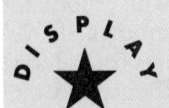

Verbs Used for Developing Behavioral Objectives

Cognitive Domain	Psychomotor Domain	Affective Domain
Describes	Displays	Asks
Defines	Demonstrates	Chooses
Explains	Reacts	Selects
Distinguishes	Assembles	Discusses
Predicts	Organizes	Describes
Differentiates	Mixes	Initiates
Compares and contrasts	Selects	Adheres
Summarizes	Constructs	Defends
Identifies	Prepares	Displays

Content and Teaching Strategies

Once the behavioral objectives are identified, content and teaching strategies can be identified for each objective.

Content. The content of the teaching plan should reflect the objectives identified. The nurse should provide the information needed for a child and parent to master the objective. If the plan is developed in a columnar format, content is shown across from the objective. The sample teaching plan uses a columnar format. For example, the content that addresses the normal blood components would include a discussion of red and white blood cells, platelets, and plasma and perhaps a discussion on how each is formed. Teaching strategies might include diagrams and booklets that show different blood cells.

Strategies. The research on teaching and learning in various situations addresses the importance of using a variety of teaching strategies. People remember 10% of what they read, 20% of what they hear, 30% of what they see, 50% of what they see and hear, and 80% of what they see, hear, and do.[40] This supports the previous discussion on planning patient education to complement the person's learning style. Table 6-5 provides examples of various teaching strategies that can be combined for teaching children and families.

Play can be an important tool for teaching young children. Puppets, dolls, and hospital equipment can be used in the instructions. This activity allows the nurse to define the terms for the child. The nurse may first show a child the x-ray machine and describe the procedure. A toy x-ray machine and doll can then be used by the child and nurse to discuss the procedure again. Children enjoy telling their parents and siblings about the procedure using dolls. (This allows the nurse to evaluate the child's learning.) Anatomical models also can be effective tools for teaching younger children. Children enjoy taking the models apart and putting them back together. Coloring books can be used effectively to teach children about certain procedures and diseases. Some of these products are available commercially, and others may be fashioned from available materials.

Group teaching can be effective for adolescents, who often benefit from discussing their concerns with peers (Fig. 6-9). They often discover that their fears and anxieties are not unique. Teenagers may be more willing to try a technique that another adolescent has found useful, rather than trying suggestions from adults. Group teaching also can be helpful for families experiencing similar problems. Another effective strategy is role playing. The secret to role playing is providing the participants with enough information to play the role. The nurse may want to play the "patient" role with a patient being the nurse. Alternatively, two nurses may demonstrate the process and then have groups of patients play various roles. Group teaching should be followed by individualized teaching sessions.

Print media (booklets, flyers) can be helpful for teaching adults. The nurse should always read the material before giving it to the family. The nurse marks through sections that do not apply or places a note beside the information explaining why it does not apply. When the parent and child are given printed material, the nurse

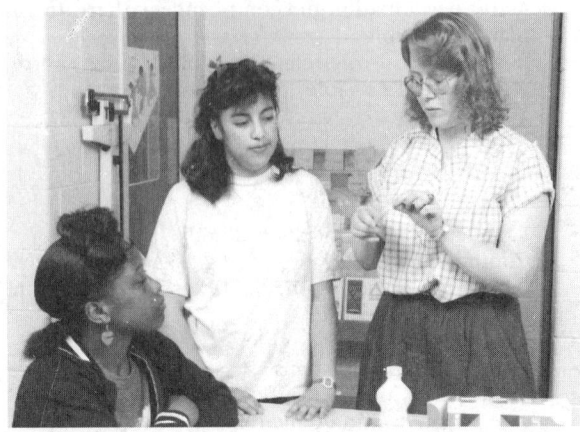

FIGURE 6-9
Adolescents respect each other's attitudes. Teaching adolescents in small peer groups can help to get a message across. (Courtesy of School of Nursing, University of Washington, Seattle, WA.)

should take time to review the material with them before and after the family reads it.

The readability of print material should be considered, and the reading level should be noted. Redman[33] reported that more than 23 million Americans are considered functionally illiterate. She stated that 20% of the population reads at a fifth-grade level or lower. The level of readability of material can be computed by several formulas. This chapter does not prepare nurses to conduct readability levels; however, it is important that nurses review material and ask whether or not children and parents can comprehend the content of booklets that hospitals routinely make available. The accompanying display provides a sample of material rewritten at the fourth-grade level.

The teaching of specific skills requires time for demonstrations and practice. Gagné's theory is an excellent base for developing teaching strategies for learning health care skills. The first step should be to outline the component tasks that a person needs to be able to accomplish to learn the skill. After the nurse assesses the skills that the child and family can perform, he or she can structure a teaching-learning opportunity for putting the component skills together to accomplish the task. Often nurses believe that they have taught parents how to do certain procedures because they showed them the procedure in a step-by-step fashion. The child and family must have several opportunities to practice and ask questions. When the parent is performing a new procedure, the nurse often will "help" them. Unless the parent is told how the nurse "helped," they may not learn the complete procedure and may have difficulty when the nurse is not present.

When children and families are being taught how to do procedures in a step-by-step pattern, the nurse should provide a written description of the steps for the family.

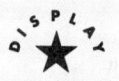

Example of Rewritten Material for Teaching

Portion of Caution Statement for Aspirin-Type Drugs

Original material, written at 11th- or 12th-grade level: If pain persists for more than 10 days or if redness is present, or in arthritic or rheumatic conditions affecting children younger than 12 years of age, consult a physician immediately.

Material rewritten at fourth-grade level: If pain lasts for more than 10 days or if skin is red, talk to a doctor right away. If children younger than 12 years of age have signs of arthritis or rheumatism, talk to a doctor right away.

Note: Sentence length was reduced and these difficult words removed: persists, redness, arthritic, rheumatic, conditions, affecting, consult, physician, immediately.

(From Pyrczak, R., & Roth, D. H. [1976]. The readability of directions on non-prescription drugs. Journal of the American Pharmaceutical Association, 16, 242–267.)

Any nurse assisting in the teaching should follow the same steps in the same order. Steps should not be combined during this time, nor should the nurse reverse steps even if the change does not make a difference. Gagné's theory of learning procedures by first learning the component steps supports the importance of following the same pattern until the final task is successfully learned and retention is verified.

Evaluation

The final section of the teaching plan is the evaluation. The behavioral objectives can be used for designing the evaluation steps. Behavioral objectives that are in the cognitive domain may be evaluated by question and answer sessions, multiple choice tests, or observation of families explaining the illness and treatment to other family members. Psychomotor skills should be evaluated by observing the caregiver performing the skill without assistance. Questions during or following the procedure can be used to ensure that the caregiver understands the rationale for the various steps in a procedure. Attitudinal objectives are the most difficult to evaluate and may require a long-term plan for observing a change in the way a child or family feels about the condition, treatment, or required activities. The verbs used in the behavioral objective should direct the nurse in designing the evaluation of the teaching plan (see the accompanying Teaching Plan).

Implementation

The implementation of the teaching plan occurs only after the plan, including the plan for evaluation, is completed. The importance of involving the learner in all phases of the teaching-learning interaction cannot be stressed enough. Teaching is much more than telling. Another important consideration in implementing the teaching plan is when and where. The setting for teaching families should be wherever the nurse is in contact with the child and family. This may be the home, outpatient clinic, or hospital. The amount of time the nurse has available for teaching will influence how much of the teaching plan can be completed.

When too much information is covered too quickly without time for reinforcement of the content or for asking questions, families may be confused. The nurse should allow for adequate time, which may mean that the teaching plan will be divided into segments. One segment may be taught each day until the teaching plan is completed. People have different attention spans, so the nurse must be aware of how much can be presented effectively at one time. People tend to lose interest or quit paying attention when they can no longer comprehend. The nurse must observe the learner's responses carefully and be prepared to stop when the child and family have reached their limit. A home referral may be necessary to complete teaching programs.

Interruptions during the teaching session can be difficult for families and nurses. When possible, nurses should try to arrange for other staff members to assist

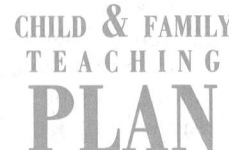

CHILD & FAMILY
T E A C H I N G
PLAN

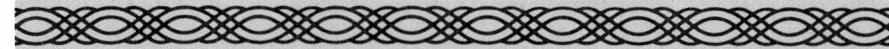

Care of a Neonate With an Ostomy

Assessment

A baby girl, 5 days old, was diagnosed with rectal atresia, and colostomy was performed at 48 hours of age.

This is the first child for these parents. The family will live with maternal grandparents in a small inner city apartment. Limited financial assistance is available. Medical supplies are available through city hospital but will be limited to distributions once a month. Parents are able to read at third-grade level. Both mother and father have good manual dexterity. The mother has been identified as the primary care provider. The father is interested but works long hours and is not readily available in the home.

Mother states that she learns best if she can see what is to be done and then practices each step. She has helped care for younger brothers and sisters.

Parents acknowledge that they do not know about colostomies, and have never seen a stoma or known anyone with an ostomy. The nursing diagnosis, anxiety related to caring for a newborn with a colostomy, was made. The nursing intervention planned included teaching the mother colostomy care.

Child and Family Objectives	Specific Content	Teaching Strategies
1. Identify the reason for performing the ostomy and the type of ostomy.	1. Explain the effects of disease on the affected organs. Define imperforate anus, rectum, atresia, bowel function. Describe the procedures that will be used in the treatment.	1. Use anatomic model if available or drawings.
2. Describe the anatomic changes following ostomy surgery.	2. Describe the appearance of the stoma, and type of drainage, and a pouching system. Answer all questions.	2. Use anatomic model that allows the nurse to bypass part of bowel and create stoma. Encourage questions and allow enough quiet time with parents so that they are able to ask questions comfortably.
3. Describe the appearance of a stoma.	3. Stoma is red and moist. Same as oral mucous membrane. No sensory nerve endings, but motor nerve endings are intact and movement seen is normal peristalsis. Size will change as swelling from surgery diminishes.	3. Following surgery, show the parents the baby's stoma, and describe the appearance of a normal stoma. Encourage questions by providing examples of some questions parents have.
4. Verbalize feelings related to infant's surgery and care needs.	4. Parents discuss feelings related to caring for the colostomy. Parents look at and touch stoma. Parents participate in care of colostomy as well as other aspects of care.	4. Encourage parents to express fears and concerns. Nurse should touch stoma and discuss how it feels and what the infant feels. Parents can identify the pace at which they are comfortable assuming care of the infant in the hospital. Begin with feeding and rocking and then add colostomy care.

(Continued)

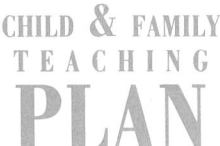

CHILD & FAMILY
T E A C H I N G
PLAN

Care of a Neonate With an Ostomy (continued)

Child and Family Objectives

5. Demonstrate the application of skin barrier and pouch.

Specific Content

5. Teach basic pouching techniques:

(1) Gather all clean equipment, warm water, washcloth, trash bag.

(2) Prepare new pouching system. Detail the system that has been selected for the individual infant.

Pattern: A paper towel can be used to trace a pattern. The pattern should hug the stoma but not ride up on it. Always label the pattern for "top" and "skin side." Consider outer dimensions of the pattern as well as stoma opening (avoid hip bone, ribs, pubic area, folds, navel).

Skin barrier: Use ½, ¼, or full wafer (4 × 4), round the corners or conform the shape to the adhesive on the pouch. Trace pattern on paper side of barrier. Cut a hole on pattern line. Smooth sides of the opening with your finger.

Pouch: Pouch opening is slightly larger than opening in skin barrier. Draw pattern on pouch paper side, and cut opening larger than the line of the pattern. Edges should be smooth. Remove paper backing from the pouch and center the opening on the top of the skin barrier, and press the two together. Use tape, tissue, or powder to cover any exposed adhesive on the pouch. Make up extra pouching systems, and have them handy.

(3) Remove old system, and cleanse the skin gently and pat dry. Observe the skin for any signs of breakdown.

(4) Apply clean system: Warm the skin barrier in your hands. Remove the backing (save this paper, it can serve as your pattern next time). Center the opening with the stoma; press and seal to skin. If any skin is visible, go up through the bottom with stomahesive or karaya powder and sprinkle around the stoma and skin.

Teaching Strategies

5. Show the parents each step on several occasions, and allow them opportunities to practice.

Parents can pratice making new pouching systems when the nurse is not available. This practice is helpful, and it provides completed pouching systems when the pouch needs changing (once a day).

Allow parents to practice on a stoma model so that they can become accustomed to centering the opening on a stoma.

(Continued)

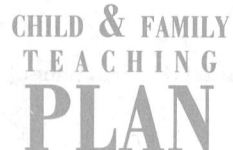

CHILD & FAMILY
T E A C H I N G
PLAN

Care of a Neonate With an Ostomy (continued)

Child and Family Objectives	Specific Content	Teaching Strategies
	(5) Check supplies and reorder as necessary.	
6. Identifies signs and symptoms of diarrhea and dehydration.	6. Define diarrhea, dehydration, vomiting.	6. Have parents identify signs and symptoms of diarrhea and dehydration. Find examples of the symptoms from their past experiences and relate to their infant.
	When diarrhea starts, stop formula or solid foods. Begin feeding clear liquids. Pedialyte, a special solution, is available at the drug store. It is important to provide liquids, so do not stop all feedings. If the amount of stool slows down, continue clear liquids. Check with your doctor if diarrhea does not stop in 18 to 24 hours.	Provide written instructions and explanations. Keep wording simple.
	Call physician or bring to clinic when your infant or child has diarrhea and listlessness (not as active as usual), fever, foul-smelling stools, vomiting and diarrhea, and abdominal distention (full belly).	Provide phone numbers of clinic, doctors, and home health nurses.

Evaluation

- Parents identify that the rationale for performing the ostomy is to allow for bowel movements and to allow the baby to grow before the definitive surgery is completed and that a loop colostomy was the type of ostomy.
- Parents describe the bypass of the rectal segment and discharge of stool through the colostomy stoma.
- Parents describe the stoma as red, moist, and without sensory nerve endings. The normal motion of the stoma is peristalsis.
- Parents express their concerns and fears about caring for the infant.
- Parents demonstrate correct procedures for changing the pouch, protecting the skin, emptying the pouch, and recognizing skin irritation.
- Parents describe the appropriate steps for managing diarrhea.
- Parents demonstrate the ability to read written instructions provided, to state where they can obtain new equipment, and to determine the type of equipment needed.
- Parents state the resources available in the community and identify appropriate names and numbers from a printed list.

with their assigned patients while they are teaching a family. Even 15 minutes of uninterrupted time can be an effective teaching session. Families are more relaxed when they do not feel that the nurse is rushed and has time for their questions.

The nurse can assist the child and family by providing written instructions for them to take home. The written material should be as specific as possible. For example, if teaching families about medications, provide the name, time, and amount of dosage. If a family has difficulty read-

ing, tape a pill to a card, then draw a clock face(s) with the time(s) noted. If the child will need equipment, write down the names and order numbers of the equipment needed and where it can be ordered.

The availability of a contact person following discharge from the hospital and clinic is important. When a home referral is not indicated, the family should feel comfortable calling the physician's office, clinical nurse specialist, or patient educator. The name, phone number, and hours should be provided in writing.

Qualities of Effective Teachers

The nurse as a patient educator should possess certain qualities. The nurse should be able to break tasks into simple steps that he or she can easily explain and demonstrate. The nurse should be comfortable providing instruction and translating complex medical terms into lay terms.[11] Nurse educators routinely use terminology that the child and family understand, or they define the terms used. Abbreviations or letters should be avoided until the family is comfortable with their meanings. For example, ALL for acute lymphocytic leukemia may be correct and reflect the diagnosis, but it may have no meaning for the family.

Effective nurse educators tend to encourage children and families to try tasks without making it seem difficult. Another quality is the ability to relate the skills to common, daily tasks. For example, preparing an ostomy pouch requires the use of a pattern. A mother who sews is accustomed to using patterns and may make the transition easily if the comparison is pointed out.

An important quality of effective nurse educators is organization. All supplies and equipment are gathered before the instruction is started. The nurse knows what is needed, comes prepared, and presents an organized, simplified approach to teaching the child and family.

Managing the questions of children and families requires confidence and patience. Nurses should feel knowledgeable about the subject matter being taught and should be able to manage questions. Nurses should feel comfortable referring questions to physicians when appropriate or seeking answers that they do not have. Because everyone learns at a different pace, nurse educators need to have patience and repeat the content until the family feels confident in their abilities. This implies that a new nurse will learn with personal experience the confidence needed to be an effective teacher and the knowledge about the disease, treatment, and teaching needs required by families.

Documentation

The teaching session should be documented in the nursing notes or on a flow sheet. It is important to communicate what has been taught and what is planned for the next session. This specificity allows the staff to support the teaching program by reinforcing content already presented and supporting the family in trying the skills they have been taught.

Evaluation

The evaluation phase of the instructional design system is planned before the implementation. The evaluation described in the planning section is summative evaluation; that is, it occurs after the teaching plan is completed. During the teaching process formative evaluation can be conducted. Formative evaluation allows the teacher to evaluate the teaching daily and make changes in the teaching plan based on feedback at each stage of instruction. If a family is unable to learn a component of the task, the plan is altered to help them master the com-

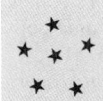

Ideas for Nursing Research

Nurses teaching families about health and health care have a unique opportunity to conduct research to identify successful teaching strategies for various age groups and to explore the long-term impact on the family of chronic illnesses. The following areas need to be explored:

- Comparison of adolescents' management of their self-care routines when parents are involved in the teaching directly and when parents are in a supportive role only.
- Most effective strategies for nurses to use to evaluate the outcome of patient teaching.
- The nurse's role in health education provided by the school system.
- Time at which children and adolescents are most receptive to health education, including nutrition, safety, exercise, and disease prevention strategies.

ponent. Changes may be made in the teaching strategies to help people, or additional content or material may be used.

Once the plan for evaluation is implemented, the results are reported in the chart. The evaluation criteria, or the outcome criteria, are used by hospitals in chart audits to assess patient teaching. Nurses can use the information obtained during the evaluation to change the teaching plan so that the next child and family can benefit from what the nurse learned during the implementation phase.

Summary

A systematic planned approach to patient teaching based on a sound theoretical foundation of learning allows nurses to ensure that each family receives all the content and skills needed to effectively care for their child and that attitudinal changes are planned that relate to the physical, emotional, and spiritual needs of the child. It is easier to adjust and individualize a written teaching plan than it is to create a new one. Nurses learn by teaching families. These experiences can be used to revise and improve teaching plans. Children and families share experiences of what they needed to know and how they learned. This information can be useful for other families undergoing similar experiences.

References

1. Armstrong, M. L. (1989). *Orchestrating the process of patient education: Methods and approaches. Nursing Clinics of North America, 24*(3), 597–604.
2. Bartlett, E. E. (1985). At least a definiton. *Patient Education and Counseling, 7*, 323–324.

3. Becker, M. H., Haefner, D. P., Kasl, C. V., et al. (1974). A new approach to explaining sick-role behaviors in low income populations. *American Journal of Public Health, 64*, 205–216.

4. Bell-Gredler, M. E. (1986). *Learning and instruction: Theory into practice.* New York: MacMillan.

5. Benner, P. (1984). *From novice to expert: Excellence and powers in clinical practice.* Menlo Park, CA: Addison-Wesley.

6. Bigge, M. L. (1982). *Learning theories for teachers* (4th ed.). New York: Harper and Row.

7. Caffrella, R. S. (1981). Hospital-based education programs for patients: Views of health care professionals in Maine. *Public Health Report, 98*, 560–567.

8. Close, A. (1988). Patient education: A literature review. *Journal of Advanced Nursing, 13*, 203–213.

9. Dennison, P. D. & Keeling, A. W. (1989). Clinical support for eliminating the nursing diagnosis of knowledge deficit. *Image: Journal of Nursing Scholarship, 21*(3), 142–144.

10. DiFlorio, I. A. & Duncan, P. A. (1986). Design for successful patient teaching. *American Journal of Maternal Child Health, 11*(4), 246–249.

11. Elsberry, N. L., & Sorensen, M. E. (1986). Using analogies in patient teaching. *American Journal of Nursing, 86*(10), 1171–1172.

12. Foster, K. E. (1985). Involving Blue Cross plans in patient education. *Patient Education Newsletter*, April, 3–4.

13. Gagné, R. M. (1962). Military training and principles of learning. *American Psychologist, 17*, 83–91.

14. Gagné, R. M. (1968). Contributions of learning to human development. *Psychological Review, 75*(3), 177–191.

15. Gagné, R. M. (1974). *Essentials of learning for instruction.* Hinsdale, IL: Dryden Press.

16. Gagné, R. M. (1977). Conditions of learning (3rd ed.). New York: Holt, Rinehart and Winston.

17. Gagné, R. M., & Biggs, L. J. (1979). *Principles of instructional design* (2nd ed.). New York: Holt, Rinehart and Winston.

18. Garity, J. (1985). Learning styles: Basis for creative teaching and learning. *Nurse Educator, 10*(2), 12–16.

19. Gronlund, N. E. (1985). *Stating objectives for classroom instruction* (3rd ed.). New York: MacMillan.

20. Janz, N. K., & Beckes, M. H. (1984). The health belief model: A decade later. *Health Education Quarterly, 2*, 1–47.

21. Jenny, J. L. (1987). Knowledge deficit: Not a nursing diagnosis. *Image, 19*(4), 184–185.

22. Karam, J. A., Sundre, S., & Smith, G. A. (1986). Cost-benefit analysis of patient education. *Hospital and Health Services Administration, 31*(4), 82–90.

23. King, I. M. (1986). *Curriculum and instruction in nursing.* Norwalk, CT: Appleton-Century-Crofts.

24. Kolb, D. A. (1984). *Experiental learning: Experience as the source of learning and development.* Englewood Cliffs, NJ: Prentice-Hall.

25. Lipetz, M. J., Bussigel, M. N., Bannerman, J., & Risley, B. (1990). What is wrong with patient education programs? *Nursing Outlook, 38*(4), 184–189.

26. McCowen, C., Court, S., Hackett, A. F., & Parkin, J. M. (1988). An evaluation of multiple choice questionnaires for the assessment of knowledge in diabetic children and their families. *Diabetic Medical, 5*(5), 474–488.

27. Oberst, M. T. (1989). Perspectives on research in patient education. *Nursing Clinics of North America, 24*(3), 621–628.

28. Piaget, J. (1951). *Play, dreams and imitation in children.* New York: W.W. Norton.

29. Piaget, J. (1985). *The moral judgment of the child.* New York: Free Press.

30. Pender, N. J. (1987). *Health promotion in nursing practice* (2nd ed.). New York: Appleton-Century-Crofts.

31. Pre-op education cut LOS and cost, aid PPS delivery. (1985). *Hospitals, 59*(4), 78.

32. Priest, A. R. (1989). The CNS as educator. In Hamric, A. B. & Spross, J. (Ed.). *Clinical nurse specialist in theory and practice* (pp. 147–167) (2nd ed.). Philadelphia: W.B. Saunders.

33. Redman, B. K. (1988). *The process of patient education* (6th ed.). St. Louis: C.V. Mosby.

34. Rogers, C. (1969). *Freedom to learn.* Columbus, OH: Charles E. Merrill.

35. Ruzicki, D. A. (1989). Realistically meeting the educational needs of hospitalized acute and short-stay patients. *Nursing Clinics of North America, 24*(3), 629–637.

36. Skinner, B. F. (1953). *Science and human behavior.* New York: MacMillan.

37. Skinner, B. F. (1969). *Contingencies of reinforcement.* New York: Appleton-Century-Crofts.

38. Smith, C. E. (1989). Overview of patient education opportunities and challenges for the twenty-first century. *Nursing Clinics of North America, 24*(3), 583–587.

39. Stafford, M. G. (1985). The clinical nurse specialist's faculty role. In K. E. Barnard & G. R. Smith (Eds.). *Faculty practice in action: Second annual symposium of nursing faculty practice.* Kansas City: Academy of Nursing.

40. Thomas, K. J. (1990). *Selection of patient education media.* Lecture. Atlanta, GA: Emory University.

41. Vanetzian, E. (1988). Force field analysis: A person-centered approach to behavior change. *Rehabilitation Nursing, 13*(1), 23–25.

2 UNIT

Health Assessment, Promotion, and Maintenance

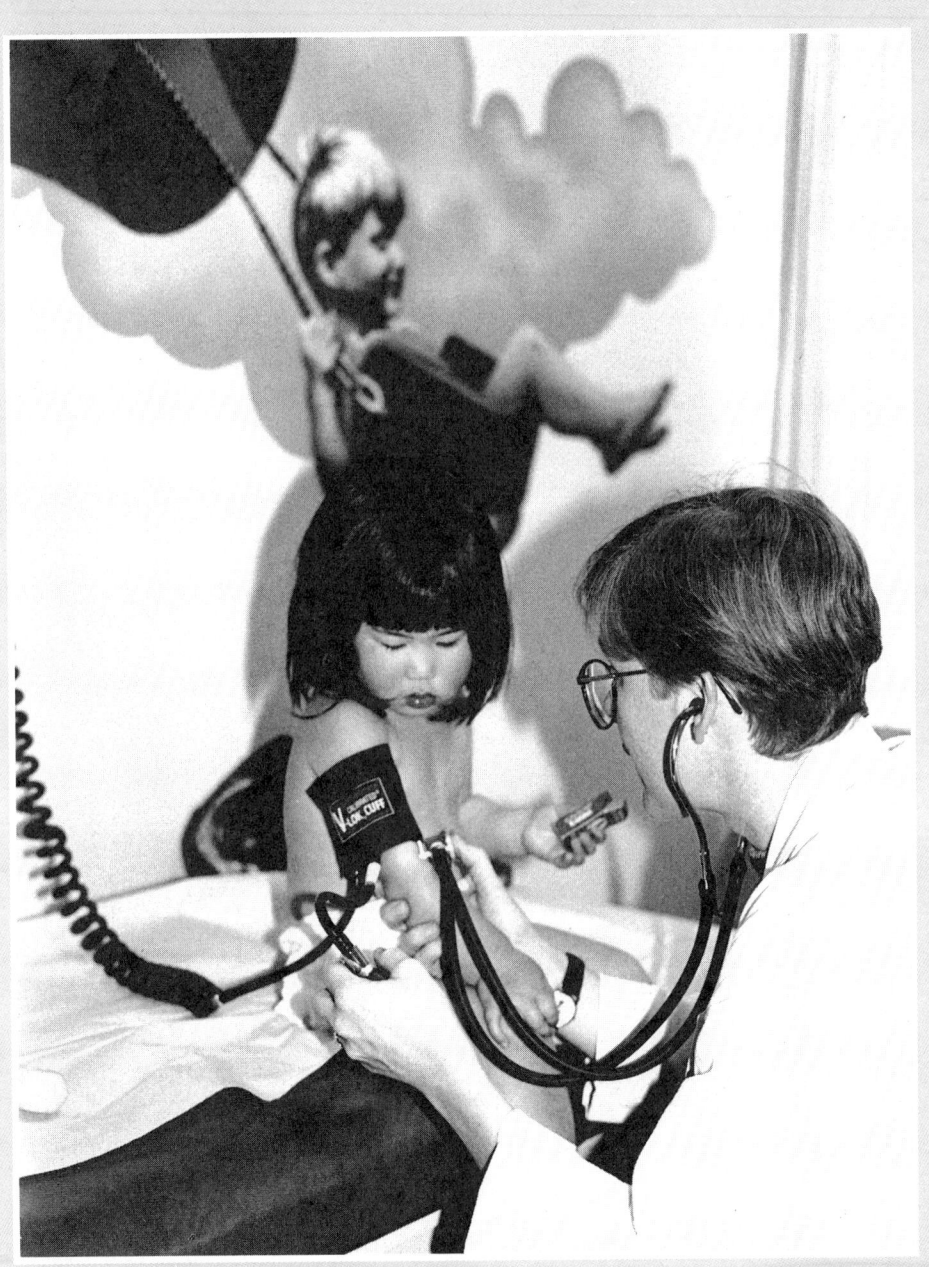

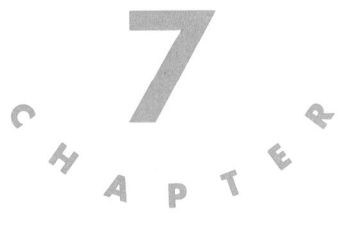

7 CHAPTER

Health Promotion and Maintenance

BEHAVIORAL OBJECTIVES

Compare historic views of health.

Define *health, health promotion,* and *health behaviors.*

Discuss factors that influence acceptance and use of health behaviors.

Identify advantages of Project Health PACT.

Explain nursing process in relationship to health promotion and maintenance.

Evolution of the concepts of health and health promotion has proceeded at a relatively slow pace. Early references to health and health promotion can be found in the Code of Hammurabi, Mosaic Law, and the Bible. It was not until about 1000 A.D., however, that the word *health* appeared in writing.[32] Although the term *health* was originally derived from the Old English word *hoelth,* meaning sound and whole of body, common use of the word implied simply the freedom from disease. Contemporary use of the terms *health* and *health promotion* is inconsistent, and they do not convey the same meaning to all people.

Florence Nightingale's view of nursing as "care that puts a person in the best possible condition for nature to either restore or preserve health to prevent or cure disease or injury" reflected an early concern within nursing for health and its promotion.[27] However, as nursing developed, it sometimes imitated medicine and focused more on the prevention and treatment of disease. Renewed emphasis on health promotion and maintenance has been evident within the profession.

Several phenomena have converged to generate the present societal concern about health promotion for the general population. First has been the recognition that the majority of diseases affecting the population are those of choice rather than chance; therefore, many conditions are controllable. Second, the spiraling cost of illness care has resulted in a need for massive cost containment efforts; health promotion is less expensive than illness care. Finally, consumers have increasingly demanded greater participation in their health care and have displayed willingness to accept responsibility for health-promoting behaviors.

National support for the development of health promotion/risk reduction programs was evident as early as 1979 when the United States Surgeon General published the report entitled *Healthy People.*[34] This report asserted that major health gains could be achieved not from improved illness care, but from advances in physical fitness, nutrition, personal lifestyle, immunizations, and changes in the environment. The need to begin these activities during childhood was emphasized.

107

Despite national interest and multiple calls for major changes in health behaviors, current estimates suggest that about half of the annual deaths in the United States result from the selection of health-damaging lifestyle choices made in childhood and carried into adolescence and adulthood.[20] For example, fewer than 50% of children get enough exercise to promote the development of healthy cardiorespiratory systems, 98% have at least one risk factor for heart disease, and 75% consume diets that contain excess amounts of fat.[13] Suicide is on the rise and constitutes the second leading cause of death among the adolescent population of the United States.[21] These figures starkly present the urgent need to help children make choices that contribute to a lifetime of physical, emotional, and psychosocial health.

In the diversity of their roles and responsibilities, nurses have countless opportunities to promote health in children. The concepts of health promotion and maintenance are major themes of this text. This chapter clarifies terms and explores factors that influence children and families to accept and use healthy behaviors. Application of the nursing process to health promotion and maintenance for children is also examined.

Health, Health Promotion, Health Behaviors: What Are They?

There is little consistency in the way health, health promotion, and related concepts are defined.[23,26] Confusion over terminology reflects both rapid social changes and philosophical differences among health care providers.[12] The following discussion of health and related subconcepts will help orient the reader to their usage in this text.

Health

The definition offered by the World Health Organization in 1974 stated that health is "a state of complete physical, mental, and social well-being, not merely the absence of disease or infirmity."[36] This definition has stood for many years, but it does not address degrees or levels of health that people may attain. The term *health* needs further exploration.

Smith observed that four different perspectives or models have been used to describe the concept of health.[31] The *clinical model* views health simply as the absence of signs and symptoms of physical or psychosocial illness. Such a perspective places health and illness at opposite ends of a continuum and fails to address people who, in spite of chronic illness or disability, achieve a positive health status. The *role performance model,* determining whether people are able to execute their prescribed social functions, appeals to common sense. However, this perspective is narrow and does not speak to emotional or psychosocial well-being. The *adaptive model* is more expansive and describes health as a result of a person's effective interaction with the physical and social environment. Finally, the *eudaemonistic model* of health focuses on the person's general well-being and self-realization, a view congruent with contemporary humanistic values. These models of health are progressively inclusive, with the eudaemonistic model embracing all the others and serving as the basis for contemporary definitions.

To clarify the term for nursing, Pender[27] defined health as "the actualization of inherent and acquired human potential through satisfying relationships with others, goal directed behavior, and competent personal care while adjustments are made as needed to maintain a level of stability compatible with system integrity." Pender observed that health and wellness are terms that may be used interchangeably and that optimal health and high-level wellness are conceptually similar. This view of health has gained wide acceptance among health care practitioners.

Health Promotion

Health promotion is the organized application of educational, social, and environmental resources enabling people to adopt and maintain behaviors that reduce the risk of disease and enhance wellness.[28] This definition assumes acceptance of *health maintenance* as those activities aimed at conserving a stable health state and *disease prevention* as those activities aimed at avoiding specific illnesses. Activities that encourage the alteration of personal habits or the environment to achieve increasing levels of wellness are accepted and pursued.[3]

Health Behaviors

Health behaviors are those activities undertaken by people who believe themselves to be well for the purpose of preventing or detecting disease or promoting health.[20] Examples of health behaviors include having children immunized, making sure that all people in a car wear seat belts or are in approved car seats, and walking, rather than riding, whenever possible (Fig. 7-1).

Factors That Affect Acceptance and Use of Health Behaviors

The acceptance and use of behaviors that promote and maintain health depend on many variables including the child's developmental level, a person's definition of health, perception of one's locus of control, the environment, and socioeconomic status. Although discussed separately, these variables occur simultaneously and interact in a complex manner. Other factors such as health-promoting options available, interactions with health care providers, and perceived cues to action versus barriers to progress must also be considered.[26] The way in which

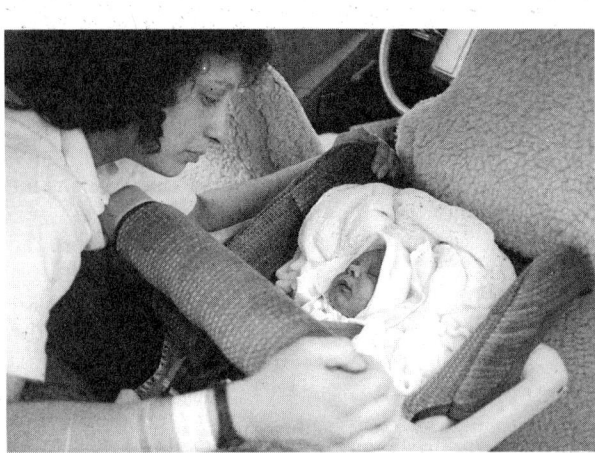
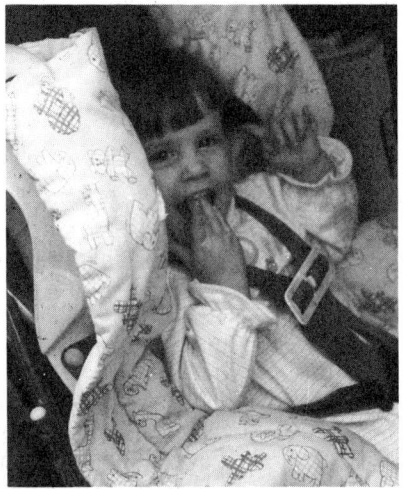
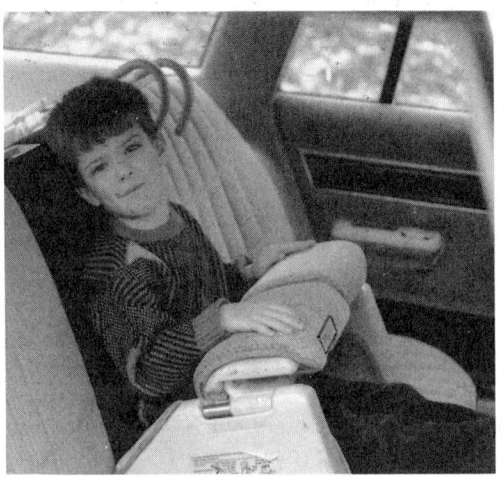
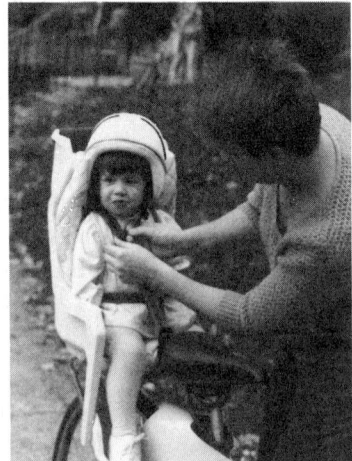
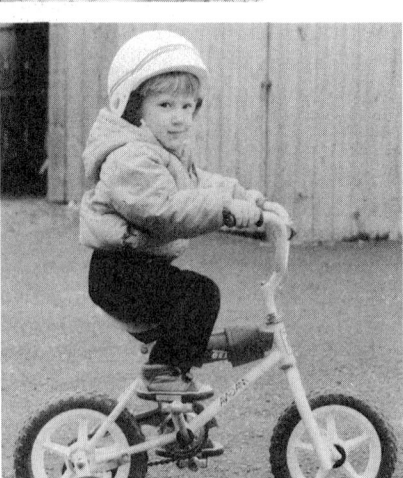

FIGURE 7-1
The family that institutes health behaviors when the newborn is brought home from the hospital and through the early childhood years will help individual members practice health behaviors as they grow older.

these factors are expressed is unique to a particular child and family. Nurses must be aware of these complex interactions and their potential effect on health promotion and maintenance behaviors.

Developmental Level

Nurses in child health care must have a comprehensive knowledge of childhood developmental theories to influence health behaviors successfully.[4] An understanding of the child's developmental level and its associated tasks provides the nurse with a means by which to encourage the incorporation of health-promoting behaviors into the child's and family's daily life experiences. For example, an understanding of the toddler's developmental need to achieve autonomy and to avoid the development of feelings of shame and doubt enables the nurse to encourage parents to capitalize on the child's desire to do things without assistance. By demonstrating health-promoting activities such as exercise and dental hygiene, parents may be

able to get a child to engage in new and beneficial behaviors. The child's developmental level, not chronologic age, should guide nursing actions.

View of Health

Research on children's views of health is limited. A recent study confirmed that children generally perceive health as a multidimensional construct.[14] Dimensions of health described by school-age children include activity-exercise, personal grooming, physical health, nutrition, emotional health, and sleep.[18,22,24,29] Less consistent support has been confirmed for children's inclusion of other health dimensions including dental care, social support systems, and personal behavior.

Children who do not perceive health as a multidimensional construct require assistance in understanding how such things as sleep and physical activity, for example, are related to their health. Nurses can be most effective when they are aware of how a child views his or her health. This information may be obtained if functional health patterns are systematically used to establish the comprehensive database in a health history.[11]

Locus of Control

How people view their ability to control circumstances affecting their lives is known as locus of control. This concept may be viewed on a continuum that ranges from internal to external control. People with internal locus of control believe that their personal actions can influence their health. They are more likely to be oriented toward health and to engage in health promotion and maintenance activities than those with an external locus of control. People with an external locus of control believe that health events occur in random fashion and cannot be changed. They are less likely to engage in health promotion and maintenance behaviors.[15]

Children are often encouraged to remain passive participants in an adult-dominated process until a certain unspecified point in their development. The same adults who have held control suddenly expect them to assume responsibility for their own health behaviors.[19] To develop internal control and to assume responsibility for carrying out health-promoting behaviors, children must be given the opportunity to practice these skills in settings that provide both support and corrective feedback. Because parents are known to influence strongly the child's adoption of health related behaviors, it is helpful if they can be the ones to provide the necessary role modeling.[7,15] In some cases, the nurse may need to identify other significant adults, such as grandparents or teachers, to carry out this vital role.

The work of Richmond and Kotelchuck[30] on locus of control suggests that children who have experienced frequent childhood illnesses may develop an inappropriate belief that chance is the major determinant of health outcomes. The development of positive childhood health behaviors, resulting in a decrease in both the number and severity of health problems may, therefore, be important in assisting the child to develop a sense of control over his or her health in adulthood.

Project Health PACT (Participatory and Assertive Consumer Training) is aimed at assisting school-age children to become active participants in their own care.[16,17] They are taught to ask questions, communicate information about themselves to health care providers, ask for specific instructions related to health care, participate in decision making, and clarify personal responsibilities for care. Programs such as Health PACT appear to be adaptable to a variety of settings including clinics and physicians' offices; they may offer a viable approach to involving children in the decision-making process while providing necessary support.

Environment

Social Influences

Any plan for the promotion of health behaviors in a particular child must take into consideration the influence of social groups and media on the child at different ages. If nurses are to make effective use of the child's social environment to promote healthy lifestyle choices, they must understand at what age and to what degree these different groups exert their influences on the child.

From a traditional perspective, parents are the earliest and strongest influence on the development of the child. Although parental influence decreases as interactions with peers and nonfamily acquaintances increase, parents continue to play an important role throughout childhood. Dissemination of health promotion information to parents from school-based programs has several advantages. Both parents and children can benefit from the information, and parents can provide guidance and support to the child while new habits are being formed. Attitudes and practices are more likely to be adopted permanently if they are incorporated into the lifestyle of the entire family rather than just the child's.[6]

Peer influence begins when the child enters school and is dominant in adolescence. The nurse can make maximum use of the adolescent's normal tendency to turn to peers for information. Peer support groups under the direction of a nurse, for example, can provide accurate and essential health promotion information.[10]

The traditional picture of home, school, and peers as major influences on health behaviors becomes blurred as societal changes occur. Fewer households are headed by two parents and, in those that are, the proportion in which both parents work is increasing each year. As more mothers enter the work force, more young children are cared for in day-care settings or homes other than their own. Likewise, a growing number of children are caring for themselves after school until an adult returns from work. Many children are growing up in blended families or living in settings with more than one generation of family members. Children in these situations are at increased risk for receiving inadequate or inconsistent emphasis on the development of healthy lifestyle activities.

The nurse faces increasing challenges in promoting health in the presence of ongoing changes. Parents may not serve as appropriate role models because they may not be practicing healthy behaviors. There also may be conflict between members of different generations in the home as to what constitutes appropriate health care practices. Peers may play an earlier and greater role in the adoption of practices affecting health care. Schools facing cutbacks in funding of programs may be unable or unwilling to commit scarce financial resources to health promotion programs.

Child health nurses also need to understand the control that media exerts on children in relation to health promotion and maintenance behaviors. Involvement with media, most specifically television, begins in early childhood and continues unabated through adolescence.[7] Television continues to show the use of alcohol, violence, drugs, and casual sexual contact as appropriate methods of coping with the stressors encountered in a complex world. The behaviors are in obvious conflict with the concept of health maintenance. Children need assistance in clarifying desirable behaviors that contribute to long-term health.

Culture and Religion

Both cultural and religious beliefs play an important role in how the child and family view and implement health-promoting behaviors. To provide care for children and families from different cultures nurses must have knowledge about major cultural beliefs and customs, accepted health care practices, language, and dietary patterns. Pressure from the nurse on the child and family to adopt specific health behaviors that are at variance with cultural beliefs causes conflict and is to be avoided.

Religious beliefs, practices, and taboos are often interwoven with cultural beliefs and practices, and nurses need to understand these relationships. However, such understanding alone is not enough. Families within a particular culture or religious group may vary widely in their acceptance and practice of particular behaviors of the larger group. The locus of decision making in some cultures, for example, may reside with someone other than the biologic parents. People within families may also differ significantly in their belief and use of cultural and religious practices. The nurse may find that as the child matures, his or her acceptance of religious and cultural beliefs and practices may be different from those of parents, thus leading to increased stress in the family unit. The nurse should be aware of this potential problem and attempt to support the child and family without bias.[9]

Minority Group Membership

Membership in some minority groups (e.g., African American, Hispanic, or Native American) increases the person's potential for illness or death from cancer, cardiovascular disease, infant mortality, violence, diabetes, and chemical dependency.[33] Health promotion strategies that have reduced morbidity and mortality from these diseases in the larger American society have either not reached these groups or not effected changes in health care practices. Damberg[8] suggests that a major reason for the lack of progress is that health promotion programs offered to minority groups are insensitive to ethnic and cultural characteristics, beliefs, and practices (Fig. 7-2). Chapter 4 provides more information about ethnic groups.

Socioeconomic Status

When immediate needs such as employment, food, and adequate housing are unmet, family members may be unable to accept or use health promotion and maintenance behaviors. Acceptance and use of health-oriented activities demand that the child and family be able to visualize their lives in the future. When results of the practice of health behaviors are not immediately apparent, their value may be unrecognized.[15]

The Nursing Process in Health Promotion and Maintenance

Application of the nursing process to health promotion and maintenance for specific age groups is discussed in

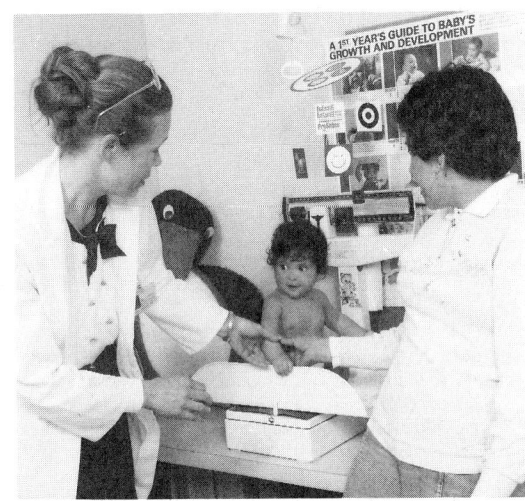

FIGURE 7-2
The nurse's sensitivity to the family's cultural and religious background affects how the family will relate to health care workers and facilities in the future. Here the nurse discusses a Hispanic child's health with the mother. (Photo courtesy of the University of Washington School of Nursing.)

other chapters of this Unit. The material presented below is applicable to use of the nursing process for any age group. The nurse takes into consideration factors that affect the acceptance and use of health promotion and maintenance behaviors when providing care for the child and family.

Assessment

Functional health and nursing process was discussed in Chapter 2. One of the patterns of functional health—health perception and health maintenance—addresses how the child and family perceive and manage health. Compliance with recommendations and the ability of the child and family to perceive relationships between personal behavior and current health status must be assessed.

Subjective data are collected about the child's and family's perceptions of health and illness, health habits, and compliance with suggested or prescribed activities, treatments and medications. Table 7-1 lists examples of questions that nurse may ask when assessing health perception and health maintenance. The child's history and health care records also yield important information. Objective data about the child's actual health practices are more difficult to obtain, but the nurse can observe general appearance, posture, and expression during the interview. Measurement of height, weight, and vital signs also provides pertinent information. Additional objective data are collected during the physical examination.

Nursing Diagnoses

Analysis of the database may reveal health promotion or maintenance concerns that may be treated independently by nurses or may require collaboration with other health professionals.[11] Two nursing diagnoses accepted

TABLE 7-1
Nursing Assessment: Questions for Assessing Health Maintenance and Health Promotion

Questions to Ask Parents*	Questions to Ask Child†
• What do you think it means to be healthy?	• What does it mean to you to be healthy?
• How would you describe your child's health?	• Do you think that what you do or don't do can help you stay or get healthy?
• On a scale of 1 to 10 (10 is excellent), how would you rate your child's health?	• How would you describe your health?
• Describe any health problems you see in your child.	• On a scale of 1 to 10 (10 is excellent), how would you rate your health?
• What events or activities do you feel affect your child's health in a positive way? In a negative way?	• Describe any health problems you think you have.
• What do you feel you can do to keep your child healthy?	• What events or activities do you feel affect your health in a positive way? In a negative way?
• What do you do for your child when he or she has a health problem?	• What do you feel you can do to keep yourself healthy?
• How often do you take your child for well-child visits (health promotion) at the physician's office or clinic?	• What do you do for yourself when you have a health problem?
• When was the child's last: immunization (are they up to date?), dental check, developmental assessment, vision/hearing screening, physical examination? What do you know about the results?	• When was your last: immunization (are they up to date?), dental check, developmental assessment, vision/hearing screening, physical examination? What do you know about the results?
• What safety hazards are present in your home? Environment? Do you take any precautions for your child? Yourself?	• What safety hazards are present in your home? Environment? Do you take any precautions for yourself?
• Do you feel you are included in the development of a health promotion plan for your child?	• Do you feel you are included in the development of a health promotion plan for yourself?
• Are you able to follow the plan? If not, what do you think interferes?	• Are you able to follow the plan? If not, what do you think interferes?

* Examples of questions nurses may ask parents until children are able to answer questions for themselves.
† Examples of questions children may be asked when they are old enough to answer.

by the North American Nursing Diagnosis Association (NANDA) specifically address health perception and health maintenance: Health-Seeking Behaviors and Altered Health Maintenance.

Health-seeking behavior is defined as "the state in which an individual in stable health actively seeks ways to alter personal health habits and/or the environment to move toward a higher level of wellness."[5] Stable health is achieved when age-appropriate illness prevention measures are employed, the client reports good or excellent health, and signs and symptoms of disease, if present, are controlled. This diagnostic category would generally be used to describe a child without symptoms but could also be used for a child with a chronic condition who wishes to achieve a higher level of wellness.

Altered health maintenance is defined as "the state in which an individual or group experiences or is at risk of experiencing a disruption in health because of an unhealthy lifestyle or lack of knowledge to manage a condition."[5] This diagnostic category could be used to describe a child or family wishing to make changes in unhealthy lifestyles or in need of teaching about a disease or condition so that they can manage their own care.

Assessment of other aspects of functional health also may provide additional data to support nursing diagnoses for which interventions that promote health are appropriate. The nurse must identify relevant cues and make inferences from a complete database.

The development of additional wellness diagnoses remains a challenge to nursing.[1,27] The inclusion of Health-Seeking Behaviors as a diagnostic category in the NANDA classification system is a significant addition addressing wellness. Increasing the number of wellness diagnoses would support nurses' work in health promotion and illness prevention, thereby helping to reduce health care costs and improve the quality of life.

Planning

Although the goal of nursing is to promote health, it is the child and family, not the nurse, who manage health.[11] The child and family must be involved in decisions about desired outcomes and in determining priorities. An appropriate model the nurse can use for decision making, applicable to both children and their families, is humanism. Humanism is a philosophical view that takes into consideration the values of the nurse or other health care provider and the child and family members. All are coparticipants in decisions affecting health care. The nurse assists the child and family in developing a plan rather than imposing one.[2]

Intervention

A major difference in the intervention step in the area of health promotion and maintenance is that many, if not all, of the interventions developed will be implemented by the child and family while the nurse remains available to provide further education, consultation, and support (Fig. 7-3).

Nurses may have difficulty in relinquishing control over the interventions. Concern may develop about the ability and willingness of the child and family to comply with the plan. While nurses may find it easy to continue to work with the compliant child and family, they may find it difficult to work with those who are noncompliant

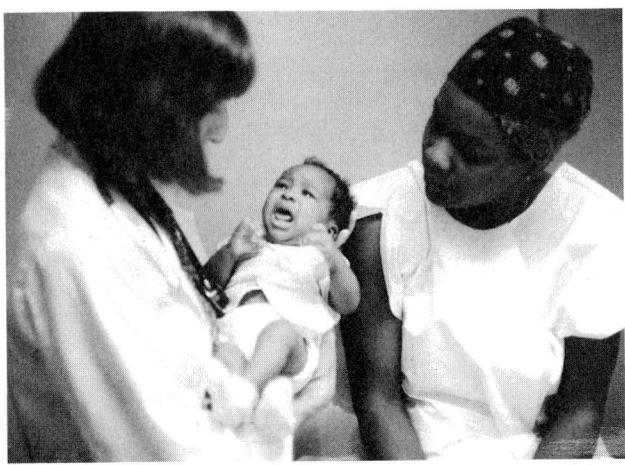

FIGURE 7-3
The nurse and mother of the newborn discuss health care, immunizations, and follow-up visits. The nurse must accept the family as responsible for well-care visits, while the nurse remains available for education, support, and counseling. (Courtesy of the former Booth Maternity Center, Philadelphia.)

with the plan. Nevertheless, the acceptance of the child and family for the responsibility of the health care plan is essential to its ultimate success.

Evaluation

The child and family and the nurse must remember that the establishment of positive health behaviors may take a long time, that lapses are not uncommon, and that factors affecting health behavior choices may undergo frequent change. Evaluation should actively include the child and family. Reviewing achievement of goals provides an opportunity for further education, clarification of questions or concerns, and reinforcement of positive health behaviors. Development of additional plans to achieve health goals may be necessary.

Summary

A strong emphasis on health promotion and maintenance by the nurse providing care to children and their families is essential for comprehensive care. The nurse must take the many complex factors that play a part in the acceptance and use of health behaviors into consideration during the use of the nursing process. The care plan may require several modifications to achieve the goals of health promotion and maintenance.

The demands on the finite human and financial resources of the health care system continue to grow. Informed decisions about use of these dwindling resources must be made based on knowledge of social, political, and economic issues. Certainly, efforts aimed at preventing the development of disease or disability while promoting health are most cost-effective.

The learning and practice of health promotion and maintenance behaviors must take place in a broad variety

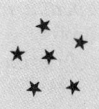

Ideas for Nursing Research

There is a need for nursing research in health promotion and maintenance in children. The nurse is responsible for using the nursing process in working with the child and family to help identify and achieve goals. Because it is the child and family, not the nurse, who will carry out interventions, new approaches to the development and delivery of programs aimed at wellness in childhood are needed if adults are to be healthier in the future. The following areas need to be explored:

- Long-term outcomes of health promotion and maintenance interventions in childhood.
- Development of effective health promotion and maintenance programs using children's views of health at different ages.
- Types of mass media approaches to use in fostering positive health behaviors in children.
- Comparison of gender differences in response to learning positive health behaviors.
- Means to maximize parental involvement in health promotion for children.
- Development of wellness diagnoses to be used in the promotion of wellness in children.

of settings to be most effective. Homes, schools, community groups, churches, places of employment, hospitals, doctor's offices, and nursing centers are all appropriate settings for the nurse to engage in assisting the child and family. Rather than waiting for settings and opportunities to present themselves, nurses can take a creative approach in designing health promotion strategies.

References

1. Allen, C. J. (1989). Incorporating a wellness perspective for nursing diagnosis in practice. In R. M. Carroll-Johnson (Ed.), *Classification of nursing diagnoses.* Philadelphia: Lippincott.
2. Bille, D. A. (1987). Locus of decision making in patient and family education: Its effect on promoting wellness. *Nursing Administration Quarterly, 11*(3), 62–65.
3. Brubaker, B. H. (1983). Health promotion: A linguistic analysis. *Advances in Nursing Science, 5,* 1–14.
4. Bruhn, J. G., Cordova, F. D. (1977). A developmental approach to learning wellness behavior, part 1: Infancy to early adolescence. *Health Values: Achieving High Level Wellness, 1,* 246–254.
5. Carpenito, L. J. (1992). *Nursing diagnosis: Application to clinical practice* (4th ed.). Philadelphia: Lippincott.
6. Crockett, S. J. (1987). The family team approach to fitness: A proposal. *Public Health Reports, 102,* 546–551.
7. Crooks C. E., Iammarino, N. K., & Weinberg, A. D. (1987). The family's role in health promotion. *Health Values, 11*(2), 7–12.
8. Damberg, C. (1986). Strategies for promoting the health of minorities: The school-age population. *Health Values, 10*(3), 29–33.

9. Evans, M. L., Hansen B. D. (1985). *A clinical guide to pediatric nursing* (2nd ed.). Norwalk, CT: Appleton-Century-Crofts.

10. Gillis, A. (1988). Promoting health among teenagers. *International Nursing Review, 35,* 10–12.

11. Gordon, M. (1991). *Manual of nursing diagnosis.* St. Louis: Mosby.

12. Grasser, C., & Craft, B. J. G. (1984). The patient's approach to wellness. *Nursing Clinics of North America, 9,* 207–216.

13. Haydon, D. F. (1987). The family and health/fitness. *Health Values, 11*(2), 36–39.

14. Hester, N. (1987). Health perceptions of school-age children. *Issues in Comprehensive Pediatric Nursing, 10,* 149–159.

15. Hussey, L., & Gilliland, K. (1989). Compliance, low literacy, and locus of control. *Nursing Clinics of North America, 24,* 605–611.

16. Igoe, J. (1983). PACT full of health. *Nursing Times, 79*(7), 53–56.

17. Igoe, J. (1984). Project Health PACT in action. *American Journal of Nursing, 80,* 2016–2021.

18. Kalnins, I., & Love, R. (1982). Children's concepts of health and illness—and implications for health education: An overview. *Health Education Quarterly, 9,* 104–115.

19. Lewis C. E., & Lewis, M. A. (1982). Children's health related decision making. *Health Education Quarterly, 9,* 225–237.

20. Longenecker, G. D. K., & Woods, N. F. (1991). Health and illness: The human experience. In W. J. Phipps, C. Long, & N. F. Woods (Eds.): *Medical-surgical nursing: Concepts and clinical practice* (4th ed.). St. Louis: Mosby.

21. Maglacas, A. M. (1988). Health for all: Nursing's role. *Nursing Outlook, 36*(2), 66–71.

22. Mickalide, A. D. (1986). Children's understanding of health and illness: Implications for health promotion. *Health Values, 10*(3), 5–21.

23. Moore, P. V., Williamson, G. C. (1984). Health promotion: Evolution of a concept. *Nursing Clinics of North America, 19,* 195–207.

24. Natapoff, J. N. (1978). Children's views of health: A developmental study. *American Journal of Public Health, 68,* 995–1000.

25. Nightingale, F. (1946). *Notes on nursing.* Philadelphia: Lippincott.

26. Pender, N. J. (1987). *Health promotion in nursing practice* (2nd ed.). Norwalk, CT: Appleton & Lange.

27. Pender, N. J. (1989). Languaging a health perspective for NANDA taxonomy on research and theory. In R. M. Carroll-Johnson (Ed.): *Classification of nursing diagnoses.* Philadelphia: Lippincott.

28. Petosa, R. (1986). Emerging trends in adolescent health promotion. *Health Values, 10*(3), 22–28.

29. Rashkis, S. R. (1965). Child's understanding of health. *Archives of General Psychiatry, 12,* 10–17.

30. Richmond, J. B., & Kotelchuck, M. (1984). Personal health maintenance for children. *Western Journal of Medicine, 141,* 816–823.

31. Smith, J. A. (1981). The idea of health: A philosophical inquiry. *Advances in Nursing Science, 3*(3), 43–50.

32. Sorochon, W. (1983). Health concepts as a basis for orthobiosis. In E. Hart & W. Sechrist (Eds.). *The dynamics of wellness.* Belmont, CA: Wadsworth.

33. U.S. Department of Health and Human Services. (1985). *Report of the Secretary's task force on black and minority health.* Washington, DC: Government Printing Office, 1985.

34. U.S. Department of Health, Education and Welfare. (1979). *Healthy people: The Surgeon General's report on health promotion and disease prevention.* Washington, DC: Government Printing Office.

35. Weber, J. (1988). *Nurses' handbook of health assessment.* Philadelphia: Lippincott.

36. World Health Organization. (1947). Constitution of the world health organization. *Chronicle of World Health Organization, 1,* 31.

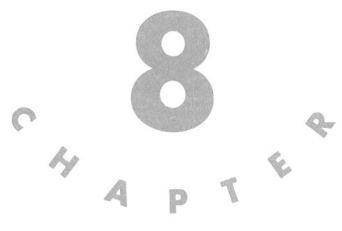

8

Growth and Development of Children

BEHAVIORAL OBJECTIVES

Differentiate among the terms *growth*, *development*, and *maturation*.

Explain how child development is used in the nursing process.

Identify major internal and external factors that influence a child's growth and development.

State basic principles of growth and development related to *direction*, *sequence*, *timeliness*, and *pace*.

Summarize theoretical views on aspects of child development, including personality, psychosexual, psychosocial, cognitive, and moral reasoning.

The study of child development is a relatively young science that has attracted scholars from a wide range of academic and professional disciplines. At the turn of the 20th century the study of child development was considered important because it enhanced understanding of adult behavior. That purpose remains valid, but scientists now recognize that knowledge from child development studies provides a rich reservoir of information about children. Knowledge of developmental processes, such as thinking, feeling, perceiving, and interacting with others, leads to a better understanding of what can be expected of children at different ages. Furthermore, the effect of conditions in which children live and the social trends that affect their lives can be better understood.

Although the growth and development of children has fascinated scientists for many years, much is still unknown and more is only poorly understood. The complexity of human nature presents an endless variety of opportunities for investigation, but the study of children holds special challenges. As physical competencies evolve, so do social, emotional, and cognitive characteristics and abilities. The interplay between these ever changing facets of development produce children who are unique but also similar to their peers.

The goal of research on child development is to gain greater insight into the processes and influences that account for changes in behavior that occur from birth to adulthood. Children do not grow and develop in a vacuum but with other people in a society and environment. Thus, not only are children studied as individuals, but also their families and others who interact with and influence them. This chapter provides a discussion of some of the dimensions of child development research and some of the principles and theories that have resulted.

Clarification of Terms

Any serious discussion of child development inevitably raises questions about some commonly used terms. Growth, maturation, and development are words that often are used interchangeably, and indeed they are closely related. Nevertheless, distinctions may be made among them, and the student of child development should clearly understand those differences.

The term *growth* refers to an increase in physical attributes, such as length, weight, or strength of the whole body or any of its parts, and is the result of biologic changes. The multiplication of cells is necessary for an increase in size and differentiation of cells for the large variety of tissues and organ systems in the body. Growth may be objectively evaluated in quantitative measures, such as centimeters or kilograms. An individual's potential for growth is genetically determined, but reaching full growth potential may be impeded by influences including nutrition, environmental conditions, and illness.

Another physical process determined by genetic inheritance is *maturation*, which refers to qualitative changes brought about by aging. Maturation typically parallels growth and theoretically may occur in the absence of learning, which requires interaction with the environment. Rare instances of maturation without growth or development may be described. A child who has progeria, for example, experiences rapid maturation of the skin, skeleton, and other body systems without accompanying changes in growth or development. Because maturation is almost invariably linked with learning, the term development may be considered inclusive. Thus, when the phrase "growth and development" is used, maturation and learning also may be assumed to occur.

Development is a dynamic phenomenon, and the term refers to progress in skill and complexity of functioning. Development occurs as a result of growth, maturation, and learning and thus requires interaction of the child with the environment. The development of an individual embraces all the physical, psychological, intellectual, and social changes that occur throughout the life span. As an example of the interaction among the concepts of growth, maturation, and development, consider the child who plays the piano. The child must physically be able to strike the keys and control the muscles of the arms and fingers, but these physical capacities must be accompanied by an understanding of the relationship between these movements and the production of a melody. Growth and maturation produce the physical abilities, but learning through experimenting and possibly instruction are necessary for the development of skills required to produce music.

Growth and development may be conceptualized in many ways, but often changes in characteristics and behaviors are linked to ages at which differences are noted. Authors in this text often speak of periods of development in terms that may be only vaguely familiar to the new student of child development. Definitions of terms used in this text's age-related framework for growth and development are the following:

- Prenatal—conception to birth
- Neonatal—birth through 1 month
- Infancy—first year
- Toddler—1 to 3 years
- Preschool—3 to 6 years
- School-age—6 to 11 or 12 years
- Adolescent—11 or 12 to 19 years

Application of Knowledge to the Nursing Process

Nurses who care for children need to understand dimensions of growth and development to use the nursing process effectively. When a child's characteristics and behaviors are assessed by the nurse during the first phase of the nursing process, the data are cognitively compared to the nurse's existing knowledge base about a typical child at that age. Analysis of the assessment data demands a knowledge of norms so that deviations may be recognized. In a similar way familiarity with different theoretical views of child development assists the nurse in understanding and explaining the behavior that has been observed.

Nursing diagnoses of actual or potential health problems result from this comparison of what is assessed and what is known about developmental processes in "normal" children. The nursing diagnosis "Altered Growth and Development" indicates that an individual "has, or is at risk for, impaired ability to perform tasks of his/her age group."[10] A child may lag behind others of a similar age in physical growth or may have difficulty performing any number of skills, including motor, personal, social, cognitive, or language. Other characteristics may include a child's inability to perform self-care or self-control activities appropriate for a given age group or signs and symptoms of disturbed social or emotional responses. Objective and subjective data obtained through the assessment process and screened through the nurse's bank of knowledge will likely yield an accurate nursing diagnosis, but the nurse needs to continue to investigate the clinical and personal situations that have caused or contributed to the existing alteration in functional health.

Carpenito[10] has suggested that the etiologic, contributing, or risk factors in altered growth and development may have a pathophysiologic, situational, maturational, or treatment-related basis. Focused assessment of the child, family, and environment is necessary to understand the complex nature of the child's problem. Once the scope of the difficulty is understood, nurses must be able to set goals mutually acceptable to the parents and child. The nurse again draws from the existing reservoir of knowledge and understanding of human growth and development, as well as other knowledge of pathologic conditions, to determine suitable actions for a particular child and family. Nursing care can then be planned and provided to assist the child in obtaining or maintaining optimum health functioning.

When a potential or actual alteration in growth and development has been identified and the etiologic, contributing, or risk factors understood, nursing interventions are then directed at reducing or eliminating these factors. Referral of the child and family to a developmental clinic, a school health nurse, a community health nurse, or other health care provider may be necessary. Thus, clear, concise, and accurate communication of the assessment data and the resulting nursing diagnosis is essential. Actual interventions may include parental education and guidance on age-related developmental tasks, opportunities provided to the ill child to meet age-related developmental tasks, or initiation of health teaching and referrals.[10]

Nursing follow-up is necessary to evaluate the plan of care and the patient's progress toward reaching the stated goals. Follow-up may not be provided by the same nurse who was involved in diagnosing the health problem, but a nurse who actively provides nursing interventions is responsible for evaluating the child's and family's progress toward reaching the goals that had been set and determining whether the alteration in growth and development has been resolved. When reviewing the problem and interventions the nurse should determine whether the plan of care needs to be continued as designed, revised, or discontinued.[10] Ongoing evaluation also may be appropriate to assess for the return of a developmental problem that had been resolved earlier.

Influences Affecting Growth and Development

Several major factors influence an individual's growth and development from the fetal period throughout the entire life span. These influences may be conceptualized as originating from inside or outside of the child, but in fact they often interact to produce unique effects on individual children. A brief overview of some of these important internal and external influences is presented below, and many are explored in more depth in other chapters of this text.

Internal Influences

Heredity

Heredity is the term used to refer to genetic characteristics that are transmitted from parent to child. Biologic inheritance is an active influence on human development throughout life. Each individual's unique heredity will guide the development of all physical characteristics, but its effect is not necessarily simple and obvious (Fig. 8-1). Environmental influences, such as nutrition, disease, or social deprivation, may influence whether a child's full potential for development of physical characteristics, abilities, and tendencies will be met. Likewise, how much behavior and personality differences may be attributed to genetic inheritance is unclear, but there is general agreement that the interaction of heredity and environment play a part in determining all aspects of growth, maturation, and development of a child. Chapter 10 should be consulted for detailed information about genetic influences on health promotion and maintenance.

Gender

Differences in the abilities and behaviors of members of both sexes have been the subject of intense investigation for the last 2 decades. In a review of literature on gender differences in behavior at birth, Jacklin & Maccoby[30] note that boys and girls seem very much alike. Studies on phenomena such as muscle strength and activity often have conflicting results. If differences exist between the sexes at birth, the magnitude of the differences seems very small. Remarkable, however, is the evidence that parents tend to stereotype their newborns according to gender. Parents tend to view girls as delicate

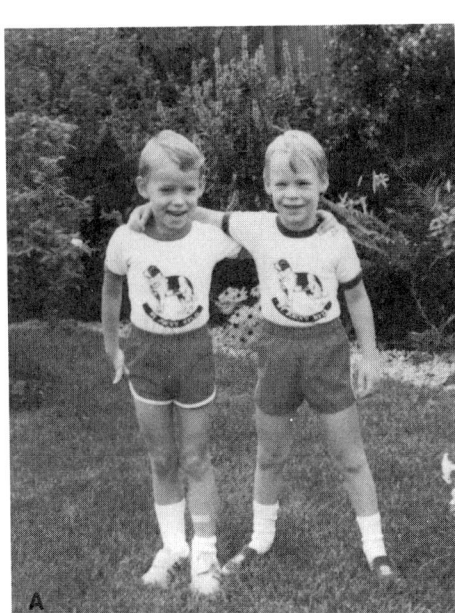 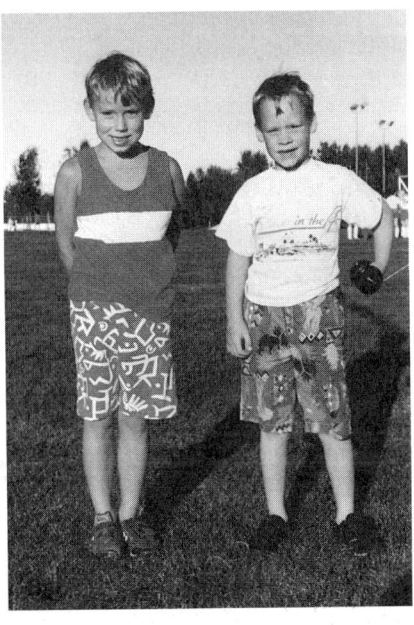

FIGURE 8-1
Genetic influences on growth. (A) Photograph of two first cousins who could easily be taken for twins. The boy on the left is 4 years and 3 months old, while the boy on the right is 5 years and 6 months old. (B) The same boys 2 years later. The cousin on the left is now 8 cm taller than the one on the right.

and small and boys as big and robust, even when infants are the same size.

Gender differences also are suspected to exist during the toddler and preschool years. Girls are thought to mature faster than boys, an assumption that would account for alleged differences. Jacklin and Maccoby[30] report that girls do show more rapid bone development and are toilet trained earlier. With well-designed research, however, no differences have been found between boys and girls in sleep patterns, in reaching sensorimotor developmental milestones, or in verbal ability. Until the prepubertal growth spurt, gender differences in maturation are thus relatively minor.

Differences in temperament between boys and girls also have been questioned, but few have been substantiated. Studies of crying and irritability studies and levels of timidity, for example, may suggest somewhat higher irritability in boys and somewhat more timidity in girls. Likewise, boys are sometimes found to be more active than girls. Often, however, analysis of the methodologic issues and statistical procedures used in these studies reveals deficiencies that may account for the findings of the studies.[30]

Investigations of gender differences in play behavior do suggest that boys and girls are not alike. Boys consistently display more peer-directed aggression, especially in the presence of male patterns, and rough-and-tumble play is seen in boys more frequently.[30] How much of this difference in play behavior is attributable to biologic factors rather than the tendency of care providers, peers, and others in society to reinforce stereotyped play remains open to question. The same question haunts similar investigations into alleged differences in verbal abilities, mathematical abilities, and visual-spatial abilities that have been investigated in school-age children.

Although biologic factors may contribute to some gender differences in behavior, these differences seem to be very small. Jacklin and Maccoby[30] conclude that predicting an individual's ability on the basis of gender alone is impossible. Environmental factors must be taken into account for sex differences that are reported, because neither a biologic nor a social explanation is entirely sufficient. As the "nature versus nurture" debate wanes, more attention will be placed on the similarities of the sexes rather than on the differences.

Race

Membership in a group that draws from the same genetic pool determines an individual's race. There are three human races: Caucasian, Negro, and Mongolian. Often ethnicity is used as a synonym for race, but ethnicity refers to an individual belonging to and identifying with a group of people who have common cultural traditions, belief systems, genetic history, and language. An individual's ethnic background may actually draw from two racial groups. The ethnic group of Puerto Ricans, for example, draws from both the Caucasian and Negro racial groups.

Sometimes differences among children are attributed to racial characteristics. Physical differences, such as facial features, skin color, hair texture, and other characteristics, may be fully explained by race. Differences in physical and motor development among children also require in-

vestigation as to racial influence. Flake-Hobson, et al[19] caution that norms stated for children generally do not reflect racial differences. In fact the American Academy of Pediatrics has called for separate norms for African American and white babies, but these are not yet available.

Racial differences in cognitive, psychological, emotional, and other nonphysical features in children have been a source of concern for some child development scholars. The question concerning genetic differences in intelligence has been particularly controversial, but most agree that although a child's genetic makeup determines intellectual potential, the extent that the potential will be realized depends on environmental factors.[69]

Caution should be taken concerning the degree to which growth percentile charts are used. Because most such charts have used white, full-term infants to produce percentiles, they are of little use in assessing gestational or racial differences. Research indicates that African American infants are, on average, longer and heavier than white infants of a comparable socioeconomic status.[5] Research also indicates that Asian children are shorter and lighter than white children.[5] More growth percentile charts for nonwhite groups are needed. Chapter 4 provides further insight into the cultural influences on the growth and development of children.

Genes

Genes are sometimes responsible for certain diseases and abnormalities in children. In most cases the disorders are linked to recessive rather than dominant genes and occur when the individual inherits a given recessive gene from each of the parents. While the presence of two recessive genes will almost invariably manifest the abnormality, individuals who are carriers of a single recessive gene for some defect may not give any evidence of the abnormality. Two common childhood conditions that are caused by genetic defects are sickle cell anemia and Down's syndrome. These and other conditions attributed to genetic defects are discussed in later chapters.

External Influences

The environment is more pervasive than many realize, because it includes all the influences that surround and affect an individual. There has been a tendency in recent years to also consider influences that originate within the person as part of the total environment, but this section presents major influences on child growth and development that originate from outside the child.

Cultural Patterns

Groups of people who share common traditions, beliefs, values, and activities and who speak the same language share a common culture. Because cultures differ, attitudes toward children and childrearing practices also must differ. Therefore, behavior of children cannot be analyzed outside of the cultural context.

The lifestyles of many North Americans have produced a significant number of overweight individuals. One researcher has documented that 5% to 16% of North

American children are obese.[45] Once adipose cells have been produced, they cannot be eliminated, only reduced in size. This places the obese child at greater risk for obesity in later developmental stages. Television is a major influence in the development of a sedentary lifestyle and obesity. A large longitudinal study reported in 1985 cites excessive television watching as directly correlated to obesity in children.[16] If families use food as a means of reward or of expressing warmth, comfort, and love, food takes on a symbolic value inconsistent with actual growth need.

Physical exercise promotes physical development. The President's Council on Physical Fitness and Sports reported that one of every six children from middle childhood through adolescence was physically underdeveloped.[21] This and other such reports have resulted in active lobbying to encourage more awareness of physical fitness for all ages and both sexes. In Canada a federally funded fitness awareness program called "Participation" has been aggressively pursued in the last several years with some encouraging results.

The North American "ideal" body image, as depicted on television and in advertising, has had a particularly deleterious effect on female adolescent physical development. The media obsession with "thinness" as the ideal has provoked a significant increase in the serious development disorder anorexia nervosa. The disorder, most common in adolescent girls, affects 10% to 15% of young women between the ages of 12 and 25 years.[55] (Anorexia nervosa is a complex condition discussed in detail in Chapter 19. It is examined here only in the context of physical development.) The anorexic, preoccupied with food and compulsive dieting to the point of starvation, has a number of alterations in normal physical development. Among the more significant are muscle wasting, organic dysfunction, and amenorrhea.

Socioeconomic Status

The socioeconomic level of a family depends on the income, education, and social status of its members. Children who grow up in a family whose parents are frequently unemployed, for example, are considered disadvantaged. The differences between growing up in an advantaged home and in a disadvantaged home are obvious. In disadvantaged homes where parents are continually struggling to survive, children often receive less attention; they may even be ignored or abused. Undernutrition is often a problem for children in families of low socioeconomic status, and health problems are frequently left untreated or are undertreated. Although disadvantaged homes may be noisier and more crowded than advantaged homes, children often receive less intellectual stimulation. However, many children in disadvantaged families thrive in spite of the deprived conditions because their caregivers provide the much needed love and affection.

The recorded observations of men and women maintained over the years have indicated an interesting trend in the rate and age of maturation. In developed countries people are taller and are reaching adult height and sexual maturity earlier than their ancestors.[47] Because this trend has not occurred in underdeveloped countries, it is as-

sumed that better standards of nutrition and standards of living in developed countries are the major reasons for the change. Questions have been raised about food production, particularly the use of hormones in cattle and whether the hormones are passed from cattle to children, influencing maturation. (See Chapter 4 for more information on the economic influences on child development.)

Family Structure

The structure of the American family is in a state of transition. In the past 2 decades, attitudes toward marriage and childrearing have changed dramatically. If current trends continue, approximately 40% of present marriages will end in divorce. Due to divorce and unmarried parenthood, close to 60% of American children younger than 10 years will spend some time in a single-parent home.[46] The majority of these homes are headed by a woman. Although more divorced fathers are gaining custody of their children than ever before, this happens in only 10% of cases.[26] The effects on children of divorce and being reared in a single-parent home are being studied intently, but the findings are not always clear cut. Evidence exists that behavior problems among these children, especially boys, are more frequent than in two-parent families. Families are discussed in Chapters 3 and 5.

Family Functioning

The progressive influx of women into the labor force has been phenomenal in the last decade. Whereas in 1975 about 45% of married women with children younger than 18 were in the labor force, in 1985 it was more than 63%.[65] Women have joined the work force for the personal satisfaction it provides, but principally because they have to earn money to meet their family's financial needs.[41] Research on the two-provider family has focused on the effects of the mother's employment on their children's development as well as on the family's well-being. The effects of having both parents employed vary according to the age and gender of the child and depend on many factors that vary from family to family.[35] One such factor is how the mother feels about her work, because if mothers enjoy working, children are likely to benefit more than children whose mothers are dissatisfied.

Nutrition

Another major influence of growth and development is nutrition. Nutrition influences physical development, intellectual ability, and adaptive bahavior, and all may be irreversibly impaired by undernutrition early in life.[52] The dietary requirements of nutrients have been studied for years, but precise needs are not yet fully known. Individual variations in use of nutrients make the development of an optimal diet for children virtually impossible. Likewise, situational factors such as illness also can alter nutritional needs.

The most significant result of inadequate nutrition in the prenatal and infancy stages is a decrease in brain size. The number of brain cells increases steadily throughout the prenatal period. This growth in brain cell numbers increases, although more slowly, from birth to approximately 6 months of age. From 6 months until early toddlerhood, growth in brain cell numbers continues but is limited. From 12 to 18 months the total complement of brain cells is complete. From toddlerhood to adulthood increase in brain mass is a result of growth in the size of the given number of brain cells already established. Papalia and Olds[47] cite research indicating that the brains of malnourished fetuses and infants contained up to 60% less of the total number of brain cells than fetuses and infants of equivalent age who were adequately nourished. Pipes[48A] further supports the relationship between nutrition and brain size by stating that malnourishment in infancy decreases the total number of brain cells, while malnourishment in childhood decreases brain cell size. The implications of inadequate brain mass are obvious: There is a decrease in intelligence and overall cognitive capacity.

Adequate nutrition can be a concern of parents who are unsure how much the infant or child needs to eat, particularly if the child is a "picky" eater. Table 8-1 identifies the amount of calories required at various ages for growth. The USDA in 1992 presented its Food Guide Pyramid, which goes beyond the previously used basic four food groups. The pyramid represents the USDA's research-based food guidance system. The pyramid appears on the inside cover of the book. Table 8-2 illustrates the breakdown of servings for calorie needs. Studies have shown that when earlier nutritional difficulties are improved in later childhood, the losses in growth potential may never be fully recovered; therefore, parents should be helped to provide adequate nutrition.[55]

Other Influences

External developmental influences are too numerous to list. The impact of school, interactions with teachers and caregivers, church and religious training in the home, opportunities to travel, mass media, and loss of loved ones are just a few of the many influences that could be considered. Many of these important influences in childhood are discussed elsewhere in this text.

TABLE 8-1
Calories Required for Growth by Age

Age	Calories/Kilogram of Body Weight	
0–6 mo	108	
6 mo–1 y	98	
1–3 y	102	
4–6 y	90	
7–10 y	70	
	Males	Females
11–14 y	55	47
15–18 y	45	40

(National Academy of Sciences. [1989]. *Recommended dietary allowances.* (10th rev. ed.). Washington, DC: National Academy of Sciences.)

Characteristics of Growth and Development

Although the growth and development of children are complicated processes and impossible to completely describe, general patterns and trends may be discussed. These principles of growth and development are useful guidelines in assessing, predicting, or evaluating a child's progression in all areas of growth and development, including physical, psychological, social, emotional, cognitive, moral, and spiritual.

Directional Patterns

Growth and development of children are progressive, systematic, and sequential. The principle of directionality is evidenced in several ways. First, progression in growth and development moves from general to specific. In physical growth, for example, general tissue types appear in the embryonic stage and differentiate into tissues that have specific functions. Likewise, in emotional development a general feeling of trust in infancy may develop into an intense attachment directed toward a specific individual in childhood.

Directionality also is expressed by the progression in growth and development from simple to more complex behaviors and abilities. In motor development, for example, simple grasping of objects with the infant's fist soon gives way to use the pincer grasp using only the thumb and first finger to pick up small objects. In language development the toddler demonstrates the ability to gradually pronounce more complex words. Whatever aspect of growth and development, the interested observer may trace progression from a more general action or behavior to the more complex.

Another aspect of directionality that is observed especially in physical growth and development is the progression in cephalocaudal and proximodistal directions (Fig. 8-2). *Cephalocaudal* progression refers to the head-to-toe direction of development, while *proximodistal* refers to the progression from midline to the periphery of the body. Cephalocaudal maturation of the nervous system permits infants to progress from controlling their head movements to sitting, crawling, and finally walking; proximodistal maturation allows the infant to first master total body movements, such as rolling over, to controlling individual body limbs and digits. Although the terms cephalocaudal and proximodistal are generally used when referring to motor development, the same general directional patterns can be seen in other aspects of development as children move from a self-centered existence to a broad social world.

Timeliness

The fact that growth and development are orderly, systematic processes suggests that development of new characteristics, skills, and behaviors may be noticed at certain times. Some child development scientists have

TABLE 8-2
Approximate Food Group Servings Per Day Based on Three Levels of Calorie Needs

Food Group	Source	Number of Servings at Lower Calorie Level: 1600*	Number of Servings at Moderate Calorie Level: 2200†	Number of Servings at Higher Calorie Level: 2800‡
Bread	Bread (contains fiber), ready-to-eat and cooked cereal (iron fortified), rice, spaghetti, noodles, bagel, muffin, biscuit, waffle, pancakes	6	9	11
Vegetable	Vitamin C: asparagus, broccoli, brussels sprouts, cabbage, cauliflower, greens, spinach, tomatoes	3	4	5
	Vitamin A: broccoli, carrots, greens, spinach, sweet potatoes, tomatoes, winter squash			
Fruit	Vitamin C: cantaloupe, grapefruit, honeydew, orange, papaya, strawberries, tangerine	2	3	4
	Vitamin A: apricot, cantaloupe, nectarine, papaya, peach, tangerine, watermelon			
Milk	Milk, cheese, yogurt, soup made with milk	2–3§	2–3§	2–3§
Meat (ounces)	Cooked fish, chicken, turkey, beef, pork, lamb, or liver; cooked beans, peas; peanut butter, cottage cheese; eggs	5	6	7
Total fat (grams)	Fats provide many calories but few nutrients	53	73	93
Total added sugars (teaspoons)	Sweets provide calories but few nutrients	6	12	18

(Data from USDA's Food Guide Pyramid. Prepared by Human Nutrition Information Service, USDA, Home and Garden Bulletin #249, April 1992. Sources from a variety of sources. Details on the previous information may be obtained from the Bulletin.)

* Although they need the same variety as other family members, some preschool children may need less than 1600 calories per day.

† 2200 calories per day are needed for most children and adolescent girls. Pregnant or breast-feeding women may need somewhat more.

‡ 2800 calories per day are needed for adolescent boys.

§ Pregnant or breast-feeding women and adolescents need three servings.

Example of food group servings:

Bread, cereal, rice, and pasta: 1 slice bread; 1 cup ready-to-eat cereal; ½ cup cooked cereal, rice, or pasta

Vegetable: 1 cup raw leafy vegetables; ½ cup other vegetables (cooked or chopped raw); ¾ cup vegetable juice

Fruit: 1 medium apple, banana, or orange; ½ cup chopped cooked or canned fruit; ¾ cup fruit juice

Milk, yogurt, and cheese: 1 cup milk or yogurt; 1½ oz natural cheese; 2 oz processed cheese

Meat, poultry, fish, dry beans, eggs, and nuts: 2–3 oz cooked lean meat, poultry, or fish; ½ cup cooked dry beans (1 egg or 2 tablespoons peanut butter count as 1 oz lean meat)

questioned whether child development is characterized by the presence of *critical periods*, time periods in which an organism is ready for certain activities; if circumstances delay the opportunity for the action to occur, future growth and development are jeopardized. The concept of critical periods has been confirmed in animal studies. Lorenz's[37] study of imprinting, for example, demonstrates that attachment of young ducks and geese to a moving object occurs only during a given period of the bird's early life and is essential to the bird's ability to survive.

Critical periods are known to exist for development of physical features in children, especially in the prenatal period. If, for example, the embryo is exposed to certain teratogens before the 12th week of gestation, the child is at great risk for birth defects. If exposure to the same teratogens occurs after the 12th week when the major body systems have already been differentiated, those birth defects are unlikely. Although other aspects of physical development are markedly affected by nutrition, nurturing, and a host of other influences, specific critical periods are not known to exist.

Although critical periods in the clinical sense have been difficult to confirm in children, agreement does exist that there are sensitive periods in the development of children during which optimum growth and development may be promoted or impeded. When a certain point of growth and maturation has been reached, the child needs interaction with the environment for development to occur. This period of sensitivity may be illustrated in a child's language development. Physical readiness for language must be supplemented by social interactions so that the child can hear sounds and experiment with imitating those sounds. If a child lives in deprived circumstances in which there are no opportunities to imitate and prac-

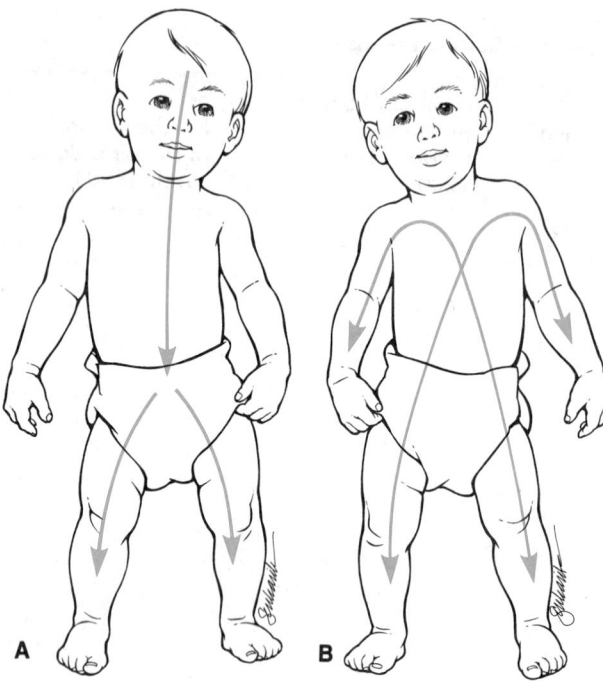

FIGURE 8-2
Principles of growth. (**A**) Cephalocaudal. Growth proceeds from the head to toe or tail. (**B**) Proximodistal. Growth proceeds from the center outward.

tice, language development may be permanently affected adversely. Furthermore, social skills, intellectual skills, and other aspects of development may be threatened, because the deficits are cumulative. A comprehensive knowledge of the growth and development process in children is thus invaluable for recognizing these periods of readiness to learn and providing what is necessary to promote optimal growth and development.

The growth and development of children are predictable and occur in an orderly sequence. Although the precise ages for the development of abilities cannot be given, general norms are recognized. For example social smiles in infants may be expected around 2 months of age, walking around 1 year, and the ability to read around 6 years. General time frames for the sequential appearance of these *developmental milestones* have been established through countless studies of child development and are an essential component of the knowledge base of those who provide care for children.

Pace

Although sequential patterns of many aspects of growth and development are known, the process is hardly consistent in pace. At times children give evidence of tremendous spurts in development, and at other times plateaus occur when little change is apparent. Cycles of behavior also may be noticed, particularly in the emotional development of children. The comparisons between the behavior of 2 year olds and adolescents in attempting to gain independence will reveal similarities, for example. Human growth occurs steadily with the rate very rapid during the first 2 years, slower but steady dur-

ing early childhood, slowest in middle childhood (lagging), and advancing rapidly during early adolescence (spurting).

Growth rates are more logical indicators of growth sensitivity than the concept of critical growth periods. The "spurt" and "lag" aspects of growth can be correlated directly with the rate of organ growth. Each body system, lymphoid, neural, skeletal, and reproductive, has specific rates and peaks of growth. There appears to be only two specific times when all systems tend to peak or spurt together. These times are birth to 2 years and early adolescence. Adolescence is the only period actually described as having a growth "spurt." Although there is a wide range of normality, the apex of the adolescent growth spurt occurs on average for girls at age 11½ years and for boys at age 14 years.[21]

Individual Differences

Development of characteristics or abilities occurs within widely varying time frames, and individual differences are to be expected. The pace of growth and development is specific for each child, governed by internal and external influences unique to the individual. Assessment of aspects of a child's growth and development should therefore focus not on one specific ability or characteristic, but on several aspects of development. More important than whether the child fits standard tables of norms is whether the child's own pattern of development is consistent. A child who has shown normal or precocious development and who subsequently begins to lag behind, for example, is giving evidence of disrupted development.

Catch-Up Growth

Catch-up growth occurs when deficits (e.g., inadequate nutrition) to growth are corrected. It is literally a time when the child grows more quickly to "catch-up" to the growth phase that would have been apparent had the deficit not been present. Catch-up growth can occur any time in childhood but may be most visible, for example, in the premature infant. In such an infant growth and developmental delays appear to be directly related to the level of prematurity. For example an infant who is 8 weeks premature may be expected to be developmentally delayed by approximately 2 months. After the first year the lag time in development lessens, and by the preschool years most premature infants without other insults reach the normal growth curve. Most children born prematurely without significant problems will catch up (Fig. 8-3). Catch-up growth at any stage of development does have upper limits. If the deficit is severe and prolonged, particularly during peak developmental phases, permanent growth impairment may occur.

Interrelatedness of Developmental Components

Human development is an extremely complex process that occurs throughout the life span. Processes reg-

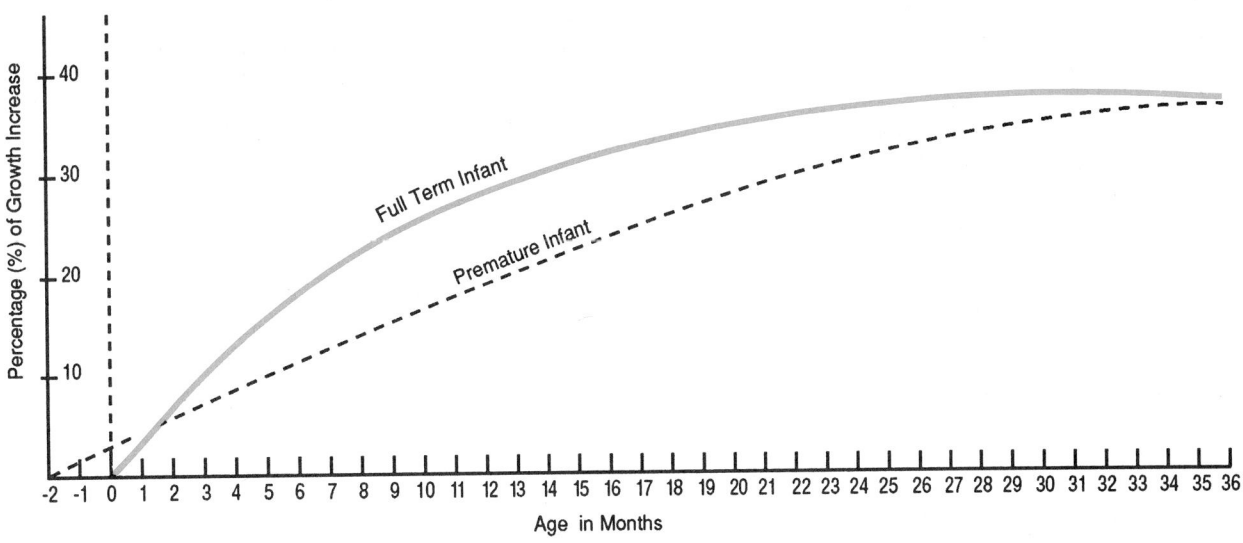

FIGURE 8-3
Catch-up growth. The preterm infant's growth rate slowly increases so that by approximately age 3, the child has caught up to the full-term infant.

ulating physical growth and development are somewhat better understood than other aspects simply because many facets can be studied with physical evidence in the laboratory. The processes of cognitive, emotional, social, and other aspects of development are not as accessible for study and thus are less well understood. Nevertheless, the processes of growth and development are interdependent, and disturbance in one area of development gives rise to the risk that other aspects of growth and development will be affected.

Theoretical Approaches to Child Development

The scientific study of children has attracted scholars from many of the biologic, social, and behavioral sciences. Science cannot provide absolute and enduring truth about the development of all children, but it can provide evidence that promotes understanding of the developmental process. Theories of child development can be used to explain and predict behavior in children. No one theory, however, can provide a comprehensive view of child development; typically, each theory concentrates on only one aspect of development. Thus, several theoretical views of the developing child need to be considered. The following sections present a brief synopsis of common approaches to the study of human development from social, mental, moral, spiritual, and self-esteem perspectives.

Psychosocial Development

Freud's Theory

The founder of psychoanalytic theory, Sigmund Freud (1856 to 1939), advanced his belief that human behavior is motivated by forces deep within the individual's mind that are usually unconscious. Biologic drives and instincts

prompt individuals to action, and through experiences in the external environment, the personality develops and contributes to psychosexual and psychosocial development. The psychoanalytic approach, then, is the examination of mental phenomena, especially the emotions, to discover the origins and meanings of overt behavior.

Study of *personality development* was one of Freud's central interests.[64] Although difficult to define, personality may be considered the core of individual traits and characteristics that are consistent and stable with time. Freud described three components of the human personality, each having separate functions: the id, ego, and superego. The *id* is evident at birth and is made up of all the innate biologic urges or instincts to seek pleasure. Observation of infants reveals that their most powerful urge is to seek immediate satisfaction of impulses such as hunger or discomfort. Unlike the process of the id, which is unconscious, the *ego* emerges out of a realization of what is possible and what is not. The ego is the conscious and rational component of the personality. Formed during the first year of life, the infant's ego tests the limits of the real world. Infants who are mentally retarded fail to develop a properly functioning ego and must be protected from the dangers that the id impulses may induce. Normally evidence of the third personality component, the *superego*, appears in early childhood and encompasses all the internalized values and rules of behavior that are formed through the child's interaction with parents and others. Development of the superego enables growing children to exert internal control over their own behavior instead of relying exclusively on external controls. Presence of the superego creates feelings of guilt when the internal moral code is broken; likewise, feelings of pride are generated when that code is followed.

Freud taught that these three forces, the id, ego, and superego, operate in every child's personality and that a healthy balance among the components is necessary for the development of socially acceptable behaviors. This description of the personality, however, is incomplete without mention of *ego defenses*. These unconscious mechanisms are irrational but help individuals cope with the feelings of anxiety created by the ongoing struggle between the id and the superego. Created by the ego, defense mechanisms assist the personality to operate in an apparently healthy manner, but their excessive use may be considered unhealthy. Because these mechanisms frequently are used by children when coping with environmental change, common ego defenses are described further in Chapter 17.

Another of Freud's primary interests was *psychosexual development*.[64] Psychoanalytic theory explains that personality development is closely related to the psychological aspects of sexual development. From infancy into adolescence, innate energy or tensions are manifested, and individuals seek gratification in a succession of targeted body areas. Each area represents a stage of the child's life and is the focus of pleasurable sensation during that period of time. The developing ego and superego thus occur as psychosexual development progresses through a sequence of five stages. Each stage, described in Table 8-3, builds on and elaborates previous stages, but the transition from one stage to another may be blurred and may occur in variable time frames that reflect a child's individuality.

Freud's Theory Critiqued. The psychoanalytic approach to development has had far-reaching impact on our understanding of human behavior. Freud's elaborate and complex theory supplied the concepts and terms needed to explain the process of development, and it has been responsible for heightening sensitivity to the influence of early childhood experiences on later outcomes. Although Freud may be considered one of the most influential of all social thinkers and theorists, the theory itself is open to serious criticism.

A fundamental flaw in Freud's theory is that it is based on a very limited number of observations, most of which were collected by Freud on individuals who suffered from various forms of mental illness. The rigors of scientific investigation were not applied to the development of his theory; rather, an intuitive approach was taken. Rothstein[53] and others therefore claim that Freud's theory must be considered weak from a scientific point of view.

Another deficit in Freud's theory is that different, and sometimes directly opposed, predictions of human be-

TABLE 8-4
Erikson's Stages of Psychosocial Development

Approximate Age	Primary Conflict
Birth–1 y	Trust versus mistrust
1–3 y	Autonomy versus shame and doubt
4–5 y	Initiative versus guilt
6–11 y	Industry versus inferiority
12–18 y	Identity versus identity diffusion
Young adult	Intimacy versus isolation
Adult	Generativity versus stagnation
Older adult	Ego integrity versus despair

havior can be based on it. Consideration also should be given to the fact that the theory relies heavily on hypothetical unconscious processes that are not directly measurable. When measurable aspects of Freud's theory have been subjected to well-designed research, they have not always been supported.

The aspect of Freud's theory that has generated the most criticism concerns his excessive emphasis on sexual and aggressive impulses as the principal determining forces in the development of personality. Although Freud's preoccupation with sexual repression and male domination might be explained in light of the Victorian era in which the theory was developed, many today find his views offensive. The concept most vigorously challenged is that of penis envy, which suggests that girls are inferior because of the absence of male genitalia. Freud's[23] description of mature women as masochistic, passive, narcissistic, and victims of an "anatomic tragedy," has been strongly criticized by innumerable scholars.

Erikson's Theory

In an extension of psychoanalytic theory, Erik Erikson downplayed the role of sexuality and instead placed new emphasis on the environment in human development.[17,18] He believed that not only do biologic forces shape human development, but also social, historic, and cultural influences. Furthermore, Erikson envisioned the persistence of psychosocial development throughout the life span, while Freud's stages of psychosexual development ended at adolescence. Erikson described eight age-related stages that may be characterized by a dominant psychological conflict. The crises are brought about primarily by the person's need to adapt to the social environment, and a particular type of personality development must occur to resolve each crisis. The crisis of one stage must be resolved if the next stage is to be successfully achieved, but evidence of earlier or later conflicts may be recognized at any stage of development. The conflicts that dominate each stage of psychosocial development are listed in Table 8-4 and described below.

During infancy a conflict begins between the tendency to mistrust a world that is poorly understood and the opposite tendency to develop a trusting attitude toward that world. Erikson believed that trust is the most basic component of a healthy personality and that the

TABLE 8-3
Freud's Stages of Psychosexual Development

Stage	Age	Activities
Oral	Birth–2 y	Pleasure obtained from exploration of objects with mouth and sucking.
Anal	2–3 y	Control of elimination of body wastes.
Phallic	3–6 y	Exploration of genitalia. Attraction for opposite-sex parent and hostility for same-sex parent.
Latent	6–12 y	Dormant sexual feelings. Identification with same-sex parent.
Genital	12–18 y	Pleasure from elimination and masturbation. Development of heterosexual relationships.

infant is presented with multiple opportunities to experience the conflict of *trust versus mistrust*. The role of the care provider in infancy thus cannot be underestimated, because trust is built on the sense that people in the infant's world can be counted on to provide comfort and care. If the infant's world is chaotic and unpredictable and the affection of the caregivers is absent, the infant develops a sense of mistrust, feeling anxious and insecure in social interactions.

The second stage of psychosocial development evolves from the conflicting feelings of *autonomy versus shame and doubt*. During infancy children react to the surrounding world, but in the toddler years children begin to realize that they are able to initiate many of their own actions; often they can control the course of events. The ability to gain control over body functions (especially bowel and bladder) serves as a prototype of control over inner urges and feelings. Although these feelings of autonomy begin to develop, toddlers also are threatened by violent emotions and an inclination not to accept responsibility for their actions. If care providers overprotect children, stifle their attempts to explore the environment, or offer criticism and punishment instead of praise, then children develop shame, doubt, and uncertainty about themselves and their abilities. If, however, care providers nurture with guidance and affection a child's attempts to exert independence, then feelings of competence and self-confidence begin to develop.

During the preschool years children experience conflicting feelings of *initiative versus guilt*. With increased exploration of their environment children develop a sense of initiative in their behaviors, becoming more responsible for their own actions. They enjoy being active and will plan and execute tasks of their own design, often using role play to explore social functions of adults. Care providers who encourage a child to explore, plan, and work toward goals are promoting a sense of purpose and direction and ultimately the development of feelings of moral responsibility. In contrast, care providers who are unsupportive of a child's activities and restrict exploration of the environment foster feelings of guilt for making those attempts.

The fourth stage of psychosocial development is characterized by feelings of *industry versus inferiority*. During the school years children realize what can be accomplished through their own efforts. They replace the vagaries of play with the ability to complete productive situations, often in settings of formal instruction. If the child's industry is supported and encouraged, positive feelings of self-esteem and accomplishment result. On the other hand a lack of support and encouragement is likely to result in the child's withdrawal from attempts to learn new skills and the development of feelings of inadequacy and inferiority.

The fifth stage of psychosocial development occurs during adolescence. In the transition from childhood to adulthood adolescents experience many changes in physical and intellectual development, and these changes are accompanied by the desire to redefine themselves not only in terms of who they are, but also in terms of what they will become. The struggle between the attempts to establish a *personal identity versus role confusion* demands the integration of past learning, inner feelings, and future expectations. In the face of many choices and a wide range of societal expectations, the adolescent must begin to establish a sense of self, make decisions about friendships, determine what kind of lifestyle is desired, and explore the possibilities for life work. Adolescents may over identify with popular heroes if they are having difficulty clarifying their own identity, but nurturing and understanding caregivers and friends can provide security, guidance, and support, thus facilitating psychosocial development through these confusing years.

The remaining three stages of psychosocial development described by Erikson occur during the adult years, each presenting a new psychological crisis that must be confronted and resolved. Erikson's theory thus describes optimal development of the healthy personality throughout a lifetime of continuous change. With less than optimum development, however, the theory allows for old developmental conflicts to be confronted again. The person may then make new attempts to resolve the crisis, thereby achieving a better balance between the opposing personality forces.

Erikson's Theory Critiqued. In contrast to Freud's exploration of maladjusted personalities, Erikson's observations were used to develop a theory that describes the development of a healthy personality. His appealing and somewhat idealized view of human development over the life span is tempered by the recognition that, like's Freud's work, the theory is difficult to validate experimentally. Another general criticism of Erikson's work is that the chronologic ages assigned for each stage can only suggest a general sequence of events, especially during adulthood. The social and physical changes of childhood are more predictable in children. Erikson's theory of psychosocial development has provided greater insight into the process of human development, and his work has been widely used in the behavioral sciences.

In spite of the criticism of psychoanalytic theory, it remains a rich reservoir for ideas that promote an understanding of children and the development of their personalities. The observations and theories originally presented by Freud and extended by others like Erikson have spawned much research and discussion in academic and clinical arenas, and new theories of child development have resulted.

Temperament

People who have had an opportunity to work with newborns often comment on how each baby is different and responds to the environment in different ways. Some babies are "good" babies, and some are "difficult." Thomas and Chess[63] began the New York Longitudinal Studies (NYLS) in 1956 when they became interested in the behavioral individuality of children in the first weeks of life. Their work has been the cornerstone of examining and studying temperament in children. Temperament is defined as "the manner of thinking, behaving, or reacting characteristic of an individual."[12] Temperament is not a qualitative judgment, but a description of how an infant and later child and adult interacts with his or her environment and how the people within that environment respond. The importance of examining the temperament

TABLE 8-5
Temperament Characteristics of Infants

Characteristic	Infant
Activity level	The motor activity present during bathing, eating, playing, dressing, handling; the proportion of active and inactive periods.
Rhythmicity (regularity)	Predictability in the timing of basic functions such as eating, sleeping, and elimination. School-age students are assessed on predictability by examining the quality of organization.
Approach/withdrawal	Initial response to a new stimulus. Approach responses are positive (smiling, moving toward an object). Withdrawal responses are negative (crying, fussing, moving away).
Adaptability	The ease of accepting new situations and the ease with which initial responses are adjusted or modified.
Threshold of responsiveness	The level of intensity required to evoke a discernible response.
Intensity of reaction	The energy level of the response, irrespective of quality or direction.
Quality of mood	The amount of pleasant, joyful, and friendly behavior as compared to unpleasant, crying, and unfriendly behavior.
Distractibility	Effectiveness of extraneous environmental stimuli in altering the direction of the ongoing behavior.
Attention span and persistence	Attention span is the length of time the child is engaged in an activity. Persistence is the continuation of an activity in the face of obstacles.

(Adapted from Thomas, A. & Chess, A. [1977]. *Temperament and development.* New York: Brunner and Mazel; and Hegvik, et al. [1982]. The middle childhood temperament questionnaire. *Journal of Developmental and Behavioral Pediatrics, 3*(4), 197–200.)

of infants is to begin to assess the parent–infant interaction. Temperament theory asserts that children respond to novel situations in predictable manners.[40] Chess and Thomas[12] refer to the "goodness of fit" in describing these relationships. Goodness of fit postulates that healthy functioning and development occur when the abilities

and characteristics of the child are compatible with the expectations and demands of the environment. Thus, a nurse in a well-baby clinic can begin to assess babies and their environments and help parents cope with situations in which there is a poor fit. To understand the concept of goodness of fit, one begins by exploring how temperament is assessed and categorized.

Table 8-5 defines the nine characteristics that are assessed when determining a child's temperament. Activity level, rhythmicity, approach–withdrawal, adaptability, threshold of responsiveness, intensity of reaction, quality of mood, distractability, attention span, and persistence are used to form temperament constellations. The three temperament constellations are the easy child, the difficult child, and the slow to warm up child, as summarized in the accompanying display. The easy child has regular or predictable sleep–wake cycles, approaches new situations easily and positively, and adapts readily to changes.

The importance of studying temperament is to assist parents in understanding their baby's or child's reactions to new situations or changes. The parent can help the slow to warm up child have a positive rather than negative response by understanding that the child needs time to adjust to new friends, a new baby-sitter, a new playground, a new way home from school, and so forth. The difficult child may need even more support from a parent to handle changes in his or her world. The parents should know that the child is not trying to be difficult, negative, or hard to manage but is is reacting to change in his or her own way.

Multiple strategies have been developed for assessing children's temperaments. Although most parents and nurses will not use the formal method of identifying temperament, the nurse should be aware that such methods are available.

Cognitive Approaches

Piaget's Theory

Psychoanalytic theories are concerned primarily with aspects of personality development, but others have ex-

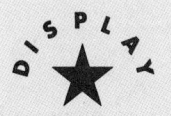

Temperament Constellations

EASY CHILD

Regularity of biologic functions (predictable)
Positive approach responses to new experiences
High adaptability to change
Mild or moderately intense mood (mostly positive)

DIFFICULT CHILD

Irregularity in biologic functions (unpredictable)
Negative withdrawal responses to new stimuli
Slow adaptability to change
Intense mood expressions (negative)

SLOW TO WARM UP CHILD

Displays a combination of behaviors
Active
Mild negative responses to new stimuli
Slow adaptability (repeated contacts help)
Less irregularity of biologic function than the difficult child
Some negative moods
Develops gradually, quiet and positive interest and involvement

plored the cognitive (intellectual) development of children. The theory presented by the Swiss biologist Jean Piaget (1896 to 1980) describes child development as the emergence of progressively more logical forms of thinking.[64] The ability to think, reason, and understand may be traced through stages of childhood as the child adapts to the environment.

Although cognitive development is considered a continuous process, Piaget's theory divides childhood into four major periods. Transitions from one stage to another are not abrupt but occur gradually with time as children adapt to their environment. For Piaget the mental representation of a behavior is known as a *scheme*, and some are present at birth. The sucking scheme, for example, is derived from a basic reflexive action. The mental processes of *assimilation* and *accommodation* interact to assist in the adaptation process. Assimilation involves using activities that are already known, while accommodation requires that behavior already learned be modified to fit present needs and demands. Each stage of cognitive development is characterized by a distinctly different way of viewing the world and adapting to it. Table 8-6 summarizes the stages and characteristics of Piaget's theory.

During the first 2 years of life a child is in the *sensorimotor period*, when he or she understands the world primarily through immediate sensation and action. During this stage the concept of object permanence is developed. At first infants have no understanding that when objects disappear, they may still exist. Toward the age of 2 years, however, they realize that objects have a permanence and an identity of their own. The toddler also begins to acquire language, thereby moving toward symbolic thinking.

The *preoperational period* emerges at approximately 2 years and lasts until the child is about 7 years. The increasing use of representational thought characterizes this stage of development when words and other symbols are used as substitutes for the actual object or action. At this age children also begin to recall past events and solve problems, but they rely more on their own perception of circumstances rather than logical reasoning. For example the same amount of water poured into different-shaped containers will not be equal in the child's eye. The period of *concrete operations* lasts from about 7 until about 11 or 12 years of age. During this stage children develop the ability to think operationally. In Piaget's theory an operation is a mental action performed on ideas according to certain rules of logic. The school-age child's logic, however, is bound to real, concrete objects and events.

They have difficulty thinking abstractly about hypothetical situations or events.

The fourth stage of cognitive development is characterized by *formal operations*. From age 11 or 12 to adulthood, children develop the ability to manipulate abstract ideas. Thinking becomes as logical as it will ever become, and adolescents are able to solve increasingly complex verbal problems. Cognitive development is considered essentially complete at this time.

Piaget's Theory Critiqued. Because Piaget's theory makes specific predictions about how average children function intellectually at different age levels, a great number of these predictions have been tested through well-designed research. Although the order of Piaget's stages of cognitive development has been confirmed, much variation has been noted in the age ranges in which these events occur, and findings suggest that the theory may underestimate the reasoning abilities of young children but overestimate the reasoning abilities of adolescents.[11] Piaget's theory therefore has limited usefulness in explaining individual differences among children. Likewise, Piaget's theory fails to suggest how cognitive development can be promoted in children.

In spite of criticisms now addressed to Piaget's theory, it remains useful in providing a basic understanding of how children think. His approach to cognitive development has raised important questions that are still being explored today about the thinking abilities of infants and young children. Like Freud's psychoanalytic theory, Piaget's theory has been the stepping stone for additional research and the development of new theories.

Information Processing Theory

In the past 2 decades Piaget's exploration of the phenomenon of cognition has taken a new turn through the inquiry of several developmental psychologists. The most popular approach to studying children's thinking today is called *information processing* theory, and this approach describes how ideas are organized, stored, and used.[60] The term processing refers to mental activities, such as sorting, analyzing, rehearsing, summarizing, and other similar strategies that children use to learn about their environment. Age and experience are strongly correlated with the child's development of these cognitive skills.

Information Processing Critiqued. A serious comparison of the Piagetian and information processing views on cognitive development would reveal similarities. Both attempt to describe the cognitive abilities of children at various points in development and to explain how children become able to understand concepts. Both approaches also emphasize the importance that existing understandings have on children's ability to acquire new understandings.[60] Differences in the two approaches also are apparent. Information processing theory places more emphasis on describing in detail the mechanisms that cause thinking to change than the Piagetian approach. Likewise, information processing theories value knowing how adults think to achieve a clearer understanding of the progressive development of thinking abilities in children.

TABLE 8-6
Piaget's Cognitive Theory

Stage	Age	Characteristics
Sensorimotor, six substages	Birth–2 y	Development of senses, motor activity
Preoperational, two substages	2–7 y	Beginning of intellectual ability
Concrete operations	7–11 y	Reasoning, organizing, relationships
Formal operations	11 y–death	Abstract thinking, deductive reasoning

Although information processing has become a popular way of studying cognitive development, that approach has been subject to criticism on the grounds that it too is inadequate to completely explain the complexities of cognitive development.

Case[11] acknowledged the value of the previous theories and cited the need for a new theory that would incorporate the strengths of previous theories that dealt with the structure and processes of cognition and eliminate their weaknesses. Thinking of children as problem solvers using mental procedures called executive strategies was proposed as an alternative to other approaches. The significance of this complex model in the evolution of cognitive development research remains to be seen.

Behavioristic Approaches

Skinner's Theory

While psychoanalytic and cognitive approaches to child development focus on the internal processes of feeling and thinking, behavioristic approaches are primarily interested in observable actions.[64] Foundations of behaviorism were introduced by a psychologist named Edward L. Thorndike, who did experiments with cats, and were later popularized by John B. Watson. However, behaviorism as an approach to human development flourished under the intense investigation of B. F. Skinner (1904 to 1991), an American psychologist. The central tenet underlying behaviorism is that the behavior of humans is lawful and follows rigid rules of cause and effect. Thus, human behavior is perfectly predictable but only if all the laws about behavior are understood and if the environment is completely controlled.

Skinner developed an elaborate theoretical model on the concept of conditioning. Unlike Pavlov's interest in *classical conditioning* (achieving the desired response by substituting one stimulus for another, such as dogs salivating at the sound of a bell instead of the appearance of food), Skinner was intrigued by the concept of *operant conditioning*, in which behavior is changed by altering the environmental antecedents and consequences. Behaviors that are rewarded (reinforced) are repeated, and those that are not reinforced or are punished are extinguished. With reinforcement children can learn to perform complicated actions that would not have been learned otherwise.

Behavior modification is a method of controlling behavior that applies principles of conditioning and has been used extensively with children. Any actions considered undesirable are either negatively reinforced or punished. For example a child who hits a care provider may be given negative reinforcement (e.g., ignored) or punished (e.g., sent to an empty room for "time out"). In contrast any action that moves toward desirable behavior is positively reinforced. Increasing the appeal of the reward allows behavior to be shaped until it reaches the desired level.

Skinner's Theory Critiqued.
Skinner's emphasis on environmental influences in shaping human personalities and behaviors has contrasted sharply with other theories that emphasize the biologic aspects of development. The notions that behavior can always be explained by identifying the objective stimulus conditions in which it occurs and that all learning depends on reinforcement may be considered a denial of innate influences that also may exert control. The assumed absence of innate drives and instincts renders the individual as simply a reactor to environmental stimuli and not the initiator of actions, a mechanistic view that many child development scholars find distasteful.

Another criticism is that Skinner's theory cannot explain the development of conceptual processes, such as analyzing, problem solving, and evaluating. Rather, the behavioristic approach is most useful for explaining actual behavior and some types of learning, including the learning of emotional responses, and for explaining the effectiveness of rewards and punishments. Additionally, behavior modification techniques have been extremely useful in a wide variety of settings.

Bandura's Theory

Another American psychologist interested in human learning processes is Albert Bandura (1925), who applied behaviorism to child development in an approach known as *social learning theory*.[4] This view of child development supports the idea that much of human behavior is acquired by observing the behavior of others and sometimes imitating it. Imitative behavior does depend on reinforcement but not necessarily to oneself. Watching other people and seeing what happens when they do something provides instruction to individuals about what is desirable behavior for them. Rewards for learning do not have to be concrete, but they may be social responses, such as attention, affection, and praise. Bandura differentiated between the acquisition of new responses and the performance of them. What is learned is not a response but an idea.

Bandura's Theory Critiqued.
Although Bandura's[4] theory of social learning extends the scholarship of Skinner and other behaviorists, it remains heavily dependent on the concept of operant conditioning and thereby is subject to the criticism mentioned previously. Social learning theory does not systematically describe a sequence of stages, but explains that similarities among children in development are attributable to environmental regulation and the learning process. This view of development provides an alternative explanation for how learning occurs, but it leaves unexplained phenomena such as creativity and the development of other conceptual processes.

Humanistic Approach

Maslow's Theory

Humanistic psychologists emphasize the uniqueness of the individual child and the importance of perceiving the world as the child experiences it. Abraham Maslow's (1908 to 1970) work represents this approach to human development.

Maslow was primarily concerned with the development of the healthy personality, and he believed that two systems of needs motivate behavior.

Basic needs are both physiologic (e.g., food and drink) and psychological (including security, love, and esteem), and deficiencies in these areas must be met before other needs can be considered. *Metaneeds* are at a higher level than basic needs and include the individual's desire to know, to appreciate beauty and truth, and to become self-actualized or fulfilled as a person. Figure 8-4 presents this hierarchy of human needs. Humanists place much stress on environmental conditions that stimulate the full development of a person's potential, and the individual is viewed as fully participating in the developmental process.

Maslow's Theory Critiqued. The humanist approach to studying human development does not readily lend itself to the formation of theories that need to be very specific but also widely applicable. However, Maslow's theory is valuable in that it can illuminate aspects of development that are not easily explained by any other theories. His view of self-actualization as an essentially positive and self-directed process that guides the direction of development is an appealing contrast to the more mechanistic, less inner-directed theories described by others.

Moral Development

As part of the study of cognitive development in children Piaget studied the phenomenon of moral reasoning in children. Moral behavior has been defined as behavior that is intended to be good, just, and fair.[57]

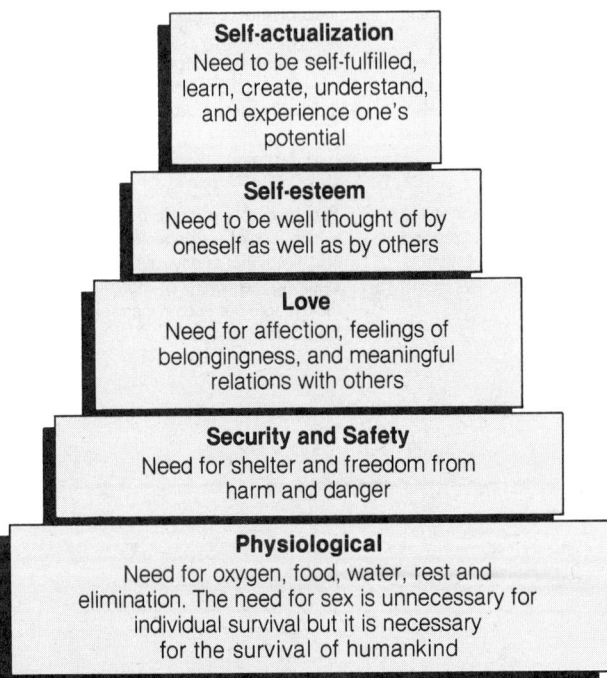

FIGURE 8-4
Maslow's hierarchy of needs.

Kohlberg's Theory

The American psychologist Lawrence Kohlberg (1927 to 1987) greatly extended Piaget's work.[77] Kohlberg believed that moral behavior is a matter of the person's ability to make decisions rather than strength of conscience. As children learn to internalize rules of behavior, their morality develops in a progression of three levels. Table 8-7 outlines the stages of moral development, the consequences of action, and the social implications of the stage. In addition to internalizing parental or societal rules or standards, moral behavior includes developing empathic reactions and acquiring personal standards.[57]

In the first level of moral development children younger than age 9 are considered *preconventional* or premoral. At this level children are concerned primarily with the possibility of "getting caught" in questionable activities, and they judge right and wrong on the basis of the likely outcome. Activity that would be punished is considered wrong, and that which is obedient to the given rules is considered good. Likewise, what gives the child personal pleasure is right, while that which brings undesirable consequences is considered bad.

In the second level of moral development, the *conventional* level, children seek approval from significant people, including parents, teachers, and peers. After the age of 9 years or so, children have a desire to conform to social rules of behavior. They have respect for a higher authority who defines what is right or wrong. Kohlberg believed that most Americans remain at this second level of morality all their lives.

At the highest *postconventional level* of moral development, children are able to view right and wrong in terms of individual rights and as ideals or principles. The approval of others or the possibility of negative consequence is overshadowed by personal feelings of what is good or right behavior.

Kohlberg's Theory Critiqued. Intense research on Kohlberg's theory has resulted in criticism of several points of his views on moral development. Longitudinal studies, for example, have not always supported Kohlberg's claim that the three levels of moral development are achieved in invariable sequence. Individuals at times are observed to regress from a higher to a lower level of development. Other studies have shown wide discrepancies between what individuals say about hypothetical situations and their behavior when faced with the actual situation. Finally, Carol Gilligan[25] has challenged the validity of Kohlberg's stages of moral development for women. Her research suggests that women are more concerned with relationships and responsibilities than men, and women therefore make moral decisions with these considerations. In contrast men are more concerned with legal rights and rules than women. Because Kohlberg's theory was structured around rules and the data collected were initially from 10- to 16-year-old boys, Gilligan[25] contends that the stages of moral development described in Kohlberg's theory are not a valid standard by which to judge moral reasoning in women.

Kohlberg[49] has continued his work in moral development and has applied his theory to moral education in the form of cluster schools. These schools are based on

TABLE 8-7
Kohlberg's Six Stages of Moral Judgment

Level and Stage	Content of Stage		
	What is Right	Reasons for Doing Right	Social Perspective of Stage
LEVEL I. Preconventional Stage 1: Heteronomous morality	Avoiding breaking rules backed by punishment; obedience for its own sake; avoiding physical damage to persons and property.	Avoidance of punishment and the superior power of authorities.	*Egocentric point of view.* Doesn't consider the interests of others or recognize that they differ from the actor's; doesn't relate two points of view. Actions are considered physically rather than in terms of psychological interests of others. Confusion of authority's perspective with one's own.
Stage 2: Individualism, instrumental purpose, and exchange	Following rules only when it is to someone's immediate interest; acting to meet own interests and needs and letting others do the same. Right is also what's fair, an equal exchange, a deal, an agreement.	Serving own needs or interests in a world where other people have their interests too.	*Concrete individualistic perspective.* Aware that everybody has his or her own interest to pursue and these conflict, so right is relative (in the concrete individualistic sense).
LEVEL II. Conventional Stage 3: Mutual interpersonal expectations, relationships, and interpersonal conformity	Living up to what is expected by people close to you or what people generally expect of people in your role as son, brother, friend, and so forth. "Being good" is important and means having good motives, showing concern about others. It also means keeping mutual relationships, such as trust, loyalty, respect, and gratitude.	Needing to be a good person in own eyes and those of others. Caring for others. Belief in the golden rule. Desire to maintain rules and authority that support stereotypically good behavior.	*Perspective of the individual in relationships with other individuals.* Aware of shared feelings, agreements, and expectations that take priority over individual interests. Relates points of view through the concrete golden rule, putting yourself in the other person's shoes. Does not yet consider generalized system perspective.
Stage 4: Social system and conscience	Fulfilling the actual duties to which you have agreed. Laws are to be upheld except in extreme cases when they conflict with other fixed social duties. Right is also contributing to society, the group, or institution.	Keeping the institution going as a whole; avoiding the breakdown in the system "if everyone did it" or the imperative of conscience to meet defined obligations (easily confused with stage 3 belief in rules and authority).	*Differentiation of societal points of view from interpersonal agreement or motives.* Takes the point of view of the system that defines roles and rules. Considers individual relations in terms of place in the system.
LEVEL III. Postconventional or principled Stage 5: Social contract or utility and individual rights	Being aware that people hold a variety of values and opinions, that most values and rules are relative to your group. These relative rules should usually be upheld, however, in the interest of impartiality and because they are the social contract. Some nonrelative values and rights like *life* and *liberty*, however, must be upheld in any society and regardless of majority opinion.	A sense of obligation to law because of social contract to make and abide by laws for the welfare of all and for the protection of all people's rights. A feeling of contractual commitment, freely entered upon, to family, friendship, trust, and work obligation. Concern that laws and duties are based on rational calculation of overall utility, "the greatest good for the greatest number."	*Prior-to-society perspective.* Perspective of a rational individual aware of values and rights prior to social attachments and contracts. Integrates perspectives by formal mechanisms of agreements, contract, objective impartiality, and due process. Considers moral and legal points of view; recognizes that they sometimes conflict and finds it difficult to integrate them.
Stage 6: Universal ethical principles	Following self-chosen ethical principles. Particular laws or social agreements are usually valid because they rest on such principles. When laws violate these principles, one acts in accordance with the principle. Principles are universal principles of justice: the equality of human rights and respect for the dignity of human beings as individuals.	The belief as a rational person in the validity of universal moral principles and a sense of personal commitment to them.	*Perspective of a moral point of view from which social arrangements derive.* Perspective is that of any rational individual recognizing the nature of morality or the fact that people are ends in themselves and must be treated as such.

(Source: Kohlberg, L. [1984]. *Essays on moral development* (Vol. 2). San Francisco: Harper & Row.)

the premise that moral development is learned, and therefore environmental and educational activities can be used to influence a child's ability to make moral judgments.[49]

Spiritual Development

Spirituality refers to a person's beliefs about a larger meaning of life, a divine being, and the "natural" goodness of people.

Fowler's Theory

James Fowler[26] described developmental stages associated with creating conceptions of ultimate reality and answering questions such as "What is the meaning of life?" Fowler's work is based on that of Piaget, Kohlberg, and Erikson. Fowler[22] defined faith as a way of seeing life in holistic images. An image is an inner representation and one's feelings about a state of affairs. Fowler describes the stages as dynamic and connected in a spiral, with each stage linking and adding to the previous one. "The *contents* of the individual's faith (as opposed to its structure) consist of centers of value (those concerns of greatest worth), images of power (that which sustains the individual in difficult times), and master stories (our interpretive stories about events that affect our lives)."[52]

Undifferentiated faith (infancy) is a prestage in which the groundwork for positive emotions (love and trust) are formed and the environment is safe. Infants have no concept of right or wrong and have no beliefs. The infant does not fear abandonment or deprivation, and this beginning of trust through the relationships with parents and caregivers provides the foundation for faith. The first stage emerges with the acquisition of language.

Stage 1, intuitive-projective faith (early childhood), is "a fantasy-filled imitative phase in which the child can be permanently influenced" by the faith of the parents.[61] Children begin to imitate their parents and accept their beliefs and values without understanding the meanings.

Stage 2, mythic-literal faith, occurs during the school years. As the child's cognitive development continues, the child is able to acquire beliefs from experiences in the community, church or synagogue, or school. The existence of a deity is accepted, and children may expect rewards for good behavior. At the same time children may feel that they have "caused" bad things to happen to others through wishing or asking for something to happen. The child with a sick sibling or parent may be worried about being responsible for the illness. Children begin to feel bad when they have misbehaved; a conscience is developing.

Stage 3, synthetic-conventional faith, is a time when adolescents synthesize values and information from divergent sources (e.g., school, work, peers, media, and religious groups) to form a sense of identity and a perspective on life. As adolescents begin to reason and question the beliefs of others, they may experience spiritual dissonance. The transition to the next stage of spiritual development may be precipitated by the contradictions between religious authority and personal experiences that lead the adolescent to reflect and question his or her beliefs and values.

Stage 4, individual-reflective faith (young adulthood), is reflective of the change in identity; the young adult's self-identity is differentiated from others. The young adult distinguishes between his or her viewpoints and others, translates symbols into conceptual means, and seeks to eliminate myths. The young adult is making personal decisions about his or her faith, beliefs, and patterns.

The last two stages are not part of childhood and adolescence, but are a part of a person's continuing growth and development.

Stage 5, conjunctive faith (midlife and beyond), is characterized by the individual's ability to examine the deeper self and to perceive the significant meanings of the spiritual experiences.

Stage 6, universalizing faith, is a stage in which individuals are able to be open and respect other people's faiths. Love and justice are the overriding values of this stage.

Fowler's Theory Critiqued. Fowler's sample in his study was not random and was overrepresented by some religious groups and underrepresented by others. Fowler reports that no research has been conducted with Eastern religions and traditions. Some theologians challenge his distinction between faith, religion, and belief, as well as his stipulative definition of faith. In spite of the weaknesses Fowler has attempted to outline the spiritual development of individuals using the theories of Erikson, Piaget, and Kohlberg. Functional health assessments regarding values and beliefs are addressed in Chapters 10 through 16.

Development of Self-Concept

Self-concept is a frame of reference that describes how a person sees himself or herself. Self-concept is a complex and dynamic process that involves body image, self-esteem, roles, and identity. Erikson and Piaget are two of the most useful theorists concerned with how children develop and evolve with a sense of self and self-worth. The following is a brief discussion of the major components of self-concept.

Body image is an individual's perception of his or her body, including feelings and attitudes about physical characteristics and abilities. Thus, body image is the mental representation that a person has of his or her body and is not dependent on the actual physical characteristics. Normal changes in growth and development, such as puberty, and changes related to illness, injury, or surgery affect body image. However, young girls often see themselves as overweight when in fact they are thin and possibly sick (anorexia). The individual's self-perception is influenced by societal and cultural attitudes and values. The American media emphasizes youth, beauty, and wholeness.

Self-esteem is defined as an individual's sense of self-worth. The individual evaluates himself or herself based on a set of internal and external criteria. Self-esteem is related to how well a person feels he or she is doing at school, home, and work. The constant feedback that people have in their daily lives is part of this self-evaluation. Are young toddlers told they are bad when they do normal toddler activities? Are preschool children encouraged to be creative? Are teachers giving positive or negative feedback? An individual has an image of an ideal self (aspirations, goals, values, and standards of behavior that a person strives to attain) and evaluates himself or herself against this ideal self. The closer the self is to the ideal self, the higher the self-esteem.[8]

A *role* is a set of behaviors by which a person participates in a social group. Every person has multiple roles. A young child may be a daughter *and* a sister. As we grow and mature and move into society, we assume more and more roles. Roles involve expectations or standards of behavior that have been sanctioned by society.

A young child learns about roles through a process called *socialization.* Socialization is the "acquisition of the requisite orientation for satisfactory functioning in a role."[48] The process of socialization begins at birth and is part of a values orientation. The five methods by which infants learn behaviors that are sanctioned or approved by society are through reinforcement-extinction, inhibition, substitution, imitation, and identification.

Identity implies a consciousness of being oneself with persistent and consistent behaviors distinct and separate from others.[9] Erikson's fifth stage of development is focused on identity. From the time of toddlerhood children progress toward independence, autonomy, and a separateness that leads to an identity unique to the individual.

Thus, self-concept is composed of how a person sees himself or herself as related to body image, self-esteem, roles, and identity. In each of the subsequent chapters in this unit, self-perception and role and relationship are presented as a development of functional health patterns.

Development of Sexuality

Sexuality is more than being born male or female. Sex roles are learned through play and social interactions from a early age. Girls play with dolls, and boys play with guns. Are boys really better at math and science than girls, or is this socialization and learning? These questions are different from the development of sexuality but at the same time are inherently linked to sexuality. The Sex Information and Education Council of the United States[59] has defined sexuality in holistic terms as "a function of the total personality. . . concerned with the biological, psychological, sociological, spiritual and cultural variables of life which, by their effects on personality development and interpersonal relations, can in turn affect social structure."

The biologic differences between boys and girls are determined at conception with the XX (female) or XY (male) chromosome. This is referred to as gender identity. By the time a child is 3 years old she or he has an awareness of self as male or female. The toddler also is able to identify mother as a woman, father as a man, and brother as a boy. The awareness of self as female or male is then combined with experiences within the environ-

ment. This refers to gender role behavior, the way people act as women and men. Children respond to these environmental stimuli by assuming characteristics associated with the gender through such processes as imitation, identification, and reinforcement. Thus, the child learns behaviors consistent with the gender role, that is feminity or masculinity.

Sexuality and sexual activities are related but not the same. A person's sexual orientation is part of sexuality and self-concept. Sexual orientation is the persistent, erotic preference for a person of one sex or the other.[8] The origins of sexual orientation are not well understood. Whether or not a person is heterosexual or homosexual may be determined by genetics, learning experiences, and cognitive processes.[8] When a person's inner sense of sexual identity is inconsistent with the biologic gender, a person is referred to as homosexual.

Physical sexual development is discussed with each group in this chapter under "Stages of Physical Development." In Chapters 11 through 16 sexuality–reproduction as functional health pattern is presented.

Development of Language

The development of language skills and speech articulation is of considerable interest to researchers. Prior to the development of verbal skills, children appear to be able to understand or comprehend the verbal communications with parents and care providers. Infants have different crying sounds to indicate hunger versus pain. Parents are able to decipher the meanings of these sounds. A toddler is able to follow simple directions and commands, indicating an ability to understand and act on the spoken language. Parents are able to "understand" the early meaning of words or sounds of their infants and toddlers. At the same time children often repeat the words that they hear without understanding the meaning or the concept of the word. At different ages a child may or may not understand even what they say.[34] The development of language is an interaction between language, thought, and social interaction. Various theorists approach language development by emphasizing cognitive or social interaction. As a child develops before language acquisition the behavior is characterized by a gradually more complex organization of means and ends.[20] Children's use of language, according to Piagetian concepts, is based on the organization of concepts through cognitive development. According to Vygotsky, language development is the motor development associated with the child's interactions with the world.[66]

Empiricist/behavioral theory suggests that language acquisition is the result of operant conditioning. With positive reinforcement the infant repeats sounds, and as maturation occurs the repetition of sounds becomes more sophisticated. Lack of positive reinforcement for articulation results in retarded speech development.[61]

Linguistic/innate theory purports that universal linguistic schemata are innate to all humans. Infants are preprogrammed with the ability to determine syntax regardless of the language being learned. With cognitive maturation and social interaction the infant's natural speech production skills will be stimulated.[14] Chomsky suggested that an innate language structure, named language acquisition device, enables infants and toddlers to process what is heard and to understand and process speech. In biologic theory language development is based on maturation of the central nervous system. Development of language skills occurs in a regular, fixed order and at a similar rate in children.[36]

There are certain prerequisites to adequate speech production. These prerequisites can be placed into five categories:

- *Intact structures for the physical production of sound.* This includes larynx, respiratory structures, oral cavity structures, and nasal cavity structures.
- *Functioning structures for the physical reception of sound.* This includes a discriminating auditory apparatus and receptive speech center.
- *Maturation of the central nervous system.* This involves myelination of major neural pathways, growth in functional capacity of the cerebral cortex, and a functioning speech control center in the cerebral cortex.
- *Cognitive Maturation.* This includes adequate intellectual ability and the ability to process thoughts.
- *Psychological Stimulation.* This includes verbal and nonverbal human interaction and adequate environmental stimulation.

Table 8-8 describes the stages of language development. As children develop language and move from the babbling phase of infancy to words, they want to know that others understand their communication. For example one 30-month-old child wants her mother to repeat her sentences to clarify that the mother has understood her. She will tell her mother, "Say it." This is also an example of telegraphic speech in this age group. The process of language development through each stage of development is discussed in Chapters 12 through 16, including assessment strategies and suggestions for parents and caregivers for stimulating and encouraging language development.

TABLE 8-8
Stages of Language Development

Stage	Age	Activities
Prelinguistic	0–2 mo	Crying, cooing
	2–6 mo	Babbling, repeating sounds
Holophrastic	12–18 mo	First words; one word used to denote phrase or sentence
Telegraphic	18 mo–3 yr	Rapid vocabulary acquisition; open and pivotal content words; omits articles, prepositions, etc.
Preschool	3–5 y	Steady word acquisition; multiword sentences
School-age	6–12 y	Complex sentences; mastery of language

TABLE 8-9
Theorists' Interpretation of Play: A Major Role in Child Development

Theorist	Theory	Interpretation to Play
Psychoanalytic		
Freud	Cathartic	Play is an opportunity for children to repeat activities that make an impression on them and to express feelings.
Erikson	Ego mastery	Play is an attempt for a child to bring into harmony the desires of self and social norms and roles gaining mastery.
Behavioral		
Hull	Drive reduction	Play is an opportunity for children to satisfy the need for achievement, affiliation, and independence.
Miller and Dollard	Imitative learning	Play is an opportunity for children to imitate adult behaviors and to learn through imitation play.
Berlyne	Arousal seeking	Play is a time for exploring and investigating the environment. Curiosity and uncertainty about a new situation lead to exploration, which helps to reduce fears associated with new experiences or situations.
Cognitive		
Piaget	Cognitive development	Play and imitation are ways that a child assimilates reality. Play varies throughout the stages of cognitive development. Sensorimotor—practice games Preoperational—make-believe play Concrete operations—games with rules

Role of Play

Play is an important part of a child's development. Various forms of play occur at different ages and provide fun opportunities for children to learn about the world, about themselves, and about interacting with others. Table 8-9 identifies common theorists and their interpretation of play and play activities. Through cognitive play children practice language, and social and moral decision making. Children's creativity is seen from early ages, as when 3 year olds "read" stories to their stuffed animals or to mother or dad at bedtime. Physical activities support the development of muscles and coordination and are a fun way of exercising. Team or group activities allow children to learn to play with others, to follow rules, and to learn social skills.

Opportunities for unplanned, unstructured play with inexpensive toys that encourage creative play are important. Children should be allowed time to play without the activity leading to some adult standard. Specific suggestions for parents and care providers in promoting play for each age group are discussed in Chapters 12 through

16. The importance of play as a teaching methodology for sick children is discussed in Chapter 23.

Assessment of Growth and Development

The discussion of the assessment of growth and development in this chapter is a brief summary of what a nurse would assess. The skills for performing these assessments are discussed in Chapter 9 and in the following health promotion chapter for each age group (see Chaps. 10 through 16).

The Apgar Scoring System

The Apgar scoring system, named for Virginia Apgar, MD, who designed the tool, measures a newborn's overall state of health and thus is an indirect measure of the functional maturation of vital organs.[2] The Apgar scoring system rates the newborn in five general areas: appearance (i.e., color), pulse (i.e., apical heart rate), grimace (i.e., reflex action), activity (i.e., muscle tone), and respirations (i.e., breathing pattern). The infant is graded 0, 1, or 2 in each of the five categories (see Table 11-1). A rating is done at 1 and 5 minutes after birth. Ninety percent of newborns score 7 or better.[58] A score between 4 and 7 suggests that some assistance with extrauterine adaptation is required by the infant. Such a score certainly necessitates close monitoring in the ensuing hours after birth. A score below 4 necessitates intensive medical intervention to facilitate survival. Such a low score suggests developmental difficulties in major organ systems.

Head Circumference

Head circumference is a common measurement used to assess growth in the first 36 months of life. Head circumference directly measures skeletal (i.e., skull) growth and indirectly measures cerebral growth (see Chap. 12). Head growth proceeds in a predictable manner in the healthy child. Although the head circumference of female

TABLE 8-10
Proportion of Body Length to Head

Age	Proportion of Body Length to Head
2-month fetus	$\frac{1}{2}$
5-month fetus	$\frac{1}{3}$
Newborn	$\frac{1}{4}$
Age 2 years	$\frac{1}{5}$
Age 6 years	$\frac{1}{6}$
Age 12 years	$\frac{1}{7}$
Adulthood	$\frac{1}{8}$

(Data from Papilia, D. E., Olds, S. W. [1986]. *Human development* [3rd ed.]. New York: McGraw-Hill.)

TABLE 8-11
Ratio of Head-to-Chest Circumference

Age	Ratio
Birth	Head circumference is larger than chest circumference by approximately 2 cm.
1–1½ y	Head circumference and chest circumference are relatively equal.
2–3 y	Head circumference is slightly smaller than chest circumference.
3 y and older	Head circumference is smaller than chest circumference by 5–7 cm.

newborns is, on average, 1 cm smaller than that of male newborns, the rate of head growth for both sexes is essentially the same. The proportion of body length taken up by the head at various ages of childhood is presented in Table 8-10.

Chest Circumference

Chest circumference can be used as a complementary growth measure to head circumference. Its usefulness lies in how it compares to head circumference. Table 8-11 provides a ratio of head to chest measurements that can be used for assessment. Chest circumference is measured across the nipple line and should be taken between inspiration and expiration.

Head-to-Body Ratio, Height, and Weight

While not an exact tool for growth measurement, body proportions do change markedly from conception to adulthood. The male infant is, on average, 2 to 3 cm longer at birth than the female. During the first year of life the infant growing normally should increase his/her height by 25 to 30 cm. By age 2 the child should be an average of 12.5 cm taller. Most toddlers have reached approximately half their adult height.[5] By age 3 an additional 6 to 8 cm will be added to linear growth. The rate of height increase should continue at a rate of 5 cm per year until the adolescent growth spurt. During the adolescent growth spurt height will increase by 7.5 to 15 cm per year until the adult height is reached in late adolescence. (For growth percentile measuring in boys and girls see the Appendix).

The average newborn boy weighs approximately 3400 g, while the average girl weighs 3200 g. An infant will approximately double his or her birthweight by age 5 months. By 1 year of age the birthweight usually triples to approximately 10 kg. The average weight gain during the second year of life is approximately 2 to 3 kg. This yearly 2 to 3 kg weight gain increases until the adolescent growth spurt. The growth spurt will produce an average weight gain of 17.5 kg in girls and 23.7 in boys. (Comparative weight percentiles are available in the Appendix.)

Percentiles as Valued Indicators of Growth

Growth percentiles can be useful tools in assessing height, weight, and head circumference compared with the norm. Because nutritionally deprived children tend to be in the lower percentile, such a measurement may be a raw indicator of a nutritionally related growth abnormality. Care must be taken with the degree to which growth percentile charts are used.

The Brazelton Neonatal Behavioral Assessment Scale

The Brazelton assessment[8] is conducted on newborns to determine their response and adaptation to the extrauterine environment. The evaluation of neurologic, motor, and overall physical development of the newborn is obtained.[7] A more in-depth description of the use of the Brazelton assessment is included in "Behaviors" in Chapter 11.

Denver II

The Denver Developmental Screening Test (DDST and DDST-Revised) is used to detect developmental delays during infancy and preschool years. A major revision and restandardization of the DDST and DDST-R has resulted in a new form, the Denver II. The advantages of the Denver II include well-constructed and evaluated items, clear pictorial charts, and the modification or elimination of previously difficult-to-administer items. The Denver II is simple to administer, score, and interpret (see Appendix D). With instruction and practice, the Denver II can be administered in approximately 15 minutes. The assessment tool consists of 125 items in four categories: gross motor function, language, fine motor-adaptive, and personal–social. Each item has been validated and tested for reliability. Items with significant differences related to ethnicity, maternal education, place of residence, and sex are discussed in the technical manual. Norms for subpopulations, which assist the examiner in evaluating developmental delays related to sociocultural and environmental differences, are provided.

The results of the Denver II are classified as:

- *Advanced:* Passed an item completely to the right of the age line (passed by 25% of children at an age older than the child)
- *OK:* Passed, failed, or refused an item intersected by the age line between the 25th and 75th percentile
- *Caution:* Failed or refused items intersected by the age line between the 75th and 90th percentile
- *Delay:* Failed an item completely to the left of the age line; refusals to the left of the age line may be considered delays, since the refusal may be related to an inability to perform the task.

During the procedure, the nurse records the observations on the Denver II form, and over time the nurse can document a pattern of development. The time sequence for conducting a Denver II corresponds to the American Academy of Pediatrics recommended well-baby and well-child visits.

The Denver II test kit includes a red skein of yarn; raisins; a rattle with a narrow handle; a small clear bottle with a ⅝-inch opening; eight one-inch square blocks in red, blue, yellow and green; a small bell; a tennis ball; a pencil; a doll; a feeding bottle; and a cup. An instruction manual and forms are available from Denver Developmental Materials, Inc., P.O. Box 6919, Denver, CO 80206.

Each item on the Denver II appears in a bar or box that is coded by the percent of children capable of performing the skill at each age. The nurse selects appropriate items for assessment by following the age located at the top and bottom of the grid. To identify areas of concern, all items intersected by the age line are administered. To screen for only developmental delays, the items to left of the age line are assessed. To determine advanced development, items to the right of the line are tested. Approximately 20 items are assessed at each age to determine whether the child can perform the majority of tasks passed by 90% of the normative sample. On the scoring form, the nurse is referred to specific instructions for clarification. The nurse also documents testing behaviors of the child, such as compliance, interest in surroundings, fearfulness, and attention span.

Nursing Implications. A common practice in physician offices is to ask the parent or guardian about the child's development rather than taking time to conduct a Denver II. Parents are good observers of their child's behaviors, but may not know what behaviors are expected at each developmental stage. Parents may overestimate or underestimate certain areas. The nurse in well-child settings is encouraged to learn to use the Denver II and routinely assess young children. The developmental screening instruments are not designed as predictive tests (such as IQ tests), but are used to assess developmental function expected at a given age. The nurse should consider intervening variables such as predisposing biological factors, chronic infections, repeated hospitalizations, family dynamics, current physical status, prematurity, and so forth in interpreting the results of the assessment.

The nurse can discuss with parents the purpose of the Denver II prior to beginning the assessments. Parents should understand that the nurse will review the results when the Denver II is completed rather than during the procedure. The nurse will need time to record, score, and interpret the findings before reporting the results to the parents. Toddlers and preschoolers will cooperate more easily if the assessment is presented as a game or a fun activity rather than a "test." The nurse can use the nonthreatening assessment as a means of developing a relationship with the child and parents. Experience conducting the Denver II will provide a novice nurse with skills in moving from one section of the assesssment to another, and removing one set of toys to another.

Parents can validate their child's performance with his or her activities at home, including the child's co-operation and compliance. The results are presented to parents by discussing the successfully completed areas first and then identifying items that were failed. The nurse may use this time to teach parents about normal childhood development and activities that they can use to stimulate their child's development (see Chapters 11 to 16 for specific suggestions).

When a child shows signs of a developmental delay, the nurse and parents discuss an appropriate time for repeating the Denver II. If a developmental delay is identified, further studies are indicated for diagnosis and treatment. For example, a language delay is followed by otological and hearing evaluations.

Denver Articulation Screening Exam

The Denver Articulation Screening Exam (DASE) is used to assess language skills from age 2½ to six. The DASE allows the nurse to assess the ability of the child to imitate words and sound elements. During the procedure, the child repeats 22 words that include 30 sound elements. The nurse records the number of correctly pronounced sound elements, not just the words. The raw score is compared to the percentile rank of children in a comparable age group. Intelligibility is ranked according to one of four categories: easy to understand, understandable half the time, not understandable, or cannot evaluate. The DASE can be completed in 10 minutes and is an initial screening for language development. Some practice is required for the nurse to be able to accurately evaluate the sound elements, and initially, the nurse may ask a speech therapist to evaluate and validate the results obtained (see Appendix C).

Stages of Physical Development

Prenatal Development

The genetic blueprint for the physical characteristics of each human being is mapped at fertilization. The orderly development of the zygote, from a single-cell organism to a human infant capable of surviving independently in the extrauterine environment, occurs in three distinct stages. While pregnancy lasts for approximately 9 calendar months, for purposes of isolating physical development it is usually discussed in terms of weeks or lunar months (1 lunar month = 4 weeks). A full pregnancy is 10 lunar months.

The Pre-Embryonic Stage (0 to 3 Weeks).   Several major developmental activities occur during the pre-embryonic stage. These include rapid cellular division of the zygote to form a blastocyst, the appearance of the embryonic disk on the outer edge of the blastocyst, movement of the zygote/blastocyst along the fallopian tube to the uterus, and implantation of the blastocyst in the uterine wall by approximately 6 days postfertilization. The differentiation of the embryonic disk into the ectoderm and endoderm occurs in this stage. The ectoderm will eventually form the nervous system, including the brain and spinal cord, skin, hair, and nails. The endoderm will eventually form the digestive system and accessory organs and the respiratory system.

This differentiation occurs at approximately the end of the first week in the pre-embryonic phase. The beginning of the development of the placenta, amniotic sac, and umbilical cord takes place. By the end of the pre-embryonic stage the mesodermal layer will appear. This layer will eventually develop into the body's structural supports—skeletal system, muscles, cartilage, and connective tissue—and the circulatory, reproductive, urinary, and lymphatic systems.

Embryonic Stage (4 to 8 Weeks).   Developmental occurrences of primary significance during the embryonic stage include rapid differentiation of the germ layers into the major body organs and systems (organogenesis), the completion of placenta and umbilical cord development, and the beginning of bone ossification.[39]

Fetal Stage (9 Weeks to Birth).   During this final stage of prenatal development the fetus continues to mature until it is capable of surviving outside the uterus. A major concern is lung development. Birth will occur sometime between the 240th and 300th gestational day.

Human gender is determined at conception. The female ovum carries X sex chromosomes only. Half of the male sperm carry X sex chromosomes, the other half Y sex chromosomes. If at conception an X chromosome ovum joins with an X chromosome sperm, the zygote will have two X chromosomes (XX) and will become a female infant. If the X chromosome ovum joins with a Y chromosome sperm, the zygote will have an X and a Y chromosome (XY) and will become a male infant.

During the sixth week after conception the "indifferent gonad" appears. This indifferent gonad is a cluster of cells with the potential to develop into either a male or female infant.[31] If the developing infant is male (XY), genes on the Y chromosome send a biochemical signal that tells the indifferent gonad to develop into male sex organs. The testes begin to develop first at about 7 weeks. The remainder of the male sex organs develop in the early fetal period. If the embryo is female (XX), no signal is sent, and female genital organs develop.[6] By the fourth lunar month after conception, the external male and female organs are fully formed.[43]

Newborn

The infant is classified as a newborn for the first month of life. Most newborns adjust readily to extrauterine life. Their physiologic development and functional abilities are sound. The functional health and growth and development of the newborn are discussed and illustrated in Chapter 11. A normal alert neonate is shown in Figure 11-7.

Transition to Extrauterine Life.   Although several physiologic changes occur immediately at birth, the two most profound are changes in the circulatory path and changes in respiratory function. When the infant is born and takes a breath, his or her lungs begin to function, and placental circulation ceases. The following five structures, which had significant circulatory responsibilities prior to birth, are obliterated: umbilical cord, umbilical arteries, ductus venosus, ductus arteriosus, and foramen ovale. The following four structures alter their function considerably to adjust to extrauterine life: lungs, pulmonary arteries, aorta, and inferior vena cava. If these expected physiologic alterations in function do not occur or if the newborn's respiratory or circulatory system has anomalies in structure or function, extrauterine life will be severely compromised.

Body Proportions. The weight range of the normal newborn is 1500 to 4300 g. Two thirds of all full-term infants weigh between 2700 and 3800 g. The average female infant weighs 3200 g and the average male, 3400 g. A weight loss up to 8% to 9% is normal during the first few days of life. The weight lost is readily regained.

The average length for newborns is 46 to 54 cm. The average female infant is 48 cm long and the average male, 50 cm. The normal range of head circumference is 33 to 37 cm. The average female head circumference is 34 cm and the average male head circumference, 35 cm.

Respiratory System. Physical, chemical, and sensory stimuli initiate respirations at birth. The newborn's respirations are irregular in rate, rhythm, and depth. The rate can range from 40 to 80 per minute. Normally, respirations are quite shallow and diaphragmatic. An adequate degree of crying is usually necessary to allow for satisfactory lung expansion. Mucus is present in the respiratory passages, particularly in the newborn of a cesarean delivery.

Cardiovascular System. Until the medulla is fully functioning the pulse rate is irregular, ranging from 100 to 160 beats per minute. Crying increases the rate and degree of irregularity. The blood pressure is usually low, highly variable, and difficult to assess. The systolic average is 60 to 70 mmHg. Blood volume is approximately 10% of body weight. At birth red blood cells range from 4.0 to 6.5 million/mm^3; hemoglobin ranges from 14 to 23 g/dl; and hematocrit ranges from 48% to 70%. These readings drop when improved vascular oxygenation occurs. Because vitamin K is synthesized in the bowel, its levels must be increased artificially until bowel function is adequate. Physiologic jaundice occurs in 50% to 60% of newborns around the third day. This decreases as the liver becomes functional.

Skeletal System. At birth most bones are soft and made primarily of cartilage. Symmetry of the gluteal folds and extremities usually indicates normal skeletal structures underneath. The normal back is straight and flat. The legs are short and curve outward, while the feet tend to turn inward. The arms are relatively short. There is normal range of motion in the joints. The skull is the only skeletal structure with a significant degree of ossification at birth. The skull is composed of eight separate bones joined together at the suture lines. The fontanels are openings in the skull structure at major bone union points. The posterior fontanel will close by 2 to 2½ months. The anterior fontanel will not fully close until approximately 18 months.

Integumentary System. In the normal newborn the skin is elastic and smooth, and the tissue turgor is firm.

Lanugo is scant in the full-term infant, primarily in body folds. Milia are common on the nose and chin. Skin pigmentation varies according to race: white infants are pink or red; African American infants are black with a reddish hue; Oriental infants are dusty rose; and Native American infants are reddish-brown.

The umbilicus should dry up slowly and change from yellow-brown to black. It usually falls off by the sixth day but may last as long 2 weeks. Swelling of breast tissue in male and female infants is common and is a result of maternal hormones in the infant's bloodstream. This swelling subsides as the maternal hormones are excreted. The following are common temporary discolorations.

Mongolian spots are a dark, blue-gray discoloration on the lower back of African American, Oriental, Native American, and Mediterranean neonates. Mongolian spots do not require treatment and disappear on their own in late toddlerhood or early in the preschool years. Stork bites, more properly called telangiectatic nevi, are flat, red areas occurring primarily on the eyelids and nose; they disappear spontaneously in toddlerhood. Acrocyanosis is cyanosis of the hands and feet; this disappears with full circulatory function. Cutis marmorata is a bluish mottling when the infant is cold.

Gastrointestinal System. The mouth of the normal newborn is fully formed (except for dentition). The gums appear rough, and tooth buds may be visible. The healthy newborn's hard palate is closed over and may have several small white cysts, called Epstein's pearls, on its surface. These cysts are common and disappear on their own. The salivary glands do not begin to function until around the second month of life. The digestive capabilities of the newborn are limited to glucose, water, and colostrum. As the digestive tract becomes more functional at approximately 3 days, breast milk and formula become digestible; breast milk is the most digestible. At birth the infant's stomach likely has a capacity of 30 to 60 ml. This gradually increases. This low volume capacity, combined with the immature cardiac sphincter, make regurgitation common.

Intestinal elimination is involuntary, and eliminated contents change in characteristics. The initial stool, called meconium, is an odorless dark-green sticky substance produced from intrauterine digestion of amniotic fluid and other materials. The transition phase produces stool that is primarily brown with streaking. Once normal bowel function is established, the stool color varies according to whether the infant is breast-fed or bottle-fed. The breast-fed newborn produces bright golden-yellow, sweet-smelling, and frequent stools. It is not uncommon for a breast-fed infant to have half a dozen stools per day. The stool of the bottle-fed infant is pasty-yellow in color. Bowel movements occur less often in the bottle-fed infant, perhaps one to two times a day, and the stool has an odor more akin to an adult stool. Once hepatic function is established, after about 4 to 5 days, physiologic jaundice disappears. Digestion occurs very quickly in the newborn; thus, caregivers must be alert to dehydration.

Dentition. On occasion a neonate is born with one or more supernumerary teeth. Because these teeth are not part of regular dentition and are rootless, they are usually extracted. Calcification of deciduous teeth begins at about 6 months' gestation. It is not unusual for the calcification of the earliest permanent teeth to begin in late gestation. Most newborns, however, present with no obvious dentition.

Genitourinary System. The kidneys' ability to concentrate urine at birth is limited, and urine is pale yellow. The color becomes more straw-like as the kidneys' concentration abilities increase. Uric acid crystal may give the diaper a ruddy streak on the first few diaper changes. The normal newborn will urinate during the first few hours after birth. A delay in urination of more than 48 hours indicates dehydration.

The exterior genital structures of newborns appear proportionately large compared to the rest of the body. The testicles of the boy usually descend in the late prenatal period. The scrotum is deeply rugated and darker than the rest of the body. Transient edema is common and subsides within a couple of days. The foreskin usually is tightly adhered to the glans. The urinary meatus should be visible. The female infant has prominent labia and may have a hymenal tag. This tag, however, should not be imperforate because vaginal mucus can accumulate behind it.

Reproductive and Sexual Development. The sexual organs of the newborn infant are proportionately larger than other parts of the body. Some of this largeness is related to birth trauma and resulting swelling; the rest is innate. Female hormones from the mother, which cross the placenta, may cause transient swelling of breast tissue in male and female infants. Female infants also may pass blood-tinged mucus, called pseudomenstruation, from the vagina. Pseudomenstruation is also transient and caused by maternal hormones that have crossed the placenta.

Thermoregulatory System. The normal temperature range for the newborn is 36.5° to 37.5° C. The stability of temperature is quite fragile. The evaporation of amniotic fluid from the skin, coupled with the atmospheric temperature in the delivery room, results in an immediate drop in temperature for the newborn. A lack of shivering ability, limited subcutaneous fat, and a metabolic rate twice that of an adult adds to this labile thermoregulating mechanism.

Neuromuscular System. Muscle cell production is almost complete at birth. Further growth of muscles is generally based on increased growth of muscular cells as opposed to an increase in the total number of cells. The muscle tone in the normal newborn is sound. Because the tone in flexor muscles is stronger than that in extensor muscles, the healthy newborn will usually lie with limbs flexed and fists clenched. There is resistance to passive muscle movement and to pressure on a muscle. Muscles, even at this age, should feel slightly hard on palpation. Muscular strength in the neck is very weak. In the prone position the newborn can lift his or her head for a few seconds, but for the first few months external support must be provided for the neck and head.

Neurologic Function and Reflexes. The normal newborn resists restraint, pulls away from pain, and cries when uncomfortable; nonetheless, most early neuromuscular responses are purposeless and random. Neurologic immaturity may result in facial tremors, a common occurrence in the neonate, which disappear shortly. Neurologic normality can best be determined by the presence of several reflexes. Such reflexes may be divided into three categories (see Unit 13 for more definitive information on neurologic reflexes):

- Survival reflexes are altered with maturity. These reflexes include rooting, sucking, and extrusion of the tongue and are essential to infant survival until neurologic maturity offers a selection of alternative behaviors to meet basic needs.
- Primitive subcortical reflexes disappear with maturity. Most of the reflexes in this category may have had some purpose in the evolution of humans, particularly because their neurologic basis is in the subcortical area. As the higher brain or cerebral cortex matures, these reflexes are inhibited. Subcortical reflexes include Moro's, startle, palmar grasp, plantar grasp, tonic neck, Babinski's, walking, crawling, placing, Perez, Galant, and doll's eye.
- Protective reflexes persist to adulthood. These reflexes have protective purposes necessary throughout life and include sneezing, coughing, yawning, gagging, blinking, pupillary, glabellar, and withdrawal.

Special Senses.

Vision. The eyes of all newborns are slate-gray. True eye color may not be distinguishable until the infant is 1 year old. Visual acuity varies from 20/100 to 20/800 depending on the type of test used. The immaturity of the ciliary muscles limits accommodation and fixation to a few seconds. The fixation and focusing skills that the neonate has are best at approximately 20 cm. Researchers believe this is an evolutionary development allowing for attachment to the mother. A distance of 20 cm is approximately the distance between the breast and the mother's face. The evolutionary nature of this focusing distance is further supported by the fact that its intensity is acute during the first few hours of life and then deteriorates for a period of time. Even the very young infant can follow a moving object for a short time.

Distinct visual preferences are evident in the newborn, as shown in Figure 8-5. Ludington-Hoe[39] indicates the following:

- Black and white are preferred over medium colors (yellow, pink, and green), which are preferred over strong colors (red, orange, and blue)
- Shiny items are preferred over dull
- Contrasting colors are preferred over plain
- Geometric shapes are preferred to lines and blanks

It also is clearly evident that neonates have a strong affinity for the human face. This affinity becomes even more exacting with age. For example after a few weeks the eyes on the face most capture the infant's attention. Research also has shown that ocular abilities may be used as accurate predictors of overall neurologic functioning. A group of infants, considered high-risk for neurologic damage, were given visual tests that examined their ability to distinguish patterns and geometric shapes. On the basis

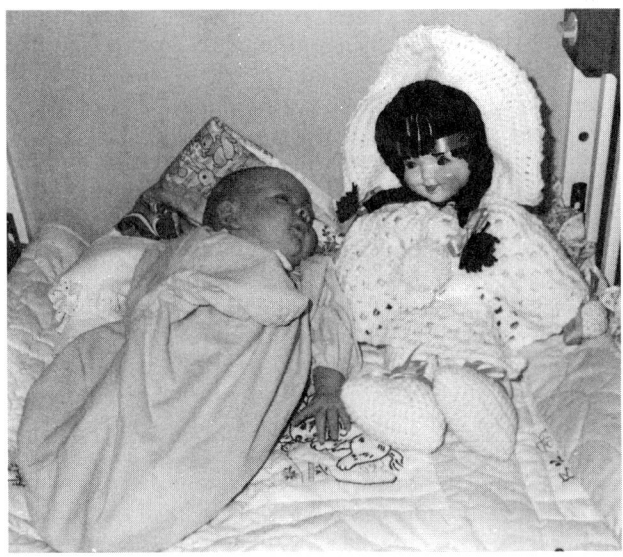

FIGURE 8-5
Neonatal visual preferences. A 2-week-old infant is interested in the doll and her face. The doll has a shiny finish on its face.

of these test results the infants were classified as having "normal," "suspect," or "abnormal" neurologic functioning. The infants were then subjected to standard newborn neurologic tests. When IQ tests were administered to these children at age 4, the correlation between the visual testing and later neurologic/intellectual ability was much higher than the correlation between standard newborn neurologic tests and later IQ.[42]

Hearing. Hearing is well developed, even *in utero*. Gentle, high-pitched sounds are preferred to shrill, harsh, or loud sounds. The human voice, particularly the female voice, is preferred to other sounds, and the infant soon recognizes and prefers the mother's voice to that of other women. Bimodal perception (the functioning of hearing and vision as one perceptual unit) begins in the neonatal period and becomes perfected with time. The ability of the infant to move his or her eyes toward a sound is the simplest example of bimodal perception.

Taste. The sense of taste is well developed at birth. An early preference for the sweet taste is evident.[67] Experiments conducted in the 1940s suggest that the taste differentiation is well developed *in utero*. When saccharin was added to the amniotic fluid, increased swallowing by the fetuses was observed.[68]

Smell. Several experiments conducted in the 1960s and early 1970s provide evidence that newborns are capable of differentiating smells. Of particular significance is research indicating that neonates can distinguish their mother's milk from the milk of other women.[54]

Touch. Tactile sensation is very well developed in the neonate. A sensitivity to touch is useful for self-preservation and the development of attachment behaviors.

Sleep–Wake Patterns. Considerable research has been conducted recently on neonatal sleep patterns. Prechtl and colleagues[50] described newborns as having six sleep–wake patterns: quiet sleep, active sleep, quiet alert, active alert, crying, and transition phase.

Coons and Guilleminault[15] report that 50% to 80% of the newborn's sleep time is spent in active sleep. (Active sleep can be equated with adult rapid eye movement, or REM sleep.) The normal newborn sleeps an average of 18 h/24 h in 3- to 5-hour stretches. Wake periods of longer than 2 hours are unusual in early infancy.

Infancy

Tremendous changes in development and growth occur during the first 12 months of life. Infancy is discussed and illustrated in Chapter 12.

Body Proportions. Infants will double their birthweight by 5 months and triple it by 1 year. By age 1 year the average female infant weighs 9.6 kg and the average male, 10.2 kg. By the end of the first year the infant will increase its length by about 50% making the average 1-year-old girl 72 cm and the average boy 74 cm. By 1 year the head circumference of the average girl is 46 cm and the average boy, 47 cm. Weight proportion gradually shifts, so muscle production is favored over fat production by the end of the first year. This shift in weight proportion results from two important physiologic changes: the body's thermoregulatory mechanisms are more mature, and its reliance on fat for warmth is reduced. Also, the need for motor competence increases.

Respiratory System. The respiratory rate by 1 year ranges from 20 to 40 per minute. This fairly rapid respiratory rate is necessary to fill the rapidly enlarging lung capacity. Breathing is primarily nasal until 5 to 6 months when mouth breathing begins to be a useful alternative.

Cardiovascular System. The heart rate slows to a range of 90 to 140 beats per minute by 12 months. The overall increase in size of the heart and the efficiency of the left ventricle at pumping blood to the systemic circulation results in an increased average systolic blood pressure of 70 to 80 mmHg. Body fluid and vascular volume begin to approximate adult proportions by 12 months. Red blood cell production decreases at approximately age 3 months in response to unusually high levels of fetal hemoglobin remaining in the infant's blood. As the transition to nonfetal iron begins around age 3 months erythropoiesis rejuvenates. White blood cell counts reach adult proportions in late infancy.

Skeletal System. Ossification of bones is a slow, steady process. Centers of ossification appear in the wrists at approximately 4 to 6 months, and x-rays of the wrists can be excellent indicators of growth. The skull continues to develop, and by 2 to 2½ months the posterior fontanel should be closed over. The anterior fontanel will become smaller but will not close over before toddlerhood.

Integumentary System. More sebum excretion produces skin in infancy that is less susceptible to peeling and less sensitive to topical irritants. Lanugo present at birth and scalp hair usually are shed. New downy hair, which may differ in color from birth hair, begins to grow on the scalp. The infant's nails are soft and grow very rapidly.

Gastrointestinal System. Rapid growth of the stomach increases its capacity to 200 to 350 ml by 12 months. This increased capacity delays emptying time, and, consequently, the time between feedings can be lengthened. The liver doubles its weight by 1 year but is one of the slower maturing digestive organs. The liver's slow development of glycogen storage capacity makes the infant susceptible to hypoglycemia. Susceptibility to gastrointestinal infections decreases with maturation and with the production of digestive enzymes and normal gastrointestinal flora. Swallowing becomes voluntary after 3 to 4 months of age. As chewing ability begins and salivation increases, solid food can be eaten by 5 to 6 months of age.

Improved absorption from the large intestine increases the consistency of stool. As the cardiac sphincter matures regurgitation decreases. The anal sphincter muscles develop in the process of the infant becoming upright. This allows for more predictability of defecation by the end of the first year. Predictability of defecation, however, should not be confused with voluntary control, which is not possible until 18 to 24 months. Simpler carbohydrates and fats are easiest to digest in early infancy, followed later by complex carbohydrates and protein.

Dentition. The first tooth, a lower central incisor, usually arrives between 4 and 7 months, although some infants do not get their first teeth until as late as 10 or 11 months. Range of teething in the first year is found in Chapter 12.

Genitourinary System. Kidney function, particularly tubular reabsorption, improves slowly. This slow maturation of kidney function makes dehydration and overhydration potential threats. As with bowel function kidney maturation and increased bladder capacity begin to produce some predictability of urination by the end of the first year. The reproductive organs are dormant in infancy. Reflex erection of the penis or clitoris may occur, but this is a physical, not psychosexual, response.

Thermoregulatory System. By approximately 2 to 3 months the infant begins to perspire, and this assists with thermoregulation. Thermoregulatory ability becomes more stable in late infancy due to reduced metabolic rate and vasoconstrictor and vasodilator ability in peripheral blood vessels.

Neuromuscular System. Cerebral growth continues rapidly during the first year. The brainstem, which is responsible for basic, unconscious, physiologic functions like respiration, is fully mature by 12 months. Nerve myelination continues; the complexity of nerve synapse structures increases; and nerve conduction time becomes more rapid. Overall, improved neurologic function, along with bone and muscle growth, results in improved motor abilities. The development of gross motor function follows the proximodistal principle. The development of motor ability is described in Table 8-12 (see page 142).

Special Senses. Improvement of vision in the infant is related to physical changes that are occurring. The eyeball of the infant is less spherical than that of the adult. Tracking, staring, range of peripheral vision, and hand–eye coordination become more mature and sophisticated with increased ciliary muscle control in the second half of the first year. Macular function is usually well established by 5 to 6 months, thus allowing for depth perception. Classic experiments conducted in 1960 involving a "visual cliff" clearly substantiated that by 6 months depth perception is well established.[24] Further experimentation with the visual cliff determined that infants as young as 2 months had some ability to perceive depth.[9] Binocular fixation usually is established no later than 4 months,[27] as illustrated in Figure 8-6. Vision reaches 20/40 to 20/50 by 12 months.

Hearing continues to become more discriminatory. By 4 months infants can clearly distinguish the most familiar voices in their lives. Taste and smell continue to become more discriminatory. Sensitivity to touch continues to be strong. The sense of touch also is used more adeptly for environmental exploration.

Sleep Patterns. By the time the infant reaches 3 months total sleep hours may be down to 18 hours per day. By 6 months average sleep will likely be 15 to 16 hours per day. As stomach emptying time slows the infant is able to consolidate sleep into larger blocks. Somewhere between 3 to 6 months most infants are able to give up their night feeding. Older babies tend to have sleeping patterns more like those of an adult. Non-REM sleep time increases, and by 12 months the infant is usually able to fall asleep easier and awake more smoothly than in earlier months.

Toddlerhood

Toddler refers to a child age 1 to 3. The toddler years are an exciting time for parents. The toddler is mobile and each day can do new and exciting things. Parents

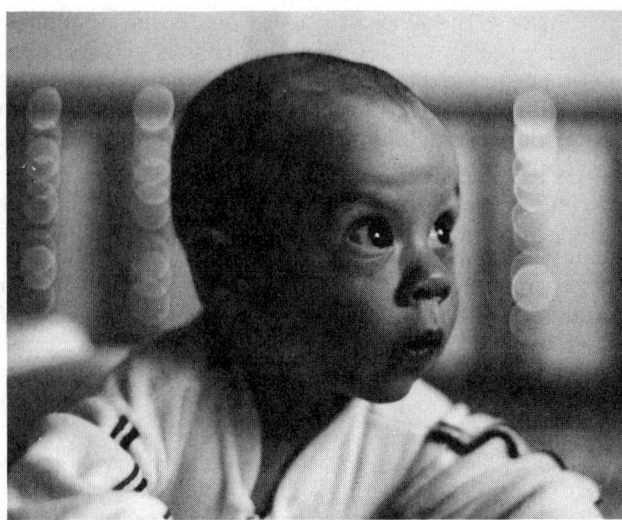

FIGURE 8-6
This 3½-month-old boy evidences sound binocular vision and fixation.

must be aware of the ever-changing need to child proof the house at new heights. Toddlers are discussed and illustrated in Chapter 13.

Body Proportions. Because the head incorporates one fifth of the total body mass, the toddler is usually chubby. Weak abdominal muscles produce a pot-bellied appearance (Fig. 8-7). The toddler, by age 2, weighs 14 to 18 kg, approximately four times the birthweight. Also by age 2 the toddler is about 80 to 95 cm tall, close to half the expected adult height. At the beginning of toddlerhood the circumference of the head and chest are approximately equal. By the end the head is somewhat smaller than the chest. General growth rate slows at approximately the middle of the toddler period.

Respiratory System. As the thoracic volume increases the respiratory rate of the toddler drops to 20 to 30 per minute. Because the lungs and chest cavity are still growing, breathing remains abdominal through most of toddlerhood.

Cardiovascular System. While the heart continues a steady growth in toddlerhood, its rate of growth is lower than other organ and systems. As the heart becomes a more efficient pump and the cardiac output and stroke volume increase, the blood pressure rises to an average of 95/65 mmHg, and the pulse rate drops to an average of 90 to 110 per minute by age 3.

Skeletal Systems. Ossification points in bone tissue increase to about 25 by age 3. Long bones grow rapidly during this stage. The vertebral column begins to harden and the adult-like *S*-shaped spine becomes more visible.

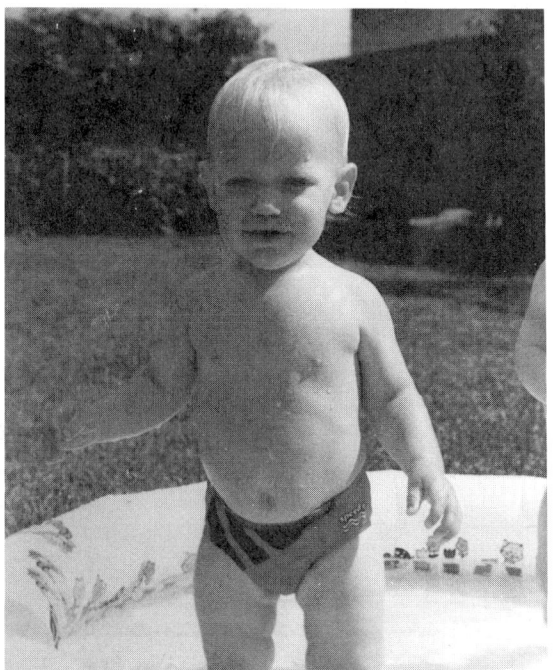

FIGURE 8-7
Body proportions of the toddler. This 15-month-old boy clearly illustrates the chubby, pot-bellied appearance characteristic of the toddler.

As with infancy, growth of bone tissue from cartilage is most obvious on x-rays of the wrists and ankles. Also, some smaller bones join together to form larger ones. Two thirds of the toddler's height increase results from long bone growth of the leg. As the cerebrum reaches 90% of its maximum capacity in toddlerhood, suture lines begin to knit, and the anterior fontanel closes over.

Integumentary System. Decreased fluid content in the epithelium encourages the epidermis and dermis to adhere more closely. This allows the epidermis to become a more resilient and less sensitive structure. Infant-like hair gives way to hair that is usually thicker and darker. Body hair appears as a fuzz on the lower arms and legs.

Gastrointestinal System. Stomach capacity continues to increase so that meals can be spaced 4 to 6 hours apart with small snacks in between. Stomach acidity increases, thus maturing overall digestive ability. Chewing improves because of increased dentition, and this allows for better use of salivary digestive enzymes. Increased myelination of nerves to the anal sphincter allows for physiologic voluntary control of bowel function, usually around the middle of toddlerhood. As the composition of intestinal flora becomes more adult-like and stomach acidity increases, gastrointestinal infections become much less common.

Dentition. All 20 deciduous teeth should be present by the end of toddlerhood.

Genitourinary System. The genital organs remain functionally dormant in toddlerhood, except for unconscious reflex activity. Three major changes in the urinary system allow for voluntary bladder control during this stage:

- Increase in the ability of the kidneys to concentrate urine,
- Growth and increased capacity of the bladder, and
- Myelination of nerves leading to the urethral sphincter.

Daytime bladder control is usually achieved after bowel control and before nighttime bladder control. By the end of toddlerhood a bladder retention time of up to 3 hours is not uncommon.

Reproductive and Sexual Development. The sexual organs of the infant and toddler remain dormant in terms of mature functioning and reproductive ability. The sex organs are, however, capable of producing physiologic pleasure sensation. Infants and toddlers of both sexes attempt to reproduce accidental stimulation of the penis and clitoris. Reflex erections are quite common in male infants. Jones[33] suggests that one in three toddlers is physiologically capable of experiencing a sexual orgasm.

Thermoregulatory System. Thermoregulatory stability is much more prevalent in toddlerhood due to the decreased water content of the skin and thus decreased water loss through the skin; functioning eccrine glands that react more smoothly to temperature changes; in-

TABLE 8-12
Motor Development of the Infant

Age	Gross Motor Skill	Fine Motor Skill
1 month	Lies primarily in a flexed position Demonstrates cervical curve as head is momentarily lifted Has slight ability to move elevated head from side to side	Has a hand-to-mouth tendency Makes swiping action when object is seen Has involuntary grasp reflex Drops objects from grasp without notice
2 months	Can hold head erect reasonably well when held upright Has less flexion when body is prone Holds head primarily in the side position Turns head from side to side when prone Can hold head at 45-degree angle for 20–30 seconds when prone	Can become excited by the sight of an object but unable to grasp it unless placed in hand Shakes a rattle involuntarily for a brief moment Releases palmar clench occasionally
3 months	Can sit with support but tends to lean forward because back is rounded Can raise head and upper chest when prone Holds head at 90 degrees Has minimal head lag Holds head steady for some time Has more symmetry to body movements Prefers a sitting or reclining position	Use of palmar grasp declines rapidly Holds hands more loosely Looks at hands Can begin to hold an object purposefully Begins reaching movements Can follow an object of interest for 180 degrees
4 months	Holds head and full chest at 90 degrees for some time when prone Holds a standing position momentarily when upper body supported Rolls from front to back	Holds hands open Activates hand for purposeful reach Attempts apposition of the thumb Tries to pick up objects with two hands Plays with fingers Hands come together at the midline
5 months	Rolls from back to front Demonstrates no head lag when pulled to a stand Sits well with only slight support Prefers upright position	Has improved thumb apposition Regards hands less often Looks at and reaches toes Grasps objects well Alters hand to accommodate object size Can reach for a second object in other hand while maintaining grasp on original object
6 months	Bears weight on legs fairly well when pulled up Can turn over 360 degrees Can pull self to a sitting position Sits alone reasonably well	Can manipulate fingers well enough to handle small objects and finger foods Can manipulate an object somewhat, move it from one hand to another, turn it over Might hold bottle for a short time
7 months	Sits alone with back reasonably straight May begin crawling If held downward reaches out in "parachute reflex" to brace a fall	May prefer one hand over other May hold a cup but likely needs assistance Can initiate some motor acts Will "scratch" or "rake" to grab a small object on a flat surface

3 months

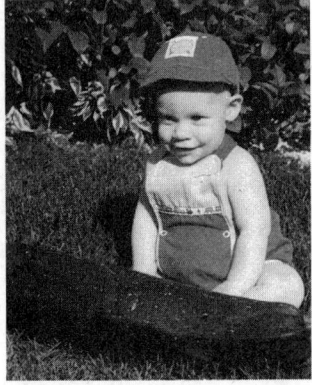

7 months

(Continued)

TABLE 8-12
(Continued)

Age	Gross Motor Skill	Fine Motor Skill
8 months	Pulls self to a firm stand Sits upright for long periods	Begins to use pincer grasp Turns wrist to look at objects in hand Lets objects go intentionally
9 months	Has well-established crawling May begin creeping Can pull self to a stand and move along in a sideways position, holding on May begin walking Can reach a proper sitting position alone	Can hold eating instruments but does not reach mouth with much sophistication Drinks from a cup reasonably well Pokes and bangs objects
10 months	Can sit for long periods Can pull self onto some items Establishes creeping ability May begin walking If falls, can right self	Has sophisticated pincer grasp Demonstrates hand dominance Eats with instruments, but crudely
11 months	Stands erect without support Moves sideways quite well May be walking	May begin placement of objects inside other items and then retrieve them Can make gross stroking movements with a large coloring instrument
12 months	Walks with a broad base Falls while walking	Eats quite well with fingers and drinks well from a cup Can make quite sophisticated finger movements such as pointing

10 months

11½ months

creased shivering ability, which allows for increased heat production when needed; and increased ability of the peripheral capillaries to dilate or constrict in response to atmospheric temperature changes and thus conserve a stable core temperature. The average temperature range is 37.2° to 37.5° C.

Neuromuscular System. Rapid muscle fiber growth and innervation of muscles allow for considerable improvement in the gross and fine motor skills of the tod-dler. The transition of gross and fine motor performance from the beginning to the end of toddlerhood is described and illustrated in Figure 8-8.

Special Senses. Binocular vision and accommodation are well developed in toddlerhood. Visual acuity is approximately 20/40 by age 3. hyperopia, or far-sightedness, is common in toddlerhood because lens refractiveness is slow. Persistent strabismus at this age seriously affects vision, and professional evaluation is

Beginning ━━━━━━━━━━━━━━━━━━━━▶ End

GROSS MOTOR SKILLS

Stands broadly but steadily ──────▶ Can stand alone on one foot for several seconds

Walks with a wide-stanced, toddling gait ──────▶ Runs with a few falls

Jumps crudely in one spot and usually falls ──────▶ Can jump from a low step or stool to the floor without falling

Climbs up stairs slowly, often losing balance ──────▶ Climbs stairs up and down, holding railing, one foot at a time and alternating

Pulls or pushes large toy ──────▶ Manipulates pedal or walker car (A)

Climbs onto items and often falls off ──────▶ May climb into cupboards, boxes, and so forth (B)

Enjoys activities like throwing a large ball but often falls ──────▶ May enjoy sliding or climbing on monkey bars with parental supervision (C)

Throws overhand and usually falls ──────▶ Throws overhand accurately about 6 feet

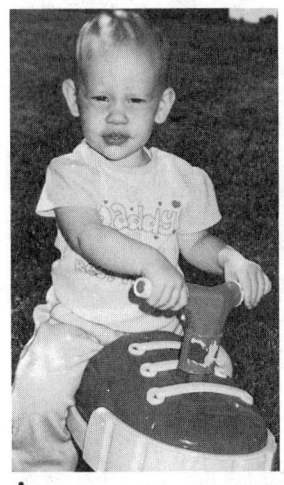
A
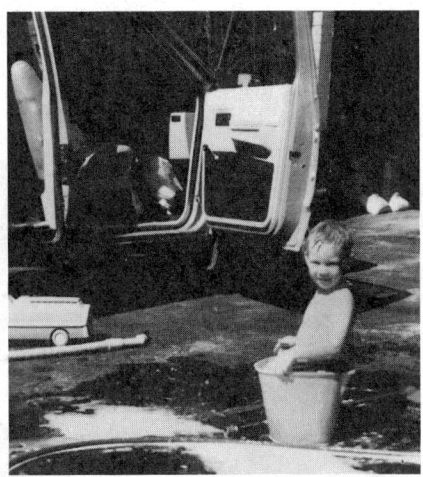
B
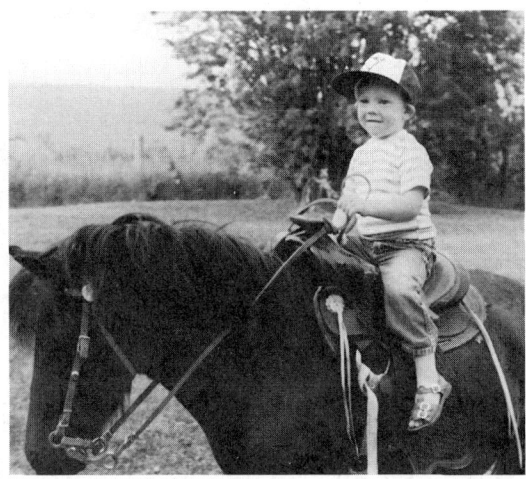
C

Beginning ━━━━━━━━━━━━━━━━━━━━▶ End

FINE MOTOR SKILLS

Builds towers two to three blocks high ──────▶ Builds block trains, towers eight or nine blocks high, constructs with large interlocking blocks

Scribbles or makes broad strokes ──────▶ Can make an enclosed circle intentionally

Holds large crayon or paint brush with whole hand ──────▶ Holds coloring instrument with fingers instead of whole hand

Pats pages in a book ──────▶ Can turn book pages one at a time

Crudely manipulates feeding tools with much spillage ──────▶ Pours from a small pitcher and can use a fork reasonably well

FIGURE 8-8
Transition of gross and fine motor performance from the beginning to the end of toddlerhood.

warranted. Convergence should occur quite smoothly during this time. Two abilities indicating a fusion of cognitive and visual performance in this stage are recognition of geometric shapes and recollection of visual images.

Adult hearing abilities usually are present in toddlerhood. Sound localization occurs in all planes. Recurrent infections in the short, straight eustachian tubes may compromise hearing and thus should receive prompt treatment. Cephalocaudal development of the nervous system increases sensitivity to touch (e.g., tickling) in the lower limbs. All the senses work together in a more sophisticated manner in the toddler years.

Sleep Patterns.   Toddlers require 12 to 15 hours of sleep per day. They take longer to fall asleep than infants but often are able to entertain themselves quietly until sleep overtakes them. At least one afternoon nap is common.

Preschool

Preschool children are 3 to 5 years of age. Preschoolers are discussed and illustrated in Chapter 14. These children may be involved in formal preschool programs that prepare children cognitively for school using play and formal structure.

Body Proportions.   Genetic influences in body measurements may become apparent by the end of the preschool years. Weight by age 5 will be approximately double the weight at 1 year. The average girl weighs 19 to 20 kg by age 5 and the average boy, 20 to 21 kg. Birth length is approximately doubled by age 5. The average girl is 96 to 100 cm tall and the average boy, 100 to 110 cm tall. Average head circumference by age 5 for girls and boys is 50 cm and 51 cm, respectively. The pot-bellied toddler gives way to the leaner, more well-proportioned preschooler.

Respiratory System.   By about age 5 chest breathing overtakes abdominal breathing as the major respiratory style. The chest appearance becomes more adult-like by the end of the preschool years, with the transverse diameter of the chest becoming larger than the anteroposterior diameter. The respiratory rate ranges from 20 to 25 breaths per minute.

Cardiovascular System.   Cardiovascular growth continues at a steady rate. The pulse rate ranges from 90 to 95 beats per minute; the average blood pressure is 100/60 mmHg. Physiologic cardiac murmurs are heard in 50% of preschoolers due to the thinness of the chest wall and changing anatomic relationships between cardiac and thoracic structures.[62] Such murmurs disappear on their own and are of no medical significance.

Skeletal System.   Ossification and calcification of bones continue at a slow, steady pace in the preschool years. The amount of red bone marrow decreases, with the only remaining hematopoietic centers in the sternum, ribs, vertebrae, and pelvis. Some ossification centers fuse in the preschool years. There are gender differences in

fusion milestones. For example the bony center of the patella appears at approximately age 3 in girls and between ages 4 and 5 in boys.[3] The earlier forward tilt of the pelvis straightens out in the preschool years, allowing for a more erect posture.

Integumentary System.   Sebum is produced in small amounts during the preschool years, and dry skin is common. The skin's resilience continues to improve. Hair continues to get darker and more coarse. It has likely reached a length where a first hair cut or trim is necessary.

Gastrointestinal System.   The preschooler's digestive tract is functionally mature. Gastric acidity increases, and the preschooler can tolerate most adult foods. Swallowing becomes adult-like (i.e., without protruding tongue movements). This, along with a more smooth-functioning epiglottis, reduces some of the earlier risk of food aspiration. Digestive enzymes begin to reach adult levels. Bowel control should be well established.

Dentition.   All 20 deciduous teeth are present at age 3. A few children lose their first deciduous teeth at age 5. A visit to the dentist by age 3 to 3½ allows for an assessment of the progress of dentition (Fig. 8-9).

Genitourinary System.   The sexual organs continue to grow but remain functionally dormant. Kidney function is well differentiated. Specific gravity and other characteristics of urine should be similar to adult norms.[34] From 3 to 5 years of age the length, weight, and filtration capacity of the kidneys increases slightly. During stress this ability is decreased, and the child's renal system takes longer to reestablish homeostasis than does the adult's.[8] Day and night bladder control should be the norm by the middle of the preschool years.

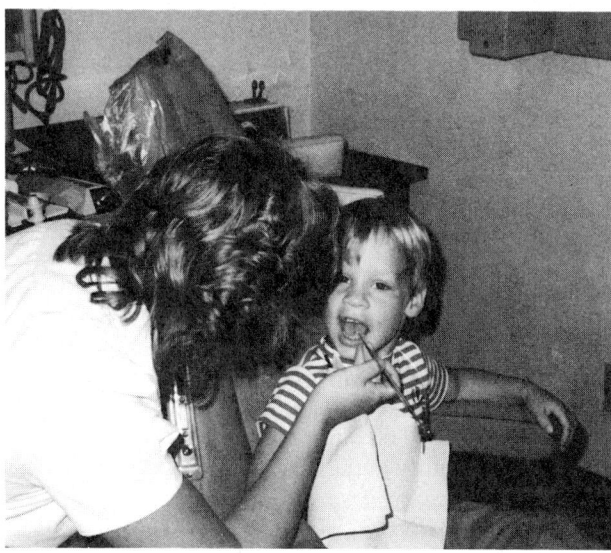

FIGURE 8-9
Dental hygiene in the preschool years. A visit to the dentist is recommended by age 3 to 3½ to assess the progress of dentition and to reinforce good dental hygiene habits.

Reproductive and Sexual Development. Mature sexual development is still dormant in this age group. The size of the sexual organs increases only in relation to overall body growth. Many preschoolers actively pursue masturbation for physiologic pleasure. One study suggests the percentage might be as high as 60%.[33] Such activity, of course, is innocent and not psychosexual in the adult sense.

Thermoregulatory System. Thermoregulatory control is similar to that of the adult except in two aspects: eccrine glands still produce only minimal amounts of perspiration, and apocrine glands are nonsecretory at this age.

Neuromuscular System. Nerve myelination is complete, and muscles continue to grow in size and strength with use. The preschooler is much more competent in motor activity than the toddler. The ability to perform more complex motor tasks increases. Hand dominance is clearly distinguished by the preschool years. Gross motor accomplishments include such skills as the following:

- Pedaling a tricycle (and by age 5 a two-wheeler with training wheels)
- Running well
- Walking backward
- Walking up and down stairs without the use of a handrail
- Dancing (quite rhythmically by age 5)
- Jumping and climbing well
- Skipping well by age 5

Fine motor accomplishments include such skills as the following:

- Using fingers to catch a ball
- Using paint and crayons well
- Cutting out paper
- Stringing large beads by age 3 and small beads by age 5
- Washing hands
- Buttoning well by age 5
- Brushing teeth
- Making recognizable letters and numbers by age 4 to 5
- Doing puzzles (24 pieces by age 3, 60 to 75 pieces by age 5)
- Hitting a nail accurately by age 5

Special Senses. The tendency toward hyperopia continues in the preschool years. Acuity of 20/20 should be reached by age 5. The lacrimal glands are fully mature by age 4. Depth perception is fully functional by the end of the preschool years. Except for very subtle shading, color vision should be quite precise. All other senses are fully discriminatory in the healthy preschooler.

Sleeping Patterns. The preschooler sleeps an average of 11 to 13 hours per day. Most still need an afternoon nap at age 3, but by age 5 most are beginning kindergarten and no longer nap. Bedtime rituals become trying at times for parents. Nightmares are common and normal in the preschool years.

School-Age

The school-age child is between the ages of 5 and 12. The role of the family as the center of the child's life is beginning to lessen as the child develops friendships at school. The school-age child is discussed and illustrated in Chapter 15.

Body Proportions. Genetic influences on height, weight, and body proportions are clearly evident in the school-age child. Between the ages of 5 and 12 the child's height increases an average of 5 to 7 cm a year, and the child's weight increases by an average of 1.5 to 3 kg a year. In the early middle years boys tend to be slightly taller and heavier than girls. Even at this young age girls tend to carry a bit more body fat proportionately than boys. Toward the end of the middle years, girls begin their adolescent growth spurt (as early as 10 years but on average 11 years), about 1 to 2 years ahead of boys. Thus, in later middle childhood many girls are taller and more physically mature than their male counterparts. The general growth rate is slower in the early two thirds of the middle years than at any other time in childhood.

Respiratory System. The respiratory rate declines to 18 to 22 breaths per minute in the school-age years. The vital capacity of the lungs increases to 2600 ml for girls and 2800 ml for boys by age 12.[32]

Cardiovascular System. By the end of the school-age years the heart is six times its birth size. At age 5 years the child's pulse rate is, on average, 85 to 95 beats per minute. By the end of this period, at age 12, the pulse range is usually 70 to 90 beats per minute. The mean blood pressure during middle childhood is 105/60 by age 5 to 8 and 110/60 by age 8 to 12.[38] Blood values approximate adult levels.

Skeletal System. Bones continue to lengthen and harden during the middle years. Toward the end of the middle years and into early adolescence skeletal growth may overtake muscular growth and development, resulting in a gangling appearance. The "S" curve of the spine should be well established. Overall posture becomes more adult-like.

Integumentary System. The integumentary system is unremarkable in the school-age child. It is functionally mature and the epidermis is tough and resilient.

Gastrointestinal System. By the end of the middle years the child's stomach assumes the "bagpipe" shape of the adult's stomach.[28] Appetite and caloric requirements usually slow down until the late middle (preadolescent) years. The gastrointestinal tract is functionally mature.

Dentition. Between the ages of 5 and 12 the deciduous teeth are lost, and all the permanent teeth (except the third molars) are likely to be present. Dentition during this time is not an instantaneous occurrence. Several months may pass from the beginning to the end of permanent dentition. The four general phases in the process of permanent dentition, in chronologic order, follow:

- Deciduous tooth is shed
- Permanent tooth pierces alveolar bone
- Permanent tooth pierces gingival tissue
- Permanent tooth makes contact with teeth on the opposite jaw

Genitourinary System. The genital–reproductive organs remain dormant through most of the school-age years. With girls in particular, however, reproductive changes (including menstruation) may begin as early as 9 years of age. The urinary system is functionally mature. The ability of the kidneys to rebound from physiologic insult improves with age. The kidneys' ability to concentrate urine continues to increase.

Reproductive and Sexual Development. Sexual development, in the physiologic sense, remains dormant until the preadolescent years (9 to 11 years). Masturbation remains a common practice. The psychosocial aspects are still vague to the child, although curiosity begins to focus on adult sexuality.

Thermoregulation and Endocrine Function. The school-age child's average body temperature is 36.5° to 37° C. Thermoregulatory function is mature. All endocrine functions, except those related to reproductive development, are mature. This results in an increase in the ability of the school-age child to maintain or regain homeostasis during stress.

Neuromuscular System. Cerebral growth reaches approximately 95% of its adult potential by the end of the middle years. Increasing myelination and development of complex pathways within the cerebral cortex increase cognitive ability. Improvement in voluntary control of gross and fine motor skills makes the school-age child quite neuromuscularly competent.

Examples of gross motor skills acquired during this age include the following:

- Bicycling without training wheels, often by age 6
- Roller skating
- Skateboarding
- Bicycle trick riding, in the middle years
- Running progressively faster
- Jumping progressively higher

Examples of fine motor skills acquired during this age include the following:

- Printing in early school-age and writing in later school-age years
- Performing crafts requiring increasing dexterity
- Playing games (e.g., video games) requiring increasing dexterity
- Computer competence

The combination of cognitive, gross motor, and fine motor skills allows the school-age child to begin devel-

oping competence in individual sports like swimming, track and field, golf, and team sports like baseball, basketball, soccer, and hockey (Fig. 8-10).

Special Senses. All special senses should be functionally mature. Increasing sensory discrimination is a result of increased cognitive ability and environmental experience.

Sleep Patterns. The 5 year old requires 10 to 12 hours of sleep per night. By age 12, 10 hours of sleep are usually sufficient for the average child.

Adolescence

The adolescent is between the ages of 12 and 18. Many researchers divide this stage into preadolescence, 12 to 13 years, and adolescence, 14 to 18 years. Certainly, the needs and interests of preadolescents are different from older adolescents. Adolescence is a time of physical and emotional changes related to growth and development. Life choices are an integral part of this stage of development. Adolescents are discussed in Chapter 16.

Body Proportions. Twenty percent of adult height and 30% to 50% of adult weight are achieved during adolescence. While girls usually reach adult body proportions by age 15 to 16, boys may be in their early 20's before reaching maximum adult body proportions. If the

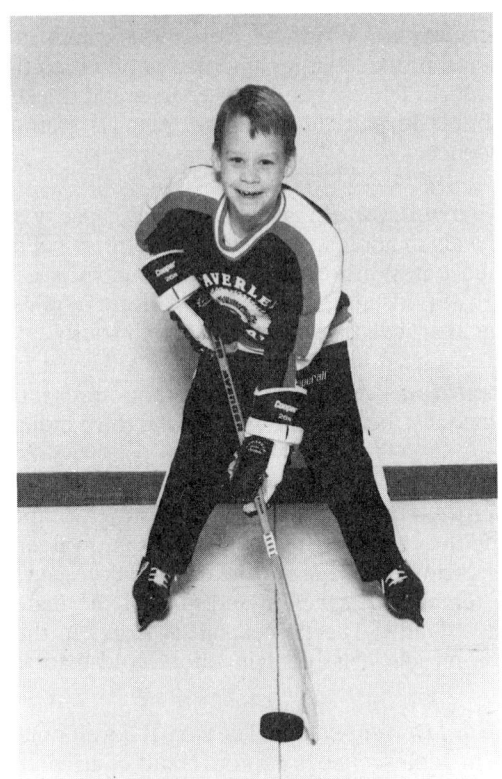

FIGURE 8-10
Complex motor abilities of the school-age child. The school-age child joins groups or teams and begins to combine gross and fine motor skills with rules and structure and team play.

adolescent growth spurt occurs early, adult height will likely be less than if the growth spurt occurs later.

Respiratory System. Adult lung capacity is achieved in both sexes around 17 to 18 years. The vital capacity of males becomes and remains greater than that of females. Adult respiratory rate of 16 to 20 breaths per minute is reached by mid to late adolescence.

Cardiovascular System. By about age 18 the heart's size and its electrocardiogram pattern are at adult levels. The male heart becomes and remains larger than the female heart. The pulse rate continues to decline, reaching adult levels in late adolescence. The male pulse rate is approximately 10% less than the female's, primarily because of the larger blood-pumping capacity of the male heart. The pulse rate ranges from 60 to 85 beats per minute for both sexes. The blood pressure by the end of adolescence should be approximately 120/70 mmHg.

Skeletal System. Growth occurs in the length, weight, and density of bones. Leg length accelerates first, followed by hip width, chest width, shoulder width, trunk length, and chest depth. Distal limb growth is more prevalent than proximal growth in adolescence. The ratio of trunk length to leg length increases in adolescence.[28] Ossification and epiphyseal fusion occur earlier in girls than in boys. This later ossification in boys accounts for the larger bone size and greater overall average height in boys.

Integumentary System. Sebaceous glands increase in size and produce larger amounts of oily secretions in adolescence. The skin becomes coarser and thicker, and facial pores in particular enlarge. Acne is common in adolescence.

Gastrointestinal System. Stomach capacity reaches adult levels in adolescence. The gastrointestinal musculature becomes thicker and stronger, thus increasing the strength of peristaltic movement.[29] Caloric requirements are high, particularly during the growth spurt.

Dentition. All permanent teeth are present in adolescence. By the end of this stage the third molars may appear.

Genitourinary System. Kidney structure and function and the characteristics of urine are equivalent to the adult's during this stage. By the end of adolescence 50% of the female body weight and 60% of the male body weight is fluid.[13] The percentage is larger in the male because muscle mass contains more fluid than adipose tissue.

Sexual Development. The sexual development that occurs in adolescence is a direct result of an increase in the amounts of and relationships among several hormones described in detail in Unit 18.

This hormonal activity develops the adolescent into a sexually mature adult. Sexual development in adolescence occurs in three distinct stages: prepubescence, pu-

bescence, and postpubescence. During prepubescence growth in the overall body increases, especially the reproductive organs. The secondary sex characteristics also begin to appear. The reproductive organs, however, are not fully functional. During pubescence secondary sex characteristics continue to develop and ovulation and spermatogenesis begin. During postpubescence full reproductive maturity is reached. The average female postpubescent period occurs between 15 and 18 years; the average male postpubescent period occurs between 16 and 20 years. Full body growth and reproductive fertility are completed during this stage.

Sexual development in adolescence usually follows a predictable pattern. There are exceptions, however, in both timing and sequence. The rapid pace of physiologic change and significant data related to it are discussed in Chapters 66 and 67.

Thermoregulation and Endocrine Function. The adolescent's average body temperature is 36.8° to 37.2° C. Thermoregulatory function is fully mature. The apocrine and eccrine glands are especially active in boys during adolescence. Endocrine function related to reproduction is covered in Chapter 66.

Neuromuscular System. The central nervous system is functionally mature by the end of adolescence. Muscle growth expands rapidly but not as rapidly as skeletal growth. The clumsiness and disproportionate appearance of many adolescents, particularly boys, is a result of this uneven skeletal and muscular growth rate. By late adolescence male muscle mass is close to twice that of the female's.

Special Senses. All senses are functionally mature and continue to influence cognitive development.

Sleep Patterns. Because of his or her high activity level, it is often difficult for the adolescent to obtain adequate rest. Sleep requirements, on average, are 8 to 10 hours per night.

Immunoregulatory Function

The functions and responses of the body's immune system and the production of immunoglobulin as part of the developmental process are described in Chapter 27. Reference here is to the growth of immune system organs and the developmental aspects of immunoglobulin production.

The elements of general circulation that play a major role in immune responses are the primary leukocytes (lymphocytes) and the secondary leukocytes (monocytes, neutrophils, eosinophils, and basophils). Adequate levels of leukocytes usually are present early in childhood. The tonsils and adenoids play a major role in immunoregulation and usually reach peak development by early school-age years. The growth of these two organs results from general tissue growth and the stimulation of re-

Ideas for Nursing Research

Research conducted by professional nurses interested in the growth and development of children can lead to an improvement in the quality of care provided for children in all health-oriented settings. Nursing interventions best suited for children whose patterns of behavior have been disrupted by disease, illness, or dysfunction, as well as healthy infants and children, can be examined. The following areas need to be explored:

- Effectiveness of behavior modification in assisting preadolescents to overcome problems with bedwetting during long-term hospitalization
- Comparison of the presence or absence of parents in the recovery room on the preschool child's immediate postoperative response
- Effect of peer interaction in mealtime groups on eating patterns of school-age children
- Effectiveness of parental rooming-in with a preterm infant prior to discharge on the parents' sensitivity to their infant's cues for physiologic and emotional needs
- Effectiveness of rewards for positive and caring behavior on moral development in structured environments
- Differences in the rate of growth and development of low-birthweight infants who are breastfed and those who are bottle-fed
- Result of teaching a new mother to provide tactile, verbal, and visual stimulation for her new infant on the potential for, rate of, and degree of maternal–infant attachments

peated infection. The lymphatic system peaks in growth at approximately age 10.

Summary

In the future, the study of child development and relationships will continue to yield new discoveries to support and discount some current beliefs; this is the nature of theory development. Essential to the nurse is a working knowledge of the basic concepts and principles related to child development investigation and an appreciation of the value of interdisciplinary investigation and practice. Additionally, a familiarity with current theoretical approaches to the study of child development will enable the nurse to explain facets of behavior observed in children and to plan more effective nursing interventions.

In the remaining chapters in this unit, the application of these theories related to cognitive, psychosocial, language, moral, and physical development is addressed. This chapter should be used as an introduction and foundation on which the reader can build more specific nursing applications throughout the textbook.

References

1. American Academy of Pediatrics Committee Statement. The ten-state nutrition survey: A pediatric perspective. *Pediatrics, 51,* 1095–1099.
2. Apgar, V. (1953). A proposal for a new method of evaluation in the newborn infant. *Anesthesia and Analgesia, 52,* 260–267.
3. Baer, M. J. (1973). *Growth and maturation: An introduction to physical development.* Cambridge, MA: Howard Drake.
4. Bandura, A. (1977). *Social learning theory.* Englewood Cliffs, NJ: Prentice-Hall.
5. Bee, H. (1985). *The developing child* (4th ed.). New York: Harper and Row.
6. Berger, K. S. (1988). *The developing person through the lifespan* (2nd ed.). New York: Worth Publishers.
7. Brazelton, T. B. (1984). *Neonatal behavioral assessment scale.* (2nd ed.) Philadelphia: J.B. Lippincott.
8. Broadwell, D. (1987). Psychosocial factors in health. In P. A. Potter & A. G. Perry (Eds.). *Basic nursing: Theory and practice* (pp. 271–295). St. Louis: C.V. Mosby.
9. Campos, J. J., et al. (1970). Cardiac responses on the visual cliff in prelocomotor human infants. *Science, 170,* 196–197.
10. Carpenito, L. J. (1992). *Nursing diagnosis: Application to clinical practice* (3rd ed.). Philadelphia: J.B. Lippincott.
11. Case, R. (1985). *Intellectual development: Birth to adulthood.* Orlando: Academic Press.
12. Chess, S., & Thomas, A. (1986). *Temperament in clinical practice.* New York: The Guilford Press.
13. Chinn, P. (1979). *Child health maintenance* (2nd ed.). St. Louis: C.V. Mosby.
14. Chomsky, N. (1957). *Syntactic structures.* The Hague: Mouton.
15. Coons, S., & Guilleminault, C. (1982). Development of sleep-wake patterns and non-rapid eye movement sleep stages during the first six months of life in normal infants. *Pediatrics, 75,* 807–812.
16. Dietz, W. H., & Gortmaker, S. L. (1985). Do we fatten our children at the television set? Obesity and television viewing in children and adolescents. *Pediatrics, 75,* 807–812.
17. Erikson, E. H. (1959). *Identity and the life cycle: Selected papers. From psychological issues, I* (Monograph series, No. 1). New York: International Universities Press.
18. Erikson, E. (1963). *Childhood and society* (2nd ed.). New York: Norton.
19. Flake-Hobson, C., Robinson, B. E., & Skeen, P. (1983). *Child development and relationships.* Reading, MA: Addison-Wesley.
20. Fletcher, P., & Garman, M. (1986). *Language acquisition* (2nd ed). Cambridge: Cambridge University Press.
21. Fogel, A., & Melsone, G. F. (1980). Delayed menarche and amenorrhea in ballet dancers. *New England Journal of Medicine, 303,* 17–19.
22. Fowler, J. W. (1981). *Stages of faith: The psychology of human development and the quest for meaning.* San Francisco: Harper and Row.
23. Freud, S. (1927). Some psychological consequences of the anatomical distinction between the sexes. *International Journal of Psychoanalysis, 8,* 133–142.
24. Gibson, E. J., & Walk, R. D. (1960). The "visual cliff." *Scientific American, 202,* 64–71.
25. Gilligan, C. (1982) *In a different voice: Psychological theory and women's development.* Cambridge, MA: Harvard University Press.
26. Harris, J. R., & Liebert, R. M. (1984). *The child: Development from birth through adolescence.* Englewood Cliffs, NJ: Prentice Hall.
27. Held, R. (1985). Binocular vision-behavioral and neuronal development. In J. Mehler & R. Fox (Eds.). *Neonate cognition: Beyond the blooming buzzing confusion* (pp. 37–44). Hillsdale, NJ: Erlbaum.

28. Hill, P. M., & Humphrey, P. (Eds.). (1982). *Human growth and development throughout life: A nursing perspective.* New York: Wiley.

29. Hurlock, E. (1973). *Adolescent development* (4th ed.). New York: McGraw-Hill.

30. Jacklin, C. N., & Maccoby, E. E. (1983). Issues of gender differentiation. In M. D. Levine, et al (Eds.). *Developmental-behavioral pediatrics* (pp. 175–184). Philadelphia: W.B. Saunders.

31. Jirasek, J. E. (1976). Principles of reproductive embryology. In J. L. Simpson (Ed.). *Disorders of sexual differentiation: Etiology and clinical delineation* (pp.). New York: Academic Press.

32. Johnson, T. R., Moore, & Jeffries. (1978). *Children are different: Developmental physiology* (2nd ed.). Columbus, OH: Ross Laboratories.

33. Jones, R. E. (1984). *Human reproduction and sexual behavior.* Englewood Cliffs, NJ: Prentice-Hall.

34. Kuczaj, S. (1982). *Language development (vol 1): Syntax and semantics.* Hillsdale, NJ: Lawrence Erlbaum Associates.

35. Lamb M. (1982). Maternal employment and child development: A review. In M. E. Lamb (Ed.). *Nontraditional families: Parenting and Childrearing* (pp. 45–70). Hillsdale, NJ: Erlbaum.

36. Lenniberg, E. (1967). *Biological foundation of language.* New York: Wiley.

37. Lorenz, K. (1952). *King Solomon's ring.* London: Methuen.

38. Lowry, G. H. (1975). *Growth and development of children* (6th ed.). Chicago: Yearbook Medical Publishers.

39. Ludington-Hoe, S. M. (1983). What can newborns really see? *American Journal of Nursing, 9,* 1286–1289.

40. McClowry, S. G. (1990). The relationship of temperament to pre- and posthospitalization behavioral responses of school-age children. *Nursing Research, 39,* 30–35.

41. Moen, P. (1982). The two-provider family: Problems and potentials. In M. E. Lamb (Ed.). *Nontraditional families: Parenting and child development* (pp. 13–44). Hillsdale, NJ: Erlbaum.

42. Miranda, S. B., Hack, M., Fantz, R. L., Fandroff, A. A., & Klaus, M. H. (1977). Neonatal pattern of vision: Predictor of future mental performance? *Journal of Pediatrics, 91,* 642–647.

43. Moore, K. L. (1982). *The developing human: Clinically oriented embryology* (3rd ed.). Philadelphia: W.B. Saunders.

44. Nelms, B. C., & Mullins, R. G. (1982). *Growth and development: A primary health care approach.* Englewood Cliffs, NJ: Prentice-Hall.

45. Neuman, C. G. (1977). Obesity in pediatric practice: Obesity in the preschool and schoolage child. *Pediatric Clinics of North America, 24,* 117–122.

46. Norton, H. A., & Glick, P. C. (1986). One-parent families: A social and economic profile. *Family Relations, 35,* 9–16.

47. Papilia, D. E., & Olds, S. W. (1986). *Human development* (3rd ed.). New York: McGraw-Hill.

48. Parsons, T. (1951). Illness and the role of physician: A sociological perspective. *American Journal of Orthopsychiatry, 21,* 452–460.

48A. Pipes, P. L. (1981). Nutrition in infancy and childhood. (2nd ed.). St. Louis: Mosby.

49. Power, C. F., Higgins, A., & Kohlberg, L. (1989). *Lawrence Kohlberg's approach to moral education.* New York: Columbia University Press.

50. Prechtl, H. F. R., et al. (1973). Behavioral state cycles in abnormal infants. *Developmental Medicine and Child Neurology, 15,* 606.

51. Rheingold, H. (1980). The significance of speech to newborns. *Developmental Psychology, 16,* 397–403.

52. Rich, J. M., & DeVitis, J. L. (1985). Theories of moral development. Springfield, IL: Charles C. Thomas.

53. Rothstein, E. (1980). The scar and Sigmund Freud. *New York Review of Books, October 9,* 14–20.

54. Russell, M. J. (1976). Human olfactory communication. *Nature, 260,* 520–522.

55. Salkind, N. J., & Ambron, S. R. (1987). *Child development* (5th ed.). New York: Holt, Rinehart, and Winston.

56. Saunders, R., Miller, B., & Cates, K. (1989). Pediatric family care: An interdisciplinary team approach. *Children's Health Care, 18*(1), 53–58.

57. Schulman, M., & Mekler, E. (1985). *Bringing up a moral child.* Reading, MA: Addison-Wesley.

58. Self, P., & Horowitz, F. (1987). The behavioral assessment of the neonate: An overview. In J. D. Osofsky (Ed.). *Handbook of infant development* (2nd ed.). (pp. 126–164). New York: Wiley.

59. Sex Information and Education Council of the United States. (1980). The SIECUS/New York University/Uppsala principles basic to education for sexuality. *SIECUS report, 8,* 8.

60. Siegler, R. S. (1986). *Children's thinking.* Englewood Cliffs, NJ: Prentice-Hall.

61. Skinner, B. F. (1957). *Verbal behavior.* New York: Appleton-Century-Crofts.

62. Smith, D., & Bierman, E. (1978). *The biological ages of man.* Philadelphia: W.B. Saunders.

63. Thomas, A., & Chess, S. (1977). *Temperament and development.* New York: Brunner and Mazel.

64. Thomas, R. M. (1985). *Comparing theories of child development* (2nd ed.). Belmont, CA: Wadsworth.

65. U.S. Department of Labor, Bureau of Labor Statistics. *Monthly Labor Review.* December.

66. Vygotsky, L. S. (1981). The genesis of higher mental functions. In J. V. Wertsch (Ed.). *The concept of activity in Soviet psychology* (pp. 12–14). Armonk, NY: M.E. Sharp.

67. Weiffenbach, J., & Thach, B. (1975). Taste receptors on the tongue of newborn human: Behavioral evidence. A paper presented at the biennial meeting of the Society for Research in Child Development. Denver.

68. Windle, W. F. (1940). *Physiology of the fetus: Origin and extent of function in prenatal life.* Philadelphia: W.B. Saunders.

69. Zigler, E. F., & Finn-Stevenson, M. (1987). *Children: Development and social issues.* Lexington, MA: Heath.

Health Supervision of Children

BEHAVIORAL OBJECTIVES

Describe the importance of well-child health supervision as part of primary prevention.

Explain the importance of anticipatory guidance in primary prevention.

Describe essentials of the health history.

Describe preparation and approach in physical examination.

Describe the physical examination for a well-child checkup.

Identify risks and benefits of immunizations.

Childhood is a time of rapid growth and development with body characteristics demonstrating increasing maturation. It is important, therefore, for children to be examined on a regular schedule so that deviations from normal can be identified early and interventions can be devised.[15] In addition to examination of body systems and performing related laboratory studies, health supervision visits for children provide an opportunity for evaluating developmental milestones, for giving immunizations against communicable diseases, and for teaching parents about health and developmental needs of their children.

An integration of the science and art of physical examination of children is emphasized in this chapter. Once the principles described are applied in a variety of situations, each nurse develops particular approaches that are unique while still applying the underlying knowledge. The sequence of any examination may be modified to accommodate the examiner's preference and the child's condition.

Well-Child Health Supervision

The health supervision visit is an example of the primary level of prevention of disease (discussed in Chap. 3). Primary prevention refers to *screening*, the process of examining large population groups to identify those people with deviations from normal.[36] The purpose of such visits is to identify those children who exhibit abnormalities, to plan further assessments if necessary, and to provide interventions that promote normal growth and development. These visits are discussed in more detail related to various developmental levels at the ends of Chapters 11 through 16.

The American Academy of Pediatrics (AAP), through its Committee on Psychosocial Aspects of Child and Family Health, has established guidelines for recommended health supervision of children (Table 9-1). The recommendations for timing of assessments refer to healthy children without unusual psychosocial stresses. The schedule may need to be altered if, for example, an abnormality is identified in some body system, the family unit is experiencing stress or change, or the child manifests a variation in developmental level.

Many of the principles discussed here can be applied in a variety of settings. Health supervision visits are usually performed in physician and nurse practitioner offices, in clinics, and sometimes in schools. However, some parts of the examination are performed in hospitals and other settings. For example, a community health nurse or hospital nurse may decide to perform a vision test on a child who appears to be squinting or may perform a heart and lung examination on a child who is breathless after mild exercise or who is recovering from surgery. Although the approaches to the child need to consider developmental level and prior experiences, such examinations differ from health supervision visits in purpose. They are concerned with a particular body system or developmental state rather than being part of an integrated examination. They are performed on children who are at particular risk or who manifest certain characteristics rather than on all children.

TABLE 9-1
Guidelines for Health Supervision

Item	Infancy						Early Childhood					Late Childhood					Adolescence[1]			
Age[2]	By 1 mo	2 mo	4 mo	6 mo	9 mo	12 mo	15 mo	16 mo	24 mo	3 y	4 y	5 y	6 y	8 y	10 y	12 y	14 y	16 y	18 y	20+ y
History																				
Initial/interval	●	●	●	●	●	●	●	●	●	●	●	●	●	●	●	●	●	●	●	●
Measurements																				
Height and weight	●	●	●	●	●	●	●	●	●	●	●	●	●	●	●	●	●	●	●	●
Head circumference	●	●	●	●	●	●														
Blood pressure										●	●	●	●	●	●	●	●	●	●	●
Sensory screening																				
Vision	S	S	S	S	S	S	S	S	S	S	O	O	O	O	S	O	O	S	O	O
Hearing	S	S	S	S	S	S	S	S	S	S	O	O	S³	S³	S³	O	S	S	O	S
Development/Behavior Assessment[4]	●	●	●	●	●	●	●	●	●	●	●	●	●	●	●	●	●	●	●	●
Physical Examination[5]	●	●	●	●	●	●	●	●	●	●	●	●	●	●	●	●	●	●	●	●
Procedures[6]																				
Hereditary/metabolic[7] screening	●																			
Immunization[8]		●	●	●			●	●				●					●			
Tuberculin test[9]						●			●				●							
Hematocrit or hemoglobin[10]				●					●				●							
Urinalysis[11]					●				●				●							
Anticipatory Guidance[12]	●	●	●	●	●	●	●	●	●	●	●	●	●	●	●	●	●	●	●	●
Initial Dental Referral[13]										●										

Key: = ● to be performed: S = subjective, by history: O = objective, by a standard testing method; arrows indicate that the test should be performed once within that period.

[1] Adolescent related issues (e.g., psychosocial, emotional, substance usage, and reproductive health) may necessitate more frequent health supervision.

[2] If a child comes under care for the first time at any point on the schedule, or if any items are not accomplished at the suggested age, the schedule should be brought up to date at the earliest possible time.

[3] At these points, history may suffice: if problem suggested, a standard testing method should be employed.

[4] By history and appropriate physical examination: if suspicious, by specific objective developmental testing.

[5] At each visit, a complete physical examination is essential, with infant totally unclothed, older child undressed and suitably draped.

[6] These may be modified, depending on entry point into schedule and individual need.

[7] Metabolic screening (e.g., thyroid, PKU, galactosemia) should be done according to state law.

[8] Schedule(s) per Report of Committee on Infectious Disease, 1986 Red Book.

[9] For low-risk groups, the Committee on Infectious Diseases recommends the following options: ① no routine testing or ② testing at three times—infancy, preschool, and adolescence. For high-risk groups, annual TB skin testing is recommended.

[10] Present medical evidence suggests the need for reevaluation of the frequency and timing of hemoglobin or hematocrit tests. One determination is therefore suggested during each time period. Performance of additional tests is left to the individual practice experience.

[11] Present medical evidence suggests the need for reevaluation of the frequency and timing of urinalysis. One determination is therefore suggested during each time period. Performance of additional tests is left to the individual practice experience.

[12] Appropriate discussion and counseling should be an integral part of each visit for care.

[13] Subsequent examinations as prescribed by dentist.

N.B.: **Special chemical, immunologic, and endocrine testing** are usually carried out upon specific indications. Testing other than newborn (e.g., inborn errors of metabolism, sickle disease, lead) are discretionary with the physician.

From Committee on Psychosocial Aspects of Child and Family Health. (1987). Guidelines for health supervision II. Elk Grove Village, IL: American Academy of Pediatrics.

Nurses play many roles in health supervision visits. Pediatric nurse practitioners are prepared to perform thorough physical examinations on children and do so in a variety of settings. Often physicians perform such examinations and registered nurses assist by taking histories, giving immunizations, performing parts of the examination (e.g., vision screening), and doing anticipatory guidance with parents.[21] Some specially trained community health nurses are prepared to perform examinations of children in health department settings and schools. All pediatric nurses apply parts of the physical examination in contacts with children. For example, a hospital nurse must adeptly examine the cardiac and pulmonary function of a child after surgery. Even though the information presented here can be used in many settings, the focus of this chapter is the integrated physical examination performed at regular intervals on children to identify those at risk and to promote wellness.

Anticipatory Guidance

Anticipatory guidance is a type of health teaching that considers the next expected developmental accomplishments of the child and prepares parents to deal with them and to prevent problems. This process is an essential component of each health supervision visit and can be included during history taking, throughout the examination, or in a special session before terminating the visit.

Anticipatory guidance requires application of knowledge about developmental norms. For example, when the baby is 4 months of age, topics to be discussed include introduction of solid foods, safety needs, and sleep patterns. The examiner prepares the parent for the coming developmental milestones, offers advice and suggests resources to assist in their management. As children grow older, they can be included in anticipatory guidance by teaching them about such topics as wise snack choices, importance of exercise, and bicycle safety practices. Chapters 11 through 16 contain detailed discussions about health maintenance and promotion topics for each developmental level. Anticipatory guidance is discussed, and tables highlight the information. Chapter 6 provides further information related to child and family teaching.

Health History

A history of the child provides many clues to guide the examiner during the physical assessment. Although the comprehensiveness and content of the history vary depending on the amount of information available in the record and on the child's age, it is an essential element of each health supervision visit. The history should precede the physical examination so that the information gained can guide the order and depth of the examination.[26]

Some of the history data may be collected by having the parent (or the child if old enough) complete the answers to written questions. However, in such cases, the examiner reviews the history, asks further questions to clarify certain areas, and provides a forum for parents or children to raise questions and concerns.

The history should have an organizational basis for ease of data collection and interpretation.[8] Examples of organizational frameworks for histories include the use of body systems or of functional health areas (see Chap. 2). Tools have been developed to gather such data easily. An example of a tool using functional health is given in the accompanying display on nursing assessment.

Preparation and General Guidelines

The examiner wishes to obtain accurate history data. To do so, the data should be collected in a nonjudgmental manner. When parents or children fear they will be "scolded" for certain behaviors, they are unlikely to be candid in responses to questions. Although teaching is often performed in conjunction with history taking, the examiner must be certain to avoid authoritarian approaches, to use understanding, and to provide information in a helpful manner.

History is best collected in a calm setting and with a relaxed approach. This is an additional reason to precede the examination with history when the young child is generally quiet and most rested. After an examination, a child may be crying or tired, making it difficult for a parent to concentrate on questions or responses.

Although every child's chart should provide thorough background information, such data are not all included at one visit, nor are prior data recollected unless it is pertinent at a later date. An overall history profile may be obtained before a first visit by having a parent complete a form before coming to the office or while in the waiting room. The examiner may wish to clarify information pertinent for the individual child during the visit. A newborn's parents, for example, may be asked some specific questions regarding diet, sleep, and adjustment to the new baby. The parents of an 18-month-old child may be asked about diet, developmental milestones, and plans for initiation of toilet training. The chart, when looked at in totality, provides a picture over time of all pertinent history areas.

A contrasting example would be when a 6-year-old child is found to have some developmental delays. The examiner may wish to ask questions about birth history, stressors, and other topics that might provide clues to contributing factors for the present situation. Thus, just as history can guide physical examination, the examination may suggest areas to be more fully explored in history.

Similarly, the biologic system history is guided both by the examiner's knowledge of pertinent issues at a particular age and by findings of physical examination. Questions regarding incidence of ear infections are always pertinent in the first years of life during the time when such infections are most frequent. A history finding of frequent infections guides the examiner to perform hearing assessment on the child. Likewise, if an older child is found to have a hearing deficit, the examiner asks questions about past ear infections, presence of infectious disease in the mother during pregnancy, and other potential contributing factors.

In addition to usual history content, the child's history should contain additional questions pertinent for the

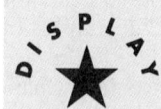

Nursing Assessment: Tool for Recording the Child Health Database Using Functional Health

Functional Health Status

Nursing History/Examination—Children

Date: _____ Time: _____ Name: _____ Source of Information: _____
Admitting Diagnosis: _____ Age: _____
Reason for Admission: _____

I. Health Perception and Health Management = Subjective Data	Objective Data
A. What is the problem? Why did you seek help today? Describe the problem. How has the problem been managed at home?	
B. Current health Preventive and safety practices Health today as related to past months, years Family/parent health	General appearance Child/parents

C. Past health
  1. Birth history
  Prenatal: Planned pregnancy	

C. Past health
  1. Birth history
  Prenatal: Planned pregnancy

Emotional response	Wt. gain
Complications	Alcohol use; medication

  Natal: Length of labor   Spontaneous/induced
  Vaginal/cesarean   Anesthesia
  Complications
  Bonding   Support person
  Neonatal: Wt.: _____ Length: _____
  Head circ.: _____
    Apgar
    Nursery course:

  2. Immunizations: DPT   Polio   Measles   Mumps
              Rubella   TB test   Flu   Hib
  3. Growth and development:
    Motor: Rolling over _____
            Sitting _____
            Crawling _____
            Standing _____
            Walking _____
            Sports _____
    Social-cognitive:
            Smiling _____
            First Word _____
            Sentences _____
            Playing _____
            School _____
    Early behavior patterns as viewed by parents
  4. Frequency of health assessments and checkups—date of last visit
  5. Hospitalizations: Date, reason, length, diagnosis
  6. Accidents or injuries: Time, place, reactions, physical response
  7. Allergies/reactions: Drugs, foods, contactants, inhalants
D. Family history: Familial, inherited, genetic disorders
  (use back of sheet to illustrate)

Parents	Heart
Sibilngs	Hypertension
Aunts, uncles (maternal, paternal)	Arteriosclerosis
Cousins	Coronary artery

disease

Maternal grandparents	Blood disorders
Paternal grandparents	Renal disease

(Continued)

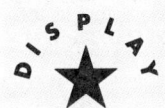

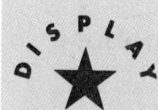

Nursing Assessment: Tool for Recording the Child Health Database Using Functional Health (continued)

VII. *Self-Perception–Self-Concept Patterns*
    Outstanding personality trait
    Overall behavior
    Interests
    What causes fears, strong emotions   How handled?
    Sense of humor

Body posture/movement
Eye contact
Behavior changes
Self-confidence

VIII. *Role Relationship*
    Usual caregiver/parent–child interaction
    Siblings:
    Sibling–child relationship
    Grandparents
    Peer interactions
    Favorite person
    Security objects
    Additional members of household
    Response to separation
    Dependency
    School adjustment

Observed interaction with significant others

IX. *Sexuality-Reproductive Patterns*
    Knows if she/he is a girl/boy (feelings of maleness, femaleness)
    Basic language for body parts and functions
    Direct teaching regarding sexuality
    Response to questions
    Best friend
    Menarche

Testicles examination
Breast examination
Genitalia

X. *Coping-Stress Tolerance Patterns*
    Response to stress changes
        New environment/people
        Illness
        Hospitalization
    Frequent illness(es)
    Experience of separation from parents
    Occurrence of dependent behavior
    Method of discipline
        Reaction
    Response to criticism, correction
    Family stressors
    Community resources used by the famlily

Problem solving/coping observed

XI. *Value-Belief Patterns*
    Goals for future
    What qualities are important in life
        Parents/child
    Is religious belief important/supportive to family?
        Religion   Sunday school

Varied health practices

Other Diagnostic Screening Tests   *Other Laboratory Tests*
Denver II
Preschool Readiness: Experimental Screening Scale
Draw-a-Person
Neonatal Perception Inventory
Anticipatory Guidance Need
Others

Summary Statement: (Cluster cues—Nursing diagnosis)

This form was developed for use in acute care settings but could be adapted to other health care settings.
(Developed by Marita Hoffart, Assistant Professor of Nursing, Minot State University, Minot, ND.)
From Fuller, J. & Shaller-Ayers, J. (1990). *Health Assessment: A Nursing Approach.* Philadelphia: Lippincott.

given age group. Some of the areas that are similar for adults and children include demographic data, reason for present visit, a detailed analysis of any health problems, and a review of biologic systems. Areas specific to children or that require different data from adults include past health history, developmental landmarks, family history, and nutritional status. These are explained more fully below.

Past Health History

The past health history includes information related to the child's conception, birth, early life, significant diseases, surgeries, immunizations, allergies, and accidents. Initially, the mother's and father's health is examined. Any parental chronic or acute diseases, maternal obstetric history, prenatal care, psychological state during pregnancy, environmental exposure of parents (including radiation, illicit drugs, medication, alcohol, tobacco smoke, and other potentially harmful agents), and maternal health state during pregnancy are questioned.

Next, the child's birth history is obtained. Information includes the length of labor, maternal complications of labor or postpartum, medications during labor, type of delivery, child's Apgar score, birthweight, and gestational age.

The postnatal history includes information concerning condition in the first month of life, presence of any complications, feeding history, anomalies, maternal recovery and psychological state, parental bonding with the baby, and reactions of siblings to the newborn. This background begins to put the child in a family context for the nurse and alerts the nurse to potential problems that need further exploration.

Family History

Data significant to the health of close family members are collected. Parents, siblings, grandparents, aunts, and uncles are specifically included, although the presence of diseases or conditions in cousins may also be important (e.g., cystic fibrosis). The age and cause of death for deceased members are included. Questions are directed to family members' health states. Examples of the types of conditions to be mentioned are diabetes, heart disease, high blood pressure, cancer, thyroid disease, respiratory conditions, birth defects, and surgeries. When indicated, all disease conditions are explored in depth. A family tree may be used to indicate health problems recurrent in various family members (Fig. 9-1).

A psychosocial history of the family is also taken and includes information on the age, sex, and family roles (e.g., parent, sibling) of family members. The marital status of parents, as well as history of divorce and remarriage is included. Details about the child's school and other activities, such as grade level, school performance, friendships, and after-school activities are collected. (High-risk families are discussed in Chap. 5.)

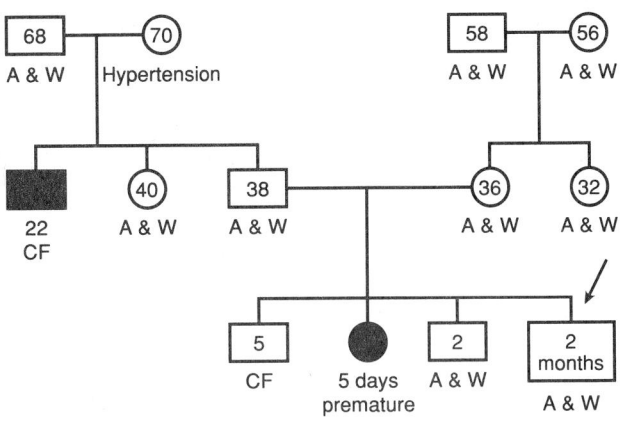

□ = Male
○ = Female
■ ● = Deceased
A & W = Alive and well
CF = Cystic fibrosis
→ = Child of interest in particular family health history
FIGURE 9-1
Family tree shows health problems of relatives of 2-month-old boy.

Assessment of Developmental Landmarks

Questions regarding developmental landmarks are included in each history just as the assessment of developmental progression is performed throughout childhood at each physical examination.[9] The questions to be asked depend on the age of the child and the data already present in the record. For young children, data regarding gross motor skills, fine motor skills, and use of language are included. For example, the ages when the baby could roll over, sit, pull to standing, and walk unassisted illustrate large motor skills. Fine motor skills are indicated by ability to hold rattles, bang blocks, and feed self. History regarding presence of coos and babbles and age at emergence of words and sentences should be included. Developmental test results become part of the record. For example, normal performance on a Denver Developmental Screening Test (now called the Denver II) as well as any delays on task performance are part of the history (see Chap. 8 for discussion of the Denver II).

Additional data are included in the developmental history of older children. For example, gross motor skills may include age of skipping, running, hopping on one foot, or enrollment and performance in sports. Fine motor skills may include buttoning, typing, art work, and writing. Language and cognitive skills may be shown by school performance and ability to communicate.

Other areas to include in a developmental history are age of urinary and bowel training, ability to dress self, attendance at day care or preschool, grade level in school, age of sleeping through the night, occurrence of any sleep problems, or presence of behavioral problems. As with all histories, the examiner focuses on landmarks and asks more specific questions related to any deviations from expected norms.

Assessment of Nutritional Status

Because good nutrition is so critical in fostering normal growth and development, this area is generally considered as a separate and essential area during history taking. Feeding problems are frequent during early childhood. Feeding sessions are infrequently observed; therefore, asking clear and comprehensive questions of the parents is important.

During each health care visit, information is sought about the amount, type, frequency, and length of time of feedings. For example, for a bottle-fed newborn, the examiner asks what type of formula is fed, how often, how much the baby eats, how long the feeding takes, if the baby eats eagerly or has trouble sucking or tires easily. Do the parents use ready-to-feed, concentrate, or powdered formula? A review of preparation methods is needed to identify any errors in cleanliness or formula strength. Does the baby sleep longer at night or awake equally frequently during day and night hours? Is there spitting or vomiting? What is the consistency and frequency of stools? How often does the baby have wet diapers? Is the baby held for feedings or are bottles propped? Are bottles given to assist the baby to go to sleep?

Likewise, the breast-fed baby's intake is questioned. Although the amount consumed during feedings is not known, signs of satisfaction, ability to suck and cause a letdown reflex, and the mother's description of her milk supply are elicited. The use of supplements such as vitamins and fluoride is questioned.

Once the child is taking solid foods, data regarding type, amount, consistency, baby's reactions, and method of introducing new foods are collected. By the end of the first year, information on finger foods and regular table foods must usually be included. Numbers of feedings per day and type and amount of milk intake are considered. As the child progresses into toddler and preschool years, a 1-day diet recall is a good method to gather information on diet.[33] If problems with intake or growth are noted, a more detailed 3-day or 1-week diet history may be needed.

The growing independence of school-age children contributes to a further need for regular dietary analysis. Use of school lunch programs, breakfast patterns, and snack habits are all examined. Diet frequently takes on added importance related to body image adaptations and independence of actions as the child reaches adolescence. It is, therefore, important to address nutritional intake as well as to assess dietary knowledge during the teen years. Nutritional needs of each developmental level are explored in the remaining chapters of Unit II.

Physical Examination

A primary objective of the periodic health supervision visits for young children is the performance of a physical examination. Other aspects of the assessment (history, developmental exam, assessment for anticipatory guidance, and so forth) may be integrated throughout the physical examination, but, for clarity, they are explored in other parts of this chapter.

Physical examination of children requires a combination of both *science* and *art*. The *science* of physical examination includes application of knowledge related to physical assessment, to physical development parameters during childhood, and to cognitive and psychological development of children. For example, the nurse must know how to inspect, palpate, percuss, and auscultate and must identify the expected as well as abnormal outcomes in each body system. The physical findings that vary due to the biologic maturity of the child must be considered (e.g., a positive Babinski's reflex under 1 year of age is an expected finding). And finally, children's developmental levels must be identified so that their understanding of the examination and dependence on parents are recognized.

The *art* of physical examination requires that the nurse use all of the various pieces of knowledge to integrate an examination for the most effective approach to an individual child. For example, the best place for conducting a physical examination on a 10-month-old child is the mother's lap because the separation anxiety evident at this stage frequently leads to loss of cooperation in an infant who is taken from the mother and placed on an examination table. In addition, skills such as auscultation are nearly impossible to carry out on a loudly crying baby, and the nurse can either delay that portion of the examination or use a strategy to gain the child's quiet cooperation.

This section provides an overview of the physical examination for children with suggestions for managing age differences. A text on physical assessment should be consulted for more detailed information about techniques, and later chapters on assessment and diagnosis of disorders in body systems provide guidelines for examining children who present with symptoms.

Preparation and General Guidelines

Data gathering of physical information is a continual process, beginning with a perusal of the record before calling the child into the examining room. This review provides clues for areas of potential need for the present visit. If feeding problems were evident in the past, for example, growth measures and dietary intake may need emphasis. If gross motor delays were evident, developmental testing and musculoskeletal assessment are important.

When the child is called in, observation of the parent–child interaction is begun. Are the parent and child socializing? Is the young infant or toddler held close and comforted if insecure? Is the preschooler or school-age child included in the conversation? Does the parent have developmentally appropriate expectations of the child's behavior?

General observations of the child include general size, coloring, presence of developmental landmarks, coordinated movements, and awareness of people and environment. Such observations can guide the examination. For example, a baby who does not turn toward sounds may need further hearing assessment, and a 1-year-old child who uses only two words should have language evaluation. Likewise, an overweight, pale, listless, 18-

month-old child needs dietary assessment and laboratory studies for potential anemia.

The examination of a young child must be carefully planned and well organized to gain the trust and cooperation of the child. Effective approaches and a timely manner assist in working with the child who, due to developmental level, perceives the examiner as a stranger and who has a short attention span (Fig. 9-2).

The wise examiner begins the interaction with the child slowly and by talking first with the parent. A young child is more likely to accept interaction with a stranger if that person has obviously been accepted by the parent, as demonstrated by friendly interchanges. This introductory time is ideal for taking the history, clarifying parental concerns, and explaining what will take place. The examiner might have an interesting instrument in hand such as stethoscope, tongue blade, or otoscope. The child may reach out to touch it; handling can lessen fears of such instruments. When the child seems happy and receptive, the examiner talks to and perhaps reaches over to touch the child. Before physically examining the child, the examiner's hands are washed and warmed to preserve aseptic technique and the child's comfort. Measurements that are generally performed at the beginning of the examination include pulse, blood pressure, height, weight, chest circumference, and head circumference. Temperature may also be taken. See Table 9-1 for the general measurements and ages at which these measurements are performed. Chapter 25 provides guidance for taking vital signs; normal values for vital signs in children of different ages may be reviewed in the Appendix.

Approaches

Approaches for children of various ages are described here. Figure 9-3 also illustrates some approaches.

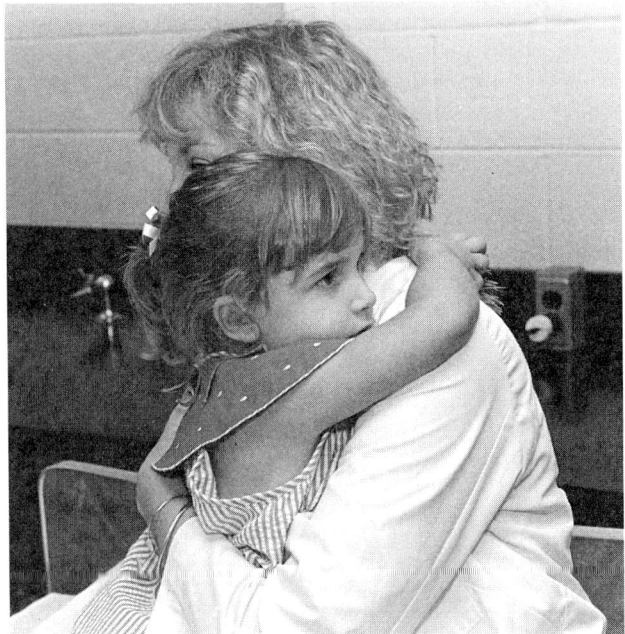

FIGURE 9-2
If the nurse gains the child's trust and cooperation, the child may see the nurse as a friend.

Infants

Privacy is not a concern at this age; however, the possibility of causing hypothermia by undressing the child for prolonged periods should be considered. Newborns are particularly ill equipped to regulate internal temperatures during external variations. The room should be kept warm; some pediatric examination rooms have heating lights over the examination table. The young infant who is undressed on entry to the room should be wrapped in blankets until examined. Parents can hold the infant to promote warmth.

The examination may appear threatening to infants. To the infant under 6 months of age, leaving the warmth of a parent's arms for the cold table may be uncomfortable. The parent can accompany the baby to the table, and a blanket can be used on the hard surface. For the infant between 6 and 12 months of age, stranger anxiety leads to a fear of the examiner, especially when taken from the arms of the parent. If such anxiety seems evident, the baby can remain in the parent's arms; nearly the whole examination can be completed there (see Fig. 9-3A).

The usual order of examination can be altered with infants. If the baby is happy and cooperative initially, it is wise to listen to heart and lung sounds. If the baby seems guarded, a look at extremities coupled with some playful "toe tickling" may lead to smiles and cooperation. The head, mouth, and ear examinations are done last because they are most likely to result in crying.

Diapers can remain in place for most of the examination, being removed for weight and assessment of abdomen and genitalia. The diaper should be kept close so that it can be used if the baby urinates during examinations.

Toddlers

The child from 1 to 3 years generally remains dependent on the parent for comfort and encouragement. Increased interest in manipulating instruments may occur and should be encouraged because familiarity with the equipment can decrease fears (see Fig. 9-3B). The examiner talks with toddlers, explaining what is happening and playing games throughout, taking advantage of opportunities for data gathering. For example, the child should be observed while walking into the examining room, because she or he may refuse to walk for gait assessment later. Some toddlers are eager to climb onto the examination table, whereas others prefer to remain close to the parent. A sitting position is least threatening to the child; therefore, parts of the examination requiring the supine position should be left until the end.

Preschoolers

Preschool-age children have an interest in the body and how it works. This interest, together with well-developed language skills, can be used to advantage during physical examination. Many questions during the history can be directed to the child. Do you go to preschool? What is your favorite toy? What games do you like to play? What do you like to eat?

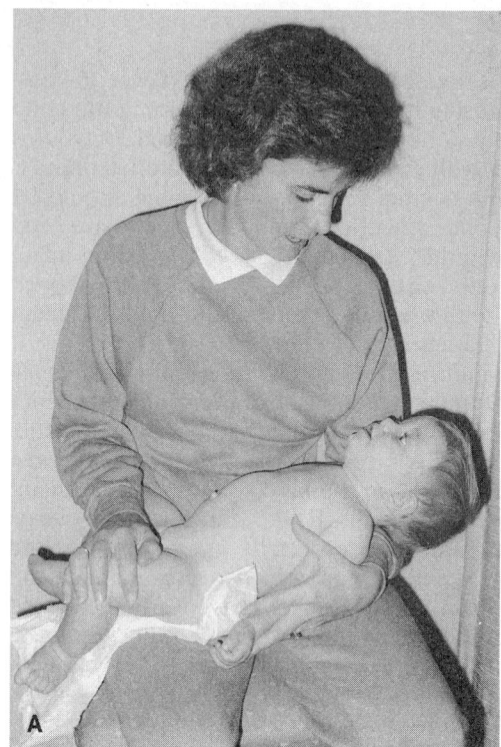
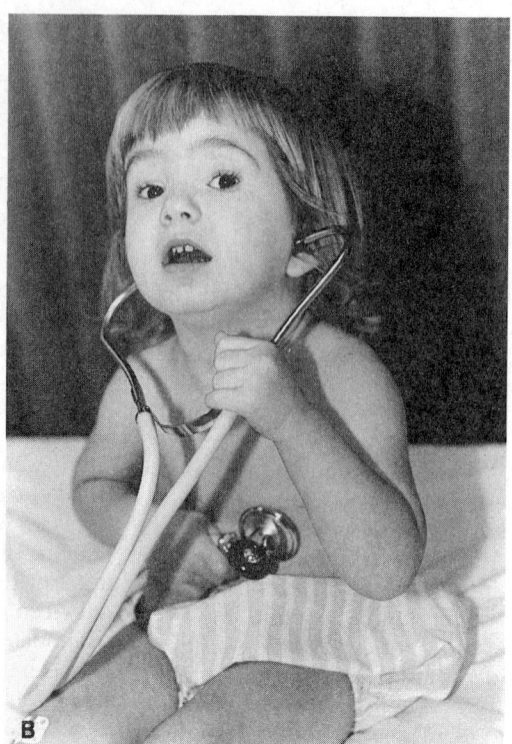
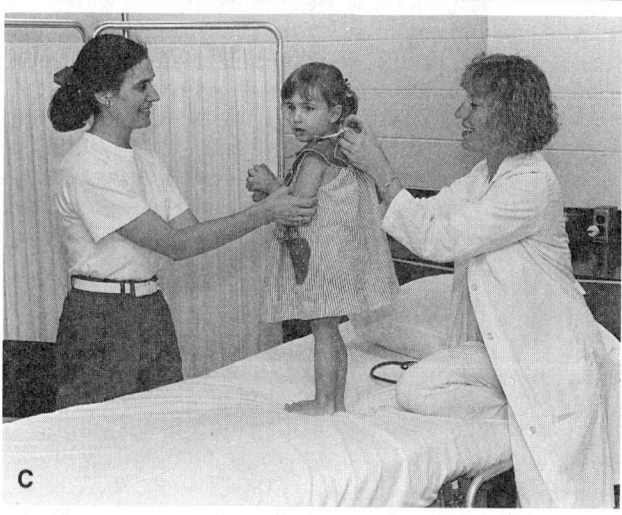

FIGURE 9-3

Approaches to children vary at different ages. (**A**) For instance, the infant may feel more comfortable being held on the mother's lap during the examination. (**B**) If the toddler manipulates the instruments before the examination, he or she may not fear their use by the nurse. (**C**) Once rapport has been established between the nurse and the preschooler, the preschooler may be willing to get on the examining table and have clothing removed or help with removing clothing. The mother is near for security.

Examination equipment can be shown and explained. Allowing the preschooler to touch, manipulate, and even try out such instruments on the examiner (e.g., stethoscope, otoscope) can allay fears and increase cooperation. A hurried approach to beginning the examination may heighten the child's feelings of fear, anxiety, and mistrust.

Once rapport has been established, the preschooler generally is willing to climb onto the examination table (see Fig. 9-3C). Most preschoolers do not object to removing a shirt. Sometimes pants are more problematic, and they can be left on until the leg and genitalia exams are performed. The examiner's hands should be warm and the touch should be gentle but firm to decrease tickling sensations. When a preschooler is relaxed and cooperative, the eye and mouth examination may not be threatening and can be done when the examiner desires. For an apprehensive preschooler, they may be left for later.

Although the preschooler is interested in body functioning and receptive to health and body teaching, the use of preoperational thought limits the understanding of some concepts. Most procedures that require entering the body are viewed as intrusive and potentially mutilating. Preschoolers think it is easy to change the body and even one's gender. Procedures such as rectal temperatures, drawing blood, and immunization injections are frightening and best left until the end of the examination. Explanations of what will be done are given directly before the procedure, and assurance is given that there will be no alteration in the body. "I will quickly push this lancet into your finger. You will feel a prick. I will get out a few drops of blood and put a Band-Aid on. Your body stops the bleeding right away, and the Band-Aid also keeps any more blood from coming out. You can cry if the prick hurts; just try to hold still so I can do it quickly. Your mother will help hold your hand still for me." Preschoolers often fear that once the skin is punctured, the body contents can flow out, somewhat like a balloon. This reasoning explains why Band-Aids are so reassuring at this age. To summarize, preschool is an age to allay fears, to provide some teaching that increases body knowledge, and to begin integrating the child more actively into the examination process.

School-Age Children

The school-age child is generally cooperative during physical examination, but some special approaches can make it a more positive experience. Emerging sensitivity about the body necessitates an offer of a gown when requesting the child to undress. Particularly during the later school years when pubertal changes occur, the child may be sensitive and self-conscious about the body. For this reason, it is best to ask the child if he or she wishes to have the parent present during the examination. Some children definitely wish the parents to be present, whereas others feel differently. Any concerns or questions of the parents can be learned during a preliminary interview with the parents and child or at a separate discussion with the parent. Parents may need sensitive handling and an explanation that children of this age often prefer to attend examinations independently.

The school-age child is in the stage of concrete operational thought, which is characterized by a new ability to reason and to solve problems when concrete experiences provide the background for new learning.[17] School-age children are interested in the body and how it functions.[6,14] For this reason, the examiner should explain what is being done and what the findings are. Health teaching is easy to integrate throughout the visit.

When the school-age child is quiet during the history and examination, open-ended questions can encourage sharing of information. For example, "What are the three favorite foods you might choose for a snack after school?" "What do you like to do on weekends?" This information gives the nurse greater insight into the child's cognitive, emotional, and psychosocial development.

Adolescents

Adolescent health care is often considered an independent field because adolescence is a time of greater maturity, therefore requiring different approaches from health care during childhood. At the same time, some of the concerns of adolescents and approaches for health care differ from those of adults. Pubertal changes bring an interest in and need for teaching related to sexuality. Body changes may lead to discussions of sports and other physical activity. Information regarding safety should be geared to risks for adolescence, such as those related to motor vehicles, drugs, firearms, and water sports.

Adolescents come for health care infrequently. A common reason for health supervision visits is a sports physical. The time health care providers spend with them must be used to greatest advantage to provide comprehensive examination and teaching. The examiner must be aware of adolescent health risks to teach preventive practice.[33]

Increasing body maturity contributes to a need for sensitivity and provision of privacy. Interviews must be conducted when the adolescent is fully clothed, and drapes are provided for examination. Explanations of the examination and findings are essential. The adolescent should be given an opportunity to raise questions and concerns about areas such as menstruation, dieting, sexual intercourse, and contraceptives. Statements such as "Many teens have questions about. . . How about you?" make the adolescent feel less unusual and more apt to discuss pertinent topics. They should be assured that their concerns and questions will be kept confidential.

Parents should generally not be present for adolescent health supervision visits. If they do accompany the adolescent, the examiner should give them an opportunity to express concerns, then state that they can wait outside where results will be summarized for them. Occasionally, an adolescent wishes to have a parent present; an adolescent girl, for example, may wish her mother to be there for a first pelvic examination. Sensitivity to the feelings of the adolescent and parent requires skills in identification and intervention.[17]

The adolescent uses the mature, cognitive thought of formal operations, so approaches used with younger children are inappropriate. Adolescents should learn about the examination, the body's functioning, and health supervision concerns such as safety when driving and the effects of alcohol. Even topics taught at a younger age may need repeating now that they are old enough to use mature thought processes.

Equipment Required

Whereas the adult client may be silently displeased when an examiner has to search for an instrument or has cold hands, the child overtly shows displeasure by crying and manifesting other uncooperative behavior. Such behavior may make the examination difficult. Therefore, all equipment should be clean and ready before use. The equipment listed below is required. Procedures for using some of the equipment are discussed in Chapter 25.

The *scale* is used for height and weight. A recumbent balance scale is used for children until about 2 years of age; a standing balance scale is used thereafter. Infants are generally weighed nude; older children may have underwear on. *Growth grids* are used to record height, weight, and head circumference to elicit child's percentiles. Examples are given in the Appendix.

A *sphygmomanometer* is used to take blood pressure on children 3 years of age and over. The blood pressure cuff must cover 75% of the arm from shoulder to elbow and must completely encircle the arm without overlapping, so several sizes should be available for different ages of children. Traditional devices in addition to newer ultrasound methods are available. Blood pressure cuff sizes and the procedure for taking blood pressure in children are discussed in Chapter 25.

The *stethoscope* is used in measuring blood pressure as well as listening to sounds of the heart, lung, and bowel. It is helpful to have a pediatric stethoscope with a smaller diaphragm and bell for use with young children.

An *ophthalmoscope* is used to perform fundoscopic

examination of the eye; an *otoscope* is used to examine the structures of the ear canal and middle ear. Generally, the same base in used for the ophthalmoscope and otoscope, with the proper head inserted for the particular part of the examination. A variety of speculum sizes is needed for the ears of children. The otoscope may also be used for a nasal speculum.

Thermometers are used for temperature measurement. Although traditional oral or rectal mercury thermometers may be used, some prefer less invasive techniques for children. Axillary temperatures, electronic and digital thermometers, skin thermometers, and tympanic membrane sensor thermometers are all popular alternatives.

A *wooden tongue blade* is used to depress the tongue to visualize the pharynx. It may not be needed for children who can open their mouths wide. A *pen light* is useful for checking extraocular movements, light reflex, and pupillary response. A *dental mirror* may be useful for counting and assessing teeth and performing other parts of the oral exam. A *reflex hammer* is used to elicit deep tendon reflexes. A *tuning fork* may be used to perform Rinne and Weber's tests during hearing assessment.

Gloves are used when the examiner will come into contact with bodily secretions from the child such as during examination of the mouth and genitalia and during blood drawing.

Head-to-Toe Examination

The physical examination must be conducted in an organized way. One of the methods is head-to-toe, used here.

Somatic Measures

Somatic growth measurement is performed during each regularly scheduled health supervision visit and provides valuable information about the child's state of health. Height or length and weight are performed on all children. Occipital-frontal circumference (OFC) of the head and sometimes chest circumference are measured in children 2 years of age and under and may be performed at older ages if indicated. Additional measurements such as skin fold thickness and crown to rump may be assessed in special circumstances. The child's data for each measurement are plotted on a percentile chart and analyzed. Although each percentile is important, the examiner also compares percentiles for various measures. For example, are height and weight proportional, or is one in a low percentile while the other is high? Is the head circumference in approximately the same percentile as other growth measures? These findings may indicate a need for closer examination of family history (particularly family size), remeasurement, dietary counseling, or further diagnostic testing.

Procedures for assessment are discussed in Chapter 25. These include body temperature, pulse, respirations, blood pressure, and methods for collecting specimens.

Length and Height.   Recumbent length is measured until a child is 2 years of age. Examination tables may be equipped with a headboard and a movable footboard for ease in measurement. In this case, the head is held flat against the board with neck and body straight, knees extended, heels on table, and the foot is flexed upward to form a right angle with the leg. The footboard is placed flat against the feet, and length is measured.

When a measuring table is not available, the child is placed on a piece of paper covering a flat surface such as the examining table. An assistant holds the head in alignment, and the examiner straightens the knees and flexes feet upward to maintain heels on the surface. A pen is placed at a right angle to the surface, and the examiner marks the head and heel points. The distance between the two marks is measured (see Fig. 12-3). It is advisable to have an assistant (who could be the parent) and to proceed quickly to minimize the effects of the child's movement in causing inaccuracy of data.

The length is plotted on a growth grid for birth to 36 months, specific for the particular sex of the child.

Standing height is usually assessed in children over 2 years of age. The child stands on a platform scale with shoes removed and posture straight. The upper lever is placed on the top of the child's head and kept parallel to the floor and perpendicular to the scale (Fig. 9-4).

When no scale is available, the child stands on a flat floor with back to a wall, maintaining heels, buttocks, shoulders, and head touching the wall. The child looks straight ahead, and a book or other object is placed on the uppermost part of the head, held parallel to the floor and perpendicular to the wall. A mark is made on the wall, and the distance from the floor to the mark is measured.

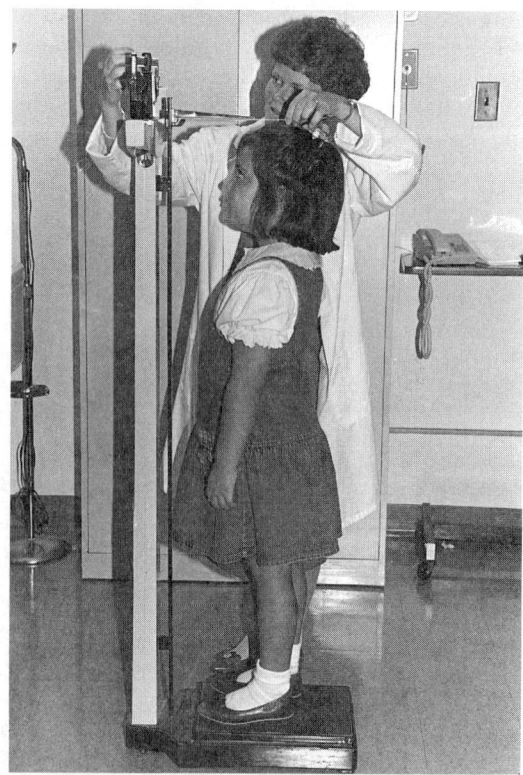

FIGURE 9-4
Standing height is measured in the child over age 2. Usually the shoes are removed for the measurement.

Height is plotted on a growth grid for children 2 to 18 or 2 to 11 years of age, specific for the particular sex of the child. Children from 2 to 3 years who are measured for standing height must be plotted on the growth grid for this type of measurement, not on the birth to 36-month grid, which is intended only for recumbent length. Growth grids appear in the Appendix.

Weight. Weight is measured on a balance beam scale, with a small scale for lying or sitting with infants and toddlers, or a standing scale for older children (see Fig. 12-3). Before weighing each child, the examiner should check to be certain that the scale is balanced and should make adjustments as needed.

Infants are weighed without clothes, and readings are taken to the nearest 1/2 ounce. To ensure safety, the examiner's hand is kept directly above the baby without touching. Babies may be frightened when placed on the scale due to its movement. Comfort measures such as talking can help the procedure to progress smoothly. The infant lies on the scale; the toddler may sit and hold onto the sides.

Children generally are weighed on a standing scale with underwear or light clothing. Coat, shoes, sweater, and other heavy clothing should be removed before weighing. The reading is made to the nearest ¼ lb. Many standing scales have a post the child can hold onto for stability.

Weight is plotted on a growth grid to elicit the child's percentile. Comparison with height percentile is made. Growth grids appear in the Appendix.

Occipital-Frontal Circumference. The occipital-frontal or head circumference is measured in children up to approximately 2 years of age. A metal or paper tape measure is placed just over the largest part of the occiput and brought above the eyebrows. The circumference is measured in the nearest tenth of a centimeter. The examiner may wish to take three measures on each child and average them for greatest accuracy. The OFC is recorded on a growth grid, and the percentile is compared to those for height and weight and to percentile measurements on previous visits. Referral is made for changes in percentile readings or lack of congruence with other body percentiles.

Chest Circumference. Although chest circumference may not be performed routinely on all children, it provides valuable data when growth patterns appear abnormal. The OFC is greater than the chest circumference in children under 1 year of age. The two dimensions are roughly equivalent at that age, and then the chest begins to exceed OFC. The tape measure is placed around the baby from front to back at the nipple level.

Skin

The skin is examined early in the visit as well as throughout. Inspection is the major technique used with observation of color, texture, lesions, and edema. Palpation of the skin is performed for temperature, moisture or hydration, texture, edema, and turgor. Some frequent abnormalities include pallor resulting from anemia, le-

sions due to communicable disease, infection, or skin rash, and turgor or hydration variations due to disease causing fluid imbalance. The examiner should develop skill in identifying normal variations in skin color and texture related to various cultural groups. Parts of the body with least melanin such as palms of hands, soles of feet, nail beds, lips, and conjunctiva can be the most reliable locations.

The hair is inspected for color, texture, distribution, hygiene, and for the presence of dandruff or lice. Abnormal occurrence of hair on any body part is noted, as are areas of scalp baldness. Hair growth in the axillary and genital regions helps to establish stage of puberty. Palpation of the hair is used to describe texture and quality.

Nails are examined for color, shape, texture, and condition. Palpation to cause blanching and counting of time for color return provides clues to circulatory status. A more extensive examination of the skin and accessory structures may be necessary if anomalies are suspected. These are discussed in Chapter 64.

Head and Neck

Although the assessment of head and associated structures is routinely performed first in adult examination, it is often performed last when examining children because they usually view this as an intrusive and uncomfortable experience.

Head. The head is inspected for symmetry and shape. Any lesions, protuberances, or indentations are noted. The amount of head lag is noted when a baby is pulled to the sitting position. Head control when sitting is observed in the young child. The head is palpated for lesions, skull suture lines, and fontanels, and the hair palpation is performed as described above. Head circumference is measured until 1 year of age. Detailed examination of the head and neck is described in Chapter 34.

Face. The face is inspected for symmetry of structures such as eyes, nose, mouth, and ears (Fig. 9-5). Shape

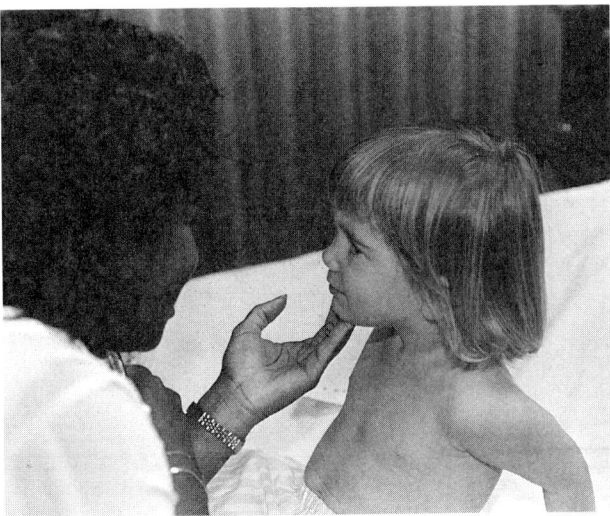

FIGURE 9-5
The nurse examines the child's face for symmetry, contour, and relationship of structures.

of the face, contour, relationship of structures, lesions, and edema are noted. The face is palpated for tenderness such as in the sinus area and for edema.

Eyes. Eyes are carefully observed for ability to focus on near and far objects, reaction of pupils to light and accommodation, ability to follow objects to all quadrants, coordination of movement, color of iris, color of sclera and conjunctiva, presence of tears, distance between eyes and presence of epicanthal folds, symmetry of eyelids and their movement, and pattern of eyebrow and eyelash hair (Fig. 9-6).

Color vision is assessed, particularly among male children, who most commonly manifest the disorder. A family history of color blindness is a risk factor to be considered. Although some tests can be done with younger children, color blindness testing is usually performed during the school years. Ishihara's test, a series of cards with a number concealed in a background, is a common test used.

Visual acuity is of obvious importance. Whereas the infant's ability to focus on and follow objects is noted, a number of more sophisticated tests are used in preschool and school-age children. Many states mandate vision screening for certain grade levels and set minimum standards for passing. Generally, children who are 3 to 5 years old should read 20/40 or better; children 5 years and over should read 20/30 or better. Failure to meet this standard or a one line difference between eyes is reason for referral. The most commonly administered vision test is Snellen's test. The child stands 20 feet from the chart and covers each eye alternately. One more than half the symbols on a line must be read correctly to pass the line.

Letters or an E chart may be used. A variety of other tests are available and may be used in specific settings. A list of vision screening tests is given in the accompanying display. Vision testing is also discussed in Chapter 34.

Ears. Ears are closely inspected for the level of placement on head, degree of backwards tilt, and cartilage configuration. The presence of skin tags or sinuses in the ear area is noted. The tragus is palpated for tenderness, and the external ear is palpated for lesions. An otoscope is used to examine the external canal for color, intactness, cerumen, and lesions. The middle ear structures are identified. The umbo and cone of light should be visible in normal locations; tympanic membrane should be pearly gray, clear, and movable when a puff of air is directed at it by way of a pneumatic otoscope. Auditory acuity is assessed. The examiner observes an infant's ability to alert and turn to noises as well as the presence of coos and other vocalizations. Older children are assessed with ticking watches, Rinne and Weber's tests, and audiometry. See the accompanying display for a list of hearing screening tests. Figures pertaining to ear structure and further discussion of testing are in Chapter 34.

Positioning of the child for otoscopic examination is important. The examiner's hand is securely placed on the child's head before the speculum is inserted. The hands and legs of young children may need to be restrained by a helper or parent for safe otoscopy. This may be done with the child on the examining table or on the mother's lap. The pinna of the ear is pulled down and back to examine children under about 6 years of age, and up and back for older children due to the differing angle of the canal.

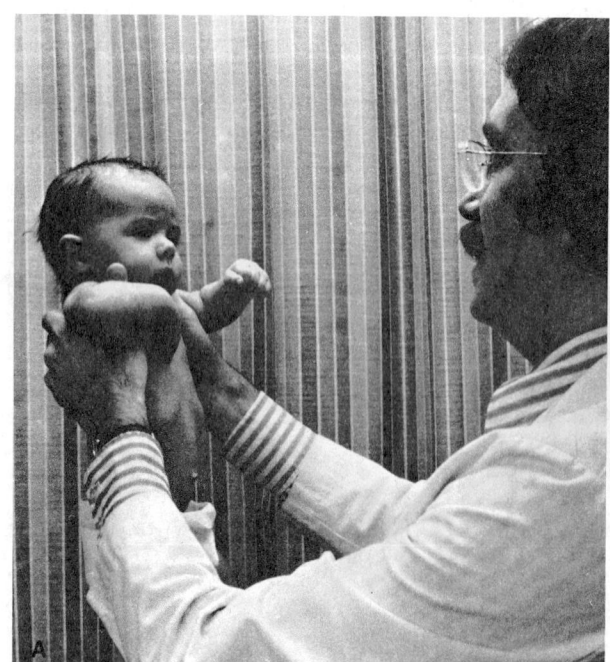 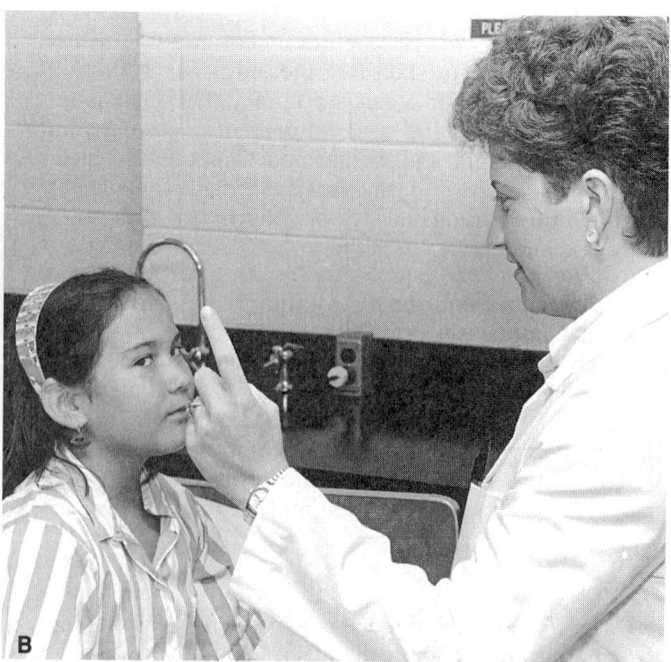

FIGURE 9-6

General examination of eyes. (A) The neonate is held up with the examiner's thumbs at side of face. This should open the baby's eyes. (B) The child's eyes follow the movement of the examiner's finger across and up and down. (Source for A: Bates, B.: A Guide to Physical Examination and History Taking, 5th ed. Philadelphia: J. B. Lippincott, 1991.)

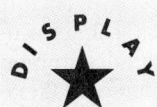

Vision Screening Tests

Doll's eye test—Used during first 10 days of life to test for blindness

Hirschberg test—Used in early childhood to detect esotropia and exotropia

Cover test—Used in early childhood to detect frank strabismus

Miniature toy test—Used in early childhood to test visual acuity at 10 ft

Worth's test—Used in early childhood to detect visual acuity

Snellen symbol—Used in very young children to test visual acuity at 10 ft

Snellen E—Used in cooperative children over age 3 for visual acuity

Snellen letter—Used in children who can recognize alphabet to test visual acuity

Ishihara's test—Usually performed during school years to test for color blindness

Auditory testing should begin in infancy and be performed several times during childhood. Whereas the infant can be evaluated for alerting to sound, some specialized machinery is available to measure infant activity level or tympanic membrane movement in response to sound. For older children, the Rinne and Weber's tests provide clues to sound conduction. In the Rinne test, a tuning fork is struck and placed on the child's mastoid bone. When the sound is no longer heard, the tuning fork is quickly moved in front of the ear. The sound should still be audible there, air conduction being roughly twice as long as bone conduction. In Weber's test, a tuning fork is struck and placed in mid forehead. The sound should be heard equally in both ears; lateralization to one side is abnormal.

Pure tone audiometry is widely used and is mandated in some states for use on school-age children at particular years. Sounds, usually between 500 and 4000 Hz are delivered to the child by way of earphones at 20 to 25 dB, and a response is elicited. If the child does not respond to sounds at the screening level, the decibel level can be raised to find out where the child does hear. Bone conduction testing can be performed to learn if the loss is only by air conduction (conductive loss) or also by bone conduction (sensorineural loss). Children with identified deficits are retested in 2 weeks and referred if the screening is not passed at that time.

The tympanometer is a device being used increasingly often to provide data about ear function. In this procedure, a sound is delivered to the ear and a machine reads the compliance of the tympanic membrane.

Nose. The nose is inspected for symmetry, patency, and drainage. A speculum is used, and the head is tilted back to examine for color of nasal mucous membranes, exudate, and edema of membranes and sinuses. Ability

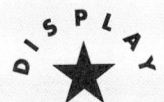

Hearing Screening Tests

Clinical tests—crude tests used in infancy to evaluate sound:
- After first week of life, infant will blink at sound at side of head (acoustic blink reflex)
- Around 2 weeks of life, infant responds to sound by throwing arms out at side (startle reflex)
- Around 10 weeks, infant will cease body movement momentarily on hearing sound
- 3–4 months—eyes and head turn toward sound

Voice/whisper test—gross screening of hearing acuity, especially high frequency sounds

Watch-tick test—gross screening of hearing acuity, especially high-frequency sounds

Weber's test—tuning fork is used to test perception of sound from midline on older child

Rinne test—tuning fork is used to test bone conduction versus air conduction in older child

Schwabach test—tuning fork is used to compare child's perception of sound conduction with examiner's perception

Pure tone audiometry—used before beginning school or during early school years to test severity of hearing loss (may be used in delayed speech, but it is preferable to send the child to a hearing or speech center for testing)

Tympanometry—easier to use in the older child to detect disease or abnormalities to smell is bilaterally measured in children old enough to respond.

Mouth and Neck. The mouth is inspected for size, color, and condition of the lips. Internal inspection includes number and condition of teeth, presence of caries and fillings, condition of gums, color and consistency and mobility of tongue, color of floor of mouth, buccal mucosa, ability to salivate, and presence of lesions (Fig. 9-7). The palate is examined for intactness and lesions. Presence and strength of sucking and rooting reflexes are observed in neonates. Tonsillar size and color are noted. This examination can be performed by having the cooperative child open wide while a tongue blade is used to depress the tongue for better visualization.

The examination of the head is concluded with inspection and palpation of the neck. Range of motion and presence of masses are observed. The symmetry, size, and configuration of the neck are noted. The trachea is palpated with thumb and index finger for placement in midline and presence of masses. The thyroid area is palpated, when swallowing if possible, for masses.

The lymph nodes are palpated by pressing firmly along the lymph node chains, noting the presence of any nodes, their mobility, temperature, and size (see Fig. 9-7*B* and *C*). The child is asked if there is any tenderness on palpation. The nodes palpated in the neck include the anterior and posterior chains, submental, submaxillary, tonsillary, and cervical nodes (see Chap. 33). The cranial nerve examination is generally integrated at appropriate points during the physical examination (see Chap. 52).

Upper Extremities

The arms are inspected for symmetry and general alignment on the body. The fingers are counted, and size is observed. Range of motion of shoulders, elbows, wrists, and fingers is performed. If not previously palpated, radial and antecubital pulses are assessed for strength, rhythm, and regularity. Strength of hand, biceps, and triceps muscles is measured by having the child bilaterally squeeze fingers, push and pull with arms. Deep tendon reflexes of the triceps and brachioradialis are performed. If body weight does not appear normal, triceps skin fold measurement may be included.

In the newborn, additional neurologic tests such as the grasp reflex, Moro's reaction, and tonic neck reflex are included; fine motor control and sitting ability are assessed in infants. These assessments are described in Chapter 11.

Chest

The chest is inspected for symmetry, bulging, or indentations. During infancy, the anteroposterior diameter is equal to the transverse diameter. Such a shape (1:1 diameter) gradually approaches 2:1 during childhood. The intercostal angle is noted and is about 45 degrees. Chest circumference often is measured until 1 year of age. Rate, rhythm, and depth of respirations are observed. Abnormalities of respiration are noted, such as retractions, difficult breathing, wheezing, or rapid or slow breathing.

The heart is examined first. Palpation of all areas of the heart is carefully performed with both fingertips and the ball of the palm at the following areas: aortic (second right intercostal space at sternal border), pulmonic (second left intercostal space at sternal border), tricuspid (fourth left intercostal space at sternal border), and mitral (fifth left intercostal space in midclavicular line). Any thrills and bounding are noted. The point of maximum impulse (PMI) is felt at the heart's apex. This PMI is generally readily palpated in children and is also visible. The apex of the heart varies in location with the age of the child, being higher (at the fourth intercostal space) in infancy and young childhood. Percussion may be done to estimate the heart borders and to rule out cardiomegaly, although, if cardiac enlargement is suspected, further studies are done.

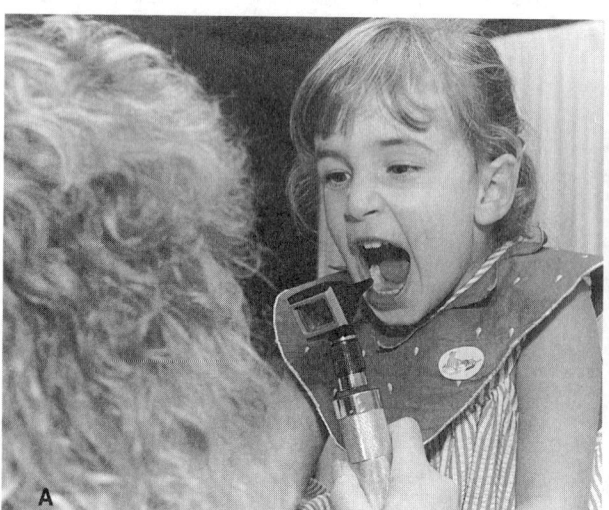 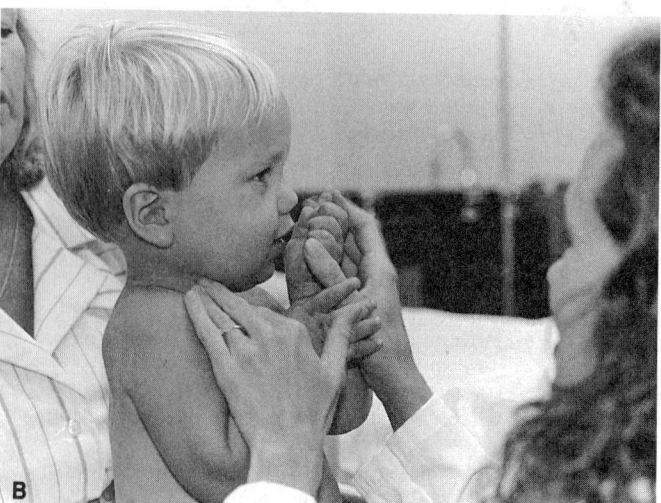

FIGURE 9-7
Assessment of the mouth and neck. (**A**) The teeth and inside of the mouth are examined. (**B**) A younger child may not be cooperative, and the nurse has to distract his hands.

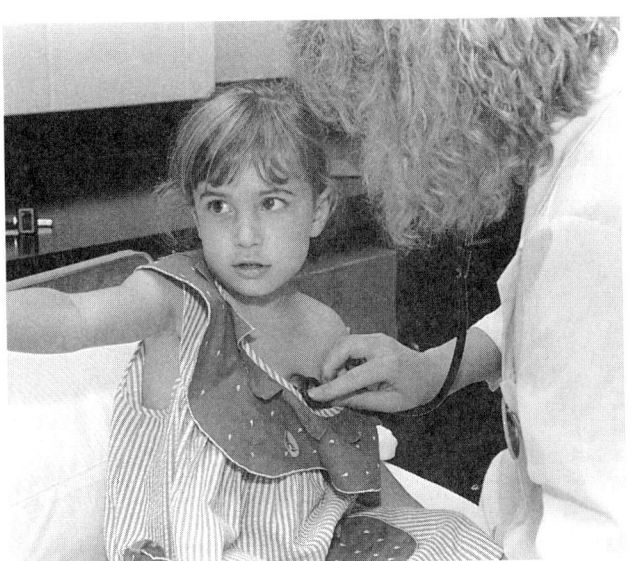

FIGURE 9-8
The nurse auscultates for heart sounds.

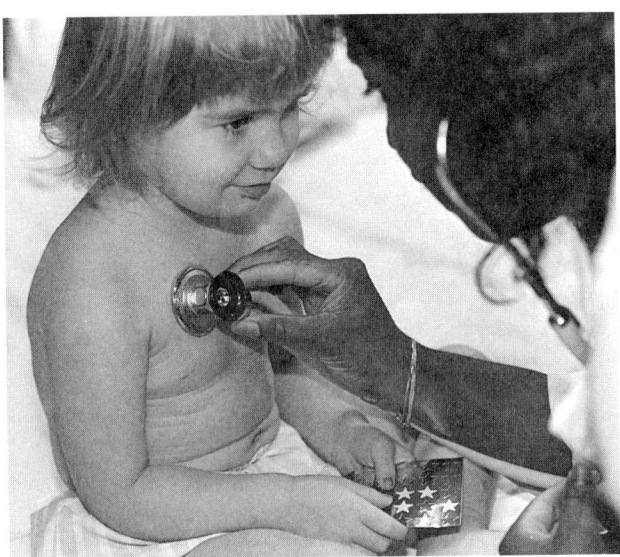

FIGURE 9-9
The nurse auscultates for lung sounds.

Auscultation is performed with the stethoscope, noting heart sounds (S) at each area described above under palpation and illustrated in Figure 9-8. S_1 (the closure tricuspid and mitral valves) and S_2 (the closure of pulmonic and aortic valves) are heard at each site. Loudness and clarity of S_1 and S_2, rate and rhythm, and any sounds in the intervals between them are noted. S_3 (the sound of the ventricles filling) is frequently heard in young children. S_4 (atrial contraction) is always considered abnormal. Murmurs are described in terms of location, loudness, relation to S_1 and S_2, and variation with position change because they may be normal or indicate pathology, depending on findings. Chapter 40 provides more detail about cardiac assessment.

The lungs are assessed by palpating the chest for equal expansion. Tactile fremitus is rarely palpated in the screening examination on young children. Percussion is carried out to listen for resonance over all lung fields. Auscultation with the stethoscope over all lung fields establishes clear breath sounds, lung expansion, and any abnormal, adventitious sounds (Fig. 9-9). Bronchial sounds (expiration longer than inspiration) are normally heard only over the trachea, bronchovesicular sounds (inspiration and expiration of equal length) are heard over bronchi, and vesicular sounds (inspiration longer than expiration) are heard over all peripheral lung fields. Chapter 37 should be consulted for more information about assessment of lung sounds.

Abdomen

The abdomen is often examined close to the finish of the examination, just before eye, ear, and mouth examination for young children, because examination of the abdomen can be viewed as intrusive. The child needs to recline, usually on the examining table; however, the parent's lap may be used for a frightened child. With the child's knees flexed, the abdomen is first inspected for color and characteristics of the skin, for contour, symmetry, peristalsis, and other movements. The umbilicus

is inspected for placement and shape; the cord should be inspected for drainage in the newborn who still has an umbilical stump or who has just lost it. Because umbilical hernias are relatively common and may need surgical correction, the size of any protuberance is carefully described. Rolling a small section of abdominal skin between thumb and finger is done to measure skin turgor.

The abdomen is auscultated next so that percussion and palpation do not interfere with normal peristalsis before its evaluation. The diaphragm of the stethoscope is placed lightly on each quadrant, and number of bowel sounds per minute are counted (Fig. 9-10A). Bruits near midline or other unusual sounds are noted. Assessment of the abdomen with relation to gastrointestinal disorders is described in Chapter 58.

Percussion is performed to establish the size of the liver and spleen and to note tympany over normal intestines (see Fig. 9-10B and C). Palpation is performed to find any tenderness, masses, or unusual muscle tone in any quadrant. The liver is palpated in the right upper quadrant (see Fig. 9-10D). It is normal to palpate the liver about 2 cm below the costal margin in children. Spleen palpation is attempted and may be possible in young children. Kidneys and bladder palpation may be performed (see Fig. 9-10E). Inguinal nodes are palpated. Small, nontender, mobile nodes may be present normally. Palpation for femoral hernias is performed, and femoral pulses are noted (see Fig. 9-10F).

Lower Extremities and Back

The legs are inspected for symmetry and general alignment. Toes are counted, and size is observed. Range of motion of hips, knees, and ankles is performed[23] (Fig. 9-11). Hip alignment and movement is performed with infants to rule out congenital dislocation of the hips. Strength of quadriceps and hamstrings is assessed by having the child extend and flex the legs against the examiner's hand. Gait assessment is performed on all children who walk. Neurologic testing, such as Babinski's reflex

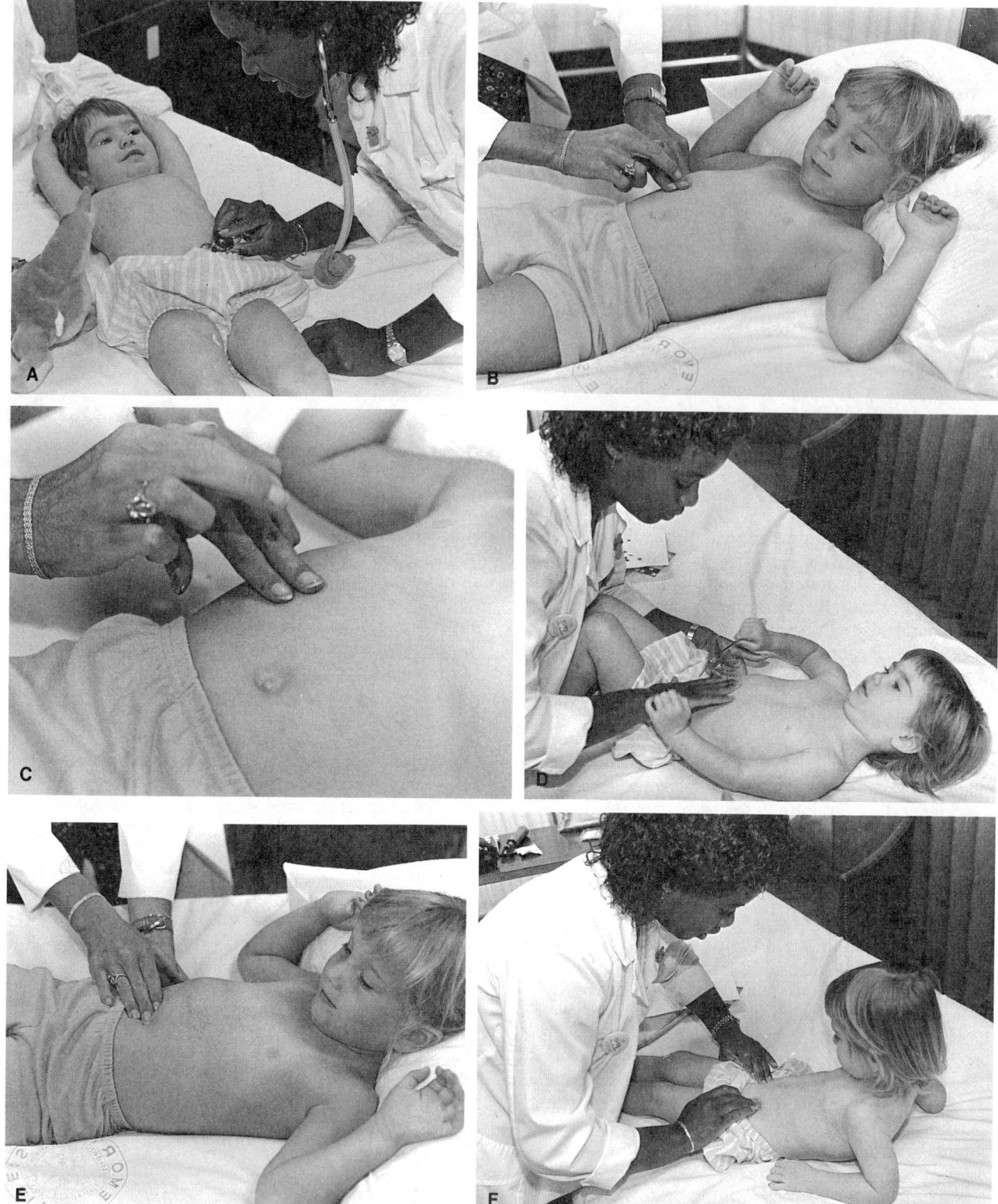

FIGURE 9-10

Assessment of the abdomen. (**A**) Auscultation is performed on each quadrant. (**B and C**) Percussion is performed to determine size of liver and spleen and to note tympany over the intestine. (**D**) The liver is palpated bimanually in the right upper quadrant. (**E**) The kidney is palpated manually. (**F**) Femoral pulses are noted, and assessment is made for presence of femoral hernias.

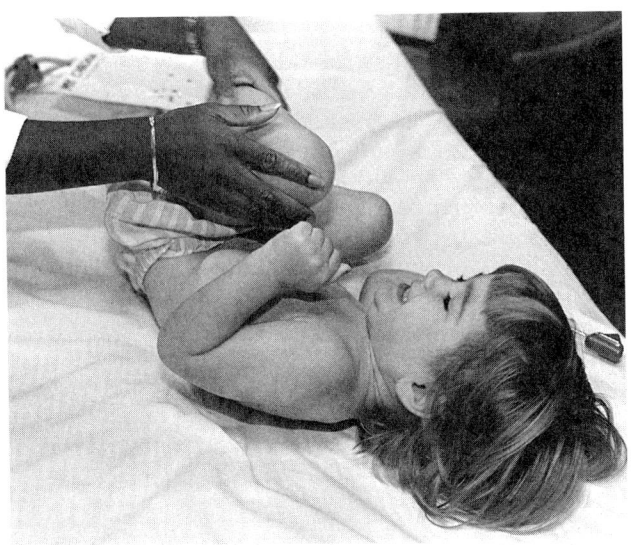

FIGURE 9-11
The nurse performs range of motion movements as part of the assessment of the lower extremities.

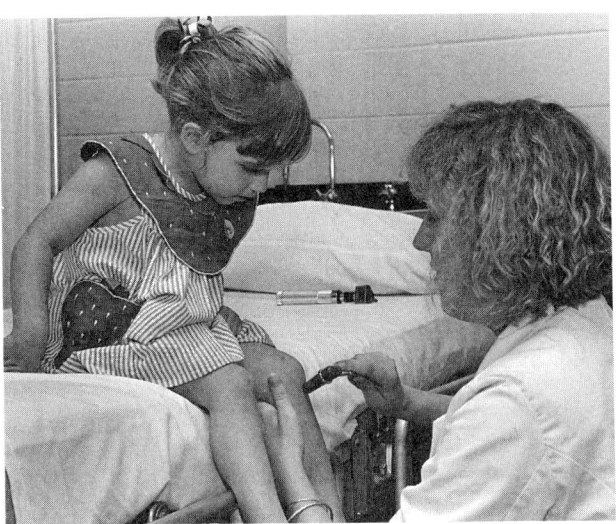

FIGURE 9-12
Reflexes are tested by the nurse.

and deep tendon reflexes at the knee (patellar) and ankle, is performed (Fig. 9-12). Tests of cerebellar function, such as the Romberg and heel to shin tests, may be administered. Additional neurologic responses such as the walking reflex are assessed in neonates. Standing and walking are evaluated once children have accomplished these tasks. In-depth neurologic examination is described in Chapter 52, and the musculoskeletal examination is described in Chapter 61.

The back is assessed for symmetry and straightness. Intactness of the spine, dimples, or hair tufts over the spine are observed. In the child about 10 to 13 years of age when scoliosis is a risk, symmetry of shoulders, clavicles, and flank is observed when the child stands and bends over. Distance between arms and waist and hip levels is assessed.

Genitalia

The genital examination usually is performed after the abdominal assessment when the child is supine. The nurse should ask the parent's permission to remove the child's underclothes. The hips are abducted in the child less than 3 years old. The genitals and perineum are inspected for lesions and rashes. The anal area is examined for position and rectal opening, redness, and dimpling.

In infant girls, the labia minora are more prominent than the labia majora. They quickly atrophy and become almost nonexistent until puberty. Normally, there is no redness or discharge.

Erections are common in boys during infancy. Presence or absence of foreskin is noted. The foreskin may be retracted in older males but may not be retractable in boys under 3 years of age. The location of the urethra is important. The scrotum may appear enlarged or asymmetric.

The stage of pubertal development is assessed using Tanner staging (see Chap. 66). Other aspects of examination of the reproductive organs are discussed in Chapter 67.

Developmental Milestones Data

A specific developmental test such as the Denver II (see the Appendix) may be performed simultaneously with the physical examination or at an separately scheduled visit. Data regarding development are also integrated into every physical examination of a child. For example, gross motor skills such as sitting, standing, and walking are observed during the examination of the child in the first year of life. Fine motor skills such as the ability to reach for objects, or later to button, are important. Language development proceeding from quality of the cry to coos and babbles to words and then sentences can be assessed throughout the examination. Many sections of the neurologic examination give clues to the developmental status and are also integrated throughout the examination.

Laboratory Studies

Blood

The most commonly performed blood studies during childhood are the hematocrit and hemoglobin, primarily used to detect anemia at times when children are at highest risk for that disorder. The hematocrit is generally measured at about 9 to 12 months of age. By then, the infant's iron stores acquired in the uterus from the mother have been exhausted for a few months. Intake of iron-fortified cereals and meats is increasing and should provide for an adequate iron intake. Occasionally, an infant shuns this solid food intake and drinks large amounts of formula or milk. Caloric intake is high but iron intake is low, leading to an overweight but anemic baby.

Hematocrit or hemoglobin is also measured one time during preschool years (2 to 5 years of age), once during school years (6 to 12 years of age), and once during adolescence (13 to 18 years of age). More frequent measures are taken if the examination indicates abnormalities such as lethargy, weakness, pallor, or poor dietary intake.

Other blood studies may be done in special circumstances, for example, when frequent bruising or infections are present. These studies, such as a complete blood count (CBC), red blood cell count (RBC), white blood cell count (WBC), or blood glucose are not routinely performed during health supervision visits (see Chap. 43 for more information). Finally, increasing numbers of health care providers believe in the importance of blood cholesterol and lipid level testing at some point in early childhood.[37] Values for all laboratory studies are presented in the Appendix.

Urine

Urinalysis is done about the same time as hematocrit testing, that is, once in the first year, once in preschool, once during school years, and once in adolescence. Procedures for collecting urine specimens are described in Chapter 25. Asymptomatic urinary tract infections can occur in childhood, so this periodic testing is a valuable screening procedure. Tests done to assess renal and urinary function are discussed in Chapters 46 and 49, respectively.

Immunizations

Immunizations are usually administered at the end of a health supervision visit so that the history and examination can rule out contraindications. Furthermore, crying caused by the injection can be avoided during the examination.

A number of immunizations against communicable diseases are available and strongly encouraged for young children. Such practices have been instrumental in eradicating smallpox from the world and in decreasing the incidence of diseases such as measles from 481,530 in 1962 to 6,273 cases in 1986 in the United States.[10] Unfortunately, when fewer children are immunized, illness and death rates from these diseases increase, a trend happening with measles in the United States. Many young parents have not seen the life-threatening illness caused by communicable diseases[24] and are not frightened by the possible outcomes. Some parents are opposed to immunization on religious or philosophic grounds, desiring to avoid use of these biologic products. Other parents are frightened by the stories of children severely injured after being immunized. Such stories have been available in the media, particularly in regards to pertussis vaccine. Although side-effects to all immunizations do occur, nearly all are mild and easily managed. Severe side-effects with life-threatening results or permanent sequelae are rare. The risk of acquiring the disease is always greater than the risks of immunization.

Explanations about the risks of communicable diseases and the risks and benefits of immunizations should be given to parents to enable them to make informed decisions about the care of their children. Providing such information is mandated by the National Childhood Vaccine Injury Act.[28] Analysis of current controversies and

media exposure is necessary before informed consent can be given. State law should be reviewed because numerous states require some immunizations for school enrollment. Parents need to understand common side-effects and what can be done to promote comfort. They should also be able to identify severe side-effects and have an emergency plan to follow if any occur.

Two groups that study immunization practices and make recommendations for immunization schedules in the United States are the Committee on Infectious Diseases of the AAP and the Advisory Committee on Immunization Practices (ACIP) of the Public Health Services. Table 9-2 presents the schedule for immunizations. The AAP publishes its recommendations in the *Report of the Committee on Infectious Diseases*, commonly called

TABLE 9-2
Recommended Schedule for Immunization of Healthy Infants and Children*

Recommended Age†	Immunizations‡	Comments
2 mo	DTP, HbCV,§ OPV	DTP and OPV can be initiated as early as 4 wk after birth in areas of high endemicity or during epidemics
4 mo	DTP, HbCV,§ OPV	2-mo interval (minimum of 6 wk) desired for OPV to avoid interference from previous dose
6 mo	DTP, HbCV§	Third dose of OPV is not indicated in the U.S. but is desirable in other geographic areas where polio is endemic
15 mo	MMR,‖ HbCV¶	Tuberculin testing may be done at the same visit
15–18 mo	DTP,**,†† OPV#	(See footnotes)
4–6 y	DTP,§§ OPV, MMR¶¶	At or before school entry
11–12 y	MMR	At entry to middle school or junior high school
14–16 y	Td	Repeat every 10 y throughout life

* For all products used, consult manufacturer's package insert for instructions for storage, handling, dosage, and administration. Biologics prepared by different manufacturers may vary, and package inserts of the same manufacturer may change from time to time.

† These recommended ages should not be construed as absolute. For example, 2 months can be 6 to 10 weeks. However, MMR usually should not be given to children younger than 12 months. (If measles vaccination is indicated, monovalent measles vaccine is recommended, and MMR should be given subsequently, at 15 months.)

‡ DTP = diphtheria and tetanus toxoids with pertussis vaccine; HbCV = *Hemophilus b* conjugate vaccine; OPV = oral poliovirus vaccine containing attenuated poliovirus types 1, 2, and 3; MMR = live measles, mumps, and rubella viruses in a combined vaccine; Td = adult tetanus toxoid (full dose) and diphtheria toxoid (reduced dose) for adult use.

§ As of October 1990, only one HbCV (HbOC) is approved for use in children younger than 15 months.

‖ May be given at 12 months of age in areas with recurrent measles transmission.

¶ Any licensed *Hemophilus b* conjugate vaccine may be given.

** Should be given 6 to 12 months after the third dose.

†† May be given simultaneously with MMR at 15 months.

May be given simultaneously with MMR and HbCV at 15 months or at any time between 12 and 24 months; priority should be given to administering MMR.

§§ Can be given up to the seventh birthday.

¶¶ Many states require MMR before school admission.

From Committee on Infectious Diseases. (1991). Report of the Committee for Infectious Diseases. Elk Grove Village, IL: American Academy of Pediatrics.

the "Red Book"; the ACIP recommendations are found in the weekly publication *MMWR—Morbidity and Mortality Weekly Reports.* Both groups generally have the same recommendations, but occasional differences do occur. As new vaccines are available, disease patterns are studied, and other factors are considered, health care providers must always consult package inserts for administration information and study published data from the two groups described above. The information below discusses data available at the time of this book's publication; however, some changes are predicted for the near future. As an example, an immunization against chickenpox may become available in the future.[31]

Careful storage and preparation are needed to ensure vaccine efficacy. Manufacturer recommendations for storage should be followed carefully, and vaccines should be placed in the body of the refrigerator rather than on the door where temperature variations are greater. Other items such as lunches and laboratory specimens should not be stored in the same location, and keeping a refrigerator thermometer in place helps to ensure proper temperature. Contact with the live polio virus should be avoided, and used immunization containers should be discarded with necessary precaution.

Accurate recording in the child's chart of date, route, site, the vaccine manufacturer and lot number, as well as the name, address, and title of the person who administered the immunization is required by the National Childhood Vaccine Injury Act.[23,28] Certain events indicating reactions to immunization must be reported to the state health department or Food and Drug Administration (Table 9-3). The guidelines specify not only what symptoms must be reported but also the procedure that must be followed when the report is made (Table 9-4).

Terminology

The following terminology needs to be clarified when discussing immunizations.

- Toxoid—A toxoid is a poisonous substance produced by a microorganism that has been treated so that it does not cause illness but can still induce the human body to form antibodies to a disease.
- Vaccine—A vaccine is a collection of infectious material obtained from an organism. It may contain live infectious organisms or dead organisms, or it may contain material extracted from the organism, which evokes immunologic response in the body.
- Attenuated—Attenuated means weakened. Attenuation is used to weaken live organisms used in vaccines so they can induce human antibody formation but cannot generally cause disease.

Diphtheria and Tetanus Toxoids and Pertussis Vaccine (DTP)

DTP is given to children at 2, 4, 6, and 18 months and 4 to 6 years of age for a total of five doses. It is given intramuscularly (0.5 ml) into the lateral thigh or into the deltoid for the 4- to 6-year dose.

Risk of Disease

Diphtheria causes infection of the respiratory tract and skin and may cause complications including myocarditis and neuritis. *Tetanus* is a serious disease caused by the bacillus *Clostridium tetani* that affects muscles of the head and neck. There is a 44% to 55% mortality rate in children who have tetanus, and the rate is even higher (60%) in neonates.[5] Because the tetanus spores live in dust, soil, and animal intestinal tracts, transmission of the disease does not depend on exposure to someone with the disease. *Pertussis* or whooping cough is a respiratory infection caused by *Bordetella pertussis,* a hemolytic gram-negative coccobacillus. Although it is a mild disease when acquired by older children and adults, pertussis is severe in young children. A 50% mortality rate in infancy, generally due to pneumonia and dehydration, has been reported.

Risk of Immunization

The reaction to DTP is usually mild with redness, nodule, or pain at the injection site, low-grade fever, fussiness, and anorexia being the most common side-effects. Severe reactions such as high fever, persistent crying, insomnolence, and seizures are rare; most have an incidence of 1 in 1750 children who receive DTP immunization.[37] Such reactions are generally thought to be due to the pertussis component of the immunization. Parents should be instructed to report side-effects, because these severe reactions indicate contraindication to further pertussis vaccine. There are reports that in about 1 in 310,000 cases of pertussis vaccine, permanent neurologic damage or ongoing seizures have occurred.[19] However, newer analysis has demonstrated that this estimate is too high and that pertussis vaccine does not appear to be responsible for causing permanent neurologic problems in children without prior neurologic disease.[2,19]

Nursing Considerations and Teaching

The health care provider must precede DTP immunization with a careful history. What was the reaction to prior doses of DTP? Does the child have a neurologic condition? If so, is it static (such as well-controlled seizures) or developing? Has the child ever had seizures? When? What type? Do any family members have a history of seizures? Contraindications to pertussis immunization include the presence of a developing or undiagnosed neurologic condition or any of the above severe reactions to prior immunization, and the DTP vaccine is not given after 7 years of age because of increasing reactions to pertussis vaccine in older children and adults. Static neurologic conditions are not a contraindication because the vaccine is unlikely to cause serious side-effects, and these children need to be protected from the diseases. Although seizures after pertussis vaccine occur more commonly in the child with a family member who has had seizures, this is not a contraindication to receiving the vaccine. Parents should be instructed to administer acetaminophen to reduce fever should it occur.[7]

When pertussis is contraindicated, the child is given DT or diphtheria tetanus toxoids (pediatric type). This

TABLE 9-3
Vaccination Events That Must Be Reported

Vaccine/ Toxoid	Event	Interval from Vaccination
DTP, P, DTP/polio combined	A. Anaphylaxis or anaphylactic shock	24 h
	B. Encephalopathy (or encephalitis)*	7 days
	C. Shock-collapse or hypotonic-hyporesponsive collapse*	7 days
	D. Residual seizure disorder*	(See Aids to Interpretation*)
	E. Any acute complication or sequela (including death) of above events	No limit
	F. Events in vaccinees described in manufacturer's package insert as contraindications to additional doses of vaccine* (such as convulsions)	(See package insert)
Measles, mumps, and rubella; DT, td, tetanus toxoid	A. Anaphylaxis or anaphylactic shock	24 h
	B. Encephalopathy (or encephalitis)*	15 days for measles, mumps, and rubella vaccines; 7 days for DT, Td, and T toxoids
	C. Residual seizure disorder*	(See Aids to Interpretation*)
	D. Any acute complication or sequela (including death) of above events	No limit
	E. Events in vaccinees described in manufacturer's package insert as contraindications to additional doses of vaccine†	(See package insert)
Oral polio vaccine	A. Paralytic poliomyelitis	
	• in a nonimmunodeficient recipient	30 days
	• in an immunodeficient recipient	6 mo
	• in a vaccine-associated community case	No limit
	B. Any acute complication or sequela (including death) of above events	No limit
	C. Events in vaccinees described in manufacturer's package insert as contraindications to additional doses of vaccine†	(See package insert)
Inactivated polio vaccine	A. Anaphylaxis or anaphylactic shock	24 h
	B. Any acute complication or sequela (including death) of above event	No limit
	C. Events in vaccinees described in manufacturer's package insert as contraindications to additional doses of vaccine†	(See package insert)

* Aids to Interpretation:
Shock-collapse or hypotonic-hyporesponsive collapse may be evidenced by signs or symptoms such as decrease in or loss of muscle tone, paralysis (partial or complete), hemiplegia, hemiparesis, loss of color or turning pale white or blue, unresponsiveness to environmental stimuli, depression of or loss of consciousness, prolonged sleeping with difficulty arousing, or cardiovascular or respiratory arrest.
   Residual seizure disorder may be considered to have occurred if no other seizure or convulsion unaccompanied by fever or accompanied by a fever of less than 102°F occurred before the first seizure or convulsion after the administration of the vaccine involved.
And, if in the case of measles, mumps, or rubella-containing vaccines, the first seizure or convulsion occurred within 15 days after vaccination or in the case of any other vaccine, the first seizure or convulsion occurred within 3 days after vaccination.
And, if two or more seizures or convulsions unaccompanied by fever or accompanied by a fever of less than 102°F occurred within 1 year after vaccination.
   The terms seizure and convulsion include grand mal, petit mal, absence, myoclonic, tonic-clonic, and focal motor seizures and signs. Encephalopathy means any significant acquired abnormality of, injury to, or impairment of function of the brain. Among the frequent manifestations of encephalopathy are focal and diffuse neurologic signs, increased intracranial pressure, or changes lasting at least 6 hours in level of consciousness, with or without convulsions. The neurologic signs and symptoms of encephalopathy may be temporary with complete recovery, or they may result in various degrees of permanent impairment. Signs and symptoms such as high-pitched and unusual screaming, persistent unconsolable crying, and bulging fontanel are compatible with an encephalopathy, but in and of themselves are not conclusive evidence of encephalopathy. Encephalopathy usually can be documented by slow wave activity on an electroencephalogram.

† The health care provider must refer to the Contraindication section of the manufacturer's package insert for each vaccine.

From "National childhood vaccine injury act: Requirements for permanent records and for reporting of selected events after vaccination." (1988). Morbidity and Mortality Weekly Report, 37(13), 198.

TABLE 9-4
Guidelines for Reporting Events Occurring After Vaccination

	Vaccine Purchased With Public Money	Vaccine Purchased With Private Money
Who reports:	Health care provider who administered the vaccine	Health care provider who administered the vaccine
What products to report:	DTP, P, measles, mumps, rubella, DT, Td, T, OPV, IPV, and DTP/polio combined	DTP, P, measles, mumps, rubella, DT, Td, T, OPV, IPV, and DTP/polio combined
What reactions to report:	Events listed in Table 9-3 including contraindicating reactions specified in manufacturers' package inserts	Events listed in Table 9-3 including contraindicating reactions specified in manufacturers' package inserts
How to report:	Initial report taken by local, county, or state health department. State health department completes CDC form 71.19	Health care provider completes Adverse Reaction Report-FDA form 1639 (include interval from vaccination, manufacturer, and lot number on form)
Where to report:	State health departments send CDC form 71.19 to: MSAEFI/IM (E05) Centers for Disease Control Atlanta, GA 30333	Completed FDA form 1639 is sent to: Food and Drug Administration (HFN-730) Rockville, MD 20857
Where to obtain forms:	State health departments	FDA and publications such as *FDA Drug Bulletin*

From "National childhood vaccine injury act: Requirements for permanent records and for reporting of selected events after vaccination." (1988). *Morbidity and Mortality Weekly Report 37*(13), 199.

solution is distinguished carefully from Td or tetanus and diphtheria toxoids (adult type) to be used in people over 7 years of age. Recommendations for scheduling immunizations for children not immunized in their first 7 years of life are presented in Table 9-5. DT and Td are contraindicated in people who have had prior anaphylactic reaction to such immunizations.

Parents are instructed to watch for both mild and the severe side-effects. Health care should be sought for severe effects, and the reaction should be reported before future DTP doses. Instruction in proper acetaminophen dosage for age can help parents to decrease the child's fever and discomfort. An immunization record is given to the parent, and it should be brought to future visits to record additional doses. The record is also necessary for the child's school entry.

Epinephrine 1:1000, its doses written for child age groups and weights, and resuscitative drugs and equipment should always be available during administration of immunizations. Parents should remain in the office with the child for 20 to 30 minutes after immunization in case of anaphylaxis.

Vaccine Storage

DTP is kept refrigerated between 35°F and 46°F (2°C and 8°C). It should be kept in the interior of the refrigerator and is not to be frozen. It should be well-shaken before withdrawal, but a cloudy appearance of the solution is normal.

Tetanus and Diphtheria Toxoids (Td)

Tetanus and diphtheria are described above. The risks of immunization include mild local reactions such as pain,

swelling or redness, and low-grade fever. Severe reaction such as anaphylaxis is extremely rare.

Td is given every 10 years; the child with an initial DTP series, therefore, requires a Td booster about age 15 years. A wound necessitates reimmunization after 5 years, and guidelines differ if the child has received more or less than three previous injections (Table 9-6). Td is given intramuscularly (0.5 ml) generally into a deltoid. The previous section on DTP should be consulted for information about teaching and storage.

Trivalent Oral Polio Vaccine (TOPV)

Live polio vaccine is given orally at 2, 4, and 18 months and 4 to 6 years of age for a total of four doses. Generally, two drops or the entire content of a single dose dispenser is given. The package insert should be consulted for correct dosage for the specific product. Oral polio vaccine (OPV) is distinguished from inactivated polio vaccine (IPV), which is not a live virus and is given by injection when TOPV is contraindicated or when immunizing adults who have not received prior TOPV.

Risk of Disease

Polio is a potentially serious viral disease that can affect muscle groups throughout the body. Temporary or permanent paralysis, inability to breathe, and death can occur.

Risk of Immunization

Side-effects from oral polio vaccine are extremely rare. There is a slight chance (1 in 7.8 million) of a child's

TABLE 9-5
Recommended Immunization Schedules for Children Not Immunized in First Year of Life

Recommended Time	Immunization(s)	Comments
Less Than 7 Years Old		
First visit	DTP, OPV, MMR	MMR if child ≥15 mo old; tuberculin testing may be done at same visit
Interval after first visit:		
1 mo	PRP-D	For children aged 18–60 mo; can be given concurrently with DTP (at separate sites) and other vaccines*
2 mo	DTP, OPV	
4 mo	DTP	A third dose of OPV is not indicated in the U.S. but is desirable in geographic areas where polio is endemic
10–16 mo	DTP, OPV	OPV is not given if third dose was given earlier
4–6 y (at or before school entry)	DTP, OPV	DTP is not necessary if the fourth dose was given after the fourth birthday; OPV is not necessary if recommended OPV dose at 10–16 mo following first visit was given after the fourth birthday
10 y later	Td	Repeat every 10 y throughout life
7 Years Old and Older		
First visit	Td, OPV, MMR	
Interval after first visit:		
2 mo	Td, OPV	
8–14 mo	Td, OPV	
10 y later	Td	Repeat every 10 y throughout life

* The initial three doses of DTP can be given at 1- to 2-month intervals; so, for the child in whom immunization is initiated at age 24 months or older, one visit could be eliminated by giving DTP, OPV, and MMR at the first visit; DTP and PRP-D at the second visit (1 month later); and DTP and OPV at the third visit (2 months after the first visit). Subsequent DTP and OPV 10 to 16 months after the first visit are still indicated. PRP-D, MMR, DTP, and OPV can be given simultaneously at separate sites if return of vaccine recipient for future immunizations is doubtful.

From Committee on Infectious Diseases. (1991). Report of the Committee on Infectious Diseases. Elk Grove Village, IL: American Academy of Pediatrics.

TABLE 9-6
Guidelines for Tetanus Prophylaxis in Wound Management*

History of Tetanus Immunization (doses)	Clean, Minor Wounds		All Other Wounds†	
	Td	TIG	Td	TIG
Uncertain or less than 3	Yes	No	Yes	Yes
3 or more‡	No§	No	No¶	No

* Td = adult type tetanus and diphtheria toxoids. If the patient is less than 7 years old, DT or DTP is given. TIG = tetanus immune globulin.
† Including but not limited to wounds contaminated with dirt, feces, soil, saliva; puncture wounds, avulsions; and wounds resulting from missiles, crushing, burns, and frostbite.
‡ If only three doses of *fluid* toxoid have been received, a fourth dose of toxoid, preferably an adsorbed toxoid, should be given.
§ Yes, if more than 10 years since the last dose.
¶ Yes, if more than 5 years since the last dose.

From Committee on Infectious Diseases. (1991). Report of the Committee on Infectious Diseases. Elk Grove Village, IL: American Academy of Pediatrics.

is not ill but a family member is, IPV (the inactivated polio vaccine) injection is used so that the child is immunized but the immunosuppressed family member is protected. TOPV immunization is delayed in children who have received immune serum globulin within the last 90 days, as well as those with acute febrile illness. TOPV is not given to people over 18 years of age, especially those who have never received the oral vaccine, because the incidence of vaccine-induced disease is slightly higher in adults than children.[12] If parents have not been immunized against polio, IPV may be given to them before TOPV administration to their baby to provide disease immunity and prevent oral vaccine associated disease in the parents.

Parents must be told about the slight risk of polio disease to the child and to caretakers who have contact with the child's feces. They are instructed to wash their hands well and to dispose of the diapers carefully for 4 weeks to avoid fecal–oral spread of the live vaccine excreted in the stool. The child receiving the booster at 4 to 6 years is taught to wash hands well after toileting.

Vaccine Storage

TOPV is maintained in the freezer at 14°F (−10°C). Once thawed, the vaccine can be refrozen if it did not exceed 46°F (8°C) during the thaw period. A maximum of ten thaw–freeze cycles are acceptable; containers should be labeled and dated each time they are thawed and refrozen. If not opened, a thawed container may be kept refrigerated at 35°F to 46°F (2°C to 8°C) for 30 days. If opened, containers can be refrigerated for only 7 days. Containers must be clearly labeled and dated.

Measles-Mumps-Rubella Vaccine (MMR)

MMR is given at 15 months of age and once during childhood by way of subcutaneous injection into the up-

contracting polio from the vaccine and a somewhat greater chance (1 in 5.5 million) that a nonimmune family member will contract polio when the virus is inadvertently transmitted to them from the feces of the immunized child.[12]

Nursing Considerations and Teaching

People at greatest risk of contracting polio are those who are immunosuppressed. The history should focus on identifying children who are immunosuppressed as well as those who have immunosuppressed family members. TOPV is contraindicated in these cases. If the child per outer arm. Single-dose vials of the powdered vaccine are mixed with diluent provided by the manufacturer, and the entire amount is administered. For a number of years, only one dose of MMR was recommended; however, recent increases in the incidence of measles and related deaths, in addition to findings of inadequate titers in some children, and inadequate documentation of immunization history, have prompted the recommendation for a second dose.[20] The AAP recommends that a second dose be given during middle school (about 12 years of age); the ACIP recommends the age of 4 to 6 years for the second dose.[1,29] Health care providers may decide on the particular timing based on the characteristics of their practices (i.e., whether there are cases of the diseases in the community and whether children are likely to be seen for health care at 12 years of age). However, some states have mandated the age when the second vaccine is required for school attendance.

Risk of Disease

Measles, mumps, and rubella were prevalent in this country before the late 1960s when vaccines became available. *Measles* is usually a mild viral disease causing a rash, anorexia, and malaise. However, it can develop into complications such as otitis media, pneumonia, and encephalitis; the latter can lead to permanent disability or death. The *mumps* virus affects glands such as the parotids as well as ovaries and epididymis. Although usually characterized by mild symptoms, mumps can lead to serious complications such as deafness and sterility in both males and females. *Rubella* or German measles is a viral disease leading to rash, fever, malaise, and lymphadenopathy. Although it is usually mild when acquired by children, pregnant women infected with rubella are at high risk for having an infant with congenital rubella syndrome, which is characterized by symptoms such as deafness, blindness, and mental retardation in the newborn.

Risk of Immunization

Side-effects from MMR are usually mild and generally occur within 7 to 10 days after immunization. Low-grade fever, tenderness at the injection site, and a measleslike noncontagious rash can occur. Rare side-effects include joint pain, anaphylaxis, encephalitis, and seizures.

Nursing Considerations and Teaching

History should identify past MMR doses or the incidence of these diseases. Allergy to neomycin is a contraindication to the vaccine, because the vaccine contains minute amounts of neomycin. The vaccine is also contraindicated in children who are allergic to eggs because measles and mumps vaccines are grown on chick embryo tissue cultures. Children who are immunosuppressed, who have received immune serum globulin within the last 90 days, or who have acute febrile illness should not be immunized. Pregnant women are not immunized, so girls of childbearing age should be asked if they could be pregnant; suspicion of pregnancy warrants withholding the vaccine. Immunized females are instructed to avoid pregnancy for three months. There is no risk to the vac-

cinee or to nonimmunized contacts of acquiring the diseases even though live attenuated viruses are given.

Parents are taught the side-effects of the vaccine and instructed to give acetaminophen for relief of mild discomfort. Children with a history of seizures have a slightly increased chance of seizure after immunization, but the risk is slight and outweighed by risks of the diseases. A record of immunization is given to parents. Epinephrine 1:1000, its doses written for child age groups and weights, and resuscitative drugs and equipment should always be available during administration of immunizations. Parents should remain in the office with the child for 20 to 30 minutes after immunization in case of anaphylaxis.

Vaccine Storage

Vials are stored in the dark in the body of a refrigerator (not on the door) at 35°F to 46°F (2°C to 8°C). The vials may be wrapped in aluminum foil if taken from the box to protect them from light; the diluent can be kept at room temperature. Once reconstituted with diluent, the vaccine must be kept in the dark, refrigerated, and used within 8 hours.

Hemophilus Influenzae-B *(HiB)*

One of the newest vaccines available for the general public is against *Hemophilus influenzae* bacteria.[35] Several formulations of HiB vaccine are available and administered subcutaneously or intramuscularly, depending on the particular preparation. Whereas most were previously given at 15 months of age, one (Hib-TITER or HbOC) has been approved for doses at 2, 4, and 6 months and a booster at 15 months (four doses total). It is given at a different site from the DTP. A second vaccine (Pedvax HiB) is approved for administration at 2 and 4 months of age with a booster at 12 months (three doses total).[28,31] Due to the ongoing research on this vaccine, published data and package inserts should be carefully studied so that recommended practices are followed.

Risk of Disease

Hemophilus influenzae-b causes a number of diseases, such as otitis media, osteomyelitis, bronchitis, meningitis, and others. Although it rarely causes serious disease in older children and adults, HiB causes serious, life-threatening disease in infants.

Risk of Immunization

HiB vaccine is one of the safest vaccines; only mild effects of redness or tenderness at the injection site are common. The incidence of anaphylaxis after HiB vaccination is extremely rare.

Nursing Considerations and Teaching

Prior *Hemophilus influenzae-b* disease does not necessarily create immunity; such children should still be immunized. A history of prior HiB injections should be assessed, and package inserts should be consulted to establish appropriate immunization plans for the present visit. The HiB vaccine is not usually given to children over 5 years of age because there is little risk of serious disease from the bacteria in older age groups.

Immunization is delayed if the child has an acute febrile illness so that the illness does not interfere with immunologic response. It is also contraindicated if the child is hypersensitive to any vaccine component, including mercury (due to thimerosal, a mercury derivative used as preservative) or diphtheria toxoid (used in one type of the vaccine). Package inserts need to be read for specific history questions regarding allergies that should be asked.

Parents are informed about side-effects and when to return for a visit. A written record of the immunization is provided for the parents and should specify which type of HiB vaccine was used. Epinephrine 1:1000, its doses written for child age groups and weights, and resuscitative drugs and equipment should always be available during administration of immunizations. Parents should remain in the office with the child for 20 to 30 minutes after immunization in case of anaphylaxis.

Vaccine Storage

The vaccine and reconstituted unused solutions are refrigerated at 35°F to 46°F (2°C to 8°C) in the body of the refrigerator (not on the door).

Tuberculin Test

A skin test for tuberculosis is generally performed once in infancy, once in preschool, and once in adolescence. If there is a high risk of the disease, annual testing is recommended. Two types of tuberculin preparations are available: old tuberculin (OT) and purified protein derivative (PPD) of tuberculin. The TB test is administered intradermally, usually by applying a multiple puncture device to the forearm for 1 second (Tine test, Monovacetest, Applitest, Sclavotest); this device may contain either OT or PPD. The test may also be performed by injecting 5 tuberculin units (TU) of PPD in 0.1 ml solution intradermally (Mantoux test).

Risk of Disease

The bacillus *Mycobacterium tuberculosis* generally affects the respiratory system and leads to cough, hemoptysis, and other symptoms. Other body areas such as bones, kidneys, and brain can also become infected.

Risk of TB Test

The most common side-effect of the TB test is a hypersensitive reaction at the test site in those children with a previously known positive reaction to the test. Systemic anaphylaxis is a rare complication.

Nursing Considerations and Teaching

A history of former tuberculosis disease or bacillus Calmette Guérin (BCG) vaccination, or positive reaction

to the tuberculin test is assessed because these are contraindications to future skin testing. BCG vaccine is developed from *Mycobacterium bovis* and is used in some countries, and occasionally in the United States, for prevention of tuberculosis, particularly in groups where the disease is endemic.

Parents are instructed in the rare side-effects of the test and when to return for the test to be read. Reliable caregivers may read the test, but they are given instructions for reporting the results to health care providers. For the multiple puncture test, reading is done at 48 to 72 hours. Vesiculation or induration of 2 mm or greater is a positive result to the tine test and is followed by a Mantoux test. The Mantoux test is also read at 48 to 72 hours, with under 5 mm induration viewed as negative, 5 to 9 mm questionable, and 10 mm significant. Significant and possibly questionable results are followed by another Mantoux test, physical examination, and chest x-ray. Written results of the test are given to parents. Drug therapy and other care may be indicated.

Epinephrine 1:1000, its doses written for child age groups and weights, and resuscitative drugs and equipment should always be available during adminstration of immunizations. Parents should remain in the office with the child for 20 to 30 minutes after immunization in case of anaphylaxis.

Test Storage

Multiple puncture devices are stored at room temperature not exceeding 86°F (30°C). TB test solutions are refrigerated at 35°F to 46°F (2°C to 8°C).

Hepatitis B Vaccine

Risk of Disease

Hepatitis B virus can cause asymptomatic or mild disease such as nausea, anorexia, acrodermatitis, malaise, and jaundice, or it can lead to serious fatal illness such as hepatitis, cirrhosis, or liver cancer.[12]

Hepatitis B vaccine is given to population groups in which the infection is endemic, to those exposed to someone with the disease, to those who are at risk of contracting the disease through exposure (i.e. hemophiliacs receiving blood products, staff and residents at institutions for developmentally disabled, dialysis patients, those with multiple sex partners, health care workers with occupational exposure to blood), and to infants of mothers who are HBsAg positive (hepatitis B surface antigen positive). Generally, a 0.5-ml intramuscular injection is given to infants three times with the second injection 1 month after the first, and the third 6 months after the first. The deltoid muscle is the site of choice in older children and adults; the anterolateral thigh is used in infants. The dose is generally 1.0 ml in adults but may be altered in those with immunosuppression (Table 9-7).

Risk of Immunization

Local tenderness or redness at the injection site may occur. Occasional hypersensitivity reactions to yeast or

TABLE 9-7
Recommended Doses (Given Intramuscularly) and Schedules of Currently Licensed Hepatitis B Vaccines*

Group	Vaccine†·‡		
	Heptavax-B§ (MSD‖) Dose (μg) (ml)	Recombivax HB (MSD‖) Dose (μg) (ml)	Engerix-B¶ (SK**) Dose (μg) (ml)
Infants of HBV carrier mothers	10 (0.5)	5 (0.5)	10 (0.5)
Other infants and children < 11 y	10 (0.5)	2.5 (0.25)	10 (0.5)
Children and adolescents 11–19 y	20 (1.0)	5 (0.5)	20 (1.0)
Adults > 19 y	20 (1.0)	10 (1.0)	20 (1.0)
Dialysis patients and other immunocompromised persons	40 (2.0)††	40 (1.0)#	40 (2.0)††·§§

* From Centers for Disease Control (1990). Protection against viral hepatitis: Recommendations of the Immunization Practices Advisory Committee (ACIP). *MMWR,* 39(No. RR-2), 11.

† Vaccines should be stored at 2°C to 8°C. Freezing destroys effectiveness.

‡ Usual schedule for each vaccine is three doses, given at 0, 1, and 6 months.

§ Available in U.S. only for hemodialysis and other immunocompromised patients and for persons with known allergy to yeast.

‖ Merck, Sharp & Dohme.

¶ Alternative schedule: four doses at 0, 1, 2, and 12 months.

** SmithKline Biologicals.

†† Given as two 1.0-ml doses at different sites.

\# Special formulation for dialysis patients.

§§ Four-dose schedule recommended at 0, 1, 2, and 12 months.

the mercury-based preservative thimerosal used in the vaccine have occurred.[7]

Nursing Considerations and Teaching

It is recommended that all pregnant women be tested to identify hepatitis B virus carriers due to the high risk of transmitting the disease to their offspring. These children can be immunized with hepatitis B vaccine, 0.5 ml within 7 days, preferably 12 hours, after birth. They also are given 0.5 ml of hepatitis B immune globulin intramuscularly within 12 hours after birth. Follow-up visits for the second and third doses of hepatitis B vaccine should be established, and reminders should be provided. These infants are also tested at 9 months of age for HBsAg and anti-HBsAg. If test results are negative, a fourth booster dose of hepatitis B vaccine is given. In endemic populations, such as Alaskan natives and Pacific Islanders, or if testing is not feasible, hepatitis B vaccine can be routinely administered. Breast-feeding is allowed for the infant with a mother who is HBsAg positive when the infant has started receiving hepatitis B vaccine.

Parents are taught the common side-effect of site tenderness, and a history is taken before immunization to rule out allergy to yeast and mercury compounds. Epinephrine 1:1000, its doses written for child age groups and weights, and resuscitative drugs and equipment should always be available during administration of immunizations. Parents should remain in the health facility with the child for 20 to 30 minutes after immunization in case of anaphylaxis.

Vaccine Storage

Hepatitis B vaccine is kept refrigerated between 35°F and 46°F (2°C and 8°C); it should not be frozen. It should be well-shaken before withdrawal and will be a slightly opaque, white suspension.

Summary

The child health supervision visit is an example of the primary level of disease prevention. The health care provider is instrumental in preventing the occurrence of disease in young children and in detecting early any deviations from normal. The American Academy of Pediatrics has established guidelines for recommendations for health supervision of children. Principles of health supervision can be applied in a variety of settings, and nurses may play various roles in health supervision. To be effective, the examiner brings an understanding of physical norms and developmental progression. This knowledge is applied and integrated with specific approaches to enhance the effectiveness of data gathering, physical examination, and teaching. Anticipatory guidance, an essential component of each well-child visit, is a type of teaching that considers the next expected developmental accomplishments, prepares parents to deal with them, and prevents problems. Both the science (knowledge base) and the art (techniques) of examination are merged to enhance the interaction with the child and family. A head-to-toe examination is one of the methods of con-

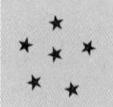

Ideas for Nursing Research

The nurse who sees the same children over a period of years for well-child visits is ideally situated to study aspects of the growth and development of children longitudinally. Information obtained through systematic observations in a conceptual framework could be used to improve the effectiveness of nursing interventions. Potential topics for exploration are innumerable. The following areas need to be explored:

- Identify specific cues that indicate parental readiness for anticipatory guidance related to developmental changes in children.
- Identify the characteristics of the nurse's approach and the environment that are most likely to result in positive interactions with the parents and child and yield the most comprehensive data base.
- Perform reliability checks for assistants who obtain somatic measures to improve accuracy in measurement and documentation on growth grids.
- Effectiveness of administering acetaminophen routinely to children receiving immunizations.

ducting a physical examination. A number of immunizations against communicable diseases are available and encouraged. Such practices have been instrumental in eradicating or decreasing the occurrence of specific diseases. There are risks, however, to immunizations, and explanations of these should be part of the information given to parents before they consent to immunizations.

References

1. American Academy of Pediatrics. (1989). Measles: Reassessment of the current immunization policy. *Pediatrics, 89,* 1110.
2. Baraff, L., Shields, D., Beckwith, L., Strome, G., Marcy, S., Cherry, J., & Mandark, C. (1988). Infants and children with convulsions and hypotonic-hyporesponsive episodes following diphtheria-tetanus-pertussis immunization: Follow-up evaluation. *Pediatrics, 81*(6), 789–794.
3. Barnes, L. (1991). Teaching self-care to children. *MCN: American Journal of Maternal Child Nursing, 16*(2), 101.
4. Bates, B. (1991). *A guide to physical examination and history taking* (5th ed.). Philadelphia: Lippincott.
5. Behrman, R., & Vaughan, V. (1992). *Nelson textbook of pediatrics* (14th ed.). Philadelphia: Saunders.
6. Bibace, R., & Walsh, M. (1981). Children's conceptions of illness. In Bibace, R., & Walsh, M. (Eds.) *Children's conceptions of health, illness, and bodily function.* San Francisco: Jossey Bass.
7. Bindler, R., & Howry, L. (1991). Pediatric drugs and nursing implications. E. Norwalk, CT: Appleton-Lange.
8. Block, G., & Nolan, J. (1986). *Health assessment for professional nursing: A developmental approach.* E. Norwalk, CT: Appleton-Lange.
9. Bowers, A., & Thompson, J. (1988). *Clinical manual of health assessment.* St. Louis: Mosby.
10. Brunell, P. (1988). Measles vaccine—One or two doses? *Pediatrics, 81*(5), 722–724.
11. Committee on Infectious Diseases. (1987). Family history of convulsions in candidates for immunization with pertussis containing vaccines (diphtheria, tetanus, pertussis). *Pediatrics, 80*(5), 743–744.
12. Committee on Infectious Diseases. (1991). *Report of the committee on infectious diseases.* Elk Grove Village, IL: American Academy of Pediatrics.
13. Committee on Psychosocial Aspects of Child and Family Health. (1988). *Guidelines for health supervision.* Elk Grove Village, IL: American Academy of Pediatrics.
14. Crider, C. (1981). Children's conceptions of the body interior. In Bibace, R., & Walsh, M. (Eds.). *Children's conceptions of health, illness, and bodily function.* San Francisco: Jossey Bass.
15. Edelman, C., & Mandle, C. (1990). *Health promotion throughout the life span.* St. Louis: Mosby.
16. Edwards, K., & Karzon, D. (1990). Pertussis vaccines. *Pediatric Clinics of North America, 37*(3), 549–566.
17. Flavell, J. (1963). *The developmental psychology of Jean Piaget.* New York: Van Nostrand.
18. Fuller, J., & Schaller-Ayers, J. (1990). *Health assessment: A nursing approach.* Philadelphia: Lippincott.
19. Griffith, A. (1989). Permanent brain damage and pertussis vaccination: Is the end of the saga in sight? *Vaccine, 7,* 199–210.
20. Hull, H., Montes, J., Hays, P., & Lucero, R. (1985). Risk factors for measles vaccine failure among immunized students. *Pediatrics, 76*(4), 518–523.
21. Jones, D., Lepley, M., & Baker, B. (1984). *Health assessment across the life span.* New York: McGraw-Hill.
22. Killam, P. (1989). Orthopedic assessment of young children: Developmental variations. *Nurse Practitioner, 14*(7), 27–36.
23. Landwirth, J. (1990). Medical-legal aspects of immunization. *Pediatric Clinics of North America, 37*(3), 771–784.
24. Lochhead, Y. (1991). Failure to immunize children under 5 years: A literature review. *Journal of Advanced Nursing, 16,* 130–137.
25. Lowrey, G. (1986). *Growth and development of children.* Chicago: Year Book Medical.
26. Mahoney, E., & Verdisco, L. (1982). *How to collect and record a health history.* Philadelphia: Lippincott.
27. Medical letter. (1991). *H. influenzae* vaccine for infants. *Medical Letter, 33*(836), 5–7.
28. MMWR. (1988). National childhood vaccine injury act. *MMWR. Morbidity and Mortality Weekly Report, 37*(13), 197–200.
29. MMWR. (1989). Measles prevention: Recommendations of the immunization practices advisory committee. *MMWR. Morbidity and Mortality Weekly Report, 38,* 5–9.
30. MMWR. (1990). Second haemophilus b conjugate vaccine approved for infants. *MMWR. Morbidity and Mortality Weekly Report, 39*(50), 925–926.
31. Phillips, C. (1991). Keeping up with the changing immunization schedule. *Contemporary Pediatrics, 8,* 20.
32. Pipes, P. (1989). *Nutrition in infancy and childhood.* St. Louis: Mosby.
33. Schubiner, H. (1989). Preventive health screening in adolescent patients. *Primary Care, 16*(1), 211–230.
34. Shapiro, E., & Berg, A. (1990). Protective efficacy of *Haemophilus influenzae* type b polysaccharide vaccine. *Pediatrics, 85*(4), 643–653.
35. Stangler, S., Huber, C., & Routh, D. (1980). *Screening growth and development of preschool children: A guide for test selection.* New York: McGraw-Hill.
36. Strong, W. B., & Dennison, B. A. (1988). Pediatric preventive cardiology: Atherosclerosis and coronary heart disease. *Pediatric Review, 9,* 303–314.
37. Walker, A., Jick, H., Perera, D., Knauss, T., & Thompson R. (1988). Neurologic events following diphtheria-tetanus-pertussis immunization. *Pediatrics, 81*(3), 345–349.

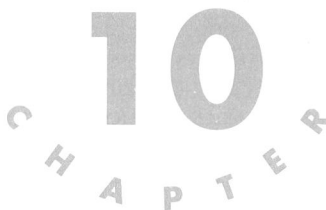

10

C H A P T E R

Health Assessment, Promotion, and Maintenance for the Prenatal Period

BEHAVIORAL OBJECTIVES

Identify preconception health patterns that affect subsequent fetal and newborn health.

Describe the developmental tasks of pregnancy.

Discuss the impact of nutrition on the healthy outcome of pregnancy.

Describe the influence of culture on childbearing.

Describe selected factors that place the mother and fetus at risk.

Identify the role of the nurse in promoting health during childbearing.

Comprehensive care during pregnancy is the one major factor that can reduce infant mortality in the United States. Many other developed nations provide care to all expectant mothers as a routine part of health policy. Although this nation has many excellent facilities and community health programs, these are not available to all women. Factors such as poverty, lack of transportation to a clinic, or difficulty in finding a reliable person to care for other children are often identified as problems that limit access to health care. Noncompliance may be related to lack of family support, a knowledge deficit, or cultural differences in the view toward preventive health care. Statistics on the high numbers of premature and low birthweight infants delivered in this nation are evidence of inadequate prenatal care. The March of Dimes and the National Commission to Prevent Infant Mortality are actively involved in trying to reverse this trend.[24]

This chapter identifies selected influences on fetal development that may foster functional health in infancy and childhood or lead to subsequent problems. The role of the nurse is integrated throughout the chapter with suggestions for assessments and interventions that improve maternal health and fetal outcome.

Normal Reproduction

Even before puberty, young boys and girls prepare their bodies for procreation. Health maintenance patterns established early in life often influence the outcome of subsequent pregnancies. Factors such as health practices, rest and exercise, nutrition, and stress management either contribute to a healthy gene pool or compromise reproduction. The impact of culture, socioeconomic status, support systems, and developmental level on childbearing and childrearing provide the basis for many research studies. Exposure to teratogens, substances that affect embryo-fetal organ development, may affect health in infancy and childhood.

Although the man's physical and psychological states directly influence embryo-fetal development, this chapter focuses on the impact of preconceptual and prenatal health of the woman. Emphasis is placed on a healthy lifestyle and identification of personal strengths and risk factors.

As the young woman develops physically, influenced by hormonal spurts, secondary sex organ changes become evident. The adolescent girl should be well-nourished, in good functional health, and of optimal weight for stature when the hypothalamus and pituitary glands trigger ovum development and the beginning of the menstrual cycle. The adolescent girl's hips widen, with evident fat deposits. The pelvic bones calcify and provide an adequate passageway for birth.[4] Anatomy, physiology, and assessment of reproductive function are further discussed in Unit 18.

The developmental stage at which a young woman becomes pregnant influences parenting abilities. A review of developmental tasks of school age and adolescence (see Chaps. 15 and 16) reveals many cognitive, perceptual, emotional and interactional factors that affect the ability to nurture and care for a child. Developmental theorists suggest that prolonged adolescence in today's society delays the independence of many young women from their families. Although intimate relationships may occur, the ability to give oneself empathetically to a child (Erickson's stage of generativity) does not occur until adulthood.

Fetal Development

After fertilization, the newly formed cell undergoes a series of divisions through a process called mitosis. The growing cluster of cells is called the morula. Continuing the process of growth through repeated divisions, the morula travels down the fallopian tube to the uterus. In about 7 days, the fertilized ovum implants in the uterus. While the embryo-fetus grows and develops, maternal factors may enhance health or threaten its survival. An overview of fetal development is presented in the display. A more detailed presentation of development is found in the first chapters of each unit on systems.

Antepartal Care

The physical and emotional states of the woman beginning a pregnancy provide a baseline assessment for the 38 to 40 weeks of gestation. Ideally, the pregnant client maintained consistently good health patterns before conception.

Visits to the physician, nurse-midwife, or nurse practitioner should begin as early as possible once pregnancy is suspected. The woman often reports that a self-performed urine test is positive, usually after a menstrual period is missed and mild morning sickness occurs. The woman seeks confirmation that she is pregnant. The practitioner may repeat the urine test for the presence of human chorionic gonadotropin (HCG). However, positive confirmation of pregnancy depends on hearing a heart beat, observing fetal movement, or viewing an ultrasound or x-ray image.

Prenatal Testing

Most women do not need to undergo prenatal testing. Those who may need to include women who are at risk due to: age (over 35), prior birth anomalies, family history, multiple births, and some chronic illnesses. In other cases, placental gas exchange may be compromised by postmaturity, infections, or hypertension. For women who do have these tests, it is important that the nurse explain the procedures (the risks and the benefits) and support them during the test, in the interval before the test results are known, and as they explore options should any abnormality be detected. Refer to Table 10-1 for a summary of tests of fetal well-being.

Nursing Implications for Functional Health

The nurse should take a thorough history, including vital information about past health patterns, illnesses, and prior pregnancies. The nurse should allow sufficient time to establish rapport with the woman, interview her, listen carefully to responses, and ask additional questions to clarify data. Cues to the client's emotional state, social situation, and family relationships are often detected during an initial interview.

At the initial visit and the subsequent monthly appointments, the nurse assesses vital signs and weight and performs a urinalysis. Changes that suggest potential problems over time must be evaluated and documented. For example, a weight gain pattern of 2 lb a month that suddenly increases to 8 lb suggests that further assessment is needed. The presence of edema must be noted. Changes in eating patterns should be identified. Blood pressure must be closely monitored.

In addition to a pelvic examination and Pap smear, blood is drawn for laboratory studies. Generally, these tests include blood type, Rh, and a complete blood count. Later in the pregnancy, tests for sexually transmitted diseases and other potential problems are performed. If the woman is Rh-negative, an antibody titer is drawn to identify early antigen–antibody responses. This blood test (indirect Coombs') may be repeated. If no antibodies are found, Rhogam may be given to the woman during the third trimester to block subsequent antibody formation, which could occur as a result of exposure to fetal Rh-

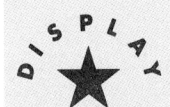

Fetal Development

1st LUNAR MONTH

The fetus is 0.75 to 1 cm in length.
Trophoblasts embed in decidua.
Chorionic villi form.
Foundations for nervous system, genitourinary system, skin, bones, and lungs are formed.
Buds of arms and legs begin to form.
Rudiments of eyes, ears, and nose appear.

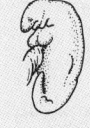

4 weeks

2nd LUNAR MONTH

The fetus is 2.5 cm in length and weighs 4 g.
Fetus is markedly bent.
Head is disproportionately large, owing to brain development.
Sex differentiation begins.
Centers of bone begin to ossify.

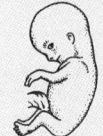

8 weeks

3rd LUNAR MONTH

The fetus is 7 to 9 cm in length and weighs 28 g.
Fingers and toes are distinct.
Placenta is complete.
Fetal circulation is complete.

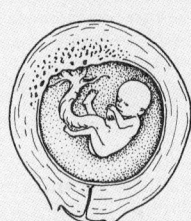

3 months

4th LUNAR MONTH

The fetus is 10 to 17 cm in length and weighs 55 to 120 g.
Sex is differentiated.
Rudimentary kidneys secrete urine.
Heartbeat is present.
Nasal septum and palate close.

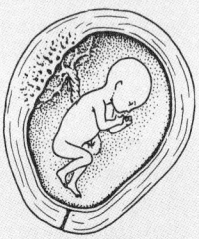

4 months

5th LUNAR MONTH

The fetus is 25 cm in length and weighs 223 g.
Lanugo covers entire body.
Fetal movements are felt by mother.
Heart sounds are perceptible by auscultation.

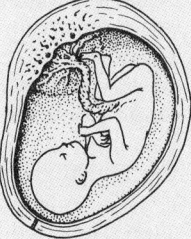

5 months

6th LUNAR MONTH

The fetus is 28 to 36 cm in length and weighs 680 g.
Skin appears wrinkled.
Vernix caseosa appears.
Eyebrows and fingernails develop.

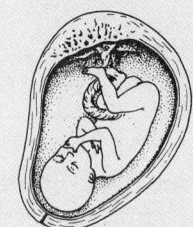

6 months

7th LUNAR MONTH

The fetus is 35 to 38 cm in length and weighs 1200 g.
Skin is red.
Pupillary membrane disappears from eyes.
The fetus has an excellent chance of survival.

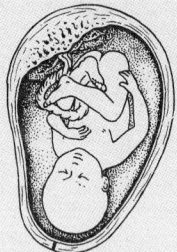

7 months

8th LUNAR MONTH

The fetus is 38 to 43 cm in length and weighs 2.7 kg.
Fetus is viable.
Eyelids open.
Fingerprints are set.
Vigorous fetal movement occurs.

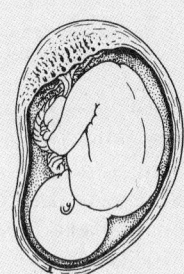

8 months

9th LUNAR MONTH

The fetus is 42 to 49 cm in length and weighs 1900 to 2700 g.
Face and body have a loose wrinkled appearance because of subcutaneous fat deposit.
Lanugo disappears.
Amniotic fluid decreases.

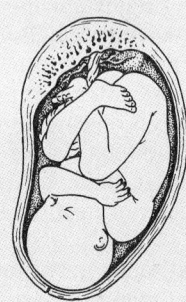

9 months

10th LUNAR MONTH

The fetus is 48 to 52 cm in length and weighs 3000 g.
Skin is smooth.
Eyes are uniformly slate colored.
Bones of skull are ossified and nearly together at sutures.

Reeder, S. J., Martin, L. L., & Koniak, D. (1992). Maternity nursing: Family, newborn, and women's health care (17th ed.). Philadelphia: Lippincott.

TABLE 10-1
Tests of Fetal Well-Being

Test	Test Description	Data Provided	Risks
Ultrasound (timing varies)	To visualize the embryo-fetus placenta and amniotic fluid by use of sound waves	Location of placenta confirms tubal pregnancy, fetal growth, multiple gestation, certain defects (i.e., SGA, hydrocephalus)	Painless for the mother. No known risk to fetus
Amniocentesis (after 15th week)	Aspiration of amniotic fluid for analysis	Chromosomal abnormalities (e.g., Down's syndrome), genetic disorders (e.g., sickle cell anemia, cystic fibrosis), fetal sex, fetal lung maturity	Relatively painless for the mother. Small risk to fetus; slight risk to mother
α-fetoprotein (16th–18th week)	Venous blood sample analysis for the presence of the fetal protein (α-fetoprotein)	Abnormally high levels indicate fetus may have a neural tube defect. Low levels have been linked to Down's syndrome[13]	Only risk lies in false-positive results. To prevent this, an abnormal outcome is followed by amniocentesis and/or ultrasound
Chorionic villus sampling (9th–10th week)	Gentle suctioning to remove cells from the chorion by way of a tube inserted through the cervix into the placenta	Same as amniocentesis but earlier in pregnancy	Greater risk to fetus than an amniocentesis. Requires very skilled practitioner
Non-stress test (after 32nd week)	Measurement of fetal heart rate in response to fetal movement by way of an external monitor on the mother's abdomen	Well-oxygenated fetus shows increased heart rate with activity	Risk only in false-positive reading
Daily fetal movement count (third trimester)	Self-monitoring of fetal activity at home	Adequate placental gas exchange as demonstrated by consistent activity	No risk
Contraction stress test (third trimester)	Measurement of fetal heart rate after stimulation of contractions (may be induced with dilute pitocin)	Differentiates between fetal well-being and distress	Premature labor may ensue

Note: This chart suggests data provided and possible outcomes for tests. Nurses must recognize that ethical decisions often occur when test results are confirmed. However, this chapter does not discuss such issues, because they are resolved before infant's birth.

positive cells. The cord blood of the newborn is tested through a direct Coombs' test to identify its blood type and Rh, and to detect antibodies that may lead to hyperbilirubinemia and red blood cell destruction.

Risk factors are assessed at the initial and regular monthly visits. For example, it is accepted practice to test every pregnant woman between the 24th and 28th weeks of pregnancy for gestational diabetes. Blood samples are drawn after ingestion of a glucose beverage or a test meal (glucose tolerance test or a postprandial blood sugar). Although the incidence of gestational diabetes is fairly low, the fetal risk can be great. The woman's hyperglycemia stimulates the fetal pancreas to secrete large amounts of insulin. This results in a newborn of larger than average size, increasing the risk of birth trauma. Hyperglycemia over time also leads to increased fetal mortality, higher incidence of anomalies and risks for hypoglycemia, respiratory distress and jaundice in the newborn. Home blood sugar monitoring and periodic testing of glycosated hemoglobin levels have improved the diabetic management that includes diet, exercise, and insulin.[32]

Health Perception and Health Management

Health practices vary among school-age girls, adolescents, and adult women. Many females are aware of the importance of health and exhibit positive health man-

agement patterns in daily living. They practice good personal hygiene, follow guidelines for tampon selection and use, and regularly perform self breast examinations. These young women keep appointments for regular gynecologic checkups and Pap smears. Problems identified by the young woman are reported to the physician and nurse and become a part of the database for ongoing care.

Unfortunately, even among educated young women, there are many who fail to manage personal health adequately. Improper handwashing before meals and sharing a common soda can are common careless behaviors. Surveys of female college students indicate that, although many are aware of the importance of the self breast exam, they fail to carry out the assessment regularly. Some young women complain of frequent incapacity from premenstrual tension or dysmenorrhea, yet do not seek relief of symptoms from the health care provider. "I don't think the doctor listens to me!" is a frequent comment. Others report that they have no opportunity to see one consistent clinic physician or nurse practitioner, limiting the opportunity for confidential discussion of gynecologic or reproductive concerns.

The role of the nurse in recognizing the impact of altered health practices is to assess those factors that place the young woman at risk psychologically or physically, and to teach and reinforce positive health management patterns. Dysfunctional health patterns may initially affect only the well-being of the young woman, but early intervention that leads to positive change promotes a better outcome for subsequent children as well.

During the health assessment, the nurse should ob-

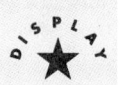

Patient Teaching: Topics to Discuss With Young Women Before Conception

Personal involvement in health promotion
Normal reproductive function
Healthy nutrition/exercise/rest patterns
Stress management and coping patterns
Common gynecologic problems and available treatments
Reportable signs of health alteration
Decision making about childbearing
Community resources for education and counseling
Consultation with healthcare providers

serve the young woman and make note of her general appearance, energy level, and skin tone. Interview questions should address rest and activity patterns, health practices, and patterns of behavior. Time should be provided to demonstrate the self breast examination and reinforce that knowledge at later visits. Films and pamphlets may be appropriate learning aids. If at all possible, a consistent caregiver should be assigned to foster an open and trusting relationship that allows for free discussion of health concerns. The nurse should avoid negative judgments about dysfunctional health patterns; instead, positive changes might be suggested, with the benefits clearly explained. Suggested topics for discussion are given in the patient teaching display.

Substance Abuse

The young woman who avoids tobacco, alcohol, and drugs is preparing herself for childbearing. Unfortunately, many young girls are unaware that substance experimentation may affect the future development of their children. The nurse working with young people has an excellent opportunity to identify drug problems and provide early intervention. Programs that begin early to focus on personal strengths, self-esteem, and independent decision making are gaining increasing attention from families, educators, and health care professionals. Such programs may focus on preventing or altering destructive lifestyles, avoiding environments with pressure for drug use, or offering alternatives. Many school- or community-based programs use peer support to help youngsters make choices and avoid drug and alcohol dependency.

Drug use during pregnancy affects the fetus. The nurse must help the pregnant woman understand that the placenta is not a filter. Drugs taken by the mother cross the placenta and enter the body of the fetus. Although any abused substance can be harmful to the fetus, specific drugs affect the growing baby differently.

Cocaine. The placenta does not protect the fetus from the effects of cocaine. In fact, due to liver immaturity, cocaine remains in the body of the fetus or newborn longer than it does in the adult. Cocaine causes vasoconstriction and increased blood pressure. Pregnant women who use cocaine are more likely to suffer first trimester

abortions, possibly due to constriction of the blood vessels of the placenta. These women are also more likely to have a sudden onset of premature labor shortly after cocaine use. In addition, there is an increased chance of placental abruption within 1 hour after cocaine use, probably due to the sudden increase in blood pressure. The elevation in fetal blood pressure can result in a cerebral vascular hemorrhage and fetal death. The fetal heart rate also is elevated after cocaine use.

If the woman does not miscarry or suffer hemorrhage, she will deliver a baby who tends to be irritable, experiences tremors, and has labile emotions. These children are being studied and are considered at risk for developmental and learning disabilities. In addition, babies born to mothers who use cocaine are more prone to die from sudden infant death syndrome (SIDS). Unlike many other habit-forming drugs, there is no predicting how much cocaine is dangerous. One cocaine trip can induce premature labor, abruptio placentae, or miscarriage.[14]

Because cocaine use is a major problem in our society, it is part of the nurse's role to ask pregnant women about drug use and to assess the patient carefully for any signs of cocaine abuse. Patient teaching is critical and must include the location of support services available.

PCP and Heroin. The infants of women addicted to these drugs tend to be restless and irritable in the newborn period. They are born addicted to the drug and must go through withdrawal during the first weeks of life, during which time they tend to be emotionally distant. Long-term studies are being conducted, and it is felt that these children may have subsequent learning problems.[22]

Marijuana. Babies born to mothers who smoke marijuana are not physically addicted to the drug. Studies are underway to determine whether these children suffer long-term emotional and learning problems. Studies with animals indicate that heavy marijuana use during pregnancy may cause central nervous system abnormalities in the baby.[31]

Cigarettes. According to the March of Dimes Birth Defects Foundation, "cigarette smoking during pregnancy is clearly associated with an increase in stillbirth, miscarriage, prematurity, low birthweight, and neonatal death."[23] In addition, children of smoking parents have more respiratory problems than those of nonsmoking parents. The incidence of bronchitis and pneumonia in infancy is twice as high in children of smoking parents when compared to children whose parents do not smoke.[41]

Women who smoke during pregnancy have twice the chance of having a low-birthweight baby or a premature baby as do their nonsmoking counterparts. Nicotine causes vasoconstriction, diminishing the amount of oxygen and nutrients available to the fetus. In addition, smoking exposes the fetus to carbon monoxide, which further limits the oxygen supply for the growing organs and tissues. The effects of nicotine and carbon monoxide are responsible for fetal growth retardation.

Changes in uterine blood vessels brought on by smoking may also be the reason for the increased risk of placenta previa and abruptio placentae in women who smoke. These complications put both the mother and fetus at a higher risk for hemorrhage and death.

Long-term studies indicate that smoking during pregnancy may result in learning problems and hyperactivity. The children of women who smoked during pregnancy may have more problems with spelling and reading than those of mothers who did not smoke.[23]

The effects of smoking on the fetus are directly related to the number of cigarettes smoked each day and the length of time the mother smoked. Women who stop smoking early in the pregnancy decrease the risk of having a low birthweight baby to almost that of a nonsmoker. However, women who stop or cut back later in pregnancy can still reduce the risks. The nurse should urge women to stop smoking before becoming pregnant; if they cannot stop, they must be encouraged to cut down the number of cigarettes, particularly during the second half of pregnancy.

Alcohol. Drinking during pregnancy increases the risks of stillbirth, spontaneous abortion, and birth defects. Children born to heavy drinkers may be affected with fetal alcohol syndrome (FAS), a condition that includes growth deficiency, mental retardation, and facial and organ anomalies. Children with FAS may have some or all of the defects associated with the syndrome. No one knows how much alcohol causes damage to the fetus. Women who drink heavily bear the highest risk, but children born to mothers who drink moderate amounts of alcohol (between two and five drinks daily) can also have some fetal alcohol effects. In addition to FAS, women who drink heavily during pregnancy have a two to four times higher risk of having a miscarriage and a two to three times greater risk of losing their babies during the perinatal period than do nondrinking women.

Because researchers do not know how much alcohol is tolerable to the fetus and cannot explain why some women who only drink a small amount during pregnancy can still have an affected baby, the nurse should counsel any woman planning a pregnancy to stop drinking and to abstain throughout the pregnancy and breast-feeding period. If the woman is still drinking after conception, she should be encouraged to stop as soon as the pregnancy is confirmed.[21]

Caffeine. Caffeine is a stimulant that crosses the placenta. Although no toxic effects to the human fetus have been proven, large doses of caffeine given to laboratory animals have resulted in defective animal fetuses. Because any drug that crosses the placenta may be harmful to the fetus, pregnant women are advised to cut down on caffeine intake.[18] It is important that the nurse help the pregnant woman identify the numerous sources of caffeine. It is the nurse's role to counsel and explore caffeine use and alternatives with the client. In addition to coffee, caffeine is contained in tea, cola, chocolate, and many over-the-counter drugs, such as cold remedies (which may not be approved for use during pregnancy). The nurse should assess the alternative drinks chosen by the woman. Many of the herbal teas available are attractive because they are caffeine-free. However, overconsumption of some herbs may also be detrimental. Several of these teas contain toxins and may cause diarrhea, vom-

iting, allergic reactions, heart palpitations, and alterations in blood pressure.[10]

Toxic Substances

A pregnant woman is exposed to many environmental hazards, whether in the home, outdoors, or in the workplace. Although exposure during the first trimester poses the greatest danger to the developing baby, contact later in pregnancy may also compromise fetal outcome. Table 10-2 identifies selected teratogenic hazards. The nurse must teach the young woman to recognize potential environmental problems in the home or workplace that may affect fertility or embryo-fetal health.[36] Unsafe conditions must be reported, altered, or avoided, especially during the critical first trimester. Education remains the primary prevention for many teratogenic problems; the nurse is often the key health professional in recognizing and reducing such potential hazards.

Nutrition and Metabolism

Nutrition patterns are established early in life and are key elements in physical growth and in preparing for healthy reproduction. Assessment of nutrition status should be part of regular pediatric examinations. Teaching the value of a balanced diet begins within the family and should be included in the curriculum from elementary school through college.

The convenience of fast food service results in overindulgence in foods high in sodium, fat, and carbohydrates by many young women. Peer pressure and concerns over body image often lead a group of friends to limit some meals to diet soda and salad. A deficiency in protein is common among some young women. The nurse's teaching should emphasize changing needs during times of growth, the basic four food groups, and healthy eating habits.

Nutritional alterations common in our society may impact on the health of the adolescent and young adult. Among these problems are long-term patterns of underweight and overweight, anorexia, bulimia, sudden changes in weight due to appetite changes or dental problems such as gum deterioration, decay, or temporomandibular joint syndrome (TMJ).

The nurse has an excellent opportunity to identify potential and actual nutritional and metabolic problems when encountering healthy school-age, adolescent, and young adult women. Early intervention and health teaching may prevent these problems from becoming a life threat or seriously impairing future childbearing.

For the young woman who has established a healthy nutrition pattern, and even more so for the woman who has nutritional deficiencies, pregnancy places additional demands on the body's metabolic stores. The nurse must impress on the woman the necessity of ingesting the right amount of nutrients for both herself and the growing fetus.

The first question many women ask is "How much weight should I gain during pregnancy?" Although there is no definite answer, most physicians recommend a gain of at least 25 lb to ensure adequate fetal nutrition. Most of this gain should occur during the latter half of preg-

TABLE 10-2
Selected Teratogenic Hazards: Exposure May Compromise Fetal Development

Teratogen	Avenue of Exposure	Nursing Interventions
Rubella	Virus contracted by mother, especially harmful during first trimester, but still dangerous in later stages of pregnancy. May cause rubella syndrome in the baby (CNS, cardiac, and sensory abnormalities).	Encourage routine childhood immunizations. Assess maternal rubella titers early in pregnancy. If maternal titer is negative, have woman avoid exposure to anyone with rubella throughout pregnancy. Do not give vaccines to pregnant clients. Give vaccine after the baby is born and avoid a subsequent pregnancy for 3 months.
Streptococcus	Bacteria contracted by mother. Often found in vagina of pregnant woman. May result in miscarriage or stillbirth.	Explain importance of avoiding risk factors and practicing good hygiene. Toxoplasmosis protozoan infection transmitted through uncooked meat and feline intestinal waste. May result in miscarriage, stillbirth, or CNS damage to the fetus. Cook all meats thoroughly. Tell client to have other family members empty kitty litter box or wear rubber gloves when changing it.
Carbon monoxide	Inhaled in areas of heavy traffic, in tunnels, or near highways or airports. Causes a decrease in fetal oxygen supply and an increased risk of mental retardation or cerebral palsy.	Advise client to avoid areas of traffic congestion. Advise client to close car windows. Advise client to avoid second-hand smoke.
Inhalation anesthesia	Exposure to waste gases while working in a hospital operating room. Results in reduced fertility and increased rate of miscarriage. Increased rate of birth defects in offspring of exposed mother and father have been identified.	Counsel client on considering a job transfer or ask for a change in tasks.
Radiation	Exposure while working in the medical or dental fields or through diagnostic x-rays.	Counsel client on changing jobs or tasks. Avoid unnecessary x-rays. Provide a special lead apron to shield the uterus if an x-ray is unavoidable.
Lead	Exposure to heavy metal in arts and craft industry or eating or drinking from improperly fired china or ceramics. May cause prematurity, birth defects, or mental retardation in offspring.	Counsel client on asking for a job transfer. Tell client to avoid cooking and serving in dishes that may be improperly fired.
Vinyl chloride	Exposure to industrial chemical especially in plastic companies. Linked with birth defects.	Have client explore feasibility of job transfer or change of task.
PCBs (polychlorinated biphenyls)	Linked with growth retardation and skull abnormalities in fetus.	Advise client to avoid consumption of PCB. Decrease on-the-job exposure or explore change of task or job transfer.
Heptachlor and chlordane	Pesticides used in gardening. Exposure in utero increases risk of childhood cancer.	Explain importance of reading labels of gardening sprays and fertilizers. Advise client to be aware of community spraying projects and avoid areas where spraying is in progress.
Medications		
Tetracycline	Antibiotic. Causes bone and teeth abnormalities in fetus.	Tell client to inform physician of pregnancy and request a different antibiotic.
Dilantin	Anticonvulsant taken by epileptics. Causes fetal phenytoin syndrome (abnormal facial features, growth retardation, finger and toe abnormalities).	Make sure client seeks medical help to develop an alternative medical protocol.
Diethylstilbestrol (DES)	Hormone, formerly used to prevent miscarriages. Causes cancer in many female children exposed to drug in utero.	Tell client to avoid hormone treatment during pregnancy.
Steroids	Used to treat inflammatory conditions and increasingly used by young people for body building.	Tell client to avoid steroid treatment.
Vaccinations	May be given before traveling or after exposure to a communicable disease. Crosses placenta and may cause active disease in fetus.	Advise client to avoid all live vaccines. Limit any vaccination to use if exposure cannot be avoided.

nancy. Fewer pounds gained may result in a smaller baby. Babies who weigh less than 5½ lb have a greater risk of developing metabolic, nutritional, and neurologic disorders.[30]

Eating for the baby means not only that the woman increases the amount of food she eats (calories) but also that she follows a well-balanced diet. In general, a preg-nant woman should add about 300 calories and 30 g of protein a day to her regular diet. She should also divide her daily intake among the basic food groups as follows:

Milk, yogurt, and cheese—four servings
Meat, poultry, fish, dry beans, eggs, and nuts—two to three servings

Vegetable protein—three to five servings
Bread, cereal, rice, and pasta—six to eleven servings
Fruit—two to four servings

In addition, the physician prescribes a prenatal vitamin supplement, particularly one containing iron and folic acid. Megavitamins should be avoided because they can harm the fetus. Adequate amounts of vitamins and minerals are always necessary for optimal body functioning. However, during pregnancy, certain elements are of particular concern.

Minerals

Because of its role in the production of hemoglobin, adequate *iron* is essential for good fetal development. Many pregnant woman have depleted iron stores due to menstruation and poor diet. In addition, iron needs increase during pregnancy. For this reason, iron supplementation of 30 to 60 mg is recommended. The infant born to an iron-deficient mother has limited iron stores and suffers from anemia in infancy. Because iron is best absorbed in an acid medium and in the presence of vitamin C, the nurse should advise the client to take the iron with orange juice or some citrus fruit juice.

Calcium is needed for bone growth and nerve and muscle activity. Its absorption increases during pregnancy. *Phosphorus*, likewise, plays a role in bone development. It also enhances calcium absorption, glucose conversion, fat transportation, and vitamin B functioning. Intake of 1200 milligrams per day of both minerals is necessary for fetal development. Four glasses of milk a day provide this amount. Because both calcium and phosphorous absorption are enhanced by vitamin D, milk is the best source of these minerals. Calcium and phosphorous need to be in balance. An increase in phosphorous alone may cause leg cramping in the latter stages of pregnancy.

Deficiency of *zinc* has been linked to fetal growth retardation. Because the human body does not store zinc, a good dietary intake is necessary. Zinc is found mostly in animal protein sources. The recommended dose is 20 milligrams per day.

Megadoses of these minerals in supplementary forms can harm the fetus. Many minerals work in balance with others, so an increase in one may affect the functioning of another. Too much calcium, for instance, can reduce iron and zinc uptake. High zinc levels are linked to nausea and to premature birth. Large doses of some trace metals may be poisonous. The nurse should advise pregnant women to eat a well-balanced diet and to avoid all supplements unless prescribed by the physician.[10]

Vitamins

Vitamin supplements are not a substitute for good nutrition. Foods that provide the necessary vitamins are essential. There are thirteen vitamins, and all are necessary for fetal development.

Fat-Soluble Vitamins.   *Vitamin A* is called retinol in its animal form and carotene in its vegetable form. It plays a role in epithelial cell development, infection resistance, and dim light vision. High doses of retinol can be toxic to the fetus, resulting in birth defects. Pregnant women, particularly adolescents, may take an acne drug that contains retinol. These drugs must be discontinued before conception. The Food and Drug Administration (FDA) requires strict warnings and prescription protocols to warn consumers of the danger these drugs pose to a fetus. Megadoses of retinol in over-the-counter vitamin supplements must also be avoided. The required amount of vitamin A is 1000 RE (retinol equivalents.)[2]

Vitamin D, necessary for the absorption of calcium and phosphorous, also plays an important role in the development of bone and teeth. Both over- and underdoses may be harmful to the fetus. Excessive doses may cause abnormal mental and physical development in the fetus. Maternal deficiency may result in rickets or seizures in the newborn.

Vitamin E helps in normal red blood cell development and enhances vitamins A and C and polyunsaturated fat utilization. No ill effects to the fetus from overdose or deficiency have been identified.

Vitamin K is an essential vitamin for blood clotting. Overdoses may cause birth defects.

Because vitamins A, D, E, and K are fat-soluble, they can be stored in the body. For this reason, megadoses can remain in the fetus and build to toxic levels. It is important that the nurse stress the fact that no vitamin should be taken indiscriminately, and that fat-soluble vitamins are especially dangerous.[10]

Water-Soluble Vitamins.   Essential for the development of bones, teeth, blood cells and blood vessels, *vitamin C* also helps in the formation of collagen, increases the absorption of iron, and enhances the healing process. It must be consumed daily. Low maternal intake has been linked to increased infant mortality. Women who smoke have an increased need for vitamin C.

Vitamin B_1, thiamine, enhances both carbohydrate metabolism and the function of the nervous system. Women who consume large amounts of alcohol are susceptible to thiamine deficiency. Some studies indicate that thiamine may relieve the nausea common in early pregnancy.

Vitamin B_2, riboflavin, helps the body release energy from carbohydrates, fats, and proteins. A deficiency in this vitamin may lead to bone and organ anomalies in the fetus.

Vitamin B_3, niacin, helps convert glucose to energy and is important for fetal growth and development. Deficiencies may occur in women who are alcoholics.

Vitamin B_6, pyridoxine, aids in fat and protein utilization and is important for fetal brain and nerve tissue development. Women who were taking oral contraceptives just before conception may be deficient in vitamin B_6. Megadoses of this vitamin may lead to withdrawal problems in the newborn.

Vitamin B_{12} is essential for red blood cell formation, cell division, and nervous system development. Low vitamin B_{12} levels are associated with premature birth. Women who drink heavily or who have been on long-term antibiotics may be deficient. Vitamin B_{12} supplements may be prescribed for some pregnant vegetarians.

Folacin is necessary for cell division, blood cell and enzyme production, and amino acid metabolism. Pregnancy doubles the need for this vitamin, thus prenatal vitamin supplements have higher levels of folacin than regular multivitamins. Folacin deficiency has been linked with neural tube deformities in the fetus.

Pantothenic acid aids in the metabolism of carbohydrates, fats, and proteins, and in hormone production. Because canning may destroy some pantothenic acid, fresh or frozen sources may be preferable. Deficiencies are rare.

Biotin aids in the production of fatty acids and enhances energy release from carbohydrates. There are no known risks to the fetus from excess.

With the exception of vitamin B_{12}, water-soluble vitamins are not stored in the body. Megadoses of these vitamins are still not recommended.[6,10,39,40]

The nurse must be aware of current research on vitamin and mineral needs during pregnancy, risks of overdosing, and hazards in following trendy diets or fads. Nutritional assessment of young women before and during pregnancy should lead to appropriate diet teaching for her height, weight, and health status.

Elimination

For many active young women a pattern of poor nutrition and rushed meals leads to poor elimination habits that further jeopardize general fitness. The work or school environment may not be conducive to optimal or frequent emptying of the bladder, or defecation when the need is evident. Preconception patterns may be exaggerated further during pregnancy as uterine growth increases the pressure on the stomach, gallbladder, large and small intestines, and ureters. Altered elimination patterns may result in minor discomforts to the pregnant woman, such as frequency of urination during the first and third trimesters, heartburn, constipation, and hemorrhoids. The fetal risk is increased with self-medication to remedy these problems, because many over-the-counter remedies for nausea and constipation may have teratogenic effects.

Of great concern are those changes in elimination patterns that result in dehydration or bladder and kidney infection.

The nurse should teach all young women the importance of regular emptying of the bladder to prevent infection, and defecating in response to the urge to do so to prevent subsequent problems. The pregnant woman should be taught normal elimination changes that occur during each trimester. Emphasis must be placed on early reporting of alterations in elimination patterns and the avoidance of self-medication.

Activity and Exercise

A regular exercise program helps improve muscle tone and strength, increases endurance, and enhances cardiovascular output. Additional benefits of exercise include socialization, emotional and physical well-being, and increased cognitive function. Walking, swimming, biking, tennis, jogging, and aerobics are forms of exercise enjoyed by many adolescent and young adult women. However, many young people do not maintain optimal body tone through sensible exercise. Nursing assessment

and intervention before conception should focus on helping young women form healthy exercise patterns for optimal conditioning.

For the pregnant woman, a regular exercise program has many benefits, but may also pose some risks. For this reason, the woman should consult her physician, midwife, or nurse practitioner before embarking on an exercise routine. For the pregnant woman, the benefits of exercising are similar to those for the nonpregnant woman: improved cardiovascular output, muscle strengthening and endurance, increased flexibility, and improved coordination. The risks include: increases in body temperature, which may be harmful to the fetus (a temperature above 102.4°F may be detrimental); the diversion of blood flow and thus oxygen away from the abdominal organs (and uterus); a constriction of blood flow through the vena cava; or a rise in fetal heart rate. Pregnant women are also more susceptible to joint injury because pregnancy hormones relax the connective tissue. Generally speaking, women who have already established an exercise program should be able to continue. Pregnancy is not a good time to embark on a new, strenuous routine.

Swimming, walking, and low-intensity aerobics are considered good exercises for pregnant women provided they are accompanied by a warming up and cooling down routine. Jogging is acceptable if the woman is used to this exercise and has good muscle tone. She should take care to consider environmental hazards and avoid jogging during times when there are pollution alerts. High-intensity aerobics, long distance running, and contact sports are not recommended for pregnant women because of the rise in heart rate, body temperature, or danger of contact injuries. Hot tubs and saunas are also not recommended due to the rise in body temperature resulting from their use.

Although exercise is generally recommended for pregnant women, there are some exceptions. Exercising may be hazardous for women with a history of vaginal bleeding, incompetent cervix, or premature labor. Women who have heart disease, hypertension, or diabetes should exercise only under careful supervision.

Guidelines for safe exercise during pregnancy have been established by the American College of Obstetricians and Gynecologists. Some of their recommendations include:

- Regular exercise (at least three times a week) is better than intermittent exercise.
- Heart rate should be measured periodically and should not exceed 140 per minute.
- Exercise sessions should be no longer than 15 minutes, excluding warming up and cooling down periods.
- Liquids should be taken liberally before and after exercise.
- Jerky, bouncy motions should be avoided.
- Deep bending or extension of joints and activities that require jarring motions, rapid changes in direction, or jumping should be avoided.
- Stop exercising and consult the physician if any unusual symptoms appear.[9,16]

The nurse must be aware of the woman's usual exercise patterns and her ability to tolerate these during

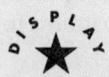

Patient Teaching: Kegel Exercises

Tightening and relaxing the pubococcygeal muscle keeps the vagina toned, increases the strength of the perineum, and helps prevent or control hemorrhoids. This contributes to the strength of the pelvic sling in supporting the fetus, increases sexual pleasure, and enhances urinary control.

The muscle that is used to stop the flow of urine is the pubococcygeal muscle. Practice stopping urine by squeezing this muscle several times to become familiar with it. When lying down, insert one finger into the vagina and contract the pubococcygeal muscle; note the feeling of the contraction around your finger.

EXERCISES

1. Squeeze the pubococcygeal muscle for 3 seconds, relax for 3 seconds, and squeeze again. Begin with 10 three-second squeezes per day, and increase gradually until you are doing 100 twice daily.
2. Squeeze and release, then squeeze and release alternately as rapidly as you can. This is called the "flutter" exercise.
3. Bear down as during a bowel movement, but concentrate on the vagina instead of the rectum. Hold for 3 seconds.

Kegel's exercises can be done anywhere and anytime. The increased control gained over the pubococcygeal muscle is useful throughout pregnancy, during labor, during intercourse, and to prevent loss of vaginal tone with aging. This exercise, done regularly, is useful for the rest of your life.

Reeder, S., & Martin, L. L., (1991). Maternity nursing: Family, newborn, and women's health care. *Philadelphia: Lippincott.*

uterus. A consistent rest/sleep/activity plan should be adopted by the pregnant woman, considering the demands of school or employment, and needs of other small children within the family. Women who are at increased risk during pregnancy because of chronic or acute health problems need to plan additional rest periods.

The nurse should assess the unusual rest and sleep patterns of the young woman, and emphasize the need for adequate rest and sleep, especially during pregnancy. Interventions should include individualized teaching based on the woman's health, work situation, and family demands. The woman should be urged to avoid self-medication to promote sleep or relaxation because many of these drugs have teratogenic effects on the embryo-fetus. A warm glass of milk before bedtime, avoidance of caffeine beverages in the evening, and balancing activity and rest periods may improve rest patterns.

Cognition and Perception

Cognitive functioning varies with developmental level, intelligence, and the environment. Many young women entering pregnancy have some basic awareness of bodily functions and the need for health maintenance and promotion. Others have deficits that result in poor nutrition, risk-taking behaviors, and inadequate preparation for parenting. Perceptions of one's own abilities, strengths, and limitations also vary significantly. With the responsibilities that accompany parenting, such perceptions may affect safe caregiving.

The nurse must assess the cognitive and perceptual abilities of each young woman, ideally before and during the pregnancy. Enrolling in childbirth preparation classes may help the couple anticipate the birth process and begin to plan for newborn care. After the birth, the couple may benefit from parenting classes, a list of telephone resources including the numbers of community hot lines, parent support organizations, and the La Leche League.

pregnancy. Teaching should focus on activities that promote maternal and fetal health, with minimal potential risk.

It is important that the pregnant woman strengthen those muscles that are involved in delivery. The nurse should teach specific prenatal exercises such as the Kegel perineal exercise (see display) and encourage daily practice.

Sleep and Rest

Inadequate sleep and rest patterns are the norm for many students and active adults. Balancing classroom or work responsibilities, social and leisure activities, and family life increases stress and lowers resistance to infection. Young women who develop inconsistent sleep and rest patterns may enter pregnancy with low energy and increased risk.

The need for regular periods of rest and a full night's sleep increase during pregnancy, as increased hormone levels increase fatigue and the fetus grows within the

Roles and Relationships

The quality of a newborn's life is greatly enhanced by the parent–child bond that begins even before birth (Fig. 10-1). The unborn child may be a long-anticipated and joyfully welcomed being, or may represent an unplanned event in the lives of a couple. As the pregnant woman perceives movement, hears the fetal heart beat, and prepares for birth with false labor contractions, she often struggles with common conflicts. For example, it is normal for the woman in the early weeks of pregnancy to express uncertainty and ambivalence. This is usually followed by an understanding that the unborn child is a real and separate person. Through the abdominal wall, the fetus may be spoken to and exposed to the parents' musical preferences. The bond may be strengthened by viewing an ultrasound image or hearing the fetal heart beat during a routine prenatal examination.

By the due date, it is hoped that the couple is ready to take on the parenting role. Ideally, the expectant parents await the birth of the child with some knowledge of the process, are prepared for the reality of lifestyle

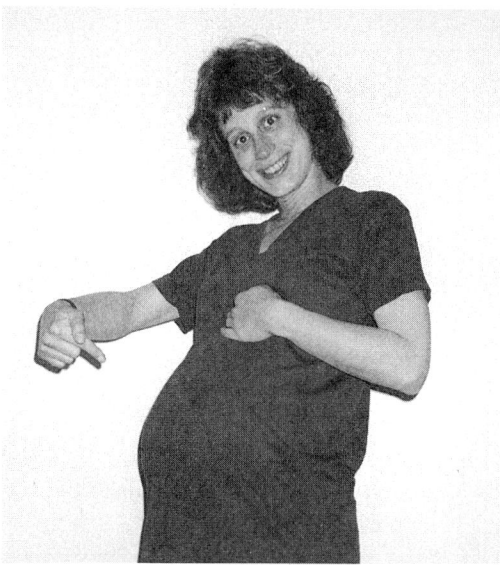

FIGURE 10-1
Pregnancy can be an exciting time for a woman as she develops her first relationship with the fetus.

changes, and are able to give safe and nurturing care.[33] The nurse may contribute to role transition through allowing time for discussion of feelings, assessing adaptive changes throughout the pregnancy, and supporting role transition.

Sexuality and Reproduction

Family planning and reproductive patterns directly affect the woman's concept of sexuality. The nurse needs to assess fertility and infertility history that precedes childbearing. In some situations, birth control measures used previously may affect the ability to conceive or the health of the fetus. The client who continues to take prescribed oral contraceptives, unaware that she has conceived, may deliver an infant with teratogenic defects from high estrogen levels. The woman who has used an intrauterine device (IUD) for several years may have difficulty conceiving because of repeated infections. In other situations, the treatment for infertility problems may lead to preterm birth of multiple babies with poor survival rates.

Lack of knowledge of family planning may result in pregnancy for the young adolescent who has experienced just one or two menstrual cycles, or closely spaced pregnancies for a woman unable to provide for several children. The nurse must be aware that a sexually active adolescent may know about birth control, but may avoid advance planning because she values spontaneity. Or the teen may feel that pregnancy is something that cannot happen to her! Discussion groups in school-based clinics are one answer to the needs of this group.

In addition to serving as a resource person on family planning, the nurse can share information on advances in fertility and ovulation test kits. These products are increasingly reliable, and add autonomy to the couple's decision to conceive or to delay parenting. If a couple is concerned about reproductive risks because of a woman's

age or the couple's history, the appropriate genetic screening referral should be made.

Unprotected sexual activity continues to be common among young people, despite a general awareness of acquired immunodeficiency syndrome (AIDS) as a major health problem. In fact, the growing incidence of AIDS and other sexually transmitted diseases among adolescents has greatly concerned public health officials. The behaviors that lead to increased potential for infection affect the safety of the young women, their sexual partners, and infants conceived during unprotected intercourse.[31]

Coping and Stress Tolerance

Emotions, coping behaviors, and stress tolerance influence health. The exact nature of this interaction is not known, but current research indicates that stress affects the immune process, blood pressure, and cardiac function. Specific effects of stress on a fetus are under investigation. Research findings suggest that moderate stress in labor promotes oxygen uptake and may be adaptive for the full-term fetus.[38] Other studies have linked severe maternal stress with fetal hypoxia and neonatal problems such as respiratory distress and hypothermia.

Everyone is subject to multiple stressors throughout life. As identity crises are resolved, young women form intimate relationships and undergo many role transitions. Life span theorists have explored the predictable and unexpected changes that occur in our current society. In addition to beginning a family, the young female may be combining education or career with caring for elderly family members. Poverty may affect her nutritional state, physical health, and emotional well-being. If the young girl is adolescent, the stress of a pregnancy and ensuing parental responsibility may interrupt school, social life, and plans for the future.

The relationship with the partner or spouse may be supportive or strained. Friendships may ease the transition to the parenting role or fade because of geographic separation or changing interests.

Although some degree of stress promotes adaptation and can lead to growth, the nurse needs to be aware of the childbearing woman's ability to tolerate stress. If her self-esteem diminishes as a result of maladaptive coping with multiple problems, the nurse should help the client and her family identify internal and external sources of stress. Strategies that strengthen the young woman's self-perception and self-concept can enable her to reach her fullest potential.[25]

Relaxation and exercise may be important factors in managing stress during daily life. Environmental modifications that may reduce anxiety in the home or workplace should be suggested. The nurse should identify risk-taking behaviors that may place the client or fetus in jeopardy (Fig. 10-2). Norris suggests that, although these actions are common among adolescents, adults of childbearing age may also use poor judgment because of knowledge deficit.[29] Cognitive approaches can be effective in altering dysfunctional problem-solving patterns, regardless of age.

The young woman may need help to resolve family crises that often accompany pregnancy. With assistance,

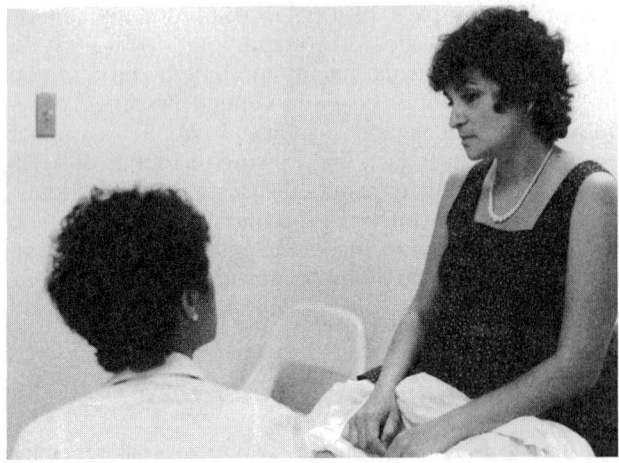

FIGURE 10-2
The nurse assesses and counsels the woman. Some women may find pregnancy stressful and may have trouble with their coping mechanisms. (Courtesy of the former Booth Maternity Center, Philadelphia.)

she may be able to evaluate existing support systems and to explore alternative resources such as teen or parent outreach groups.

If the young woman is at social risk due to poverty, divorce, or abuse, alcohol and drug use may become a problem. The nurse should assist the young woman to assess her situation, make informed choices, and change behaviors. With help, she can anticipate situations that make her life more difficult, and consult with mental health professionals as needed. Suicide prevention programs may become a critical part of the health promotion plan for some young women who are experiencing depressive episodes.[26]

Values and Beliefs

Culture, emotions, and coping patterns influence the choice of a life partner, the decision to become pregnant, and compliance with prenatal health practices during pregnancy. Priorities vary for persons, families, and groups; the approach to health teaching must match what the client perceives as significant. Because childbirth and childbearing experiences are subject to varied beliefs and rituals, the nurse functions more effectively by first exploring with the client unique aspects of the culture. Rather than labeling a woman as "noncompliant" for failing to keep clinic appointments during pregnancy, the nurse should investigate what value is placed on health promotion in her group.

Among the common beliefs across cultures is the view that birth and caring for a newborn are life crises, causing a period of vulnerability for the woman and her infant. However, social interactions and the immediate environment differ in importance among cultures.[15] In the last decade, anthropologists, sociologists, and nurses have added much to the body of knowledge of birth across cultures.

Western societies emphasize the medical aspects of childbirth. This biologic view causes much strain for the couple with traditional values and beliefs. Although token

changes have occurred in response to consumer demands for some control, the soft colors of a birthing room have not diminished the technological emphasis or medical management of birth. For example, consider the response that might occur as a recent Southeast Asian immigrant delivers in an urban American hospital. The lack of maternal control of birth, use of advanced technology, and care by unfamiliar attendants who do not speak her language lead to disharmony and a birth experience filled with fear. To remedy this situation, in an uncomplicated labor, continuous fetal monitoring might be replaced with intermittent auscultation with a fetoscope (following recent guidelines of the American College of Obstetrics and Gynecologists).[27] The presence of a birth attendant who speaks her language might ease the strangeness of the situation and promote a birth that is culturally "right."

Even among families from Western cultures, many different beliefs surround childbearing. The role of the lay midwife for home birth is well-accepted in some developed countries. Noninterference, or allowing nature to take its course in birth, is emphasized in some European countries. In the United States, labor induction, forceps deliveries, and a high cesarean section rate are often accepted as the medical norm. Second-generation American families and couples with cross-cultural marriages may experience conflicts, as traditional values and beliefs are frustrated in a hospital environment. The new emphasis on fetal rights has resulted in ethical dilemmas and parental stress. Adaptation patterns to these dilemmas vary among people from diverse cultures.

The initial contact with the newborn is a significant event for all new parents. Early in labor, the nurse should allow the client and family to verbalize their preferences for early breast-feeding, contact with the newborn, or a time for the woman to rest. The health care team should be aware of rituals or symbols that are important in the culture. Warm or cold beverages or perineal compresses, which may be desired after birth, should be permitted if at all possible. Spiritual beliefs should be respected.

Fong[8] urges health care workers to avoid stereotyping people or responding to clients based on their own culture. As a first step, she suggests that the nurse must be aware of personal values, beliefs, and cultural influences. Through open communication, the caregivers can improve the birth experience for families of diverse cultures; in the process, they can learn more about the factors that enrich biologic reproduction.

The nurse must assess each client, her family, and their culture in terms of what is ideal for their birth experience. Discussion of preferred support people, place for birth, appropriate position, warm or cold nourishment, pain relief measures, and privacy may contribute to a harmonious birth plan. Individualizing the birth experience may be simple because specific artifacts may have special meaning. Allowing the woman to use a favorite stool to support labor squatting may be as helpful as encouraging a Lamaze-trained couple to focus on a favorite wall hanging. Other environmental adaptations can often be made without breaking sterile technique or inconveniencing staff in uncomplicated labor and birth situations. The positive effect of meeting special needs may contribute to a culturally appropriate birth experience.

Anticipatory Guidance

Prenatal visits offer an opportunity for anticipatory guidance throughout the pregnancy. The concerns of the woman, her partner, and family are also addressed as the nurse functions as teacher and counselor.

Women must cope with many discomforts during pregnancy. As the pregnancy progresses and common minor problems arise, the nurse should help the woman identify measures that can prevent or alleviate the discomforts. The nurse has an excellent opportunity to relieve some of the stress these discomforts cause through anticipatory guidance. While conducting a thorough interview, the nurse assesses the woman's normal health and activity patterns, coping strategies, and support systems. Table 10-3 shows some of the common discomforts of pregnant women, the reason they occur, and some symptom-relieving steps the woman can take.

Traveling

For most women, traveling during pregnancy presents no harm to the fetus. When riding in an automobile, both shoulder and lap seat belts should be worn, with the lap belt placed low over the abdomen. For long trips, loose clothing, pillows for support, and frequent stops to walk and stretch help avoid discomforts.

If the woman travels to other countries, it is wise to carry a copy of her prenatal records with her. She should also take normal precautions to avoid diarrhea (drinking bottled water and avoiding unwashed foods and undercooked meats), eat regular meals, rest, empty her bladder frequently, and avoid carrying heavy luggage.[11]

Working

Most women can work throughout their pregnancies with no danger to the baby. It is important that the nurse encourage the woman in a sedentary job to stand up and move around during the day to aid circulation and lessen muscle strain. Frequent changes in position and chair height may also be helpful. Rest periods should be programmed into the work schedule, as should a regular lunch period. Heavy lifting should be avoided.

Some jobs may have special hazards, so the nurse and physician should be aware of the woman's employment to assess potential risks. Jobs that expose the woman to radiation, gases, pesticides, organic mercury, polychlorinated biphenyls (PCBs), high levels of noise, or second-hand smoke may need to be evaluated. Researchers are studying the effects of working at a computer terminal during pregnancy, although, to date, no harmful effects have been proven.[1] If the woman's job requires her to perform hazardous tasks or to work in an area where she is exposed to substances potentially toxic to the fetus, she should consult with her employer or union representative. The right to a safe and healthful workplace is guaranteed to all employees under the Occupational Safety and Health Act (OSHA). Many employers arrange for a woman to transfer to another job area during pregnancy.

Childbirth Preparation

Childbirth education is an important area of health promotion available through hospitals, schools, and community agencies. Recognizing that each parent brings a unique personal history and expectations to a pregnancy, the childbirth educator prepares the couple for the birth process. A major focus of prenatal teaching is physiologic and psychological adaptation to the growing embryo-fetus throughout pregnancy, labor, and birth. The woman and her support person are prepared to work as a team to promote relaxation and comfort (Fig. 10-3). Information on nutrition, rest, and exercise are shared in a group setting. An important goal of prenatal classes is to enhance the self-concept of women during a period of great change. Positive coping mechanisms are reinforced, and ways to deal with discomforts are suggested.

In the class setting, values may be explored, myths clarified, and consumers' rights identified. The nurse teaching prenatal classes has an opportunity to assist couples to formulate a birth plan that meets unique needs of a cultural group or of an individual woman. Referrals may be made to a nutritionist, social worker, physician, or other health care providers.

Types of classes vary with the philosophy of the educator, policy of the agency, and the needs of expectant parents. The Lamaze psychoprophylactic method uses conscious application of conditioning (stimulus–response), with cues or a focal point in the environment. As tension is reduced, relaxation occurs. Specific breathing patterns are practiced during pregnancy and used to increase comfort during labor. Although the couple may learn specific patterns of breathing, such as rapid chest breathing, there is a trend toward paced breathing. Visualization, the use of touch and voice, are increasingly emphasized in the Lamaze classes.

In some areas of the United States, application of the principles of Grantley Dick-Read may be used to interrupt the fear–tension–pain cycle.[5] The English physician felt that the "illness orientation" to birth resulted in needless anxiety and discomfort. The Gamper method, developed by the pioneer American nurse-educator, uses this approach.[5] The important focus in this method is natural, abdominal breathing, much like that observed in a puppy at rest. The couple are taught to work with the labor, focusing on uterine contractions within as productive for birth.

The Bradley approach suggests no specific exercises or breathing patterns.[5] Rather, the method is woman-centered, with responses of her body guided by knowledge of the birth process. The husband as coach is a critical element for success. The major goal is unmedicated "natural birth."[5]

The nurse referring a couple for classes should be aware of special courses available within the community and investigate the availability of classes for people with specific needs. There are programs in some areas for adolescent girls, high-risk women, siblings, and couples anticipating a cesarean birth or vaginal birth after a cesarean (VBAC). If a client has a disability, she should be referred to the course which best meets her needs.

TABLE 10-3
Nursing Interventions for Altered Function

Altered Function	Cause of Alteration	Suggestions to Client for Relief
Altered Health Perception and Health Maintenance		
Varicose veins	Pressure from both increased blood volume and enlarging uterus, which slows venous return Prolonged standing Family predisposition	Take frequent breaks to stand and walk if job is sedentary. Prop up legs as often as possible. Avoid tight knee socks or garters. Wear support stockings. Do not cross legs. Elevate legs at a 90-degree angle to the body twice a day.
Altered Nutrition and Metabolism		
Nausea and vomiting, ''morning sickness'' (particularly during 4th through 12th weeks)	Slowing of the gastrointestinal (GI) system due to hormonal influence	Eat dry carbohydrate foods, particularly before getting up in the morning. Consume smaller more frequent meals and snacks. Avoid spicy or greasy foods. Stay well-hydrated. Avoid over-the-counter antiemetics.
Heartburn	Gastric reflex due to relaxation of smooth muscles of GI tract and cardiac sphincter (influenced by progesterone) Decrease in gastric hydrochloric acid due to estrogen Pressure of enlarging uterus	Eat small frequent meals. Avoid spicy or greasy foods. Sit upright after eating. Drink milk. Wear loose clothing around the waist. Avoid antacids with sodium or aspirin.
Altered Elimination		
Frequent urination	Compression of bladder due to enlarging uterus usually experienced in first and third trimester, with no signs of infection	Void frequently to avoid distention. Continue to drink adequate fluids during the day. Possibly decrease fluid intake at night. Limit caffeine intake. Do Kegel exercises.
Constipation	Decreased peristalsis due to progesterone Increased extraction of water from stools Uterine pressure	Increase fluid intake. Eat fruits, raw vegetables, whole grain cereals and bread. Take pitted prunes as snacks. Chew thoroughly. Drink adequate amounts of fluids. Exercise. Avoid harsh laxatives and mineral oil.
Hemorrhoids	Constipation Pressure of uterus Straining during bowel movements	Avoid constipation (see above). Avoid straining during bowel movements. Take warm tub baths. Practice good perineal hygiene. Apply cool witch hazel compresses (such as Tucks). Perform Kegel exercises. Avoid over-the-counter preparations unless approved by birth attendant.

(Continued)

TABLE 10-3
(Continued)

Altered Function	Cause of Alteration	Suggestions to Client for Relief
Altered Activity and Exercise		
Backache	Weight of growing uterus	Wear low-heeled shoes.
	Lax muscles due to hormonal influence	Avoid heavy lifting.
	Fatigue	Bend from the knees when lifting.
	Muscle tension	Refrain from overexertion.
		Perform exercises (such as pelvic tilt).
		Use heating pad or massage.
Leg cramps	Muscle strain	Exercise.
	Uterine pressure on nerves	Elevate legs.
	Calcium–phosphorus imbalance	Keep legs warm.
		Flex the toes.
		Do not point the toes when stretching.
		Increase milk consumption to 1 qt a day.
		With birth attendant's approval, take aluminum hydroxide gel to decrease phosphorus uptake from milk consumption.
		When the cramp occurs, force toes upward and put pressure on knee to straighten leg.
Swollen ankles	Decreased venous return due to uterine pressure	Elevate legs.
	Increased salt and water retention due to hormones	Rest during the day.
		Avoid salty snacks.
Difficulty breathing	Enlarging uterus compromises lung expansion and compresses vena cava	Rest with upper body and head elevated on pillows.
		Keep on left side.
		Avoid overexertion.
Dizziness	Changes in circulatory pattern and blood volume	Rise slowly.
	Nausea and vomiting	Lie on left side when dizziness occurs.
	Decreased blood pressure (second trimester)	
Altered Sleep and Rest		
Fatigue (particularly during first and third trimesters)	May be due to changes in hormonal level (particularly progesterone and relaxin)	Get adequate sleep (8 h/night).
	Increase in basal metabolic rate	Take frequent naps or rest periods.
	Increase in cardiac output in last trimester	Exercise regularly.
	Anemia	Get assistance with care of home or other children.
	Psychologic causes	Avoid overexertion.
Altered Self Concept		
Stretch marks	Enlarging uterus	Apply lanolin-based cream, cocoa butter, baby oil.
Altered Coping Tolerance		
Food cravings	Increased caloric needs	Eat a well-balanced diet.
	Stress	Use vitamin supplements as prescribed.
	Pica	Avoid nonfood substances.
		If craving is harmless and not excessive, allow it.[28,34]
Altered Sexuality		
Vaginal secretions	Increased blood and glucose supply to the area	Keep perineal area clean and dry.
	Increased cervical secretions in absence of infection	Wear cotton underwear, loose underclothes.
		If secretions become odorous or if itching is severe, consult physician to rule out a yeast infection.

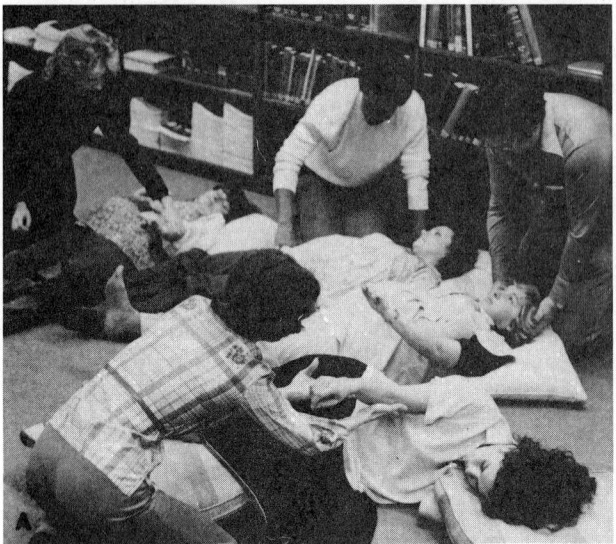

FIGURE 10-3
Couples practice muscle relaxation for labor during childbirth classes.

The labor room nurse should evaluate the couple's ability to apply breathing techniques and exercises learned during prenatal classes. The couple should be assisted in a spirit of cooperation as they adapt the environment to promote comfort and apply previously learned relaxation responses. If the nurse is unfamiliar with the program completed by the couple, they should be asked to describe the approach briefly, and tell the nurse their expectations for support.

If a couple has not attended classes, simple breathing techniques can be taught during labor. As the cervix dilates and thins and the fetus descends, an ongoing explanation of progress should be given. The presence of a consistent caregiver can promote relaxation, which may

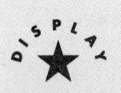

Expected Behaviors Reflecting a Pregnant Woman's Ability to Take on a Parenting Role

Achieves some independence from own parents
Develops a sense of identity
Establishes an intimate relationship
Seeks early prenatal care
Balances a healthy diet and exercise
Changes behaviors that could place fetus at risk
Avoids environmental hazards that affect health
Identifies fetus as a separate being
Bonds with fetus
Attends childbirth preparation classes
Learns about infant development
Prepares for the parenting role
Conveys empathy

Adapted from Young, M. (1988). Parenting during mid-adolescence: A review of developmental theories and parenting behaviors. Maternal-Child Nursing Journal, 17(1), 1–12.

improve fetal oxygenation. Thus, the ultimate benefit of prenatal classes may be to the infant, although research in this area is limited. Perhaps the psychological well-being of parents who are able to work together to relax throughout labor contributes to initial attachment with the infant. In any case, satisfied parents frequently share their positive feelings about childbirth education programs and often repeat classes during a subsequent pregnancy. The display suggests behavior patterns that may be evident during prenatal visits or childbirth classes.

Factors Affecting Pregnancy Outcomes

Reproduction is affected by many factors. Some of them are discussed here. The display on Nursing Assessment on the next page suggests questions the nurse might ask the pregnant client to establish how various factors are affecting the pregnancy. From the responses, problems or risk are identified and interventions can be planned.

Poverty

Poor women and minorities experience disproportionately high infant morbidity and mortality. Because many poor women are unable to afford an adequate diet and often have little or no prenatal care, they are at risk for delivering a low-birthweight baby. Many of these babies suffer severe complications, which result in lifelong disabilities. Many poor pregnant clients are young and single, and they face additional emotional stress and isolation. Many of these young women drop out of school and raise their children in poverty.

Nurses must reach out to these women both in the schools and the community. They have the opportunity to help these mothers identify available prenatal care facilities and support programs.

Age and Parity

Women who become pregnant when they are 17 years of age or younger face risks to both themselves and their babies. Complications for the mother may occur during gestation or at birth, whereas effects on the baby may be lifelong.

Many adolescents are anemic due to growth demands and food fads common in that age group. Pregnancy places an additional strain on the body of the poorly nourished adolescent, predisposing her to fatigue and infection. The young primipara is more likely to develop pregnancy-induced hypertension (preeclampsia). This condition may prove life-threatening to both mother and baby.

Labor may present further danger to the young adolescent mother. The physical development of the pelvis is not completed until the latter part of adolescence. The small pelvis may be too narrow to accommodate the fetal head as it passes into the birth canal, thus increasing the

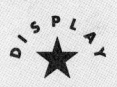

Nursing Assessment: Questions for Assessing Health Behaviors in Pregnant Women

What does a healthy pregnancy mean to you?

Have you any experience caring for young children?

Describe a typical 24-h eating pattern.

What is your usual exercise program?

How do you deal with stress?

Are you aware of problems in the environment at home or work that could affect your unborn baby?

What do women of your culture value in the child-birth experience?

What lifestyle changes could you make that would improve the health of your fetus?

What do you need to learn about childbirth?

How can the nurse and physician help you adapt to changes during pregnancy?

Do you have any medical problems that require supervision?

Describe your plans for health care for the baby.

chance that the young mother will have to have a cesarean delivery.

The baby of the young mother has a greater chance of being born prematurely and small for age. These low-birthweight babies have an increased incidence of hypothermia, hypoglycemia, birth anomalies, and developmental disabilities.[19,20]

The nurse who works with pregnant adolescents has an excellent opportunity to assess nutrition and lifestyle patterns. The Teaching Plan for Adolescent Nutritional Care During Pregnancy is an example of the nurse's promotion of a healthy outcome. The young woman should be given an opportunity to discuss emotional and financial support systems. Opportunities available to help the young mother continue her education should be explored. Finally, the nurse should strongly encourage the mother to schedule and keep regular prenatal appointments.

Women who become pregnant after age 35 have an increased risk of an ectopic pregnancy, a risk that becomes even higher if there is a history of IUD use. They are also more likely to have pregnancy-induced hypertension than women in their twenties. The older mother who is a multipara has an increased chance of developing placenta previa.

Women over age 35 have a greater chance of bearing a child with a congenital defect. Chromosomal aberrations such as Down's syndrome are more common in the older childbearing years. Current research is re-examining the risk of "elderly primiparas," but statistics still support a high risk.

The nurse has an excellent opportunity to provide counsel and support to the older pregnant patient. Many of these women have delayed childbearing to pursue careers. They tend to be financially secure and well-educated as a group. Nevertheless, they have many concerns about the baby and their ability to handle the many changes that will occur in their lives. For those women

who undergo prenatal screening, the nurse has the chance to provide both information and support.[28]

Acute Health Problems

Acute health alterations during a pregnancy may affect the life or well-being of the woman and the fetus or newborn. Examples of nursing diagnoses for some of these problems include: High Risk for Injury related to altered gas exchange across the placenta caused by hemorrhage or pregnancy-induced hypertension, and High Risk for Infection related to premature ruptured membranes. These complications account for the highest incidence of deaths related to pregnancy.[3] Health promotion, prevention, and detection of problems can make a significant difference in maternal well-being and fetal/newborn outcome. The woman is encouraged to report promptly all problems and symptoms to the physician for further evaluation. Among these reportable signs that can affect maternal–fetal well-being are bleeding, leaking fluid, edema, infection, and trauma.

Hemorrhage

Hemorrhagic conditions that occur in the third trimester, or final 3 months of a pregnancy, are often life-threatening. Although the fetus may be viable after about the 22nd week, its survival often depends on the early detection and treatment of maternal blood loss.

The condition of placenta previa, malposition of the placenta with partial or complete blockage of the cervix, is manifested by painless bleeding in the last 12 weeks of pregnancy. (Earlier bleeding may indicate a miscarriage or abortion.) The immediate care of the woman includes absolute bedrest with ongoing assessment for blood loss and signs of labor. If the uterus contracts and the cervix dilates, delivery of the placenta may precede birth of the infant. Oxygen and nutrient delivery across the placenta ceases to provide for the fetal needs; survival of the newborn depends on an immediate cesarean delivery. Even with emergency delivery, the newborn may remain at risk due to prematurity and the effects of fluid volume deficit.

A second serious condition due to hemorrhage late in pregnancy is abruptio placentae. Women who have a hypertensive history are among those at risk for this complication. Symptoms include bleeding with abdominal pain or tenderness as the placenta prematurely separates from the uterine wall. For some women, the bleeding is concealed within the uterus, although signs of shock are evident. To prevent fetal death, blood is replaced rapidly, oxygen is administered to the mother, and an immediate cesarean birth is performed. The woman is at great risk for subsequent disseminated intravascular coagulation (DIC), a condition in which uncontrolled hemorrhage and multiple thrombi may occur. The newborn may not survive the fetal injury, may be premature with complications from hypoxia, or may experience problems related to fluid volume deficit. Both mother and newborn require intensive care in the immediate post-birth period.

The nurse assisting in the clinic, emergency room, or labor and delivery setting plays a critical role in pre-

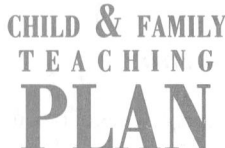

CHILD & FAMILY
T E A C H I N G
PLAN

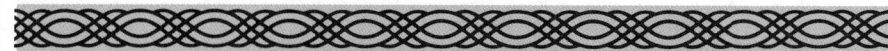

Adolescent Nutritional Care During Pregnancy

Assessment

Kim Johnson, 17, comes to the clinic with the following history: Last menstrual period was 7 months ago. She appears pale and tired. She states she eats one main meal daily, the school lunch, but does not like the milk or fruit. She says her family is poor; there is never enough to eat toward the end of the month. She reports that she smokes and uses marijuana occasionally, but denies alcohol or other drug use.

Her only complaint is occasional difficulty breathing while sleeping on her back, and a sudden gain in weight in the last 2 weeks. "All of a sudden I can't get my rings on my fingers!" She is still attending school, but otherwise leads an inactive life, watching TV until midnight. "If I'm upset, I just go to bed and skip school."

Kim states she's happy to be pregnant; "I'll do things different than how I was raised! I'll hold the baby all the time and tell him how good he is!" Family consists of Kim, her mother who works nights, and an older brother who is presently unemployed. Her boyfriend is in the Army and doesn't know she is pregnant. "I haven't told anyone; I really don't have many friends."

There were no significant problems at her last school physical 1 year ago. Her weight at that visit was 85 lb. Today she weighs 95 lb for a height of 5'6". The estimated weeks of gestation by dates is 24 weeks. Her hands and ankles are swollen. Fundal height is approximately 20 weeks, and fetus seems small for dates. Fetal heart rate is 146.

Child and Family Objectives	*Specific Content*	*Teaching Strategies*
1. Identify nutritional patterns.	1. A 48-h diet recall. Have her return the completed form in 24 h.	1. Explain 48-h diet recall exercise. Explore the diet recall with the client pointing out which foods/meals supply the necessary nutrients and which do not.
2. Identify the basic food groups.	2. Basic food groups and the number of servings she should consume from each group:	2. Use audiovisual aids to identify the basic food groups (charts, simulated food servings).
	Milk, Yogurt, and Cheese The pregnant woman should consume four servings of this group each day (four or more for the breast-feeding mother). In addition to milk, requirements can be met by eating yogurt, ice cream, cottage cheese, cheese, and soybean milk.	Various sample diets. Nutrient analysis sheets for common/favorite foods. Encourage Kim to join a group diet class. Provide simulated food servings.
	Meat, Poultry, Fish, Dry Beans, Eggs, and Nuts Both the pregnant and breast-feeding woman should consume two to three servings of meat, fish or fowl, or other protein sources.	Provide simulated food servings.
	Fruits and Vegetables Three to five servings of vegetables and two to four servings of fruit a day are necessary to fulfill the	Provide simulated food servings. Review likes and dislikes and identify sources acceptable to her.

(Continued)

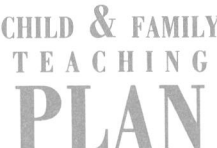

CHILD & FAMILY
T E A C H I N G
PLAN

Adolescent Nutritional Care During Pregnancy (continued)

Child and Family Objectives	*Specific Content*	*Teaching Strategies*
	requirement for both the pregnant and breast-feeding woman. These servings should include both vitamin C-rich fruits and vegetables such as tomatoes, green peppers, orange, grapefruit, and leafy green vegetables or yellow vegetables, which supply vitamins A and B.	
	Bread, Cereal, Rice, and Pasta Both pregnant and breast-feeding mothers need six to eleven servings a day. Potatoes, noodles, rice, cereals, crackers, tortillas meet this requirement.	Provide simulated food servings.
	Fats, Oils, and Sweets Limit fats and sweets; avoid alcohol.	
	Water—Several glasses of water a day are required.	
3. Identify specific nutrients whose requirements increase during pregnancy.	3. **Iron** An increase of 30 to 60 mg a day is recommended. Because teenagers are often deficient in this vitamin, diet and supplementary sources need to be explored.	3. Review nutritional needs during adolescence using audiovisual aids, group discussion.
	Folic Acid Pregnancy doubles the need for this vitamin. Because cooking destroys its potency, a vitamin supplement is usually ordered.	
	Vitamin D Teenagers who do not drink milk need to be introduced to alternative sources.	Review teen's likes and dislikes and identify sources acceptable to her.
	Vitamin C Sources need to be emphasized if the teen smokes.	Review those vitamins that are depleted by smoking.
	Prenatal vitamins are prescribed.	
4. Identify dietary modifications that alleviate some of the discomforts of pregnancy.	4. *Morning sickness* may be alleviated by eating a dry cracker before getting up in the morning, taking smaller more frequent meals, avoiding greasy or spicy foods, and drinking water.	4. Supply information sheet listing interventions for discomforts of pregnancy.
	Heartburn is decreased by sitting upright after eating, drinking milk, eating smaller meals, and eating nongreasy or nonspicy foods.	

(Continued)

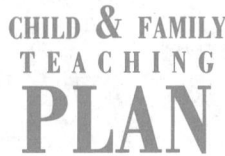

CHILD & FAMILY
T E A C H I N G
PLAN

Adolescent Nutritional Care During Pregnancy (continued)

Child and Family Objectives	*Specific Content*	*Teaching Strategies*
	Constipation is relieved and normal bowel movements are achieved by increasing fluid intake; eating fruits, raw vegetables, and whole grain foods; chewing thoroughly; and, if necessary, eating pitted prunes.	
	Hemorrhoids may be alleviated by avoiding constipation, refraining from straining during defecation, and taking a warm bath daily.	
	Leg cramps often are alleviated by increasing milk consumption.	
5. Identify ways to meet nutritional needs on a limited budget.	5. WIC Program, school lunch, generic foods, bulk foods, less expensive meats, fish, vegetables.	5. Use sample labels to help client identify nutrient values in brand and generic food. Teach client about newspaper ads, coupons, ways to store bulk foods, and WIC referral forms.
6. Identify exercise as a way to stabilize nutritional needs.	6. Exercise aids digestion and prevents constipation. It may also increase the appetite.	6. Provide films, poster, pamphlets, return demonstration.

Evaluation

- Kim identifies her nutritional patterns.
- Kim demonstrates improved diet on second 48-h diet recall.
- Kim describes food groups and her preferred choices of each.
- Kim describes her changing habits to acquire needed nutrients.
- Kim states she has not smoked cigarettes or marijuana since her last appointment.
- Kim expresses less discomfort from pregnancy.
- Kim identifies resources she has used since last appointment.
- Kim states she is exercising daily.

serving the optimal health of mother and fetus when hemorrhage is experienced. Careful, frequent assessment of the woman provides information as to the blood volume lost and the physiologic response to shock. The health care team is alerted to expect a possible cesarean delivery. Before birth of the fetus, adequate fluid and blood replacement must be maintained. Oxygen is frequently administered to benefit both mother and fetus. The presence of a calm nurse, supporting the woman and her family, is critical to reduce anxiety and fear.

Fetal responses to the blood volume loss are observed closely through electronic fetal monitoring. Changes in the heart rate pattern or baseline may be the initial warn-

ing that the fetus is at great risk because of reduced placental gas exchange. The pediatrician, anesthesiologist, and respiratory therapist are alerted to attend the delivery of a premature newborn.

Hypertension

Hypertensive disorders during pregnancy may lead to acute problems for the fetus and mother. Preexisting hypertension may be related to cardiovascular or kidney disease. Rising blood pressure levels diminish placental blood flow and decrease gas exchange for the developing fetus. This may result in chronic hypoxia and growth retardation or an acute problem of fetal distress. The condition identified as pregnancy-induced hypertension (also called PIH or preeclampsia) often affects adolescents or women over 35 during a first pregnancy. Although the exact cause is unknown, there appears to be a strong relationship among inadequate prenatal care, nutritional deficits, and the development of hypertension during late pregnancy.

The nurse plays a key role in prevention, early detection, and treatment. Encouraging regular antepartal care for all pregnant women is a first step in prevention of this and other problems. The routine assessments of weight, urine, and blood pressure take on major importance as changes in these parameters are early warnings of pregnancy-induced hypertension. The woman may report the first changes: her ring no longer fits and shoes are not comfortable because of swollen feet. On assessing the client, significant changes in the baseline readings of vital signs and a rising diastolic pressure are apparent. The presence of protein in the urine indicates that vasoconstriction has altered kidney function.

The goal of care is to maintain a stable blood pressure. The woman is encouraged to rest in a left lateral position as much as possible. Health status is closely monitored. If the diet is inadequate, increased protein may be suggested. Should the client's blood pressure continue to rise, she may be advised to reduce salt. Many women respond to conservative home treatment. Family support is critical, especially if care responsibilities include other small children.

Fetal growth is closely monitored because vasoconstriction and vasospasm affect placental gas exchange. The pregnancy is usually allowed to continue until the fetal lungs are mature, as indicated on amniotic fluid analysis, (i.e., lecithin-sphingomyelin [L/S] ratio). If the woman's condition remains stable, medication may not be necessary. If her condition worsens, magnesium sulfate is often prescribed to prevent eclamptic seizures. The use of magnesium sulfate requires continuous nursing surveillance because the medication acts as a central nervous system depressant and may decrease respiratory rate. This change directly reduces fetal oxygenation.

When the physician feels that the woman is stable and fetal lungs are mature, labor may be induced with pitocin stimulation. In some cases, a premature delivery is necessary to prevent further risk of maternal or fetal injury. A vaginal delivery is preferred to cesarean birth because the stress of surgery may cause further vascular problems for the woman. Although the newborn may experience no obvious problems as a result of pregnancy-induced hypertension, health care team members must evaluate the baby carefully for effects of diminished placental blood flow.[35]

Infection

Infection during pregnancy can affect the fetal outcome. Early in development, the embryo may be aborted as a result of infections such as syphilis or rubella. Serious organ formation defects may occur as a result of maternal infections, such as cytomegalovirus (CMV) or toxoplasmosis. Sexually transmitted diseases may affect fetal well-being in utero or during the birth process, as with herpes

II. Hepatitis and the AIDS virus cross the placenta and cause serious problems for the fetus, resulting in high infant mortality. Prevention of infection is the primary focus of health teaching. Screening of couples at risk for AIDS may identify women who should not conceive. The nurse should be aware of exposure to any infection during pregnancy and should urge the woman to alter risk behaviors and comply with prescribed therapy.

In advanced pregnancy, the most frequent cause of fetal injury is related to preterm labor and premature rupture of the protective membranes. The optimal environment for the fetus is disturbed when a tear in the fragile amnion and chorion allows some of the 1000 ml of clear amniotic fluid to escape. Although the exact cause of premature ruptured membranes is often unknown, the event puts both mother and fetus at great risk for infection.

If the fetus has neared maturity when the membranes rupture, treatment consists of careful assessment of maternal temperature and fetal heart rate, and analysis of objective data including culture and sensitivity. The birth may be induced within 12 to 24 hours to prevent possible serious effects of infection.

Should the membranes rupture some time before fetal lungs have matured, the woman is maintained on bedrest and is monitored closely. Aseptic technique is enforced; antibiotics may be administered. Fetal heart rate changes are reported immediately. The nurse must be alert to signs of developing maternal infection or beginning premature labor. If premature birth occurs, the newborn may be at risk because of immature lungs and may experience physical injury related to exposure to organisms. Usually the infant is considered septic until cultures are negative. Antibiotics are often prescribed for mother and newborn, with isolation of mother and newborn a part of the treatment. This separation seriously delays initial attachment and bonding, considered important in transition to the parenting role.

Chronic Health Problems

Chronic health problems may complicate the pregnancy and place the mother and the fetus or newborn at risk. These problems include some preexisting conditions that may be well-regulated before conception but which may worsen during pregnancy. The medications prescribed as treatment may have severe teratogenic effects. For example, the young woman may be a well-controlled epileptic who continues to take anticonvulsant medications without informing the obstetrician of her problem. An insulin-dependent diabetic who has experienced few serious problems since diagnosis in late childhood may find that she has frequent episodes of hypoglycemia or recurring vaginal infection. The young woman with a chronic cardiac condition may have adapted well and may continue to follow prescribed diet, exercise, and medication regimen. However, the increased circulatory blood volume of pregnancy that provides for fetal-placental needs may lead to further congestive heart damage.

One population of women with special needs is disabled pregnant women. Little research on their health needs during childbearing appears in the literature. Kopala reports some negative perceptions of mobility-impaired women toward the assistance given by health care professionals. Advice some of these women would share with nurses includes: learn more about disabilities; work with the woman and her knowledge of own limitations; and ask how the environment might be modified during labor and birth.[17] Nurses are challenged to learn from these women about their unique adaptive health patterns that evolved as they coped.

When working with clients with chronic health problems, health promotion becomes a challenge for the nurse, client, and family. Therapy is often changed, and more frequent visits to the physician are required. Previously effective coping patterns may no longer relieve stress. The woman needs to be aware of reportable signs that her condition is worsening or medication is ineffective. Teaching should be reinforced at every visit. Fetal development must be monitored closely; frequent tests of fetal well-being may be necessary.

Summary

The maternity and child health nurse must recognize that many factors influence fetal and newborn health. It is critical to be aware of the couple's preconceptual health patterns. Because the health status of a woman before and during pregnancy directly affects fetal-placental well-being, the nurse working with a pregnant client and her family must be skilled in assessment, differentiating between normal changes and potential problems. When a problem is identified, the situation is analyzed and appropriate intervention or teaching is carried out early to minimize the risks and promote a healthy outcome.

Caring for women during the childbearing cycle requires much of a nurse. Maternity nursing practice demands a sound knowledge base of physiologic and psychological changes that affect the woman's health and fetal development. The client needs to be directed to early and comprehensive prenatal care, so that she anticipates common problems and reports unusual incidents. Nutrition assessment and education must be integrated in each clinic visit to promote optimal fetal growth. The woman must be informed of environmental hazards that could damage the unborn child. The couple should be referred for prenatal classes so that the birth is anticipated with an understanding of the process and with minimal fear. The nurse must be aware of stress management patterns and must promote positive coping styles in the woman and her family.

Healthy behaviors never eliminate all potential problems for the pregnant woman and her child. However, the efforts pay off in reduced fetal and infant mortality and a better outcome for surviving children.

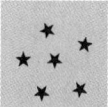

Ideas for Nursing Research

Implications for research into ensuring optimal fetal outcome by promoting health before conception and during pregnancy are many. Maternity and child health nurses have many opportunities to assess strengths and limitations, identify potential and actual problems, and plan interventions that foster health promotion and maintenance before birth. The following areas need to be explored:

- Factors that motivate young school-age and adolescent girls to develop positive health patterns before conception.
- Relationship between awareness of health practices and adoption of positive health behavior by nonpregnant women.
- Nursing interventions effective in promoting positive health patterns for young women before conception.
- Factors contributing to optimal health during pregnancy.
- Variables that influence early and consistent prenatal care.
- Relationship between support systems and positive health patterns.
- Impact of childbirth education on fetal well-being.
- Nursing measures that promote a positive birth experience for families from culturally diverse populations.
- Fetal level of tolerance to various environmental hazards.
- Autonomy of the mother in health decision making.

References

1. Blackwell, R., & Chang, A. (1988, May). Video display terminals and pregnancy. A review. *British Journal of Obstetrics and Gynecology, 95,* 446–453.
2. Committee on Obstetrics: Maternal and Fetal Medicine. (1987, July). *Maternal and fetal medicine: Vitamin A supplementation during pregnancy.* American College of Obstetricians and Gynecologists Committee Opinion. No. 52.
3. Cunningham, F., MacDonald, P., & Gant, N. (1989). *Williams Obstetrics* (18th ed.). Norwalk, CT: Appleton-Century-Crofts.
4. Davis, B., Holtz, N., & Davis, J. (1985). *Conceptual human physiology.* Columbus: Merrill.
5. Edwards, M., & Waldorf, M. (1984). *Reclaiming birth: History and heroines of American childbirth reform.* Trumansburg, NY: Crossing Press.
6. Finn, S. C. (1988, February). A, B₆, C, E. . .Unscrambling the vitamin alphabet. *American Baby, 1,* 70–83.
7. Fogel, C., & Woods, N. F. (1981). *Health care of women: A nursing perspective.* St. Louis: Mosby.
8. Fong, C. (1985). Ethnicity in nursing practice. *Topics in Clinical Nursing 7*(3): 1–10.
9. Gause, R. W. (1988, July). Exercise during pregnancy. *American Baby, 1,* 56–78.
10. Hess, M. A., & Hunt, A. E. (1982). *Pickles and ice cream: The complete guide to nutrition during pregnancy.* New York: McGraw-Hill.
11. Hillard, P. A. (1985). Traveling while you're pregnant. *Parents, 60*(12): 157–158.
12. Hillard, P. A. (1987). Environmental hazards. *Parents, 62*(2): 140–143.
13. Hillard, P. A. (1987). Screening for neural tube defects. *Parents, 62*(9): 194–197.
14. Hillard, P. A. (1988). Recreational drugs: Cocaine. *Parents 63*(1): 134–136.
15. Jordan, B. (1978). *Birth in four cultures.* St. Albans Vt: Eden Press.

16. Kaslman, R. (1988, January 27). Exercise during pregnancy: Good for mom and baby. *Loyola University Medical Center News Release.*

17. Kopala, B. (1989). Mothers with impaired mobility speak out. *MCN: American Journal of Maternal Child Nursing, 14*(3), 115–119.

18. March of Dimes Birth Defects Foundation. (1980, September). *Science Information. Caffeine and Birth Defects.*

19. March of Dimes Birth Defects Foundation. (1984). *Facts you should know about teen-age pregnancy.*

20. March of Dimes Birth Defects Foundation. (1986, October). *Public Health Information Sheet: Low Birth Weight.* 09-285-00.

21. March of Dimes Birth Defects Foundation. (1988). *Background paper on drinking alcohol during pregnancy.*

22. March of Dimes Birth Defects Foundation. (1988). *Background paper on drug use during pregnancy.*

23. March of Dimes Birth Defects Foundation. (1988). *Background paper on smoking during pregnancy.*

24. March of Dimes Birth Defects Foundation & National Commission to Prevent Infant Mortality. (1988). *NAACOG Newsletter 15*(7), 1.

25. Mercer, R., May, K., & DeJoseph, J. (1986). Theoretical models for studying the effects of antepartum stress on the family. *Nursing Research, 35*(6), 339–345.

26. Moleti, C. (1988). Caring for socially high-risk pregnant women. *MCN: American Journal of Maternal Child Nursing, 13*(1), 24–27.

27. NAACOG. (1988). *Nursing responsibilities in implementing fetal heart rate monitoring.* NAACOG Statement.

28. May, K. A., & Mahlmeister, L. R. (1990). *Comprehensive maternity nursing: Nursing process and the childbearing family* (2nd ed.). Philadelphia: J. B. Lippincott.

29. Norris, A. (1988). Cognitive analysis of contraceptive behavior. *Image 2d*(3), 135–139.

30. Office of Research Reporting, National Institute of Child Health and Human Development. (1977). *Little babies, born too soon, born too small.* Bethesda, MD: DHEW, Publication No. (NIH) 77-1079.

31. Reeder, S. J., Martin, L. L., & Koniak, D. (1992). *Maternity nursing: Family, newborn, and women's health care* (17th ed.). Philadelphia: Lippincott.

32. Robertson, C. (1987). When your pregnant patient has diabetes. *RN 50*(7): 33–35.

33. Rubin, R. (1975). Maternal tasks in pregnancy. *MCN: American Journal of Maternal Child Nursing, 4*(3): 143–153.

34. Schulman, H. (1982). Growing pains: Common discomforts of pregnancy. *Childbirth Educator,* Spring, 1: 11–12.

35. Shannon, D. (1986). HELPP syndrome: A severe consequence of pregnancy-induced hypertension. *Journal of Obstetric, Gynecologic, and Neonatal Nursing 16*(6): 395–402.

36. Shepard, T. H. (1986). *Catalog of teratogenic agents* (p. 600). Baltimore: Johns Hopkins University Press.

37. Shephard, J. (1987). Today's prenatal testing. *McCalls 114*(88).

38. Simkin, P. (1986). Stress, pain and catecholamines in labor: Part 1: A review. *Birth 13*(4): 227–232.

39. Udall, J. (1983). Dietary adjustments that benefit mother and fetus. *Consultant,* July, 170–181.

40. Whelan, E. M. (1979). Pregnancy basics. Washington, DC: Office of Research Reportings, National Institute of Child Health and Human Development.

41. World Health Organization. (1975). *Smoking and its effects on health: A report of a WHO expert committee.* World Health Organization Technical Report Series No. 568. Geneva, Switzerland (cited in Hess & Hunt [1982]).

11

C H A P T E R

Health Assessment, Promotion, and Maintenance for the Neonate

BEHAVIORAL OBJECTIVES

Identify interventions that facilitate the neonate's transition from an intrauterine to an extrauterine life.

Identify normal physical characteristics and behavior of the neonate.

Describe characteristics of neonate, mother, and nurse that promote attachment or bonding.

Identify infant care skills needed by the mother and father.

Identify nursing actions that facilitate maternal–neonatal bonding.

Describe psychosocial factors that influence the mother's and family's adjustment to a new baby.

Describe the nursing role in the hospital and home.

Describe societal attitudes that promote the health and well-being of the young family.

irth through the first 29 days of life is generally referred to as the neonatal period. Birth is a normal maturational event for which the fetus is well prepared, but it is an event that requires rapid adaptations in life processes. These adaptations are dramatic and herald new life. Profound physical changes are also experienced by the mother, and the new role of parenthood assumed by a couple is sudden and stressful. Essential nursing roles during this period are to promote the adaptation and maturation of the neonate, to foster attachment between the newborn and mother, to assist the mother in achieving physical and emotional adjustment, and to aid the parents in adjusting to their new roles and developing confidence in their ability to care for the newborn.

Assessments of the Neonate

Extrauterine adaptations in the first 24 hours critically affect the newborn's survival. Systematic assessments of the newborn are made to facilitate prompt interventions for problems.

Immediate Assessment

The focus of nursing care at birth and immediately after is to observe the neonate's condition and to make early identification of actual problems or newborns at risk (Fig. 11-1).

Neonates with a history of maternal or delivery risk factors are kept under special observation. The systems most altered as the fetus moves from an intrauterine to extrauterine life are the respiratory and cardiovascular systems. Because these systems provide essential oxygen for the baby, observations that signal their successful adaptation are essential. Five observations are made at 1- and 5-minute intervals about the neonate's color, heart rate, reflex responses, muscle tone, and respiratory effort. This is referred to as the Apgar score (Table 11-1). During the following hours, the neonate is assessed for subnormal or elevated temperature and for the ability to ingest food and eliminate wastes.

Respirations. At birth, air must replace the fluid that fills the respiratory tract. The newborn's nose and mouth are suctioned even before birth, and after the cord is clamped and cut, the neonate begins to breathe and cry. Normally only a few breaths are required to expand the lungs well. After breathing is established, respirations are shallow and irregular, ranging from 30 to 60 breaths/min, with short periods of apnea (less than 15 seconds). Apneic breathing (periodic breathing) is characteristic of the newborn. It occurs most often during the active sleep cycle (rapid eye movement, REM) and decreases in frequency and duration with age.

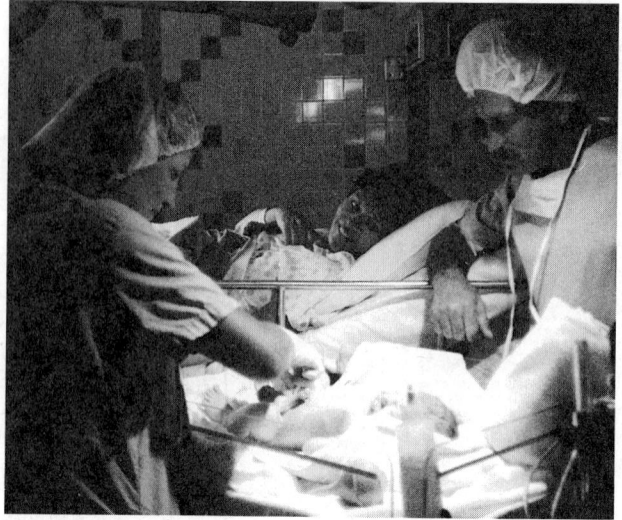

FIGURE 11-1
While the nurse makes immediate assessments, she also helps the parents in their bonding. The father is encouraged to stand nearby and watch as the nurse makes her assessment. The examining table should be placed near the mother so she can also watch the assessment. (Courtesy of the former Booth Maternity Center, Philadelphia.)

Circulation. With the neonate's first breath and inflation of the lungs, there is a reduction in pulmonary blood flow and pressure. As pressure in the right atrium decreases, the increased pulmonary blood flow to the left side of the heart increases the pressure in the left atrium. These pressure changes cause the foramen ovale (between the atria) to close; complete anatomic closure, however, may take several weeks to a year. The ductus arteriosus constricts almost immediately after birth but may not close anatomically for 1 to 3 months. As the umbilical cord is clamped and severed, the umbilical vein and ductus venosus close immediately. The assessments of the neonate to evaluate oxygenation are reviewed in the accompanying display.

TABLE 11-1
Apgar Score

Observation	0	1	2
Heart rate	Absent	Slow (Below 100)	Over 100
Respiratory rate	Absent, hypoventilation	Weak cry	Good
Muscle tone	Limp	Some flexion of extremities	Well flexed
Reflex response			
1. Response to catheter in nostril	No response	Grimace	Cough or sneeze
2. Tangential foot slap	No response	Grimace	Cry and withdrawal of foot
Color	Blue, pale	Body pink, extremities blue	Completely pink

Scoring: The infant is first scored at 1 min and 5 min; some examiners use a third score taken at 10 min. The score at 1 min suggests the degree of acidosis; the score at 5 min usually predicts mortality and morbidity. Scores below 6 are abnormal and demand immediate attention.

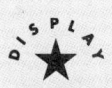

Oxygenation Assessments

Physiologic remnants of life in utero (related to
    oxygenation)
   Rales in lungs: amniotic fluid
   Heart murmurs*: delay in closure of patent ductus
    arteriosus or foramen ovale
Respiratory rate: respiratory ease—no retractions,
   nasal flaring, grunting; see-saw respirations are
   not normal
Apical pulse
Skin color
Alertness, responsiveness

*Most heart murmurs during the neonatal period have no
pathologic significance, and more than half disappear.*

Newborn Physical Assessment

The delivery room nurse reports significant findings
to the nursery room nurse who continues newborn assessments, including general observations, samples for
laboratory tests, and evaluation of gestational age.

The assessment of the neonate continues until the
time of discharge from the hospital, and resumes in the
home, physician's office, or outpatient clinic.[19] The purpose of a physical examination is to identify, not only the
infant's current health status, but to provide a basis on
which future changes can be understood. Descriptions
of newborn responses are time-dependent, for a normal
response at 5 minutes may not be a normal response at
1 day of age.

Information regarding the mother's pregnancy, labor
and delivery, and health status are essential components
of the newborn assessment. The infant's appearance and
behavior may be affected, for example, by the type or
dosage of maternal analgesics, and these need to be assessed accurately. During the neonatal period, assessments of parental interactions also contribute valuable
information on the infant's potential growth and
development.

Providing adequate lighting and a warm environment
to maintain the infant's temperature are important components of the physical examination. A major portion of
the examination should take place unobtrusively, before
the infant is undressed. Undressing the infant is saved
until the end of the examination to minimize distress.
Manipulating the baby often invokes crying, which
impedes and makes the examination more difficult. Although the physical examination of the newborn is best
done in a systematic head to toe order, this is not always
possible. Palpation of the fontanels, observation of respirations, or auscultation of the heart can be done on a
quiet or sleeping infant. As the nurse observes the infant's
face, the general tone and symmetry of movements, the
breathing patterns, the color, and response to stimuli,

she has learned a great deal. Tests that disturb the infant
should be done last.

A physical examination of the newborn should be
performed in the presence of the parents before the infant's discharge from the hospital. Performed in a relaxed
and unhurried manner, this assessment provides the nurse
with the opportunity to discuss the uniqueness and special
needs of the infant, as well as to identify actual or potential
problems. Plans for follow-up care can be addressed with
the parents. Table 11-2 summarizes the normal findings
of the physical examination of the neonate.

The Head

The head circumference of the normal newborn is
generally between 33 and 37 cm, 2 cm larger than the
chest circumference. The head is one fourth of a newborn's body length, whereas an adult's head is one eighth
of the total body length.[19] The neonate's head is disproportionately large in relation to the body because brain
growth is rapid during this period. Muscle control begins
from the infant's head and moves gradually downward to
the rest of the body. The head circumference is measured
with a tape measure, encircling the infant's head at the
frontal and occipital bones.

Six bones compose the skull of the neonate: frontal,
occipital, two parietal, and two temporal bones. These
bones are unconnected at the time of birth and held together by narrow bands of connective tissue called sutures. The major sutures of the skull are the coronal,
lambdoid, and sagittal sutures. The unfused skull bones
allow the head to overlap and to change shape, permitting
the head to be pushed and molded during the delivery
process.

Fontanels. Between the cranial bones of the newborn's head are two spaces or soft spots, known as fontanels. The anterior fontanel is located above the infant's
forehead, between the frontal and two parietal bones.
Diamond-shaped, the anterior fontanel measures approximately 2 to 3 cm in width and 3 to 4 cm in length,
and if one watches closely, pulses can be detected with
each heartbeat. The posterior fontanel, approximately 1

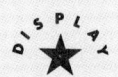

Universal Precautions

Because medical history and examination cannot
identify all patients infected with HIV or other
bloodborne pathogens, *blood and body-fluid precautions should be used for ALL clients.* Gloves
should be worn for touching blood, body fluids, and
mucous membranes, or for handling items or surfaces soiled with blood or body fluids. Gloves should
be changed after contact with each patient.[49] Universal precautions are on the inside back cover of
this book.

TABLE 11-2
Physical Assessment of the Neonate

Organ	Normal Findings	Normal Variations	Clinical Implications
Measurements	Weight 3400 g (7 lb, 8 oz)	2500–4000 g (5 lb, 8 oz–8 lb, 13 oz)	
	Length 50 cm (20 in)	45–55 cm (18–22 in)	Measure from head to heel; difficult due to incomplete extension
	Head circumference 33–35 cm (13–14 in)	Head circumference is 2–3 cm larger than chest circumference	Measure head at greatest diameter
	Chest circumference 30–33 cm (12–13 in)		Measure chest at nipple line
Head			
Appearance	Asymmetric due to molding, forceps, or difficult labor	Molding (overriding of cranial bones during delivery)	May decrease head circumference; remeasure after several days
		Caput succedaneum (palpable, edematous, soft purple mass after prolonged or difficult labor)	Edema gradually absorbed, disappearing within a few days without treatment; explain causes and reassure parents
		Cephalhematoma (collection of blood between the skull bone and the periosteum)	Appears after several hours or after first day; resolves 3–6 wk; support parents and reassure them of temporary nature of disfigurement
		Cradle cap (yellow-orange greasy scalp patches)	
		Craniotabes (softening of the skull bones due to pressure against bony pelvis in utero)	Disappears in 1–2 mo
Fontanel ("soft spot")	*Anterior* (diamond-shaped); closes around 18 mo. *Posterior* (triangular); closes around 12 wk, but may be closed at birth	Anterior fontanel 0.6–3.6 cm; pulsates with each heartbeat	Palpate fontanels. Explain purpose to parents (protects and allows for growth of brain); no danger in touching soft spot, membrane is tough as canvas
Face	Symmetric, makes facial grimaces, features small in comparison to size of head	Temporary facial changes if fetus packed tightly in utero	
Eyes	Visual acuity, 20/500; nearsighted at birth; blink reflex present; reacts to light and touch		Responds to patterns, shapes, and colored objects; objects seen clearly at 8–10 in
		Swollen from physical trauma of birth	Swelling decreases and resolves in 1–2 wk
	Symmetric in size, shape; moves eyes in all directions	Pseudostrabismus	Reassure parents will disappear spontaneously as muscles of eye strengthen; may persist 3–4 mo
	Iris: white infants, blue gray; African American infants, brown gray		Eye color of white infant may change several times before setting by 3–6 mo; all irises gradually darken
	Cornea: clear	Subconjunctival hemorrhage (rupture of capillaries during birth)	Reassure parents eyes will not be impaired; usually disappears in 2–3 wk
	Sclera: Slightly blue in color from thin sclera		
	Pupils: equal and round	Epicanthal folds in Asian babies and 20% of white babies; eyes appear malaligned	Causes pseudostrabismus; when present with other signs may indicate chromosomal disorders
	Eyelids: present		
	Discharge: none	Chemical conjunctivitis (instillation of silver nitrate—onset first 24 h)	Demonstrate cleansing of eyes and reassure parents of no damage to eyes; subsides in 2–4 days
	Absence of tears until 4–6 wk (a few shed tears from birth)	Blocked nasolacrimal duct	Not injurious to eye; may last 1–2 mo
Nose	Smelling acuity, distinguishes and identifies odors; nares patent bilaterally (obligatory nose breathers); sneezes to clear nose; even placement	Nasal discharge	May cause stuffiness or visible runny nose with discharge
		Nose may appear flattened or bruised from passage through birth canal	
Mouth	Identifies different tastes; discriminates sweet from bitter and salty	Mucus for 1–2 days after delivery	Remove excessive mucus with bulb syringe. Reassure parents cysts are common and will disappear
	Soft and hard palate intact	Epstein's pearls (small, shiny, white retention cysts)	
	Short frenulum		

(Continued)

TABLE 11-2
(Continued)

Organ	Normal Findings	Normal Variations	Clinical Implications
	Presence of reflexes: Extrusion, rooting, swallowing, and gag		
	Sucking reflex strong and coordinated	Sucking blisters on upper lip	Indicates avid sucker; vanishes between feedings
	Lips hypersensitive to touch; symmetric		
	Tongue, noncoated	Thrush (white, cheese-adhering appearance; on cheeks and tongue; organism responsible is *Candida albicans*)	Can be painful and interfere with feeding. Assess diaper area because organism responsible for thrush may manifest as monilial diaper rash
Ears	Hearing acuity distinguishes types of sounds, loudness, pitch, and direction	No response to sound	May indicate deafness; observe head movement in direction of sound
	Position of ears: upper part of ear on same plane as angle of eye; set at same level on both sides of head	Positional deformity (bent ear as outcome of crowding in uterus)	Positional deformity will return to normal; deformed ears may indicate chromosomal or kidney disorders
		Low placement or deformed ears	
Skin	*Touch:* responds to pressure, pain, and changes in temperature		
	Texture: dry and flaky; wrinkled and blotchy at birth	Physiologic epidermal desquamation (hands and feet peel or flake); mottling (general circulation lability)	Encourage good skin care, avoiding lotions, powders, and oils; instruct parents to keep infant warm; mottling occurs if baby is exposed to decreased temperatures; improves as circulation improves
	Color: at birth, reddish pink color	Acrocyanosis (cyanosis of hands and feet for several hours after delivery)	Reassure parents this harmless situation will improve as circulation improves
	Hydration	Normal weight loss after birth up to 10% of birthweight	Weigh infants routinely; explain weight loss to parents
		Normal physiologic jaundice (appears yellowish in color); 3–4 days after birth	Usually requires no treatment; may be treated with bililight (protect infant's eyes); increase fluids to prevent loss due to evaporation
	Coverings: Vernix caseosa, lanugo, milia neonatorum (rash of yellowish, white pinpoint size lesions located on chin, cheeks, and bridge of nose)	Miliaria (seen on first day of life; tiny, pinpoint water-filled blisters)	Instruct parents that vernix caseosa will flake off; lanugo will disappear in 2–4 wk; milia neonatorum requires no treatment and disappears in 1–2 wk; miliaria rubra more common in summer, but can develop if infant is too bundled in winter; toxic erythema short-lived; benign and disappears without treatment
		Miliaria rubra (small discrete red, raised areas containing pinpoint blisters)	
		Toxic erythema (newborn rash; red blotches with light center on face)	
	Diaper rash (red papules and patches of rough, red skin)	Yeast or monilial (bright red spots that come together to form a solid red area; small papules can be seen; as it heals crusty and scaly areas are seen)	Responds to treatment of Nystatin ointment; over-the-counter Lotrimin is effective
		Seborrheic (worse in folds than on prominences; pustules present; infant may have increased temperature)	May respond to steroid or antibiotic treatment
	Birth marks	Mongolian spots (large dark bluish areas mostly over sacrum)	Reassure parents that it will disappear by 4 y of age; seen in infants of Hispanic, African, or Asian origin
		Stork bites (irregular pink spots on nape of neck, forehead, or eyelids present at birth)	Lesions usually fade by 4 y of age with no treatment
		Strawberry hemangiomas (begin to develop by 3–4 wk)	May grow for a while, fade to pearly gray; 90% disappear by 5–10 y of age; occasionally treatment will be indicated (compression and massage; steroids; surgery; or laser therapy may be used)
		Port wine stain or nevus flammeus (purplish red marks composed of dilated mature capillaries)	May fade, but do not disappear; laser therapy may be effective in removing them

(Continued)

TABLE 11-2
(Continued)

Organ	Normal Findings	Normal Variations	Clinical Implications
Neck	Short, thick, usually surrounded by skin folds; can be turned 80 degrees, to right and left; can be bent 40 degrees toward either shoulder; Tonic neck reflex present	Torticollis	
Chest	Minor asymmetry		
	Breasts	1% to 5% of infants born with extra breast enlargement	No medical or cosmetic significance; may remain swollen for 3–5 days due to maternal and infant hormones; fades by 6 mo
		Supernumerary nipples	
		Swollen breasts for males and females	
		Secretion of milk substance from breasts	Do not attempt to squeeze milk from nipples
Heart	Rate 90–150 beats/min Point of Maximum Impulse (PIM) (auscultated at third to fourth intercostal space, lateral to the midsternal border)		Influenced by physical activity; 180 beats when crying and 70–90 when sleeping
	Quality: sharp and clear; 1st sound (closure of mitral/tricuspid valves); 2nd sound (closure of aortic and pulmonary valves)	Murmurs (90% are transient and considered normal)	Auscultate for 1 full minute to detect irregularities
		Sinus arrhythmias	
	Blood pressure 75/50	Transient cyanosis when crying or straining	Reassure parents; heart may appear to be racing
	Chest wall thin	Mottling	
Lungs	Respiratory rate 30–50/min	Momentary apneic spells common	Count respirations for full 1 minute to detect irregularities
	Respirations mostly abdominal	Nasal flaring	
	Breathes through nose unless crying	Difficulty with inspiration or expiration	
	Cough reflex present 1–2 days after birth	Stuffy nose	Sneezes to clear nasal passages; sneezes dry
	Hiccups		Hiccups are harmless; feeding slowly may help
	Mucus (fluid from lung or amniotic fluid)		Suction excessive mucus; disappears first week
Abdomen	Round bellies; abdominal muscles weak; trunk of newborn 75% of body		
	Umbilicus: blue-white at birth; yellow-brown at 24 hr; black-brown until drops off, end of second week		Keep cord dry, clean, and observe for signs of infection
		Umbilical hernia (swelling close to navel when infant cries)	Size of baby determines when it resolves—few weeks to first year
		Umbilical granuloma (slow-growing pink mound of tissue producing clear discharge)	Physician will treat with silver nitate
Hips	Symmetry of gluteal folds; hip abduction to 60–70 degrees	50% of infants have symmetric thigh creases	Observe and evaluate hip stability (Ortolani's test)
Back	Spine intact		
	No openings, masses, or prominent curves		
Extremities	Symmetry of extremities, full range of motion possible, equal muscle tone	Often assumes position maintained in utero	May take several weeks to assume normal posture
	Arms and hands: hands clenched in fists; arms abducted, flexed and externally rotated; arms equal in length and longer than legs		
	Legs and feet: feet flat and soles well-aligned, both legs equal in length	Feet appear to be turned in but can be externally rotated	
Genitalia			
Female	Labia and clitoris edematous, appear larger in proportion to their bodies because of infusion of maternal hormones; labia minora larger than labia majora	Bruising, edema, ecchymosis of genitalia and buttocks in breech presentation	
		Vaginal or hymenal tags	Disappears in 1–2 wk

(Continued)

TABLE 11-2
(Continued)

Organ	Normal Findings	Normal Variations	Clinical Implications
	Voids within 24 h (urine is pale and acidic)	Urates may cause pink staining	Observe and record voiding
	Discharge, vernix caseosa between labia	Mucoid vaginal discharge (milky white); may be tinged with blood (pseudomenstruation)	Reassure parents this occurrence is normal in first week of life due to maternal hormones passing to infant before birth
Male	Genitalia increased in size (due to birth process and maternal hormones)	Edema, ecchymosis if breech presentation	
	Penis 3–4 cm long		
	Urethral opening on tip of penis		
	Circumcised penis: swelling and yellow scab at healing site		Instruct parents on care of circumcised penis
	Uncircumcised penis: penis and foreskin fused at birth		Instruct parents not to retract the foreskin; 90% of foreskins will be retractable by 3 y of age
	Testes: usually descended in scrotum and palpable	Undescended testes	Most will descend by 3 mo; treatment if undescended by 1 y
	Scrotum	Physiologic hydroceles (round, fluid-filled sac in scrotum)	Usually disappears within 3 mo
		Pigmented with rugae	
	Discharge	Smegma (yellow, cheesy material that gets trapped in foreskin)	
	Voids within 24 h	Urates in urine may cause pink staining	Observe and record voiding
	Erections		Reassure parents erections are normal and often occur with a full bladder
Anus and rectum	Patent anal opening; passes meconium within 24–36 h; greenish-black sticky substance which fills intestine in utero	Blood in stool 1–2 days after birth may be from swallowing mother's blood during delivery	Put baby to breast and ensure adequate fluid intake to promote passage of meconium and decrease the risk of elevated bilirubin levels
			Record the passage of meconium
	Transition stool: 3–4 days after birth		
	Breast-fed babies: bright mustard color, seedy, watery to soft, little odor		
	Bottle-fed babies: yellowish-green, more formed and odoriferous		
	Breast-fed babies tend to have more stools per day but the number is highly individual		

cm in length and 1 cm in width, is triangular and located between the occipital and parietal bones.[19] The anterior fontanel usually closes between 18 months and 3 years, whereas the posterior fontanel closes between 1 month and 3 months, but may be closed at birth. Because an enlarged or depressed fontanel may indicate certain diseases, careful measurement is important.

The infant's head is observed for symmetry and for the presence or absence of edema. The anterior and posterior fontanels are palpated for fullness, depression, or overriding. A bulging fontanel is a sign of increased intracranial pressure, whereas a depressed fontanel is a sign of decreased intravascular volume (dehydration).[19] Pulsations often are observed in the anterior fontanel when an infant is crying or feeding. An infant's head is often distorted and out of shape at birth. Many factors, as follows, produce alterations in a newborn's head shape.

Caput Succedaneum. Caput succedaneum is a palpable, edematous, soft, occasionally purple mass of the scalp. A common condition found in newborns, it may involve more than one area of the head. The swelling is usually located over the vertex and is more obvious after a prolonged labor or a difficult delivery. Although the edema is gradually absorbed, disappearing within a few days without treatment, the associated bruise may last somewhat longer.

Molding. A mother's pelvis is usually an inch narrower than the circumference of a baby's head. To accommodate for this narrowness, the bones of the skull overlap at the suture line to allow passage of the newborn's head through the birth canal. This process is known as molding. In most vaginal deliveries, infants experience some amount of molding, causing the head to appear asymmetric and to have a duncelike appearance. The head circumference may be affected by this condition, making it impossible to obtain an accurate head measurement. After a few days, the head measurement may be repeated when the head has shifted back to its unmolded shape.

Cephalhematoma. Cephalhematomas are tense, cystic feeling, swollen areas of the head, occurring in up to 1% of deliveries. Cephalhematomas occur more often in boys and three times more often on the right side of the head.[36] These swollen areas are usually located between the surface of the cranial bones and the surface of the overlying periosteal membrane.[19] They may be unilateral or bilateral. Filled with collections of blood from vessels that have ruptured, they are thought to occur from the veins of the scalp tearing from the to and fro movements of uterine contractions.[17] Cephalhematomas are observed within the first 24 hours of life, growing larger each day for 2 to 5 days. After 1 to 2 months, the swelling subsides, leaving no disfigurement of the head. A large cephalhematoma may cause excessive jaundice in the newborn because it is a significant source of additional bilirubin.[36]

Craniotabes. Craniotabes are soft areas usually located near the back of the skull close to the posterior fontanel. Pressure of the fetus's head against the mother's bony pelvis while in utero causes craniotabes. These areas are softer than the rest of the skull, disappearing in 1 to 2 months.

Scalp Scars. Fetal monitoring instruments, placed on the infant's scalp during labor, may cause small bruises or small patches of baldness.

The Face

Facial features are small compared to head size, with the facial contour unique in each newborn. At birth, cramping in the womb or passing through the birth canal causes the face to appear temporarily asymmetric. A difficult forceps delivery or compression of the infant's face against the mother's sacrum may cause damage to the facial nerve, resulting in an infant who moves only one side of the face. This outcome, however, is usually favorable.

Eyes. At birth, the eyes are fully developed. Newborns respond to patterns and shapes, to black, white and colored objects, with red and yellow colors especially appealing to infants. A mother's face, however, is the most interesting thing in the world to a newborn infant. Although nearsighted at birth, the normal newborn has approximately 20/500 vision, seeing objects clearly 8 to 10 in away, and it is at this distance that the infant views his or her mother while feeding.

The eyes are observed for shape, position, size, appearance of pupils, symmetry, and presence of discharge, hemorrhage, or edema. The visual acuity of the infant is indirectly assessed by the presence or absence of visual reflexes at birth. Newborns, sensitive to light, close their eyes or blink in response to a bright light or to a sudden noise (blink reflex). The pupils should be equal and should react to light. Consensual pupillary constriction is elicited by shining a light first in one eye and then in the other. As the light is brought down from the infant's forehead or in from the side of the head, the pupils should constrict.[19]

The eyes are best examined and observed when they open voluntarily. Because the eyes are usually closed in the early days of life, holding an infant in an upright position, gently moving him back and forth, encourages him to open his eyes. At the time of birth, the iris is normally blue or gray in light-skinned infants and brown in dark-skinned infants. The pigment of the iris is evident at about 3 months, but its final color develops over the first year of life, as pigmentation continues to increase. The sclera of the newborn is relatively thin, allowing the color of the choroid to show through, resulting in the sclera having a slightly bluish color. The cornea is clear, and the size of the cornea is proportionate to an adult's. Enlarged corneas may indicate congenital glaucoma. Newborns usually cry without tears for the first 4 to 6 weeks of life.

Swollen Eyelids. The swelling of a newborn's eyelids, usually caused by the physical trauma of delivery, subsides in 1 to 2 weeks.

Pseudostrabismus. Many infants appear cross-eyed (pseudostrabismus) during the newborn period. Enhancing this appearance is the wideness and flatness of the nose or the fold of skin that some newborns have on their upper lids (epicanthic folds), creating the illusion that the eye is turned inward. Parents need reassurance that this lack of coordination of the eyes is normal and may persist up to 3 months after birth.

Subconjunctival Hemorrhage. During the birth process, small capillaries in the sclera may rupture, causing a red spot on the sclera or redness of the entire eye. Known as subconjunctival hemorrhage, this phenomenon usually disappears spontaneously, resolving within 2 to 3 weeks. Forty percent of newborns have blood spots on their eyes.[36]

Chemical Conjunctivitis. Silver nitrate installation in the eyes of newborns to prevent gonococcus infection may cause chemical conjunctivitis. A crusty yellow discharge with redness and swelling appears within 3 to 6 hours of installing silver nitrate and disappears within 48 hours. Any discharge developing 2 or 3 days after delivery requires medical attention. *Chlamydia trachomatis* causes neonatal conjunctivitis and appears 3 to 4 days after birth. Tetracycline or erythromycin is employed in many hospitals today in place of silver nitrate, because these medications treat both the gonococcus and the *Chlamydia* bacteria.

The Nose. The newborn infant distinguishes and identifies odors, especially the smell of breast milk. As the result of the delivery process, the nose may appear flattened or bruised. In the neonatal period, it is common for newborns to sneeze. Sneezing clears the nasal passages, providing a clear airway for the infant. The newborn's nasal passages are observed for patency bilaterally and for the presence of discharge. Some discharge or visible runniness is normal in the newborn. Newborns are obligatory nose breathers, except when crying.

The Mouth. The large number of touch receptors on the lips makes the lips of newborns hypersensitive. In the first month of life, newborns, unable to reach for objects, use their mouths to learn about their world. Touching the lips of an infant elicits an immediate sucking reflex.

The sense of taste, highly developed in newborns, permits identification and differentiation of different tastes. Research studies indicate sucking responses increase with sweet tastes and decrease with salty or bitter tastes. The external appearance of the lips is observed for symmetry and color. Asymmetry of the mouth is more apparent when a newborn is feeding or crying, and may be caused by a minor abnormality of the depressor anguli oris muscle. When an infant cries, one side of the mouth does not move downward and outward as well as the other side.[36]

A yawn or cry offers an opportunity to observe the tongue, throat, and internal mouth of the newborn. If the infant's chin is gently pressed down, the mouth opens for internal inspection. All newborns have mucus in their mouths for 1 to 2 days after delivery, excessive amounts of which may be removed with a bulb syringe.

Tongue. The tongue is short in newborns, with the frenulum extending to the tip of the tongue. In the past, an infant's frenulum was often cut by midwives and physicians in the hope of preventing speech problems. This procedure is not performed routinely today because of the risk of hemorrhage and infection to the infant and because this phenomenon rarely interferes with speech. The tongue is gently depressed to observe the internal mouth and palate.

Epstein's Pearls. Eighty-five percent of infants are born with small, yellow-white swellings on both sides of the hard plate of the mouth. These epithelial cysts are thought to be the result of an overload of calcium deposited in the uterus. They disappear by 1 to 3 months of age and are often mistaken for tooth buds or thrush. The white deposit of thrush firmly covers the mouth and can be removed, whereas Epstein's pearls cannot.

Thrush. Thrush is a fungal infection caused by *Candida albicans,* manifesting as white, cheeselike patches, adhering firmly to the sides of the cheeks and of the tongue. The covering behind the patches often is swollen and red, bleeding easily if attempts are made to scrape it off. Thrush is transmitted to the newborn from the mother's vaginal canal during the birth process. The mother, if breast-feeding, may also transmit *Candida albicans* through her milk. As the infant ingests the mother's milk, the fungus in the milk travels through the digestive tract, revealing itself as a monilial diaper rash. Nystatin drops to the mouth or nystatin ointment to the diaper area is the recommended treatment for these conditions.

Sucking Blisters. Infants who are avid suckers often develop blisters on the lips. The blisters peel and re-form again. Sucking blisters differ from the blister of herpes; herpes blisters are not confined to the upper lip.[36]

The Ears. At birth, the nerve tracts and bony structures of the ears are completely mature with the cartilage formed to retain the shape of the ears. Hearing is well developed early; newborns adeptly distinguish types of sounds, their loudness and pitch, and the direction from which sound emanates. High-pitched sounds are preferred by newborns, and mothers, especially, use high-pitched voices when speaking to their infants (baby talk).[21] Research studies indicate that mothers speak to their infants in high-pitched voices and in nonsense syllables, regardless of their native languages.

Hearing acuity is evaluated by observing the infant's response to sound. A sudden noise, eliciting a startle reflex, may be a reaction to a vibration and not a true test of hearing ability. A preferable indicator of an infant's hearing acuity is the movement of an infant's head in the direction of a sound. Acoustic responses, difficult to elicit in newborns, need to be assessed over time for accurate interpretation. Hearing is more acute several days after birth as the eustachian tubes become aerated and mucus disappears from the middle ear.

The general shape, size, and position of the ears are observed. The placement of a newborn's ears is important. The upper part of the ear should be on the same plane as the angle of the newborn's eye. Low-set or malformed ears are often associated with congenital or chromosomal abnormalities, particularly renal agenesis. Ears folded inward at birth may be the result of compression of the fetus in a tightly packed womb, and they unfold shortly after birth. After a forceps delivery, the ears are also inspected for injury or damage.

The Skin

Various skin conditions are noted at birth (Table 11-3). The sense of touch is well-developed in the newborn infant. Pressure, pain, and changes in temperature elicit responses, with cold eliciting faster reactions than heat.[17] Although the entire body of a newborn is sensitive to touch, the lips and hands assist the infant in discovering surroundings. Warmth and closeness ease the infant's entry into the world, and no amount of holding or cuddling

TABLE 11-3
Skin Conditions in the Neonate

Skin Condition	Description	Cause
Petechiae	Minute hemorrhages on the surface of the skin	Capillary fragility due to increased venous pressure during labor and delivery
Milia	Tiny, white, benign papules on the nose, cheeks, and forehead; disappear in 2–4 wk	Plugged sebaceous glands
Telangiectatic nevi	Flat, red or purple localized areas on nose, upper lip, eyelids, nape of the neck	Capillary dilitation
Erythema toxicum	Transient, papular or vesicular rash, surrounded by a mild erythema on back or buttocks	Appears soon after birth, benign, and disappears in 2–3 days

can spoil an infant during the neonatal period. Such treatment only offers an infant a sense of security.

During the neonatal period, the skin serves as the largest sensory organ of the body and provides protection as well. Changes observed in the skin are often the first clues to an underlying illness. The newborn's skin is observed for the following.

Texture. Most infants have ruddy complexions. At birth, newborns are wrinkled and blotchy, with mottling of the skin due to general circulation lability. Dry and flaky skin is normal; the infant's hands and feet often peel. This condition, known as desquamation, is caused by the contrast of the dry air environment out of utero to the warm, lubricating amniotic fluid in utero. Abrasions observed on the skin may be caused by the use of forceps or the pressure of the mother's pelvis on the infant's skin during the delivery process. These abrasions usually disappear in 2 to 3 days.

Lanugo. At birth, the skin of the newborn may be covered with fine, soft downy hair known as lanugo. The lanugo, covering the shoulders, back, and upper arms, wears away and disappears in 1 to 2 weeks. Lanugo, common in premature infants, is rarely seen in post-mature infants (greater than 42 week gestation).

Vernix Caseosa. Newborns are also covered with vernix caseosa, a white, cream-cheeselike, waxy substance. Concentrated in the folds of the skin, the vernix need not be removed because it dries up and fades away. Vernix serves as a protective covering and lubricant, easing the infant's passage through the birth canal.

Color. At birth, skin color is determined by the amount of subcutaneous fat present on the infant.[13] After only a few hours of life, a healthy newborn's skin is a reddish pink color. A preterm infant's skin is transparent and appears reddened because the blood vessels are visible. If meconium has been passed before the birth, the infant's skin may have a greenish color.

Jaundice. During the first few days of life, infants may have a yellow hue to their skin, known as jaundice. Jaundice in the first day of life is abnormal, usually the result of blood incompatibility. In the first 3 to 4 days of life, however, 50% of newborn infants experience normal physiologic jaundice. Many newborns produce excessive amounts of bilirubin, which their immature livers cannot process. As bilirubin builds in the bloodstream, a yellowish color to the skin results, known as normal physiologic jaundice. As the level of bilirubin rises, jaundice appears on the head and face first, then the trunk and extremities, and finally on the sclera of the eye.[2] Gently depressing the bridge of the nose and noting the color of the skin as the pressure is released reveals jaundice.[15] Treatment is usually not necessary for normal physiologic jaundice, but severe cases can be managed with phototherapy. Normal physiologic jaundice usually diminishes in 7 to 10 days, lasting longer in premature infants. Breast-fed infants may have increased blood levels of bilirubin, which remain elevated for up to 6 weeks of life.[8]

Acrocyanosis. In the infant's first 48 hours of life, the hands and feet may appear cyanotic. Poor peripheral circulation present at birth results in this common condition, referred to as acrocyanosis.

Birth Marks. Large dark bluish areas, mainly over the sacrum, but also present on the thighs, dorsum of the hands and feet, buccal mucosa, shoulders, and forehead, are known as mongolian spots.[17] These spots are frequently seen in Asian and African American infants; they resolve by 4 years of age. Stork bites or nevus simplex are salmon patches seen on the forehead, nose, mouth, upper eyelids, or the nape of the neck. During the first 2 years of life, 95% of stork bites completely fade away. The nevus simplex is the routine birthmark of the light-complexioned newborn, in contrast to the mongolian spots observed in dark-complexioned infants.[36] Strawberry hemangiomas are soft, raised, red birthmarks, composed of immature vascular materials that break away from the circulatory system during fetal development.[8] This common birthmark occurs in one of ten newborns, developing at 3 to 4 weeks of age and disappearing about 5 to 10 years of age, with no treatment necessary or blemish remaining.

The Chest

The chest of the newborn is observed for shape, breast swelling, and accessory nipples. The circumference of the chest is measured by placing the tape measure at the level of the nipples midway between inspiration and expiration. Accessory nipples occur in 1 in 500 males or females.[17] Eighty percent of full-term babies have some degree of breast enlargement, beginning after 2 to 3 days of birth and peaking in the second week of life.[17] The cause of this swelling is not fully understood, but it is thought to be related to ovary and pituitary gland secretions.

The Heart

Heart Rate. The heart rate of an infant, at birth, may be as rapid as 180 beats/min as the neonate struggles to initiate respirations. During and after the transition period, the heart rate fluctuates. The normal heart rate ranges from 120 to 150 beats/min, affected by activity changes and sleep and wake states. For example, an infant's heart rate in deep sleep is 100 beats/min, whereas, in the crying state, it may rise to 160 beats/min.[19] If the infant's rate is out of the normal range, the infant's activity state is charted. The heart rate is auscultated for one full minute at the PMI (point of maximum impulse), located lateral to the nipple line at the fourth intercostal space. For an accurate assessment of the heart rate, auscultation should be done on a quiet infant. The blood pressure of the normal newborn infant is on the average 74/47 mmHg and is assessed using the Doppler technique or a 1- to 2-in cuff and a pediatric stethoscope over the brachial artery.

Arrhythmias. It is not unusual to hear murmurs while auscultating the heart in the neonatal period because the sinus node of the newborn infant is easily distracted because of the infant's immature nervous system. Eighty to ninety percent of these murmurs are transient and disappear in the first year of life.[33]

The Lungs. The respiratory and cardiovascular systems of the newborn infant are impossible to separate.

Adaptations to postnatal life are intertwined between these two systems; disorders of one system closely mimic or are consequences of the other system.[33]

The average respiratory rate of the newborn is between 30 and 60 breaths/min. At birth, the respiratory rate may be as high as 80 breaths/min, often irregular and shallow. Fast breathing in an infant may indicate pneumonia or heart failure, but many babies breathe fast due to a harmless condition known as transient tachypnea. Infants experiencing stressful deliveries or oversedated mothers during labor tend to have transient tachypnea, with boys more susceptible than girls. The infant with this condition does not appear to be laboring for breaths, rather the infant appears to be huffing and puffing with each breath. This condition is caused by the poor quality of the pumping mechanism of the left ventricle in the first few days of life.[36]

Brief Sleep Apnea. During the sleep state, all babies are sometimes breathless as a result of their immature nervous and respiratory systems. Because an infant is unable to fine tune its rate of breathing to its changing body chemistry, a baby's respiratory pattern makes pauses, known as periodic apnea.[36] These pauses should be differentiated from apneic spells, which last 20 seconds or longer, resulting in the slowing of the heart rate and loss of color.[36] Periodic apnea spells last only a few seconds.

Assessment of the respiratory system begins with inspection and observation of the neonate in the resting state. The respiratory rate, like the heart rate, is influenced by emotion, crying, and hunger. The bell of the stethoscope is placed in front of the nose of a quiet infant to count the respirations, because newborn infants are obligatory nose breathers. The rate, regularity, and depth of respirations are assessed. Newborns breathe using their diaphragmatic and abdominal muscles, and the abdomen is observed for rising on inhalation and falling on expiration with little thoracic movement.[19] The presence or absence of retractions, the degree of respiratory effort by the infant, and the use of accessory muscles to aid breathing are assessed.

Mucus. Newborn mucus is fluid secreted from the lungs or a blend of fetal lung secretions and amniotic fluid. During the labor process, the fetus's chest squeezes abundant amounts of mucus out through the nose and mouth. Immediately after delivery and throughout the first few days of life, remaining amounts of mucus are suctioned with a bulb syringe.

Hiccups. All babies hiccup. The sudden contraction of the diaphragm muscle creates a vacuum, sucking air into the windpipe, causing a abrupt closure of the vocal cords, resulting in a hiccup.[36] Newborns who feed ravenously, swallowing air as they feed, are apt to hiccup more.

The Abdomen. Newborn infants have round bellies. Weak abdominal muscles and distended stomachs, filled with milk and air, give a lopsided appearance to the newborn's abdomen. The abdomen is auscultated for the presence of bowel sounds; bowel sounds can be heard 1 hour after birth.

The umbilical stump begins to shrink and dry up after delivery and separates from the infant's abdomen during the second week of life. As the navel begins to heal, an opening in the deep muscles of the abdomen sometimes remains. If a small part of the intestines protrude through this opening, an umbilical hernia occurs. African American babies and premature infants often have umbilical herniations. Umbilical hernias normally require no intervention and disappear early in childhood.

Genitalia

Female Genitalia. The labia majora and labia minora are inspected. In female newborns, the labia minora are often more prominent than the labia majora, and separation of the labia usually reveals large amounts of vernix caseosa. The labia of the female newborn are observed for adhesions, which usually resolve by 18 months of life, requiring no treatment. Tissue from the hymen or labia minora, known as vaginal or hymenal tags, may also be present at birth and disappears within the first weeks of life. At birth, the genitalia may be swollen. This swelling is caused by transference of maternal hormones to the newborn or by a breech delivery. Bruising and ecchymosis of the genitalia and buttocks also occur in breech presentations.

In female infants, a milk-white discharge may be present for several days after delivery. Occasionally, this discharge is tinged with blood, referred to as *pseudomenstruation.* It is thought to occur as the result of the withdrawal of maternally derived estrogen.

Male Genitalia. The genitalia of the male newborn consists of a large scrotum and a small penis, usually 3 cm in size. The scrotum is inspected for size and symmetry, and the scrotal sac is palpated to verify the presence of two testes of equal size. Occasionally, the testes are not present in the scrotal sac at birth. Although the majority descend in 3 months, surgery may be required if they do not descend by 1 year of age.[36] At birth, the scrotum of the newborn may also be swollen due to a breech delivery or to the influence of maternal hormones. The scrotum may contain bilateral fluid, known as a hydrocele, which usually subsides spontaneously as the fluid is absorbed.

The head of the penis, or glans, is inspected for the location of the urethral opening. The external meatus is located at the center of the tip of the glans penis, but occasionally is located elsewhere. If the opening is on the ventral side of the penis, it is known as hypospadias; if the opening is on the dorsal side, it is known as epispadias. The infant with either hypospadias or epispadias is not circumcised because the infant's foreskin is needed for future surgical repair.

The shaft and the glans of the penis are covered by foreskin, known as the prepuce. The foreskin is usually nonretractable at birth and remains that way until the child is 1 or 2 years of age. By the second year of life, nine out of ten uncircumcised infants' foreskins can be retracted from the glans.[8] Erections occur in the normal male newborn, especially when the bladder is full or the infant urinates.

The Hips. The stability of the infant's hips is evaluated by a procedure known as Ortolani's test (illustrated in Fig. 61-5). The infant is placed in a supine position, and the hips and knees are flexed at right angles. Both

TABLE 11-4
Protective Reflexes in the Newborn

Protective Reflexes	Purpose
Coughing	Clears the respiratory passages and provides a clear airway
Sneezing	Helps to clear airway
Gagging	Aids in spitting up food that goes down the wrong way or in spitting up mucus from mother's womb after delivery
Blinking	Protects eyes from objects that come too close
Yawning	Helps the infant draw in oxygen
Crying	Allows withdrawal from painful stimuli; aids in bonding process
Extrusion	Aids extrusion of any substance placed on tongue; protects infant from swallowing inedible substances

hips should abduct as they lie flat against the bed. A clicking sound may be noted if the joint is unstable.

Anus and Rectum.   At birth, the infant's intestines are filled with a tarry greenish-black substance, known as meconium. The passage of meconium indicates that the bowels are unobstructed. After the meconium has been passed, transitional stools begin. The first stools of the infant may contain traces of blood, because some newborns swallow their mother's blood during delivery. After 3 to 4 days of transitional stools, the breast-fed infant's stools are a mustard color, loose, and sometimes a seedy or mushy consistency. The stools of the bottle-fed infant are more formed than the breast-fed infant's stool and range in color from pale yellow to brown green, depending on the type of formula prescribed for the infant. Iron-fortified formula or iron vitamin drops make the stools appear greenish or dark brown in color. A newborn infant may have a bowel movement after each feeding, especially if the infant is breast-fed. Frequent bowel movements result from the stimulation of the lower intestines as the stomach fills with food and is known as the gastrocolic reflex.

Reflexes.   Reflexes are automatic observable responses, whose presence, absence, and time of appearance or disappearance are important indicators of the health status of the neonate. Reflexes protect the newborn infant, as well as stimulate interaction between parents and infants (Table 11-4). The following reflexes should be present and tested in the newborn infant:[19]

Babinski's Reflex.   Babinski's reflex, a sign of spinal cord integrity, is elicited by gently stroking the lateral plantar surface of the foot from heel to toe. The toes flare (hyperextend) as the foot turns in. This reflex disappears by the end of the first year, after which the toes curl downward.

Grasp Reflex.   The grasp or palmar reflex is a primitive reflex, diminishing by 3 months of age. Some scientists believe the palmar reflex to be an evolutionary adaptation when newborns cling to their mothers for

safety. This reflex is elicited by placing pressure with a finger or an object on the palm of the infant's hand. The infant responds by flexing the hand in an attempt to grasp the finger or object.

Landau Reflex.   When a newborn infant is held in a prone position, with a hand supporting the trunk, the infant attempts to hold the spine in a horizontal position (Fig. 11-2). Sagging into an inverted U position indicates extremely poor muscle tone, and referral for follow-up is necessary.

Moro's Reflex.   Moro's reflex is elicited when the infant is startled suddenly by a loud noise, by the jarring of a crib, or by a bright light. It is also elicited by pulling the infant by both arms and allowing its head to drop back abruptly about 30 degrees. The infant's response is to abduct and extend the arms and legs, placing the fingers in a C position (all digits extend except the thumb and index finger) arching the back while bringing the arms into an embracing position. Moro's reflex is a sign of an intact nervous system in the neonatal period and usually disappears by 4 to 5 months.

Rooting Reflex.   Stroking an infant's cheek elicits the rooting reflex; the infant responds by turning in the direction of the stroking, opening its mouth as if to suck. This reflex aids the newborn to find its food source and disappears in about 6 weeks. As the infant's eyes mature, he or she is able to focus more clearly to see the source of food.

Stepping Reflex.   The stepping reflex is elicited by holding the infant in a standing position on a hard surface and gently pressing the feet on that surface. The infant draws up each foot as if walking. The existence of the stepping reflex does not forecast early walking; it disappears around 3 months of age and reappears 1 year later as the complex art of walking.

Sucking Reflex.   Newborns love to suck, not only for food, but to comfort themselves. In the early weeks

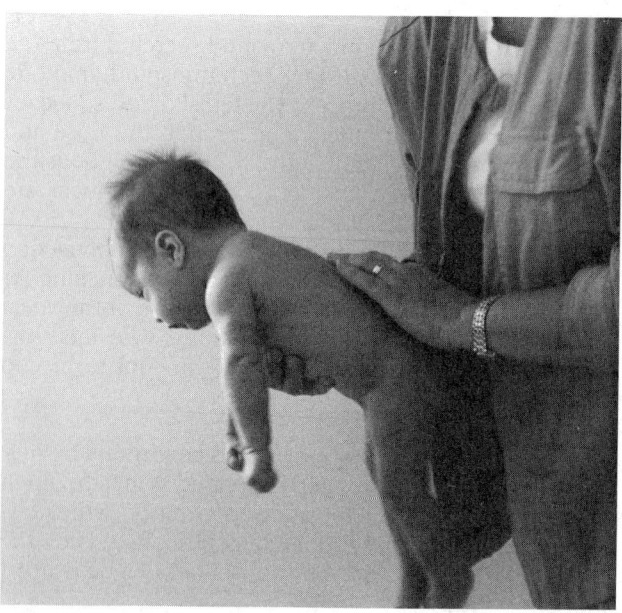

FIGURE 11-2
The Landau reflex is demonstrated with this newborn.

of life, this reflex is elicited by placing a finger between the lips of the infant, causing vigorous sucking.

Tonic Neck Reflex. The tonic neck reflex is elicited by placing the infant on his back where he assumes a fencing position. As the infant turns his head to one side, he extends the arms and leg on that side and flexes the opposite arm and leg (Fig. 11-3). This reflex is also known as the fencing reflex and disappears by 3 to 4 months of age.

Laboratory Tests

Hyperbilirubinemia

For the first month of life, the neonate has a higher red blood cell count (polycythemia) than the adult. This is a normal condition for the neonate because extra red blood cells are needed in utero to compensate for the fetus' lower oxygen supply. As the normal life of neonatal red blood cells ends (80 to 100 days as compared to 120 days for the adult), the cells die, break down, and release bilirubin. The breakdown of the red blood cells, coupled with mild dehydration, results in bilirubin, which the newborn's immature liver cannot metabolize. As the plasma bilirubin rises during the first 3 days of life, it becomes visible in the skin. This condition, called normal physiologic hyperbilirubinemia, results in jaundice, a yellow pigment in the skin.[24] Bilirubin, which is unconjugated (with the glucoronide radical) and unbound (to the albumin in the plasma), is able to invade skin and unmyelinated nerve tissues. When this quantity is excessive, damage to central nervous system tissue occurs and the infant is subject to permanent effects from kernicterus. Hyperbilirubinemia is treated when serum bilirubin concentrations exceed a level of 12 to 12.9 mg/dL.[24]

The fetal hemoglobin present in the red blood cells of the neonate is specially adapted to supply the needs of the fetus in utero. Fetal hemoglobin can carry 20% to 30% more oxygen than adult hemoglobin and may account for the neonate's ability to withstand longer periods of oxygen deprivation than an adult.

State Mandated Testing

Blood tests mandated in many states identify health problems in neonates who appear normal; early treatment of these conditions may prevent mental retardation and other adverse effects.

Phenylketonuria (PKU). This test measures serum phenylalanine levels, an essential amino acid found only in food. To measure the level, a neonate must have ingested breast milk or formula for 1 to 4 days. Blood for PKU is taken for testing (the Guthrie test) on the fourth day of life.

PKU is a disorder of amino acid metabolism; it results from the inability of the liver to convert the amino acid phenylalanine to tyrosine. The frequency of PKU is about 1 in 12,000 births. A diet that restricts phenylalanine intake must be started in the first months of life to permit normal development. The affected child often has lighter pigmentation including blond hair, blue eyes, and light skin. Mental deficiency is common among untreated children.

Thyroxine (T$_4$). Thyroxine levels in the blood are tested at the same time as the PKU. The fetal thyroid begins to produce T$_4$ and other thyroid hormones by the end of the third month of gestation; subsequently, the fetus is largely dependent on its own thyroid. Not enough maternal thyroxine crosses the placenta to ensure adequate supplies if the fetus is not making its own, affecting the development of the brain and other organ systems. However, it is after birth that the hypothyroid infant is at greatest risk. During these early months, normal brain development depends on the presence of adequate thyroid hormones; permanent defects in brain structure and function may occur if the infant is hypothyroid during this time. Treatment with thyroxine is started as soon as the diagnosis is suspected. The frequency of thyroid dysfunction is approximately 1 in 4500 live births.

Other Tests

Biotinidase deficiency may occur in 1 out of every 40,000 births.[38] It is an enzyme deficiency that causes the inefficient use of vitamin B. If left untreated, an infant may experience hair loss, skin lesions, hearing loss, poor muscle tone, and developmental delay. After biotinidase deficiency is diagnosed, the treatment is to administer biotin orally.

Congenital adrenal hyperplasia is a genetic disorder that may occur in 1 out of every 15,000 births.[38] The condition causes a lack of the sugar-producing hormone, cortisol, and may also cause a lack of the salt-retaining hormone aldosterone. The affected newborn may develop severe dehydration and fail to gain weight. Treatment consists of giving cortisol and aldosterone.

Galactosemia may occur in 1 out of every 25,000 newborns.[38] If a baby has galactosemia, the body is unable to use a part of milk sugar called galactose. The resulting accumulation of galactose in the system can cause many

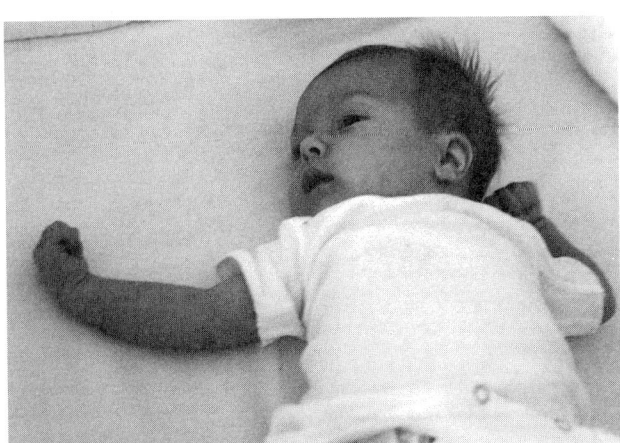

FIGURE 11-3
The tonic neck reflex of the newborn.

problems, including liver and brain damage. Treatment consists of a special diet.

Some states screen for the most common hemoglobin disorder, *sickle cell disease.* Sickle cell is a blood disease that causes pain and can damage vital organs. Early detection of sickle cell disease is the first step toward comprehensive health care, which includes treatment with an antibiotic, immunizations, and counseling. The treatment has prolonged and improved the quality of life for infants born with this disease.

The *PCR or polymerase chain reaction (HIV test)* is able to differentiate between antibody-positive neonates who do *not* have the immune deficiency virus (HIV) from neonates who do have the virus. Maternal HIV antibodies from a mother with HIV may persist in an infant's blood up to 15 months and obscure the diagnosis of human immunodeficiency infection.[28,44]

Assessment of Gestational Age

The size of a newborn does not necessarily reflect gestational age. A newborn is considered large for gestational age (LGA) if his or her weight is greater than the 90th percentile, and small for gestational age (SGA) if his or her weight is less than the 10th percentile for newborns of the same number of weeks' gestation at birth. A neonate is appropriate for gestational age if he or she falls within the 10th and 90th percentile. Premature refers to an neonate of less than 38 weeks' gestation, full-term refers to a neonate of 38 to 42 weeks, and post-term refers to one of greater than 42 weeks.

An infant's maturation and, therefore, his behavior, are a function of age, not just size. Clinical problems differ in infants of comparable weight but different gestational maturity. Preterm infants with normal weight for their gestational age may have problems such as respiratory and temperature control difficulties, feeding problems, and immature enzyme systems. Infants who are small for gestational age but full-term may have problems such as hypoglycemia, polycythemia, and hyperirritability.[27]

In 1977, Dubowitz and Dubowitz developed a gestational scale based on two categories: external characteristics and neurologic signs.[7] External characteristics include edema, skin texture, skin color, skin opacity, lanugo, sole creases, nipple formation, breast size, ear form, ear firmness, and genitalia. Some of the neurologic signs are posture, square window, ankle dorsiflexion, leg and arm recoil, popliteal angle, heel to ear, scarf sign, head lag, and ventral suspension. The nurse who studies these characteristics of the newborn gains skill in recognizing developmental differences in normal newborns.

The assessment produces the most accurate and reliable results when completed within the first 5 days of life. After the neurologic criteria and external criteria are scored, the total is added and plotted on a graph to determine the gestational age in weeks. Five criteria are considered especially useful and of value in estimating gestational age. They are assessments of the breasts, ears, genitalia, sole creases, and posture.

Special Procedures

Care of the Umbilical Stump

The clamp on the cord is usually removed within 24 to 36 hours. After the clamp has been removed, the stump is painted with triple dye or liberally soaked with 70% alcohol on a regular basis to promote drying. This can be done at each diaper change using a cotton ball saturated with alcohol. At the same time, the base of the stump should be cleaned with a cotton-tipped applicator soaked in alcohol.

Administration of Required Medication

Certain prophylactic medications are given to all neonates.

Eye Medication

A legal requirement for all newborns is to have a prophylactic drug instilled in their conjunctiva to prevent gonococcal or chlamydial eye infections (Fig. 11-4). These infections, called ophthalmia neonatorum, may cause blindness and are transmitted to the baby from the birth canal of infected mothers. Erythromycin or tetracycline ophthalmic products are used in place of silver nitrate because silver nitrate does not prevent chlamydial infections. Prophylactic eye care should be given shortly after birth. A delay of up to 1 hour is acceptable to allow the visual interaction between mother and baby known to facilitate mother–infant bonding. After the drug is instilled, there should be no attempt to clean the eyes for several hours.

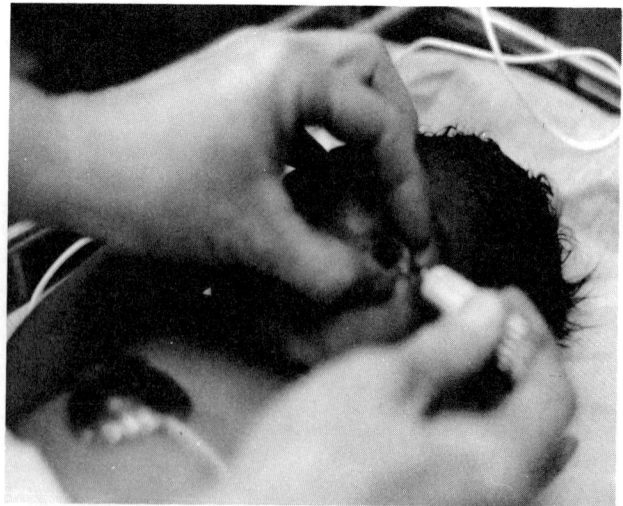

FIGURE 11-4
Ointment is applied to the newborn's eyes to prevent infection. (Reeder, S. J., Martin, L. L., & Koniak, D. (1992). *Maternity nursing: Family, newborn, and women's health care* (17th ed., p. 571). Philadelphia: J.B. Lippincott.)

Vitamin K—Bleeding Disorders

Newborns are susceptible to bleeding disorders because they lack adequate supplies of vitamin K during the first 3 to 4 days of life. Vitamin K is normally produced by bacterial action in the large bowel, but is absent in the newborn because the bowel is sterile. A single dose of vitamin K preparation is given within hours after birth in the anterolateral aspect of the baby's thigh (Fig. 11-5).

Identification Procedures

In the hospital, every mother and baby must be properly identified. Matching identification bands, which include the mother's full name and hospital number, the infant's sex, the date and time of birth, and a code number, are applied to the mother and infant. Some hospitals take a footprint and handprint of the baby to provide positive identification of the infant, because the arrangement of ridges on the prints is unique.

Registration of Birth

The registration of the baby's birth should be done before the infant leaves the hospital. The law requires that the birth attendant submit notification of the birth to the local registrar, with specified information about the infant's name, date of birth, and parents. Each state has its own certificate standard, and these records are legal documents filed with the state bureau of vital statistics.

Circumcision Procedures

A controversy remains concerning circumcision. The American Academy of Pediatrics stated in 1989[8] that some medical benefits and advantages do support the circumcision of male infants. Uncircumcised boys have a ten times greater risk of urinary tract infections.[8]

Epidemiologic studies have indicated that "an intact foreskin may predispose men to infection by human immunodeficiency virus-type 1 (HIV-1)."[42] An anatomic link between HIV-1 transmission and the foreskin has been identified in rhesus monkeys. Although all the research is certainly not completed at this time, it is suggested that the foreskin keeps the underlying skin on the penis a "fragile mucous membrane." When the foreskin is removed, the skin becomes keratinized and more resistant to trauma.[42]

The parents should discuss their feelings and collect data about the procedure before delivery. The decision regarding circumcision is a personal one each family must make. Some newborns are circumcised at home as part of a religious observance. Other parents feel circumcision is not necessary and do not want their child to experience the pain. Also, no surgical procedure is without potential complications.

The two major procedures are Gomco and Plastibell. A clamp is used in the *Gomco procedure*. A cut is made in the foreskin, exposing the glans. The foreskin is stretched over a circular metal cap that has been applied between the glans and the foreskin. It is tied, and the foreskin and glans are pulled through a hole at the end of a rectangular plate, compressing the foreskin against the inner metal cap. A screw-type device at the other end of the rectangular faceplate applies pressure to the foreskin causing it to be ischemic. The ischemic foreskin is removed with a scalpel. The device is removed in 3 to 5 minutes.

In the *Plastibell technique,* a Plastibell ring is applied over the glans after a cut in the foreskin. The foreskin is pulled back over the ring and a string is tied tightly over the foreskin and around the ring, acting as a tourniquet. Excess foreskin is trimmed. The handle of the ring is removed, leaving the string and ring in place. The foreskin extending beyond the string should sclerose and drop off within 10 days.

A *Freehand technique* is used when circumcision is performed after the neonatal period. The procedure involves surgical removal of the foreskin under general anesthesia. For physical and psychological reasons, elective circumcision is best performed between 12 and 18 months.

Nursing Implications

Before delivery, the nurse should be available to the parents to provide information that can help them make an informed choice. The nurse prepares the newborn for the procedure on a special restraining form (Fig. 11-6A).

After circumcision, the glans will be red, raw-looking, and sensitive until healed. If the Plastibell procedure has been used, the nurse regularly checks the operative site for signs of glans constriction such as unusual swelling or for cellulitis caused by a retained ring. In any procedure, the nurse provides the following care after circumcision (Fig. 11-6B).

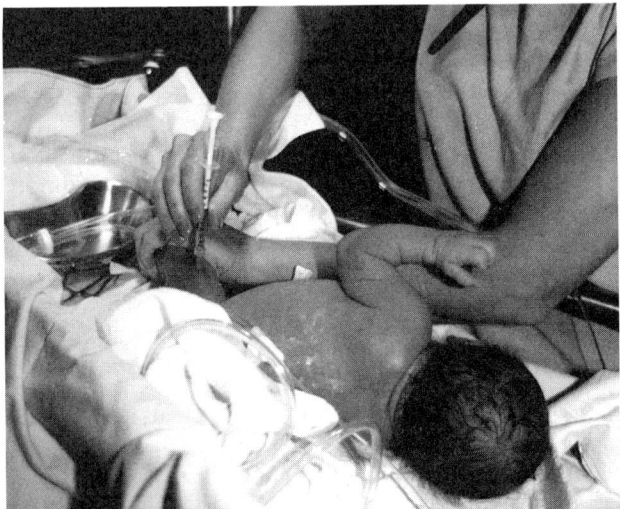

FIGURE 11-5
A vitamin K preparation is given to the newborn to prevent bleeding disorders. (Courtesy of the former Booth Maternity Center, Philadelphia.)

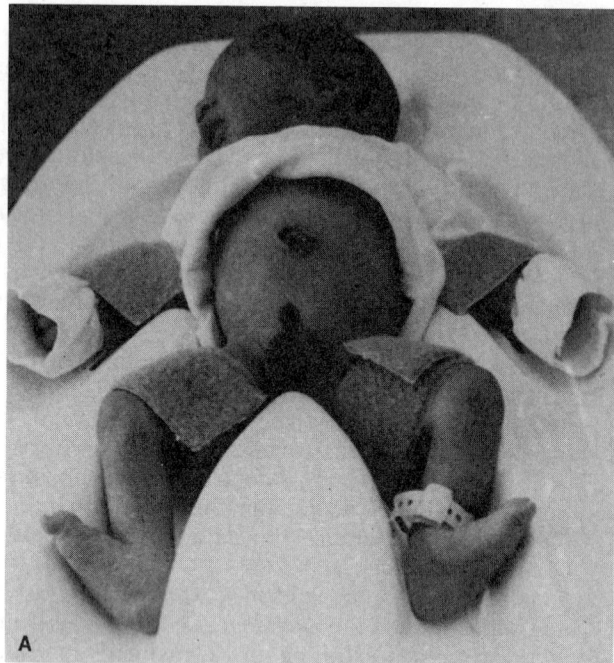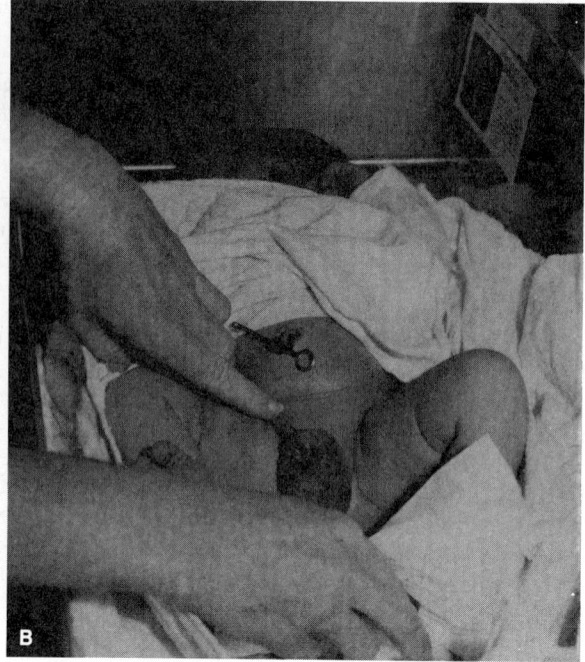

FIGURE 11-6

Nursing care for circumcision procedures. (**A**) The nurse places the newborn in a special restraint board in preparation for the procedure. (**B**) The nurse inspects the postcircumcised newborn regularly for hemorrhage, swelling, and infection. (Reeder, S. J., Martin, L. L., & Koniak, D. (1992). *Maternity nursing: Family, newborn, and women's health care* (17th ed., pp. 700–701). Philadelphia: J.B. Lippincott.)

- Keep the area clean and dry.
- Observe for hemorrhage or infection.
- Change the petroleum jelly dressing, as needed, maintaining it as a pressure dressing if that is its purpose.
- Keep the infant supine or side-lying for the first 12 to 18 hours.
- Change the diaper immediately after each voiding or defecation.
- Observe the infant's urinary pattern, particularly frequency, volume, force of stream, and pain or discomfort on voiding, for the first 2 to 3 days after the procedure.

Assessing, Promoting, and Maintaining Optimal Nutrition and Metabolism

Metabolism

The metabolic rate of the newborn is about twice that of the adult; this accounts for a cardiac output and respiratory rate that are twice the adult rate. The newborn is more vulnerable to heat loss because the body surface per unit weight is about three times greater than that of adults. Shortly after birth, the newborn's temperature falls several degrees because body temperature regulatory mechanisms are poor initially (immature hypothalamus, inability to shiver and perspire) and marked deviations in temperature occur.

The neonate passes through phases of instability in the first 6 to 8 hours after birth. The first phase lasts up to 30 minutes after birth, and the second phase occurs about the fourth to eighth hour after birth. During these periods, the infant is awake and responsive. During the second phase, there is usually gagging with regurgitation of mucus and maternal blood from the birth canal. A meconium stool is often passed, and the infant appears hungry and ready to suck.

Feeding

The newborn's first feeding is sterile water between 1 and 6 hours after birth. Water is given in case the feeding is aspirated, because water is readily absorbed by the lung tissue. Feeding the neonate when he is alert and responsive is important in facilitating a good intake and promoting elimination and the passage of meconium; in the normal newborn, this reduces the risk of hyperbilirubinemia. When the bilirubin in meconium is not excreted as stools, it may be reabsorbed in the circulatory system and may cause elevated bilirubin levels.

Breast-feeding is the recommended method of feeding for all babies. The Teaching Plan illustrates a nurse's participation in helping new parents adjust to breast-feeding. Breast-feeding should begin as soon after delivery as possible. Some babies go to breast easily, and others do not. The entire body of the baby should be turned toward the mother's breast with the mouth adjacent to the nipple. The baby must be awake, alert, hungry, and able to suck. In the initial hours and sometimes days after

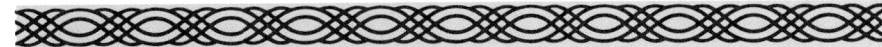

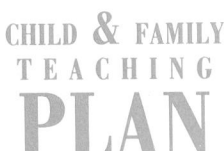

CHILD & FAMILY
TEACHING
PLAN

Breast-Feeding for New Parents

Assessment

The Stevens family consists of a 39-year-old mother, 40-year-old father, a newborn, and two sets of grandparents. This is the first grandchild for the maternal grandparents. The mother's pregnancy was complicated with low progesterone levels during the first trimester, gestational diabetes, pregnancy-induced hypertension and preeclampsia. The labor was long (19 hours), and medication was required to treat the hypertension. A vaginal delivery was possible, and the parents spent 1 hour with the newborn before she was sent to the nursery. The newborn weighed 6 lb, 9 oz at birth and was 19½ in long.

The newborn was healthy. The family used the rooming-in available on the maternity unit. The parents have decided to breast-feed the baby and have asked for help in learning how to breast-feed.

This teaching plan was developed as a strategy to address the nursing diagnosis, Anxiety related to lack of knowledge about breast-feeding.

Child and Family Objectives	Specific Content	Teaching Strategies
1. Discuss general concerns of families in the 1990s.	1. Content related to mother's roles, possible concerns guilt in working versus nonworking; changing roles of husband and wife; support groups available.	1. Allow parents an opportunity to discuss issues of concern to them as they prepare to take the baby home from the hospital.
2. Identify the selected method of newborn feeding.	2. Breast-feeding versus bottle-feeding. Allow time to explore concerns about the decision made. Include issues that will come up after discharge: • Breast milk appears thin and watery, and if it sits in a bottle the fat will separate. • Breast milk is easy to digest, and babies eat more often (1–1½ h). • Mother needs to eat a well-balanced diet and drink lots of fluids. • The amount of milk produced is related to the baby's need. The more the baby nurses, the more milk is produced.	2. Help the mother and father as needed in making an informed choice. Mothers need support during the early weeks of breast-feeding.
3. Apply demonstrated placement of baby for breast-feeding.	3. Positions for breast-feeding including the football hold and side to side. Assist mother in using her free hand to place the nipple in the baby's mouth.	3. Assist the mother in placing the baby to the breast; observe her method. Follow-up with each subsequent feeding.
4. Use demonstrated method for expressing milk from the breast.	4. Manual milk expression and use of a breast pump. Include information about storage of milk for later feedings when she is out or returns to work. Breast milk can be frozen (plastic bottles) and warmed when needed. Microwaving should not be used to thaw breast milk, because it destroys the immunity factors.	4. Use diagrams, models, and pumps to demonstrate hand expression of milk and the use of a breast pump.

(Continued)

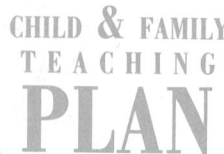

CHILD & FAMILY
T E A C H I N G
PLAN

Breast-Feeding for New Parents (continued)

Child and Family Objectives	Specific Content	Teaching Strategies
5. Discuss common concerns about breast-feeding.	5. Explore common myths and misconceptions about breast-feeding. Provide resource phone numbers for problems or questions that develop after discharge. Let the mother know that it takes time for the mother and baby to become an effective breast-feeding team.	5. Provide written information for the mother including phone numbers and names of local groups.
6. Recognize importance of support system in neonatal period.	6. Explore ways in which husband and maternal grandparents can offer assistance. Father can give supplemental feedings when mother is tired. Let mother know it is important to let others help.	6. Help support persons understand physical and social changes mother is experiencing: need for rest, time to bond with baby, ability to develop as a family unit.
7. Discuss use of birth control while breast-feeding.	7. Discuss the fact that breast-feeding does not prevent conception. Discuss couple's choice of birth control method.	7. Supply list or table of various contraceptive methods. Health care workers often do not recommend using the pill while breast-feeding. Women may want to continue using the pill. The 1981 American Academy of Pediatrics approved the use of oral contraceptives in lactating women after effective lactation is well established (by 4–6 wk). Although both estrogen and progestin may be found in breast milk, no significant adverse effects on infants have been shown with low-dose birth control pills. If the pill is the breast-feeding woman's choice, it appears to be appropriate to permit use.[14]

Evaluation

- Couple discusses issues that may affect family dynamics and create family tensions.
- Mother correctly places baby to breast.
- Couple discusses common myths and misconceptions about breast-feeding.
- Mother identifies community resources for breast-feeding.
- Mother uses a breast pump to express milk.
- Mother identifies support that would be helpful in making adjustments in neonatal period.
- Couple verbalize importance of using birth control while the mother breast-feeds.
- Couple select a birth control method.

birth, this may be difficult. Patience is important. Both the baby and mother can learn. During the first day or two, the breasts produce colostrum, a high protein milk that is a laxative and assists in the expulsion of meconium. Breast-feeding is discussed further in Chapter 12.

At birth, the newborn is usually in good nutritional balance if the mother has had an adequate diet. Nutritional needs are high, however, because of the newborn's rapid metabolic rate and growth (weight doubles in 4 to 5 months). Important growth also takes place in brain mass, which is reflected in a rapidly increasing head circumference. The head circumferences of malnourished infants have been found to be smaller than those who are well-nourished.

TABLE 11-5
Daily Fluid/Nutrient Requirements According to Age

Requirements	Age	Weight	24 Hours
Fluid	3 days	3.0 kg	80–100 cc/kg of body weight
	10 days	3.2 kg	125–150 cc/kg of body weight
	3 months	5.4 kg	140–160 cc/kg of body weight
Calorie	Birth to 6 months		115/kcal/kg of body weight
Protein	Birth to 6 months		2.2 g/kg of body weight

* Most formulas provide 20 kcal/oz.

For his size, the neonate requires more fluid, calories, and protein than an adult. By the end of a week or 10 days of life, the infant needs 80 calories per kilogram of body weight to gain well and often requires 100 to 120 calories per kilogram. Based on size, the greatest number of calories are needed between ages 14 and 28 days, a time often described as the "hungry period." The neonate requires more fluid because of a proportionately larger surface-to-volume ratio and a limited ability to form concentrated urine (Table 11-5).

Mothers in good physical condition (minimal problems during labor and delivery) who have positive feelings toward their babies and are experienced in infant care are more successful with feeding. These mothers probably have a heightened awareness of their newborn's individuality. The baby who sucks well and grows well makes the mother feel confident in her role as mother. If she breast-feeds her infant, she often concludes that her baby likes her milk and, by extension, likes or loves her. Not all babies are easily understood, however, and it is wrong to leave mothers feeling incompetent when they experience difficulties in caring for their baby.

Neonates show distinct individuality in temperament in the first weeks of life; this is independent of the parents' handling or their personality style. In addition, some neonates appear to have a smoother biologic transition than others. Undetectable differences in gastrointestinal function may cause discomfort for some in the process of digestion or the passage of stools.

Nursing Implications

Body Temperature

An essential nursing responsibility is helping the neonate maintain a normal body temperature. After delivery, the baby should be wiped dry but not bathed until his or her body temperature is stable; this takes about 6 to 8 hours. Overhead radiant heaters are useful in providing additional heat when needed.

Feeding

Developing a workable feeding situation is a shared search by both mother and infant. The nurse helps the new mother in this process. Feeding involves holding and positioning the neonate, making sure the baby is sucking adequately, knowing when the baby has had enough, and encouraging the mother to burp the baby during and after the feeding.

The baby's status at birth influences the ability to suck and feed. Not all infants are able to suck well at birth. Often a period of 3 or 4 days is needed for the infant and mother to develop a method for feeding. Forty percent of 600 infants studied had to be taught to suck in the following manner: the mouth was opened by the nurse or mother, the nipple inserted well inside the mouth cavity, and the chin of the baby worked rhythmically up and down. Infants also have individual patterns of sucking that include periods or "bursts" of sucking followed by pauses or rest periods.[11]

Both human milk and infant formula supply approximately 20 kilocalories per ounce. The baby should have an adequate intake, but not too much. The baby's general appearance and weight are valid indicators of intake.[37] Babies who are *not* gaining well appear dehydrated (depressed fontanel, poor skin turgor) and are listless, fussy, and irritable (see Nutritional Profile).

The newborn is weighed at birth and every day afterward (in the hospital) at the same time. A normal newborn loses 5% to 10% of birthweight in the first days after birth. This weight loss occurs because the infant is no longer influenced by maternal hormones (salt and fluid-retaining); the infant is also voiding, passing stools, and has a relatively low nutritional intake.

How does a mother know her baby is getting a sufficient intake of milk? In a study of breast-feeding women (N=88), approximately 32% of unsuccessful breast-feeders stated they had insufficient milk.[12] As long as the baby is wetting four to six diapers a day, sleeping adequately, and gaining at a steady rate, he or she is probably getting enough milk. Table 11-6 provides a guide for feeding and weight gain for the neonate.

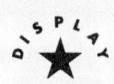

Developmental Nutritional Profiles of the Full-Term Neonate

Peristalsis and swallowing unstable
Hiccups after burping
Vigorous sucking elicited only when hungry, preceded by rooting movements; may stop sucking, rest, and even sleep for brief periods during a feeding
Definitely feels hunger and satiation
Crying and rooting movement indicates desire for food
Steady weight gain after first 4–5 days
Danger signals that may be organic or reactional to adult tensions are referable to GI tract (i.e., anorexia, failure to suck, vomiting, diarrhea)

Adapted from Kennedy-Caldwell, C., & Caldwell, M. (1986). Pediatric Enteral Nutrition. In J. Rombeau & M. Caldwell (ed) Parental Nutrition: Clinical Nutrition, Vol II, Philadelphia, WB Saunders, 434–479.

TABLE 11-6
Guide for Feeding and Weight Gain

Age	Amount of Each Feeding	Expected Weight Change
First 3 days	1 oz/day of life (sterile water is given for first feeding)	5% to 10% weight loss
10–14 days	2–3 oz/lb of body weight (if infant weighs 7 lb, takes 14–21 oz)	Regain birth weight
3–4 weeks	Approximately 3–4 oz/lb of body weight	Gain approximately 2 lb/mo

Spitting Up

The mother should be reassured that spitting up or regurgitating predigested milk is common in the early months. A large percentage of both breast- and bottle-fed babies spit up after nearly every feeding, but they gain weight and progress well in spite of it.[5] An immature gastric sphincter, too rapid ingestion of milk, or reverse peristalsis are common causes. For the bottle-fed baby, the nipple may be too soft or the hole too large; for the breast-fed baby a large amount of milk may be "let down" all at once, causing an episode of choking.

After feeding, young infants are placed on their right sides to permit breast milk/formula to flow toward the pyloric sphincter and to allow swallowed air to rise above the fluid and be released through the esophagus.

When feeding, the bottle-fed baby should always be held to provide closeness and avoid the risks of bottle propping. A bottle-fed baby ingests more air while sucking than does the breast-fed baby; the nipple of the bottle should be full of liquid at all times to avoid ingesting unnecessary air.

The baby may be burped *before* the feeding especially if he or she has been crying, halfway through the feeding, and at the end of the feeding. The baby is burped by placing him in a sitting position on the caretaker's lap or holding the baby upright, looking over the caregiver's shoulder, and massaging his back.

Broussard developed a neonatal perception inventory for the nurse to use in assessing the mother's concerns.[9] Below are questions that are worded to allow the mother to describe how much "bother" the baby causes.

- How much crying has your baby done?
- How much trouble has your baby had feeding?
- How much spitting up or vomiting has your baby done?
- How much difficulty has your baby had in sleeping?
- How much difficulty has your baby had with bowel movements?
- How much trouble has your baby had in settling down to a predictable pattern of eating and sleeping?

The nurse should avoid advising the mother to "not worry." If a mother rates her infant as having difficulty in any of these areas, further information should be obtained. The mother who identifies difficulties with feeding can be asked to keep records of the infant's feeding pattern for 3 days, noting the difficulties she experiences, the difficulties the infant experiences, how often they occur, how long the difficulties last, and what she does to alleviate the situation.[9]

Observing a feeding is also helpful. To prevent spitting up, the baby may be propped in a semi-upright position such as an infant seat *before* burping to allow the milk to settle. Frequent burping also helps to prevent spitting up; the bottle-fed baby should be burped after every ounce of formula, and the breast-feeding mother can hand-express the initial rush of milk so the breasts "let down" more evenly.

Assessing, Promoting, and Maintaining Optimal Elimination

Voiding and Stools

The infant's first void occurs within 12 to 24 hours after birth. After that, voiding may occur as often as 18 times a day. Meconium is passed within 24 hours in over 90% of babies; the passage of meconium occurs later for the baby who does not nurse or go to breast readily, the cesarean section baby, and the baby whose mother had pregnancy-induced hypertension (PIH). As a result, these babies are at greater risk for developing hyperbilirubinemia.

Stools

The number of stools varies during the first week. Transitional stools (thin, slimy, and brown to green because of the continued presence of meconium) are passed from the third to sixth day. Thereafter, the stools of breast-fed and bottle-fed babies differ. The stools of the breast-fed baby are loose, unformed, golden yellow, and non-irritating to the infant's skin. The bottle-fed baby has stools that are formed but soft, pale yellow, and irritating to the infant's skin. Babies on iron-enriched formula have stools with a greenish color and often have problems with constipation. The number of stools decreases in the first 2 weeks from five or six each day (after every feeding) to one or two per day.

Fluid Balance

Newborns require more fluid intake relative to their size than adults because of their proportionately larger surface-to-volume ratio and their relative inability to form concentrated urine during the first month of life. The rate of fluid intake and fluid excretion in the infant is seven times as great in relation to weight as in the adult, which means that even a slight alteration in fluid balance can cause rapidly developing abnormalities. The immaturity of the kidneys and large fluid turnover place the infant at risk for dehydration.

Diapers

Diapers come in two types: disposable and reusable cloth (e.g., flannel). Disposable diapers have the advantage of being more sanitary and more convenient than cloth diapers. However, they are relatively expensive, often unnecessarily perfumed, and considered an environmental hazard because they are not biodegradable. Cloth diapers are reusable, but care must be taken to launder them well. Some hospitals use disposable diapers, but many still use cloth.

Nursing Implications

One observation the nurse makes of the neonate is for signs of a functional gastrointestinal and urinary tracts. Is the infant voiding and passing stools?

Diaper Care. Diapers should be changed as soon as possible after an infant has voided or defecated to reduce the risk of perineal skin irritation or diaper rash. After voiding, the perineum should be cleansed with clear water. If feces are present, the area should be cleansed first with tissues. After fecal matter is removed, the perineum and buttocks should be cleansed with a soft cloth, soap, and water or commercial baby wipes. The clean area should be dried.

Applying lotions, creams, or powder before putting on a clean diaper is an individual decision. If the perineum and buttocks are clean, dry, and not red or irritated, such items are not necessary. Some hospitals routinely apply petroleum jelly or zinc ointment as a prophylactic measure.

Disposable diapers are applied using the attached sticky tabs. The most common techniques for applying cloth diapers are the triangular diaper method and the rectangular diaper method. To apply or remove a diaper, the infant should be placed supine on a flat surface protected with a plastic pad, or on a change table. A cloth diaper is removed by detaching the two safety pins, reclosing them, and placing them out of the infant's reach. The infant's lower body is raised off the surface by grasping both ankles in one hand and lifting up. The soiled diaper is removed, and the infant is laid back down. After cleansing, the infant should be relifted and a new diaper is applied. Diaper covers are available that eliminate the need for safety pins making them easy and safe for families to use.

Once the infant is safely rediapered and returned to the crib or infant seat, the dirty diaper should be discarded. Any large pieces of fecal matter on the diaper should be flushed down the toilet. Some disposable diapers have biodegradable inner liners to accommodate this type of disposal. The remainder of the disposable diaper should be rolled together and placed in a sealed garbage bag with other disposable diapers to reduce odor. Cloth diapers should be placed in a laundry bag used exclusively for diapers.

Diaper Rash. Diaper rash is caused by irritation. Diapers should be changed soon after soiling, and the diaper area should be cleansed (as above). The application of ointments at each diaper change or exposing the area to air aids healing. Cloth diapers must be washed in a mild soap and rinsed well. If irritation is caused by disposable diapers, a number of different brands may have to be tried. If the baby's bottom is extremely irritated, a bath may be comforting. Warm water may be used to cleanse the skin of any stool. Commercial wipes may sting and hurt, and wash cloths may be rough against the tender irritated skin. Lotrimin or other antifungal agents may be needed for severe diaper rash or yeast infections. The most severe type of diaper rash occurs when the area becomes infected, indurated (hardened), and tender. This type of rash requires medical advice and a specially prescribed ointment such as nystatin.

Assessing, Promoting, and Maintaining Optimal Activity and Rest

The newborn infant responds to touch and the environment according to his or her level of wakefulness or sleep. A newborn infant gestures, moves, cries, sleeps, and responds to parents with definite patterns and meanings. Gestures and movements were once thought to be without meaning, but research has shown that babies' movements have patterns. The amount of movement varies with each infant. Not only do infants show individuality in their movements and responses, but cultural practices and racial backgrounds affect the movements of the neonate. In the Russian culture, when infants are swaddled, they become quiet and exhibit little movement. Research on the activity levels show that Asian infants are less active at birth than other racial groups, and African American infants are generally more active.[22]

Sleeping Behaviors

Apparently unrelated activities of the newborn can be arranged into behavioral groups[5,9] and classified into six different states of consciousness.

Quiet Alert State. In the quiet alert state, the infant rarely moves, and the eyes are wide open, bright, and shiny (Fig. 11-7). Immediately after birth, the infant is in this state for an average of 40 minutes, a time when mutual gazing between mother and infant facilitates bonding. "Motor activity is suppressed and the baby's energy seems to be channeled into seeing and hearing—as though the mother and infant rehearsed for this meeting."[22 (p.9)]

Infants are in this state about 10% of the time during their first week of life.

Active Alert State. In the active alert state, the infant looks around with his eyes, moves his body and face in an active manner, and breathes irregularly. The infant in this state is easily disturbed by stimuli such as hunger pangs, noise, or being handled too much. Before feeding or at fussy times, an infant moves his arms and legs for a few minutes. Parents need to understand that many babies

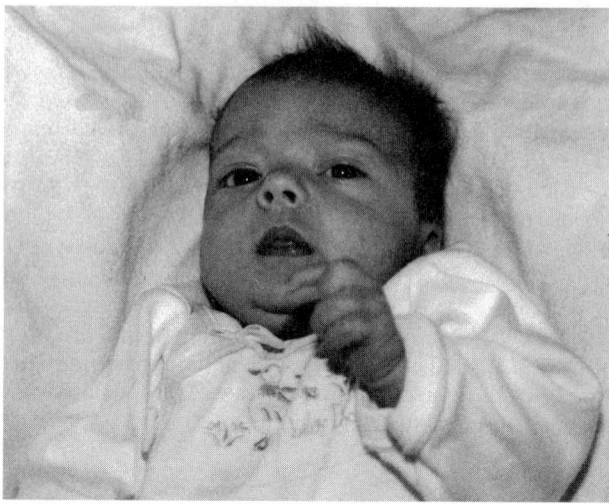

FIGURE 11-7
The quiet alert state of the neonate is characterized by the wide-open eyes.

console themselves if left alone, whereas others may need parental interventions.

Crying State. In the crying state, an infant's eyes may be tightly closed, his face contorted and red, his arms and legs moving actively, and breathing is irregular.

Drowsy State. In the drowsy state, the infant is either waking up or falling off to sleep. The infant sometimes smiles, frowns, and moves. The eyes are dull, glazed, and not focused, and the eyelids appear heavy. In this state, infants often fall asleep while feeding.

Quiet Sleep State. In the quiet sleep state, the infant's face is relaxed and still. The eyelids are closed, there are no body movements, and the pattern of breathing is regular. The infant is difficult to arouse in the quiet sleep state.

Active Sleep State. In this state, the infant's eyelids are closed, but a fluttering movement may be visible under the lids (rapid eye movement). The infant makes funny faces, smiles, makes sounds, or chomps his mouth as if nursing. The two sleep stages alternate about every 30 minutes.

Sleep Pattern

The typical newborn sleeps about 16 hours in a 24-hour period.

In the first weeks of life, infants awaken several times during the night to be fed. Most infants drop their nighttime feeding by 10 to 12 weeks of age. However, there are great differences in temperament and adaptive status of babies.

Nursing Implications

Knowledge of the activity levels of newborns helps parents understand and recognize when an infant is hun-

gry, overstimulated, or ready for play. Parents can be assisted to correlate their caregiving activities with their infants' sleep or wake states. For example, a whimpering infant in active sleep often returns to quiet sleep if left alone. Parents do not need to rush to feed or change an infant everytime the infant stirs.

Nurses should reassure parents that few infants are predictable in their sleeping patterns in the early weeks of life. As they mature, infants sleep for longer periods and a more predictable pattern emerges.

Massage

Massage offers a special kind of caring touching and is used with infants in many cultures.

Field[10] conducted a study of infant massage comparing preterm newborns receiving massage with a control group. Preterm newborns received massage three times a day. Despite almost identical milk intakes, the stimulated infants averaged 47% more weight gain per day than did the control infants.

Long gentle stroking motions should be used to massage a baby under 4 weeks of age; the massage flows from top to toe, starting at the head and flowing onto the face, neck, shoulders, arms, chest, belly, legs, and feet. A vegetable oil may be used on the baby's body (not the head); the oil is poured into the hand, held briefly to warm it, and smoothed onto the baby's body. Massage for about 10 minutes (more for older infants).

Assessing, Promoting, and Maintaining Optimal Role Relationships

The New Family

Going home with a new baby is a major hurdle. The changes in a couple's relationship and lifestyle are seldom anticipated before the baby's arrival. In addition to the rewards of caring for a new baby, there are also overwhelming feelings of being out of touch with the rest of the world. This is especially true for the first-time mother.[30] Some families may lack adequate support systems or lack the competencies necessary for the parental role. Others may face additional stresses because of unique situational demands such as low socioeconomic or inadequate support systems (see display).

The Mother

Whereas the rest of the family adapts psychologically, the mother has both psychological and physical adjustments to make. Rubin,[35] an early maternity nurse clinical researcher, determined there are three phases in maternal behavior, as outlined in the display.

As a mother practices her role, her image of herself depends heavily on her husband's estimation of her worth in her new role. If the husband does not value his wife as a mother, or competes with the children to be

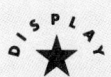

Parental Adjustments to the Neonate

Perception of Newborn

Planned or unplanned baby—wanted or unwanted
 baby
Appearance and physical condition of baby
Temperament of baby—difficult versus easy
Amount of "bother" caused by baby

Coping Ability

Self-esteem—own nurturing as a child
Marital status, relatives, friends, neighbors
Number of other children
Risk factors:
 Preexisting health problem (e.g., mental retar-
  dation)
 Poverty (e.g., inability to comply with health care)
 Role changes or conflicts (e.g., change in lifestyle)
 Situational crisis (e.g., teen pregnancy, single
  mother)
 Dysfunctional behavior (e.g., anxiety, depression,
  abuse)

Environmental Conditions

Housing interior and exterior facilities, condition
Community: services, transportation, safety

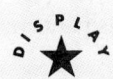

Rubin's Maternal Phases

Taking In: A Period of Dependent Behavior

- Focus on self
- Verbalization of need for sleep and food
- Reliving of birth experience
- Passive and dependent behavior

Taking Hold: Moving Between Dependence and Independence

- Widening of focus to include infant
- Independence in self-care activities
- Verbalized concern about body functions of self
  and infant
- Openness to teaching on care of self and infant
- Lack of confidence (mother is easily discour-
  aged about caretaking skills)

Letting Go: Taking on New Role Responsibilities

- Increasing independence in care of self and
  infant
- Recognition of infant as separate from self
- Grief work for relinquished roles, expectations
- Adjustments of family relationships to accom-
  modate infant

May, K. A., & Mahlmeister, L. R. (1990). Comprehensive maternity
nursing: Nursing process and the childbearing family *(2nd ed.),*
p. 865. Philadelphia: Lippincott. 1990.

mothered instead of giving her support in her relationship
with the children, the situation is more difficult.[20]

Mothers may choose to function between two extremes of mothering styles. In one, the mother lives relatively independently of the newborn baby, and sees the
baby as having an existence separate from hers; the
mother continues her life with few changes. On the other
hand, there is the mother whose baby physically and
emotionally becomes securely attached to her; the
mother's body and life become intertwined with the
baby's; she becomes the baby nourisher and the baby
comforter.

There are, of course, many points along the continuum between these two extremes. Each mother may feel
guilty or anxious that she is not mothering in the "right"
way. The woman who goes back to work, leaving the
baby with caretakers, may feel guilty about not breast-
feeding and caring for the baby herself. But, the mother
who immerses herself totally in motherhood may feel
frustrated and deprived of her former life. The concerns
of mothers during the puerperium (6 weeks after delivery) are varied and relate to the mother's body image,
role, psychological and social well-being.

The Father

"Most men feel both gratified and burdened by parenthood. Participation in childbirth classes and the birth

may be positive experiences for the father, but they do
not adequately prepare him for the level of reorganization
and adjustment required once the couple is home with
their new baby."[25] The father worries about financial matters and alternates between feeling exhilarated and overwhelmed by his new responsibilities. He often feels left
out by his wife's readjustment and her attention to the
baby. His own relationship with the new baby may still
be distant. He may be afraid to hold the baby; it "may
break."

His initial response to the baby depends on the part
he played in the birth experience, but little is known
about his response in the remaining neonatal period.
More research needs to focus on the father's adaptation
to parenthood.

The Siblings

Older children must adapt to feeling displaced while
the parents make a place in the family for the newborn.
Parents are often disappointed if an older child does not
delight in the baby. Although parents may explain the
differences between being a baby or being "big," a child
seldom is prepared for a new baby's functional level.

Noting the attention the baby requires and receives, the child may regress to infant behavior and wet his pants or demand to drink from a bottle.

An older child may harm the baby through play or "rough" handling; he may appear to love the baby excessively or show hostility toward his mother through direct physical or verbal attacks. He may be disappointed with the sex of his new sibling, feeling his choice was ignored.

Societal Attitudes

Being a mother is a full-time occupation that demands all one's intelligence, emotional resources, and capacity for speedy adjustment to new challenges. Brazelton[5] states a mother or father should be at home and in charge of his or her baby for at least the first 4 months, as an absolute minimum to feel the sense of self-esteem that comes from having made it through this early difficult period. But Brazelton[5] also recognizes that not all mothers and fathers are able to be on leave for 3 to 4 months. Several consumer groups are working to lengthen and strengthen maternity and paternity leave policies that support the family.

Cultural Differences

The general pattern in preindustrial societies is for the baby to be with and close to the mother, and to remain with her, day and night, for the postpartum weeks. The baby is often fixed to her body in one way or another, bound by shawls, slung in a net or special carrier, or wound into a strip of cloth that may actually also be her own dress, frequently in flesh-to-flesh contact.[6] In other societies, the new mother and baby are segregated from the rest of society; this pattern of seclusion of mother and baby is an important factor both for survival of the newborn and their "tuning in" to each other and their emotional bonding.

Nursing Implications

Nursing support of the new family should address personal, environmental, and social factors as well as give family-centered care. Mothers especially need help in identifying and resolving conflicts caused by their new role. They appreciate assistance such as exercises for getting their figures back into shape, help devising a schedule that provides free time and nap time, advice about nutritional needs for herself and the baby, and learning about when and how to start family planning.

The nurse facilitates sibling acceptance of the newborn if the hospital allows sibling visits. Under supervision, the sibling can hold the newborn (Fig. 11-8).

Siblings experiencing stress after the arrival of a new brother or sister should never be ridiculed for behavior that signals anxiety and feelings of displacement. Parents should focus on the older child as well as the baby and include him in caregiving activities. Both girls and boys seem to enjoy helping in the care of a substitute baby (doll). If a new activity is planned for the older child, (e.g., nursery school, toilet training), it should begin be-

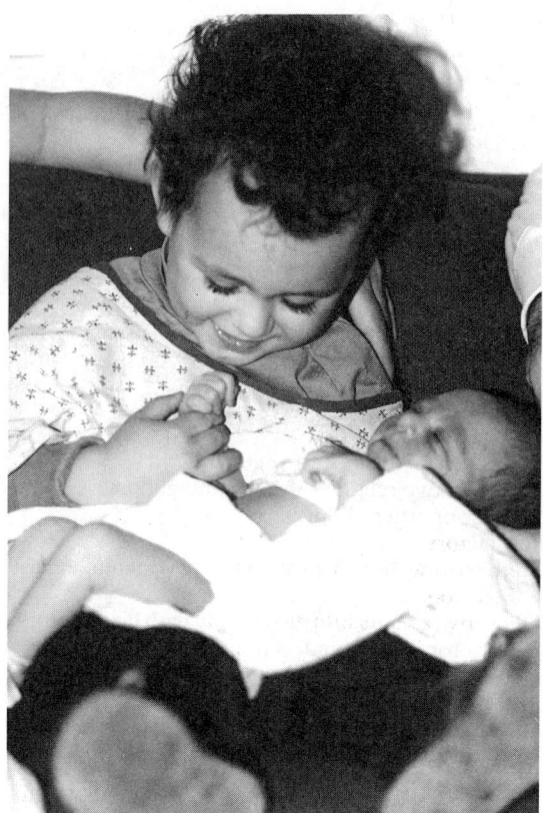

FIGURE 11-8
The older sibling will feel a special closeness to the newborn if allowed to hold and examine the newborn. (Courtesy of the former Booth Maternity Center, Philadelphia.)

fore the new baby is born or not until several months after the birth when the child has had a chance to adapt to the new baby.

The nurse may help siblings identify the mixed feelings they are experiencing. "Sometimes you will wish the baby wasn't here. You may wish the baby didn't take so much of your Mom's or Dad's time." Libraries offer excellent stories for young children with a new baby in the family. Sibling rivalry is also discussed in Chapter 14.

The nurse can link families with needed services such as counseling, nutrition, and childcare through local community programs (see display). Low-income families should always be assessed for basic assistance programs such as WIC (Women, Infant, Child Feeding Program) and food stamps. Many hospitals provide parenting classes or new baby groups for mothers and babies.[39]

Early hospital discharge (48 hours or less after delivery) has moved care for many new mothers and their babies into the home and the community for cost-containment reasons. This movement of care from the hospital into the home offers an opportunity for pediatric and community health nurses to expand their roles.[23] It provides an opportunity for involvement with new mothers and babies in the early days and weeks after discharge when most mothers and babies are "lost" to the health care system.[23,43] These mothers and babies usually have no health supervision until their first well-baby visit at 2 months or until the mother has her 6-week checkup.

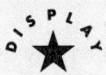

Resources for Support of Expanding Families

Nutrition

- WIC (supplemental food program for women, infants, children): Provides formula, food, and education to participants identified to be nutritionally at risk because of inadequate income or nutrition.
- Food Stamps: Provides direct assistance to low-income households by supplementing their food-purchasing ability.

Child Development

- Headstart: Offers comprehensive health, educational, nutritional, social services to children 3 years to school age and families who are economically disadvantaged.
- Adolescent Pregnancy Schools: Provides continuing education for mother, health care, and social services.

Home visiting permits the nurse to assess a family's housing status. Safety factors, cleanliness, size of the home in relation to family needs, and lack of basic facilities, such as working plumbing or refrigeration, can be identified. The nurse's definition of a "clean" home must often be reevaluated: a spotless environment is a clean home, but a cluttered home may be clean also. Concerns about the environment should focus on factors such as whether there are conditions producing health hazards (e.g., insects, rodents, inadequate facilities for hygiene, safety risks).

In summary, the types of assistance many families need and can be provided by visiting nurses include information and assistance for the following:

- Making the home a safe and nurturing environment for the infant.
- Providing nutritional guidance for the new mother and infant.
- Providing basic health services (physical and developmental assessments, immunizations).
- Linking the pregnant mother and family with an ongoing source of health care and social services as necessary.
- Teaching basic health care.
- Assisting families needing help integrating an infant into a family's structure and lifestyle.
- Identifying families at special risk and in need of services.
- Enhancing the parents' ability to stimulate the infant's social and cognitive development.
- Personalizing health care in ways not easily accomplished in the usual health care setting.

At a national level, nurses must advocate for parents and assure them of the importance of their early relationship with their baby. To do this, nurses must be certain businesses and professions don't penalize parents for family leaves.

The Attachment Process

The neonate's ability to adapt and grow depends on the responsiveness of the parents, especially the mother, in fostering an environment conducive to meeting his or her needs. The mother's ability to attach or bond to her newborn depends on her own state of health and well-being, her age, her desire for this child, and experiences in her own childhood. Physical and hormonal changes occurring within a mother's body also affect her responsiveness to her infant.[21]

The process of attachment is intricate and complex. Even before an infant is born, the attachment process may begin. For some mothers, the first movements of the fetus initiate feelings of attachment, which continue to develop throughout birth and the events surrounding delivery. Although no studies have been conducted, the increased use of ultrasound examinations during pregnancy may also be associated with earlier bonding. As mothers and fathers are informed earlier in the pregnancy regarding the sex of the child, the family is able to relate to the baby as "he" or "she" or by name.

Most literature considers birth and several days after birth as the critical time-limited sensitive period when a mother is particularly open to forming a relationship with her infant.[33] Immediate physical contact of mother and neonate is the most effective means of facilitating attachment, if their condition permits (Fig. 11-9). Grasping a parent's finger is one of the infant's earliest responses to the touch of his mother or father. Initial contact immediately after delivery finds the eyes of the mother and infant unconsciously trying to align themselves with each other (enface position). Gazing at one another is the first dialogue between mother and infant. This visual dialogue has a profound effect on the mother, making her feel closeness and affection for her newborn infant. These periods of visual attention occur throughout the neonatal period and help to draw parents to their infant.

The newborn's unique characteristics play an important role in fostering interaction between infant and parent. Crying is an infant behavior that some believe fosters the bonding process. Research studies demonstrate increases in the blood flow to the mother's breast when her infant is crying, indicating a biologic preparation for nursing.[16] If an infant cries excessively or refuses to suck, however, the mother experiences increased anxiety when still physically depleted and least able to tolerate this behavior.[17]

Some parents miss the early sensitive periods with their infants, and some do not experience immediate love for their infant. Almost all parents, however, become attached to their children. Their love does not occur immediately, but grows through caring, daily contact, and familiarity with their newborn infant. A variety of behav-

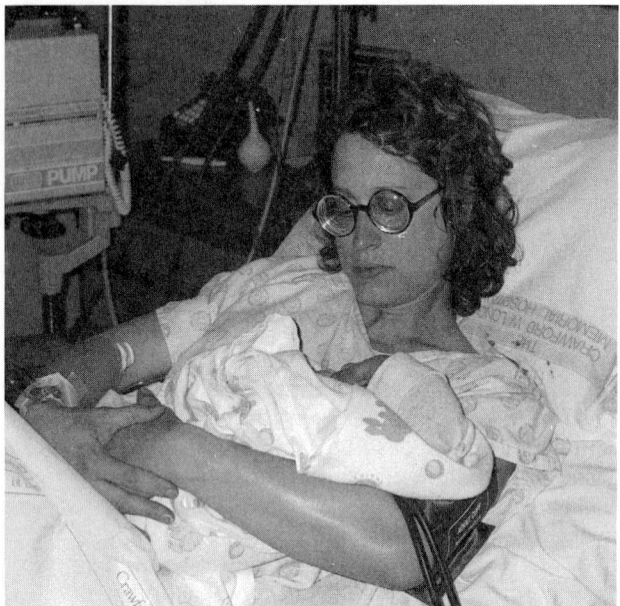

FIGURE 11-9
Mother–infant bonding is enhanced by early interactions between mother and newborn, but continues to develop over time. (Courtesy of the former Booth Maternity Center, Philadelphia.)

iors foster bonding between the infant and mother. Maternal behaviors include talking, touching, maternal heart sounds, breast-feeding, love language, and maternal odor. Infant behaviors include quiet alert state, crying, grasp reflex, startle reflex, and dependency state.[16]

The woman who is able to adapt to the mothering role, grow in her experiences, and whose infant does well has certain characteristics. They include the following:

- Past experience in caring for, and positive feelings about infants.
- A supportive mate and family members.
- A mother able to acknowledge her capabilities and independence.
- A level of hostility that is not excessive.
- A cognitive level of functioning that permits recognition of and understanding of her infant's behavior.
- An emotional level of maturity sufficient to delay her own gratification for the gratification of her infant.
- Perception that her infant is above average in comparison to other infants.[26]

Nursing Implications

The nurse facilities attachments by providing an opportunity for the mother, father, and newborn to be alone in a quiet environment after birth. The nurse can point out the individuality of their newborn, interpret signals for them, and encourage early physical contact. The nurse is in a unique position to foster and promote this bond by encouraging parents to touch, explore, and sense the wonder of this child who is theirs.

Because many mothers and normal newborns are discharged within 48 hours of delivery, it is important for the nurse to involve parents in caring for their baby as soon as possible. The nurse can offer general information about the behaviors and capabilities of infants as well as the unique characteristics and responses of the individual infant.

The nurse can teach the father by demonstrating care or by having him observe the mother in her care provision. The father can be encouraged to hold the baby properly under supervision. The father can cuddle the baby while giving a bottle feeding (Fig. 11-10). The nurse continues to assess each father and support him according to his individual needs.

Assessing, Promoting, and Maintaining Optimal Coping and Stress Tolerance

Behaviors

A systematic approach for assessing and rating infant behaviors has been developed by T. Berry Brazelton.[4] The Brazelton Neonatal Behavioral Assessment Scale requires observation and testing of a newborn, full-term infant. The main focus of the scale is on the observation and rating of an infant's interactive behavior. In addition, it helps to structure approaches for observing the subtle responses of the infant, how successful he is, the features he has that affect the response of others, and how he attempts to control his own environment. A neurologic component of the examination provides guidelines for observing and recording selected newborn reflexes. How does the infant's environment affect him and how does

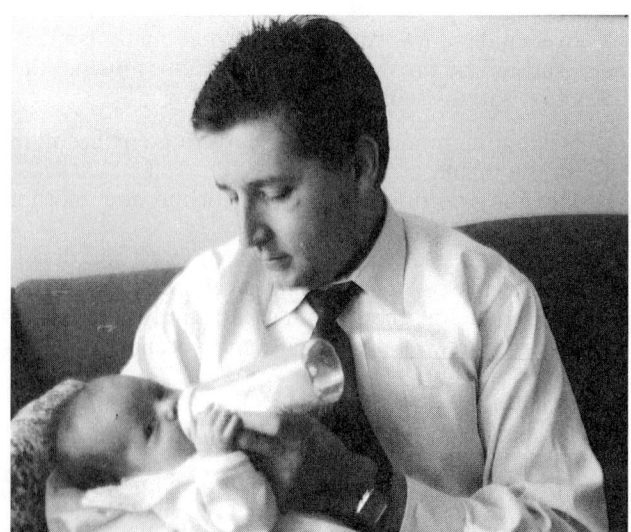

FIGURE 11-10
The relationship between father and newborn can be enhanced by the interactions promoted during contact between nurses and families in a variety of settings.

the infant respond? Most newborns habituate to repeated stimuli, especially disturbing ones. The infant who becomes more alert or agitated by disturbing stimuli probably needs further observations.

Repeated assessments using the scale up to the age of 1 month are considered to be more valuable than a single assessment; these observations provide information about how the infant is developing and adapting to meet his or her own needs. An assessment takes 20 or 30 minutes.[9] The scale includes items that require the repeated introduction of stimuli to an infant (e.g., response to rattle or light). To administer and score the scale accurately, an examiner must obtain special training.

All of the assessments for behavioral items are administered according to the infant's state or level of consciousness. The infant is observed as being able to console himself without assistance or as able to console himself only with the assistance of another person. Brazelton[5] suggests graduated approaches for consoling a fussy infant such as presenting the face alone; adding the voice; placing a hand on the abdomen; holding both of the baby's hands to limit his response; putting clothes or blankets on to minimize motor activity of hands and feet; picking up, rocking, and talking to see if the infant quiets down and stops crying; and using a pacifier after the previous measures have been initiated.

The Neonatal Behavioral Assessment Scale measures a set of infant behaviors that can be organized into six general categories.

- *Habituation.* Observations are made of how soon the infant diminishes responses to stimuli from light, sound, and a pinprick to the heel.
- *Orientation.* Auditory and visual items are presented to determine how much the infant attends to, focuses on, and responds to animate or inanimate stimuli.
- *Motor maturity.* Several items provide assessments of the degree of the infant's motor coordination and control over motor activities during the examination.
- *Variation.* Selected items assess the infant's rate and amount of change, as well as observations of his or her states, color, activity, and peaks of excitement.
- *Self-quieting abilities.* Items assess how much, how soon, and how effectively the infant is able to console himself when upset or distressed. This category includes the graduated intervention of the caregiver to quiet the infant.
- *Social behaviors.* Items assess the infant's smiling and amount of cuddling.

As a result of the work of Brazelton and others,[5,9] it is known that infants have the following abilities:

- They can shut out noxious sounds and stimuli they do not like.
- They can maintain attention for relatively long periods of time.
- They can coordinate certain motor movements.
- They can initiate activity and adapt to most situations.
- They can sense their needs and try to communicate them.
- They can quiet and console themselves in a stressful environment.

Crying

Excessive crying is especially disruptive to family patterns. When mothers are unable to console their crying infants, they may feel inadequate. Crying strongly affects parents physiologically. When they have to listen to persistent crying, their blood pressure rises, their breathing increases, and their palms sweat.[18]

Some mothers feel there is a danger of spoiling the infant, either by fussing over him too much or by indiscriminately "giving in" to demands for attention. But, some also believe some children are constitutionally difficult and especially demanding from birth. There is an impression of great inconsistency as parents make and break resolutions to not spoil an infant. Most health care providers agree that a newborn cannot be spoiled and that the newborn's cries indicate needs to be met through touch, food, or diapering.

Colic

Infants with colic cry for periods that total more than 2 hours a day because of abdominal pain or gas, or for unknown reasons. Milk-based formula may not be well-tolerated and a change to one containing hydrolyzed casein (Nutramigen) or soybean-base (Isomil) may facilitate digestion and decrease gastric discomfort.

Physiologically, gastric acidity and the enzyme pepsin are necessary to begin the digestion of milk before it enters the small intestine. At birth, the infant's level of gastric acidity is similar to the adult's, but within a week it decreases and may remain reduced for 2 to 3 months. This decreased gastric acidity may cause the disturbing symptoms of colic, which babies often outgrow by 3 months.

Nursing Implications

The nurse, although not specially trained with the Brazelton Scale, may use selected items, such as cuddliness and self-quieting, when discussing the behavior of a newborn with a mother; the nurse can help the mother understand the unique responses of her baby, her own reactions to the baby's behavior, and the feelings this behavior evokes.

Attempts to deal with a baby who cries excessively include changing the formula or, if the mother is breast-feeding, counseling her about reducing milk and dairy products in her diet or other potentially gas-producing foods; assessing intake for adequacy, excessiveness, or solid food; and offering advice about the behavioral reasons that babies cry. Crying is the infant's communication method. Newborns cry when they are hungry, tired, over-stimulated, or in pain. Crying is a sign of distress from the infant. The basis of trust develops at this time if the infant receives a positive response to his call. Table 11-7 lists actions the nurse can teach for consoling.

Infants are sensitive to touch and pressure. Skin contact and warmth, especially from the mother's body, are their most potent stimulation in the first few months of life. A baby soaks in feelings from handling; he can sense rough, inappropriate, or insufficient handling, and he ap-

TABLE 11-7
Parent Teaching: Crying and Consoling Actions

Interventions	Rationale
Rocking • Rock infant in arms, a rocker, a cradle, or hammock • Take the crying infant for a car ride	Infants like swinging movement.
Swaddling • Wrap the infant's arms tightly against the body with a receiving blanket	Infants feel secure with firm, steady pressure.
Sucking • Allow the infant to put hands in mouth and suck	Infants console themselves by sucking.
Talking softly • Speak softly and gaze into infant's eyes	Newborns love the sound of the human voice and enjoy viewing the human face.
Carrying • Carry infant in a sling or carrier	Infants cry less when held and carried often during the day. Holding an infant does not spoil him.
Changing positions • Change infant's position • Place a familiar object in front of baby	The baby may be uncomfortable from a piece of clothing or a new environment.
Seeking help • Seek help from family and neighbors	Parent needs to obtain relief from crying infant.

preciates touch suited to his needs. Many fussing or crying babies become quiet, alert, and interested when a hand is placed on their abdomens or their foot is firmly restrained. Swaddling is even more effective because it combines the quieting, soothing feeling of touch with firm, steady pressure.

Assessing, Promoting, and Maintaining Newborn Safety

Any caregiver with a skin infection, mucocutaneous (especially herpes) lesions, or a respiratory or intestinal infection is a threat to the health of the newborn. Protective care in the hospital or at home should include individual supplies, gowning or protection clothing, and handwashing before and after giving care. Handwashing should be routine after a diaper change, after using the toilet, or after touching any part of one's body, including face, hair, nose, mouth, or skin.

Immunity

The neonate at birth encounters a new environment and potentially dangerous pathogens. Antibodies that fight infection may be present in the neonate by diffusing from mother's blood by way of the placenta into the fetus, by developing as the response of exposure to organisms, or by being transferred from the mother to the neonate by breast-feeding. Infection during the neonatal period is different from infection during late infancy and child-

hood. Organisms that do not cause illness later in life may be pathogenic for the newborn. Nonspecific behavior such as hypothermia, lethargy, irritability, and disinterest in feeding may be the only signs of illness.

The most frequent causes of neonatal infections are the bacteria that comprise the normal flora of the mother's intestinal and genital tracts. Once an organism invades the neonate's system, a rapid progression occurs that often results in serious illness. The inflammatory response is less vigorous in the neonate than in children and adults because phagocytes (neutrophils, monocytes) cannot be mobilized in full strength.

The neonate's ability to produce an antibody immune response does provide protection against some bacteria such as pneumococci, streptococci, and staphylococci, and *Hemophilus influenzae.* No protection, however, is available for the enteric gram-negative agent, *Escherichia coli,* which often infects the neonate.

Safety Teaching

First-time parents need to be taught, and experienced mothers need a review, about newborn safety. The following are some of the concerns. A baby should never be left alone on any surface (including a sofa or bed) or in a wash basin or tub. Babies on flat surfaces should be held secure by a hand. Room temperature should be warm and draft-free. It is recommended that parents check the temperature of the hot water heater and keep the thermostat at 120°F. Cold water should be flushed through the tap after using the hot water to prevent a burn.

Concerns about a baby smothering are often inappropriate. The neonate can move his head from side to side to remove an object covering the nose and mouth, and can cross an arm over his face to push an object away. A nurse can demonstrate the baby's skills to the parents during the hospital stay or during a home visit.

Car Seats

A car seat is required equipment. Hospitals do not allow babies to be discharged unless a car seat is available. Most hospitals have programs that rent infant seats at reasonable rates. The seat should be positioned to face the rear of the car until the baby is a year old or weighs 20 lb. See Chapter 12 for additional information.

Assessing, Promoting, and Maintaining Health Perception and Health Management

Health Care

Bathing

A newborn infant is given a sponge bath until the umbilical cord falls off and heals. This usually occurs between 7 and 10 days. To prepare for the bath, the caregiver should gather the needed supplies: a mild soap, a clean washcloth, cotton balls, alcohol (for umbilicus), and a towel. Soap is never used on the face. The scalp is washed daily with soap and rinsed well to prevent cradle cap. A fine-toothed comb or brush helps to remove scales. Nurses can demonstrate bathing and ask the parents to return the demonstration. The nurse helps parents understand that bathtime is a special time when they can play (talk, sing, touch) with the baby as well as inspect and massage the baby.

Eyes. The eyes are cleansed with cotton balls, one for each eye. The cotton balls are dipped in clean water (no soap) and wiped from the inner to outer canthus in one stroke. The cotton ball is discarded, and the procedure is repeated on the other eye using a fresh cotton ball. As the infant gets older, the eyes can be cleaned with the corners of a clean washcloth. The principle of inner to outer canthus is followed, using a fresh corner of the washcloth for each eye.

Ears and Nose. Regular care of the ears and nose does not require special techniques. Ears can be cleansed with a cotton ball or clean washcloth. Only the external ear folds are washed. Cotton-tipped applicators (Q-tips) should *never* be inserted into the aural canal for cleansing or removal of wax because there is a risk of perforating the eardrum. Regular cleansing of the aural canal is unnecessary. If there is reason to suspect excessive wax accumulation, the ear should be examined by a physician. No regular hygiene practices are necessary for the nose. The sneezing reflex is present at birth and, barring upper respiratory infections, it is sufficient for maintaining a clear nasal passage. If slight crusting occurs, a cotton swab, twisted and moistened with water, can be used to clear the lower nasal passage. Cotton-tipped applicators (Q-tips) should never be inserted into the nose.

Genitals and Perineum. Both male and female newborns have a cheeselike sebaceous gland secretion called smegma in the creases and folds of the genitalia. Smegma appears in the labia of the female and under the prepuce of the penis in uncircumcised males. Smegma is removed from the labia by wiping the creases with a moist cotton ball, wiping from front to back, using a new cotton ball for each stroke. As retraction of the prepuce is usually contraindicated until the preschool years, doing so to remove smegma should only occur if the amount is substantial and causing irritation.

Rashes

A red rash may develop on the infant's face from rubbing the face against the sheets, especially if regurgitated stomach contents are not washed off promptly. Miliaria or "prickly heat" occurs in warm weather or when babies are overdressed or sleeping in an overheated room. This rash has clusters of pinpoint reddened papules with occasional vesicles and pustules; it is surrounded by a reddened area or erythema, which often appears on the neck first. The rash spreads upward to the ears and the face, or down onto the trunk. Helpful measures for infants with miliaria or "prickly heat" are bathing the infant twice a day during hot weather and adding a small amount of

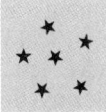

Ideas for Nursing Research

The nurse who interacts with new parents and newborns during the first month of life has an opportunity to explore a number of concerns with mothers, fathers, siblings, and other family members. The following areas need to be explored:

- Factors that are most beneficial in promoting beast-feeding for first-time mothers.
- Long-term impact of early discharge on newborn (and infant) care when mothers and babies leave the hospital between 12 and 48 hours after delivery.
- Comparison of adapting to a newborn between the older first-time mother (over 35) and a younger mother.
- Comparison of nursing strategies that promote learning in group sessions versus learning in individual teaching.
- Measurement of effects of institutions that offer home visiting to young families.
- Response of health care system to the problem of infant mortality.
- Comparison to maternal child benefits in other countries and their influence on health status.

baking soda to the bath water. The temperature of the room may also be reduced, and excessive clothing worn by the infant should be removed. Diaper rashes were discussed earlier in the chapter.

Care of the Umbilical Stump

The stump falls off within a week or 10 days, although a tenacious stump may hang on longer. Until the stump falls off, diapers should be folded down to expose the area and the infant should not be submerged in bathwater. Once the cord falls off, debris may be cleansed away for a day or two with a cotton ball or applicator soaked in alcohol. From then on, no special hygiene measures are necessary. If the area appears inflamed, or has a foul odor or exudate, a physician should be consulted.

Hispanic or African American mothers may place a coin or marble over the stump and wrap a binder around the baby to hold the object in place. They believe this practice prevents development of an umbilical hernia. Until the umbilical stump heals, covering the area with an object or binder should be discouraged to prevent potential infection. After the area is clean and dry, there is no risk with the mother using a belly-binder.

Summary

Birth is a natural maturational event. However, many adaptations must be made by the newborn in the first 24 hours and by the family during the neonatal period. As soon as the neonate establishes respirations, immediate assessments are made. More detailed assessments are made when the newborn is stable. These are critical to establishing which newborns are at risk or have actual problems. The support provided by nurses during this time helps new parents prepare for the months and years ahead. Parents may need help learning parenting skills and in developing family lifestyles. They need information about safety and resources available in the community.

References

1. Anderson, O. W. (1989). *The health services continuum in democratic states.* Ann Arbor, MI: Health Administration Press.

2. Avery, M. E., & Taeusch, H. W. (1984). *Schaffer's diseases of the newborn* (2nd ed.). Philadelphia: Saunders.

3. Boston Women's Health Book Collective. (1978). *Ourselves and our children. A book by and for parents.* New York: Random House.

4. Brazelton, T. B. (1973). The neonatal behavioral assessment scale. London: William Heinemann, Ltd., and Philadelphia: Lippincott.

5. Brazelton, T. B. (1981). *On becoming a family. The growth of attachment.* New York: Delacorte Press/Seymour Lawrence.

6. Dickenson-Hazard, N. (1992). The first through sixth years of life. In M. Stanhope & J. Lancaster (Eds.), *Community health nursing, process and practice for promoting health* (3rd ed., pp. 485–512). St. Louis: Mosby.

7. Dubowitz, L., & Dubowitz, V. (1977). *Gestational age of the newborn.* Reading, MA: Addison-Wesley.

8. Elsenberg, A., Murkoff, H., & Hathaway, S. (1989). *What to expect the first year.* New York: Workman.

9. Erickson, M. L. (1976). *Assessment and management of developmental changes in children.* St. Louis: Mosby.

10. Field, T. (1988). Simple soothers for LBW infants. *Pediatric Nursing, 13*(6), 385–387.

11. Grassley, J., & Davis, K. (1982, November/December). Common concerns of mothers who breast-feed. *American Journal of Maternal Child Nursing, 3*(6), 347–351.

12. Gulick, E. (1982, November/December). Informational correlates of successful breast-feeding. *American Journal of Maternal Child Nursing, 7*(6), 370–375.

13. Gundy, J. H. (1984). *Assessment of the child in primary health care.* New York: McGraw-Hill.

14. Hillard, P. J. (1991, August). Institute of Medicine Committee completes comprehensive review of available data on breast cancer and oral contraceptives. *Emron, Inc.: The Contraception Report, 2*(3), 11–12.

15. Hoekelman, R. A. (1992). *Primary pediatric care* (2nd ed.). St. Louis: Mosby.

16. Horowitz, J. A., Hughes, C. B., & Perdue, B. J. (1982). *Parents reassessed—A nursing perspective.* Englewood Cliffs, New Jersey: Prentice-Hall.

17. Illingworth, R. S. (1987). *The normal child.* London: Churchill Livingstone.

18. Jones, S. (1983). *Crying baby, sleepless nights.* New York: Warner Communications Company.

19. Judd, J. (1985). Assessing the newborn. *Nursing 85, 15*(2), 34–41.

20. Kitzinger, S. (1980). *Women as mothers.* New York: Vintage Books.

21. Klaus, M. H., & Kennell, J. H. (1976). *Maternal-infant bonding.* St. Louis: Mosby.

22. Klaus, M. H., & Klaus, P. H. (1985). *The amazing newborn.* Reading, Massachusetts: Wesley.

23. Luker, K., & Orr, J. (1985). *Health visiting.* Oxford: Blackwell.

24. Maisels, M. J., Gifford, K., Antie, C. E., & Leib, G. R. (1988, April). Jaundice in the healthy newborn infant: A new approach to an old problem. *Pediatrics, 81*(4), 505–510.

25. May K. A., & Mahlmeister, L. R. (1990). *Comprehensive maternity nursing: Nursing process and the childbearing family* (2nd ed., pp. 11–79). Philadelphia: Lippincott.

26. Mercer, R. T. (1977). *Nursing care for parents at risk.* Thorofare, New Jersey: Slack.

27. Miller, C. A., Fine, A., Adams-Taylor, S., & Schorr, L. B. (1986). *Monitoring children's health. Key indicators. Low birth weight infants* (p. 26). Washington, DC: American Public Health Association.

28. PCR: A new test for HIV. Clinical news. (1988). *American Journal of Nursing, 88*(9), 1172.

29. Petze, C. F. (1984). Health promotion for the well family. *Nursing Clinics of North America, 19*, 2.

30. Pridham, K. F. (1987, Summer). The meaning for mothers of a new infant: Relationship to maternal experience. *Maternal-Child Nursing Journal, 16*(2). Pittsburgh: Graduate Programs of Maternity Nursing and Nursing Care Children at the University of Pittsburgh.

31. Pringle, S. M., & Ramsey, B. E. (1982). *Promoting the health of children, a guide for caretakers and health care professionals.* St. Louis: Mosby.

32. Report of the Select Panel for the Promotion of Child Health (to the U.S. Congress and the Secretary of Health and Human Services). (1981). *Better health for our children: A national strategy,* Vol. 1. Washington, DC: U.S. Department of Health and Human Services.

33. Roberton, N. R. (1986). *Textbook of neonatology.* Edinburgh: Churchill Livingstone.

34. Ross Laboratories. (1987). *The first year caring for your baby.* Columbus, OH: Ross Growth and Development Series, Division of Abbott Laboratories.

35. Rubin, R. (1961, November). Basic maternal behavior. *Nursing Outlook, 9*(11), 683–686.

36. Simon, G., & Cohen, M. (1985). *The parent's pediatric companion.* New York: William Morrow.

37. Stahl, M. D. P., & Guida, D. (1984, March/April). Slow weight gain in the breast-fed infant: Management options. *Pediatric Nursing, 10*(2), 117–120, 164.

38. State of Illinois. (1988, June). *Checkup for life: Screen your newborn,* pp. 4-5. Springfield, IL: The Newborn Screening Program, Division of Family Health, Illinois Department of Public Health.

39. Stockwell, E. G., Swanson, D. A., & Wicks, J. W. (1988, March–April). Economic status differences in infant mortality by cause of death. *Public Health Reports, 103*(2), 135–142.

40. Tanner, J. M. (1978). *Foetus into man: Physical growth from conception to maturity.* London: Open Books.

41. Taubman, B. (1988, June). Parental counseling compared with elimination of cow's milk or soy milk protein for the treatment of infant colic syndrome: A randomized trial. *Pediatrics, 81*(6), 756–761.

42. Touchette, N. (1991). HIV-1 link prompts circumspection on circumcision. *Journal of NIH Research, 3*(7), 44, 46.

43. Trause, M. A. (1981). Extra postpartum contact: An assessment of the intervention and its effects. In V. L. Smeriglio (Ed.), *Newborns and parents* (pp. 65–87). Hillsdale, New Jersey: Lawrence Erlbaum.

44. U.S. Department of Health and Human Services. (August 21, 1987). Recommendations for prevention of HIV transmission in health-care settings. *MMWR. Morbidity and Mortality Weekly Report* [*Suppl.*], *36*(2S).

Health Assessment, Promotion, and Maintenance for Infants

BEHAVIORAL OBJECTIVES

Describe patterns of development of infants related to nutrition, elimination, sleep, psychosocial development, cognitive and language development, play and safety.

Identify common concerns of parents related to infant development.

Describe nursing assessment approaches with infants and parents related to development.

Describe nursing interventions to assist parents in promoting optimal development of infants.

Identify teaching needs of parents related to promoting optimal development of infants.

Discuss health maintenance needs of infants.

Infancy is defined as the first year of life. It is a time of dramatic growth and development. Optimal growth and development during infancy demand a nurturing, predictable, and consistent environment. Ideally, the environment includes supportive care providers who are sensitive to the infant's changing needs. These care providers are most commonly the infant's parents; however, in a changing society, the nurse encounters other primary care providers including but not limited to grandparents, foster parents, aunts, and uncles.

The needs of the infant can be discussed in relation to functional health. This approach provides the nurse with an organizing framework. This framework is beneficial in directing the assessments of infants and parents. These assessments provide the supporting data for actual and potential nursing diagnoses related to normal development. This framework can also be used to provide anticipatory guidance for parents on an ongoing basis. This chapter uses functional health as the basis for discussion of the role of the nurse in promoting optimal growth and development patterns during infancy.

Goals for optimal infant development during the first year include:

- Physical growth through the development of progressively sophisticated feeding patterns.
- Development of sleep patterns that reflect progressive neurophysiologic development.
- Development of consistent patterns of elimination.
- Development of a sense of trust.
- Development of relationships and attachments with parents and primary care providers.
- Development of interest in and interactions with the environment.
- Development of the ability for expression through crying, smiling, gesturing, pointing, and early verbalization.
- Refinement of motor skills from reflexive behaviors to purposeful movements, mobility, sitting, crawling, standing, reaching, grasping.

These developmental goals of infancy are best fostered by care providers who are aware of the specific needs of the infant and who interact with the infant in a reciprocal and affectionate way. Care providers should provide meaningful, varied, and developmentally appropriate experiences in their attempts to foster each area of growth and development. In some cases, the infant is placed in a day care center. This alternative is discussed in Chapter 14.

Parental responsibilities during the first year include:

- Promoting physical growth through provision of age-appropriate nutrition.
- Meeting infant needs related to elimination.
- Assisting the infant to develop healthy sleep patterns.
- Developing an affectionate relationship and attachment to the infant.
- Providing a variety of experiences and activities to foster psychosocial, cognitive, and motor development of the infant.
- Providing a safe, consistent, enriched environment for the infant.
- Initiating health promotion behaviors on behalf of the infant.

In their efforts to promote healthy infant development, parents have questions and concerns about the specific needs of the infant. Child health nurses need to be prepared to answer parents' questions and provide support and anticipatory guidance in a variety of settings including clinics, doctors, offices, health departments, homeless shelters, day care centers, and hospitals. The nurse must take the initiative in discussing development with parents and be ready to assist parents with concerns and questions for optimal infant development.

Assessing, Promoting, and Maintaining Optimal Nutrition

One of the first major decisions new parents make is how to provide nutrients for the newborn. In an effort to make the best choices for the child, parents seek information from nurses. Optimally, discussion of infant nutrition should begin in the prenatal period, giving parents an opportunity to discuss options for infant feeding and express concerns they may have. A discussion of the importance of nutrition for growth and development is an ideal starting point.

In the first month, parents may have many concerns and some parents experience difficulty in meeting their infant's nutritional needs. Even if a mother leaves the hospital breast-feeding an infant, there is no assurance that success will continue. Parents encounter problems and concerns at home that they had not considered while in the hospital. As early discharge increasingly becomes a reality, parents do not have as many opportunities to discuss their concerns or even identify their problems before discharge. Lactation specialists may provide mothers with phone support after discharge and refer parents to community groups for continued support in breast-feeding efforts. However, not all institutions employ lactation specialists and parents may go home without the support services they need. Parents who choose a commercially prepared formula are also frequently on their own after discharge. It is important, therefore, for the child health nurse to be prepared to discuss all aspects of nutrition.

Nutrition in the first year of life is critical in promoting optimal physical growth. During this time, the infant's birthweight triples. The infant must receive adequate nutrients to promote optimal development of all organ systems (see Developmental Nutritional Profile of the Infant). Lack of essential nutrients can result in reduced cognitive functioning, decreased motor abilities, and failure to master early developmental tasks.[18]

Feeding in the First 6 Months

For the first 6 months, the infant's diet should consist of either breast milk or commercially prepared formula that meets nutritional needs of the infant and is appropriate for the neurophysiologic level of development. The sucking and swallowing reflexes already present at birth are well-developed. When the infant's cheek or lips are touched, the rooting reflex is elicited, enabling the infant to find the nipple (Fig. 12-1). These reflexes are present for the first 3 months and are followed by continued neurophysiologic development in preparation for solids.

Choosing Breast-Feeding or Bottle-Feeding

The parents' choice to breast-feed or bottle-feed their newborn should be made only after they have an opportunity to explore the nutritional value of each method as well as the non-nutritional considerations that may impact on their decision. Nurses must be prepared to provide parents with the information and support they need to make this choice. Child health nurses must also be able to assist parents with concerns that arise related to feeding after the newborn period.

Nutritional Considerations. The nutritional needs of infants in the first 6 months can be provided by either human milk or modified cow's milk formula. However,

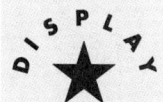

Developmental Nutritional Profile of the Infant

Infant at 1 Month

- Gain of 1 lb over birthweight
- Sucking when hungry still preceded by rooting movements; remains vigorous until hunger is appeased and is no longer interrupted by short catnaps
- Sucking desire present when not hungry; will accept pacifier
- Hunger constitutes powerful demand for attention
- Periodicity of need for food becoming regular
- Sensation of warmth and body contact enjoyed while eating

SAMPLE MENU: 2½ TO 4 OZ, SIX TO EIGHT FEEDINGS (IN 24 H)

5:00 A.M.	3 oz breast milk or formula
8:00 A.M.	3 oz
11:00 A.M.	3 oz
2:00 P.M.	3 oz
5:00 P.M.	3 oz
8:00 P.M.	3 oz
11:00 P.M.	3 oz
2:00 A.M.	3 oz
TOTAL	24 oz breast milk or formula

Infant at 4 Months

- Gain in weight rapid
- Peristalsis is usually in right direction and a little slower (less spitting up, stools less frequent, firmer)
- Sucking is strong and vigorous and is no longer preceded by rooting movements
- Sucks and "mouths" fingers and anything held in hands
- Shows excitement at sight of food
- Considerable spluttering with spoonfed food
- Comfort in being held when sucking milk

SAMPLE MENU

6:00 A.M.	6 oz breast milk or formula
10:00 A.M.	1 oz breast milk or formula mixed with 2 tablespoons (T) rice cereal (spoon fed)
	6 oz breast milk or formula
2:00 P.M.	1 oz breast milk or formula mixed with 2 T rice cereal (spoon-fed)
	6 oz breast milk or formula
6:00 P.M.	1 oz breast milk or formula mixed with 2 T rice cereal (spoon-fed)
	6 oz breast milk or formula
10:00 P.M.	5 oz breast milk or formula
TOTAL	32 oz breast milk or formula
	6 T rice cereal

Infant at 7 Months

- Weight gain in infant's own channel of growth
- Vigorous sucking, enjoys sucking milk but also sucks fingers and anything baby can put into mouth
- Constant drooling and chewing
- Taste preferences and will spit out food not liked
- Finger foods
- Interest in trying to hold bottle
- Both hands used to dive into bowl of food
- Few sips of water or juice taken from cup*
- Food put into mouth with fingers is chewed but may object to lumps in spoon-fed food

SAMPLE MENU

Breakfast	2 oz strained juice
	¼ white dry toast
	4½ T jar strained fruit
	4 oz breast milk or formula
	1 teething biscuit
Snack	1 teething biscuit
	2 oz strained juice
Lunch	2 T strained meat
	4½ T jar strained vegetable
	4½ T jar strained fruit
	6 oz breast milk or formula
Snack	4 oz breast milk or formula
Dinner	4 T strained meat
	4½2 T jar strained vegetable
	4½2 T jar strained fruit
	6 oz breast milk or formula
Bedtime	7 oz breast milk or formula
TOTAL	27 oz breast milk or formula
	9 T strained vegetables
	13½ T strained fruit
	6 T strained meat
	4 oz strained juice
	2 teething biscuits
	¼ white dry toast

* The baby is introduced to the cup between 5 and 6 months of age.

Infant at 9 Months

- Weight gain in own channel of growth
- Vigorous sucking
- Holds own bottle
- Interested in feeding self with hands
- Interested in chewing
- Interested in cup for water or juice

SAMPLE MENU

Breakfast	½ dry toast
	½ mashed banana
	6 oz breast milk or formula
Snack	2 oz strained juice
	2 salt-free saltines
Lunch	2½ T strained meat (beef)
	5 T strained or jr. vegetable (green beans)
	5 T strained or jr. vegetable (carrots)
	5 T strained or jr. fruit (pears)
	6 oz breast milk or formula
Snack	2 oz strained fruit juice
	4 T Cheerios

(Continued)

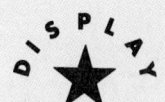

Developmental Nutritional Profile of the Infant (continued)

Dinner	2½ T strained meat (chicken)
	5 T strained or jr. vegetable (peas)
	2 T mashed potatoes
	5 T strained or jr. fruit
	6 oz breast milk or formula
Bedtime	6 oz breast milk or formula
TOTAL	24 oz breast milk or formula
	15 T strained or jr. vegetables
	4 oz strained fruit juice
	2 salt-free saltines
	5 T strained meat
	10 T strained or jr. fruit
	4 T Cheerios
	2 T mashed potato
	½ banana
	½ toast

Infant at 1 Year

- Triple birthweight
- Sucking is fading
- Anticipation on sight and smell of food; many also associate sounds with food
- Definite food preference
- Eats spoon-fed food well
- Wants to feed self with fingers
- Chews soft lumps in food

- Enjoys sucking and may insist on holding own bottle
- Prefers water or juice from cup and takes some swallows of milk from cup

SAMPLE MENU

Breakfast	6 T cereal/fruit combination
	½ dry toast
	8 oz breast milk or formula
Snack	2 oz strained fruit juice
Lunch	1/1 sandwich: 1 slice bread and ½ oz cheese
	6 T vegetable (carrots)
	½ mashed banana
	8 oz breast milk or formula
Snack	2 oz of strained fruit juice
Dinner	5 T jr. meat (turkey)
	6 T jr. vegetables (carrots)
	2 T rice
	1 apple wedge
	8 oz breast milk or formula
TOTAL	24 oz breast milk or formula
	1½ slice of bread and ½ oz cheese
	5 T jr. meat
	12 T jr. vegetables
	4 oz strained fruit juice
	6 T jr. cereal/fruit
	½ banana
	2 T rice
	1 apple wedge

Adapted from Kennedy-Caldwell, C., & Caldwell, M. (1986). Pediatric enteral nutrition. In Rombeau, J. & Caldwell, M. (ed.) Parenteral Nutrition: Clinical Nutrition. Vol. II. Philadelphia: W. B. Saunders, p. 434–479.
Sample menus adopted from Guide to Feeding Your Baby (1981). Nutrition Graphics. Cowallis, OR.

human milk is considered the ideal food because it is species-specific and is more uniquely suited for the infant's needs. The American Academy of Pediatrics[2] recommends breast-feeding for all full-term infants unless there are other problems including maternal illness such as tuberculosis or illnesses requiring chemotherapeutic agents. It is also discouraged in mothers who are on lithium or Valium, and mothers who abuse addictive drugs.

Human milk contains a host of immunologic components that protect the breast-feeding infant against infections.[28] In 1961, Hanson[30] identified the secretory form of IgA (SIgA) in human milk. The SIgA plays a role in the immunologic protection of mucous membranes of the human organism.[35] SIgA has also been found to provide immunologic protection of intestinal mucosa against bacterial and viral infection and the prevention of antigen penetration across the epithelial barrier.[35] Infants do not develop allergy to breast milk because SIgA in breast milk binds allergens and prevents their absorption. Breast milk, if free from contaminating bacteria, is readily available and maintained at an appropriate temperature. Breast milk

has been found to be nutritionally superior to commercially prepared formulas and more specific to infant needs. Further, the breast-fed infant is less likely to be overfed because milk intake is generally determined by the infant, whereas the formula-fed infant may be coaxed into finishing a bottle or taking a little more.

Commercially prepared formula is considered the substitute for human milk when breast-feeding is not chosen, unsuccessful, inappropriate, or stopped early. The American Academy of Pediatrics[2] in 1976 set standards for infant formulas to reflect the composition of human milk and avoid any undesirable nutrient-to-nutrient interaction. An iron-fortified commercially prepared formula offers all the nutrients the infant requires for the first 6 months. Formulas prepared for full-term infants provide 20 calories per ounce. Prepared formula does not provide immunologic protection and is more difficult to digest than breast milk. Because there is no SIgA, the infant does not have immunologic protection against viral and bacterial infection and has an increased risk of developing an allergy to formula.

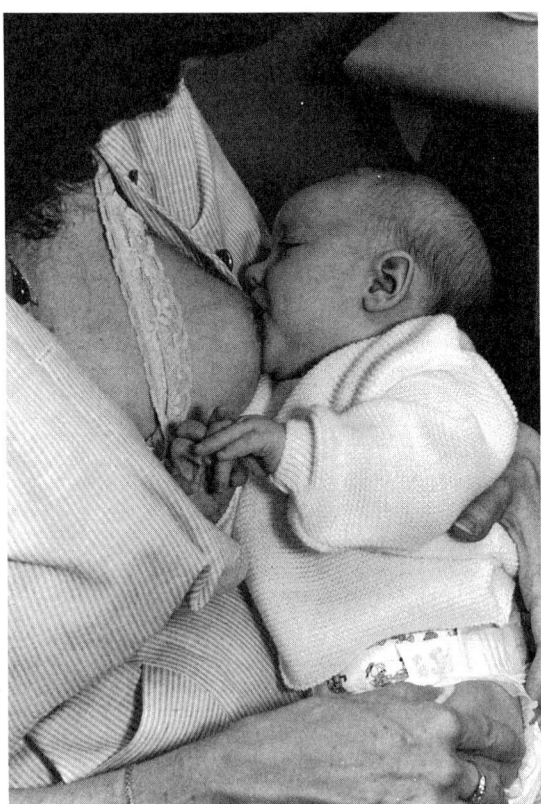

FIGURE 12-1
The rooting reflex enables the infant to find the nipple. Sucking and swallowing reflexes are well developed at birth.

A wide variety of infant formulas are available. Formulas may be based on modified cow's milk (SMA, Similac, Similac with Iron, and Enfamil with Iron) or on soybean isolate for infants who are allergic to cow's milk (Nursoy, Isomil, Prosobee, and I-Soyalac). Table 12-1 lists current infant formulas.

Specific formulas have been developed for infants with medical needs or inborn errors of metabolism (Progestimil and Nutramigen). Formulas for preterm infants contain more calories per ounce, most commonly 24 calories per ounce compared to the standard 20 calories per ounce found in formula for full-term infants.

Evaporated milk is concentrated cow milk and must be diluted before use. The traditional dilution is 13 oz evaporated milk and 19 oz water. Two tablespoonfuls of corn syrup (not honey) is added as an additional carbohydrate. When prepared properly, evaporated milk meets the nutritional needs of the infant.

Whole milk, skim milk, and 2% milk are always inappropriate for infants in the first 6 months. They do not meet the nutritional needs of the infant until a diet containing solid food is well established. Although the American Academy of Pediatrics Committee on Nutrition in 1983 found no harmful effects associated with the introduction of whole cow's milk after 6 months, more recent research has demonstrated significantly lower levels of serum ferritin values at 1 year of age in infants on whole milk compared to infants on iron-fortified formula.[57]

Non-nutritional Considerations. Breast milk is more economic than commercially prepared formulas with the only increased expense being the increased nutritional needs of the breast-feeding mother. Additionally, a working mother may also need to purchase or rent equipment including a breast pump, storage cooler, and infant bottles. Other considerations of the working mother who chooses to breast-feed include the conduciveness of the work environment to foster successful breast-feeding. Does the mother have a private area where she can pump her breasts? Is the mother allowed the time for this or is she expected to do this on her lunch break instead of eating? Is the mother willing to invest the extra time and planning it takes to work and breast-feed?

Prepared infant formulas can be costly in the ready-to-use form. However, they are less expensive in powder form and can be prepared by parents for a 24-hour period. Overconcentration and overdilution are common errors that can cause illness in the infant.[54] The need for preparation can be disadvantage for parents who have difficulty following directions. Formula preparation also requires a clean environment with equipment available to wash bottles and prepare formula without bacterial contamination.

If infant formulas are used, fathers, siblings, and grandparents can play a more active role in feeding the infant (Fig. 12-2). For the working mother, no changes are necessary in the work environment.

Evaporated milk is the least expensive infant formula available. However, preparation is more involved because of the need to add water and corn syrup in correct amounts. Low-income families for whom cost would be a major consideration are assisted by the Supplemental Food Program for Women, Infants and Children (WIC), which provides commercially prepared formula at little or no cost. Child health nurses who encounter parents using evaporated milk because of financial constraints or parents who are diluting formula to make it go further can assist parents in getting assistance through WIC. This program has been found to be beneficial to those enrolled; however, according to a recent national evaluation of the program, many children who would benefit from the program are not enrolled.[51]

Need for Supplements

Iron. Breast milk provides iron that is readily absorbed by the intestine. At birth, the infant has iron stores that are used during the first 4 months of life. Once these iron stores are depleted, the American Academy of Pediatrics[3] recommends iron supplementation of 1 mg/kg/day not to exceed 15 mg/day from the fourth month. This iron can be provided with infant vitamin preparations or by way of iron-fortified infant cereals.[1] A review of more recent research by Fomon[25] indicates that the bioavailability of iron in dried infant cereals is uncertain because of its exposure to oxygen. Based on this review, Fomon[25] recommends that wet-packed cereal and fruit combinations are the best choice once tolerance for individual ingredients is determined. These cereal and fruit com-

TABLE 12-1
Infant Formulas

Product	Manufacturer*	Kcal/ml	Osmolarity, mOsm/l	Renal Solute Load, mOsm/l	Protein, g/ml; Source
Milk-Based Formulas (for routine infant feeding)					
Breast milk		0.67	300	80	0.012; lactalbumin, casein
Similac 20 with Fe	Ross	0.67	290	108	0.015; skim milk
Enfamil 20 with Fe	Mead J	0.67	300	100	0.015; lactalbumin, skim milk
SMA 20	Wyeth	0.67	300	128	0.015; skim milk, demineralized whey
Similac Spec Care 20	Ross	0.67	250	129	0.018; lactalbumin, whey
Soy-Based Formulas (for lactose intolerance and galactosemia)					
Isomil	Ross	0.67	260	125	0.018; soy
Isomil SF	Ross	0.67	150	131	0.020; soy
ProSobee	Mead J	0.67	200	130	0.020; soy
Nursoy 20	Wyeth	0.67	296	172	0.021; soy
Special Formulas					
Pregestimil Hypoallergenic Intractable diarrhea	Mead J	0.67	350	120	0.019; casein hydrolysate
Nutramigen Hypoallergenic	Mead J	0.67	480	130	0.019; casein hydrolysate
Portagen Pancreatic insufficiency Hepatic insufficiency	Mead J	0.67	220	150	0.023; casein
Similac 24 with Fe Higher calorie	Ross	0.80	360	152	0.022; skim milk
SMA 24 Higher calorie Lower sodium	Wyeth	0.80	364	153	0.018; lactalbumin, casein
Similac 27† Higher calorie	Ross	0.90	410	170	0.025; skim milk
SMA 27† Higher calorie	Wyeth	0.90	416	123	0.020; lactalbumin casein
Similac PM 60/40 Low electrolyte/ low mineral	Ross	0.67	260	90	0.016; lactalbumin; casein
Formulas for Very Low Birthweight Infants					
Similac Special Care 24	Ross	0.80	300	156	0.022; lactalbumin
Enfamil Premature 24	Mead J	0.80	300	130	0.024; lactalbumin, skim milk
SMA 24 Preemie	Wyeth	0.80	268	175	0.020; lactalbumin, casein

MCT, medium-chain triglycerides; Na^+, sodium; K^+, potassium; Ca^{++}, calcium; phos, phosphorus; Fe, iron.
* Mead Johnson & Co, Evansville, IN: Ross Laboratories, Columbus, OH; Wyeth Laboratories, Philadelphia, PA.
† Protein content is higher than some infants can tolerate.
Weinsier, R. L., Heimburger, D. C., & Butterworth, C. E., Jr. (1989). *Handbook of clinical nutrition* (2nd ed.). St Louis: Mosby.

binations are not exposed to oxygen until they are opened, and the ascorbic acid added to these products actually enhances iron absorption.

Vitamin D.   Until recently, it was thought that breast-fed infants required vitamin D supplements daily because of the inadequate amount found in human milk. Vitamin D has been found to be present in breast milk as a water-soluble conjugate and in quantities sufficient for the infant.[29]

Fluoride.   Fluoride is supplemented in all infants because of its role in maintaining both enamel and resistance against tooth decay. Supplementation is in the form of infant drops or can be supplied by preparing formula with fluorinated water. The American Academy of

Carbohydrate, g/ml; Source	Fat, g/ml; Source	Na$^+$, mEq/ml	K$^+$, mEq/ml	Ca^{++}, mg/ml	Phos, mg/ml
0.070; lactose	0.038; human milk fat	0.007	0.014	0.68	0.28
0.072; lactose	0.036; coconut, soy	0.010	0.021	0.51	0.39
0.069; lactose	0.038; coconut, soy	0.008	0.018	0.46	0.31
0.072; lactose	0.036; coconut, oleo, safflower, soy	0.007	0.014	0.44	0.32
0.072; lactose, glucose polymers	0.037; MCT, soy, coconut	0.015	0.024	1.2	0.61
0.068; corn syrup, sucrose	0.037; soy, coconut	0.014	0.024	0.71	0.51
0.068; glucose polymers	0.036; soy, coconut	0.014	0.020	0.71	0.51
0.066; glucose polymers	0.035; soy, coconut	0.010	0.021	0.62	0.49
0.069; sucrose	0.036; oleo, coconut, safflower, soy	0.009	0.017	0.62	0.44
0.090; glucose polymers	0.027; corn 60%, MCT 40%	0.014	0.019	0.62	0.42
0.090; glucose polymers	0.026; corn	0.014	0.019	0.62	0.42
0.077; glucose polymers, lactose, sucrose	0.031; MCT 85%, corn	0.014	0.021	0.62	0.47
0.085; lactose	0.043; soy, coconut	0.015	0.028	0.73	0.57
0.086; lactose	0.043; oleo, coconut, safflower, soy	0.008	0.017	0.52	0.39
0.096; lactose	0.048; soy, coconut	0.017	0.032	0.82	0.64
0.097; lactose	0.048; oleo, coconut, sunflower, soy	0.009	0.019	0.59	0.44
0.069; lactose	0.037; soy, coconut	0.007	0.015	0.38	0.19
0.086; lactose, glucose polymers	0.044; MCT 50%, soy	0.018	0.029	1.46	0.73
0.089; lactose, glucose polymers	0.041; MCT 40%, coconut, soy	0.014	0.023	0.94	0.47
0.086; lactose, glucose polymers	0.044; MCT 10%, soy, coconut, oleo	0.014	0.020	0.78	0.42

Pediatrics[4] offers a schedule to be used for supplementation (Table 12-2). It is important for parents to discontinue fluoride drops when the child is drinking fluorinated water or when infant foods are prepared with fluorinated water.[26] Parents can find out if their water supply is fluorinated by contacting their local health department. Infants receiving iron-fortified formula need fluoride supplementation if their parents use premixed formula. If formula concentrate or powdered formula is prepared with fluorinated water, no supplement is necessary.

Promoting Successful Feeding Experiences: Nursing Implications

Because feeding is equated with perceived adequacy of the maternal role, mothers need to experience success

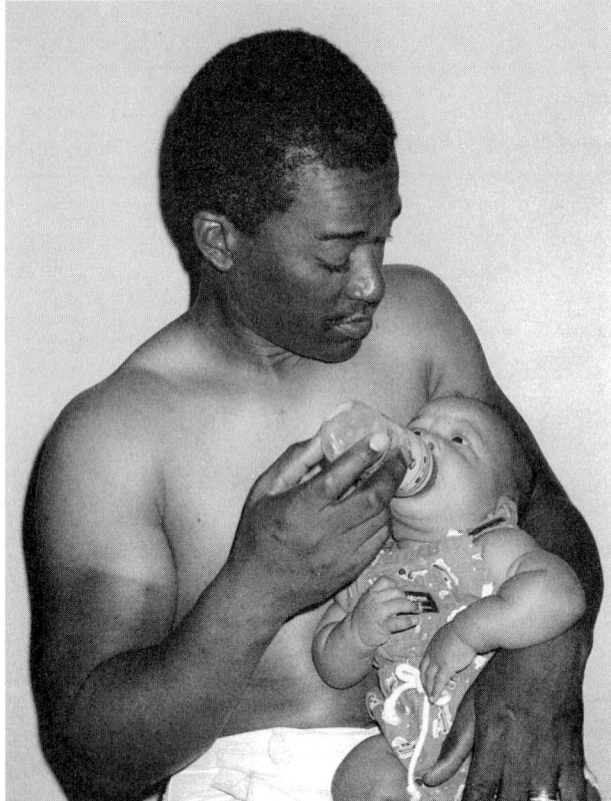

FIGURE 12-2
Father feeding his infant son.

with feeding. Increasingly, nurses with a special expertise or certification as lactation specialists are being introduced into the health care system. However, any nurse working with mothers and infants can play a crucial role in assisting mothers with appropriate feeding practices. Systematic observations of mothers' behaviors during initial feeding attempts can assist the nurse in identifying potential feeding problems and planning nursing interventions to promote positive feeding experiences. Observations of mothers during early feeding experiences should include the following:

*   Comfort in holding the infant.
*   Ability to insert the nipple.
*   Problem-solving efforts of the mother.

TABLE 12-2
Supplemental Fluoride Dosage Schedule

Age	Concentration of Fluoride in Drinking Water (ppm), Mg of Fluoride Per Day		
	<0.3	0.3–0.7	>0.7
2 weeks–2 years	0.25	0	0
2–3 years	0.50	0.25	0
3–16 years	1.00	0.50	0

With permission from American Academy of Pediatrics Committee on Nutrition. (1979). Fluoride Supplementation: Revised dosage schedule. *Pediatrics, 63,* 151.

*   Maternal satisfaction with the feeding experience.
*   Mother's ability to observe infant's state changes, readiness for feeding, time for termination.

If the mother demonstrates difficulties in her ability to feed, the nurse can discuss the mother's feelings of frustration and lack of success, and can assist the mother in identifying what the difficulties are and offer suggestions for their resolution. The nurse must discuss with parents assessments of the mother–infant feeding situation, and discuss methods that have been known to promote successful feeding experiences. Discussion alone may decrease maternal anxiety and facilitate a more successful experience. More specific instruction may be needed in relation to nipple insertion, position of infant, or comfort measures of the breast-feeding mother. Instruction in this area is most beneficial if, in addition to describing techniques to the mother, the nurse supports the mother in several feeding attempts until maternal skill and confidence are gained.

Mothers who elect to breast-feed may also experience concerns related to adequacy of their diet, loss of independence, concerns about adequate milk production, or dilemmas of continuing with breast-feeding while going back to work. The nurse should be prepared to listen to a mother's concerns and focus on her priority concern. A problem-solving approach related to maternal concerns is a key factor to continued efforts for success. Before offering concrete advice, nurses should respond to the mother with empathy, focusing on how the mother feels about what she is experiencing. Nurses need to collect data on what the mother has thought of, what has worked for her, and what she thinks is the best solution to her unique concern. The nurse must determine the amount and quality of the mother's support systems. Who does the mother consider to be most helpful when she experiences feelings of inadequacy, uncertainty, or is faced with problems?

The nurse is in a strategic position to promote and facilitate successful feeding. The key roles of the nurse include assessment, education, and support. Issues related to nutrition are part of prenatal care, postpartum care, and infant care throughout the first year. Parents come in contact with a variety of nurses during these three phases of parenting, and nutrition concerns are an ongoing part of the nurse's responsibility.

Assessing the extent of parental agreement regarding feeding allows for early intervention for parents who may have different beliefs regarding childrearing issues. Was the father involved in the choice of breast- versus bottle-feeding? How do the parents think feeding is progressing? Do the parents discuss the infant's progress? Do both parents initiate questions or ask for advice? What are the parents' overall perceptions of the feeding experience? Does the father feel an important role in the progress that is being made? Are there clues that he feels left out or included in the experience? Intervening early with parents who disagree about feeding procedures is not only important in the feeding of their infant but may be of help in future parenting decisions they make.

It is valuable for the nurse to interview and discuss with parents the infant's progress with feeding. Sharing with parents changes in infant height, weight, and head circumference gives the nurse an opportunity to explore with parents their beliefs as to what they expect and feel is optimal (Fig. 12-3). This early assessment of parents' perceptions can aid in health promotion. It also serves as the basis for prevention of problems associated with overfeeding or underfeeding. Parents can offer valuable clues associated with the risk for infant malnutrition or obesity. An example of such a clue is a set of parents who believe that a fat baby is a healthy baby. On the other extreme, nurses are seeing increasing numbers of parents who apply recommendations for decreased fat intake and decreased caloric intake in adults to the young infant. For

example, parents who are aware of the need to decrease their own fat intake may restrict the fat intake of an infant by feeding the infant skim milk rather than formula. Or parents who are concerned about obesity may overly restrict the infant's intake. Research[44,45] has documented this emerging trend toward nonorganic failure to thrive and parental health beliefs. Although the motive of the parents is to promote optimal health through nutrition, the result can be detrimental to the infant's well-being.

The nurse has a responsibility to assess physical parameters of nutrition through careful height, weight, and head circumference measurements. Charting of this in-

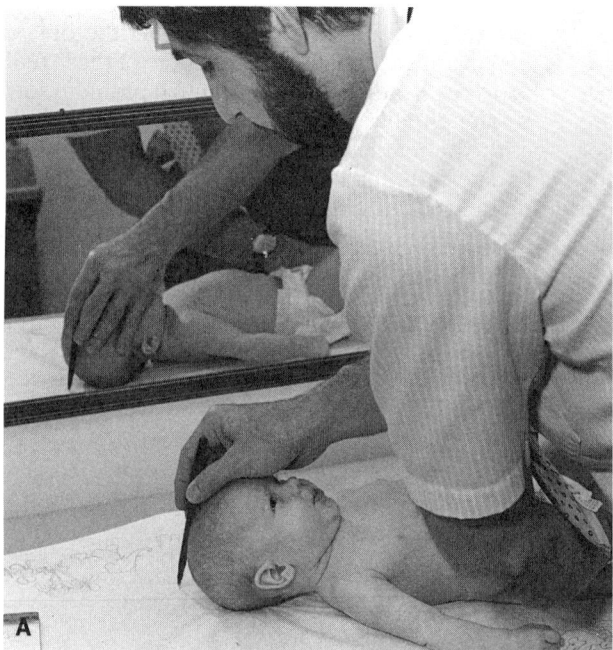

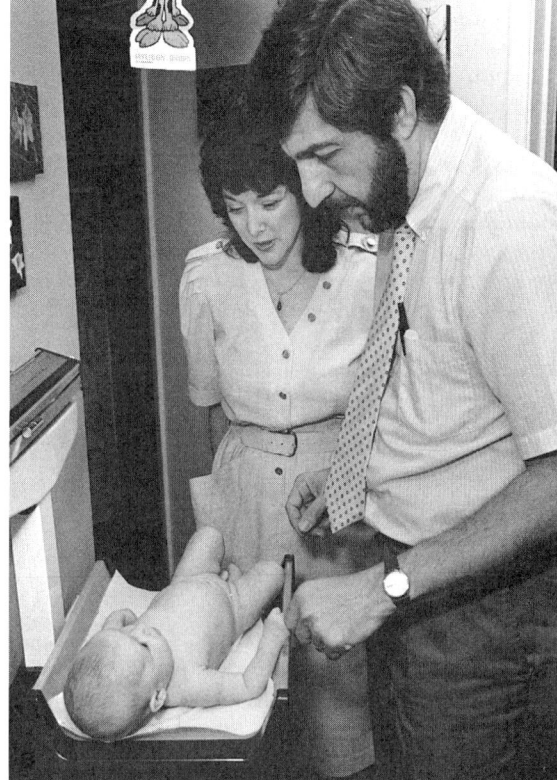

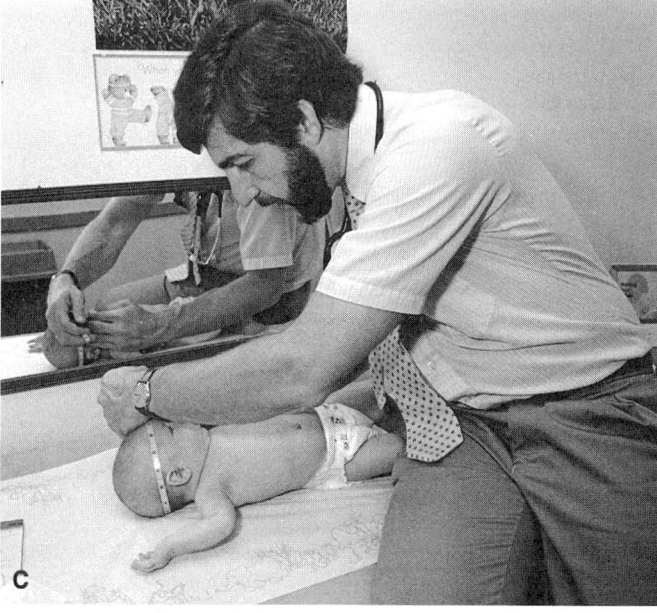

FIGURE 12-3

Measurements of height, weight, and head circumference are indices of growth and can be used to validate parental concerns about feedings. (**A**) Height is often measured by marking a surface area at the infant's head and heel, and then measuring the distance. (**B**) The infant is weighed without diapers. Note that the mother is involved during the data collection. (**C**) Head circumference should be measured at each well-baby visit.

formation is vital for repeated evaluation of growth on a serial basis. An essential component of the nurse's role is to educate parents about nutritional needs of infants and normal patterns and typical rates of physical growth. The nurse can share the infant's recorded height and weight and emphasize what is normally expected for an infant of a specific age. The nurse can explain height and weight in relationship to established norms of other infants. Nurses need to become accustomed to discussing height and weight in terms of percentiles and the significance of each physical parameter that is measured. Increasingly, nurses are providing individual height and weight forms so that parents can be objectively informed as to the infant's steady progress. (See Appendix—Growth Charts for Boys and Girls, Birth to 36 Months.)

Discussion of ongoing nutritional needs provides the nurse with an indication of the amount of support and education the parents need as the infant's nutritional needs change. (Questions for Nursing Assessment are listed in Table 12-3.) It also allows for investigation of parents' problem-solving skills and identification of any unrealistic expectations related to the frequency and amount of infant intake. Based on assessment data, the nurse and parents can develop a plan to resolve any identified problem or prevent potential problems. A time for a follow-up appointment or phone call should be made for parents so that the nurse can evaluate the effectiveness of the proposed plan. Parental feelings about the success of the plan and the identification of progress or unforeseen problems should be the focus of discussion. Ongoing support of parents, early identification of problems, and willingness to try alternative approaches by the nurse increase the chances of parental success.

Promoting Successful Breast-Feeding. Assessment of the mother's knowledge of breast-feeding, her attitudes toward breast-feeding, and her rationale for choosing breast-feeding should be completed. Optimally, this assessment should be performed during the prenatal period, after delivery, and again at the first visit with the pediatrician and child health nurse. Early detection of ambivalent feelings gives the nurse the opportunity to explore with the mother the source of these feelings and provides an atmosphere for mutual problem solving. Ambivalent feelings may be related to misinformation such as the belief that small breasts are unable to produce adequate milk, or it may be the result of more complex feelings such as the mother who is uncomfortable with breast-feeding because of the emphasis on the sexual nature of the breast in our culture. Whatever the cause of ambivalence, the success of breast-feeding depends on the nurse's skills in assessment and support to mothers.

TABLE 12-3
Nursing Assessment: Questions for Assessing Patterns of Nutrition in the First 6 Months

Area of Assessment	Key Questions
Parental expressions of satisfaction with choice of feeding method chosen	What led you to choose breast/formula feeding and how is it going?
Parents expressions of satisfaction with present feeding behaviors of their infant	Tell me, how is _____ doing with feeding?
Extent of parental agreement of the best approaches to meet nutritional needs of the infant	How does _____'s father feel the feeding is going?
Adequacy of parental knowledge regarding ongoing nutritional needs of their infant	Do you anticipate any changes in _____'s nutritional needs in the near future?
Parents' perception of adequacy of nutrition provided by other caregivers	How does _____ react when fed by other caregivers?
Parental perception of infant's height, and weight (overweight, underweight, optimal weight)	What do you think of _____'s height and weight today?
Maternal ability to recognize cues of hunger	How does _____ let you know when he is hungry?
Maternal ability to recognize cues of satiation	How does _____ let you know when he has had enough?
Mother's awareness of infant's ability to regulate intake	Does _____'s intake vary from feeding to feeding?
Scheduled or demand feeding	How often does _____ eat? Is he on a particular schedule?
Identification of parental concerns related to infant feeding	Do you have any concerns about _____'s feeding behavior?
Parental problem-solving efforts for identified areas of concern	You have mentioned _____ as a concern. What have you tried so far and how has it worked?
Parental expectations of changes in infant feeding behaviors	Do you anticipate any changes in feeding in the near future?
Maternal estimate of adequacy of nutritional status to meet nutritional needs of infant	How satisfied are you with your own diet in meeting needs for successful breast-feeding?
Evaluation of adequacy of maternal diet for successful breast-feeding	Would you give me an example of your diet by telling me everything you ate and drank yesterday?
Parental descriptions of infant's social responses during feeding (eye contact, alertness, smiling, responsiveness)	Would you describe for me the way _____ indicates pleasure during feedings?
Parental description of infant temperament during feeding	Some infants are easier to feed than others. What are some of _____'s behaviors? (fussy, irritable)
Assessment of support to mother	Most mothers want to do the best they can in feeding their infants and seek others for advice. Who has been the most support to you during your feeding experiences with _____?

Even in situations where parents have a strong commitment to breast-feeding, success is not guaranteed. Early discharge after delivery does not allow for the time it takes for a mother to become truly comfortable with breast-feeding. Often, problems arise shortly after the mother goes home, resulting in the discontinuance of breast-feeding. The child health nurse must be sensitive to parental expressions of satisfaction with breast-feeding and also alert to potential problems that may arise that are specific to the mother. A discussion of the proper care of the breast and how to deal with sore or cracked nipples is frequently done during the postpartum stay. Because this is a time when parents are learning so much about their infant, this information may not be absorbed. Topics including nipple care, sore nipples, and cracked nipples should be addressed again during the first well-care visit for the infant.

Nipple care involves cleansing with plain water, avoiding ointments, and using both breasts in every feeding experience. Even with proper care, sore nipples are a frequent concern of mothers.

Sore Nipples. It is common in the first few days of nursing for the mother to experience some discomfort when the nipple is initially grasped and sucked. As lactation becomes established, this discomfort decreases. Sore nipples may also be a result of improper positioning during feeding. The mother should support her breast with her hand, and the infant should be squarely facing the breast. When soreness is due to tender tissue, dry heat between feedings may help. Dry heat can be applied through the use of an electric lamp with a 60-W bulb, 18 inches from the breast for 15 to 20 minutes. A hairdryer on low or warm setting has also been found to bring comfort when held 6 to 10 inches from the breast.

Cracked Nipples. Cracked nipples can also be of concern to the breast-feeding mother. When a mother complains of pain, the nipples should be inspected under adequate light to observe for cracks or subepithelial petechiae, which may be a precursor of cracking. A history of the mother's present breast care regimen is important to identify self-prescribed treatments. As with sore nipples, an observation of the feeding position is helpful. In the precracked stage dry heat, as described above, is most effective. If the nipples are cracked, treatment must be instituted. Recommended treatment includes feeding the infant on the unaffected side first, allowing for let-down to occur automatically in the affected breast. While the infant is nursing on the unaffected side, the affected side should be exposed to air. Heat treatments are useful in promoting healing. Ointments that must be removed before feeding are contraindicated due to the likelihood of increased trauma.

Along with interviewing, direct observation is extremely valuable in assessing mother–infant feeding interactions. Behaviors to observe are listed in Table 12-4. Through observation, the nurse can validate what the parents have reported and can identify contributing factors to problems parents have described. Observation is only useful if the nurse knows what to look for and the significance of the behaviors of both mother and infant.

The key to observation is a planned, objective, and systematic approach. Observation should include mother's responsiveness to infant's cues of hunger, the

TABLE 12-4
Nursing Assessment: Observation of Infant Feeding

Parental Behavior	Infant Behavior
Social interactions with infant	Readiness for feeding
En face position	Rooting, sucking, and mouthing movements
Eye contact	Alert state
Smiling	Searching with eyes
Talking to infant	Observes mother
Rocking	Social interactions
Touching	Makes eye contact
Caressing	Smiles
Maternal levels of comfort	Feeding behavior
Relaxed position	Accepts nipple
Contact of infant to mother's body	Sucks vigorously
Rhythmic, unhurried manner	Pauses during sucks
Relaxed facial expression	Remains alert
Changes feeding sides	Termination of feeding
Responsiveness to infant	State change of alertness
Observes infant's readiness to eat—feeds infant when rooting	Turns head away
Changes pace according to infant rhythm	Decreases suck
Stops feeding if infant rejects efforts	Smiles, content
• Looks away	Body relaxes
• Stop sucking	
• Spits out food	
Burps infant at regular intervals	

quality of mother–infant interaction, and the responsiveness of the infant to the mother (Fig. 12-4). Discrepancies between parents' perceptions and nurse's observations should be noted and discussed. Parents find it helpful if the nurse begins by making reference to positive behaviors that were noted, rather than focusing on negative traits or deficits that were seen.

Assessment must be an ongoing process because making a decision to breast-feed and initiating breast-feeding does not ensure continued success. The nurse must continue to assess the progress, problems, and feelings the parents experience. The nurse has a direct influence on the success a mother has by the information provided, how it is provided, and the quality of support offered. Offering anticipatory guidance as well as ongoing support to breast-feeding mothers facilitates success. See Table 12-5 for ideas for anticipatory guidance. Child health nurses must also assume responsibility in this process.

Maternal comfort in seeking assistance rather than giving up is directly related to the third role of the nurse, support. Emotional support offered by the nurse is vital to the mother. The nurse who encourages mothers and actively helps them solve the problems of breast-feeding may enhance maternal self-confidence in feeding. The amount and type of support necessary for each individual mother depend on assessment of maternal comfort with her choice to breast-feed, her ability to respond to problems that arise, and the availability and quality of other support people such as husband, mother, or friend. The amount of support necessary can vary from an occasional

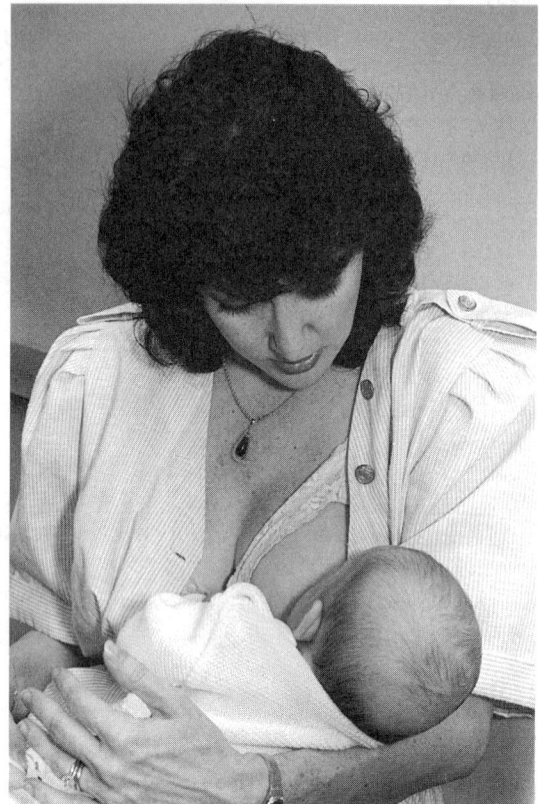

FIGURE 12-4
Observation of mother–infant feeding situations is important in validating behaviors and in identifying problems.

phone call to frequent visits and coaching in the breast-feeding process.

Early Discontinuance of Breast-Feeding. Although there are increasing numbers of women choosing to breast-feed their infants, many stop breast-feeding a short time after delivery. Chapman and coworkers[17] reported concerns described by breast-feeding mothers that are common from birth to 4 months. These concerns were divided into three categories including breast concerns, infant concerns, and postpartum concerns. Breast concerns were related to adequacy of milk, sore nipples, frequency of breast-feeding, infant developing a preference for one breast, and expressing and saving milk. Infant concerns centered around behaviors such as fussiness, sleepiness, day–night confusion, rashes, too rapid or too slow weight gain, and upper respiratory problems. Postpartum concerns expressed were fatigue, adjustment of siblings, adjustment involved in returning to work or school, lack of weight loss, and upper respiratory infections.

These concerns may increase maternal anxiety beginning a cycle that is difficult to break. Mothers may discontinue breast-feeding and begin feeding the infant commercially prepared formula. To decrease the incidence of early discontinuance of breast-feeding, the nurse must be alert to those concerns that influence the mother's decision. Early intervention includes adequate preparation of mothers who choose to breast-feed, discussion of common concerns described by others who have breast-

TABLE 12-5
Nursing Intervention: Anticipatory Guidance for Breast-Feeding Mothers

Beginning to breast-feed	Depending on mother's condition may begin shortly after delivery. The newborn is usually awake and alert for the first hour.
	Mother must be comfortable.
	Infant placed at level of breast.
	Milk production depends on nipple stimulation. Infant should be fed frequently until milk production is well established.
Feeding schedule	Optimally, infant should be fed when they indicate hunger. Initially, 5 min on each breast, alternating the breast used to begin feeding.
	By second or third day, time should be increased to 10–15 min on first breast and second breast until satiated.
Indicators of adequate intake	Wetting diapers regularly. Sleeping 2–3 h between feeding. Gaining weight.
Weight loss	Normal in first week and not related to adequacy of milk
Storing breast milk	Discard initial 5–10 cc. Place in sterile bottle in refrigerator for 24 h. Breast milk may be frozen and kept for 3 mo in deep freezer or 2 wk in freezer compartment of the refrigerator.
	Do not refreeze breast milk.
	Thaw gradually in cool to warm water.
	Discard unused milk after feeding.
	Never microwave breast milk.
Caring for nipples	Wash with plain water.
	Do not apply ointments.
	Change breast during feeding.
Burping	Burp infant when changing sides and at end of feeding.
Weaning	Indicators include: • Easily distracted during feeding • Decreased time sucking • Introduction of solids at 6 mo • Offer cup gradually, one feeding at a time
Maternal needs	Adequate intake of all foods. 500 calories more than if not breast-feeding. Increased protein, calcium, phosphorus. Increased rest.

fed, discussion of solutions to common concerns, and direct support and intervention when concerns are identified.

For the majority of mothers, there are no reasons other than the mother's personal preferences to prevent breast-feeding. However, there are some situations in which breast-feeding is absolutely contraindicated, including the following:

- Maternal tuberculosis and treatment with isoniazid (INH).
- Mental illness and the use of psychotropic drugs including Valium, lithium, and Nardil.
- The use of other drugs including combination oral contraceptives, chloramphenicol, tetracycline if given for longer than 10 days, anticancer drugs, and any addictive drugs with the exception of prescribed postpartum pain medications.
- Inborn errors of metabolism requiring special formula for the infant.
- Maternal HIV-positive blood result (this is not an absolute and is under study).[60,61]

Women who are forced to give up breast-feeding or women who are unable to even try to breast-feed may suffer prolonged mourning and suffering. Richards[47] found that women in these situations expressed grief reactions similar to those of mothers who experienced the death of an infant or had a loss of another kind. When describing the support they received in dealing with these feelings, few mothers spoke of professionals and, indeed, several commented that professionals did not understand at all what they felt.

Clearly, the nurse needs to be aware of the trauma women experience and be sensitive to their needs for support during the time of grief and mourning. Through understanding and support, the nurse can help the mother rebuild her confidence in her ability to care for the infant.

Promoting Successful Feeding With Commercially Prepared Formula: Nursing Implications

As with the parents of the breast-fed infant, the nurse's role in meeting the needs of parents using commercially prepared formula also includes assessment, education, and provision of appropriate support. Parents who are using commercially prepared formulas have questions related to which formula to use, preparation, storage, and amount and frequency of feedings.

Assessment of why parents chose to use commercial formula and the parents' understanding of the theoretical and practical aspects of formula-feeding helps the nurse identify the specific needs of the parents related to infant feeding. Early identification of a mother who preferred to breast-feed but was unable for any reason is crucial for immediate assessment and intervention, which would include providing an opportunity for the mother to express feelings and also to provide information on other factors that promote healthy growth and development.

Assessment of the parents and infant who is fed formula must include all areas of concern previously discussed in Table 12-3. Observation of the feeding situation,

with special attention to parental ability to identify and respond to infant cues of hunger and satiation, is also necessary.

Preparation and Storage of Formula. Education for parents must include proper preparation and storage of formula to prevent illness in the infant. Although there is a trend toward the use of clean technique for formula preparation, some health professionals still recommend the use of terminal heating or aseptic technique in formula preparation.[24,52] The nurse can assist parents in choosing a method based on individual needs and environmental conditions. The goal of all methods is to decrease the risk of bacterial contamination of formula.

Clean Technique. Parents begin by washing their hands with hot soapy water and drying hands with a clean towel. The surface to be used for bottle cleaning and formula preparation must also be free of bacteria. If bottles are to be washed by hand, the sink should be cleaned with detergent and rinsed with clean hot water. A sink can be contaminated with *Salmonella* or botulinum spores after general food preparation. Because the sink is frequently moist through tap water use, it is an excellent environment for bacterial growth. The use of a dishwasher is optimal for bottle cleaning when available. All items to be used in formula preparation need to be washed. This includes can opener, top of formula can, and measuring cups. Ideally, a single bottle method of preparation should be followed. This means that, although bottles can be cleaned all at once, only one bottle is filled with formula just before each feeding.

Terminal Heating. In terminal heating, clean bottles are filled with formula and placed in boiling water for 25 minutes. They are allowed to cool over a period of 2 hours and can be kept in the refrigerator for 24 hours.

Aseptic Technique. The aseptic method involves boiling in a covered pot for 20 minutes the bottles, nipples, and all preparation equipment. The bottles, nipples, and equipment are placed on a clean cloth or paper towel. Parents should be careful not to contaminate the sterile items when adding formula to them. Parents should be instructed carefully on the concept of sterile technique. If tap water is to be used in preparing formula, it should be boiled for 5 minutes. Sterile water may also be used. It is important that prepared formula be stored in the refrigerator until it is used. An open can of concentrated formula may be kept in the refrigerator for 24 hours. Any formula left after a feeding should be discarded.

Types of Nipples. There are a wide variety of infant nipples on the market. There is no evidence to suggest that one nipple is better than another. However, it is best to use a consistent nipple type. Mothers who breast-feed and supplement with a bottle should use a nipple that resembles the breast nipple.

Amount and Frequency of Feeding. The amount of formula an infant requires is based on energy requirements as well as other nutrient requirements. An estimate of caloric requirements can be obtained by multiplying the infant's weight in kilograms by the Recommended Daily Allowance (RDA) for energy in an infant of that age. For example, an infant weighing 3 kg requires 3

× 115 calories per day or 345 calories per day. Infant formula containing 20 calories per ounce would meet this requirement if the infant is fed 17 or 18 ounces per day or 3 ounces every 4 hours. Most newborns require six to eight feedings per day, and by 12 to 16 weeks some infants may be able to sleep through the night feeding.[40]

Parents need to be aware of the variations that exist between individual infants. If allowed, the infant demonstrates self-regulation, which is facilitated by demand feeding rather than scheduled feedings. A bottle containing 3 to 4 oz of formula should be offered at each feeding, and the infant should be allowed to stop voluntarily. Leaving a small amount at the end of the feeding provides parents with a feeling of security that the infant is getting as much as desired, and parents should not attempt to force feed the rest (Table 12-6).

Two common parental concerns of both breast-fed and formula-fed infants include colic and the use of pacifiers. Nurses must be prepared to discuss these concerns with parents. (See discussions in this chapter under Health Care.)

Feeding in the Second 6 Months

The second half of the first year brings new eating and feeding experiences for infants and parents. The concept of weaning becomes a major issue for infants and parents. *Weaning* is defined as any change from one form of feeding to another. This includes changing from liquids to solids, from breast to bottle or cup, and from bottle to cup.

Promoting Successful Weaning

Weaning usually begins around the sixth month. It is associated with the loss of early feeding reflexes and the emergence of new abilities related to neuromuscular development. The infant should be sitting without support, have hand-to-mouth motions, and have established head and neck control. Other indicators of infant readi-

ness for weaning include easy distractibility during breast- or bottle-feeding and decreased interest in breast milk or formula.

Cultural beliefs, socioeconomic factors, and maternal knowledge play a role in how and when an infant is introduced to solid foods. A study of low-income mothers and infants demonstrated that lack of knowledge was a major factor in the decision to introduce solids early.[19] These mothers felt that they had been given adequate information on breast- versus bottle-feeding but none related to the introduction of solids. Mothers expressed desire for information related to the introduction to solid foods.

Introduction of Solids. Introducing solid food is usually the first step in weaning. Iron-fortified cereals commercially prepared for infants should be introduced first. Rice cereal is the least allergenic and most easily digested. Introduction between the fourth and sixth month may provide the added iron the infant needs at this time.[6] Current recommendations[25] suggest that the use of jarred cereals may be more beneficial in providing iron than dry cereal preparations.

Learning to Use the Spoon. The infant should be fed with a spoon that has been chosen for this purpose. It should be small enough to fit in the back of the mouth, decreasing the amount of food pushed out by the tongue. Through practice, the infant learns to eat from the spoon and eventually learns self-feeding. Allowing the infant to hold one spoon while the parent feeds with another should be encouraged.

Once cereals are well established in the diet, other foods can be introduced. Ideally, new foods are introduced one at a time with 5 days between each new food. This allows for detection of any food allergies. Adequacy of nutritional intake depends on the introduction of solids and a balance of all four food groups. Exposing the infant to a wide variety of foods to establish tastes promotes lifelong habits that ensure good nutrition. Honey should not be given to an infant because it has been known to cause

TABLE 12-6
Nursing Intervention: Anticipatory Guidance for Mothers Feeding Infant Formula

Choosing a formula	Many commercial formulas are avaialble. Parents often continue to use brand the infant had in the hospital. Full-term infants should receive iron-fortified formula 20 Kcal/oz.
Feeding schedule	Optimally, infants should be fed when they indicate hunger. Feeding schedules vary. Infants generally eat every 3–4 h, less often as the infant gets older.
How much to feed	Need to be alert to infant's cues of satiation. • Turning away • Sleeping • Decreased sucking • Spitting out formula Do not push infant to finish bottle
Indicators of adequate intake	Wetting diapers regularly. Sleeping 2–3 h between feeding. Steady weight gain.
Preparing formula	Careful attention to directions for dilution. A clean environment is necessary. Parents may sterilize bottles for the first month. Prepare 24 h at a time or one at a time if using clean technique.
Unused formula	If making one bottle at a time, keep concentrate in the refrigerator covered for not more than 24 h. Dispose of any formula after the feeding is over.
Burping	Every 2 oz or as infant indicates.
Weaning	When introducing solid food at 6 mo, substitute cup for one bottle feeding at a time or serve formula in a cup with meals.

botulism.[9] Egg whites should be avoided until the child is 1 year old because of the high incidence of allergic reactions among infants. Although there is no prescribed order for the introduction of foods after cereal, the most commonly seen pattern is fruits and vegetables followed by meats. Juices can be offered at 5 to 6 months. As long as the infant is taking sufficient quantities of breast milk or formula, adequate amounts of vitamin C are ingested. If the introduction of juice is deferred until it can be offered in a cup, this decreases the risk of nursing bottle caries.[1,32,37]

New Textures. The transition to solid foods also involves the addition of new textures. The first texture is cereal mixed with formula, the second is strained foods. The infant is given mashed table foods such as mashed potatoes, mashed vegetables, and ground meat sometime between the seventh and ninth month. Finger foods should be offered once the infant can sit alone and demonstrate hand–eye coordination. Finger foods provide the infant with opportunities for self-feeding and exploration of textures. Food that can be easily picked up, such as toast or a zwieback cookie, provides the infant with the first self-feeding opportunity and pleasure in the exploration of a new object. Small food items such as raisins, berries, or nuts should not be given to the infant because they are commonly the cause of aspiration in infants and children.

Commercial Versus Home-Prepared Foods. Public pressure has brought about changes in the preparation of commercial foods. Many products are made without the addition of sugar and salt, and they contain fewer additives. By reading the label, parents can determine the nutritional value of individual products. Ingredients are listed on the label in decreasing order by weight. A label whose first ingredient is water is significantly different from a label whose first ingredient is meat.

Home-prepared food is an alternative to commercial food. It is less costly but not necessarily better. Nutritional value depends on how it is prepared. Parents should be encouraged to avoid the use of added salt or sugar when preparing infant food. Fresh foods are usually the best choice because they contain less salt and sugar than canned foods. Blenderizing home cooked meats, vegetables, and fruits with water they were cooked in adds to nutritional value and provides the liquids necessary to obtain the desired consistency.

Weaning From Breast or Bottle to Cup: A Major Transition. The infant can approximate his lips to the rim of the cup by the fifth month, demonstrating readiness to make the transition to the cup. The breast-fed infant can be weaned directly to the cup if weaning takes place after 6 months. However, parents may choose to wean to a bottle first. Weaning from the breast before the sixth month requires a transition to the bottle first and, when ready, transition to the cup.

Weaning begins with the substitution of the cup for one feeding each day. Gradually, the cup replaces all feedings. Many times, it is the bedtime feeding that the infant is most reluctant to give up. The infant who is just learning to drink from a cup may regress to earlier feeding

behaviors during times of separation or illness. Caregivers need to be sensitive during these stressful times and allow for temporary regressive behavior until the infant regains a sense of security.

Introducing Whole Milk. Ideally, infants should continue to receive breast milk or formula until 12 months of age.[57] Whole milk can be introduced after 6 months if a mixed diet is well-tolerated. Unlike breast milk and infant formulas, whole milk does not supply all essential nutrients. Caregivers need to be aware that whole milk intake without adequate intake of solids leads to malnutrition, anemia, and possible gastrointestinal disturbances including diarrhea.

During the first year of life, at least 30% of calories should come from fat. The American Academy of Pediatrics[5] recommends that fat not be restricted in this age group. After the second year, 2% milk and skim milk are acceptable.

Promoting Independent Feeding Behaviors in Infants. Infants should be allowed to attempt self-feeding through opportunities with finger foods and handling their spoon. Parents should be discouraged from adding food to an infant's bottle because it deprives the infant of important oral–sensory–motor experiences necessary for self-feeding and the development of appropriate eating habits. The nurse can help parents recognize an infant's need to explore food including looking at, touching, holding, manipulating, and controlling the food offered. This process can be messy, and parents need support in being patient with the mess that often results (Fig. 12-5).

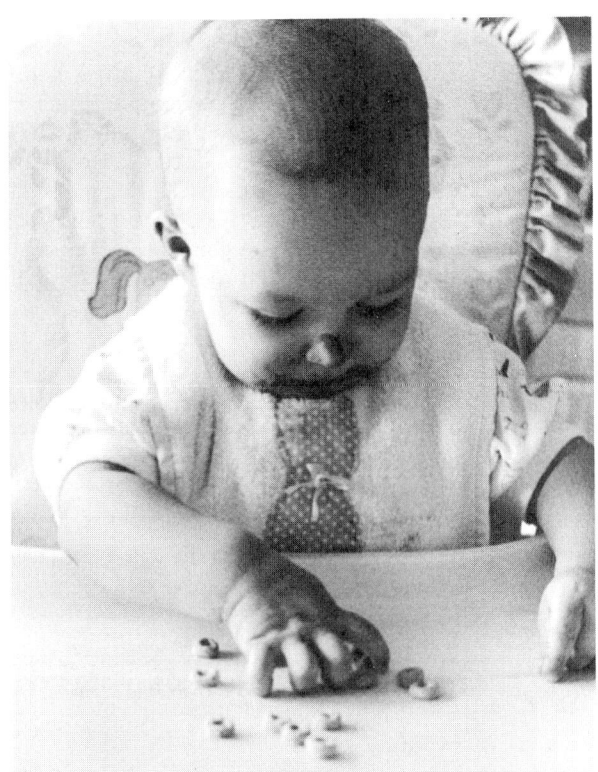

FIGURE 12-5
An infant learning to feed herself is often a messy affair.

Nursing Implications.   Although simple in theory, the transition to solid food and the elimination of the breast or bottle is complex and may present major child-rearing concerns for parents. The nurse is one member of the health care team who can use assessment, observational, and supportive skills in responding to parents involved in the weaning process. A principal goal of the nurse is to assist infants and parents in the transition. The nurse uses a systematic process that begins with assessment of parental beliefs and perceptions about an infant's readiness for something new, such as solid food. The nurse also must be sensitive to the cues of parental readiness to adapt to developmental changes in infants. Infants give many behavioral clues as to their readiness to explore new stimuli. Infants actively attempt to reach and hold the bottle and explore foods with their hands and mouths. Progressively, infants attempt to take a spoon from the parent and investigate it with their eyes and mouths. The infant must not be denied these opportunities for mastery of early fine motor skills. The nurse can help parents support this natural process of development that is enhanced by active participation of the infant.

The nurse needs to consider ways to include both parents in infant feeding and weaning methods. The nurse can include parents in discussions about how and when weaning should be implemented for each infant. Initially, parents can be asked to identify any internal or external factors that might affect successful outcomes with weaning.

The nurse can next assess parents' readiness for allowing infants greater independence, an increase in exploratory behavior, and more autonomy in feeding. The assessment of parental readiness to allow the infant increased autonomy in touching, holding, or exploring of food is essential to identification of potential parent–infant feeding conflicts.

It may be difficult for some parents to observe, identify, recognize, and accept the increasing abilities and desires of the infant to participate in the feeding process. If the nurse discovers that a parent or caregiver is experiencing distress, conflict, or difficulty in allowing an infant increased participation in feeding behaviors, the focus must shift toward supporting the parent. The nurse can allow the mother or father to express feelings of giving up a nurturing action associated with holding the infant and breast- or bottle-feeding. The nurse can be empathic and supportive and can diminish pressures that a parent may be experiencing. The nurse should determine at what point the parent believes the infant should participate in the feeding process. If the nurse determines that parents have unrealistic expectations of the infant's ability to be more self-sufficient, the nurse needs to concentrate attention on the parents' perceptions of other feeding, play, and self-help skills. If parents have unrealistic expectations of infants, the nurse can encourage parents to discuss their feelings of disappointment or surprise and be supportive to parents in their observation and problem-solving skills. When parents are observed to show signs of inappropriate readiness for the infant to master new tasks or demonstrate unrealistic expectations, the nurse must explore feelings with parents and support them as they respond to changing infant needs and behaviors. Suggestions concerning parental weaning practices are given in Table 12-7.

The nurse's knowledge of current research and trends in weaning is necessary to correct parental misperceptions and myths related to weaning practices. Although the American Academy of Pediatrics[5] has recommended approaches for the weaning process, discrepancies are apparent in the literature.[1,25,45] Discrepancies are the result of a century of transitions in feeding practices.[59] Parents are often advised and instructed by the child's grandparents in weaning practices. This information may have been state-of-the-art when grandparents were raising their children, but it has been replaced with new recommendations. Parental deviation from these sources of advice can cause conflict, dilemmas, and parental stress.

Lack of information and socioeconomic factors may also prevent parents from following current recommendations for weaning. Parents may choose to give their 3-month-old child powdered cow's milk because it is cheaper than formula and three older siblings are drinking it. These parents may know it is not the best choice but the only one they can manage at the time. The nurse would agree that the choice is not optimal and, in addition, can assist them in finding supplemental financial support to purchase formula. Another set of parents may be feeding their 1-month-old child all types of solids be-

TABLE 12-7
Nursing Assessment: Questions for Assessing Parental Weaning Practices

Areas of Assessment	Key Questions
Parents' beliefs about weaning practices, myths, and facts	What do you believe is important in weaning?
Parents' ability to identify readiness of their child for solids and participation in feeding process	Describe for me any changes you have noticed in _____'s behavior.
Maternal feelings related to infant's changing needs	Many mothers feel sad when their infant changes and does not seem to want to be fed and held in the same way as the early months. What feelings have you experienced with changing behavior?
Parents' ability to choose: appropriate amounts of food, a variety of food, foods from each of four food groups	Tell me what _____ ate yesterday?
Parents' perceptions of adequacy of diet	Are you satisfied with what _____ eats? Explain.
Identification of areas of concern for parents	What do you consider to be the most difficult part of weaning?

cause they believe solids are necessary for growth. These parents may eliminate solids if they are provided with information. If the nurse believes that these parents intend to continue feeding solids, the goal may be to limit solids to cereal. Nurses must be sensitive to the needs of individual parents and find ways to provide information or to work within cultural or socioeconomic restraints. Nurses should be accepting of parental decisions rather than judgmental. Unless the infant's physical well-being is threatened, minor variations in weaning practices should be tolerated. The nurse must be willing to take the time to discuss parental beliefs about the choices they are making before they offer advice. This approach indicates to parents that the nurse is truly interested in helping them rather than just telling them what to do.

Recommendations for weaning are based on developmental readiness of the infant. At 3 to 4 months, the protrusion reflex disappears, and, by 5 months, the infant can approximate the rim of a cup to lips. When weaning is in progress, usually by the sixth month, the infant has head and neck control, hand-to-mouth motion, and is beginning to sit alone. The order and timing of the introduction of new foods are determined by the nutritional needs of the infant and knowledge of foods that are well-tolerated as well as foods known to be associated with illness and allergy. Anticipatory guidance for weaning is discussed in Table 12-8.

The new feeding experiences of the infant promote physical growth and fine motor development. Weaning requires extra time and patience on the part of parents. However, if parents have an opportunity to discuss personal experiences, the pleasure of observing their child develop and master new skills is evident. Sensitive, nurturing, supportive approaches designed to meet the needs of parents during the unique period of infancy can facilitate optimal feeding practices and assist in the special challenges presented in the next stage of the toddler years.

Assessing, Promoting, and Maintaining Optimal Elimination

There is a wide range of normal in the elimination patterns of infants. Infants who are breast-fed may stool each time they are fed, or they may stool three times a day. Their stools are usually soft and yellow and have minimal odor. Diarrhea is uncommon in breast-fed infants, although to someone unfamiliar with this typical pattern of elimination there would be concern that the infant did have diarrhea.

The elimination patterns of infants fed formula is different from that of the breast-fed infant. Infants fed formula usually have firmer stools either once or several times a day. Some infants on formula experience constipation (see discussion in this chapter under Health Care). If their formula is iron-fortified, the stool is brown and has more of an odor than those of the breast-fed infant.

Parents generally have some initial questions about the elimination patterns of the infant, especially if the infant is having a loose stool with each feeding. Once

TABLE 12-8
Nursing Intervention: Anticipatory Guidance for Weaning During the Second 6 Months

Developmental readiness

3–4 mo

Disappearance of protrusion reflex

5 mo

Can approximate rim of cup to lips

6 mo

Suck, swallow reflex wanes

Sits unsupported

Hand-to-mouth motion

Head and neck control

Utensils

Small spoon to fit infant's mouth

Order of food introduction

Iron-fortified infant cereal, 4–6 mo

After well-tolerated, give strained foods

One new food every 5 days

Include vegetables, meat, fruit

Finger foods, soft and low in sugar

Advance texture to mashed table food, 7–9 mo

Substitute the cup for one feeding at a time

Foods deferred until the end of the first year

Egg whites

Honey

Formula should be continued until the end of the first year; however, whole milk may be given if child has well-established, mixed diet

Suggestions for promoting development

Allow infant to explore food with hands

Allow infant to attempt self-feeding with spoon

Offer finger foods with each meal

Anticipatory guidance for regressive behaviors

Allow infant to progress and regress throughout the weaning process

Attempt methods other than offering the bottle for comforting the infant; holding, rocking, rubbing back

Observe for infant behaviors that indicate hunger and respond by prompt feeding

Allow additional time for feeding

parents are informed of the normalcy of the child's elimination patterns, they may become more comfortable. Parents who are aware of the infant's typical elimination patterns are able to identify variations from the infant's normal patterns including diarrhea or constipation.

Bladder capacity of the infant is small, about 15 ml, and the infant can have up to 20 voids in 24 hours. Infant's urine is generally colorless and odorless. The widespread use of disposable diapers and the increasing ability of the diaper to absorb fluid can make it difficult for parents to assess urine output. After one void, the infant's diaper may appear dry. If parents have concerns about urine output, the nurse can recommend that they remove the diaper and check for urine by pulling the first layer off the diaper.

Assessing, Promoting, and Maintaining Optimal Sleep

During the first 3 months of life, sleep patterns of infants undergo tremendous change. The newborn does not have the ability to sleep through the night, and sleep periods may range from 20 minutes to 6 hours.[23] By the time the infant is 3 months old, sleep occurs at night.[23,40] The ability to sleep through the night generally occurs by the sixth month[23] (Table 12-9). Active versus quiet sleep also changes with age. Parmelee and Stern[41] describe the sleep of premature infants as mainly REM (rapid eye movement) sleep. Term infants have equal REM and NREM (non-rapid eye movement) sleep cycles, and, by 8 months, quiet sleep occurs twice as long as active sleep. These differences in sleep patterns have been related to the maturation of the central nervous system. Quiet sleep is a highly controlled state requiring a mature nervous system.

Naps or daytime sleeping occurs throughout the first year. As much as 8 hours of sleep occurs during daytime hours in the first week, decreasing to 2¼ hours at 1 year. Napping both in the morning and in the afternoon is common in the first 6 months. Gradually, the morning nap is eliminated, and the older infant takes only an afternoon nap.

Sleeping Through the Night

For most parents, the first concern related to sleep behavior is when to expect the infant to sleep through the night. Sleeping through the night is a significant development that is more in tune with parental sleep cycles. Other changes parents note in sleeping behaviors is the infant's ability to find self-comforting methods to enhance falling asleep, such as thumb sucking or rocking in the crib. In the first months after birth, when the infant awakens during the night it is usually from hunger. Some parents find it easier to have the infant in their room so that the infant can be fed with minimal household disruption. By the fourth month, most infants are able to go through the night without a feeding. However, it is not uncommon for the infant to awaken at various times and go back to sleep.[23] These night awakenings are related to the infant's physiologic sleep patterns. When infants do awaken during the night, they may play and entertain themselves and go back to sleep without parents knowing they were awake. Some infants, however, cry and need assistance in getting back to sleep. The infants may need parental comforting or a feeding before they are able to get back to sleep. A recent study found that scheduled awakenings and systematic ignoring as methods to decrease nocturnal awakenings were equally effective.[48] This information is especially helpful for parents who are unable to ignore any cries of the infant. However, scheduled awakenings need to be specific and consistent to be effective in reducing the frequency of awakenings. Parents who bring the infant back to their bed, play with the infant, or sleep in the infant's room have difficulty in reducing the frequency of night awakenings. These behaviors can be indicative of parental overanxiety related to parental personality, advancing maternal age, difficulties in becoming pregnant or maintaining pregnancy, first-time parents who are aware of SIDS, or an infant who has had other problems.[33] Anxious parents may have difficulty allowing the infant to discover and use self-comforting behaviors. Ferber[22] has found that infants and children who are unable to go back to sleep without intervention may have developed associations with falling asleep that are not present when they awaken during the night. For example, the infant who is breast-fed until asleep may associate suckling with sleep and after a night awakening may not be able to go back to sleep without suckling even in the absence of hunger. Although this is not true for all infants, it should be considered when a parent describes frequent awakenings that require specific interventions before the infant can get back to sleep. Ferber[22] recommends that infants be given opportunities to develop healthy sleep behaviors. An infant who is placed in the crib while still awake learns to fall asleep without assistance. This ability to sleep without intervention carries into childhood. Ferber's work suggests that the infant should be allowed to fall asleep alone in the crib and should be placed on a consistent schedule of naps and bedtime that facilitates the development of the infant's own circadian rhythms.

An infant who is ill may need to be soothed and helped back to sleep. As the infant feels better, parents need to recognize the readiness for discontinuance of this behavior. If parental interventions are discontinued, the infant can rely on self-comforting behaviors to fall asleep.

Nursing Implications

Nurses must discuss with parents sleep patterns of infants at each well-child visit. Assessment of sleep patterns and behaviors should include parental description of sleep patterns, including the length of time the infant sleeps, where the infant sleeps, and whether the infant's sleep patterns meet parental expectations. Assessment should also include parental response to infant crying when the infant is put to bed or after awakening during the night, as well as parental observation of the infant's ability to use self-comforting measures (Table 12-10).

TABLE 12-9
Typical Sleep Requirements of Infants

Age	Hours of Sleep/24 h	Hours of Nighttime Sleep	Hours of Daytime Sleep
1 wk	16½	8½	8
1 mo	15½	8¾	6¾
3 mo	15	9½	5½
6 mo	14¼	11	3¼
9 mo	14	11¼	2¾
12 mo	13¾	11½	2¼

Adapted from Ferber, R. (1987). Sleeplessness, night awakening, and night crying in the infant and toddler. *Pediatrics in Review*, 9 (3), 76.

TABLE 12-10
Nursing Assessment: Questions for Assessing Patterns of Infant Sleep

Areas of Assessment	Key Questions
Sleeping environment—is it separate from parents' bedroom?	Where does _____ sleep?
Normal sleeping patterns for age	How long does _____ sleep at a time?
	Does _____ sleep through the night (if infant 16 wk and still waking at night, further assessment may be necessary)
Parental ability to allow infant to entertain himself when he awakens	What does _____ do when he awakens?
	What is your reaction to this behavior (i.e., crying—does parent go to him immediately; playing—does parent allow him to play)?
Parental ability to identify infant preferences	In what position does _____ like to sleep?
Early identification of parental anxiety or fear related to sleep	Do you find yourself checking _____ while he sleeps?
	How often?
	What do you fear?
Relationship of infant patterns to parental well-being	How do you meet your own needs for sleep when you need to get up during the night with _____?

Nurses need to support and reassure parents as they adjust to the sleep patterns of the infant. Anxiety and frustration caused by an infant who has difficulty going to sleep or staying asleep lead to parental insecurity in their role as parents. Further, parents may be experiencing sleep deprivation, which decreases the effectiveness of their problem-solving efforts.

Nurses should discuss with parents normal patterns of infant sleep as well as the uniqueness of an individual infant's sleep behaviors. By decreasing parental feelings of inadequacy, the nurse can assist parents in finding ways to cope with infants who have difficulty with sleep.

Parents find it helpful if the nurse provides anticipatory guidance related to sleep behaviors, what to expect in the future, and suggestions for dealing with common sleep concerns (Table 12-11).

Assessing, Promoting, and Maintaining Optimal Psychosocial Development

Psychosocial development is directly related to the infant's attachment to parents and resulting sense of trust in the environment. Attachments and trust develop over a period of time and are influenced by both the child and the parents. Behaviors such as crying, smiling, cooing, eating, sleeping, and playing are brought to the relationship by the child. The parental response to these behaviors affects the overall psychosocial development of the child.

Developing a Sense of Trust

Erik Erikson[21] described the development of a sense of trust as the first task of ego development. A sense of mistrust can occur during the first year and a half and interfere with healthy ego development.

Erikson emphasized that establishing a sense of trust is the most significant task of maternal care. The infant's parental relationships must assist the infant to depend on others to meet physical and emotional needs. Merely meeting the infant's physical needs for food, warmth, and comfort is not sufficient for trust to develop. The infant needs consistency, continuity, and sameness of experience such that feelings of "inner goodness" are associated with familiar and predictable caregivers.[21] Those who care for the infant must be trustworthy and reliable. The infant must be able to rely on consistent responses from primary caregivers to develop trust.

TABLE 12-11
Nursing Intervention: Anticipatory Guidance for Infant Sleep

Environment
- Infant should sleep in room separate from parents.
- Environment should be quiet, but infant also needs to adjust to normal noise levels.
- Infant crib should have railings up and side pads to prevent head or extremities from being caught in the rail.
- Infant should have items to look at and play with during periods of wakefulness (mobile, rattle). These toys should be safe without strings or small pieces.
- Infant crib can be moved periodically to offer variety of stimuli.
- During extended waking periods, infant should be placed in portable crib or infant seat and allowed to be with family and exposed to different stimuli.

Helping the Infant Go to Sleep
- After the infant has been fed, changed, cuddled, and rocked, he can be placed in his crib.
- The cries of a newborn should be attended to promptly.
- The older infant (after 6 mo) should be given an opportunity to comfort himself but should not be allowed to cry for extended periods of time.
- If the infant awakens during the night and is unable to get back to sleep, rock or soothe him but try not to bring the infant to parent's bed.
- Parents should not have to be overly quiet when the infant is sleeping
- Allow the infant to become accustomed to normal noises.
- Infant may experience increased periods of fussiness during the fourth or fifth week of life related to brain maturation.

A parent who is unpredictable in feeding, bathing, dressing, comforting, and responding to an infant's care needs or who is inattentive may create a sense of mistrust in the infant.[21] Providing care, consoling, attending to, and responding in different ways prevents the infant from experiencing reliable responses to behaviors and needs.

In promoting a sense of trust, parents should respond to infant crying without undue delay. Parents should interact with the infant in caring ways through holding, rocking, talking to, and maintaining eye-to-eye contact during interactions. Parents can be encouraged to spend time with the infant that is not related to caregiving activities. Parents promote trust through the development of routines the child can depend on over time. These include routines for feeding, bathing, sleeping, and playing.

Nursing Implications

Assessment of the infant's developing sense of trust is based on observations of the infant's behaviors, physical responses, and interactions with care providers. The nurse can evaluate the infants progress toward development of trust by assessing the relationships between parents and infant and the quality of the infant's experiences within the environment (Table 12-12).

Do parents respond to infant crying without undue delay? Do parents interact with the infant through touching, holding, rocking, talking to the infant, and engaging in eye-to-eye contact? Do parents spend time with the infant when not providing caregiving activities? Do they describe positive qualities of the infant? In addition to making systematic observations of interactions between parents and infants, the nurse needs to be prepared to respond to parental concerns and offer anticipatory guidance for parents related to the promotion of infant trust. Parents should be encouraged to respond to the infant in a consistent caring manner. Optimally, the infant should have a daily routine for eating, bathing, sleeping, and playing. Parents should spend time holding, rocking, cuddling, and soothing the infant. Parents should respond to infant-initiated interactions, such as cooing or smiling. These responses come naturally when parents take opportunities to have fun with their infant.

Parental Concern: Infant Crying

One of the most common parental concerns related to the developing sense of trust is related to infant crying. Parents often do not feel secure in deciding how and when to respond to an infant who cries after being held, fed, changed, and played with. Parents express fear of spoiling the infant by responding to every cry but at the same time may be feeling that the infant would not cry unless there was something wrong.

All infants cry, and the nature of the cry varies with the need of the infant. Research[11] has shown that mothers are able to identify the cry of their infant within 48 hours of birth. Identifying the cause of the crying may be more difficult for some parents, and inability to comfort the infant may cause stress, frustration, anxiety, and feelings of parental inadequacy.

Anticipatory Guidance

Parents must be given information regarding crying, especially the wide variety of causes.[34] They also need guidance in determining how to deal with a crying infant.

Hunger. Hunger is a common cause of crying in infancy. The infant, like adults, experiences discomfort when hungry, and crying is one way to express this need to parents. Infants develop more tolerance for waiting for attention, feeding, or comforting as they get older. An infant who stops crying when picked up may not be hungry but may be communicating other needs for attention, love, caring, or affection. Parents should be discouraged from offering food each time the infant cries. If the infant has been fed before crying, other causes should be considered.

TABLE 12-12
Nursing Assessment: Guidelines for Assessing Developing Trust

Infant Behaviors That Demonstrate Trust	Parental Behaviors That Facilitate Trust	Infant Behaviors That Demonstrate Mistrust	Parental Behaviors That Facilitate Mistrust
Regular sleep patterns	Responds to infant cries without undue delay	Excessive crying	Unresponsive or delayed response to infant cries
Regular feeding patterns and weight gain	Interacts with, sensitive to infant needs, touching, holding, rocking, talking, singing, eye-to-eye contact	Fretful sleep	Leaves infant in crib for extended periods without interacting with him or her
Increasing tolerance for frustration, including hunger, loneliness	Responds to infant-initiated interaction, babbling, smiling	Poor eating and lack of weight gain	Scolding the infant for crying, soiling, or spitting up
Ability to anticipate maternal behaviors—mother coming to feed or pick-up	Spends time with infant not related to caregiving activities	Decreased social interactions	Delegates majority of care tasks to multiple caregivers including siblings, sitters, relatives, even though available
Smiles, babbles, plays	Parent identifies positive qualities of infant	Anxious, fretful	Personally provides care on an irregular basis
Calms and consoles self	Parental handling demonstrates love and confidence	Less interactive, few smiles, less babbling, and decreased interest in play	Describes infant in negative terms
			Demonstrates hostility and impatience, is rough with infant

Pain. Pain from gas, illness, teething, or other physical discomfort elicits crying in the infant. This crying starts suddenly and is arrhythmical. Parents usually respond promptly to infant's cries of pain or distress. This crying often requires physical comforting such as rocking, holding, or a gentle backrub.

Temperature. Infants require similar amounts of clothing and coverings as adults. Infants who are improperly clothed and are too hot or too cold cry from distress associated with physiologic discomfort.

Boredom. As the infant becomes more interested in the environment, being placed in the crib and deprived of stimuli may cause crying. This crying might be decreased by changing the infant's position or environment or by presenting animate or inanimate visual and auditory stimuli.

Fatigue. Just like adults, infants may become irritable when overtired. The infant may not be easily soothed. Infants may cry when put down or when held, and infants may refuse to eat. Often, infants who are fatigued cry until they sleep from exhaustion. Parents who are able to anticipate fatigue place the infant in the crib for rest and sleep when they recognize early signs of fatigue. Providing the infant with a regular daily schedule decreases crying from fatigue.

Loneliness. The desire for love also results in crying. Infants need to be held, rocked, and cuddled and, at times, have increased need for the closeness of their mother and father. Parents may underestimate these cries if the infant has been fed and changed and is safe because they have fears of spoiling the infant. Although it is expected that infants cry briefly before going to sleep, any prolonged crying should received appropriate attention from parents. Parents need to trust their own instincts in responding to infant crying. If the infant needs love, attention, and affection, it can be given freely and generously because most parents have an abundant supply of smiles, love, and caring to offer infants.

Generally, parents should be encouraged to respond to the newborn without excessive delay. As the infant gets older, opportunities should be given to the infant to develop self-comforting behaviors. A 1-week-old infant who cries after being put in the crib should be attended to by a parent if crying persists beyond a few minutes. On the other hand, an 8-month-old infant who cries when put in the crib should be allowed an opportunity to comfort himself.

Before responding to parental concerns about crying, the nurse should obtain information regarding frequency, duration, and timing of crying as well as parental response to crying. Parents should be informed of the wide range of factors that may cause crying and methods for comforting the infant. It is not uncommon for parents to believe that infant crying is abnormal except when the infant needs feeding or changing.[38] These parents may attribute all other crying episodes to colic or may ignore the infant's cries in an effort not to spoil the infant. Brazelton,[12] in a study of crying behavior of infants, found that in the first 7 weeks an infant spends an average of 2¼ hours crying with no apparent cause. This crying appears to serve as an outlet for accumulated tension in the infant rather than an indication of a spoiled infant. Parents should be encouraged to respond to the infant's cries for the first 3 to 4 months. Beyond 3 or 4 months of age, the infant's cry becomes a less accurate indicator of genuine needs. Older infants may begin to use their cry in a manipulative way, and the application of behavior modification techniques becomes appropriate to prevent the development of true spoiling.[38] Offering support to parents and decreasing parental feelings of responsibility each time the infant cries are beneficial. The nurse should reassure parents that responding to infant cries and meeting infant needs in the first 3 to 4 months of life do not result in a spoiled child.

Promoting the Development of Attachments

The infant's ability to develop an attachment to parents and primary caregivers is a critical task of infancy. Research[42] indicates that the establishment of secure attachment of the infant and primary care providers is correlated with later development. The securely attached infant at 2 years of age demonstrates increased attention span in problem-solving tasks, less frustration, more positive affect, and is able to use parent's help effectively.

Because of the significance of attachment as the foundation for later relationships, it is imperative that nurses observe, assess, and plan interventions with parents that facilitate early, healthy attachments. The reciprocal nature of the parent–infant interaction leads to attachment. John Bowlby[11] defines *attachment* as an affectional tie that the infant forms to another specific person which binds them together and endures over time. It is a relationship that develops gradually in a continuum of phases.

Phases of Infant Attachment[11]

Phase I. 0 to 1 month: In the first phase, the infant behaves in characteristic ways to adults but is unable to discriminate one person from another.

Phase II. 1 to 6 months: The infant continues to respond to people but does so in a more specific way to his mother-figure. Differential responsiveness to auditory stimuli is observed after the fourth week, and responsiveness to visual stimuli is observed after the tenth week.

Phase III. 6 to 24 months: In this phase, the infant has become increasingly discriminating and demonstrates more responses including following his mother as she departs, greeting her when she returns, and using her as a base from which to explore. Strangers are treated with increasing caution and alarm.

Phase IV. 24 to 36 months: The mother has become an independent object and, by observing her, the child is acquiring ability to distinguish differences in his mother's feelings and motives. His picture of the world is broadened, and he is more flexible, allowing more complex relationships such as a partnership to develop.

Developing Attachments

Both the infant and mother play a role in the development of a secure maternal–infant attachment. Each brings behaviors to the relationship that initiate and maintain proximity between mother and infant (Table 12-13).

Initially, the infant exhibits attachment behaviors such as crying, smiling, babbling, gazing, sucking, and clinging. These behaviors elicit behaviors in the parent including touching, smiling at, talking to, holding, rocking, hugging, kissing, and comforting the infant. Gradually, the infant begins to respond to the parent in a discriminating manner and is able to recognize the parent's voice, touch, and presence (Fig. 12-6). As the infant develops, increasing social and motor skills, more complex attachment behaviors emerge and earlier ones diminish. In the second 6 months, attachment behaviors include crawling, climbing, reaching to be picked up, and an increased anxiety when strangers are present. Robson and Moss[50] state that "if new reinforcements were not forthcoming throughout infancy and childhood, the extended parental attachments that our species require would not be sustained." The reciprocal relationship between parent and child continues over time with the development of increasingly more sophisticated behaviors, especially language.

Factors That Influence Attachment

Many factors may influence parental interactions with the infant. These factors include past experiences, such as parental relationships with their own parents; parental feelings about the pregnancy and whether it was planned or unplanned, easy or difficult. Is the infant what parents hoped for or is he the wrong sex? Is the infant healthy and perfect in relation to parental standards? Multiple variables influence a parent's ability to attach to the infant

as well as the timing and degree of attachment that develops.

In studying 54 primiparous mothers, Robson and Moss[50] found that it was not until the second month when infants began to exhibit visual fixation and the smiling response that maternal feelings intensified. The infant was viewed as a person with unique characteristics. Those mothers who experienced immediate intense attachments were extremely invested in having their babies. The mothers who attached late or developed no attachment at all did not want a child or they felt their infant was "difficult."

The research of Ainsworth and colleagues[8] also has important implications for nurses. These researchers found that mothers who were responsive to their infant's cries also tended to engage their infants in more playful interactions and fed their infants when infants indicated hunger. These mothers correctly and promptly responded to infant communications. They accepted their infants but were also able temporarily to restrict the infant's activities, and cooperated rather than interfered in the infant's ongoing activities. Mothers who were unresponsive did not react quickly or at all to the cries of the infant. They spent more time in caretaking activities than in playful face-to-face interactions, and they fed their infants on a schedule regardless of infant hunger or lack of hunger. These mothers resented their infants and tended to be controlling regardless of infant mood or wishes. Most mothers fall between the extremes of these reactions that Ainsworth[8] described as sensitivity/insensitivity, cooperation/interference, and acceptance/rejection.

Parental progressive attachment to the infant influences how parents interact with the infant. Parental attachment also influences the ability of parents to promote growth and development and be sensitive to the infant's unique developmental needs. The infant's attachment to parents and other primary caregivers influences the infant's ability to develop affectionate relationships, dem-

TABLE 12-13
Nursing Assessment: Attachment Behaviors of Parents and Infants

Infant's Age	Attachment Behaviors of Infants	Attachment Behaviors of Parents
0–3 mo	Crying, smiling, babbling, gazing, sucking, and clinging	Touches
		Looks at
3–6 mo	Recognizes and responds to parent's voice, touch, and presence in discriminating way; follows parent when she moves; greets parent when she returns	Smiles at
		Talks to
		Rocks
6–12 mo	Crawling, climbing, reaching to be picked up. Anxious with stranger	Hugs
		Kisses
12 mo–3 y	Walking and speech. Uses parent as a base from which to explore	Uses en face position
		Comforts cries
		Responds to infant attachment behaviors
		Initiates social interactions with infant
		Available to child as he or she explores
		Plays games such as peak-a-boo
		Provides opportunities to learn to tolerate brief separations

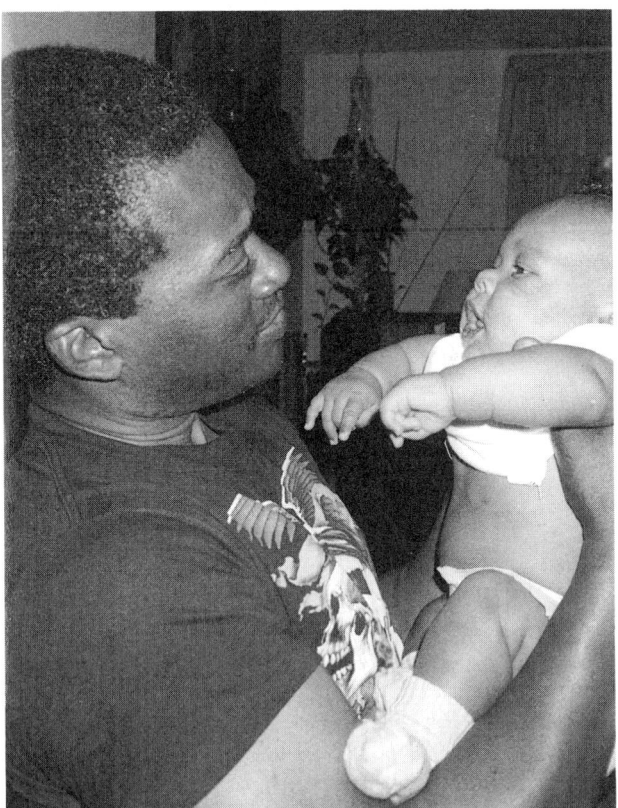

FIGURE 12-6
Parental interactions are important to cognitive, motor, and psychosocial development of the infant.

onstrate appropriate social behaviors, and interact in relationships with others.

Infant Temperament and Attachment

It has been demonstrated that the infant's temperament plays an important role in attachment. Brazelton[13] stresses the need to be aware of the individual differences of infants. He describes the infant at birth as a unique individual already possessing unlearned skills that foster and shape the parent–infant interaction. The neonate has the ability to organize and control reflexes, the ability to quiet himself when distressed, as well as a need for and attention to stimulation. The Brazelton Neonatal Assessment Tool is a tool for infant assessment that can also be used for teaching parents.

Thomas and Chess[56] found that even in the early months of life there are differences in temperament among infants, which influence their response to the environment and the response of others to them. These researchers define nine categories of temperament that assist in observation and assessment of temperamental characteristics in children who may be identified as "easy," "difficult," or "slow to warm up."

Carey[16] developed a questionnaire designed to obtain data on an infant's temperament. The questionnaire consists of 70 statements to be answered by the parent. Each statement has three options from which the one most descriptive of the infant is selected. Statements relate to feeding, sleeping, eliminating, daily care activities, responses to people, and play. The questionnaire is self-administered and serves as a framework for anticipatory guidance for parents.

Each child is unique, and not all children fit precisely into categories described by Carey. It is evident, however, that consideration and assessment of the infant's temperament are necessary for promotion of attachment. When parental concerns are presented, the nurse cannot assume that the problem is a result of inadequate parenting but may be a reflection of the infant's unique temperament. Observations and assessment of infant and parental behaviors must be planned and evaluated. Once observations have been completed on the infant's behaviors, interactions and temperament, and parental concerns have been identified, shared and validated, the nurse should formulate goals for altering patterns of infant care and decreasing feelings of parental inadequacy.

For example, the easily distracted infant may need specific interventions for developing a feeding environment that is quiet and away from the main activities of the household. An infant who has difficulty adjusting to changes in sleep and feeding schedules should be placed on a schedule that is consistent and one that can be followed by parents with minimal alterations. An infant who is sensitive to stimuli including light, noise, or touch may need decreased amounts of stimuli occurring at one time. Anticipatory guidance, problem solving, and emotional support may be appropriate for parents who are experiencing difficulties or concerns with infants who exhibit a behavioral style of "difficult" or "slow to warm up."

Parents promote attachment between the infant and themselves by providing an environment that is consistent and responsive to infant needs. Parents promote attachment through interacting with the infant in affectionate ways. Responding to infant-initiated interactions and demonstrating love and caring by holding, cuddling, and rocking the infant also promote enduring attachments.

Attachment is a gradual process that requires a caring relationship over a period of time. Parents who love their infant and enjoy their presence should have little difficulty forming attachments.

Nursing Implications

Nurses must assess the parent–infant relationship for evidence that attachment behaviors are present and for cues that attachments are developing. Do parents observe and describe the infant in positive terms? Do they call the infant by name? Do they hold and interact with the infant? Do they ask questions related to infant care? Do they appear comfortable in caring for the infant? Does the infant respond to parental interactions by smiling, cooing, or relaxing when held? Does the infant have extended periods of crying or become rigid when held? Does the older infant have anxiety related to strangers? Examples of assessing maternal and paternal attachment are given in Tables 12-14 and 12-15.

Nurses need to consider the multiple factors that influence mother–infant and father–infant relationships. Some of these variables exist before delivery and even

TABLE 12-14
Nursing Assessment: Guidelines for Observing Maternal Attachment Behaviors

Critical Attachment Tasks	Criteria of Attachment Indicators	Observed Behaviors (✓)
Observes Infant's Appearance	Spends time looking at baby, other than when providing care.	☐
	Inspects or reviews head, trunk, and extremities.	☐
	Partially unwraps or undresses baby to observe body features.	☐
	Comments on baby's features (e.g., size, sex, hair)	☑
Observes Infant's Behaviors	Talks to baby or smiles in response to infant's movements.	☑
	Comments on baby's behavior (e.g., opening eyes, grasping with hand).	☐
	Comments on infant's bodily functions (e.g., wetting, sucking, burping).	☐
Identifies Infant's Physical Condition	Makes realistic statements about condition, "Her eyes are not so puffy today." Or, "He looks so pale."	☐
	Asks questions about condition (e.g., "What is the mark on her head?" Or, "Is he getting better?").	☐
Sees Infant as Another Human Being	Has selected a name for the baby.	☐
	Uses given or affectionate name when talking to or about baby.	☐
	Associates infant's characteristics with human characteristics (e.g., "He looks like a football player." Or, "She looks like a real baby now.").	☑
Includes Infant in the Family	Attempts to associate infant's characteristics with those of other family members (e.g., "She has her daddy's eyes." Or, "He doesn't look like anyone else in the family.").	☐
Talks to Infant	Talks or sings to infant.	☑
Establishes Eye Contact	Uses en face position.	☑
	Changes own position or that of infant to establish eye contact.	☑
	Stimulates infant to open eyes by shielding them from the light or by using other maneuvers.	☐
Demonstrates Physical Closeness	When handed infant, reaches out to receive baby	☑
	Uses fingertips on head and extremities.	☑
	Uses palms on infant's trunk.	☐
	Enfolds infant in arms and holds against her body.	☐
	If infant hospitalized after mother discharged, visits a minimum of twice a week, for not less than 30 min per visit.	☐
Changes Behaviors in Response to Infant's Behavior	When infant is fussy, attempts to soothe by patting, cuddling, rocking, or talking to baby.	☐
	Does not continue behaviors that upset infant, or behaviors to which infant does not respond.	☐
	When infant is quiet and alert, makes eye contact and talks to baby.	☑
	Meets infant's needs before her own (e.g., "I'll feed him now and have breakfast later.").	☐
Recognizes Infant's Needs and Provides Appropriate Care	Readily participates in care when asked.	☐
	Recognizes baby's needs and attempts to meet them or communicate them to someone who can (e.g., changes shirt after baby spits up, or changes wet diaper).	☐
	Handles baby in a manner that is comfortable for infant (e.g., infant's head and body are well supported and infant is handled gently with smooth rather than jerky movements).	☐
Plans for Ways to Care for Infant at Home	Has obtained basic supplies for infant's care before infant's discharge.	☐
	Asks questions about care (e.g., feeding schedule, formula preparation, cord care).	☐
	Has made plans for or asks assistance with plans for well-baby care.	☐
Perception of Infant	Comments about baby are predominantly positive.	☑
	Smiles frequently when looking at infant or when talking to or about baby.	☑
Perception of Self	Comments about self are predominantly positive.	☐
	Expresses satisfaction with mothering role.	☐
Total Number of Behaviors Observed		11

Date _____ 8-9-77 _____   Time _____ 4 P.M. _____
Situation First interaction with infant following delivery

Johnson S. (1986). *Nursing assessment and strategies for the family at risk: High risk parenting* (2nd edition, pp. 30–31). Philadelphia: Lippincott.

TABLE 12-15
Nursing Assessment: Paternal Attachment

Time Situation	Adaptive	Maladaptive
Touches child	Freely, uses whole hand, gentle	Infrequent, uses fingertips, rough
Holds child	Holds close to body, relaxed posture	Holds distant from body, unrelaxed
Talks to child	Positive manner, tone; uses appropriate language, speed, content	Uses curt, loud, inappropriate language or content
Facial expression	Makes eye contact, expresses spectrum of emotions	Makes limited eye contact, little change in expression
Listens to child	Active listener, gives feedback	Is inattentive or ignores child
Demonstrates concern for child's needs	Active, involves others, seeks information	Indifferent, asks few questions
Aware of own needs	Expresses feelings about self in relation to child	Gives no expression about self
Responds to child's cues	Responds promptly to verbal, nonverbal cues	Has limited awareness and response
Relaxed with child	Posture, muscle tone relaxed	Posture rigid, tense, fidgets
Disciplines child	Initiates reasonable, appropriate discipline	Does not initiate or uses measures too severe or too lax
Spends time with, visits child	Routinely, uses time so that child is involved	Has no routine, no emphasis on child during time spent
Plays with child	Uses appropriate level of play, active, both enjoy	Uses inappropriate play, no obvious enjoyment
Gratification after interaction with child	Father states, appears gratified	Gives no statement of display of gratification
Initiates activity with child	Frequently	Infrequently
Seeks information and asks questions about child	Concerned, asks frequent, appropriate questions	Asks few questions, needs prompting
Responds to teaching	Positive, reinforces instructor, seeks more information	Has low interest
Knowledge of child's habits	Is knowledgeable	Has little knowledge
Participates in physical care	Feeds, bathes, dresses child	Allows others to perform tasks
Protects child	Aware of environmental hazards, actively protects	Protective behaviors not exhibited
Reinforces child	Gives verbal/nonverbal responses to child's positive behaviors	Does not notice or acknowledge child's behaviors
Teaches child	Initiates teaching	No teaching
Verbally communicates with mother about child	Uses positive, frequent verbal encounter	Gives negative, infrequent communication
Verbally and nonverbally supports mother	Demonstrates support—reassures, touches, guides	Support not obvious
Mother supports father, father responds	Gives positive response	Responds negatively, no response
Speaks of other children	Responds when asked, initiates, shows interest	Shows no interest, no initiation

Johnson S. (1986). Nursing assessment and strategies for the family at risk: High risk parenting (2nd edition, pp 30–31). Philadelphia: Lippincott.

before pregnancy. The nurse must plan to listen to parents as they describe their experiences in having an infant and their perceptions of the infant as compared to what they expected. The nurse must provide support to parents as they attempt to establish affectionate relationships with their infant and assist them in expressing feelings about the infant. Having the mother and father describe the infant in terms of feeding, sleeping, socializing, and crying gives the nurse valuable information about the parents' expectations and the extent to which their expectations are consistent with their perceptions of the infant.

Parents may initially spend more time describing concerns to health care professionals than describing the positive aspects of their child's behavior. They want to do what is best for their child and seek guidance in areas they feel the child or they are having difficulty. To reassure parents and promote self-confidence in the parenting role, nurses must assist parents in describing the positive aspects of the child as well as the positive aspects of themselves as parents. Pointing out an infant's response to a parental behavior, such as the infant's smile when the

parent speaks, may seem simple but is most helpful to parents if they are concerned about the frequency of the infant's crying.

Most parents benefit from an explanation of the attachment process and how both parents and child participate. Pointing out examples of the positive interactions observed gives parents a sense of pride in their parenting role. Allowing parents to express feelings of frustration, anxiety, or anger related to infant behaviors provides the nurse with the opportunity to explain that these feelings are normal and assist parents in coping with them. The nurse must first work with parents to define the behavior they have difficulty with, review what has already been tried to change the behavior, and offer suggestions for alternative ways of dealing with the problem. Parents who express feelings of frustration, anxiety, or anger may need assistance in finding time for themselves for rest and relaxation to deal more effectively with the infant. Parents who are having difficulty attaching to their infant because of infant temperament, parental anxiety, or parental feelings of inadequacy may need more specialized assistance and support.

Parental Concern: Stranger Anxiety

Associated with the attachment process is an increased fear or anxiety of the infant when a stranger is near. Stranger anxiety can be observed as early as 3 months of age, is common at 5 to 6 months, and peaks about at 12 to 18 months.[53] The infant who has developed an attachment to parents cries or wants to be held when a stranger is present. The severity of stranger anxiety varies from infant to infant even within the same family.

Parents should be reassured that this behavior is a result of the strong attachment the infant has developed to parents. Parents should be given methods for dealing with stranger anxiety that are helpful to the infant and themselves. Some infants may need parents present on several different occasions as a new person is introduced. Other infants who demonstrate anxiety when a parent leaves the room may benefit from hearing the parent's voice coming from the other room. Having a familiar person care for the infant, such as relative or regular baby-sitter, is necessary to give parents an opportunity for some time alone. Parents need reassurance that stranger anxiety passes and responding to the infant's need for close contact does not result in a spoiled child.

The amount of anxiety demonstrated by infants is a reflection of their individual personalities and adaptive behaviors. Preparing parents for this normal and temporary behavior before its development can be helpful in decreasing parental concerns. Although there are no methods of preventing this tension in the infant, parents who are prepared are able to give the infant a sense of security as this stage of development is reached and passed.

Assessing, Promoting, and Maintaining Optimal Cognitive Development

The infant's cognitive abilities increase as a result of interactions with parents and siblings and experiences within the environment. The infant is endowed with a variety of reflexes that gradually, through repeated use, become increasingly refined. These progressive changes are the building blocks of cognitive growth.[43]

The rate and timing of cognitive development are related to physical maturation and environmental influences. Parents are often interested in finding specific ways to foster the child's cognitive development. Some parents are extremely invested in promoting cognitive development, whereas others may feel learning takes place when the child goes to school. A parent's desire to promote cognitive growth is related to their educational background, knowledge of child development, cultural background, and environmental influences including financial resources, support systems, and the ability to meet the infant's basic needs for food, warmth, and comfort.

Because success in our society is often related to intellectual abilities, parents seek information regarding how their infant compares to others. Parents are concerned when the infant does not demonstrate a developmental task at the "normal" time. Parents ask nurses for information regarding the when, how, and what aspects of development. Nurses must be prepared to provide parents with information related to cognitive abilities and offer suggestions for fostering cognitive development throughout infancy.

Progression of Cognitive Abilities

In the first month, infants need opportunities to use basic reflexes such as sucking through repeated experiences with nipples, pacifiers, and thumb. The ability to fixate with their eyes is fostered when the human face is presented, which is interesting to the young infant. The infant also learns by observing the human face as expressions change from smiling, to frowning, to laughing, to talking.

From 1 to 4 months, the infant has more specific abilities due to the combining of various schemes. The infant grasps an object and proceeds to suck on it or sees an object and grasps it. Moving the infant around the house and taking the infant outside provides new and varied stimuli. All the sights and sounds we have become accustomed to are new learning experiences for the infant (Fig. 12-7). The feel of the wind on the infant's face brings a look of surprise and a hand to investigate. The infant looks to see where the sound of the vacuum cleaner is coming from or the sound of running water. At this stage, providing the infant with objects that have a variety of textures provides visual stimuli and tactile experiences. These objects should include but are not limited to such things as a sponge, a soft ball, a hard plastic object, a fluffy stuffed animal, a comb or brush, a fluid-filled container, or any object that offers the infant a new experience.

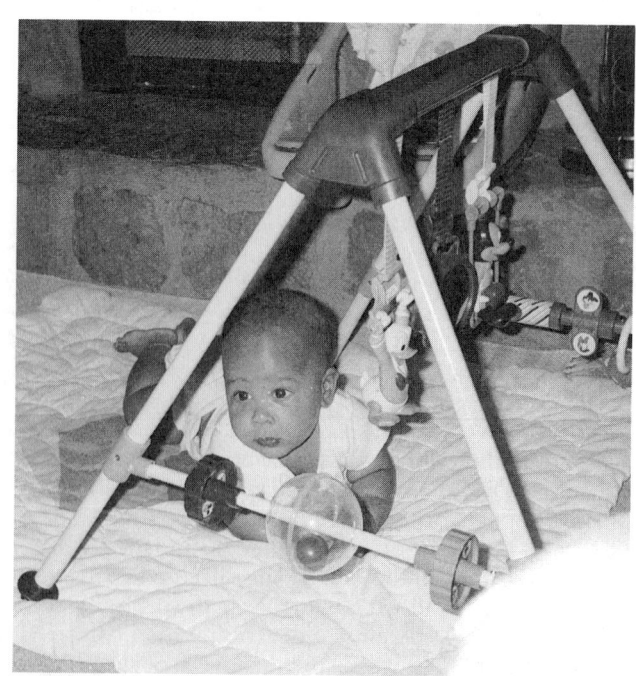

FIGURE 12-7
Play is an important part of learning during infancy.

Between the fourth and eighth month, the infant becomes increasingly interested in the effects of action on objects. A wide variety of objects that can be dropped, thrown, banged, or rolled should be available. Objects that can fit one into another allow for some early problem solving. A busy box that makes sound or motion when manipulated provides an early experience with cause and effect. Bath time is more interesting as the infant splashes in the water and pushes objects under water, watching them pop up.

By the end of the first year, the infant's increased mobility encourages exploration of the environment by allowing the infant to crawl to objects that are out of reach, push and pull objects, and retrieve objects that have gotten away. Objects within the household offer great pleasure, including pots and pans, spoons, plastic containers, and any number of lightweight objects that can be manipulated.

Self-exploration is also part of the infant's learning experience. Playing with toes, looking at hands, and smiling in the mirror all foster the infant's discovery of being a separate person. Learning games such as patty-cake occur during the end of the first year. The infant claps hands together and repeats the behavior if the behavior is mimicked immediately by parents, siblings, or other play partners.

Developing Object Permanence

The development of object permanency also occurs in the first year and continues into the second year. It is the ability to maintain a mental representation of an object once out of sight.[43] For the young infant, once an object is out of sight, it no longer exists. Gradually through experience, the infant follows the object as it moves and ultimately can retrieve a hidden object.

At each stage of developing object concept, the infant can be provided with opportunities to practice new skills. In the first 4 months, the infant should be provided with visual stimulation. This should include objects that can be tracked by the infant. Such objects as moving mobiles or an object that interests the infant can be manually moved from side to side in front of the infant.

From 4 to 8 months, the infant can be provided with objects that can be dropped from the high chair and followed by the infant's eyes. Partially hiding a favorite object under a cover provides the infant with an opportunity to reach for an object almost out of sight. By the end of the first year, parents can play hide and retrieve games with objects first hiding and retrieving the object for the infant and later allowing the infant to retrieve the object without assistance. Games such as peek-a-boo aid in the development of object permanency. The infant learns through repetition that people still exist when they go away and come back.

Parental Role in Cognitive Development

Parents promote cognitive development by the variety of objects and experiences they provide for the child as well as through interactions with the child. Although

developmentally appropriate objects including busy boxes, mobiles, toy keys, and other objects known to interest infants are available commercially, it is not necessary that parents purchase these toys. Infants can learn through the manipulation of many common household items. The key to promoting cognitive development lies in the parents' ability to provide different objects for the infant. Changing the infant's environment so that the infant can see a variety of rooms and the kinds of things that go in the kitchen, bathroom, family room, or basement provide new learning experiences for the infant. Trips outside introduce the infant to temperature changes, wind, grass, trees, and animals. Talking to the infant and explaining what you are doing, for example, "Mommy is washing Tommy's face," also are valuable in fostering cognitive development (Table 12-16).

Language Development

Much of the infant's learning about language occurs long before speech begins. The infant learns to pay attention to others' speech and listens for changes in sound and attends to the rhythm of speech long before the words are understood.

The infant needs exposure to a wide variety of noises that occur in everyday experiences as well as the complex sounds made by adults talking directly to him. Within a few days of birth, infants are highly responsive to speech or other sounds similar to the pitch of the human voice. From the beginning, infants are able to discriminate speech from nonspeech, and they pay particular attention to speech.

By the third or fourth month, the infant begins to babble sounds that approximate speech. A steady increase in babbling occurs until 9 to 12 months when the infant produces the first understandable words. Some infants cease to babble at this time; others continue.

Language acquisition is facilitated through the interactions between the child and parents. In the first year, these interactions involve the child's use of hand and body gestures and direction of gaze to draw attention to an object. At the same time, the infant begins to interpret adult gestures. The infant begins to understand when a response is required and when it is not expected.

Parental Role in Language Development

The quality of language and amount of time parents spend talking to their infant is an important factor in the infant's developing language skills. In the first months, the infant observes parents as they speak and may respond with a smile or change in activity. Parents can talk to the infant and smile, hold, and interact frequently with the infant during feedings or when the infant is alert after waking up.

As the infant gets older, the response to language increases. The infant turns to the sound coming from behind. The infant may raise arms when parents reach down and say "come up." Parents should look at the infant and smile when talking. When the infant makes sounds, parents can repeat these sounds for the infant. Parents can

TABLE 12-16
Nursing Intervention: Anticipatory Guidance for Promoting Cognitive Skills in the Infant

Age	Cognitive Abilities	Appropriate Experiences
Birth–6 wk	Basic reflexes	Allow sucking
		Nipple hard-soft
		Thumb
		Pacifier
	Infants tend to look to right rather than straight ahead when on their back	Talk to infant
		Face-to-face contact
		Hold, rock, cuddle
		Mobile placed to right or left of baby about 12 in from eyes
	Interest in upper portion of human face	Bold contrasting colors
		Crude facial features of upper face
1–4 mo	Increasing ability to: combine various schemes	Move infant around house to see various objects
	Increasing interest in objects	Take out in stroller
	Grasping–sucking	Provide objects he can handle and examine with eyes and mouth
	Sucking–grasping	Variety of textures:
	Seeing–grasping	Sponge
	Grasping–seeing	Wood spoon
		Plastic rattle
		Soft cloth
		Squeezable rubber
		Cold teething ring
		Place objects where infants can see and reach them
		Allow infant to choose object
		Very interested in own hands
	Hearing-looking	Music box
		Your voice, talking, singing
		Wind chimes
		Sound of passing cars
		Mirror
4–8 mo	Increasing interest in effect of actions on objects	Offer items to drop, throw, bang, kick, bat
		Cradle gym
		Weight toys
		Any object he can safely drop, throw, or bang
		Objects that can be placed inside other objects (nesting cups) or household objects
	Beginning imitation	Repeat action of infant immediately after he performs actions
		Repeat infant sounds
		Make sounds for infant to imitate
		Reinforce success to facilitate continued imitative attempts
8–12 mo	Means–end behavior	Continue to offer objects to explore
	Performs a behavior for an intended result	
	Learning characteristics of objects	Introduce objects that have working parts that when activated produce a result
		Surprise box
		Busy bath
		Balls of various shapes and sizes
		Toys that produce sound when pushed pulled
	Learning characteristics of object	Variety of texture
		Doll with detailed eyes, fingers, ears, toes
		Objects that fit into each other
		Pots and pans in kitchen
		Objects that open and close:
		Cabinet door
		Hard page book
		Container with lid

talk to the infant during bath time, bedtime, and when feeding or providing other daily activities.

By the end of the first year, the infant stops an activity when parents say "no-no" or when the infant's name is called. The infant may give an object to a parent if the parent requests it and makes a gesture with their hands. Mama and dada are words the infant can say, and the infant can imitate speech sounds such as lip smacking or tongue clicking. Parents need to provide the infant with simple commands that are accompanied by physical gestures. (Refer to Chap. 8 for more discussion of language development patterns.)

Cognitive and Language Development: Nursing Implications

In assessing cognitive and language development, the nurse must assess the quality of the infant's environment. One assessment tool that is suitable for observation of the quality and quantity of an infant's environment is the HOME Tool.[15] The HOME Tool, developed to be used with children from birth to 3 years, is helpful to the nurse in gathering data on the parents' emotional and verbal responsivity to the infant, the parents' use of restriction or punishment, the opportunities the infant has or changes in the environment, provision of appropriate play materials, parents' involvement with the child, and opportunities for variety in daily stimulation. Elardo and colleagues[20] conducted research using the HOME Tool and found that infants whose parents provided a variety of toys at 12 months of age demonstrated significantly better cognitive scores at 3 years of age (see Chap. 17).

Once an assessment of the infant's environment is completed, the nurse can use observations in discussing development with parents. Providing positive reinforcement for parents who are providing the infant with a variety of experience builds parental confidence and makes them feel good about their parenting. Early identification of parental inability to provide experiences due to lack of knowledge or difficulty dealing with an increasingly independent infant, provides an opportunity for early intervention. The nurse can assist parents by providing the infant with a new object and helping parents observe the infant's interest in and interactions with the object. Some parents simply need to have the infant's abilities and opportunities for learning that occur on a daily basis pointed out. Families of all income levels benefit from a discussion on how everyday experiences and objects as well as age-appropriate toys in the home foster cognitive, language, and motor development.

Assessing, Promoting, and Maintaining Optimal Activity Levels

Motor development during the first year reflects the infant's rapidly developing central nervous system and the increasing strength and coordination of the muscularskeletal system. This development can be promoted or hindered by opportunities or lack of opportunities provided for the infant.

Patterns of Motor Development

Initially, the infant requires the assistance of others to move from one place to another or from one position to another. The infant, however, can move both arms and legs if they are left unrestricted. Dressing the infant in a sleeper rather than swaddling in a blanket provides the freedom the infant needs to move extremities. The infant should also be placed in the prone position so that he or she can move the head from side to side or lift it momentarily off the bed. When pulling the young infant to a sitting position, the head needs to be supported as long as head lag is present. The infant holds and releases an object such as a rattle when it is placed in the palm of the hand. At this point, an infant does not reach for an object or grasp it without it being placed in the hand. Placing the infant in a seat that provides head support provides for a variety of stimuli and encourages the infant in maintaining a sitting position.

By the fourth month, the infant can lift both head and chest off the bed when placed prone. The infant should be placed in the prone position and provided with interesting visual stimuli when the head is lifted from the bed (Fig. 12-8). Parents should observe the infant's line of vision when the head is lifted and place a mirror, picture of the human face, or colored object at this spot. The infant should be given opportunities to practice sitting. Parents can pull the infant to the sitting position and maintain this position by holding the infant's hands. This offers the infant some experience with head control.

Once the infant is able to sit alone, the infant can be placed in a high chair, swing, or walker and can be given objects to manipulate (Fig. 12-9). Placing the infant on the floor provides the added opportunity to balance and reach for an object not immediately available. Objects can be held for longer periods of time, and the infant should be given a choice of several objects, both large and small, to grasp with one or both hands.

By nine months, the infant begins crawling. Once

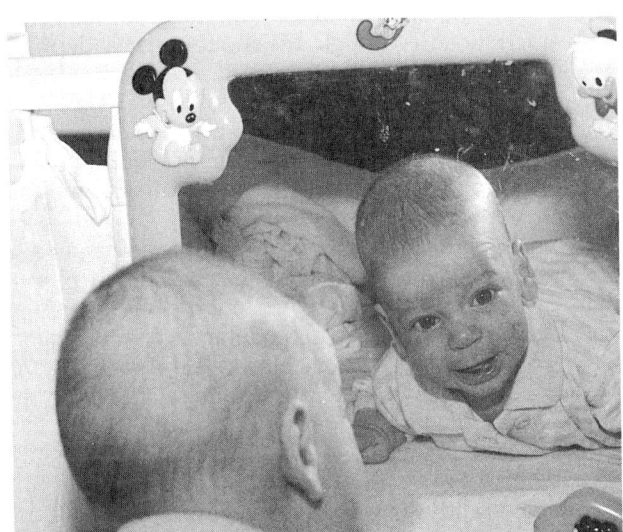

FIGURE 12-8
Provide infants with opportunities to encourage head lifting.

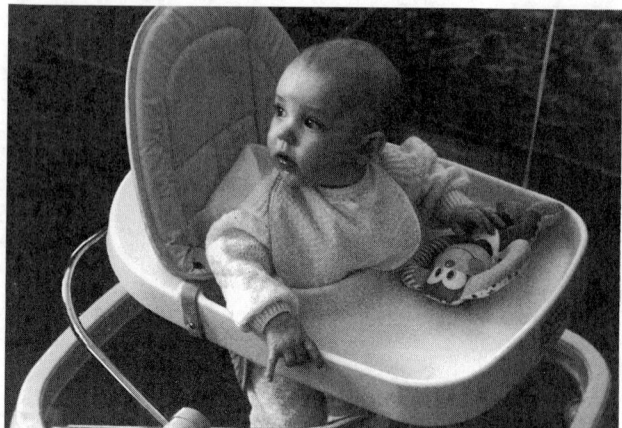

FIGURE 12-9
Once the infant can sit alone, provide interesting toys for her to manipulate.

TABLE 12-17
Nursing Intervention: Anticipatory Guidance for Promoting Motor Development

Age	Activities
1–2 mo	Place infant in prone position.
	Support head until lag decreases. Pull to sitting position.
	Place objects such as rattle in hand.
	Place in infant seat with head support.
4 mo	Continue to place in prone position.
	Place something in crib he can see when he lifts his head up off bed.
	Allow infant to sit up in high chair.
	Place interesting objects in reach.
5–8 mo	Pull to sitting position.
	Allow to sit in high chair.
	Provide firm surface (covered floor) for infant to practice sitting.
	Offer objects to pick up, large and small.
9–12 mo	Make room for crawling.
	Allow infant (with supervision) to pull himself up and walk holding onto furniture.
	Hold infant by both hands and allow him to practice walking.
	Provide container that infant can put objects into and dump objects out of.

the infant realizes the potential of this new ability, the environment is actively explored. Because the infant needs one-to-one supervision when left free to crawl, parents tend to place the infant in a confined area such as a playpen while they are busy. However, parents should be encouraged to allow the infant to crawl in an open area several times each day. If the room is childproofed, parents do not have to interfere with the child's movement and exploration. Placing interesting objects in different places encourages the infant to crawl from one place to another.

Toward the end of the first year, the infant pulls up to a sitting or standing position and begins to walk holding onto furniture. The infant also practices walking if hands are held by parents or siblings. Parents should be sure that furniture is stable and not allow the infant to hold onto an object that may fall. Again, the infant needs opportunities to walk even though this new behavior requires more parental time.

Parents promote motor development by the opportunities they provide for the infant to move about with increasing independence. It is important that parents allow the infant to try newly gained skills even if it entails some falls or bumps. Running to the infant's rescue each time a fall looks as though it is about to occur deprives the infant of valuable experiences. If an infant is in a safe environment on a soft carpet or grass, parents should sit back and observe the infant using new-found motor skills. Reassuring parents that the older infant falling on his or her bottom does not cause any harm may reduce overprotectiveness.

Providing the young infant with objects attached to the crib encourages reaching and grasping. These objects must be securely attached to the crib on short cords so that there is no safety risk to the infant. The older infant needs opportunities to move physically by crawling and walking as the environment is explored. Allowing the infant out of the playpen encourages active mobility. Parents may also participate in activities with the infant such as rolling a ball, playing "gonna get you," and assisting the infant in early crawling and walking experiences. Anticipatory guidance for motor development is discussed in Table 12-17.

Infant Exercise

As the adult population has become increasingly health conscious, there had been a steady rise in the advertisement and availability of structured exercise programs and equipment. This new enthusiasm for exercise is also seen in the infant section of the toy department. Such items as infant gym equipment and infant exercise pads, which include exercise instructions, are becoming popular among toy manufacturers. Many parents, especially those who exercise themselves, have questions about these new items. Are they necessary, are they safe, and does my infant need to specifically do exercises to facilitate the development of a particular muscle or physical skill? Should I enroll my infant in an exercise program?

No data suggest that structured programs or advanced skills provide any long-term benefits to normal infants.[10] Additionally, the bones of infants are more prone to trauma than those of children and adults. Based on the above information, the American Academy of Pediatrics makes the following recommendation: "(1) Structured infant exercise programs should not be promoted as being therapeutically beneficial for the development of healthy infants and (2) parents should be encouraged to provide a safe, nurturing and minimally structured play environment for their infant."[7]

Infant swim programs have been available for a longer period of time. These programs, in addition to providing physical activity, begin to teach the infant water safety skills. The quality of these programs varies, and it is important that parents investigate the program they choose and determine if it meets their expectations and beliefs about infant learning style and parental involvement. Parents may ask the nurse if they think they should begin these classes. Rather than answering this question directly, the nurse should assess further the parents' rationale for wanting to provide this for their child, what their concerns are, and what are their options. Additionally, if a parent decides on beginning the classes, they should be encouraged to observe their infant's response to these classes and progress at a rate appropriate for the infant.

Using Play to Promote Development

The purpose of play is to gratify the basic psychological, cognitive, and psychomotor needs of infancy. Through play, the infant processes information; learns to relate in socially pleasurable ways with others; begins to explore, manipulate, and master body movements as well as the environment; and benefits from a variety of sensory–motor–perceptual and kinesthetic stimuli. Infants use play to express satisfaction and gratification of their experiences and relationships with significant care providers in a variety of settings.

Throughout the first year, the infant becomes increasingly involved in playful interactions with parents and other care providers. During the first 6 months, play centers on the infant's body and then the parent's body. By exploring his hands and feet and mother's mouth and father's face, the infant continues to discover separateness.

The infant becomes actively involved in play by first attending visually to play activities. The infant begins to express verbal and bodily responses of pleasure with playful activities. Initially, parents play both roles in games for the pleasure of the infant, who receives pleasure from watching and listening.

During the second 6 months, the infant becomes more actively involved in play by following the rhythm of the game. The infant demonstrates active pleasure when toys disappear and reappear.

By the end of the first year, the infant actively participates through touching, reaching, grasping, releasing small objects, and by pointing, searching, knocking down toys or blocks, and pulling a cover over eyes to play peek-a-boo. The infant initiates games.

Play provides the infant with pleasurable experiences, offers opportunities to learn about objects, and provides opportunities to practice separation. Thoughtfully chosen toys, games, and activities can enhance the infant's development. The ultimate goal is to provide an infant with pleasurable experiences that help the infant begin to explore, manipulate, and gain mastery over the body and the environment. Play can occur during bathing, dressing, and other daily care activities. Playing with an infant in the bath, splashing water, kicking feet, and manipulating objects is an example of play as part of a daily experience (Fig. 12-10). Allowing the infant to work at getting one object out of another without interfering provides the infant with a feeling of success. Taking the infant outside to explore offers a wide range of experiences, sights, and sounds.

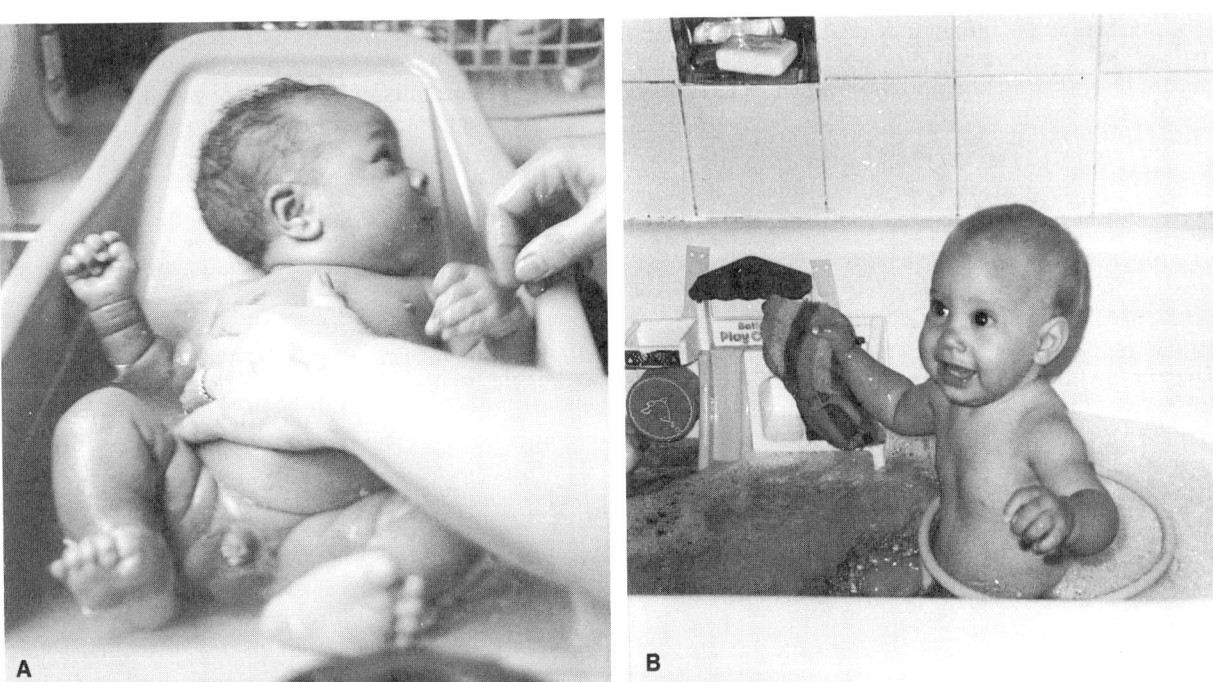

FIGURE 12-10
Bath time can be fun for infants and parents. (**A**) Infants are initially sponged or bathed in an infant bath. (**B**) The older infant enjoys playful splashing, kicking and manipulation of objects in the bath. At both ages, bath safety is very important and a safety ring may be used. Infants and children should never be left alone in the water.

Nursing Implications in Assessing and Promoting Optimal Play Experience in Infancy

A primary goal of a nursing assessment of an infant's play is to make systematic observations of the infant's play behaviors, play interactions with others, and to determine the number, variety, and types of toys and play activities that are provided for the infant during the first year of life.

The nurse needs to incorporate play as a major topic in the interview with parents. The nurse can question parents about the frequency of play with the infant and obtain information on parents' perceptions of the need for play, and their expectations of the infant's play behaviors.

Nursing intervention begins with the nurse sharing the assessment of infant play behaviors. This assessment can reinforce parental skill in providing age-appropriate toys and play experiences and also serve as a springboard for anticipatory guidance. Anticipatory guidance should include suggestions for appropriate activities during each stage of infant development.

The infant's ability to become involved in play and the pleasure that comes from play increase for both the infant and parents. Parents may benefit from a discussion of the changing needs of the infant throughout the first year. For example, in the first few months, babies enjoy listening to parents speak to them, sucking on objects, and being held and rocked. With increasing abilities, the older infant needs more stimulation and opportunities to manipulate objects and explore independently. These changing needs require different toys, including nesting cups, finger foods, blocks, and toys that can be pushed and pulled. Safety is always an important consideration in choosing toys and planning activities and should always be part of any discussion related to infant care. Safety issues are discussed in detail in the following section.

Assessing, Promoting, and Maintaining Infant Safety

Safety concerns during the first year of life need to be addressed in the perinatal period and reinforced throughout the first year. The initial concerns center around the provision of a safe environment. In preparing a place for the infant in the home, parents must consider many things. Whether the infant is going to have a nursery or share a room with a sibling, parents must take time to plan space that provides a safe environment when the infant is young and relatively immobile and one that continues to be safe as the infant develops.

Parents who plan an elaborate nursery or just clean and prepare a small space in the home for the new infant have to consider the following.

Environmental Safety

Cribs

The infant's crib must have no more than 2 3/8 inches of space between slats. Because this is required (by the Consumer Products Safety Commission [CPSC]) of all crib manufacturers, this is a concern only for parents who are using an older crib. Additionally, cornerposts should be less than 5/8 in high.[27] Mattresses should fit securely; the space between the mattress and frame should not allow more than two fingers to be inserted. Placement of the crib should be away from any hazards such as windows and blinds with cords that hang down. Once the infant can sit up, items should never be hung from the railing of the crib or strung across the crib because this places the infant at risk for strangulation. If parents want a protective covering for the mattress, they should be instructed to use one designed for that purpose and not use a plastic bag or thin plastic covering from the drycleaners. If bumper pads are used, they should fit securely around the crib and have at least six straps to secure them. They should only be used until the infant can pull to a standing position. A child who is 35 inches or taller has outgrown the crib and should begin sleeping in a bed.

Changing Tables

The CPSC projects an estimate of 1400 injuries requiring hospital emergency treatment annually related to the use of changing tables.[27] The majority of these injuries are due to falls. To avoid the potential for falls, parents should be instructed to purchase a table with a safety strap. The restraint strap should be used even for short periods of time, and, more importantly, parents should keep one hand on the infant at all times. If a parent needs to leave the room even for a moment while changing the baby, they should not leave the baby on the table even with the safety strap on. All items for baby care such as powder, pins, and ointment should be out of the infant's reach. In addition to changing tables, parents must be aware of the potential for falls from a variety of places including beds, sofas, infant seats, stairs, and walkers. One study[49] found falls to be the most common cause of accidental injuries (47%) in infants under 1 year of age.

Car Safety Seats

Every state requires the use of car seats even for newborns. Many hospitals provide parents who cannot afford a car seat the use of one for free or a nominal fee. Some hospitals give parents a car seat as a baby gift. The Public Health Department of most cities also have car seats available for those who cannot afford one. Information on loaner programs can be obtained by writing to the National Child Passenger Safety Association, Suite 300, 1705 DeSales Street N.W., Washington, DC 20036. Car seats manufactured after January 1, 1981, should be purchased because these seats must meet federal regulations and have passed a simulated crash test.

Since the institution of laws requiring car seats for infants and young children, there has been a decline in mortality related to car accidents. However, motor vehicle accidents continue to be the major cause of accidental deaths in infants.[58] This is a result of the improper use of the car seat. Researchers[14] observed the use of car restraints and found that, of the 618 observed, 459 were misused. The common misuses included improper use of harness strap, failure to secure the seat with a seat belt, nonuse of tether strap, and incorrect positioning of the infant.

Parents should be instructed to place the infant in a car seat in the center of the back seat with the infant facing the rear of the car. The positioning provides for the absorption of an impact to spread evenly across the infant's back and decreases the risk of head and neck injury. The infant should be placed in this position if less than 26 inches long and weighing less than 21 lb. Parents may express dissatisfaction with this position because it is difficult to attend to the infant who is fussing or in some distress. In these situations, it is important for the nurse to explain to parents that attending to an infant at the same time they are trying to drive poses a risk for an automobile accident. If an infant needs attention, the parent should stop the car and attend to the infant.

Pacifiers

Pacifiers pose the risk of strangulation to infants if they are attached to the infant with a ribbon or cord. Parents may not consider this risk and generally attach the pacifier to the infant to prevent it from falling on the floor. Since 1977, the CPSC requires that all pacifiers be strong enough to prevent breaking into small pieces, that they have a shield that prevents the aspiration of the nipple, and that the shields have ventilation holes.

Walkers

Infant walkers are also responsible for over 15,000 injuries a year.[27] Most of these injuries are from tipping over, falling down stairs, and finger entrapment. Infants should never be left unattended in a walker. Walkers should never be used on stairs or uneven surfaces. When purchasing a walker, parents should be instructed to look for a walker with a wide base and one free of sharp edges. Parents should be informed that walkers do not promote early walking as is commonly believed.

Smoke Detectors

The installation of smoke detectors are advantageous for everyone. However, the birth of a child provides an opportunity for the nurse to encourage parents to install them if they do not have them. Additionally, parents should be reminded to test the smoke detector every 3 months for proper functioning.

Tap Water

Water heaters should be regulated such that the hot water temperature does not exceed 120°F.[36] Although this does not prevent burns, it does require a longer period of exposure for a burn to occur.

Nursing Implications

Nurses are in a position to assist parents by addressing the issue of safety at each well-care visit. Ideally, this education of parents should begin during pregnancy. Childbirth classes may be an appropriate time to discuss safe environments; however, the timing of these classes is during the last trimester and parents may have already invested in infant products. Ideally, nurses working with mothers during early prenatal visits should emphasize the importance of product safety in preparing for the new family member. This nursing responsibility must continue to be a priority of the pediatric nurse throughout the child's growing years. Explaining to parents an infant's current level of development as well as what to expect in coming months provides an optimal opportunity to discuss safety issues. For example, Sue is able to sit by herself and soon she will be crawling. Therefore, you need to be sure that your home is safe for this experience by placing unsafe objects out of reach, keeping cords out of reach, covering electric outlets, keeping doors closed, placing gates at the top and bottom of stairs, keeping small objects and sharp objects out of reach, and so forth.

In spite of national efforts to prevent the manufacturing of unsafe products to be used with infants, unsafe products are still on the market. It is extremely difficult for parents to sort through all of the products available, keeping in mind all of the potential risks.

Safety During Activities of Daily Living

Bath

Giving an infant a bath requires planning and uninterrupted concentration. The baby bath is routinely a topic of newborn education classes in the hospital. However, a parent who feels comfortable in the hospital may feel differently at home. A nurse seeing parents at the infant's first well-care visit should ask if they have any concerns or difficulties in bathing the baby. The most common concerns are related to an infant who does not like being bathed and the difficulty of holding the infant while trying to wash him. Parents benefit from reassurance from the nurse that bathing an infant can be difficult and frightening. There are products on the market to assist in this process and decrease the risk of accidents (see Fig. 12-10). However, these products cost money and, therefore, are not available to everyone. Nurses can help parents by offering suggestions that do not require additional financial resources. These suggestions include, but are not limited to, having two people present for the bath so that one can hold and one can bathe the infant. The infant should be bathed in a small basin in the crib, or a rubber mat can be placed in the sink filled with only a few inches of water to reduce the risk of the infant's bottom slipping.

Water temperature should be tested before the infant is placed in the bath, and the infant should be removed from the bath if additional water is to be turned on for rinsing until correct temperature can be assured. At no time should an infant be left during a bath even if the infant is able to sit alone or is in a bath seat. Bubble baths are not recommended for infants because the detergent base of many of these products strip the infant's skin of natural oils and can cause rashes and irritation.

Feeding

Infant formulas should be prepared according to manufacturers' instructions. Infant formula should never be warmed in a microwave oven. Infants have been burned due to "hot spots" that can occur with the use of a microwave. Infants should be placed on their abdomen or side after eating to prevent aspiration if milk is spit up.

When finger foods are introduced, small food items such as hard candies, raisins, popcorn, peanuts, Vienna sausages, or regular wieners should never be given to the infant. These foods and foods of similar size and shape pose great risk for aspiration.

Nursing Implications

Although all of the information provided above appears to be basic common sense, infant deaths and hospital admissions related to these behaviors continue to be a problem. Nurses working with parents and infants must take responsibility to talk continually to parents about these issues. A nonthreatening, nondemeaning approach to the discussion of these topics may prevent an accidental injury of an infant whose "parent probably knows these things." For example, the nurse can approach the issue of finger foods by saying, "Now that Tim is eating finger foods, we like to remind all parents of the foods that can cause choking. These foods include. . . ." Nurses should also include anticipatory guidance for safety as a part of each well-care visit. Information should include preventive measures related to falls, burns, choking, aspiration, and child care equipment.

Assessing, Promoting, and Maintaining Health Perception and Health Management

The birth of an infant brings new responsibilities for parents in seeking and maintaining health care for the infant. The infant is generally introduced into the health care system at birth when a complete physical assessment is done by a pediatrician. In rural areas, the physical examination may be done by a nurse practitioner or midwife. Health care visits from this point on become the responsibility of the parents who choose a physician or clinic for the ongoing health needs of their newborn. A teaching plan for a 15-year-old mother of an infant is given here.

Although health care is considered a basic right of all people there is a wide gap in the availability and quality of health care within our society. Infant morbidity and mortality rates reflect this discrepancy between what we believe and what is occurring. It is important to keep in mind that the following is a presentation of what is considered to be the ideal health care practices and ones that should be pursued, not ones that exist for all people.

Choosing A Care Provider

As with every other aspect of parenting, there are choices to be made in the selection of a health care provider. It has become increasingly common in metropolitan areas for parents to interview a number of pediatri-

cians before choosing one to care for their child. Books, articles, and videotapes are also available to assist parents in this process. Parents are encouraged to ask questions of the pediatrician related to hours, availability of the physician during non-office hours, hospitals at which the physician has admitting privileges, and physical set-up of waiting area to accommodate the well-child separate from acutely ill children.

Additionally, parents are encouraged to ask what kind of phone information services are available. Can parents call the office and speak with a nurse or physician about a concern or for some advice in handling such things as colic or teething? Parents may also want to know the pediatrician's philosophy of handling children to decrease fear and anxiety, the amount of time allotted for a visit, and the willingness of the pediatrician to explain what to expect at the current visit as well as upcoming visits (Fig. 12-11).

In a recent study done in Tennessee, researchers[31] found that parents choose involvement of parents in decision making as the most important consideration in selecting a physician. Other frequently cited considerations included the importance of having phone calls returned quickly and a warm personality.

Parents who must rely on health clinics for well-child care due to lack of insurance or lack of access to a private physician also have questions and rights in the selection of a health care system. Although their choices are limited, it is important that the nurse working with them provide them with the same information a parent would obtain during the interview of a pediatrician. A positive, supportive introduction to the health care system increases the likelihood that the child will be brought back for scheduled visits.

Typical Schedule of Well-Care Visits

Well-care visits occur regularly throughout the first year. Six visits are recommended. (More information and a schedule for immunizations are provided in Chap. 9.)

Visit 1

The first visit after birth is generally at 2 weeks or 1 month of age. This visit is as much for the benefit of the parents as it is for the infant. New parents, especially first-time parents, can be easily overwhelmed by the amount of time and energy a newborn requires. Parents often have insecurities about what they are doing and are concerned with the progress the infant is making in height, weight, and general development. This visit provides the nurse with an opportunity to assess how the parents are doing, address concerns, and demonstrate through weighing and measuring the infant that he is making progress. It is important that the nurse reassure the parents and also assess and discuss the parents' needs for nutrition, rest, and time away from the infant.

The infant is weighed, measured, and given a general physical examination. Measurements are charted on growth charts, and the information is shared with the parents. Parents should be given ample opportunity to ask questions and voice concerns. Some parents may need

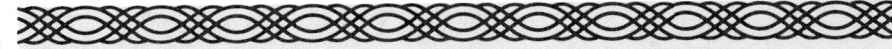

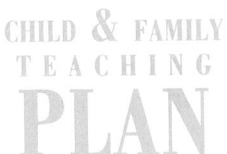

CHILD & FAMILY
TEACHING
PLAN

Infant Care During the First 3 Months

Assessment

Ms. Smith is 15 years old. She brings her 6-week-old daughter, Susie, to the clinic with the complaint, "She never stops crying. She wakes up during the night, even if I give her cereal before putting her down. I think there is something wrong with her."

Ms. Smith has had minimal experience in newborn care. She received no prenatal care and did not attend any type of prenatal classes. Her delivery was uncomplicated, and she had a short hospital stay. During her hospital stay, she attended a baby bath class and found it very helpful. "Susie loves to have her bath."

Ms. Smith was discharged from the hospital with Susie 48 hours after delivery. She completed the ninth grade but left school to care for Susie. She does not have a job and rarely sees her friends anymore. She lives with her mother in a two-bedroom apartment.

Susie weighed 6 lb, 6 oz at birth and was 18 in long; she now weighs 6 lb and is 18 in long.

Ms. Smith verbalizes approaches to nutrition that can be the cause of the infant's weight loss including overdiluting formula, attempting to feed the infant solids, and feeding the infant infrequently. She is concerned about her infant and is seeking help. Based on the nursing assessments, the nursing diagnosis, Knowledge deficit related to infant nutritional needs, was made. The teaching plan was developed to address this problem.

Child and Family Objectives	*Specific Content*	*Teaching Strategies*
1. Identify the needs of the infant related to nutrition	1. The role of formula in meeting all of the infant's nutritional requirements.	1. Use verbal explanation and encourage questions.
	Delaying the introduction of solids until 4–6 mo.	Demonstrate the extrusion reflex. Point out the infant's lack of teeth and inability to handle solids. Explain that research has not shown that cereal helps the infant sleep through the night.
	Formula preparation including proper dilution and clean technique.	Demonstrate preparation of a bottle using clean technique. Emphasize the need for measuring accurate amounts of formula and water. Have mother do a return demonstration. Encourage questions. Provide positive reinforcement.
	Feeding schedules and amount to be offered.	Outline a feeding schedule on paper 10 A.M., 2 P.M., 6 P.M., 10 P.M., 2 A.M., 6 A.M.
	5–6 oz every 4 h	Demonstrate 5–6 oz in a bottle.
	Six feedings per day	
	Burping infant one to two times during feeding and after feeding.	Demonstrate proper holding and burping on Susie, providing support to the head and gently rubbing or patting the infant's back.
	Placing the infant on abdomen or side after feedings.	Demonstrate the position of the infant on side or abdomen.

(Continued)

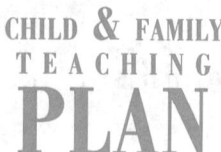

CHILD & FAMILY
T E A C H I N G
PLAN

Infant Care During the First 3 Months
(continued)

Child and Family Objectives	Specific Content	Teaching Strategies
2. Identify the needs of the infant related to safety.	Fall prevention. Never leave the infant unattended on changing table, bed, or sofa. Rapid rate of motor development in infancy. • Lifting head • Pushing up with arms when prone • Rolling over Infants should not be given small objects. Objects should not hang from string or ribbon on the crib. Crib safety Do not tie pacifier around infant's neck Discuss potential for burns or injury during bathing. Water safety. Do not turn water on while infant is in the tub or sink. Keep one hand on the infant at all times.	Demonstrate infant's ability to pick up head off the exam table when prone. Explain the increasing abilities of the infant as she develops. Discuss the potential hazards. Show photos. Have the mother describe any safety concerns she has. Provide a written handout on safety. Discussion of issues and written handout.
3. Identify importance of maternal and infant attachment.	Role of the mother in the attachment process: • Holding the infant • Talking to the infant • Responding to infant cries Role of the infant in the attachment process: • Looking at mother • Calming when held • Comfort of her feeding	Point out positive maternal behaviors Ms. Smith demonstrates and reinforce. Point out positive infant behaviors and reinforce.

Evaluation

• Ms. Smith demonstrates proper formula preparation using the clean technique.
• Ms. Smith verbalizes Susie's need for formula five to six times a day.
• Ms. Smith verbalizes safety issues in a young infant.
• Ms. Smith continues to practice good maternal behaviors for attachment.
• Ms. Smith returns for follow-up visits.

encouragement to ask questions. They may fear that asking questions indicates to the nurse that they are not able to care for their infant. The nurse should always be aware of the response to a parent's concern or question. A response that indicates frustration, annoyance, or lack of understanding may result in a parent's decision to stop asking questions or to stay away from the health care system. Nurses must be aware of the teaching needs parents have related to instructions for home care. For example, it is not enough to tell parents to take the infant's tem-

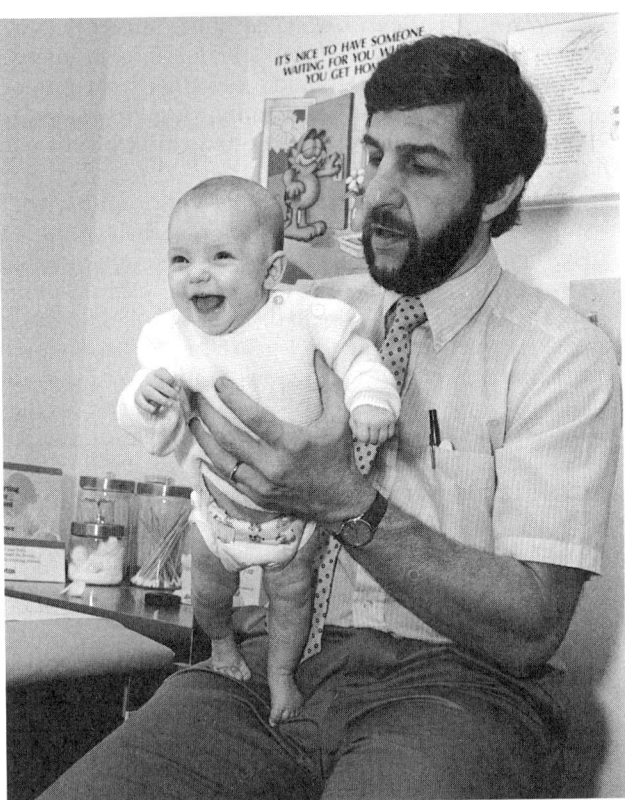

FIGURE 12-11
The pediatrician, whether in private practice or a health clinic, plays an important role in providing consistent care and teaching for parents. Parents should be comfortable asking questions about their baby and feel that the doctor cares.

perature if they suspect a fever. The nurse must be certain that the parents know how to take a temperature correctly. The nurse must use communication skills that allow for the parents to feel safe in saying that they cannot read a thermometer. Such a statement might be: "Mrs. Jones, we would like you to take Tim's temperature if he feels warm to you. Has anyone ever shown you how to take a rectal temperature or read a thermometer? I am glad to go over this with you as it can sometimes be difficult." This approach is more likely to make parents comfortable in saying they do not know how to take a temperature than if they were asked "Do you know how to take a temperature?" Topics appropriate for discussion during the first visit include nutrition, sleep, crying, and safety.

Visit 2

At 2 months, the infant returns to the health care system for head circumference, height, and weight measurements and for the first set of immunizations, which include DTP (diphtheria, tetanus toxoids, and pertussis vaccine), OPV (oral polio vaccine), and HiB (hemophilus influenzae type B; Fig. 12-12). The DTP can cause a local or systemic reaction, and acetaminophen is increasingly given before or at the time of injection to decrease the response (see Fig. 12-12). Parents are informed what to watch for and what measures to take should the infant have a reaction. For minor local reactions, acetaminophen can be given every 4 hours around the clock in a dose

prescribed by the pediatrician. A more severe reaction or any indication of neurologic involvement should be brought to the attention of the pediatrician immediately. No significant side effects to OPV or HiB have been reported (see Chap. 9).

The nursing assessment should include discussion of the infant's feeding patterns, parents' concerns related to feeding the infant, problems associated with feeding such as spitting up and maternal satisfaction with feeding. Sleep–wake patterns, elimination patterns, and motor and cognitive development should be assessed and discussed.

Visit 3

At 4 months, the infant returns for immunizations. The second set of DTP, OPV, and HiB immunizations is given. Before administering these, the nurse should take a careful history as to the response of the infant to the last set. Any time a serious reaction is described, the nurse should consult the physician before giving the injection. Once the immunizations are given, the nurse should review with the parents what side effects to watch for and what to do to minimize these effects (see visit 2).

Because many mothers have gone back to work at this time, it is important for the nurse to ask mothers about the transition. Mothers often have feelings of guilt when they first have to leave their newborn in the care of another person. The nurse can talk to mothers about their feelings and reassure them that these feelings are normal and a result of her attachment to her infant. A mother who is breast-feeding should be given an opportunity to talk about the experience and any difficulties she may be experiencing. Positive reinforcement at this time may serve to maintain breast-feeding longer.

Visit 4

At 6 months, the infant returns for a general physical assessment, height, weight and head circumference mea-

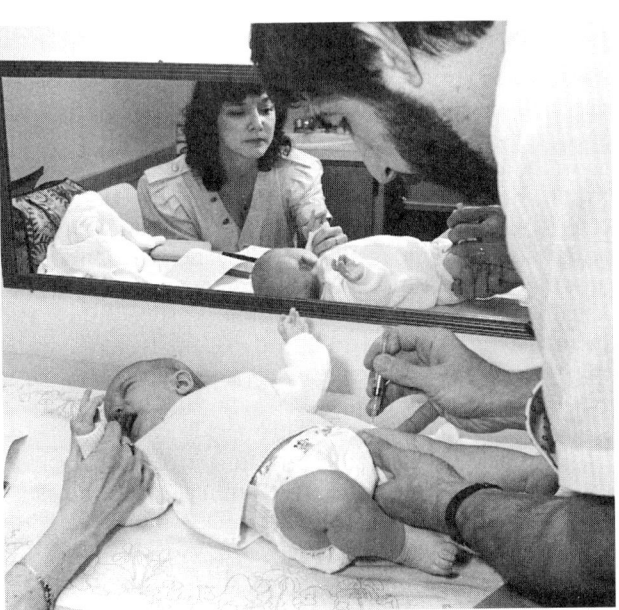

FIGURE 12-12
Immunizations are begun at 2 months with the DTP injection and oral polio vaccine.

surements, and the third set of DPT, OPV, and HiB immunizations. A developmental assessment is done at this time. The nurse continues to be supportive of the parents, encourages questions, and offers anticipatory guidance related to future developmental expectations. This visit should include a review of safety concerns that arise from the infant's progressing mobility.

Visit 5

This occurs sometime during the eighth to tenth month and is for a general physical assessment, developmental assessment, and measurement of growth. Parents should be asked about all areas of development including sleep–wake patterns, elimination patterns, feeding patterns, and activity patterns. Safety issues should be addressed.

Visit 6

The 1-year visit can be an exciting time for parents because their infant has made considerable progress in so many areas. The infant is given a physical assessment, weighed and measured, and assessed for progress in development in all areas. Parents should be provided positive reinforcement for their parental role. It is often helpful to talk to parents about their overall impressions of the past year. Parents should be asked if there are any concerns related to any area of development as well as their expectations for the coming year. A discussion of safety issues is vital as the infant moves into the toddler years. This visit is also an ideal time to offer anticipatory guidance concerning toilet training, negativism, and decreased appetite so that parents can begin to discuss approaches to these typical concerns of toddlerhood.

Health Care

Colic

Colic is frequently a concern that arises during the second or third well-care visit. Colic is caused by the spasmodic contractions of smooth muscles in the gastrointestinal tract, which cause the infant to cry for prolonged periods of time. The infant assumes a position with legs drawn up as if in pain. It is not uncommon for an infant to cry for 3 to 4 hours or more at a time. Episodes usually occur in the late afternoon or early evening. The infant may cry hard and is difficult to calm. Holding, walking, rocking, or rubbing the infant's back may bring some comfort to the infant. However, when this activity is stopped, the infant begins to cry again.

A colicky infant can cause a great deal of distress, concern, and frustration for parents. Maternal self-confidence is shaken, and new parents wonder why they cannot calm the infant.

Colic usually subsides by the third month of life. It occurs with equal frequency in breast-fed and bottle-fed infants. All infants have episodes of crying, and this should be differentiated from true colic.

Nursing Implications. The nurse must first reassure parents that they are not to blame for the infant's distress. A careful history should be obtained to determine the frequency, duration, and timing of colic episodes. Other conditions must be ruled out, including otitis media, a hernia, or anal fissure.

The nurse must support parents' efforts and various treatments. These may include changing the formula or changing the mother's diet for a breast-fed infant. Holding, walking, or rocking the infant may help, and parents should be reassured that doing this during colicky periods does not spoil the infant. Taubman[55] found that both parental counseling to assist parents in interpreting cause of infant crying and changing formula or maternal diet resulted in decreased crying episodes. However, the parental counseling decreased episodes of crying more quickly. Parents need to be encouraged to spend some time away from the infant without feeling guilty. Parents who are frustrated and overtired have more difficulty dealing with these episodes.

Pacifiers

The infant's sucking needs are greatest in the first 3 to 4 months of life. Even after feeding, the infant may have a need to continue sucking. These non-nutritive sucking needs should not be confused with hunger but rather must be met through other means.

Parents frequently ask for advice regarding the use of pacifiers or thumb-sucking behavior. They are concerned about the effect of these on dentition. The use of pacifiers or thumb sucking generally does not cause malocclusion if they are given up before the age of 5.

By providing a pacifier for the infant, parents decrease the likelihood of him developing thumb-sucking behaviors. The pacifier is less readily available for the infant, providing opportunities for him to develop other self-comforting activities. In discussing the use of pacifiers with parents, the nurse should discourage the use of pacifiers as the sole method for calming an infant. The pacifier should not be used to satisfy the need to be held, cuddled, or rocked. Pacifiers should not be dipped in sweet solutions because of the damage caused by sugar on the teeth.

A common practice in hospitals is to make pacifiers out of bottle nipples by stuffing them with gauze or cotton. This practice is unsafe and may result in aspiration and death of infants. A request has been sent to the American Academy of Pediatrics for a Policy Statement on safe pacifiers. Parents should be informed of this potential danger and encouraged to purchase one-piece pacifiers.[39] Hospitals should be encouraged to provide one-piece pacifiers.

Teething

The eruption of teeth in infants begins at about 6 months, and the child has all deciduous teeth by about 30 months (Table 12-18). Getting teeth is frequently the rationale most parents use for fussiness, restlessness, irritability, increased drooling, fever, diaper rash, runny nose, diarrhea, decreased appetite, and chewing on hard

TABLE 12-18
Tooth Development and Function

	Primary		Permanent		
	Average Age at Eruption (mo)	No.	Average Age at Eruption (y)	No.	Function
Central incisors	6–9	4	6–8	4	Shear, cut
Lateral incisors	7–10	4	7–9	4	Shear, cut
Canines	16–20	4	9–12	4	Tear
First premolars			9–10	4	Grind, chew
Second premolars			10–12	4	Grind, chew
First molars	15–21	4	6–7	4	Grind, chew
Second molars	20–24	4	11–13	4	Grind, chew
Third molars (wisdom teeth)			17–25	4	Grind, chew
Total		20		32	

objects. There is continued controversy related to what symptoms are directly related to teething among both the medical and nursing professions. There is consensus that infection or symptoms of illness such as fever, diarrhea, or vomiting should not be readily ascribed to teething.

The treatment of the symptoms that are a result of teething include the application of topical analgesics, systemic analgesics, and provision of hard or cold objects to bite.

Nursing Implications. Nurses should inform parents of the symptoms that may be associated with teething. More importantly, the nurse should inform parents of the symptoms often associated with teething that, in fact, are an indication of an illness. Beliefs about teething and the interventions recommended vary among cultures. It is important that the nurse provide parents with correct information and at the same time respect cultural beliefs. Rather than telling parents that grandparents are giving them incorrect information, a more appropriate approach would be to tell parents that new information is available that was not available to their parents. Any treatment or cultural remedy for teething that does not jeopardize the infant should be allowed.

When recommending treatment for teething, the nurse should include the following items in the discussion. The use of topical analgesics should be used in strict accordance with manufacturers' instruction. Overuse can result in depression of the gag and cough reflexes. Systemic analgesics should also be used with caution and only as prescribed. Acetaminophen is the usual drug of choice with infants and children due to the association of aspirin and Reye's syndrome during infectious illness. At each well-care visit, the nurse should provide the parents with the appropriate dose of acetaminophen based on the infant's weight. The nurse should be sure that the parents are able to measure correctly the dose of this medication or any medication prescribed. Cold or hard objects may also be helpful for the infant. Teething biscuits may soothe the infant and provide an opportunity for self-feeding.

Teething provides the nurse with an opportunity to discuss with parents their beliefs about dental care and

their plans for dental care for the infant. Although most dentists do not see a need for a dental visit in the first year, they do recommend fluoride drops if the drinking water is not fluorinated. Dental care should include cleaning the teeth with a washcloth or soft toothbrush. At 8 months, the desire to imitate parents provides a perfect opportunity to begin introducing the toothbrush.

Spitting Up

Bottle-fed and breast-fed babies swallow air when eating. This causes the baby discomfort and requires burping. Parents should hold the infant up in their lap or up on their shoulder to burp. Two burps during feeding and one after feeding are usually sufficient; however, as with all aspects of infant behavior, this can vary from infant to infant. If an infant does not burp after several minutes, feeding can be resumed.

Spitting up when a child is burped is common. It should not cause any concern as long as the infant is gaining weight. For reasons unknown, some babies spit up more than others or spit up a large amount of a feeding. The usual recommendation for parents is to burp the infant more frequently, sit the infant up after feedings, and decrease the amount of physical handling after feedings. However, these interventions do not always work, causing parents considerable stress. When these interventions are unsuccessful, it is generally related to the immaturity of the pyloric sphincter. Parents should be told that the spitting up decreases as the infant grows. Any projectile vomiting or vomiting resulting in weight loss or dehydration requires emergency intervention.

Loose Stools and Constipation

Loose stools are not uncommon during infancy, especially in the breast-fed infant. Loose stools should not be confused with diarrhea, which can be serious in the infant. Generally, parents are aware of the infant's usual stools and patterns of elimination, and, therefore, it is important for the nurse to listen to their concerns related to any change in this pattern. An assessment by the nurse should include a description of the stool, frequency, and associated symptoms. The nurse should also ask parents about the introduction of any new foods, an increase in the intake of vegetables or fruits, or a change in the maternal diet of a breast-fed infant. If the problem can be associated with one of these factors, the parents should be encouraged to temporarily eliminate the new food or change the maternal diet to see if there is an improvement. Diarrhea that persists may be a result of an infection, and medical attention should be sought.

Constipation is also seen in infants, especially in infants fed iron-fortified formulas. Parents may express concerns related to decreased frequency of stools or hard stools. A decrease in the frequency of stooling does not necessarily mean the infant is constipated. The pattern of elimination in the infant changes with the maturation of the gastrointestinal system and changes in diet. If parents describe the infant as having constipation, the nursing assessment should include questions about the consistency of the stool. Constipation is a dry, hard stool. If parents describe the stool as being soft but occurring much less frequently than usual, there should be little concern. If parents describe hard stools that cause the infant distress when passing, assessment should include additional information related to diet changes, a decrease in fluid intake, decrease in intake of fruits and vegetables, or a change in maternal diet. As with loose stools, the problem may be readily resolved with dietary changes. Dietary management of constipation includes increasing fluid intake or the addition of 1 teaspoon to 1 tablespoon of corn syrup or prune juice to an 8-oz bottle of formula. An infant taking solid foods can be given increased fluids and additional cereal, fruit, and vegetables.[46] Enemas and laxatives are not recommended for infants without direct supervision of the physician.

Diaper Rash

Diaper rash is a common occurrence in the infant. It is the result of bacteria formed by the heat and moisture that builds up in a wet or soiled diaper. There are several types of rashes that, if recognized and treated promptly, are easily resolved.

The most common type of diaper rash is the result of irritation of the buttocks and lower abdomen through contact with urine. This type of rash responds well to increasing the frequency of diaper changes and leaving the diaper area open to air when possible.

Red and raw rashes in the folds of the skin frequently result from heat and friction. This type of rash resolves if rubber pants are temporarily removed to decrease the amount of heat in the pants. Parents can be instructed to double diaper the infant to prevent urine from soaking through.

Red sore areas confined to the rectum and genital area usually result from loose stools. This may clear without treatment or application of petroleum jelly after cleaning and drying the area.

Ointments such as zinc oxide should not be used on irritated skin but may be used after the rash is gone to prevent reoccurrence. Baby powder should be used sparingly, and the use of cornstarch should be avoided because it can be a culture medium for bacteria. Any rashes that have blistering or drainage should be evaluated by a physician.

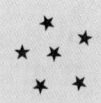

Ideas for Nursing Research

The child health nurse has an unique opportunity in well-child care to observe infants with their parents. This time can be used to study what works in positive infant–parent relationships, the roles the nurse may play in enhancing positive infant–parent relationships, and the impact of well-care and health promotion in general. The following areas need to be explored:

- Relationship between nursing intervention and maternal feelings of competence in breast-feeding.
- Relationship between early and repeated supportive interventions by nurses and the length of time a mother chooses to breast-feed.
- Presence of physiologic symptoms in addition to pain related to teething.
- Effectiveness of interventions related to colic as reported by mothers.
- Types of services provided by nurses used by parents in promoting optimal development of their infant.
- Correct use of infant car seats by parents with whom nurses have worked.

Summary

The first year is an eventful one as both the infant and parents grow and develop through the experiences they share. Nurses play an important role in assisting parents to promote optimal health patterns for the infant through assessment, identification of possible or actual problems, planning and instituting interventions with parents, and evaluating the effectiveness of interventions.

Nurses encounter parents and infants in many environments including well-care clinics, pediatricians' offices, hospitals, child care centers, and homeless shelters. Each interaction between the child health nurse and parents provides an opportunity for the nurse to assist parents in meeting the multiple needs of the infant and to foster confidence in their role as parents.

Parental success in problem solving during the first year and feelings of confidence in their role as parent provide a solid foundation for handling the new challenges of the toddler years. Parents who have positive experiences with a child health nurse during the first year continue to use the child health nurse for information, support, and problem-solving skills.

References

1. Ainsworth, M., Bell, S., & Stayton, D. (1972). Individual differences in the development of some attachment behaviors. *Merrill-Palmer Quarterly, 18*(2): 123–143.
2. American Academy of Pediatrics. (1985). Pediatric nutrition

handbook. Forbes, G. (Ed.). Elk Grove: American Academy of Pediatrics.

3. American Academy of Pediatrics Committee on Nutrition. (1976). Commentary on breast feeding and infant formulas, including proposed standards for infant formulas. *Pediatrics, 57,* 278.

4. American Academy of Pediatrics Committee on Nutrition. (1976). Iron supplementation for infants. *Pediatrics, 58,* 746.

5. American Academy of Pediatrics Committee on Nutrition. (1979). Fluoride supplementation: Revised dosage schedule. *Pediatrics, 63,* 150.

6. American Academy of Pediatrics Committee on Nutrition. (1979). *Pediatric nutrition handbook.* Elk Grove: American Academy of Pediatrics.

7. American Academy of Pediatrics Committee on Nutrition. (1980). On the feeding of supplemental foods to infants. *Pediatrics, 65,* 1178.

8. American Academy of Pediatrics Committee on Sports Medicine. (1988). Infant exercise programs. *Pediatrics, 82*(5), 800.

9. Arnon, S., Midura, J., Damus, K., Thompson, B., Wood, R., & Chin, J. (1979). Honey and other environmental risk factors for infant botulism. *Journal of Pediatrics, 94,* 311.

10. Baldwin, K. (1984). Muscle development: Neonatal to adult. *Exercise and Sports Sciences Reviews, 12,* 1–19.

11. Bowlby, J. (1969). *Attachment and loss,* Vol. I. New York: Basic Books.

12. Brazelton, T. B. (1962). Crying in infancy. *Pediatrics, 29,* 579–588.

13. Brazelton, T. B. (1973). *The neonatal behavioral assessment scale.* Philadelphia: Lippincott.

14. Bull, M., Stroup, K., & Gerhart, S. (1988). Misuse of car safety seats. *Pediatrics, 81*(1), 98–101.

15. Caldwell, B. (1970). *Instruction manual inventory for infants (home observation for measurement of the environment).* Little Rock, Arkansas.

16. Carey, W. (1978). Revision of the infant temperament questionnaire. *Pediatrics, 61,* 735.

17. Chapman, J., Macey, M., Keegan, M., Baum, P., & Bennett, S. (1985). Concerns of breast feeding mother from birth to 4 months. *Nursing Research, 34*(6), 374.

18. Dobbing, J. (Ed.). (1987). *Early nutrition and later development.* London: Academic Press.

19. Doucet, H., & Berry, R. (1988). Feeding practices of low income infants: A New Orleans Health Department study. *Journal of the Louisiana State Medical Society, 140*(3), 16–20.

20. Elardo, R., Bradley, R., & Caldwell, B. (1975). The relation of infant's home environments to mental test performance from six to thirty months: A longitudinal analysis. *Child Development, 46,* 71–76.

21. Erikson, E. (1963). Childhood and society. New York: W. W. Norton.

22. Ferber, R. (1986). *Solve your child's sleep problems.* New York: Simon and Schuster.

23. Ferber, R. (1987, September). Sleeplessness, night awakening, and night crying in infants and toddlers. *Pediatrics in Review, 9*(3).

24. Fomon, S. (1974). *Infant nutrition* (2nd ed.). Philadelphia: Saunders.

25. Fomon, S. (1987). Reflections of infant feeding in the 1970s and 1980s. *American Journal of Clinical Nutrition, 46*(1 suppl), 171–182 (review).

26. Geopferd, S. (1987). Infant oral health: A protocol. *Pediatric Dentistry, 9*(1), 9–12.

27. Gillis, J., & Fise, M. (1986). *The childwise catalog: A consumer guide to buying the safest and best products for your children.* New York: Pocket Books.

28. Goldman, A., Garza, C., Nichols, B., & Goldblum, R. (1982). Immunologic factors in human milk during the first year of lactation. *Journal of Pediatrics, 100*(4), 563–567.

29. Hakdawlala, D., & Widdowson, E. (1977). Vitamin D in human milk. *Lancet, 22,* 167.

30. Hanson, L. A. (1961). Comparative immunological studies of the immune globulins of human milk and blood serum. *International Archives of Allergy and Applied Immunology, 181,* 241–267.

31. Hickson, G., et al. (1988). First step in obtaining child health care: Selecting a physician. *Pediatrics, 81*(3).

32. Howard, R., & Winter, H. (1984). *Nutrition and feeding of infants and toddlers.* Boston: Little, Brown.

33. Illingworth, R. (1966). Sleep problems of children. *Clinical Pediatrics, 5,* 45–48.

34. Illingworth, R. (1983). *The development of the infant and young child.* London: Churchill Livingstone.

35. Jatsyk, G., Kuvaeva, I., & Gribakin, S. (1985). Immunological protection of the neonatal gastrointestinal tract: The importance of breast-feeding. *ACTA Paediatrica Scandinavica, 74,* 246–249.

36. Maley, M., & Achauer, B. (1987). Prevention of tap water scald burns. *Journal of Burn Care and Rehabilitation, 8*(1).

37. Marino, R., Bomze, K., Scholl, T., & Anhalt, H. (1989). Nursing bottle caries: Characteristics of children at risk. *Clinical Pediatrics, 28*(3), 129–131.

38. McIntosh, B. (1989). Spoiled child syndrome. *Pediatrics, 83*(1), 108–115.

39. Millunchik, E., & McArtor, R. (1986). Fatal aspiration of makeshift pacifier. *Pediatrics, 74,* 171.

40. Parmelee, A., Wenner, W., & Schultz, H. (1964). Infant sleep patterns from birth to 16 weeks of age. *Journal of Pediatrics, 65,* 839–848.

41. Parmelee, A., & Stenn, E. (1972). Development of sleep states in infants. In C. Clemente, Purpura, D., & Mayor, F. (Eds.), *Sleep and the maturing nervous system.* New York: Academic Press.

42. Pfeiffer, S. (Ed.). (1985). *Clinical child psychology: An introduction to theory, research and practice.* New York: Grune & Stratton.

43. Piaget, J. (1969). The theory of stages of cognitive development. New York: McGraw-Hill.

44. Pugliese, M., Weyman-Daum, M., & Lifschitz, F. (1987). Parental health beliefs as a cause of non organic failure to thrive. *Pediatrics, 80,* 175–182.

45. Parental health beliefs may cause failure to thrive. (1988) *Nutrition Reviews, 46*(6), 217–219 (review).

46. Queen, P., & Wilson, S. (1987). Growth and nutrient requirements of infants. In R. Grand, et al. (Eds.), *Pediatric nutrition: Theory and practice.* Boston: Butterworths.

47. Richards, M. (1982). Breast feeding and the mother–infant relationship. *ACTA Paediatricia Scandinavica (Suppl), 299,* 33–37.

48. Rickert, V., & Johnson, M. (1988). Reducing nocturnal awakening and crying episodes in infants and young children: A comparison between scheduled awakenings and systematic ignoring. *Pediatrics, 81*(2).

49. Rivara, F., Kamitsuka, M., & Quan, L. (1988). Injuries to children younger than one year of age. *Pediatrics, 81*(1), 93–97.

50. Robson, K., & Moss, H. (1970). Patterns and determinants of maternal attachment. *Journal of Pediatrics, 77,* 976.

51. Rush, D., Leighton, J., Sloan, N., Alvir, J., & Horvitz, D. (1988). The national WIC evaluation: Evaluation of the special supplemental food program for women, infants and children. VI. Study of infants and children. *American Journal of Clinical Nutrition, 48*(2 suppl), 484–511.

52. Satter, E. (1986). *Child of mine: Feeding with love and good sense.* Palo Alto, CA: Bull.

53. Schuster, C., & Ashburn, S. (1992). *The process of human development* (3rd ed.). Philadelphia: J. B. Lippincott.

54. Taitz, L. S., & Byers, H. D. (1972). High calorie/osmolar feeding

and hypertonic dehydration. *Archives of Disease in Childhood, 47,* 257–260.

55. Taubman, B. (1988). Infant colic syndrome treatment. *Pediatrics, 81,* 756.

56. Thomas, A., & Chess, S. (1977). *Temperament and development.* New York: Brunner and Mazel.

57. Tunnessen, W. (1987). Consequences of starting whole cow milk at 6 months of age. *Journal of Pediatrics, 111,* 813–816.

58. U.S. Department of Health and Human Services, Public Health Service. (1984). *State from National Center of Health Statistics.*

59. Weigley, E. (1990). Changing patterns of offering solids to infants. *Pediatric Nursing,* 16(5), 439–441.

60. World Health Organization. (1987). Breast-feeding/breast milk and human immunodeficiency virus. *Weekly Epidemiological Record, 33,* 345–346.

61. Ziegler, J., Cooper, D., Johnson, R., & Gold, J. (1985). Postnatal transmission of AIDS—associated retrovirus from mother to infant. *Lancet,* 896–897.

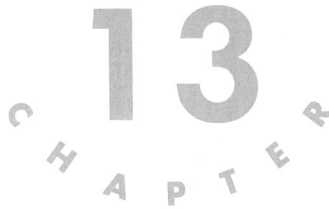

13

C H A P T E R

Health Assessment, Promotion, and Maintenance for Toddlers

BEHAVIORAL OBJECTIVES

Describe patterns of development of toddlers related to nutrition, elimination, sleep, psychosocial development, cognitive and language development, play, and safety.

Identify common concerns of parents related to toddler development.

Describe nursing assessment approaches with toddlers and parents related to development.

Describe nursing interventions to assist parents in promoting optimal development of toddlers.

Identify teaching needs of parents related to promoting optimal development of toddlers.

Discuss health maintenance needs of toddlers.

The beginnings of early childhood are reflected in the dramatic transition from infancy to toddlerhood. A toddler is a child who is 1 to 3 years of age. The psychosocial, cognitive, and psychomotor development of the toddler focuses on gaining independence, establishing a sense of self-awareness, actively exploring the environment, and achieving a sense of self-worth and autonomy.

Developmental theorists conceptualize and emphasize the toddler period as one in which the young child becomes more mobile, develops a greater sense of curiosity, and actively seeks to explore, manipulate, and achieve control over the immediate environment. The toddler shows more initiative in exploration such as touching, pushing, pulling, throwing, climbing, and dropping objects than was observed during infancy.

Goals for optimal toddler development include the following:

- Physical growth through a variety of foods and the development of self-feeding skills.
- Development of control of body functions—toilet training.
- Development of a sense of autonomy.
- Development of a sense of self-awareness.
- Improvement in motor skills.
- Use of language to communicate.
- Adoption of appropriate social behaviors.
- Toleration of separation from parents.

The toddler years present special and demanding challenges for parents. The independence and willfulness of the child may be new to parents and unexpected after a year of cuddling, holding, protecting, and meeting the dependency needs of the infant. Protecting the toddler during explorations of the environment and simultaneously encouraging emerging learning needs and curiosity pose new challenges for parents. Parental questions and concerns center on how to respond to the variety of new behaviors that emerge. Concerns that frequently arise correspond with the toddler's level of development. Parental concerns include changing nutrition patterns, struggles for independence, negativism, discipline, toilet training, and child safety. The toddler years are accompanied by specific goals for parents that include the following:

- Fostering optimal growth patterns through introduction of new foods and self-feeding skills.
- Beginning and promoting toilet training.
- Allowing for increasing autonomy.
- Enhancing cognitive and language development.
- Providing opportunities to develop psychomotor skills.
- Creating an environment that is safe and fosters development.
- Providing for health care needs.
- Incorporating health promotion behavior into daily activities.

During the toddler years parents need support and time for themselves away from the toddler. Knowing that new and sometimes difficult behavior is related to normal development does not help a parent who is tired and frustrated. Finding opportunities to take breaks is vital for the well-being of both toddler and parent. Parents can be asked about the outlets they have and how they regain their energy. Parents benefit from the nurse who offers anticipatory guidance in relation to the typical toddler behaviors that cause parental concern. Parents also need positive reinforcement in their parenting role and should be praised for their success.

Assessing, Promoting, and Maintaining Optimal Nutrition

As the rate of growth slows during the second year so does the toddler's appetite. Yet adequate growth and development depends on adequate intake of all nutrients (see Developmental Nutritional Profile). The increased activity levels of the toddler increase energy needs. Protein, calcium, ascorbic acid, and iron are especially important to growth in the toddler years (see RDA tables in Appendix). To meet the nutritional needs of the toddler, food must be chosen carefully so that the toddler's small appetite is satisfied with foods of high nutritional value. Food intake should include all four food groups in amounts appropriate for the toddler (see Chap. 8).

Milk intake should decrease during the toddler years as solid food intake increases. Energy needs should be met by solid food rather than milk because whole milk is deficient in vitamin C and iron.[34] Milk intake at the expense of solids will lead to iron deficiency anemia. The toddler who prefers milk to solids should be served milk at the end of the meal and juice between meals to prevent satiation before sufficient solids have been taken. Milk intake should not exceed 1/4 to 1/3 daily caloric intake or 32 ounces per day, unless appetite for solids is adequate and the toddler is not overweight.[1]

Preparing Foods for Toddlers

Optimally, toddler's food should be prepared without added salt or sugar. Food should be cut into small pieces the toddler can chew and served at room temperature. New and varied foods should be introduced. Research[6,7,11] has indicated that children are least likely to accept foods that are unfamiliar and foods that their parents dislike. Serving new food in small amounts along with familiar foods increases the chances that the toddler will try a new food. Additionally, toddlers need to become familiar with new foods before tasting them for the first time. Looking at, touching, and smelling a new food prior to tasting it is common. The acceptance of unfamiliar food increases with exposure to the food.[7] A toddler who refuses a food or spits it out after tasting it should, over time, have additional opportunities with the food.

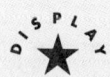
Developmental Nutritional Profile of the Toddler

- Slow but steady gain in weight
- Sphincter control developing
- Abandons bottle (varies with age)
- Feeds self and resents any help except when unusually tired
- Dining pleasures consist of getting food in mouth; conversation at meals more often a distraction
- Table manners rudimentary; frequently uses fingers instead of conventional tools
- Food consumption small

Adapted from Kennedy-Caldwell, C. & Caldwell, M. (1986). Pediatric enteral nutrition. In Rombeau, J., & Caldwell, M. (eds.). Parenteral nutrition: Clinical nutrition, Vol II, Philadelphia: Saunders, 434–479.

Developmental Considerations in Feeding Toddlers

Changes in eating behaviors during the toddler years are related to the toddler's desire for control over the environment, ability to elicit attention from parents, and ability and desire to explore the environment independently. Developing a sense of autonomy and "doing it myself" is critical to the developing toddler. Mastery of self-feeding provides the toddler with positive experiences and a sense of accomplishment. These developmental needs can be met or thwarted depending on opportunities that are provided and parental responses to toddler behaviors at mealtime.

Toddlers should be allowed to feed themselves. Through repeated practice they can master the skills necessary for getting food from the plate to their mouth without spills. Toddler skill in self-feeding is enhanced by having a child-sized spoon and fork and by having a dish or bowl with sides that are rounded up (Fig. 13-1). Drinking from a cup that is half full will increase their chances for success.

The toddler can experience a sense of accomplishment by eating all of the food if portions are small. Regularly introducing new foods with familiar foods provides many opportunities for experimentation with a variety of tastes and textures. However, parents need reassurance that the toddler may eat everything one day and next to little or nothing the next. The toddler should not be forced to eat. Over time the toddler will get all necessary nutrients if a variety of foods are offered at regular intervals.[1]

The toddler, who enjoys being involved, can begin to learn about social behaviors related to eating through imitation and mimicry. A positive experience is provided when the toddler is allowed to help set the table and sit with the family for meals.

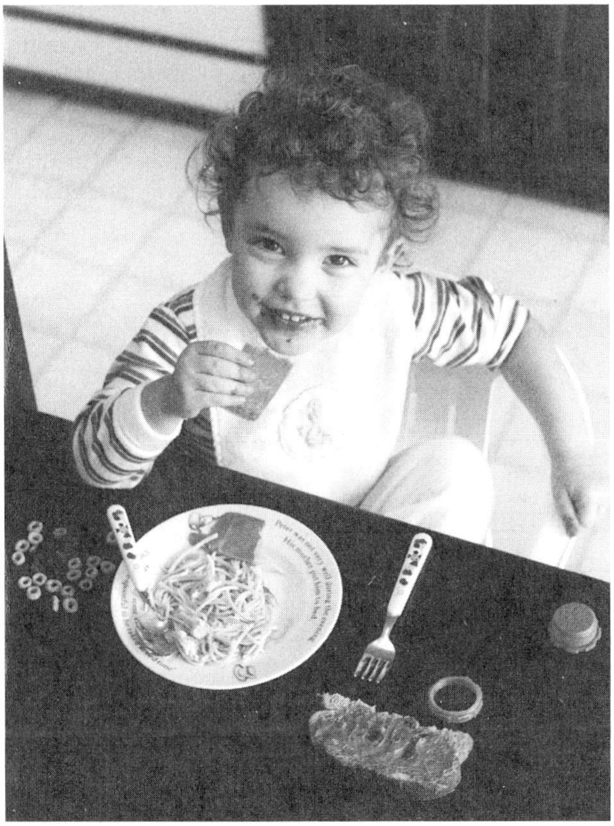

Parental Responses to Toddler Eating Behavior

For parents, the toddler is very different from the infant they have been raising. Changes in eating behavior cause many parents a great deal of stress. They may feel as though they are losing control, a feeling that is reinforced by the toddler's "no, no, no" response to offerings of food. Out of frustration, parents may frantically offer every food they have available until they find one the toddler accepts, or they may attempt to force feed the toddler. In both instances, parents are expressing concern for the toddler's physical growth. Parents who have had limited experience in problem solving with each other may not agree about the most appropriate ways to respond to these new and challenging behaviors.

Feeding toddlers requires a calm, relaxed manner. The ability to ignore negative behavior and reinforce positive behaviors is the key to the development of appropriate eating habits.

Continued Need for the Bottle

The toddler is at high risk for dental caries if the bottle is continued into the toddler years as a security object, especially at bedtime.[29] A child who needs the bottle to get to sleep has an increased potential for tooth decay due to the stagnation of milk or juice on the teeth. If parents have difficulty weaning the toddler from the bottle, they should be encouraged to give water in the bottle. Rather than going from whole milk to water in one step, parents can gradually make the transition by diluting the milk with increasing amounts of water until the transition to plain water is complete. Other ways to offer comfort, such as holding, rocking, or talking to the toddler, can be encouraged.

Typical Toddler Behaviors That Cause Parental Concern

Rejection of Foods. The toddler is able to refuse food by keeping the mouth tightly shut or spitting out disliked food. These behaviors can be very frustrating for parents. Parents need to know that this behavior is common and even the foods the toddler liked as an infant may be rejected. Offering small amounts of these foods along with accepted foods may help. Further, what a toddler rejects one day may be eaten with enthusiasm a few days later.

FIGURE 13-1
A toddler's skill in self-feeding is enhanced by using child-sized forks and spoons.

Food Jags. It is also common for the toddler to develop "food jags." This occurs when the toddler will only eat certain foods such as a peanut butter sandwich or grilled cheese. These food jags can cause considerable alarm in parents who fear the toddler is not getting adequate nutrients. Reassuring parents at this time that these behaviors are temporary and normal will prevent battles over food consumption between parent and toddler. Offering small amounts of other foods along with the desired food may be beneficial.

Food Rituals. Toddlers begin to develop rituals in eating behavior. They make a dish, cup, and utensils their own and refuse to eat with alternate utensils. The presentation of food also becomes ritualistic, such as cutting sandwiches square, not on an angle. These rituals will pass and should not be of concern to parents. Parents must be aware that these rituals should be shared with other caregivers to maintain the toddler's sense of security, especially in the absence of parents.

Food Routines. Toddlers also need routines. Meals are best eaten if served on a regular schedule. Toddlers often refuse to eat when they are tired or out of their normal routine. Routines should be shared with other caregivers, and parents need to consider routines when traveling to decrease frustration of both the toddler and parents.

Promoting Optimal Nutrition Patterns of Toddlers: Nursing Implications

Parents need an empathic, knowledgeable counselor to listen to their concerns about the adequacy of nutrition and feelings of frustration in feeding the toddler. Nursing assessment should include how parents handled weaning

during the first year, including the amount of independence they allowed the infant, parental knowledge of the developmental needs of toddlers for autonomy, and the extent of parental communication and agreement related to toddler eating behaviors.

Assessment should include all common areas of concern related to toddler eating behaviors (Table 13-1). Assessing which behaviors the toddler exhibits, including food jags, rituals, food refusals, and normal routines as well as the parents' responses to these behaviors provides the information necessary for planning interventions. Allowing parents to talk about their experiences with toddler self-feeding and the amount of food they think is adequate will facilitate the early identification of unrealistic expectations. Parents benefit from anticipatory guidance in relation to the typical toddler behaviors known to cause parental concern (Table 13-2). Knowing what behaviors a child may exhibit prior to their occurrence can prevent parental anxiety and parental overreaction to developmentally appropriate behaviors.

Assessing, Promoting, and Maintaining Optimal Elimination

Toilet training is a major developmental accomplishment that takes place during the toddler years. Toilet training requires parental patience and parental encouragement of the toddler. Based on a 10-year study of 1170 children, Brazelton[8] found that most children are trained by 27 to 29 months. However 40% of children were wetting the bed at age 4 and 30% at age 5.[8]

The decision to begin toilet training must take into consideration the child's readiness to begin and the parents' willingness to implement training. Parents may express concerns regarding toilet training practices. They may be confused about when to begin and how much pressure to exert. Parents may attempt to train the child

TABLE 13-1
Nursing Assessment: Questions for Assessing Patterns of Nutrition in Toddlers

Areas of Assessment	Key Questions*
Offers clues to parents' perception of feeding behavior.	How has _____ appetite been?
Are parents helping the toddler to develop eating skills through practice?	Does _____ feed himself or do you feed him?
Do parents have realistic expectations of eating abilities of the toddler?	How does _____ do when feeding himself?
Parents' feelings about adequacy of nutrition in their absence.	Does _____ eat well at the day care center?
Are parents aware of the ritualistic behavior of toddlers?	Does _____ have his own dish and utensils?
Are parents giving the child opportunities to learn through imitation and mimicry?	Does _____ eat meals with the rest of the family?
Do parents understand need for routines?	Does _____ eat on a regular schedule?
Have parents developed a feeding routine?	What is _____ regular routine? How does he react when routine is disrupted?

* State child's name.

TABLE 13-2
Nursing Intervention: Anticipatory Guidance for Toddler Nutrition Patterns

"Food jags"	Offer small amounts of other foods along with food the child will eat. Do not force the child to eat.
Foods offered	All four food groups should be offered. Children may eat a food previously rejected if served several times without comment. Toddlers enjoy finger foods.
Food environment	The toddler should be allowed to sit at the family table and begin to learn social eating behavior.
Utensils	The toddler should have a fork and spoon that are small and easily handled. Plates and bowls should have rounded sides to facilitate getting food on the spoon.
Maintain routines	The toddler does best when a routine for meal and snack time is established. Routines should be considered when traveling, and anyone caring for the child should be aware of the child's routines.
Milk consumption	Increased milk intake often results in a decreased appetite for foods. If intake of solids is poor, milk should be held until the end of the meal.
Introducing new foods	New foods should be introduced one at a time. Offering new foods along with familiar foods is helpful in getting a child to taste a new food.
Positive reinforcement	Toddlers benefit from positive reinforcement of appropriate eating behaviors. Negative behaviors such as spitting out food, dropping food, or throwing food should be ignored, which will decrease these behaviors.

before the child is physically ready. Some parents may have unrealistic expectations related to how long training should take and an intolerance of accidents. A survey of seemingly well-informed parents found that 50% of the parents studied planned to begin toilet training before the child was 16 months old, and 84% of those studied expected toilet training to be completed by the second birthday.[42] Listening to parents discuss toilet training concerns is an important role of the nurse in well-child care. Asking parents about their feelings and ideas regarding toilet training, when they plan to start and how they plan to proceed, should be done as early as the 12-month well-care visit. Early discussions of toilet training may facilitate a more relaxed, unpressured approach because parents will have an opportunity to observe for signs of the child's readiness, plan how to begin, obtain necessary equipment, and anticipate how to respond to the child's achievements and setbacks. Assessing for indications of the child's physical and physiologic readiness is an important part of the process.

Agreement exists among child health experts[8,17,33,39] that determination of a child's readiness for toilet training should include an assessment of motor skills that indicate neurologic readiness and of behavioral cues that indicate emotional readiness. The child is physically ready if the following behaviors are present. The child should be able to walk forward and backward and to sit comfortably on a toilet or potty chair without assistance. The child should be able to remove trousers and underclothing that have elastic waistbands and be able to stay dry for at least 2 hours.

Behavioral cues that indicate the child's emotional readiness include behavioral changes parents notice be-

fore and after the child wets or soils. The child may become quieter or seek attention; the child may shift body weight or have a facial color change. The child may have a word, gesture, or symbol indicating a need to eliminate.

Once the child exhibits physical and emotional cues of readiness, toilet training can begin. In most children such readiness emerges when the child is between 18 and 30 months of age.[8] In addition to the child's readiness, parents must evaluate their own readiness to begin toilet training. Parents should avoid toilet training just before or after a move, after an illness or hospitalization, just after the birth of a sibling, or during times when separations are more frequent. Adding the developmental crisis of toilet training to other stressful situations in the child's life increases the risk for frustration and failure in toilet training.[10,24,33,40]

Once the decision to begin toilet training has been made, parents need to choose a method to follow. A variety of toilet training approaches are available in child health and parenting literature. These approaches range from toilet training in 1 day[3] to more gradual training over several months.[8,14,16,27,33,40]

The decision to begin bowel training before bladder training is often reflective of the child's age. A younger child, 18 to 24 months, is more aware of the sensation to defecate and therefore more likely to gain control of defecation initially. If toilet training is started later, after the second birthday, the child may be trained for both bowel and bladder control simultaneously.[3,27]

Child care experts[8,14,16,17,27,33,40] recommend a gradual, child-centered approach to toilet training. The success of this approach depends on child readiness, parental readiness, and positive reinforcements for the child. The child is introduced to the potty chair at 18 months of age through observation of parents, siblings, or peers. It is acceptable for a child to observe others in the bathroom at an earlier age; however, actual toilet training should not begin earlier (Fig. 13-2). The child can be encouraged to sit on the potty fully clothed while in the bathroom with others. Parents may remove a soiled diaper while the child is sitting on the potty chair and drop the stool into the potty chair. After sitting on the potty chair clothed for several weeks, the child can sit on the potty chair without a diaper. Parents who can identify usual patterns of defecation may place the child on the potty chair at these times. If the child does not do anything, the child can be wiped and praised for the effort. A regular schedule of trips to the potty for bladder training can be helpful. This schedule may be when getting up in the morning, before breakfast, mid morning, after snacks, after lunch, mid afternoon, before and after dinner, and at bedtime. Parents should allow the child as much independence in the process as desired, helping only when necessary. All successes of the child should be praised through verbal expressions and physical displays of affection such as smiling, clapping, and hugging. Positive reinforcements for success with toilet training can be geared to the individual child's desires. These may include having a story read, going to the park, and so on.

Accidents should be expected throughout the training period and may occur even after training is completed. Parents should be encouraged to respond sympathetically rather than scold or punish the child.[40]

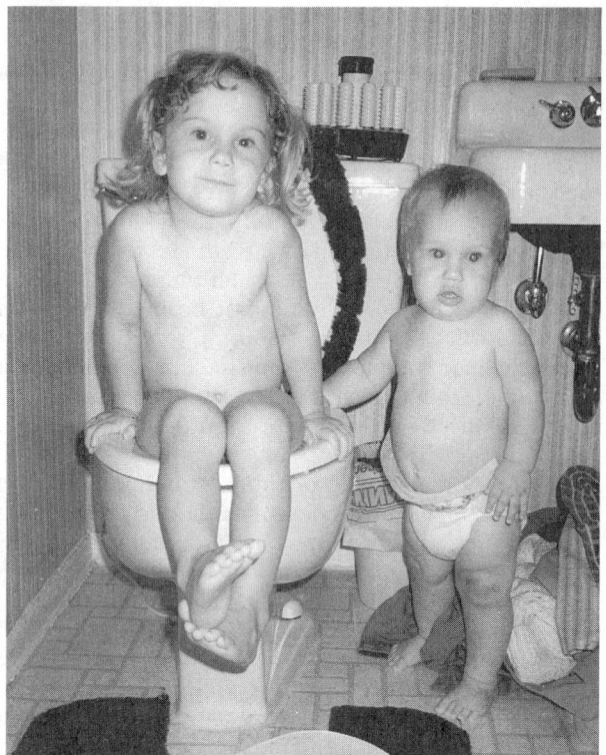

FIGURE 13-2
Sometimes toddlers learn about toilet training by observing older siblings.

A child who does not respond to or protests training efforts may not be ready for toilet training. Parents should temporarily discontinue training for several weeks and then try again.[33,40]

Assessing, Promoting, and Maintaining Optimal Sleep

By the second year a distinctive pattern of sleep behaviors emerges. At 1 year most children are sleeping 14 hours a day—this may include both a morning and afternoon nap.[19] The toddler usually sleeps 13 hours a day by the second year, with a 1- to 2-hour nap after lunch.[19] Parents need to determine a sleep schedule for the toddler because the toddler, if allowed to choose a bedtime, will stay up until he or she falls asleep on the spot. Because of the strong attachment to parents, the toddler may have some difficulty with the separation involved in bedtime. Common behaviors include a few or many post-bedtime demands, all of which seem reasonable in themselves.[41] These demands include needing a glass of water, needing to go to the bathroom, needing to put something away, and so forth. Parents can misinterpret this behavior and believe the child is being naughty, or they may feel it is indicative of a need for increased attention. If parents are prepared for this change in behavior, they will be better prepared to deal with it. This is a normal stage in the developing toddler, and parental accommodation to these demands is appropriate as long as parents are able to set reasonable limits on the toddler's behavior.

As the toddler gets older, going to bed becomes more difficult and bedtime rituals develop (Fig. 13-3). The increased difficulty in going to bed is related to a decreased tolerance of separation as well as a desire to exert independence. Rituals assist the child in coping with separation at bedtime because they reinforce the familiar and consistent patterns of parental behavior. Further, rituals give the child some sense of control because they are child centered. Rituals include setting animals in special places on the bed, turning on a night light, reading particular stories, and kissing everyone goodnight. Parents who are aware of this developmental phase prior to its occurrence can allow for rituals and at the same time keep rituals from becoming too complex. Parents may also choose to introduce the child to bedtime prayers as part of the bedtime ritual. Rituals provide the toddler with a sense of security and reflect the need for routines in daily activities. All rituals should be shared with other care providers to minimize disruption of the toddler's routines when parents are unavailable. Preparing the toddler for bedtime can be a special time for the toddler and father or mother who has been at work all day.

Fears of separation at bedtime can be decreased by allowing the child to take a favorite teddy, blanket, or toy to bed. This approach is more helpful in the long run than one that avoids separation, such as one parent lying down with the child until the child is asleep or bringing the child into the parents' bed until the child is asleep. Children develop sleep associations through rituals and routines that become familiar and dependable. If a child awakens during the night and sleep associations familiar to the child are present, the child may be able to go back to sleep without parental intervention. For example, if the bedtime ritual includes mother or father lying down with the child until the child is asleep, the child may find it difficult to go back to sleep during the night without

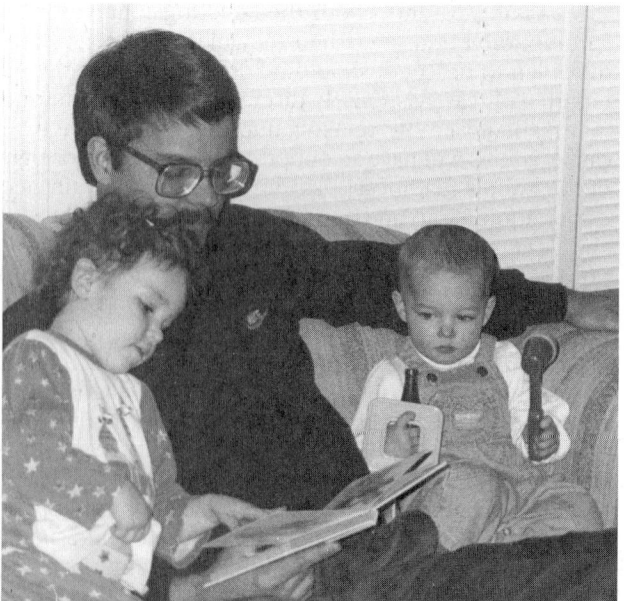

FIGURE 13-3
Bedtime rituals may include the use of stuffed animals, bedtime stories, or other activities.

the presence of parents. If instead the child goes to sleep with a special object such as a teddy, the teddy will still be there when the child awakens and the child can go back to sleep in an environment that is comfortable and familiar. However, not all children need environmental circumstances to be the same to be able to go back to sleep without assistance after a night awakening.

Nursing Implications

Nurses who work with parents need to assess the sleeping behaviors of toddlers by interviewing parents regarding sleep. Naptime and bedtime rituals are topics that need to be addressed. During the discussion of toddler sleep behaviors, the nurse can also assess parental ability to identify when the toddler is in need of sleep, avoiding increased irritability, fussiness, negativism, or temper tantrums (Table 13-3). By providing anticipatory guidance, nurses can prepare parents for typical toddler sleep behaviors. Anticipatory guidance specifically in relation to rituals also helps parents accept and enjoy the bedtime experiences (Table 13-4).

Cosleeping

Child health care professionals frequently advise parents not to sleep with their children.[4,9,20,25,41] However, in other cultures, including families in Latin America and Asia, infants and children sleeping with other family members is common practice. In our own culture cosleeping between parents and children was a routine practice until the twentieth century.[43] Specific concerns about the potential ill effects of cosleeping are that it may interfere with the child's development of independence, it may become a habit that is difficult to break, or it may interfere with the parental relationship and cause anxiety for the child because of the increased likelihood of witnessing sexual intercourse. These concerns have not been empirically studied, but the relationship between cosleeping and sleep disturbance has been studied. Lozoff et al.[26] studied urban families with children between the ages of 6 months and 4 years. They found cosleeping to be a routine practice in 70% of black families and 35% of white families. Sleep problems were more common in the white population, with more than half of the children sleeping with parents having a disruptive overall sleep problem. Among black children there was no association between cosleeping and sleep problems. Instead, there was a nonsignificant increase in the number of black children with sleep disturbances who did not sleep with other family members.

The authors suggest that the reason for these findings may be related to the acceptance of cosleeping patterns within a subculture. They suggest that cosleeping must be considered in its cultural context, and consideration of the reasons that motivate the practice must be examined before judgment is made. Rigorous study of the relationship between cosleeping and other concerns described by child health care professionals is still needed.

Nursing Implications

Nurses are in a position to discuss sleep patterns with parents. The nurse should be aware of the variety of sleep arrangements that exist due to cultural, socioeconomic, and individual differences in parenting. The assessment of the child and family's satisfaction with sleep patterns, the identification of any sleep problems, and the overall well-being of the child can be discussed.

If sleep disturbances are identified, a discussion of sleeping arrangements, bedtime rituals, specific sleep behaviors, and parental response to disturbances described must be pursued. The nurse can then assist parents in identifying underlying cause of the sleep disturbance and offer suggestions for their resolution.

TABLE 13-3
Nursing Assessment: Questions for Assessing Toddler Sleep Patterns

Areas of Assessment	Key Questions*
Parents' awareness of sleep needs of toddlers.	Tell me about _____ sleeping patterns.
	Naps _____
	Time to bed _____
	Time up _____
Parents' ability to observe behaviors indicating need for sleep.	How do you know when _____ is getting ready for bed?
Behaviors associated with going to bed.	Does _____ have a bedtime routine?
	Describe.
Parents' perception of factors that interfere with toddler's normal routines.	Under what circumstances does _____ have difficulty going to bed?
Parents' ability to deal with these factors.	What do you do to help _____ in these situations?
Night waking and parents' response.	Does _____ wake up during the night?
	How do you handle this?

* State child's name.

TABLE 13-4
Nursing Intervention: Anticipatory Guidance for Promoting Healthy Sleep Patterns

Environment	The toddler should sleep in a separate room from parents. The crib should be placed away from any hazards such as cords on blinds, windows, or electrical outlets. The mattress should be in the lowest position. A favorite toy or blanket should be available.
Prebedtime activities	Parents can spend some quiet time with the toddler prior to bedtime.
	Toddler benefits from a routine related to bedtime such as having dinner, then a bath followed by a story, and then going to bed.
	The toddler will have less difficulty with sleep if regular hours are followed for naps and bedtime.
	All bedtime rituals and routines should be shared with other caregivers.
Night waking	It is normal for toddlers to awaken during the night. Awakenings are generally short, and the toddler should be able to go back to sleep on his or her own. If a toddler needs parental assistance, parents should consider possible sleep associations that interfere with the toddler's ability to go back to sleep alone. Parents can assist the child in developing self-comforting skills by gradually delaying intervention every time the child cries and and by avoiding bringing the child to the parents' bed.

Assessing, Promoting, and Maintaining Optimal Psychosocial Development

Psychosocial development is a major focus of the toddler years. The toddler is developing a sense of autonomy and self-awareness at the same time as dealing with separation anxiety, learning acceptable social behaviors to cope with frustration, and developing increasing self-control. These needs should be considered when selecting a day care center (see Chap. 14).

Developing Autonomy

According to Erikson's[18] scheme, toddlerhood is a time to develop a sense of autonomy and a corresponding sense of self-worth. A sense of shame or doubt, which can lower the child's sense of self-esteem, is the potential negative outcome of this phase of development.

Autonomy is promoted when there is a secure, nurturing, supportive, and positive relationship between parents and toddler. A toddler who did not develop a sense of trust in the first year may need to experience a more secure, trusting relationship with primary care providers to achieve a sense of autonomy. The child's comfort in exploring the environment depends on a sense of trust that parents are available and will protect the child. Trust must continue to be nurtured during the toddler years. A child who does not trust will not try new experiences and may cling to parents or become withdrawn. The toddler's psychosocial development can be encouraged and reinforced by parents who are aware of the need to set consistent limits, provide support and reassurance,

communicate in positive and more complex ways, and create a growth-fostering, trusting environment that shapes a toddler's positive self-image.

Parental Role

A safe environment where the toddler is free to explore is optimal as the child develops autonomy. The toddler needs a variety of experiences inside the home as well as outside. These experiences may include opportunities to manipulate household objects such as pots and pans. They may also include trips to the store, park, or zoo. Autonomy can be supported by allowing extra time for the toddler to participate in self-care activities, including eating, dressing, bathing, and picking up play things (Fig. 13-4). The toddler should be allowed to make simple choices between two alternatives, such as what to wear and eat or in what activity to participate. Giving the toddler more than two choices may be overwhelming. As the child develops autonomy, consistent, reasonable limit setting is beneficial for the toddler. These limits will be tested and need to be maintained if the toddler is to learn self-control.

Nursing Implications

The nurse can assess the toddler for evidence of developing autonomy (Table 13-5). A toddler demonstrating autonomy will be observed actively exploring the environment, seeking parental approval when a task is mastered, and moving away from parents to explore. The au-

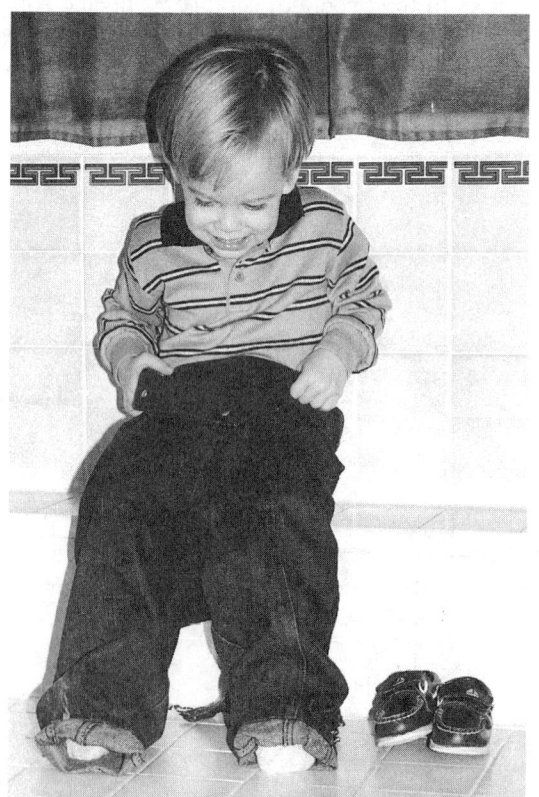

FIGURE 13-4
Allowing toddlers opportunities to help dress themselves can promote autonomy.

TABLE 13-5
Nursing Assessment: Observation of Developing Autonomy

Toddler Behaviors That Demonstrate Autonomy

- Actively explores the environment.
- Seeks parental approval when he or she has mastered a task.
- Willing to explore away from mother or father.
- Exerts independence during feeding, dressing, and toileting.
- Initiates social interchange with parents.
- Smiles, talks, and shows mother objects from a distance.
- Able to wait until mother is done with something to have needs met.

Parental Behaviors That Foster Autonomy

- Present when the toddler explores toys and objects but does not inappropriately interfere.
- Provides varied experiences that are developmentally appropriate for the child's level of skill.
- Provides immediate, positive reinforcement when the child is successful with goals and tasks.
- Allows the toddler independence in activities of daily living, including dressing, eating, and toileting.
- Allows child to play with a variety of toys.
- Permits child to practice rituals.
- Answers child's questions in appropriate, positive ways.
- Provides child with opportunities to interact with other children and environments away from home.

Toddler Behaviors That Demonstrate Shame and Doubt

- Does not explore toys, objects, spaces, and home environment.
- Unable to tolerate separation from mother or father.
- Does not smile or express needs to mother.
- Does not initiate interactions with parents.
- Does not attempt to participate in feeding, dressing, and toileting.
- Does not engage in parallel play with other children.

Parental Behaviors That Lead to Shame and Doubt

- Keeps child in playpen or crib and does not allow exploration.
- Does not provide any stimulating experiences or objects or provides objects that are too complex.
- Continues to keep child dependent by feeding, playing for, and not allowing exploration.
- Overly concerned about neatness of the house.
- Discourages rituals.
- Focuses on failure to master a new task.
- Fails to reinforce successful experiences.
- Fails to answer child's questions.
- Views exploratory behavior as being bad and perceives child as always getting into things.

tonomous child will also exert independence in feeding, dressing, and bathing, interacting with parents and being tolerant of short waiting periods for parental attention.

The nurse can also assess parental ability to promote autonomy and assess parental comfort with the toddler's demands for independence. A parent fostering developing autonomy will be present for the child but not interfere with the child's explorations. The parent will provide a variety of experiences that are appropriate for the toddler's level of skill. For example, a parent would provide a toddler a five-piece wooden puzzle to master rather than a 50-piece puzzle. The parent will reinforce the child's success by giving verbal praise when a task is mastered. Parents who understand the toddler's need for increasing independence will allow the toddler to participate in daily self-care activities. This may include self-feeding with a spoon, removing clothes after they have been unbuttoned and partially removed, and washing one's tummy in the bathtub with the washcloth as a parent washes other areas (Fig. 13-5). Parents who allow the child to interact with other children and experience environments away from home are fostering autonomy.

Parents need positive reinforcement for their successful attempts at promoting autonomy. Parents also need an opportunity to be given information that may be helpful in the ongoing experience with an increasingly independent toddler (Table 13-6). Discussing with parents that the transition from dependent infant to independent toddler can be difficult is an ideal place to begin. Explaining to parents that conflicts can be reduced by allowing the toddler to make simple choices will provide

parents with a starting point. For example, parents might allow the toddler a choice between a snack of apple slices or orange sections.

Parents who respect the toddler's choices will increase the toddler's self-confidence in making choices. Parents must also be aware that a toddler may persist in an activity the parent wants stopped in an effort to get attention. Most importantly, nurses must stress that promoting autonomy and at the same time setting limits requires much parental thought and patience. Parents will

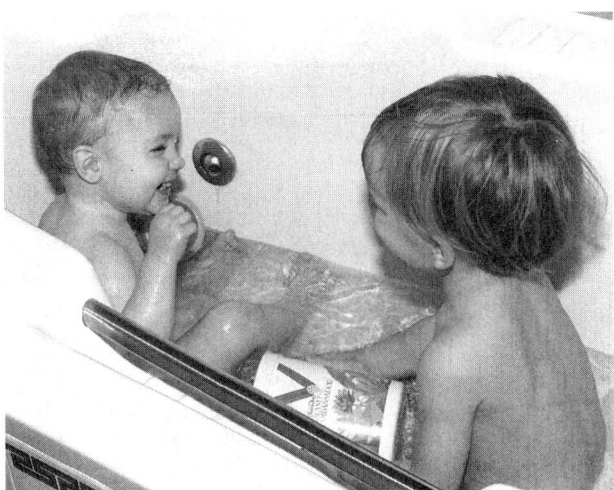

FIGURE 13-5
Bath time can be fun and is an opportunity to learn how to bathe oneself.

TABLE 13-6
Nursing Intervention: Anticipatory Guidance
for Promoting Autonomy

- Provide a safe environment where the toddler can explore.
- Set reasonable and consistent limits.
- Provide varied experiences for toddler both inside and outside the home, including kitchen play with pots and pans, outdoor play with water or sand.
- Praise toddler when he or she seeks approval and is successful with new tasks.
- Acknowledge the child's sense of self-control and ability to tolerate frustration.
- Be available to the toddler but do not interfere in play unless the toddler requests participation or assistance.
- Allow extra time for independence in feeding and dressing.
- Allow the child small measures of control.
- Anticipate that child will test limit-seeking behaviors.
- Follow through on limits that have been established for the child.

not always have the patience necessary when confronted with multiple demands for their time and energy. However, by offering anticipatory guidance for promoting autonomy, the nurse can provide parents with concrete suggestions that will make the experience a positive one.

In working with parents who are having difficulty with developing autonomy, the nurse will often find that the problem is related to parents' lack of knowledge regarding this developmental stage. Helping parents to understand that the child is not intentionally trying to misbehave but rather is going through a developmental phase may allay some anxiety. However, some parents may need direct support and assistance in coping with toddler independence (see the Parent Teaching display).

Developing Self-Awareness

By the end of the first year the infant begins to have an awareness of being a separate individual. This is a major developmental milestone and involves a healthy process of separation-individuation. The toddler moves away from the total protection of parents. Parents who provide a safe and caring atmosphere for exploration promote the child's sense of self as a separate and unique person.

This sense of self-awareness can be promoted by parents who provide the child with opportunities to explore the environment. Initially they must be in sight when the toddler ventures away to provide a sense of security. As the toddler gets more comfortable in explorations, parents will be less frequently summoned. Allowing the toddler to assist with dressing and undressing provides opportunities to experience the difference between self and objects such as clothing, shoes, and hats. A mirror provides opportunities for toddlers to see themselves as separate from parents or siblings, especially when all participate in the activity. Teaching the toddler names of body parts, including eyes, toes, fingers, nose, an so forth, and associating them with the child, for example, "Tommy's nose," also fosters a sense of self. Playing simple games such as peek-a-boo and saying "where's Tommy" when eyes are covered brings expressions of delight and a vigorous "here I am!" A game of modified hide-and-seek when a parent or child only partially hides fosters the toddler's understanding of separate individuals and a sense of self.

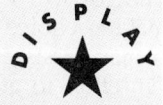

Parent Teaching: Topics to Assist in Resolving Conflicts and Concerns Related to Autonomy

- Many parents find it difficult and confusing to go through the transition from the child's total dependence to wanting to do some things for and by self.
- Many parents experience that frictions tend to be reduced when the young child who is struggling for autonomy is allowed to make some decisions about himself or herself that involve simple choices.
- Some children who are allowed to make simple choices when they are ready seem to become independent earlier, e.g., dressing, self-feeding, picking up own toys.
- Some of the child's first verbalizations, like "me do it," "no," and "mine" indicate that the child is beginning to have a sense of self and is ready to make some choices.
- Sometimes children persist in doing something the parent does not want them to do to get attention.
- Many parents find it easier to anticipate troublesome situations with their child and try to prevent them rather than react strongly after the child has gotten into trouble.

- Setting limits requires a great deal of thought, and helping the young child learn requires much adult patience.
- Parents can prepare their child to make reasonable choices later by acknowledging the child's likes and dislikes verbally, e.g., "I guess you really like pudding," or "I can see that you don't like this little doll as well as you like this little ball."
- Most young children can handle only simple choices between two alternatives, e.g., "Do you want to wear the red sweater or yellow sweater today?
- The child will gain confidence and the ability to make choices if the parent is able to respect the child's choices and acknowledge them.
- Making choices for himself or herself in the early years may help the child to be more self-reliant and responsible in later years.

Adapted from Bromwich, R. (1981). Working with parents and infants: An interactional approach (pp. 224–225). Austin, TX: Pro-Ed Inc.

Parental Concerns Related to Psychosocial Development

Directly related to the toddler's developing sense of autonomy and self are behaviors that cause parental concern. These behaviors include separation anxiety, negativism, and temper tantrums and reflect ambivalence on the part of the toddler for increased autonomy and a continued desire to be cared for by parents. How parents deal with these concerns can affect the child's coping skills and development of appropriate social behavior.

Separation Anxiety

Separation anxiety is a frequent concern of parents during the toddler years. Children experience separation anxiety in varying degrees, but it most commonly peaks first at about 8 to 10 months and again from 18 to 24 months. A child's reaction to separation is related to the following variables[36]:

- The degree of attachment with mother or father.
- The age of the child.
- Past experiences with separation.
- Duration of separation.
- Circumstances surrounding separation.

Many parents ask for guidance in dealing with separation anxiety. However, all parents should be prepared for this developmental phase.

Parental Role

Parents can help children cope with separation through playing games such as peek-a-boo and later hide-and-seek. These games help the child to realize that mother can be out of sight yet still exist. Providing opportunities for the child to experience separation early and avoiding first separations when separation anxiety is at its peak may lessen the anxiety and distress for the child. Repeated, short separations help to prepare the child for longer ones. If a parent knows a child will be going to day care in the fall, the child can be given frequent opportunities during the summer with a sitter or relative. As the fall draws near, separations can be daily for short periods or as frequently as they are to occur when day care is begun.

Ideally, a child should be exposed gradually to a new caregiver. Parents can facilitate this by having a new caregiver come to the house and interact with parents and child. This experience allows the child to become comfortable while parents are available. If a child is going to day care, a parent can accompany the child and stay at the day care the first few times. Each day the parent may increase distance from the child, encouraging the child to become involved with activities. Establishing a routine for saying "good-bye," such as walking the parent to the door, giving a hug and kiss, or waving out the window, can be reassuring to the child. Parents should tell the child when they will return in terms the child can relate to. For example, rather than saying "I will be back at 2 o'clock" say "I will be back after you eat your lunch."

Having a favorite toy or something that belongs to the parent may help the child tolerate separation away from home. Practicing separation through age-appropriate games can be beneficial. A 12-month-old child can learn about going away and coming back through peek-a-boo; an 18-month-old can be sent on an errand to other rooms in the house; the 2- and 3-year-old can play hide-and-seek.[39]

Nursing Implications

Collecting data about an individual toddler is necessary before the nurse can develop specific interventions to decrease separation anxiety. Assessment can be approached by a discussion of the variables known to increase separation anxiety. In assessing the degree of attachment to parents, the nurse can collect information related to the frequency of crying and clinging behaviors, how long the child cries after parents leave, and the child's response to parents when they return. Because separation anxiety is more pronounced from 18 to 24 months of age, knowing the child's age and when parents first noted changes in the child's reaction to separation may be used to reassure parents that this is a normal phase for the child. Past experience with separation and the length of past separations may have an impact on the child's tolerance for separation. A child who has been going to day care since infancy will have less difficulty going as a toddler than a child who has never gone to day care.

When circumstances surrounding separation are due to illness of child or parent or family disharmony, the reaction of the child will be more intense.

Nurses must work with parents to develop specific interventions for each child (Table 13-7). The suggestions offered earlier must be tailored to each individual family situation.

Parents also may have difficulty coping with the separation. This may be due to feelings of guilt related to leaving the child, especially if the child has a strong reaction. Helping parents deal with the child's response will increase parental self-confidence and decrease feelings of guilt.

Negativism

In the desire to become autonomous, the toddler may exhibit behaviors that alarm parents and make them feel inadequate in their parenting abilities. Why else would Tommy behave so badly and be so stubborn? This "negativism" is expected to occur in all toddlers in varying degrees between the ages of 18 months and 2 1/2 years. This phase of negativism is considered a normal aspect of early child development. Behavioral manifestations of negativism include the frequent emphatic "no" by the toddler to any request or the use of nonverbal expressions such as running away, dawdling, refusing to lie down at bedtime, or refusing to stop a specific action. At times this seeming negativism is just an exercise in testing parents' limit-setting behaviors. All children pass through this stage in varying degrees depending on their temperament and how parents respond to their behaviors. Any child who is overtired, hungry, or ill may be more inclined toward the use of negativism.

TABLE 13-7
Nursing Intervention: Suggestions to Assist Parents in Helping Child Cope With Separation

- Emphasize that repeated brief separations help to prepare a child for longer ones.
- Discuss that first staying with friends and relatives with whom the child is familiar will help child adjust later to other caregivers.
- Explore how useful it might be to have the child become familiar with a new caregiver while parents are present.
- Emphasize that it helps the child to realize that the parent "likes" the new caregiver as the child observes them talk with each other in a friendly manner.
- Suggest that after the child has enjoyed playing with the new caregiver once or twice in the parent's presence, the child might find it easier to accept and enjoy the caregiver.
- Stress that some children exhibit more anxiety and stress associated with separation during certain stages of development.
- Suggest that it is easier for the child physically to move away from the parent than to be "left" by the parent.
- Discuss that the parent's leaving may be less difficult for the child if he or she can practice a routine for saying good-bye, e.g., waving at the window, handing the mother her purse, driving around the block with the parent.

- Emphasize that it might make it easier for the child to cope with separation if the caregiver accepts the child's feelings upon the parents' leaving, e.g., "Yes, I know you are angry and unhappy that Mommy is going out . . ."
- Discuss that it may help the child to be told when the parent will be back in terms of a sequence of routine events with which the child is familiar, e.g., "Mommy will be back after you eat your lunch, take your nap, and play for a while, and she will be home in time to bathe you and place you in bed tonight."
- Stress that some children respond better to separation if they remain in familiar surroundings or if they can hold on to something belonging to the parent or some favorite toy when away from own home.
- Explain that not only young children but their parents, too, experience separation as a difficult process.
- Support parents by stressing that it is not unusual for young children and parents to feel anxious about the first few separations and that these feelings are a reflection of the strength of their mutual attachment.

Adapted from Bromwich, R. (1981). *Working with parents and infants: An interactional approach* (pp. 189–190). Austin, TX: Pro-Ed Inc.

Parental response to this negative behavior is an important variable in reducing or resolving undesirable behaviors or verbalizations. Parents who accept negativism as a normal behavior are more likely to be tolerant and patient and to respond in a regular and consistent manner. Parents who are able to tolerate frustration will get through this phase without undue problems. Parents benefit from suggestions on how to decrease the frequency and intensity of this behavior. The nurse can recommend that parents keep directions and rules to a minimum, avoid unnecessary demands and keep safety the priority concern. When choices do not exist, it is helpful for parents to present a request in a positive way, "Let's take you for your bath and then have a story" instead of "You have to take your bath now or you will not be read a story." Further, children benefit from some transition time when engaged in a pleasurable activity. If parents tell the child, "You have a few more minutes to play and then we will be having dinner," the child knows what to expect. Parents who insist on breaking the child's will, use physical force, or perceive and treat the child as bad and naughty may elicit more extreme behaviors such as temper tantrums, kicking, biting, and throwing.

Temper Tantrums

Temper tantrums may be observed between 18 months and 3 years. "A temper tantrum is an intense outpouring of anger and frustration which is frightening to both a parent and a child."[30] Temper tantrums can be a result of the normal developmental phase of negativism during the toddler years. Although parents can minimize the amount of confrontations by providing the toddler some independence and choice, not all conflicts can be avoided. At some point a toddler will confront parental limit setting that thwarts the toddler's desires, and a temper tantrum may be the result. Temper tantrums are likely to occur if the child is overtired, hungry, jealous, or insecure or when parents are excessively strict. The child may scream, drop to the floor, kick, bite, throw objects, hit out at parents, or hold his or her breath to the point of turning blue or passing out.

Parental Role

Children require appropriate, consistent limit setting from parents to help them diminish and cope with such behavioral expressions, which are counterproductive to developing a sense of control and self-worth. Limit setting is the establishment of boundaries of behavior that will and will not be accepted. Limit setting requires that the consequences of not staying within limits will be dealt with in a predetermined manner and followed consistently. Limit setting will be discussed further in the section on discipline.

As parents deal with temper tantrums, they must first realize that attempts to reason with the child, hitting the child, or scolding the child only serve to increase this behavior. Parents who attempt to stop the tantrum by giving into the child are rewarding the child's behavior and increase the chances of the behavior being repeated.

Ignoring temper tantrums is the most frequently suggested method for decreasing or eliminating temper tantrums.[10,17,30,39] In addition, making an effort to give the child attention for positive behaviors is necessary to decrease temper tantrums. This attention can be in the form of a verbal praise or a physical pat on the back, a hug, or a kiss. However, parents often find it difficult to ignore temper tantrums in a public place. They are embarrassed by the child's behavior and may be willing to give in to the child just to avoid a scene. In this situation it would be more helpful for the child if the parent physically removed the child from the situation, explaining that the child's behavior is unacceptable. The parent can then take the child to a private area where any continuance of the behavior can be ignored. Shaming, criticizing, and humiliating the child should be avoided at all costs. These responses serve only to degrade the child and diminish feelings of self-worth. Parents may feel guilty, inadequate, and powerless in their actions when these methods of dealing with temper tantrums are used. Instead, the child should be given love, attention, praise, and desired objects when not exhibiting temper tantrum behaviors. Parents should explain to the child after the tantrum is over that they understand how the child feels but they want to help the child to express feelings in a different way.

Modifying a child's behavior often requires a change in parent-child interaction patterns and consistency in the method chosen to change behavior. Frequently parents will try various approaches to changing a child's behavior. Often the frequency with which they try a different approach does not allow for the consistency factor so important in helping a child learn new behavioral patterns.[30] Initially, parents need to identify the child's behaviors that are distressing to them. This goal can be accomplished by keeping a record of the child's behaviors and parental responses to undesirable behaviors. Parents can then be assisted to identify the precise behaviors they want to change in the child. Once ineffective behavioral responses are identified, alternative behaviors can be used to facilitate change. The use of techniques of behavior modification is appropriate for parents and children.

Behavioral modification involves changing the parent's behavior, which in turn modifies the child's behavior.[22] Behavior modification requires the initial identification of behaviors to be changed and keeping an ongoing record of progress made toward this goal. The combination of ignoring negative behavior and reinforcing desired behavior takes time and consistency (see the following section on discipline and limit setting). Parents must be willing to observe, record, and systematically reinforce desirable behaviors in children. Parents need support during the behavioral change process and the benefit of evaluation and feedback from health care professionals if they are to be successful in their new parenting interactions.

Nursing Implications

Anticipatory guidance for the parents when the infant is 12 months old may decrease the frequency of temper tantrum behavior. Nurses must be supportive of parents as the child passes through the stage of negativism and offer assistance in developing strategies to prevent temper tantrums. The nurse can emphasize that temper tantrums are difficult for parents in their relationship with their child. Prior to offering suggestions to deal with temper tantrums, the nurse must explain to parents that temper tantrums may be a reflection of the child's attempts to become a separate person, or they may be an expression of anger or frustration that the child is unable to cope with in more positive ways.

The nurse can then work with parents to identify behaviors that are distressing to parents. This can be done by asking parents to keep a record of the child's behavior and their responses to undesirable behaviors for a 7- to 10-day period. Once temper tantrum behaviors and precipitating factors are identified, specific interventions can be developed (Table 13-8). If temper tantrums are the result of the parents not allowing the child any choices or participation in activities of daily living such as eating, dressing, bathing, or selection of play activities, parents may simply need this pointed out. Providing the child with simple choices gives the child a sense of control and decreases temper tantrum behavior. Choices should be offered in areas that are flexible so that when decisions must be made related to child safety or at other times when the child must do as parents ask, the child will be more willing to comply without issue. If parents identify

---

TABLE 13-8
Nursing Intervention: Suggestions to Assist Parents in Responding to Child's Temper Tantrum Behaviors

- Emphasize that most parents experience temper tantrums as a difficult time in their relationship with their children.
- Emphasize that assertiveness, which is an aspect of the temper tantrums, reflects that the child is establishing himself or herself as a separate person.
- Explain that young children use their bodies to express anger and frustration before they are able to express feelings in a meaningful way.
- Reinforce that temper tantrums are difficult to live with, but they are a developmental step in the child's gradual learning of how to cope with negative feelings.
- Remind parents that some confrontations can be avoided by recognizing that toddlers want to do things by themselves and in their own way, e.g., ''I guess you want to put the toothpaste on all by yourself.''
- Discuss that ways can be found to avoid some situations that lead to temper tantrums, especially at certain times of the day when the parent's and the child's tolerance level is low, e.g., late afternoon and before dinner when both are tired.
- Discuss that allowing the child simple choices when possible may avoid a temper tantrum, e.g., ''Do you want to wear this blouse or that blouse?''
- Discuss which limits the parents are willing to be flexible about and which cannot be, such as safety issues versus less critical issues. Staying in the car seat while riding in the car and not playing in the street might be inflexible, whereas wearing boots on a warm day, playing with food, or eating another ice cream cone might be flexible.

- Explore if the child knows clearly what limits are and whether these limits are enforced, and that tantrums tend to decrease because having a tantrum is one way a child can test parental limits.
- Remind parents that as the child grows in self-control, the tantrum behavior will gradually decrease.
- Discuss that some children have a much more difficult time than others in learning and practicing self-control and that such children are more trying for their parents because the children need more help and the parents need to exercise more patience, yet will require more support from family and friends.
- Share with parents that it helps the child if the parent can accept the child's feelings but, at the same time, let the child know that his or her behavior is not acceptable, e.g., ''I know you are angry at me, but I will not let you hit me.''
- Share with parents that some infants and toddlers get over their tantrums more quickly when they are distracted by something interesting to do, e.g., ''I know you are upset, but why don't we read a story?''
- Remind parents that, knowing their children and themselves best, they ultimately must be the judge of what works best for both of them (parent and child). For example, some parents have learned that a child's temper tantrums are shorter and less intense when the child doesn't have a captive audience; others find that their child tends to calm down more quickly when the parent remains in the same room with the child.

Adapted from Bromwich, R. (1981). *Working with parents and infants: An interactional approach* (pp. 202–203). Austin, TX: Pro-Ed Inc.

temper tantrum behaviors as occurring at specific times of the day, especially when the child is tired, changing daily routines may help. Extending the child's naptime or having a quiet activity available for the child before dinner, such as reading a story, may provide extra attention at a time when the child is especially vulnerable. Parents must also understand that as the child develops increasing self-control, temper tantrums will decrease.

Discipline and Limit Setting

The young child needs assistance from parents and care providers to control impulses and learn socially acceptable behavior. Through experience the child will learn self-control of impulses and urges. Parents are responsible for promoting the development of self-control in the child through the appropriate use of discipline and limit setting. A variety of factors influence parental discipline practices. These include cultural background, religious beliefs, educational level, race, social class, and parental beliefs about the nature of power.[37] Parents who are unsure of how to discipline their child will generally follow cultural patterns or manage the child as they were managed. It is not uncommon for two parents to differ in opinion as to the best approach for discipline. A discussion of discipline and limit-setting practices is an important part of promoting healthy child development and should be part of well-child care.

Parents generally follow one of three childrearing philosophies.[37]

Restrictive Style. Emphasis is placed on having a child be obedient, respectful, and well mannered. Individuality and creativity are less valued attributes. Corporal punishment may be used if necessary. Limit setting is an important aspect of a restrictive parenting style, emphasizing the need for guidance and a consistent predictable environment.

Permissive Style. Emphasis is placed on autonomy and creativity. Strict limit setting through physical or psychological means is avoided. Rather than directing the child, parents use verbal interactions attempting to accommodate the child's impulses and desires, reason with the child, and suggest alternative behaviors for the child.

Authoritative Style. A combination of permissive and restrictive styles is employed. These parents emphasize their authority and set limits for the child more vigorously than permissive parents. However, they also encourage verbal interactions examining the reasons for a child's behavior and offering an explanation for their response to that behavior.

Although parenting styles may be quite different, no consistent differences were found in the incidence of behavioral problems among two groups of children reared by restrictive versus permissive parents.[12] A more important factor found to influence child behavior was maternal warmth, seen by the use of praise, the quality of time spent with the child, and the frequency of physical displays of affection, hugging, and kissing.

Teaching Discipline. The word *discipline* refers to teaching. Through discipline parents instill desirable values and a discipline based on those values into the

minds of children.[5] Children learn as they admire and emulate those they love.

The toddler who developed a sense of trust and attachment to parents has a desire to gain parental approval. Parental disapproval will influence the child's conduct. However, there are times when the child's desire to explore or to do something the parent does not wish the child to do is stronger than the desire for parental approval. For example, a child may have a stronger urge to investigate the flashing lights and multiple buttons and knobs of the stereo than to gain parental approval by not going near the stereo when parents say "no." The child is not deliberately trying to misbehave but rather is acting on the natural urge to explore the environment.

During the toddler years parents may have to make temporary changes in the environment so that the child is not constantly being told "no, don't touch that." It is especially helpful if the child has a room that is safe for exploration and contains minimal forbidden objects.

At times the child's impulses can be redirected by substituting an appropriate activity for a desired activity that is not allowed. In the case of the stereo, the child can be given a busy box with knobs and cranks and doors. If a substitution is not effective and the child's urges are strong, physical removal from the room may be necessary. See Table 13-9 for discussion questions to guide parents in practicing discipline.

Discipline that is excessive or inadequate may result in a child who is unable to control impulses or learn acceptable patterns of behavior. Discipline is excessive if it demands more than the child is capable of doing. If a child is expected to be perfectly obedient, always clean and tidy, and have perfect manners, frustration and self-doubt will result. It is also unrealistic to expect a toddler to be able to control impulses to explore in a room filled with interesting objects that are off-limits.

On the other hand, a toddler allowed to follow desires without restraint will gain no self-control and become undisciplined and out of control. Parents must find a medium between these extremes. This entails setting limits that are appropriate for the developmental level of the child. For example, a young toddler may need to be removed from a situation as well as being told "no." Limits must be enforced calmly and firmly many times before the child is able to internalize them. Parents must consistently follow up on limits set and enforce them. Priority limits should be set first with gradual introduction and enforcement of other limits because the young child cannot respond adequately to too many demands. Limits must be re-evaluated as the child gets older to be sure they are still appropriate.

Methods Used for Discipline. Parents use various techniques to enforce the limits they have set. The choices they make are based on their childrearing philosophy. The use of corporal punishment (spanking) continues to be a part of American child rearing. The philosophy of "spare the rod, spoil the child" is still held by many parents.[44,39] However, child health professionals and professional organizations have taken a position against the use of corporal punishment as a method of discipline.[2,5,13,31,32,35] Instead, the goal is to assist parents in using practical, effective alternatives to corporal punish-

TABLE 13-9
Nursing Intervention: Suggesions to Assist Parents With Discipline

- Share with parents that some problems can be avoided by putting valuable objects out of reach until the child gets older.
- Discuss that toddlers may react to the tone of "no" and stop what they are doing but that they do not really understand what is being prohibited and therefore may not remember the limit later.
- Discuss with parents that it is helpful to remove a toddler from a situation and take away an object in addition to saying "no."
- Share with parents that as children grow older and change, it is desirable to re-evaluate limits set for them to make sure the limits are still developmentally appropriate.
- Discuss with parents that it is important to convey a clear message to the child about what is allowed and what is not permissible.
- Share with parents that high-priority limits should be set first, i.e., those essential to the child's safety, and that other limits should be introduced and enforced gradually because the young child cannot respond adequately to too many limits at one time.
- Discuss with parents that the child learns verbal limits when they are combined with actions that clearly define them, e.g., saying, "No, you cannot have these scissors," while removing them from the child's hands.

- Share with parents that the child is more likely to respond to limits if the adult is physically close and gets down to the child's level while talking to the child.
- Remind parents that it may be necessary to enforce limits calmly and firmly many times before the child learns to limit and internalizes the message.
- Share theat children need the security of knowing that the parents will follow up on the limits they set and enforce them.
- Discuss that it may help to offer the child an alternative activity when he or she has been stopped from doing something unacceptable, e.g., "You can't play with this cup, but here are some spoons to play with."
- Share that children will learn more quickly and adapt to limits more easily if parents set and enforce reasonable expectations.
- Emphasize that the child is likely to feel a sense of self-worth when he or she is able to meet parents' reasonable expectations.
- Encourage parents to try alternative methods for setting and enforcing limits and to describe which methods they are most comfortable with and which seem to work the best.

Adapted from Bromwich, R. (1981). *Working with parents and infants: An interactional approach.* Austin, TX: Pro-Ed Inc.

ment and support them during the time of transition. The purpose of punishment is not to hurt a child but to teach the child limits of acceptable behavior. Consistency of discipline rather than severity is what helps children learn. It is difficult for parents to spank the child for every misdeed, and the inconsistency is confusing for the child.

Physical punishment is considered the least effective method of teaching discipline over time. Although a child may initially respond to a slap on the hand, over time more aggressive hitting will be necessary to stop a behavior. Further, using an aggressive approach to discipline teaches the child that it is all right to hit someone to control them. Even when parents know that spanking a child may not be the best choice, many parents will at some time slap a child's hand or spank the child's bottom. For this reason some professionals[30,37,39] recommend that parents who are unwilling to give up this method of discipline be given guidelines for safe physical punishment (see the Parent Teaching display).

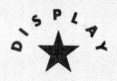

Parent Teaching: Restrictions on Physical Punishment (If eliminating it is impossible)

- Spank with an open hand: never use a paddle or belt.
- Only hit the buttocks or hand, never the face.
- Don't swat more than once.
- Don't spank children before they have learned to walk.
- Don't spank more than once a day.
- Don't spank for aggressive misbehavior.
- Don't shake children for punishment.
- Use time-out and other types of discipline.

From Schmitt, B. (1987). Seven deadly sins of childhood. Advising parents about difficult developmental phases. Child Abuse and Neglect, 11(3), 423.

Extinction or ignoring is considered one of the simplest methods currently recommended for eliminating troublesome behaviors. However, it requires a systematic evaluation of the child's behavior and parental responses to behavior and consistency when instituted. Extinction involves a systematic withdrawal of attention. Extinction has two phases: a baseline phase and the extinction phase itself. The baseline phase focuses on data collection by parents of the child's undesirable behavior and parental response to these behaviors. The data serve two purposes: (1) they validate whether the behavior is occurring as often as parents report; and (2) they provide baseline data for parents to evaluate the effectiveness of the extinction procedure. One of the most frequent problems with extinction is lack of consistency in using this approach—unacceptable behavior must be ignored each time that it occurs. Parents should be warned that extinction may initially increase the frequency of the undesirable behavior as the child tests the parents' stamina. For example, a child who exhibits temper tantrums two to three times a day may initially increase the number to three or four times a day. Parents who are aware of this are more likely to continue systematic ignoring, the result being a positive change in the child's behavior.

Time-Out. Time-out involves putting the child in a specific quiet but nonfrightening environment following the occurrence of unacceptable behavior. This may mean sitting in a chair in the corner of a room. Generally the time the child spends in time-out is 1 minute per year of age up to 5 minutes. A timer can be used so the child knows when the time is up and so parents do not leave the child for extended periods.

Ideally a specific, consistent place should be available. The child should be made aware of the procedure to be followed. Parents should not wait until a child misbehaves before explaining the time-out procedure. The child should be told in advance what the procedure will be so that he or she is able to listen to the explanation. Parents may practice a time-out so the child knows what to expect. It is very important that parents agree on what behaviors will result in a time-out and provide the child with this information. "If you hit Mommy, you are going to have a time-out." Each time the child misbehaves as predetermined, the time-out should occur. Consistency is the key to effectiveness. The child should be told the reason for the time-out and how long it is to last. "You hit Mommy. Now you have to go to time-out for 3 minutes." After the time-out the child should be allowed to start over without comments or reminders of the misbehavior.

Consistency is a vital component of teaching discipline. The child who is disciplined one day for biting a sibling and not the next day will become confused. The consistency required for effective discipline is a major factor in the degree of success parents will experience. No method of discipline will be beneficial unless the child is given a chance to learn. This means that regardless of the approach used, parents need to talk to the child about the unacceptable behavior and offer suggestions for more appropriate behavior.

Nursing Implications.   During the childrearing interview it is crucial that the nurse encourage parents to describe their methods of discipline. Such questions and observations are given in Table 13-10. The nurse must assess usual discipline approaches and who is responsible for establishing limits for the child. The frequency of discipline and the use of verbal and physical methods should be determined. With this information the nurse can begin to determine if discipline is appropriate to the child's level of development and if it is used consistently and reasonably. By having parents describe acceptable behaviors of the child and how these behaviors are rewarded, the nurse can assess the amount and quality of positive reinforcement given to the child.

If parents express concerns about limit setting or discipline, it is expected that the nurse will obtain information as to what has worked in the past, how have they tried to resolve specific problems, and if they plan to alter their responses or disciplinary methods with a child. The nurse must determine if the parents are realistic in their expectations of their child, if the child understands the parents' limit-setting goals, and if the disciplinary methods are actually appropriate for the child's developmental accomplishments.

This assessment is concluded through an interview and discussion of parental practices. Information provided by parents can be further validated by observing the parent-child interaction at the time of the visit. Do the parents have reasonable expectations of the toddler's behavior? How do they use discipline and limit setting when the child attempts to touch something in the room? How do they respond when the child continues a behavior after they have said "don't touch that"? By observing the interaction between parents and child, the nurse can identify discrepancies between parental beliefs about discipline and the practices they use. These observations should be shared with parents.

Parents can benefit from a nurse who will listen empathically to their concerns, validate what is distressing

---

TABLE 13-10
Nursing Assessment: Guidelines for Assessing Parental Discipline and Limit Setting

Aspects of Childbearing Practices

- It is important to assess how discipline is exercised and who is responsible for establishing limits for the child.
- It is valuable to determine how often the child is disciplined.
- It is helpful to gain information on the parents' use of verbal or physical methods of discipline (or a combination of both).
- It is necessary to determine if rules are realistic for the toddler.
- It is helpful to have parents describe how the child's acceptable behaviors are rewarded.
- It is useful to obtain information on how the child is expected to learn in life, i.e., by example, role modeling, experimentation, or trial and error. Do these methods appear reasonable and appropriate for the child's developmental level and cognitive understanding?
- It is vital to assess the parents' description of the child. What do parents cite as the best aspects of their child's personality? Is there any aspect they would change?

Key Questions*

- What limits do you wish to set for _____?
- What are your priorities (areas) for limit setting?
- What limits have you already set for _____?
- How is _____ responding to the limits that have been set?
- How have you tried to enforce limits?
- Which behaviors of _____ do you wish to change?
- Do you think _____ understands what is expected?
- How does _____ respond when punished?
- Do you consider your methods of disciplining to be effective?
- What alternative methods of limit setting have you considered?
- What are your perceptions of the child's positive attributes and strengths?

General Guidelines for Discussion and Observations of Parents and Toddler

- Are parents realistic in expectations of their child and self?
- Do parents seem reasonable in rules and discipline for a toddler?
- Are parents responding to child's behaviors in appropriate ways?
- Is there too much emphasis on discipline? Is discipline consistent? How much does the mother talk about discipline?
- What is the degree of permissiveness or rigidity of rules?
- Are parents overreactive to the child's behaviors?
- How much argument is there between the mother and father on the best way to approach a problem?
- How much child-care reading is parent doing? Do parents attend parent groups and seek other kinds of resources?
- How predictive is the parenting environment for the child? (How much can the child count on? Are there differences from day to day? Does the child appear secure and confident?)
- What are the parents' characteristic problem-solving approaches to the child?
- What do parents expect from the child, and how do they think they will respond to new behaviors or changes in the child?

* State child's name.

to the parents, and offer support as they attempt to formulate effective childrearing approaches with the toddler. Parents find it helpful for the nurse to comment positively on their appropriate decisions and gain immeasurably from a nurse who can offer anticipatory guidance about what to expect next in the child's developmental achievements.

Nurses find it helpful for parents to describe a toddler's positive traits and strengths while discussing negative aspects of development. Eliciting positive parental perceptions about a toddler and their expectations of new changes is an appropriate and rewarding way to terminate a problem-solving discussion during a well-child visit.

Assessing, Promoting, and Maintaining Cognitive Development

The toddler has gained new cognitive abilities through the variety of experiences offered in the first year. According to Piaget, the toddler is making the transition from learning through sensory-motor experiences to using symbolic-representational thought (see Chap. 8). The toddler is curious and motivated to explore, experiment, and manipulate the outside world. The toddler exerts more effort in trying a variety of approaches to reach a goal. For example, a toddler who wants to remove one object from another will try dumping it, pulling it, banging it, or throwing it. Through trial and error the toddler gains new skills. The toddler is also now capable of imitating behaviors seen in others.

Fostering Cognitive Development

Parents promote cognitive development by providing the toddler with a variety of toys and objects that challenge the toddler. These may include large objects that fit together and can be taken apart. Blocks to build and knock over as well as objects to be pushed and pulled offer learning experiences for the toddler. The toddler needs a variety of experiences both in the home and outside. Going to feed the ducks, seeing animals in the pet store, or going to the park all provide learning experiences that are fun and promote physical activity as well. Allowing the toddler opportunities to observe parents in their daily activities and encouraging imitation enhances learning. For example, allowing the toddler to push his or her popper while a parent vacuums or cuts the grass helps the child understand everyday activities (Fig. 13-6).

Toddlers learn from verbal interactions with parents. Although toddlers may not be able to carry on a conversation, they take in a great deal of information through observation and listening to others talk about people and events. For example, a toddler who rides the bus with a parent will observe many people and activities. This provides an opportunity for the parent to talk to the child about what is going on.

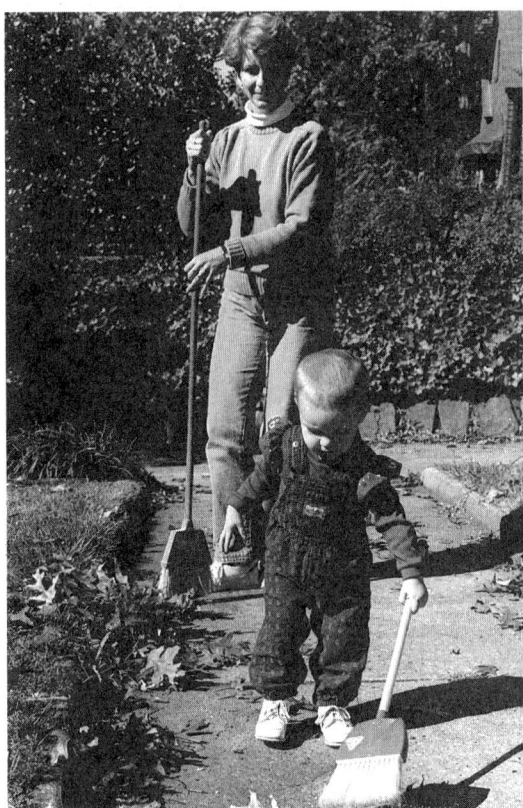

FIGURE 13-6
Toddlers learn by imitating adult activities.

Language Development of the Toddler

Language progressively develops during the toddler years and is dependent on physical maturation, exposure to language, and reinforcement for language expression. The transition from babbling to the use of specific words reflects a change from playing with sound to actually planning and expressing self through controlled speech. A child's first words represent the objects and events that are most familiar such as daddy, mommy, cookie, juice, or bath or anything the child associates with regular experiences. The toddler learns names of animals even though at first all four-legged animals may be called dogs. The toddler learns and uses words to regulate the environment, such as up, down, open, and out. Language development is promoted when parents incorporate learning into daily routines. For example, during the bath the mother can say, "Tommy is going into the water," "Here is the soap to wash Tommy," or "Here is the towel to dry Tommy." If Tommy has an opportunity to hear the names of objects at the same time as they are being used, Tommy will begin to learn new words. Feeding time is also a good time to present the names of utensils and foods. Learning the names of body parts and different articles of clothing can be done when the child gets dressed. The use of books with colorful pictures and common objects provides another opportunity for the toddler to learn vocabulary. The toddler should also be encouraged to use words to ask for something. This can be accomplished if the parent asks the child to vocalize a request rather than anticipating the child's desires. Having the child repeat words the parent uses promotes the use of language through imitation.

Nursing Implications

During well-child care the nurse can assess progress in cognitive and language development by asking parents questions about the child's curiosity and use of language. The nurse can also observe the child for use of language and assess the amount of encouragement given by parents. Do the parents give the child a chance to express needs, or do they anticipate or interpret the child's behavior and respond to a need before the child verbally expresses it? The nurse should be supportive of parental attempts to promote cognition and language development and offer suggestions for future needs. Parents may not always have the resources to purchase books or take a child on an outing. This, however, does not mean the child cannot gain skills. Instead, everyday experiences can be used for learning. Although talking to a child does not cost money, it does require parental patience and parental understanding of the importance of language development. This becomes an important factor for working parents who are very tired and stressed. The nurse can emphasize the need as being one of quality interactions rather than just the amount of time spent with the child. Parental willingness to set aside even a short time each day to talk with the child, read a book, or tell a story can be extremely beneficial.

Assessing, Promoting, and Maintaining Optimal Activity Levels

The toddler appears to be in constant motion as motor skills are used for exploration and self-satisfaction. The toddler moves about in the upright position, first holding onto furniture and soon thereafter walking unaided. Gross motor skills become increasingly refined through repeated practice. By the third year the toddler can be observed climbing stairs, running, jumping, and riding a tricycle. Fine motor skills are also improving, and the toddler develops the ability to hold and use objects purposefully, such as a crayon for scribbling.

The toddler needs opportunities to practice walking, climbing stairs, and getting on and off chairs. Skill in walking can be promoted by providing the child with push-pull toys that encourage walking. The toddler needs space to walk and run where falls will not cause physical injury. Early experiences with fine motor skills can be provided by large crayons and large pieces of paper on which the toddler can scribble. The older toddler may attempt to imitate simple shapes drawn by parents. Coordination is promoted through the use of a tricycle or similar pedal toy.

Using Play to Promote Development

Play during the toddler years reflects social, cognitive, language, and motor development. In fact, play contributes to each area of development and promotes the development of new skills.

It is often difficult to get from one place to another when traveling with a toddler. The toddler has a desire to stop and explore along the way. Objects hold a new challenge for the toddler, who spends extended periods exploring their potential. The experimentation with objects enhances creative problem-solving skills. The trial and error and persistence of the toddler to get an object to do something, such as getting a drawer open or closing a door, reflects creativity and problem-solving skills. The pleasure of mastery is seen in facial expressions as parents are shown the accomplishment.

The value of play in promoting development should be stressed to parents. Parents can promote growth through play by choosing appropriate and varied toys for the toddler.

The child's play environment both indoors and outside should include a variety of developmentally appropriate toys and activities (Table 13-11). These toys do not have to be store bought—many objects within the house can serve as toys that encourage manipulation, cause-and-effect experiences, and satisfaction through exploration. However, it is very important that the items the child is allowed to play with be safe. Inside the home the child can have a small table and chair, a bucket to carry toys in, and a shelf for storing toys that the toddler can reach. Toys that require supervision or contain small pieces should be placed on a shelf out of the child's reach. By keeping toys in different rooms, the child can follow parents and at the same time have something to play with. Having a special cupboard in the kitchen for the child's play pots and pans can be helpful while parents prepare dinner. Some parents may find it helpful to have a special toy put away by the phone that can be given to the child when the parent is on the phone. This toy can then be returned to its storage space until the next phone call.

Outside the home a safe environment that is enclosed is optimal. The outdoor area can include such items as a sand box, climbing equipment, balls, and water play. The child should have opportunities to run, jump, climb, and explore. A swing set or jungle gym will be enjoyed by the older toddler. Because not all families can provide this environment for the child, alternatives can be suggested. Many neighborhoods, schools, and churches have playgrounds for children (Fig. 13-7).

Nursing Implications

The nurse must assist parents in choosing appropriate toys and play experiences for the toddler. The nurse must also assess the child's use of play and may observe child play by having toys available in the office or clinic. Pointing out the association between play and development and encouraging parents to observe their child's play will promote increased parental enjoyment of the developmental process.

TABLE 13-11
Nursing Intervention: Play Activities That Promote Development of the Toddler

Large Motor

- Climbing, sliding: ramps; furniture; small jungle gym
- Jumping: table leaf with phone books 8″ off floor
- Crawling: cut-out large cartons
- Ride-on vehicles: Tyke Bike; ATV Explorer; jumphorse (Wonder Horse)
- Pull-toys: small wagon; those that are pulled by a string
- Walkers: pushing furniture, etc.; toy corn popper
- Running
- Building: (mostly knocking down)

Small Motor

- Throwing: ball (Nerf or whiffle); foam blocks; bean-bag
- Put together: pots and pans: simple puzzle; ball inside ball; take-apart pop-it beads; Legos; coffee pot; lock and key; little dolls that fit in round holes
- Nesting: cans; bowls; round cups
- Filling and dumping: junk mail into oatmeal carton; large ice cream container; carrying basket or pail of things; emptying drawers
- Pounding: pounding board (plastic hammer)
- Stacking: rings on wooden dowel; round cans
- Building: 1″ blocks
- Noisy toys: turning switches; small cars and trucks with wheels
- Screwing lids: lid on jars (baby food jars)
- Sorting: shape-sorting box

Messy Play

- Sand: pail, shovel, or spoon; cups; later, a dump truck; use cornmeal in winter
- Water: sprinkler can outside; tub, sink inside
- Dirt

Surprise Toys (the unexpected happens)

- Surprise box
- Telephone pop-up
- Jack-in-the-box (music box also)
- Toys with strings where something happens when you pull them
- Flashlight; bells; buzzers

Imitation Social Play

- Dress-up: hats (soft, with brim); beads; goggles or glasses; gloves
- Help in kitchen: mop, broom, etc.; setting table; cooking
- Toy telephone
- Dolls; stroller; stick horse
- Plastic tools
- Working in the yard: using a hose or watering can
- Putting things back in their place

Dance, Music

- Rhythm instruments
- Listening to music; dancing
- Songs such as ''Ring Around the Rosy,'' ''Pop Goes the Weasel''

Crafts (table and chairs)

- Play-dough
- Crayons
- Chalk (outside)

Concentration/Language Activities (lots of relating with parents)

- Reading: catalogs; books (if child holds them, use cardboard or cloth); may try to take out picture or not recognize it; scrapbooks
- Talking: about opposites; quality of objects; hot-cold, slow-fast; time words; parts of body; what they're doing; uses of objects
- Singing
- Playing games: pat-a-cake; this little piggy

Security Objects

- Blankets, cuddly animals or dolls; bottles

From Rothenberg, A., Hitchcock, S., Harrison, M., & Graham, M. (1983). *Parent-making: A practical handbook for teaching parent classes about babies and toddler* (pp. 235–236). (Postoffice Box 7326) Menlo Park, CA 94025: Banster Press.

Assessing, Promoting, and Maintaining Toddler Safety

Toddlers, with their rapid rate of motor development and concurrent fascination with the environment, are extremely prone to all types of accidents. The rate of injuries is highest in children between the ages of 1 and 2 years. It is common to hear from parents, "He did it so fast. I only turned my back for a minute," or "I didn't think she could reach or do that" (Fig. 13-8). These comments reinforce the need for anticipatory guidance and preparation for the increasing abilities and curiosity of the toddler.

Discussion of safety during the toddler years cannot be started too early or reinforced too often. Although parents may have an awareness of the potential for injuries, they all benefit from specific information related to prevention. Education related to safety should include specific information in relation to the environmental changes parents will have to make. Increasing mobility places the toddler at risk for a wide range of potential accidents.

The toddler now is invested in exploring with all senses. They will reach for any object they can see; they will reach up to a countertop even if they cannot see what is there. They will put any object into their mouth, and they are especially fascinated with putting objects into objects. They want to run, jump, and climb on anything from a chair to a bookcase.

Making the environment safe can be a very difficult task for the first-time parent as well as a parents who have other children because each has to take into consideration factors they may not have realized.

First-time parents are generally amazed at the newfound skills of the toddler. They can be alternately delighted and frustrated by the toddler's behavior. They discover what potential hazards exist by observing the toddler doing something they had not considered when they "childproofed" their home. There are risks lurking around every corner, and short of living in an empty room it is impossible to provide a completely safe environment. However, there are some basic steps parents can take to protect the toddler (see the Parent Teaching display).

In addition to the recommendations given in the Par-

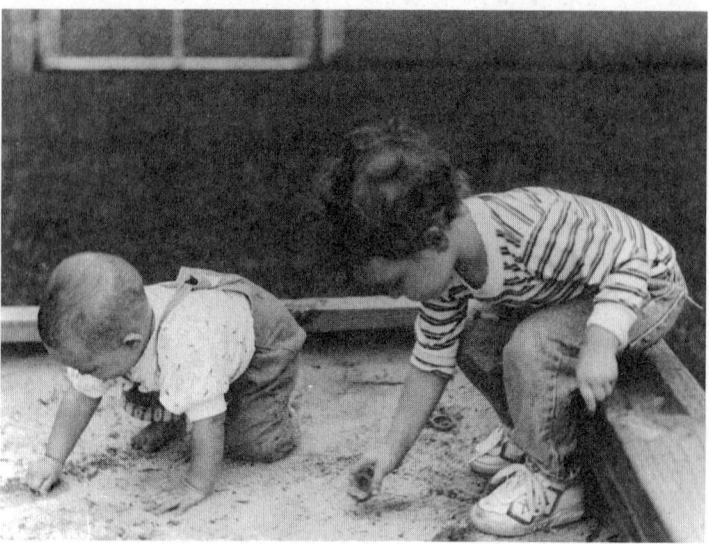

FIGURE 13-7

Playground activities allow toddlers opportunities for developing motor skills while playing. Most play is parallel play with other children at this age.

ent Teaching display, parents who have an older child in the house should be informed of the potential additional hazards this provides.

- The older child will have toys that can be potentially threatening to the young child. Any small pieces of toys or games should be kept away from the toddler. Any items that can potentially cause a puncture wound, such as scissors, should be kept away from the toddler and only used by the older child under supervision.
- The older child should be told about the potential dangers associated with the toddler. Assisting the older child in keeping toys together in one place and out of the hands of the toddler will provide safety as well as respect for the older child's belongings.
- The older child may need assistance in determining what activities are appropriate for the toddler. This may decrease the risk of the toddler becoming in-

volved in an activity that is beyond the toddler's capability.

Nursing Implications

Parents benefit from a discussion of preventive measures during the well-care visit. Parents should be provided with information that includes the developmental abilities that make the toddler prone to these types of injuries, the actual factors involved in the injury, and the preventive measures that will decrease the risk of occurrence of these injuries. See the Teaching Plan for nursing actions in safety promotion.

Additionally, nurses who work with children can provide information related to accident prevention through participation in community educational programs, education of child care center personnel, and preparation and distribution of information pamphlets.

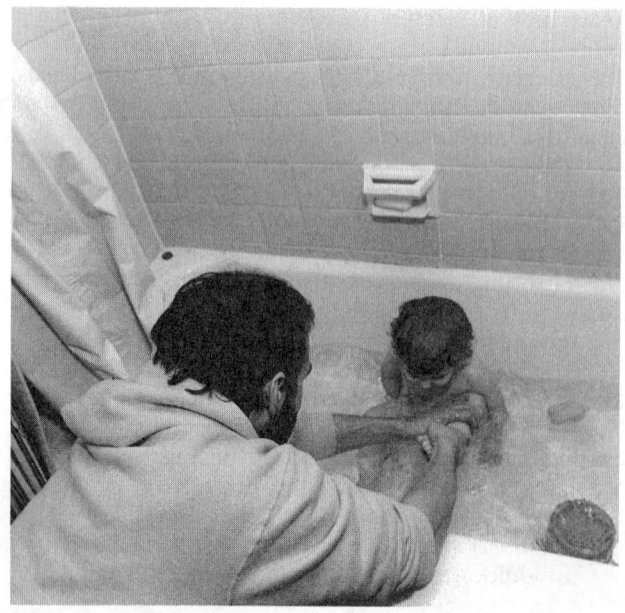

FIGURE 13-8

Safety is a major problem for parents of toddlers, who cannot be left unsupervised. Young children should never be left unattended during bath time.

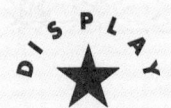

Parent Teaching: Basic Steps Parents Can Take to Protect the Toddler

- Do not leave the toddler unattended for even short periods. This is one of the most difficult tasks because keeping up with an active toddler interferes with the normal activities of parents. Parents frequently complain, "I can't get anything done while my toddler is awake."

- Crawl around on the floor—discover what the toddler sees and eliminate any potential risks. This will include covering electrical outlets, removing electrical cords, and securing anything in the toddler's reach that could be pulled onto the toddler. Freestanding bookcsases can be very hazardous and should be secured to the wall. In the kitchen, pots should be placed on back burners with the handle turned toward the wall. Counters should be clear of all knives or sharp cooking utensils. Cords from all appliances should be coiled up and out of reach.

- Go through cupboards and closets to find potential poisons and hazardous substances. All unlabeled containers should be discarded. All containers that do not have childproof caps should be replaced or placed in a locked container. All potentially hazardous materials should be placed out of the toddler's reach and preferably locked. It is best to discard any medications or prescriptions not needed by family members. Use nonlead paints, and remove any lead-based paints from surfaces the child might chew.

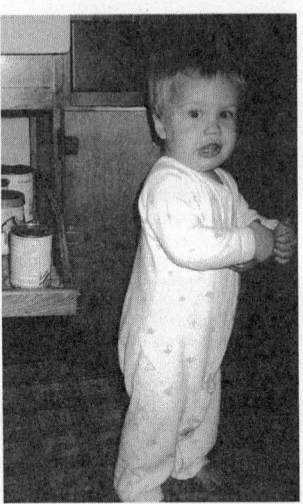

- Toddlers have the highest rate of asphyxiation by foods during childhood.[23] Foods posing the highest risk are hot dogs, nuts, grapes, and candy.[23] Many childhood deaths related to asphyxiation are preventable. Parents can decrease the chance of choking by providing supervision while a child is eating, by having the child sit to eat rather than eating on the run or while playing, and by avoiding foods known to pose risks of aspiration. Some high-risk foods can be altered to decrease the risk of choking. This includes cutting hot dogs lengthwise in thin strips, avoiding peanuts except in butter form, and steaming or cooking vegetables to soften them.

- Decrease the risk of falls by placing safety gates at the top of stairs. Purchase high chairs and strollers that have a wide base and low center of gravity. Secure the toddler with a safety strap when he or she is in the stroller or the high chair. Provide continual supervision when the toddler is in the bathtub or playing on swings and other playground equipment. Keep furniture that the child can climb on away from windows.

- Decrease the risk of burns by keeping household hot water temperature at 120° F.[28] Keep matches and lighters out of reach. Purchase matches that have the strike bar on the opposite side of the opening. Protect child from burns in the kitchen (see the second suggestion above). Dress child in fire-retardant clothing and wash clothing according to manufacturer's directions.

- Decrease the risk of injury during travel by consistently using child safety seat. Use seat according to manufacturer's instructions. Purchasing car seats manufactured after January 1981 ensures that the seat meets federal regulations. When using bicylcemounted child seats, always have the child wear appropriate bicycle helmets.[38] The carriers should be secured according to manufacturer's directions. When purchasing a bicycle seat, parents should look for a seat that has leg protectors, no sharp edges, an easy-to-use safety strap, and a high back to protect the child from head and neck injuries. Helmets should be fitted to the child and worn consistently. When traveling by plane, parents must inform the airline that they will be traveling with a child on their lap so that an additional oxygen mask will be available. Once the child reaches the age of 2 and a separate seat must be purchased, parents can place the child in a car seat if it is approved for both car and plane travel.

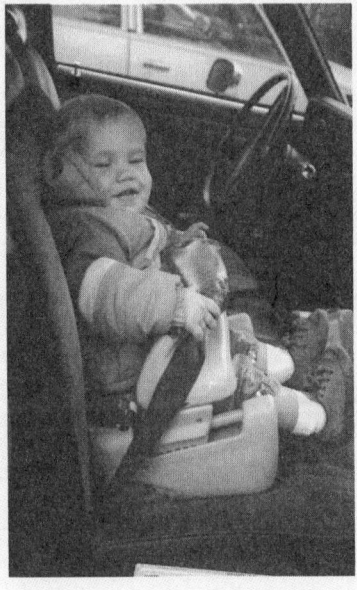

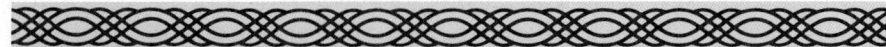

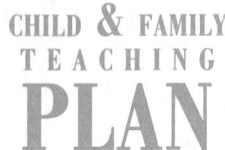

CHILD & FAMILY
T E A C H I N G
PLAN

Safety for a 2-Year-Old Toddler

Assessment

Tim is 2 years old and has come to the clinic with his parents for his well-care visit. He lives in a single-family home with his parents. Both parents work, and Tim is cared for by a sitter who comes to his house. Tim's parents describe him as "very active and into everything." They express concern that his increasing curiosity has put him at risk for injury.

Tim is developmentally prone to injury. He is unable to determine what is safe and what is unsafe. He actively explores the environment and takes opportunities to try his new skills. He is able to open cupboards and bottle caps, and he climbs onto counters and tables. He has curiosity about objects and attempts to explore new objects. His mother caught him taking a knife from the counter. He actively explores the clinic examination room. The teaching plan was developed as an intervention for the nursing diagnosis, Knowledge deficit related to safety.

Child and Family Objectives	Specific Content	Teaching Strategies
1. Decrease risk of trauma related to increased mobility and curiosity.	1. *Climbing.* Secure bookcases or furniture that would fall over on the child if he attempts to climb on it.	1. Have parents describe potential risks they have considered and add to their information.
	Dangerous objects (including knives, matches, lighters, scissors) should be placed out of the child's reach. Because Tim likes to climb, putting these objects in the cupboard above the counter is not sufficient. He can climb onto the counter and open the cupboard.	Provide a written handout of potential hazards for children.
	Cooking. Use back burners for cooking and turn handles toward the wall.	Have parents consider activities that may be helpful in entertaining Tim while dinner is being prepared. For example, do they have a low cupboard that is away from the stove, with pots and pans Tim can play with?
	Small appliances are kept out of reach and unplugged. Keep electrical cords coiled.	Ask parents to describe their kitchen. What appliances are on their counter? Do they pose a risk, e.g. sharp blades?
	Cover electrical outlets and do not allow Tim to have objects that would fit into the pocket.	Tell parents where covers can be purchased.
	Tim's desire to experiment with cause/effect. "Mom puts that cord in the wall and the vacuum comes on."	Explain how caretaker should not use electrical equipment in front of Tim. He is likely to want to imitate this behavior.
2. Provide safe bath time.	2. Tim is to be supervised at all times during the bath. His desire to be on the move may encourage him to stand up or turn on the faucet.	2. Point out how Tim's motor skills can increase his risk for accidents in the tub.

(Continued)

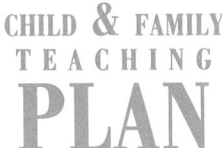

Safety for a 2-Year-Old Toddler (continued)

Child and Family Objectives	Specific Content	Teaching Strategies
3. Provide safe play.	3. Keep play equipment in good repair. Place play equipment on soft surfaces such as grass. Riding toys, including tricylces, sit-on toys, and wagons, should be well balanced with a wide base and low to the ground. The use of any ride-on toys should be restricted to flat areas away from stairs, sharp objects such as garden tools, and the street.	3. Discuss with parents the types of play equipment Tim has and any potential risks. Encourage questions.
4. Provide safety in the car.	4. Tim should be in his car seat at all times when riding in the car.	4. Ask parents if they use the car seat as instructed by the manufacturer. Assess how often the car seat is used and how Tim tolerates being in the car seat.
5. Decrease risk of poisoning related to increased mobility, curiosity, and ability to open closets and remove bottle caps.	5. *Medications.* Discard all medications not used by family members. All potential poisons should be labeled and kept out of Tim's reach. These items should be placed in a locked cabinet or closet. Avoid putting poisonous substances in alternate containers, e.g., bleach in a small juice blottle.	5. Identify what risks exist for poisoning and how parents can limit the risk.
6. Decrease risk of suffocation related to mobility and desire to put substances into mouth.	6. Develop habit of sitting for meals and snacks. Prepare high-risk foods such as grapes and hot dogs by cutting them lengthwise.	6. Explain how a small round object can become lodged in a small child's throat.

Evaluation

- Parents identify potential risks for accidental injuries in their home.
- Parents verbalize methods to decrease accidental injury of Tim.

Assessing, Promoting, and Maintaining Health Perception and Health Management

Typical Schedule of Well-Care Visits

Ideally the toddler should continue to have regular well-care visits during the toddler years (see Chap. 9). These visits are necessary for the continuation of im- munizations, as well as opportunities to assess develop- mental progress and nutritional habits and assist parents in dealing with common and sometimes trying behaviors.

15 Months

The well-care visit at 15 months should include a physical assessment; serial height, weight, and head cir- cumference measurement; immunization; and develop- mental assessment. Parents may have many questions about new and difficult behaviors, including separation anxiety, negativism, temper tantrums, and eating patterns. Nurses should listen to parents' concerns, provide them with information as to the normalcy of these behaviors, and assist them in planning interventions (see discussion of each of the topics in this chapter).

The toddler is given the measles, mumps, and rubella (MMR) and *Hemophilus influenzae-b* (HiB) vaccines at this visit. Prior to its administration the nurse should assess the child for history of febrile illness, immunodeficiency or immunosuppression therapy, or history of anaphylactic reaction to eggs. The presence of any of these factors precludes the administration of the immunization. After the injection parents need to be informed of the types of potential reactions. Parents should be informed not to expect a reaction until 7 to 10 days after the administration of the immunization. The child may have no reaction or may have local irritation at the injection site, irritability, or fever. Acetaminophen may be given for any mild reaction up to every 4 hours in a dose appropriate for the child's weight. Medicating the child just before or after the MMR with acetaminophen is not necessary because the potential reaction to the immunization is delayed. (Many states require a second measles vaccine before admission to school.)

18 Months

The 18-month visit includes a physical examination, serial height and weight, and developmental assessment. The nurse should review the child's record before seeing the parents so that concerns that were brought up at the last visit can be discussed. Parents should be asked about the child's behavior, toilet training, and the effectiveness of any interventions previously suggested.

The child will also receive the fourth and final dose of diphtheria-pertussis-tetanus and the third dose of oral poliovirus vaccine (OPV). A review of potential reactions should be shared as well as suggestions for decreasing the response, including local heat application to a sore injection site and acetaminophen for fever.

24 Months

The 24-month visit includes all of the interventions of previous visits. Because this is the last frequent well child visit (from the second birthday visits are scheduled yearly), the nurse should review all developmental areas and common parental concerns.

At this visit the child will receive the final HiB vaccine.

Health Care

Dental Care

During the second year the child continues to need fluoride through the administration of drops or the use of fluorinated water. The child can begin to be involved in personal dental care by using a toothbrush after meals and snacks. The toddler will need assistance in dental cleaning. A visit to the dentist is appropriate. The first visit may be used to introduce the child to the environment and the people who work in the office.

Nutrition is very important to healthy teeth. Nurses can discuss with parents nutritional patterns of the toddler. Nurses should discourage foods high in sugar content and encourage nutritious snacks such as cut-up fruits and vegetables.

Colds

Viruses are the primary cause of colds in children. The child may have symptoms that include nasal congestion, rhinorrhea, and sneezing. There may also be fever, coughing, and sore throat. These symptoms can last for 1 to 2 weeks. After 2 weeks continued symptoms indicate the need to seek health care for evaluation.

A parent may call the office for information regarding the home care of a young child with a cold. Prior to giving advice the nurse should obtain information about the child's symptoms, state of hydration, responsiveness, and what the parent has already done for the child. Parents should then be instructed to encourage liquids. Milk intake may be temporarily decreased and replaced with clear liquids. The child should be allowed to play and continue daily activities as tolerated. Children usually restrict their own activity level when ill. Cold remedies currently on the market are not known to be effective.

Parents should be instructed to come to the office if the child spikes a fever, is unable or unwilling to drink fluids, or has no improvement in symptoms within 2 weeks.

Diarrhea

Diarrhea is defined as an excessive loss of fluids and electrolytes in the stool. Acute diarrhea is generally self-limiting and lasts from a few days to a week. Diarrhea that lasts longer than 3 weeks is more likely related to conditions such as malabsorption.

Acute diarrhea is caused by viruses (human rotavirus), bacteria (*Escherichia coli, Shigella, Salmonellae*), or parasites (*Giardia lamblia*).

Although most children with diarrhea can be managed at home, a thorough history is necessary before recommending treatment. Information about the child's diet and dietary changes is a good starting point. Also a history of travel, other family members experiencing gastrointestinal disturbances, and attendance at a day care center are helpful. A careful history of stool should include a description of number of stools, consistency, odor, and presence of mucous or blood. Associated symptoms, including fever, vomiting, or abdominal cramps, may assist in the determination of a causative agent. In addition, the child's hydration status can be evaluated by eliciting information related to intake of fluids and urine output.

The goals of treatment are to restore and maintain adequate hydration and electrolyte balance, recovery of the intestine, and maintenance and restoration of the child's nutritional status. These goals are best met through the provision of fluids and foods. Antidiarrheal agents should be avoided.

Treatment involves giving appropriate oral hydration fluids frequently and in small amounts. The oral solution can be an electrolyte solution such as Pedialyte or Lytren. Household beverages including fruit juice, soft drinks, or gelatin water can also be used if mixed one part beverage to two parts water. Full-strength beverages are hyperosmolar and can worsen the diarrhea.[21] Commercially prepared soups are contraindicated because of the high salt content. Parents need to monitor hydration status throughout the treatment period. Oral fluids may continue even in the presence of some vomiting. If the child's condition worsens, medical care may become necessary.

Current recommendations support the early reestablishment of nutrition. The tendency to submit children to varying periods of fasting may still be seen in spite of evidence validating the safety of early feeding.[15,21] After 24 hours with oral solutions the child can be gradually returned to solids, ensuring that fats and protein (meats and cereals) are given. One common diet known as the BRAT diet includes bananas, rice cereal, applesauce, and toast (dry). Foods high in carbohydrates, such as fruits and sweet desserts, should be avoided. The child should be allowed to determine amount of intake. After solids have been re-established, milk or formula can be restarted. For a day or two milk or formula should be half strength progressing to full strength as tolerated. A child who does not tolerate milk or formula can be given a lactose-free substitute. Once the child has recovered, extra foods should be available to the child to ensure recovery of any nutritional deficiencies resulting from the acute illness.

Vomiting

Vomiting is a common complaint during childhood. It is a symptom with a wide variety of causes. It can indicate either a minor or major illness. Vomiting is frequently associated with gastroenteritis, pneumonia, and otitis media. It is also a symptom of peptic ulcers, diabetes, meningitis, appendicitis, Reye's syndrome, increased intracranial pressure, and hepatitis.[15]

Vomiting may be the result of an inflamed gastrointestinal tract (gastroenteritis); stretching of an organ or membrane (otitis media, bowel obstruction); vestibular reflex (seasickness); stimulation of chemoreceptor trigger zone (diabetes, radiation therapy); and increased intracranial pressure (brain tumor, meningitis).[15]

Treatment of vomiting involves initial evaluation of concurrent symptoms and level of hydration. A child is likely to have some vomiting with diarrhea or gastroenteritis, whereas fever may indicate a more systemic disease. Any change in the child's level of consciousness can indicate a serious problem. Abdominal pain associated with vomiting may indicate appendicitis.[15]

Initially, vomiting, especially when associated with diarrhea, can be treated with oral rehydration. The approach is similar to the one described earlier for diarrhea. Parents need to be instructed to bring the child to the office or clinic if vomiting persists for more than 24 hours, if fever persists more than 24 hours, or if the child has a change in level of consciousness or increasing dehydration.

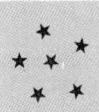

Ideas for Nursing Research

The nurse involved with parents and toddlers has a unique opportunity to explore the behaviors and responses that promote the toddler's independence and autonomy and reduce parent's stress. The following areas need to be explored:

- Parental behaviors that assist children in successfully coping with "temper tantrums."
- Play activities that encourage toddlers to develop both language and gross motor skills.
- Value of educational programs for parents on safety for toddlers.

Summary

The toddler years are very busy years for parents and toddlers. Major changes occur in the child's ability to interact with the environment and with those around him or her. There is a shift from dependency on parents to self-determination in toileting, nutrition, and daily activities. The toddler must also begin to gain control of impulses and be taught discipline.

The road to independence is not without ambivalence, and such things as separation anxiety and the need to control impulses and delay gratification can be frightening to the child and parents.

The nurse has an important role in working with parents and toddlers. By listening to parental concerns, providing anticipatory guidance, and assisting parents in problem-solving approaches, the nurse can help the family develop in positive ways during these exciting, yet sometimes difficult years.

References

1. American Academy of Pediatrics. (1985). *Pediatric nutrition handbook* (2nd ed.). Elk Grove, IL: Author.
2. American Academy of Pediatrics, Committee on Psychosocial Aspects of Child and Family Health. (1983). The pediatrician's role in discipline. *Pediatrics, 42,* 373–374.
3. Azrin, N. H., & Foxx, R. M. (1974). *Toilet training in less than a day.* New York: Pocket Books.
4. Behrman, R., & Vaughan, V. (Eds.). (1992). *Nelson's textbook of pediatrics* (14th ed). Philadelphia: W. B. Saunders.
5. Bettelheim, B. (1985). Punishment vs discipline. *Atlantic Monthly, 256,* 51–59.
6. Birch, L. (1980). The relationship between children's food preferences and those of their parents. *Journal of Nutrition Education, 12,* 14–18.
7. Birch, L., & Martin, D. (1982). I don't like it; I never tried it: Effects of exposure on two-year-old children's food preferences. *Appetite, 3,* 353–360.
8. Brazelton, T. B. (1962). A child-oriented approach to toilet training. *Pediatrics, 29,* 121–128.
9. Brazelton, T. B. (1959). *Infants and mothers: Individual differences in development.* New York: Charles Scribner and Sons.

10. Brazelton, T. B. (1974). *Toddlers and parents: A declaration of independence.* Lawrence, NY: Delacorete Press.
11. Burt, J., & Hertzter, A. (1978). Parental influence on the child's food preference. *Journal of Nutrition Education, 10,* 127.
12. Chamberlin, R. (1978). Relationship between child-rearing styles and child behavior over time. *American Journal of Diseases of Children, 132,* 155–160.
13. Christophersen, E. (1982). Incorporating behavioral pediatrics into primary care. *Pediatric Clinics of North America, 29,* 261–296.
14. Cole, J. (1983). Parents' book of toilet training. New York: Ballantine.
15. Dershewitz, R. (Ed.). (1988). *Ambulatory pediatric care.* Philadelphia: J. B. Lippincott.
16. Doleys, D., & Dolce, J. (1982). Toilet training and enuresis. *Pediatric Clinics of North America, 29,* 297–307.
17. Dworkin, P. (1988). The preschool child: Developmental themes and clinical issues. *Current Problems in Pediatrics, 18,* 79–134.
18. Erikson, E. (1963). *Childhood and society.* New York: W. W. Norton.
19. Ferber, R. (1987). Sleeplessness, night awakening, and night crying in the infant and toddler. *Pediatrics in Review, 9,* 69.
20. Ferber, R. (1986). *Solve your child's sleep problems.* New York: Simon and Schuster.
21. Hamilton, J. (1985). Treatment of acute diarrhea. *Pediatric Clinics of North America, 32,* 419–427.
22. Harper, R. (1975). Behavioral modification in pediatric practice. *Clinical Pediatrics, 14,* 962–967.
23. Harris, C., Baker, S., Smith, G., & Harris, R. (1984). Childhood asphyxiation by food: A national analysis and overlook. *Journal of the American Medical Association, 251,* 2231–2235.
24. Horner, M., & McClellan, M. (1981). Toilet training ready or not? *Pediatric Nursing, 7,* 15–18.
25. U.S. Department of Health, Education, and Welfare, Human Development Services. (1980). *Infant care* (DHHS Publication No. OHDS 80-300 15). Washington, DC: U.S. Government Printing Office.
26. Lozoff, B., Wolf, A., & Davis, N. (1984). Cosleeping in urban families with young children in the United States. *Pediatrics, 74,* 171.
27. Mack, A. (1983). Toilet learning: The picture book technique for both children and parents. Boston: Little, Brown.
28. Maley, M., & Achauer, B. (1987). Prevention of tap water scald burns. *Journal of Burn Care Rehabilitation, 8,* 62.
29. Marino, R., Bomze, K., Scholl, T., & Anhalt, H. (1989). Nursing bottle caries: Characteristics of children at risk. *Clinical Pediatrics, 28,* 129–131.
30. McIntosh, B. (1989). Spoiled child syndrome. *Pediatrics, 83,* 108–121.
31. Policy resolution of the Governing Council of the American Public Health Association. (1980). *American Journal of Public Health, 70,* 308.
32. Policy statement of the American Psychological Association. (1975). *American Psychologist, 30,* 632.
33. Powell, M. (1981). *Assessment and management of developmental changes and problems in children* (2nd ed.). St. Louis: C. V. Mosby.
34. Queen, P., & Wilson, E. (1987). Growth and nutrient requirements of young children. In R. Grand, J. Sutphen, & W. Dietz (Eds.). Pediatric nutrition: Theory and practice. Boston: Butterworth-Heinemann, 341–349.
35. Report of the Task force on Corporal Punishment, National Education Association. (1972). Washington, DC: Author.
36. Robertson, J. (1958). *Young children in hospitals.* London: Favistock.
37. Rosenfeed, A., & Levine, D. (1987). Discipline and permissiveness. *Pediatrics in Review, 8,* 209–215.
38. Sargent, J., Peck, M., & Weitzman, M. (1988). Bicycle-mounted child seats: Injury risk and prevention. *American Journal of Diseases of Children, 142,* 765.
39. Schmitt, B. (1987). Seven deadly sins of childhood: Advising parents about difficult developmental phases. *Child Abuse and Neglect, 11,* 421–432.
40. Schmitt, B. (1987). *Your child's health: A pediatric guide for parents.* New York: Bantam Books.
41. Spock, B. (1976). *Baby and child care.* New York: Basic Books.
42. Stephens, J. A., & Silber, D. C. (1974). Parental expectations vs outcome in toilet training. *Pediatrics, 54,* 493–495.
43. Thevenin, T. (1976). The family bed. Minneapolis: Thevenin.
44. Wessel, M. (1980). The pediatrician and corporal punishment. *Pediatrics, 66,* 639–641.

Health Assessment, Promotion, and Maintenance for Preschool Children

BEHAVIORAL OBJECTIVES

Describe patterns of development of preschool children related to nutrition, elimination, sleep, psychosocial development, cognitive and language development, play and safety.

Identify common concerns of parents related to preschool development.

Describe nursing assessment approaches with preschoolers and parents related to development.

Describe nursing interventions to assist parents in promoting optimal development of preschool children.

Identify teaching needs of parents related to promoting optimal development of preschool children.

Identify concerns and needs in day care programs.

Discuss health maintenance needs of preschool children.

The preschool years are special years for both the child and parents. The preschooler demonstrates greater independence in daily care activities, including eating, bathing, dressing, and toileting. There is a marked decrease in the negativism that was so prominent during the toddler years, and the preschooler is able to communicate needs through verbal expression.

The preschooler has an insatiable curiosity to explore the unknown and seeks explanations for that which is not understood. The preschooler's vivid imagination and expression of fantasy offer insights into the preschooler's perception of the world and perception of people they meet. Through play the preschooler learns about the world, its people, customs, and social behavior, and has an opportunity to work out frustrations, fears, and difficult experiences. At the end of the preschool years the child is ready for school and formal learning.

Goals for optimal development of preschoolers include the following:

- Maintenance of a balanced diet and learning about nutrition.
- Maintenance of sleep patterns related to physiologic needs.
- Development of a sense of initiative.
- Development of a positive self-concept and sex role identification.
- Maintenance of activity levels to refine gross and fine motor skills.
- Development of increasingly sophisticated cognitive and language skills.
- Development of social skills: sharing, cooperation, and coping with frustration.
- Preparation for entry into school.

The preschool years bring changes in the parent-child relationship. The preschooler continues to have needs for love and affection from parents. Parents continue to be the primary teachers, protectors, and supporters of the child as the child develops new skills and discovers his or her uniqueness.

Parental goals during the preschool years are as follows:

- Providing a well-balanced diet for growth and offering opportunities for learning about nutrition.
- Assisting the child in maintaining sleep patterns necessary for optimal functioning.
- Fostering the child's sense of initiative.
- Fostering the development of a positive self-concept and sex role identification.
- Fostering the development of optimal activity levels.
- Promoting increasingly sophisticated cognitive and language skills.
- Promoting the development of social skills through role modeling and teaching.
- Providing opportunities for the child to learn skills necessary for school entry: colors, numbers, name, phone number, and address.
- Promoting a safe environment and educating the child in safety issues.
- Maintaining well-child care and including the child in health care issues.

Assessing, Promoting, and Maintaining Optimal Nutrition

The preschooler has mastered the basic skills necessary for self-feeding. Assistance is still needed with such tasks as cutting meat and spreading butter. As the preschooler grows, earlier motor skills become refined and new abilities emerge. The preschooler's fine and gross motor skills develop rapidly through constant activity and exploration of the environment. The preschool years are a time of initiative, and the preschooler wants to participate actively in all family activities, including those related to food and nutrition. Food purchasing, preparation, and serving and the social interactions at the dinner table are all opportunities for parents to introduce the preschooler to the importance of nutrition. Children can learn about foods and how food is important for health and growth.

Preschoolers food preferences can be influenced by

peers,[6] parents,[27] social-affective variables,[8] and contingencies.[7] Preschoolers are likely to try a food they observe a peer eating even if it is refused at home.[6] One research study[8] found that children developed preferences for foods that were presented as rewards as well as for foods presented in conjunction with adult attention. Foods that are presented at regular snack time or in a nonsocial context did not increase the preschooler's preference for these foods. Attempts to get a child to eat by making another activity contingent on consumption, for example, "Eat your vegetable and then you can go outside," or "Eat your meat and you can have a cookie," can have a negative impact in children's food preferences.[7] This practice enhances the preference for sweet foods and reinforces to the children the belief that if they have to eat meat to get a cookie, meat must taste bad.

Preschoolers' desire to imitate their parents and other adults who serve as care providers makes them extremely receptive to learning appropriate eating habits. Likewise, poor eating habits may be imitated and adopted if role modeled by parents.

Parents are responsible for the provision of nutritious foods in the home as well as seeing that foods offered in the day care setting meet the child's needs (see Developmental Nutritional Profile). Parents should plan activities, rest, and meals to promote good appetites and normal growth. Parents have an extremely important role in education. Preschoolers can be educated about nutrition and be involved in food planning. Preschoolers require guidance in distinguishing reliable information from promotional information in many of the commercials they see. Parents can begin to help the preschooler understand the need to eat in moderation and eat a balanced diet in an effort to decrease the child's risk of obesity and heart disease later in life. Most importantly, parents must role model appropriate eating habits for their preschoolers. This includes eating a variety of foods, eating meals on a regular schedule, and eating nutritious snacks rather than junk foods. This may require an evaluation of the parents' own eating patterns and the development of new habits when necessary.

The nurse should be available to assist parents in their self-evaluation. By asking key questions that will

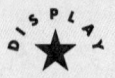

Developmental Nutritional Profile of the Preschooler

- Weight gain slow and steady.
- Has mastered art of getting food into mouth.
- Drinks completely from cup or glass.
- Chews easily; eats what family eats.
- Table manners reasonably acceptable.
- Interested in companionship at mealtime.
- Actual food consumption small.

Adapted from Kennedy-Caldwell, C., and Caldwell, M. (1986). Pediatric enteral nutrition. In Rombeau, J., & Caldwell, M. (Ed.). Parenteral nutrition: Clinical nutrition (Vol II). Philadelphia: Saunders, 434–479.

help parents assess their own eating behaviors, parents may be able to identify eating habits that they do not want to pass on to the child. (See Table 14-1 for key questions to ask.) Asking parents what foods they like and dislike will help parents identify specific food groups that they must consciously provide for the child. For example, parents who do not eat fruit routinely are less likely to offer a variety of fruits to the child. A discussion of the relationship between food and health for the child may encourage parents to be concerned about their own health as well as the child's. Parents should be given positive reinforcement for their healthy nutritional practices. If areas for change are identified, the nurse supports parents in the problem-solving process. Optimally, both parents should be involved so that they can discuss, assess, problem-solve, and plan together. Parents will also need support while attempting to change lifelong eating habits. If parents find it difficult to change their eating habits or choose not to change their habits, the nurse should assist them in finding ways to promote healthy dietary habits in the child. Setting the child up for success is a key intervention. This can be done by providing foods disliked by parents in a nonbiased manner. For example, rather than saying, "Here are your peas. I know that they don't taste good but they are good for you," parents can say, "Here are your peas. I think you are going to like them."

Nutritional requirements during the preschool years do not change drastically from the toddler years (see Chap. 61). Portions continue to be small, with emphasis on variety of foods offered from all food groups. Because appetites continue to vary on a day-to-day basis, parents may have concerns about the adequacy of the preschooler's food consumption. However, as with the toddler, the preschooler generally eats adequate amounts of all nutrients over time if a variety of foods are offered. The preschooler should not be forced to eat. More importantly, the child should be offered food in an unbiased manner, and foods not eaten should be removed without

TABLE 14-1
Nursing Assessment: Questions for Assessing Parental Eating Habits and Preschooler's Eating Behaviors

Focus of Concern	Key Questions*
Assessing Parental Eating Habits	
Typical eating behaviors and patterns of parents (3 meals, skipped meals, snacking).	Can you tell me all you ate yesterday and times you ate?
Foods parents are apt to eliminate from child's diet. Are they significant?	Are there foods you really dislike and do not purchase?
Parental perception of importance of meal planning and their ability to incorporate it into a busy day.	Now that so many mothers work it is very difficult for them to plan and prepare meals. Can you tell about your experience with this? And how you have dealt with it?
Reliance on fast foods for nutrition.	How often do you go out to dinner or pick up a prepared dinner? What kind of food?
Parental perception of nutrition and their health.	How important do you feel nutrition is for you and your health?
Parents' ability to identify the behaviors they have that they want children to acquire and behaviors they would not want their children to learn.	When evaluating your own nutritional health, are there behaviors or eating habits you would like your children to learn from you? Are there behaviors or eating habits you would like your children to avoid?
Parents' perceptions of how they can incorporate good eating behaviors and avoid poor eating habits.	What do you feel you can do to help _____ develop good nutrition patterns and avoid poor eating habits?
Typical daily food intake. This may require recall of more than one day for adequate information.	Can you tell me what _____ ate yesterday? (If daily intake is adequate or lacking essential food groups, get history of another day.)
Assessing Preschooler's Eating Behaviors	
Parents' knowledge of child's food preferences.	What are _____ favorite foods? What does _____ dislike?
Parents' perception of preschooler's eating behaviors.	How do you feel _____ is doing in terms of diet and eating?
Parents' perception of preschooler's eating skills.	Describe for me what help _____ needs in eating?
Parents' perception of appropriate portions of food for child.	How much of each food (in tablespoons) do you feel _____ needs with each meal.
Use of food as reward for good behavior or as method of keeping child quiet.	How do you reward _____ for doing something good such as putting toys away or behaving in a public situation?
Relationship of eating to boredom.	Does _____ tend to eat when bored?
Opportunities for child to learn social behavior associated with mealtime.	Does _____ eat with the family? Does _____ participate in preparing or serving food?
Child's influence in food purchased.	Some parents have a hard time in the grocery store because their preschooler wants to buy such things as cereals with prizes or things advertised on TV. How do you deal with this?
Parents' perception of how child's eating behaviors have changed.	What are the changes you have noticed in _____ eating behaviors over the past year?

* Use child's name in blank space.

comment.[32,38] Preschoolers need exposure to a variety of foods. What a preschooler will not eat one day may be accepted another day.

Activities to Teach Nutrition

The preschooler's natural curiosity and ability for make-believe play provide opportunities for teaching nutrition. During make-believe play preschoolers frequently play out such roles as keeping house, shopping, cooking, and serving food. Parents can set up a play experience that reinforces good nutrition. For example, a parent may provide the child with pictures of fruit, vegetables, meats, breads, and milk and have the child serve these foods to dolls or playmates. During play parents can tell the child how important it is to give the doll some of each type of food.

Preschoolers can also begin to learn which foods belong to which food groups. Cutting with scissors is a new skill that preschoolers enjoy. Cutting out pictures of meats, fruits, vegetables and dairy products and sorting them into groups encourages the child to learn food groups and reinforces the need for all food groups in their diets.

Preschoolers learn best through active participation. Making food preparation a fun experience is one way to encourage preschoolers to eat foods they may dislike (Fig. 14-1). This can be accomplished by using a children's cookbook that has easy-to-follow directions, offers only recipes of nutritional value, and introduces the child to

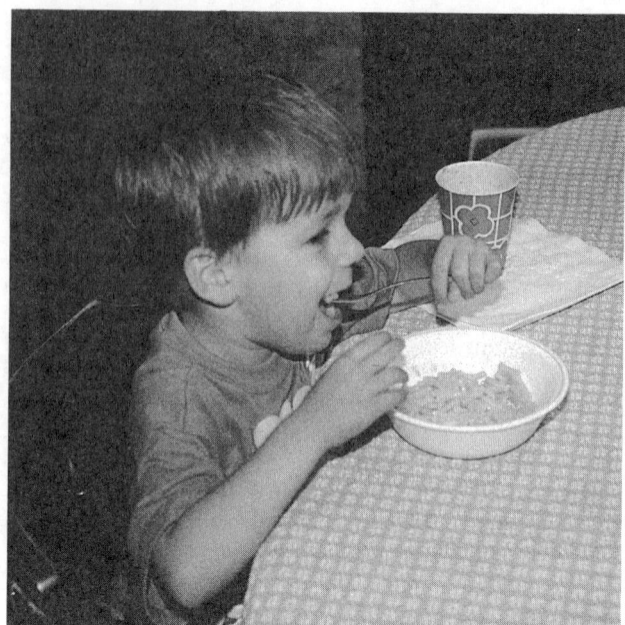

FIGURE 14-2
The eating habits of preschoolers will be formed as they begin to emulate parental eating behaviors.

a disliked food with a new approach. The accompanying display lists several children's cookbooks. Allowing the preschooler to serve food and using appropriate-sized utensils and pitchers provides another opportunity to learn through active participation. The preschooler's great desire to imitate adult behaviors should be used to teach nutrition, positive eating behaviors, and social skills associated with eating (Fig. 14-2). Including the preschooler in food-related activities such as purchasing, preparing, serving, and cleaning up prepares children for the move away from the family in the school years when they begin to make their own food choices in the school cafeteria.

Nursing Implications

The nurse should do a thorough assessment of the preschooler's eating patterns as well as an assessment of the environments in which long-term behaviors will develop. This includes an assessment of parental beliefs and practices related to nutrition and an assessment of nutritional practices in the day care environment. As with all children the nurse will first assess physical parameters, including serial height and weight. This is done by comparing the child's present height and weight with data obtained from previous well-care visits. The nurse can then evaluate whether growth is occurring in a steady pattern over time. Additionally, the nurse should assess intake for type, amount, and frequency. Parents should be given an explanation of how the child is doing in relation to the expected norms for growth and food intake. Even if the nurse notes optimal physical growth, other areas of the child's dietary status need to be addressed if the nurse is to promote continued growth and development. Assessment of the preschooler's opportunities for learning about nutrition, exposure to positive role models, and ability in self-feeding all serve to give the nurse clues

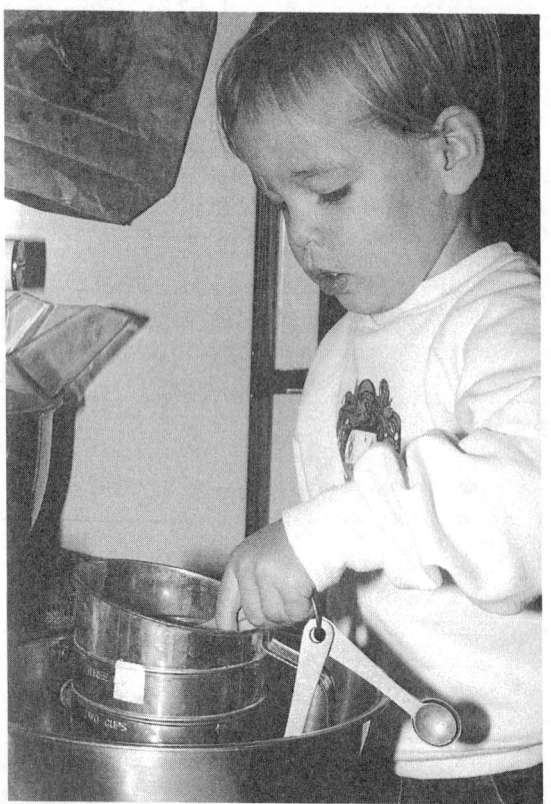

FIGURE 14-1
Preschoolers enjoy eating foods they can help prepare.

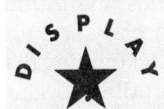

Selected Books for Preschoolers

CHILDRENS COOKBOOKS

Kinder-Krunchies: Healthy Snack Recipes for Children by K. Jenkins; Discovery Toys, 1982.
The Little Gardener's Cookbook by K. Bullock; Best Sellers Publications, 1987.
What a Good Lunch by S. Watanabe; (I Can Do It All by Myself books) Putnam Publisher Group, 1981.
Crunchy Bananas and Other Great Recipes Kids Can Cook by B. Wilms; Gibbs Smith Publishers, 1984.
I'll Eat Anything If I Can Make It Myself by M. Stori; Chicago Review, 1980.

BEDTIME

Bedtime for Frances by R. Hoban; Harper and Row, 1960.
The Bad Dream by J. Aylesworth; Albert Whitman and Company, 1985.
There's a Monster Under My Bed by J. Howe; Atheneum, 1986.
When Monsters Seem Real by F. Rogers; Random House, 1988.

LEARNING ABOUT YOURSELF

If We Were All the Same by F. Rogers; Random House, 1988.
People by P. Spier; Doubleday, 1988.
Quick as a Cricket by A. Wood; Child's Play, 1982.
Feelings by Aliki; Greenwillow Books, 1984.
My Book About Me by Dr. Seuss and R. McKie; Random House, 1969.

NEW BABY AND SIBLINGS

A Baby for Max K. Lasky; Macmillan Company, 1984.
Mom and Dad and I Are Having a Baby by M. Malecki; Penny Press, 1982.
The New Baby by F. Rogers; Random House, 1985.
No One Can Ever Take Your Place by F. Rogers; Random House, 1988.
How You Were Born by J Cole; Morrow Junior Books, 1985.
Before You Were Born by M. Sheffield; Knopf, 1983.
Baby Brother Blues by M. Polushkin; Bradbury Press, 1987.

DAY CARE

A Parent's Guide to Day Care. (1980) U.S. Department of Health and Human Services Administration for Children, Youth and Families. Day Care Division. DHHS Publication #(OHDS) 80-30254.

---

as to areas where parents may need education or reinforcement. By reviewing earlier eating patterns, especially during the toddler years, the nurse can explore with parents how they have dealt with problems such as food jags, food dislikes, refusal to eat, and dawdling in the past and their perception and satisfaction with their child's present eating patterns. Parents benefit from concrete suggestions that encourage preschoolers to eat a variety of nutritious foods.

Nurses can ask the preschooler directly about food preferences. Preschoolers are able to give reliable information about what they like and dislike.[5] The nurse can reinforce to the child foods that are nutritionally valuable and foods that should be eaten in moderation. "I am glad you like to eat chicken because chicken is very good for you." "I know that soda pop tastes good but it will not help your bones become strong like milk will. So you be sure and drink milk every day."

Parental Concern: Dawdling

Preschoolers are very active exploring the environment and observing what is going on around them. During mealtime their attention can be easily distracted from eating to watch something going on across the room, lis-

ten to someone speak, or just drift off into a fantasy of their own. Parents may find themselves continually bringing the child's attention back to the meal. Dawdling behavior draws out the time spent at the table with the preschooler sitting in front of a half-full plate long after everyone else is finished. Dawdling is frustrating for parents who are concerned about nutritional needs but are unable to get the child to eat their meal.

Parents must be reassured that dawdling is common during the preschool years. They should be assisted in finding ways to deal with dawdling without making mealtime a scene of conflict. Parents should be discouraged from using approaches such as making the child sit at the table for extended periods. If the child has not eaten after a reasonable time, removing the food and offering a nutritious food at the regularly scheduled snack time will provide the nutrients and avoid a battle. Presenting the child with food refused at one meal for the next meal should also be discouraged. Instead, parents can be assisted to deal with dawdling by decreasing stimuli at mealtime, including turning off the television, removing toys from the eating area, and setting a time goal with the child.

Regular times for meals and snacks can be useful in helping the child regulate intake. A child who eats off and on throughout the day may not have an appetite for regular meals. Between-meal snacks, if carefully chosen and including such foods as raw fruits and vegetables, can contribute positively to the child's overall nutrition. Preschoolers should be served small portions that are warm rather than hot and bland rather than spicy (Table 14-2).

Assessing, Promoting, and Maintaining Optimal Elimination

During the preschool years toileting becomes a more independent activity, and the child assumes increasing responsibility for the hygiene measures associated with toileting. Girls should be taught to wipe front to back to decrease the risk of urinary tract infections. Boys need to learn to raise and lower the toilet seat if they stand to void. All children need to learn to wash their hands after toileting. However, the preschooler will need consistent reminding of these measures if they are to incorporate them into routine behavior.

Most preschoolers are able to control bowel and bladder functions during the day. Accidents, especially wet pants, that do occur are generally related to illness, anxiety, or intense involvement in play activities. For some preschoolers nighttime wetting continues. Approximately 15% of all 5-year-old children and 5% of all 10-year-old children wet the bed.[11,19] Boys are more likely to have enuresis than girls.[44] The continuation of bed-wetting can be related to physiologic, psychological, or environmental factors.[19] Physiologic factors include organic pathology, urinary tract infection, small bladder capacity, genetic predisposition, or maturational lag (see Chap. 50).[19] Psychological aspects include divorce, family

death, birth of a sibling, moving, illness, hospitalization, or a result of initiating toilet training too early and too aggressively.[9,12] Brazelton[9] suggests that toilet training that is begun too early leaves the child susceptible to later breakdowns. Children who develop night control of urine at their own pace are likely to have continued bladder control. A child-centered approach to toilet training that allows the child to develop at his or her own pace may decrease the risk of the child developing nocturnal enuresis.[12] (See Chap. 13 for discussion of toilet training.) Environmental factors may include inadequate lighting from the bedroom to the bathroom, the need to share a communal bathroom with another family, or lack of adequate heat in the house or apartment.[11]

Nursing Implications

During well-care visits the nurse should discuss the child's elimination patterns with parents and identify problems, including bedwetting, accidents during the day, or difficulty of the preschooler in assuming responsibility for toilet-related hygiene. Once problems are discussed and potential causes identified, the nurse can assist parents in developing approaches to deal with the problem. Solutions may include spending extra time with the child who has started preschool or who has a new sibling. It may require an opportunity for the child to talk about feelings after stressful events, such as divorce or a move. A child who frequently has wet pants when involved in play may benefit from behavior modification techniques. Parents can make a star chart and give the child a star after successfully staying dry and using the toilet during the day. After earning a set number of stars the child will be given a reward. This method may motivate the child to stop an activity and go to the bathroom. Over time the child will be able to do this without the assistance of a chart.

If the problem is enuresis related to functional bladder capacity or the child's inability to respond to signals indicating bladder fullness when asleep, bladder training and conditioning techniques such as bedwetting alarms and dry bed training have been found to be successful.[11,19] Other methods frequently tried by parents, including restriction of fluids and periodic wakening of the child at night for toileting, have not proven to be successful over the long term. Instead of developing an ability to hold urine or awaken to urinate by themselves, they rely on parents to keep them from wetting the bed.[11] So in fact parents are trained to get up and wake the child. It is important that the nurse encourage the parents not to scold the child for bedwetting because the problem is not one the child can control without intervention.

TABLE 14-2
Nursing Intervention: Guidelines for Parents to Promote Optimal Nutrition of Preschool Children

Serving foods to preschoolers.	Preschooler's portions should be smaller than adult portions—rule of thumb is 1 tablespoon per year of age of each food.
	Preschoolers generally prefer food warm rather than hot.
	Preschoolers prefer raw to cooked vegetables.
	Preschoolers enjoy finger foods.
	Preschoolers do not like food mixed on a plate; each food must have its own place.
	Reintroduce in smaller portions those foods rejected earlier.
	Have nutritious snacks readily available such as cut-up fruit and vegetables.
Promoting development of positive food-related behaviors.	Role model eating behaviors you want child to learn.
	Include child in buying, preparing, and serving food.
	Allow child opportunities to learn social skills through participation in family meals.
	Allow increasing independence for child in serving self; feeding self; preparing some foods, such as cereal in the morning.

Assessing, Promoting, and Maintaining Optimal Sleep and Rest

Preschoolers continue to have some difficulty getting into bed and falling asleep.[3] Bedtime routines lasting more than 30 minutes are typical during the preschool years.[3] Once in bed many preschoolers remain awake for up to

30 minutes.[3] Typical sleep requirements for the 3-year-old child is 12 hours, decreasing to 11 hours for the 5-year-old child.[19]

Naps during the day may be eliminated or take the form of quiet time during which the preschooler is either sleeping or involved in quiet activities (Fig. 14-3).

Sleep Concerns

The most common sleep concerns during the preschool years include nighttime awakening, bedtime fears, nightmares, and night terrors.[3,15,19,23] Parental concerns related to sleep intensify if the child's sleep disturbance interferes with parental sleep or family functioning.

Night Waking

Night waking is common during the preschool years. The child awakens during the night and may stay awake for varying lengths of time. The child who stays in bed and does not cry out for parents will not cause parental concern; in fact, parents may not even realize the child is awake. The child who cries out and needs parental assistance to get back to sleep can cause much parental anxiety. These behaviors often lead parents to seek assistance from health care professionals. Because night awakenings are a part of normal sleep patterns at all ages, the focus of care needs to be on helping the child develop the ability to go back to sleep without parental assistance.[19,23] The child who awakens and is unable to go back to sleep may have developed sleep associations that are not readily available during night awakenings, such as being rocked, fed, held by parents, or, in some instances, even being taken in the car.[3] Parents benefit from a discussion of normal sleep patterns, why awakening occurs, and how parents reinforce awakenings. Parents can then be assisted in changing the child's behavior by setting up new sleep routines. This means having the child go to bed with conditions that will be present when the child awakens during the night. The child can be put

down for bedtime alone in the crib with a treasured object, without a bottle, without being carried till asleep or rocked to sleep. As the child learns to fall asleep under these new conditions, going back to sleep after night awakenings will also be possible. Gradually decreasing parental intervention at night allows the parent to provide some support during the learning phase. The parents are told to return briefly to the child who awakens after giving the child progressively longer time to develop self-comforting measures. This type of program can be difficult for parents, and they need reassurance that assisting the child in this way will not cause psychological harm. Parents should have close follow-up and access to the health care professional during the transition.

Bedtime Fears

Bedtime fears are a frequent occurrence during the preschool years. It is during the preschool and early school years that children develop the greatest number of new fears in general.[36] Some of the most common sources of fear include animals, dark, monsters, storms, doctors and dentists, nightmares, school, water, and death.[35] These fears may be the result of a frightening experience such as being chased or bitten by a dog, hearing about another child's frightening experience, seeing something frightening on television, or hearing scary stories.[35] The child's vivid imagination and egocentric thinking can lead to the development of fears. Children may fear going down the drain when the bath plug is pulled or going down the toilet if the trip is pulled while the child is still sitting on the seat. These fears are a normal result of the child's limited cognitive skills. The child's imagination and animism create monsters that are real for the child. In a dark room the child can see monsters and animals in the shadows.

Helping a child overcome fears is most successful if attempts are made to decrease fears from becoming too strong or preventing them altogether. Helping children develop a strong self-concept will increase their confidence in their ability to control events and challenges in their lives. Children who have a strong positive self-concept are less vulnerable to fear because they have confidence in their ability to master and control events.[35] If fears develop, parents can discuss them with the child. Children need to know that being afraid is a normal feeling, and all people at one time or another have fears.

In dealing with children's fears, Sarafino[35] describes methods that can make fears worse. Parents should not force the child in contact with the fear, for example, making the child pet a dog that frightens him. Ridicule and shaming a child, because a fear seems silly to the adult, will not decrease the child's fear but rather decrease the child's self-esteem. Punishment or scolding—"Stop crying! There is nothing to be afraid of"—does not decrease fear but instead is another unpleasant experience for the child. Overprotection may increase fears because the child has little opportunity to cope with threatening experiences. Ignoring fears will not make them go away.

According to Ferber,[19] bedtime fears occur throughout childhood and adolescence and may reflect emotional conflict the child experiences during the day. For the preschool child these bedtime fears may be related to

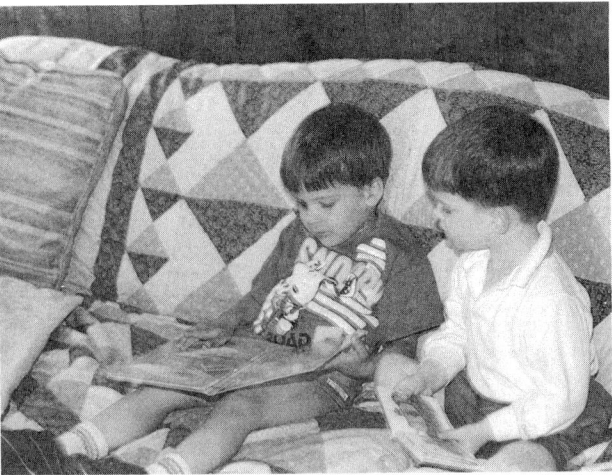

FIGURE 14-3
Nap time for preschoolers may be replaced by more quiet time or quiet activities.

developmental issues that arise, such as a resurgence of separation fears once school is started, a fear of soiling after toilet training, or anxiety caused by sexual impulses or genital play. Other causes of bedtime fears can include a recent death in the family, a new sibling, or experience of being lost or ill. Fears that arise at bedtime, such as darkness, monsters, and ghosts may require a night light or leaving the child's door open. These are temporary fears and will pass. Parents should be discouraged from going to extremes in showing the child that there are no monsters. They can provide verbal reassurance. There are also many books available to help the preschooler with fears (see Selected Books for Preschoolers).

Nightmares

A nightmare is a frightening dream that awakens the child from sleep. Nightmares usually occur at the end of the night during rapid-eye-movement sleep.[19] Once the child recognizes that the environment is familiar and safe and reassurance from parents is given, the child can usually go back to sleep. The preschooler may need physical comforting as well as verbal reassurance that everything is alright. If nightmares are frequent, parents must try to explore where these feelings are coming from. This is best done during the day by observing the child for situations or experiences that cause stress. Parents can then help the child cope with these conflicts or fears. At one time or another all children experience nightmares.

Night Terrors

Night terrors are different from nightmares. Night terrors occur early in the night during the deep sleep phase.[19] A child who has a night terror will not fully awaken but will scream, cry, or moan.[19] The child will not recognize parents and may become agitated if parents try to provide physical comfort measures.[19] Even if the child does awaken there is no recollection of the episode

and the child will not remember it in the morning. Night terrors will resolve on their own and, unlike nightmares, the child does not need the assistance and comforting of parents because the child is not awake. Because a night terror is not a result of a bad dream, there is not reason to wake the child up but rather allow sleep to continue. Frequent nightmares or night terrors that do not disappear with time indicate a need for investigation of the child's emotional state and an evaluation of what is occurring in the environment.

Nursing Implications

Sleep patterns should be assessed by the nurse during routine well-care visits (Table 14-3). Parental concerns should be investigated by assessment of the child's behavior prior to bedtime, during the night, and on awakening. The nurse should obtain more specific information, including the frequency of the behavior, the parental response, and the usual outcome. Parents can be reassured that these behaviors are a normal part of development. However, if a child has frequent sleep problems that are disruptive to the family, individualized interventions should be planned. Assisting the parents in determining whether the child is experiencing nightmares or night terrors and providing them with information on how to deal with the specific one their child is experiencing will help prevent further problems (Table 14-4).

Assessing, Promoting, and Maintaining Optimal Psychosocial Development

Psychosocial development in the preschool years includes the development of a sense of initiative, a positive self-concept, and sex role identification. The preschooler must also develop social skills, learn to control aggressive impulses, and share the attention of adults.

TABLE 14-3
Nursing Assessment: Questions for Assessing Sleep During the Preschool Years

Areas of Assessment	Key Questions*
Are child's sleeping behaviors appropriate for stage of development?	Describe for me _____ sleeping patterns.
Parental awareness of sleep needs.	What time does _____ go to bed?
Any environmental conditions that promote or interfere with sleep.	Where does _____ sleep?
Night awakenings and causes.	Does _____ awaken at night? What is usually the cause of the awakening (hunger, bathroom, no specific reason)?
Sleep associations.	What do you have to do to get _____ back to sleep?
Behaviors of child when he or she awakens at night.	If _____ wakes up during the night, what does he/she do?
Parental reactions to behavior during night wakenings.	What do you do when _____ exhibits this behavior?
Presence and frequency of nightmares or night terrors.	Does _____ have nightmares or cry out in his/her sleep? How often?

* Use child's name in blank space.

TABLE 14-4
Nursing Intervention: Anticipatory Guidance for Promoting Optimal Sleep Patterns

Developing a normal sleep routine.	Provide a consistent bedtime. Set bedtime so that the child goes to bed before becoming overly tired.
Naptime.	Provide quiet time in the afternoon. The child may read books or play alone in his or her room. The child may sleep. Most children need and enjoy this time alone.
Night awakenings.	It is normal for children to awaken during the night. If the child needs parental assistance to go back to sleep, determine the type of intervention necessary. If the child needs the parent to be in the room, gradually stay for shorter periods and provide a stuffed animal for the child. Expect the time of transition to be difficult.
Difficulty going to bed.	Develop a routine for bedtime. Do not allow routines to become too elaborate. Behavior modification such as the use of a star chart may be helpful.
Child who wants to go to parents' bed.	Sleeping with parents should be discouraged. If this behavior is avoided early, it should not become a problem. Provide a night light for the child. Leave the child's door open. Tell the child he or she can come to your room when the sun comes up.
Nightmares and night terrors.	Normal during this stage. Provide quiet, pleasant activities before bedtime. Avoid viewing of television shows that display violence or aggression. Reassure child when frightened. Allow a child who is having a night terror to continue to sleep.

Developing a Sense of Initiative

Erikson[18] describes the major psychosocial conflict of the preschool years as initiative versus guilt. Initiative is the ability to undertake new activities, planning, and 'attacking' a task for the sake of being active and on the move.[18] The child derives pleasure in conquest and fantasizes about being powerful. Intrusion is the primary mode at this stage. The preschooler's developing physical and mental abilities moves the child forward into a variety of activities. "These include the intrusion into others bodies by physical attack; the intrusion into other people's ears and minds by aggressive talking; the intrusion into space by vigorous locomotion; and intrusion into the unknown by consuming curiosity."[18] The child with a sense of initiative makes plans, sets goals, and persists at attaining them. Initiative brings the child into contact with others, and the child makes self-discoveries by trying on adult roles. Initiative that is supported by parents and other adults has a positive influence on self-concept, body image, and psychosexual development of the child.

An overwhelming sense of guilt is the potential negative outcome of the preschool years. The preschool child has begun to incorporate adult expectations of behavior. Preschoolers are less dependent on parents to control behavior because of an increasing ability of the children to direct their own actions. The child internalizes social prohibitions through the development of the superego, which serves to keep impulses in check. The conscience of the preschooler can be cruel and uncompromising and can result in an overwhelming sense of guilt when rules are broken or the child's curiosity is impeded.

Parental Role

Parents promote initiative by responding positively to the child's curiosity, enthusiasm, and excitement in learning about people, places, objects, and adult roles. By showing enthusiasm and pleasure for the preschooler's initiative, parents promote the preschooler's desire to learn. Taking the time to answer questions and explain events, as well as praising the child's questions, portrays to the child that parents value the child's desire for knowledge. Casual learning through everyday experiences demonstrates that learning can be fun and occurs in both formal and informal settings. Initiative is fostered when parents allow the child opportunities to role play and participate in family activities. Chores around the house, such as helping with meal preparation, laundry, and yard work, foster a sense of initiative and positive feelings about one's abilities. Praise for a job well done or for an earnest attempt and helping when assistance is needed builds confidence in the performance of newly learned skills.

Initiative is encouraged when parents allow preschoolers the extra time it may take to do something on their own, such as tie their shoes or button their coats. Parents can provide opportunities that expose the child to new experiences such as going to the zoo, fire station, museum, aquarium, swimming class, or duck pond. Being patient with the child who stops to explore and allowing the child to interact with other children and adults are all behaviors that foster initiative.

Nursing Implications

When working with preschool children, the nurse should assess for indications of a developing sense of initiative. A child who demonstrates excitement and enthusiasm for new experiences and one who is actively involved in exploration of the physical and social world through verbal questioning and active participation is demonstrating initiative. A child's curiosity about events, people, and adult roles such as firemen, policemen, and nurses indicates a growing curiosity and desire to learn. Children experience guilt when rules are broken, explorations and questions are viewed as bothersome, or the child's curiosity is not rewarded. A child who is fearful of new situations and who is withdrawn when around adults and other children may be exhibiting signs of a developing sense of guilt. Other symptoms of guilt may include an overdependency on parents or self-reference as "bad boy" or "bad girl."

The nurse can use the assessment to support a diagnosis of healthy psychosocial development or one of potential problems in this area (Table 14-5). When a nurse

TABLE 14-5
Nursing Assessment: Guidelines for Assessing Initiative

Child Behaviors That Demonstrate Initiative	Parental Behaviors That Foster Initiative
Demonstrates excitement when given opportunities for new experiences.	Gives the child an opportunity to talk about his or her day.
Involved in exploration of the physical and social world through active exploration and verbal questioning.	Provides varied and enriched experiences such as going to the zoo, shopping, park.
	Is patient with frequent questions.
Interacts with peers and is comfortable with adults other than parents.	Takes time to answer questions and explain events and social behaviors the child experiences.
Demonstrates curiosity about events, sex, and roles of various adults such as police and firemen.	Provides positive reinforcement for child's independence, curiosity, social interaction, and role imitation.
Energetic, enthusiastic, and curious.	Allows child to express disagreement.
Child Behaviors That Demonstrate Guilt	**Parental Behaviors That Lead to Guilt**
Child is excessively fearful of new situations, events, or interactions.	Does not allow child to talk about experiences.
Does not actively explore environment or socialize with others.	Does not provide a variety of experiences to stimulate the child's curiosity.
Dependent on parents and does not interact with peers or other adults.	Becomes angered by child's frequent questions.
Does not express curiosity about events, sex, and adult roles.	Does not take time to explain expected behavior; rather, uses power to control behavior.
Apathetic and withdrawn.	Does not allow child to express disagreement.
Calls himself or herself bad boy or bad girl.	Does not provide positive reinforcement for child's success in activities.

observes a child demonstrating initiative through exploratory behavior and verbal curiosity, the nurse can share these observations with parents. Positive reinforcement for parents is provided by explaining how parental interactions and patience with the preschooler has fostered the child's initiative.

A child who appears to be overly dependent on parents and does not show any curiosity about what is going on during the interview or physical examination should alert the nurse to a potential problem. Because the child's lack of interest may be a result of anxiety related to the health care visit, it is important that the nurse discuss with parents the child's behavior when in a more familiar and comfortable environment.

Parents who report feelings of annoyance with the child's insatiable curiosity about the how and why of everyday experiences need an explanation of the normalcy of this behavior. Pointing out to parents that this curiosity and desire to learn is beneficial for the child's develop-

TABLE 14-6
Nursing Intervention: Anticipatory Guidance for Fostering Initiative

- Provide positive reinforcement for children's curiosity, enthusiasm, and excitement in learning about people, places, objects, and adult roles.
- Provide children with a variety of experiences where they can learn about the society they live in and can observe the diversity of adult roles (shopping, going to the park, zoo, museum, church, etc.).
- Provide opportunities for children to interact with other adults and peers by attending nursery school or playing with other children in the neighborhood.
- Answer children's questions about events, social behaviors, sexuality, and everyday events as the questions arise and at a level they can comprehend.
- If preschoolers ask questions when parents do not have time to answer, tell them you will talk about it later and make a point of answering questions when you can.
- When helping preschoolers control their behavior, explain reasons for your actions and allow the child to express feelings without giving up parental control.

ment may help parents to be more responsive to the child's questions and exploratory behavior. Sharing with parents ideas of how to foster initiative and role modeling for parents though the nurse's interactions with the child are important interventions (Table 14-6). The nurse can foster a sense of initiative by taking the time to talk with the child, asking about new experiences, school, or play activities. The nurse should also allow the child independence in undressing and dressing for a physical examination. The nurse must also talk directly to the preschooler, be alert to questions preschoolers may have, and take the time to let preschoolers listen to their hearts and assist with parts of the examination. The natural curiosity of preschoolers provides many opportunities for teaching.

Developing a Positive Self-Concept and Body Image

During the preschool years the child develops a self-concept based on interactions with significant persons and the child's own perceptions of the body and its functions. Parents and other adults have an important role in helping the child develop a positive self-concept.

The preschooler's increasing competence in mastering and functioning in the environment adds to the developing self-concept. Mastering a new skill such as learning to tie shoelaces, skip, or put a puzzle together promotes a positive self-concept. A child who does not experience success in attempts to master new skills will not develop a positive self-concept. The child needs the support of parents to try again after a failure. Preschoolers begin to view themselves as being unique, special, valued, and loved or the opposite, being inadequate, disliked, and unloved, based on the responses they receive from parents and other significant adults. These feelings become part of the self-concept and affect the child's interactions with others.[31]

Parental Role

Parents have a significant impact on the preschooler's developing self-concept. Parents verbal, nonverbal, and physical interactions with the young child reflect their feelings toward the child and influence the developing self-concept. The child who consistently experiences negative reactions to behavior, is ignored, or does not receive positive reinforcement for the mastery of new skills will not have feelings of being a valued person. The child develops feelings of self-worth by the positive reactions of parents to the mastery of new skills, being hugged and kissed, being included in family activities, and being supported when unsuccessful or feeling rejected. These initial self-perceptions become especially important in the years ahead when the child leaves the security of the home and begins to be evaluated by peers, teachers, and other persons. A child who does not have a positive self-concept may experience greater difficulty in school performance and peer relationships.[30,31]

Children who perceive themselves as lacking positive qualities such as being smart, being likeable, being skillful in an activity or sport often feel powerless, easily frustrated and avoid situations that provoke anxiety.[31] However, self-concept is responsive to outside influences which affect self-perceptions throughout the life cycle. Early identification of a child who appears to have a negative self-concept provides opportunity for intervention.

Nursing Implications

Assessing the child's self-concept is a major role of the nurse in promoting healthy development. Through systemic observations of the child's interactions with parents, attempts to master new skills, ability to perform activities of daily living, ability to cope with frustration, and expressions of self-pride at the mastery of new skills, the nurse can begin to evaluate the child's self-concept. In the interview with parents the nurse can elicit information of parents' abilities and progress in fostering a positive self-concept in the preschool child. By having parents describe their perceptions of the child, including both positive and negative qualities, the nurse can assess the types of messages the child may be receiving from parents that may be incorporated into the developing self-concept (Table 14-7).

The nurse can also observe parental interactions with the child. Do the parents praise the child for successful experiences? Do parents hug, kiss, or playfully interact with the child? Do parents express positive verbal de-

TABLE 14-7
Nursing Assessment: Questions for Assessing the Development of a Positive Self-Concept

- What do parents like best about the child?
- How do parents interact with the child?
- How do parents describe the child?
- What do parents dislike about the child and why?
- How do parents feel the child compares to siblings or other children the same age?
- How do parents express positive feelings toward the child (e.g., physical contact, hugging, kissing, holding, or verbal expressions of pride and pleasure)?

TABLE 14-8
Nursing Intervention: Anticipatory Guidance for Promoting a Positive Self-Concept

- Children need opportunities to master new skills.
- Children benefit from parents who verbally express positive attributes of the child.
- Children benefit from parents who physically express positive feelings toward the child, including hugging, kissing, and engaging in playful activities.
- When a child does something wrong, it is helpful if parents explain that it is the behavior, not the child, they are upset about.
- Children incorporate values, attitudes, and behaviors that are role modeled by their parents.
- Children need support when they experience failure or feelings of rejection.

scriptions of the child such as smart, sensitive, fun, talented, playful, or wonderful, or do they refer to the child as stupid, slow, bratty, messy, or lazy? Through discussion of the nurse's observations and parental verbal reports, the nurse can help parents understand how their interactions and perceptions of the child influence the child's self-concept. The nurse can offer guidance for parents in their attempts to foster a healthy self-concept in the child. Based on an assessment, the nurse can discuss with parents how daily interactions with the child become incorporated into the child's self-concept. Some parents may need encouragement and an explanation of the importance of focusing on the child's positive qualities rather than negative qualities (Table 14-8).

Nurses also add to the child's self-concept by the physical and verbal interactions that occur during a health visit. Incorporating the child into the conversation during the visit and asking the child about daily activities and special interests give the child a feeling of being important. Sharing with the child an admiration for the mastery of new skills or the learning of a new game promotes a positive self-concept. When a child is unable to describe any new accomplishments or successful experiences, it is important that the nurse point out to the child strengths observed by the nurse or reported by parents.

Developing a Positive Body Image

Preschool children are becoming more aware of themselves as separate, unique individuals. They have an interest in their own body as well as the bodies of others and are curious about how they resemble and differ from others. As preschoolers become increasingly aware of the differences of boys and girls, they may play "doctor" or demonstrate curiosity and a desire to see other children of both sexes. Through interactions with others, the child begins to develop a body image. The preschooler learns personal characteristics such as being pretty, strong, tall, handsome, thin, or fat. They learn the color of their eyes, hair, and skin and watch with amazement as they lose their first tooth and a new one comes in.

Parental Role

Parents contribute to the child's developing body image from the earliest interactions with the newborn. Parents who find the infant unattractive or significantly different from their expectations may, without realizing it, hold the infant less, interact with the infant less, or may even repeatedly vocalize their displeasure.[28] On the other hand, most parents are able to identify quickly the positive qualities of the child, such as pretty eyes, a cute nose, or a family characteristic, and the infant feels the closeness and attachment. Through vocal expressions, facial expressions, and physical expressions of parents, the child begins to develop a body image. By the preschooler years the child is able to verbalize personal attributes of themselves which are reinforced by parents. There is a special interest in being weighed and measured. By keeping markings on the wall, door, or height chart in the child's room, the child can watch the physical changes that are taking place. Growing taller is a positive experience for preschoolers, who want to show everyone how much they have grown (Fig. 14-4). Preschoolers want to show their strength and their ability to use their bodies for new challenges such as swinging high on the swing set or climbing to the top of the jungle gym. Preschoolers need opportunities to use new physical skills; they also need praise for their abilities.

Preschool children are ready to learn the proper names and functions of various body parts. The child benefits from opportunities to look in the mirror. The preschooler wants some say in what clothes are worn, and he or she usually has favorites. Parents can also read books to the preschooler that describe feelings and discuss physical attributes (see Selected Books for Preschoolers).

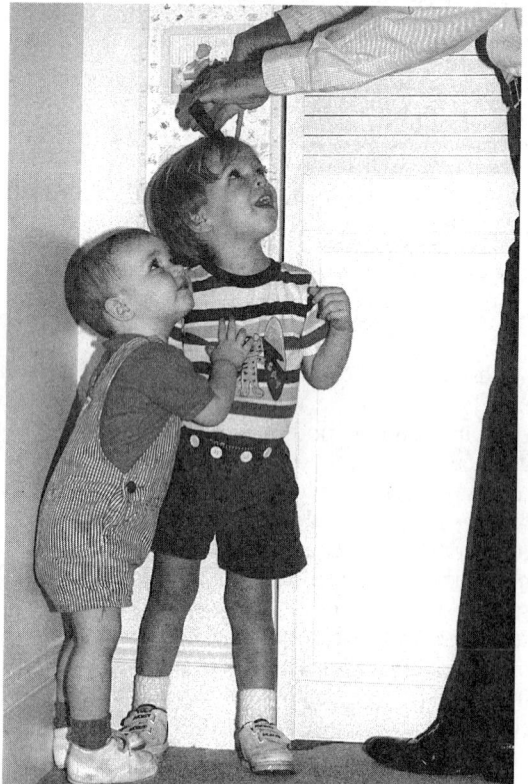

FIGURE 14-4
Preschoolers enjoy having special attention given to their growth. Keeping a chart at home can be fun for children and parents.

TABLE 14-9
Nursing Assessment: Questions for Assessing the Development of a Positive Body Image

• Are parents comfortable discussing body parts and body functions with the child?
• Do the parents verbally describe the child's changes in physical development? ("You are getting tall.")
• Do parents allow the child some control over what to wear?

Nursing Implications

Nurses can help parents promote a positive body image of the child by discussing with them how the body image develops and how parental interactions with the child contribute to the child's self-perceptions. Nurses can explore with parents what messages parents feel they are conveying to the child (Tables 14-9 and 14-10). When a child is handicapped, it is especially important to help parents evaluate how often their interactions focus on the handicap and how often the focus is on other attributes of the child. Identifying a child's strengths is especially important for a child with a physical handicap. By identifying and focusing on the strengths, the handicap will not become the central focus of the child's body image.

In direct contacts with the child, the nurse can evaluate the child's self-perceptions and enhance the development of a positive body image. The nurse can elicit the child's self-perceptions by encouraging verbal descriptions of what the child thinks about present physical growth and physical characteristics. "Have you grown since I last saw you?" "Have you gotten stronger?" "Tell me something you can do now that you could not do when you were little." The nurse may also have the child draw a self-portrait while doing a favorite activity. In explaining the self-portrait, the child will express positive as well as negative qualities that have been incorporated into the body image. Verbal, facial, and tactile expressions by the nurse must be positive.

Promoting Psychosexual Development

The preschooler's curiosity focuses on all aspects of life, including the reasons why girls and boys are anatomically different. This interest in genitals occurs at the same time as Freud's oedipal stage. Typically the child attempts to win the attentions of the parent of the opposite sex

TABLE 14-10
Nursing Intervention: Anticipatory Guidance for Promoting a Positive Body Image

• Preschool children are ready to learn the names and functions of various body parts.
• Children should be given opportunities to look at themselves in the mirror.
• Children enjoy being measured for increasing height and weight and are proud of their growth.
• Preschoolers benefit from books read to them that describe feelings and physical attributes with which they can identify.
• Preschoolers like to choose what clothes to wear.

while developing feelings of rivalry for the parent of the same sex. The child is learning what it means to be a boy or girl (gender identity) and, at the same time, appropriate sex roles or behaviors.

Preschoolers observe, imitate, and incorporate behaviors of others, especially their parents. The parent of the same sex is usually the person the preschooler will identify with and imitate most frequently. Through the identification process with parents, preschoolers begin to learn and adopt behaviors, values, attitudes, and interests that form sex roles within the culture. These behaviors are incorporated into and become part of the self-concept. Preschoolers begin to evaluate self-worth in terms of how well they are meeting the role expectations of parents.

Through self-exploration, the child experiences sensations and pleasurable feelings associated with touching the genitals. Preschool children often engage in some form of self-stimulation.[20,24,39] If not excessive, this behavior is a natural way of learning about one's body. Sexual curiosity also develops and centers around issues including "where do babies come from?" "how do they get inside mommy?" and "how do they get out?" The preschooler is not interested in a full description of sexuality but is demonstrating curiosity that is reflective of his or her developmental level. How parents react to these behaviors and questions posed by the preschooler can affect the child's self-image and sexual development.[20]

Parental Role

Before responding to a child's questions, parents can determine what the child believes and correct misconceptions. Children benefit from honest, simple answers to their questions about sexuality. If parents answer a child's question simply and honestly, the child is usually satisfied. Parents may misinterpret a simple question and assume the child wants to know everything about sexuality. In this instance parents may react by giving the child more information than can be understood by the child or not giving the child any information at all. There are many books available that address parental concerns and offer suggestions for approaches to the topic of sexuality. There are also books parents can read to children to help the child begin to understand relationships, reproduction, and sexuality (see Selected Books for Preschoolers). Parents also may express concern regarding self-stimulation during the early years. Most importantly, parents need to be aware that self-stimulation by young children is a normal part of body exploration. This behavior may be more frequent when a child is bored or upset. If parents find an increase in self-stimulation behavior as a result of boredom, they can assist the child in finding other activities. Parents who are able to deal with self-stimulation casually and calmly will prevent the development of guilt feelings in the child.

Nursing Implications

Nurses should discuss psychosexual development with parents. Parents may be uncomfortable discussing this topic not only with the child but also with health care workers. The nurse may be the one to approach the topic by asking parents if the child has been asking questions and how parents have responded. Explaining to parents that this is a normal part of development may reassure them that there is not something wrong with their child. Parents especially benefit by hearing that the questions require simple answers rather than in-depth detail.

Closely associated with psychosocial development are two common parental concerns that arise during the preschool years: aggression and sibling rivalry. Parents who are prepared for these behaviors can reduce the severity by early intervention.

Dealing With Aggressive Behavior

Aggressive behavior during the preschool years is frequently verbal expression through name calling and swearing or some physical expression, including biting, hitting people, and throwing toys or other objects. The frequency and degree of aggressive behavior that a child exhibits depend on many factors, including the following[4]:

- Intensity of the hostility.
- Level of the environmental frustration experienced.
- Rewards obtained for the aggressive behavior.
- Exposure to and imitation of aggressive models.
- Anxiety and guilt caused by expressions of aggression.

Aggression can be a reaction to frustration. Frustration can occur when a person is unable to attain a goal, is deprived of a personal desire, or experiences a threat to self-esteem.

Children are confronted with potentially frustrating experiences every day. For example, a child who is engrossed in a play activity may experience frustration when a parent tells him to stop and come to dinner. A child who is building with blocks will feel frustration if someone accidently knocks over the blocks. Preschool children may also have a desire to have something that belongs to another child. How a child will react to experiences that cause frustration depends on the child's temperament, ability to tolerate frustration, and the frequency and intensity of frustrating experiences. The amount of help from parents the child has received in controlling aggressive behavior influences the continuation or discontinuation of the behavior. Aggression, like other behaviors, can be influenced by rewards or punishments. If aggression results in the desired outcome, that is, the child gets the toy she wants, the child will use this approach again. Aggressive behavior can also be learned by observation or by being the recipient of aggressive acts. A child who views aggression on television or observes aggressive behaviors of parents or peers will be more inclined toward aggression. Parents who rely on physical punishment to discipline a child are teaching the child that aggression can be used to control others.

Nursing Implications

In an effort to decrease or eliminate aggressive behavior, nurses should work with parents in identifying contributing factors such as frustrating experiences, exposure to violence on television, or parental use of aggression. It is helpful to determine situations or events that precipitate aggressive behavior. Is aggressive behavior more frequent or intense during certain times of the day? Can parents anticipate aggressive behavior? How have parents dealt with aggressive behavior, and has their method worked? Which behaviors of the child do parents find especially difficult? The answers to these questions provide the information necessary to develop interventions such as monitoring television viewing, increasing transition time from play activities to mealtime or bedtime, and talking to the child about feelings.

Together parents and the nurse can plan interventions based on the specific needs of the child. Some general interventions known to decrease aggressive behaviors can be shared with parents. These interventions can then be adapted to the child's situation.

Initially, the nurse should discuss with parents that it is not easy for the child to handle conflicts verbally, but, with time and role modeling by parents and other significant people, the child will gradually learn positive coping mechanisms. Increased language skills can be used to teach the child to deal with frustration by expressing feelings of anger, hurt, or rejection: "Tell me how you feel"; "I know you want to have that toy, but Sue is playing with it right now"; "Why don't you ask her nicely if you can try it?" or "Wait a few minutes and then ask her for a turn." However, when the child becomes overwhelmed by emotions, verbal attempts to deal with the frustration often give way to physical methods, and parents have to intervene by physically removing the child briefly.

In planning interventions, the nurse should emphasize that the young child needs help from parents in controlling behavior. Because television has been found to convey aggression as a method of conflict resolution, parents should be encouraged to monitor what the child watches on television.[1,46] A child who is being aggressive in group play may need to be removed from the situation until calm. Removal should be for a short period, 1 to 2 minutes, so that the child has an opportunity to go back to the situation and use other methods of coping, such as finding another toy to play with or asking to use the desired toy. Parents and nurses should accept the child's feelings and at the same time let the child know the behavior is not acceptable, for example, "I know you are angry but you cannot bite Billy."

A hospitalized child may show an increase in aggressive behavior, especially if subjected to invasive procedures, including injections, surgery, or catheterization. Talking to the child and validating feelings of anger, fear, and frustration are helpful in this situation. The child may have a need to express feelings physically by pounding clay or playing out the experience with a doll. Children with enforced immobility may need to be given other outlets for frustration, including banging and pounding toys and throwing games.

Handling Sibling Rivalry

The arrival of a second child presents unique challenges to parental childrearing methods (Fig. 14-5). The preschool child responds to the presence of a new sibling in ways that reflect the lack of experience in sharing the attention of parents. Parents can benefit from a nurse who offers anticipatory counseling related to expected behavior changes of an older sibling when a new infant is brought home.

When the new infant is brought home, the older child may feel deprived of a parent's love. The infant needs considerable time from the mother during feeding, bathing, diapering, rocking, cuddling, and other displays of affection. The older child observes the attention given to the infant and experiences feelings of deprivation and loss of attention, love, and affection. Parents must be alert to behavioral manifestations that signal the older child's need for appropriate parental attention. The accompanying display lists behavior that may be manifested. Powell[33] offers the following examples of the wide variety of responses seen among children who are attempting to cope with the arrival of a new sibling: regression, aggression, irritability, and negativism.

The nurse should explore parental readiness for dealing with these behaviors and provide guidance that will make the adjustment easier for both child and parents. Child care professionals can assist parents in preparing the older child for the birth of a new sibling by sharing information of common reactions and suggesting activities to decrease the intensity of feelings. Parents can talk to the child about what babies are like and what special needs they have. Books that deal with feelings an older child has when a sibling is born can be read to the child (see Selected Books for Preschoolers). Any changes that the older child will be expected to make, such as moving to a new room or going to nursery school, should be planned and done several months in advance. Even the child who is prepared in advance for the arrival of a new sibling may have difficulty when the occurrence becomes a reality. Parents should be aware of and anticipate changes in behavior of the older child even if the child is prepared for the arrival before birth (see Fig. 14-5).

If parents identify changes in behavior of the older child, they should pay close attention to behavior patterns between the older child and younger infant. Parents should also be aware of how they respond to these behaviors. Do they scold or spank the child? Do they tell the child they are bad or acting like a baby? These types of reactions may be reinforcing some undesirable behaviors. If an older sibling reacts aggressively toward a new infant, the older child may be aware that this behavior will bring prompt parental attention. If this pattern is allowed to become established, the older child will continue to act aggressively toward the infant. Parents who are aware that they may be reinforcing undesirable behavior can change their responses to the child. Parents can be encouraged to respond to the older child in positive ways. Powell[33] recommends planned attention by parents to help the older child change behavior patterns. Parents can give the child attention and praise when the child is playing quietly or being independent in self-care activities rather than during episodes of crying, whining, or reverting to earlier, less mature developmental habits. A simple smile, hug, or touch will convey parental approval to the child. Setting special time aside for the older child who is allowed to choose an activity for this time is helpful. Realistically, this may be a period of 10 to 15

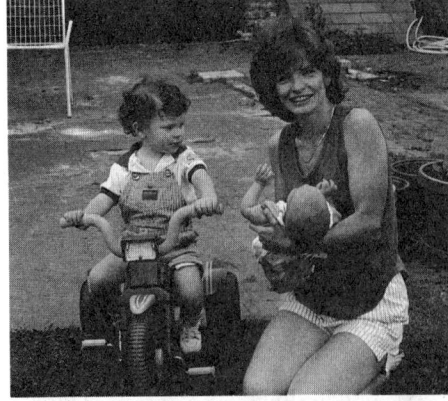
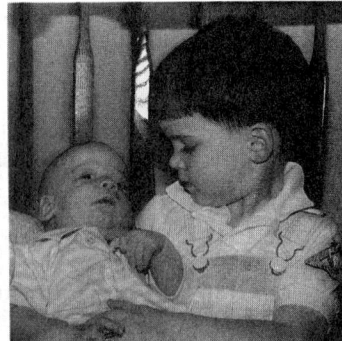
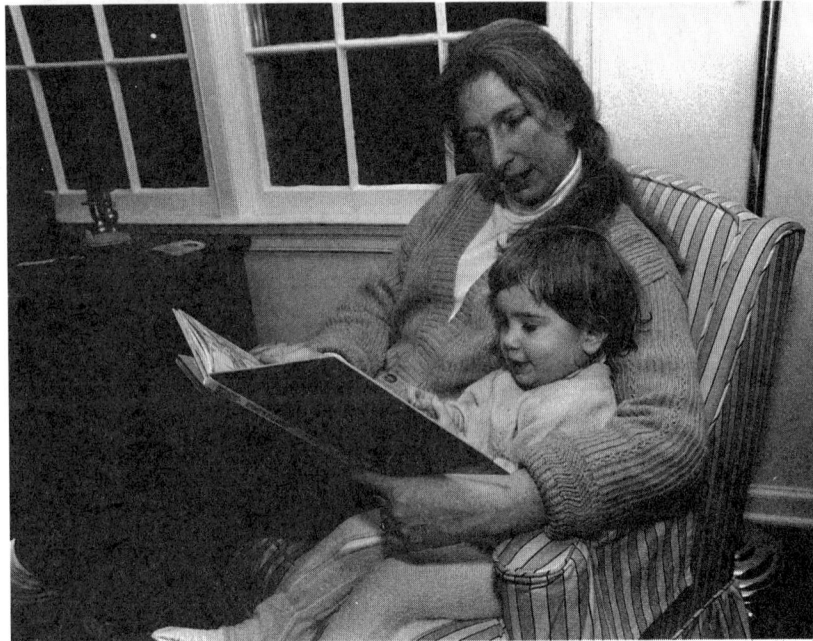

FIGURE 14-5
Parents can help in the transition to a new baby by
involving the older sibling, allowing the child to hold the
new baby, and by providing a special time between
parents and children to promote affection and cuddling.

minutes. This experience will help children learn to share
parental attention just as they learned to share toys. Parents should praise the child during the day for positive
behavior even if it is a behavior that was previously taken
for granted. A teaching plan for addressing sibling rivalry
in a preschooler accompanies this section.

Powell[33] stresses the importance of avoiding instant
advice. Parents are often told to give equal attention to
both the infant and older child, give equal time to both
the infant and older child, or have the older child help
care for the infant. Each of these options is unrealistic
and does not meet the needs of the parents or the older
child. A 3-year-old child is unable to provide care for a
newborn. The newborn requires extended time from the
mother, and she will be unable to divide time equally
between children. Instead, parents must be assisted in
finding ways to give the older child extra attention during
the times that are planned in advance and planned with
the child's participation. For example, a parent can explain to the older child that "While the baby is napping,
Mommy is going to read you a story. Why don't you pick
out which book you want Mommy to read just to you?"
Physical displays of affection and cuddling during these
times provide the older child reinforcement of parental
feelings of love (see Fig. 14-5). Having activities planned

for the older child during the time the baby is being
bathed or fed can decrease problems. This may include
having a special coloring book or toy blocks the child
uses at this time to make something for mommy or daddy.

Assessing, Promoting, and Maintaining Optimal Cognitive Development

The preschooler's cognitive development is characterized
by egocentrism and animism. Preschoolers perceive the
world from their own viewpoint. If something happens,
such as the sun comes up, they perceive it occurred to
keep them warm. Preschool-age children focus on one
aspect of the situation rather than on all aspects. Their
reasoning appears to be illogical and a reflection of their
own limited viewpoint. "I got a thorn in my finger because
the rose bush didn't want me to pick the flower." Animism, or the attribution of life to inanimate objects, is a
normal response to everyday occurrences. The preschooler believes that everything has a cause and will
respond with "Why?" to each and every explanation.
"Why did Daddy go to work?" "To earn money." "Why

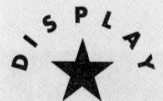

Behaviors Observed in Children Adjusting to the Arrival of a New Sibling

- Increasing attempts at gaining mother's and father's attention, whether the new infant is present in the same room or absent.
- Tendency to whine, fret, and cry when asked to do a task that is routinely carried out in a positive way.
- Increased requests for help in undressing, dressing, bathing, and self-care activities.
- Requests for help in getting ready for bed.
- Tendency to resist bedtime preparation; attempts at prolonging rituals preceding bedtime; getting out of bed.
- Tendency to suck thumb even though habit may have stopped.
- Clinging behaviors, such as pulling at mother's skirt or physically trying to direct her attention.
- Increased attempts at climbing into mother's lap or seeking affection.
- Increased use of "I can't" when asked to do something and more "why's."
- Increased use of "no" even after the stage of accentuated negative responses.
- Shyness with family members, friends, and sometimes playmates.
- Changes in eating patterns.
- Regression in toilet-training habits.
- Imitative behaviors with dolls that replicate parents behaviors with new infant.

- Increased display of nurturing behaviors when playing with dolls.
- Overt signs of trying to get physically closer to mother when she is engaged in care giving activities with the infant.
- Increase in spilling food.
- Tendency to revert to baby talk or jargon.
- Evidence of wanting to eat when the new infant is being fed.
- Outbursts of crying with tears when mother is observed to display overt signs of kissing, smiling at, laughing at, and talking baby talk with the new infant.
- General increase in dependency.
- Prolonging of time to complete a task.
- Unusual interest in playing with the new infant's toys.
- Attempts at sucking at the baby's bottle.
- Changes in play habits, toy preferences, attention span to toys, and reduced pleasure in playing alone.
- Increased requests for mother and father to play.
- Reference to self as "a baby" or "I'm little."
- Expressions of questions that imply the child's need for reassurance.
- Reduction of exploratory behaviors.

From Powell, M. (1981). Assessment and management of developmental changes and problems in children, *2nd Ed. St. Louis: C. V. Mosby.*

does he have to earn money?" "To buy food and clothes and pay the rent." "Why does he have to buy food and clothes and pay the rent?" "Because. . . ."

Through questioning why things are the way they are or why things happen, the preschooler learns. Although cognitive abilities are in part related to genetic endowment, the quality of the child's environment is an important factor in the development of potential abilities.

Parental Role

Throughout this section on promoting development of the preschool child, there are many recurring themes, such as the child needs opportunities to learn about the world and people; the child needs a variety of experiences; the child needs adults that will listen and answer questions; the child needs to learn specific ways of behaving appropriate to the society. In this sense, all areas of development can foster cognitive development and give the child a desire to learn. Parental enthusiasm for learning can be an extremely positive force in the child's developing attitude toward learning and school. Informally, parents can promote cognitive ability by answering questions, defining words, and conversing with the child about everyday experiences.

Parents can also help the child gain the basic knowledge necessary for school entry through everyday ex-

periences. This includes learning colors, numbers, and letters; learning opposites such as up and down, hot and cold; and learning days of the week and holidays.

Using songs, stories, and rhymes will help the child learn colors, numbers, and letters. Games such as identifying a color for the day ("today's color is yellow") reinforce learning in a fun way. Playing Simon-says promotes ability to follow directions and listen carefully. A calendar that has days of the week, weather, and activity patches can be a fun way to learn days, holidays, and eventually months. Calendars such as these can be purchased or made at home. Teaching the child their name, address, and phone number is a cognitive skill necessary not only for school but for the child's safety on a daily basis. Included in the teaching should be a discussion of how to deal with strangers and who is there to help you, including the policeman, teacher, or relative.

Child development experts[17,40] emphasize the need to allow the preschooler to learn through experiences and interaction in the environment. There is increasing concern that attempts to teach the preschooler using the methods appropriate for the older child, that is, teacher-directed learning, decreases the child's desire to learn. Young children learn from activity, exploring real objects, talking with people, and solving real problems such as how to balance a stack of blocks or how to negotiate a zipper. Young children learn from practical experiments

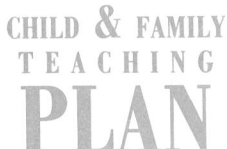

Sibling Rivalry in a 3-Year-Old Child

Assessment

Kathy is a 3-year-old child who has been coming to the clinic regularly since birth for well-child care. Her parents have had little difficulty over the past 3 years meeting her developmental needs and dealing with the common concerns related to nutrition, sleep, activity, and safety. Kathy now has a sibling, Tim, who is 4 weeks' old. Kathy's mother complains that she is having a great deal of difficulty with Kathy, who is being aggressive toward Tim. "She takes his rattle and pacifier away from him and throws them on the floor. She has hit him and gets angry and acts out every time I feed him or when I am giving him a bath. I know that this is sibling rivalry and we spent a lot of time with Kathy and talked about the arrival of a new sibling throughout my pregnancy. Right now I am at my wit's end with her behavior."

Mother is able to provide the following information: Kathy gets most upset when mother is feeding and bathing Tim: "She refuses to eat if I give her a meal to feed herself while I feed Tim." Kathy takes away Tim's pacifier when he is quietly sitting in his infant seat and mother is nearby looking at a magazine or watching television. Parents have tried a variety of methods to decrease Kathy's aggressive behavior; they state that none of these approaches work.

Further questioning reveals that, in fact, there are times when Kathy is loving toward Tim and may talk to him or give him his pacifier if it falls out of his mouth. Kathy's parents ask for help in finding ways to cope with this new behavior and help Kathy accept her new brother. Based on the nursing assessments, the nursing diagnosis, Parenting, Altered, is selected. The Teaching Plan is developed to address this problem.

Child and Family Objectives	Specific Content	Teaching Strategies
1. Accept the fact that sibling rivalry is normal.	1. Kathy's behavior is indicative of sibling rivalry; she can be assisted to cope with her new brother in positive ways. Preparation for the arrival of a new sibling does not assure an easy transition, especially for a child who has not had to share the attention of parents for 3 years.	1. Offer pamphlets, books on subject. Offer support to parents by verbalizing an understanding of how difficult it must be for them to see Kathy behave this way.
2. Help Kathy deal with the arrival of new sibling.	2. Kathy needs reassurance that her parents have not stopped loving her. Plan interventions to help Kathy deal with rivalry.	2. Involve parents actively in planning because they will be expected to implement the plan. Offer suggestions on how to reassure Kathy. Allow parents an opportunity to add to these suggestions based on their relationship with Kathy. For example; "Since Kathy gets so upset when you feed Tim while she is eating, can her mealtime be a time when you focus on her?" A parent may respond: "I could probably wait to feed her lunch when Tim finishes his feeding and is sleeping. Then we could have a picnic like we used to before Tim was born."

(Continued)

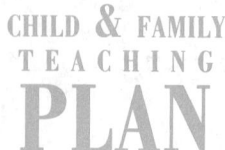

Sibling Rivalry in a 3-Year-Old Child (continued)

Child and Family Objectives	*Specific Content*	*Teaching Strategies*
3. Plan specific times for intervention.	3. Behavior modification requires consistency to be successful. Kathy will benefit most from a consistent pattern of "special time" so that she can look forward to it, depend on it, and be reminded by parents that it is planned when they are involved with the infant. Allow Kathy to determine what she would like to do during her "special time." Changing Kathy's behavior will take time and patience, and consistency is the most important factor in being successful.	3. Discuss and determine a time parents can spend focusing their attention on Kathy. Explain that this special time should be consistent. Assist parents in developing a plan to decrease Kathy's aggressive behavior toward Tim.
4. Develop a reward system.	4. Parental approval of behavior increases the chances that the behavior will be repeated. Minor acts of aggression that do not get parental response may cease more quickly if ignored. Behaviors that cannot be ignored, such as hitting, may require the use of a "when-then" contingency statement. "When you can treat Tim nicely, you can come back in the room with us."	4. Encourage parents to reward Kathy for any positive behavior toward her younger sibling. Tell parents to ignore vocalizations such as "I don't like him" or "Are you feeding him again?"
5. Plan for "time out."	5. If other steps are ineffective, parents can issue a warning: "If you don't leave Tim alone and play with your own toys, you are going to have a time out." Parents should choose in advance a place for time out. It should be a place away from positive reinforcement. There should be no toys and no interactions with parents but it should not be dark or frightening. Time out should be used each time Kathy acts aggressively toward Tim. After time out, parents should not discuss the incident further.	5. Use role play. Explain to parents that the initial use of behavior modification techniques may result in an increase in the undesired behavior as the child tests parents' limits. Other careproviders, including relatives and sitters should have an explanation of the approach parents are using and follow the same plan.
6. Continue to receive support from health care personnel.	6. Parents may need support, reassurance, or information as they attempt to implement the plan. Evaluation of progress allows for reinforcement of success and continued problem solving if difficulties arise.	6. Provide phone number of clinic for questions or concerns during implementation of the plan. Set up a follow-up appointment for 2 or 3 weeks to review progress and make necessary revisions of the plan.

(Continued)

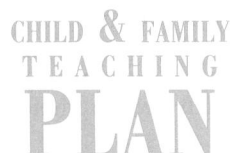

CHILD & FAMILY
T E A C H I N G
PLAN

Sibling Rivalry in a 3-Year-Old Child (continued)

Evaluation

- Parents state they understand sibling rivalry is normal.
- Parents state Kathy seems to be adapting to baby brother.
- Parents describe their initial plans and schedule they will use.
- Parents demonstrate their time-out technique.
- Parents express their feeling that the family is "growing closer."

such as trying a picture puzzle, making mistakes, and trying again, until they can say to themselves, "I did it!"[17]

Language Development

Speech during the early preschool years is egocentric and self-satisfying. There is a gradual transition to more socialized speaking, including requests, commands, questions, and answers. Vocabulary grows rapidly during these years, expanding the child's communication ability. A 2-year-old child has a vocabulary of about 300 words; this increases to 1000 words by the age of 3 years.

Listening is an important aspect of language development. A child learns language by listening to models they encounter.[14a] The egocentric preschooler may need assistance in developing listening skills.

Factors Affecting Language Development

The child's home environment, including socioeconomic status, influences language development. Children from a lower socioeconomic class have a smaller vocabulary than their middle-class peers. Children in the upper class have exposure to more language experiences through travel, exploration, and interactions with parents who themselves are experienced linguistically. A home environment that is warm and nurturing enhances language development. Families in which members have affectionate relationships in nurturing environments encourage language activities. Children who have exposure to toys, books, and other learning opportunities have varied language experiences. Parents who encourage language and correct speech foster development.[2a]

Parental Role

Parents can have a great deal of influence on the child's language development. Parents should be encouraged to gain the child's attention before speaking, repeat and rephase speech when conversing, as well as expand the child's short sentences.[41] For example, a parent can respond to "I play ball" with "Oh, you are playing ball outside in the yard?"

Parents can promote language skills by reading familiar stories to the child.[25] Parents can build a child's vocabulary by using words that may have been previously changed or deleted from the story because of the child's limited ability to understand and shorter attention span. Books that are illustrated help the child associate words with objects and actions they represent. Encouraging the child to talk about a drawing or to tell a story provides an opportunity for verbal expression and the development of complex sentence structure. Asking a child to "tell me about your picture" will encourage verbal expression.

The preschooler benefits from reinforcement to use language that is associated with common courtesy. The child should be encouraged to use "please" and "thank you" as well as wait his or her turn to speak in a group.

Groups of children can act out stories or play games that involve naming pictures or identifying colors. Most importantly, parents, nurses, and child care workers can facilitate language development by taking the time to converse with children and provide activities and projects that facilitate conversation before, during, and especially after participating in them.[21] Research has shown that day care programs can also be an effective means of language intervention for culturally and economically disadvantaged children.[29]

Nursing Implications

Cognitive and language development are an important part of the preschool years because each has an impact on school readiness and school performance.[21] Nurses must be aware of expected levels of development and assess children for normal patterns of development in each area. Talking directly to the child provides opportunities for assessment of language skills and indicates the nurse's desire to hear what the child has to say. Nurses can talk to parents about the relationship of development to school entry and offer suggestions for facilitating optimal language and cognitive development. Nurses should also discuss with parents that the child's reaction to school and learning is in part a reflection of parental beliefs in this area. Explain to parents that their enthusiasm for the child's growing knowledge and increasing skills will give the child positive feelings about self and a willingness and desire to try new experiences.

Preschool

Attending preschool can promote growth and development and expose children to peers from different backgrounds. A preschool provides supervision, meals, and activities that are directed at preparing the child for school entry.

Parents send their children to preschool for a variety of reasons. These include care for the child when parents work, opportunity for an only child to interact with agemates when there are few in the neighborhood, and the opportunity to learn skills prior to school entry.

Preschools can provide the child with many experiences that promote growth and development. Social development is fostered by learning to share the attention of adults and interact with agemates. Participating in preparing for and cleaning up after snack time, lunch time, and play time and in group activities promotes the development of social skills.

Cognitive development is fostered through playing group games, learning colors, and telling and listening to stories. The child must use language to communicate needs and has opportunities to talk about feelings, activities, and home. These activities are often the focus of preschool activities. Motor skills are refined through outdoor activities, running, jumping, climbing, and quiet activities such as drawing, cutting and pasting, and helping to serve snacks and lunch (Fig. 14-6). Attending preschool can help the child tolerate separation from parents and experience a more structured environment. In preschool the child is expected to focus attention on specific activities for increasing lengths of time, which may help the child in the first school experience.

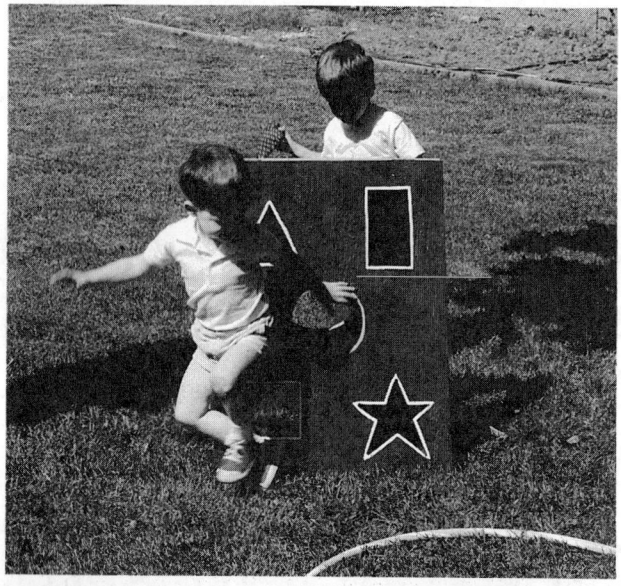

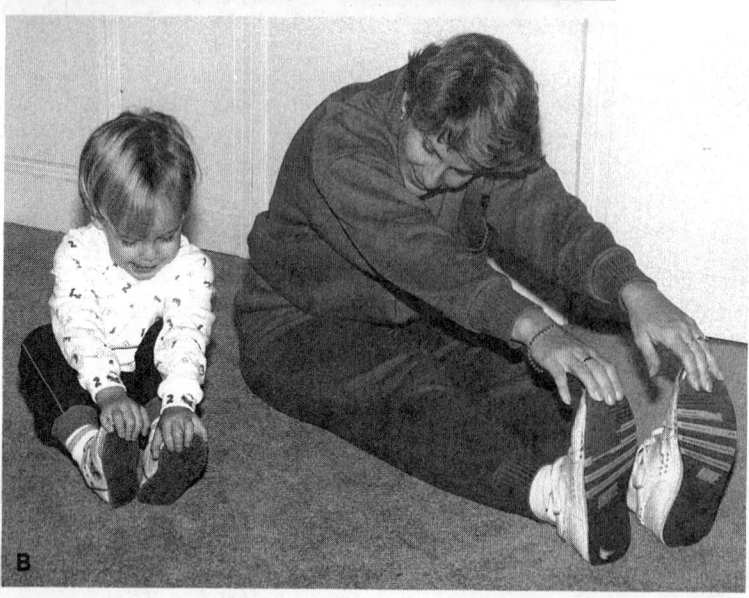

FIGURE 14-6

Physical activity should be encouraged. (**A**) Motor skills are refined through outdoor activities such as running, jumping, and climbing. (**B**) Preschoolers can be included in family exercise programs.

Not all preschools meet the needs of the developing child. Parents often seek guidance in selecting a preschool. Common concerns include determining an appropriate time to enroll the child and preparing the child for the new experience. Age is one variable that should be considered when deciding to begin preschool. Most preschools require that the child be 3 years old. Other factors that should be considered include the child's experience with separation, level of maturity, and ability to direct attention for short periods.

In assisting parents in choosing a preschool, the nurse can reinforce the child's natural desire to learn and encourage a setting where this is supported and nurtured. Parents can be encouraged to look for a school that has a variety of age-appropriate activities and learning experiences. Preschools where stories are read out loud and children are involved in indoor, outdoor, and dramatic play are optimal. The preschool "should be an outward extension of the home rather than a downward extension of the school."[17]

School Readiness

Determination of school readiness should begin in the preschool years. The early identification of a child who may experience difficulty with academic performance during the school years provides opportunity for intervention prior to school entry. Early intervention can decrease the potential for a child to enter school with a low self-esteem or lack of self-confidence.

The evaluation of a preschool child for school readiness should focus not on long-term potential but rather on the child's ability to succeed in the next phase of education. For example, the preschooler should be evaluated to determine whether he or she has the skills for kindergarten. The kindergarten child should be assessed for skills necessary for entry into first grade. The type of classroom setting the child is entering, that is, open or traditional, should also be considered in the evaluation. A comprehensive evaluation, including strengths and weaknesses of the child, will be necessary in planning an individual child's educational curriculum.

Preschool screening and assessment require much more than a preschool test. Assessment should include general health, physical development, neuromaturation, gross and fine motor skills, visual processing, spatial orientation–body awareness, auditory-language skills, sequential organization–memory, cognitive development, temperament, and school behavior.[16]

An interdisciplinary approach to assessment is optimal. Observations of a child by a variety of professionals, including preschool teachers, pediatricians, nurses, and others, provides a more reliable assessment. A child who has difficulty with one area of a readiness test given by a school system can be further evaluated by communication with the pediatrician, nurse, or preschool teacher to validate findings or determine the need for further assessment or repeat testing. Dworkin and Levine offer the following examples of observations and tasks that can be used in the assessment of a child entering school[16]:

- Increasing abilities during the preschool years (Table 14-11).
- Gross and fine motor skills (Table 14-12).
- Visual processing tasks (Table 14-12).
- Spatial orientation and body awareness skills (Table 14-12).
- Language function (Table 14-12).
- General areas of function (Table 14-13).

Assessing, Promoting, and Maintaining Optimal Activity Levels

The refinement of fine and gross motor skills during the preschool years prepare the child for entry into kinder-

TABLE 14-11
Examples of a Child's Increasing Abilities During the Preschool Years

Area of Function	2 Years	3 Years	4 Years	5 Years
Gross motor	Running Kicking a ball	Walking up stairs by alternating feet Pedalling a tricycle	Performing a standing broad jump	Skipping smoothly Balancing on one foot for 20 seconds
Fine motor	Turning pages of a book Holding a glass securely Building a tower of 6 blocks	Pouring from a pitcher Scribbling with a crayon Building a tower of 9 to 10 blocks	Buttoning clothes Lacing shoes	Brushing teeth Combing hair Washing face
Visual processing	Imitating a circular stroke while drawing	Copying a circle	Copying a cross Drawing a man with two parts	Copying a triangle Drawing a recognizable man
Auditory–Language	Using I, me, and you, although not necessarily correctly Verbalizing immediate experiences	Using an active vocabulary of 1000 words Speaking so strangers can understand	Engaging in long narratives	Speaking using adult sentence structure

From Dworkin, P., and Levine, M. (1980). The preschool child: Prediction and prescription. In A. Scheiner and I. Abroms (eds.), *The practical management of the developmentally disabled child*, (p. 346). St. Louis: C. V. Mosby.

TABLE 14-12
Examples of Skills and Tasks That May Be Used in Assessing the Preschooler for School Readiness

Task	Description	Observations
Gross and Fine Motor Skills		
Heel walking	The child is asked to walk across the room on his heels.	Does the child walk well on the heels for 2 min without faltering?
Standing on one foot	The child is asked to imitate the examiner; the child stands up; one foot is placed in the popliteal fossa of the other leg while the eyes are kept open for 15 seconds.	Is the child able to maintain the position without faltering more than once?
Tandem gait	The child is asked to walk in a straight line as if walking on a tightrope and to put his heel right in front of his toe each time.	Is the child able to walk well without faltering for 2 min?
Sequential finger opposition	The child tries to imitate the examiner; first, the thumb and forefinger are opposed, and then, one by one, the remaining fingers on the hand.	Does the child perform the task without more than one or two errors, or only minor difficulty getting started?
Pencil grasp and utilization	The child is asked to write his name on a blank piece of lined paper.	Does the child properly grip the pencil with the first three fingers of the hand? Is the grip fairly distal? Does he demonstrate a fist-like grasp?
Rhythm tapping	The examiner asks the child to imitate from memory a series of rhythm taps, such as two taps with the left and one with the right hand.	Is the child able to successfully imitate two of three sequences?
Visual Processing Tasks		
Copying figures	The child is asked to copy a series of figures. Examples are:	How accurate are the drawings from the standpoint of orientation, relative size of various parts, relative position of various parts, quality?
Block construction	The child is asked to construct, by direct imitation, some stairs made with six blocks, like so: The child is asked to construct from memory a three-block bridge, like so:	Does the child copy the staircase accurately? Is the child able to reproduce the bridge in 10 seconds?
Object span	Four items (key, pencil, penny, block) are placed before the child. The examiner points to each one in a certain order, and the child is asked to point to each in the same order after the examiner finishes.	This is a test of visual sequential memory. Is the child able to correctly repeat two or three sequences?
Matching figures	The child is asked to match identical figures on a card, like so:	Is the child able to correctly match letters within 10 seconds?
Body parts	The child is asked to point to his nose, then knee, then heel, then waist.	Is the child able to correctly identify three of four body parts?
Simple laterality	The child is asked to show his right hand, then his left foot, then his left hand, then his right foot.	This is not usually attained by preschool children. Does the child cross the midline with his responses?
Graphesthesia	The child is shown a card with each of the following: The child is asked to name each shape. While he views the cards, the examiner takes the child's hand behind his back and traces one of the shapes on the child's palm. The child is asked to point to the one the examiner has drawn.	Is the child able to correctly identify three shapes?
Stereognosis	Four shapes are put in front of the child while identical shapes are held by the examiner.	Is the child able to correctly identify three shapes?

(Continued)

TABLE 14-12
(Continued)

Task	Description	Observations
	One of each shape is placed in the child's hand, out of view, and he is asked to point to the identical shape in front of him.	
Language Skills		
Sound memory	The examiner presents to the child a series of phonemes, repeating each set twice. The child is asked to then repeat the set. Examples are ''laudy-tu-dum,'' ''above and below,'' ''behind and ahead,'' ''quack duck quack.''	Is the child able to repeat the sounds accurately with only one or two errors, requiring assistance only once or twice?
Sentence memory	Similar to sound memory, a series of sentences or phrases are read to the child, and the child is asked to repeat each one immediately, ''my big black dog,'' ''please pass the meat and peas,'' ''we had lots of fun playing at the park.''	Similar to sound memory.
Serial command	The child is asked by the examiner to do some things, but to wait until he has finished with all the instructions. He is asked to do exactly what he is told in the right order, ''I want you to put the pencil on the chair, and then open the door, and then come back here and give me a block, and sit down.''	Auditory sequential memory and patterned motor output are involved. Is the child able to perform the command without more than one mistake?
Object naming	The child is told, ''Bread and meat are good to eat. Tell me other things you can eat. Name as many as you can, as fast as you can.''	Is the child able to name six foods in 30 seconds?
Definitions	The child is asked to define words, such as ''What is a ball? . . . river? . . . street?''	Is the child able to define word in terms of use, shape, composition, or general category?

From Dworkin, P., and Levine, M. (1980). The preschool child: Prediction and prescription. In A. Scheiner and I. Abroms (eds.). *The practical management of the developmentally disabled child*, (pp. 347–349). St. Louis: C. V. Mosby.

garten. Prior to entry into kindergarten, the child must be able to attend to toileting, wash hands, button and unbutton clothing, and be able to put on a coat and hat. Coordination should be increasing, allowing the child to manipulate objects such as scissors and crayons or pencil. Each of these skills is a reflection of the maturation of the central nervous system. In addition to specific skill development, health benefits of physical activity is becoming an increasingly important concern starting in the early years.[2,42] Studies show that physical activity among children is decreasing.[34] Two thirds of preschool children were found to have inadequate levels of physical activity.[37] Preschool children were found to be inactive even in situations where they could choose their own activity level.[34] Child activity patterns were found to be related to parental activity patterns.[34]

Parental Role

Motor development is enhanced through a wide variety of opportunities that reflect increasing abilities. The preschooler needs opportunities to manipulate objects that require coordination. This can be done by allowing the child to hand-mix cake batter or cookie dough. Encouraging the child to button and unbutton shirt and trousers and manipulate puzzles also promotes development of fine motor skills. Total-body and hand-eye coordination can be enhanced by exercising to music, playing ball, or bowling with plastic pins. Preschoolers can practice early writing skills through opportunities to draw, copy, or write their names. One activity that can be fun for a group of children involves taping a long sheet of brown paper to the bottom of the play room wall the children can then use this to draw a picture of their own.

Vigorous physical activity and the use of large muscles should be encouraged (see Fig. 14-6A). Swings, jungle gyms, and pedal toys continue to be valuable in promoting the use of large muscles. The preschooler can learn to play games, such as hide-and-seek, tag, and relay races, that encourage running and promote an increased heart rate over time. Preschoolers may also be included in family exercise with parents by learning to do pull-ups, sit-ups, and jumping jacks (see Fig. 14-6B). When choosing a day care facility, parents can be encouraged to investigate the types of physical activities the child will be involved in.

Play and Development

Play during the preschool years is rich and varied and promotes development in all areas. Through play, preschool children gain increased control and coordination of their bodies, try on adult roles, learn to cooperate and share with peers, have an opportunity to express themselves creatively, and derive pleasure and a positive sense of self in their ability to master new skills. Several forms of play, including associative, cooperative, and sociodramatic play, are observable during the preschool years and reflect the preschooler's increasing social development.

In the early preschool years, parallel play predominates. Children play side by side but not together. In the latter part of the preschool years, children engage in more associative play, borrowing and loaning toys to each other but each child acting independently (Fig. 14-7A).

Cooperative play gradually emerges. Cooperative play includes the assigning of roles and discussion of

TABLE 14-13
Examples of Questions That May Be Asked of the Preschool Teacher to Survey Various Areas of Function

Area of Function	Sample Questions
Gross motor skills	Is the child always tripping and falling?
	Is the child clumsy and awkward?
	Does the child appear to have poor balance?
Fine motor skills	Is the child able to pour liquids into containers without spillage?
	Does the child have difficulty using scissors?
	Is the child's pencil or crayon grasp awkward?
	Is the child able to tie shoelaces?
	Is the child able to manipulate zippers and buttons?
Visual processing ability	Is the child able to match shapes or forms?
	Is the child able to differentiate larger from smaller?
	Is the child able to copy simple figures or letters?
	Is the child able to draw a circle? a cross? a square?
Language	Does the child often ask to have words repeated?
	Does the child have difficulty understanding what is being said?
	Is the child able to follow directions?
	Is the child able to answer questions about stories read to him?
	Is the child's speech often difficult to understand?
	Is the child's expressive vocabulary limited?
Spatial orientation—body awareness	Does the child often get lost in the school or playground?
	Does the child have difficulty orienting himself relative to surroundings?
Sequencing organization—memory	Does the child have difficulty remembering words to nursery rhymes or songs?
	Does the child seem to have poorly developed time concepts?
	Does the child have difficulty remembering the order of things?
Attention—activity	Is the child in constant motion?
	Is the child easily distracted?
	Does the child seem to "tune out?"
	Is the child very impulsive?
Social—emotional status	Is the child usually quiet and withdrawn? sad?
	Does the child get upset easily?
	Does the child appear to have little self-confidence?
	Is the child disliked or rejected by peers?

From Dworkin, P., and Levine, M. (1980). The preschool child: Prediction and prescription. In A. Scheiner and I. Abroms (eds.). *The practical management of the developmentally disabled child* (p. 352). St. Louis: C. V. Mosby.

activities—"I'll be the doctor, you be the patient, and I will give you a shot."

Dramatic play, or "let's pretend," is a frequent play activity in the preschool years. Dramatic play fosters learning about oneself and fosters identification with adults (Fig. 14-7B). Common themes include house, fireman, nurse, doctor, policeman, and prince and princess. The ability to use fantasy allows children to try on adult roles and feel in control of situations that have threatened or overwhelmed them, and provides them with the opportunity to relive an experience that gave them pleasure. Children like to dress up for dramatic play to look like the person they are trying to be (Fig. 14-7C). Household objects such as pots, pans, old clothes, and shoes help them play their parts.

Play also provides opportunities for mastering fine and gross motor skills. The preschooler can learn to ride a bicycle, climb a jungle gym, and lift and move objects. Opportunities to use scissors to cut and paste shapes and pictures, to draw with crayons, or to paint a picture promote fine motor skills. Preschool children like to use their skills to create things from materials such as popsicle sticks, clay, and construction paper. Quiet activities are also important such as listening to music, being read to, or just observing the surroundings.

Children begin to develop a self-concept through the mastery of skills and the learning experiences of their play activities. Play provides a feeling of pleasure and mastery of new skills, which helps children feel good about themselves.

Parental Role

Parents can make available materials for dramatic play, including the household items, adult clothes and shoes, and old baby items. Traditional toys such as dolls, trucks, baby carriage, doll house, and fire hat also encourage dramatic play and should be available to both boys and girls. Children should be allowed to choose their own roles and play activities. Changing roles such as being daddy, then being mommy, and then being baby give the child opportunities to try different roles.

Cognitive skills can be developed through puzzles, games for learning colors, books about nature, people, and events, and matching and sorting games. Parents can participate in these activities with the child.

Motor skills are enhanced by providing a ball, wagon, jungle gym, or tricycle that requires the use of large muscles and helps in the development of coordination.

In speaking with parents about play, emphasis should be placed on the child's need for a variety of stimulating play experiences in the home and at day care. In performing a developmental assessment, the nurse should make observations of children's play, play interactions with peers, and the play materials available to the child. The use of the HOME Tool (see Appendix) may be helpful in assessing the play environment.

Assessing, Promoting, and Maintaining Preschool Safety

The preschooler's cognitive abilities and language skills have an impact on safety issues. Unlike the toddler, the preschooler has a better understanding of what words such as "hot," "dangerous," "slippery," and "sharp"

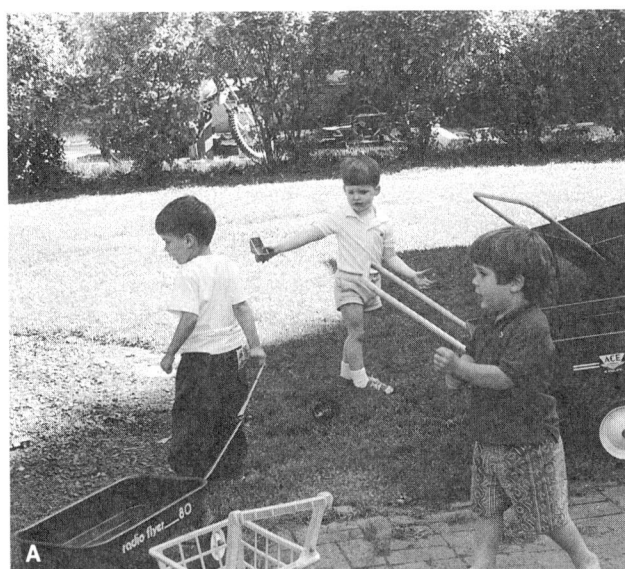
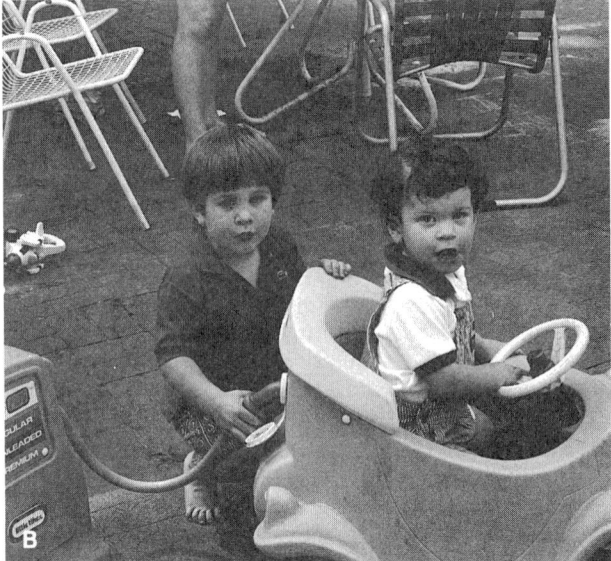
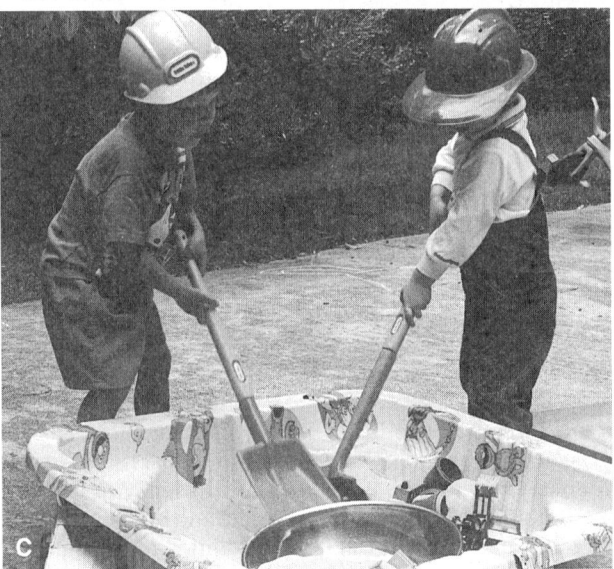

FIGURE 14-7
Children in the latter stages of preschool years engage in associative and dramatic play. (**A**) They may act independently.
(**B**) They identify with adults. (**C**) They enjoy dressing up to look like the people they are playing.

mean. Developmental issues that increase the risk for accidents in toddlers continue into the preschool years, but the preschooler is less likely to do such things as reach up to pull a pot off the stove. However, preschoolers are still curious, and accidents occur when they attempt to do something they are not capable of doing. For example, the toddler, when around an iron, may reflexively try to pull it down to investigate it, causing a serious burn. On the other hand, preschoolers will burn themselves by trying to iron doll clothes just as they saw a parent ironing because of lack of coordination or inability to handle the weight of the iron. Because the safety concerns of the preschool years are a reflection of the child's developmental progress, parents need to be aware of potential hazards that are related to new abilities and desires.[22]

The preschooler does not require the constant supervision the toddler needed. Preschoolers may play in one room while parents cook, wash, or clean in another room. They still need supervision, and parents should check on them periodically. Preschoolers are less likely to play with electrical outlets or put an electrical cord in their mouth, but they are more likely to try and plug in an appliance. Parents now need to explain to the child about the dangers of electricity and how to handle electrical equipment properly in an effort to assist the preschooler in learning about safety. The preschooler learns a great deal by observing parents. Parents who consider safety measures when doing daily activities teach their children without even realizing it. Putting equipment away when not in use can be an excellent example in teaching a child to put away toys. Turning off and unplugging electrical equipment before working on it, such as the toaster when a slice of bread is stuck inside, teaches the child safety through modeling.

As parents involve the child in activities of daily living such as cooking, parents can use the experience to teach safety in the kitchen. Parents should be reminded that the preschooler should not be allowed to cook unsupervised.

The preschooler is more prone to accidents outside the home, especially on playground equipment and bicycles. Playground equipment should be sturdy and placed over a soft surface such as a grassed area. Children should be shown how to use equipment and what will not be acceptable. Bicycles should be the right size for the child and kept in good condition. Bicycle safety should be the first step in teaching a child to ride a bicycle. Bicycle helmet use can be introduced early, and it should be worn consistently. Bicycles for older children and other outdoor wheel objects such as skateboards and roller skates are not appropriate for this age group and should be discouraged.

The preschooler's fascination with the roles adults play in society, such as policeman, fireman, nurse, construction worker, or cook, provides many opportunities to teach safety. The preschooler is able to learn what to do in a fire, the phone number of the fire department, and how to prevent fires. In addition to teaching the preschooler these things, taking him or her to a fire station reinforces the learning experience. Preschoolers need to learn their own address and phone number and appropriate responses to strangers.

Nursing Implications

The nurse should assess the preschooler's knowledge about safety and parents' beliefs about safety teaching. Parents can be told of the many valuable opportunities to teach and role model safety on a daily basis. The nurse can also reinforce teaching during the health care visit. For example, a child who tells the nurse that she has a new bike can be asked, "You are getting very grown up. What things do you need to remember so you won't get hurt when riding your new bike?" After the child gives a response, the nurse can add any additional information.

Assessing, Promoting, and Maintaining Health Perception and Health Management

Day Care

As increasing numbers of mothers enter the work force, issues related to day care need to be addressed by child health professionals. It is estimated that 50% to 75% of mothers work full- or part-time outside the home.[45] Although a great deal of research exists on the effects of day care on child development, there is still concern about the effects of day care on children.[45] It is important, however, to realize that the effect day care will have on an individual child depends on a number of factors related to the child as well as the day care setting. This is an area of concern that impacts children, parents, and society in general.[26]

Day care options fall into three general categories: in-home care, day care centers, and family day care. The parents' decision to use one type of care over another is largely based on cost and distance from home.[45] In addition to these considerations, many other factors need to be evaluated when choosing child care. Child care, regardless of setting, should provide for the child's physical needs, provide age-appropriate stimulation, promote cognitive language and motor development, and provide nurturing caregivers who have knowledge of child development.

Not all child care options meet the needs of an individual child and family. Parents often seek guidance in choosing child care from health professionals. Ultimately, parents must make the decision based on the needs of the child and family. The nurse can assist in this process by offering guidelines for parents as they evaluate alternatives (see the Day Care Checklist). Parents need to know that evaluating and choosing child care take time and patience. If parents make a decision hastily without adequate information, they may not feel comfortable with the choice they make.

Parents should first investigate the philosophy and purpose of the child care center or family day care. If in-home care is chosen, parents should talk to perspective care providers about their philosophy of child care. By comparing the philosophy with personal expectations, parents can narrow their choices. Once an environment is found that is philosophically what parents are seeking, a visit should be planned so that parents can observe the day care when in session. Parents should note the indoor and outdoor facilities and the types of toys and play activities available. Parents should observe if these toys and activities are safe and age appropriate. Is the supervision adequate and the adults caring and responsive to the specific needs of individual children? Talking to other parents who use the day care can also offer insight.

Other issues that should be discussed are the center's or individual caregiver's philosophy about discipline and how misbehavior is handled. What types of meals are offered, and do they meet the nutritional needs of the child? In addition to asking about these issues, parents can make observations while at the center or home. Because children have different needs at different ages, parents may find it helpful to consider what they expect from child care prior to evaluating different alternatives.

Because the incidence of viral infections is increased among children attending day care, parents need to observe for hygienic measures taken by care providers. Do care providers wash their hands after changing a diaper, assisting a child with toileting, or wiping a child's nose? Are toys and equipment washed regularly at least two to three times a week? What are the policies related to health concerns? When does a child have to stay home, and how are emergencies handled?

Once a day care has been chosen, parents should prepare the child in advance for the new experience, beginning with a discussion that emphasizes the pleasant aspects. The child should be shown the center and visit with parents present. Leaving the child for a few hours initially; gradually building up to a full day may decrease anxiety. Some children also benefit by having something from home with them. Parents should share with the care providers the child's rituals in eating, toileting, and napping as well as some details of the home environment, such as siblings and pets.

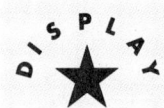

A Day Care Checklist for Parents

This checklist is designed to help you decide what things about a day care arrangement are most important to you and your family. It can also help you make sure your child's arrangement offers the things you believe are important. Read through the checklist and circle those items you want the arrangement to provide. Then, when you talk to a possible caregiver or visit a home or center, decide whether the arrangement offers those things. Just check "yes" or "no." Use the checked-off list to help you make a decision. Remember, this checklist tries to be as complete as possible. Not everything will apply to your family's situation. Look at the headlines in the lefthand column to see what you should read and what you can skip.

DOES YOUR CHILD'S CAREGIVER:

	Yes	No
For All Children		
Appear to be warm and friendly?	_____	_____
Seem calm and gentle?	_____	_____
Seem to have a sense of humor?	_____	_____
Seem to be someone with whom you can develop a relaxed, sharing relationsip?	_____	_____
Seem to be someone your child will enjoy being with?	_____	_____
Seem to feel good about herself and her job?	_____	_____
Have childbearing attitudes and methods that are similar to your own?	_____	_____
Treat each child as a special person?	_____	_____
Understand what children can and want to do at different stages of growth?	_____	_____
Have the right materials and equipment on hand to help them learn and grow mentally and physically?	_____	_____
Patiently help children solve their problems?	_____	_____
Provide activities that encourage children to think things through?	_____	_____
Encourage good health habits, such as washing hands before eating?	_____	_____
Talk to the children and encourage them to express themselves through words?	_____	_____
Encourage children to express themselves in creative ways?	_____	_____
Have art and music supplies suited to the ages of all children in care?	_____	_____
Seem to have enough time to look after all the children in her care?	_____	_____
Help your child to know, accept, and feel good about him or herself?	_____	_____
Help your child become independent in ways you approve?	_____	_____
Help your child learn to get along with and to respect other people, no matter what their backgrounds are?	_____	_____
Provide a routine and rules the children can understand and follow?	_____	_____
Accept and respect your family's cultural values?	_____	_____
Take time to discuss your child with you regularly?	_____	_____
Have previous experience or training in working with children?	_____	_____
Have a yearly physical exam and TB test?	_____	_____
And If You Have an Infant or Toddler (Birth to Age 3)	Yes	No
Seem to enjoy cuddling your baby?	_____	_____
Care for your baby's physical needs such as feeding and diapering?	_____	_____
Spend time holding, playing with, talking to your baby?	_____	_____
Provide stimulation by pointing out things to look at, touch, and listen to?	_____	_____
Provide care you can count on so your baby can learn to trust her and feel important?	_____	_____
Cooperate with your efforts to toilet train your toddler?	_____	_____
"Child proof" the setting so your toddler can crawl or walk safely and freely?	_____	_____
Realize that toddlers want to do things for themselves and help your child to learn to feed and dress him or herself, go to the bathroom, and pick up his or her own toys?	_____	_____
Help your child learn the language by talking with him or her, naming things, reading aloud, describing what she is doing, and responding to your child's words?	_____	_____
And If Your Child is a Preschooler (Aged 3 to 5 or 6)	Yes	No
Plan many different activities for your child?	_____	_____
Join in activities herself?	_____	_____
Set consistent limits which help your child gradually learn to make his or her own choices?	_____	_____

(Continued)

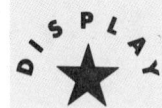

A Day Care Checklist for Parents (continued)

Recognize the value of play and encourage your child to be creative and use his or her imagination?

Help your child feel good about him or herself by being attentive, patient, positive, warm, and accepting?

Allow your child to do things for him or herself because she understands children can learn from their mistakes?

Help your child increase his or her vocabulary by talking with him or her, reading aloud, and answering questions?

	Yes	No
And If Your Child is School Age (Aged 6 to 14)		
Give your child supervision and security but also understand his or her growing need for independence?		
Set reasonable and consistent limits?		
At the same time, allow your child to make choices and gradually take responsibility?		
Understand the conflict and confusion that growing children sometimes feel?		
Help your child follow through on projects, help with homework, and suggest interesting things to do?		
Listen to your child's problems and experiences?		
Respect your child when he or she expresses new ideas, values, or opinions?		
Cooperate with you to set clear limits and expectations about behavior?		
Understand the conflicts and confusion older school-age children feel about sex, identity, and pressure to conform?		
Provide your child with a good adult image to admire and copy?		

DOES THE DAY CARE HOME OR CENTER HAVE . . .

	Yes	No
For All Children		
An up-to-date license, if one is required?		
A clean and comfortable look?		
Enough space indoors and out so all the children can move freely and safely?		
Enough caregivers to give attention to all of the children in care?		
Enough furniture, play things, and other equipment for all the children in care?		
Equipment that is safe and in good repair?		
Equipment and materials that are suitable for the ages of the children in care?		
Enough room and cots and cribs so the children can take naps?		
Enough clean bathrooms for all the children in care?		
Safety caps on electrical outlets?		
A safe place to store medicines, household cleansers, poisons, matches, sharp instruments, and other dangerous items?		
An alternate exit in case of fire?		
A safety plan to follow in emergencies?		
An outdoor play area that is safe, fenced, and free of litter?		
Enough heat, light, and ventilation?		
Nutritious meals and snacks made with the kinds of food you want your child to eat?		
A separate place to care for sick children where they can be watched?		
A first aid kit?		
Fire extinguishers?		
Smoke detectors?		
Covered radiators and protected heaters?		
Strong screens or bars on windows above the first floor?		
And If You Have an Infant or Toddler (Birth to Age 3)	Yes	No
Gates at tops and bottoms of stairs?		
A potty chair or special toilet seat in the bathroom?		
A clean and safe place to change diapers?		
Cribs with firm mattresses covered in heavy plastic?		
Separate crib sheets for each baby in care?		

(Continued)

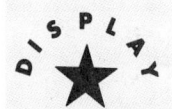

A Day Care Checklist for Parents (continued)

	Yes	No
And If Your Child Is A Preschooler (Aged 3 to 5 or 6)	Yes	No
A stepstool in the bathroom so your preschooler can reach the sink and toilet?		
And If Your Child Is School Age (Aged 6 to 14)	Yes	No
A quiet place to do homework?		
Places to store personal belongings?		

ARE THERE OPPORTUNITIES . . .

	Yes	No
For All Children	Yes	No
To play quietly and actively, indoors and out?		
To play alone at times and with friends at other times?		
To follow a schedule that meets young children's need for routine but that is flexible enough to meet the needs of each child?		
To use materials and equipment that help children learn new physical skills and control and exercise their muscles?		
To learn to get along, to share, and to respect themselves and others?		
To learn about their own and others' cultures through art, music, books, songs, games, and other activities?		
To speak both English and their family's native language?		
To watch special programs on television that have been approved by you?		
And If You Have An Infant or Toddler (Birth to Age 3)	Yes	No
To crawl and explore safely?		
To play with objects and toys that help infants to develop their senses of touch, sight, and hearing (for example, mobiles, mirrors, cradle gyms, crib toys, rattles, things to squeeze and roll, pots and pans, nesting cups, different sizes boxes)?		
To take part in a variety of activities that are suited to toddlers' short attention spans (for example, puzzles, cars, books, outdoor play equipment for active play, modeling clay, clocks, boxes, containers, for creative play)?		
And If Your Child Is A Preschooler (Aged 3 to 5 or 6)	Yes	No
To play with many different toys and equipment that enable preschoolers to use their imaginations (for example, books, musical instruments, costumes)?		
To choose their own activities, for at least part of the day?		
To visit nearby places of interest, such as the park, the library, the fire house, a museum?		
And If Your Child Is School Age (Aged 6 to 14)	Yes	No
To practice their skills (for example, sports equipment, musical instruments, drama activities, craft projects)?		
To be with their own friends after school?		
To do homework?		
To use a variety of materials and equipment, including: art materials, table games, sports equipment, books, films, and records?		
To use community facilities such as a baseball field, a swimming pool, a recreation center?		

From A parent's guide to day care. *(1980). U.S. Department of Health and Human Services Administration for Children, Young, and Family Day Care Division. DHHS Pub. #(OHDS) 80-30254.*

Health Care

During the preschool years health visits become less frequent, and an otherwise healthy child may be seen only once a year. Health visits include serial heights, weights, blood pressure, and physical assessment. The child now should have routine vision and hearing screening during each visit. There continues to be some controversy as to the effectiveness of hearing and vision screening in this age group.[43] However, the potential benefits of early screening and early detection of any actual or potential problem indicate the need for early and regular screening. Researchers[10] have found that young children who are afraid of the equipment have more accurate results if they first have time to familiarize themselves with the equipment.

The health visit should also include a review of the child's nutrition; elimination patterns; sleep patterns; social development; adaptation to preschool or kindergarten; cognitive, language, and motor skills; and parental concerns related to all or any of these areas. Because the frequency of visits has decreased, it is especially important for the nurse to talk with parents about common concerns that may arise during this stage of development. It may be helpful for the nurse to offer anticipatory guidance in each area rather than simply to address concerns identified by parents (see other sections for common concerns related to development). Many states require a second measles injection before school admission.

Dental Care

The preschooler should now be seeing the dentist every 6 months for routine examination and cleaning. The preschooler can be expected to maintain personal oral hygiene but continues to require reminding and review of proper brushing techniques. In areas where the water is not fluorinated, supplements should continue (see Table 12-2 in Chap. 12).

Thumb Sucking

Parents may express concern about continued thumb-sucking behavior in the preschool years. This behavior may cause concern that the teeth will be permanently displaced forward.

Parents should be informed that it is not abnormal for a child to thumb suck until the age of 3 years. After this age, further assessment is required to determine the frequency of the behavior, the relationship of thumb sucking to other activities, and what parents have tried to decrease the behavior. Some children may have an increase in this behavior with the birth of a sibling, a recent illness, increased amount of time separated from parents, or problems within the family. In these instances the nurse can recommend that the parents spend some additional time with the child. Parents can be instructed to remove the child's thumb or fingers from the mouth after the child is asleep. Parents should be discouraged from constantly telling the child to remove the thumb or removing it themselves. Products on the market that have an unpleasant taste and are meant to be used on the thumb to discourage thumb sucking should be avoided, especially if the thumb sucking is related to emotional problems, because the use of these products will only serve to exacerbate the problem. Encouraging parents to consult their dentist about thumb sucking can also serve to decrease anxiety. Dentists can provide the child with a special mouth appliance to wear to decrease thumb pressure on the front teeth. Parents benefit from reassurance that permanent damage will not occur if the behavior is given up by the age of 6 years.[13]

A child who is using thumb sucking as a coping mechanism to deal with an emotional conflict such as parental death, divorce, or separation needs more supportive responses from parents rather than punishment. The child may perceive parental attempts to stop thumb sucking as punishment.

Common Childhood Diseases

Most parents are concerned with common childhood diseases. Chicken pox, or varicella, is an excellent example of a common and generally mild disease.[14] The

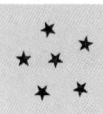

Ideas for Nursing Research

The nurse during the preschooler years has an opportunity to explore positive health promotion activities that become the groundwork for healthy living throughout childhood and beyond. The following areas need to be explored:

- Relationship between the preschooler's exposure to a variety of experiences and school readiness.
- Relationship between involvement of preschoolers in food purchasing and preparation and the preschooler's eating patterns.
- Relationship between planned preschooler exercise class and later exercise as a health promotion behavior.

pathology of many viral childhood diseases is covered in detail in Chapter 9. The major role of the nurse is in assisting parents in identifying the disease, protecting other children in the family when possible, and managing the symptoms associated with the disease. The antiviral drug, acyclovir, is now being used with children 2 to 12 years of age to reduce the effects of chicken pox.

Summary

The preschool years can be exciting years for the child and parents. The newfound independence in activities of daily living, the rapid development of language skills, and the insatiable curiosity and desire to learn provide the foundation for optimal development of the child. The preschool child is receptive to learning about health promotion, including safety, nutrition, exercise, and self-responsibility. Everyday experiences can provide the child with valuable learning experiences. The willingness of parents and other adults to answer questions and communicate with the preschooler assists in the development of effective communication skills that will be valuable throughout childhood and adolescence.

Nurses are in an optimal position to foster healthy development of preschoolers and parent-child relationships during the preschool years. By using the nursing process, the nurse can reinforce positive aspects of developmental progress, provide parents with information to support their efforts in promoting development, and assist parents in identifying and dealing with common concerns. The nurse can also become involved directly with preschoolers not only during the health visit but through community programs such as health fairs, preschool programs, and church activities.

References

1. American Academy of Pediatrics Policy Statement. (1984). Children, adolescents and television. *Pediatrics, 74,* 114.

2. American Academy of Pediatrics. (1976). Fitness in preschool children. *Pediatrics, 58*(1), 88–89.

2a. Ashburn, S., Schuster, C., Grimm, W., & Goff, S. (1992). Language development during childhood. In Schuster, C., & Ashburn, S. (Eds.). *The processes of human development: A holistic life span approach.* (3rd ed.). Philadelphia: J. B. Lippincott.

3. Beltramini, A., & Hertzig, M. (1983). Sleep and bedtime behavior of preschool aged children. *Pediatrics, 71*(2), 153–158.

4. Berkowitz, L. (1974). Control of aggression. In B. Caldwell & H. Ricciuti (Eds.). *Review of child development research* (Vol. 3). Chicago: University of Chicago Press.

5. Birch, L. (1979). Dimensions of preschool children's food preferences. *Journal of Nutrition Education, 11,* 77–80.

6. Birch, L. (1980). Effects of peer models' food choices and eating behaviors on preschooler's food preferences. *Child Development, 51,* 489–496.

7. Birch, L., Birch, D., Marlin, D., & Kramer, L. (1982). Effects of instrumental consumption on children's food preference. *Appetite, 3,* 125–134.

8. Birch, L., Zimmerman, S., & Hind, H. (1980). The influence of social-affective context on the formation of children's food preferences. *Child Development, 51,* 856–861.

9. Brazelton, T. B. (1973). Is enuresis preventable? In I. Koluin, R. MacKeith, & S. Meadows (Eds.). *Bladder control and enuresis.* London: Heinemann.

10. Brown, M., & Collar, M. (1982). Effects of prior preparation on the preschooler's vision and hearing screening. *American Journal of Maternal Child Health, 7,* 323.

11. Butler, R. (1987). Nocturnal enuresis. In *Psychological perspectives.* Bristol: Wright.

12. Christmanson, L., & Hisper, H. (1982). Parent behaviors related to bedwetting and toilet training as etiological factors in primary enuresis. *Scandinavian Journal of Behavior Therapy 11,* 29–37.

13. Curson, M. (1974). Dental implications of thumb sucking. *Pediatrics, 54,* 196.

14. Dershewitz, R. (Ed.). (1988). *Ambulatory pediatric care.* Philadelphia: J.B. Lippincott.

14a. Dumtsch, J. (1988). Recognizing language development and delay in early childhood. *Young Children, 42,* 16–24.

15. Dworkin, P. (1988). The preschool child: Developmental themes and clinical issues. *Current Problems in Pediatrics, 18,* 79–134.

16. Dworkin, P., & Levine, M. (1980). The preschool child: Prediction and prescription. In A. Scheiner & I. Abroms (Eds.). *The practical management of the developmentally disabled child.* St. Louis: C.V. Mosby.

17. Elkind, D. (1987). Superbaby syndrome can lead to elementary school burnout. *Young Children, 42,* 14.

18. Erikson, E. (1963). *Childhood and society.* New York: W.W. Norton.

19. Ferber, R. (1986). *Solve your child's sleep problems.* New York: Simon and Schuster.

20. Gallo, A. (1979). Early childhood masturbation: A developmental approach. *Pediatric Nursing, 5,* 47–49.

21. Garrard, K. (1987). Helping young children develop mature speech patterns. *Young Children, 42,* 16–21.

22. Greensher, J., & Mofenson, H. (1985). Injuries at play. *Pediatric Clinics of North America, 32,* 127.

23. Guilleminault, C. (Ed.). (1987). *Sleep and its disorders in children.* New York: Raven Press.

24. Heagarty, M., Glass, G., & King, H. (1974). Sex and the preschool child. *American Journal of Nursing, 74*(8), 1479–1482.

25. Joels, R. (1987). Picture books that bring comprehension to life. *Childhood Education, 63,* 362–365.

26. Lerner, J., & Galambos, N. (1991). Employed mothers and their children. New York: Garland Publishers.

27. Lowenberg, M. (1989). Development of food patterns in young children. In P. Pipes (Ed.). *Nutrition in infancy and childhood* (4th ed.). St. Louis: Times Mirror/Mosby.

28. Maccoby, E., & Martin, J. (1983). Socialization in the context of the family: Parent-child interaction. In Mussen, P. H. (Ed.). *Handbook of Child Psychology: Socialization, personality, and social development* (Vol. 4). New York: John Wiley.

29. McCortney, K., & Scarr, S. (1984). Daycare as language intervention. *First Language, 5,* 75–77.

30. Morrison, R. (1978). Self-esteem, need for approval and self estimates of academic performance. *Psychological Reports, 43,* 503–507.

31. Owens, K. (1987). *The world of the child.* New York: Holt, Rinehart and Winston.

32. Pipes, P. (1989). *Nutrition in infancy and childhood* (4th ed.). St. Louis: Times Mirror/Mosby.

33. Powell, M. (1981). *Assessment and management of developmental changes and problems in children* (2nd ed.). St. Louis: C.V. Mosby.

34. Sallis, J. (1988). Family variables and physical activity in preschool children. *Journal of Developmental and Behavioral Pediatrics, 9,* 57–61.

35. Sarafino, E. (1986). *The fears of childhood: A guide to recognizing and reducing fearful states in children.* New York: Human Sciences Press.

36. Sarafino, E., & Armstrong, J. (1986). *Child and adolescent development.* St Paul: West Publishing.

37. Saris, W., Binkhorst, R., & Cramwinckel, A. (1980). The relationship between working performance, daily physical activity, fatness, blood lipids, and nutrition in school children. In K. Berg & B. Ericksson (Eds.). *Children and exercise.* (Vol. 4, pp. 166–174). Baltimore: University Park Press.

38. Satter, E. (1987). *How to get your kid to eat . . . but not too much.* Palo Alto, CA: Bull.

39. Satterfield, S. (1975). Common sexual problems of children and adolescents. *Pediatric Clinics of North America, 22*(3), 643–652.

40. Sava, S. (1987). Development no academics. *Young Children, 42,* 15.

41. Schachter, F., & Strage, A. (1982). Adults' talk and children's language development. In Moore, S., Moore, G., & Cooper, C. R. (Eds.). *The young child: Reviews of research* (Vol. 3). Washington, DC: National Association for the Education of Young Children.

42. Shephard, R. (1984). Physical activity and child health. *Sports Medicine, 1,* 205–233.

43. Sullivan, L. (1988). How effective is preschool vision, hearing, and developmental screening? *Pediatric Nursing, 14,* 181.

44. Verhulst, F. C., Van Der Lee, J. H., Akkerhuis, G. W., Sanders-Woudstra, J. A., Timmer, F. C., & Donkhorst, I. D. (1985). The presence of nocturnal enuresis: Do DSM III criteria need to be changed? *Journal of Child Psychology and Psychiatry, 26,* 989–993.

45. Zigler, E., & Hall, N. (1988). Daycare and its effect on children: An overview for pediatric health professionals. *Developmental and Behavioral Pediatrics, 9*(1), 38–45.

46. Zuckerman, D., & Zuckerman, M. (1985). Television's impact on children. *Pediatrics, 75*(2), 233–240.

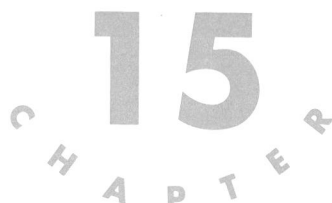

15

CHAPTER

Health Assessment, Promotion, and Maintenance for School-Age Children

BEHAVIORAL OBJECTIVES

Describe typical patterns of school-age children's development related to nutrition, elimination, sleep, exercise, school, and peers.

Identify needs for nursing assessment during the school years.

Consider the role of school on the development of the school-age child.

Discuss teaching needs of the school-age child related to the development of healthy lifestyle patterns.

Describe the role of the nurse in primary, secondary, and tertiary prevention.

The school years, or middle childhood, refers to children between the ages of 6 and 12 years. The school years tend to be the healthiest years in the life cycle and "health issues are best defined in the context of the developmental tasks of this period."[45] The development of lifestyle patterns is a major focus of concern during the school years. It is during the school years that children develop patterns of behavior that can impact on health throughout the life cycle. The school years bring new challenges for children, parents, and child health professionals. A major focus of the school years is on formal learning. The child will spend a significant amount of time in school. In addition to educational goals, school can influence all aspects of a child's development. School provides opportunities to develop a sense of industry and to develop social skills. School provides experience with developing new relationships with peers as well as teachers and other adults. The child is exposed to new ideas, new experiences, and, to a limited extent, children from varying cultural and socioeconomic backgrounds. The development of healthy lifestyle patterns is an important part of education both in school and in the community. The school years are an ideal time for the child health nurse to focus on health promotion through health assessment, health teaching, and direct intervention in assisting school-age children to become responsible for promoting their own health.

Nurses working in primary care and acute care settings will have opportunities to work with school-age children. However, most health promotion education will be done in the school and community setting. Child health nurses working with school-age children need to be in the community and need to understand the developmental goals of the school years.

Developmental goals during the school years include the following:

- Maintenance of optimal physical growth through nutrition and exercise.
- Development of a sense of industry.
- Development of relationships outside the home with peers, teachers, and other adults.
- Development of new cognitive and social skills in the classroom setting.
- Development of a positive self-concept.
- Identification of the moral standards of the family and society.
- Incorporation of safety measures in daily activities.
- Development of lifestyle patterns that can promote health throughout the life cycle.
- Active participation in health promotion activities.

Parents and other adults, including teachers, nurses, and youth workers, have many opportunities during the school years to promote successful attainment of the developmental tasks of the child. Parents and other adults have a significant impact on the child's physical growth, self-esteem, and cognitive, moral, and social development. Additionally, parents and other adults can assist the school-age child in learning preventive safety measures related to common activities as well as assisting the child to be an active participant in health promotion activities.

Parental goals during the school years include the following:

- Promoting physical growth through provision of optimal nutrition.
- Fostering the development of a sense of industry.
- Encouraging peership and participation in peer group activities.
- Encouraging and supporting school activities.
- Discussing and modeling moral standards of the culture.
- Fostering the development of a positive self-concept.
- Teaching safety measures related to daily activities.
- Fostering the development of lifestyle patterns that form the basis for health throughout the life cycle.
- Fostering the development of health promotion behaviors.

Assessing, Promoting, and Maintaining Optimal Nutrition of School-Age Children

Nutrition continues to be a major focus of health promotion during the school years. In the early school years the child has a steady rate of growth and, subsequently, increased appetite and intake of food.[5,38] Nutrient re-

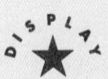

Developmental Nutritional Profile of the School-Age Child

- Growth is steady.
- Usually accepts family food patterns.
- Desires companionship at dining.
- Desires after-school snacks.

Adapted from Kennedy-Caldwell, C., and Caldwell, M. (1986). Pediatric Enteral Nutrition. In Rombeau, J., Caldwell, M. (Ed.). Parenteral nutrition: Clinical nutrition (Vol II.). Philadelphia: Saunders, 434–479.

quirements (see Chap. 8) should be met with foods of high nutrient density. Inadequate nutrition during the school years can result in decreased attention span, irritability, lack of physical energy, and poor growth.[38] Poor nutrition habits may precipitate long-range problems, including obesity, hypertension, and atherosclerosis.[17] See the accompanying display for a developmental nutritional profile.

Obesity among school-age children is a growing concern. Nationwide surveys demonstrate that obesity rose by 54% among children aged 6 to 11 years between the mid 1960s and late 1970s.[25] Obese children are at greater risk for hypertension, psychosocial dysfunction, respiratory disease, diabetes, and some orthopedic conditions[25] (see Chap. 56 for discussion of obesity).

The school-age child is an active child who is more independent of the family and spends more time with peers than the younger child. The many activities in which school-age children become involved can interfere with regular mealtimes. Rushing to school, they miss breakfast or, anxious to get into the playground, they rush through lunch. After school they are hungry and consume snacks that may or may not provide the nutrients they need and may also interfere with dinner appetites. The potential for dietary problems during the school years include (1) small, poorly chosen, or omitted breakfasts; (2) inadequate lunches; (3) food choices being left to the child without adult guidance; (4) failure to eat enough foods from each food group; and (5) expenditure of school lunch money on foods such as candy, chips, and soft drinks.[7]

In most states the goals of school lunch programs are to meet the nutritional needs of children by providing nutritionally adequate and acceptable meals at a reasonable price and to reinforce health and nutrition education by allowing students to practice food behaviors consistent with classroom instruction.[22]

Aware of the importance of nutrition in children, the U.S. government subsidizes the National School Lunch Program. School lunches are served to 60% of children in U.S. public schools and account for 25% to 33% of total daily nutrition.[36] Students are required to take only three of five lunch components: milk, vegetables, protein, fruit, and bread.[20] A variety of foods that are offered within each food group encourages a child to take the full meal.[22] School breakfast programs are also available on a smaller

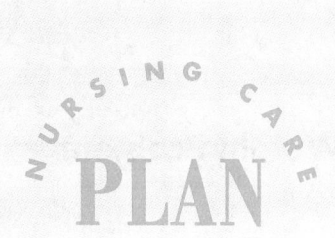

A 9-Year-Old Child With a Weight Problem

Assessment

Case Study Description

Peter is 9 years old and is having his annual well-care visit. He has had no health problems during his childhood. He lives with his parents and one brother aged 6. Both his parents appear obese, and Peter also looks as though he may be overweight. His mother describes him as being inactive and always snacking. Peter tells the nurse that he does not want to be fat but he is hungry all of the time.

Assessment Data

Peter weighs 92 lb and is at greater than 95% for weight. He is 4'6" tall, placing him in the 40th percentile for height. Twenty-four-hour recall of food intake includes:
- Breakfast—waffles, syrup, and butter; chocolate-covered donut; orange juice.
- Morning snack during recess—chocolate cupcake.
- Lunch—2 slices of pizza; cake; ½ carton of milk.
- After-school snack—½ dozen cookies; small bag potato chips; soda.
- Dinner—Cheeseburger, french fries; soda; apple pie.
- Evening—3 more cookies; another bag of chips; soda.

Activity includes the following. Peter plays games during recess, such as tag, dodge ball, and cops and robbers. After school, he hangs out with friends, plays video games, and watches TV. After dinner, he does homework and watches TV or plays video games. In the morning, he does his paper route but his mother drives him. Mother states, "He complains of being tired if he does the paper route on his bike."

Nursing Diagnosis	*Intervention*	*Rationale*
1. Nutrition, altered: high risk for more than body requirements.	Ask Peter what he thinks his ideal weight should be.	It is important to determine what Peter's goals are related to weight.
Supporting Data: • Diet not balanced • Diet contains many foods of minimal nutritional value and high in fat, sugar, and sodium • Family history of obesity • Sedentary lifestyle	Have Peter describe what he believes causes obesity.	By evaluating Peter's knowledge the nurse can correct misinformation and provide factual information.
	Review with Peter and his parents what factors predispose a person to weight gain. Include: • dietary factors • heredity factors • environmental factors • physiologic factors • psychological factors	It is important for Peter and his family to understand the many variables associated with obesity.
	Have Peter look at his 24-hour diet history and identify the foods that: • are good for him • are not good for him and what other foods he likes could serve as alternatives.	This will help the nurse evaluate Peter's knowledge as well as demonstrate to Peter that many of the foods are not good for him.
	Review basic food groups and ask Peter to identify which ones were missing from his 24-hour dietary intake.	School-age children learn from active participation.

(Continued)

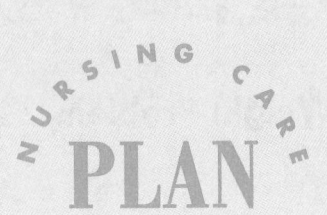

A 9-Year-Old Child With a Weight Problem
(continued)

Nursing Diagnosis	Intervention	Rationale
	Ask Peter to name some foods he likes that are part of the food groups missing from his diet.	This involves Peter in the planning process and provides the nurse with information on likes and dislikes.
	Assist Peter's mother in making environmental changes. • Eliminate or decrease non-nutritious foods from family food supply, including cookies, potato chips, cake. • Make nutritious foods available that require minimal preparation for Peter (i.e., cut up fruits, cut up raw vegetables, juice).	Peter's attempts to change his diet depends on support from parents and availability of alternative foods.
	Set up an appointment for parents with a dietitian who can assist them in planning low calorie, nutritious meals.	Parents may need assistance in planning easy to prepare low calorie meals.
	Provide Peter with a food diary and show him how to keep a record of food intake.	This encourages active participation.
	Tell him to bring the diary to a follow-up visit to see how he is doing.	This provides motivation to keep the diary up.
	Help Peter set realistic short term goals: • decrease consumption of junk foods • eat fruits or vegetables for after school snacks • limit food consumption while watching TV	Unrealistic goals can result in frustration and giving up.
	Involve the family by encouraging all of them to work toward the same goals.	It is difficult to change behavior if other family members are not supportive or are eating what you are trying to avoid.
	Provide reinforcement by calling Peter a few days or a week after the visit.	Provides motivation and indicates to Peter a commitment to help him.
	Have Peter return in 2 weeks to review food diary and be weighed.	Provides an opportunity for reinforcement and discussion of problems encountered.
	Identify to Peter ways to increase caloric expenditure. • Exercise or riding his bike to school. • Riding his bike for his paper route (this may be done gradually by having him do half of it riding his bike and half with the assistance of his parents).	Exercise is an important factor in weight control. This allows Peter a period of time to adjust to new activity patterns.
	Show parents exercises learned in physical education class and involve family in daily exercise.	
	Encourage family activities that involve activity (i.e., playing ball, riding bikes, walking or hiking).	Group activities are more successful than individual.

(Continued)

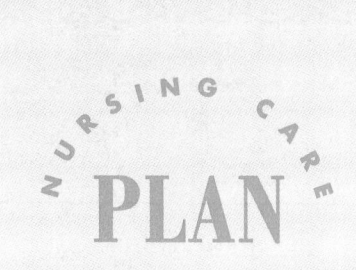

A 9-Year-Old Child With a Weight Problem
(continued)

Evaluation
- Peter identifies contributing factors of his weight gain.
- Peter demonstrates his active involvement in controlling his weight gain.
- Peter uses a food diary.
  Peter identifies positive and negative aspects of daily food intake.
- Peter states that he is more physically active.

Expected Outcomes
- Parents demonstrate support for Peter's attempts to control his weight gain.
- Parents exhibit their support of family activities that enhance optimal patterns of nutrition and patterns of activity.

---

basis. In 1986 Congress increased funding for breakfast programs to improve the quality of foods served.[20] Currently, school breakfast programs serve children who live in low-income areas or who travel long distances to school.[5] School breakfast is not common in schools that serve middle- and upper-middle-class families where skipping breakfast is becoming more of a concern.[5] School breakfast and lunch programs alone cannot promote optimal nutritional intake of children. Children must be assisted in choosing appropriate foods and educated about nutrition and health, especially in the early school years.

School-age children should learn about nutrition from parents, teachers, and nurses and be prepared to make appropriate food choices. A Nursing Care Plan and a teaching plan concerning nutrition and weight balance are presented here. For the child who, in the early years, had opportunities to try a variety of foods and who was gradually taught about nutrition, the continuation of good eating habits is likely. The child who has not had these experiences will have a more difficult time choosing nutritious foods. A child who has difficulty eating the foods served at school may need to bring a lunch from home that meets nutritional needs and reflects the child's likes, cultural food preferences, or both.

Skipping Breakfast

The changing lifestyles of many families has resulted in the development of more casual eating patterns. School-age children may be left to prepare their breakfast if both parents work. It is estimated that 8% to 29% of children do not eat breakfast.[34] The impact of skipping breakfast on cognitive functioning and school performance requires further study.[39] However, a study of well-nourished 9- to 11- year-old children who stopped breakfast demonstrated more errors on cognitive tests such as matching familiar figures.[40] In another study, skipping breakfast improved immediate recall in short-term mem-

ory.[39] The substitution of meals with continuous snacking can adversely affect the nutritional level of school children, especially if the snacks chosen are of low nutrient density such as soft drinks, candies, and cakes. If, on the other hand, a wide variety of nutritious foods such as fresh fruit are readily available in the home, between-meal snacking can have a positive impact on overall nutrition.[32] Snacks have been found to provide up to 18% of the school-age child's total energy intake.[32]

Nutrition and Development

The school years are a time of industry. The school-age child needs opportunities to develop a sense of industry and avoid feelings of inferiority. Adequate nutrition is necessary for the school-age child to master school work and to participate in sport and recreational activities with peers. Inadequate nutrition can interfere with these activities and increase a child's sense of inferiority. The child who feels good enjoys learning new skills and takes on new challenges. School-age children's desire to fit into the group and their sense of industry make them receptive to nutrition education if it is taught in a developmentally appropriate way.

Nursing Implications

The nurse working with school-age children must be aware of the importance of nutrition on development during the school years. The nursing assessment of nutrition will include serial heights and weights in relation to national norms, the child's school performance, the child's understanding of nutrition, and parental influence of the child's diet.

Obtaining information regarding dietary intake for even 24 hours becomes more difficult now that the child does not eat all meals at home and is a likely to eat many between-meal snacks. However, at this age, if the child is given a specific task to accomplish and the responsibility

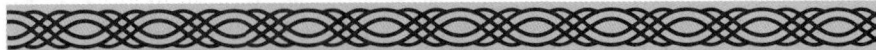

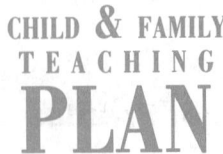

CHILD & FAMILY
T E A C H I N G
PLAN

Weight Regulation for a 9-Year-Old Child

Assessment

Peter is 9 years old and is being treated for potential obesity. He is 4'6'' and weighs 92 lb. Both his parents appear obese. Peter needs help in understanding the adjustments to be made in his dietary habits and how to exercise more. The reader is referred to the Nursing Care Plan developed earlier in the chapter. The nursing diagnosis, Knowledge Deficit related to altered nutrition, was identified during the initial interactions with the family.

Child and Family Objectives	*Specific Content*	*Teaching Strategies*
1. Determine understanding of weight gain.	1. Determine Peter's goals related to weight. Misinformation to be corrected. Peter and his family understand the many variables associated with obesity.	1. Ask Peter what he thinks his ideal weight should be. Have Peter describe what he believes causes obesity. Provide factual information. Review with Peter and his parents what factors predispose a person to weight gain. Include: • Dietary factors • Heredity factors • Environmental factors • Physiologic factors • Psychological factors
2. Review four food groups and nutritional information.	2. The nurse evaluates Peter's knowledge as well as demonstrates to Peter that many of the foods are not good for him. Peter's mother's involvement: • Eliminate or decrease non-nutritious foods from family food supply, including cookies, potato chips, soda. • Make nutritious foods available that require minimal preparation for Peter, e.g., cut-up fruits, cut-up raw vegetables, juice.	2. Have Peter look at his 24-hour diet history and identify: • Foods that are good for him • Foods that are not good for him • What other foods he likes that could serve as alternatives Use diagrams to review four food groups. Ask Peter to identify which ones were missing from his 24-hour dietary intake. Involve Peter in the planning process. Ask Peter to name some foods he likes that are part of the food groups missing from his diet. Assist Peter's mother in making environmental changes.

(Continued)

CHILD & FAMILY
T E A C H I N G
PLAN

Weight Regulation
for a 9-Year-Old Child (continued)

Nursing Diagnosis	Intervention	Rationale
3. Use various support systems and methods to support Peter and family in changing eating habits.	3. Parents may need assistance in planning easy-to-prepare low-calorie meals.	3. Set up an appointment for parents with a dietician who can assist them in planning low-calorie, nutritious meals.
	Food diary food personal evaluation.	Provide Peter with a food diary and show him how to keep a record of food intake.
		Tell him to bring the diary to a follow-up visit to see how he is doing.
	Unrealistic goals can result in frustration and giving up. Set realistic goals: • Decrease consumption of junk foods. • Eat fruits or vegetables for after-school snacks. • Limit food consumption while watching TV.	Help Peter set realistic short-term goals. Involve the family by encouraging all of them to work toward the same goals. Provide reinforcement by calling Peter a few days or a week after the visit.
	Reinforcement and discussion of problems encountered.	Have Peter return in 2 weeks to review food diary and be weighed.
4. Initiate personal and family activities to increase caloric expenditure.	4. Exercise is an important factor in weight control. Peter plans for increased activity level: • Exercise or riding his bike to school. • Ride his bike for his paper route (this may be done gradually by having him do ½ of it riding his bike and half with the assistance of his parents).	4. Use handouts to identify methods of increasing caloric expenditure. Help Peter write goals and plan activities.
	Family activities that involve activity, e.g., playing ball, riding bikes, walking, or hiking.	Show parents exercises learned in physical education class and involve family in daily exercise. Discuss group activities and when they could be scheduled.

Evaluation

• Peter identifies factors contributing to his weight gain.
• Peter becomes actively involved in controlling weight gain.
• Peter identifies positive and negative aspects of daily food intake by keeping a food diary.
• Peter states he has become more physically active.
• Parents exhibit support of Peter in his attempts to control his weight gain.
• Parents participate in planning and carrying out patterns of activity.

to complete the task, an accurate history can be obtained. Information related to school lunch intake may have to be obtained from school teachers if a child is not growing as expected. Similarly, information concerning school performance, alertness, and participation in the classroom requires teacher input. If nutrition and growth concerns are identified, the nurse working in the primary care setting may have to involve the school nurse or public health nurse in obtaining dietary information. Because school teachers, school nurses, and public health nurses see many children, obtaining information may be difficult. Rather than having information available at the time of the health visit, the nurse may have to request the information and follow-up with parents after the teacher and/or school nurse can gather information over several days or weeks. As with all children, the nurse should discuss with parents their beliefs about nutritional needs and how they can best be met. Parental understanding of the relationship of nutrition to school performance, dietary concerns of parents, nutritional status of the child, and actions undertaken by parents are vital information for the nurse concerned with health promotion. In many communities school lunch menus are posted in the local newspaper. Parents should be encouraged to review these menus and provide a lunch for the child when menu items will not be eaten by the child for religious, cultural, or other reasons.

The nurse also needs to talk with the child. As children get into the school years, they are ready to learn and gradually take responsibility for their own health. The nurse must ascertain what the child knows about food and growth (Table 15-1). By asking the children directly what was eaten in the past 24 hours, the nurse indicates to them the belief that they have the ability to remember and report this information. Further, the nurse can ask children their perceptions of the quality of intake and

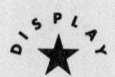

Goals of Nutrition Education

- Becoming a knowledgeable consumer.
- Developing an understanding of nutrition concepts that can be used in individual problem solving.
- Forming positive attitudes toward nutrition.
- Selecting and consuming nutritious foods.
- Applying students' understanding of the principles of nutrition to evaluate nutrition controversies and select healthy meals in a variety of settings.
- Being motivated to continue the learning process.

From Weiss, S., & Kein, L. (1987). A synthesis of research on nutrition education at the elementary school level. Journal of School Health, 57(1), 8–13. Copyright 1987. American School Health Association, P.O. Box 708, Kent, OH 44240; reprinted with permission.

TABLE 15-1
Nursing Assessment: Questions for Assessing Eating Behaviors of School-Age Children

Area of Assessment	Questions to be Asked of the Child*
Adequacy of meal in meeting nutrient requirements.	What did you eat for breakfast, lunch, and dinner yesterday?
Changes in eating behavior.	Do you eat more, less, or the same as last year? Do you generally eat the same things you ate last year?
What foods are missing from the diet, and are daily requirements met with substitutions?	Are there any foods you won't eat? Do you eat _____? (name some foods that would serve as a substitute)
Types of foods offered at school.	Give me an example of some of your school lunches. How much do you usually eat at lunch?
Broad assessment of school performance.	How are you doing in school? Do you find it harder to concentrate on days when you don't have a good breakfast and/or lunch?
Assessment of physical activities.	What physical activities are you involved in? How often are you involved in physical activities? Do you enjoy physical education class? How often do you have it?
Child's awareness of the relationship between food and growth.	Can you tell me why it is important for us to eat food?
Child's awareness of specific need for a variety of foods.	What foods are especially important for us and why?
Child's ability to identify low-nutrient foods.	What foods do you or your friends eat that are not good for you?
Child's awareness of life-style patterns and long-term health.	Do you think that the foods you eat now will affect you as you get older? How?

* Questions should be directed to the child. Parents may add additional information.

which foods eaten in the last 24 hours were healthy and which ones had minimal nutritional value. The nurse can then explore with them how and why food choices were made. This type of interaction between the child and nurse provides information about the child's decision-making ability related to food choice, the influence of peers on food selection, and the availability of foods in the home and at school.

Teaching Nutrition to School-Age Children

Research has shown that school programs for nutrition education are effective in developing knowledgeable consumers, creating positive attitudes, and promoting healthy eating behaviors.[48] The goals of nutrition education in the school years focus on comprehension of basic nutrition concepts and provision of a theoretical and practical foundation for selecting a diet based on current and future information.[48] The display lists goals of nutrition education. Children learn best by seeing and doing. Nurses can work with teachers in deciding what should be taught and how to best present the material. The school nurse may be given responsibility for this content and therefore is in a critical position that requires creativity and commitment to helping children learn about food and their health.

Teaching should influence behavior rather than simply provide information. Eating behaviors can be changed through experiences in actual eating situations and through group activities that allow for the evaluation of eating habits[48] (Fig. 15-1). Passive intake of information by lecture should be replaced by student involvement in the learning process. For example, rather than telling students what a good diet is as compared to a poor diet, teachers can include students by having them analyze their own diets.[29] School-age children learn through and

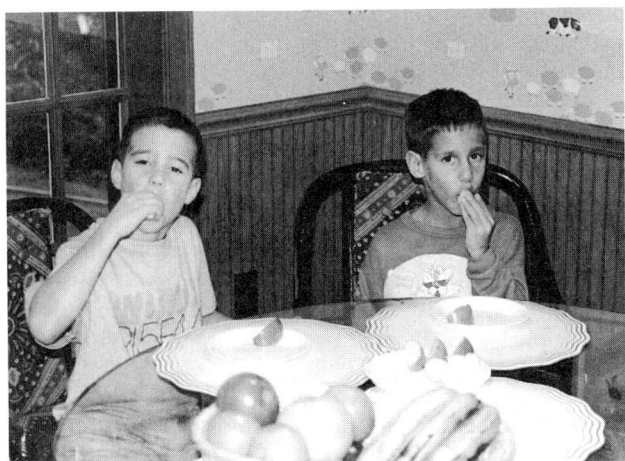

FIGURE 15-1
Eating behaviors can be changed through experiences in actual eating situations and group activities.

enjoy doing experiments and group activities. Growing plants or keeping small animals in the classroom provides a basis for discussion of nutritional needs of living organisms. Through the use of creativity, the nurse can provide age-appropriate information during a time children are especially eager to learn. By being available at lunch time, teachers and school nurses can help children choose foods from each of the basic food groups, make substitutions, and encourage them to eat all the food provided since it provides only the minimal required nutrients.

Assessing, Promoting, and Maintaining Optimal Elimination

Elimination patterns are well established during the school years, and it is uncommon for the school-age child to have loss of bowel or bladder control during the day. Bedwetting can still be a problem. Approximately 5% of all 10-year-old children still wet their beds.[19] The causes of enuresis and treatment are the same as those for the preschooler (see Chaps. 14 and 50).

The school-age child no longer wants assistance in the bathroom. They want to function independently and have developed modesty related to toileting activities. It continues to be important for parents to occasionally remind the child about handwashing. Parents should also be aware of any difficulties with constipation and diarrhea. Asking the child about elimination patterns is important so that any changes can be identified early.

Assessing, Promoting, and Maintaining Optimal Sleep

Sleep is extremely important during the school years because of the effects of sleep deprivation on school performance and physical growth. The amount of time spent sleeping shows a steady decrease during the school years. Typically, children aged 6 and 7 years sleep for 9 to 9.5 hours; children aged 8 to 9 sleep for 8.5 hours; and chil-

dren aged 10 to 11 sleep 7.5 hours.[11] Difficulty getting the school-age child up in time for breakfast before leaving for school may indicate a late or delayed sleep phase. Late bedtimes followed by "catch-up" morning sleep, which occur during vacations, holidays, and periods of illness, as well as bedtime struggles that lead to later sleep onset are frequent causes of delayed morning awakening times.[18] Parents can unwittingly allow the development of a delayed sleep phase by allowing the child to catch up on sleep in the morning or with naps.[18] Treatment for delayed sleep phase is straightforward. The child is allowed to start with the late bedtime to decrease bedtime arguments and struggles. The waking time in the morning is predetermined and should be consistently enforced, including weekends. This need to awaken the child on weekends can be difficult for parents but is a necessary part of moving the child's sleep phase. Bedtime is shifted back gradually about 15 minutes per day until a desired schedule is obtained[18] (Table 15-2).

Sleep Walking, Sleep Talking, and Night Terrors

Sleep disturbances are less frequent in the school years and are most commonly related to partial wakenings in the deep sleep phase. These disturbances may include sleep walking, sleep talking, and night terrors in the early hours of sleep. Sleep disturbances in the school years are more often a response to an emotional concern rather than a developmental issue. These emotional concerns are usually minor and may be the child's way of expressing feelings such as hate, anger, and guilt when the child is uncomfortable expressing these outwardly. Occasional occurrence of sleep walking or night terrors should not cause concern. However, frequent and more intense episodes may indicate that the child is experiencing some emotional distress.

TABLE 15-2
Nursing Assessment: Questions for Assessing Sleep Patterns During the School Years

Area of Assessment	Questions to Be Asked of the Child and Parents*
Child and parental concerns related to sleep patterns.	Do you have any trouble sleeping?
Child and parental responsibility for meeting the sleep needs of the child.	What time do you usually go to bed? Who decides on your bedtime? Do you generally go to bed when you are told?
Child and parental awareness of altered sleep cycles.	Do you get up easily in the morning? Do you wake up during the night? If yes, do you have trouble getting back to sleep?
Child and parental awareness of relationship between school performance and sleep deprivation.	Do you have any difficulty in school, (concentration, memory, sleepiness) when you stay up late?
Child and parental ability to recognize indicators of sleep deprivation.	How do you feel when you are overtired?

* Questions should be directed toward the child. Parents can then provide additional information or validation.

Because these sleep disturbances occur during partial wakenings, the child will not remember them. Again, waking the child will not help. If left alone, the child will return to sleep.

In dealing with sleep walking, parents should be told to speak calmly to the child and they may be able to instruct the child to go back to bed without waking the child. The child may need to stop at the bathroom along the way. If the child fully awakens after the episodes, feelings of embarrassment are common. It is important not to make any negative or teasing remarks. The environment should be made safe to prevent accidental injury. Leaving a light on in the hall and removing obstacles from the floor may prevent falls. For younger children a gate may be necessary at the top of the stairs. A lock above the child's reach will prevent sleep walking outside the house. If this behavior is frequent or causing parental concern, a referral is indicated.

Nursing Implications

During the school years the school nurse assesses sleep patterns and the parent's ability to maintain regular sleep times on school nights (see Table 15-2). School performance as well as parental recognition of behaviors exhibited by the child when deprived of adequate sleep should also be discussed. Children who are reluctant to go to bed and are then difficult to wake up may need assistance in changing their sleep cycle.

Assessing, Promoting, and Maintaining Optimal Psychosocial Development

Psychosocial development during the school years focuses on the development of a sense of industry and the development of peer relationships. Each of these, in turn, will affect the developing self-concept.

Developing a Sense of Industry

Erikson[16] describes the major psychosocial task of the school years as industry versus inferiority. The school-age child learns to earn recognition by producing things and by being successful. School offers opportunities for developing industry through academic achievements (Fig. 15-2*A*). Learning to read and write is essential for functioning in our society and is therefore critical to a sense of industry.

Skill acquisition during the school years includes not only classroom skills but also activities, games, and sports (Fig. 15-2*B*). A variety of activities brings the child in contact with peers and adults, and the child has an opportunity to develop social skills. Developing friendships, belonging to a group or club, and gaining competence in social interactions all foster a sense of industry and a positive sense of self. Feeling inferior is the potential danger of this stage of development. According to Erikson,[16] this may occur if the child is unable to separate psychologically from the primary caregiver. The dependent school-age child who uses energies to maintain contact with mother does not have sufficient energies left to invest in social peer relations or academic tasks. Inferiority may also result if the child sets goals too high or if adults, whose opinions the child values, are too frequently critical. The school-age child must balance the mastery of both social and technical skills. Inadequate development of either will lead to a sense of inferiority, incompetency, and poor self-esteem.

Parental Role

Parents can foster a sense of industry by taking an active interest in the child's day-to-day experiences. Par-

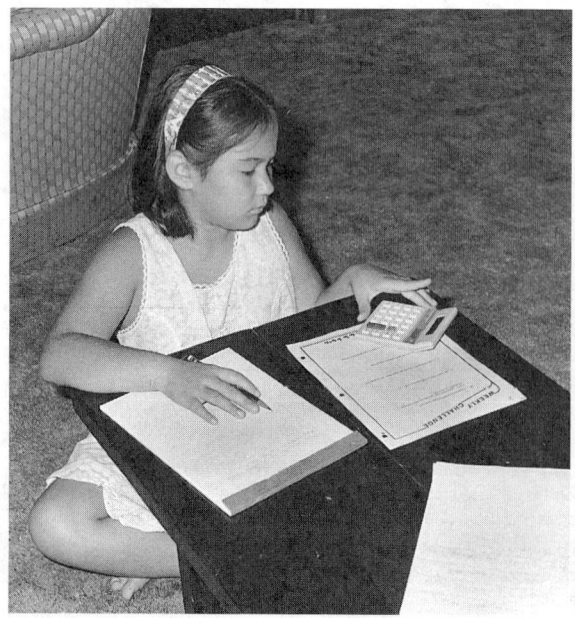
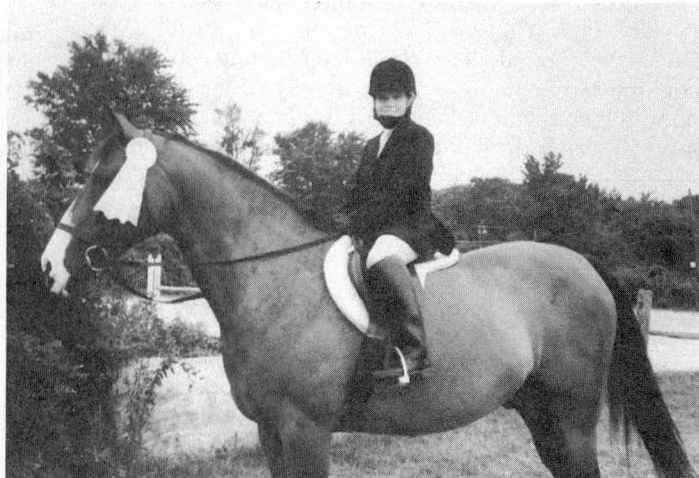

FIGURE 15-2
School-age children learn to be industrious in academic studies and in sports and activities.

ents promote a sense of industry when they provide positive reinforcement for the mastery of new technical skills, such as reading, writing, and math, and also for development of social skills, such as being a team member or being kind to a friend. Positive reinforcement can be a verbal expression of pride or encouragement. It can also be a more active reinforcer, such as attending a sports event, attending a science fair, or in any way actively participating in the child's activities.

Parents can also help a child set goals that are realistic and attainable. If goals are always set beyond the child's ability, feelings of inferiority may develop. Parents must learn to balance their roles in encouraging independence and helping the child to master new skills. This is clearly seen in the following examples.

John, a sixth grader, is preparing for the school science fair. He tells his parents that he plans to build a model of the workings of a telephone. His parents say "that sounds nice" and have no further involvement. John encounters many problems building the project, but his parents feel that this is his project and they should not interfere. John does what he can but loses interest. At the time of the science fair, John is frustrated and ashamed to exhibit his project.

Tom is a sixth grader preparing for the school science fair. He tells his parents of his plans to build a model of the workings of a telephone. His parents become very excited and tell Tom that they want to help him with his project. Tom's mother buys a kit at the hobby shop of a working telephone model, but it is too advanced for Tom. Tom's father therefore builds it for Tom. At the time of the science fair, Tom's parents are very proud of their son, but Tom feels he had no part in the project.

Both of these situations are extreme examples of how parents can negatively influence a child's sense of industry. A more beneficial approach by parents requires an appropriate amount of involvement to assist a child in learning new skills. To feel a sense of accomplishment, a child needs to participate actively in reaching a goal and at the same time have support and assistance when difficulties arise. In the cases of Tom and John, the parents could have assisted them by talking about the idea of building a phone; obtaining Tom's and John's perception of the project; encouraging them to do the parts they were able to do; and assisting them in completing the project using a teaching approach.

Parents have many opportunities to promote industry even if they make a few errors along the way. Parents should be encouraged to take time to talk to the child about school and take an interest in the child's homework and school activities. Regular communication with the teacher indicates to the child parental commitment and interest in the child's life. Parents should also encourage peer interaction and activities. Parents can help the child manage time to allow for both homework and extracurricular activities. Playing with the child is also important, and the parents can help a child learn and enjoy a new sport or master a skill through practice.

Nursing Implications

The nurse has a role in assessing a child's developing sense of industry. This assessment is based on observations of the child's behaviors, interactions with parents, peers and siblings, and school performance. Information in each area must be obtained from both the child and parents (Table 15-3).

The child's self-perceptions in relation to school, peership, and physical and social skills are important variables in building self-esteem. Early identification of any unrealistic goals that the parents or child may have set can be a topic of discussion. Some parents may need assistance in changing their interaction patterns when it is found that they are overly involved in the child's activities or not involved at all with the child's activities.

Because many parental errors are a result of their deep desire to help a child, a discussion of the potential undesired effects of their efforts may be sufficient to change their behavior. In other instances, parents may not be able to change their intense desire to have a child meet expectations that may be unrealistic and unattainable. Parents should be encouraged to respond to the

TABLE 15-3
Nursing Assessment: Guidelines for Observation of Industry

Child Behaviors That Demonstrate a Sense of Industry	Parental Behaviors That Foster a Sense of Industry	Child Behaviors That Indicate Feelings of Inferiority	Parental Behaviors That Promote Sense of Inferiority
• Generally enjoys school and is successful in learning new skills. • Does not give up when initially unsuccessful with a new task. • Interacts and spends time with peers in constructive activities (playing ball, jumping rope, girl scouts, boy scouts). • Actively seeks new challenges. • Talks about activities and feels proud of accomplishments.	• Provides positive reinforcement for mastery of new tasks. • Supports efforts when goals are not realized. • Takes time to help child master new skills (homework, social activities, girl scouts, boy scouts). • Verbally expresses positive feelings about the child. • Has realistic expectations of the child's abilities.	• Loss of interest in school work. • Gives up attempts to master a task after minimal effort. • Consistently gives up projects before they are complete. • Avoids playing with other children. • Doing well in one area of development such as sports but doing poorly in academics or vice versa. • Exhibits destructive behavior or socializes with a peer group that spends time in nonconstructive activities.	• Highly critical of child and has unrealistic perception of child's abilities. • Refers to child in negative terms (dumb, stupid, clumsy). • Does not take time to support and help child master developmental tasks. • Encourages mastery of one area of development at the expense of another, e.g., child not allowed after school activities or peer play, all attention must focus on academic achievement.

successes the child experiences and at the same time assist the child in coping with failures.

Parents can be asked to describe positive and negative attributes and abilities of the child, their expectations of the child's performance in school, sports, and peer relations, and their perceptions of the child's ability to live up to these expectations.

Nurses must also reinforce parent's positive perceptions of the child, evaluate further negative descriptions, and discuss parental perceptions of why the child is unable to meet expectations. Parents may need assistance in setting more realistic goals for the child, accepting the child as a unique individual, and responding appropriately to positive qualities in the child.

Promoting Psychosocial Development Through Peer Relationships

The development of peer relations is an important task of the school-age child. As the child moves away from home and into the school environment, more and more time is spent with peers who influence the child's development. Peer interactions serve many socializing functions and influence the developing self-concept. Through peer experiences in the neighborhood and school environment children, develop more mature and mutually satisfying relationships with friends.

Initially, friends are chosen based on what toys they have or where they live in the neighborhood. In the early school years, egocentrism continues to be seen in peer relationships. "To be my friend you have to do what I want to do." As the child gains increased experience in peer relationships, the meaning of friendships changes and more personal, mutually rewarding friendships develop (Fig. 15-3).

Children aged 9 or 10 expect mutual respect and affection from their friends. Peership influences the development of respect for others, an understanding of others' needs for affection, and the importance of consideration for others' feelings. Loyalty is considered a critical factor in maintaining friendships, and best friends are the friends you can trust with your feelings. Trusting someone outside the family helps the child learn to share feelings. Friends empathize with each other, spend time talking, and share experiences. A friend who goes to another school or moves away is missed, but new friends are found because of the important role friendships play in the developing child's life.

Gangs

The development of groups or "gangs" is also part of the social experience during the school years. The child's participation in group activities is a major socializing agent during the school years. The child learns to be a group member and may learn to be a group leader. Initially these gangs are organized loosely and develop in neighborhoods or school playgrounds. Children meet for a mutual goal such as playing ball, riding bikes, or playing with dolls. Membership changes rapidly, and new

children are allowed to join. The group promotes cooperation and sharing, and children become less egocentric.

In the middle school years, gangs become more formal. Secret clubs are formed with specific rules, secret codes, and rituals. Identification with a club gives the child a sense of belonging and a sense of self-worth. These clubs are more organized and have recognized leaders, and each member is assigned a particular position in the hierarchy. Club rules and new memberships are discussed and voted on, giving members an opportunity to govern themselves and their activities. Formal clubs run by adults, such as Boy Scouts, Girl Scouts, and Little League, also have an important role in development. Children have opportunities to learn specific skills. Self-esteem is fostered by the chance to earn merit badges or by contribution to a team effort.

Through peer group interactions children learn that others experience many of the same feelings, fears, and frustrations about home, school, or their own abilities. Being part of a group promotes the child's feelings of being important and valued by others. A child's self-concept is influenced by peer interactions. Children who have difficulty fitting in with their peer group or who are rejected by their peers may develop a sense of inferiority and loneliness.

In addition to the "gangs" that are a part of the typical developmental phase of the school-age child, there is an alarming increase in the development of gangs involved in illegal and destructive activities. The young school-age child often becomes involved in these gangs through older siblings. An increasing number of destructive gangs are seen in urban areas. These gangs are frequently involved in drugs and drug-related crime. The result has been an alarming incidence of gunshot wounds in children under the age of 10.[35]

Parental Role

Parents can encourage peer interactions and developing relationships of the child. If allowed, most children will interact with peers and develop friendships. It is more difficult for the child who has many home chores or who is expected to care for younger siblings after school and on Saturdays. Parents should set expectations for household chores that allow free time for peer interactions. The child must also feel comfortable bringing other children home to play and be allowed to go to the homes of peers.

Children who have difficulty developing peer relationships may benefit from a more structured peer group. Parents should consider the interests of the child when choosing a group activity. A child who does not enjoy playing ball will not benefit from Little League. A shy child may be more comfortable interacting with another child who feels similar discomfort in interacting with peers. Parents can discuss the child's shyness with teachers and ask about children who may have similar feelings. Parents can then help the child to invite another child with a similar personality home to play.

In areas where there are fewer adult-sponsored youth groups and less financial resources, such as the inner city or rural community, parents have to be more creative. However, it is usually these same parents that have many

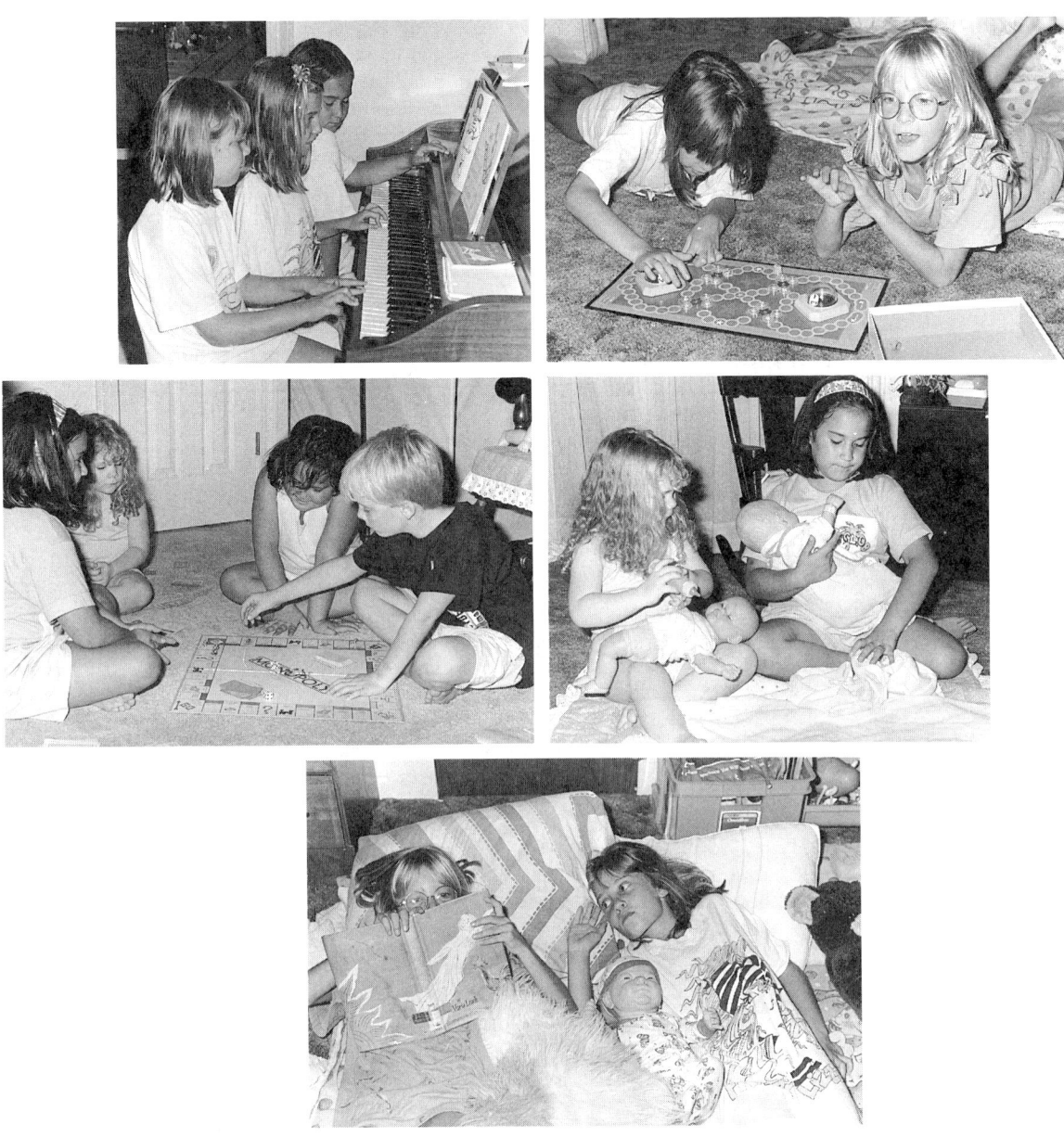

FIGURE 15-3
Friendships develop during the school years and provide an opportunity for children to expand their worlds.

daily stresses and the child's peer interactions may not be a realistic priority. In this instance, the nurse or teacher can take a more active role in helping the child develop friendships. In most cities there are a variety of groups open to all children, including summer camps, sports teams, and activities sponsored by the public library and local museums. Parents may need assistance in getting a child enrolled in these types of programs.

Nursing Implications

Discussion of peer relations is an important part of the nurse's role in promoting healthy development in school-age children. Nurses should talk to both the child and parents regarding participation in group activities and interactions with friends. Nurses can offer support to the child who is having difficulty in interacting with peers and developing friendships. It is important to identify

factors that may be contributing to the child's difficulty, such as parental overprotectiveness; lack of other children in the neighborhood; living a long distance away from school, which decreases opportunities for after-school activities; or the child's particular personality type.

Parents who express concern about the child's choice of friends need an opportunity to discuss their concerns. The child can be involved in this discussion so that parental feelings are shared with the child. Parents can be asked why they do not feel a child or group of children are appropriate friends for their own child.

Through discussion of the role of peer interaction in the child's development of self-concept, industry, and feelings of self-worth, nurses can assist parents in promoting peer relationships. The parents and child may be asked to describe what activities the child enjoys and what special abilities the child has developed. If the child is having difficulty interacting with the peer group, a more organized group run by adults may be beneficial. This information is also beneficial for the nurse working in an acute care setting or long-term care facility. Children of school age should be placed in rooms with age mates. Because peer relations have an important influence on self-concept and self-confidence, peership must be supported in all environments. A child with a poor self-image is at greater risk for becoming involved in gang activity.

Promoting a Positive Self-Concept

Until the school years, the child's self-concept, either positive or negative, is predominately a reflection of the perceptions of the child and the child's family. School now brings the child in contact with peers, teachers, and other adults who will also influence the child's self-concept. Even for the child who begins school with a positive self-concept, fostered by caring parents who provided positive reinforcement for the child, the self-concept is developed further, incorporating the perceptions of peers, teachers, and other adults. Nurses provide help for parents in promoting the child's adjustments to school (Table 15-4).

School entry exposes the child to new people, new expectations, and new challenges. The child's attempts to meet these challenges result in exposure to positive and negative responses from those with whom the child interacts. The child may also experience concern about personal capability and acceptability when evaluated in relation to peers and parental and personal expectations. Negative feelings such as "I'm no good" or "Nobody likes me" may surface. These feelings are not passed off lightly, and for a time the child may lose confidence and not attempt to pursue goals that appear to be difficult to obtain.

Parental Role

School-age children need supportive, caring, empathic adults to assist them as they redefine their self-concepts. They require support from others to keep small failures and disappointments in perspective. They need praise for their accomplishments, encouragement to do things for themselves, and reassurance that they are trusted and loved.

Negative self-concept may develop from interactions with those who embarrass or humiliate a child who has

TABLE 15-4
Nursing Intervention: Anticipatory Guidance for Promoting Adjustment to New School or First Grade

- Prepare child for school entry by talking about school activities prior to the beginning of school.
- Show the child the school, school bus, or school route prior to the beginning of school.
- Take the child to any school orientation activities that are offered.
- Take the child to school and pick the child up after school the first day.
- Introduce the child to the teacher.
- Talk to the child about school and school activities he or she enjoys.
- Schedule regular appointments with the teacher if the child does not adapt well to the new situation. This may be demonstrated by the child in several ways, including not wanting to go to school, complaining of illness, lack of interest in talking about school, or mood changes from school days to weekends.

failed to live up to teacher, parent, or peer expectations. Feelings of inadequacy in school, sports, school activities, or peer interactions lead to the development of a poor self-concept. Parents, teachers, and child-care professionals must treat the school-age child as an individual person with unique qualities. It is difficult for the child to live up to unrealistic expectations or to be always compared with an older sibling or peer who has qualities or abilities valued by parents and teachers.

School-age children need adults to support them, encourage them, and help them reach desired goals. If parents or teachers view the children as failures, these feelings will become a part of the children's self-concept. Before a child can set realistic goals, parents must set realistic expectations for the child. All children benefit from adults who point out strengths of the child while helping them overcome weaknesses.

Nursing Implications

Parents need guidance and support in their attempts to help the school-age child develop a healthy, positive self-concept. The nurse can share with parents the fact that school-age children develop their self-concept by interacting with others and observing the response of peers, teachers, and parents to them and their abilities. Explain that it is common for the child to feel inadequate or less valued when he or she leaves the security of home and must interact with many children and other adults. This knowledge may help a parent deal with a child's sudden lack of confidence. Prepare parents for the fact that a child may give up a task or goal he or she feels unable to obtain.

During the well-child visit, the nurse has many opportunities to assess the child's self-concept as well as parental perceptions of the child. When discussing school performance, peer relationships, and progress toward meeting developmental tasks with the child, the nurse must be alert to cues of insecurity, disinterest, emphasis on negative feelings, and apathy in talking about everyday experiences. A child who shrugs in response to inquiries of school or states "I don't have any friends" or says "Tim does everything better" is expressing very real feelings. The child may need the nurse's assistance in describing positive feelings. The child may be asked to describe his favorite activities, activities he is successful at and what he is able to do that pleases himself, his parents, his teachers, and his peers. "Tommy, tell me about your favorite activities and what you do best?" "Tommy, is there anything you wish you could do better?" What is keeping him from being successful, and how does he plan to work at improvement? When the nurse has a perception of the child's self-concept, the information can be used to reinforce positive attributes and qualities of the child. The nurse may provide guidance when expectations are unrealistic or unattainable and help the child define more realistic goals (Table 15-5).

Promoting Moral Development

The child's moral development occurs over time and develops in specific stages (see Chap. 8). During the school years parents foster moral development by assist-

TABLE 15-5
Nursing Intervention: Anticipatory Guidance for Promoting a Positive Self-Concept

- The nurse can share with parents that school-age children develop their self-concept by interacting with others and observing the response of peers, teachers, and parents to them and their abilities.
- The nurse explains that it is common for school-age children to feel inadequate or less valued when they leave the security of the home and interact with many children and other adults.
- Discuss with parents that children may give up a task or goal if they feel unable to attain it.
- School-age children need adults to support them, encourage them, and help them reach desired goals.
- Children will view themselves as a failure if parents and/or teachers view them this way.
- Parents need to set realistic expectations for children and help them set realistic goals for themselves.
- Children benefit from adults who point out strengths of a child while helping them overcome a weakness.

ing the child in developing a tolerance for different viewpoints and respecting others. This requires a tolerance on the part of parents for many questions about why something is different and why something is right or wrong. Simply telling a child what is right or wrong is not sufficient for teaching morality. The child needs opportunities to explore alternatives to a moral dilemma and to be allowed to express feelings. Children need opportunities to see lifestyles different from their own. School, extracurricular activities, and athletics provide opportunities for this when the child leaves the neighborhood school to attend a junior high that serves many neighborhoods.

In the home environment, parents can create an environment of mutual respect by admitting when they are wrong. Parents should listen to and consider the opinions of their children and can help children by considering others. Parents should encourage children to think of how a decision one person makes might affect other members of the family or friends. Most importantly, parents should be role models for their children.

Discipline During the School Years

Discipline continues to be a concern during the school years. Children need parental assistance in learning to control behavior and developing self-discipline. The methods for teaching discipline are different from those used in the toddler and preschool years. Effective methods of discipline reflect the school-age child's increased ability to discuss issues with parents (Table 15-6).

In the early school years, behavior modification techniques such as "time out" continue to be effective.[10] Other methods appropriate for the school-age child include "using deprivation of privileges, appeals to the child's self-esteem or sense of humor, arousal of the child's sense of guilt, and reminders that children are responsible for what happens to them."[31]

Discipline during the school years, as in earlier years, requires consistency to be effective. The child needs to be aware of what behavior is acceptable and what behavior

is unacceptable. Consistent expectations and consequences result in children who are more motivated to control their behavior and who develop positive self-concepts.[12]

In addition, follow-through is very important. Once parents determine reasonable consequences for unacceptable behavior, these consequences must be carried out. It is important that parents consider carefully the consequences they are using. If consequences are unreasonable or unrealistic—"You will never be allowed out of the house again"—they will be ineffective because parents will be unable to follow through.

Parental modeling becomes an important aspect of discipline during the school years. The school-age child is able to discuss issues with parents and will frequently argue parental unfairness and point to a parent's inconsistencies. For example, a child who is deprived of watching her favorite television program because she lied about where she was after school may respond with "Well, you lied last night when you told Dad to tell Mrs. Smith you were not at home." Parents who want a child to incorporate values, morals, and beliefs must model these themselves.

Parental Concerns: Lying and Stealing

Lying and stealing are common behaviors of school-age children. Children will frequently tell lies to cover up for a misdeed, or they may lie to make themselves superior to their peers. For example, a school-age child

TABLE 15-6
Basic Principles of Discipline

Principle	Description
Consistency	Rules are applied as uniformly as possible.
Follow-through	Reasonable consequences are carried out; no escape for child.
Pacing	Expectations are consistently based on justice and freedom but adapted to the child's developmental level.
Modeling	Adults and parents monitor their own behavior so children learn approved behavior by imitating and identifying with them.
Immediate feedback	Consequences of behavior are felt as soon as possible after it occurs or just before it takes place.
Truthfulness	Parents are truthful about their reasons for their expectations.
Trust	Adults verbally express trust in, and act trustingly toward, their children until such trust is broken by the children.
Logical outcomes	Consequences of behavior are logical results of the behavior.
Self-disclosure	Parents are not afraid to disclose their own feelings and mistakes to children.
Genuine love	The key to all effective discipline is genuine unearned love.

From Wise, F. (1986). Development of self-discipline. In C. Schuster and S. Ashburn (Eds.). *The process of human development: A holistic life-span approach* (2nd ed.; p. 373). Boston: Little, Brown.

who hears a friend boast about the size of a collection of coins may respond with "mine is twice that size." Chronic and excessive lying may indicate an underlying problem or may be the child's most effective method of gaining parental attention. How parents handle lying will influence whether the behavior continues. Ideally, parents should confront the child when the child is lying and ask why he or she told the lie. Parents can reinforce the importance of telling the truth.

Stealing is another behavior that may be seen in this age group. Children want many things and can be very impulsive. They see something they want but cannot afford and so they steal it. Parents need to deal with this behavior each time it occurs. The child should be told the behavior is unacceptable and the stolen object must be returned. Parents should supervise the return. The child will then have an opportunity to observe how they have embarrassed their parent. Punishment in addition to returning the stolen item is not recommended. "The child's sense of guilt usually centers more on the pain he has caused than on the misdeed itself. For this reason punishment is a weak deterrent; it makes the offender so angry at those who inflict it that his sense of guilt is diminished."[6] Sometimes stealing occurs because the child is attempting to impress peers or fit into a group. It is important that stealing done for this reason be identified and dealt with early. A child with a poor self-concept or a child struggling to find a place with peers is at high risk for developing aberrant behaviors to fit in somewhere.

Assessing, Promoting, and Maintaining Optimal Cognitive Development

Entering First Grade

Most children look forward to starting school and are anxious to bring home their books and demonstrate their newly learned skills. However, beginning school brings special challenges, including adjusting to a new environment, new adult figures, many children, and new behavior patterns. Many children have opportunities such as preschool, play groups, or day care experiences that help them tolerate separation from parents and home. Children who have no experience with separation or who are intolerant of separation may find first grade a frightening experience. Even children who look forward to starting school may have some anxiety initially.

Children in the first year of school need to know how to share with peers, share the attention of the teacher, and wait their turn. The child is now expected to sit for varying periods and attend to a specific task. The child who has not had an opportunity to practice this will find school stressful.

Through systematic assessment of a child prior to school entry, nurses can identify factors that may affect school adjustment or school performance (see Chap. 14 for discussion of school readiness). In addition to assessing indications of school readiness, nurses should talk with the child about school entry and how the child feels about the new experience. Parents should be asked about the child's past adaptation to change and reactions to new experiences such as preschool or day care.

Information regarding parental expectations of school adjustment and performance as well as the value they place on academic and social achievements are important prior to school entry and throughout the school years. Nurses can assist parents in setting realistic goals and support them in their problem-solving efforts throughout the school years.

Promoting Development in the School Environment

About half of the school-age child's waking hours are spent in school or in school-related activities. School can and does play an important role in the development of cognitive, language and writing, math and science, as well as social skills. School does not promote or hinder development in isolation but is one factor among many that all together influence a child's development. The child, parents, teachers, and school environment each have a significant role in fostering optimal development.

Role of the Child in School

There is a great deal of variation among children in their response to the school environment and level of school performance. All children do not respond in the same way to similar environmental situations. Some children readily adapt to the classroom setting, whereas others have difficulty adjusting.

Leaving home or preschool to begin formal education is a major transition for the 6-year-old child. A child who has difficulty adjusting to the new environment or new expectations of behavior will have little energy to invest in the learning process.

A child's response to school is partly a reflection of the child's unique temperament. Researchers[8,9] have demonstrated a relationship between temperament and academic achievement. In describing a child's temperament, Carey et al.[8] look at characteristics of the child's behavior. The goal is to identify the child's ability to adapt to new situations, the child's attention span, the child's activity level, the child's response to stimulation, and the child's persistence in doing a task or activity. A combination of these variables provides valuable information on how a child might respond to school and what type of school program is best for the child. Information regarding a child's temperament may also provide insight into possible causes of poor school performance.

Carey et al.[8] have developed a questionnaire for school-age children ages 8 to 12 called "The Middle Childhood Temperament Questionnaire." The questionnaire is completed by parents in approximately 20 minutes, then scoring takes about 15 minutes. The questionnaire has been tested for reliability and validity.

In addition to a unique temperament, the child also brings to the school environment self-perceptions about abilities and an estimation of self-worth. A child's attitudes toward school and learning reflect the attitudes of parents. Most children begin school with enthusiasm and a desire to succeed, but after the first years some lose their enthusiasm whereas others continue to grow. This change in attitude toward school in the middle-school years is the result of a range of variables. It may be in response to frequent failures, lack of parental involvement, or teacher-related variables such as a teaching method that does not reflect the individual child's best method for learning. The nurse should do a systematic assessment of all these variables when a child has lost interest or is not performing to potential.

Role of the School Environment

Because all children are not the same and do not respond to similar situations in the same way, it would be inappropriate to have only one type of learning environment. However, in American culture, the educational system mostly operates as traditional schools.

The philosophy of the traditional school is based in part on underlying assumptions that do not reflect what is known about how children learn. The first assumption is that children of the same age should learn the same material deemed to be necessary in a given amount of time and by the same method. The method most frequently used in the traditional classroom is verbal explanation and the use of written texts. The second assumption is that the teacher must be in charge of the learning process. This is based on the fear that a child who is left to select their own topics and methods for learning would waste time and fail to master basic skills. The third assumption implies that communication between children in the classroom is disruptive to the learning process.

In the traditional school it is therefore not surprising to find a specific curriculum that outlines what must be taught and how much should be mastered at each level. The teacher is there to provide lessons and determine whether learning has taken place. The environment is structured to maintain discipline and control by the teacher. The chairs are placed in rows facing the teacher, and children are expected to sit quietly as the teacher gives the lesson.

The traditional classroom meets the learning needs of many children; however, it does not meet the needs of all children. As discussed earlier, each child has a unique temperament that influences the child's best method of learning. The major flaw in the traditional classroom is the inability to address the individual learning needs of each child.

An alternative type of school environment that is becoming more popular in the United States is the open classroom. The open classroom stresses the role of both the child and teacher in the learning process. It is built on the underlying philosophy that the child has a natural desire to learn socially valued skills. The open classroom attempts to tap this natural desire by providing the child with a variety of interesting choices for learning. This requires that the classroom be arranged so that each child moves at a pace that is self-determined. The teacher becomes a facilitator of the child's learning. The child develops new skills by involvement with concrete materials and everyday problems. The child in this school develops skill in the formal school areas of reading, writing, math, geography, and science but is much more active in the learning process. The child has more opportunities to express feelings and creativity.

Each of these school environments has pros and cons, and one is not necessarily better than the other. What is important is that one may be better than the other for a particular child. In some instances, a child may do best in a school that uses a combination of these two environments.

Role of the Teacher

The child's teacher can and will influence the child's response to school, school performance, and overall development. Each teacher brings to the classroom a unique personality and beliefs about learning and past experiences that influence how the class and individual child will be approached. Each child will also respond to the teacher in a unique way. A child comes to school from a home environment that has become predictable. The child knows the response parents will have to particular behaviors. If the child's first teacher is similar to the parents, the child will find adjustment easier. If the teacher is quite different from the parents, the child may go through a time of self-doubt. The child must readjust to new teachers each year, and leaving a teacher the child has become attached to can be difficult.

Optimally, every teacher should be warm and encouraging, helping a child to become involved in learning and dealing with failures. The teacher should encourage individual initiative, self-esteem, and social responsibility through guidance, direction, and an ability to set standards and goals.

It has been hypothesized that a teacher's expectations, either high or low, may influence a child's performance independent of ability. Although this hypothesis has some support, it does not take into account all of the multiple variables that can and do influence school performance.[15] The teacher has an important role in school performance but should not be expected to foster learning in isolation of other variables. The teacher will be successful only if given support from the parents and school system.

Parental Role

Parents play a vital role in the educational development of the child. It is the parents who have a major influence on the child's emerging self-concept and self-esteem before school entry. The family, especially parents, have been the dominant influence in the child's life and will continue to be a vital force in the school years.

The home environment, including parent's income and educational level, is the most important factor in predicting the child's academic success. Also important are school-related variables, including curriculum, teachers, and organization of programs.

Along with parental income and educational level, the parents' actual behavior with the child influences school performance. Children sense parental evaluation of their abilities and try to live up to these expectations, whether they be high or low. Parents give messages to the child by their interest or lack of interest in school activities. A child who has a parent who takes the time to listen to a new experience or problem will do better than a child who gets no response. Children need positive reinforcement for their efforts.

Parents can help the child divide time between school activities and play. Initially, parents may require completion of school work before play. As the child develops a regular routine and becomes aware of the time needed for schoolwork, play may precede homework. Children spend less time doing homework than they do viewing television. The average television viewing time is 2 hours a day during the week and over 3 hours on weekends.

Optimal school performance requires adequate and regular sleep hours. Parents can maintain regular hours for meals and sleep based on the child's individual needs. Most importantly, parents need to stay informed about their child's progress by attending parent-teacher meetings and school activities.

The child's educational success depends on parental ability to provide encouragement, support, and guidance throughout the school years. This is a difficult task, especially for parents who have many stresses in their own lives. However, most parents have a desire to see their children succeed and, if given guidance, will do what is necessary to encourage this success (Fig. 15-4).

Parental guidance should include the need to help the child develop disciplined study habits. This can be accomplished by setting aside a specific area and time for this purpose. The parents should be available to assist the child as needed and review the child's work. Positive reinforcement is an important factor. Even in environments where there is limited space as well as limited quiet, private areas, parents can help the child develop study habits. This may require that the kitchen table be free for the child to use daily during specific times. The television should be off and disruptions kept to a minimum. Although all parents may not be able to provide an ideal physical environment for the development of study skills, they can provide consistent, reasonable expectations for the child related to school work.

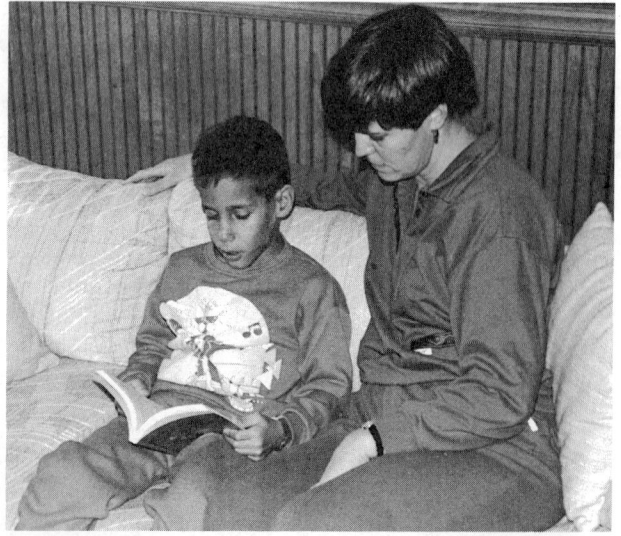

FIGURE 15-4
Parental involvement in school activities and homework is related positively to the child's educational success.

Nursing Implications

Assessing the child's adjustment to school and school performance requires an assessment of the multiple variables involved. Initially, parents and child may be asked how school is going. The nurse should be alert for both the parents' and child's response. Do they exhibit an interest and enthusiasm for school? Do they describe positive qualities of the classroom setting or teacher? Is there a desire to express areas of success? Do parents have an awareness of how the child is doing?

If school concerns are brought up or identified, a more in-depth evaluation is necessary as part of the problem-solving process. This evaluation should include determination of the child's temperament, presence of any learning disabilities, and subjective feelings about school and school performance. The evaluation can also involve parental involvement in school work, parental expectations, and parental attitudes toward school. The teacher and particular school environment should be evaluated in relation to the individual needs of the child.

Once the specific factors leading to poor school performance are identified, the nurse can assist parents in making the necessary changes that will promote optimal school performance. Parents may need assistance in finding a school program that meets the needs of the individual child. Parents may need assistance in redefining expectations or increasing involvement in school-related activities. Some children may need more concrete rewards for performance and concrete evidence of parental involvement. This may take the form of a chart on the refrigerator for encouragement of a specific activity. For example, a child who is having difficulty getting homework assignments done may get a star on a chart whenever homework is successfully completed. A predetermined number of stars can be rewarded. This system requires not only improvement by the child but also parental involvement through reviewing homework done.

Parents frequently reward children for good grades, which demonstrates the value parents place on success in the classroom. For some children this serves as a motivation to work hard. However, because the reward is so far removed from the work necessary to get the grade, small rewards for progress may be more helpful in motivating a child over time.

In planning strategies to improve school performance, the nurse must be aware of the importance of involving the child, parents, and teachers. The child, parents, and teacher must all be aware of the goals that are set and the method to be used to obtain the desired goals.

Promoting Cognitive Development Outside the Classroom

The child has many opportunities to use and develop cognitive skills outside the classroom. The school-age child is in Piaget's stage of concrete operations. The child learns best by seeing and doing. Through concrete experiences the child develops the concepts of reversibility, seriation, and classification.

The child needs opportunities to take things apart and put them together. This can be promoted by letting an older child take apart a broken clock and see the parts. Also, many hobby stores have kits for building and rebuilding working machines.

Classification abilities are promoted by starting a collection of stamps, coins, bottle caps, baseball cards, or dolls. Collections are very popular during the school years, and encouraging the child in this area is a way of fostering a natural desire.

Table games such as checkers, Monopoly, Chance, and others encourage decision-making skills and skill at developing strategies based on more than one piece of information. Allowing the child to be banker reinforces math skills. Following directions for a game is a pleasant way to learn how to follow directions.

Most activities the child is involved in will in some way enhance cognitive skills. Parents can play with the child or direct the child into an activity when bored. Long periods of television viewing instead of activities should be discouraged.

Language Development

Language continues to develop at a rapid pace throughout the school years. Sentence structures become more complex, and children use more adjectives and adverbs. They become skilled in opposites and realize that one word can have several meanings depending on how it is used. There is also an increase in the use of culturally specific words.

Reading is one of the most effective ways to promote language skills. Reading out loud to the child or having the child read to parents provides opportunities for the child to try new words and ask about their meanings. Introducing the child to the library early and taking the time to help the child select books is an important part of making learning a positive and enjoyable experience. During the school years the child can learn how to use a library and find books of specific interest, such as finding the collection related to hobbies.

Assessing, Promoting, and Maintaining Optimal Activity Levels

The benefits of activity during childhood are optimal growth, decreased risk of obesity, and decreased risk of cardiovascular disease.[4] Even though children tend to be more active than adults, evidence is accumulating that most children do not engage in activity of sufficient intensity, duration, or frequency to produce a protective effect against cardiovascular disease.[4]

According to a study by the U.S. Department of Health and Human Services, children in the United States are not developing the fitness skills necessary to maintain healthy bodies and healthy cardiorespiratory systems in adulthood.[28]

In a study of third to sixth grade children, researchers found that children were not involved in aerobic activity. The common belief that children are very active by nature is questionable. Children were found to be active but for short spurts rather than over a period of time necessary to have an aerobic effect.[4]

The increasingly sedentary lifestyles adopted by young children is a reflection of changes that have been occurring over the years: children ride the bus to school instead of walking; they watch television and play video games rather than participate in physical activities. School physical education programs focus on learning sports rather than skills that can be continued later in life. In fact, children may spend as little as 2 minutes of a physical education class engaging in physical exercise.

Now, more than ever, it is important that parents be assisted in providing or seeing that their children are involved in physical activities, both at school and at home. These activities must be adequate for the development of healthy bodies. They must start at an early age and continue throughout childhood and adolescence in such a manner that exercise will become a lifetime habit.

Parents may believe that children are meeting their activity needs through daily activities and school physical education programs. Because this is not the case, nurses must work with parents by providing information related to exercise needs and offer guidance in how these needs can be met. Haskell et al.[27] recommend that children's physical activity include an emphasis on the use of large muscles, dynamic exercise, moving the body over distance and against gravity, and developing flexibility. The intensity should be moderate to vigorous for 30 minutes a day in one or more sessions.

During the early school years the child can be taught games such as hide-and-seek, tag, dodge ball, and jump rope that encourage the use of large muscles and promote an increased heart rate for a period of time. Cycling, swimming, and climbing are also beneficial. A family team approach to fitness has been recommended.[13] This program involves both children and parents. This approach is based on the belief that children require parental support if they are to change eating and exercise patterns. Parents can benefit from health information in making behavior changes themselves, especially when they are trying to promote healthy activity patterns in children. Changes that occur are likely to be maintained longer if the whole family is involved.

Throughout the school year children should be encouraged to participate in some physical activity after school rather than watching television. Walking or riding bicycles to activity programs is better than being driven by parents (Fig. 15-5). Schools must also take responsibility for developing physical fitness skills. At a Senate hearing, Dr. Richard Schieken, a pediatric cardiologist, made the following statement:

More emphasis should be placed on learning the skills of sports that people will continue as life-long activities. There are after all only 40 kids in a school, sometimes of 5000, that are on the football team, and that leaves a lot of kids out in the stands sitting and watching, rather than participating in a sport that they can enjoy and that they can continue in later life.[28]

Play in the School Years

Play during the school years becomes more cooperative and facilitates the development of a sense of industry, self-esteem, improved coordination, and peer in-

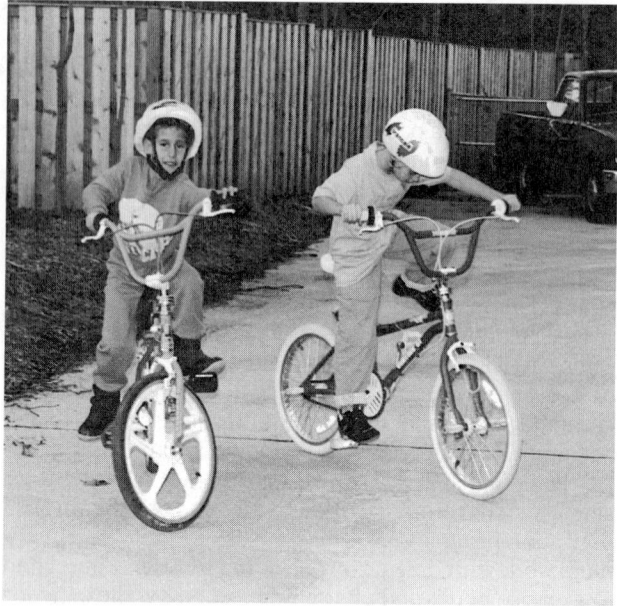

FIGURE 15-5
Outdoor activities that encourage physical activity are recommended for school-age children. Helmets are an important part of bike safety.

teractions. The school-age child's participation in a wide variety of activities is a reflection of the rapid developments occurring in all areas of growth. In the early school years children continue to enjoy playing with dolls, trucks, and cars and begin to prefer same-sex playmates. Motor development and coordination have progressed, and the child can begin to ride a bike, play kickball, or start dance lessons.

Middle-school–age children enjoy activities that reflect a growing sense of industry. They enjoy arts and crafts and making things for themselves and their parents and teachers. Cooking, woodworking, sewing, and building tree houses provide opportunities to use creativity and fine motor skills and to enjoy a sense of accomplishment.

Group activities that involve skill and competition promote cooperation, team effort, and group relationships. Activities such as baseball, kickball, and volleyball are enjoyed equally by boys and girls. Opportunity for physical activity is important after sitting in the classroom and is a constructive way of releasing anxiety and tension. Group sports activities improve coordination and refine both fine motor and gross skills. Children learn to deal with winning, losing, taking turns, being the best, and being the worst.

Learning to play an instrument or taking dance lessons, among other activities, promotes self-discipline and teaches the child that success is the result of hard work and practice. Play is an important factor in the development of school-age children and is therefore an important part of the nursing assessment.

Nurses should interview both children and parents regarding activities in which they participate. Parents benefit from a discussion of the relationship between play and development. The following questions related to play activities may be asked: What are the child's favorite activities? How often does the child engage in these activ-

ities? Do parents feel the amount of time spent in play activities is adequate or inadequate? In what school sports does the child participate?

Based on this assessment, the nurse can encourage parents to involve their child in age-appropriate activities that will foster development. A child who is unable to participate in more common activities because of size or physical disability may need assistance in finding those activities that provide opportunity for the development of a positive self-concept, motor skills, and peer relationships.

Competitive Sports During the School Years

Competitive sports during the school years have often been a concern of parents and health care professionals. The American Academy of Pediatrics makes the following recommendations concerning contact sports[2]:

Boxing has no place in programs for children of elementary school age because its goal is injury and because the educational benefits attributed to it can be realized through other sports. Sports with varying degrees of collision risk include baseball, basketball, ice hockey, soccer, softball, and wrestling. The hazards of such competition are debatable. The risks are usually associated with the conditions under which play and practice are conducted and the quality of supervision offered the participants.

Unless the school or community can provide exemplary supervision, medical and educational, it should not undertake a program of competitive sports, especially collision sports at the preadolescent level.

Well-designed sports programs can be valuable and enjoyable for school children. However, parents and other adults need to be aware that there are potentially inappropriate behaviors associated with sports.[46] See the display on the young athlete's bill of rights. Child health care professionals must consistently evaluate the child's exposure to sound programs of physical fitness. Physical exercise and fitness have known benefits for decreasing the risk of obesity, back problems, and cardiovascular disease.

Assessing, Promoting, and Maintaining School-Age Safety

The issue of safety during the school years continues to be important. The safety concerns that arise are a reflection of developmental changes that are occurring and the developmental tasks of this age group. The school-age child's developing sense of industry results in a desire to do such things as woodworking, chemistry experiments, carving, pottery, cooking, and other activities that involve the use of equipment that, if misused, can result in injury.

Although it is important that school-age children be given opportunities to try new and complex tasks, it is equally important that they receive adequate instruction and supervision. Ideally, parents should set aside specific times when the child can try one of these new activities

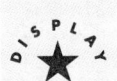

The Young Athlete's Bill of Rights

1. The right to have the opportunity to participate in sports regardless of one's ability level.
2. The right to participate at a level commensurate with the child's developmental level.
3. The right to have qualified adult leadership.
4. The right to participate in a safe and healthy environment.
5. The right of each child to share leadership and decision making.
6. The right to play as a child and not as an adult.
7. The right to proper preparation for participation in sports.
8. The right to equal opportunity to strive for success.
9. The right to be treated with dignity by all involved.
10. The right to have fun through sports.

From Strong, W. (1988). So what's good about sports? American Journal of Diseases of Children, 142, 143.

with direct supervision. Parents can use these opportunities to teach the child about the appropriate uses of equipment, how to store equipment, what precautions to take when using equipment, and the potential dangers associated with the equipment.

Additionally, the school-age child is ready to learn some basic first aid skills that may be necessary should an accident occur. For example, parents can instruct a child working with a chemistry set that the spillage of any substance on their clothes or skin should be washed off immediately with a stream of running water. A parent who takes opportunities to assist the child in their early attempts at new and complex tasks will feel more comfortable in allowing increasing independence as the child develops good safety habits.

The school-age child spend more time with peers and therefore less time in the home and with family. This transition to increasing independence brings with it potential risks for injury. Peer pressure in the form of taunts such "don't be a chicken" or "everyone else is going to do it" may influence a child to engage in a high-risk activity even though they are aware of the potential danger. Parents can talk to children about the difficult aspects of peer pressure and reinforce the need to stand up to peers when safety is the major concern. Parents can suggest to children that they use parental disapproval or lack of parental permission to avoid getting involved in an activity they feel uncomfortable about.

The school-age child frequently rides a bike to visit friends or deliver papers. Bicycle accidents account for a great number of injuries in this age group.[50] In one study, researchers[44] collected data on bicycle-related injuries among children seen in a children's hospital emergency department. In a 6-month period, 520 children were seen for bicycle-related injuries, accounting for 10% of trauma visits. Eighty percent of those seen were be-

tween the ages of 5 and 14. Most of the injuries occurred between 4:00 PM and 8:00 PM in clear weather conditions.[44] School-age children need to develop safe biking habits that optimally begin in the preschool years. Bike safety education of the school-age child should focus on riding in traffic, crossing streets, wearing appropriate clothing that can be seen at dawn and dusk, and wearing a helmet (see the display on safe bicycling). Prior to the school years the child generally does not have much experience with biking outside the driveway or without supervision. Many communities and local police stations offer bike safety courses. These courses are a valuable service and, when available, should be highly recommended to all parents. When purchasing a bike for the child, parents should choose one that is the right size and that the child can ride easily. Bikes should be well maintained. The following guidelines are recommended by the American Academy of Pediatrics[50]:

- The intended driver should be present so the bike can be properly sized.
- The child should be able to grasp the handbrake levers comfortably and easily apply sufficient pressure to brake the bike.
- The rider should be able to place the balls of both feet on the ground when seated on the bicycle.
- There should be approximately 1″ of clearance between the crotch and the center bar when the child straddles the bike with both feet on the ground.

The school-age child is also ready for and expected to learn how to behave during an emergency situation, including fires, tornadoes, hurricanes, and other disasters. Often these behaviors are taught in the school. It is important for parents to take the time to listen to the child who comes home from school and wants to share what has been learned. By listening to the child, parents give the child a message that they believe what has been learned is important. Further, they can reinforce the teaching by applying what the child has learned in the home environment. For example, the parent can ask the child which place in the house is safest during a tornado or what exits are available if a fire occurs.

Assessing, Promoting, and Maintaining Health Perception and Health Management

Many of parent's questions during the school years center around school performance and how to motivate the child in school. School is a very complex issue and involves many people, including parents, teachers, the child, peers, and various other people involved in the operation and decision-making process of schools. The first and most important step for the nurse in discussing school problems with parents is to encourage and allow parents to verbalize what their perception of the problem is: what they feel are underlying causes or associated factors related to the problem; what they have tried already in attempting to solve the problem; and their perceptions of why it has not worked. A thorough and systematic assessment of the situation is a necessity for the nurse to

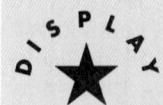

Safe Bicycling Starts Early

When a child receives his or her first bicycle, a lifelong pattern of vehicle operation is begun. A bike is not just a toy, but a vehicle that is a speedy means of transportation, subject to the same laws as motor vehicles.

TRAINING CHILDREN IN PROPER USE OF THEIR BICYCLES

1. Parents should set limits on where children may ride, depending on their age and maturity. Most serious injuries occur when the bicyclist is hit by a motor vehicle.
   a. Under age 8, children should ride only with adult supervision and off the street.
   b. The decision to allow older children to ride in the street should depend on traffic patterns, individual maturity, and an adequate knowledge and ability to follow the rules of the road.
2. Children must be provided with helmets (approved by ANSI or Snell) and taught to wear them on every ride, starting when they get their first bike.
3. The most important rules of the road for them to learn are:
   a. Ride with traffic.
   b. Stop and look both ways before entering the street.
   c. Stop at all intersections, marked and unmarked.
   d. Before turning, use hand signals and look all ways.
4. Children should be taught never to ride at dusk or in the dark. This is extremely risky, even for adults. Your child should be told to call home for a ride.
5. Children who ignore safety rules should be disciplined appropriately, such as by temporarily denying the use of the bike, to establish the significance of the misbehavior.
6. Children should learn how to keep their bikes in good repair, with the parents checking tires, brakes, seat and handlebar height annually.

From TIPP: The injury treatment program. *Copyright 1990, American Academy of Pediatrics.*

assist parents in the problem-solving process. By having parents go through the assessment process, the nurse will often find that they look at the problem in a new way or feel that the issues are clearer. Once the actual problem is identified, the nurse will be in a better position to offer parents advice or, if necessary, refer them for more specialized help.

Well-Care Visits

Health care visits continue annually during the school years. Parents will generally schedule these visits prior to the beginning of school or perhaps in the summer if the child goes to camp. Health visits during the school years should focus on all aspects of the child's physical and psychosocial development, school performance, nutrition and sleep, elimination, and activity patterns. Parents need opportunities to discuss concerns and any problems they identify.

The nurse should involve the child as an active participant in the assessment process. Questions about school, activities, nutrition, sleep, elimination, and exercise can be asked directly to the child. By involving children in the interview process, the nurse is encouraging children to think about health issues and their own health status. A child who states, "I do not exercise," may be asked if exercise is important for a child his or her age. This type of interaction provides an opportunity for the child to consider health promotion issues as well as an occasion for the nurse to provide information or correct misinformation. Parents may need encouragement to allow the child to attempt to answer questions before answering for them. Parents can then be given an opportunity to clarify the child's history and bring up concerns of their own. Increasing the child's responsibility for providing information and answering questions can be enhanced by seeing the 10- to 14-year-old child alone while parents are in the waiting area. This facilitates the transition to independent health care visits in the adolescent years.

Health Care

Health care needs during the school years center on health promotion and health education of children and families to enhance the development of life-long behaviors that result in optimal levels of wellness. Because well-care visits are infrequent during the school years, and the school-age child is relatively healthy, nurses need to go beyond the primary and acute care setting to have an impact on children's health.

The School Nurse

The role of the school nurse has changed considerably since the first school nurse, Lina Rogers Struthers, was placed in a New York City school in 1902.[51] The initial role of the school nurse was to prevent and control the spread of communicable disease. Eventually the role broadened to include early case finding, disease prevention, and promotion of health behaviors through education.[51,52] The purpose of school nursing today is "to enhance the educational process by the modification or removal of health related barriers to learning and by promotion of an optimal level of wellness."[3] School nursing is community based and family centered, and focuses on all levels of prevention.[14]

Ideally, the role of the school nurse should go beyond the tasks of providing first aid, controlling the spread of communicable disease, and teaching hygiene to include a variety of services that promote the optimal well-being of children, families, and school personnel. Rustia's[43] school health promotion model demonstrates an expanded role for nurses in meeting the complex health care needs of children within a school health program. This model emphasizes the need for an interdisciplinary approach, coordinated by a nurse who is knowledgeable of health and developmental needs of children and skilled in assessment, communication, program planning and evaluation, policy formation, and research. The model is presented in Figure 15-6.

Although the need for educated and specialized school nurses has increased, considerable variation still exists in school health services offered and educational requirements of school nurses.[1,51,52] The role of the school nurse in health management, health counseling, health education, program planning, and community liaison is an integral component of fostering optimal levels of wellness among school-age children. Nurses working in child health clinics, hospitals, and private offices need to be aware of the specific school health programs available to individual clients. When services are not available, the child health nurse can assume responsibility for the provision of the needs of individual children, families, and communities. For example, a nurse working in an acute care setting can discuss with parents the child's need to maintain school work and return to school as soon as possible. The nurse can work with teachers who have children with chronic illness in the classroom or meet the needs of a child following an acute illness. Child health nurses can serve as consultants to schools and offer educational programs related to health promotion for both children and staff. Nurses can support local and national efforts to mandate quality health programs within schools and to establish educational and certification requirements for school nurses or school nurse practitioners.

Dental Health

The first tooth is lost sometime around age 6, and permanent teeth come in at a rate of about four a year until the child is 12 or 13. Regular dental check-ups should occur every 6 months. Children who live in an area without fluorinated water should continue to take fluoride supplements (see Table 12-2 in Chap. 12). School-age children are able to assume responsibility for daily care of the teeth. Brushing after meals and snacks and flossing daily should be encouraged.

Latch Key Children

Between 2 and 5 million children aged 6 to 13 are at home alone and caring for themselves before and/or after school and during school holidays and vacations.[21]

Children who are home alone for all or part of the day are referred to as "latch-key" children. Another term, considered to be less stigmatizing is "self-care." The latch-key phenomenon is a reflection of a changing American society. Parents who work outside the home go to work before the child leaves for school and return home several hours after school is dismissed.

Although professionals have expressed concern about the welfare of latch-key children, few studies have been done to support or refute any negative effects of self-care.[53]

Studies[23,41] of children in rural areas demonstrated no differences among self-care children and their adult-care peers in academic achievement, school adjustment, fear of going outside, self-esteem, social adjustment, and interpersonal relations. Long and Long,[30] in studying children in a urban setting found latch-key children more fearful, more lonely and having more trouble with peer relationships and schoolwork than their adult-care peers. A more recent study[47] of suburban children in one of four after-school arrangements (home with mother, home alone, in a day care, or with a sitter) demonstrated no differences between latch-key and mother-care children in peer relationships, academic grades, test scores, conduct, and teacher ratings of social, emotional, and academic functioning. Children in day care or with sitters had more problems with peer relations and lower test scores. The researchers suggested that the children in day care may have been placed there because they were having difficulties rather than the day care precipitating the problems.[47] Day care issues are discussed in Chapter 14.

Hypothesized benefits of self-care include increased maturity, self-reliance, decision making, freedom, and responsibility.[24] There is a continued need for research related to children in self-care. Areas to be addressed are safety and emergency preparedness, age of the child and risk of injury or victimization, the availability of neighbors, and the effects of environment including urban, suburban, and rural areas.[55]

Current Alternatives for Latch-Key Children

There are an increasing number of nonacademic after-school programs for school-age children within school facilities. Some of these programs are free to everyone, whereas others charge a fee, making them more accessible to middle- and upper-class families.[53] More than 100 cities have instituted telephone call-in services for children at home in self-care.[26,49] Most calls made to these services by children have been related to boredom or loneliness; other issues include fear, homework, minor medical problems, and personal issues, such as getting along with siblings and school mates.[26,49] One program under study is a family day care check-in program.[33] This

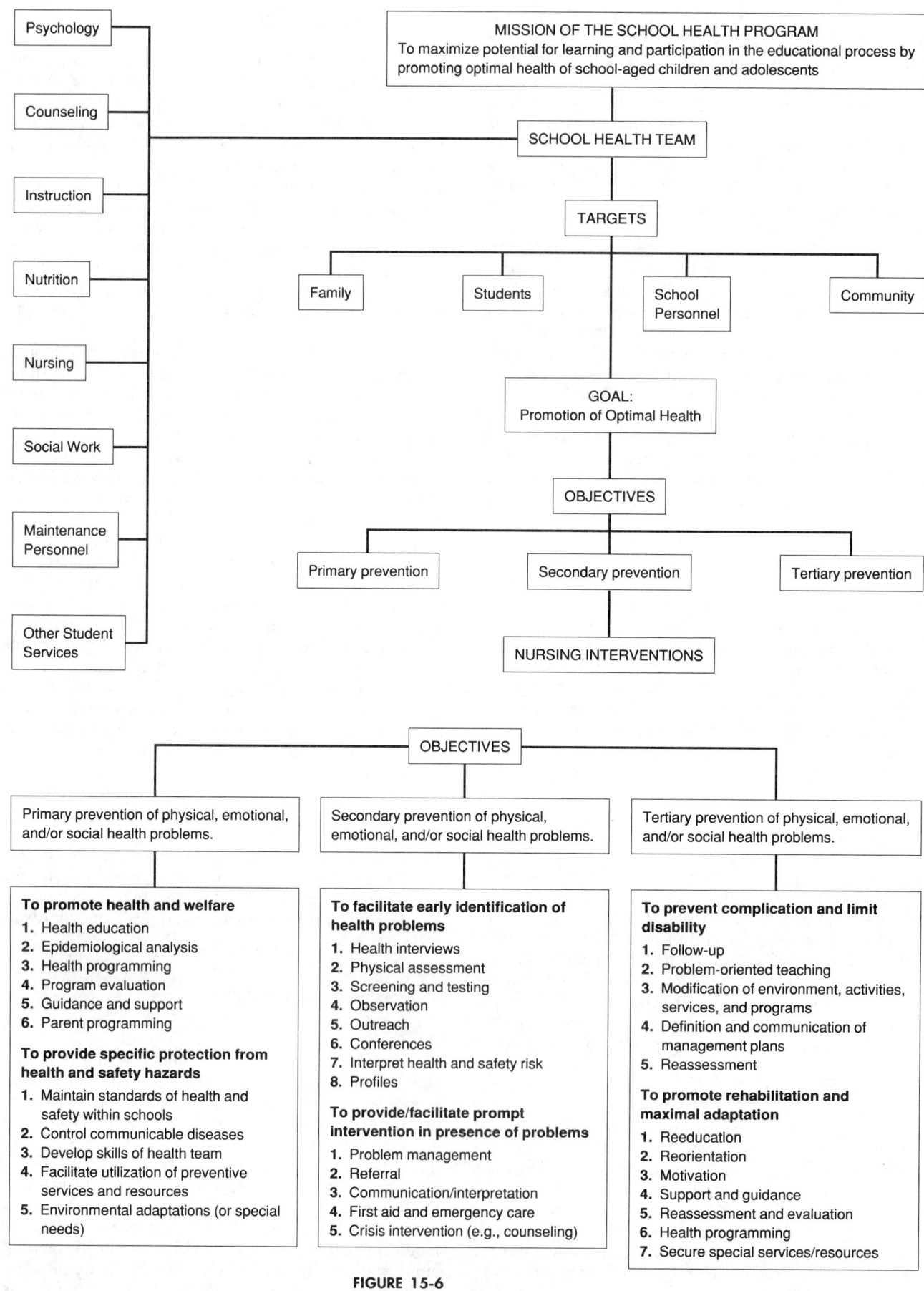

FIGURE 15-6
Rustia's school health promotion model.

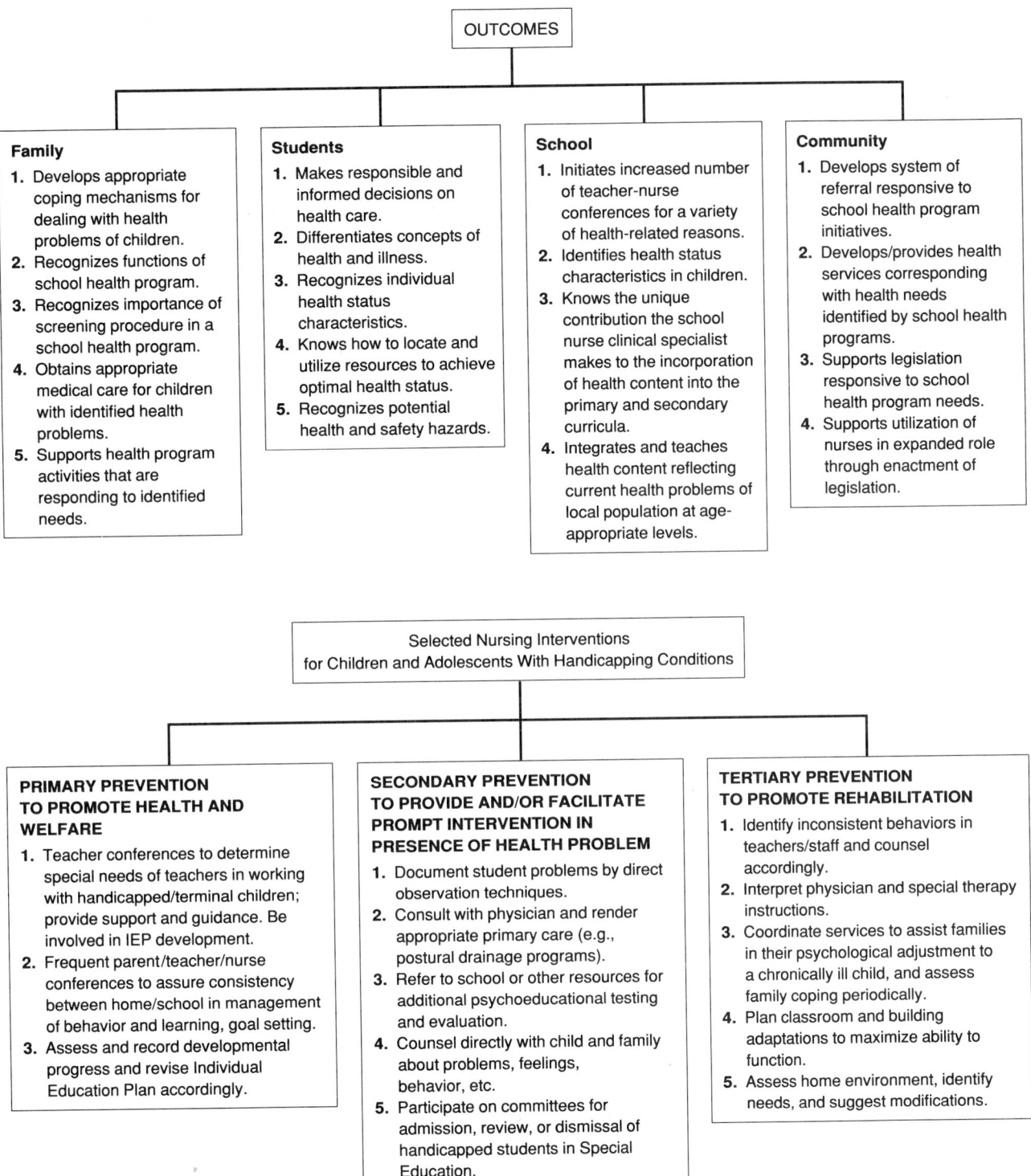

OUTCOMES

Family

1. Develops appropriate coping mechanisms for dealing with health problems of children.
2. Recognizes functions of school health program.
3. Recognizes importance of screening procedure in a school health program.
4. Obtains appropriate medical care for children with identified health problems.
5. Supports health program activities that are responding to identified needs.

Students

1. Makes responsible and informed decisions on health care.
2. Differentiates concepts of health and illness.
3. Recognizes individual health status characteristics.
4. Knows how to locate and utilize resources to achieve optimal health status.
5. Recognizes potential health and safety hazards.

School

1. Initiates increased number of teacher-nurse conferences for a variety of health-related reasons.
2. Identifies health status characteristics in children.
3. Knows the unique contribution the school nurse clinical specialist makes to the incorporation of health content into the primary and secondary curricula.
4. Integrates and teaches health content reflecting current health problems of local population at age-appropriate levels.

Community

1. Develops system of referral responsive to school health program initiatives.
2. Develops/provides health services corresponding with health needs identified by school health programs.
3. Supports legislation responsive to school health program needs.
4. Supports utilization of nurses in expanded role through enactment of legislation.

Selected Nursing Interventions for Children and Adolescents With Handicapping Conditions

PRIMARY PREVENTION TO PROMOTE HEALTH AND WELFARE

1. Teacher conferences to determine special needs of teachers in working with handicapped/terminal children; provide support and guidance. Be involved in IEP development.
2. Frequent parent/teacher/nurse conferences to assure consistency between home/school in management of behavior and learning, goal setting.
3. Assess and record developmental progress and revise Individual Education Plan accordingly.

SECONDARY PREVENTION TO PROVIDE AND/OR FACILITATE PROMPT INTERVENTION IN PRESENCE OF HEALTH PROBLEM

1. Document student problems by direct observation techniques.
2. Consult with physician and render appropriate primary care (e.g., postural drainage programs).
3. Refer to school or other resources for additional psychoeducational testing and evaluation.
4. Counsel directly with child and family about problems, feelings, behavior, etc.
5. Participate on committees for admission, review, or dismissal of handicapped students in Special Education.

TERTIARY PREVENTION TO PROMOTE REHABILITATION

1. Identify inconsistent behaviors in teachers/staff and counsel accordingly.
2. Interpret physician and special therapy instructions.
3. Coordinate services to assist families in their psychological adjustment to a chronically ill child, and assess family coping periodically.
4. Plan classroom and building adaptations to maximize ability to function.
5. Assess home environment, identify needs, and suggest modifications.

FIGURE 15-6 (Continued)

program provides for the after-school needs of the child but, in addition, allows for the child to visit with friends, spend time alone at home, as well as the family care center. This type of program is ideal for the child in upper elementary and junior high schools. These children may not need to be under constant observation of an adult, but like their peers who have parents home, they do need guidance, supervision, and an adult to turn to. A designated family care center within the neighborhood offers

such supervision. The child and parents determine what the child can do in advance and, after checking in at the family care center, the child may go to the library, playground, friend's house, or other predetermined activity. The child is free to return to the family care center at any time.

For children who are at home in self-care, efforts have been made to provide training programs related to emergencies, including cuts, fires, and weather; dealing with strangers, including answering the phone and door when alone; and safe daily habits after school, including choosing nutritious snacks and safety issues in food preparation.[37] Training programs require support from parents as well as reinforcement over time, especially in the area of emergencies.

Nursing Implications

Nurses should discuss with parents the school-age child's care after school. Parents who express concern for the child who is home alone benefits from a discussion of factors to consider when contemplating leaving a child alone. Parents need to first consider the maturity level of the child and how much time the child can handle alone. The environment needs to be safe, and the child should have phone access to a neighbor or friend in addition to parents. Before a child is left alone, he or she should demonstrate some basic skill in handling emergencies, including being able to describe what should be done in case of fire, tornado, or accident. The child should be able to remember 911 or the phone numbers for fire, police, and medical assistance. It is important that the child know what information to give in an emergency, including name, address, and nature of the problem. Personal safety can be enhanced by teaching the child how to answer the phone or door when alone. The child can be taught to say that parents are unable to come to the phone rather than saying parents are not at home. Children at home benefit from a plan of activities during the time they are alone. This may include chores, homework, or selected activities with friends in the neighborhood.

The nurse can also assist parents in finding alternative care arrangements by providing a list of after-school programs in the area.

Television Viewing During the School Years

American children spend more time in front of a television than in the classroom.[54] In a review of research findings of television's impact on children, Zuckerman and Zuckerman[54] found several areas of concern. The most frequently stated concern relates to violence on television and its relationship to children's aggressive behavior. According to the Neilsen Index, a child watches 18,000 murders on television before graduating from high school.[42] Children are also frequently watching other violent activities, including bombings, beatings, and torture. Research has consistently demonstrated that violence on television has a negative impact on children.[54] Another area of concern is the child's exposure to prejudice and stereotypes on television. Minority groups and women are frequently portrayed in stereotypic roles.[54] For example, nonwhite characters tend to be depicted as criminals and victims and dominated by whites. Women tend to be dominated by men, and women in traditional roles are depicted more favorably than women in nontraditional roles, for example, employed women are more often portrayed as villains than are homemakers. This type of

television portrayal can have implications for the child's developing attitudes toward minority groups and women as well as on the child's developing self-esteem if they are a member of one of these groups.[54]

Concern has also been focused on the impact of television on children's school performance and reading skills. This area has not been studied as much as violence has, and preliminary findings suggest that television does not have an impact on these areas.[54]

The relationship between television advertising and health behaviors is a major concern. Even though the school-age child develops in ability to understand commercials, most children believe the commercials they watch provide accurate information.[54] Studies on the impact of television commercials generally support the concern that children's attitudes toward food, health products, and medicine are influenced by television.[54]

Children's television viewing plays a role in development of lifestyle patterns and health behaviors. Although television can have a positive impact on children, current prime time programming reflects more negative behaviors.

Child health professionals should address the issue of television and its impact on children with individual parents as well as in the community. Zuckerman and Zuckerman[54] suggest that parents be encouraged to limit the number and kinds of programs children watch and become selective viewers themselves. Parents can also discuss alternative plots with children that demonstrate effective problem solving and alternatives to violence. Programs that emphasize cooperation, such as "Mr. Rogers," and Saturday morning programs that demonstrate positive problem-solving behaviors, including helping or assertive nonaggressive behaviors, can influence children's behavior in positive ways.[54]

Summary

The school years bring many changes for the child. The child's world expands as a result of entry into school and the development of relationships with peers, teachers, and other adults. Cognitive abilities expand, and the school-age child is receptive to learning skills in areas such as reading, writing, math, history, and science. In addition, the child is developing a lifestyle that will impact the quality of health throughout the life cycle. The child has increasing control in food selection, activity, personal safety, and daily behavior patterns that influence health. Opportunities for nurses to influence the healthy development of the child are predominately in the community environment. The emphasis of nursing during the school years is on health promotion.

The school years are important years for the development of lifestyle patterns that maintain and promote health. Decreasing the multiple risk factors associated with common adult diseases is a major goal of child health professionals during the school years.

Child health nurses can become involved in health promotion of school children by becoming involved in school and community programs. Nurses can become involved in the development of after-school, health pro-

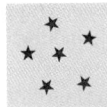

Ideas for Nursing Research

The nurse who is involved with school-age children has an opportunity to explore a variety of well-child concern with both the children and their parents. This is an exciting time of growth and maturation beyond the family. The following areas need to be explored.

- Where school-age children learn about factors that influence the development of healthy lifestyle patterns.
- Reliability of the school-age child as a historian concerning developmental issues.
- Risk of latch-key children for injury compared to their peers whose parents are at home.
- Perception of child health nurses as to their role, including health education in the school and community setting.

motion, and fitness programs for school-age children. Groups geared toward the school-age child such as Girl Scouts, Boy Scouts, sports teams, and school clubs provide a forum for nurses to discuss health behaviors with children, parents, and youth workers.

References

1. American Academy of Pediatrics, Committee on School Health. (1987). Qualifications and utilization of nursing personnel delivery: Health services in schools. *Pediatrics, 79*(4), 647–648.
2. American Academy of Pediatrics. (1977). *Standards of child health care* (3rd ed.). Elk Grove, IL: Author.
3. American Nurses Association. (1983). *Standards of school nursing practice.* Kansas City, MO: Author.
4. Baranowski, T., Tsong, Y., Cieslek, C., & Nader, P. (1987). Aerobic physical activity among third-to-sixth-grade children. *Journal of Developmental and Behavioral Pediatrics, 8,* 203–206.
5. Beal, V. (1980). *Nutrition in the life span.* New York: John Wiley & Sons.
6. Bettelheim, B. (1985). Punishment vs discipline. *Atlantic Monthly, 256,* 51–59.
7. Burton, B., & Foster, W. (1988). *Human nutrition* (4th ed.). New York: McGraw-Hill.
8. Carey, W. B., Fox, M., & McDevitt, S. (1977). Temperament as a factor in early school adjustment. *Pediatrics, 60,* 621.
9. Chess, S. (1968). Temperament and learning ability of school children. *American Journal of Public Health, 58,* 2231.
10. Christophersen, E. (1982). Incorporating behavioral pediatrics into primary care. *Pediatric Clinics of North America, 29*(2), 261–296.
11. Coble, P., Kupfer, D., Reynolds, C., & Houck, P. (1987). EEG sleep of healthy children 6 to 12 years of age. In C. Guilleminault (Ed.). *Sleep and its disorders in children.* New York: Raven Press.
12. Coopersmith, S. (1981). *The antecedents of self-esteem.* Palo Alto, CA: Consulting Psychologist Press.
13. Crockett, S. (1987). The family team approach to fitness: A proposal. *Public Health Reports, 102*(5), 546–551.
14. Edwards, L. (1987). The school nurse's role in school-based clinics. *Journal of School Health, 54*(4), 157–159.
15. Epps, E., & Smith, S. (1984). School and children: The middle childhood years. In Collins, A. (Ed.). *Development during middle childhood: The years from six to twelve.* Washington, DC: National Academic Press.
16. Erikson, E. (1963). *Childhood and society.* New York: W. W. Norton.
17. Evans, M., & Cronin, F. (1986). Diets of school-age children and teenagers. *Family Economics Review, 3,* 14–21.
18. Ferber, R. (1987). Circadian and schedule disturbances. In C. Guilleminault (Ed.). *Sleep and its disorders in children.* New York: Raven Press.
19. Ferber, R. (1985). *Solve your child's sleep problems.* New York: Simon and Schuster.
20. Food and Nutrition Service. (1986). Code of regulations: 7 parts (Report No. 210–299, p. 18). Washington, DC: US Department of Agriculture.
21. Fosanelli, P. (1984). Latch key children. *Journal of Developmental and Behavioral Pediatrics, 5,* 173–177.
22. Frank, A., Vaden, A., & Martin, J. (1987). School health promotion: Child nutrition programs. Journal of School Health 57(10), 451–460.
23. Galambos, N., & Garbarino, J. (1983). Identifying the missing links in the study of latch key children. *Children Today, 12,* 2–4; 40–41.
24. Garbarino, J. (1980). Latch key children: Getting the short end of the stick. *Vital Issues, 30*(3), 1–4.
25. Gortmaker, S., Dietz, W., Sobol, A., & Wehler, C. (1987). Increasing pediatric obesity in the United States. *American Journal of Diseases of Children, 141,* 535–540.
26. Guerey, L., & Moore, L. (1983). Phone friend: A prevention-oriented service for latch key children. *Children Today, 12,* 5–10.
27. Haskell, W., Montoge, H., & Orenstein, D. (1985). Physical activity and exercise to achieve health-related physical fitness components. *Public Health Reports, 100*(2), 202–211.
28. Hearing on Child Health and Fitness. (1985). Senate Labor and Human Resource Committee (99th Congress): Selected Hearings Nos. 251–296 (p. 3). Washington, DC: US Government Printing Office.
29. Johnson, D., & Johnson, R. (1985). Nutrition educator: A model for effectiveness, a synthesis of research. *Journal of Nutrition Education, 17*(2), 51–544.
30. Long, T., & Long, L. (1982). *Latch key children: The child's view of self care.* Washington, DC: Catholic University. (ERIC Document Reproduction Service No. ED 211 229).
31. Maccoby, E. (1984). Middle childhood in the context of the family. In A. Collins (Ed.). *Development during middle childhood: The Years from Six to Twelve.* Washington, DC: National Academic Press.
32. McBean, L. (1988). Nutrition and the school age child. *Dairy Council Digest, 59*(2), 7–11.
33. McKnight, J., & Shelsby, B. (1984). Checking-in: An alternative for latch key kids. *Children Today, 13,* 23–25.
34. Morgan, K., Zabik, M., & Leveille, G. (1981). The role of breakfast in nutrient intake of 5 to 12 year-old children. *American Journal of Clinical Nutrition, 34,* 1418.
35. Ordog, G., Wasserberger, J., Schatz, I., Owens-Collins, D., English, K., Balasubramanian, S., & Schlater, T. (1988). Gunshot wounds in children under 10 years of age. *American Journal of Diseases of Children, 142,* 618–622.
36. Parcel, G., Simons-Morton, B., O'Hara, N., Baranowski, T., Kolbe, L., & Bee, D. (1987). School promotion of healthful diet and exercise behavior: An integration of organizational change and social learning theory interventions. *Journal of School Health, 57*(4), 150–156.
37. Petterson, L. (1984). The "safe at home" game: Training comprehensive prevention skills in latch key children. *Behavior Modification, 8*(4), 474–494.

38. Pipes, P. (1989). *Nutrition in infancy and childhood* (4th ed.). St. Louis: Times Mirror/Mosby.

39. Pollitt, E., Leibel, R. L., & Greenfield, D. (1981). Brief fasting, stress, and cognition in children. *American Journal of Clinical Nutrition, 35,* 1526.

40. Pollitt, E., Lewis, N. L., Garza, C., & Shulman, R. J. (1982/1983). Fasting and cognitive function. *Journal of Psychiatric Research, 17,* 169.

41. Rodman, H., Pratto, D., & Nelson, R. (1985). Child care arrangements and children's functioning: A comparison of self-care and adult-care children. *Developmental Psychology, 21*(3), 413–418.

42. Rothenberg, M. (1975). Effects of television violence on children and youth. *Journal of the American Medical Association, 234,* 1043–1046.

43. Rustia, J. (1982). Rustia school health promotion model. *Journal of School Health, 52*(2), 108–114.

44. Selbst, S., Alexander, D., & Ruddy, R. (1987). Bicycle related injuries. *American Journal of Diseases of Children, 141,* 140–144.

45. Shonkoff, J. (1984). The biological substrate of physical health in middle childhood. In A. Collins (Ed.), *Development during middle childhood: The years from six to twelve.* Washington, DC: National Academy Press.

46. Strong, W. (1988). So what's good about sports? *American Journal of Diseases of Children, 127,* 143.

47. Vandell, D., & Corasaniti, A. (1988). The relation between third graders after-school care and social, academic, and emotional functioning. *Child Development, 59,* 868–875.

48. Weiss, E., & Kien, L. (1987). A synthesis of research on nutrition education at the elementary school level. *Journal of School Health, 57*(1), 8–12.

49. Williams, R., & Fosarelli, P. (1987). Telephone call-in services for children in self-care. *American Journal of Diseases of Children, 141,* 965–968.

50. Wishon, P., & Oreskovich, M. (1986). Bicycles, roller skates and skateboards: Safety promotion and accident prevention. *Children Today, 15,* 11–15.

51. Wold, S. (1981). *School nursing: A framework for practice.* St. Louis: C.V. Mosby.

52. Zanga, J., & Oda, D. (1987). School health services. *Journal of School Health, 57*(10), 413–416.

53. Zigler, E., & Hall, N. (1988). Day care and its effect on children: An overview for pediatric health professionals. *Journal of Developmental and Behavioral Pediatrics, 9*(1), 38–45.

54. Zuckerman, D., & Zuckerman, B. (1985). Television's impact on children. *Pediatrics, 75*(2), 233–240.

55. Zylke, J. (1988). Among latch key children problems: Insufficient day-care facilities, data on possible harm. *Journal of the Aerican Medical Association, 260*(23), 3399–3400.

16

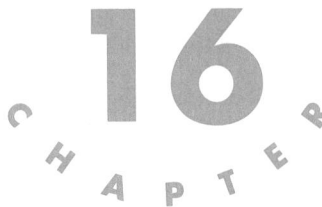

Health Assessment, Promotion, and Maintenance for Adolescents

FEATURES OF THIS CHAPTER

Nursing Assessment: Observation of Behaviors That Reflect a Developing Sense of Identity, Table 16-1

Nursing Assessment: Questions for Assessing the Adolescent's Attainment of Developmental Tasks, Table 16-2

Teaching Plan: Sexuality Concerns of a 14-Year-Old Female Client

Ideas for Nursing Research

BEHAVIORAL OBJECTIVES

Describe patterns of development of adolescents related to nutrition, sleep, elimination, psychosocial development, cognitive development, and safety.

Identify common concerns of adolescents related to development.

Identify common concerns of parents related to adolescent development.

Describe nursing assessment approaches with adolescents and parents.

Describe nursing interventions to assist adolescents in attaining optimal development.

Describe nursing interventions to assist parents of adolescents deal with common concerns.

Discuss risk-taking behaviors of the adolescent.

Describe the role of the nurse in interviewing, counseling, and teaching the adolescent and parents.

The adolescent years span from the age of 11 or 12 through age 19 or into the 20's for some youths. These age ranges are arbitrary and may vary among cultures.[13] The extension of adolescence into the 20's may be the result of advanced education, including graduate school or professional training, that continues familial economic dependence and postponement of career decisions.

The adolescent years are eventful years in development that may bring about concerns and problems for the individual adolescent and family. Because adolescence can span a period of 10 years, it is important to realize that a 14-year-old adolescent has very different needs than a 17-year-old. The concept of developmental phases during the adolescent years is important because it emphasizes the differences between the older and young adolescent. The adolescent years are frequently divided into three distinct phases: early adolescence (ages 11 to 14 years), middle adolescence (ages 15 to 17 years), and late adolescence (ages 17 to 19 or later). This delineation by chronologic age only serves as a guideline, and there is much overlap between phases. For example, one 15-year-old person may clearly still be in early adolescence, whereas another 15-year-old may be in late adolescence.

Each phase brings new challenges to the adolescent and parents. There are some specific developmental tasks for the adolescent during each phase. Keep in mind that although a developmental task is prominent at one time does not mean it does not continue on another level throughout the adolescent years.

Tasks of the adolescent years include the following:

- Maintaining adequate nutrition, sleep, and activity to support rapid rate of physical growth.
- Developing a personal identity.
- Accepting and achieving comfort with body image.
- Achieving independence from parents.
- Developing a personal value system.
- Developing a relationships with peers.
- Achieving control and expression of sexual drives.
- Preparing for a productive role in society.
- Avoiding potentially self-destructive behaviors.
- Actively participating in health promotion behaviors.

During the adolescent years, parents may feel more isolated or alienated from their offspring. However, parents continue to have an important role in promoting development. Parents often anticipate the adolescent years with anxiety and concern about how they will be able to deal with a child who is going through some significant developmental changes. As with previous stages of development, parents should first be aware of the tasks facing the adolescent. Parents also should be aware of their role in assisting the adolescent in forming a personal identity, in supporting the adolescent's coping with a rapidly changing body image, and in fostering the development of a personal value system. Parents must also allow for increasing independence, and support the adolescent's pursuit of educational or work goals, or both. Parents may be confronted with difficult situations related to sexuality, independence, and a developing value system. Both parents and adolescents need support, encouragement, and, at times, assistance from a person outside the situation as they cope with the multiple issues that can arise during the adolescent years. These issues are discussed throughout this chapter.

Parental responsibilities during adolescence include the following:

- Identifying personal beliefs about adolescence.
- Identifying fears and concerns related to adolescent development.
- Determining parental expectations of the adolescent.
- Using effective communication skills with the adolescent.
- Assisting the adolescent in meeting developmental tasks.
- Anticipating potential areas of conflict before they arise.
- Deciding on methods to be used to deal with conflicts.
- Discussing approaches to deal with common parental concerns.

- Identifying resources to assist parents or adolescents with problems that arise.

Parents may need support in dealing with an adolescent who seems suddenly to be so different from the child they knew. Parents may wonder why the adolescent spends so much time with peers, demands independence, or is critical of parental beliefs or lifestyle. Parents benefit from anticipatory guidance in relation to adolescent development and suggestions on how to increase the adolescent's sense of responsibility for personal well-being while maintaining some influence over their development. As adolescents grow, they still need parents to help them set limits, offer support, and praise them for their successes.

Assessing, Promoting, and Maintaining Optimal Nutrition

The adolescent years bring changes in physical, social, emotional, and cognitive spheres, all of which impact on dietary practices of adolescents. Since birth, the infant and then the child gains increasing control over food consumption. The adolescent years bring an increasing desire for independence, and food habits reflect decreasing parental influence over food choices and food consumption. The adolescent may be spending more time away from home, and more meals are eaten outside the home.

Nutrition and Adolescent Growth

The rate of growth during adolescence is second only to infancy (see display for nutritional profile). Failure to consume necessary requirements for this period of rapid growth can potentially retard growth and delay sexual maturity. Significant increases in most nutrients are necessary during rapid growth (see Chap. 8). Energy and nutrient requirements need to be assessed for each adolescent. Energy requirements are recommended in ranges by the Food and Nutrition Board of the National Academy of Sciences, National Research Council, to account for this variation in growth rates (see RDA tables in Appendix).

Assessing Adolescent Growth

Assessing adequacy of growth during adolescence is more difficult than in previous years. Chronologic age is a poor reference point because of the variability of growth among adolescents of the same age. This variability among adolescents also decreases the usefulness of the National Center for Health Statistics growth grids (see Appendix: Growth Charts). Skeletal age determinations are the most accurate means of evaluating maturation. However, this requires radiographs that are expensive and not always available. Tanner,[31] using mixed longitudinal studies, developed a classification of maturity based on secondary sex characteristics. Changes in secondary sex characteristics coincide with skeletal age and are of great value in assessing adolescent growth. Regardless of early

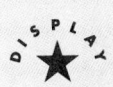

Developmental Nutritional Profile of the Adolescent

PUBERTY–EARLY ADOLESCENT

- Rapid growth, boys gain more weight and height than girls.
- Constantly hungry.
- Companionship desired with meals.

LATE ADOLESCENT

- Growth has subsided.
- Full stature almost attained.
- Food requirements approaching adult level.
- Companionship desired with meals.

Adapted from Kennedy-Caldwell, C., & Caldwell, M. (1986). Pediatric Enteral Nutrition. In Rombeau, J., & Caldwell, M. (Ed.). Parenteral nutrition: Clinical nutrition (Vol II.). Philadelphia: Saunders, 443–479.

or late development, the sequence of events is closely adhered to, and there is a close relationship between growth in height and organ development (see Chap. 66).

Regular assessments of secondary sex characteristics are most valuable when repeated over time, allowing the nurse to observe changes from one stage to another. However, assessment of sex characteristics is useful even if the child is seen only once. Other parameters, including measurement of skin folds, hematocrit, and hemoglobin, are also useful in the nutritional assessment of adolescents.

Eating Patterns of Adolescents

Meal skipping, between-meal snacking, and eating outside the home are typical adolescent eating behaviors. These food habits are related to the adolescent's increased involvement in activities outside the home. Adolescent involvement in work, school, and social activities may increase the number of fast foods they consume.

Snacking. Snacking is a major characteristic of adolescent eating behavior. Adolescents appear to be eating constantly, and a common concern is that between-meal snacking will decrease appetite for regular meals. In fact, between-meal snacking makes a significant contribution to the total nutritional needs of adolescents, if food items are chosen carefully. Snack food choices are important— selecting cheese, raw vegetables, fresh fruit, or yogurt rather than cookies, donuts, candy, and potato chips will meet the energy and nutritional needs of a rapidly growing adolescent. Because most of the foods consumed by the adolescent continue to come from the home food supply,[8] parents have an opportunity to influence the quality of the adolescent's diet. Parents who provide foods that contribute nutrients and are low in fat, sugar, and sodium provide a high-quality diet for the adolescent. Having nutritious snacks readily available will increase the likelihood that they will be chosen. If carrots and

celery are already cut up in the refrigerator, the adolescent may choose them. However, if they must prepare these foods themselves, they may instead select cookies.

Fast Foods. A study done by Shannon and Parks[27] found that most people do not frequent fast food restaurants enough to influence their diet significantly. They found that fast foods have nutrient inadequacies and caloric excess due to both limited menu choice and customer selection. Nutritious alternatives are increasing with the introduction of salad bars in many fast food restaurants. The addition of a salad to a typical fast food meal of hamburger, french fries, and soda increases nutritional value. Likewise, the introduction of breakfast foods has improved overall nutritional value of fast food menus. Even adolescents with specific dietary restrictions related to diabetes can sometimes opt for fast food if the meal is chosen carefully.[9] Helping adolescents select foods of nutritional value rather than trying to keep them out of fast food chains should be the goal of nutritional education (Fig. 16-1). Information is available to nurses to supply authoritative data on the nutritional value of individual foods.[21]

Body Image and Adolescent Nutrition

Body image is the picture of our body formed in our mind. Body image changes as adolescents go through rapid and dramatic growth in their physical, emotional, and social selves. Adolescents are extremely concerned with the normalcy of their physical status. They are concerned with how they appear in the eyes of others and endlessly compare themselves with their peers. A study of 326 adolescent girls found an exaggerated concern with obesity regardless of their body weight or knowledge of nutrition.[18] Underweight, overweight, and normal-weight subjects reported dieting to lose weight and frequent self-weighing behavior. As many as 51% of the girls that were underweight expressed fear of becoming overweight.[18] Searching for the ''body beautiful,'' the body that fits their ideal body image, makes adolescents easy prey for many useless products and harmful body-building and weight-loss programs. Promises of quick weight reduction or enhanced muscle development are difficult for adolescents to resist. In addition, such behaviors as binging and vomiting may lead to significant health risks (see Chap. 19 for a discussion of anorexia and bulimia).

The time spent with peers frequently centers around eating and is an important part of the socialization process. Peers have an important role in influencing the adolescent. The peer group defines what is socially acceptable and sets standards. Being like others and fitting into the group influence dietary practices of adolescents. If peers are going to a fast food restaurant, staying behind or bringing a nutritious lunch may not enhance one's position in the group. Even adolescents who have developed healthy nutritional practices may change habits when with peers.[29] For example, an adolescent who drinks milk at home may choose a soft drink when with peers.

Nursing Implications

Allowing the adolescent to express concerns related to growth or lack of growth is vital to the nurse who

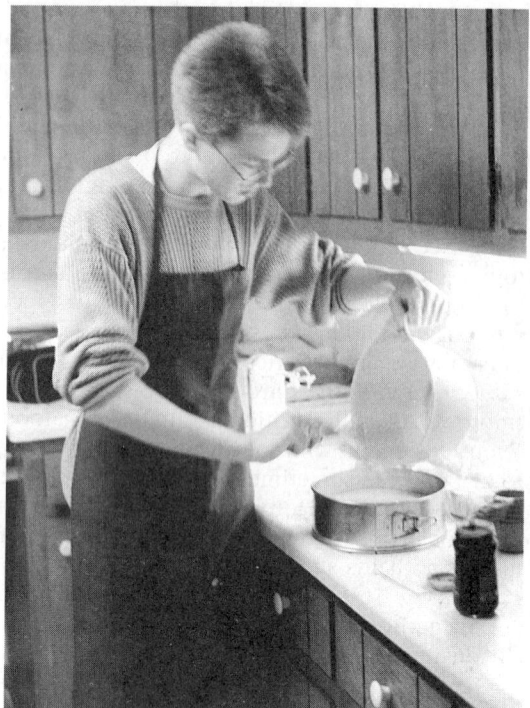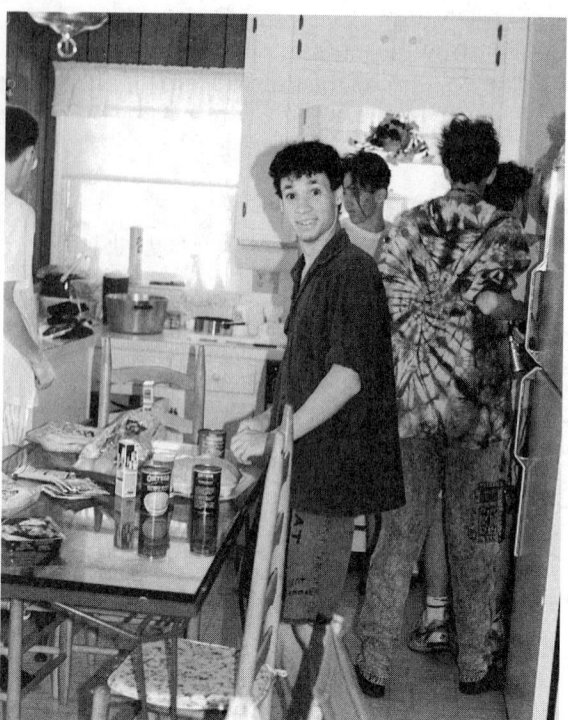

FIGURE 16-1
Young people learn about nutrition by cooking for themselves. When nutritional foods are supplied, adolescents will have fun together preparing wholesome meals.

chooses to work with adolescents. Telling late-developing adolescents that they need not worry, they will "catch up," does not address the concerns the adolescent has about being like peers. An approach of being sensitive to these feelings and not passing them off as foolish worries is needed for a relationship to develop.

Assessment is the first step in promoting healthy eating patterns during adolescence. The nurse who interviews the adolescent should have a sincere and concerned attitude that is nonjudgmental. Adolescents quickly pick up responses and reactions of others to their personal concerns and will quickly shut off communication if they feel the person they are speaking with does not care, ignores what they are saying, or appears to have little understanding of their concerns.

Assessment should include the adolescent's perception of present diet, body weight, height, and stage of pubertal development. This assessment will identify areas of concern for the adolescent. Even though these concerns may seem foolish to the nurse, they must be taken seriously because they have a major impact on adolescent behavior. Assessment should also include adolescent eating patterns, food choices, the relationship of food to health and growth, and how the adolescent deals with concerns that may include obesity, short stature, or early or late pubertal development. Smoking, alcohol, and drug behaviors are important to nutrition during the adolescent years and should be evaluated even if the adolescent does not "appear" to engage in them.

After the assessment the nurse must take time to sit with the adolescent in a private area and talk about concerns. Simply telling an adolescent that fears are un-founded, that he or she is perfectly normal, will not necessarily relieve fears. Acknowledging that fears are normal and that most adolescents have them will decrease feeling of being different or abnormal. Sharing information about patterns of development, showing the adolescent where he or she is in relation to norms, and telling the adolescent what to expect in the future may help allay some fears.

The adolescent who is at risk for inadequate nutritional intake owing to the use of fad diets or useless gadgets needs to have an explanation of why these products should not be used; more importantly, the adolescent must be given a substitute method of obtaining the goal they seek. Using the nursing process to help the adolescent meet personal goals through healthy dietary practices requires assessment, goal setting, the development of a plan to meet goals, and a preestablished method for evaluating progress. However, the success of this approach depends on the nurse's ability to involve the adolescent in every part of the process. For example, an obese adolescent who desires to lose weight will need assistance in assessing current dietary practices as well as setting goals and planning strategies for a healthy weight reduction program. Helping the adolescent set realistic goals and providing support as the adolescent attempts to obtain goals requires the support of not only the nurse but also parents.

Parental Role

Parents must also have an opportunity to talk with the nurse and express their concerns. These concerns may include unhealthy eating patterns, consumption of junk foods, frequent eating at fast food restaurants, and binge dieting, as well as binging and vomiting. Parental support will be necessary in helping the adolescent obtain goals or cope with feelings of insecurity or being different as puberty develops. Parents should be involved in supporting the obese adolescent's efforts at weight loss or the adolescent's attempts to improve nutritional patterns. For example, after initial discussion and goal setting with the adolescent for weight reduction, the parent should be involved in planning how these goals can be met. Because the home continues to be the main source of food, parents may need to change food-purchasing activities to assist the adolescent in reaching desired goals. The adolescent will also need parental support in following the diet plan and reaching goals through positive reinforcement.

Assessing, Promoting, and Maintaining Optimal Elimination

Elimination patterns during adolescence are well established. The adolescent has few problems with bowel and bladder function but may have complaints of constipation. Constipation during adolescence is frequently related to inadequate fluid intake, inadequate intake of dietary roughage, frequent ignoring of defecating urge, and irregular stooling patterns.[14] When an adolescent complains of constipation, these factors should be evaluated, and education of the adolescent in changing behaviors to promote normal elimination patterns should follow. More serious conditions related to elimination, including Crohn's disease and ulcerative colitis, often have their onset during adolescence[14] (see Chap. 59 for discussion of these conditions).

Assessing, Promoting, and Maintaining Optimal Sleep

During the adolescent years, sleep patterns continue to mature and the adolescent develops adult sleep cycles. Parents note increasing sleepiness during the day, increased difficulty in waking the adolescent in the morning, and the adolescent's preference for staying up late at night.

Sleep Disturbances

Difficulty getting to sleep and periods of wakefulness during the night emerge in the adolescent years and may continue into the adult years. In a study of 639 adolescents, researchers found that 49.8% of the sample had no reported sleep disturbances, 37.6% experienced occasional sleep disturbances, and 12.6% reported chronic or severe sleep disturbances.[23] Students who reported sleep disturbances more frequently described themselves in negative terms. They reported feeling tired, moody, grumpy, and tense. Most poor sleepers attributed their sleep problems to worry, tension, and personal, family, or school problems.

Anders et al.[2] believe that the changes in adolescent sleep patterns and sleep disturbances during adolescence "reflect an interaction between increasing social demands that restrict nighttime sleep and changing neuroendocrine relationships as the secretion of certain pituitary hormones become linked to specific nighttime sleep stages."

The fact that adolescents experience sleep disturbance that may continue into their adult lives clearly indicates the need for health care professionals to address sleep habits when working with adolescents. Adolescents should be asked about their typical sleep patterns, difficulty going to sleep, problem with night wakening, and how they have dealt with these disturbances. The nurse should assist adolescents in identifying the cause of sleep disturbances and help them in their problem-solving efforts.

Assessing, Promoting, and Maintaining Optimal Psychosocial Development

Erikson[7] describes the major issue of the adolescent years as the resolution of the crises of personal identity. Personal identity is partly a product of past experiences and a reflection of the adolescent's ability to become comfortable with a rapidly changing body, to develop relationships with the opposite sex, to gain independence from parents, and to define educational and occupational goals.

Developing a sense of identity is an evolving process that reflects increasing cognitive, emotional, and social development. A sense of personal identity is gradually formed as the adolescent confronts and masters developmental tasks. Self-perceptions may change, and the adolescent may sometimes struggle with identity formation. Further, the personal identity of each individual is continually subjected to scrutiny and refined throughout the adult years. An adolescent who has developed a sense of identity can set goals for the future and plan strategies to meet these goals.

The potential negative outcome of this developmental crises is role confusion. Role confusion is demonstrated in the adolescent who is unable to "find a place" in the adult world. All adolescents may exhibit some role confusion as they develop an identity. However, an adolescent who does not have a positive sense of self, a sense of belonging, or goals for the future is at risk for being unable to fit into the adult world. Delinquent behavior may result as the adolescent searches for a place to fit.

Identity formation is a process that reflects previous developmental patterns as well as new developmental challenges. Each developmental task during adolescence will influence identity formation.

Nursing Implications

Assessment of a developing sense of identity during the adolescent years is a critical role of the nurse who works with adolescents and their parents. Systematic ob-

TABLE 16-1
Nursing Assessment: Observation of Behaviors That Reflect a Developing Sense of Identity

Adolescent Behaviors That Reflect Positive Identity Formation	Adult Behaviors That Foster Identity Formation	Adolescent Behaviors That Reflect Role Confusion	Adult Behaviors That May Result in Role Confusion
• Gradually becomes comfortable with body changes and body image.	• Understands the increased concern of the adolescent related to body image.	• Unable to accept changing body.	• Intolerant of adolescent's need to be like peers.
• Develops friendships with peers.	• Allows and encourages peer relationships.	• Difficulty functioning in school.	
• Discusses personal and social values and ideals and can define what is important to him or her.	• Allows the adolescent to express and discuss values and ideologies that may be different from parents.	• May be involved in delinquent behavior.	• Does not have interest in adolescent's daily life.
• Is able to handle increasing independence and self-responsibility.	• Allows increasing independence and helps the adolescent set limits on behavior.	• Unable to communicate with parents.	• Allows either total independence or no independence of the adolescent.
• Makes responsible decisions related to sexual behavior.	• Discusses issues related to sexual behavior and responsibility.	• Unable to plan future goals.	• Does not communicate with adolescent about feelings, goals, values.
• Discusses alternative educational or vocational goals.	• Discusses future plans with the adolescent.	• Exhibits anger and hostility toward parents and society.	• Describes the adolescent in negative terms such as delinquent, stupid, immature.
• Develops adult-to-adult relationships with parents and other adults.	• Allows for changing parent-child relationship.		

servations of adolescent and parent interactions (Table 16-1), as well as individual interviews with the adolescent, the parent, and a combined interview with both are often necessary to obtain adequate data of adolescent progress in meeting developmental tasks. Assessment of each developmental task appropriate for the adolescent's stage of development should be done because they are all vital to identity formation.

Parental Role

Prior to adolescence and throughout the adolescent years, parents as well as other adults and peers influence identity formation through interactions with the adolescent. It is important for parents to realize that adolescent behavior during these years reflects the adolescent's search for a personal identity. Parents should also be aware that the process of identity formation may temporarily result in extreme behaviors or behaviors that do not reflect parental expectations.

Although the parent-child relationship will undergo changes, parents should not give up their role as parents. Parents need to continue to teach, to be role models, and to provide support for the adolescent throughout this developmental stage. The adolescent continues to need limit setting and discipline while experiencing new ideas and trying on new roles. Limit setting can be especially difficult for parents when the adolescent begins to question parental standards of behavior. The multiple influences outside the home, including peers, school, and society, expose the adolescent to a variety of value systems and lifestyles. Parents who are able to evaluate personal beliefs and determine where they can be flexible and where they must stand firm are more likely to give the adolescent room to grow while at the same time to provide structure and support (Fig. 16-2). Research has dem-

onstrated that how parents feel about their children has a considerable impact on the type of adult the child becomes. Genuine parental love resulted in the highest levels of social and moral maturity.[17]

Developmental Tasks That Influence Identity Formation

Identity formation is an ongoing process reflective of the many developmental tasks of adolescence. Assessment of each developmental task is necessary; anticipatory guidance to avoid and/or cope with frequently encountered conflicts is also required (Table 16-2).

Promoting the Development of a Positive Body Image

The developmental task of developing acceptance and comfort with one's body image is a major task of early adolescence (ages 11 to 14). Early adolescence is characterized by pubertal development and rapid physical growth. The body becomes the focus of concern as the adolescent must cope with new sensations, changing physical appearance, and alterations in coordination. The adolescent may often have concerns that there is something wrong. The adolescent's main concern during these early years is the normalcy of growth and body function.

Body image is defined as the "image of our body that we form in our mind."[25] During adolescence the perception of self is intensified because of the radical physical changes that occur. In an effort to incorporate new physical characteristics and body sensations into the existing perception of oneself, the adolescent becomes greatly interested in and concerned with physical appearance. Because of the wide variation in the age at which puberty

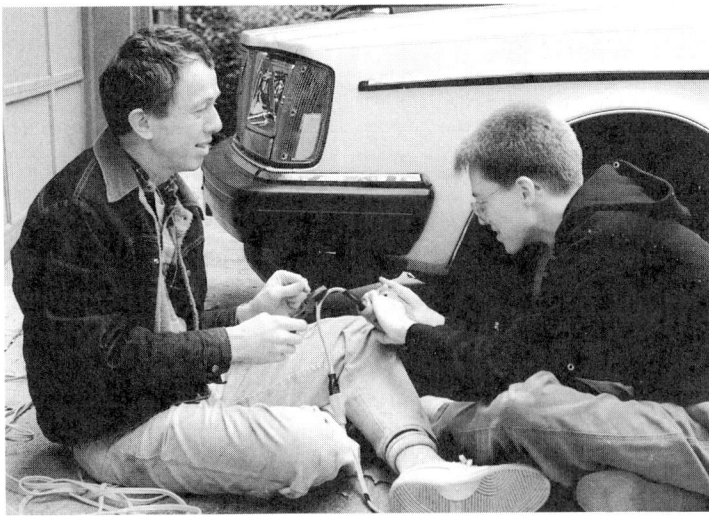

FIGURE 16-2
Parents serve as role models for their children.

begins and the rate of physical growth, adolescents experience increased anxiety concerning any perceived deviation. As adolescents adjust to their changing appearance, they go through a period of narcissism characterized by irritability, self-absorption, and an overdramatized self-perception, often at the expense of reality. They spend a great deal of time in front of the mirror defining what they like and dislike about their bodies (Fig. 16-3A). They also are concerned with how they appear in the eyes of others, especially their peers, and compare themselves with peers of the same sex (Fig. 16-3B).

Adolescents also have an ideal body image or view of how they would like to look.[26] This ideal body image develops as the adolescent makes comparisons between himself or herself and others. Media, including television and teen magazines, influence the ideal body image and often overemphasize unrealistic standards of what is beautiful and what is deviant. Being like everyone else is extremely important, and adolescents begin to dress alike and wear similar hair styles in an effort to proclaim their normalcy.

Parental Role

In an effort to help an adolescent cope with a rapidly changing body, parents should first understand the significant physical, physiologic, emotional, and social implications of puberty. Second, parents need to understand the adolescent's need to "fit in" as all of these changes are occurring. Adolescent concerns may seem unreasonable or invalid to parents but are very real to the adolescent. Parents, therefore, must be careful not to dismiss the adolescent's concerns too quickly or demand that the adolescent meet parental expectations for appearance. Instead, parents should be supportive of the adolescent's need to be like peers. At the same time, parents can help the adolescent make realistic appraisals of self and peers. Parents need not accommodate the adolescent's every desire but instead should be flexible and compromising. For example, Jane may desire to be like peers by wearing worn and dirty blue jeans to school. Her parents may find this objectionable but are able to find a compromise by letting Jane wear blue jeans but ones that are clean.

Each new generation of adolescents demonstrates through their appearance a desire to be different from the status quo. This is seen throughout history in such areas as styles of dress and hair, jewelry, and ear piercing. Parents may find it easier to tolerate the adolescent's desire to be different if asked to look back on their own adolescent years. Parents also need reassurance that most of the expressions of individuality such as clothing styles, hair styles, including multicolored hair or partial shaving of the head, are not permanent. The desire for a permanent alteration such as a tattoo should be discouraged during the adolescent years.

Parents also assist the adolescent in developing a positive body image by taking the time to talk through issues that arise. Rather than just saying "no" to a request, parents should explain why they are doing so. This process of communication serves two purposes. First, when parents are willing to explain their view of a situation to the adolescent, they must first think through their decision and the rationale for the choice they made. This process may reinforce their feelings or make them realize that the adolescent's request is not all that unreasonable. Second, the adolescent benefits from knowing why parents responded in the way they did. This may or may not make the adolescent more accepting of the decision, but it may provide the adolescent with information that was not considered, as well as reinforce parental willingness to communicate.

Nursing Implications

The nurse also has a role in helping the adolescent adjust to a rapidly changing body. The nurse should be aware of common adolescent concerns, such as not developing normally, being different from peers, and coping with new and intensified emotions. The nursing history should include questions that focus on the adolescent's perception of progress in growth. The adolescent also needs opportunities to express concerns. Evaluating the adolescent's self-perceptions or body image can be done

TABLE 16-2
Nursing Assessment: Questions for Assessing the Adolescent's Attainment of Developmental Tasks

Area of Assessment	Key Questions for the Adolescent*	Key Questions for Parents
Adaptation to a changing body	• Describe yourself. • What do you like most about yourself? • Is there anything about you that you would change if you could? • Do you feel you are overweight, underweight, or optimal weight? • How are you like your peers? • How are you different from your peers? • Do you have any questions about the physical changes of your body?	• Describe _____ for me. • What physical changes have you noticed in _____? • How do you feel _____ is dealing with physical changes? • Do you have any concerns regarding _____ physical development? • Do you feel _____ has concerns about his/her physical development?
Developing relationships with peers	• Do you have a close friend? • Tell me about your activities with your friends outside of school. • Do you feel that you can talk to your friends about personal feelings and concerns? • Do your parents like your friends? • Do you ever feel lonely?	• Does _____ have a close friend? • What types of activities does _____ enjoy with peers? • Do you like _____ friends? • Do you think _____ ever feels lonely? • Do you have any concerns about _____ friendships?
Developing responsible sexual behavior	• Have you dated? • Do you currently have a girlfriend/boyfriend? • What are your feelings about teenagers having sex? • Do your peers feel the same way? • What do you feel are the responsibilities of the boy if he has sex with a girl partner? What are the responsibilities of the girl? • What do you/would you consider before becoming sexually involved with someone? • What information have you been given related to contraception, sexually transmitted disease, human reproduction? • Who provided this information? • How have you used this information? • Have you ever had sex with someone of the same sex? opposite sex? • Would you feel comfortable saying ''no'' to sex if you did not want to have sex with someone? • Are you currently having sex with someone? • Are you using birth control? Do you have any concerns or problems using birth control? How does your partner feel about the birth control you are using? • Have you ever been pregnant/the father of a baby? What happened to the pregnancy? How do you feel about it? • Have you ever had a sexually transmitted disease? Have you asked your boyfriend/girlfriend if they have? • How many different people have you had sex with? • Have you ever had oral/anal sex? • Who would you go to if you had any questions about sex? • Do you have any questions or concerns related to sex that you would like to discuss now?	• What are your feelings about teenage sexuality? • Have you discussed sexuality with _____? • Are you comfortable discussing sexuality? • What information have you given to _____? • What other sources of information related to sexuality does _____ have? • Do you have any questions related to helping _____ develop in this area?

(Continued)

TABLE 16-2
(Continued)

Area of Assessment	Key Questions for the Adolescent*	Key Questions for Parents
Developing independence from parents and self-responsibility	• Can you tell me how you demonstrate your ability to be responsible for yourself? • How would you describe your parents' expectations of you? • How would you describe your expectations of yourself? • What do you like most about your parents? • What causes conflict between you and your parents? • How do you deal with conflict? • What do you feel your parents can do to decrease conflicts? • What do you feel you can do to decrease conflicts?	• What expectations do you have of _____ in school, home, socially? • How well do you think _____ is meeting these expectations? • What expectations does _____ have of himself/herself? • What causes conflict between you and _____? • How do you deal with conflict between you and _____? • What do you feel _____ can do to decrease conflict? • What do you feel you can do to decrease conflict?
Preparing for a productive role in society	• What are your goals for the future? • How do you plan to reach these goals? • Have you shared these goals with your parents? • How do your parents feel about your goals? • Do you feel your parents are supportive of your choices for your future? • What concerns do you have about reaching your goals?	• What are _____ goals for the future? • Do you feel these goals are realistic? • How can you help _____ reach these goals? • What concerns do you have related to _____ ability to reach goals?

* Not all questions are appropriate for each adolescent. The nurse must choose areas of assessment depending on the age and needs of each individual.

by asking questions such as, "What do you like about your physical appearance?" "What would you like to change about your appearance?" "Do you feel you are overweight? underweight?" "Do you feel you are like others your age?" (see Table 16-2).

Although reassuring the adolescent does not decrease anxiety, pointing out signs of impending development may help allay some fear. Early identification of extreme distortions of self-concept or unrealistic expectations can facilitate intervention. Such problems as bulimia, anorexia, unhealthy dieting, and the use of drugs for body building may be avoided (see Chap. 19 for discussion of these topics). Teaching the adolescent about the physical and emotional changes that occur during puberty can reassure the adolescent that the concern felt about development is not a unique experience. Teaching can be done on an individual basis or in groups. Individual teaching may provide a more comfortable environment for the expression of individual fears and concerns, whereas group discussions may be more beneficial in helping an adolescent realize that anxieties, fears, and concerns are also experienced by peers.

The nurse must also work with parents and help them understand the normalcy of the adolescent's behavior. Parents can also provide information of any extreme changes in behavior that may indicate a problem. Parents may need some assistance in allowing the adolescent to be like peers. This requires compromise, and parents are generally able to resolve this issue when given time to

discuss their concerns with a person removed from the situation.

Development of Peer Relationships

The adolescent peer group arises from the need of adolescents to compare themselves with members of their own sex. Through peer group interactions, adolescents can evaluate their normalcy in terms of how others react to them and whether others accept or reject them (Fig. 16-4A). In the early adolescent years relationships often are developed with peers of the same gender. The establishment of an intense mutual friendship with one friend is common. Establishing a close friendship gives the adolescent an opportunity to understand and accept himself or herself. A friend who is valued and trustworthy can listen as the adolescent expresses feelings that may be difficult to share with parents, other adults, and peers. A mutual friendship provides reassurance that someone else experiences similar feelings and provides comfort and support during times of insecurity. Dating may begin during early adolescence but tends to be more group oriented rather than individual couples. Older adolescents date more seriously in preparation for determining qualities in a future mate (Fig. 16-4B). Young adolescent girls who date older boys are at risk for the early initiation of sexual activity and subsequent pregnancy. Older males are most frequently the fathers in cases of pregnant teens under the age of 15.[11]

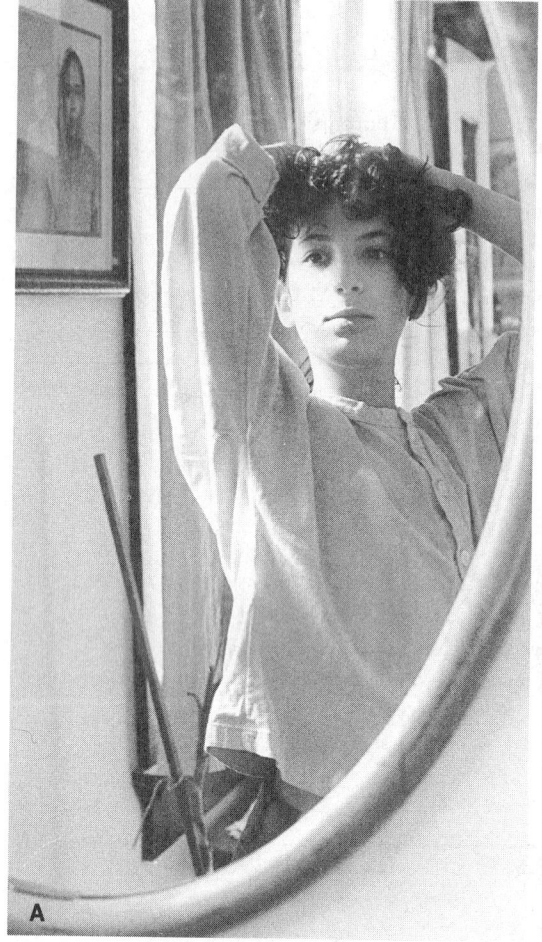
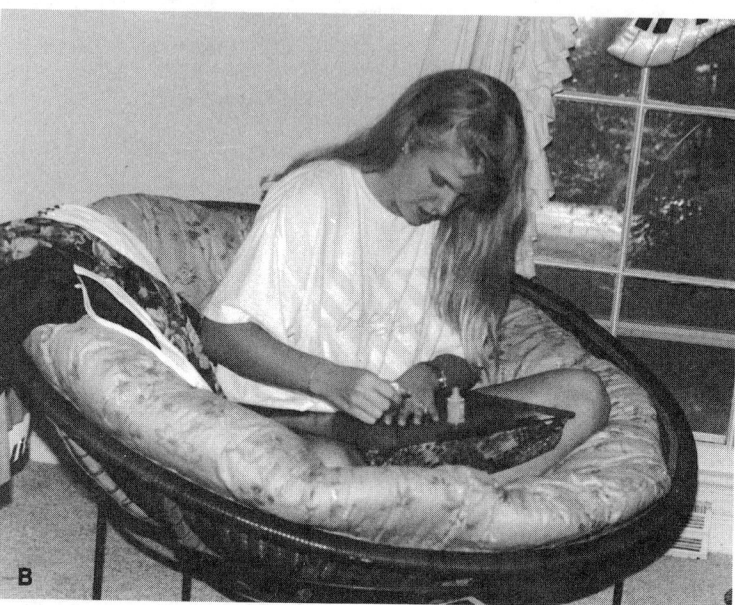

FIGURE 16-3

Adolescents are developing a body image. (**A**) They are concerned about their appearances and compare themselves to others. (**B**) They spend time trying to be "normal," which means conforming to the standards set by their peers. ([**A**] Photo courtesy of Kathy Sloane.)

Parental Role

Parents should be supportive of the adolescent's need to develop friendships and peer relationships. The adolescent's need to spend long periods of time with friends, both outside the home and on the phone, may initially seem unreasonable to parents. Parents may feel as though they are losing control and the best friend is controlling the adolescent's life. Parents who are able to allow the adolescent time for friendships and peer interactions are facilitating the adolescent's ability to deal with developmental changes. At the same time, parents should help the adolescent set limits on behavior that may affect development. Limiting the frequency and duration of phone calls and of being with friends at the expense of other obligations provides the adolescent with some direction in keeping school, home, and peer responsibilities balanced.

Parents should encourage adolescents to bring friends home and become familiar with the friends the adolescent spends time with on a regular basis. Parents should be encouraged to become attuned to observing the adolescent's friends in relation to age, common in-terests, family responsibilities, and similarity in rules and expectations of behavior.

Nursing Implications

The nurse should assess the development of peer relationships during the well-care visit. The adolescent may be more comfortable discussing peers with the nurse than with parents, especially if parents do not approve of the teen's choice of friends. In the assessment the nurse should explore the presence or lack of friends or friendships parents find inappropriate or objectionable (see Table 16-2).

The nurse should be alert to potential problems such as young adolescents spending most of their time with older adolescents, adolescents who suddenly drop all their interests to be with a specific group, adolescents who suddenly find their friends to be inadequate, or adolescents who demonstrate negative changes in attitudes or behavior after giving up old friendships for new ones. By asking the adolescent questions about these changes, the nurse has an opportunity to evaluate the situation

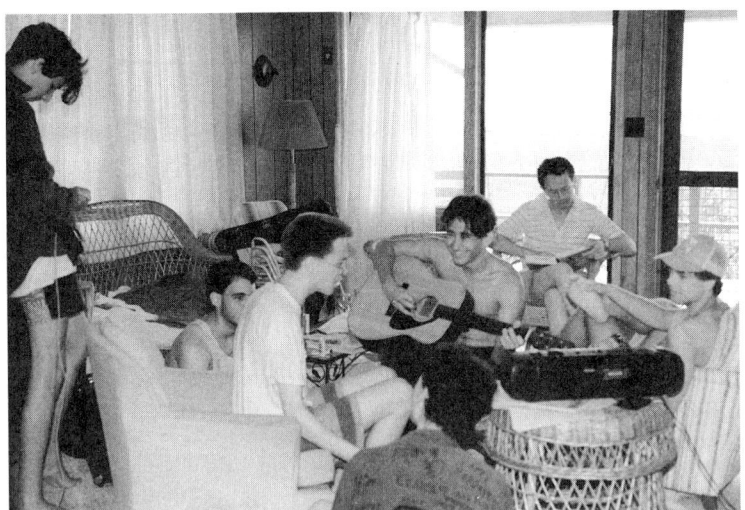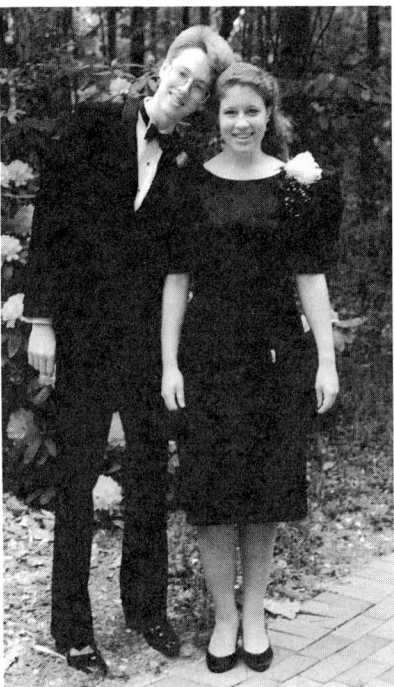

FIGURE 16-4
Development of peer relationships. *Left,* Peer relationships develop around mutual interests and hobbies. *Right,* The high school prom is a big event for both males and females.

more objectively. The response of the adolescent to questions will alert the nurse to actual and potential problems.

Achieving Control and Expression of Sexual Drives

During middle adolescence (ages 15 to 17) the desire to begin dating brings special challenges to the adolescent-parent relationship. The adolescent is concerned with asking or being asked out, being popular, dating a particular person, and meeting the social expectations of the peer group. For some teens, dating can be a traumatic time, especially if they are unable to live up to self- or peer expectations. Having a steady date can be beneficial in building self-confidence and acceptance. Dating can also be an area of concern if relationships become too intimate or lead to sexual activity that the adolescent is not yet ready to handle.

Parents, too, are concerned about the adolescent's ability to fit in with the peer group, date, and be invited to attend social events. However, parents are also concerned with the growing number of teen pregnancies, sexually transmitted diseases, including acquired immunodeficiency syndrome (AIDS), as well as the adolescent's ability to stand up to peer pressure. Parents may have double standards for their sons and daughters. Sons may be given more freedom in dating, whereas fear of pregnancy may cause parents to be less flexible in their rules for the daughter's dating experiences.

Adolescent sexuality is also a major concern of society. An increasing number of adolescents are initiating sexual intercourse before adulthood and before marriage. Between 1971 and 1982, the percentage of never-married women age 15 to 19 who lived in metropolitan areas and had sexual intercourse rose from 28% to 42%.[12] In the United States the average age for first sexual intercourse is 17.2 years for women and 16.5 years for men.[38] Estimates indicate that by the age of 20, three out of four women and five out of six men have had sexual intercourse at least once.[4]

Sexually transmitted diseases, including gonorrhea, chlamydia, herpes simplex virus, human papillomavirus, and syphilis, are of increasing concern in the adolescent population, with one in seven teenagers contracting a sexually transmitted disease each year.[4]

The Centers for Disease Control (CDC) in February 1992 reported 797 13- to 19-year-olds were diagnosed with AIDS. In the 20- to 24-year-old range, 8265 cases were reported, many of whom contracted the disease as adolescents.[4a] These cases support the concern of a rapidly increasing incidence of AIDS among teens. Because AIDS has a latency period of up to 10 years, few people will actually develop the disease during their adolescent years. The tendency of adolescent girls to have sexual intercourse with older men (in their 20's) rather than with males their same age places them at greater risk for acquiring AIDS.[4]

Health care professionals have a critical role in working with parents and adolescents as the adolescent develops relationships with the opposite sex and develops a functional sexual role. A teaching plan related to sexuality is provided here. The issues that arise during adolescence related to sexual development, functioning, and responsibility impact not only on adolescent devel-

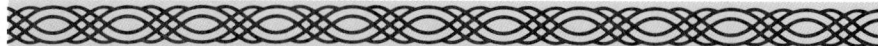

CHILD & FAMILY TEACHING PLAN

Sexuality Concerns of a 14-Year-Old Female Client

Assessment

Paula is a 14-year-old girl who has come to the clinic for a physical examination prior to entering the tenth grade at the high school. She has been healthy for the past 3 years, and her last health care visit was when she was 10 years old and entering middle school. She is accompanied by her mother. The nurse explains to her and her mother that she would like to speak with each of them after the physical. The nurse explains the importance of Paula assuming increasing responsibility for her own health during the adolescent years. Both Paula and her mother agree to meet with the nurse individually.

Paula feels she is like her peers and has lots of friends at school. She is an A to B student, plans to attend college after high school, and become a lawyer. Paula states that her mother generally lets her buy the clothes she wants but sometimes won't let her wear things that are too short or too tight. She feels she gets along with her parents pretty well but that she doesn't tell them as much as she used to because she knows they are a little old fashioned and would keep her at home.

During the individual interview with Paula the following information was obtained. Paula has a boyfriend who is 17 years old and already goes to the high school. She met him through a friend, and they have been seeing each other after school a couple of times a week for the past 2 months. Her mother has not met him, and Paula has not mentioned him because, "She doesn't think I am old enough to have a boyfriend until I am 16 or 17 years old. I only see him on Friday or Saturday night if my friends and I meet him and his friends at the movies or something."

First menstrual period: 6 months prior to visit; has had a total of four periods since this time. Last period 2 weeks prior to visit.

Sexual activity: Involves mostly kissing and petting, but has had sexual intercourse once 3 weeks ago. Did not use contraceptive. Rationale: "Tim said we didn't need it because he wouldn't 'come' inside me. Besides, we only had sex once, and we probably won't do it very often."

Feelings about teenage sexuality: "All my friends think it is okay if you really like each other." "Tim thinks it is the best way to show him I really care about him." "I guess it is okay because everyone is doing it." "I guess I don't want to do it all the time but once in a while it is okay."

Interest in using contraceptives: "If I get birth control and my parents find out, they will think I plan to have sex, and I don't. It is just something that might happen sometimes."

During the interview with Paula's mother the following information was obtained. In response to questions about how she and her husband are dealing with their daughter becoming an adolescent: "We are a little afraid of her going to the high school since there is so much happening today with drugs and alcohol and sex. We just keep telling her that drugs and alcohol can ruin her life and her future, and that if we find out she is using them we will take away all of her privileges. . . . I hope the high school has a good sex education program so she won't get involved in that either. I don't think she should get into any of that until she is married. We have already told her she could not date until she was 17, so I guess we have a few years before we have to worry about that. Her father thinks we should just provide her with information and access to birth control when she starts to date, but I feel like that is the same as saying it is okay to have sex."

(Continued)

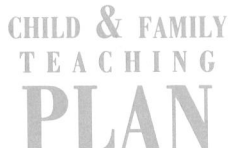

Sexuality Concerns of a 14-Year-Old Female Client (continued)

Child and Family Objectives	*Specific Content*	*Teaching Strategies*
1. (Paula) obtain knowledge related to risk of pregnancy with unprotected sexual intercourse and methods for contraception.	1. Paula's risk-taking behavior due to incorrect information puts her at risk for pregnancy. Provide basic information in concrete terms of the potential for pregnancy with one unprotected sexual intercourse. Misinformation related to reliability of withdrawal as a birth control method is corrected. Misinformation related to frequency of intercourse and potential for pregnancy is corrected. Paula needs more information and support. Over-the-counter birth control will give Paula adequate protection and is readily available. Even when using birth control, failure may result if used incorrectly. Until Paula makes a decision she is comfortable with, abstinence is the best option.	1. Use audiovisual aids and models. Provide Paula with resources (booklets or packets of information) that will give her correct information. She should be given some literature at the time of the visit. Such information will reinforce teaching and provide more indepth information. The short clinic visit does not allow for the teaching needs of Paula. Refer Paula to school or community family planning clinic. Provide Paula with information about over-the-counter birth control (foam, sponge, condoms). Give her samples. Instruct Paula on the correct method for using each form of over-the-counter birth control. Reinforce the option of abstinence.
2. (Paula) resolve decisional conflict about sexual behavior related to peer pressure.	2. Adolescents need reassurance that peers are not always the best source of advice or information. Paula needs help in using the decision-making process.	2. Point out that peers seem to be influencing her decision to have sex before she feels ready. Ask her to think of ways she would deal with peer pressure if she were asked to be involved in something she was really against. Have her list the pros and cons of having sex at this time.
3. (Parents) discuss issues about today's adolescent and sexuality and how to maintain open communication with Paula.	3. Parents need to be aware of the adolescent's need to deal with sex-related issues. Parents need to understand the significance of peer pressure and misinformation or lack of information related to sexuality on the decision to engage in or abstain from sexual activity. Parental agreement on developmental issues is an important first step in setting expectations for the adolescent. Communication is necessary if parents want to have an impact on the adolescent related to sexual decision making.	3. Explain normal adolescent desire to relate to the opposite sex and the sexual experimentation (often unplanned) that this may involve. Provide mother with information related to adolescent sexuality, including the rate of teen pregnancy, peer pressure, insufficient or incorrect information provided by peers, and misconception that information leads to early initiation of sex. Encourage mother to discuss issues related to Paula's sexual development with her husband and come to an agreement in handling issues.

(Continued)

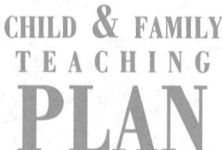

Sexuality Concerns of a 14-Year-Old Female Client (continued)

Child and Family Objectives	Specific Content	Teaching Strategies
	Mother needs help in finding a place to begin and direction to take.	Reinforce the need to talk about sexuality with Paula. Emphasize the opportunities this provides for parents to share their beliefs and values as well as hear what Paula is being exposed to outside the home.
		Recommend that mother obtain information on the sex education program at the high school and follow up the topics discussed at school with a discussion at home.
		Provide mother with information related to talking to the adolescent about sexuality.
		Written material may increase parental sense of confidence and serve as a reference for specific information.
		Role play.
4. (Paula & mother) participate in a discussion regarding the importance of communication within families.	4. The changing roles that emerge as adolescents grow are identified.	4. During the joint meeting with Paula and her mother the nurse should emphasize the importance of communication between parents and teenagers as they both experience many changes. The nurse can point out that they both seem to have some concerns related to sexuality during the teen years and reinforce the need to talk about this issue with each other so that problems do not arise. Reassurance should also be provided that the nurse will be available if either has concerns or questions in the future.

Evaluation

- Paula verbalizes risks of unprotected intercourse.
- Paula identifies over-the-counter contraception available and correct usage of these methods.
- Paula increases confidence in her ability to stand up to peers and share with her boyfriend her reluctance to engage in sexual intercourse at this time.
- Paula's mother verbalizes the need to discuss the issue of sexuality with Paula.

opment but also on the teen's future ability to bear and raise children.

The problems of teenage sexuality and teen pregnancy have far-reaching implications for the individual, family, and society. The teenager is confronted with mixed messages regarding sexuality. The media bombard them with sexual imagery and offer little, if any, role models for abstinence. Peer pressure often encourages sexual activity. Parents who try to counter the multiple influences that induce their children to engage in early sexual activity do not have adequate support from the community.[4]

Parental Role

Parents have a vital role in sex education and value formation of their children, but they cannot deal with these issues unless they have support outside the home. Parental messages require reinforcement from the community, including the schools, religious organizations, community organizations, the media, and health professionals. Parental support and parental communication have been found to delay the initiation of sexual activity and minimize the possibility of unintended pregnancy.[11]

How a parent handles the issue of sexuality is influenced by many factors. Parents need to be aware of their own sexuality. A parent who is uncomfortable or dissatisfied with their sexuality will have more difficulty in helping the adolescent develop positive feelings. Religious background also greatly influences parental beliefs about sexuality and is an important factor in how sexuality of the adolescent is handled. Parental comfort in discussing sexuality will influence the amount and kind of dialogue that takes place between parent and teen. Parental awareness of adolescent behaviors common in our society and ability to see the potential situations their own child can become involved in will help them avoid denial.

There are no absolute methods for dealing with adolescent sexuality that can guarantee the adolescent will develop a healthy sexual role without difficulty. However, parents can and do play an important role in this part of the adolescent's development.

Ideally, the concept of sexuality should be introduced early in childrearing along with other issues, including responsibility, accountability, self-esteem, self-confidence, and an open communication between parent and child. In our society, sexuality is frequently considered a taboo topic, especially with young children. Instead, parents may wait until adolescence to discuss sexuality, and some parents are never able to discuss the topic. This leaves the adolescent open to misinformation and feelings of insecurity or guilt related to new sexual feelings. Some parents fear a discussion of sexuality may encourage the adolescent to become sexually active. Others believe that if they provide the adolescent with contraception, their worries are over. However, because pregnancy is no longer the only potential hazard of sexual behavior, birth control is not the only answer.

Parents need to evaluate how they as individuals feel about their sexuality and how they as a couple want the child to develop sexually. Most parents want their children to develop normal, healthy relationships with the members of the opposite sex but are unsure of how to go about facilitating this. Open communication is a primary factor in how parents and children develop and problem-solve. Parents should begin by identifying blocks to communication and attempting to overcome these blocks. One frequently seen block to communication is parental inability to discuss an issue with an adolescent. Instead, parents tell the adolescent how they want the adolescent to think and feel. This approach may have been used in earlier years when parents taught children by telling them what was acceptable behavior and what was not acceptable behavior. Now, the adolescent, armed with information and opinions that differ from his or her parents must have an opportunity to express himself or herself and discuss varying opinions as they problem-solve together. Adolescents also need information specific to sex, reproduction, and disease. Parents cannot depend solely on the school to provide this information but should be involved in this part of the child's education. By taking an active part in sex education, parental values

and moral beliefs can be included in the educational process. Parents should also assist the adolescent in developing self-esteem and comfort in making choices that may conflict with the peer group. Ideally, parents should promote decision making throughout early childhood, but even if this has not occurred, adolescents can make choices for themselves with support. To do this, parents must allow the adolescent to make choices at home, some of which may not reflect parental desires.

Another necessary component of communication is parental interest in the adolescent's life. Parents can and should ask the adolescent about school, friends, teachers, concerns, and fears. Adolescents need to feel comfortable talking to parents about everyday experiences before they will be comfortable discussing more personal feelings about sexuality.

Nursing Implications

During the adolescent years nurses must assume a role in helping adolescents and parents deal with issues related to sexuality. Through discussions of issues related to sexuality, the nurse assesses parental and adolescent's perceptions of how this phase of development is progressing (see Table 16-2). It is important that nurses interview the adolescent and parents separately. In the assessment the nurse should be alert to cues that indicate potential or actual problems in sexual development. Some findings that may reflect a potential problem include parental expression of discomfort in discussing the topic of sexuality with the adolescent or parents' belief that there is no need for discussion of sexuality with their child. Adolescents who believe that they are somehow protected from the possible hazards of sexual activity, that they have feelings of being different from peers, or that they are unable to attract a member of the opposite sex are at risk. Any adolescent involved in other risk-taking behaviors, such as alcohol or drug use, is at high risk for early sexual activity.

Through discussion of issues related to adolescent sexuality with parents, the nurse can reinforce the need for parents to be involved in this part of development. The nurse can give parents suggestions for topics to discuss with the adolescent, including but not limited to sexuality, and at the same time reinforce the need to discuss rather than lecture. Topics chosen should include such factors as the adolescent's goals for the future and how they plan to reach these goals and the adolescent's approach to problem solving or decision making about peers, school, and other activities. Through listening to the adolescent describe his or her decision-making process, the parent can gain some insight into the adolescent's ability to problem-solve and deal with the mixed messages he or she may be receiving related to risk-taking behavior.

In discussing sexuality with adolescents, the nurse must also discuss the multiple issues facing the adolescent rather than focus only on sexuality. The nurse can then foster the adolescents' ability to define appropriate sexual behavior for themselves. Once specific information is provided related to the multiple issues involved in the early initiation of sexual activity, the nurse needs to engage the adolescent in discussion of the multiple issues that they have encountered related to sexuality. Through the use of values clarification, the nurse can assist the adolescent in determining present values related to sexuality and/or develop a set of values based on scientific information, personal beliefs, and values. Decision-making skills are also effective in helping the adolescent make choices about sexuality and birth control. Rather than being told what to do, the adolescent can be assisted to make choices based on a discussion of issues, sharing of knowledge, and active participation in the decision-making process. Tauer[32] has adapted several exercises that can be used to counsel individual adolescents or groups of adolescents (see the accompanying display). These exercises encourage the exploration of personal beliefs, request the adolescent to give a rationale for why one choice is better than another, and reinforce that even among the peer group there are varying opinions and beliefs about sexuality. In addition to dealing with the general topic of sexuality and sexual decision making, the nurse should obtain a sexual history from the adolescent. As the incidence of sexually transmitted disease increases in the adolescent population, more specific questions about sexual activity need to be addressed.[10] Before obtaining this history, the nurse should give the adolescent time to become comfortable by asking questions related to less personal topics such as school, activities, and nutrition (see Chap. 67). Another approach recommended by some adolescent specialists involves history taking to be done in private by filling out a questionnaire or answering questions through the use of a simple computer program.[22] These methods are believed to be less threatening for the adolescent than direct questioning, and the information can then be reviewed and areas of concern discussed with the adolescent. Computer games have also been found to be beneficial in the education of adolescents in relation to sexual behavior.[22]

Programs Aimed at Decreasing Adolescent Sexuality and Pregnancy

The nurse should be aware of programs that are aimed at the prevention of unintended pregnancy and should be aware of the strengths and limitations of these programs. After talking with the adolescent and parents, the nurse may choose to recommend a program or group to assist the adolescent and family in dealing with issues related to sexuality.

Most programs are one of three types: (1) those that impart knowledge or influence attitudes; (2) those that provide access to contraception; and (3) those that enhance life options.[6] The majority of programs are education or service oriented and represent the traditional approach. They are aimed at educating adolescents and providing access to services to prevent unintended pregnancy. Education alone has not proven to be a successful method of decreasing the incidence of early sexual activity or teen pregnancy.[16,30] Programs that train the adolescent in assertiveness skills and decision making have been found to have some positive effects; however, data are limited and more rigorous studies need to be done. There is some evidence that family planning clinics that have a strong educational component may improve contraceptive use among sexually active adolescents without

encouraging sexual intercourse among those adolescents who are not personally ready for such involvement.[37] These types of programs are especially beneficial for motivated teenagers who want to make informed decisions about their sexual behavior and receive the services to control fertility. However, educational and service programs do not have an impact on adolescents who are not motivated to avoid pregnancy. The third approach, programs that enhance life options, have been established to enhance the adolescent's sense of future, sense of self-worth, understanding of the value of education, and awareness of work and career options.[11] These programs include such aspects as mentoring and role modeling, improving school performance, developing skills for employment, and involving the adolescent in groups that look at life choices, life goals, and what it will take to meet goals. The success of these programs is also hard to establish due to lack of data; however, studies are underway to evaluate the effectiveness of all programs.[6]

Nurses, health professionals, parents, and community organizations need to become involved in all of these programs to enhance their effectiveness. In addition, the nurse needs to be aware of the programs available as well as the purpose, focus, and method used in the programs so that referral can be made that will meet the unique needs of the individual adolescent and/or family.

Developing Increasing Independence

Independence from parents is a necessary component of developing a personal identity. The adolescent's relationship with parents undergoes change during the adolescent years. No longer are parental standards and parental authority accepted without question. The adolescent evaluates parents in relation to others and society and openly criticizes any flaws that are found. This thought process is necessary as the adolescent breaks away and takes on self-responsibility. However, the emancipation process frequently causes some level of conflict. In fact, developing independence is the aspect of adolescent development that most frequently leads to struggles between the adolescent and parents (Fig. 16-5).

Arguments over using the car, staying out late, going out during the week, and telling parents what the teen plans to do while out are just a few of the areas of conflict that arise. Adolescents often view their parents as being old fashioned and out of touch with present reality. Teens may feel that parents do not understand the importance of each request and often view not being allowed to go out or drive the car as a major crisis that will subsequently ruin their life.

Parental Role

Allowing the adolescent increasing independence can be difficult for parents. Parents frequently have ambivalent feelings related to independence issues. On the one hand, parents want the adolescent to become independent and be responsible for themselves; on the other hand, they fear the adolescent may not be able to handle the responsibility to make appropriate decisions. Some parents are unable to give the adolescent any increased self-responsibility or more liberal privileges out of fear that something might happen to the child. Other parents

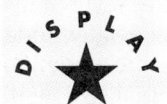

Exercises for Counseling Adolescents in Sexuality

FORCED CHOICE EXERCISES

Objectives
- To experience choosing in an either-or situation.
- To recognize that different people can make the same choice for different reasons.
- To recognize that to make choices, the adolescent must think about his or her values.

Procedure
1. Leader asks participants to stand so that there is a wide path from one side of the room to the other.
2. Leader then asks an either-or question. For example, "Would you rather be a Volkswagen or a Cadillac?"
3. Leader indicates by pointing that those that identify more with Volkswagens are to go to one side of the room and those who identify more with Cadillacs are to go to the other.
4. Leader then asks participants on each side to share some of the reasons for their choice. If anyone is standing alone or just with a few people, ask how it feels to be in the minority.
5. Everyone returns to center of room. Then the leader gives another either-or, or forced choice.

Questions
1. Would you rather:
   a. Have your mother buy all your clothes at any time, but only ones she likes, *or*
   b. Get a clothing allowance of half as much, but you have approval of choices?
2. Would you rather:
   a. Have to be home at 9:00 PM on Friday nights and 11:00 PM on Saturday nights, *or*
   b. Have to be home by 10:00 PM on both Friday and Saturday nights?
3. If you are doing this exercise with older teenagers, here are some other examples of forced choice items.
   a. Hammer *or* nail.
   b. Live alone all your life *or* live in a commune.
   c. Choose a life partner at 18 *or* remain single for life.
   d. All teenagers have sex *or* no teenagers have sex.
   e. Have an unwanted child *or* have a dangerous abortion.
   f. Be a parent at 16 *or* never have children.

Process Points
1. What kinds of things did you consider when making your choice?
2. How does it feel to only have two choices? Point out that sometimes people are faced with two very difficult choices and may not feel that they have an in-between alternative.

VALUES CHOICE EXERCISE

To choose one alternative and reject others, the teens have to examine their feeling and their values. This process helps individuals to clarify what is really important to them. Having to justify a choice forces a person to look carefully at the decision and evaluate it clearly.

Procedure
1. Introduce the exercise to the entire group: We are going to do an exercise called values choice, and in the process we will break into small groups. I will read a set of statements. Each of you is to choose which statement is the most important in your life and which is the least important. Then we will discuss the reasons for your choice.
2. It is important that people do not take a great deal of time to make their decisions, but rather trust their initial response. After discussing their choices with the group, they may discover that they would have chosen differently if they had taken other factors into account, or they may find that they can trust their initial reactions.
3. Read the first set of statements:
   The method of birth control I would choose would be:
   a. No sex
   b. The pill
   c. Diaphragm
   d. IUD
   e. Foam and rubbers
   f. Other
   Of the possible side effects of the pill, which one would keep me from using it as a birth control method?
   a. Weight gain
   b. Breakthrough bleeding
   c. Skipped periods
   d. Moodiness
   The worst thing I could find out about my boyfriend/girlfriend is that he or she:
   a. Has a venereal disease
   b. Is sterile
   c. Is having sex with another person
   If my parents discovered I was using birth control I would:
   a. Feel good that we could be more honest with each other
   b. Stop using birth control
   c. Be afraid of being punished
4. Give 5 to 10 minutes for sharing each time you present a set of statements. Encourage the group to think about questions such as "What made me choose this statement rather than the others?" "What does that tell me about myself?" Suggest that they not be judgmental toward those who have different reasons for their choices and try to understand what others are trying to communicate.

From Tauer, K. (1983). Promoting effective decision-making in sexually active adolescents. Nursing Clinics of North America, 15, *275.*

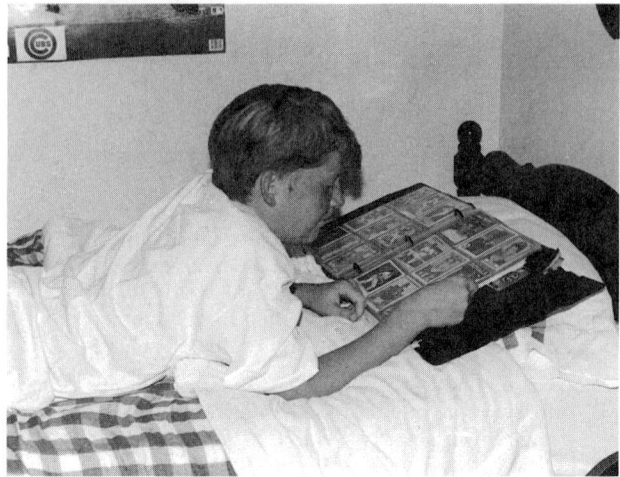

FIGURE 16-5
As adolescents struggle for independence, their room often becomes "off-limits" to other family members.

may give an adolescent total freedom without direction or support. Yet, most parents fall somewhere in between these extremes and constantly evaluate and adjust their approach as the adolescent develops.

Ideally, parents should discuss with each other their feelings about such issues as driving, dating, and social activities prior to the adolescent years. Parents who have prepared for this stage of development will have less conflict among themselves and subsequently will be better able to communicate feelings to the adolescent. Parents who are unable to agree on these issues set themselves up for conflict and arguments and place the adolescent in the middle.

Another advantage of discussing independence issues prior to adolescence is an early and paced introduction of the child to self-responsibility. It is more beneficial for the child gradually to take on increased responsibility rather than suddenly be given more responsibility than can be handled. This introduction begins in the early years. Parents can expect that the young child will pick up toys when finished playing or that the older child will take responsibility for school work, some specific household chores, and keeping one's room clean. By early adolescence parents can expect the child to help with younger children by baby sitting or helping them with a new task.

It is important that parents do not give double messages to the adolescent. For example, Jane is 16 years old. Her mother expects her to be able to sit with her two younger siblings, aged 6 and 10, when the parents want a night out. Her mother expects that she will be able to serve the younger children dinner, get them ready for bed and know what to do should an emergency arise. These expectations tell Jane that her mother feels she is responsible and has the ability to make decisions on her own. Later, when Jane asks to go out with her friends, her mother says "no" because she fears Jane will not be able to make the right choice should her friends want to do something they should not be doing. In this example the parent is expecting a certain level of responsibility in one situation but is telling the adolescent that she is not ready for responsibility in the other.

Parents should be aware of their child's level of maturity and comfort in making choices, especially under peer pressure. Maturity should determine the amount of freedom and timing of new privileges. Open communication between parent and child is required. Through open communication, both parents and teens can negotiate together and come to mutual agreement. Parents who are able to give increased independence are preparing the adolescent for their introduction into society and the expectations society holds for each member.

Nursing Implications

Working with adolescents and parents during middle adolescence is a challenging and demanding task. Parents may expect the health care professional to assume an authoritative role and reinforce to the adolescent the need to adhere to parental demands and expectations. In contrast, adolescents may expect the health care professional to take their side and tell parents that they are too controlling or unfair in their expectations of what the adolescent can and cannot do. The nurse cannot assume either of these roles but must, instead, work with both the adolescent and parents to help them find the best solution for them as a family.

Problem solving will involve a systematic assessment of the adolescent, the parents, and the problem. The nurse, through assessment, should determine the adolescent's level of maturity, self-esteem, expectations of self and of parents, and perception of the problem, its causes, and its possible solutions. The nurse should also assess parental perception of the adolescent's level of maturity, their own expectations of the adolescent, and their perception of the problem, its cause, and options for resolution. In doing this assessment, the nurse must use well-developed communication and interviewing skills and demonstrate respect for both the adolescent and parents (see Table 16-2).

Through discussion of each person's expectations and how each perceives factors that have contributed to the conflict, both the adolescent and parents may be able to view the situation from the other's perspective. Depending on the level of communication between parents and adolescent, this can be done as a group or may need to be done separately prior to group discussion with the nurse as moderator.

Once typical problems are identified and clearly defined, mutual problem solving can begin and strategies for dealing with conflict can be discussed. This process should be used by nurses working with adolescents and parents even if conflicts are not obvious or causing a great deal of stress. Through communication, the relationship can be strengthened and potential conflicts anticipated. When parents and adolescents are unable to communicate or problem solve together, and if major problems exist, they should be referred to a specialist in family counseling.

Preparation for a Productive Role in Society

Toward the end of the adolescent years, old conflicts subside and new challenges appear. Concerns of body image, sex role relationships, and emancipation from parents lose prominence and the adolescent's main concern centers around finding a place in the adult world. The adolescent is confronted with making choices regarding educational pursuits, job possibilities, marriage and children, and community involvement.

In the later part of adolescence, peer relationships are based on mutual enjoyment and understanding rather than on the need to test one's ability to relate to the opposite sex. Although most adolescents, in western culture, do not marry at this time, adolescents are more likely to be involved with one person for a period of time.[13] Intimacy involves a sense of commitment rather than the experimentation and fantasy of the younger adolescent.[14]

The peer group becomes less significant as members go separate ways to seek personal opportunities in college or vocation. Conformity is less important as people form their own personal identities. The adolescent who has not developed a personal identity may continue to depend on a peer group and may have difficulty mastering additional developmental tasks.

As with any stage of development, not all adolescents will develop in all areas at the same rate. Among late adolescents, one person may focus on one aspect of life more intently than another. Some late adolescents focus a great deal of time and energy on relationships, whereas others focus on the pursuit of a career or job opportunity. The emphasis on choosing a life-long career during late adolescence is not as critical as it was in the past. Adolescents today are aware of the options available to them and the possibility that although they may choose one vocation or occupation, they may change occupations in the future.[24] Another change in our society is the increased number of women seeking careers and combining marriage, children, and career.[24] It is important to keep in mind that although an individual adolescent may not have a commitment to a life-long vocation, this alone does not indicate developmental failure. Instead, the ability to set goals for oneself in searching for a place in the work world and to take the necessary steps to meet these goals indicates the adolescent's progress in meeting this task.

The adolescent is now making more of his or her own decisions. Family relationships are becoming smoother, and the adolescent communicates on a more adult level with parents. The older adolescent can listen to parental advice and then make personal decisions about what to do. Conflicts may continue to surface if vocational or educational goals differ between parents and adolescent, but these can be resolved through communication.

Choosing A Career

As the adolescent makes progress toward mastering developmental tasks and makes personal choices regarding a career, education, relationship, or job, the adolescent has a more clearly defined personal identity. Reaching these goals provides the adolescent with an opportunity to use skills, be identified as successful, and develop increased self-esteem.

Choosing a career is a difficult task. The adolescent must weigh alternative possibilities with respect to financial, educational, or intellectual resources and to level of commitment. Additionally, the adolescent must consider

the needs of society and the discrepancy between personal goals, personal abilities, and job availability. Career choice may be influenced by parents as well as peers and role models the adolescent encounters outside the home. Role models include teachers, adults in the community, people the adolescent comes in contact with while working at a parttime job, and role models in the media. The availability of role models vary, especially among high- and low-socioeconomic groups.[24] Most parents hope that their children will rise above their own status, and many sacrifice to help their child achieve this goal. However, when role models are not visible to the adolescent, the adolescent may feel trapped with few life options.

Some adolescents are confronted with a wide variety of opportunities, whereas others are limited by education, finances, and communication skills. The possibility of higher education, vocational training, family business, or on-the-job training are all potential options (Fig. 16-6). Some adolescents choose to follow in their parents' footsteps. Others may not be aware of options or may not have found something they want to pursue as a career. Not knowing what direction to choose can cause the adolescent a great deal of stress. The adolescent may feel inadequate compared with peers who have made choices. The adolescent may try several options, such as taking a job or starting college, but may fail because of lack of true commitment. They may try several different jobs before they find the place where they fit.

Parental Role

For parents who have adolescents who know what direction they want their lives to take, this time is enjoyable. Parents feel a certain amount of relief that they have successfully raised a child who is finding a place in society.

Parents who have a confused adolescent who is unsure of what direction to take need to be patient and help the adolescent find a role in society. Parents may need

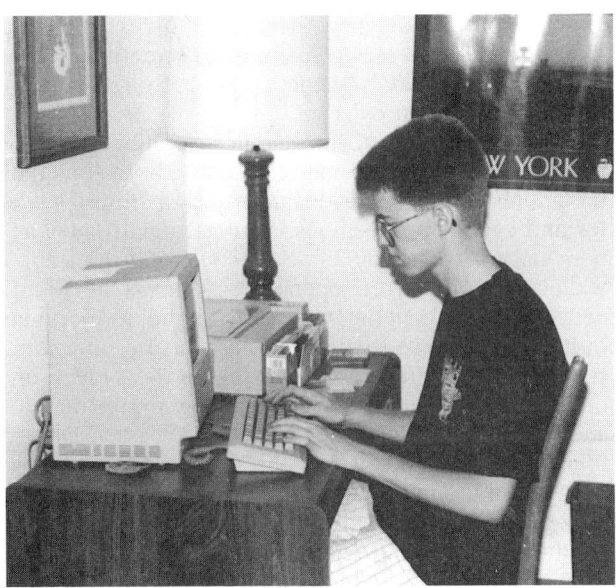

FIGURE 16-6
Computers can be used for schoolwork and for play.

support during this time because they may fear their child will not make it in the adult world.

Communication, again, is a valuable tool for parents. Talking to the adolescent about dreams and aspirations reinforces to the adolescent that parents do believe they have the potential to succeed. Also, parents may need to allow the adolescent to try out ideas even though parents can see many limitations, for example, allowing the adolescent to take a job after high school rather than pursuing higher education. At this stage of development the child can benefit from making mistakes. Parents should allow older adolescents opportunities to make personal decisions and be careful not to protect them from learning through trial and error.

Nursing Implications

The nurse and other health professionals can serve as role models for the adolescent and, in addition, support the adolescent in this aspect of development. Throughout the adolescent years, the nurse should talk to the individual teen about his or her goals for the future. The nurse can stimulate the adolescent to think about options available and may identify an adolescent who, because of limited role models or resources, is at risk for failure (see Table 16-2). Even though the nurse is not trained to work with adolescents and families in this area, early identification of potential problems and referral to a school counselor, career counselor, or family counselor is part of the health promotion role of the nurse.

Assessing, Promoting, and Maintaining Optimal Cognitive Development

Piaget's formal operative thought is the last stage of cognitive growth. This stage usually begins at about 12 years but may be delayed, partially developed, or not developed at all. Formal operative thought includes the ability to generate or consider hypotheses and to reason deductively. These processes constitute the scientific method whereby factors are systematically controlled and observed to test a particular set of propositions.

The adolescent becomes a reflective thinker with the ability to think about thought. Thinking in this manner, the adolescent can consider different possibilities both for and against propositions, such as social issues and personal goals. The younger child could only think about what is real in concrete operations, whereas the adolescent can think about the possible. With the development of formal operative thought, adolescents become introspective and interested in themselves, their ideas, and their fantasies. They realize that they can think one thing and say another. For example, if a peer asks "Do you think this looks good on me?" the adolescent can respond "yes" even though he or she may think that it does not look good. At the same time adolescents realize this ability, they realize that others are capable of the same thing. This results in the frequent need for reassurance: "Are you sure it looks good?"

The adolescent with new cognitive abilities is now able to evaluate events from more than one perspective. The adolescent now begins to examine personal beliefs and to search for inconsistency. The adolescent compares childhood beliefs and values with what is experienced in the world. Conflicts between old beliefs and new values may arise, causing confusion and anger. For example, "All men are created equal. Poor people do not have sufficient resources to live. If all men are equal, why is there so much inequality." The adolescent has an idealistic view of the world and is likely to embrace new ideologies, reject the status quo, and fantasize about changing the world. At this stage there is much verbal criticism of what could be or might have been, but at the same time the adolescent is aware of personal limitations for changing society. Later the adolescent realizes that change takes cooperation and effort and begins to work constructively with others within the society.

The ability to use formal operative thought does not permeate all aspects of the adolescent's life. Adolescents' concurrent narcissism, impulsiveness, desire to enjoy the "here and now," and feelings of being indestructible frequently result in their lack of consideration of the potential negative outcomes related to their behavior. This is demonstrated in risk-taking behaviors, such as driving while drinking, having sexual intercourse without the use of contraceptives, or experimenting with drugs.

Parental Role

Parents facilitate cognitive functioning by encouraging the adolescent to express new ideas and question old beliefs. Through discussion the adolescent not only expresses beliefs but is provided with another opinion or way of looking at things. The more input adolescents have when going through the process of evaluating beliefs, the more successful they will be in setting values and goals for themselves. Parents should be careful not to just quickly dismiss adolescent opinions or matter of factly state they are wrong. This response does not provide the adolescent with an opportunity to learn and grow. Parents also need to be aware of the fact that many times an adolescent may verbally express an opinion that contradicts parental values but does not act on this opinion. Instead, they are simply trying to understand why people believe what they believe.

Confrontations over beliefs and values between parent and adolescent may cause parental distress. Yet, it is these very confrontations that promote cognitive development and assist the adolescent in making independent personal decisions. The long discussions or arguments at the dinner table are, in fact, very valuable experiences.

Nursing Implications

The nurse must also encourage adolescents to express their views on issues related to their individual health, sexuality, risk-taking behaviors, and health promotion. Adolescents who are allowed to express their opinion are more willing to listen to the opinion of others. Additionally, the nurse has an opportunity to evaluate how the adolescent views the risks associated with specific behaviors and any misinformation the adolescent has related to health issues. The nurse should assist the adolescent in looking at long-term consequences of behavior and at the same time keep in mind the need for presenting information in concrete terms that will be meaningful for the adolescent.

Assessing, Promoting, and Maintaining Optimal Activity

School sports activities and physical fitness programs are the main organized physical activity experiences of the adolescent. The adolescent who is busy with school, friends, parttime jobs, and social activities has little time left for such things as a daily exercise routine or jogging (Fig. 16-7). A study, "Perceived Barriers to Exercise Among Adolescents,"[33] documents the following findings. In general, perceived barriers included wanting to do other things with free time, lack of interest, unsuitable weather, school work, lack of equipment or facilities, and job responsibilities. Males described the most significant barriers to include having a girlfriend and the use of alcohol and other drugs. The most significant barrier described by females was wanting to do other things with their time.

The combination of the many facets of adolescence that potentially can result in a lack of health promotion behaviors reinforces the need for regular, consistent, and well-designed activity patterns. Factors that put the adolescent at risk for illness and long-term poor health practices include inadequate nutrition; poor sleep; use of substances, including alcohol, drugs, and tobacco; and generalized feelings of being invincible. The adolescent who experiences these problems is the adolescent who is most likely to also have ineffective activity patterns.

Aside from forced participation in gym, adolescent's activity patterns are dependent on their beliefs about activity and well-being. An adolescent who is unwilling to exercise for health reasons may be willing to exercise for an improved body shape or physical skills. Parents and health professionals must use creativity in their approach to the adolescent who has inadequate activity patterns. By focusing on the adolescent's priorities they may be able to assist the adolescent to incorporate exercise in everyday activities.

Assessing, Promoting, and Maintaining Adolescent Safety

Safety issues during adolescence center around the adolescent's risk-taking behavior. Adolescents with limited or no experience engage in potentially destructive behaviors without considering the immediate or long-term consequences of their actions. These behaviors that impact on the adolescent's health and well-being include sexual activity, substance use, and reckless driving (Fig. 16-8).

Adolescents and young adults were the only age groups to experience a rise in mortality rates over the last 20 years.[19] The increase is largely related to violent events, of which injuries are the leading cause.[20] Unintentional injuries, homicide, and suicide account for 80% of all deaths in these age groups[3] (see Chap. 19 for a discussion of adolescent suicide). Motor vehicle accidents alone account for 37% of adolescent deaths.[15] Researchers[15] have found a correlation between the adolescent's involvement in one type of risk-taking behavior and other areas of risk

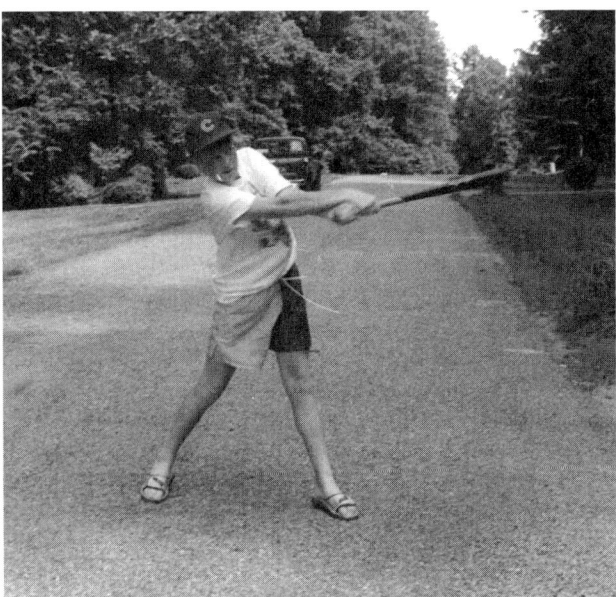

FIGURE 16-7
Most sports are part of organized school programs, and adolescents continue to need encouragement to be physically active.

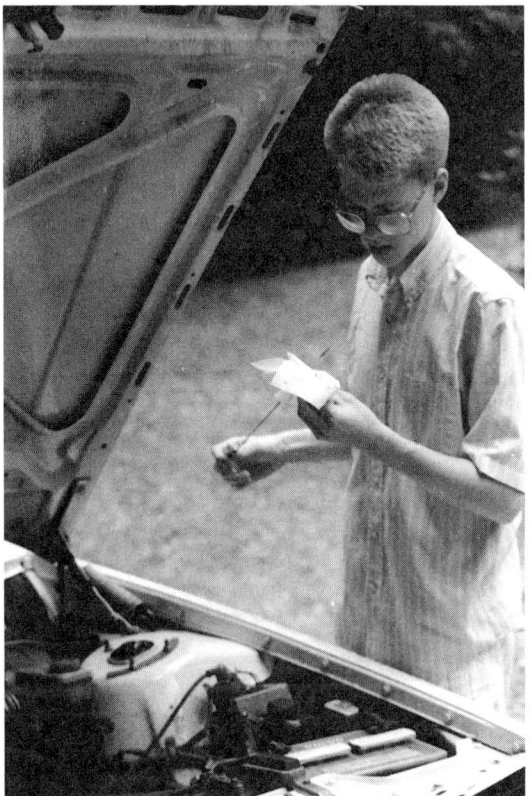

FIGURE 16-8
Automobiles are important to adolescents. Safety education regarding driving, speeding, and drinking is extremely important.

taking. For example, adolescents involved with substance use initiate sexual activity earlier and use less effective means of contraception. A link between the use of alcohol and motor vehicle accidents has been well documented. Additionally, other accidents, such as drowning, falls, and burns, are associated with substance use.

Adolescent risk-taking behavior is associated with the process of normal development. Emancipation from parents results in peer group association, with the potential for peer pressure to engage in risk-taking behaviors. In early adolescence behaviors such as smoking, experimenting with drugs, handling guns, or operating recreational vehicles place them at risk for injury as well as the development of habits that will have long-term negative consequences for their health.

The adolescent may have the cognitive skills to think abstractly, to consider possibilities, and to examine the long-term effects of behavior, but these abilities may be negated by the adolescent's impulsiveness The adolescent's egocentrism and feelings of invulnerability encourages experimentation and defiance of limits.

The timing and onset of puberty independent of the adolescents chronologic age may increase the incidence of and timing of risk-taking behaviors.[15] The adolescent who develops early may become involved in sexual activity earlier and therefore be at risk for pregnancy and sexually transmitted diseases. The late-developing adolescent may be at risk for developing risk-taking behaviors such as substance use.

The identification of the potential health and safety risks during the adolescent years is well established. Unfortunately, statistics indicate that decreasing the potential and actual negative outcome for adolescents has made little progress. However, some recommendations have been made that reflect the multiple factors involved.[15]

First, those persons who choose to work with adolescents should have an understanding of the unique development issues of adolescence in physical, psychosocial, and cognitive development. Second, early identification of one type of risk-taking behavior would indicate the need to look for other behaviors or the potential for the development of other behaviors. Third, attempts to delay the onset of the initial risk-taking behavior will decrease the likelihood of a second behavior from developing. Role modeling by parents and other adults throughout childhood is optimal. Parents who practice health-promoting rather than health-damaging behaviors before the onset of adolescence may decrease the incidence of risk-taking behaviors by the adolescent. Fourth, the professional should try to assist the adolescent in finding appropriate ways to accomplish what the negative behavior is providing the adolescent. For example, an adolescent who drinks alcohol to decrease feelings of insecurity needs assistance in developing other methods for improving self-esteem. Fifth, Because it is impossible to protect the adolescent from all potential hazardous behaviors, emphasis may sometimes need to be placed on preventing the most potentially dangerous outcomes. This is seen in the contracts adolescents sign with their parents stating that if they do drink, they will not drive.

Additionally, parents can be encouraged to use the services available in the community to assist them in providing safety in the daily life of their adolescent. These community programs center around prevention and generally are developed with the unique needs of the adolescent in mind. These community programs include driver education, water safety, and group programs such as Mother's Against Drunk Driving (MADD) and Students Against Drunk Driving (SADD).

Nurses who work with adolescents in schools and clinics also need to become involved in these programs. Additionally, they need to assess risk-taking behaviors or the potential for their development when seeing an adolescent in the well-care clinic.

Assessing Promoting, and Maintaining Health Perception and Health Management

Physical illness is not a major concern during the adolescent years. The adolescent is relatively healthy and may not seek health care unless he or she has a specific problem. Health care commonly focuses on problems related to developmental issues such as concerns about physical development, illness, injury related to risk-taking behavior, or sexuality.

Each time the adolescent seeks assistance from a health care professional, the adolescent should be given opportunities to participate actively in the assessment and the planning of interventions to foster optimal growth and development. The nurse, as an objective outside person, is in an ideal position to work with the adolescent. Unlike the adolescent's parents and teachers, the nurse is not evaluating the adolescent on a daily basis. The nurse can be a resource person for the adolescent as well as a person the adolescent can use when working through a problem. The adolescent may feel safer confiding feelings to the nurse when the adolescent has control over how the relationship develops.

The nurse working with adolescents must also develop skill in working with parents. It is not uncommon for the nurse to be in a situation where intervention is required to assist an adolescent and parents in resolving a conflict. However, it is optimal for the nurse to prevent conflicts from developing by anticipating potential areas of conflict and avoiding them through education, understanding, and support. The nurse should systematically evaluate where the adolescent is developmentally and determine on which developmental task the adolescent is presently focusing. By doing this, the nurse will be able to give more specific assistance rather than generalized assurances to both the adolescent and parents.

Adolescent Health Visits

Optimally, the adolescent health visit should occur annually, with additional follow-ups between visits as necessary.[13] The American Academy of Pediatrics recommends biannual visits for health screening but emphasizes the need for more frequent visits for other adolescent issues, including substance use and reproductive, psychosocial, and emotional issues.[1]

The nurse's communication skills, approach with the adolescent, and ability to listen will influence the adolescent's decision to return for future health care visits.

The nurse-client relationship with adolescents is facilitated by a nurse who is aware of the needs of the adolescent. The adolescent needs to be approached in an unhurried manner. The adolescent can and does participate in health care decisions. It is important that the nurse treat the adolescent as an individual. It is important that the nurse directly involve the adolescent and obtain the history and physical without the presence of parents. If parents object to this, the nurse can explain to them that adolescents need opportunities to take responsibility for their own health and that this is a good starting point. During the interview the nurse should start with less threatening topics and move to more difficult topics, including substance use and sexual activity. The most important skill the nurse should use is listening. The nurse who listens carefully to the adolescent will pick up cues as to what issues are important to the adolescent. These issues may be quite different from what the nurse or parents perceive the issues to be. If the nurse does not speak to the issues described by the adolescent or dismisses them, there is a risk that the adolescent will not to make further attempts to express concerns or ask questions.

If problems are identified, the nurse should express them openly to the adolescent so that he or she can discuss the concerns and begin to problem solve. The adolescent should also be given an opportunity to express how the health visit has or has not met individual needs.

Parents should be seen by the nurse also. Parents can provide information related to changes in behavior, school performance, sleep, nutrition, and activity. It is helpful to get parental perceptions of how the adolescent is doing and any concerns they have related to development and behavior.

In some instances the nurse may want to bring the adolescent and parents together to discuss issues that are causing problems. Both parties can express feelings and mutual problem solving can occur with the assistance of the nurse.

Health Care

Acne Vulgaris

Acne is defined as a chronic inflammatory disorder of the pilosebaceous follicles.[28] Acne vulgaris is the most common skin disorder during adolescence. The incidence of acne among adolescents is as high as 90%, but the degree of involvement varies from very minor problems to severe scarring and hypertrophic scars. Lesions are either inflammatory or noninflammatory. Comedonal lesions are noninflammatory and are either open comedones (blackheads), which are composed of an epithelium-lined sac filled with keratin, lipid, and organisms and have widespread dilated orifices; and closed comedones (whiteheads), in which openings are microscopic, preventing keratin and sebum from escaping. Inflammatory lesions are generally that result of closed lesions. Acne lesions consist of papules, pustules, cysts, nodules, and scars. The most common sites of acne are areas where the sebaceous glands are well developed including the face, back, chest, and upper arms.

The exact cause of acne is unknown. However, factors including hormonal factors, menstruation, diet, stress, climate, and bacteria have been implicated.[28] Dietary causes of acne continue to be an area of much debate.

Treatment for acne should be individualized to meet the specific needs of each adolescent. Topical therapies are the most common and include benzoyl peroxide and retinoic acid. Antibiotics include tetracycline hydrochloride, erythromycin, clindamycin, and minocycline. The effectiveness of treatment frequently depends on the adolescent's compliance with a treatment plan. Tunnessen[34] describes the following common pitfalls to treatment and recommends emphasis on education of the adolescent at the time of initial treatment:

- Compliance is a frequent cause for lack of success in treating acne. The adolescent needs very specific instructions related to the treatment prescribed and the necessity to follow directions. Follow-up appointments will also increase compliance.
- The concept that if a little topical medication works more will work even better causes the adolescent to experience erythema and peeling. Adolescents may stop using the medication if their face becomes red and scaly, blaming the medication rather than the overuse of the medication.
- One of the most common causes of topical medication failure is the adolescent's dabbing medication on lesions rather than on the entire surface of the face, back, or chest. Treating individual lesions will work, but unless medication is applied to unaffected areas, new lesions will continue to appear.
- The desire for instant response to topical medication encourages the adolescent to give up a treatment plan before it has time to work. It takes 4 to 6 weeks of daily use before an initial response is seen. Adolescent need to be aware of the amount of time it will take to have a response to treatment.
- Adolescents may vigorously scrub the face and attempt to remove pimples by breaking them. These behaviors are frequently the result of misinformation regarding the formation of acne. Acne is not caused by dirt, and vigorous scrubbing can actually break blocked pilosebaceous units below the skin surface, promoting new lesions. Popping pimples may result in scarring. Adolescents should be taught to wash with mild soap and water.

Because of acne's potential negative affect on self-image, it is an important topic for discussion at routine adolescent health visits. The impact acne has on a particular adolescent will depend not on the extent of the condition but on the adolescent's perception of the problem and the adolescent's comfort with his or her body image. Adolescents benefit from knowledge regarding the cause, treatment, and common reasons for failure to respond to treatment. The emphasis of treatment should center on control rather than cure. Adolescents need to be instructed in the proper use of any treatment regime and assisted in finding the best approach to ensuring compliance.

Dysmenorrhea

Dysmenorrhea is a common problem among adolescent girls.[35] However, many adolescents may not identify dysmenorrhea as a problem unless specifically asked. Adolescent girls may believe that menstrual cramps are a normal female experience even when accompanied by severe pain, nausea, vomiting, diarrhea, headache, dizziness, and fatigue.[35] Even if dysmenorrhea is considered a problem, adolescents may not be aware that therapy can relieve their distress and therefore do not identify the problem at the health care visit.[35]

Most adolescents with menstrual pain have primary dysmenorrhea, a condition that does not have an organic cause for symptoms.[5] Primary dysmenorrhea is thought to be caused by the production and release of prostaglandin by the uterus during menstruation. The adolescent may experience mild or moderate to severe symptoms. Dysmenorrhea can indicate a serious disease of the reproductive organs, including endometriosis, uterine anomaly, or pelvic infection. It is important that dysmenorrhea with an underlying medical problem be detected and treated early to prevent long-term reproductive problems (see Chap. 68).

Primary dysmenorrhea can have a significant impact on adolescent development. School absenteeism, lack of concentration, and poor school performance have been related to dysmenorrhea. One study found dysmenorrhea to be the leading cause of short-term school absenteeism.[36]

Nursing Implications.   During the health care visit the nurse should obtain a complete menstrual history with presence of dysmenorrhea, treatments used to decrease symptoms, and effectiveness of therapies used to manage symptoms. The adolescent benefits from education related to the cause of dysmenorrhea as well as a plan for the management of symptoms.

A biopsychosocial model for management of dysmenorrhea has been found to be effective with adolescent girls.[35] Initially, the adolescent needs information describing dysmenorrhea, with emphasis on the fact that dysmenorrhea may be decreased through self-help measures and/or medical treatment. In addition to education, the adolescent should be given information regarding self-help lifestyle changes, including aerobic exercise for 20 to 30 minutes a day; a well-balanced diet free of alcohol, caffeine, excessive simple carbohydrates, or salt; and the avoidance of fasting. Heat, adequate rest, and over-the-counter analgesics and ibuprofen are helpful in decreasing discomfort. Medical management may include antiprostaglandins or oral contraceptives. Regardless of treatment, recommended follow-up is necessary to evaluate its effectiveness.

Dental Care

The adolescent continues to need routine dental care every 6 months. Fluoride supplements continue until the age of 16 in areas where water is not fluorinated (see Table 12-2 in Chap. 12 for supplemental fluoride dosage schedule).

Summary

Adolescence is a time for dramatic changes in the lives of youths as they make the transition from childhood to

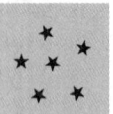

Ideas for Nursing Research

Adolescents experience many exciting changes as they grow and develop through early to late adolescence. Nurses have an opportunity to explore many issues related to the three stages of adolescence. The following areas need to be explored:

- Relationship between adolescent health promotion behaviors and parental health promotion behaviors.
- Relationship between school performance and risk-taking behaviors of adolescents.
- Most effective approaches to obtaining a health history from an adolescent.
- Adolescent use of health services developed specifically for them as compared to use of general health services.

adulthood. The transition is not always smooth, and adolescents may encounter obstacles as they adjust to rapid physical changes, deal with strong emotional feelings, seek independence, and find a place in the adult world.

Parents also experience fear and concern as the adolescent struggles to master developmental tasks. Parents must balance the adolescent's need to make the transition to adulthood with the need for parental support and assistance in avoiding failure.

The adolescent years can be very exciting for the adolescent and parents and need not be feared. In a society that focuses on the negative aspects of adolescent behavior, it is common for parents, teachers, and health care workers to focus only on the problems, losing the ability to see the strengths. Nurses who work with adolescents in health promotion have a unique opportunity to emphasize the positive aspects of this period of development. Nurses can assist both the parent and adolescent in avoiding or dealing with common problems through anticipatory guidance, early identification of potential problems, and assistance with problem-solving efforts to deal with identified concerns.

References

1. American Academy of Pediatrics, Committee on Practice and Ambulatory Medicine. (1988). Recommendations for preventive pediatric health care. *Pediatrics, 81,* 466.
2. Anders, T., Carskadon, M., & Dement, W. (1980). Sleep and sleepiness in children and adolescents. *Pediatric Clinics of North America, 27,* 29.
3. Bass, J., Gallagher, S., & Kishor, M. (1985). Injuries to adolescents and young adults. *Pediatric Clinics of North America, 32,* 31.
4. Bundis, C., & Jeremy, R. (1988). *Adolescent pregnancy and parenting in California: A strategic plan for action.* San Francisco: Sutter Publishing.
4a. Centers for Disease Control (CDC) (Feb. 1992). *HIV/AIDS Surveillance Report,* Feb, 1–18.

5. Dershewitz, R. (Ed.). (1988). *Ambulatory pediatric care.* Philadelphia: J.B. Lippincott.
6. Dryfoos, J. (1983). *Review of interventions in the field of prevention of adolescent pregnancy: Preliminary report to the Rockefeller Foundation.* New York: Rockefeller Foundation.
7. Erikson, E. (1963). *Childhood and society.* New York: W.W. Norton.
8. Evans, M., and Cronin, F. (1986). Diets of school-age children and teenagers. *Family Economics Review, 3,* 14.
9. Franz, M. (1986, Spring). Life in the fast food lane. *Diabetes: The Newsletter for People Who Live with Diabetes,* 1–4.
10. Grant, L., & Demetriou, E. (1988). Adolescent sexuality. *Pediatric Clinics of North America, 35,* 1271.
11. Hayes, C. (Ed.). (1987). *Risking the future: Adolescent sexuality, pregnancy, and childbearing.* Washington, DC: National Academy Press.
12. Hofferth, S., and Hayes, C. (Eds.). (1987). *Risking the future: Adolescent sexuality, pregnancy, and childbearing* (statistical appendixes). Washington, DC: National Academy Press.
13. Hofmann, A., Becker, R., & Gabriel, H. (1976). The hospitalized adolescent: A guide to managing the ill and injured youth. London: Free Press.
14. Hofmann, A., and Greydanus, D. (Eds.). (1983). Adolescent medicine. Boston: Addison Wesley.
15. Irwin, C., and Millstein, S. (1986). Biopsychosocial correlates of risk-taking behaviors during adolescence. *Journal of Adolescent Health Care, 7,* 82S.
16. Marsiglio, W., & Mott, F. (1986). The impact of sex education on sexual activity, contraceptive use and premarital pregnancy among American teenagers. *Family Planning Perspectives, 18,* 151.
17. McClelland, D., Constantian, C., Regalado, D., & Stone, C. (1978). Making it to maturity. *Psychology Today, 12,* 42.
18. Moses, N., Banilivy, M., & Lifshitz, F. (1989). Fear of obesity among adolescent girls. *Pediatrics, 83,* 393.
19. National Center for Health Statistics. (1982, December). *Health: United States 1982* (DHHA Publication No. PHS 83–1232). Washington, DC: U.S. Government Printing Office.
20. National Safety Council. (1982). *Accident facts.* Chicago, IL: National Safety Council.
21. Pennington, J. (Ed.). (1992). *Bowe's and Church's food values of foods commonly used* (16th ed.). Philadelphia: J.B. Lippincott.
22. Paperny, D., & Starn, J. (1989). Adolescent pregnancy prevention by health education computer games: Computer assisted instruction of knowledge and adapted. *Pediatrics, 83,* 742.
23. Price, V., Coates, T., Thorensen, C., & Grinstead, O. (1978). Prevalence and correlates of poor sleep among adolescents. *American Journal of Diseases of Children, 132,* 583.
24. Rogers, D. (1985). *Adolescents and youth* (5th ed.). Englewood Cliffs, NJ: Prentice-Hall.
25. Schilder, P. (1964). *The image and appearance of the human body* (Science Eds.). New York: John Wiley & Sons.
26. Schonfeld, W. (1969). The body and body image in adolescence. In S. Lebovici, *Adolescence: Psychosocial perspectives* (pp. 27–53). New York: Basic Books.
27. Shannon, B., and Parks, S. (1980). Fast foods: A perspective on their nutritional impact. *Journal of the American Dietetic Association, 76,* 242.
28. Shearin, R., and Wientzen, R. (1983). *Clinical adolescent medicine.* Boston: G.K. Hall.
29. Story, M. (1989). A perspective on adolescent lifestyle and eating behavior. *Nutrition News, 52,* 1.
30. Stout, J., Frederick, P., & Rivara, M. (1989). Schools and sex education: Does it work? *Pediatrics, 83,* 375.
31. Tanner, J. (1962). *Growth at adolescence* (2nd ed.). Oxford: Blackwell Scientific Publications.
32. Tauer, K. (1983). Promoting effective decision making in sexually active adolescents. *Nursing Clinics of North America, 15,* 275.
33. Tappe, M., Duda, J., & Ehrnwald, P. (1989). Perceived barriers to exercise among adolescents. *Journal of School Health, 59,* 153.
34. Tunnessen, W. (1989). Acne vulgaris: Preventing treatment pitfalls. *Pediatric Currents, 38(1),* 3–4.
35. Wilson, C., & Keye, W. (1989). A survey of adolescent dysmenorrhea and premenstrual symptom frequency: A model program for prevention, detection, and treatment. *Journal of Adolescent Health Care, 10,* 317.
36. Yliklorkala, O., & Dawood, M. (1978). New concepts in dysmenorrhea. *American Journal of Obstetrics and Gynecology, 130,* 733.
37. Zabin, L., Hirsh, M., Smith, E., Strett, R., & Hardy, J. (1986). Evaluation of a pregnancy prevention program for urban teenagers. *Family Planning Perspectives, 18,* 119–126.
38. Zelnik, M., & Kantner, J. (1980). Sexual activity, contraceptive use, and pregnancy among metropolitan area teenagers: 1971–1979. *Family Planning Perspectives, 10,* 230.

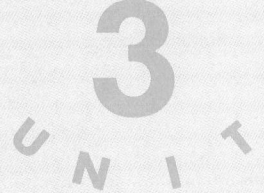

3 UNIT

Emotional and Psychosocial Considerations of the Child and Family

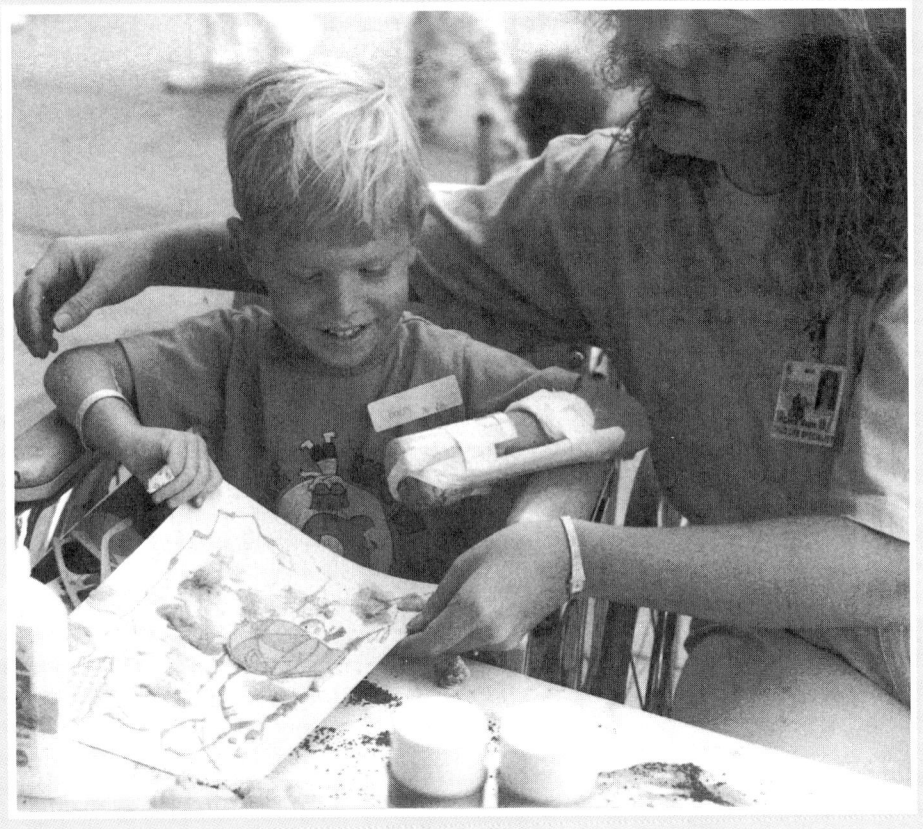

17

Coping With Change

BEHAVIORAL OBJECTIVES

Define coping as part of the adaptation process.

Identify factors that may influence a child's coping ability.

Identify common changes or stressors that occur during childhood.

Describe selected behavioral responses to changes or stressors

as they occur across developmental levels.

Discuss the nurse's role in maintaining or enhancing the child's and family's ability to cope with change.

Describe selected assessment tools available to assess the coping ability of the child and family.

FEATURES OF THIS CHAPTER

Nursing Care Plan: A Toddler Using Regression as a Defense Mechanism

Teaching Plan: Dealing With Separation Anxiety in a 3-Year-Old Child

Ideas for Nursing Research

Nursing Interventions: Developmental Coping Methods, Table 17-1

Children are expected to cope with normal changes inherent to everyday life. At each developmental level, the child encounters new challenges that require adaptation and a certain degree of mastery. Infants have their initial experiences with stress and frustration while attempting to have their basic needs met. The toddler and preschooler often experience feelings of conflict as limits are placed on their newly found sense of autonomy. The school-age child competes with peers in the classroom as well as on the playground; this competition will result in experiences of success as well as failure. The adolescent, not unlike the toddler, re-experiences the thrill of independence. However, the process of independence and self-identification is often associated with periods of self-doubt and confusion. These are normal developmental conflicts.

The child growing up in the 1990s must also deal with other confounding issues. Changes in the nuclear family configuration, the increase in the number of children who live in poverty, the increased availability of drugs in school, the increase in sexual activities at earlier ages, and the AIDS epidemic are just a few of the factors that effect the child's ability to cope with the normal challenges of everyday life.

Nurses are in a unique position to assess the child's and family's coping abilities and to determine appropriate interventions that can maintain or enhance the family's existing coping patterns. The purpose of this chapter is to examine the child's ability to cope with normal developmental changes. The activity of coping is described as part of the overall process of adaptation. Factors that may influence a child's ability to cope as well as some methods to assist the child and family to cope effectively with developmental changes are discussed. Selected assessment tools to identify child and family coping abilities are reviewed, and nursing interventions are summarized. Specific needs are addressed in other chapters in this unit.

389

The Coping Process

Theoretical Overview of Coping as an Adaptive Process

Coping can be viewed as part of the overall process of adaptation. Through the activities of coping, the goal of adaptation is reached. *Adaptation* is an adjustment to environmental conditions. The goal of adaptation is to maintain a steady state between the organism and the environment. The organism's adjustment to the environment is necessary for survival, reproduction, and the process of natural selection.

Neuman describes coping and adaptation as interventions that help individuals to maintain their basic structure.[26] Neuman defines health as a state of equilibrium on a continuum of wellness to illness. In a state of health, the person's normal lines of defense are intact and the system's needs are being met. When the lines of defense are penetrated by stressors, the person's equilibrium is affected and a reduced state of wellness may occur.

Adaptation has been described in the literature as both a physiologic and a psychological phenomenon. One of the foremost theories regarding human adaptation to change and stress was developed by the physiologist Hans Selye. Selye[34] defines *stress* as a nonspecific response of the body to any demands made on it from its external or internal environment. The *general adaptation syndrome*, termed by Selye, describes the body's physiologic response to a stressor, which occurs in three stages. In the first stage, the alarm reaction, the individual recognizes the stressor and the pituitary adrenal cortical system responds by producing hormones to either fight or take flight from the stressor. The body's physical response includes an increase in heart rate and blood sugar, dilation of the pupils, and a slowed digestion. In the stage of resistance, the second stage, the body begins to repair the effects of the stressors. The stage of exhaustion occurs when the body can no longer respond to the stress and failure ensues. It is through their innate and acquired mechanisms that humans cope with their continually changing environment.[32] Stress theory and the general adaptation theory are discussed more fully in Chapter 18.

Several authors portray coping as a positive reaction to one or more environmental stressors. Although some stressors are situation specific, others are the result of life and growth and development.[21] The developmental theories of Freud, Erikson, Piaget, and others describe the child's ability to adapt to and cope with environmental stressors. Mastery or adequate adaptation in one stage must be achieved before moving on to the next stage. In coping with a stressor, loss of control has been identified as one of the underlying threats to the individual. Mastery of the situation becomes the desired outcome. Successful coping results when a person perceives control of the situation through persistent efforts to master the situational threats posed according to developmental level.

Another outcome of effective coping is competence. Murphy[22] describes competence as the collection of skills resulting from cumulative mastery achievement. Effective coping behaviors will be called on again when people are faced with what they consider to be a similar situation. Tiedeman[40] describes coping as routine, accustomed patterns of behavior used to deal with daily situations as well as to the production of new ways of behaving when drastic changes defy familiar responses. There are situations in which one's usual coping efforts may not be effective. A strategy that has worked in the past may not be successful in another situation. In addition, new strategies may not always be effective. Ineffective coping strategies can increase the existing level of stress and may result in abnormal or aberrant coping behaviors.

Coping strategies are learned, deliberate, and purposeful emotional and behavioral responses to stressors and are used to adapt to or change the stressors.[17]

Two forms of coping strategies described by Lazarus[17] are direct-action tendencies and defensive adjustment. Direct-action tendencies describe coping efforts as being aimed at the elimination of the initial condition or stressor. The goal is to change the situation so that the person will no longer be in danger. In contrast, defensive adjustment involves the use of defense mechanisms.

Freud[12] described a defense mechanism as an "unconscious" psychological process aimed at self-deception about the presence of possible dangers. Some of the more commonly used defense mechanisms include denial of reality, repression, rationalization, regression, displacement, reaction formation, sublimation, projection, and intellectualization. The use of defense mechanisms can be regarded as a coping strategy because it is a psychological method of dealing with threat and frustration.[16,17] However, prolonged or inappropriate use of defense mechanisms can result in an individual not dealing with the threat or danger and not taking the appropriate steps to maintain integrity.

The literature on coping in children is sparse. The bulk of work done in this area examines the concept of coping styles rather than coping strategies. Moos[21] differentiates between the terms *coping styles* and *coping strategies*. Coping styles are inherent patterns of responding to stressors that are global traits and that persist over time. Coping strategies are the actual behaviors that are used to cope with stress, which are learned, vary over time, and can be changed.

Coping is a dynamic response to the changes and stressors in one's daily life. Successful coping occurs when the person has maintained and equilibrium between the internal and external environment.

Factors Influencing a Child's Ability to Cope

Coping capacities will vary from child to child and depend on the interaction of a number of factors within the environment. Growth and development levels, physical health, psychological and emotional health and self-esteem, support systems, and previous coping experiences are some of the contributing factors that should be examined when assessing a child's ability to cope with any change or stressor.

Growth and Development Level

Achieving appropriate growth and development levels is critical to a child's ability to respond to change and stress. As children develop they achieve certain cognitive as well as psychosocial abilities. Coping ability includes the use of cognitive function (perception, speech, judgment), motor activity, emotional expression, and psychological defenses.[18,21]

Coping activities are cultivated from birth. When infants' needs are consistently met, they develop a sense of trust in their main caretaker. The infants begin to trust that their demonstration of certain cues will elicit a positive response from their caretakers and that needs will be met. Observed coping behaviors in the infant include increased motor activities such as restlessness, crying, moving away from negative stimuli, habituation, sucking, and hand-to-mouth activities.

The toddler and preschooler have identified themselves as being separate from their mother. Enthralled with the idea of self, the young child is constantly testing his or her individual capabilities. Egocentric thinking and fantasy are used as methods by this age group to explain how and why things happen. Coping behaviors demonstrated during this period may include regression, temper tantrums, clinging, whining, increased motor activity, and bed wetting. Comforting measures that may be employed by the young child include thumb sucking, holding a special blanket or toy, and moving in a continuous rocking motion (Fig. 17-1).

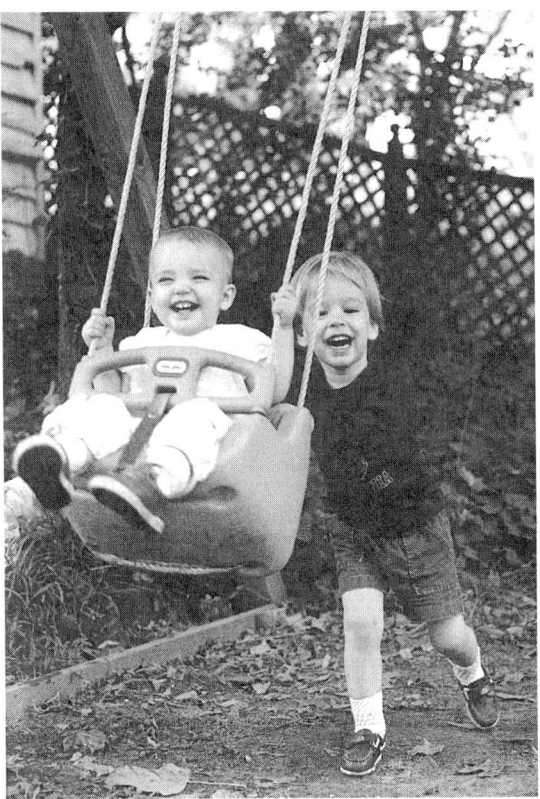

FIGURE 17-2
Physical activities can help children to develop coping strategies. Older siblings can be encouraged to help younger siblings as a way of learning to cope with the addition to the family, which has created changes in their lives.

As a result of cognitive maturation and previous life experiences, the school-age child has a better array of coping behaviors from which to choose than a younger counterpart. Self-care, school attendance, and socialization with peers are essential life experiences that foster self-esteem and appropriate social skills. Some coping strategies used by the school-age child include controlling behaviors (strict adherence to the rules), humor, increased motor activity, and withdrawal (Fig. 17-2). Some aberrant coping strategies at this age would include compulsive lying, truancy, alcohol and drug abuse, and stealing.

The adolescent struggles with a new and different sense of autonomy. One of the main tasks during this period of development is to achieve a sense of balance between dependence on parents, peers, and self. Coping strategies used by the adolescent may include defense mechanisms such as rationalization, intellectualization, and sublimation; controlling behaviors; and increased motor activity. Aberrant coping behaviors would include truancy, eating disorders, alcohol and drug use, suicide, and gang-related activities.

Physical Health

A healthy child will have more energy available to deal with stressors than a child whose energies have been depleted due to illness. Any alteration in health, whether

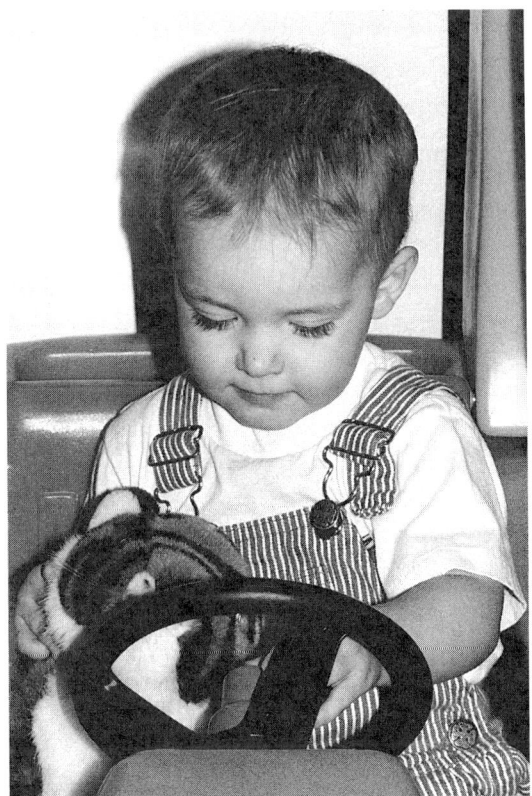

FIGURE 17-1
Special blankets and toys can serve as a comforting measure for toddlers.

it be an acute or chronic episode, can result in the child's use of regression as a coping strategy. Regression allows a child to revert temporarily to an earlier, previously abandoned developmental stage to regain mastery of a stressful, anxiety-producing, or frustrating experience.[1] Regression helps the child feel a sense of protection. During regression, less demands are made on the child; therefore, the child's energies can be directed toward dealing with the change or stressor. Although temporary regression may be a viable coping method, efforts should be made to promote and maintain the child's age-appropriate growth and development level, particularly for the child with a long-term or chronic illness.

For the ill, hospitalized child, separation from family and the unfamiliar hospital environment are the major stressors that must be faced. When possible, a tour of the hospital before admission will help the child to become familiar with the environment. In addition, much has been written in the literature regarding specific methods to help the child cope with painful procedures. It has been suggested that preparation prior to a procedure will help a child cope more effectively with the stress associated with that procedure.[9,31,42]

Age and the amount of information given to prepare a child are two of the variables that have been studied in relation to children's coping ability. La Montagne[15] determined that as age increased, children were given more preoperative information, which, in turn, related to more active coping. In addition, children who received more detailed information about their surgery used more active coping strategies compared with children who received either general or less information.

An aspect of coping that has been more recently studied is that of healthy siblings' response to their ill siblings' illness. Common elements of concern that surfaced included loss of both quality and quantity of family relationships, particularly between healthy siblings and parents, and changes in family routines and activities, which generally resulted in siblings feeling excluded from the vital flow of family life in the midst of crises. Ultimately, an increase in the sharing of the burden resulted when siblings realized or gained a more total appreciation of the illness. Coping with illness and hospitalization is further discussed in Chapter 23.

Psychological-Emotional Health and Self-Esteem

Psychological-emotional health is equally as important as physical health in contributing to a child's coping ability. Murphy[23] has cited the following factors as ones that are important determinants of positive coping resources in children: a positive outgoing attitude toward life including self-pride; courage to face challenge and difficulty; and resilience and capacity to mobilize resources after frustration and disappointment.

Positive self-esteem has been cited frequently as an essential condition for satisfactory adaptive behavior. For a child to continue with the effort required to cope and succeed in a given situation, positive reinforcements are needed throughout the experience. Parents can foster self-care and self-esteem in their children by providing a supportive atmosphere in which a child can try different coping mechanisms.

Support Systems

Success in coping with change or stress depends partly on the child's available support systems. Initially, parents are the child's major resources or support system. One can assess the "degree of fit" between the parents and the child or the amount of emotional support that is provided to the child who is faced with a new or changing situation.[41] Respect and encouragement of the child's capabilities is essential for the development of the child's sense of competency. Parents, family members, and, eventually, peers may serve as buffers between the child and the stressor until the child has developed a level of self-esteem and coping skills sufficient to meet the challenges.

The influence of parental coping styles should also be examined. The child's framework for understanding, accepting, and mastering stressful situations depends to a large extent on the parents' ability to cope successfully. Parents who fail to develop such psychosocial coping skills may affect the child's ability to learn these skills. In addition to parental coping style, many other factors may affect a family's ability to serve as a support system for their child. Concurrent family stressors that may have an impact the family's ability to support the child, such as illness of another family member, divorce, and job loss, are discussed in Chapter 5.

Previous Coping Experiences and Perception

Successful coping in previous situations encourages the child to explore and deal with new challenges. Cognitive maturation determines the child's ability to recall previous experiences and the perceptions of those experiences.[41] Children who have received gratification from previous accomplishments can recall this feeling and are likely to use coping skills that were successful in the past. A child is more likely to perceive a new situation positively and approach it more confidently with a past history of successful coping experiences.

It is also important to examine the child's interpretation or perception of the situational threat. Lazarus and Launier[19] state that response to change or stress is a personal experience. The experience reflects a process that occurs between a person and a situation. The following factors contribute to the assessment of the change-stressor and will determine response strategies: (1) the child's previous opportunities for autonomy and independent exploration; (2) the amount of age-appropriate sensory stimulation provided to meet the child's needs; and (3) exposure to challenging situations or circumstances developing mastery and enhancing self-esteem. Other environmental aspects that affect perception include those determined by the child's cultural background. What may be considered a stressor in one culture may not be considered one in another.

Common Childhood Changes and Stressors

Throughout development, there are certain inevitable maturational changes that confront the child. How successfully the child copes with these "normal" changes will lay the foundation for an ability to cope with situational or unexpected changes.

Developmental-Related Fears

Fears usually develop owing to a state of anxiety regarding impending danger, pain, or loss. Fears can be categorized as specific or general and real or imagined. An example of a specific fear would be fear of women with dark hair as opposed to a generalized fear, such as fear of flying. Real fears would include fear of an actual object or situation, such as fear of all white dogs, because the child was bitten by one, whereas an imagined fear would refer to a fear of something that cannot be observed, for example, fear of monsters or the boogieman.

Dibrell and Yamotto[6] interviewed 36 children between the ages of 4 and 10 years to determine what experiences made the children feel upset or sad. Themes that were repeated by the children included (1) parental quarreling and fighting; (2) being lost or abandoned; and (3) physical harm.

The children's concerns regarding abandonment and powerlessness revealed an underlying sense of vulnerability and dependence.

Most childhood fears are predictable and are related to developmental levels. Children between the ages of 2 and 6 years have a higher incidence of fears than any other age group. It is unclear whether infants generally have the cognitive capacity to understand and develop fears. Separation from mother or father is the most important concern for the infant. Toddlers also fear separation from mother or father and association with unfamiliar people.

Among the preschooler's fears are fear of the dark and imaginary creatures such as monsters. A young child's thinking process includes aspects of fantasy and magic; therefore, the child may fear harm from imagined creatures that may seem real to them. Fears related to body integrity and body mutilation are also dominant in this age range. Preschoolers have a vague and often incorrect understanding of how their bodies work. They begin to fantasize about inner body function and may have misconceptions about these functions. In an early study, Gellert[13] studied large groups of children and their knowledge of body function. She gave children an outline of a body and asked them to draw in a certain part. Tools such as Gellert's can be used not only to assess knowledge base but also to teach about body function as well as nursing and medical procedures.

Fears in the school-age range are more grounded in reality than in the preschool years. Fear of separation from parents decreases for the child who is becoming increasingly more dependent on self and less dependent on parents. The school-age child may continue to fear body mu-tilation, injury, or death of themselves or a family member. A prominent fear in this age group is related to school performance. The school-age child may feel pressured to meet their parents' or teacher's expectations. Therefore, the child may fear failure in the classroom as well as the retribution it may incur at home.

The adolescent continues to carry some of the same fears of earlier years in relation to death and physical danger. However, fear of lack of acceptance in a peer group seems to outweigh all other fears. It is the submission to peer pressure that serves as one of the motivating forces for experimentation with drugs and other illegal or unhealthy behaviors.

Fears can serve a useful purpose, for example, some fears may help a child avoid danger. However, if a child's fear becomes irrational and persistent, appropriate consultation should be recommended.

Separation

Separation can be viewed as a normal experience for children as they move from the symbiotic relationship with mother to a gradual independence from mother. However, for most children, separation from mother, father, or main caretaker is a primary fear and source of stress. The negative effects associated with separation of the mother and child have been widely documented by classic studies of institutionalized children.[2,3,11,28,29,38] Maternal deprivation has been associated with an increase in infant mortality, susceptibility to disease, growth retardation, and failure to achieve developmental milestones. This was first demonstrated in the early studies by Spitz.[37,38] These studies demonstrated the need for an ongoing, sustained relationship between the mother and/or father and the child for optimal physical as well as psychosocial development of the child. The findings from these as well as other studies have helped to change traditional views of parental involvement in the care of their hospitalized child.[10,27,31] For example, more liberal visiting hours and parents' participation in their ill child's care are encouraged.

A child's response to separation depends partly on age, cognitive development, degree of attachment to the person or object, previous separation experiences, duration of the separation, and preparation of the child for the separation. It is believed that the child is most vulnerable to the effects of separation between the ages of 6 months and 4 years. Stranger anxiety occurs at around 6 to 7 months of age due to the infant's ability to distinguish family members from strangers. As toddlers increase their understanding of object permanence, they learn that their mothers may leave but that they will not disappear and will eventually return. One of the main tasks of toddlerhood is to master separation from parents for brief periods. Playing games such as peek-a-boo helps the toddler to learn object permanence and allows them to be in control of the loss. Separation anxiety usually lessens with increasing age of the child.

If the infant or toddler has never been cared for by anyone other than mother, father, or grandparent, the initial separation experience, however brief, may be a difficult one for both the child and parent. The child who has experienced previous separations with a positive outcome is more likely to approach subsequent separations with a similar outlook (Fig. 17-3).

It has been documented in the literature that prolonged separation can cause risk to a child's psychological stability. In a classic work on separation, Bowlby and Robertson[3] describe three phases of the child's response to separation: protest, despair, and detachment or denial. In the stage of *protest*, the child actively demonstrates his or her separation from the attachment. Behavior in this stage includes crying, biting, kicking, temper tantrums, and resistance to comforting measures by others. The child calls for the mother and visually searches for her. Although the length of this stage is variable, it usually does not extend beyond 2 or 3 days. In the second stage of separation, *despair*, the child becomes withdrawn and passive and is often described as being "apathetic." In mourning the loss of the mother, the child shows little interest in the environment and refuses to eat. Behavior during this stage is often misleading as the child's lack of resistance to treatments and procedures may be seen as an initial adjustment to the separation. Regressive and self-stimulating behaviors are usually seen in this stage. The stage of despair may last between 1 to 3 weeks.

In the last stage of separation, *denial-detachment*, the child may seem to have adjusted to the situation as some participation in day-to-day activities may occur. For the child, however, this minimal participation merely signals a resignation to the separation. When parents come to visit, the child may have a delayed response to them. When parents leave, the child shows little if any signs of protest. Bowlby[2] states that in this stage the love object

is not forgotten, but an emotional gulf is created between the child and the love object. This stage lasts for the duration of the separation and can continue for awhile after the separation.

Prolonged separation from parents may have long-term, deleterious effects on the child's emotional development. It is thought that children who sustain prolonged separation from their parents may have difficulty forming meaningful relationships in the future. Coping strategies for the hospitalized child are discussed in Chapter 23.

Loss and Death

Experiences of loss and death are common in all families. Losses can also be classified as maturational or situational. *Maturational losses* are those that occur by virtue of growth and development, that is, the loss of a favorite toy or blanket; the loss of a relationship, whether it is real or fantasy (the loss of belief in Santa Claus); a friend moving; or the death of a pet. A *situational* or *accidental loss* is a result of an unusual or unexpected experience, for example, the unexpected death of a parent or other family member or the divorce of parents. Losses may be further categorized in terms of what is lost. These categories include loss of a significant person; loss of some aspect of self; loss of an external object; and loss that occurs in the process of human growth and development.[37] A loss in any category can be devastating, depending on the person and his or her particular situation.

A person's response to a loss depends on the significance of the loss to that person. Reactions to the loss can be manifested by a variety of psychological and

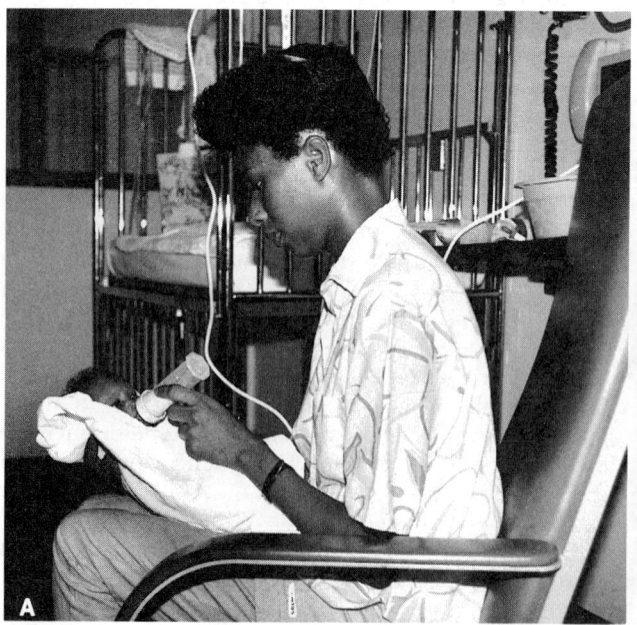 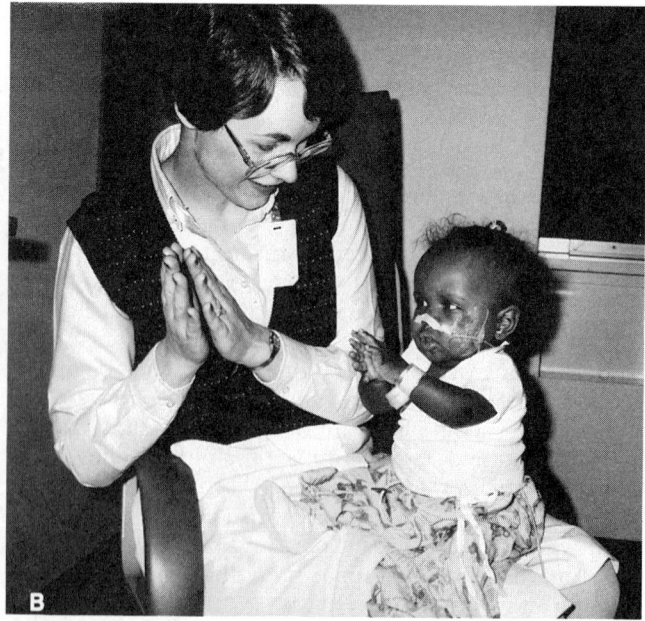

FIGURE 17-3

Two methods to cope with separation. (**A**) Mothers can be encouraged to participate in their infants' care. Separation can be difficult for both the mother and the infant. (**B**) Primary nursing care can help toddlers cope with hospitalization, particularly when parents are unable to stay at the hospital for prolonged periods. (Photograph submitted by S. Allen, Children's Medical Center, Dallas, TX.)

sometimes physical states that may include anxiety, grief, anger, depression, guilt, and mourning.[27] The infant and young child's experiences with separation and loss are essential to their understanding of death. Maturational as well as situational losses help prepare the child to deal with death. Death and dying are discussed in Chapter 32.

Nagy[24] was one of the first authors to describe the stages of the child's understanding of death. In Nagy's study,[24] Budapest children between the ages of 3 to 10 years were asked to express their feelings about death through words and pictures. The children's responses were categorized based on developmental stages. It is believed that the infant and toddler have no realistic understanding of the concept of death. For that age group, death and separation are synonymous. In the preschool period, death is seen as a temporary and reversible state. The dead person may continue to live, eat, and become alive again. This understanding of death is similar in the preschooler's mind to the process of being asleep and waking up.

In the early school age child (5 to 9 years) there is a realization that death is inevitable but that it is usually only old people who die. In the later school-age years (10 to 12 years), the child realizes that death is inevitable for all living things. Feelings of guilt and punishment often occur when a family member or friend has died. Children may feel that because of anger or ill wishes they may have caused the person's death. Similarly, preschool and school-age children who are ill may feel that their own illness is a punishment for something that they have done. It is not until the school-age period that a dying child can understand the prognosis.

The adolescent's cognitive understanding of death should be the same level as that of an adult. The adolescent's concept of death is influenced by previous experiences with loss and death, culture, and religious beliefs. Although the adolescent understands the concept of death, it is seen as something in the distant future. Most adolescents see themselves as invincible, which may lead to dangerous behaviors, such as experimentation with drugs or reckless driving.

It is important that children experience loss and death in a supportive and positive environment. How previous losses in early childhood are resolved will impact how a child copes with subsequent losses throughout life. Regardless of the type or degree of loss, a period of adjustment following a loss or death is necessary for the child. A child may use ritualistic practices to work through the loss or death experience. For example, a child may insist on writing letters to the dead person. Although parents may comply with the child's wishes, it must be stressed that the dead person will not return or write back and that the family is allowing this activity only in memory of the loved one.

The young child needs constant reinforcement that death is a permanent state. Parents can read stories or books to children about death. A successful resolution to the loss or death is critical to the child's future development. Depending on the meaning of the loss, a child and family may benefit from counseling to resolve the loss. The nursing management of a child who is terminally ill is discussed in Chapter 32.

The Child's Behavioral Response

The child's behavioral response to a change or stress depends on many factors, including the type of change (maturational or situational), perception of the change, growth and development level, previous reactions to change, and parental support, among others. Some common childhood responses to change and stress are discussed here. The subject is also the major content of Chapter 18.

Aggression

Aggressive behavior is often the result of feelings of anger that usually involves the intent to harm or cause injury to another.[14] The child's behavioral response to anger are be affected by temperament and to a large extent by the way his or her family responds to anger. For example, if shouting and arguing are the family's main methods of responding to stress and anger, then the child will probably use similar behavioral responses.

Aggression is not a behavior that can be clearly delineated during infancy. Crying and fussy behavior may indicate the infant's frustration in attempts to get basic needs met. Overt aggressive behavior is more clearly demonstrated by the toddler. A toddler's cognitive development does not include an understanding of cause and effect. A low tolerance for frustration, combined with an inability to verbally express that frustration, often leads to the display of a temper tantrum. Temper tantrums are most commonly seen between the ages of 18 months and 3 years. During this age range, young children have difficulty controlling their emotions and have not yet learned the socially acceptable norms for displaying anger. A temper tantrum usually occurs in response to something that toddlers cannot physically accomplish or something that they are told they should not attempt. The toddler's behavioral response to this limit setting may include shouting, screaming, kicking, and breath holding. Temper tantrums are discussed in Chapter 13.

The preschooler may also exhibit temper tantrums, although not as frequently as in the toddler period. A child who continues to have temper tantrums past the age of 5 may be displaying signs of depression or poor self-esteem, or may be living in a family in which emotional problems exist.[30] In these cases, referral to appropriate counseling services may be necessary.

Other aggressive behaviors that may occur in the preschool and school-age period include biting, hitting, and grabbing. These behaviors are socially unacceptable, and parents and teachers should try to determine the motivation that may underlie them. In general, school-age children become increasingly more capable of controlling their emotions. With an increase in verbal abilities, the school-age child tends to use more verbal and less physical methods to communicate anger. Verbal methods of expressing anger may include the use of sarcasm, arguing, and talking back.

It is important for parents to spend time teaching their child age-appropriate ways to handle stress, such as time out or walking away from the situation, and providing age-appropriate physical activities as a release. These methods of stress reduction should be consistent with the parents' own pattern of coping behaviors. An abnormal level of aggressive behavior may be associated with other forms of dysfunctional behaviors, such as substance abuse. The child who frequently displays aggressive behavior should be referred for evaluation.

Television Violence and Aggressive Behavior

There has been a great deal of controversy concerning the relationship between viewing violence on television and the development of aggressive behaviors. A longitudinal study conducted by Eron et al.[7] documented that a preference for violent television programs in young boys was related to both concurrent and subsequent aggression. Singer et al.[36] demonstrated that intensive television viewing at an early age is associated with less self-control and more aggressive behavior than at a later age.

A landmark report from the National Institute of Mental Health[25] stated that the consensus among most of the research community is that violence on television does lead to aggressive behavior by children and adolescents who watch certain programs. Cartoons and crime shows, for example, tend to be more violent than situational comedies. A young child may believe that aggressive behavior is an acceptable solution to provocation if they see cartoon violence that is depicted as morally justified.[36]

Because regulatory action of violence on television has not occurred, and the exact nature of the impact of television is controversial, parents should be advised to screen and limit the types of programs that their children watch. Parents may want to watch potentially violent shows with their children and discuss what has been viewed.[20] The nurse may want to consider taking a child's "television history" regarding the amount and type of television watched, particularly in the child who exhibits a behavioral problem.

Fantasy

Fantasy is a type of play in which the child develops a particular situation and then acts it out. Fantasy may be used by the child to role play an experience or situation in which the child was frustrated, upset, angry, or confused, for example, a child who has been scolded for doing something wrong. With role playing, the child may work through problems using the imaginary situation as an outlet for their frustration and tension. The child may talk with imaginary playmates or may take the role of father, mother, teacher, or doctor and relive the particular experience. Fantasy play enhances the process of identification and the learning of social roles through the imitation of adults. Fantasy may also be used to relive a positive experience. That same positive experience or memory may be recalled by the child to help him or her get through a stressful time, such as bedtime or after a nightmare.

During the preschool and early school-age period, "pretend games" are most noticeable. Girls may become absorbed in playing with Barbie or baby dolls or acting out family roles. For boys, aggressive play involving mastery over the enemy is prominent. Pretend games may include cops and robbers, aliens and humans, or assuming the role of a character such as Spiderman, Ninja Turtles, Superman, or Superwoman. During the late school-age and adolescent period, fantasy may take on the form of "hero worship." The child may try to dress like or act like a particular television or movie star or sports hero. Hero worship may be an important step in making the transition from dependence on family members to interdependence on non-family members. The use of fantasy and other expressive behaviors reveals efforts to master the anxieties associated with normal growth and development as well as critical experiences such as illness and hospitalization.

Dramatic play with puppets or dolls may be a particularly helpful activity for the ill or hospitalized child. Unidirectional play, or the repetition of a particular theme in play, is a clue to the observer that the child is working on a particular issue.[26] As with previously cited coping behaviors, long-term use of fantasy or the inability to bridge fantasy with reality should be considered an abnormal use of this coping mechanism.

Defense Mechanisms

Freud[11] saw defense mechanisms as unconscious coping strategies, contrived by the ego for distorting awareness to reduce stress. The use of defense mechanisms enables the child or adult to ward off threats to one's self-esteem and should be viewed as a positive, healthy coping strategy. Due to cognitive maturation, specific defense mechanisms will be employed by certain age groups. A description of some of the more commonly used defense mechanisms is found in the display.

The use of defense mechanisms cannot be easily observed until the toddler and preschool periods. Regression, denial, repression, and projection are the defense mechanisms most commonly used in this age group. As a result of a sense of industry and competition, school-age children may use defense mechanisms to help them bridge the gap between what they are capable of doing or what others would like them to do. The school-age child most often uses the defense mechanisms of sublimation and reaction formation. Owing to an increased vocabulary, combined with an ability to think abstractly, the adolescent has the largest repertoire of defense mechanisms. The adolescent is cognitively capable of using rationalization, intellectualization, as well as all previously mentioned defense mechanisms.

It is important for the nurse to help parents to understand and accept the child's use of defense mechanisms. Although defense mechanisms may be used as part of an overall coping strategy, their use may not always result in adaptation. As with any coping behavior, if the use of defense mechanisms becomes excessive, then referral to an appropriate counselor should be sought.

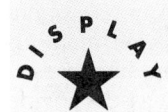

Commonly Used Defense Mechanisms

Regression: A temporary return to an earlier level of development in an attempt to cope with a threatening or frustrating experience. Regression due to illness or hospitalization is often seen in the areas of toilet training, communication, and feeding and an increased need for transitional objects such as a security blanket. A common example of regression is the newly toilet-trained child who becomes incontinent during an admission to the hospital. For the younger child, regression usually occurs due to fears of separation and abandonment. The older child and the adolescent may employ other defense mechanisms, such as displacement, denial, and projection, as methods of coping.

Denial of reality: The ability to ignore any thoughts or feelings that might be painful, e.g., the child whose parents frequently fight but she acts as if everything is fine.

Repression: The ability to render painful memories as unavailable to the conscious mind, e.g., the child who still speaks about a dead sibling as if the sibling is still alive.

Projection: The ability to transfer negative emotions, thoughts, or feelings to others, while denying they exist in oneself. This defense mechanism protects the

individual against unfavorable self-evaluations, e.g., child who takes candy from store but says that another child told him that it was all right to do it.

Displacement: The redirection of pent-up hostilities or feelings to an object or a person that is less dangerous than to the one who originally aroused the emotion, e.g., a child spanks a doll after getting a shot from a nurse.

Sublimation: Finding socially acceptable outlets for aggressive impulses, e.g., a child hits a punching bag instead of hitting his new sibling.

Reaction formation: Repression of an impulse and replacing it with opposite characteristic, e.g., a diabetic school-age girl who is afraid of shots but boasts her lack of fear when giving the injections.

Rationalization: False justification for one's behavior to hide an anxiety-producing situation, e.g., the anorexic teenage girl who will not eat because she thinks she is overweight.

Intellectualization: A method for displacing aggression and in reducing tension, e.g., the adolescent who uses her aggressive energies to plunge into academic and intellectual affairs, which earns her recognition and respect.

School Phobia

School phobia, which may also be referred to as school refusal, is an unwillingness to attend school. School phobia crosses socioeconomic levels and is most prevalent among children who are seen as "good students" but are also characterized as overprotected, passive, and dependent. The child affected by school phobia may display any of the symptoms associated with an anxiety reaction, such as stomachache, headache, nausea, vomiting, diarrhea, sore throat, anorexia, palpitations, bone or joint pain, insomnia, oversleeping, and dysmenorrhea. The child may even run a low-grade fever. The symptoms begin to abate when the child is given permission to stay home. These symptoms are rarely seen on the weekend. Physical complaints may begin to surface again on Sunday evening or toward the end of a vacation.

School phobia can occur concurrently with a maturational event, such as the beginning of school, the birth of a sibling, or a situational event like a recent illness, a move to a new school, parental divorce, or death of a loved one. Although there may be contributing factors to this disorder, it is believed that there is a basic anxiety that underlies school phobia. The anxiety can be related to fear of separation from mother, with attendance at school being seen as a forced separation. In some instances, the mother may be overprotective, making it more difficult for the child to leave. The anxiety may also

be related to the fear of not meeting the teacher's, parent's, or their own academic achievement standards.

It is important not to overlook the fact that the child's refusal to attend school may be related to a more tangible concern, such as a problem with a particular teacher or a certain child (bully) at school. The child's teacher should be consulted to determine if there are any stressors that the child is experiencing in school. School phobia is discussed in Chapter 18.

★ ASSESSMENT

Nurses interact with children and their families in a wide variety of settings. Well-child visits, school health screenings, clinic appointments, home visits, and hospitalizations due to an acute or chronic illness all present opportunities for the nurse to assess the child's and family's ability to cope with maturational and situational changes.

Functional health can be used as a way to organize assessment data and identify nursing diagnoses. The term *pattern* refers to a sequence of behavior across time. During the data collection phase a health pattern should begin to emerge from the client's descriptions and the nurses' observations.

Function refers to a client's strengths, whereas dysfunction can lead to alterations in health. Information concerning the child's functional health is obtained during the health history from the parent or guardian. As communication skills develop, information should also be obtained from the child.

SELF-PERCEPTION AND SELF-CONCEPT

A positive perception or concept of self was cited earlier as an important determinant of effective coping. A negative evaluation of self or perceptions of one's abilities can impact other function, i.e. nutrition, health management. Change and loss are factors that commonly impinge on self-concept. Information that will help the nurse to assess self-concept include the child's temperament, behavior, sense of worth, identity, number of friends, history of fears or anxieties, discipline problems (history of temper tantrums), and school adjustment.

Specific questions to elicit this information include the following:

* Is your child generally happy?
* How does your child feel about herself/himself?
* How does your child handle anger?
* Does your child play with friends outside of your family?
* Does your child have any fears or anxieties? (e.g., fear of the dark, of animals, of school)
* How does your child feel about school?

COPING AND STRESS TOLERANCE

The more effective a child's coping patterns, the greater the sense of control that the child can exert over the threat to integrity. Stress tolerance is described as the amount of stress a client can handle effectively. Information to be obtained during the history includes the child's usual coping pattern to change and stress; methods of handling stress, the child's perceived ability to control and manage situations; and available family support systems.

Questions that will elicit information on coping and stress tolerance include some of the following:

* How does your child usually handle stress?
* What activities does your child engage in to deal with stress?
* How well do you think your child manages stress?
* Are there any stressors in the family (e.g., separation or divorce, illness, difficulty with school)?

Because the parents' patterns of function greatly influence the child's development, the nurse should determine the parents' strategies for dealing with change and stress. Parents can teach their child to use positive coping behaviors. It would also be helpful to know if there are any concurrent or existing life stressors or family stressors.

If analysis of data collected during the assessment phase reveals that the child and family are coping effectively, this information should be shared with families in an effort to support the maintenance of existing coping strategies. When the child or family is not coping effectively, the nurse and family members need to meet and determine a plan that will enhance their coping abilities.

ASSESSMENT TOOLS

Assessment tools and screening strategies may help the nurse by supplying another framework from which data can be organized and analyzed. Assessment tools may also be used before and after any intervention to determine the effectiveness of the intervention. Any assessment tool should be used in conjunction with other methods of data collection to determine the nursing diagnoses.

There are numerous tools available to assess a wide range of areas, such as growth and development levels, intelligence, school adjustment, temperament, and family coping. The following provides descriptions of several tools that are available to assess the child's self-esteem and the child's and family's ability to adapt to maturational or situational changes. The description and psychometric evaluation of each tool discussed are included.

THE SEPARATION ANXIETY BEHAVIORAL INDEX: THE YOUNG CHILD'S REACTION TO MOTHER-CHILD SEPARATION

AUTHOR: PHYLLIS J. SHANLEY, RN, EDD

Tool Description

The purpose of the Separation Anxiety Behavioral Index (SABI)[35] is to assess the response of a young child (15 to 48 months of age) when separated from the mother. The separation experience may be brief or extensive in duration, arising from a situation such as day care or hospitalization. The SABI is an observational schedule that includes seven behavioral subsets (mother-child interaction, separation anxiety, eating behavior, play activity, autoerotic behavior, sleep behavior, and elimination). Each subset explicates a specific behavior. Items are coded positively if they represent more developmentally appropriate behavior and negatively if they represent less developmentally appropriate behavior. Administration of the tool should take the observer approximately 30 minutes to complete.

Psychometric Evaluation

Reliability of the SABI has been established for internal consistency (0.91 to 0.98), test-retest ($r = 0.75$ to 0.99) and interobserver agreement (0.83 and 1.00). Content validity was established by a panel of experts. Shanley[35] suggests that the SABI, used in conjunction with other assessment data, may be useful in assessing a child's behavioral reaction to separation from the mother. The SABI may also be used to assess a child's adjustment to a new environment such as day care.

Further information or a copy of the tool can be obtained by writing to Phyllis Shanley, RN, EdD, Associate Professor of Nursing, Seton Hall University, South Orange, NJ 07079.

PIERS-HARRIS CHILDREN'S SELF-CONCEPT SCALE: THE WAY I FEEL ABOUT MYSELF

AUTHORS: ELLEN V. PIERS AND DALE B. HARRIS

Tool Description

The Piers-Harris (P-H)[29] measures self-concept for children between the ages of 8 to 12 years of age. The P-H consists of 80 first-person declarative statements to which the child responds "yes" or "no" (for example, "I am happy"; "I am an important member of my family"). The instrument provides scores on behavior, happiness-satisfaction, intellectual and school status, physical appearance, anxiety, and popularity, as well as an overall score. This instrument should take approximately 15 to 20 minutes for the child to complete.

Psychometric Evaluation

The P-H scale was standardized on 1183 children in grades 4 through 12. Criterion validity correlations with similar self-concept tools are in the mid 60s, and peer validity coefficients are around 70; stability, reliability, test-retest reliability ranges from 0.71 to 0.77; internal consistency reliability of the scale ranges from 0.78 to 0.93.

Further information or a copy of the tool and manual can be obtained by writing to Ellen Piers-Harris and Dale B. Harris, The Piers-Harris Children's Self-Concept Scale Manual, Counselor Recordings and Tests, Nashville, TN

THE SCHOOL-AGER'S COPING STRATEGIES INVENTORY

AUTHOR: NANCY M. RYAN, RN, PHD

Tool Description

The School-Agers' Coping Strategy Inventory (SCSI)[33] is a 25-item self-report instrument to measure frequency and effectiveness of children's stress-coping strategies. Children are asked to think about when they feel stressed, nervous, or worried and then to circle how often they do any of the 25 listed coping strategies before, during, or after the stressful event. Examples of the items include "Bite my nails or crack my knuckles," "Cry or feel sad," and "Talk to someone." The items are rated on a scale of 0 to 3, with 0 = never; 1 = once in awhile; 2 = a lot; and 3 = most of the time. The same scale can be used to ask the child the effectiveness of the strategies or how much each thing helps him or her feel better when he or she feels stressed, nervous, or worried.

Psychometric Evaluation

The SCSI has an internal consistency of 0.79, test-retest correlation of 0.73 to 0.81, and interrater reliability of scoring of 100%. The author cautions that the SCSI items were developed and validated on primarily white children from lower- to upper-middle- class environments and should only be used with similar populations until further studies can validate its use with other cultural or ethnic groups.

Further information or a copy of the tool may be obtained by contacting Nancy Muir Ryan, PhD, RN, College of Nursing, Ohio State University, 1585 Neil Avenue, Columbus, OH, 43210.

HOME OBSERVATION FOR MEASUREMENT OF THE ENVIRONMENT

AUTHORS: BETTYE M. CALDWELL, PHD, AND ROBERT H. BRADLEY, PHD

Tool Description

The Home Observation for Measurement of the Environment (HOME)[4] is a standardized observation-interview technique used to measure the quality and quantity of cognitive, social, and emotional support for development available in a child's home environment. The HOME assesses the impact of both animate and inanimate aspects of the child's development that either foster or impede growth and development. The goal of the HOME inventory is to observe natural behavior between parent and child and to get full, candid information regarding events that typically occur at home.

There are three versions of the HOME inventory. One is designed for families of infants, birth to age 3 (45 items). The second is for preschoolers, ages 3 to 6 years (55 items). The third is for the early school-age child, 6 to 10 years (59 items). Each version of the inventory measures certain subscales (see following).

All items are scored "yes" or "no" for each subscale. Subscale scores are then summed to get a total HOME score.

The information for the inventory is obtained through observations and verbal communication with the child and mother. The appropriate version is administered by a moderately skilled interviewer in the child's home. Administration requires approximately 1 hour.

Calloway[5] suggests that the HOME inventory provides data that

may be used to counsel parents about ways that they regulate the child's environment and how to effect changes in the environment to facilitate a child's growth and development. The HOME inventory may also be useful in situations where there is some question about the child's environment. It has been used to examine health outcomes in children who have developmental delays, low birth weight, malnutrition, lead burden, nonorganic failure to thrive, and child abuse.

Psychometric Evaluation

Full psychometric information on the HOME inventory is available in the technical manual for the instrument.[6] Internal consistency for each subscale on each of the three versions was estimated using the alpha coefficient: for the Infant version, alpha coefficients ranged from 0.44 to 0.89; for the Preschool version, the range was 0.53 to 0.93; and for the Elementary version, the range was from 0.52 to 0.90. Traditional test-retest reliability estimates have not been done for the HOME inventory because of the cost to readminister the scale and because of the "artificiality" of talking about the same things with parents less than a month after the original visit. Interobserver agreement for the scales averages about 90%.

The authors recommend that scores from the HOME inventory not be used in isolation to make decisions about children and families but that they be used in conjunction with other information about the child and family as part of a more complete assessment. The HOME manual may be obtained from authors for a fee at the Center for Child Development and Education, the University of Arkansas at Little Rock, 33rd and University Avenue, Little Rock, Arkansas, 77204.

Sample Items From the Home Inventory

- Infant Version
  - Emotional and Verbal Responsivity of Parents
    - Parent responds to the child's vocalizations with verbal response.
    - Parent caresses or kisses child at least once during visit.
  - Acceptance of Child
    - Parent does not shout at child during visit.
    - Parent does not interfere with child's actions or restrict child's movements more than three times during visit.
  - Organization of the Physical and Temporal Environment
    - When parent is away, care is provided by one of three regular substitutes.
    - Someone takes child to grocery store at least once a week.
  - Provision of Appropriate Play Materials
    - Child has some muscle-activity toys or equipment.
    - Parent provides toys or some interesting activities for child during visit.
  - Parental Involvement With Child
    - Parent consciously encourages developmental advance.
    - Parent structures child's play periods.
  - Opportunities for Variety in Daily Stimulation
    - Father provides some caretaking every day.
    - Family visits or receives visits from relatives once a month.
- Preschool Version
  - Stimulation Through Toys, Games, and Reading Materials
    - Child has record player and at least five children's records.
    - Family buys a newspaper daily and reads it.
  - Stimulation for Communicative Competence
    - Parent teaches child some simple manners: to say "please," "thank you," "I'm sorry."
    - Parent uses correct grammar and pronunciation.
  - Physical Environment—Safe, Clean, and Conducive to Development
    - Building has no potential structural or health defects.
    - There is at least 100 square feet of living space per person in the house.

- Pride, Affection, and Warmth
  - Parent holds child close at least 10 to 15 minutes a day.
  - Parent spontaneously praises child's qualities or behavior at least twice during visit.
- Stimulation of Academic Behavior
  - Child is encouraged to learn colors.
  - Child is encouraged to learn to read a few words.
- Modeling and Encouragement of Social Maturity
  - Some delay of food gratification is demanded of child.
  - Child is permitted to hit parent without harsh reprisal.
- Variety of Stimulation
  - Child was taken by a family member to a scientific, historical, or art museum within the past year.
  - Child eats at least one meal per day on most days with mother (or mother figure) and father (or father figure).
- Physical Punishment
  - Parent does not use physical restraint, shake, grab, or pinch child during visit.
  - No more than one instance of physical punishment occurred during the last week.
- Elementary Version
  - Emotional and Verbal Responsivity of Parent
    - Parent sometimes yields to child's fears or rituals.
    - Parent responds to child's questions during interview.
  - Encouragement and Maturity
    - Family requires child to keep living and play areas reasonably clean and neat.
    - Parent introduces interviewer to child.
  - Emotional Climate
    - Parent has not lost temper with child more than once during previous week.
    - Parent uses some term of endearment or some diminutive for the child's name when talking about child at least twice during visit.
  - Growth-Fostering Materials and Experiences
    - Child has access to at least 10 appropriate books.
    - House has at least two pictures or other types of art work on the walls.
  - Provision for Active Stimulation
    - Family encourages child to develop or sustain hobbies.
    - Child has access to library card, and family arranges for child to go to library at least once a month.
  - Family Participation in Developmentally Stimulating Experiences
    - Family member has taken child, or arranged for child to go, on a trip of more than 50 miles from his or her home.
    - Parents discuss television programs with child.
  - Paternal Involvement
    - Father (or father substitute) regularly engages in outdoor recreation with child.
    - Child eats at least one meal per day, on most days, with mother (or mother figure) and father (or father figure).
  - Aspects of the Physical Environment
    - The interior of the house or apartment is not dark or perceptually monotonous.
    - Building has no potentially dangerous structural or health defects.

THE FEETHAM FAMILY FUNCTIONING SURVEY

AUTHOR: SUZANNE L. FEETHAM, RN, PHD

Tool Description

The Feetham Family Functioning Survey[8] was originally formulated for the purpose of measuring the effect on families of a child with myelodysplasia. This instrument has been used for research purposes and is not designed for clinical use. It is of value to clinicians because of its relevant content; its strength is in the way the questions are asked. The questions are designed to give guidance in problems to look for leading to appropriate interventions.

There are 23 questions in the self-report survey that assess family functioning in the following six areas: household tasks, child care, sexual and marital relations, interactions with friends and family, community involvement, and sources of emotional support. The respondent is asked to rate "what is" and "what should be" in each area on a scale from 1 (little) to 7 (much). The discrepancy between these two ratings, together with the degree of importance the respondent places on each item, contributes to the assessment of the family functioning. Clinical use indicates that a high discrepant score on selected items and a high importance rating on the same items is a basis for further assessment and possible intervention with the family.

Psychometric Evaluation

The reliability alpha coefficients for the total score of (1) "how much there is" = 0.66; (2) "how much there should be" = 0.75; and (3) the discrepancy between A and B = 0.81. Test-retest reliability was 0.85. The original instrument was reviewed by a panel of experts for content validity. A copy of the revised scale and manual may be obtained by writing to the Department of Nursing Research and Development, Children's National Medical Center, 111 Michigan Avenue N.W., Washington, DC 20010.

★ NURSING DIAGNOSES AND PLANNING

Nursing diagnoses associated with ineffective coping may include the following:

- Self-Esteem Disturbance related to separation anxiety.
- Chronic Low Self-Esteem related to inexperience in using defense mechanisms.
- Anxiety related to separation from family.
- Family Coping: Potential for Growth related to parents' desire for family growth.
- Ineffective Family Coping: Compromised related to situational crises.
- Ineffective Family Coping: Disabling related to ambivalent family relationships.
- Ineffective Individual Coping related to situational crises.
- Dysfunctional Grieving related to lack of previous experience in loss.

An example of nursing diagnoses, interventions, and outcomes is demonstrated in the Nursing Care Plan and Teaching Plan.

★ INTERVENTIONS: COLLABORATIVE AND INDEPENDENT

The nurse can help parents and children manage behavioral responses, as illustrated in the nursing care plan and teaching plan displays. As children are taught socially acceptable ways of coping, the parents will need to set realistic limits on undesirable behaviors. Children are then provided with opportunities to express their feelings in controlled situations, such as puppet play, drawing pictures, and physical activities.[39] The activities should be selected according to the age of the child.

Nursing interventions that promote coping will vary with each child and family. The nurse's role is to assist children and families to use coping mechanisms that are positive and that facilitate growth and development. Par-

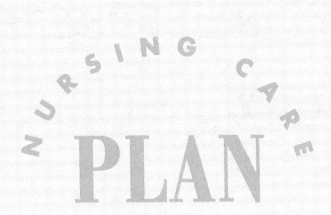

NURSING CARE
PLAN

A Toddler Using Regression as a Defense Mechanism

Assessment

Case Study Description

Anne Fay, aged 3, has recently started preschool. For the first 2 months of school Anne has cried every morning and has had two accidental episodes of urinary incontinence per week. This has required Mrs. Fay to pack a spare pair of clothes every day. Anne told her mother that when she comes back to the classroom in different clothes, the other children make fun of her and call her a baby. Mrs. Fay is concerned about Anne's reaction to school and asks the pediatric nurse for guidance. On taking a history, the nurse learns that Mrs. Fay has a 6-week-old infant and that Anne completed toilet training only 3 weeks before starting school.

Mrs. Fay describes Anne's behavior at home as "demanding and whiny." Mrs. Fay states that Anne was a happy and social child before beginning school. Mrs. Fay is concerned that Anne may be too young for preschool.

Assessment Data

Anne cries every day when leaving for school.

Anne has had urinary incontinence at school approximately 16 times in a period of 8 weeks.

Anne demonstrates regressive behavior at home.

Anne has a 6-week-old baby brother.

Nursing Diagnosis	Interventions	Rationale
1. Ineffective individual coping Supporting Data: • Change in coping related to preschool activities • Crying • Incontinence • Regressive behavior	Collect information about Anne's usual coping pattern to change and stress. Determine usual methods of handling stress. Assess available family support systems. Determine parents' usual coping strategies.	Determine the child and family's stress tolerance and coping pattern.
	Use the Separation Anxiety Behavioral Index[35] as an assessment tool.	Increase the nurses' understanding of the situation and the child and family's abilities and resources.
2. Self-esteem disturbance	Discuss with parent the child's temperament, sense of worth, identity, number of friends, and history of fears, anxieties, and school adjustments. Include questions related to the birth of the new baby and family changes that are related to the addition of a new member.	Determine factors that may be affecting the child's self-concept or perception of her abilities, because an altered self-esteem can impact other areas of the child's functioning.

Evaluation

- Mrs. Fay identifies family coping strategies.
- Mrs. Fay identifies family support systems.
- Mrs. Fay discusses family changes related to birth of new baby.

The nurse develops a teaching plan and discusses it with Anne and her parents and teachers. Please refer to the teaching plan in this chapter that continues this care plan.

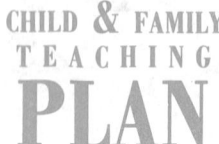

CHILD & FAMILY
T E A C H I N G
PLAN

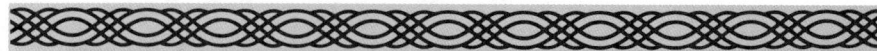

Dealing With Separation Anxiety in a 3-Year-Old Child

Assessment

Three-year-old Anne Fay seems to be displaying regressive behavior that may be related to the recent birth of a sibling. She is also unwilling to attend preschool, probably due to fear of separation from her mother. She cries and has accidents requiring changes in clothes. Additional assessment data are found in the preceding Nursing Care Plan. The Teaching Plan is a strategy for addressing the problems identified in the care plan.

Child and Family Objectives	Specific Content	Teaching Strategies
1. Identify common changes encountered by the preschooler.	1. Separation, beginning school, birth of a sibling. Discuss with parents that separation is a prominent fear for the preschooler and how this fear is being impacted by the start of school and the birth of a sibling.	1. Discussion and reference to books that can be read to Anne, e.g., *A Baby Sister for Henry*.
2. Describe some common coping strategies used by preschoolers to respond to change and stress.	2. Defense mechanisms; in particular, regressive behaviors. Describe positive effects that regression may have for Anne.	2. Discussion; use of a chart listing defense mechanisms.
3. Identify interventions to promote effective coping strategies.	3. The addition of a baby brother and going to preschool are normal changes that occur with which a child will need to learn to cope.	3. Discussion of interventions: playing with dolls; letting Anne participate in care of the baby.
	Parents should view Anne's use of regression as a temporary mechanism and move Anne toward more age-appropriate coping mechanisms, e.g., fantasy "trying on the experience." Parents should try to provide opportunities for Anne's self-expression. A baby doll may allow Anne to work out some of her fears about separation and the birth of the sibling. When the parents feel comfortable, they can let Anne participate in the care of the baby, e.g., helping with the bath, getting diapers, etc.	
	Mr. and Mrs. Fay should each try to provide special times for Anne without the baby being present so that she still sees herself as an important member of the family.	
	A behavior modification program may be initiated to reward Anne for each day that she does not have an accident at school. This program should be devised with Anne, her parents, and her teacher.	Discuss with the parents and teachers; develop a specific plan of action for Anne. Include Anne in the discussions.

(Continued)

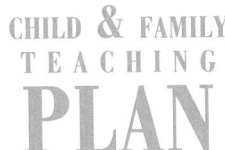

CHILD & FAMILY TEACHING PLAN

Dealing With Separation Anxiety in a 3-Year-Old Child (continued)

Evaluation

- The parents identify some of the common changes and stressors that the preschooler may encounter.
- The parents describe some of the common coping strategies used by the preschooler to respond to change and stress.
- The parents discuss methods to promote positive coping behaviors for Anne.
- Anne exhibits adjustment to school as evidenced by lack of accidents and a positive outlook on school attendance.
- Anne participates in age-appropriate care of the baby.

ents may need guidance as to what are considered age-appropriate responses to change and stress as well as ways to support positive behavioral responses in their child. Specific coping strategies for various age groups and nursing interventions to promote developmentally appropriate coping methods are depicted in Table 17-1. After completing a thorough assessment of the child and family, the nursing interventions are selected and implemented.

★ EVALUATION

The nurse and family periodically evaluate the outcomes of care given. Example of outcomes for the child with coping problems are given in Table 17-1 and the Nursing Care Plan.

Summary

Coping, as part of the overall process of adaptation, is an individual process that begins at birth and continues until death. Throughout childhood there are some common changes or stressors that the child will encounter. Some of the more common childhood changes or stressors are developmental-related fears, separation, and experiences of loss and death.

Coping strategies and capacities will vary from child to child and are dependent on the interaction of a number of factors. Factors that may influence a child's ability to cope include growth and development level, physical health, psychological-emotional health, available support systems, and previous coping experiences, among others. Ability to cope increases with age and cognitive development.

No one coping strategy is considered inherently better than another. The goodness of fit of any strategy is determined only by its effect on any given situation as well as its effects in the long term.[19] A strategy can be considered effective if it results in growth, greater auton-

omy, and an increase in self-esteem. A combination of regressive, defensive, and progressive coping behaviors may be used by the child to maintain integrity while mastering the situational threat. The nurse can facilitate effective coping through assessment of the child's and family's usual coping patterns. This information can be obtained through specific questions asked during the health history as well as data collected through the use of coping-related assessment tools. The nurse can make a diagnosis and then determine methods that can maintain or enhance the child and family's coping strategies.

Information about usual coping patterns is helpful to the parent and child. If parents are knowledgeable

Ideas for Nursing Research

Nurses play an important role in assisting children to cope with situational as well as maturational changes and stressors. Children should be encouraged to use existing positive coping strategies that have been successful for them in the past. The nurse helps parents find ways to help their children cope effectively. The following areas need to be explored:

- Assessment of coping strategies of children in all age ranges (few studies have been done with the infant, toddler, or preschool population).
- Determination of interventions that help the child and family to cope effectively with situational and maturational crises, e.g., birth of a sibling, separation, illness of the child or a family member, divorce of parents.
- Ways in which coping strategies change during hospitalization and illness.
- How selected coping strategies (e.g., relaxation techniques) can be taught to children.

TABLE 17-1
Nursing Interventions: Developmental Coping Methods

Coping Strategies	Nursing Interventions	Evaluation
Infant		
Motor Activity		
• Changes in position • Restlessness • Body rocking • Toy manipulation • Locomotion • Turning away from undesirable stimuli • Generalized gross motor response	Sit infant up in seat. Change infant's position when lying in the crib. Rock the infant. Stroll the infant or put in infant swing. Provide room for exploration in the crib, playpen, or on a pad on the floor.	The infant exhibits comfort responses to changes in position and physical contact.
	Provide for stimulation and play through colorful mobiles, music boxes, squeeze toys, soft cuddly toys, rattles, mirrors, contact with other babies, pictures on the crib or the wall, and large, safe objects to explore, such as plastic blocks and balls, large plastic beads, stacking rings.	The infant makes appropriate responses to periods of increased stimulation and appropriate periods of decreased stimulation.
Crying/Fussing Behavior *Sucking/Hand-Mouth Activity*	Accept that infants usually cry for a reason and that their crying should be responded to and the reason for crying investigated. Assess infant's other needs as reasons for crying, such as hunger, wet diapers. Observe first to see if the infant can comfort self through either listening to a soothing voice, seeing a familiar face, through own movement, or by putting fingers into mouth. Initiate self-quieting measures, such as holding the infant's arms folded close to body or bringing the infant's fingers into his or her mouth to suck. Stroke the infant or hold and cuddle.	The infants exhibit appropriate response to physical needs being met consistently.
Toddler/Preschooler		
Defense Mechanisms		
• Regression • Denial • Repression • Projection	Accept child's use of defense mechanisms as temporary healthy coping responses, yet recognizing and providing for child to move to more age-appropriate responses *when ready*. Help parents to understand and accept child's use of defense mechanisms as constructive way for child to deal with overwhelming threat until able to mobilize other coping resources.	The toddler/preschooler uses age-appropriate coping responses with direction and support from parents.
Aggression *Protest Behavior/Temper Tantrums*	Accept this behavior as healthy response. Set realistic limits on undesirable behavior. Provide for self-expression, role reversal, and opportunities to control situation through use of puppet play and dolls, drawing pictures, and aggression-release activities, such as hammering pegs, Play-Doh, throwing ball, water play.	Parents demonstrate ability to help the child to act out aggression in socially acceptable ways.
Fantasy *"Trying on the Experience"*	Accept that use of fantasy is normal and healthy in these age groups. Provide opportunities for self-expression. Provide opportunities for practicing for potentially stressful events, for example, birth of a sibling, hospitalization, going to the dentist, starting nursery school. Make reality-oriented statements concerning child's fears, assuring the child that nursing or medical procedures are done for a specific reason and not as punishment for a misdeed.	The child uses a variety of methods to effectively cope with change and stress.
Controlling/Restructuring	Maintain rituals, such as night light, reading books, special blanket. Provide for autonomy, i.e., give simple choices; feed and dress self within capabilities; allow to help with simple household chores.	The child verbalizes feeling comfortable with the maintenance of routines and rituals.
Exploration	Encourage exploration of environment within safe limits. Provide opportunities for diversional play, such as push-pull toys, wooden blocks, simple puzzles, picture books, paper and crayons, finger paintings, dress-up clothes, punching bag.	
School-Age Child		
Defense Mechanisms		
• Regression • Denial • Repression	See Toddler/Preschooler.	

(Continued)

**TABLE 17-1
(Continued)**

Coping Strategies	Nursing Interventions	Evaluation
• Projection/displacement • Sublimation • Reaction formation		
Cognitive Mastery (problem solving/ communication)	Encourage the child to verbalize feelings about situation, and help the child deal with them in a reality-oriented manner. Ask the child to tell you what he or she knows about the situation and encourage questions. Clarify misconceptions with honest, simple explanations. Use books and games to work through feelings.	The parent participates with the child in accurately assessing the stressful situation.
Controlling Behaviors	Help the child prepare ahead for stressful events by recalling what has helped in past situations. Give the child positive reinforcement for helpful behaviors that will increase self-esteem. Let child be responsible for own self-care and dress. Set consistent age-appropriate limits.	The schoolage child uses age-appropriate and socially acceptable methods for dealing with change and stress.
Use of Humor	Be a good listener! (School-age children enjoy telling jokes and asking riddles.) Be a good sport! (School-age children enjoy playing jokes on others.) Share anecdotes and cartoons with child that may relieve tension.	
Aggression	Accept this behavior within reasonable limits. Provide for aggression-release activities, such as action-oriented activities.	
Adolescent		
Defense Mechanisms		
• Regression • Denial • Repression • Projection/displacement • Sublimation • Reaction formation • Rationalization • Intellectualization	See Toddler/Preschooler.	
Cognitive Mastery (abstract thinking/introspection)	Ask adolescents to tell you what they know about their situation and why they think they have this particular problem. Clarify misconceptions and discuss specifics of the situation. Consider that the adolescents' intellectualization and use of sophisticated terminology does not necessarily mean they understand the total picture. Help adolescents interpret normal body changes from the abnormal and anticipate future body changes that will occur. Encourage them to talk about their feelings. Honestly reflect their feelings, for example, "You really sound furious," and help them focus on their concerns in a reality-oriented way. Encourage self-expression by their sharing thoughts and feelings with peers and through music, drawings, poetry, arts and crafts. Emphasize the adolescents' strengths and help them find ways to make these strengths work for them.	The parent exhibits skills in assisting the adolescent to accurately assess the stressful situation.
Conformity	Help adolescents verbalize feelings about how they compare with peers, being left out, and dealing with peer pressure. Respect adolescents' need to conform to peer standards and help parent gain better understanding about this need. Encourage positive role modeling, e.g., famous persons who have achieved success.	
Motor Activity	Explore usual means of dealing with stress and facilitate its use. Set consistent, reasonable limits on behavior with rationale. Encourage optimal activity, such as sports, leisure activities, dancing, lifting weights, watching television programs with action themes. Promote self-responsibility in health care.	The adolescent uses age-appropriate and socially acceptable methods for dealing with change and stress.

Adapted from Vipperman, J. F., & Rager, P. M. (1980). Childhood coping: How nurses can help. *Pediatric Nursing*, 6(2), 11–18.

about age-appropriate coping strategies, effective coping can be encouraged, while ineffective coping should be discouraged. In addition, when children are aware of their coping abilities and limitations, they can determine in which situations they may need some assistance. When children are supported during times of change or stress, they are more likely to develop effective coping strategies. In general, the greater the child's array of successful coping strategies, the greater his or her chance to master change and stress as it is encountered.

References

1. Audette, M. S. (1979; Spring). The significance of regressive behavior for the hospitalized child. *Maternal-Child Nursing Journal, 3,* 31–40.
2. Bowlby, J. (1973). *Attachment and loss* (Vol. 2). New York: Basic Books.
3. Bowlby, J., & Robertson, J. (1958). The nature of the child's tie to his mother. *International Journal of Psychoanalysis, 39,* 350–373.
4. Bradley, R. M., & Caldwell, B.M. (1988). Using the home inventory to assess the family environment. *Pediatric Nursing,* 14(2), 97–103.
5. Calloway, S. (1982). Home observation for measurement of the environment. In S. Humenick (Ed.), *Analysis of current assessment strategies in the health care of children and childbearing families.* Norwalk, CT: Appleton Century 252–258.
6. Dibrell, L., & Yamotto, K. (1988). In their own words: Concerns of young children. *Child Psychiatry and Human Development,* 19(1) 14–25.
7. Eron, L. D., Huesman L. R., Lefkowitz M. M., & Walder, L. O. (1972). Does television violence cause aggression? *American Psychologist, 27,* 253–263.
8. Feetham, S. B., & Humenick, S. (1982). The Feetham family functioning survey. In S. Humenick (Ed.), *Analysis of current assessment strategies in the health care of young children and childbearing families.* Norwalk, CT: Appleton Century 259–268.
9. Ferguson, C. K. (1984). Children coping adaptive behavior during intensive care hospitalization. *Critical Care Quarterly, 4,* 81–94.
10. Flint, N. S. (1988). Visiting policies in pediatrics: Parent's perceptions and preferences. *Journal of Pediatric Nursing, 3*(4), 237–246.
11. Freud, A. (1966). *The ego and the mechanisms of defense.* New York: International Universities Press.
12. Freud, S. (1920). *Beyond the pleasure principle* (J. S. Strachy, Trans.). New York: Liveright Publishing.
13. Gellert, E. (1962). Children's conceptions of the content and functions of the human body. *Genetic Psychology Monographs, 65,* 293–411.
14. Harter, S. (1981). A model of intrinsic mastery motivation in children: Individual differences and developmental change. In W. A. Collins (Ed.), *Minnesota symposium on child psychology* (Vol. 14; pp. 215–255). Hillsdale, NJ: L. Elbaum.
15. La Montagne, L. L. (1984). Children's locus of control beliefs as predictors of their pre-operative coping behavior. *Nursing Research, 33*(2), 76 85.
16. La Montagne, L. L. (1987). Adopting a process approach to assess children's coping. *Journal of Pediatric Nursing, 3*(3), 159–163.
17. Lazarus, R. S. (1969). *Patterns of adjustment and human effectiveness.* New York: McGraw-Hill.
18. Lazarus, R. S., & Folkman, S. (1984). *Stress, appraisal and coping.* New York: Springer.
19. Lazarus, R. S., & Launier, R. (1978). Stress-related transactions between person and environment. In L. A. Pervin & M. Lewis (Eds.). *Perspectives in interactional psychology* (pp. 287–322). New York: Plenum.
20. Liebert, R., & Sprafkin, J. (1992). Television and the family. In R. Hoelkelman (Ed.), *Primary pediatric care* (2nd ed.). St. Louis, C.V. Mosby.
21. Moos, R. (Ed.). (1976). *Human adaptation: Coping with life crisis.* Lexington, MA: Heath.
22. Murphy, L. B. (1962). *The widening world of childhood: Paths toward mastery.* New York: Basic Books.
23. Murphy, L. B., & Moriarity, A. E. (1976). *Vulnerability, coping and growth: From infancy to adolescence.* New Haven, Yale University.
24. Nagy, M. H. (1959). The child's view of death. In H. Feifel (Ed.), *The meaning of death.* New York: McGraw-Hill.
25. National Institute of Mental Health. (1982). Television and behavior: Ten years of scientific progress and implications for the eighties (DHHS Publication No. ADM 82–1195). Washington, DC: U.S. Government Printing Office.
26. Neuman, B. (1982). *The Neuman systems model: Application to nursing education and practice,* East Norwalk, CT: Appleton Century Crofts.
27. Oremland, E. (1988). Mastering developmental and critical experiences through play and other expressive behaviors in childhood. *Children's Health Care, 16*(3):150–156.
28. Peretz, D. (1970). Development, object-relationships, and loss. In B. Schoenbert, A. C. Carr, D. Peretz, & A. H. Kutscher (Eds.), *Loss and grief: Psychological management in medical practice.* New York: Columbia University Press 3–19.
29. Piers, E., & Harris, D. (1969). *The Piers-Harris children's self-concept scale manual:* Nashville: Counselor Recording and Tests.
30. Prazar, G. (1992). Lying and stealing. In R. Hoekelman (Ed.), *Primary pediatric care* (2nd ed.). St. Louis: C.V. Mosby.
31. Proctor, D. L. (1987). Relationship between visitation policy in a pediatric intensive care unit and parental anxiety. *Children's Health Care, 16*(1), 13–17.
32. Roy, C. (1984). The Roy adaptational model of nursing. In C. Roy (Ed.), *Introduction to nursing: An adaptational model* (2nd ed.). Englewood Cliffs, NJ: Prentice-Hall 27–41.
33. Ryan, N. (1989). Stress-coping strategies identified from school age children's perspective. *Research in Nursing and Health, 12,* 111–122.
34. Selye, H. (1974). *Stress without distress.* Philadelphia: J.B. Lippincott.
35. Shanley, P. (1982). Separation anxiety behavioral index: The young child's reaction to mother-child separation. In S. Humenick (Ed.). *Analysis of current assessment strategies in the health care of young children and childbearing families.* Norwalk, CT: Appleton Century.
36. Singer, J. L., Singer, D. G., & Rapaczynski, W. S. (1984). Family patterns and television viewing as predictors of children's beliefs and aggression. *Journal of Communications, 34*(2):73–89.
37. Spitz, R. A. (1945). Hospitalism: An inquiry into the genesis of psychiatric conditions in early childhood. In *Psychoanalytic study of the child* (Vol. 1). New York: International University Press 53–74.
38. Spitz, R. A. (1946). Hospitalism: A follow-up report. In *Psychoanalytic study of the child* (Vol. 2). New York: International University Press 113–117.
39. Taylor, M. M., & Williams, H. A. (1980). Use of therapeutic play in the ambulatory pediatric hematology clinic. *Cancer Nursing, 3,* 433–437.
40. Tiedeman, M. E. (1989). The Roy adaptational model. In J. J. Fitzpatrick & A. L. Whall (Eds.), *Conceptual models of nursing: Analysis and application* (2nd ed.) (pp 185–204). Norwalk; Connecticut: Appleton & Lange.
41. Vipperman, J. F., & Rager, P. M. (1980). Childhood coping: How nurses can help. *Pediatric Nursing, 6*(2), 11–18.
42. Wolf, J. A., & Visintainer, M. (1979). Psychological preparation for tonsillectomy patients: Effects on children's and parent's adjustment. *Pediatrics, 64,* 646–655.

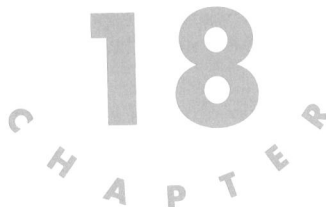

Behavioral and Emotional Responses to Life Stress

BEHAVIORAL OBJECTIVES

Describe stress in childhood as a biopsychosocial factor potentially affecting children's health and well-being.

Identify the relationship between life stress and the child's behavior and emotional responses.

Explain different approaches in classifying selected emotional and behavioral problems in children and discuss their impact on nursing assessment in these situations.

Describe the nursing management of common behavioral and emotional problems.

In contrast to the extensive empirical research on life stress in adults and its impact on physical and psychological health, little research has been done on the impact of life stress on children and adolescents. In fact, it was not until about 1980 that childhood stress started to attract researchers' attention.[32] Even then, reports on the comparative stressfulness of life events depended on clinicians', teachers', or parents' judgments.

Limited normative information is available on children's reactions to stress. This has been due mostly to the difficulty in obtaining data, whether because research methods might be invasive or because they might require cooperation beyond a young child's ability. Adults have sometimes supplied their observations, but observations of the impact of stress on a child cannot have the same immediacy or accuracy as direct reports from the child would provide.

Stress in Life's Continuum

Stress is not unique to adults. Despite their tender years, many children experience tremendous amounts of life stress. Their lack of experience and inability to express themselves only increase the magnitude of their stress. Children's lack of maturity constitutes a stressor that is unique to children and that may partly explain the fears, irrationality, and faulty logic that interfere with children's ability to perceive a situation clearly and respond or react appropriately.

407

Depending on their stage of development and the stressfulness of life events, children may react by developing a variety of emotional and behavioral problems. Some might react by "acting out" (e.g., fighting, cursing, stealing), whereas others might show their emotional pain by internalizing problems (e.g., suffering physical symptoms, sleeping poorly, or being withdrawn, too quiet and depressed).

A lack of social skills and limited expressive abilities may hide the true suffering that is at the root of children's or adolescents' emotional and behavioral problems. When unresolved, these problems are carried over into adulthood, with damaging consequences.

Stress Theory

Stress is neither good nor bad and can produce both positive and negative effects. As part of everyday life, stress challenges us and enables us to grow and develop into capable and healthy human beings. However, stress (especially in young children) can sometimes exceed the ability to cope and therefore can negatively affect health.

Hans Selye[24] defined stress as a state manifested by a specific syndrome consisting of many changes within a biologic system. Because Selye linked stress to a specific pattern of physiologic events, his theory was soon challenged. Many researchers demonstrated that psychological factors also played a major role in the stress syndrome.

Since 1940, when Selye first coined the term, "stress" has often been defined as a stimulus or as a response to a stressor. More recently, some researchers have conceptualized stress as neither stimulus nor response, but as a construct that intervenes between a threatening stimulus and the response to it. According to Harris and Hastings,[13 (p.54)] putting the emphasis on stress as a construct that comes between a stimulus (stressor) and a response (stress response) offers

"ways to pose questions about what creates stress, how stress affects health, and how humans can actively cope with stress. Central to this way of looking at stress is the importance of interpretation and the idea that all ways of responding—physiologic response, cognition, emotion, and action—are parts of coping with the stress."

To cope with stress effectively requires adaptation. That is, the organism "must either change itself to achieve harmony with its surroundings or alter the environment so it is synchronous with the organism."[9] Effective coping through adaptation allows the achievement and promotion of a state of health, growth, and accomplishment of the various developmental tasks at the appropriate stages of life, and the building up of energy resources to meet life goals. If, on the other hand, coping is ineffective, maladaptation occurs, resulting in lack of growth, internal disharmony (illness), or disharmony between the child and the environment (social disruption).

Stressors

A stressor can be anything that stimulates an imbalance between the demands of the child and the child's ability to cope.[18a] Physical, biologic, and psychosocial stressors arise from the environment outside oneself (poverty, emotionally disturbed parent) or within oneself (poor nutrition, self-critical thoughts). Developmental tasks, when not accomplished in the appropriate stage of life, can also represent stressors in later periods.[13] The accompanying display outlines some of those life cycle stressors.

Interpretation

Interpretation refers to the subjective meaning each person gives to events in his or her life. According to Harris and Hastings' model of stress, the interpretation

---

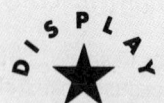

Life Cycle Stressors

Early childhood
  Prematurity
  Malnutrition
  Separation from caregivers
  Social deprivation
  Parental incompetence/inconsistency
  Disruption of diurnal rhythm
  Lack of parental acceptance
Preschool years
  Inadequate parental support
  Lack of peer acceptance
  Authoritarianism
  Inconsistency

Later childhood
  Lack of peer acceptance
  Inadequate parental support
  School pressures
Adolescence
  Social isolation
  Peer pressure
  Failure to separate from parents
  Failure to integrate socially
  Failure to prepare for work
  Hypochondriasis
  Lack of adult acceptance

*(Harris, J. S., & Hastings, J. E. [1987]. Coping with stress. In D. P. Sheridan & J. R. Winogrord [Eds.], **The preventive approach to patient care** [pp. 354–374]. New York: Elsevier Science.)*

of a given event determines whether or not that event causes a stress response in a person's life.[13] Some stressors need little or even no interpretation. However, most stressors—especially the psychosocial ones—are subject to personal interpretation.

The physiology that accounts for the interpretation of a stimulus is well understood. Our knowledge is based on research studies dealing with adults, because little has been done to analyze the interpretation and appraisal process of stress in children. However, it is expected that, as children mature, the interpretation of stressors would follow a pattern similar to that of adults. When a person encounters a stimulus, the information received is processed in one of two ways: through the thalamus or cortical system.

The pathway through the *thalamus* is used by stimuli that require little or no interpretation. Because of their often harmful nature, stressors like physicochemical stimuli (noise, heat, cold, pressure) usually cause a stress response without immediate conscious interpretation.

The *cortical system* pathway is used to process stressors that are of a more psychosocial nature. Harris and Hastings[13] (p.357) suggest that "information processed from sensory receptors through the corresponding cortical area to associative areas is checked to determine if it was previously a threat. If, because of previous experience, symbols, values, beliefs, logical analogy, or unpleasant physical sensations constitute a threat, the endocrine, reticular activating, and sympathetic nervous systems are activated. The limbic system generates unpleasant emotions, and the situation is perceived as stressful."

Many researchers agree that, to understand the development of children's emotional and behavioral problems, information is needed not only about their stressors and their coping skills but also about the way the two interact. One model proposes that children develop behavioral problems if they have low coping skills in relation to both their actual environmental stressors and their "protectors."[10]

In early childhood, when children are not yet physiologically mature, many factors appear to influence the interpretation of potentially stressful stimuli and the ability to cope. Factors are:

- Physical condition
- Personality and temperament
- Family situation and social support
- Culture and environment
- Actual event
- Spiritual beliefs
- Developmental level
- Gender (girls more resilient than boys)
- Ability to perform well academically
- Inherited differences in intelligence and ability to handle stress

Different kinds of appraisals take place almost simultaneously throughout the interpretation of stressors. *Primary appraisal* determines consciously and deliberately the nature of the stressor. Does it represent a harm, a loss, the threat of a future harm or loss, or, on the contrary, a challenge or an opportunity for growth? *Secondary appraisal* examines whether one can handle the stress.

It allows revision of the primary appraisal by assessing previous experience with the stressor. For instance, a primary appraisal of threat (e.g., failing an examination and hence the threat of staying back a grade at school) may be reinterpreted as a challenge because of success in passing exams in the past. Or a defensive reappraisal may allow one to extract some good from a stressor (e.g., "If I fail and am not promoted to high school, I can still be a part of the Junior hockey team"). An accurate interpretation triggers an appropriate response to a stressor, whereas an inaccurate interpretation leads to inadequate coping or to a response that wastes energy.

Protectors

A number of protective factors can reduce the effects of stressors on a person. These "environmental protectors" can buffer a person from the negative effects of a stressful situation.[26] For example, strong family ties can help a child cope with a move to a new school or town. Some children appear to be untouched by enduring stressors; these are referred to as *invulnerable* or *resilient children.* These "superkids" conquer the most difficult circumstances and go on to succeed in life. Examples of resilient children include emotionally healthy offspring of schizophrenic parents, abused children who develop successful intimate relationships, and youngsters living in the ghetto who turn out to be distinguished professionals. Against persistent "corrosive" stressors, two protectors are especially worthy of mention:

- Child's personality—the child has a positive attitude within the situation. He or she is able to adapt to change, has a healthy self-concept, and is independent, friendly, and attentive to others.
- Child's family—the child has a positive relationship with at least one supportive parent or with mutually supportive parents.

Responses to Stress

Selye has used the term *general adaptation syndrome* (GAS) to describe the response of the body to life challenges. He demonstrated experimentally a triphasic response to stressors that starts with the stage of alarm (the ergotropic function), proceeds to a stage of heightened function (resistance), and ends with a stage of chronically impaired function (exhaustion). This is illustrated in Figure 18-1.

These stress responses, also called coping, have been defined as efforts to meet the demands of a stress, whether or not those responses are purposeful or successful. Over time, every child develops coping patterns to maintain a sense of equilibrium when faced with positive or negative stressful situations. These coping behaviors could be adaptive or maladaptive (see Chap. 17). However, on a physiologic and biochemical level, the body does not distinguish between positive stressors (e.g., new home, vacation, or graduation) and negative stressors (e.g., parental divorce, new sibling, or academic failure). Both elicit the same responses, and both can have positive or

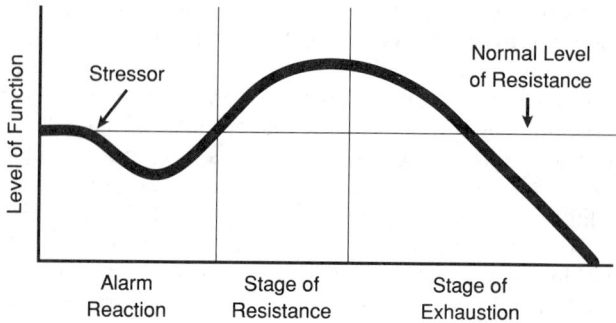

FIGURE 18-1

The general adaptation syndrome. (Selye, H. [1976]. *The stress of life.*
New York: McGraw-Hill.)

negative consequences. Negative stressors often are more intense and more demanding; they are usually more harmful, too, because the arousal associated with them has a tendency to be prolonged (e.g., feeling angry and upset long after losing a class election).

A person has many levels of response to stress. These include physiologic, emotional, cognitive, and behavioral responses.

Physiologic Responses

Physiologic responses comprise reactions of three major systems that are affected once a sensory input has been mediated through the hypothalamus. First, the *sympathetic nervous system* is stimulated directly, affecting the skeletal and visceral muscles, salivary glands, pancreas, and the adrenal medulla. A second system affected by stress is the *endocrine system.* A third group of physiologic responses involves the *immune system.* Responses of these systems are listed in the display.

Emotional Responses

Activated through the *limbic system,* immediate emotional responses to stress include fear, anxiety, anger,

rage, or, on the other hand, joy or elation. Fear triggers the flight response to remove people from danger. Conversely, anger encourages a person to fight—another behavioral response that enables people to combat a stressful situation directly. These two emotions—fear and anger—correspond to the resistance stage of GAS. Depression is another emotional response to stress; it coincides with the exhaustion stage of the syndrome.[13]

Cognitive Responses

Cognitive responses involve conscious thoughts, such as planning an escape or avoiding a given situation, as well as angry and aggressive thoughts. Other types of cognitive responses include more purposeful thoughts, such as examining assumptions or beliefs, or developing solutions to the problems the stressors impose.

Behavioral Responses

Behavioral responses include complex human behavior such as aggression or anxiety-reducing rituals. Behavioral responses can be directed appropriately at the stressor or inappropriately at a less threatening target. Obsessions, compulsions, and phobias can reduce anxiety by enabling people to avoid stressful stimuli. Other adaptive responses may be employed; taking drugs, smoking, and overeating are a few common ones. Finally, especially during the exhaustion stage, inactivity and social withdrawal are responses to stress.[13]

General Guidelines for Care in Common Childhood Emotional and Behavioral Problems

The nursing care of children and adolescents with emotional and behavioral problems requires special clinical skills and a solid background in child mental health issues. Efficient collaboration with other health profession-

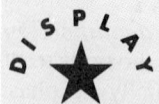

Physiologic Responses to Stress

SYMPATHETIC NERVOUS SYSTEM RESPONSES

- Increased muscle tone (joint pain, headache, back pain)
- Increased neural tone (dry mouth, tachycardia, sweating)
- Perceptual inaccuracies (prone to accidents, changes in time sense, memory alteration)

Sympathetic Adrenal Responses
- Increased cardiac output and rate
- Increased blood pressure
- Dilation of pupils
- Cool, pale skin

ENDOCRINE SYSTEM RESPONSES

- Decreased thymic factor (resulting in decreased cell-mediated immunity)
- Increased thyroid-stimulating hormone (leading to increased metabolic rate)

IMMUNE SYSTEM RESPONSES

- Interferon production
- Suppression of thymic factors
- Increased prostaglandins
- Failure of lymphocyte activity

(Adapted from: Harris, J. S. [1984]. Stress and Stressors in critical care. Crit Care Nurse 4 [1]: 6.)

als and an advocacy role on behalf of the child are particularly necessary tasks of the child health nurse.

★ NURSING ASSESSMENT

Nursing assessment provides data for planning intervention(s) to prevent or manage children's emotional and behavioral problems. Children's developmental differences make nursing assessment a difficult task. Moreover, depending on the age of the child and the given situation, the child health nurse may have to rely on the parents or caregivers (and hence on the validity of their reports), as well as other indirect methods of assessment: history-taking, reports, checklists or ratings by teachers, or self-reports by older children or adolescents. More direct methods involve observation, physical examination, and behavioral assessment.

Not all problematic childhood behavior is related to stressful situations that create overtaxing demands. Other factors such as diseases (brain tumors), toxic products (lead poisoning), or substance abuse (drugs, alcohol) can also lead to dysfunctional behavior. Moreover, some problematic behaviors resolve over time.

The child health nurse should perform a thorough initial screening, as well as a more specific in-depth assessment. Both the screening and specific assessment are conceptually based on the overall structure recommended by Gordon (1987),[9a] which combines three main dimensions: the client–environment focus, the developmental focus, and the functional focus or integrative function of the whole person.

The following guidelines borrow from a practical guide to the assessment and management of the emo-

tional and behavioral problems in children. Herbert[14] recommends four steps:

- Construct a problem profile by asking specific questions.
- Develop a functional analysis of the problem behavior by using a basic equation, the ABC analysis (Fig. 18-2).
- Assess the child's strengths.
- Obtain information from other sources regarding the child's overall physical and psychosocial assessment.

The *problem profile* is constructed by asking specific questions. What is (are) the problem(s)? How is each problem defined by the parents and the child? What is the level of agreement or disagreement between parents and child about what the particular problem(s) is (are) and how they would like things to be different? In what setting does the problem occur? Who is pressing for change in the situation, and what are the implications of change?

A *functional analysis of the problem behavior* is developed by using the following basic equation ("the ABC analysis"):

$$\text{Antecedent Events} \rightarrow \text{Behavior} \rightarrow \text{Consequences}$$

This analysis stresses that changes in a person's behavior create changes in the environment, and vice versa. The analysis provides a description of the elements of a situation and of their relationships (e.g., the behavior is affected by the antecedent events as well as by its consequences). Another way to refer to the ABC sequence is the "three-term contingency" (see Fig. 18-2). The nurse may find out what events (setting events) are associated with the behavior. Also, the parameters of the problem behavior need to be explored. The acronym FINDS[15] has

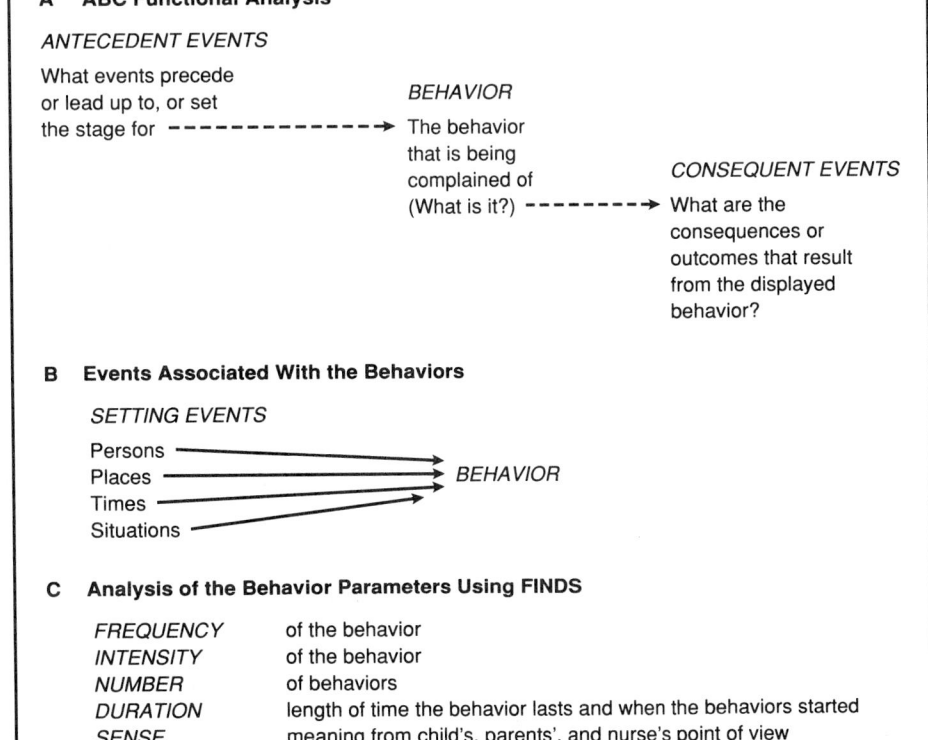

FIGURE 18-2

Three-term contingency for analysis of behavioral problems. (**A**) The ABC sequence of analysis refers to antecedent events, behavior, and consequent events. (**B**) An in-depth analysis of the behavior includes events associated with the behavior. (**C**) The parameters of the behavior are described by the acronym FINDS. (*From: Herbert, M. [1981]. Behav. treatment of problem children—A practice manual.* London: Acad. Press.)

A   ABC Functional Analysis

ANTECEDENT EVENTS

What events precede or lead up to, or set the stage for - - - - - - - - - →

BEHAVIOR

The behavior that is being complained of (What is it?) - - - - - - →

CONSEQUENT EVENTS

What are the consequences or outcomes that result from the displayed behavior?

B   Events Associated With the Behaviors

SETTING EVENTS

Persons
Places
Times
Situations

BEHAVIOR

C   Analysis of the Behavior Parameters Using FINDS

FREQUENCY	of the behavior
INTENSITY	of the behavior
NUMBER	of behaviors
DURATION	length of time the behavior lasts and when the behaviors started
SENSE	meaning from child's, parents', and nurse's point of view

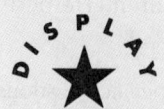

Specific Emotional and Behavioral Problems

Anxiety
  Avoidant disorder
  Overanxious disorder
  Separation anxiety disorder
  School phobia
Conduct disorders
  Noncompliance
  Oppositional disorders
  Truancy
  Running away
  Drug/alcohol experimentation
Eating disorders
  Anorexia nervosa
  Bulimia nervosa

Elimination disorders
  Enuresis
  Functional encopresis
Sleep disorders
  Sleep-walking
  Sleep terror
Exacerbation of chronic illness
  Recurrent abdominal pain
  Headache
  Hyperventilation

been used to describe the dimensions of the problem behavior: Frequency, Intensity, Number, Duration (both actual duration and time since onset), and Sense (from the child's, family's, and nurse's point of view).

A child's *strengths* are identified to counterbalance the efforts to improve the emotional or behavioral problem. Moreover, if parents learn to focus on the child's positive behavior, such behavior is likely to increase. Finally, the nurse needs to identify reinforcers or rewards that the child and the parents find pleasurable.

Information is obtained from *other sources* regarding the child's overall physical and psychosocial assessment. This is described in later sections of the chapter dealing with each separate emotional and behavioral problems. Specific emotional and behavioral disorders are listed in the accompanying display. (Eating disorders, including anorexia nervosa and bulimia nervosa, are discussed in Chapter 19.)

★ NURSING DIAGNOSES AND PLANNING

Nursing diagnoses associated with behavioral and emotional problems may include the following signs and symptoms:

- Anxiety.
- Constipation.
- Diarrhea.
- Fear.
- Pain.
- Sleep Pattern Disturbance.
- Stress Incontinence.

During this phase of the nursing process, interventions and goals or expected client outcomes are planned. A written or verbal contract can be initiated with the child and parent. This is a formal agreement between the nurse and the child and/or the parent(s). The contract is based on the principles of behavior modification in which the primary goal is to increase the frequency of desirable behavior. Such contracts provide a mechanism for clear communications among all those involved in the child's

care, as well as a means for evaluating accurately and reliably the progress made by the child.

★ INTERVENTIONS: COLLABORATIVE AND INDEPENDENT

Selection of interventions depends on whether the child's problem is one of excess (needs to decrease or extinguish behavior), or of deficit (needs to increase or acquire a new behavior). Changes can be encouraged not only by positive and negative reinforcement, but also by role modeling.

Reinforcers vary widely and depend on the individual child's age and preference. The display on the following page lists behavioral programs including methods for altering behaviors and reducing behaviors. Essentially, all these methods of behavior modification constitute an educational process involving persuasion, instruction, demonstration, training, and monitoring.

The nurse and parents must find ways to motivate the child. If age permits, the child is involved in the intervention. The parents' collaboration is crucial to the success of any intervention. Practical help for the parents, such as day care services, could promote their participation in the therapeutic intervention. Grandparents or siblings can also be used as a valuable resource.

Anxiety and Phobic Disorders

Anxiety and fear are appropriate responses in a variety of situations (e.g., fear of a hot stove after being burned). Yet, some emotional problems of childhood associated with anxieties and phobias do not seem to be related to physical danger.

Anxiety has been defined by NANDA as "a vague uneasy feeling whose source is often nonspecific or unknown to the individual."[20] *Fears* are specific, often physical reactions to clear stimuli, whereas anxieties are considered more diffuse reactions to sometimes less concrete stimuli. *Phobias* are fears that are illogical and

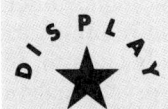

Behavioral Programs Including Methods for Altering Behaviors and Reducing Behaviors

METHODS FOR ALTERING BEHAVIOR

Tangible Reinforcers

Objects: Stars, stamps, small toys, books, comics, marbles, stickers, puzzles, favorite food or drinks, notebooks, pencils, baseball cards, records

Activities: Watching television, visits from friends, games (Monopoly and so forth), drawing, painting, playing computer games

Privileges: Extra pocket money, special outing, going to the movies or hockey match, staying up late, choice of meal

Intangible Reinforcers

Smiles, hugs, encouragement

Self-praise, self-appreciation
Parental role modeling of behaviors

METHODS FOR REDUCING BEHAVIOR

Punishment (mild, occasional, for example, isolation, withdrawal of privilege)

Gradual exposure to aversive stimuli (desensitization)

Cognitive restructuring for older children and adolescents (encouraging the child to talk about past experiences and reevaluate potentially distressing experiences)

---

disproportionate to the actual situation and are not able to be mediated cognitively.

Anxiety Disorders

The classification of the American Psychiatric Association[1a] in its *Diagnostic and Statistical Manual,* 3rd edition, revised (DSM-III-R) is discussed in Chapter 19. It lists separation anxiety disorder (SAD), avoidant disorder, and overanxious disorders (OAD) as subtypes of anxiety disorders. There is some controversy over the diagnostic reliability and independent use of each of these subtypes. Quay and Werry (1986)[21a] suggest there is little empirical evidence to support such a classification. They propose that anxiety be considered a "symptom" that encompasses fears of people, objects, events, or situations, all of which may "reflect a generalized tendency to react to a wide variety of environmental stimuli as a signal of impending pain or punishment or as novel events giving rise to the inhibition of behavior." Anxiety in children is generally accompanied by symptoms of social withdrawal and dysphoria, which Quay and Werry call the "anxiety-withdrawal-dysphoria" syndrome.

Only recently have childhood anxiety disorders become a focus of clinical and research efforts. A study at the University of Pittsburgh School of Medicine appears to offer some support to the DSM-III-R distinction between separation anxiety disorder and overanxious disorder. Of the 91 children between the ages of 5 and 18 years examined at the Child and Adolescent Anxiety Disorder Clinic, a total of 69 children (76%) met criteria for SAD (N = 22), or both SAD and OAD (N = 21). Children with SAD were observed to be younger and from lower socioeconomic status than children with OAD. Children with OAD were more likely to present with an additional anxiety disorder such as simple phobia or panic disorder.[16]

Another recent study appears to support the idea that anxiety and depression are associated. Strauss and coworkers[28] investigated the peer social status of sixteen 6- to 13-year-old children diagnosed with such a condition. They found that among these 16 children referred to the University of Georgia Children's Center for Psychological Assessment, about 31% (N = 5) were codiagnosed with depression and almost 12% (N = 12) manifested simple phobia. Despite their relatively small sample, their findings also indicate that when childhood anxiety disorders coexist with depression, they are associated with diminished peer popularity.

Although the etiology of childhood anxiety disorders is not always known, one theory believes that these behaviors are learned in much the same way that appropriate fears are learned.[5] However, other factors could be implicated in the different types of anxiety (e.g., hereditary or familial factors, such as introverted parents or closely knit families).

The subtypes of anxiety disorders are presented here in the order that corresponds to the earliest age of onset.

Avoidant Disorder

Avoidant disorder includes the avoidance of contact with strangers to the degree that social functioning with peers is impaired. According to the DSM-III-R, this diagnosis must be of at least 6 months' duration and is not diagnosed before 2.5 years of age. Relationships with family members and other familiar people are normal. The child's shyness and withdrawal are not usually manifested until he or she starts nursery school. Parental concern often diminishes as the child progresses on to school, because such behavior does not interfere with the school program. In fact, most teachers fail to notice the child's inappropriate behavior, noticing instead other children's more disruptive or aggressive behavior. It is usually during adolescence that the low rate of typical adolescent social activities becomes a concern to parents.

Overanxious Disorder (OAD)

Overanxious disorder involves excessive anxiety concerning future situations. Although not focused on a particular event, the anxiety usually deals with evaluation by others (e.g., in relation to school or athletic performance or social events). The child or adolescent may seem unable to relax, needs excessive reassurance, and may also experience nausea, headache, a lump in the throat, or digestive problems. DSM-III-R reports that overanxious disorder occurs more often in boys, especially older ones belonging to small families in which there is a concern about performance. The disorder is relatively common and would not usually come to the health professional's attention. It may persist into adulthood.

Separation Anxiety Disorder (SAD)

In separation anxiety disorder there is excessive anxiety associated with separation from family members or familiar surroundings. Affected children may refuse to stay in a room or at other people's houses by themselves. They may have problems going to sleep or even have nightmares. They may also experience fears of animals, burglars, accidents, or even death. These fears usually focus on danger to themselves or to their families. Often SAD affects children who have become rather dependent on family members after a major life stress such as illness of the child or the family member, moving, changing school, or death of a pet or a close relative. SAD may occur in preschool children, with the development of a pattern of chronic anxiety related to a situation of anticipated separations. This disorder may persist into adulthood. Deltito and coworkers (1986) hypothesize that childhood anxiety—especially SAD accompanied by school phobia—predisposes a person to agoraphobia (fear of open spaces).

School Phobia

One particular form of anxiety, school phobia, is especially common among children. Because it may have serious and potentially long-lasting educational, psychological, and even legal implications, school phobia is discussed in some detail here. Like all phobias, school phobia has emotional, physical, and behavioral manifestations. Phobias are defined as fears that are disproportionate to the demands of a situation and cannot be reasoned away.[3] Emotionally, there is intense anxiety, feelings of dread, worry, and even panic. Physically, the child may manifest tremors, diaphoresis, nausea, hyperventilation, palpitations, or tachycardia. Behaviorally, the phobic child avoids the feared situation.

School phobia has been defined as refusal to attend school because the child is afraid. It is different from truancy, in which fear is not the major problem. The DSM-III-R further emphasizes that school phobia refers to the child's being fearful of the school situation, whereas school avoidance (persistent reluctance or refusal to go to school because of the fear of leaving home or the parents) is one of the criteria for establishing the diagnosis of SAD.[1,5]

Although there has been no evidence that biologic and constitutional variables can be implicated in the etiology of school phobia, the issue of biologic vulnerability has been suggested as a possible contributing variable. Basically, two theories are commonly cited to explain why school phobias develop.[5] The psychoanalytic theory emphasizes the psychological factors and attributes school phobia to a disturbed personality or disturbed family interactions (e.g., the child has assumed the caretaker role for a sick parent); hence, school phobia may be a form of SAD.

The cognitive theory proposes that school phobia is the product of environmental factors. According to this view, and based on the principles of classic and operant conditioning, the school environment may be paired with an aversive stimulus that has triggered some fear, anxiety, or other strong emotions in the child. The operant component may come into effect if the parents or significant others reinforce the child's negative statements about the school or encourage staying home from school. In addition, the child's previous experiences may be influential. Children who are punished physically at home may be more liable to suffer from school phobia. The school environment may play a critical role (e.g., a quiet, timid student might have special difficulty adjusting to a large classroom). Therefore, in diagnosing school phobia, a thorough assessment is essential, with particular attention to the patterns and timing of the child's symptoms.

★ NURSING ASSESSMENT

Appropriate assessment methods can assist in selecting suitable intervention strategies. It is essential to assess manifestations of the three facets of this syndrome: the physiologic, emotional, and behavioral.

PHYSIOLOGIC ASSESSMENT

Interviews with the child, the parents and other caretakers, and teachers or other relevant school personnel are most commonly used to establish a history. The following areas should be included:

- Child's emotional history and development
- Type and quality of interactions between parent(s) and child
- Child's current situation and environment, especially with regard to school
- Timing and description of symptoms
- Other important factors the child cannot verbalize (obtained with such tools as the child's drawings and paintings, projective picture test, and stories).

Throughout data collection, the nurse should observe and record the content and process, as well as the verbal and nonverbal communication between parents and child. A genogram may help to establish the therapeutic relationship, to reduce the parents' anxiety, and to create a beginning picture of the "setting events."

A complete physical examination often is needed to identify any related physiologic problem(s) that might account for the signs and symptoms manifested by the child (Table 18-1). Sometimes, depending on the reason(s) for seeking health care, the following diagnostic tests are performed: blood counts, throat swab cultures, auditory evaluations, stool analysis, urine analysis, and vision screening.

TABLE 18-1
Physical Manifestations of School Phobia

System	Manifestation
Musculoskeletal	Rigid tense muscles
	Muscular tremors
	Increased weakness
	Inability to move
Cardiovascular	Hyperventilation
	Palpitations
	Tachycardia
	Increased blood pressure
	Diaphoresis
	Cold hands and feet
Gastrointestinal	Nausea
	Abdominal pain or cramps
	Vomiting
	Anorexia
Other	Sleep disturbances
	Urinary urgency
	Urinary frequency
	General malaise
	Headache
	Low-grade fever

EMOTIONAL ASSESSMENT

Emotional evaluation constitutes an important aspect of the child's assessment in cases of school phobia. In addition to some of the tools described in the chapter on developmental and behavioral assessment (see Chap. 8), self-reports are among the most common diagnostic methods used. Self-report methods are of two types:

- Those focusing on anxiety as a generalized trait, such as the Children's Manifest Anxiety Scale developed by Castaneda, McCandless and Palermo,[2] which is designed to measure the child's tendency to experience a general or a chronic state of anxiety across a variety of situations
- Those measuring specific fears, such as the Fear Survey Schedule for Children,[23] an 80-item scale related to the specific areas of school, home, social, physical, animal, and other fears.

BEHAVIORAL ASSESSMENT

Three common categories of behavioral measures of children's fears are as follows:

- Observational codes: The Observer Rating Scale of Anxiety, designed by Melamed and Siegel,[19] is an observational code that includes 29 behaviors to be observed for their presence or absence using a time-sampling procedure.
- Behavioral checklists: Particularly helpful in research and screening programs, these involve a standard set of specific behaviors that are to be rated by someone familiar with the child.
- Global behavioral ratings: These involve making a global rating of the child's fear-related behavior in the anxiety-producing situation. They should be used in combina-

tion with other methods, because they are sometimes rather subjective.[5,15]

★ NURSING DIAGNOSES AND PLANNING

Nursing diagnoses associated with school phobia may include the following:

- Anxiety related to anticipation of separation from parent(s).
- Fear of School related to potential cognitive distortion associated with problematic child–parent relationship.
- Social Isolation (Self-Imposed) related to interrupted school attendance.
- Impaired Social Interaction related to insufficient contact with peer group.
- Sleep Pattern Disturbance related to worrying about attending school.
- Ineffective Individual Coping related to avoidance of attendance at school.
- Ineffective Family Coping: Compromised related to altered ability to manage regular child's attendance at school.

The immediate goals are to alleviate the child's distress and assist the child to return to school. The long-term goals are to provide the child with an alternative means of coping with his or her fear of school; to alter the family environment, and, if possible, the school environment so that the problem does not recur; and, finally, to avoid long-term anxiety disorders.

Outcome criteria may involve the following:

- Child discusses fears about school.
- Parents report success in using reinforcement with the child.

★ INTERVENTIONS: COLLABORATIVE AND INDEPENDENT

Ideally, the best nursing intervention is promotion of school readiness and continued school attendance. Prevention of school phobia often can be achieved by anticipatory guidance and adequate parenting programs. However, if school phobia does develop, it is essential that it be properly and promptly addressed. Its prognosis is usually good in preadolescent children, but relatively poor in older ones.[17] Therefore, an early intervention program must be established in cooperation with the parents and child. Research has indicated that when treatment was initiated immediately after the onset of symptoms, results were more rapid and successful than when treatment was delayed for weeks or months.

The following strategies are recommended as useful in the management and evaluation of a child with school phobia:

- Therapeutic play, talking with the child about his or her fears, as well as other cognitive behavioral approaches.
- Behavioral modification using positive reinforcers, particularly desensitization, in which the child is exposed to increasing contacts with the school.
- Age-appropriate stress management skills (e.g., relaxation) and social skills training.
- Cognitive restructuring for parents, including counseling and teaching parenting skills.

- Environmental restructuring, arranging for environmental contingencies that reinforced the child for going to school.
- Follow-up for guidance and support, especially because both the child and the family will be trying to modify their behavior over a long-term period.

When the child's situation is a complex one, or when there are additional familial or marital problems, a referral to a pediatric clinical nurse specialist, or to a child psychiatric or mental health nurse is recommended. Individual psychotherapy, or family or marriage counseling may be needed. However, nursing strategies can usually be developed in collaboration with the parents, teachers, counselors, school administrators, and other health professionals.

Conduct Disorders

Conduct disorders are defined as "a repetitive and persistent pattern of conduct in which either the basic rights of others or major age appropriate societal norms or rules are violated."[1a (p.58)] The behaviors in conduct disorders are more serious and repetitive than ordinary childhood and adolescent mischief and pranks. Conduct disorders are classified into four subtypes: undersocialized aggressive, undersocialized nonaggressive, socialized aggressive, and socialized nonaggressive (Table 18-2). Socialized refers to the presence (or absence) of social bonds. In undersocialized children, the child is unable to estab-

lish warm and affectionate relationships with others. The child does not display concerns for others or appropriate guilt and remorse for behaviors.[18] The presence (or absence) of aggressive behavior is characterized by a repetitive pattern of physical violence against others or thefts outside the home involving confrontation with others. Both types of aggressive behavior violate the rights of others. The nonaggressive subtypes are characterized by antisocial behaviors that violate rules or basic rights of others, such as truancy, running away, lying, and stealing (without confrontation).

Conduct disorders are estimated to be found in 9% of males and 2% of females under the age of 18,[32] and they are the major admission diagnosis of males to psychiatric clinics. Numerous theories have been put forth to explain the occurrence of conduct disorder, but no single theory explains the behavior. No one factor, but a combination of events predisposes children to conduct disorders.

A higher prevalence is found in males from a low socioeconomic status. Other factors, such as parental rejection, the presence of an alcoholic father, inconsistent and harsh discipline, and associations with delinquent subgroups have been found to be related to conduct disorders.[7]

Etiology and Diagnosis

Conduct disorders are distinguished by the presence or absence of social behaviors and aggressive behavior.

TABLE 18-2
Classifications of Conduct Disorders

Conduct Disorder	Undersocialized Aggressive	Undersocialized Nonaggressive	Socialized Aggressive	Socialized Nonaggressive
Essential features	Failure to establish warm satisfactory relationships with others, including peers	Failure to establish warm satisfactory relationships with others, including peers	Evidence of satisfactory relationships with others, including peers	Evidence of satisfactory relationships with others, including peers
	Repetitive and persistent pattern of antisocial behavior, which includes either physical violence against persons or property or thefts outside home involving confrontation with victim	Repetitive and persistent pattern of nonaggressive antisocial behavior in which societal norms or rules are broken and basic rights of others are violated	Repetitive and persistent pattern of antisocial behavior, which includes either physical violence against persons or property or thefts outside home involving confrontation with victim	Repetitive and persistent patterns of nonaggressive antisocial behavior in which societal norms or rules are broken and basic rights of others are violated
Associated features	Behavior difficulties at home and at school	Behavior difficulties at home and at school, such as running away and truancy	Behavior difficulties at home and at school	Behavior difficulties at home and at school, such as running away and truancy
	Early smoking, drinking, drug abuse, and sexual activity	Shy or withdrawn	Early smoking, drinking, drug abuse, and sexual activity	Poor school performance
	Poor school performance	Poor school performance	Poor school performance	Poor self-esteem
	Poor self-esteem	Poor self-esteem	Involvement with police	Irritability and low frustration tolerance
	Irritability and low frustration tolerance	Irritability and low frustration tolerance	Irritability and low frustration tolerance	
Minimal duration of symptoms	Six months	Six months	Six months	Six months

(Adapted from: American Psychiatric Association. [1987]. *Diagnostic and statistical manual of mental disorders* [Revised 3rd ed.]. Washington, DC: American Psychiatric Association, and Levine, M. D., Carey, W. B., Crocker, A. C., & Gross, R. T. [1983]. *Developmental-behavioral pediatrics* [p. 665]. Philadelphia: W. B. Saunders.)

Early experiences and bonding during the first 3 years of life play an important role in the development of conduct disorders. When an infant and toddler are not provided with an opportunity to form an attachment and bond, he or she is likely to develop a personality characterized by a lack of guilt and an inability to form a lasting relationship.[22,31] This failure of early bonding is associated with antisocial tendencies. Family discord and disharmony, which may precede a divorce or separation, is associated strongly with antisocial behavior in children.[22] The process by which the bonding and attachment issues and marital discord led to conduct disorders has been explored in multiple research studies. Marital discord has been associated with a lack of parental supervision, inconsistent discipline, and role modeling of aggressive behaviors.[15,31] Although no clear and definitive mechanisms are identified, the research does support the importance of these areas in the development of conduct disorders. Other parental behaviors associated with the development of conduct disorders include harsh and punitive discipline, rejecting or critical attitudes and behaviors, and poor supervision.[18]

A diagnosis of conduct disorder requires the physician to rule out the possibility of an emotional disorder such as anxiety, sadness, fear, worry, or misery.[18] An adjustment disorder is classified according to the impairment of social functioning or maladaptive behavioral reactions that have occurred within 3 months of a known psychosocial stressor. Therefore, the difference between a conduct disorder and an adjustment diagnosis is an identifiable environmental stimulus in adjustment disorder.[7]

A conduct disorder is diagnosed when a disturbance of conduct lasting at least 6 months has three of the following present:

- Stealing or forgery on more than one occasion
- Running away from home at least twice (or once without returning)
- Lying
- Fire-setting
- Truancy from school
- Breaking and entering
- Destroying other's property
- Physically cruel to animals
- Forcing someone to engage in sexual activity
- Using weapons

- Starts physical fights often
- Mugging, purse-snatching, extortion, and so forth
- Physically cruel to people[12]

Common Behaviors in Conduct Disorders

Noncompliance is defined as disobedience and opposition to authority figures.[21] All children at some point in time may display signs of noncompliance. The sporadic behavior may not be a sign of impending problems. When the behavior becomes frequent, severe, and persistent, the diagnosis of conduct disorder may be warranted. When parents identify their child as "difficult" or as having a difficult temperament at an early age, this may increase the risk for conduct disorders. A difficult temperament is characterized as being difficult to comfort, having irregular sleeping and eating patterns, high intensity with negative attitudes, and slow to adapt to new situations (see Chap. 8). What part labeling of children as difficult and then expecting difficulty plays in the development of conduct disorders has been identified by Levine and coworkers.[18] Children with conduct disorders display their behaviors in all environments (home, school, community). Physical aggression, as previously noted, is common, as is covert stealing, shoplifting, breaking and entering, and cheating even in children's games. These children and adolescents are often apprehended by the police and may have been disciplined by the court system. These children may be labeled as "delinquent."

The "run away" experience, common in many social–emotional disorders, is another behavior pattern associated with conduct disorders. However, not all "run away" children and adolescents have conduct disorders; motivation and extending circumstances need to be assessed before the diagnosis is applied.

Regular use of illicit drugs, alcohol, and tobacco, and early sexual behaviors are commonly found among children with conduct disorders. Of special note is that these behaviors begin in preadolescence.

Academic performance is usually poor, because these children suffer from impulsive behavior and a low frustration tolerance. Several factors should be considered with the child with conduct disorders and learning (Fig. 18-3). First, do learning problems develop as a result of antisocial behaviors, which interfere with the classroom dynamics or with the child missing classes because of

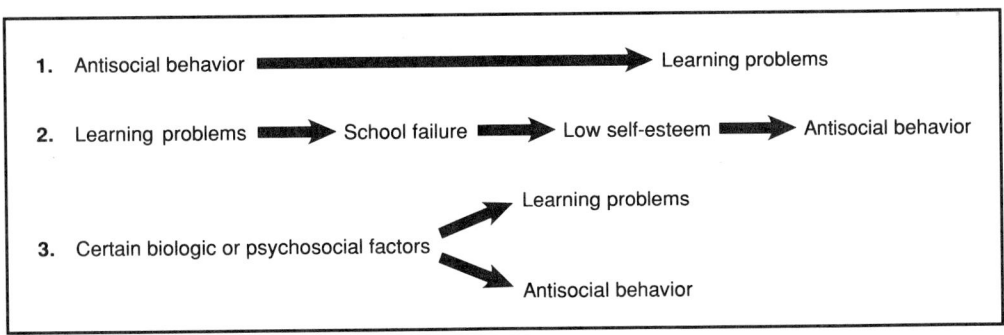

FIGURE 18-3
Hypothesized relationships between learning problems and antisocial behavior. (*From:* Levine, M. D., Carey, W. B., Crocker, A. C., and Gross, R. T. [1983]. *Developmental-Behavioral Pediatrics* [p. 673]. Philadelphia: W. B. Saunders.)

behavioral problems (i.e., being sent to the principal's office). Second, does the child have a learning disability that goes undetected, leading to low self-esteem and failure and ultimately leading to antisocial behavior? Or, third, do biologic and psychosocial dimensions of the child lead to both learning problems and antisocial behaviors independently? These are illustrated in Figure 18-3.

Truancy from school is a frequent occurrence because these children and adolescents engage in these destructive behaviors. The antisocial nature of the behaviors means that they experience no feeling of remorse for breaking the law or hurting others.

★ NURSING ASSESSMENT

The nursing assessment of a child with a conduct disorder is based on nursing interviews, behavioral questionnaires, and behavioral observations. Nursing interviews should focus on identifying high-risk families (see Chap. 5) who lack social support and financial resources, and who have many family crises. Assessment includes asking specifically about alcohol and drug abuse, financial problems, and marital instability. The interview should also include specific questions concerning the child's school history, peer relationships, and social interactions.[30]

If the interview identifies the family as high-risk, the nurse can examine the child's behaviors in more detail. Areas to be explored include:

- Types of behavior that lead to conflict
- Whether both parents see the behavior as a problem
- Frequency and severity of the problem behavior
- Circumstances that precede and follow the problem behaviors
- Approaches the parents have used in the past to deal with the behaviors[29]

Questionnaires or behavioral checklists may also be of help in assessing the presence of a conduct disorder. A sample outline for a behavioral interview is given in the accompanying display. Checklists such as the Eyberg Child Behavior Inventory, a 36-item survey, provide normative data on the behavior problems of 2- to 16-year-old children.[6] This helps determine whether the child is displaying a normal or abnormal amount of aggression. The questionnaires are filled out by parents, teachers, or day care providers. This helps to determine whether the behaviors are different in any given situation.[29] Parents may feel that their child is presenting signs of overaggression, which, in fact, may be normal behavior for a 2-year-old child, but abnormal behavior for a 7-year-old child.

The nurse may assess parent–child interactions as another source of data collection. The areas that should be observed include attention, communication, acceptance, nonacceptance, control, and submissiveness (Fig. 18-4). Hanf[11] suggests that parents and children be allowed to play a parent game followed by a child game. During the child's time, he or she selects the nature and rules of the play activities. After 5 minutes, the leader switches and the parent selects the activity. The nurse observes the parents for the amount of praise and enthusiasm or criticism of the play ideas, the parents commands, and frequency of commands. The nurse observes the child for deviant behaviors and observes the parent's responses to the child's behaviors. During the parent's game, the child is observed for noncompliant behaviors, and, again, parental response to the child's behavior is noted. The nursing assessment includes not only the behavior, but also the interaction between parents and child. Both are important to the development of nursing interventions.

The child's strengths should be identified as well.

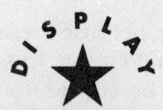

Nursing Assessment: A Structured Assessment Interview Guide for Conduct Disorders

SEVERITY OF EACH PROBLEM BEHAVIOR

- How often does it occur?
- How severe is it?
- How long does it last in each instance?

SITUATIONAL CONTEXT

- When does it occur?
- Where does it occur?
- Around whom does it occur?
- What was happening just before it occurred?

CONSEQUENCES OF PROBLEM BEHAVIOR

- Parental response
  Attention (sympathy, reassurance, scolding, hitting, criticism)

Discipline (type, frequency, effects, consistency with previous discipline, person who usually handles discipline)
- Inconsistencies in positive or negative consequences

DESIRABLE BEHAVIOR

- Behaviors to take place of undesirable behaviors
- Incompatible desirable behaviors

(Webster-Stratton, C. [1983]. Recognizing and assessing conduct disorders in children. American Journal of Maternal Child Nursing, 8, 332.)

Attention
Do parents and child play together, or do they work on their own activity independently and ignore the other's activity? Do parents and child attend to and watch each other?

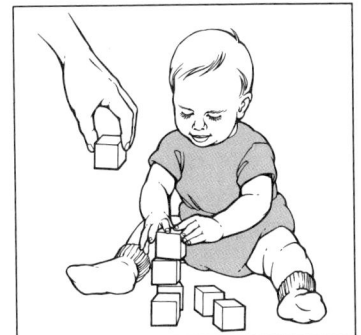
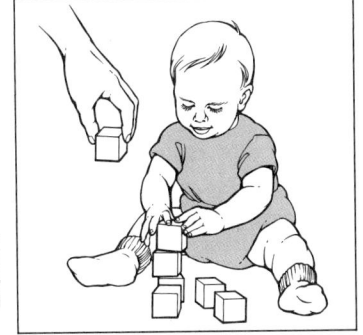

Nonacceptance
How much negative commenting, correcting, punishing, judging, explicit refusals, and criticism occur? Does the child or either parent seem not to accept himself?

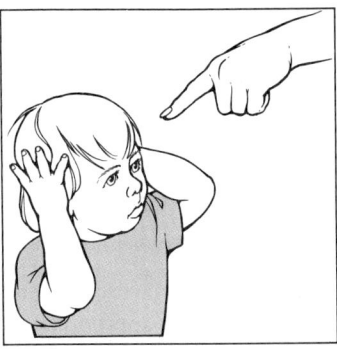

Communication
Do parents and child share in conversation together, or is there silence or one-sided talking? How clear and effective are the parents in communicating or setting rules?

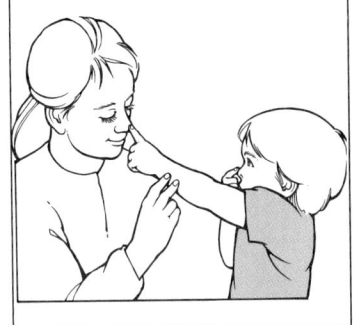

Control
How much ordering or competition for control is there? Who usually takes the lead, gives commands, or initiates suggestions for play?

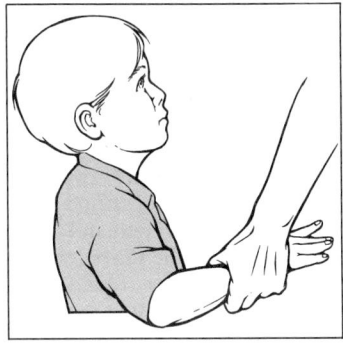

Acceptance
How much praise, warmth, affection, and positive acceptance is given by parents to child and child to parents?

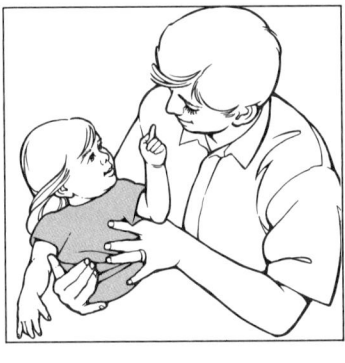

Submissiveness
Does the child or either parent constantly ask for approval from the other? Does the child or either parent accept and go along with rules set by the other?

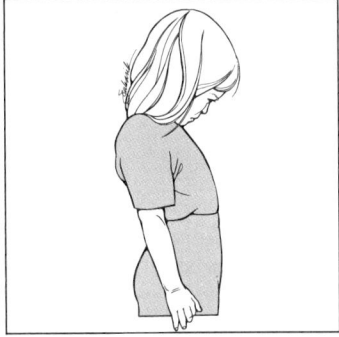

FIGURE 18-4
Parent–child observational assessment. All items are checked for both parent and child. (*From:* Webster-Stratton, C. [1983]. Recognizing and assessing conduct disorders in children. *American Journal of Maternal Child Nursing, 8,* 334.)

This helps the child and parents to identify areas of achievement and success that can be promoted.

★ **NURSING DIAGNOSES AND PLANNING**

After the data have been gathered from the various sources, nurses formulate nursing diagnoses. Nursing diagnoses associated with a conduct disorder may include the following:

- High Risk for Violence: Self-Directed or Directed at Others related to retarded ego development, poor impulse control.
- Altered Family Processes evidenced by aggressive body language, overt and aggressive acts, self-destructive behavior, hostile and threatening verbalizations, rage, possession of destructive means, and increased motor activity.
- Chronic Low Self-Esteem related to poor academic and social achievement.
- Impaired Social Interaction as evidenced by cheating, lying, stealing, and so forth.

Possible outcome criteria include the following.

- Parents express need for help in rearing child.
- Parents describe reward and punishment methods they will use.
- Parents describe a decrease in the number of negative behaviors.

★ **INTERVENTIONS: COLLABORATIVE AND INDEPENDENT**

The most effective treatment of conduct disorders among children has been the training of parents in effective child rearing practices. As such, the parents become a part of the treatment team. When the parents become involved in learning a new way to interact with the child, they begin to feel more hopeful and competent as parents. Thus, the child–parent relationship improves and the negative cycle of punishment can be broken.[29] Examples of disciplinary methods are given in the accompanying display.

The skills needed by parents center around play

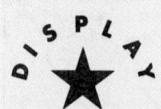

Parent Teaching: Disciplinary Methods for Children With Conduct Disorders

RULES AND LIMIT SETTING

- Identify what household rules are most important.
- Give clear, specific demands for the desired behavior.
- Make age-appropriate demands.
- Reduce the number of commands to those that are most important.

BASIC COMPONENTS OF IGNORING

- Look away from the child; no eye contact or non-verbal cues.
- Move away from the child; no physical contact.
- Neutral facial expression.
- Ignore all of child's verbalization, no verbal contact.
- Ignore immediately when misbehavior starts.
- Ignore the misbehavior *every time* it occurs.

USING TIME OUT

- Remain calm, firm, and consistent.
- Make sure rules and consequences and rationales have been stated before misbehavior occurs.

- When child noncomplies, restate rule and consequence.
- Ignore subsequent verbalizations and excuses. Do not nag, debate, or argue with child.
- Follow through with time out quickly. Do not push, shove, or drag child to time out. Do not provide a rationale while taking child to time out or while child is in time out.
- Do not scold child after time out is over. Watch for appropriate behavior to praise. Repeat original command with which child did not comply.
- Use time out for only one or two deviant behaviors to begin with until that behavior is under control and then try on other behavior.

(Data from: *Webster-Stratton, C. [1983]. Intervention approaches to conduct disorders in young children. Nurse Practitioner, 13[2], 23–24, 29, 33–34.*)

techniques, reward and reinforcing methods, and punishment techniques. These skills are taught in a particular order, which should be carefully followed for good results. Effective play and reward techniques are taught before punishment methods. This increases the chance of positive behavior from the child and less need for the use of punishment.

Parents are encouraged to play with their children and taught how to follow the child's lead. Independence is encouraged by teaching the parents to let the child work out their own ideas without interference or criticism. Such play activity increases the chance of a positive interaction and decreases the chance of a negative reaction of child and parent.[29]

Rewarding the child is also important. Parents are taught to label the behavior and be specific with praise. They are also instructed to praise the child immediately after the desired behavior and to do it every time it occurs. Praising the child in front of other people also increases the child's feeling of self-worth.

The nurse helps the parents understand the differences among normal behavior, mischief, and conduct disorder. What is acceptable as normal curiosity or development at one age is not acceptable as the child grows older.

Punishment methods are designed to decrease the aggressive behaviors of the child. In families with children who have conduct disorders, usually the problems surrounding punishment are extreme. Either the parents are extremely harsh or extremely lax. Families may also combine the two extremes where one parent is strict and

the other is lax. Effective disciplinary methods focus on two main components: limit setting and compliance training.[30]

★ **EVALUATION**

Children with conduct disorders are difficult to treat. Therefore, evaluation of the effectiveness of the treatment plan is based on sometimes small improvements in the child's behavior. The ability of the parents to feel in control of the situation is one of the greatest goals of treatment. Parents should be given as much praise by the health care worker for each situation they are able to handle successfully. As the parents begin to feel in control of the situation, the tension within the family setting should decrease. Often, progress is not of a smooth and steady kind, but more of a three steps forward and two steps back variety. It is important to continue to encourage the parents in their struggle to gain control of their situation.

Elimination Disorders

Enuresis

Enuresis is defined as involuntary urination that occurs beyond the expected age for bladder control. Most authorities agree that by 5 years of age, a child should have accomplished diurnal and nocturnal bladder control.

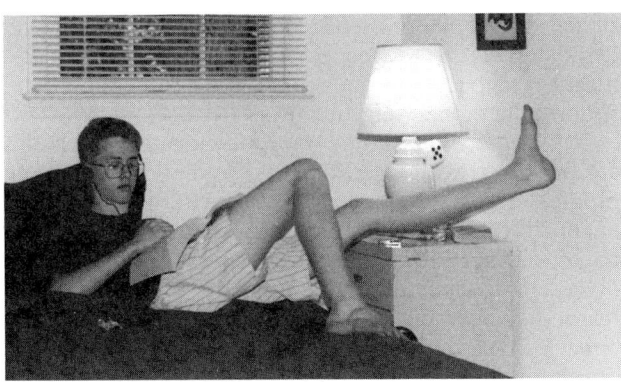

FIGURE 18-5
Distinguishing between normal behaviors and conduct behaviors requires patience and careful assessment on the part of the nurse and parents. For example, adolescents normally like time alone, and this is not necessarily a sign of antisocial behavior.

Primary enuresis is a condition in which a child has never had a prolonged period of being dry. *Secondary enuresis* describes recurring wetness in a child who has been dry for at least 6 months. Although both are distressing disorders, this is a self-limiting disorder. The reader is referred to Chapter 48 for a discussion on the physiologic development of continence and to Chapters 49 and 50 for the physiologic disorders that are associated with enuresis and that must be ruled out or diagnosed and treated before other etiologies of enuresis are assumed.

The incidence of enuresis is higher among those of lower socioeconomic status, with greater frequency in boys and predominantly in black children. The majority of cases are primary and nocturnal. Often referred to as "bedwetting," enuresis appears to be a hereditary condition. Environmental factors also have significance when exploring the etiology of poor bladder control. A lack of cleanliness, difficult toilet training, inaccessible toileting facilities, and cold weather appear to increase the prevalence of enuresis in children.

The familial tendency linked to enuresis suggests a physiologic factor, which involves maturational delay of neurologic mechanisms linked to bladder control. Whether this maturational delay is triggered genetically or by the environment, the development of bladder control is retarded.[5]

In the past, the diagnoses of sleepwalking, nightmares, and enuresis were thought to be related. However, recent studies have brought into question the relationship between enuresis and sleepwalking and nightmares.[18]

Diagnostic Studies. Urine cultures are important to rule out infective processes, which may trigger enuresis. Metabolic disorders, neurologic tests, and renal scans and other radiologic exams may also be required. A bladder capacity test involves asking the older child to withhold from urinating until discomfort and urgency reach peak discomfort. At that time, the child is asked to void into a graduated receptacle to determine bladder capacity. (Expected volume is 300 to 350 ml of urine.)

★ NURSING ASSESSMENT

Due to the many factors involved in enuresis, nursing assessment should involve a comprehensive history, physical assessment, and careful evaluation of potential organic causes.

A careful history from parents is essential in determining primary versus secondary enuresis. In addition, it is important to ascertain if loss of bladder control occurs diurnally or nocturnally. Parents should be asked to examine carefully if there is a pattern to enuresis. Does it occur around stressful events or are there emotional factors involved in the wetting occurrence? Any previous disorders, such as urinary tract infections, epilepsy, and diabetes, should be documented.

Careful physical assessment of bladder discomfort, flank pain, or burning on urination should be assessed. The color and amount of urine with each void, as well as fluid intake for each day, are essential to evaluate.

★ NURSING DIAGNOSES AND PLANNING

Nursing diagnoses associated with enuresis may include the following:

* Altered Urinary Elimination related to lack of bladder control.
* Sleep Pattern Disturbance related to bedwetting during the night.
* Impaired Skin Integrity related to urinary incontinence.
* Impaired Social Interaction related to inadequate bladder control.
* Self-Care Toileting Deficit related to inability to control urination patterns.

Enuresis is a family problem. Therefore, any intervention involves family response and adaptation. Children need to be given the sense of control over their incontinence problem, and families need to understand the feelings of shame and guilt that may occur. This may require family therapy, because many times parents feel responsible for the child's symptoms, and the child may suffer a poor self-concept.

★ INTERVENTIONS: COLLABORATIVE
  AND INDEPENDENT

Various methods are used to assist the child with enuresis. Usually more than one method is prescribed. The traditional methods of withholding fluids, awakening the child to void, or punitive measures have not been found to be effective treatments.

One method of treatment uses an electrical device to condition the child to awaken when the urge to void occurs. An electrically wired pad attached to a buzzer, which alarms when urine hits a sensor, awakens the child. In this situation, the child is conditioned to get out of bed to use the toilet and void. This plan requires that the child cooperates with the placement and setting of the device.

Medication may be used. In the past, the tricyclic antidepressants, which inhibit urination by an anticholinergic action, have been prescribed. New studies support the idea that children with enuresis may have lower secretion levels of antidiuretic hormone at night, leading to a higher urine output (see Chap. 50). One promising treatment is the use of desmopressin. Desmopressin, an analogue of the antidiuretic hormone vasopressin, has been found to be extremely effective in the treatment of enuresis.

★ EVALUATION

Validation that families understand the plan of treatment and are capable of home-care is essential. Support and encouragement are necessary throughout all phases of treatment to instill the independence and confidence that many of these children lack.

Functional Encopresis

Functional encopresis has been defined as the repeated voluntary or involuntary passage of feces of normal or near-normal consistency in inappropriate places. Encopresis occurs over the age of 4 years with a frequency of at least once a month, and it is not related to a physical disorder. Encopresis is differentiated into two types: *primary,* in which bowel control has never been achieved; and *secondary,* in which control has been achieved for a period of months.

It has been estimated that 1% of 5-year-old children have this disorder, and the tendency decreases slowly as a function of age. Encopresis is more common in boys, particularly in low socioeconomic classes. Encopresis appears to be associated with functional enuresis in about 25% of the cases.

There is no single, agreed-upon explanation of the etiology of this elimination disorder. Each theory has its own set of implications for nursing assessment and management. The nurse must understand that, for a given encopretic child, the etiology could be one or a combination of several of these theories.

The DSM-III-R definition of encopresis includes retention with overflow or constipation-type encopresis,[1a] whereas pediatric texts exclude these from their definitions. When encopresis is voluntary, it is usually associated with other psychological problems.[5] When it is involuntary, it can be either retentive or nonretentive.

In *retentive encopresis,* the child has constant leaking of fecal-stained fluid from the rectum. The child's rectum and sometimes the colon become distended by hard stools. This distention weakens and ultimately may impair the anal reflex. Abdominal pain of a chronic, intermittent, or severe nature is a frequent complaint. Nausea, vomiting, and stomach problems are often reported, too. Controversial explanations for the etiology of such retention have been presented by health professionals. Pediatricians commonly favor physical factors, such as constipation developing in late infancy causing pain on defecation. Abnormal defecation dynamics have been implicated as possible etiologic factors.

A genetic predisposition has also been proposed, which suggests an abnormal or increased water absorption from the stool in transit through the colon. Psychiatrists, on the other hand, argue that retention is caused by a "distortion of the normal anal-retentive phase of psycho-

sexual development or disturbance of parent–child relationships."[21a (p.265)] Encopresis is thus interpreted as a means of defying parental control or as regression in response to a threatening situation.

In *nonretentive encopresis,* fully formed, soft stools are produced without evidence of retention. Three etiologic theories have been suggested. In the first theory, encopresis is believed to be associated with anxiety about coercive toilet training. In the second, it is a simple case of lack of proper toilet training; the child has never learned or been taught the socially acceptable toileting behavior. The third possibility is urgency, which may be physiologically based. Although there is no consensus about the frequency of retentive versus nonretentive types of encopresis, it is possible that stool retention is a factor in the majority of cases. In fact, some studies show retention exists in 80% to 100% of encopretic children.[21a]

The nature of the relationship between behavior problems and encopresis is subject to debate. Some studies have reported that physiologic abnormalities of the bowel are consistently associated with encopresis. They have found a high incidence of social and behavioral problems in their study population (among girls with abnormal defecation dynamics in particular). However, they have also found that, whereas treatment failure was related to the inability to defecate and to relax the external sphincter during defecation attempts, failure was not related to behavioral or social competence scores on the Child Behavioral Checklist.[6] Other studies have yielded opposite findings about the psychopathology of encopretic children linking persistent encopresis with aggressive behavior and social withdrawal, as well as with a tendency toward a lack of self-assertion, a low tolerance for demands, and difficulty in handling aggression.[21a] Such psychopathologic features may be either primary or secondary to the encopresis. This elimination disorder can be distressing socially, triggering further emotional and behavioral disturbances.

Diagnostic Studies. Other explanations for the child's soiling are excluded before a diagnosis is made. Techniques used include direct examination of the gastrointestinal tract with endoscopy (upper tract), sigmoidoscopy (lower colon, anus, and rectum), or proctoscopy (anus and rectum). Stool analysis helps rule out ova and parasites.

★ NURSING ASSESSMENT

Because of the various theoretical perspectives, the nursing assessment should be multidimensional. In addition to the suggested general guidelines, the following approach is recommended:

A history should include information on diet, toilet training, and elimination patterns. Organic causes are ruled out by identifying any nutritional deficiencies or food intolerance. Limited fluids, lack of vegetables and fruits, excessive consumption of junk foods, and irregular mealtimes can contribute to constipation. Toilet training methods are assessed, especially in relation to the child's age and the parents' approach. Was the child too young? Was a coercive or traumatic training technique used? Was the parental approach inconsistent?

Have the parents describe the frequency, volume, consistency, and color of stools. The nurse must clarify what these terms mean to the parents. The nurse must determine whether there is any history of constipation, diarrhea, or fecal soiling, how parents and child have responded to the encopresis, whether there has been any attempt by the child to conceal fecal soiling (i.e., hiding soiled clothes or bedding), or whether the child defecates in the tub, in closets, or behind doors.

Initial assessment of the anal reflex (gentle pricking/scratching the anal sphincter) is essential, and not a routine assessment procedure once the reflex has been elicited. The presence of bowel sounds or of any fecal material distending the colon (abdominal distention) or accumulated around or in the anus needs to be assessed. Careful description of the abdominal assessment should include qualifiers such as soft, firm, or rigid on palpation. Presence or absence of abdominal pain is also important to document.

★ NURSING DIAGNOSES AND PLANNING

Nursing diagnoses associated with encopresis may include the following:

- Bowel Incontinence related to voluntary or involuntary passage of feces.
- Impaired Social Interaction related to incontinent bowel elimination.
- Self-Esteem Disturbance related to inability to control elimination patterns.
- Ineffective Individual Coping related to poor elimination control.
- Ineffective Family Coping: Comprised related to altered ability to manage the child with elimination problems.
- Self-Care Deficit: Toileting related to poor elimination patterns.

The following are examples of expected outcomes:

- Child demonstrates squeezing and relaxing of anal sphincter.
- Parents describe schedule for having child sit on the toilet.

★ INTERVENTIONS: COLLABORATIVE AND INDEPENDENT

Management of most encopretic children should consist of counseling and education about the problem, medications and diet, retraining, monitoring, and follow-up. If retentive encopresis with fecal impaction is the problem, catharsis is the first approach; enemas, laxatives, and stool softeners are used until the bowels are clear. Depending on the pediatrician and the family, this can be done either at home or in the hospital. An example of a cleanout program and maintenance treatment are outlined in Table 18-3. The child's fluid and electrolyte balance during this treatment must be monitored.

Once the bowels are cleared, bowel retraining can be initiated to establish a regular pattern of elimination. Oral laxatives and mineral oil are given daily. Because in many cases the inability to relax or squeeze the external sphincter appropriately seems to be the result of an unconscious volitional act, these children are taught external

TABLE 18-3
Typical Programs Used to Treat Functional Encopresis

Treatment	Comment
A Typical "Cleanout" Program	
Day 1—hypophosphate (Fleet) enema bid	May be given once a day in mild-to-moderate stool retention
Day 2—bisacodyl (Dulcolax) suppository bid	May be given once a day in mild-to-moderate stool retention
Day 3—bisacodyl (Dulcolax) tablet qid	Usually best given in the afternoon after school—never before school or before bedtime
Repeat cycle four times.	
Maintenance Treatment	
Light mineral oil (2 tablespoons bid)	Only average dose may be reduced if leakage into underwear
	Slowly titrate to bowel habits
	Vitamins to compensate for poor absorption (A, D, E, & K vitamins most important)
Senacot (1 tablet or 1 tsp) qid	May need bid initially
	Titrate to bowel habits. Dulcolax bisacodyl may be needed for severe cases.
Child sits on toilet for 10 min (5 min for children under 8) after every meal.	Timer may prove useful
	May read, listen to radio, and so forth.
Increased roughage in diet	Bran, vegetables, popcorn, raisins helpful
Maintenance of frequent telephone contact	Scheduled calls very helpful for these problems
Follow-up every 1–2 months as needed	

(Landman, G. B. [1990]. Disorders of elimination: Encopresis and enuresis. In: F. A. Oski, [Ed.], *Principles and practice of pediatrics* [pp. 693–694]. Philadelphia: J.B. Lippincott.)

relaxation and squeeze. (Children are more likely to recover if they are able to relax the external sphincter during defecation attempts.)

Parents must remind the child to use the toilet regularly after meals. Regular bowel habits and use of the toilet as soon as an urge to defecate is felt are essential. Some pediatricians expect the child to sit on the toilet at regular times during the day (i.e., for 10 minutes after meals). An adequate foot support is needed so that the child can strain, squeeze, and push.

A high-residue diet with lots of fluids is encouraged. The family (including the siblings) needs to be involved in that diet and to encourage the child. Exercise is also suggested.

Behavioral techniques are used concurrently with the regimen above. These aim at eliminating anxiety associated with toileting, as well as praising and rewarding the child. No punishment is used. Family therapy is often needed to alter existing family dynamics.

★ EVALUATION

The program is evaluated every 6 weeks. Cathartics are gradually discontinued. With child and family compliance, a regular elimination pattern can usually be established within 6 months. After that, follow-up should continue at lengthier intervals.

Sleep Disorders

An estimated 10% to 20% of children have some sleep disorder. Most occur during the early childhood years and decrease as the child gets older. The cause of such disorders is not known but is thought to be related to the immaturity of the central nervous system (CNS) in children.

During infancy, sleep disorders related to organic problems are predominantly found in babies with colic. A baby with colic experiences inconsolable crying. Parents, particularly mothers, often feel responsible for the baby's crying and upset over their inability to comfort the newborn. Colic has been associated with the mother's diet (when breast-feeding), overstimulation, and other factors. A discussion of colic is found in Chapter 12.

Infants over the age of 4 months can suffer from night crying whenever their bedtime routine is disrupted. If infants are rocked to sleep or suck a bottle or breast until asleep, they may have difficulty falling back to sleep during the night if they awaken. If infants routinely fall asleep in a place other than their crib, then when brought to their usual sleeping place and awaken, they cry until their nighttime ritual is resumed (riding in a car, infant swings). Some of the nighttime rituals begin as the parents' way to cope with a baby with colic or baby who has difficulty falling to sleep on his or her own. The pattern that is developed is difficult to change and requires time and effort on the part of both parents and caregivers (sitters, day care personnel).

As children approach toddlerhood, it is common for them to experience night crying once put to bed. However, ritualistic behaviors (e.g., taking a stuffed animal to bed with them) usually manage this type of problem. Parents need to be careful what rituals they initiate and whether these rituals are something they want to continue. If a child awakens and cries at night and the parent reads a story to the child at 2 AM, a pattern may develop. A story at 8 PM may be reasonable, but in the middle of the night other comfort measures should be recommended. More information on sleep patterns and parental strategies may be found in Chapter 13.

During the preschool years, children are prone to *night terrors*. This does not necessarily point to serious pathology but is associated with prolonged non-REM (rapid eye movement) sleep during age 3 to 4. These children may improve with the use of nightlights or a ritual that involves helping the child "wind down" (e.g., a bedtime story). Although 12 hours of sleep is the expected average for preschoolers, there is evidence that children with sleep disturbances sleep less. Night terrors are also found in other age groups, particularly after traumatic/stressful events (e.g., surgery).

Somnambulism (sleep-walking) occurs more frequently in boys and predominantly during the years of 5 to 12. Safety is the issue of concern for these children because somnambulism is a self-limiting disorder.

In a study by Fisher and Wilson,[8] sleep-walking and nightmares were found to be strongly associated with one another. They also found an association with a family history of sleep-walking. Contrary to what other studies report, Fisher and Wilson found no relationship between socioeconomic levels or sex and sleep disturbances. The treatment of sleep-walking is limited to the prevention of self-injury. Parents should be instructed to lock doors and windows and remove dangerous objects.[25]

Adolescent insomnia has received more attention because 10% to 20% of adolescents complain of disturbed nocturnal sleep and complain of "feeling tired" most of the time.[27] There is suggestion that adolescent insomnia may be associated with depression. A constant period of 2 to 5 hours of sleep with decreased amounts of non-REM sleep is common. In addition, there is a shorter interval from falling asleep to the first REM period. Premature awakening occurs, as does daytime napping.

A second type of adolescent insomnia involves delayed sleep, sleep onset insomnia, with adequate sleep maintenance once begun. This area of insomnia is emerging as an interesting phenomenon during adolescence and may indeed refer to biorhythmic disruption.

★ **NURSING ASSESSMENT**

A careful history is essential in ascertaining the type of sleep disturbance that is occurring. Most parents are able to explain activities before bedtime, eating patterns at night, bedtime rituals, characteristics of the sleep disturbance, and duration of symptoms as well as of onset. Descriptions of involuntary movements, verbalizations, and methods used to reduce each occurrence are critical in formulating management plans. An assessment of the child's life stresses and traumas is also crucial.

★ **NURSING DIAGNOSES AND PLANNING**

Nursing diagnoses associated with sleep disorders may include the following:

- High-Risk for Injury related to involuntary movements during sleep.
- Fear related to disorientation upon awaking from a nightmare or sleep-walking.
- Sleep Pattern Disturbance related to interrupted night rest periods and loss of sleep.
- Ineffective Family Coping related to overconcern and overprotectiveness of child with a sleeping disorder.
- Anxiety related to misunderstanding of sleep disorders and child's lack of control over episodes.

Regardless of the age of the child or related stress, management is similar. The child may need extra support or special consideration for bedtime preparation. Expected outcomes may include the following:

- Parents express relief that condition is self-limiting.
- Parents describe methods for providing safety for the child who sleep-walks.

★ **INTERVENTIONS: COLLABORATIVE AND INDEPENDENT**

Management of children with sleep disorders involves parent teaching with regard to the nature of the sleep disturbance, growth and developmental expectations, and prevention of injury. Reassurance that most disturbances are self-limiting is helpful to anxious parents or those concerned about long-term effects.

Behavioral techniques such as instituting rituals at bedtime (storytelling, transitional objects) that calm the child and promote relaxation are helpful. Avoiding excessive fatigue by encouraging naps and helping the child to prepare for bedtime often assist families through these transient problems.

Although medications such as diazepam and imipramine are effective in controlling some sleep disturbances, they are restricted to use only when the child's waking behavior is seriously compromised. Some authorities advocate the use of dietary management, which includes a high-protein intake and the age-old "warm milk" before retiring (the amino acid L-tryptophan has been associated with effective sleeping).[25]

★ EVALUATION

Because this is considered a self-limiting disorder, periodic evaluation is helpful. Effective safety precautions (placing a safety gate at the top or bottom of stairs, locking windows, removing obstacles in potential pathway) need to be reassessed and evaluated as episodes occur. If behavioral management is ineffective, alternative plans should be considered and medication may be necessary. Careful follow-up with drug levels would be essential for those children managed on medications.

Physical Symptoms of Stress Response

Somatic complaints that occur in childhood need to be evaluated in a comprehensive manner to rule out organic causes. Recurrent abdominal pain, headaches, and hyperventilation are disorders that frequently have psychogenic etiology, but require careful assessment.

Abdominal pain has many organic causes (see Chaps. 58 and 59), but *recurrent abdominal pain* is triggered during stressful times. These stresses can include typical childhood events (fighting with a friend, teasing, and so forth) or can be a traumatic event (death of a loved one). Most of these children have experienced abdominal pain at least three times during a 3-month period. Characteristically, these children suppress their anger and are uncomfortable with authoritative figures who express anger or argue. Some children who suffer from school phobia may demonstrate recurrent abdominal pain, because school can aggravate their symptoms.

Headaches or *migraines* can also have an emotional component to their etiologies. Typically, children do not experience headaches, and when this symptom appears it warrants immediate evaluation. Classically, migraines are heralded by visual disturbances, and it is not uncommon to experience nausea and vomiting during the course of the severe headache.

A family history of migraines is found in over half of the patients who have this documented disorder. Boys have a higher incidence than females, and these symptoms can occur as early as 5 years of age. Typically, migraines occur early in the day and are terminated by sleep. The personality style of most children with migraines includes compulsiveness and a strong desire to please parents. Additionally, they do not easily vent anger, rather "holding" their discontent to themselves.

Hyperventilation is another example of a physical symptom usually associated with emotional states. Usually it manifests as shortness of breath, inability to inspire deeply, and "tightness" in the chest. Additionally, numbness or tingling in the fingers and toes, rapid heart rate, and abdominal pain may result from the primary symptom of hyperventilation, which creates respiratory alkalosis. Children are usually unaware of "overbreathing" and respond well to rebreathing techniques. These children often have a history of chronic fatigue and weakness. Underlying anxieties are highly correlated with this symptom, with resultant treatment aimed at determining the influential anxiety source.

★ NURSING ASSESSMENT

A careful assessment as to the frequency, symptoms, duration, and corresponding stressors is essential in determining the etiology and subsequent treatment of somatic complaints. A family history of similar symptoms and the nature of the child's relationships with peers, parents, and siblings assists in identifying factors that may contribute to their symptoms. Because many symptoms involve suppressed angers, questions pertaining to family interactions and any evidence of depression should be validated.

A complete physical assessment is essential in somatic complaints. A complete review of systems with emphasis on the primary affected system is required (see chapters on altered function).

★ NURSING DIAGNOSES AND PLANNING

Nursing diagnoses associated with somatic complaints related to life stressors may include the following:

- Pain related to recurrent abdominal pain or headaches.
- Sensory-Perceptual Alteration: Visual related to symptoms of migraines.
- Anxiety related to repeated episodes of symptoms that compromise daily activities.
- Powerlessness related to lack of control over emotional responses.
- Ineffective Family Coping related to dealing with a child who has somatic complaints.

The major emphasis of planning and nursing intervention should be directed toward further assessment of the underlying causes that precipitate these events. Expected outcomes may include the following:

- Child practices relaxation techniques.
- Child discusses possible sources of stress.

★ INTERVENTIONS: COLLABORATIVE AND INDEPENDENT

Management of stress-related disorders can be difficult. Hospitalization may be required to establish pain man-

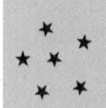

Ideas for Nursing Research

The dynamics of emotional and behavioral problems in children and adolescents are complex and difficult to change. Nurses are in a unique position to identify children and adolescents at risk in school settings, physician offices, and homes. The following areas need to be explored:

- Assessment strategies that are most useful in identifying children at risk for school phobia.
- The most successful interventions or combinations (therapeutic play, behavioral modification, stress management skills, or environmental restructuring) for school phobia in young children.
- Many intervention programs for emotional and behavioral problems suggest that parents learn new disciplinary skills. Disciplinary techniques most appropriate for each age group, and method for teaching parents.

agement, rule out organic etiologies, and identify aggravating factors that precipitate symptoms.

The child with recurrent abdominal pain is often treated medically as a "spastic colon," and may be given antispasmodic medications. Usually, dietary restrictions apply to "irritable" bowel symptoms (see Chap. 59).

Headaches or migraines can be treated with medication as well. The usual over-the-counter medicines are available (aspirin is no longer prescribed for children without careful medical monitoring), but a vasoconstrictor (ergotamine tartrate) may be necessary for severe migraines.

Hyperventilation usually responds to rebreathing maneuvers (breathing into a paper bag). However, if the child is prone to bronchospasm, further treatment with medications that relax the bronchial may be necessary. Psychotherapy, family therapy, or stress reduction techniques can be helpful to families who have a child with stress-related complaints. Consultation and referral to a social worker, psychiatrist, and psychiatric liaison nurse provide the best comprehensive approach to these children.

★ EVALUATION

Often the offending stressors cannot be removed; therefore, follow-up care is important. Alternative responses to stress can be learned. Support and encouragement are essential for these families, with community resources a vital component for successful management.

Summary

Stressors and stress responses in the childhood context take into consideration the biologic, psychological, and social maturation that result from growth and life expe-

riences. This life content approach allows the nurse to understand the relationship of a child's specific problem to broader issues. For instance, when an adolescent describes a given situation (e.g., "insomnia"), the nurse must understand its relationship to developmental issues such as peer group acceptance. The life context approach also promotes an overall vision of the continuity of the child's life. Previous growth and development patterns and accompanying exposure to various kinds and degrees of life stress, as well as the child's future potential and reaction to stress, are essential components of the nursing process. Nurses have a unique opportunity to design and evaluate effective strategies for children with emotional and behavioral problems.

References

1. Casat, C. D., Ross, B. A., Scardina, R., Sarno, C., & Smith, K. E. (1987). Separation anxiety and mitral valve prolapse in a 12-year-old girl. *Journal of the American Academy of Child and Adolescent Psychiatry, 26*(3), 444–446.

1a. American Psychiatric Association. (1987). *Diagnostic and statistical manual of mental disorders* (Revised 3rd ed.). Washington, DC: American Psychiatric Association.

2. Castaneda, A., McCandless, B. R., & Palermo, D. S. (1956). The children's form of the Manifest Anxiety Scale. *Child Development, 27*(3), 317–326.

3. Chisholm, M. (1988). Anxiety. In C. M. Beck, R. P. Rawlings, & S. R. Williams (Eds.), *Mental health-psychiatric nursing. A holistic life-cycle approach* (2nd ed., pp. 203–227). St. Louis: Mosby.

4. Deltito, J. A., Perugi, G., Maremmani, I., et al. (1986). The importance of separation anxiety in the differentiation of panic disorder from agoraphobia. *Psychiatric Developments, 3,* 227–236.

5. Erickson, M. T. (1987). *Behavior disorders of children and adolescents* (pp. 1–10, 261–307). Englewood Cliffs, NJ: Prentice-Hall.

6. Eyberg, S. M. (1980). Eyberg Child Behavior Inventory. *Journal of Clinical Child Psychology, 9*(1), 29.

7. Faulstich, M., Moore, J. R., Carey, M., Ruggiero, L., & Gresham, F. (1986). Prevalence of DSM-III conduct and disorders for adolescent psychiatric inpatients. *Adolescence, 21*(82), 333–337.

8. Fisher, B., & Wilson, A. (1987). Selected sleep disturbances in school children reported by parents: Prevalence, interrelationship, behavioral correlates and parental attributions. *Perceptual and Motor Skills, 64*(3), 1147–1157.

9. Frain, M., & Valiga, T. M. (1982). The multiple dimensions of stress. In: D. C. Sutterley & G. F. Donnelly (Eds.), *Coping with stress—A nursing perspective* (pp. 59–68). Rockville, MD: Aspen Systems.

9a. Gordon, M. (1987). *Nursing diagnosis: Process and application* (2nd ed.). New York: McGraw-Hill.

10. Gunnar, M. R. (1987). Psychobiological studies of stress and coping: An introduction. *Child Development, 58,* 1403–1407.

11. Hanf, C. (1970). *Shaping mothers to shape their children's behaviors.* Unpublished manuscript, University of Oregon Medical School, Eugene, OR.

12. Harnett, N. (1989). Conduct disorder in childhood and adolescence: An update. *Journal of Child and Adolescent Psychiatric Mental Health Nursing, 2*(2), 74–76.

13. Harris, J. S., & Hastings, J. E. (1987). Coping with stress. In: D. P. Sheridan & J. R. Winogrord (Eds.), *The preventive approach to patient care* (pp. 357–374). New York: Elsevier.

14. Herbert, M. (1981). *Behavioral treatment of problem children—A practice manual* (p. 93). London: Academic Press.

15. Johnson, P. L., & O'Leary, K. D. (1987). Parental behavior patterns and conduct disorders in girls. *Journal of Abnormal Child Psychology, 15*(4), 573–581.

16. Last, C. G., Hersen, M., Kazdin, A. E., Francis, G., & Grubb, H. G. (1987). Comparison of DSM-III separation anxiety and overanxious disorders: Demographic characteristics and patterns of comorbidity. *Journal of the American Academy of Child and Adolescent Psychiatry 26*(4), 527–531.

17. Leung, A. K. (1989). School phobias. Sometimes a child or teenager has a good reason. *Postgraduate Medicine, 85*(1), 281–282, 287–289.

18. Levine, M. D., Carey, W. B., Crocker, A. C., & Gross, R. T. (1992). *Developmental-behavioral pediatrics.* (2nd ed.). Philadelphia: W. B. Saunders.

18a. Massten, A. S., Garmezy, N., Tellegen, A., et al. Competence and stress in school children: moderating effects of individual and family qualities. *Journal of Child Psychology and Psychiatry and Allied Principles, 29(6),* 747–764.

19. Melamed, B. G., & Siegel, L. J. (1975). Reduction of anxiety in children facing hospitalization and surgery by use of filmed modeling. *Journal of Consulting and Clinical Psychology, 43*(4), 511–521.

20. NANDA—North American Nursing Diagnosis Association. (1990). *Taxonomy I revised—1990: With official nursing diagnoses.* St. Louis: North American Nursing Diagnoses Association.

21. Patterson, G. R. (1980). *Coercive family processes.* Eugene, OR: Castalia.

21a. Quay, H. C., & Werry, J. S. (Eds.). *Psychopathological disorders of childhood* (3rd ed.). New York: John Wiley & Sons.

22. Rutter, M. (1979). Maternal deprivation, 1972–1978, new findings, new concepts, new approaches. *Child Development, 50*(2), 283–305.

23. Scherer, N. W., & Nakamura, C. Y. (1968). A fear survey schedule for children (FSS-SC): A factor analytic comparison with manifest anxiety (CMAS). *Behaviour Research and Therapy, 6,* 173–182.

24. Selye, H. (1976). *The stress of life.* New York: McGraw-Hill.

25. Siegel, F. (1982). Eating and sleeping difficulties in young children. *Consultant, 2,* 95–107.

26. Stiffman, A. R., Jung, K. E., & Feldman, R. A. (1986). A multivariate risk model for childhood behaviour problems. *American Journal of Orthopsychiatry 56*(2), 204–211.

27. Strauch, L., Dubral, I., & Struchholtz, C. (1973). Sleep behavior in adolescents in relation to personality variables. In Javanovic, V. J. (Ed.). *The nature of sleep* (pp. 121–123). Stüttgart, Germany: Fisher-Verlag.

28. Strauss, C. C., Lahey, B. B., Frick, P., et al. (1988). Peer social status of children with anxiety disorders. *Journal of Consulting and Clinical Psychology, 56*(1), 137–141.

29. Webster-Stratton, C. (1983). Intervention approaches to conduct disorders in young children. *Nurse Practitioner, 8*(5), 23–24, 29, 33–34.

30. Webster-Stratton, C. (1983). Recognizing and assessing conduct disorders in children. *American Journal of Maternal Child Nursing, 8,* 330–335.

31. Webster-Stratton, C. (1985). Comparison of behavior transactions between conduct-disordered children and their mothers in the clinic and at home. *Journal of Abnormal Child Psychology, 13*(2), 169–183.

32. Yamamoto, K., Soliman, A., Parsons, J., & Davies, O. L., Jr. (1987). Voices in unison: Stressful events in the lives of children in six countries. *Journal of Child Psychology and Psychiatry and Allied Disciplines 28*(6), 885–864.

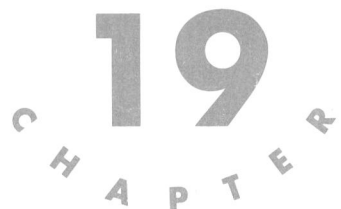

19
CHAPTER

Mental Health Issues in Childhood and Adolescence

BEHAVIORAL OBJECTIVES

Explain how the three levels of health prevention apply to child mental health/psychiatric nursing.

Recognize the impact of various family factors on a child's experience and developmental progress.

Describe the key elements of a child's psychiatric assessment.

Explain the use of play to assess children's thoughts and concerns.

Describe the cause of the various diagnoses described.

Identify the role of nursing in mental health issues of childhood and adolescence.

Approximately 17% of the U.S. population younger than the age of 18 needs some type of psychiatric mental health service. Only 7% of those who need help receive the necessary services, these 7% representing the most severely disordered children.[3] Children with mental health problems remain the most underserved population in the health care arena. Little hope exists that these dismal statistics will change in the 1990s because of cost trimming and cutbacks in service.[22]

The nursing specialty that focuses on the care of children with mental health disorders is child psychiatric nursing, a small specialty within the psychiatric nursing specialty. The disorders described in this chapter are some of the most difficult and emotionally exhausting disorders that confront children, families, and child health nurses. The ability of the nurse to use therapeutic techniques to assist the child/adolescent and family is an essential component of the intervention programs. The child and family are involved in all therapeutic strategies.

*Overview of Mental Health Issues
in Childhood and Adolescence*

History of Child Psychiatry

Concern for the mental health of children gained momentum in the 1890s, about 100 years after the start of treatment for mentally ill adults. Any problems that children might have were thought to be miniature versions of adult problems.

At the turn of the century, few theories existed about child development, and children were a low priority. Most often children were viewed as commodities of the family, to be used to help in the family's economic survival. Treatments for children with mental health problems were the same as those provided for adults. No developmental considerations were used in altering the treatment plans.[22] In 1908, the National Committee for Mental Hygiene established the first child guidance clinics to provide treatment for children. In 1944, Bruno Bettelheim founded the Orthogenic School for the treatment of severely disturbed children.[22]

With the advent of the community mental health services in the 1960s, the treatment of children moved from inpatient treatment centers to outpatient services.[23] Children remained in their homes while receiving treatment for their mental health disorders. Community services and care were believed to decrease the severity of the illnesses. Community mental health care was predicted to decrease the need for institutionalization. Further, the access to mental health care was to increase for those children who were emotionally disturbed under the program changes. The reality of the situation is somewhat different, and mental health care in the community has proven as successful in meeting the needs of the patient population as proposed.

Primary, Secondary, and Tertiary Prevention

In 1978, the President's Commission on Mental Health called for a renewed effort to focus on primary and secondary prevention of mental disorders in children. The President's commission emphasized the need for primary prevention for children at risk of pathologic development. Also stressed was the need for early case finding and intervention, or secondary prevention, of those children already displaying symptoms.[22] Research into the incidence of psychiatric disturbances in children has identified six risk factors that are correlated with the emergence of psychiatric disorders.[10] These risk factors, listed in the accompanying display, are associated with family problems including marital distress, socioeconomic factors, and parenting styles.

Primary prevention in child psychiatric disorders focuses on preventing illness from occurring. Nurses provide primary prevention when they teach parenting skills, increase the self-esteem of a child, or do anything that promotes a positive growth experience. Early identification of high-risk families (see Chap. 5) and early inter-

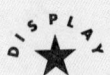

Family Risk Factors Correlated With Psychiatric Disorders

* Severe marital distress
* Low social status
* Overcrowding or large family size
* Paternal criminality
* Maternal psychiatric disorder
* Admissions of children into foster home placement

(Source: *Johnson, B. S.* [*1989*]. Psychiatric mental health nursing: Adaptation and growth. [*2nd ed.*]. *Philadelphia: J.B. Lippincott.*)

vention with families may prove very helpful in the management of potential and actual mental health problems. Assessing the presence of these risk factors is part of the primary prevention role of the nurse. Primary prevention is a part of well-child assessments a nurse conducts. Signs of impending problems may be identified by careful and attentive listening to the family describe the newborn or toddler. Are parental expectations appropriate to the age of the child? Are parents comfortable with their parenting roles? Observation strategies that can be used are presented in Chapter 18. Early primary prevention in a hospital setting includes preventing stress from hospitalization. Helping children deal with the stress of surgery or body image changes are important primary prevention techniques. Techniques that may be used include role playing with dolls or drawings or games that the child develops.

Secondary prevention in child psychiatric disorders focuses on early detection of problems in children. Nurses who work in public schools or clinics are in a good position to do assessment of child disorders. Because these nurses have access to high-risk children, they must be able to identify behaviors that indicate the need for further treatment. The behaviors related to specific mental health problems will be described later in this chapter. Secondary interventions include developmental counseling, support of children and parents in crisis, and anticipatory guidance.

The following types of programs could be considered either primary or secondary prevention:

* Preventive programs at birth and infancy. This includes parent education programs, prevention or early treatment of perinatal injuries, and promotion of mother-child bonding.
* Crisis intervention in the preschool years, such as developmental screening, and concerns about child abuse and neglect.
* Programs dealing with physical illness as a crisis in the home and at the hospital.
* Intervention programs for teenage pregnancy, children of alcoholic parents, and children with school difficulties.[15]

Tertiary prevention remains the focus of most child psychiatric nurses. These nurses work with children who have already been labeled as having emotional or behavioral problems. Most of these children are seen in settings where the emphasis is on helping the children and families move toward higher improved mental health and functioning. The remainder of the chapter will focus on tertiary prevention of identified mental health problems in children.

Standards of Practice

As a specialty area, child psychiatric nurses follow the American Nurses Association Standards of Psychiatric and Mental Health Nursing Practice. The purpose of the standards is to "fulfill the profession's obligation to provide a means of improving the quality of care. The standards represent agreed-upon levels of practice. They have been developed to characterize, to measure, and to provide guidance in achieving excellence in care."[1]

Developmental Aspects of Mental Health

The developmental stages of childhood are discussed in detail in Chapter 8. A summary of the issues that should be considered in mental health assessments and interventions are described here. The three primary areas of development that affect mental health are cognitive, moral, and psychosocial.

Cognitive Development

Cognitive development affects the child's perception of the world and his or her behavior. Consequently, the nurse must have an understanding about the age-appropriate reasoning abilities of the child. Piaget's stages of cognitive development are: sensorimotor (birth to 2 years), preoperational (2 to 7 years), concrete operations (7 to 12 years), and formal operations (12 to 15 years).[16] For example, a 4-year old boy whose blanket is an important transitional object and who has named it "blankie," may not understand why blankie will not be sad if left at home. Preoperational thinking is a time when children learn through actions, magical thinking, and imaginative play. When assessing children at various ages, the assessment strategies need to reflect the cognitive development.

Moral Development

Closely linked to cognitive development is the moral development of children. Kohlberg's work delineates six stages of development in the understanding of right and wrong behaviors (see Table 8-7). These stages are summarized here:

Level I: Pre-Conventional
   Stage 1: avoidance of punishment and obedience because of the power others have over your behaviors

   Stage 2: doing the "right" thing, what is fair and an equal exchange between self and others
Level II: Conventional
   Stage 3: interpersonal conformity, or living up to others' expectations, a belief in rules and authority
   Stage 4: ability to differentiate between interpersonal motives and societal obligations
Level III: Post-Conventional
   Stage 5: recognition of the moral and legal points of views in making social contracts or formal agreements
   Stage 6: belief in the universal moral principles and the value of individuals, or universal ethical principles[12]

Although the stages are not age specific, one must go through the earlier stages before reaching a more mature level of understanding. Thus, children are not able to grasp the idea of a higher ideal that makes rules not applicable in certain situations. The classic moral dilemma used to illustrate this is the man who had no money to buy the medicine for his dying wife and so stole the medicine from a drug store.[11] Children who are told this story are asked what should happen to the man. The age of the child will determine the answer that is provided. At stage 1, most are unable to get past the idea that the man is guilty of stealing, and therefore should go to jail: the notion of punishment and the need to be obedient. At stage 2, children will suggest "deals" that could be made between the man and the druggist. By stage 6, the adolescent may be able to discuss the rights of both the man and his wife to health care services, and societal responsibilities to assist these individuals without affecting the rights of the druggist.

The moral development of a child may be assessed when children present with mental health problems or emotional and behavioral problems. The antisocial behaviors that often are observed include a lack of compassion or empathy, a lack of concern about the rights of others, a disinterest in the needs of others, physical aggression such as hitting or biting, and verbal abusive language.

Psychological Development

Erikson's theory about the stages of psychological development of children is helpful in understanding children's behavior. The tasks set for each stage provide expectations for each child's behavior, abilities, and activities that can promote psychosocial development. During the early years, infants and toddlers have three major tasks to master: gaining a certain sense of trust that the world will meet their needs (trust versus mistrust); gaining control over their bodily functions and separation from mother (autonomy versus shame and doubt); and controlling their impulsive behaviors (initiative versus guilt). If young children are able to meet these challenges, they are ready to begin school and find pleasure in reaching goals based on their ability to perform (industry versus inferiority). Successfully meeting the challenge during the school years prepares the child to move on to the adolescent (identity versus identity diffusion) and young adult (intimacy versus isolation) stages of psychological development. Conversely, if the psychological tasks of childhood are not met or only partially met, the child will be ill equipped to face the challenges of adolescence and adulthood. The behavior of the child often reflects the developmental milestones that have not been successfully completed. The maladaptive behavior then is seen as a disorder that requires intervention. For example, during the first 3 years of life, if the toddler is unable to feel trust and a sense of attachment and bonding to a parent or caregiver, antisocial behaviors are more common during childhood and adolescent.[13]

Classification of Childhood Psychiatric Disorders

The complex nature of children's behavior makes describing and measuring behavioral problems difficult. Indeed, little agreement exists about what childhood disorders exist and even less agreement on the need for a diagnostic classification. Erikson[1] said that "no one label can adequately describe all the nuances of a particular child's behavior or environment." Certainly, classification systems ought to be used cautiously by nurses, to prevent labeling children inaccurately when no adequate label is available in the system. Still, in the last decade, child health professionals have recognized the need for a classification system of behavioral problems that would (1) facilitate communication among professionals; (2) offer a basis for description, assessment, and management of the behavioral problems; and (3) provide a theoretical framework for research purposes.[24]

One of the advantages of classification systems is their objectivity, which permits a more reliable measurement of the degree to which a child manifests a particular behavior. With such quantitative measures, the methods of data collection and the situation in which the behavior is observed can affect the results. From the thousands of children and adolescents studied empirically, however, major disorders common to both sexes and common to all ages, with the exception of the "socialized conduct disorder" in very young children, have been identified. Further comparison shows that, whether classified according to the categorical or dimensional model, the prevalence of most childhood and adolescent disorders varies with gender.

Another important feature of the multivariate studies is their cross-cultural generality. Both in the various subcultures of the United States and in other countries around the world, some common patterns of behavior disorders in children and adolescents have emerged, indicating that the biopsychosocial factors that precipitate those disorders are not limited to the North American culture.

Current Classifications

Three types of clinically derived classification systems are currently being used: (1) the DSM-III-R, contained in the *Diagnostic and Statistical Manual* (3rd ed., revised), published by the American Psychiatric Association; (2) the WHO Multiaxial Classification, developed for the World Health Organization in 1975 by Rutter, Shaffer, and Sheperd; and (3) the IDC-9 or International Disease Classification. Although there are some common elements among these three classification systems, they do differ in general concerning how to separate some behavioral disorders. For instance, in the DSM-III-R, "hyperactivity" is considered under attention deficit disorder, which is subdivided into whether hyperactivity is present or not. In contrast, the WHO system classifies hyperactivity as a subcategory of the developmental disorders, and the IDC-9 acknowledges three separate hyperkinetic syndromes (DSM-III-R).

Diagnostic and Statistical Manual-III-R The official classification system used in the United States is the *Diagnostic and Statistical Manual of Mental Disorders,* 3rd ed., revised (DSM-III-R). The purpose of the manual is to provide descriptive and observable criteria for diagnosis. Child psychiatric disorders are included in the DSM-III-R. According to this system, the child's problem is to be classified along five axes:

Axis 1: descriptions and diagnostic criteria of major syndromes
Axis 2: descriptions and diagnostic criteria of minor (personality and specific developmental) disorders
Axis 3: concomitant physical disorders
Axis 4: associated stresses
Axis 5: premorbid level of functioning[24]

A major criticism of the DSM-III-R classification system concerns disagreement in use of diagnostic criteria, especially when using the system for child referrals. Several studies have indicated that, in general, there was a less than 50% agreement between "experts" and ordinary raters who used the DSM-III for child referral. This falls far short of the minimum expected for reliable instruments.

WHO Multiaxial Classification The WHO classification deals with behavioral problems by examining the nature of the problem and the "intellectual level, biological factors, and associated or etiological psychosocial influences."[18]

International Disease Classification (IDC-)9 The IDC-9 does not offer a classification that is specific to particular age groups, but it does provide five categories of disorders that are relevant to children and adolescents.

Care Settings

The care of children with psychiatric disorders occurs in a variety of settings. Ideally, the least restrictive setting is preferred in treating children with mental health problems. Most children are able to stay with their families and receive psychiatric care through mental health services in the community. If the child's behavior becomes a threat to himself or others, the child may be hospitalized in an acute care setting. Acute care environments may include a psychiatric hospital with a children's unit or in a children's hospital with a psychiatric unit. If the child does not respond to inpatient acute treatment, he or she may be transferred to a long-term care facility. Such a transfer is done only as a last resort. A careful evaluation with documentation from psychiatrists, nurse therapists, social workers, pediatricians, and psychologist is stringently required before children can be placed outside their family.

Pervasive Developmental Disorders Emerging in Infancy

Of all the psychiatric disorders that occur in children and adolescents, those that begin during infancy and early childhood are seen as the most difficult to treat. Fortunately, such disorders are rare. Estimates are that pervasive developmental disorders affect 10 to 15 in every 10,000 children.[3] The cause of pervasive developmental disorders is not known. They do appear in boys, however, at four times the rate as in girls.

The term "pervasive developmental disorder" is used to categorize several types of pathology seen in the infant or very young child. Such disorders as early infantile autism, symbiotic infantile psychosis, and childhood schizophrenia are found in this category.

There is a great deal of controversy over the exact definition of each of the diseases found within the category of pervasive developmental disorder. Primarily, differential diagnosis is based on the age of onset and the degree of impairment of social interactions. Table 19-1 gives a summary of the clinical picture of childhood schizophrenia, infantile autism, and infantile psychosis. Schizophrenia is further discussed in the section on Psychosis in Adolescence in this chapter.

Numerous theories have been proposed about the cause of pervasive developmental disorders. Some view the disorders as the child's response to severe stress from the environment. The child retreats into a fantasy world because he or she is unable to cope with reality. Other theories support the premise that the cause is a neurologic defect. Most clinicians agree that although the cause may be biologic in nature, the treatment of the behaviors associated with the disorder is based on trying to entice the child to leave his or her fantasy world.

★ NURSING ASSESSMENT

Children with pervasive developmental disorder have several characteristic responses to the environment around them. They are unable to respond to others, or respond inappropriately. If someone tries to hold them or cuddle them, they will not respond at all, or will begin to scream in terror. The child acts as if they inhabit a world with no one else in it. Another characteristic is the lack of meaningful communication skills. The child has repetitive movements of the body, such as rocking or twirling. Often, they will engage in self-damaging behavior such as head banging or body slamming.

TABLE 19-1
Summary of Clinical Manifestations for Three Childhood Psychoses

Clinical Picture	Childhood Schizophrenia	Early Infantile Autism	Symbiotic Infantile Psychoses
Onset	Gradual between age 2 to 11 after period of normal development	Gradual from birth	Between 2½ to 5 years after normal development
Social and interpersonal	Decreased interest in external world, withdrawal, loss of contact, impaired relations with others	Failure to show anticipatory postural movements; extreme aloneness; insistence on sameness	Unable to tolerate briefest separation from mother; clinging and incapable of delineating self
Intellectual and cognitive	Thought disturbance; perceptual problems; distorted time and space orientation; below average IQ	High spatial ability; good memory; low I.Q. but good intellectual potential	Bizarre ideation; loss of contact; thought disturbance
Language	Disturbances in speech; mutism, and if speech is present, it is not used for communication	Disturbances in speech; mutism, and if speech is present it is not used for communication. Very literal; delayed echolalia; pronoun reversal; I and You are absent till age 6	
Affect	Defect in emotional responsiveness and rapport; decreased, distorted, and/or inappropriate affect	Inaccessible and emotionally unresponsive to humans	Severe anxiety and panic over separation from mother; low frustration tolerance; withdrawn and seclusive as psychosis persists
Motor	Bizarre body movements; repetitive and stereotyped motions; motor awkwardness; distortion in mobility	Head banging and body rocking; remarkable agility and dexterity; preoccupied with mechanical objects	
Physical and developmental patterns	Unevenness of somatic growth; disturbances of normal rhythmic patterns; abnormal EEG	Peculiar eating habits and food preferences; normal EEG	Disturbed normal rhythmic patterns
Family	High incidence of mental illness	Aloof, obsessive, and emotionally cold; high intelligence and educational and occupational levels; low divorce rate and incidence of mental illness	Pathological mother who fosters the symbiosis

(Source: Knopf, I. J. [1984]. *Childhood psychopathology: A developmental approach.* [2nd ed.]. [p. 240]. Englewood Cliffs, NJ: Prentice-Hall. Adapted by permission.)

★ NURSING DIAGNOSES AND PLANNING

Nursing diagnoses often used with the patient and families with a child with a pervasive developmental disorder are:

- Social Isolation related to inability to interact with others.
- Impaired Verbal Communication related to language confusion or distortion.
- Ineffective Individual Coping related to need for sameness in environment.
- High Risk for Injury related to self-mutilating behaviors and sensory deficits.
- Self-Care Deficits in Activities of Daily Living related to cognitive and affective impairments.
- Ineffective Compromised Family Coping related to increased stress.

The focus for planning and intervention for the child is on the management of behavior and maintenance of safety. Family support in its struggle to deal with the behavior and its attempt to return to social activity is an important consideration. Expected outcomes might include the following:

- Child uses gesture to indicate thirst.
- Parents discuss need for respite care.

★ NURSING INTERVENTIONS

Emphasis is placed on helping the child learn to attend to the outside environment. Teaching the child to use nonverbal behaviors to communicate is the first step. The child is encouraged to touch, mimic facial expressions, and use gestures. After the child has begun to master the basic skills, all normal behaviors must be taught in the same general manner. Things that normal children do automatically, such as play, feed themselves, etc., must be taught to the pervasive developmental disordered child. Reinforcement techniques are used to teach appropriate behavior. Families are taught basic behavior modification techniques to accomplish this.

Families need a great deal of emotional support in handling children with pervasive developmental disorders. The enormity of the stress on the families should be recognized and acknowledged by the nurse. Families are often reluctant to leave the child in the hands of a sitter to relax and get away. Nurses should inform families of resources available in the community to provide respite care. Home care infant stimulation programs, community health nurses, and various community resources are critical when treating these families.

★ EVALUATION

The prognosis for the child is poor, even with rigorous treatment. There is some evidence, however, that early diagnosis and treatment does improve the prognosis. Yearly psychological assessments and appropriate educational placements provide the best prognosis for these children.

Evaluation focuses on a decrease in the child's destructive behaviors and the ability of the family to cope.

Evaluation needs to be ongoing. Follow-up care involves changes in day care programs based on the child's and family's changing needs.

Infantile Autism

Infantile autism was first described by the child psychiatrist Leo Kanner in 1943. It is an organic brain disorder that becomes apparent in the early years of life and is characterized by atypical social or mental behaviors. Approximately 1 in 2000 to 3000 has this disorder, and boys are affected four times as often as girls.[31] Distribution shows that the upper socioeconomic group may have a somewhat higher incidence, but this may be due to the availability of better health care and more accurate diagnosis for this segment of the population.

The word "autism" means "morbid self-absorption." A child with this disorder characteristically demonstrates difficulty forming meaningful social relationships, is especially resistant to body contact, and has a powerful need to be left undisturbed.

Other typical characteristics include ritualistic and repetitive behavior such as rocking back and forth and self-stimulation or mutilation such as head banging. Affected children demonstrate inappropriate attachments to or preoccupation with mechanical objects. Some have an excellent rote memory or irregular sleep patterns. Researchers have suggested that as many as 70% to 90% of children with autism have accompanying mental retardation.[20]

Language development is nonexistent, delayed, or inappropriate. Echolalia, the repetition of words or phrases, or delayed echolalia, where the repetition occurs days or even weeks later, may be present. This attempt at language may be a precursor to the development of meaningful speech and has a positive prognostic value for the child. Indeed, if some form of language development has not been achieved by school-age years, the prognosis for the acquisition of language skills is poor.

The cause of autism remains unknown despite continued research. Two to five percent of siblings of children with autism are also autistic, so genetic transmission has been investigated.[31] Prenatal factors, infant biochemical imbalances, and environmental factors have been explored. One hypothesis suggested that professional parents who were cool in nature and lacked "warmheartedness" were the root of the autistic child's problems. This theory has been discounted and now is considered a myth.[31]

★ NURSING ASSESSMENT

Autism is difficult to diagnose because of the range of presenting symptomatology (see the accompanying display on autistic disorder diagnostic criteria). All children with autism do not exhibit all of the described behaviors. Some display signs early in infancy, and others apparently develop normally until 18 to 24 months and then regress or develop slower from that time forward. A thorough developmental history is imperative to rule out other disorders such as visual or hearing impairments, developmental language disorders, mental retardation, and

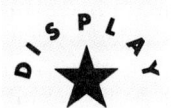

Diagnostic Criteria for Autistic Disorder

At least eight of the following 16 items are present, these to include at least two items from A, one from B, and one from C.

Note: Consider a criterion to be met *only* if the behavior is abnormal for the person's developmental level.

A. Qualitative impairment in reciprocal social interaction as manifested by the following:
(The examples within parentheses are arranged so that those first mentioned are more likely to apply to younger or more handicapped, and the later ones, to older or less handicapped, persons with this disorder.)
   (1) marked lack of awareness of the existence or feelings of others (e.g., treats a person as if he or she were a piece of furniture; does not notice another person's distress; apparently has no concept of the need of others for privacy)
   (2) no or abnormal seeking of comfort at times of distress (e.g., does not come for comfort even when ill, hurt, or tired; seeks comfort in a stereotyped way, e.g., says "cheese, cheese, cheese" whenever hurt)
   (3) no or impaired imitation (e.g., does not wave bye-bye; does not copy mother's domestic activities; mechanical imitation of others' actions out of context)
   (4) no or abnormal social play (e.g., does not actively participate in simple games; prefers solitary play activities; involves other children in play only as "mechanical aids")
   (5) gross impairment in ability to make peer friendships (e.g., no interest in making peer friendships; despite interest in making friends, demonstrates lack of understanding of conventions of social interaction, for example, reads phone book to uninterested peer)
B. Qualitative impairment in verbal- and nonverbal communication, and in imaginative activity, as manifested by the following:
(The numbered items are arranged so that those first listed are more likely to apply to younger or more handicapped, and the later ones, to older or less handicapped, persons with this disorder.)
   (1) no mode of communication, such as communicative babbling, facial expression, gesture, mime, or spoken language
   (2) markedly abnormal nonverbal communication, as in the use of eye-to-eye gaze, facial expression, body posture, or gestures to initiate or modulate social interaction (e.g., does not anticipate being held, stiffens when held, does not look at the person or smile when making a social approach, does not greet parents or visitors, has a fixed stare in social situations)

   (3) absence of imaginative activity, such as play-acting of adult roles, fantasy characters, or animals; lack of interest in stories about imaginary events
   (4) marked abnormalities in the production of speech, including volume, pitch, stress, rate, rhythm, and intonation (e.g., monotonous tone, questionlike melody, or high pitch)
   (5) marked abnormalities in the form or content of speech, including stereotyped and repetitive use of speech (e.g., immediate echolalia or mechanical repetition of television commercial); use of "you" when "I" is meant (e.g., using "You want cookie?" to mean "I want a cookie"); idiosyncratic use of words or phrases (e.g., "Go on green riding" to mean "I want to go on the swing"); or frequent irrelevant remarks (e.g., starts talking about train schedules during a conversation about sports)
   (6) marked impairment in the ability to initiate or sustain a conversation with others, despite adequate speech (e.g., indulging in lengthy monologues on one subject regardless of interjections from others)
C. Markedly restricted repertoire of activities and interests, as manifested by the following:
   (1) stereotyped body movements, e.g., hand-flicking or -twisting, spinning, head-banging, complex whole-body movements
   (2) persistent preoccupation with parts of objects (e.g., sniffing or smelling objects, repetitive feeling of texture of materials, spinning wheels of toy cars) or attachment to unusual objects (e.g., insists on carrying around a piece of string)
   (3) marked distress over changes in trivial aspects of environment, e.g., when a vase is moved from usual position
   (4) unreasonable insistence on following routines in precise detail, e.g., insisting that exactly the same route always be followed when shopping
   (5) markedly restricted range of interests and a preoccupation with one narrow interest, e.g., interested only in lining up objects, in amassing facts about meteorology, or in pretending to be a fantasy character
D. Onset during infancy or childhood.

Specify if childhood onset (after 36 months of age).

(American Psychiatric Association. (1987). Diagnostic and statistical manual of mental health, *[revised ed. 3]. Washington, D.C.: American Psychiatric Association.)*

schizophrenia. The earlier autism is identified, the better the prognosis becomes. In general, prognosis for autism is poor, with IQ and language ability being the most useful predictors of adult adjustment.

The major characteristic behaviors of infantile autism are the lack of interaction with the environment, the lack of meaningful language, and the repetitious movements of the body. If a parent tries to hold or cuddle the child, the child may not respond at all or may scream in terror. The child probably will not be able to sit still for any length of time and will not participate objectively in the assessment. A family history and parental concerns will help the nurse obtain objective data. Observations will supply information for subjective data.

The needs of the family are an important issue. The families of these children are under great stress. Because the child's behavior is unpredictable, most families stay at home and interact with few others. They often become isolated. Most of these children are maintained in their homes, with institutionalization used only as a last resort. Research into the stress of the families with severely disturbed children shows that the amount of stress is related to the child's inability to care for themselves and the inability to communicate with the child.

★ NURSING DIAGNOSES AND PLANNING

Examples of nursing diagnoses for the autistic child are the same as those given in the previous section.

Initially the nurse caring for a child with autism helps the family understand the meaning of the mutual diagnosis.

The goals for management include 1) modifying behaviors that are most disturbing or destructive to the child to help him or her become an acceptable member of society, 2) teaching everyday survival skills so that the child can become self-sufficient and independent, and 3) providing order to the child's chaotic world. The nurse teaches strategies to parents and the child to help the child become a functional member of society. Realistic goals are tailored individually.

★ NURSING INTERVENTIONS

Pharmacologic agents are the primary form of medical treatment, but major behavioral changes as a result of medication are rare. Anticonvulsants are indicated in at least 25% of children with autism who have accompanying seizures.[8] Amphetamines may reduce hyperactivity, and hypnotics may be necessary if sleeping disorders are involved. All pharmacologic agents should be monitored carefully, because children with autism may respond atypically to medication.

Emphasizing the positive and focusing on skills possessed by the child are essential. The nurse teaches parents principles of behavior modification and gives them encouragement to reinforce their efforts. It is not uncommon for parents to feel unsuccessful because their child's inappropriate behavior continues. Parents are taught to give immediate feedback so the child can associate cause and effect. The nurse educates parents about safety factors such as using helmets if head banging occurs. Because communication skills are tremendously difficult for these

children, the nurse teaches parents to monitor body language closely. Parents are strongly encouraged to continue social interactions with the child even when met with unresponsiveness. When a child shuns tactile stimuli, the parent's tendency is to withdraw. Different forms of communication, including tickling, holding, and cuddling, give a child with autism experiences similar to those of other children. The nurse may need to demonstrate to parents how to teach a child to mold his or her arms in an embrace, or to kiss, or to shake hands. Being this specific with activities that generally are taken for granted can be extremely difficult and emotionally upsetting for some parents.

Speaking in short sentences and simplifying commands enable the child to understand the world better. Parents are taught to maintain daily routines because this provides the child with a sense of predictability and allows him or her to feel safe in this unsure, chaotic world. Eliminating unnecessary change reduces confusion. A consistent, firm approach is necessary, especially when coupled with caring, loving attitudes. The nurse gives parents ample emotional support because no definitive cure currently exists for autism.

Institutionalization is an option, but this is occurring less frequently today than in the past. Educationally, these children are mainstreamed whenever feasible. Educational programs must provide a structured, consistent environment, and use behavior modification principles consistent with those used in the home environment.

★ NURSING EVALUATION

A behaviorally oriented educational approach to treatment will help children with autism to make gains in communication, social, self-help, and academic skills. Early intervention, intelligence (IQ level), degree of language impairment, and involvement in structured treatment programs are important considerations in establishing evaluation criteria for individual children. Parental support, community-based programs, and special education are needed for children to develop to their full potential.

Psychosis In Adolescence: Schizophrenia

Psychotic illnesses are defined as those disturbances of such magnitude and intensity that there is personality destruction and loss of reality orientation. Schizophrenia is a major psychotic disorder in which the person has disordered thinking, a poor perception of reality, limited ability to relate to others, and little control of affect and behavior. Schizophrenia usually has its onset during the adolescent or early adult years of life. Although there is no known cause for schizophrenia, there are certain behaviors that are used to distinguish schizophrenia from other psychoses.

The diagnosis of schizophrenia is given when the person shows signs of delusions, hallucinations, loose associations, and inappropriate affect. All of these symptoms may be found in the adolescent schizophrenic. Weiner[28] describes the characteristic behavior of adolescent schizophrenia in the following manner:

- Bizarre cognition: the adolescent confuses personal pronouns, using his name instead of "I" when referring to himself. Speech is often disconnected or incoherent. Often the adolescent reports hearing voices or other types of hallucinations.
- Bizarre action: the adolescent has odd facial expressions, such as grimaces or movements. The adolescent puts inedible things into the mouth, such as cigarette butts, garbage, etc. Often he or she rocks back and forth while sitting or eating.
- Schizoid withdrawal: the adolescent has a faraway look in the eyes. Often, the adolescent will sit and stare for no apparent reason or talk to himself or herself, carrying on complete conversations.
- Emotional detachment: the adolescent keeps his or her distance with others, particularly with adults. Often, the adolescent has a fixed, flat facial expression that does not change with the situation.
- Poor emotional control: the adolescent gets very upset if things do not go the way he or she expected. The adolescent is easily upset by peers and is unable to control angry impulses.

These behaviors are extremely disturbing to parents and friends and can be dangerous to the adolescent, as well as to the others around them.

The cause of this mental disorder has been described by many different theories, including psychological, family, and biologic or genetic. Most clinicians do agree that the onset of illness is either in childhood or adolescence. Onset occurs earlier for men than women. Women and men are equally affected, at least in the Western civilizations. Early-onset cases have more disorganized features and a poorer prognosis than late onset. Schizophrenia in children and adolescents is divided between prepubertal onset and pubertal onset. The earliest reported cases of schizophrenia are in children 4 to 5 years old. During the early school years, children presenting with schizophrenia show evidence of undifferentiated subtypes. Organic brain disease and neurologic signs are indicative of the severity of the disorder in the very young.[13] A familial history of schizophrenia or related diagnoses is related positively to schizophrenia in children and adolescents.

★ NURSING ASSESSMENT

Nursing assessment of the adolescent with schizophrenia centers around the adolescent's behavior. The key features of this disorder are delusions, noneffective auditory hallucinations, or thought disorder. The accompanying display outlines the diagnostic criteria for schizophrenia disorder. Three phases of the disease process are the prodromal phase, in which there is a clear deterioration in functioning; the active phase of the illness; and residual phase.[16] Functional deterioration is associated with social isolation, poor scholastic performance, bizarre behavior, poor personal hygiene, flat affect, odd ideas, unusual perceptual experience, and over-elaborate speech.

DISTURBANCES IN THINKING

Adolescents with schizophrenia have difficulty expressing their thoughts. Often their thinking is very concrete. The term "loose association" is used to describe a schizo-phrenic way of thinking in which the thought patterns are not logical, and shift from one topic to another without any apparent connection. The adolescent is unaware that his or her comments have very little to do with the subject of the conversation. A loose association response to the question, "How was your day today?", might go like this: "Today's day was blue like your dress." Such comments may have symbolic meaning to the person, but little relevance to others.

Often, schizophrenics feel as if they have magical control over those around them, thinking that they can control events and behaviors outside of themselves. Although such thinking is often found in preschool children, magical thinking is not appropriate in adolescence. Beliefs concerning the ability to control another person's thoughts through mind control are often present in schizophrenia.

Delusions, or fixed, false beliefs, are part of the disturbance of thinking. In schizophrenia, the delusions are characteristically bizarre with no basis in fact.[3] The delusions may center on thoughts of persecution, such as someone is out to get them. Another common delusion is the delusion of grandeur, or thinking that they have powers that no one else has. Delusions cannot be reasoned away, and it is ineffective to try to reason with a delusional schizoid patient.[10]

Hallucinations are false sensory perceptions. That is, the person sees, hears, smells, or tastes something that is not there. Auditory hallucinations are the most common, followed by visual. Hallucinations can be very frightening to the person who is experiencing them.

DISTURBANCES IN FEELINGS

Affect is used to describe the mood or feeling tone of a person. Often, the schizophrenic adolescent is characterized by a flat affect. That is, the adolescent is unable to respond to the environment. The face is blank, and the voice expressionless. An inappropriate affect indicates that the expressions are inappropriate or incongruent with the content of the speech or ideas. When given sad news, the adolescent may laugh, or when told a joke, cry. A blunted affect refers to a marked reduction in the intensity of the response or expression.[13]

DISTURBANCES IN BEHAVIOR

Unusual or bizarre behavior is often the reason an adolescent is brought in for evaluation of schizophrenia. Mannerisms, echopraxia (involuntary imitation of others' movements), and catatonia may be observed during acute and chronic forms of schizophrenia. Often, the adolescent will become fascinated with an object such as a clock and will spend hours watching it. The adolescent may invest hours into a project such as drawing a fantasy universe and naming the planets. These projects are not play or fun, but very serious work.

Communication is used to express private thoughts, not to build relationships. Sexual identity is of great concern to the adolescent with schizophrenia. Often their behavior reflects their obsession with sexual identity. Masturbation and inappropriate sexual language and behavior often are observed.

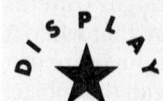

Diagnostic Criteria for Schizophrenia

A. Presence of characteristic psychotic symptoms in the active phase: either (1), (2), or (3) for at least 1 week (unless the symptoms are successfully treated):
 (1) Two of the following:
 (*a*) Delusions
 (*b*) Prominent hallucinations (throughout the day for several days or several times a week for several weeks, each hallucinatory experience not being limited to a few brief moments)
 (*c*) Incoherence or marked loosening of associations
 (*d*) Catatonic behavior
 (*e*) Flat or grossly inappropriate affect
 (2) Bizarre delusions (i.e., involving a phenomenon that the person's culture would regard as totally implausible, e.g., thought broadcasting, being controlled by a dead person)
 (3) Prominent hallucinations [as defined in (1)(*b*) above] of a voice with content having no apparent relation to depression or elation, or a voice keeping up a running commentary on the person's behavior or thoughts, or two or more voices conversing with each other
B. During the course of the disturbance, functioning in such areas as work, social relations, and self-care is markedly below the highest level achieved before onset of the disturbance (or, when the onset is in childhood or adolescence, failure to achieve expected level of social development).

C. Schizoaffective Disorder and Mood Disorder with Psychotic Features have been ruled out, that is, if a Major Depressive or Manic Syndrome has ever been present during an active phase of the disturbance, the total duration of all episodes of a mood syndrome has been brief relative to the total duration of the active and residual phases of the disturbance.
D. Continuous signs of the disturbance for at least 6 months. The 6-month period must include an active phase (of at least 1 week, or less if symptoms have been successfully treated), during which there were psychotic symptoms characteristic of Schizophrenia (symptoms in A), with or without a prodromal or residual phase, as defined below.
Prodromal phase: A clear deterioration in functioning before the active phase of the disturbance that is not due to a disturbance in mood or to a Psychoactive Substance Use Disorder and that involves at least two of the symptoms listed below.
Residual phase: After the active phase of the disturbance, persistence of at least two of the symptoms noted below, these not being due to a disturbance in mood or to a Psychoactive Substance Use Disorder.

There are additional Prodromal and Residual Symptoms and a Classification of Course in the full Diagnostic Criteria.
(*American Psychiatric Association.* [*1987*]. Diagnostic and statistical manual of mental health. [*revised 3rd ed.*]. *Washington, D.C.: American Psychiatric Association.*)

★ NURSING DIAGNOSES AND PLANNING

The following are examples of possible nursing diagnoses for the adolescent with schizophrenia[9]:

- Sensory/Perceptual Alterations related to hearing voices, sounds; seeing images, etc.
- Altered Thought Processes related to non–reality-based ideas.
- Social Isolation related to irrational behavior; disruptive behaviors.
- Impaired Verbal Communication related to nonreality base of functioning.

Nursing interventions focus on providing for basic needs, functions, and safety and on supporting the adolescent's relationships with peers, health care workers, and family members. Expected outcomes for the children and adolescents with schizophrenia may include the following based on reality participation.

- Child or adolescent demonstrates interest in events by reading newspaper and joining in discussion.
- Child or adolescent participates in relaxation techniques before bedtime.

★ NURSING INTERVENTIONS

The basic needs of the actively schizophrenic individual must be monitored by the nurse. Inappropriate eating behaviors, such as rummaging in garbage cans or eating cigarette butts, calls for observation and encouragement to eat normally. Often the adolescent with schizophrenia is restless and has difficulty sleeping. The nurse can help by administering medications as ordered, encouraging relaxation before bedtime, and limiting caffeine intake. Exercise should be encouraged, primarily activities that use the large muscle groups. Activities such as puzzles or craft work are often frustrating in schizophrenia, because of the adolescent's inability to concentrate on tasks for long periods.

Because of the distortions found in the schizophrenic thinking, as well as the presence of hallucinations and delusions, safety is a primary area of concern. Adolescents must be safeguarded from attempting life-threatening behaviors that auditory or visual hallucinations prompt them to initiate. Nurses need to monitor the presence or absence of hallucinations and be aware of the adolescents' behaviors that indicates they are experiencing hallucinations. If the adolescent is seen carrying on a conversation when there is no one there, or seems to be listening to a conversation when no one else is around, the nurse should suspect that the adolescent is responding to internal voices, or hallucinations. Intervention is based on trying to get the adolescent back in touch with reality. The nurse encourages the adolescent to listen to what the nurse is saying instead of what the voices are saying.

Simple activities of daily living need to be monitored by the nurse if the adolescent is actively hallucinating. Activities such as shaving or showering must be monitored in case the voices tell the adolescent to harm himself by cutting his throat or drowning.

Interactions between the adolescent and peers and family should be encouraged. Often adolescents with schizophrenia are withdrawn and unwilling to communicate with others. Activities that encourage direct communication are helpful.

Time spent with adolescents with schizophrenia should focus on helping them relate to the environment outside of themselves. Activities such as reading the newspaper, talking about daily events, and interacting with a group support the learning of appropriate social behaviors. It is critical to include family members in these activities as much as possible. Family members may need teaching family programs about the symptoms of schizophrenia. Specific methods of dealing with the frustration felt by those close to the adolescent are also important aspects of family care.

Psychotropic medications known as antipsychotic medications are given to relieve symptoms of schizophrenia. Although it is not known exactly how these medications work, they do provide relief from the hallucinations and bizarre thinking experienced by the schizophrenic. These medications are extremely potent, and the nurse must monitor the adolescents for side effects. The accompanying display on phenothiazines gives examples of the antipsychotic medications used in treating adolescents and associated nursing interventions.

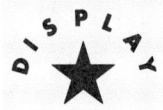

Antipsychotic Medication: Phenothiazines

Therapeutic Uses
Used to treat acute or chronic psychoses and for sedation. **Trifluopromazine, prochlorperazine, chlorpromazine** are used as antiemetics. **Chlorpromazine and thioridazine** can be used to control combativeness and hyperexcitability in children with behavior problems.

Contraindications
Contraindicated in hypersensitivity, severe toxic CNS depression, persons in a coma, or those with subcortical brain damage, bone marrow depression, or those receiving L-dopa therapy. **Trifluopromazine** is contraindicated in children and adolescents with suspected Reye's syndrome.

Precautions
Should be used cautiously in persons with seizure disorders or those receiving anticonvulsants; those with cardiovascular disorders; those exposed to high environmental temperatures; the debilitated; those with hepatic or renal disorders, glaucoma, prostatic hypertrophy, chronic respiratory conditions, and hypocalcemia; and those persons who have a severe reaction to insulin or electroconvulsive therapy. Some preparations of **trifluperazine, perphenazine,** and **chlorpromazine** contain sulfites and should be used cautiously in persons with sulfite sensitivity to prevent possible allergic reaction. Some preparations of **mesoridazine** and **promazine** contain tartrazine and should be used cautiously in persons who have a sensitivity to tartrazine.

Nursing Considerations
Instruct client in disease, treatment, regimen, compliance, and signs and symptoms of adverse reactions; avoid direct contact of drug with skin; obtain baseline information about the overt signs of emotional disturbance, anxiety level, depression, suicidal ideation; obtain baseline information about vital signs and usual patterns of elimination; monitor vital signs frequently during therapy; assess intake and output for signs of urinary retention; obtain blood studies, including CBC, platelet counts, and liver function studies; evaluate emotional status for changes and institute safety and suicide precautions as necessary; assess neuromuscular status for involuntary movements; instruct client not to withdraw or stop taking the drug suddenly; instruct client to avoid beverages and over-the-counter drugs containing alcohol; warn client to avoid activities requiring mental alertness and coordination until effects of drug are known; administer with milk or foods to minimize GI upset; instruct client that excessive exposure to sunlight may cause photosensitivity reactions; teach client to avoid extreme heat or cold temperatures because of risk of hypothermia and hyperthermia; suggest measures to relieve dry mouth such as ice chips, gum, hard candy; warn client that urine may become discolored; dilute concentrate with 2–4 ounces of liquid such as water, carbonated drinks, fruit juice, tomato juice, milk, or puddings; avoid using apple juice or caffeine containing products.

Administer IM **chlorpromazine, fluphenazine, mesoridazine, perphenazine** and **promazine** deep into the upper outer quadrant of the buttocks and massage afterwards to prevent abscess formation; protect liquid concentration from light. When giving **promethazine** by IV drip, wrap solution container in foil to protect from light. Monitor the client's blood pressure closely, sitting, standing, and lying, when giving promazine IV.

(Adapted from: *Spencer, R. T., Nichols, L. W., and Lipkin, G. B., et al.* [*1993*]. Clinical pharmacology and nursing management [*ed. 4*]. *Philadelphia: J.B. Lippincott.*)

★ EVALUATION

Evaluation of adolescent schizophrenia involves not only the child but the family. The adolescent must be evaluated on his or her ability to function in the environment. Consequently, the family is an integral part of the team. The presence or absence of family support is part of the decision as to the type of treatment facility that will best meet the needs of the client.

Affective Disorders in Childhood and Adolescence

Affective disorders range from manic to depressive on a continuum of emotional response. The range determines the severity of the disorder. This section centers on depression and the impact of depression on the infant, child, or adolescent.[17]

Nonorganic Failure to Thrive

The term "failure to thrive" is used when an infant's or child's growth rate falls below the third percentile for age, or declines from a previously normal rate for weight on the standard growth chart. Failure to thrive is also diagnosed when an infant or small child presents with an acute weight loss. When this happens, a complex set of symptoms results that require medical intervention. The seriousness of failure to thrive cannot be underestimated given the rapid physiologic changes that can occur in infants. Failure to thrive is a chronic, potentially life-threatening disorder affecting 10% of the rural outpatient population and 3% to 5% of all infants admitted to medical teaching hospitals.[13]

There are two types of failure to thrive: organic and nonorganic. Organic failure to thrive is attributed to physiologic reasons; nonorganic is related to the dysfunctional families and poor nurturing situations.[30] Nonorganic failure to thrive is sometimes equated with *anaclitic depression in infants.*[30] Anaclitic depression occurs in infants who have lost contact with a significant other. Anaclitic depression was first described by Spitz in relation to the behavior seen in infants placed in orphanages during World War II who typically had a three-phase reaction to the separation from mothers: angry protest, resignation and depression, and detachment and reorganization.[13] Regardless of the cause, organic or nonorganic, the infant has insufficient nutrition to sustain growth.

The symptoms of nonorganic failure to thrive are not limited to height and weight deficiency. These infants suffer from social, motor, adaptive, and language delays. Diagnosis of the infant with failure to thrive begins with a determination of whether the problem is physical or psychological in nature. The diagnosis is not made easily, and often takes time.

★ NURSING ASSESSMENT

A complete history of the child is taken. Table 19-2 provides an outline for conducting the nursing assessment

**TABLE 19-2
Nursing Assessment: Guidelines for Assessing Failure To Thrive**

Prenatal History

Was the pregnancy planned?

What were the parents' feelings about the pregnancy?

Was the pregnancy normal?

Was an abortion considered, or were there attempts to obtain an abortion?

Did the mother have unrealistic expectations about "the joys of motherhood?"

What were the parents' expectation about this infant?

Did the mother experience any emotional upset, such as illness, lack of support, or the deaths of significant others?

During the pregnancy, did the mother have any medical problems, such as high blood pressure, bleeding, or infections?

Did the mother use any medications?

Did the mother use alcohol, drugs, or cigarettes?

Birth History

What was the child's gestational age?

What were the child's height and weight at birth?

What were the child's APGAR scores?

What were the length and perceived difficulty of labor?

What was the type of delivery? What medications were used?

Were there any complications for either mother or child?

Did the child have any congenital anomalies?

What were the parents' initial perceptions of the infant?

Past Medical History

What illness or injuries has the child experienced?

Has the child had frequent infections?

Does the child have any allergies?

Has the child been hospitalized previously?

What growth data for the child can the parents provide?

Family History

What are the ages and health status of other family members?

Do any illnesses run in the family?

What are the height and weights of the parents, grandparents, siblings, and members of the extended family?

Nutritional History

How is the child fed?

How do the parents prepare food?

What kind of foods are commonly eaten by the child? (Obtain a 24-hour recall of food intake, and do a calorie count and evaluation of the distribution of calories among fats, proteins, and carbohydrates.)

What are the child's eating habits and meal patterns?

What are mealtimes like for the family?

Social History

Is the father currently unemployed?

Is the mother employed outside the home?

How do the mother and father interact? Are the parents experiencing marital instability?

Has the child been abused?

Does the family have enough money for food and the basics of existence?

Developmental History

When were major developmental milestones achieved by the child?

How does the child's development compare with siblings or with what the parents expected?

(From: Yoos, L. (1984). Taking another look at failure to thrive. *American Journal of Maternal Child Nursing, 9,* 32–36.)

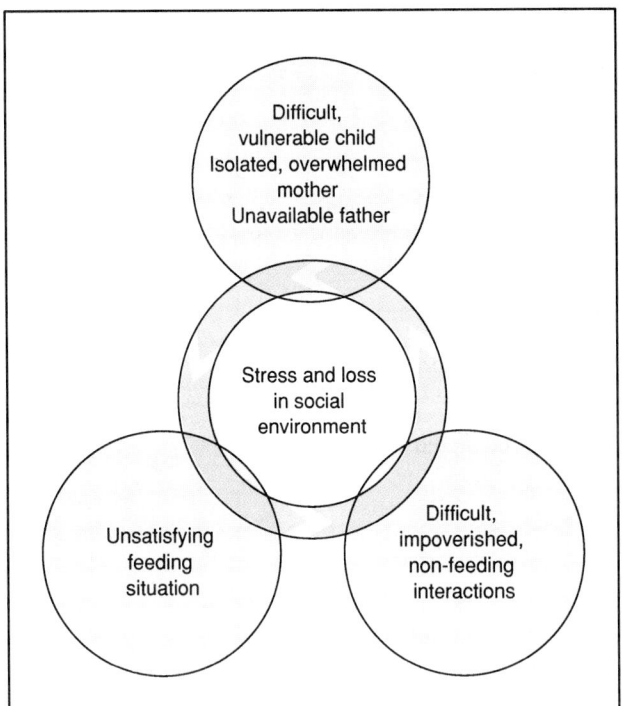

FIGURE 19-1
Nonorganic risk factors in failure to thrive. (Redrawn from: Levine, M. D., Carey, W. B., Crocker, A. C., et al. [1983]. *Developmental behavioral pediatrics.* Philadelphia: W. B. Saunders.)

of the family and infant with failure to thrive. The major areas of family functioning which are assessed include: temperament and sickliness of the child and parental difficulties; feeding behaviors and interactions; non-feeding interactions; and psychosocial stressors. Figure 19-1 demonstrates the relationship between these areas of family functioning and the development of nonorganic failure to thrive. In addition to the interview, the nurse can observe the parent-infant feeding behaviors, parent-infant interactions, developmental assessments, and history and physical examination. The reader is referred to Chapter 8 for a discussion on temperament and techniques for assessing temperament of infants and children.

★ NURSING DIAGNOSES AND PLANNING

If a medical diagnosis of failure to thrive is made, the care plan is determined by an interdisciplinary team, of which the nurse plays an integral part. The nurse primarily acts as an advocate for the child and the family. Hospitalization is used only as a last resort, because hospitalization can further communicate to the parents that they are inadequate. Physical deterioration of the infant, however, may necessitate an admission and can be used positively to promote parental education on parenting skills and basic infant care.

The following are examples of possible nursing diagnoses for the family and infant with failure to thrive:

- Ineffective Individual Coping related to vulnerability.
- Altered Nutrition: Less Than Body Requirements related to refusal to feed.
- Altered Parenting related to interrupted binding process.

Nursing care is addressed in such actions as the following:

- Parents identify infant's dietary needs.
- Parents communicate with eye contact with the infant during feeding.

★ NURSING INTERVENTIONS

Often, infants and children with failure to thrive are difficult to feed. They will refuse the bottle or stiffen and refuse to eat. After the nurse asks for a very detailed description of the child's diet, parents are taught about the appropriate diet for the child's age, as well as amounts of food. A very specific feeding schedule is developed, and the child's weight is checked frequently.

A fixed feeding schedule with a calm structured approach is essential. Modeling a calm approach, with toys and distractions removed from the room, is beneficial to feeding efforts. Ideally only one person (nurse or mother) should be interacting with the infant during feeding. The nutritional needs of the infant or child will be carefully calculated to provide more than normal caloric intake to help the child initiate and maintain growth.

Another important nursing intervention is emotional support of the parents, especially the mother. Life stresses in the mother are assessed, and suggestions for decreasing the stresses are made where appropriate. The mother of infants with failure to thrive often reports feeling overwhelmed and socially isolated. The father may be absent or not involved in the family life. Marital discord or stress, financial difficulties, and other family problems may be present. A referral for counseling and family support may be an important intervention. A list of social risk factors associated with failure to thrive is found in the accompanying display.

Observations of the interaction between the child and parents are made with suggestions and role modeling used to modify the parents' behaviors. Encouragement and praise is given to the parents for incorporating positive parenting skills into their routine.[30] The accompanying Nursing Assessment display provides an outline for evaluating the feeding and nonfeeding interactions between the mother and infant.

Hospitalization is indicated if a child presents with severe dehydration or malnutrition. Evidence of child abuse also may indicate a need for hospitalization to assess the situation more carefully and to protect the infant. Infants who are not responding to therapy as an outpatient may be hospitalized. On occasion, the infant will be hospitalized because of the extreme parental anxiety and fears over helping their child improve.[13] If the child must be hospitalized, the treatment focuses on these areas: nutritional intake, the child's eating behaviors, apathy, developmental delays, parental education, and counseling. Effort is made to interact with the child during feedings. Positive eating behaviors are taught to parents and modeled. Continuity of care is extremely important in failure to thrive infants. Therefore, effort should be made to have the same nurses care for the infant during the hospitalization.

Infant stimulation programs may benefit failure to thrive infants both during hospitalization and at home.

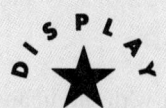

Social Assessment or Risk Factors in Failure to Thrive

Multiproblem family
  Marital stress, dissatisfaction
  Financial stress, layoffs
  Disorganized life styles
  Highly dependent relationships
  Chronic illness
Social isolation
  Mothers isolated from family, neighborhood
  Fathers unable or unwilling to help
  Help rejecting style with caregivers
  Ineffective or nonuse of medical and community
    support

Unplanned, difficult pregnancy
  Maternal illness, depression, or loss
  Lack of birth control
  Adolescence
  Expectation of "damaged" child
History of loss
  Death or abandonment in family
  Loss of sense of self (e.g., adolescent pregnancy,
    illness)
  Loss of "expected child"

(From: Levine, M. D., Carey, W. B., Crocker, A. C., & Gross, R. T. [1983]. [p. 567]. Developmental–behavioral pediatrics. Philadelphia: W.B. Saunders.)

Many times these children suffer from physical and emotional developmental delays. A developmental evaluation may be necessary to validate the need for special community services once the child is discharged.

★ NURSING EVALUATION

Careful monitoring of feeding sessions, with evidence of parental competence and infant weight gain, is essential. Both parents may require therapy in managing the psychosocial stressors present in the home. Much support and continued encouragement on a daily basis is needed from nurses, physicians, and family members. Assessing adaptability to various feeding techniques, as well as suc-

cess with repeated efforts is important in determining the parent's ability to feed the infant beyond the hospital environment.

Mood Disorders in Childhood and Adolescence

According to the DSM-III-R, mood disorders are grouped into the two major patterns of disturbance: mania and depression. Mood is an emotional reaction that is sufficiently intense to affect a person's entire psychic state and is not due to any other physical or mental problem.[2] Mood disorders are determined by the pattern of mood episodes.[2] The mood disorders are further classified as bipolar and depressive disorders. *Bipolar Disorder* is identified by exaggerated mood swings, bizarre behavior, and grandiose delusions. The patient experiences at least one manic episode, followed by one or more depressive episodes. The patient's mood is extremely elevated or irritable, followed by a deep depression. Although uncommon in prepubertal children, the child with bipolar depression will present with extreme mood swings of short duration. The usual age at onset is in the early 20s.[2] A strong family history in close biologic relatives has been reported.

Depression

Major depressive disorder or unipolar disorder describes the situation in which the patient has cycles of depression followed by a return to normal levels of energy. The major feature of major depressive episodes is a depressed or irritable mood or loss of interest or pleasure in most activities. The symptoms may persist for 2 weeks to 6 months. Dysthymia is a chronic, milder depressive disturbance with a duration of at least 2 years.[2] Such periods of depression may not be linked to events occurring in the individual's life. The age of onset for

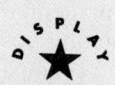

Nursing Assessment: Observation* of Mother–Infant Interaction in Failure to Thrive

Observe pair for:

• Richness of interaction
• Amount of eye and physical contact
• Sense of mutual pleasure
• Warmth and affection
• Consistency of response

Observe each for:

• Responsivity
• Self-regulatory capacity
• Tolerance level

Also assess:

• Appropriateness of mother's expectations
• "Burdensomeness" of infant's demands

* Observe in feeding and nonfeeding situations.
(Adapted from: Levine, M. D., Carey, W. B., Crocker, A. C., & Gross, R. T. [1983]. [p. 566]. Developmental–behavioral pediatrics. Philadelphia: W.B. Saunders.)

major depressive disorders is in the late 20s, but may begin at any age, including infancy.[2]

There may be a familial pattern to depression.[2] An imbalance in one or more neurotransmitters in the brain or receptors has been associated with depression and explains the benefits of most antidepressant agents that are used to manage depression.

Only recently, the presence of depression in children and adolescents has been recognized. Adults may have difficulty realizing that the "best years of life" are not always the carefree and happy times of childhood. Another reason that depression in children and adolescents has been ignored is that depressed children do not exhibit the same symptoms as adults, making depression difficult to recognize. Acting out behaviors are common in childhood depression. Wide mood swings, along with isolation from friends and family, should be clues that the child is experiencing depression. Because these behaviors are seen during normal adolescence, persistence of the behaviors may indicate a depression.

In young children, depression is manifested by listlessness, anorexia, psychomotor retardation, feeding problems, and sad facial expressions that continue over time. Toddlers may be hyperactive, withdrawn, or have discipline problems. Depression in very young children or in infants results from being taken away from someone with whom they have had a relationship or strong attachment.

Older children also may be affected by the loss of someone through death or divorce. Often, the child blames himself or herself for the loss of the person. Such thinking produces guilt in the child. Children with alcoholic or drug-addicted parents also are at risk for depression. Because their parents do not function adequately in their roles as parents, the child often takes on adult responsibilities that are unrealistic. Therefore, they are often not able to accomplish the tasks and feel inadequate.

Most depressions that occur in children and adolescents are thought to be situational in nature. That is, the depression is a reaction to a situation in which the child or adolescent experiences some type of loss, changes, traumatic experience, or achievement failure, and therefore is referred to as situational depressional, or may be considered a form of separation anxiety, in which the child is depressed until the mother or significant others returns. A depressive mood is strongly associated with separation anxiety disorder[13] (see Chapter 18 for SAD).

In adolescents, failure or perceived failure to meet the expectations of peers and family often results in low self-esteem and depression. An adolescent may believe that normal challenges of adolescence are impossible. Precipitating events may not be noticed by adults surrounding the adolescent. Often the precipitation event is associated with not being able to "make the grade" with peers or not being able to meet the parental expectations.

Major depressive disorder may be associated with hallucinations and delusions and depressive symptoms. A careful diagnosis is needed to distinguish between depressive hallucinations and schizophrenia.

Traditionally, the diagnosis of depressive disorder has not been made until early adulthood, but the trend is to make the diagnosis in early adolescence or childhood.[11] The diagnosis is sometimes difficult to make in adolescence, especially if the teenager has been involved in drug or alcohol abuse. This is because drug use, especially marijuana use, has a depressive effect[9] and alcohol or drug use may be an attempt to alleviate the depression.[13]

Adolescents with major depressive disorders should be under the care of a psychiatrist who is familiar with the medications available to treat the depression. Often, other family members may suffer from similar symptoms, and as such, may ignore the child's depression as a personality style.

★ NURSING ASSESSMENT

The assessment process in depression is often a lengthy one. Symptoms of childhood depression are not the same as in adults. The major symptoms in depression are a persistent depressive mood and a pervasive loss of interest or pleasure in usual activities.[13] When assessing children about feelings of depression, use a variety of words to desire the feelings being asked, such as sad, depressed, low, down, down in the dumps, empty, blue, very unhappy, or "bad feeling inside."[13] The child's behavior needs to be assessed in different situations, such as school, home, and social activities. Changes in behavior over time are the greatest indication that something is not right with the child. The accompanying display on diagnostic criteria for major depressive episodes provides the diagnostic criteria for depression in children and adolescents.

The mood changes are associated with a least four of eight commonly present physical symptoms:

- Change in appetite, either increased or decreased;
- Sleep disturbance such as difficulty going to sleep, waking up at night, early morning awakening, or sleeping too much;
- Loss of energy, fatigability or tiredness;
- Psychomotor agitation or retardation, such as an inability to sit still, pacing, temper tantrums, or visible slowing down of physical movements, speech, or a sluggishness;
- Feelings of excessive or inappropriate guilt for minor failings that seem exaggerated;
- Loss of interest or enjoyment in activities;
- Difficulty concentrating or thinking; and
- Thoughts of death or suicide.[13]

★ NURSING DIAGNOSES AND PLANNING

Nursing diagnoses that may be used in cases of depression disorders among children and adolescents include:

- Altered Nutrition: Less Than Body Requirements related to loss of interest in eating.
- Impaired Social Interaction related to self-concept disturbance.
- Ineffective Individual Coping related to situational crises.
- Hopelessness related to isolation.
- High Risk for Injury related to disinterest in environment.
- Self-Esteem Disturbance related to feelings of guilt.
- Social Isolation related to loss of interest in others.

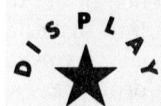

Diagnostic Criteria for Major Depressive Episode

Note: A "Major Depressive Syndrome" is defined as criterion A below.

A. At least five of the following symptoms have been present during the same 2-week period and represent a change from previous functioning; at least one of the symptoms is either (1) depressed mood, or (2) loss of interest or pleasure (do not include symptoms that are clearly due to a physical condition, mood-incongruent delusions or hallucinations, incoherence, or marked loosening of associations):

  (1) Depressed mood (or can be irritable mood in children and adolescents) most of the day, nearly every day, as indicated either by subjective account or observation by others

  (2) Markedly diminished interest or pleasure in all, or almost all, activities most of the day, nearly every day (as indicated either by subjective account or observation by others of apathy most of the time)

  (3) Significant weight loss or weight gain when not dieting (e.g., more than 5% of body weight in a month), or decrease or increase in appetite nearly every day (in children, consider failure to make expected weight gains)

  (4) Insomnia or hypersomnia nearly every day

  (5) Psychomotor agitation or retardation nearly every day (observable by others, not merely subjective feelings of restlessness or being slowed down)

  (6) Fatigue or loss of energy nearly every day

  (7) Feelings of worthlessness or excessive or inappropriate guilt (which may be delusional) nearly every day (not merely self-reproach or guilt about being sick)

  (8) Diminished ability to think or concentrate, or indecisiveness, nearly every day (either by subjective account or as observed by others)

  (9) Recurrent thoughts of death (not just fear of dying), recurrent suicidal ideation without a specific plan, or a suicide attempt or a specific plan for committing suicide

B. (1) It cannot be established that an organic factor initiated and maintained the disturbance

  (2) The disturbance is not a normal reaction to the death of a loved one (Uncomplicated Bereavement)

  Note: Morbid preoccupation with worthlessness, suicidal ideation, marked functional impairment or psychomotor retardation, or prolonged duration suggest bereavement complicated by Major Depression.

C. At no time during the disturbance have there been delusions or hallucinations for as long as 2 weeks in the absence of prominent mood symptoms (i.e., before the mood symptoms developed or after they have remitted).

D. Not superimposed on Schizophrenia, Schizophreniform Disorder, Delusional Disorder, or Psychotic Disorder NOS.

(American Psychiatric Association. [1987]. Diagnostic and statistical manual of mental health [revised 3rd ed.]. Washington D.C.: American Psychiatric Association.)

Possible outcomes may be the following:

- Child expresses feelings during play.
- All family members participate actively in therapy sessions.
- Adolescents and parents demonstrate understanding of medication regimen and outcomes.

★ NURSING INTERVENTIONS

The interventions used in managing depression are not the same for children as for adolescents and adults. This is because children, especially younger children, have a limited ability to express themselves verbally. The precautions necessary for suicide prevention are the same, however, focusing on physical safety.

Most therapeutic interactions with the child use the medium of play. All types of material—clay, toys, punching base, doll houses—are used to help the child express the thoughts and feelings inside that they cannot express verbally. The nurse begins to build a trusting, comfortable relationship in which the child feels free to express what is troubling him or her. Adolescents should be able to express their feelings more openly, be able to find alternative solutions to problems, and increase their feelings of control and self-esteem.

The most effective intervention technique for dealing with depression in children is family therapy. Nurses with special training may conduct family therapy sessions. Staff nurses can support the therapy goals by emphasizing the importance of the family sessions to the parents.

Antidepressant medications such as the tricyclics are prescribed by the physician to counteract the depression. The nurse is responsible for administering medications and knowing the dosages, side effects, and adverse effects of the antidepressants. Antidepressant medications are listed in the accompanying display. Patient teaching with regard to medication is vital. Accurate dosage and compliance are critical. Parents may need to regulate the administration of medications at certain times, and therapeutic blood levels should be evaluated on a routine basis.

★ NURSING EVALUATION

The symptoms that signalled the problem of depression should decrease. The child should be able to interact

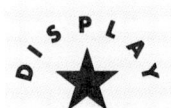

Anti-Depressant Medications

MAO Inhibitors
These drugs nonselectively inhibit the enzyme mono-amine oxidase, which metabolizes neurotransmitters at receptor sites:

> Isocarboxazid (Marplan)
> Phenelzine sulfate (Nardil)
> Tranylcypromine sulfate (Parnate)

Tricyclic Antidepressants
These drugs increase neurotransmitter concentrations of norepinephrine, serotonin, or both, reducing the signs and symptoms of depression:

> Amitriptyline hydrochloride (Elavil, Emitrip, Endep)
> Clomipramine (Anafranil)
> Desipramine hydrochloride (Norpraamin, Pertofrane)
> Doxepin hydrochloride (Adapin, Sinequan)

Imipramine hydrochloride (Janimine, Sk-Pramine, Tofranil)
Nortriptyline hydrochloride (Aventyl, Pamelor)
Protriptyline hydrochloride (Vivactil)
Trimipramine maleate (Surmontil)

Second-Generation Antidepressants
Drugs developed to treat depression with fewer side effects and inhibit reuptake of neurotransmitters norepinephrine or serotonin or both;

> Amoxapine (Asendin)
> Bupropion hydrochloride (Wellbatrin)
> Fluoxetine hydrochloride (Prozac)
> Maprotiline hydrochloride (Ludiomil)
> Trazodone hydrochloride (Desyrel)

(Adapted from material found in: *Baer, C. L., & Williams, B. R. [1992]*. Clinical pharmacology and nursing. *[2nd ed.]. Springhouse, PA: Springhouse Corp.*)

---

with the environment around them. Their affect should brighten and their activity level return to normal. If applicable, parents should be able to recognize the impending symptoms or problems or event that precipitated the child's depression. The behaviors observed in the depression, such as acting out or temper tantrums, should decrease.

Suicide

The rates of suicide in the United States are on the rise. Suicide accounts for the third most common cause of death among teenagers. For every successful suicide, it is estimated that another 150 to 200 attempts were made. Seventy percent of those attempting suicide have a history of depression. Most people have normal mood swings, and occasionally feel sad. If the depressed mood lingers for longer than a 2-week period, however, serious depression could be emerging. Drug overdose is the most common form of suicide attempt. Girls attempt suicide more often than boys, but the boys complete the act more often than girls. Death in boys is more violent, such as hanging or shooting.[9]

Depressed people have a higher rate of suicide. A second group of children at risk for suicide attempts are children with conduct disorders and depression who are facing a disciplinary action.[13] The major consideration is that suicide is a symptom of a variety of disorders. When the adolescent believes there is no other solution to current problems, suicide is perceived as the final option. Other risk factors involved in suicide attempts include:

- A history of suicide within the family or close friends, making it an acceptable means of problem-solving
- Past suicide attempts

- Frequent drug and alcohol abuse
- Social isolation

★ NURSING ASSESSMENT

The greatest obstacle in assessing suicidal ideation in any client is the health professional's ideas about suicide. One of the most lethal myths is the myth that if one asks a person whether they are considering suicide, one will give them the idea to commit suicide. Asking about suicidal intention, however, is often preventative in and of itself. By asking the person whether they are considering suicide, one acknowledges the pain and despair the person is experiencing. The nurse should assess suicidal tendencies in any person that expresses self-destructive thoughts.

The first step in assessment is to ascertain the seriousness of the intent. Has the adolescent taken steps to obtain access to a gun, or a stockpile of pills? Have they recently given away prized possessions? Secondly, do they have a detailed plan on how they intend to commit suicide? Is the plan feasible? Investigation of the intent of the adolescent or child is vital in determining the intervention necessary. Table 19-3 summarizes factors useful in assessing suicide risk.

★ NURSING DIAGNOSES

The following list of nursing diagnoses could be applied to suicidal patients:

- High Risk for Injury related to feelings of aloneness, hopelessness, or rejection.
- Sleep Pattern Disturbance related to inability to sleep, waking early, or sleeping more.

TABLE 19-3
Nursing Assessment: Guidelines for Assessing Risk Status for Patients Who Attempt Suicide

Factor	Minimal Risk	Moderate Risk	High Risk
Method used in attempt	Few pills (e.g., aspirin)	Moderate number of pills Superficial wrist slash	Entire bottle of pills Use of gun or hanging
Associated events	None or an argument	Disciplinary action Failing grades Family illness	Relationship breakup Death of a loved one Pregnancy
Suicidal plan	None	Vague possibilities	Specific
Purpose of act	None or not clear	Relief of shame or guilt To punish others To get attention	Wants to die Escape to join deceased
Prior adjustment	Effective Good grades in school Close friends No prior suicide attempt	Moody Variable grades Some friends Prior suicidal thoughts	Depressed Poor grades Few or no close friends/withdrawn Prior attempt
Family's reaction and structure	Supportive Intact family Good coping and mental health No history of suicide	Mixed reaction Divorced/separated Usually copes and understands	Angry and unsupportive Disorganized Rigid/abusive Prior history of suicide in family

- Hopelessness related to feelings of loss of control, power, or rejection.
- Social Isolation related to withdrawal from friends, peers, and family.
- High-Risk for Self-Directed Violence related to lack of perceived alternative actions.

Nursing interventions used in the treatment of adolescents with suicidal tendencies are similar to those used with adults. The goals of nursing management focus on physical safety, increased self-esteem, expression of emotional pain, and increased feelings of self-determination and control.

Examples of expected outcomes may include:

- Adolescent demonstrates ability to perform assigned tasks.
- Adolescent demonstrates self-esteem by taking more interest in hygiene and grooming.
- Adolescent discusses alternative actions for solving problems.

★ NURSING INTERVENTIONS

As long as the adolescent is at risk for suicide, physical safety is the primary focus. All sharp objects are kept away from the adolescent. This includes not only razors and knifes, but also simple things such as metal coat hangers, belt buckles, and glass or ceramic flower vases. Medication overdose is a popular method of suicide attempt among adolescents. Therefore, the nurse must check to see that any medication given is not hoarded. This may include periodic inspections of the adolescent's belongings and room. Psychiatric units have specific protocols for implementing suicide precautions. The nurse must be familiar with the established protocols.

Along with maintaining a safe environment, the nurse uses herself in a therapeutic manner to help the adolescent increase his or her self-esteem and discuss the pain and isolation of the depression. Praise is given for all small steps taken by the adolescent toward health. This includes being responsible for any tasks assigned, taking an interest in activities, or joining in a conversation with peers or staff. Group therapy session also may be used to help the adolescent deal with his or her feelings. Because most people who are depressed or thinking about suicide will not talk about their feelings, the emergence of verbalization and expression of emotions is critical to therapeutic intervention. Reassurance of help and encouragement that depression and suicidal tendencies can be treated is essential.

★ NURSING EVALUATION

The adolescent may sign a contract agreeing to participate in a care plan. Evaluation involves monitoring for compliance with use of antidepressants and attendance of psychotherapy sessions. Reinforcement from the family and health care professional is essential.

Selected Psychiatric Problems Emerging in Adolescence

Adolescence is recognized as period of extreme vulnerability to outside influence. Adolescents wish to separate themselves from the family and to be accepted by peers. Normal development crises of identity place demands on egos not yet firmly grounded. If their earlier developmental tasks have not been met, adolescents face the task

TABLE 19-4
Comparison of Anorexia Nervosa and Bulimia Nervosa

	Differences	
Similarities	Anorexia Nervosa	Bulimia Nervosa
Eating disorder	Encourages others to eat her food	Eats others' food
Etiology not fully understood	Weight loss	Weight fluctuations
Primary occurrence in women	Amenorrhea	Menstrual disturbances only
Fear of being fat	Denies hunger	Admits strong appetite
Intrapsychic conflicts	Childhood compliance ("model child")	Childhood defiance (possibility of other behavioral problems)

[*Data from:* Futrell, J. A., & Collison, C. R. [1987]. Intervening with families of adolescents with bulimia. In: M. Leaky & L. Wright. *Families and psychosocial problems.* Springhouse, PA: Springhouse Corp., pp. 194–215; and Gelazis, R. S., & Kempe, A. [1988]. Therapy with clients with eating disorders. In: C. K. Beck, S. Rawlings, & Williams [eds.]. *Mental health-psychiatric nursing. A holistic-life cycle approach.* [2nd ed.]. St. Louis: Mosby, pp. 669–679.]

of forming identities without necessary ego strength. Thus, problems that may have not been recognized earlier may now come to the forefront of the adolescent's personality. There are three psychiatric problems that usually are identified as adolescent issues. They are: eating disorders, substance use disorders, and cult involvement.

Eating Disorders

From infancy through adolescence, food and eating behavior can acquire new meanings and significance. Eating disorders often arise from individual and family problems that create stress. Such disorders are a form of maladaptive coping.

Types of Disorders

An eating disorder is the misuse, or perceived misuse, of eating in an attempt to solve or camouflage problems of living that seem otherwise unsolvable. Hence, an eating disorder is by definition symptomatic of emotional and social disturbance. Anorexia nervosa and bulimia are two extreme types of eating disorders of adolescence. Although they are two distinct entities, anorexia nervosa and bulimia nervosa have much in common, with the primary motivation being fear of being fat (Table 19-4).

Anorexia Nervosa Anorexia nervosa is a life-threatening psychiatric disorder characterized by self-induced starvation. The anorexic adolescent has a distorted body image and is fearful of becoming obese. Despite a marked preoccupation with food and food preparation, there is a refusal to eat and a denial of hunger.

There is a major debate in the literature about whether the incidence of anorexia nervosa has increased in the last 45 years.[4] This eating disorder has recently been estimated to occur in 1 of 100 American adolescents, mostly girls (female:male ratio of 9:1). Anorexia nervosa

is common between the ages of 13 and 18 years, with two peaks at 13 to 14 years and 17 to 18 years. Only 50% of treated cases recover. Death occurs in 15% to 21% of the diagnostic cases.[4] Most reports of anorexia nervosa have involved the Caucasian population in the Western world. Only within the past decade has it been reported in other races, both in the United States and in Africa.[4]

Bulimia Nervosa In *bulimia nervosa* (also called bulimarexia, the gorge-purge syndrome, or dietary chaos syndrome), periods of craving for food result in binges and purging. During binging, the person consumes a high number of calories (an average of 3415 calories per binge).[5] The binge is followed by self-induced vomiting; purging with laxatives, diuretics, or enemas; or vigorous exercise. Until recently, the incidence of bulimia nervosa was not known. Currently, the only country to provide statistics about estimated rates of this disorder is the United States. Estimates about bulimia nervosa are especially uncertain, because some studies fail to differentiate between binge eating, which is not unusual among young women, and bulimia.

Etiologic Theories

Five theoretical approaches to anorexia and bulimia are presented in this chapter. Figure 19-2 demonstrates the inter-relationship between the multiple factors associated with anorexia nervous, including biologic, psychological, and social. A similar model could be proposed for bulimia.

Psychoanalytic Theory According to psychoanalytic theorists, eating disorders are a form of regression to prepuberty. Anorectic and bulimic behaviors are maladaptive responses to dealing with life stresses, especially with the transition into adolescence and with sexuality.

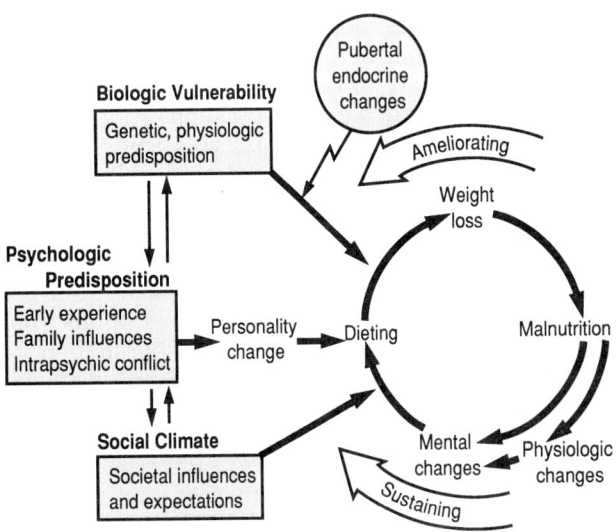

FIGURE 19-2
A theoretical model for understanding the multiple factors associated with anorexia nervosa. Such a model could be similarly constructed for bulimia. (*Reprinted with permission from:* Lucas, A. R. [1981]. Toward the understanding of anorexia nervosa as a disease entity. *Mayo Clin Proc,* 56, 258.)

Cognitive Theory Cognitive theorists believe that perceptual disturbances contribute to these two conditions. Distorted body image and irrational thoughts result in a paradoxical obsession with having food and the simultaneous need to get rid of it by abstaining, exercising excessively, or eliminating it through vomiting, diuretics, purges, or enemas.

Developmental/Family Systems Theory Developmental and family systems theorists attribute the eating disorders to intrafamilial conflicts. Early familial interaction involving parents who have high expectations and who are overly controlling, overprotective, and rigid often results in disturbed family dynamics. Such dynamics result in a dependent child who cannot adequately cope with the normal, stressful adolescent developmental tasks of separation, self-mastery, and control. In this context, anorexia may be the way in which an overly compliant adolescent struggles for autonomy and self-control. In contrast, bulimic children are defiant rather than compliant and experience more obvious family conflict. Thus, bulimia may be another form of rebellion and disobedience.

Cultural Theory Another approach suggests that anorectic and bulimic children suffer from a cultural obsession with thinness. Eating disorders almost exclusively affect middle or upper class young women. A continuum may exist from normal female adolescent development to the development of eating disorders, in which thinness and dieting become symbolically tied to autonomous career development and a denial of the need for interpersonal relationships. Studies of Japanese-American, English, and Irish girls further corroborate this theory. These studies support the pioneer research of Douvan and Adelson,[6] who proposed a reversal of Erikson's stages of identity and intimacy for adolescent girls: the developmental task of the girl is first to achieve intimacy through close relationships; that of the boy is to achieve identity. In follow-up studies,[27] high school girls were concerned with self-concept and interdependence or relationship issues; male students were concerned with role function (school grades, new job, etc.). Hence, in a culture emphasizing perfection, we find obsessions with physical appearance and thinness and the possible genesis of body image distortions and eating disorders.

Organic/Neurologic Theory Futrell and Collison[8] suggest that anorexia nervosa and bulimia could result from a disturbance in the appetite center in the hypothalamus. Other theories posit that bulimia results from neurologic dysfunction (much like parkinsonism) or from endocrine dysfunction. Recent research has documented low levels of cholecystokinin (CCK). The low level of CCK has been related to a lack of satisfaction after a meal, so that the adolescent continues to eat to feel satisfied. The current question is whether the low level of CCK is the cause of bulimia or the result of the repeated binge-purge cycles.[25]

★ NURSING ASSESSMENT

The nursing assessment of eating disorders includes an individual and family history, physical assessments, diagnostic studies and psychosocial assessments (Table 19-5). A multidisciplinary team is beneficial in completing the assessment of eating disorders and initiating the planning and goal setting for the adolescent and family.

ANOREXIA NERVOSA

Table 19-6 lists clinical manifestations of anorexia nervosa. The clinical assessment for anorexia nervosa includes severe weight loss in the absence of organic disease. The adolescent with anorexia nervosa has cessation of menses, dry skin, stringy hair, sunken abdomen, and no fat so that every bone is visible.[13] Physiologic symptoms include low blood pressure, slow pulse, low basal metabolism, anemia, and sleep disturbances.[13] A psychiatric assessment is also needed to confirm the diagnosis and to establish a baseline for psychotherapy and family therapy. A clear distinguishing factor in anorexia nervosa is the adolescent's refusal to eat. The adolescent does not have a loss of appetite, but does not eat because of an unrealistic view of her weight. Common traits of adolescents with anorexia nervosa include:[13]

- Denial of illness
- Active refusal of food or binge eating and vomiting–purging
- Overactivity and perfectionism
- Disturbance of body image

TABLE 19-5
Nursing Assessment: Guidelines for Assessing Eating Disorders

History
 Individual

- Eating patterns, daily calorie intake
- Patterns of elimination (bulimia nervosa)
- Level of physical activity
- Menstrual history
- School performance and other parental expectation(s)
- Any drugs used
- Social activities, leisure time
- Developmental history to date and length or chronicity of condition

 Family

- Genogram of parent–child relationships
- Relationships with siblings and outside acquaintances (friends, schoolmates)
- Marital relationship (discussion should not be held in the presence of the child)
- Decision-making and conflict resolution patterns
- Family members' own perceptions of the problem(s)
- Related family history

Physical Examination

- General appearance, screening for signs of malnutrition in skin, hair, eyes, mouth, teeth, nails
- Weight and height with comparison to the growth chart norms
- Cardiac and renal systems screening, including vital signs

Diagnostic Studies

- Serum electrolyte studies and complete blood count
- Urinalysis
- Hormone studies
- Radiological and barium studies (in bulimia nervosa)

Psychosocial Assessment

- Family communications: clues to enmeshed family (sitting arrangement, parent speaking for adolescent)
- Predominant emotions, moodiness

TABLE 19-6
Clinical Manifestations of Eating Disorders

Manifestation	Anorexia Nervosa	Bulimia Nervosa
Physical	Disturbed body image	Recurrent episodes of rapid consumption of large amounts of high-calorie food, usually in less than 2 hours
	Weight loss of at least 15% of original weight	Inconspicuous eating
	Absence of known physical illness	Termination of eating episodes by sleep, social interruption, or abdominal pain or self-induced vomiting
	Absence of three consecutive menstrual cycles	Repeated attempts to reduce weight by severe, restricted diets, self-induced vomiting, or use of cathartics or diuretics
	Yellow-tinged skin (hypercarotenemia)	Frequent weight fluctuations of more than 10 pounds coinciding with binges and fasts
	Lanugo (fine body hair) possibly due to prolonged malnutrition	No known physical illness
	Deterioration of teeth, mucous membranes, hair, nails, loss of muscle mass, and dependent edema	
	Fatigue, hypotension, and bradycardia, as weight continues to drop	
Emotional	Intense fear of becoming obese	Fear of not being able to stop eating voluntarily
	Feelings of fatness even when emaciated	Before binge eating: anxiety, helplessness, anger, depression, sense of futility, inability to meet others' expectations, or elation and joy
	Coldness, indifference, anxiety, anger, and withdrawal	During and after the binge-purge behavior: guilt, repulsion, self-disgust, or excitement, increased energy, and stimulation
	Being out of touch with own emotions	Tension (the Antecedent) drives bulimic adolescents to the Behavior of binging and purging, which relieves the tension and produces euphoria or an almost sexual release followed by calmness and a sense of relaxation (Consequence) (See Chap. 18, Fig. 18-2.)
	Fear of sexual maturity, feeling of incompetence in dealing with a changing body and new social and emotional requirements	
Cognitive	Constant preoccupation with food, and refusal to maintain body weight above a minimum for age and height	Self-deprecating thoughts after binge eating
	Negative attitude about self and own achievements	Refusal to acknowledge inner stress or adjustment difficulties
	Irrational beliefs (e.g., must be perfect in everything)	Denial of underlying emotional problem(s)
	Attempts to be in control of all aspects of own life	
Social	Low self-esteem	Low self-esteem
	Isolation and alienation from significant others	Family dynamics that involve power struggles, dependence, enmeshed roles, or identities
	Other behavior including excessive exercising, compulsive weighing of oneself, and food rituals	History of other impulsive behavior (e.g., shoplifting, alcohol or drug abuse, suicide attempts, and self-mutilation)

(Data from a variety of sources.)

- Inaccurate perception of hunger and other bodily sensations
- Deficit in sense of identity and effectiveness

BULIMIA

Table 19-6 lists clinical manifestations of bulimia. The assessment of the adolescent for bulimia nervosa should include careful observations of the eating habits. The adolescent with bulimia consumes 5000 or more calories in a single binge, and follows the binge with some form of purging. Strict dieting, fasting, or vigorous exercise programs to maintain weight may be a sign of a problem. Health problems are related to the purge activities and include abnormal blood chemistries, severe abdominal pain, inflammation of the salivary glands, gastritis or esophagitis, fatigue, weakness, and seizures.

★ NURSING DIAGNOSES AND PLANNING

Possible nursing diagnoses in eating disorders include the following:

- Altered Nutrition: Less Than Body Requirements related to fear of obesity.
- Bowel Incontinence related to use of laxatives.
- Fluid Volume Deficit related to self-induced vomiting.
- Ineffective Individual Coping related to inability to accept self and own limitations.
- Ineffective Familial Coping: Compromised related to overly rigid parental expectations.
- Social Isolation related to role conflict.
- Hopelessness related to repeated binge-purge behavior.

Immediate goals are to correct the adolescent's nutritional deficiencies and to restore the nutritional status to normal, using a holistic approach (i.e., addressing the mind, body, and spirit as a unit). The long-term goals are to maintain the adolescent's appropriate weight, to create a supportive environment to facilitate communication between the client and the family (especially to encourage the adolescent to express personal needs, concerns, and feelings and to manage them appropriately) and to teach effective family stress management and control. Examples of outcome criteria are the following:

- Adolescent discusses dietary needs.
- Adolescent participates in an exercise program.
- Adolescent lists relaxation techniques for bedtime.

★ NURSING INTERVENTIONS

The adolescent with an eating disorder often misunderstands bodily functions. Patient teaching centers on presenting a clear and accurate description of the systems, particularly digestive and reproductive. Pamphlets, models, and diagrams are often extremely helpful.

Girls with an eating disorder have difficulties with accepting their body image and sexuality. Most are frightened by the changes occurring during adolescence, and confuse the ability to control weight with the ability to be happy and successful. Interventions focus on helping the individuals become comfortable with themselves and accepting change. Because of their concrete thinking, adolescents with eating disorders tend to have poor problem solving, stress, and coping skills with which to face the world. A major focus of intervention is teaching the adolescent new and better ways of making decisions.

The crucial aspect of nursing intervention in eating disorders is the ability of the nurse to establish and maintain a therapeutic relationship with the adolescent. This task is often more easily said than done, because of the nature of the adolescent's behavior. The nurse must have extreme patience and be able to handle the adolescent's tendency to try to manipulate the staff.[19]

MANAGEMENT OF THE ADOLESCENT WITH ANOREXIA NERVOSA

Depending on the adolescent's condition, hospitalization often is needed to allow nutritional rehabilitation. This generally is initiated slowly through a balanced 1200-calorie, salt-limited diet, which may be blended to prevent the client from discarding any particular food. Calories and size of feeding are increased gradually. A weekly weight gain of about 2 pounds is sought. Potential problems (abdominal distention, constipation, diarrhea, and edema) must be monitored. Rest and a specified regimen of daily exercise are encouraged. A daily monitoring of fluid and calorie intake, urine output, elimination, serum electrolytes, and other blood values is necessary. Pharmacotherapy may be used during hospitalization, when the adolescent may suffer from concurrent anxiety or depression.

The nurse must be sensitive and supportive, yet firm and consistent, in encouraging consumption of food during mealtimes. Power struggles must be avoided, because although weight gain and nutritional improvement are

necessary, they are not in themselves sufficient for recovery. The anorectic adolescent must be guided by the nurse toward these ultimate goals:

- Overcome fear of being fat and of gaining weight.
- Gain insight into the seriousness of the eating problem and its effect on her health.
- Be aware of her compulsion to control the environment through maladaptive eating pattern.
- Provide reality orientation (replacing her irrational thinking and distorted perceptions with more healthful ideas) about accepting her imperfections, developing mutually supportive relationships, and accepting responsibility for making mistakes.

The adolescent should be involved in her own care. The nurse can help her establish some mutually agreed-on goals with graded, realistic targets for weight gain. Principles of behavior modification must be applied. Positive reinforcers (visiting privileges, recreational or school-related activities, new clothes, records) should be selected carefully and need to be contingent on progress toward the selected goals. The use of negative reinforcers (tube feeding or hyperalimentation, bed rest) are indicated only if the adolescent is severely ill and refuses all oral intake or regurgitates food.

Management is challenging, because these adolescents are proficient with manipulative behaviors. The nurse needs to anticipate frustrations and be empathetic while understanding that the patient feels safe within the bounds of her maladaptive behavior and may probably resist treatment. The need to involve the family in intervention strategies is paramount. It is not unusual, however, for family members to object to family therapy sessions, because they believe the anorectic adolescent is the only one who needs help. In this situation the nurse must act as advocate for the anorectic client to help everyone recognize the importance of the whole family's involvement and support. The nurse should understand that some parents feel guilty, even desperate, about their child's condition; this may be reflected in their manner with the health care staff. Also, the nurse should be prepared and prepare the parents for possible complaints by the adolescent about the "strict" or even "cruel" nursing care; such a response is quite common when confronting and enforcing a change in behavior.

A multidisciplinary perspective is essential if the interventions are to be successful. Collaboration with the pediatrician or family physician, dietitian, psychiatrist or psychiatric nurse, school or community health nurse, and teacher is required both in the hospital and in the community. In addition, the involvement of support persons (a sibling or friend, or a pastor or priest) who may act as coach or mediator should be encouraged. The referral to self-help support groups—available through national organizations and usually listed in the telephone or community services directories—can contribute to the recovery process, as well as to the prevention of further serious deterioration from this form of self-destructive behavior.

MANAGEMENT OF THE ADOLESCENT WITH BULIMIA NERVOSA

Basically, the bulimic client is aware of her abnormal eating behavior and of her lack of control. She may feel guilty, frustrated, and angry and become involved in dysfunctional behavior (e.g., drug abuse, sexual promiscuity). Therefore, both regulation of her physiologic status and assistance with cognitive and behavioral changes are necessary. The nurse monitors serum electrolytes, monitors a strict weight assessment, and encourages adequate, balanced oral intake.

A combination of self-monitoring and contracts is initiated to encourage the adolescent to stop using laxatives, diuretics, and induced vomiting. Close observation by a support person or coach is needed, especially after meals. It may be helpful to plan the number, size, and frequency of meals, and to have the client keep a diary of binges. Reinforcement techniques can help the bulimic client gain control. Efforts should be made to help the adolescent recognize and manage her stress and tension more productively. Physical activity, relaxation techniques, and talking to others are some ways of diffusing tension.

Psychotherapy and family counseling are also recommended. It is essential to help the bulimic adolescent improve her self-concept; she can do this by participating in worthwhile projects, having meaningful relationships, developing a sense of humor, and learning to give herself positive messages. Alternate methods of managing family stress should be explored in family sessions, to increase positive family coping.

★ NURSING EVALUATION

Evidence of weight gain and laboratory values within normal ranges indicate that the adolescent has complied with the prescribed nutritional regimen. Improved problem-solving skills and evidence of better coping mechanisms are essential for long-term therapy. Because many theorists believe that suppressed fear is at the crux of the eating disorders, ventilation of anger is a sign that an alternative avenue for coping is open.

Substance Use Disorders

Although not strictly a problem of adolescence, substance abuse and dependency often begins during the adolescent period. Substance use disorders are separated into two categories: abuse and dependency. Substance abusers continue to use drugs or alcohol in spite of knowing that it is harmful, and they use the substance in situations where it is dangerous. Dependency occurs when the person has to have more of the substance to

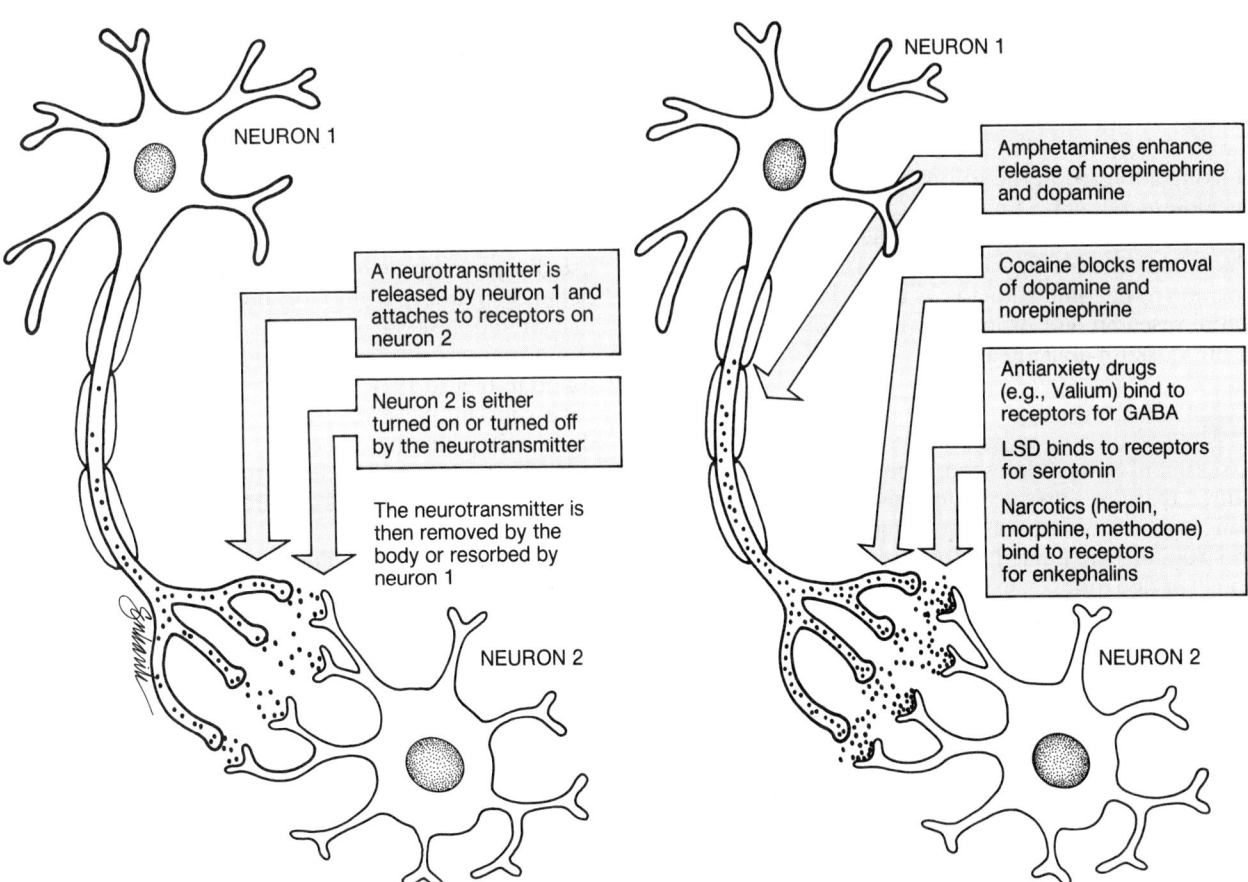

FIGURE 19-3
How drugs affect brain chemistry. (A) Brain activity depends on neurotransmitters, chemical messages that either inhibit or excite neurons. Dopamine excites neurons. Norepinephrine and acetylcholine may be either, depending on the receptors. (B) Drugs affect both neurotransmitters and receptors. (*Redrawn from:* Hales, D. [1992]. *An invitation to health.* [5th ed]. [p. 342]. Redwood City, CA: Benjamin/Cummings.)

acquire the same effect and the person has no control over the desire for the substance. When this happens, obtaining and using the substance is the most important thing happening in the person's life.

There are almost as many theories regarding the cause of substance use disorders as there are abused substances. The problem of dependency and abuse crosses race, sex, and economic lines. There is no "typical drug abuser" that helps identify those who are at risk. Adolescents in general are at risk for abuse and dependency because of two factors: 1) peer pressure with a need to be accepted by the group, and 2) the adolescent's belief of infallibility, or "it can't happen to me" belief. These two factors can influence the adolescent to use drugs and alcohol in an experimental mode, and can ultimately lead to the dependency of the adolescent on the substance. What is known about the adolescent substance user is that drug use is correlated with early anti-authority and antisocial behavior.[21]

Commonly used substances are alcohol, marijuana, cocaine, opiates, hallucinogens, inhalants, sedative-hypnotics, and nicotine.[3] Although not all drugs are addictive physically, all are related to psychological addiction. The use of one of the above seriously increases the odds that other substances, or multiple substances, are abused. Figure 19-3 demonstrates the effects of the drug on the central nervous system.

Unlike other disorders, abusers fall into no particular stereotypic risk group. Incidence rates are misleading, because a large percentage of abusers are "enabled" or kept out of the health care system unless serious physiologic consequences have emerged. To illustrate the differences between adult substance abuse and that of the abusing adolescent, the following comparison is made: an adolescent can become an alcoholic in 6 to 18 months, whereas it takes 5 to 15 years for the adult to become an alcoholic.[3] The biologic implications and genetic predisposition to become addictive is an important avenue for future research. For example, children of alcoholics are at high risk for abusing alcohol.

★ **NURSING ASSESSMENT**

Assessment of the adolescent who abuses substances requires that the nurse examine his or her own feelings concerning substance use. A nonjudgmental attitude is the best tool the nurse has for assessing the presence of abuse or dependency in an adolescent. Persons who use and abuse drugs and alcohol are extremely sensitive to nonverbal clues given by others. They often use this information to manipulate the situation to their own advantage. In abuse and dependency situations, this includes the tendency to deny the problem and or to place the blame elsewhere.

One of the universal signs of abuse in adolescence is a change in behavior. This includes the time spent at home, as well as the time at school. Kids who were outgoing, friendly, and well mannered become withdrawn, angry, and disruptive. The exact behaviors will depend on the substance that is being abused. Table 19-7 provides an outline of mild to severe specific signs and symptoms of various drugs.

Because the main symptom of abuse is denial of a problem, it is often difficult to assess substance use disorder. This is especially true if the assessment takes place as a one-time encounter, unless the setting is an emergency room. Assessment must include careful observation of the adolescent, as well as an interview with both family and school personnel who can give an account of the adolescent's behavior. Indications of drug/alcohol abuse are provided in the accompanying Nursing Assessment display. The nurse is encouraged to ask for consultation from other health professionals, particularly drug counselors, in assessment of substance use disorders. There are also nurses who are Certified Addictions Registered Nurses (CARN), who have been identified by the National Nurses Society on Addictions (NNSA).

★ **NURSING DIAGNOSES AND PLANNING**

The following are potential diagnoses that can be applied to patients involved in substance abuse:

- Ineffective Individual Coping related to abusing substances.
- Self-Esteem Disturbance related to destructive behaviors.
- Social Isolation related to reliance on drugs to alter situations.
- High Risk for Injury related to altered levels of awareness.

Possible outcome criteria are the following:

- Patient contrasts experiences when on drugs versus drug-free.
- Patient participates in a drug rehabilitation program.

★ **NURSING INTERVENTION**

The interventions discussed here for use in substance use disorders are of a general nature. Specific protocols depend on the type, amount, and nature of the substance that the adolescent is abusing. The long-term physical manifestations of marijuana and codeine use/abuse are found in Figure 19-4. Intervention with adolescents who have substance use disorders are primarily handled by those who have expertise in the field. A primary intervention of the nurse is referral to the appropriate agency. Some community resources are listed in the accompanying display.

One of the most difficult problems associated with intervention is the denial of the problem by the person who is abusing the substance. Often, it is not until a crisis has emerged that the person is willing to come for help. Again, the nurse's main intervention is the ability to establish a therapeutic relationship with the adolescent. Trust and belief in others is often lacking in their history, making it very difficult for the person to ask for help.

Intervention focuses first on getting the adolescent physically free from drugs. Detoxification protocols vary with the substance being abused. The psychological freeing of the adolescent from the need for substances then becomes the primary focus for intervention. The need for the substance, and what problems the substance is supposed to cure, are discussed and confronted. Finally, new ways of coping that do not include substances are introduced.

TABLE 19-7
Effects of Abuse of Various Substances

Drug and Method of Administration	Physical and Possible Psychological Dependence (Phys)	(Psych)	Effect of Intoxication	Risks With Long-Term Use	Withdrawal Effect
Opiates					
Opium*†	↑	↑	Euphoria; emotional lability; drowsiness; clouding of consciousness; psychomotor retardation; slow and shallow breathing; nausea; constricted pupils; decreased muscle tone, with circulatory collapse and cyanosis; dilated pupils; coma; possible death	Physical dependence; malnutrition; lowered immunity; infections of the heart lining and valves; skin abscesses; congested lungs; tetanus; hepatitis; liver disease; HIV infection from sharing needles; overdose; death	Runny nose; watery eyes; severe anxiety to panic; gooseflesh; chills and sweating; yawning; irritability; loss of appetite; muscle cramps; tremors; tachycardia; hypertension; increased respirations and temperature; insomnia; nausea and vomiting; diarrhea and dehydration
Morphine‡†	↑	↑			
Diacetylmorphine (heroin)‡#	↑	↑			
Meperidine (Demerol)*‡	↑	↑			
Codeine*‡	→	↑			
Methadone*‡	↑	↑			
Depressants					
Sedative-hypnotics					
Barbiturates					
Amobarbital (Amytal)*‡	↑	↑	Slurred speech; irritability; impaired attention, memory, and judgment; emotional lability; talkativeness; lack of coordination; disorientation; tremors; cold and clammy skin; dilated pupils (with barbiturates, constricted pupils); drunken behavior without alcohol odor	Disrupted sleep; dangerously impaired vision; increased risk of fatal overdose as higher dosage required; birth defects	Nausea and vomiting; weakness; hypertension; tachycardia; orthostatic hypotension; gross tremors; agitation; disorientation; anxiety; nightmares; insomnia; visual hallucinations; hyperthermia; delirium; convulsions; coma; possible death
Pentobarbital (Nembutal)*‡	↑	↑			
Secobarbital (Seconal)*‡	↑	↑			
Miscellaneous					
Meprobamate (Equinal, Miltown)*	→	→		Physical and psychological dependence; overdose	
Diazepam (Valium)*	→	→			
Glutethimide (Doriden)*	↑	↑			
Chloral hydrate (Noctec)*	↑	↑			
Alcohol*			Slurred speech; lack of coordination; unsteady gait; impaired attention; talkativeness; euphoria or depression; emotional lability	Stupor to coma; physical dependence; liver damage; malnutrition; fetal damage (fetal alcohol syndrome)	Hyperactivity; tremors; psychomotor agitation; hypertension; tachycardia; irritability or depression; impaired attention; memory loss; auditory or visual hallucinations; disorientation; delusions; delirium; orthostatic hypotension; convulsions
Stimulants					
Cocaine‡#	→	↑	Increased alertness; excitation; psychomotor agitation; increased pulse rate and BP; dilated pupils; perspiration and chills; impaired judgment; psychotic symptoms; loss of appetite; insomnia; tremors; confusion; convulsions; possible death	Damage to nose (if snorted), blood vessels, and heart; chest pain; disruptions in heart rhythm; stroke; liver and lung damage; possible hepatitis and HIV infection; malnutrition; miscarriage; impaired fetus	Fatigue; depression; long periods of sleep or disturbed sleep; apathy; cravings; irritability; disorientation
Amphetamine (Benzedrine, Dexedrine)*‡	↓	↑			
Methylphenidate (Ritalin)*	↓	↑			
Phenmetrazine (Preludin)*					
Hallucinogens					
Lysergic acid diethylamide (LSD)*	0	?	Dilated pupils; tachycardia; hypertension; hyperthermia; hyperreflexia; nausea; visual hallucinations; extreme emotional lability; poor time perception; feeling of depersonalization; psychic numbness; psychosis; violent outbursts; amnesia; convulsions; possible death	LSD: disturbing flashbacks; psychological dependence PCP: stupor; increased heart rate and blood pressure; convulsions; coma; ruptured cerebral blood vessels; cardiopulmonary failure; death	Not reported; however, in PCP use, flashbacks may occur for 5 or more days with unpredictable behavior
Phencyclidine (PCP)*‡†	0	?			
Mescaline*‡	0	?			

(Continued)

TABLE 19-7
(Continued)

Drug and Method of Administration	Physical and Possible Psychological Dependence (Phys)	(Psych)	Effect of Intoxication	Risks With Long-Term Use	Withdrawal Effect
Cannabis sativa					
Marijuana, hashish, hashish oil*†	?	→	Euphoria; disorientation; hallucinations; delusions; panic; depression; flashbacks; psychosis; apathy; impaired attention and judgment; increased appetite	Malnutrition; skin disorders; ulcers; lack of sleep; depression; vitamin deficiencies; brain damage; high blood pressure; stroke; heart failure; hyperthermia; violent behavior; fatal overdose	Irritability; insomnia; hyperactivity; tremors; perspiration; nausea; loss of appetite in some users

Key for Method of Administration:
*Oral
†Smoked
‡Injected
#Sniffed.

Key for Dependence:
↑ High
→ Moderate
↓ Possible
? Degree unknown
0 None.

Data for this table are from a variety of sources.

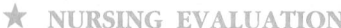

★ NURSING EVALUATION

Often the process of intervening in substance use disorders is slow and frustrating for the health professional. The physical detoxification of the adolescent is relatively easy. The psychological healing is not. The nurse needs to be aware that successful handling of substance use disorders rarely occur the first time the adolescent is admitted for treatment, and repeated episodes are expected.

Cult Involvement

Concern over adolescents and cults has increased in the last decade, because there has been a reported increase in numbers of adolescents involved in cults, particularly satanism. Involvement in a cult, whether Satanism or a religious group such as the Hari Krishna, is primarily a youth phenomenon. Those who are drawn to such organizations are usually dissatisfied with their life,

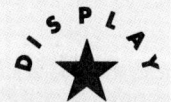

Nursing Assessment: Guidelines for Observation of Substance Abuse in Adolescents

DRUGS

- An abrupt change in attitude, including a lack of interest in activities once enjoyed
- Frequent vague, withdrawn moods
- A sudden resistance to discipline or criticism
- Secret telephone calls and meetings, and a demand for greater privacy concerning personal possessions
- Increased frustration levels
- Changes in sleeping and eating habits
- A sudden weight loss
- Evidence of drug use (smell of marijuana, drug paraphernalia)
- Frequent borrowing of money
- Stealing
- Disregard of personal appearance
- Impaired relationships with family and friends
- Ignoring deadlines, curfews, or other regulations
- Unusual flare-ups of temper
- New friends, especially known drug users, and strong allegiance to these friends

ALCOHOL

- Experiencing the following symptoms after drinking: frequent headaches, nausea, stomach pain, heartburn, gas, fatigue, weakness, muscle cramps, or irregular rapid heartbeats
- Needing a drink at specific times in the day (for example, to start the day)
- Denying having any problem with alcohol
- Doing things while drinking that are regretted afterwards
- Dramatic mood swings, from anger to laughter to anxiety
- Sleep problems
- Depression and paranoia
- Forgetting what happened during a drinking episode
- Changing brands or going on the wagon to control drinking
- Having five or more drinks a day

(Data from: *Hales, D.* [1992]. *An invitation to health.* [5th ed.]. [pp. 348, 390]. *Redwood, CA: Benjamin/Cummings.*)

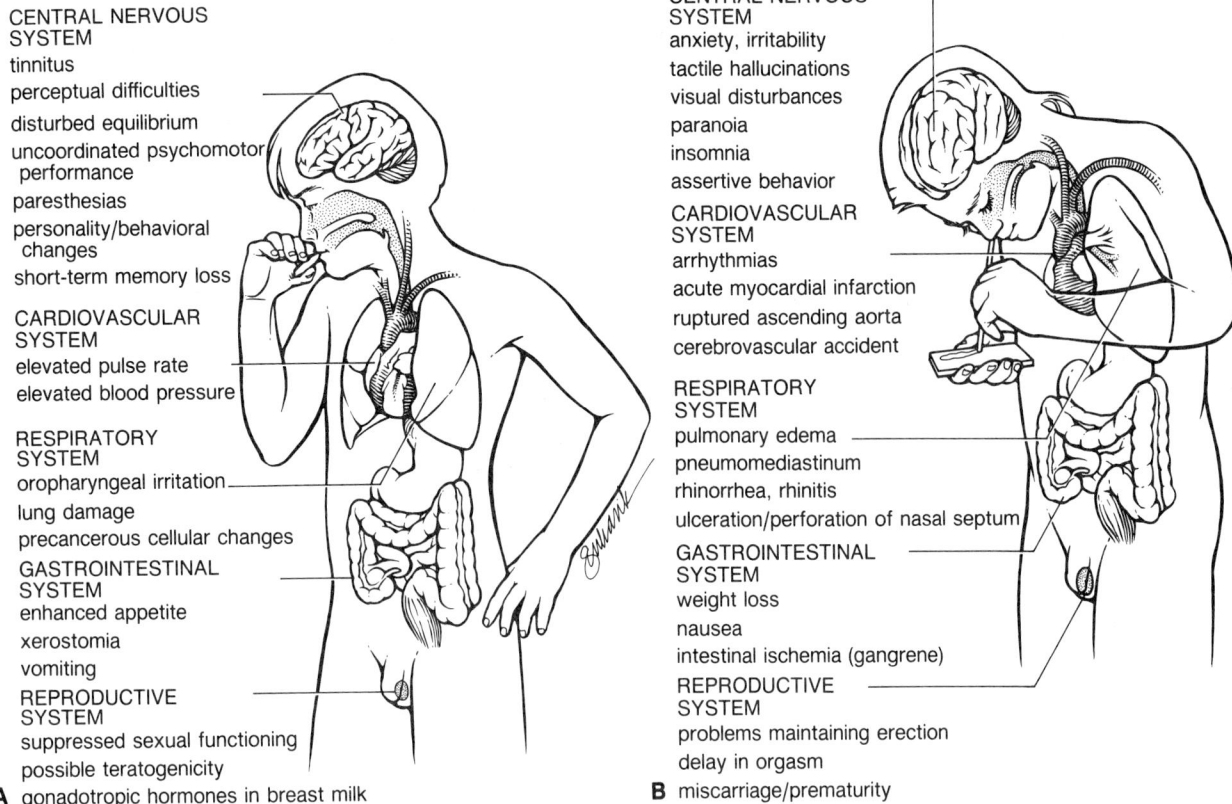

CENTRAL NERVOUS
SYSTEM
tinnitus
perceptual difficulties
disturbed equilibrium
uncoordinated psychomotor
  performance
paresthesias
personality/behavioral
  changes
short-term memory loss

CARDIOVASCULAR
SYSTEM
elevated pulse rate
elevated blood pressure

RESPIRATORY
SYSTEM
oropharyngeal irritation
lung damage
precancerous cellular changes

GASTROINTESTINAL
SYSTEM
enhanced appetite
xerostomia
vomiting

REPRODUCTIVE
SYSTEM
suppressed sexual functioning
possible teratogenicity
A gonadotropic hormones in breast milk

CENTRAL NERVOUS
SYSTEM
anxiety, irritability
tactile hallucinations
visual disturbances
paranoia
insomnia
assertive behavior

CARDIOVASCULAR
SYSTEM
arrhythmias
acute myocardial infarction
ruptured ascending aorta
cerebrovascular accident

RESPIRATORY
SYSTEM
pulmonary edema
pneumomediastinum
rhinorrhea, rhinitis
ulceration/perforation of nasal septum

GASTROINTESTINAL
SYSTEM
weight loss
nausea
intestinal ischemia (gangrene)

REPRODUCTIVE
SYSTEM
problems maintaining erection
delay in orgasm
B miscarriage/prematurity

FIGURE 19-4
Effects of chronic drug use on the body. (**A**) Effects of chronic marijuana use. Psychic and perceptual effects may vary widely, depending on mental status, mood, previous experience, expectations, environment, and particular circumstances. Chronic use may result in psychologic dependence but physical dependence is rare. (**B**) Effects of chronic cocaine use. Repeated use can lead to an overwhelming psychologic dependence, which is characterized by extreme involvement in procuring and using the drug daily. There is also a true physical dependence. (*Data from:* Malseed, R.T. [1990]. *Pharmacology: Drug therapy and nursing considerations* [3rd ed]. [pp. 838, 840]. Philadelphia: J. B. Lippincott.)

or are not willing to take on the traditional roles of adulthood. The lure of the cult for the adolescent is "the promise of acceptance by others, security, and freedom from unwanted responsibility and decision making."[21]

Common personality characteristics of adolescents involved in satanism have been identified. These adolescents usually describe themselves as loners, feel as if they do not fit in, and are the black sheep of the family. Most are angry, depressed, and paranoid. They are not interested in the normal peer group activities. Alcohol and drug abuse are almost always present.[29]

★ NURSING ASSESSMENT

Assessment of the adolescent suspected of cult involvement requires that the nurse have at least some knowledge about the cult that is in question. In assessing involvement, one must be aware of the activities and symbols associated with the cult. Knowledge of a few of the symbols, however, does not necessarily imply that the adolescent is involved in the cult. One also must be able to ascertain the depth of knowledge. Adolescents who are involved in the satanic cults are reported to be involved in the following activities:

- Use of tarot cards or ouija boards
- Meetings of covens on a regular basis to worship Satan
- Conducting seances to request Satan's presence
- Chanting used to unify Satan worshipers
- Conducting "black weddings" to signify marriage to Satan
- Sacrificing animals and drinking animal blood
- Conducting ceremonies in cemeteries and focusing on death
- Reading books on Satanism
- Listening to heavy metal rock music
- Selling one's soul to Satan in return for power[29]

★ NURSING DIAGNOSES AND PLANNING

Nursing diagnoses useful in adolescent cult disorders includes the following:

- Ineffective Individual Coping.
- Social Isolation.
- Self-Esteem Disturbance.
- High Risk for Injury.
- High Risk for Self-Directed Violence.

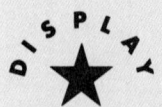

Resources for Adolescents and Families With Substance Abuse

Alcohol and Drug Abuse Problems Association
of America, Inc.
444 North Capitol Street, N.W., Suite 181
Washington, DC 20001

Alcohol, Drug Abuse, and Mental Health
Administration
5600 Fishers Lane
Rockville, Maryland 20857

American Academy of Psychiatrists in Alcoholism
and Addictions
PO Box 376
Greenbelt, Maryland 20770

American Council for Drug Education
204 Monroe Street
Rockville, Maryland 20850

American Medical Society on Alcoholism and
Other Drug Dependencies
6525 West North Avenue, #204
Oak Park, Illinois 60302

Association for Medical Education and Research
in Substance Abuse
Brown University, Box G
Providence, Rhode Island 02912

Committee on Problems of Drug Dependence, Inc.
3420 N. Broad Street
Philadelphia, Pennsylvania 19140

National Clearinghouse for Alcohol and Drug
Information
PO Box 2345
Rockville, Maryland 20852

National Council on Alcoholism, Inc.
12 West 21st Street
New York, New York 10010

National Federation of Parents for Drug-Free
Youth
8730 Georgia Avenue, Suite 200
Silver Spring, Maryland 20910

National Institute on Alcohol Abuse and
Alcoholism
5600 Fishers Lane, Room 16-105
Rockville, Maryland 20857

National Institute on Drug Abuse
5600 Fishers Lane, Room 10-05
Rockville, Maryland 20587

National Self-Help Clearinghouse
33 West 42nd Street
New York, New York 10036

(American Psychiatric Association Joint Commission on Public Affairs and the Division of Public Affairs. [1988]. Washington, D.C.: American Psychiatric Association.)

Outcome criteria may include the following:

- Adolescent discusses importance of cult to his self-esteem
- Adolescent participates in school activities on a regular basis.

★ NURSING INTERVENTIONS

Interventions with adolescents involved in cults focus on substituting something more attractive and meaningful to the adolescent for cult involvement. Often, the adolescent is removed from the situation, and all things associated with the cult are removed from the environment. The goal is to decrease the negative reinforcement of the cult and replace it with positive reinforcement of activities unrelated to cult activities. Insight is developed into why the cult involvement was so attractive to the adolescent. Verbalization of needs is encouraged, and acting out behavior is discouraged.[29]

★ NURSING EVALUATION

The ability of the family to incorporate the adolescent and make changes in their way of functioning is probably the most reliable measurement for evaluation. No matter

how successful the treatment program, if the adolescent returns to the same family situation, the chances of maintaining the success are extremely slim. If the family is able to support the adolescent, however, the chances increase dramatically that the changes made during the treatment will last.

Summary

The mental health issues of childhood and adolescence require the nurse to be aware of the needs of the child from a cognitive, moral, and psychosocial developmental viewpoints. Whether a mental health problem is related to an organic or nonorganic origin, the key to effective treatment programs is family and child therapy. The disorders suffered by children and adolescents require specific treatment plans, which include psychiatric, medical, and nursing interventions. The nurse plays a major role in the early case finding of children having difficulties. Through the National Institutes of Mental Health, nurse researchers have an opportunity to contribute to the improvement of care and treatment of children and adolescents with mental health problems.

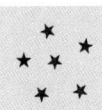

Ideas for Nursing Research

Nurses who work with children and adolescents with mental health problems have been at the forefront of nursing theory development and nursing research. Because of the tradition of research, new avenues have developed for nurse research into the role of the child psychiatric nurse through the National Institutes of Mental Health. The following are ideas for future research:

- Benefits of therapeutic interaction with autistic children
- Types of nursing interventions needed by families with developmentally delayed children
- Relationship between adolescent and adult substance abuse
- Effectiveness of the child psychiatric nurse as a case manager in the general/acute care hospital

References

1. American Nurses Association (1982). *Standards of Psychiatric Mental Health Nursing Practice.* Kansas City, MO: ANA.
2. American Psychiatric Association (1987). *Diagnostic and Statistical Manual of Mental Disorders* (Revised 3rd ed.). Washington, D.C.: American Psychiatric Association.
3. American Psychiatric Association Joint Commission on Public Affairs and the Division of Public Affairs (1988). Washington, D.C.: American Psychiatric Association.
4. Anderson, A. E. (1988). Anorexia nervosa: Who are you? Where are you? *Mayo Clinic Proceedings 63,* 511–513.
5. Decker, S. (1993). Eating disorders. In B. S. Johnson (Ed.). *Psychiatric-Mental Health Nursing: Adaptation and Growth* (3rd ed.). Philadelphia: J.B. Lippincott.
6. Douvan, E. & Adelson, J. (1966). *The Adolescent Experience.* New York: John Wiley & Sons.
7. Erikson, M. T. (1987). *Behavior Disorders of Children and Adolescents.* New Jersey: Prentice-Hall.
8. Futrell, J. A, & Collison, C. R. (1987). Intervening with families of adolescents with bulimia. In: M. Leaky & L. M. Wright (Eds.), *Families and Psychosocial Problems.* (pp. 194–215). Springhouse, PA: Springhouse Corp.
9. Greene, J. & Keown, M. (1986). Depression and suicide in children and adolescents. *Comprehensive Therapy, 12*(1), 38–43.
10. Johnson, B. S. (1993). *Psychiatric-mental health nursing: Adaptation and growth* (3rd ed.). (pp. 313–343, 463–494). Philadelphia: J.B. Lippincott.
11. Kerbeshian, J. & Burd, L. (1989). Tourette disorder and Bipolar symptomatology in childhood and adolescence. *Canadian Journal of Psychiatry, 34,* 230–233.
12. Kohlberg, L. (1981). *The philosophy of moral development.* Philadelphia: Harper & Row.
13. Levine, M. D., Carey, W. B., Crocker, A. C., & Gross, R. T. (1992). *Developmental Behavioral Pediatrics* (2nd ed.). Philadelphia: W.B. Saunders.
14. McBride, A. (1988). Coming of age: Child psychiatric nursing. *Archives of Psychiatric Nursing, 2*(2), 57–64.
15. McConville, B. (1982). Secondary prevention in child psychiatry: An overview with ideas for action. *Canada's Mental Health, 30*(4), 4–7.
16. McWeeney, M. (1988). Life span growth and development: A review and application to nursing diagnosis. *Journal of Enterostomal Therapy, 15*(2), 81–86.
17. Miller, D. (1986). Affective disorders and violence in adolescents. *Hospital and Community Psychiatry, 37*(6), 591–596.
18. Minshew, N. J., & Payton, J. B. (1988). New perspectives in autism: Part II: The differential diagnosis and neurobiology of autism. *Current Problems in Pediatrics, 18*(11), 613–694.
19. Muscari, M. (1988). Effective nursing strategies for adolescents with anorexia nervosa and bulimia nervosa. *Pediatric Nursing, 14*(6), 475–482.
20. Myers, B. A. (1989). Misleading cues in the diagnosis of mental retardation and infant autism in the preschool child. *Mental Retardation, 17*(2), 85–90.
21. Nubel, A., & Solomon, L. (1988). Addicted adolescent girls. *Journal of Psychosocial Nursing, 26*(1), 32–35.
22. Poster, E. C., & Delaney, K. (1989). Mental health counseling of children. In: L. M. Birkhead (Ed.), *Psychiatric mental health nursing*: The therapeutic use of self. (pp. 489–509.). Philadelphia: J.B. Lippincott.
23. Pothier, P. (1984). Child psychiatric nursing. *Journal of Psychosocial Nursing, 22*(3), 11–21.
24. Quay, H.C. (1986). Classification. In H. C. Quay & J. S. Werry (Eds.), *Psychopathological disorders of childhood* (3rd ed.). (pp. 1–34). New York: John Wiley & Sons.
25. Rosenfeld, A. (1989). New treatment for bulimia. *Psychology Today, 23,* 28 March.
26. Schwartz, L., & Kaslow, F. (1981). The cult phenomenon: Historical, sociological, and familial factors contributing to their development and appeal. *Marriage and Family Review, 4,* 3–30.
27. Thomas, S. P., Shoffner, D. H., & Groer, M. W. (1988). Adolescent stress factors: Implications for the nurse practitioner. *Nurse Practitioner, 13*(6), 20–29.
28. Weiner, I. (1970). *Psychological disturbance in adolescence.* New York: Wiley.
29. Wheeler, B., Wood, S., & Hatch, R. (1988). Assessment and intervention with adolescents involved in Satanism. *Social Work, 23*(6), 547–550.
30. Yoos, L. (1984). Taking another look at failure to thrive. *American Journal of Maternal and Child Nursing, 9,* 32–36.
31. Zoltak, B. B. (1986). Autism: Recognition and management. *Pediatric Nurse, 12*(2), 90–94.

The Child With Special Needs

BEHAVIORAL OBJECTIVES

Explore strategies for assisting families with a child who has special needs.

Discuss the role of the pediatric nurse in facilitating normal growth and development for a child who has a developmental disability.

Recognize factors that place a child at risk for experiencing developmental disabilities or delays.

Explain the impact of recent legislation and current public policy in planning for early intervention programs and long-term care of children with special needs.

"Special needs" is an all-inclusive term. When used in reference to a child, the term implies that something is unique about that child. Numerous words exist in the media to convey the same idea. Examples include handicapped, disabled, delayed, crippled, deficient, impaired, disadvantaged, and exceptional. These labels invoke stereotypic images. Less stigma is attached to the child with "special needs." The nurse focuses on the child as an individual within a family who happens to need special consideration in day-to-day living.

This chapter addresses the population of children with special needs of a developmental, physical, sensory, and cognitive nature. Some are gifted with creativity and special talents. Most of these children experience developmental stages and emotions similar to other children without "special needs."

All of these children have fears and anxieties, hopes and dreams, but challenges and obstacles exist that may prevent them from achieving their full potential. The knowledgeable nurse develops and implements nursing interventions 1) to promote early identification of children at risk, 2) to enhance the quality of life, and 3) to increase the likelihood of positive outcomes for the family.

Impact of Increasing Numbers of Developmentally Delayed Individuals

The availability of quality nursing care to families of children with special needs has become a major challenge to child health nurses. As more preterm infants survive and neonatal technology continues to develop, an entire population of children with special needs emerges. These children and families have complex multiple needs that require a multidisciplinary approach. Nurses, as case managers, will need to respond to individual's needs and families' needs as well as organize services at all levels, incorporating community programs. Public Law 99-457 (The Education of the Handicapped Act Amendment of 1986) calls for further expansion of services to infants and preschoolers who are at high risk for developmental disorders. Therefore, nurses will expand their roles in the area of child health as early assessment, identification, and interventions are legally mandated.

Current Trends in Care

On November 29, 1975, President Gerald R. Ford signed The Education for all Handicapped Children Act of 1975, which created public law (PL) 94-142. This law mandates that children with disabilities 3 to 21 years of age are guaranteed tax-supported, appropriate, free education and related services. Congress reaffirmed its position through this act that handicapped individuals can enjoy the same freedoms and rights as any other American citizen. The key is that these children have a legal right to a free and appropriate education in the least restrictive environment possible. Thus, "special education" became a reality for all children.

Public Law 94-142 had a profound impact on the educational system. Public school districts throughout the United States had to assume the responsibility of complying with and enacting the law. If they were unable to meet the child's needs within the district, the responsibility of payment for the child's private education remained with the public school district so that parents would not shoulder the additional financial burden.

Mainstreaming, or the integration of developmentally delayed children with those who are developing normally, came into existence. With the increase in numbers of handicapped children in the classroom, teachers were forced to assume a broader role in these children's lives. Advantages of mainstreaming are that, educationally, all children are treated equally. Those with disabilities are not singled out and labeled as different. All children learn to feel more comfortable with those who are intellectually and physically different from themselves. As the younger generation matures, less stereotyping, prejudice, and discrimination inevitably will surround individuals with disabilities.

As mandated by law, local school officials must develop, in conjunction with the parents (or guardian), an *individualized educational plan (IEP)* for each identified student. The IEP is reviewed and updated annually and is the educational equivalent to a nursing care plan. The IEP is the written plan identifying both short-term and long-term educational objectives and services that must be provided for that child. Requiring parents to participate in this process has placed a potential, additional burden on them. As advocates for their child, parents may have to initiate steps and be assertive to insure that guarantees are fulfilled. This is stressful for many parents, and time-consuming for all.

In 1986, the Education of Handicapped Act Amendments (PL 99-457) expanded the population of potentially "at-risk" individuals to include those from birth to age 3. This act also expanded the IEP to include the total family, thus making it an *Individual Family Service Plan* (IFSP).

The Americans with Disabilities Act was passed in 1990, which makes it unlawful to discriminate against a qualified individual with a disability in the work place. As children and adolescents mature, they will need to be well-informed about their rights in the work force.

Society is attempting to overcome restrictive attitudes of handicapism by enacting laws to prevent discrimination against individuals with disabilities. Thus, adults with disabilities have competitive employment opportunities and access buildings that were once unavailable to them because of physical barriers.

Why is it necessary for the nurse to know about various laws and the educational system's involvement in rehabilitation? First, the need for early assessment and intervention has a profound impact on nursing practice, because services expand as mandated by law. The nurse must possess knowledge and skills to assess children and to plan appropriate interventions. Second, the nurse serves as a positive role model to help educators overcome possible negative attitudes toward students with special needs. When a child with a disability is mainstreamed, teachers may feel uncomfortable because of knowledge deficits about the specific nature of the problem or problems. The nurse bridges this gap by providing a better understanding of the child's physical and emotional limitations as well as of the dynamics of the family. By empowering the educators with more knowledge, teachers enhance the child's self-esteem and self-confidence. The nurse may plan and implement health teaching plans in the school system. Third, the nurse assists parents to become their child's advocate. Not only is the nurse a role model for parents, but the nurse teaches assertiveness skills that prepare parents for dealing with large bureaucratic systems. The nurse provides encouragement and support to parents so that they feel confident in their endeavors. The National Committee for Citizens in Education is a group that answers questions about parents' rights in the public school system and refers parents to local child advocacy groups or other legal organizations. In summary, parents, teachers, and nurses must work collaboratively in an effort to maximize the child's abilities. Funding and information is available through a variety of national and local organizations. Some of these are listed in the accompanying display on resources for children and families with developmental disorders.

Normalization does not mean that children will be "cured" or "normal." Normalization does, however, challenge society to determine ways to provide accessibility to services and environments where all individuals may lead productive lives. The important goal in normalization is to increase the quality of life for these children and their families. The stereotyping, prejudice, and discrimination of handicapism is slowly being erased as this normalization movement increases.

"Normalization" begins with early identification. Accessibility for special developmental services includes family training, counseling, home health services, medical

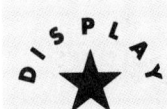

Resources for Children and Families With Developmental Disorders

Auditory Disorders
Alexander Graham Bell Association for the Deaf (AGBAD)
3417 Volta Place, N.W.
Washington, DC 20007

American Society for Deaf Children (ASDC)
814 Thayer Avenue
Silver Spring, MD 20910

National Association of the Deaf (NAD)
814 Thayer Avenue
Silver Spring, MD 20910

National Association for Hearing and Speech Action
(NAHSA)
10801 Rockville Pike
Rockville, MD 20852

National Hearing Aid Society (NHAS)
20361 Middlebelt Road
Livonia, MI 48152

Autism
Autism Society of America (ASA)
1234 Massachusetts Ave., N.W.
Suite C-1017
Washington, DC 20005

Cerebral Palsy
United Cerebral Palsy Association (UCPA)
66 East 34th Street
New York, NY 10016

Communication Disorders
American Speech-Language-Hearing Association (ASHA)
10801 Rockville Pike
Rockville, MD 20852

Dyslexia
The Orton Dyslexia Society (ODS)
724 York Road
Baltimore, MD 21204

Education
National Committee for Citizens in Education (NCCE)
10840 Little Patuxent Parkway, Suite 301
Columbia, MD 21044

Epilepsy
Epilepsy Foundation of America (EFA)
4351 Garden City Drive
Landover, MD 20785

Gifted and Talented Children
American Association for Gifted Children (AAGC)
% Anne Inpellizeri
New York City Partnership
200 Madison Avenue
New York, NY 10016

Council for Exceptional Children (CEC)
Talented and Gifted Children
TAG Division
1920 Association Drive
Reston, VA 22091

Gifted Child Society (GCS)
190 Rock Road
Glen Rock, NJ 07452

National Association for Gifted Children (NAGC)
4175 Lovell Road, Suite 140
Circle Pines, MN 55014

The National/State Leadership Training Institute on the
Gifted and Talented (N/S-LTI-G/T)
One Wilshire Bldg.
624 S. Grand Avenue, Suite 1007
Los Angeles, CA 90017

U.S. Department of Education
Office for Gifted and Talented
400 Maryland Ave., S.W.
Washington, DC 20202

World Council for Gifted and Talented Children
(WCGTC)
HMS Rm. 414
University of South Florida
Tampa, FL 33620

Handicapped
ICD—International Center for the Disabled
340 East 24th Street
New York, NY 10010

National Information Center for Children & Youth With
Handicaps (NICCYH)
P.O. Box 1492
Washington, DC 20013

TASH: The Association for Persons with Severe Handicaps
(TASH)
7010 Roosevelt Way NE
Seattle, WA 98115

Learning Disabilities
Association for Children and Adults with Learning
Disabilities (ACLD)
4156 Library Road
Pittsburgh, PA 15234

Mental Illness
American Association on Mental Retardation (AAMR)
1719 Kalorama Road, N.W.
Washington, DC 20009

Association for Children with Retarded Mental Development (A/CRMD)
162 Fifth Avenue, 11th Fl.
New York, NY 10010

Association for Retarded Citizens (ARC)
P.O. Box 6109
Arlington, TX 76005

National Down Syndrome Society (NDSS)
141 Fifth Avenue
New York, NY 10010

(Continued)

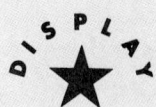

Resources for Children and Families With Developmental Disorders

National Fragile X Foundation
1441 York St.
Suite 215
Denver, CO 80206

National Institute of Mental Health
5600 Fishers Lane
Rockville, MD 20852

Parents of Down Syndrome Children (PODSC)
% Montgomery County Assn. for Retarded Citizens
11600 Nebel Street
Rockville, MD 20852

Retarded Infants Services (RIS)
386 Park Avenue South
New York, New York 10016

Multiple Sclerosis
National Multiple Sclerosis Society (NMSS)
205 East 42nd Street
New York, NY 10017

Muscular Dystrophy
Muscular Dystrophy Association (MDA)
810 Seventh Avenue
New York, NY 10019

Orthopedics
Arthritis Foundation (AF)
1314 Spring Street, N.W.
Atlanta, GA 30309

National Easter Seal Society (NESS)
70 East Lake Street
Chicago, IL 60601

National Scoliosis Foundation (NSF)
93 Concord Avenue
P.O. Box 547
Belmont, MA 02178

Self-help Groups
Parents Anonymous (PA)
6733 S. Sepulveda, Suite 270
Los Angeles, CA 90045

Parents Without Partners (PWP)
8807 Colesville Road
Silver Spring, MD 20910

Sibling Support Groups
Sibling Information Network (SIN)
Connecticut's University Affiliated Program on Developmental Disabilities
991 Main Street
East Hartford, CT 06108

Spina Bifida
Spina Bifida Association of America (SBAA)
1700 Rockville Pike, Suite 540
Rockville, MD 20852

Technologically Dependent Children
Center for Special Education Technology (CSET)
1920 Association Drive
Reston, VA 22091

SKIP: Sick Kids Need Involved People
216 Newport Drive
Severna Park, MD 21146

Visually Impaired
American Council of Blind Parents (ACBP)
Adelphia House, M-5
1229 Chestnut St.
Philadelphia, PA 19107

American Foundation for the Blind (AFB)
15 West 16th Street
New York, NY 10011

Helen Keller National Center for Deaf-Blind Youths & Adults (HKNCDBYA)
111 Middle Neck Road
Sands Point, NY 11050

The Library of Congress
Division for the Blind and Physically Handicapped
1291 Taylor, NW
Washington, DC 20042

National Association for Parents of the Visually Impaired (NAPVI)
PO Box 562
Camden, NJ 13316

National Association for the Visually Handicapped (NAVH)
22 W. 21st St.
New York, NY 10010

National Society to Prevent Blindness (NSPB)
500 E. Remington Road
Schaumburg, IL 60173

services, nursing, nutrition, etc. The State of Maryland alone estimates that at full implementation, approximately 7000 infants and toddlers, plus their families, or 3.5% of the total population of Maryland from birth through age 2 will be participating in Early Intervention Services (EIS).[28]

Ethical Issues

In times of financial concerns and constraints, validating essential expenditures and costs has emerged as a top priority. Viability of the handicapped child as a contributing member of society creates many discussions and raises ethical issues that historically were nonexistent. Technology-dependent children, severely brain-damaged infants, and chronically ill children require a significant portion of our health care funding and will continue to do so (see Chap. 21). Religious, moral, and ethical issues will face the nurse and society as fewer dollars become available for increasing treatment and services.

A number of children at risk have no way to access programs or enter the health care system early. This merely compounds their problems. These children require emotional support, counseling and assistance in daily living in order to live a quality life. Children at high-risk may require foster home placement or adoption to provide the safest and healthiest of environments, which poses another dilemma for society.

Genetic Screening Early interventions and treatments begin with genetic screening. The science of genetics has increased the ability to identify chromosomal abnormalities from blood samples as well as from amniocentesis. Although these are expensive laboratory tests, the cost can far outweigh the long-term expenditures to the family and society. Certain chronic illnesses, such as cystic fibrosis, sickle cell anemia, hemophilia, and Tay-Sachs disease, can be addressed early, as carriers are identified. The ethical dilemma that ensues involves the decision to remain nonreproductive and childless, to abort a fetus with single or multiple birth defects, or to prepare for early interventions in the delivery room.

Prenatal Diagnosis Tests available for prenatal identification of diseases and defects are summarized in Table 10-1. Fetoscopy enables the physician to view the fetus and obtain tissue and blood samples. DNA studies and other information also can be done with this test. Early attempts at surgical intervention through fetoscopy are being conducted. Newborn screens are also helpful in detecting abnormalities, and in many states are mandatory (see Chap. 11). Phenylketonuria (PKU) testing in the newborn period is an example.

Funding of Case-Findings Funding health care is always an issue. Public Law 99-457 passed in October 1986, provided a 5-year phase-in schedule for planning, developing, and implementing a system of early intervention. This law provided for a full range of multidisciplinary services to be rendered under public supervision, administered at no cost to the family except where Federal or State law has an established payment system (e.g., sliding fees). Funding allocations for each state are derived from data obtained from the Census Bureau for the number of infants and toddlers residing in a state.[28] Eligibility for programs is defined by the state. Another source of funding is through Crippled Children's Services which provides a significant amount of funding for children with a wide range of disabilities.

Corrective or Cosmetic Surgery Corrective or cosmetic surgery also raises ethical issues. Many individuals believe that if there is a potential benefit to the child, treatment must occur. Others of a different philosophy suggest that painful and expensive procedures are cruel and inhumane when the prognosis is limited regardless of the interventions. Defining who is appropriate for such interventions is a difficult religious, moral, and social issue to debate.

Depending on the type of disability involved, orthopedic surgery to improve locomotion, plastic surgery to assist with daily activities, and ophthalmic procedures to promote improved sensory functions are a few examples of interventions that may be required.

Developmental Disorders

An array of developmental disorders exists within the pediatric setting. The Developmental Disabilities Act of 1984 defines disability as "one that is attributed to mental and/or physical impairments; begins before age 22 years; is likely to continue indefinitely; and results in limitations in at least three of seven activities of daily living."[30] Developmental disorders may be categorized under physical or mental disorders. Oftentimes there is considerable overlap between physical and mental disabilities, and when this occurs, the child is said to be "multihandicapped." Regardless of the disorders, the overall goal for all children is to promote wellness despite the developmental disability.

Scope of Problems

Developmental disorders are a result of biologic and environmental factors (see the accompanying display on differences among developmental disorders). Approximately 20% are biologically or organically caused and include genetic, prenatal, perinatal, and postnatal conditions.[32] Chromosomal disorders (i.e., Down syndrome)

Differences Among Developmental Disorders

Delayed Development: development that has stopped at some point with behavior specific to the phase in which this occurred (e.g., mental retardation)

Deviant Development: development that is inappropriate or unstable (e.g., schizophrenia)

Single Versus Multiple: development in one modality is affected versus multiple system disabilities (e.g., blindness versus cerebral palsy with mental retardation)

Secondary Disability: development in modality if not recognized leads to a secondary disability (e.g., child with ADHD develops reading disorder.)

Chronic Illness: A condition that interferes with daily functioning for more than 3 months in a year, causes hospitalization of more than 1 month in a year, or is likely to do either of these. (Chronic illness is discussed in Chapter 21.)

and inborn errors of metabolism (i.e., Tay-Sachs disease) are examples of genetic abnormalities. Approximately 80% of developmental delays are caused by environmental elements.[32] A complex relationship exists between cognitive development and psychosocial factors. Environment risks include lack of infant stimulation, nutritional deficits, and emotional and social deprivation.

Statistics of developmental disabilities are difficult to estimate or project because research uses various definitions and populations. The number of children with long-term illnesses, developmental disabilities, and congenital disorders has required this nation to respond by instituting numerous and accessible early intervention services across the United States.

Case-findings extend from the prenatal period, when known problem exist, to the newborn nursery with identification of abnormal assessment findings, to pediatricians' offices and clinics, to community health programs and to schools. During emergency room admissions, children can be identified for select developmental interventions. Nurses practicing throughout all areas, are ideal health professionals to initiate referrals.

Variables Associated With Disorders

Prenatal factors influence the outcome of the fetus and include maternal infections (i.e., rubella or German measles), maternal ingestion of drugs including alcohol, malnutrition, predisposing maternal chronic illness, and maternal age. Any of the variables can effect the fetus, with a combination of the above factors creating higher risk for fetal damage. Intrapartal and postnatal factors which contribute to a high risk of developmental disabilities include hypoxia, weight at birth, prematurity nutritional intake, birth injuries, and acquired infections (e.g., sepsis). *Neonatal infections* also are involved in contributing to developmental disabilities. Specifically, neurologic insults may develop from untreated meningitis. Similarly throughout childhood, untreated infections, trauma, or exposure to neurotoxins (e.g., lead) may lead to developmental deficits.

The Affected Child

The child with a developmental disorder has emotional needs as well as physical care needs that cannot be ignored. The nurse helps the family anticipate developmental periods that may be particularly arduous. For example, the first realization that "I'm different" can be extremely agonizing for the child. Growing up involves incorporating body image into one's self-concept. By focusing on positive aspects instead of deficits, the child's self-esteem is enhanced. Encouraging play with dolls that have disabilities or handicaps (Fig. 20-1) allows the child to feel less unique and different.

Younger children overlook many differences in others. They also help the less physically mobile explore the environment, and facilitate learning that may be precluded by a physical defect. School-age children are aware of physical deviances and can be cruel and insensitive to the needs of others, especially to a handicapped child. Adolescence is exceptionally stressful for the child with

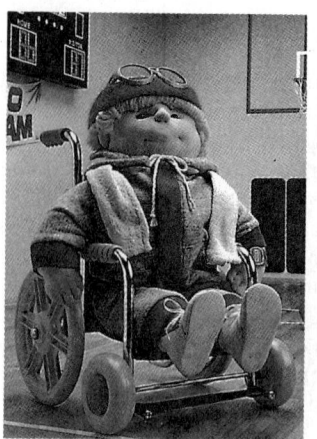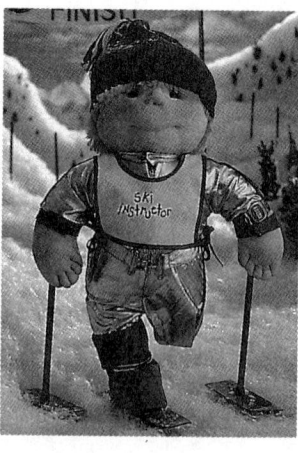

FIGURE 20-1

"Hal's Pals: I'm Glad to be Me." Dolls with disabilities help the child gain self-esteem. (Reprinted with permission from © SAInc., 1985.)

special needs. Physical independence may be difficult to achieve, because many of these children require a great amount of assistance with activities of daily living. Body image takes on varying degrees of importance throughout development, but adolescents are highly sensitive to physical differences. Conforming to the norm and looking like everyone else becomes tremendously important during this stage.

Coping mechanisms used by the affected child depend on gender, age, personality, mental reasoning abilities, and support systems available to the child. Typically, a healthy adaptation by parents facilitates a positive adjustment in the child, regardless of the extent of the disability.

The type and characteristics of the disorder also impact the child's response to a disability. Those conditions that are visible and tangible (i.e. cerebral palsy) are a constant reminder to the child and society that they are different. Less obvious conditions such as sickle cell anemia or diabetes may make it easier for the child and family to deny the problem. Continual assessment of adaptation to the condition and prospective planning for the future is critical for the child to lead a healthy and productive life.

The Parents and Family

The diagnosis of a developmental disorder is universally a difficult period for parents. When the diagnosis occurs at birth, parents may be surprised by the suddenness of the situation and need help grieving for the loss of their less than perfect child. When lag time ensues between sensing something is not quite right and confirming a definitive diagnosis, parents still need time to grieve for the loss of their idealized child.

The search for "why" a disability occurs can be present throughout many years. It is most intense during the first few months, however, with parents questioning "what did I do wrong?" Emotional support is necessary during the period of uncertainty. In some instance, parents may even question or doubt their parenting skills in an attempt to blame themselves for the problem rather than believe something is wrong with their child.

After a developmental disorder is confirmed, a time of adjustment is required when hopes and aspirations are redefined and realistic goals based on the child's capabilities are planned. The impact of the diagnosis raises questions and concerns for the future. What kind of ramifications does the diagnosis have for the family? What kind of financial burden will this impose? What kind of physical care will be required? Will my child achieve academically? Will my child be self-sufficient and independent? How will my job or career be affected? How will the extended family react? How will society react? Will there be time for social activities? These worries and many more tend to be constant and place incredible emotional strain on parents. Critical times throughout the life span of the child impact the family's ability to cope with the child who has special needs.[8]

Olshansky discusses the concept of chronic sorrow in his classic article entitled "Chronic sorrow: A response to having a mentally defective child."[22] Olshansky believes that there are times throughout the child's life when parental sorrow and grief surface, and that these emotions are not limited merely to the time of diagnosis. Especially vulnerable times for parents are times when their child fails to reach developmental milestones and when the child is excluded from peer activities. The nurse helps parents anticipate these times, is sensitive to their feelings when this occurs, and helps them refocus on their child's positive attributes.

The long-term dependence of a child with special needs is physically draining for parents. Parents need time to be able to give attention to their spouse and other children, and to become revitalized themselves, both emotionally and physically. Some hospitals allow parents to admit the child with special needs to the pediatric floor if empty beds are available to provide a short break for the parents. Such "respite care" may facilitate parental rejuvenation.

Impact on the Family

Vulnerable Child Syndrome

The steps in the vulnerable child syndrome may occur in families who have a handicapped child (Fig. 20-2). When a traumatic event is experienced in which a fatal outcome for a child is expected but survival results, emotional upheaval is endured by the parents. The potential or threatened loss of the child affects the parents so greatly that they have difficulty "letting go." An example of this phenomenon is the premature infant who survives after an extremely precarious beginning. Parents are excessively anxious, overly protective, and have difficulty separating from the child.

Both parents and child demonstrate specific symptomatology in this syndrome. Parents worry excessively about minute details of the child's health and seek medical attention for minor ailments. Parents are undeniably overprotective, overindulgent, and oversolicitous. They are unable to leave their child in the care of others, are unable to set limits and tend to "baby" the child. Parents are consumed by continual fear for their child's life. This exaggerated concern transfers to the child, who often

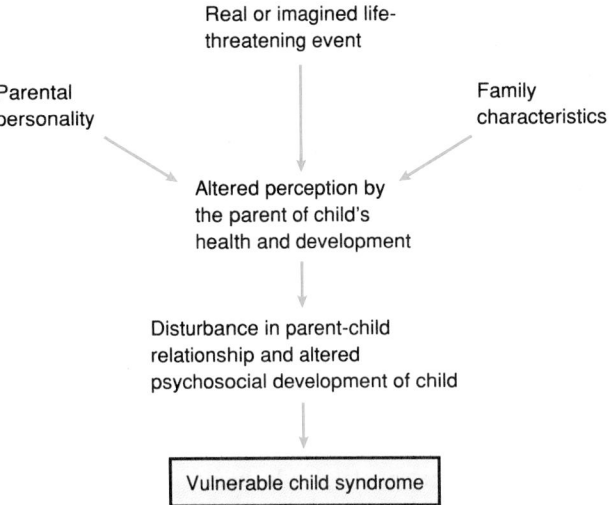

FIGURE 20-2
Vulnerable child syndrome. (*Reprinted with permission from:* Culley, B., Perrin, E., & Chaberski, M. [1989]. Parental perceptions of vulnerability of formerly premature infants. *J. Pediatr Health Care,* 3[5], 238.)

voices similar complaints. The child becomes hypochondriacal, is extremely dependent, disobedient, irritable, argumentative, and uncooperative.

At the time of any traumatic episode, the nurse can help parents work through and verbalize feelings of grief and potential loss. With appropriate nursing interventions at the time of the traumatic episode, this syndrome may be prevented or decreased. Once the syndrome is established, the nurse intervenes by encouraging independence for both parents and child, by helping parents establish consistent guidelines for discipline, and by encouraging participation in support groups. The display earlier in this chapter identifies support groups and resources available for a variety of different developmental disorders.

Unaffected Siblings

Parents are not the only members of the family affected by having a child with special needs residing within the same environment. "Unaffected" siblings increasingly are gaining attention in the literature.[17,18] The health care system needs to understand, support, and include siblings in the plan of care, as well as help families provide a nurturing environment for all family members. Because parents may be absorbed totally by the child with special requirements, the nurse may remind parents that unaffected siblings also have needs that cannot be dismissed or forgotten. Concerns of and interventions with the unaffected sibling are discussed in Chapter 21.

Both positive and negative consequences result for unaffected siblings. As they experience first-hand problems unique to individuals with special needs, these unaffected children have an unusual opportunity for growth. Positive outcomes include developing a mature outlook on life, establishing a strong sense of family solidarity, and developing the ability to handle increased responsibility. These children tend to model their parent's attitudes and demonstrate sensitivity and compassion to all individuals with special needs.

Negative outcomes relate to the unaffected sibling feeling overburdened. Physical assistance in housekeeping chores are often required of them, and increased pressure for academic achievement may be applied. These siblings may harbor guilt because they are not the one with the disability. Sometimes they even fantasize about becoming defective like their brother or sister in an attempt to overcome this guilt or to demand more parental attention. These children may feel isolated because parents tend to be preoccupied with the other child. Anger and resentment can build and may be directed toward either the parents or the affected sibling, or may be manifested as behavioral or social problems at school. The nurse should plan to inform unaffected siblings about the nature of their sibling's disability and actively listen to concerns and frustrations. Encouraging open family discussions of the special needs demystifies the situation and may allay any fears and anxieties (see Chap. 21).

Nursing Implications

When working with families, nurse is encouraged to avoid professional jargon, to validate what parents have heard, and to provide written information that can be reviewed again at home. The label of developmental delay may have a self-fulfilling prophecy, as parents expect less of the child and therefore decrease interactions and stimulations. The nurse may help families set realistic goals.

Prevention

The nurse plays a key role in the prevention of developmental disorders by providing families with educational information about the importance of excellent prenatal care, infant stimulation, sound nutritional practices, and emotional nurturing. The nurse also participates in early screening programs to identify children at risk so that interventions are instituted before problems multiply.

★ NURSING ASSESSMENT

Nursing assessment of the child with developmental delays involves a comprehensive interview of the parents and observations of the child. The nurse assesses dynamics of the family and discovers vital information about their level of functioning by asking questions and gathering data, as outlined in the accompanying display on assessing family dynamics. A history is essential to document the child's developmental milestones, growth patterns, and parents' impressions of the child's capabilities.

Physical assessment includes growth measurements and use of growth charts to identifying deviance in developmental expectations. Many parents keep records of growth patterns and immunization schedules that can assist in a complete and accurate history. A complete physical examination, including a complete review of systems, is necessary to determine absence or loss of certain physical abilities.

Mental assessment, formal psychological assessment of mental abilities, is usually done by a psychologist who specializes in pediatric development. There are, however,

a variety of screening instruments available to assess developmental delays, as listed in Table 20-1. Numerous factors such as age of the child, reliability and validity of instrument, and qualifications of administrator determine which instrument is selected. Two of the most common tools used are The Brazelton Neonatal Behavior Assessment Scale (see Chap. 11) and the Denver II (see Appendix). These tools compare abilities and behavior with established norms, but have no predictive value. Denver II is used on children from birth to 6 years of age and assesses four broad areas: personal-social, fine motor adaptive, gross motor, and language; The Brazelton Neonatal Behavior Assessment Scale measures various aspects of infant interactive behavior only.

Developmental charts chronologically describe behaviors and capabilities of children that can be used in routine assessments of children. Child Life Workers are also available to assist the nurse in collaboratively screening children in the midst of medical procedures, as well as during play.

★ NURSING INTERVENTION

Interventions that may be important and appropriate for one family may not be for another family, so plans are individualized. Continual reassessment over time is essential, because of the ever-changing nature of families and the child's progress.

The nurse assists parents in focusing continually on positive aspects and emphasizing strengths that increase the child's self-esteem and confidence. The nurse demonstrates empathy for the family's situation, establishes a therapeutic relationship, and forms a collaborative partnership with parents. This collaborative partnership is developed by recognizing parents' expertise. Because parents live daily with their situation, they are in the best position to identify what "works" for their child. The nurse working in the hospital setting should be careful not to undermine this expertise when the child is rehospitalized for ongoing medical treatment.

Nursing plans include teaching the family how to manage the daily physical tasks at home, and different strategies to cope with the additional stresses of having a child with special needs. Families need to be encouraged to maintain as much normalcy as possible while coping with additional stresses. Anticipatory guidance allows parents to know what to expect at various periods. Stages of normal growth and development occur, but the time frame may be different or delayed for their child. Depending on the child's diagnosis, puberty may be a particularly difficult phase. Adolescents typically seek independence at this time, and sexual arousal emerges. Achieving independence may pose a dilemma if numerous physical tasks need to be performed by someone else. Encouraging problem-solving skills increases the child's self-confidence and self-esteem and helps him or her feel more independent. Physical maturation may occur even if behavior does not correlate with age. Interest in sex may tend to be on an immature level. Masturbation may be a problem because of lack of social sense. The nurse teaches parents to handle this problem in a matter of act manner, with statements such as "we don't do this now or here."

TABLE 20-1
Assessment Tools Frequently Used by Nurses

Instrument	Ages	Description	Where to Obtain
Denver II	1 month–6 years	Concise, easy to administer, systematic approach to assessing preschool child; tests areas of personal-social skills, fine-motor adaptive skills, language skills, and gross-motor skills	LADOCA, Project & Publishing Foundation, Inc., E. 51st Avenue and Lincoln Street, Denver, Colorado 80216
Washington Guide to Promoting Development in the Young Child	1–52 months	Assists in systematically observing the child in areas of feeding, sleep, play, language, discipline, toileting, dressing; expected tasks are presented, with activities suggested to provide for enhancement of growth and development	In Teaching children with developmental problems: A family care approach, by K. Barnard and M. Erickson. St. Louis: Mosby, 1976
Developmental Profile (Alpern-Boll)	Birth to preadolescence	Screens a child's development in physical, self-help, social, academic, and communication areas; a questionnaire administered to parent or teacher	Psychological Development Publications, 7150 Lakeside Drive, Indianapolis, Indiana 46273
Neonatal Behavioral Assessment Scale (Brazelton)	First month	Behavioral assessment scale and psychological scale for the newborn infant; valuable in the detection of abnormality as well as developing insight about infant's repertoire of behavior	T. Berry Brazelton: The National Behavioral Assessment Scale. London, William Heinemann Ltd. 1973 (Philadelphia, J. B. Lippincott Co., 1972).
Nursing Child Assessment Feeding Scales	Birth to 1 year	Assesses parent-child interactions during feeding; subscales address parent characteristics and infant characteristics; requires observation of the entire feeding	NCAST, T-436 Health Sciences Building, SC-74, University of Washington, Seattle, Washington 98195
Nursing Child Assessment Teaching Scales	Birth to 3 years	Assesses parent-child interactions during teaching; subscales address parent characteristics and infant characteristics	NCAST, T-436 Health Sciences Building, SC-74, University of Washington, Seattle, Washington 98195
Caldwell Home Inventory	1. Birth to 3 years 2. 3–6 years	Home observation for measurement of environment in areas of social, emotional, and cognitive supports	Center for Early Development and Education, University of Arkansas, 814 Sherman, Little Rock, Arkansas 72202

(Source: Levine, M. D., Carey, W. B., Crocker, A. C., & Gross, R. T. [1983]. *Developmental-behavioral pediatrics.* Philadelphia: W. B. Saunders, p. 1002.)

The nurse plays a significant role in helping parents become their child's advocate. Learning to negotiate the maze of services is not always an easy task for parents because bureaucratic systems are large, complex, and overwhelming. The nurse teaches parents management skills, assertive skills, and negotiation skills so that they can access the systems earlier and receive maximal support for their child. The nurse should be knowledgeable about public policies to inform parents of their legal rights under current laws.

Support systems available to the family are critical for providing physical care and relief as well as emotional support. The nurse should be alert for risks of parental stress or burnout because the plight of caring for a child with special needs is relentless. Potentially, mothers may be at greater risk than fathers for parental breakdown, depending on the delegation of responsibilities as primary care providers. Therefore, fathers are incorporated in the plans and encouraged to participate continually. This establishes a mutual state of parental cooperation and decreases the chance of marital discord. As dual partnership for financial stability escalates in our society, so must the partnership for sharing the burden of child care.

Networking, both informally and formally, is another invaluable source of support for parents. Someone who has literally "walked in my shoes" can truly empathize and lend emotional support to parents experiencing similar situations. Numerous national, state, and local agencies are available, and all parents should be offered the

address and phone number of the appropriate local support group. Organizations were listed near the beginning of the chapter.

Special programs, e.g., Head Start, support groups (Down Syndrome Society), and events (Special Olympics) assist the handicapped child in living a full life. Childhood is the time to explore and enjoy the wonders of the world. Society is committed to making this an accessible goal regardless of physical or mental limitations.

The value of literature is enormous for both the child and family. Often overlooked, the use of literature can be therapeutic in forming positive attitudes toward the disabled and providing good role models for those with disabilities. The nurse may suggest classic and current literature, remembering that books must be age appropriate. Preschoolers, for example, enjoy stories that are presented in illustration format. Doctor's office, pediatric clinics, and hospital units might incorporate a small library with stories about children with developmental disabilities into waiting areas. Other strategies to encourage may be art and music therapy, and use of creative writing. Many individuals are able to express in writing feelings that they are unable to express verbally.

The financial ramifications involved in the management of a child with special needs are potentially monumental for parents and society in general. Parents lose employment days because local services often are unavailable and travel is required to receive necessary services. Parents also lose work simply because services are not coordinated. The best model of health care delivery

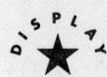

Nursing Assessment: Guidelines for Assessing Family Dynamics

- How are the members of the family communicating?
- What support systems, both physically and emotionally, are available to the family?
- What is the educational background of the parents? Do they understand the information given to them about the diagnosis and the importance of the treatment plan?
- What kind of organizational pattern does the family exhibit?
- Are spouses sharing the burden of care for their child? Is there lack of marital harmony because one spouse is "carrying the load"?
- What are the family's priorities that may help or hinder their ability, wilingness, or desire to help the child?
- What are the financial resources available to the family?
- Are the parents "getting away from it all" on occasion? Do they have some form of "respite care" so that they can become rejuvenated emotionally and physically?

to compensate for this problem is "case management," in which services are coordinated by the case manager.

Financial resources are not extensive for families. Private health insurance coverage varies widely, but for those with income below the poverty level, accessibility is nonexistent. Some insurance carriers penalize families by not covering expenses for preexisting conditions. Federal monies allocated through individual states include Medicaid and Crippled Children's Services (CCS).

Physical Disorders: Cerebral Palsy

Physical disorders, as discussed in this chapter, involve skeletal/motor problems. Cerebral palsy (CP) is the most common motor disorder of infants and children, and occurs in 2 per 1,000 live births.[27] Terminology and classification of cerebral palsy has undergone much change over the past 20 years. The agreed-on definition of CP is "a disorder of movement and posture due to a static defect or lesion of the immature brain."[27] The clinical manifestations of the disease vary according to etiology, associated defects (communication disorder, mental retardation), topographic characteristics (number of limbs involved), functional capacity, neuroanatomic factors, and therapeutic factors.

Although early diagnosis is beneficial, cerebral palsy is difficult to diagnosis during infancy because motor dysfunctions are subtle in infants. Prematurity and hypoxia (along with a host of other variables) complicate the early clinical assessment that would delineate clearly this specific disorder. Some of the neurologic findings associated with cerebral palsy are disordered movements, tonal abnormalities (hypertonies, hypotonus), sustained clonus of stretch reflexes, and asymmetrical signs.

Approximately 50% to 60% of children with CP have associated defects including developmental delays, such as language and perceptual problems, attention deficit hyperactivity disorder, seizure disorders, and a degree of mental retardation.

Identifying the exact cause of this disorder is complicated because many prenatal, perinatal, and postnatal factors are thought to contribute. Although neurologic handicap is a frequent outcome of prematurity, most extremely preterm babies do not have cerebral palsy (see Chap. 53).[1]

Nursing Implications

Regardless of the orthopedic or neurologic disability, common but unique problems exist for the child and his or her parents. Whether it be cerebral palsy, spina bifida, muscular dystrophy, juvenile rheumatoid arthritis, or multiple sclerosis, mechanical difficulties emerge as a primary issue. For children who are compromised by severe motor defects, as well as sensory disorders, the health care team must collaborate extensively to determine the best avenue for learning and communication.

Equipment Specialized equipment is required to facilitate body control and locomotion. The current market is replete with appliances to facilitate aspects of daily living, as shown in Figure 20-3. Parents need to be wise consumers when purchasing equipment for a physically dependent child, because the financial burden escalates rapidly with additional purchases. The nurse helps parents discern what equipment is essential and investigates the resources available in the child's community. Rental equipment is often a good option, but cost may be the major concern.

The nurse educates parents on important aspects to consider before purchasing equipment. For a child who lacks fine motor coordination, dishes with nonskid bases and scooped rims are helpful. Cups weighted to prevent spills and having large, flexible handles that bend into different shapes facilitate holding while drinking. Multigrip utensils are advantageous for those with grasping difficulties. Velcro is commonly used for stabilizing objects effectively.

Postural alignment is another consideration. Various models of standing frames are designed to accommodate children who bear some weight but lack total control (see Fig. 20-3). These frames facilitate crutchless standing so that upper limbs are free for activities. Children whose movement is severely restricted need extra support straps for chest, buttocks, or knees. Wheelchairs, as with other equipment, range from basic to deluxe models and are priced accordingly. Before purchasing, the nurse assists parents in deciding what is best for their particular situation. Are safety belts, handrims for self-propelling, and cushions standard equipment? The chair's functional ability to accommodate different heights and its ability to collapse with ease for transport are other important features to contemplate. For the severely handicapped child, leg abductor wedges and adjustable scoliosis pads may

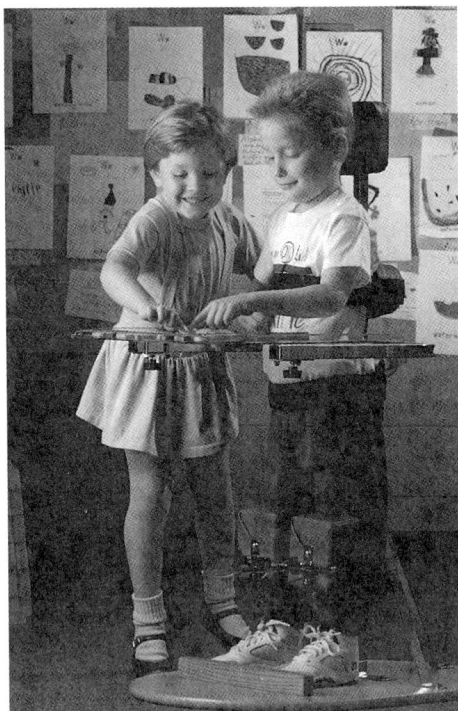

FIGURE 20-3
Special equipment is available to facilitate body control, locomotion, and postural alignment. The upright standing frame is one example and provides the child with the opportunity to participate in play activities. (Courtesy of Ortho-Kinetics, Inc., Waukesha, WI.)

be necessary for proper positioning. Often the social worker can assist with financial arrangements through public or private organizations.

Toys Toys play a prominent role in helping children learn developmental skills. The nurse should recommend a selection of toys that are both age appropriate and developmentally appropriate. For a child paralyzed from the waist down, toys using upper body movement and cognitive abilities are ideal. For a child with poor fine motor coordination, large toys that rely on gross motor skills should be used. For a child with poor total body balance, equipment is available that provides body support structures so that an ordinary childhood activity such as bike riding may become a reality. The goal is to have fun and be challenged with toys, but not discouraged or frustrated by them. As a child experiences success with toys, a sense of mastery accumulates, enhancing self-confidence.

Anticipatory Guidance Mechanical difficulties are not the only problems encountered by parents who have a child with skeletal or motor disorders. Anticipatory guidance helps parents recognize what to expect as the child matures. As previously mentioned, normal stages of growth and development may occur, but the time frame may be different or delayed.

Toilet training often poses problems for parents because the child may have difficulty achieving sphincter control. Constipation occurs because of neuromuscular abnormalities as well as decreased physical activity. Den-

tal problems may be encountered because of slow eruption, malocclusion, poor nutritional intake, or poor hygienic care. Parents need help to determine the age at which to begin toilet training, discuss ways to increase fiber and fluid content in the child's diet, and learn methods to prevent dental caries. Often, behavioral psychology can institute toilet training programs to assist parents in particularly difficult cases.

Sensory Disorders

Impairment of the auditory and visual senses radically influences a child's ability to explore the environment and hence acquire knowledge about it. Auditory sensation is essential for language development; initial vocalization is made through parroting sounds and noises. Likewise, exploration of the environment occurs through the visual sense. Communication disorders affect the child's ability to process or to give information. Without these senses the child is limited in experiences and delayed in acquisition of knowledge about the world around him or her. Sensory disorders are often related to dysfunction of the cranial nerves. The reader is referred to Chapter 51 for a description and review of the functions of the cranial nerves.

Visual Impairments

Visual impairments are a significant problem. The most frequent causes of blindness in children are prenatal cataracts due to heredity or maternal rubella, optic nerve atrophy, and retrolental fibroplasia resulting from oxygen toxicity in the newborn period. Other causes of visual impairments include congenital glaucoma, retinoblastoma, myopia, strabismus, and trauma due to accidents. Each year, 160,000 school-age children are estimated to sustain eye injuries in sports-related accidents or from hazardous products such as cigarettes, pencils, metal objects, and glass. For in-depth discussion of visual impairments, see Chapter 35.

Nursing Implications

When assessing the eye, there are primarily two areas of concern: visual acuity and visual field. *Visual acuity* refers to the eye's refractive powers and *visual field* refers to the area within which objects may be seen when the eye is stationary. The main refractive error in the pediatric population is myopia or nearsightedness. Close objects are seen more clearly than far, distant objects. This becomes especially significant as the child enters school. Academic standing may be compromised if writing on the blackboard at the front of the classroom is indistinguishable. To test for myopia, the Snellen chart is used. The chart, which has letters graduating in size, is placed 20 feet away from the viewer and letters are identified. Children who wear glasses should be tested with their glasses on. The result is reported as a ratio of 20 over the number of the last line read correctly. Normal acuity is considered 20/20. A score of 20/60 indicates for example that a child was able to read at a distance of 20 feet what a person with normal vision could read at 60 feet. Any child with 20/40 or less in either eye should be referred for further evaluation. The term *legally blind* is defined by a visual acuity score of 20/200 or worse in the good eye after correction, or a visual field of less than 20 degrees in the better eye after correction. Visual field is tested by moving an object (e.g., pencil) from the periphery to the center of the face as the child fixates on something directly in front of him. The child states at what point the object is first seen. Normal visual field is considered to be 50 degrees upward, 70 degrees downward, and 90 degrees outward. Each eye should be tested individually. Again, if the visual field is less than 20 degrees in the better eye after correction, tunnel vision is produced and the person is considered legally blind.

Early detection of visual disorders is essential to prevent visual impairments. Routine eye examinations are recommended shortly after birth, again at 6 months of age, once during preschool years, and periodically thereafter. Once a child is enrolled in school, screening programs typically are conducted by the school nurse, and referral is made to either an optometrist or an ophthalmologist. For children with multiple disorders, it is vital to assess each problem (e.g., vision) on a yearly basis (see Chaps. 34, 53).

Two main goals of treatment for a child with visual difficulties are: 1) to help remove limitation in the surrounding environment and 2) to help achieve independent function. For a child with partial sight, numerous aids such as clocks with large numbers, calendars with large letters, and books with large print are available to reduce frustrations within the environment. Parents may need to relocate furniture in the home environment to allow the child to move independently with assurance and confidence.

For an infant with complete visual impairment, a delicate balance between encouraging normal exploration and safety precautions must be achieved. For the older child, learning both to read and write in Braille is advantageous. This system relies on the tactile skill of feeling embossed dots that represent letters, words, and numbers. Knowledge of this system enables the child to function independently. The Library of Congress is the largest distributor of books, magazines, and various other resources such as cassette tapes and players for the blind. In our highly technological society, a blind child can be taught computer training, daily living skills, and recreational activities such as skiing and bowling.

Because 90% eye accidents can be prevented, education for the prevention of eye injuries is paramount.[14] The nurse teaches parents to be alert for hazardous play objects and the importance of teaching children to play safely.

Hospitalized Child   Special strategies should be used for the hospitalized child who is visually impaired. The nurse must understand that the use of verbal cues is critical in orienting the child to place and time. Insuring safety in the unfamiliar environment is essential. Both the patient and the family need ample support and reassurance throughout the hospitalization. A multidisciplinary follow-up ensures the comprehensive care of these children and is essential to habilitation.

Auditory Impairments

Auditory disorders represent a significant problem in pediatrics. Approximately 1000 babies are born deaf each year in the United States and another one million children from birth to age 21 are hearing impaired.[14]

Auditory disorders may be incomplete or complete, unilateral or bilateral, and are broadly classified as conductive or sensorineural impairments. Conductive (also referred to as peripheral) hearing disorders are those in which the transmission of sound waves through the external or middle ear is impaired. This may be due to congenital malformations of the middle ear, obstruction of the external canal by foreign bodies or cerumen, or by a perforated tympanic membrane. The most common cause of conductive hearing loss in children, however, is chronic serous otitis media. Therefore, it is essential that the nurse educate parents to the importance of seeking prompt medical help for ear infections and, when placed on antibiotics, to complete each course of antibiotics to decrease the potential for permanent hearing loss. If recurrent otitis media persists, a myringotomy or placement of pressure-equalizer tubes may be required to equalize pressure in the middle ear (see Chap. 35).

Sensorineural or nerve deafness results from damage to auditory neurons or to the hair cells inside the cochlea. Sensorineural loss may be caused by genetic disorders or maternal infections, or may be acquired from head trauma, infections (especially meningitis), recurrent exposure to extremely loud noises, and exposure to ototoxic drugs (i.e., aminoglycosides).

Nursing Implications

Every child needs continual audiologic assessments. For the infant, absence of the startle reflex to a loud sound or failure to turn the head toward loud noises may be suggestive of hearing impairment. Advances in diagnostic techniques allow the detection of hearing impairments during the first few months of life, making early intervention possible. The primary clue to a potential hearing deficit is failure for an infant to make babbling sounds after about 6 months of age. For the older child, two main indicators of hearing impairment are: 1) lack of response to any form of noise and 2) requests to have statements or questions repeated. Referrals for further evaluation should occur any time hearing is questioned. An audiologist is trained to detect and assist in diagnosis of hearing problems; an otorhinolaryngologist is a physician specializing in ear, nose, and throat disorders.

The major goal of treatment for any child with hearing impairment is to help him develop the ability to communicate with others. Treatment may include hearing aids, alternative forms of communication, or speech training. If hearing aids are recommended, the type of auditory disorder dictates the kind of hearing aid to be worn. Children with conductive hearing loss who have some residual hearing abilities benefit the most from hearing aids. It is possible to fit a child as young as 8 to 10 months of age with hearing devices. Parents must be aware that hearing aids never restore hearing completely, nor do they distinguish or make sounds more intelligible.

They merely amplify all environmental sounds by making them louder (see Chap. 34).

A child with substantial hearing loss may use different language systems for communication. Oral communication employs lip reading. The main advantage to this system is that the child lives in an oral society. However, because many sounds look alike, lip reading is difficult. Only 30% of the English language is visible on the lips.[14] Therefore, the vocabulary acquired by the deaf child does not increase as rapidly as other children's vocabulary. Manual communication involves American sign language (ASL) and finger spelling. American sign language uses hand gestures to convey words and concepts. Finger spelling spells out each word separately and is therefore a slower method than ASL. Vocabulary may be built quicker with manual communication, but the child can communicate only with those individuals who also sign. As the child becomes increasingly independent, this may pose a substantial problem. Children who combine oral and manual systems of communication have the greatest advantage.

Hospitalized Child   Special strategies must be used for the hospitalized child who is hearing impaired. The nurse must understand that the use of touch and eye contact are extremely important before attempting verbal communication. Visual aids are beneficial, and if the child is old enough to express himself or herself in writing, the use of chalk boards may be indispensable. Methods to enhance lip reading include facing the child directly, speaking clearly and slowly, and keeping sentences short and to the point. Interpreters may be necessary to communicate with the child who uses sign language when parents are unavailable. The nurse must be the child's advocate by actively including the child in care and by helping other health team members to communicate in a uniform fashion.

Communication Disorders

Communication disorders encompass a wide spectrum of problems. Regardless of the nature of the problem, however, the impact for any child with a language disorder is significant, because language influences the emotional, social, and academic life of the individual. Logopedics is the science dealing with the study of speech and language pathology and treatment of these communication disabilities.

The five most common conditions associated with communication disorders are hearing impairments, cerebral palsy, autism, craniofacial anomalies, and mental retardation.

Communication disorders are categorized under two broad headings: oral-motor disabilities (speech disorders) and communication delays/disabilities. *Oral-motor disabilities* result from neuromuscular deficits or structural abnormalities that impair movement of the oral muscles and prevent proper formation of sounds and words. Speech disorders are listed in the accompanying display. These problems are usually a result of birth defects or severe brain dysfunction. Surgical intervention is the treatment of choice for structural problems. Historically,

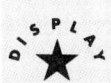

Possible Manifestations of Speech Disorders

Disorders of Respiration
Insufficient respiratory support for speech
Abnormal breath pattern: clavicular breathing, forced inspiration–expiration, audible inspiration

Disorders of Phonation
Abnormalities in loudness: monoloudness, excess loudness variation, inappropriate loudness
Abnormalities in pitch: pitch breaks, monopitch, inappropriate pitch
Abnormalities in voice quality: breathy, harsh, hoarse, strain-strangled, tremor, voice stoppages, aphonia

Disorders of Resonance
Hypernasality
Hyponasality
Nasal emission
Vowel distortion

Disorders of Articulation
Distortion of speech sounds
Omission of speech sounds
Imprecision of speech sounds
Irregular articulatory breakdowns

Disorders of Prosody
Abnormalities in rate of speech: short rushes of speech, variable rate, increase in rate of sound segments, increase in overall rate
Abnormalities in rhythm of speech: excessive and equal stress, reduced stress, prolonged intervals, inappropriate silences
Prolonged phonemes
Repeated phonemes

(Source: Oski, F. A., DeAngelis, C. D., Feigin, R. D., & Warshaw, J. B. (Eds.). (1990). [p. 626.] Principles and practice of pediatrics. Philadelphia: J. B. Lippincott.

other forms of treatment focused on exercises to strengthen the specific muscles of speech, but recently, sign language and synthetic speech are augmenting the traditional approach. Because articulation, fluency, and voice are involved in speech production, a team approach including dentist and speech pathologist must be used.

Communication delays/disabilities are caused by the same array of factors that cause any developmental disorders. Language development is the domain of the left hemisphere, and any insult or damage to this area of the brain may result in some form of language difficulties.

Communication is a complex process involving both receptive and expressive language. *Receptive language* is the process of receiving a message and attempting to decode, decipher, and comprehend it. An estimated 3% to 10% of school-age children have a developmental receptive language disorder.[2] A receptive language disorder typically appears before the age of 4 years, and with educational interventions normal language skills may be acquired.

Expressive language is the process of sending a message. A child has difficulty with encoding when there is a problem with expressive language. The child may have a limited vocabulary or limited variety of sentence structures on which to depend. Words may be omitted or substituted incorrectly, and sounds or syllables may be transposed. Another 3 to 10% of school-age children are estimated to have developmental expressive language disorders.[2] Minimal brain dysfunction may cause this, but the major factor involved is limited exposure to environmental or educational stimuli. Poor expressive communication among all individuals correlates most significantly with low socioeconomic status.[11] Compared to children of higher socioeconomic levels, children of low socioeconomic status unfortunately are not exposed to a variety or wealth of experiences. Lack of these experiences leads to a dearth of communication skills, delayed academic performance, and poor social interactions. The nurse must educate parents to the importance of verbal stimulation. Because an association exists between language disabilities and abused or neglected children, the nurse also must assess the parent-child dyad for possible signs of abusive behavior (see Chap. 5). Severely neglected and emotionally traumatized children show the lowest scores on all areas of language development.[11]

Terminology used to describe specific language problems includes lisping, articulation problems, and fluency difficulties. Lisping occurs when the sounds of "s" or "z" are substituted for the "th" sound. Articulation is the ability to produce or sequence speech appropriately. The use of tat for cat or bo for boat is an example of articulation problems. Fluency refers to the rate, rhythm, or general flow of speech. Examples of difficulties with fluency include hesitations, repetitions, prolongations, and stuttering.

Stuttering, synonymous with stammering, typically begins during the course of speech and language development, with a peak onset at age 5. Approximately 5% of children stutter, with a 3:1 male:female ratio.[2] Recent research suggests genetic factors may be involved in the cause. Stuttering has an insidious onset, but when recognized, may exacerbate during periods of stress and anxiety. Eighty percent of those children who stutter recover totally, usually after the age of 16. Sixty percent of this group recovers spontaneously without any form of treatment.[2] The nurse provides emotional support to the child and encourages parents to have patience. The nurse reassures parents by explaining that additional pressure for the child to correct the speech impediment may make the child self-conscious and indeed intensify the problem.

Nursing Implications

The nurse takes every opportunity to assess children for communication disorders. Is the child speaking spontaneously? Are sentences age-appropriate, short or long, simple or sophisticated? A comprehensive workup is required whenever possible language problems are recognized. Initially an auditory assessment is requested to rule out audiologic difficulties that may not have been identified previously. Indications for referral are listed in the accompanying display on guidelines for referral of an infant.

Treatment for communication disorders is dictated by the underlying cause, but the overriding goal is to help the child communicate more effectively. Prevention when possible is optimal. Treatment focuses on remediation or compensation. Remediation refers to work that corrects or counteracts problems, typically with assistance from a speech pathologist. Compensation refers to augmentational efforts that allow the child to counterbalance deficits. Nonverbal communication may rely on eye blinks or sophisticated electronic devices tailored individually to the user (i.e., light-pointing equipment that selects locations on a manual communication board). Figure 20-4 is an example of such computerized technology. These options have significantly improved the quality of these children's lives. As industry continues to cooperate in the endeavor to supply equipment for synthetic speech, those with multihandicaps will be able to communicate in some form.

Selected Cognitive Disorders

A distinction must be made between mental, along with developmental delay, and deviant development. The former refers to development that has stopped at some point with behavior specific to the phase in which this occurred (e.g., mental retardation). The latter refers to development that is inappropriate or unstable. Examples of deviant development are neurosis, schizophrenia, and psychotic states and are addressed in Chapter 19. Cognitive disorders addressed in this chapter include mental retardation and learning disorders.

Mental Retardation

According to the American Association on Mental Retardation, mental retardation is defined as "significantly subaverage general intellectual functioning existing concurrently with deficits in adaptive behavior and manifested during the developmental period."[13] The list of variables that are correlated with mental retardation include infection, prenatal substance abuse, trauma, poor prenatal nutrition, or endocrine disorders, brain disorders, genetic abnormalities, and environmental factors (see Table 20-2 for a more complete list of causes). Severe mental retardation is associated with genetic, biochemical, viral, or developmental factors. Environment factors are associated with moderate mental retardation.

An individual is diagnosed with mental retardation before 18 years of age and scores a minimum of two standard deviations below the average for his/her age group on a standardized intelligence test. People with mental retardation are grouped according to their IQ test results (Table 20-3). Seventy-five to 85% of individuals with mental retardation are categorized in the mild group and have the potential to perform activities of daily living.

The prognosis for children with mental retardation has increased because institutional care is no longer recommended. These children are mainstreamed whenever feasible and are taught survival skills. A multidimensional orientation is used when working with children with mental retardation, considering their physiologic, cog-

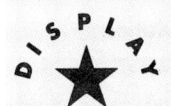

Nursing Assessment: Guidelines for Referral for Audiologic Speech-Language Evaluation

Interaction-Communication
1. Excessive crying after 3 months of age.
2. Lack of crying, or crying that is perceived as abnormal in infancy.
3. Lack of eye contact or of smiling after 3 months of age.
4. Lack of cooing vocalizations or response to smiling adults from 3 to 6 months of age.
5. Expressions of dislike at being held (squirming, crying, consistent tenseness that is relieved by placing child in infant seat) in first 6 months.
6. Failure of appearance of laughter, or lack of laughter in interactive situations, by 6 months of age.
7. Failure to respond in interactive peek-a-boo and patty cake games by 1 year of age.
8. Failure to indicate communicative intention nonverbally by 1 year of age.

Reception-Comprehension
1. Failure to respond to environmental sounds.
2. Failure to quiet to mother's voice when infant's fussing or crying and when mother is out of immediate line of sight and not in contact with infant.
3. Difficulty in localizing a sound source correctly after 9 to 12 months.
4. Failure to respond to voices of family members in the second 6 months of life, when these persons return after an absence and are still out of immediate line of sight and not in contact with infant.
5. Failure to understand common words or commands by age 18 months.
6. Failure to indicate one or two familiar objects or people when these are named with gesture in the second year of life.
7. Failure to indicate one or two familiar objects or people when these are named (without accompanying gesture toward or gaze at object-person) early in the third year of life.
8. Failure to understand simple discussions of past or future events by age 3.
9. Report that a child does not understand what is said to him, "takes no notice" of what is said to him, or "takes a long time to catch on" to what is said in the third year of life.

Expression-Production
1. Failure to produce any consonantal sounds (raspberries, nasals, and stops) in the first year of life.
2. Failure to produce consonantal sounds toward front of mouth in second 6 months of life.
3. Failure to produce high front /v/, back /a/, and rounded vowels /u/ by 15 months of age.
4. Failure to produce prolonged vocalic or consonantal sounds, to combine primitive consonantal and vocalic elements in a single segment, or to produce series of segments or syllables in noncry in the first 12 months of life.
5. Failure to produce reduplicated babbling by 9 to 10 months of age.
6. Lack of or use of an excessive amount of expressive jargon after 18 months of age.
7. Failure to produce recognizable words by age 2.
8. Failure to use several recognizable two-word combinations that combine two ideas by age 2 years 6 months; e.g., "more juice."
9. Lack of multiword utterances (phrases, sentences) by age 3.
10. Lack of intelligible speech by age 3.
11. Many initial consonants omitted at age 3. Lack of final consonants by age 4.
12. Continuing substitution of easy sounds for more difficult sounds after age 5.
13. Persisting faults of speech articulation after age 7.
14. Decrease in amount of speech produced, instead of steady increase, at any age from 3 to 7 years.
15. Sentences that are poorly formed, confused, marked by word reversals or telegraphic style after age 4 (dialectal variations not to be considered in this category).
16. Noticeable stuttering or other types of abnormality of rhythm or rate (rapid speech, cluttering) after age 4.
17. Monotonous, unusually loud, hoarse, harsh, or inaudible voice.
18. Pitch that is not appropriate to child's age and sex.
19. Noticeable hypernasality or lack of normal resonance.
20. Embarrassment or disturbed feelings about his speech on the part of the child at any age.

(Source: *Levine, M. D., Carey, W. B., Crocker, A. C., & Gross, R. T. 1983. [p. 853]. Developmental-behavioral pediatrics. Philadelphia: W. B. Saunders.*)

nitive, social, and emotional development. Emotional development tends to lag behind the other areas. Specific causes of mental retardation are complex.

★ NURSING ASSESSMENT

The nursing assessment of a child with mental retardation includes careful review of a recent psychological evaluation and physical examination. Psychometric testing such

as the Stanford-Binet Test and Wechsler Intelligence Scale for Children-Revised, categorizes the child's level of disability and dictates options available to the child. Early infant behaviors that may indicate a cognitive disability include nonresponsiveness to contact, poor eye contact during feeding, slow feeding, diminished spontaneous activity, decreased responsiveness to surroundings, decreased alertness to voice or movement, and irritability.[17] Because these children may not understand why a phys-

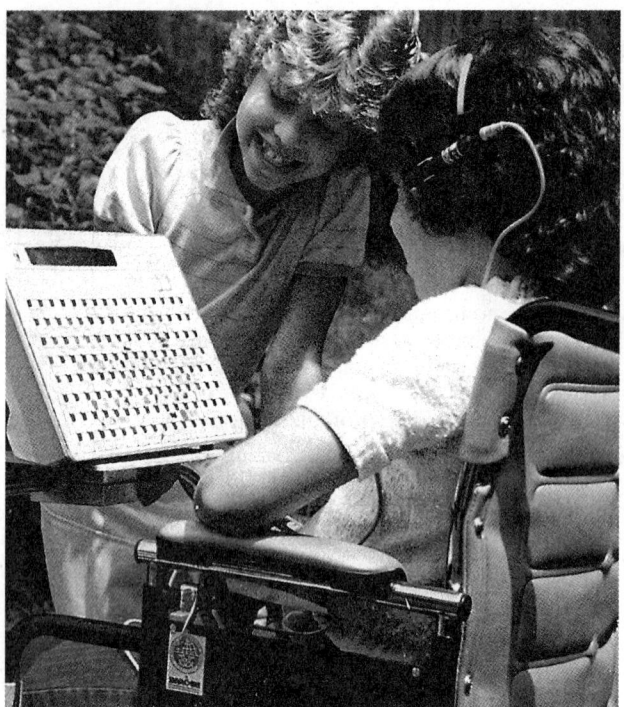

FIGURE 20-4
Touch Talker and Light Talker, computerized equipment that responds to touch, light, and a control switch. (Courtesy of Prentke Romich Co.)

TABLE 20-2
Etiologies Associated With Mental Retardation

Hereditary Disorders (preconceptual origin; variable expression, multiple somatic effects, frequently a progressive course)

- Inborn errors of metabolism (e.g., Tay-Sachs disease, Hurler disease, phenylketonuria)
- Other single-gene abnormalities (e.g., muscular dystrophy, neurofibromatosis, tuberous sclerosis)
- Chromosomal aberrations, including translocation
- Polygenic familial syndromes

Early Alterations of Embryonic Development (sporadic events affecting embryogenesis; phenotypic changes, usually a stable developmental handicap)

- Chromosomal changes, including trisomy (e.g., Down syndrome)
- Prenatal influence syndromes (e.g., intrauterine infections, drugs, unknown forces)

Other Pregnancy Problems and Perinatal Morbidity (impingement on progress of fetus during last two trimesters or newborn; neurologic abnormalities frequent, handicap stable or occasionally with increasing problems)

- Fetal malnutrition—placental insufficiency
- Perinatal difficulties (e.g., prematurity, hypoxia, trauma)

Acquired Childhood Diseases (acute modification of developmental status; variable potential for functional recovery)

- Infection (e.g., encephalitis, meningitis)
- Cranial trauma
- Other (e.g., cardiac arrest, intoxications)

Environmental and Behavioral Problems (dynamic influences, operational throughout development; commonly combined with other handicaps)

- Deprivation
- Parental neurosis, psychosis
- Childhood neurosis
- Childhood psychosis, including autism

Unknown Causes (no definite hereditary, gestational, perinatal, acquired, or environmental issues; or else multiple elements present)

(Adapted with permission from: Crocker, A. C. In: Thompson, G. H., et al. [Eds.]. [1983]. Comprehensive management of cerebral palsy. New York: Grune & Stratton, Inc.)

ical assessment is necessary and may even fear evaluation by nursing personnel, a nonthreatening approach with the help of the parent or caretaker is essential.

In addition to the physical assessment, documentation of daily living skills are important. Evaluations with the Vineland Social Maturity Scale and the AAMR Adaptive Behavior Scale are helpful in determining age levels at which the child functions. A careful family assessment also provides information on the family's response to the child with mental deficits, if there are other members with impaired cognition, the degree of independence encouraged at home, and the stability of the family unit.

★ **NURSING DIAGNOSIS AND PLANNING**

The following nursing diagnoses may be applied to children with mental retardation:

- Altered Growth and Development related to limited cognition.
- Knowledge Deficit related to inability to consistently problem-solve.
- Altered Family Processes related to consistent dependent family member.

The long-term goals for children with mental retardation are highly individualized and are dependent on the level of mental retardation (mild to profound). Parents should be involved in establishing realistic goals for their child. Examples of long-term goals may include:

- The child dresses himself or herself
- The child maintains continence of stool and urine
- The child demonstrates acceptable social behaviors.
- The adolescent participates in a structured work program

★ **NURSING INTERVENTIONS**

Early intervention programs are essential for children with mental retardation to maximize the children's potential development. This necessitates early recognition and referral. Nurses have an opportunity to evaluate children in the nursery, in the clinic during well-child health care, in schools, and during acute management. The potential of each child will vary according to the degree of mental retardation (Table 20-4). The key for success is that the child's strengths and potential abilities are emphasized rather than deficits.

The goal of early intervention programs is to promote optimum development. This includes programs that teach infant stimulation, activities of daily living, and independent self-care skills. In addition, learning social skills and adaptive behaviors assist the child in building a positive self-image. For older children and adolescents, assistance is needed to prepare individuals who are mentally retarded for a productive work life.

Sexuality becomes a major concern as these children mature. Some individuals who are mentally retarded may

TABLE 20-3
Classification of Levels of Mental Retardation Assessed by Standardized Intelligence Tests as Recommended by the AAMR*

	Obtained Intelligence Quotient	
Levels	Stanford-Binet and Cattell ($\sigma = 16$)	Wechsler Scales ($\sigma = 15$)
Mild (Educable)	67–52	69–55
Moderate (Trainable)	51–36	54–40
Severe (Dependent Retarded)	35–20	39–25 (Extrapolated)
Profound (Life Support)	19 and below	24 and below (Extrapolated)

* American Association on Mental Retardation

form emotional attachments to those of the opposite sex and normal sexual desires. However, their decision-making skills are limited. Teaching contraceptive methods are important to emphasize with both the child and family. Decisions regarding sterilization are highly controversial, and presents society with a moral and ethical dilemma.

Down Syndrome

Down syndrome (DS), or trisomy 21, involves mental retardation. In Down syndrome, the child is born with an extra chromosome number 21. The incidence of trisomy 21 is 1:1000 live births, with equal representation for males and females. Because the risk of trisomy 21 increases with maternal age, pregnant women older than age 35 are recommended to undergo amniocentesis to karyotype fetal cells.

Typical phenotypic features for a child with trisomy 21 include: short, stocky stature; flat head with flat facial features; short, broad, stubby hands with a simian crease (a single transverse palmar crease); upward-slanting eyes with prominent epicanthal folds, small oral cavity accompanied by a large, protruding tongue; low-set ears; and hypotonia. Other characteristics include a short neck, a short nose with depressed nasal bridge due to an underdeveloped nasal bone, extra wide spacing between first and second fingers and toes, speckled iris (Brushfield spots), and dental and visual abnormalities. Because of these typical features, children with trisomy 21 are diagnosed with mental retardation earlier than those children with mild retardation of unknown cause. Children with trisomy 21 have an increase in congenital cardiac defects, and leukemia occurs more frequently compared with the general population.

TABLE 20-4
Behavioral Manifestations of Mild, Moderate, Severe, and Profound Levels of Mental Retardation

Activity of Daily Living (ADL) Skills	Social/Interpersonal Skills	Educational Skills/ Problem-solving Skills	Motor/Coordination Skills
Mild Retardation			
Can be taught independent activities of daily living. Can be taught to live independently	Can develop social skills. Can develop ability to verbalize rather than act out feelings and needs	Can succeed in reading, math, and spelling skills. Can succeed in vocational education. Limited abilities for abstract thinking	Has gross and fine motor abilities—can often do semiskilled manual labor—can do unskilled manual labor
Moderate Retardation			
Requires some assistance with activities of daily living. Requires some structure in living arrangements (e.g., halfway house)	Simple work mastery. Some ability to act out versus verbalization of feelings and needs	Can learn words, numbers, and signs that facilitate basic survival. Poor abilities for abstract thinking	Follows simple two- to three-word instructions. Poor fine motor skills, good gross motor skills. Can participate in unskilled labor requiring repetitive tasks
Severe Retardation			
Possibility of teaching some ADL skills with long-term consistent behavior modification. Requires great deal of assistance. Requires structured living arrangements	Some expressive skills; says a few words. Strong nonverbal acting out of needs/feelings	Rarely can learn to read, write, spell, or use math. No ability to abstract	Poor gross and fine motor skills; uncoordinated
Profound Retardation			
Unable to complete ADLs independently. Typically requires institutional placement and full-time care	Unable to relate verbally to others	No success in academic skills. No ability to abstract	No fine or gross skills

(Developed from a variety of sources. *Printed with permission from:* McFarland, G. K., and Thomas, M. D. [1991]. [p. 502]. *Psychiatric mental health nursing: Application of the nursing process.* Philadelphia: J. B. Lippincott.)

These children require a multidisciplinary approach to care. Considering the many physiologic problems, cognitive impairments, and social needs, planning involves early intervention, close follow-up, and prospective planning.

The care plan for children and families with Down syndrome is similar to the care plan for other children with mental retardation. The nurse needs to be aware of the developmental delays seen in children with Down syndrome and assist parents in modifying their expectations of when certain behaviors can occur. The nurse may help parents set realistic goals by identifying the strengths and special talents of their child. Table 20-5 provides a comparison of developmental milestones and self-care activities of children with Down syndrome with "normal" children. Children with Down syndrome seem to benefit from early intervention programs and environmental enrichment and stimulation at home. Those children with congenital heart problems have an improved prognosis for intellectual development.[17] In planning care, nurses should consider that children with Down syndrome are sensitive to unfamiliar situations, separation from mothers, and the presence of new people.[17] Children with Down syndrome seem to be sensitive to the needs and feelings of others and have adequate social abilities.[17]

Fragile X Syndrome

A significant cytogenetic advancement has been the identification of the fragile X chromosome. The fragile X syndrome is an X-linked pattern of inheritance associated with mental retardation. The discovery of the fragile X chromosome was made in the 1960s, but changes in the culture medium used to detect chromosomes occurred in the 1970s, and in the new medium the fragile site on the X chromosome went undetected.[17] The discovery of the influence of the culture medium on identification of fragile X has lead to improved diagnosis of the chromosomal abnormality. It is estimated that fragile X syndrome occurs in 1 in 1000 male births.[17] Fragile X syndrome is the second leading cytogenic cause of mental retardation, second to Down syndrome.[17]

★ **NURSING ASSESSMENT**

Affected males with fragile X syndrome have the following characteristics: short stature, normal-to-increased head circumference, long face, prominent forehead, large ears, midfacial hypoplasia, prominent symphysis of the mandible, large hands and feet, and large testes. Males with fragile X syndrome are often developmentally delayed and will have mild-to-moderate mental retardation. However, borderline intelligence to severe mental retardation have been reported. Learning disabilities and speech difficulties such as apraxia have been reported. The child may present with rapid speech, stuttering, and repetition of words that are characteristic speech pattern noted in males with fragile X syndrome.[17] Temper tantrums and autistic behaviors have been associated with fragile X.

TABLE 20-5
Developmental Milestones and Self-Care Skills of Children With Down Syndrome Compared With "Normal" Children

	Children With Down Syndrome	"Normal" Children
	Average	Average
Smiling	2 months	1 month
Rolling over	8 months	5 months
Sitting alone	10 months	7 months
Crawling	12 months	8 months
Creeping	15 months	10 months
Standing	20 months	11 months
Walking	24 months	13 months
Talking, words	16 months	10 months
Talking, sentences	28 months	21 months
Eating		
Finger feeding	12 months	8 months
Using spoon and fork	20 months	13 months
Toilet training		
Bladder	48 months	32 months
Bowel	42 months	29 months
Dressing		
Undressing	40 months	32 months
Putting clothes on	58 months	47 months

(Source: Levine, M. D., Carey, W. B., Crocker, A. C., & Gross, R. T. [1983]. [pp. 358–359]. *Developmental-behavioral pediatrics.* Philadelphia: W. B. Saunders.)

Classic infantile autism may be the presenting diagnosis reported in some males with fragile X chromosome.

The expression of fragile X in heterozygous women has been reported, but is not common. The identification of the asymptomatic fragile X carriers is difficult to determine. Both affected women and affected men are capable of transmitting the fragile X condition.[17]

Screening techniques to diagnose fragile X syndrome are recommended for a family once a child is diagnosed in order to plan genetic counseling and teaching programs for future pregnancies as well as to identify carriers in female children.

★ **NURSING DIAGNOSIS, PLANNING, INTERVENTION, AND EVALUATION**

The reader is referred to those discussions of children with Down syndrome. The nursing diagnoses, goals, and outcomes for children with mental retardation remain the same regardless of the primary etiology.

The treatment for fragile X syndrome does not include a cure. Medical treatments include phenothiazines to control behavioral problems and central nervous system stimulants to manage the attention-deficit hyperactivity disorder, which is often associated with fragile X. Early speech and language therapy is important as well as special education programs, which help children learn basic skills for activities of daily living.

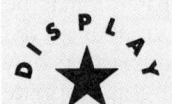

Types of Fetal Disorders Associated With Maternal Alcohol Consumption

Fetal Alcohol Syndrome (FAS)
(a) Prenatal or postnatal growth retardation (below the 10th percentile)
(b) Central nervous system disturbances including tremulousness, poor sucking reflexes, abnormal muscle tone, hyperactivity, attention disorders, or mental retardation
(c) At least two characteristic facial anomalies, including narrow eye width, ptosis, thin upper lip, short upturned nose with underdeveloped groove, hypoplasia of midfascial area[33]

Clinodactyly
Small distal phalanges
Small fifth fingernails
Short stature
Hypotonia
Fine motor dysfunction
Cardiac murmurs: VSD,
  ASD usually gone by
  age 1 year

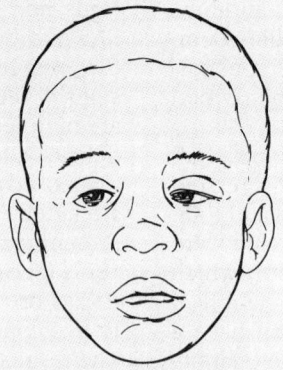

Fetal Alcohol Syndrome

Key Figures
Mild to moderate microcephaly
Short palpebral fissures
Smooth philtrum
Thin vermillion border of upper lip

Other Findings
Maxillary hypoplasia
Short, upturned nose
Cleft lip and/or palate
Short neck
Posteriorly rotated, prominent ears

Alcohol-Related Birth Deficits (ARBD)
Complications of pregnancy or birth defects attributed to alcohol

Fetal Alcohol Effects (FAE)
Range of congenital abnormalities associated with maternal drinking such as eye and ear defects, heart murmurs, genitourinary deficits, hemangiomas, and finger print and palm crease abnormalities.[24]

(Illustration from: Oski, F. A., DeAngelis, C. D., Feigin, R. D., & Warshaw, J. B. [Eds.]. [1990]. Principles and practice of pediatrics. Philadelphia: J. B. Lippincott.)

Fetal Alcohol Syndrome

The effects of alcohol on the developing fetus have been reported in the literature since the 18th century.[33] Fetal alcohol syndrome (FAS) refers the presence of growth retardation, mental retardation, developmental delays, neurologic abnormalities, and facial deformity associated with heavy maternal alcohol consumption during pregnancy. Heavy alcohol consumption has been defined as 8 ounces or more of liquor or 8 glasses or more of wine per day.[34] The term "fetal alcohol syndrome" has been reserved for children who present characteristic findings in the three areas of central nervous system disturbances, growth retardation, and facial features of FAS (see the accompanying display on types of disorders associated with maternal alcohol abuse).

The term fetal alcohol effects (FAE) is used to classify children who have a variety of fetal problems associated with moderate maternal alcohol use. Moderate amounts of maternal alcohol consumption are associated with stillbirths, midtrimester abortions, congenital abnormalities, growth retardation, and physical and mental delays.[34]

The incidence of fetal alcohol syndrome is 1.9 per 1000 live births.[33,34] Alcohol use during pregnancy is considered the third known cause of birth defects. Fetal alcohol syndrome is the leading known cause of mental retardation, ranking ahead of Down syndrome and spina bifida.[24,33,34] The rate of FAS may be significantly higher in certain populations including the North American Indians, who are known to consume alcohol excessively. The Southwest Plains Indians have an incidence of 9.8 per 1000 live births.[23] Pueblo and Navajo Indians' incidence of FAS is equal to that of the general population, at 1.9/1000. Global statistics for FAS include: 1/1000 live births in France; 1/6000 in Sweden, to 1/750 in Seattle, Washington.[34]

In addition to persistent exposure to alcohol, FAS and alcohol-related birth defects (ARBD) increase the following risk factors: frequent beer drinking, low prepregnancy weight, low maternal weight gain, and low socioeconomic status.

Cause and Pathophysiology Three mechanisms have been proposed in an attempt to understanding the effects of alcohol on the developing fetus: secondary effect hypothesis, dosage hypothesis, and segregation hypothesis. The various hypotheses have been developed to explain the relationships between cognitive and behavioral deficits of FAS and FAE, and the physical defects.[16]

The secondary effect hypothesis suggests that the physical effects of FAS are secondary to direct and specific intake of alcohol during critical fetal growth periods and that the cognitive and behavioral developmental delays are related to nutritional deficiencies induced by prenatal alcohol and by impaired postnatal maternal behaviors.[16] Alcohol appears to impair the maternal absorption of nutrients into the blood or across the placenta to the fetus. Maternal weight curves and nutritional habits of mothers are being studied by researchers. Recent studies demonstrating the effects of alcohol on the fetal nervous system development support the theory that the behavioral deficits are not the result of poor mothering.[16]

The dosage hypothesis states that the amount of alcohol consumed and over what period of time is related to the risk and severity of the symptoms of FAS and FAE. Sheriff[7] found that the fetal abnormalities in mice were related to the maternal blood levels of alcohol, which would involve not only the amount, but the metabolism rate of the mother. Thus, binge drinking may have a greater negative impact than drinking the same quantity of alcohol over an extended period of time. Binge drinking associated with maternal smoking was found to be more harmful than binge drinking by the nonsmoker.[34]

The segregation hypothesis proposes that the susceptibility of the fetus to the teratogenic effects of alcohol varies with fetal developmental. For example, a teratogen inflicted during the gestational period from day 20 to day 55 results in gross structural defects or death. A teratogen ingested during the second half of pregnancy causes growth retardation and functional deficits.[16] The teratogenic effects of alcohol include direct alcohol toxicity, fetal hypoxia, and acetaldehyde toxicity.[33]

In summary, research studies are continuing to investigate the effects of alcohol fetal development, and the relationship between volume and timing of that consumption. The teratogenic effects of alcohol are a societal concern, and warning labels have been placed on all alcoholic beverages and in various locales (bars, grocery stores, alcoholic beverage stores) where alcohol is sold.

★ NURSING ASSESSMENT

Mothers are the most important factor in preventing FAS. Therefore, it is essential to know if a prior history of alcoholism exists so that appropriate intervention may occur. During the pregnancy, the mother is evaluated for alcohol consumption and given appropriate information about the effects of alcohol on the fetus. Alcohol-dependent women may underestimate the amount they drink. Some women may feel guilty about drinking and therefore under-report use of alcohol or even a history of alcoholism.[24] Some women may also find it difficult to admit they smoke, compounding their problems. Techniques for discussing prenatal concerns are described in Chapter 10.

Roman[24] suggests that health care professionals be cautious in considering the prevention of FAS as the woman's sole responsibility: difficulties and barriers may impede or prevent women from accessing appropriate assistance for alcohol problems. Drinking behaviors of women are influenced by the spouses or partners. Roman,[24] therefore, believes that males have a major responsibility in reducing or eliminating their alcohol intake when their partner is pregnant.

The newborn who has been exposed to alcohol prenatally may have significant alterations in reflexive behaviors. The newborn has less mature motor behaviors and increased activity levels.[24] The newborn presenting with characteristic facial features, altered neurologic signs, and low birth weight would signal FAS. Although FAS may be diagnosed in the neonatal or infant period, the long-term implications are significant. Neurologic signs of fetal alcohol syndrome throughout the lifespan are outlined in the accompanying display on neurologic deficits. Children with fetal alcohol effects may not be diagnosed until motor or language developmental delays are noted. The nurse may use a variety of developmental screening techniques, including growth charts and Denver II (see Chap. 9) to assess children for developmental delays or deficits. IQ testing of children with FAS and FAE is commonly administered during preschool years. The results of IQ tests of children with FAS and FAE are stable from childhod to adolescence.[31]

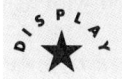

Neurologic Deficits Associated With Fetal Alcohol Syndrome

Neonate:	Poor sucking
	Disrupted sleep states
	Low levels of arousal
	Tremulousness
	Unusual body orientation
	Excessive mouthing
	Abnormal reflexes
	Hypertonia
	Poor adjustment to repetitive stimuli
Infancy:	Disrupted sleep-wake patterns
	Poor visual recognition memory
	Decrements in mental and motor development, spoken language, and verbal comprehension
Preschooler:	Attention deficit disorder
	Delayed reaction times
	Decrements in fine and gross motor performance
Adolescent:	Psychosocial problems
	Overt psychopathology
Adults:	Adaptative living
	Self-sufficiency lacking

(Adapted from: *Warren, K. R., & Bast, R. J. (1988). Alcohol-related birth defects: An update.* Public Health Reports, 103(6), 638–642.)

★ NURSING DIAGNOSES AND PLANNING

Based on the findings from the nursing assessments, history, physical examination, and other related studies, the following nursing diagnoses may be appropriate:

- Ineffective Family Coping (Disabling) related to maternal alcoholism.
- Altered Growth and Development, related to fetal exposure to alcohol.
- Sensory-Perceptual Alterations related to fetal alcohol syndrome.
- Sleep Pattern Disturbance related to fetal alcohol syndrome.

The parents, child, and nurse plan nursing interventions to help the child develop to his or her full potential. The nurse assists the family in meeting the needs of both the child and family. The following are examples of goals:

- The child participates in self-care activities: dressing, feeding, toileting
- The child receives appropriate academic challenges
- The family identifies community support programs to assist them in day-to-day care of their child

★ NURSING INTERVENTIONS

Prevention of fetal alcohol syndrome occurs prior to conception. The nurse has an obligation to educate women of childbearing age about the dangers of alcohol consumption during pregnancy. Adolescent females in particular need to be counselled about these hazards. The nursing interventions are aimed at improving the growth and development of the child both cognitively and physically. Fetal alcohol syndrome is a complex, multifaceted problem. The child with sensory and auditory problems may require prostheses (glasses, hearing aids). Motor development varies according to the severity of the involvement. The presence of mental retardation may be measured in the preschool years, and long-range plans are developed to include educational, vocational, and housing needs. Special education opportunities may vary slightly from community to community.[31] The educational goals should stress life skills.

Attention-deficit hyperactivity disorder is associated with FAS probably because of neurologic abnormalities. Other maladaptive behaviors observed in FAS and FAE, include problems with concentration, attention, impulsivity, and bullying. Adolescents may be sullen or stubborn. Lying, stealing, and cheating have been observed in FAS and FAE.[31] The number of psychosexual or behavioral problems creates new problems as the child ages. Strategies for disciplining children with behavioral problems may be ineffective because of the degree of mental retardation.[31] The inability of the adolescent (or later adult) to learn socially acceptable behaviors may lead to placement outside the home. Waterson and Murray-Lyon[34] suggest that FAS-related mental retardation accounts for 11% of the annual cost for institutionalizing people with mental retardation.

★ EVALUATION

The prognosis of children with FAS and FAE is not positive. The children do not appear to "catch up" developmentally. The family and child need to be re-evaluated on a regular basis to promote continued involvement in special education programs, appropriate treatment for medical problems, and referrals to support services. Preventing FAS through public education, media campaigns, and support programs for women with drinking problems is the best solution.

Attention-Deficit Hyperactivity Disorder

Attention-deficit hyperactivity disorder (ADHD) is a learning disorder with behavioral overtones. In 1987 the DSM-III-R (third revised edition of the *Diagnostic and Statistical Manual for Mental Disorders*) expanded the criteria for attention deficit disorder (ADD) to give the symptom of hyperactivity more significance.[2] Thus it became ADHD. This condition, usually identified by the age of 3, may be diagnosed any time during the school-age years. Boys are affected 4 to 10 times more often than girls, with a prevalence in the total population estimated at 1.2% to 20%, depending on the criteria used for diagnosis.[4] Diagnostic criteria for ADHD are listed in the accompanying display.

The cause of ADHD is not known. Neurotransmitters have been an area of much speculation, but research has not identified any specific abnormality. The Attention Deficit Disorder Association states that the disorder is a neurologic and biochemical condition that makes it difficult for people to concentrate.[12] External substances including toxins (i.e., lead, prenatal alcohol) and food additives (i.e., artificial color and flavors) have been suggested as possible culprits, but research has failed to provide conclusive support for a definitive relationship. Psychosocial factors such as inconsistent parental discipline, deviant parental role models, and disorganized, chaotic environments may produce signs and symptoms of ADHD, making diagnosis extremely difficult.

Three characteristics most common to ADHD are inattentiveness, impulsiveness, and motor hyperactivity, as listed in the diagnostic criteria. The child has an extremely short attention span, is easily distracted, and is unable to attend to tasks at hand. The child calls out in class frequently, has difficulty awaiting turns in group situations, and demonstrates poor cooperative play.

Hyperactivity permeates throughout the child's day. The child fails to follow through with parental or teacher requests; movements are haphazard, random, and purposeless, and activity is not goal directed. Parents are frustrated easily and daily because of this hyperactivity.

★ NURSING ASSESSMENT

An excellent developmental history is imperative. Attention-deficit hyperactivity disorder is traced usually to early childhood, with common threads of recurring behavior apparent throughout the child's life. Numerous tests can

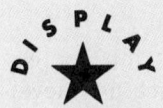

Diagnostic Criteria for Attention-Deficit Hyperactivity Disorder

Note: Consider a criterion met only if the behavior is considerably more frequent than that of most people of the same mental age.

A. A disturbance of at least 6 months during which at least eight of the following are present:

   (1) Often fidgets with hands or feet or squirms in seat (in adolescents, may be limited to subjective feelings of restlessness)
   (2) Has difficulty remaining seated when required to do so
   (3) Is easily distracted by extraneous stimuli
   (4) Has difficulty awaiting turn in games or group situations
   (5) Often blurts out answers to questions before they have been completed
   (6) Has difficulty following through on instructions from others (not due to oppositional behavior or failure of comprehension), e.g., fails to finish chores
   (7) Has difficulty sustaining attention in tasks or play activities
   (8) Often shifts from one uncompleted activity to another
   (9) Has difficulty playing quietly
   (10) Often talks excessively
   (11) Often interrupts or intrudes on others, e.g., butts into other children's games
   (12) Often does not seem to listen to what is being said to him or her
   (13) Often loses things necessary for tasks or activities at school or at home (e.g., toys, pencils, books, assignments)
   (14) Often engages in physically dangerous activities without considering possible consequences (not for the purpose of thrill-seeking), e.g., runs into street without looking

Note: The above items are listed in descending order of discriminating power based on data from a national field trial of the DSM-III-R criteria for Disruptive Behavior Disorders.

B. Onset before the age of 7.
C. Does not meet the criteria for a Pervasive Developmental Disorder.

Criteria for severity of Attention-Deficit Hyperactivity disorder:
Mild: Few, if any, symptoms in excess of those required to make the diagnosis and only minimal or no impairment in school and social functioning.
Moderate: Symptoms or functional impairment intermediate between "mild" and "severe."
Severe: Many symptoms in excess of those required to make the diagnosis and significant and pervasive impairment in functioning at home and school and with peers.

(Source: *American Psychiatric Association.* [*1987*]. Diagnostic and statistical manual of mental health [*revised 3rd ed.*]. *Washington, D.C.: American Psychiatric Association.*)

be used by various professionals in an attempt to diagnose ADHD. The nurse should be aware that no one single test confirms a diagnosis of ADHD and that controversy of diagnosis is a reflection of the difficulties of objective measurements with these tests. The nurse should provide parents with emotional support, particularly during the difficult diagnostic period. The nurse helps the parents understand the diagnosis and encourages them to verbalize frustrations.

Interviews with the parents focusing on the description of the child's behavior are a critical part of the assessment process. Examples of the frequency, severity, and context of the behavior are needed. This is important because what one family may consider hyperactivity may be seen as normal in another family. Included in the family interview is a detailed history. Because parents of children with ADHD often have a history of ADHD themselves, the nurse must obtain information on each of the parents concerning problems in their own childhood. This includes obtaining information about alcoholism and antisocial personality disorders in the family.

The observations of the parents, teachers, significant others in the child's life, and the child himself are used in diagnosing ADHD. In addition, educators have a battery of tests to aid in the diagnosis of ADHD. The interview of the child is usually done by the physician. The nurse plays an important role in coordinating and gathering information.

As with any specific learning disabilities, a comprehensive workup is necessary to rule out other conditions or to ascertain whether lack of academic performance is due to poor motivation. Attention-deficit hyperactivity disorder is especially difficult to diagnose because considerable overlap exists between hyperactivity and other disorders.

★ NURSING DIAGNOSES AND PLANNING

The following are nursing diagnoses that may apply to a child with ADHD.

- Sleep Pattern Disturbance related to inability to rest or to nap.
- Altered Growth and Development related to poor continuous and selective attention functions.
- Ineffective Family Coping related to disruptive and inconsolable behaviors in the affected child.

Because of the multifaceted behavior problems associated with ADHD, a multimodal treatment plan is most effective. Intervention incorporates a combination of family involvement, manipulation of the environment, academic remediation, and medication. Examples of goals are:

- The family identifies coping strategies for managing disruptive behaviors
- The child and family discuss their feelings related to the disorder
- The child identifies activities that bring success

★ NURSING INTERVENTIONS

Family involvement is an important part of the treatment of ADHD. The nurse often is the liaison for the family and the rest of the health team. The nurse interviews the family for health histories, provide information regarding the disorder and suggest reference material for them to read. Information given to the family includes a description of the syndrome, the symptoms, and the likely outcomes if treatment is not begun.[5] The nurse also educates parents that no "magical cures" exist for ADHD. Because of media hype, parents may want to experiment with something that is not scientifically valid. Parents need to understand what ADHD and that symptoms may vary from mild to severe.

ENVIRONMENTAL MANIPULATION

To help increase the child's learning capabilities, the nurse teaches parents to minimize environmental stimuli, to discipline and set limits as they would for other children, and to use consistent approaches for all situations. These strategies help improve the child's behaviors. Decreasing stress producing situations and encouraging physical exercise are beneficial techniques in managing hyperactive behavior.[5] Cognitive behavior therapy that includes use of positive reinforcement and positive role modeling may be used. Parents need support to be consistent and to focus on positive behaviors. If necessary, individual or group psychotherapy may be recommended to address behavioral issues.

ACADEMIC REMEDIATION

Because most ADHD children have some type of learning or communication disorder, academic remediation is important. Activities for preschoolers need to be provided constantly to keep the child occupied and out of trouble. As the child matures and enters school, academic performance becomes a major issue. Because there is an inability to focus on topics or to attend to tasks at hand, academic performance declines and other problems such as reading delays or language disabilities develop. As peers continue to achieve academically, the child with ADHD increasingly falls behind and a low self-image emerges. A vicious cycle ensues in which failure rather than successes become the norm. Without interventions, continual academic failures increase the risk for school dropout and antisocial behavior.

Academically, a child with ADHD is mainstreamed but prospers in a smaller classroom setting where stimuli is minimized and close attention is paid to special needs.

Referrals should be made to educational specialists for appropriate testing and academic treatment plans.[5] Specific strategies such as study skills can be taught by educators to help the individual compensate for attention deficits. Research suggests that interventions that initially focus on academic difficulties rather than behavioral problems have a positive effect on both the behavioral and academic aspects of the disorder.[13]

EDUCATION REGARDING MEDICATION

The most common treatment of ADHD is the use of psychotropic medication. Typically, a stimulant is prescribed such as methylphenidate, magnesium pemoline, or an amphetamine. When the child does not respond to the stimulants, tricyclic antidepressants such as imipramine are used. The nurse documents the child's response to the medication and teaches the family about the side effects found with particular medications[55] (Table 20-6).

The drug of choice currently is methylphenidate hydrochloride (Ritalin). Similar to amphetamine, this central nervous system stimulant has a marked effect on mental rather than motor activities. The dose must be tailored individually and is administered in a flexible fashion. For example, a certain dose may be required during school hours when attention is essential, whereas a lower dose may be used for sports and other activities when attention is less critical. Because of this scheduling mode, compliance is an issue for some families.

The nurse teaches parents the importance of the medication regimen. The nurse explores attitudes of the family that may impede compliance. Do parents feel that they are "drugging" their child by giving medications? Do they feel that giving the medication subdues typical "boyish," behavior?

Antidepressants (such as imipramine) are the second drug of choice and have several advantages. Antidepressants are less apt to disturb sleep patterns, are not associated with growth retardation or suppression (as stimulants may be), and reduce risks of abuse and dependency. The duration of action is longer and therefore administration is typically once per day. If compliance is an issue, this medication is the preferred choice.

★ EVALUATION

Evaluation of the effectiveness of the interventions focuses on the cessation of the behaviors associated with the diagnosis. For children with attention-deficit disorder, the goal is to increase the child's ability to concentrate. Improving academic performance, decreasing outbursts, and decreasing tension at home are all positive signs that the intervention plan is working. Close attention should be paid to the medications the child is receiving. Side effects and therapeutic effects need to be monitored closely by the physician and nurse.

Gifted, Creative, and Talented Children

Approximately 5% or 2.6 million elementary and secondary school children are gifted, creative and talented.[19] The Marland Report of 1972, commissioned by the U.S. Office

TABLE 20-6
Medications Used in ADHD

Medication	Examples	Uses
Psychostimulants	methylphenidate (Ritalin); pemoline (Cylert)	Acts by increasing alertness, concentration, motor activity; decreasing fatigue and sleepiness; suppressing appetite
		Management of hyperactive behavior in conjunction with parental counseling
		Antidepressant in adolescents
		Treatment for hyperactivity, hyperaggressivity, hyperdistractability
Antidepressants	imipramine (Tofranil); amitriptyline (Elavil); nortriptyline (Aventyl); trazodone (Desyrel); doxepin (Sinequan)	Acts by elevating mood and improving sleep and appetite patterns; by treating enuresis
		Treatment of depression (with or without anxiety) in children
		Imipramine is sometimes more effective in treatment of attention deficit disorders in children than CNS stimulants
Anticonvulsants	diphenylhydantoin (Dilantin); carbamazepine (Tegretol)	Management of childhood behavior disorders with or without associated convulsions
		Treatment of hyperactive children with organic impairment

of Education, broadly defines this term to include potential abilities in intellect, creative or productive thinking, leadership, psychomotor, or visual and performing arts.[20] Identification of these children, therefore, is not based merely on IQ test results and includes a quest and zest for learning and intellectual curiosity. The accompanying display lists some common characteristics of gifted, creative, and talented children.

Educational and psychosocial factors are important aspects in the development of these children. In the educational arena, major concerns relate to the identification

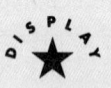

Common Characteristics of Gifted, Creative, and Talented Children

- Demonstrate a quest and zest for learning
- Grasp concepts and ideas quickly
- Exhibit a wide range of interests
- Demonstrate intellectual curiosity
- Work well independently
- Memorize quickly
- Ask complex questions
- Demonstrate superior powers of reasoning
- Think abstractly
- Exhibit a broad attention span
- Are self-critical
- Tend to be more physically active than the average child
- Enjoy associating with adults
- Possess unusual imagination

process and to teaching methodology. School districts use different guidelines to qualify individuals for enrichment services. Parents often worry that once identified, the child may not be properly challenged. Psychosocially, these children perceive themselves as different, similar to the emotions experienced by children with disabilities. Feelings of frustration, isolation, or boredom are not uncommon. Peers may resent gifted children for their exceptional abilities. This becomes especially significant for the adolescent who yearns to be like everyone else. The adolescent may even undermine capabilities at this point to appear like his or her friends.

A child who is gifted and talented should be recognized first and foremost as an individual. The nurse can help parents understand this concept by teaching them not to focus continually on achievements. A child raised in such an atmosphere may believe that his or her worth is based solely on accomplishments, impeding the development of healthy self-esteem. Parents also may be under the delusion that all facets of the child's personality are superior when only one area is exceptional. The nurse teaches parents that a child may remain emotionally at his or her developmental age even though intellectually, he has surpassed his chronologic age. Precocious intellect is not synonymous with maturity. Therefore, the nurse assists parents in setting realistic and age-appropriate expectations. Parents benefit by meeting other parents in similar situations so that mutual feelings and concerns can be shared. Numerous magazines available to parents of gifted children may also be suggested by the nurse.

A child who is gifted and talented needs security and emotional support, as well as encouragement to reach his or her potential. When interacting with such a child, the nurse must demonstrate sensitivity for his or her particular needs. The nurse should not assume the child un-

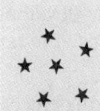

Ideas for Nursing Research

The special needs of children vary from minor to severe disorders and from positive, gifted children to situations requiring more intense help for families from professionals. The nurse who works with these families has an opportunity to explore the effectiveness of nursing interventions. The following are areas for further study:

- Nursing interventions that increase family stability (decrease parental discord) when caring for a child with special needs.
- Strategies that actively and effectively involve fathers of children who have developmental disabilities.
- Nursing interventions that focus on the functional strengths of a child who has a developmental disorder.
- Long-term impact of unaffected sibling's adjustments to growing up with a child who has special needs.
- Longitudinal screening programs and effective follow-up care.

derstands everything that is occurring just because of his or her exceptional status. In summation, the nurse works in collaboration with parents to help the child establish a healthy self-esteem while cultivating his or her unique gifts.

Summary

A child may have special needs because of a variety of reasons. The developmental disorders, mental retardation, and attention deficit disorders are typically the first conditions that come to mind. The nurse is in a unique position to identify those children with less observable disorders who also may need appropriate interventions. This chapter discusses important nursing assessment skills and interventions for children with special needs and their families including considerations for gifted children, physical, emotional, and mental problems only compound the unique needs of children and adolescents.

References

1. Allen, M. & Capute, A. (1989). Neonatal neurodevelopmental examination as a predictor of neuromotor outcome in premature infants. *Pediatrics, 83*(4), 498–506.
2. American Psychiatric Association. *Diagnostic and statistical manual of mental disorders* (3rd ed.). Washington, D.C.: American Psychiatric Association, 1987.
3. Blondis, T. A., Accardo, P. J., & Snow, J. H. (1989). Measures of attention deficit. Part II: Clinical perspectives and test interpretation. *Clinical Pediatrics 28*(6), 268–276.
4. Bond, W. S. (1987). Recognition and treatment of attention deficit disorder. *Clinical Pharmacology, 6*(8), 617–624.
5. Cantwell, D., & Baker, L. (1987). Attention deficit disorder in children: The role of the nurse practitioner. *Nurse Practitioner 12*(7), 42–54.
6. Chalfant, J. C. (1989). Learning disabilities: Policy issues and promising approaches. *American Psychology, 44*(2), 392–398.
7. Chernoff, G. F. (1980). The fetal alcohol syndrome in mice: Maternal variables. *Teratology, 22*, 67–71.
8. Clements, D., Copeland, L., & Loftus, M. (1990). Critical times for families with a chronically ill child. *Pediatric Nursing, 16*(2), 157–161.
9. Culley, B. S., Perrin, E. C., & Chaberski, M. J. (1989). Parental perceptions of vulnerability of formerly premature infants. *Journal of Pediatric Health Care, 3*(5), 237–245.
10. Dosen, A. (1989). Diagnosis and treatment of mental illness in mentally retarded children: A developmental model. *Child Psychiatry and Human Development, 20*(1), 73–84.
11. Fox, L., Long, S., & Langlois, A. (1988). Patterns of language comprehension deficit in abused and neglected children. *Journal of Speech Hearing Disorders, 53*(3), 239–244.
12. Learning disability: A neurological disorder. (1992). *The Greenville News,* Health/National/International section, Wednesday, June 10, page 2A.
13. Grossman, H. J. (Ed.). (1977). *Manual on terminology and classification in mental retardation.* Washington, D.C.: American Association on Mental Deficiency.
14. Jackson, C. B. (1989). Primary health care for deaf children. *Journal of Pediatric Health Care, 3*(6), 316–318.
15. Jacobs, P., & McDermott, S. (1989). Family caregiver costs of chronically ill and handicapped children: Method and literature review. *Public Health Rep 104*(2), 158–163.
16. Lenzer, I. I., Hourihan, C. M., & Ryan, C. I. (1982). Relation between behavioral and physical abnormalities associated with prenatal exposure to alcohol: Present speculations. *Perceptual and Motor Skills, 55*, 903–912.
17. Levine, M. D., Carey, W. B., Crocker, A. C., & Gross, R. T. (1992). Developmental Behavioral pediatrics. (2nd ed.) Philadelphia: W. B. Saunders.
18. McGee, R., & Share, D. (1988). Attention deficit disorder-hyperactivity and academic failure: Which comes first and what should be treated? *J Am Acad Child Adolesc Psychiatry, 27*(3), 318–325.
19. Miller, B. S., & Price, M. (Eds.). *The gifted child, the family and the community.* New York: Walker and Company by the American Association for Gifted Children.
20. Miller, M. W. (1988). Effect of prenatal exposure to ethanol on the development of cerebral cortex: 1. Neuronal generation. *Alcoholism, 12*, 440–449.
21. Munoz-Millan, R. J., & Casteel, C. R. (1989). Attention-deficit hyperactivity disorder: Recent literature. *Hospital Community Psychiatry 40*(7), 699–707.
22. Olshansky, S. (1962). Chronic sorrow: A response to having a mentally defective child. *Social Casework 43*(4), 190–193.
23. Reis, S. M. (1989). Reflections on policy affecting the education of gifted and talented students: Past and future perspectives. *Am Psychol 44*(2), 399–408.
24. Roman, P. M. (1988). Biological features of women's alcohol use: A review. *Public Health Reports, 103*(6), 628–637.
25. Rothery, S. A. (1987). Understanding and supporting special siblings. *Journal of Pediatric Health Care, 1*, 21–25.
26. Seligman, M. (1987). Adaptation of children to a chronic illness or mentally handicapped sibling. *Canadian Medical Association Journal, 135*(12), 1249–1252.
27. Shapiro, B., Palmer, F., & Capute, A. (1987). Cerebral palsy: History and state of the art. In J. Williams (Ed.) *Textbook of developmental pediatrics* (pp. 11–25). New York: Plenum Publishing.
28. State of Maryland Office of Special Secretary. (1989). *Estimated*

impact of early intervention services in Maryland. Maryland Infants and Toddlers Program Interagency Coordinating Council, October.

29. Steele, S. (1988). Preschool children with developmental delays: Nursing intervention. *J Pediatr Health Care, 2,* 245–252.

30. Steele, S. (1989). Values and persons with developmental disabilities. *Journal of Pediatric Health Care 3*(3), 113–114.

31. Streissguth, A.P., Randels, S.P., & Smith, D.F. (1991). A test-retest study of intelligence in patients with fetal alcohol syndrome: Implications for care. *Journal of the American Academy of Child and Adolescent Psychiatry, 30,* 584–587.

32. Yoos, L. (1985). Assessment and management of the developmentally delayed infant in primary care. *Nurse Practitioner 10*(11), 24–36.

33. Warren, K. R., & Bast, R. J. (1988). Alcohol-related birth defects: An update. *Public Health Reports, 103*(6), 638–642.

34. Waterson, E. J., & Murray-Lyon, I. M. (1990). Preventing alcohol related birth damage: a review. *Social Science Medicine, 30*(3), 349–364.

35. Wintz, L. (1987). Private initiatives: A focus on the Easter Seal Society. *Pediatric Nursing 13*(2), 84–88.

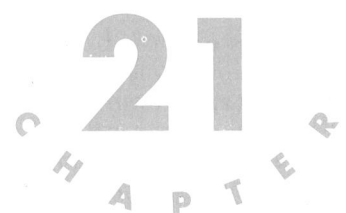

21

CHAPTER

Impact of Chronic Illness on Children and Families

OBJECTIVES

Define *chronic illness.*

Compare acute and chronic illness.

Describe the impact of chronic illness on children and families.

Consider major issues, problems and stressors of children with chronic illness and their families.

Describe steps in the nursing process in the care of children with chronic illness and their families.

Describe family-centered care for families with chronic illness.

Chronic illness is one of the most widespread health care problems affecting children and their families today. The child with a chronic illness presents many serious challenges to parents, families, and health care professionals. A chronic illness may interfere with the vital physical, cognitive, and psychosocial tasks that are achieved in infancy, childhood, and adolescence. Family functioning may be affected by the unique demands and burdens associated with a chronic illness. Children and their family members may be required to develop different, more effective coping strategies in order to maintain optimal functioning. Nurses have many exciting opportunities for leadership in prevention, early casefinding, health promotion, and management of quality care for children and their families on a lifelong basis. The primary goals for nurses are to assist children to become more independent, develop adaptive behaviors, learn appropriate coping methods, develop mastery with successive developmental tasks, and live happy, healthy, and harmonious lives.

This chapter discusses the significance of chronic illness for children and their families. The extent of the problem and predictable stressors for parents and other family members are included. The nurse's roles in family-centered care are highlighted. Nursing assessments for planning appropriate interventions for the ill child, well siblings, parents, and extended family members are included. Nurses increasingly are aware of the need to conceptualize care for children with chronic illness as being lifelong. Such a perspective ensures more comprehensive care and services

485

that are preventive, developmentally-focused, family-centered, and promote health throughout the different ages and stages of a child's development. Actual health care delivery systems are addressed in Unit 4.

Significance of the Problem

A chronic illness is defined as a condition that interferes with daily functioning for more than 3 months in a year, causes hospitalization for more than 1 month in a year, or (at time of diagnosis) is likely to do either of these.[28]

There are distinct differences between acute and chronic illness. With acute illness, usually treated in the hospital, the goal is complete elimination of acute symptoms. With chronic illness there usually is not a cure, and the goals are to support and nurture the child from one crisis to another. Prevention of crises is a foremost nursing priority for the child and family. Chronic illnesses are treated in a combination of hospital, clinic, office, special pediatric centers, and the home.

With chronic illness assessments may seem unending with intermittent and lifelong follow-up care. A definite diagnosis of the illness may never be determined; in fact, there will probably be interrelated diseases and pathophysiologic problems. Serious handicaps may result. The prognosis may be highly unpredictable. Family counseling may be needed during subsequent periods of crisis.[33]

In acute illness one physician usually provides the care; in chronic illness interdisciplinary expertise will be needed, and the family ultimately becomes case manager for the child's illness. The family crisis may be brief in an acute illness, but extensive and unforeseen adjustment problems may occur with chronic illness.

Nurses play important roles in case finding, screening, and lifetime management for children and their families with chronic illnesses. Therefore, nurses need to be familiar with the unique characteristics of chronic illness, as listed in the accompanying display, so they can respond in sensitive and caring ways to help meet the changing needs for education, support, and guidance.

Although precise numbers of children with chronic illness and disabilities are difficult to identify, the absolute numbers of disabled and chronically ill children are increasing as children survive longer.[1] National surveys indicate that the proportion of children with a reported major activity limitation has increased considerably in recent years.

One million children and adolescents have been estimated to have a severe form of chronic illness that interferes with activities of daily living and growth and development. Another 10 million children are reported to have less serious forms of chronic illnesses.[14] Overall, an estimated 10% to 20% of children and adolescents have chronic illnesses.[14] This growth may be due in part to changes in survey methodologies, but the increase also may be due to families' increased awareness of illness and increased survival rates of children with certain chronic illness, such as cystic fibrosis and spina bifida. In addition, new technologies and advances in systems of care are resulting in larger numbers of children who survive birth or trauma but who are diagnosed with long-term disabilities[1] (Fig. 21-1).

Of great importance is the rising and alarming incidence of acquired immunodeficiency syndrome (AIDS). AIDS is predicted to continue to spread in infants and children.[8] The diseases of AIDS are likely to increase the number of children receiving prolonged intravenous drug therapy, nutritional support, and intensive nursing care. Some hospitals have reported sharp increases in the number of infants with AIDS and the number of those infants who are now growing up in hospitals.[3] Another group of infants who are at increased risk for developmental problems and chronic conditions is the rapidly growing number of neonates born to mothers who are substance abusers.

Family Issues

The chief issues and difficulties for children and their families may range from long-term survivorship, costs, pain of treatment, conflicting advice, difficulty mastering developmental tasks, changes in roles and relationships, and death. Often illness imposes burdens of increased tasks and time commitments, such as providing special diets, daily or weekly therapy, 24-hour monitoring of high-technology equipment, appointments with medical facilities, and hospitalizations resulting in forced family separations. The accompanying display lists issues of chronic illness faced by children and families.

Developmental Tasks

Recent data suggest that children with chronic illnesses are living longer and survive into adulthood. They too, need opportunities to grow, develop, change, gain competence, become independent, and master problems and issues associated with chronic illnesses. These children can be positively encouraged to live successful and productive lives.

Although the majority of chronic illnesses are not life-threatening in nature, some may interrupt a child's ability to master cognitive, social, emotional, physical, and physiologic developmental tasks. Some children may experience early problems with feeding and sleeping. Others may have difficulties in socialization because of separations from peers and siblings, while others may experience delayed language development or fine motor

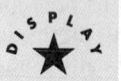

Unique Characteristics of Chronic Illness

- Irreversible pathologic alteration
- Lengthy periods of supervision
- Permanency
- Residual disability
- Need for special rehabilitative training
- Multiple causes
- Diverse manifestations
- Irreversibility
- Long duration

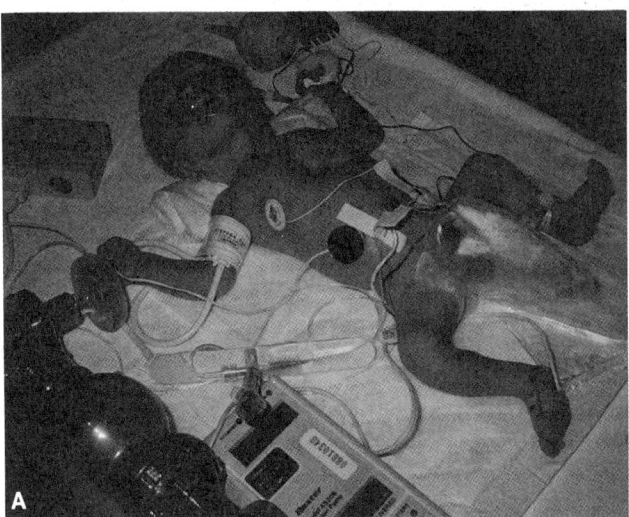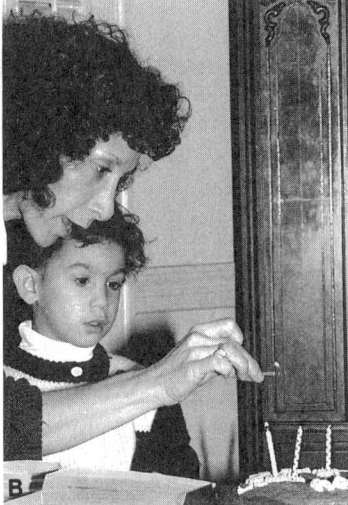

FIGURE 21-1

Advanced technology has increased survival rates. (**A**) Low-birthweight neonates who would not have lived 10 years ago are treated successfully in neonatal intensive care units. (**B**) Children with chronic respiratory problems associated with premature delivery may need lifelong care by their families and the health care system.

skills. The child may be confronted with pain, intrusive procedures, uncertainty, hospitalizations, numerous medical regimens, special diets, and separation from caring family members. Some conditions may impede a child's cognitive mastery and success in school. Children may suffer from being separated from parents, siblings, and other loving family members.

In contrast, however, most children with chronic illnesses develop coping and adaptive skills that allow them to master all their developmental tasks, in spite of the stressors and burdens that they face. The majority of children with chronic illnesses are independent, demonstrate adaptive behaviors, are industrious, strive for competence, and live out lives characterized by success, achievement, productivity, and happiness at home, at school, and in their communities. Much of what they accomplish will depend on the quality of care they receive and health care professionals' sensitivity, support, and commitment to their well-being.

Roles and Relationships

Because a child with a chronic illness is a member of a family unit, the child's illness may present a number of issues that directly affect family members' feelings and ways of functioning. Pressure, tension, and stress may be increased between parents and between parents and well siblings, and undue strain may occur between parents and the child who is ill. The child's illness may lead to extensive worrying by parents and siblings, and an increase in intrafamily tension and conflict may occur. Some illnesses may lead to modifications in family activities and goals, such as restricted options for family vacations, reduced flexibility in the use of leisure time, fewer opportunities for both parents to pursue careers, and parental worry and uncertainty as to whether to have more children when the illness is associated with genetic factors.

According to Patterson and McCubbin[27] the family has major roles in managing the child's care and treatment throughout the child's lifetime. Because the child generally lives at home, the chronic illness may be a source of stress and may result in many hardships for the family. Strained family relationships may occur and may be manifested in overprotectiveness of the ill child and development of coalitions between the primary caregiver (usually mother) and the child, with other family members feeling left out.

Financial

Families may experience additional financial burdens due to special medical consultations, hospitalizations, medications, equipment needs, and various therapies. Amount of insurance coverage will affect direct costs to families. Some families may have to arrange for special housing adaptations and fitting the home with special features such as a ramp for a wheelchair.

Social Isolation

Families may experience different degrees of social isolation because of friends' or relatives' responses to and expectations regarding the child with a chronic illness. Some families may experience increased social isolation because of embarrassment of the visibility of a physical abnormality. Other families may suffer from limited mobility of the child with an illness. Some families may not have access to adequate child care; others may fear accidents or exposure to infection, which might exacerbate a child's illness.

Health Management

Family members may experience lifelong concerns related to obtaining competent medical care; some families may have ongoing concerns related to their understanding of the child's illness; some may experience compliance problems with prescribed home and school

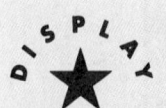

Issues of Chronic Illness Affecting Children and Their Families

LIVING WITH CHRONIC ILLNESS

- Chronic illness is no longer limited to adults and elderly.
- No child is too young to be afflicted.
- Survival rates are increasing.
- Children are now reaching adulthood.
- Numbers are expected to increase.
- Many diseases require treatments that are arduous, painful, and embarrassing and result in the question of whether a prolonged life is worth it.
- Chronic illness is constant (a "constant shadow" is cast).

SOCIETAL TRENDS

- Children with chronic conditions and family members may be neglected by society.
- Society is organized to take care of *some* handicapped individuals.

FINANCIAL CONCERNS

- Overall costs are high.
- Many visits to physicians are required.
- Repeated hospitalizations are expensive.
- Prescribed medical regimens are lifelong.
- Home care equipment is needed.
- Days are lost in school.

FAMILY CONCERNS

- Burdens of families are high, and greater attention to meet is needed.
- Uncertainty of future course creates psychological problems for children and family members.
- Problems of adjustment can be exacerbated during normally difficult periods of development.

HEALTH CARE SYSTEM

- Children and families interact with many health providers for an extended period of time.
- Treatment regimens are often complex and at times conflicting.
- Children and families have difficulty in making sense out of conflicting advice.
- Cures for the majority of chronic illnesses are not available.
- Prevention, care, and treatment receive primary emphasis.
- Poor children are likely to have more illness and more severe illness than nonpoor children.
- Families require access to specialty medical and surgical services of high quality not required by other children.
- Children in rural areas have special unmet needs.
- Traditional roles of medicine and nursing are not sufficient to meet the complex needs of children and families.

RECURRENT EXPERIENCES OF THE CHILD WITH A CHRONIC ILLNESS

- Pain (anticipated and actual)
- Repeated medical procedures
- Boredom of waiting for health care professionals, information and instructions, progress, and healing
- Feelings of anger against indifferent health care professionals
- Sense of gratitude for those who care in special ways
- Fear of death in the midst of a frightening, unpredictable crisis
- Being different from other children; making friends
- Relief when symptoms abate
- Despair when pain begins again
- Uncertainty versus security
- Mastery and success with challenges

treatment regimens. Families may have concerns about a child's compliance and how to help a child minimize or endure painful procedures, and many families are beset with worries and uncertainties regarding the child's immediate and future prognoses. Families may experience concerns about meeting a child's special needs in school or providing education in the child's home environment.

Coping

Grieving, mourning, and chronic sorrow are often associated with lifelong responses of parents and family members to a child with a chronic illness. Often parents must cope with developmental delays, abnormalities, or restricted life opportunities for a child, and for some families anticipation or actual experiencing of a premature or painful death must be endured and accepted by members of the family.

Predictable Stressors

Levine et al.,[21] in addition to the previous discussion, identified predictable stressors in the course of chronic illness in children. By knowing which stressors are likely to affect families, nurses can provide anticipatory guidance for coping with each specific event.

The first predictable stressor is the onset and diagnosis of an illness. Often the diagnosis can be devastating, and family members' reactions range from shock, anger, guilt, disbelief, denial, helplessness, and powerlessness to grief and mourning. An individual's responses may not be to the actual diagnosis, but to an actual perception of what the illness is. The family member's own perceptions, understanding, or preconceived notions may cause the most stress. Some conditions may cause more emotional distress than others. A cardiac problem may not be as devastating as a physical congenital defect that is highly visible to everyone.

Hospitalization may serve as a major stressor. Parents and siblings may experience stress because of forced separation from a child, their own adaptation to the hospital environment, adjustment to multiple caregivers for a child, seeing other sick children, and ideas about a child's submission to machines, anesthesia, or surgery. Hospitalization of a child may reinforce family members' worst fears about an illness.

Another predictable stressor for family members is the appearance of an unexpected major complication. Parents and the child who is ill also may be confronted with significant therapeutic choices in which they are asked for their own personal preferences. Some parents may be tempted to turn to choices that are not endorsed by the medical community. The failure of an expected therapeutic response may be very stressful to parents and other family members. Sometimes medications fail to produce the desired results or a treatment doesn't have the effect it was supposed to have produced. Obviously, the threat of imminent death is a crucial stressor to parents, siblings, and other members of the family, and nurses and other health care professionals must respond in a skillful, supportive manner.

Health Care Needs

The Office of Technology Assessment[32] has estimated that the medically stable, technology-dependent child population is made up of four alternative groups, including children with acute medical and surgical problems, children with terminal illnesses, children who are severely intellectually disabled, and children with chronic conditions such as respiratory problems, malabsorption, or central nervous system problems. These four groups are discussed in Table 21-1.

This population has complicated, extensive, and special needs requiring comprehensive care by *many* health care disciplines. Children with long-term illnesses may require many services that are scattered over considerable geographical distances. Interprofessional teamwork is essential to bring diverse services to the aid of

TABLE 21-1
The Population of Children Currently Served in Programs Emphasizing Alternative to Hospital Care

Categories	Description	Services	Sample Diagnoses
Children with acute medical/surgical problems	Children with acute medical/surgical problems who are discharged early from the hospital but who continue to need individualized technical care for limited periods of time	These children may receive medications, unusual feedings, monitoring of vital signs, and certain forms of technical treatment.	Severe infectious diseases, postoperative conditions, acquired immune deficiency syndrome
Children with terminal illness	Children requiring technical care for a terminal illness that is expected to result in death within 6 months	These children may, for a period of time, require oxygen, assistance, or medication for comfort.	Renal failure, terminal cancer
Children with several intellectually disabling conditions	Children who, as the result of an illness, trauma, congenital anomaly, or hereditary disease, are severely intellectually disabled so that they cannot and will not be able to care for themselves	These children require varying degrees of assistance in feeding, defecating, urinating, positioning, and other personal care.	Severe microcephaly, severe postmeningitis, severe hydrocephalus
Children with chronic medical problems	Children who will have chronic medical problems for long periods of time and are dependent on technical care	These children may require complex alimentation, certain medications, suctioning, catheterization, intravenous therapy, tracheostomies, equipment monitoring, prescribed therapy regimens, or colostomies/illeostomies.	Chronic malabsorption syndrome, severe cystic fibrosis, multiple congenital anomalies, severe seizure disorders, dystrophies, myasthenia, chronic aspiration syndrome, short gut syndrome
Children who have chronic respiratory problems	Children who will be oxygen dependent for relatively long periods of time. Children who need ventilation assistance for periods of time; children who are completely ventilator dependent	These children will require oxygen and may require suctioning or cardiopulmonary monitoring. These children will require ventilator care and bronchial suctioning. They may require cardiopulmonary monitoring and gastrostomy feeding.	Chronic bronchopulmonary dysplasia (BPD) Postencephalitis, progressive CNS disease, tracheobronchial malacia, Ondine's curse
Children who have central nervous system (CNS) dysfunction	Children who have CNS problems, either the result of trauma or CNS disease so that they will not be able to care for themselves	These children may require assistance in physical positioning, feeding, defecating, or urinating. Some may be ventilator dependent.	Progressive CNS disease, spinal cord trauma

(MacQueen, J. [1987]. Alternatives to Hospital Care. In: U.S. Congress, Office of Technology Assessment. *Technology-Dependent Children: Hospital V Home Care: A technical memorandum*, OTA-TM-H-38 [p. 16]. [1988]. Washington, D.C.: U.S. Government Printing Office.)

individual infants, children, and their families. Health care professionals continue to express concerns about families of chronically ill children who need to see and interact with a variety of team professionals. Some families receive most or all of their care from specialists, others from primary care providers, and others from a combination of specialty and primary care plus other services in the community; the result is often fragmented care with an overemphasis on the child's impairment and functioning.

Hymovich[16] also described the growing trend of caring for children in their homes rather than in institutions. This changing trend requires that health care professionals be available to families when they require assistance.

The trend of earlier discharge also suggests that more children and families are at home attempting to cope with chronic illness, increased care needs, concomitant knowledge deficits, health risks, and comfort problems. At the same time that acute care is increasing in complexity because of advanced technology, chronic illness requires complex and intense adaptations to be made in the home.

Nursing Implications

MacQueen,[22] Cook and Forsman,[6] Gittler,[12] Rose and Thomas[26] and Hymovich[16] observed that nurses are in positions to assume leadership roles in individualization of care. Nurses, more than other health care professionals, have the knowledge, expertise, and abilities to assume key positions in coordinating and managing hospital care, ambulatory care, and home care. Nurses strive to coordinate comprehensive care for a child and family members; prevent dysfunction; promote adaptation for the child, his or her siblings, parents, and family; facilitate support mechanisms for all family members; and promote quality of life. Nurses as care managers play pivotal and progressive roles in the ongoing monitoring and care of children throughout their lives.

Most of the care for children and families will be implemented in community health settings, such as day care centers and schools. Because of Public Law 94-142 called the "Education for all Handicapped Children Act,"[30] passed by the 94th Congress in 1975, each state has established priorities for providing free, appropriate public education for all handicapped children. Such a law assures that children with chronic conditions, regardless of diagnosis or severity of limitations, have the right to education and related services. Nurses have therefore assumed expanding roles in the coordination of children's care in schools.

Home health care agencies, community ambulatory clinics, health departments, special pediatric centers, and children's foster homes, family homes, and homeless shelters are other settings in which nurses provide care to children and families. To be successful in planning, implementing, and evaluating care for children, nurses need an in-depth knowledge of the pathophysiology, diagnoses, and treatments required for special chronic illnesses. Moreover, nurses must be able to apply extensive knowledge of normal growth, family systems, theories of development, and concepts of vulnerability, coping, and

adaptation to ensure the most favorable outcomes for children and their families.

Nursing plans for children ideally reflect a comprehensive physical, psychosocial, cognitive, and developmental assessment. In addition, family members and their interactions, relationships, dynamics, and available support require assessment for comprehensive care.

Increasingly nurses are integrating positive and innovative approaches in direct care, education, and case management of children and their families. Most importantly, nurses are involving children and family members as active participants of care, rather than as passive recipients of care, thus assuring the integrity of the family and the most optimal outcomes for children.

Nurses are assuming expanded roles in encouraging family members to be resourceful in their problem-solving efforts with infants and children. Parents and family members are increasingly being acknowledged for their creativity, resourcefulness, and strengths. In short nurses are treating parents and family members in a more collegial manner, reflecting that respect for a family is a priority. A major goal for nurses is to assist and encourage family members to become case managers of their own children.[15]

Instead of relying on trial and error when planning and evaluating care, nurses are using more systematic methods of problem solving in the best interests of children. Nurses are reluctant to provide superficial answers to parents and instead are focusing on performing earlier, more thorough assessments; collecting data; and obtaining complete information from parents, the child, and extended family members. Nurses are incorporating a holistic approach to care by integrating concepts of development, principles of family-centered care, and innovative, individualized plans for children and their family members on a lifetime, rather than episodic, basis.

Nurses are clearly making vital contributions to the care of children with chronic illnesses by concentrating on planning lifetime goals rather than planning short-term goals. Nurses apply knowledge of family dynamics and provide anticipatory guidance and support before known crises develop, thus demonstrating commitment of caring for children and their families.

Families are also benefiting from the expertise of nurses' case management skills, therapeutic communication skills, supportive techniques, and counseling approaches. Nurses are serving as exemplary role models for comprehensive, coordinated family-centered health care for millions of children who suffer from a variety of chronic conditions. Because of nurses' leadership skills and insightful planning, fragmentation, duplication, and gaps in children's services are being reduced.

★ NURSING ASSESSMENT

A thorough assessment of the parents and family members and their adaptive responses to a chronic condition is essential. This assessment may occur in a series of visits with the parents and families and is ideally completed by convening the entire family. Such a family conference is helpful at the time of initial diagnosis of the illness or during an initial hospitalization.

TABLE 21-2
Nursing Assessment: Questions for Assessing Needs of Parents, Family Members, and Children With Chronic Illness

Parents

Parents' Understanding of the Meaning of the Child's Illness

Initial Understanding Appropriate in Newborn Period to First 6 Months

1. Describe your infant to me so I can get a picture of him or her.
2. Was this child planned or unexpected?
3. What was the pregnancy and delivery like?
4. What do you recall about the birth of this child?
5. When did you first see your child?
6. What were your first observations of your child?
7. How soon were you informed that something was wrong, and how were you told?
8. Who told you?
9. Did you know this person?
10. Who was with you when you were told?
11. How did you react to this information?
12. Did you talk to each other about the child's illness? What were each of you first told about your child?
13. Did you feel any sense of responsibility for your infant's illness?
14. How do you feel now?
15. What did you tell your parents about the infant and his or her condition?
16. What were your parents', friends', and relatives' reactions?
17. How soon did you hold your infant?
18. How soon did you feed the infant?
19. How soon did you begin to care for the infant?
20. How easy was it for you to distinguish the infant's cry and what the infant wanted?
21. How soon did you name the infant?
22. Did you send out birth announcements?
23. Did you take the infant home with you from the hospital?
24. How long was the infant in the hospital after you left?
25. What were some positive features of the infant that you recall?
26. What is special about your infant?
27. Describe a typical day with your infant and the family.

Subsequent Course of the Illness Appropriate for Parents of an Older Infant or Child

1. Have you ever had any experiences with any chronic illness?
2. Describe the kind of symptoms your child had in early infancy.
3. What were the treatments the child needed when he or she was younger?
4. How much of your time was required?
5. Who performed the treatments for the child?
6. What kinds of medications did you give to the child?
7. What were your reactions to any major medical events when he or she was younger, such as hospitalization or surgery?
8. Were there any changes in the diagnosis or prognosis?
9. Did you experience any changes in your thoughts or feelings about your child's illness?
10. Tell me about these changes.
11. What has it been like providing care for your child over the last several years?
12. Has the care been different (better or worse) than your original expectations?
13. What has been your biggest worry or concern about your child or his or her care?
14. How has your child's illness affected your own life, your relationships with your spouse and other family members?
15. What has helped you the most in adjusting to your child, his or her needs, and the care required over the years?
16. Have there been any major changes in your child's medical status or in treatments or medications?
17. Has your child changed his or her behavior or general responses?
18. Which agencies, groups, or people have been most supportive to you?

Parents' Concerns

Concerns About the Future

1. Do you have any concerns about changes in the child's illness in the future?
2. Do you think that you will be able to manage any problems that may arise in the future?
3. Do you have any questions about your child's growth and development in the future?
4. Do you have any concerns about the cost of care in the future?
5. What do you think the future will be like for your child?
6. What do you think the future will be like for you as a family?
7. What do you think the future will be like for you as a parent?

Parenting Skills for the Ill Child

1. Describe your child to me.
2. What kind of a personality does your child have?
3. What do you like most about your child?
4. What do you like least about your child?
5. Who does your child remind you of?
6. How do you think your child feels about himself or herself?
7. Please define your child's illness to me.
8. How does your child define his or her illness?
9. What have you told your child about his or her illness?
10. Do you allow your child to visit a friend's home or stay overnight?
11. How far away do you allow your child to go when at home?
12. What was it like when your child first went to day care?
13. What was it like when your child went to preschool?
14. What was the first day of school like for you and your child?
15. What kinds of responsibilities does your child have in feeding, toileting, dressing, giving medications, or treatments?
16. What do you expect of your child in regard to household chores?
17. How well does your child mind you?
18. How do you set limits on your child's behaviors?
19. Have you had any concerns about discipline?
20. Have you had to manage any behavioral problems of your child?
21. Do you think that you have been able to manage your child's physical care in a way that is satisfactory to you?
22. How much of your time is devoted to actual planning or giving care to your child?
23. Do you feel you have been able to manage your child's emotional needs in a way that is satisfactory to you?
24. Are there any concerns about the child's physical care or ways to best meet his or her emotional needs?
25. Who helps you the most in making decisions to best meet your child's needs and your own needs?
26. How much assistance do you receive from your family members in regard to your decisions about childrearing?
27. Have you received any assistance from health care professionals about your parenting responsibilities?
28. What concerns do you have now that your child is becoming a toddler, preschooler, school-age child, or adolescent?

Roles and Relationships

Parents as Individuals

1. In what ways has your child's illness affected you?
2. Has your child's illness affected your being able to work?
3. Are you working (full or part-time)?
4. Has your child's illness affected your own physical stamina?
5. Are you getting enough rest?
6. Do you ever have time just for yourself?
7. Are you able to see friends?
8. Do you have any time as a couple to be alone or get out together?

(Continued)

TABLE 21-2
(Continued)

Marital Relationship of Parents

1. Who makes the major decisions in your family about the children?
2. How are these decisions made?
3. Who is responsible for specific tasks regarding the child?
4. How much flexibility is involved in sharing parental tasks?
5. How would you describe your relationship with your husband or wife?
6. Are you satisfied with the way you and your husband or wife communicate with each other?
7. Do you receive enough attention from your husband or wife?
8. How do you and your husband or wife resolve your differences or disagreements?
9. Does your marriage allow you to be as independent as you wish to be?
10. Do you and your husband or wife talk about your concerns for the child and his or her future?
11. Have you discussed the possibility of having more children?
12. Do you share in important decisions regarding your child's care and what and when to talk to the child about his or her illness?
13. Do you discuss the best way to prepare your child for medical procedures, treatments, surgery, or hospitalization, or does one parent make all the decisions?
14. How involved is the father or mother in the child's care?
15. How much time do you spend in activities with the child that don't involve medical or nursing care?

Family Members

Parents' Communication With Other Family Members

1. Have other members of your family been informed about _____'s illness?
2. What specifically have they been told?
3. How have they responded so far?
4. If concerns related to _____'s illness arise, which affect other members of the family, how is it resolved?
5. Have your relationships with your family members changed because of _____'s illness?

Siblings

Siblings Responses to the Child With a Chronic Illness

1. How do _____'s siblings view themselves in this family?
2. How are _____'s brothers and sisters doing in their growth and development?
3. How do _____'s siblings view _____?
4. Have _____'s brothers and sisters been told about _____'s illness?
5. If yes, what, and if not, is there a reason for not sharing this information?
6. How does each of the children define _____'s illness?
7. How do _____'s siblings act toward _____?
8. Do the sibling's ever feel left out because of the amount of time or care you have to devote to _____'s care?
9. To what extent are _____'s sibling's involved in _____'s care?
10. In general how well do you think _____'s siblings have adjusted to his or her special needs?
11. Do you feel satisfied with the amount of time you can spend with _____'s siblings?
12. Do you feel that there is extra pressure on _____'s siblings?
13. Are you ever concerned that _____'s siblings will become ill?

Parent's Responses to the Child's Illness

1. Please explain _____'s current medical status to me.
2. Are you satisfied with the information you have received about _____'s illness?
3. Do you feel that your understanding of _____'s illness is realistic?
4. Are you interested in learning new information about the illness?
5. Who has been most helpful in explaining your child's current medical status?
6. Who are the primary health care professionals that you see?
7. Have you thought of joining any organizations to increase your contact with other parents?
8. What literature do you read to become better informed about _____'s illness?
9. Are you satisfied with the professional health care providers that you see?

10. Do you feel they are genuinely supportive and interested in you and your child?
11. Do you feel that you have been able to adjust to the feelings you have about _____'s illness or do you think you still have some adjusting to do?
12. How visible is _____'s condition?
13. Do you consider _____'s condition to be visible to all, invisible to all, invisible to social others, or visible to the family and others who are aware of such a condition?
14. To what extent do you think the visibility of _____'s condition influences others' reactions to him or her, such as members of the family, friends, school teachers, and peers at school?

Family Members' Understanding of the Illness

1. Are you satisfied with the information you have received so far about _____'s illness?
2. What new information do you think would be helpful to you?
3. What kind of literature have you read that helps you to understand _____'s illness?
4. Who has assisted you the most in explaining _____'s current health status to you?
5. How would you define _____'s illness?
6. To what extent do _____'s grandparents understand _____'s illness?
7. Are you satisfied with other family members' understanding of _____'s illness?
8. What else do they need to know?

Day-to-Day Management of the Child Who is Ill

1. Who provides daily care to _____?
2. Who gives _____ medications?
3. Who prepares special meals?
4. Who decides to call the physician about a problem?
5. Who takes _____ to his or her clinic appointments?
6. How satisfied are you with the care _____ receives?
7. Do you have any concerns about _____'s care?
8. Are there any reasons that _____ is not receiving the care, medications, or treatment he or she requires?

Support Systems

Parents' Relationships With Health Care Professionals

1. Do health care professionals ask for your opinions, ideas, and suggestions about _____'s care?
2. To what extent do health care professionals incorporate your ideas or recommendations about _____'s care?
3. Are you satisfied with the extent to which you receive regular feedback from health care professionals?
4. Do health care professionals include you in active decision making that is required for any changes in _____'s care?
5. Do you feel that your ideas about _____'s care are valued by health care professionals?
6. Are you able to speak up about how you feel regarding _____'s progress, changes in care, or concerns?
7. If you are not satisfied with health care professional's responses to your input, what have you thought of to help others listen to what you are saying?

Adaptations in Family Living

1. Has _____'s illness resulted in any changes or interferences, such as vacations, family celebrations, or traditions?
2. Have any financial problems resulted because of _____'s illness?
3. Has _____'s illness placed any burdens on where the family must live?
4. What special arrangements have had to be made in the home because of _____'s illness?

Available Support Systems

1. Do you discuss your feelings and reactions with anyone?
2. If yes, who, and to what degree is this helpful to you?

(Continued)

TABLE 21-2
(Continued)

Available Support Systems (*continued*)

3. To whom else can you turn for help with the stresses of _____'s illness (family members, friends, neighbors, community or religious agencies, health care professionals)?
4. Who is generally available and helpful when you feel sad, discouraged, or overwhelmed?
5. Is there anyone with whom you discuss your successes in caring for _____?
6. To whom can you turn when you need financial assistance?
7. Who is helpful when you need transportation to the hospital, clinic, school, or camp?
8. Who is available to help with administering medications or treatments or checking home health care equipment?
9. On whom do you rely to care for _____ so that you and your spouse can go out together?

Communication With School Personnel

1. How often do you talk with _____'s teacher about his or her illness?
2. What has _____'s teacher been told about _____'s illness?
3. Does the teacher have any concerns about his or her condition?
4. Are you able to discuss _____'s growth and development with _____'s teacher?
5. Are you able to discuss psychosocial problems with _____'s teacher?
6. How often does _____'s teacher discuss _____'s academic performance with you?
7. Does _____'s teacher inform you about _____'s relationships with friends and peers at school?
8. Does _____'s teacher have a realistic picture of _____'s capabilities and strengths?

9. Is there any information that _____'s teacher needs about managing _____'s care at school?

School-Age Child and Adolescent

1. What have your parents told you about your illness?
2. What did your doctor tell you about your illness?
3. What did your nurse tell you about your illness?
4. What have you told your brother, sister, or grandparents about your illness?
5. Point to where you are sick.
6. Draw me a picture of where you are hurt.
7. What have you told your friends about your illness?
8. Tell me what you do to care for yourself.
9. Do you need any help from anyone in caring for yourself?
10. Do you go to school every day? (If you miss school, how do you catch up?)
11. What do you enjoy most at school?
12. Who do you like to play with at school?
13. What do you and your friends like to do together at school?
14. What is easiest for you at school?
15. What is hardest for you at school?
16. Who helps you the most when things are hard for you at school?
17. What do you think you do best at school?
18. What do you think other children with your illness fear the most?
19. If you ever are afraid, who do you talk to?
20. If you are ever sad, lonely, or angry, who do you talk to?
21. If you had three wishes about yourself, what would they be?

Goals for the child and family and individualized interventions will be based on thorough assessments of the parents', family members', and children's needs. The assessment questions in Table 21-2 are designed to be asked during early and later infancy as well as early and later childhood. The emphasis of the assessment shifts from the parents' feelings and their roles and relationships with the ill child to that of the well siblings' relationship with the child. In addition the assessment focuses on important questions related to the day-to-day management of an illness, parents' relationships with health care professionals, and support systems for the family. The last part of the assessment relates to questions that are appropriate for a school-age child or adolescent. The questions in Table 21-2 are used with a comprehensive physical examination and history of the newborn, infant, child, or adolescent.

★ **NURSING DIAGNOSIS OF FUNCTION**

The attitudes and responses adopted at the time of the initial diagnosis may shape family members' future perceptions of the illness and the child. Nurses can support parents and other family members in their responses and let them know their responses are normal. Success or failure of early coping efforts have a great influence on the family's and child's outcomes in later stages and may determine the pattern of lifelong adaptation to an illness. Repeated coping failures may lead to impaired psychosocial development and a more difficult course of illness. On the other hand growth and positive changes during such a life crisis as the diagnosis of an illness also can

occur. The nurse observes for signs of hopelessness and helplessness and even temporary immobility. Members of the family may respond with anger or hostility toward health care professionals. Some members of the family may respond with denial, leading to an inability to grasp the seriousness of the situation.

The nurse initially assesses a family's prior experiences and competence in handling the stress of illnesses or crisis. A family's prior coping skills may reflect its ability to respond to the present crisis of a chronic illness. The nurse also determines if other life stressors are operating within the family.

The nurse should encourage the parents to be together at the time the medical diagnosis is shared. Both parents need to hear the same information together, so that one parent does not have to bear the stress of the diagnosis alone; also the parents can be supportive for each other when important and difficult information is being conveyed about a child. If the parents are together at the time of the diagnosis, they may be better prepared to support their child as he or she learns of an illness. If the parents are not told together, marital strain may be increased. If parents are told along with other family members, it can be beneficial because all can share the grief, shock, and feelings of despair, resulting in shared feelings and support. Parents and other family members also can be encouraged by the nurse to express positive reactions and ideas about how the illness will affect the family and what each can contribute to make life easier for the child and other members of the family.

Using Gordon's[13] system for organizing a nursing assessment based on function, the nurse can collect essen-

TABLE 21-3
Nursing Diagnoses for Children With Chronic Illness and Their Families

Functional Health Patterns	Potential Nursing Diagnosis
Health Perception and Health Management	Altered Growth and Development
	Altered Health Maintenance
	Health-Seeking Behaviors
	Noncompliance
Cognition and Perception	Altered Comfort
	Pain
	Chronic Pain
	Decisional Conflict
	Knowledge Deficit (specify)
Self-Perception	Anxiety
	Fatigue
	Fear
	Hopelessness
	Powerlessness
	Self-Concept Disturbance
	Body Image Disturbance
	Personal Identity Disturbance
	Self-Esteem Disturbance
	Increased Chronic Low Self-Esteem
	Increased Situational Low Self-Esteem
Roles and Relationships	Impaired Verbal Communication
	Altered Family Processes
	Grieving
	Anticipatory Grieving
	Altered Parenting
	Parenting Role Conflict
	Altered Role Performance
	Impaired Social Interaction
	Social Isolation
Coping and Stress Tolerance	Impaired Adjustment
	Ineffective Individual Coping
	Ineffective Disabling, Family Coping
	Ineffective Compromised Family Coping
	Family Coping: Potential for Growth
Values and Beliefs	Spiritual Distress

tial data to determine the child's and family's health status and function. Table 21-3 demonstrates the categories that the nurse, parents, and family may consider to determine and promote more positive functioning of the child and family.

★ NURSING INTERVENTIONS

The nurse initially provides support to family members as they attempt to cope with the diagnosis of a chronic illness. Next, the nurse encourages each member to progress in personal developmental tasks while helping the family to complete developmental life cycle tasks (see Chap. 3). The nurse plays significant roles in providing information and education to the family members and child with a specific illness. The nurse helps families use

their own strengths and resources while appropriately using available community resources. The nurse assists the family in the daily management of the child's illness while encouraging open, honest communication among family members.

The nurse can be especially helpful in encouraging all family members to learn specific skills involved in the child's care. The nurse encourages the ill child to express how other family members can help. Most importantly, the nurse helps the family and child to be in charge of the child's illness and to become case managers for the ill child throughout his or her lifetime. The nurse plays a valuable role in helping the family develop an appropriate balance between the needs of the ill child and the need for continued growth and development of the ill child and all other family members. The nurse also has a role in identifying families who are not progressing well or are dysfunctional by referring these families to appropriate health care professionals.

TEACHING

Nurses are assuming greater responsibility in educating parents about chronic illness. Assessments can reveal the parents' prior experience and competence in handling illness and other crises and can help determine if other major life stressors are being experienced by family members.

Providing information about a child's chronic illness requires skill. The amount of medical information may be overwhelming. If parents are experiencing anxiety, information processing may be difficult. Initially, there may be a risk of information overload. Therefore, the nurse must first find out what the parents have been told or what they understand to be wrong with their child. Because misunderstanding and forgetting can occur, the nurse needs to provide highly specific but brief amounts of information. Written materials may enhance parental comprehension.

The nurse assists the family to develop a cognitive understanding of the illness: its course, prognosis, potential complications, routines, and rationale of treatment. Nurses play valuable roles by being supportive to family members who must revise their impressions of the child's physical health and learn how the illness affects the child's daily life. A vital goal for every family is to learn which areas of the child's life are not affected by illness and plan for as much normalcy as possible. In addition the family can assign management tasks to the child that are commensurate with the child's age and developmental status. Simultaneously, the family assumes responsibility for monitoring the child's physical condition and performance with activities of daily living.

Nurses play a valuable role by providing simple, repeated explanations that give basic information about the child's condition and the nature of the illness. It is helpful for the parents to repeat what they understood from the nurse in their own words. Complications of an illness and details of the longer course of the illness may take time to comprehend and understand fully. The initial period of diagnosis and onset of disease may *not* be the most appropriate time to undertake a definitive discussion of these matters.

Some families become information seekers and experts about the child's illness. Others may avoid information, continuing to deny the illness of their child. Each family may require assistance and additional support. The nurse's primary goal is to help the family, parents, and children direct their energies at anticipatory coping. If nurses provide adequate and appropriate anticipatory guidance, children and parents are likely to manage better and have better outcomes.

PSYCHOSOCIAL SUPPORT

The nurse can be instrumental in helping the parents to accept their inability to guarantee the child's health. Family members may need to acknowledge their feelings of inadequacy, anxiety caused by the uncertainty of the illness, and fears that the child's condition may worsen. Feelings of guilt, blame, and helplessness must be assessed and responded to appropriately. The nurse's major responsibility is to help all members of the family "normalize" their feelings. Nurses can assure parents that their responses are normal.

Children can be taught to respond to control by others as well as their own increased dependency. They may experience changes in body function and self-esteem. Some may require extra support in accepting and restrictions imposed by illness (Fig. 21-2). At the same time children need to be acknowledged for their strengths, ability to change, and unique abilities to cope with stressors. Family members are entitled to feedback from nurses on their capacities to assist their children and the expertise they have developed to meet their children's needs.

The nurse may assist the family to integrate treatment regimens into preexisting family routines. In spite of the child's illness, the family has to achieve and preserve important family functions and carry out essential tasks. Families can create an atmosphere that maintains a child's self-esteem and provides for continuing development of competence and mastery. The family also is expected to encourage the child's participation with peers. Finally, the family must develop collaborative relationships with child health care providers, school personnel, and community agencies that are providing care.

SUPPORT OF THE MOTHER

The mother of an infant diagnosed with a chronic illness may experience awkwardness, anxiety, and feelings of failure as she attempts to develop and attain her maternal role. The infant may require a high degree of technical skill. The mother may feel that she will never be able to adequately meet the infant's needs. An infant with chronic illness may not provide distinct and clear behavioral cues for the mother, which makes it even more difficult for the mother to identify and respond to the infant's different cries, distressful behaviors, sleep and awake states, cues of hunger and satiety, fatigue, or illness.

All mothers have the task of restructuring the family system to include the new infant. The infant's personality and special needs must be recognized and accepted into the family's patterns of living. For the mother to be successful in restructuring the family, she requires a clear understanding of the infant's needs and behaviors. The mother's comprehension of the infant's needs may be delayed because of repeated hospitalizations and unclear behavioral cues from the ill infant. Mothers of ill infants may experience repeated periods of adaptation and reorganization that the mother of a well infant does not experience.

Kaplan and Mason[18] researched parental reactions to the birth of a premature infant. They found that mothers have to complete four psychological tasks to successfully establish a sound and healthy parent-infant relationship. The first task at delivery is to prepare for the fact that the premature infant might die; thus, mothers have to grieve and mourn this potential loss. The second task for the mother is to accept the fact that she has not produced a normal infant. This issue of maternal failure has to be resolved if the third task is to be initiated and accomplished.

In the third task the mother is required to relate to the ill infant to establish a relationship. This third task is often difficult because the mother has to work through her disappointment while responding to a sick infant who may require medical treatment and may look different. When the mother resolves this third task, she may better understand how the infant differs from a normal, well infant specifically in regard to his or her unique needs and growth patterns.

To be successful with the fourth task, the mother has to perceive that the infant has special needs and characteristics. At this time the mother needs a cognitive understanding of prematurity as well as the ability to develop an emotional acceptance of the infant. Both are required if the mother is to achieve her roles of providing appropriate caregiving and mothering to her infant (Fig. 21-3).

The nursing implications of Kaplan and Mason's[18] research are that nurses observe for anticipatory grief and provide emotional support and reassurance when mothers are expressing feelings of maternal failure. When mothers are observed to be making statements of guilt or inadequacy, the nurse becomes an active listener, providing empathic statements. Nurses also can correct mothers'

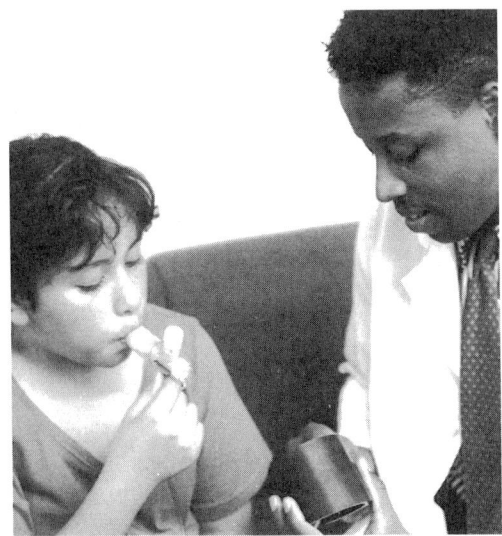

FIGURE 21-2
Older children learn to accept the requirements of their condition and manage their care. Support from the nurse and parents helps the child cope.

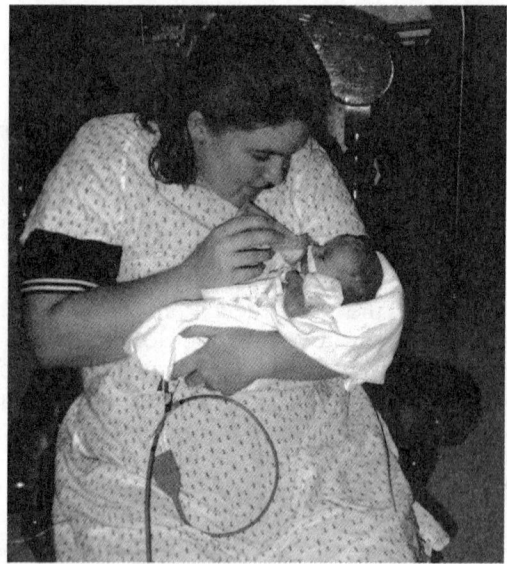

FIGURE 21-3

A mother needs time and support to adjust to a newborn who is ill and who will need long-term care to grow and develop. Just learning to hold and feed her baby is a new experience.

misinformation and discourage distortions of reality. It is appropriate for nurses to assist mothers in the attachment process with their infants. Nurses carry out special roles in helping mothers to become acquainted with and to identify infants' unique needs for feeding, sleeping, consoling, playing, and interacting with the mother.

Drotar et al.[9] described the sequence of stages that parents move through in response to a congenital malformation. The first stage for parents is shock and denial, in which parents may withdraw from their infant. This stage is followed by sadness, grief, anger, anxiety, and guilt. During this second stage parents experience ambivalent feelings about the infant, fears of abnormal development, and fears of death. Parents may feel disappointed and confused and may avoid caregiving of the infant during this period. During the third stage of adaptation parents experience growing feelings of confidence in caring for their infant and begin to recognize their infant's special characteristics. The fourth and last stage, reorganization, is one in which parents begin to plan for the child to be included in the family and begin to establish long-term goals.

During the first stage of shock and denial, it is important that the nurse be present, offer support, and reassure parents that their feelings are normal and expected. During the second stage of parental sadness, the parents should be encouraged to talk to each other as well as health care professionals. Parents can be encouraged to vent their feelings of grief, anger, or anxiety. Nurses can make special contributions to parents during the third stage of adaptation by encouraging parents to hold their infant, identify the infant's positive traits, and learn to identify behavioral cues, such as states of alertness, crying, hunger, and distress. Positive traits of the infant need to be reinforced at all stages of adaptation. Finally, during the fourth stage of reorganization, it is important for the nurse to focus on mother's and father's perceptions of the infant, encourage mutual support of parents, and en-

courage both parents to plan for the infant's special place in the family.

The nurse's most valuable roles are those of assessing parental feelings, adaptation, and goals. The nurse can provide support through each of the four complex stages and demonstrate the infant's strengths and needs. The nurse plays a pivotal role in teaching parents about infant care and what to expect from the infant and helping them focus on successful attachment and bonding for the benefit of infant and parents.

Holaday[15] investigated how mothers learn to interpret the meaning of a chronically ill infant's cry. In her research she described the sequences that are involved as a mother moves from an inadequate conceptual set to a more sophisticated conceptual set. Holaday visited mothers and infants in their homes for 3 months until the infant reached 6 months of age. Holaday described four stages that mothers progressed through in developing a conceptual set of an infant's cry. She found that as mothers considered more complex reasons for an infant's cry, they were better able to consider a wider range of choices for consoling infants. As mothers increased their alternatives before action was taken to console an infant who was crying, they also decreased the number of different actions taken in response to one cry. As a result Holaday[15] saw more abstract reasoning rather than fixed deterministic reasoning by the mothers.

Holaday's paradigm has use in assessing parental adaptation to the birth of an infant with chronic illness. Nurses can be effective in assisting mothers to assess an infant's cry before the infant goes home from the hospital. The nurse can assess if there are differences in the clarity of the infant's cries. How clear is one cry from another? The nurse can also encourage mothers to record their infant's cries (when, how often, how long, and how it affects the mother). The nurse also can support the mother in problem solving about the best and most appropriate time to console the infant. The mother and nurse together can observe if the infant is able to console himself or herself and settle down, and they can determine the best action to reduce crying. The nurse can be especially helpful to mothers as they attempt to refrain from responding immediately to an infant's first cries.

SUPPORT OF THE FATHER

Much of the research on fathers indicates a sense of inferiority when they have a child with a chronic illness. Cummings'[7] research suggests that fathers are more depressed than mothers and may experience less meaningful relationships with family members when a child is diagnosed with a chronic illness. Research findings also indicate that fathers feel less of a sense of parental competence and do not feel they are as involved in the child's care as the mother. Frequently the father is left out and he may become less involved than the mother in the child's daily care.

Gallagher's[11] and McKeever's[23] research data on fathers of infants who are chronically ill indicate that fathers have few helpful ways to contribute to the well-being of their children, have limited opportunities to share their feelings with other fathers, and often have little opportunity to progress through the mourning process. The nurse can make vital contributions to the parent-child

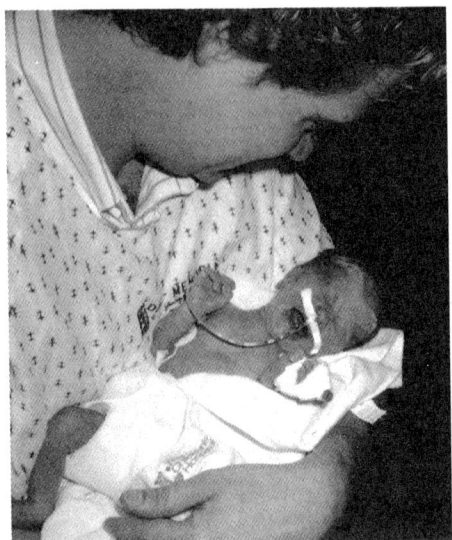 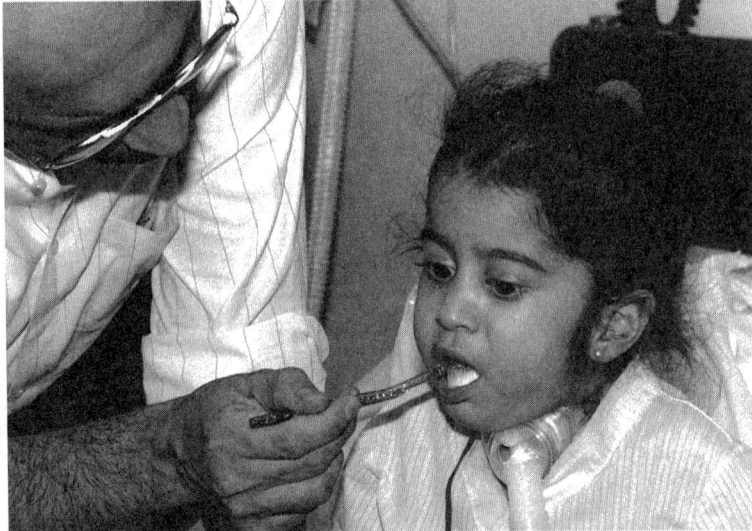

FIGURE 21-4
Fathers are important care providers for infants and children who have chronic illness. Early involvement in the baby's care can establish a lifelong pattern of a helping relationship.

relationship by assuring that both parents understand the nature of the illness and how they are expected to manage the child's illness (Fig. 21-4). Because the father's needs may be overlooked, the nurse should plan to include the father when assessing a child, making home visits, or demonstrating care techniques in a hospital setting.

The father can be actively involved in discharge planning, and the nurse can reinforce that the father's observations, ideas, and care are valuable. In order to include the father as an active participant in the child's care early on, the nurse plans child care conferences when the father can be present, arranges home health care visits that are convenient for fathers, and shares diagnostic information, goal setting, care planning, and evaluation with fathers. The nurse can demonstrate nurturance and sensitivity to the needs of fathers by referring them to discussion groups for support and providing appropriate literature for fathers to become better informed about a child's specific illness.

Before a nurse includes fathers in care planning and problem solving, he or she should elicit the father's perceptions of an illness and what it means to a father. Nurses can be effective in supporting the feelings that fathers have regarding the child with an illness. The nurse can make himself or herself available and encourage fathers to discuss their feelings as they move through progressive stages of shock, denial, anger, grief, sadness, sorrow, and adaptation to infants and children with chronic illness.

Nurses have essential roles to play in assisting fathers to become actively involved in the attachment process when an infant with a chronic illness is born. Nurses can implement interventions to be certain that fathers, like mothers, can identify desirable traits of infants; describe specific behavioral cues of crying, alert, awake, and sleep states; and recognize the most optimal times to interact with the baby.

SUPPORT OF WELL SIBLINGS

In order to provide quality care, nurses recognize the need to assess, plan, and implement care for well siblings too. Well siblings clearly have special needs for information, warmth, support, and attention to their own unique growth and development. Thoughtful and well-planned interventions for well siblings can often make significant differences in assisting families to function more optimally and to maintain healthy, nurturing roles and relationships.

Little is known about the dynamics of sibling relationships in general. Therefore, it is difficult to differentiate the effects of illness or handicaps from the intensity and ambivalence that already exists between siblings (Fig. 21-5).

Most of what we know about siblings who have a sister or brother with a chronic illness is based on parental perceptions. Siblings have not always spoken for themselves, and most data about siblings have been obtained through secondary or incidental findings in family studies. In addition the majority of studies have focused on siblings who have brothers or sisters who were mentally retarded, handicapped, terminally ill, or born with birth defects. In general the sample sizes of children were small, and children studied ranged in age from 3 to 18 with the greatest number being older than age 7.

Sibling research has been plagued with conflicting conclusions as well. Therefore, siblings and their chronically ill brothers and sisters need more attention paid to them. The magnitude of children with chronic illness makes it incumbent to focus on the needs of well siblings.

Research indicates that the sibling subsystem as a whole is affected by an ill or handicapped child. Altered roles and relationships may stimulate or hinder personal development and interaction over the length of the illness. Several researchers have found that well siblings experience a variety of negative and positive responses to ill siblings, which are are listed in the accompanying display.

The most noteworthy research findings are that children who have been given frequent and complete information about a sibling's illness and who were included in a sibling's care had more positive dimensions in

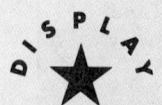

Well Siblings' Negative and Positive Responses to Ill Siblings

NEGATIVE RESPONSES

- Fear
- Resentment
- Anger
- Jealousy
- Anxiety
- Poor school achievement
- Sibling rivalry
- Attention-seeking behaviors
- Behavioral problems
- Development of physical symptoms
- Withdrawal
- Isolation
- Deprivation
- Inadequate knowledge of illness
- Inferiority
- Prone to failure
- Increased competition
- Egocentricity
- Guilt conflict
- Self-blame
- Communication

POSITIVE RESPONSES

- Empathy
- Nurturing
- Cooperation
- Sensitivity
- Compassion
- Maturity
- Self-esteem
- Cognitive mastery
- Ability to assume responsibilities
- Tolerance
- Appreciation of family bonds
- Idealism
- Sense of family pride
- Sense of family loyalty
- Coping skills
- Problem-solving skills
- Appreciation of own health

their own development. Those well children consistently made remarks that their experiences had been growth experiences.

Simeon[31] formulated common questions that siblings of children with chronic illness ask regarding the cause and prognosis of a sibling's illness (see the accompanying display on common questions asked by siblings of children with chronic illness).

This display identifies questions that siblings ask about their own health, the unfairness of the illness, feelings, the future of brothers and sisters, questions about a child's own future, and responsibilities assumed by well siblings.

Because siblings may be expected to educate peers about a sick brother or sister, much of their energy may be taken up in explaining and answering others' questions. Nurses can help assist them in this role. More than ever before, nurses also have leading roles to play in educating school personnel about siblings and their unique needs and keeping teachers informed as to a child's condition and progress.

Nurses are in a strategic position to encourage siblings to join sibling support groups where they can share their feelings with their peers. Nurses also play a valuable role in establishing bereavement programs for parents and siblings when a brother or sister dies.

By using a family systems approach, the nurse can plan comprehensive, family-centered assessment and interventions. The cornerstone of achieving success naturally rests on systematic observations and assessments of siblings with particular attention to how siblings responded before a brother or sister became ill. A major

focus then shifts to supporting, educating, and providing anticipatory guidance to family members.

Nurses make a substantial contribution to the quality of the siblings' lives by keeping children informed on the progress of the sick sibling. Well siblings need to feel special and have appropriate attention and support, particularly when a sick sibling is in crisis or in pain.

Nurses can meet siblings' educational and emotional needs in many creative ways. The accompanying display focuses on emerging trends of planning care in meeting well siblings' needs.

Simeon[31] also outlined some prevention–intervention strategies for parents of children with chronic illness. Simeon presents a number of strategies that are helpful in assisting parents to meet the needs of well siblings. These strategies are listed in the accompanying display.

SUPPORT OF THE ILL CHILD

Children's care needs are based on their developmental stages and attainments. The effects of a chronic illness will be different for each child because of the developmental levels and tasks the child is attempting to master. Thus, the nurse is expected to apply theories and principles of growth and development to plan sound nursing interventions for children with chronic illness. Children's growth and development may be affected in a variety of ways by a specific chronic illness.

Certain chronic illnesses will limit a child's ability to achieve expected and successive developmental skills and to master their environments. A developmental framework can assist children to move successfully from dependency to increased autonomy, mastery, and a secure

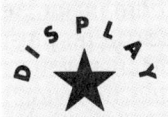

Common Questions of Siblings of Children With Chronic Illness

ABOUT CAUSATION OR PROGNOSIS

What caused my brother or sister's illness disability?
Will it get worse?
Will he or she ever get well?
Will he or she die?
Will I catch what my brother or sister has?
Has my own health been bought at the cost of my brother or sister's health?
Is my brother or sister somehow defective or less of a person?
Why didn't my parents stop this from happening?
How can I explain this to other people?

ABOUT THEIR OWN HEALTH

Am I ill or handicapped, too?
How many of my brother or sister's characteristics do I share?
Will the same thing happen to me sometime, or am I safe?

ABOUT THE UNFAIRNESS

Why did this happen to our family?
What did we do to deserve this?
Why should I have to live with this when my friends don't?
Why are there different rules for my brother or sister than for me?
Am I not as important as my brother or sister?

ABOUT FEELINGS

Do I have the right to be mad at someone who is ill or helpless?
How come all the money (time, love, etc.) goes to my brother or sister?
Doesn't anyone know that what I need is important, too?
How can I help my brother or sister and still make other kids like me?
Do I have to love him or her when he or she makes me so unhappy?
Whom do my parents love most?

ABOUT FUTURE OF BROTHER OR SISTER

I hear a lot about ill and handicapped children, but I never hear about adults.
What happens to ill or handicapped children when they grow up?
Do ill or handicapped children grow up at all?

ABOUT OWN FUTURE

Will I be able to have my own children?
Do I carry a defective gene that I will pass on to other generations?
Will I have a defective child?
Will some accident or disease strike my life unexpectedly as it did with my parents?
Will this sister or brother compromise what I want to do with my own grown-up life?

ABOUT RESPONSIBILITY

How much do I owe my brother or sister?
How much can I leave to others?
Where does ultimate responsibility lie for my brother or sister?
Will I be responsible for my brother or sister when he or she grows up?
Do my parents expect me to take charge when they no longer can?
Will I be able to do a good job in caring for my brother or sister?
Will I find a spouse who will want to share this job?
How much of what I need and want am I supposed to give up so my brother or sister can be happy, included, well?
Do I have to achieve twice as much to make up for what my brother or sister lacks?
Am I responsible for care of my parents, to support and comfort them?

(From: Siemon, M. [1984]. Siblings of the chronically ill child. Nursing Clinics of North America, 19, 302.)

sense of self. It is useful for the nurse to consider each child's particular stage of development to fully understand and assess the extent to which it impacts on the way children cope with illnesses. Stages of development were discussed in Chapter 8. Developmental tasks are discussed further in the remaining sections of this chapter.

To plan individualized, comprehensive care, the nurse considers the following:

- The child's concept of illness
- The child's responses to procedures, treatments, home care, school, and hospitalization
- Age-related psychosocial, cognitive, and developmental tasks

Yoos[34] has addressed the effects of chronic illness on children of different ages and the developmental tasks that must be mastered at successive stages. Yoos[34] also formulated several creative intervention strategies to promote the most optimal developmental outcomes. Table 21-4 presents the stages of childhood, developmental tasks that must be achieved by children, the effects of chronic illness, and intervention strategies that are developmentally focused for children with chronic illness. Developmental tasks for each stage and appropriate family-centered nursing care are discussed further in the remaining sections of this chapter.

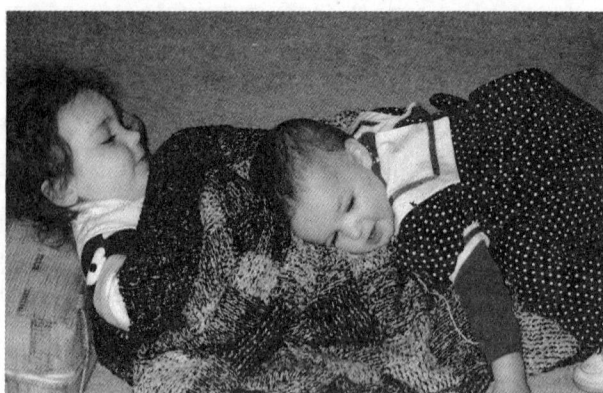

FIGURE 21-5
The special relationships between siblings can be supported by parents and nurses when a child develops a chronic illness and requires more attention.

Developmental Considerations

The Newborn

Developmental tasks of the neonate include the following:

- Achieve physiological stability.
- Establish biophysical and psychosocial patterns of sleep–awake states, feeding, and elimination.
- Develop attachment to parents.
- Develop a sense of trust versus mistrust.

The neonate is entirely dependent on the parents and other caregivers. The nurse encourages parents to express their feelings of grief and loss and experience them as normal.[24,34] Nurses plan care that takes into consideration the need for parental attachment with the infant.

The primary goals of interventions are to reduce any interferences with the attachment process. Parents ideally are included in the caregiving of the newborn infant. As the infant achieves physiologic stability, the parents must be allowed to touch, see, and hold the infant as well as identify the infant's unique characteristics, behavioral cues, and strengths. If the newborn is hospitalized, the parents can be encouraged to console infants appropriately when they cry, identify and respond to their feeding needs, identify their different awake and sleep states, provide appropriate animate and inanimate stimuli when the infant is most alert, and provide appropriate toys and sensory experiences to enrich the infant's hospital environment.

During the neonatal period, parents' anxiety and need for information are best addressed early and immediately. A wise nurse will plan several sessions to answer parents' questions about the illness, the outcome, and the development of the neonate. Parents need repeated reassurance and anticipatory guidance about what to expect from the newborn. The nurse may use home visits to assess the quality of parent-infant relationships, parental contact with the infant, and parental implementation of care provider and parenting roles.

A principal need of the parents is to achieve a sense of competence and mastery of their parenting skills in feeding, bathing, dressing, comforting, and providing necessary treatments and medications. The parents can be viewed as vital sources of appropriate stimulation for the infant and can be acknowledged as experts in the care of their own newborn; nurses can acknowledge their creative problem solving, decision making, and resourcefulness in adapting to a newborn infant with many complex needs.

The nurse plays a key role in helping parents to perceive the infant as a newborn rather than concentrating on the diagnosis. The nurse who interacts with the sick neonate in affectionate and nurturing ways shows acceptance and serves as a role model for the family. The nurse is unique in his or her roles of concentrating on the in-

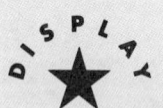

Nursing Interventions: Guidelines for Planning Family-Centered Care for Well Siblings of Children With Chronic Illness

- Concentrate on well child's social, emotional, cognitive, and physical needs.
- Assess well sibling for physical symptoms, quality of relationships with family members, social behaviors with peers, communication abilities, and progress in school.
- Assess learning needs of well child, and develop appropriate teaching strategies.
- Delegate health care tasks to well sibling commensurate with age, cognitive abilities, and developmental stages.
- Keep well child informed as to sick child's status.
- Thoroughly observe well child for behavior manifestations of bed wetting, thumb sucking, heightened separation anxiety, nightmares, or other clues of regression in development.

- Monitor well child's academic performance, and observe for poor grades, underachievement or overachievement, or behavioral problems in school.
- Ask specific questions of well child's understanding of the ill sibling's condition and how doctors make siblings better. Respond to teachers' needs for information on illness, medications, treatments, and health care regimen.
- Invite well and sick siblings to join support groups (e.g., diabetic or oncology support groups).
- Meet with well sibling, and elicit perceptions of well child's understanding of sick child's illness and the meaning assigned to it by the well child. Answer questions about child's future and responsibilities.
- Encourage well and sick siblings to speak for themselves.

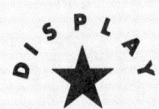

Parental Teaching: Intervention Strategies to Help Siblings of Children With Chronic Illness

- Relay information to siblings so they feel like a part of the family.
- Use family conferences to provide an open setting for siblings to ask questions and acknowledge feelings.
- Recognize and admit what is happening, expressing feelings and concerns honestly.
- Keep care routines (bed, meals) as consistent as possible.
- Have a consistent caregiver in parental absences.
- Prepare siblings for changes in home life before they actually occur.
- Understand that each child has different needs; allow siblings to set their own pace for learning and involvement.
- Help siblings to develop their own identities, seeing the differences and similarities between themselves and a child with special needs, and achieving successes without guilt.
- Legitimate reasonable anger. Even ill or disabled children behave badly sometimes.
- Respect sibling's reluctance to be with or include a child with special needs in their activities. It is not a failure on parents' part to instill proper love.
- "Dethrone" an ill or disabled child, putting him or her back in perspective and in the proper place in the family rather than as the focus of the family around whom all else revolves.
- Weigh the cost of actions to all children against the benefit to one. It may be a mistake to devote all time and attention to one child, even one who is terminal.

- Work to balance the facets of family life so that tasks of care do not dominate.
- Find ways to include siblings realistically into care and treatment of a brother or sister.
- Find manageable ways to spend quality time individually with siblings.
- Seek professional help for decisions that involve consideration of other children (e.g., rooming-in).
- Recognize that lengthy explanations designed to anticipate every question work no better for illness or disability than for sex education.
- Recognize that children mature, and relationships change. No attitude endures forever. Through all the changes flows the continuity of belonging to each other.
- Do not take problems as "whole." Break them into manageable parts.
- Recognize own need for extra help and care. Accept support offered by others.
- Use extended family to provide substitutes for siblings of parental involvement.
- Let teachers know what is happening so they can be understanding and helpful to school children.
- Maintain balance in family life through the use of professional and informal support systems.
- Acknowledge the personal strengths siblings have and their ability to cope with stress successfully.

(From: *Siemon, M.* [*1984*]. *Siblings of the chronically ill or disabled child.* Nursing Clinics of North America, 19, *304.*)

fant's strengths, positive features, and unique traits, rather than focusing on negative traits or deficits. Nurses can reinforce the normalcy of the acutely sick neonate and his or her care routines.

It is important that the nurse inquire about siblings' concerns about parents and the neonate. Because parents often spend more time with newborns, siblings may feel neglected. The nurse is in an excellent position to offer anticipatory guidance about sibling rivalry (see Chap. 13) and encourage parents to spend appropriate time with siblings. It is desirable for the nurse to inquire as to what parents have told siblings regarding the infant's illness, their responses, and whether the siblings have assumed any major roles and responsibilities. The nurse can encourage siblings to visit the newborn, to become acquainted, and to initiate and preserve the natural sibling bond that will develop. The nurse also can inquire as to how parents are responding to grandparents' needs and determine if grandparents are a source of stress. Nurses find including grandparents in conferences that are planned to meet the infant's ongoing and lifelong needs are rewarding and helpful for the family.

To be successful in implementing nursing care strategies, the nurse will include the parents in a mutual par-

ticipation model, in which the parents perceive their own uniqueness, competencies, and significant contributions for ensuring their infant's optimal growth and development. Parents can begin to master their own developmental tasks for successful parenting of an infant with lifelong health care needs.

The Infant

Developmental tasks of infancy include the following:

- Continue to develop attachment with parents and primary care givers.
- Experience a consistent, safe environment.
- Acquire a sense of trust versus mistrust.
- Experience repetition of the cause-effect sequence.
- Learn through sensorimotor explorations.

Infants may experience an inconsistent environment because of pain and discomfort from an illness or treatments and repeated hospitalizations. Forced separations from parents may interfere in the attachment process, which is critical for the development of trust and later

TABLE 21-4
Effects of Chronic Illness on Developmental Tasks and Intervention Strategies

Stage of Childhood	Developmental Task	Effect of Chronic Illness	Intervention Strategy
Neonate	1. Achieving physiologic stability	Chronic illness may decrease infant's access to environmental inputs if all of his or her energy is needed to survive. Body rhythmicity may be disturbed. Physiologic stability is essential for development in all other major areas.	Help caretaker become aware of and cope with the infant's pattern of sleep, feeding, and elimination. Infant's adjustment to extrauterine life needs to be assessed, and parents need to be taught important symptoms.
	2. Developing bonding and attachment	Parental guilt, grief, or anger may interfere with attachment process as may the infant's ability to respond. Parents may withdraw. Attachment requires time to develop. Prolonged hospitalization may disrupt early relationship.	Encourage parents to express feelings and identify them as normal. Give factual information about what is known about the child's problem. Guide parents in establishing physical and emotional contact with the infant. Help parents develop a sense of competence.
Infancy	1. Continuing to develop with the primary caregiver	Major separation from parents when attachment is just being formed may interfere with process. Infant's social responsiveness may be decreased, thereby diminishing parents' attachment.	Help families to maintain a consistent presence in infant's life during hospitalization. Maximize opportunities for parents to participate in care. Help parents learn about their infant's characteristics and behaviors. Teach when and how to stimulate infant and when to decrease the intensity of the interaction.
	2. Acquiring a sense of trust	Developing trust depends on having needs met in a consistent manner, which is difficult to achieve in a hospital setting. Illness may violate expectations of a nurturing, pain-free environment. Inconsistent care and separations from parents may lead to mistrust.	Meet expectations about the environment whenever possible. Facilitate consistent care through communicating infant's characteristics with other care providers. Maximize parents' opportunities to provide their infant with care.
	3. Developing an initial sense of individuality	May decrease the infant's sense of control and effect on his or her environment. Illness may lead to a sense of helplessness.	Encourage parents to give infant as much opportunity for exploration and mastery as possible.
	4. Learning through sensorimotor exploration	Opportunities for exploration and manipulation of objects may be diminished.	Help parents use age-appropriate toys and activities adapted to child's needs. Help parents with creating useful play experiences and how to best approximate those experiences.
Toddler	1. Developing autonomy	Autonomy is aided by opportunities for exploration and independence. Illness may hamper exploring and using motor skills. Parents may overprotect and be reluctant to set limits.	Help parents devise some measurements so a child can move independently if possible and some opportunities to play independently. Give child simple choices when possible. Help parents confront their guilt that may be preventing them from setting appropriate limits.
	2. Mastering new skills in body control, hand use, and speech	May not have the opportunity to engage in tasks requiring eye–hand coordination, assembling and categorizing objects. Some conditions affect ability to control bowel and bladder functions.	Help parents to be creative in providing play experiences. Tasks involving successful toileting should be broken down into small specific behaviors.
Preschooler	1. Mastering self-care skills	Parents may overprotect. Regression occurs in most children during illness.	Help parents verbalize concerns; suggest parents' strengths. Help parents to encourage independence and self-reliance.
	2. Developing initiative and purpose	May lack exposure to new experiences. Parents may try to buffer interactions with the environment and peers and limit the child's opportunity to develop coping mechanisms. Initiative may be discouraged.	Explore possibilities for preschool experiences for child with parents. Also may need to work with school regarding the nature of child's illness, limitations, etc. Arrange for orientation or observation visit to preschool.
	3. Using mental symbolization (although still has egocentric thought, and focuses attention on only one part of an event)	Illness may be defined in terms of single external symptom. Illness cause may be attributed to punishment for bad behavior or something they did not do.	Encourage play to help child explore experiences and feelings about illness. Help child prepare for procedures by repeating facts playing out procedures.
Middle Childhood	1. Using concrete operations	Achieving this task is enriched by school, hobbies, and interactions with peers. May have diminished opportunities for learning and irregular school attendance.	Encourage and facilitate regular attendance. Nurse practitioner may need to act as liaison between school and family and advocate for the child. Educate teachers and healthy peers about chronic illness. Be creative when school is missed. Use computer hook-up or home VCR.

(Continued)

TABLE 21-4
(Continued)

Stage of Childhood	Developmental Task	Effect of Chronic Illness	Intervention Strategy
	2. Developing industry and initiative; "I can do" (comes about primarily through mastering social interactional situations and concrete skills)	May have decreased interactions with peers. May feel different from peers. May miss out on experiences that lead to the normal development of self-esteem and a sense of mastery. May show a pattern of underachievement when compared to tested abilities.[29a]	Encourage enhancing peer relationships through participating in clubs and sports. The importance of normalized school and life experiences cannot be overemphasized. Health care providers need to collaborate with school personnel (Magrab, 1985). School-age children should participate as much as possible in their own care and decisions affecting their treatment. Children need factual, honest information about their disabilities. Allow children to have control over diet or medications as child's ability to handle these situations develops.
Adolescence	1. Establishing independence	Disease management may make independence difficult. Complying to medical regimen may become a problem. Relationships with parents and health care providers may become increasingly hostile. Job and career choice may be diminished.	Identify feelings of anger as normal, and offer support. Encourage families to find areas in adolescent's life in which they can have independence. Assist parents in facing some of the complexities of possible living arrangements. Help develop skills for self-care. Referrals to vocational rehabilitation services may be appropriate.
	2. Becoming comfortable with one's body	Preoccupation with bodily functions and changes are normal for all teens, accentuated for adolescents with a chronic illness. Physical illness manifestations may make them feel markedly different from peers. Adolescents with visible physical defect experience sadness, grief, and anger.	Respect need for privacy. Assist in finding support groups. Acknowledge feelings; facilitate family sharing feelings. Teenagers need to understand the specifics about their physiologic condition and the treatment they are receiving. The ability to look at and care for one's own body, including those parts that are different, is necessary for the eventual acceptance of that body.[25]
	3. Establishing sexual identity and building new and meaningful relationships	May have decreased opportunity to be part of a peer group. May have decreased access to peers with whom they can discuss sexual questions.	Help parents understand that an adolescent with a disability is as much a sexual being as any other person. Encourage adolescent to participate in activities and initiate friendships. Provide information about birth control.
	4. Developing formal operational thought	Deficit in previous stages may prevent this. Developing adolescent's cognitive abilities is aided by interaction and cooperation with others.[29] Ill adolescents may have fewer opportunities for confrontation with peers.	Encourage opportunities for adolescents to be faced with opinions, values, and beliefs that may differ from their own. Promote advocacy within school system.

(*From:* Yoos, L. [1987]. Chronic childhood illnesses: Developmental illness. *Pediatric Nursing, 13* [1], 25–28.)

exploration by the child. The infant also may be placed in an intensive care nursery, which may be excessively overstimulating due to lights, noises, and multiple procedures. Because the infant's care is provided by multiple caregivers, there is the possibility of overstimulation. Therefore, the infant's early environment may be experienced as unsafe, undependable, distressful, and lacking in consistency.

Parents may experience fear of an infant who is visibly deformed or acutely sick. Parents may be discouraged by an infant who doesn't respond to their smiles, touches, and consoling efforts. The infant may be demanding and may have a cry that is irritable, high pitched, or negative. Parents can feel defeated and inadequate. If the infant is physically unable to respond or too weak or fatigued to provide feedback, parents may become discouraged and withdraw, thereby compromising early attachment.

The infant needs to achieve attachment with parents to gain trust, and in turn, parents need to attach to their infant to develop a sense of parental competency and mastery. If parents are overwhelmed with grief or fear after learning the diagnosis, it may influence increased withdrawal from the infant and may result in inconsistent physical care.

The primary goals of intervention are to maximize the attachment process between the parents and infant and promote a consistent caregiving environment. Nurses can assist parents to identify and interpret behavioral cues accurately so they will feel more adequate and consistent in their caregiving responses. Parents can learn their infant's best times to be held, comforted, consoled, or fed. Most importantly, parents can learn the best times to interact socially with the infant. Although parents may need to initiate interactions when an infant is ill, fatigued, or in discomfort, they also can learn from the observations of the nurse when the infant may be signaling them or attempting to initiate interactions with them.

Parents respond to encouragement to visit or stay with the infant during hospitalizations or forced separations. Parents can be reinforced for their efforts in providing care and getting to know their infant better. (Fig. 21-6). Above all, parents need to learn skills and competencies of caring that will reinforce their sense of parental competency. Care solely by the parents fosters a consistent

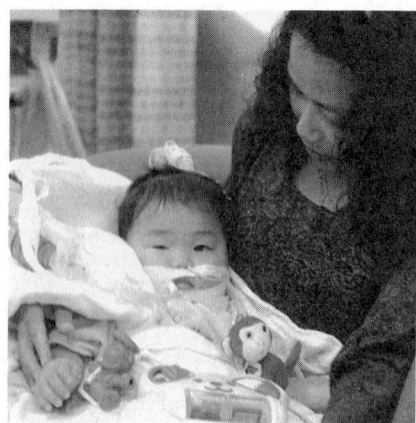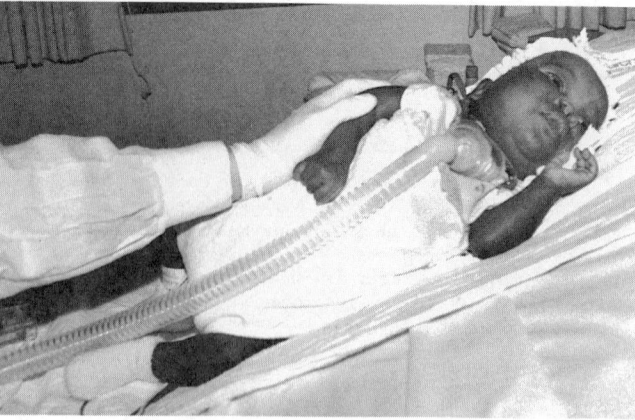

FIGURE 21-6
Parents should be encouraged to spend as much time as possible in the hospital with the infant, providing care when possible. Children should be held and cuddled. If therapy does not allow for the infant to be held, the parents can touch and stroke the child.

caregiving environment in which greater trust is provided for the infant.

Fathers also need guidance from the nurse to help them read cues, promote attachment, be consistent in their approaches, and participate in the complex care regimens. Fathers and mothers need opportunities to share their feelings and concerns with other fathers and mothers who are experiencing the challenges of parenting an infant who is ill. The nurse plays a pivotal role in referring both parents to appropriate parent support groups for infants diagnosed with a chronic condition.

The Toddler

Developmental tasks of the toddler include the following:

- Develop autonomy versus shame and doubt.
- Master new skills of body control and fine-motor coordination.
- Acquire language skills.
- Emergence of abilities to use mental combinations.
- Increase testing of social limits.

During the toddler period children have begun to experience themselves as separate from their parents.[24,34] They are attempting to master and develop autonomy. They are striving to master and refine new skills in body movement, coordination, and control. Because of their unique developmental and psychosocial characteristics, young children with chronic illnesses are attempting to master the normal developmental tasks of autonomy, becoming separate by exploring, and independently engaging and initiating coherent activities and ideas. At the same time they are preserving an attachment to their parents.[24,34] The development of autonomy by toddlers and subsequent separation from parents can be impeded by a chronic illness.

Therefore, the primary goals of interventions are to assist the toddler to develop a sense of autonomy and self-control through active exploration of the environment (Fig. 21-7). While helping young children to master developmental tasks, nurses also need to be supportive of

parents who may be overprotective or fail to set realistic limits.[4] The nurse encourages parents to establish age-appropriate limits and to provide suitable opportunities to play independently.

Parents can be reinforced in their efforts at providing children with simple choices in playing, eating, and toileting. It may be helpful for parents to discuss any feelings of guilt that prevent them from setting appropriate limits.[34] If parents are concerned about beginning toilet learning, the nurse assesses the parent's readiness to begin training and the child's physiologic and physical readiness. The parents need to be comfortable with the steps of the training process and show a commitment for a positive, relaxed approach to learning.

The Preschooler

Developmental tasks of the preschooler include the following:

- Develop initiative versus guilt.
- Master self-care skills.
- Emergence of preoperational thought.
- Learn rules and expectations of others.
- Play in interactive ways.
- Imitate sex role.

During the preschool years children are faced with the process of incorporating the knowledge of an illness into an emerging sense of self.[13] Young children characteristically view experiences in an egocentric or intuitive manner, relying on very primitive logic.[20,31] Children at this developmental level do not completely differentiate between themselves and the world.[24]

Many experts in the field of child development have indicated that young children view illness as a punishment for bad behavior and believe that parents or other significant adults could cure an illness if they so desired.[24] Further, children view treatments and procedures as punishment for wrong or bad behavior or something they failed to do.[24,34] Children may experience anxiety and fear abandonment if they are subjected to repeated or prolonged hospitalizations for a chronic illness. Because the most common basis for anxiety in children younger than 4 years is separation from parents and family members,[24] children may be at risk for losing confidence in their parents and may experience decreased security if forced separations occur.[24]

The primary goals of intervention are to achieve a balance between encouragement of initiative and appropriate limit setting characterized by consistency. Nurses can encourage parents to allow children to begin taking responsibility for themselves. Parents can establish realistic goals for children and allow them to initiate activities on their own. Above all else, children need to have success rather than repeated discouragement, defeat, and lack of goals. The parents can be supported in their ideas about how to encourage greater independence for their child, enrich the child's developmental environment, and provide activities that help foster the child's initiative. It is important that the nurse explore the child's preschool experiences with the parents.[34]

The nurse should help the parents to recognize that young children need repeated assurances that they are loved and will not be abandoned and that illness is not a form of punishment for wrongdoing or bad behavior. Above all, children need to know that parents will be available to them if they are hospitalized. Parents and health care professionals can be helpful by providing simple explanations of the illness to children to eliminate or decrease the fears they may be experiencing. Parents should plan to spend extra time with hospitalized children, provide care, and reassure their love and affection. Nurses may need to encourage parents to allow the child to have appropriate experiences with activities requiring eye-hand coordination.[34] Through a variety of creative experiences, children can learn greater self-control and achieve the tasks of their peers.

Because of the child's chronic illness, parents may tend to overprotect the child and limit exposure to varying environmental stimuli, new experiences, activities, toys, peers, and even family members. The child may become passive and discouraged from developing appropriate and necessary coping mechanisms. The parents also may not encourage the child to develop initiative. The child may regress to earlier, less acceptable forms of behavior during periods of a chronic illness.[34] The nurse can foster positive growth and development of the child while acknowledging parental strengths, needs, and competence in parenting a preschool-age child.

When providing direct care for the child, the nurse can use play to assist the child to express his or her feelings about the illness or procedures or treatments that must be administered to the child. The child can be prepared for procedures by playing out and mastering them. The nurse, parents, and other health care professionals must repeat facts for the child and provide simple, brief explanations.[24,34]

The School-Age Child

Developmental tasks of the school-age child include the following:

- Develop industry versus inferiority.
- Use concrete operations (logical thinking with ability to serialize, reverse, and conserve mental images).
- Decenter self-other and part-whole thinking.
- Develop greater understanding of self and others.
- Sustain efforts to master tasks and produce.
- Acquire and master skills.
- Become more involved with peers, and seek peer approval.
- Develop concerns about fairness.

Throughout the school years children are faced with developing a greater sense of mastery over their environment, achieving new skills and knowledge, formulating moral attitudes and values, and developing rewarding relationships with peers.[24] The school-age child has more capacities to reason in rational and logical ways and has made major developmental strides in abilities to differentiate between self and the world.[24] They can focus and respond to external, real events. Although children of early school years (ages 6 through 11) may view illness as punishment or the result of wrong behavior or disobedience, they no longer think of parents and other adults as being omnipotent.[24] Children of this age are capable of concrete operations and strive to develop control and achieve industry. Achieving these developmental tasks is enhanced by regularly attending school, interacting with peers who accept them, and establishing meaningful hobbies.

Repeated illnesses and hospitalizations of school-age children may result in increased school absences, making it difficult to succeed with school assignments. Peers and teachers may experience fear of a child with a chronic condition and may avoid him or her. Teachers may react to a child's illness by becoming overprotective or reducing their expectations of the child's performance. Magrab[24] reported several studies that found lower academic achievement among children with chronic illnesses (who had normal cognitive abilities). The cognitive, motor, or sensory limitations imposed by a chronic condition may interfere significantly with the mastery of tasks for this age group and thereby result in lowered self-confidence, decreased self-esteem, and a sense of inferiority rather than industry.

A chronic illness may lead to decreased interactions with family members and especially peers. Acceptance by one's peer groups is critical for a child's social development and skills. The child may feel different from his or her peers, worry about being different, and try to hide or withdraw out of fear of rejection. As a result the child might miss out on experiences with others that would lead to the normal development of self-esteem and a sense of mastery.

The primary goals of intervention are to help the school-age child achieve a sense of industry by producing things using skill acquisition and reaching goals. When providing care for school-age children, the nurse provides simple, honest, and specific information about a child's illness. Because children of this age can use information about origin, causation, diagnosis, and treatment of their illness, nurses and parents need to be consistent and persevering in their efforts to provide essential information.[24] The nurse and others can help the child cope by labeling the illness and discussing its symptoms with the child. The nurse can determine how much the child is processing and encourage the child to express questions, fears, negative feelings, and positive views of themselves as they cope with their illness. The nurse can provide sustaining, supportive, nurturing, and empathic reassurance that the child is not alone in his or her coping and adjusting.

The nurse reinforces the need for normalized school and life experiences for the child and family.[24,34] The nurse encourages regular school attendance[24] and may meet with the child's teachers to explain the illness and answer questions. The nurse can be supportive to teachers who are anxious or have fears about a child attending school. The nurse first determines the teacher's knowledge levels and comprehension of the illness and then provides simple, clear explanations. Effective and ongoing communication among parents, school personnel, and community agencies is facilitated by nurses. Children with chronic conditions or developmental disabilities are encouraged by nurses and others to acquire social skills. Some children may benefit from learning how to relate to their peers in more socially acceptable ways, such as not interrupting while another is talking. The nurse can role model positive interactions for the child to gain greater social acceptance. Participation in clubs, sports, and camps for children with special health needs are beneficial.

School-age children should participate as fully as possible in their own care at home and school, be responsible for health care decisions that will affect their treatment, and be allowed appropriate control over diet, medications, and treatment regimens. This will allow them a greater sense of control and mastery.[24,34]

The Adolescent

Developmental tasks to be achieved by adolescents include the following:

- Develop formal operational thought.
- Achieve identity versus role confusion.
- Develop deductive reasoning.
- Apply knowledge to solve problems.
- Evaluate one's own thinking.
- Have sense of confidence in one's personality.
- Make career choices.
- Develop social maturity and comfort with the same and opposite sex.
- Become comfortable with one's body.
- Establish beliefs and values.
- Establish greater independence from parents.

During the developmental period of adolescence, teenagers are absorbed and preoccupied with establishing independence, becoming comfortable with their own body, establishing a sexual identity, and building new and meaningful relationships.[24] An additional developmental task is developing formal operational thought. The complex period of adolescence is compounded by a serious chronic condition, which may add doubts about the ability to obtain a job, complete school, have sexual relationships, and have normal relationships with peers. The foremost task of adolescence, developing independence from the family, may become a significant obstacle because of the dependency and need for help from others.[24]

The primary goals of intervention are to encourage adolescents to discover their identity and separate from their parents while undergoing major physiologic, psychological, and social changes and stresses associated with a chronic illness. Because adolescents tend to live intensely in the present and are greatly influenced by peer pressure, they may experience feelings of heightened difference from their peers.[24] Adolescents with more visible physical defects may experience sadness, grief, and anger.[34] Because of a chronic illness, they may have reduced opportunities to be involved with their peer group or may withdraw because of fear of social rejection. Hence, the adolescent may have limited access to peers with whom to discuss sexual questions or concerns.

The nurse provides anticipatory guidance regarding adolescents' relationships. Adolescents may demonstrate anger, rebellion or bitterness about their condition to family members. While family members strive to nurture and protect an adolescent who has a decreased need for such dependency on well-intentioned family members, adolescents may become hostile.[24] Sensitivity to adolescents' individual needs, strengths, and competencies can help the adolescent experience success with peers, parents, and others.

Identifying feelings of anger as being normal,[34] the nurse intervenes if anger becomes maladaptive and interferes with daily functioning or compliance with medications and treatments. In addition families can identify areas in an adolescent's life in which they can experience independence.[24,34] The nurse also plays a pivotal role in encouraging family members to respect an adolescent's needs for privacy.[34] Above all else, adolescents need privacy, information about their illness and procedures, truth, respect, and dignity in their life.[34]

A primary goal for the adolescent is to develop skills for self-care.[24] The nurse helps parents understand the adolescent's needs as a sexual being, encourages adolescents to participate in activities and discuss feelings, and provides factual information about birth control.[34] In addition nurses encourage adolescents to confront opinions, values, beliefs, and philosophies that differ from their own[34]; serve as an advocate within the school system; and inject a realistic sense of hope for the future.[24,34]

Evaluation

Systematic, objective, and ongoing evaluations on the progress of children and families are essential. The nurse initially observes the adolescent to determine if physical pain and suffering are reduced. In addition the nurse observes if the child worries less and has decreased fears and uncertainty about the chronic illness. The nurse evaluates the child's increased knowledge about the illness, medications, treatments, and necessary care procedures. The nurse discovers from a variety of sources whether the child has become more independent in his or her functioning regarding activities of daily living; has become more active and mobile; has mastered developmental tasks at the proper time; is achieving in school and attending regularly; has positive relationships with parents, siblings, family members, peers, and friends; and has a healthy positive self-esteem. The child is observed directly to determine the presence of behavioral problems, appropriate responses to discipline and limit setting, and compliance with medical and health promotion behaviors. Principally, the nurse gathers observational data to determine that the child with a chronic illness is living a quality life and is making positive adjustments and realistic, healthy adaptations to any problems imposed by the illness.

Is the family experiencing less suffering and decreased overall burdens? How much time are family members committing to the ill child? The nurse is concerned about the extent of worries and fears about the illness, its course, and future outcomes. The nurse focuses on the extent of disruption of family routines, daily functioning of the family, and changes in roles and relationships. The nurse also assesses the extent of family support available for each member, whether members are experiencing social isolation, and the degree to which family members are adapting to various changes and using internal and external resources. The nurse also evaluates if problem-solving skills, decision-making skills, and family goals are appropriate and realistic in light of the child's condition.

Nurses analyze the family members' communication, roles, and relationships and whether the family has achieved an overall successful equilibrium while meeting the needs of a sick member. The nurse also judges the quality of the relationship between the parents and whether they are experiencing any or less depression, stress, strain, or difficulty in their marriage. The nurse analyzes the amount of caregiving by the mother and father as well as time and responsibilities invested by the child's grandparents. In addition the nurse observes for any concerns the parents express about siblings and the type and extent of sibling problems as well as successes. The nurse evaluates how well the parents have engaged in problem solving and the future goals for the well siblings in the family.

Summary

Children with chronic illnesses and their families are confronted with a variety of complex problems, concerns, and issues. Nurses are in a strategic position to meet the vast and multidimensional needs of this at risk population. Because of their expanding roles, nurses are assuming increased responsibilities in assessment, prevention, health promotion, and case management of common problems associated with chronic illnesses.

By using a family-centered care approach to children and their needs, nurses plan, implement, and evaluate interventions that are developmentally focused. Such interventions, based on a sound, normalizing framework of growth and development, can assist children and families to cope in more positive, optimal ways to the challenges of chronic illness.

Nurses are increasingly sensitive to the effects of chronic illness on all family members, especially to the needs of fathers, siblings, and grandparents.

Chronic illness imposes additional stresses on chil-

Ideas for Nursing Research

The advances in medical technology have resulted in more preterm, low birthweight babies surviving chronic illnesses such as the newborn period, more children with serious illness living longer, and more children surviving cancer. These are positive changes in the success stories of medical care. The long-term impact is that children now have a chronic illness that must be managed by the family. In addition children who were once treated in hospitals and institutions are now cared for by families at home with and without assistance. Nurses have varied opportunities to explore these changes in relation to the care and expertise that are needed by families, children with chronic illness, and nurses involved in their care.

- Cost/benefit ratios of caring for children with chronic illness in the home
- Most effective preparation nurses can give parents and siblings for caring for a child on a respirator in the home
- Most effective instructional methodologies in teaching children and parents about diabetes, the long-term concerns with diabetes mellitus, management of the diet and insulin needs, and management of complications
- Methods nurses should use to monitor long-term progress with chronic illness, medication compliance, and potential complications

dren and family members, and nurses play increasingly vital roles throughout the child's lifetime in a variety of health care and home settings.

In accordance with the guidelines for health care professionals by Drotar et al.,[10] nurses provide care that is characterized by continuity of relationships with children and families, active participation by professional caregivers, mutual participation of the child and his or her family as case managers of the child's illness, advocacy, and an emphasis on coping and competence. In addition, nurses provide care that is based on a developmental framework and a commitment to family-centered quality care throughout a child's lifetime.

References

1. Avery, M. E., Tooley, W., Keller, J. B., et al. (1987). Is chronic lung disease in low birth weight infants preventable? A survey of eight centers. *Pediatrics, 79*(1), 26–30.
2. Barnes, C. M. (1985). Training nurses to care for chronically ill children. In N. Hobbs & J. M. Perrin (Eds.). *Issues in the care of children with chronic illness* (pp. 498–513). San Francisco: Jossey-Bass.
3. Boodman, S. G. (1987). Born dying: AIDS 2nd generation. *Washington Post,* Al, A8.
4. Cerreto, M. (1986). Developmental issues in chronic illness: Implications and applications. *Topics in Early Childhood Special Education, 5(4),* 23–25.

5. Colbert, A. P., & Schock, N. C. (1985). Respirator use in progressive neuromuscular diseases. *Archives of Physical Medicine and Rehabilitation, 66,* 760–762.

6. Cook, C. L., & Forsman, I. (1986). Looking to the future. In *Monograph: A collection of papers of contemporary leadership in state maternal child health/crippled children program.* Region IV MCH project 969. Lexington, KY: University of Kentucky, pp 140–147.

7. Cummings, S. T. (1976). The impact of the child deficiency on the father: A study of fathers of mentally retarded and chronically ill children. *American Journal of Orthopsychiatry, 46,* 246–255.

8. Curran, J. W., Morgan, W. M., Hardy, A. M., et al. (1985). The epidemiology of AIDS: Current status and future prospects. *Science, 229,* 1352–1357.

9. Drotar, D., Baskiewicz, A., Irvin, N., Kennell, J., & Klaus, M. (1975). The adaptation of parents to the birth of an infant with a congenital malformation: A hypothetical model. *Pediatrics, 56,* 710–717.

10. Drotar, D., Crawford, P., & Ganofsky, M. A. (1984). Prevention with chronically ill children. In: M. C. Roberts & L. Peterson (Eds.). *Prevention of problems in childhood.* (pp. 232–265). New York: John Wiley & Sons.

11. Gallagher, J. J. (1981). Parental adaptation to a young handicapped child: The father's role. *Journal of Diseases of Early Childhood, 3,* 3–4.

12. Gittler, J. (1988). *Community-based systems of comprehensive services for children with special health care needs and their families.* National Maternal Child Health Resource Center, U.S. Department of Health and Human Services, Public Health Service, HRSA, BHCDA, Division of Maternal and Child Health, pp 1–17.

13. Gordon, M. (1982). Historical perspective: The national group for classification of nursing diagnoses. In M. J. Kim & D. A. Moritz (Eds.). *Classification of nursing diagnoses* (p. 3). New York: McGraw-Hill.

14. Gortmaker, S. L., & Sappenfield, W. (1984). Chronic childhood disorders: Prevalence and impact. *Pediatric Clinics of North America, 31,* 3–18.

15. Holaday, B. (1982). Maternal conceptual set development: Identifying patterns of maternal response to chronically ill infant crying. *Maternal-Child Nursing, 11,* 47–59.

16. Hymovich, D. P. (1985). Nursing services. In N. Hobbs & J. M. Perrin (Eds.). *Issues in the care of children with chronic illness* (pp. 478–497). San Francisco: Jossey-Bass.

17. Kaufman, J. (1988). Executive director for coordinating center for home and community care. Baltimore, MD. Personal Communication.

18. Kaplan, D. M., & Mason, E. A. (1960). Maternal reactions to premature birth viewed as an acute emotional disorder. *American Journal of Orthopsychiatry, 30,* 539–552.

19. Koop C. E. (1987). *Surgeon General's report: Children with special health care needs, campaign '87.* U.S. Department of Health and Human Services, Public Health Service, U.S. Government Printing Office, 184-020/65654, pp 1–40.

20. Leventhal, J. M. (1984). Psychosocial assessment of children with chronic physical disease. *Pediatric Clinics of North America, 31,* 71–86.

21. Levine, M. D. (1983). Chronic illness. In M. D. Levine, W. B. Carey, A. C. Crocker, & R. T. Gross (Eds.). *Developmental behavioral pediatrics* (p. 455). Philadelphia: W.B. Saunders.

22. MacQueen, J. C. (1987). The population of children currently served in programs emphasizing alternatives to hospital care. In *technology v. home care: A technical memorandum.* U.S. Congress, Office of Technology Assessment OTA-TM-H-38. Washington, D.C., U.S. Government Printing Office.

23. McKeever, P. T. (1981). Fathering the chronically ill child. *American Journal of Maternal Child Nursing, 6,* 124–128.

24. Magrab, P. R. (1985). Psychosocial development of chronically ill children. In N. Hobbs & J. M. Perrin (Eds.). *Issues in the care of children with chronic illness.* (pp. 698–716). San Francisco, CA: Jossey-Bass.

25. Miezo, P. (1983). *Parenting children with disabilties.* New York: Marcel Dekker, Inc.

26. Rose, M. H., & Thomas, R. B. (Eds.). (1987). *Children with chronic conditions: Nursing in a family and community context.* New York: Grune and Stratton.

27. Patterson, J. M., & McCubbin, H. I. (1983). Chronic illness: family stress and coping. In C. R. Figley & H. I. McCubbin (Eds.). *Stress and the family.* New York: Brunner/Mazel.

28. Perrin, J. M., Ireys, H. T., Hobbs, N., et al. (1985). Introduction. In N. Hobbs & J. M. Perrin (Eds.). *Issues in the care of children with chronic illnesses* (pp. 1–2, 913–921). San Francisco: Jossey-Bass.

29. Piaget, J. (1950). *The Psychology of intelligence.* London: Routlege and Kegan Paul, Ltd.

29a. Pless, I. B., & Pinkerton, P. (1975). *Chronic childhood disorder: promoting patterns of adjustment.* Chicago: Yearbook Medical Publishers.

30. Public Law 94-142, 94th Congress. (1975). *United States Statutes at Large Containing Public Laws 91–696, 93–650, 93–651, and the Laws and Concurrent Resolutions Enacted During the First Session of the Ninety-fourth Congress of the United States of America,* (Vol. 89). Washington, D.C.: United States Government Printing Office.

31. Simeon, M. (1984). Siblings of the chronically ill or disabled child. *Nursing Clinics of North America, 19,* 302–304.

32. U.S. Congress, Office of Technology Assessment. (1987). *Technology-dependent children: Hospital vs. home care—a technical memorandum.* (OTA–TM–H–38). Washington: D.C.: U.S. Govt. Printing Office.

33. Waechter, E. H., Phillips, J., & Holiday, B. (1985). *Nursing care of children.* Philadelphia: J.B. Lippincott.

34. Yoos, L. (1987). Chronic childhood illness: Developmental issues. *Pediatric Nursing, 13*(1), 25–28.

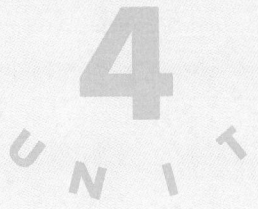

UNIT 4

Health Care Delivery Systems for the Family

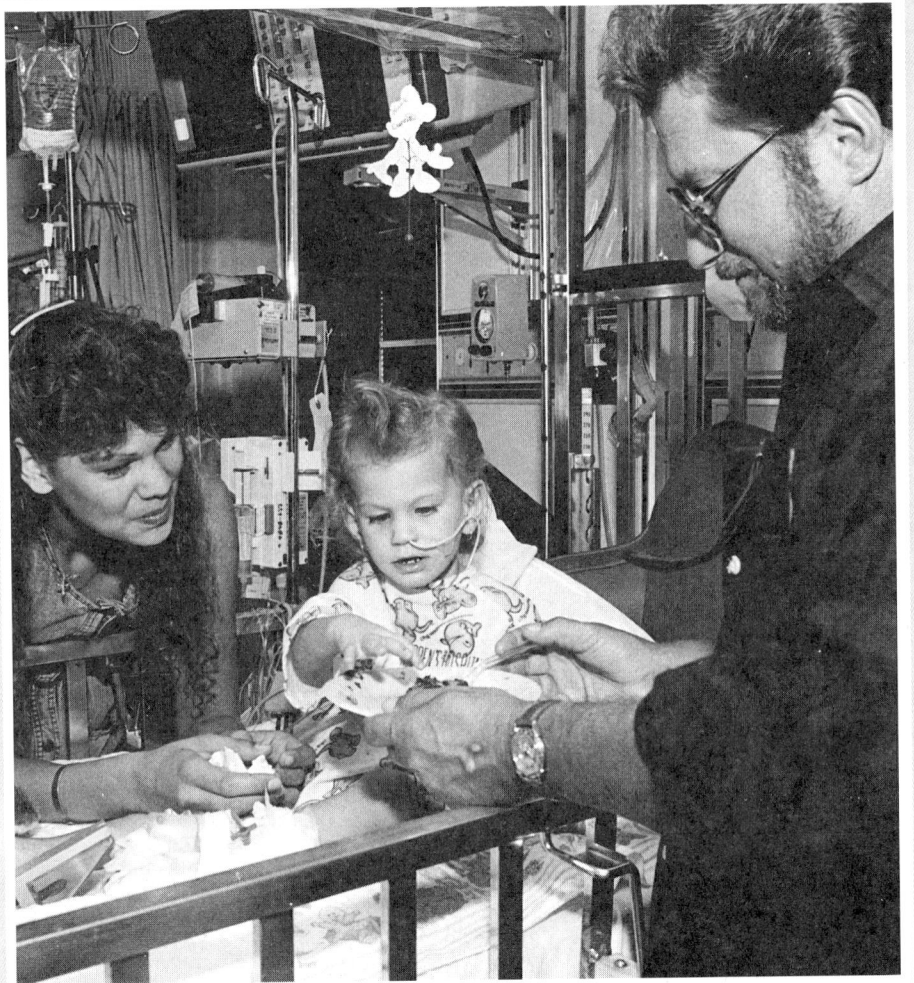

22

Ambulatory Care
for Children

BEHAVIORAL OBJECTIVES

Describe what is meant by the term *ambulatory care*, potential settings for its delivery, and the population it serves.

Discuss the evolution of ambulatory care in the United States.

Contrast the three levels of prevention in health care.

Differentiate primary care from ambulatory care.

Describe the activities included in the domain of ambulatory nursing practice.

Describe the role of the pediatric nurse practitioner in ambulatory care.

Discuss the range of nursing interventions provided in ambulatory care.

The cost of health care has spiraled out of control. To contain health care costs, the care of patients has shifted in recent years from hospitals to alternative settings whenever feasible. The numbers of children who receive health care in ambulatory settings has increased. Growth in the variety of settings where ambulatory care is available for children has been matched by the expansion of potential roles for nurses. Nurses need to become more knowledgeable about current trends and issues related to ambulatory care of children and to capture the opportunities available to clarify nursing's areas of expertise.

Ambulatory Care Described

Ambulatory care is different from inpatient care (Table 22-1). However, describing ambulatory care is difficult because standard terminology has not been adopted. Ambulatory care has been defined as care delivered within a health care facility to patients who do not stay overnight.[21] For a pediatric population, however, this definition excludes children who may receive care outside of health facilities. Some infants, for example, may be followed by health care providers at home. Likewise, professional health care may be provided for children in schools, but a school would not be called a "health care facility."

Another definition of ambulatory care suggests that the type of patients seen in these settings are vertical or upright, as opposed to horizontal or bedridden.[12] If

511

TABLE 22-1
Differences Between Inpatient and Ambulatory Care Nursing

Element	Inpatient Settings	Ambulatory Care Settings
Episode of care	Hospital admission	Visit or phone encounter
Treatment period	Continuous	Episodic
	Well-defined boundaries (admission and discharge)	Unclear boundaries
Requirement for nursing	Universal and continuous	Unclear and variable
Workload capacity	Limited to bed capacity	Theoretically limited but easily bypassed by walk-ins
Control of timing	By provider	By patient
Organizational position of nursing	Separate department	May not be separate organizationally
Major service	Nurse managed	May not be nurse managed

Hastings, C. E. (1987). Classification issues in ambulatory care nursing. *Journal of Ambulatory Care Management, 10,* 50–64.

taken literally, this definition would exclude all infants because they are developmentally unable to be "vertical." Other essentially healthy children who are unable to walk or sit because of permanent disabilities would also be excluded.

With sensitivity to the difficulties inherent in these descriptions, another definition has been proposed: "An ambulatory patient is an individual seeking personal health services who is not currently admitted to any health care institution. . . ."[39] This definition is comprehensive enough to include the diversity of children who are provided health services in a wide variety of care settings, and it is used as the focus of this chapter.

Nurses who work in ambulatory settings potentially provide care not only for individual children but also for families and communities. The community focus for nurses can take such forms as health education, screening, or planning in neighborhoods, towns, or cities. Ambulatory care nurses with a community focus using good data collection and thorough assessment skills can also be instrumental in influencing public policy on many levels.

Levels of Prevention

The spectrum of health care provided for ambulatory patients is generally health oriented and includes all three levels of prevention: primary, secondary, and tertiary. *Primary prevention* has two components: health promotion and disease prevention. Health promotion is often accomplished through education of parents and children and through counseling in such areas as exercise, hygiene, diet, and lifestyle.[49] Disease prevention refers to those activities that help to avoid the occurrence or spread of illness. Fluoridation for dental health protection and im-

munization programs are examples of disease prevention programs. The goal of primary prevention is to remove or decrease risk factors that impinge on a child's, family's, or community's health.

Secondary prevention involves screening and education to identify people with disease at the earliest possible stage.[45] Screenings for impaired vision or hearing, hypertension, scoliosis, scabies, or lice are examples of the diversity of care provided at the secondary prevention level. Although immediate care may be provided for these children in ambulatory care settings, they may be sent to an acute care setting for comprehensive treatment of the disease or disability.

Tertiary prevention is performed "when a defect or disability is fixed, stabilized or irreversible."[49] This care helps the person obtain an optimal level of functioning within the constraints of the disability. When acute care is no longer necessary or beneficial, some children receive tertiary care in ambulatory care settings.

For many families, ambulatory care is their initial (and sometimes only) contact with the health care system. Ambulatory care encourages children and families to maintain high levels of wellness and to prevent illness or injury. For ill people, ambulatory care centers may serve as a site for immediate care or for referral to other types or sites of care. During recuperation, ambulatory care providers can monitor follow-up needs.

Ambulatory Care in the Health Care System

The explosive growth of ambulatory care services provides a wide range of options to clients entering the health care system. The origin of ambulatory care nursing, however, is not recent. Examining the historic development of ambulatory care helps nurses see the forces that continue to shape nursing's role in the health care of children.

History

In Colonial times, the rapid growth of new American cities and the compression of population in limited spaces spawned a variety of illnesses and health problems. Wealthy families could afford medical care, which was provided in patient homes or private offices. Free-standing clinics for the poor were established in 1780 in Philadelphia, and this inaugurated modern ambulatory care in the United States. Throughout the 1800s, however, health care for the poor was a growing public concern.

During the 1890s, private philanthropies in New York supplied "milk stations" for poor mothers who were unable to breast-feed their infants. Before this time, infants often became ill because the milk available was unpasteurized, unclean, and unrefrigerated. This service expanded to include general infant care and formed the beginnings of the Department of Public Health. The goal of this public health movement was to "prevent disease secondary to the unsanitary environment and to limit the spread of communicable disease."[46] Nurses were at the forefront in providing new services for children.

As attendance in public schools became the norm, large numbers of children were forced into close contact with each other. At the turn of the century, school medical officers were appointed in some of the larger school systems to help quell the transmission of communicable diseases. "Medical inspection" to check for contagion was the initial task assigned to the officers, but nurses soon were employed full time, not only to assist with prevention of communicable diseases, but also to investigate other health conditions that would impede children's education.

Between 1900 and 1920, public health departments and voluntary health agencies became firmly established. Their primary goal was to establish some clinics for well babies and others for children with specific diseases. Milk was still supplied for infants, but education on illness prevention was also disseminated.[10] In 1921, the Sheppard-Towner Act was passed, and the federal government assumed responsibility for improving maternal–child health.[3] The monies granted by this act allowed states to establish services to decrease infant and maternal mortality.[35]

During the 1920s, federal involvement in child health care was such a radical idea that Congress repealed the Sheppard-Towner Act in 1929.[3] Unfortunately, this cutback was poorly timed; the economic problems of the early 1930s created hardships for many children and their families. In 1935, however, the federal government stepped in again, this time with the Social Security Act, including Aid for Dependent Children. This new act helped states provide ambulatory services such as well-baby clinics, immunizations, and school health care.[3]

In the following years, hospitals and private medical practices proliferated. In the socially conscious 1960s, neighborhood health centers were set up by the U.S. Office of Economic Opportunity to provide health care to the urban poor. In 1965, programs to prepare community health nurses for the new pediatric nurse practitioner role were begun.[15] The introduction of these nurses into the health care system encouraged the expansion of health services to greater numbers of children.

Another milestone in 1965 was the implementation of Medicaid (Medical Assistance or MA), which provided health care funding for poor families. Although MA ensured better access to health care for the poor, several problems arose due to its scope. The MA program became so expansive that many older, well-established health programs and agencies were eliminated. In addition, MA payment policies caused a dramatic increase in the federal government's health care bill.[46] Consequently, legislators began to explore ways to curb spiraling health care costs.

Following the lead of private insurance companies, the government sought a way to pay a single fixed annual rate for each MA client served.[14] The Health Maintenance Act of 1973 provided federal grants to investigate the development and feasibility of a prepaid system.[46] Slowly, health maintenance organizations (HMOs) emerged, but not for the poor. Instead, HMOs were embraced as a means of providing health care and insurance coverage to working families. This type of "prospective payment" system has become a driving force in today's health care climate. It was not until the early 1980s, however, that the original intent, to provide prepaid fixed cost health care for those eligible for Medical Assistance, was reached.

The rapidly rising costs of health care also stimulated the development of a new kind of center, the ambulatory care center (ACC), sometimes called urgent care center. Originally called "free-standing emergency centers," the name was soon changed to avoid regulations related to emergency care. These centers were designed to handle urgent problems that could be treated more inexpensively than in a hospital emergency department. Although minor surgery may be performed in some ACCs, they should not be confused with surgicenters, in which outpatient surgery is provided almost exclusively.

This historic perspective has revealed that ambulatory care in the United States began in the last century as a social response to health problems.[47] However, the economics of health care has been the impetus in the recent proliferation of new ambulatory care services. The availability of multiple types of settings for ambulatory care means that populations of children whose health needs were previously unmet may be provided.

Settings for Practice

Well-child care is necessary to ensure that children reach their full potential during the years of rapid growth and development. The American Academy of Pediatrics has developed a preventive care schedule of regular periodic visits to provide immunizations and screening tests for the developing child. These regular visits and the treatment of minor acute problems constitute a well-child practice. In 1989, approximately 29% of the visits made to pediatric offices involved health assessment or health maintenance activities; the remainder were made because of acute illness, primarily of the upper respiratory tract or ears.[41] Children with chronic illnesses are also seen in these settings.

The type of care just described is known as *primary health care*. The American Nurses' Association defines primary health care as "care the client receives within the health care system at the first point of contact to resolve a presenting problem. It is continuous and comprehensive care and includes all services necessary for the promotion of health, the prevention of disease, and the early detection and treatment of illness."[2]

Whereas primary care is often administered in ambulatory care settings, not all ambulatory care is primary care. Verran[52] observed that "primary care is the newest responsibility to be added to the domain of ambulatory care nursing and includes those activities usually thought of as part of the extended nursing role." Children may receive primary care in a variety of settings, all of which have a common goal: to maximize the well-being of children (Fig. 22-1). The source of payment is a major difference.

Public Health Clinics

Public health clinics often attract families from lower socioeconomic strata. Historically clinics have been designed for the poor, and many clinics still orient themselves to poorer clientele.[46] Organizations such as county

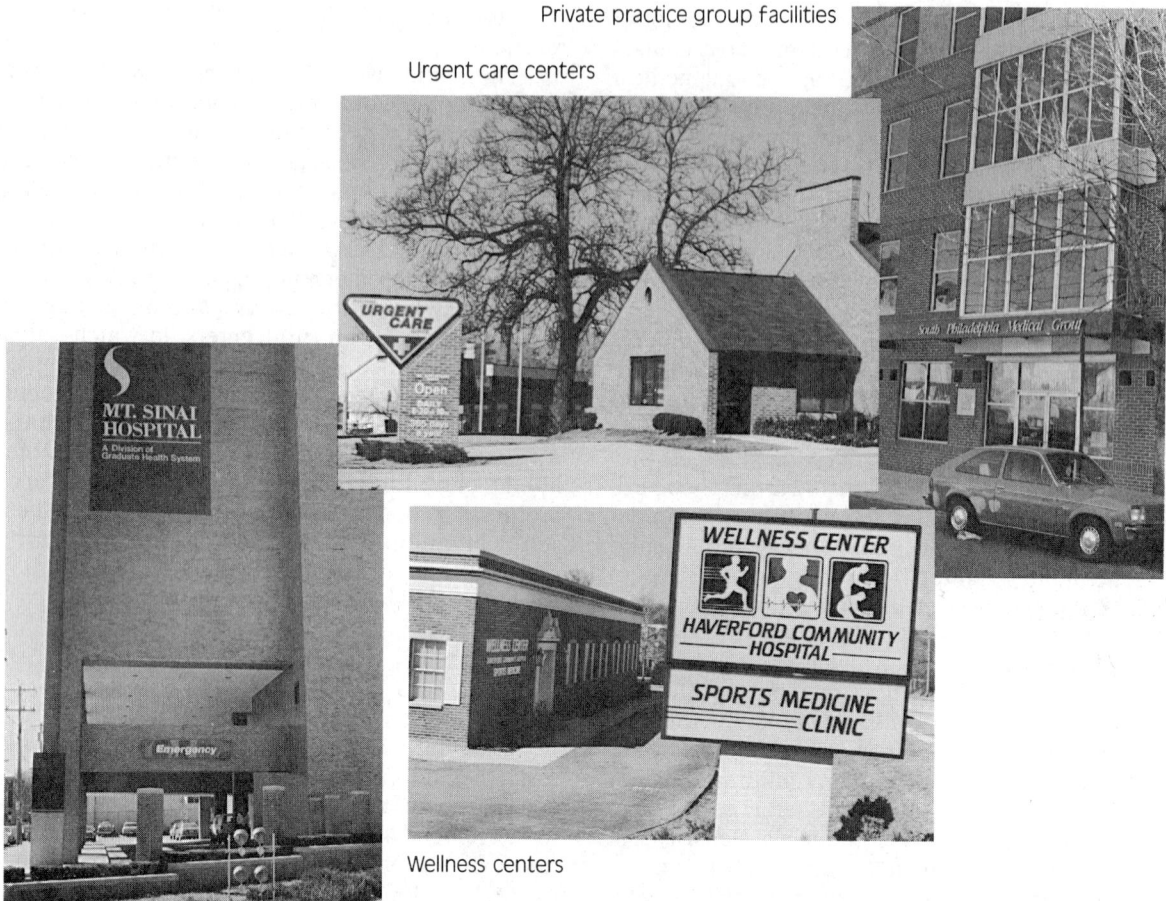

Private practice group facilities

Urgent care centers

Wellness centers

Multi-facility health-care systems

FIGURE 22-1

The number and variety of health care settings have increased dramatically. (Photo by Tracy Baldwin.)

health departments or visiting nurse associations may offer clinics to provide all children in their jurisdiction with essential health care services. Some supply only well-child care such as immunizations and screening, and refer to other providers for acute care. Families may receive free care, pay for care on a sliding scale, or receive Medical Assistance.

Health Maintenance Organizations (HMOs)

HMOs are prospective payment systems. Consumers pay only a set monthly fee and receive all of the health services they require to meet their needs. The philosophy of HMOs is that preventive care avoids expensive illnesses later in life. Their goal is to reduce long-term health care costs. In HMOs, a family commits to a specific provider or group of providers for all of their health care needs. The providers charge a fixed yearly fee, called a capitation fee, for services including primary care and the coordination of any specialist or emergency services that may be needed.

The HMO provider has a financial incentive to keep the child and family healthy because payment for *any* extra services (hospitalization or referrals, for example) comes from the capitation fee. Providing care for less than the capitation fee allows the practice to generate

profits. Because hospital care is far more expensive than ambulatory care, HMO's have been a primary impetus in the expansion of ambulatory services.

The concept of the HMO was originally developed as a means of stabilizing the government's cost of providing health care to Medicaid-eligible families.[14] Unfortunately, HMO care has often been unavailable to the poor and unemployed. Only a small fraction of Medical Assistance recipients use a prepaid insurance program. In addition to being unable to pay capitation fees, MA families have not joined HMOs for the following reasons:

Recipients of state Medicaid programs lack understanding of HMOs; Medicaid HMO reimbursement rates are low; considerable paperwork is required; bureaucratic controls are excessive; marketing of HMOs to Medicaid recipients is limited; and patient turnover rates are high due to changing eligibility for Medicaid.[16 (p.30)]

In some cities, HMOs for the economically needy exist with the "premiums" paid by Medical Assistance. The benefits include increased continuity of care and decreased costs for the taxpayer.

Private Practices

Physicians or groups of physicians and/or pediatric nurse practitioners own and operate private practices.

Families usually pay for this care out of pocket, occasionally on a sliding scale. Insurance companies rarely cover preventive care. If an ill child is seen in a private practice, the insurance company may pay for the "sick visit" and diagnostic laboratory services, depending on the family's health insurance coverage.

A small number of private practices accept patients who have Medical Assistance as their sole means of health insurance coverage. In most states, the Medical Assistance reimbursement to the practice from the government is so low that the practice loses money. A desire to ensure that all children receive adequate health care, rather than financial remuneration, is the motive for physicians in private practice to provide care to families on MA.

Large HMO corporations also enlist private practices to provide care. The practices receive a capitation fee, and the patients pay a small deductible or copayment (often in the range of $2 to $5) at each regular office visit. Using private practices makes it easier for families to find a practice conveniently located and congruent with their own philosophy on health care.

Hospital Emergency Departments

Today's hospitals offer a variety of pediatric ambulatory services. This diversity of services is often combined under the term "outpatient services." The primary goal of the emergency department is to provide 24-hour, urgent care. Unfortunately, many families have either no primary health care provider or find themselves unable to wait hours or days other settings may require for treatment of problems. These families turn to the emergency department for care.

Treating nonurgent problems in the emergency department is a misuse of services. As a solution, many hospitals have set up "walk-in clinics." Children with nonurgent problems are triaged to an area with facilities and staff more suitable for their situation. This arrangement frees emergency department personnel to handle true emergencies and allows the hospital to provide care at a lower cost than in the emergency department.

There are disadvantages to receiving care through a hospital walk-in clinic. The child and family still are subject to long waits, and continuity of health care is lacking. Each time the child has a problem, a different physician or nurse sees the child. In addition, the care is episodic in nature with important primary care needs often unmet.[56]

Hospital Outpatient Clinics

Outpatient clinics are another type of ambulatory care service. These are different from "walk-in clinics" because a child has an assigned appointment and often may see the same provider or group of providers for each visit. In many children's hospitals or large pediatric services, residents and teaching staff establish and operate outpatient clinics to provide primary care to medically needy populations. Although at times the wait may be long and the visit brief, the child receives more consistent care than in the "walk-in clinic." Monitoring of concerns such as adequate immunization status is more likely.

A child may also be referred to a specialty clinic such as orthopedics or neurology. The referral is for a specific pediatric problem requiring special expertise. Often the child has a chronic illness and needs more comprehensive care than can be obtained closer to home. At times, the family travels long distances to bring their child to the specialty team for care.

Hospital Short Stay Units

The number of short stay or day surgery units has grown rapidly since the 1960s. A shortage of beds for children forced hospitals to find better ways to accommodate children with simple surgical needs.[31] Formerly, some types of diagnostic procedures or surgery required one or more days of hospitalization. It is more financially advantageous and still medically sound to conduct these procedures on a "day surgery" or "short procedure" unit.

Instead of hospitalizing the child for 1 to 2 days, laboratory work, histories, physical examinations, and preparatory teaching are all done in one or two outpatient visits. At some hospitals, the children are allowed to manipulate equipment that they might see on the day of their surgery.[28] This activity helps nurses to identify fears before the procedure. Parents are encouraged to be active participants in the emotional support of their child throughout the entire visit.

On the day of the surgery, the child is admitted to the hospital through the day surgery unit. Generally, the child recovers in this unit (often with the parent available as soon as the child is stable) and is discharged to home before the day is over. Outpatient surgery nurses have an important role in maintaining telephone follow-up of these patients within 24 hours to answer questions and to help resolve problems.[28]

The benefits of day surgery units are less hospitalization time for the child and, therefore, less financial cost to the insurance company and family. More important to the child and family is that the psychological impact of hospitalization may be diminished.[31] The only disadvantage may be the short amount of time available for family preparation and teaching. As more day surgery units are being built, nurses have an important role in suggesting structural designs that facilitate more family involvement in the care of the child.[28]

Ambulatory Care Centers (ACC)

Although the first ACCs were established in the early 1970s, the concept was not well-known even in 1980.[55] Yet, today some 4500 facilities are thought to exist.[24] One of the reasons for the proliferation of these centers is convenience. A typical location of an ACC might be a shopping center, open 12 to 14 hours a day, 7 days a week; no appointment is necessary. Children and other family members may receive health care quickly and at a reasonable cost.

ACCs have disadvantages that should be noted. For example, the back-up services commonly available in a hospital are rarely located on site in an ACC. Therefore, if a child needs major surgery or intensive care, stabilization in the ACC is followed by rapid transfer to a hospital. Another problem results when families use the ACC only for urgent, episodic care. This type of use decreases opportunities for the development of a relationship with a primary care provider and increases the likelihood that health care is fragmented.

Strategies to improve continuity and comprehensiveness of care in ACCs have been suggested.[24] For example, nurse practitioners may be employed to provide family-centered care and follow-up independently, whereas the physician provides emergency care and consultation for the nurse practitioner. This arrangement emphasizes the complementarity of the physician and nurse practitioner roles and ultimately benefits children and families who receive health care in the ACC.

Schools and Camps

Schools and camps supply an ideal location for ambulatory care because of the large numbers of children congregated in one area. On the most basic level, first aid for injuries and care for minor acute problems can be provided. Triage to hospitals or other health professionals is available for more serious problems. In the ideal setting, however, more than just first aid and emergency care is available.

For some children, due to family circumstances or economics, contact with nurses and other health providers at school or camp may be the only form of health care they receive. To aid all children optimally, it is ideal that nurses in schools and camps be prepared to provide nursing care at all three levels of prevention: primary, secondary, and tertiary.

The scope of nursing practice and the population served in schools and camps depend on factors such as the nurse's education and experience, the numbers of children in a nurse's caseload, state mandates, and an understanding of the nurse's role by agency administrators. Increasing numbers of school nurses are certified as school nurse practitioners, and this credential enables them to provide a broader range of health care than is possible otherwise.

In schools and camps, primary prevention can occur through health promotion, maintenance, and education activities. For example, the nurse may coordinate a program to teach children about fire or water safety. Health teaching may occur in groups, but individualized instruction may also be given when a child comes in for illness care or counseling. Personal attention helps the child become a responsible health consumer.

Secondary prevention in the form of screening to diagnose disease and provide treatment at the earliest possible state is also provided in schools and some camps.[59] The scope of secondary prevention can range from blood pressure screening to rule out hypertension to assessing those at risk for teenage pregnancy or substance abuse. Some states mandate that nurses in schools also screen children for impairments such as hearing and vision.

Handicapped or chronically ill children may receive tertiary prevention through schools and camps. In 1975, the Education for All Handicapped Children Act was enacted, mandating that children who are mentally retarded, hard of hearing, speech impaired, visually handicapped, seriously emotionally disturbed, or who have specific learning disabilities, certain orthopedic problems, or other health impairments may not be segregated from their classmates. Today, these children are educated with their peers (or "mainstreamed") to the maximum extent possible.

Because these children have been mainstreamed into public schools, there is an increased need of health services for them. The goal is to maintain or improve their level of functioning. The school must provide someone to perform health services such as administration of medications or procedures, to teach the teachers and staff about the specific illness or disability, to provide emergency care (e.g., insulin reactions, seizures), and to provide counseling to the child, family, and staff about the child's disability.

Many regular camps do not accept children with chronic diseases because of the additional nursing care required, yet these children are often capable of participating in many of the same types of camping activities that other children enjoy. In response to this need, special camps for children are offered to "foster independence and emphasize what the children can do rather than what they can not do."[51 (p.30)] Other goals of a chronic illness camp are to promote positive peer relationships and to enhance the ill child's self-image. Clearly, the role of the nurse in such settings is broad, and many opportunities exist to provide holistic health care.

Homes

Ambulatory care can also include the assessment of young children and families in their home. In contrast to the technical or hospice services generally required of a family with an ill child, these families require mainly teaching and support for brief periods. For example, many families leave the hospital as soon as 24 hours after childbirth, and a home visit by a nurse follows soon afterwards.

In the home setting, nurses can answer the family's questions about issues such as newborn care, breast-feeding, or sleep patterns. Maternal and infant assessment also may be performed. Finally, some forms of medical intervention, such as phototherapy for elevated levels of bilirubin, may be managed at home if an ambulatory care nurse is available to assist the family. (Home care for ill children is discussed in Chapter 24.)

Nursing Implications

What is the scope of roles and responsibilities for today's ambulatory nurse? The trend toward more care being offered in ambulatory settings necessitates nurses becoming more independent and highly skilled beyond the requirement of traditional roles. Being a "traffic director, manager of appointments, and technical assistant to the physician" is no longer adequate.[21, p.142] Nine areas of nursing responsibility in ambulatory nursing have been identified:

- Health status assessment
- Planning (e.g., nursing diagnosis, problem lists, and care planning)
- Patient counseling and support including advocacy
- Patient education
- Therapeutic care—direct physical care or specific

nursing procedures such as medications and respiratory treatments

- Communication—referrals, coordinating and imparting information to family members and other health professionals
- Documentation
- Normative care such as directing, chaperoning, or transporting
- Non-client centered care (e.g., continuing education, student training, administrative duties).

Although additional study is needed to determine which responsibilities could be delegated to others, these nine areas of provide a preliminary taxonomy of ambulatory clinic nursing activities.

How nurses carry out the responsibilities required in ambulatory care depends on their education, experience, and the scope of practice permitted under their state practice act. Certification in ambulatory care nursing may be obtained to recognize a specialized knowledge base and practice. Graduate education for clinical specialists or pediatric nurse practitioners (PNPs) is also possible. These nurses practice with a greater degree of autonomy than others with less preparation.

Nursing Assessment

Collecting a nursing history and patient assessment are integral parts of ambulatory nursing. The amount and depth of information collected depend on the setting and the urgency of the situation. A nurse in private practice might ask basic questions about the reason for the visit and areas of concern before taking vital signs, recording anthropomorphic measurements, and assessing parental child care abilities. All of this would be done in preparation for a more in-depth history and physical examination by a PNP or physician. In other settings, the nurse may be responsible for assembling a comprehensive database including a review of functional health patterns and a head-to-toe physical examination. Further investigation is needed to clarify the ambulatory nurse's role in assessment and to develop strategies to improve the effectiveness and efficiency of nursing assessment methods.

Specific screening tests may also be part of the nurse's assessment of children in the ambulatory setting. Screening is so important that, in 1967, as an adjunct to Medicaid, the Early and Periodic Screening for Diagnoses and Treatment (EPSDT) program was federally funded to provide screening services to Medicaid-eligible children and reimbursement to providers. Areas assessed include past medical history; family history; a complete physical examination; nutrition; laboratory tests such as lead screening, hematocrit, urinalysis; screening for dental, hearing, vision, and developmental problems; and immunization status. The program is available to all children less than 21 years of age eligible for Medical Assistance. All of these assessments are used to identify nursing problems and, ultimately, to plan care to address them.

Nursing Diagnoses

The use of nursing diagnosis has become widespread for nurses in inpatient settings. Although ambulatory nurses assess patients and develop plans of care, they may not be documenting their nursing diagnoses. Hastings explains that nursing diagnoses "have been primarily developed and studied in inpatient settings; there is not yet clear understanding of their applicability and adaptability to ambulatory care"[21, p.146] Others argue that use of nursing diagnoses may be even more important for the rapidly expanding area of ambulatory nursing. Nursing diagnoses provide a framework for the development of nursing standards in ambulatory nursing.[50]

Research has begun on generating clinically useful nursing diagnoses for application in pediatric ambulatory care settings.[7,37] The Omaha[38] system, for example, is used by many community health nurses for clients of all ages. The taxonomy of diagnoses developed by Burns,[6] however, is used only in the care of children and is presented in the accompanying display. Three domains of diagnoses are identified: developmental problems, diseases, and daily living problems. Although some object to a category of "disease" being included in a taxonomy of *nursing* diagnoses, it does encompass conditions that are frequently identified by nurses in expanded roles. Including this category ensures that important teaching opportunities are not missed.

Using Burns'[6] taxonomy, some examples of nursing diagnoses related to developmental problems and daily living problems are presented below. Brief descriptions of a potential situation with the child and family are included.

Language Delay—3-year-old male with a vocabulary of less than 50 words and no sentences due to a lack of verbal stimulation in the home.

Gross Motor Delay—10-month-old boy born at 28 weeks who is unable to sit without support.

High Risk for Infection—sibling of a 5-year-old just diagnosed with strep throat.

Health Perception: Adjustment Impaired—single mother of a newborn having difficulty adapting to parenthood.

Knowledge Deficit: Behavior Expectations—mother of 2-year-old who insists her child is "bad." Mother does not understand the need for independence and exploration in this age group.

Altered Nutrition: Less Than Body Requirements—adolescent mother diluting the formula of her infant due to lack of funds.

Impaired Verbal Communication—family of an adolescent who complains of "always fighting" with the child.

Planning

Involving the child and family in planning care is essential in ambulatory settings. Once children leave the clinical site, their health care needs are generally professionally unsupervised until the next visit. Children and parents must have adequate preparation to provide the care needed.

At what age can children begin self-care activities? A school-age child (approximately 6 to 11 years old) has attained Piaget's level of concrete operations. Because of this ability, Koster[33] believes that school-age children are

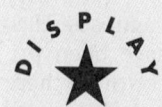

Integrated Classification of Diagnoses for Use by Pediatric Nurse Practitioners

I. Developmental problem diagnoses
  Cognitive development
    Cognitive delay
    Learning disability
    Other cognitive development problems
  Language development
    Language delay
    Speech delay
    Other language development problems
  Motor development
    Gross motor delays
    Fine motor delays
    Other motor development problems
  Social development
    Social development delay
II. Pediatric diseases
  Infectious and parasitic diseases
  Endocrine, nutritional, and metabolic diseases and immunity disorders
  Diseases of the blood and blood organs
  Diseases of the nervous system
  Diseases of the circulatory system
  Diseases of the respiratory system
  Diseases of the digestive system and dental disorders
  Diseases of the genitourinary system
  Diseases of the skin and subcutaneous tissue
  Diseases of the musculoskeletal system and connective tissue
  Congenital anomalies
  Conditions of the perinatal period
  Symptoms, signs, and ill-defined conditions
  Injury and poisoning
III. Daily living problems
  Health perception and health management
    Adjustment impaired
    Health maintenance alteration
    Home management impaired
    Home care resources inadequate
    Knowledge deficit (specify lifestyle area)
    Noncompliance
    Self-care deficit
  Nutrition and metabolism
    Anorexia
    Colic
    Nausea
    Nutrition alteration (specify)
    Other nutritional-metabolic pattern problem
  Elimination
    Encopresis
    Enuresis
    Other elimination pattern problem

Activity and exercise and sleep and rest
  Activity intolerance
  Diversional activity deficit
  Mobility impaired
  Sleep pattern alteration
  Other activity-exercise pattern or sleep-rest pattern problem
Cognition and perception
  Attention deficit disorder
  Neglect, unilateral
  Sensory-perceptual alteration
  Thought process alteration
  Other cognitive-perceptual pattern problem
Self-perception and self-concept
  Depression
  Self-concept disturbance
  Other self-perception/self-concept pattern problem
Role and relationships
  Abuse, child/adult
  Breast-feeding, asynchronous
  Communication impaired: verbal
  Coping, family
  Family process alteration
  Parenting alteration
  Social isolation
  Other role-relationship pattern problems
Sexuality
  Pregnancy
  Sexual dysfunction
  Sexual patterns, altered
  Other sexuality pattern problems
Coping and stress
  Anxiety
  Comfort alteration
  Coping, individual
  Fear
  Grieving
  Hopelessness
  Powerlessness
  Substance misuse
  Violence, potential for, self-directed or toward others
  Other coping-stress tolerance problems
Values and beliefs
  Spiritual distress
  Other value-belief pattern problems

Adapted from Burns, C. (1991). Development and content validity testing of a comprehensive classification of diagnoses for pediatric nurse practitioners. *Nursing Diagnosis, 2,* 93–104.

"cognitively capable for taking responsibility for their own health care." Yet, preparation for self-care should begin at an earlier age. For example, nurses can take the time to communicate with the child during the well-child visit. Health care providers often channel all of their questions to the parent or caretaker, speaking as though the child is invisible. As soon as children are able to communicate, they can respond to questions such as, "How are you feeling?" "Where does it hurt?" Significant concerns and health perceptions arise when a 3- or 4-year-old is asked, "Why do you think you are sick?" "What will make you feel better?" "What makes you grow?"

Given options, a child can make personal decisions about lifestyle choices. Not only does the child become an educated health consumer but self-reliance increases.[33] Behaviors developed in childhood set the patterns for a lifetime of habits.[22,23] Igoe[27] believes that children who have a more assertive role in their own health are not only better able to follow healthful habits, but also are better able to maintain their own daily health.

Aside from having the nurse, child, and family be collaborators in determining the goals of care, planning in ambulatory settings involves the same principles as in other settings. Documentation of plans for care is critical to ensure continuity and to measure progress, because care is often sporadic, and multiple care providers are involved.

Nursing Interventions

Self-care and health promotion activities are the major thrust of nursing interventions, but ambulatory nurses provide a variety of different interventions based on their setting and practice location. Counseling, education, therapeutic care, and communication with others are commonly required nursing interventions in the ambulatory setting.

Counseling

Counseling involves helping a family to explore alternative solutions to a problem and to make the final decision based on their own needs. Chow suggests health counseling involves a "mutual exchange of ideas and advice on how to achieve optimal physical/psychological and social well-being."[9 (p.523)] Criticism has been directed at staff in clinics for too often providing directive advice to patients as opposed to allowing them to make informed choices. Further research is needed to investigate this charge and to determine what type of counseling is appropriate for the ambulatory population.

Education

Education is a major component of health promotion and a fundamental nursing responsibility. Families with children receiving care in ambulatory settings require comprehensive teaching because they, not the nurse, are the primary caregivers. Teaching can involve pre- and postoperative instructions for day surgery, signs and symptoms of worsening conditions in the emergency department, health maintenance activities, and countless

other topics. Because children usually are not seriously ill when they visit the ambulatory care site, they and their families are better able to focus on health promotion and illness prevention topics.

Health promotion involves teaching lifestyle alterations that help to ensure optimal health, and includes such issues as safety, exercise, and nutrition. For example, an ambulatory nurse might instruct a child in good hand-washing techniques. The nurse may discuss the likely characteristics of a classmate with a upper respiratory infection to encourage disease avoidance. Another example of teaching about prevention of illness would be emphasizing to families the importance of maintaining current immunization records.

Nurses should recognize that their personal actions also influence children's future feelings about health care. For many children, ambulatory settings are their initial introduction to the health care system. Negative experiences can color children's views on health care for the rest of their lives. Considerations for a child's feelings and privacy, allowing the child decision-making opportunities whenever possible, and communicating fully about procedures can make health care encounters positive.

In ambulatory care, *anticipatory guidance* is an extremely important form of teaching. Parents are better able to cope with their children and can develop better parenting skills if they understand the range of normal behaviors expected for their child's next developmental phase. Anticipatory guidance helps parents to develop confidence in their parenting capabilities because they can confirm that their expectations for their child are typical for our society. For example, parents consider infants to be "good eaters" because they are experiencing a period of rapid growth. For many children, as they approach 1 year to 18 months, their growth decelerates and their new found mobility makes them interested in everything but food. Parents who are aware of this are less likely to make mealtimes a battleground. They learn to accept the fact that as long as the fluid and junk food intake is kept reasonable, toddlers will eat if hungry.

Another valuable teaching strategy for nurses is to *validate positive behaviors* observed in family interactions. This reinforcement can help increase parental self-confidence and nurse–family rapport. "Look at how that baby quiets down as soon as you pick him up—he really knows you." "I am glad to see that your infant is only wearing socks—expensive shoes are not necessary until he starts to walk well." "How nice to see you offering your baby 100% juice rather than fruit punch, because juice is more nutritious." Parental esteem and confidence are enhanced by such confirmation bestowed by a respected professional.

It is important for nurses not to deflate a parent's self-confidence by taking over when a behavior snag occurs. Instead, *modeling appropriate behavior* is a useful teaching method. "Watching your child in this room, I can understand your frustration at his behavior. Can I show you a 'time out' procedure that will be more effective in the long run than yelling?" "I know it seems silly to talk to a 15-month-old child, but look at how he mimics me when I point out interesting things in this window."

Family education is a vitally important component of

an ambulatory nurse's role, but sometimes it is difficult to find the necessary teaching time. Some clinics have such a large volume of children that individual teaching becomes a problem. Nurses need to be creative in finding the best way to impart information.

Offering new parents a 15- to 30-minute class on infant care in the waiting room not only helps to pass their waiting time, but may foster supportive relationships with other parents who have children at the same developmental level. If a nurse is not available to teach in person, showing carefully selected videos in the waiting room might be an alternative. Although not an ideal form of teaching, the video's usefulness can be enhanced by discussing it with the parents during the interview and exam.

Written materials are best used to reinforce previous teaching, not to provide an original presentation of information. However, nurses in high-volume clinics may be unable to provide other types of education. It is imperative that nurses select written materials that match the education and reading level of the parent. Ideally, ambulatory nurses make the time to review and highlight the handouts with children and their families to increase their effectiveness in teaching.

Therapeutic Care

Therapeutic measures include physical care, treatments, and monitoring that are often medically delegated. These tasks may be performed by the professional nurse or assigned by nurses to be performed by the support staff (such as respiratory or intravenous therapists).[21] Far fewer therapeutic activities are provided in an ambulatory setting than in the hospital arena. Those provided are usually on a one-time basis (e.g., emergency treatment in the emergency department) or on a periodic basis (e.g., weekly intravenous chemotherapy for oncology patients or immunizations for well children).

Prescriptive and protocol functions are limited by state practice acts. Some states require that nurses in advanced practice follow specific protocols or work in conjunction with a consulting physician. Each state's regulations are listed in an article by Labar.[34]

Communication With Others

One aspect of communication important for ambulatory nurses is *referrals*. After an assessment, a nurse may identify additional services that would benefit the family or child. For example, analysis of data may indicate that a family needs counseling in the form of intensive weekly care beyond the scope of the ambulatory care setting. Ambulatory nurses must be knowledgeable about available community resources and must know how to use the referral system efficiently.

Another aspect of communication is required in the ambulatory nurse's role as *case manager*. In the past, an episode of illness would be managed from beginning to end in an acute care setting. Today, attempts to provide efficient health care and contain costs have resulted in care that is often fragmented.[25] Ambulatory nurses are in excellent positions to help coordinate care and services.

Coordination of services through case management is "a strategic method used by nurses and underwritten by employers to manage complex, costly care and to as-

sure quality care for high-risk patients."[11 (p.55)] Case management is particularly beneficial for chronically ill children. For example, a child with cancer may receive weekly chemotherapy treatments, yet be well enough to attend school. The oncology clinic nurse, acting as case manager, may teach the school nurse how to manage emergencies related to the treatments and thereby facilitate the child's integration into normal school life. During the child's hospitalizations, the oncology clinic nurse could provide background information so that inpatient staff can provide better care. The outpatient nurse could also attend daily rounds and discharge planning sessions.

Case management is similar to the concept of primary nursing in that one nurse is accountable for a child's care. But a case manager is less responsible for direct care than for coordination of ongoing care, possibly over a period of months or years. Case management can not only improve the quality of care that a child receives, but it can also help contain costs.[58]

Another aspect of communication is required in *telephone contacts* with children or their families. One fifth of all family contacts with the health care system occur by telephone, and these calls may require over 11 minutes each.[30,44] Effective handling of the telephone call can help parents develop strategies and confidence in the care of their children, decrease unnecessary visits, and promote positive public relations. Mismanagement, however, can lead to improper care of the child's illness or behavior problems, legal liabilities, and parental dissatisfaction.

Ambulatory settings that receive many telephone calls should have established protocols so that each provider obtains adequate information and gives the same advice for similar problems. To establish rapport, the nurse should identify himself or herself and briefly state his or her credentials. The name, sex, and age of the child should be identified. The nature of the problem dictates the information that needs to be gathered but usually includes the exact nature of the symptoms and their duration, whether other family members have similar problems, and chief parental concerns. The ability of the caller or caretaker to handle the situation should also be assessed; their responses help determine a plan of action.

A published manual of protocols such as *Pediatric Telephone Advice* may be used to guide responses.[48] Some situations can readily be managed over the phone, whereas others may require a visit. The care center may establish limits for the length of telephone consultations; likewise, specific hours may be posted for telephone consultations. These procedures may reduce the number of interruptions during the ambulatory nurse's day.

In giving advice over the telephone, the nurse should ensure accuracy by having the parent repeat the instructions. The nurse should also outline signs of worsening that warrant a return call or visit. Documentation of the information exchanged is essential to promote continuity of care and to provide protection should a liability issue later arise.

Nursing Evaluation

The process of evaluating nursing care in ambulatory settings is less direct than evaluation of hospital care. In inpatient settings, an "episode of care" is demarcated by admission and discharge, but in ambulatory settings, the period of care to be evaluated is not as easily delineated. Hastings[19] suggests three possible organizational methods to define what constitutes an episode of care. These are listed below with examples.

Clinic session—the care administered by three nurses to all of the children in an oncology clinic on Tuesday from 9:00 to 12:00.
Single visit—nursing administered to one child during an appointment.
Problem-solving episode—nursing care provided to a family to resolve a child's behavior problem.

Although inpatients can be evaluated continuously until discharge, ambulatory families may leave the care setting never to return. This prospect is even more likely if families were unhappy with the care; an entire segment of an evaluation population thus may be lost. One method of follow-up is to call families and determine how well the child responded to the planned care. Even better is to place the responsibility for the call on the child and family with an instruction such as, "I'd like to hear from you between 9:00 and 10:00 A.M. tomorrow at this number to know if the condition is improving."

The Joint Commission on the Accreditation of Hospitals has developed the *Ambulatory Health Care Standards Manual* to clarify "an organization's responsibilities for monitoring and evaluating" patient care quality.[29] (p.26) Standards of ambulatory nursing practice developed by the American Academy of Ambulatory Nursing Administration are also useful in developing expected outcomes.[1]

After examining their responsibilities, it is clear that today's ambulatory care nurses truly have an important role in the health care system. The opportunity exists for these nurses to function both independently and in collaboration with other health professionals. Koerner believes ambulatory nurses must understand their role in ambulatory care, redefining their job descriptions as necessary, to prevent role encroachment by non-nurses. It is only through an understanding of these roles that nurses flourish in today's economically driven ambulatory care market.[32]

Current Issues and Trends

Access to Care

Obtaining access to health care can be difficult when the decision-making burden is placed on the parent or family member. Not only must the person have enough health knowledge to determine if the child needs care, but a decision as to which ambulatory service is most appropriate must be made. Some ambulatory care centers have developed plans specifically tailored to facilitate the family's entry into the health system.[13]

Once the child is in the system, other deterrents to families seeking care in an ambulatory setting may be identified. Long waiting times, inconvenient hours, lack of continuity of care, and lack of privacy discourage some families from returning.[42] For many families, however,

the major barrier to ambulatory care access is financial. It is estimated that 11 million children younger than age 18 (one in every six children, and one in every three poor children) are not covered by medical insurance.[8] Perhaps even more disturbing is the fact that two thirds of uninsured children live in families in which at least one parent works full time.[8] Many of these uninsured parents cannot afford individual policies and have employers who do not offer health insurance.[57]

Research has shown that children who receive comprehensive primary and preventive benefits under Medicaid have annual health costs 10% less than children who do not.[8] (p.4) Yet, methods previously used to shift costs from nonpaying clients to those who can pay have been detrimentally affected by recent changes in the health system to reduce costs. Finding ways to provide adequate health care for all children is a national issue in which ambulatory nurses can take an active role.

Cost Containment

Administrators look for ways to cut costs in ambulatory settings. Nurses need to conduct research to demonstrate the importance and economic value of their services. Particularly at risk are those services that others see as "nonessential" such as teaching and counseling. Examination of nursing responsibilities to determine which can be provided by less expensive staff without sacrificing quality of care must occur. Similarly, families may assume even more responsibility for their child's health care within the health care system. For example, parents may be taught to weigh and measure their children at a well-child visit.

Homeless Families

Today, families with children represent more than one third of the nation's homeless population.[8] The main reason that families are homeless is due to economic forces. Government support has not kept pace with rising costs, so there is an increase in family poverty. In addition, there is a decrease in the availability of affordable housing.[18]

What is the nurse's role in caring for these homeless children? The nurse should recognize that the family's basic priorities may be different than the health care provider's. These families are concerned with day-to-day survival, and often little energy is left for needs such as health care. Homeless children often arrive at an ambulatory care facility because of a need to be treated for a acute health problem, and they generally receive only sporadic preventive care. Therefore, while the ambulatory nurse gives care for the chief complaint and helps the family find such basics as food and shelter, there may also be an opportunity to perform a complete health assessment. Wood[60] recommends that the following areas be assessed: nutrition, immunization, academics, development, behavior, abuse, and medical status. These are discussed in the accompanying display on nursing assessment.

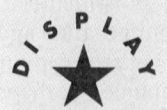

Nursing Assessment: Guidelines for Assessing Homeless Children

Nutritional Status—Children are at high risk for failure to thrive, delayed growth, or obesity. Investigators in one study found three fourths of the homeless girls over age 10 were overweight.[40] Another study found anemia rates in homeless children double that of the "general" pediatric population.[62]

Immunization Status—Immunizations are often not up to date or no record may exist due to frequent moves. Homeless children also should be screened annually for tuberculosis because they are at high risk.

Academic Achievement—Absenteeism and school failure are common in homeless children. Frequent moves, level of energy needed for survival, and even denial of school admission due to lack of immunization records or a stable address contribute to the problem.

Developmental Status—Developmental delays in homeless children may go unnoticed due to infrequent contact with the health care system. One study found developmental problems at a rate three times greater than

in other poor children.[5] Many shelters lack play areas indoors (space constraints) and outdoors (poor neighborhood safety). These children may spend their leisure time watching television.[49a]

Behavior—Mood and affect should be assessed. "Pseudomaturity," when children act in a manner much older than their developmental age, is a maladaptive behavior found in children who are forced into a level of responsibility that they are unprepared to handle. Depression is a frequent symptom, especially in school-aged children.[5]

Sexual or Physical Abuse—Child abuse is common in homeless families. In one study, three fourths of the homeless mothers reported being abused in the past.[4] Parents who have been abused are at risk to abuse their own children.

Medical Status—A careful physical examination including screening tests is important. Discovery of untreated acute conditions is not uncommon.

Outpatient and Community Nursing Centers

The concept of a nurse-managed center emerged as early as 1962, but few centers were established until the late 1980s when the Community Nursing Center Act was passed.[36,43] This legislation stimulated the development of outpatient community nursing centers to provide independent nursing services. These centers are especially designed to promote wellness and manage with the demands of self-care placed on families caused by increasingly shorter hospital stays.[17,43] Although many of these centers have been formed to meet the needs of elderly clients, the model is easily adaptable to the pediatric population. The counseling, health teaching, and other nursing services provided by these centers are applicable to all populations, including children.

Patient Classification Systems

One area receiving intense investigation is the effort to develop a patient classification system applicable to ambulatory care settings.[20,26,40,44,53,54] The purpose of this research is to explore the hours of nursing care needed in consideration of the complexity of the care required by the variety of ambulatory patients. The long-term goal is to develop a tool to help ambulatory care managers match nursing resources to child and family needs.

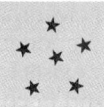

Ideas for Nursing Research

Because ambulatory nursing is a relatively new area of practice for nurses, the field is open for research in many areas. Several needs have been suggested in the content of this chapter. Other areas to be explored are the following:

- Investigation of formats to do comprehensive but quick nursing documentation.
- Examine methods to evaluate nursing care in ambulatory settings.
- Study the long-term effectiveness of school-based programs designed to decrease lifestyle risk factors.
- Investigation of methods families use to access care and barriers to care.
- Discover nursing interventions to reduce "no show" appointments.
- Find ways to research information about families that do not identify themselves as needing health care (ones that do not come).
- Continue research on the long-term economic benefits of prevention.
- Research parents' and children's ability to perform accurately some screening activities (weight, height, urinalysis).

Summary

The recent changes in the health care system imply that nurses, now more than ever, need expert assessment, diagnostic, planning, intervention, and evaluation skills to practice competently in ambulatory settings. These skills enable them to provide comprehensive, holistic nursing care to children and their families in a variety of settings. Further research is crucial to document nursing's role accurately so that other health professionals are aware of the value of nursing in today's ambulatory health care climate.

References

1. American Academy of Ambulatory Nursing Administration. (1987). *Ambulatory care nursing administration and practice standards.* Pitman, NJ: Jannetti.

2. American Nurses' Association. (1987). *The standards of practice for the primary health care nurse practitioner.* Kansas City: American Nurses' Association.

3. Arnold, L., Brecht, M., Hockett, A., Amspacher, K., & Grad, R. (1989). Lessons from the past. *MCN: American Journal of Maternal Child Nursing, 14,* 75, 78, 80, 82.

4. Bassuk, E., & Rosenberg L. (1988). Why does family homelessness occur? A case control study. *American Journal of Public Health, 78,* 783–788.

5. Bassuk, E., Rubin, L., & Lauriat, A. S. (1986). Characteristics of sheltered homeless families. *American Journal of Public Health, 76,* 1097–1101.

6. Burns, C. (1991). Development and content validity testing of a comprehensive classification of diagnoses for pediatric nurse practitioner. *Nursing Diagnoses, 2,* 93–104.

7. Burns, C., & Thompson, M. K. (1984). Developing a nursing diagnosis classification system for PNPs. *Pediatric Nursing, 19,* 411–414.

8. Children's Defense Fund. (1988). *A call for action to make our nation safe for children: A briefing book on the state of American children in 1988.* Washington, DC: Children's Defense Fund.

9. Chow, M., Durano, B., Feldmen, M., & Mills, M. (1984). *Handbook of pediatric primary care* (2nd ed.). New York: Wiley.

10. Cone, T. E. (1979). *History of American pediatrics.* Boston: Little, Brown.

11. Conti, R. (1989). The nurse as case manager. *Nursing Connections, 2,* 55–58.

12. Daugherty, L. G., & Buchanan, G. J. (1981). Nursing role in ambulatory care. In L. L. Jarvis (Ed.), *Community health nursing: Keeping the public healthy* (pp. 113–122). Philadelphia: Davis.

13. Dodwell, A. B., & Oas, K. H. (1988). Assessment of issues related to access to ambulatory care services at The Children's Hospital of Boston. *Journal of Pediatric Nursing, 3,* 222–228.

14. Finch R. H. (1981). Statement on Medicare and Medicaid reforms. March 25, 1970. Unpublished document as cited in M. Roemer. *Ambulatory health services in America. Past, present, future.* Rockville, MD: Aspen.

15. Ford, L., & Silver, H. (1967). The expanded role of the nurse in child care. *Nursing Outlook, 9,* 43–45.

16. Gordon, T., DeAngelis, C., & Peterson, R. (1986). Capitation reimbursement for pediatric primary care. *Pediatrics, 77,* 29–34.

17. Gresham-Kenton, L., & Wisby, M. (1987). Development and implementation of nurse-managed health programs: A problem oriented approach. *Journal of Ambulatory Care Management, 10,* 20–29.

18. Hartman, C. (1983). *America's housing crisis: What is to be done?* Boston: Routledge & Kegan.

19. Hastings, C. (1987). Measuring quality in ambulatory care nursing. *Journal of Nursing Administration, 17,* 12–20, 1987.

20. Hastings, C. E. (1987). Classification issues in ambulatory care nursing. *Journal of Ambulatory Care Management, 10,* 50–64.

21. Hastings, C., & Muir-Nash, J. (1989). Validation of a taxonomy of ambulatory nursing practice. *Nursing Economics, 7,* 142–149.

22. Hayman, L. L., Weill, V. A., Tobias, N., Stashinko, E., & Meninger, J. (1988). Which child is at risk for heart disease? Part I. *MCN: American Journal of Maternal Child Nursing, 13,* 328–333.

23. Hayman, L. L., Weill, V. A., Tobias, N., Stashinko, E., & Meninger, J. (1988). Reducing risk for heart disease in children. Part II. *MCN: American Journal of Maternal Child Nursing, 13,* 442–448.

24. Henne, S. J., Warner, N. E., & Frank, K. J. (1988). Ambulatory care centers: A unique opportunity for nurse practitioners. *Nurse Practitioner, 13,* 43, 46–47, 50–51, 55.

25. Hicks, M. (1986). Outpatient nursing: Getting ready for a growing field. *Nursing Management, 17,* 26–30.

26. Hoffman, F., & Wakefield, D. S. (1986). Ambulatory care patient classification. *Journal of Nursing Administration, 16,* 23–30.

27. Igoe, J. B. (1980). Project Health Pact in action. *American Journal of Nursing, 80,* 2016–2021.

28. Issacs, P. J. (1989). Crisis prevention in an outpatient surgery center. *MCN: American Journal of Maternal Child Nursing, 14,* 352–354.

29. Joint Commission on the Accreditation of Hospitals. (1987, January). Monitoring and evaluation of the quality and appropriateness of care: An ambulatory health care example. *Quality Review Bulletin, 13,* 26–30.

30. Katz, H. P. (1982). *Telephone manual of pediatric care.* New York: Wiley.

31. Kirkpatrick, S. B. (1989). Pediatric nurse practitioners develop ambulatory surgery cardiac program. *Journal of Pediatric Health Care, 3,* 88–92.

32. Koerner, B. L. (1987). Clarifying the role of nursing in ambulatory care. *Journal of Ambulatory Care Management, 10,* 1–7.

33. Koster, M. K. (1983). Self care: Health behavior for the school-age child. *Topics in Clinical Nursing, (April),* 29–40.

34. Labar, C. (1986). Filling in the blanks on prescription writing. *American Journal of Nursing, 86,* 31–33.

35. Lesser, A. J. (1985). The origin and development of maternal and child health programs in the United States. *Journal of Public Health, 75,* 590–598.

36. Lewis, C., & Resnick, B. (1962). Nurse clinics and progressive ambulatory patient care. *New England Journal of Medicine, 277,* 1236–1241.

37. Lyons, J. F., & Hester, N. O. (1987). Research generated nursing diagnosis for healthy school age children. *Issues in Comprehensive Pediatric Nursing, 10,* 149–159.

38. Martin, K., & Scheet, N. (1992). The Omaha system: Applications for community health nursing. Philadelphia: W. B. Saunders.

39. McLemore, T., & De Lozier, J. (1987, January 23). 1985 Summary: National ambulatory medical care survey. *National Center for Health Statistics Advance Data 128.*

40. Miller, D. K. (1985). Classifying patients for ambulatory surgical care. *Nursing Management, 16,* 33–36.

41. Miller, D., & Lin, E. (1988). Sheltered homeless families. *Pediatrics, 81,* 668–674.

42. Orr, S. T., Charney, E., & Straus, J. (1988). Use of health services by black children according to payment mechanism. *Medical Care, 26,* 939–947.

43. Pappas, C. A., & Van Scoy-Mosher, C. (1988). Establishing a profitable outpatient community nursing center. *Journal of Nursing Administration, 18,* 31–33.

44. Parrinello, K., Brenner, P., & Vallone, B. (1988). Refining and testing a nursing patient classification instrument in ambulatory care. *Nursing Administration Quarterly, 13,* 54–65.

45. Pender, N. (1987). *Health promotion in nursing practice* (2nd ed.). Norwalk, CT: Appleton & Lange.

46. Roemer, M. I. (1981). *Ambulatory health services in America. Past, present, future.* Rockville, MD: Aspen.

47. Roemer, M. I. (1986). *An introduction to the health care system* (2nd ed.). New York: Springer.

48. Schmitt, B. D. (1980). *Pediatric telephone advice.* Boston: Little, Brown.

49. Shamansky, S. L., & Clausen, C. L. (1980, February). Levels of prevention: Examination of the concept. *Nursing Outlook, 28,* 104–108.

49a. Shulsinger, E. (1990). Needs of sheltered homeless children. *Journal of Pediatric Health Care, 4,* 136–140.

50. Swehia, M. (1988). Nursing diagnosis as a standard methodology for identifying and validating diagnoses in an ambulatory care setting. *Nursing Administration Quarterly, 12,* 18–23.

51. Swensen, T. G. (1988). A dose of Camp Dost: Meeting the psychosocial needs of children with cancer. *Issues in Comprehensive Pediatric Nursing, 11,* 29–34.

52. Verran, J. A. (1981). Delineation of ambulatory care nursing practice. *Journal of Ambulatory Care Management, 4,* 1–13.

53. Verran, J. A. (1986). Patient classification in ambulatory care. *Nursing Economics, 4,* 247–251.

54. Verran, J. A. (1986). Testing a classification instrument for the ambulatory care setting. *Research in Nursing and Health, 9,* 279–287.

55. Walters, S. A. (1985). What it's really like to work in an ambulatory care center. *RN, 28,* 51–53.

56. Weir, R., Rideout, E., & Crook, J. (1989). Pediatric use of emergency departments. *Journal of Pediatric Health Care, 3,* 204–210.

57. Wilensky, G. R. (1987). Viable strategies for dealing with the uninsured. *Health Affairs, 6,* 33–46.

58. Winder, P. G. (1988, July). Case management by nurses at a county facility. *Quality Review Bulletin, 14,* 215–219.

59. Wold, S. J. (1981). *School nursing—A framework for practice* (pp. 49–60). St. Louis: Mosby.

60. Wood, D. (1989). Homeless children: Their evaluation and treatment. *Journal of Pediatric Health Care, 3,* 194–199.

61. Woodwell, D. (1992). Office visits to pediatric specialists, 1989. Advance data from Vital and Health Statistics, #208. National Center for Health Statistics. Hyattsville, MD.

62. Wright, J. D. (1990). Homelessness is not healthy for children and other living things. *Child and Youth Services, 14,* 65–88.

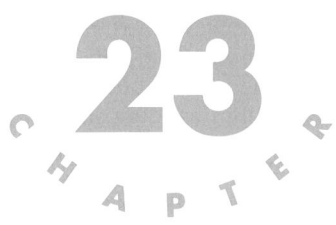

Hospital Care for Children

CHAPTER 23

FEATURES OF THIS CHAPTER

Nursing Intervention: Actions to Address Responses to Hospitalization, Table 23-2

Nursing Assessment: Coping Strategies Used During Hospitalization

Nursing Interventions: Role-Related Activities, Table 23-3

Nursing Intervention: Anticipatory Guidance for Hospital Admission, Table 23-4

Ideas for Nursing Research

BEHAVIORAL OBJECTIVES

Describe roles of the nurse in the care of the hospitalized child.

Describe the general response of children, adolescents, parents, and siblings to hospitalization.

Summarize strategies that facilitate adaptation and coping.

Identify strategies for preparing children, parents, and siblings for a scheduled admission.

Describe preparation of the child for procedures in the hospital setting using principles of growth and development.

Describe physiologic and psychological preparation of the child and family for surgery using principles of growth and development and concepts of preparation.

Describe the effects of admission to the intensive care unit (ICU) on both the child and the family.

In recent years, at least 3.2 million children less than 15 years of age have been hospitalized annually.[34] These children were hospitalized for a variety of reasons including respiratory illnesses; ear, nose, and throat problems; and congenital anomalies. The leading causes of hospitalization for both males and females less than 15 years of age, not including newborns, are listed in Table 23-1.[33] Many of these children were scheduled for hospitalization, but others were admitted for emergencies.

Hospitalization is a difficult time for families. The amount of stress experienced depends on many factors:

- Whether the admission was scheduled or an emergency.
- Severity of the illness/injury.
- Age and developmental level of the child.
- Prior experience with hospitalization.
- Coping skills of both the child and the family.
- Strength of the available support systems.

Much study has been devoted to the reactions of children and their families to hospitalization and has led to an increased understanding of their needs.

525

Response to Hospitalization

The Child's Response

Hospitalization can be a threatening experience for the child who is striving to achieve the appropriate developmental tasks. (See Chapter 8 for developmental tasks for each age group.) The child's response to hospitalization depends on such influences as developmental level and coping mechanisms, the parent–child relationship, cultural and ethnic influences, previous experiences with hospitalization, the nature of the illness, and the child's perception and knowledge of the event.[20,37,53]

Hospitalization imposes at least five threats to children of all ages[53]:

- Physical harm or bodily injury.
- Separation from parents and the absence of trusted adults.
- The strange and unknown.
- Uncertainty about limits and expected acceptable behavior.
- Loss of control, autonomy, and competence.

These threats have a variety of meanings for children at different developmental stages. The fear of separation, physical harm or bodily injury, and loss of control are discussed in detail as they apply to each age group. Fear of the strange and the unknown and uncertainty about limits are included in the discussion on coping. Table 23-2 lists specific behaviors that might be observed in the child and suggests possible nursing interventions. This information can serve as a guideline for nursing assessment and plan of care.

TABLE 23-1
Leading Causes of Hospitalization for Children Under 15*

Diagnosis	Percentage of Hospitalizations
Males	
Pneumonia, all forms	7.0
Acute respiratory infection	6.1
Bronchitis, emphysema, and asthma	6.1
Chronic disease of tonsils and adenoids	6.0
Congenital anomalies	5.7
Fracture, all sites	5.6
Otitis media and eustachian tube disorders	4.4
Females	
Chronic disease of tonsils and adenoids	7.8
Acute respiratory infection	6.3
Noninfectious enteritis and colitis	6.0
Pneumonia, all forms	5.7
Bronchitis, emphysema, and asthma	4.8
Congenital anomalies	4.5
Otitis media and eustachian tube disorders	4.1

* Data are based on a sample of hospital records and reflect discharges from non-Federal short-stay hospitals in 1984; does not include newborns.
Data from *Health United States*, (1986). DHHS Publication Number (PHS) 87-1232.

Infancy

At 0 to 5 months of age, the infant has not yet attached strongly to the primary caretaker; however, stress due to a change in caregivers or in the number of caregivers, and change in the environment can be detected through altered sleeping, feeding, and elimination patterns.[37] Stranger anxiety surfaces between 5 and 7 months of age when the infant shows displeasure at the approach of unfamiliar people.[37] Separation anxiety appears between 7 and 9 months of age.[37] By this time, the infant has attached to the primary caregiver and is upset when separated.

Early Childhood

Separation. Separation anxiety peaks around 18 months of age,[23] but the effects of separation are a major threat to hospitalized children through the preschool years. Separation from parents can be extremely traumatic for toddlers and preschoolers. The amount of separation anxiety experienced by the child depends on development, previous experience with separation, and the amount of social contacts outside the family.[36] Separation from parents or the primary caregiver threatens the feelings of autonomy and sense of initiative that the child is trying to achieve.[14,37]

Robertson described three stages that children might progress through if separated from mother: protest, despair, and denial.[38] Table 23-2 outlines specific behaviors in each stage. Some children who are hospitalized for only a short period of time do not advance beyond the stage of protest, but others reach the stage of despair. Children hospitalized for a long period of time, who are cared for by several different nurses may progress to the stage of denial.[38]

Although Robertson's research focused on separation from mothers, the presence of the father is important. Maccoby's[23] research has demonstrated that, although separation from the mother is more intense, the child begins to respond to separation from the father around 15 months of age.

Physical Harm or Bodily Injury. Toddlers and preschoolers are unable to understand the reason for hospitalization and generally view it as punishment for wrongdoing. Procedures are threatening to the child who has no control over what is being done. Children in the preschool period can misunderstand or misinterpret the meaning of procedures. A child of this age is prone to fantasies of mutilation. The child especially fears harm to body parts that are developmentally important, such as the genitals, and to sensitive areas such as the eyes and ear.[37]

Loss of Control. Hospitalization threatens the feelings of mastery over basic tasks that children accomplish at each developmental age. Children who are placed in an unfamiliar environment with strangers are likely to regress to earlier stages of development to cope with the stress. The child usually gives up the most recently learned behavior such as toilet training or drinking from

TABLE 23-2
Nursing Intervention: Actions to Address Responses to Hospitalization

Response	Expected Behavior	Nursing Interventions
Infancy—5 to 12 Months		
Stranger anxiety	Cries when approached by nursing staff and physicians	Allow parents to remain present during procedures
	Clings to parents	Provide consistent caregivers
Separation anxiety	Cries when parents leave	Encourage ''rooming-in''
	May reject attempts to comfort	Liberal visiting hours
Early Childhood—1 to 5 Years		
Separation	**Protest**	Encourage ''rooming-in''
	Cries loudly when mother leaves	Liberal visiting hours
	May continue to cry for several minutes or hours	Suggest ways that parents can spend more time at hospital, if appropriate
	Throws self about in bed	Allow child to bring toys, stuffed animals, blankets from home
	Rejects attempts to comfort	
	Despair	Have parents leave something of theirs each time they leave
	Appears to have settled in, but really has increased hopelessness that parent will return	Keep pictures of family at bedside
	Less active	Encourage family to make tapes with parents and siblings talking to child, singing favorite songs
	Cries intermittently	
	Makes no demands on environment	Provide consistent caregivers
	If parent returns, may cry loudly, releasing anger	Careful assessment of child's response to separation through therapeutic play
	Denial	Spend extra time with the child who is alone
	Hopeless of parent's return	Encourage play with other children on unit
	More interest in environment	
	Plays, smiles	
	Does not cry if parents return and leave again	
Physical harm and bodily injury	Kicks, screams, and pulls away during procedures	Explain all procedures carefully to children old enough to understand simple explanations
	May become upset and cry if the procedure is mentioned	Be truthful about whether or not the procedure is painful
		Explain to child why he must hold still and how to do so
		Allow parents to be present during procedure to provide comfort, not to hold child down
		Demonstrate procedure on dolls
		When surgery is anticipated, tell child that he or she will be operated on only the problem area
Loss of control	Regresses to earlier stage of development (e.g., bottle, pacifier, bedwetting)	Allow control when possible (e.g., choice about which leg for injection, which pill to take first)
	Protests attempts to perform procedure	Allow child to wear underpants to surgery if possible
Middle Childhood—6 to 8 Years and Preadolescents—7 to 12 Years		
Separation	May be sad when parents leave	Encourage family and friends to visit
	Cheerful when family and friends visit	Allow frequent phone calls, assist if needed
	Talks to friends on phone	Plan activities on the unit that encourage interactions with other patients
	May request roommate	Assign to room with same age, same sex patient, if feasible
Physical harm or bodily injury	May become upset during procedures	Assess understanding of all procedures
	Expresses concern about what will happen to body, especially during surgery	Clarify misconceptions
		Explain exactly what body part will be affected and what it will look like afterwards
		Use models, pictures, body outlines, dolls with tubing, dressings
		Provide opportunity for therapeutic play
Loss of control	May regress to earlier stage of development (e.g., increased dependency on parents)	Allow child to participate in decision making and self-care
		Assess feelings about hospitalization and surgery through therapeutic play

(Continued)

TABLE 23-2
(Continued)

Response	Expected Behavior	Nursing Interventions
	Expresses fears related to anesthesia, may ask about waking up during surgery, saying things while under anesthesia	Explain anesthesia as a special sleep and assure child that he will not wake up during surgery
		Explain purpose of side rails, dietary changes
Adolescence—13 to 18 Years		
Separation	Asks to see friends	Allow friends to visit frequently
	Cheerful when friends visit	Encourage phone calls and assist if needed
	Talks on phone to friends	Plan group activities for adolescent patients
	Verbalizes missing friends, activities, wants to go home	
Physical harm or bodily injury	Expresses concern about how the procedure will alter appearance, especially about how he will appear to others	Assess understanding of procedures by having adolescent explain what will happen. Use body diagrams and pictures to show how body parts will be affected
		Have another adolescent with similar operation or condition talk with him or her
Loss of control	May regress to earlier stage of development (e.g., increased dependency on others for self-care)	Encourage participation in decision making and self-care
		Explain what will happen during operation
	Expresses fear of dying during surgery, concern about talking while under anesthesia	Answer all questions and offer reassurance

a cup. Children may react to attempts to restrain them by kicking, screaming, and pulling away. Staff who do not understand what is happening tend to increase physical restraint to perform a procedure, but more restraint leads to more intense rebellion, and a no-win cycle is established.

Middle Childhood

Separation.   During the early school-age years, the child develops relationships with people outside the family. Although separation anxiety is not as obvious in this age group as in early childhood, separation from family, friends, and the usual environment poses a threat to the independence and new relationships the child has begun to establish. Regression to an earlier stage of development is also common in this age group.

Physical Harm or Bodily Injury.   School-age children are cognitively able to understand about their illness. The depth of understanding, however, is limited, frequently leading to misconceptions and the view that hospitalization is a result of their own actions. These children are afraid of what will happen to their bodies in situations in which they are not in control, such as during surgery when they are under anesthesia or during a major procedure when they are heavily sedated.[37]

Loss of Control.   Fear of loss of control intensifies in middle childhood.[37] As the child's sense of independence has increased with new experiences, so has the sense of control over the environment. Hospitalization threatens the child's mastery. The young school-age child fears loss of control in situations such as surgery and anesthesia. For example, the child may be afraid of what he or she might say while under anesthesia.

Preadolescence

Separation.   Separation from parents is generally not detrimental to children in this age group. Preadolescents are less dependent on parents and are also able to understand that parents will return. The presence of parents in the hospital setting, however, at least part of the time, helps to decrease the stress associated with hospitalization. Separation from peers is a greater concern for children at this age, because this is the time when contacts outside of the home are steadily increasing and their independence is increasing.

Physical Harm or Bodily Injury.   Preadolescents are able to understand more about their illness than the younger child; however, they still have many fantasies, misconceptions, and fears about illness that are similar to those experienced by the school-age child.[20] These children are concerned about what is going to happen to their bodies.[30]

Loss of Control.   The sense of loss of control experienced by the preadolescent is similar to that of the school-age child. These feelings are intensified by the fact that the child is becoming increasingly independent as relationships with people outside of the home increase. Sudden dependence on both family and strangers interferes with the sense of accomplishment that preadolescents are trying to achieve.

Adolescence

Separation.   Hospitalization separates the adolescent from peer relationships that are vitally important during this stage of development. Maintaining contact with peers is just as important as maintaining contact with family. Adolescents may even prefer friends to family as they try to establish their own identity.

Physical Harm or Bodily Injury. Adolescents are generally preoccupied with their appearance; therefore, the many procedures that take place during hospitalization may be threatening. Adolescents are concerned about what will happen to their bodies and whether they will look different to others when they recover. This fear is particularly applicable to those who are undergoing a surgical procedure that may alter their appearance.

Loss of Control. Hospitalization of the adolescent threatens the sense of independence that has been established recently. They often feel as if they have little control over their environment and at times regress to being dependent on others for self-care.[29] The nurse's challenge is to "minimize the adoption of the 'sick role' by the adolescent and to maximize attention toward maintaining normal adolescent development during this potentially stressful period."[29]

Parental Response

Reactions of parents to the hospitalization of their child are unique. Individual personalities and coping styles, cultural differences, previous experience in similar situations, the nature of the illness, and the parents' knowledge and understanding of the hospitalization all influence responses. Additionally, current life stressors play a large role in their reactions, suggesting that the same parent might react differently on separate occasions. For example, a mother might show much more emotion and difficulty with the hospitalization when her support people are unavailable than when they are able to accompany her to the hospital. Recent illness or death in the family, change in the family structure, and financial difficulties are other examples of stressors that might affect how parents respond to the hospitalization of a child. The nurse must assess parents' reactions during each hospital admission and avoid preconceived notions regarding how they will respond.

Whether the admission is scheduled or not, most parents exhibit a certain amount of anxiety when their child is hospitalized. Some behaviors that might be observed include: crying, nervousness, asking numerous questions, impatience, aggression, and anger. Emergency admissions, life-threatening illnesses, or hospitalizations for which the parent may feel some responsibility (e.g., accidents) generally increase parental anxiety. These reactions, however, are individualized, and a parent whose child is hospitalized for elective surgery might exhibit just as much anxiety as another whose child has emergency surgery. The nurse must assess all parents individually and provide emotional support and teaching as indicated in each situation.

The number of other children in the home can also affect the amount of anxiety experienced by the parents. When parents are concerned about providing for the needs of other children, there is increased stress. Parents may feel torn between wanting to stay with the hospitalized child and needing to be at home with the other chil-

dren.[1] Parents who are not willing to leave their hospitalized child alone often find someone, such as grandparents or friends, to stay with the child for awhile so they can spend some time at home with the other children. The mother and father often take turns staying with the hospitalized child while the other one spends time at home. When parents do leave the hospital to spend time with the other children, the nurse should be supportive of this decision and reassure them that care will be provided for the hospitalized child.

On the other hand, admission of an only child to the hospital can also be anxiety-producing. Parents may fear that they will lose their only child, adding to the normal stressors of hospitalization.[52]

Sibling Response

The usual routines of other family members are disrupted when a child is hospitalized. Sometimes other children in the family are given added responsibility at home while their parents are spending more time with the hospitalized child.

Siblings are frequently separated from parents, especially from the mother, who often stays with the ill child.[9] The toddler and preschooler can experience some of the same effects of separation as the hospitalized child if placed in unfamiliar surroundings and separated from parents. The age of the siblings determines the focus of their concerns and are somewhat similar to the concerns of the hospitalized child.

The display lists 12 behavior and feeling changes that can take place in siblings of hospitalized children.[9,10] The amount of change each sibling experiences is individualized. Craft et al.[10] identified several factors that intensify the effects of hospitalization on siblings: those who have a close relationship with the hospitalized child, those who are afraid of getting the illness, and those who stay in someone else's home during their sibling's hospitalization. Siblings who receive limited explanations or no ex-

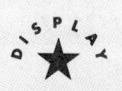

Feelings and Behavior Changes in Siblings of Hospitalized Children

Getting mad
Trouble concentrating in school
Difficulty sleeping
Nervousness
Fighting with kids
Nightmares
Nail biting
Wanting to be alone
Wanting to spend time at home with parents
Health perception
Sadness or depression
Food intake

Perceived Change Scale. Copyright Martha J. Craft, PhD, RN. Used with permission.

planation about the hospitalization are affected more than those who receive thorough explanations.

Parents may not realize that siblings are affected by the hospitalization. The nurse should alert the parents to potential behavior changes and suggest ways that these effects can be minimized. For example, sibling visitation should be encouraged, especially for those children who have a close relationship with the hospitalized child. The nurse might also suggest that one parent stay with the hospitalized child while the other spends time at home. Parents should also be aware of the importance of educating siblings about the child's hospitalization.

Coping With Hospitalization

Coping is defined as "one's ability to deal with new situations and stressful experiences."[50] Coping strategies are those mechanisms, conscious or unconscious, that a person uses to manage stressful situations. Unconscious coping strategies also are referred to as defense mechanisms. The hospitalized child copes with the trauma of hospitalization in a variety of ways depending on age and prior experience with similar stressors. Examples of coping strategies characteristic of hospitalized children in each age group are listed in the accompanying display on nursing assessment. Parents also use a variety of coping mechanisms to deal with the hospitalization of their child. The manner in which they cope depends on the same factors that influence their reaction to hospitalization. Many parents use denial as a means of coping. For example, they may seek another opinion or express disbelief of the diagnosis.

Anger and frustration are observed in some parents. This behavior may be directed toward the hospital staff

---

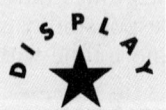

Nursing Assessment: Coping Strategies Used During Hospitalization

Infancy—0 to 12 Months

Increased motor activity, restlessness
Crying, fussing, and screaming
Sucking
Hand–mouth activity

Early Childhood—1 to 5 Years

Regression*	Resistance	Familiarization
Displacement*	Making requests	Motor activity
Denial*	Information seeking	Play
Aggression	Temper tantrums	Clinging, comfort-seeking
Protest	Fantasy	Attempts to control and restructure
Striking out	Withdrawal, hiding	
Pushing away	Trial and error experimentation	

Middle Childhood—6 to 8 Years and Preadolescence—9 to 12 Years

Avoidance	Support seeking	Sleeping, rejection of others
Active participation	Fantasy	Cooperation
Information seeking	Denial*	Attempts to control and restructure
Cognitive mastery	Sublimation*	Diversional thinking
Orientation	Repression*	Humor
Rehearsal	Aggression	Crying
Repetition	Protest	Regression*
Problem solving	Resistance	Displacement*
Motor activity	Withdrawal, quiet behavior	Reaction formation*

Adolescence—13 to 18 Years

Information seeking	Repression*	Motor activity
Cognitive mastery	Sublimation*	Withdrawal, quiet behavior
Orientation	Rationalization*	Denial*
Fantasy	Diversional thinking	Displacement*
Sleeping	Conformity	Reaction formation*
Regression*	Controlling behaviors	Intellectualization*

Psychological Defense Mechanisms
Source: Compiled from a variety of sources.

as they attempt to collect information or care for the child. Often, parents direct their negative feelings toward each other, especially if one parent blames the other for the illness or injury. Parents who react in this manner might be labeled as "difficult," but nurses should look beyond the behavior to recognize the underlying cause. The nurse can help parents manage their stress by giving them an opportunity to express how they feel about the hospitalization. Educating the parents about the illness, answering questions, and clarifying misconceptions frequently help decrease the anxiety associated with the hospitalization.

Many parents cope better with their child's hospitalization by staying with the child and actively participating in their care. Others stay with the child but assume a more passive role, often observing the staff care for the child. There are also parents who choose not to stay with their child; being away from the situation is thereby a coping mechanism. Frequently, however, the parent wants to stay with the child but is unable to for a variety of reasons. For example, the single parent with other children at home may be unable to find or afford child care, or parents may be unable to miss work because of financial responsibilities. Families sometimes live a long distance from the hospital and find it difficult to visit frequently, especially if transportation is limited. Nurses must be careful not to label parents as noncaring when they do not stay with their child. They should encourage the parents to visit as often as possible, but also assure the parents that their child will be cared for in their absence.

Nursing Implications

Nursing Roles

Nurses have the opportunity to fulfill a variety of interrelated roles while caring for the hospitalized child. Nurses not only serve as caregivers, offering both physical and emotional support, but they also act as advocates and educators. The amount of time spent in each of these roles varies considerably with the age of the child, severity of illness, and whether the parents are present.

As a *caregiver,* the nurse uses a wide range of knowledge, techniques, and skills to provide the physical aspects of care essential during a child's hospitalization. The nurse may be called on to provide daily needs such as feeding, bathing, and diapering, as well as collaborative measures such as giving medications, monitoring IVs, vital signs, and dressing changes. Just as important, however, is the ability to provide effective emotional care for the child and family. Emotional support, for example, helps to calm the fears of the child and the family.

In the child health setting, the nurse has an excellent opportunity to serve as an *advocate* for the child and family. Nursing advocacy may be demonstrated through efforts to reduce unnecessary interruptions of the infant or child who is sleeping, to promote optimal nutrition for the child, to promote normal growth and development of the child, and to minimize separation from family and friends. The nurse also may identify cues that indicate the need for the family to have an opportunity to talk with the physician or other health team members. Acting as

an advocate, the nurse can facilitate this communication by contacting the appropriate people and making them aware of family needs.[40]

The role of *educator* is incorporated into comprehensive nursing care throughout the child's hospital stay. The nurse faces the challenge of teaching people whose level of understanding varies a great deal. Principles of teaching and learning, as well as those of growth and development, must be incorporated into the nurses' teaching efforts. Table 23-3 gives some specific examples of how the nurse functions in providing emotional support, advocacy, and education.

Facilitating Adaptation and Coping

Nurses help children and their parents adapt to and cope effectively with hospitalization. The trend is to allow at least one parent to be with the child at all times and to offer liberal and flexible visiting privileges. "Rooming-in" is generally effective in decreasing anxiety and facilitating coping and adaptation in both parents and children (Fig. 23-1). When at least one parent stays with the child, the effects of separation are minimized. Limiting separation is especially important in the younger child.

Rooming-in also allows parents to participate in the care of the child, especially with the daily physical needs such as bathing, feeding, and comforting. Parental participation in care helps to minimize the effects of the

TABLE 23-3
Nursing Interventions: Role-Related Activities

Role	Specific Activities
Provider of emotional support	Hold infant or young child who is separated from parents
	Stay with the child during a painful procedure
	Listen attentively to parents who are upset because of their child's illness
	Keep parents informed when surgery is delayed
Advocate	Facilitate communication between family and health care workers
	Plan care to avoid frequent interruptions of the sleeping infant or child
	Provide foods that the child likes
	Provide toys or diversional activities
	Encourage parents to stay with the child
	Encourage sibling visitation
	Allow friends to visit
Educator	Orient child and family to the unit
	Explain the policies of the unit
	Provide teaching about child's illness and answer related questions
	Explain procedures and answer questions
	Pre- and postoperative teaching for the child and family
	Discharge teaching that includes caring for the child at home, signs of complications, and how to handle potential behavior problems that might occur after discharge

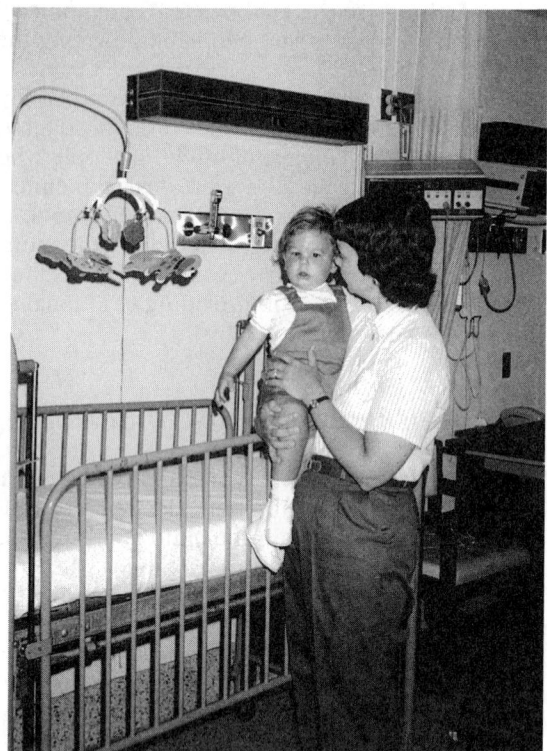

FIGURE 23-1
Presence of a parent helps toddler cope during hospitalization.

strange environment and often decreases the fear of loss of control and bodily harm or injury. Parents usually welcome the chance to participate actively and make choices regarding their child's care. The nurse should communicate to parents that they are allowed to participate in their child's care and assess their desire to do so.[2,43] Parents know their child better than anyone else and can offer helpful suggestions regarding techniques for medication administration, food preferences, and other aspects of care. They feel more in control when they are allowed to make decisions regarding, for example, waking the child and timing of vital signs and procedures. Allowing parents to participate in decision making is important; however, the nurse must remember that the child's health is the first priority. When parents are under stress, they may not be able to make the best decision without assistance or without detailed information.

Allowing both the child and parents to have some choices (when there are some) decreases the sense of loss of control or helplessness. During painful procedures, an approach that gives the child some control is generally best. For example, when appropriate, the child can decide which leg the injection will be given in. Uncertainty about limits and acceptable behavior is also a major threat of hospitalization.[53] The child should be told before the procedure what is expected and what the limits are. For example, during venipuncture, the child should be told that it is okay to cry and scream, but that holding still is essential.

Maintaining parental discipline consistent with that at home increases the sense of security in children during hospitalization. Changes in discipline, especially when parents become more lenient, often increases the child's

feeling that the condition is serious. Knowing that parents are still in control often helps the child cope more effectively with painful procedures. Some parents might find it difficult to discipline the sick child, but the nurse can encourage parents to continue to discipline the child as they do at home as much as possible.

For preadolescents and adolescents, peer visitation is effective in facilitating coping and adaptation to the hospital setting. Visits from peers enable the patient to maintain the contacts that are so important.

Fear of the unknown also is one of the major threats of hospitalization.[53] Not knowing what to expect produces anxiety in both the child and family. The "unknown" should be explained as much as possible to facilitate coping and adaptation. Education regarding admission, disease/condition, procedures, surgery, and discharge that offers a clear explanation of the event is vital (see sections entitled "Admission," "Preparation for Procedures," "Surgery," and "Discharge").

The environment also affects childhood coping. Most pediatric units are decorated with bright colors, murals, and pictures. Special areas such as an aquarium, a playroom, and a teen room should be provided.

Use of Play

Play is essential in the child's development. Through play, the child achieves language skills, develops gross and fine motor skills, learns about the environment, expresses fears and fantasies, uses imagination, and solves problems. Therapeutic play is an aspect of play through which the child can attain a sense of mastery and competency during hospitalization.[7,36] Therapeutic play is used to asses the child's physical, emotional, and developmental status; to assess the child's understanding of hospitalization and procedures; to teach the child concepts and procedures; to provide diversional activities for the child; and to provide an outlet for expression of feelings.[17] Therapeutic play should not be referred to as play therapy, which is an entirely different concept used with emotionally disturbed children (see Chap. 18).[17]

Many hospitals have child life specialists whose responsibility is to provide supportive services to the child and family to facilitate coping.[49] The child life specialist works with children in the playroom, the teen lounge, and at the bedside. Care is based on individual needs. Nurses are also involved in providing developmentally appropriate activities for children, especially those that teach the child about the hospital experience.

Playing with hospital equipment or miniature replicas allows the child to establish familiarity, to act out feelings, and to demonstrate what is understood about the equipment and associated procedures (Fig. 23-2). Doll houses and dolls can be used to investigate the child's feelings about separation from the family. Children often enjoy bandaging their dolls or stuffed animals and "performing procedures" or "surgery." Any misconceptions revealed during play should be clarified by the nurse or child life specialist.

Several other techniques are used for expression of feelings related to hospitalization and procedures. For example, children may be asked to draw a picture about what has happened to them. Baretich et al.[4] used drawings

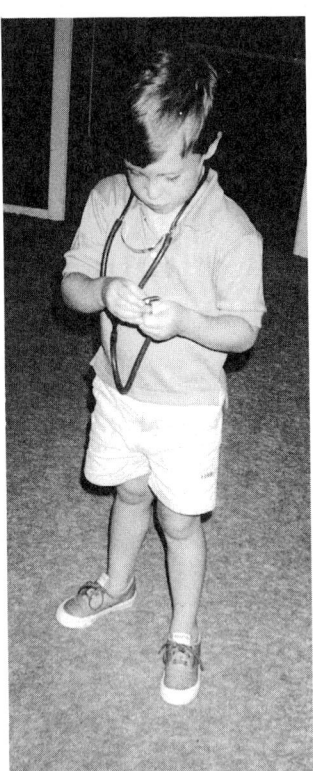

FIGURE 23-2
Playing with hospital equipment allows the child to become familiar with it and decreases some aspects of the unknown.

to assess children's perceptions of visits to the physician's office. The drawings frequently depicted a small child figure with small or missing body parts. Drawings may also show medical equipment drawn out of proportion and inaccurate use of objects, especially those depicting intrusive procedures. Other pictures may show the child alone in the room surrounded by equipment. Drawings such as these can indicate feelings of insecurity, inadequacy, fear, or a misunderstanding of the event.[4]

Children can use puppets to verbalize feelings through nonthreatening means. For example, the child can be asked to tell a story about a child's visit to the hospital using the puppets. Nurses can also use puppets for telling a story about the hospital and to clarify misconceptions about specific procedures.

The use of needle play *under supervision* is encouraged if the child has adequate motor skills, because it allows the child to act out the procedure often dreaded most by the child.[13,36] Needle play should be conducted by the nurse or child life specialist individually or with small groups of children with *adequate* supervision. In a study of chronically ill children, a majority of time spent in play focused on injections. Children who experienced more injections and venipunctures spent more time in injection play.[13] Children have been observed giving injections in both appropriate and inappropriate places, using varying degrees of force.

The playroom is an essential component of the pediatric unit and should be a "safe place" for the child. Procedures, including administering medications, should not take place in the playroom. The child often thinks of the playroom as a fun place to go, and visits there help

to decrease some of the anxiety associated with hospitalization. For the school-age child, play decreases boredom often associated with hospitalization. Video and computer games are popular in this age group. For the older preadolescent and the adolescent, a teen lounge is a place that facilitates interactions with peers and provides age-appropriate activities. When the child is unable to go to the playroom or teen lounge, appropriate materials can be brought to the bedside.

Admission

Scheduled Admission

The hospitalized child has been the focus of much research in the past several years. Many of these studies have focused on decreasing anxiety in the hospitalized child, but some have looked at preparation of the child before admission to the hospital.[15,16,24,25,45,51,53] Tours of the hospital that include an opportunity for the child to see and handle equipment and to ask questions, videotaped puppet shows, booklets, hospital kits, and information sessions have been suggested as means to prepare the child for planned admission to the hospital.[25,48,51,54]

Preparation of the child *before* a planned admission to the hospital decreases anxiety and fear of the unknown associated with hospitalization. A variety of methods are effective in preparing the child for admission. Timing, appropriate information to include, and the selection of strategies depend on the developmental age of the child and are outlined in Table 23-4. These guidelines must be adapted for each individual child.

Parents often experience intense anxiety over the anticipated admission of their child. Reduction of parental anxiety is important because it can be communicated to the child. The following guidelines can be used in parental preparation[35]:

- Review of the child's view of illness based on developmental stages.
- Preadmission tour, informal interview, and information session.
- Presentation of preadmission parent–child guidelines.
- Printed resources for both parents and children.

Parents are often the ones who provide information to the child before admission and should therefore receive appropriate information and educational materials.

Because hospitalization of a child also affects siblings, they also should be prepared adequately for this experience. Age-appropriate teaching similar to that described in Table 23-4 is important. When talking to siblings, it is important to emphasize:

- That they are not to blame for their brother's or sister's hospitalization.
- What arrangements have been made for their care.
- When they will be able to see their brother or sister.

Parents usually are the ones who provide information to siblings and should therefore receive appropriate guidelines and materials.

TABLE 23-4
Nursing Interventions: Anticipatory Guidance for Hospital Admission

Timing	Information to Include	Strategies
Early Childhood		
1–3 days before admission	Reason for hospitalization	Simple verbal explanations (Stress presence of parents, if appropriate, and reason for hospitalization)
	Part of body that will be affected	Show child where parents will be waiting during the operation
	Limits and expected behavior	Avoid use of words such as "dye" and "put to sleep"
	Participation in care	Play with dolls, puppets, medical equipment or replicas
	Presence of parents during hospitalization	Booklets, simple pictures
	Playroom visits	
Middle Childhood		
1 week before admission	Same as for early childhood	Verbal explanations
	Also include anticipated length of stay, activity limits, and diversional activities (e.g., playroom)	Clarify misconceptions after assessing how child perceives what will happen
		Play with puppets and medical equipment
		Books, pictures, films, videotapes, models, body outlines
		Provide opportunity to ask questions
Preadolescence		
1–2 weeks before admission	Reason for hospitalization	Verbal explanations
	Types of procedures, treatments, and surgery	Clarify misconceptions after assessing how child perceives what will happen
	Participation in care	Books, films, videotapes, diagrams with minimal detail, body outlines
	Anticipated changes in appearance	Opportunity to handle equipment
	Anticipated length of stay, activity limits, and diversional activities	Opportunity to ask questions
	Visiting hours; family and friends	
Adolescence		
As soon as scheduled	Same as for preadolescent	Verbal explanations
	Include more detail	Books, diagrams, with full detail
	Use correct medical terms	Body outlines
		Provide opportunity to ask questions after assessing adolescent's perceptions

Unscheduled Admission

Many children are hospitalized each year because of accidents or acute illness. Emergency admissions are extremely stressful to the child and family. The amount of stress depends somewhat on the child's condition on admission. The fact that there is no opportunity for preadmission preparation increases the stressors associated with fear of the unknown.

The stressors the child and family experience are generally intensified when the admission is unscheduled, especially if the child is in critical condition and spends much time in the emergency department or is admitted directly to the ICU. The child and family need emotional support during this time. Educating the family and child (if age and condition permit) about what has happened and what is anticipated in the next few hours is vital to increase their ability to cope. Both parents and child should be encouraged to talk about what has occurred. Misconceptions should be clarified as appropriate.

Admission Procedures

The actual admission has been identified as one of the most stressful times during the child's hospitaliza-

tion.[53] The number of people involved and procedures the child undergoes varies. The following are essential components of all admissions.

- Nursing history (including questions about what the child knows, fears, routines, sleeping habits, favorite foods, toys, toilet training, immunizations, and history of chickenpox or recent exposure to the illness).
- Physical examination.
- Developmental assessment.
- Orientation to the environment (particularly the child's room and the playroom).
- Explanation of policies and procedures (especially regarding rooming-in and visitation).

The child benefits if at least one parent remains during the admission procedures, not only to provide information and clarification but also to provide emotional support for the child (Fig. 23-3).

Preparation for Procedures

Preparation of the Child

Any procedure, no matter how minor it may seem, should be explained to the child.[22] The general fears and

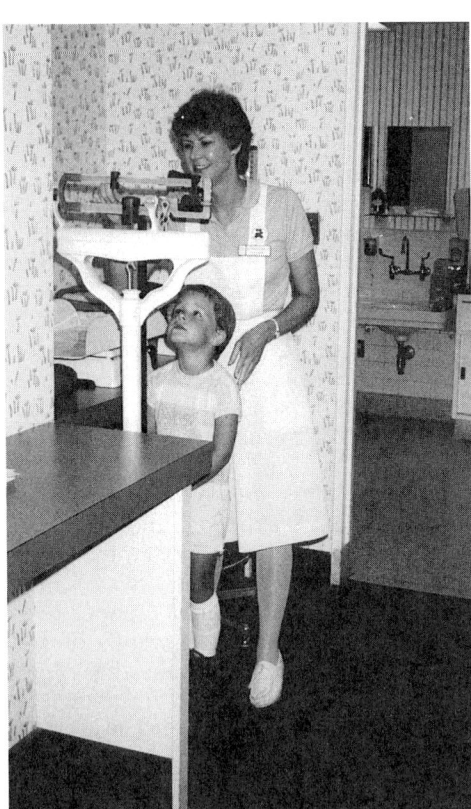 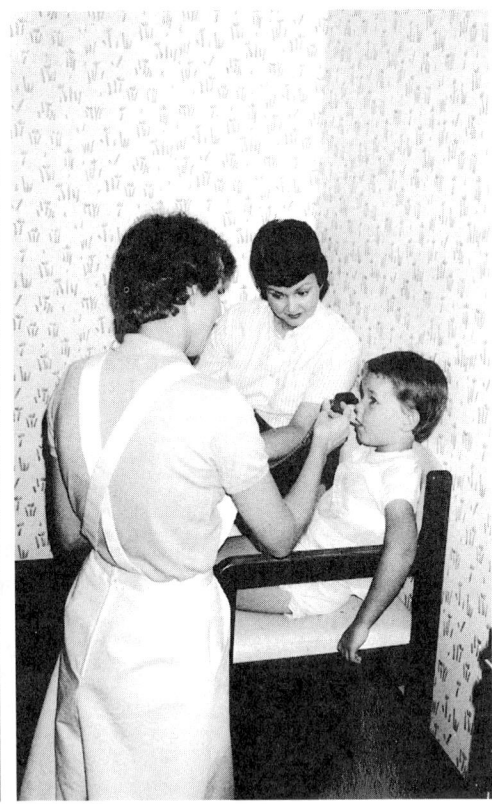

FIGURE 23-3
On admission, the child is exposed to a variety of procedures. A parent's presence during admission procedures provides support for the child.

reactions of the child should be considered. The nurse should:

- Assess the child's level of development and coping skills.
- Find out what the child knows about the procedure.
- Explain the procedure in terms of what the child will see, hear, feel, smell, and taste.[18]
- Tell the child how he can help during the procedure and what the limits are.
- Use age-appropriate terminology.

The same strategies identified in Table 23-4 can be followed. Timing of preparation should be based on the age of the child. Hansen and Evans[18] offer the following guidelines: The child ages 2 to 5 should be prepared for a minor procedure such as an injection just before its occurrence. For major procedures, such as IV insertion, casting, or x-rays, the child should be prepared 2 to 3 hours in advance, if possible. The explanation of when the event is to occur should be related to the child's routine activities, such as "after lunch" or "after your nap." Children ages 6 through adolescence should be told about the procedure as soon as it is scheduled.

After the procedure, the child should be encouraged to express feelings about the procedure and to ask questions. For the young child, drawing a picture or reenacting the procedure through play is appropriate (Fig. 23-4). Any misconceptions should be clarified.[6] Approaches to Nursing Procedures is discussed in Chapter 25. Preparation for procedures is only briefly discussed here.

Preparation of Parents

Parents also have a need for adequate preparation. Parental consent is required for many procedures such as lumbar punctures, cardiac catheterizations, and intravenous pyelograms. The physician is legally responsible for making sure that parents give informed consent. Before parents are asked to give their consent, they should be given a full explanation that includes benefits and possible complications. The use of diagrams, pictures, or models in addition to verbal explanations is helpful. The nurse's role is to clarify and to explain portions of the content not understood by the parents. If parents continue to have questions, the physician should be notified and asked to provide additional information.

Surgery

Each year, many children are hospitalized for elective or emergency surgery. Current trends in pediatric surgery have led to many operations being performed on an outpatient basis, especially myringotomies and hernia repairs. Other operations such as tonsillectomies and adenoidectomies are performed the morning the child is admitted to the hospital, thereby frequently decreasing the length of hospital stay to one night.

In addition to general concerns and fears of each age group discussed earlier in this chapter, specific fears related to surgery and anesthesia are listed below:[30,47]

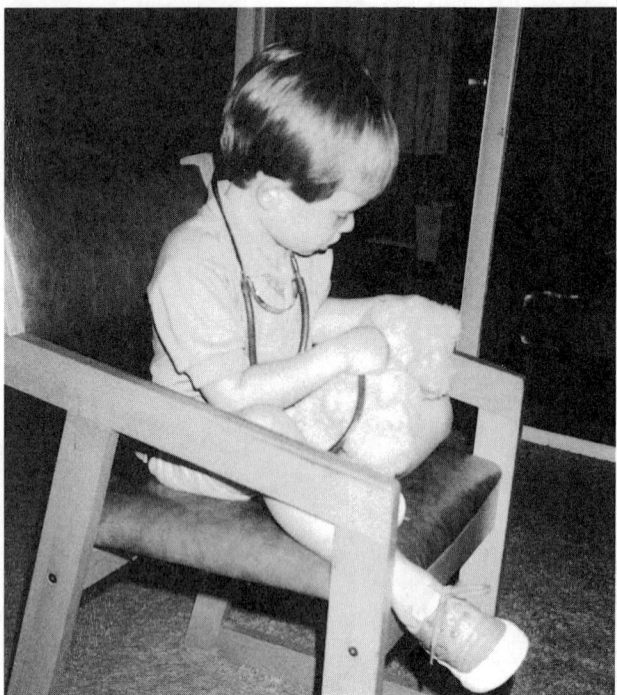

FIGURE 23-4
After a procedure, the young child can express feelings through play.

- Early childhood—Separation from family, unfamiliar environment.
- Middle childhood—Fear of the operation, mutilation.
- Preadolescence—Loss of control while under anesthesia, death.
- Adolescence—Loss of control while under anesthesia, death.

Preparation for Surgery

Preparation of the child for surgery is extremely important and has been the focus of much research.[45] Preparation for elective surgery follows the guidelines presented in Table 23-4 with specific information added for the particular operation. Preparation should be started in the physician's office by the physician or the nurse and continued at home by parents. Preoperative assessment of the child's knowledge should be done by the nurse when the child is admitted to the hospital. The child admitted the day of surgery must go to the hospital or clinic the day before admission for laboratory work and anesthesia evaluation. At this time, the nurse can assess the child's knowledge and provide clarification and additional information as needed.

Preoperative medical orders for the pediatric patient vary depending on age and body size. Orders related to fluid intake may vary. Betts and Downs recommend the following:[5]

- No milk or solids be given within 12 hours of induction of anesthesia.
- Clear liquids with glucose be given up until 4 hours before induction in infants 0 to 6 months, 6 hours for children 6 months to 3 years, and 8 hours for those over 3 years of age.

If surgery is delayed, intravenous (IV) fluids should be started on infants to decrease the possibility of dehydration.

Oral fluid restriction can be particularly difficult for infants and their parents. An infant's cries due to hunger can be extremely distressing. The parents should understand the rationale for the restriction of fluids. The nurse can suggest alternative comfort measures such as holding, rocking, and walking. In instances where parents are frustrated, the nurse can offer to hold the child for awhile to give the parents a break.

Whenever possible, children, especially infants and toddlers, are scheduled for surgery early during the day to decrease the amount of time the child must remain NPO (nothing by mouth). The nurse can serve as an advocate by ensuring that the child is scheduled early if this is possible. When the child is not taken to the operating room as soon as expected, the nurse can try to find out why there is a delay and when the child is expected to go to surgery.

The type and amount of preoperative medication depend not only on age and weight of the child, but also on the preference of the anesthesiologist. The current trend is to give either no medication[42] or medication by mouth instead of injection.[5] Because injections are usually remembered as the most traumatic experience of hospitalization, they should be eliminated as much as possible. When preoperative sedation is given, the following protocols[5] are recommended:

- 0 to 6 months—Belladonna.
- 6 to 12 months—Belladonna and sedative.
- >12 months—Belladonna, sedative, and narcotic.

Agents used are atropine or scopolamine (belladonna derivatives); pentobarbital or Valium (sedatives); and morphine or Demerol (narcotics) given intramuscularly or by mouth, depending on the medication and the physician's orders. When preparing the preoperative medication, the nurse must validate the order and calculations with another nurse to decrease the possibility of over- or undermedication of the child before surgery.

Preps, procedures that prepare a certain body part for surgery, are rarely ordered for children unless bowel surgery or bone surgery is scheduled. Examples of preps used in children include enemas and irrigations for bowel surgery, and scrubs, showers, or baths with special soaps for bone surgery. When preps are included in preoperative care, both the child and parents must receive appropriate explanations.

Parental consent is necessary for all pediatric surgical procedures. If parents are not present in the hospital, they must be contacted by telephone, following hospital policy for obtaining consent. The legal responsibility for making sure that the parents are giving informed consent is the responsibility of the physician. If the child is in someone else's custody (e.g., Social Services), consent must be obtained from the legal guardian.

The Intraoperative Period

Regardless of the type of surgical procedure, certain considerations should be taken into account for the infant or child having surgery. Differences in body size, weight, respiratory anatomy and physiology, central nervous system, cardiovascular system, energy metabolism, liver and kidney function, fluid and electrolyte metabolism, and temperature regulation must be considered in the infant or child placed under anesthesia.[42] In general, smaller body size, immature systems, and rapid rate of metabolism make the young child vulnerable to complications from even minor operations. Close monitoring of vital signs and body functions decreases the chance of complications.

Immediately before surgery, the child is subjected to several procedures including vital signs, dressing in a hospital gown, voiding, and, sometimes, preoperative medication. Continued education and presence of parents can help to alleviate associated anxiety.

Transport to the operating room is a stressful time for the child.[53] Parents are generally allowed to accompany their child as far as the doors of the operating room, but toddlers and preschoolers benefit from parents staying with them until anesthesia is induced. Many hospital policies, however, do not permit parents into the operating rooms. Allowing the child to take a favorite toy such as a doll or stuffed animal to the holding room often provides some security. The toy should have an identification band on, to decrease the possibility that it will get lost. Transport can also be made less frightening by allowing parents to carry the child, or having the child ride in a wagon instead of using a stretcher.

Induction of anesthesia can be frightening for children. Inhalation anesthesia by way of mask is generally used for toddlers and preschoolers. The anesthesia can be blown into the child's face until the child is asleep, or the mask can be placed on the child's face while he or she is still awake. A clear plastic mask or a decorative one with a pleasant smell is generally more acceptable to the child than a solid black one.[42] An IV infusion is started after the child is asleep. In older children, the IV is usually started while the child is awake and is the means by which anesthesia is induced.

While the child is in surgery, parents need information about the child's progress. Some hospitals have a surgical liaison nurse who communicates with them and operating room personnel, provides emotional support, and arranges for a visit to the recovery room.[31] If the hospital does not have someone designated as surgical liaison, the nurse can voluntarily call the operating room to obtain information for the parents. This intervention helps to decrease parental anxiety and often helps them to support the child more effectively in the postoperative period.

The Postoperative Period

In the recovery room, the child's vital signs are monitored closely during recovery from anesthesia. Special attention is given to respiratory status, including respiratory effort, rate, and breath sounds, because children often encounter respiratory difficulty postoperatively.[42] Other problems that are frequently encountered include unstable temperature, nausea and vomiting, pain, excitement, and delayed awakening.[42] The recovery room nurse must be aware of these potential problems and approach

them in relation to the age of the child and the surgical procedure.

The child is returned to the pediatric unit when partially awake and stable, but transport from the recovery room can be stressful.[53] Although groggy, the child is usually aware of the environment, but if parents are allowed to accompany their child from the recovery room or at least are present when the child arrives on the unit, the child is comforted.

Once the child returns to the room, the nurse should assess vital signs at frequent intervals until stable. Attention should also be given to frequency of voiding, fluid intake (if allowed), IV monitoring, and presence of pain, nausea, vomiting, or bleeding. Other assessments particular to the type of surgery should be included (e.g., dressings, drains, tubes). Continued assessment of the child's progress should be made through the remainder of the hospital stay. Parents should be involved in care and taught how to care for their child after discharge.

The Child in the Intensive Care Unit

Admission to ICU

Planned Admission

Admission of a child to the ICU is an extremely stressful experience for both the child and the family. In some cases, admission to the ICU is planned to follow a major surgical procedure. Planned admission allows for advanced preparation of the child, parents, and siblings.

Preparation of the child for ICU follows principles of preparation discussed earlier. Specific emphasis should be placed on what the child will see and hear. For example, IV tubing, nasogastric tubes, catheters, and endotracheal tubes can be shown to the child with simple explanations of the purpose of each piece of equipment. Pictures of the ICU can also be shown with explanations about activities that might be going on around the child, such as people talking, nurses taking care of other patients, and sounds of monitors and ventilators. The child should also be told how frequently their parents will be allowed to visit.

Parents must also be prepared for admission of a child to the ICU. Preparation should include information about what they will see and hear, and procedures that will be performed. For example, parents should be told what type of equipment will be used to monitor their child. In some institutions, parents are allowed to tour the ICU and are given an opportunity to meet some of the staff who will be caring for their child.[12] The shock of seeing strange equipment and hearing unfamiliar noises when their child is admitted is thereby diminished.

Emergency Admission

Emergency admission of the child to the ICU is more stressful than a planned admission and is the result of sudden acute illness, complication of an illness, or trauma.[12] The child may be critically ill, and the prognosis may be unknown. The alert child should be prepared for the flurry of events surrounding him. Often, however, the child is not alert, and the focus of preparation is the family.

Nurses play an important role in reducing the stressors experienced by the family. The nurse should talk with parents before they visit the child in the ICU to prepare them for their child's appearance and to explain equipment that is being used. The nurse can also offer emotional support to parents by spending time with them, answering questions, and clarifying misconceptions. Behaviors that parents might observe in the child such as confusion, unresponsiveness, and aggressive behavior should also be discussed.

Sibling visitation can decrease fears, increase understanding, and give them an opportunity to share in the family's situation.[41] Like parents, siblings should be prepared for the child's appearance and for sights and sounds in the unit.

Stressors in the Intensive Care Unit

Invasive procedures that cause pain and discomfort have been identified as the worst stressors experienced by children in the ICU. Other stressors involve physical factors such as sleep deprivation; environmental factors such as exposure to equipment, seeing other patients, noise, lights, and health care worker activities; social stressors such as separation from family and friends; and psychological factors such as lack of knowledge and understanding, lack of privacy, and parental behavior.[32,46]

Sensory overload is also a problem for the child in the ICU. The ICU is a complex and active environment. Factors such as lighting, crowding, unpleasant smells, painful touch, and noise contribute to sensory overload.[3] Sensory overload intensifies stressors and can lead to ineffective coping.

Stressors cannot be eliminated completely; however, nurses can decrease the amount of stimuli by reducing noise around patients and dimming lights, especially at night. Other nursing interventions that focus on decreasing the stressors of the ICU include liberal parental visitation, including the child in medical conversations at the bedside or removing these conversations from the bedside, and providing for the child's privacy and control.[32]

The child in the ICU can also develop *sensory deprivation* as a result of care that focuses on machines and procedures.[37] When the child is attached to several monitoring devices (e.g., cardiac, respiratory, central venous pressure), has tubes inserted into several body orifices (e.g., nasogastric tubes, urinary catheters, IV lines, chest tubes), and needs procedures performed frequently (e.g., chest physiotherapy, suctioning, blood tests), emotional needs may be overlooked. While performing procedures and monitoring body functions, the nurse should incorporate aspects of emotional care such as talking to, touching, and holding the child. A consistent caregiver who focuses on the emotional needs as well as the physical needs of the child, can reduce the likelihood of sensory deprivation.

Several research studies by Miles and others have focused on parental reactions to ICU. Their conceptual framework categorizes stressors affecting parents as sit-uational, personal, and environmental.[27] One investigation identified sources of environmental stress.[27] Seventy-nine stressors were identified and grouped into eight dimensions: sights and sounds, child's appearance, procedures, child's behavior, child's emotions, staff communication, staff behaviors, and parental role deprivation. The results of this study were used in developing the Parental Stressor Scale: Pediatric Intensive Care Unit (PSS:PICU) to assess parents' perceptions of stressors in the ICU.

The instrument was used in a later study to compare the amount of stress experienced by mothers and fathers of children in the ICU. Results of the study indicated that mothers and fathers found the experience equally stressful.[26] Further research compared the amount of stress experienced by parents with planned admission of a child to the ICU and those who experienced an unexpected admission of their child. Those who experienced an unexpected admission demonstrated significantly higher stress levels than those who knew in advance that their child would be admitted.[12]

The intensity of the stressors experienced by parents can be diminished by providing ongoing information about the child's condition, treatments, and how the child is responding to care. The nurse can also provide emotional support to the parents and explain how they can help their child.[28]

Discharge

Discharge planning should begin early during the hospital stay. The amount of planning required depends on the illness and the resources available to the family. Essential components of discharge planning include:

- Arrangements for follow-up health care (e.g., physician, outpatient clinic, health department, visiting nurse association, rehabilitation services).
- Facilitating contact with community resources as needed (e.g., social services for financial support, developmental center for evaluation).
- Discharge teaching about medications, diet, activity, signs of complications, anticipatory guidance for well-child care, post-hospital adjustment, and needs specific to the illness/injury.

Post-Hospitalization Adjustment

The child's behavior after hospitalization depends on many factors including age, personality, and the ability to cope with the experience. Research also suggests that the amount of preparation the child receives and whether parents stay with the child during hospitalization affect how the child responds after discharge.[45]

Regressive behavior after discharge is frequently related to the separation from family and the home environment while hospitalized.[37] Children may also have nightmares or difficulty sleeping.[48]

The nurse should include information about post-hospital adjustment in preparation of parents before admission of the child or early during the hospital stay, and

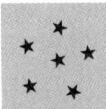

Ideas for Nursing Research

Hospitalization is difficult for both the child and the family, and stress is felt by all. Much research has been done on responses of various age groups and coping mechanisms, but more needs to be done so that the needs of children and their families can be met. The following areas should be explored:

- Compare perceptions of the role of the child health nurse as viewed by parents of hospitalized children and child health nurses.
- Compare responses of children hospitalized for the first time with those who have had previous hospitalizations.
- Identify stressors of children hospitalized on the pediatric unit.
- Identify stressors of parents of children hospitalized on the pediatric unit.
- Compare responses to hospitalization of children whose admission was scheduled to those who had an emergency admission.
- Evaluate effects of hospital orientation programs for well children.
- Compare posthospitalization responses in children who received advanced preparation for hospitalization with those who did not.

during preparation for discharge. Parents should be encouraged to help their child return to normal activities as soon as possible.[37] They should also be encouraged to let the child act out feelings about the hospitalization through role playing, drawings, play with equipment, and play with dolls. Not all children have difficulty after they return home; however, if parents are informed before discharge that their child may have some difficulty readjusting to the home environment and how they can help, they can assist the child more effectively.

Summary

Hospitalization of the child can be a stressful experience for the child, parents, and siblings. The nurse in the child health setting is in a unique position to provide the psychosocial support, advocacy, and education needed by the family. Some of the trauma generally associated with admission, procedures, surgery, and intensive care can be alleviated by using a family-centered developmental approach that prepares the child, parents, and siblings for the experience.

References

1. Alexander, D., White, M. & Powell, G. (1986). Anxiety of non-rooming-in parents of hospitalized children. *Child Health Care, 15,* 14–20.
2. Algren, C. L. (1985). Role perception of mothers who have hospitalized children. *Child Health Care, 14,* 6–9.
3. Baker, C. F. (1984). Sensory overload and noise in the ICU: Sources of environmental stress. *Critical Care Quarterly, 6*(4), 66–80.
4. Baretich, D. M., Stephenson, P. A., & Igoe, J. B. (1989). Using art to understand children's perceptions of roles in physician's office visits. *Pediatric Nursing, 15,* 355–360.
5. Betts, E. K., & Downes, J. J. (1986). Anesthesia. In K. J. Welch, J. G. Randolph, M. M. Ravitch, J. A. O'Neill, Jr & M. I. Rowe (Eds.) *Pediatric surgery* (4th ed., pp. 50–67). Chicago: Year Book.
6. Betz, C. L. (1982). After the operation—Postprocedural sessions to allay anxiety. *MCN: American Journal of Maternal Child Nursing, 7,* 260–263.
7. Betz, C. L., & Poster, E. C. (1984). Incorporating play into the care of the hospitalized child. *Issues in Comprehensive Pediatric Nursing, 7,* 343–355.
8. Byers, M. L. (1987). Same day surgery: A preschooler's experience. *Maternal Child Nursing Journal, 16,* 277–282.
9. Craft, M. J., & Wyatt, N. (1986). Effect of visitation upon siblings of hospitalized children. *Maternal Child Nursing Journal, 15,* 47–59.
10. Craft, M. J., Wyatt, N., & Sandell, B. (1985). Behavior and feeling changes in siblings of hospitalized children. *Clinical Pediatrics, 24,* 374–378.
11. Curry, S. L., & Russ, S. W. (1985). Identifying coping strategies in children. *Journal of Clinical Child Psychology, 14,* 61–69.
12. Eberly, T. W., Miles, M. S., Carter, M. C., Hennessey, J., & Riddle, I. (1985). Parental stress after the unexpected admission of a child to the intensive care unit. *Critical Care Quarterly, 8*(1), 57–65.
13. Ellerton, M. L., Caty, S., & Ritchie, J. A. (1985). Helping young children master intrusive procedures through play. *Child Health Care, 13,* 167–173.
14. Erickson, E. H. (1968). *Identity youth and crisis.* New York: Norton.
15. Fassler, D. (1980). Reducing preoperative anxiety in children: Information vs. support. *Patient Counseling and Health Education, 2,* 130–134.
16. Ferguson, B. F. (1979). Preparing young children for hospitalization: A comparison of two methods. *Pediatrics, 64,* 656–664.
17. Gilman, C. M., & Frauman, A. C. (1987). Use of play with the child with chronic illness. *American Nephrology Nurses Association Journal, 14,* 259–261.
18. Hansen, B. D., & Evans, M. L. (1981). Preparing a child for procedures. *MCN: American Journal of Maternal Child Nursing, 6,* 392–397.
19. Hyson, M. C. (1983). Going to the doctor: A developmental study of stress and coping. *Journal of Child Psychology and Psychiatry and Allied Disciplines, 24,* 247–259.
20. Lambert, S. A. (1984). Variables that affect the school-age child's reaction to hospitalization. *Maternal Child Nursing Journal, 13,* 1–18.
21. La Montagne, L. L. (1984). Three coping strategies used by school-age children. *Pediatric Nursing, 10,* 25–28.
22. Luciano, K., & Shumsky, C. J. (1975). Pediatric procedures: The explanation should always come first. *Nursing, 5*(1), 49–52.
23. Maccoby, E. E. (1980). *Social development: Psychological growth and parent–child relationship.* New York: Harcourt Brace Jovanovich.
24. Melamed, B. G., & Siegel, L. J. (1975). Reduction of anxiety in children facing hospitalization and surgery by use of filmed modeling. *Journal of Consulting and Clinical Psychology, 43,* 511–521.
25. Meng, A. L. (1980). Parents' and children's reactions toward impending hospitalization and surgery. *Maternal Child Nursing Journal, 9,* 83–98.
26. Miles, M. S., Carter, M. C., Spicher, C., & Hassanein, R. S. (1984). Maternal and parental stress reactions when child is hospitalized

in a pediatric intensive care unit. *Issues in Comprehensive Pediatric Nursing, 7,* 333–342.

27. Miles, M. S., & Carter, M. C. (1982). Sources of parental stress in pediatric intensive care units. *Child Health Care, 11,* 65–69.

28. Miles, M. S., & Carter, M. C. (1983). Assessing parental stress in intensive care units. *MCN: American Journal of Maternal Child Nursing, 8,* 354–359.

29. Miller, S. A. (1987). Promoting self-esteem in the hospitalized adolescent: Clinical interventions. *Issues in Comprehensive Pediatric Nursing, 10,* 187–194.

30. Miller, S. R. (1979). Children's fears: A review of the literature with implications for nursing research and practice. *Nursing Research, 28,* 217–223.

31. Mitiguy, J. S. (1986). A surgical liaison program: Making the wait more bearable. *MCN: American Journal of Maternal Child Nursing, 11,* 388–392.

32. Munn, V. A., & Tichy, A. M. (1987). Nurses' perceptions of stressors in pediatric intensive care. *Journal of Pediatric Nursing, 2,* 405–411.

33. National Center for Health Statistics. (1986). *Health, U.S. 1986.* DHHS Pub No (PHS) 87-1232. Public Health Service, Washington, DC: U.S. Government Printing Office.

34. National Center for Health Statistics. (1986). E. J. Graves. *Utilization of short-stay hospitals, U.S., 1984 Annual Summary, Vital and Health Statistics,* Series 13 84, DHHS Pub No (PHS) 86-1745. Public Health Service, Washington, DC: U.S. Government Printing Office.

35. Pass, M. D., & Pass, C. M. (1987). Anticipatory guidance for parents of hospitalized children. *Journal of Pediatric Nursing, 2,* 250–258.

36. Petrillo, M., & Sanger, S. (1980). *Emotional care of hospitalized children* (2nd ed.). Philadelphia: Lippincott.

37. Prugh, D. G. (1983). *The psychosocial aspects of pediatrics.* Philadelphia: Lea & Febiger.

38. Robertson, J. (1970). *Young children in hospital* (2nd ed.). London: Tavistock.

39. Rose, M. H. (1972). The effects of hospitalization on the coping behaviors of children. In M. V. Batey (Ed.), *Communicating nursing research.* Boulder: Western Interstate Commission for Higher Education.

40. Savedra, M., Tesler, M., & Ritchie, J. (1987). Parents' waiting: Is it an inevitable part of the hospital experience? *Journal of Pediatric Nursing, 2,* 328–332.

41. Shonkwiler, M. A. (1985). Sibling visits in the pediatric intensive care unit. *Critical Care Quarterly, 8*(1), 67–72.

42. Smith, R. M. (1980). *Anesthesia for infants and children* (4th ed.). St. Louis: Mosby.

43. Stull, M. K., & Deatrick, J. A. (1986). Measuring parental participation: Part 1. *Issues in Comprehensive Pediatric Nursing, 9,* 157–165.

44. Tesler, M., & Savedra, M. (1981). Coping with hospitalization: A study of school-age children. *Pediatric Nursing, 7*(2), 35–38.

45. Thompson, R. H. (1985). *Psychosocial research on pediatric hospitalization and health care.* Springfield: Thomas.

46. Tichy, A. M., Braam, C. M., Meyer, T. A., & Rattan, N. S. (1988). Stressors in pediatric intensive care units. *Pediatric Nursing, 14,* 40–42.

47. Timmerman, R. R. (1983). Preoperative fears of older children. *AORN Journal, 38,* 827, 830–832.

48. Trouten, F. (1981). Psychological preparation of children for surgery. *Dimensions in Health Service, 58*(3), 9–12.

49. Vanek, E. P., & Yanda, C. P. (1981). Academic programming for child life education: A case study. *Child Health Care, 10,* 53–57.

50. Vipperman, J. F., & Rager, P. M. (1980). Childhood coping—How nurses can help. *Pediatric Nurs, 6*(2), 11–18.

51. Visintainer, M. (1977). The effects of preadmission psychological preparation on children's stress responses and adjustment during and following hospitalization for minor surgery. *Nursing Research Report, 12,* 305–307.

52. Vulcan, B. M., & Nikulich-Barrett, M. (1988). The effect of selected information on mothers' anxiety levels during their children's hospitalization. *Pediatric Nursing, 3,* 97–102.

53. Wolfer, J. A., & Visintainer, M. (1975). Pediatric surgical patients' and parents' stress responses and adjustment. *Nursing Research, 24,* 244–255.

54. Zweig, C. D. (1986). Reducing stress when a child is admitted to the hospital. *MCN: American Journal of Maternal Child Nursing, 11,* 24–25.

24

Home Care for Ill Children

BEHAVIORAL OBJECTIVES

Describe the population of children receiving home care.

Distinguish between professional and technical home care.

Describe the major roles of the nurse who provides home care to ill children.

Outline the primary nursing competencies necessary to promote optimal home care.

Identify significant issues that will affect the continued evolution of home care for children.

FEATURES OF THIS CHAPTER

The American Nurses' Association Home Care Nursing Standards

Home Care Bill of Rights

Ideas for Nursing Research

Care of ill children in their home is not a new concept. Historically, families delivered health care to their children at home under the guidance of a local physician. Hospitalization was required only if the illness became life-threatening or if surgery was necessary. However, home care of ill children today is much more complex, involving high-tech equipment, coordination of multidisciplinary care, and creative approaches to financing. Simultaneously, home care of children considers developmental needs of the child and family.

In this chapter the term *home health care* is used to describe the broad spectrum of professional and technical services delivered in the home to chronically or terminally ill children. Factors that have had an impact on the evolution of home care of children and those issues that continue to influence its development are discussed. Additionally, nursing roles and competencies needed within a home care delivery system are described. The chapter focuses on the home care delivery system and not on specific types of interventions. Attention is given to care of ill children and not to child health maintenance or preventive health care activities, which also may be provided in home care delivery systems.

Evolution of Home Care

Home health care in the United States began in the late 1800s after its conception in England under the guidance of Florence Nightingale. The first visiting nurse associations (district nurse associations) were established in Boston and Philadelphia in 1865.[9] Public health nursing agencies were formed in the late 1800s. From the early 1900s to the 1960s, community health care systems consisted primarily of these two types of nursing service agencies. The chief responsibility of visiting nurse associations was care of the sick at home, and these agencies were privately funded. In contrast, public health nursing agencies were supported by public funds and focused on public health activities such as infection control, health maintenance, and disease prevention. If nurses in public health agencies provided care for the sick at home, their role was to teach the patient or extended family direct care (self-care) versus provision of direct care.[9]

The first multidisciplinary home health program in the United States began in 1946 when Montefiore Hospital in New York developed its "hospital without walls."[2] This was an acute care program for patients after hospitalization, and its opening signified the beginning of convalescent home care.

The evolution of home care was enhanced when insurance companies began to include home nursing as a covered service. This coverage was first offered by Metropolitan Life in 1909, and by the 1920s, many insurance companies had followed suit. Title XVIII (Medicare) and Title XIX (Medicaid) of the Social Security Act of 1965 have had the most significant impact on development of home care in the United States. Medicare, a national program of health insurance for the aged or disabled, and Medicaid, a medical assistance program to states, became primary sources of reimbursement for home health care services.

Legislators have been inspired by the belief that home and community care systems could reduce long-term care expenditures if appropriately substituted for institutional care. Consequently, they have enacted several amendments to the original legislation to increase the scope and accessibility of services offered under Medicare and Medicaid. For example, Congress added Section 2176, the Medicaid and Home Community Based Waiver Program, as part of PL 97-35, the Omnibus Budget Reconciliation Act of 1981 (OBRA).[16] Enactment of this waiver program closely followed national publicity on the case of Katie Beckett, a 3-year-old child who survived encephalitis but, as a result, was left ventilator-dependent. Discharge from the hospital would have resulted in her losing Medicaid coverage for necessary home care. A review board was subsequently established to consider special requests to waive the Supplemental Security Income (Titles XVI, State Crippled Children's Program) requirements, thereby providing Medicaid funding for home-based care.[10]

Home care services for children have drawn increasing attention nationally as advances in medical knowledge and technology have increased survival rates of children with special health care needs. Greater numbers of these children with chronic illness have not only affected health care costs but have also increased awareness of both parents and professionals that a lifetime of hospitalization is not in the best interest of the child or family.[3] Children and families have a better chance of achieving optimal psychosocial growth and development when the child is able to reside at home rather than in an institution.[8] The home environment provides more stable routines and normal social interaction; both are interrupted during hospitalization and may result in developmental regression for the child.

Advanced technology with availability of ventilators, infusion pumps, monitors, and other equipment that can be used by trained personnel in the home environment has increased delivery of services in the home. Ill-child home care is also cost-effective when compared to hospital care. The average cost of caring for a ventilator-dependent child at home, for example, has been reported to be 87% less than in a hospital setting.[7] Studies have demonstrated that overall home care costs are 70% less than hospital costs for other high-tech needs.[7] The indirect but significant savings when home care services prevent more serious complications or the need for rehospitalization cannot be ignored.

The Surgeon General's workshop on "Children With Handicaps and Their Families" in 1982 provided a basic framework for planning comprehensive services needed by children with special health care needs.[15] Recommendations from this workshop include defining the scope of the problem, developing standards, developing systems of care, improving financing of care, incorporating principles of care into training for health professionals, and supporting research.

Demographics of Home Care

Populations Receiving Care

Approximately 10 million children in the United States are considered chronically ill.[7] The National Center for Health Statistics 1985 National Health Interview Survey showed that 3.7% of children under 18 years of age are either unable to engage in major usual activities or are limited in the amount or kind of usual activities. Smaller numbers are estimated to be dependent on technology for sustaining life.[14] The number of chronically ill children has steadily increased over the past two decades due to advances in medical and surgical technology that permit survival of children who would have previously succumbed.

Children with chronic illness include those born prematurely or of low birthweight who develop chronic lung disease or neurologic impairment due to complications encountered in the perinatal period, children born with life-threatening congenital defects that are surgically corrected, and children with cancer, cystic fibrosis, diabetes, or other health conditions that are diagnosed in later childhood. Chronic illnesses range from mild, which have a minimal impact on the child's function, to others more severe that result in a child considered "medically fragile." The medically fragile child requires routine use of a medical device to sustain life (i.e., ventilator) and daily, ongoing care by trained personnel. This population of children, as well as children with a terminal illness such as AIDS, are able to receive much of their health care in the home.

The Office of Technology and Assessment (OTA), a research department of the U.S. Congress, defined four populations of children that might reasonably be considered candidates for home care services. These clinical populations considered for home care are defined in the accompanying display.

Providers of Care

Concurrent with the increase in populations of children receiving medical care in the home, the number of home care providers has also increased. The accompanying display on Pediatric Home Care Services lists the types of home care services that exist for ill children. Differences between "professional home care" and "technical home care" have been explained as well as the boundaries of practice that exist between these two types of care.[6] *Professional home care* is based on scientific principles with professional standards of care. The providers have received formal instruction with licensure, certification, or documented qualifications to provide quality home care. Nurses, social workers, allied health professionals including occupational, physical, speech/language, and respiratory therapists, and paraprofessionals including home health aides are examples of personnel who provide professional home care.

Technical home care is product-driven with the emphasis on monetary profits to the providers. Care delivery is based primarily on reimbursement guidelines with no standards or regulations on how home care is provided. Examples of providers in this category include durable medical equipment providers, oxygen vendors, and other home equipment providers.

Central to the success of home health care is the role parents and other family members play in providing care to their children. "While professionals can offer expertise of their discipline and knowledge gained from working with a number of children, parents are the only ones who can contribute information on their particular child in all settings."[15] Parent–professional collaboration with recognition of the family as an important constant in the child's life is critical to the optimal outcomes of care in the home delivery system.

Financial Considerations

Care of children with complex medical needs is costly in any setting. Generally, services provided in hospital settings have been well covered by private and public funding. However, community-based services including physician and nursing services, social work, nutrition services, physical and occupational therapy, respite care, and family counseling are not well covered, resulting in excessive out-of-pocket expenses for families. These costs exceed resources of even the wealthiest of families. According to the Surgeon General's report, "inadequate insurance, limitations on benefits, deductibles, copayments, lack of coverage of certain types of services, and limits on maximum lifetime benefits all place significant hardships on families caring for children with special health care needs."[12]

The lack of funding is a major impediment to successful home care. In the home, private insurance companies and Supplemental Security Income provide the majority of funding for technology-assisted children. Title XIX Medicaid Model Waivers is a more recent funding mechanism that allows for services, such as high tech ventilators, not already covered by Medicaid that are usually covered in the hospital but not paid for in the home. When financial eligibility of the family is considered, requirements take into account family income but adjust for medical expenses. To qualify for assistance, families must provide documentation that the cost of services delivered in the home does not exceed institutional costs.

Nursing Implications

Figure 24-1 provides a conceptual model of the factors that must be considered in home health care and the role of nursing. This model is based on a systems theory in which all components are related and a change in one area consequently affects the entire system. Central to

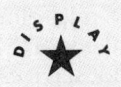

Clinical Populations Considered for Home Care

I. Children dependent at least part of each day on mechanical ventilators.
II. Children requiring prolonged intravenous administration of nutritional substances or drugs (such as children with AIDS).
III. Children with daily dependence on other devices for nutritional or respiratory support including tracheostomy care, oxygen support, or tube feedings.
IV. Children with prolonged dependence on other medical devices that compensate for vital body functions and require daily or near daily nursing care. This group includes: infants that require cardiac and apnea monitoring; children requiring renal dialysis; or children requiring other medical devices such as urinary catheters or colostomy pouches as well as substantial nursing care in connection with their disabilities.

Technical Memorandum, U.S. Congress, p. 17, 1987.

Pediatric Home Care Services

Medical care and supervision
Nursing care and supervision
Social work services
Physical therapy
Occupational therapy
Speech therapy and language therapy
Nutritional support
Laboratory services
Inhalation therapy
Appliance, equipment, and sterile supply services
Pharmaceutical services
Transportation for patient and equipment
Homemaker and home health aide services

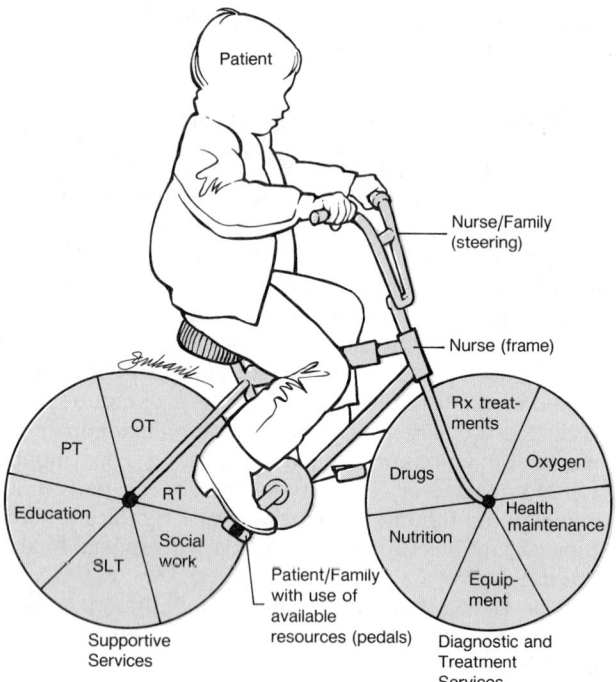

FIGURE 24-1

Conceptual model depicting the interrelationships among components of the home health care system. RT = recreational therapy, OT = occupational therapy, PT = physical therapy, and SLT = speech and language therapy.

this model is the patient and family. They provide the basis for home care, collaborating with the nurse to provide direction to the care system (steering). They control the speed and efficiency in which the system operates through their knowledge and use of available resources (including financial; pedals). The nurse provides the basic unit of support (frame), uniting diagnostic- and treatment-related factors and support services to meet the patient and family needs. Nursing draws from both biologic and psychological sciences, providing the nurse with an adequate knowledge base to serve in the supportive and guiding role.

The role of the nurse in home care is comprehensive, involving coordination and liaison activities, provision of direct patient care, education of the family regarding technical aspects of care and developmental needs of the child, and determination of financial coverage for services. In this section, each of the home nurse's roles is discussed further. The following section discusses nursing competencies necessary for these roles to be satisfactorily conducted.

Liaison and Coordination

The goal of providing home care is to promote optimal physical, emotional, and developmental functioning of the child. To achieve this goal, coordination of services in the home health care system is critical. Early identification of the child as a candidate for home care and use of appropriate medical and allied health resources in the hospital and community settings decrease fragmentation of services once the child is discharged to home. Therefore, nurses working in home care systems must have

liaison roles with inpatient hospital settings. Communication among inpatient providers must occur early in the discharge planning process. Establishing priorities, identifying necessary home-based services, and identifying barriers to services are part of this liaison and coordination role. According to the Surgeon General's report,[12]

Children with special health care needs and their families require a wide variety of services from many agencies and professionals. These services are provided in different settings usually referred to as primary, secondary or tertiary levels of care. These children need basic health care (primary care), usually provided by pediatricians, family doctors or local health clinics. They also require a variety of health, education, mental and social services provided at the community level (secondary care). These community based services must be integrated to be responsive to the needs of the families and coordinated to prevent fragmentation, gaps in service, or duplication. . . . more sophisticated care (tertiary care) is provided in children's hospitals, large medical centers and teaching hospitals. Strong linkages between the more sophisticated tertiary care and community services providers enhance continuity of care and help insure cost effective quality care within coordinated systems.[16]

The nurse must work collaboratively with the family to help balance professional recommendations with family priorities so that the program of care meets the long-term needs of the family rather than immediate needs of the child. Without this balance, unrealistic demands may be placed on the family, setting the family up for failure. Inability to meet demands results in feelings of guilt and frustration on the part of the family and may result in future distrust of health care systems. Case conferences arranged by nurses provide a means to facilitate this coordination of services among providers and with families.

Direct Care Provision

Direct care includes actual nursing interventions delivered in a home care setting. Activities such as assessing the child and family needs, formulating nursing diagnoses, developing and implementing a plan of care for the child and family, identifying resources necessary for comprehensive care, and ongoing evaluation of the child's status are included. Direct care is based on the nursing process. Using the nursing process benefits the child and family by encouraging their active participation in care. It also facilitates communication among care providers, provides legal documentation of care, and justifies coverage to third-party payers.[7]

Because home care is usually provided at intermittent, short-term visits, direct care activities must involve the child's family so that ongoing necessary care is provided in the nurse's absence. In cases where continual nursing coverage is provided, the family members need to participate at a minimum in the child's personal care needs such as bathing, grooming, or dressing. These personal care activities are not a routine nursing function, and if they exceed the family's capabilities, the need for a home health aide or alternate source of assistance must be considered.

Education of the child and family regarding the diagnoses, prescribed treatments (including medications), and means to facilitate the ongoing development of the child are also components of direct care in home nursing. Direct training of the family regarding the use of monitors and complex equipment (e.g., ventilators) is usually provided by a team of experts following a rigid training protocol in an acute care facility before home discharge. Nurses in the inpatient setting are responsible for documenting the knowledge and skill of parents in use of equipment before discharge. If parental limitations impede the ability to use this equipment safely, alternative placement (outside the home) would likely be considered. The home health nurse is responsible for ongoing documentation of the family's appropriate use of the equipment (i.e. response to alarms) in the home. The child's ongoing safety must be considered the highest priority.

Due to the complex medical conditions of many children receiving home care, little attention may be given to the emotional and developmental needs of the child or other family members. Parents desire information and support in meeting these developmental and emotional needs. The home nurse can be pivotal by

- Assessing and providing feedback regarding the developmental level of the child with attention to the child's capabilities (strengths) versus focusing on deficits
- Giving parents permission to be a "parent" to the child versus a therapist or nurse
- Identifying (in collaboration with parents) sources of respite so that they can provide for the ongoing emotional and developmental needs of siblings and themselves. Healthy family functioning is promoted by enabling the family to meet normal developmental tasks.

Another direct care function of the home health care nurse is parent education regarding community resources and negotiation for services for their child. An example is PL 94–142, which mandates every state to provide a free and appropriate education to children ages 6 to 17. This law has far-reaching implications for medically complex children, and parents need to understand how to obtain necessary educational services for their children. "It is a rare parent who has even the slightest knowledge of where to go or how to obtain the necessary resources to help his youngster."[4]

Primary health care of children requiring home care services often is overlooked, and suggests another direct care activity for the nurse. The nurse should ensure that parents (1) have a primary health care provider identified, (2) make arrangements for the child to receive immunizations on schedule, and (3) arrange for routine screening and preventive health measures such as audiology, ophthalmology, and dentistry.

Necessary Nursing Competencies

Home health nursing as it exists today blends community health nursing knowledge with acute care skills in a home setting. It requires knowledge and skill in biomedical and psychosocial management of chronically ill children

and their families, and coordination of multispecialty providers. Nursing competencies that promote optimal home-based care of children are discussed in the following sections.

Knowledge and Skills

The nurse providing home care to chronically ill children must possess a strong background in the pathophysiology of disease processes and interventions necessary for treatment, cure, palliations, or rehabilitation. Familiarity with pathophysiology of each organ system and related diagnoses ensures optimal monitoring of home care patients, thereby minimizing complications. Knowledge of medications used for chronic illnesses, including their function, side-effects, drug interactions, and route of metabolism is also necessary to promote safe care. The nurse must possess strong physical and neurologic assessment skills so that a change in the child's condition can be identified early, permitting more immediate interventions to minimize complications and possibly prevent rehospitalization of the child.

The nurse must also possess knowledge and skills in using a variety of methods for nutritional support of children. These include hyperalimentation and the care of central venous catheters and enteral feedings by way of gastrostomy tubes, gastrostomy tube buttons, jejunal feeding devices, naso- or orogastric feedings, and feeding infusion pumps (Fig. 24-2). Knowledge of caloric needs of children and the large variety of nutritional supplements on the market today further enhances home care nursing of children.

Continued technological advancements have made increasingly sophisticated equipment available for home care. The nurse needs training in specialized equipment such as ventilators, intravenous pumps, and monitors. Updates by the nursing agency regarding orientation to new equipment and changes in the use of old equipment should be provided regularly with training protocols to ensure proper use.

In addition to the acute medical needs, the nurse must possess knowledge about normal growth and development of children and must recognize variances. The ability to assess developmental functioning of children with chronic illness systematically, identifying strengths as well as areas of deficit, provides direction for management and also allows documentation of gains that may result from the interventions. Regression, which signifies a deterioration in the child's condition, will also be possible. Awareness of the untoward effects of chronic illness, family stress, and hospitalization of children on the emotional development of children must also be considered by the nurse, and interventions to support more optimal emotional development must be implemented. The nurse should also be aware of the effect of the child's illness on siblings and the parents so that a plan to facilitate their most optimal development can be devised.

Availability of community resources and how to gain their access, the role of allied health professionals including, for example, occupational and physical therapists and speech and language therapists, and the role of paraprofessionals (including home health aides) and sources

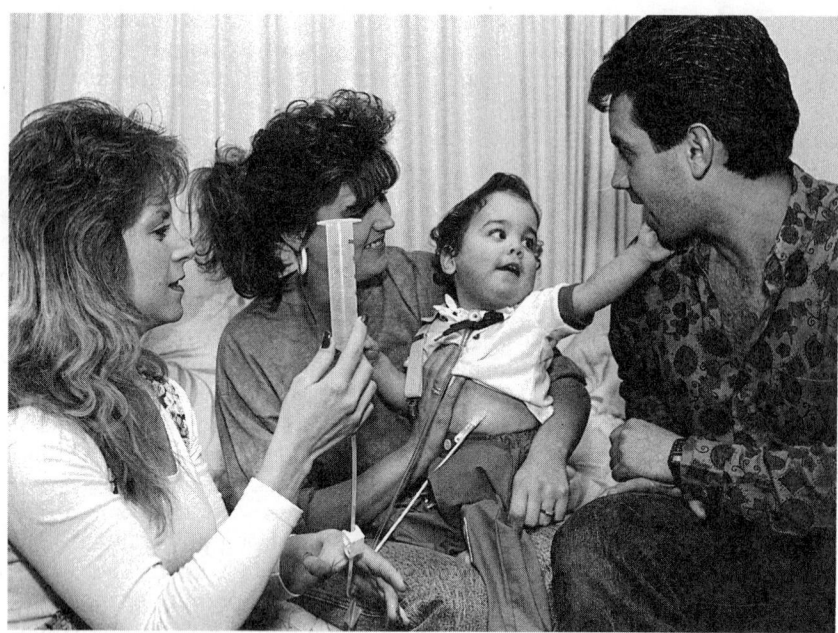

FIGURE 24-2
The nurse needs knowledge and skills to perform procedures and to teach parents to perform procedures. (Photo by Kathy Sloane.)

of funding for home care services should also be understood by the home health nurse. Use of the nursing process encourages systematic, comprehensive, and ongoing evaluation of the child's condition, with revisions in administration of care made accordingly. The nurse participating in home care of children must therefore demonstrate the ability to use the nursing process in health care delivery.

Interpersonal Communication

In addition to the knowledge and skills the home health nurse must possess in the biomedical realm of patient care, the ability to communicate with the child, the family, and other care providers is critical for success of home-based care. This ability requires the nurse's awareness of cultural and socioeconomic variance. ". . . before a partnership can genuinely exist, there must be give and take, mutual respect, and something like moral and cultural equality. Both the parent and professional must attempt to understand the other's point of view. . . ."[5] The ability to establish partnerships also requires awareness by the nurse of his or her own values and beliefs, and how these are communicated. Exercises in values clarification to increase this awareness may serve as a catalyst.

Interpersonal communication skills may also relate to the developmental level and "nursing maturity" of the home care nurse. Three developmental levels that occur in perinatal nurses have been defined.[14] These levels can reasonably be applied to nurses in other areas of child health nursing practice. These levels occur in a sequential progression: (1) technician, (2) surrogate parent, and (3) contracted clinician. The technician focuses on acquisition of technical competency with little awareness (if any) of emotional aspects in the process of providing care. In the surrogate parent stage, the nurse's orientation is on the individual patient with limited ability to deal with parents or other health team members. The nurse dictates

to others how to provide care and views himself or herself as the authority and expert. Little collaboration or mutual goal setting occurs. In the final stage, the contracted clinician, the nurse incorporates the values of others and has awareness of his or her own values and beliefs and how they affect care. Collaboration and optimal patient care occur.

Communication in home care also occurs by way of written documentation. The documentation of care given to the child and family in the home is as important as the quality of care delivered.[7] It serves as justification for third-party reimbursement and is key to the nurse's and agency's protection from liability. The accompanying display lists guidelines for effective documentation.

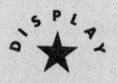 **Guidelines for Effective Documentation**

I. Maintain accurate and updated records regarding all diagnoses, prescribed treatments, and medications.
II. Content of the patient's record should contain concrete, measurable data (objective) rather than casual observations and subjective data.
III. Documentation of the patient's initial and ongoing status, and all nursing interventions (including notification of a change in status) must be included in the record.
IV. Documentation of patient's and family's education and evaluative statements related to their understanding that would support their ability to monitor properly and care for the patient should be clearly recorded.
V. Errors in documentation should be clearly corrected by drawing a single line through the entry and initialing above.

Home care agencies should offer guidelines regarding appropriate documentation of sensitive areas of practice such as child abuse, questionable practice by another member of the health team, or unsafe care delivered by a person in the family home who is not employed by the home care agency.[7] The nurse, however, remains accountable for delivery of care at well-defined standards and must take necessary action to ensure the ongoing safety and well-being of the patient.

Confidentiality is another issue of communication that must be considered by the home health nurse. The American Nurses' Association code for nurses says that the "rights, well being, and safety of the individual client should be the determining factors" in making judgments about what information is discussed "to those who are directly concerned with the client's care.[1] The nurse safeguards the client's right to privacy by judicially protecting information of a confidential nature." Various state and federal laws also protect confidentiality of patients with regulations regarding release of information in patient records.

Standards of Nursing Care

The essential component of home care nursing that differentiates it from technically based home care is that nursing practice is based on professional standards of care.

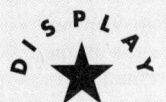

The American Nurses' Association Home Care Nursing Standards

Standard I. Organization of Home Health Services

All home health services are planned, organized, and directed by a master's-prepared professional nurse with experience in community health and administration.

Standard II. Theory

The nurse applies theoretical concepts as a basis for decisions in practice.

Standard III. Data Collection

The nurse continuously collects and records data that are comprehensive, accurate, and systematic.

Standard IV. Diagnosis

The nurse uses health assessment data to determine nursing diagnoses.

Standard V. Planning

The nurse develops care plans that establish goals. The care plan is based on nursing diagnoses and incorporates therapeutic, preventive, and rehabilitative nursing actions.

Standard VI. Intervention

The nurse, guided by the care plan, intervenes to provide comfort, to restore, improve, and promote health, to prevent complications and sequelae of illness, and to effect rehabilitation.

Standard VII. Evaluation

The nurse continually evaluates the client's and family's responses to interventions in order to determine progress toward goal attainment and to revise the data base, nursing diagnosis, and plan of care.

Standard VIII. Continuity of Care

The nurse is responsible for the client's appropriate and uninterrupted care along the health care continuum, and therefore uses discharge planning, case management, and coordination of community resources.

Standard IX. Interdisciplinary Collaboration

The nurse initiates and maintains a liaison relationship with all appropriate health care providers to assure that all efforts effectively complement one another.

Standard X. Professional Development

The nurse assumes responsibility for professional development and contributes to the professional growth of others.

Standard XI. Research

The nurse participates in research activities that contribute to the profession's continuing development of knowledge of home health care.

Standard XII. Ethics

The nurse uses the code for nurses established by the American Nurses' Association as a guide for ethical decision making in practice.

Standards of Home Health Nursing Practice. (1986). Kansas City, MO: American Nurses' Association.

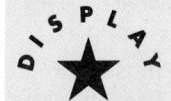

Home Care Bill of Rights*

Home care consumers (clients) have a right to be notified in writing of their rights and obligations before treatment is begun. The client's family or guardian may exercise the client's rights when the client has been judged incompetent. Home care providers have an obligation to protect and promote the rights of their clients, including the following rights.

Clients and Providers Have a Right to Dignity and Respect

Home care clients and their formal caregivers have a right to mutual respect and dignity. Caregivers are prohibited from accepting personal gifts and borrowing from clients. Clients have the right:

- To have relationships with home care providers that are based on honesty and ethical standards of conduct;
- To be informed of the procedure they can follow to lodge complaints with the home care provider about the care that is, or fails to be, furnished, and regarding a lack of respect from property (to lodge complaints with us call _____).
- To know about the disposition of such complaints;
- To voice their grievances without fear of discrimination or reprisal for having done this; and
- To be advised of the telephone number and hours of operation of the state's home health comment line. The hours are _____ and the number is _____ .

Decisionmaking

Clients have the right:

- To be notified in writing of the care that is to be furnished, the types (disciplines) of the caregivers who will furnish the care, and the frequency of the visits that are proposed to be furnished;
- To be advised of any change in the plan of care before the change is made;
- To participate in the planning of the care and in planning changes in the care, and to be advised that they have the right to do so; and
- To refuse services or request a change in caregiver without fear of reprisal or discrimination.

The home care provider or the client's physician may be forced to refer the client to another source of care if the client's refusal to comply with the plan of care threatens to compromise the provider's commitment to quality care.

Privacy

Clients have the right:

- To confidentiality with regard to information about their health, social and financial circumstances, and about what takes place in the home; and

- To expect the home care provider to release information only as required by law or authorized by the client.

Financial Information

Clients have the right:

- To be informed of the extent to which payment may be expected from Medicare, Medicaid or any other payor known to the home care provider;
- To be informed of the charges that will not be covered by Medicare;
- To be informed of the charges for which the client may be liable;
- To receive this information, orally and in writing, within fifteen working days of the date the home care provider becomes aware of any changes in charges; and
- To have access, upon request, to all bills for service the client has received regardless of whether they are paid out-of-pocket or by another party.

Quality of Care

Clients have the right:

- To receive care of the highest quality;
- In general, to be admitted by a home care provider only if it has the resources needed to provide the care safely, and at the required level of intensity, as determined by a professional assessment; however, a provider with less than optimal resources may nevertheless admit the client if a more appropriate provider is not available, but only after fully informing the client of its limitations and the lack of suitable alternative arrangements; and
- To be told what to do in the case of an emergency.

Quality of Care

The home care provider shall assure that:

- All medically related home care is provided in accordance with the physicians' orders and that a plan of care specifies the services to be provided and their frequency and duration; and
- All medically related personal care is provided by an appropriately trained homemaker-home health aide who is supervised by a nurse or other qualified home care professional.

* In 1982, the National Association for Home Care adopted a comprehensive Code of Ethics to which all members subscribed. Among the elements in this Code was a clients' Bill of Rights similar to the righs outlined in this document. In 1987, Congress enacted a provision requiring home care agencies to inform clients of these rights. National Association for Home Care. (1990).

These standards are based on current knowledge of best practice and offer concrete guidelines for the provision and evaluation of quality patient care. The American Nurses' Association Home Care Nursing Standards can be found in the accompanying display.

Home care nursing must also incorporate the Home Care Bill of Rights established by the National Association for Home Care and given in the accompanying display. These guidelines provide ethical standards that guarantee rights of consumers and protect the quality of home care they receive.

The Future of Home Care for Ill Children

Home care delivery systems for ill children continue to evolve and change, influenced by technological advances, demands by consumers of home health care, and changes in reimbursement mechanisms. The nursing profession, with its foundation in the biologic and psychosocial sciences, plays a critical role in this evolution. Without professional, scientific-based home care, the future of children and families requiring these services is tenuous.

Innovative mechanisms for financing home care services must be explored. Expansion of private health insurance plans, identification of impediments to access of available public funds for home care, and continuation of the Medicaid Waiver programs are examples. Of equal importance is further documentation of the relative costs of hospital and home care for technology-dependent children because concrete data in this area are not readily available.

Developing standards of care that are based on best practices supported through research offers quality assurance in home care delivery systems. These standards should promote consistent, comprehensive, and safe care to children receiving home care services.

Identification of gaps in current home care delivery systems offers direction for development of more comprehensive, coordinated home care in the future. The Task Force on Technology Dependent Children stated that "an effective coordinating system, available to all technology dependent children and their families is critical to overcome barriers to appropriate care and services."[10 (p.35)] This report further emphasized the overlap and contradictory mandates that exist in the various state agencies that serve children. These problems also need to be resolved.

Models of family-centered care that address service needs, supports, education and training needs, coping strategies used by families of children requiring home care, and parent–professional collaboration enhance satisfaction and positive outcomes for the child and family requiring home care services. "There is little known in nursing and other health related sciences about how families adapt to care giving demands in ways that maintain and enhance the health of the individual family members and a family as a whole."[13] Studies to date have focused on the negative impact versus the positive experiences families encounter with medically complex children.

As home care delivery in child care expands, the number of nurses providing this care will likewise in-

crease. The nurse must possess knowledge in acute care, community health, mental health, management, and pediatric acute and chronic illnesses. Nursing curricula must be developed to facilitate adequate preparation of nurses.

Summary

The population of children receiving home-based nursing care has increased dramatically over the past decade due to advancements in technology resulting in increased survival of children with chronic illness, and the availability of medical equipment that can be used in the home setting. Concurrently, changes in health care financing have allowed for the provision of care by skilled nurses in the home as a covered service.

The home environment has many advantages over the hospital environment in promoting optimal emotional-developmental outcomes for infants and young children with chronic illness. However, the entourage of multiple health care providers who may have limited knowledge of the growth and developmental needs of children and their families, and poorly defined roles for these providers, may negate the benefits of home-based care for some children. Close monitoring of the home care delivery process, adhering to well-defined professional standards of care, and comprehensive training of home health care providers are necessary to render optimal outcomes.

Nursing, with its base in the biologic and psychosocial sciences, is the discipline that must take the lead in furthering the study and development of home-based care and providing direction for the continued growth of home health care services for children.

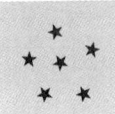

Ideas for Nursing Research

Superior nursing care is critical for optimal functioning of children with chronic or complex health care needs and their families. Research will contribute significantly to quality, standardized home care delivery systems in the future. The following areas need to be explored

- Impact of home care on family function: the unit as a whole and on individual family members.
- Models for coordination of home care services.
- Developmental outcomes of children receiving home care versus those maintained in hospital settings.
- Models of education and training of home care providers including those in supervisory positions.
- Creative approaches to financing home care.
- Alternatives to the natural home for meeting needs of children who have complex medical needs.
- Curriculum development at graduate level regarding home care of ill children.

References

1. American Nurses' Association. (1985). *Code for nurses with interpretive statements*. ANA Pub. No. G-56, ANA, Kansas City: American Nurses' Association.

2. Bullough, B., & Bullough, V. (1990). *Nursing in the community*. St. Louis: Mosby.

3. Feetham, S. L. (1986, September–October). Hospital and home care: Inseparable in the 80s. *Pediatric Nursing, 12*(5), 383–386.

4. Gallagher, J. J., & Gallagher, G. C. (1978). Family adaptation to the handicapped child and essential professionals. In A. Turnball & R. Turnball (Eds.), *Parents speak out: Views from the other side of a two way mirror*. Columbus, OH: Merrill.

5. Gleidman, J., & Roth, W. (1980). *The unexpected minority: Handicapped children in America*. New York: Harcourt Brace Jovanovich.

6. Humphrey, C. J. (1988). The home as a setting for care—Clarifying the boundaries of practice. *Nursing Clinics of North America, 223,* 305–314.

7. Humphrey, C. J., & Milone-Nuzzo, P. (1991). *Home care nursing: An orientation to practice*. Norwalk, CT: Appleton & Lange.

8. Kaufman, J., & Hardy-Ribakow, D. (1987, August). Home care: A model of a comprehensive approach for technology assisted chronically ill children. *Journal of Pediatric Nursing, 2*(4), 244–249.

9. Keating, S. B., & Kelman, G. B. (1988). *Home health care nursing concepts and practice*. Philadelphia: Lippincott.

10. Kettrick, R. D. (1988). *Report to Congress and the Secretary by the Task Force on Technology Dependent Children* (Vol. 2). Department of Health and Human Services, Washington, DC. HCFA Pub. No. 88–02171.

11. Kettrick, R. D. (1983). *Report of the Surgeon General's Workshop on Children With Handicaps and Their Families. Case example: The Ventilator Dependent Child.* (DHHS Publication #83–50194) Washington, DC; U.S. Government Printing Office.

12. Koop, C. E. (1987). *Surgeon General's Report of Children With Special Health Care Needs: Commitment to Family-Centered, Community-Based, Coordinated Care*. Rockville, MD; U.S. Department of Health & Human Services.

13. Patterson, J. M. (1988). *Chronic illness and disability*. Chronic Illness in Children and the Impact on Families in Trouble series, Vol. 2. Newbury Park, CA: Sage.

14. Perez, R. H. (1981). *Protocols for perinatal nursing practice*. St. Louis: Mosby.

15. Shelton, T. L., Jeppson, E., & Johnson, B. (1987). *Family centered care for children with special health care needs* (2nd ed.). Washington, DC: Association for Care of Children's Health.

16. U.S. Congress Office of Technology Assessment. (1987). *Technology dependent children: Hospital vs. home care—A technical memorandum,* OT-TM-H-38. Washington, DC: U.S. Government Printing Office.

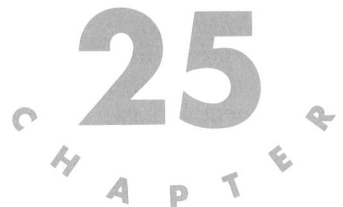

Approaches to Nursing Procedures

BEHAVIORAL OBJECTIVES

Describe the general concepts that
should be addressed when performing
procedures on children.

Explain how the nurse can reduce
anxiety related to painful or invasive
procedures in children.

Identify the general differences
between performing nursing
procedures on children and on adults.

Describe the specific techniques
required in selected procedures that
assess or restore the health of
children.

Although the scope of nursing practice has broadened in recent years, "hands-
on" procedural activities are still a critical component of nursing practice. Earlier
emphasis on rote memorization of procedural steps has given way to the conceptual understanding of the scientific principles underlying particular nursing actions and the application of these principles to practice. In addition, the holistic
approach to patient care emphasizes the integration of physical, emotional, spiritual,
and cognitive needs of the patient when practicing professional nursing.

Concepts Related to Procedures for Children

Some general concepts should be considered when the nurse performs procedures
for children. These concepts can be applied to the activities described in this chapter
and to interventions throughout the book.

Informed Consent

Consent for treatment must be obtained for all patients, regardless of age or
mental state, prior to interventions, except in emergencies. A general admission
consent is signed at the time of admission to the hospital. Many of the procedures
in this chapter are included within that general admission consent. Separate consent
may be needed for the release of information or records to another health care
facility, an insurance company, or legal practitioner; surgical treatment; some therapies that would place the child at risk; and autopsies. The term "informed" implies
that the following have been provided:

- Explanation of the purpose of the procedure
- Explanation of the expected benefits and consequences
- Explanation of the potential risks
- Description of all the alternatives
- Description of the equipment and steps involved
- Opportunity to ask questions

Because children are considered minors, the parent or legal guardian must provide informed consent for any procedure performed on a child. Parents have legal control over their children. Although informed consent is ultimately provided by the parent or guardian, older children and adolescents can provide mutual consent if an effort is made to seek their opinion.

Teaching

The parent-child relationship is a contributory factor to the child's response to a procedure. The amount of parental support that is beneficial to the child, as well as the contagion of the parents' own fears, should be assessed. Recognizing the child's cognitive capabilities and level of developmental understanding is critical. In addition, coping styles, ability to cooperate, personal fears and anxieties, level of adjustment to the health care environment, and expected degree of physical resistance are important assessment criteria.

Accurate explanations need to be provided to the child and guardian. Ideally, the explanation of a procedure should be given when the child is rested, alert, and comfortable. Developmentally appropriate approaches to preprocedural teaching (e.g., doll play, diagrams, etc.) and the use of clear terminology are critical to successful preparation. Telling what they will hear, see, smell, taste, and feel helps children of all ages. Correcting fantasies and accepting fears by allowing children to express emotions are also therapeutic interventions. Finally, as with any teaching session, children should be encouraged to ask questions and provide feedback to assess the accuracy of their understanding. These nursing actions should ultimately lead to mutual consent, which in many instances decreases the sense of powerlessness felt by the child and parent.

Behavioral Response and Coping

Nature provides humans with an innate desire to avoid pain; fear of the possibility of experiencing pain during a procedure is logical. As a child becomes cognitively aware of his or her own self as a unique physical being, an additional fear related to procedures is added—that of body invasion.

The child who is younger than 5 years of age does not have the sense of self-power, reasoning ability, coping strategies, life experience, or patience to handle anxiety or fear comfortably or the ability to process time accurately. Although possessing more experience, reasoning ability, and coping strategies, the older child is still plagued with a sense of powerlessness and fear of the unknown when preparing to undergo a test or procedure

in the hospital. Because of their more advanced social skills, older children and adolescents are also likely to fear embarrassing themselves during a procedure by crying out or demonstrating a loss of control.

Each age group has unique expressions of anxiety and fear, as listed in Table 25-9, which is placed at the end of the chapter. These developmentally based expressions must be clearly understood by the nurse and used as a rationale for selecting appropriate nursing actions.

There are several strategies a nurse can employ or suggest to reduce stress on the child during a procedure. These strategies use internal and external resources.

Internal resources are those coping strategies generated from within the child. Examples of such strategies include the following (the older child may participate in the strategies):

- Use play as a means of working out coping behaviors.
- Use distraction produced through such activities as focusing, "thought-stopping," imagery, verbal repetition, counting, or self-coaxing.
- Activate alternative motor behaviors that do not interfere with the procedure itself.
- Use muscle relaxation techniques.
- Employ desensitizing techniques (particularly useful for procedures expected to be repetitive over long periods).

External resources are those not generated from within the child. Examples of such resources include the following:

- Assure parental involvement in, or support during, a procedure.
- Provide a controlled physical environment in which the presence of stimuli is reduced.
- Encourage participation of the child in the procedure, for example, holding scissors, opening packages.

Table 25-9 describes not only common behaviors and emotions but also appropriate nursing interventions and rationale.

In most circumstances parents are excellent comforters and supporters of children undergoing procedures. When it is clear that parental involvement is not beneficial, the nurse needs to encourage the parents tactfully to reduce their role during a procedure without leaving them feeling inadequate. Frankness may be appropriate in some circumstances. In such instances, it may be best for the nurse to emphasize the importance of the parent's comfort and reassurance to the child after the procedure is completed.

Safety

Safety implies a wide range of activities used to protect children from harm. During procedures, safety principles related to asepsis, restraints, and transportation are extremely important.

Asepsis

Handwashing and gloving are of critical importance during procedures. Hands should be washed before and after all procedures, and hands should be washed between each patient. Health care providers should follow universal precautions by wearing gloves when handling any body fluids, including blood, urine, stool, and sputum. The use of medical or surgical asepsis has more ramifications for the infant with an immature immune system than for the adult.

Restraints

The skeletal system of the young child is soft and vulnerable; thus, protection against mechanical injury requires vigilance during any procedure. Anxiety, fear, pain, or simply the inability to understand the reason for a procedure place the child at risk for self-injury. The judicious use of restraints often is a requirement during pediatric procedures. There is no absolutely risk-free environment. At least three circumstances in the pediatric setting require partial or total restraint of the child, including the following:

- Temporary restraint for the purpose of performing a diagnostic or therapeutic procedure
- Restraint for the purpose of preventing disruption of therapy (e.g., dislodging an intravenous [IV] line or pulling off a dressing)
- Restraint for the purpose of preventing injury to the child (e.g., falling out of a crib)

Although restraints do have a legitimate place in the nursing care of children, the use of restraints is, legally, a basic infringement of human rights. In the United States restraint contravenes the basic tenets of freedom implied in the Constitution. Most states have specific laws governing the use of restraint. In Canada, restraints contradict the principle of inviolability of the person and the rights and freedoms recognized under the Civil Code, the Criminal Code, the federal and provincial Charters of Rights and Freedoms, and the Canadian Nurses Association Code of Ethics.[9]

The ethical decision to restrain can best be evaluated by the nurse through answering the following two questions:

Has the need for controlling specific movements been properly explained to the child and parents? Explanation of the need for reduced mobility is known to reduce the need for restraints in older children. With younger children, explaining the need for reduced mobility to parents can elicit their help in monitoring movement and providing the protection needed in lieu of restraints.

Are restraints being considered as an easy correction of a behavioral problem resulting from a need for more observation or attention? In some circumstances the child may need to be moved closer to the nursing station for easier observation. At other times the child is bored and needs some appropriate diversional activities. Parents can often be enlisted to comfort and entertain the child, thus precluding the need for restraints.

After all alternatives have been considered, if it is determined that restraints are needed, the nurse must then proceed to apply the restraints correctly. When restraints are used, the nurse should be concerned about helping the child maintain normal function. Information presented in the accompanying display on nursing interventions to maintain healthy function during the use of restraints will be helpful for the nurse who is using restraints for a child.

The types of restraints commonly used with children are described in the following paragraphs, and the most common restraints used are illustrated in Figure 25-1. However, restraints must never be used to replace personal attention or adequate supervision. Neither should restraints be used for punishment or negative reinforcement of inappropriate behavior or as a "convenience" for the nursing staff.[9]

Safety Strap. Safety straps secure the child by producing a T-binder hammock that can be secured at the back, thus keeping the child stationary but allowing free movement of the limbs. The safety strap is used primarily to prevent children from falling out of high chairs, infant seats, feeding tables, and so forth.

Mitts. Mitts prevent the use of the hand while allowing movement of the arm (see Fig. 25-1A). The mitt restraint allows the child limb movement while protecting the upper torso and head from finger activity that can tear a dressing, remove nasal prongs, or dislodge a scalp vein IV. The mitt should be removed every 12 to 24 hours to exercise the wrist and fingers.

Elbow Restraint. The elbow joint can be immobilized so that it cannot be flexed. The elbow restraint is used when the head and neck area must be protected. Elbow restraints prevent the child from pulling out gastric tubes or scalp vein IVs, from dislodging facial or eye dressings, or from scratching the face. The elbow restraint is usually made of flannel or muslin with several immobilizing blades sewn into pockets. It is wrapped around the elbow joint and secured with a closed-top safety pin (see Fig. 25-1B).

Jacket Restraint. The jacket restraint immobilizes movement of the upper torso and keeps the child supine in bed or upright in a chair or wheelchair. The jacket restraint prevents the child from falling out of a bed or chair while at the same time allowing for free movements of the upper limbs. It can prevent the dislodging of an upper abdominal or chest dressing or drainage tube. The jacket restraint is sleeveless, ties at the back, and is anchored in place by securing the ties to the bed frame on either side of the bed (see Fig. 25-1C).

Clove Hitch Restraint. Arms or legs may be immobilized by attaching a clove hitch tie at the wrist or ankle (see Fig. 25-1D). Such restraints are used primarily to prevent dislodging of IVs from sites in the given limb. An ankle or wrist restraint may be a ready-made restraining pad with attached ties, or it may be prepared using gauze pads, abdominal pads, washcloths, or other items secured with rolled gauze or Kerlix and tied down with cotton ties attached with a clove hitch.

Abdominal Restraint. The child with an abdominal restraint is immobilized in the supine position from the lower chest to the lower abdomen. The abdominal restraint is used primarily to immobilize the abdominal area

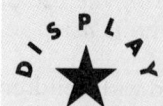

Nursing Interventions for Retaining Functional Health When Restraints Are Used

- Maintain movement of all parts of the body not restrained.
- Release the child from the restraint every 3–4 hours and exercise the restrained area for 5–10 minutes, or supervise release time.
- Explain the purpose of the restraint to the child and parents to:

  Reduce fear and vigorous physical protesting by the younger child.

  Enlist the assistance and cooperation of the older child in maintaining rather than resisting the restraint.

  Enlist the assistance and cooperation of the parents in observing and maintaining the restraint.

- Apply proper restraint considering the size, nature of the child, and area to be restrained.
- Pad restraints before securing into place.
- Ensure that the restraint is secured snugly (do not hamper circulation).
- Check the restraint every 1–2 hours.
- Ensure that the restraint can be removed readily in an emergency.
- Allow for mobility of the restrained area and improved circulation to the skin under the restraint on a routine schedule.
- Secure restraint to the bed or crib frame and not the siderails or cribrails. If a restraint is attached to other than a crib or bed, ensure that it is tied to a secure, *immovable* part.

- Provide stimulation (e.g., mobiles, pictures on the ceiling or crib sides, stuffed animals, radio, record player, or tape deck or even singing to the child).
- Encourage age-appropriate games that do not require use or movement of the restrained body part.
- Encourage parents and visitors to come as often as is feasible to provide interaction, entertainment, and diversion.
- Apply the restraint with sufficient padding to prevent chafing.
- Secure the restraint so as not to impede circulation to the area.
- Remove the restraint daily to wash, dry, and stimulate the skin.
- Apply clean restraints daily.
- Explain the purpose for the restraint to the child and the parents.
- Allow the child to have some element of choice in other aspects of care to compensate for the powerlessness of the restraint.
- Encourage the expression of frustration in other ways, such as drawing for an older child, gross motor activities like pegboard hammering for a younger child, and vocalization of feelings.
- Encourage coping by placing a child's beloved security objects within reach or vision.

---

to prevent dislodging of large dressings or drains in the region. An abdominal restraint is secured from the lower chest to the lower abdomen with safety pins. The ties are then secured to the bed frame (see Fig. 25-1*E*). Care must be taken not to secure the binder so tight as to hamper breathing.

Mummy Restraint.   A mummy restraint immobilizes the total body, leaving only the head and neck mobile. The mummy restraint is used primarily for temporarily restraining a child for examination of the head or neck or for performance of procedures involving the head or neck. The mummy restraint involves the wrapping of the infant or child in a draw sheet or flannelette blanket (see Fig. 25-1*F*). The blanket is placed flat on the bed and folded in half. The child is placed supine on the center of the blanket with his or her neck at the edge of the fold. The side of the blanket on the child's right side is pulled firmly over the child's right shoulder, and the remainder of that part of the blanket is tucked under the child's left side of the body. The procedure is repeated with the other side of the blanket. The bottom portion of the blanket is separated and pulled up toward the

child's neck, tucking both sides of the blanket under the child's body. The blanket is secured in the back by tucking in the excess or by pinning the blanket in place.

Bed Cradle.   The bed cradle protects the lower part of the body by lifting linen off and allows free movement of the lower limbs. It removes pressure and irritation by linen and protects the lower body from the child's hands. Thus, the child cannot scratch or dislodge dressings from the lower body. The cradle is usually made of a metal framework. The frame is padded with a sheet or bath blanket and secured with pins. The cradle is then covered with the top bed linen and secured snugly in place by tucking the top linens under the mattress at both sides.

Crib Cover Restraint.   The crib cover is used primarily as a preventive device against injuries incurred from the child trying to crawl over the crib sides while allowing for free movements within the crib's confines. A crib net covers the entire top, sides, and ends of the crib and is tied securely to the bed frame and legs of the crib. A Plexiglas dome or bubble allows the child total freedom of movement within the confines of the crib and

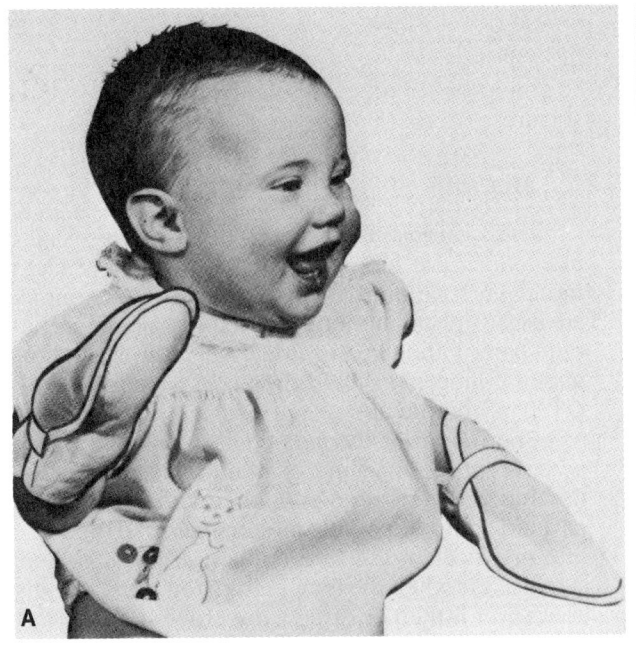

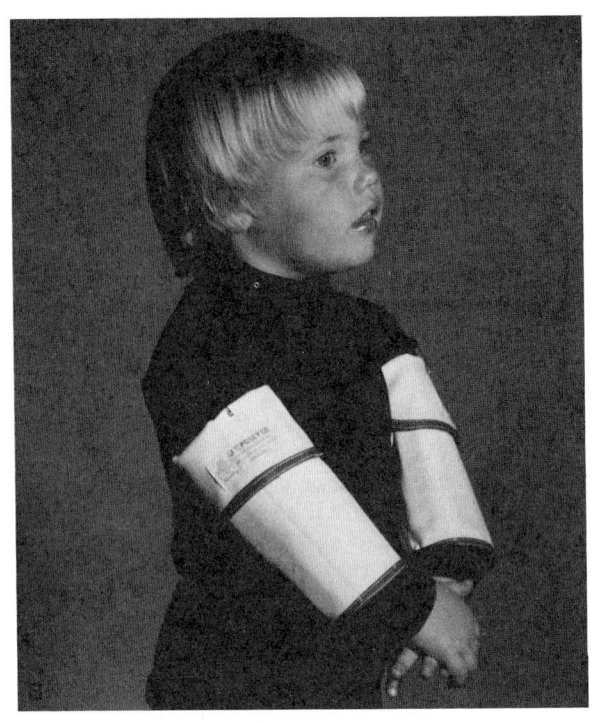

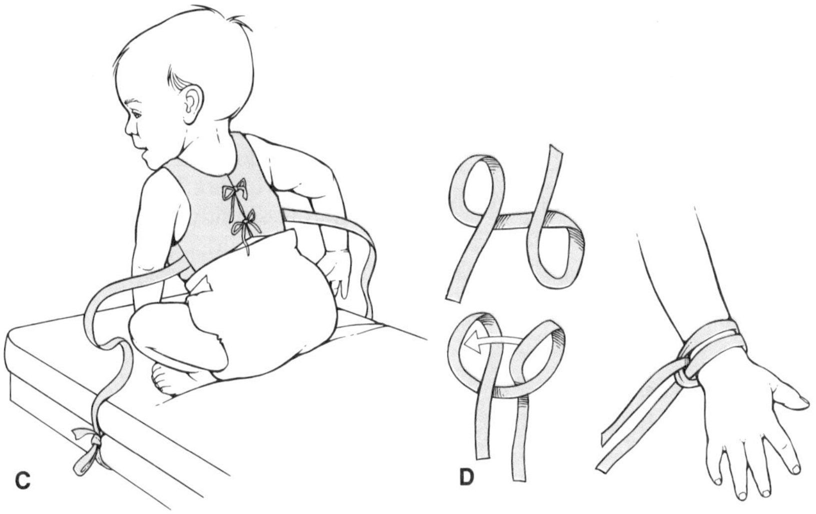

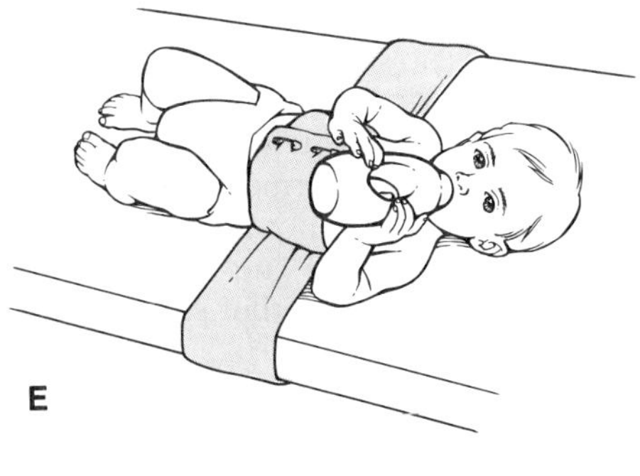

FIGURE 25-1

Safety restraints. (**A**) Mitts. (**B**) Elbow restraints. (**C**) Jacket restraint. (**D**) Clove hitch restraint, which is made by making a figure ''8'' with the tie. Both loops are picked up with the fingers and drawn together, allowing ends to hang down. The loops are slipped over the child's hand or foot. Each end is alternately pulled and tied to the bed frame. (**E**) Abdominal restraint. (**F**) Mummy restraint. (Steps for wrapping the child are provided in the text.) (Sources: **A** and **B** courtesy of J. T. Posey Company, Arcadia, CA.)

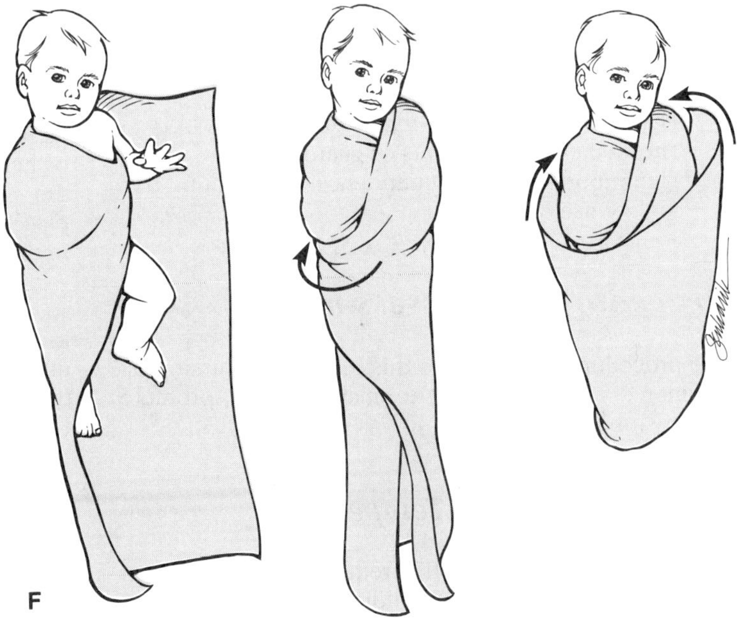

provides the child with an unobstructed view of the environment.

Transportation of Children

The principles underlying the transportation of children do not differ from those for the transporting of adults. Such principles are discussed in most fundamental texts. The main consideration in all age groups is that patients are transported *safely* and *securely* to and from their destination.

Infants.   Infants can be safely carried within a nursing unit. An infant should be carried with the head and neck resting in the crux of the carrier's elbow. If infants are being transferred to another part of an institution, they should be transported in a bassinet, crib, or stroller with safety belts securely attached.

Small Children.   The choice of transport mode for young children must be based on the child's general level of health and mobility and whether the child can walk. For example, a healthy preschooler who is hospitalized for diagnostic tests can walk to a laboratory accompanied by a nurse who is holding the child's hand. Carrying young children for long distances is unwise and unsafe for the following reasons:

- The nurse may risk a back injury.
- The nurse may be unable to control a resistant child, and both could be injured.

Small children can be transported in cribs, beds, small wheelchairs, or gurneys with side rails up and appropriate safety belts on.

Older Children and Adolescents.   Older children and adolescents are transported in the same manner, and with the same consideration, as adults. The nurse must occasionally decide on the advisability of an older child or adolescent leaving the unit independently. Many hospitals require a physician's order for such privileges. Consideration should be given to the following:

- The general health and mobility of the patient
- The general maturity of the person
- The wishes of the parents or guardians
- The importance of independence to the young person's sense of control

Procedures for Assessment

The procedures discussed in this section are nursing assessments made primarily to maintain and promote healthy function.

Assessing Body Temperature

Many factors influence the frequency of temperature assessment in hospitalized children, but two universal principles must be considered: (1) the younger the child, the more unstable the thermoregulatory mechanisms; and

(2) the younger the child, the greater the risk of febrile seizures.

Methods

Glass thermometers come in two styles: oral thermometers have long, slender tips, whereas rectal thermometers have short, rounded tips. Rectal thermometers are usually distinguished from oral thermometers by their blue base. Either type can be used at the axilla site. The glass thermometer should always be shaken down to 35.5° C (90° F) before use.

The *electronic thermometer* is a rechargeable device with two probe attachments: one with a blue end for oral use and one with a red end for rectal use. The probe is covered with a disposable plastic shield and then inserted into or placed at the selected site. A visual or auditory signal alters when the temperature registers. The disposable cover is then discarded, the probe is reinserted into the unit (effectively turning off the device), and the unit is returned to the rechargeable base.

In using the *tympanic membrane thermometer*, a disposable plastic cover is placed over the probe of the electric thermometer and unobtrusively inserted into the ear canal. An auditory alert sounds when the temperature registers. Care should be taken to avoid use of this type of thermometer in the child who has otitis media because of the discomfort it would cause.[36]

Convenient *topical thermometers* in the form of temperature-sensitive strips are available. They can be placed over the child's forehead. Depending on the manufacturer, either an actual numeric reading appears or a color change occurs that indicates a fever. However, inaccuracies can occur due to perspiration or poor circulation.

Sites

A child's temperature can be assessed orally, rectally, at the axillary space, at the tympanic membrane, or topically.

Oral.   There is no substantial difference in the technique of measuring oral temperature for children and adults. The nurse must be certain, however, that the child has the ability to hold the thermometer in place with his or her mouth closed and is not likely to bite the tip off the instrument (Fig. 25-2). The oral thermometer is placed under the tongue on either side of the frenulum in the sublingual pocket.

Axillary.   The axillary site can be used with the child in a sitting or lying position. The thermometer is placed in the middle of the axilla and held in place by holding the child's upper arm securely against the thermometer (see Fig. 25-2).

Rectal.   The rectal site can be safely accessed in four positions: supine with hips flexed (most common); prone with knees flexed; left-side lying; and prone across the lap of a seated adult. Regardless of position, the thermometer should be lubricated with a water-soluble jelly and inserted no further than 2.5 cm (approximately 1 in.) into the rectum. The thermometer should be held firmly

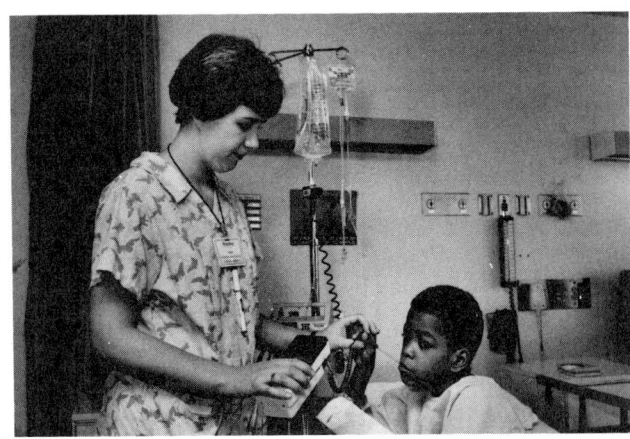
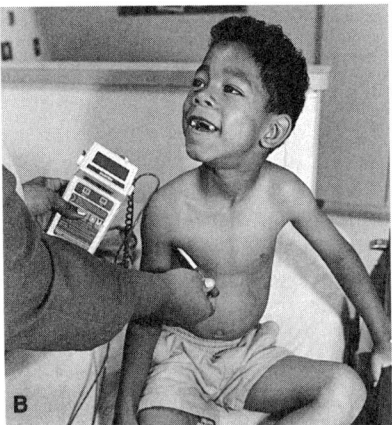
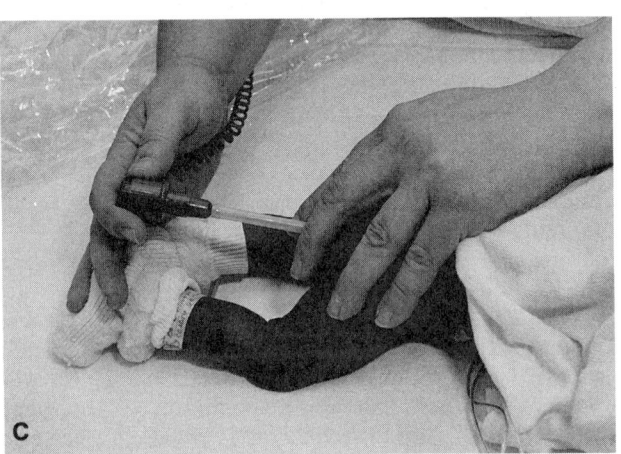

FIGURE 25-2

Sites for temperature assessment. (**A**) Oral temperature used with the older child when the child is developed enough to understand how to hold the thermometer in his mouth without biting on the thermometer. (**B**) Axillary site used with the child sitting or lying. Applicable for any age. (**C**) One position used for rectal temperature. The child and thermometer are held securely so that the child will not be hurt. Rectal assessments are inappropriate before age of 6 weeks and embarrassing when used with adolescents. (Source of **A** and **C**: Skale, N. [1992]. *Manual of pediatric nursing procedures.* Philadelphia: J. B. Lippincott; **B**: Photo by Kathy Sloane, Courtesy of Children's Hospital, Oakland, CA.)

in place and never forced against any resistance in the rectum (see Fig. 25-2).

Site Selection

There are three major factors that influence the selection of an appropriate site for taking the temperature, as follows:

- *The child's age and developmental level*—The oral site is safe if the child is capable of holding the thermometer in place in the mouth and is not at risk of biting the thermometer. Use of the rectal site is often embarrassing to older children and adolescents and should be a last resort for these age groups. The rectal site is inappropriate before age 6 weeks due to the fragility of the rectal mucosa.
- *The status of the site itself*—Such disruptions as trauma, perspiratory irritation, infection, or surgical intervention require nursing judgment in the selection of a site to assess the temperature.
- *The length of time needed for temperature reading*—This factor is only of significance if a glass thermometer is used. With the advent of electronic thermometers, readings from all three sites can be obtained in less than 60 seconds.

Factors Affecting Accurate Readings

The recommended time range for an accurate reading at each site with a glass thermometer is the following:

Oral—3 to 7 minutes
Rectal—3 to 5 minutes
Axilla—5 to 10 minutes

Normal temperature ranges according to age group are shown in the front of this book.

Factors affecting temperature in children vary. Regardless of the site selected, vigorous activity and crying increase the metabolic rate and consequently inflate core body temperature artificially. Each site can be influenced by site-specific factors. A reading from the oral site, for example, can be influenced by the temperature of food or fluids recently ingested, the presence of oxygen therapy (particularly by nasal cannula or face mask), and the predominance of mouth breathing by the child. Likewise, the presence of stool in the rectum can alter the accuracy of a rectal reading.

Continuous Temperature Monitoring of the Newborn

When a neonate requires continuous temperature assessment, a skin temperature probe (connected to an electronic monitor) is attached to the abdomen (see Chapter 11).

Assessing Pulse

The pulse is carefully measured and noted for its rate, regularity, rhythm, and quality. Normal pulse rates for children are given in the front of the book. Pulses can be palpated and auscultated in several areas.

In infants, the apical pulse is located lateral to the left midclavicular line at the third and fourth intercostal space (Fig. 25-3A). As the child grows, the apical pulse is lower and medial to the midclavicular line at the fourth and fifth intercostal space. In young children the most reliable assessment of heart rate is taken at the heart apex (apical rate). Apical pulse is usually auscultated for 1 full minute to determine regularity, rhythm, and quality. Apical pulse is correlated with peripheral pulses and should share the exact rate, rhythm, and quality. In a thin child, the apical pulse may also be viewed as a pulsation on the chest wall.

Other locations for palpating pulses include the carotid, temporal dorsal pedalis, femoral, radial, brachial, and popliteal areas (see Fig. 25-3B).

Although the radial pulse is reasonably reliable after 2 years of age, the apical pulse remains the most consistent choice until age 3 or 4 years. The apical rate is also the most appropriate choice when a child has a known cardiac disorder. Apical-peripheral pulse comparisons (e.g., apical-femoral, apical-radial) are helpful in assessing the degree of circulatory impairment caused by a particular cardiac anomaly.

Crying and vigorous activity cause a short-term increase in the pulse. Thus, the most consistently accurate reading is obtained when the child is quiet and resting. Respirations also can affect the pulse rate; a slight decrease in the rate occurs at maximum expiration. For the most part, these differences resulting from respiratory pattern are negligible and are not taken into consideration in assessing the overall rate.

Normal pulse ranges for age groups can be directly correlated with heart size (as measured by weight).[15] The greater the weight of the heart, the slower the average heart rate. With preterm or ill neonates whose pulse may be weak or difficult to detect, monitoring may be done with an ultrasonic stethoscope or a continuous electronic pulse monitor.

Assessing Respirations

The manner in which respirations are assessed varies according to the age of the child. Infants are abdominal breathers and often have irregular respiratory patterns. Thus, greater accuracy is achieved when determining the respiratory rate of an infant if the rise and fall of the abdominal wall is observed for 1 full minute. Abdominal breathing remains prominent until age 4 or 5 years. Once chest breathing begins, respirations are measured in the same manner as with adults. It is important to assess the rhythm, depth, and quality of respirations, as well as the rate (Table 25-1).

Assessing Blood Pressure

Proper equipment and technique is essential for accurate blood pressure reading. An appropriate-size blood pressure cuff size is a width about 2/3 the length of the upper arm or thigh. A cuff that is too narrow produces a falsely high reading; conversely, a cuff that is too wide produces a falsely low reading. Cuffs are labeled as newborn, infants, child, small adult, and large adult (Table 25-2). However, cuff size should not be selected on the

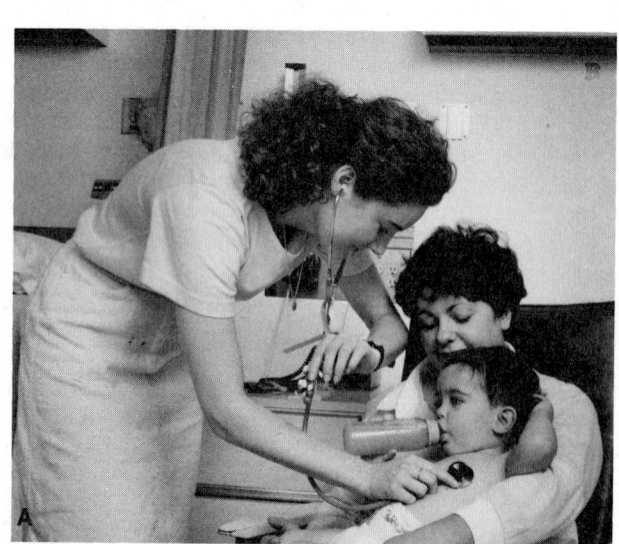 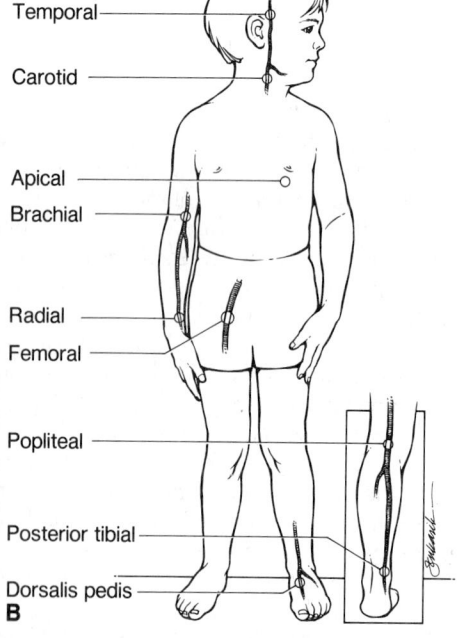

FIGURE 25-3

Location of the pulses. (A) In an infant and young child, the apical rate is taken by placing the stethoscope between the left nipple and sternum. (B) Other locations of the pulse. (Source of photo for A: Skale, N. [1992]. *Manual of pediatric nursing procedures.* Philadelphia: J. B. Lippincott.)

TABLE 25-1
Respirations in the Healthy Child

Age	Rate Range Per Minute	Rhythm	Depth	Quality and Characteristics
Neonate	40–80 and variable	Primarily regular	Irregular but primarily shallow	Diaphragmatic and occasionally labored
Infant	20–40	Often irregular	Becoming deeper	Diaphragmatic and, until about 6 months, nasal
Toddler	20–30	Primarily irregular	Primarily deep	Diaphragmatic; able to use both nose and mouth to breathe
Preschooler	20–25	Regular	Deep	Chest by age 5 and effortless
School-age	18–22	Regular	Deep	Chest and effortless
Adolescent	16–20	Regular	Deep	Chest and effortless

basis of age; rather, it should be appropriate for the size of the arm.

During examination, the environment should be quiet and the child reassured. The child should be placed in a position for comfort. The arm is fully exposed and resting on a supporting surface at heart level. Infants should be supine and children seated for the measurement. Normal blood pressure values for children are listed in the front of the book.

Methods for Taking Blood Pressure

Auscultation. The auscultation method of measuring blood pressure is the same for children as for adults (Fig. 25-4).

Palpation. When a stethoscope or electronic measuring device is unavailable, the less precise palpation method can be used to obtain a reading. The cuff is put in place as with the auscultation method, and the pulse site is located. With the arm, the brachial pulse is felt best, but the radial pulse can be used. The cuff is initially inflated until the pulse can no longer be palpated and then a further 20 to 30 mmHg. The cuff is slowly deflated, and the point at which the pulse can again be palpated is noted. The palpation technique used in older children

TABLE 25-2
Recommended Bladder Dimensions for Blood Pressure Cuffs for Children

Arm Circumference at Midpoint* (cm)	Cuff Name	Bladder Width (cm)	Bladder Length (cm)
5–7.5	Newborn	3	5
7.5–13	Infant	5	8
13–20	Child	8	13
24–32	Adult	13	24

* Midpoint of arm is defined as half the distance from acromion to olecranon. Use nonstretchable metal tape.

Source: Adapted from American Heart Association. (1987). *Recommendations for human blood pressure determination by sphygmomanometers: Report of a Special Task Force.* Dallas, AHA.

requires lightly pressing on the radial artery during cuff deflation; the pressure reading when the first pulse is felt approximates systolic blood pressure. When documenting, a "P" may be placed beside the reading to indicate it was measured by palpation, for example, 102/P.

There are differing views on what is being measured when the palpatation method is used. Some authors identify the reading as the systolic pressure, whereas others suggest that it is a mean pressure (the average of the systolic and diastolic reading). It is agreed that palpation is an imprecise measurement and provides only a rough figure.

Electronic and Oscillation Methods. The oscillation method of blood pressure measurement requires the use of an instrument powered by electricity (either direct outlet or battery) that, through a transducer, detects the movement of red blood cells through the blood vessel.

Blood pressures are often inaudible in children under the age of 2 years. For these children, a battery-operated ultrasonic stethoscope (Doppler) can provide an adequate measurement (Fig. 25-5). A standard pressure cuff is correctly placed, and the pulse site is located. Transmission gel (not K-Y jelly) is applied to the transmission probe at the narrow end of the encased transducer or directly over the skin over the pulse site. The procedure continues as in the manner used with a standard stethoscope. The transducer translates the ultrasonic frequency changes produced by blood movement into audible sounds. These sounds are picked up by the stethoscope headset. The nurse notes the gauge reading at systole and diastole (if the model allows for diastolic measurement—many models allow for only systolic measurement). The measurement is charted with a notation that it was taken by an ultrasonic stethoscope.

As this device is battery operated, it is common practice to label the transducer casement with the date of the most recent battery change. These batteries have a 5- to 6-month functional life.

Intermittent readings can also be obtained with the use of an oscillometer (Doppler instrument), in which an audible sound is produced through a transducer in the blood pressure cuff itself.

When frequent measurements of blood pressure are

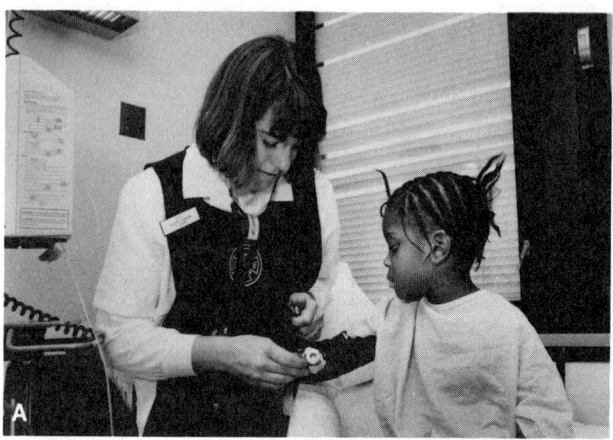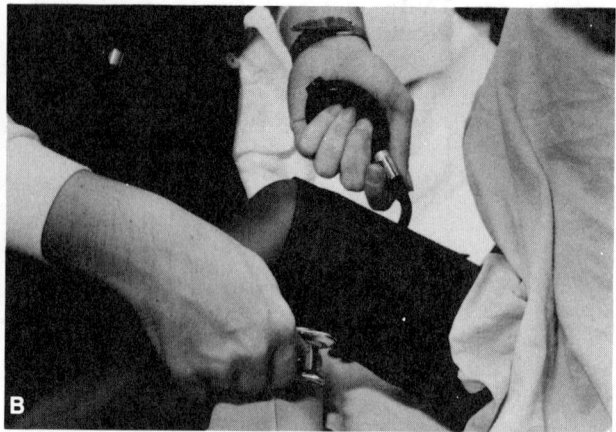

FIGURE 25-4
Auscultation of pulses. **(A)** On the arm at the brachial artery. **(B)** On the thigh at the popliteal artery. (Source: Skale, N. [1992]. *Manual of pediatric nursing procedures.* Philadelphia: J. B. Lippincott.)

required, the electronic sphygmomanometer is used. The cuff routinely inflates at regular intervals, and systolic and diastolic readings are translated into numeric values and displayed on a digital screen.

Intra-Arterial Blood Pressure. Because significant changes in the clinical status of the ill neonate may be evident in blood pressure changes prior to behavioral changes, continuous intra-arterial blood pressure monitoring is common in neonatal intensive care. The umbilical artery is usually the preferred site.[14]

Factors Affecting Accurate Readings

Except for blood pressure measurements taken by palpation, the American Heart Association recommends pediatric blood pressure readings be assessed as follows:

- Systole: Korotkoff sound phase 1—first tapping sound
- Diastole: Korotkoff sound phase 4—first muffled sound

If a particular institution wishes, a third measure where the sound disappears entirely (Korotkoff sound

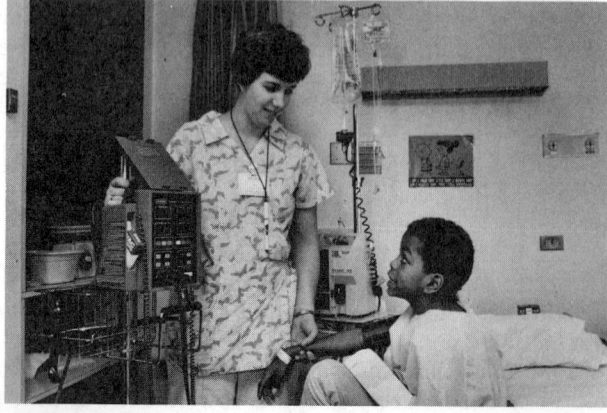

FIGURE 25-5
Doppler method of measuring the pulse. (Source: Skale, N. [1992]. *Manual of pediatric nursing procedures.* Philadelphia: J. B. Lippincott.)

phase 5) can be taken. However, current thinking suggests that this third reading has no particular significance in children.

General Considerations

The following are general considerations in assessing blood pressure in children:

- Both systolic and diastolic blood pressure rise steadily throughout childhood as a direct result of an increase in the size and muscle strength of the heart.[15]
- After the age of approximately 14 years, the systolic blood pressure levels off in girls. The systolic pressure in boys, however, continues to rise until around age 16 or 17 years.
- A reasonable estimate of the average systolic blood pressure at a specific age can be made by using the following formula:

$$83 + (2.5 \times \text{age in years})$$

This formula can be used from age 5 years in both sexes to age 16 in girls or age 18 in boys.

- Blood pressure should be a routine part of a yearly health examination by age 3 years.
- Children at risk for, or with a family history of, hypertension or circulatory disorders should have their blood pressure checked regularly (two to three times a year).
- Thigh measurements of systolic blood pressure should range from 10 to 20 mmHg higher than arm systolic measurements.
- Children who have systolic blood pressure readings below the 5th and above the 95th percentile should have a sequence of blood pressure measurements taken to test the validity of the original measurement. If these measurements remain, and there is no associated medical state that might affect blood pressure, the child is said to have low-normal or high-normal blood pressure, not hypotension or hypertension.
- Anxiety increases blood pressure; therefore, the child should be as calm as possible when blood pressure is measured.

Assessing Intake and Output

Measurement of intake and output is necessary whenever a disruption in fluid and electrolyte balance is suspected (see Chapter 26). Children have less total body mass, fluid compartment area, and total body fluid than adults. Therefore, fluid and electrolyte imbalances can occur rapidly in children and can escalate to life-threatening states.

Intake

Intake measurement includes all fluids (including IVs) taken into the body. Fluids should be measured in milliliters and recorded on a daily fluid balance record. Occasionally, the child health nurse may be called on to assess the fluid intake of an infant who is being breast-fed. This can be accomplished by accurately weighing the baby (in milligrams) immediately before and immediately after breast-feeding, tallying the difference between prenursing and postnursing weights, and translating that amount into milliliters (1 mg = 1 ml). This process is usually referred to as "ac and pc weights."

Output

Output includes urine, liquid feces, vomitus, fluids extracted by suction or from drainage tubes, drainage from fistulas or wound sites, and perspiration. Urine and liquid feces can be measured in two ways. First, collection bags can be attached over the appropriate orifice, and the resulting contents can be measured in a calibrated container. The second approach is to weigh the dry diaper before putting it on the infant, weigh the same diaper once soiled, subtract the weight difference, and translate that weight difference into milliliters. As dry diapers vary in weight, the dry weight should be marked on the diaper before placing it on the infant. The weight can be marked with a felt marker on a disposable diaper or onto a strip of masking tape attached to a cloth diaper. Output that drains onto clothing or bed linen can be reasonably estimated by pouring water from a calibrated container onto a piece of dry cloth until an area is saturated as close to the actual size of the output loss as possible. The amount of water used to produce the relatively equivalent saturated area can be recorded as the output. As perspiration can be visualized, but not accurately measured, it should be recorded on the fluid balance record with descriptors indicating degree (e.g., slight, moderate, or profuse).

Collecting Specimens

Nurses must be able to collect specimens for routine laboratory tests. This section discusses the methods for such collections: urine, sputum, respiratory secretions, stool, and blood. Regardless of source, any specimen collection should be labeled with the child's name, room number, physician's name, test to be conducted, as well as the date and time of collection.

Urine Specimens

Collection of urine specimens is common both in the health care facility and in the well child clinic. Collection of the first morning void is preferable but not always possible. Of more importance is the fact that the urine specimen is fresh. A midstream specimen is routinely requested, and it should be examined within 1 hour of voiding. Specimens may be obtained from young children in a potty chair, urinal, or bedpan. Collection devices may be applied to infants and toddlers who are not yet potty trained. With adequate explanation and privacy, adolescents and school-age children can usually provide urine specimens independently.

Adolescent and school-age children must be advised of the purpose of the procedure and the necessary aseptic practices to be used during the collection process. They need to be provided with the appropriate collection receptacle and given privacy.

Preparation. Prior to any urine collection, handwashing and the application of gloves are essential. If the parents are going to assist, they also should wash their hands before and after the procedure.

Urine specimens are collected after careful cleansing. The child should be placed on the back with the genitalia exposed. A parent or second nurse may be needed to comfort the child and to help maintain the position. In routine collections, the perineum should be washed well with soap and water, rinsed, and thoroughly dried. Washing should proceed from anterior to posterior, especially with female children.

If a sterile catch is to be collected, sterile soap and water are used. Cotton balls are used for one stroke and then discarded. In female children, cleansing proceeds with strokes moving from above the clitoris toward the anus. The first stroke goes across the meatus, and subsequent strokes move outward from the meatus. For male children, the meatus and glans are cleansed well, the foreskin is retracted, and the glans underneath is cleansed if retraction can be done without force being used. The perineum is rinsed with antiseptic solution and then sterile water. The perineum is then patted dry with sterile sponges.

Method of Collection. A pediatric urine collection bag may be used in infants and toddlers who are not toilet trained. Older children can void into a bedpan, potty, or urinal. Some older preschool boys may be able to void into a clean specimen container.

Midstream sterile specimens may be obtained through straight catheterization. If the older child is able to stop and start the stream, he or she should void into a clean receptacle, stop the stream, and then void into the sterile receptacle.

A urine collection bag is commonly used for children who cannot control the urine stream voluntarily. Following cleansing of the perineum, the adhesive strips on the bag are removed. Application varies with the sex of the child. In the female child, the perineum is stretched taut laterally. The lower edge of the bag is attached first (avoiding the anus). The bag can then be attached upward, with the labia fitting inside the bag. The upper edge

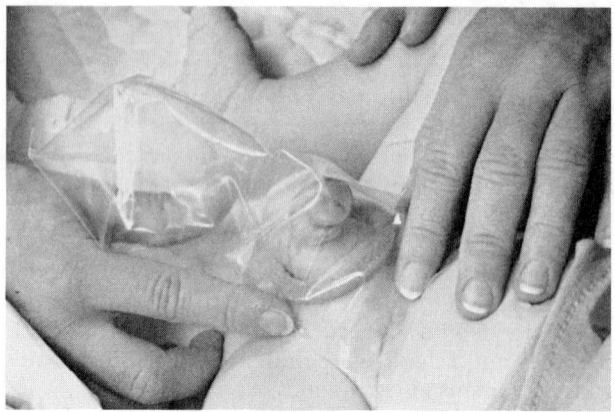

FIGURE 25-6
Disposable urine collection devices are available for infants and small children who have not yet achieved voluntary bladder control.

of the adhesive should then be attached to the perineum above the clitoral hood. In the male infant or toddler, application begins at the lower edge, with special caution to avoid the anus. The bag should be applied upward to include the penis and the scrotum (Fig. 25-6).

The bag should be removed carefully to avoid contamination of the specimen. When the collection bag has been removed, it can be sealed shut by pressing the adhesive surfaces together and using the collection bag as a collection receptacle. In other circumstances, the urine may need to be transferred to a specimen container.

A clean-catch sterile specimen is obtained in the same manner, except the bag and specimen container need to be sterile. Urine is placed in the sterile specimen container by the nurse from the straight catheter or from a midstream "catch" for children able to assist in specimen collection.

24-Hour Urine Collection. When a 24-hour urine specimen is needed the first voiding is discarded, and timing begins with the next voiding. Many 24-hour urine specimens require a special additive to the collection receptacle, so care should be taken to seek advice from the laboratory on specific directives.

Saving 24-hour urine collections from infants and toddlers who are not toilet trained may require some creativity on the part of the nurse. Several methods may be used. Urine collection bags with attached tubing that drains into a collection receptacle at the foot of the crib is the ideal technique from an aseptic and safety viewpoint.

The undiapered child lies in the center of the bed, and urine drains into the receptacle. The disadvantage of this technique is that the child must be restrained. The need for restraint can be reduced by using a collection bag with a drainage tube that is securely capped or clamped and coiled inside the diaper away from the child's hands. In such instances care must be taken to empty the bag in a manner that maintains asepsis, and the bag must be drained often enough to prevent backflow and pull on the adhesive hold.

In some circumstances sufficient urine may be collected from a wet diaper to conduct common tests on

nonsterile urine. Such urine is collected by the following methods:

- Using gloved hands to squeeze the urine from the wet portion of the diaper into a specimen container
- Placing a portion of the wet diaper into a syringe barrel and squeezing out a sufficient volume of urine with the plunger

Sputum Specimens

Older children and adolescents can cough up sputum specimens independently. Such specimens are best collected in the morning, as secretions are most apt to pool in the lungs during sleep. The contents of the first cough are discarded to prevent acquiring saliva and mucus from the back of the throat.

The second cough should be as deep as possible so as to acquire sputum from the body of the lung. The sputum should be expectorated into a sterile container, labeled, and sent immediately for laboratory analysis.

Sputum specimens from infants and young children who are unable to comprehend instructions or to perform deep coughing on command must be collected by means of a sputum trap. Gagging is to be expected during this procedure, so the child should be placed in an upright or side-lying position to reduce the risk of aspiration of gastric contents. The catheter tube is directed into the nasopharynx, automatically stimulating the cough reflex. The second tube provides the source of suction. Suction can be provided orally by the nurse or by mechanical suction apparatus. Suctioning provided orally by the nurse is likely to be gentler than mechanical suction, but the risk of specimen contamination is always present. Mechanical suctioning provides no microbial risk, but caution must be applied to prevent excessive suctioning pressure, which can damage fragile mucous membrane. Once suction is applied, sputum is drawn into the mucus chamber and trapped there. The specimen may be sealed right in the trap or transferred to a sterile container for laboratory transport.

Swab Cultures of Respiratory Secretions

Swab cultures are necessary at times to collect respiratory secretions. They may be of three types: nasal, nasopharyngeal, and oropharyngeal. The entry sites for these swabs are shown in Figure 25-7.

A *nasal swab* requires that the nasopharynx and adenoids are cultured. Specifically, the swab enters through the nares, and cultures of the outer nasal passages are obtained.

Nasopharyngeal cultures can be obtained in two ways: either through the nasal entry, whereby a flexible swab enters through the nares, bypasses the adenoids, and swabs the nasopharynx; or through the mouth entry, whereby a swab enters the mouth, curves up and around the uvula and adenoids, and swabs the nasopharynx.

Oropharyngeal cultures are obtained by entering the mouth and swabbing the upper tracheal and oropharyngeal area, as well as the tonsils.

Regardless of the type of swab sought, the following are common guidelines for the procedure:

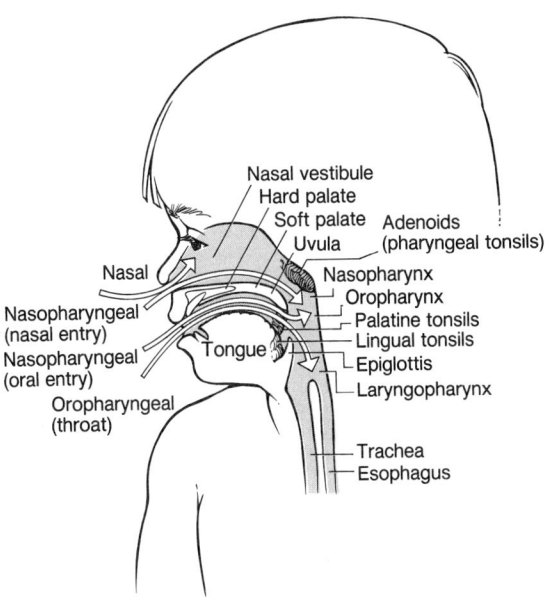

FIGURE 25-7
Swab cultures of respiratory secretions may be made at several entry sites. *Nasal entry:* Swab enters the nares and cultures the outer nasal passages. *Nasopharyngeal with nasal entry:* Flexible swab enters the nares, bypasses the adenoids, and swabs the nasopharynx. *Nasopharyngeal with oral entry:* Flexible swab enters mouth, curves up and around the uvula and adenoids, and swabs the nasopharynx. *Oropharyngeal entry:* Swab enters the mouth and cultures the upper tracheal and oropharyngeal area and the tonsils.

- Apply the swab to the appropriate tissue *on exit.*
- Avoid touching the tongue on entry or exit through the mouth.
- Use a twisting motion to saturate the swab.
- Purposely swab visual areas of redness or purulence at the selected site.
- Transport the swab to the laboratory in a medium that prevents the culture from drying.

Stool Specimens

The bowel is not a sterile cavity; therefore, medical asepsis rather than sterile technique should be followed during the collection of stool specimens. Stool specimens that have not been contaminated with urine are ideal, even though acquiring urine-free stool is difficult, if not impossible, in the very young. Urine-free stool specimens are especially important when trying to distinguish organisms that may be resident in the one form of excreta but pathogenic in the other. For example, *Escherichia coli* is expected in stool but may be pathogenic in urine.

When stool specimens are difficult or impossible to obtain, a rectal swab is an acceptable alternative even though it is less precise. A cotton-tipped applicator is inserted a maximum of 2.5 cm into the rectum and then slowly withdrawn in a twisting motion. This twisting motion ensures saturation of the swab with mucosal moisture. Rectal swabs have limited value, because most bowel organisms remain exclusively in fecal matter.

The procedure for collecting stool from older children and adolescents is the same as for adults. The child should defecate into a bedpan or a collection pan placed

under the toilet seat. A small sample of the stool is extracted with a clean tongue depressor and placed in a stool specimen cup. With newly toilet-trained toddlers and preschooler children, a training potty for the sake of can be used for the child's comfort and anxiety. Stool specimens can be obtained from infants by scraping a small amount of feces off the diaper with a tongue depressor.

When a child has diarrhea, it is often imperative to determine the organism responsible. In such instances a tongue depressor is used to collect some semi-solid stool from the receptacle or diaper. The end of the tongue depressor is used to extract the loose stool from the receptacle and should be broken off and included with the specimen. Although little stool is needed to make an accurate pathogenic assessment, placing the stool-saturated end of the tongue depressor into the specimen container helps ensure a sufficient amount.

Because many organisms in stool specimens have limited viability, stool specimens must be delivered to the laboratory quickly after collection or be refrigerated until taken to the laboratory. Many tests require a collection of stool over the course of a few days (e.g., fecal fat). These types of stool collections require that fresh specimens be placed in a metal can that is refrigerated until the test is completed.

Blood Samples

In many institutions blood samples are taken by laboratory technicians. In others, or in specialized areas, the nurse may be called on to obtain blood samples. There are common elements to blood sampling procedures, regardless of the type of procedure or site used. These elements and their nursing considerations are discussed in the following paragraphs.

Blood sampling involves breaking the body's skin barrier and thus places the child at risk for infection. Care must be taken to ensure that adequate *medical asepsis* is used do the following:

- Cleanse the nurse or technician's hands prior to preparing equipment.
- Cleanse the sampling site prior to puncture.

Adequate *surgical asepsis* is used to ensure the sterility of those parts of the equipment that either break the skin barrier or come into contact with the child's bloodstream.

Blood sampling places the nurse or technician at risk for coming into direct contact with the child's blood. Universal precautions require nurses or technicians to take precautions to prevent inadvertently pricking themselves with contaminated needles. They must also wear gloves during the procedure and use care in handling samples afterward. Mouth pipetting of capillary samples is contraindicated.[6]

A child's fears related to the procedure can be reduced or controlled with appropriate teaching and reassurance. Children should be assured that blood loss is not permanent and that the human body is constantly replacing "old" blood with "new."

The risk of localized vessel collapse and tissue fibrosis or necrosis increases with repetitive use of the same sam-

TABLE 25-3
Venous and Capillary Blood Sampling

Site Selection and Considerations	Positioning	Restraint Needed	Preparation	Site-Specific Procedural Considerations
			All sites should be swabbed with alcohol or povidine-iodine before the needle or lancet enters it.	Needles should be 21 gauge or smaller. Needle should enter site at 15- to 30-degree angle.
Venous Sites				
Antecubital Fossa Appropriate for child older than 2 years of age.	Child's arm held extended on flat surface with palm up.	Young children should be restrained. Older children may keep arm or leg immobile. Some children may need, or ask for, the security of being held or cradled.	Tourniquet may be secured *above* site to distend and visualize veins.	Skin at sites pulled taut and stabilized. Helps to visualize and locate veins. Once specimen obtained, tourniquet is removed immediately.
Extremities Dorsum of hands and feet for older children, and, occasionally, younger children. Difficult to locate in infants and toddlers.	Child's hand or foot on flat surface: hand is held palm down, foot is placed flat.			
External Jugular Vein Appropriate for infants and toddlers when peripheral veins are unavailable.	Child is supine on examining table. Shoulders remain on table while the head and neck are held and supported securely off table. Head is turned to one side a maximum of 60 degrees from the midline.	Mummy restraint. It is critical that the child be immobile.	Sternocleidomastoid muscle stretched to expose vein. Care must be taken not to overstretch neck area and disrupt ventilation.	Secure immobilization of head and neck critical. Crying encouraged because it helps distend and visualize vein.
Femoral Vein Appropriate for infants and toddlers. Contraindicated when child is immobile or on bedrest because of the risk of thrombophlebitis and emboli.	Child supine on examining table. Person standing at child's head secures child's upper body with the upper arms. The lower arms and hands secure child's knees so they are flexed and abducted (frog-leg position).	Upper body and knees firmly restrained. It is critical that the child be immobile.	Genital area covered to prevent urinary contamination of site.	Skin below site should be pulled taut and stabilized.
Scalp Vein Appropriate for infants and toddlers. Scalp veins are smaller than external jugular or femoral veins; thus, blood flow will be slow. Site will need to be shaved.	Child's head secured in a side-lying position with the scalp area unobstructed.	Mummy restraint.	Small tourniquet may be placed around the head *below* the site to distend and visualize veins.	Head held securely and traction provided at site. Needle should puncture vein against flow; helps speed entry of blood into receptacle. Once specimen is obtained, tourniquet removed immediately.
Internal Jugular Vein Used when other sites have failed. Risky because vein cannot be visualized and must be entered blindly. A nurse would not select this site without expert assistance.				

(Continued)

TABLE 25-3
(Continued)

Site Selection and Considerations	Positioning	Restraint Needed	Preparation	Site-Specific Procedural Considerations
Peripheral Capillary Sites				
Heel				
Appropriate for child younger than 2 years	Distal third of the foot is held securely around the toes, exposing the bottom outer aspect of heel.	Firm grasp of foot, heel, or great toe needed. For finger sites, hand needs to be held securely. Additional restraint dependent on child and circumstances. Goal of additional restraint is to prevent sudden movement or grabbing for lancet.	Warm compress applied to site for 5 to 10 minutes will produce vessel dilation.	Lance must be sharp. Lancet should strike site only once with quick sharp stab. To prevent complication involving bones close to site, lancet should go no deeper than 2 mm in a finger site or 2.5 mm in a heel or great toe site. Tissue should never be squeezed or "milked"; such activities decrease blood flow. Blood should be extracted by pipette or placed on slide or filter paper for transport to laboratory.
Middle Three Fingers				
Appropriate for child older than 2 years.	Finger is held securely at its base. Lancet should strike padded part of fingertip.			
Earlobe				
Appropriate for child older than 2 years.	Upper part of earlobe is held securely. Lancet should strike bottom of earlobe.			
Great Toe				
Appropriate for child older than 2 years if finger and earlobe sites cannot be used.	Great toe should be separated and held securely at base. Lancet should strike pad on underside of toe.			

pling site. When successive samples of blood must be taken, sites (or different aspects of the same site) should be rotated.

Venous and Capillary Sampling. Table 25-3 outlines site selection, necessary restraints, positioning, preparation at site, and specific considerations. Positioning for major sites are shown in Figure 25-8. After the blood sample has been obtained and the needle or lancet has been removed, pressure should be applied to the site with a gauze pad. Alcohol swabs or cotton balls are inappropriate: alcohol swabs produce unnecessary pain, and cotton balls can stick to the site. Pressure should be applied to sites as follows:

- Antecubital fossa, extremities, scalp vein—2 to 5 minutes
- External jugular and femoral veins—5 to 10 minutes
- Peripheral capillaries—up to 2 minutes

Once bleeding has subsided, the site should be covered with a Band-Aid. Venous sites should be observed regularly for bleeding and hematomas for about an hour after completion of the procedure. Pain at capillary sites can be reduced somewhat with the application of warm compresses.

Arterial Blood Sampling. Extracting arterial blood samples requires specialized training and would not be within the realm of responsibility of the bedside child health nurse. The nurse would be responsible, however, for observing an arterial sampling site for postprocedural complications, such as hemorrhage or hematomas. Arterial sampling sites used for children include the radial, brachial, dorsalis pedis, and temporal artery sites. Because of the risk of hemorrhage and arterial collapse, arterial sampling is used primarily when capillary sampling produces inexact results (e.g., blood gas analysis). In most

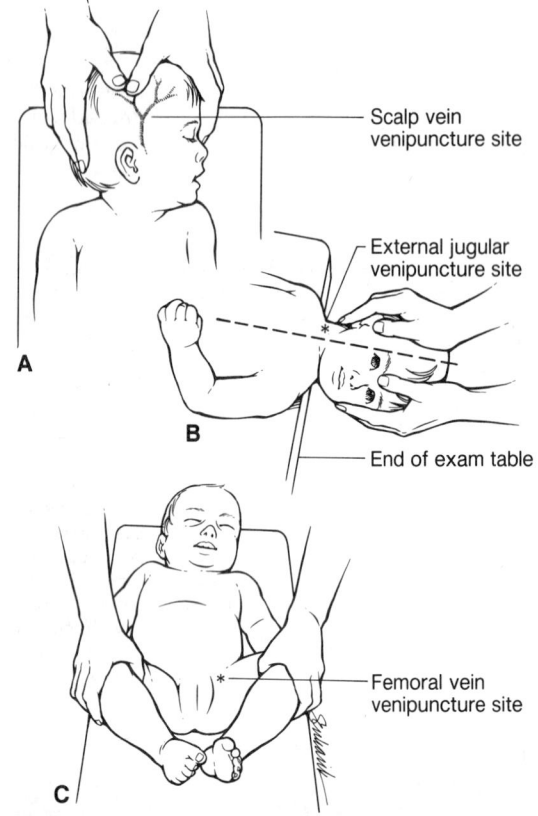

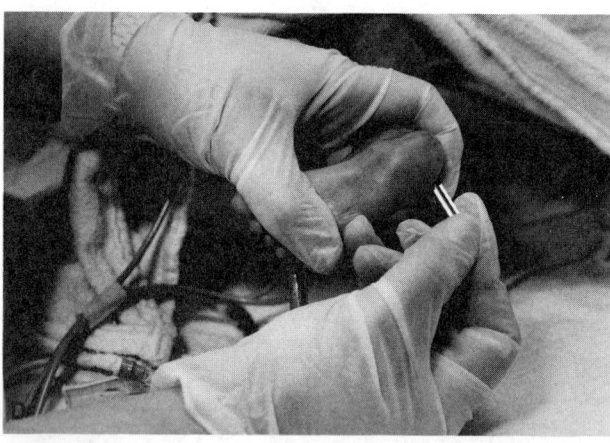

FIGURE 25-8
Positioning and sites for venipuncture and capillary blood sampling in infants and young children. (**A**) Scalp vein venipuncture site. (**B**) External jugular vein venipuncture site. (**C**) Femoral vein venipuncture site. (**D**) Capillary (heel stick) puncture site. (Source of **D**: Skale, N. [1992]. *Manual of pediatric nursing procedures*. Philadelphia: J. B. Lippincott.)

instances, however, capillary blood, which has been extracted correctly and analyzed quickly, produces satisfactory laboratory results.

Procedures Involving Therapeutic Intervention

The ill child requires a variety of therapies. In many instances, the bedside nurse is the one who manages the child's care during the therapy. Such therapies require responsible actions on the nurse's part. The procedures in this section include medication therapy, IV therapy, blood transfusion, thermoregulation, oxygenation, and procedures involving immunoregulation.

Administering Medications in the Pediatric Setting

An understanding of the actions of drugs in children, developmental issues, and correct calculations are necessary for safe administration of medications to children. The general principles of medication delivery and procedural steps, rationale, and measurement techniques can be obtained from any nursing fundamentals or pharmacology book. The physician is responsible for the determination of a therapeutic dose of medications; the nurse is responsible for evaluating the accuracy of the dose prior to administration and determining the safest method for administration.[6]

Pharmacotherapeutics and Children

Careful consideration of the manner in which medication is absorbed, distributed, metabolized, and excreted is essential to therapeutic response in the delivery of medications to children. General and systemic developmental issues related to drug therapy in children must be addressed.

Absorption. Gastric *p*H is more alkaline in infants. Levels of acidity approximating those of an adult are not usually reached until the preschool years or later.[1] Thus, medications that react positively to an alkaline environment (e.g., penicillin) are more readily absorbed in infants and toddlers. Medications that react unfavorably to an alkaline environment (e.g., phenobarbital) are absorbed poorly in those same infants and toddlers.

Inadequate production of intestinal flora in the neonate and very young infant reduces the digestion and absorption of drugs dependent on such flora. Neonates and young infants have fewer intestinal enzymes that are essential for the absorption of some drugs. Additionally, intestinal motility is decreased in infancy, suggesting that absorption time should be longer than with older children and adults. However, decreased intestinal motility is more than compensated for by a relatively short intestinal tract and faster transit time. The overall effect is decreased intestinal absorption.

Subcutaneous and intramuscular absorption of medications is unpredictable in infants and young children due to peripheral vasomotor instability and decreased muscle tone. Thus, the IV route is often preferable.[1]

Topical drugs are absorbed by children at the same rate as adults. However, because children have a greater surface area relative to total body mass, topical drugs are absorbed more completely.[1]

Distribution. Incomplete myelinization renders the blood-brain barrier ineffective in preventing drugs from reaching the brain in young children. Neonates and infants are especially susceptible to increased respiratory depressant effects of narcotics and general anesthetics.[10]

Immaturity of enzyme systems and individual specific enzymes affect the distribution of drugs that use enzymes as "carriers." Some enzyme receptors in children have an increased affinity for drugs, whereas others have a decreased affinity.[6]

Infants produce fewer plasma proteins to which drugs can bind. Because only unbound drugs produce a pharmacologic effect, infants are exposed to an increased risk of toxicity when given drugs with a protein-binding affinity. Neonates are at greater risk of developing kernicterus when given drugs with a high protein-binding affinity.[1] Such drugs compete with bilirubin for protein-binding sites, leaving the neonate susceptible to excessive free bilirubin in the bloodstream.

A larger percentage of total body weight is fluid in infants and children, and more of this fluid is in the extracellular compartment. Consequently, water-soluble drugs are diluted more rapidly in children, making them less effective. This rapid dilution suggests that for water-soluble drugs, loading doses for the desired plasma concentration may need to be higher in infants and young children. Body fluid composition makes young children prone to dehydration during illness. The risk of drug toxicity is increased in these circumstances.[10]

Fat distribution increases with age. Thus, infants and young children are at greater risk for poor distribution of fat-soluble drugs.

Metabolism. In the neonatal period, liver immaturity results in poor metabolism of drugs. As the liver matures, the opposite state becomes more prevalent. The liver is twice the percentage of total body weight in infants and young children than it is in adults. Thus, infants and young children metabolize some drugs more rapidly. Children also metabolize drugs requiring oxidation more rapidly than adults.

Excretion. The liver has a role in drug excretion and thus its maturity has implications for this process. However, the major organ responsible for drug excretion is the kidney. The rate and success of such excretion is dependent on the glomerular filtration rate, the tubular reabsorption rate, and the tubular secretion rate. The ability to concentrate urine at close to adult levels does not occur until somewhere between 3 and 7 months of age. Adult functional maturity, including adult urine volume levels, does not occur until 3 to 4 years of age. Thus, considerable care must be taken to prevent drug toxicity, particularly in the first 3 months of life.

Developmental Considerations

Some medications have serious effects on growth and development. For example, tetracycline binds readily to calcium and can decrease bone growth from the prenatal period up to approximately 8 years of age.[43] The drug can cause permanent discoloration of developing teeth during that same period. Corticosteroids suppress overall growth, so care must be taken with the use of these drugs in children, particularly long-term use for chronic health problems. Care must be taken with regard to the types of drugs given, amounts of drugs given, sites of drug delivery, spacing of drug doses, and observations for side effects and toxicity. Developmental considerations are listed in Table 25-4.

Calculating Dosages for Children

Until recently, formulas for determining pediatric dosages were based on computations involving a child's mass or age and the "average" adult dose (i.e., Clark's rule, Fried's rule, Young's rule). With advances in pediatric pharmacology, it became clear that such formulas neglected the most useful measure for calculating pediatric dosages: body surface area (BSA). BSA correlates with several important physiologic factors affecting drug dosages, including blood volume, basal metabolic rate, cardiac output, and glomerular filtration.[11]

A child's BSA is first estimated using a nomogram (see Appendix for nomogram). The pediatric dose is then calculated using the following formula:

$$\text{Child's BSA} \times \text{usual adult dose} = \text{child's dose}$$

Devices for Measuring Medications

There are various methods for measuring medications, as shown in Figure 25-9. The most accurate device for measuring liquid medications in the pediatric setting is a calibrated syringe. If the amount required is less than 1 ml, a tuberculin syringe can be used. Dosages greater than 10 ml can be accurately measured in a clear plastic (or glass) calibrated medication cup, using the bottom of the liquid meniscus as the measuring point. The thumbnail is placed at the desired calibration on the medication cup, and held at eye level. The medication is poured and when the bottom of the meniscus made by the medication reaches the calibration marked by the thumbnail, the correct amount has been poured.

When a parent is to give medication at home, amounts are often given in household measure (e.g., 1 tsp). However, household teaspoons can vary as much as 2 ml in accuracy (1 tsp = 5 ml). To ensure accuracy, parents can be instructed to use one of the following methods:

- Measure the medication accurately with a syringe first, and then place the medication in a household teaspoon.
- Use a specially designed medication teaspoon (available in most pharmacies).
- Use a calibrated dropper; the meniscus of the medication should rest on the mark for the dose desired.

Administering Oral Medications

Decisions regarding the delivery of oral medications are based on the child's ability to suck, swallow, drink, and chew. As efficient chewing is the last of these skills to be acquired, oral liquids are the preferred form of medication until about 5 years of age. After about age 2½, most children can take a chewable tablet with supervision. Swallowing whole tablets is difficult, if not impossible, for all children, including the adolescent.

If the medication is not available in alternate forms, most tablets can be crushed or capsules emptied for easier administration. A pharmacist should be consulted before advising parents in the process. Some medications may

TABLE 25-4
Developmental Considerations and Nursing Interventions in Medication Administration

Age	Behaviors	Nursing Interventions
Birth–3 months	1. Reaches randomly toward mouth and has a strong reflex to grasp objects	1. The infant's hands must be held to prevent spilling of medications.
	2. Poor head control	2. The infant's head must be supported while medications are being given.
	3. Tongue movement may force medication out of mouth	3. A syringe or dropper should be placed along the side of the mouth.
	4. Sucks as a reflex with stimulation	4. Use this natural sucking desire by placing oral medications into a nipple and allowing the infant to suck.
	5. Stops sucking when full	5. Administer medications before feeding when infant is hungry. Be aware that some medications' absorption will be affected by food.
	6. Infant responds to tactile stimulation	6. Increase the likelihood that the medication will be taken by holding the infant in a feeding position.
3–12 months	7. Begins to develop fine muscle control and advances from sitting to crawling	7. Medication must be kept out of reach to avoid accidental ingestion.
	8. Tongue may protrude when swallowing	8. Administer medication with a syringe.
	9. Responds to tactile stimuli	9. Physical comfort (holding) given after a medication will be helpful.
12–30 months	10. Advances from independent walking to running without falling	10. Allow the toddler to choose position for taking a medication.
	11. Advances from messy self-feeding to proficient feeding with minimal spilling	11. Allow the toddler to take medicine from a cup or spoon.
	12. Has voluntary tongue control. Begins to drink from a cup.	12. Disguise medication in a small amount of food to decrease incidence of spitting out medication.
	13. Develops second molars	13. Chewable tablets may be an alternative.
	14. Exhibits independence and self-assertiveness	14. Allow as much freedom as possible. Use games to gain confidence. Use a consistent firm approach. Give immediate praise for cooperation.
	15. Responds to sense of time and simple direction	15. Give directions to "Drink this now" and "Open your mouth."
	16. Responds to and participates in routines of daily living	16. Obtain information about toddler's daily activities.
	17. Expresses feelings easily	17. Allow for expression through play.
30 months–6 years	18. Knows full name	18. Ask the child his or her name before giving the medicine.
	19. Is easily influenced by others when responding to new foods or tastes	19. Approach the child in a calm, positive manner when giving medications.
	20. Has a good sense of time and a tolerance of frustration	20. Use immediate rewards for the young child and delayed gratification for the older child.
	21. Enjoys making decisions	21. Give choices when possible.
	22. Has many fantasies. Has fear of mutilation	22. Give simple explanations. Stress that the medication is not being given because the child is bad.
	23. Is more coordinated	23. Can hold cup and may be able to master pill-taking.
	24. Begins to lose teeth	24. Chewable tablets may be inappropriate because of loose teeth.
6–12 years	25. Strives for independence	25. Give acceptable choices. Respect the need for regression during hospitalization.

(Continued)

TABLE 25-4
(Continued)

Age	Behaviors	Nursing Interventions
	26. Has concern for bodily mutilation	26. Give reassurance that medication given, especially injectables, will not cause harm. Reinforce that medications should only be taken when given by nurse or parent.
	27. Can tell time	27. Include the child in planning daily schedule for medication. Make the child a poster of medications and time due so he or she can be involved in care.
	28. Is concerned with body image and privacy	28. Provide private area for administration of medication, especially injections.
	29. Peer support and interaction are important	29. Allow child to share experiences with others.
12+ years	30. Strives for independence	30. Write a contract with the adolescent, spelling out expectations for self-medication.
	31. Is able to understand abstract theories	31. Explain why medications are given and how they work.
	32. Decisions are influenced by peers	32. Encourage teens to talk with their peers in a support group. Work with teens to plan medication schedule around their activities. Differentiate pill-taking from drug-taking.
	33. Questions authority figures	33. Be honest and provide medication information in writing.
	34. Is concerned with sex and sexuality	34. Explain relationship between illness, medications, and sexuality. For example, emphasize that "This medication will not react with your birth control pills."

Source: Skale, N. (1992). *Manual of pediatric nursing procedures.* Philadelphia: J. B. Lippincott.

be mixed with a palatable vehicle such as jam, jelly, or syrup. When mixing in a vehicle, the following points should be considered:

- Use only a small amount of the vehicle to ensure that the entire medication is consumed in one or two swallows.

- Use an artificially sweetened vehicle when carbohydrate control is essential, such as with the diabetic child.
- Be certain that the vehicle used does not cause an adverse pharmacologic reaction when mixed with the medication.
- Do not use essential or favorite food items (e.g., milk, juice, or formula) as vehicles. Such combinations may cause a negative association between favorite or essential food items and discomfort.

Enteric-coated tablets cannot be crushed. The nurse must either assist the child with swallowing (e.g., use a "pill glass") or advise the pharmacist or physician that another form of the medication must be provided.

Occasionally a medication is not unpalatable when swallowed but leaves an unpleasant aftertaste. In such instances, a "chaser" of milk, juice, or formula can provide relief. If such an aftertaste produces nausea, carbonated beverages are sometimes helpful.

Medications should be kept out of the reach of young children. Even if a child takes his or her medication independently, some supervision is recommended.

Crying increases the risk of aspiration, so the more secure and comfortable the child is while receiving medication, the better. Parents may be permitted to comfort the child and deliver the medication in the nurse's pres-

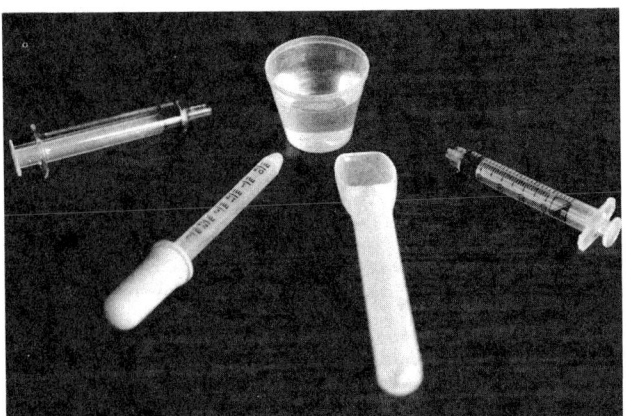

FIGURE 25-9
Devices for accurate measuring of liquid medications. (*left to right*) Oral syringe; dropper; clear medication cup; medication teaspoon; injection syringe without needle.

ence. From toddlerhood on, appropriate explanation should be given to the child. Even if a drug is mixed in a pleasant-tasting vehicle, the older child should understand that a medication is being administered.

Positioning for Oral Delivery.   Older children can be placed upright in a chair or bed. If the child needs to be flat in bed, the nurse can cradle the child's head and shoulders to facilitate swallowing.

Ideally, the infant should be cradled securely in a semi-sitting position on the nurse's lap. The infant's arms should be held away from the face, the head supported and kept immobile, and the body held firmly against the nurse (see Fig. 25-10 for positioning.) This same position can be used to secure the frightened or uncooperative toddler. Because the toddler is larger and more vigorous than the infant, two persons (e.g., two nurses or a nurse and a parent) may need to be involved in giving medications to this age group. One person can secure the child while the other delivers the medication. Medications given to infants and toddlers by syringe should be placed about halfway down the tongue and to the side of the oral cavity. Correct placement of the syringe and slow delivery (about 1 to 1½ ml per "squirt") reduce the risk of aspiration. Medication delivered by spoon should be placed similarly. Because of the natural tongue-thrusting movements of the young infant, spooned medication placed on the tip or front of the tongue is automatically spit out. Even with careful placement, some medication is likely to be pushed out onto the lips and chin. The medication should be carefully scraped up and reinserted. A pleasant-tasting liquid medication can sometimes be placed in an empty bottle nipple. The infant can then suck the medication from the nipple. An unpleasant medication should not be given this way, as it may cause the infant to associate suckling with discomfort. To assist the infant who is resistant to swallowing, the

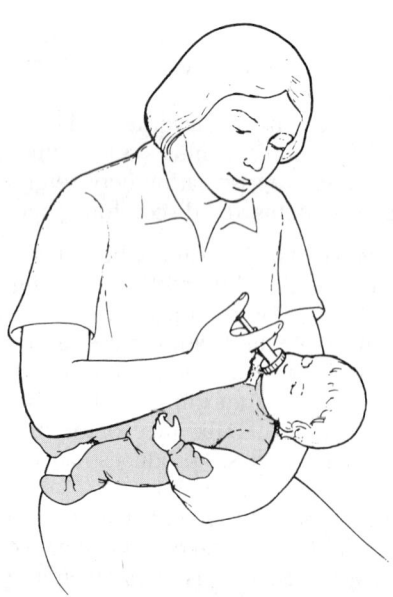

FIGURE 25-10
Holding the infant firmly in a cradle position, the nurse allows the infant to suck the medication through a nipple. (Source: Skale, N. [1992]. *Manual of pediatric nursing procedures.* Philadelphia: J. B. Lippincott.)

mouth is held closed and the chin is lifted, or the side of the throat is stroked gently.

The use of force in delivering oral medications to very young children is dangerous, frightening, and anxiety provoking. Patience, reassurance, and gentle firmness meets with success in most circumstances. Older children usually cannot be forced, and attempts to do so can produce hostility and subversive attempts to thwart care. Older children need to be given some degree of independence in the act of taking medication to support their sense of control.

Administering Rectal Medications

The rectal route for administering medications to children may be selected for the following reasons:

- The oral route is contraindicated (e.g., nausea, difficulty swallowing, NPO, or oral surgery).
- The only alternative is an injection route.

Several medications are absorbed satisfactorily through the rectum, including antipyretics, antiemetics, and sedatives. Although the absorption rate through the rectal mucosa can be unpredictable, once absorption has occurred, therapeutic blood levels can be obtained rapidly because the drug does not pass through the liver prior to entering the systemic circulation.[5]

When preparing to administer a rectal medication, developmental concerns associated with the rectal area in childhood should be considered. Of particular concern are the toddler and preschool stages.

The psychoanalyst Sigmund Freud suggested that toddlers are in the anal stage of development and are becoming consciously aware of bowel sensation and function (see Chap. 8). Mastery over bowel habits is in process, and fixation on bowel activity is common. Rectal medications are usually perceived as an assault. Such an intrusion may be vigorously protested, and attempts to expel the medication are common. With this knowledge in mind, the nurse's approach in giving rectal medication to the toddler should include a short, clear explanation; the assistance of a second person to hold the child; a calm, firm approach; quick completion of the procedure; and comfort and praise for compliance.

The preschool child is more focused on the genitals. As the rectum shares the perineum with external genital structures, the child can easily perceive rectal intrusion as a genital assault or physical punishment for wrongdoing. Care must be taken to reassure the preschooler that the procedure is for therapeutic purposes and is not a punishment. Postprocedural praise for cooperation after the procedure helps build the child's self-esteem.

Older children and adolescents are more likely to be embarrassed by the procedure. Privacy is appropriate at all ages but essential with older children. Many adolescents prefer to insert the medication themselves.

Positioning for Rectal Delivery.   The infant or young toddler can be positioned supine with the knees flexed. Beyond older infancy, the most appropriate attitude is the left-lateral Sims' position. This position places the sigmoid colon lower than the rectum and reduces the risk of spontaneous expulsion of medication.[8] Prone with the knee flexed or any side-lying position is acceptable if the left-lateral Sims' position is not possible.

Insertion. Rectal medications come primarily in suppository form. Suppositories are usually bullet shaped, with a blunt end and a rounded tip. The lubrication of suppositories before insertion is a controversial practice. If lubrication is needed, water or water-soluble lubricant is usually all that is required. Oil-based lubricants interfere with drug absorption. With the use of a gloved finger or cot (a single-finger glove that looks like a small condom), the suppository is inserted past the internal anal sphincter and deposited in the body of the rectum. If fecal matter is encountered, the child should be allowed to expel the feces before leaving the suppository, as fecal matter in the rectum delays absorption. The actual distance of insertion varies, but an average guide would be the following:

- For infants and young toddlers, insert 2.5 to 3 cm (1 to 1½ in.).
- For older toddlers and preschoolers, insert 5 to 7.5 cm (2 to 3 in.).
- For school-age children and adolescents, insert 7.5 to 10 cm (3 to 4 in.).

The little finger is the best digit for insertion into infants and young toddlers. Past those ages, the index finger is more appropriate. Encouraging the child to take a deep breath helps relax the sphincters.

Once the suppository is inserted, the nurse's primary concern is preventing expulsion of the suppository prior to its dissolution. With very young children, the nurse should try to hold the buttocks tightly together for several minutes (10 minutes is ideal, 5 is realistic). Taping the buttocks together might be tolerated by infants but not older children. Parental comfort and other distractions usually are more helpful in such circumstances.

If inability to retain the suppository becomes a consistent impediment to success, the following approaches also can occasionally be used:

- Split the suppository longitudinally, and insert one half at a time. The major disadvantage of this technique is that because of split insertion, overall absorption time is longer, and lower blood levels result.
- Insert the suppository blunt-end first. With contraction of the internal anal sphincter, the suppository automatically will be propelled further into the rectum. In such circumstances the suppository must be well lubricated, and care must be taken to prevent mucosal injury during insertion.

Administering Nasal Medications

Nose drops are most often used to shrink swollen mucous membranes and reduce nasal congestion. Nasal congestion and swelling are particularly disruptive when children are too young to blow their own noses. Effective instillation of nose drops implies the following:

- The dropper will not come into direct contact with the nares or internal mucosa.
- The medication will fall directly on the nasal mucosa.

- The medication will flow toward the nasopharynx by gravitational pull
- The medication will not land directly on the pharynx.

In preparation for the procedure, the drops should be at room temperature, to reduce the risk of the child being startled and jerking out of position during instillation. Prior to instillation, the infant's nose should be gently cleared of excessive discharge with a manual bulb syringe. Older children can be assisted in blowing their noses.

Because nasal congestion disrupts the ability to smell and taste in all children and interferes with the ability to suck in young infants, nose drops are probably most effective if given 15 to 20 minutes before meals or feedings. Sleep is more restful if decongestant nose drops are given within 30 minutes of bedtime.

Positioning the Infant. Instillation of nose drops can best be accomplished by placing the infant in one of the following three positions. First, the infant can be held in an adapted football hold. The nurse's supporting arm must cradle the infant's body, block movement of the infant's hands and arms, and support the infant's head extended, slightly lateral and immobile. Second, the infant can be cradled in a manner similar to that shown in Figure 25-10; however, the baby must be tipped downward so that the head is extended, turned slightly lateral, and then immobilized in position between the side of the nurse's body and the crook of the supporting arm. Third, if the infant cannot be removed from the crib, the head can be extended by placing a rolled towel under the neck; the baby's head can then be turned slightly lateral and immobilized by the nurse's nondominant arm. The nurse can use the upper part of his or her dominant arm to immobilize the infant's upper limbs, leaving the lower arm and hand free to instill the drops. If none of the three positions can be maintained by the nurse alone, seeking an assistant or using a mummy restraint is appropriate.

Positioning the Older Child. Unless the older child is uncooperative, the use of enforced immobilization is unnecessary. Instilling nasal drops into an uncooperative older child should be done with assistance. The cooperative older child can be positioned similarly to the second step described earlier. Adapting the second position would require the older child to sit in the nurse's lap with the head extended over the nurse's supporting arm. The third position requires the rolled blanket or pillow to be placed under the older child's shoulders. Children who are too big to sit in the nurse's lap can sit in a chair and tip their head back for nasal instillation. If the child is not to sit up, lying across the bed with head extended over the edge is acceptable. The nurse can face the top of the child's head, cradling the head with one hand and instilling the drops with the other. The child can be instructed to turn the head slightly to the left for instillation into the left nares and slightly to the right for instillation into the other side.

Extension and slight lateral turning of the head ensures instillation in both infants and children. The nasal opening can be widened by placing gentle pressure on the tip of the nose.

Once nose drops are instilled, the head should be maintained below the shoulders for 2 to 3 minutes to allow the medication to be pulled by gravity into the nasopharynx. The older child should be warned to expect a taste of the medication, especially if the urge to sniff cannot be contained. If the child begins to cough, reposition the child to a sitting position immediately.

Some older children can insert their own nasal drops. If medication can be provided in a nasal spray, self-administration is even easier for the child. Nasal sprays are not appropriate for infants or young children because inspiration cannot be voluntarily coordinated with propulsion of the spray, and it is difficult to control the force of propulsion, which increases risk of mucosal irritation and choking.

Administering Ear Medications

Otic medications are given to children to relieve inflammation or infection in the ear and the pain that often accompanies these conditions. If necessary, the external ear can be cleansed with a damp cotton ball prior to beginning the procedure. The infant or young child can be placed in a sidelying or supine position, either on an adult's lap or in a crib. Whichever position is chosen, the head must be immobilized and turned to place the affected ear in the superior position. Older children may lie supine with their head turned so that the affected ear is accessible, or they can sit upright with the head tilted toward the shoulder on the unaffected side. If the older child desires a greater sense of security, the head can be held immobile by the nurse. Unless older children are uncooperative, however, the choice of position should be theirs.

The medication should be at room temperature or warmed to prevent startling the child and risking disrupted positioning, vertigo, dizziness, or nausea. Instillation of ear drops requires that in children younger than 3 years of age, the external auditory canal is straightened by pulling the lobe of the pinna down and back (Fig. 25-11A). In children older than 3 years of age, the external auditory canal is straightened by pulling the upper helix of the pinna up and back (see Fig. 25-11B). Ear drops are directed against the wall of the external auditory canal,

never directly against the tympanic membrane. After instillation, gentle massage in front of the ear near the tragus helps propel the drops toward the eardrum.

Unless there is a suspected break in the tympanic membrane and, therefore, direct access to inner ear structures, the medication should be clean, but sterility is not essential. The drops should be instilled one at a time onto the wall of the external auditory canal from a point approximately 1 cm (1/2 in.) above the canal's meatus. Placing drops in this manner prevents startling the child and risking possible ear trauma; dizziness, vertigo, or nausea may result from sudden jarring of the inner ear or forcing an unknown occlusion further in the auditory canal.

The child should remain in position for 3 to 5 minutes after instillation to allow gravity to move the drops inward. A cotton ball can be placed loosely against the meatus of the external auditory canal of older children for 15 minutes. This helps absorb excess medication that flows outward when the head is righted. The nurse should watch for dizziness, vertigo, and nausea in the older child for the first 30 minutes after the instillation of ear drops.

Administering Eye Medications

Because eye tissue is among the most sensitive to external manipulation, it is almost impossible to instill eye medications in infants and young children without the assistance of a second person to secure the child. In preparation for the procedure, the medication should be warmed or kept at room temperature. Cleansing of the eye with a clean, damp face cloth from inner to outer canthus helps remove any obvious foreign matter or encrustations.

The child should be positioned supine with a support device—a rolled towel under the neck and shoulders—to extend the head. If able, the older child can sit in a chair and extend the head independently. It is best to deliver eye medication to an infant in the crib, unless the person providing the restraint is able fully to secure the baby in an arm-cradling position.

Eye Drops.   Placement of the hands when delivering eye drops (Fig. 25-12) should be as follows:

• The hand holding the medication dropper should rest on the forehead above the affected eye.

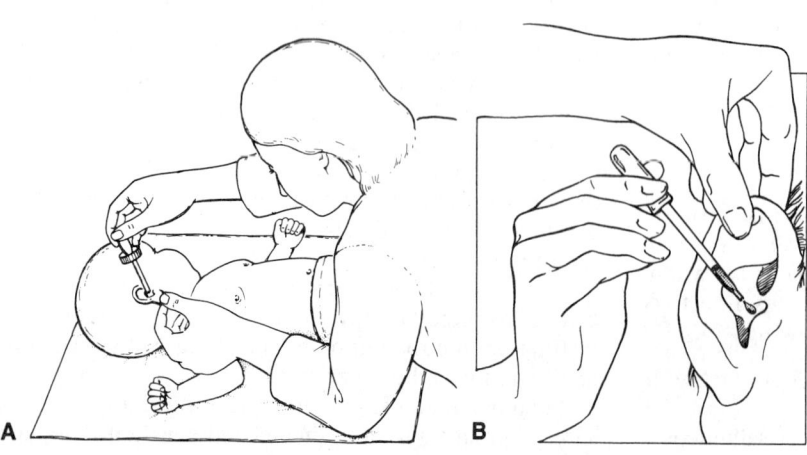

FIGURE 25-11
Administration of ear drops. (A) Child younger than 3 years of age. (From Skale, N. [1992]. *Manual of pediatric nursing procedures.* Philadelphia: J. B. Lippincott.) (B) Child older than 3 years of age. (Source: Ellis, J. R., Nowlis, E. A., & Bentz, P. M. [1992]. *Modules for basic nursing skills,* Vol. 2, 5th ed. Philadelphia: J. B. Lippincott.)

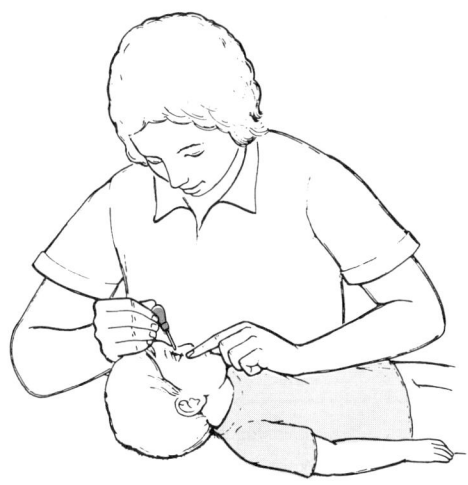

FIGURE 25-12
Administration of eye drops. A young child may have to be restrained by a second person. (Source: Skale, N. [1992]. *Manual of pediatric nursing procedures*. Philadelphia: J. B. Lippincott.)

- The other hand should rest below the affected eye in a manner that allows the index finger to pull the lower eyelid downward and pouch out the conjunctival sac.

Once the child is positioned, and the nurse's hands are in place, the drops should be instilled one at a time in the lower conjunctival sac, toward the outer canthus. Drops should never be placed directly on the cornea. Drops placed too close to the inner canthus risk being lost through the nasolacrimal duct. The older child can facilitate dispersion by rolling the eyeball upward before the drops are instilled. As the eyelid automatically blinks in response to the instillation, the eyeball rolls back into place naturally, dispersing the drops across its surface. Encouraging the child to keep the eyes shut also facilitates dispersion. Loss of medication through the nasolacrimal duct can be prevented by placing firm pressure against the inner canthus for a few seconds. If for some reason the eye cannot be opened, the drops can be placed on the inner corner of the eye and allowed to seep in between the closed lids.

Eye Ointment. When the eye ointment is instilled, the thumb is used to hold open the lower lid, and the index finger of the same hand that holds open the upper lid provides sufficient traction to prevent blinking during instillation. The ointment is then applied in a quick stroke from the inner to outer canthus in an even bead. The child should close the eyes and disperse the ointment by rolling the eyeball in all directions. Excess ointment can be wiped off, from inner to outer canthus, once dispersion is complete. If the instillation of eye ointment is hampered significantly by an uncooperative child, the procedure can often be successfully performed when the child is sleeping.

Medication to be administered once a day should be instilled at night, when the inherent effects on visual acuity are least disruptive.

Administering Topical Medications

Because infants and small children have a thin epidermis and large BSA, their absorption of topical medication is more efficient.[2] The nurse's responsibilities in administering to topical medications include applying the medications as thinly as possible, restricting the area of application to the affected site only, and maintaining vigilance in observing for adverse and toxic affects.

Administering Medications by Injection

Because injections are both painful and invasive, the choice to use them in children must be weighed against the therapeutic value expected as compared with other routes of administration and the emotional and physical distress likely to be engendered in the child. The procedural steps and the principles underlying these steps in intramuscular, subcutaneous, and intradermal injections are the same for children as for adults.

Factors Affecting Technique. Alterations in technique for children are related to physical growth and development, body mass, and tissue size. Such alterations specifically affect the following factors: site selection and location, needle length and gauge, and type and volume of medications.

Site Selection and Location. Subcutaneous and intradermal sites are essentially the same for children and adults. However, all sites, including intramuscular sites, should be selected with consideration of tissue size and mass, as well as the chronologic age of the child. Table 25-5 identifies the five intramuscular sites commonly used in the pediatric setting, as well as their location, age appropriateness, delivery technique, advantages, and disadvantages.

Needle Length and Gauge. Choice of the needle length to be used for a child's injection is a nursing judgment. The needle must be long enough to pierce the tissue and deposit medication within the muscle but not too long to extend beyond the proper injection site. Gauges also vary with the site, age of the child, and length of the needle. Table 25-6 identifies the most common needle lengths and gauges for the three injection types in the pediatric setting.

Type and Volume of Medication. Table 25-7 describes the maximum volume of medication to inject into a child according to age, type of medication, and site of injection.

Restraint. A restraint is needed in certain circumstances to protect the safety of the child and nurse.

Risks. In a large research study on complications of intramuscular injections in a pediatric setting, the following provocative results were discovered[2]:

- Thigh sites and the dorsogluteal site suffered the most complications.
- Most complications occurred in children from birth to 5 years of age.
- Most of the nurses had not been taught to use the ventrogluteal site, although they had received their nursing education within the last 10 years.

TABLE 25-5
Intramuscular Injection Sites

Vastus Lateralis

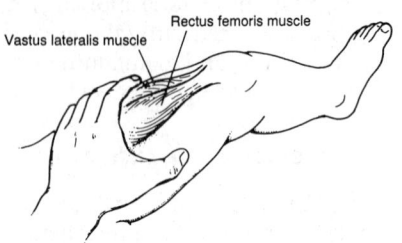

Age Appropriateness

Preferred site for infants and children under 3. Barring individual contraindications, can be used up to 6–8 years of age.

Location: Vastus lateralis. Divide the *lateral* aspect of the thigh, between the knee joint and the greater trochanter, into thirds. The injection site is located in the middle third.

Delivery Technique

Grasp the thigh and compress the muscle. Insert the needle at a 90° angle or pointing slightly toward the anterior thigh. In some situations with infants, the needle may be held at a 45–60° angle and pointed in the direction of the knee.

Advantages

- Muscle mass well developed at birth
- No major nerves or blood vessels located close by
- Can hold a reasonable volume of fluid
- Easily accessed, mapped, and located

Disadvantages

- Muscle actively used by child so injection may cause residual pain
- Child can easily view the procedure
- Not recommended for children older than 6–8 years

Ventrogluteal

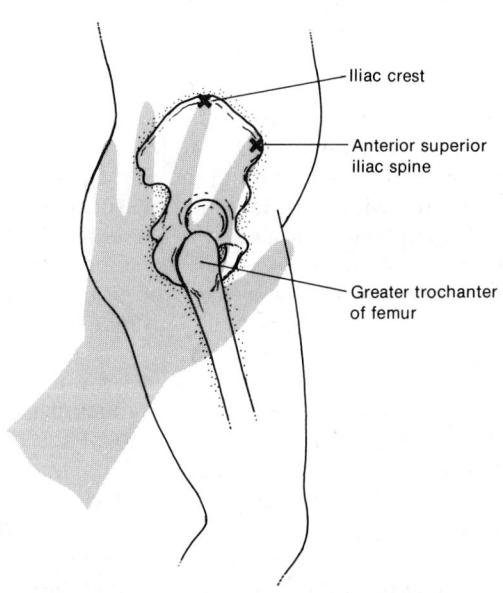

Iliac crest

Anterior superior iliac spine

Greater trochanter of femur

Age Appropriateness

Good site for children over age 3. Preferred site for older school-age children and adolescents.

Location: Ventrogluteal. Using the nurse's right hand and the child's left leg, place the heel of the hand on the greater trochanter, the index finger on the anterior superior iliac spine, and the middle finger posteriorly as far along the iliac crest as possible. Inject into the center of the **V** formed by the index and middle fingers.

Delivery Technique

Muscle is pressed taut. Needle is inserted at a 90° angle or bent slightly toward the iliac crest.

Advantages

- Landmarks are easily located
- Muscle mass is close to surface and not heavily padded with fat
- No major nerves or blood vessels located close by
- Can hold a large volume of fluid
- Can be accessed from almost all positions.
- Buttock or perineal area need not be exposed

Disadvantages

- Usually not recommended in children under age 3
- Advantages of the site recently discovered, and many nurses unsure of mapping

(Continued)

TABLE 25-5
(Continued)

Dorsogluteal

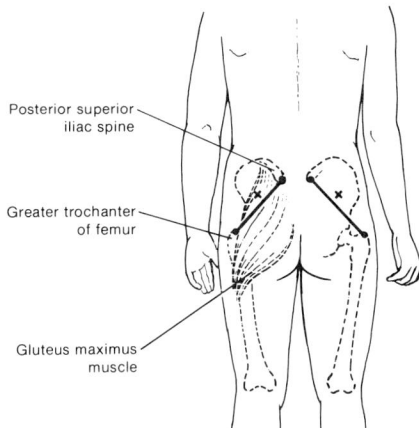

Posterior superior iliac spine

Greater trochanter of femur

Gluteus maximus muscle

Age Appropriateness
Should be avoided if any other suitable sites are available. Should not be used unless a child has been walking for at least a year. Not recommended for children under age 6.

Location: Dorsogluteal. Draw an imaginary line between the posterior superior iliac spine and the greater trochanter of the femur. The site is located lateral and superior about halfway along this imaginary line.

Delivery Technique
Press area taut and insert the needle at a 90° angle.

Advantages
• Large muscle mass can hold large volume of fluid
• Easily accessible in supine or lateral positions
• Out of child's line of vision
• Increases potential sites for older children

Disadvantages
• Unsafe site unless child has been walking for at least one year
• Not recommended for children under age 6
• Large fat padding of buttocks makes landmarks (and thus, site) difficult to locate
• Sciatic nerve is closer than with ventrogluteal site
• Exposes the buttocks, which may embarrass the older child

Deltoid

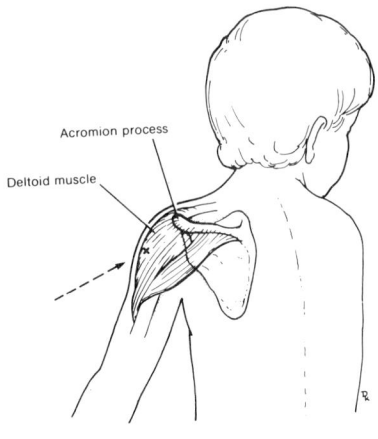

Acromion process

Deltoid muscle

Age Appropriateness
Not preferred site for any age. Can be used for children over 6 who are receiving small amounts of medication.

Location: Deltoid. The site is located in the upper third of the muscle. Inject into the area located below two adult fingerbreadths from the acromium process but not lower than the point opposite the axilla junction.

Delivery Technique
Bunching the muscle mass prior to injection can be helpful with children. The needle is inserted at a 90° angle or slightly toward the shoulder.

Advantages
• Rate of absorption faster than gluteal or thigh sites
• Easily accessed, mapped, and located
• No need to expose normally covered areas of the body
• Can be accessed standing, sitting, or lying

Disadvantages
• Not recommended for children under age 6
• Maximum volume recommended for injection is 1 ml
• Brachial artery and radial nerve are close by
• Child can view procedure

(Continued)

**TABLE 25-5
(Continued)**

Rectus Femoris

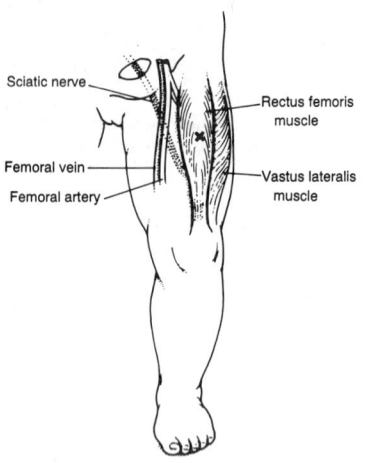

Age Appropriateness

Acceptable but not preferred site for any age. Most useful for older children giving their own intramuscular injections.

Location: Rectus femoris. Divide the *anterior* surface of the thigh into thirds. The injection site is located in the middle third.

Delivery Technique	*Advantages*	*Disadvantages*
Muscle should be bunched. Needle should be inserted at a 45° angle with the point of the needle toward the knee.	• Muscle mass well developed at birth • Can hold a reasonable volume of fluid • Easily accessed, mapped, and located • Can be used with infants when vastus lateralis site is contraindicated	• Seems to produce even more residual pain than vastus lateralis site • Child can easily view the procedure • Closer to femoral artery, vein, and sciatic nerve than vastus lateralis site • Not recommended for older children

• The most commonly reported causes of complications involved techniques, including choosing inappropriate needle length; injecting excessive fluid volume; giving multiple injections in a single site; patient movement and inadequate restraint; and inadequate mapping or inappropriate site selection.

The most notable recommendations from the study[2] were the following:

**TABLE 25-6
Needle Length and Gauge for Pediatric Injections**

Age	Length (inch)	Gauge
Infant		
Intramuscular	⅝	25–26
Subcutaneous	⅜–½	26–27
Intradermal	⅜	26–27
Young Children		
Intramuscular	1	22–24
Subcutaneous	⅝	25
Intradermal	⅜–½	25–26
Older Children and Adolescents		
Intramuscular	1–1½	21–22
Subcutaneous	⅝	25
Intradermal	⅜–½	25–26

Data source: Baer, C. L., & Williams, B. R. (1988). *Clinical pharmacology and therapeutics.* Springhouse, PA: Springhouse.

• The ventrogluteal site should be evaluated as a primary site for injection in children 12 years old and older.
• Care must be taken to map sites accurately.
• The dorsogluteal site should be avoided in infants and young children.
• Needles longer than 1 inch should not be used in infants and small children.
• More care must be taken with selecting appropriate injection equipment, rotating injection sites, matching volume of medication with sites, and adequately restraining children.

Intravenous Therapy in Children

Children receive IV therapy for the following reasons, which are the same as those for adults:

• To restore or maintain fluid balance
• To provide a route for rapid and efficient drug administration

Factors Affecting IV Therapy

The unique aspects of IV therapy in children relate primarily to the child's coping mechanisms, sites, equipment, restraint, rate of flow, and risks.

Coping and Stress Tolerance. Parents often view the initiation of IV therapy as a sign that the child's illness is becoming more serious. This may be true, but IV therapy often is used as an adjunct to other therapies or as an

TABLE 25-7
Recommended Maximum Volume of Medication to Inject According to Age and Type and Site of Injection

Age	Type and Site of Injection	Recommended Maximum Volume (ml)
Young infant	Intradermal—all sites	Not recommended or commonly used
	Subcutaneous—all sites	0.2
	Intramuscular	
	Vastus lateralis	0.5
	Ventrogluteal	Not a recommended site
	Dorsogluteal	Not a recommended site
	Rectus femoris	0.5
Older infant and toddler	Intradermal—all sites	Not recommended or commonly used
	Subcutaneous—all sites	0.3
	Intramuscular	
	Vastus lateralis	1.0
	Ventrogluteal	Not a recommended site
	Dorsogluteal	Not a recommended site
	Deltoid	Not a recommended site
	Rectus femoris	1.0
Preschooler to young school-age	Intradermal—all sites	Not commonly used, 0.1
	Subcutaneous—all sites	0.5
	Intramuscular	
	Vastus lateralis	1.5
	Ventrogluteal	1.5
	Dorsogluteal	Not a recommended site
	Deltoid	Not a recommended site
	Rectus femoris	1.5
Older school age to adolescent	Intradermal—all sites	0.1
	Subcutaneous—all sites	0.5–0.75
	Intramuscular	
	Vastus lateralis	1.5–2
	Ventrogluteal	1.5–2
	Dorsogluteal	1.5–2
	Deltoid	0.5
	Rectus femoris	1.5–2
Older adolescent	Intradermal—all sites	0.1
	Subcutaneous—all sites	1.0
	Intramuscular	
	Vastus lateralis	1.5–2, but not a preferred site
	Ventrogluteal	2–2.5
	Dorsogluteal	2–2.5
	Deltoid	1.0
	Rectus femoris	1.5–2, but not a preferred site

efficient method of delivering medications. Useful nursing approaches for meeting the emotional needs of children and their parents can be obtained from Table 25-9 at the end of the chapter.

One helpful guideline is to start an IV in the treatment room; in this way, the child's bed or crib is not associated with the discomfort and fear of IV insertion.

Site Selection. Site selection is based primarily on the age and condition of the child, as shown in Figure 25-13. The umbilical vein is an appropriate infusion site for a neonate. Scalp veins are the most commonly used sites for infants and have several advantages, including the following:

- They are easily visible below the skin surface.
- They have no valves, so the IV needle can be placed in either direction.

Some nurses and physicians prefer to insert the scalp vein needle so that it follows the natural blood flow. In most instances, large scalp veins flow toward the neck. Care must be taken to clean the site well and to use scrupulous aseptic technique during insertion, as scalp veins are directly connected to the sinuses in the cerebral dura. If possible, frontal scalp veins should be selected so that the infant's head turning need not be restricted.

Hand sites can be used for all ages. Parents often find hand sites more aesthetically pleasing than scalp sites for infants, particularly because there is no need to shave off any hair. Hand sites are preferred to foot sites when the child is walking. However, hand sites require restraints when used with infants and young toddlers. Veins on the hand are often more difficult to find in infants because of fat padding over the sites. Care should be taken to avoid using the dominant hand for placement of the IV needle.

Foot sites can be used for all ages but are most pre-

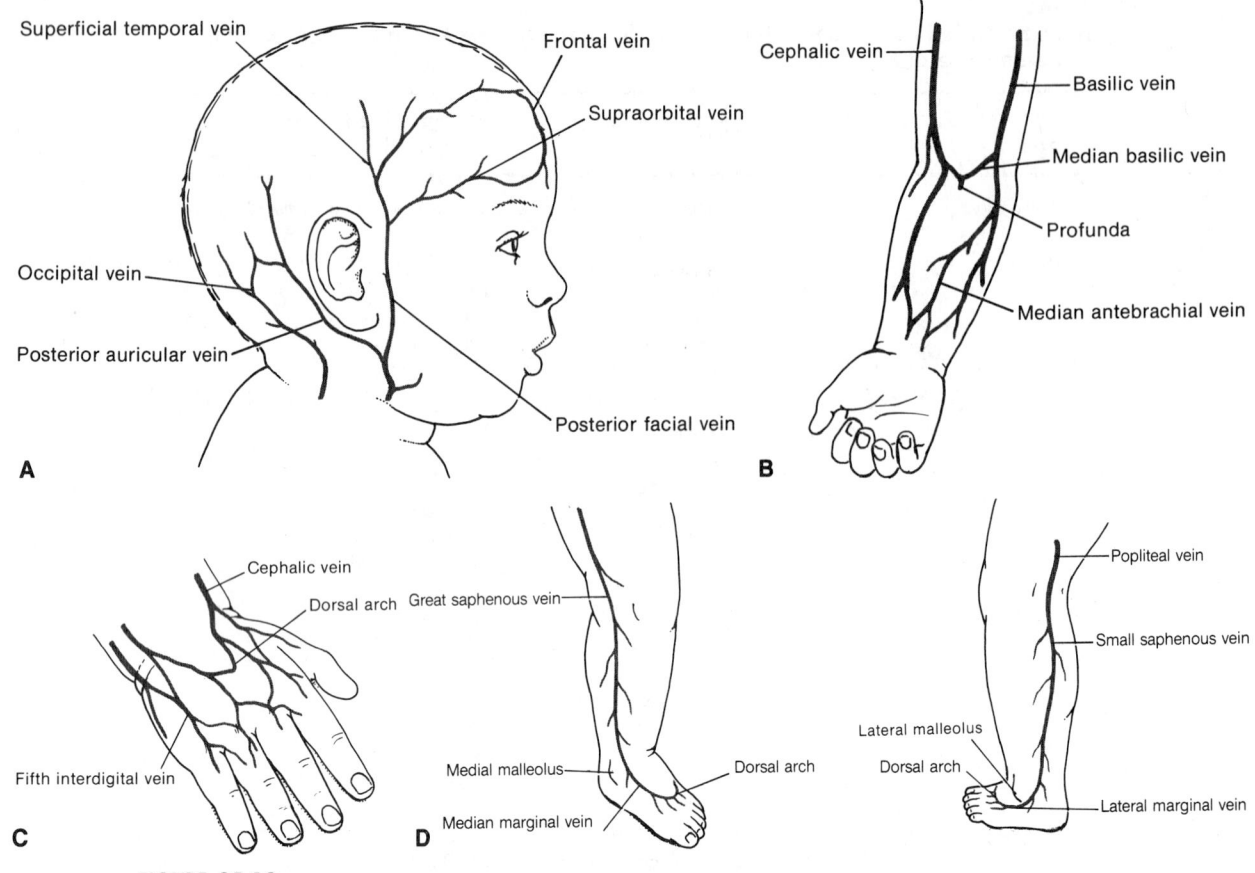

FIGURE 25-13

Commonly used intravenous sites in children. (**A**) Six scalp vein sites used primarily in infants. (**B**) Arm sites used for older children. (**C**) Hand sites used for all ages. (**D**) Median and lateral veins of foot used for all children. (Source: Skale, N. [1992]. *Manual of pediatric nursing procedures*. Philadelphia: J. B. Lippincott.)

ferred when the child is nonambulatory. Arm, leg, and other sites can be used with older children.

Equipment. Various IV needles may be used. IV needles, such as the butterfly or scalp vein, have the advantage of being easier to insert and less prone to producing site infections than IV catheters. Plastic catheters, however, are more malleable, and risk infiltration problems less often. Cutdown catheters may be inserted for long-term therapy. Catheter and needle gauges used for pediatric IVs can be as small as 27-gauge. Although tiny lumens are easier to insert, they clog more readily. Control of volume, and thus the risk of circulatory overload, is essential in caring for children. Strict volume control requires the use of the following:

- *The microdrip or minidrip*: The microdrip attachment reduces the actual size of the drops so that 1 ml of IV fluid is equal to 60 drops instead of the usual 10 to 15 drops. The smaller drip allows for easier rate calculation, rate monitoring, and overall volume control.
- *The controlled fluid administration set (e.g., Buretrol, Pediatrol, Soluset)*: These devices have highly accurate calibrations, limited volume capacity, and automatic shut-off valves. All of these features help control the volume infused. As these devices work on gravity, difficulties are sometimes encountered

when small volumes of fluid are used. For example, sometimes 25 to 30 ml of fluid does not produce sufficient hydrostatic pressure against a vein to maintain the rate of flow. The lower the fluid level becomes, the slower the rate will be.

- *Infusion pumps*: Infusion pumps come in two types. Peristaltic pumps such as the IVAC or the IMED put pressure on the IV tubing. Piston pumps, like the Harvard pump, push the fluid through a syringe. Both types of machines allow for preset and very minute rates of flow. They usually come equipped with alarms that sound when mechanical difficulties occur or the solution runs dry.
- *Site locks*: Site locks, such as the heparin lock, are used for intermittent IV infusion. They are discussed later in this section.

Restraint. Restraints are usually required for infants and young children during IV insertion (Fig. 25-14). Once established, the IV sites themselves need to be protected and immobilized. Scalp vein sites require the least immobilization; however, the young child's hands often need to be restrained to prevent scalp vein IVs from being accidentally or intentionally pulled out. Older children usually require less restraint but may need frequent reminders. Information provided earlier in this chapter can be used to determine the appropriate restraints to use

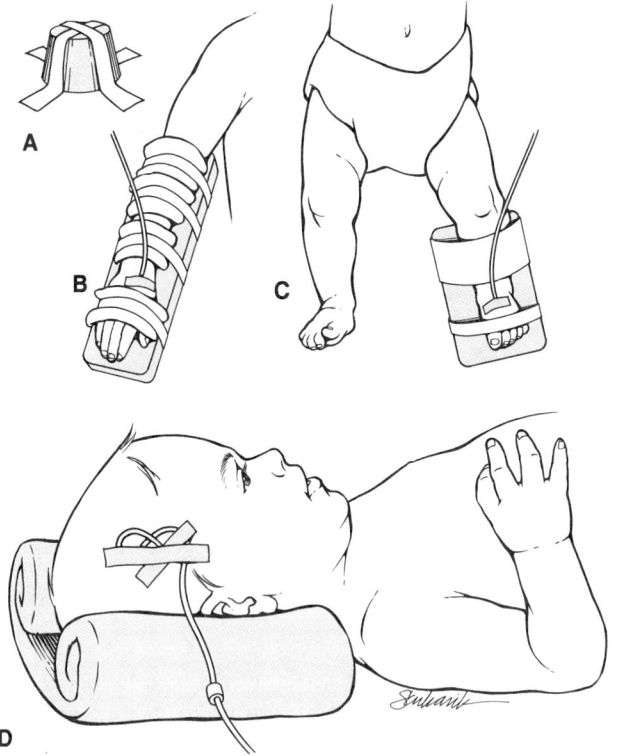

FIGURE 25-14
Protection of intravenous sites in children. (**A**) Paper cup taped over
venipuncture site. (**B**) Arm restraint for protecting hand intravenous site.
(**C**) Leg restraint for protecting foot intravenous site. (**D**) Positioning and
protection of scalp vein site.

during both the insertion and maintenance phases of IV
therapy.

Risks.   The most serious IV complication in the pediatric setting is circulatory overload. The younger the
child, the faster the complication can occur, and the more
dangerous the complication can become. Inadequate attention to the potential for excessive volume infusion is
unsafe nursing practice.

The smaller lumens in IV needles and catheters increase the risk of clotting and blockage at the site. Small
lumens are more easily blocked by medication residue.
Pediatric IV systems should be equipped with membranes
to filter out undissolved drug residue. Flushing the IV
site after medication delivery also helps reduce drug residue. Older children can be taught to watch for problems
with both the system and the site. Particularly responsible
older children can even be taught some safe manipulation
techniques to disrupt or prevent problems. Table 25-8
describes common IV complications in pediatrics, their
supportive data, and appropriate nursing interventions.

Rate of Flow.   Virtually all manually monitored flow
rates in pediatrics use a minidrip or microdrip system.
Flow rates are simple to calculate:

number of ml/hour = number of drops/minute

If a physician's order is given as a total volume over
a number of hours, for example, 400 ml per 8 hours, the
nurse simply determines the number of milliliters per
hour as follows:

$$400/8 = 50 \text{ ml}$$

The rate, then, is 50 drops per minute. If standard IV
administrations systems (e.g., 1 ml = 10 drops) are used
for older adolescents, appropriate calculation formulas
are used.

Maintenance of the IV System

The accompanying display describes a checklist for
IV administration.

Intermittent IV Infusion

Many children have IVs for the purpose of intermittent drug administration. A site lock system (e.g., heparin
lock) may be used so that the IV need only be connected
when the medication is administered. The site lock has
a rubber chamber into which the IV needle is inserted at
the time of drug administration. Once the drug is totally
infused, the IV system is removed, but the lock maintains
the site open until the next drug dose is needed. Site
locks are usually flushed with a heparinized saline solution to prevent clotting in the needle between infusions.
Recent research has questioned the necessity of heparinized saline solutions for such purposes and suggests that
normal saline is superior to heparinized saline for flushing
infusion devices.[17] Site locks are ideal for short-term IV
drug therapy, and they allow older children the opportunity to maintain such therapy independently at home.

Adding Medication to the IV

Adding medications to an IV for a child is similar to
adding medications to an IV for an adult. Special emphasis
is placed on the more serious potential for complications
in the young. The basic procedure and what the nurse
must determine are as follows:

- The compatibility of the IV medication with the IV
  solution itself and other medications (if any) in the
  IV—If incompatibilities exist, the pharmaceutical directions given to circumvent them must be followed.
- The appropriateness of the dosage ordered for the
  age and size of the child.
- The minimum amount of IV dilution required, that
  is, how much IV solution must be used to dilute safely
  the amount of medication to be given. This concern
  is of particular importance for children when the
  medication virtually always goes in the controlled
  infusion chamber. Consider the following example:
  The minimum dilution for cloxacillin is 50 mg/ml.
  Thus, for every 50 mg of cloxacillin to be added to
  an IV, there must be 1 ml of IV solution. The minimum amount of IV solution you would require for a
  child who is to receive 200 mg of cloxacillin by IV
  is:

$$200 \text{ mg}/50 \text{ mg} \times 1 \text{ ml} = 4 \text{ ml}$$

A minimum dilution is usually indicated to prevent unnecessary irritation at the vein site because a

TABLE 25-8
Complications of IV Therapy

Problem and Cause	Supportive Data	Nursing Interventions
Infiltration Caused by: • Needle or catheter displacement • Blood leakage from vein	• Site swelling (scalp vein puffing) • Cool skin at site • Lack of blood backflow	• Stop flow and remove needle or catheter • If noted within 20–30 minutes of infiltration, apply ice to swelling • If noted after 30 minutes, apply warm compresses to encourage absorption *Restarting* • Stabilize site adequately • Use a catheter rather than a needle
Phlebitis Injury to the vein caused by: • Movement of needle, or improper stabilization • Too slow rate • Overuse of the vein • Irritating additive	• Sluggish flow • Site warm, red • Some swelling • Hardness along the vein site • Pain or tenderness at site • Possible mild fever	• Stop flow and remove needle or catheter • Apply warm, moist compresses *Restarting* • Select a larger vein site for subsequent infusion • Alternate sites • Dilute additives more to maintain an adequate flow rate
Circulatory Overload Caused by: • Too fast a flow rate • Too large a volume infiltrated	• Elevated blood pressure • Tachycardia • Increased urine output • Possible distension of neck veins • Periorbital edema • Bulging fontanelle • Dyspnea, rales • Cough • Frothy sputum	• Slow infusion to "to keep open" (TKO) rate • Raise child to semi- or high Fowler's position • Give oxygen as needed • Notify physician • Monitor edema • Monitor urine specific gravity • Monitor vital signs, especially blood pressure and respirations
Air Embolism* Caused by: • Using system with no automatic shut-off allowing IV to run dry • Tubing improperly cleared of air	• Cyanosis • Drop in BP • Weak, rapid pulse • Loss of consciousness • Data indicative of shock	• Turn child on left side • Give oxygen as necessary • Inspect system for air leaks and correct • Notify physician immediately
Infection (Local at Site, or General) Caused by: • Improper aseptic technique during initiation of IV • Subsequent maintenance	• Swelling at site • Foul-smelling discharge • Elevated temperature • Chills • Blood culture positive for pathogens	• Discontinue IV • Seek local or systemic therapy for infection *Restarting* • Maintain strict aseptic technique during initiation and maintenance
Clotting at Site Caused by: • Too small a lumen or vein • Too sluggish a drip rate • IV running dry	• No IV flow • No blood backflow • Infiltration	• Discontinue IV, restart in larger vein, and monitor more closely
Skin Irritation Injury to the skin caused by: • Taping • Restraints • Infiltration • Pressure	• Redness at site • Raised, irritated areas • Itching and burning around tape	• Under careful supervision, remove irritant, and reapply dressing over insertion site (hypoallergenic tape is available)

* No current research exists that suggests how much air in the system is dangerous. The standard of no more than 10 ml of air for an adult suggests that for young children, 3–5 ml could be excessive, and for infants, as little as 1 ml could cause problems.

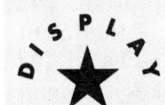

Intravenous Checklist

— *The right solution*: the tonicity, electrolyte, and sugar content must be compatible with child's age and condition

— *The right size bag*: 150- or 250-ml bags prevent wastage with young children receiving small amounts of IV fluids

— * *The correct rate of flow*: circulatory overload can occur more quickly and with more serious effects in young children

— *The right equipment*: tubing, needle, and control sets

— * *The right labeling*: includes fluid levels/hour, medication tags if drugs added

— *The date, time bottle and tubing were hung*: most tubing is changed every 24–48 hours

— * *Patency of the tubing*: check for kinks, blocks, air, blood, leaks, and flattening

— * *Height of bottle and effect on flow*

— * *Infusion pump is functional,* if used

— * *Tubing correctly attached to infusion pump*

— * *Clamps are properly open or closed*: the air valve clamp should be open. If a controlled infusion set is being used, the clamp connecting it to the main IV bag should *always be clamped,* unless control unit is being filled

— * *Clamps are out of young child's reach*

— * *The child is properly restrained*: check that restraints are correctly and safely maintained

— * *System alarms are functional*

* *Check the site for:*

— Pain

— Swelling or puffiness

— Warmth or coolness

— Tenderness

— Blanching

— Redness

— Vein hardness

— Wetness

— * *Patency of overall system, including site*

— *The child's vital signs*: alterations can indicate IV complications

— *Urine output*

— *Visible edema*

— *Cough, frothy sputum*: could be indicative of fluid overload

— * *General appearance of the child*

— * *Fluid balance record*: should be current for hourly and running volume totals

* *Items marked with an asterisk should be assessed each time the IV is checked, which may be as often as every 15–30 minutes with an infant or young child and a minimum of every 60 minutes with older children. Other items should be checked at least once a shift or at the change of shift.*

---

drug is too concentrated. Cloxacillin has a reputation for being particularly irritating. The maximum dilution is often left to the discretion of the nurse after all the variables have been considered. For children, the least volume possible is usually best.

- The minimum and maximum delivery time. This information is necessary to determine the drip rate of the IV during medication delivery. Other facts to consider when determining the drip rate include fluid restrictions for the child (if any), the length of time that the drug is stable in solution, and the side effects and toxic effects of the drug.

After the medication is added, the nurse must do the following:

- Label the controlled fluid set indicating the name of drug, dose, date, and time of addition to IV, and signature of the nurse who added the drug.
- Monitor the IV carefully during drug administration, particularly watching for side effects and allergic reactions.

Procedures Involving the Bloodstream

Blood Transfusions

The administration of blood engenders a natural fear in both children and their parents for the following reasons:

- Blood transfusions are an intrusive and painful procedure.
- Blood has many psychological and spiritual meanings.
- Blood transfusions often mean a worsening of the child's condition.

The general principles underlying blood transfusions for infants and children are the same as for adults. The correct procedure for delivering blood transfusions to infants and children in a step-by-step fashion is described in Chapter 44. Some of the differences in delivering blood transfusions involve the points discussed in the following paragraphs.

Neonatal Transfusions. Most transfusions given to neonates result from the following:

- *Blood loss:* A loss of 5% to 10% of total blood in less than 48 hours usually necessitates a transfusion.
- *Nonphysiologic anemia:* Anemia occurring prior to 3 weeks of age must be considered pathologic. The need for a blood transfusion is based on the severity of symptoms.

Grouping and Cross-Matching. If a neonate is less than 6 days of age, grouping and cross-matching for transfusion can be done against the mother's serum rather than the infant's. If the infant is older than 6 days or has already received an initial transfusion, the grouping and cross-matching must be done on the infant's own serum. The group and cross-match should be repeated every 48 hours.[7]

Universal Donor Blood. Multiple transfusions from a single unit of blood (a cost-saving factor) can be accomplished by routinely administering O-negative (universal donor), saline-washed red blood cells to infants less than 4 months of age. The risk of transfusion reactions in infants less than 4 months of age is negligible, because the infant's immune system is still not fully developed.

Volume to Be Administered. The volume of blood to be administered to children is based on milliliter per kilogram of body weight. Standard volumes for various components are given in Chapter 43. Special small pediatric units can be prepared to prevent blood wastage. Examples are the Pedipack, which equals 250 ml, and the Aliquot, which are specially prepared packs containing from a few milliliters up to the Pedipack size.

Saline Flush. Because of the much greater risk for circulatory overload, saline flushes accompanying blood transfusions must be calculated with care. A 1-ml saline barrier is sufficient in most pediatric situations.

Rate of Transfusion Flow. The rate of transfusion flow is based in the viability of the product and the cardiopulmonary and hemodynamic status of the child. To assess for hemolytic transfusion reaction, the initial rate of flow for products containing red blood cells is slower than the ordered rate. In the care of children, this initial flow rate is determined by calculating 5% of the total product to be given and delivering this calculated amount over the first 15 minutes. If no reaction occurs after 15 minutes, the ordered flow rate can be initiated.

Equipment. Needles as small as 27-gauge can be used safely with some blood products. Microaggregate filters should be used with all blood products in the pediatric setting. Microaggregate filters remove small particles that, although harmless to adults, have the potential to become emboli in very young infants. Pump infusions are recommended, as they produce a safe, steady rate of flow.

Warmth of Blood Product. Infants and young children have immature thermoregulatory mechanisms. Care must be taken to ensure that blood products are administered to children at room temperature, or in some instances, body temperature.

Exchange Transfusions

Exchange transfusions are performed on neonates primarily to treat kernicterus and Rh incompatibilities. However, severe anemia, retarded liver function, and other hemopoietic conditions can necessitate a transfusion in some circumstances.

Such exchanges are usually administered through the umbilical vein, which remains reasonably patent for several days after birth. The volume of blood used for the exchange is twice the estimated volume of the infant's blood. The infant's blood is removed and replaced, 10 to 20 ml at a time, and the entire procedure takes 45 minutes to 1 1/2 hours. The process usually replaces 90% to 95% of the neonate's blood. The nurse is responsible for keeping the infant warm; assessing vital signs regularly; and keeping an accurate, running account of the amount of blood removed and replaced.

Exchange transfusions can take place in utero between 28 and 34 weeks' gestation. Such exchanges are usually performed when the risk of hydrops fetalis is high. Adult red blood cells are injected into the peritoneal cavity of the fetus through the abdominal wall of the mother and the amniotic sac. If hydrops fetalis is already established in utero, exchange transfusion is of little aid.

Nonreaction Transfusion Risks

Circulatory overload, air emboli, and infiltration are blood transfusion risks in the same manner that they are IV infusion risks. They should be prevented and treated similarly. If the risk of circulatory overload is great, packed cells should be favored over whole blood. Most metabolic derangements such as acidosis or alkalosis, hyperkalemia, and hypocalcemia can be minimized by using fresh blood, no older than 4 to 5 days.

Procedures Involving Thermoregulation

Ineffective thermoregulation in neonates may result from an immature thermoregulatory mechanism or illness. Older infants and children have thermoregulatory difficulties primarily caused by illness. Immediately after birth, a cap is placed on the neonates, and they are wrapped securely. Mitts may be placed on their hands and feet.

The Closed Incubator

The closed incubator (or Isolette) provides a controlled thermal environment (Fig. 25-15A). The inside of the incubator is, for the most part, free of external influences. Infants in a closed incubator system are in a "neutral thermal environment." Such an environment can best be described as one that maintains the infant's body temperature between 36.5° and 37° C without the expense of excessive use of brown fat and glycogen stores and the excessive consumption of oxygen. A neutral thermal environment prevents the use of body energy to maintain body heat that is maintained through a feedback system called *servocontrol*. A temperature probe attached to the abdomen (on the lower right quadrant) feeds the infant's temperature reading to the heating mechanism in the incubator. This heating mechanism is set to respond to any change in infant temperature from a preprogrammed measurement.

If a change in the infant's temperature occurs, heat is automatically increased or decreased in the incubator until the infant's temperature returns to the preset norm.

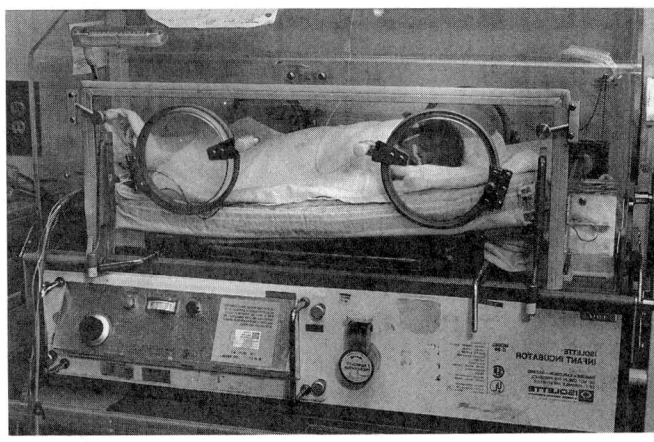
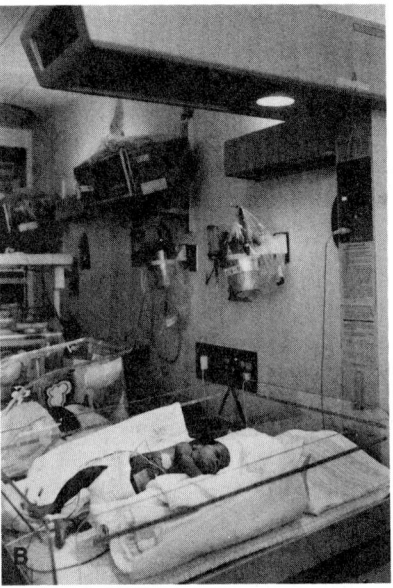

FIGURE 25-15
Thermoregulation units. (**A**) Closed incubator (Isolette). (**B**) Radiant warmer (open incubator). (Source: Skale, N. [1992]. *Manual of pediatric nursing procedures.* Philadelphia: J. B. Lippincott.)

Radiant heat loss through the outer walls of the incubator can be reduced with a double-walled hood. The "greenhouse effect" can be diminished by maintaining the environmental temperature outside the incubator comfortable but not excessively warm.

Nursing responsibilities related to the infant in thermal incubation include the following:

- Observing the incubator hood temperature often and taking special note of a gradient rise or drop over time—Gradient alterations in hood temperature may be indicative of hypothermic or hyperthermic illness in the infant.
- Maintaining the thermal probe on an open area of the skin exposed to circulating incubator air—If the probe risks being blocked because of the infant's position, the probe should be moved to a more suitable site.
- Opening the incubator portholes only when essential.
- Ensuring that all items coming in contact with the infant (e.g., stethoscope) are prewarmed.
- Avoiding removal of the infant from the closed incubator unless absolutely necessary—When infants must be removed, they should be well covered, especially the head. If infants must be exposed or kept out of the closed incubator for more than a few minutes, a radiant warmer should be used. Infants should be transported in a portable closed incubator.
- Weaning of the infant from the incubator—Such weaning can begin when the infant's probe temperature has remained between 36° and 37° C without assistance from the servocontrol system for 48 hours.

The Radiant Warmer (Open Incubator)

More stable infants may be cared for under a radiant warmer (or open incubator; see Fig. 25-15*B*). Although the skin probe and servocontrol mechanism are also used with radiant warmers, the bassinet environment is still exposed to external influences. Because of this exposure, the infant who is under a radiant warmer for extended

periods is more susceptible to fluid loss. This loss must be compensated with additional oral or IV fluids. The body temperature probe should be covered with a cotton ball and tape when the infant is under the radiant warmer. This prevents the probe temperature reading from being influenced by heat moving directly downward from the radiant hood.

Other Thermal Support Equipment

Concave heat shields or thermal bubble blankets can be used to conserve body heat in an open or closed incubator when it is necessary for the infant to remain visually exposed. An electronic thermal blanket with a wide temperature range can accommodate cooling of the hyperthermic child (temperature is set at about 5° C) or warming of the hypothermic child (temperature set at about 40° C).

The Tepid Sponge Bath

The cooling bath has been used as a means of reducing body temperature for decades. Recent evaluation of the tepid sponge bath has produced some interesting facts, such as the following:

- Some research suggests that tepid sponging does not have an antipyretic effect.
- Some evidence suggests tepid sponging has a therapeutic effect primarily when fever is the result of excessive heat production, when the body's set point has remained normal. Although the recommended temperature range for the tepid sponge bath is usually 29.5° to 32.5° C for infants and children, there is evidence to suggest that a tepid sponge bath at 37° C (normal body temperature) can be just as effective.

The principle underlying the use of the tepid sponge bath is that the evaporation of water from the skin's surface produces cooling. Evidence suggesting that a tepid sponge bath is more effective than immersion in tepid water lends credence to this rationale. Care must be taken not to use cold water because water much lower than 27° C usually produces surface vasoconstriction and shivering, both of which increase core body temperature. Water cooler than 27° C is contraindicated unless the child's temperature is excessively high (>41° C), thus producing a risk of febrile seizures or cerebral dysfunction.

Because of the relative instability of thermoregulation in infancy, a tepid sponge bath for an infant should not exceed 10 to 15 minutes in length. Older children may be sponged for 20 to 40 minutes, depending on the circumstances. The child's temperature should be monitored regularly during the bath and for 1 to 2 hours after it. A temperature drop greater than 0.5° C per hour is contraindicated as it may produce shock or thermoregulatory mismanagement by the body. The alcohol sponge bath, once considered an appropriate technique for reducing body temperature, is no longer encouraged because of the following reasons:

- Alcohol produces a too rapid heat loss (up to 1° to 1.5° C per hour).
- Alcohol is absorbed through the skin.
- Alcohol has a drying effect on the skin.

With each degree Celsius rise in body temperature, the child experiences a 10% to 13% fluid loss. The nurse must ensure adequate fluid intake as well as employ techniques to reduce body temperature.

Procedures Involving Oxygenation

Because breathing is vital to life, a common nursing responsibility is to help the child receive adequate oxygenation.

Oxygen Therapy

The pathophysiologic conditions requiring oxygen therapy in children are numerous. However, the physiologic alterations requiring such therapy fall into two categories: *hypoxemia,* which leads to *hypoxia.* Hypoxic states can occur quickly in children, and oxygen therapy accomplishes two purposes: (1) it increases the oxygen tension of blood plasma; and (2) it restores the oxyhemoglobin in the red blood cells to normal proportions. When a child needs oxygen therapy, a physician's order must be written specifying the method or type of delivery, the concentration to be given, and the duration of delivery (continuous or intermittent).

Pure oxygen is cool and dry. Both of these characteristics can cause problems for children. Thermoregulatory mechanisms are unstable in the young child, and the use of unwarmed oxygen can lead to hypothermia. Children suffering from infectious conditions are usually febrile, and they respond to excessive cooling by shivering uncontrollably. Unhumidified oxygen can lead to bronchoconstriction and excessive drying of mucous membranes in the mouth, throat, and respiratory organs.

Equipment. The following paragraphs describe the most common types of oxygen equipment and their delivery concentrations, maximum flow rates, advantages, and disadvantages.

Nasal Cannula (Prongs). The nasal cannula is illustrated in Figure 25-16A.

Oxygen concentration delivered by nasal prong as much as 45% to 50%. Maximum flow rate is 5 to 6 liters per minute. The advantages of using nasal prongs include the following:

- The prongs allow considerable mobility.
- The equipment does not distort the child's visual field.

Disadvantages of the use of nasal prongs include the following:

- Young children often resist cannulas.
- Restraints may be needed.
- The oxygen can be irritating to the nares and nasal mucosa.
- Oxygen concentration is difficult to measure.

Blow-By (Offset) Cannula. An adaptation of nasal prongs, an offset cannula may be a regular nasal cannula with the prongs cut off or a narrow oxygen catheter containing small perforations through which oxygen can flow. Its openings may be placed under the child's nose or anchored on the face in such a way as to direct the oxygen flow toward the nose.

The oxygen concentration delivered by a cannula is approximately 25% to 30%. The maximum flow rate is 5 to 6 liters per minute. The advantages include the following:

- The cannula allows for considerable mobility.
- Children tolerate the cannula more readily than prongs.
- Nasal mucous membranes are not irritated by cannula.
- The cannula does not distort the child's visual field.

The disadvantages include the following:

- Restraints may be needed.
- The concentration of oxygen actually reaching the child is variable and difficult to control or measure.

Nasal Catheter. The nasal catheter delivers oxygen in as much as a 50% concentration. The maximum flow rate is 5 to 6 liters per minute. The advantages include the following:

- The catheter allows considerable mobility without risk of dislodgement.
- The child can be discharged on home oxygen therapy using a nasal catheter.

The disadvantages include the following:

- Oxygen concentration cannot be measured accurately.
- The catheter must be moved to alternate nares every 8 to 12 hours to prevent mucosal irritation.

Face Mask. Oxygen may be delivered by the mask (see Fig. 25-16B), and the oxygen concentration delivered, depending on the type of mask, is the following:

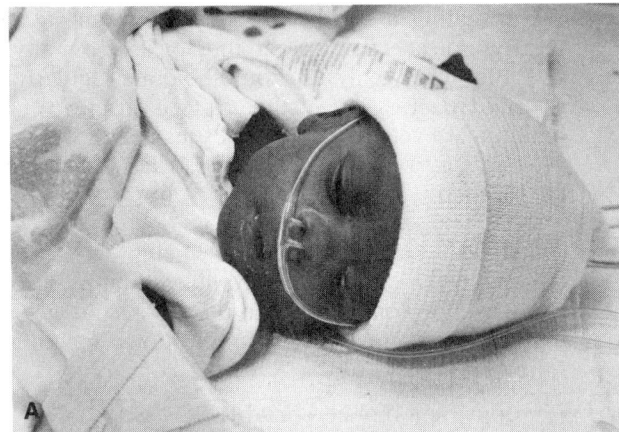

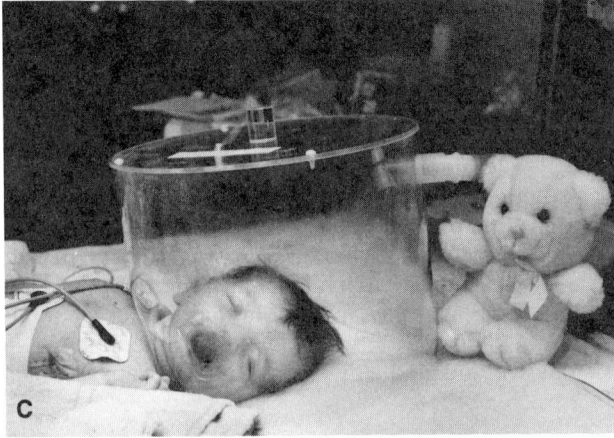

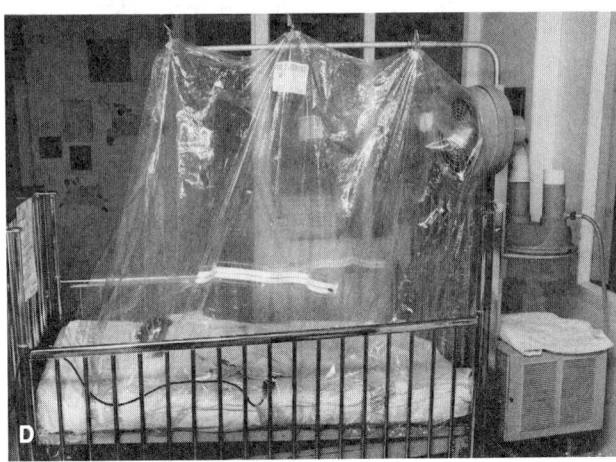

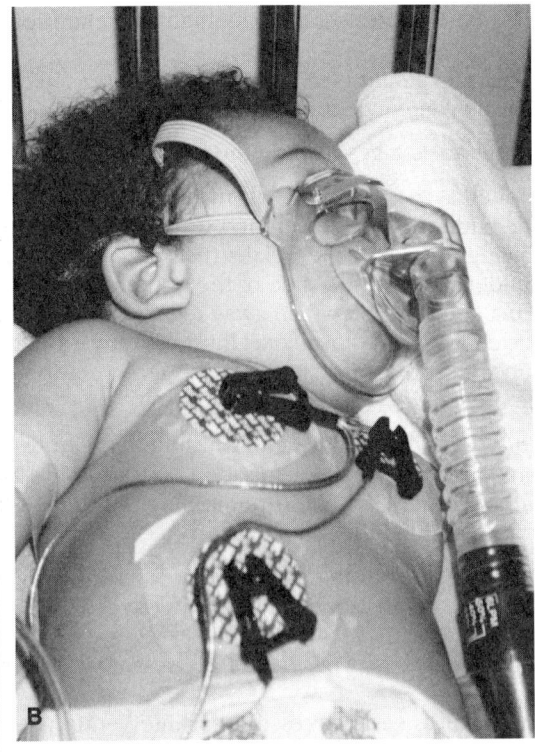

FIGURE 25-16
Several types of oxygen therapy for children. (A) Nasal cannula. (B) Face mask. (C) Oxygen hood. (D) Mist tent. (Source: Skale, N. *Manual of pediatric nursing procedures.* Philadelphia: J. B. Lippincott.)

- *Venturi*—25% to 50%
- *Non-rebreathing*—50% to 95%
- *Partial rebreathing*—40% to 60%

The maximum flow rate is 5 to 10 liters per minute but should not be more than 4 to 5 liters for an infant. Advantages include the following:

- A high concentration of oxygen is delivered effectively.
- The concentration of oxygen is easy to measure.
- The mask can be used to deliver aerosol therapy.

The disadvantages include the following:

- Children may not tolerate a face mask well because it covers both the mouth and the nose and can feel restricting.
- The oxygen concentration is dependent on the security of mask and size of air intake holes.
- The mask is not well tolerated for long-term therapy because it can be irritating to facial tissue.

Oxygen Hood. The oxygen hood is illustrated in Figure 25-16C. Oxygen concentration delivered is 40% to almost 100%. The maximum flow rate is 10 liters per minute. The advantages include the following:

- The hood can deliver a stable, high concentration of oxygen.
- Facial movement is not restricted.
- The oxygen concentration can be readily assessed.

The disadvantages include the following:

- Limited access to head is allowed.
- The child must be positioned so that oxygen is not flowing directly at the facial structures.
- Condensation on the side of the hood has a cooling effect and must be wiped away regularly.
- The child's head movements must be watched so that skin abrasions caused by rubbing against equipment are prevented.

Isolette. The open isolette illustrated in Figure 25-15*B* can deliver oxygen concentration at 40% to 85%. The maximum flow rate is 10 liters per minute. Advantages of the isolette include the following:

- Mobility is not restricted.
- A steady, even concentration of oxygen can be maintained.
- The infant is easily observed for assessment from all angles.
- The infant is easily accessible for interventions.
- Oxygen concentration is easily measured.

The disadvantages include the following:

- An oxygen hood must be placed inside the Isolette to achieve concentrations of oxygen higher than 85%.
- Sensory stimulation may be needed because the infant is totally enclosed.

Mist Tent (Croupette). The mist tent is illustrated in Figure 25-16*D*. The oxygen concentration delivered averages 35% to 40%. If the flow rate is not kept at 10 liters per minute or greater, an oxygen concentration of 40% is difficult to maintain.[3]

The advantages of mist tent use include the following:

- The tent allows the older child considerable freedom of mobility.
- It allows oxygen to be delivered with high moisture content when needed.
- Some aerosol medications can be delivered by mist tent.

The disadvantages include the following:

- Adequate oxygen concentration levels are difficult to maintain; oxygen leaks out under a loose canopy.
- Vision and hearing are distorted by the tent.
- The child can feel trapped and isolated.

Effectiveness. Oxygen therapy should be guided by the following principle: Give the lowest concentration for the shortest period to produce the desired results. Oxygen concentration can be measured readily with face masks, hoods, and Isolettes. Measurement of delivered concentration is difficult, and at best inaccurate, with nasal prongs, blow-bys, and nasal catheters. Measurements of oxygen concentration should be conducted close to the child's face every 4 to 6 hours.

The most important measure of therapeutic success is the PaO_2 level in the circulating blood. Blood gas analysis revealing a steady PaO_2 rate between 58 and 62 mmHg indicates that oxygen therapy is essentially effective. Blood gas analyses should be done regularly when the child receives oxygen therapy (see Chapter 37). When children are very ill, blood gases may be drawn as often as every 15 to 30 minutes until satisfactory PaO_2 levels are reached.

Risks. Care must be taken when providing oxygen therapy to the child with chronic respiratory disorders. Excessive, prolonged oxygen therapy results in oxygen toxicity, producing many complications, including the following:

- Constriction of cerebral blood vessels
- Bronchodysplasia
- ''Lung burn'', resulting in decreased mucus production, alveolar impairment, surfactant inactivation
- Interstitial fibrosis
- Atelectasis
- Pulmonary edema (possibly leading to death)

Retinopathy of prematurity (ROP) was, until recently, thought to result from high concentrations of oxygen given to preterm infants. Recent research, however, suggests that ROP has multiple causative factors. In fact, some studies indicate that high concentrations of oxygen were not implicated in any way in the development of ROP.[4] As with many drugs, oxygen therapy should be withdrawn slowly and gradually unless complications are suspected.

Postural Drainage, Percussion, and Vibration

Postural drainage, percussion, and vibration are chest therapy techniques used for the following reasons:

- Prevent the accumulation of secretions in the lungs
- Assist the force of gravity and natural ciliary activity of the bronchial tree to move secretions upward
- Provide an opportunity for effective coughing

Postural Drainage. Postural drainage may be accompanied by percussion, vibration, or both. These two activities mechanically assist with dislodging and moving secretions toward the trachea for expulsion. Postural drainage can be performed once a day or as often as four times a day, depending on the extent of lung congestion. When postural drainage is performed once a day, it is best done in the morning before breakfast, thus removing all secretions that have collected overnight. Usually, the most effective schedule for postural drainage is four times a day: early morning, 1 to 1½ hours before lunch and supper, and before bedtime. Bedtime sessions clear the lungs for a restful sleep and reduce the volume of secretions accumulating overnight.

Positioning. Positions selected for postural drainage are determined primarily by information obtained from chest x-rays and auscultation of the chest. In most large institutions a physiotherapist does the initial chest assessment and postural drainage plan. The physiotherapist may then orient the nursing staff to the plan so that they can carry out the activity if necessary. Infants can be held in the lap or positioned in the crib over pillows (Fig.

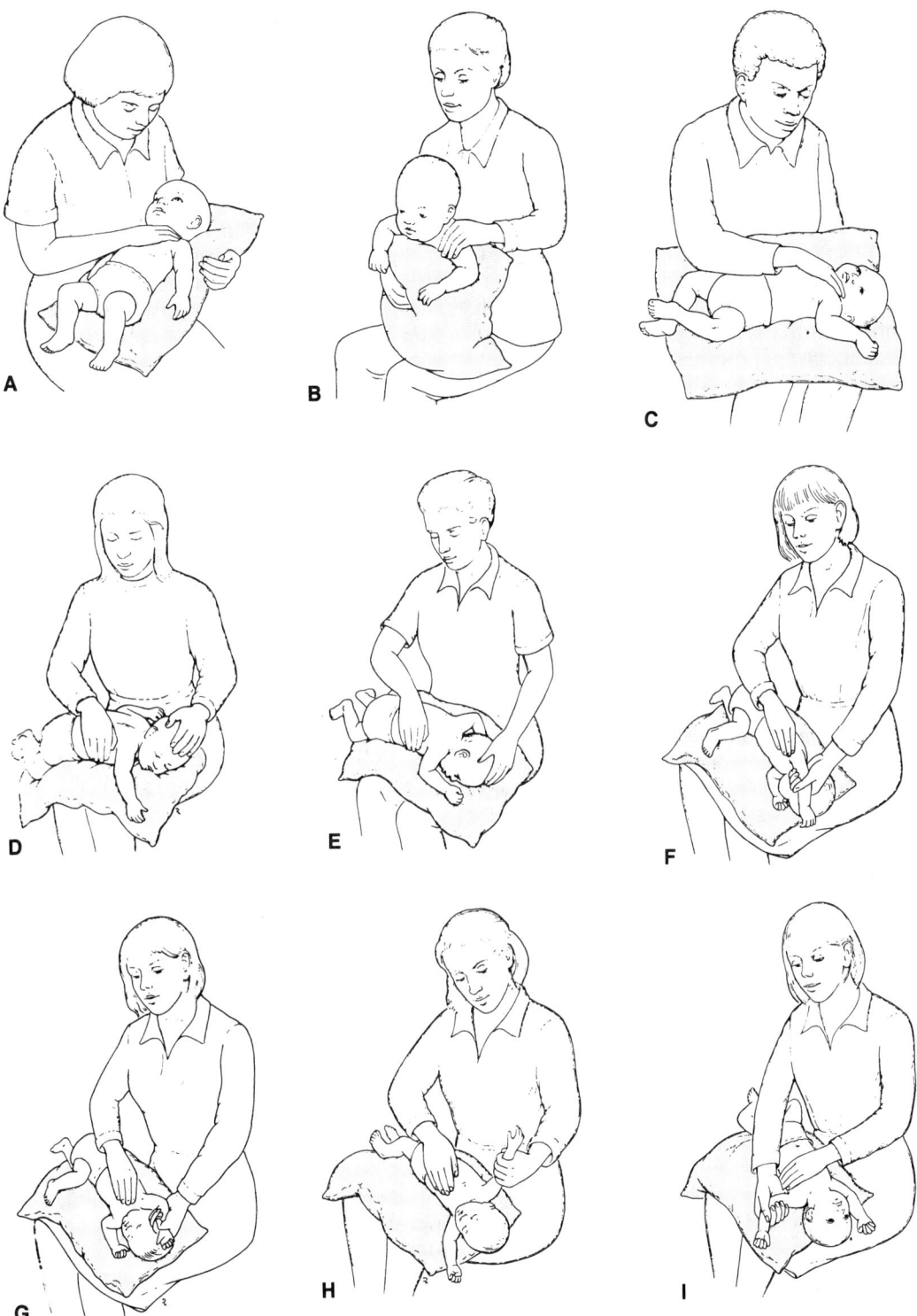

FIGURE 25-17
Bronchial drainage positions for the main segments of all lobes in infants. (**A**) Apical segment of left lower lobe. (**B**) Posterior segment of left lower lobe. (**C**) Anterior segment of left upper lobe. (**D**) Superior segment of right lower lobe. (**E**) Posterior segment of right lower lobe. (**F**) Lateral segment of right lower lobe. (**G**) Anterior basal segment of lower lobe. (**H**) Right middle lobe. (**I**) Lingular segments of left upper lobe. (Source: Skale, N. [1992]. *Manual of pediatric nursing procedures.* Philadelphia: J. B. Lippincott.)

25-17). Older children may be positioned over the knees or in bed, with appropriate adjustments made to the bed's position (Fig. 25-18).

Thirty minutes is the maximum time a child should receive postural drainage. Positions may be held from 2 to 10 minutes, with four to six positions being the maximum number that can usually be tolerated at one session. Infants can often only tolerate 10 to 15 minutes. Infants in Isolettes can be positioned by using small towels or washcloths for positioning, or the Isolette can be tipped.

Coughing should be encouraged but not forced during postural drainage. Deep diaphragmatic breathing with a full cough on the third expiration tends to be the most effective. The sequence of postures usually follows gravitational pull (i.e., lower to middle to upper lobes), although this sequence can vary.

Percussion.

The correct technique for performing percussion includes the following three directives:

- Hands are cupped and held in that shape.
- The arms are relaxed.
- The hands are moved up and down at the wrist. A hollow sound is produced as the cupped hand is drummed over the area being percussed.

With older children, percussing is done at a rate of two to three cups per second for 1- to 2-minute stretches. Infants may be unable to tolerate more than 30 to 60 seconds at a time. Total percussion time should not exceed 20 to 30 minutes for an older child or 10 to 15 minutes for an infant. If the hands are too large to percuss an infant safely, adaptations can be made to small aerosol face masks or feeding nipples so that they can be used as percussion instruments. Mechanical percussors are also available.

Vibration.

Vibration may be performed after, or in place of, percussion and is sometimes used on infants. There are many hand-held vibrators but a covered electric toothbrush is an effective vibrating device for young infants. The technique for performing vibrations manually requires the following directives:

- One hand is placed over top of the other to form one unit shaped like a V.
- Both arms are locked stiff at the elbow and shoulders.
- The heel of the bottom hand is propelled forward with a quivering motion.

If the hands are too large to provide vibration for an infant, an adapted version using the balls of the index and middle finger together can be used. Vibrations are performed in rapid succession on expiration. All unforced efforts to cough should be encouraged.

Aerosol Medications.

If bronchodilator or mucolytic aerosol medications are ordered by the physician, they should be given about 20 minutes before postural drainage, percussion, and vibration procedures begin. The medication helps stimulate productive coughing during the procedures. If a child is unable to cough productively or expel sputum, suctioning may be necessary.

General Considerations.

Percussion and vibrations should never be performed over bare skin and should be confined to the area needing treatment. Neither technique should be directed over the sternum, stomach, flank, or spinal column. The procedures are contraindicated if the child has acute asthma, pulmonary hemorrhage (or at risk for hemorrhage), bronchospasms, seizures (or risk of seizures), risk for pathologic fractures, chest pain, or pulmonary embolus. Once the procedures have been completed, the chest should be reassessed by auscultation to determine the effectiveness of the activities. Charting of chest therapy procedures should include the following:

- Area(s) of the lung drained
- Actual techniques used
- Length of time of procedures
- Tolerance of procedures
- Effectiveness of procedures
- Amount and characteristics of sputum

Suctioning

Suctioning of the mouth, pharynx, and nares is performed to accomplish the following:

- Remove excess secretions that may hamper breathing
- Remove secretions that the infants or children may be unable to remove on their own
- Collect a sputum specimen for diagnostic purposes, when infants or children are unable to provide such a specimen independently

Suctioning the Neonate.

Except in special circumstances, neonatal suctioning is performed manually with a bulb syringe. Mechanical suction is usually unnecessary and may, in fact, provide a level of suction pressure harmful to delicate mucosa. The mouth and pharynx are cleared first, and the nares last. This sequence prevents sneezing or gasping caused by stimulation of the nares. Such responses can cause aspiration. The most critical step in bulb suctioning is to squeeze the bulb *before* placing the syringe in the mouth or nares. Squeezing the bulb after insertion can drive mucus further down the throat or cause aspiration.

Suctioning the Child.

Suctioning is carried out under sterile conditions. Equipment includes a sterile suction catheter, Y-connector to suction, sterile gloves, and sterile normal saline. The catheter depends on the size of the child, as follows:

- Small infant: 6 to 8 French
- Older infant to preschooler: 8 French
- Older than preschooler: 10 French

The procedure for *oropharyngeal suctioning* the child includes the following:

- Wash hands and gloves.
- Attach catheter to suction system.
- Dip the catheter in saline for lubrication.
- Leaving the Y-connector tip OPEN, insert the catheter along one side of the oral cavity to the back of the pharynx.

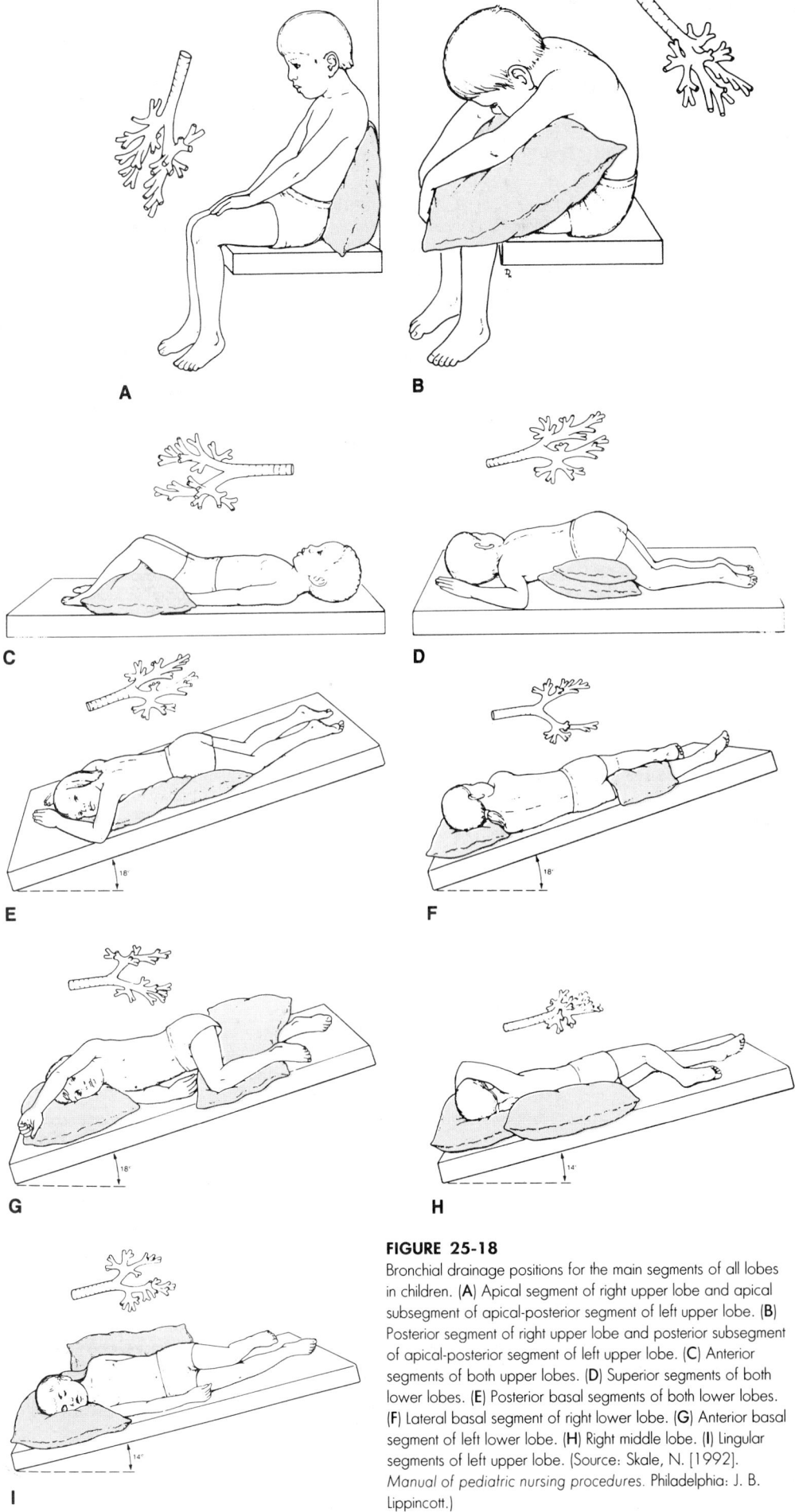

FIGURE 25-18

Bronchial drainage positions for the main segments of all lobes in children. (**A**) Apical segment of right upper lobe and apical subsegment of apical-posterior segment of left upper lobe. (**B**) Posterior segment of right upper lobe and posterior subsegment of apical-posterior segment of left upper lobe. (**C**) Anterior segments of both upper lobes. (**D**) Superior segments of both lower lobes. (**E**) Posterior basal segments of both lower lobes. (**F**) Lateral basal segment of right lower lobe. (**G**) Anterior basal segment of left lower lobe. (**H**) Right middle lobe. (**I**) Lingular segments of left upper lobe. (Source: Skale, N. [1992]. *Manual of pediatric nursing procedures.* Philadelphia: J. B. Lippincott.)

TABLE 25-9
Nursing Interventions for Anxiety and Fear Related to Painful or Invasive Procedures

Emotional Response	Nursing Interventions	Rationale
Infants		
Loud crying and withdrawal behavior when physically hurt	Interact (hold, play, and talk) with the infant before performing a procedure.	Infants are primarily concerned with the development of trusting relationships.
Vigorous crying and general physical activity when restraint attempted	Give a brief, nonthreatening explanation in anticipation of discomfort, e.g., ''You're going to feel a little prick'' (injection).	Although it is clear that the infant cannot fully understand what is being explained, such ''preparation'' may allow the infant a feeling of not being ''attacked.'' It also helps to prevent a wary suspiciousness toward all nurse-infant interactions.
Inconsolable if tension-producing circumstances are prolonged	Distract the infant during the procedure with a toy, picture, or interaction with a nonthreatening third party (e.g., parents).	Infants have a short attention span and are easily distracted. This activity also may produce a side benefit by making parents feel more useful and less anxious. *Caution:* Use discretion as the infant should not associate long, painful procedures with the parent.
	Complete the procedure as quickly, efficiently, and painlessly as possible (e.g., collect all preparatory equipment prior to the procedure).	Infants have a low tolerance for prolonged stress and a limited repertoire of self-initiated tension-reducing behaviors.
	Provide the infant with immediate physical and verbal comforting as soon as the procedure is completed (e.g., offer security object or return infant to parents).	Invasive or painful procedures violate the infant's sense of trust. If this violation is to produce only short-term, situational stress, the sense of trust must be reinforced as soon as possible after a procedure is completed.
Toddlers		
Fear of strangers or health professionals (especially dressed in white)	Explain the procedure in relation to the toddler's senses, e.g., ''this will feel like a mosquito bite'' (subcutaneous injection) or ''this medicine tastes like bubble gum'' (flavored amoxicillin).	Toddlers are egocentric and view the world through their senses.
Fear of separation from the parent produces considerable crying and acting out		
Toddlers sometimes imagine that a procedure will cause the body to fall apart (e.g., parts of body might come out an injection site)	Use words that do not promote fantasizing. Words and phrases like ''fix,'' ''help you feel better,'' and ''take away the hurt'' imply helpful, nonthreatening intervention. Words like ''cut,'' ''blood,'' ''break,'' and ''poke,'' imply injury and feelings of threat to body integrity.	Toddlers' fantasies are based on: Limited perceptions of body boundaries Inability to conceptualize cause and effect A concrete understanding of words A fear of words implying body threat
Fear of injury or pain can produce acting-out behaviors like temper tantrums	Present information to the toddler in simple words and short sentences.	Toddlers' understanding of language is limited.
Regressive behavior is common (e.g., a toilet-trained toddler begins wetting)	Present small amounts of information at a time.	Toddlers have a short attention span.
An increase in self-comforting behaviors like thumb sucking or clutching of security objects	Have the child tell you what will happen during a procedure and clarify misconceptions.	The explanation allows the nurse to evaluate how much incorrect fantasizing about a procedure has occurred.
	If appropriate and time allows, let the child play with equipment to be used during a procedure.	The toddler learns primarily through sensory-motor interaction.
	Time the explanation according to the trauma it will produce. Traumatic procedures, such as injections, should be explained *just before* they are performed.	The toddler's conception of time is limited, as are coping strategies.
	Offer choices within the toddler's ability to grasp.	A sense of autonomy and beginning independence are important to the toddler. Choices must be kept within the toddler's concept of causality.
	Allow the child a short opportunity to be angry and protest before beginning a procedure.	Allowing the initial expression of natural responses to fear will help toddlers initiate their own rudimentary psychological defenses. Because these defenses are limited in scope, the expression of anger and protest must have a limited time frame.
	Encourage the parents to participate in the procedure by supporting and comforting the child whenever possible.	Separation anxiety is a major fear in toddlerhood.
	Allow the child to hold (or be near) a treasured security object during a procedure.	Such objects support attempts to self-comfort and promote a sense of control.
	Encourage the toddler to use helpful behaviors that will please parents.	Most toddlers are eager to please loved ones or other significant persons and enjoy hearing, ''You were so helpful.''

(Continued)

TABLE 25-9
(Continued)

Emotional Response	Nursing Interventions	Rationale
	Toddlers' desire for autonomy makes them proud of even the simplest accomplishment.	Encourage toddlers to play afterward. Equipment used during a procedure can be offered if appropriate.
	Hold the child firmly (when necessary), be consistent with expected behavior, and complete the procedure as quickly as possible.	Firm physical holding and consistency of expectations can help the toddler feel secure and reduce the fear of loss of limited self-control. Completing the procedure quickly reduces the time that the toddler's own limited coping strategies need to be functional.
	Distract rather than restrain the child when appropriate.	Toddlers are easily distracted and fear undue restraint.
	Sanction the expression of emotions, such as crying, during a procedure.	The toddler's coping strategies are limited, and crying is an effective tension reducer.
	Allow the toddler to take part in the procedure in any way reasonable, e.g., holding a Band-Aid.	Encourage autonomy and independence.
	Comfort and console the child after the procedure.	Sense of trust and desire for security and love are prominent in toddlerhood as well as infancy.
Preschoolers		
Castration fears evident when procedures involve the penis or perineal area	Use words of explanation that will prepare the child for the sensation that can be expected during the procedure.	The preschooler still relates to the world primarily through the senses.
Fear of pain is prominent because the child has had some experience with pain	Supplement verbal explanations with demonstrations that allow the child to use the visual, auditory, and tactile senses (e.g., use of dolls and puppets, or practice trials with real equipment).	Although more verbally competent than the toddler, the preschooler still relates better through sensory interaction.
As with castration fears, a general fear of body mutilation is at its peak	Tell the child exactly what body parts will be involved in the procedure, and reassure that privacy will be maintained.	Fear of castration and body mutilation are strong in the preschooler. Imagination and fantasy are still prominent. This is the time when privacy is important, and drapes are appreciated.
The child may invent bizarre scenarios related to the procedure	Demonstrate actual equipment to be used when explaining whenever it is feasible.	Preschooler needs to see or touch the equipment to alleviate fears.
As language understanding progresses, preschoolers can express fears with more verbal finesse than toddlers	Use time frames that relate to the activities of the child's day, e.g., ''just after breakfast,'' ''before 'Sesame Street' comes on,'' or ''before you go to bed.''	Although the preschooler's time perception is better than the toddler's, it still tends to revolve around the child's boundaries of daily living.
Separation anxiety with loud crying may still be a prominent reaction	Allow the preschooler to make limited choices related to the procedure when feasible.	Preschoolers are trying to master their environment, and opportunities to exercise self-determination are useful in this achievement process.
	Separate complicated explanations by conducting two or three shorter sessions.	The preschooler has an attention span of approximately 15 minutes.
	Clarify any misconceptions the child has about the procedure ahead of time.	The preschooler has a vivid imagination, and explanations can reduce unnecessary anxiety.
	Make it clear to the child that the procedure is not a punishment for wrongdoing.	The preschooler is beginning to develop a conscience and may perceive a procedure, particularly a painful one, as punishment.
	Encourage the preschooler to ask questions about the procedure and answer such questions simply and honestly.	The preschooler is naturally inquisitive. Encouraging this activity assists the child in understanding activities in the immediate world.
	Offer the preschooler clear direction as to ways he or she can be helpful during the procedure.	Preschoolers are learning norms of behavior and are usually anxious to conform to the expectations of others.
	Encourage the preschooler to help in any way that is reasonable during a procedure.	Helping can promote the child's sense of mastery.
	After a procedure is completed, verbally praise the child and reward in concrete ways, e.g., stickers.	Preschoolers respond well to praise and concrete rewards for appropriate behavior.
	With any procedure that invades body integrity (e.g., injection or blood sample), offer the child a Band-Aid.	Fear of body mutilation is high, and this alleviates the child's fears.
	Offer toys or equipment for postprocedure acting-out.	Although preschoolers have better language understanding than toddlers, they still have difficulty expressing their emotions verbally.

(Continued)

TABLE 25-9
(Continued)

Emotional Response	Nursing Interventions	Rationale
	Include parents in all aspects of the procedure (if appropriate). Especially encourage them to comfort the child once the procedure is complete.	Separation anxiety is still a common fear and, in most instances, parents are still the best comforters.
School-Age Children Fear of loss of control over situation Fear of pain or injury Fear of body mutilation Fear of "losing face" with adults or fear of "losing status" with peers.	Prepare the child in a private setting. The older school-age child may prefer not to have parents present.	Peer group relations are important, and the child may not want to risk asking a "dumb" question in front of others. The older school-age child may wish to maintain status as an independent person by preparing for and undergoing a procedure without the presence of parents.
	Explain the procedures verbally with the assistance of diagrams, pictures, and other items.	The school-age child is verbally competent and, by the late school years, has a reasonably broad vocabulary. Visual skills are usually well developed; therefore, using diagrams and pictures is appropriate.
	Use correct terminology during the explanation. Medical terminology can be used within reason.	The child's vocabulary is increasing. Scientific terminology is presented in school, and using language that is too simplistic or "babyish" can be insulting.
	Use anatomically correct drawings and teaching dolls to explain procedures.	The school-age child is aware of parts and can be anxious when body integrity may be disrupted. Using visual aids ensures that the child has a concrete grasp of what will happen. Abstract thinking is too complex, and concrete explanations are best.
	Encourage the discussion of feelings and the verbalization of fears. Discuss concerns about privacy needs.	Although the school-age child is intent on mastering situations and maintaining control, unsubstantiated fears often cause regression in mastery behaviors. An underlying fear of revealing body parts is also a concern.
	Have the child describe the procedure to clarify misconceptions about the process, body parts involved, or expectation of results.	Fears of mutilation are still intense in the school-age child, who knows his or her own physical structure reasonably well and is reluctant to risk a disruption of its integrity.
	Give the school-age child a broader range of choice than the preschooler when possible, e.g., time for a procedure to be performed, selecting a site for an injection, and other situations.	The desire for situation mastery is strong in the school-age child. Their general knowledge of cause and effect and ability to reason indicate that school-aged children are probably able to make sensible choices in circumstances they understand.
	Begin to prepare the child for a procedure as soon as possible.	The school-age child has a more realistic concept of time. Advance information gives the child time to mobilize some of the defenses needed to maintain self-control during a procedure.
	Expect cooperation from the child, but assure the child that crying is acceptable and usually helpful, particularly when a procedure is painful.	The school-age child is capable of cooperation. However, excessive self-restraint may be harmful as emotional mastery is still in its early stages. Crying as an emotional release can provide the child with the strength to reinforce other aspects of self-control, e.g., staying still or not crying out.
	Provide as much opportunity as possible for the child to participate in the procedure.	Situational mastery is important to the school-age child and may prevent regressive behavior after the procedure.
	Praise the child liberally once the procedure is completed. Particularly emphasize the cooperative and assisting behaviors the child exhibited.	Positive feedback produces a pride in accomplishment. This contributes to a general sense of environmental mastery and fosters the desire to be responsible in other circumstances.
Adolescents Fear of loss of independence Fear of loss of control Intense fear of body mutilation Concern about the invasion of privacy Disruption of body image identity	Prepare the adolescent in privacy, preferably without the parents.	The adolescent values privacy and may prefer to make decisions independently.
	Prepare the adolescent well in advance as much as possible.	Advance preparation allows the adolescent to use problem-solving skills to prepare the necessary coping strategies.

(Continued)

TABLE 25-9
(Continued)

Emotional Response	Nursing Interventions	Rationale
	Explain the procedure using scientific terms and body diagrams to reinforce explanations, and provide rationale for treatment.	Adolescents can think in more sophisticated terms than younger children. Although most are concerned about how the procedure will affect the body, they also need to know of any lasting residual effects that can be expected.
	Explain that the feelings engendered by the procedure are common and that other adolescents undergoing the procedure have the same types of feelings.	The need to feel a ''sameness'' with the peer group or not to be unlike the others is intense during adolescence.
	Reinforce teaching by having another adolescent who has undergone the procedure talk to the patient.	A peer can be seen as a confidant and reinforce feelings of ''sameness.'' It may be easier for adolescents to express feelings to a peer because appearing dependent in the presence of an adult threatens autonomy.
	Give the adolescent as much control as possible over elements such as time and place for a procedure and who can be present.	The desire for self-control and independence is intense in adolescence.
	Reassure the adolescent that privacy will be maintained as much as possible.	The adolescent's need to maintain control in front of others makes the need for privacy acute.
	Provide an opportunity for the patient to talk to another adolescent who has been in similar circumstances after the procedure is completed. The ideal situation would be to have the patient talk to the same adolescent who was helpful before undergoing the procedure.	The opportunity to share in retrospect provides both adolescents with reinforcement for their normality and ''sameness.''

- Once the catheter is in place, apply gentle suction by occluding the Y-connector outlet with the thumb.
- Draw the catheter out using a smooth motion along the side of the oral cavity.
- The catheter should be rolled constantly as it is being withdrawn. This motion helps prevent mucosal tissue from being sucked against the catheter opening.
- The withdrawal process should take about 5 to 10 seconds for an infant and about 15 to 20 seconds for an older child.
- The withdrawal stroke should be one smooth motion outward. Back and forth stroking is inappropriate.
- Once the suctioning stroke is completed, the catheter should be rinsed with normal saline.
- After allowing the child to rest for 1 to 3 minutes, the process can be repeated along the other side of the mouth.
- Suctioning can continue, with alternating of the sides of the mouth until the oropharynx is clear or the child is fatigued.

The procedure for *nasopharyngeal suctioning* is identical to that of oropharyngeal suctioning, with the exception of the following:

- The distance for catheter insertion is determined by measuring the distance from the tip of the nose to the earlobe. The catheter is inserted the number of centimeters indicated by that measure.
- Suctioning is performed by alternating nares.

Once the procedure is completed, the catheter and gloves are discarded, the remaining equipment is properly disposed, required specimens are collected, and the procedure is charted. Documentation should include notations regarding the child's tolerance of the procedure and the characteristics of suctioned sputum. It is not uncommon for the infant or small child to be given an oxygen flush prior to suctioning. This procedure is especially useful when obstructive respiratory conditions, coronary conditions, or pulmonary edema are present.

Procedures Involving Immunoregulation

Isolation

Isolation should always be considered an undesirable option in pediatrics and, when required, should be as brief as possible. Most childhood isolation consists of one of the following methods:

- Contact precautions—for acute respiratory infections
- Respiratory precautions—for communicable diseases
- Enteric precautions—for gastroenteritis or diarrhea

These precautions are known as *category specific*, meaning that the precautions are based on the mode of transmission of the infectious agent. *Disease-specific* precautions are developed on the basis of the mode of transmission of the organism responsible for the disease. Such isolation may require a private room, use of gowns and masks, and proper disposal of articles used by or for the patient.

Extreme forms of isolation include the laminar flow hood and plastic bubble. The laminar flow hood is an enclosure that separates air flowing through it into layers. Each layer is then cleansed of microorganisms. These items are commonly used for children with compromised immune systems or during chemotherapy. The plastic bubble is a completely enclosed, germ-free environment for the child with immunodeficiency disease. It is rarely used.

Risks. When used with children, isolation causes some particular psychosocial concerns including the following:

- Exaggeration of normal separation anxiety in infants and toddlers
- Risk of isolation being perceived as a punishment by preschoolers and young school-age children
- Sensory anxiety and deprivation
- Parental resistance
- Disruption of vital tactile comforting in children
- Exaggeration of the pain and loss associated with severe illness such as burns, acquired immunodeficiency syndrome, and leukemia
- Regression in general development related to anxiety and sensory deprivation
- Distorted perceptions and fantasizing because of the nature of isolation clothing, that is, the masks, gowns, caps, gloves
- Regression of communication skills because significant facial body language of caregivers may be blocked by masks

Reduced sensory deprivation that accompanies isolation can generally be helped by consulting with a child life therapist and ensuring that age-specific play materials are provided for the child. Parents need to be encouraged to spend as much time comforting and playing with their children as circumstances allow. The nurse also should make an effort to comfort and play with the child outside of visits to perform procedures.

Parental resistance is usually based on the natural desire of parents to comfort and touch their ill child. Resistance can also be caused by a lack of understanding of reasons for, and procedures involved in, the particular type of isolation precautions their child is experiencing. Parental resistance can usually be overcome with teaching and encouragement.

The purpose and procedures involved in isolation precautions should also be explained to the child at his or her level of understanding. For the preschooler and young school-age child, *Meehan's Coloring Book* is a helpful teaching aid.

Summary

The child is a unique person who requires specialized nursing care based on evolving cognitive capabilities, developing social awareness, maturing physiology, and varying coping mechanisms. The integration of these factors is the critical element in implementing all procedures, whether the nurse relies on hospital procedure manuals or textbooks.

Basic concepts in procedural approaches consider informed consent, teaching related to procedures to be

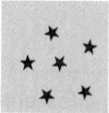

Ideas for Nursing Research

The large number of procedures performed on children for diagnostic and treatment purposes make this a rich area for investigation. Procedures are sometimes modified without adequate empirical confirmation that the change is beneficial. Likewise, some procedures remain unchanged because no scholarship has provided evidence of the need for change. The following areas need to be explored:

- Comparison of the length of the emotional recovery period after a painful procedure between children who had beloved security objects with them during the procedure and children who had no security objects with them.
- Expression of powerlessness during and after a procedure when children's mutual consent for the procedure has been sought and obtained and when it has not been sought and obtained.
- Comparison of the number of expressions of behavior indicative of inner ear disturbance (i.e., vertigo, nausea, and others) between children whose ear medications were given at room temperature and children whose ear medications were given warmed.
- Comparison of the rate of infiltration between scalp vein IVs infusing with the flow of blood and IVs infusing against the flow of blood.
- Comparison of findings of tests for specific gravity and fractional urine when urine is obtained from disposable versus cloth diapers.

performed, behavioral responses and coping mechanisms, and safety. The nurse's understanding of developmental goals and milestones aids in planning interventions for unique needs. Safety includes aseptic practices, judicious use of restraints, and movement of the child within the hospital environment.

General concepts introduced in this chapter help the student apply common procedures and nursing interventions in the assessment and maintenance of children's functional health and in nursing interventions to restore function.

References

1. Baer, C. L., & Williams, B. R. (1988). *Clinical pharmacology and nursing.* Springhouse, PA: Springhouse.
2. Beecroft, P. C., & Redick, S. (1989). Possible complications of intramuscular injections on the pediatric unit. *Pediatric Nursing, 15*(4), 333–336.
3. Clarke, P. H., & Deeds, N. C. (1988). The child in a mist tent. *Pediatric Nursing, 14*(6), 446–450.
4. George, D. S., Stephen, S., Fellows, R. R., & Bremer, D. L. (1988). The latest on retinopathy of prematurity. *MCN, 13,* 254–258.
5. Gerald, M. C., & O'Bannon, F. V. (1988). *Nursing pharmacology and therapeutics* (2nd ed.). Norwalk, CT: Appleton-Lange.
6. Hogue, E. E. (1988). Informed consent: Implications for critical care nurses. *Pediatric Nurse, 14*(4), 315–316.

7. Kelting, S., & Johnson, C. (1987). Erythropoiesis and neonatal blood transfusions. *MCN, 12,* 172–177.

8. Kozier, B., & Erb, G. (1989). *Techniques in clinical nursing* (3rd ed.). Menlo Park, CA: Addison-Wesley.

9. Manitoba Association of Registered Nurses. (May 11, 1988). *Position statement on the use of restraints.* Winnipeg, Manitoba, Canada: MARN.

10. Mathewson, M. K. (1991). *Pharmacotherapeutics: A nursing process approach* (2nd ed.). Philadelphia: F. A. Davis.

11. Osis, M. (1986). *Dosage calculations in SI units.* St. Louis: C. V. Mosby.

12. O'Brien, E. (1988). Clinical thermometry: In need of nursing research. *Journal of Pediatric Nursing, 3*(3), 207–208.

13. American Heart Association. (1987). *Recommendations for human blood pressure determination by sphygmomanometers: Report of a special task force.* Dallas, AHA.

14. Reeder, S. J., Martin, L. I., & Koniak, D. (1992). *Maternity nursing: Family, newborn, and women's health care* (17th ed.). Philadelphia: J. B. Lippincott.

15. Ross Laboratories. (1970). *Children are different: Relation of age to physiologic function.* Columbus, OH: Ross Laboratories.

16. Spencer, R. T., Nichols, L. W., Lipkin, G. B., Sabo, H. M., & West, F. M. (1993). *Clinical pharmacology and nursing management* (4th ed.). Philadelphia: J. B. Lippincott.

17. Taylor, N., Hutchison, E., Milliken, W., & Larson, E. (1989). Comparison of normal versus heparinized saline for flushing infusion devices. *Journal of Quality Assurance, 3*(4), 49–55.

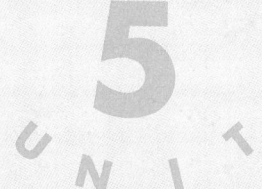

Physiologic and Pathophysiologic Foundations of Child Care

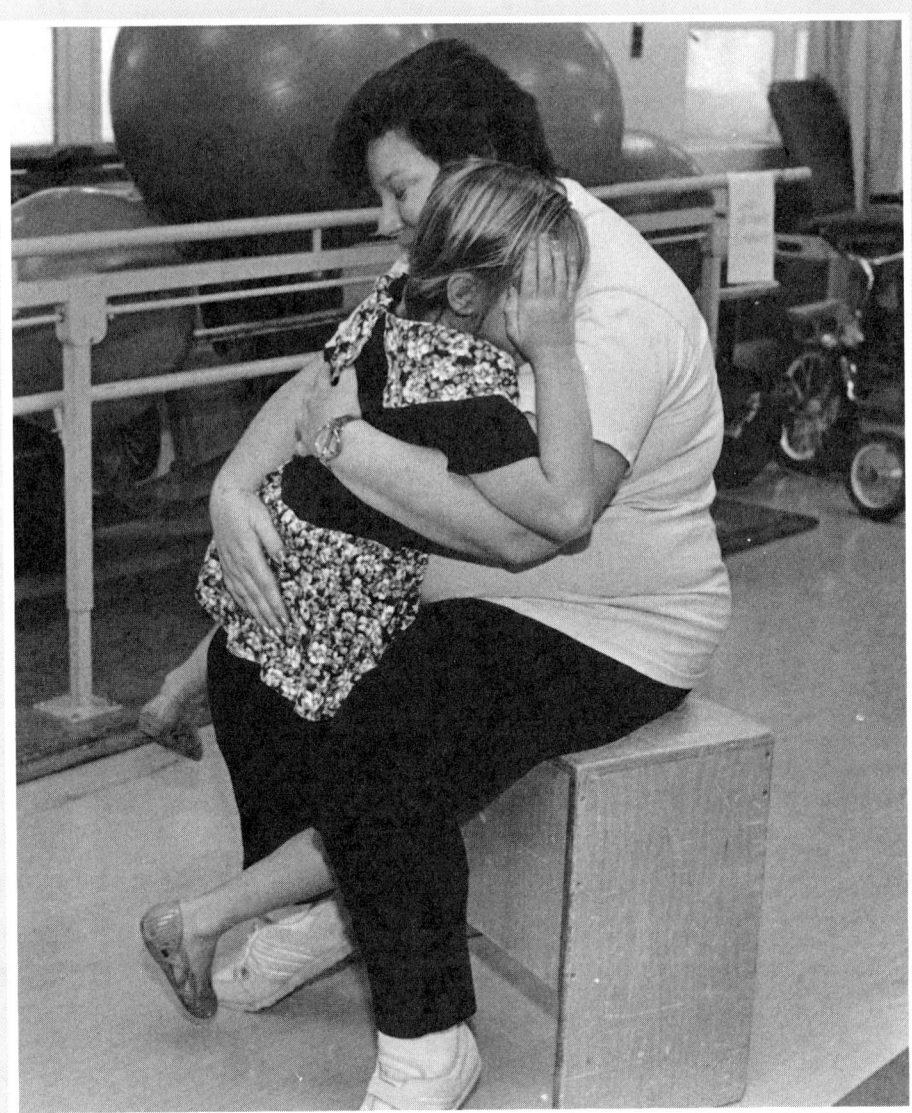

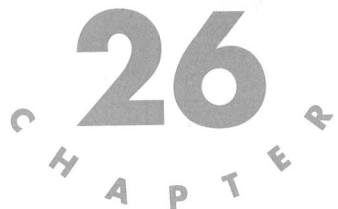

26
CHAPTER

Homeostatic Mechanisms and Responses

BEHAVIORAL OBJECTIVES

Describe the mechanisms that move water within the body's fluid compartments.

Discuss the primary physiologic processes that regulate acid–base balance.

Describe invasive and noninvasive methods of determining blood gas values.

Identify clinical features that might be expected in a child with a fluid deficit or increase.

Describe assessment factors and interventions that might be anticipated for a child with an altered electrolyte concentration.

Distinguish between *respiratory* and *metabolic acidosis* and *alkalosis,* emphasizing pathophysiological processes and major clinical signs.

Discuss nursing implications for the child with an altered acid–base balance.

Distinguish between *isotonic, hypotonic,* and *hypertonic* solutions and the primary objectives of their use in parenteral therapy.

The human body is an intricate combination of systems and countersystems designed to maintain dynamic equilibrium and normal function of the entire organism, even when under physiologic stress. The process of maintaining a relatively stable internal environment is called *homeostasis*. Children are extremely vulnerable to physiologic stress, but their resistance is remarkably strong. Threats that would upset the delicate balance between strength and vulnerability sometimes are unrecognized because the homeostatic mechanisms work so well.

This chapter provides a review of some of the mechanisms that regulate homeostasis in children. A discussion of fluid and electrolyte and acid–base regulation opens the chapter, because these fundamental mechanisms are influenced by so many illnesses. Various alterations in fluid-electrolyte balance and acid–base status

599

follow. The chapter concludes with a review of fluid therapy for children. Throughout the chapter special emphasis is given to differences between homeostatic responses of adults and children.

Homeostatic Mechanisms

Fluid and Electrolyte Regulation

Body Fluids

The primary constituent of body fluid is water. Although a person may live many days without food, the body will survive only a few days without water. Water serves many functions, but one of its primary functions is to supply nutrients to the cells and to remove wastes as necessary. Cells, the basic operating units of the human organism, require this stable environment.

Total body water (TBW) comprises approximately 60% of body weight in an adult and approximately 65% to 85% of body weight in a child and infant, depending largely on the age of the child. The younger the child, the greater the proportion of body weight that is attributable to water. About 90% of a preterm infant's weight is water.[12]

Water Distribution.   Body water is distributed into two major fluid compartments: the extracellular fluid (ECF) space and the intracellular fluid (ICF) space. The ICF is contained *within* the cell walls, while the ECF remains *outside* the cells. The ECF is further subdivided into interstitial water (*between* the cells) and intravascular water (plasma in the vascular bed).

Because the body requires water to function, it attempts to protect itself by keeping its vital fluids in a more protected, less exposed compartment: the intracellular fluid space. In adolescents and adults, the ICF comprises approximately two-thirds of TBW (40–50% of body weight) and the ECF comprises the remaining one third of TBW (20%–30% of body weight). The remainder of body weight is due to solid matter (Fig. 26–1).

Infants and children, have proportionately more water in the ECF space than do adults. Over half of the newborn's TBW is in the ECF space. Growth processes, especially during the first 6 months, cause loss of extracellular fluid. By the end of the second year, the toddler's TBW is about the same as the adult's, but slightly more fluid is kept in the ECF than in the ICF until a child reaches puberty.[12] The significance of this distribution is that water in the ECF space is less protected from depletion than water stored in the ICF space. Infants and children are therefore more vulnerable to fluid volume deficit than adolescents and adults.

The volume of body fluid in the intravascular bed is relatively small, but it is the only directly accessible source for laboratory analysis of the body's fluid and electrolyte status. Analysis of the plasma is therefore useful to determine cellular functioning of the body.

Water Movement.   The physical laws regulating the movement of water within the body of a child are similar to those affecting adults. Living human cells are in a dy-

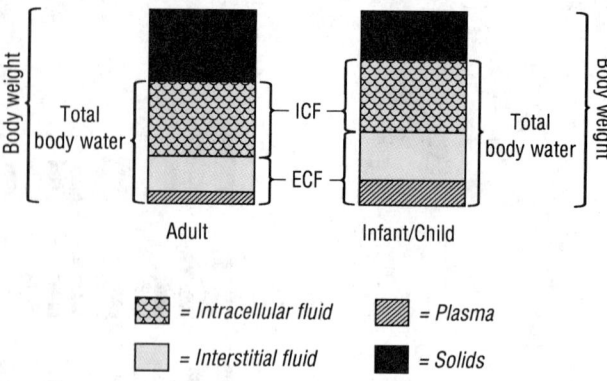

FIGURE 26-1

Body water distribution. Children have a proportionately higher total of body water than adults, and children have more extracellular fluid. Extracellular fluid is composed of intrastitial fluid and plasma. Plasma is a component of intravascular fluid. (ECF, extracellular fluid; ICF, intracellular fluid.)

namic state requiring actions and counteractions to maintain a state of equilibrium. The ICF and the ECF are separated by a semipermeable membrane that is impermeable to most solutes but freely permeable to water. Movement of water between these two compartments must be maintained in equilibrium.

The movement of water in the body is governed by several principles: the law of electroneutrality, the law of osmolality, active ion pump mechanism, and pressure gradients.

The law of electroneutrality affects the movement of water and electrolytes into and out of cells, so a particle of one charge (either positively charged cations or negatively charged anions) must be balanced by a particle of equal and opposite charge. The types of cations are different between the ICF and the ECF, but the numbers are approximately equal.

Osmolality is the number of particles contained in body fluids and is measured by milliosmoles per kilogram (mOsm/kg) of water. *The law of osmolality* refers to the pull or attraction of water that results from the concentration of solutes across a semipermeable membrane, creating osmotic pressure. The side of the semipermeable membrane with the greater solute concentration has greater osmolality and therefore greater attraction for water. Water continues to move in greater amounts in the direction of greater concentration until the solute concentration is essentially equal on both sides of the semipermeable membrane, as shown in Figure 26-2. Solutions that have the same effective osmolality as body fluids are considered isotonic. Those with greater osmolality are hypertonic and those with less are hypotonic.[8]

The active ion pump mechanism regulates the disparity in the types of cations concentrated in the ICF as compared to the ECF and thus determines the osmotic content of each compartment. Because this mechanism is energy consuming, oxygen and sugar are needed. When deprived of these nutrients, the active ion pump mechanism does not function and cannot effectively regulate the movement of water. Evidence of cellular dysfunction and inadequate water regulation appears when a child is deprived of oxygen or glucose during anoxia, ischemia, or severe hypoglycemia.

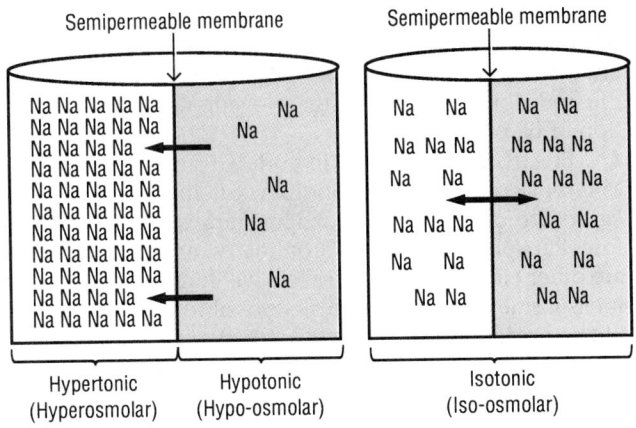

Semipermeable membrane   Semipermeable membrane

Hypertonic   Hypotonic   Isotonic
(Hyperosmolar)   (Hypo-osmolar)   (Iso-osmolar)

FIGURE 26-2

Solute concentration and water movement. Solutions of greater osmolarity attract more water until the solute concentration is equal on both sides of the semipermeable membrane. (Arrows denote water movement.) Hypertonic fluids have greater osmolality than body fluids, and hypotonic fluids have less. Fluids that have the same effective osmolality as body fluids are isotonic.

Pressure gradients also greatly influence fluid movement within the body. *Hydrostatic pressure* is the force or pressure caused by the weight of fluid against a surface. Factors that may influence hydrostatic pressure include the volume of fluid, the type of fluid, and the forces operating on the fluid. *Atmospheric pressure* is the force caused by the weight of air against a surface, and its influence may promote or prevent the movement of water in a certain direction within the body.

Water moves predominantly in relation to the concentration of the cation sodium (Na^+) in the ECF, and it is maintained by the concentration of potassium (K^+) inside the cell. The active transport of sodium is the chief process responsible for generating an osmotic gradient that leads to the movement of water. There is also a slight gradient (i.e., difference in concentration) between the ECF and the ICF, with the ICF containing a larger total number of cations and their balancing anions. The gradient is one of the cell's protective mechanisms to guard against what might be a fatal loss of water.

Pressure gradients help maintain the fluid equilibrium of the body (Fig. 26-3). The active pumping of the heart creates a pressure gradient (hydrostatic pressure) between the arterial bed and venous bed that favors movement of water out of the arterial side of the capillary network and into the tissues. Once the fluid moves into the tissues, another gradient is established to move fluid back into the venous bed. This time the concentration of protein molecules (oncotic pressure) in the venous system creates the pressure gradient. Albumin is the principle solute responsible for oncotic pressure and for regulating net water movement across capillary walls. Fluid is taken from the tissue into the venous vascular bed.[16]

Fluid Homeostasis. Fluid homeostasis is maintained by three primary mechanisms: osmolality (which has already been discussed), osmoreceptor activity, and pressoreceptor activity. The *osmoreceptors,* located in the posterior pituitary and the hypothalamus, normally maintain serum osmolality in the very narrow normal range

of 285 to 295 mOsm/kg.[16] They are highly sensitive to small changes in serum osmolality, which trigger or inhibit secretion of antidiuretic hormone (ADH), which in turn regulates loss of fluid (urine output) and concentration of solutes (i.e., electrolytes) and maintains serum osmolality in the safe range.

Pressoreceptors are located primarily in the kidneys and the aortic arch and are very sensitive to both intravascular volume and pressure. When either volume or pressure is low, the kidneys are stimulated to release renin, which ultimately is converted into angiotensin II, a very potent vasoconstrictor. Vasoconstriction of the vessels reduces the space in which the volume is contained and causes increased blood pressure. The adrenal glands also are stimulated to release aldosterone. Aldosterone subsequently stimulates sodium conservation in the kidneys and results in the retention of water.

Normal Fluid Loss. Fluid movement throughout the body is an essential process required for the physiologic function. Certain fluid losses are essential for normal body functioning and can be classified as either *sensible or insensible losses.* Sensible losses, such as loss through urine or stool, are visible and measurable. Insensible losses are not directly measurable but are evaporative and occur primarily through the skin as a byproduct of metabolism and heat regulation and through the lungs during respiration.

For infants and children normal fluid loss in the stool varies with age, but under normal circumstances it is an inconsequential loss compared with that of urine. Because of the infant's and child's higher basal metabolic rate (BMR) and kidney immaturity, the relative daily urine losses vary significantly with age. In the adult, the average range of hourly urine output is 40 to 80 ml but in the child, urine output ranges from 0.5 to 2 ml/kg/hr.[7]

Water that is lost as a consequence of evaporative processes is essentially free of electrolytes and is called *free water.* Children have a greater daily free water turnover than adults because of their increased BMR with concomitant increased evaporative losses and an elevated

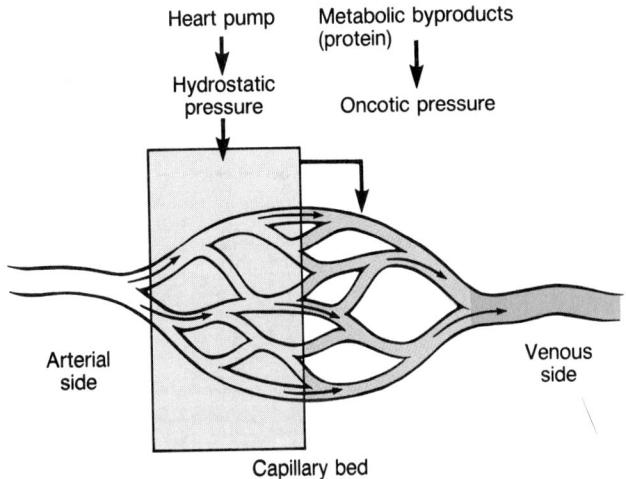

Heart pump   Metabolic byproducts
                  (protein)

Hydrostatic
pressure   Oncotic pressure

Arterial   Venous
side   side

Capillary bed

FIGURE 26-3

Hydrostatic pressure moves water out of the arterial side of capillary networks and into tissues, but the oncotic pressure on the venous side encourages the uptake of fluid to maintain fluid equilibrium.

resting respiratory rate that compounds their vaporization losses.

In some situations the daily turnover of water in infants and children exceeds that which is expected, such as with vomiting, diarrhea, wound losses, and nasogastric losses. Such losses often lead to a disturbed state. In some cases the signs of abnormal water loss are less obvious and initially may go undetected, such as with polyuria (excess urine output), diaphoresis (excess perspiration), and salivation, drooling, or suctioning, or with tachypnea or fever. Other causes of intravascular volume depletion in children include trauma, anaphylaxis, sepsis, and nephrotic syndrome. (These conditions are discussed in other chapters.)

Normal Fluid Intake. The normal amount of fluid intake is usually provided in the daily intake of food and drink that is stimulated by hunger and thirst. Water requirements at various ages are listed in Table 26-1. In disease states the normal mechanisms of intake through the gastrointestinal (GI) tract may be altered, necessitating the parenteral administration of essential fluids.

Maintenance fluid refers to that required for normal body functioning, taking into consideration the anticipated obligatory losses, both sensible and insensible. These requirements vary with age and size of children. Calculations of maintenance fluid requirements are based on the kilogram weight of the child as shown in the display on the fluid maintenance formula.

Electrolytes

Electrolytes are solutes that separate into electrically charged particles when dissolved in a solvent and are measured by their capacity to combine with each other (milliequivalents/liter—mEq/L). Positively charged particles are called *cations*, and negatively charged particles are called *anions*. The law of electroneutrality, discussed previously, requires that particles of one charge must be balanced by particles of equal and opposite charge. This law not only influences the movement of water within the body, but also governs the movement and concentration of electrolytes.

Electrolytes are found in both ICF and ECF, albeit in different concentrations. Sodium, calcium, chloride, bicarbonate, potassium, and magnesium are discussed below. Phosphates, sulfates, proteinates, and organic acids are other electrolytes that are less well understood. Direct measurement of electrolytes is possible only in plasma, but an understanding of the law of electroneutrality permits estimations of intracellular electrolyte activity. The influence of intracellular electrolytes on body function is based on their extracellular concentrations and the body's reaction to those concentrations.

Because electrolytes are absorbed by the GI tract and regulated by the kidneys, GI or renal problems can greatly affect electrolyte balance. However, hormones also influence the rate and efficiency of the absorption and elimination of electrolytes. Plasma electrolyte concentrations vary little among infants, children, and adults.[12]

Sodium. The primary cation of the extracellular space is sodium (Na^+), found in normal concentrations of 135 to 145 mEq/L. Sodium is best known for its ability to affect the movement of water within the body. However, sodium also has an important role in maintaining irritability and conduction of nerve and muscle tissue, and in helping to regulate acid–base balance. The normal daily requirement is 2 to 4 mEq/kg and is available in most foods.

Because Na^+ is the major cation of ECF, the normal serum sodium value is used as a standard for osmolality.[8] Two terms used to describe sodium values or the child's sodium status are hyponatremia and hypernatremia. *Hyponatremia* refers to a state in which the child's current level of sodium is less than normal, and *hypernatremia* exists when serum sodium exceeds accepted normal values.

Renal regulation of sodium relies on conservation in the distal renal tubules. The law of electroneutrality in-

TABLE 26-1
Range of Average Water Requirements of Children at Different Ages Under Ordinary Conditions

Age	Average Body Weight (kg)	Total Water in 24 h (ml)	Water per kg Body Weight in 24 h (ml)
3 d	3.0	250–300	80–100
10 d	3.2	400–500	125–150
3 mo	5.4	750–800	140–160
6 mo	7.3	950–1100	130–155
9 mo	8.6	1100–1250	125–145
1 y	9.5	1150–1300	120–135
2 y	11.8	1350–1500	115–125
4 y	16.2	1600–1800	100–110
6 y	20.0	1800–2000	90–100
10 y	28.7	2000–2500	70–85

(Source: Metheny, N. M. [1992]. *Fluid and electrolyte balance: Nursing considerations* [2nd ed.] Philadelphia: J. B. Lippincott; Adapted from Behman, R. E. & Vaughn, V. C. [1987]. *Nelson textbook of pediatrics.* [13th ed.]. Philadelphia: W. B. Saunders.)

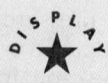

Fluid Maintenance Formula

100 ml/kg per 24 h for first 10 kg (1 to 10 kg)
50 ml/kg per 24 h for second 10 kg (11 to 20 kg)
20 ml/kg per 24 h for each kg > 20 kg

Example: Child weighing 17 kg

100×10 kg = 1000 ml/24 h
$\underline{50 \times 7}$ kg = $\underline{350}$ ml/24 h
17 kg   1350 ml/24 h
(~56 ml/h)

This formula may be used to calculate the amount of fluids needed to maintain normal body functioning. Requirements vary with age.

fluences an exchange of Na^+ for equivalent cations. Because water follows sodium and because water is essential for normal cellular function, the body's homeostatic influences conserve sodium at the expense of other important cations (particularly potassium). The conservation of sodium is directly influenced by the level of aldosterone released into the system by the adrenal cortex. Sodium increases as the level of the steroid increases.

Calcium. Calcium (Ca^{++}) plays an essential role in determining cellular excitability and hence influences muscle contraction. Calcium is the primary physiologic determinant of *threshold potential* (TP), the point at which electrical stimulation is sufficient to cause rapid depolarization of the cell and subsequent muscle contraction. The higher the TP, the greater the stimulation required to cause depolarization.

The calcium in ECF is only a small fraction of the total amount found in the body. The normal serum level of Ca^{++} in children is 8.7 to 10.2 mg/dL, and the range is slightly higher in infants (11 to 13 mg/dL) who have immature calcium-regulating mechanisms. *Hypercalcemia* and *hypocalcemia,* are terms used to indicate that the serum level, is higher or lower, respectively, than normal. Of the total plasma calcium only 50% is ionized under normal circumstances; the other 50% is protein bound. The ionized calcium is active in blood coagulation, membrane permeability, and function of muscles and nerves. Protein-bound Ca^{++} is unavailable for these purposes; the availability of Ca^{++} is therefore influenced by the plasma concentration of protein.

Parathormone, a hormone secreted by the parathyroid glands, has direct influence over Ca^{++} regulation in the body. Parathormone raises the ionized plasma Ca^{++} concentration. As plasma Ca^{++} levels rise, phosphate (HPO_4^{--}) levels decrease; conversely, as HPO_4^{--} levels rise, Ca^{++} is eliminated in the urine. Because Ca^{++} and HPO_4^{--} cannot subsist together in high concentrations, renal regulation becomes important in maintaining an appropriate difference in relative plasma concentrations. Parathormone also increases the rate of Ca^{++} absorption from the intestines, and further acts on the renal tubular cells, causing Ca^{++} to be saved and HPO_4^{--} to be lost. Therefore, high levels of parathormone usually result in hypercalcemia.

Chloride and Bicarbonate. The primary extracellular anions include chloride (Cl^-) and bicarbonate (HCO_3^-). Together they comprise approximately 80% of the extracellular anion concentration. So essential is their contribution to this anion pool that the depletion of one usually results in the relative increase in the other. For example, as chloride concentration falls, bicarbonate concentration rises by a commensurate amount. Both chloride and bicarbonate rely primarily on renal regulation for maintenance of normal balance. Chloride is present in the ECF in large amounts, exerting an important influence on acid–base balance and osmotic pressure. The normal blood concentration Cl^- is 100 mEq/L.[8]

The serum bicarbonate level is directly influenced by kidney regulation, but it is also eliminated in small amounts in stool. Diarrhea may result in excessive loss of HCO_3^-. The effect of HCO_3^- on acid–base balance is discussed later in the chapter.

Potassium. Potassium (K^+) is present in large quantities and is the major cation in ICF functioning similarly to sodium in the ECF in determining osmotic pressure and influencing acid–base balance. Potassium also is the primary physiologic determinant of the electrical resting point to which cells return and remain until the next excitation and depolarization occur; this state is called the resting membrane potential (RMP). Potassium's normal influence over muscle performance relies on a normal concentration ratio between intracellular and extracellular potassium concentrations.

Normal serum K^+ range is 3.5 to 5.5 mEq/L, while intracellular K^+ concentration equals 150 mEq/L. Therefore, a normal concentration ratio is 1:30 or more. Serious muscle performance problems occur when the K^+ ratio of ICF to ECF is less than 1:30 or significantly more than 1:40. With potassium balance myocardial performance is affected adversely and may be life-threatening.

Intracellular potassium concentration cannot be directly influenced. For an intracellular K^+ depletion to be recovered, cellular and body processes must work together to provide for intracellular uptake of available extracellular K^+. This process takes time and requires that both cellular and body processes are effective enough to facilitate recovery.

A daily requirement of 1 to 2 mEq/kg of K^+ is easily accomplished by GI absorption because potassium is available in abundance in a variety of foods. In fact the daily intake of K^+ for most individuals exceeds the requirement. The body, therefore, must rely on normal kidney function to maintain K^+ homeostasis by excretion of the excess. By contrast, the renal mechanisms for the conservation of K^+ are not as efficient. In addition GI wastage accounts for the majority of extrarenal potassium loss. *Hypokalemia* and *hyperkalemia* are terms referring to low or high serum K^+ levels.

Magnesium. Magnesium (Mg^{++}), the other major cation in the ICF, is present in substantially smaller quantities (~40 mEq/L) than K^+. The influence of Mg^{++} on extracellular or intracellular processes is poorly understood. As with the other electrolytes, the body relies primarily on daily absorption of magnesium through the GI tract to supply daily requirements, and renal function provides homeostatic maintenance. Consequently, problems involving GI or renal performance can result in alterations of the Mg^{++} level in the body. Inadequate or overabundant amounts of Mg^{++} in the body ("*hypomagnesia*" or "*hypermagnesia*") can lead to neurologic dysfunction, including coma. Furthermore, the presence of hypomagnesemia may prevent the symptoms of hypokalemia or hypocalcemia from being corrected until normal amounts of Mg^{++} have been restored.

Acid–Base Regulation

In addition to regulating fluid and electrolytes, the body also must regulate acids and bases in the internal environment. An *acid* is a substance that can donate hydrogen ions (H^+). Many substances may contain hydrogen in their molecular structure, but only those that can liberate it as an ion are known as acids. A *base* is a substance that readily accepts hydrogen ions. All bases are alkaline substances and are negatively charged ions (anions). An example of a base is OH^-, which can combine with H^+ to form water (H_2O).

The *p*H is a measurement of the hydrogen ion concentration and essentially expresses the relationship between the concentration of base (usually bicarbonate) to acid (H^+) in mathematical terms.

An inverse relationship exists between the *p*H and the H^+ concentration. Thus, the fewer the H^+ present, the higher the *p*H.

Normal *p*H is 7.40, but the body's cells continue to work when the *p*H is maintained in the range of 7.35 to 7.45. The ratio of base to acid required to maintain a normal *p*H is 20 to 1, that is, 20 times more base than acid. If *p*H values fall below 7.40, the solution is acid (acidosis), and values above 7.40 indicate alkalinity (alkalosis). Acidosis and alkalosis may occur simultaneously, and the body's systems can compensate and reach re-equilibrium.

Physiologic Mechanisms

Chemical Buffers. Buffers help to maintain a constant *p*H by removing or releasing hydrogen ions. Acids are generated continuously as a result of cellular metabolism, but chemical buffers limit the number of free H^+, thereby diminishing the effect a strong acid or base would have on the body's *p*H. Buffers are present in all body fluids and act immediately to correct an abnormal *p*H. Newborns and preterm infants have less buffering capacity than do older children and adults.[12]

Bicarbonate is the body's major buffer system, and it operates in the ECF. To maintain a normal *p*H, the 20:1 ratio of bicarbonate (HCO_3^-) to carbonic acid (H_2CO_3) must be maintained. In normal circumstances, the ratio is preserved by the kidneys, which increase or decrease bicarbonate, and the lungs, which increase or decrease carbonic acid. Newborns and preterm infants have a tendency toward a bicarbonate deficit (a slightly lower *p*H) due to high metabolic acid production and renal immaturity.[10]

Other buffer systems are less important. The primary intracellular buffers are proteins, organic and inorganic phosphates, and hemoglobin. Bone carbonate also contributes to the buffering of acid or base loads.

Respiratory Processes. Carbonic acid (H_2CO_3), the most common acid in the body, easily releases its H^+ ions, and its amount in the body then significantly affects the acid–base status of the patient. Carbonic acid can be broken down into water (H_2O) and carbon dioxide (CO_2) and eliminated during respiration. In normal conditions the lungs can readily rid the body of compounds before carbonic acid forms. Elimination is relatively fast and can effectively achieve re-equilibration within 15 to 20 minutes. An acid that can be eliminated through the lungs is called a *volatile acid*. The efficiency of the respiratory processes in acid control makes it the most important method of acid–base regulation available to the body.

Metabolic Processes. The body also has available a nonrespiratory or metabolic process for eliminating unwanted acids. The H^+ of carbonic acid can be excreted by the kidneys in the form of ammonium ions (NH_4^+) or in the form of carbonic acid (H_2CO_3) broken down into bicarbonate (HCO_3^-) and H^+. Bicarbonate is the primary base of the body and thus provides the body's primary buffering system by assisting in the neutralization of metabolic acids, converting them into the more volatile acids that can be easily and rapidly eliminated through the lungs. During this process the kidneys can eliminate or retain bicarbonate as a buffering agent when needed. This *metabolic process* is much slower than the *respiratory process*. The process of metabolically re-establishing equilibrium in some cases may take up to several hours or even days.

If the respiratory and renal systems function as they should, a failure in one system will be countered by mechanisms in the opposing system. Thus, a balance exists between metabolic and respiratory processes and allows for attempts at re-equilibration by one mechanism when the other fails. Metabolic compensatory mechanisms are much slower than respiratory processes but can be effective over time.

Analysis of Acid–Base Balance

Arterial Blood Gases. The best method of assessing acid–base balance and the quality of blood oxygenation is to measure arterial blood gases (ABGs). Samples of arterial blood are obtained using an indwelling catheter or arteriopuncture. Venous blood gives inaccurate information and is not used alone as an indicator of blood oxygenation. A more comprehensive evaluation of body tissue oxygenation is possible, however, by a comparison of arterial and venous blood gas values.

Analysis of an ABG sample reveals details of the child's acid–base status, including the respiratory and the metabolic components. Information about the originating site of an acid–base problem and factors contributing to the child's current physiologic state also may be ascertained through analysis of ABGs.[14] The procedure used to perform ABGs on children is described in Chapter 37.

The tension or pressure that O_2 and CO_2 exert by occupying space in blood is measured in "torr" units; one torr equals one mmHg. The PaO_2 (also referred to as PO_2) value represents the tension or pressure of oxygen in the arterial blood. This pressure drives oxygen from the arterial circulation into the tissues. The accompanying display lists normal ABG values.

Older people and newborns tend to have lower normal PaO_2 values, but children tend to have high normal values.[17] To calculate the normal PaO_2 value for a child, the following formula may be used:

$$103 - (0.4 \times \text{child's age in years})$$

The $PaCO_2$ (also called PCO_2) is a measure of the pressure (tension) of dissolved CO_2 in the arterial blood. This value is influenced only by respiratory processes. As a result of metabolism, food is normally converted by body tissues to H_2O and CO_2. In plasma excess amounts of CO_2, that is $PaCO_2$ values >40 mmHg, may combine with H_2O to form carbonic acid.

Normal Values for Arterial Blood Gases

PaO_2 = 80 to 100 mmHg

$PaCO_2$ = 35 to 45 mmHg

pH = 7.35 to 7.45

HCO_3^- = 22 to 26 m Eq/L

Base Excess = ± 2 m Eq/L

Oxygen Saturation = 95%–100%

Noninvasive Monitoring. With recent advances in technology many new tools for patient evaluation have become available to the nurse. Two important pieces of equipment provide a noninvasive approach to blood gas determination and assessments in children. These tools include the pulse oximeter, an instrument designed to provide continuous and immediate reflection of the patient's hemoglobin (Hb) oxygen saturation, and the transcutaneous O_2 and CO_2 monitor, an instrument designed to reflect continuous information regarding gas exchange across the skin barrier.

Each of these machines has advantages and disadvantages. One of the primary advantages of both is that they can provide moment-to-moment information about internal physiologic changes without requiring invasive procedures. Another advantage is that both provide immediate feedback regarding the patient's physiologic response to a variety of stressors or interventions, allowing for rapid alterations in care. Both devices also are relatively inexpensive forms of blood gas assessment. However, each has components that affect their accuracy, and these are considered separately.

The information obtained from the *pulse oximeter* frequently is misinterpreted. Its accuracy is directly affected by the child's perfusion status. Locally or systemically compromised perfusion presents the oxisensor with acutely desaturated blood, which may not accurately reflect the child's current systemic oxygen status. The oxisensor also is motion sensitive and may provide inaccurate information if motion disturbs the sensor's ability to track pulsatile blood flow.

In ideal operating conditions, the pulse oximeter provides "beat-to-beat" information on the amount of oxygen carried by the hemoglobin (Hgb). The instrument can be invaluable for assessing immediate changes in the child's oxygen status. The O_2 saturation value (O_2 sat.), however, is commonly misinterpreted as representative of arterial PaO_2. There is a significant correlation between the two indicators, but decreases of one are not linearly related to decreases of the other.

A child with a normal PaO_2 of 80 to 100 mmHg (and a normal body pH of 7.40) would have an O_2 sat. value of 98% to 100%. However, a gradual decline in oxygen saturation values reflects a precipitous fall in oxygen availability. An O_2 sat. value of 93% represents hypoxemia with a PaO_2 value in the low 70s, and an O_2 sat. value of

85% reflects serious hypoxemia with correlating PaO_2 values in the 40 to 50 range.

When assessing the importance of any of these values, it is essential to consider all aspects of oxygen availability and oxygen delivery, any one of which could result in inadequate tissue oxygenation. Tissue oxygenation relies on the level of Hgb in the body, the amount of oxygen that is carried on each unit of Hgb (O_2 saturation), cardiac output (CO), the mechanism by which oxygenated blood is delivered to the tissues, and the PaO_2. If any of these aspects of oxygen provision is compromised, the system will be oxygen deprived to some degree.

Transcutaneous oxygen (TCO_2) and carbon dioxide ($TCCO_2$) monitors measure *gas exchange* at the skin surface, which has been roughly correlated to gas exchange in the arterial–alveolar circulation. Absolute correlation between skin gas exchange and alveolar gas exchange is impossible. Therefore, the information obtained using the TCO_2/$TCCO_2$ monitor should be interpreted with caution.

Another consideration is that although transcutaneous gas exchange has been studied in the neonatal population, the investigations have not been as extensive in pediatric and adult patient populations; therefore, their accuracy in these populations may not be as reliable. In the neonatal population the correlation between the $TCCO_2$ and the arterial $PaCO_2$ values is fairly reliable in a wide range of $PaCO_2$ values. This correlation also follows for $PaCO_2$ values obtained from capillary blood gases. Transcutaneous analysis of CO_2 can therefore be used to accurately estimate changes in arterial or capillary $PaCO_2$ values.[20]

Correlation between TCO_2 values and arterial PaO_2 values, however, is not strong. Using the TCO_2 value as a reflection of the child's arterial PaO_2 is dangerously misleading. The TCO_2 value should be used only for evaluating PaO_2 changes within a narrow range. In neonates the range within which some comparative values can be demonstrated is limited to TCO_2 values of 33 to 50 mmHg, which only roughly correlate to arterial PaO_2 values of 35 to 70 mmHg.[20] The TCO_2 value also correlates roughly to the capillary PaO_2 value and may be useful in identifying situations that need intervention. However, neither value is useful for determining the degree of intervention required. In summary, monitoring TCO_2 changes on a child may be useful to indicate trends and situations that might require intervention, but precise analysis requires analysis of a sample obtained directly from arterial blood.

Altered Fluid-Electrolyte Balance

Fluid Volume Imbalances

Alterations in fluid and electrolyte balance are intricately related, and alterations in one influence the status of the other. In this section, however, the disturbances in fluid balance are discussed separately. A broad discussion of diminished fluid volume is followed by a focused presentation on dehydration seen in children. Likewise, the discussion of fluid volume excess is followed by more in-depth descriptions of edema and water intoxication.

Nursing assessments appropriate for children with fluid volume disturbances close the section.

Hypovolemia

A reduction in the volume of ECF is called fluid volume deficit or *hypovolemia*. In children, hypovolemia results primarily from loss of body fluids, but a diminished intake also can contribute to the problem. As noted earlier, children have a relatively greater total body water content, but a greater percentage is stored in the extracellular compartment than intracellular spaces and is therefore more vulnerable to loss. Additionally, the daily turnover of free water is also greater in infants and children than adults because of their higher BMR, immature renal function, and a relatively large body surface area relative to weight.

Hypovolemia in children is chiefly related to *absolute fluid* losses from one or more possible routes. The loss of gastrointestinal fluids may occur through vomiting, diarrhea, nasogastric suction, intestinal drainage, or from the abuse of laxatives or enemas. Excessive urine output (polyuria) may be due to use of hyperosmolar tube feedings, diuretics, renal disease, adrenal insufficiency, or to hyperglycemia. An elevated body temperature and perspiration, burns, and hemorrhage may also result in diminished amounts of body fluids.

Relative fluid losses are different than absolute losses because they occur from a redistribution of fluid within the body. Fluid shifts out of the vascular bed and into other spaces where it is inaccessible to meet the body's demand for increased fluid volume for tissue perfusion. This alteration in fluid volume is called the "third-space phenomenon," because fluid accumulates in areas other than ECF and ICF, the two compartments in which body fluids are normally distributed. Examples of third-space shifts include pericardial and pleural effusions (leakage of serous fluid into the pericardium or pleurae), ascites (leakage of serous fluid into the abdominal cavity), and fluid compartmentalization as a result of a crushing injury (inflammatory exudate). Fluid trapped in these spaces may eventually be absorbed, or it may be removed mechanically.

Hypovolemia is seldom caused by insufficient fluid intake. Except for abusive or accidental circumstances, unavailability of fluids is rare in children. However, the fact that infants are unable to express their thirst except through crying makes them vulnerable to a care provider's sensitivity to their fluid needs.

When a deficit in body fluid occurs, homeostatic processes maintain the organs essential for survival, such as the brain and heart, and sacrifice the tissue beds that are not immediately essential, such as the skin. This condition is commonly seen in children as mattled coloring. As with all compensatory mechanisms, there is a point at which this compensation fails to satisfy the needs and may promote further harm to the body. For example vasoconstriction can cause such a severe reduction in vessel size that perfusion is inadequate to meet the metabolic demands, and the child may experience shock. The signs and symptoms of primary organ dysfunction include diminishing central and peripheral pulses, changes in level of consciousness, and finally shock (see Chap. 29). Fortunately, early diagnosis and interventions can restore normal fluid volume in most cases.

Dehydration and Its Severity

Dehydration refers to the loss of body water alone, a condition that leaves the person with excessive sodium.[12] A common cause of dehydration in childhood is diarrhea. Passing of a large amount of liquid stools rapidly depletes normal ECF volume, especially if it is accompanied by vomiting. Dehydration from diarrhea is a major cause of infant and child mortality in developing countries, and it is a significant cause for emergency room visits and hospitalization in this country.

In traditional use of the word, dehydration has been said to exist when at least 6% of the body's weight has been lost during an acute illness. Although any weight loss is roughly equal to the amount of fluid loss, the amount of fluid in a child's body varies with age, size, and amount of adipose tissue. Therefore, identical weight losses would not have equivalent effects on children of different sizes. Estimates of dehydration would be more accurate if expressed in milliliters per kilogram of body weight rather than a percentage.[5]

Current clinical practice may persist in classifying the severity of dehydration based on percent of weight loss. A 5% loss is considered mild and 20% dehydration is considered life-threatening. Table 26-2 presents the clinical manifestations of four levels of dehydration.

The presenting signs and symptoms of dehydration reflect the degree of deficiency in the infant or child, especially when combined with a supporting history. The nurse must be skilled at detecting subtle changes and appreciating their significance. Typically, the criteria used to indicate dehydration in an adult are of little value when applied to a child. When identifying dehydration in the child, familiarity with the age-variable norms for vital signs is essential. Findings that are outside the accepted norms must be evaluated for their potential to be life-threatening.

A change in weight that accompanies all forms and all degrees of dehydration is an essential component of assessment. At 10% dehydration a loss of 10% of body weight in water is implied and represents a significant amount of fluid deficiency. An evaluation of the percentage of weight loss is essential for determining risk and the amount of fluid replacement required to achieve normovolemia. Regardless of the clinical presentation of the child, weight loss remains the true representation of the amount of deficit suffered. When available, a history of the child's weight before the onset of illness contrasted with current weight provides invaluable information.

With 5% dehydration most of the clinical indicators show minimal changes, and without a supporting history they might not immediately indicate a problem. Most infants and children can tolerate 5% dehydration without experiencing significant physiologic compromise, and many can be managed at home successfully with oral fluid rehydration if the dehydration is assessed to be minimal and ongoing significant losses are not anticipated. Younger children, however, are at increased risk because they have limited absolute water stores and greater free-water

TABLE 26-2
Changes in Clinical Manifestations With Increasing Dehydration

Clinical Manifestations	Degree of Deficit			
	5%	10%	15%	20%
Heart rate	Normal range	Compensatory tachycardia	Noncompensatory tachycardia	Morbid tachycardia Bradycardia
Blood pressure	Normal range	Normal range	Low normal	↓ Blood pressure
Quality of pulses	Normal	2+ peripheral 3+ central	1+ peripheral 2+ central	0 peripheral 1+ central
Capillary refill	2–3 sec.	>3 sec.	>4 sec.	>5 sec.
Urinary output	<2 ml/kg/h	<1 ml/kg/h	<0.5 ml/kg/h	None
Level of consciousness	Irritable	Irritable/lethargic	Obtunded	Obtunded/coma
Color/temperature	Pink/warm	Pale/cool	Cyanotic/cold	Ashen/cold
Mucous membranes	Moist	Dry	Dry	Parched
Fontanel	Flat	Slightly depressed	Sunken	Sunken
Weight	↓ 5%	↓ 10%	↓ 15%	↓ 20%

turnover each day. Infants and young children can progress from 5% to 10% deficit in hours and thus may require hospitalization.

With *10% dehydration* a consistently elevated heart rate is typical and classified as compensated tachycardia. The heart rate will usually drop back into the normal range when the infant is quiet and unstimulated. With time a decrease in urine output may be expected, but this information may be unavailable initially. Other clinical indicators of 10% deficiency include dry mucous membranes and a decrease in skin turgor, noted as a decrease in fullness of tone and elasticity. The central nervous system (CNS) also begins to be affected, and the infant or child typically becomes irritable. However, the stress of hospitalization is very difficult to differentiate from irritability caused by dehydration or by some other external stimulus. An older child who has previously experienced the sensation and who has verbal competence to describe it may complain of dizziness at this time. Thirst also may be demonstrated.

With *15% dehydration* the elevated heart rate usually does not return to normal when the child is quiet and urine output falls significantly. Pulses are weak to "obliteratable" in the periphery (indicative of serious functional hypotension). Level of consciousness frequently descends to lethargy at this point, and the skin becomes cool and mottled. Capillary refill time prolongs to >4 to 5 seconds. Mucous membranes are dry, no tears can be made, and the skin tents over the abdomen when turgor is tested.

With *20% dehydration* the heart rate fails to provide compensation, and myocardial performance begins to show subtle signs of deterioration. All the characteristics of alterations in perfusion seen at 15% are exaggerated at 20%. A child presenting in this condition is on the brink of total circulatory collapse. Without rapid intervention, cardiac arrest is likely.

Types of Dehydration. Because a variety of forces cause dehydration, it is best classified as three types: isotonic (water and electrolytes are lost proportionately), hypertonic (water lost in excess of electrolytes), and hypotonic (electrolytes lost in excess of water).[12] Sodium is the primary solute in ECF, and its deficit or excess is a primary determinant of the clinical manifestations.

Isotonic Dehydration. In isotonic dehydration both compartments lose fluids and electrolytes in proportionately equal amounts, so no gradient is established between the ECF and ICF. Isotonic disturbances commonly occur in children who experience large quantities of liquid stools, fever, excessive vomiting, hemorrhage, or burns. Clinical manifestations include thirst, acute weight loss, dry skin and mucous membranes, sunken eyeballs, cold extremities, depressed body temperature, lethargy, oliguria, longitudinal furrows on the tongue, and signs of hypovolemia. If 15% of the body weight is lost in 1 to 2 days, a moribund or near-moribund state is produced.[4]

Hypertonic Dehydration. Hypertonic dehydration (hypernatremia) occurs when the measured concentration of sodium is greater than normal. This condition results from a net loss of water in excess of salt or as a result of excessive solute intake. This condition establishes an osmotic gradient between the ECF and the ICF. The greater sodium concentration in the ECF encourages water movement *out* of the cells and into the ECF (i.e., the interstitial and intravascular spaces).

Common causes of hypertonic dehydration in children include gastroenteritis in infants who are fed high-solute replacement fluids (such as whole milk or boiled skim milk) or incorrectly prepared condensed formula. Hypertonic dehydration also occurs in children who have fever with hyperventilation, particularly in small infants. In contrast, diabetes mellitus, which results not in excess sodium concentration, but in glucose concentration in the blood, has a similar effect and may result in hypertonic (or more accurately, hyperosmolar) dehydration. The osmotic gradient caused by excess amounts of glucose in the plasma influences water movement out of the cells and into the ECF.

The clinical features of hypertonic dehydration are based on the alteration in fluid homeostasis and the consequent effects on cellular performance resulting from intracellular dehydration. These characteristics are listed under "Hypernatremia" in Table 26-3. Although this is a dehydration syndrome, the evidence of circulatory disturbance may be absent initially because the intravascular volume is conserved at the expense of intracellular water.

The primary risk of hypernatremic dehydration is intracellular dehydration, which results in early evidence of cellular dysfunction in the central nervous system (CNS). Altered CNS status can lead to seizures, coma, and intracranial bleeding. Approximately 10% of infants and young children with this derangement demonstrate intracranial bleeding, but it rarely occurs in adults.

Hypotonic Dehydration. Hypotonic dehydration occurs when electrolytes are lost in greater amounts than water. Because sodium is the chief electrolyte in ECF, its deficit is the primary cause of symptoms. In hypotonic dehydration, the child's serum sodium falls below 130 mEq/L. A greater net loss of sodium than water from the ECF results in an osmotic gradient between the ECF and the ICF. This gradient encourages the movement of water *into* the cell at the expense of the ECF in an attempt to re-establish equality of ion concentrations across the semipermeable membrane.

The common causes of hypotonic dehydration in children include diarrheal disorders (especially when electrolyte-free solutions are given for volume replacement), the syndrome of inappropriate ADH, and excessive amounts of salt-poor solutions given in the presence of impaired renal function.

Clinical features of hypotonic dehydration are listed in Table 26-3 under the heading "Hyponatremia." The primary risk is for intravascular volume (IV) depletion and intracellular (IC) overhydration. IV volume depletion can result in cardiovascular dysfunction and inadequacy of tissue perfusion resulting in shock, while IC overhydration has devastating effects on the CNS and may lead to seizures and coma.

Nursing Assessment. If the child is suspected or is at risk for having a fluid deficit, assessment includes a review of history and laboratory data and a systematic physical examination. A history from the parents usually reveals a decreased appetite, less activity, and irritability.[12] Large losses of fluid through diarrhea or vomiting may be reported. Metheny[12] suggests the following assessments in a systematic approach: comparison of total fluid intake and output, urine volume and concentration, skin and tongue turgor, degree of moisture in oral cavity, body weight, thirst, tearing and salivation, appearance and temperature of skin, facial appearance, edema, vital signs, neck and head vein filling, central venous pressure, and neuromuscular irritability. The following provides specific guidelines for assessing children.

Weight. A comparison is made between baseline weight and present data. Rapid weight loss is characteristic of fluid volume deficit. The child should be weighed at the same time, without clothing (or with the same clothing), on the same scales, and under the same circumstances (for example, before eating and after voiding) at each weighing.

Tissue Turgor. Abdominal areas and the medial aspects of the thigh are the best areas to palpate for tissue turgor. In a well child pinched skin will return to normal; the skin may remain raised for a brief time in a child with fluid volume deficit (Fig. 26-4). When water loss exceeds sodium loss, the skin has a firm, thick feeling.

Body Temperature. Because of reduced energy output, a subnormal temperature often is associated with fluid volume deficit. However, fever may accompany fluid volume deficit, depending on the underlying cause.

Heart Rate and Respirations. Assessment of pulse rate and volume and respiratory rate, rhythm, and depth is critical. Hypervolemia may cause dyspnea and a bounding pulse. Hypovolemia may be manifested by a rapid, weak, and thready pulse.

Mucous Membranes. Feeling the mucous membrane of the mouth reveals a variety of information. For instance, a dry and sticky mucous membrane indicates sodium excess, and a smaller-than-normal tongue indicates fluid depletion.

TABLE 26-3
Clinical Features of Sodium Derangement

Hyponatremia	Hypernatremia
Seizures, coma	Marked lethargy
Dry, sticky, mucous membranes	Extreme hyperirritability with stimulation
↓ Urine output	↓ Urine output
Rapid, thready pulse	Initial absence of circulatory disturbance
Hypotension	↓ Skin turgor (thick & firm)
Shock	Weight loss
Doughy skin	Avid thirst
Weight loss	Muscle rigidity
Na < 130, BUN ↑, K ↔ ↑, Cl ↓	Na > 150, BUN ↑, K ↔ ↓, Cl ↑

Key: ↑, increased; ↓, decreased; ↔, normal range; BUN, blood urea nitrogen; Na, sodium; K, potassium; Cl, chloride.

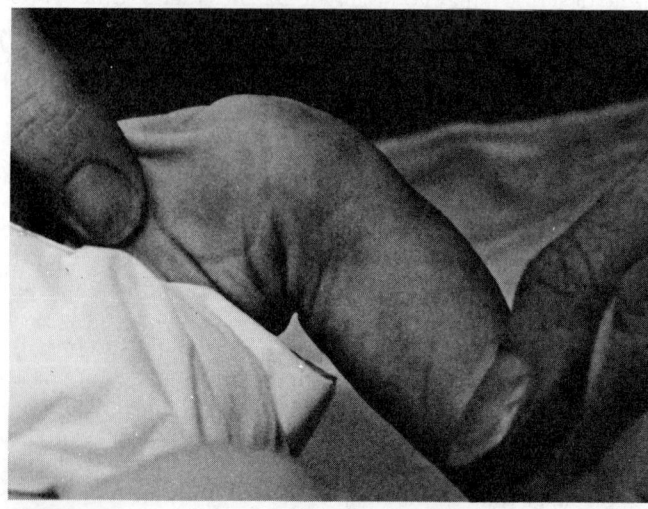

FIGURE 26-4
Poor skin turgor in an infant.

Fluid Intake and Output. Measurements should be taken of all intake and output, if possible. As a general rule normal urinary output is about 1 mL/kg of body weight per hour.[13] Devices and the procedures for assessing urinary output are described in Chapter 25.

Computations of Fluid Requirements. Normal water requirements for infants and children are listed in Table 26-1. Requirements are based on caloric consumption and expenditure.[12]

The nurse should conduct a computation of the child's fluid requirements to make informed judgments regarding the appropriateness of the fluid orders. An evaluation of appropriateness of the ordered volume is impossible without first calculating normal maintenance requirements (see the display on fluid maintenance formula) and the degree of deficit and ongoing loss using 1 kg of acute weight loss to represent 1 L (1000 ml) of fluid loss. Primary deficit recovery usually occurs during the first 24 hours of hospitalization and may be satisfactorily accomplished using the normal hourly maintenance requirements for the child to calculate the total estimated amount of deficit (see the accompanying display on computation of fluid deficit by weight loss).

Nursing Interventions. Normal fluid volume and accompanying alterations in electrolyte or acid–base balance must be restored. Fluids may be administered orally or parenterally. The types of fluids available and guidelines for their administration are found in the last major section of this chapter.

Hypervolemia

Hypervolemia is a state of overhydration in which an abnormal increase in ECF volume exists. The fluid excess may be distributed throughout the body tissues, as with the excessive administration of IV fluids or abnormal renal function (acute or chronic renal failure with oliguria). Sodium and water also are retained throughout the body with heart failure, cirrhosis, nephrotic syndrome, and excessive administration of glucocorticosteroids.[8] Sometimes, the excess ECF is carried in the intravascular space (IVS) alone, the most common cause being iatrogenic.

Weight gain is the one true characteristic of hypervolemia, revealing an elevation commensurate with the amount of excess volume. Other signs and symptoms vary depending on the actual distribution of the fluid, the competency of the system in dealing with the overload, and to some extent the length of time the imbalance has existed. Edema is expected if enough time has lapsed for fluid to be deposited in the interstitial spaces. An increase in urine output is expected if the renal function remains relatively normal, and the peripheral vascular bed may be distended if substantial amounts of fluid remain in the IVS.

The response of the cardiovascular system varies depending on its preexisting condition. An elevation in blood pressure may accompany a decreased heart rate with full and bounding pulses. Infants may have more difficulty managing additional intravascular volume and may experience an increase rather than a decrease in heart rate. Rales or ronchi and respiratory distress as a consequence of fluid overload are late signs. In adults excess fluid moves first into peripheral and dependent tissues, but in children fluid is first sequestered in the liver. Hepatomegaly thus becomes one of the hallmarks of chronic fluid overload in children.

Nursing Assessment. A history of the child's illness reveals risk factors of conditions that contribute to the hypervolemic status of the child. Assessment for shortness of breath or orthopnea determines respiratory compromise. Ongoing assessment of weight gain, edema, and vital signs is necessary to monitor for changes in physical status. As with any fluid imbalance, intake and output and urine specific gravity are monitored closely.

Nursing Interventions. Hypervolemia in children is much rarer than hypovolemia, and its treatment depends upon both the cause and the effect. If an infant or child has competent renal function, then treating hypervolemia generally is not a problem. Limitation of sodium and water intake may be necessary. If renal function is compromised, alternative forms of fluid removal, such as dialysis, may have to be used. An assessment of the adequacy of intravascular volume is of greater concern than that of TBW. If volume in the intravascular compartment is compromised, the treatment of choice is to deliver volume to that compartment even though the other evidence

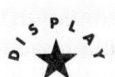

Computation of Fluid Deficit by Weight Loss

Fluid loss can be calculated according to the weight loss of the child. For example the weight loss of a child weighing 10 kg suffering 10% dehydration would equal 1 kg. Each kg of weight loss is equal to 1000 ml of fluid loss.

10 kg infant, 10% dehydrated

10% of 10 kg = 1 kg

1 kg = 1000 g = 1000 ml

Example of Calculations Used to Determine Fluid Replacement Needs in a 10-kg Infant With 10% Dehydration

Maintenance requirements = 100 ml × 10 kg
= 1000 ml/24 h or
42 ml/h

Total estimated deficit = 10% of 10 kg
= 1000 g = 1000 ml

½ deficit = 500 ml replacement over 8 h or 62 ml/h

IV rate for first 8 hr = 104 ml/h + any ongoing loss

Remaining ½ deficit = 500 ml replacement over 16 h or 31 ml/h

IV rate for next 16 h = 73 ml/h + any ongoing loss

might suggest TBW overload. Only after circulation is stabilized are interventions to remove excess water from the tissues appropriate.

Edema

Fluid expansion of the interstitial fluid space (IFS) frequently is an effect of hypervolemia, although the exact cause may vary. Edema results when alterations in the equilibrium occur between hydrostatic and oncotic pressures in the tissue bed. Increases in hydrostatic pressure in the capillary network can cause excessive pressure in the arterial and venous beds and can override the attempts of oncotic pressure to retrieve those fluids. Increases in hydrostatic pressure can result from volume overload or defects in kidney filtration, perfusion, or excretion. An increased gradient between the IFS and the IVS can be caused by nephrosis. Another situation that may result in edema is sepsis, which results in increased capillary membrane permeability. The lymphatic system is responsible for the retrieval of the slight excess of fluid in the tissues that is not recovered by oncotic venous pressure. This system is responsible for recovery of 2% to 4% of interstitial fluid daily. Therefore, edema also could result with time in the presence of lymphatic obstruction.

Edema may be generalized or localized.[8] Generalized edema initiated by renal or cardiac failure is most evident in dependent areas such as the ankles or pre-tibial areas of the legs. However, edema around the eyes (periorbital), in the fingers, and other body parts may be evident in more severe cases. Edema of the extremities or sacral area is assessed by pressing the index finger firmly into the tissues for several seconds. The site is observed as the finger is withdrawn to determine if an indentation was left in the area. Barely visible edema is documented as +1 and a deep, persistent pit is rated +4. Less severe degrees of edema are rated +2 and +3.

Treatment for edema is aimed at treating the primary problem. The edema may be mobilized out of tissues pharmacologically with diuretic therapy or with conservative measures such as bed rest, supportive hose, and dietary restriction of sodium and fluids. Severe generalized edema is called *anasarca* and may necessitate the use of paracentesis or renal dialysis (see Chap. 47). Cerebral edema is considered life threatening.

Water Intoxication

Water intoxication may occur when children take in large amounts of fluid without corresponding electrolytes. Causes of water intoxication include the administration of inappropriate hypotonic solutions,[16] too rapid renal dialysis, tap water enemas,[10] infant formula overdiluted with water,[11] too vigorous hydration to reduce fever, and swallowing large amounts of water while swimming.[2] These causes are accidental, but parental abuse by forcing children to drink large amounts of water also occurs.

As intake of fluids continues, the serum concentration of sodium decreases, urine output increases, and vomiting and diarrhea occur. The movement of water into brain tissue causes irritability, and the child may become somnolent. Severe headache may be followed by generalized seizures, coma, and death if the condition is untreated.

Treatment includes restricting water intake and carefully elevating serum sodium level.[16] The prognosis is good if skilled care is given.

Electrolyte Imbalances

Electrolyte concentration and regulation in the body are not substantially different for children and adults. Differences do exist, however, in the causes of electrolyte imbalances, clinical presentation, and management of these derangements.

Hypokalemia

Hypokalemia occurs when the serum potassium value falls much below 3.5 mEq/L. A significant deviation below normal usually reflects depletion of K^+, which can have serious metabolic consequences. Derangement in children is rare except during hospitalization. Common causes of K^+ depletion include diuretic therapy, especially for chronic diarrhea, poor dietary habits, perspiration with chronic fever, and endocrine system abnormalities—especially diabetes mellitus and conditions involving the adrenals.

Hyponatremia may accelerate the rate of renal loss of K^+ in favor of the Na^+ conservation; thus, hypokalemia may be further augmented. The presence of hypomagnesemia also can result in the persistence of symptoms of hypokalemia (even when K^+ supplementation has resulted in the correction of the hypokalemic condition). Until Mg^{++} levels have been corrected, K^+ supplementation alone will not correct the hypokalemic condition.

Hypokalemia is predominately recognized in poor muscle performance (Table 26-4). Because the primary risk of this condition is the generation of lethal cardiac dysrhythmias, management requires frequent and careful electrocardiogram (EKG) assessment, looking particularly for evidence of the dysrhythmias listed in Table 26-4.

Interventions. Replacement of potassium is ideally through the oral route because the GI tract is especially designed for K^+ absorption. However, high concentrations of oral K^+ solution, especially >70 mEq/L may not be well tolerated. Hospitalized children may refuse to

TABLE 26-4
Clinical Features of Potassium (K^+) Derangement

Hypokalemia	Hyperkalemia
Muscle weakness and cramps	Ascending muscle weakness
Paralytic ileus	Flaccid paralysis
Nausea, vomiting	Respiratory paralysis
Cardiac arrythmias:	Cardiac arrhythmias:
T-wave notching/T-wave inversion	Peaked T-waves
ST depression	Prolonged PR interval
Serum K^+ <3.5	Bradycardia
	Ventricular tachycardia
	Serum K^+ > 5.5

swallow the K^+ solution even though it is flavored. However, they may respond to creative strategies with storytelling or play. K^+ can be given parenterally if children experience nausea and vomiting.

Parenteral recovery of a potassium deficit requires careful administration. Rapid intracellular K^+ replenishment is impossible, and rapid delivery of potassium into the extracellular compartment (the IVS) may have fatal consequences. Administration precautions include the following.

Maximum Concentration. Generally, parenteral solutions of K^+ should contain <80 mEq/L, with continuous EKG monitoring for any solutions with K^+ concentration ≥ 35 mEq/L. If a concentration of 100 mEq/L (equal to 1 mEq/10 ml) is required due to fluid restrictions or other considerations, the potential risk to the child must be weighed against the potential benefit. Concentrations in excess of 100 mEq/L are *not* recommended.

Rate of Infusion. A reasonably diluted dose (i.e., not >1 mEq/10 ml) should be delivered in no less than 1 hour. An even safer approach would be in a minimum of 2 hours, especially if higher concentrations are used. An excess of K^+ in the ECF cannot be rapidly absorbed into the ICF, and the extracellular concentration of K^+ alters the ratio to the ICF concentrations, creating a potentially lethal hyperkalemic situation.

Site of Infusion. Because K^+ is irritating to tissues and causes pain and possibly phlebitis, the best site for its administration is controversial. Some suggest that concentrated K^+ is better tolerated if infused through a central venous line, because increased blood volume dilutes the K^+ solution and reduces discomfort. The countering argument is that infusion through a peripheral vessel is safer. The K^+ infusion is diluted by blood as it returns through the venous system to the right side of the heart. Peripheral infusion route reduces the risk of a potentially lethal concentration of potassium being delivered to the myocardium. Some clinicians consider the risk of pain and phlebitis much less significant than that of a lethal dysrhythmia and therefore recommend peripheral sites. If a child requires repeated, concentrated potassium infusions, a reasonable approach is to add the K^+ to the continually infusing solution, thereby providing for maximal dilution and avoiding the risk of large fluctuations in K^+ concentration in the ECF.

Hyperkalemia

Hyperkalemia occurs when serum potassium values exceed 5.5 mEq/L and is usually lethal when serum levels reach >7.5 mEq/L. Because potassium regulation primarily depends on GI absorption and renal excretion, disturbances in these systems can alter potassium levels. Common causes of hyperkalemia include renal failure, iatrogenic parenteral administration, excessive oral intake (particularly in the presence of any renal impairment), and Addison disease (hypoaldosteronism). Potassium-sparing diuretics (such as spironolactone) rarely cause hyperkalemia except with excessive oral intake. (KCl, which is commonly substituted for NaCl in low-sodium diets, can be a source of significant potassium intake.)

Because of potassium's essential role in establishing

cellular RMP, many of the consequences related to alterations of potassium concentration result in dysfunctional muscle performance. The more prominent symptoms are listed in Table 26-4.

Interventions. Because the most life-threatening consequence of hyperkalemia is the generation of lethal cardiac dysrhythmias, comprehensive management requires early recognition of children at risk, continuous EKG monitoring, regular serum potassium evaluation, and a plan for immediate intervention if symptoms arise. When a serious elevation in serum potassium (i.e., >5.5 mEq/L) is confirmed, continuous EKG monitoring must be used. If evidence of electrical disturbance occurs, therapy is begun to reduce the dangerously high concentration of potassium. That reduction, however, depends primarily on renal excretion, which takes time. If the child is already symptomatic, and renal performance is in question, there may be inadequate time for the recovery of homeostasis; institution of emergency measures may be appropriate.

Emergency interventions for hyperkalemia rely on the redistribution of potassium in the body and the reestablishment of a normal ratio between ICF and ECF potassium concentrations, but they do nothing to relieve the body of its excessive potassium load. The success of these measures is a result of the following:

- A bolus of calcium alters the TP for the cells, attempting to re-establish the gradient between the RMP and the TP on which normal electrical stimulation and depolarization of the cells depends. The electrical alterations in myocardial performance are thereby reduced.

- A bolus of sodium bicarbonate encourages cellular uptake of K^+ in exchange for H^+ by presenting the ECF compartment with an alkalotic condition and relying on potassium's responsiveness to changes in *p*H.

- Glucose with or without insulin also encourages intracellular uptake of potassium, which normally occurs as glucose is metabolized and taken up by the cells.

In the absence of normally functioning kidneys some interventions that may encourage the elimination of potassium from the body include a Kayexalate enema, a cation exchange resin that relies on the exchange of Na^+ for K^+ in the GI tract, requires time, and may result in hypernatremia; peritoneal dialysis, relying on elimination of K^+ by osmosis through the vast capillary network of the peritoneal cavity; or hemodialysis, actual blood filtration to remove K^+ and other potential toxins from the blood in substitution for the kidneys. Hemodialysis usually is reserved for the most serious or less responsive conditions because the hazards of therapy often outweigh potential benefits for most children suffering from transient hyperkalemia (see Chap. 47).

Hypocalcemia

Hypocalcemia occurs when serum calcium falls below 8.7 mg/dL or when there is an acute reduction in ionized Ca (as with alkalosis). This condition results in a reduction of calcium available for use in blood coagulation, membrane permeability, and most importantly, the function of the heart, other muscles, and nerves.

As with the other electrolytes, calcium derangement generally occurs as a result of renal and GI disturbances. Common causes of hypocalcemia include hypoparathyroidism, malabsorption syndromes, rickets, and diuretic therapy. Other conditions that cause an increase in the binding of calcium to other molecules resulting in low calcium levels include (1) respiratory alkalosis in which calcium binds to protein molecules and (2) delivery of large-volume blood transfusions, causing calcium to bind to citrate, a preservative added to banked blood. Hypomagnesemia can potentiate the effects of hypocalcemia, causing unresponsiveness to therapy until the magnesium deficit has been corrected. Hyperphosphatemia also leads to hypocalcemia by increasing the renal wasting of calcium.

The primary risk of hypocalcemia is myocardial dysfunction which is indicated by electrocardiogram (ECG) changes in which the QT interval is prolonged, and the QRS is widened. These changes cause symptoms of cardiogenic shock. Other clinical effects of hypocalcemia are listed in Table 26-5.

Interventions. The underlying cause of hypocalcemia ultimately must be addressed, but in life-threatening hypocalcemia (especially if confirmed by laboratory analysis) the primary treatment is the immediate reconstitution of calcium ions to the circulating blood volume. Calcium chloride (CaCl) is given parenterally by IV volutrol or slow IV push *to a central IV only*. Calcium gluconate (CaGluc) also may be given parenterally by IV volutrol to peripheral or central IV sites.

In life-threatening situations CaCl given by slow IV push is preferred because it immediately dissociates in the serum and liberates Ca^{++} into the circulation. In contrast CaGluc requires metabolism of the gluconate by the liver to liberate the calcium ion, a relatively slow process that results in only one-third the amount of Ca^{++} being released compared to an equivalent dose of CaCl. Calcium gluconate, however, has a safety advantage because it delivers Ca^{++} much more slowly into the system, thereby avoiding the risk of hypercalcemia and tissue necrosis. This approach to therapy is more commonly used in neonates and in situations that do not require life-saving maneuvers.

TABLE 26-5
Clinical Features of Calcium (Ca^{++}) Derangement

Hypocalcemia	Hypercalcemia
	Nausea and vomiting
	Thirst
Extremity numbness/tingling	Renal calculi
Muscle cramping	Bradycardia
Palpitations	Cardiac arrhythmias:
Irritability	Widened, round T-waves
Hypotension	Shortened Q-T interval
Serum Ca^{++} < 8.7	Serum Ca^{++} > 10.2

Hypercalcemia

Hypercalcemia occurs when the serum calcium level is >10.2 mg/dL. Common causes include hypophosphatemia (usually due to hyperparathyroidism), diuretic therapy using thiazide diuretics, and unintentional parenteral overdose (iatrogenic).

The primary risk of hypercalcemia is related to cardiac effects. The EKG should be evaluated for widening and rounding of the T-wave and shortening of the QT interval. Ultimately, bradycardia and finally asystole could cause life-threatening effects. Other common clinical characteristics of hypercalcemia are listed in Table 26-5.

Interventions. The obvious approach to therapy is first to restrict further delivery of calcium and to rely on the body's own mechanisms to eliminate the excess calcium. This process might be augmented by administering parenteral fluids (ideally 5% albumin) and fostering calcium's elimination using the classification of drugs known as loop diuretics.

In some cases the child may have a low serum calcium combined with a low serum protein or a high serum calcium with a high serum protein and have a functionally normal calcium picture. No signs of hypocalcemia or hypercalcemia, respectively, would be exhibited.

Altered Acid–Base Balance

When the buffering systems cannot prevent further acidosis, acidemia results (*p*H levels less than 7.35) or when further alkalosis cannot be buffered, alkalemia results (*p*H levels more than 7.45). Assessing the *p*H often can indicate whether a body's system has more tendency toward acidity or alkalinity in acid–base imbalance. Acid-base events are rarely as straightforward as presented here. Multiple problems often occur simultaneously, and as with other examples of multiple system dysfunction, dysfunction in the acid–base regulating systems can lead rapidly to severe alterations in ABG values.

Respiratory Acidosis

Respiratory acidosis results from a dysfunctional respiratory apparatus in which carbon dioxide is not efficiently or effectively eliminated by the lungs. An elevated $PaCO_2$ (hypercapnia) precipitates a rise in extracellular bicarbonate (HCO_3^-). If the resultant action of buffers is insufficient, the pH of the blood declines (acidemia).

Respiratory acidosis may be acute or chronic, although the acute condition is much more common in children. Causes of acute respiratory acidosis include severe lung disease such as pneumonia, cardiac arrest, asphyxia, drug overdose with depression of the respiratory center, chest wall trauma, and other conditions in which CO_2 is not excreted from the body adequately.[8] Children who are in pain or who have restrictive dressings, for example, may hypoventilate, allowing CO_2 to accumulate. Clinical manifestations of acute respiratory acidosis include tachycardia and tachypnea, dyspnea, restlessness, altered sensorium, diaphoresis, and cyanosis in extreme cases.

Chronic respiratory acidosis is typically attributed to a chronic respiratory disease such as cystic fibrosis, bronchial asthma, or advanced multiple sclerosis. Patients with these conditions gradually accumulate CO_2, and the body's compensatory mechanisms are given time to operate. Children with chronic respiratory acidosis may have few symptoms, but headache and weakness are possible.

Interventions. Comprehensive management of this condition requires correcting the major physiologic problem contributing to respiratory acidosis and increasing alveolar ventilation. Deep breathing exercises, chest vibration, and percussion may be instituted to increase ventilation. Intubation and mechanical ventilation may be necessary.

Respiratory Alkalosis

When too much CO_2 is eliminated by the lungs, it results in an extra amount of unmatched base remaining in the body, resulting in an alkalotic state. Hyperventilation is the major cause of respiratory alkalosis; however, it also may occur with meningitis or salicylate poisoning.

Anxiety and fear may contribute to the development of hyperventilation and subsequent respiratory alkalosis in a child. Rapid, deep breathing is present as well as tingling of the face and extremities. Dizziness also may be present.

Interventions. Management of this condition is directed toward correcting the major physiologic problem causing hyperventilation. Inhaling CO_2 through rebreathing techniques (such as a paper bag) and voluntary slowing of respirations may alleviate symptoms.

Metabolic Acidosis

Any accumulation of acids (from other than respiratory causes) or loss of bicarbonate leads to an acid state from metabolic causes or *metabolic acidosis*. The bicarbonate value (HCO_3^-) represents the amount of available base in the body to buffer acid. Greater amounts of base cause the pH to rise, and lesser amounts decrease the pH. Bicarbonate values are influenced by metabolic processes only.

The presence of metabolic acidosis generally is linked to other diseases and illnesses such as diabetic ketoacidosis, diarrhea, renal failure, and lactic acidosis. It also may be caused by ingestion of salicylates. Newborns and preterm infants tend toward metabolic acidosis with pH averages slightly lower than normal (7.30 to 7.35).[7] This mild metabolic acidosis probably is related to high metabolic acid production and renal insufficiency.[12]

The child in metabolic acidosis has increased respirations and may experience anorexia, nausea, and vomiting. Lethargy may develop and lead to drowsiness and coma.

Interventions. Management of metabolic acidosis is aimed at correcting the major physiologic problem. When adequate ventilation has been established and is likely to be maintained, IV sodium bicarbonate may be used to temporarily increase the pH level. This intervention must be monitored carefully by measurement of blood gases.

Metabolic Alkalosis

Metabolic alkalosis results from an increase in bicarbonate or a loss of nonvolatile acids. Common causes of this condition include excessive bicarbonate ingestion, excessive vomiting, or gastric suctioning.

Children with metabolic alkalosis experience irritability, numbness and tingling of the extremities, weakened muscles, and carpopedal spasm. The body compensates for metabolic alkalosis through kidney excretion of bicarbonate and depressed respirations.

Interventions. Management of metabolic alkalosis involves limiting bicarbonate ingestion and replacing lost fluids and electrolytes.

Fluid Therapy

The type of intervention needed for alterations in fluid-electrolyte balance is determined by the type of homeostatic dysfunction. Interventions include dietary planning, medication administration (such as diuretics), decreasing or increasing fluid intake, blood transfusion, and parenteral therapy. Many of these are discussed throughout this text. The following section briefly discusses the use of oral rehydration and parenteral fluid therapy.

Oral Rehydration

Oral replacement of fluids is preferred over parenteral replacement because oral fluids are absorbed slowly, there is less risk of fluid overload, and the child is not confined as with parenteral therapy.[12] Oral rehydration therapy is the only treatment available in many developing countries, and it has provided a significant reduction in the mortality rate from acute diarrhea.[16]

Oral administration of a glucose–electrolyte solution is preferred. Glucose facilitates sodium transport across the intestinal wall.[16] The composition of oral rehydration solutions used by the World Health Organization and several commercial products are presented in Table 26-6. The administration, amount, and rate are calculated by the degree of volume depletion and weight of the child. Vomiting is not necessarily a contraindication to oral rehydration therapy.[1]

Although "force fluids" is common hospital terminology, it is not an accurate description of replacement therapy in children. Forcing fluids initiates a negative response from children. The nurse must develop methods for encouraging children to take fluids. The accompanying display provides guidelines for encouraging infants and children to take fluids.

Parenteral Fluid Therapy

In cases such as impending hypovolemic shock, severe nausea, or inability to drink, parenteral therapy must

TABLE 26-6
Commercial Oral Electrolyte Solutions: Concentration When Diluted

Product	Na (mEq/L)	K (mEq/L)	Cl (mEq/L)	Base (mEq/L)	Glucose g/L
Rehydration					
ORS (WHO)	90	20	80	30	20
Rehydralyte (Ross)	75	20	65	30	25
Maintenance					
Infalyte (Penwalt)	50	20	40	30	20
Lytren (Mead Johnson)	50	25	45	30	20
Pedialyte (Ross)	45	20	35	30	25
Resol (Wyeth)	50	20	50	34	34

(Source: Metheny, N. M. [1992]. *Fluid and electrolyte balance: Nursing considerations* [2nd ed.]. Philadelphia: J. B. Lippincott; Adapted from Feld, L. G., Kaskel, F. J. & Schoeneman, M. J. [1988]. The approach to fluid and electrolyte therapy in pediatrics. In L. A. Barness [Ed.]. *Advances in pediatrics* [vol. 35]. Chicago: Year Book Medical Publishers.)

be used. Because of their immature homeostatic regulating mechanisms, young children must be given special considerations when planning replacement therapy. Renal output, acid–base balance, body surface, calcium-phosphate regulation, and electrolyte concentrations must be taken into consideration.

Parenteral fluid therapy is categorized according to need:

- *Maintenance therapy* to maintain a state of hydration until oral feedings or fluids can be reinstituted.
- *Deficit therapy* to replace losses of salt and water occurring prior to the physician's examination.
- *Replacement therapy* to replace ongoing losses after the patient has entered a therapeutic program.[16]

Three basic rules for fluid intervention follow:

- Replace (as closely as is reasonably possible) the type of fluid being lost. For example, if whole blood is being lost, such as in the case of hemorrhage from trauma, then whole-blood replacement is the ideal fluid intervention.
- When the patient is in shock, use isotonic solutions for initial management. Thus, if the child is in shock as a consequence of acute blood loss, although whole blood is ideal and isotonic, it is often not immediately available. Appropriate isotonic substitutes include isotonic solutions such as normal saline, Ringer's lactate, or 5% albumin.
- Once the child's shock state has been stabilized, replace fluids in approximately the same length of time in which they were lost.

Procedures for administering IV fluids are discussed in Chapter 25.

Nutrients may be given through a peripheral vein in relatively dilute concentrations or in stronger concentrations through a central vein. Total parenteral nutrition (TPN), also known as hyperalimentation, is able to sustain growth for 60 days or longer.[16] Information about TPN, discharge planning and family teaching related to it, and a teaching plan for home TPN are included in Chapter 59.

Types of Parenteral Fluids

Two types of fluids are available for volume expansion: colloids and crystalloids (Table 26-7). *Colloids* are protein-based products and are therefore typically blood or blood products. In contrast, *crystalloids* are solutions of water and electrolytes in varying combinations and concentrations. Because the protein molecule typically is larger than the countering crystalline molecule, colloid products have the advantage of being less likely to pass through a semipermeable membrane. They may therefore have a greater tendency to remain in the vascular bed where initial fluid management is directed. This property is believed to make colloids more valuable for recovery of intravascular volume.

However, this reasoning may not always be true, especially in situations in which a "capillary leak" is demonstrated, such as in sepsis. In these cases the loss of integrity of the capillary network may allow or promote translocation of fluid outside the vascular space. If the fluid that leaks out is proteinaceous, an increase in extravascular oncotic pressure occurs, which may cause the fluid to be attracted to places where it is not easily retrievable and where its presence may cause additional problems, such as with pulmonary edema.

Parenteral fluids are described as hypotonic, isotonic, and hypertonic (Table 26-8).

Hypotonic Solutions. Solutions that have an effective osmolarity less than body fluids are considered hypotonic.[8] Hypotonic solutions such as D$_5$ plus .22% NaCl and D$_5$ plus .3% NaCl are often used as maintenance solutions for children. These fluids are more diluted than those typically given to adults, and they allow the delivery of additional free water. Because children have a greater daily free water turnover than adults, more additional free water must be available for restoration.

Isotonic Solutions. Solutions that have the same effective osmolarity as body fluids (approximately 280 to 300 mOsm/kg) are called isotonic.[8] Isotonic solutions include normal saline, Ringer's lactate, fresh frozen

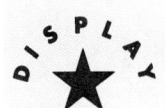

Nursing Interventions: Guidelines for Encouraging Infants and Children to Take Oral Fluids

- Talk with the child's parents, and learn about the child's usual experience in taking fluids at home. What type of fluids does the child usually drink? What amount? What temperature? How often? What method (bottle, cup, or special glass)? What are favorite fluids?
- Plan with the parents to meet the child's fluid needs, and involve them in encouraging fluids, measuring amounts, and recording the intake accurately.
- Offer small amounts of favorite fluids in small containers at frequent intervals (at least every hour).
- Use measured containers for precise determination of intake, and record the intake accurately.
- Promote the child's comfort before offering fluids. Make certain the child is clean and dry and the upper airway is clear of mucus. (A rubber syringe can be used to remove mucus from the nares.)
- Continue to offer fluids on a regular schedule, even though the infant or child may refuse to drink.

- Hold infants before and after offering fluids. Toddlers and preschool children may prefer to sit on the nurse's lap and hold the cup or glass.
- Toddlers may respond positively to a routine, such as offering a drink to a stuffed animal before offering the child a drink. Toddlers might also respond to the opportunity to feed themselves bite-sized pieces of frozen Popsicle, soda, or fruit juice.
- Young children like stories and may respond to the power of suggestion in stories about thirsty boys or girls who are looking for a drink.
- Some young children will drink if they have some solid food to hold or mouth, such as a saltine cracker or a vanilla wafer.
- Infants and children who are required to fast before surgery or diagnostic tests should have extra fluids just before the period of fasting to prevent dehydration. A pacifier helps relieve the distress that infants experience while oral feedings are withheld.

(Metheny, N. M. [1992] Fluid and electrolyte balance: Nursing considerations (2nd ed.). Philadelphia: J. B. Lippincott.)

plasma, and albumin. Normal saline and Ringer's lactate are crystalloids, but fresh frozen plasma and albumin are colloids. Synthetic plasma-replacing products are considered isotonic and include dextran, hetastarch, and Plasmanate. These fluids have not been well studied for the effect of rapid- and large-volume infusion in children; they may prove less than ideal.

Hypertonic Solutions. Solutions with a higher osmotic pressure than body fluids are hypertonic.[19] Hypertonic solutions are used with extreme caution because

they can be lethal if infused carelessly.[12] They can cause tetany, seizures, and cardiac arrhythmias. Hypertonic solution in the form of sodium bicarbonate is used to treat severe metabolic acidosis. Sodium bicarbonate is available as a 5% solution, furnishing 595 mEq/L each of sodium and bicarbonate.[13] The general recommendation is that parenteral bicarbonate should cease when pH reaches 7.2.[3]

Half of the total estimated deficit is then replaced along with the hourly maintenance during the next 8 hours. The remaining half of the deficit is similarly replaced during the next 16 hours. Any appreciable ongoing losses should be added to the hourly intake of fluid. This process may result in a significant but appropriate volume of fluid being administered to the child. Selection of the type of fluid is based on the type lost as well as normal fluid and electrolyte requirements. This formula is presented in the previous display.

Any ongoing measurable losses, such as those encountered with excessive urine output, diarrhea, and vomiting, should be tracked. Risk of additional loss from nonmeasurable sources must also be recognized and appreciated. Infants and very young children are particularly prone to substantial free water losses from elevated respiratory rates and fevers; in fact, an additional 12% insensible volume loss is incurred for every degree above 37.5° C, which is sustained for each 24 hours.

The computation of need in shock states is somewhat different, and continuation of therapy is based on the child's response to the interventions and to the supporting history. Fluids used to treat shock usually are not considered in the overall deficit recovery numbers. For example, if a 10-kg infant receives 200 ml to remedy a shock situation but also is determined to be 15% dehydrated, the

TABLE 26-7
Types of Parenteral Fluids Typically Used to Build Intravascular Volume According to Disorder That Caused the Loss

Disorders of Volume Loss	Recovery Fluid Types

Gastroenteritis (Vomiting or Diarrhea); diabetes mellitus; diabetes insipidus; gastric suction	Crystalloid:
	   Isotonic: NS, LR
	   Hypotonic: D_5 & 0.2 NaCl
	                D_5 & 0.3 NaCl
	   Hypertonic: 3% saline

Burns; Anaphylaxis	Colloid:
	   Plasma
	   Albumin
	   Plasmanate

Trauma; Gastrointestinal Bleeding; Hemorrhage	Blood:
	   Whole blood
	   Packed red blood cells

TABLE 26-8
Types of Parenteral Fluids and Their Electrolyte Components

| Types | \multicolumn{7}{c|}{Electrolyte Concentrations in mEq/L} |
	Na+	K+	Ca++	Mg	Cl−	HCO₃−	HPO₄−−
Isotonic							
Plasma	141	5	5	3	103	27	3
0.9% NaCl	154				154		
Lactated Ringers	130	4	2.7		109	28	
5% albumin	145	1			120	trace	
Hypotonic							
0.45% NaCl	77				77		
0.22% NaCl	38.5				38.5		
Hypertonic							
3% NaCl	513				513		
5% NaCl	855				855		

200 ml typically will *not* be subtracted from the 1500-ml calculation of fluids necessary for deficit recovery.

Summary

This overview of the major physiological mechanisms that regulate homeostasis reveals a complex interaction of all the body's systems. However, the basic operating unit of the human organism is the cell, and its function depends on a stable environment. A constant supply of nutrients and continuous removal of metabolic wastes are neces-sary. The delivery system on which the cells depend is the circulating blood volume.

Almost all illnesses affect fluid and electrolyte balance or acid–base balance, and children are especially vul-nerable to these changes. Compared to adults children have a higher proportion of body water, much of which is in extracellular spaces and therefore readily lost. Ad-ditionally, some aspects of the physiologic mechanisms needed to maintain homeostasis in children are immature.

To provide competent care to ill children, nurses need intimate knowledge of the physiologic mechanisms that regulate homeostasis. Early recognition of signs and symptoms of impending disorders or worsening condi-tions is vital to prompt and effective intervention. Nursing care is thus directed on restoring homeostasis and pre-venting further disequilibrium.

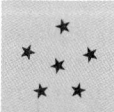

Ideas for Nursing Research

In the area of assessment of fluid balance distur-bances in children nurses often can make a crucial difference in the outcome of a child's illness. Most existing research concerning fluid and electrolyte balance focuses on acutely ill adults. Yet, it is known that major physiologic differences exist between adults and young children. The following areas need to be explored:

- Determination of reliable noninvasive indicators of isotonic, hypotonic, and hypertonic "dehy-dration" in children younger than 2 years.
- Correlation of weight changes with invasive in-dicators of fluid volume status in acutely hy-povolemic children.
- Useful methods of encouraging young children to drink when they have little desire for oral fluids.
- Factors affecting the accuracy of weight mea-surements in acutely ill infants.
- Factors affecting the accuracy of fluid intake and output measurements in acutely ill infants.

References

1. American Academy of Pediatrics Committee on Nutrition. (1985). Use of oral fluid therapy and posttreatment feeding fol-lowing enteritis in children in a developed country. *Pediatrics, 75*, 358.
2. Bennett, J., Wagner, T., & Fields, A. (1983). Acute hyponatremia and seizures in an infant after a swimming lesson. *Pediatrics, 73*, 125.
3. Dunagan, W., & Ridner, M. (1989). *Manual of medical thera-peutics* (26th ed.). Boston: Little, Brown.
4. Feld, L., Kaskel, F., & Schoeneman, M. (1988). The approach to fluid and electrolyte therapy in pediatrics. In Barness (Eds.). *Advances in Pediatrics* (Vol. 35). Chicago: Year Book Medical Publishers.
5. Finberg, L. (1990). Assessing the clinical clues to dehydration. *Contemporary Pediatrics 7*(4), 45–57.
6. Gahart, B. (1990). *The handbook of intravenous medications* (6th ed.). St. Louis: C.V. Mosby.
7. Hazinski, M. F. (1988). Understanding fluid balance in the se-riously ill child. *Pediatric Nursing, 14*(3), 231–263.
8. Horne, M. M., & Swearingen, P. L. (1989). *Pocket guide to fluid and electrolytes.* St. Louis: C.V. Mosby.
9. Ichikawa, I., Narins, R., & Harris, H., Jr. (1990). Regulation of

acid–base homeostasis. In I. Ichikawa (Ed.). *Pediatric textbook of fluids and electrolytes* (pp. 84). Baltimore: Williams & Wilkins.

10. Kokko, J., & Tannen, R. (1990). *Fluids and electrolytes* (2nd ed.). Philadelphia: W.B. Saunders.

11. Medani, C. (1987). Seizures and hypothermia due to dietary water intoxication in infants. *Southern Medical Journal, 80,* 421.

12. Metheny, N. M. (1992). *Fluid and electrolyte balance: Nursing considerations* (2nd ed.). Philadelphia: J.B. Lippincott.

13. Pestana, C. (1989). *Fluids and electrolytes in the surgical patient* (4th ed.). Baltimore: Williams & Wilkins.

14. Raffin, T. (1986). Indications for arterial blood gas analysis. *Annals of Internal Medicine, 105,* 3, 390–398.

15. Rimar, J. (1988). Recognizing shock syndromes in infants & children. *MCN American Journal of Maternal Child Nursing, 13,* 32–37.

16. Robson, A. (1987). Parenteral fluid therapy. In R. Behrman & V. Vaughan (Eds.). *Nelson textbook of pediatrics* (13th ed.). (pp. 202). Philadelphia: W.B. Saunders.

17. Dong, S-H., et. al. (1985). Arterialized capillary blood gasses and acid–base studies in normal individuals from 29 days to 24 years of age. *American Journal of Diseases of Children, 139,* 1019–1022.

18. Siegel, N. J., Carpenter, T., & Gaudio, K. M. (1990). The pathophysiology of body fluids. In F. A. Oski, C. D. DeAngelis, R. D. Feigin, & J. B. Warshaw (Eds.). *Principles and practice of pediatrics.* Philadelphia: J.B. Lippincott.

19. Thomas, C. L. (Ed.). (1989). *Taber's cyclopedic medical dictionary* (16th ed.). Philadelphia: F.A. Davis.

20. VanKessel, A., Ariagno, R., & Robin, E. (1985). *Clinical application of capillary and transcutaneous gas measurements in prematurely born infants,* Submitted for publication. Stanford: Stanford University Hospital.

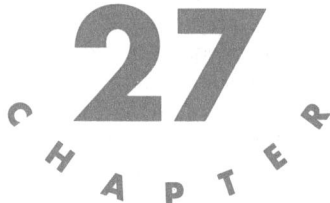

27 Immune Responses

CHAPTER 27

BEHAVIORAL OBJECTIVES

Discuss the differences between the *nonimmune defense system* and the *immune defense system.*

Describe the development of *immunity.*

Describe the *inflammatory process.*

Discuss the four types of *hypersensitivity* reactions.

Explain the concept of *autoimmunity.*

Conduct a nursing assessment of a child with an immunologic problem using key concepts.

Describe the pathophysiology, clinical manifestations, medical management, and nursing intervention of selected immunologic problems in children.

Acquired immunodeficiency syndrome (AIDS) has received widespread attention in the media in the last 10 years, and it is perhaps the most well-known immune dysfunction today. Pediatric AIDS is the 9th leading cause of death among children aged 1 to 4 years and the 12th in young people aged 5 to 24 years. Minority children are disproportionately represented in pediatric AIDS, comprising approximately 77%.[6] Yet immune disorders constitute a vast array of health-related problems, ranging from the simple annoyance of allergic rhinitis (hay fever) to life-threatening conditions such as AIDS.

Historically, the immune response was recognized as early as the fifth century BC when the Greeks noticed that a person who recovered from an illness seldom contracted the illness a second time. In 1798, Dr. Edward Jenner performed the first immunologic experiment when he inoculated the arm of a young boy with material from a milkmaid infected with cowpox (a disease closely related to smallpox). He subsequently injected material from a smallpox pustule into the boy, performing the first *vaccination* on record.

Knowledge about the immune system and immunity has become more sophisticated in the last 2 decades, resulting in an understanding of major immune problems. The increased use of transplantation has added impetus to the study of immunology, including histocompatibility, which is the quality of tolerance between tissues, allowing effective grafting of such tissues.

This chapter provides an overview of the immune system and mechanisms related to immune response. This overview is followed by a discussion of information the nurse needs to assess a child with possible immune problems. The major diseases of altered immunity are presented.

The Immune System

"The immune system is a complex network of specialized organs and cells that protects the body from destruction by foreign agents and microbial pathogens, degrades and removes damaged or dead cells, and exerts a surveillance function to prevent the development and growth of malignant cells."[35] The immune system is composed of immune cells and central and peripheral lymphoid structures. The immune cells move throughout the body, searching for and destroying foreign substances but avoiding cells regarded as self.

The Body's Defense Systems

The body uses defense systems to combat insults to health and life. These basic defense mechanisms are explained in Table 27-1 and can be broken down into nonimmune and immune responses.

Nonimmune Defense System

The *nonimmune* or *protective defense system* is present and effective at birth and does not require previous exposure to a substance to be effective.[41] These represent the body's first line of defense. The protective defense system is nonspecific in its action but is directed against any potentially harmful insult to the body. The level of response tends to be fairly constant, rather than increasing in severity with repeated assaults.

One example of nonimmune defense is the integumentary system, which presents a natural barrier to invasion through the skin. Other examples include tearing in the eyes and the ciliary action in the respiratory tract. Tearing washes away foreign objects and weakens or destroys pathogens through the bacteriostatic property of lysozyme, which is present in tears. Cilia in the respiratory tract move particles and organisms that are trapped in the normal mucous secretions of the respiratory tract up to the oropharynx where they can be expelled or swallowed. These actions prevent harmful substances from entering the individual's internal environment.[38]

Another example of a nonspecific defense mechanism is phagocytosis, the *inflammatory response*, which is discussed in greater detail in a later section.

Immune Defense System

The *immune defense system*, while present at birth, is not effective until exposure to specific substance(s) has occurred.[37] The immune response often has been identified as the body's ability to distinguish "self" from "nonself."[21,38] Substances that are foreign to the body (nonself) and that elicit a defensive response are called *antigens*. Examples of antigens include substances such as pollen, dust, chemicals, and drugs or organisms such as viruses, bacteria, fungi, or parasites. Antigen responses are specific in their action and demonstrate memory because responses tend to be more rapid and severe with repeated exposures to the antigens. A desired immune response occurs whenever the offending antigen is identified and destroyed.

The immune system consists of primary lymphoid organs and secondary lymphoid organs. Primary lymphoid organs include the bone marrow and thymus, sites of immune cell production.[35] The bone marrow of ribs, sternum, and long bones produces stem cells, some of which then travel to the thymus where they multiply and mature into T cells (Fig. 27-1). Other stem cells mature into B cells. The secondary lymphoid organs include the lymph nodes, spleen, tonsils, and submucosal areas of the gastrointestinal (GI) tract.[22] Their functions are storage of lymphoid cells and filtration.

The immune response consists of physiologic and biochemical interactions between B lymphocytes (B cells), and T lymphocytes (T cells), both of which are *immunocytes* or *immunocompetent cells*. These two types of cells act in specific ways to neutralize and destroy antigens. First, they offer protection against specific antigens (nonself) in the following way: The B cells produce antibodies that neutralize the antigen, and the T cells attack the antigen directly. Second, some of these cells (memory cells) demonstrate "memory" for a specific antigen. Exposure of the antigen on subsequent occasions triggers more rapid responses each time. The capability demonstrated in the immune system relative to specificity and memory is what in turn produces long-lasting protection against specific antigens. This process is known as *immunity*.[38,40]

Development of Immunity

Natural Versus Acquired Immunity

Natural immunity is not produced by the immune response. This type of immunity is present at birth and appears to be present in all members of a species. For

TABLE 27-1
Defense Mechanisms Against Illness

Type of Defense	Characteristics	Examples
Nonimmune or protective defense mechanisms	Nonspecific in action Present at birth Constant level of response	Skin, tears, cilia in respiratory tract, mucous membranes
Phagocytosis (a nonimmune response)	May be acute or chronic	Inflammatory response
Immune response	Specific in action Not effective until exposure to antigen	Cell-mediated: T cells, lymphokines
	Response increases in severity with repeated exposures	Humoral: B cells, plasma cells, immunoglobins

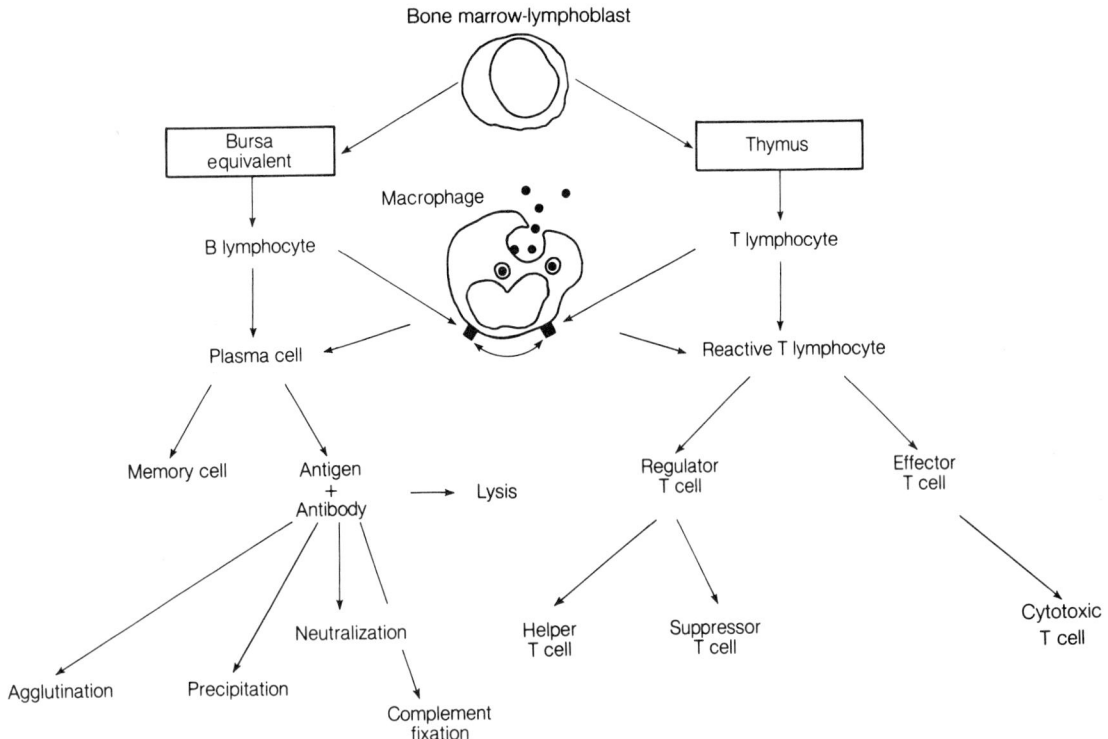

FIGURE 27-1

The development of cellular and humoral immunity. (Porth, C. M. [1990]. *Pathophysiology: Concepts of altered health states* [3rd ed.]. Philadelphia: J. B. Lippincott.)

example, humans are naturally immune to some agents that cause illness in other species, such as canine parvovirus or cowpox. Another type of natural immunity appears to be related to an individual's characteristics (i.e., presence or absence of risk factors), which have some relationship to the subsequent development of certain diseases.[38]

Acquired immunity develops after birth as a result of exposure to an antigen, thereby activating the immune response. Acquired immunity can be either active or passive, depending on whether the immune response took place in the host or a donor. *Active acquired immunity* is produced by the individual (host) after a natural exposure to an antigen or an immunization with a weakened form of the antigen. *Passive acquired immunity* is not a result of an elicited immune response. Instead, preformed antibodies or T cells are transferred to the recipient, either through the transplacental shift from mother to infant or as a result of clinical treatment with immune serum that contains antibodies. Clinical treatments to produce passive immunity are used in emergency situations, such as snakebites or rabies exposure. Passive immunity is temporary.[15,38]

The immune response may be affected by endogenous (internal) and exogenous (external) factors. Endogenous factors include age, sex, nutritional status, genetic background, and reproductive status. These factors may put the individual "at risk" for an altered or suppressed immune reaction to an antigen. Exogenous factors, such as surgery, trauma, radiation, disease, or drugs, also may have a significant effect on the individual's immune system.[9,15,38]

Specific Immune Mechanisms

Specific immune responses are seen when the body demonstrates an ability to recognize an antigen and to respond selectively. Specific immunity may be either humoral immunity or cell-mediated immunity. Both the B cells and T cells are involved in these types of immunity.

Humoral Immunity

Humoral immunity develops outside the cell in the following way: Stem cells (lymphocyte precursors) originate in the liver and spleen of the fetus and in the bone marrow of the child or adult. These migrate to lymphoid tissue in various parts of the body, maturing into either B lymphocytes or T lymphocytes. Each B cell is preprogrammed to react to a specific type of antigen and displays the type of antibody it is capable of producing on its cell surface (receptor site). When activated by an antigen, B cells divide and differentiate into *plasma cells*. The plasma cells produce and secrete large quantities of antibodies that are specific to the antigen.[22,23,27]

Antibodies are immunoglobulins (Ig) that are specific for particular antigens. Five classes of antibodies may be produced in this manner: IgG, IgA, IgM, IgE, and IgD (Table 27-2). These antibodies are released directly into the circulation, where an antigen–antibody reaction results.

The *primary immune response* occurs when B cells begin to produce predominantly IgM within the first 2 to 3 days after exposure to the antigen. A second exposure to the same antigen creates a *secondary immune re-*

TABLE 27-2
Major Classes and Functions of Immunoglobulins

Immunoglobulin	Normal Values	Function
IgG	0.8–1.6 g/dl	Major immunoglobulin in humans
		Circulates in blood and tissue
		Can cross placenta
		Active against many bacteria, viruses, parasites, and some fungi
		Activates complement
IgM	0.06–0.2 g/dl	Kills bacteria in bloodstream
		Activates complement
IgA	0.15–0.4 g/dl	Concentrates in body fluids and secretions
		Protects entrances of body (gastrointestinal and respiratory tracts)
		Activates complement
IgE	Trace	Major antibody in allergic response
		Attaches to mast cells and basophils and causes them to release contents after contact with an antigen
IgD	Trace	Regulates activation of B cells from within cell membrane

Adapted from Gurka, A. M. (1989). The immune system: Implications for critical care nursing. *Critical Care Quarterly, 9*, 25–26.

sponse. To protect the individual, antibodies are produced even more quickly and in larger amounts than during the first exposure. This is due to the presence of memory cells that more quickly identify the antigen as nonself than occurred during the first exposure. In addition to IgM production, large quantities of IgG are produced during this response. The primary and secondary responses confer active acquired immunity. Antibodies bind with the antigens to weaken and or kill the offending antigen, thus eliminating the threat to the organism. Antibodies also may aid in phagocytosis of the antigen. In phagocytosis, the macrophage (see Fig. 27-1) ingests and digests the foreign substance and then moves the antigen fragments to the surface of the cell. Once the antigen is destroyed, antibody production falls.[15,27,38]

Cell-Mediated Immunity

Cell-mediated immunity takes place within the cell. In the thymus gland under the influence of thymic hormones, lymphoid stem cells mature into T cells that are capable of responses against antigens. Certain antigens have no specific place on their cell surfaces for antibody binding. These cells must be destroyed directly by T cells. There are five types of mature T cells, each with a different function. These include memory cells, which produce the secondary immune response; cytotoxic (Tc) cells; lymphokinine-producing cells (Td cells), which are responsible for delayed hypersensitivity reactions; and helper (Th) and suppressor (Ts) cells, which control both humoral and cell-mediated immune responses. Antigens can cause large numbers of T cells to be produced, which are capable of acting against the same antigen in a variety of ways.[27,38]

Complement System

The complement system is the primary mediator in the humoral immune response. It assists the body in initiating inflammation and in supporting the localization of an infectious agent.[35] The complement system consists of a series of at least 10 proteins that commonly circulate in the blood. When activated, complement initiates a series of reactions known as the complement cascade. Each step must be completed before a subsequent interaction can take place. Complement is a nonspecific type of self-defense that plays a key role in the inflammatory reaction. For example, complement may weaken bacteria so that they may be destroyed more easily by phagocytes (opsonization). Complement action also may damage bacterial cell walls. In addition, chemicals that facilitate the inflammatory process may be secreted as part of the complement activation.[15,27,38] Complement-mediated immune responses are listed in Table 27-3.

Differences in Immune Systems of Children and Adults

The normal human infant has no fully active immune system at birth because of immaturity. It relies instead on passively transferred antibodies from the mother. This maternal antibody slowly decreases in concentration and for all practical purposes, has waned by 1 year. The infant's own production of antibody begins to be meaningful at 7 or 8 months. There is in effect a "low point" age near 4 to 6 months of age when the total of maternal and infant antibody is low. One has waned and the other is not up to full strength. This is the age when many of the infec-

TABLE 27-3
Complement-Mediated Immune Responses

Response	Effect
Cytolysis	Destruction of cell membrane of body cells or pathogens
Adherence of immune cells	Adhesion of antigen–antibody complexes to the inert surfaces of cells, or tissues, such as the reticuloendothelial cells that line the blood vessels and have the capacity for phagocytosis
Chemotaxis	Chemical attraction of phagocytic cells to foreign agents
Anaphylaxis	Degranulation of mast cells with release of histamine and other inflammatory mediators
Opsonization	Modification of the antigen so that it can be easily digested by a phagocytic cell

Porth, C. M. (1990). *Pathophysiology: Concepts of altered health states* (3rd ed.). Philadelphia: J. B. Lippincott, p. 188.

tious disease processes of infancy begin (e.g., otitis media, pneumonia).

In newborns, complement activity, antibody production, and phagocytic activity are not present. However, the potential for competent immune response is present, even though active immunity is lacking. As has been previously noted, to protect the child during the first few months of life, passive immunity is received transplacentally from maternal IgG. At birth, total IgG levels in umbilical cord blood are near adult levels. Immediately after birth, these levels begin to drop due to catabolism. At the same time, neonatal production of IgG begins. By 6 months of age, total IgG levels produced by the infant enable the immune system to begin to assume its defensive role.[38]

Through breast milk, breast-fed babies receive IgA and other substances, which provide additional disease-fighting abilities. Children may acquire immunity in all of the ways previously described, that is, naturally and artificially, passively and actively. Immunizations against and exposure to childhood infectious diseases produce active acquired immunity.

Active immunity develops after exposure to antigens that stimulate the antigen–antibody response previously described. Normally children will experience a higher than usual number of illnesses and infections during the first few years of exposure to other children or adults, such as day care or school. As active immunity develops, the number and severity of such episodes decrease, resulting in relatively healthy outcomes by late middle school and high school years.

Pathophysiology

Inflammatory Response

At times, protective defense mechanisms are ineffective. When this occurs, harmful substances, such as chemicals, foreign bodies, or pathogenic organisms may enter the cells and tissues. The *inflammatory response* is triggered immediately after the invasion occurs. Inflammation is a nonimmune defense response. In contrast

to the immune response, inflammation is nonspecific. The same series of events occurs no matter what triggers the reaction. It does not increase in severity or rapidity of reactions upon subsequent exposure to the offending element.[37]

Inflammation is the body's attempt to mobilize forces to rid itself of the offending agent. It may be divided into two types: acute and chronic (Fig. 27-2). The acute inflammatory response usually lasts 8 to 10 days. If the inflammatory response continues for longer than 2 weeks, it is considered chronic. Characteristic signs of inflammation are redness, heat, swelling, pain, and loss of function.[37]

During an inflammatory response, injured cells or tissues release complement-activating hydrolases. Complement not only assists the inflammatory response, but also may directly attack offending cells such as bacteria. Vasodilation and increased capillary permeability cause edema and an increase in plasma and blood cells at the site (swelling and pain from increased pressure). Phagocytes are attracted to the area to engulf the foreign agent. Death of phagocytes attracts more phagocytes to the area. Circulation is increased, causing the redness and heat. The affected cells or tissues are surrounded by phagocytic cells (neutrophils and monocytes) and fluids that are equipped to destroy and remove the invader, thereby promoting healing. Fibrinogen from the serum in the affected area leads to the formation of a fibrin network, which acts as a trap to hold foreign particles for phagocytosis. This network also helps to wall off the injured area from nonaffected tissue to prevent further injury. If the inflammation cannot be contained and destroyed, further tissue destruction or even tissue death can occur.[37] The inflammatory response, like the first-line defenses previously discussed, is present at birth and helps to protect the infant while the immune response is being developed.

Infection

Infection is the result of invasion of the body by microorganisms. These may be bacteria, viruses, fungi, or

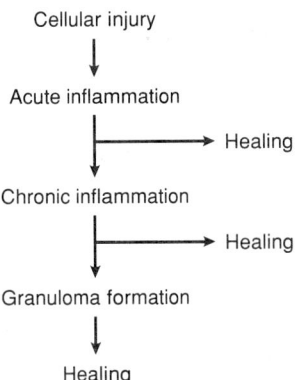

FIGURE 27-2
The inflammatory process. (Rote, N. S. (1990). Inflammation. In K. L. McCance, S. E. Heuther (Eds.), *Pathophysiology: The biologic basis for disease in adults and children* (p. 218). St. Louis: C.V. Mosby Co.

parasites. Organisms that are able to survive and grow in the human body may cause injury to cells and tissues. The disease-producing potential of a microorganism depends on its ability to (1) enter and incapacitate cells, (2) produce toxins, and (3) produce hypersensitivity reactions. All infections produce inflammatory reactions. Infections that begin as localized areas of injury, if unresolved by the inflammatory process, may progress to encompass larger tissue groups, organs, and eventually the entire body; this results in overwhelming sepsis and ultimately death. Systemic manifestations of inflammation include fever, leukocytosis, and an increase in circulating plasma proteins. The fever is believed to be a result of the interaction of endogenous pyrogen (interleukin 1, a product of T cells), which acts directly on the hypothalamus to reset the body's thermostat to a higher than usual temperature. Fever decreases activity of microorganisms, which are temperature sensitive. Leukocytosis occurs as a result of the inflammatory process. Plasma proteins increase for the same reason. Acute systemic inflammation can be perceived through hematologic tests.[37] In addition to the body's natural defense seen in the inflammatory response, infections may be lessened or eradicated with medications specific for the causative organism as with the administration of penicillin for streptococcus.

Hypersensitivity

Sometimes in otherwise healthy individuals, the immune system may produce an undesirable outcome. For example, the body may mistakenly identify a harmless substance as an antigen and produce a hypersensitive reaction.

Hypersensitivity reactions are classified according to the source of the antigen that stimulated the hypersensitivity response. These include type I, immediate hypersensitivity or IgE mediated allergic responses; type II, cytotoxic or tissue-specific hypersensitivity; type III, immune complex hypersensitivity; and type IV, delayed type or cell-mediated hypersensitivity.[23] Each of these is described in Table 27-4 and in the following discussion.

Type I

Type I, IgE-mediated hypersensitivity, is the hypersensitivity response that is elicited as a result of exposure to environmental antigens. This is commonly called *allergy*. The offending antigen is called an allergen. Examples include inhalants (animal dander), dust, chemicals, injectants (bee stings), and ingestants (food). The severity of the response depends on the challenge dose and the previous exposure to the allergen. Allergic reactions may be localized (e.g. allergic rhinitis), or they may be systemic (e.g., anaphylaxis).[23,36]

After initial exposure to an allergen, antigen-specific IgE is produced by certain B cells and attaches to the surface of mast cells. With re-exposure to an antigen such as cat dander, histamine and other chemical substances are released, and tissue swelling and itching enhance the subsequent inflammatory reaction. Repeated exposure to relatively large doses generally must take place before sensitization occurs.[36]

Clinical manifestations of IgE-mediated hypersensitivity reactions are primarily a result of histamine production, which causes swelling, increased circulation, and in some instances, increased mucus production in the affected area. IgE-mediated reactions may be found in the GI tract, in the respiratory tract, or on the skin. Symptoms include vomiting, diarrhea, abdominal pain, rhinitis, conjunctivitis, swelling of the hands or other body parts (angioedema), wheezing, dyspnea, hives, and urticaria. Examples of type I conditions include hay fever, eczema, food and drug intolerance, and anaphylaxis.[23,36]

There appears to be a genetic predisposition to allergies, known as *atopy*. Atopic individuals produce higher than normal amounts of IgE and have more available receptors on their mast cells. The skin and airways of atopic individuals appear to be more reactive to external stimuli than the skin and airways of nonatopic individuals. Children of atopic parents tend to be much more likely to develop allergies, including hay fever, asthma, and eczema, than those of nonaffected parents.[23,36]

Treatment of type I hypersensitivity reactions includes identification and removal of the offending aller-

TABLE 27-4
Types of Hypersensitivity Reactions

Type	Description	Example
Type I (immediate hypersensitivity or IgE-mediated hypersensitivity)	Elicited as a result to exposure to environmental antigen	Hay fever Anaphylaxis (B cells)
Type II (tissue-specific hypersensitivity)	Found only on tissue or organs with specific antigens	ABO incompatibility (B cells)
Type III (immune complex mediated)	Immune complexes are formed in circulation and then deposited in tissues, stimulating complement reaction	Glomerulonephritis (B and T cells)
Type IV (cell-mediated delay type)	Does not involve antibody; controlled by specific T cells	Tuberculin skin test Contact dermatitis (poison ivy) (T cells)

gen and avoidance of future contact. Medications, particularly antihistamines, which are blocking medications, may also offer some symptomatic relief. Other types of allergies, especially respiratory allergies, may be treated by desensitization. In desensitization, minute amounts of the allergen are administered subcutaneously over a period of months or years to increase immune system tolerance to the allergen.[36]

The Nursing Care Plan and Teaching Plan apply to the child with allergies.

Anaphylaxis. The most life-threatening reaction to type I allergies is known as anaphylaxis. For this to occur, the individual must have had previous exposure to the offending allergen. *Anaphylaxis* is a generalized hypersensitivity reaction in an affected individual. The most common causes of human anaphylactic reactions are drugs, food, and insect venoms.[7,12,23,39]

Once the allergen is in the body, an immediate and widespread immune and inflammatory response is triggered. The effects of this response include vasodilation and increased vascular permeability, which causes peripheral pooling and tissue edema. The resulting hypovolemia causes a decrease in tissue perfusion, which in turn impairs cellular metabolism. In addition, severe respiratory difficulty occurs due to extravascular smooth muscle constriction.[23,36]

The onset of anaphylaxis usually occurs within seconds or minutes of exposure to the allergen; the more suddenly the clinical symptoms appear after exposure, the more severe the reaction will be. Death can occur within minutes of the onset of symptoms.

Symptoms include flushed skin, rash, swelling, anxiety, difficulty breathing, GI cramps, hives, and a burning sensation on the skin. As the reaction progresses, blood pressure drops dramatically and mental confusion may occur. Angioedema may be observed in the eyelids, lips, tongue, hands, feet, and genitalia. Symptoms of airway obstruction follow. Pulmonary edema, laryngeal edema, and shock also may be seen.[7,12,23,39]

Management of anaphylaxis depends on rapid recognition of the condition and aggressive treatment to stop the allergic reaction. The first step is to remove the antigen if possible. Airway and respiratory distress are managed with high-flow oxygen, an oral airway, and ventilation as indicated. Epinephrine is the drug of choice to reverse the vasodilation and airway constriction. Volume expanders may be given to combat the hypovolemia, and antihistamines also may be given to stop the inflammatory reaction. A severely allergic person may be advised to wear medical identification at all times to share information about allergies in case of future exposures.[7,12,39]

Type II

Type II, tissue-specific hypersensitivity reactions, are found only on tissues or organs that have particular antigens. Antigens on the target cell bind with antibodies and either are prevented from functioning or are destroyed. An example of this type of reaction is an ABO transfusion reaction with hemolysis.[12,39]

Type III

Type III, immune complex-mediated injury, occurs when immune complexes are formed in the circulation and later deposited in blood vessels or other healthy tissue, thereby stimulating the complement reaction. Type III reactions are not specific to any organ; symptoms are unrelated to the antigenic target of the antibody. Examples of type III reactions are serum sickness and glomerulonephritis.[12,23,36]

Type IV

Type IV, cell-mediated delay type hypersensitivity, reactions are controlled by specifically sensitized T cells and do not involve antibody. Type IV reactions occur either as a result of cytotoxic T cells or of T cells that recruit and activate phagocytic cells to the inflammatory site. Examples of type IV reactions are tuberculin skin test reactions, graft rejection, and contact dermatitis from agents such as poison ivy or metals.[18,23,36]

Autoimmunity

Sometimes the immune system mistakenly identifies self as nonself. In *autoimmunity,* the body begins to make antibodies (autoantibodies) against its own normal, healthy cells (autoantigens) or otherwise inhibits cell function without cell destruction. These autoantibodies attach to the individual's own cells or to extracellular proteins.[23,36]

The pathophysiology of autoimmune reactions includes the development of immune complexes, which are then deposited in tissues such as skin, joints, and kidneys, resulting in tissue damage. Complement is also activated, which destroys self cells and may result in damage to organs. Predisposing factors appear to be related to genetics, certain drugs, and viruses.[23,36] Examples of autoimmune disorders in children include juvenile-onset diabetes mellitus (see Chap. 56), rheumatic fever (see Chap. 41), and systemic lupus erythematosus (SLE). SLE will be discussed in greater detail in a later section of this chapter.

Transplantation and Rejection

The immune system also may cause rejection of transplanted organs (nonself) in the host (self). For this reason, host tissues and donor tissues are matched for antigenic compatibility, also known as histocompatibility. Immunosuppression through medication may delay or prevent rejection of donor tissues or organs.[23,36]

Nursing Assessment

Nursing assessment of a child with an immunologic problem includes a comprehensive history, physical examination, and examination of laboratory test results. It is also important to obtain information about any behavioral manifestations. Signs and symptoms may be con-

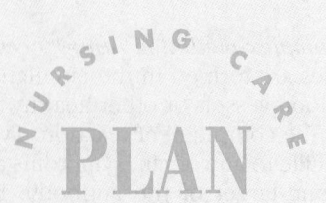

An 8-Year-Old Child With Allergies

Assessment

Case Study Description

John S. is an 8-year-old white boy who is visiting the well child clinic for a routine checkup today. His mother asks if perhaps the nurse thinks he might be sick, because he has a "runny nose" and slight cough. She also reports that he complains frequently of being tired. He prefers lying on the couch and watching television to active sports outside. He has a 6-year-old sister who has asthma. He lives with his mother and sister in a frame house in a rural area of the southeastern United States. Family pets include two cats who sleep on his bed at night.

Assessment Data

Family History.

Mother has hay fever and asthma. Sister has asthma. Maternal grandfather has "skin problems" and asthma. Aunt and grandmother on paternal side had diabetes. Other family history unremarkable.

Overall Appearance.

Slightly thin white boy in no apparent distress; obvious mouth breather.

Eyes, Ears, Nose & Throat (EENT).

Clear watery discharge from both nares; bluish coloring under both eyes ("allergic shiners"); transverse crease across bridge of nose ("allergic salute"); mucous membranes of nose pale gray and slightly swollen; posterior pharyngeal area reddened with drainage evident; respiratory rate 22; no rales, occasional rhonchi; breathing audible at 10 feet; frequent dry, nonproductive hacking cough.

Nursing Diagnosis	Intervention	Rationale
1. Ineffective airway clearance related to increased tracheobronchial secretions Supporting Data: • Ineffective cough • Increased secretions secondary to allergic response	Increase fluid intake.	Fluids help keep secretions thin so they can be expelled more easily.
	Instruct mother to administer antihistamines and cough medicine as ordered by physician.	Antihistamines help to suppress allergic response, and cough suppressant helps to quiet cough reflex.
	Advise mother to keep child indoors during periods of high pollen counts.	Common allergens include grasses and plants; frequent exposure may worsen symptoms.

Evaluation

John's symptoms continue, and he is referred to a pediatric allergist for testing. He is found to be allergic to animal dander, ragweed, grasses, dust mites, and oak trees. Desensitization shots are ordered. The physician also recommends that the home be modified to minimize exposure to allergens, including installing air conditioning, removing the carpet and draperies in John's room, and getting rid of the family pets. John's mother says to the nurse, "I'm really worried about how I can afford to do all these things. John's dad walked out 2 years ago, so I am all alone. He's really attached to his cats, too. His dad bought them for him just before he left. Do you think that if he takes the allergy shots, that will be enough to help him?"

(Continued)

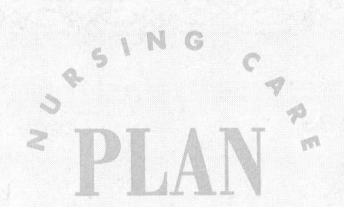

An 8-Year-Old Child With Allergies (continued)

Nursing Diagnosis	Intervention	Rationale
2. Altered health maintenance related to lack of material resources and reported impairment of personal support system Supporting Data: • Reported lack of financial or other resources • Reported impairment of personal support system	Explore availability of allergy shot administration in public health clinic rather than private physician's office. Assist mother in exploration of alternative personal and material support sources (e.g., church, extended family, neighbors).	Cost may be considerably lower if administered in public health setting rather than in private physician office. Cultural practices common to the rural Southeast often are centered in church members assisting each other as needed. Support systems would help to decrease the sense of isolation and helplessness a single parent in a rural area might be experiencing.

Evaluation — Mother keeps most, but not all, appointments for allergy shots. Mother can identify some alternative support systems and describe how they can help. Long-term evaluation focuses on the extent to which these have been used and the mother's perception of how helpful they were.

Nursing Diagnosis	Intervention	Rationale
3. Knowledge deficit related to lack of exposure to allergen removal measures and information misinterpretation Supporting Data: • Inaccurate follow through of instructions	Develop and implement teaching plan relative to management of allergies.	Understanding of the relationship between exposure to allergens, immune response, and subsequent symptoms is needed to assist mother and child in implementation of appropriate measures.

Evaluation — Mother and child describe appropriate measures to reduce exposure to allergens; measures are implemented in home environment. Mother is able to verbalize reason for allergy shots and follows regimen for allergy shots.

---

fusing or frightening to the child and his or her parents. Carefully directed questions should be used to elicit accurate information that may be used in establishing the diagnosis.

Historical Data

In addition to the usual information obtained in a history, the nurse should obtain a description of the illness, beginning with its onset and continuing to the present. Data on the age of the child, the number of previous illnesses in the last year, the type and number of medications used to treat any illnesses, the presence of a rash or sore throat, and frequency and amount of fever should be included. The nurse also should ask how many times a health care provider was seen during the last year for the problems described, how many days were missed from school, and if others in the family have had similar symptoms or problems. Any exposure to drugs or toxic

chemicals prior to the onset of symptoms also should be determined.

Reported allergies of any type should be fully described as well as any unusual reactions to a substance. Symptoms to ask about include an unexplained rash, runny nose without symptoms of a cold, wheezing, persistent headache, or dry hacking cough without any other sign of infection. If the child is receiving or has received desensitization treatments (allergy shots), this also should be noted.

The child's immunization status should be assessed. In addition, any reactions to immunizations must be noted and described in detail. Immunizations are discussed in Chapter 9.

Physical Data

A physical assessment should be conducted in a systematic manner so that important signs and symptoms

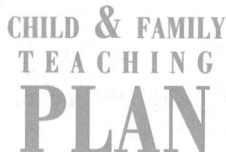

CHILD & FAMILY
T E A C H I N G
PLAN

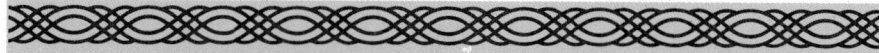

Care of a Child With Allergies

Assessment

John S. is an 8-year-old child recently diagnosed as allergic to grasses, dust mites, oak trees, and animal dander.

Desensitization shots and allergen removal measures for home were ordered by physician. This is the youngest child in a family of three that includes the mother and a sister. Mother is the sole support of the family. She has a high school education. Mother states that a lot of her family have allergies, and they just "put up with it." No family members have been treated by an allergist other than her son.

Child and Family Objectives	*Specific Content*	*Teaching Strategies*
1. Describe the allergic process.	1. A hypersensitivity response occurs when the body identifies a harmless substance as harmful and reacts to protect itself. Repeated exposure to the substance (allergen) creates the response. Severity of response depends on the dose and the previous exposure to the allergen. Symptoms of hypersensitivity reactions include increased mucous production, swelling, running nose, difficulty breathing, and itching. Hay fever is an example of this type reaction.	1. Use diagram to show allergic response.
2. Describe the way desensitization shots can help allergies.	2. Desensitization shots, also known as allergy shots, help to teach the body that it does not need to react against the allergen. This is done by injecting very tiny amounts of the allergen under the skin over a period of months or years to gradually increase the body's tolerance for that substance. The amount of the allergen is increased very slowly and carefully as the body adjusts to the allergen. In time, the hypersensitivity reaction becomes much weaker than it was before the desensitization shots. Individuals who receive allergy shots must remain in the health care setting for 30 minutes following the shot in case of a severe allergic reaction. If this were to happen, appropriate medication could be given.	2. Use analogy of "teaching" body not to react by giving repeated "reminders" (shots) that the allergen is "okay." Encourage parent and child to ask questions.
3. Describe common measures used to reduce environmental allergens.	3. Common measures that help to reduce allergies include removing carpet and curtains from the bedroom of the person with an allergy to reduce the amount of dust	3. Provide written materials in pamphlet or list form in addition to verbal instruction. Reinforce rationale for measures that are ordered.

(Continued)

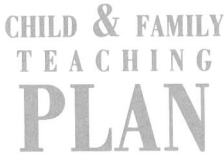

Care of a Child With Allergies (continued)

Child and Family Objectives	Specific Content	Teaching Strategies
	in the environment. Venetian blinds or shades are recommended instead of draperies. Floors should be damp mopped daily or several times a week to minimize dust accumulation. Keep windows and doors closed and use air conditioning to decrease pollen that is airborne. Keep pets outside to reduce exposure to animal dander.	
4. Identify resources and medications available to assist in allergen management.	4. Allergy shots may be administered by nurses in a clinic or at the public health department. Many health insurance plans cover medicines for allergies, including the substances used in the allergy shots. Sometimes the physician also will order over-the-counter or prescription medications to help relieve symptoms. These include pills, liquids, or inhalants. Inhalants may be used if ordered before vigorous outside exercise. Avoid mixing types of medicine without checking with the doctor or pharmacist first. Always take only the amount prescribed at the times specified.	4. Determine what measures have been used in the past; incorporate these in instruction if appropriate. Allow time for parent and child to ask questions.
5. Verbalize feelings about changes in environment necessitated by presence of allergens.	5. Parent and child discuss feelings related to changes in environment, including removal of indoor pets.	5. Encourage child and parent to express feelings about changes in house, including removal of pets. Reinforce rationale for changes needed. Explore alternative pets, such as fish, which could remain in house.

Evaluation

- Parent and child describe the allergic process, including common allergens and examples of hypersensitivity response.
- Parent and child describe how desensitization shots help allergic response.
- Parent and child describe common measures that reduce environmental allergens in the home.
- Parent and child identify resources and medications avilable to assist in allergen management.
- Parent and child express feelings about changes in environment that have been necessitated by presence of allergens.

are not overlooked. The order of the examination may be modified somewhat depending on the developmental level. A young child is frequently more cooperative if the mother holds the child's hand and assists with the examination.

In addition to the usual physical assessment, the nurse should look for evidence related to the symptoms reported during the history. Examples include a reddened or swollen throat with lymph node enlargement (history of sore throat and fever), dark circles under the eyes

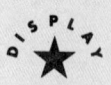

("allergic shiners"), weeping lesions on exposed areas (exposure to poison ivy), a rash in a butterfly pattern on the cheek and bridge of the nose (possibly suggestive of SLE), joint pain and tenderness (history of morning joint pain), wheezing, dyspnea, or barrel-shaped chest (history of respiratory problems). Other physical findings related to specific immune disorders will be discussed in greater detail in sections under each disease category.

Behavioral Data

Assessment of behavioral changes is another significant area for nurses. Children with immune-related disorders may exhibit a variety of different behaviors, ranging from extreme anxiety and clinging to parents to lethargy and apparent indifference to their surroundings. The symptoms that arise from immunologic disturbances, including nonspecific malaise, may be quite frightening to the child and the child's parents, resulting in overdependency and overprotectiveness. Other children may appear to be unaffected by their conditions.

Children who exhibit hypersensitivity to allergens may have episodes of acute onset that are triggered by allergens and that demand dramatic attention. After the acute episode subsides, both children and their parents need help verbalizing their fears and understanding what has happened.

Autoimmune disorders tend to be long-term chronic illnesses that may interfere with normal development because of changes in health status. Affected children and their parents may need assistance in promoting normalcy and may need opportunities for verbalizing fears and questions related to the child's condition. Nursing assessment should always include observation and docu-

mentation of behavioral data so that appropriate interventions can be included in the plan of care.

Laboratory Data

Laboratory studies for immune disorders involve a variety of serologic studies. The *humoral response* is evaluated by measuring immunoglobulins and by studying antigen–antibody reactions using a number of tests. Elevated levels of IgE suggest an allergic reaction. Decreased levels of IgG, IgM, and IgA may denote an increased susceptibility to infection. Examples of antigen–antibody tests include radioimmunoassays, precipitation tests, agglutination tests, and complement fixation tests. These tests help to identify the presence of antigens or antigen–antibody reactions that may indicate a specific disease process.

Children of all ages generally dislike having their blood drawn because of the discomfort involved and the fear and anxiety associated with needles and the withdrawal of body substances. The nurse should offer age-appropriate explanations about the procedure and then obtain the specimen with as little fanfare as possible. It is important to remember to spend time with a child after performing such a procedure to decrease the resulting negative association the child might have about the nurse.

The *cell-mediated response* is evaluated most often by using skin tests for which a minute amount of allergen(s) is introduced intradermally. Reaction to the specific allergen is observed. Although not extremely painful, skin tests can be quite uncomfortable and threatening to the child. In addition, a reaction such as itching or burning may frighten the child. With skin tests, there is also the possibility of a severe hypersensitivity reaction (anaphylaxis), which could quickly become life-threatening.[40] For these reasons, it is important that the nurse stay in close proximity to the child for approximately 30 minutes after administering a skin test.

Immunodeficiency Disorders

An immunodeficiency disorder occurs when the normal function of one or more components of the immune response (B cells, T cells, phagocytes, or complement) is disturbed. A summary of these major categories is given in the accompanying display on immunodeficiency states. *Congenital (primary) immunodeficiency* is the result of a genetic dysfunction; *acquired (secondary) immunodeficiency* is the result of diseases such as human immunodeficiency virus (HIV) or cancer. Lymphocyte malfunction is the primary cause of immunodeficiency. The primary clinical manifestation of an immunodeficiency disorder is the tendency to develop unusual prolonged or repeated severe infections.[37] In children, six to 12 relatively mild upper respiratory infections per year are considered to be the norm. Usually these are either upper respiratory tract viral infections or pharyngitis due to streptococcal infection. Children with immunodeficiency disorders, however, are susceptible to repeated bouts of chronic prolonged infections, such as pneumonia, bronchitis, or meningitis, or infections caused by organisms that are not usually pathogenic (e.g., *Pneumocystis carinii*).[23,36]

Congenital Immunodeficiency

Severe Combined Immunodeficiency

Severe combined immunodeficiency (SCID) is the most severe form of primary immunodeficiency. Both T lymphocytes and B lymphocytes are affected. It affects only infants and young children, and survival beyond childhood depends on treatment outcomes.

Diagnostic Criteria. Within the first 2 months of life, children with SCID present with severe infections; failure to thrive; fungal (candidal) infections of the skin, mouth, and upper GI tract; and chronic otitis media. Lymph nodes, tonsils, and the thymus are either undersized or absent. Immunoglobulin levels are low or absent. T lymphocytes are never present; B cells may be absent as well but in some instances, are present in normal numbers.[23,36]

Medical Management. Bone marrow transplants are the treatment of choice for SCID. The major problem is that the bone marrow must be histocompatible to be successful. The best means of achieving this is with a sibling donation; cure rates approach 70% in this instance.[23] Children with SCID will not reject mismatched donated bone marrow because they are deficient in their immune capacity; however, they are at risk of suffering from graft versus host reaction if the bone marrow is not histocompatible. When this occurs, little can be done to offset the problem.

Nursing Diagnoses. The following nursing diagnoses are applicable for a child with SCID:

* High Risk for Infection related to inadequate secondary defenses
* Knowledge Deficit regarding bone marrow transplant
* Altered Family Processes related to life-threatening illness in child

Nursing Intervention. Nursing management of a child with SCID is directed toward prevention of infection and enhancement of growth through adequate nutrition, rest, and exercise within the limitations allowed. The child with SCID is prone not only to the usual infections, but also frequently to opportunistic infections, despite careful adherence to prescribed regimens.

Parents of a child with SCID need consistent information and support. If a bone marrow transplant is ordered, the child and family need to be taught what to expect with this procedure. Parents need to be instructed to contact the health care provider at the earliest signs of infection. They also need an opportunity to express their fears, hopes, anger, and sadness over the child's condition.

Evaluation. Evaluation of nursing care outcomes is focused on the following areas:

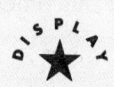

Immunodeficiency States*

ANTIBODY (B CELL) IMMUNODEFICIENCY

Primary
Transient hypogammaglobulinemia of infancy
Common variable immunodeficiency
X-linked hypogammaglobulinemia
Selective deficiency of IgG, IgA, IgM

Secondary
Decreased synthesis of immunoglobulins (lymphomas)
Increased loss of immunoglobulins (nephrotic syndrome)
Production of defective immunoglobulins (multiple myeloma)

CELLULAR (T CELL) IMMUNODEFICIENCY

Primary
Congenital thymic aplasia (DiGeorge syndrome)
Abnormal T-cell production (Nezelof syndrome)

Secondary
Malignant disease (Hodgkin's disease and others)
Transient suppression of T-cell production and function due to an acute viral infection such as measles
AIDS

COMBINED ANTIBODY (B CELL) AND CELLULAR (T CELL) IMMUNODEFICIENCY

Primary
Severe combined immunodeficiency (autosomal or sex-linked recessive)
Wiskott-Aldrich syndrome (immunodeficiency, thrombocytopenia, and eczema)
Immunodeficiency with ataxia and telangiectasia

Secondary
X-radiation
Immune suppressant and cytotoxic drugs
Aging

COMPLEMENT ABNORMALITY

Primary
Selective deficiency in a complement component
Angioneurotic edema (complement-1 inactivator deficiency)

Secondary
Acquired disorders in which complement is used

PHAGOCYTIC DYSFUNCTION

Primary
Chronic granulomatous disease
Glucose-6-phosphate dehydrogenase deficiency
Job syndrome

Secondary
Drug induced (e.g., corticosteroid and immunosuppressive therapy)
Diabetes

* *Examples are not inclusive.*
Porth, C. M. (1990). Pathophysiology: Concepts of altered health states (3rd ed.). Philadelphia: J. B. Lippincott.

- Frequency and severity of infections
- Assessment of knowledge relative to bone marrow transplants, including what to expect with the procedure and associated risks and benefits
- Assessment of family members' ability to maintain usual roles within the family
- Assessment of family relationships and family ability to support and assist each other
- Assessment of the extent to which family members verbalize their feelings about the child's condition

Wiskott-Aldrich Syndrome

Wiskott-Aldrich syndrome is an X-linked recessive disorder that is nearly as severe as SCID.[23] It not only affects the cellular and humoral immune systems, but also has other manifestations as well. IgM antibody production is generally very low; therefore, recurrent bacterial infections are seen. Symptoms usually are seen between 6 months and 1 year of age.

Diagnostic Criteria. Diagnostic criteria for Wiskott-Aldrich syndrome include the presence of a triad of symptoms: recurrent infections caused by all classes of microorganisms, thrombocytopenia, and eczema of the skin. The recurrent infections usually are not seen until 6 months of age. Meningitis, pneumonia, sepsis, otitis media, and systemic fungal infections may occur. Thrombocytopenia may cause bleeding in the brain, leading to death in 20% of affected children. Eczema is seen by 1 year of age and is similar to that found in allergic children. Children with Wiskott-Aldrich syndrome are also at risk of developing autoimmune disease and malignant tumors; up to 25% of children with this disease develop lymphomas.[23]

Medical Management. The treatment of choice for Wiskott-Aldrich is bone marrow transplant if a histocompatible donor can be identified. Splenectomy may be ordered to control the thrombocytopenia.[23] Prophylactic antibiotics are indicated to prevent and control infections.

Nursing Diagnoses. The following nursing diagnoses are applicable for a child with Wiskott-Aldrich syndrome:

- High Risk for Infection related to inadequate secondary defenses
- Impaired Skin Integrity related to chemical irritants
- Vascular Fluid Volume Deficit related to bleeding
- Knowledge Deficit related to prevention of infection and management of bleeding episodes

Nursing Intervention. Nursing management of a child with Wiskott-Aldrich syndrome includes careful attention to measures for preventing infection, including strict handwashing; avoidance of crowds, particularly when communicable diseases are more common (flu season); and administration of antibiotics as ordered. Nursing measures to prevent bleeding are similar to those indicated for hemophilia (see Chap. 44). Nursing measures for the care of a child with eczema are found in Chapter 65.

Evaluation. Evaluation of nursing care outcomes is focused on the following areas:

- Frequency and severity of infections
- Frequency and severity of bleeding episodes
- Condition of the skin in all body areas, including those with eczema
- Assessment of parental knowledge about prevention of infection and management of eczema and bleeding episodes

Humoral Deficiency

Humoral deficiency is manifested in the form of either *aggammaglobulinemia* (immunoglobulins are absent or nearly absent) or *hypogammaglobulinemia* (immunoglobulins are present but in inadequate numbers).[36]

Diagnostic Criteria. The child with a humoral deficiency will present with severe chronic infections caused by staphylococcus, streptococcus, and *Haemophilus influenzae*. Because of the protective effect of maternal antibodies, these generally are not seen until 9 months to 2 years of age. Generally, children with repeated bouts of pneumonia or skin infections are tested for agammaglobulinemia. Laboratory studies will reveal low or nearly absent levels of IgG. Plasma cells will be lower than normal. T cell levels will be normal.

Medical Management. Infections are treated with vigorous antibiotic therapy. Intravenous infusions of gamma globulin are given on a regular schedule, most often biweekly or monthly after the initial administration. Recent clinical studies have indicated that this can be administered effectively by parents or by an older child in a home setting, rather than requiring the child to travel to a hospital or health care center as in the past.[24]

Nursing Diagnoses. The following nursing diagnoses are applicable for a child with humoral deficiency:

- High Risk for Infection related to inadequate secondary defenses
- Knowledge Deficit regarding home administration of intravenous immunoglobulin

Nursing Intervention. Nursing management of a child with a humoral deficiency is focused on teaching the parents (and the child if age-appropriate) how to avoid infections. Careful handwashing and avoidance of crowds, particularly during high-risk periods (flu season) should be stressed. Parents need to be instructed to contact the health care provider at the earliest signs of infection.

If a child is on a home-administered regimen of intravenous immunoglobulin, the nurse needs to teach the parents and children the principles of intravenous (IV) administration and care, how to handle the immunoglobulin preparation, and how to recognize and manage adverse reactions. It is also important to plan for regular review sessions and observations of technique to assure protocols are being followed.[24]

Evaluation. Evaluation of nursing care outcomes is focused on the following areas:

- Frequency and severity of infections
- Assessment of knowledge related to home administration of IV gamma globulin

Complement Deficiency Diseases

Complement deficiency diseases also may lead to increased infections. If the complement defect is in the early pathway, infections will be mild; defects in the late pathway are associated with recurrent severe infections.[36]

AIDS

AIDS is probably the most familiar form of immunodeficiency that develops after birth. It is a result of infection with HIV type 1 (HIV-1). Although HIV-1 virus has been isolated in all body fluids, including blood, semen, vaginal secretions, tears, saliva, breast milk, cerebrospinal fluid, and urine,[11] transmission appears to be possible only as a result of contact with infected blood, breast-feeding, and intimate sexual contact. The primary risk factor for pediatric AIDS appears to be exposure to an HIV-infected mother, either transplacentally or during delivery[2] (Table 27-5). Postpartum, HIV infection may be transmitted through breast-feeding.[10] Adolescent AIDS is linked to intravenous drug experimentation and to sexual experimentation, including sexual abuse and promiscuity.[3]

HIV is a retrovirus that primarily invades T-helper cells. Once activated, the virus may lie dormant for years while the individual remains asymptomatic. If viral growth occurs, the infected cells will be destroyed, and other T-helper cells will be attacked and killed. This infection also diminishes the function of other parts of the immune system (Tc lymphocytes, B lymphocytes, and macrophages). The result is a widespread dysfunction in immune response.[23,27]

Diagnostic Criteria. There is no definitive test for HIV. The enzyme-linked immunosorbent assay (ELISA or EIA) is used to determine antibody response to the virus. The Western Blot Analysis also is used to confirm the presence of HIV antibodies.[25]

Diagnosis of AIDS in infants is difficult for the following reason: All infants born to HIV-infected mothers will have positive ELISA *and* Western Blot tests in most instances for up to 15 months due to the transmission of

TABLE 27-5
Pediatric AIDS Cases by Transmission Categories*

Category	Cases	Percent
Parent with or at risk of AIDS	2184	83
Hemophilia or coagulation disorder	132	5
Transfusion or blood components	243	9
Other, undetermined	69	3
TOTAL	2628	100

* Includes children 13 years of age at the time of diagnosis.
Centers for Disease Control. (1990). HIV/AIDS Surveillance through September. These data are provisional.

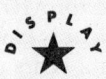

Clinical Manifestations of Pediatric AIDS

Failure to thrive (weight loss, diarrhea)
Frequent fevers, diaphoresis
Hepatosplenomegaly
Chronic cough
Persistent recurrent oral thrush and chronic otitis media
HIV encephalopathy: Neurological and developmental deficits
Lymphocytic interstitial pneumonitis and *Pneumocystis Carinii* pneumonia
Renal disease (nephrotic syndrome) usually after age 2
Kaposi's sarcoma usually *does not* develop

maternal antibodies, whether or not they are infected.[11,25] However, passively acquired HIV antibody levels will begin falling rather than progressively rising as the infant matures, decreasing to undetectable levels usually between 12 and 15 months of age. Infected infants, on the other hand, will have persistent or rising antibody titers to HIV.[2] Other diagnostic tests that are being used in limited studies include isolation of the virus itself (viral culture), viral antigen detection, and molecular detection of HIV-1 DNA.[25,43]

Clinical manifestations of pediatric AIDS differ somewhat from those seen in adults (see the accompanying display on clinical manifestations of pediatric AIDS). Symptoms may be seen as early as 2 months of age if acquired early in gestation and usually are seen before 2 years.[4] If the mother is severely debilitated with HIV, the infant may be very ill shortly after birth. Clinical manifestations include symptoms of failure to thrive (weight loss, diarrhea), developmental delays, frequent fevers, diaphoresis, hepatosplenomegaly, and chronic cough. Marked lymphadenopathy (enlarged lymph nodes) may be seen. Enlarged lymph nodes are not generally found in other congenital immunodeficiency disorders. Persistent recurrent episodes of oral thrush, chronic otitis media, and pneumonia also may be seen.[5,16,34]

The most significant manifestations of pediatric AIDS are associated with the brain and the lungs. HIV encephalopathy (changes in the brain) is associated with developmental and neurological deficits. Previously attained developmental milestones may be lost. The child with AIDS also may develop lymphocytic interstitial pneumonitis (LIP) and *P. carinii* pneumonia (PCP). LIP is found in approximately 25% of infected children and generally is associated with a better prognosis than PCP. Median survival for a child with LIP is 8 years; median survival following PCP is 14 months.[3] Children with HIV infections also develop renal disease (nephropathy) as frequently as adult victims.[42] Unlike adults with HIV infections, however, children with HIV generally do not develop Kaposi's sarcoma.[3]

Medical Management. There is no cure for AIDS. So far, approximately 50% of pediatric AIDS victims have died. The majority of the deaths occur within 2 years of diagnosis. Early central nervous system (CNS) involvement and development of symptoms within the first 2 months of life are linked with a rapidly progressing fatal outcome. Children who have not demonstrated CNS involvement and severe infections such as PCP have survived without symptoms for a decade or more and are of great interest.[3]

Treatment of pediatric AIDS focuses on general supportive care, treatment for infection, support of immune system function, and specific medications. Each of these is discussed briefly. Currently the only drug licensed in the United States for treatment of AIDS is zidovudine (AZT), which works by inhibiting the replication of HIV DNA within the host cells. While not a cure for AIDS, AZT does help to slow the progression of the disease. Clinical improvements seen after administration of AZT include improvement of IQ scores, weight gain, reduction in hepatosplenomegaly, and improvement in immune system function.[14,26]

Prevention of infection is an important aim of treatment. Prophylaxis for PCP may be given in the form of trimethoprim and sulfamethoxazole (Bactrim, Septra) by mouth three times a week. Monthly administration of gamma globulin may help to prevent bacterial infections. Home oxygen therapy may be ordered for a child with LIP. If oral nutritional intake is inadequate, parenteral hyperalimentation and feedings by gastric tube may be indicated.

Immunizations for an HIV-infected child should be given according to the usual guidelines. (This includes immunization against measles, mumps, and rubella). The only exception is to administer inactivated polio virus (IPV) instead of oral polio virus (OPV) to the child and all close contacts. Vaccines against pneumonia should be given at age 2; influenza vaccinations are recommended at age 6 months and yearly thereafter. If active chicken pox appears, intravenous acyclovir should be administered.[1,5,8]

Nursing Diagnoses. The following diagnosis are applicable for a child with AIDS:

- High Risk for Infection related to inadequate secondary defenses
- Altered Nutrition: Less Than Body Requirements related to increased metabolism and inability to ingest or absorb nutrients
- Altered Growth and Development related to neurodevelopmental deficits
- Altered Family Processes related to life-threatening illness in child
- Anticipatory Grieving related to potentially fatal illness

Nursing Intervention. Nursing management of the child with HIV infection requires collaboration with a multidisciplinary team. The plan of care must address the specific needs related to the HIV infection, but it must also consider the child's and family's developmental stage and needs as well.[44] Many HIV-infected children spend a large portion of their lives in hospitals because of the severity of their illness and the inadequacy of home care alternatives available to them. It is generally agreed, however, that optimally, children with HIV infection should be treated at home.[4] The nurse can play a key role in coordinating resources to make home care a reality. Universal blood and body fluid precautions as recommended by the Centers for Disease Control should be followed by all care providers to protect themselves against exposure to HIV. A summary of these precautions is given on the inside back cover of this book.

Infections present a constant grave threat to the child with HIV. The nurse can assist the child and family in dealing with this threat by teaching them the importance of careful hygiene, including thorough handwashing and avoidance of contact with ill individuals. Children with AIDS also should avoid exposure to common infectious diseases, such as chickenpox and other viral illnesses.

Parents should be taught the importance of adherence to prescribed regimens of prophylactic antibiotics such as Bactrim or Septra. They also should be instructed to notify the health care provider immediately if any signs of infection are noticed. If the child is on a home-administered regimen of IV immunoglobulin, the nurse needs to teach the parents and child the principles of IV administration and care, how to handle the immunoglobulin preparation, and how to recognize and manage adverse reactions. Also, it is important to plan for regular review sessions and observations of techniques to assure protocols are followed.[24]

Caloric needs for the HIV-infected child are double those of a nonaffected child. Maintenance of adequate caloric intake poses a great challenge to caretakers. Calorically dense small frequent feedings need to be offered at regular intervals. If oral lesions are present, a bland soft diet at room temperature may be accepted more readily. The child who is unable to take in adequate calories by mouth may need to be fed by hyperalimentation or enterally using a nasogastric tube.[34]

Developmental deficits are commonly seen in HIV-infected children as previously discussed. Nursing management should include careful assessment of developmental milestones at regular intervals; documentation of progress or deterioration is essential. Regardless of the extent of neuropathy, opportunities for developmentally appropriate play and interaction should be available to the child within the limitations of the illness. Parents also

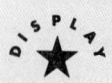

Prevention of Transmission of Human Immunodeficiency Virus (HIV)

Because health care workers are at risk for exposure to HIV during any circumstances in which they potentially come in contact with the blood or body fluids of a child infected with HIV, they must observe universal precautions (see inside back cover of this text).

should be given anticipatory guidance and should be encouraged to foster development through offering stimulation and interaction with the child. Parents should be encouraged to look for signs of improvement in development if the child has been given AZT.

Generally, school age children are permitted to attend school. Exclusion from school with home-bound instruction may be indicated if an outbreak of an illness such as measles or chickenpox occurs in the school. It is generally not necessary to inform school officials that a child has an HIV infection, nor is it recommended because of the social isolation the child might face as a result. Exclusion may be indicated for a child who lacks control over body secretions or whose behavior (such as biting) poses some risk.[3,20]

Evaluation.   Evaluation of nursing care outcomes is focused on the following areas:

- Frequency and severity of infections
- Weight gain
- Assessment of developmental milestones
- Assessment of family relationships and family ability to support and assist each other
- Assessment of family members' ability to maintain usual roles within the family
- Assessment of the extent to which family members verbalize their feelings about the child's condition.

Rheumatic and Connective Tissue Diseases

Inflammation of connective tissue is seen in a group of autoimmune disorders. These include juvenile rheumatoid arthritis (JRA), systemic lupus erythematosus (SLE), dermatomyositis, scleroderma, and mixed connective tissue disease, as identified in Table 27-6.

Juvenile Rheumatoid Arthritis

JRA is an autoimmune disease involving connective tissue in the joints. The etiology of rheumatoid arthritis is not understood fully; however, it is believed to be related to an inappropriate immune response to an unidentified antigen. Normal antibodies turn into autoantibodies after long-term exposure to the antigen and attack the body's own tissues. Autoantibodies that are present in individuals with rheumatoid arthritis are called rheumatoid factors (RFs). Immune complexes are formed when RFs bind with target self-antigens in the blood and synovial membrane. These trigger the production of complement, resulting in symptoms of inflammation. Inflammation begins in the synovial membrane, then spreads to surrounding areas in the joint, causing pain, deformity, and loss of function.[19,29]

JRA comprises approximately 5% of all arthritis cases. The symptoms begin at two peak time periods: ages 1 to 3 and 8 to 11 years. Girls are more often affected than boys. Symptoms of JRA develop more abruptly than in the adult form. There are three types: systemic, pauciarticular (arthritis in less than five joints), and polyarticular (arthritis in more than five joints). (See the accompanying display on the subtypes of JRA.) All three types have the following characteristics in common: symptoms that vary in severity from mild to severe, stiffness in the morning or after inactivity, and intermittent joint pain or swelling.[29,32]

Children with systemic onset have symptoms including fever, rash, malaise, pericarditis, myocarditis, pleuritis, hepatosplenomegaly, and abdominal pain. Joint pain may not appear for weeks, months, or years after the other symptoms.[29]

Children with pauciarticular JRA, the most common type, are at risk of inflammatory eye disease, which can result in functional blindness. Only one joint is affected in approximately one half of the children with this type. Children with polyarticular JRA are at greatest risk of permanent disability.[29,31]

Overall, children with JRA are less apt to be disabled than adults with rheumatoid arthritis. However, they may have leg length discrepancies, short stature, and failure to thrive as a result of the disease. Permanent visual impairment may be caused by inflammatory eye disease. Some children have a spontaneous remission after having symptoms for 1 to 2 years. Others, if not diagnosed early and treated, will progress to permanent disability due to the joint destruction.[29]

Diagnostic Criteria.   Diagnosis of JRA is based on symptoms of joint pain and stiffness along with radiological findings of joint effusion and destruction. Serologic

TABLE 27-6
Incidence of Connective Tissue Diseases in Children

Disease	Sex Ratio (Female:Male)	Race Ratio (White:Black)	Peak Age at Risk (Year)	Childhood Onset (Percent)
Juvenile rheumatoid arthritis	3:1	Equal	Increases with age (20–50)	5
Systemic lupus erythematosus	8:1	1:4	15–45	18
Dermatomyositis	2:1	1:3	45–65	20
Scleroderma	3:1	Equal	Increases with age (30–50)	3

Andrews M. M., Mooney, K. H. (1990). Alterations in musculoskeletal function. In K. L. McLance, S. E. Heuther (Eds.), *Pathophysiology: The biological basis for disease in adults and children* (p. 1373). St. Louis: C. V. Mosby Co.

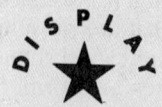

Subtypes of Juvenile Rheumatoid Arthritis

SYSTEMIC ONSET (20% TO 30% OF CASES)

Systemic Symptoms
Rheumatoid rash
Polyarthritis
ANA (−), RF (−) = 25% to 40% permanent deformity

POLYARTICULAR (25% TO 40% OF CASES)

Mild or absent systemic symptoms
Five or more joints involved
RF (+) = 50% permanent deformity
RF (−) = 10% to 15% permanent deformity
ANA (−)

PAUCIARTICULAR (30% TO 40% OF CASES)

Less than five joints involved
ANA (+), RF (−)
Uveitis 10% blindness
60% expected remission

(ANA, antinuclear antibodies; RF, Rheumatoid factor.)
Page-Goertz, S. (1989). Juvenile rhematoid arthritis. Pediatric Nursing 15, *12.*

tests are used to confirm the presence of antinuclear antibodies (ANAs). Speiser et al.[41] noted that rheumatoid factor is detectable in only 2% to 10% of children with JRA. Erythrocyte sedimentation rate (ESR) or C-reactive protein will indicate an inflammatory process somewhere in the body but are nonspecific for JRA.[17]

Medical Management. There is no cure for JRA. Treatment aims are supportive and directed toward relief of pain, reduction of the inflammatory process, and prevention of deformity to the extent possible. Medications that are commonly ordered include nonsteroidal anti-inflammatory drugs (NSAIDs). High doses of salicylates (aspirin in doses of 80 to 120 mg/kg per day) are most often used. The only other NASIDs that are approved by the Food and Drug Administration for use in children younger than age 12 are Tolectin and Naprosyn. Slow-acting antirheumatic drugs, such as gold, hydroxychloroquinine, and d-penicillamine, may be used when NSAIDs are ineffective. Corticosteroids are used only when life-threatening complications of JRA such as pericarditis occur. Cytotoxic agents such as methotrexate or cyclophosphamide may be given if the JRA does not respond to the usual medical regimen or if life-threatening complications are seen.[29,31,32]

Physical therapy and a regular program of exercise often are ordered to promote mobility and function. Many times heat is used to improve circulation and relieve pain and stiffness in the joints. Treatment also is directed toward stress management, because many times, the disease worsens in times of high stress.

Nursing Diagnoses. The following nursing diagnoses are appropriate for a child with JRA:

* Pain related to arthritic process
* Impaired Mobility related to activity intolerance and discomfort
* Ineffective Family Coping related to chronic illness
* Altered Growth and Development related to effects of physical disability

Nursing Intervention. Nursing care of a child with JRA is directed toward helping the child and his or her family cope with the acute manifestations and the long-term effects of the disease. Pain management is achieved through administration of medications, heat or cold as ordered, and rest. Morning stiffness can be helped by instructing the child to do gentle limbering exercises when awakening. A warm bath or shower when getting up also may help to relieve the discomfort. Anti-inflammatory medications should be taken with a snack upon awakening. Other suggestions include having the child sleep in footed pajamas or a sleeping bag or use a heated water bed or electric blanket.[29]

The child and parents should be instructed in exercises that are ordered and in the judicious use of heat prior to exercise. A physical therapist may come into the home to assist with exercise as ordered. A child with JRA may avoid participating in normal activities because of the discomfort that may result. The parents and the child need the opportunity to plan activities that promote normalcy and that are acceptable given the limitations of the disease. Recommended activities include bicycle riding, swimming, and piano playing.[29]

All family members of a child with JRA need an opportunity to verbalize feelings and concerns about the illness. The nurse is in a primary position to be the liaison between the family and other members of the health care team, acting as a referral agent, collaborator, and resource person.

Evaluation. Evaluation of nursing care outcomes is focused on the following areas:

* Level of comfort as measured by verbal and nonverbal indicators
* Assessment of mobility and level of activity
* Assessment of developmental milestones
* Assessment of family members' ability to deal with effects of chronic illness

Systemic Lupus Erythematosus

SLE is a chronic inflammatory immune disorder. Young women most often are affected by the disease. However, it can be found during early adolescence and later adulthood as well. Approximately 18% of SLE cases begins with a childhood onset. It affects black people four times as often as white people.[13]

The autoimmune reaction seen in SLE causes tissue inflammation and injury wherever the immune complexes activate complement. Multiple body systems frequently are affected in children, resulting in organ damage. Children with SLE often are very ill at initial diagnosis, in contrast to adults with SLE who more often have a gradual onset and less common multisystem problems.[13]

Clinical manifestations vary widely, depending on the body systems involved. Characteristic symptoms include a butterfly-shaped rash on the cheeks and bridge of the nose, weight loss, anorexia, fatigue, fever, malaise, and joint pain. Oral ulcers, glomerulonephritis, nephrotic syndrome, pericarditis, endocarditis, and splenomegaly are some of the systemic manifestations that may be seen. If the CNS is involved, the patient may have seizures or psychosis. Hemolytic anemia, thrombocytopenia, or leukopenia also may occur. Progressive retinopathy may lead to blindness.[13,32]

Diagnostic Criteria. Diagnosis of SLE is based on signs and symptoms presented and serologic findings. These include low complement levels, the presence of ANAs, anti-DNA antibodies, and deposits of immunoglobulin and complement at the dermoepidermal junction. C-reactive protein and erythrocyte sedimentation rates frequently are elevated with SLE but are nonspecific for the disease.[13,18,32]

Medical Management. There is no cure for SLE. Treatment aims are supportive and are directed at the organ systems that are affected by the disease. Aspirin is ordered for joint pain relief and for its anti-inflammatory effect. Steroids also are frequently ordered for their anti-inflammatory effect. Antimalarial drugs are used for cutaneous involvement. Immunosuppresant drugs have been used in limited instances.[13,32]

Sunlight appears to exacerbate the disease, so it must be carefully avoided. Stress also seems to negatively affect the course of the illness. The patient needs to be taught to recognize personal stress levels and to use appropriate stress management techniques.

The prognosis of the disease depends on the extent and degree of organ involvement. Death usually is a result of damage to the kidneys, which results in kidney failure.

Nursing Diagnoses. The following nursing diagnoses are appropriate for a person with SLE:

- Impaired Skin Integrity related to immunologic disturbance
- Pain related to joint or other tissue group involvement
- Altered Growth and Development related to effects of physical disability
- Ineffective Individual Coping related to personal vulnerability

- Body Image Disturbance related to actual or perceived change in body function

Nursing Intervention. Nursing management of a child with SLE is directed toward helping the individual maintain as normal a lifestyle as possible within the constraints of the illness. The child needs to be taught to wear a sunscreen or protective clothing any time he or she is in daylight. Side effects and dosages of medications need to be monitored carefully. If undesirable physical aftereffects occur with medications ("moon face" from steroids, alopecia from immunosuppresant drugs), the patient needs support and assistance in dealing with the change in body image.

Because the disease most often occurs at a time developmentally when independence is highly sought and valued, nurses must offer opportunities for independence in decision making whenever possible. Sometimes an SLE patient will refuse treatment regimens as a way of rebellion; rationale for every treatment ordered should be incorporated into nursing care so that the patient can assist with appropriate decision making.

The patient also needs time to express feelings about the illness and its impact on the present and future life plans. Today, many of the symptoms of SLE may be controlled, and affected people can live full lives into adulthood. However, any patient who is considering pregnancy needs to know that pregnancy may cause a flare-up of symptoms either during pregnancy or postpartum. Also, the infant may be born with SLE-associated problems.[13,32]

Evaluation. Evaluation of nursing care outcomes is focused on the following areas:

- Avoidance of direct exposure to sunlight
- Level of comfort as evidenced by verbal and nonverbal indicators
- Developmental level (dependence versus independence)
- Assessment of personal coping with chronic illness
- Assessment of self-concept, including body image

Dermatomyositis

Dermatomyositis is a generalized muscle inflammation accompanied by skin lesions. It is believed to be related to an autoimmune disorder, produced by cell-mediated or humoral immune factors. Symptoms include those seen in other inflammatory processes: fever, malaise, muscle swelling, pain, and tenderness. Symmetrical body weakness, manifested in difficulty climbing stairs or getting in and out of chairs, may be the first sign of a problem. Other body systems may be involved, creating additional clinical manifestations, such as dysphagia, reduced esophageal motility, vasculitis, Raynaud's phenomenon, cardiomyopathy, and interstitial pulmonary fibrosis. A purple skin rash (heliotrope rash) covering the upper eyelids, face, chest, and extensor surface of the extremities is also seen.[19,28,32]

Diagnostic Criteria. Diagnosis is by muscle biopsy, which shows inflammatory cells grouped around blood vessels and perifascicular atrophy in the muscle.

Electromyography abnormalities are also seen. The ESR may be elevated, as are muscle enzyme levels (transaminase, aldolase, and creatine).[19,32]

Medical Management. Treatment includes immunosuppressant drugs and corticosteroids. Individuals with muscle weakness also may need a prescribed program of exercise to maximize function.[19,32]

Nursing Diagnoses. The following nursing diagnoses are appropriate for a child with dermatomyositis:

- Impaired Physical Mobility related to muscle weakness
- Pain related to inflammatory process

Nursing Intervention

Nursing Management is directed toward supportive care. Provision of a nutritious diet and adequate rest should be included in the care plan. Medications ordered for a child with dermatomyositis need to be carefully monitored for side effects and expected results. Parents may need assistance in providing exercises that are ordered to maintain function and prevent contractures. Play can be incorporated into the planned exercise, encouraging participation and at the same time assisting in promotion of normalcy.

Evaluation. Evaluation of nursing care outcomes is based on the following areas:

- Mobility and level of activity
- Level of comfort as evidenced by verbal and nonverbal indicators

Summary

Immune disorders comprise a vast array of health-related problems, ranging from the simple annoyance of allergic rhinitis to life-threatening illnesses such as AIDS. The body's first line of defense against infection is through nonimmune or protective mechanisms, such as skin, tears, and mucous membranes. The immune response is sometimes described as the body's ability to distinguish "self" from "nonself." Natural immunity is present at birth, while acquired immunity develops after or as a result of exposure to an antigen, thereby activating the immune response. Acquired immunity may be active or passive. Active acquired immunity is provided by the individual after a natural exposure to an antigen or an immunization. Passive acquired immunity is temporary and occurs through the transplacental shift from mother to infant or as a result of clinical treatment.

When protective defense mechanisms are ineffective and harmful substances enter cells and tissues, the inflammatory response is triggered. Inflammation is nonspecific to invading organisms; the same series of events occurs in response. An inflammatory response may be acute (usually lasting 8 to 10 days) or chronic.

If the body mistakes a harmless substance as an antigen, hypersensitivity occurs. The most life-threatening

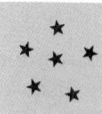

Ideas for Nursing Research

Nursing care of children with immunologic problems has the potential for many researchable ideas. Nurses are key figures in the management of health problems in children; therefore, they are able to identify areas to explore in an effort to improve care. Some areas for research that need to be explored are the following:

- Behavioral interventions that could be used to decrease anxiety associated with repeated needle sticks, such as allergy shots
- Investigation into the "lived experience" of a family with HIV to develop nursing interventions to improve quality of life
- Assessment of strategies used to enhance nutritional intake in HIV affected children
- Management of pain, including behavioral techniques and medication
- Interventions that are effective in promoting normalcy in a child with a chronic immunologic problem
- Examination of self-concept and body image of a child with an immunologic disorder
- Effectiveness of self-care teaching in home administration of intravenous gamma globulin
- Coping methods used by the affected child, siblings, and parents of an immunologically dysfunctional child

hypersensitivity is anaphylaxis. In autoimmunity, the immune system mistakenly identifies self as nonself and the body begins to make antibodies against its own normal healthy cells or otherwise inhibits cell function without cell destruction. The immune system also may reject transplanted organs; therefore, host tissues and donor tissues are matched for antigenic compatibility (histocompatibility).

References

1. AIDS Update (1988). Measles vaccine may be safe for children with AIDS. *Nursing 88, 18,* 30–31.
2. American Academy of Pediatrics (1988). Policy statement on perinatal HIV infection (AIDS). September, 1988.
3. Bernstein, L. J., MacKenzie, R. G., Oleske, J. M., & Pizzo, P. A. (1989). AIDS in children and adolescents. *Patient Care, Nov 15,* 80–114.
4. Berry, R. K. (1988). Home care of the child with AIDS. *Pediatric Nursing 88, 14,* 314–344.
5. Burroughs, M. H., & Edelson, P. J. (1991). Medical care of the HIV-infected child. *Pediatric Clinics of North America, 38,* 45–67.
6. Caldwell, M. B., & Rogers, M.F. (1991) Epidemiology of pediatric HIV infection. *Pediatric Clinics of North America, 38,* 1–16.
7. Cason, D. (1989). Anaphylactic shock. *Journal of Emergency Medical Services, 14,* 42–6, 51–2.
8. Centers for Disease Control. (1990). HIV/AIDS surveillance through September, 1990.

9. Cerrato, P. L. (1990). Does diet affect the immune system? *RN*, *85*, 67–70.

10. Claxton, R. (1989). Looking after the children. *Nursing Times*, *85*, 42–43.

11. Cruz, L. (1988). Children with AIDS: Diagnosis, symptoms, care. *AORN Journal, 48*, 893–910.

12. Dickerson, M. (1988). Anaphylaxis and anaphylactic shock. *Critical Care Quarterly, 11*, 68–74.

13. Emery, H. (1986). Clinical aspects of systemic lupus erythematosus in childhood. *Pediatric Clinics of North America, 33*, 1177–1190.

14. Engel, N. S. (1989). AZT for children with AIDS. *MCN: American Journal of Maternal Child Nursing, 14*, 121.

15. Gurka, A.M. (1989). The immune system: Implications for critical care nursing. *Critical Care Quarterly, 9*, 24–35.

16. Harrison, T. (1989). Children with AIDS. *Nursing Times, 85*, 64–65.

17. Haugen, M., & Lynch, P. A. (1987). Diagnostic tests in pediatric rheumatology: Application for nurses. *Pediatric Nursing, 13*, 389–393.

18. Heuther, S. E., & Kravitz, M. (1990). Structure, function and disorder of the integumentary. In K. L. McCance, S. E. Huether (Eds.), *Pathophysiology: The biological basis for disease in adults and children* (pp. 1402). St. Louis: C.V. Mosby Co.

19. Hoare, K., & Donohoe, K. M. (1990). Alterations of musculoskeletal function. In K. L. McCance, S. E. Huether (Eds.), *Pathophysiology: The biological basis for disease in adults and children* (pp. 1342–1346). St. Louis: C.V. Mosby Co.

20. Hughes, R. B., & Bailey, F. K. (1987). AIDS from a school health perspective. *Pediatric Nursing, 13*, 155–156, 191.

21. Karr, C. K. (1986). Autoimmunity: Then and now. *Journal of Medical Technology, 3*, 273–279.

22. Kemp, D. (1986). Development of the immune system. *Critical Care Quarterly, 9*, 1–6.

23. Klein, J. (1990). *Immunology*. Boston: Blackwell Scientific Publications.

24. Kobayashi, R. H., Kobayashi, A. D., Lee, N., Fischer, S., & Ochs, H. D. (1990). Home self administration of intravenous immunoglobulin therapy in children. *Pediatrics, 85*, 705–709.

25. Krasinski, K., & Borkowsky, W. (1991). Laboratory diagnosis of HIV infection. *Pediatric Clinics of North America, 38*, 17–35.

26. McKinney, R. E. (1991). Antiviral therapy for human immunodeficiency virus infection in children. *Pediatric Clinics of North America, 38*, 133–151.

27. Noel, G. J. (1991). Host defense abnormalities associated with HIV infection. *Pediatric Clinics of North America, 38*, 37–43.

28. Pachman, L. M. (1986). Juvenile dermatomyositis. *Pediatric Clinics of North America, 33*, 1097–1117.

29. Page-Goertz, S. S. (1989). Even children have arthritis. *Pediatric Nursing 89, 15*, 11–16, 30.

30. Parker-Cohen, P. D., Richardson, S. J., & Haak, S. Alterations in cardiovascular function. In K. L. McCance, S. E. Huether (Eds.), *Pathophysiology: The biological basis for disease in adults and children* (pp. 980–984). St. Louis: C.V. Mosby Co.

31. Person, D. A. (1986). Juvenile rheumatoid arthritis. *AORN Journal, 44*, 428–436.

32. Pigg, J. S., Driscoll, P. W., & Caniff, R. (1985). *Rheumatology nursing: A problem oriented approach*. New York: John Wiley & Sons.

33. Pepper, G. A. (1987). OTCs vs Rx for allergic rhinits. *Nurse Practitioner, 12*, 58–59.

34. Porcher, F. K. (1991). Pediatric HIV infection. Unpublished notes from presentation, Feb, 1991.

35. Porth C. M. (1990). *Pathophysiology: Concepts of Altered Health States* (3rd ed.). Philadelphia: J.B. Lippincott.

36. Rote, N. S. (1990). Alterations in immunity and inflammation. In K. L. McCance, S. E. Huether (Eds.), *Pathophysiology: The biological basis for disease in adults and children* (pp. 249–278). St. Louis: C.V. Mosby Co.

37. Rote, N. S. (1990). Inflammation. In K. L. McCance, S. E. Huether (Eds.), *Pathophysiology: The biological basis for disease in adults and children* (pp. 217–248). St. Louis: C.V. Mosby Co.

38. Rote, N. S. (1990). Immunity. In K. L. McCance, S. E. Huether (Eds.), *Pathophysiology: The biological basis for disease in adults and children* (pp. 191–215). St. Louis: C.V. Mosby Co.

39. Roth, R. (1990). Allergic response. *Emergency, 22*, 28–32.

40. Smith, S. L. (1986). Physiology of the immune system. *Critical Care Quarterly, 9*, 7–13.

41. Speiser, J. C., Moore, T. L., Weiss, T. D., Baldassare, A. R., Ross, S. C., Osborn, T. G., Dorner, R. W., & Zucker, J. (1985). Hidden 19S IgM rheumatoid factors in adults with juvenile rheumatoid onset. *Rheumatic Diseases, 44*, 294–8.

42. Strauss, J. (1989). Renal disease in children with the acquired immune deficiency syndrome. *New England Journal of Medicine, 321*, 625–630.

43. Wilbur, J. (1988). Research methods for studying HIV infection. *Focus: A Guide to AIDS Research 3*, 3.

44. Williams, A. D. (1989). Nursing management of the child with AIDS. *Pediatric Nursing, 13*, 259–261.

28

Children With Pain

BEHAVIORAL OBJECTIVES

Describe the differences in pain assessment and management in children and adults.

Identify assessment methods and tools developed for use with children in pain.

Identify appropriate nursing goals for relief of pain in the child.

Identify pharmacologic analgesic agents and adjuvant drugs used in pain management.

Identify new delivery systems for administering analgesic agents.

Identify nonpharmacologic *interventions* for children experiencing pain.

A pioneering study by Eland in 1974 followed 25 children between the ages of 5 and 8 years undergoing surgical procedures. It found that less than 50% received analgesics, and many of the doses were inadequate. Some of the diagnoses of the 13 children who received no analgesics postoperatively included spinal fusion, nephrectomy, open heart surgery, fractured femur, and amputation of a foot. When Eland matched the children with an adult sample undergoing the same surgery, adults received 26 times the amount of medication.[25] The data collected by Schroeder are even more disturbing. Schroeder[93] studied 23 consecutive admissions of severely burned children at a regional burn center and found that only two children were given analgesics for relief of their pain. Each child was given a single dose of acetaminophen. In 1983, Beyer et al.[10] matched 50 adults and 50 children undergoing cardiac surgery and found that adults received 70% of the postoperative analgesics while their pediatric counterparts received 30%. Recent research indicates that these inadequacies continue to be a problem in the management of pain in children.[33,92]

Since the early 1980s, many nursing researchers, including Hester, Beyer, Svedera, Tesler, and Jeans, have independently developed multiple-focused research projects pertaining to children's pain. Nurses can be proud that nursing research has lead the health profession in developing reliable and valid assessment tools for the measurement of children's pain and that it is engaged in the study of interventions.

Why are children undermedicated when compared to their adult counterparts? Why is there a problem with the assessment and management of pain in children? The answers are complex but can be partially explained by examining the myths surrounding children's pain.

Myths Surrounding Children's Pain

In some practice settings, none of the myths surrounding the topic of children's pain are in operation, while in other settings, children and health professionals are plagued by them daily. The following is a collection of most of the practice myths a nurse may encounter and the data to refute them.

Children's Nerves Aren't the Same as Adults. It would be wonderful if ill children did not feel pain or felt it with less intensity than their adult counterparts, but this simply is not the case. The fact that they are not neurologically defective has been known since the late 1960s.[97] Recent research by Williamson and Williamson[104] that monitored physiologic indicators during circumcision in newborn boys and by Fuller and Horii[32] that monitored infants' cries have scientifically documented what anyone who has ever watched a circumcision already knows: The infants are in pain.

If You Give Narcotics to Children, They Will Become Addicted. If health professionals knew more about the actual risk of addiction, their practice of prescribing analgesics would change dramatically. In a study by Porter and Jick,[88] *four* hospitalized patients (adults and children) out of 11,882 became addicted to narcotics during acute illness episodes. The risk of addiction (0.00033%) is actually far less than the risk of anaphylaxis to penicillin (0.15 to 0.04%).[58] McCaffery and Hart[68] and Marks and Sachar[62] feel that undertreatment of pain with narcotic analgesics may increase the chances of addiction because inadequate pain relief may cause the patient to focus on pain and on the drug itself.

Narcotics Depress Respiration. It is a physiologic fact that narcotics can depress respiration, but it is also a physiologic fact that antibiotics can cause anaphylaxis and insulin can cause an insulin reaction in certain people. Caution is always indicated whenever giving *any* medicine to a child, but caution does not prevent children from receiving antibiotics or insulin. However, in some cases, caution does prevent children from receiving the analgesics they need. Once again, the myth is refuted when the facts are examined. Miller and Jick[76] found only three out of 3263 hospitalized adult patients developed clinically significant respiratory depression, and all were due to meperidine. No data have been collected that indicate children have a greater susceptibly to respiratory depression than their adult counterparts.

Children Cannot Say Where They Hurt. Adults use 144 words to communicate the sensory, evaluative, and affective components of the pain they are experiencing.[75] Additionally, adults have an advantage because they know the names of body parts and often can identify an-

atomically where their pain is located. Young children have a limited vocabulary, do not know the names of body parts, and are still attempting to learn the variety of sensations that make up the sensation of pain. However, when asked in ways they understand, children can locate the source(s) of their pain and communicate pain intensity. (The reader is referred to the section entitled Assessment of Pain.)

Active Children Cannot Hurt. Many adults will remain inactive when in pain, but the nursing research of Primm,[89] Calamaris and Sullivan,[13] Lukens,[56] and Vorchol[99] found that children do not necessarily know that immobility means less pain. Additionally, if one thinks as a child, it is easy to understand why children remain active when in pain.

After 16 years of researching and observing the pain behaviors of hospitalized young children, Eland believes that some children think if they keep moving, they will not be found and pain will be avoided. Children who remain in their hospital rooms soon find out that the room is where they are examined, painful body parts are probed, they are "stuck" for blood, intravenous (IV) procedures are started on them, people take them to other places where painful procedures take place, and they must cough on demand even though it may be painful. *No one* (adult or child) voluntarily stays in a location where they believe harm will come to them, so the credo of the experienced hospitalized child is "stay out of your room and keep moving!"

Children Tell the Truth About Pain. Initially, children will tell the truth about pain when asked in a language they understand and will continue to tell the truth as long as there is no painful consequence from doing so. If the nurse's response to a child's report of pain is an intramuscular injection, the child will stop telling the truth because admission of pain has resulted in more pain. Eland asked 186 hospitalized children in a tertiary setting what had hurt them the worst in the hospital. Forty-eight percent of the children answered, "shot or needle." Interestingly, six of these children had undergone 25 surgeries each, and all of them answered "shot or needle."[25]

Intramuscular injections of analgesics seem inappropriate when a great majority of drugs given to ill children are given intravenously. To deny intravenous analgesics to children because of the risk involved is inappropriate and should be changed. (The reader is referred to the section entitled Pharmacologic Management of Pain.)

Children Cry When Restrained. When pain is a part of a procedure and a child begins to cry, physicians have for years told the nurses assisting with the procedure, "He can't feel that, he's crying because he is restrained." During procedures, children cry because they are in pain or are being held in painful positions for long periods of time. They *do not* cry, initially, because they are restrained. Experienced hospitalized children may cry when restrained because they know that restraint often precedes pain. Children who have been restrained to prevent them from removing IVs or other tubes sometimes cry because they have been in one position for a long period of time.

Parents Know All the Answers About Their Child's Pain. If a child is unable to communicate information about pain, the parents are the most accurate source of information about the child's pain. Nurses, however, must remember that the parent may not always be reliable because they may be seeing their child in the current situation for the first time, or they may be dealing with their own stresses over the ill child and other events surrounding the hospitalization. Parents whose children have been hospitalized on numerous occasions are excellent sources of information on how their child behaves when in pain and what *interventions* are most likely to relieve the pain.

Pain Defined

Fields defines pain as an unpleasant sensation that is perceived as arising from a specific region of the body and is commonly produced from processes that damage or are capable of damaging body tissue.[29] McCaffery says that pain is "whatever the experiencing person says it is and exists whenever he says it does."[67] The authors believe that children's pain can best be addressed by combining the two definitions. Pain is caused by tissue damage that leads to a release of pain-causing chemicals, and it exists when the child experiencing it "says" so. The word "says" does not necessarily mean a verbalization of one or more of the 144 words identified by Melzack and Torgerson.[75] "Says" in pediatrics may be a cry, body position, a painful look in the eyes, a fearful look in the eyes of a child whenever anyone approaches them, or an articulate response from a school-age child or adolescent.

Assessment of Pain

In many clinical settings, nurses continue to focus on the child's behavior as the sole basis of pain assessment, but this is the least objective measure of pain and is subject to diverse interpretation. The authors are not attempting to discredit pain expression but wish to point out that behavior is only one part of assessment. A wide variety of expressions can sometimes be confused with pain, including sadness, fear, anger, and rage.

The sensation of pain can be confusing and is a difficult concept for a child to learn. When a child is in the process of learning other concepts, they consistently have outside help to reinforce the learning of the concept. A child who is developing a vocabulary soon learns with repeated reinforcement what a green bean is or what a dog is and how to distinguish a dog from a cat. The concept is reinforced when someone who knows the concept says, "No, that's not a doggie. That's a kitty." The concept of nausea also has (on many occasions) the objective consequence of vomiting, which aids adults in their efforts to assist the child's learning, including not to vomit on a new couch. Pain has *no* objective consequence and consists of several distinct types of sensation. Pain can be the stinging of a scrape, the lightning-like pain of nerve impingement, the throbbing of an ischemic hand, the spasm of an obstructed bowel, or the dull ache of a muscle after a spasm. Unfortunately, pain cannot be objectively measured from a blood or urine sample, as can many other concepts involving illness, which makes the assessment

of pain more difficult. Assessment of pain in pediatrics consists of three parts:

- The nature of the pain-producing pathology involved
- The physiologic parameters that change with pain
- The child's behaviors

Pain Pathology

Health professionals would do well to remember the first part of the pediatric pain definition and focus on the pathologic cause(s) of pain. The *cause* of pain is tissue damage and the release of painful chemicals. A child who was struck by a car and has a fractured femur requiring surgical intervention hurts in the postoperative period because the skin, nerves, and blood vessels have been cut; the bone has been broken; muscles have been damaged at the time of injury and from the surgery, which causes them to spasm and the tissue to swell. Additionally, the child has pain from the soft-tissue injury associated with the car striking and the fall to the pavement. All of these things cause pain—there is no question that a child who has fractured a femur is experiencing pain because of the *pathology*.

The nature of the pain-producing pathology needs to identified. The nurse caring for a child should ask what physiologic damage has been done; why adults hurt with this condition or type of surgery; what structures are involved; whether the blood supply is impaired; if the nerves have been crushed; if the muscles have been damaged; and if they are spasming, whether the skin integrity has been interrupted or structures, such as bowel, ureter, or stomach, compressed?

Autonomic Responses

The physiologic changes associated with *acute* pain include diaphoresis, blood pressure and pulse rate change, pupillary dilation, and increased or decreased respiratory rate.[15] All of the indicators do not have to be present in an acute pain state.

Autonomic indicators of acute pain are identified in the accompanying display. In chronic pain, the physiologic changes may or may not be present because with time, the stress response exhausts itself.

Children's Behaviors

As stated earlier, assessment of pain in children should never be made *only* on the basis of a child's behavior. A child's behavior is subject to diverse interpretation because the communication about pain may be a combination of crying, guarding a body part, withdrawing, a painful look in the child's eyes, and no verbalizing. The emotional response of a child also may be influenced by the fact that they do not want to be in the hospital, are angry about a parent's departure, or are missing a playmate's birthday party. The following are some observations of infants, toddlers, and school-age children and their reactions to pain. These observations are not intended to be all-inclusive or complete. The reader is challenged to watch ill children's behaviors and interpret

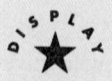

Autonomic Indicators of Acute Pain

Heart rate
Respiration
pO_2
Sweating
Endorphins
Blood pressure
Hormonal–metabolic changes

them in light of what has happened to these children during their hospitalization.

Reactions of Infants in Pain

Healthy newborn infants wake for loud noises, meals, and a soiled diaper, but otherwise, they are pretty quiet. If an infant is fussy, feeding or a diaper change combined with holding and rocking usually results in the child lying quietly or falling asleep. Infants who are ill often do not respond to the usual comfort measures and may cry until they fall asleep from exhaustion.

The reactions of sick newborns are easily explained. Sick infants go from their home in a dark, warm, quiet womb to a world full of bright light, cold, interrupted sleep, pain from diagnostic tests and therapeutic intervention, and noise levels equal to the decibel levels of rock music concerts.[105] They have been x-rayed on cold, hard surfaces, had holes poked in them innumerable times for blood or IV insertion, and some have even required major surgical intervention. They often are in a state of hyperalertness and will scream at any stimuli because they have been hurt so many times. Other newborns may be totally exhausted from the energy expenditures imposed by their pathology and the measures to correct it that they do not respond to any painful stimuli. A superficial evaluation might lead to the conclusion that the infant is not experiencing pain, when the real message from the infant is "I'm totally exhausted and don't have any fight left. I don't even have the energy to tell you to stop what you are doing."

Reactions of Toddlers in Pain

Toddlers in the hospital are often outraged that anyone or anything has interfered with their subconscious goal in life to be egocentric and always busy. These magical thinkers believe that if they stay active and out of their room, no one will find them and they will not be hurt.

Some toddlers become almost hyperactive when in pain and behave as though they, by virtue of their accelerated activity, can escape pain. They often protest loudly to all intrusions that restrict them in any way. Fear makes pain worse and a toddler who is discovering what is real and not real can be frightened badly in a hospital. To a toddler, x-ray machines look like something that an evil monster lies on in a scary movie. The toddler is put under this very scary machine and is expected to hold still. When they cannot, they are strapped down (just like the monster) and then everyone leaves the room.

A venipuncture is met with screams and howls that seem inordinately loud to the person performing the venipuncture and disproportionate to the amount of pain inflicted. A toddler's screams are truly expressing their pain and outrage. The usual response of health professionals in such a situation is to do anything to keep the child quiet because the screaming bothers them. Actually, the toddler and infant may be the healthiest of all age groups in their response to pain; they are serving notice to the world that they are being hurt and they aren't going to hold still for it. They want absolutely no part of it. They openly express these emotions and often feel better for having done so.

Reactions of School-Age Children in Pain

By the time a child reaches school age, pain assessment is easier. This child has words that represent pain and has more cognitive control than the toddler, which helps them be less afraid. As previously mentioned, a school-age child will tell the truth about pain if the response to the truth is not painful. School-age children also are capable of understanding why a procedure must be done, even though understanding may be at a limited level. A number of assessment tools have been developed by nurses to assist school-age children in their communication of pain. The Hester Poker Chip tool uses four poker chips and allows the child to show the caregiver how much they hurt by using the chips to represent pieces of hurt.[40] The Oucher developed by Beyer[6,7] is a combination of a numerical scale from 0 to 100 and a picture scale that consists of photographs of a child's face in increasing amounts of pain. McGrath has successfully used a tool consisting of five line drawings of a face in increasing intensities of pain.[69] The Eland Color Tool uses body outlines and colored markers. Children color where they hurt with a color identified by the child as representing the worst, middle, little, or no hurt. The protocol for using the Eland Color Tool is listed in the accompanying display. All four methods work, and no one tool is superior to another. Nurses caring for ill children should use the tool that works best for each child.

If a child can comprehend a five- or 10-point scale, numbers are a useful way to convey pain intensity. An explanation such as the following is given to the child: "If zero is no pain and five is the worst pain you've ever had—how much pain, zero, one, two, three, four, or five, do you have right now?" The advantage of using a numerical scale is that it is quick, easy, and requires no special equipment of any kind. Older children may prefer to use a zero- to 10-point scale or a zero- to 100-point scale to represent their pain.

Reactions of Adolescents in Pain

Unfortunately no one has undertaken a program of established research specifically to assess adolescent pain or investigated their reactions to pain. As with the toddler and school-age child, the adolescent who has had multiple experiences with the health care system may have developed their own special language for pain intensity,

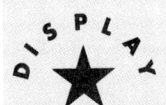

Eland Color Tool Protocol

1. Present eight markers to the child in a random order.
2. Ask the child, "Of these colors, which color is like . . . ?" (the event identified by the child as having hurt them the most).
3. Place the marker away from the other markers. (Represents severe pain.)
4. Ask the child, "Which color is like a hurt, but not quite as much as . . . ?" (the event identified by the child as having hurt them the most).
5. Place the marker with the marker chosen to represent severe pain.
6. Ask the child, "Which color is like something that hurts just a little?"
7. Place the marker with the other colors.
8. Ask the child, "Which color is like no hurt at all?"
9. Show the four marker choices to the child in order from the worst to the no hurt color.
10. Ask the child to show on the body outlines where they hurt, using the markers they have chosen.
11. After the child has colored the hurts, ask if they are current hurts or hurts from the past.
12. Ask if the child knows why the area hurts if it is not clear to you why it does.

and efforts should be made by health care providers to understand each individual's pain language. Most adolescents use a combination of sensory, affective, and evaluative words to convey their pain. Stabbing, throbbing, burning, and aching are sensory words that describe pain in terms of temporal, spatial, thermal, pressure, and other properties. Affective words convey tension, fear, and feelings about pain. Exhausting, frightful, terrifying, and killing are examples of affective words. Evaluative words describe the overall pain experience, sum up the entire experience, and include such words as miserable, intense, unbearable, and troublesome.[75]

Numerical scales (described under school-age children) often are helpful in quantifying the pain experience and evaluating specific interventions for pain relief. Adolescents who may not know the name of inner body structures or the feeling states associated with them or who are embarrassed may use body outlines to indicate where their pain is located.

Goals for Pain Relief

In an ideal situation, all pain could be eliminated, but in some clinical conditions, this is impossible. Nonetheless, the overall goal for pain relief in children should be based on the same three components as the assessment of pain: (1) alteration in pathology, (2) decrease in autonomic changes (in acute pain), and (3) absence of pain behaviors. The nurse should strive to decrease the child's pain to the lowest level indicated by whatever method he or she is using to communicate pain. The nurse is reminded to assess and reassess pain after appropriate nursing interventions. If pain relief has not been achieved, the nurse should revise the plan, intervene again, and reassess.

Alteration of Pathology

With time, the pathology causing pain may change and result in a decrease in pain intensity. In the case of a child with a fractured femur, immobility stabilizes the

fracture, the muscles stop spasming, and the painful chemicals that were produced are removed from the area. An infant recovering from surgical intervention for a bowel obstruction feels better because the cause of the bowel pain was alleviated, the surgical incision is healing, and associated painful chemicals are removed from the area. However, in a child with uncontrolled advancing cancer, the pathology causing pain will be everchanging. Recognition of this fact and ongoing assessment will enable the health care team to keep pain under control.

Change in Autonomic Signs

A child in *acute* pain has a predictable increase in pulse rate, blood pressure, respiratory rate, and other autonomic signs listed previously in this chapter. Children in chronic pain may have some or none of the autonomic changes associated with acute pain. When pain is relieved, the vital sign indicators return to baseline levels. Unfortunately, some nurses become unnecessarily alarmed when there is a slight drop in the pulse, blood pressure, and respiratory rate after medicating a child with a narcotic analgesic. These nurses believe they are seeing an adverse reaction to the narcotic analgesic when they are really seeing a decrease in pain reflected by the return of the child's vital signs to their baseline levels.

Absence of Pain Behaviors

Probably the first question to ask in this area is, "Is the child behaving as a normal child for his or her age would be behaving within the limitations of the condition?" Has the child returned to prepain personality? Is the child talkative and active or withdrawn, quiet, fearful, and tearful?

If pain intervention has been successful, the child should report the following:

- "One" or "no" pieces of hurt using the Hester Poker Chip
- "Ten" or less on the least painful picture using the Beyer Oucher

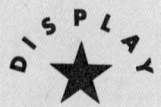

Requesting a Change of Analgesics Orders From a Physician

BEFORE NOTIFYING

Be certain the current analgesics have been given

- At the prescribed interval
- Around the clock, with no doses omitted
- Have remained in the body long enough to be effective (i.e., vomiting, diarrhea)
- Tried for an appropriate number of days (see Fig. 28-1)
- Documented as ineffective using a flow sheet

COMMUNICATION SHOULD IDENTIFY

- The patient
- Period of time drug has been tried

- The current drug(s) amount, frequency of administration, last change in dosage
- Rating scale being used
- 24-hour average pain rating—highest rating and lowest in that 24 hours
- If narcotics—the respiratory rate, level of awareness, whether the child can sleep or rest
- Drug side effects child is currently experiencing at this dosage
- Nondrug measures currently being used for pain relief
- Whether physician has suggestions for more effective use of current drugs; if he or she has no suggestions, **suggest** what to do

- The face that represents little or no pain using McGrath's faces
- The little or no pain color from the Eland Color Tool
- "Zero" or "one" on a numerical scale

Communication of Information About Pain

Nurses are with hospitalized children 24 hours a day and often are the most frequent contact person with children who are ill in the community. Nurses often contact the physician on behalf of the child in pain. Unfortunately, much of the communication conveys a limited amount of objective information about the child in pain.

The communication often is something similar to "Doctor, you must do something about Jamie Jones' pain," or "Why don't you order something stronger for Jamie Jones' pain?" Such communication gives a physician little objective information on which to base a responsible decision.

In the hospital, physicians who make early morning rounds often ask sleepy children and their sleepy parents, "How are you?" believing that this is a *pain* question. Often the child or parent responds "fine" to what they think is a *social* question. The physician believes the answer indicates that pain is under control. Later in the day if a nurse contacts the physician about inadequate pain relief, the physician is confused because the child or parent told them that things were "fine."

The nurse's communication also may relay a limited amount of information about the intensity and duration of pain or about the interventions that have been attempted and the frequency and degree of their success. Is it any wonder then that the physician is reluctant to alter the analgesic regimen?

When requesting a change in analgesics orders from a physician, the information listed in the accompanying display should be included. When this amount of information is accumulated, the nursing staff can be sure that their interventions have been implemented without suc-

cess. The communication also gives a clear and organized message to the physician about the child's pain and that the nurses have done their "homework."

When uncontrolled pain is a significant problem, a pain flow sheet, such as the one developed by McCaffery (Fig. 28-1) can be used. Flow sheets such as this conveys objective information about pain and gives the physician several hours or days worth of data on which to base a decision.

Theories of Pain

The purpose of pain theories is to attempt to describe or explain the phenomenon of pain. To guide intervention selection and provide rationale for nursing action, an understanding of the explanations for pain is necessary.

Early Theories

Early theories of pain included the specificity theory and the pattern theory. Briefly, the *specificity theory* proposes that the pain sensation, activated by noxious sub-

Pain Flowsheet

Name: Jessica Jones

RX: Small cell sarcoma, mets

Analgesic Order: MS 8 mg q 1 h, 2 mg bolus q 1 h

Pain Rating Scale Used: 1–10

Time	Pain Rating	Analgesic	R	P	BP	Level of Arousal	Plan
10 am	8	MS 8 mg	20	100	120/80	alert	
12 pm	10	MS 8 mg	20	100	124/90	crying	2 mg bo
2 pm	8	MS 8 mg	20	98	116/84	restless	2 mg bo
4 pm	8	MS 8 mg	20	98	100/88	crying	2 mg bo

FIGURE 28-1

Example of the McCaffery pain flowsheet. The patient, Jessica Jones, is discussed in the teaching plan later in this chapter.

stances produced during the pain experience, is transmitted by way of pain fibers and lateral spinothalamic tracts to specific pain centers in the brain.[78] Pain intensity would be proportional to the extent of tissue damage. The pattern theory proposes that there are temporal and spatial patterns of nerve impulses that evoke pain based on stimulus intensity and central summation.[20]

These two early theories of pain had the following major weaknesses:

- They did not explain why two people given the same stimulus may interpret noxious sensations differently.
- They focused only on physiologic pain with inadequate or no explanation of psychological factors.
- They were not applicable to a variety of situations and not usable in practice.

These inadequacies in theory led to the need for a more comprehensive study to develop theory that would incorporate psychological principles, be applicable in a variety of situations, and provide rationale for pain control intervention.

Gate Control Theory

In 1965, the gate control theory was proposed by Melzack and Wall. This is the most commonly accepted and used pain theory. The *gate control theory* of pain proposes that pain impulses, as well as other sensory impulses, travel from the nerve receptor to synapses in the dorsal horn of the spinal cord (substantia gelatinosa). These synapses are assumed to act like gates, which can open to allow nerve impulses to reach the brain or close to prevent or decrease impulse transmission. Pain signals from the body are modulated by other concurrent somatic inputs and by descending influences from the brain.[74,101]

Modulating Cord Input

Transmission of nerve impulses is affected by the kinds of sensory impulses that are simultaneously bombarding the gates. The theory suggests that a predominance of large-diameter, cutaneous afferent nerve (C fibers) inputs, which detect touch and pressure, tend to close the synaptic gates. Small-diameter, excitatory fiber (A delta) inputs, which detect irritation, generally open it. Pain impulses reach the brain when impulses on small fibers predominate and open the gates.

Interventions for pain control should be directed at increasing input from large, rapidly conducting fibers decreasing input from small fibers. These efforts will affect the child's response to the painful stimulus. Examples of actions to increase large-fiber input include rubbing the child's back or unaffected extremity, applying vibration to an affected area, and applying transcutaneous nerve stimulation (TENS). Actions that may decrease small-fiber input range from removing wrinkles in the linens and repositioning the child to using anesthetic nerve blocks.

Altering Cognitive Processing

All pain researchers agree that the brain plays an important role in mediating and inhibiting pain impulses after they pass the dorsal horn synapse. Gate theory supporters believe that past experience, emotional state, motivation, and other psychological variables influence how an individual will react to painful stimuli through descending impulses mediated in the substantia gelatinosa. Interventions directed at altering thoughts and emotions (such as centrally acting narcotics, relaxation therapy, hypnosis, distraction) contribute to the pain experience by modulating the perception and interpretation of the sensory input.

In summary, the sensory input from the body can be modulated by sensory and central neural factors.[73,74] Therefore, the brain receives messages about injury by way of a gate-controlled system that is influenced by injury signals, other types of afferent impulse, and descending controls. Although the gate control theory does not completely explain pain transmission, it provides direction for practitioners to select interventions with a rational base of action.

Current Theory Development

In addition to continued refinement and revision of the gate control theory, recent research is focusing on demonstration of pain suppression with opiate action on specific opiate-receptor sites in the nervous system. These are sites located in the nervous system and throughout the body to which opiates form chemical attachments, producing analgesia. They are thought to be connected to neural pathways that transmit pain to higher brain centers.[95] *Endorphins*, which are endogenous morphine or "morphine within," are thought to be produced by the body under certain modes of stimulation. The endorphins apparently combine with specific receptors to produce analgesic activity similar to that of morphine. Tissue massage, TENS, and placebo drugs have been shown to cause the release of endorphins, providing partial explanation for their effectiveness in pain control.

Other factors being studied include the impact of neurotransmitters, such as H+ ions, serotonin, histamine, bradykinin, prostaglandins, and substance P on pain relief. The action of these neurotransmitters may provide an explanation for the effectiveness of medications that interfere with the production of these substances.

Theories of Pain and Children

The major problem with pain theories is that they have been based on pain experiences of adults and do not account for the growth and developmental stages of a young child.[95] Difficulty communicating the physiologic sensations of pain and age-related levels of psychological and experiential factors have a serious impact on the understanding of pain perception and interpretation in children.

The age at which a child perceives pain as unpleasant is unknown and controversial. It was previously thought that infants feel no pain, and pain-inducing procedures, such as circumcision and chest tube insertion, were conducted without analgesia or anesthesia. Current research suggests that the process of myelination (necessary for the transmission of pain impulses) begins *in utero*, and myelination of sensory roots begins at birth.[98] Studies show that infants do exhibit behaviors and physiologic responses indicative of pain.[31,81,100] Therefore, it is essential that nurses operate under the assumption that children of all ages may perceive unpleasant stimuli, even if current research has not clarified the exact mechanism by which it occurs.

The work of Piaget[86] suggests that the level of cognitive development of an older child has a significant impact on the perception of the painful experience. Factors such as anxiety, fear, and separation can influence the experience.[95] Many researchers have illustrated changes in behavioral response to painful stimuli based on the child's level of concrete and abstract thinking.[4,47,52]

The nurse must be continually cognizant of the effect the child's age, cognitive and physiologic development, and experiences have on pain perception and response. The theoretical background of pain management provides a basis for selection of interventions to relieve pain in children.

The professional nurse has a critical role in the management of pain for the child. The nurse is responsible for evaluating the child for the presence of pain and for determining interventions. Many nursing actions, such as backrubs, repositioning, teaching relaxation, and other coping techniques, are initiated and carried out independently. Interventions may include the administration of analgesics, which requires many decisions of an astute nurse.

Choosing an appropriate intervention is significantly easier when a complete assessment of a child's pain is made. As discussed previously, this must include knowledge related to the etiology of pain. These biological, chemical, physical, and psychological causes of pain must be understood in relation to the three components of the pain experience—sensation, motivation, and cognition.

Pharmacologic Management of Pain

Several important aspects must be considered in appropriate pharmacologic management of pain. Prior to selection and administration of any analgesic, a comprehensive assessment is needed. (The reader is referred to the section entitled Assessment of Pain.) Noninvasive pain control measures should be evaluated and used when appropriate. When nonpharmacological measures have failed to relieve a child's pain, administration of analgesics may be the primary mode of treatment. Often pharmacological measures in combination with other noninvasive techniques provide the most effective means of controlling the child's pain. General guidelines for appropriate pharmacologic management of pain in children follow.

Drug Selection

Rationale for selection of analgesic drugs used to treat pain in children is important for the nurse to understand. As discussed previously, pain sensations originate from different sources, and the types of pain vary, which necessitates multiple treatment approaches.

The selection of a drug should be based on its site and method of action, duration, potency, and side effects. Three classes of analgesic drugs currently used have different sites and modes of action:

- *Non-narcotic analgesics* act on peripheral nerve endings at the site of injury
- *Narcotic analgesics* act by binding to opiate receptors in peripheral and central nervous systems (CNS)
- *Adjuvant analgesics* may potentiate the effects of narcotic analgesics or have independent analgesic effects[2]

Familiarity with each group of analgesic agents, particularly its actions, advantages and disadvantages, and side effects, is essential. Discussion in this text is limited to information on the three major classes of analgesic drugs used in the treatment of pain in children. Specific comparative information about drugs in each group is provided with accompanying tables. For complete pharmacokinetic information and complete nursing implications, the reader is referred to current pharmacology reference texts.

Non-Narcotic Drugs

The non-narcotic drugs are the first choice for pain relief in children and are predominantly used for mild pain. Their action is hypothesized to be, in part, due to their ability to inhibit prostaglandin synthesis, which prevents stimulation of the pain receptors. This action works best for pain associated with inflammatory conditions and is most effective against continuous, aching pain, rather than pain that is sudden and sharp.[61] Drugs included in this category are aspirin, acetaminophen (Tylenol), choline magnesium trisalicylate (Trilisate), and the nonsteroidal anti-inflammatory drugs (NSAIDS). Examples of NSAIDS are fenoprofen (Nalfon), ibuprofen (Motrin, Advil), diflunisal (Dolobid), and naproxen (Naprosyn). Ta-

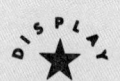

Aspirin and Reye's Syndrome

A relationship between aspirin and Reye's syndrome is suspected in the presence of viral influenza and chickenpox. It is not known whether this association extends to aspirin use in other childhood diseases. Current labeling on aspirin products, in agreement with the American Academy of Pediatrics and the Centers for Disease Control, is limited to caution against the use of this drug without physician consultation in children and teenagers suffering from viral influenza or chickenpox.

From: Rahwan, G. L., & Rahwan, R. G. (1986). Aspirin Reye's syndrome: The change in prescribing habits of health professionals. Drug Intelligence and Clinical Pharmacy, 20, 43–145.

ble 28-1 provides information on the analgesics used for treatment of mild-to-moderate pain.

Only a small number of NSAIDS are approved for use in children (ASA, naproxen, ibuprofen, diclofenac, tolmetin, and benorylate).[103] Their use must be carefully monitored, and titration of dosage should be based on extrapolation from the recommended adult dosages and careful observation of the child's response to the drug.

The four major pharmacologic properties of this class of drugs are analgesic, antipyretic, antiplatelet, and anti-inflammatory.[18] Two agents in this category do not exhibit all four properties. Acetaminophen has no anti-inflammatory or antiplatelet effects, making it a good non-narcotic analgesic for use with children. Choline magnesium trisalicylate has properties similar to aspirin but lacks its antiplatelet effects.[51] All drugs in this class have been

TABLE 28-1
Analgesics Commonly Used for Mild to Moderate Pain*

Name	Equianalgesic Dose† (mg)	Starting Oral Dose Range (mg)	Comments	Precautions and Contraindications
Non-Narcotics				
Aspirin	650	650	Often used in combination with narcotic analgesics	Chronic excessive use may cause papillary necrosis and interstitial nephritis; avoid during pregnancy, in hemostatic disorders, and in combination with steroids
Acetaminophen	650	650	Like aspirin but no anti-inflammatory effects; does not affect platelet function	
Ibuprofen (Motrin)	ND	200–400	Probably more effective than aspirin	Like aspirin
Fenoprofen (Nalfon)	ND	200–400	Like ibuprofen	Like aspirin
Diflunisal (Dolobid)	ND	500–1000	Like ibuprofen, but with longer duration of action	Like aspirin
Naproxen (Naprosyn)	ND	250–500	Like diflunisal	Like aspirin
Choline magnesium trisallcylate (Trillsate)	ND	1500	Does not affect platelet function	
Morphine-like Agonists				
Codeine	32–65	32–65	Often used in combination with non-narcotic analgesics; biotransformed, in part, to morphine	Impaired ventilation, bronchial asthma; use with caution in patients with increased intracranial pressure
Oxycodone	5	5–10	Shorter acting; also used in combination with non-narcotic analgesics (Percodan, Percocet) which limits dose escalation; oxycodone in three Percocet (15 mg) = 5 mg morphine IM	Like codeine
Meperidine (Demerol)	50	50–100	Shorter acting; biotransformed to normeperidine, a toxic metabolite	Normeperidine accumulates with repetitive dosing causing CNS excitation; not for patients with impaired renal function or receiving monoamine oxidase inhibitors
Propoxyphene HCl (Darvon) Propoxyphene napsylate (Darvon-N)	65–130	65–130	Low analgesic efficacy; often used in combination with non-narcotic analgesics; biotransformed to potentially toxic metabolite (norpropoxyphene)	Propoxyphene and metabolite accumulate with repetitive dosing; overdose complicated by convulsions
Mixed Agonist–Antagonist				
Pentazocine (Talwin)	50	50–100	Prepared in combination with naloxone to discourage parenteral abuse	May cause psychotomimetic effects; may precipitate withdrawal in narcotic-dependent patients

For these equianalgesic doses (see also comments) the time to peak analgesia ranges from 1.5 to 2 hours and the duration from 4 to 6 hours. Oxycodone and meperidine are shorter acting (3 to 5 hours) and diflunisal, naproxen, and choline magnesium trisalicylate are longer acting (8 to 12 hours).

* Note: Adult doses for use in extrapolating by age.
† These doses are recommended starting doses from which the optimal dose for each patient is determined by titration.
(ND, not determined; CNS, central nervous system.)

shown to be equal to or more effective than aspirin in controlled studies. Individual pharmacokinetics and duration of analgesia account for the differences between agents.[2]

The non-narcotics are well absorbed from the gastrointestinal (GI) tract, most within 30 minutes. Biotransformation and detoxification occur through the liver, with the main by-products excreted by the kidneys. Consideration of liver and renal function is important when selecting non-narcotics for use in children. The following list concerns the the use of non-narcotics in children:

Advantages
    Readily available orally
    Relatively safe
    Inexpensive (ASA and acetaminophen)
    Available without prescription (ASA and acetaminophen)
    Do not produce CNS manifestations, such as somnolence, mood changes, euphoria
    Do not demonstrate tolerance or dependence
    Appropriate for combination therapy
Disadvantages
    Relatively mild analgesics
    Expensive (NSAIDS)
    May be associated with serious side effects, especially in long-term therapy (ASA and NSAIDS)
Side effects
    GI hypersensitivity with irritation, leading to ulceration (ASA and NSAIDS)[45]
    Hematologic effects—prolonged bleeding time (ASA and NSAIDS)[45]
    Hypersensitivity (ASA and NSAIDS)
    Impaired renal function with chronic therapy (NSAIDS)[1]
    Hepatotoxicity at large doses (acetaminophen)

The non-narcotics exhibit a ceiling effect, which means there is a dose beyond which increments fail to provide additional analgesia. If one agent does not work or becomes ineffective because of the ceiling dose, clinical experience has shown that a drug in a different class may be effective.

Narcotics and Combination Drugs

The use of narcotic analgesics in children remains controversial because little is known about their effects on pain relief in children. However, current research has shown that children with moderate-to-severe pain can be treated safely and effectively with narcotics.[55,79]

Narcotic analgesics, consisting of the opiate and opioid compounds, are used primarily to manage severe acute pain and chronic cancer-related pain; they are the most commonly used agents for pain relief. Although their mechanism of action is uncertain, it appears that they alter the perception and interpretation of the painful stimuli at the level of the CNS. Opiates bind to receptor sites in the CNS that block multiple neurotransmitter systems from transmitting the pain sensation.

Opiate and opioid compounds can be divided into narcotic agonists (drugs that relieve pain by binding at specific opiate receptor sites—examples are morphine, codeine, and meperidine) and narcotic agonists–antagonists (drugs that have agonist properties, but when given with another agonist act as antagonists—examples are buprenorphine, pentazocine, butorphanol, and nalbuphine). When given together, the agonist–antagonist's properties can counter the analgesic effects of the agonist agent, potentially eliciting withdrawal symptoms. It is important to remember never to give different types of narcotics concurrently to the same patient.

The main differences in individual narcotic agents occur in their potency, onset, and duration of analgesia (Table 28-2). Differences in potency are not significant, because doses of equivalent analgesia can be determined.

The onset of analgesia depends largely on the route of administration: IV produces immediate, predictable results; intramuscular (IM) has a slower onset and predictable results; oral produces the slowest, most variable results because of first-pass metabolism.[60]

Narcotics (except morphine) tend to be absorbed well from the GI tract and are rapidly distributed throughout the body. Orally administered narcotics are absorbed in the stomach, taken by the portal vein to the liver and detoxified. This process is called *first-pass metabolism*. The main by-products are excreted by the kidneys. The duration of action of each drug coincides with its rate of metabolism. Exceptions are codeine, which is metabolized to an active morphine, and meperidine, which is metabolized to normeperidine, a toxic substance.[54] The following list concerns the use of narcotics in children:

Advantages
    Effective analgesic for moderate and severe pain
    Potency ranges are variable
    Beneficial sedation properties
Disadvantages
    Development of tolerance and dependence
    Unwanted sedating effect
Side effects
    Drowsiness, changes in mood, confusion, sedation
    Respiratory depression, orthostatic hypotension
    Nausea and vomiting, dry mouth, urinary retention, and constipation

Because of the frequency of side effects, it is important for the nurse to institute interventions for the prevention and management of side effects. Table 28-3 presents suitable interventions for dealing with the common side effects of narcotic use.

Although meperidine is the most frequently prescribed parenteral narcotic, clinical research has shown that its use should be limited to acute and postoperative pain of short duration. Meperidine is a poor choice for chronic pain because its duration of action is short (2 to 3 hours); it has low analgesic potency when given by mouth; and it may produce CNS excitation, irritability, or convulsions with repeated large doses (due to the accumulation of a toxic metabolite, normeperidine). The hyperexcitability produced is not reversible with naloxone and may be exacerbated.[2,13,50,51,64]

Combinations of analgesics, a narcotic, non-narcotic, or other agent possessing different mechanisms of action may have additive effects. Combination drugs allow for lower total narcotic requirement. Studies have shown that combinations of narcotics, non-narcotics, and psycho-

TABLE 28-2
Narcotic Analgesics Commonly Used for Severe Pain*

Name	Equianalgesic IM Dose† (mg)	IM/PO Potency	Starting Oral Dose Range (mg)	Comments	Precautions
Morphine-like Agonists					
Morphine	10	3	30–60	Standard of comparison for narcotic analgesics	Caution in patients with impaired ventilation, bronchial asthma, increased intracranial pressure, liver failure
Hydromorphone (Dilaudid)	1.5	5	4–8	Slightly shorter duration than morphine	Like morphine
Methadone (Dolophine)	10	2	5–20	Good oral potency; long plasma half-life (24–36 hours)	Like morphine; may accumulate with repetitive dosing, causing excessive sedation (on days 2–5)
Levorphanol (Levo-Dromoran)	2	2	2–4	Long plasma half-life (12–16 hours)	Like methadone; may accumulate on days 2–3
Oxymorphone (Numorphan)	—See comments—			Not available orally; 5 mg rectal suppository = 10 mg morphine IM	Like IM morphine
Heroin	5	(6–10)	Not recommended	Slightly shorter acting than morphine; not available in the United States	Like morphine
Meperidine (Demerol)	75	4	Not recommended	Slightly shorter acting than morphine	Normeperidine (toxic metabolite) accumulates with repetitive dosing, causing CNS excitation; avoid in patients with impaired renal function or receiving monoamine oxidase inhibitors‡
Codeine	130	1.5	See comments	Used orally for less severe pain	Like morphine
Mixed Agonist-Antagonists					
Pentazocine (Talwin)	60	3	See comments	Used orally for less severe pain; mixed agonist–antagonist; less abuse liability than morphine; included in Schedule IV of Controlled Substances Act	May cause psychotomimetic effects; may precipitate withdrawal in narcotic dependent patients; contra-indicated in myocardial infarction‡
Nalbuphine (Nubain)	10	—See comments—		Not available orally; like IM pentazocine but not scheduled	Incidence of psychotomimetic effects lower than with pentazocine
Butorphanol (Stadol)	2	—See comments—		Not available orally; like IM nalbuphine	Like IM pentazocine
Partial Agonists					
Buprenorphine (Temgesic)	0.4	—See comments—		Not available orally; sublingual preparation not yet in United States; less abuse liability than morphine; does not produce psychotomimetic effects	May precipitate withdrawal in narcotic dependent patients

For IM doses, the time to peak analgesia ranges from 0.5 to 1 hour and the duration from 4 to 6 hours. The peak analgesic effect is delayed and the duration prolonged after oral administration.

* Note: Adult doses for use in extrapolating by age.

† These doses are recommended starting IM doses from which the optimal dose for each patient is determined by titration and the maximal dose limited by adverse effects. Equianalgesic doses are based on single-dose studies in which an intra-muscular dose of each drug listed was compared with morphine to establish relative potency.

‡ Irritating to tissues with repeated IM injection.

(IM, intramuscular; PO, oral.)

tropic agents can be an effective means of providing highly satisfactory pain control rapidly, safely, and conveniently.[35,91]

Major problems with the use of narcotics in pediatrics involve the misconceptions of many practicing nurses, physicians, and children's families. Two main fears usually cited include the fear of possible addiction and of respiratory depression or arrest resulting from overmedication. According to the literature on adult patients, these un-

toward effects are rare.[62] However, there is little research on children's responses to narcotic treatment.

Fears of overmedication lead to undertreatment.[3] Research illustrates that children receive significantly fewer narcotics than adults with similar pathophysiologic processes.[10,25,92] Health professionals are reluctant to treat children effectively for fear of overmedication, even when the order for medication is available.[8] An understanding of the expected patterns of tolerance, dependency, and

TABLE 28-3
Nursing Interventions: Managing Common Side Effects of Narcotics

Side Effect	Nursing Interventions
Constipation	Promote adequate amounts of fluid.
	Encourage foods that promote bowel movements (i.e., vegetables, fresh fruits, nuts, whole grain bread and cereals, cookies with raisins).
	Encourage regular time to try to move bowels.
	Encourage daily exercise, even if short walks or exercising in bed.
	Administer stool softener daily.
	Administer bulk agent if fluid intake is adequate, such as Metamucil, if needed.
	Avoid enemas if possible
Sedation	Adjust dosage if needed to maintain appropriate level of interaction. For some children, sleepiness is a reaction to finally obtaining pain relief and catching up on much needed rest.
Drowsiness	Inform family that it usually decreases after 48–72 hours.
	May need to decrease dosage slightly.
	Have child take extra naps first few days.
	Evaluate other medications being taken.
	May initiate a stimulant such as caffeine.
	Assess for sudden changes in level of alertness.
Orthostatic/Hypotension	Have child rise out of bed slowly, allowing feet to dangle at side of bed first.
	Have child change positions slowly.
	Maintain a safe environment.
Dry Mouth	Use popsicles, shakes, sugarless gums, hard candy to counteract dry mouth.
	Promote plenty of fluids.
	Rinse child's mouth frequently.
	Good oral care is necessary to prevent cavities.
	Artificial saliva is available if severe.
Nausea/Vomiting	Administer antiemetic medication if needed.
	Give liquids 1 hour after mealtimes.
	Try small frequent feedings.
	Perform frequent oral care.
	Avoid excessive movement, have child rest quietly.
Urinary Retention	Allow opportunities for voiding.
	Use running water; offer plenty of fluids.
	Catheterization may be necessary.
Confusion/Mental Effects	If nightmares, confusion, or hallucinations occur, a different drug may be necessary.
Respiratory Changes	Decreased rate and quality of breathing often occurs after sedation or frequent falling asleep. If it is marked, adjustment in dosage may be necessary
	Encourage deep breathing, coughing, and turning.
	Treatment with naloxone may be necessary for severe respiratory depression.

Adapted from Howard-Ruben, J. Managing pain medications at home. *Oncology Nursing Forum, 12,* 78–82. (1985).

addiction and respiratory depression or arrest is essential for the nurse and the family to support an effective pharmacologic program for pain control in the child. The teaching plan on the use of a narcotic analgesia for pain in a child with cancer shows how the nurse can educate parents regarding the use of narcotic analgesics.

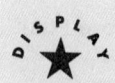

Limitations of Meperidine

The use of meperidine should be limited to short-term treatment of acute and postoperative pain because of the following:

* Its short duration of action
* Its low oral potency
* Its potential to produce central nervous system excitation, irritability, or convulsions

Tolerance, Dependency, and Addiction. Tolerance occurs when a dose of a drug produces a decreasing effect or when a larger dose is required to maintain the same effect.[30] Tolerance develops to all narcotics at varying rates. The earliest sign is the observation of decreased duration of effectiveness. It is necessary to increase the frequency of administration or increase the dose to continue pain relief. Tolerance develops more slowly with the oral route and most rapidly with IV and intrathecal routes. Tolerance also develops to the drug's side effects (such as sedation and respiratory depression). As the dose of narcotic is increased to maintain comfort, the child does not experience increased risk of respiratory depression.

Physical dependence is an altered physiologic state produced by the repeated administration of an opiate drug. It is *expected* and a result of long-term opiate use. Continuous administration is required to prevent the withdrawal syndrome (lacrimation, rhinhorrhea, diaphoresis, yawning, irritability, insomnia, dilated pupils, gooseflesh, sneezing, general malaise, chills and hot flashes, nausea, vomiting, diarrhea, muscle and bone pains, and muscle spasms).[18] The withdrawal syndrome can be precipitated when a narcotic antagonist such as naloxone is administered to a physically dependent child. Narcotics should not be stopped abruptly in anyone who has been receiving them on a regular basis for longer than 7 days. The drug dose should be decreased slowly

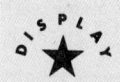

Fear of Narcotics

Fear of addiction and fear of respiratory depression and arrest lead to undertreatment of pain. Tolerance to the effects of a narcotic and physical dependence on the drug are expected consequences of long-term opiate therapy. These effects do not indicate addiction to the drug. Addiction is rare. Data show the occurrence of respiratory depression and arrest also is rare.

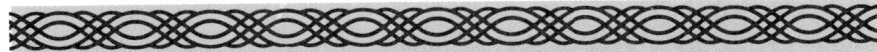

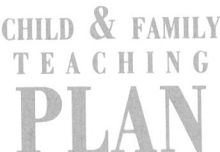

CHILD & FAMILY
T E A C H I N G
PLAN

Use of Narcotic Analgesia for Pain in a Child With Cancer

Assessment

Jessica Jones, age 8, has advanced cancer that will require morphine and multiple non-narcotic analgesics until her death. Mr. and Mrs. Jones have expressed concerns about their daughter taking "drugs" (in direct reference to the narcotic analgesic). Her parents need basic information about narcotics and their appropriateness for long-term use.

Child and Family Objectives

1. Identify the importance of Jessica's taking narcotic analgesics at this time.

Specific Content

1. "Say no to drugs" is a good slogan regarding "street drugs." However, Jessica needs pain medication as much as she needs air and water.

   Some people believe if they are taking morphine they will die soon. The staff does not believe that will happen to Jessica. In fact, once her pain is controlled, she may be her "old self" again and be able to do things she likes to do, such as play dolls with her friends or go to her grandfather's farm.

   Some people also think that if you take morphine you will get "hooked" or "high" like an addict. This does not happen to people who need morphine because they have pain.

   If you have been in pain for a long time and have not slept much, when your pain is under control you might sleep for awhile. Once you are caught up on your sleep, you will feel better.

   Jessica needs to take the morphine all the time and take all the doses. If her cancer goes away, she can stop taking the drug, but the physician and nurses would take her off the drug slowly just like they have tapered her off her steroids in the past.

   You may not want to tell everyone she's on morphine. That's okay.

Teaching Strategies

1. Use one-to-one discussion with Jessica and her parents. Both parents should be present.

   Give parents a booklet to read. One of the following would be appropriate: "Myths About Morphine," from Purdue Frederick Labs, or "Oral Morphine for Advanced Cancer," from Roxane Labs.

   After parents have read the material, plan another discussion with them. Use this time to review their questions and reinforce the information given previously.

Evaluation

- Parents verbalize their degree of comfort concerning their daughter's needs for narcotic analgesic.
- Parents state that they have read literature.
- Jessica states that she understands how the medicine will help her feel better.
- Parents describe their compliance with medication at home.

for days. Even though tolerance and dependence develop, withdrawal from the drug can be accomplished if the painful stimulus is no longer present.[87]

Many children taking narcotics will develop dependence on a drug's effects, but few become addicted. Addiction is a behavioral pattern of compulsive drug use, characterized by overwhelming involvement with the use of a drug, the securing of its supply, and a high tendency to relapse after withdrawal.[46] Addiction is rare. In one study, only four of 11,882 patients (children and adults) who received narcotics during acute illness episodes developed any drug dependence.[88]

Respiratory Depression and Arrest. Respiratory depression is another fear that has been highly overpublicized. The reported clinically significant respiratory depression in more than 11,000 patients was less than one per 1000 or .01%.[88] With careful observation during drug initiation and treatment, the cases of respiratory depression that do occur can be managed effectively.

A pure narcotic antagonist, naloxone, binds competitively to the opioid receptor sites and acts to reverse the analgesia, respiratory depression, and other effects of morphine-like drugs. It is used in the treatment of narcotic overdose resulting in respiratory depression and arrest.[21]

Pediatric dosing for administration of naloxone is 0.01 mg/kg per dose at 3-minute intervals until the desired response is obtained.[106] Onset of naloxone is 1 to 2 minutes IV and 5 to 10 minutes IM. A positive response is indicated by widened pupils, increased respiratory rate, and increased alertness. The drug may need to be given at frequent intervals because of its brief duration of action. Naloxone can precipitate withdrawal and severe pain.

When the health care team is concerned about the adverse effects of narcotics, such as respiratory depression, the use of a flowsheet may be helpful.[72] A flowsheet can be used to document initial and respective assessments, vital signs before and after analgesic administration, and changes in the level of pain. The document provides a quick summary of the child's response to the narcotic and any changes in respiration or other vital signs can be quickly identified. Naloxone also can be kept at the bedside, facilitating a quick response if a problem were to arise.

Educating families of children receiving narcotic analgesics on the difference between tolerance, dependence, and addiction; expected behavior; and evidence of the rarity of addiction is an important nursing responsibility. It may be helpful to discuss with reluctant families how receiving narcotics is not like "taking street drugs" and that the child will not get "high" or "hooked." The nurse should explain the purpose of narcotics and the expected responses of the child. Assurance that the child will be able to stop taking the medicine when the pain is gone may be helpful. The family can be told that pain is a potent respiratory stimulant, and the risk that their child will stop breathing is low. If it were to occur, treatment is available.

Pain Control in the Home. Many children can be maintained successfully on oral narcotics, which facilitate management of the child in the home setting. With the advent of newer delivery systems, such as the implanted infusion pump for continuous IV, SQ, and spinal narcotics, the option of caring for the child in severe pain at home is much more feasible.

Care of the child at home may be a desirable and rewarding experience for the family of a seriously ill child. Cooperative efforts by physicians, nurses, family services staff, social workers, and home health care or independent practicing nurse specialists is essential to provide education, supplies, and support for successful home management of the child in pain. The time required of family members to provide needed care, amount of assistance needed outside the family, availability of visiting nurses, cost and insurance coverage for home care equipment and nursing visitation, and availability of emotional support for the child and family are a few of the subjects that need discussion and resolution prior to implementing home management of the child in pain.

Adjuvant Drugs

Many drugs are considered adjuvant drugs and may enhance the effects of narcotics or non-narcotics or may have some analgesic properties independently.[30] The adjuvant drugs are most widely used for severe pain of advancing cancer. This group of drugs includes antianxiety–antiemetic agents, tricyclic antidepressants, steroids, and anticonvulsants.

Psychotropic agents are used primarily to manage the psychological effects of chronic pain and may potentiate analgesic activity and produce a sedating or calming effect.[54] Decreasing the child's anxiety may allow for decreased dosing of narcotic analgesics. Many of the calming agents, such as prochlorperazine (Compazine), hydroxyzine (Vistaril), and promethazine (Phenergan), often are ordered concomitantly with parenteral narcotics. They are not given to potentiate the analgesic, but their additive effects produce sedation and CNS depression and may help decrease the nausea and vomiting, which are common side effects of narcotics.

Tricyclic antidepressants may decrease pain by treating the mood disturbance associated with the disease. It is unknown whether they function as analgesics, potentiate the analgesic effects of other drugs, depress arousal, modify the perception of sensory input, or merely function as mood elevators.[91] Tricyclics often are not used in children. Because of their toxicity and potent adverse reactions, cautious use is suggested.

Corticosteroids (particularly dexamethasone) are used to treat pain through reduction of inflammatory processes. Steroids are used commonly for joint involvement and advanced cancer pain, bone metastasis, increased intracranial pressure, nerve pressure pain, hepatomegaly, head and neck tumors, joint pain, and edema. Steroids also may produce euphoria and increased appetite. They may have beneficial effects with short-term use, but serious adverse side effects occur with long-term therapy.[27] Adverse effects are related to dose, dosing interval, and duration of therapy. Children are no more susceptible to side effects than adults.

Anticonvulsants (such as phenytoin and carbamazepine) have been effective when used in trigeminal neuralgias. Their use also has been extrapolated for treatment of other brief lancinating pain.[2,51]

Careful consideration of the variety of adjuvant drugs available may lead to more effective pharmacologic management of the child's pain. It is the nurse's responsibility to monitor the child's response to the drug therapies selected and report significant side effects when identified. Dosing of the drug may need to be titrated, depending on the child's response. For example, oversedation may occur with antiemetics, requiring a decrease in dose or selection of an alternate drug.

Dose

Critical factors to consider when selecting appropriate dosing for the child are age and weight. Weight is thought to be the most effective measure becasue it takes into consideration the variance in children's size at the same age. If weight can be taken, it should be used to determine drug dose. Most drug references provide weight-based drug dosages.

The American Pain Society endorses dosing based on age, for children without prior extensive exposure to opiates, as follows:[2]

Younger than 2 years of age: 0.1 mg/kg per dose
Between 2 and 6 years: 20% to 25% of adult dose
Between 7 and 12 years: 50% of adult dose
Older than 12 years: entire adult dose

These are starting doses, and therapeutic doses must be individually titrated based on the child's response, the relief obtained, and the severity of adverse effects observed.[66] Refer to Tables 28-1 and 28-2 for *adult* doses for the common non-narcotics and narcotics. Extrapolation of doses for children can be completed using these values and the guidelines discussed previously.

A significant consideration when evaluating the dosage selected for narcotic analgesics is first-pass metabolism. Much of the drug dose is lost during this first-pass metabolism; therefore, it is important to administer an equianalgesic dose compared with the IM or IV route. For example, oral morphine is approximately one third to one sixth as effective as parenteral administration. Table 28-4 lists equianalgesic doses for narcotics.

Frequency

Frequency of dosage administration usually is established and stated in any current drug reference. Although standards for dosage times are identified, it is essential that analgesia administration times be individualized for each child. Frequent reassessment of the child's level of comfort and response to the type and dose of drug is essential to determine if the medication dose and frequency are effective. Most analgesics are prescribed on an as-needed (PRN) basis. Much research supports around-the-clock (ATC) administration as a more effective means of administering pain-relieving drugs. ATC administration provides a consistent blood level of the analgesic, which should eliminate the peaks and troughs that occur with PRN dosing. Figure 28-2 illustrates the difference in blood level of drugs between the two methods of administration. A consistent blood level usually can be maintained with a lower dose of narcotic and fewer side effects. A PRN order for additional narcotics between regular doses may be needed to control severe pain breakthrough resulting from activities such as turning, ambulation, or painful procedures.

PRN dosing is particularly ineffective in children for injectable analgesic therapy. Children's fears about injections and their difficulty communicating their discomfort to the nurse are two factors that interfere with determination of the need for PRN dosing and lead to inadequate pain management.

Route

The most desired route of administration, if appropriate, is the oral route. Many forms of oral medication are available and are conducive for use in all ages. These are elixirs, chewable tablets, and drops. Many analgesics can be crushed and put into ice cream or pudding. It is important to be aware which medications can be crushed because GI irritation or alteration of effective dose may occur.

Recent development of controlled-release morphine (MS Contin, Roxanol SR) has added another oral option that provides 8 to 12 hours of analgesia. Decreased frequency of administration is useful in children who resist oral medication. Nursing judgment plays an important part in determining if an alternate form of medication would be beneficial and initiating the change. When switching from another oral narcotic, it is important to calculate the 24-hour total dose of the original oral agent, then divide by two or three to determine an appropriate dose of the controlled-release agent.[83]

In some instances, the oral route is not possible or is ineffective, such as malabsorption syndromes, GI obstruction, difficulty breathing, and altered states of alertness. Often young children refuse to take oral medication. It is then essential to select an alternate route that can deliver analgesics effectively to the child.

Rectal suppositories are available for some narcotics, such as oxymorphone, hydromorphone, and oxycodone, and they should be considered before parenteral administration.[14] Two additional methods of administering opioids are being developed and tested. Sublingual administration has the potential for rapid absorption because of the rich blood and lymphatic supply in the area. If the child is old enough to understand and follow directions, this is advantageous for children because of the avoidance of needles. The newest method of opioid delivery being developed is continuous transdermal delivery. Its major advantage is the ease of self-administration. Effectiveness depends on the properties of the child's epidermis. The potent agent, fentanyl, is being tested for transdermal delivery.[9,44] As newer methods are approved, the nurse will have more options for routes of analgesic administration.

Because children find injections frightening and painful, alternative medication routes should be used when possible. It is appropriate for nurses to encourage physicians to order analgesics in effective doses and in forms less traumatic than IM. Eland and Anderson[25] strongly urge avoidance of injections in children. This is particularly true in long-term therapy when sites become

TABLE 28-4
Equianalgesic Drug Chart

Analgesic	IM Route (mg)	PO Route* (mg)	Nursing Considerations
Morphine	10	60 (30)†	Both IM and PO doses of morphine have a duration of action of about 4 to 6 hours. Sustained-release tablets and rectal suppositories are also available. The PO dose is 3 or 6 times the IM dose. The lower PO dose is suggested by several clinicians; it may be appropriate for some patients, especially elderly patients with chronic cancer pain, but it is based on anecdotal evidence, not experimental research. All other IM and PO doses in this chart are considered equivalent to 10 mg of IM morphine in analgesic effect.
Buprenorphine (Buprenex, Norwich Eaton)	0.4 (0.3)	—	A narcotic agonist–antagonist that may precipitate withdrawal in patients very physically dependent on narcotics. Dose for the sublingual form (not available in the United States) is 0.8 mg. Compared with morphine, this drug is longer acting and more likely to produce nausea and vomiting. Respiratory depression is rare but serious, because it is not readily reversed by naloxone. Not available in Canada.
Butorphanol (Stadol, Bristol)	2	—	A narcotic agonist–antagonist that may produce withdrawal in patients physically dependent on narcotics. May also produce psychotomimetic effects such as hallucinations. Not available in Canada.
Codeine	130	200	Relatively more toxic in high doses than morphine, causing more nausea and vomiting and considerable constipation. The PO dose is about 1.5 times the IM dose.
Fentanyl (Sublimaze, Janssen)	0.05	—	Most common use is for anesthesia, given IV. Onset of action when given IM is about 15 minutes; duration of action, about 90 minutes. Analgesic effect is not significantly increased by droperidol. Has been used as a substitute for high-dose IV morphine in terminally ill patients when morphine caused excitation.
Hydromorphone (Dilaudid, Knoll)	1.5	7.5	Somewhat shorter acting. Also available as rectal suppository and in high-potency injectable form (10 mg/ml). The PO dose is 5 times the IM dose.
Levorphanol (Levo-Dromoran, Roche)	2	4	Longer acting than morphine when given in repeated, regular doses. Useful alternative to PO methadone. Careful titration required because drug accumulates; both dose and interval must be adjusted. Onset of action with PO dose occurs within 1½ hours. Because drug accumulates, analgesic effect may increase with repeated doses. Initial PO dose is twice the injectable dose. (The subcutaneous route is recommended over the IM route.)
Meperidine (Demerol, Winthrop-Breon)	75	300	Shorter acting (2 to 4 hours). Watch for toxic effects on the CNS caused by accumulation of the active metabolite normeperidine, which produces neuroexcitability. Use with caution in patients with renal disease. Because of the risk to the CNS, 300 mg PO is not recommended. Because normeperidine has a long half-life (15 hours or longer), decreasing the dose in patients exhibiting a toxic reaction may increase CNS excitability, causing seizures. Effects of normeperidine are increased (not reversed) by naloxone. The PO dose is 4 times the IM dose.
Methadone (Dolophine, Lilly)	10	20	Longer acting with repeated, regular doses. Careful titration required because drug accumulates: both dose and interval must be adjusted. Onset with PO dose occurs within 1 hour. Because drug accumulates, analgesic effect may increase with repeated doses. Initial PO dose is twice the IM dose.
Methotrimeprazine (Levoprome, Lederle)	20	—	A phenothiazine (nonnarcotic) drug. Duration of action is 4 to 5 hours. Common adverse effect is hypotension; not recommended for ambulatory patients.
Nalbuphine (Nubain, Du Pont)	10 (20)	—	A narcotic agonist–antagonist that may produce withdrawal in patients physically dependent on narcotics. Longer acting and less likely to cause hypotension than morphine. In doses beyond 10 mg/70 kg, it causes no additional respiratory depression, so patient may be started on a high dose.
Opium (Pantopon, Roche; opium tincture)	20 (13.3)	(6 ml)	Infrequently used. Pantopon is the injectable form; opium tincture, the oral form. Pantopon, 20 mg, equals 10 mg of IM morphine or 15 mg of IM morphine. Opium tincture contains 1% morphine; that is, 0.6 ml equals 6 mg of PO morphine. Therefore, 6 ml equals 60 mg of PO morphine.
Oxycodone (Roxane)	15	30 (15)	Has faster onset and higher peak effect than most PO narcotics; duration of action is up to 6 hours. In one study of postoperative pain, a preparation similar to the old formulation of Percodan (containing oxycodone, aspirin, phenacetin, and caffeine) was more effective and caused fewer adverse reactions than 90 mg of PO codeine or 75 mg of PO pentazocine, and was almost equivalent to 12.5 mg of IM morphine. The PO dose is 1 or 2 times the IM dose.
Oxymorphone (Numorphan, Du Pont)	1 (1.5)	—	Also available as rectal suppository; 10 mg given rectally equals 10 mg of IM morphine. Up to 15 mg IM is now recommended as equal to 10 mg of IM morphine.
Pentazocine (Talwin, Winthrop-Breon)	60	180	Narcotic agonist–antagonist that may produce withdrawal in patients physically dependent on narcotics. Could produce psychotomimetic effects. The PO dose is 3 times the IM dose.

(Continued)

TABLE 28-4
(Continued)

Analgesic	IM Route (mg)	PO Route* (mg)	Nursing Considerations
Propoxyphene HCl (Darvon, Lilly)	—	500	The one recognized use is for mild to moderate pain unrelieved by nonnarcotics. *Never give as much as 500 mg PO; only low PO doses (65 to 130 mg) are recommended.* The IM form is not available in the United States.

* Initial PO doses are usually lower than those listed here, especially for mild to moderate pain.
† Values in parentheses refer to differences of opinion among clinicians.
(IM, intramuscular; PO, oral; IV, intravenous; CNS, central nervous system.)
Source: McCaffery, M. A practical "postable" chart of equianalgesic doses. *Nursing87, 8, 56–57.*
The equianalgesic doses in this chart are based primarily on data distributed by the Analgesic Study Section, Sloan-Kettering Institute for Cancer Research, New York. A complete list of references is available on request.

scarce, tissue absorption is altered causing peaks and troughs, and duration of action is shorter.

If intramuscular injection is necessary, consideration of principles of development, preparation of children for painful procedures, and use of the correct technique for various age groups are essential. Evans and Hansen[28] provide some guidelines that could contribute to a more positive injection experience in children. Their recommendations, with some adaptations, include the following:

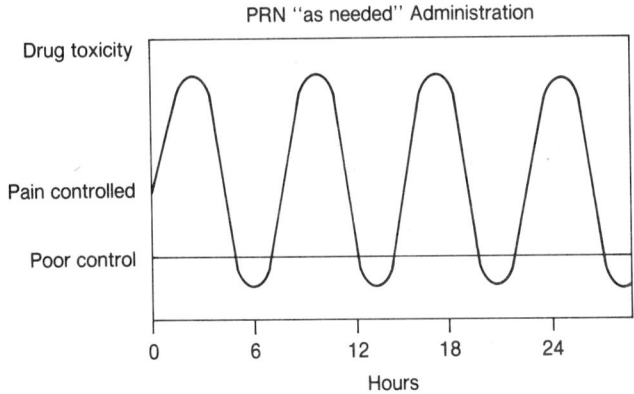

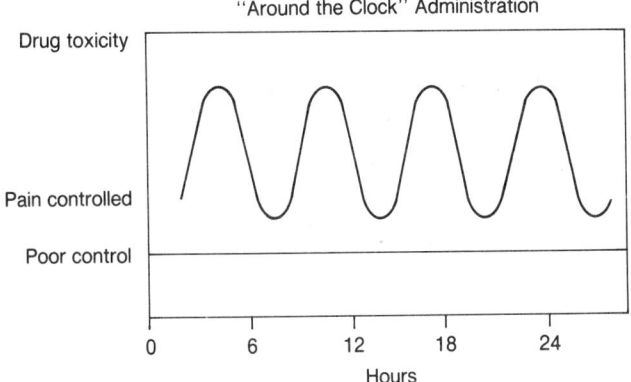

FIGURE 28-2
PRN (as needed) versus "around-the-clock" administration of medications.

- Establish a trusting relationship with the child by taking time to get to know him or her and by telling the truth about an injection.
  - For a young child, tell him or her about the injection shortly before to decrease time for fantasizing and increasing anxiety.
  - For an older child, inform him or her about the injection as a part of the preparation for the procedure and a part of the discussion of the overall plan of care.
- Do not allow delays in administration of injection (except for requests to use the bathroom). Children will try to talk you out of the medication by assuring you they no longer feel discomfort or pleading that they don't need the shot.
- Explain the rationale for IM to the child's family. If possible, do not have the parents restrain the child during injection. Children cannot understand why the parent is not preventing this painful experience. However, young children cannot differentiate between a parent who stands and does nothing to prevent the experience and one who holds him or her during the experience. The child may be comforted by the closeness and touch of a parent.
- Explain the reason for the medication (shot), and follow up with reinforcement that it worked. This helps the child understand that the pain of the injection is responsible for the child feeling better.[39,70]
- Use play therapy to prepare for injection. Demonstrate drawing up of medication from a vial, selecting and preparing a site, and administering the medication. Have the child practice the procedures demonstrated on a cloth doll with sterile water. Explain the purpose of the medication, how it is given, and why certain actions are done.[39] If the child is in severe enough pain to require analgesia, they may not have the energy or ability to play before the procedure. Opportunity to play after the procedure would be a productive alternative.

IV administration is another effective alternative when oral administration is not possible. Children who have IVs in place for fluid and antibiotic administration are

TABLE 28-5
Comparison of Morphine Peak Analgesia and Respiratory Depression by Route of Administration

Route	Peak Analgesia of Morphine	Maximum Respiratory Depression
SQ	50–90 minutes	Within 90 minutes
IM	30–60 minutes	Within 30 minutes
IV	20 minutes	Within 7 minutes

(SQ, subcutaneous; IM, intramuscular; IV, intravenous.)
Data from Boyer, M. (1982). *Continuous Drip Morphine. American Journal of Nursing, 82,* 602–604; and Stimmel, B. (1983) *Pain, analgesia and addiction: The pharmacologic treatment of pain.* New York: Raven Press.

perfect candidates for this nonpainful method of administering analgesia. IV routes often are necessary for a child in severe pain.

As with IV administration of any drugs, there are risks with IV administration of narcotics, such as increased risk of respiratory depression. Risks are assumed with other categories of drugs administered IV that have far more serious side effects. For example, IV antibiotics are not withheld because of the risk of anaphylaxis, and IV glucose is not withheld because of the risk of hyperglycemic coma. IV administration of narcotics is an appropriate and often necessary method of analgesia. It requires astute nursing assessment and monitoring of the child's status.

Knowing the peak effect of narcotics based on the route of administration should provide the nurse with guidelines for establishing time frames when monitoring adverse effects. For example, narcotics administered IV peak within 7 minutes, so the most critical time for observation of respiratory depression is during the first 15 minutes. Table 28-5 lists peak effect times based on route of administration.

Delivery Options

Many delivery options for administration of narcotics have become available for the pediatric client during recent years. These options, including continuous infusion (CI), continuous spinal opioid infusion (CSOI), continuous subcutaneous infusion (CSCI), intraventricular infusion, and patient-controlled analgesia (PCA), are most likely to be used for the delivery of opioids for chronic pain due to cancer. Continuous or repeated administration of an opioid analgesic when injections and oral dosing must be avoided can be provided by alternate delivery methods.[44] Indications for the use of alternate modes of administering narcotic analgesics include the following:

- Severe pain not controlled by around-the-clock oral and parenteral narcotics
- Vomiting, GI block, and difficulty breathing, which prevent oral administration
- Bleeding disorders, decreased platelet count, decreased muscle mass, or inadequate absorption, which make IM or SQ injection impractical
- Inability to swallow oral medications
- Contraindication to rectal analgesia[12,71]

Each of the alternate methods for administering narcotics to the child in severe pain is discussed below. References are provided for more in-depth reading on each mode of delivery.

Continuous Intravenous Infusion

This method of narcotic administration involves the continuous infusion of narcotics through an intravenous line. Research has shown that patients receiving CI morphine generally are less lethargic, more coherent, less short of breath, and less anxious than patients receiving conventional narcotic regimens.[12] CI morphine has been found to be an excellent pain relief method and is safe

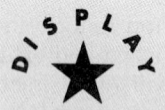

Procedure for Administering Continuous Intravenous Narcotics

1. Establish an IV line with a volume control set and an infusion pump with an alarm.
2. Begin by putting 25 ml of IV fluid into volume set and adding a 1-hour dose of the narcotic. Run this mixture through the pump at 25 ml/h. Repeat the procedure for the second hour. (Hourly dosing intially allows for adjustment of the dose according to the child's response)
3. When the child is comfortable, begin infusing the narcotic on a 4-hour schedule rather than a 1-hour schedule by instilling 100 ml in the infusion control set and adding a 4-hour dose of the narcotic. Run this at 25 ml/h.

4. Assess the child's comfort level at least every 30 minutes during the 1-hour infusions. Respiratory rate should be assessed every 5 minutes for the first 15 minutes (maximum respiratory depression with IV narcotics occurs within 7 minutes), then every 30 minutes during the 1-hour infusions. When stable, assess once every 4 hours. Dose can be titrated by the child's response.

(IV, intravenous.)
Adapted from McGuire, L., & Dizard, S. (1982). Managing pain in the young patient. Nursing84, *12, 52, 54–55.*

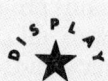

Converting From Oral Route to Continuous Infusion

1. Determine the total PO narcotic dose that the child receives in 24 hours.
2. Convert the PO dose to an IM dose by using an equianalgesic table.
3. Divide that 24-hour IM dose by 2 to arrive at the total IV dose (IV dose is usually ½ the IM dose).
4. Divide that total IV dose by 24 to arrive at the hourly dose.

(PO, oral; IM, intramuscular; IV, intravenous).
Adapted from McGuire, L., & Wright, A. (1984) Continuous narcotic infusion—It's not just for cancer patients. Nursing 84, 14, 50–55.

and efficacious with children in the terminal stages of cancer.[77] CI allows more uniform pain control using lower doses and causing fewer side effects. Dose adjustment is facilitated simply by increasing or decreasing the infusion rate.

Because of the potential side effect of respiratory depression, close monitoring of vital signs is essential along with titration of morphine, or any IV narcotic, to balance pain relief with a degree of sedation.[80] The specific starting dose is contingent on the child's previous pain medication, level of tolerance, and intensity of pain. The dosing strategy goal is to reach effective plasma concentrations and maintain a steady state plasma level. Determination of the child's normal respiratory rate and pattern is essential before initiating CI morphine. Because of individual differences, changes in respiratory rate should be evaluated against the patient's own baseline to determine when IV rate needs to be decreased.

When switching from oral administration to CI, use the guidelines in the accompanying display on converting from the oral route to CI to determine equianalgesic dosage. This conversion may not be the effective dose needed. The child's pain level and response to the dosage administered must be evaluated to determine the titration necessary to arrive at the dosing that will keep the child comfortable with the least side effects. Response to CI varies and incomplete relief of pain may occur. However, ineffective CI with one drug may be followed by success with another.

Continuous Spinal Opioid Infusion

CSOI is the introduction of opioids into the epidural or intrathecal space for the management of acute or chronic pain. The discovery of spinal opiate receptors in the late 1970s led researchers to investigate this mode of morphine administration. Major benefits of intraspinal morphine are increased quality of pain relief, longer duration of relief from a single dose (8 to 36 hours), rapidity of onset (15 to 45 minutes),[82,85] and decreased frequency of undesirable side effects because of lower doses of narcotic.[85] Equianalgesic doses can be decreased to $\frac{1}{10}$ the

equivalent IV dose for the epidural route and to $\frac{1}{100}$ the dose for intrathecal administration.[63]

Long-term epidural catheters and totally implanted systems (Infusaid) for CSOI have been developed and are showing positive results in providing relief with a decrease in opioid requirements.[17] The implantable pump should be considered in any child who will need repeated venous access,[38] and it allows for treatment of severe, chronic pain in the home setting. The reader is referred to Pageau et al.[82] and Harris et al.[38] for detailed information on implementation of totally implanted administration systems. Figure 28-3 illustrates a typical implantable infusion pump device.

Studies in children receiving epidural morphine have shown no complications or serious side effects from placement of the catheter, and postoperative requirements for narcotics are significantly less in the children who receive morphine epidurally than in those who receive narcotics parenterally. Urinary retention requiring a catheter was the most disturbing side effect.[16,36]

A potential complication of intraspinal narcotic buildup leading to CNS and respiratory depression exists. Nursing intervention should include careful monitoring of vital signs and assessing for signs of respiratory depression or decreased mental alertness every ½ hour for the first 12 hours, then every 4 hours. Naloxone, an opiate antagonist, should be kept at bedside.

Ambulatory infusion pumps allow children ongoing pain relief and the opportunity to return to the family and home environment. Depending on the age of the child,

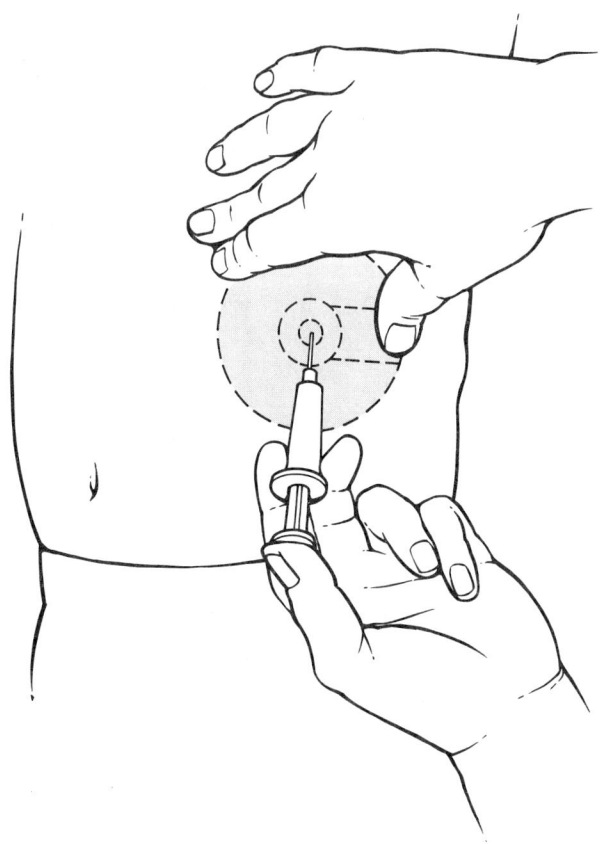

FIGURE 28-3
Schematic representation of an implanted infusion pump.

safety is a consideration. Pumps with no accessible external controls should be used with children.[22] The family caring for the child at home with an implanted infusion pump should be taught how to care for the infusion device, how to recognize respiratory and CNS depression, and how to reverse them by administering IM naloxone (Narcan). Additionally, instruction for monitoring for signs of temperature fluctuation, which can affect infusion flow rate, should be given. Health professionals must evaluate the patient's response to therapy, adjust dosage, and refill the infusion device.[82,84]

Continuous Subcutaneous Infusion

CSCI involves insertion of a needle into subcutaneous tissue of the chest wall, abdomen, or thigh. Site selection is determined by the distribution of subcutaneous tissue, mobility, and preference of the child and family. Portable infusion pumps, attached to a 27-gauge butterfly needle, have been used to infuse opioids subcutaneously in the management of pain in cancer patients.[19] Figure 28-4 illustrates a continuous subcutaneous infusion system and a young girl receiving a pain medication through a continuous infusion system.

CSCI has been shown to be relatively simple, safe, and effective for use in children with pain. Most opioid analgesics may be administered using this mode (exceptions are meperidine and pentazocine, which are irritating to the tissues). Subcutaneous infusions are rapidly absorbed and maximum concentration is reached in plasma in 10 to 30 minutes. The major determinant of absorption is the total surface area over which absorption can occur. Major advantages include even analgesia, increased mobility, less nausea and vomiting, and decreased fear from repeated needle injections. Major problems found with this method are pain breakthrough due to poor absorption at a particular site (can be managed by changing infusion site) and local irritation at the site of administration (ro-

tating sites of infusion frequently can decrease this problem; adding 0.05 mg of dexamethasone for every ml of analgesic also may help). The need for a clinical nurse specialist to assist in home management is often another problem these families face.[44]

CSCI of narcotics is an effective method of managing the patient in the home and requires instruction for the child (depending on age) and the family. The child's family can be taught to clean the skin site, insert a new needle, and cover the area with a wound dressing. The site should be changed at least weekly and observed for irritation at least twice daily. The reader is referred to Coyle et al.[19] for further information on CSCI.

Intraventricular Infusion

The procedure for this method of intraventricular opiate administration requires the implantation of an Ommaya reservoir with a catheter placed in the ventricles for delivery of the narcotic. This mode of delivery is limited because of the significant risk of respiratory depression and the complexity of the procedure.[83] For a select few, continuous intraventricular monitoring may be indicated. Paice[83] provides the reader with more detailed information on this delivery option.

Patient-Controlled Analgesia

PCA is an analgesic administration system that involves IV self-administration of analgesics. PCA has been found to be an effective pain control method for 11- to 18-year-old postoperative patients.[102] Its use in children younger than age 12 is questioned because they seem to be influenced easily by the opinions of others.[9]

IV PCA is conducted by the child who uses a device specifically designed for this purpose. PCA is most effective with continuous IV infusion plus the self-administration of boluses when needed. The infusion pump is ac-

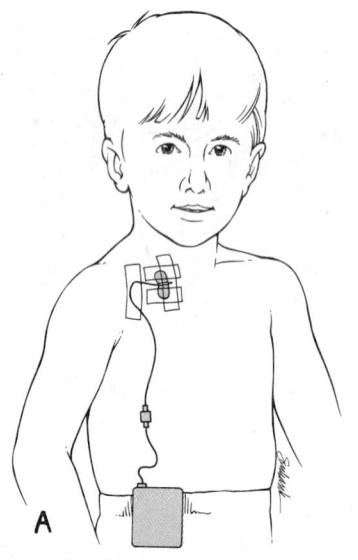
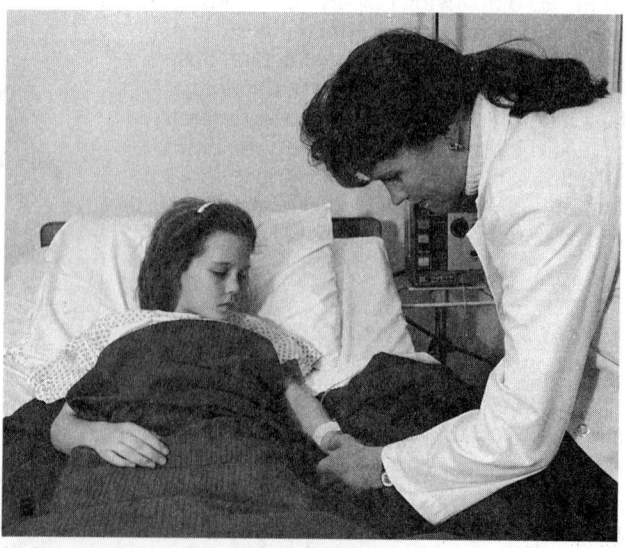

FIGURE 28-4
Continuous subcutaneous infusion. (**A**) Schematic representation of the infusion system. (**B**) A young girl uses a continuous subcutaneous infusion pump for pain management.

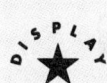

Advantages of Patient-Controlled Analgesia

- The child can determine the need for drug depending on change in intensity of pain without delay
- Decreases the child's anxiety about not obtaining relief from pain when needed
- Fewer side effects, probably due to lower total dose administered and stable serum level
- Increased pulmonary function tests and fewer pulmonary complications in postoperative patients
- Gives the child control over his or her pain

Adapted from Graves, D. A., Foster, T. S., Batenhorst, R. L., Bennett, R. L., & Baumann, T. J. (1983). Patient-controlled analgesia. Annals of Internal Medicine, 99, 360–366.

tivated by a hand-held button. A predetermined dose of narcotic is administered through the IV line. Boluses are preset with a lockout interval and a preset number of doses (in mg per hour) to prevent overdosing of the drug. Recommendations have been made for a lockout interval of 6 or more minutes.[65] The lockout intervals and doses are established by controls that are kept locked in the pump and can only be accessed by the nurse with narcotic keys. Because the nurse has ultimate control of the dosing of narcotics, PCA is considered safe for use in children. Studies are underway to determine if parents can be taught to use PCA safely for young children.

Procedures and Pain in the Child

During the early years, children often are exposed to procedures that cause them pain at varying levels. Circumcision, immunizations, and laceration repair are common procedures many children experience. Consideration of actions that may decrease the pain perceived by the child are a priority for the innovative professional nurse.

Dorsal penile nerve blocks and caudal blocks have been found to be effective for relieving pain following circumcision.[57,104] Spraying of a cooling agent (Frigiderm) to the skin site prior to injection has been shown to decrease reported pain in children.[23] Other cutaneous stimulation (such as rubbing, massaging, applying heat or cold, or using vibrators) may provide pain relief for some children receiving injections.[66] Dripping a local anesthetic into lacerations followed by slow anesthetic injection before suturing minor lacerations has been recommended.[5] Another suggestion to decrease the pain of laceration repair is the use of TAC, a solution of tetracaine, adrenalin, and cocaine, prior to laceration repair. A sterile gauze pad is soaked with TAC and placed in the open wound prior to suturing or additional local anesthetic injection.[26] Additional interventions using nonpharmacologic ap-

proaches, such as music and distraction, also should be evaluated for improving the experience of painful procedures. (The reader is referred to the section entitled Nonpharmacological Management of Pain.) Although these measures have not been thoroughly tested with children, they hold promise for the future. It is a nursing responsibility to keep current on the research in the field of pediatric pain management to identify innovative treatments and intervention approaches that may be effective in decreasing the child's pain.

Nonpharmacologic Management of Pain

A great deal of information is available on the pharmacologic management of pain because pediatric nurses have been able to borrow and extrapolate information from research with adults. In the area of nonpharmacologic interventions, much is known from the day-to-day experience of practicing nurses, but very little pediatric pain research has been completed to validate specific nursing interventions or identify what specific types of pain would most likely be alleviated by specific interventions. In spite of the absence of research-based information, practicing nurses are faced daily with the reality of providing nonpharmacologic interventions for comfort and pain relief. This section provides a brief summary of several of these methods. The Nursing Care Plan presents care of a child who first receives a medication but, after the major pain period, is also managed by nonpharmacologic care.

Provision of Information

Children and their parents who are anxious and fearful benefit from the simple process of receiving information. Johnson's extensive research in this area[48,49] has shown than when individuals are provided with information about the sensations likely to be experienced in a given situation, the amount of pain perceived and the distress associated with pain are reduced. Telling a child who is immediately postoperative that he or she must cough usually will not be welcomed. However, explaining to a child that the nurse will help him or her cough by giving medicine and holding a stuffed animal or pillow over the incision to make the hurt less may help. The nurse also may say that if the child does not cough, he or she will become sicker and have to stay in the hospital longer.

Use of Parents

Parents as an intervention for pain relief are probably the most powerful nonpharmacologic pain relief intervention known (Fig. 28-5). The majority of parents love their children and comfort them better than anyone else. Although there is no support in the research literature, one could hypothesize that when a supportive, concerned parent is comforting a child, the child releases endorphin.

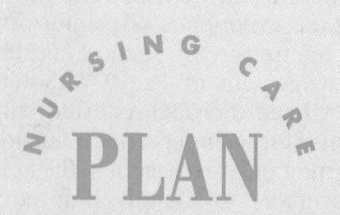

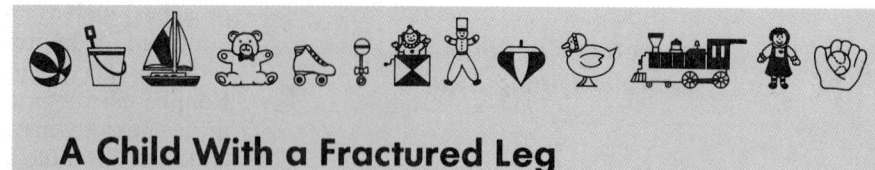

A Child With a Fractured Leg

Assessment

Case Study Description

On 9/23/92, Timothy Moss, a 7-year-old first grader, was struck by a car on the way home from school. He sustained a fractured right femur and various scrapes. Timothy was admitted to the emergency room. X-rays revealed a midshaft fracture in the right femur. Disposition: Admit for 6 weeks of traction and then cast. Upon admission to the inpatient unit, Timothy had traction applied to the extremity by the orthopedist. Medical orders include 20 mg of meperidine IM every q 3 to 4 hours and Trilisate 600 mg PO PRN pain. Both parents are present and seem appropriately concerned about their son.

Assessment Data

Timothy lies quietly in bed with leg in traction. He cries softly at times and appears fearful. Timothy was given no analgesics in the emergency room. Timothy becomes fearful when approached or leg or traction examined.

Nursing Diagnosis

1. Pain related to fracture
   Supporting Data:
   - Rates his pain with three poker chips on a four-point scale
   - Lies *very* still in bed
   - Consistently looks at his leg
   - Is not easily distracted by television or talking to parents
   - Cries softly at times
   - Facial mask of pain
   - Diaphoretic at times
   - Blood pressure, pulse, and respiratory rate increased
     - Femur is fractured resulting in:
     - Hemorrhage into the muscle from marrow
     - Interruption of periosteum
     - Pain from bone displacement and bone splinters into tissue
     - Muscle spasms, thigh is rigid
   - Interruption of arterial and venous blood supply to leg
   - Nerves have been pinched or crushed

Intervention

Administer both meperidine and Trilisate around the clock for 48 hours, inform the child and family when drugs will work and why drugs are being given around the clock. Do patient teaching regarding narcotics.

Request that the physician change the meperidine order to PO (anticipate the order will be increased due to first-pass metabolism).

Request an order for Colace or Senokot to maintain bowel function.

Request an order for a TENS unit, apply TENS unit for 30 minutes t.i.d. along right side the spinal cord at the level of lumbar vertebrae two to three, using conventional settings.

Massage lower back q.i.d.

Rationale

The major pain of the injury will be in the first 48 hours. It is virtually impossible for the child to be pain-free during this time because of the tissue damage involved. ATC administration will keep ahead of the pain and decrease the child's fear and anxiety.

There is absolutely no reason to give the drug IM. Often physicians order IM analgesics out of habit. The child has gastrointestinal function and will appreciate pain relief without the needle.

ATC administration of the narcotic will cause constipation. The immobility imposed by the traction also will influence bowel function. There is absolutely no reason why the child should suffer the pain and discomfort of constipation in addition to the existing pain. A bowel program begun at the time of admission will avoid this.

A TENS unit will either stimulate large fiber input at the level of the cord or stimulate endorphin release in the brain.

Children who have a leg in traction will become stiff in the lower back. They are not as likely to develop pressure ulcers as the elderly, but the stiffness can be unpleasant.

(Continued)

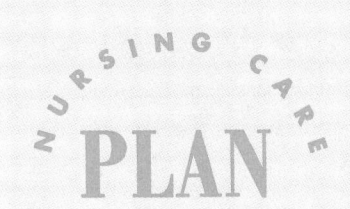

A Child With a Fractured Leg (continued)

Provide distraction: television, video games, cassette tapes, and books from patient library.

Children are perfect candidates for distraction. They are used to television, video games, cassettes, and often enjoy stories being read to them or reading stories to others.

Suggest that parents bring favorite stuffed toy and other personal items from home. Encourage a parent to spend the first two nights of the hospitalization with the child.

Familiar items from home will make the surroundings of the hospital seem less strange. Allowing a parent to spend the night will ease the child's distress and anxiety and therefore decrease pain.

Initiate therapeutic play with doll in traction twice a week or until child no longer wants to play.

Play is a child's work. Playing with a doll in traction will allow the child to express the various feelings he or she is having that he might not otherwise be able to express.

Evaluation

- Previous pain behaviors are absent.
- Timothy demonstrates return to baseline vital signs.
- Pain from the fracture recedes as leg heals.

Expected Outcomes

- Timothy identifies pain rate as zero or one poker chip.
- Timothy exhibits self-confidence when anyone enters the room.
- Timothy participates in activities as much as traction will allow.
- Timothy exhibits easy distraction by watching television or talking to his parents.

As stated in the assessment section, parents are second only to the child in providing information about pain assessment, and the same is true in the area of intervention. Parents can identify what pain relief interventions have previously been successful and unsuccessful and make suggestions to the health care team about interventions that they believe would help their child. Additionally, informed parents can assist with the implementation of many of the nonpharmacologic techniques, such as imagery, TENS, or self-hypnosis.

Play and Activity

Because children often lack the vocabulary to express their feelings, play allows them to "tell" their caregivers what is bothering them and to work through their emo-

tions and feelings. The reader is referred to Chapter 23, which includes an extensive section on play for hospitalized children. Play can also be a powerful teaching tool for the nurse. When young children do not understand the explanations about a procedure, a therapeutic rehearsal of it can provide the child with the necessary information they need to be less fearful and cooperate more fully (Fig. 28-6). During the play session, the health care team member can act out one or more of the roles in the situation and provide explanations as to why the procedure had to be done. In an emergency when there is no time for rehearsal, children can replay the emergency situation as often as needed until they become more comfortable with the event. Such sessions are important for adjusting to the present situation and for coping with the nightmares that often follow particularly frightening procedures or hospitalizations.

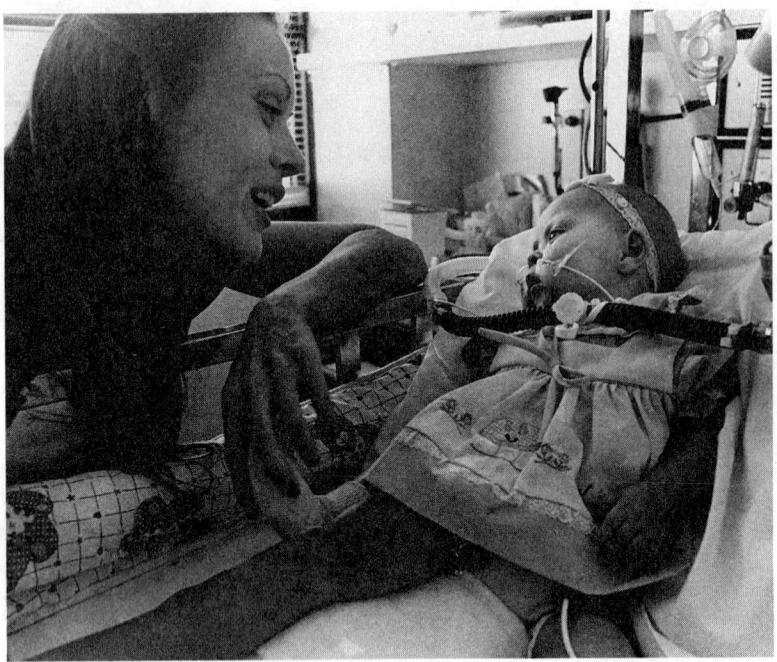

FIGURE 28-5

A mother's presence and touch give pain relief to a seriously ill child. (Photo by Kathy Sloane. Courtesy of Children's Hospital, Oakland, CA.)

Touch

The majority of children who are ill, excluding some premature neonates, need to be touched, stroked, and held. The amount of equipment attached to a child may overwhelm a parent. Parents need to be shown how to safely pick up and hold their children with the various pieces of therapeutic equipment attached (Fig. 28-7). If it is virtually impossible for a child to be held, a chair needs to be moved next to the child so that the parent can be comfortable while remaining at the bedside and maintaining close physical contact with the child. Some parents need to be told that it is completely appropriate to touch and stroke the skin of their ill child and that it will help the child's recovery.

Use of Music and Other Distractions

The authors believe that distraction is a powerful pain relief intervention that children are accustomed to using. Television or music often can be the focus of a child's attention rather than the pain they are experiencing. However, distraction should not be confused with total relief of pain. Distraction is the ability to focus attention on something other than pain and does not mean that the pain is "gone." McCaffery states that singing, counting, and tapping to the beat of a song are particularly helpful distractions for a person in pain.[67] If appropriate suggestions are made, children also can use music to relax and relieve any muscle tension they are experiencing. Children experiencing severe pain often cannot be distracted. A child who previously could be distracted but can no longer be distracted needs reassessment of his or her pain to determine what has changed about it and what interventions may be required.

Reading a child's favorite story or cassette recordings of a favorite story by significant individuals in the child's life, such as a grandparent or a parent, can be very comforting to the child. When significant others cannot be present, a familiar voice recorded on a cassette tape also can be an effective distraction. This is particularly true in the middle of the night when the number of distractions in a hospital is greatly reduced and the child is in pain or frightened by the darkness, the hospital setting, and the absence of a significant other.

Relaxation

Simple forms of relaxation may be adequate for episodes of acute pain. Instructing the child to take several slow deep breaths and to think about something they like to do refocuses the child's attention and reduces anxiety. This is often enough to reduce the muscle tension that aggravates the pain experience. Bobey and Davidson[11] in an experimental study found that relaxation techniques are the most effective methods for controlling painful stressors.

Children have an active imagination, which can be a powerful adjuvant in pain control. A child who is tense can be assisted in relaxation by suggestions. One such example is included in the following paragraph, but the reader is encouraged to provide their own scripts.

"Imagine you are floating on a cloud in the sky. It's a beautiful day that's not too hot and not too cold. You're just floating along and having a really great time. When you look down, you can see your favorite place, and if you want to, you can go there. What is your favorite place? Do you want to go visit there? You can, you know. All you have to do is close your eyes, and you'll be there. Will you tell me about your favorite place?"

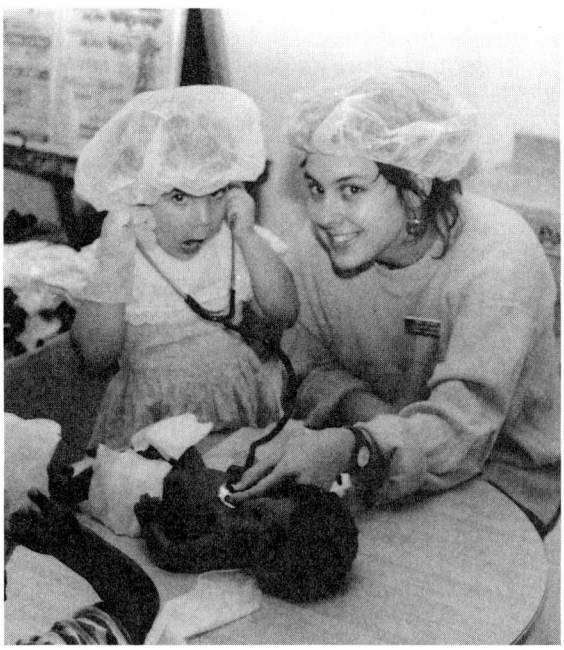
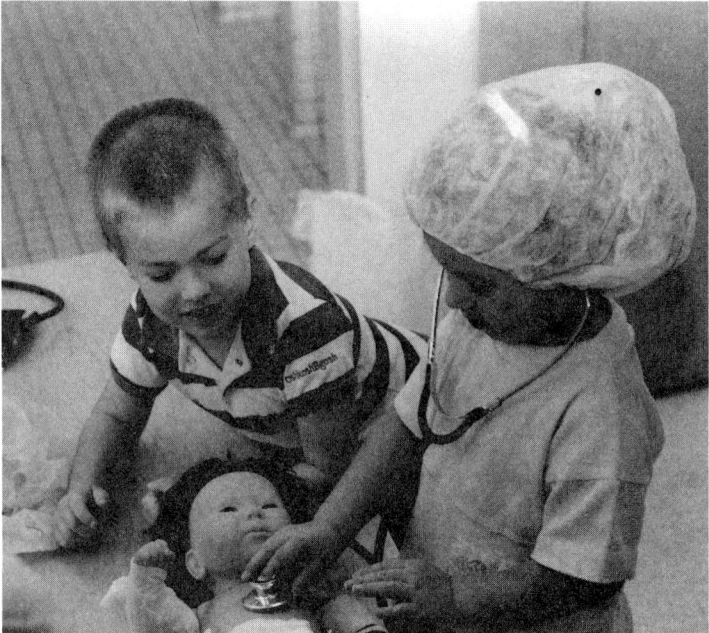
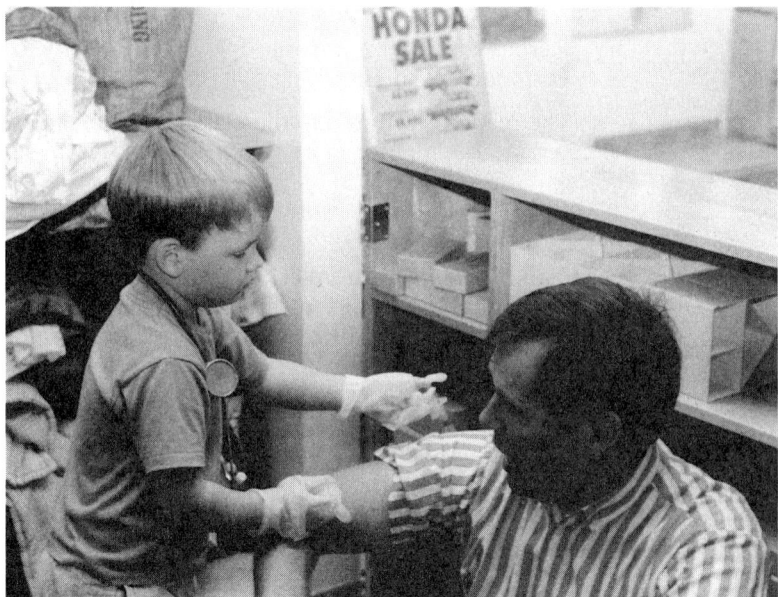

FIGURE 28-6
Play is an important nonpharmacologic method of pain relief.

Kuttner has researched the effectiveness of favorite stories and found them to be a beneficial intervention for children with cancer.[53] A videotape by Dr. Leona Kuttner entitled "No Fears, No Tears" has excellent examples with children and their parents of imagery and other relaxation techniques for children. It is available at a nominal cost from Canadian Cancer Society of Vancouver BC, BC/Yukon Division, 955 W. Broadway, Vancouver, BC, V5Z 1E5, Canada.

Hypnosis

The work of Gardner and Olness,[34] Spinetta and Deasy-Spinetta,[94] Hilgard and LeBaron,[41] and Hockenberry and Contach[42] have clearly demonstrated that hyp-

nosis is another powerful treatment modality for children who are in pain and are nauseated from the effects of chemotherapy. A textbook on child health nursing is not an appropriate place to teach these techniques, but the reader is encouraged to refer children to those in their health care setting who are trained in hypnosis and to pursue the topic further, particularly if the nurse is working with children who have chronic illnesses.

Heat and Cold

The value of application of heat or cold placed between the brain and the source of pain often is underestimated and depending on the setting, may require a physician's order. Heat promotes vasodilitation, thereby

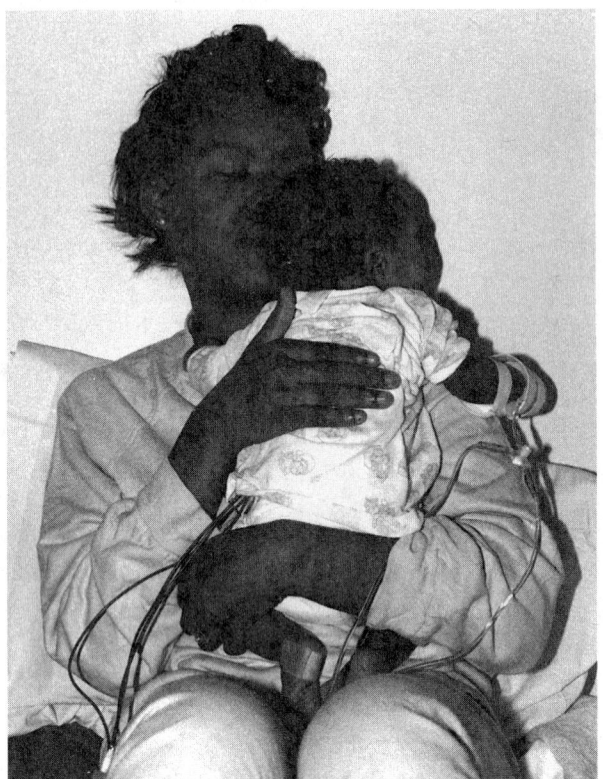

FIGURE 28-7
Touch is especially important to newborns who are attached to special equipment. Many parents have to be taught how to hold and cuddle such neonates.

increasing the blood supply to the area and allowing the removal of the by-products of cell breakdown. Children who are going to have blood samples drawn benefit from the application of a warm pack 15 minutes prior to the procedure because the pack will dilate the vessel and make entry into the vessel easier. (The temperature of a warm washcloth or heating pad must be carefully monitored to prevent accidental thermal injury to the child).

The mechanism by which cold relieves pain is not completely known; however, it is thought that the cold actually slows the ability of the pain fiber to transmit pain impulses. Application of cold also must be carefully monitored because it is possible to injure the skin.

Stimulation of Acupressure Points

Myofascial pain is muscle pain and stiffness, and it is often associated with bedrest. It is characterized by muscles that are stiff, sore, achy, and have "knots" in them. Areas that are frequently affected are between the shoulder blades (trapezious muscle), the neck muscles as they extend up into the base of the skull (trapezious), the lower back, sometimes down the legs, and the heel cord (due to physiologic shortening of the muscle fiber).

Most myofascial pain can be alleviated by one or more of the following interventions, which have as their focus stimulations of acupressure points with heat and cold alternating every 20 minutes, warm baths with muscle and

backrubs afterwards, TENS on acupuncturelike settings for no longer than 20 minutes followed by conventional TENS settings, and active or passive range of motion.[24] Muscle relaxants usually are not needed when myofascial pain is relieved using one of these methods.

TENS Units

A TENS unit consists of a small plastic box approximately $2 \times 1 \times 3$ inches that has two or four electrodes attached to the box by wires. The TENS unit delivers small amounts of electrical energy to the skin by way of the electrodes. It is thought that TENS works through either modulation of painful input into the spinal cord or through endorphin release.[59]

The authors believe TENS is an underused nursing intervention and encourage its use for a variety of conditions, including the following:

- Myofascial pain and stiffness
- Pain associated with denuded skin, including scrapes
- Infusion of painful intravenous infusions, such as amphotericin
- Bone metastasis
- Herpes zoster inflammation
- Postoperative incisional pain

The reader is referred to the classic work by Mannheimer and Lampe[59] for more information in this area.

Summary

Pain control begins with a thorough assessment of all of a child's pains. Fortunately, many of the myths surrounding pain assessment and interventions have been elimi-

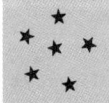 **Ideas for Nursing Research**

The future holds great possibilities for nursing research in the nursing care of children who have pain. Nurses are responsible for helping children manage pain by a variety of pharmacological and nonpharmacological interventions. Understanding the action of pain medications in all age groups and understanding the responses of infants, toddlers, school-age children, and adolescents to pain are of great importance in nursing. The following areas need to be explored:

- Application of gate control theory in children
- Effect of developmental age, cognitive level, emotions, and experience on pain perception
- Validation of effectiveness of newer pain medication delivery systems with children
- Techniques of use, cost and benefits; contraindications of newer pain medication delivery systems for children
- Study of long-term effects of a child's pain on the child and family

nated, but some myths still remain that hamper pain control in some settings. Ongoing assessment of pain is an essential part of pain management because pathology and other mitigating factors change in clinical situations.

Information in the area of analgesics and their administration has virtually "exploded" in the past 5 years. The knowledge for research-based nursing intervention is less evident in the area of nonpharmacologic interventions, but current research will result in more specific nursing interventions for children in pain.

It is an exciting time in pediatric pain research for all of the health sciences. It has been estimated that the knowledge base concerning pain control in children changes drastically every 3 years. What has been included in this chapter is current information at the time it was written. However, readers are encouraged to read current references to see what is new in the everchanging tapestry of pain relief.

References

1. Allen R. C., Petty, R. E., Lireman, D. S., Malleson, P. N., & Laxer, R. M. (1986). Renal papillary necrosis in children with chronic arthritis. *American Journal of Diseases of Children, 140*, 20–22.
2. American Pain Society. (1986). *Principles of analgesic use in the treatment of acute pain and chronic cancer pain—A concise guide to medical practice*. Washington, DC: Author.
3. Angell, M. (1982). The quality of mercy. *New England Journal of Medicine, 306*, 98–99.
4. Beales, J. F., Keen, J. H., & Holt, P. J. (1983). The child's perception of the disease and the experience of pain in juvenile chronic arthritis. *Journal of Rheumatology, 10*, 61–65.
5. Beckemeyer, P., & Bahr, J. (1980). Helping toddlers and preschoolers cope while suturing their minor lacerations. *MCN American Journal of Maternal Child Nursing, 5*, 326–330.
6. Beyer, J. E. (1984). *The oucher: A user's manual and technical report*. Evanston, IL: The Hospital Play Equipment Co.
7. Beyer, J. E., & Aradine, C. R. (1986). Content validity of an instrument to measure young children's perceptions of the intensity of their pain. *Journal of Pediatric Nursing, 1*, 386–395.
8. Beyer, J. E., & Byers, M. L. (1985). Knowledge of pediatric pain: The state of the art. *Child Health Nursing, 13*, 150–159.
9. Beyer, J. E., & Levin, C. R. (1987). Issues and advances in pain control in children. *Nursing Clinics of North America, 22*, 661–676.
10. Beyer, J. E., DeGood, D. E., Ashley, L. C., & Russell, G. A. (1983). Patterns of postoperative analgesic use with adults and children following cardiac surgery. *Pain 17*, 71–81.
11. Bobey, M. J., & Davidson, P. O. (1970). Psychological factors affecting pain tolerance. *Journal of Psychosomatic Research, 14*, 371–376.
12. Boyer, M. W. (1982). Continuous drip morphine. *American Journal of Nursing, 82*, 602–604.
13. Calamaris, D. M., & Sullivan, C. L. (1980). *The importance of pediatric pain cues as perceived by nurses*. Unpublished thesis, University of Virginia.
14. (1987). *Cancer pain: A monograph of the management of cancer pain. A report of the Expert Advisory Committee on the Management of Severe Chronic Pain in Cancer Patients*. Canada: Minister of Supply and Services.
15. (1987). Classification of nursing diagnoses. In A. M. McLane (Ed.), *Proceedings of the seventh conference*. St. Louis: CV Mosby.
16. Coombs, D. W., Saunders, R. L., Gaylor, M. S., Block, A. R.,

17. Colton, T., Harbaugh, R., Pageau, M. G., & Mroz, W. (1984). Outcomes and complications of continuous intraspinal narcotic analgesia for cancer pain control. *Journal of Clinical Oncology, 2*, 1414–1420.
17. Cousins, M. J., & Mather, L. E. (1984). Intrathecal and epidural administration of opioids. *Anesthesiology, 61*, 276–310.
18. Coyle, N. Analgesics and pain: Current concepts. *Nursing Clinics of North America, 22*, 727–741.
19. Coyle, N., Mauskop, A., Maggard, J., & Foley, K. (1986). Continuous subcutaneous infusions of opiates in cancer patients with pain. *Oncology Nursing, 13*, 53–57.
20. Crue, B. L., & Carregel, E. J. (1975). Pain begins in the dorsal horn—With a proposed classification of the primary senses. In B. L. Crue (Ed.), *Pain: Research and treatment* (pp. 35–68). Orlando, FL: Academic Press.
21. Cuddy, P. G. (1982). Management of acute opioid intoxination. *Critical Care Quarterly, 4*, 65–73.
22. Dennis, E. M. (1984). An ambulatory infusion pump for pain control: A nursing approach for home care. *Cancer Nursing, 7*, 309–313.
23. Eland, J. M. (1981). Minimizing pain associated with prekindergarten intramuscular injections. *Issues Comp Pediatr Nurs, 5*, 361–372.
24. Eland, J. M. Issues in Comprehensive Pediatric Nursing (1989). Pharmacologic management of pain. In K. Ruccione (Ed.), *Pediatric hospice manual* (pp.). Los Angeles: Children's Hospital of Los Angeles.
25. Eland, J.M., & Anderson, J. E. (1977). The experience of pain in children. In A. Jacox (Ed.), *Pain: A sourcebook for nurses and other health professionals* (pp. 453–473). Boston: Little, Brown and Company.
26. Eland, J. M., & Herr, K. A. (1988). Does suturing have to hurt so much? *Children's Nurse, 5(6)*: 1–2.
27. Ellis, E. F. (1984). Corticosteroid regimens in pediatric practice. *Hospital Practice, 19*, 143–47, 150–51.
28. Evans, M. L., & Hansen, B. D. (1981). Administering injections to different-aged children. *MCN American Journal of Maternal Child Nursing, 6*, 194–199.
29. Fields, H. L. (1987). *Pain*. New York: McGraw-Hill.
30. Foley, K. M. (1985). The treatment of cancer pain. *New England Journal of Medicine, 313*, 84–95.
31. Franck, L. S. (1986). A new method to quantitatively describe pain behavior in infants. *Nursing Research, 35*, 28–31.
32. Fuller, B., Horii, Y., & Conner, D. (1988). Acoustic assessment of infant pain and arousal. In. *Key aspects of comfort: Pain, fatigue and nausea* (pp. 46–51): Springer.
33. Gadish, H. S., Gonzales, J. L., & Hayes, J. S. (1988). Factors affecting nurses' decisions to administer pediatric pain medication postoperatively. *Journal of Pediatric Nursing, 3*, 383–390.
34. Gardner, G. G., & Olness, K. (1981). *Hypnosis and Hypnotherapy with Children*. Orlando: Grune and Stratton.
35. Gertzbein, S. D., Tile, M., McMurty, R. Y., Kellom, J. F., Hunter, G. A., Keith, R. G., Harsanyi, Z., & Luffman, J. (1986). Analysis of the analgesic efficacy of acetaminophen 1000 mg, codeine phosphate 60 mg, and the combination of acetaminophen 1000 mg and codeine phosphate 60 mg in the relief of postoperative pain. *Pharmacotherapy, 6*, 104–107.
36. Glenski, J. A., Wainer, M. A., Dawson, B., & Kaufman, B. (1984). Postoperative use of epidurally administered morphine in children and adolescents. *Mayo Clinic Proceedings, 59*, 530–533.
37. Graves, D. A., Foster, T. S., Batenhorst, R. L., Bennett, R. L., & Baumann, T. J. (1983). Patient-controlled analgesia. *Annals of Internal Medicine, 99*, 360–366.
38. Harris, L. C., Rushton, C. H., & Hale, S. J. (1987). Implantable infusion devices in the pediatric patient: A viable alternative. *Journal of Pediatric Nursing, 3*, 174–183.

39. Hawley, D. D. (1984). Postoperative pain in children: Misconceptions, descriptions and interventions. *Pediatric Nursing, 10,* 20–23.

40. Hester, N. K. (1979). The preoperational child's reaction to immunization. *Nursing Research, 28,* 250–252.

41. Hilgard, J. R., & LeBaron, S. (1984). *Hypnotherapy of pain in children with cancer.* Los Altos, CA: William Kaufman.

42. Hockenberry, M., & Contach, P. (1985). Hypnosis as antiemetic therapy applications unique to children. *Nursing Clinics of North America, 20,* 105–107.

43. Howard-Ruben, J. (1985). Managing pain medications at home. *Oncology Nursing Forum, 12,* 78–82.

44. Inturrisi, C. E. (1987). Newer methods of opioid drug delivery. In *Refresher courses on pain management, book of abstracts* (pp. 27–39). Houston: International Association for the Study of Pain.

45. Ivey, K. J. (1983). Gastrointestinal effects of antipyretic analgesics. *American Journal of Medicine, 75,* 53–64.

46. Jaffe, J. H. (1975). Drug addiction and drug abuse. In L. S. Goodman, & A. Gilman (Eds.), *The pharmacologic basis of therapeutics* (5th ed.) (pp. 245–283). New York: Macmillan.

47. Jay, S. M., Ozolms, M., Elliot, C. H., & Caldwell, S. (1983). Assessment of children's distress during painful medical procedures. *Journal of Health Psychiatry, 2,* 133–147.

48. Johnson, J. E., & Rice, V. H. (1974). Sensory and distress components of pain: Implications for the study of clinical pain. *Nursing Research, 23,* 203–209.

49. Johnson, J. E. (1972). Effects of structuring patients expectations on their reactions to threatening events. *Nursing Research, 21,* 489–491.

50. Kaiko, R. F., Foley, K. M., Grabinski, P. U., Heidrich, G., Rogers, A., Intrussi, C. E., & Reidenberg, M. M. (1982). Central nervous system excitatory effects of meperidine in cancer patients. *Annals of Neurology, 13,* 180–185.

51. Kanner, R. M. (1987). Pharmacological management of pain and symptom control in cancer. *Journal of Pain Symptom Management, 2:* 19–22.

52. Katz, E. R., Kellerman, J., & Seigel, S. E. (1980). Behavioral distress in children undergoing medical procedures: Developmental considerations. *Journal of Consulting and Clinical Psychology, 48,* 356–365.

53. Kuttner, L. (1988). Favorite stories: a hypnotic pain-reduction technique for children in acute pain. *American Journal of Clinical Hypnosis, 30,* 289–295.

54. Lacouture, P. G., Gaudicault, P., & Lovejoy, F. H. (1984). Chronic pain of childhood: A pharmacologic approach. *Pediatric Clinics of North America, 31,* 1133–1151.

55. Lukacsko, P. (1987). A Guide to the parenteral management of moderate to severe pain. *Hospital Pharmacy, 22,* 361–364, 412.

56. Lukens, M. M. (1982). *The identification of criteria used by nurses in the assessment of pain in children.* Unpublished theses. University of Cincinnati.

57. Lunn, L. (1979). Postoperative analgesia after circumcision: A randomized comparison between caudal analgesia and IM morphine in boys. *Anaesthesia, 34,* 552–554.

58. Mandell, G. L., & Sande, M. A. (1980). Antimicrobial agents. In L. S. Goodman, A. G. Gilman, & A. Gilman (Eds.), *The pharmacological basis of therapeutics.* New York: MacMillan Publishing.

59. Mannheimer, J. S., & Lampe, G. N. (1984). *Clinical transcutaneous electrical nerve stimulation.* Philadelphia: F.A. Davis.

60. Mar, D. D. (1981). The narcotic analgesics. *American Journal of Nursing, 81,* 1364–1365.

61. Mar, D. D. (1981). The "simple" analgesics. *American Journal of Nursing, 81:* 1206–1208.

62. Marks, K. M., & Sachar, E. J. (1973). Undertreatment of medical in-patients with narcotic analgesics. *Annals of Internal Medicine, 78,* 173–181.

63. McCaffery, M. (1987). A practical "postable" chart of equianalgesic doses. *Nursing 87, 8,* 56–57.

64. McCaffery, M. (1987). Giving meperidine for pain—Should it be so mechanical? *Nursing 87, 4,* 61–64.

65. McCaffery, M. (1987). Patient-controlled analgesia—More than a machine. *Nursing 87, 1,* 63–64.

66. McCaffery, M. (1977). Pain relief for the child. *Pediatric Nursing, 3,* 11–16.

67. McCaffery, M. (1972). *Nursing management of the patient in pain.* Philadelphia: J.B. Lippincott.

68. McCaffery, M., & Hart, L. L. (1976). Undertreatment of acute pain with narcotics. *American Journal of Nursing, 76,* 1586–1591.

69. McGrath, P. A., DeVeber, L. L., & Hearn, M. T. (1985). Multidimensional pain assessment in children. In H.L. Fields, R. Dubner, & F. Cervero (Eds.), *Advances in pain research and therapy* (pp. 387–393). New York: Raven Press.

70. McGuire, L., & Dizard, S. (1982). Managing pain in the young patient. *Nursing 82, 12,* 52, 54–55.

71. McGuire, L., & Wright, A. (1984). Continuous narcotic infusion. *Nursing 84, 14,* 50–55.

72. Meinhart, N. T., & McCaffery, M. (1983). *Pain: A nursing approach to assessment and analysis.* Norwalk: Appleton-Century-Crofts.

73. Melzack, R. (1982). Recent concepts of pain. *Journal of Medicine, 13,* 147–160.

74. Melzack, R., & Wall, P. (1965). Pain mechanisms: A new theory. *Science, 150,* 971–979.

75. Melzack, R. L., & Torgeson, W. S. (1971). On the language of pain. *Anesthesiology, 34,* 50–55.

76. Miller, R. R., & Jick, H. (1978). Clinical effect of meperidine in hospitalized medical patients. *Journal of Clinical Pharmacology, 18,* 180–189.

77. Miser, A. W., Miser, J. S., & Clark, B. S. (1980). Continuous intravenous infusion of morphine sulfate for control of severe pain in children with terminal malignancy. *Journal of Pediatrics, 96,* 930–932.

78. Mountcastle, V. B. (1975). Pain and temperature sensibilities. In V. B. Mountcastle (Ed.), *Medical physiology.* St. Louis: C. V. Mosby.

79. National Institutes of Health. (1986). *The integrated approach to the management of pain: Consensus development statement.* Washington, D.C.: U.S. Government Printing Office.

80. O'Donnell, L., & Papciak, B. (1981). Continuous morphine infusion for controlling intractable pain. *Nursing 81, 11,* 69–72.

81. Owens, M. E., & Todd, E. H. (1984). Pain in infancy: Neonatal reaction to a heel lance. *Pain, 20,* 77–86.

82. Pageau, M. G., Mroz, W. T., & Coombs, D. W. (1985). New analgesic therapy: Relieves cancer pain without oversedation. *Nursing 85, 15,* 47–49.

83. Paice, J. A. (1987). New delivery systems in pain management. *Nursing Clinics of North America, 22,* 715–726.

84. Paice, J. A. (1986). Intrathecal morphine infusion for intractable cancer pain: A new use for implanted pumps. *Oncology Nursing Forum, 13,* 41–47.

85. Paice, J. A. (1984). Intrathecal morphine sulfate for intractable cancer pain. *Journal of Neurosurgical Nursing, 16,* 237–240.

86. Piaget, J. (1969). *The early growth and logic in the child.* New York: Norton.

87. Portenoy, R. K., & Foley, K. M. Chronic use of opioid analgesics in nonmalignant pain: Report of 38 cases. *Pain, 25,* 171–186.

88. Porter, J., & Jick, H. (1980). Addiction rare in patients treated with narcotics. *New England Journal of Medicine, 302,* 123.

89. Primm, P. L. (1971). *Identification of criteria used by nurses in the assessment of pain in children.* Unpublished thesis, University of Iowa.

90. Rahwan, G. L., & Rahwan, R. G. (1986). Aspirin and Reye's syndrome: The change in prescribing habits of health profes-

sionals. *Drug Intelligence and Clinical Pharmacy, 20*, 43–145.

91. Richlin, D. M., et al. (1987). Cancer pain control with a combination of methadone, amitriptyline, and non-narcotic analgesic therapy: A case series analysis. *Journal of Pain and Symptom Management, 2*, 89–94.

92. Schechter, N., Schecter, N., Hansen, K., & Allen, D. (1986). Status of pediatric pain control: A comparison of hospital analgesic usage in children and adults. *Pediatrics, 77*, 11–15.

93. Schroeder, P. (1983). *A descriptive study of pain associated with therapeutic procedures in the burned school-age child.* Unpublished thesis, University of Cincinnati.

94. Spinetta, J., & Deasy-Spinetta, P. (1981). *Living with childhood cancer.* St. Louis: CV Mosby.

95. Stevens, B., Hunsberger, M., & Browne, G. Pain in children: Theoretical, research, and practical dilemmas. *Journal of Pediatric Nursing, 2*, 154–165.

96. Stimmel, B. (1983). *Pain, analgesia and addiction: The pharmacologic treatment of pain.* New York: Raven Press.

97. Swafford, L. I., & Allen, D. (1968). Pain relief in the pediatric patient. *Medical Clinics of North America, 48*, 131–133.

98. Volpe, J. (1987). *Neurology of the newborn* (2nd ed.). Philadelphia: WB Saunders.

99. Vorchol, D. A. (1983). *The relationship between nurses' and children's perceptions of pain in the acute and chronic pain experiences of children.* Unpublished thesis, University of Cincinnati.

100. Wachter-Shikora, N. L. (1981). Pain theories and their relevance to the pediatric population. *Issues in Comprehensive Pediatric Nursing, 5*, 321–326.

101. Wall, P. D. (1978). The gate control theory of pain mechanisms: A reexamination and re-statement. *Brain, 101*, 1–18.

102. Webb, C. (1987). *Self-administration of pain medications by children.* Presented at the meeting of the Association for the Care of Children's Health. Halifax: Nova Scotia.

103. Williams, P. L., Ansell, B. M., Bell, A., Cain, A. R., Chamberlain, M. A., Clarke, A. K., Craft, A. W., Hollingworth, P., Keegan, D., and Roberts, S. D. (1986). Multicenter study of piroxican versus naproxen in juvenile chronic arthritis, with special reference to problem areas in clinical trials of nonsteroidal anti-inflammatory drugs in childhood. *British Journal of Rheumatology, 25*, 67–71.

104. Williamson, P., & Williamson, M. (1983). Physiological stress reduction by a local anesthetic during newborn circumcision. *Pediatrics, 71*, 36–40.

105. Wincek, J. (1988). The effects of auditory control measures on the physiological responses of children with cerebral edema. Personal communication.

106. Zollo, M. (1984). Management of pain in critically ill children. *MCN American Journal of Maternal Child Nursing, 9*, 258–261.

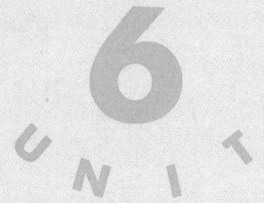

Nursing Care of Children in Life-Threatening Situations

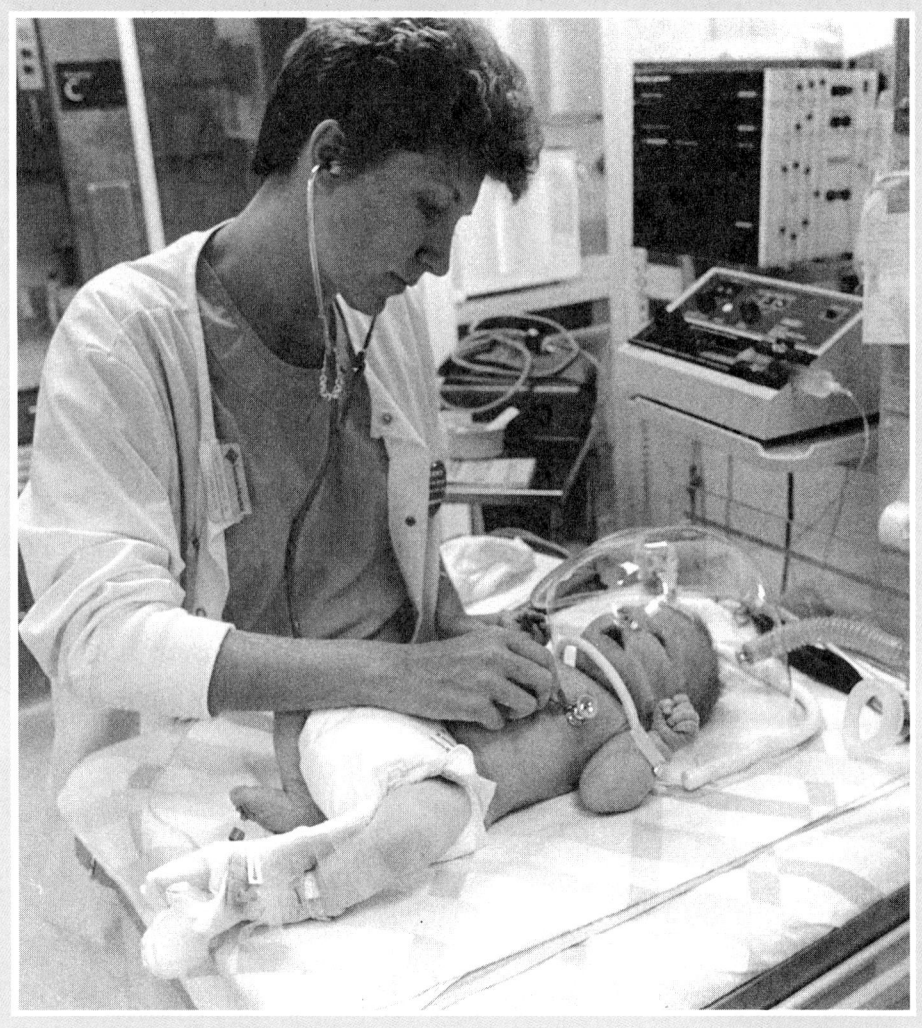

29 Childhood Emergencies

CHAPTER

BEHAVIORAL OBJECTIVES

Describe the roles of the nurse in emergency care and prevention.

List possible causes of fever in a child.

Describe nursing management of a child who is having a seizure.

Describe the different types of shock and priorities of care.

Describe recommendations for treating the child with an airway obstruction.

Identify the steps in performing cardiopulmonary resuscitation in the infant and child.

Identify ways to support the family of the child who dies of SIDS.

List common types of poisonings in children.

Describe important factors in monitoring vital signs in a child who is a near drowning victim.

Childhood emergencies account for at least 16 million emergency department (ED) visits per year, about 20% of all emergency room visits.[23] Although the majority of these visits are due to minor illnesses or emergencies, those that are due to life-threatening conditions are almost always caused by an accidental injury that could have been prevented. Accidents account for nearly half of all childhood deaths between ages 1 and 14 and cause thousands of children to be permanently disabled yearly.[24]

The type of pediatric patients seen in the ED has changed over the years. Different insurance reimbursement plans and diagnostic-related groups (DRGs) keep children who previously may have been hospitalized, out of the hospital. Many children are on home care programs and come to the ED for needed care. Therefore, children seen in the ED may be sicker and may require more care than in the past. Parents are also more knowledgeable and participate more in the decision-making process.

This chapter discusses the various roles of the nurse in caring for the child in the ED (Fig. 29-1). The nursing process is evident in all of these roles. Common childhood emergencies and the initial nursing assessment and care of children in the ED are presented in this chapter.

Roles of the ED Nurse

The roles of ED nurses are varied and include using assessment skills (triage); providing nursing care, coordinating this care, and evaluating care for various illnesses and injuries; and also providing emotional support and teaching. In addition to teaching children and parents, the ED nurse also has a teaching role with pre-hospital careproviders and other colleagues who may not routinely deal with children.

673

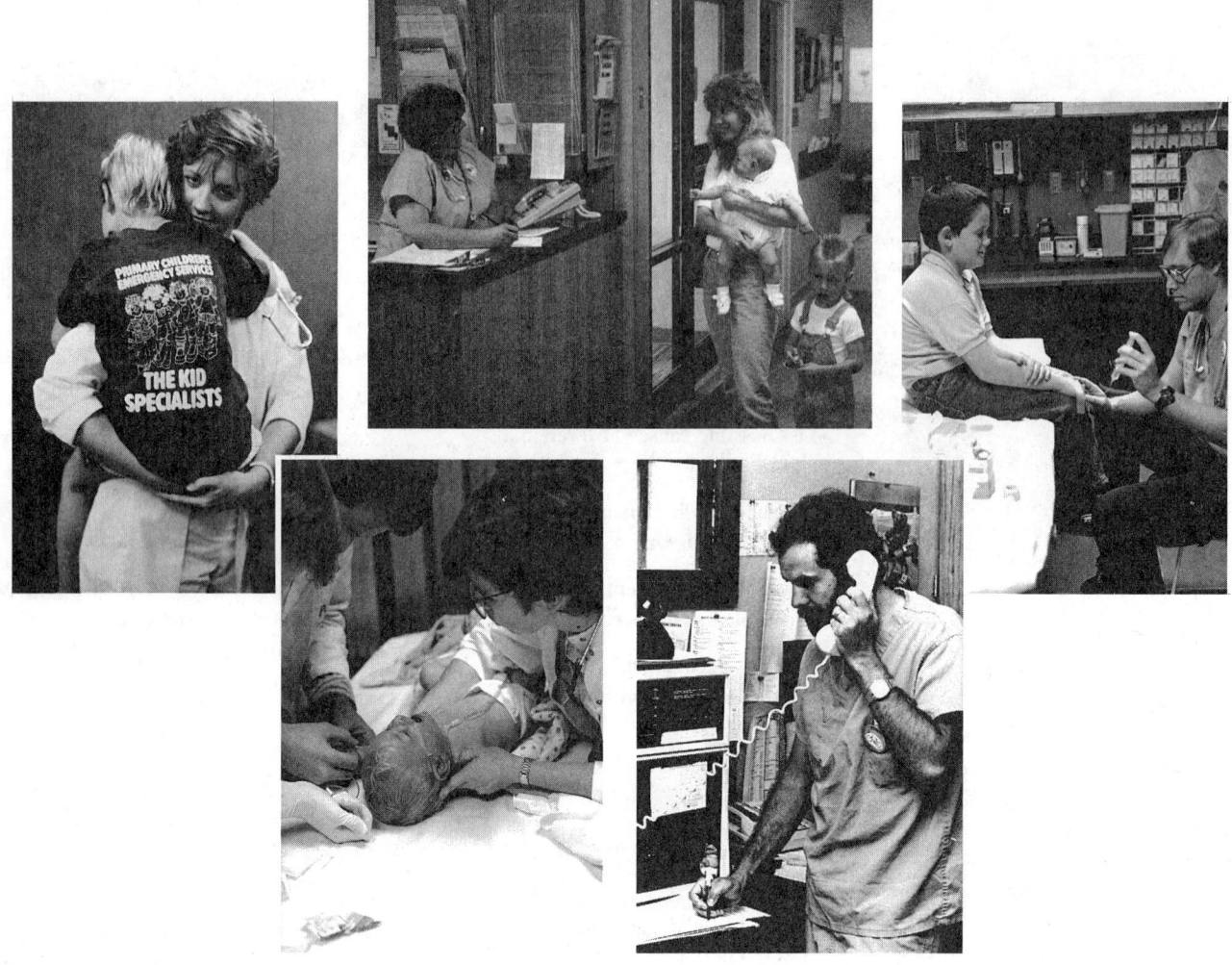

FIGURE 29-1

The emergency department nurse fills various roles. She remains calm as she initiates care in the ED and sets the tone for the visit. She gives emotional support and comfort. He provides hands-on interventions for minor and major emergencies. He coordinates care and communicates with nursing units, other departments, and other agencies. Gloves are now required for all procedures involving body substances. (Photo credits: *Top left,* Brad Husberg; *Right top and bottom,* Laurel Campbell; *Bottom left and center,* Primary Children's Medical Center, Salt Lake City, UT).

Assessment: Triage

Patient assessment in the ED usually begins with the triage nurse. Triage means "to sort." The triage nurse's role involves the immediate assessment of the child upon arrival and determination of the need for care. Ideally, the triage nurse is the first person to greet the family. The triage assessment always focuses first on airway, breathing, and circulation (the ABCs). (These are discussed in the section on Cardiopulmonary Arrest and in Chap. 30.) The triage nurse also assesses the child on the basis of the chief complaint and takes a brief history. The history should include the following:

- History of present illness and associated signs and symptoms
- Care given at home (antipyretics, other medications)
- Mechanism of injury, if applicable
- Past medical history, including the child's baseline condition, any medications child is taking
- Allergies and immunization status
- Usual source of medical care

The triage nurse must have experience in child health assessment and a knowledge of those conditions requiring immediate care. The accompanying display lists an approach to assessment of children. The primary assessment, consisting of evaluation of the ABCs and the neurologic exam, is usually completed in the triage area. Based on the findings of this examination and the history, the child is given a priority rating. Table 29-1 lists a common priority rating system used in EDs and examples of conditions for each. The secondary assessment consists of a head-to-toe examination and is completed once the child is taken to an examination room.

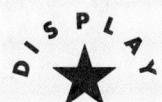

Nursing Assessment: Assessment Parameters for Physical Examination of Children in the Emergency Department*

Primary Assessment

General appearance:
  Grooming
  Activity level for age
  Interaction between parent and child
Airway and breathing: consider cervical spine injuries and maintain precautions where indicated
Signs and symptoms of respiratory distress

- Color: pale, mottled, or cyanotic
- Respiratory effort: use of accessory muscles, presence of nasal flaring or retractions
- Breath sounds: wheezing, rales, rhonchi, stridor
- Respiratory rate

Circulation
Signs and symptoms of compromised circulation

- Skin color and capillary refill time†
- Peripheral pulses
- Heart rate and blood pressure

Signs and symptoms of dehydration

- Sunken anterior fontanel
- Skin and mucous membrane turgor: moist or dry
- Presence of vomiting or diarrhea

Neurologic exam
  Pupillary responses
  Response to pain
  Movement of extremities
  Presence of seizure activity
  Vital signs: temperature, pulse, respiration (TPR), and blood pressure (BP). May be deferred to secondary assessment

Secondary Assessment

Head
  Presence of injuries
  Presence of pain or tenderness
Eyes
  Pupils: size and reaction to light
  Presence of tears
  Movement of eyes
  Drainage or periorbital swelling
  Presence of injuries
Ears
  Drainage
  Presence of pain
  Bruising behind ears (may indicate basal skull fracture)
Nose
  Nasal flaring (may indicate increased respiratory effort)
  Drainage
  Odor (foul odor may indicate presence of foreign body)
Throat: do not attempt to examine if the child is in severe respiratory distress
  Swelling or exudates in pharynx
  Swelling of cervical lymph nodes
Mouth
  Color of oral mucosa
  Lesions present
  Moistness of lips and mucous membranes
  Odor of breath
Chest
  Respiratory status as listed under primary assessment
  Presence of rashes or bruising
  Presence of tenderness
Abdomen
  Distention
  Bowel sounds
  Tenderness
Genitalia and rectum
  Diaper rash
  Vaginal discharge, irritation, or odor
  Rectal bleeding or tears
  Discharge from penis, presence of trauma
Skin and extremities: examine and compare extremities bilaterally
  Presence of swelling, deformities, or pain
  Movement
  Sensation
  Color
  Pulses
  Presence of rashes or bruising

* Although a primary assessment should be done on all children, the secondary assessment may be abbreviated depending on the child's chief complaint. The secondary examination is usually focused on the area of concern.
† Capillary refill time is measured by pressing on the child's forehead, or nailbeds of the fingers or toes to cause blanching, and observing how rapidly normal color returns (normal is less than 2 seconds).

The triage nurse may institute treatment, or diagnostic tests if protocols permit. For example, the nurse may give antipyretics to a febrile child, order an x-ray of a possible fracture, or collect urine for analysis in a child who has signs and symptoms of a urinary tract infection.

The triage nurse may be the first health care profes-
sional the child and family interact with in the hospital. The nurse needs to be calm and accepting and serve as a "public relations specialist," because this interaction sets the tone for the rest of the ED visit (see Fig. 29-1). If waiting is involved, the triage nurse must frequently reassess the child's condition and expedite care if nec-

TABLE 29-1
Triage Categories for Children in the Emergency Department

Category/Definition	Examples
Priority I—Emergent	
Children who have a condition that may result in loss of life or limb if not treated immediately	Bleeding
	Cardiopulmonary arrest
	Coma
Priority II—Urgent	
Children who require prompt care, but who will not be in danger of death or severe impairment if left untreated for a period of time, usually a few hours	Lacerations with no active bleeding
	Nondisplaced fractures without neurologic impairment
Priority III—Nonurgent	
Children who require treatment, but time is not a critical factor	Sore throat
	Flu symptoms
	Minor sprains

essary, or provide reassurance to the family that they have not been forgotten.

Provision and Coordination of Care

After a child is assessed by the triage nurse, he or she is taken to a treatment room. The patient care nurse does a complete assessment, which includes vital signs: temperature, pulse, respirations (TPR), and blood pressure (BP). These vital signs are an important part of the baseline assessment. All children need to be weighed, because dosages of medications and intravenous (IV) fluids are given on the basis of the child's weight. The weight of the child may need to be estimated if the child's condition makes it impossible to actually weigh him or her.

The nurse is involved in performing various procedures. These can range from routine tasks, such as giving injections, to life-saving measures, such as starting IVs and performing cardiopulmonary resuscitation (CPR). Although the nurse works in collaboration with the ED physician, he or she may need to recognize and initiate emergency care.

Examination and procedures have to be done in a way that takes into account the child's age and development. The nurse needs to explain all tests and procedures to the parents and encourage them to remain with the child as much as possible. The parents should not be asked to help restrain a child for a painful procedure, but should be encouraged to comfort the child while the procedure is being done. The nurse should also take a moment to comfort the child and help calm him or her (see Fig. 29-1).

The ED nurse is responsible for coordinating care of the child and family with other departments in the hospital, such as the laboratory, radiology, and pharmacy; and agencies outside the hospital, including prehospital careproviders, support groups, other hospitals, police or the department of family services (see Fig. 29-1). The

ED nurse may also communicate with inpatient nursing units to arrange admission to the hospital.

Provision of Emotional Support and Teaching

Emotional Support

Because there is usually little time to prepare a child for an ED visit, the ED nurse is faced with the challenge of dealing with a frightened child and distraught parents. Although the interaction may be brief, it affects the reactions of the parents and child to any future hospitalizations that may be necessary. Every child needs to be treated as an individual based on his or her stage of growth and development.

The nurse needs to include the parent as much as possible in the care of the child. The nurse also needs to listen to the parent, because he or she usually knows the child better than anyone else. Anything that affects the child affects the parent, and vice versa.

Especially in the midst of the clinical care, machines, and specialists, emotional needs of both the child and parent are overlooked. A busy ED is a frightening place to a small child. Offering a security object such as a familiar toy (Fig. 29-2) can do much to comfort the child. During a crisis situation, a social worker can be helpful in providing the parents with immediate support and acting as a liaison between them and the nursing and medical personnel. Often, referrals may be made to outside agencies to provide continued support after discharge.

Teaching

An important role of the ED nurse is child and parent teaching. Teaching in the ED setting may be difficult for

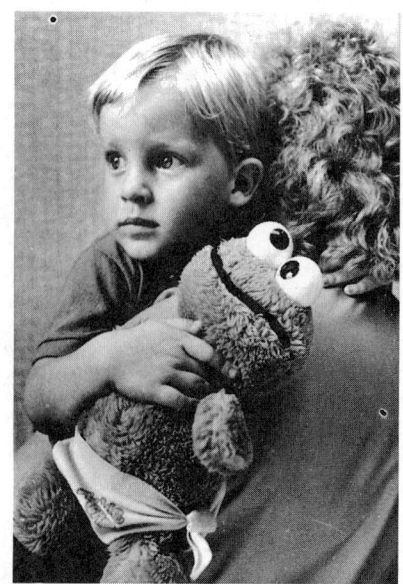

FIGURE 29-2
If a child has brought a favorite toy from home, let him keep it with him. If he does not have one, let him select a security object from the ED supply. (Photo courtesy of Primary Children's Medical Center, Salt Lake City, UT.)

several reasons. Parents are often anxious and experiencing a great deal of stress. Teaching may not be as effective, and the parents may not absorb the necessary information. Also, because of other patients, the nurse may be hurried. Because the time spent in the ED is short, there is often not enough time to develop the same nurse–patient relationship that can occur on inpatient units.

Teaching in the ED exists in several forms, including instructions about follow-up care for the present problem, general health care teaching, and anticipatory guidance.

Instructions for Follow-Up Care. Instructions for follow-up care are important. Many emergency patients have no source of routine medical care and may use the ED as their source of primary care. The nurse needs to assess the educational background of the parent and focus the teaching to this level (see Chap. 6).

The nurse should provide clear verbal instructions and give the parents a written copy of instructions to take home. The instructions should provide the hospital's phone number and the parents should be encouraged to call back if they have any concerns. In the pediatric population, noncompliance with prescribed medications has been documented to be 46%.[17,37] Many reasons may contribute to this lack of compliance, but one may be because parents are not given thorough instructions on the medication regimen. Because of liability involved in the ED, the nurse must thoroughly document all teaching on the nurse's notes.

General Health Care Teaching. During the history and physical assessment, the nurse has many opportunities to assess the need for and provide general health care teaching. For example, while taking a temperature, the nurse can give the mother instructions on how to use a thermometer (if appropriate) and methods of fever control. The nurse can also provide information on feeding and immunizations. Teaching before discharge, after the child has been treated, may be more appropriate because the parents may be calmer and more responsive.

Anticipatory Guidance. Anticipatory guidance is an important role of the ED nurse and must include discussing injury prevention. Parents often feel a sense of guilt and are often eager to learn how to prevent future injuries. Teaching is based on the current level of development of the child and the parent's level of understanding.

Fever

Fever is usually defined as an elevation in normal body temperature, which is generally 97°F to 99°F. (36°C to 37.2°C) orally and one degree higher rectally. Fever is included in this chapter because it is one of the most common chief complaints of parents bringing a child to the ED.

Pathophysiology

Body temperature is regulated by the hypothalamus. When temperature changes occur, centrally and periph-

erally located receptors relay information to the hypothalamus, which either increases or decreases heat production to maintain a constant "set point" temperature. During an infection, pyrogenic substances cause an increase in the body's normal set point. The hypothalamus increases heat production until the core temperature reaches the new set point.

Although children can develop fever for a variety of reasons, most fevers are caused by a viral infection, such as upper respiratory infections, gastroenteritis, croup, cytomegalovirus, and aseptic meningitis.

Fevers over 104°F (40°C) are more likely to be caused by a bacterial infection, especially if the child is younger than 3 months of age. *Bacterial infections* include bacteremia, cellulitis, meningitis, osteomyelitis, otitis media, pneumonia, pyelonephritis, shigellosis, and urinary tract infections.

Other less common causes of fever may be *collagen vascular diseases*, such as Schönlein-Henoch purpura, juvenile rheumatoid arthritis, lupus erythematosus, and rheumatic fever; *drug intoxication (accidental or intentional)* by amphetamines, atropine, phenothiazines, PCP, or salicylates; or *malignancies*, such as Hodgkin's lymphoma, leukemia, neuroblastoma, or sarcoma.

Fever in children younger than 3 months of age is of greater concern because these children may have no other signs and symptoms of illness, have decreased immunities, and are difficult to assess. The fever may be the only symptom of a serious illness. If other symptoms are present, they may be nonspecific, such as irritability or decreased appetite.

Although the fever is not harmful to the child, it does have some adverse effects that make fever reduction desirable. Table 29-2 lists these effects and nursing implications.

Nursing Assessment and Intervention

The nurse should take a thorough history to determine any change in activity, elimination, eating habits, exposure to illness, and recent immunizations. The nurse should also assess activity level, hydration status, and the presence of other signs and symptoms such as vomiting, diarrhea, lethargy, rashes, cough, congestion, or increased irritability.

Nursing care of a child with fever as discussed in the Nursing Care Plan includes fever reduction methods, helping to determine the cause of the fever, and ruling out serious causes such as meningitis or sepsis. Independent nursing functions to reduce fever include promoting fluid intake, undressing the child, or giving a tepid sponge bath. Collaborative care may include administering IV fluids to replace losses; assisting with laboratory procedures such as drawing blood for complete blood count (CBC), electrolytes and blood cultures; and lumbar puncture to rule out meningitis. Diagnostic tests are performed on the basis of the child's age, appearance, and symptoms. In general, all children younger than 3 months of age with a fever have a lumbar puncture done to rule out meningitis, because fever may be the only symptom of a more serious condition. Antipyretics are usually ordered to reduce the fever. Acetaminophen is the drug of choice because of aspirin's association with Reye's syn-

TABLE 29-2
Effects of Fever on the Child

Effect	Implications	Nursing Interventions

Increased metaboilc rate
  Increased heart rate
  Increased respiratory rate
  Increased fluid and caloric requirements
	The child already has a higher metabolic rate than an adult. The further increase causes increased water loss due to the increased respiratory rate. Therefore, there is an increased chance of dehydration.	Encourage fluids
		Assess for signs and symptoms of dehydration
		Give antipyretics as ordered by physician to reduce fever
		Undress child
		Give tepid sponge bath for fever > 104°F (40°C)

Decreased seizure threshold	Increased likelihood of febrile seizures in some children	Anticipate possibility of seizures Discuss any family history of seizures If seizure occurs: Protect from injury Loosen clothing Turn on side to prevent aspiration Provide oxygen by mask
Increased irritability	The child may be more difficult to assess due to the effects of the fever	Administer antipyretics as ordered

drome. The usual dose of acetaminophen is 15 mg/kg. Liquid preparations of ibuprofen are available and used for children who do not respond to acetaminophen.

Sponging with tepid water may be used for temperatures above 104°F (40°C). Shivering should be avoided because it represents the body's effort to conserve heat and may result in a further increase in temperature. Parents should be encouraged not to use alcohol sponge baths because alcohol intoxication caused by absorption and inhalation may result.

Anticipatory Guidance

The nurse needs to provide instruction to the parent about fever control and the use of a thermometer, and to evaluate the understanding of these instructions. Parents should also be questioned about their understanding of the fever, because they may have misconceptions about fever and its effects on the child. For example, parents may believe that the fever is harmful to the child and will cause brain damage, blindness, or even sterility. Parents need to be reassured that the fever is not harmful unless it is above 106°F (41°C) for prolonged periods of time. See the Teaching Plan for teaching a parent how to care for a child with a fever.

Seizures

Seizures are among the most common neurologic problems in children seen in the ED. Between 4% and 6% of all children have at least one seizure in the first 16 years of life.[27]

Seizures are defined as a paroxysmal disturbance in nerve cells resulting in abnormalities in motor, sensory, autonomic, or psychic function. Causes of seizures in children are listed in Table 29-3.

Because febrile seizures are the most common cause of seizures seen in the ED, they are discussed in detail in this chapter. For a discussion of other causes and clas-

sifications of seizures and seizure disorders, see Chapter 53.

Febrile Seizures

Febrile seizures are usually defined as seizures associated with fever and without evidence of intracranial infection or a known seizure disorder.[14] Febrile seizures occur in 3% to 5% of all children between the ages of 3 months and 6 years, but most commonly occur between the ages of 1 and 3 years. The incidence of febrile seizures is twice as high in males as in females, and genetic factors are thought to be involved.

Pathophysiology

The causes of febrile seizures are unknown, but are thought to be related to the immaturity of the child's central nervous system. The height and rapidity of the rise in temperature seem to be factors, as well as a positive family history. The younger the child is at the time of the seizure, the greater the possibility of future problems, such as recurrence of the seizure. About one third of all children have a recurrence of the seizure in a subsequent illness.[29] Factors that put a child at risk for a recurring seizure include:[29]

- Previous abnormal neurologic status
- Complex seizure
  - Duration over 15 minutes
  - Focal (involving one side or area of the body)
  - Recurrent within 24 hours
- Family history of seizures
- Age at onset less than 6 months

Nursing Assessment and Intervention

Most febrile seizures are brief in duration, and the child is no longer having seizure activity upon arrival to the ED. The nursing history should include the following:

(text continued on page 682)

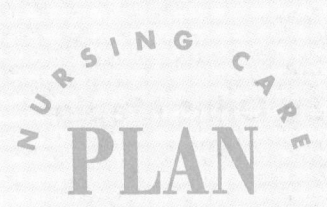

A Child With Fever Caused by Otitis Media

Assessment

Case Study Description

Sharon H. is a 10-month-old female brought to the Emergency Department with a reported rectal temperature of 40.0°C (104°F). According to Sharon's mother, a single parent with two other children, the baby has been irritable and refusing fluids. She has been up all night crying. Ms. H. first noted the temperature at 0300. Sharon has no other medical problems and has not begun her immunizations. She is on no medications. Sharon has had no other signs and symptoms of illness. Ms. H. has not given the baby any antipyretics. She expresses concern that the baby will be damaged by the fever and "take seizures." Her oldest daughter experienced a febrile seizure at age 18 months.

Ms. H. is unemployed, does not have a regular source of medical care for her children, and is on public assistance. She appears tired and admits having no close support system to help with her children. The father of the children lives out of the state and does not provide child support.

Assessment Data

On exam, Sharon is asleep, her color is pink, and she is tachypneic. She is clean and appears well-cared for.

Vital signs are: Temperature 39°C, rectally, pulse 160, respiratory rate 60, BP 98/60.

Her anterior fontanel is soft, and her skin is warm and dry to touch. No rashes are noted on the skin, and the skin turgor is normal. Her lips and mucous membranes are moist to touch.

Baby Sharon responds to the exam by awakening, pulling away, crying, and clinging to her mother.

Nursing Diagnosis	Intervention	Rationale
1. Altered body temperature 2. Discomfort related to fever 3. High risk for injury related to possibility of febrile seizures *Supporting Data:* • Rectal temperature is 39°C • History given by mother indicates temperature has been elevated for at least 24 hr • Sharon appears uncomfortable and irritable • Family history of febrile seizures	Give child 15 mg/kg of acetaminophen (collaborative action—usually requires physician's order, unless standing orders exist)	Reducing the fever will allow the baby to be examined easier. Because there is a history of febrile seizures in this child's family, the temperature should be reduced. Reducing the temperature will also reduce the child's metabolic oxygen requirements and lower the heart and respiratory rate. Because the increased respiratory rate also contributes to increased water loss, lowering the temperature may help to prevent dehydration. The analgesic effect of the acetaminophen will help to make the child more comfortable, also.
	Remove all clothing except for diaper. If the child's fever was above 40°C, sponging with tepid water might reduce fever	Removing clothing allows body heat to evaporate
	Observe Baby Sharon for any seizure activity. Don't leave her unattended	Although febrile seizures occur with increased temperatures, they usually occur during the initial rise in temperature. Mother needs reassurance that the nursing staff are aware of her concerns.

(Continued)

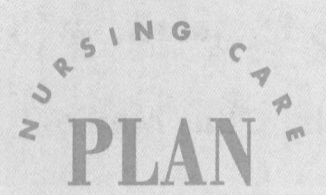

A Child With Fever Caused by Otitis Media
(continued)

Nursing Diagnosis	*Intervention*	*Rationale*
4. High risk for fluid volume deficit *Supporting Data:* • Sharon has had decreased intake of fluids for more than 24 h • Fever also increases fluid losses through evaporation and water loss through increased respiratory rate.	Provide oral fluids in the form of an electrolyte solution Encourage intake	The child does not appear dehydrated, so encouraging PO fluids will help replace fluid losses. An electrolyte solution (Gatorade, Pedialyte) is best to replace losses. If clinical dehydration was present, intravenous replacement as ordered by physician, may be necessary.

Thirty minutes after receiving 15 mg/kg of acetaminophen, Sharon's temperature dropped to 38°C, rectally. She eagerly took 8 oz of an electrolyte solution and became much more interactive. Her respiratory rate was 36, and her heart rate was 128. Examination by physician revealed an acute otitis media, and the child was given a prescription for amoxicillin. A routine complete blood count was done, which was normal. Because of her response to the antipyretic and her lack of neurologic symptoms indicating possible meningitis, the physician elected to not perform a lumbar puncture.

5. Knowledge deficit regarding fever control and meaning of fever *Supporting Data:* • Mother does not know measures for reducing fever. • Mother worries that her child will be injured by the fever. • Mother states concern about the possibility of her child having a seizure.	Provide teaching about fever control and febrile seizures (see Teaching Plan in this chapter) Arrange for follow-up care at ED clinic or other clinic Make appointment for mother, and make sure she understands importance of follow-up, as well as written instructions indicating time and place	
6. High risk for altered parenting *Supporting Data:* • Mother at risk because she has no support system and is a single parent. • Mother is tired and has no help with her three children. • Mother currently unemployed and on medical assistance.	Provide names of agencies for mother to call if she feels she needs to "get away" from her children for a while. Many communities offer a child care service for mothers in such a situation. Spend time discussing her concerns and explore other ways (support groups, neighbors, and so forth) that she may find help. Refer mother to pediatrics clinic for low-income families.	ED should have written instructions to give to families about treatment of common childhood injuries. These should be reviewed with family and given to them to take home. Teaching needs to be geared to the mother's concerns, questions, and level of understanding. Mother does not have a regular source of medical care. This child has not had immunizations, and they need to be started. The mother needs a regular source of medical care and one that she can afford.

Sharon's mother returned to the ED clinic for a recheck. Sharon's ears were completely healed, and she appeared healthy. Ms. H. stated that she has an appointment at the health department to obtain immunizations for Sharon. Mother also has become involved in a support group for single mothers and is looking for employment. She plans to obtain future medical care at the ED clinic.

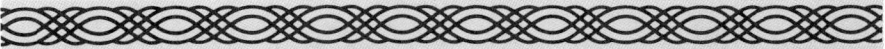

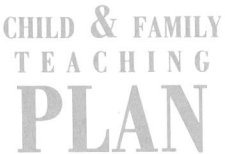

CHILD & FAMILY
T E A C H I N G
PLAN

Care During Childhood Fever

Assessment:

Ten-month-old Sharon diagnosed with acute otitis media. Has had fever for 24 h. She has no other known illnesses. Mother has not used antipyretics and does not seem to understand the meaning of fever and measures used to reduce it.

This mother is a single parent with two other children. She has no family living near her to help. She is on public asssistance. She has a high school education and says she does know how to read a thermometer "unless it is in centigrade."

This mother acknowledges that she does not know how to use fever control measures and thinks that she might have some aspirin at home. An older child experienced a febrile seizure, and while the mom is concerned about this, she is not able to give a good explanation to the nurse about the cause of the seizure, or what to do if another one should occur either in the same child or in Sharon.

Child and Family Objectives	*Specific Content*	*Teaching Strategies*
1. Discuss the meaning of fever.	1. Fever definition and its effects on the body, both behavioral and physiologic. Describe the meaning of fever and its relationship to infection.	1. Use written material—"What is a Fever?"
2. Demonstrate the use of a thermometer.	2. Taking a rectal temperature using a rectal thermometer.	2. Demonstrate technique on baby; have mother repeat the demonstration.
	Difference between rectal and oral thermometer.	
	Lubrication (K-Y, Vaseline).	
	Demonstrate how far to insert thermometer.	
	Show how to restrain baby while taking temperature.	
	Instruct on amount of time to keep thermometer in rectum	
	Demonstrate reading of both Centigrade and Fahrenheit thermometers.	Use drawings or actual thermometer to demonstrate readings. Provide mother with conversion chart: Centigrade to Fahrenheit.
3. Describe methods of fever control.	3. Undress child and bathe if temperature over 104°F; discuss proper temperature of bath water.	3. Demonstrate how to bathe child properly for fever control.
	Encourage fluids.	
	Acetaminophen—discuss proper dose with mother and discuss various preparations. Discourage use of aspirin.	Use written handout.

(Continued)

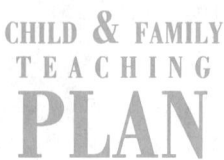

CHILD & FAMILY TEACHING PLAN

Care During Childhood Fever (continued)

Child and Family Objectives	*Specific Content*	*Teaching Strategies*
4. Describe conditions that require taking the child to see a physician.	4. Conditions requiring physician's care: • Child appears ill, cries constantly, or seems to be in pain. • Child has fever above 104°F that will not go down. • Child has frequent or forceful vomiting. • Child refuses to drink and looks dehydrated. • Child has difficulty breathing. • Child has a febrile seizure. • Child has a fever of more than 101°F and is less than 6 mo of age.	4. Use written handout. Encourage mother to call physician whenever she is concerned about child. Give Emergency department number.
5. Define febrile seizure.	5. How child acts in a seizure. Causes of a febrile seizure.	5. Discuss febrile seizures and allow mother to ask questions. Use handouts.
6. Discuss interventions for a febrile seizure.	6. Actions: • Put child on stomach with head turned to one side. • Don't put anything in child's mouth. • Call physician if seizure lasts more than 5 or 10 min. Call paramedics if the child is not breathing.	6. Use handout and allow mother to ask questions. Reassure mother that the seizures rarely will damage the brain. Encourage mother to call the ED or clinic if she has questions.

Evaluation:

- Sharon's mother defines fever and febrile seizure.
- Mother demonstrates use and reading of the thermometer.
- Mother states correct dosage of acetaminophen for her children.
- Mother demonstrates use of other methods of fever control.
- Mother identifies the correct interventions to take if her child has a febrile seizure.
- Mother recalls emergency phone numbers to call for help.
- Mother returns for follow-up.

- Events preceding the seizure: change in facial expression, cry
- Body movement: focal (affecting only one side of the body) or generalized (affecting the entire body)
- Color: presence of cyanosis
- Eyes: pupillary changes
- Respiratory changes: apnea, gasping
- Incontinence of urine or stool

If the child is still experiencing a seizure upon arrival to the ED, the nurse should also observe for the above criteria. Nursing interventions focus on maintaining airway, breathing, and circulation, and protecting the child from injury during the seizure activity. Table 29-4 lists nursing diagnoses and appropriate nursing interventions for the child who is experiencing a seizure.

Seizures that are prolonged (greater than 15 to 30 minutes) are termed *status epilepticus*. The physician may order an anticonvulsant drug to stop the seizure. Drugs commonly used to treat status epilepticus are listed in Table 29-5. Most of these drugs can cause respiratory depression, so the nurse must have airway equipment (oxygen, bag-mask, intubation equipment, suction) ready to assist with ventilation.

TABLE 29-3
Common Causes of Seizures in Different Age Groups

Neonatal (Birth to 28 Days)	Infancy (1 Month to 3 Years)	Childhood and Adolescence
Asphyxia	Chronic conditions continuing from neonatal period	Chronic conditions continuing from earlier age group
Intracranial hemorrhage		
Electrolyte disorders	Infections	Infections
Hypocalcemia	Meningitis	Meningitis
Hypomagnesemia	Encephalitis	Encephalitis
Hypoglycemia	Trauma	Trauma
Hyponatremia/hypernatremia	Neoplasms	Neoplasms
Infection	Drug overdose: Tricyclic antidepressants, lidocaine	Degenerative disorders
Intrauterine		Poisonings
Postnatal	Degenerative disorders	Genetic disorders
Congenital central nervous system disorders	Breath-holding spells	Idiopathic
	Idiopathic	
Inborn errors of metabolism		
Drug withdrawal		
Accidental injection of anesthetic		

Adapted from Holmes, G. (1987). *Diagnosis and management of seizures in children*, p. 5. Philadelphia: Saunders.

In all children, the possibility of serious infection, such as meningitis, needs to be ruled out. The physician orders appropriate diagnostic tests to help determine the cause of the seizure. The majority of fevers that cause seizures result from a viral infection.[32]

Anticipatory Guidance

A seizure is a frightening occurrence to parents. The nurse needs to provide them with information on recurrence and antipyretic therapy, as well as measures to take if the seizure recurs. The physician may prescribe continued anticonvulsant therapy based on the type and duration of the seizure and other factors that would put the child at risk for a recurrence. The nurse needs to evaluate the family's understanding of the medication, its side-effects, and any follow-up care that is necessary. This may include consultation with a neurologist and an electroencephalogram (EEG). The importance of this follow-up needs to be stressed.

Parents need to be reassured that their child can lead a normal, productive life. Parents also need to be instructed on safety measures, such as preventing injury during seizures and supervising the child while he or she bathes or is near any water.

Shock

Shock is a clinical syndrome of acute failure to perfuse tissues due to a complex state of circulatory dysfunction. Shock is generally categorized into three different types, based on etiology. These types are listed and defined in Table 29-6.

Pathophysiology

Just as in adults, the cardiac output in a child is determined by the heart rate and stroke volume (cardiac output equals heart rate times the stroke volume) or the volume of blood available at end diastole for the next contraction. Therefore, anything that affects the heart rate and stroke volume also affects cardiac output. A decrease in heart rate, most commonly caused by hypoxia in the child, or a decrease in stroke volume caused by blood or fluid loss decreases cardiac output.

TABLE 29-4
Nursing Diagnoses and Nursing Interventions for the Child Experiencing a Seizure

Nursing Diagnosis	Nursing Intervention
High Risk for injury	Protect child
	Remove restrictive clothing
	Remove objects
	Place child on floor if sitting
	Don't put objects in child's mouth
Ineffective Airway Clearance	Position child on side to prevent aspiration
High Risk for Aspiration	Have suction equipment available
Ineffective Breathing Pattern	Assess respiratory status during seizure
	Provide oxygen by mask
Altered Cerebral Tissue Perfusion	As above: observe for color changes
Altered Body Temperature: Hyperthermia	Give antipyretics, as directed by physician, after seizure has stopped

TABLE 29-5
Drugs Used to Stop Seizure Activity

Drug and Initial Dose/Route	Precautions/Nursing Implications*
Phenobarbital 10–20 mg/kg IV	Observe for hypotension and respiratory depression
	Dilute with an equal amount of IV fluid; rate not to exceed 1 mg/kg min
Diazepam (Valium) 0.1–0.2 mg/kg	Observe for respiratory depression
	Give slow IV push
	Have bag and mask ready to provide respiratory support if needed
	Very caustic, avoid infiltration
	Make sure IV is patent before administering
Lorazepam (Ativan) 0.05–0.1 mg/kg IV	Same precautions as Valium
	May be preferred over Valium because less caustic to tissue, greater duration of action than Valium
Phenytoin (Dilantin) 15 mg/kg IV up to 1 g	May cause venous irritation, hypotension
	Give at a rate of 50 mg/min
	Hot packs to infusion site may reduce irritation after infusion
	Will precipitate when infused with glucose solution
Paraldehyde 0.3 ml/kg in oil, rectally	Do not give IV
	May cause respiratory depression

* General precautions for administering all anticonvulsant drugs include:
• Don't mix medications: dilute with normal saline. Don't give as a continuous infusion.
• Be ready for respiratory depression: have necessary equipment to support the airway at the child's bedside (oxygen, bag, mask, intubation equipment).
• Place child on cardiac monitor and oxygen saturation monitor.
• Monitor vital signs before and after administration of medication.

Data from Ferry, P., Banner, W., & Wolf, R. (1986). *Seizure disorders in children*, pp. 176–190. Philadelphia: Lippincott.

When cardiac output drops, many physiologic compensatory mechanisms take over. In early stages of shock, the child experiences tachycardia due to depressed vagal activity and increased sympathetic activity. This increased sympathetic activity also causes vasoconstriction, which increases peripheral vascular resistance and increases diastolic pressure.

In an effort to conserve body fluids, large amounts of catecholamines, antidiuretic hormone, adrenocorticoids, and aldosterone are released. Available blood is shunted away from the skin, kidneys, muscles, and splanchnic beds to maintain blood flow to the brain and heart. Therefore, other symptoms that may be apparent in early stages of shock are decreased capillary refill and cool, pale, extremities. Oliguria, or decreased urine output, is generally a late sign of shock due to the ability of a child's kidneys to compensate for extended periods of time. Anxiety and irritability due to hypoxia and decreased perfusion to the brain may be apparent.

As shock progresses, oxygen depletion causes the body to resort to anaerobic metabolism, which leads to lactic acidosis. At this stage, tachypnea may be present because the lungs try to compensate by blowing off excess carbon dioxide. The child may appear stuporous or confused due to increasing hypoxia.

In late or uncompensated shock, compensatory mechanisms may fail and hypotension may be apparent for the first time. Blood volume may be further depleted as plasma fluid enters the tissues. In this stage of shock, the child may be comatose and may require mechanical ventilation.

Circulatory alterations occur in all types of shock, but may be slightly different in distributive shock caused by anaphylaxis, sepsis, and spinal cord injury (neurogenic shock). In anaphylaxis and neurogenic shock, vascular tone is interrupted either by the antigen–antibody reactions or injury. This loss of vascular tone produces widespread vasodilation, pooling of blood, and loss of effective circulating blood volume. Due to the vasodilation, the child's skin feels warm instead of cold and clammy. In septic shock, the alteration in vascular tone and increased permeability is caused by bacterial endotoxins. In early stages of septic shock, cardiac output may be normal or increased because of vasodilation in infected tissues and the increased basal metabolic rate caused by the fever. In later stages, cardiac output cannot be maintained. Disseminated intravascular coagulation (DIC) can develop because of degenerating tissues or bacterial toxins. Signs and symptoms of DIC include bleeding from various sites such as venipunctures and body orifices, and the presence of a petechial rash. A petechial rash consists of small, pinpoint, reddish-purple lesions that look like bruises, and always indicates a serious condition.

Because children can compensate for longer periods of time in the stages of early shock, they may not appear

TABLE 29-6
Types of Shock and Causes

Causes	Examples
Hypovolemic Shock	
Blood loss	Trauma (external or internal) with uncontrolled bleeding
	Nontraumatic GI or GU bleeding
Fluid/electrolyte loss	Vomiting, diarrhea, diabetic ketoacidosis, heat stroke
Plasma loss: "capillary leak"	Sepsis, burns, peritonitis, acidosis, anaphylaxis, hypoxia, hypothermia
Distributive Shock	
Abnormalities in the distribution of blood flow	Sepsis (early), drug ingestions
Neurogenic shock—reduced vascular resistance and pooling of blood resulting in interruption of mechanisms that control vascular tone	Spinal cord or major brainstem injury
Cardiogenic Shock	
Abnormalities in cardiac function that result in failure of the cardiovascular system to meet metabolic needs	Myocarditis, cardiomyopathy, drugs, congenital heart disease, myocardial infarction, chronic anemia
Inflow and outflow obstructions. This type of shock is often classified as "obstructive shock"	Tension pneumothorax, cardiac tamponade due to trauma or infections. Pericarditis, pulmonary or air embolism

Data from American Heart Association. (1986). Standards and guidelines for cardiopulmonary ressuscitation and emergency cardiac care. *Journal of the American Medical Association, 255*, 2961; and Perry, A., & Potter, P. (1983). *Shock—Comprehensive/nursing management*. St Louis: Mosby.

to be seriously ill initially. The accompanying display reviews the differences between children and adults that need to be considered when assessing a child for shock.

Types of Shock Seen in the ED

Hypovolemic Shock

Hypovolemic shock is the most common type of shock seen in the pediatric patient. Traumatic injury and internal bleeding are the main causes. The internal abdominal organs are not as well protected as in an adult and are often injured. Trauma is discussed in detail in Chapter 30.

Children have a larger blood volume per kilogram of body weight, but less total volume than an adult. Therefore, a child may develop hypovolemic shock from a seemingly minor injury such as a bleeding scalp laceration that would not be significant in an adult. Children also have increased extracellular fluid, and a greater percentage of their total body weight is water. They can quickly develop shock from increased fluid losses from vomiting and diarrhea.

Septic Shock

Septic shock is a serious and fairly common disease in both children and adults. About 100,000 deaths occur annually due to this rapidly progressive type of shock.[33]

Septic shock is usually caused by a gram-negative endotoxin. Impaired cellular metabolism occurs early, and the invasive organism triggers many different patient responses, which may lead to widely deranged cellular and metabolic function and circulatory collapse. Septic shock often occurs in immunocompromised children, including neonates and those with diseases such as leukemia and congenital heart disease. Children with extensive burns and multiple traumas may develop septic shock later in the course of their illness. However, septic shock can develop in children who were previously healthy and can rapidly progress to death.

Anaphylactic Shock

Anaphylactic shock results from the interaction of an allergen and a patient who is hypersensitive to it.[38] The symptoms result from the antigen–antibody reaction, which releases chemical mediators that influence target organ systems. The primary mediator is histamine, which causes vasodilation, bronchoconstriction, and increased capillary permeability. Shock can result from the vasodilation, which creates a sudden inadequacy of circulating volume to meet metabolic needs. Increased capillary permeability causes further loss of volume into the interstitial space. Anaphylactic shock can be rapidly fatal if not recognized and treated. Anaphylaxis in the form of urticaria or hives frequently presents in the ED. Laryngeal edema may be present and can rapidly progress to respiratory distress and cardiac arrest.

Anaphylaxis can be caused by injections of drugs such as penicillin, analgesics, anesthetics (particularly lidocaine, which is used commonly in the ED), or vaccines. Radiologic contrast media, usually iodine-based, are used to enhance a computed tomography (CT) scan, and can also cause anaphylaxis in sensitive people. Reactions caused by this type of agent often occur in hospitals and may be avoided by asking parents if their child has had any prior reactions to such agents.

Ingestions of drugs, particularly antibiotics, and foods such as citrus fruits, milk products, sesame seeds, shellfish, bananas, egg whites, and nuts are also common causes of anaphylaxis. Bites and stings are causes of anaphylaxis usually seen in warm climates and during summer months. Types of bites depend on the geographic location and include bees, wasps, and hornets.

Signs and symptoms of anaphylactic shock are listed in Table 29-7. Signs and symptoms can occur within minutes of the exposure. Usually, the earlier the onset of symptoms is, the more severe the reaction.

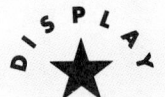

Nursing Assessment: Differences Between Children and Adults in Shock

- The basal metabolic rate (BMR) is higher in a child; therefore there already are increased oxygen, caloric, and glucose requirements.
- Vital signs vary considerably with the age of the child.
- The cardiovascular system in a child is generally more healthy and better able to compensate and maintain perfusion to the central circulation. The cardiac reserve in an infant and young child is less than that of a healthy adult; even in the absence of stress, the young heart must function near peak performance just to satisfy normal metabolic demands.

- Early signs and symptoms of shock may be harder to recognize in the child because children compensate better and may not be able to verbalize.
- The most common causes of shock in the child are trauma, hypoxia, and infection: in the adult, the most common causes are myocardial infarction and trauma.
- Drug therapy is more complex due to dosing based on weight.

Data from Pediatric advanced life support manual. *(1988). Salt Lake City, UT: Primary Children's Medical Center.*

TABLE 29-7
Nursing Assessment: Signs and Symptoms of Shock in the Child

Signs and Symptoms	Cause of Symptom	Signs and Symptoms	Cause of Symptom
Early Hypovolemic Shock		**Late Septic Shock**	
Tachycardia	Earliest sign of shock in the child	Tachypnea	Late signs and symptoms are related to cardiac insufficiency, acidosis
	Indicates the heart's attempt to increase cardiac output by increasing rate of contractions	Respiratory depression	
		Hypothermia	
		Cool, pale extremities	
Increased capillary refill time (measured by applying pressure to the nailbeds, releasing, and timing the return of circulation). Normal is 2–3 s.	Due to shunting of blood away from skin to heart and brain	Decreased peripheral pulses	
		Prolonged capillary refill	
		Hypotension	
Cool, pale extremities	Same as above	Oliguria	
Thready, weak peripheral pulses		Lethargy or coma	
Anxiety, irritability	Due to hypoxia. Also hard to distinguish from child's fear and reaction to strange environment	**Anaphylactic Shock**	
		Localized signs and symptoms:	Result from increased capillary permeability and movement of fluid from the vascular to the extravascular space
		Apprehension	
Progressive Hypovolemic Shock (Decompensating)		Light-headedness	
Tachypnea	Metabolic acidosis due to anaerobic metabolism	Edema of lips, tongue, eyes	
		Urticaria/hives	
	Lung's attempt to rid the body of increased carbon dioxide	Respiratory symptoms:	Due to bronchospasm and laryngeal edema
		Wheezing	
Confusion, Stupor	Due to increasing hypoxia	Dyspnea, air hunger	
		Cardiovascular symptoms:	
Uncompensated Hypovolemic Shock (Frank Shock)		Hypotension	Due to vasodilation and increased capillary permeability leading to decreased circulating blood volume
Hypotension	May be the earliest phase at which a decrease in systolic blood pressure is detectable. By this time, child may have lost 30%–50% of blood volume.		
		Gastrointestinal symptoms:	
		Cramping, abdominal pain	Due to smooth muscle contractions
		Vomiting	
Coma	Some children may still be able to maintain CNS perfusion and still be talking, despite decrease in blood pressure	Diarrhea	
		Urinary incontinence	
		Central nervous system:	
Marked tachypnea or dysfunctional respirations	Child requires intubation and mechanical ventilation	Decreased LOC	Due to decreased circulation to the brain and hypoxia
		Seizures	
Distributive Shock: Early Septic Shock		**Cardiogenic Shock**	
		Absent or poor peripheral pulses	Due to decreased cardiac output
Tachycardia tachypnea	Related to fever, hypoxia	Cold, clammy skin	
Warm extremities	Due to vasodilation	Decreased blood pressure	
Normal capillary refill time	Due to vasodilation	Decreased urine output	
Normal or elevated systolic blood pressure, wide pulse pressure	Initially, vital organs are able to continue functioning	Obstructive shock presents with the same signs and symptoms as above; other signs and symptoms are related to the injury, such as cardiac tamponade, tension pneumothorax	
Adequate urine output			
Mild mental confusion			

Data from Perry, A., & Potter, P. (1983). *Shock—Comprehensive nursing management*. St. Louis: Mosby.

Cardiogenic Shock

Although cardiogenic shock caused by myocardial infarction is common in adults, this form of shock is not common in children, where it is caused by primary pump failure and may be seen with congenital heart disease, myocarditis, and overdoses of certain drugs such as digitalis, beta blockers, and tricyclic antidepressants.

Obstructive shock is often categorized under cardiogenic shock. It results from the inability of the heart to fill adequately due to an inflow or outflow obstruction, causing decreased cardiac output. Usual causes in children are trauma to the chest resulting in cardiac tamponade, tension pneumothorax or hemothorax (see Chap. 30), and pericarditis.

Nursing Assessment and Intervention

The signs and symptoms of shock in the pediatric patient may be subtle or obvious. Table 29-7 lists the signs and symptoms of various types of shock. The potential for shock should be considered when the nurse is taking a history, especially if the history or chief complaint includes trauma, major burns, severe vomiting and diarrhea, infection, or uncontrolled external bleeding.

Although the vital signs in a child are important, they are not reliable indicators of shock. Because of the excellent ability of the child's body to compensate, by the time a child is hypotensive, he or she may have lost a large percentage of blood volume. The blood pressure needs to be taken as an initial baseline assessment. The proper sized cuff should be used. A cuff that is too large gives a false low reading, whereas one that is too small gives a false high reading. The blood pressure cuff should be approximately two thirds of the width of the upper arm.

The nurse should be suspicious of shock when tachycardia, increased capillary refill time (greater than 2 seconds), and cold pale extremities are present. These early signs often go unnoticed because of difficulty in assessing a child.

The first intervention in treating any type of shock is recognizing that it exists. Treatment is geared toward the ABCs. Supplemental oxygen should always be provided even though the child may not appear to be hypoxic. If a child is in late shock, intubation may be necessary to restore effective ventilation and help correct acidosis.

Any uncontrolled bleeding must be stopped, and an IV infusion using a large-bore catheter is ordered by the physician. IV access may be difficult in children, and a cutdown of the saphenous vein may be necessary. However, the use of intraosseous infusions, usually using the tibia, is becoming a quicker and easier route when peripheral access is not successful.[28] Intraosseous infusions involve inserting a bone marrow needle into the anterior medial aspect of the tibia, 2 to 3 cm below the proximal tibial tuberosity. This line serves as a temporary access for fluids and medications until a peripheral or central line can be obtained. Fluids and medications are rapidly absorbed by the extensive network of venous sinusoids and rapidly enter the systemic circulation.[22] See Figure 30-4 for an illustration of the use of an intraosseous needle. An arterial line may be initiated to monitor blood pressure and obtain serial arterial blood gases (ABGs).

Restoring fluid volume is the mainstay of treating shock. IV fluid and/or blood products are ordered depending on the type of fluid loss. An initial dose of 20 ml/kg of lactated Ringer's solution is usually given, and the child's response is evaluated. This volume may need to be repeated if the child's blood pressure does not increase and pulse improves. Large volumes of fluids should be warmed, using a blood or fluid warmer, before administration to prevent hypothermia.

Urinary output should be monitored with an indwelling Foley catheter. Vital signs, including temperature, should also be continuously monitored to evaluate response to treatment. The child should be placed on a cardiac monitor. Once the child is moved to an intensive care unit (ICU), central venous measurements of right atrial pressure and pulmonary wedge pressure may help guide fluid therapy.

Vasopressors (drugs used to maintain arterial pressures) may be ordered to treat cases of cardiogenic or distributive shock. A common vasopressor used in the ED is dopamine. Dopamine is a sympathomimetic amine that is preferred because it can also improve renal perfusion. Epinephrine or dobutamine may be used. Because these drugs are potent and have serious side-effects, they must be given using a volumetric syringe pump, and the child must be constantly monitored.

IV antibiotics are ordered by the physician whenever septic shock is suspected. Steroids have been recommended in the past, but current literature suggests that they are not useful.[8] Epinephrine is used to treat anaphylactic shock. This drug is given either IV or subcutaneously (sub Q) depending on the severity of the child's condition. Antihistamines, such as Benadryl, may be ordered to decrease circulating histamines and itching related to hives. Steroids may also be ordered to reduce the inflammatory response.

Laboratory studies are ordered, including ABGs, to monitor response to therapy. Coagulation studies are monitored to assess for the presence of DIC that may occur in septic shock. Renal function studies may be ordered if renal impairment is suspected or evident.

Children who present in severe shock are transferred to the ICU, where further care and monitoring are done. In rural settings, the ED nurse may need to assist in preparing a child for transport to another hospital that is equipped to care for a critically ill child.

The parents must be kept informed of the child's progress in the ED and plans for transfer to the ICU or another facility. A social worker or clergyperson should be called to be with the family to serve as a liaison between them and the ED team. As soon as the child is stabilized, the parents should be allowed to see him or her.

Anticipatory Guidance

Although some forms of shock cannot be anticipated or prevented, accidents and injuries can. However, the ED is not the place to chastise families whose child is critically ill or dying. ED nurses can help educate families on how to prevent injuries and how to provide first aid for bleeding control.

Anaphylactic shock may be prevented by avoiding the allergens that provoke the reactions. The child should be wearing a bracelet or necklace identifying the allergens. Nurses need to get in the habit of looking for these tags and asking parents about allergies before giving medications. Parents can be taught how to use an emergency kit containing epinephrine for a child allergic to various insect bites (bees, wasps, and hornets).

Respiratory Emergencies

Respiratory distress is a common condition affecting children in an ED setting. The distress may be mild (due to simple nasal congestion) or severe (due to a bacterial or viral infection or an obstruction). The ED nurse must do a rapid assessment of the child who appears to be in respiratory distress because early recognition and intervention may prevent the progression to respiratory failure and cardiac arrest.[25]

Causes of respiratory distress in the child are listed in Table 29-8. Some of these causes are discussed in Chapter 38. The next section of this chapter deals with respiratory distress involving airway obstruction caused by a foreign object.

Foreign Body Aspiration

Children are, by nature, curious. This curiosity often leads them to explore foreign objects by putting them in their mouths. The objects are often inhaled during the course of the child's exploration, causing an obstruction to the airway that may be partial or complete. Inhalation of food can also be a cause of airway obstruction.

Accidental inhalation or ingestion is the cause of death of 500 children annually in the United States.[24] More than 90% of these deaths occur in children younger than 5 years of age, and 65% of these children are infants.[1]

Pathophysiology

Food materials cause more than 90% of all foreign body obstructions.[6] These foods usually include nuts, seeds, raisins, hard candy, raw carrots, or sausage-shaped meats such as hot dogs. Nonfood objects include pieces of toys, marbles, pieces of balloons, screws, pins, nuts and bolts, and small batteries used in watches and hearing aids.

The effect of the foreign body in the airway and on respiration depends on its size and shape and location in the airway. Laryngotracheal foreign bodies may produce an acute obstruction, whereas bronchial foreign bodies produce a more chronic course of inflammation and irritation or abscess formation. Laryngotracheal foreign bodies require immediate intervention due to the possibility of complete airway obstruction.

Nursing Assessment and Intervention

The nursing assessment of a child in acute respiratory distress is obvious: the child may be coughing, gagging,

wheezing, drooling, and unable to swallow. Cyanosis is a late sign of severe respiratory distress and is a true emergency. Stridor is common with objects partially obstructing the upper airway, and the use of chest accessory muscles and sternal retractions may also be present. The child may be unconscious and not breathing at all.

What is not always so obvious is the cause of the obstruction. The nurse should suspect a foreign body obstruction based on the history, especially if the respiratory distress occurred while the child was eating or playing with small objects or toys. The ingestion may have been witnessed by a parent or sibling.

Regardless of the cause of respiratory distress, the nursing priority is to open the airway and maintain respirations. Manual attempts at clearing the airway should be considered for:[1]

- Children whose aspiration is witnessed or strongly suspected
- Unconscious, nonbreathing children whose airways remain obstructed despite the usual maneuvers to open them

Controversy continues concerning the best way to relieve suspected foreign body obstruction in children. The accompanying display describes the current recommendations for treatment of a child with airway obstruction, which consist of a combination of back blows and chest thrusts and the Heimlich maneuver. The Heimlich maneuver is not recommended for children 1 year of age or younger because of the risk of injury to the abdominal organs. After these maneuvers are attempted, the airway is opened using the head tilt/chin lift maneuver. If spontaneous breathing is absent, rescue breathing is performed. If the chest does not rise, the head is repositioned, the airway is opened, and rescue breathing is performed. If the chest does not rise, the head is repositioned, the airway is opened, and rescue breathing is attempted again. If this is still unsuccessful, maneuvers to remove the foreign body should be repeated. After breathing is restored, the child should be seen by a physician to rule out complications.

Anticipatory Guidance

Because foreign body aspiration is a common childhood event that may result in death, parents need to be aware of a young child's curiosity and tendency to explore objects with the mouth. They should also be instructed not to feed children small hard foods until they are old enough to chew them thoroughly (generally around age 3, but this may vary from child to child). All foods such as hot dogs, sausages, and so forth, should be cut into small pieces. Parents should also check toys for small removable parts that can easily be ingested. The Consumer Product Safety Commission also has guidelines available on different types of toys for different age groups. This agency can be contacted at the following address:

Consumer Product Safety Commission
PO Box 91236
Los Angeles, CA 90009

Parents should be instructed to "baby-proof" their homes so that small objects are kept out of reach. Because

TABLE 29-8
Causes of Respiratory Distress in Children

Upper Airway	Lower Airway
Bacterial/viral infections	Foreign body aspiration
Croup	Bacterial/viral infections
Epiglottiditis	Pneumonia
Tracheitis	Pertussis
Peritonsillar abscesses	Bronchiolitis
Foreign body aspiration	Asthma
Food	Congenital anomalies
Toy or parts of toys	Mechanical obstructions
Batteries (from watches or hearing aids)	Pulmonary edema
Trauma	Pneumothorax
Burns/ smoke inhalation	Botulism
Blood in airway due to facial injuries	Polio
Congenital anomalies	

children are great mimickers and learn by example, parents should not put small objects (straight pins, sewing needles) in their mouths. Classes are taught in most communities on recommended techniques for emergency treatment of the choking victim. Parents should be encouraged to participate in these courses.

Cardiopulmonary Arrest

Cardiopulmonary arrest in the child, unlike that in the adult population, is rarely caused by a primary cardiac condition. More than 90% of all pediatric arrests are caused by a respiratory problem. Because cardiac arrests in children are usually caused by prolonged hypoxia, the outcome of CPR in the child who has suffered a cardiac arrest has been poor.[31] However, if the child's respiratory condition is corrected before the development of a cardiac arrest, the outcome is much better.[21] ED nurses must recognize the signs and symptoms of respiratory distress and intervene before this condition progresses to a cardiac arrest.

Pathophysiology

The major causes of cardiac arrest are the following: injuries (motor vehicle accidents, drowning, firearms,

---

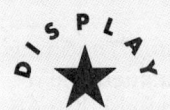

Emergency Treatment of the Child With a Suspected Airway Obstruction

Infant

1. Hold infant face down with head lower than trunk. Support head by firmly holding the jaw.
2. Rest supporting arm on thigh and deliver five back blows forcefully with the heel of the hand between the infant's shoulder blades (see figure).
3. Place free hand on infant's back so infant is sandwiched between two hands—one supporting the neck, jaw, and chest; the other supporting the back.
4. Turn infant, place on thigh with head lower than trunk.
5. Do five quick downward chest thrusts. Same location as external chest compressions, but at a slower rate (see figure). *Note:* An alternate method is to lay the infant face down in lap with head lower than trunk and firmly supported. Apply back blows, turn infant, and apply up to five chest thrusts.
6. Remove the foreign body if it is visualized.
7. Open the airway and attempt rescue breathing.

Child: Heimlich Maneuver With Victim Standing or Sitting

1. Stand behind victim, arms directly under the victim's axillae encircling victim's chest, with one hand made into a fist.
2. Rest thumb side of fist against the victim's abdomen in the midline slightly above the navel and well below the tip of the xiphoid process.
3. Grasp fist with other hand and exert a series of up to five quick, upward thrusts.
4. Repeat if necessary. Each thrust should be a separate and distinct movement.

Heimlich Maneuver With Victim Lying (Conscious or Unconscious)

1. Position child face up on back, kneel beside the child or straddle the victim's hips.
2. Place heel of one hand on the child's abdomen in the midline slightly above navel and well below rib cage.
3. Place other hand on top of the first and press into abdomen with a quick, upward thrust. Direct thrusts upward in midline and not to sides. If necessary, a series of five thrusts is performed.

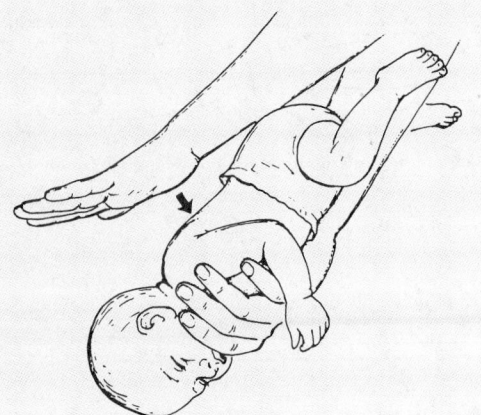

Step 2. Back blow in an infant.

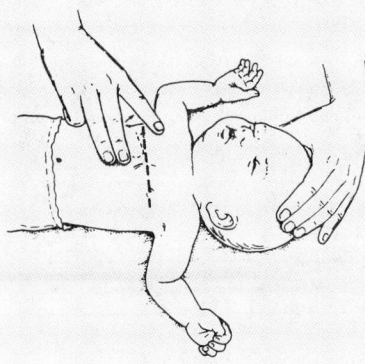

Step 4. Locating finger position for chest compression in an infant.

Data from American Medical Association. (1992). Pediatric basic life support. Journal of the American Medical Association; 268, 2258–2260. Figures from Skale, N. (1992). Manual of pediatric nursing procedures. Philadelphia: Lippincott.

burns, poisoning. These cause 44% of all deaths in children between the ages of 1 and 14); suffocation caused by foreign bodies; smoke inhalation; sudden infant death syndrome (SIDS); and infections (especially those affecting the respiratory system). Many of these causes are preventable. Because the outcome of children requiring CPR is poor, time spent aimed at prevention may be more useful in preventing deaths caused by cardiac arrests than teaching CPR techniques.

Pediatric Basic Life Support Techniques

The following sequence of CPR is from the current recommendations by the American Medical Association.[1]

1. *Determine responsiveness.* This is done by tapping the child or speaking loudly. If there is head or neck trauma, do not move or shake the child.
2. *Call for help.* After determining unresponsiveness or respiratory difficulty, the rescuer should call for help. If the rescuer is alone and the child is obviously not breathing, CPR should be performed for 1 minute before calling for help.
3. *Position the child.* If CPR is to be effective, the child needs to be on his or her back on a flat surface. The circumstances in which a child is found provide clues to the possibility of neck injury. If trauma is involved, there is an increased likelihood of spinal injury. The child should be turned as a unit, with firm support of the head and neck.
4. *Open the airway.* The small airway of a child can easily be obstructed by vomitus or blood. In addition, the child has a large tongue that can fall back and obstruct the airway. The airway should be opened using the head tilt/chin lift maneuver. If there is a possible neck injury, the jaw thrust maneuver should be used. These maneuvers are shown and illustrated in the accompanying display.
5. *Determine whether the child is breathing.* The airway is opened, and, while patency is maintained, the rescuer places his or her ear close to the child's nose

---

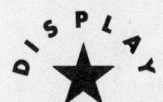

Techniques for Opening the Child's Airway

Head-Tilt/Chin-Lift

1. Place hand closest to child's head on the forehead and tilt the head gently back into a neutral or slightly extended position. Avoid overextension.
2. To augment head tilt, lift the chin, with its attached structures, including the tongue, from the airway.
3. Place the fingers (but not the thumb) of the hand away from the victim's head, under the bony part of the lower jaw at the chin.
4. Lift the chin upward. Do not close mouth completely or push on soft parts under chin.
5. Continue to tilt head back with other hand (except in cases of suspected cervical spine injuries).

Jaw-Thrust

1. Place two or three fingers under each side of the lower jaw at its angle.
2. Lift jaw upward and outward. Rest elbows on surface on which victim is lying.

Note: If the jaw thrust alone does not open the airway, jaw thrust may be accomplished by slight head tilt when neck injury is not evident.

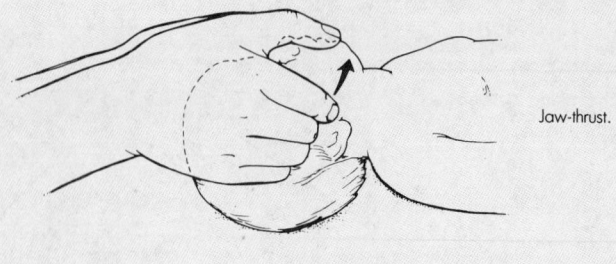

Jaw-thrust.

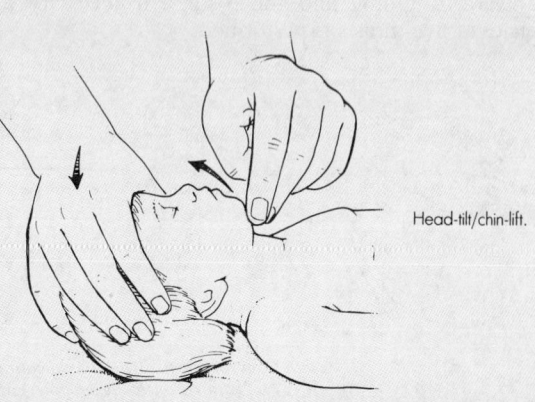

Head-tilt/chin-lift.

Figures from Skale, N. (1992). Manual of pediatric nursing procedures. Philadelphia: Lippincott.

and mouth, listening and feeling for exhaled air flow, while looking at the chest and abdomen for movement (Fig. 29-3*A*).

6. *Breathe for the child.* Rescue breathing must be done if the child is not breathing. Breathing is done using mouth-to-mouth technique in a child (Fig. 29-3*B*), or mouth-to-mouth-and-nose in an infant (Fig. 29-3*C*). Two slow breaths are given with a pause between for the rescuer to take a breath. There are three things to remember with rescue breathing:

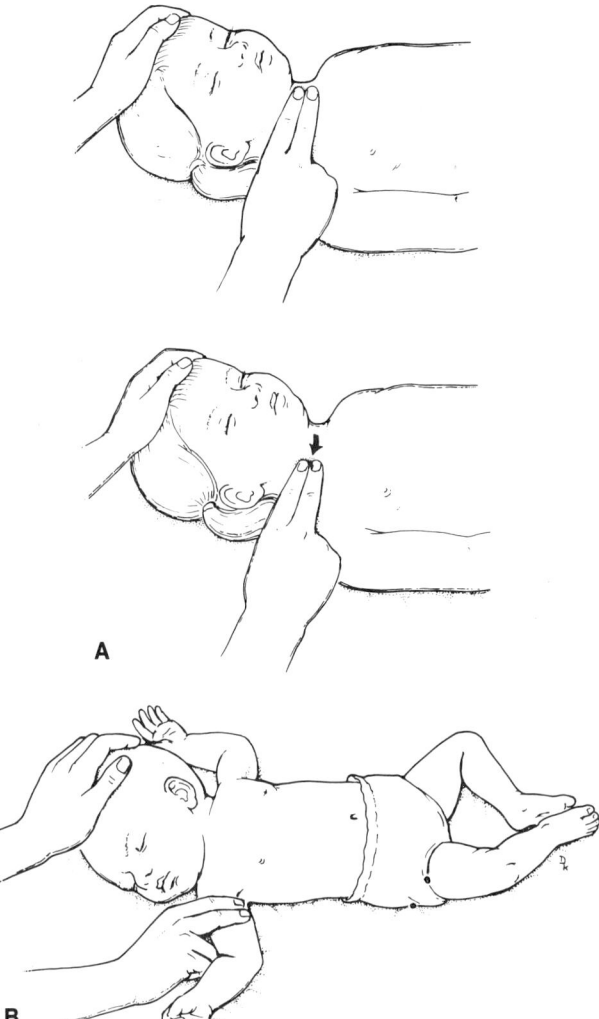

FIGURE 29-4
Checking the pulse for circulation. (**A**) Locating and checking the carotid artery in a child. (**B**) Locating the brachial artery in an infant. (Skale, N. [1992]. *Manual of pediatric nursing procedures.* Philadelphia: Lippincott.)

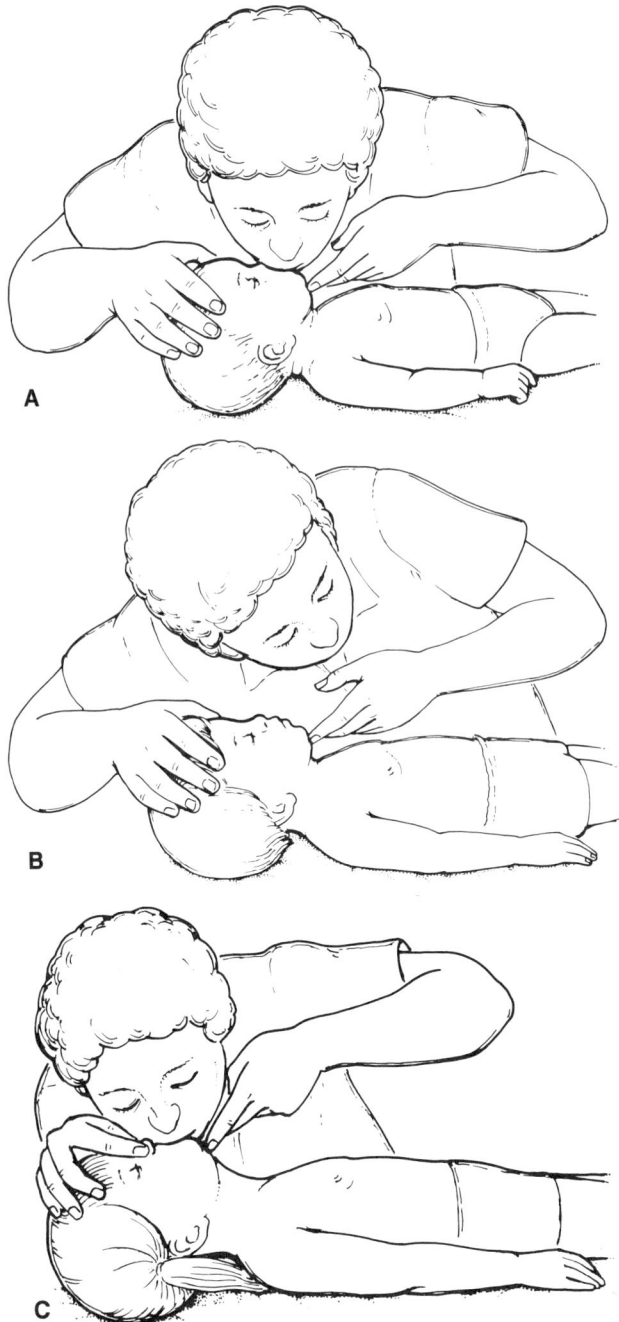

FIGURE 29-3
Rescue breathing. (**A**) Look and listen for exhaled airflow. If the child is not breathing, (**B**) mouth-to-mouth technique is used in a child; (**C**) mouth-to-mouth-and-nose is used in an infant. (Skale, N. [1992]. *Manual of pediatric nursing procedures.* Philadelphia: Lippincott.)

Rescue breaths are the single most important maneuver in assisting a nonbreathing child.
An appropriate volume is that which makes the chest rise and fall.
By giving the breaths slowly, an adequate volume is provided at the lowest possible pressure and gastric distention is avoided.

7. *Circulation—check the pulse.* In a child older than 1 year, the carotid is the most accessible and central artery for assessing the pulse (Fig. 29-4*A*). In an infant younger than 1 year, the short, chubby neck makes the carotid difficult to palpate, and the branchial artery is recommended (Fig. 29-4*B*). If a pulse is not present, chest compressions must be begun and coordinated with rescue breathing.

8. *Activate the Emergency Medical Services (EMS).* This step is included for those arrests occurring outside the hospital setting.

External chest compressions consist of serial, rhythmic compressions of the chest by which blood is circulated to vital organs to keep them viable until advanced life support can be done. Chest compressions are always accompanied by rescue breathing. Position, depth, and rate of compressions in infants and children are described in the accompanying display.

Anticipatory Guidance

Because many of the conditions leading to cardiopulmonary arrest in children are preventable, steps should be taken to educate parents to prevent trauma by encouraging the use of seat belts, classes in swimming, and fire safety. Parents need to be taught about the dangers of aspiration in toddlers. They need to be aware of their child's developmental level and what age-related injuries are common in that age group.

The EMS, as well as nursing personnel, need to be able to recognize respiratory emergencies quickly and to intervene properly to prevent cardiac arrest. Most hospitals require that nursing personnel be certified in Basic Life Support and be recertified on a yearly basis. In addition, hospitals should have appropriate emergency equipment for treating children. This equipment should be checked on each shift. ED nurses should also be cer-

tified in Advanced Pediatric Life Support. Certification involves knowledge of cardiac drugs, defibrillation procedures, and equipment. Courses are available that are taught by medical personnel skilled in dealing with children.

Sudden Infant Death Syndrome

Sudden infant death syndrome (SIDS) is defined as the unexpected death of an apparently healthy infant between the ages of 1 month and 1 year for which a thorough autopsy fails to demonstrate an adequate cause of death.[39] SIDS is the leading cause of death in children between the ages of 1 week and 1 year and claims the lives of 7 to 8000 babies each year.

Pathophysiology

SIDS has been described in the medical and lay literature since biblical times. Despite numerous theories, the cause is still not known. In earlier times, SIDS was blamed on neglect of the mother and on infanticide; al-

---

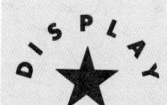

Techniques for Chest Compressions in Infants and Children

Infants

Position

1. Locate imaginary line beween nipples over breastbone.
2. Place index finger of hand farthest from infant's head under the intermammary line where it intersects the sternum.
3. Area of compression is one finger's width below this intersection at location of middle ring finger.

Depth	Rate
0.5–1 in	100/min

Position

Children (younger than 8 years of age)

1. With middle and index fingers, locate lower margin of rib cage on the side next to rescuer.
2. Follow margin of rib cage with the middle finger to notch where ribs and breastbone meet.

3. Place middle finger on this notch. Place index finger next to middle finger.
4. Place heel of hand next to index finger, with the long axis of the heel parallel to that of the sternum.
5. Compressions are done with the heel of one hand.

Depth	Rate
1.0–1.5 in	80–100/min

Children (older than 8 years of age)

1. Locate position the same as for a child less than 8 y.
2. Compressions are done with the heel of both hands, one over the other.

Depth	Rate
1.5–2 in	80–100/min

Note. In both the infant and the child, the compressions should be smooth and not jerky. In the child, care should be taken to keep the fingers off the ribs. If the child is older than approximately 8 y, the techniques recommended for adult CPR should be used. The ratio of chest compressions to ventilations in both the infant and the child is 5 to 1. The two-man rescue is only used by medical personnel and is not taught to the general public. Reassess the patient after 10 cycles (1 min) and every few minutes thereafter.

Data from *American Medical Association. (1992). Pediatric basic life support.* Journal of the American Medical Association; *268,* 2256, 2257.

though these factors may contribute to unexplained infant deaths, they are not the cause of SIDS. Another SIDS theory that has been disproved is the relationship to the diphtheria-tetanus-pertussis vaccine. An autopsy must be done to rule out other causes of death; SIDS is only diagnosed after an autopsy shows no other conditions that would be lethal.

Current theories being researched relate SIDS to a cardiovascular condition or a form of prolonged apnea. Cardiovascular conditions being studied include prolonged periods of bradycardia and abnormal prolonged QT intervals in the conduction system. Apnea appears to be a more likely theory, because autopsy findings in infants suspected of dying of SIDS indicate that circulation persists after respirations have ceased.[16] Many of the characteristics of infants who die of SIDS are related to the respiratory system: prematurity, history of recent upper respiratory infection, and time of year when SIDS is the most prevalent (winter months, when there is a greater incidence of respiratory infections). Theories relating SIDS to apnea and dysrhythmias continue to be researched. Current research is focused on problems *in utero*.[39]

Despite the unclear etiology of SIDS, there are some common characteristics of babies dying from SIDS. These are listed in Table 29-9.

Some of the conditions that put infants at risk for SIDS, such as low socioeconomic conditions and younger mothers, are also risk factors for child abuse and neglect.

TABLE 29-9
Characteristics of Infants Who Die of Sudden Infant Death Syndrome

Sex/race	Higher percentage of males
	Greater incidence in African Americans
Age	2–4 mo, peak age is 4 mo
	90% die before the age of 6 mo
Time of death	During sleep
Time of year	Primarily in winter months
Birth factors	Higher incidence in:
	Premature infants
	Low birthweight infants
	Multiple births
	Infants with CNS problems
Maternal factors	Breast-feeding does not decrease risk
	Maternal smoking increases risk
	Younger mothers
	Any condition that places the mother at risk during pregnancy increases the risk of SIDS in the infant
Siblings	May not be at as great a risk as previously thought
History before death	Healthy, may have had mild upper respiratory symptoms
	May have recently visited doctor
Appearance when found	Apneic, blue, lifeless, with frothy, blood-tinged fluid in nose and mouth

Data from Beckwith, J. (1984). Discussion of terminology and definition of sudden infant death syndrome. In A. Bergman (Ed.), *Proceedings of the Second International Conference on Causes of Sudden Death in Infants*. Seattle: University of Washington Press; and Guntheroth, W. (1989). *Crib death. The sudden infant death syndrome* (2nd ed.). Mount Kisco, NY: Futura.

Therefore, child abuse needs to be considered as a cause of death, especially if there are obvious injuries such as external bruising or burns. Often, no external causes of abuse are found on examination. Child abuse as a cause of death is usually verified on autopsy. One study suggests that child abuse should be considered in all children who die unexpectedly or are in a high-risk group identified as children younger than 1 year of age who die unexpectedly and those who are dead on arrival to the ED.[12] In this study, 9 out of 43 unexpected deaths were found to be related to child abuse and neglect.

Nursing Assessment and Intervention

A child who is thought to have died from SIDS is usually brought to the ED by prehospital personnel, who are still performing CPR. However, depending on local EMS protocols, the decision not to attempt resuscitative methods may occur in the home. The child is usually unable to be resuscitated and is pronounced dead in the ED.

The parents of the child thus become the "patients." How they are dealt with by prehospital care personnel and the ED staff affects their grieving process. One essential component of care is to avoid implying that parents are at fault in the death. Although the possibility of child abuse has to be considered, it must be investigated in a sensitive way that the family does not construe as accusations.

Sometimes the parents may arrive during the resuscitative efforts. A nurse or social worker should serve as a liaison between the parents and medical staff to keep them informed. A physician should talk with the family as soon as possible. Many parents want to see the child during the resuscitation. This situation needs to be managed on an individual basis, but many parents feel that this is their last chance to say goodbye and to comfort the baby. To them, as long as the resuscitation is in progress, the baby is still alive.

If the child is pronounced dead before the parents arrive, they should be taken to a quiet room and told that the baby has died. They should be allowed to see their child and hold and touch him or her to say goodbye. However, parents need to be prepared as to what to expect. The parents should be told about endotracheal tubes and IV lines that may need to remain in place for the medical examiner. The baby should be cleaned and wrapped in a blanket. A nurse or a social worker should remain with the family unless the family requests otherwise.

In most states, an autopsy is required by law on all unexplained deaths. Parents may have questions about the procedure that need to be answered. An autopsy may help alleviate parental feelings of guilt. In some areas, the medical examiner visits the family and discusses autopsy findings. Parents may wish to have their child be an organ donor. Because of the unknown cause of SIDS, many organs cannot be used. Heart valves often can be used. The opportunity to be an organ donor should be an option offered to the parents, but the subject needs to be approached in a sensitive manner according to hospital protocols.

Anticipatory Guidance

SIDS has far-reaching effects on all family members, including grandparents and siblings, as well as babysitters. Nurses can play an active role in reducing the stress. The accompanying display gives some guidelines for counseling family members in the ED. Many EDs have follow-up programs in which nurses call or visit the family to offer support and answer questions about the death and what was done.

All families whose babies are suspected of dying of SIDS should be referred to a SIDS support group. Most communities have a local chapter that often includes other parents who have had the same experience. Parents may benefit from a visit by a SIDS group member. Parents can also be referred to the National Foundation for Sudden Infant Death Syndrome. This foundation is the major parent support group in the United States. The address is:

National Foundation for Sudden Infant Death Syndrome
8240 Professional Place
Landover, MD 20785-2246

The death of a healthy infant is also stressful on nursing staff. Time should be taken to discuss the resuscitation and to allow staff to express their feelings. Many nurses find participation in a local SIDS chapter a therapeutic experience.

SIDS cannot be prevented because the actual cause is unknown. Risk factors that predispose a baby to SIDS are known, and steps can be taken to identify mothers and babies at risk. Improving overall prenatal care would decrease risk factors in infants.

Accidental Poisoning

Accidental poisoning accounts for 7% to 10% of all ED visits.[4] Of these visits, 85% are children.[2] Poisoning can include ingested, inhaled, or absorbed substances. This section discusses the emergency treatment of ingested poisonings. Smoke inhalation and carbon monoxide poisoning are discussed in Chapter 33.

Pathophysiology

Characteristics of childhood poisoning cases are listed in Table 29-10. In children less than 1 year of age, poisoning usually results from unintentional parental misuse of a drug. In the toddler, poisoning is more often a result of curiosity and the tendency to explore objects with the mouth.

Although the majority of poisonings occur in the home, incidents may occur anywhere medications and toxic substances are stored. Table 29-11 lists some common household products that contribute to accidental poisoning. These products contribute to poisoning in children because (1) they are kept in old bottles or cans instead of the original containers; (2) they are removed from their usual storage places; (3) the storage place is unlocked and easily accessible to children; (4) 75% are "in sight" and therefore sought; and (5) parents fail to reapply safety closures properly or parents purchase household products for homes in which small children reside, that are not in chip-proof containers.[2]

Nursing Assessment and Intervention

Table 29-12 lists common signs and symptoms for various ingestions. Any unconscious child without a history of injury or illness should be suspected of drug intoxication and should be treated immediately. The first priority in the assessment is always the ABCs.

After the assessment of the ABCs, the nurse should obtain a complete history. This may need to be done by someone else while the child is being cared for. Many times, a parent is aware that an ingestion has occurred and can identify the substance. If the ingestion is known, the nurse should question the parents about the type of medication or substance, possible amount, time of ingestion, and any treatment initiated before arrival at the hospital. Because many drugs are secreted in breast milk, nursing mothers should be questioned on their use of drugs, particularly "recreational" drugs. For example, mothers who use cocaine may not perceive it as a danger because they are inhaling it instead of ingesting it.

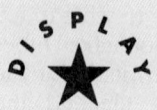

Nursing Guidelines for Counseling a Family Whose Baby Has Died of SIDS

- Say you are sorry.
- Give the family time to hold and say goodbye to the baby.
- Offer to make necessary phone calls.
- Answer any questions concerning the resuscitation or funeral arrangements. Many families are concerned that an autopsy means a viewing is not possible.
- Give information about Sudden Infant Death Syndrome chapter and provide parents with phone numbers.

- Give information about the grief process or refer them to someone who can answer their questions.
- Walk with the family to their car when they leave the ED.
- Don't say you "know how they feel."
- Don't imply that they are guilty in any way.
- Don't tell them they can "always have another baby."

Data from *Thomas, D. (1991). Quick reference to pediatric emergency nursing (p. 268). Rockville, MD: Aspen.*

If the ingested substance is unknown, the nurse should question the parents about any medications in the home, including those in the form of skin patches (scopolamine, nitroglycerine, some antihypertensives, estrogen) because there have been cases of poisoning caused by their ingestions.[11] Because therapeutic overdoses of acetaminophen and salicylates are common in the younger age group, parents should be questioned about any over-the-counter medications given, and their dosages, especially those containing acetaminophen or salicylates.

The principles of management for the poisoned child include:

- Initial stabilization: the ABCs
- Identifying the poison: history, physical examination, laboratory diagnosis
- Decreasing absorption of the poison
- Hastening elimination of the poison
- Providing symptomatic care
- Giving appropriate antidote
- Anticipatory guidance (preventing reoccurrence)

Initial Stabilization. Initial nursing management focuses on the ABCs. The comatose child should always receive supplemental oxygen. Children with severe hypoxia and respiratory depression may need intubation. An IV is ordered to support the circulation and to give medications if necessary. Laboratory studies may be ordered for toxicologic examination at the same time as the IV is started. A complete set of vital signs should be obtained, and the child should be placed on a cardiac monitor to observe for dysrhythmias. The child may be catheterized, and the urine should be sent for a drug screen. After the ABCs are stabilized, efforts are focused on identi-

TABLE 29-10
Characteristics of Childhood Poisoning Cases

Age	12.6% older than 5 y
	72.4% younger than 5 y
	Peak incidence at 2 y
Recurrence	25% chance of similar incident within 1 y
Most common type	*Pharmaceuticals:* analgesics (acetaminophen, aspirin), vitamins (especially those with iron), topical preparations (diaper care products)
	Sedatives (tricyclic antidepressants, benzodiazepines)
	Hypnotics
	Nonpharmaceuticals: plants, cleaning substances, cosmetics, hydrocarbons, alcohols
Location of poisons	Kitchen—41%
	Bathroom—21%
	Bedroom—12%
	Other—26%
Outcome	Majority of poisonings can be handled on an outpatient basis or require short hospitalizations

Data from Arena, J. M. (1986). *Poisoning. Toxicology, symptoms, treatment* (4th ed.). Springfield, IL: Charles C. Thomas; Bayer, M. J., Rumack, B. H., & Wanke, L. (1984). *Toxicologic emergencies.* Bowie, MD: Robert J. Brady; Lacroix, J., Gaudreault, P., & Gauthier, M. (1989). Admission to a pediatric intensive care unit for poisoning: A review of 105 cases. *Critical Care Medicine, 17,* 748–750; and Veltri, J., & Litovitz, T. (1984). 1983 Report of the American Association of Poison Control Center's national data collection systems, *American Journal of Emergency Medicine, 2,* 420–443.

TABLE 29-11
Some Potentially Poisonous Substances Found in or Around the Home

Substance	Examples
Polishes and waxes (furniture)	Kerosene, mineral seed oil, naphtha, turpentine
Paint solvents and related compounds	Acetone, methanol, naphthalene, toluene
Cleaning, polishing, and bleaching agents	Dry cleaning fluids, detergents for dishes or laundry, metal cleaners and polishes
Cosmetic preparations	Skin tonics and lotions, permanent wave solutions, hair dyes, tints, shampoos, nail preparations
Other household products/chemicals	Antifreeze, carburetor cleaners, deodorizing tablets, brake fluids, shoe cleaners and polishes, some inks, fire extinguishing fluids, plastic menders, glue (nail repair), Christmas tree bubbling lights, drain cleaners, salt substitutes, thermometer fluid
Plants	Bird of Paradise, elephant ear, dumb cane, English ivy, holly, Jack-in-the-pulpit, Jerusalem cherry, mistletoe, rhubarb, peach and cherry pits, wild mushrooms, lily of the valley

Data from Arena, J. (1986). *Poisoning. Toxicology, symptoms, treatment* (4th ed.). Springfield, IL: Charles C. Thomas; and Dreisbach, R., & Robertson, W. (1987). *Handbook of poisoning.* Norwalk, CT: Appleton and Lange.

fying the poison, decreasing absorption, and increasing elimination.

Decreasing Absorption. Absorption of drugs is minimized by stimulating vomiting with syrup of ipecac. Ipecac is not given to unconscious children, those with a decreased level of consciousness, or in children younger than 6 months of age because of the danger of aspiration of vomitus due to a decreased gag reflex. Ipecac is also contraindicated in children who have ingested an acid, alkali, or a hydrocarbon that does not contain camphor, aromatic products, or pesticides. Inducing emesis in these cases may be harmful because the caustic acids may cause further damage to the esophagus during emesis. Inducing vomiting for hydrocarbon ingestions puts the child at risk for aspiration pneumonia.

Ipecac is given in a dose of 15 to 30 ml. The effectiveness of ipecac is not increased with forcing fluids or with ambulation, as was previously thought.[35] Ipecac usually takes effect in 15 to 20 minutes. If there is no response in this time, the dose may be repeated in children older than 1 year of age. The child should be closely observed and positioned on the left side to prevent aspiration. Any vomitus should be inspected to see if pill fragments are present.

If a child is unconscious, lavage is ordered.[30A] This procedure is contraindicated for caustic or acid ingestions. Lavage involves placing a large-bore orogastric tube (28 to 36 Fr) and instilling saline and repeating until the returns are clear. Checking tube placement before instillation is essential to avoid accidental aspiration. Lavage should be done with the child on the left side. If the child is unconscious, intubation is usually done by the physician to protect the airway. Gastric lavage is a fright-

TABLE 29-12
Some Symptoms of Drug Intoxications

Symptom	Drug(s)
Dysrhythmias	Amphetamines, anticholinergics, beta-blockers, carbon monoxide, chloral hydrate, digitalis, phenothiazines, sympathomimetics, tricyclic antidepressants, theophylline
Cyanosis not responding to oxygen	Anesthetics (local), nitrates, nitrites, phenacetin, sulfonamides
Vital sign changes:	
• Increased blood pressure	Amphetamines, anticholinergics, sympathomimetics, nicotine
• Decreased blood pressure	Cyanide, narcotics, sedative/hypnotics, tricyclic antidepressants
• Increased heart rate	Alcohol, amphetamines, anticholinergics, sympathomimetics, theophylline
• Decreased heart rate	Barbiturates, digitalis, narcotics, sedatives/hypnotics
• Increased respiratory rate	Amphetamines, anticholinergics, hydrocarbons, salicylates
• Decreased respiratory rate	Alcohols, barbiturates, narcotics, sedatives/hypnotics
• Increased temperature	Amphetamines, anticholinergics, atropine, beta-blockers, phenothiazines, salicylates, sympathomimetics, tricyclic antidepressants
• Decreased temperature	Alcohol, anesthetics (general), barbiturates, carbon monoxide, narcotics, phenothiazines, sedatives/hypnotics, tricyclic antidepressants
Neurologic changes:	
• Coma	Amphetamines, anticholinergics, barbiturates, benzodiazepines, carbamazepine, carbon monoxide, chloral hydrate, cocaine, ethanol, isopropyl, haloperidol, narcotics, phencyclidine, phenytoin, salicylates, sedative/hypnotics
• Seizures	Camphor, carbon monoxide, caffeine, cocaine, cyanide, aminophylline, amphetamine, lidocaine, anticholinergics, aspirin, pesticides, phencyclidine, phenol, propoxyphene, tricyclic antidepressants
• Headache	Carbon monoxide, phenol, benzene, nitrobenzene, nitrates, nitrites, aniline, lead, acetone, caffeine, cyanide
Gastrointestinal changes:	
• Nausea, vomiting, diarrhea	Heavy metal salts, corrosive acids and alkalis, cathartics, nicotine, botulism, local anesthetics, salicylates, xanthines, lead
• Burning throat and stomach	Camphor, picrotoxin, iodine, arsenicals, antimony compounds
Behavior disorders:	
• Toxic psychosis	Hallucinogens (LSD), phencyclidine, sympathomimetics, heavy metals
• Paranoid, violent reactions	Phencyclidine
• Depression, paranoid hallucinations, emotional liability	Sympathomimetics
• Hallucinations, delirium, anxiety	Hallucinogens, anticholinergics
Movement disorders:	
• Choreoathetosis, orofacial dyskinesis, nystagmus, ataxia	Phenytoin (Dilantin)
• Extrapyramidal symptoms	Anticholinergics, phenothiazines, haloperidol
• Choreoathetoid movements	Tricyclic antidepressants
• Ataxia	Heavy metals
• Nystagmus	Phenytoin, carbamazepine, primidone, phencyclidine, carbon monoxide
Pupillary reactions:	
• Constricted pupils (miosis)	Barbiturates, cholinergics, narcotics (except meperidine), organophosphates
• Dilated pupils (mydriasis)	Alcohol, anticholinergics, antihistamines, barbiturates, meperidine, phenytoin, sympathomimetics

Data from Arena, J. (1986). *Poisoning. Toxicology, symptoms, treatment* (4th ed.), pp. 15–19. Springfield, IL: Charles C. Thomas; and Barkin, R., & Rosen, P. (1986). *Emergency pediatrics* (2nd ed.), p. 268. St Louis: Mosby.

ening experience to children who are awake, and they should be comforted as much as possible. Children sometimes believe they are being punished for their behavior, and the nurse needs to talk calmly to the child and explain as much as possible.

In many institutions, gastric lavage has replaced Ipecac as the initial treatment, because administration of Ipecac may delay administration of activated charcoal due to Ipecac's emetic effect. Lavage allows activated charcoal to be given sooner to further decrease absorption. Activated charcoal may be ordered after lavage or about 30 to 60 minutes after induced emesis. Activated charcoal absorbs most organic and inorganic substances. The usual dose is 1 g/kg orally, mixed with water or a flavored syrup. Many premixed preparations are available; unfortunately, none of them completely disguises the gritty taste of the charcoal. Most children do not voluntarily drink this preparation, and it usually must be given by nasogastric or orogastric tube. Parents need to be told that the charcoal will cause the child's stools to be black.

Hastening Elimination. A cathartic such as magnesium sulfate is ordered at the same time as the charcoal to hasten elimination of the drug. Shortening the elimination time of some drugs (phenobarbital, salicylates) must be accomplished by promoting diuresis and increased urinary excretion. Elimination usually occurs over a period of time in the ICU, but may be begun in the emergency room. Dialysis may be required in life-threatening situations when there are marked elevations in serum drug levels of drugs such as phenobarbital, salicylates, theophylline, methanol, ethylene glycol, and lithium.

Providing Symptomatic Care and Nursing Evaluation. The nurse in the ED must constantly monitor the poisoned child by taking vital signs, assessing level of consciousness, and measuring urinary output. The parents need to be kept informed of what is going on. They usually have a sense of guilt because the ingestion could have been prevented. Fortunately, the majority of children who ingest medications are discharged home.[19] Those requiring hospitalization usually go to the ICU where they can receive appropriate care and monitoring while the poison is eliminated.

Giving Appropriate Antidote. Specific antidotes are not available for every poison. Nurses should always contact the poison control center in their area for specific guidelines. Acetaminophen is one commonly ingested drug that does have an antidote. Acetaminophen is being used more frequently in many preparations and is a common cause of poisoning in children. *N*-acetlycysteine (NAC; Mucomyst) is the antidote used in serious cases. NAC detoxifies acetaminophen metabolites to prevent liver damage. Its usage is guided by determination of serum levels of acetaminophen. If NAC is to be given, activated charcoal should not be used because it will absorb the NAC.

Naloxone is the antidote for narcotic overdoses. This drug works to reverse the effects of the narcotic, but other methods to decrease absorption of the drug need to be applied as well. This includes gastric lavage or inducing emesis, depending on the child's level of consciousness.

Although all cases of poisoning in children follow the same general guidelines, specific treatment may vary depending on the drug ingested. Table 29-13 lists examples of specific treatment for some common poisonings seen in children.

Anticipatory Guidance

The solution to the problem of childhood poisonings lies in prevention. The nurse in the ED can discuss various preventive measures with parents after their child is out of danger. These measures include:

- Store all cleaning solutions out of the reach of children. Put safety locks on all cabinets.
- Keep all medications out of the reach of children. Do not store any medications in purse.
- Keep all medications and cleaning products in original containers.
- Do not refer to medicine as candy.
- Check to be sure household plants are not poisonous.
- Check garage and basements to be sure all paints, solvents, and fertilizers are out of the reach of children.
- Have syrup of ipecac available.
- Know the number for the local poison control center.

Many emergency departments have a policy that requires a public health nurse to inspect the home of any child who has been seen for a poisoning incident. The nurse should consider the possibility of child abuse in repeated cases.

Although the overall death rate due to poisoning has almost doubled between 1955 and 1985, the death rate for the 0 to 4-year-old age group has decreased dramatically.[24] This can be attributed in part to education of the public and the manufacturing of child-proof caps for medications. Overdose of narcotics and opiates in the 25 to 44-year-old age group has contributed the most to the overall increase.

Drowning and Near Drowning

Drowning accidents account for about 5000 deaths per year in the United States and are the second most common cause of accidental death in children. Drowning is the third leading cause of death in children between the ages of 1 and 14.[26] The two age groups at greatest risk are adolescent boys and toddlers. Adolescent boys drown when their ability to swim is exceeded or when they are under the influence of alcohol. Toddlers drown when they are left unsupervised around any source of water, usually a private swimming pool.

Drowning is usually defined as death by suffocation after submersion in liquid. Near drowning is survival or temporary survival greater than 24 hours after a submersion episode. A new category of drowning that has recently been defined is ice water drowning or ice water near drowning, which involves prolonged submersions in cold water.[26]

Pathophysiology

The complications of drowning are directly related to anoxia and to the volume and composition of the water that is aspirated. Salt water has three times the osmolarity of normal extracellular body fluid, but both salt water and fresh water damage the alveoli, destroy surfactant, and cause pulmonary edema.

Animal studies of fresh water versus salt water drownings have documented differences in the physiologic response to each type of water. Although the initial response is different, the end result is the same in humans. Fresh water, being hypotonic, moves quickly through the alveoli, across the alveolar-capillary basement membrane and into the intravascular space. Salt water, being hypertonic, moves from the intravascular space into the alveo-

TABLE 29-13
Treatment of Specific Poisonings in Children

Drug	Toxic Dose	Signs and Symptoms	Treatment and Nursing Care
Acetaminophen	Between 70–140 mg/kg *Example:* 18 80-mg tablets in a 10-kg toddler	*Early* (up to 24 h after ingestion): Nausea, vomiting, diaphoresis, anorexia *Late* (72–96 h after ingestion): Hepatic necrosis, oliguria, jaundice, encephalopathy	*Initial stabilization:* Assess ABCs *If dose taken less than 140 mg/kg:* Ipecac will be ordered. Check emesis for pill fragments. Charcoal and cathartic per nasogastric tube to decrease absorption and hasten elimination. *If dose greater than 140 mg/kg:* Induce emesis or lavage. Do not give charcoal unless ingestion occurred within 2 h of admission to ED, or if other drugs are involved Draw blood for acetaminophen levels (must be obtained at least 4 h after ingestion) N-acetylcysteine may be ordered IV or PO *Parent Teaching:* Which over-the-counter drugs contain acetaminophen
Tricyclic antidepressants: Imipramine, trimipramine, Desipramine	*Potentially lethal:* 30 mg/kg	*Anticholinergic symptoms:* Dry mouth, flushing, hyperthermia, tachycardia, dilated pupils *Cardiac symptoms:* Dysrhythmias, prolonged QRS interval *Neurologic symptoms:* Lethargy, disorientation, coma, seizures	Support ABCs Cardiac monitor to observe for dysrhythmias Gastric lavage and charcoal—no ipecac due to decreased level of consciousness. Start IV sodium bicarbonate to reduce pH, increase protein binding of toxin Treat dysrhythmias Treat seizures Treat hypotension Teach parents about dangers of these drugs: Imipramine commonly used in children to treat enuresis
Iron: children's vitamins, prenatal vitamins	*Mild to moderate:* 20–60 mg/kg *Severe:* 60 mg/kg	*Gastrointestinal (GI) symptoms:* Vomiting, diarrhea, abdominal pain, GI bleeding, may progress to shock	Support ABCs Ipecac or lavage depending on age, level of consciousness Treat for shock if present Abdominal x-ray to observe for pills Blood studies for iron levels Deferoxamine, a drug that binds with iron, is ordered in severe cases and is usually given IV or IM—may cause hypotension if given too rapidly
Salicylates: Children's chewable aspirin, oil of wintergreen	*Mild to moderate:* 150–300 mg/kg *Potentially severe:* Greater than 300 mg/kg *Potentially lethal:* Greater than 500 mg/kg	Deep respirations Decreased level of consciousness Dehydration Metabolic acidosis Tinnitus	Ipecac, charcoal Obtain salicylate level Monitor blood gases Treat for shock, as necessary

Data from Arena, J. (1986). Poisoning, toxicology, symptoms, treatment (4th ed.). Springfield, IL: Charles C. Thomas; Bayer, M., Rumack, B., & Wanke, L. (1984). Toxicologic emergencies. Bowie, MD: Robert J. Brady; and Dreisbach, R., & Robertson, W. (1987). Handbook of poisoning. Norwalk, CT: Appleton and Lange, 1987.

lus. Because of the high concentration of electrolytes in sea water, sodium, chloride, and magnesium move into the intravascular space. When salt water enters an alveolar space, it destroys surfactant, damages the alveolar basement membrane, and produces alveolitis. The end result in both types of drowning is noncardiogenic pulmonary edema, hypoxemia, and acidosis.

The response to unexpected submersion has been defined in three stages,[26] as shown in Table 29-14.

The majority of morbidity and mortality associated with submersion accidents occurs from damage to the central nervous system due to hypoxia. The outcome and degree of damage depend on the child's age and preexisting health, the water temperature, and duration of the

TABLE 29-14
Stages of Submersion Responses in Drowning

Stage	Description
I	A small amount of water is aspirated, causing laryngospasm. Lasts for 2 min of submersion
II	Child panics, becomes increasingly hypoxic, and begins to swallow water.
III	One of two situations occurs: • *Dry drowning:* Severe laryngospasm occurs again and this time persists to severe hypoxia and death (occurs in 10%–15% of all cases). • *Wet drowning:* Laryngospasm relaxes secondary to hypoxia, and large volumes of water are aspirated. (occurs in 85%–90% of all cases).

Data from Orlowski, J. (1987). Drowning, near drowning, and ice-water submersions. Pediatric Clinics of North America, 34(1), 75–92.

child's submersion, as well as how soon after submersion resuscitation was started. The child's outcome also can be related to the initial presentation in the ED.

Nursing Assessment and Intervention

The nursing assessment includes airway, breathing, circulation, level of consciousness, purposeful movement, and response to stimuli. Based on this assessment, the initial presentation of the child has been classified[13] as shown in Table 24-15.

All of the children in category C need varying degrees of advanced life support measures.

Nursing care depends on the child's initial condition. Usually resuscitative measures have been started at the scene. Later, nursing care is aimed at supporting respirations and circulatory status, preventing increased intracranial pressure and complications such as aspiration of stomach contents. Rewarming may also be a big part of the treatment, if hypothermia is present. Care must be taken if a cervical spine injury is suspected. Cervical spine injury commonly occurs in diving injuries. The child's neck should always be stabilized during the initial assessment of the airway.

Children who can be classified in category A or B may require supplemental oxygen, chest x-ray, and ABGs. Minor rewarming using warmed IV or oral (PO) fluids and warm blankets may be required. The unconscious child should have a nasogastric tube placed to prevent aspiration. Vital signs, as well as neurologic status, should be monitored continuously to evaluate the child's improvement in response to interventions. These children are admitted to the hospital for 24 to 48 hours for observation and usually do well.

Category C children require more aggressive treatment, including mechanical ventilation and aggressive rewarming techniques. They are managed in the ICU, and the prognosis is best for those children who are classified as C1 or C2.

Children who present in full cardiac arrest are a special problem if the drowning occurred in cold water. The medical literature reports cases of survival after up to 66 minutes of submersion.[7] These children may have good

outcomes when aggressive rewarming is attempted. Rewarming may be done with warmed IV fluids, peritoneal lavage, and even by extracorporeal warming using cardiopulmonary bypass. Children who appear dead after prolonged exposure to cold temperatures should not be considered dead until they have a near normal body temperature and are still unresponsive to CPR. Therefore, nurses need to be familiar with rewarming techniques and know of the nearest facility that can perform extracorporeal rewarming, even though all drowning victims are not candidates for this procedure. The decision to use extracorporeal rewarming needs to be based on the temperature of the water, length of submersion time, and initial blood gases of the child.

Anticipatory Guidance

Because most drownings could have been prevented, parents feel a great sense of guilt. A nurse or a social worker should remain with the family. They need to be told that everything is being done that can be done, without giving them a false sense of hope. Even if the child survives in the ED, there is still an increased chance of severe brain damage and death due to lung complications. The grief of the parents is compounded by their guilt. Sometimes a support group can be beneficial in helping parents deal with these feelings. Hospital social workers would be a good resource for referrals to these groups.

Prevention

All children should be taught water safety measures, beginning as soon as the child is able to comprehend such instruction. Children of all ages should never be left unsupervised near any bodies of water. Fences should be placed around neighborhood pools. Children with seizure disorders are at even greater risk and should always be supervised in water, no matter what their age. They should be taught to take showers instead of baths to minimize the likelihood of drowning in a bathtub during a seizure.

Parents whose children arrive in the ED awake and without symptoms are amenable to water safety teaching. Nurses are in a good position to provide this teaching as

TABLE 29-15
Initial Presentation of the Near Drowning Victim

Category	Description
A	Child awake and alert with minimal injury.
B	Child unconscious but has normal respirations, normal pupillary response, and purposeful movement to pain.
C	Child comatose and has more severe brain injury and respiratory impairment. Further divided into four stages, each with a progressively poorer prognosis. These stages all exhibit respiratory and circulatory impairment. C1: Comatose, nonpurposeful response to pain, all reflexes intact C2: Comatose, no withdrawal to pain, most reflexes intact C3: Comatose, most or all reflexes absent C4: Comatose, absent reflexes, apneic, asystolic

Data from Conn, A. (1979). Cerebral resuscitation in near drowning. Pediatric Clinics of North America, 26(3), 691–701.

part of anticipatory guidance during any routine visits. The basic lesson is that young children should never be left alone in or near water of any kind, including pools, hot tubs, buckets of water, or bathtubs.

Other Pediatric Emergencies

Many types of pediatric problems are encountered in the ED. These problems range from life-threatening to minor

childhood diseases. Table 29-16 summarizes other common conditions and nursing interventions. Some of these conditions are discussed in respective interventions chapters in the latter part of the book.

Summary

Childhood emergencies cause many deaths and disabilities in children each year. Nurses need to be aware of

TABLE 29-16
Common Pediatric Complaints or Conditions Seen in the Emergency Department

Category/Nursing Diagnosis and Examples	Nursing Interventions
Altered respiratory function	Assist with diagnosis
Example:	Assess need for immediate intervention, such as oxygen or airway support
Minor colds, asthma, croup, pneumonia	Evaluate interventions, family's need for information concerning disease process and prescribed treatment
Altered gastrointestinal function	Assess for signs and symptoms of dehydration
Example:	Assist with fluid replacement (IV or by mouth)
Vomiting/diarrhea, dehydration, intussusception, bowel obstructions, abdominal trauma	Prepare for possible hospitalization/surgery
	Provide teaching on home care if discharged
	Evaluate interventions
Altered skin integrity	Control bleeding by direct pressure dressing
Example:	Assess function of injured area: motor, neurologic, sensory, clean wound
Lacerations (most common in this category), contusions (bruising), abrasions	Evaluate for other related injuries
	Assist with repair of laceration, as needed
	Provide family with instructions on wound care, suture removal, signs and symptoms of infection
	Provide tetanus prophylaxis, as needed
	Discuss measures for pain relief, as necessary
Rashes	Evaluate child for other signs and symptoms of illness
	Isolate child from others if rash is thought to be contagious (chickenpox, measles, and so forth)
	Evaluate rash: color, size, distribution, presence of itching, response to pressure (blanching)
	Any rash associated with respiratory distress, or one that resembles bruising (purpura or petechiae) may indicate a serious condition and warrants immediate evaluation by physician
Altered neurologic function (actual or potential)	Assess neurologic status: level of consciousness
Example:	Assist with and prepare child for x-ray, CT scan, as needed
"Minor" head trauma (no evidence of intracranial bleeding, no loss of consciousness, child is awake, alert, oriented)	Observe child for changes in level of consciousness
	Teach family about signs and symptoms to observe for deteriorating condition
	Provide follow-up information
Pain	Provide comfort measures as ordered: topical anesthetic drops for ear pain
Example:	Assess for related signs and symptoms: shock, airway obstruction, fever, vomiting and diarrhea, history of trauma
Ear pain (otitis media), throat pain (streptococcal pharyngitis, tonsilitis, viral sore throat)	Provide necessary teaching for medications, treatment or follow-up
Abdominal pain: gastroenteritis possible appendicitis, abdominal obstruction, trauma	
Skeletal or joint pain, headaches, chest pain (rarely a cause of heart disease in children)	
Altered parenting; altered family processes; Ineffective family coping	Identify children at risk
Example:	Provide any needed interventions related to injury
Child abuse: types of injuries often related to abuse include cigarette burns, other circumferential burns, submersion burns, unusual bruising, bruises in various stages of healing, fractures in various stages of healing, rib fractures, human bites, belt marks	Report to proper authority
	Refer family for counseling
Evidence of sexual abuse: rectal or vaginal trauma	

Additional information may be found throughout the text.

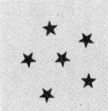

Ideas for Nursing Research

Trauma or emergency situations can have a lasting effect on the child. Health careproviders need to find ways to minimize these effects. Because prevention is the only sure method to reduce the number of children killed and injured each year, more research needs to be done in the field of emergency nursing care. The following areas need to be explored:

- Family factors that may contribute to injuries: number of children, socioeconomic status, geographic location.
- Effectiveness of written instructions and verbal instructions in emergency prevention.
- Methods of teaching prevention to families without a regular source of medical attention.
- Factors influencing how a child in the ED responds to pain.
- Child's emotional response to emergencies and trauma with consideration of emotional support in providing care.

the risks involved for children of all ages and developmental levels, and be able to teach parents ways to avoid accidental injury and death.

Caring for children and families in the ED is a many faceted role. The emergency nurse must be a generalist, possessing knowledge of minor childhood illnesses and complaints, as well as a specialist in treating critically ill or injured children. The ED interaction among the nurse, parent, and child is brief; the nurse must deal with the family as well as the child and do it in a way that meets both the physical and emotional needs of each. Emergency nursing is an expanded role and requires advanced knowledge of the nursing process: assessment, planning, intervention, and evaluation.

The nurse must be aware of the differences in the pediatric patient that require specialized care. The nurse is also responsible for keeping up to date on current methods of caring for the child in an emergency situation, because advances are continually being made.

Nurses are in a good position to assess a family's understanding of growth and development and to teach them good safety habits to prevent death and injury. Prevention is the key to reducing death and injuries.

References

1. American Medical Association. (1992). Pediatric basic life support for cardiopulmonary resuscitation and emergency cardiac care. *Journal of the American Medical Association, 268,* 2251–2261.
2. Arena, J. (1986). *Poisoning. Toxicology, symptoms, treatment* (4th ed.). Springfield, IL: Charles C. Thomas.
3. Baker, D., Fosareli, P., & Carpenter, R. (1987). Childhood fever. Correlation of diagnosis with temperature response to acetaminophen. *Pediatrics, 80,* 315.
4. Bayer, M., et al. (1984). *Toxicologic emergencies.* Bowie, MD: Robert J. Brady.
5. Beckwith, J. (1984). Discussion of terminology and definition of sudden infant death syndrome. In A. Bergman (Ed.), *Proceedings of the Second International Conference on Causes of Sudden Death in Infants.* Seattle: University of Washington Press.
6. Blazer, S., et al. (1980). Foreign body in the airway. A review of 200 cases. *American Journal of Diseases of Children, 134,* 68–71.
7. Bolte, B., et al. (1988). The use of extracorporeal rewarming in a child submerged for 66 minutes. *Journal of the American Medical Association, 260,* 377–379.
8. Bone, R., et al. (1987). A controlled clinical trial of high dose methylprednisone in the treatment of severe sepsis and septic shock. *New England Journal of Medicine, 317,* 653–658.
9. Briening, E. (1988, September). Septic shock: Tough cases that teach the most. *RN, 36.*
10. Buschbacher, V., & Delcampo, R. (1987). Parent's response to sudden infant death syndrome. *Journal of Pediatric Health Care, 1,* 85.
11. Caravati, M., & Bennett, D. (1988). Clonidine transdermal patch poisoning. *Annals of Emergency Medicine, 17,* 175–176.
12. Christoffel, K. (1985). Should child abuse and neglect be considered when a child dies unexpectedly? *American Journal of Diseases of Children, 139,* 876–880.
13. Conn, A. (1979). Cerebral resuscitation in near drowning. *Pediatric Clinics of North America, 26*(3), 691–701.
14. Consensus Development Conference on Febrile Seizures. (1981). *Epilepsia, 22,* 377–381.
15. Dymoski, J., & Vehara, D. (1987). Common household poisoning. *Pediatric Emergency Care, 3,* 261.
16. Guntheroth, W. (1989). Crib death. The sudden infant death syndrome (2nd ed.). Mount Kisco, NY: Futura.
17. Jones, J. (1983). Compliance with pediatric therapy. *Clinical Pediatrics, 22,* 262–265.
18. Kelley, S. (1988). *Pediatric emergency nursing.* Norwalk, CT: Appleton and Lange.
19. Lacroix, J., et al. (1989). Admission to a pediatric intensive care unit for poisoning: A review of 105 cases. *Critical Care Medicine, 17,* 748–750.
20. Lorin, M. (1987). Fever: Pathogenesis and treatment. In R. Feigin & J. Cherry (Eds.). *Textbook of pediatric infectious diseases* (pp. 148–154). Philadelphia: W.B. Saunders.
21. Ludwig, S., et al. (1984). Pediatric cardiopulmonary resuscitation. *Clinical Pediatrics, 23,* 71.
22. Manley, L., Haley, K., & Dick, M. (1988). Intraosseous infusion: Rapid vascular access for critically ill or injured infants and children. *Journal of Emergency Nursing, 14,* 63–69.
23. Meier, E. (1981). The pediatric emergency patient. *Emergency Medicine, 13,* 29.
24. National Safety Council. (1990). *Accident facts.* Chicago: Author.
25. Ogle, K. (1988). Problems in the management of respiratory distress. In R. Luten (Ed.). *Problems in pediatric emergency medicine* (pp. 219–241). New York: Churchill Livingston.
26. Orlowski, J. (1987). Drowning, near drowning, and ice-water submersions. *Pediatric Clinics of North America, 34*(1), 75–92.
27. Packer, R., & Berman, P. (1988). Neurologic emergencies. In G. Fleisher & S. Ludwig (Eds.), *Textbook of pediatric emergency care* (pp. 391–412). Baltimore: Williams & Wilkins.
28. Rosetti, V., et al. (1985). Intraosseous infusion: An alternate route of pediatric intravascular access. *Annals of Emergency Medicine, 14*(9), 885–887.
29. Strange, G. (1987). Febrile seizures: Evaluation and management. In R. Barkin (Ed.). *The emergently ill child* (pp. 201–216). Rockville, MD: Aspen.
30. Thomas, D. (1988). The ABCs of pediatric triage. *Journal of Emergency Nursing,* 14, 154.

30a. Thomas, D. (1991). *Quick reference to pediatric emergency nursing.* (pp. 233–234). Rockville, MD: Aspen.

31. Torphy, D., et al. (1984). Cardiorespiratory arrest and resuscitation of children. *American Journal of Diseases of Children, 138,* 1099.

32. Wallace, S. (1988). *The child with febrile seizures.* London: Wright.

33. Wetzel, R. (1987). Shock. In Mark C. Rogers (Ed.). *Textbook of pediatric intensive care,* Vol. 2. Baltimore: Williams & Wilkins.

34. Wintemute, G., Kraus, J., Teret, S., & Wright, M. (1987). Drowning in childhood and adolescence. A population based study. *American Journal of Public Health, 77,* 830.

35. Wong, D. (1988). Dispelling some myths about ipecac. *American Journal of Nursing, 88*(7), 952.

36. Woolsey, S. (1988). Support after sudden infant death. *American Journal of Nursing, 88,* 1348.

37. Yoos, L. (1984, March/April). Factors influencing maternal compliance to antibiotic regimens. *Pediatric Nursing,* 141–147.

38. Zimmerman, S. (1985). Anaphylaxis. In S. Zimmerman & J. Gildea (Eds.), *Critical care pediatrics.* Philadelphia: W.B. Saunders.

39. Zylke, J. (1989). Sudden infant death syndrome: Resurgent research offers hope. *Journal of the American Medical Association, 262,* 1565–1566.

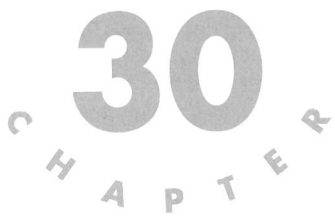

30

CHAPTER

Multiple Trauma in Children

BEHAVIORAL OBJECTIVES

Discuss the nurse's role in prevention of trauma.

Discuss seasonal and age-related factors as causes of childhood trauma.

Discuss the nurse's role in dealing with the psychosocial care of the child and family in traumatic injuries.

List the priorities of emergency assessment and resuscitation for the child with multiple injuries.

Describe the anatomic and physiologic differences in children, as related to injury and nursing intervention.

Describe the nurse's role in dealing with trauma to body systems.

Traumatic injury is the number one killer of children, a threat four times greater than childhood cancer. Each year traumatic injuries to children are responsible for 8,000 deaths, 50,000 permanent disabilities, and 2 million temporarily incapacitating conditions or disabilities.[8]

This peak in child morbidity from trauma is a direct reflection of two societal factors. First, the industrialization and mechanization of our society have increased the scope of opportunities for trauma to occur, as well as the magnitude of the resulting injuries. Second, although our nation has, through immunization and medical advances, successfully decreased the death rate from childhood illnesses, traumatic injury to children continues to receive proportionally little attention and financing for programs of research, awareness, and education.

The main tenet of childhood trauma care is that children are not just small adults. Due to developmental differences, they are injured by mechanisms that may differ from how adults are injured. Because of their small size and the resulting dissipation of energy, children often incur multiple system injuries when adults may receive an isolated injury. Children have specific anatomic and physiologic characteristics that affect how injuries are manifested. In addition, children have unique emotional and psychological needs that vary with developmental stages. These differences are addressed throughout this chapter.

Epidemiology

Motor vehicle accidents, falls, drownings, burns, and firearms are the major causes of morbidity and mortality in children. The causes of trauma in children are both seasonal and age related. Table 30-1 outlines age-related causes of injury and children's emotional responses. During the winter, fires are commonly responsible for trauma admissions, whereas, in the summer, motor vehicles and falls are the major mechanisms. Over all age groups, head injury and fractures are the most common diagnoses, as shown in Fig. 30-1*A*, whereas gunshot wounds incur the highest percentage of deaths,[34] as shown in Figure 30-1*B*.

In infancy, the leading causes of death are asphyxiation and motor vehicles. Burns, drownings, and falls are also frequently responsible for infant and toddler mortality. In children under the age of 5, motor vehicle crashes, house fires, and drownings are the leading causes of death; falls and poisonings are the leading cause of nonfatal injuries. The school-age child, with increasing independence and peer influence, is most susceptible to bicycle and pedestrian motor vehicle crashes. In the adolescent age group, the highest percentage of deaths are due to passenger motor vehicle crashes, drownings, and firearms.[4]

The epidemiology of injury also indicates that boys are injured more often than girls.[34] Specific characteristics may identify a child at high risk for injury. These include impulsiveness, risk-taking behavior, extroverted and physically active personality, poor locomotion abilities,

TABLE 30-1
Developmental Characteristics of Children That Cause Injury and Developmental Level Reactions

	Characteristics	Injury	Fears	Coping
Infant	*Creeper*			
0–3 m	Poor head control	30% respiratory		
3–6 mo	Rolls back-to-front	20% motor vehicle accidents	Separation	Parents
	Hand-to-mouth activity	Falls	Unknown	Swaddle
6–12 mo	Creeps	Burns		Pacifier
	Stands and cruises	Child abuse		
Toddler	*Cruiser*			
	Can walk, climb, run	MVA as passenger, pedestrian	Separation	Parents
	Tests reality	Falls	Strangers	Blanket
	Short memory	Burns—electrical	Loss of control	Motion
	Limited language	Poisons	Loss of special object	Demonstrate all actions
		Drowning		
		Child abuse		
Preschooler	*Climber, curious*			
	Imaginative	MVA as passenger, pedestrian	Separation	Parents
	"I'll do it"	Falls	Loss of control	Motion
	Developing verbal skills	Poisoning	Punishment	Explanations
	In constant motion	Child abuse	Body image	Band-aids
	Private zones			Play
School age	*Creator, explorer*			
	Growth spurts	MVA as passenger, pedestrian	Separation	Parents
	Communicates well	Bicycles	Punishment	Explanations with repetition
	Tests all limits	Sports	Pain	Help with treatment
	Peer influence	Water injuries	Body image	Play
	Modest	Tools	Body integrity	
			Death	
Adolescent	*Dreamer*			
	Good historian	MVA as passenger, pedestrian, driver, motorcycles	Separation	Parent/peer
	Magical thinker	Sports	Pain	Inform of choices
	Modest	Water injuries	Death	Give privacy
	Peer pressure	Firearms	Disfigurement	
	Hysterical reaction	Drugs, alcohol	Disability	

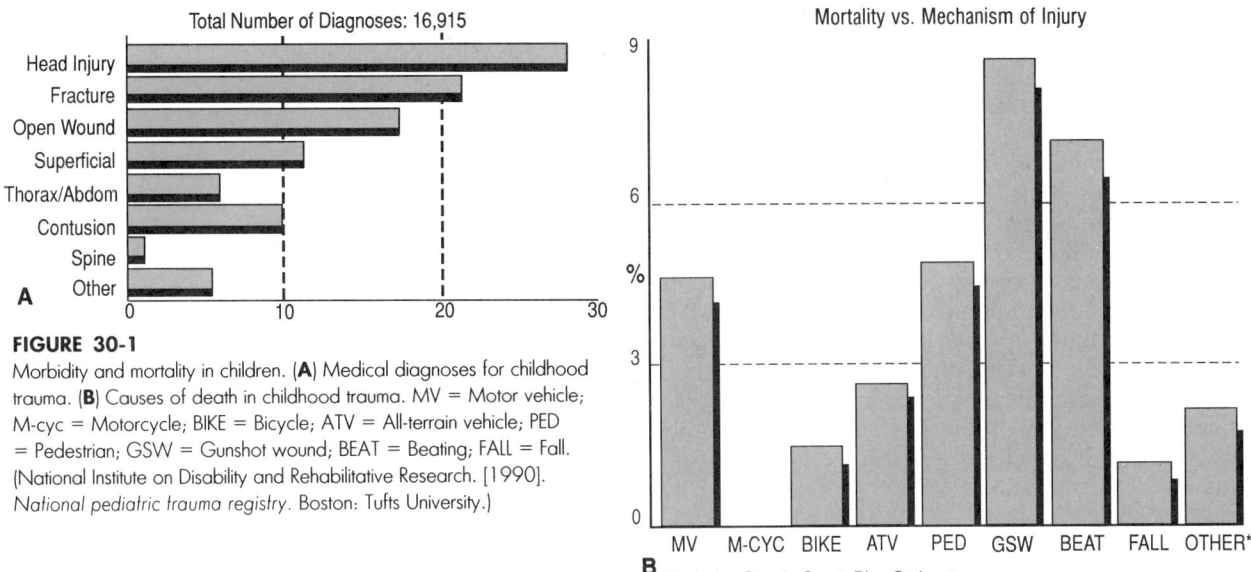

FIGURE 30-1

Morbidity and mortality in children. (**A**) Medical diagnoses for childhood trauma. (**B**) Causes of death in childhood trauma. MV = Motor vehicle; M-cyc = Motorcycle; BIKE = Bicycle; ATV = All-terrain vehicle; PED = Pedestrian; GSW = Gunshot wound; BEAT = Beating; FALL = Fall. (National Institute on Disability and Rehabilitative Research. [1990]. *National pediatric trauma registry*. Boston: Tufts University.)

poor visual and perceptual abilities, developmental delays, increased incidence of illness, and drugs or alcohol use.[5]

Trauma Care

Prevention

The first line of defense against trauma is prevention, commonly referred to as injury control. Injury control occurs at three levels:

Primary—prohibition (e.g., installation of gates on stairs and fences around swimming pools)
Secondary—protection (e.g., the use of helmets and goggles)
Tertiary—treatment (e.g., acute care of head injury)

To maintain an effective injury control program, the health care system must work at all three levels. Legislative efforts, public education, and system development are essential components of such a program. Health promotion and health management are discussed in Chapter 7. Anticipatory guidance for emergency prevention is summarized in Chapter 29.

Continuum of Care

Advances in the knowledge of traumatic injury patterns and the child's physiologic response to multiple injuries has dramatically improved the care injured children receive. With the implementation of regionalized care, critically injured children are being transported to specialty centers for definitive tertiary care. Unfortunately, this high level of care is not universal throughout the country. Injured children are cared for in a variety of settings, from small community hospitals in rural areas to university-affiliated pediatric centers.

The key concept in decreasing morbidity and mortality is that the right child is treated by the right team of professionals, at the right center with the right resources and commitment, in the critical time frame of the "Golden Hour" of trauma care. National and state organizations have developed standards of care, criteria for trauma center designation, protocols for triage and treatment of injured children and adults, and guidelines for trauma system design to promote the regionalization of emergency care and tertiary trauma care for all injured people. The success of these efforts varies widely across the country due to the nature of medical and governmental organizations and the politics associated. Access to specialized trauma care remains a problem in many areas.

The continuum of trauma care can be conceptualized as a timeline, as shown in Figure 30-2. The event that

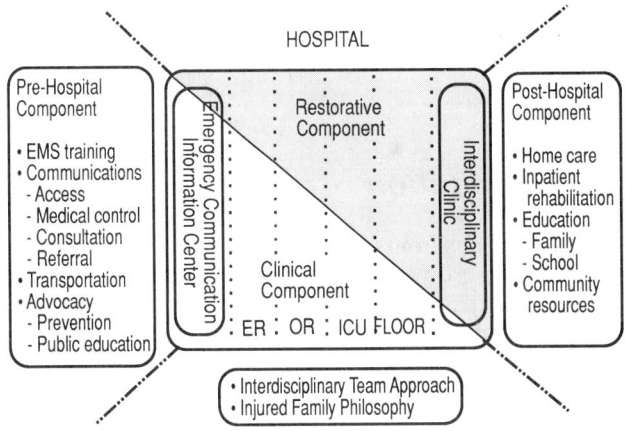

Note: Horizontal axis indicates time, Vertical axis indicates resource utilization

FIGURE 30-2

The continuum of pediatric trauma care spans prehospital, inpatient, and postdischarge components. (Redrawn from Evans, D. W., & Eichelberger, M. R. [1988]. The pediatric trauma center: A commitment to the continuum. In M. R. Eichelberger & G. S. Pratsch [Eds.], *Pediatric trauma care*. Rockville, MD: Aspen.)

causes the traumatic injury occurs in seconds, the pre-hospital emergency care and resuscitation on the scene is completed within minutes, and the trauma response team's assessment and stabilization should take less than an hour. Management of vital functions during this critical time period, commonly referred to as the "Golden Hour," often determines ultimate outcome for the injured child. The care of the injured child is continued in specialty care areas, including radiology, operating rooms, intensive care units, and specialty pediatric units over hours, days, and weeks. The child's recovery to a stable medical status may be followed by weeks and months of rehabilitation both in the hospital and at home. For the child, the delivery of each phase of care is critical and has a lasting impact on how he or she interacts with family, peers, community, and the health care system in the future.

Systems Approach

Successful pediatric trauma care requires a systems approach, which begins with components of access, communication, training of initial responders, triage, and transportation[10] before the injured child even arrives at the hospital. Although their capabilities differ depending on level of training and geographic location, emergency medical technicians (EMTs) and paramedics perform a rapid on-scene assessment and initiate life-saving or first aid measures. However, their goal is to minimize scene time and transport the child as rapidly as possible to a definitive care center.

In the emergency department (ED), the inner core trauma team normally consists of a group of specialized interdisciplinary caregivers, including nurses, surgeons, respiratory therapists, and anesthesiologists. Outside the resuscitation bay are other essential team members, including social workers, laboratory and x-ray personnel, and coordinators. Clearly delineated roles and responsibilities enable the evaluation and treatment of the patient to progress smoothly. Equipment and supplies are readily available in the full range of pediatric sizes. The roles of the nurse in childhood emergencies are discussed in Chapter 29.

Resuscitation

Most deaths from trauma occur in the first hour after injury as the result of airway complications, hemorrhagic shock, or irreparable central nervous damage.[17] The goal of early resuscitation is to reverse the pathophysiology before changes become irreversible.

Primary Survey and Management

The initial assessment of the pediatric trauma patient takes place according to the ABCs (airway, breathing, circulation) or the ABCDE mnemonic, which addresses airway, breathing, circulation, disability, and exposure. This initial assessment, or primary survey, ensures that all po-tentially life-threatening injuries are discovered and treated as rapidly as possible.[17]

A: Airway

Hypoxia is the final common pathway by which the three main killers in trauma—airway obstruction, hypovolemic shock, and central nervous system injury—affect the injured child (Fig. 30-3). Thus, immediate attention to oxygenation is essential. The airway is first assessed for patency. Because infants are obligate nasal breathers, any obstruction to the nares such as blood or mucus can result in airway compromise. The child's relatively large tongue and abundant lymphoid tissue can also be a source of obstruction, especially when the child is obtunded (not fully conscious). The jaw thrust maneuver aids in relieving this type of blockage. This is accomplished by grasping the mandible at the angle of the jaw and lifting upwards, without tilting the head (see Chap. 29). An oral airway may be used if the child is unconscious, but this causes gagging and coughing if the child is awake. Suctioning may be required if secretions or blood are present.

If a patient arrives in the ED without neck immobilization, protection against potential cervical spine injury must be addressed simultaneously with airway management. For the child approximately 3 years and older, commercial cervical collars are available to fit and should be applied. For the younger child and infant, the use of towel rolls, combined with securing the head in a midline position with tape, is an alternative. The entire spinal column must also be protected against movement. Straps and taping are commonly used. Many new devices— "high tech" boards—have been placed on the market for immobilization, but few accommodate the varying heights and weights of all children. Further research is needed to ensure the safety of these boards.

Most pediatric trauma victims who are having difficulty breathing are easily treated by suctioning and positioning, but if dyspnea persists, bag-mask ventilation or endotracheal intubation may be necessary. Bag-mask ventilation requires an appropriately sized bag and mask, along with a tight seal of the mask over the mouth and nose. The bag should be compressed until the child's

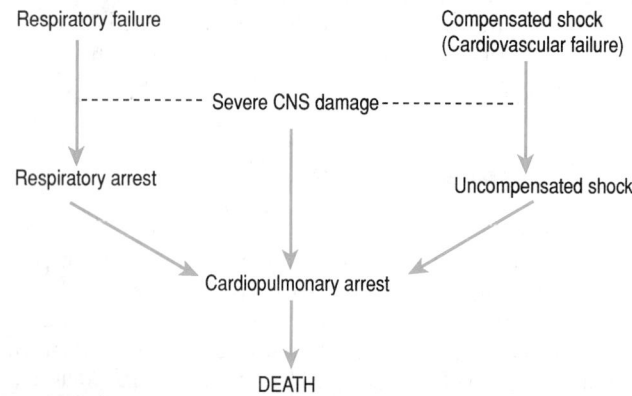

FIGURE 30-3

Respiratory failure, CNS injury, and hypovolemic shock can lead to a final common pathway in the injured child. Adapted from Ramenofsky, M. L., Jurkovich, G. J., & Dierking, B. H. [1987]. *Advanced pediatric life support.*]

chest rises. The four general indications for intubation are:

- Control of ventilation, such as when respiratory effort is inadequate or hyperventilation is required
- Oxygenation
- Airway protection, such as when long distance transport is necessary
- Long-term pulmonary hygiene[39]

The size of the endotracheal tube may be approximated by the size of the child's "pinky" finger. The formula

16 + age in years ÷ 4 = internal diameter in mm

may also be used.[1] Uncuffed endotracheal tubes are generally used in children up to the age of about 8 years to minimize the potential for subglottic ulceration; also, the narrowest aspect of the trachea is at the level of the cricoid cartilage, which forms a natural "cuff." Orotracheal tubes are generally preferred unless oral trauma is present. The tube is anchored securely with tape, and breath sounds are auscultated. In infants, breath sounds can be readily transmitted despite lack of ventilation in one lobe or lung. For this reason, a chest x-ray is always done after intubation to ascertain correct placement. If endotracheal intubation is unsuccessful due to massive airway trauma or low obstruction, needle cricothyroidotomy may be used as a temporary measure. Tracheostomy is a complex, risky procedure in the child with a compromised airway and should only be attempted in the controlled setting of the operating room. However, such surgical procedures are rarely required for the child's airway.[32]

B: Breathing

Breathing is assessed for rate, quality, and depth of respirations. Retractions are a "see-saw" movement of the chest and abdomen that indicate respiratory distress. Children are diaphragmatic breathers, and any compro-mise of diaphragm excursion limits the child's ability to ventilate. The most common source of such compromise is gastric distention due to air swallowing (aerophagia). Thus, a naso- or orogastric tube is mandatory. All childhood trauma patients should be provided with supplemental oxygen initially. If the child has been transported with an oxygen mask or cannula, this should be connected to a source of humidification as soon as possible. Nonhumidified oxygen is extremely drying and can lead to mucous plugs or airway irritation.

C: Circulation

Shock must be recognized and treated rapidly in the pediatric trauma patient. Because of the child's small circulating blood volume, a blood loss of as little as 20 ml/kg may precipitate shock in the child. The child in early hypovolemic shock may have a normal blood pressure due to extremely effective compensatory mechanisms. More reliable indicators of shock include tachycardia, change in level of consciousness, capillary refill time greater than 2 seconds, poor peripheral pulses, and pale/mottled and cool extremities.[1]

Initial treatment of shock includes control of hemorrhage and fluid replacement. Most external bleeding can be controlled by direct pressure. Intravenous access can be difficult in the child, who may present with small veins, hypovolemia, and vasoconstriction. Antecubital or saphenous veins are generally preferred. Cutdowns are avoided during resuscitation due to the specialized technique and time required for the procedure. Neck veins may be cannulated but may make airway and chest procedures more difficult. If IV access cannot be obtained in a relatively short period of time, intraosseous infusion is an alternative in the child less than 5 years old. In this procedure, a needle with stylet is inserted directly into the bone marrow, preferably at the anterior tibial plateau, as shown in Figure 30-4. Because of the rich network of venous sinusoids in the marrow of long bones, drugs,

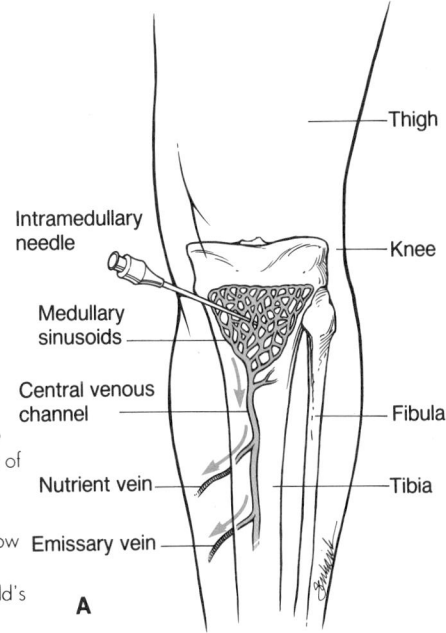
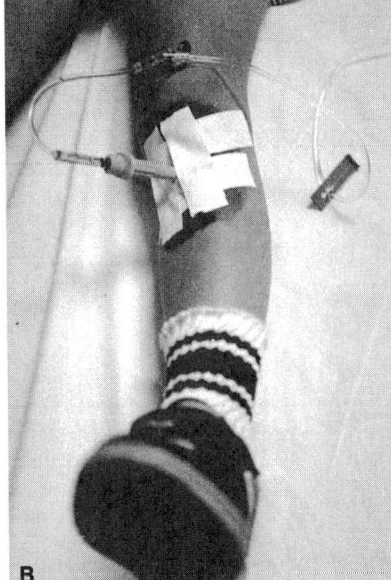

FIGURE 30-4

Intraosseous infusion is an emergency alternative to venous access in the young child. The rich network of venous sinusoids within long bones allows rapid infusion into the central circulation. (**A**) Schematic diagram illustrating venous drainage from the marrow of a long bone with an intramedullary needle in place. (**B**) An intraosseous needle in place in a child's leg. (Photo courtesy of Brad Husberg.)

Labels in Figure 30-4A: Intramedullary needle, Medullary sinusoids, Central venous channel, Nutrient vein, Emissary vein, Thigh, Knee, Fibula, Tibia fluids, and blood are readily absorbed. Complications are rare but may include extravasation and osteomyelitis.[30]

Once intravenous access is obtained, crystalloid solution is given in 20-ml/kg boluses. Response should be monitored, including increasing level of consciousness, return to normal heart rate and blood pressure, and urine output. Boluses may be repeated one or two times. If no response is seen to replacement of 40 ml/kg, ongoing internal hemorrhage is likely; blood transfusion and surgery may be indicated.[38]

D: Disability (Neurologic Injury)

To ascertain the presence of neurologic injury, which may be life threatening, a brief neurologic examination is performed at this point. Because level of consciousness is the most sensitive indicator of neurologic status in children,[18] responses should be assessed for developmental appropriateness. For example, a young child would be expected to cry during painful procedures such as blood drawing. The modified Glasgow Coma Scale (GCS), as shown in the accompanying display, should be calculated on a serial basis.

A score of 15 for all three categories is normal; 7 or less indicates coma; 3—the lowest possible score—generally points to brain death.

Ability to move all extremities, sensation, and pupillary reflexes should be documented. Effective cerebral resuscitation depends on adequate cerebral perfusion, so attention to airway, oxygenation, and adequate fluid replacement is essential to outcome.

E: Exposure

The injured child should be exposed, or undressed, to allow for examination of the entire body. This helps to ensure that no injuries are missed (Fig. 30-5). However, the high ratio of body surface area to mass, a higher met-

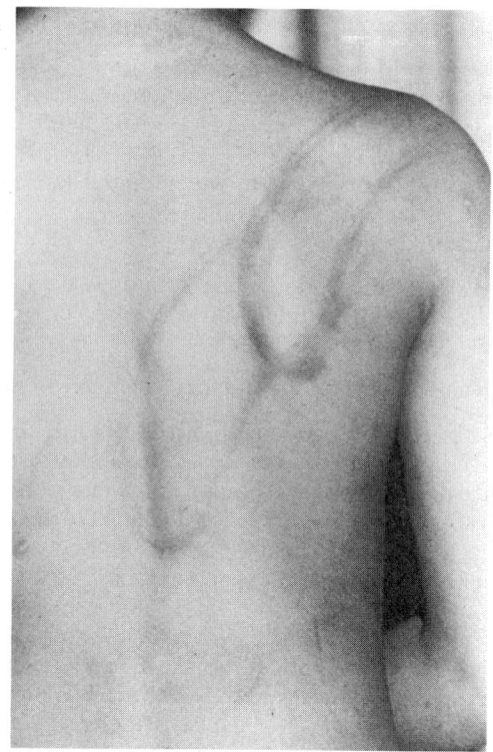

FIGURE 30-5
Clothing may conceal some injuries, so the trauma victim should be undressed for examination. Patterns of injury may be significant in identifying child abuse. These contusions resulted from whipping with a looped cord.

abolic rate, the small glycogen stores in the liver, and the lack of substantial body fat predispose the child to heat loss and resulting hypothermic stress. Hypothermia can cause shivering and stimulate the release of catecholamines, which can, in turn, render a child refractory to attempts at controlling shock.[15] The emergency room should have warming lights or thermostatic control of room temperature available for the injured child. In addition, large volumes of IV fluid or blood should be warmed before administration.

Secondary Survey and Management

After the ABCs have been assessed, a more complete exam, or secondary survey, is performed. This includes blood work and radiologic studies, as well as a thorough head-to-toe assessment of each body system. A nasogastric (NG) tube should be inserted after the integrity of the cribriform plate is confirmed; a Foley catheter is placed once urinary tract disruption is ruled out.[26]

Psychosocial Care

Trauma is a sudden, unexpected threat to life that usually requires more coping ability than is available. Beyond the impact of the injury on the physiologic systems of the child, the psychological impact on both the child and family is sudden and complex. The child and family

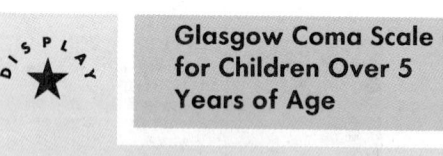

Glasgow Coma Scale (GCS) for Children Over 5 Years of Age		
Eye opening response	Spontaneous	4
	To voice	3
	To pain	2
	None	1
Best verbal response	Oriented	5
	Confused	
	Inappropriate words	4
	Incomprehensible sounds	3
		2
	None	1
Best motor response	Obeys commands	6
	Localizes pain	5
	Withdraws (pain)	4
	Abnormal flexion	3
	Flexion (pain)	2
	None	1

do not have an opportunity to prepare for the event and subsequent hospitalization.

The Child

The child who is hospitalized for trauma leaves the comfort and security of home and encounters a strange and unknown environment filled with unfamiliar equipment, frightening sights and sounds, painful procedures, and new people. The child may be disoriented due to his physical condition. The child's ability to eat, speak, play, or even move around may be compromised by tubes and restraints. Enforced dependence may thwart an evolving sense of independence. Ability to understand these changes may be limited due to both the child's developmental level and the suddenness with which they occurred.

Throughout resuscitation, the team must remember that the patient is a child undergoing an overwhelming crisis. Every effort should be made to explain to the child what is happening, even if the child's awareness is questionable. One team member should be assigned to provide psychosocial care for the child, including reassurances and brief preparation for procedures.

The Parents

Injury to a child never occurs in isolation, and the health care system must be prepared to treat the injured family as well as the injured child.[8] The manner in which parents are able to relate to and support the child after a traumatic injury has a great influence on the child's reaction and ability to cope with the experience.

The child senses and reacts to the parents' emotions and actions; thus, the extent of parental knowledge and anxiety has a profound effect on the child's perception and adjustment. Parents need emotional support through reassurance and reliability, tangible support of services and supplies, and informational support, including factual data about their child's injuries and treatment. Regular feedback from consistent caregivers and anticipatory guidance about how they and their child will psychologically respond to the injury are keys to successful coping and adaptation.

As soon as the child's condition allows, parents should be allowed to visit with their child in the emergency room. Such family-centered care recognizes the holistic nature of pediatric trauma care and begins the process of allowing the child and family to participate in recovery.

The Siblings

The siblings of injured children experience many of the same feelings and fears as parents—those related to separation, the unknown, death, and guilt. Siblings need simple, honest information about their injured brother or sister, the care being provided, and the environmental surroundings. Siblings frequently feel alone and abandoned by both parents and the injured child. To assist brothers and sisters to become a part of the team, nursing interventions include preparation for visitation and consistent visitation policies, suggestions of items to bring from home, orientation to the surroundings, suggestions on what to say to a child who is not completely awake, and opportunities for diversional activities in a quiet area close by the injured child and parents.

Discharge

Discharge from the hospital is a stressful time for the child and family. At home, the professional staff is no longer available for questions and constant support. Reactions of friends and the community must be dealt with. Changes in home lifestyle, even temporary, that need to be made for the injured child impact all members of the family. Preparation for discharge needs to begin early, allowing the family to get ready psychologically as well as logistically.

Nutritional Considerations

Provision of adequate nutrition is a critical aspect of recovery from trauma. After injury, the body enters a hypermetabolic state, which can persist for up to 10 days. During this period, up to twice the normal number of calories may be required. In addition, children require adequate calorie and protein intake to continue the ongoing process of growth and development. However, due to physiologic changes that occur after trauma and resuscitation, measurement of the usual objective indicators of nutritional status (weight, skinfold thickness, urine urea nitrogen, serum proteins, and so forth) may not be accurate.[23] Thus, calculation of nutritional needs can be difficult; there are no methods available that are specific to the needs of the multiply-injured child.

Head Trauma

Head injuries in children are a leading cause of death and disability from trauma. Children's susceptibility to head injury is related to both anatomic characteristics and developmental stages. The child's head is proportionally much larger than his body. At birth, the brain is 15% of adult size, whereas the body at birth is 5% of adult size. The infant and young child's skull has more ability to expand and tolerate increases in intracranial pressure due to the open anterior fontanel (before 18 months) and the lack of fused suture lines. Infants have little muscle support for their heads and, therefore, are at great risk for injuries from poor head control and from "shaken baby syndrome."

As children begin to creep, crawl, and walk, they lead with their heads and thus sustain many minor bruises and bumps to the head. More serious injuries to the head and brain occur from the energy involved in a fall or blow from another object. External injuries to the head are often significant because of bleeding from the highly vascularized scalp. Internal injuries to the brain include blunt contusions, intracerebral bleeding, and shearing injury to the base of the brain.

The growing child continues to be at high risk for head and brain injury. Motor vehicles, falls, and bicycles (motorbikes) are the leading cause of head injury for the young, school-age, and adolescent child. An example of nursing care of a child with injuries from a bike or motor vehicle accident is given in the Nursing Care Plan. Although children have a lower incidence of intracranial hematomas than adults, the incidence of contusions, fractures, and increased intracranial pressure is higher than in adults.[24]

Classification of Head Injuries

The classification of head injury into mild, moderate, and severe relates to level of consciousness at the time of the injury and immediately afterwards, the type of brain injury sustained, and the long-term prognosis for recovery and return to the home, school, and community.[24]

Mild Injury

A mild head injury has an initial GCS of 13 to 15 and includes concussions with or without posttraumatic seizures, as well as linear skull fractures without disruption of the cranium. Concussion occurs when the brain receives a brief blow or jar from an external source that results in a mild degree of back and forth movement. There may or may not be a brief period of loss of consciousness associated. There is no structural injury to the brain that can be seen with computed tomography (CT) scan or magnetic resonance imaging (MRI). After a concussion, children typically have some loss of memory surrounding the injury (posttraumatic amnesia), mild headaches, confusion, and nausea. Typically, these symptoms decrease in frequency within a day or two and disappear within 2 weeks.[49]

Scalp lacerations and hematomas are often associated with mild head injuries. Blunt injury to the head may result in a subgaleal hematoma occurring in the scalp, which swells for few days and then slowly reabsorbs.

Skull fractures are classified into three types: linear, depressed, and basilar. Linear skull fractures are seen frequently in children, most often without associated brain injury. Typically, these fractures require no special care and heal within 6 months in infants or 12 months in older children. Depressed fractures in children most commonly occur in the parietal area and frontal region from a direct blow, causing the bone to fracture inward. Surgical intervention is generally needed if the fracture is deeper than the thickness of the skull or if it is associated with open scalp injury.

Basilar skull fractures occur after a direct forceful blow to the head or a high-speed impact with a solid surface (ground, car, wall). Classic signs of basilar skull fractures include:

- Blood in external auditory canal or behind tympanic membrane
- Cerebral spinal fluid (CSF) draining from ear or nose
- Bruise on mastoid bone behind ear (Battle's sign)
- Periorbital discoloration (raccoon eyes)[12]

Children exhibit posttraumatic seizures more frequently than adults. Typically, the seizure is a one-time occurrence within an hour of the injury; it is self-limiting,

and the child remains free from deficits or sequelae. No specific pharmacologic treatment is needed after the initial resuscitation as long as the child remains free from further seizure activity. Follow-up evaluations should be established within a month of injury.

Moderate Injury

A child with a moderate head injury presents with a GCS of 9 to 12. This level of injury includes open skull fractures, depressed skull fractures, and contusions. Contusions result from more force or energy to the brain and cause bruising, which can usually be seen on CT scan. Contusions are associated with specific deficits related to the area of the brain affected, which may vary in duration. Resulting motor deficits may include hemiparesis, loss of oral motor coordination, and difficulties in balance. Cognitive deficits include disorders of memory, attention, language processing, problem solving, and impulse control.[24,49]

Severe Injury

Children with severe head injuries present with a GCS of 8 or less. This level of injury includes epidural and subdural hematomas, intracranial hematomas, brain laceration, and herniation. Epidural hematomas in children most frequently occur in the temporal region of the brain. Subdural hematomas occur more frequently in children than epidural hematomas and result from shearing of veins or damage to cortical surface arteries. These may occur with brain contusions or lacerations. The blood spreads widely through the subdural space.[31] Intracerebral hematomas in children most frequently occur in the temporal lobe from a direct blow to the area or from shearing forces during a high energy impact.

Assessment

The emergent and immediate care for children with all types of head injuries starts with the assessment and stabilization of the ABCs. The establishment of a secure airway is especially important for the child with a severe injury because neurologic status may change quickly, leading to shallow breathing or hypoventilation. Oxygenated blood in adequate volumes must reach the injured brain to prevent further injury and long-term disability or death. The primary injury to the brain occurs at the time of impact, but secondary injury can occur if appropriate care is not initiated to minimize edema and hypoxia. Blood loss from other injuries can have a detrimental effect on the injured brain; thus, early recognition and treatment for shock are imperative.

Once the respiratory and cardiovascular status is stabilized, the neurologic assessment and intervention proceed. A quick neurologic check can be completed during the primary survey within the first minutes of care. The Glasgow Coma Score[48] has become the national standard for both initial and ongoing assessment of level of consciousness after a head injury. The Glasgow Coma Score can easily be applied to children of all ages by professionals who recognize the normal behaviors for specific

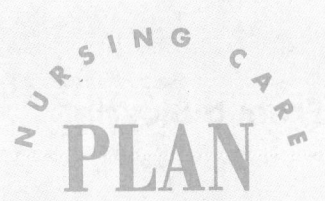

A 7-Year-Old Child Thrown From a Bicycle

Assessment

Case Study Description

Tony C. is a 7-year-old male involved in a motor vehicle crash while riding on his bicycle. Car was going approximately 35 mph, and Tony was not wearing a helmet. Tony was thrown 8 feet and landed on sidewalk. Witness described brief (about 3 s) loss of consciousness, multiple abrasions, and crying. Paramedic evaluated patient with GCS = 15, lethargic, P = 140, BP = 75/P, tender abdomen, intact reflexes. Child transported to trauma center.

Assessment Data

On arrival in ER: Tony was quiet yet responded to questions about age, name; GCS = 15; no recall of injury or car, normal neurologic examination. Facial abrasions on left side, with 3 cm deep laceration VS: P = 135, R = 30, BP = 75/P, capillary refill 3 s. Abdomen tender to palpation in RUQ. Abrasions on left lateral calf, intact neurovascular status to both upper and lower extremities.

Parents arrived within 20 min, anxious and crying. Full medical history given with no previous illnesses or injuries. Up-to-date on all immunizations.

CT scan showed a liver laceration. Trauma x-ray series of cervical spine, pelvis, chest were negative. Facial CT and facial flat plates were negative.

Tony tearful with procedures, responding with age-appropriate answers, no recall of injury, street, or preceding 15–20 min. Full recall of school and home.

Nursing Diagnosis	Intervention	Rationale
1. Fluid volume deficit related to hemorrhage secondary to blunt injury	Establish intravenous access and administer fluid bolus per protocol or order.	Volume resuscitation must occur within first hour of care and be continually reassessed.
	Ensure patient remains on bedrest with minimal movement.	Patient immobility essential for 5–7 days to allow for stabilization.
	During next 24 h, reassess: Vital signs every 4 h with level of consciousness, liver function studies, hemoglobin and hematocrit, and intake and output.	Frequent assessment to determine if liver continues to hemorrhage; surgery or transfusion may be indicated.
	Maintain venous access, administer fluid volume as ordered. Maintain strict intake and output.	
2. Altered thought processes secondary to blunt injury	Assessment of level of consciousness, neurologic examination, GCS every 15 min until stable, every 2 h for 12 h, then every 4 h.	Brief loss of consciousness can be associated with delayed response to head injury, and frequently results in temporary memory loss. Child and parents need reassurance that this response is expected.
	Reassess memory of event and emergency room experience at 12 and 24 h.	
	Provide written and oral information to child and parents about head injury and posttraumatic amnesia.	Family may need frequent repetition and reference of information given, due to stress of situation. Planning follow-up will alleviate parental anxiety and enhance compliance.

(Continued)

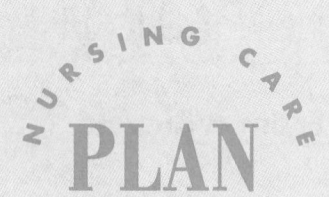

A 7-Year-Old Child Thrown From a Bicycle
(continued)

| | Ensure follow-up care arranged with neurosurgery before discharge. | |
| | Provide information for school teacher on concussion and posttraumatic amnesia | Parents need oral and written information to assist their child and teacher. |

Nursing Diagnosis	*Intervention*	*Rationale*
3. Diversional activity deficit secondary to bedrest for 5–7 days	Establish daily routine for AM and PM care, rest, playroom, school work: • Post calendar • Written schedule • Develop team plan	School-age child placed on bedrest for 5–7 days has experienced great loss of control and independence.
	Provide new activities during playroom time: • New hobbies • Books about hospitals • Craft projects • Reward program for assisting with activities of daily living	Personalization of daily routines and the development of new activities assist with both primary and secondary coping skills.
	Involve siblings with selection of toys, crafts. Provide parents with written activity restrictions for first week, and next 3 mo.	Family participation with schedule and activities help parents with meeting the needs of all family members and in enforcing activity restrictions.

Evaluation

Emergency Care

- Tony exhibits return to hemodynamic stability.
- Tony verbalizes orientation to all procedures and surroundings.
- Parents are reunited with Tony as soon as history is obtained and Tony is physiologically stable.
- Parents accompany Tony to CT scan and to room.

Inpatient Care

- Tony remains on bedrest for 5 days.
- Tony verbalizes orientation to nursing unit and playroom.
- Tony participates in development of daily schedule and calendar.
- Parents demonstrate knowledge of care at home for both liver injury restrictions and for concussion.
- Parents report they have contacted school and arranged for alternative activites during gym class.

Follow-Up Care

- Parents demonstrate knowledge of emergency care in case of sudden change in child's neurologic status.
- Tony reports he is maintaining restricted activity.
- Tony and family relate any difficulties with sleep, dreams, personality, attention, to concussion during first week home.
- Tony and siblings share with their class and neighborhood the importance of helmets in bicycle riding.

ages. The neurologic assessment also includes evaluation of pupil size, symmetry, and response to light; cranial nerve function, motor strength, reflexes, and symmetry in all extremities; and sensory components of visual acuity, auditory function, proprioception, and balance.

The most serious complication of increased intracranial pressure (ICP), herniation, is the displacement of part of the brain from one compartment to another. Signs of herniation include rapid decrease in level of consciousness, cranial nerve deficit, bilateral or unilateral motor extension and then flexion, brainstem dysfunction, and changes in vital signs and respiratory status. Herniation is a surgical emergency requiring rapid decompression of the cranial vault. (ICP and herniation are discussed in Chap. 53.)

Nursing Interventions: Collaborative and Independent

Intracranial pressure (ICP) is measured in millimeters of mercury (mmHg). The neurosurgical team places an intracranial monitoring device through the use of an external ventriculostomy, subarachnoid bolt, or intracranial catheter. The normal ICP for a child is 0 to 15 mmHg. Monitoring the ICP after brain injury requires notation of baseline values, patterns of pressure waves and associated stimuli, and careful documentation of ICP over 24 hours.[24] Specific nursing interventions are directly related to the degree of increased ICP. Immediate nursing interventions are listed in the accompanying display.

Recovery after a head injury in children varies widely with both the severity of injury and the child and family's understanding of the recovery process.

Treatment after a concussion, laceration, or external hematoma includes limitation of vigorous activity, anal-

gesia for headaches, and observation for infection. The parents are able to take the child home once he or she is oriented at an age-appropriate level, can tolerate a regular diet, and has a normal neurologic exam.

Nursing care following surgery for a depressed skull fracture or hematoma focuses on the repeated neurologic assessment and prevention of infection. Of greatest concern to the child may be the altered body image secondary to the new haircut, sutures, and Betadine used by the neurosurgeon.

Initial management of basilar skull fractures includes prevention of further injury, identification of any underlying intracranial lesion, and prevention of infection. An NG tube should not be inserted, and only one physician should examine the child's ears and nose due to the possibility of introducing infection or further injury.[24] Close neurologic assessment is needed for 24 hours and until the child returns to a normal state. Antibiotic therapy will most likely be prescribed for any child with a dural tear and associated cerebral spinal fluid drainage from the nose or ears. The child and family can return home with specific activity restrictions and close neurosurgical follow-up.

Teaching

Parents should be given written and verbal instructions on specific signs for concern. The accompanying display is an example of a handout for parents after their child has sustained a minor head injury.

Even children who sustain only a mild injury such as a concussion may have changes in their personality, circadian rhythm, recurrent headaches, and problems with attention and motivation for a period of weeks to months. Research indicates that children and their families should be given specific anticipatory guidance related to the

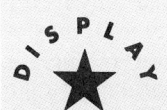

Nursing Intervention: Immediate Care Related to the Degree of Increased Intracranial Pressure (ICP)

Mild increase ICP (15–20)

- Decrease extraneous noise and stimuli
- Elevate head of bed to 30 degrees
- Maintain head in midline position
- Maintain patent airway
- Restrict fluid and maintain strict intake and output
- Administer mild sedation/analgesia as ordered for pain control
- Cluster interventions to promote periods of rest and decreased stimuli

Moderate ICP (20–30)

- Provide above interventions, with specific attention to airway, elevation, and stabilization of head
- Provide hyperventilation before any procedures
- Provide hyperventilation to maintain pCO_2 between 25–30 mm Hg

- Sedate as prescribed with serial neurologic assessment
- Control pain
- Use diuretics cautiously, if prescribed
- Structure and limit duration and variety of stimuli

Severe ICP (>40)

- Provide above interventions with constant hyperventilation by machine and manual intervention with peaks
- Limit all unnecessary stimuli
- Provide sedation/analgesia as ordered for agitation and pain control
- Administer diuretics as prescribed with strict I & O
- Provide osmotic therapy, as prescribed
- Maintain barbiturate coma, as prescribed
- Reassess and prepare for imaging and/or surgery

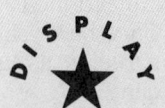

Family Teaching: Your Child Has a Head Injury

After your child hits his head he may:

- Become very upset and excited
- Vomit
- Become sleepy

Treatment of Head Injuries at Home

- Wake baby every 4 h for feeding
- Wake older child every 4 h to see how he is feeling
- Give only sips of clear fluids such as water, fruit juices, and ice pops for the first 8 h after your child hits his head

Call the Doctor

If baby is:

- Very hard to wake up or if he will not wake up
- Vomiting 8 h after he hit his head
- Irritable (very fussy)
- Having convulsions (fits)

If child:

- Is very hard to wake up or if he will not wake up
- Is vomiting 8 h after he hit his head
- Has a bad headache 8 h after he hit his head
- Seems confused; does not know who he is or where he is
- Has convulsions (fits)

From *Children's National Medical Center, Washington, DC.*

---

cognitive and behavioral changes that may occur. Too frequently, these children look normal and can go through daily activities of living, yet are unable to function at school or with groups of people. The National Head Injury Foundation has coined the phrase the "silent epidemic" or the "walking wounded."[29,50]

Rehabilitation

Mild head injury rehabilitation includes close monitoring by a knowledgeable team of health careproviders. Primary care physicians and nurse specialists/practitioners need to assess for subtle changes in behavior, personality reports from parents, and difficulties at school. Any problems should be referred to the neurotrauma team for specific cognitive and psychological assessment. Specific recommendations for family and school can prevent the slow self-perpetuating sequence of events seen after "mild" or "minor" head injury.

The child who has sustained a moderate-to-severe injury needs a specialized rehabilitation program related to specific areas of disability. Recovery for head injury can also be guided using the Ranchos Los Amigos Cognitive Scales, which describe specific stages of recovery. As outlined in Table 30-2, specific nursing interventions are recommended for each level of recovery. In some areas of the country, outpatient services and school services can be combined to assist the child with a mild hemiparesis or a specific linguistic deficit (e.g., short-term memory loss or expressive aphasia). But, in most circumstances, the child who has a temporary deficit that prevents him or her from returning to school and a former level of independence should receive intensive rehabilitation services in an acute pediatric head injury program.

Maxillofacial Trauma

Unless it involves significant airway injury, maxillofacial trauma is not likely to kill its victims. However, the potential for disfigurement, along with damage to sensory organs, make these injuries important in terms of psychosocial and developmental impact. The goal of the trauma team is to maintain or restore function while providing for optimal cosmetic outcome.

Maxillofacial injuries include abrasions, lacerations, and fractures, as well as penetrating trauma. The pediatric facial skeleton is lighter and more protected by its relatively large cranium than is the adult skeleton; thus, injuries to this area are less frequent in children. The most common mechanisms for pediatric maxillofacial injury are incidents involving motor vehicles (with victim as occupant or pedestrian) and falls. A significant decrease in mid- and upper-face fractures has been noted, probably due to the impact of seat belt and car seat use.[40]

Zygomatic fractures may occur at any of the attachments to the frontal, maxillary, sphenoid, or temporal bones. These fractures are usually produced by deceleration forces and are frequently accompanied by other facial fractures. The child often has flatness of the affected cheekbone (although this may be masked by edema), tenderness of the orbital rim, with periorbital edema and ecchymosis. A change in the child's gaze pattern may also be noted. Trismus, or the inability to open the mouth, may indicate that a zygomatic fracture is displaced.[22]

A blow-out fracture of the orbital floor is sustained as a result of blunt trauma, when a sudden increase in intraorbital pressure takes the path of least resistance and ruptures the bottom of the orbital socket. Hallmarks of this injury are diplopia and displacement of the globe

TABLE 30-2
Ranchos Los Amigos Scales and Interventions to Plan Nursing Care During Different Stages of Recovery from Head Injury

No.	Level	Description	Interventions
I	No response	Unresponsive to any stimulus	Talk and touch; turn on lights
II	Generalized response	Limited, inconsistent, nonpurposeful responses, often to pain only	Use photos and calendar, familiar tapes
III	Localized response	Purposeful responses; may follow simple commands; may focus on presented object, responses are inconsistent, may be delayed	Reinforce names; use simple commands and explanations; Repeat all input
IV	Confused, agitated	Heightened state of activity, confusion, disorientation, aggressive behavior; unable to do self-care; unaware of present events; agitation related to internal confusion; often emotional	Provide a structure-oriented program (channel, compensate)
V	Confused, inappropriate, nonagitated	Appears alert; responds to commands; highly distractable doesn't concentrate on task; agitated responses may continue; verbally inappropriate; difficulty with new information	Increase attention, memory, and organization
VI	Confused, appropriate	Good directed behavior, needs cueing; can relearn old skills of activities of daily living; memory problems; some awareness of self/others	Use schedules, notebook, and rewards
VII	Automatic, appropriate	Robotlike appropriate behavior, minimal confusion; shallow recall; poor insight into condition; initiates tasks, but needs structure; poor judgment, problem solving and planning skills	Provide a community-oriented program; decrease structuring; increase independence and contact with home
VIII	Purposeful, appropriate	Alert, oriented; recalls and integrates past events; learns new activities and can continue without supervision; independent in home and living skills; capable of driving; problems with stress tolerance, judgment, abstract reasoning persist	Encourage use of a journal, making choices, adapting a new schedule

Adapted from Ranchos Los Amigos Scales. Copyright 1990 C. J. Wright, MSN, RNC.

downward.[3] Entrapment of muscles and nerves by bone fragments can lead to the need for surgical intervention.

Mandibular fractures often occur in pairs because the U-shaped mandibular structure transmits force from one side to the other. The mandibular condyle is the major growth center of the mandible; fractures during the first 3 years of life can predispose the child to long-term problems.[13] The strong muscles of mastication present in the jaw can reduce or further displace the fracture, depending on the site and angle of muscle attachment. Evidence of this injury commonly includes malocclusion, with pain and limited range of jaw movement.

Nasal fractures are the most common facial fracture in children. In childhood, the midline suture in the nasal bone is a weak point, which makes the bone vulnerable to fracture after a direct blow. These are reduced early, before the onset of edema, to avoid the need for surgical intervention.

Eye injuries are generally painful and anxiety-provoking, regardless of the severity of injury. Hyphema, the presence of blood in the eye's anterior chamber, occurs as the result of blunt force or the child's being poked in the eye with an object. The usual duration of uncomplicated hyphema is approximately 5 to 7 days. Therapy is focused on preventing ocular hypertension and promoting eye rest. Complications that may occur include reoccurrence of bleeding and damage to the eye tissue.[16] Other injuries to the eye include foreign bodies and chemical burns, as well as abrasions and lacerations.

Trauma to the ear can cause hearing loss, vertigo, and pain. Ear injuries commonly occur in combination with other head injuries. For example, a temporal bone fracture can cross the middle ear and disrupt the tympanic membrane. Otorrhea, hemotympanum, and Battle's sign (ecchymosis of the mastoid bone) may be indications of basilar skull fracture and should be carefully followed.

Assessment

The primary objective in early assessment and management of the child with maxillofacial trauma is to secure a stable airway. Loose teeth, blood, vomitus, edema, or loss of support of the tongue can contribute to airway obstruction (Fig. 30-6). Because of instability of the face and neck structures, airway management can be challenging in the patient with maxillofacial injuries. An artificial airway may be required, yet orotracheal intubation is generally contraindicated in the presence of assumed cervical spine injury, and attempts at nasotracheal intubation may damage brain structures in the case of massive midface trauma. However, a stable airway must be ensured before further assessment and treatment. In planning airway management of these children, assessment includes the mechanism of injury, the patient's condition, and the existence of other injuries.[26] Options may include orotracheal intubation, nasotracheal intubation, tracheostomy, or cricothyroidotomy. Cervical spine control must be addressed simultaneously with the airway (see "Resuscitation" in this chapter), and any major bleeding should be stopped. The face and scalp of a child are highly vascular and can bleed profusely.

Because facial injuries are often the result of a direct blow, they often occur concurrently with cervical spine

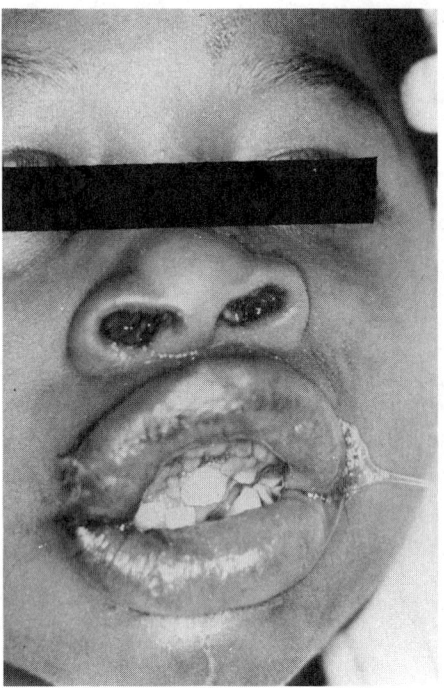

FIGURE 30-6
Edema and bony instability resulting from maxillofacial trauma can lead to airway obstruction.

or closed head injury. Thus, neurologic function should be assessed as part of the initial survey.

On inspection, symmetry of the face and any muscular weakness of the facial muscles should be noted. The intraoral examination includes inspection of the teeth, gums, and tongue, and evaluation of occlusion. Discoloration of the oral mucosa should be noted—a hematoma in the mouth suggests a fracture.[3]

Any drainage, clear or bloody, from the nose, ears, or eyes is noted. Extraocular movements (EOMs) are assessed by asking the child to gaze up, down, and to each side. Pupillary shape, size, and reaction are noted. Gross visual acuity is evaluated by using objects in the room or holding up fingers. A fluorescein examination using a Wood's lamp may be performed to rule out corneal abrasion. Contact lenses should be removed.

The entire face is gently palpated, feeling for step-offs and noting any tenderness. The eyes are not palpated if there is an obvious injury or penetrating object, because this increases intraocular pressure.

Nursing Interventions: Collaborative and Independent

For general maxillofacial trauma, suction and emergency airway equipment should be set up at the child's bedside. If the patient's cardiovascular status is stable, the head of the bed should be elevated to minimize edema. Ice compresses may also be effective in limiting edema and pain.

Any chemical injuries to the eye should be copiously irrigated with normal saline. The child may require sedation or topical anesthetic to obtain cooperation. In cases of hyphema and open eye injuries, the eye may need to

be protected from further injury by an eye shield or patch. Drug therapy, including cycloplegics, hemostatic agents, and mydriatics, may be used in treatment of eye injuries.

Lacerations and abrasions should be cleaned thoroughly to prevent infection and improve cosmetic results. Debris such as dirt or gravel that remains in a wound leaves a "tattoo," which causes an unsightly scar. A convenient method of cleaning lacerations is to attach a 20-gauge IV catheter to a large syringe and use this for irrigation.

Careful monitoring of the airway should continue throughout hospitalization for any child who has sustained major maxillofacial trauma. If jaw wiring has been required, wire cutters must be kept with the patient for opening the airway in the event of vomiting or choking. Goals for continuing nursing care include preventing infection, monitoring of neuromuscular status, assisting the patient to adapt to either temporary or permanent body image changes, and providing adequate nutrition. Patients with intermandibular fixation and other surgical procedures may require a liquid or blenderized diet for a period of days or weeks. Particularly with the young child, creativity is required to make mealtime appealing and ensure adequate nutrition.

Spinal Cord Trauma

Spinal cord injuries (SCIs) are uncommon in children, representing less than 10% of spinal injuries in all age groups.[45] Although the incidence in children is low, these injuries tend to be devastating, requiring drastic alterations in the child and family's lifestyle. In addition, SCIs that occur in childhood impact many more life-years than when these injuries occur in adulthood. Aggressive early intervention, combined with intensive rehabilitative care, can do much to minimize the extent of disability.

SCI has a predictable pattern of occurrence related to developmental age. Infants sustain SCIs when they are unrestrained or inappropriately restrained during motor vehicle crashes. During the toddler and preschool years, most SCIs are the result of pedestrian accidents. School-age children sustain SCIs from pedestrian accidents, falls, and the lap belt complex seen when young children wear only lap belt restraints. The adolescent population has the highest incidence of SCI from motor vehicle crashes, sports injuries, diving, and penetrating injuries.

State laws and educational efforts have increased the use of restraints in rear seat passengers, especially children. The older preschool-age child and the young school-age child who have "outgrown" their car seats are frequently restrained in a lap belt only. Research has shown that children in this age group are at risk to sustain the "seat belt syndrome" or the lap belt complex of injuries.[35,42] The infant and child's underdeveloped musculoskeletal structure make proper fitting of a lap belt impossible, and most shield-type toddler restraint devices do not accommodate a child over 4 to 5 years old. Because of their weight distribution, children in lap belts sustain the force of the energy at the middle abdomen and against the spinal column on impact. In contrast, the adult frame allows for the focal point of impact to be at the pelvic girdle, spreading the impact across the strongest bones.[35]

During deceleration, the lap belt acts as a fulcrum on which the child's body pivots and snaps back into extension. The lap belt complex of injuries can include:

- Ecchymosis across pelvis and abdomen
- Hematuria
- Lumbar spinal column fracture and/or subluxation
- Lumbar spinal cord injury (typically incomplete)
- Abdominal injury to hollow organs (bowel perforation)
- Abdominal injury to solid organs (spleen/liver)
- Perforation of the intestinal viscera
- Bladder hematoma or rupture
- Mild-to-moderate head injuries[35]

Early recognition of this injury complex and the potential risk of permanent injury starts with prehospital care. The lap belt complex should be suspected until the child has been evaluated for thoracic and lumbar injuries, abdominal injuries, and neurologic deficits. X-ray procedures usually include a lateral view of the thoraciclumbar spine, abdominal CT scan, and flat abdominal film. Careful nursing history and serial evaluations of neurologic, cardiovascular, gastrointestinal, and genitourinary status are critical to the identification of delayed signs of injury. The use of lap belts is preferable to no restraint, yet better technology is needed to protect adequately the preschool- and school-age child.

Because of the child's elastic vertebral ligaments and immaturity of bony structures, momentary subluxation of the vertebral column can occur, leaving the spinal cord vulnerable to injury. Such injuries are not evident on x-ray and may be referred to as SCIWORA (spinal cord injury without radiographic abnormality).[37] The resulting injury may range from minor, transient motor or sensory deficits to complete cord transection.

Hyperextension injuries are frequently the result of falls and occur when the spinal cord is stretched and contused on the dorsal aspect. Although hyperflexion injuries are frequently the result of diving into shallow water or the deceleration of a motor vehicle crash, both column and cord injuries are seen with these mechanisms of injury.[20] After any traumatic injury that involves motion (falls, motor vehicles, diving, child abuse), injury to the cervical spine should be suspected. As with other injuries, the emergency priorities of care are the ABCs and immobilization.

After traumatic injury, the spinal cord may sustain injury through a number of mechanisms. Transection of the cord caused by a penetrating object results in incomplete or complete lesion at the level of the penetrating injury (see Fig. 53-7). Physiologic transection, usually complete, occurs when the vascular system to the cord is compromised from blunt force and hemodynamic changes. The spinal cord may suffer an incomplete lesion from bruising or contusion to the cord from blunt force or shaking. Functional classification of the extent of cord injury has been developed for ongoing assessment and prognosis (Table 30-3).

After initial stabilization and resuscitation, the child with a cervical spinal cord injury is placed in a temporary immobilization device. Usually the "halo vest" is used. Pins are surgically placed in the skull and attached to a

TABLE 30-3
Frankel Grades Used to Describe Extent of Spinal Cord Injury

Grades	Description
A	Complete transection.
B	Incomplete—preservation of sensation. No voluntary motion.
C	Incomplete—preservation of motor, yet nonfunctional. Sensory function may be present.
D	Incomplete—preservation of motor function that can be useful.
E	Complete recovery—full return of sensory and motor function; abnormal reflexes may persist.

ring that secures to a vest, which is strapped on securely. The child wears this halo vest for 3 to 4 months until the injury stabilizes with callus. Surgical stabilization with wires and bone chips is sometimes the treatment of choice for early mobilization.

The nursing assessment for the child with a spinal cord injury should include the parameters for an immobilized child's physiologic and psychological needs. Skin integrity, bowel and bladder management, changing body image, and dependency are of primary concern for the child and family. Routine attention to respiratory and cardiovascular status is critical for the immobilized child.

The ideal plan of care for a child with a spinal cord injury who is free from other injuries and complications should target transfer to a pediatric rehabilitation center within 2 weeks of injury. Consistent interdisciplinary team planning should begin in the ED and continue throughout the rehabilitation, outpatient, and home care phases. Involvement of parents and siblings in the early days after injury is a critical component of the plan of care for all children, especially those with permanent disabilities. Although the specific level of spinal cord injury has the most significant impact on the child's potential level of independence, continual advances in rehabilitative technology offer the child and family an ever-increasing array of assistive devices (see Chap. 53).

Thoracic Trauma

The thorax is a common site of injury in children, with up to 30% of pediatric trauma victims suffering thoracic injury.[8] Injuries to the thoracic structures can alter airway function, ventilation, chest wall integrity, CNS function, and cardiac function. Due to their proximity, thoracic injuries often occur concomitantly with abdominal injuries. Early recognition and prompt treatment of these potentially life-threatening injuries are essential to successful outcome.

Although trauma to the chest is usually blunt, penetrating injuries do occur in children as a result of shattered glass, gunshots, and stabbings. Chest trauma may also result from a rib or clavicle fracture. Blunt chest trauma may present with few external signs, but any child with a history of a significant general blow or impact should be examined with a high index of suspicion for internal injuries. Due to the pliability of the child's rib cage, energy is easily transmitted inward toward vital structures. The child's mediastinum is mobile and, if distorted, can lead to dislocation or angulation of the great vessels or heart and compression of the lungs and trachea.[15]

Loss of airway is the most common direct cause of death in pediatric trauma.[34] Because of the small size of airway structures, the airway can be easily compromised by obstruction from blood, secretions, vomitus, or teeth. In addition, the child's large tongue tends to relax and cover the glottic opening in the obtunded or unconscious child.

Types of Injury

Pulmonary Injury

Pneumothorax is the most common consequence of injury to the chest region.[12] Pneumothorax consists of an accumulation of air in the pleural space, which leads to either partial or complete lung collapse. It can occur as a result of penetrating injury, esophageal perforation, or secondary to disrupted lung parenchyma. Whereas pneumothorax frequently occurs with fractured ribs in adults, it often occurs without rib fracture in children. The child may be asymptomatic or may have signs ranging from dyspnea and pain radiating to the shoulder to decreased breath sounds and bradycardia. Abrasions and hyperresonance heard on percussion may suggest the injury, along with decreased breath sounds or a tracheal shift. Pneumothorax may be managed with the insertion of a thoracostomy tube, or if the patient is not in acute distress and pneumothorax involves less than 15% of the lung volume, the patient may simply be observed. Spontaneous reabsorption of the air may occur after a period of hours or days.

Tension pneumothorax occurs when an injury allows air to enter the thoracic cavity with inspiration but not escape on expiration. The ipsilateral lung collapses and a shift of the mediastinum compresses the heart, major vessels, trachea, and the contralateral lung. Venous return is compromised, and cardiac output decreases. This is a medical emergency and is treated by needle aspiration. In the child, a needle is inserted in the fourth or fifth intercostal space at the mid-axillary line.

Pulmonary contusion occurs as a result of a high-speed impact; a recent study estimated that 90% of pulmonary contusions in children were related to motor vehicle accidents.[2] Thus, pulmonary contusion is frequently associated with injury to other body systems. There are frequently no early presenting signs; tachypnea and abnormal breath sounds may or may not be present. The injury is manifested by parenchymal hemorrhage and edema to the alveoli. With this disruption at the alveolar–capillary interface, ventilation-perfusion shunting occurs and can lead to progressive respiratory insufficiency and hypoxia. The degree of respiratory insufficiency that occurs is relative to the size of the contusion.[12] Care is basically supportive, providing supplemental oxygen as needed, and encouraging deep breathing, coughing, and turning to mobilize secretions and expand the lungs.

Fluids are often restricted, because excess fluids may add to the degree of pulmonary edema.[8]

Hemothorax is usually associated with penetrating injury and can represent a major source of bleeding. The presence of blood in the thoracic cavity impairs ventilation and restricts cardiac output. Hemothorax is evacuated by means of a thoracostomy tube. Fluid resuscitation must take place before or simultaneous with the evacuation of blood, or hypovolemic shock may be precipitated.

In assessing the tracheobronchial tree, the examiner should keep in mind that a child's pliable ribs may allow compression of a bronchus on the vertebral column. A crush injury to the larynx or trachea may occur as a result of blunt trauma to the neck, such as a "clothesline injury" or contact with a car dashboard. These types of injury may cause symptoms of pneumothorax as well as hoarseness, retractions, and dyspnea.

Although rib fractures are uncommon in the pediatric trauma victim, the fracture of a rib in more than one place produces a flail chest. The resulting paradoxical movement and respiratory insufficiency are often compounded by pulmonary contusion.[8] Internal stabilization of flail chest is usually achieved by means of analgesia, intubation, and mechanical ventilation.

Cardiovascular Injury

The cardiovascular system is also vulnerable to injury as a result of thoracic trauma. Although children are usually not victims of the "steering wheel syndrome" and therefore suffer a lower incidence of chest trauma than do adults, Eshel et al[9] note that evidence of cardiac injury occurs in 10% to 75% of all chest trauma. However, the diagnosis of these injuries is frequently delayed due to the trauma team's focus on more severe or visible injuries and the fact that there is frequently no evidence of thoracic injury.[7] The consequences of cardiac injury may manifest gradually, so a careful baseline assessment is important.

The effect of trauma to the heart may be functional, as manifested by rhythm or conduction changes, or organic, as with penetrating injury to the heart muscle, coronary arteries, or major vessels.[9] Pericardial injury is usually due to blunt force to the heart. Hemopericardium can be sudden, as with a major laceration to the heart wall, or may be a slow oozing, which may reabsorb spontaneously. In the case of pericardial tamponade, blood accumulating in the pericardial cavity after a myocardial injury leads to a decrease in venous return and restriction of myocardial contraction, resulting in compromised cardiac output. Although the etiology of these symptoms can be difficult to diagnose, the findings of jugular venous distention, increased central venous pressure, and persistent hypotension after fluid resuscitation may indicate tamponade. Pericardiocentesis, or the needle aspiration of blood from the pericardial sac, usually results in immediate improvement.

Assessment and Nursing Interventions

A history of high-impact blows to the chest or rapid deceleration should raise the index of suspicion for myocardial contusion. Associated injuries to the ribs, sternum, or clavicle are also typically seen with myocardial contusion. Myocardial contusion may produce nonspecific ST segment or T wave abnormalities, as well as creatine phosphokinase (CPK) or MB band elevations, although in many cases these are normal.[7]

Patients suffering thoracic injury require prompt and continuous attention to the ABCs. The airway should be assessed for patency and tracheal position. Respirations should be monitored for rate, depth, retractions, and nasal flaring. Observation of the child's color provides information about respiratory as well as cardiovascular status; circumoral pallor or cyanosis tends to reflect respiratory distress, whereas peripheral cyanosis tends to indicate poor perfusion and is a late sign. The patient's level of consciousness is monitored because restlessness or confusion can be an early sign of hypoxia or poor perfusion. Symmetry of the chest wall should be noted, as well as equality of breath sounds on auscultation.

Vesicular, bronchial, and bronchovesicular sounds are normal only when they are in their correct locations (e.g., bronchial sounds heard over the lung periphery may indicate consolidation). Breath sounds are easily transmitted throughout the chest wall of the child, and assessment of location is a skill that requires practice. In palpating the chest wall, subcutaneous emphysema ("crackles"), tenderness, or deformities should be noted.

The child in respiratory distress is generally most comfortable in a semi-Fowler's position, which allows optimal excursion of the diaphragm and full lung expansion. The nurse should ensure aggressive respiratory therapy, with attention to deep breathing, coughing, and early activity. Although pain management is essential, pain medications must be monitored for their respiratory depressant effect. Nonpharmacologic pain relief measures, such as massage, music, reading, or repositioning, may be preferred to or used in conjunction with drug therapy.

Chest x-rays are followed closely in the child with a respiratory system injury. Arterial blood gases (ABGs) are also monitored, although the advent of pulse oximetry has decreased the need for such invasive measures in monitoring. Fiberoptic bronchoscopy may be used in assessing degree and character of injury to specific respiratory structures.

In assessing circulation, the heart rate and rhythm should be monitored. Sinus tachycardia is a normal compensatory response to stress or hypovolemia and should be assessed in terms of age-related norms. The child should be placed on an electrocardiogram (ECG) monitor. Any complaints of chest pain should be noted. Quality of heart sounds, including the presence of murmurs or friction rubs, are documented. The quality and strength of peripheral pulses are noted along with the temperature and color of extremities.

Diagnostic studies used in the assessment of the cardiac trauma patient include serial ECGs and chest x-rays, echocardiography, and monitoring of isoenzymes. Ejection fraction, which is the percentage of total ventricular volume ejected with each heart beat, is assessed by radionuclide and echocardiography studies. In decreased cardiac function, this value is lowered. Aortography may be used to assess for integrity of the aorta.

Nursing care is primarily supportive, including oxygen supplementation, the provision of bedrest with progressive activity, and analgesia. Generally, the child with a cardiac injury should not be given anticoagulants.

Abdominal Trauma

Abdominal injuries are frequent sequelae of major trauma. Several physiologic and anatomic factors make the child's abdomen vulnerable to injury. The abdominal wall and musculature are thin, affording little protection from blunt forces. The pliable rib cage does not cover the protuberant abdomen, and the child's pelvic girdle is small and underdeveloped. Thus, the child is susceptible to blood loss from damage to highly vascular and vital organs such as the liver and spleen.

Bearing in mind that a relatively small volume blood loss can lead to shock in the young child, rapid assessment and management of abdominal injuries can positively influence outcome in the trauma patient. In addition, it must be recognized that blood loss from an abdominal injury can lead to worsening of other system injuries.[46] For example, hypovolemia combined with head injury can lead to decreased brain perfusion and anoxia, hampering efforts to optimize cerebral resuscitation.

Because of the increasing incidence of violent crime in the adolescent population reported from stab and gunshot wounds, penetrating injuries are infrequent. Eighty to ninety percent of abdominal injuries in children are blunt, resulting primarily from motor vehicle accidents, bicycle accidents, and falls.[34] With the advent of mandatory seat belt legislation in all 50 states, an increase in seat belt related injuries has been noted (see "Spinal Cord Trauma" in this chapter).

An infrequent but often lethal mechanism of abdominal injury is child abuse.[6] Because of the obscure history surrounding the incident, diagnosis may be difficult and treatment delayed. The child may present with symptoms similar to those of acute illness, such as fever, tachycardia, decreased hematocrit, and poor perfusion. Mortality may be related to hypovolemic shock and sepsis.

Types of Injury

Spleen Injury

Because it is a large organ that is not adequately protected by the rib cage in children, the spleen is especially vulnerable to blunt trauma. A common source of splenic trauma is the impact of handlebars as a child is thrown from a bicycle.

Initial signs of splenic injury may range from minor pain to hypovolemic shock. The combination of left upper quadrant and left shoulder pain constitutes Kehr's sign and is characteristic of splenic injury.[36] Abdominal distention may be present.

In the past, splenic trauma was frequently treated with removal of the organ. Because of the high incidence of sepsis later in life among children who have undergone splenectomy, the current philosophy is toward nonoperative management of these injuries whenever possible. The nurse may be responsible for obtaining and monitoring serial hemoglobin/hematocrit determinations, as well as monitoring for signs of shock, which may indicate continued bleeding and the possible need for surgical intervention. Fluid resuscitation is critical for these patients and may include administration of blood. Bedrest is enforced during hospitalization, and both child and family must be taught the importance of contact sports restriction in the months after discharge.

Liver Injury

Like the spleen, the liver is a highly vascular organ that is susceptible to trauma in the child. Principles of assessment and treatment are similar, with the addition of monitoring hepatic enzymes.

Hemoperitoneum may or may not produce peritonitis. Although whole blood is not a peritoneal irritant, the lysis of red blood cells may produce a chemical peritonitis, which can lead to secondary bacterial infection. The increased blood flow and capillary permeability that result can lead to third spacing of fluids, causing increased distention.[33]

Pancreas Injury

When the pancreas is damaged by blunt or penetrating trauma, pancreatic enzymes may be released into surrounding tissue. These enzymes can have devastating effects. As digestion and necrosis of tissue occur, vasoactive substances are released. These cause increased vasodilation and fluid sequestering in the area, which can precipitate shock.[21]

Massive bleeding does not occur frequently with pancreatic injury, but pancreatitis may result from the impact, pharmacologic therapy, or ischemia secondary to shock.[21] The child may experience pain, nausea and vomiting, an increase in heart or respiratory rate, and moderate abdominal distention. The serum amylase is generally elevated and should be monitored. Patients with pancreatic injury are kept on bedrest with a restricted diet until the amylase normalizes and symptoms subside.

Hollow Viscus Injury

Injuries to the hollow viscus organs (gallbladder, stomach, and intestines) are uncommon in children, but can result from three basic mechanisms:

- A direct blow, causing a sudden increase in intraluminal pressure
- A shearing injury at the point of intestinal fixation to the abdominal wall
- Crushing of organs against the vertebrae.[45] Signs of such injury include decreased bowel sounds, severe pain, and symptoms of peritonitis.

Stomach injuries in children are usually the result of blunt force after a recent meal. Intramural duodenal hematoma is frequently seen with blunt gastric injury. The trauma disrupts duodenal vasculature, and the resulting hematoma causes intestinal obstruction. The patient may complain of epigastric or right upper quadrant pain and may have vomiting and an elevated amylase. Healing may take 10 days to 3 weeks.

Small bowel rupture is a common result of seat belt injury. Symptoms may appear gradually, and peritonitis may begin to appear by the time the patient seeks medical care. Treatment of hollow viscus injuries generally includes NG suction and total parenteral nutrition until gastrointestinal function returns to normal.

Colon or anorectal injuries are uncommon in children and are most often the result of abuse or deviant sexual activity.[15] Such injuries may be inflicted under the guise of "discipline" for toilet training mishaps.

Assessment and Nursing Interventions

Assessment of the abdomen may be difficult in children. Gastric distention is caused by aerophagia, or air swallowing, and may be exacerbated by ileus (lack of intestinal peristalsis), which frequently accompanies major injury. Bag-mask ventilation techniques may also force air into the stomach and cause distention.[15] Such distention may mimic acute bleeding. Apprehension and pain may cause children to tighten their abdominal muscles, making palpation difficult.

On initial examination, inspection of the abdomen may reveal obvious findings, such as tire tracks, abrasions, or ecchymosis. The presence or absence of bowel sounds and their location provides information about the functioning of the gastrointestinal tract. Because children are diaphragmatic breathers, abdominal pain such as that caused by peritoneal irritation may cause alterations in breathing patterns. Any tenderness to palpation or on rebound should be noted. A rectal examination is performed and includes testing for the presence of heme in the stool. Although abdominal girth measurements may be of limited value, serial measurements should be made to assess for progressive distention.

After initial examination, diagnostic tests may be used to enhance evaluation of the injury. Radiography may be used, but is generally of limited value. A CT scan is extremely useful in the hemodynamically stable child. Abnormal fluid collections, masses, and organ structures can be identified. Disadvantages of CT scanning are the considerable expense and the time required to perform the test, which make it unsuitable for the unstable child. Diagnostic peritoneal lavage is useful for the child with multiple injuries who requires surgery for nonabdominal problems. In this test, a small incision is made near the umbilicus and sterile isotonic fluid is instilled. The fluid is returned and examined for evidence of blood, enzymes, or food fibers, which could indicate organ or intestinal injury.

Once it has been established that the cribriform plate is intact, an NG tube should be inserted in any child suspected of having an abdominal injury. Decompression of the stomach is essential in preventing vomiting/aspiration and respiratory embarrassment due to limited diaphragmatic excursion. Once the stomach has been evacuated, the NG tube can be connected to low intermittent suction.

Genitourinary Trauma

Genitourinary injuries are frequently associated with pelvic trauma. Although these injuries are rarely lethal, they can result in long-term morbidity if not appropriately managed in the early stages.[26]

The child's kidney is vulnerable to injury as a result of direct blows or shearing forces. It is proportionately larger than the adult kidney in relation to the abdominal cavity, and is less well protected by fat and muscle. The child's pliable rib cage also affords little protection from blunt forces. Preexisting renal abnormalities are sometimes discovered for the first time during the trauma assessment, complicating management. The kidney is not fixed to retroperitoneal structures, so a blow to the lower abdomen or flank can cause a renal laceration or contusion from contact with other organs or the spine.[26] However, contusion is the most common type of renal injury.

Hematuria is the hallmark of renal injury, occurring in 80% to 90% of affected children. Although the degree of hematuria does not correlate with the severity of injury, assessment of urine for gross or microscopic blood is an important factor in evaluation. The presence of flank tenderness or ecchymosis or a high-riding prostate in males are clues to kidney injury, but may not always be present.

Bladder contusion or rupture may result from a direct blow to the lower abdomen or trunk. Little force is required to rupture a full bladder at its weakest point, the dome. Penetrating injury to the bladder can also be related to pelvic fracture, in which case high mortality has been reported.[26] Signs of bladder injury include an inability to void, lower abdominal tenderness or flank pain, and anuria. Peritoneal signs may also be present, such as rebound tenderness, distention, or rigidity.

Urethral trauma is often associated with pelvic fractures, but may also occur as a result of straddle injuries in girls. Bladder distention and blood at the urinary meatus are contraindications to catheterization, which could convert a partial urethral tear to a full tear (Fig. 30-7).

Radiographic evaluation may consist of a combination of tests. An intravenous pyelogram (IVP) or excretory urogram is generally the initial study performed. This, along with the more sensitive renal scan, can identify urinary extravasation. Ultrasonography may demonstrate the size and location of perirenal fluid collection. Retrograde urethrography may be used to identify urethral injury. CT scanning is a valuable diagnostic test because it can be used to check for other abdominal injuries at the same time.

The majority of renal system injuries are managed nonoperatively. Bedrest is usually an early requirement, along with frequent testing for hematuria. The nurse must closely monitor vital signs, especially blood pressure, as well as balance of intake and output. If surgery is performed, a variety of drainage devices, including suprapubic catheters and cystostomies, may be used. The young child often requires extra support and explanation to deal with this change in body function and image. Long-term follow-up includes monitoring for hypertension, which can be a complication of renal injury.

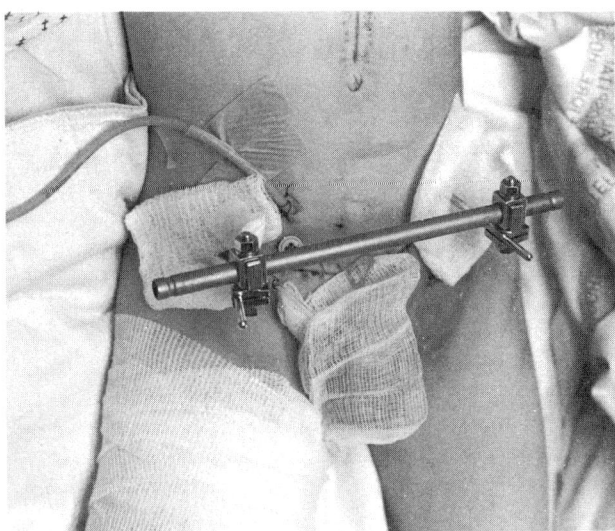

FIGURE 30-7
External pelvic fixation, suprapubic cystostomy, and urethral stenting were used in treating this child's pelvic fracture with a urethral tear. This 9-year-old boy was run over by a car (note the hematoma on the left groin).

Orthopedic Trauma

Mechanism and types of orthopedic injuries in children can be related to both developmental age and seasonal changes. The table of orthopedic injuries related to age outlines each age group's risk areas (Table 30-4).

As with all injured children, the primary and secondary survey provide the priority for assessing and treating injuries. The assessment for orthopedic injuries in children is typically part of the secondary assessment. Pelvic and vascular injuries in children should be considered during assessment and treatment for hypovolemic shock. Unlike adults, children who sustain a fractured femur do not lose enough blood to become hypovolemic. A child with signs of hypovolemia should be carefully assessed for other injuries. Knowledge of the mechanism of injury is extremely important during both the primary and secondary assessments.

Musculoskeletal injuries are infrequently life-threatening in the first hour of care, yet the early identification and plan for treatment are essential for the child's long-term recovery. The unique features of orthopedic injuries in children necessitate careful assessment of all body parts and management to prevent permanent disability. The bones of children are more porous and flexible than adults' and thus manifest different patterns of injury. The bones of a child bend and splinter during stress and energy impact from injury. Children are more likely to sustain greenstick, bend, and buckle fractures, therefore increasing the risk for soft tissue, vascular, and nerve damage. The child's ligaments and tendons are much stronger than the developing bone, leading to a low incidence of strains and sprains. If a child complains of pain in a joint after injury, a fracture should be suspected. The growth plate is a frequent site of fractures in children and must be diagnosed by special positioning during x-rays. Injury to the growth plate can lead to permanent disturbances in growth and result in deformities and dis-

TABLE 30-4
Orthopedic Injuries Related to Children's Developmental Stage

Age Group	Mechanism of Injury	Types of Injuries
Infant 6–12 mo		
Rolls over	MVA: passenger	Brain injury
Creeps	Falls: high chair, crib, tables, stairs	Fractures: skull, extremity
Crawls		
Toddler 1–3 y		
Walking	MVA: passenger, pedestrian	Brain injury
		Fractures: skull, extremity
Climbing	Falls: stairs, tables, playgrounds, windows	Soft tissue injury
		Nursemaid's elbow
	Held up, pulled, or lifted up by one arm	
Preschooler 3–6 y		
Growth spurts	MVA: pedestrian, passenger, bike, and big wheel	Brain injury
Very active		Fractures: skull, pelvis, extremity
Very curious	Falls: playground, windows, bikes, big wheel	Soft tissue injury
	Lawnmower	
School Age 6–12 y		
Growth spurts	MVA: pedestrian, passenger, bike	Brain injury
Peer pressure		C-spine injury
Accepts dares	Falls: bike, skateboard	Fractures: skull, pelvis, extremity
	Sports	Subluxation L1-2, dislocation
		Soft tissue injuries
Adolescent 12–16 y		
Peer pressure	MVA: passenger, pedestrian, driver	Brain injury
		C-spine injury
	Falls: motor bikes	Soft tissue injury
	Sports: contact and water	Fractures: skull, pelvic, facial, extremities

Copyright 1990 C. J. Wright, MSN, RNC.

abilities. Long bone length discrepancies and joint deformities can result after a growth plate injury.

Assessment

An orthopedic assessment includes a head-to-toe survey. Inspection and observation can provide key information. Guidelines for a pediatric orthopedic assessment are given in the accompanying display. *Before* touching the child, the nurse should watch the child's voluntary movements and observe for symmetry, strength, and coordination in all extremities. Frequently, the child immobilizes an injured extremity by the instinctive reaction to decrease pain. The nurse should always examine the uninjured extremity first. Each extremity should be assessed for swelling, deformity, open wounds, and neurovascular status. The neurovascular assessment on a child must be objective and done without the child's visualization of which toe or finger is being touched. The injured child is frightened, and an accurate assessment of sensation is a technique perfected by repeated experience.

Fractures

Immobilization of a bone or joint limits pain and prevents further tissue and nerve damage. Principles of immobilization are listed in the accompanying display. Immobilization presents a challenge to the prehospital careproviders, the emergency room nurse, the orthopedic surgeon, and the orthopedic and intensive care nurse. Frequently, standard equipment does not fit the infant and young child. During the initial immobilization, at the scene and for transport, pillows, blankets, and IV boards can be adapted for use as splints. The two key principles for immobilization of the child are:

- Make the equipment fit the child, not the child fit the equipment
- Immobilize above and below the joint

The child's musculoskeletal system is highly vascularized and constantly developing. Fractures heal faster in young children than in adolescents. Many fracture deformities in young children correct themselves over time through the process of remodeling. Bone healing starts within minutes of injury with the formation of a hematoma, which creates the framework for the granulation over the next few days.

Specific fractures require surgical intervention. All open wounds associated with a fracture must be taken to the operating room for debridement and irrigation as soon as the life-threatening injuries are stabilized. Preparation of the child for surgery includes:

- Baseline orthopedic assessment
- Establishment of IV access
- Administration of prescribed antibiotics
- Strict maintenance of NPO status
- Neurovascular assessment every hour with vital signs
- Preparation of the child and family for the operating room and procedure
- Initiation of nursing database and care plan

Fractures which frequently require surgical correction include the following: epiphyscal injuries, spinal column fractures, distal fractures of the radius and ulna, supracondylar fractures, wrist fractures and femoral neck fractures, long bone fractures with severe angulation, and placement of skeletal traction. Surgery may be required for devices such as Steinman pins for femur fractures. External fixation devices provide rigid immobilization of the fracture while allowing mobilization of patient from bed, direct access for wound care and adjustment of alignment without repeated surgery. Severe open frac-

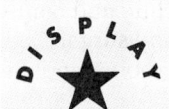

Guidelines for Pediatric Orthopedic Assessment

- Make preoperative and preprocedural assessment for a baseline.
- Monitor neurovascular status every 30 min to 1 h for the first 24 h after application of cast or traction or after surgery, then every 4 h for the duration of the therapy.
- Check all five digits of each extremity.
- Compare bilateral symmetry.
- Increase frequency of assessment if the neurovascular status changes (and notify physician).
- Check neurovascular status 30 min after you do skin care and reapply skin traction.
- Use a pin or pinch to assess sensation and motion in an infant.

- Make a game out of neurovascular assessment with toddlers.
- Obtain proof of neurovascular status for all children less than 10 y of age.
- Listen to what parents and children say.
- Assess pain and effect of pain medication. Irritability may indicate pain in a child.
- Document findings and note conditions or changes.
- Elevate casted or splinted extremity above the level of the heart.

Copyright 1990 C. J. Wright, MSN, RNC. Children's National Medical Center, Washington, DC. Trauma Service.

tures, fracture with burns, fractures with major skin disruption requiring grafts or flaps, unstable pelvic fractures, and fractures associated with vascular repair/nerve repair are frequently managed with external fixation devices.

Compartment Syndrome

Complications from orthopedic injuries include the immediate or delayed onset of hypovolemic shock, infection from contaminated wounds, vascular and nerve damage from the injury, and compartment syndrome. Compartment syndrome results from an increasing pressure within the closed space of a muscle and, if untreated,

leads to progressive vascular compromise resulting in the death of soft tissue and nerves.[41] Compartment syndrome may be caused by hemorrhage within the compartment, vascular injury to a major arterial supply, or external compression from a cast or splint. The forearm and lower leg are the most common sites for compartment syndrome. After direct trauma or external compression, the edema and venous obstruction within the compartment, along with increased capillary permeability, lead to an increasing intramuscular pressure. Ultimately, the pressure causes arterial occlusion and hypoxia to the tissues resulting in death of soft tissue. The death of muscle and nerve cells releases toxins, which increase the capillary permeability, and the cycle repeats itself. The primary

Principles of Immobilization

- Control severe bleeding *first!*
- Assess neurovascular status before you apply splint or traction.
- Keep broken bone ends and adjacent bones from moving.
- Immobilize above and below the injury.
- Immobilize the joint above and below the injury.
- Note specific injures in which you "splint them where they lie."
- Fixation: immobilizes the area
  Traction: relieves muscle spasms, prevents overriding bone injuries
- Apply traction only until you see a sign of relief

and then maintain that degree of traction. Do not let go!
- Use the noninjured leg or the chest to immobilize a fractured leg or arm if supplies are not available or are the wrong size for the child.
- Assess neurovascular status after you apply splint or traction and compare to your previous findings.
- When in doubt—splint.

Goals: to prevent further damage
to decrease pain
to decrease chance of shock
to prevent further fear and panic.

Copyright 1990 C. J. Wright, MSN, RNC. Trauma Service, Children's National Medical Center, Washington, DC.

sign of compartment syndrome is extreme pain on passive range of motion. Compartment syndrome is a surgical emergency requiring rapid preparation and transport of the injured child to the operating room. The surgical team performs a fasciotomy to relieve the pressure and prevent further cell death (Fig. 30-8).

Postoperative care of the child after fasciotomy begins with a new baseline assessment of neurovascular status and repeated assessments every hour until stabilized. The specific type of wound care is determined by the extent of injury and tissue damage. Pain control and maintenance of fluid hydration are critical postoperative care interventions. After the edema subsides, the child returns to the operating room for closure of the open wound. Preparation for primary closure or skin graft is determined during the recovery period.

Amputation

Traumatic amputation and avulsions in children are most often the result of crushing injury or contact with machinery. Common sources of injury include escalators, car doors, lawn mowers, railroad cars, bicycle chains, or pedestrian motor vehicle crashes in which the child's extremity is caught under the wheel and carried for a distance. The emergency treatment must follow the primary and secondary assessment and stabilization. Although the extremity injury is the visual focal point, the trauma team must ensure adequate oxygenation and volume resuscitation. Additional priorities after the primary and secondary survey include: antibiotic coverage, identification of surgical special teams and transportation to the operating room or other facility, aggressive irrigation and debridement in the operating room, and a team approach to the reconstruction or reimplantation. If an amputated extremity is brought along to the ED, it should be cleaned gently with sterile saline, wrapped in a sterile saline-soaked dressing, and placed in a plastic bag over ice. Proper care of the amputated part and rapid mobilization of the surgical team are crucial to the success of reimplantation.

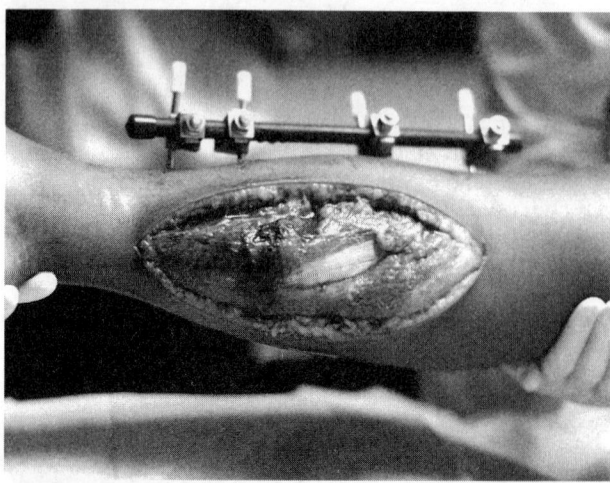

FIGURE 30-8
Fasciotomy may be required to prevent neurovascular and tissue damage resulting from compartment syndrome.

Other nursing interventions for the child and family focus on the preparation for procedures and surgery, education about the operating and recovery rooms, and initiation of a database and care plan.

Throughout the perioperative and postoperative phases of care, assessment of the child's level of consciousness, neurovascular status, and pain control is critical to successful recovery. The child may be placed on anticoagulants after microvascular surgery and should be watched for bleeding. The operated limb should be elevated to aid venous return, and circulatory checks (including extremity temperature) should be performed frequently.

Hospitalization after a traumatic avulsion or amputation can be prolonged by reconstructive surgeries, a high rate of infection, and repeated skin grafting procedures. The early establishment of an individualized plan of care and daily schedule for the child and family facilitates adjustment to the hospitalization and positive coping mechanisms.

Burns

Over 60,000 children annually are hospitalized for burn injury.[14] Children are developmentally vulnerable to burns because they have a decreased perception of danger, little control over elements in their environment, and a limited ability to react effectively in a fire or burn situation. House fires are responsible for 84% of pediatric burn deaths, with most of these resulting from smoke inhalation rather than flame injury.[33]

Classifications

Burns are classified according to source and depth. Thermal burns include flame and scald injuries. Electrical burns may result from power sources or lightning. Chemical burns can occur due to contact with or ingestion of caustic substances. The prevailing mechanisms of burn injuries change with the growth and developmental level of children. Because infants are dependent on caretakers, they are at risk for scald injuries resulting from spills of hot liquids, bath water that is inappropriately hot, or swallowing hot liquid from a microwaved bottle. Toddlers are mobile and inquisitive, and are prone to pulling hot food or drinks onto themselves, to touch hot surfaces, and to chew on or play with electrical cords. Preschoolers may be burned while experimenting with matches, lighters, and so forth. Adolescent burn injuries commonly involve electricity or gasoline and matches.[33] Child abuse accounts for approximately 5% of burn admissions, with caretakers inappropriately using hot surfaces or liquids in disciplinary situations.

Burn depth is classified according to degree or thickness. Superficial, or first-degree burns, result from injury to the epidermis alone. These are red and painful, and heal in 3 to 5 days. Sunburn is an example. In partial-thickness, or second-degree burns, injury to the dermis occurs. These burns may be red, pink, or whitish. The capability of regenerating skin is retained, because epithelial cells are contained in the lower layers of dermis.

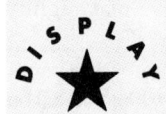

Lund and Browder Chart for Determining Extent of Burns

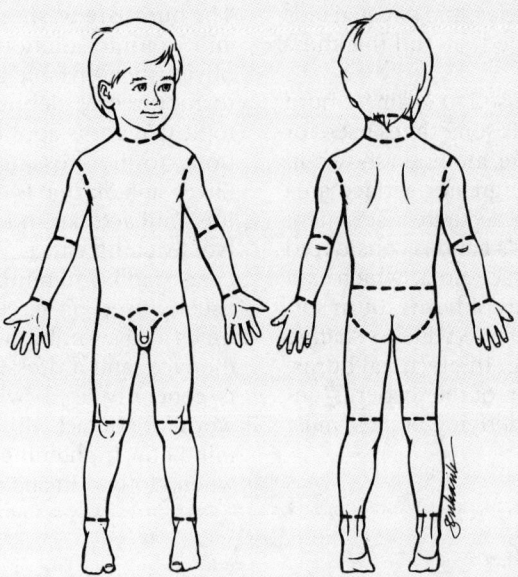

Age-Years

Area	0-1	1-4	5-9	10-15	Adult	%2	%3	%Total
Head	19	17	13	10	7			
Neck	2	2	2	2	2			
Ant. Trunk	13	13	13	13	13			
Post. Trunk	13	13	13	13	13			
R. Buttock	2	2	2	2	2			
L. Buttock	2	2	2	2	2			
Genitalia	1	1	1	1	1			
R. U. Arm	4	4	4	4	4			
L. U. Arm	4	4	4	4	4			
R. L. Arm	3	3	3	3	3			
L. L. Arm	3	3	3	3	3			
R. Hand	2	2	2	2	2			
L. Hand	2	2	2	2	2			
R. Thigh	5	6	8	8	9			
L. Thigh	5	6	8	8	9			
R. Leg	5	5	5	6	7			
L. Leg	5	5	5	6	7			
R. Foot	3	3	3	3	3			
L. Foot	3	3	3	3	3			
					Total			

Adapted with permission from *Franklin H. Martin Memorial Foundation. (1944).* Surgery, Gynecology, and Obstetrics, 79, *352.*

Healing is slower than with superficial burns, sometimes requiring weeks. Burns extending into the subcutaneous tissue are referred to as full-thickness, or third-degree burns. These have a waxy or leathery appearance and require grafting because the epithelial cell layer has been destroyed. Nerves, muscle, hair follicles, and sweat glands may also be destroyed or damaged in full-thickness burns.[19]

In adults, the Rule of Nines is used to estimate burn surface area. Although this method is sometimes used for children also, the Lund and Browder method (shown in the display) takes into account the greater surface area of the child's head and gives a more accurate assessment based on age. The palm of the child's hand is considered to represent 1% of total body surface area, which is a helpful fact in estimating small areas of burns. Burn surface area may be initially underestimated due to change in appearance of the burn over time. In electrical burns, visible wounds may be only the "tip of the iceberg," indicating progressive damage to underlying nerves, muscle, bone, and tissue.

Initial Assessment and Nursing Interventions

The first priority of management is to stop the burning process. On the scene, smothering flames, running cool water over an extremity burn or chemical burn, and applying cool compresses to a burn covering less than 20% of the body surface area minimizes damage and relieves pain. Ice should never be used because it may worsen the injury. A child with severe burns should be transported in a clean, dry sheet, because cold water can cause a drop in body temperature and precipitate shock.

Assessment of the burned child begins with attention to the airway. When smoke or hot air is inhaled, the combination of airway edema and the child's small airway structures can easily result in obstruction. In addition, carbon monoxide released during the burning process can cause toxicity. ABGs and carboxyhemoglobin levels should be obtained. The child is placed in a semi-Fowler's position and provided with supplemental oxygen in cool mist. The airway must be continually monitored for changes in the hours after injury.[14] Sooty sputum and the development of hoarseness or stridor are danger signals.

Within the circulatory system, massive fluid shifts after burn injury can lead to shock. It is important to obtain an accurate weight of the child to calculate fluid needs. Various methods may be used; the Parkland formula calls for 4 ml of Ringer's lactate per percent of burned area times the child's weight in kilograms, to be given over the first 24 hours. Half of this total is given in the first 8 hours, and the other half is given during the next 16 hours. The child is monitored for signs of adequate response, such as normalization of vital signs, adequate pulses, and urine output of 1 ml/kg/h or more. The child must also be assessed for signs of fluid overload, because inhalation injury may predispose the child to pulmonary edema or adult respiratory distress syndrome (ARDS). Circulation to the extremities is monitored if there has been a circumferential burn. When edema occurs underneath hard,

inelastic eschar, neurovascular compromise may signify the need for escharotomy.[14]

After the initial resuscitation, the burn wounds are cleaned and debrided. If the child's condition allows, the procedure is usually done in a tub or on a shower table. The burns are washed gently with a mild cleansing agent and isotonic solution, using a wet gauze pad. Areas of obviously nonviable tissue and blisters that appear ready to rupture are debrided; firm blisters are left intact. A topical agent is applied to the burns or, in some institutions, to the dressings, which are applied to the burns. Silver sulfadiazine is commonly used in children because it is antibacterial and soothing, and has minimal electrolyte leaching effect.[14] Dressings limit contamination, decrease pain, and minimize fluid and heat loss, so they are usually used on large burns and changed two or three times a day. Antibiotic ointment is commonly applied to the face, and a dressing is eliminated. Clean technique is generally used, with gown, mask, and gloves being worn for contact with open wounds. It should be kept in mind how frightening caregivers must appear to the child when clothed in such garments.

Nursing Interventions: Collaborative and Independent

With a burn injury, the body has lost the integrity of its primary barrier against infection. This factor, combined with the physiologic stress of injury, makes the burned child a compromised host. The threat of infection must be kept in mind constantly, and precautions must be taken during dressing changes, invasive procedures, and care of lines and tubes.

Pain may be an issue for the burn patient from admission through rehabilitation. Pain can be especially excruciating in partial-thickness burns due to exposed nerve endings in burned tissue. Positioning and physical therapy can be painful as tissues are moved and muscles and joints are placed in position of function. The child's perception of pain is heightened by fear and anxiety. (See Chap. 28 for a discussion of pain.)

Indicators of pain in children must be critically assessed before giving medication, because some of the same signs that indicate pain (restlessness, tachycardia, tachypnea) may be caused by hypoxia or shock.[19] Medications are given IV during the first 3 days post burn because of the erratic absorption from the tissues related to fluid shifts. In addition to an effective schedule of pain medication, limiting exposure of wounds to air and minimizing unnecessary stimulation of wounds help to minimize pain.

Elements of physical therapy (PT) and positioning begin almost at admission. The goals of PT are to preserve function by preventing scar contracture and muscle atrophy. Basic principles of positioning for burned areas include placing the neck in slight extension (no pillow); 90 degree abduction of the shoulder; and keeping the trunk straight without hip flexion.[11] Splints are often used over dressings to maintain functional positioning. Activity is encouraged as the child's condition stabilizes. Exercise and physical therapy can be provided in the form of play, as in encouraging the child to reach for a toy, providing riding toys, and tossing a ball back and forth.

Compression dressings, such as Jobst garments and Ace wraps, are applied to healed tissue to prevent scar hypertrophy. These are worn 24 hours a day and must be refitted as the child grows (Fig. 30-9).

Discharge from the hospital is not the endpoint of care for the burned child. Rehabilitation extends far beyond the hospitalization, and parents are often given a large share of responsibility for the process. Discharge teaching must address wound care, guidelines for exercise and activity, nutritional needs, the importance of compliance with pressure garment regimens, and the need for continued physical and psychological follow-up. When the child leaves the hospital, he or she must begin to deal with the difficulties of functioning in the real world and with the reactions of others to any scarring or disfigurement. The family should be prepared for potential behavior changes and be given resources for help in dealing with them.

Traumatic Death and Organ Donation

Occasionally, cardiovascular status is resuscitated without the return of brain function. In such cases, brain death is diagnosed by physical examination and confirmed with diagnostic tests. Criteria for brain death are listed in the accompanying display.

Due to the advent in recent years of improved surgical techniques and immunosuppressant therapy, organ transplantation is a viable, successful means of treatment for many patients in end-stage organ failure. Although the traumatic death of a child is one of the most difficult

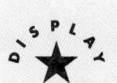

Criteria for Brain Death

Complete reversal of muscle relaxants and narcotics, anticonvulsant levels of barbiturates, normal electrolytes, normothermia

No spontaneous movement

No response to deep pain

No spontaneous respirations with po_2 greater than 100 mmHg and pco_2 greater than 60 mmHg

No brainstem reflexes:

- Dilated pupils fixed to light stimulation
- No corneal reflexes
- No oculocephalic reflexes
- No gag or cough reflexes
- No vestibular response to cold caloric stimulation

Neurologic opinion that damage involves the whole brain, that recovery is improbable, and that the condition is not reversible

From *Johnson, D. L. (1988). Head injury, In M. R. Eichelberger & G. L. Pratsch (Eds.)*, Pediatric trauma care. *Rockville, MD: Aspen.*

kinds of loss, the opportunity for the family to permit their child's organs to be used to sustain another life may help alleviate some of their grief.

All areas of the country have access to a regional donor center, which handles coordination of organ donation and transplantation needs. Once brain death has been established, the child's family is sensitively approached by a nurse, physician, or other professional for permission to use the child's organs. The organ procurement coordinator collaborates with the attending physician and nursing staff to order necessary blood work, medications, and any other required measures. The child remains in the intensive care unit and is cared for as any critically ill patient until the time of surgery. Nursing documentation should include the time of brain death declaration, interventions provided for the child and family, and time of transfer to the operating room.

The family should be allowed to say goodbye at the bedside. The sense of denial of death may be strong at this time because the child may have no outward signs of trauma. Support by a primary nurse, social worker, or chaplain during this time is essential.

Approximately 25 types of tissues and organs can be successfully transplanted, yet the number of organs available falls far short of the need.[28] There are few absolute donor exclusions, but sepsis, most malignancies, transmittable diseases, and end-organ dysfunction may preclude use of a donor organ.[47] Pediatric trauma victims are often ideal donors because they usually have no preexisting problems and are effectively resuscitated after trauma. It is rare that organ donation is requested in the emergency room; families must be given time to grieve and to come to terms with their own feelings. Families must also deal with their own doubts as well as the doubts

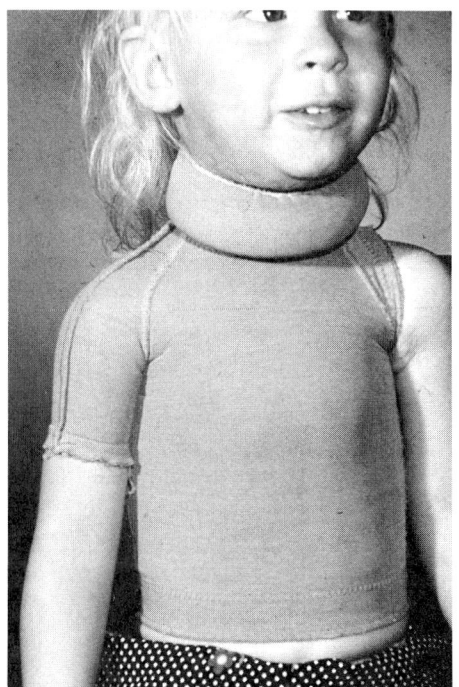

FIGURE 30-9

Compression garments help to minimize scar formation after burn injury.

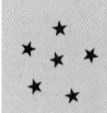

Ideas for Nursing Research

Traumatic injuries account for 8000 deaths of children and adolescents and 50,000 permanent disabilities each year. Advances in technology and advances in knowledge of traumatic injury patterns and physiologic responses have dramatically improved the care provided to injured children. Major traumatic injury is related to motor vehicle accidents, falls, drownings, burns, and firearms. The following are ideas for nursing research related to trauma using the injury control model (primary, secondary, tertiary):

- Effectiveness of health education programs on safety and accident prevention provided in the school system, in physicians' offices, and in health departments
- Proper use of carseats: Do parents use car seats and restraints correctly and consistently? Are parents aware of the dangers of inappropriate use of car seats? What problems do parents report related to car seats with infants and toddlers? How can nurses improve the safety of children in cars?
- Most helpful strategies in assisting parents and siblings in coping with a traumatic injury to a child during the initial phase of treatment

of other family members and friends. Honest, complete information provided compassionately by physicians and nurses can enhance this process and promote a favorable view of the organ donation process.

A family's religious or personal beliefs may preclude their being able to give permission for donation; these wishes should be respected and the issue should not be pressed. Although confidentiality of the organ recipient must be maintained, the donor family should be provided with resources for continued professional support and counseling in the months after the death of their child.

Summary

Children are frequently victims of injury. Recent advances in trauma care have resulted in increased survival rates and often complex care needs. This trend demands a multidisciplinary team approach, which includes careful attention to psychological needs of the injured child and family throughout the continuum of care.

Trauma nursing is a specialization incorporating a specific, complex body of knowledge. The trauma nurse must have an understanding of the physiologic response to injury, the relationship of mechanism of injury to types of injury sustained, and an awareness of the complex interrelationships among body systems in multitrauma. In addition, the pediatric trauma nurse must have a knowledge of how developmental level affects a child's perception of injury and treatment, what psychological re-

sponses to the injury and treatment are likely to occur, and how to assess and intervene in the disrupted family dynamics that occur after injury to a child.

The major challenge to health care professionals in pediatric trauma is to return a physically and psychologically healthy child and family to their home. This challenge does not begin at the moment of injury, nor does it end at discharge from the acute care hospital, but starts and continues with concepts of injury control and trauma system development.

References

1. American Heart Association. (1988). *Pediatric advanced life support.* Dallas: AHA National Center.
2. Bonadio, W. A., & Hellmich, T. (1989). Post traumatic pulmonary contusions in children. *Annals of Emergency Medicine, 18*(10), 1050–1052.
3. Boyajian, M. J. (1988). Maxillofacial injuries. In M. R. Eichelberger & G. L. Pratsch, (Eds.). *Pediatric trauma care.* Rockville, MD: Aspen.
4. Boyce, W. T., Springer, L. W., Sobolewsi, S., & Schaefer, C. (1984). Epidemiology of injuries in a large, urban school district. *Pediatrics, 74*(3), 342–349.
5. Cohen, G. J. (1983). The accident-prone child. *Clinical Proceedings, 39*(1), 5–10.
6. Cooper, A., Floyd, T., Barlow, B., et al. (1988). Major blunt abdominal trauma due to child abuse. *Journal of Trauma, 28*(10), 1483–1487.
7. Cunningham, J. L. (1987). Assessment and care of the patient with myocardial contusion. *Critical Care Nursing, 7*(2), 68–69.
8. Eichelberger, M. R., & Anderson, K. D. (1988). Sequelae of thoracic injuries in children. In M. R. Eichelberger & G. L. Pratsch, (Eds.). *Pediatric trauma care.* Rockville, MD: Aspen.
9. Eshel, G., Gross, B., Bar-Yochai, A., et al. (1987). Cardiac injuries caused by blunt chest trauma in children. *Pediatric Emergency Care, 3*(1), 96–98.
10. Evans, D. W., & Eichelberger, M. R. (1988). The pediatric trauma center: A commitment to the continuum. In M. R. Eichelberger & G. L. Pratsch (Eds.). *Pediatric trauma care.* Rockville, MD: Aspen.
11. Fader, P. (1988). Preserving function and minimizing deformity. In H. F. Carvejal & J. H. Parks (Eds.). *Burns in children: Pediatric burn management.* Chicago: Year Book.
12. Fought, S., Hall, M. M., & Larson, L. (1986). *Trauma nurse core course* (2nd ed.). Chicago: Emergency Nurses Association.
13. Gerhart, S. M. (1989). Facial trauma. In C. Joy (Ed.). *Pediatric trauma nursing.* Rockville, MD: Aspen.
14. Guzzetta, P. C., & Holihan, J. A. (1988). Burns. In M. R. Eichelberger & G. L. Pratsch, (Eds.). *Pediatric trauma care.* Rockville, MD: Aspen.
15. Haller, J. A., & Pokorny, W. J. (1988). Pediatric trauma. In K. L. Mattox, E. E. Moore, & D. V. Feliciano, (Eds.). *Trauma.* Norwalk, CT: Appleton and Lange.
16. Hankewich, M. (1986). Hyphema. *Journal of Ophthalmic Nursing and Technology, 5*(5), 169–173.
17. Harris, B. H., Latchaw, L. A., Murphy, R. E., & Schwaitzburg, S. D. (1987). The crucial hour. *Pediatric Annals, 16*(4), 301–304.
18. Hazinski, M. F. (1984). *Nursing care of the critically ill child.* St Louis: Mosby.
19. Helvig, B. (1988). Trauma to the integument: Burns. In E. Howell, L. Widra, & M. G. Hill (Eds.). *Comprehensive trauma nursing.* Glenview, IL: Scott, Foresman.
20. Hersenberg, J. E., & Hensinger, R. H. (1989). Pediatric cervical spine injuries. *Trauma Quarterly, 5*(2), 73–81.
21. Hill, M. G. (1988). Intra-abdominal trauma. In E. Howell, L.

Widra, & M. G. Hill (Eds.). *Comprehensive trauma nursing.* Glenview, IL: Scott, Foresman.

22. Howell, E., Sherer, C., & Leyden, A. (1988). Face and neck trauma. In E. Howell, L. Widra, & M. G. Hill (Eds.). *Comprehensive trauma nursing.* Glenview, IL: Scott, Foresman.

23. Jensen, T. G. (1984). Determination of nutritional status in critical care. *Perspectives in Practice, 84*(11), 1345–1348.

24. Johnson, D. L. (1988). Head injury. In M. R. Eichelberger & G. L. Pratsch (Eds.). *Pediatric trauma care.* Rockville, MD: Aspen.

25. Joy, C. (1989). *Pediatric trauma nursing.* Rockville, MD: Aspen.

26. Kass, E. J. (1988). Genitourinary injuries. In M. R. Eichelberger & G. L. Pratsch (Eds.). *Pediatric trauma care.* Rockville, MD: Aspen.

27. Keen, T. P. (1990). Nursing care of the pediatric multitrauma patient. *Nursing Clinics of North America, 25*(1), 131–141.

28. Krom, R. A. F. (1989). Organ donation—Are we moving in the right direction? *Mayo Clinic Proceedings, 64,* 705–707.

29. Lehr, E. (1990). *Psychological management of traumatic brain injuries in children and adolescents.* Rockville, MD: Aspen.

30. Manley, L., Haley, K., & Dick, M. (1988). Intraosseous infusion: Rapid vascular access for critically ill or injured infants and children. *Journal of Emergency Nursing, 14*(2), 63–68.

31. Manwarning, K. H., & Spetzler, R. F. (1986). Head and central nervous system injury in the child. In R. E. Marcus (Ed.). *Trauma in children.* Rockville, MD: Aspen.

32. McGill, W. A. (1988). Airway management. In M. R. Eichelberger & G. L. Pratsch (Eds.). *Pediatric trauma care.* Rockville, MD: Aspen.

33. McLoughlin, E. G., & McGuire, A. (1990). The causes, costs, and prevention of childhood burn injury. *American Journal of Diseases of Children, 144,* 677–682.

34. National Institute on Disability and Rehabilitative Research, U. S. Dept of Education. (1990). *Pediatric Trauma Registry, Annual Report 1990.* Grant # HI33B80009-90.

35. Newman, K. D., Bowman, L. M., Eichelberger, M. R., Gotschall, C. S., Taylor, G. A., Johnson, D. L., & Thomas, M. (1990). The lap belt complex: Intestinal and lumbar spine injury in children. *Journal of Trauma, 30*(9), 1133–1138.

36. Peckham, L. M., & Kitchen, L. A. (1989). Abdominal and genitourinary trauma. In C. Joy (Ed.). *Pediatric trauma nursing.* Rockville, MD: Aspen.

37. Pollock, I. F., Pang, D., & Sclabassi, R. (1988). Recurrent SCIWORA in children. *Journal of Neurosurgery, 69,* 177–182.

38. Ramenofsky, M. L. (1987). Pediatric abdominal trauma. *Pediatric Annals, 16*(4), 319–326.

39. Ramenofsky, M. L., Jurkovich, G. J., & Dierking, B. H. (1986). *Mini-residency in advanced pediatric life support.* Mobile: University of South Alabama.

40. Reath, D. B., Kirby, J., Lynch, M., & Maull, K. I. (1989). Patterns of maxillofacial injury in restrained and unrestrained motor vehicle crash victims. *Journal of Trauma, 29*(8), 1173–1176.

41. Reff, R. B. (1988). Musculoskeletal injuries. In M. R. Eichelberger & G. L. Pratsch (Eds.). *Pediatric trauma care.* Rockville, MD: Aspen.

42. Reid, B., Letts, R. M., & Black, G. B. (1990). Pediatric chance fractures: Association with intra-abdominal injuries and seatbelt use. *Journal of Trauma, 30*(4), 384–391.

43. Reynolds, E. A., Davidson, D. L., & Dierking, B. H. (1989). Delivering and documenting care in child abuse. *Journal of Emergency Medical Services, 14*(10), 71–76.

44. Reynolds, E. A., & Ramenofsky, M. L. (1988). The emotional impact of trauma on the toddler. *MCN: American Journal of Maternal Child Nursing, 13*(2), 106–109.

45. Ryckman, F. C., & Noseworthy, J. (1985). Multisystem trauma. *Surgical Clinics of North America, 65*(5), 1287–1300.

46. Smeltzer, S. C. O. (1988). Research in trauma nursing: State of the art and future directions. *Journal of Emergency Nursing, 14*(3), 145–153.

47. Soifer, B. E., & Gelb, A. W. (1989). The multiple organ donor: Identification and management. *Annals of Internal Medicine, 110*(10), 814–822.

48. Teasdale, G., & Jennett, B. (1974). Assessment of coma and impaired consciousness: A practical scale. *Lancet, 2,* 81–84.

49. Wright, C. J. (1990). *Mild head injury: Care of the child at home.* Washington, DC: Children's National Medical Center.

50. Ylvisaker, M. (1985). *Head injury rehabilitation: Children and adolescents.* San Diego: College-Hill Press.

Children With Cancer

BEHAVIORAL OBJECTIVES

Discuss the incidence, etiology, and
survival rates of childhood cancers.

Describe the different types of
childhood cancers by their presenting
signs and symptoms, diagnostic
studies, treatment, and prognosis.

Examine various treatment modalities
used for childhood cancer.

Identify specific nursing diagnoses
and interventions used in the care of
children with cancer.

Describe the psychological impact
cancer has on the child and family
and the nurse's role in providing
support.

Review effects of cancer therapy that
may occur months to years following
treatment for childhood cancer.

Only a few decades ago, a diagnosis of cancer meant certain death for a child. Today, with advances in the diagnosis and treatment of childhood cancers, many malignancies once considered fatal are now curable. More than 50% of all children with cancer will be long-term survivors.[22] Increasing prospects of cure in the area of pediatric oncology make it one of the most exciting and gratifying challenges in the field of cancer nursing.

Less than 5% of children with acute lymphocytic leukemia (ALL) survived their disease in 1960. By 1991, 5-year survival rates for this type of cancer were 60% or higher (Fig. 31-1). Major gains have been made in many of the malignancies of childhood. Five-year survival rates for cancers of the brain and central nervous system (CNS) approach 50% and non-Hodgkin's lymphomas (NHLs), 54%. Other success stories include survival rates of 40% to 50% for osteosarcoma and rates as high as 80% to 90% for Wilms' tumor, Hodgkin's disease, and retinoblastoma (Fig. 31-2). The mortality from childhood cancer has experienced an impressive decline from 8.3 per 100,000 in 1950 to 4.1 per 100,000 in 1983.[2]

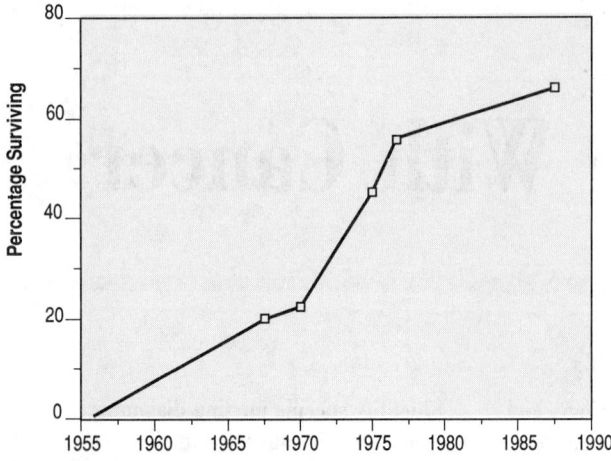

FIGURE 31-1

Five-year survival rates for children with acute lymphocytic leukemia. (Sources: American Cancer Society. [1985]. *Vital statistics of the U.S.—1980. CA—A Cancer Journal for Clinicians, 35*[1], 34. American Cancer Society. [1987]. *Cancer statistics 1987. CA—A Cancer Journal for Clinicians, 37*[1], 18–19. Sutow, W. W., Fernbach, D., & Viettio, T. [1984]. *Clinical pediatric oncology* [3rd ed.]. St Louis: C.V. Mosby.)

Much of the success in pediatric oncology can be attributed to the interdisciplinary and collaborative approaches taken by experts committed to the improvement of the lives of children. Children diagnosed with a malignancy in the United States are managed by teams of experts who participate in cooperative clinical investigations. The two major cooperative study groups for childhood cancer are the Pediatric Oncology Group and the Children's Cancer Study Group.

Incidence and Etiology

Approximately 6600 new cases of cancer occur each year in children younger than age 15, with common sites including the blood and bone marrow, CNS, bone, lymph nodes, brain, kidneys, and soft tissues.[2,7] ALL accounts for approximately 30% of the cancer diagnoses; CNS tumors, 19%; and lymphomas, 14%. Cancers of the musculoskeletal system and kidney occur in approximately 17% of children diagnosed with cancer (Fig. 31-3). Other more rare types of cancer account for the remaining 20%.

Although great strides have been made in the treatment of children with cancer, an estimated 2200 of these children will die, approximately half of them from leukemia.[2] Cancer in childhood is considered rare, yet it remains the leading cause of death by disease in children and is exceeded only by trauma as the leading killer of children between the ages of 1 and 15.[2,7]

Little is known about the causes of childhood cancer. Environmental agents have been implicated as causes of cancer in the young, and exposure during childhood to environmental pollutants may be linked to the development of a malignancy in adulthood. Data suggest that some tumors may be attributable to genetic abnormalities that predispose to tumors. Retinoblastoma, Wilms' tumor, and neuroblastoma all appear to present in hereditary and nonhereditary forms.[22] Ionizing radiation, ultraviolet radiation, asbestos, drugs, viruses, and immunodeficiency disorders are all being examined for their role in the development of pediatric malignancies.

Race, Age, and Sex

Leukemia, brain tumors, and lymphomas are the most frequent types of tumors in African-American and white children in the United States and account for greater than 60% of all cancers in children.[39] Although the cancer incidence rate for African-American children is similar to that for white children, the incidence of leukemia is greater in white than African-American children, with rates of 40% and 24%, respectively. Certain other tumors, such as Ewing's sarcoma, melanoma, and testicular cancers, are relatively rare in African-American children.[39]

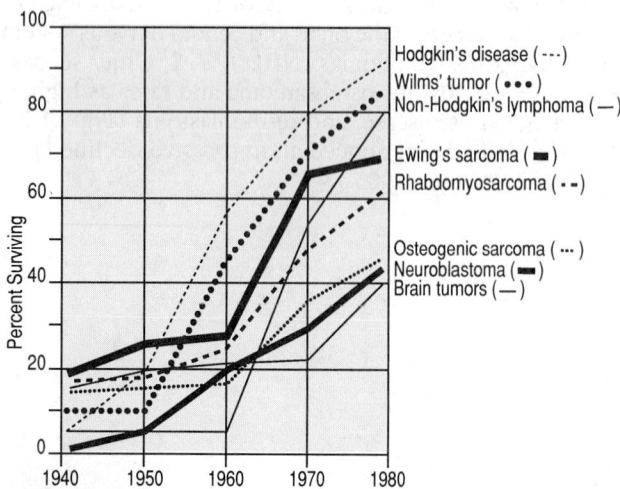

FIGURE 31-2

Survival rates for solid tumors in children. (Source: American Cancer Society. [1987]. *Cancer statistics 1987. CA—A Cancer Journal for Clinicians, 37*[1], 18–19.)

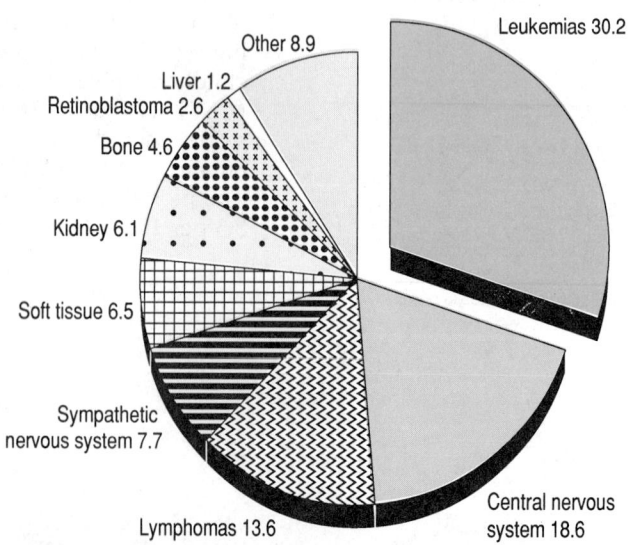

FIGURE 31-3

Frequency of specific childhood cancers. (Source: American Cancer Society. [1987]. *Cancer statistics 1987. CA—A Cancer Journal for Clinicians, 37*[1], 19–10.)

With many tumors, including acute lymphoblastic leukemia, Wilms' tumor, neuroblastoma, and retinoblastoma, the peak incidence is in children younger than 5 years of age. Lymphomas and bone tumors occur with increased frequency in children older than 10 years, while tumors of the CNS are predominant in the 5- to 10-year age group.[16]

In the United States, the overall male to female incidence of cancer is 1.2 to 1. Tumors that are more frequent in men include ALL, lymphomas, and CNS tumors.[34]

History of Management

The first successful use of a medicine for the treatment of cancer occurred in 1948, with the use of aminopterin for ALL.[36] This was followed by a number of significant advances in pediatric oncology that quickly led to increased survival rates[34]:

- Development of specific drugs that are most effective in ALL for induction, maintenance, and treatment of occult disease
- Identification of a specific therapy for a certain disease (e.g., actinomycin D for Wilms' tumor)
- Development of centers designed to implement comprehensive care for children with cancer while performing essential research to improve treatment
- Collaboration among treatment centers to place children on studies designed to provide information for the development of effective therapeutic regimens
- Initiation of supportive care through advanced technology to allow for the use of more aggressive therapeutic regimens
- Acknowledgment of the psychologic effects that childhood cancer has on the child and family

Because most early treatment successes began with children, pediatric oncology became a model for the cure of cancer. Childhood ALL has been the most important model of early work with chemotherapeutic agents. By the early 1960s, combination chemotherapy regimens were being used in children with ALL. After 1965, the therapeutic approach to children with ALL used combination therapy to induce complete remission, CNS prophylaxis to prevent overt CNS disease, and maintenance therapy to prevent disease recurrence. The prognosis changed during these years from a uniformly fatal disease to a disease with a cure rate of more than 60%.

Wilms' Tumor, a tumor of the kidney, has been treated successfully using multimodal and adjuvant therapy, establishing the concept of such treatment for other types of solid tumors. The National Wilms' Tumor Study Group, established in the 1960s, developed a comprehensive network for research centers to pool patients. Research results from the National Wilms' Tumor studies have become the model for treatment of all solid tumors.

Numerous events have led the way to increased cure for children with cancer. The organization of comprehensive oncology teams, successful research trials, improved supportive care measures, and the identification of important prognostic variables within diseases are major advances that provide an opportunity for cure.

Assessment for Signs and Symptoms

The nurse plays an important role in the management of children with cancer. The nurse's role begins with assessment for signs and symptoms of cancer.

Routine health assessments during childhood should include screening for signs and symptoms of neoplastic growth. The child and family health history may reveal etiological factors or a family history of malignancies. The seven danger signs published by the American Cancer Society should be kept in mind while asking the child or family questions. Weight loss is a common symptom of cancer. Diagnostic tests are used to confirm a medical diagnosis. These procedures include blood analysis, x-ray studies, biopsy, sonogram, and magnetic resonance screening.

Pain. Bone pain occurs in approximately 20% of children with leukemia. Presentation of pain is sometimes confused with juvenile arthritis in these children. Bone tumors may present with pain, swelling, and tenderness at the site. Some solid tumors cause pain, depending on their location and size. Headaches are associated with some brain tumors and may be accompanied by nausea and vomiting.

Fever. Fever, a frequent occurrence in children, may be caused by numerous illnesses. Fever is most commonly caused by infection, even in a child with cancer. A white blood cell differential will document neutropenia and may indicate the presence of abnormal cells in the peripheral smear.

Brusing and Pallor. Bruising most commonly occurs from a low platelet count caused by leukemia. A leukemic child will appear with numerous bruises on the extremities that occur from unknown causes. Nose bleeding may occur when the platelet count falls below 40,000. Anemia also may occur from replacement of the bone marrow with leukemia cells.

Mass. An abdominal mass is a common presentation in children with Wilms' tumor and neuroblastoma. A mass in the abdomen must be considered malignant until proven different. Any mass in an unusual location or one that is growing requires further investigation.

Lymphadenopathy. Swollen lymph nodes are common in children. However, enlarged lymph nodes in a child with fever for more than 1 week, recent weight loss, or an abnormal chest x-ray may indicate a serious disease. A biopsy should be performed if lymph nodes in an asymptomatic child increase in size after 2 weeks, fail to decrease in size after 4 to 6 weeks, or do not return to normal after 2 to 3 months.

Changes in the Eye. The presence of a white reflection as opposed to the normal orange pupil reflex in the pupil of a child's eye is the classic sign of retinoblastoma. Some children may squint or act as if they cannot see well. Any of these signs warrant an immediate ophthalmoscopic examination.

Disturbance in Gait or Personality. Brain tumors commonly occur in children with cancer, with more than half developing in the posterior fossa. Symptoms of a tumor located in this area of the brain include disturbances in gait and balance. Seizures may occur when the tumor presents in the supratentorial area. Midline tumors in the brain may produce personality changes. Commonly, the parent notices that something is different about the child but is unable to identify what is wrong.

Treatment for Childhood Cancers

Treatment for childhood cancers includes surgery, radiation therapy, chemotherapy, or bone marrow transplantation. Combinations of treatment modalities depend on the type and stage of the malignancy.

Depending on the type of cancer, treatment may continue for months to years. Visits to the hospital or clinic may be frequent. Education at the time of diagnosis is essential to prevent fewer problems in the home and to support the family in coping with diagnosis and treatment. Discussion must include a detailed review of the side effects of therapy.

The following is a brief overview of the most common types of treatment modalities used in children with cancer. These modalities and long-term side effects are summarized in Table 31-1. Specific nursing diagnoses related to side effects of treatment and nursing care interventions for children undergoing treatment for cancer follow later in this chapter.

Surgery

Surgery plays a major role in diagnosis and treatment of solid tumors in children. Cure for many childhood tumors depends on the ability to surgically remove the tumor at diagnosis. Surgery is most frequently used in combination with radiation therapy or chemotherapy. Surgery is an extremely stressful event for parents and children. Families are faced with the diagnosis of cancer and at the same time must cope with their child having an operation. It is essential for the nurse to spend time with the family to make sure all questions regarding the surgery are answered. The child and parents must be knowledgeable about the need for the operation. Time must be taken to prepare the child for the operating room. The use of play, books, or an actual visit to the operating room area can be very helpful to an anxious child and to the parents. Other interventions to prepare for hospitalization and other procedures are discussed in Chapter 23.

TABLE 31-1
Common Side Effects of Treatment for Childhood Cancer

Treatment Modality	Acute Side Effects	Long-Term Effects
Surgery	Change in function (i.e., organ, limb)	Scarring and adhesions
		Fistula formation
Chemotherapy	Myelosuppression	Second malignancy
	Infection	Liver cirrhosis
	Hemorrhage	Gonadal dysfunction
	Anemia	Chromosome aberrations
	Nausea and vomiting	Adrenal dysfunction
	Alopecia	Chronic cystitis
	Mucositis	White- and gray-matter dysfunction
	Steroid effects	
	Cardiomyopathy (anthracyclenes)	
	Neuropathy (vinca alkaloids)	
	Cystitis (Cyclophosphamide)	
	Allergic reactions (L-asparaginase)	
	Pancreatitis (L-asparaginase)	
	Pneumonitis (methotrexate, bleomycin)	
Radiation Therapy	Skin and mucosal inflammation	Second malignancy
	Tissue edema and inflammation	Soft-tissue and visceral fibrosis
	Pneumonitis	Gonadal dysfunction
	Nausea and vomiting	Endocrine dysfunction
	Enteritis	Dental problems
	Myelosuppression	Cataracts
	Alopecia	Bony growth delay
		White- and gray-matter dysfunction

Chemotherapy

Chemotherapy is the most common treatment modality for childhood cancer and is frequently combined with other types of treatment. Advanced technology allows most children to receive all or part of their treatment in an outpatient clinic. Research in cancer chemotherapy has brought forth complex and effective treatment protocols requiring highly skilled nurses to provide care. Nurses caring for these children are knowledgeable regarding chemotherapy and their side effects (see Tables 31-1 and 31-2). Nurses must be competent in the administration and management of common side effects.[18] They also are responsible for teaching parents what to observe following treatment.

Numerous chemotherapeutic agents are vesicants and pose significant clinical complications when extravasated into the subcutaneous tissue. Careful administration into a patent intravenous line is essential to prevent complications (see Table 31-8). Indwelling intravenous catheters are commonly used in patients receiving prolonged treatment. Catheters such as the Broviac or Hickman provide venous access without the need for needle access. Implanted catheters, such as the Infusaport or the Mediport, allow venous access through a port planted underneath the skin connected to a catheter that extends into the superior vena cava. Nurses must be knowledgeable regarding the different types of indwelling catheters and provide expertise for families learning how to care for these catheters when at home (see the Nursing Care Plan for more detail).

Concern has developed over the potential hazard to health professionals who are chronically exposed to chemotherapeutic agents. Protective eyewear, masks, gloves, and gowns are now used at many institutions. Gloves are highly recommended for nurses directly involved in administering chemotherapy.

Radiation Therapy

Radiation produces cellular loss of reproductive capability. Its effect on cancer cells prevents them from multiplying and spreading, which leads to the death of cancer cells. Radiation therapy plays a variable role in the treatment of childhood cancer, depending on the type of tumor, site, and stage of the disease. For some tumors, radiation is the primary treatment modality rather than an adjuvant to systemic therapy.

Nurses must be aware of the specific side effects of radiation therapy (see Table 31-1). These side effects are dependent on the part of the body that is being irradiated and the size of dose the area is receiving. For example, a young child receiving high-dose radiation therapy (greater than 2000 cGy) to the femur will have a reduced potential for growth in that extremity. Radiation therapy to the head and neck area may result in decreased saliva, irritation to the oral mucosa, and parotiditis. As more children who have had intense radiation survive, the long-term side effects of radiation become more apparent. Because radiation may damage any cells in its path, any body tissue could be affected. These long-term effects should be discussed as part of informed consent.

Bone Marrow Transplantation

Innovative approaches for high-risk malignancies using various treatment modalities followed by bone marrow transplantation are being instituted at many comprehensive cancer centers. This approach allows for higher doses of chemotherapy or radiation to be used to eradicate the disease, which is followed by bone marrow rescue. Bone marrow transplantation is hoped to improve survival for high-risk children with cancer. Three types of bone marrow transplants are used with children who have cancer:

- *Autologous*: The child's own bone marrow is harvested and reinfused after aggressive treatment.
- *Synergeneic*: The child has an identical twin who donates the marrow, which is administered after aggressive treatment.
- *Allogenic*: The child receives bone marrow from someone with a compatible human lymphocyte antigen (HLA) typing after aggressive treatment is given. The donor is usually a sibling. Recent work has been done using HLA-mismatched related donors and recipients. The bone marrow is treated with either lectin or monoclonal antibodies before infusion to prevent rejection of the bone marrow.

The actual bone marrow transplant is simple. The pretransplant treatment and post-transplant complications create complex and multidisciplinary challenges for all health care professionals involved. Profound bone marrow suppression occurs for 2 to 4 weeks after the bone marrow is infused.

As technology continues to advance and bone marrow transplantation continues to increase survival for high-risk children with cancer, nurses will be expected to play major roles in the management of the acute side effects of transplantation and the long-term follow-up of children who are cured.

Specific Childhood Cancers

The following section discusses specific types of childhood cancers by presenting the incidence, presenting signs and symptoms, diagnostic workup, treatment, and prognosis.

Leukemia

Leukemia is a malignant hematopoietic disease in which normal bone marrow elements are replaced by abnormal, poorly differentiated lymphocytes commonly called blast cells. ALL is the most common type of cancer diagnosed in children, accounting for approximately 30% of all cases of cancer in children. The incidence of leukemia in children younger than 15 years is 3.5 per 100,000.[6] It occurs more commonly in boys than girls, 1.5:1.0, and occurs more frequently in white children than in nonwhite children. The incidence of leukemia peaks between 3 to 5 years of age.[30]

TABLE 31-2
Common Chemotherapeutic Agents and Their Side Effects

Drug	Route	Nursing Implications	
		Side Effects	Specific Information
Actinomycin-D (dactinomycin, Cosmegan)	IV	Nausea, vomiting 4–5 hours after dose	Anorexia may last a few weeks
		Stomatitis	Extravasation must be avoided.
		Diarrhea	Drug reactivates inflammation at radiation therapy site.
		Alopecia, acne	
		Mental depression	
		Fever, malaise	
		Myelosuppression	
Adriamycin (doxorubicin)	IV	Nausea, vomiting	Drug causes red color in urine—may last for 12 days.
		Fever	EKG will be done periodically to observe for changes in cardiac motility.
		Stomatitis	
		Rash and hives	Total dose should not exceed 450 mg/m^2.
		Myelosuppression	
		Severe alopecia	Extravasation must be avoided.
		Cardiotoxicity after maximum dose	
5-Azacitadine	IM	Nausea, vomiting, diarrhea	Hypotension is a possibility.
	IV	Myelosuppression, stomatitis	Infusion is given slowly
Bleomycin (Blenoxane)	IM	Allergic reaction:	Pulmonary function tests will be done periodically.
	IV	Fever, hypotension, anaphylaxis, 3–5 hours after dose	
		Nausea and vomiting	
		Macular rash	
		Stomatitis	
		Alopecia	
		Pulmonary fibrosis after maximum dose	
Cis-platinum	IV	Anaphylactic reactions	Drug given with mannitol over 8 hours to prevent renal toxicity.
		Nausea, vomiting	Urine output is monitored closely.
		Renal toxicity	
		Auditory changes	
		Myelosuppression	
		Possible hypocalcemia, seizures, peripheral neuropathies, loss of taste and memory	
Cytosine arabinosine (ara-C, Cytosar)	IV	Nausea, vomiting, anorexia	Drug also used to treat CNS leukemia.
	IM	Stomatitis	
	IT	Myelosuppression 7–14 days after dose	
		Diarrhea, skin rash	
		Liver toxicity	
		Immunosuppression	
Daunomycin (daunorubicin)	IV	Nausea, vomiting, anorexia	Urine may turn red.
		Cardiac toxicity	EKG will be done periodically.
		Fever	Total dose should not exceed 450 mg/m^2.
		Stomatitis, rash	
		Alopecia	Extravasation is avoided.
		Myelosuppression	
		Abdominal pain	
		Sudden congestive heart failure after maximum dose	
DTIC (Dacarbazine)	IV	Nausea, vomiting 1–2 hours after dose	Drug may irritate veins while being injected.
		Headache, myalagia, malaise	Child may complain of pain if infused into a small peripheral vein.
		Mild liver toxicity	
		Myelosuppression	
		Facial paresthesia and flushing	

(Continued)

TABLE 31-2
(Continued)

Drug	Route	Nursing Implications	
		Side Effects	Specific Information
5-FU (fluorouracil)	IV PO	Nausea, vomiting, diarrhea Skin rash Stomatitis Myelosuppression 9–14 days after dose Some alopecia GI bleeding and ulcers	Veins may darken after prolonged use. Oral dose may be taken with carbonated beverage
L-Asparaginase (L-ASP)	IM	Nausea, vomiting in 50% Fever, tiredness Possible anaphylaxis Hyperglycemia—abdominal pain, increased thirst Liver toxicity Hypotension Convulsions Weight loss	Patient to remain in clinic ½ hour to 45 min after dose in case of anaphylaxis
6-MP (mercaptopurine, Purinethol)	PO	Myelosuppression Stomatitis Liver dysfunction—jaundice	Patient may be given reduced dose if also on allopurinol because allopurinol may interfere with 6-MP breakdown and lead to toxicity.
Methotrexate	IV IM PO IT	Nausea, vomiting, diarrhea Mouth ulcers, intestinal ulcers Stomatitis Photosensitivity Myelosuppression Osteoporosis Rashes Kidney dysfunction at high doses	Child must avoid vitamins, tetracycline, chloramphenicol, Dilantin, and alcoholic beverages.
Nitrogen mustard (Mustargen, HN2, mechlorethamine)	IV	Nausea and vomiting Immunosuppression Myelosuppression Anorexia, diarrhea Phlebitis Weakness	Extravasation must be avoided.
Prednisone (Deltasone)	PO	Increased appetite and weight gain Euphoria Body changes: Moon face, striae, trunk obesity, purpura, osteoporosis, muscle weakness, emotional changes Hypertension Heartburn, peptic ulcers Suppression of signs of infection and inflammation Increased thirst, urination, and sugar in urine	Foods should not be salted. Fried foods and foods high in salt must be avoided.
Procarbazine	PO	Nausea, vomiting Myelosuppression Mild depression, restlessness Some alopecia Stomatitis Dermatitis Lethargy	MAO inhibitors to avoid: alcohol, antihistamines, narcotics, sedatives, ripe cheese, bananas and milk. Use with caution with Dilantin.
Thioguanine (6-TG)	PO	Some nausea, vomiting Diarrhea, stomatitis Skin rash	

(Continued)

TABLE 31-2
(Continued)

Drug	Route	Nursing Implications	
		Side Effects	Specific Information
Vinblastine (Velban)	IV	Photosensitivity	Extravasation must be avoided.
		Myelosuppression	
		Immunosuppression	
		Nausea, vomiting, diarrhea	
		Myelosuppression	
		Neurotoxicity:	
		Constipation	
		Urinary retention	
		Loss of deep tendon reflexes	
		Paresthesias	
		Obstruction	
		Mental depression	
Vincristine (Oncovin)	IV	Abdominal cholic, diarrhea, constipation, nausea, vomiting	Bowel elimination must be assessed.
		Stomatitis	Stool softener may be needed while on vincristine.
		Alopecia	Extravasation must be avoided.
		Neurotoxicity:	
		Tingling in hands and feet	
		Weakness—muscle	
		Ataxia	
		Paresthesias	
		Pain in limbs, jaws, abdomen	
		Severe constipation	
		Some myelosuppression	
		Liver toxicity	
		Fever	
		Immunosuppression	
VM-26	IV	Hypotension	Infusion given over 30–60 minutes.
		Myelosuppression	Extravasation must be avoided.
		Alopecia	
		Nausea, vomiting, diarrhea	
		Anaphylaxis	
VP-16	IV	Jaw pain	Infusion given over 30–60 minutes.
		Alopecia	
		Myelosuppression	
		Nausea, vomiting, anorexia	
		Hypotension	
		Liver toxicity	
		Headache	
		Fever	

(IV, intravenous; IM, intramuscular; PO, oral; IT, intrathecal; EKG, electrocardiogram; CNS, central nervous system; GI, gastrointestinal; MAO, monoamine oxidase.)

Classification. Leukemia is classified by cell type (i.e., lymphocytic or nonlymphocytic) and by cellular differentiation (i.e., undifferentiated or primitive versus mature cells). ALL, the most common type of leukemia, is distinguished by predominantly undifferentiated white blood cells and accounts for approximately 80% of all childhood leukemia.[3] Cellular morphology, cytochemistry, and immunologic markers are used to classify childhood leukemia.

Morphology. The standard classification system for differentiation of leukemia is that described by the French-American-British (FAB) group.[24] Criteria used to distinguish between ALL and acute nonlymphocytic leukemia (ANLL) include cell size; nuclear–cytoplasmic ratio; number of nucleoli; and presence or absence of cytoplasmic vacuoles, granulocytes, and Auer rods.

Cytochemistry. Leukemia cells and their reaction to specific cytochemical stains provide a second means of differentiating lymphocytic from nonlymphocytic leukemia. In general, lymphocytic cells are positive with a periodic acid-Schiff (PAS) stain and negative with a Sudan black stain and with stains for myeloperoxidase and various esterases that are positive in nonlymphocytic cells.

Immunology. ALL can be divided into several subgroups, including T cell, B cell, pre-B cell, and non-T non-B (common) cell leukemias. Various cell markers are used to distinguish between the various leukemias. The common ALL antigen is found in patients with pre-B and non-T non-B cell types of ALL. Ia antigens are found on non-T non-B, B, and pre-B leukemic cells and some of the ANLL subgroups. B-cell leukemia is characterized by the presence on the cell surface of immunoglobulin molecules. Pre-B cells lack surface immunoglobulin, but using a fluorescent stain on fixed cells, they can be shown to contain the heavy chain of immunoglobulin M (IgM) in their cytoplasm. T cells are characterized by their ability to form rosettes with sheep erythrocytes or by the presence of T cell-specific membrane antigens recognized by several antisera or monoclonal antibodies. The diagnosis of a particular immunologic type of ALL is associated with a predictable clinical course, response to therapy, and prognosis.

Clinical Manifestations.

Almost all of the clinical signs and symptoms of leukemia result from leukemic replacement of normal bone marrow.[4] Replacement of normal bone marrow by leukemic cells results in anemia, neutropenia, and thrombocytopenia. Anemia causes fatigue, weakness, pallor, and lethargy. Neutropenia predisposes the child to infection. Thrombocytopenia results in cutaneous bruises or purpura, petechiae, epistaxis, melena, and gingival bleeding. Enlargement of the liver and spleen and lymphadenopathy are common. Leukemic infiltration expands the bone marrow and may cause bone and joint pain in many children.[22]

Diagnostic Studies.

The diagnosis of leukemia in children is confirmed by bone marrow aspiration. Classification of the specific type of leukemia is essential to ensure adequate treatment. Subtypes of both groups are now recognized by cellular morphology, cytochemistry, and immunologic markers.[24] In approximately 20% of children diagnosed with acute leukemia, cell lines other than lymphoid cells are involved. This is ANLL and occurs in children of all ages, although it is more common in older children. It occurs with equal frequency in boys and girls. The greatest difference between ANLL and ALL is the poorer prognosis for ANLL and more aggressive treatment regimen used for these types of leukemia.[34]

Treatment.

Treatment programs for all types of acute leukemia involve an induction phase, prophylactic CNS therapy, and a maintenance phase of therapy using multiple drugs. A combination of drugs is used initially to induce remission. Drugs most commonly used for ALL inductions are vincristine, prednisone, and L-asparaginase. The purpose of induction is to reduce the tumor burden to the degree that normal bone marrow function returns with resolution of clinical symptoms. Ninety-five percent of all children with ALL go into remission during induction.[34]

The induction phase of therapy for ALL is followed by CNS prophylaxis. CNS treatment is given to prevent development of CNS leukemia. CNS treatment consists of either radiation therapy with intrathecal methotrexate or intrathecal therapy alone consisting of methotrexate, cytosine anabinoside, and hydrocortisone. Specific CNS therapy depends on the type of leukemia and risk factors of the child. Presently, several approaches to CNS treatment are being studied in the different subgroups of children with leukemia to determine the most effective therapy with the least side effects.

Maintenance therapy is given for 2 to 3 years to eliminate residual leukemia cells. Maintenance therapy for ALL includes methotrexate, 6-mercaptopurine, vincristine, and prednisone. Studies are being conducted using more aggressive therapy for ALL to improve survival in high-risk children. The cure rate for childhood ALL is now reaching 60%.

Drug combinations effective in children with ALL are not effective with ANLL. Induction regimens are much more aggressive and usually consist of cytosine arabinoside and an anthracycline (doxorubicin or daunorubicin). Remissions are obtained in approximately 70% of children with ANLL, and survival rates reach 50% with the more aggressive treatment regimens.[34]

Hodgkin's Disease

Hodgkin's disease is a malignancy of the lymphoid system and is differentiated from other lymphomas by histology, cell lineage, clinical behavior, and response to treatment.[32] The annual diagnostic rate for Hodgkin's disease in the United States is 5.8 per million for white children and 6.1 per million for African-American children.[2] The incidence is rare before 5 years of age, but increases steadily thereafter and peaks at 15 to 34 years of age. Hodgkin's disease is twice as common in boys than in girls, although this difference diminishes with age.

Clinical Manifestations.

Hodgkin's disease usually arises in a single lymph node or anatomic group of lymph nodes. The majority of children with Hodgkin's disease present with painless adenopathy in the lower cervical region. Other symptoms include anorexia, weight loss, malaise, lassitude, fever, and night sweats.[31] The presence of symptoms, specifically fever, night sweats, and weight loss, is classified as "B symptoms," which indicates a poorer prognosis than children with no symptoms, classified as "A symptoms."

Diagnostic Studies.

Diagnosis of Hodgkin's disease is confirmed by lymph node biopsy. Identification of the staging of the disease is the most important factor in determining treatment and projecting prognosis. Imaging studies are essential to determine the extent of nodal involvement. Lymphangiography frequently is used to evaluate pelvic and para-aortic lymph nodes. Exploratory laparotomy with splenectomy, liver biopsy, and multiple lymph node biopsies is necessary when disease is not detected through imaging techniques to determine the extent of intra-abdominal involvement. Once the diagnostic studies are completed, the child is staged according to the criteria in Table 31-3.

Hodgkin's disease is defined histologically as a lesion containing Reed-Sternberg cells. These cells alone are not sufficient for the diagnosis of Hodgkin's disease because they can be found in disorders such as infectious mononucleosis, nodular histiocytic lymphoma, and graft-versus-host reactions.[34] There are four histologic categories of Hodgkin's disease: lymphocyte predominance, nodular sclerosing, mixed cellularity, and lymphocytic depletion.[22] Histologic categories, once thought to have significant prognostic implications, have become less significant with the use of adjuvant combination chemotherapy and radiation therapy. Nodular sclerosing Hodgkin's disease is the most common type found in children.

Treatment. The mainstay of treatment for Hodgkin's disease is radiation therapy, and the extent of therapy depends on the stage of the disease. Chemotherapy is used in combination with radiation therapy for children with more extensive disease. A combination of chemotherapy using nitrogen mustard, vincristine, procarbazine, and prednisone (MOPP), alternating with doxorubicin, bleomycin, vinblastine, and DTIC (ABVD) is used. Chemotherapy frequently is administered before radiation therapy to decrease the long-term effects of radiation therapy.

Survival rates for children with Hodgkin's disease are 90% in stages I and II and approximately 80% in stages III and IV.[31]

Non-Hodgkin's Lymphomas

The NHLs are solid tumors of the hematopoietic system in which the lymph node is diffusely involved with malignant lymphoblasts of either T- or B-cell origin. The peak incidence is between the ages of 7 and 11, with the frequency of occurrence increasing with age. The annual incidence rate is estimated to be 7.5 per million people.[34] There is a 3:1 male to female predominance. Because NHL is a malignancy of the immune system, immunodeficient patients have a high risk of developing the disease. Genetic considerations also exist, due to the evidence of chromosomal anomalies, particularly in Burkitt's lymphomas.[34] A possible viral cause is also under investigation due to the presence of the genome for the Epstein-Barr virus in the DNA of African children diagnosed with Burkitt's lymphoma. Similar association with the American Burkitt's lymphoma are uncommon.

Classification. The four types of NHL include lymphoblastic, Burkitt's, non-Burkitt's, and large cell. Staging for NHL depends on the extent of disease. Table 31-4 demonstrates one of the staging systems for childhood NHL.

Clinical Manifestations. The clinical presentation of NHL depends on the site and extent of tumor. Common sites include the abdomen, mediastinum, head and neck, and peripheral nodes. An intra-abdominal presentation leads to constipation, abdominal fullness, and cramping and often is accompanied by vomiting. More widespread involvement may lead to diffuse abdominal pain, abdominal distention, and appendicitis-like symptoms. A mediastinal presentation may lead to a cough, transient fever, and respiratory distress.

Diagnostic Studies. Diagnosis of lymphoma is confirmed by surgical biopsy. Extent of disease must be evaluated by extensive examination using scans, x-rays, bone marrow aspiration, and lumbar puncture. Rapid disease progression frequently occurs, requiring early initiation of treatment.[22]

Treatment. Combination chemotherapy is the major treatment used in children with lymphoma. Drugs effective for NHL include cyclophosphamide, vincristine, methotrexate, daunorubicin, and prednisone. Radiation therapy also may be used. Due to the propensity of these tumors to metastasize to the CNS, intrathecal chemotherapy is prophylactically given.[22] A greater than 80% remission rate is reported for children with NHL, due to the aggressive treatment programs that are now used.[15]

Central Nervous System Tumors

Tumors of the CNS include those of the brain and spinal cord. They are the second most common tumor of childhood, and the incidence rate in the United States is 2.4 per 100,000 children younger than 15 years.[2] The peak age of incidence for childhood brain tumors is between 5 and 10 years of age.

Clinical Manifestations. Each major anatomic area of the brain and spinal cord has its own symptomatology when invaded by tumor, and symptomatology results from general and focal effects.[35] General effects of lesions are caused by increased intracranial pressure, and symptoms include headaches, malaise, somnolence, irritability, personality changes, impaired vision, and projectile vomiting without preceding nausea. Cranial enlargement and a bulging fontanel are characteristic of increased intracranial pressure in infants whose sutures have not completely closed. Focal neurologic effects may include disturbances in gait and balance (cerebellar tumors), nystagmus (cerebellar tumors), visual field disturbances (midline tumors), endocrine abnormalities (midline

TABLE 31-3
Staging System for Hodgkin's Disease

Stage	Description
I	Involvement of a single lymph node region
II	Involvement of two or more lymph node regions on the same side of the diaphragm
III	Involvement of lymph nodes on both sides of the diaphragm
IV	Diffuse or disseminated involvement of one or more extralymphatic organs or tissues with or without associated lymph node enlargement

TABLE 31-4
Staging System for Childhood Non-Hodgkin's Lymphoma

Stage	Description
I	Single tumor (extranodal) or single anatomic area (nodal), with the exclusion of mediastinum or abdomen
II	Single tumor (extranodal) with regional node involvement
	Two or more nodal areas on the same side of the diaphragm
	Two single (extranodal) tumors with or without regional node involvement on the same side of the diaphragm
	Primary gastrointestinal tract tumor, usually in the ileocecal area, with or without involvement of associated mesenteric nodes only*
III	Two single tumors (extranodal) on opposite sides of the diaphragm
	Two or more nodal areas above and below the diaphragm
	All the primary intrathoracic tumors (mediastinal, pleural, thymic)
	All extensive primary intra-abdominal disease*
	All paraspinal or epidural tumors, regardless of other tumor site(s)
IV	Any of the above with initial CNS or bone marrow involvement†

* A distinction is made between apparently localized GI tract lymphoma versus more extensive intra-abdominal disease because of their quite different pattern of survival after appropriate therapy. Stage II disease typically is limited to a segment of the gut plus or minus the associated mesenteric nodes only, and the primary tumor can be completely removed grossly by segmental excision. Stage III disease typically exhibits spread to para-aortic and retroperitoneal areas by implants and plaques in mesentery or peritoneum, or by direct infiltration of structures adjacent to the primary tumor. Ascites may be present, and complete resection of all gross tumor is not possible.

† If marrow involvement is present initially, the number of abnormal cells must be 25% or less in an otherwise normal marrow aspirate with a normal peripheral blood picture.

(CNS, central nervous sytem; GI, gastrointestinal.)

From Murphy, S. B., & Donaldson, S. S. (1982). Pediatric lymphoma. In Carter (Ed.), *Principles of cancer treatment.* New York, McGraw-Hill. With permission.

tumors), paresis or paralysis (spinal tumors), and bowel or bladder dysfunction (spinal tumors).[4]

Diagnostic Studies. The diagnostic workup for a child with a possible brain tumor includes a computed tomography (CT) scan (enhanced and unenhanced), myelogram, and spinal fluid examination as well as magnetic resonance imaging (MRI) of the brain. When possible, confirmation of the specific type of tumor is established by surgical biopsy. Stereotactic biopsies are used frequently to approach lesions once considered inoperable. Through the combined used of CT scanning and careful biopsy techniques, accurate biopsies are able to be obtained, allowing for a specific pathologic diagnosis.

Treatment. The treatment of choice is complete surgical removal of the tumor. However, complete surgical removal is not always feasible without subjecting the patient to residual neurologic damage. Radiation therapy becomes a primary treatment modality in children older than 3 years whose tumors have not been completely excised. High doses of radiation are necessary (4500 to 6000 cGy) and are given in six to eight treatment periods.[4] Radiation therapy rarely is administered to children younger than 2 years due to the severe side effects of cranial radiation therapy on young children. Children younger than 2 years are at substantial risk for developing mental retardation after receiving radiation therapy.[5] Chemotherapy may be used in these young children instead of radiation therapy. Chemotherapy also is used for children in whom the tumor was not completely removed or who are at risk for reoccurrence or spread.

Survival rates for children with brain tumors depends on tumor type, degree of malignancy, and location; however, overall survival rates approximate 50% for these children.[35]

Neuroblastoma

Neuroblastoma is a tumor of the sympathetic nervous system. The primary tumor is most commonly seen in the adrenal medulla or adjacent sympathetic ganglia of the abdomen and pelvis but also can occur in the chest, neck, and head. The common sites of occurrence are shown in Figure 31-4.

Neuroblastoma is the third most common malignancy of childhood. The annual incidence rate in the United States is 9.4 per million people in white children and 6.7 per million in African-American children.[34] The median age at diagnosis is younger than 2 years, with 35% occurring before 1 year of age, 55% before 2 years, and 88% before 5 years.[34]

Clinical Manifestations. The clinical manifestations of neuroblastoma are related to the site of the primary tumor. An abdominal tumor may cause a full stomach or a distinct mass. As the tumor grows, it can cause abdominal pain, loss of appetite, and bowel or urinary problems. A tumor in the chest may cause a persistent cough, chest pain, or shortness of breath. A tumor of the head and neck may present as a mass around the eye or in the jaw. Spinal involvement may lead to paresis or paralysis of the lower extremities or bladder and bowel incontinence. The child may develop exophthalmos, ec-

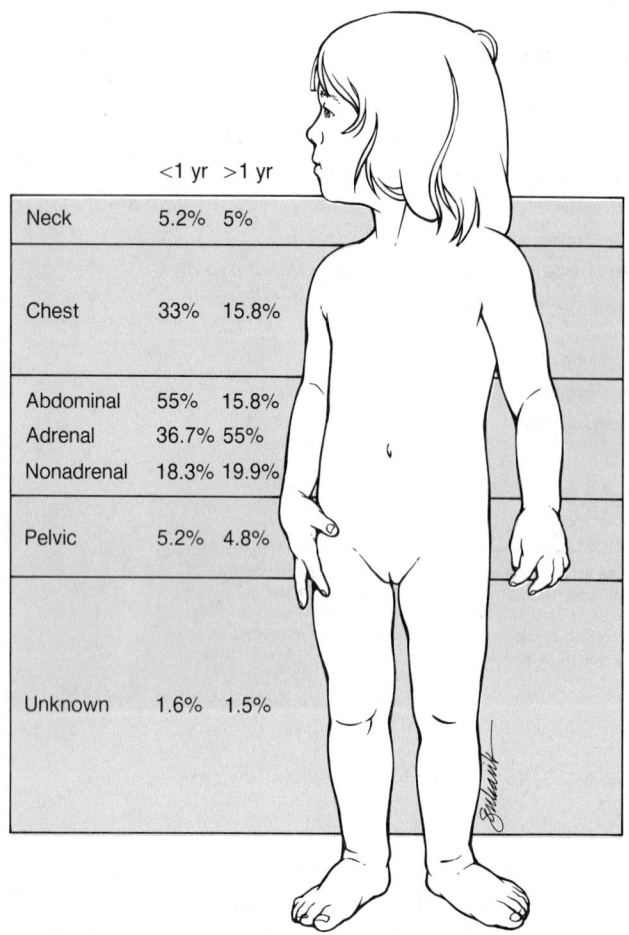

	<1 yr	>1 yr
Neck	5.2%	5%
Chest	33%	15.8%
Abdominal	55%	15.8%
Adrenal	36.7%	55%
Nonadrenal	18.3%	19.9%
Pelvic	5.2%	4.8%
Unknown	1.6%	1.5%

FIGURE 31-4
Common primary sites of occurrence for neuroblastoma at age of diagnosis. (Data from Pizzo, P. A., Poplack, D. G. (1989). *Principles and practice of pediatric oncology.* Philadelphia: J.B. Lippincott.)

chymosis, and Horner's syndrome, which includes ptosis of the eyelid, constriction of the pupil, and flushing of the affected side of the face.[38] Metastases, which often are present at diagnosis, may lead to bone and joint pain, skin and skull nodules, fever, and weight loss. Some neuroblastomas produce large amounts of catecholamine, which causes hypertension, excessive sweating, bounding pulse, pallor, polyuria, and polydipsia.

Signs and symptoms of neuroblastoma in infants include enlarged liver, subcutaneous nodules, anemia, feeding difficulties, vomiting, weight loss, and dyspnea.[2] Flaccid paralysis and urinary dysfunction, including bladder distention and dribbling, may indicate neuroblastoma.

Diagnostic Studies. Many tests are useful to confirm the diagnosis and determine the extent of disease. These include CT scans of the chest, abdomen, and pelvis; abdominal ultrasound; bone scan, bone marrow aspirate, and biopsy; and a 24-hour urine collection for catecholamines. Elevated levels of catecholamines may correlate with the extent of disease involvement.[34]

Treatment. Children with localized disease may be treated with surgery alone. Combination chemotherapy, with the most frequent drugs being cyclophosphamide,

vincristine, and DTIC, is used for children with more extensive disease. Unfortunately, survival rates have not improved with more aggressive chemotherapy regimens. Recent research has seen promise of increased survival using high doses of chemotherapy followed by autologous bone marrow transplantation in children with more extensive disease. Prognosis for children with neuroblastoma varies with the extent of disease involvement, and age of the child at diagnosis. Children younger than 2 years have a better prognosis. Children with stage I and II localized disease have much better prognoses than children with metastatic disease, who have a survival rate between 5% and 10%.[38]

Wilms' Tumor

Wilms' tumor, or nephroblastoma, is a tumor arising from the renal parenchyma. Wilms' tumor accounts for less than 10% of all malignant tumors in children, and 30% occur before 1 year of age. Seventy percent of all Wilms' tumors occur before the age of 4, and they rarely occur in children older than 7 years. There is no sexual predominance. The incidence of Wilms' tumor is 7.8 per million children between the ages of 1 and 14 years. Wilms' tumor is also discussed in Chapter 50.

Classification. Wilms' tumor is classified according to the extent of tumor spread (stages I to IV) and whether the tumor is defined as favorable or unfavorable histology. The specific stages of Wilms' tumor are established by the National Wilms' tumor study.

Clinical Manifestations. The most common presenting symptom of Wilms' tumor is a large abdominal mass. Pain, hematuria, general malaise, fever, anorexia, and weight loss also may be presenting symptoms. Mild to severe hypertension, caused by elevated plasma renin levels, is present in a majority of patients. Wilms' tumor often is associated with congenital anomalies, including hypospadias, cryptorchidism, and fusion anomalies of the kidneys.

Diagnostic Studies. Diagnosis is confirmed by surgery, with pathology confirming the diagnosis. Numerous radiographic studies are essential to evaluate the stage of disease. An ultrasound of the kidney, IV pyelogram, and abdominal and chest CT scans are essential. Arteriography sometimes is necessary to evaluate a kidney not well visualized by other methods to determine the extent of tumor involvement.

Treatment. Treatment for Wilms' tumor represents one of the first unified multimodal approaches to solid tumor therapy. Surgery is aimed at removing the tumor. Postoperative chemotherapy may include vincristine, actinomycin D, and doxorubicin. The duration of chemotherapy may range from 10 weeks to 15 months, depending on the extent of disease spread. Radiation therapy used in combination with chemotherapy depends on the stage of the tumor. Long-term survival rates for children with Wilms' tumor is 90% depending on the stage and histology of the tumor.

Rhabdomyosarcoma

Rhabdomyosarcoma is a malignancy of striated muscle cells and is the most common pediatric soft-tissue sarcoma. The peak ages of incidence for this tumor are in early childhood and late adolescence. The annual incidence in the United States is estimated to be 4.4 per million white children and 1.3 per million African-American children younger than age 15.[34] The male-to-female ratio is 1.4:1.

Rhabdomyosarcoma most often occurs in the head and neck, accounting for 38% of all cases, of which 10% are located in the orbit.[34] Other sites in order of frequency include the genitourinary system, extremities, trunk, retroperitoneum, gastrointestinal (GI) tract, and the perineum–anus region.

Clinical Manifestations. The symptoms of rhabdomyosarcoma are variable and depend on the location of the tumor as demonstrated in Table 31-5. The most common symptom of rhabdomyosarcoma is the presence of a hard, nontender mass. Orbital involvement may cause swelling, ptosis, visual disturbances, and eye movement abnormalities. Nasopharyngeal involvement may cause chronic sinusitis with nasal discharge and chronic unilateral otitis media. Genitourinary involvement may cause urinary obstruction, hematuria, dysuria, vaginal discharge, or a protruding vaginal mass.[33]

The four major histologic types of rhabdomyosarcoma are classified as embryonal, alveolar, pleomorphic, and mixed cellularity. The most common type is embryonal rhabdomyosarcoma and is seen in approximately 75% of head and neck and genitourinary tumors.[34] Rhabdomyosarcoma is staged according to the extent of disease involvement.

Diagnostic Studies. The diagnosis is confirmed by pathology through a biopsy or surgical resection of the tumor. Radiologic studies include CT scans of the chest to detect lung metastasis, bone scans to evaluate for bone metastasis, and CT scans of the primary site. Bone marrow biopsy and aspiration are necessary because of the risk of bone marrow metastasis.

Treatment. The primary treatment is surgery, requiring wide surgical excision of the tumor. When surgical removal would be functionally disabling, radiation therapy is used. Chemotherapy is essential to prevent metastasis in all patients. A combination of drugs using vincristine, actinomycin D, cyclophosphamide, and doxorubicin is the most successful in treating rhabdomyosarcoma. Radiation therapy is used in all children

TABLE 31-5
Primary Sites of Rhabdomyosarcoma With Symptoms

Site of Presentation	Associated Symptoms
Head and Neck	
Orbit	Pain, swelling, ptosis, visual disturbances, and changes in cranial nerves III, IV, VI
External auditory canal	Earache, ear drainage, hearing loss unilaterally, poor visualization of tympanic membrane with suspected foreign object (tumor)
Surface muscle primary	Swelling, mass not associated with injury, changes in cranial nerves—especially, VII—enlarged firm cervical lymph nodes with lymphatic metastasis
Nasopharyngeal	Chronic sinusitis with purulent or clear discharge, chronic unilateral otitis media unresponsive to antibiotics, dizziness, headaches, mastication or feeding difficulty, epistaxis
Central nervous system	Thirty-five percent of patients with nasopharyngeal primary rhabdomyosarcoma develop direct meningeal extension within 6 months of diagnosis; presenting symptoms may include headaches, vision changes, cranial nerve change, gross motor changes, and presence of malignant cells in spinal fluid; rhabdomyosarcoma cells in the spinal canal may also develop into ''drop'' metastasis along lower areas of the cord, causing compression with associated paralysis or neurologic symptoms such as ''shooting'' pain or numbness
Trunk	
Chest wall	Swelling, respiratory distress, pleural inflammation; usually asymptomatic until mass is very large
Retroperitoneal, pelvis, perineum	Flank or back pain, renal obstruction, constipation, hematuria (rare), hypertension with hydronephrosis and increased renin secretion
Extremity	Changes in gait, decreased use of limb, enlarged lymph node proximal to lesions, enlarging mass
Genitourinary	
Bladder, urinary tract, prostate	Urinary obstruction, hematuria, dysuria, progressive regression in toilet training, urinary tract infection
Vagina	Vaginal bleeding, vaginal drainage, protruding mass

Source: Sutow, W. W. (1981) Rhabdomyosarcoma. In W. W. Sutow (Ed.), *Malignant solid tumors in children: A review.* New York: Raven Press.

who have residual disease following surgery.[37] The most important prognostic indicator is the extent of disease spread, and children with localized disease have a 70% to 80% chance of long-term survival.[37]

Osteogenic Sarcoma

Osteogenic sarcoma, also called osteosarcoma, is a primary malignant tumor of the bone that arises from primitive bone-forming mesenchyma and is characterized by the production of osteoid and bone from a sarcomatous stroma. This is the most common bone tumor in children, and the majority of cases occur between 10 and 20 years of age. In the adolescent, it reaches a peak incidence of approximately 11 cases per million population. Osteogenic sarcoma has a peak incidence during the time the child is most rapidly growing and is slightly more common in boys than girls with a ratio of 1.5:1.[34]

The tumor generally arises in the metaphysical region of the long bones but may occur in the diaphysis. Eighty percent of all lesions occur around the knee and shoulder, and the most common site is the distal femur.

Clinical Manifestations. Pain over the area of the tumor usually is the earliest presenting symptom of osteogenic sarcoma.[29] A swollen area or a palpable mass appears over the involved bone. Tumor impingement on muscles, nerve endings, and blood vessels leads to edema of the affected extremity, increased pain, limited function, and diminished strength. As the tumor size increases, the skin over the tumor becomes stretched and glossy with an almost translucent appearance.[13]

Diagnostic Studies. The diagnosis of osteogenic sarcoma requires a pathologic confirmation by biopsy of the lesion. The diagnostic workup involves CT scans and an MRI of the involved site and a bone scan and CT scan of the chest to rule out metastasis. Serum alkaline phosphatase may be elevated in these patients due to increased bone activity caused by the tumor.[23]

Treatment. The primary treatment is surgery and chemotherapy. The surgical approach depends on tumor size, tumor location, and age of the child. Surgery involves amputation or a limb-salvage procedure.[12] Limb-salvage procedures allow for preservation of the limb by surgically removing the tumor-involved bone and replacing it with a prosthesis. Chemotherapy is essential to prevent metastases.[25] Chemotherapy most commonly used to treat osteogenic sarcoma includes high-dose methotrexate with leucovorin rescue, doxorubicin, and cisplatin. The survival rate for children with osteogenic sarcoma is approximately 60%.[23]

Ewing's Sarcoma

Ewing's sarcoma is a tumor of the bone, with a different histologic appearance and behavior than osteosarcoma. It is a rare malignancy; however, Ewing's sarcoma accounts for 30% of bone tumors in children. Ninety percent of all patients with Ewing's sarcoma present before 30 years of age, and 70% occur before 20 years of age. The ratio of occurrence in men to women is 1.6:1.[29] Ewing's sarcoma is rare in the African-American population.

Ewing's sarcoma may affect any bone of the skeleton. The most frequent sites for the primary lesion are the femur, pelvis, tibia, humerus, ribs, vertebra, fibula, scapula, and sacrum. The tumor frequently infiltrates the soft tissues around the involved bone.[27]

Clinical Manifestations. The clinical presentation of Ewing's sarcoma is similar to the presentation of osteogenic sarcoma. Pain and a soft-tissue mass are the usual presenting symptoms. Other symptoms depend on the site of the tumor, such as neurological signs secondary to spinal cord compression or a respiratory syndrome secondary to an intrathoracic rib tumor.[29]

Diagnostic Studies. Confirmation of Ewing's sarcoma is established by surgical biopsy. The diagnostic workup is similar to osteosarcoma.

Treatment. High-dose radiation therapy is an essential treatment modality for Ewing's sarcoma. Chemotherapy, with the most common drugs being vincristine, cyclophosphamide, doxorubicin, and actinomycin D, is necessary to prevent metastases. Surgery is used if total surgical resection can be performed for a tumor that is located in an expendable bone (e.g., clavicle, scapula, rib). Prognosis for Ewing's sarcoma has greatly improved with the addition of combination chemotherapy. Long-term survival is greater than 80% for patients with nonpelvic primary tumors and no metastasis at diagnosis.[27]

Retinoblastoma

Retinoblastoma is a tumor that arises from the retina of the eye and occurs most predominantly in young children. Retinoblastoma accounts for approximately 1% to 3% of all childhood malignancies.[34] The annual incidence in the United States is estimated to be 11 per million children younger than 5 years of age. There is no difference in frequency between African-American and white children.

The tumor may be bilateral or unilateral with multiple foci. Retinoblastoma can be hereditary or nonhereditary. Bilateral disease is considered hereditary, transmitted by an autosomal dominant gene.

Clinical Manifestations. The classic signs of retinoblastoma are leukokoria, a white papillary reflex, and strabismus. Leukokoria, also called the cat's eye reflex, is described as a white light in the pupil that is noticed only with certain angles or lighting. The cat's eye reflex is caused by alignment of the tumor with the dilated pupil. As the tumor increases in size, the eye may become reddened and inflamed, and glaucoma may develop.[27]

Diagnostic Studies. The diagnostic evaluation for retinoblastoma includes a careful family history and workup for metastatic disease, including CT scans, bone marrow aspiration, bone scan, and lumbar puncture. An ophthalmologic evaluation of both eyes is essential. Because of the hereditary factor associated with this tumor, a careful family history should be obtained as well as an ophthalmic evaluation of all siblings. The classic grouping of retinoblastoma, defined by Reese and Ellsworth, is seen in Table 31-6.

Treatment. Treatment is based on extent of disease at diagnosis and the potential for preserving or recovering vision. When the disease is advanced with no hope for vision recovery, the eye is enucleated. Recent advances in treatment with the use of external beam radiation therapy have decreased the frequency of enucleation. For children with advanced disease, chemotherapy consisting of cyclophosphamide and vincristine is given systemically. Tumor extension into the CNS is treated with intrathecal chemotherapy or radiation therapy. The prognosis for children with retinoblastoma is greater than 90%. Children with metastatic disease, however, are almost always incurable.[9]

Nursing Diagnoses and Planning

Children undergoing treatment for cancer frequently are more ill from the therapy than from the cancer itself. It is essential for nurses to be familiar with common side effects of cancer therapy. General side effects of chemotherapy are listed in Table 31-2, while acute and late effects of surgery, chemotherapy, and radiation therapy are noted in Table 31-1.

The list of nursing diagnoses associated with cancer therapy is too long to list here. However, the common nursing diagnoses are listed in Table 31-7 along with appropriate nursing interventions. Other examples of nurs-

TABLE 31-6
Reese-Ellsworth Staging Classification of Retinoblastoma

Group	Description
I	Very favorable
	Solitary tumor, smaller than 4 disk diameters*, at or behind the equator
	Multiple tumors, none larger than 4 disk diameters, all at or behind the equator
II	Favorable
	Solitary tumor, 4 to 10 disk diameters in size, at or behind the equator
	Multiple tumors, 4 to 10 disk diameters in size, behind the equator
III	Doubtful
	Any lesion anterior to the equator
	Solitary tumors larger than 10 disk diameters behind the equator
IV	Unfavorable
	Multiple tumors, some larger than 10 disk diameters
	Any lesion extending anteriorly to the ora serrata
V	Very unfavorable
	Tumors involving more than half the retina
	Vitreous seeding

* 1 disk diameter = 1.5 mm.

ing diagnoses, interventions, and outcomes are demonstrated in the Nursing Care Plan and Teaching Plan in the chapter.

Nursing Implications

One of the most important roles of the pediatric oncology nurse is to teach the patient and family about the disease and its treatment. Well-informed families are better able to anticipate and manage side effects. They are prepared for the side effects in the hospital and at home.

Children and parents should have written information about specific agents so that side effects and toxic reactions may be reviewed. The treatment scheme, which plots the proposed dates for specific therapies, helps the family to plan ahead. The Nursing Care Plan works through the nursing care of a 5-year-old child with ALL and his family. Teaching related to this child is discussed later in the chapter.

Management of Side Effects

A discussion of specific side effects and interventions for nursing management of cancer therapy follow.

Nausea and Vomiting

Nausea and vomiting occur as a result of a chemotherapeutic agent's effect on particular areas of the brain or as a result of radiation's effect on the small intestine.[20] Psychogenic vomiting can occur when a child is anxious about chemotherapy, and he or she begins to vomit at the thought, sight, or smell of a drug.

Several antiemetics are used to control nausea and vomiting. To ensure constant therapeutic blood levels of an antiemetic, doses are started before nausea begins and are repeated around the clock according to specific drug instructions. Relaxation techniques, including guided imagery, are being investigated as a means of reducing the severity of treatment-related nausea and vomiting.[5]

A patient with severe nausea and vomiting is observed for signs of dehydration, including sunken eyes, decreased skin turgor, and dryness of the mouth. Fluids can be replaced intravenously if necessary, and antiemetics can be continued to decrease vomiting.

Altered Nutrition: Less Than Body Requirements

A patient's ability to maintain adequate caloric intake while receiving chemotherapy is compromised by food aversions, changes in taste acuity, emetic-inducing properties of treatments, and the psychologic and metabolic effects of the disease. Children can develop aversions to familiar and preferrred foods when receiving gastrointestinally toxic therapy.[10] The tumor itself can generate anorexia, although the mechanism responsible is not well understood. Depression also may be a factor in anorexia and weight loss.

At the time of the medical diagnosis, the child should undergo a full nutritional assessment, including weight,

TABLE 31-7
Common Nursing Diagnoses and Nursing Interventions Associated With Cancer Therapy

Nursing Diagnoses	Nursing Interventions
Health Perception and Health Management	
High risk for injury	
Bone marrow suppression	Monitor blood counts.
	Teach precautions against infection and bleeding.
Neurologic complications	Evaluate for paresthesia, peripheral neuropathies, decreased tendon reflexes, and motor weakness.
Chemotherapy extravasation	Evaluate patency of IV before chemotherapy is given.
	Administer drugs slowly, observing patency of IV during infusion.
Nutrition and Metabolism	
Problem: nausea and vomiting	Administer antiemetics before chemotherapy.
	Continue antiemetics around the clock.
	Ensure adequate hydration.
	Monitor strict intake and output.
Altered nutrition: less than body requirements.	Monitor nutritional intake.
	Provide nutritional counseling.
	Stress small, frequent high-caloric meals.
Elimination	
Constipation	Monitor bowel habits.
	Stress diet rich in bulk.
	Use stool softeners as needed.
Diarrhea	Monitor hydration status.
	Evaluate severity of diarrhea (number of stools, volume, appearance).
	Evaluate for skin breakdown of buttocks.
Cognition and Perception	
Knowledge deficit	Provide written information regarding treatment, side effects, management information, etc.
	Discuss side effects of treatment.
	Review child and parental concerns for home.
Self-Perception and Self-Concept	
Body image disturbance	Provide information on wigs, scarves, hats.
	Avoid sexism.
	Stress that hair will grow back.

(IV, intravenous.)

height, anthropometric measurements, and complete dietary history. Weight should be monitored closely during chemotherapy treatments. Oral caloric supplements can be offered if the child is unable to eat solid foods. A dietician may suggest more palatable foods and smaller, more nutritious meals. If weight loss becomes severe, nasogastric or IV feedings may be required.

Constipation

Vincristine, a widely used chemotherapeutic agent, can cause severe constipation, abdominal pain, and paralytic ileus. Enemas and suppositories are avoided in the immunocompromised patient, but children with painful fecal impactions may need them. A prophylactic regimen against constipation is recommended for patients receiving vincristine. Such a regimen may include stool softeners, a high-fiber diet, and generous fluid intake.

Diarrhea

Diarrhea can be caused by various chemotherapeutic agents, radiation therapy to the large bowel, and certain antiemetics. Monitoring of fluid intake and output for children with severe diarrhea is essential. The frequency and consistency of stools should be recorded. If dehydration occurs, IV rehydration may be necessary. The dietitian can suggest alternative foods that may be helpful. If irritation of the buttocks occurs, sitz baths may offer relief.

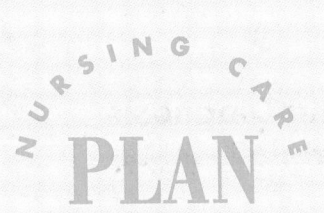

A 5-Year-Old Child Following Diagnosis of Acute Lymphocytic Leukemia

Assessment

Case Study Description

Allen Jackson, a 5-year-old African-American boy, is diagnosed with acute lymphocytic leukemia after a 2-week history of low-grade fever, weight loss, and bone pain. Bone marrow aspiration confirmed the diagnosis. The child was started on chemotherapy consisting of vincristine and prednisone. Due to the difficulty of establishing venous access, it was decided to place an implanted infusaport catheter once remission was obtained.

Assessment Data

Physical Examination:

Shoddy anterior cervical lymphadenopathy; spleen palpable 2 cm; liver 3 cm below the right costal margin. Ecchymoses on lower extremities; petechiae on upper arms.

Laboratory Findings:

White blood cell (WBC) count 2500/mm^3 with 75% blasts, 15% lymphocytes, 8% neutrophils, 2% monocytes, hemoglobin 7.9 g/dL, platelets 35,000/mm^3.

Lumbar puncture: negtive for leukemia cells.

Bone marrow aspiration: 95% blasts.

Chest radiograph: normal.

Blood chemistries: normal.

Nursing Diagnosis	Intervention	Rationale
1. Anxiety Supporting Data: • Diagnosis of cancer in a child is frightening • Immediacy of the situation may cause panic, leading to anxiety	Encourage verbalization of concerns. Recommend support groups for families.	Emotional distress is realted to the diagnosis, hospitalization, and initiation of treatment.
	Allow time for family to express feelings. Stress that it is important to talk about the situation to significant others.	Development of early coping skills adds strength to the family.
2. High risk for injury: infection Supporting Data: WBC 2500 mm^3 with neutrophil count of 8%, at extreme risk for infection.	Assess the mouth, skin, anal region, and lungs every nursing shift.	The child with a low neutrophil count has no defense against infection. Sepsis can occur quickly.
	Observe temperature every 4 hours. *Do not use a rectal thermometer.*	Do not use rectal thermometers because this can damage the rectal mucosa, resulting in an infection and abscess in the rectum.
	Report temperature higher than 38.3° C, changes in respiration (depth and rate), and changes in urine (dysuria, cloudy or foul smelling) immediately. If fever develops, obtain blood cultures, throat culture, urine culture, and chest x-ray, and begin intravenous broad-spectrum antibiotics. Administer acetaminophen for fever. Observe closely for signs of sepsis.	Any child with fever and no neutrophils should be assessed quickly, and antibiotics should be started immediately following the cultures. A child can die within 6 hours once sepsis occurs if antibiotics are not administered.

(Continued)

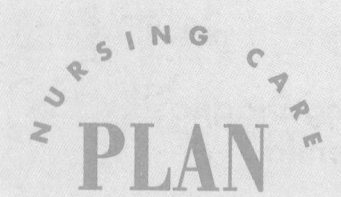

A 5-Year-Old Child Following Diagnosis of Acute Lymphocytic Leukemia (continued)

Nursing Diagnosis	Intervention	Rationale
3. High risk for injury: bleeding Supporting Data: Platelet count 35,000/mm³, ecchymoses, and petechiae on physical examination.	Use pressure on puncture sites for 5–10 minutes. Avoid intramuscular injections. Use toothettes to clean teeth and gums. Check urine, emesis, and stool for blood.	Children with platelet counts below 20,000 mm³ are most susceptible to spontaneous bleeding.
	Allow no contact sports or activity placing the child at risk for head injury when platelet count is low.	Children are at risk for an intracranial hemorrhage when head trauma occurs with a low platelet count.
	Teach parents and child the proper way to stop a nosebleed if it occurs. Place the child in an upright position and pinch just below bridge of nose for 10 minutes.	Placing the child in an upright position allows gravity to assist in stopping the nosebleed.
4. High risk for injury: kidney damage Supporting Data: Packed bone marrow with 95% leukemia cells places the child at risk for rapid breakdown of leukemia cells.	Assess for adequate hydration using 1½ times maintenance. Maintain strict I & O. Check urine for alkalinization.	Rapid destruction of leukemia cells may cause damage to the kidneys. Hydration assists in flushing the kidneys.
	Administer allopurinol on schedule. Obtain daily weights to observe for weight gain. Review electrolytes; blood, urea, and nitrogen (BUN); creatinine; and uric acid levels daily.	Allopurinol helps in breaking down uric acid, which can be increased when there is rapid breakdown of leukemia cells.
5. Ineffective individual coping Supporting Data: Five-year-old child, cognitively unable to understand the meaning of cancer.	Encourage child to play with favorite toys or games. Use a routine for the daily schedule that includes naptime, play time, and mealtimes. Try to keep the schedule similar to his home schedule. Provide stimulus at bedside: favorite toys, books, pictures, cards.	
	Tell the child what will happen before intrusive procedures take place.	The young child is afraid and not able to understand what is happening to him. Explaining what will occur before the procedure with words the child can understand gives him some control over the situation.
	Allow the child to perform procedures on dolls or stuffed animals.	Play therapy is useful in helping the child express his feelings about what is happening. It will also let staff know how the child views these intrusive procedures.

(Continued)

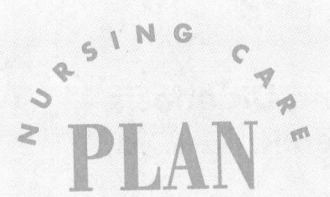

A 5-Year-Old Child Following Diagnosis of Acute Lymphocytic Leukemia (continued)

Nursing Diagnosis	*Intervention*	*Rationale*
6. Knowledge deficit regarding discharge and home management Supporting Data: Parents may be unable to care for the child at home because of fear.	Emphasize major areas of concern: fever, bleeding, change in behavior.	Parents often fear taking the child home following a diagnosis of cancer.
	Review medications to be given at home and determine whether parents understand their side effects. Written information is extremely helpful.	Reviewing the major concerns often during the hospitalization greatly reduces most fears.
	Encourage the family to allow the child to return to kindergarten as soon as the WBC count improves.	Written information can facilitate a better understanding of the major problems that can occur at home and the parents' appropriate actions.
	Assure parents that they may call when there is a concern or question. Make sure they have the appropriate phone numbers in writing.	

Evaluation

The child did well during the 4-week induction period and returned to the hospital to have an implanted catheter inserted.

7. Knowledge deficit regarding care of the implanted catheter Supporting Data: Catheter requires surgery for placement; child is at risk for infection following the procedure until the incisions heal.	Discuss placement of the central venous catheter, including the following points: • Catheter is placed during general anesthesia. • Catheter is threaded into the superior vena cava through the jugular vein. • There will be an incision under the clavicle as well as above the entry port. • The child will have a bandage on his chest to keep the incisions clean and dry. • The catheter can be used for chemotherapy, IV fluids, blood products, and blood drawing.	Implanted catheters are now used more frequently than external catheters (Broviacs) because of the decreased risk of infection and no need for home care of the catheter. The catheter enters the vein through the incision above the clavicle.
	Discuss the care of the catheter at home by emphasizing the following: • During the immediate postoperative period, the incision sites must be observed for redness or swelling. Notify the hospital immediately if this occurs. • Once the incisions have healed, there is virtually no care for the catheter at home. • The catheter is flushed once a month with heparin, usually following a chemotherapy treatment. • Thin children may bump the port, causing pain and irritation of the skin. They may wish to place a gauze pad over the port when it is not being used.	The incision site can become infected during the immediate postoperative period. Less subcutaneous tissue causes the port to protrude more profoundly, making it a target for bumps and bruises.

(Continued)

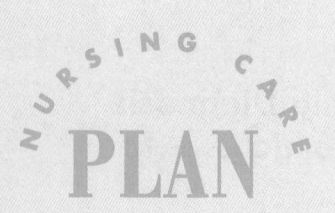

Evaluation

- Parents verbalize concerns and fears concerning diagnosis
- Parents identify ways of coping with the diagnosis.
- Parents discuss the reason the child is at risk for infection when the neutrophil count is decreased.
- Parents identify precautions necessary for the child when the platelet count is decreased.
- Child communicates at his cognitive level an understanding of the reason for treatment and hospitalization.
- Parents return and demonstrate the care required with the use of an implanted catheter.

High Risk for Injury: Infection and Bleeding

A progressive, transient decrease in the number of leukocytes and platelets in the peripheral blood often follows administration of chemotherapy. Radiation therapy to areas containing large bone marrow reserves also leads to decreased hematopoietic function.

Children with neutropenia are susceptible to infection and are encouraged to avoid large crowds of people and to maintain meticulous hygiene. Also, staff members with infections or illnesses should avoid patients with neutropenia. IV sites, skin breakdown, and oral lesions are monitored for infection, and IV tubing is changed daily. When temperature elevations occur, antipyretics are used after appropriate blood, urine, and throat cultures have been obtained. Acetaminophen is preferred over aspirin as an antipyretic because aspirin interferes with blood clotting. Often antibiotics are ordered by the physician for a child with neutropenia and fever. Taking temperatures rectally, which could lead to infection or bleeding, is avoided.

Excessive bleeding is often a problem for children with thrombocytopenia. Nosebleeds are frightening to children and their parents. If a nosebleed occurs, the child is instructed to sit upright and apply pressure below the bridge of the nose until bleeding stops for up to 10 to 15 minutes. Uncontrolled bleeding secondary to thrombocytopenia is treated by IV platelet infusion.

Anemia is a less common and less severe side effect of chemotherapy. Repeated chemotherapy courses can eventually slow red blood cell production, but their longer production cycle and life span make them less susceptible to chemotherapy-induced damage than platelets or white blood cells.

High Risk for Impaired Skin Integrity

Certain chemotherapeutic agents and radiation ther- to the mouth may cause stomatitis, an inflammation and breakdown of the buccal mucosa, gingiva, tongue, and lips. Careful observation of the oral mucosa and good oral hygiene are the keys to preventing stomatitis. Children with mucositis are instructed to clean their teeth with soft nylon toothbrushes, a toothette (styrofoam toothbrush), or gauze. Flossing is not recommended because it can contribute to gingival breakdown, and commercial mouthwash preparations are not recommended because they contain alcohol,[20] which also can cause buccal damage.

Radiation damage to salivary function may result in an increase in the viscosity of saliva and a decrease in its volume. Because saliva constitutes part of child's natural defenses against tooth decay, meticulous oral hygiene, including prophylactic fluoride treatments, is necessary.

Irritated and ulcerated tissues are highly sensitive to temperature changes and pressure. Children may have less taste acuity and more difficulty in talking, chewing, or swallowing. To ensure adequate nutrition, a bland, semisoft diet is recommended.

Numerous chemotherapeutic agents cause extravasation. Table 31-2 lists the specific drugs that cause extravasation. Children can develop extensive tissue damage from leakage of these agents into the subcutaneous tissue. Extreme caution must be taken to prevent extravasation from occurring. The site of the infusion should be observed for swelling, blood return, and pain. If any of these signs are present, the infusion should be discontinued immediately. The following guidelines should be used when an extravasation is known:

- Aspirate as much as the agent as possible through the line before discontinuing the IV. If there is an obvious bleb of extravasated drug, aspirate it with a 25-gauge needle.
- Consult the pediatric oncologist as soon as possible.
- Although its efficacy has not been proven, the site may be injected subcutaneously with Solu-Cortef 40 mg/cc. Consult a physician before administering.
- Cover the area with hydrocortisone cream and an occlusive dressing.

- Place ice on the area of infiltration and continue to use the ice pack intermittently for 20 minutes every 2 to 3 hours for 24 hours or as tolerated. For vinca alkaloid extravasation, apply heat in the same manner.

Body Image Disturbance

A bothersome adverse effect of chemotherapy for many children is loss of hair (Fig. 31-5). Children must understand that alopecia is temporary and that their hair will return when chemotherapy is completed. Younger children tend to dislike wigs because of the discomfort, so they may want to wear caps or scarves. Children in warm climates should protect their heads from sunburn by wearing hats or sunscreen. If an older child chooses to wear a wig, obtain one before the hair begins to fall out.

High Risk for Injury: Renal Complications

Certain chemotherapeutic agents can cause renal failure. The child's renal status must be evaluated before each dose of these drugs. Also, adequate hydration is essential during and after drug infusion to flush the chemicals out of the kidneys.

Hyperuricemia can occur from increased breakdown of tumor cells after chemotherapy. The kidney is unable to excrete the larger amounts of uric acid, and, if untreated, renal failure can follow. Other chemotherapeutic agents can lead to liver dysfunction; therefore, liver function tests are performed frequently in children taking these agents.

Discharge Planning

Nurses prepare the family and child for specific precautions to be taken while on treatment. This discussion is part of discharge planning. Written information rein-

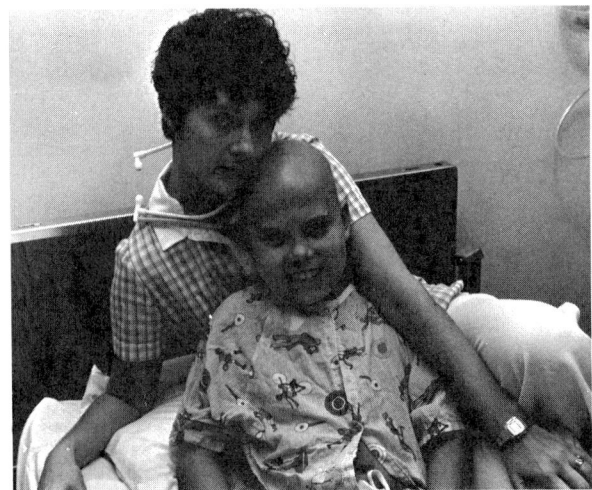

FIGURE 31-5
The staff nurse can help a child build up confidence in his or her body image by indicating that hair loss does not prevent warm interactions with people. (Courtesy of Children's Medical Center, Dayton, OH.)

forces the discharge teaching provided by the nurse and provides the family with a resource when at home. (See the Teaching Plan at the end of the chapter.) The following nursing diagnoses should be incorporated into the discharge teaching care plan.

High Risk for Injury

Infection. The family must have a basic understanding of neutropenia (less than 1000 neutrophils). Families are instructed to call the clinic or physician immediately if fever higher than 101° F and any of the following symptoms occur: cough or rapid breathing, congestion, diarrhea, stomach ache, headache, lesions or sores, earache, sore throat, or pain around the rectum. Never take rectal temperatures because rectal manipulation may lead to infection.

Bleeding. Bleeding may occur when the platelet count is low (usually below 40,000). The most common sites of bleeding are from the nose, mouth, gums, and GI tract. Dark, tarry-appearing stools are signs of upper GI tract bleeding. If a nosebleed occurs, the family should be taught to apply pressure below the bridge of the nose for 10 minutes. The family should be advised to call the hospital once the nosebleed is controlled. The child should never receive aspirin-containing products because they interfere with platelet function.

Impaired Physical Mobility

Normal activities should be encouraged when treatment permits the child to do so. Restricted activities such as going to crowded shopping centers and day care is necessary during times of severe myelosuppression (less than 500 neutrophils). Exposure to infectious diseases such as chickenpox should be discussed with the physician immediately. Children should receive varicella zoster immunoglobulin (V-ZIG) intramuscularly within 72 hours of a chickenpox exposure to prevent development of chickenpox.

Potential Problem: Reaction to Live Immunizations

No live vaccines should be administered while the child is on treatment. Diphtheria, pertussis, tetanus, and the *Haemophilus influenzae* B vaccine can be given according to the usual schedule.

Altered Nutrition: Less Than Body Requirements

Encourage high-protein, high-calorie foods. Stress the importance of small frequent meals. Eating with someone else or companionship at meals may stimulate an appetite (Fig. 31-6). Review the principles of adequate nutrition.

Self-Concept Disturbance: Role Peformance

Children should attend school. Teachers should be aware of the child's treatment and should know when to

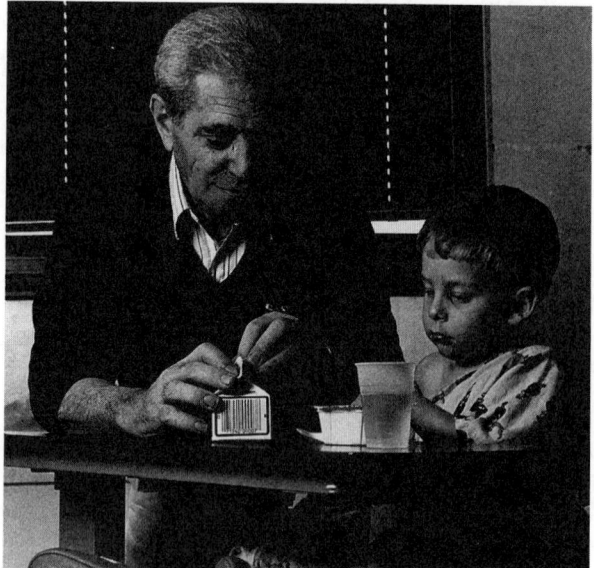

FIGURE 31-6

Decreased appetite may be a side effect of radiation or chemotherapy. Here a grandfather tries to stimulate his grandson's appetite by helping at lunchtime. (Courtesy of the Department of Medical Photography, Children's Hospital, NY.)

call. If the child has not had chickenpox, an exposure at school should be reported to the parents immediately. (See the Nursing Care Plan for more details.)

Psychosocial Support

Although survival rates for childhood cancer have dramatically improved in the past 20 years, the emotional impact from a diagnosis of childhood cancer has not. Cancer brings feelings of anxiety, fear, depression, and helplessness. The family's initial reaction includes disbelief, shock, and denial. Families may be unable to recognize the facts and accept the diagnosis. Factors affecting the family's ability to adjust vary with the nature of the disease, prognosis for the child, parental attitudes and emotional stability, adjustment of the child at diagnosis, and threats that the disease may have to the child's basic needs. How extensively cancer restricts a child's activities greatly affects the family's ability to cope.

Health care professionals must intervene early to help families cope. Supporting families through crisis periods can be the most difficult, and the most gratifying, role for a pediatric oncology nurse. Support groups designed for parents and children can provide the family with opportunities to talk about their fears and concerns with others in the same situation. Most cancer centers have organized support groups that meet routinely in the clinic or hospital setting. National organizations such as the Candlelighter's Foundation, which was founded for parents with children who have cancer, provide support through literature and group meetings.

Compassionate Friends support groups, organized for parents who have lost a child are in most states. Nurses knowledgeable regarding available professional support groups can be important advocates to the parents and child.

Impact of Cancer on the Family

Cancer affects the whole family. Family stability plays a major role in a child's acceptance and adjustment to the diagnosis of cancer. Factors affecting the parents' ability to adjust vary according to the nature of the disease, prognosis of the child, parental attitudes and emotional balance, adjustment of the child at the time of diagnosis, and threats the disease may have to the child's basic needs.

The degree to which cancer restricts a child's activities greatly affects the parents' ability to cope. Constructive exploration of feelings and fears is essential to allow for each family member to gain strength and begin to examine positive coping mechanisms. With identification of these coping skills, the family usually is able to accept the diagnosis of cancer and begin to develop ways in which to build on their previous lifestyle. Specific developmental tasks essential for families with a child who has cancer are found in Table 31-8.

TABLE 31-8
Nursing Intervention: Anticipatory Guidance to Help Families Meet Developmental Tasks When Children Have Cancer

Nursing Diagnoses	Nursing Interventions
Cognition and Perception	
Knowledge Deficit	Provide education at the parent's level regarding child's diagnosis, prognosis, treatment plan, long-term goals, alterations in lifestyle.
	Review these concepts frequently to provide parents with a knowledge base from which to cope and alter their lifestyle.
Role and Relationships	
Altered Family Processes	Assist in providing options to alter areas in which the family can no longer function because of the disease (i.e., mother can no longer work—seek help with the budget; babysitter needed—help explore options in the community).
	Identify strengths in the parents that can be used to support the entire family system.
	Reassure parents that they have needs also and must take time to meet those needs.
	Stress importance of parents' continued involvement with others. Emphasize importance of parents sharing with each other and continuing their relationships as husband and wife.
	Ensure that siblings remain active in family communications.
Coping and Stress Tolerance	
Ineffective Family Coping: Compromised	Ensure maintenance of intact family system by exploring strengths and identifying weaknesses in family (i.e., transportation, work).
	Stress importance of continued interaction with family members, especially siblings.

Communication between the parents and the child's siblings provides understanding that is essential to the child. Siblings often think they have caused the child to become ill. The sibling may fear acquiring the disease but may be unable to express this concern. Parents must be encouraged to continue their previous relationship with the other children in the family. The sibling must not feel neglected but must continually feel like a part of the family.

Impact of Cancer on the Child

Developmental levels must be taken into account when considering the impact of cancer on the patient. For instance, an infant does not have an understanding of illness, its seriousness, or its consequences. However, cancer occurring in the first year of life may alter the development of self-awareness. Normal development toward an independent person separate from the mother is disrupted. Realization of the infant's lack of perception of cancer can facilitate normal growth and development. Emphasis on meeting the child's basic needs of warmth, touch, food, and shelter will maximize the infant's ability to adjust to cancer and its treatment.

In early childhood, cancer jeopardizes the ability to become autonomous. The fear caused by procedures and treatment for cancer leads to regression. These fears are exaggerated because the toddler has no mechanism for perceiving what it means to have cancer. Support systems and the security of loved ones assist in providing emotional support to the toddler. Although toddlers are too young to understand, they can be supported through consistent behavior from others.

The school-age child is threatened by anything that may alter body image. Children aged 6 to 9 years have real fears regarding their body being mutilated. Procedures such as injections, bone marrow aspirations, and lumbar punctures may be overwhelming for these children, and they may respond by acting out. The diagnosis of cancer interferes with normal peer relationships. When hospitalized, the child is separated from friends and classmates. Alterations in appearance caused by cancer or its treatment may cause the child to withdraw and become depressed. Explanations, information, and trust in those providing care will facilitate adjustment to the changes brought on by cancer. Many children this age find it easier to express feelings through drawings, stories, or other forms of play. Allowing the child to express fears provides a therapeutic way to facilitate coping methods in the child.

The preadolescent and adolescent are able to understand their diagnosis, treatment, and prognosis. Cancer is frightening; it brings with it a realization that the adolescent's lifestyle will be altered and the future threatened. The diagnosis of cancer immediately alters goals, plans, and dreams. Autonomy, a goal that adolescents strive for as they think about the future, is challenged and altered with the onset of cancer. The adolescent may become dependent on significant others for assistance in meeting even basic needs. This dependence frequently creates strife and loss of pride. As treatment causes alterations in body image, the adolescent must struggle with accepting those changes.[11] Nurses must be sensitive to these changes and explore feelings of self-worth with the adolescent. Emphasis must be placed on the positive attributes of the individual. These children must accept alterations in lifestyle, while reorganizing their lives to continue to obtain previously identified goals.

Crises Points in Cancer

There are several crises points in the development and management of childhood cancer. They are diagnosis, treatment, discontinuation of therapy, relapse, and end-stage disease. The nurse assists families to develop coping skills for each of these phases of childhood cancer. The accompanying Teaching Plan gives information pertaining to defining the disease and treatment and discharge planning.

Medical Diagnosis. The diagnosis of cancer causes turmoil for all family members. Parents often react with disbelief, anger, guilt, and grief. Their previous methods of coping will affect their initial reactions. The crisis of the diagnostic period is further intensified by the treatment regimen and the necessity for immediate treatment.

Treatment. Families vary in resilience and ability to adapt to treatment. The initiation of treatment forces the family to think about the reality of the diagnosis. Cost of care becomes a major stress factor and must be addressed early by pursuing all available programs that may provide support for the family. There is a tendency to overprotect and isolate the child to prevent infection and bleeding. Parents need constant guidance and support to allow the child to grow, develop, and meet normal maturational needs.

Discontinuation of Therapy. The family eventually learns to adjust to changes the cancer diagnosis has placed on them. The family has experienced shock, emotional trauma, fear, and uncertainty, but treatment has become a way of life. Discontinuation of therapy initiates new fears because now the security of treatment is gone. Many parents fear discontinuing treatment more than initiating it. Preparation for cessation of therapy should begin 2 to 3 months before therapy is actually stopped. This allows time for the family members to express concerns and fears. This adaptation process prevents the family from living in constant fear of disease recurrence.

Relapse. Relapse is a word feared above all others; it causes a feeling of hopelessness. It is essential for the nurse to be honest about the situation. The child and family must reestablish a sense of control and adjust to a new set of circumstances. Parents must be assured they have done nothing to cause the disease to return. Not all children who relapse will die; many will obtain remission and have no further evidence of disease.

End-Stage Disease. At the time of diagnosis, families are confronted with the possibility of death. The return of the child's disease brings with it the reality of the diagnosis and prognosis. Although families have faced numerous crises, none is so difficult as the child's terminal illness and the family's anticipated loss. The crisis of end-

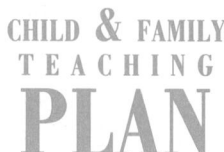

CHILD & FAMILY
T E A C H I N G
PLAN

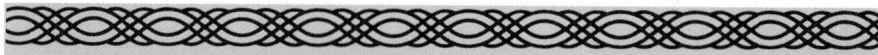

Initial Care and Discharge Planning for a 5-Year-Old Child With Acute Lymphocytic Leukemia

Assessment

Allen Jackson, the 5-year-old African-American boy diagnosed with acute lymphocytic leukemia (ALL), is presently receiving induction chemotherapy at the medical center 120 miles away from home. His mother is 23 years old, unmarried, and lives with the grandmother who assumes much of the care of the child during the day. The mother also has a 7-year-old daughter living with them. Mother works at a fast food restaurant parttime.

Mother and grandmother are staying with the child while hospitalized. The daughter is staying at home with an aunt. Mother looks to grandmother for decision-making. Grandmother wants daughter to be involved, yet feels she is too young.

Child and Family Objectives	*Specific Content*	*Teaching Strategies*
1. Describe a basic overview of leukemia and Allen's treatment plan.	1. Definition: Acute lymphocytic leukemia—replacement of bone marrow with leukemia cells inhibiting the production of normal cells that carry oxygen to the cells, stop bleeding (platelets), and fight infection (white blood cells). Signs and symptoms: Anemia-causing pallor, fatigue, decreased activity, and anorexia. Thrombocytopenia may cause petechiae, ecchymosis, epistaxis, and gingival bleeding Neutropenia may result in fever. Use the child's own data in presenting the disease process to the parent. Plan of treatment overview (protocol): • Induction, • Consolidation, • Central nervous system (CNS) prophylaxis, • Maintenance	1. Use discussion. Supply handouts on drugs and protocol plan. Distribute written information on ALL. Assess readability level of handouts for Allen's mother and grandmother.
2. Verbalize the reasons for Allen's receiving chemotherapy.	2. Review the process in which leukemia cells invade and replace the bone marrow. Define the need to destroy these cells to enable the bone marrow to begin producing normal cells again. This phase of therapy is called induction, meaning to "induce" remission, which is the absence of leukemia on the physical examination, clinical parameters	2. Begin discussion. Give handouts on drugs. Use the protocol sheet as a road map. Use a calendar with the family to indicate each time chemotherapy or examinations are needed.

(Continued)

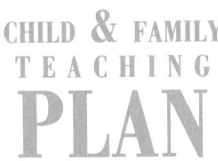

CHILD & FAMILY TEACHING PLAN

Initial Care and Discharge Planning for a 5-Year-Old Child With Acute Lymphocytic Leukemia (continued)

Child and Family Objectives	Specific Content	Teaching Strategies
	(bone marrow, lumbar puncture, laboratory blood counts), and performance (physical state of wellness). Discuss the side effects of chemotherapy.	
3. Communicate an understanding of bone marrow and spinal tap (lumbar puncture.)	3. Bone marrow transplant allows higher doses of radiation and chemotherapy to be used. Also, it may help kill remaining leukemic cells. Outline steps of procedures.	3. Introduce the subject using dolls. Invite Allen to play with the dolls. Let Allen demonstrate his perception of the procedure.
4. Identify the importance of proper nutrition during chemotherapy.	4. Chemotherapy is often better tolerated with children in good nutritional status. Explain benefits of various diet modifications related to side effects of chemotherapy. Examples: Prednisone—increased appetite, water retention, Cushingoid effect. Vincristine—constipation.	4. Discuss the importance of good nutrition for growth and development. Distribute an introductory packet: "Feeding the Sick Child," "Basic Four Food Groups." Distribute materials on "No Added Salt Diet" and "High Fiber Diet." Consult with a dietitian for appropriate materials for the family.
5. Verbalize understanding of need for continued monitoring of dietary habits and weight and height changes.	5. Dicuss present eating habits as well as recent weight and height changes.	5. Use a one-to-one discussion with Allen and family. Complete history forms, food array, and typical daily intake with dietary consultant. Chart weight and height on growth chart for future reference
6. Discuss changes Allen may undergo as a result of the disease and treatment.	6. Review Allen's, mother's, and grandmother's concerns.	6. Provide psychological support as indicated. Use leukemia coloring book from National Cancer Institute: "What Happened to Me." Refer Allen to child life worker and psychologist when needed and stress participation in groups at hospital.
7. Discuss the impact of Allen's diagnosis and treatment on 7-year-old sister.	7. Discuss stresses the diagnosis has made on the family. Encourage sibling vists to the hospital. Discuss sibling's feelings of abandonment.	7. Encourage mother and grandmother to bring sibling to the hospital. Provide ongoing psychological support as needed. Refer to other members of the mental health team as needed.
8. Identify areas of concern for discharge.	8. Review the functions of blood cells and signs and symptoms that may	8. Provide handout on functions of cells and normal counts. Provide

(Continued)

CHILD & FAMILY
T E A C H I N G
PLAN

Initial Care and Discharge Planning for a 5-Year-Old Child With Acute Lymphocytic Leukemia (continued)

Child and Family Objectives	*Specific Content*	*Teaching Strategies*
	occur at home if the counts are low. Discuss the most recent blood counts, using them as examples to explain the symptoms. Examples: • If low WBC count, look for fever (neutrophils ≤1000). If oral temperature is greater than 101°F. Call the hospital immediately. • If low WBC counts, Allen should not attend kindergarten or go anywhere there are crowds, like malls. The child should stay home until counts recover. • If low platelet counts, take precautions against falling, running into objects, bicycling, or playing rough games.	handout on "How to Take a Temperature" with a demonstration and a return demonstration by the mother. Discuss concerns.
	• If Allen develops a bloody nose or gums, call the hospital. Teach the parent how to stop a nosebleed: • Sit the child upright and pinch the nose below the bridge tightly for 10 minutes. Do not lay the child down. • If hemoglobin is low, Allen will be more tired than usual, not as energetic, appetite will be poor. Counts will be monitored and a transfusion of red cells will be given as needed.	Ask mother to demonstrate how to stop a nosebleed.
9. List precautions to take at home.	9. Never give aspirin. Never receive live immunizations while on therapy. If exposed to chickenpox, call hospital immediately.	9. Use discussion. Give handouts listing this information. Ask mother to describe these precautions.
10. Identify medications needed at home.	10. Medications taken at home include • Prednisone • Allopurinol • Tylenol, if needed Times and methods for giving each are discussed and reviewed. Methods for giving medications may include ice cream or syrup. Mother is able to state the importance of taking each	10. Provide a written schedule for each medication that includes a sample of each drug taped to the card. Prescriptions and refills are noted when given to Mother.

(Continued)

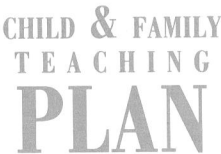

**Initial Care and Discharge Planning
for a 5-Year-Old Child With Acute
Lymphocytic Leukemia** (continued)

Child and Family Objectives	*Specific Content*	*Teaching Strategies*
	medication and states the effect of missing a dosage.	
	Financial resources for medications are discussed and assistance obtained as needed.	
Evaluation	• Family defines leukemia, method for treatment, and prognosis.	

• Family defines leukemia, method for treatment, and prognosis.
• Family states the process by which chemotherapy is able to induce remission.
• Child participates in play therapy sessions that explain bone marrow transplantation and spinal tap.
• Child and family identify foods necessary for a well-balanced diet.
• Child and family state which type of dietary modifications are necessary with the associated side effects of the drugs.
• Family uses the appropriate resources in the community and the hospital for financial assistance.
• Child and family discuss feelings regarding the changes in activity social life, body image, and pain.
• Family identifies major areas of concern for discharge.
• Family identifies medicines and medication regimen.

stage disease may last from weeks to months. The state of questioning what each day will bring creates added stress. Family involvement in the child's care is essential during this period. Involvement allows for acceptance of the impending death and gives the family a sense of being needed and making a difference. To provide appropriate support, nurses must be aware of the family's spiritual needs and attitudes toward death. Resources to facilitate families' wishes must be pursued. Where will the child die? In the hospital or at home? This question must be addressed early to allow time for plans to be established.

Families who are given permission to openly discuss their concerns and fears are better able to cope with the final days than families who do not express their concerns. Chapter 32, The Child Who Is Dying, discusses in detail specific interventions essential for the terminally ill child.

The Child's Return to School

The child should return to as normal an environment as possible following diagnosis. Because school is a major aspect of a child's life, it should remain so following a diagnosis of cancer. However, the child, family, and classroom must be prepared for the child's return to school. Teachers must be educated regarding the child's illness and treatment. The teacher's concerns must be addressed, and specific situations must be discussed. For example, teachers must be aware that children on che-

motherapy are more susceptible to infection and that parents should be notified immediately when the child does not feel well. Prepared school personnel will not fear the child's presence in the classroom but will provide an environment essential for the child's continued growth and development.

Late Effects of Cancer Therapy

By the year 2000, one in 1000 young adults will have survived childhood cancer.[17] However, cancer therapy often results in long-term complications referred to as late effects. Physical changes may be obvious, such as surgical amputation, scoliosis secondary to spinal radiation, or lack of breast development secondary to either pelvic or cranial irradiation.[1,19,26] Other physical effects may be more subtle, such as sterility secondary to radiation, surgery, or chemotherapy; impaired intellectual function caused by cranial irradiation; or mutagenesis secondary to chemotherapy.[21,26]

Children who are cured of cancer may be left with fears of disease recurrence or a second malignancy, questions about sexuality and marriage, tetratogenic effects, fears about living with disfigurement, and uncertainties regarding their future education, vocations, and ability to obtain insurance.[14,17,28] A cure should therefore extend to consider the patient's mental, emotional, and spiritual

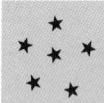

Ideas for Nursing Research

The future holds great possibilities for nursing research in the nursing care of children with cancer. Nurses are responsible for the care of children during all stages of the illness, from diagnosis to cure. Innovative approaches to nursing care are essential to assist in the pursuit of increased survival rates. The following areas need to be explored:

- Control of side effects of treatment, especially behavioral interventions to decrease nausea and vomiting.
- Pain management (pharmacologic and non-pharmacologic methods).
- Evaluation of late effects of cancer therapy (through late-effects nursing clinics)
- Development of screening tools for children at risk for late effects of cancer therapy.
- Assessment of growth and development during treatment.
- Evaluation of effective school reentry programs.
- Evaluation of the effects of a child with cancer on siblings.
- Long-term follow-up of the impact cancer has on the child's self-competence.

well-being. The quality of life for a child with cancer is no longer measured only by how well the disease is eradicated. It must also be measured by how the cancer and its treatment affect future development.[28]

Summary

Many malignancies of childhood once considered fatal are now curable. Much of the success of pediatric oncology can be attributed to an interdisciplinary and collaborative approach.

Little is known about the causes of childhood cancer; there are a variety of etiological factors. Although childhood cancer is considered rare, it remains the leading cause of death by disease in children.

Treatment includes surgery, radiation therapy, chemotherapy, or bone marrow transplantation. Treatment may continue for months or years. The child may go through several remissions or reach a cure.

Specific childhood cancers include leukemia, Hodgkin's disease, NHL, CNS tumors, neuroblastoma, Wilms' tumor, rhabdomyosarcoma, osteogenic sarcoma, Ewing's sarcoma, and retinoblastoma.

Cancer affects the whole family. Communication must be kept open with and between the patient, parents, and siblings. Developmental levels must be taken into account when considering the impact of cancer on the patient and siblings.

The nurse is the primary resource and contact for each family. The nurse remains the team leader from initial diagnosis through treatment, remission, and cure or

death. Much of his or her involvement centers around educating and preparing the family for the concerns related to the disease, treatment, and prognosis. Research improves care provided to each child and family. The future holds great possibilities for nursing research in the field of pediatric oncology.

References

1. Byrd, R. (1985). Late effects of treatment of cancer in children. *Pediatric Clinics of North America, 32*(3), 835–848.
2. Cancer Facts and Figures (1990). New York: American Cancer Society.
3. Castoria, H. A. (1986). Childhood leukemias. In M. J. Hockenberry & D. K. Coody (Eds.), *Pediatric oncology and hematology: Perspectives on care* (pp. 14–42). St. Louis: CV Mosby.
4. Coody, D., & van Eys, J. (1986). Central nervous system tumors. In M. J. Hockenberry & D. K. Coody (Eds.), *Pediatric oncology and hematology: Perspectives on care* (pp. 123–141). St. Louis: CV Mosby.
5. Cotanch, P., Hockenberry, M., & Herman, S. (1985). Self-hypnosis as anti-emetic therapy in children receiving chemotherapy. *Oncology Nursing Forum, 12*(4), 41–46.
6. Diamond, C. A., & Matthay, K. K. (1988). Childhood acute lymphoblastic leukemia. *Pediatric Annals, 17*, 156–170.
7. Fernbach, D. J., & Vietti, T. J. (1991). *Clinical Pediatric Oncology.* St. Louis: CV Mosby.
8. Gootenberg, J. E., & Pizzo, P. A. (1991). Optimal management of acute toxicities of therapy. *Pediatric Clinics of North America, 38*, 269.
9. Green, D. M. (1985). Retinoblastoma. In D. M. Green, *Diagnosis and management of malignant solid tumors in infants and children* (pp. 90–128). Boston: Martinus Nijhoff.
10. Hilton, A. (1987). Approaches for feeding the young child with anorexia. *Journal of Pediatric Nursing, 2*, 45–54.
11. Hinds, P. S., Martin, J., & Vogel, R. I. (1987). Nursing strategies to influence adolescent hopefulness during oncologic illness. *Journal of the Association of Pediatric Oncology Nurses, 4*, 14–22.
12. Hockenberry, M. J., & Lane, B. (1988). Limb salvage procedures in children with osteosarcoma. *Cancer Nursing, 11*(1), 2–8.
13. Katznelson, A., & Nerubay, J. (1982). The clinical picture of osteosarcoma. In A. Katznelson & J. Nerubay (Eds.), *Osteosarcoma, new trends in diagnosis and treatment* (pp. 15–22). New York: Alan R. Liss.
14. Koocher G., & O'Mally, J. (1981). *The Damocles syndrome: Psychological consequences of surviving childhood cancer.* New York: McGraw-Hill.
15. Kurtzberg, J., & Graham, M. L. (1991). Non-Hodgkin's lymphoma. *Pediatric Clinics of North America, 38*, 443.
16. Lenarsky, C. (1983). Etiology of childhood malignancy. In P. Lanzkowsky (Ed.), *Pediatric oncology* (pp. 1–12). New York: McGraw-Hill.
17. Meadows, A. T., Krejmas, N. L., & Belasco, J. B. (1980). The medical cost of cure: Sequelae in survivors of childhood cancer. In J. van Eys & M. P. Sullivan (Eds.), *Status of the curability of childhood cancer* (pp. 263–276). New York: Raven Press.
18. Meeske, K., & Ruccione, K. S. (1987). Cancer chemotherapy in children: Nursing issues and approaches. *Seminars in Oncology Nursing, 3*, 118.
19. Moore, J., Glasser, M. E., & Ablin, A. R. (1988). The late psychosocial consequences of childhood cancer. *Journal of Pediatric Nursing, 3*, 150–164.
20. Noyes, N. (1986). Chemotherapy. In M. J. Hockenberry & D. K. Coody (Eds.), *Pediatric oncology and hematology: Perspectives on care* (pp. 309–337). St. Louis: C.V. Mosby.
21. Peckham, V. C., Meadows, A. T., Bartel, N., & Marrero, O. (1988).

Educational late effects in long-term survivors of childhood acute lympocytic leukemia. *Pediatrics, 81,* 127–133.

22. Pizzo, P. A., & Poplack, D. G. (Eds.). (1989). Principles and practice of pediatric oncology. Philadelphia: JB Lippincott.

23. Pratt, C. B. (1984). Osteosarcoma. In V. C. Kelley (Ed.), *Practice of pediatrics* (vol. V, ch. 80 pp. 1–9). Philadelphia: Harper and Row.

24. Pullen, D. J. (1983). Pediatric Oncology Group classification protocol for ALL. In S. B. Murphy & J. R. Gilbert (Eds.), *Leukemia research advances in cell biology and treatment* (pp. 221–239). New York: Elsevier Science.

25. Rosen, G., & Nirenberg, A. (1984). Chemotherapy for primary osteogenic sarcoma: Ten year evolution and current status of preoperative chemotherapy. In S. E. Salmon & S. E. Jones (Eds.), *Adjuvant therapy of cancer IV* (pp. 593–600). New York: Grune & Stratton.

26. Ruccione, K. & Fergusson, J. (1984). Late effects of childhood cancer and its treatment. *Oncology Nursing Forum, 11*(4), 55–64.

27. Schweisguth, O. (1982). *Solid tumors in children.* New York: John Wiley and Sons.

28. Shanfield, S. B. (1980). On surviving cancer: Psychological considerations. *Comprehensive Psychiatry, 21*(2), 128–134.

29. Stanfill, P., & Pratt, C. (1986). Bone tumors. In M. J. Hockenberry & D. K. Coody (Eds.), *Pediatric oncology and hematology: Perspectives on care* (pp. 104–122). St. Louis: CV Mosby.

30. Steinherz, P. B. (1987). Acute lymphoblastic leukemia of childhood. *Hematology/Oncology Clinics of North America, 4,* 549–560.

31. Sullivan, M. P. (1987). Hodgkin's disease in children. *Hematology/Oncology Clinics of North America, 4,* 603–620.

32. Sullivan, M. P., Fuller, L. M., & Butler J. J. (1984). Hodgkin's disease. In W. W. Sutow, D. J. Fernback, & T. J. Vietti. (Eds.), *Clinical pediatric oncology* (pp. 416–451). St. Louis: CV Mosby.

33. Sutow, W. W. (1981). Childhood rhabdomysarcoma. In W. W. Sutow (Ed.), *Malignant solid tumors in children: A review* (pp. 129–147). New York: Raven Press.

34. Sutow, W. W., Fernbach, D. J., & Vietti, T. J. (1984). *Clinical pediatric oncology* (3rd ed.). St. Louis: CV Mosby.

35. van Eys, J. (1984). Malignant tumors of the central nervous system. In W. W. Sutow, D. J. Fernbach, & T. J. Vietti (Eds.), *Clinical pediatric oncology* (pp. 142–151). St. Louis: CV Mosby.

36. van Eys, J. & Sullivan, M. P. (1980). *Status of the curability of childhood cancers.* New York: Raven Press.

37. Vogel, R., & Pratt, C. (1986). Rhabdomyosarcoma. In M. J. Hockenberry & D. K. Coody (Eds.). *Pediatric oncology and hematology: Perspectives on care* (pp. 142–151). St. Louis: CV Mosby.

38. Voute, P. A. (1984). Neuroblastoma. In W. W. Sutow, D. J. Fernbach & T. J. Vietti (Eds.), *Clinical pediatric oncology* (pp. 559–587). St. Louis: CV Mosby.

39. Young, J. L. Jr., Ries, L. G., Silverberg, et al. (1986). Cancer incidence, survival, and mortality for children younger than age 15 years. *Cancer, 58,* 598–602.

The Child Who Is Dying

BEHAVIORAL OBJECTIVES

Discuss the impact of childhood mortality rates on parental expectations for their children.

Apply growth and development theory to both the content and process of discussing death with children.

Discuss the concept of death for the dying child and the surviving siblings according to developmental stages.

Apply growth and development theories to nursing interventions with children facing death and with their families.

Differentiate the impact of expected and unexpected death on the child, parents, and nurse.

Relate all phases of treatment, from diagnosis to death, to the emotional responses of the child and family.

Identify nursing interventions for each phase of grieving.

Contemporary American society has been accused of being a "death-denying" culture. Not only does the general public try to avoid the subject of death, but the pioneering research of Glaser and Strauss[8] revealed that hospital professionals also have a great deal of difficulty working with a dying patient. The professional's attitudes toward the dying patient were explored further by Kübler-Ross[14] in her work with the dying. In Kübler-Ross' early work, she found that the health professionals went so far as to deny that there were any dying patients in the hospital. When a dying patient initiated conversation on the subject of his or her own death, the health professional responded with platitudes and quickly left the room. These early studies identifying the attitudes toward the patient and the needs of dying patients have helped bring the subject into the health care professional's conscious awareness.

The role of the physician has long been to diagnose and treat the patient's disease or injury with the intention of cure. Similarly, nursing has traditionally been charged with the role of physically caring for the patient with an emphasis on promotion or restoration of health. Death was to be conquered, and when it was not, the physician and nurse typically felt a degree of *failure*. Fortunately, today's health care professionals are realistically examining their attitudes, beliefs, and roles in working with the inevitability of death.

TABLE 32-1
Major Causes and Frequency of Death in Children

Cause of Death	Younger Than 1 Year	Age 1–4	Age 5–9	Age 10–14	Age 15–19	Total
Accidents	890	2856	1995	2257	8202	16,200
Neoplasms	114	543	607	576	860	2700
Cardiovascular diseases	1085	363	178	248	544	2418
Congenital anomalies	8561	840	272	197	231	10,101
Conditions originating in prenatal period	19,068	139	9	4	5	19,225
Meningitis	257	159	21	20	13	470
Total from all causes	40,030	7339	4168	4765	15,068	71,370

Source: United States Department of Health and Human Services, National Center for Health Statistics. (1988). *Vital statistics of the United States.* Vol. II, Part B.

Professional nurses accept the challenge of caring for the dying child and the child's family. Nurses have often said that "the patient is the family." If nurses are to pay more than lip service to "family-centered care," the needs of the parents and the siblings must be addressed. Family-centered care is especially important in pediatric nursing because of the immaturity of the ill child. The child is particularly vulnerable and the family is his or her source of primary support.[49] Nursing care for the child is not limited to physical needs, but should include the psychosocial and spiritual needs of the child as well as those of the family and friends.

Few will argue that there is no more difficult death to face than that of a child. Although all deaths involve the pain of loss, a child's death takes on additional meanings. Adults are said to have "lived a long life" and to have accomplished much in their lives. The child's death is viewed as premature and tragic with a sense of a lack of fulfillment. Hopes, aspirations, and dreams for the child's future go unrealized. There appears to be no purpose, no sense of justice, and a disruption of the expected life span.

The purpose of this chapter is to identify the theoretical and experiential issues of childhood death, with the intention of providing nursing guidelines for helping the child and family cope with the crisis. There are no absolutes or definitives for how the nurse must care for these families. Individual circumstances will require nurses to use their clinical judgment. When available, research findings and extensive clinical experiences will form the scientific basis for nursing interventions. For optimal nursing care, there must be a humanistic involvement between the nurse and the family. Nurses would do well to remember the anonymous French folk saying, "To cure sometimes, to relieve often, to comfort always."

This chapter focuses on the psychosocial and spiritual needs of the child and family facing death. While some needs may be unique to a specific diagnostic disorder, the focus is the general theory of death and dying. Specific differences between an acute or sudden, unexpected death and an expected death from a chronic, long-term illness are discussed.

Incidence of Childhood Mortality

While accidents are the leading cause of death in children in the United States, cancer is the leading cause of death from *disease.* Table 32-1 identifies the major causes of death in children younger than 19 years of age. The National Center for Health Statistics records accident mortality rates. These statistics reveal that accidents account for approximately 30% of all deaths between 1 and 19 years of age.[32] Table 32-2 compares the major causes of accidental deaths in children younger than 19 years of age.

Even with modern medical technology and treatment modalities, approximately 71,000 children die in the United States every year. Every nurse who works with children will eventually encounter parents facing the potential or actual loss of their child. What does this mean for today's American family? Is the meaning different today than in the beginning of the 20th century? Are there differences within the American culture and worldwide?

By 1900, the death rate for all ages was 17.2 per 1000 population. The infant (birth to 1 year) mortality rate was much higher at 162.4 per 1000 population.[39] In 1900, due to a high maternal mortality rate, a man could expect to have two wives during his lifetime and father at least six children, with slightly more than half of the children sur-

TABLE 32-2
Major Causes and Frequencies of Accidental Deaths

Cause of Death	Younger Than 5 Years	Age 5–9	Age 10–14	Age 15–19
Motor vehicle accident	1195	1063	1256	6282
Other accidents	2551	932	1001	1920
Homicide	548	167	250	1602
Suicide	0	3	275	1849
Total	4294	2165	2782	11,653

Source: United States Department of Health and Human Services, National Center for Health Statistics. (1988). *Vital statistics of the United States.* Vol. II, Part B.

viving into adulthood.[3] Frequent causes of death during this time were pneumonia, influenza, diarrhea, and scarlet fever. The direct impact was that the experience of a child's death was relatively common to families. Improved sanitation, public health measures, and advances in medicine, such as antibiotics and immunizations, have brought many lethal conditions under control. The present infant mortality rate is 10.6 per 1000 live births with neonatal (the first 28 days of life) accounting for 7.0 deaths per 1000.[32] With a lowered childhood mortality rate, it is now uncommon for a family to experience a child's death.

As the mortality rate fell, the value of individual children has increased. With time, families have changed from expecting at least one child to die to expecting children to outlive their parents. Parents have no reason to guard their emotions at the birth of a child; therefore, they make a greater emotional investment sooner in the life of the child. The death of a child is one of the most tragic events for the parents because today the bond between children and their parents is primarily emotional. This is very different from the turn of the century when children represented financial and occupational resources for the family. In Third World countries, children still represent a significant source of labor with financial implications. This is not to imply that children are not loved in other cultures, but that they are valued for additional and different role expectations.

Meaning of Dying and Death

To the Dying Child

What does it mean to a child to be dying?

Developmental Considerations

Although each child exhibits a unique approach to dying, children's concepts of death appear to evolve developmentally.[11,21,37,50] Without the use of language, it is impossible to assess the meaning of death to an infant. A very young child does not have a sense of permanence toward death but sees it as reversible and associates it with separation and immobility. This egocentric view of death correlates with Piaget's sensorimotor and early preoperational stages of cognitive development.[43] During the early school years, children begin to understand the finality of death, but the cause of death often is viewed as punishment for wrongdoing. The concrete operational child learns through direct concrete exposure to situations. They have a heightened fear of the unknown, so they respond well to concrete explanations of their disease, treatments, drugs, and procedures. This stage corresponds to Erikson's stage of industry, in which the child seeks to attain a sense of control and understanding with the environment. When confronting death, the school-age child asks many questions regarding what happens to the body, the funeral and burial, and thereafter. Sensitive, honest communication is essential from the nurse and the parents. A study done in Hungary in 1948[31] found that children personified death as a bogeyman or an angel. Later work in the United States has not corroborated the

notion of personification.[12] This difference may be due to cultural variations[7] or to the influx of information through the media and television.

Around the age of 10, children approach a more adultlike concept of death that roughly approximates Piaget's stage of formal operations.[43] The ability for abstract thought is fundamental for understanding death in all its reality. While death is viewed as inevitable, the preadolescent and adolescent still have difficulty accepting the fact that death can happen to them or to those they love. Death interferes with their hopes, dreams, and aspirations. The existential understanding that they are alone in their encounter with death may be overwhelming. Their sense of independence and role identity is severely threatened. An awareness of the major concerns and fears regarding death at different ages can alert the nurse to appropriate interventions for relief or reduction of distress.[51] Table 32-3 presents a summary of concepts toward dying and death throughout childhood and suggests areas for nursing interventions.

Awareness of Dying and Death

Traditionally the initial approach of parents and health professionals was to try to protect the child from knowing the diagnosis of a fatal prognosis. Children were told a plausible story to explain the treatments without verbalizing the seriousness of the illness. Children were not told the truth because it was believed that they lacked the necessary cognitive abilities and defense mechanisms to cope with the truth. This belief was challenged by Waechter in 1971.[44] She found evidence that even very young children sense or learn from other sources the serious nature of their illness. "To tell or not to tell" became a major dilemma. Many people felt that by trying to hide the truth and lying to children, parents and health professionals eroded their credibility and created a situation in which the child had no one to trust or turn to. Another significant finding of the Waechter study was that children who had the opportunity to discuss the illness, treatment, and prognosis appeared less anxious. The decision not to tell may be easier at first but with time it places additional strain on the well siblings, the parents, health professionals, and virtually anyone coming in contact with the child. Waechter's research findings have been supported by numerous subsequent studies.[19,36,40]

In an exploratory study of the awareness and communication in terminally ill children, Bluebond-Langner[1] found that children acquire information about their disease in five stages (Fig. 32-1). In stage 1, children learn that this illness is serious and unlike any other previous illness. Stage 2 is characterized by the children learning the names and side effects of the medications they are taking. Although in stage 3 they understand the procedures used to administer the medications and special treatments required as a result of the side effects of the medications, it is not until the next stage that they understand the larger perspective of the disease process. By stage 4, they see the disease as a series of relapses and remissions; they see that they can get sick over and over again. It is not until stage 5 that they learn that the series of remissions and relapses ends in death. Information and experience gained in one stage are necessary

TABLE 32-3
Developmental Summary of Dying and Death

Piaget	Erikson	Major Fears and Concerns	Own Dying and Death	Nursing Interventions for Dying Child
Sensorimotor (birth to 2 years)	Trust versus mistrust (birth to 1 year) Autonomy versus shame and doubt (1–3 years)	Separation from parents Immobility–physical restrictions Distress from pain Consistent caregiver	Separation anxiety React more to immobility, pain, separation, and alterations in own routine rituals. Perceive and react to parent's emotional state.	Avoid separating child from parents as much as possible. Avoid continuous use of restraints. Assess signs of pain and treat early. Assess family rituals (time of bath, feeding, etc.) and incorporate into nursing care plan. Provide emotional support to parents Be alert to Bowlby's three stages of separation (protest, despair, and detachment).
Preoperational (2–7 years)	Initiative versus guilt (3–6 years)	Separation Immobility Darkness Body integrity and mutilation Realization of fantasies	Believe illness and treatment procedures are punishment for thoughts and actions. Death is equated with sleep or departure and is temporary. Greatest fear is separation from parents.	Be alert to passive behavior as a sign of guilt feelings. Place death in context of naturally occuring events (change of seasons) or nonpunitive events. Assess child's fear of darkness and sleep.
Concrete operational (7–11 years)	Industry versus inferiority (6–12 years)	(6–8 years) Abandonment Loss of control Punishment Pain/mutilation (9–11 years) Fears death as a reality Inability to live up to adult expectations Greater awareness of impending death	(6–8 years) Starts to fear the process of dying, being alone, and the unknown. Concrete understanding that death is the end of life, but fantasize that they can return. (9–11 years) Death is inevitable, final, and results from internal processes.	Establish consistent nursing staff and give reassurances if there are fears of abandonment. Provide honest, but sensitive, concrete answers to questions. May need to repeat explanations more than once. Encourage realistic, short-term, attainable goals. Prepare child for treatments and procedures.
Formal operations (11–15 years)	Identity versus role confusion (12–18 years)	Being alone Unrealized dreams and goals Independence/dependence from parents and other adults Being different from peers Changes in body image	Adult comprehension of death. Most difficulty in coping with own death. Death and dying threaten their developmental tasks of identity and independence from parents. Deteriorating physical condition increases feelings of being different from peers.	Provide consistent nursing staff assignments because adolescents rarely open up to strangers. Focus on what the child has accomplished in his or her life. Allow for as much independent action and personal choice as possible. Be sensitive and respect feelings about body changes (need for privacy, importance of wig or hat, etc.)

for moving into the next stage. For example, if a child is in stage 3 (knows the names of the medications and the side effects as well as the purposes of medical treatments and procedures) but does not know the disease is chronic (stage 4), the news of another child's death from the same disease does not lead the child to conclude that he or she has a fatal prognosis (stage 5).

Bluebond-Langner also described five stages reflecting changes in the child's self-concept[1] (see Fig. 32-1). Like the stages of information acquisition, the self-concept stages are successive and require certain experiences to move on to the next stage. From the point of diagnosis, they see themselves as seriously ill, primarily due to the emotional responses of adults. Once they experience a remission or an improvement in their symptoms, they enter stage 2 in which they see themselves as seriously ill but will get better. With the first relapse, the children begin to see themselves as always ill, but still with the belief that they will recover (stage 3). With additional relapses and complications, the children begin to see themselves as always ill with relapses and remissions lasting indefinitely (stage 4). Through the experience of learning of the death of another child, the children realize that the cycle is not indefinite, but rather that it ends in death (stage 5).

Today, most practitioners advocate telling the child in simple honest terms what their diagnosis is, the treatment process, and the chances of recovery. The essential issue today is not *if* the child is told, but rather *how* and *when*. The method of explaining and the message con-

Response to Death of a Sibling or Loved One	Nursing Interventions for Surviving Child
There will be a period of readjusting to absence.	Help child to express feelings.
Toddlers persist in wanting to see or talk to the dead person as if nothing has happened. Desire to maintain rituals of keeping dead person's room, belongings, and setting a place at the table for him or her.	Allow rituals, but restate that dead person will return in thoughts and memories only.
Due to fewer defense mechanisms to deal with loss, child frequently uses denial, detachment, or makes light of the situation to distance from the overwhelming impact. May believe his or her actions are the cause of the death. May fear he or she is next.	Do not force child to abandon defense mechanisms. Help child to clarify his or her feelings. Explore his or her personal view of the cause of death. Assess guilt thoughts and feelings. Explore cause of death in relation to the surviving child's probability of dying.
Very interested in postdeath services and what happens to body. May harbor guilt or resentments toward the dead person. May privately believe that illness or death was precipitated by own actions. May fear that they will die next. May resent the parents' inability to protect loved ones from death.	Provide honest, concrete answers to questions. Prepare for what to expect during funeral services. Provide a support person for postdeath services if needed. Provide information to understand the disease so as to allay fears that they will be next.
May appear undisturbed by the death, extremely angry, or silent and socially withdrawn.	Help child to identify and express feelings. Need to know they are not alone in their grief.
Some adolescents will appropriately express feelings and talk about the loss. May fear losing control at the funeral services or not knowing what is expected of them.	Prepare for what to expect at the funeral services if needed. Provide reassurances that it is acceptable to cry at services.

veyed are extremely important. The will to survive must not be destroyed by dispelling all hope. There is a tremendous difference between being cruel and blunt and being sensitive but honest. Using the medical name of the disease, describing its effect on body functioning, explaining the reason for treatment, and assuring the children that you will be there with them in their fight against the disease fosters hope, honesty, and a supportive relationship. Children should be told about their condition a few days after the parents are told to enable the parents to be supportive instead of emotionally "falling apart" in front of the child (Fig. 32-2). Hysterical parents only frighten the child more.

Nurses working with dying children must be alert and open to the language children use to reveal their thoughts and emotions concerning death. A young child does not possess the verbal language skills or the ability for abstract thought to discuss death as an adult would. Children express their concerns through symbolic language. Through stories, art work, and play the child will use symbols to express what they cannot in words. One boy who was dying of a rhabdomyosarcoma told his nurse that he was worried about his pet turtle. The turtle had not moved in quite a while, and the boy wanted to know what was happening to him. Another child drew several pictures of a family, always placing a little girl in the bottom right corner with each successive picture devoting less attention to the girl and more to the family. In her final picture she drew a box around the girl with the family members all looking on. The nurse working

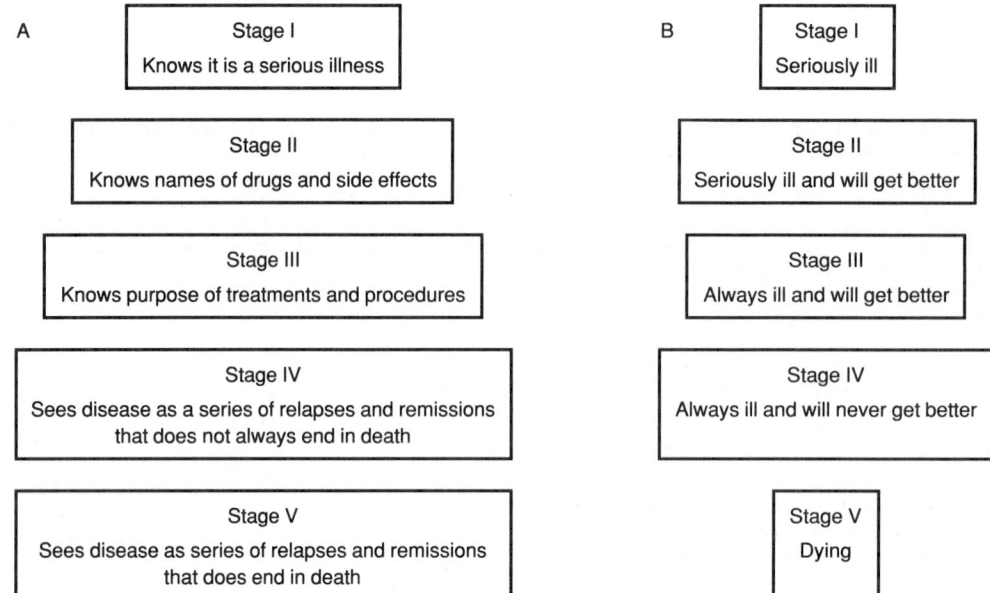

A

| Stage I |
| Knows it is a serious illness |

| Stage II |
| Knows names of drugs and side effects |

| Stage III |
| Knows purpose of treatments and procedures |

| Stage IV |
| Sees disease as a series of relapses and remissions that does not always end in death |

| Stage V |
| Sees disease as series of relapses and remissions that does end in death |

B

| Stage I |
| Seriously ill |

| Stage II |
| Seriously ill and will get better |

| Stage III |
| Always ill and will get better |

| Stage IV |
| Always ill and will never get better |

| Stage V |
| Dying |

FIGURE 32-1

Bluebond-Langner's study of death awareness and communication. (**A**) Stages of death awareness. (**B**) Stages of self-concept changes. (Adapted from Bluebond-Langner. [1978]. *The private worlds of dying children.* Princeton: Princeton University Press.)

with both of these children realized that the children were expressing their fears symbolically. The nurse was then able to initiate conversations that enabled the child to express how the turtle or the girl in the picture might feel. The children's major concerns were then identified, allowing the nurse to intervene appropriately.

Explaining the Death of Another Child

Anyone who is hospitalized frequently or for a prolonged time may be exposed to the death of another pa-

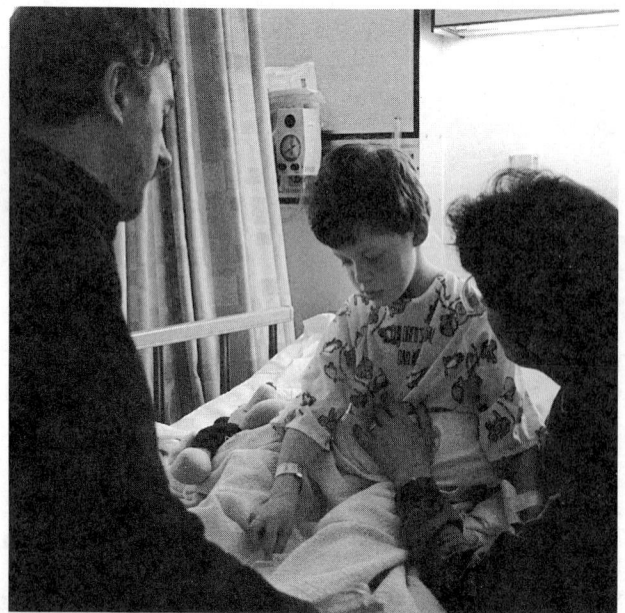

FIGURE 32-2

Children should be told about their condition a few days after the parents to enable the parents to be supportive when the child is told. (Photo by Kathy Sloane, courtesy of Children's Hospital, Oakland, CA.)

tient. Here too the "to tell or not to tell" dilemma has received much debate. It was reasoned that children, especially ill children, cannot cope with knowing that a fellow patient has died. Nurses used to shut the doors, pull curtains, and fabricate stories about where the other patient has gone. Over the years, experience has taught us that children are too intelligent, observant, and sensitive to the moods of adults not to catch on to what has happened. The nurse's failure to discuss death with children conveys the message that it is not good to talk about such matters. This policy aborted many opportunities to dispel fears and foster personal growth. What adults failed to realize is that life never completely shields anyone, even children, from death. The expression of feelings and discussion of the meaning of the loss can result in a valuable experience for coping with future personal tragedies (Fig. 32-3).

Exactly how and what to tell children about a death is a highly individual matter. However, as a guideline, the parent or nurse must always consider the child's developmental age, previous knowledge and experience with death, depth of relationship with the deceased, and the available resources for coping with the loss. Adults must have enough personal composure to avoid using the child for their own support needs.[35]

Past Experience With Death

The nurse should assess each child's past experiences with death and his or her emotional response to death. Many children have suffered the loss of a pet, seen a dead bird that hit a window, or watched a dog get hit by a car. Children also may have suffered the loss of a grandparent or other family member. Because patients with chronic, life-threatening diseases, such as cystic fibrosis, heart disease, or cancer, frequently are treated in a clinic for that specific disorder, it is not uncommon for them to have

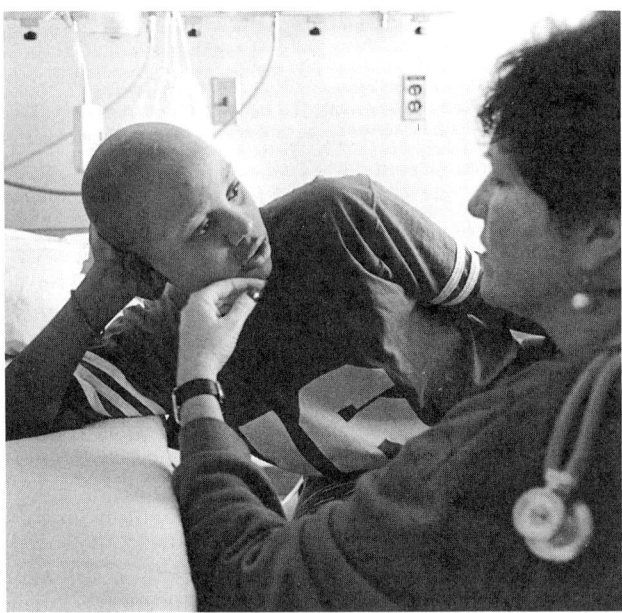

FIGURE 32-3
The nurse in the oncology unit talks with a 13-year-old boy about the death of another child on the unit. (Photo by Kathy Sloane, courtesy of Children's Hospital, Oakland, CA.)

lost a friend to a similar disease. All of these experiences impact children and influence their responses to their own impending death.

Kübler-Ross' Stages of Dying

Based on thousands of interviews with dying patients, Kübler-Ross[14] identified five stages of dying that most adult patients experience. Each patient may not pass through all the stages or may, at times, revert back to a previous stage. Although not universally accepted, these stages can help health professionals to conceptualize the behavioral reactions of the anticipatory grief involved in losing one's life. This framework may have limited application to very young children; however, it is useful with older children. Furthermore, it has been noted that the loved ones of the dying child also may experience the same stages. The sequence of the stages may differ between the children and their loved ones.

Denial. The first stage of dying is *denial*. It usually begins when the person is told the diagnosis. This is typified by the "no, not me" response of shock and disbelief. The duration of denial depends on the individual's coping mechanisms, their support systems, the responses of significant others, and sometimes the actual disease process. Complete denial would result in maladaptive behaviors because needed medical treatment would be refused. Physicians and nurses once thought that all denial was maladaptive. However, partial denial has been found to be an adaptive method of coping with the life-threatening disease.[18] Children who use denial to some degree are able to cope with the illness while continuing to have a productive attitude toward life.[33] Through the use of denial, these children appear to be able to maintain hope. The role of the nurse is to support the child or family in whatever stage they are in, not to "force" or maneuver them into another stage. The most effective means of support is through the use of empathetic active listening.

Anger. The second stage of dying is *anger*. In this stage, reality penetrates, and the response is "why me?" The person may feel anger, hostility, resentment, or envy. These feelings may be directed inward or at others (frequently hospital staff). It is important for the nurse to remember that the child needs to express these feelings without being judged, made to feel guilty, or fear retaliation. To support the child's anger, nurses must realize that the anger is not directed at them personally. Finding out where the anger originates and what it is directed toward often can point to possible interventions. If the child is angry because the illness interferes with important peer activities, the parents and nursing staff frequently can work out acceptable alternatives for the child. For example, if maintenance chemotherapy is scheduled to be given on a Monday, but the child has a school play that day, the chemotherapy may be postponed until Tuesday.

Bargaining. The stage of *bargaining* is characterized by "making a deal" either with God or another significant person. The child promises to do something in exchange for some special favor. Bargains often are difficult to assess because they are not overtly shared. One way of discovering it is to ask the child, "If you could do one more thing, what would it be?" Bargaining, often for more time, is an attempt to postpone the inevitable. Bargaining frequently is with God. "If I am very good, will you let me have one more trip home?" When a bargain is struck with God, and it fails, religious faith may be shaken.

Depression. The fourth stage is that of *depression*. Once the child can no longer deny the seriousness of their illness, expresses anger about the condition, and realizes that bargains cannot postpone the progression of the disease, he or she usually experiences depression. Kübler-Ross identified two types of depression, both the result of losses.[14] *Reactive depression* is the result of past losses, such as physical health, beauty, a sport or activity, social contacts that the activity afforded, or family recreational activities due to mounting financial constraints. In any terminal illness, many such loses are readily recognizable, and physicians, nurses, social workers, teachers, and concerned friends often can do something about them.

The second type of depression is *preparatory depression* and is in anticipation of the impending loss of all love objects. With reactive depression, concerned people often can "cheer up" the dying child. For instance, the child who can no longer play baseball may still get in uniform and participate as a team member from the dugout. With anticipatory depression, however, well-intentioned encouragements and reassurances to "look on the bright side" are not as meaningful. Children are profoundly saddened because they realize they are about to lose everything and everybody they love. This depression is a silent inner depression with little need for words to "talk things over." Children need to deal with it in their own way. The silent presence of one or two significant people is more supportive than words or many visitors. Children usually want their parents more than anyone else. Nurses need to be sensitive to this and should not intrude. This is also a time to avoid assigning a new nurse to the patient. These children need to be cared for by a person with whom they have a strong relationship that does not require talking and "getting to know each other." The child may want things to be done in a certain ritualistic way without having to explain it to a new person.

Acceptance. The final stage of dying is that of *acceptance.* Given enough time, anger and depression give way to a state of resolution. This is not a happy time but rather a time of inner peace. Many children have frequent periods of restful sleep and prefer a quiet room without bright lights. One 12-year-old boy awakened from a nap with a smile on his face. The nurse who had taken care of him during his many hospital admissions during the previous year asked if he had had a pleasant dream. Patrick had been withdrawn and depressed for several weeks, hardly speaking to anyone, but that day he asked his nurse if she knew the story of Hans Brinker and the Silver Skates. She sat in the chair at his bedside and said she knew the story well. Patrick explained that he felt he was gliding over smooth ice on silver skates and that it was very peaceful. He reached out and held his nurse's hand while reminiscing over the many happy times in his life. This is just one example of how a child might display an inner peaceful acceptance of dying.

To The Family

The Parents

Two primary roles of parenting are to protect the child from harm and foster the child's growth and development. A dying child threatens both of these roles. Different causes of death may accentuate different feelings and foster or hinder the grieving process for the parents.[38] Due to significant medical advances, many childhood cancers that were previously fatal within a short time after diagnosis are now chronic illnesses with a potentially fatal prognosis. Still with other disorders, such as cystic fibrosis, children live for many years knowing there is no cure and that at some time death is inevitable. What then are the parents' reactions to the diagnosis of a fatal disease?

When the diagnosis means certain death, the parents begin a process of anticipatory grief. Except in conditions of sudden, unexpected death, parents usually have some amount of time to work through this process. Parents who have only a few weeks or months advance knowledge will not usually be at the same stage in the grief process as parents who have had years to adjust to the loss. Although the process is similar for all parents, it is the time frame that differs. The actual death is no less painful in an expected death, but the stage of acute grief and the work of mourning after the death usually are shorter.

Although Kübler-Ross' stages of dying were developed from the perspective of the dying patient, parents go through similar stages. The diagnosis brings on a state of *shock and denial.* Parents have described the diagnosis as "unreal," "impossible," "must be wrong," and literally having their world torn apart. Often they hear nothing after the fatal or potentially fatal prognosis. Later they may ask many questions because they say that "I don't remember anything said after the word 'cancer.' It was just too much to take all at once." The initial shock occasionally makes parents want to delay the initiation of treatment. Parents are tempted to "doctor shop" in an attempt to disprove the fatal diagnosis.

Nurses must realize that denial may be a necessary defense to cope with emotions at this time. To try to break away denial prematurely leaves the parents defenseless against the effects of so great a loss. When denial is interfering with their ability to focus on solving problems, it may have more detrimental consequences, and the parent may need help in working with their denial. Lazarus refers to the use of these two types of denial as "problem-focused coping and emotion-focused coping."[18] Given time and emotional support, the parents will eventually abandon the use of emotional denial. Only when the use of denial is so great that it interferes with their ability to cope with actual problems should health professionals intervene.

Following the diagnosis, *multiple stressors* begin to exert themselves on the parents. Potential stressors are financial concerns, time demands, the needs of the ill child and other family members, rest and sleep disturbances, and the constant bombardment of new things to learn about. While most parents can successfully deal with a single stressor, the result of multiple stressors can lead to frustration, maladaptation, and possible crisis states.

As denial yields to the pressure of reality, *anger* usually surfaces. Parents are angry that their child has a fatal illness. They are angry with other parents for having healthy children. They are angry at God for allowing this to happen. They are angry at medical science for not being able to save their child. When the death is the result of accident or injury, there can be many other targets for their anger. Parents can be angry at themselves for not recognizing symptoms earlier or not preventing the accident. With so many possibilities for negative feelings, it is not surprising that anger often is directed toward hospital personnel. Because anger is not socially condoned, it is often expressed indirectly. Nurses who are unaware of the role of anger in this process perceive the parents' reaction as a personal assault and turn away from the angry parents rather than helping them to work it through.

Like the dying child, parents also may go through a *bargaining* stage, which often is a silent bargain with God. Because the bargain may be associated with guilt, it is important to explore the meanings behind the bargain with the parents.

With the threatened or actual loss of a child, parents lose a part of themselves. "To bury a child is to see a part of yourself, your eye color, your dimple, your sense of humor, being placed in the ground."[5] The depth and complexity of the parent–child relationship leads, understandably, to feelings of profound *sadness, loneliness,* and *depression.* Even when surrounded by friends and family, the parents feel alone. After the death, parents are shunned by others who see the magnitude of their loss and look away out of their own feelings of inadequacy. The parents need to talk about the child and the death, but they find few people who can listen. Nurses need to assess the type and amount of support needed by each parent. Many parents have found self-help organizations, such as Candlelighters, Compassionate Friends, and Parents of SIDS, extremely helpful in dealing with the death of their child. Nurses need to be aware of local organizations and of national organizations for families who are experiencing death, which are given in the accompanying display.

The goal for all parents should be an *acceptance* of the reality of the loss and a readjustment to living a full and complete life with that loss. With time, support, and love parents will find comfort, not pain, in their memories of the child, and they will rediscover a meaning for living.

The Siblings

Siblings attach their own personal meanings to dying and death. Much of the sibling's response to the dying child will be shaped by their own developmental stage as well as the attitudes, beliefs, and behaviors of the parents. Table 32-3 shows a developmental comparison of the well siblings' responses. Siblings can have lasting psychosocial problems as a direct result of the death of a brother or sister.[48] Because the siblings will live their entire lifetimes with the memory of the illness and death, it is essential that health care professionals concern themselves with preventing disturbed emotional reactions while promoting optimal emotional health adjustments in this high-risk population.

If one child in a family is sick, it is only natural for the parents to focus their attention on that child. When the illness is of a relatively short duration, such as having a tonsillectomy or the flu, normal family life is only temporarily interrupted and the well children are only minimally displaced. When the illness is severe with the threat of death, however, the impact is often profound. In chronic life-threatening diseases, the emotional needs of the well siblings are less adequately met than the ill child's or the parents'.[40a] The well siblings often are physically and emotionally separated from their parents. If the treatment center is geographically far from the home, the well siblings may have to live with relatives for a period of time. Even when they live close to the hospital, the parents spend many hours at the hospital with the sick child. When the parents are home, they are preoccupied with the ill child and have little emotional reserves to attend to the siblings' needs. The lack of attention to the siblings can result in feelings of anger (both at the parents and the ill child), rejection, jealousy, and guilt over privately thinking that they have caused the disease.[47] The siblings often feel that the parents are overindulgent and overprotective toward the ill child.[30,47] These children may express their feelings behaviorally by acting aggressively, developing problems with school performance or school phobia, becoming socially withdrawn or depressed, or displaying a variety of somatic complaints.[46] Siblings and their responses are further discussed in Chapter 21. In exploratory studies with siblings of cancer patients, the siblings stated that they needed more information regarding the patient's illness and treatment process and that they would like to have been more involved in the care of the ill child.[13,30,42]

Nursing can dramatically affect the impact of a terminal illness on the lives of the siblings. The needs of the *entire* family should be assessed. One research study on sibling coping found that parents are not always aware of the coping strategies used by the healthy siblings of children with cancer.[47] This study reinforces the belief that nurses need to obtain information about the healthy siblings from the siblings, rather than just from parental report. Nurses can help the parents explain the diagnosis and treatment to the siblings and alert parents to possible concerns and problem areas. Nurses also should be aware of books, pamphlets, and organizations that may help the family. Communication between all family members can be fostered by liberalizing visiting rules to include younger siblings or by encouraging telephone and written communication between the patient and the siblings at home. Many treatment centers working with life-threatening disorders sponsor family picnics, summer camps, and holiday parties that include the siblings. These functions provide an opportunity for the siblings to interact with and attain social support from other children who also are coping with the possibility of losing a brother or sister.

Many siblings express a desire to be of assistance to the ill child (Fig. 32-4). The siblings can pick up homework assignments from the school, read to the ill child, organize a fund raiser, or work for an established organization like the American Cancer Society. The possibilities are infinite, and the potential benefits for the children are enormous.

The Extended Family

Relatives experience shock and grief reactions much as the parents do. Their interactions and adjustment vary

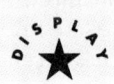

National Organizations for Families Experiencing Death

Candlelighters Foundation
(for parents of children with cancer)
  1901 Pennsylvania Avenue NW,
  Suite 1001
  Washington DC 20006
Children's Hospice International
(for care of the terminally ill)
  1101 King Street Suite 131
  Alexandria, VA 22314
Compassionate Friends, Inc. (for bereaved parents)
  P.O. Box 3696
  Oak Brook, IL 60522
Parents of Murdered Children
  1739 Bella Vista
  Cincinnati, OH 45237
SIDS (National Sudden Infant Death Syndrome
Foundation)
  Two Metro Plaza Suite 205
  8240 Professional Plaza
  Landover, MD

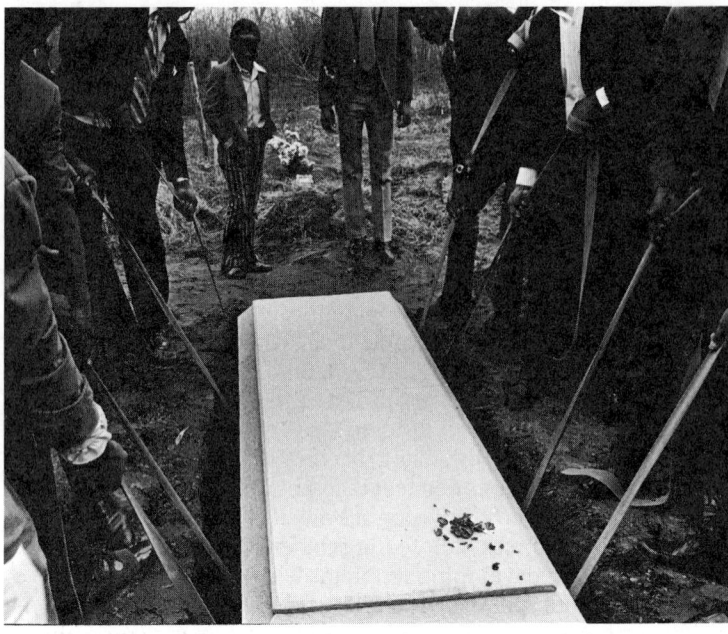

FIGURE 32-4
Children are often forgotten as adults try to cope with their own grief. The sibling may feel abandoned by both the deceased and the living. (Schuster CS, Ashburn SS: The Process of Human Development, 3rd ed. Philadelphia: JB Lippincott, 1992.)

tremendously, as does their ability to be a source of support for the family. While relatives close to the parents may provide instrumental support by helping with the care of the siblings or even helping to care for or visit the ill child, other extended family members may be only minimally involved. Unfortunately, well-meaning friends and relatives may harass the parents with suggestions to find a different physician or try alternative methods of treatment. Nurses can be instrumental in supporting the parents through these difficult situations.

The child's grandparents exhibit a dual kind of grief. They grieve not only the loss of their grandchild, but also the pain felt by their own child, the parent. Perhaps out of their own frustrations and sense of helplessness, some grandparents may offer unwanted advice and undermine the parents' attempts at control and discipline by showering the child with attention and gifts.[10,49] If there were unresolved tensions between the parents and grandparents prior to the child's illness, the stress of the illness may increase hostilities for all involved. Nurses can help redirect the grandparents' efforts to a more meaningful and constructive role. To be supportive, they need to be included in the explanations and information about the disease and treatment process.

Differences Between Unexpected and Expected Death

Death can come either unexpectedly with little or no warning, or it can be expected, the result of years with a fatal illness. While there are many similarities in the grief process, there are some notable differences. When death quickly follows an acute trauma, such as an automobile accident, burn, or drowning, there is an immediate and drastic physical change in the child. Quite literally, one day the child is normal, happy, and healthy, and the next day the child is severely injured and near death or dead. The contrast between what *is* and what *was* is profound.

From the very moment of the incident, many people mobilize to try to save the child. The child and parents quickly relinquish control to the authority figures of policemen, firemen, paramedics, emergency room staff, and finally, attending physicians and nurses. Time is of the essence for the initiation of treatment. There is no time to adjust. When asked what happened, parents frequently say, "I don't know. Everything happened so fast. I don't understand." Once the child is in the hospital, the nursing staff is extremely busy in efforts to try to save the child. There is no time to build a therapeutic relationship with the parents. Explanations, when they are made, are brief and to the point. Seldom is there time for discussion and feedback.

When heroic efforts cannot save the child's life, the medical and nursing staff often feel a sense of failure. Telling the parents that their child is dead is a difficult job. The nurse tries to comfort the parents by telling them that everything possible was done. Nurses try to be sensitive to the family's pain and anguish. However, without knowledge of the parents as individuals and without real depth to the nurse–family relationship, attempts to support the family are usually less than completely satisfactory. The family is simply in too great a state of shock.

When death comes as the expected end to a chronic illness, the circumstances are quite different. Physical changes in the child from health to diagnosis to the terminal stage occur gradually. Physical changes are less shocking because the child, family, and nurses have more time to adjust. Rather than being dramatically different extremes, the child's physical changes are likened more to a process of slowly sinking.

During the course of the illness, the child and parents have become an intricate part of the "treatment team." They are aware of, and actively involved in, the treatment, and they participate in long discussions about the pros and cons of various alternative choices. As the child approaches a terminal stage, very few decisions need to be made immediately. The physician and family have time to think and weigh the consequences of each action.

By the time a chronic illness is in a terminal stage, the family usually has lived through medical complications that severely threatened the child's life. The crisis resulting from a complication was in a sense an emotional "dress rehearsal" for the actual death. As painful as each crisis was at the time, when it was over, the family was grateful for the extension of the child's life. After the first crisis, they learn the value of each day and incorporate a philosophy of living each day to the fullest. They make a conscious effort to do an act of kindness and express affection today rather than putting it off until tomorrow. As a result, when death does come, there are fewer regrets and less unfinished business.

There are also salient differences between expected and unexpected death for the nursing staff. Ideally, the nurse caring for the dying child has known the child and the family for an extended period of time. The long-standing relationship is built on shared past experiences. The nurse was there with the family during a previous crisis. Because of the nurse's actions during a prior crisis, the family usually has a strong sense of trust in the nurse. With expected death, the nurse also has the luxury of time to explain what is happening and to validate understanding through the use of feedback. Time, experiences, trust, and rapport can significantly alter the impact of the actual death on the family and on the nurse. However, the nurse–family relationship is a two-way relationship. Just as the family is invested in the nurse, so is the nurse invested in the family. When a child dies within hours after admission, the nurse is usually less emotionally invested in the child and family than when a long-term relationship has occurred. All children's deaths are difficult, but when the child and family are intimately known to the nurse, there is a qualitative difference in the nurse's emotional response. Nurses grieve, not only for the family, but with the family. Table 32-4 compares some of the major differences in expected and unexpected deaths.

Death Trajectory With Fatal and Potentially Fatal Chronic Illnesses

In many disorders, such as Duchenne's muscular dystrophy, Tay-Sachs, hypoplastic left-heart syndrome, acquired immunodeficiency syndrome, and progeria, little supportive therapy can prolong life, and death is a certain outcome. When death will occur, however, cannot be predicted with any reasonable degree of accuracy. The parents know that their child will die, but not when. It may be weeks, months, or years.

With other diseases, such as cystic fibrosis, some forms of congenital heart disease (e.g., single ventricle), several types of blood dyscrasias (e.g., congenital pure red cell anemia and severe thalassemia major), and some immune disorders (e.g., systemic lupus erythematosus and combined immunodeficiency disease), there is a lack of curative treatment, but modern medicine often can offer supportive therapy that may significantly prolong

TABLE 32-4
Comparison of Differences Between Expected and Unexpected Deaths

	Expected	Unexpected
Physical changes in the child	Gradual	Sudden
Mobilization of medical team	Limited	Extensive
Family's coping patterns and resources	Known	Unknown
Prior experience coping with medical crisis	Likely	Unlikely
Anticipatory grief work	Yes	No
Nurse's involvement with family	Extensive	Limited

the child's life. During lengthy periods of supportive care, parents maintain hope that a medical or surgical cure will be discovered. With some of the chronic fatal illnesses, the child may respond so well to supportive therapies that the progression of symptoms is in remission. The child may be in a state of medical maintenance therapy of uncertain duration. Eventually the disease exacerbates with progressively severe symptoms, leading to a terminal stage and death. Figure 32-5 demonstrates the death trajectory of such fatal chronic illnesses and some of the associated emotions experienced.

When a child's condition is a steady progression toward death, the family increasingly anticipates the loss. What differences are there when death is *not* inevitable, but life *is* severely threatened? This is the predicament faced by families with many types of childhood cancers for which there is a strong probability for cure but also a possibility for death. The family should not completely prepare for death but should maintain hope for cure. The ambiguity of the prognosis places the cancer family in a state of limbo. Figure 32-6 illustrates the process of cancer treatment with typical psychosocial concerns associated with each phase of therapy.

Because cancer is the most common cause of death from disease in childhood, the psychosocial concerns of the child and family during each phase of cancer treatment will serve as a model for fatal illnesses in general. Although other fatal diseases such as cystic fibrosis do not have an induction, remission, cessation of therapy, or cure as treatment phases, the children and families do experience similar concerns in the remaining treatment phases. The psychosocial concerns during diagnosis, maintenance (for other fatal diseases this phase is similar to when the child's symptoms are more or less controlled), relapse (a phase of exacerbation of symptoms), terminal stage, and death and postdeath phases of treatment are similar to those experienced by families of a child with cancer.

Diagnosis and Induction

In the diagnosis and induction phase of cancer therapy, the family usually experiences feelings of shock, denial, guilt, anger, and depression. During the early phase of treatment, some parents intellectually withdraw

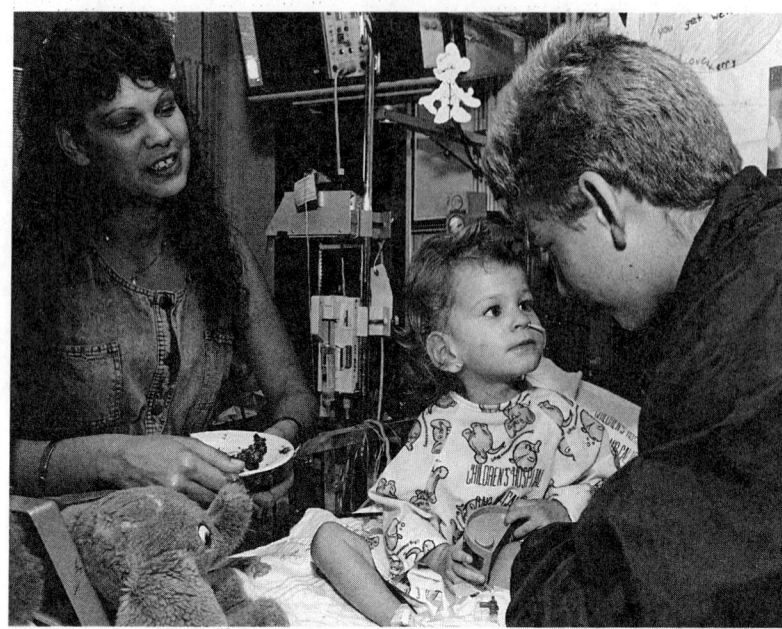

FIGURE 32-5
A sibling wants to be with, support, and play with his 2-year-old sister who is a heart patient. (Photo by Kathy Sloane, Courtesy of Children's Hospital, Oakland, CA.)

from active involvement in the treatment process in an attempt to shield themselves from additional distressing information. The nurse must recognize this reaction as a protective mechanism and not try to force the parents into an active role prematurely. Parents need time to regain confidence in their ability to care for their child. A simple thing like helping the child with a bath may appear complex to the parent when the child has an intravenous (IV) tube.

Usually the withdrawal is short lived, and the parents develop an insatiable search for knowledge about the disease, medical and nursing procedures, and cancer therapies. Sometimes this can be problematic for the hospital staff if they react to the parents' unending ques-

tions as a direct challenge to their knowledge or the quality of care. Nurses need to recognize that the parents are trying to regain control and discover their unique role as a member of the treatment team. Listening, answering questions, and teaching become major nursing functions. Occasionally parents will intellectualize in an attempt to distance themselves from extreme emotional stress. With time, support, and counseling, this defense mechanism can be effectively confronted.

From the start of induction to the attainment of remission, the child and parents frequently are angry. The child is angry over all the intrusive procedures, changes in daily lifestyle, treatments that frequently make the child feel worse than before therapy, and activity restrictions.

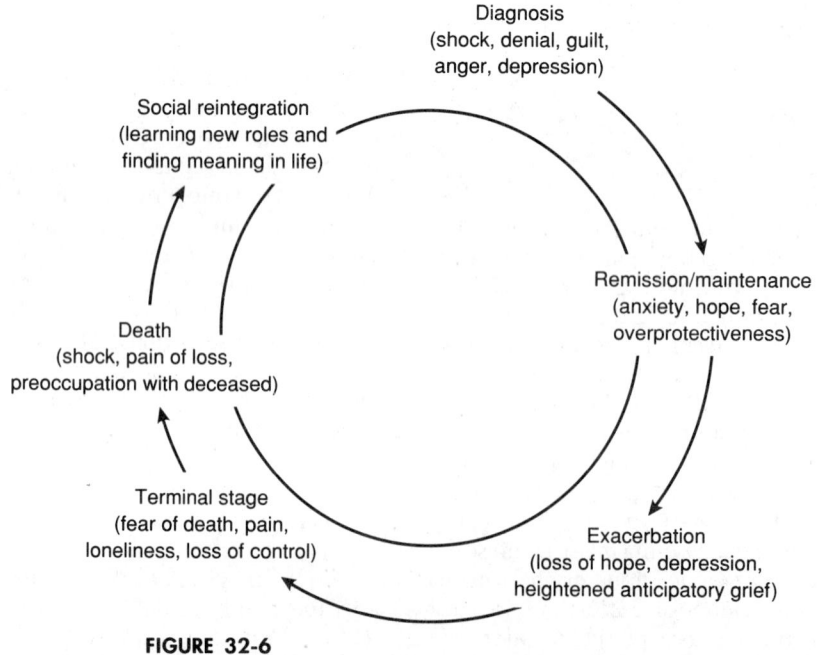

FIGURE 32-6
Death trajectory of chronic fatal illnesses and associated emotions.

A parent's anger may be directed toward self (usually tied in with guilt feelings), the spouse (resulting in arguments and a decrease in communication), the child (almost always passive anger), the physician (for not diagnosing the cancer earlier or having quicker success in attaining remission), or the nursing staff (for perceived insensitivity or inadequacies in nursing care). The nurse should allow the child and parents to vent their angry feelings. The child and parents often can provide solutions for genuine problems by talking about what makes them angry.

Remission

If remission is never attained, the family proceeds with increased anticipatory grieving. Fortunately, the majority of cancer patients will attain a remission. However, waiting for confirmation of the remission is a time of significant anxiety. Once confirmed, the elation renews hope for the child's future. Within days or a few weeks, ambivalent feelings arise regarding the "price" of remission. Many families realize that they will never be the same as before diagnosis. The impact of the physical changes in the child due to surgery, radiation, or chemotherapy are felt more intensely. Of course, there is the constant fear that the child will have a relapse. The nurse can help the family by reassuring them that these feelings are normal and a part of adjusting to the disease and to treatment.

Maintenance

Once in remission, there is usually a long period of maintenance therapy. For some cancers, it may be as short as 6 months or for others as long as several years. This is a time of hope and fear. If there are no complications, the family tends to incorporate the cancer treatment as a normal part of their lives. However, if complications from therapy occur, such as anemia, bleeding, or infections, the family will have more difficulty putting the threat of relapse and death out of their conscious awareness.

Often parents react to their own fears for the child by overprotecting and overindulging the child. The consequences of excessive protection and indulgence are detrimental to all family members. The ill child becomes dependent, undisciplined, and emotionally confused by the meaning of the special treatment from the parents. The child often will worry that such special treatment means the illness is more seriously threatening than it actually is. Children want more than anything to live a normal life. To the child, special treatment sets them apart from other children more than the cancer itself. Some children will misbehave deliberately to be disciplined like other children. Overprotection, dependency, and the lack of discipline severely hinder the child's optimal physical and emotional growth and development. Parents need to appreciate the necessity for the child to lead a normal life. Carried to the extreme, the result is a child that may have survived cancer, only to be an emotional cripple. When the parents are overprotective or overindulgent toward the ill child, the siblings frequently complain that just the opposite treatment is given to them. Lack of attention and greater discipline toward the siblings

result in anger and resentment that can be directed to the ill child or the parents. In either event, it places additional stress on the siblings.

One area of particular importance is the child's return to school. Parents are hesitant to send their child back to school because it impedes their ability to protect the child. The child also may be afraid to return to school for fear of what the schoolmates' responses will be. They may be concerned about their loss of hair, gain or loss of weight, surgical scars, radiation markers, or any number of other perceived or real limitations. Siblings also may be ashamed or embarrassed due to the additional attention focused on their family.

Nurses can assist the family in making a healthy adjustment to cancer by anticipating possible problem areas and preparing the family to deal with them. Discussing overprotection, discipline, school re-entry, and the concerns of the siblings and other family members can help the family cope with the demands of the illness.

Cessation of Therapy

When maintenance therapy is over, the child comes off all therapy. Although this is a very happy time for all

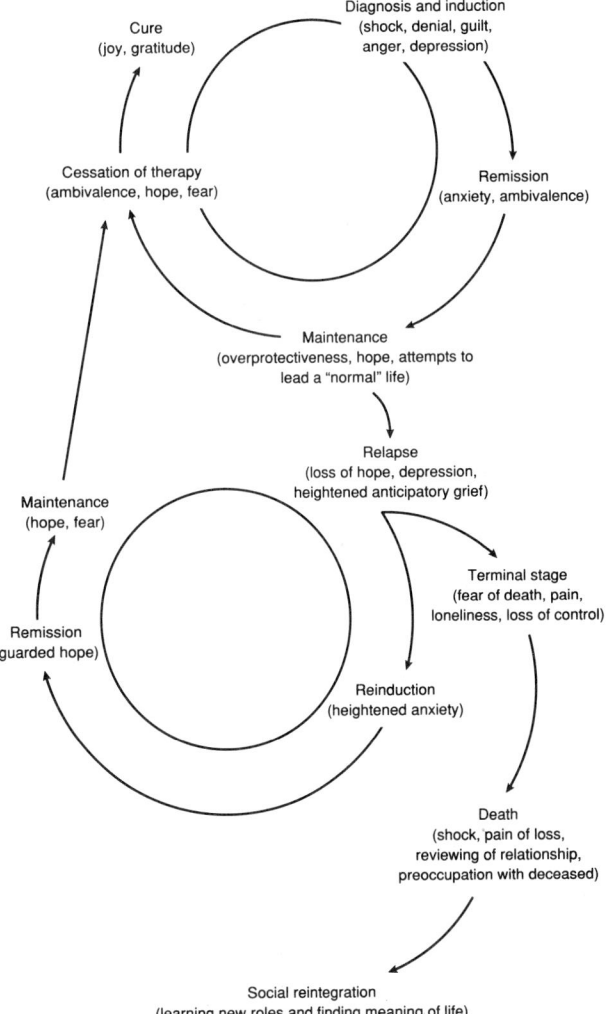

FIGURE 32-7

Family's emotional responses throughout the cancer treatment process.

concerned, it is also very stressful. The child's life has been maintained by therapy, and now there are understandable fears that without therapy, the disease will return. A sense of security developed in the routine of medications, radiation, and frequent physical examinations. Parents question whether additional treatment is needed. Hospital staff need to let the parents know that they will continue to be available to the family and encourage them to deal with their ambivalent feelings. Most parents readily accept the fact that continued medical supervision is advisable for many years. "Cure" in many types of cancers will not officially be confirmed until the child is off therapy for several years.

Relapse

Any time after the initial remission, it is possible for the disease to relapse. For some families, relapse is a more difficult time than the initial diagnosis because each relapse diminishes the hope for a cure. Relapse is also a jolting of the reality of the uncertainty of the disease. With some types of cancer, the child was admitted to the hospital for the diagnosis but has not required hospitalization for therapy, so the return to the hospital is very distressing in itself. With a relapse, even a child whose disease was classified as "low risk" at diagnosis, is now changed to a "high-risk" category. It is understandable that relapse causes an exacerbation of all the previous stages of grieving. Some parents have stated that relapse is emotionally more difficult because they "know what lies ahead" and that they have "less faith in what medical science can do."

With a relapse, the child starts a reinduction phase of therapy with the hope that different drugs will attain a second remission. Usually the new chemotherapy regimen is more intense than the first. With each relapse, there is also the fear that eventually they will run out of different drugs to try.

Relapse is often a difficult time for the nurse as well as the family because hopes for recovery are threatened. To be of assistance to the family, nurses must recognize and work through their own feelings to avoid transferring them to the child and family.

Terminal Stage

The final relapse leads into the terminal stage. As all forms of therapy fail to control the growth of the cancer, the family begins an intensification of the grieving process characterized by loss of hope, depression, fear of what the end will be like, and possibly acceptance. As the child approaches death, the child's and parents' predominant fear is of death itself. They often ask questions like, "What will happen?," "What will it be like?," "Will there be pain?," and "How will I know when my child is actually dying?" A sensitive nurse must listen to the overt content of the question and to any covert questions. For example, instead of giving a clinical answer to the question "What will it be like?," the nurse should first assess what the person *fears* it will be like. For example, if the parent fears their child will "bleed to death," they may have an image of massive hemorrhage with blood virtually pouring out. They may be very comforted to know that most hemorrhaging is internal with perhaps a nosebleed being the only visible blood. Nurses should not be too explicit, however, because no one can predict exactly how a child will die.

The fear of intractable pain often is associated with cancer deaths and feared by the child and the parents. With proper medical and nursing management, it is the exception, not the norm, for a child to die in extreme pain. Furthermore, even with the use of continuous IV morphine drips, the medication can be titrated so that pain relief is attained without heavily sedating the child. It is important to remember to try all the approaches to pain management, not just medication. Perhaps the child will be made comfortable by a darkened room, a cool cloth, music, or being positioned in a certain way. The important thing is for the nurse to reassure the family that he or she will be there to continue interventions until relief is obtained. Not all pain is physical. Sometimes the fear of abandonment is the most severe form of pain.

The fear of abandonment and isolation can be intense. Parents frequently worry that they will not be there when their child dies. Although there are no guarantees, nurses can be instrumental in alerting parents to impending death, thus giving them the opportunity to be with their child. Children, out of their own fears of being alone, often will demand that the parents stay at the bedside. If the parents do have to leave the room and the child becomes frightened at being alone, a favorite nurse will be a comfort for both the child and the parents.

Another concern is that of losing emotional or physical control at the moment of death. Again, it is not possible to predict what any individual will do at that time, but the nurse can use nonjudgmental behaviors to lessen the family's concern for maintaining control. During the terminal stage, the fears and concerns of the child and family should be the basis of the nursing care plan. Keeping the family informed of the child's changing condition greatly increases their sense of control. The Nursing Care Plan for the child with terminal cancer discusses some of the problems and needs of the family just before and after the death of the child.

Death and Postdeath

No matter how prepared the family is for the death, there is a period of acute grief. One mother expressed it this way. "I just couldn't believe that one minute he was breathing and the next it was all over. I thought I was prepared for it, but the suddenness of it still shocks me." Immediately after the death, most families want some time with the child. It is often best for the nurse to stay in the room for a few minutes with the family to assess the degree of their shock and their own personal desires. Then the nurse should ask the parents if they want to be alone with their child. The parents of a 9-year-old boy tried to hug him as he lay dead in his bed. Side rails and equipment were obviously in the way. The nurse asked the parents if they would like to hold him. They said yes, so the nurse proceeded to help them by lifting the child into their arms. For some minutes, the parents cried while

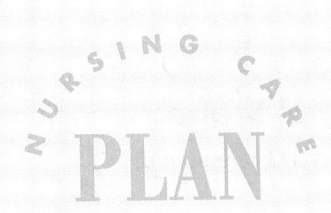

A 15-Year-Old Boy in Terminal Stage of Acute Lymphocytic Leukemia

Assessment

Case Study Description

Dave, a 15-year-old boy, was diagnosed with acute lymphocytic leukemia (ALL) 2 years prior to this admission. Initial remission was obtained within 6 weeks of diagnosis, and he went on maintenance therapy. He relapsed 7 months ago and has not responded to reinduction chemotherapy. The patient is admitted to the hospital at this time for treatment of bone pain.

The family consists of a 40-year-old father, a 38-year-old mother, the patient, and a 10-year-old sister. The family lives 100 miles from the hospital. Extended family includes both sets of grandparents and several aunts and uncles. None of the extended family lives in the same state as this family. The daughter is left in the care of friends, while the parents accompany the son to the hospital. During the course of this admission, the boy's condition has progressively deteriorated. He is on a continuous intravenous morphine drip for pain control and remains conscious. The boy is in the terminal stage of his illness.

Assessment Data

Function Assessment of Cognition and Perception

Pain tolerance—Dave is on continuous IV morphine drip, which controls his pain.

Sensory deficits—All senses are intact with noted increased sensitivity to touch and a sensation of warmth, although skin feels cold and body temperature is 97° F.

Parent/child teaching needs—Parents state they do not know what to do for their child. Parents ask many questions regarding what will happen at the end.

Self-Perception

Response to separation—patient refuses phone calls and visits from friends. Requests both parents stay in the room with him.

Fears—Patient expresses fear of abandonment, pain, and losing control.

Roles and Relationships

Change in family membership—Forthcoming loss of one member to death. Parents verbalize concern for daughter's emotional well-being and fear they will not be able to meet her needs.

Coping and Stress Tolerance

Management of hospitalization—Both parents are rooming with patient.

Awareness/understanding of diagnosis and prognosis—Patient is aware of diagnosis and impending death. Parents verbalize recognition that the end is near and request that resuscitation measures not be used.

Helpful interventions with previous stressors—Family has never experienced the death of a member before.

However, parents state that they find it helpful to talk over their problems with others who have had a similar problem.

Values and Beliefs

Religion and degree of activity—Protestants who attend church infrequently but do maintain relations with several other members of their church.

Cultural background—White, working class Americans.

(Continued)

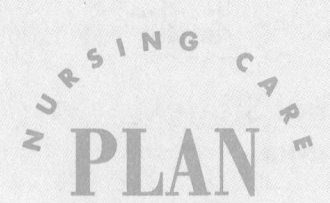

A 15-Year-Old Boy in Terminal Stage of Acute Lymphocytic Leukemia (continued)

Nursing Diagnosis	Intervention	Rationale
1. Altered parenting Supporting Data: • Feelings of inadequacy regarding care of ill child and needs of well child • Reluctance to perform caretaking activities for Dave • Fear of impact of death on the family.	Provide opportunity for parents to verbalize feelings and explore possible solutions. Explain all treatments	Expression of feelings and exploration of solutions enhance coping, facilitate adaptation, and may prevent a crisis. Parents need support and encouragement throughout all phases of the illness.
	Teach parents basic care-taking skills, such as positioning, comfort measures, working around IV lines, and physical needs of the dying. Encourage them to participate in care.	If parents are taught how to perform skills, they will feel more comfortable doing them.
	Provide anticipatory guidance regarding typical concerns of a 10-year-old who has lost a sibling. Provide anticipatory guidance regarding phases of grieving for both parents and surviving sibling.	Although grief over the loss cannot be avoided, knowledge of grief may make it more manageable and faciliate coping with the experience.
	Refer to community support group (e.g., Candlelighters)	Other people who have also lost a child provide a unique type of support.
	Assess parent's desire for presence of clergy member.	Religious needs may be heightened as a result of death.
2. Social isolation Supporting Data: • Dave has lost interest in social contacts • Dave requests parents to stay in room • Minimal communication with other people • Parents have not been home since the child was admitted.	Keep consistent nursing staff. Avoid assigning new staff person. Minimize contact with new professional staff. Facilitate any social contact for which Dave expresses desire.	Use of consistent personnel relieves patient and parents from burden of getting to know new staff and having staff try to learn this family's individual needs.
	Support parents in staying with the child. Provide parents with comfortable environment in child's room (e.g., chairs, food, drinks, sleeping arrangements).	Parents may not realize that it is acceptable for them to stay in the room. If they are comfortable, they will be better able to meet the needs of the child.
	Provide back-up relief so that parents can take breaks from the child's room.	Parents also should know that it is OK for them to leave to meet their own needs and that the staff is there to help them.
	Assist parents in maintaining contact with their family and friends (e.g., a place to make telephone calls).	Provides another measure of social support for the family.

(Continued)

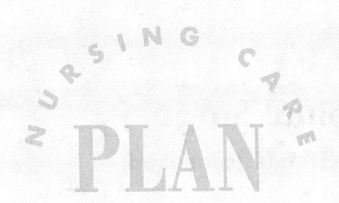

A 15-Year-Old Boy in Terminal Stage of Acute Lymphocytic Leukemia (continued)

Nursing Diagnosis	*Intervention*	*Rationale*
3. Pain Supporting Data: • Continuous IV morphine drip • Patient states that pain becomes unbearable when IV morphine is reduced • Facial grimacing when sheets or position are changed • Sensation of heat is uncomfortable despite temperature of 97°F and skin cold to the touch.	Monitor and record IV rate at least every hour. Maintain IV morphine, and report any signs of increasing pain to physician so rate can be adjusted accordingly. Position for comfort. Do not have to change position every 2 hours but rather as requested. Change sheets as needed for soiling or moisture. Provide alternative pain relief measures such as distraction (e.g., music, gentle massage, games, television, and other activities as tolerated). Subdue lighting and noise as requested by patient. Provide comfort measures for heat sensation—fan for good ventilation, cool cloth to forehead, sponge baths, cool liquids, minimal clothing, and bed linens.	As pain increases, or decreases, the IV morphine rate may need to be changed to optimize relief. Routine nursing practices may need to be altered for dying patient's comfort. The dying patient who is experiencing pain will need analgesics, but the effectiveness of the analgesics may be enhanced by alternative measures. These measures will need to be individualized for each patient according to their personal response. The dying patient's thermoregulation may be altered.

Evaluation

• Comfort and pain relief provided for Dave.
• Presence of parents supports Dave until his death.

Expected Outcomes

• Parents verbalize feelings and fears.
• Parents provide physical care and support for Dave.
• Parents discuss with Dave the fact that they will not abandon him.
• Parents identify some of the typical concerns and fears of the surviving sibling.

Change in Status: Dave's condition deteriorates. The sister is brought to the hospital. Dave subsequently dies.

4. Anxiety: acute grief, death of a child Supporting Data: • Mother crying and saying "Oh no, please no" • Father crying and shaking his head no • Parents trying to cradle dead child in their arms	Assign one nurse to stay with parents and one with the sister to assess their needs, while another nurse notifies physician Discontinue IV and other equipment after child is pronounced dead. Clean the child's body of any soiling from body fluids.	Family should not be left alone until they want to be. One nurse should support sibling as parents cannot be expected to at this time. Family should have as peaceful as possible last image of their child.

(Continued)

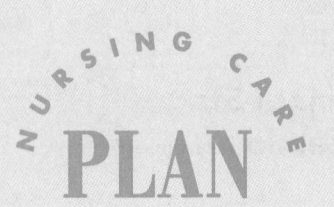

A 15-Year-Old Boy in Terminal Stage of Acute Lymphocytic Leukemia (continued)

Nursing Diagnosis	*Intervention*	*Rationale*
• Parents stating they want to stay with child "a little longer" • Sister appears fearful and is crying quietly	Assess parents' wishes regarding holding their child and being left alone with the child.	Assessment is necessary because each family may have different desires.
	Provide parents with telephone to make calls or offer to make calls for them.	Assisting parents with necessary tasks provides additional instrumental support through a difficult experience.
	Arrange for transport to the morgue after the child has been viewed by family.	
	Assist parents in gathering together child's belongings.	
	Provide parents with telephone numbers for appropriate people to provide aftercare (e.g., hospital staff, clergy, support group).	Support indicates that nursing care continues even after the child's death.

Evaluation

• Parents' desire to be with their son was met.
• Support from staff, family, friends, and clergy was available.

Expected Outcomes

• Parents state appreciation of support provided them during the postdeath experience.
• Sibling discusses her grief and needs with support person.

rocking the child. Sensing that they would like to be alone with their child, the nurse asked them. The mother replied, "No, please don't go yet." Within 3 minutes, the mother looked at the nurse and said, "I'm OK now. I would like to be alone with him for awhile, thank you." Later the mother came out of the room and said that she had been too frightened to be alone at first and appreciated the nurse's presence until she was more comfortable. Without directly asking, the nurse would have had difficulty in knowing just what the parents' desires were. It is better to ask than to try to guess.

The child's body should not be whisked out of the room immediately after death. Many times parents want a second visit or other family members may be on their way to the hospital to see the child. If necessary, the nurse should clean the body and disconnect medical equipment calmly, but quickly. Whatever the circumstances, it is important for the family that their last visual image of the child be one of peace.

Home Care for the Dying Child

When a child is in a terminal phase, and there is no hope for cure-oriented medical treatment, the family undergoes several stressors: the repeated separations of the family due to hospitalization of the child, a sense of loss of control over the family and life's events, additional nonmedical expenses, and a general sense of helplessness.[2] Providing home care for the terminally ill child has been studied as a possible way of assisting the family to cope with these stressors.

Martinson conducted a longitudinal study to provide home care for a child with cancer, which has become the model for home care programs.[23,26] In this project, terminally ill children were returned to their homes with the family acting as primary care providers and the home-care nurse functioning as the major source of direction for that care. Some of the benefits of home care are psychosocial rewards for both the parents and the child when the parents are the care givers. The children are relieved to be at home with their families, familiar furnishings, favorite foods, and the company of their siblings, friends, and pets. The study also found that there were some additional stressors for the family caring for a child in their own home. There were considerable changes in family roles and relationships, nursing skills to be learned, informational needs, additional expenses not covered by insurance, and possible loss of support from familiar hospital personnel. The availability of the home-care nurse 24 hours a day helped to offset many of these problems, while enhancing the family's ability to cope with the death. The home-care nurse provides needed psychosocial support and material resources during the terminal phase and after death.

In subsequent studies of home care for dying children, the family's psychosocial adjustment following the death of the child at home was compared to family adjustment following a child's death in the hospital.[16,17,29] Families participating in home care displayed significantly less psychosocial sequelae and a more positive adjustment sooner than the hospitalized children's families. Additional research is needed to see if different family characteristics make some families more amenable to home care than others.[22,29]

The salient contribution of home care is that, although it does not protect the family from the inevitable pain, the family can experience the sorrow fully. Furthermore, the family regains a sense of control and experiences feelings of usefulness. The parents, siblings, and extended family contribute to the well-being of the dying child and are available to each other for support.[2]

Physical Care of the Dying Child

The physical needs of a dying child vary considerably in accordance with the child's age, diagnosis, course of disease, complications from disease or treatment, type of nursing procedures used, level of consciousness, and amount of pain. This discussion does not detail pain management interventions, care of the unconscious child, or other nursing care issues that may be similar to other acutely ill children, but it explores some of the sensory responses common to the dying state. It must be remembered that no two children will experience the exact sensations nor have the same care needs. The following are suggestions that may be used for a specific child only after a thorough assessment of that child's condition.

Sense of Touch. Dying children may have an exaggerated sense of touch. Bed linens and blankets may feel unusually heavy. Although some children will be comforted by a gentle massage or light sensory stimulation, other children complain that any amount of touching increases their pain or causes discomfort. Asking the conscious child about alterations in sense of touch or observing the semiconscious child's behaviors are essential components of the nursing assessment.

Sense of Vision. Although actual visual acuity rarely is affected, many children find bright daylight or artificial lights distressing. Dimming the lights and pulling the curtains or blinds may make the room more comfortable for the child. If the room is dim and the nurse needs light to perform a task, a flashlight may be more comforting than turning on overhead lights. Nurses should be sensitive to the child's needs, however, and should not shine the flashlight directly at the child or in his or her eyes. The eyes may become sunken, bulging, or glazed.[27] A damp cloth over the eyes may provide needed moisture and may be more comfortable.

Sense of Smell. Very few children experience any unusual or heightened olfactory stimulation. Occasionally a child may complain that perfumes are noxious, however. Nurses and the child's parents may need to avoid wearing perfumes if this is the case.

Sense of Taste. Some dying children state that foods and fluids seem bland. Exactly what relation this has to the dying state rather than to their disease or weakened condition is unclear. Certainly if the child expresses a preference or an aversion for a specific food or fluid, their wishes should be respected.

Sense of Hearing. Even though speech may be difficult for the child and the family may have trouble understanding what is said, the child often is able to understand what is said. The sense of hearing is believed to be the last sense to go in the unconscious or comatose patient. There have even been reports of patients hearing operating room conversations while they were under general anesthesia. Although there is no way to determine if the semiconscious or even comatose dying patient can hear, the accepted nursing principle is to assume that the patient can hear. For this reason, conversations held at the child's bedside, in the room, or at the doorway should not cause any additional distress to the child. Family members should be encouraged to continue talking to the dying child. When a nurse entered a room and overheard a father talking to his unconscious son, the father became embarrassed and apologized for his "strange" behavior. The nurse reassured him by explaining that his son's sense of hearing may still be intact. The father was greatly relieved and said, "I just want to tell him I love him one more time." Simply being able to express their love to the child may be instrumental in the family's long-term adjustment to the death.

Sensations of Heat and Cold. The child's thermoregulation may be altered due to decreased circulation during the terminal stage. Often the child's body may be cool or even cold to touch with a subnormal temperature, and yet the child may complain of feeling warm or hot. The child's body may be covered with a damp perspiration.[27] The sensation of warmth may be so great that the child refuses bed linens and clothing. The child may even request a fan for additional air circulation. Unless there is some compelling reason not to, the child's wishes should be respected. Feeling the child's cold skin may be particularly upsetting to the family until the nurse explains this phenomenon.

Gastrointestinal Alterations. As death approaches, normal gastrointestinal movements slow down. Swallowing may become difficult, resulting in a buildup of oral secretions in the mouth and pharynx. These secretions may cause a gurgling sound in the throat, sometimes referred to as a "death rattle." Although these secretions do not appear to cause discomfort for the child, the family often is distressed by this. Positioning the child on the side or suctioning may be helpful.[27]

Respiratory Alterations. As death approaches, the rate and depth of respirations change, often displaying a Cheyne-Stokes pattern. The child experiencing dyspnea may be helped by positioning him or her in a semi-

Fowler's position or being held in the parents lap or arms. Oxygen administration may be necessary for the child experiencing "air hunger."[27]

The Grief Process

Loss

Grief is the normal psychological reaction to loss. There is an endless variety of losses. For example, one may suffer the loss of a body part or function, a social position, a love relationship, or an actual love object. Grief may be in anticipation of a loss or in relation to the actual loss. Whether the loss is perceived only by the individual experiencing it or also by others, it is no less real or painful for the individual. The nurse's empathetic response comes from identifying and accepting the personal meanings attached to the individual's loss.

Grief Symptoms

In the early 1940s, Lindemann studied the responses of people grieving the loss of a loved one.[20] He identified somatic and psychological symptoms that appeared to be characteristics of normal grief and identified symptoms of abnormal or "morbid grief." The accompanying display summarizes Lindemann's symptomatology of normal grief. These findings have important implications for nurses. By understanding the process of grieving, nurses can support the bereaved and facilitate a healthy resolution of grief. The bereaved often seek medical care, thinking that these normal symptoms are an indication that something is terribly wrong with them. Nurses can teach grievers the normal symptoms and can identify morbid symptoms for prompt psychiatric attention.

When the bereaved are the parents of a child, the normal symptoms of grief frequently cause additional problems. For example, if a man's wife dies suddenly in an automobile accident or after a long treatment for breast cancer, the husband might feel guilty for not buying new tires sooner or for not finding better medical care for her. He may need reassurance that he did all he could do, but ultimately he knows that he was not totally responsible for his wife's well-being. However, when a child dies, parents feel tremendous guilt because one of the expected roles of a parent is to protect the child from harm. Another area that is particularly difficult with the loss of child involves the need for support. If the wife were to lose an uncle, the husband usually is not as emotionally close to her relative as she is, so he can be supportive for her in her grieving. When it is their own child who dies, however, *both* the husband and wife are feeling tremendous grief and in need of support from each other. They need love, warmth, understanding, and support from each other at a time when each person is likely to have the least emotional energy. As one father aptly said, "You ask me to hold you up when I can't even hold myself up."

A third problem when parents are grievers is that they may not understand the differences in each other's grieving behavior. One parent may cry publicly while the other cries only in private. One wants to be with family and friends while the other wants to be alone. One may need to talk at a time when it is too painful for the other to talk or even listen. If the parents cannot talk about these differences, it can lead to significant problems in the marital relationship. Nurses have the real potential for supporting the parents in their grieving process, so they can grow together as a couple, rather than apart.

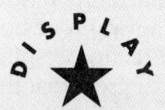

Lindemann's Normal Grief Symptoms

Physical Sensations

Tightness in the throat, sensation of choking, shortness of breath, sighing, empty feeling in abdomen, muscle weakness, intense distress described as mental pain or tension

Preoccupation With Deceased

Sees, hears, or imagines presence of dead person; sense of unreality; sense of emotional isolation from others; believes survivor is going insane

Guilt Feelings

Explores for ways of preventing death, accuses self of negligence, or minor omissions

Hostile Feelings

Irritability, anger, lack of warmth towards others, wanting to be left alone and not be bothered by others

Change in Control Pattern

Restless, unable to sit still, purposelessness moving about, searching for something to do, unable to start or maintain organized activity patterns

Data from Lindemann, E. (1944). Symptomatology and management of acute grief. American Journal of Psychiatry, 101, 141–148.

Research indicates that there is more intense symptomatology and sequelae for parents when a child dies than when a spouse or parent dies.[24,25,34] Furthermore, bereaved parents show significantly more psychological symptoms than normal, nonpatient adults and even adult psychiatric outpatients.[28] Bereaved parents may experience somatization; depression; anger; guilt; despair; marital, sleeping, and drinking problems; appetite changes; overwhelming sadness; and increased irritability.

Phases of Grieving

It was once felt that normal grief should last only a certain amount of time. Lindemann felt that normal grief should be resolved within 4 to 6 weeks.[20] Other studies of the bereaved do not confirm this, however.[4] Glick, Weiss, and Parkes[9] describe three phases of the grieving process. The first phase is from the time of death and usually lasts until several weeks after the burial. During this time, the bereaved usually have feelings of numbness, emptiness, disbelief, and profound sorrow. The second phase begins several weeks after the funeral and lasts for about 1 year. In the early part of this phase, there is frequently an obsessional review of the death, a searching for the meaning of death, and a yearning or even searching for the deceased. Usually within a few months of the death, the individual starts reorganizing life goals and activities, and functional stability returns. The second year is the beginning of the recovery or third phase. During this phase, full social functioning is resumed. Full social functioning does not imply that the bereaved will not experience times of sadness or loneliness for the lost child, but rather that those times do not significantly interfere with social functioning.

Schmidt[38] identifies three general principles in working with bereaved parents. *Principle one: Grief is a universal human phenomenon that is experienced in highly unique and individual ways.* Although grief is a universal phenomenon, like fingerprints, no two people will grieve exactly alike. Nurses must recognize this and allow for individual differences.

Principle two: Allow as much grief to be expressed at the moment as the parent is able and willing to express. Nurses working with bereaved parents must allow the parents to express what they want, when they want. The nurse must be comfortable with silence, nonstop talking, emotional outbursts, and the entirety of human emotional responses.

Principle three: Grief has its own natural timing. The nurse must recognize that grief will not follow a "textbook example" of what will happen and when. Based on clinical experience of working with bereaved parents, Schmidt has found that, in general, the first 2 months are filled with initial shock. As the shock wears off, it is replaced with constant pain between about 2 and 6 months. Somewhere between about 6 and 8 months after the death, parents hit a new low. Schmidt believes that this is the result of inadequate coping strategies. In effect, parents have no experience coping with anything even remotely similar to the loss of their child.

Table 32-5 provides examples from five patterns of

TABLE 32-5
Nursing Interventions: Working With Bereaved Parents

Functional Health	Nursing Interventions
Cognition and Perception	
Help them to accept the reality of the loss. "It's not real. It can't be true."	Talk about the child—what happened, how they found out, what they felt, the nightmare qualities as well as special memories.
Self-Perception and Self-Concept	
Assure them that they can survive the loss. "How can I continue to live without my child?"	Listen without suggesting answers. Assess suicidal thoughts. Later, explore strengths and remaining hopes for the future.
Coping and Stress Tolerance	
Help them identify and express feelings: anger, guilt, sadness, etc.	Because pain cannot be denied or avoided, help them identify and express feelings to achieve resolution. Talking, writing and activities can all be used to express emotions.
Interpret feelings and behaviors to resolve confusion. "I can't concentrate." "I think I'm losing my mind."	Assure parents that they are not losing their minds. Grief causes emotional and cognitive confusion. Parents are frightened because they can't make simple decisions.
Role and Relationships	
Find sources of continuing support. "Others cannot take away the pain, but they can share it."	Provide support during the most difficult times and refer to other sources of support (books and support groups of other bereaved parents).
Values and Beliefs	
Interpret "recovery" for them. "Incorporating the loss into their lives so they can go on living."	Reassure them that the pain will decrease first in frequency, then in intensity. Recovery takes time—much more than friends or nonexperienced professionals think.

function and their corresponding nursing interventions for working with bereaved parents. While there is still a tremendous need for additional research on the grieving process, especially with a child's death, it must be emphasized that there can be considerable variation in both the style and duration of normal grief. It also should be noted that very little research has been done on the grief process for siblings in different developmental stages.

Spiritual Needs

For the Child

When a child has a life-threatening disease, spiritual needs often are heightened. Fish and Shelly proposed three spiritual needs that correlate with children's developmental stages.[6] The first is the *need for love and relatedness* that corresponds to Erikson's stage of trust. The need for *forgiveness* appears next and parallels the child's moral development and Erikson's stages of initiative verses guilt and industry verses inferiority. It is important for the nurse to be aware of the child's need to be forgiven, even for seemingly minor transgressions. The third need is for *meaning and purpose*, which develops in early adolescence approximating the stage of identity versus role confusion. The adolescent facing death needs help in identifying attainable goals with personal meaning rather than focusing on lofty goals that could only be attained throughout a long lifetime. Recognition for actual contributions made in the lives of loved ones is more important than grandiose plans for a future that may never be.

For the Parents

Parents of seriously ill children can experience any number of spiritual needs. Because parents often have guilt feelings for their child's disease or accident, the need for forgiveness often is great. They may need to be forgiven by their spouse, family, friends, or God. Without knowing that they are forgiven, parents may lose hope, lack trust, and feel unloved. These feelings can interfere with their ability to support and love other members of the family and the ill child. If unresolved, long-standing depression may result.

Nursing Assessment

Nurses need to make a conscious assessment of the spiritual needs of the patient and family. The sources for data collection of spiritual needs include the medical chart, direct observation, other team members' observations, and specific questioning.[41] Knowing the family's religion is not enough. Nurses should assess how important religion and prayer are to the family and to whom they turn in times of need. If the family attends church, data about how involved they are and information about members of the congregation could be sources for potential social support. Parents and children may send nonverbal clues about spiritual beliefs and needs through body language, behaviors, types of reading material, radio or television programs, type of greeting cards, and even who the hospital visitors are.

Verbal clues may overtly indicate spiritual needs or actual requests for spiritual assistance. More often, they are covert messages of concern. Passing statements about beliefs and spiritual struggles frequently are made as a test to see if the nurse is willing to discuss spiritual matters. Statements like, "I don't understand how God can do this to an innocent child" can be made to test the nurse's response. The nurse who is uncomfortable discussing spiritual issues may ignore the statement or make a brief response and leave the room. An accurate assessment of the family's spiritual needs, however, requires that the nurse further explore the individual's statement. The nurse could respond by saying something like, "Yes, it seems so unfair. How has this illness changed the way you think or feel about God?" Remember that people are more likely to share deep concerns in a private, relaxed atmosphere with an empathetic listener than when they feel the constraints of time or uneasiness. In any event, nurses do not have to have the answers to the person's questions, but they should impart a genuine concern.

Rabbi Kushner[15] discusses the frequently asked question of "Why do good people suffer?" The argument, which is equally valid for most Judeo-Christian faiths, concludes by stating that sometimes there is no reason and the rest of the time the reason is known only to God. Kushner believes that asking "why" questions usually results in a sense of abandonment and isolation from God. By changing from an unanswerable question of "why" to

Ideas for Nursing Research

Families experiencing the death of a child experience many emotions and responses. The child health nurse has a unique opportunity to work with these children and their families from diagnosis through death. Exploratory, correlational, and experimental studies can be conducted to assist health care professionals in understanding their roles in helping families during these critical times. The following areas need to be explored:

- Nursing behaviors/interventions that nurses identify as facilitating coping compared to nursing behaviors/interventions that family members identify as facilitating coping.
- Identification of demographic or personality characteristics (factors) common to people who adapt (successfully or positively cope) to the death of a child and factors common to people who do not adapt.
- Correlate nursing strategies with adaptive and maladaptive outcomes with families facing life-threatening illnesses.
- Effectiveness of different modes of teaching plans for common problem areas (e.g., discipline, school concerns, sibling needs, marital concerns) for the family facing a life-threatening illness.

a statement of "when bad things happen to good people," feelings of frustration, guilt, and isolation give way to feelings of support and love.

Role of the Clergy

The child or family may expressly request that a priest, rabbi, minister, or religious leader be summoned. If they do not have one of their own, most hospitals have lists of community clergy representatives who are willing to come to the hospital on an on-call basis. When a direct request is not made, it is entirely fitting for the nurse to inform the child or family that such services are available. Once the clergy has arrived, the nurse should arrange for privacy and ask if there is anything else that they need.

Summary

Today's health care professionals are examining their attitudes toward death, the dying, and support of families involved in the dying process. In family-centered care, the needs of all, including siblings and extended family members, are considered. Physical, psychosocial, and spiritual needs are assessed and met.

Because each person is unique and families differ, there is no standard form of intervention, but each family must be assessed for its particular needs. Such an approach includes developmental considerations, personal awareness of death and dying, past experiences, and the present stage of dying. The latter have been described by Kübler-Ross as denial, anger, bargaining, depression, and acceptance.

A normal death trajectory in a serious illness involves diagnosis and induction, remission, maintenance, cessation of therapy, relapse, terminal stage, and death and postdeath. There also are salient differences between expected and unexpected death.

The physical needs of dying children vary considerably, but some sensory responses are common to all dying children. Spiritual needs often are heightened as children and families are aware of approaching death. The nurse's assessment should include these needs.

References

1. Bluebond-Langner, M. (1978). *The private worlds of dying children*. Princeton: Princeton University Press.
2. Carlson, P., Simacek, M., & Martinson, I. (1985). Helping parents cope: A model home-care program for the dying child. *Issues in Comprehensive Pediatric Nursing, 8*, 1–6, 113–127.
3. Davidson, G. W. (1985). Stillbirth, neonatal death, and sudden infant death syndrome. *Issues in Comprehensive Pediatric Nursing, 8*, 1–6, 243–257.
4. Diamond, M. (1981). Bereavement and the elderly: A critical review with implications for nursing practice and research. *Journal of Advanced Nursing, 6*, 461–470.
5. Evans, A. E., & Edin, S. (1968). If a child must die. . . *New England Journal of Medicine, 278*(3), 138–142.
6. Fish, S., & Shelly, J. A. (1978). *Spiritual care: The nurse's role*. Downers' Grove, IL: InterVarsity Press.
7. Gartley, W., & Bernasconi, M. (1967). The concept of death in children. *Journal of General Psychology, 110*, 71–85.
8. Glaser, B. G., & Strauss, A. L. (1965). *Awareness of Dying*. London: Weidenfeld and Nicolson.
9. Glick, I., Weiss, R. S., & Parkes, C. M. (1974). *The first year of bereavement*. New York: John Wiley and Sons.
10. Hall, M., Hardin, K., & Conaster, C. (1982). The challenges of psychosocial care. In D. Foctman & G. Foley (Eds.), *Nursing care of the child with cancer* (pp. 317–353). Boston: Little, Brown.
11. Irwin, C. (1986). The dying child. *Nurs RSA Verpleging, 1*(8), 24–25, 39, 42.
12. Koocher, G. P. (1974). Talking to children about death. *American Journal of Orthopsychiatry, 44*, 404–411.
13. Kramer, R. S. (1981). Living with childhood cancer: Healthy siblings' perspective. *Issues in Comprehensive Pediatric Nursing, 5*, 155–65.
14. Kübler-Ross, E. (1965). *On death and dying*. London: Weidenfeld and Nicolson.
15. Kushner, H. S. (1981). *When bad things happen to good people*. New York: Avon Books.
16. Lauer, M., & Camitta, B. (1980). Home care for dying children: A nursing model. *Journal of Pediatrics, 97*(6), 1032–1035.
17. Lauer, M., Muchern, R., Wallskog, J., & Camitta, B. (1983). A comparison study of parental adaptation following a child's death at home or in the hospital. *Pediatrics, 71*(1), 107–112.
18. Lazarus, R. (1981). The costs and benefits of denial. In J. Spinetta & P. Deasy-Spinetta (Eds.), *Living with childhood cancer* (pp. 50–67). St Louis: CV Mosby.
19. Leyn, R. (1976). Terminally ill children and their families: A study of the variety of responses to fatal illness. *Maternal-Child Nursing Journal, 5*, 179–188.
20. Lindemann, E. (1944). Symptomatology and management of acute grief. *American Journal of Psychiatry, 101*, 141–148.
21. Lonetto, R. (1980). *Children's concepts of death*. New York: Springer.
22. Martinson, I. M. (1987). The feasibility of home care for the child dying with cancer. In T. Krulik, T. B. Holaday, & I. M. Martinson (Eds.), *The Child and Family Facing Life-Threatening Illness* (pp. 313–326). Philadelphia: JB Lippincott.
23. Martinson, I. M., Armstrong, G. D., Geis, D. P., Anglim, M. A., Gronseth, E. C., MacInnis, H., Kersey, J. H., & Nesbit, M. E. (1978). Home care for children dying of cancer. *Pediatrics, 62*(1), 106–113.
24. Miles, M. (1984). Helping adults mourn the death of a child. In H. Wass & C. Carr (Eds.), *Children and death* (pp. 219–241). New York: Hemisphere.
25. Miles, M. (1985). Emotional symptoms and physical health in bereaved parents. *Nursing Research, 34*(2), 76–81.
26. Moldow, D. G., & Martinson, I. M. (1980). From research to reality—Home care for the dying child. *MCN American Journal of Maternal Child Nursing, 5*, 159–160, 162, 166.
27. Moldow, D. G., & Martinson, I. M. (1984). *Home care for seriously ill children: A model for parents*. Alexandria, VA: Children's Hospice International.
28. Moore, I. M., Gillias, C. L., & Martinson, I. M. (1988). Psychosomatic symptoms in parents 2 years after the death of a child with cancer. *Nursing Research, 37*(2), 104–107.
29. Mulhern, B., Lauer, M., & Hoffman, R. (1983). Death of a child at home or in the hospital: Subsequent psychological adjustment of the family. *Pediatrics, 71*(5), 743–747.
30. Murray, G., & Jampolsky, G. (Eds.). (1982). *Straight from the siblings: Another look at the rainbow*. Millbrae, CA: Celestrial Arts.
31. Nagy, M. (1948). The child's theories concerning death. *Journal of General Psychology, 73*, 3–27.
32. National Center for Health Statistics. (1988). *Vital statistics of the United States, 1985, Vol II*. Hyattsville, MD: United States Department of Health and Human Services.
33. O'Malley, G. E., Koocher, G., Foster, D., & Slavin, L. (1979).

Psychiatric sequelae of surviving childhood cancer. *American Journal of Orthopsychiatry, 49,* 608–616.

34. Owen, G. (1982–1983). Death at a distance: A study of family survivors. *Omega, 13,* 191–224.

35. Petix, M. (1987). Explaining death to school-age children. *Pediatric Nursing, 13*(6), 394–396.

36. Raimbault, G. (1981). Children talk about death. *Acta Paediatrica Scandinavica, 70,* 179–182.

37. Reilly, T. P., Hasazi, G. E., & Bond, L. A. (1983). Children's concepts of death and personal mortality. *Journal of Pediatric Psychology, 8,* 21–31.

38. Schmidt, L. (1987). Working with bereaved parents. In T. Krulik, B. Holaday, & I. M. Martinson (Eds.), *The child and family facing life-threatening illness* (pp. 327–344). Philadelphia: JB Lippincott.

39. Shneidman, E. S. (1976). *Death: Current perspectives.* Palo Alto CA: Mayfield Publishing.

40. Spinetta, J., Riglor, D., & Karon, M. (1972). Personal space as a measure of a dying child's sense of isolation. *Journal of Consulting and Clinical Psychology, 42*(6), 751–756.

40a. Spinetta, J. J. (1981). The siblings of the child with cancer. In J. J. Spinetta and P. Deasy-Spinetta (eds), *Living with childhood cancer* (pp. 133–141). St. Louis: CV Mosby.

41. Still, J. (1984). How to assess spiritual needs of children and their families. *Journal of Christian Nursing, 1*(1), 4–6.

42. Taylor, S. (1980). The effect of chronic childhood illnesses upon well siblings. *Maternal-Child Nursing Journal, 9,* 109–116.

43. Wadsworth, B. J. (1971). *Piaget's theory of cognitive development.* New York: Longman.

44. Waechter, E. H. (1971). Children's awareness of fatal illness. *American Journal of Nursing, 71,* 1168–1172.

45. Waechter, E. H. (1987). How families cope: Assessing and intervening. In T. Krulik, B. Holaday, & I. M. Martinson (Eds.), *The child and family facing life-threatening illness* (pp. 239–245). Philadelphia: JB Lippincott.

46. Waechter, E. H. Working with parents of children with life-threatening illness. In T. Krulik, B. Holaday, & I. M. Martinson (Eds.), *The child and family facing life-threatening illness.* Philadelphia: JB Lippincott.

47. Walker, C. L. (1988). Stress and coping in siblings of childhood cancer patients. *Nursing Research, 37*(4), 208–212.

48. Walker, C. L., Wells, L. (1990). Siblings of Children with Cancer. *Oncology Nursing Forum, 17*(3), 355–360.

49. Walker, C. L., Wells, L., Heiney, S. P., Hymovich, D., & Weekas, D. (in press). Challenges of psychosocial care. In D. Fotchman, G. Foley, and K. Mooney (eds). *Nursing Care of the Child with Cancer.* (2nd ed.) Philadelphia: W.B. Saunders.

50. Wass, H. (1985). Concepts of death: A developmental perspective. *Issues in Comprehensive Pediatric Nursing, 8*(1–6), 3–24.

51. Wass, H., & Cason, L. (1985). Fears and anxieties about death. *Issues in Comprehensive Nursing, 8*(1–6), 25–45.

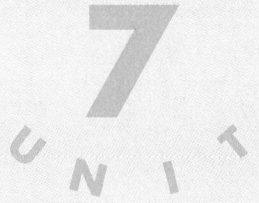

7 UNIT

Nursing Care of Children With Altered Head and Neck Function

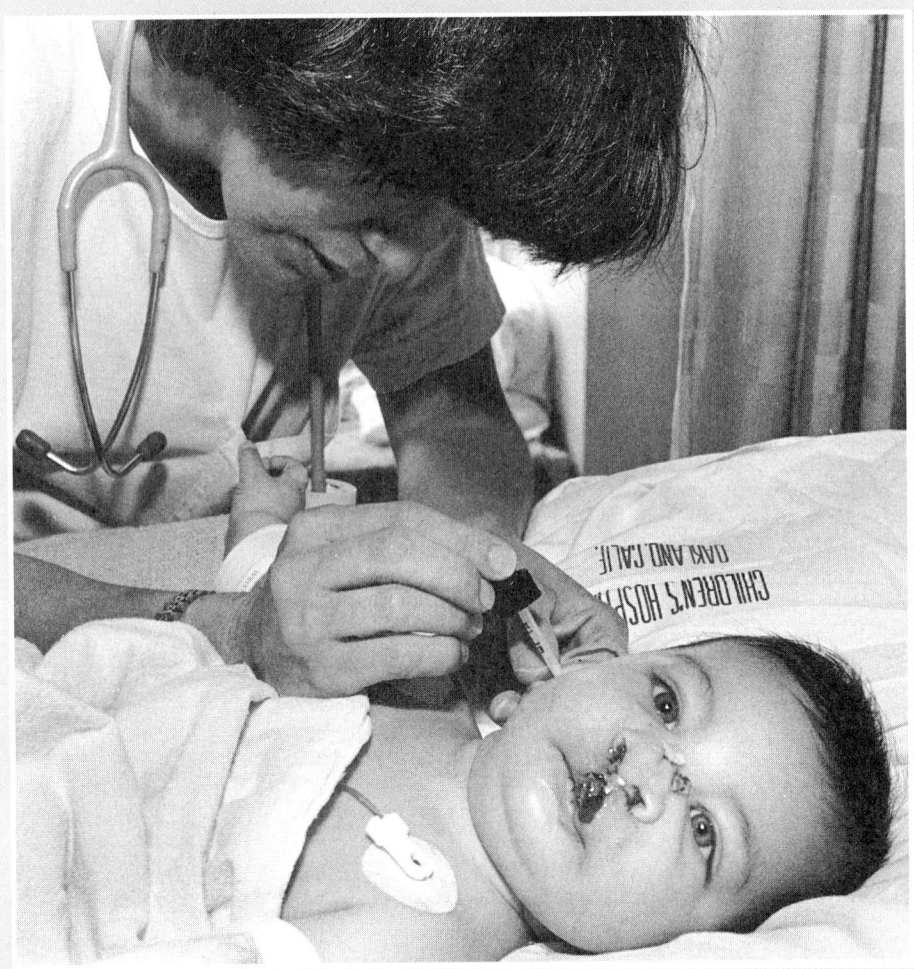

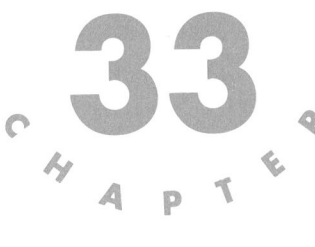

Anatomy and Physiology of the Head and Neck

BEHAVIORAL OBJECTIVES

Identify the predominant anatomic features of the head and neck.

Explain the embryogenesis of major structures in the head and neck.

Identify common abnormalities resulting from fetal maldevelopment of structures in the head and neck.

Discuss the primary functions of structures in the head and neck.

The head and neck region is a composite of highly complex and specialized tissues that are critical to a child's very existence. Four of the primary bodily senses—hearing, vision, smell, and taste—are elicited from organs located within the head. Furthermore, the external features of the head and face are unique to the individual with endless variations dependent on genetic and environmental influences. The placement and characteristics of these features help determine the child's self-concept and social acceptance. No body function escapes the influence of structures within the head and neck.

Knowledge of the anatomic and physiologic mechanisms of the head and neck structures is fundamental to accurate assessment and recognition of anomalies in children. This chapter reviews the embryonic development, structure, and function of major sensory organs, facial features, and the oral cavity. The brain and neuroendocrine functioning and the oropharynx's place in digestive and respiratory function are discussed elsewhere in the text.

Embryonic Development

Branchial Apparatus

In the human embryo, neural crest cells (derived from neuroectodermal cells involved in forming the neural tube) begin to migrate into the head and neck region around the fourth week of gestation. These cells initiate the development of six branchial arches, small ridges separated by distinct grooves.[2] Figure 33-1 elaborates on the branchial apparatus and identifies the subsequent structures that are formed through embryonic growth and development.

787

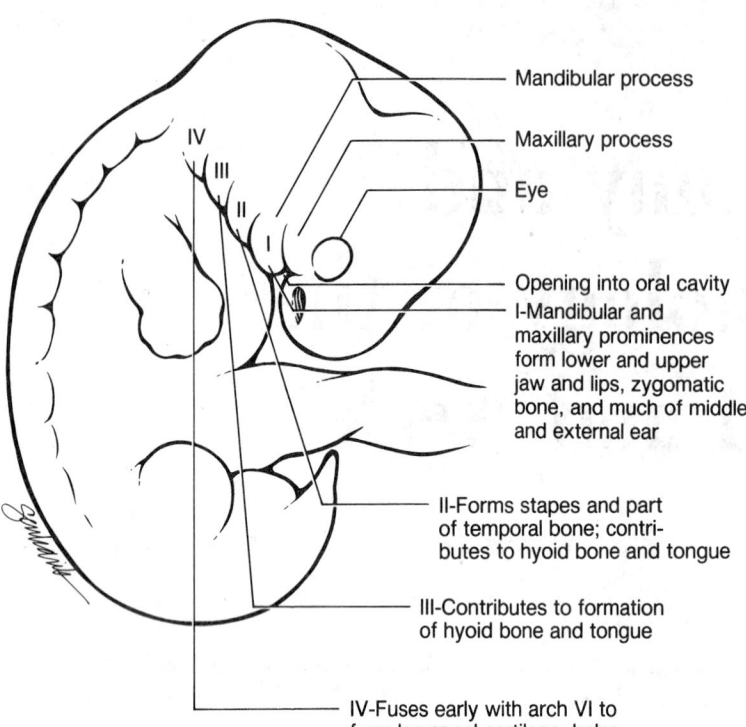

Mandibular process

Maxillary process

Eye

Opening into oral cavity

I-Mandibular and maxillary prominences form lower and upper jaw and lips, zygomatic bone, and much of middle and external ear

II-Forms stapes and part of temporal bone; contributes to hyoid bone and tongue

III-Contributes to formation of hyoid bone and tongue

IV-Fuses early with arch VI to form laryngeal cartilage; helps form tongue

FIGURE 33-1

The brachial apparatus and its derivatives. At 6 weeks, four of the six original arches can be identified as rudiments of head structures. (Arch V contributes to no definitive adult structure.)

The primitive pharynx originates from the foregut, an invagination of the yolk sac into the cranial end of the embryo. It is wide superiorly and narrow inferiorly. The endoderm of the pharynx adheres to the internal surfaces of the branchial arches and forms areas called pharyngeal pouches between the branchial arches. There are four pairs of these outgrowths in the pharyngeal wall. The first pouch forms the tympanic cavity and the mastoid antrum, which eventually coalesce to form the auditory or pharyngotympanic tube. The endodermal lining of the second pouch forms buds that develop into tonsillar crypts and eventually create the intratonsillar cleft or fossa. The third pouch is the predecessor to the inferior parathyroid gland and the thymus, and the fourth pouch develops into the superior parathyroid gland and the perifollicular cells of the thyroid gland.

Branchial membranes form in the developing embryo between the epithelia of the branchial groove and its paired pharyngeal pouch. Most of the branchial membranes disappear as mesoderm fills in between the endoderm of the pharyngeal pouches and the ectoderm of the branchial grooves. However, the first branchial membrane along with its mesodermal layer persists as the tympanic membrane.

The tongue appears in the fourth week of gestation from a medial tongue bud located on the floor of the pharynx. Next, two distal tongue buds develop, which soon fuse and override the medial tongue bud to form the anterior two thirds or oral part of the tongue. The posterior one third of the tongue is derived from parts of the second, third, and fourth branchial arches.

Tooth development arises from the ectodermal and mesodermal layers. At 6 weeks' gestation, the primary stage of deciduous (or first) tooth formation occurs with early tooth bud maturation. The root of the tooth forms after the crown is almost formed, but root development is not completed until after the tooth erupts. Primordia of permanent teeth that will eventually replace the deciduous teeth develop under the gum near the pulp of the existing teeth. Figure 33-2 illustrates the intricate layers of developing teeth.

Development of the palate begins at the end of the 5th week but is not finished until the 12th week of gestation.[7] The innermost portion of the intermaxillary segment of the maxilla prompts the formation of the primary palate or median palatine process. The secondary palate derives from the palatine processes, which are two projections extending from the maxillary prominences. With development of the jaw, the tongue drops downward in the oral cavity allowing the palatine processes to grow toward one another. These processes eventually fuse with each other and with the primary palate and nasal septum (Fig. 33-3).

Actual fusion of the palatal processes begins in the 9th week and ends in the 12th week of gestation. The palate fuses from front to back with the uvula being the last structure to form. The hard palate is comprised of the primary palate, the lateral palatine bones, and the lateral palatine processes, which all become ossified with time. The soft palate comes from the posterior part of the lateral palatine processes, which fuse together but do not make a bony structure out of this portion of the palate. The uvula is located medially in the most posterior portion of the palate and is adjacent to the soft palate.

Some of the paranasal sinuses develop late in fetal life. Small maxillary sinuses and a few ethmoidal cells are present in the neonate. Most of the growth and development of paranasal sinuses occur after birth and will be discussed later in the chapter.

The origins of the nose and other facial structures

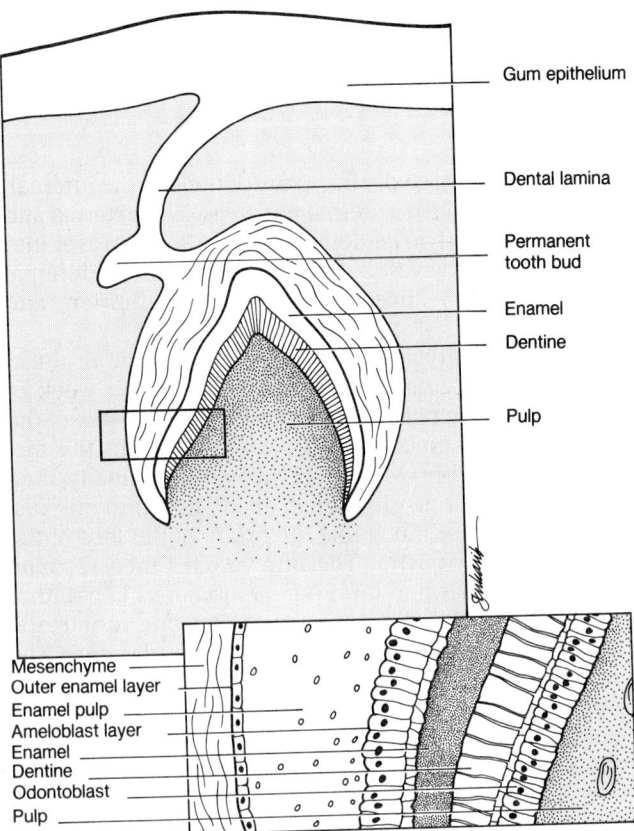

FIGURE 33-2
Developing tooth at 7 months' gestation. Detail in boxed area is sagittal section of gum and jaw.

Eyes

The three embryonic sources involved in the formation of the eyes include the neuroectoderm of the forebrain, the surface ectoderm of the head, and the mesoderm that lies between these layers. In the fourth week of gestation, a pair of optic sulci appear in the neural folds of the embryo at the cranial end. These optic sulci transform into optic vesicles, which project from the forebrain into the mesenchyma. The stems that connect these vesicles to the forebrain develop into the optic stalks, and the vesicles themselves invaginate to form the optic cups. Surface ectoderm next to the optic vesicles transforms into the lens placodes, then invaginates to form lens pits. The edges of these pits eventually merge and lead to the creation of the lens vesicles. As the lens vesicles develop, they lose connection with the ectoderm and lie in the space between the optic cup and the ectoderm. An optic fissure appears along the optic cup and stalk in each developing eye and houses the primitive hyaloid blood vessels and optic nerve. When the edges of the optic fissure fuse, these structures become an integral part of the optic cup and stalk.[7]

The retina derives from the double walls of the optic cup: the outer, thinner layer becomes the retinal pigment epithelium, and the inner thicker layer becomes the neural retina. The space between these two layers is aptly named the intraretinal space and dissipates as the layers fuse. However, this is a fragile bond, and the layers may separate or detach later in life if there is a blow to the eye. The neural retina forms the photoreceptors of the eye, which include the rods, cones, bipolar cells, and ganglion cells. This neural layer of the retina is associated

can be traced from a very early embryonic age (Fig. 33-4). Bilateral thickenings on the surface ectoderm of the frontonasal prominence, called nasal placodes, are soon ringed medially and laterally by elevations referred to as nasal prominences. Together these structures make up the nasal pits. The nasal pits develop into the nasal sacs, which eventually form the nasal cavities. The medial nasal prominences grow together to form an intermaxillary portion of the maxilla. This structure then evolves into the philtrum (the medial groove on the upper lip), the premaxillary portion of the maxilla, the gingiva or gum structures, and the primary palate. The frontonasal prominence also fashions the forehead as well as the dorsum and apex of the nose. The sides of the nose come from the lateral nasal prominences. Most of the major features of the face develop between the fifth and eighth weeks of gestation.[7]

Origins of structures in the neck, including the larynx and thyroid gland, are discussed in Chapters 36 and 54. The cervical lymph system begins to develop in the embryo shortly after the appearance of the primitive cardiovascular systems. Lymph vessels are thought to originate as capillary sprouts from the endothelium of embryonic veins. Early lymph channels are distributed along the main venous trunks, and dilations of these vessels give rise to lymph sacs, most of which become transformed into lymph nodes during the fetal period of development.

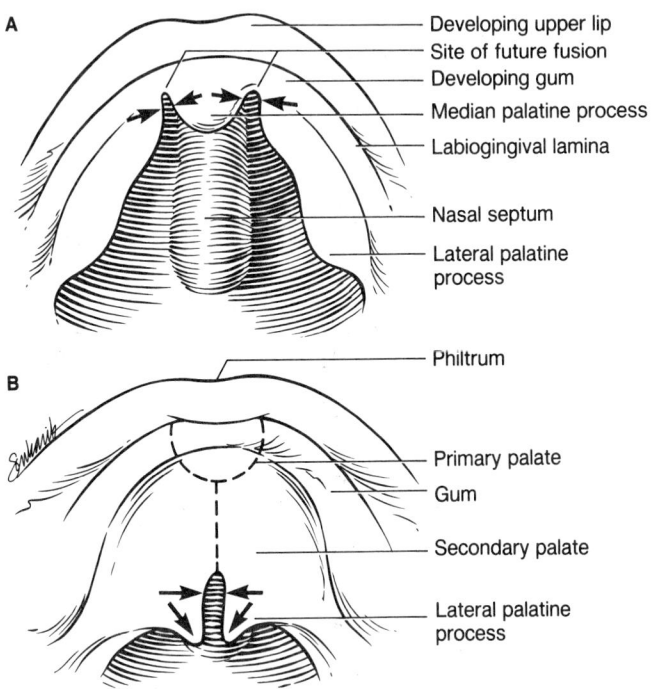

FIGURE 33-3
Development of the palate from 6 (**A**) to 10 (**B**) weeks' gestation. The broken line in **B** indicates the sites of fusion of the palatine processes. The arrows indicate medial and posterior growth of the lateral palatine process.

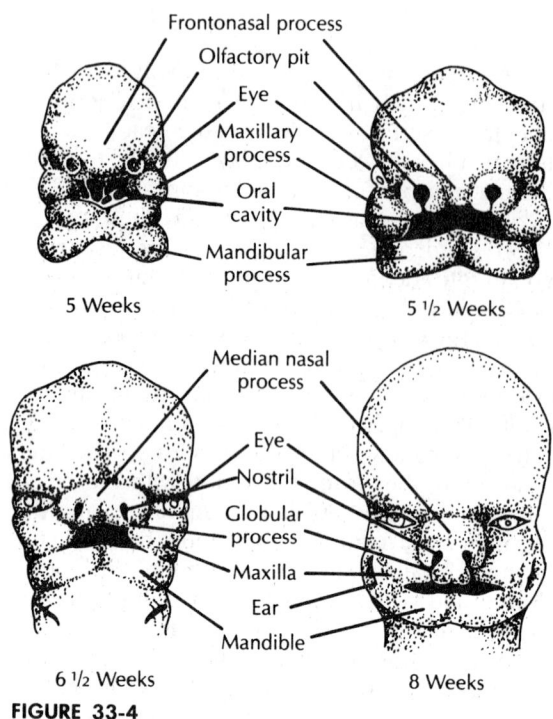

FIGURE 33-4
Development of the face from 5 to 8 weeks' gestation.

closely with the optic stalk and axons of the ganglion cells that comprise the optic nerve.[9]

The ciliary body arises from both layers of the optic cup, the retinal pigment epithelium, and the neural retina. The ciliary muscle, a smooth muscle responsible for focusing the lens, and its connective tissue derive from mesenchyma. The iris arises from the rim of the optic cup, is comprised of both layers of the optic cup, and touches the epithelium of the ciliary body and the pigmented and neural layers of the retina. The iris is bluish in the majority of infants at birth. The amount and variability of chromatophores (pigment-containing cells) in the connective tissue affects the eye color. A greater amount of melanin contributes to the brown color of some irises, and less melanin causes a blue appearance. The eye color becomes definitive in the first few months of life.

The lenses develop from the lens vesicles. The anterior wall of the lens vesicle becomes the anterior epithelium of the lens, and the cells of the posterior wall of the lens vesicle mature into the lens fibers, which eventually replace the remainder of the lens vesicle. The aqueous chambers evolve from mesenchyma while the epithelium of the cornea and the conjunctiva arise from ectoderm.

Mesenchyma surrounding the optic cup differentiates into two layers: an inner vascular layer called the choroid and an outer fibrous layer known as the sclera. The choroid generates cores of ciliary processes, which are primarily capillaries located at the edge of the optic cup. The scleral layer, which surrounds the optic cup, is continuous with the cornea anteriorly. Two surface ectodermal folds with centers of mesenchyma form the eyelids. The primitive eyelids meet and adhere in the 10th week and remain closed until the 26th week of fetal life. When the eyelids reopen, conjunctiva covers the "white" or corneal layer of the eyes and forms the inner surface of the eyelids.[8]

Ears

There are three distinct parts of the ear: the internal, the middle, and the external ear areas. The external and middle ears work in tandem to conduct sound waves into the inner ear. The vestibulocochlear organ of the internal ear performs the major functions of equilibrium and hearing.

The internal ear begins as an otic placode or thickened plate of surface ectoderm in the fourth week of gestation. These placodes are present on each side of the hindbrain (the embryonic structure that forms the medulla, pons, and cerebellum of the brain) originally, then invaginate into otic pits, which finally fuse into otic vesicles or otocysts (much like the origin of the lens of the eye noted previously). The otic vesicles then separate from the ectoderm to form the membranous labyrinth.

There are two distinct areas of each otic vesicle, the dorsal utricular part and the ventral saccular part. The utricular portion develops into the endolymphatic duct and sac, the semicircular duct, the ampulla, and the utricle. The saccular portion is the foundation for the saccule, the cochlear duct, and the cochlea. Cells of the cochlear duct specialize to form the spiral organ of Corti. Portions of the nerves of the spiral ganglion grow toward the spiral organ where they terminate on the hair cells and augment the sense of hearing. Mesenchyma surrounding the otic vesicle leads to formation of the otic capsule. Cartilage arising from the otic capsule develops into the bony labyrinth of the internal ear, and perilymph fluid, made within the otic capsule, encircles the membranous labyrinth.[8]

The structures of the middle ear evolve directly from the branchial apparatus. The tubotympanic recess of the first pharyngeal pouch grows into the tympanic cavity, while the unexpanded portion becomes the auditory tube. Ossification of the cartilages of the first two pairs of branchial arches forms the auditory ossicles: the malleus, the incus, and the stapes. Although the mastoid antrum of the tympanic cavity is present at birth, no mastoid cells are present. The mastoid processes develop during the first 2 years.

Several parts of the external ear also arise from the branchial arches. The external acoustic meatus is a remnant of the dorsal end of the first branchial groove, which is filled with a meatal plug (an accumulation of epithelial cells) during most of pregnancy. Toward the end of pregnancy, these cells die and form the meatus cavity of the external ear. The tympanic membrane develops from the first branchial membrane. Collagenic fibers within the tympanic membrane form from mesenchyma, while the external layer of skin is derived from ectoderm. Endoderm of the tubotympanic recess creates the internal epithelial lining of the tympanic membrane. Six outgrowths called auricular hillocks form around the first branchial groove and lead to the development of the auricle or pinna of the ear. The auricles originally lie in the cranial portion of the embryonic neck and migrate upward as the mandible grows.

Consequences of Abnormal Development

Several different congenital malformations of the head and neck may result from improper development of the branchial apparatus (Table 33-1). First arch syndrome, which is due to the failure of cranial neural crest cells to migrate into the first branchial arch during the fourth week of gestation, is the major abnormality arising from maldevelopment in this area. The two main manifestations of this set of symptoms include Treacher Collins syndrome and Pierre Robin syndrome, both of which are manifested in multiple anomalies of the eyes, ears, mandible, and palate.[8]

A common abnormality of tongue development is ankyloglossia or tongue-tie, in which the frenulum extends to the tip of the tongue and restricts tongue movement.[7]

Cleft lip and cleft palate are anomalies arising from maldevelopment of the face and palate (see Chap. 36).

Eye malformations are most likely to occur 22 to 50 days after fertilization. The majority of these abnormalities are a result of either genetic factors or intrauterine infections. Embryologically, most malformations arise from defects of closure of the optic fissure in the sixth week of gestation. Two of the most common eye defects are congenital cataracts and congenital glaucoma; these and other eye problems are discussed in Chapter 35.

Structure and Function

Head

The bones of the head are comprised of those forming the skull and the face (Fig. 33-5). Seven bones make up the skull: two frontal bones, two parietal bones, two temporal bones, and one occipital bone. The head of the newborn is proportionally much larger than the remainder of the body parts. The average head circumference at birth is approximately 34 to 35 cm, and the head is the same size or up to 2 cm larger than the chest in the infant.[12] This proportion changes by 2 years of age when the head is smaller than the chest.[10]

Four suture lines separate the bones of the head: coronal, sagittal, lambdoid, and frontal. The space at the suture lines gives the brain room to grow in extrauterine life. The brain expansion in turn shapes the skull bones. Sutures ordinarily feel ridged until approximately 6 months of age when the skull begins to take on a smooth, rounded appearance. Ossification of the sutures usually does not begin until brain growth ceases at about 6 years of age, and continues until adulthood.

Two fontanels or soft spots in the skull are palpable at birth. The anterior fontanel, located at the juncture of the frontal and parietal bones, measures up to 4 to 5 cm in both directions at birth. This fontanel usually closes by 18 to 24 months of age. The posterior fontanel, located between the parietal and occipital bones, is smaller than the anterior fontanel and ordinarily closes by 2 months of age.[10]

Several bones comprise the facial structure. Only the mandible is mobile. The other facial bones include the frontal, nasal, zygomatic, ethmoid, lacrimal, sphenoid, and maxillary bones. These bones as a group mostly comprise the midface and lower facial areas.

The muscles of the face are innervated by the fifth and seventh cranial nerves. Those of the midface, which control facial expression, originate on the facial bones and terminate on the soft tissues of the eyelids, nose, cheeks, and lips and are the controlled by the seventh cranial nerve. The muscles used for chewing movements lie on the floor of the mouth and are innervated by the fifth cranial nerve.[5] The tongue muscle receives its nerve impulses from the 12th cranial nerve.[1]

Nose and Paranasal Sinuses

The nose has three important functions: it conditions the air for the lower respiratory tract, produces the sense of smell, and acts as a resonating chamber for the production of speech. There are two components to the structure of the nose: the external part and the larger internal portion, which is within the skull cavity. The external nose supports a triangular frame with bone and cartilage; it is covered with skin and is lined with a mucous membrane. It is divided into two halves by the septal cartilage, with a nostril opening at the lower end. The vestibule, which is the area just inside the nostril, is covered by skin and contains a projection of coarse, stiff hairs that filter out large particles from the inspired air.

The internal nose also is divided into two halves by the nasal bones and the septal cartilage anteriorly and by the ethmoid bone and the vomer posteriorly. Superiorly, the internal nose is covered by the ethmoid bone, and inferiorly, it is separated from the mouth by the palatine bones and the maxilla of the hard palate. The internal nose is continuous with the external nose and merges with the pharynx through two openings called the internal nares or choanae.

The four paranasal sinuses and the nasolacrimal ducts open into the middle meatus and inferior meatus, respectively, of the internal nose. Three bony plates or

TABLE 33-1
Consequences of Abnormal Embryonic Development

Fetal Age (Weeks)	Structure Formed	Anomalies at Birth
4–5	Branchial apparatus	First arch syndrome
		Treacher Collins syndrome
		Pierre Robin syndrome
4	Tongue	Ankyloglossia (tongue-tie)
5–12	Hard palate, soft palate, and uvula	Cleft lip
		Cleft palate
4–7	Eye	Congenital cataracts
		Congenital glaucoma
		Eye malformations
4–5	Ear	Congenital deafness
		Anomalies of the auricle

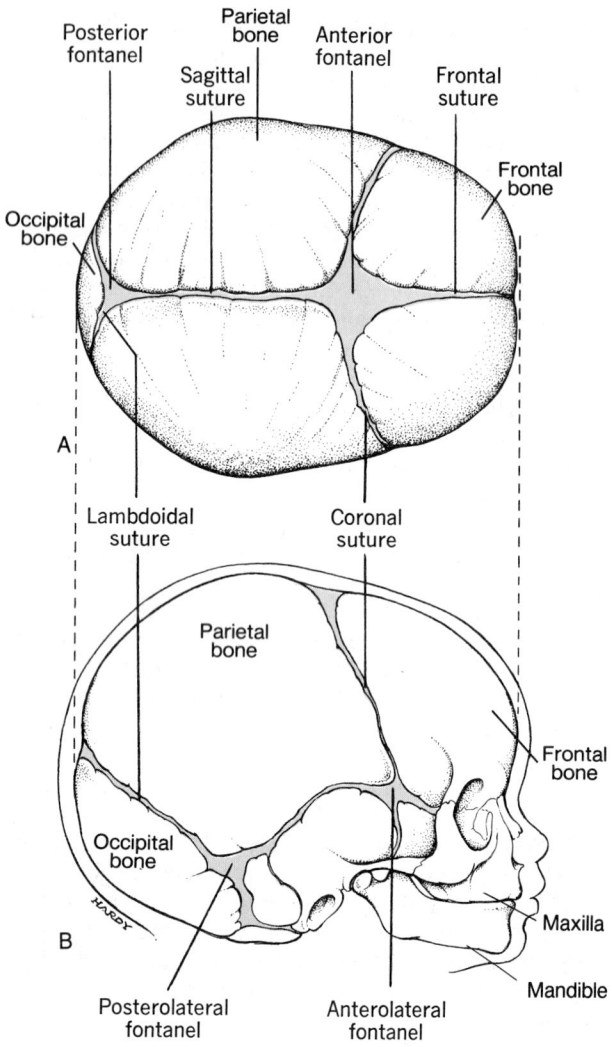

FIGURE 33-5

Lateral (A) and superior (B) views of the major bones, sutures, and fontanels in the neonatal head.

The air-filled, paired sinuses are each lined with mucous membrane and cilia.

The maxillary sinuses are positioned next to the side wall of the nasal cavity in the maxillary bone. The frontal sinus lies within the frontal bone above the nasal cavity. Positioned behind the frontal sinuses, the ethmoid sinuses are also above the nasal cavity. The sphenoid sinuses lie behind the ethmoid sinuses deep within the skull. Although present, the maxillary and ethmoid sinuses are very small at birth. The maxillary sinuses grow slowly until puberty; the ethmoid sinuses remain small until 2 years of age and do not grow extensively until 6 to 8 years of age. Even smaller in infancy are the sphenoid sinuses, which do not begin to develop until 2 years of age and do not reach their full maturity until adolescence. The frontal sinuses appear by 7 to 8 years of age.[10]

Mouth

The mouth and its associated oropharynx have the following functions: expulsion of air for vocalization or expiration, swallowing of food and liquids, beginning of digestion, and sense of taste. Several structures make up the oral cavity, including the lips, gums, palate (soft and hard), tongue, teeth, gums, salivary glands, and uvula. The two parts of the oral cavity are the vestibule, which is the area between the buccal mucosa and the outside surface of the teeth and gums, and the mouth, which encompasses the tongue, teeth, and gums. A mucous membrane covers all of the visible structures except the teeth and serves to keep the mouth hydrated, assist with digestion, and act as a mechanical and chemical barrier to trauma and infectious organisms.

The hard palate anteriorly and the soft palate posteriorly comprise the roof of the mouth, while loose tissue over the mandibular bone forms the floor of the mouth. The uvula hangs from the posterior margin of the soft palate. The tongue arises from the posterior floor of the mouth and is tethered to the anterior floor of the mouth by the frenulum. Mucous membrane covers the dorsal surface of the tongue and supports tiny projections called

shelves, called the superior, middle, and inferior turbinates, project from the lateral walls of the internal nasal cavity. Mucus secreted by the mucous membrane lining the turbinates filters out smaller particles from the incoming air, moistens the air, and warms it with the help of a dense capillary network. Thus, the internal nose conditions the inspired air by temperature control, humidity control, and filtering of dust and infectious organisms.

The sense of smell originates from the olfactory epithelium located at the top of the nasal cavity adjacent to the cribriform plate. These cells, which are bipolar neurons, receive stimulation from lipid-soluble substances in the inspired air. The axons of these neurons pass through the cribriform plate and synapse in the olfactory bulb.[4] The axons of the second neuron then carry the nerve impulse to the central nervous system for interpretation.

The four paranasal sinuses are the maxillary, frontal, ethmoid, and sphenoid sinuses (Fig. 33-6). Their main purpose is to lighten the weight of the skull, but they also drain mucus and antibodies into the nasal cavity and act as resonating chambers for the production of sound.[12]

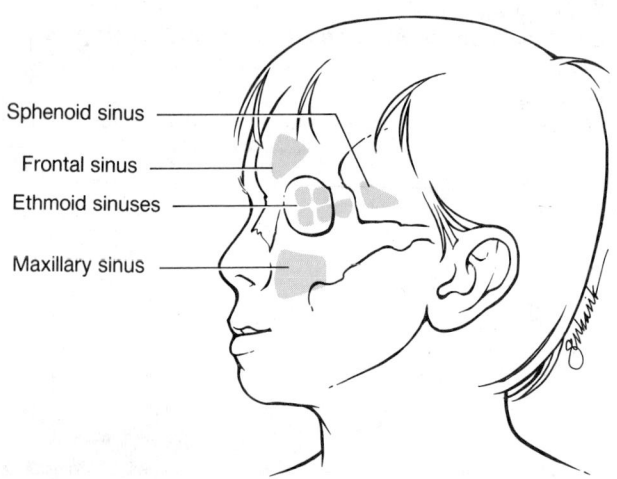

FIGURE 33-6

Location of paranasal sinuses in school-age child.

papillae. Some of these papillae at the tip of the tongue and over the posterior surface of the tongue contain taste buds. The four taste zones from front to back are sweet, salty, sour, and bitter. Taste develops as the child matures, with sweet being the first taste in the infant.

Two sets of teeth erupt at different points in life (Fig. 33-7). The deciduous or baby teeth actually start calcification at 3 months' gestation but do not erupt until they each have enough calcification to undergo the chewing maneuvers. Deciduous teeth usually begin erupting at 6 months of age and continue until all 20 teeth have come in, approximately 2 years of age. Permanent teeth, of which there are 32, start their formation in the jaw at 6 months of age but do not begin erupting until about 6 years of age.[10]

Salivary glands are located in or near the oral cavity. The parotid glands are below each ear, and the submaxillary and the sublingual glands are in the floor of the mouth. The buccal glands are in the epithelium of the cheeks and lips. Ducts extend from the salivary glands and open into the mucosa. Saliva production is regulated by the brain, which is stimulated by tastes, odors, and tactile sensations. Saliva cleanses the mucosa and provides protection from bacterial infection; it also contains enzymes that are important in the digestion of starches.

The oral cavity provides a place for food to enter the inner body and begin to convert to usable particles. Chewing and swallowing are essential digestive functions that are discussed in Chapter 57.

Eyes

The eyeball or globe is located within a bony orbit that protects it on three sides. The eyelid provides protection to the anterior portion of the eye from foreign bodies. This lid also spreads tears over the cornea and controls the amount of light reaching the eye. A membrane called the conjunctiva spreads across the cornea and beneath the eyelid providing added protection from foreign bodies and helping lubricate the eye. The lacrimal gland, located above the eyelid temporally, secretes tears that bathe and moisten the cornea of the eye continuously. Tears leave the eye at the lacrimal duct and flow into the nasal cavity. There are six extraocular muscles that insert on the sclera of the globe and allow the eye to gaze in any direction. These muscles also are responsible for keeping synchrony in the two eyes.

The internal eye structures are arranged in three coats or layers: The outer portion consists of the sclera posteriorly and the cornea anteriorly; the middle layer is made up of the choroid posteriorly and the ciliary body and iris anteriorly; and the inner part is composed of the retina (Fig. 33-8). The main purpose of the sclera is to support the globe. The sclera is an opaque structure composed primarily of connective and elastic fibers that appear as the white of the eye anteriorly. The transparent cornea, which is continuous with the sclera, occupies the anterior one sixth of the eyeball and is composed of fibrous tissue.[4] It separates the anterior chamber from the external en-

Time of eruption of deciduous teeth

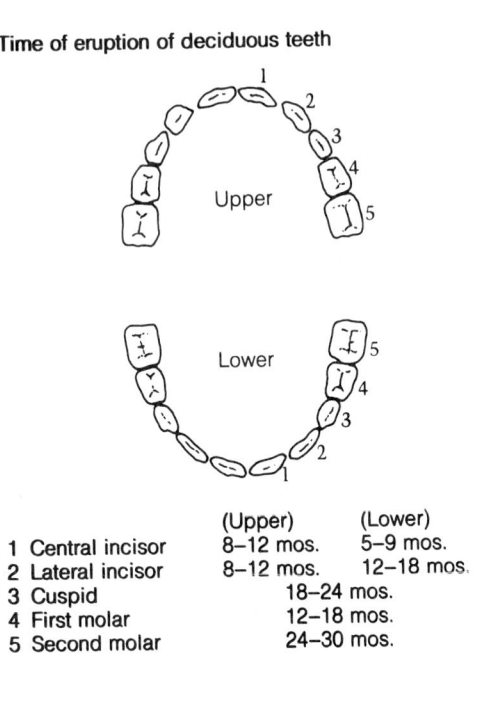

	(Upper)	(Lower)
1 Central incisor	8–12 mos.	5–9 mos.
2 Lateral incisor	8–12 mos.	12–18 mos.
3 Cuspid		18–24 mos.
4 First molar		12–18 mos.
5 Second molar		24–30 mos.

Time of eruption of permanent teeth

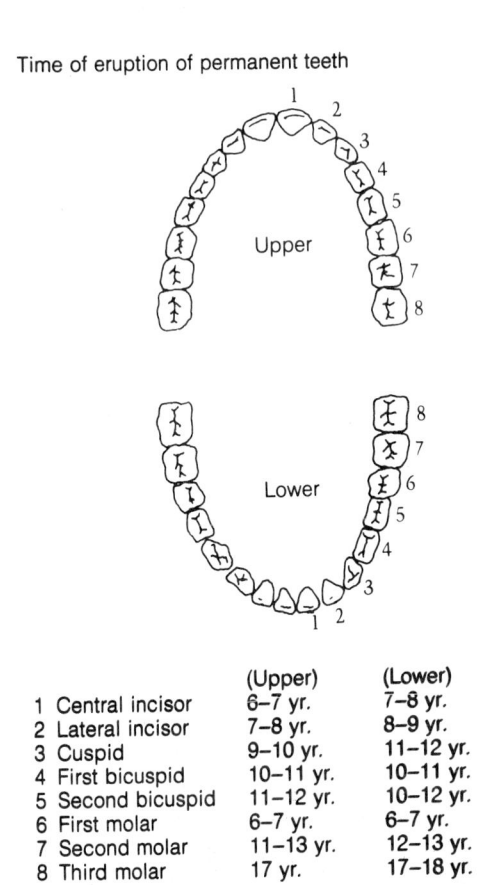

	(Upper)	(Lower)
1 Central incisor	6–7 yr.	7–8 yr.
2 Lateral incisor	7–8 yr.	8–9 yr.
3 Cuspid	9–10 yr.	11–12 yr.
4 First bicuspid	10–11 yr.	10–11 yr.
5 Second bicuspid	11–12 yr.	10–12 yr.
6 First molar	6–7 yr.	6–7 yr.
7 Second molar	11–13 yr.	12–13 yr.
8 Third molar	17 yr.	17–18 yr.

FIGURE 33-7
Pattern of tooth eruption in children. (Fuller, J., & Schaller-Ayers, J. [1990] *Health assessment: A nursing approach.* Philadelphia: J.B. Lippincott, p. 527.)

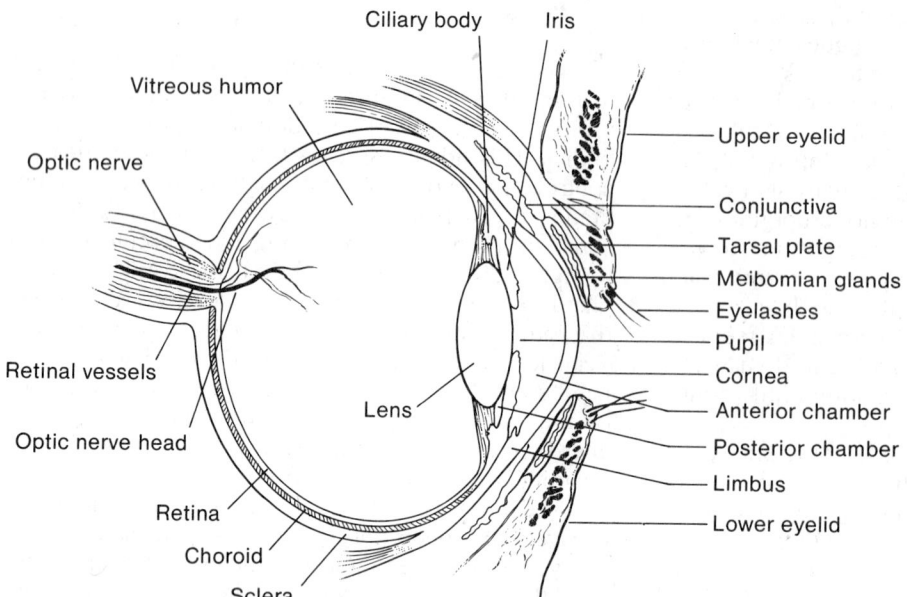

FIGURE 33-8
Cross section of the eye.

vironment and allows light to pass through its layers to the lens and retina. The cornea has pain receptors, which are important in eliciting the corneal reflex.[10]

The choroid of the middle coat is a vascular layer, which forms the inner lining of the posterior five-sixths of the sclera. The choroid separates the sclera and retina and primarily perfuses the outer portion of the retina. The ciliary body secretes the aqueous humor and regulates the shape of the lens. Fibers connect the ciliary body to the lens, thus suspending the lens and assisting with its control.

The iris, a modified version of the choroid, gives color to the eyes and shows through the cornea. Consisting of a round muscular disk, its function is to control the amount of light entering the eye by alternately constricting and dilating. Light enters the interior of the eye through the opening in the center of the iris, the pupil.

The internal, two-layered coat of the eyeball, called the retina, changes light images into nerve impulses that are transmitted through the optic nerve to the brain. The outer, pigmented layer prevents reflections from excess light. The inner, sensory layer contains photoreceptor cells—the rods and cones.

Two important landmarks on this inner layer can be visualized with an ophthalmoscope: the optic disk and the macula. The optic disk is the area of the retina where the optic nerve, retinal artery, and vein converge on their way to the brain. The optic disk has a pinkish ovoid shape and is located toward the medial nasal side of the retina. The macula is a small, yellowish spot with a depressed middle portion located in the center of the retina. This is the area with the highest concentration of cones and the greatest visual acuity.

The refracting media of the eye consist of the cornea, aqueous humor, lens, and vitreous body. The aqueous humor, a clear watery fluid, fills the cavity of the anterior chamber between the cornea and the lens and iris. The aqueous humor gives nourishment to the internal eye

parts, which do not possess a blood supply of their own. The lens allows the eye to focus on objects at different distances. The lens is transparent and biconvex, but the shape changes constantly with direction from the choroid body and due to the elasticity of the lens, which is composed of crystalline matter. The vitreous body or humor, a transparent semigelatinous material, fills the posterior four-fifths of the globe and provides support to the other eye structures. The vitreous body preserves the spheroid shape of the eye.

Vision, as with the nervous system itself, matures over the first few years of life. Infants have a visual acuity of 20/200, and most children have some degree of myopia (nearsightedness) until the eyeball gains a spherical shape around age 6. Although central vision is not fully intact at birth, peripheral vision is well developed in the newborn. Voluntary control of the eye muscles is attained by 2 to 3 months of age, and the infant is able to distinguish colors by 8 months. By 9 months of age and with further eye muscle coordination, the infant is able to focus on a single image.[4]

There are many facets to the physiology of the eye. Vision commences with the passage of light through the cornea, aqueous humor, pupil, lens, and vitreous humor. When this same light hits and forms an image on the retina, it stimulates the rods and cones, which send a message to the cerebral cortex of the brain by way of the nerves. The interpretation by the brain informs us of what we are seeing.

Four different maneuvers by the mechanism of the eye make it possible to form an image on the retina. These include refraction of light rays, accommodation of the lens, constriction of the pupil, and convergence of the eyes. *Refraction* involves the bending of light rays as they pass through the different layers of the refracting media of the eye. The various densities of the cornea, aqueous humor, lens, and vitreous body assist with this process. The ability of the lens to change its curvature (*accom-*

modation) allows the eye to focus on objects of varying distances. The ciliary muscle controls the curvature of the lens.

The amount of light coming into the eye is determined by the degree of *pupil constriction.* Muscles of the iris constrict the pupil to prevent peripheral light rays from entering the eye and blurring vision. Constriction also occurs during periods of bright light to prevent overstimulation of the retina. Because humans possess single binocular vision, the eyes move together at all times when viewing an object. When the object is very close, it is necessary for the eyes to both move medially or become "crossed." This action is referred to as *convergence.* The extrinsic eye muscles allow this medial movement of the eyes.

Images focused on the retina are upside down and a mirror reversal of their actual form. That is, light from the top of an object is registered on the retina immediately below the central fovea (the point of greatest visual acuity), and a light from the right side of the object focuses on the left side of the retina. This image is transmitted to the brain, which turns the object right-side-up and right-side-around for the individual.

The rods and cones convert the light impulses received by the retina into nerve impulses, which are then forwarded to the brain. The rods contain a substance called rhodopsin, which releases a nervous impulse when it is broken down chemically by light striking the rods. This process works best in dim light; therefore, rhodopsin is primarily responsible for night vision.

In contrast, cones function best in bright light where the photosensitive chemicals that they contain are more easily broken down. It is believed that three types of cones each contain a different visual pigment. Each of these pigments is sensitive to a single color: red, blue, or green. The combined stimulation of two or more kinds of cones is thought to account for the perception of more than 17,000 intermediate hues of color. Cones are thus the major determinant of color perception.

Impulses from the rods and cones are sent to ganglion cells by way of bipolar neurons. The ganglion cell bodies lie in the retina, but their axons exit the retina through the optic nerve. The axons then pass on to the optic chiasma where they may cross with fibers from the opposite eye and proceed to the thalamus of the brain through the optic tract. In the thalamus, a synapse occurs with other neurons whose axons deliver the impulses to the occipital lobes of the cerebral cortex for interpretation.

Ears

The ear is composed of three distinct areas: the inner, middle, and external portions (Fig. 33-9). The ear performs two important sensory functions: to recognize and interpret sound and to maintain equilibrium. Each part of the ear works in a different way to accomplish these functions.

The auricle or pinna is the visible landmark of the *external ear* position and is made up of cartilage covered by skin. Functionally, the pinna does not greatly increase the sense of hearing. Malposition of the auricle frequently occurs with congenital anomalies.

The external auditory canal or meatus is the other structure of the external ear. The meatus consists of cartilage at the external end and bone toward the inner end. The entire canal is covered by skin. However, the skin contains hairs and sebaceous and ceruminous glands in the cartilaginous portion and is thin and fragile in the bony section.[6] The meatus is *S*-shaped, but the type of curve changes from infancy to later life. In the infant, the external auditory canal has an upward curve that transforms into a downward curve by middle childhood.

The *middle ear* is housed within an air-filled space in the temporal bone and consists of the tympanic membrane and the three middle-ear ossicles: the malleus, in-

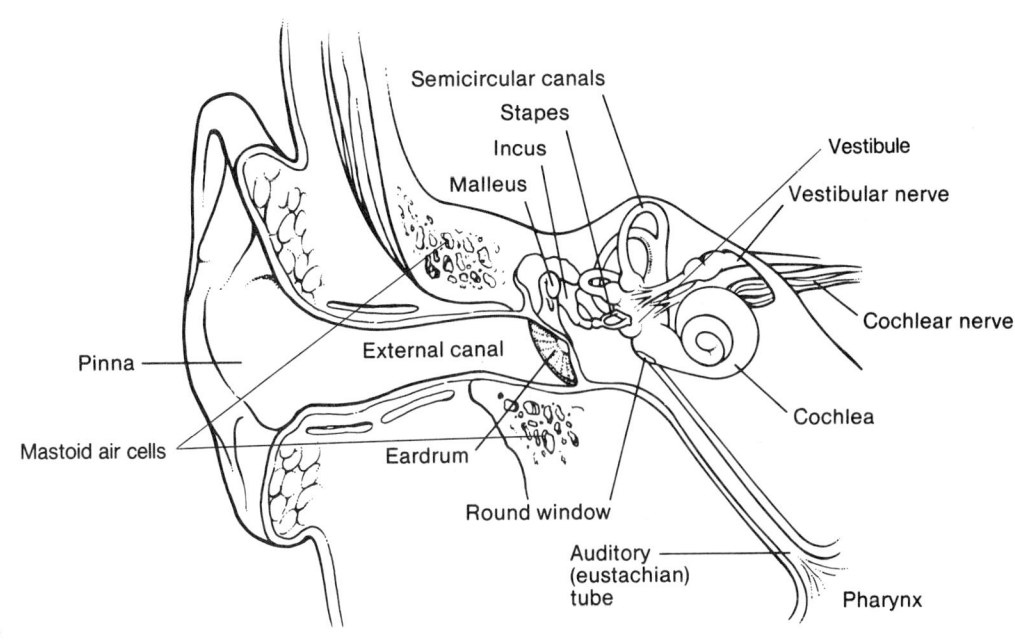

FIGURE 33-9

Structures of a mature ear.

cus, and stapes. The middle ear is in communication with the mastoid posteriorly and the nasopharynx, by means of the eustachian tube, anteriorly. The tympanic membrane or eardrum is thin and transparent, positioned at an oblique angle to separate the external canal from the middle ear. This membrane is surrounded by the annulus, a fibrous ring, and is divided into the pars flaccida, or looser superior portion, and the pars tensa, or more taut inferior portion. The malleus and middle ear space can be visualized through the tympanic membrane. A triangular light reflex usually is seen on the membrane extending from the long end of the malleus (which is attached at the center of the membrane) to the inferior anterior quadrant. The connection of the malleus to the inner surface of the tympanic membrane causes a concavity of the membrane, which is called the umbo.

The purpose of the middle ear is to conduct sound waves from the external ear to the inner ear where they can be reformulated into a nerve impulse and forwarded to the brain for interpretation. The three bones of the middle ear, the malleus, incus, and stapes, are connected to each other and transport sound vibrations from the tympanic membrane to the oval window of the inner ear. The oval window, which is the junction between the stapes and inner ear, and the round window, adjacent to the cochlea of the inner ear, are the only openings between the middle and inner ear areas.

Mucus produced by the membranes of the middle ear is cleared by the ciliary action of the eustachian tube, positioned in the posterior segment of the middle ear. The *eustachian tube* is composed of bones on its sides with cartilage in the middle. It is lined with respiratory epithelium and opens into the nasopharynx. The eustachian or auditory tube of an infant is wider, shorter, and more horizontal than that of an adult, allowing infections from the nasopharyngeal area to travel more easily to the middle ear. This structural difference accounts for the greater number of middle ear infections in infants and toddlers.[10] With age, the auditory tube becomes longer and moves to a more inferior position within the pharynx. However, anything that occludes the eustachian tube, whether it is an infection or a mechanical problem such as the position of the adenoids, may decrease aeration of the middle ear and contribute to either poor conduction or an infection of the middle ear.

The *inner ear* performs two functions: to change sound waves into nerve impulses and to maintain equilibrium. There are two divisions of the inner ear, the bony labyrinth and the membranous labyrinth. The bony labyrinth is divided into the vestibule, the cochlea, and the semicircular canals. The membranous labyrinth lies inside the bony labyrinth and essentially has its same form but is composed of several sacs and tubes. The oval central portion of the inner ear is the vestibule and houses the utricle and saccule. This is the area where the oval window connects the middle and inner ear portions and is immediately above the round window. The three semicircular canals lie above the vestibule and are in superior, posterior, and lateral positions, respectively. The utricle, saccule, and semicircular canals work together to achieve a sense of balance.[6]

The cochlea is divided into three separate chambers: the scala vestibuli, the scala tympani, and the cochlear duct. The scala vestibuli (the upper passage that terminates at the oval window) and the scala tympani (the lower route that ends at the round window) both contain perilymph fluid and at one point, are connected to each other. The basilar membrane lines the bottom, and the vestibular membrane coats the top of the cochlear duct. The organ of Corti, which is the organ of hearing, is housed within the cochlear duct. It is composed of supporting and hair cells that receive auditory sensations and transform them into nerve impulses that are mediated by the eighth cranial nerve.

Sound waves enter the ear through the external auditory canal and travel to the tympanic membrane where they cause the eardrum to vibrate. This movement transmits vibrations through the ear ossicles. The stapes, the last of the ossicles, then moves in and out against the membrane of the oval window setting up a wave of the perilymph fluid within the scali vestibuli. This wave is continued through the scali tympani. The increased pressure of perilymph fluid within the scali vestibuli also pushes in on the vestibular membrane of the cochlear duct, causing movement of the endolymph fluid against the basilar membrane, which bulges outward. The fluid of the scali tympani responds to pressure waves from both the basilar membrane and the scali vestibuli and pushes against the round window, displacing it outward into the middle ear. As the sound wave subsides, the fluid reverses its path, causing the basilar membrane to move inward into the cochlear duct. These pressure waves on the basilar membrane cause the hair cells of the organ of Corti to bend, initiating a receptor potential that energizes the neurons of the cochlear nerve, a branch of the eighth cranial nerve. The nerve impulses are then carried to the brain where the messages are interpreted.[3] This is an abbreviated explanation of the physiology of the sense of hearing.

The sense of balance is also primarily maintained by the vestibular apparatus of the inner ear. Static equilibrium, which keeps the head oriented in relation to the pull of gravity, is mediated by the saccule and utricle of the vestibule. Small calcium carbonate particles called otoliths are located in a gelatinous layer covering the sensory hairs within the membranous labyrinth of the saccule and utricle. These particles respond to downward movement of the head by moving in the direction of gravity, and in turn, they pull the gelatinous layer, which also bends the sensory hairs. Movement of the hairs stimulates dendrites at the base of the hair cells. Messages concerning the relative position of the head in space are then carried to the temporal lobe of the brain.[4] These impulses constitute the righting reflex, which works to keep the body in an upright posture.

Dynamic equilibrium is preserved by the semicircular canals of the inner ear. These canals lie in three planes at right angles to one another (frontal, sagittal, and lateral) to provide notice of an imbalance in each of the three planes. Similar to the vestibule, the ampulla or enlarged part of each semicircular canal contains a crista, which is a group of hair cells covered by gelatinous material. With head movement, the hairs bend and stimulate neurons to send impulses to the temporal lobe of the brain. These messages as well as those for static balance are mediated by the vestibular branch of the eighth cranial nerve.

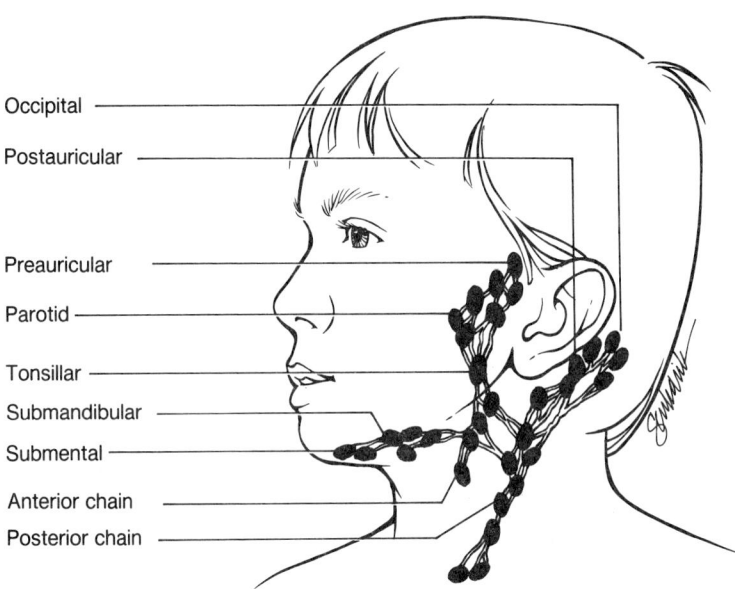

Occipital
Postauricular

Preauricular
Parotid

Tonsillar
Submandibular
Submental

Anterior chain
Posterior chain

FIGURE 33-10
Location of the cervical lymph nodes.

Neck

Structures from several body systems are located in the neck (esophagus, larynx and trachea, and the thyroid) and are discussed with the appropriate system in this text. Major muscles of the neck are the sternocleidomastoid and the trapezius. The left and right sternocleidomastoid muscles connect the temporal bone (mastoid process) with the sternum and clavicles, and each enables the head to rotate toward the opposite side. In the posterior region of the neck, a pair of trapezius muscles originates at the occiput and vertebral areas and connects to the scapula and clavicle. The trapezius muscles enable the child to raise or lower the shoulders.

The cervical lymph nodes are numerous, vary in size, and are located along the sternocleidomastoid muscles, under the chin, in front of the ear, and at various other sites (Fig. 33-10). Cervical nodes drain lymph fluid from the multiple structures of the head and neck region and return it to the bloodstream through lymphatic vessels. Lymph nodes produce lymphocytes and monocytes and act as filters in keeping particulate matter, especially bacteria, from gaining access to the bloodstream. The tonsils, which are located in the pharynx lateral to the uvula, are masses of lymph tissue that function as the lymph nodes in protecting the body from infection and aiding the formation of white blood cells.

Summary

Functioning of the sensory organs determines how the child perceives the world and influences his or her growth, development, and behavior. Many opportunities exist for anomalies to develop in the sensory organs and surrounding structures during the embryonic phase of fetal development. Knowledge of the anatomy and function of major features in the head and neck, therefore, is vital for the nurse's assessment of a child's physical and psychosocial health.

References

1. Bates, B. (1991). *A guide to physical examination and history taking* (5th ed.). Philadelphia: JB Lippincott.
2. Beck, F., Moffat, D. B., & Davies, D. P. (1985). The brachial region, mouth, palate, nose and face. In *Human embryology* (2nd ed.). Boston: Blackwell Scientific, pp. 170–194.
3. Crouch, J. E. (1985). The organs of general and special sense (receptors). In *Functional human anatomy* (4th ed.). Philadelphia: Lea & Febiger, pp. 362–389.
4. Chow, M. P., Durand, B. A., Feldman, M. N., & Mills, M. A. (1984). Child health assessment. In *Handbook of pediatric primary care* (2nd ed.). New York: John Wiley & Sons, pp. 3–46.
5. Epstein, M. H., Gann, D. S., Heese, D. W., & Ryan, J. J. (1986). The head and neck. In G. D. Zuidema (Ed.), *The Johns Hopkins atlas of human functional anatomy* (3rd ed.). Baltimore: The Johns Hopkins University Press, pp. 65–69.
6. Hall-Craggs, E. C. B. (1988). The head and neck. In *Anatomy as a basis for clinical medicine*. Baltimore: Urban & Schwarzenberg, pp. 480–627.
7. Moore, K. I. (1988). *The developing human: Clinically oriented embryology* (4th ed.). Philadelphia: WB Saunders.
8. Moore, K. L. (1989). *Before we are born* (3rd ed.). Philadelphia: WB Saunders.
9. Oppenheimer, S. B., & Lefevre, G. (1984). Organogenesis. In *Introduction to embryonic development* (2nd ed.). Boston: Allyn & Bacon, pp. 201–283.
10. Seidel, H. M., Ball, J. W., Dains, J. E., & Benedict, G. W. (1987). Head and neck. In *Mosby's guide to physical examination*. St. Louis: CV Mosby, pp. 164–188.
11. Vaughan, V. C., & Litt, I. F. (1990). The first year. In *Child and adolescent development: Clinical implications*. Philadelphia: WB Saunders, pp. 163–178.
12. Woodburne, R. T., & Burkel, W. E. (1988) The head and neck. In *Essentials of human anatomy* (8th ed.). New York: Oxford University, pp. 179–323.

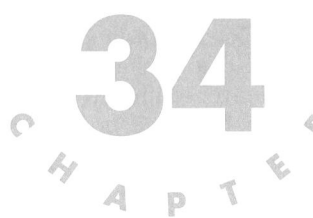

34

CHAPTER

Nursing Assessment and Diagnosis of Head and Neck Function

BEHAVIORAL OBJECTIVES

Use functional health as a guideline for assessment of the child's head and neck function.

Describe the components of a complete physical examination of the child's head and neck.

Identify deviations from the normal in physical examination of the head and neck.

Describe methods for evaluation of vision and hearing in children.

Describe diagnostic procedures used in the evaluation of a child's head and neck.

Identify nursing diagnoses that are commonly used in the care of children with dysfunctions of the head and neck.

The newborn's face and head normally enter the world first. Although new parents may objectively assess the newborn's number of fingers and toes, they examine the face more subjectively. They discuss whom the infant resembles and what name best suits the baby's appearance.

Structures of the head and neck allow a child to exchange information with environment and caregivers; alterations in the region potentially impair growth and development. Therefore, nursing skill in assessment of the head and neck is imperative to provision of comprehensive care. Application of functional health in assessing the head and neck helps the nurse to recognize the subjective significance of these parts of the anatomy while analyzing their components objectively.

Nursing Assessment

Assessment of a child's head and neck may occur as one part of a routine physical examination or as part of ongoing evaluation of illness or disability. Thorough child and family health history, identification of present patterns of behavior with regard to health, and a physical examination are the standard components of a nursing assessment. The initial contact with a child and family demands a broader base of information that, if well documented, needs not be repeated in future contacts. The following sections are a guide for gathering just such a broad range of information about the child with an anomaly of the head and neck.

799

Child and Family History

A patient history lays the groundwork for examination of the head and neck. During this phase, information is gathered regarding health problems of the head or neck that have affected the child or members of the child's immediate family. Have these health problems required medical interventions? What impact do the health problems have on the child's ability to breathe, communicate, or eat? What systems has the family used to manage the problem? Which interventions were successful or unsuccessful? Such discussion is likely to indicate the depth of understanding a patient and family have been able to achieve about an alteration in health, as well as expectations about outcomes.

Health Perception and Management

Documentation of medical assessment of the head and neck often begins with identification of a "chief complaint." Some common complaints related to the head or neck might include "swollen glands," a painful ear, nasal congestion, teething, or a sore throat. After identifying the area of concern, the nurse inquires about a family's observations related to the problem. Using the example of a sore ear, the nurse might ask about how long the symptoms have been present, how the problem was identified by the parent, and also which steps taken by the parent were successful and unsuccessful in making the child more comfortable. The nurse could also ask about the character of any drainage from the ear and whether the child drinks from a bottle. Bottle feeding while supine can encourage pooling of fluids in the nasopharynx and contribute to otitis media. Duration of the earache and extent to which a parent manages the illness independently provide indications of health perception.

Parents of infants are most likely to express concern about the head and neck as related to feeding and growth, sleeping, crying, and responsiveness. If a parent expresses concern about the shape or size of an infant's head, the nurse can ask about mode of birth, sleep positions, and history of weight and length growth parameters. The trauma of vaginal birth can significantly alter the shape of the head, and hematomas acquired in transit can be quite dramatic. A parent may perceive these findings as grossly abnormal but can be comforted by the nurse's explanations. Crying behaviors can be explored for pattern and ability to self-console. If responsiveness is of concern, the nurse may inquire about the baby's response to sounds and ability to follow objects visually. New parents may need reassurance about the limited visual field of their infant.

Nutrition and Metabolism

A thorough description of feeding behaviors of an infant or child can reveal a great deal in the assessment of health of the head and neck. An infant, whether bottle or breast fed, should be able to root and suck in a coordinated manner. Feedings should be accomplished without color change, coughing, excessive diaphoresis, or fatigue. A poor suck can indicate neurologic impairment, whereas labored breathing during feedings may alert the caregiver to some impairment of the upper respiratory tract. Reported color change, sweating, or "falling asleep" while feeding may indicate insufficiency of the cardiovascular system. Coughing, chronic congestion, or frequent emesis could alert the caregiver to impairment in swallowing. Drainage of formula from the nose with emesis may be caused by a mucous cleft in the palate or nasopharyngeal reflux.

General nutrition can be approximated by assessing fat stores and muscle mass throughout the body. The face also houses fat stores, especially in the cheeks and temporal areas. Because these areas of reserved energy are among the last to be called on to serve a desperate body, wasting of the cheeks can indicate profound nutritional deficit. If there is concern about delayed growth or weight loss, this information might be elicited from the parent by asking how long the child has been wearing the same size clothes and whether the fit of the clothing has changed. Hair texture and distribution can also be telling indicators of nutritional status. Dull, dry, or sparse hair may indicate poor nutrition, inadequate protein intake, or hypothyroidism.[10]

Elimination

The significance of head and neck findings in information gathering regarding elimination is limited. Descriptions of the character of emesis can offer clues regarding alterations in bowel function. A fondness for certain types of foods may predispose children to bowel irregularity. It is important for the examiner to keep in mind that small infants respond to any infection in a generalized way. If an infant presents with a complaint of diarrhea, the nurse should look beyond the gastrointestinal tract for a cause. Infections of the ear or upper respiratory tract or teething can cause similar complaints. Also, petechiae about the face in a fair-skinned child could be brought about by a forceful Valsalva maneuver and may result from vomiting or constipation.

Activity and Exercise

How does the child tolerate activity? Such a question may be too general to elicit needed information about a child's head and neck. When assessing a neonate, one might ask a parent about the child's appearance during crying and feeding, because these are the baby's most vigorous activities. Easy fatigue, breathing difficulties, or grayness or blueness of the mouth or nose may demonstrate an alteration in cardiac output or gas exchange. Symmetry of facial movements can also be assessed during crying or smiling; weakness or a facial droop might be noted by a parent.

Although some aspects of this assessment may hold true for the toddler and older child as well, participation in more physical activities cannot be overlooked. A propensity for swimming may leave a child at risk for ear infections, whereas biking and skateboarding without use of protective headgear bear considerable threat of head injury. In contrast, a child's visual or hearing impairment may augment perceived risk for injury and result in discouragement of athletic activities.

Sleep and Rest

An infant or child with noisy respirations during sleep may have an obstruction or abnormality involving the nasopharynx. One should elicit from the caregiver which positions are most comfortable for the child during sleep. Eased breathing in the prone position could signal abnormalities of the respiratory tract. Preference for the upright or semi-sitting position may reveal a tendency for gastroesophageal reflux, which is lessened with the help of gravity.

Hair distribution can provide clues to an infant's sleep positioning at home. Balding of the occiput, also known as *friction alopecia,* can result from rubbing the head against linens or clothing. Localized alopecia may occur as a normal variant or may reflect excessive time spent in a supine position. When unequal hair distribution is noted, the examiner should consider the implications of stagnant positioning, including decreased muscle strength in the infant and possible neglect by caregivers.

Cognition and Perception

Cognition and perception are greatly affected by sensory competencies. Because four of the primary sense organs (eyes, ears, nose, and tongue) are located in the head, assessment of their functioning is critical. In the history, each of the sensory competencies may be assessed in terms of responsiveness to stimuli and developmental ability.

Parents of even a small child should be asked about the child's vision. Does the child look at you, or do the child's eyes follow toys? Do the eyes ever wander or shake? Does the toddler attend to books? Does the child watch television? How close does the child stand to the television? Does the child feel comfortable reading a book or the blackboard at school? Can the child identify colors? Are there any particular colors that the child consistently confuses? Visual disturbances can be notable very early in a child's life, as demonstrated by lack of focusing on or following faces or objects; parents are frequently the first to discover such deficits or abnormalities of the eyes. Parents may also report unusual coloring or dullness of one eye, detected in person or in a photograph. Such dullness can represent a cataract or even a retinoblastoma.

Children with visual impairments may initially present with apparently delayed development. The motivation for infants to raise their heads is the increased visual field achieved. Without such rewards, the blind infant may not learn to support the head until as late as 10 or 12 months. Lack of the visual reinforcement of toys or parents can similarly delay crawling and walking. Use of auditory and tactile cues in place of a visual impetus can help minimize developmental delay in the visually impaired child.[18]

Auditory assessment can be equally challenging. However, a parent can report a child's reaction to household noises, how readily the infant calms to music or voice, and how the child responds to his or her name. Even the very young infant can demonstrate discriminatory hearing, expressing a preference for the mother's voice. Research reveals the neonate's ability to choose the mother's voice over other sounds through sucking in

a specific pattern.[7] A child who speaks loudly may be revealing a hearing deficit. Even a simple middle ear infection can temporarily impair a child's hearing because fluid disrupts the conduction pathway. Chronic ear infections can leave a tympanic membrane scarred and permanently diminish hearing in the affected ear.

A small infant's indifference to sounds should alert the parent to possible hearing impairment. The child may react to vibrations created by loud noises or music but respond little to the human voice. Interest in objects may exceed that in people, and frustrated tantrums are common in children who find themselves unable to communicate.[18] Even infants who have little-to-no hearing babble normally in infancy. A plateau in language development at this point should serve as a warning signal that auditory ability may be impaired.

Little is known about the gustatory sense in infants, and a common assumption is that the taste of infant formulas is of little consequence. Even neonates, however, respond to sour, sweet, bitter, and acid stimuli in distinctive ways. Some infants feed better when sweeter formulas are offered. Although cereals and fruits are commonly the first solid foods to be introduced, some pediatricians advocate the introduction of vegetables first to minimize initial acclimation to sweet tastes. The mother of an older child will likely be able to describe her child's taste preferences in great detail. Children who suffer from altered integrity of the oral mucosa may experience less taste and demonstrate little interest in food as a result.

The olfactory sense, although seldom discussed, is closely linked to long-term memory. Unlike memory of a shape or color, smell is not alterable because it is stored in a binary fashion, without size or dimension. Smells can remind one of a complex memory, especially one rich with emotion.[5] Nasal congestion and rhinorrhea can markedly impair a child's sense of smell.

Self-Perception and Self-Concept

Children perceive themselves relative to their environment. Infants play with their extremities and observe how caregivers interact with them. An abnormality of the head or face is likely to have an impact on the child's attractiveness. Children receive continual feedback on their appearance from the time they are born, and society places negative values on aberrations from normal. An unattractive appearance may result in negative feedback from parents and others, leaving the child in danger of feeling "bad" or "defective." Abnormality in a child may even alter the growth of the entire family through feelings of vulnerability projected on that child. Physical characteristics can distort perceptions of the child's aptitudes and weaknesses.[12]

There is a tendency to underestimate the intelligence of physically disabled people. Should children feel that their parents and teachers consider them inferior, they may internalize the inferiority over time. A self-fulfilling prophecy can be created: physically abnormal children are expected to demonstrate less cognitive prowess, and so they do.[2]

The impact of parents' feelings about an anomaly of the head or neck on the attitude of the affected child is paramount. An unattractive child could elicit less parental pride and a less positive attitude toward caretaking. Parents, teachers, and children alike demonstrate a preference for attractive children.[2]

Role Relationships

The appearance of an infant or child can determine early relationships with parents and others. Parents who see their children as ugly as a result of a cleft lip or other facial abnormalities may have trouble bonding with their infants.[2] A newborn's feeding, eye contact, and smiling behaviors have enormous impact on the new parents' feelings about the infant. The unattractive infant may be less able to elicit nurturance from the parent if unable to provide the smiles and verbalizations inherent to the process of bonding.[2]

Verbalizations are the earliest stage of language development, which occurs in a somewhat predictable, progressive fashion. Beginning language is cherished by the parent, because it confirms the child's recognition of that person. A specific vocabulary or an estimated number of words learned can be elicited from the parent to quantify communication skills. If a child is not exposed to language on a regular basis, such lack of opportunity can halt verbal development. A neglected child or a child of nonspeaking parents may have a delay in verbal development. Failure to verbalize also may indicate a hearing deficit in the child. Anomalies of face and mouth structure can make articulation difficult, and weakness of the airway that requires a tracheostomy tube obviates the creation of most sound.

As with any illness, medical problems affecting the head and neck can alter the parent's role in causing that parent to relinquish parts of the child's care to another. Parenting in a hospital setting can be especially stressful when the health care team takes decisionmaking on a child's behalf out of the hands of the parents.

Coping and Stress Tolerance

The newborn's suck reflex is among the most primitive of coping mechanisms. Within days of birth, new babies may find their thumbs or fists and suck on them in an effort to self-calm. Pacifiers and even bottles can take on a similar significance. Because of their impact on forming teeth, however, these methods of consolation should not be continued beyond the first year.

Parents may also be asked about children's coping behaviors and indicators of stress. A history of tooth grinding, head banging, or hair pulling not only provides insight in examination of the head but also may indicate a stressed child.

Values and Beliefs

The head and neck may hold unique significance for specific ethnic or cultural groups. Biblical references associate hair with strength, skin marking with uncleanliness, and blindness with an act of God.

Ideas concerning the spiritual significance of physical ailments may seem archaic. Caregivers must recognize, however, that anomalies may inspire emotions and reactions quite foreign to common culture in families of diverse origins. An examiner might ask whether there are any religious or spiritual beliefs that may have an impact on the care of the child or whether there are any theories about how a facial abnormality occurred.

Physical Examination

Physical examination of the infant, child, or adolescent brings special challenge. The nurse needs not only an understanding of normal anatomy and physiology but also a familiarity with growth and development. The order of examination is classically presented in the following order: inspection, auscultation, palpation, and percussion. Assessment of the head and neck does not require strict adherence to that order, because the outcome of the examination would not change. It is more logical when examining a child, however, to progress from least-invasive procedure to most-invasive procedure. This strategy preserves the child's cooperation for as long as possible.

Significant physical findings for each portion of the physical examination are listed by developmental age in Table 34-1. This information can be used in conjunction with the results of the various diagnostic tests and nursing assessment findings to determine the nursing diagnoses and begin to plan appropriate nursing interventions.

The infant's face can be examined best while the baby rests in the parent's lap. Ears can be examined with the infant's head resting on the parent's shoulder. The nurse should keep in mind that although the infant is used to being handled, being looked in the eye is new and may be frightening. The nurse's avoidance of eye contact may elicit more cooperation in the infant with separation anxiety, which usually occurs between 8 and 15 months of age.

The child will be most comfortable in the parent's lap until about the age of 5 years when separation from the parent becomes more routine. When the young child is being examined, it is important to leave probing of any orifices for last, because these procedures are likely to elicit the greatest fear. As with the infant, a minimum of equipment is used. If an otoscope or other implement is necessary, it is advisable to let the child play with and "master" the tool before it becomes part of the examination. During toddlerhood, foreign bodies become a concern in the care of the head and neck. Any unilateral nose or ear drainage, especially in the presence of foul odor, should be investigated for presence of a foreign body.

Head

The head first should be inspected for position, size, shape, and symmetry of the skull and face. Hair amount, color, texture, and distribution patterns are noted, as are skin color, pigmentation, and lesions. Palpation of the skull for suture lines and fontanels is appropriate in infants and toddlers. The parietal bone may be percussed on each side by tapping the index or middle finger directly on its surface; the "cracked-pot" (Macewen's sign) sound may be elicited in young children if the cranial sutures have not closed.[1]

Transillumination of the skull is performed routinely on infants and on older children whose heads seem en-

TABLE 34-1
Developmental Considerations in the Physical Examination of Head and Neck Function

Structure	Infant	Child	Adolescent
Head			
Inspection	Circumference 28–36 cm at 39 weeks' gestation. Increases 1.5 cm/month for 6 months, then 0.5 cm/month until 1 year. Must be evaluated relative to height and weight parameters.	Circumference increases 0.5 to 1 cm/year.	Growth continues for girls until 14–16 years and for boys until 16–18 years, with an ending measurement of 54–56 cm.
	Expect molding if neonate was born vaginally. Molding should resolve by second week of age.	Symmetrical-shaped ''tall'' appearance of the head can result from prematurity or early closure of sutures.	Symmetric shape.
	Hair distribution may be scant or may be full at birth. Spontaneous alopecia can occur normally up to 3 months of age. Hair loss in isolated areas may result from friction with bedding.	Hair thickens and lengthens with age. Shiny, full hair indicative of good nutrition. Alopecia rare in absence of disease and may result from traction (hair pulling).	Normal adult pattern of hair distribution develops. The older adolescent male may see postpubescent thinning at the temporal areas.
Palpation	The head should be firm to palpation. Softness may indicate craniotabes or may result from prematurity.	Firm, symmetric; shape determined by ethnic origin and sleeping position during infancy.	Firm, symmetric.
	Sutures may override at birth, with palpable ridges until 6 months of age.		
	Edematous or erythematous areas may result from trauma of delivery. Caput succedaneum describes an area of bruising and edema that crosses the suture lines and can be attributed to superficial birth trauma. *Cephalhematoma* describes similar findings limited to the span of a single cranial bone and may be surrounded by a bony ridge. This finding is more ominous and may indicate skull fracture.		
	Anterior fontanel feels flat when assessed with the infant supported at a 45-degree angle. Sunken fontanel indicates dehydration or malnourishment; bulging fontanel can mean hydrocephalus, infection, or hemorrhage. Closes by 12–18 months of age.	Closed	Closed
	Posterior fontanel closed by 2–3 months of age.		
	Crusting or flaking of scalp absent.	Crusting/flaking absent.	Seborrhea common after puberty.
Face			
Inspection	Round shape.	Round face. Nose is short and round. Nasal bridge is low and profile is concave. Forehead bulbous and straight. Face relatively flat with wide-set eyes. Facial features of boys and girls indistinguishable.	Facial growth slows at age 13 in girls, continues through early adulthood in boys to produce more prominent forehead and nose.
	Symmetry of movement with smile or cry.	Symmetric movement with smile, frown, ''monster face.''	Symmetric movement.
	Chvostek sign present at 1 month.		
	Skin color ruddy red at birth, becomes pale pink. African-American neonates pale at birth. Pallor, cyanosis absent. Jaundice may be present in first 10 days of life. Orange coloring related to vegetable ingestion. Erythema toxicans disappears within 7–10 days of birth.	Skin color even.	Skin color even.
	Acne neonatorum may be present up to 2 months.	Prepubescent acne on chin and forehead from age 6 to 8	Acne vulgaris common during puberty.
	Telangiectatic nevi (''angel kisses'') common.	Telangiectatic nevi fade.	
	Milia common before 2 months of age. Epicanthal folds normal in Asian children.		
	Eye placement normal, hypertelorism or hypotelorism absent as exhibited by Intercanthal index $\frac{\text{(distance between inner canthi} \times 100)}{\text{distance between outer canthi}}$	Intercanthal Index mean 38 mm for ages 6–12 years	Intercanthal Index mean 37 mm for ages 13–18
Palpation	No masses or tenderness. Fat pads in cheeks present.	No tenderness. Pain on palpation at sides of nose or over eyes may indicate sinus infection, which cannot be visualized on x-ray until 6 years of age.	No tenderness or mass. Acne may be cystic in nature.

(Continued)

TABLE 34-1
(Continued)

Structure	Infant	Child	Adolescent
Eyes			
Inspection	Placement and shape symmetric.	Placement and shape symmetric.	
	Sclera clear and white, yellow appearance with jaundice. Blue sclera can be normal variant or indicate osteogenesis imperfecta.	Sclera clear and white. Bluish hue common in African-American children.	Sclera clear and white.
	Conjunctiva have deep pink, glossy appearance.	Conjunctiva have deep pink, glossy appearance.	Conjunctiva have deep pink, glossy appearance.
	Absence of pale, deep red, or raised areas.	Absence of pale, deep red, or raised areas.	Absence of pale, deep red, or raised areas.
	Lids close completely during sleep, open symmetrically.	Lids close completely, open symmetrically on command.	Lids close completely, open symmetrically.
	Skin thin, vascular, and pale.	Skin pale and thin, free from reddened or raised areas	Skin pale and thin.
	Iris bluish in color during neonatal period.	Iris color permanent by 1 year.	Iris color uniform.
	Iris shape round and regular.	Iris shape round and regular.	Iris shape round and regular.
	Pupils constrict briskly and consensually to light.	Pupils constrict briskly and consensually to light.	Pupils constrict briskly and consensually to light.
	Eyes remain focused when body turned on side.		
	Tears present after 1 month. Excessive tearing may indicate blocked lacrimal duct, which occurs in 30% of neonates.	Tears present.	Tears present.
	Visual acuity increases gradually. Neonate keeps eyes closed, sensitive to light. Visual acuity 20/200.	Visual acuity 20/30 by 3 years of age, 20/20 by 6 years.	20/20 vision.
	At 2 weeks of age, looks at faces, large objects. Does not follow.		
	At 4–6 weeks, follows large objects to midline when held close to face.		
	At 2–3 months, follows past midline, blink response, binocular fixation, looks at own hands.		
	At 6 months, watches others in room.		
	At 9 months, observes small objects.		
	At 1 year, visual acuity 20/50.		
	Red reflex present.	Red reflex present.	Red reflex present.
	On examination of fundus, optic disc has sharp margins and is pale yellow in color. Vessels appear smooth.	On examination of fundus, optic disc has sharp margins and is pale yellow in color. Vessels appear smooth.	On examination of fundus, optic disc has sharp margins and is pale yellow in color. Vessels appear smooth.
Palpation	Slightly firm, nontender.	Moderately firm, nontender.	Moderately firm, nontender.
Ears			
Inspection	Pinna pale pink, round, pliable; rises above line of outer canthus of eye.	Pinna somewhat firm, elastic; rises above line of outer canthus of eyes.	Pinna somewhat firm, elastic; rises above line of outer canthus of eyes.
	Cerumen is waxy, light gold in color.	Waxy, light gold cerumen.	Waxy, light gold cerumen.
	Drainage absent.	Drainage absent.	Drainage absent.
	Skin tags and preauricular sinus (pit) absent.	Skin tags, preauricular sinus absent.	Skin tags, preauricular sinus absent.
	Canals obstructed by vernix in the newborn.	Canals clear and unobstructed. Color without erythema or pallor.	Canals clear and unobstructed. Color without erythema or pallor.
	Tympanic membrane not assessed in the neonate.	Tympanic membrane assessed by otoscopic examination with pinna pulled down and back for children under 3 years of age, and with pinna pulled up and back for those above 3 (see fig. 34-1).	Pinna pulled up and back for examination of tympanic membrane.
	Light reflex present.	Light reflex present.	Light reflex present.
	Tympanic membrane pearly in color. May be red with crying.	Tympanic membrane pearly in color, malleus visible.	Tympanic membrane pearly in color, malleus visible.
	Cloudy or white areas absent.	Cloudy or white areas absent.	Cloudy or white areas absent.
		Myringotomy tubes visible, if present.	
Palpation	Pinna nontender.	Pinna nontender.	Pinna nontender.
	Mastoid without mass or tenderness	Mastoid without mass or tenderness.	Mastoid without mass or tenderness.

(Continued)

TABLE 34-1
(Continued)

Structure	Infant	Child	Adolescent
Nose			
Inspection	Nares symmetric and patent.	Nares symmetric and patent.	Nares symmetric and patent.
			Notch in nasal bridge common variant, but may obstruct one nare.
	Feeding tube or other catheter passes easily through each nare.		
	Nasal mucosa appears pink.	Nasal mucosa appears pink.	Nasal mucosa appears pink.
	Drainage from nose absent.	Drainage from nose absent.	Drainage from nose absent.
		Absent creasing of nose.	Absent creasing of nose.
Palpation	Soft, compressible.	Firm.	Firm.
	Absent tenderness or edema.	Absent tenderness or edema.	Absent tenderness or edema.
Mouth			
Inspection	Lips intact, continuous, pink.	Lips intact, continuous, pink.	Lips intact, continuous, pink.
	Pallor, cyanosis absent.	Pallor, cyanosis absent.	Pallor, cyanosis absent.
	Cracking, peeling absent.	Cracking, peeling absent.	Cracking, peeling absent.
	Mucosa pink and moist.	Mucosa pink and moist. Linea alba may be present if bite is not occlusive and mucosa fits in occlusal plane.	Mucosa pink and moist. Linea alba may be present if bite is not occlusive and mucosa fits in occlusal plane.
	Tongue moist and pink, evenly covered with tiny papillae on dorsal surface.	Tongue moist and pink, evenly covered with papillae on dorsal surface. Grooves, fasciculation absent.	Tongue moist and pink, evenly covered with papillae on dorsal surface. Grooves, fasciculation absent.
	Median sulcus divides the tongue longitudinally in the midline.	Median sulcus divides tongue longitudinally in the midline.	Median sulcus divides tongue longitudinally in the midline.
	Ventral surface of tongue smooth and glossy	Ventral surface of tongue smooth and glossy.	Ventral surface of tongue smooth and glossy.
	Lingular frenulum attaches posterior ⅔ of tongue to floor of mouth. Allows extension of tongue out of mouth.	Lingular frenulum leaves anterior ⅓ of tongue free for clear speach and easy mobility. Small tags of tissue on frenulum common.	Lingular frenulum leaves anterior ⅓ of tongue free for clear speech and easy mobility. Small tags of tissue on frenulum common.
	Hard palate (anterior ⅔) and soft palate (posterior ⅓) intact.	Hard palate (anterior ⅔) and soft palate (posterior ⅓) intact.	Hard palate (anterior ⅔) and soft palate (posterior ⅓) intact.
	Uvula midline and singular, rises symmetrically with cry.	Uvula midline and singular, rises symmetrically when "Ah" elicited.	Uvula midline and singular, rises symmetrically when "Ah" elicited.
	Gums pink, firm, intact. Epstein's pearls (small white cysts) may appear in infants less than 3 months of age.	Gums pink, intact	
	First deciduous teeth appear at 6 months and one per month thereafter.	Full set of 20 deciduous teeth by 2 years of age.	Full set of 32 permanent teeth by age 22, including "wisdom teeth." Absence of wisdom teeth normal variant or from therapeutic removal.
	Foul breath absent.	Foul breath absent.	Foul breath absent.
	Throat pink, tonsils not visualized or slightly protuberant.	Throat pink, tonsils not visualized or slightly protuberant.	Throat pink, tonsils not visualized or slightly protuberant.
	Exudate absent.		
	Swallowing is accomplished easily with tongue between lips.	Swallowing accomplished with tongue pressing against palate.	
Palpation	Palate intact, suck elicited.	Palate intact.	Palate intact.
	Mucosa soft, no tenderness or mass.	Mucosa soft, no tenderness or mass.	Mucosa soft, no tenderness or mass.
	Submental glands soft and nontender.	Submental glands soft and nontender.	Submental glands soft and nontender.
Neck			
Inspection	Sternocleidomastoid muscle visible with strain or cry.	Sternocleidomastoid muscle prominent when tensed, frames sides of neck, symmetric in movement.	Sternocleidomastoid muscle prominent when tensed, frames sides of neck, symmetric in movement.
	Short, broad neck.	Slim, longer neck.	Slim, long neck.
			Larynx prominent in boys.
	Head held straight, torticollis absent.	Head held straight, torticollis absent.	Head held straight, torticollis absent.

(Continued)

TABLE 34-1
(Continued)

Palpation	Sternocleidomastoid muscle palpable and smooth bilaterally from mastoid process to jugular notch.	Larynx equal in size in boys and girls.	Larynx larger in boys after puberty.
	Thyroid notch palpable with hyoid bone above and laryngeal prominence below. Lateral sides of thyroid cartilage smooth and nontender.	No Change	No Change
	Carotid pulses, palpable above thyroid cartilage bilaterally.		
	Trachea palpated between sternocleidomastoid muscles in the jugular notch.		
	Cervical lymph nodes nonpalpable (see Fig. 33-7).		

larged. In a dark room, a flashlight that has a protective sponge or rubber collar is held against the skull from several different angles. A halo of light normally extends from the rim of the flashlight: the expected halo is 1 cm around the circumference of the flashlight in the occipital area and 2 cm in the frontoparietal region. Glowing of the entire skull or localized bright spots are not normal and should be investigated further. Transillumination of the sinuses is not routine but may be performed when sinusitis is suspected.

Nose

The nose should be in the midline with symmetrical nares, and its shape should be consistent with the child's racial heritage; creases or lesions are not expected. Patency of the nares is especially important in neonates, because they are obligate nose-breathers. Each nostril is evaluated by pressing shut one side of the nose while air movement through the other nare is felt. Inspection of the internal structures can be difficult if the child is frightened and moves during the examination. Simply raising the tip of the nose can make the vestibular region, the anterior portions of the septum, and nasal turbinates visible without use of the speculum. A penlight or otoscope with a nasal speculum may be used for better illumination. The condition of the nasal mucosa and any secretions present are evaluated.

Mouth

Inspection of the mouth begins with the lips, looking for color, symmetry, moisture, fissures, clefts, or lesions. The oral cavity may be inspected in infants while they are crying. A tongue blade may be gently inserted between the upper and lower teeth and moved toward the midline of the tongue, avoiding stimulation of the gag reflex in toddlers and older children. Unusual mouth odors are noted and need additional exploration. Using a penlight, the oral mucosa, palate, tonsils, and tooth eruption are inspected; lesions are palpated. The tongue's appearance and mobility are assessed. The normal tongue

is pink and should lay symmetrically inside the mouth. Finally, the epiglottis is visualized when the gag reflex is elicited by placing the tongue blade on the root of the tongue.

Eyes

External features of the eyes are noted, as well as movement. Each iris is inspected, and the pupil's response to light noted. A funduscopic examination should be performed, and visual acuity is assessed with the visual fields. A variety of procedures used to evaluate the eyes and their function is discussed in the section on diagnostic studies.

Ears

The position of the ears in relation to the eyes is noted. The top of the pinna should be aligned with the outer canthus of the eye. Internal ear structures are inspected with the otoscope. In the newborn and children younger than 3 years of age, the external auditory canal has an upward curvature; to visualize the structures, the auricle should be pulled down and back (Fig. 34-1). The ear is pulled upward and outward during the otoscopic examination of older children and adolescents. Examining the ear is sometimes difficult for children, because their ear canals are sensitive and they cannot see what is being done. The otoscope should be handled with care, stabilizing the examining hand on the side of the child's head. Children who resist may need gentle coaxing or restraint. Further discussion of common types of auditory assessment is found in the section on diagnostic studies.

Neck

The neck of the newborn is short, making landmarks difficult to examine. However, palpation of the neck is performed, and the head is moved through its range of motion. The cervical lymph nodes are carefully evaluated in older children and adolescents.

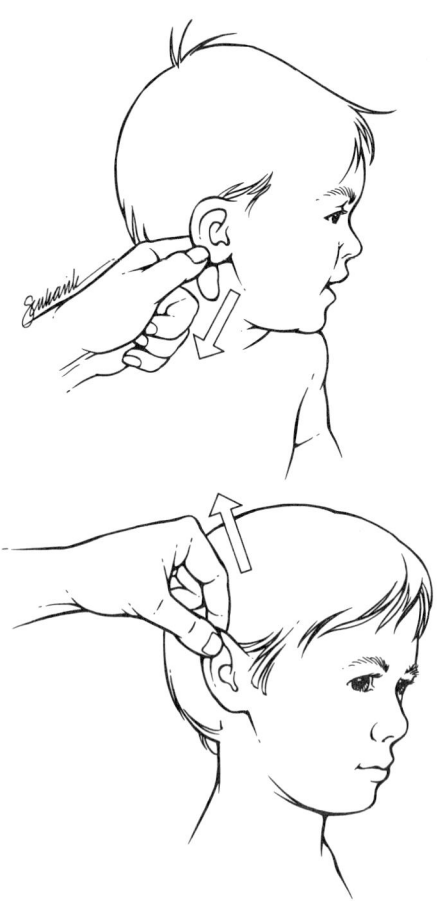

FIGURE 34-1
To straighten the auditory canal, the ear is pulled down and back in the child under 3 years and up and back if the child is older.

Diagnostic Tests

Numerous diagnostic tests are performed to evaluate normal functioning of the structures in the head and neck, and others are used when preliminary findings suggest anomalies. An overview of the laboratory studies and diagnostic procedures is presented in the following sections.

Laboratory Studies

Essentially no blood and urine studies are specific to evaluating the structure or function of the head and neck. The complete blood count provides an overview of hematologic function and screens for the presence of infection. Pallor or lymphadenopathy on physical examination may prompt interest in the complete blood count for confirmation of anemia or infection suggested by such physical findings.

Procedures

A throat culture may be necessary for symptoms of infection. In this procedure, a swabbed specimen is obtained from the nasopharynx and cultured, and an organism is identified so that targeted antibiotic therapy can begin. This procedure is discussed in Chapter 25.

The diagnostic tests used for routine screening and more intense evaluation of sensory function are presented here.

Imaging of the Head and Neck: X-Ray, Ultrasound, Computed Tomography, and Magnetic Resonance Imaging

Description/Definition

Cranial x-ray provides radiologic visualization of bony structures of the head and neck. Imaging of cranial bones, the sinuses, and the cervical spine can be accomplished by x-ray of the head.

Ultrasound of the head provides imaging of soft tissue structures for children with an open fontanel. Through transmission of sound waves, the ultrasound creates visual images of tissue density, allowing visualization of brain ventricles and brain stem.

Computed tomography (CT) scan provides x-ray imaging of thinly dissected planes, one axial plane at a time. CT scan allows detailed visualization of anatomic structures by providing sharp images. This advantage over conventional x-rays results from thinner targets for the radar beam, thereby reducing the distortion of flattening a three-dimensional image.

Like conventional x-ray and CT imaging, Magnetic Resonance Imaging (MRI) beams radiant energy into the subject and is detected as it emerges to create a visual picture. In MRI, however, radio-frequency waves are used rather than x-rays. The visual images created by MRI correlate with tissue densities, like those for CT scan. The magnetic field used for MRI provides more sensitive discrimination of tissue density to create a more detailed image.[14]

Purpose

Imaging of the head and neck may be necessary for assessment of cranial bone structure, ventricular size and integrity, lymphatics and vasculature of the neck or thyroid anatomy, or for suspicion of soft tissue mass. Decisions regarding which type of imaging to use in diagnostic evaluation of an infant or child are made according to tissue sensitivity, invasiveness, and expense. The conventional x-ray is a logical choice for evaluation of the cranial bones and sutures, the sinuses of the child over 6 years of age (Fig. 34-2), and the cervical spine, and for exploration for foreign bodies with a lateral neck view. The x-ray is the least expensive and among the less invasive options for head and neck imaging and is often the initial procedure of choice. Fluoroscopy can be used to assess airway and suck-swallow coordination, as it provides a moving x-ray image.

Ultrasound offers noninvasive visualization of neck soft tissue and head structures with an open fontanel. Ultrasound is commonly used to monitor ventricular size, subarachnoid effusions, and hemorrhages in the infant. In assessment of the neck, ultrasound can offer imaging of the thyroid, salivary glands, cervical lymph nodes, and jugular and carotid vasculature. In children, neck ultrasound examination is most commonly used in the diagnosis of thyroid lesions and neck masses.[4]

The CT scan can be used to visualize structures of the head, face, ear, eye, and neck for diagnosis of abnormalities of bony or soft tissue. MRI offers more detailed visualization of the same structures. Although CT and MRI scans are among the more expensive diagnostic options, they provide greater certitude than was previously possible. The CT scan has become more universally available and less prohibitive in cost; MRI is available at larger health care delivery centers. CT scans and MRIs may be performed with or without use of contrast materials.

Indications

- Known or suspected skull fracture.
- Altered mentation or level of consciousness.
- Fever of unknown origin.

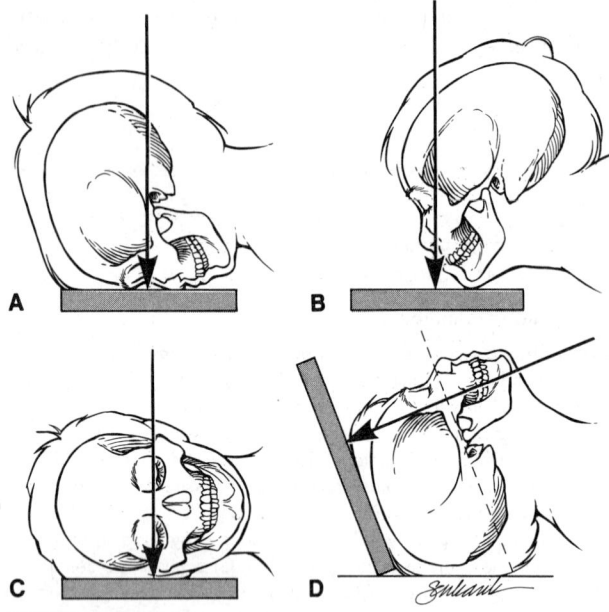

FIGURE 34-2

Paranasal sinus x-rays: (**A**) Anteroposterior view. The child's nose and forehead are placed against the film cassette. Frontal sinuses are best seen in this view. Ethmoids are also demonstrated but are superimposed over the sphenoid sinus. (**B**) Waters view: The child's nose and chin are placed against the film cassette. Maxillary sinuses are best seen in this view. (**C**) Lateral view: Provides a true lateral view of the facial bones. The sphenoid sinus is best seen in this view, and the depth of the frontal sinuses is demonstrated. (**D**) Submental-vertex view: The child is supine for this exposure, and even small amounts of pus may be seen pooling in the maxillary or sphenoid sinuses.

- Hydrocephalus.
- Head injury.
- Macrocephaly or microcephaly.
- Suspected sinus infection.
- Foreign body.
- Visual guide for biopsy.
- Suspected mass.

Contraindications

- Use of contrast materials in infants or children with known or suspected allergy.
- MRI in the presence of metals.

Preparation

Time-elapsed studies such as ultrasound, CT, and MRI require that the child remain still throughout the duration of the study. Infants and children are likely to require sedation for timely and effective accomplishment of such procedures. As always, procedures should be described to children and parents at an appropriate level of understanding for the learner. Children are not usually held NPO. Contrast materials are generally administered by those professionals conducting the study; intravenous access, however, should be obtained prior to the test. Parental consent is obtained when necessary.

Developmental Considerations

- Infant: Swaddling or use of a papoose board may be necessary to keep the infant still during the test. Sedation may be required for ultrasound, CT scan, or MRI.
- Child: Sedation may be required, especially when diagnostic testing requires separation from a parent, or appearance of equipment elicits fear.
- Adolescent: None.

Nursing Implications

Parents and children old enough to understand should be prepared for the experience of a procedure, including the appearance of equipment and sensations likely to result. Intravenous access will be required for contrasted tests. When a radioactive isotope has been used as contrast, diapers should be handled and disposed according to hospital protocol. Most hospitals advise nurses not to care for such patients while pregnant.

Hair implements, jewelry, and watches are removed prior to MRI.

Complications

Allergic reaction to contrast materials.
Respiratory depression may result from sedation.

Visual Assessment

Definition/Description

Numerous procedures are used to assess the structures of the eye and visual acuity.

FUNDUSCOPIC EXAMINATION

With an ophthalmoscope, a red reflex can be elicited from even the youngest child. More systematic evaluation of the fundus requires cooperation from the child. Such an examination begins by focusing on the optic disc, next on the retinal vessels and retina itself, and then on the macula[15] (Fig. 34-3).

AIR PUFF TONOMETRY

Used in screening for glaucoma, air puff tonometry measures the time required to flatten the cornea when a puff of air is blown on the eye. Increased time needed indicates elevated intraocular pressure, which may be caused by glaucoma.[15]

VISUAL FIELDS

Measurement of the visual field determines how far from the point of maximum acuity (the macula) the eye will continue to respond to stimulation. An isopter represents the distance between where the observer first becomes aware of a stimulus and where fixation on the stimulus would occur. The visual field, then, is defined as the area within which a subject can see a visual stimulus without altering position of gaze.[8]

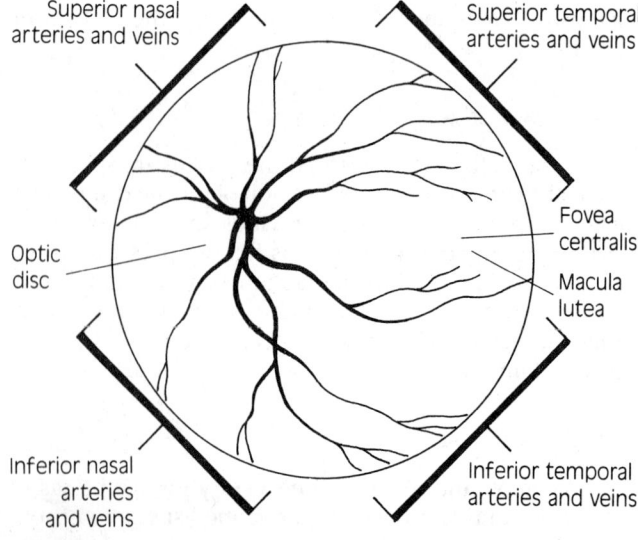

FIGURE 34-3

Retinal landmarks visualized on examination of the eye with an ophthalmoscope.

COVER TEST

An entertaining or colorful object can be used to encourage the child's interest. When visual fixation on the object occurs, one eye is covered and the other is assessed for movement. The presence of movement indicates deviation of gaze (strabismus) in that eye.[15]

VISUAL ACUITY

1. Stycar ball test: spheres of graduated sizes are introduced into the infant's or child's line of vision, and fixation on the sphere is observed. Balls of decreasing size are used until no response is obtained. This test can measure visual acuity from 6 months of age.[8]
2. Matching toys/Ffookes symbols: a child older than age 2 is shown pictures of objects at a determined distance. The child then selects the like object from a group of items nearby.
3. Allen cards: pictures of recognizable items are presented to the child of 2 years or older and the child is asked to identify the item.
4. Snellen tests: a chart with letters or symbols that become gradually smaller is presented to the child (Fig. 34-4). Standardized numbers at the end of each line of letters indicate the degree of visual acuity. The child then names the letters or indicates in which direction the symbols point on each line until they are no longer distinct. Visual acuity is recorded as a fraction, with the numerator indicating the distance of the child when the chart was read (20 feet), and the denominator indicating the distance at which a child with normal vision would be able to see the last line read.

VISUAL EVOKED RESPONSE

Electrodes are placed on skin overlying the occipital cortex, and visual stimuli are presented. Measured responses reveal integrity of the visual pathway from the optic nerve to the occipital cortex.[15]

ELECTRORETINOGRAM

Electrodes are placed on the cornea and forehead, and the eye's response to light at the neurosensory level is recorded.[15]

ELECTRO-OCULOGRAM

Electrodes are placed on the lateral lid margin and the forehead, and response of the retinal pigment epithelium to light is recorded.[18]

COLOR VISION

Plates of various colors are presented to the child, and matching of identical colors is requested. Ishiara plates and the Guy Color Vision Test provide screening for older children. Both require color discrimination for identification of numbers or objects.

Purpose

Evaluation of visual acuity, convergence, and field early in a child's life can provide the information needed for intervention and preserved visual outcomes.

Indications

- Absence of focusing behavior in the infant.
- Nystagmus.
- Strabismus.
- Chromosomal abnormality.
- Chronic head tilt.
- Frequent injuries during childhood.
- Complaints of frequent headache.

Contraindications

- Any test measuring electrical response may be altered by sedative medication.

Developmental Considerations

Assessment of vision in a small child or infant requires ingenuity on the part of the examiner. Care is taken to provide objects of visual interest for evoking responses. It is known that 20/20 vision is not achieved until 6 years of age, so parental concern over a young child sitting close to a viewed object may be unwarranted.

It may be necessary to perform chemical dilation of the pupils for funduscopic examination of the infant.

Nursing Implications

Chemical dilation of the pupils may be necessary prior to funduscopic examination. Any child who receives such medications should be protected from exposure to light.

Auditory Assessment

Definition/Description

Numerous methods of evaluating ear structures and hearing acuity are described.

OTOSCOPIC EXAMINATION

The otoscope allows lighted visualization of the ear canal and tympanic membrane. Presence of light reflex, prominence of malleus, and color and character of the tympanic membrane can be assessed (Fig. 34-5A).

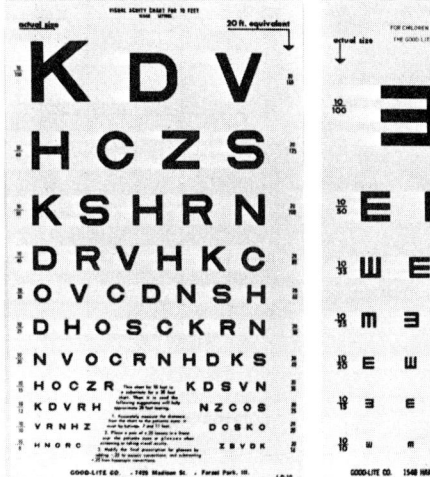
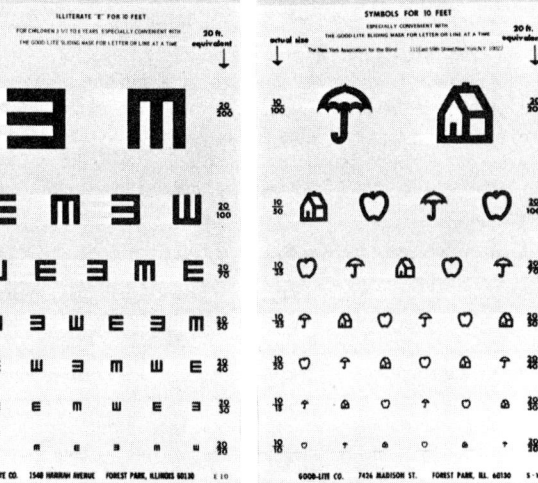

FIGURE 34-4
Various Snellen charts used to test distant vision. The charts in the center and at far right are used for very young children.

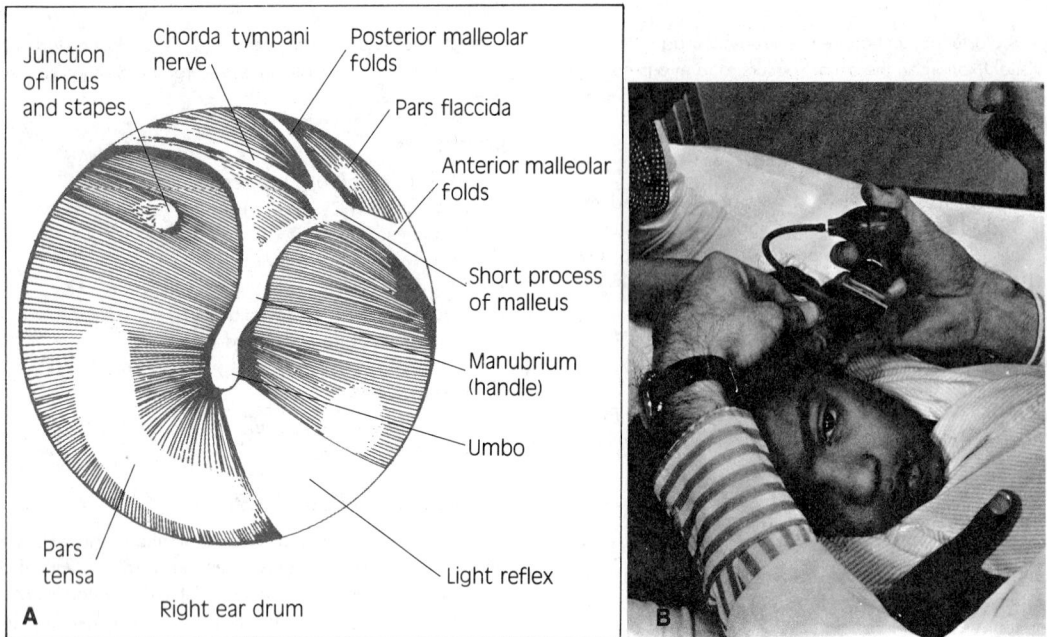

FIGURE 34-5

(**A**) Landmarks visible on otoscopic examination of the tympanic membrane. (**B**) Examination with pneumatic otoscope. (Photo from Bates B: *A guide to physical examination and history taking*, 5th ed. Philadelphia, J.B. Lippincott, 1991.)

PNEUMATOSCOPY

During otoscopic examination, air is expressed into the canal and resultant movement of the tympanic membrane is assessed (Fig. 34-5B). An immobile tympanic membrane denotes effusion or infection of the middle ear.

TYMPANOGRAM

Air is introduced in the external ear canal at a positive pressure of 200 cm H_2O, then the pressure is decreased to negative 500 cm H_2O. Compliance of the tympanic membrane should change as the pressure changes if the middle ear system is functioning normally. A graph is produced plotting air pressure against compliance. Figure 34-6 illustrates a normal tympanogram. An obstructed eustachian tube should shift the curve's peak to the left of zero. A flattened peak may result from fluid in the middle ear or scarring of the tympanic membrane, which restricts its movement.[17]

PURE TONE (CONVENTIONAL) AUDIOMETRY

Air conduction is assessed by presentation of pure tones through earphones, and bone conduction is tested by a vibrator placed on the mastoid. The hearing threshold represents the difference between the patient's reported hearing level and the standard level for normal-hearing persons. The main limitation of such testing is in its usefulness only for those old enough to report accurately and reliably what they hear, a behavior rare below the age of 3 years. The difference between air and bone conduction in a child, known as the *air-bone gap*, provides information about whether hearing loss is conductive or sensorineural.[17]

BEHAVIORAL OBSERVATION AUDIOMETRY

Observation of a young child's behavior provides information about vision and development as well as hearing. Because of its simplicity, behavioral testing is usually the initial form of hearing evaluation for children under 12 years of age. Behaviors elicited in response to sounds can be observed in children from the newborn period on and range from eye blinking and Moro's startle response to head turning and localization of sound. Full maturation of auditory behavior occurs by 13 months of age.[17]

PLAY AUDIOMETRY

By providing a play activity with hearing evaluation, children ages 2 to 4 years are more easily engaged in the testing procedure. Children are asked to place a peg in a board or point to the named object when a sound is heard. Both air and bone conduction can be assessed as listening is reinforced through play.[17]

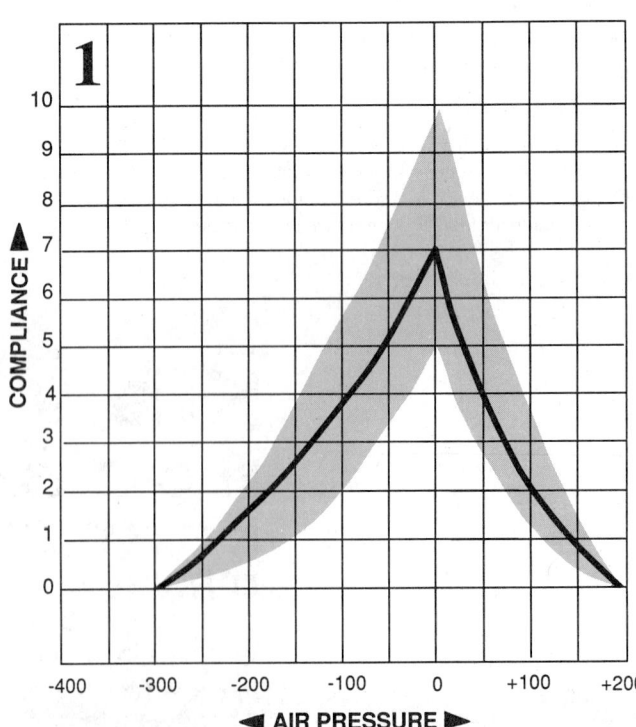

FIGURE 34-6

A normal tympanogram. (From Pappas, G. [1985]. *Diagnosis and treatment of hearing impairment in children.* San Diego, CA: College-Hill Press.)

SOUND FIELD TESTING

Hearing testing for infants over the age of 6 months can be accomplished through placement in a sound-proof booth with observation of responses to presented sounds. The helpfulness of this test is limited, in that information about individual ears cannot be obtained.

BRAIN STEM AUDITORY EVOKED RESPONSE

Scalp electrodes measure brain wave response to sound and uncover both sensorineural and conductive hearing loss in all age groups.[16]

Purpose

Examination of the ear and evaluation of hearing are crucial in the diagnosis of structural or functional anomalies of the auditory system. Such testing can distinguish congenital hearing loss from acquired loss, and conductive loss from sensorineural loss. Classification and characterization of auditory limitations provide the foundation for care and management of the hearing-impaired child.

Indications

- Chronic ear infections.
- Meningitis.
- Family history of hearing loss during childhood.
- Chromosomal abnormality.
- Misshapen external pinna.
- Inappropriate behavioral response to sound.
- Delayed progression of speech.
- Use of ototoxic medication.

Contraindications

- Sedation may alter responsiveness to sound.
- Active infection of the middle ear may alter results.

Preparation

Describe the procedure to the child in age-appropriate terms. Parents should also receive a description of the type of test conducted and the information it provides.

Developmental Considerations

Type of audiometry used should be determined by the child's capability to respond to sound stimuli and by developmental age. Written results can be described relative to the child's developmental limitations. Sedation is not recommended because it would change the child's responsiveness during the test. Toddlers and preschoolers can be expected to offer resistance to probing into ears or other orifices, regardless of painlessness.

Nursing Implications

Infants and small children need to be restrained during examination of the ears when movement could result in injury. Hearing evaluation should be scheduled when a child is rested and fed for optimal cooperation and responsiveness.

Complications

Superficial bleeding of the ear canal resulting from movement during otoscopic examination.

TABLE 34-2
Selected Nursing Diagnoses Associated With Altered Head and Neck Function

Data Analysis and Conclusions	Nursing Diagnoses
Health Perception and Management	
Verbalization of habits that encourage infection; direct observation of child experiencing ongoing risk or impaired health. *Examples:* visible tooth decay; child drinks cola from a bottle; mother describes child's need for bottle in bed at night; denial of routine dental hygiene, no formal dental care; recurrent ear infections; poor diet history; delayed growth parameters in the child.	Altered Health Maintenance related to Knowledge Deficit of nutritional requirements, dental care, causes of infection, or parental neglect Altered Growth and Development related to inadequate caretaking
Activity and Exercise	
Observed facies of "mouth breather"; "allergic salute" four times during examination, crease across bulb of nose suggests chronic use of allergic salute to clear turbinates; hospitalization in spring and fall for last 2 years; mother reports tubing for home nebulizer lost, uses over-the-counter bronchodilators; frequently misses school secondary to "colds."	Ineffective Breathing Pattern related to mouth breathing Impaired Home Maintenance Management related to insufficient family organization
Cognition and Perception	
History of chronic ear infections, mother reports that child says "Da-Da" only at 18 months of age.	Sensory-Perceptual Alteration (auditory) related to altered sensory reception
Role Relationship	
History of cleft lip and palate, reported intolerance of oral feeds, chronic nasal congestion and rhinorrhea; no vocalization except for cry; mother describes baby as "ugly," and states that the baby "doesn't like" her.	Impaired Verbal Communication related to anatomic defect and potential for hearing deficit Altered Parenting related to impaired bonding, baby's inability to feed, smile, vocalize Possible Social Isolation related to lack of parental pride
Coping and Stress Tolerance	
At birth, infant displays facies consistent with Down syndrome; mother reverses decision to "room in," declines opportunities to feed infant; parents do not accept calls from family members and friends, verbalize reluctance to bring siblings to meet newborn.	Dysfunctional Grief related to loss of perfect child. Possible Ineffective Family Coping: Disability related to feelings of guilt and despair
Values and Beliefs	
Necessity for surgery identified, potential for blood transfusion; parents' religious beliefs associate blood with one's spirit and prohibit transfusion; potential for court order allowing transfusion to ensure safety of child during procedure.	Spiritual Distress related to challenged belief and value system

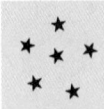

Ideas for Nursing Research

The unique and inherent challenge in caring for small children lies in their inability to communicate verbally. For this reason, understanding of perceptions and abilities of infants and children often eludes the caregiver. The following areas need to be explored:

- Assessment of gustatory and olfactory sensation in infants
- Alternative cues for the facially impaired infant to elicit parental nurturance behaviors
- Methods for preserving and accelerating the development of children with sensory impairments
- Factors that have an impact on children's definitions of attractiveness

Selected Nursing Diagnoses

After obtaining the history, performing the physical examination, reviewing results from the diagnostic tests, and tapping additional resources for information, the nurse carefully analyzes data that were obtained. Nursing diagnoses appropriate for the child with head and neck dysfunction become apparent and are used to develop a plan of care. Selected nursing diagnoses that may be appropriate for the child with head and neck dysfunction are presented by function in Table 34-2.

Summary

Just as the head and neck are generally the first part of the newborn to arrive in the outside world, they also are the first to be assessed as part of a standard head-to-toe examination. The head and neck provide countless services for the child, including protection of the brain; information about sights, smells, sounds, and tastes; humidification and warmth of air; and expression of emotion. In a similar way, examination of the head and neck provides the caregiver with volumes of information regarding function of the child's body systems and general health.

Infection status, expressive and receptive cognition, sensory integrity, and respiratory function can all be assessed through examination of the uppermost portion of the body. A thorough assessment provides the nurse with the information necessary to embark on successful use of the nursing process.

References

1. Bates, B. (1991). *A guide to physical examination and history taking* (5th ed.). Philadelphia: J.B. Lippincott.
2. Belfer, M. L. (1983). Self esteem related to bodily change in children with craniofacial deformity. In J. E. Mack & S. L. Ablon, (Eds.). *The development and sustenance of self esteem in childhood*. New York: International Universities Press.
3. Blueston, C. D., & Stool, S. E. (Eds.). (1990). *Pediatric otolaryngology* (Vol. 1, 2nd ed.). Philadelphia: W.B. Saunders.
4. Bruneton, J. N. (1987). In N. R. Raneau (Trans.), *Ultrasonography of the neck*. New York: Springer-Verlag.
5. Cann, A., & Ross, D. A. (1989). Olfactory stimuli as context cues in human memory. *American Journal of Psychology, 102*(1), 91–102.
6. Carpenito, L. J. (1992). *Nursing diagnosis: Application to clinical practice* (4th ed.). Philadelphia: Lippincott.
7. DeCasper, A. J., & Fifer, W. P. (1987).Of human bonding: Newborns prefer their mothers' voices. In J. Oates & S. Sheldon (Eds.). *Cognitive development in infancy*. London: Lawrence Erlbaum.
8. Edwards, K., & Llewellyn, R. (Eds.). (1988). *Optometry*. Boston: Butterworths.
9. Enlow, D. H. (1990). *Facial growth*. Philadelphia: W.B. Saunders.
10. Fuller, J., & Schaller-Ayers, J. (1990). *Health assessment: A nursing approach*. Philadelphia: J.B. Lippincott.
11. Gorlin, R. J., Cohen, M. M., & Levin, L. S. (1990). *Syndromes of the head and neck*. New York: Oxford University Press.
12. Harrison, A. M. (1983). Body image and self esteem. In J. E. Mack and S. L. Ablon (Eds.). *The development and sustenance of self esteem in childhood*. New York: International Universities Press.
13. Hiatt, J. L., & Gartner, L. P. (1987). *Textbook of head and neck anatomy*. Baltimore: Williams & Wilkins.
14. Lee, S. H., & Rao, K. C. (1987). *Cranial computed tomography and MRI* (2nd ed.). New York: McGraw-Hill.
15. Leitman, M. W. (1988). *Manual for eye examination and diagnosis*. Oradell, NJ: Medical Economics Books.
16. Pagana, K. D., & Pagana, T. J. (1990). *Diagnostic testing and nursing implications*. Baltimore: Mosby.
17. Pappas, G. (1985). *Diagnosis and treatment of hearing impairment in children*. San Diego, CA: College-Hill Press.
18. Zitelli, B. J., & Davis, H. W. (Eds.). (1987). *Atlas of pediatric physical diagnosis*. New York: Gower.

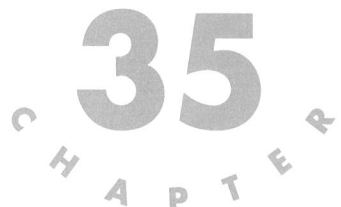

Nursing Planning, Intervention, and Evaluation for Altered Head and Neck Function

BEHAVIORAL OBJECTIVES

Describe the etiology, pathophysiology, and clinical manifestations of common disorders of the head and neck in children.

Discuss application of the nursing process in the care of the child with selected alterations of head and neck function.

Explain the special psychosocial needs of children who have impaired vision or hearing and their families.

Identify local or national agencies that may serve as resources to families of children who have alterations of the head and neck.

Although proportionately small, the head and neck contain important organs for overall functioning of the body. Five of the six senses—visual, auditory, gustatory, tactile, and olfactory—are elicited by organs located in the head. In addition the face and head are the most prominent and noticeable parts of the body; so disfigurement of this region can significantly alter self-concept. The organs of the upper respiratory system also are located in the head and neck, and contribute to a large portion of acute illnesses in children. Providing nursing care for children with altered head and neck function requires an understanding of a broad range of physiologic, developmental, and psychosocial concepts.

For children with long-term disabilities the nurse acts as a liaison between the physician and community resources to provide the child and family a comprehensive treatment plan. Continuity of care may require frequent telephone contact and even home or school visits to provide the child with optimum care. Thus, the nurse plays an essential role in ensuring the best care available for children with problems of

813

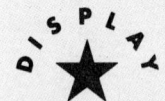

Resources for Families of Children With Vision, Hearing, and Oral Dysfunctions

Visual Impairment

American Foundation for the Blind, Inc.
15 West 16th Street
New York, NY 10011

American Printing House for the Blind, Inc.
1839 Frankfort Avenue
Louisville, KY 40200

Association for the Education of the Visually Handicapped
(The Alliance)
206 N. Washington Street
Alexandria, VA 22314

International Institute for Visually Impaired, 0-7, Inc.
1975 Rutgers Circle
East Lansing, MI 48823

Learning Disabilities Program
Bureau of Education for the Handicapped
7th and D Streets, S.W.
Washington, DC 20202

Library of Congress
Division for the Blind and Visually Handicapped
1291 Taylor Street, N.W.
Washington, DC 20542

National Association for Parents of the Visually Impaired
(NAPVI)
PO Box 180806
Austin, TX 78718

National Association for the Visually Impaired
305 East 24th Street
New York, NY 10010

National Society to Prevent Blindness
79 Madison Avenue
New York, NY 10016

Hearing Impairment

Alexander Graham Bell Association for the Deaf, Inc.
3417 Volta Place, N.W.
Washington, DC 20007

American Speech-Language-Hearing Association
10801 Rockville Pike
Rockville, MD 20852

Association for Children With Learning Disabilities
4156 Library Road
Pittsburgh, PA 15234

Conference of Executives of American Schools for the Deaf
5034 Wisconsin Avenue, N.W.
Washington, DC 20016

Council of Organizations Serving the Deaf
4201 Connecticut Avenue, N.W.
Suite 210
Washington, DC 20008

International Parents Organization
Alexander Graham Bell Association for the Deaf
3417 Volta Place, N.W.
Washington, DC 20007

National Association of the Deaf
814 Thayer Avenue
Silver Spring, MD 20910

National Association of Parents of the Deaf
814 Thayer Avenue
Silver Spring, MD 20910

The American Speech and Hearing Association
9030 Old Georgetown Road
Bethesda, MD 20014

The National Association of Hearing and Speech Action
814 Thayer Avenue
Silver Spring, MD 20910

Cleft Lip and Cleft Palate

American Cleft Palate Educational Foundation, Inc.
331 Salk Hall
University of Pittsburgh
Pittsburgh, PA 15261

The Cleft Palate Association
1218 Grandview Avenue
University of Pittsburgh
Pittsburgh, PA 15211

The Cleft Palate Foundation
1218 Grandview Avenue
University of Pittsburgh
Pittsburgh, PA 15211

the head and neck. The accompanying display lists resources for families of children with vision, hearing, and oral dysfunctions.

Disorders of the Skull and Facial Structures

Craniosynostosis

Definition and Incidence. *Craniosynostosis* refers to the premature closure and obliteration, or absence, of one or more sutures of the skull.[1] As one of the most prominent disorders involving the bones of the head, craniosynostosis occurs once in every 2000 live births. The incidence is higher in whites than in African Americans and Orientals. Approximately 63% of children with this disorder are boys.[53] Craniosynostosis usually manifests itself in the first few months of life and, if referred promptly, can be corrected by surgery.

Etiology and Pathophysiology. In 98% of affected children no clear-cut etiology can be determined for this birth defect; the other 2% result from an autosomal recessive or autosomal dominant genetic basis.[29] The hereditary forms are more likely to include stenosis of multiple sutures or other craniofacial abnormalities.

More than one classification system is used with craniosynostosis. One type distinguishes the clinical presentation as simple or compound; simple indicates stenosis of only one suture, and compound means that two or more sutures are stenosed. A second classification system divides craniosynostosis into the categories of primary, secondary, isolated, and syndromic. Primary craniosynostosis refers to closure of one or more sutures in an otherwise normal individual.[53] The term secondary craniosynostosis indicates that the sutural obliteration results from a known disorder (e.g., thalassemia, hyperthy-roidism, or microcephaly). The individual with isolated craniosynostosis has no abnormalities other than those associated with the stenosed sutures, while syndromic craniosynostosis indicates that the condition occurs in conjunction with other morphologic deviations (e.g., polysyndactyly or congenital heart defects).[13]

Previously it was thought that there was minimal risk of brain damage with simple craniosynostosis. However, Albin et al[1] cite recent studies that show increased intracranial pressure in children with single suture involvement in spite of normal physical and fundoscopic examinations. This same finding has been reported by other authors.[13,53]

Clinical Manifestations. Several configurations of the skull are possible, depending on the sutures stenosed and the order and timing at which synostosis has occurred (Fig. 35-1). The earlier in childhood the synostosis occurs, the more pronounced the effect on subsequent cranial growth and development. Conversely, the later synostosis occurs, the less effect the defect has on cranial growth and development.

Synostosis of the sagittal suture results in a long and narrow skull shape called *dolichocephaly* (also known as scaphocephaly). In *brachycephaly* the skull is shortened anteroposteriorly, and its height is increased due to premature closure of the coronal suture. Brachycephaly may be associated with depression of the orbital roof, exophthalmos, strabismus, and other eye findings if increased intracranial pressure exists. *Plagiocephaly* describes unilateral coronal or unilateral lambdoidal suture stenosis. *Trigonocephaly* presents as a triangular-shaped head with prominence of the frontal bone due to synostosis of the metopic suture. *Oxycephaly* is the defect in which all cranial sutures are closed and may be associated with severe brain involvement.

Diagnostic Studies. Physical examination of the head shape and size is the most important parameter for

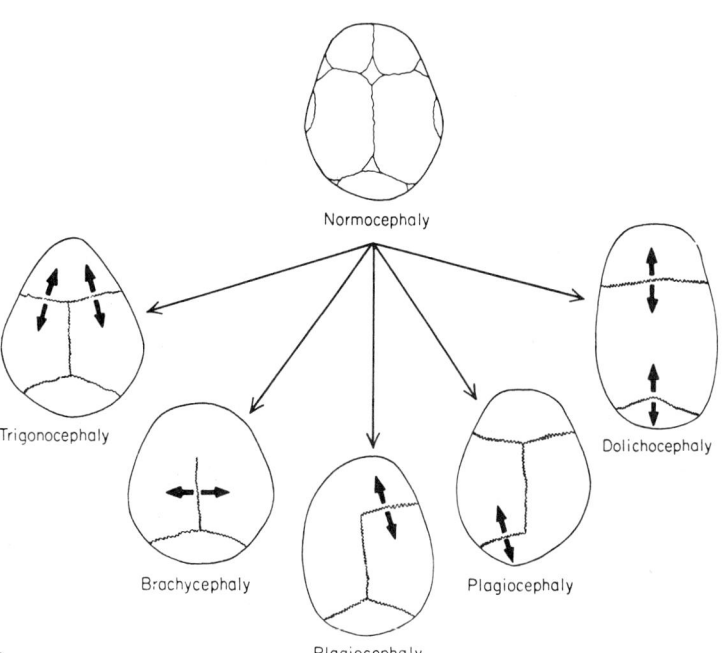

FIGURE 35-1
With craniosynostosis the shape of the skull depends on the sutures stenosed and the order and timing at which the synostosis occurred. (Courtesy of M. M. Cohen Jr., Halifax, Nova Scotia, Canada.)

screening children for craniosynostosis. Skull x-rays are the diagnostic tool of choice to confirm the diagnosis. Films should be obtained with anterior–posterior, lateral, and other views to compare and contrast the sutures at different angles. Increased density of the bone at the affected suture line may be seen on the skull x-ray of a child with craniosynostosis.[53]

A computed tomography (CT) scan also may be performed for two reasons: to determine if there is a problem with brain growth and to obtain bone windows. A CT scan performed on the brain determines if the child has primary neurologic abnormalities (e.g., microcephaly) that may affect the decision to perform surgery. Bone windows also can be obtained using a CT scan. This term refers to the mechanism for shading out the contour of the brain, thus producing a picture showing only the inner and outer contours of the skull. Bone windows can be especially useful when skull x-rays are inconclusive concerning the appearance of a particular suture or the outline of the skull.[13]

★ ASSESSMENT

The parent may be the first to notice the infant's unusual head shape. During initial inspection the nurse should note any cranial or facial asymmetry. Unilateral stenosis of the coronal suture (plagiocephaly) is especially noticeable on general facial inspection because the child displays differences in the shape and height of the orbital cavities from one side to the other.[13] Evaluation for symmetry also should include assessment of a horizontal line between the superior aspect of the external ear and the outer canthus of the lateral eye (see Fig. 52-1). Divergence of this line from a horizontal plane would warrant further investigation for a generalized syndrome.

The nurse should pay special attention to measuring and plotting the child's head circumference on the standardized growth chart. The head circumference should then be compared to height and weight parameters. Head circumference, height, and weight measurements should follow the same percentile curve on serial plotting. If there is discrepancy between the measurements, especially a head circumference much greater or smaller than the other parameters, further diagnostic tests and referral to a pediatrician or neurologist should be made.

The nurse should palpate the head, noting the size and fullness of the anterior and posterior fontanels. The anterior fontanel usually measures 2.5 × 2.5 cm, while the posterior fontanel measures about 1 × 1 cm in diameter during the first few months of life. Both fontanels should feel soft and slightly depressed to the touch. The location and mobility of the suture lines also should be determined on palpation of the head. Any ridge-like prominences over the sutures suggest craniosynostosis. Special attention should be given to palpation of the metopic, lambdoid, and even coronal sutures because these are more technically difficult to palpate than the sagittal suture.

Thorough neurologic and developmental examinations are necessary for any child suspected of having craniosynostosis to determine difficulties with brain function. Nurses often use the Denver II to quickly assess

if the child has any outstanding developmental lags. This tool assesses the developmental areas of cognitive, gross and fine motor, social and emotional, and speech and language functioning. The nurse also should assess other neurologic parameters, such as vision, motor movements, mental status, and behavior.

If the infant displays unusual head growth coupled with early fusion of the fontanels, a ridge-like prominence over one or more of the suture lines, or an asymmetry or misshapen appearance of the face or head, the child should be referred to a physician for suspected craniosynostosis. Any diagnostic tests performed also should be forwarded to the referring physician. In addition, the nurse should inform the physician about the child's developmental status and the family's perception of the child's problem.

★ NURSING DIAGNOSES AND PLANNING

Based on assessment data discussed previously and in the preceding chapter, the following nursing diagnoses may apply to the family and child with craniosynostosis:

- High Risk for Altered Growth and Development related to poor brain growth.
- Anxiety (Parental) related to knowledge deficit about the condition, its etiology, treatment, and prognosis.
- Body Image Disturbance related to misshapen appearance of the skull.
- Altered Parenting related to child's appearance.

The nurse and child (or parents) together plan effective care based on the established nursing diagnoses. Several examples of expected outcomes follow:

- The parents express diminished anxiety regarding child's condition.
- The child identifies positive aspects of self as age increases.
- The parents demonstrate appropriate attachment behaviors.
- The parents participate in the child's care.

The nurse plans for the daily care of the child based on physician's orders and nursing diagnoses. Some general nursing care goals may be the following:

- The child reaches full developmental potential.
- The family incorporates child into daily activity patterns.

★ INTERVENTIONS: COLLABORATIVE AND INDEPENDENT

The nurse should recognize the child with symptoms of craniosynostosis, collaborate with the pediatrician or neurologist in obtaining the diagnostic and developmental studies, and assist in referring the child with craniosynostosis to the neurosurgeon for corrective surgery. The referring physician and the nurse should discuss with the parents the diagnosis of craniosynostosis. They should inform the parents that there is a need for a timely referral because surgical correction is most successful when performed in the first year of life and preferably in the first 6 months.[53]

SURGICAL MANAGEMENT

Surgery generally is recommended in the first few months of life for children with simple synostosis to prevent cerebral injury and provide cosmetic repair.[1] If more than one suture is stenosed, the chance of brain damage increases significantly; the brain cannot grow properly if the skull above it does not expand. Therefore, surgery is crucial with compound craniostenosis.

The surgery, called a craniectomy, requires the removal of some of the bone on either side of the fused suture. When the bony plate adjacent to the suture also is misshaped, as the frontal bone in the child with coronal plagiocephay, the bone is also reshaped and repositioned.[1] The reason the surgery is indicated early in life is to take advantage of the maximal brain growth during this period. The enlarging brain assists in reshaping the skull once the suture has been released.

Preoperative teaching is imperative for these parents. The nurse must review what the surgeon has explained to the parents about the surgery and clarify any misperceptions the parents may have. It is especially important to explain to parents what type of equipment will be attached to the child and the location of dressings on the child's body after surgery.

The major postoperative concern of the nurse caring for the child who has had a craniectomy is the risk of bleeding or severe anemia following the surgery. As with any surgery that involves removal of bone, a great deal of blood loss usually occurs intraoperatively. More than half of the children who undergo a craniectomy require a blood transfusion during surgery.[53]

Specific measurements the nurse should carefully observe after surgery include the child's fluid intake and output, central venous pressure, serum electrolytes, hemoglobin, and hematocrit.[29] Abnormalities in these parameters, especially in fluid status, which suggests dehydration or hemoconcentration, should be reported to the physician promptly in case the child is bleeding internally. Most institutions hospitalize the child in the intensive care unit for at least the first night after surgery for close observation.

PSYCHOSOCIAL SUPPORT

The diagnosis can be anxiety-provoking for parents. Frequently the infant has been at home after birth, and the family has become attached. Most children with craniosynostosis are otherwise well and appear developmentally normal (except for children who have this disorder in conjunction with another syndrome). Therefore, advising parents that their child should undergo surgery can be quite upsetting.

The nurse can assist the parents to understand and acknowledge the child's defect by actively listening and clarifying the information presented. Kindness and sympathy on the part of the medical and nursing staff make lasting, positive impressions. Pictures of previously repaired children, both before and after surgery, may boost the parents' confidence in the surgery. Many parents of newly diagnosed children also find solace in talking with parents whose children have already undergone the procedure. Nurses can coordinate referral efforts for support groups and other services that are needed.

Older children with craniofacial anomalies may be aware of the reaction of others to the unusual facial features and expressions. Lowered self-esteem may result from the repeated reception of negative social messages. However, the severity of the defect is not always proportional to the degree of psychologic and emotional stress it generates in the child.[13] Adjustments depend to a large extent on parental attitudes, the child's personality, and the social setting. The nurse can be effective in monitoring the child's adjustment and can make referrals for additional counseling if needed.

DISCHARGE PLANNING

Discharge instructions should begin with teaching the family to keep the scalp clean and dry until the sutures or steri-strips are removed. Other appropriate teaching before discharge should include finishing any prescribed medication, keeping the head of the bed elevated, and assessing the wound daily for signs of infection (i.e., redness, swelling, or discharge from the surgical site). The nurse should tell the parents that an elevated temperature or other systemic signs of infection (i.e., poor feeding or lethargy) should be reported to the neurosurgeon promptly because infection of the bone is a common complication of this surgery.[29]

★ EVALUATION

Periodically the nurse and family evaluate the outcomes of care given. Examples of outcomes for the child and family with craniosynostosis were given under Nursing Diagnoses and Planning in this section. Have short-term goals been met? Are long-term goals still realistic? Planning for further nursing care takes into consideration complications and long-term care.

COMPLICATIONS

The most significant long-term complication is that rarely new bone does not grow back at the craniectomy site. When this situation occurs a cranioplasty can be performed. This procedure requires bone grafting to fill in the bone that is absent, but it is not performed until a reasonable length of time has passed for maximal bone growth, about 5 years postcraniectomy. The craniectomy is therefore considered successful if the child has a symmetrically shaped skull and a full growth of bone over the surgical site by 5 years of age.

LONG-TERM CARE

Most children who are diagnosed and have surgical correction early in life have a fairly normal appearing skull. Postoperatively, because of the absence of bone at the affected suture line, the child will have a soft area for varying lengths of time—usually between 1 and 3 years. New bone eventually grows back into this area.

The nurse should monitor changes in the skull at follow-up visits. Parents should be cautioned that the child must avoid head injury to prevent intracranial damage in the areas devoid of skull. Kershner and Claussen[29] suggest the use of a protective helmet for the child who has had a craniectomy. Other surgeons do not stress protective devices but limit the child's activities.

Craniofacial Dysostosis

Definition and Incidence. The most common forms of craniofacial dysostosis in children are Apert syndrome, also known as acrocephalosyndactyly, and Crouzon's disease. Less common anomalies are described in the accompanying display on rare craniofacial anomalies. The term craniofacial dysostosis implies impaired bone growth in the cranial and facial structures. Regarded as a group, craniofacial anomalies occur in 1 in 5000 to 1 in 20,000 people.

Etiology and Pathophysiology. Apert syndrome and Crouzon's disease are transmitted as an autosomal dominant hereditary trait, although 25% of the cases of Crouzon's disease occur spontaneously without previous family history of the disorder.[13] Craniosynostosis and hypoplastic facies related to maxillary hypoplasia or faciostenosis are present in both disorders.[1] Both conditions manifest a recession of the midface and abnormal skull shape due to these premature synostoses. Apert syndrome also may include fusion of all the skull sutures (oxycephaly) with associated hydrocephalus, thus causing a poor prognosis for intellectual development.[13] Significant facial deformity is especially prevalent with Crouzon's disease. Besides cosmetic considerations, these facial findings may cause difficulties with nasal breathing, eyesight, and the oral structures.

Clinical Manifestations. Apert syndrome and Crouzon's disease have craniosynostosis and hypoplastic midface, most notably an underdeveloped maxilla, as a clinical manifestation. In both syndromes the stenosis of the facial bones causes bulging eyes, hypertelorism (or wide-spaced eyes), an underbite, and an open-mouth posture (Fig. 35-2*A* and *B*). Apert syndrome also is noted for stenosis of multiple cranial sutures, syndactyly of the hands and feet, the common occurrence of hydrocephalus, the increased likelihood of mental retardation, middle ear anomalies, and the frequent occurrence of an incomplete cleft palate. Crouzon's disease has the additional features of small ear canals, middle ear anomalies, and a high incidence of optic nerve involvement. However, most children with Crouzon's disease have normal intelligence.[1]

Diagnostic Studies. A genetic workup of these disorders includes chromosome testing to determine whether the syndrome resulted from a hereditary trait or if it arose spontaneously. With this knowledge the parents can be counseled concerning the likelihood of recurrence in future offspring. Because both of these disorders are transmitted by an autosomal dominant genetic pattern, examination of the parents for clinical manifestations of the syndrome also may assist in determining if the child has the hereditary or sporadic form of the disease.

Radiographic anterior–posterior and lateral views of the skull are obtained with Apert syndrome and Crouzon's disease to confirm the presence of craniosynostosis. If brain involvement is suspected, a CT scan may be ordered to determine if other neurologic problems exist (i.e., hydrocephalus) and need correction. CT scan and perhaps magnetic resonance imaging also may be used to study facial abnormalities and assist the surgeon in planning reconstructive procedures. Other x-rays of the face may be taken for Crouzon's disease and of the hands or feet for Apert syndrome to obtain additional information about anomalies involving these areas. Such problems as malformed sinuses, small nasal cavities, and fusion of the fingers and toes may be further delineated.

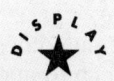

Rare Craniofacial Anomalies

Carpenter Syndrome

An autosomal recessive defect also known as acrocephalopolysyndactyly. It is characterized by a peaked head, peculiar facies, and webbed or fused fingers and toes. Children are often mentally deficient, but children with normal intelligence have been reported.

Ocular Hypertelorism

The distance between the eyes is abnormally wide, and the nose appears broad. Mild forms appear in normal children, but more pronounced forms are associated with other congenital defects or mental deficiency.

Pierre Robin Syndrome

A congenital defect of the face characterized by a small jaw and a tongue that appears large, sometimes obstructing the airway. A high-arched or cleft palate is sometimes present, as are bilateral eye defects, glaucoma, and retinal detachment.

Treacher Collins Syndrome

An autosomal dominant genetic defect characterized by deformities of the facial bones (sunken cheekbones and receding chin), palate, and pinnas. Malocclusion of the teeth and deafness are common.

★ ASSESSMENT

Nurses working in nursery and primary care settings should assess infants and young children for possible craniofacial dysostosis. Different children have various degrees of involvement; therefore, the nurse should look closely for the diagnostic symptoms unique for each syndrome. If a genetic abnormality is suspected, the nurse should gather all useful information, including head circumference measurement and plotting, accurate history concerning related health problems, and a precise description of the noted unusual facies, head shape, or associated defects before a physician referral is made.

A diagnosis of Apert syndrome or Crouzon's disease can be difficult for many families. Determining whether this anomaly was caused by a hereditary pattern or oc-

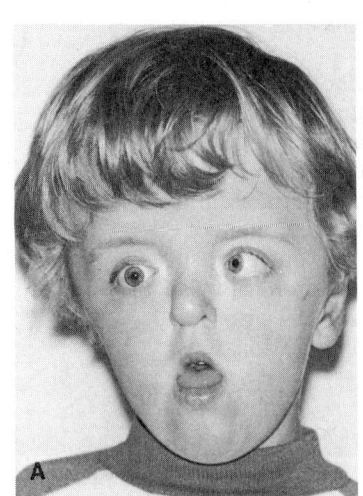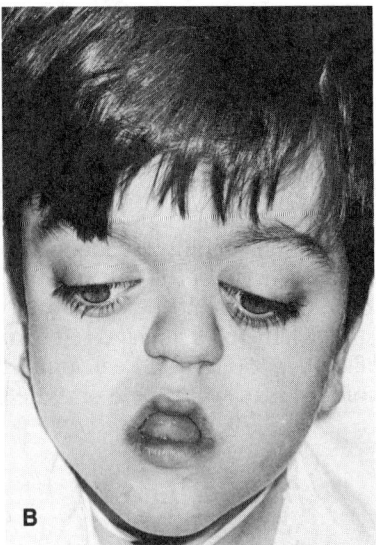

FIGURE 35-2
(**A**) Apert syndrome. (**B**) Crouzon's disease. Note the abnormal skull shape and recession of the midface. (Courtesy of M. M. Cohen Jr., Halifax, Nova Scotia, Canada.)

curred sporadically may alter the family's response to the news of the diagnosis. Because both of these disorders are inherited by autosomal dominant transmission, at least one parent must display some trait of the disease (although this may be less noticeable in an affected parent who is heterozygous, not homozygous, for the trait). Therefore, the family who already has an affected parent may accept the cosmetic deformities better than the family of a child with a spontaneous occurrence of the anomaly. However, when the child has a more serious presentation of the disease than the parent, there may be more guilt feelings on the part of the affected parent.

Nurses working with children previously diagnosed with a form of Apert, Crouzon's, or other craniofacial abnormality need to get a detailed history at each medical visit concerning symptomatology the child may be experiencing. Examples of concerns include chronic difficulties with air exchange through the nares due to recession of the midface, poor vision due to hypertelorism, and difficulty with mastication due to improper jaw closure. The nurse should offer appropriate counseling about adaptive measures that will assist the child to live with these handicaps. Physician referral may be warranted to determine indications for surgical assistance.

★ NURSING DIAGNOSES AND PLANNING

Typical nursing diagnoses are similar to those for a child with craniosynostosis. Likewise, goals and expected outcomes are similar. The section Nursing Diagnosis and Planning, developed for craniosynostosis, should be consulted and adapted to care of the child who has a craniofacial dysostosis and the family.

★ INTERVENTIONS: COLLABORATIVE AND INDEPENDENT

It is important for the nurse to offer support and information to the family of the child with craniofacial dysostosis. The initial diagnostic period can be stressful for families, especially if this is a sporadic occurrence, and no other family member has the same outward appearance. Reviewing the physical deformities associated with

each disorder with special emphasis on any functional difficulties that may be expected is appropriate. The nurse can be of special assistance to the family of the newly diagnosed child by offering concrete suggestions about how to adapt to these functional problems. Examples include the following:

- Determine the child's visual acuity, and place visual stimuli at the proper location to enhance optimum visual development.
- Assist with breathing or eating problems by placing the child in a comfortable upright position much of the time.
- Add humidity to the air to ease the child's breathing effort.
- Use soft foods and special eating utensils for children with increased difficulty chewing their food.
- Assess the child's hearing.
- Use adaptive hearing aids, or speak more directly in the child's direction.

★ EVALUATION

Periodically the nurse and family evaluate the outcomes of care given. Outcomes for the child and family with craniofacial dysostosis are similar to those listed under Nursing Diagnoses and Planning in the section on craniosynostosis.

Children who are diagnosed early and undergo appropriate surgical intervention have a better chance of improved cosmetic results and fewer functional difficulties than children who receive these interventions later in life. Because many of the operations are done by "staging" at certain ages, the nurse helps the family understand the time frame. Even when the child receives optimum surgical intervention, however, an altered facial appearance may persist. The child and parents should be told the extent of correction possible with each procedure performed.

Disorders of the Eyes

Nurses are in an excellent position to provide visual screening. This assessment may be done during the well-child visit (see Chap. 9). Nurses working in the community (schools and clinics) are in an ideal situation to assist children with visual problems to receive appropriate medical interventions.

Children who do not receive routine visual screening or who do not receive adequate treatment once a visual deficit is determined may demonstrate learning difficulties. These children also are at increased risk for injury due to their inability to adequately see certain dangers in the environment. To ensure optimal attainment of educational goals and personal safety, the nurse must be astute when observing and referring children with visual difficulties. Timely and efficient referrals to an ophthalmologist may avoid some of these complications.

Refractive Errors

Definition and Incidence. Light refraction is the bending of light rays as they pass through the lens, usually causing the light to fall directly on the retina. If the rays do not focus on the retina, the child experiences a refractive error that alters visual acuity. Refractive errors generally result from incoordination between the bending of the rays and the length of the eyeball. The most common refractive errors are myopia (near-sightedness), hyperopia (far-sightedness), and astigmatism (an irregularity in the curvature of the lens).

Approximately 75% of full-term infants are hyperopic, and about 25% are myopic. Many full-term infants also tend to have astigmatism during the first 6 months of life. Both myopia and astigmatism also are prevalent among preterm infants.[4] According to the American Academy of Pediatrics[2] approximately 20% of all children have refractive errors requiring corrective lenses before they attain full growth.

Etiology and Pathophysiology. *Myopia* is a condition in which an excessive amount of refractive power results in light rays coming to a point in front of the retina (Fig. 35-3A). This disorder causes the child to see objects close up better than at a distance and is generally due to an increased length of the eyeball. At about 8 years of age most children with this malady begin to demonstrate difficulty seeing at a distance. The myopia usually progresses through the preteen and adolescent years and reaches a plateau at about 20 years of age.[25] School-age children who complain of difficulty reading the chalkboard or whose grades decline should receive visual acuity testing to determine if they have this refractive disorder.

Several theories exist concerning the etiology of myopia. The first and most acclaimed theory is that myopia is inherited through a recessive gene. A family history typically reveals other family members who also have myopia. The use-abuse theory, which is based on the assumption that prolonged use of the eyes with close work results in excessive tension on the ciliary muscles, was discounted until recently. Some investigators now believe that the old theory may have validity in some cases of myopia.[32] Other investigators suspect vitamin deficiencies and various environmental factors as causes of myopia.

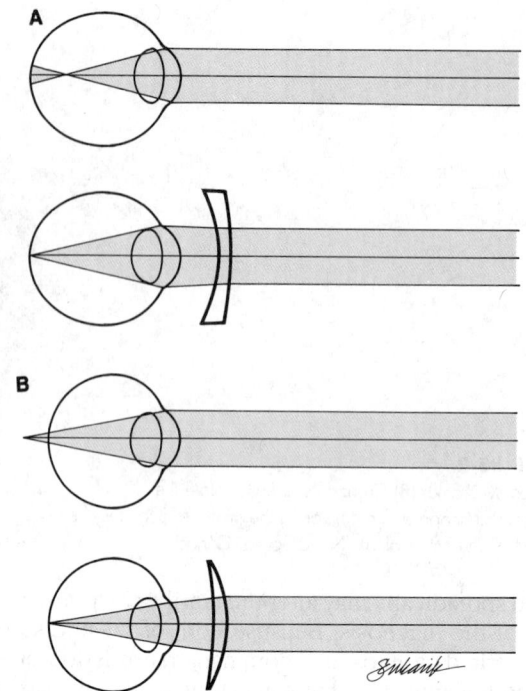

FIGURE 35-3

(**A**) Refraction in the myopic eye. Light rays come to a point in front of the retina. (**B**) Insufficient refractive power in the hyperopic eye. Point of reference is behind the retina. Note shape of lens needed for correction in each condition.

Hyperopia is the term for insufficient refractive power resulting in poor vision because the image falls behind the retina (see Fig. 35-3B). Hyperopia results in the ability to see objects at a distance better than close up. Most children have some degree of hyperopia until about 9 years of age due to a reduced depth to the eye globe. This form of hyperopia needs no correction because children generally use their accommodative powers to self-correct this problem. However, more severe and persistent forms of hyperopia requiring a corrective lens may derive from a familial pattern.[46]

Astigmatism is a refractory error in which the curvature of the cornea is not equal in all directions. Because the light rays are not focused symmetrically, images are perceived as blurred and distorted. This disorder may present by itself or along with myopia or hyperopia. Initial presentation usually occurs in late childhood. The condition may change with age because the curvature of the cornea varies with time.

Astigmatism is thought to be primarily inherited. Certain environmental factors can cause astigmatism, including damage to the cornea from overextended use of a dirty contact lens, trauma to the cornea causing malformation of the cornea and lens, tumors or other masses that push on the eye, and eye surgery.[32]

Clinical Manifestations. Each of these refractive errors results in poor visual acuity but also may cause compensatory symptoms related directly or indirectly to the inability to see clearly. Children with hyperopia exhibit symptoms that range from none to headaches, lassitude, irritated eyes, nausea, irritability from increased tension, and eye strain with close work. With prolonged undiagnosed hyperopia the child also may develop strabismus and even amblyopia (which are discussed later) due to a great deal of convergence and eye strain necessary for close work.

Classic symptoms of undiagnosed myopia include difficulty seeing the blackboard or television clearly, decreased interest in activities that require distance vision, and squinting. Mild astigmatism may present asymptomatically. However, by late childhood the symptoms as advanced hyperopia, including headaches, burning eyes, fatigue, squinting, and eye strain with close work; blurred vision, frowning, and reading problems also may be present.

Diagnostic Studies.   Visual screening tests are routinely performed by nurses in various practice settings. The majority of these tests are quick, painless, and inexpensive. However, cooperation on the part of the child is necessary. Table 34-1 describes developmental considerations when testing the eyes, and procedures are discussed in Chapters 9 and 34.

The Allen cards are routinely used for children aged 2½ to 3 years and for children who are unable to understand use of the E chart. The Allen cards contain seven pictures of easily identifiable objects. A passing score is given when the child can identify four of the seven pictures correctly.

With the E chart and Snellen screening visual acuity is recorded as a fraction. The number on the top represents the distance that the child stood away from the chart. The number on the bottom is obtained from the last line on the chart correctly read and stands for the distance at which children with normal vision can read the line. Therefore, the child who stands at a distance of 20 feet from the eye chart and is able to read down to the 30 line on the chart has a visual acuity of 20/30. These numbers imply that the child being examined can see at 20 feet what the child with normal vision can see at a distance of 30 feet.

Titmus or other desktop binocular visual screening machines are an alternative way to screen children for refractive disorders. These devices present the same E chart and Snellen chart results used with wall screenings, but they are compact because the chart is visualized by looking through binoculars into the machine. The machines are useful for mass screening because they require less space and reduce environmental distractions. They are, however, more costly than the eye charts and may frighten some children. The devices also are sometimes used to determine if a child has color vision or muscle imbalance problems.

★ ASSESSMENT

When eliciting a history from a family, the nurse seeks information concerning visual problems that the child may have. Nurses can ask leading questions, such as "Can the child correctly name objects across the room and close up? Does the child frequently squint and if so, under what conditions? Has there been a sudden decline in school grades?" On physical examination the nurse observes for signs of eye irritation, squinting, and frowning, which suggest eye strain or poor visual acuity.

Children with normal intellect should receive screening for vision beginning at 3½ years of age.[40] Testing for visual acuity is needed so that treatment for problems can be instituted at an early age. Nurses can make a great impact in the prevention of blindness by facilitating mass visual screening for preschool children.

The screening tools described previously primarily screen for distance vision and may be jointly interpreted by the following guidelines: Referral is advised if a 3 year old cannot correctly identify three of the five directions (i.e., direction of the E) of the 20/50 card or line or if a 4 to 6 year old cannot name three of six responses of the 20/40 line. Screening for near-vision problems is possible using pocket cards designed in the same format as the E chart and Snellen chart. When the cards are held 13 to 16 inches from the child, visual problems can be determined.[32] Near-vision failure using the pocket cards also merits an ophthalmology referral.

★ NURSING DIAGNOSES AND PLANNING

Based on assessment data discussed previously and in the preceding chapter, the following nursing diagnoses may apply to the family and child with refractive errors in vision:

- Altered Growth and Development related to sensory-perceptual deficit (visual).
- High-Risk for Injury related to impaired vision.
- Self-Esteem Disturbance related to wearing corrective lenses.

The nurse and child (or parents) together plan effective care based on the established nursing diagnoses. Several examples of expected outcomes follow:

- The child wears the prescribed corrective lenses as instructed.
- The child verbalizes pleasure with improved vision.
- The child verbalizes acceptance of appearance with corrective lenses.

The nurse plans for the care of the child based on physician's orders and nursing diagnoses. Some general nursing goals may be the following:

- Development is promoted.
- Self-esteem is reinforced.

★ INTERVENTIONS: COLLABORATIVE AND INDEPENDENT

The outcome of the screening examinations helps the nurse determine whether counseling or a physician referral is indicated. Prior to referral the nurse must clearly document the results of the child's screening test and previous tests. An accurate history concerning visual and school problems also should be included. This information assists the ophthalmologist in determining the length of time the child has had impaired vision and how quickly the child's visual acuity has diminished.

The nurse should encourage the parent to obtain visual screening for the child at regular intervals so that any deficits may be determined early. The fixation pattern and alignment of the infant's eyes should be determined at birth and in the first year of life to determine gross visual problems. Thereafter, the child should be screened every 2 to 3 years using the screening tools previously described.[45] If the child has normal vision for age, the nurse should instruct the parent concerning the signs that would indicate diminishing acuity, such as difficulty reading the school blackboard and increased squinting.

Children who have a visual acuity of 20/40 or worse on vision screening by 5 years of age should be referred to an ophthalmologist. A two-line difference in the visual acuity between eyes (on the eye charts) is also an indication for referral to determine if amblyopia exists.[2] A child who has a screening score of 20/30 and has related symptoms, such as eye strain, headaches, and eye pain, also should be referred to an ophthalmologist.[11]

COMPLIANCE SUPPORT

Once the child has been seen by the ophthalmologist or optometrist, the nurse also must ensure that the child is able to obtain the prescribed corrective lens. The nurse may need to assist the family in locating funds for glasses or contact lenses through private insurance or public programs. The Lion's organization is one such group. Children who use corrective lenses should be re-examined yearly to determine if their vision has changed.

Nurses can assist with compliance in wearing corrective lenses by counseling the parent on how to gain the child's confidence in wearing them. Seeking the child's input when choosing frames or contact lenses is important for encouraging compliance. Showing the child how much more can be seen and enjoyed with improved vision also is helpful. Children who complain that glasses "fall off" may be encouraged to wear the glasses more if an elastic band is attached to the earpieces bilaterally to hold the frames on the head. The use of contact lenses is an alternative for children who dislike the feel of frames. For children who have visual problems even with the use of corrective lenses, adaptive devices, such as books on tape, large print books, and preferential classroom seating, may be suggested by the nurse to encourage better school performance.

★ **EVALUATION**

Periodically the nurse and family evaluate the outcomes of care given. Examples of outcomes for the child and family with refractive errors were given under Nursing Diagnoses and Planning in this section. Have short-term goals been met? Are long-term goals still realistic?

LONG-TERM CARE

The child with poor vision should be monitored at regular intervals for satisfactory adaptation using corrective lenses and equipment. The child's needs for adaptive devices frequently change with age and new developmental milestones; the nurse should re-evaluate the child at each well-child checkup to modify the interventions as needed. As the child outgrows glasses, either by the size of the frames or by the need for new lenses, the nurse may be a resource for the family in obtaining new glasses or other corrective lenses.

Color Vision Deficit

Definition and Incidence. *Color vision deficit,* commonly called color blindness, is the condition in which the child is unable to distinguish one or more of the three primary colors: red, green, and blue. Approximately 8% of white males and 0.5% of white females are color blind.[9] The incidence of males with this disorder in other races is also increased (e.g., 2% of American Indian males, 3.7% of African American males, and 5% of Oriental males).[32]

Etiology and Pathophysiology. The etiology of the two general types of color vision deficits is congenital or acquired. Of those with congenital causation the majority arise from an X-linked recessive inheritance pattern. With X-linked disorders the woman is a carrier and passes on the defective gene for color blindness to her son. Because the male Y chromosome has no gene for color discrimination, a woman's defective X gene causes color blindness in her male offspring. This inheritance pattern accounts for the greater number of males affected with this problem.[11] The congenital form is a nonprogressive, irreversible defect, and the color deficits are usually the same in both eyes.

The acquired version occurs rarely in children and is generally a result of systemic disease or eye disorders that damage the retina or optic nerve. Acquired color vision problems may get better or worse with time. Furthermore, color deficits resulting from an acquired etiology may vary from one eye to the other.

Perception of color derives from three variables: hue, saturation, and brightness.[9] Children with color vision problems learn to discriminate colors by their saturation and degree of brightness.[25]

Clinical Manifestations. Color vision abnormalities have some implications for difficulties with school work and lifestyle but not as much as visual acuity problems. Children may have difficulty matching colors when dressing themselves and may incorrectly identify the color of traffic lights, especially if the order of the lights is altered.[11] Certain school tasks, especially in the preschool setting, use colors for learning. Most studies of children with color deficiencies, however, have shown no significant deficits in learning.[32]

Diagnostic Studies. The simplest and quickest form of mass screening is to ask a verbal child to identify several different colors.[11] If the child has difficulty with this task, several screening tests are available that may help distinguish the child's color deficiency. These tests include the pseudoisochromatic tests that are composed of lines, patterns, numbers, or letters in a variety of colors with the same level of light intensity.[25]

The pseudoisochromatic tests are the most widely used screening tools for color vision deficiencies due to their transportability and ease of administration.[32] Ishihara's plates are the leading form of the pseudoisochromatic tests used today, but they are recommended only for use with children 6 years and older because double-digit numbers are included in the test. The Hardy, Rand, and Rittler plates can be used as early as 3 years of age because they use familiar symbols, such as a triangle, circle, and cross instead of numerals. These tests do not discriminate between those with dichromatic vision and those with severe anomalous trichromatic vision, but they can determine which children have a milder type of anomalous trichromatic vision.[32]

Another color vision assessment tool is the Farnsworth-Munsell test, which uses recognition and alignment of colored buttons to determine problems. This test requires concentration and is not easily administered until the child is an adolescent. The anomaloscope, is an exact but expensive test using an optical instrument that also can be used to determine color deficit.[9,25]

★ ASSESSMENT

It is important for the nurse to determine which children need color vision screening and to implement the screening. Nurses working in the school system are well situated to observe for children with this problem who may be experiencing associated learning difficulties. Nurses working in other settings also may notice this disorder while working with the child for an unassociated problem.

If there is reason to suspect a color vision deficit in a child, one of the diagnostic tools mentioned above should be used to assess the problem. Furthermore, nurses routinely administer the pseudoisochromatic tests for color vision screening in pediatrician's offices at well-child checkups and in school during visual screening programs. Usually the examiner shows one plate at a time and asks the child to name the numeral inserted into each plate. Small children and illiterate people not familiar with the symbols may need to trace them to complete the test.

Many of the machines that test for visual acuity also have the capability for color vision screening. These machines may include several plates from Ishihara's test. However, this method has two drawbacks. The test is only a part of the larger Ishihara's test and insufficient lighting within the machine may alter the test results. Therefore, use of the complete Ishihara's or other pseudoisochromatic tests is suggested if a color vision deficiency is suspected.[32]

★ NURSING DIAGNOSES AND PLANNING

Based on assessment data discussed previously and in the preceding chapter, the following nursing diagnoses may apply to the family and child with color blindness:

- Anxiety about school performance related to impaired color perception.
- High Risk for Injury related to impaired color perception.

The nurse and child (or parents) together plan effective care based on the established nursing diagnoses. Several examples of expected outcomes follow:

- The child discusses fears and strategies planned to cope with visual deficit.
- The child and parent describe strategies used to manage the safety problems associated with color blindness.

The nurse plans for the care of the child based on physician's orders and nursing diagnoses. General nursing care goals that may be used are as follows:
- Anxiety about school performance is diminished.
- Injury is avoided.

★ INTERVENTIONS: COLLABORATIVE AND INDEPENDENT

Once the child has been screened and is found to have a color vision deficiency, the nurse should provide appropriate anticipatory guidance to the child and parent concerning this disability. The nurse needs to emphasize safety issues for the school-age and older child related to interpreting traffic light signals. The nurse can teach the child about the color sequence and meaning of the traffic signals in that community. The child also should be instructed about safety measures, including looking both ways before crossing a street.

Suggestions about how to dress with coordinated colors is also helpful. The child and parent may be taught how to mark clothes that should be worn together. Likewise, the nurse can encourage the parent to discuss the child's color vision deficit to the child's teacher. This knowledge assists the teacher in structuring assignments and tests around the child's disability.

★ EVALUATION

Periodically the nurse and family evaluate the outcomes of care given. Examples of outcomes for the child and family with color blindness were given under Nursing Diagnoses and Planning in this section.

Nurses working with children who have diagnosed color vision deficits should monitor the child's adjustment to this disability. The nurse who sees a child for routine follow-up visits can elicit this information while taking the health history. School nurses also can inquire with the teacher whether the child is better able to perform his or her schoolwork following suitable diagnosis and counseling. The need for further diagnostic testing and counseling may be recognized if the problem becomes worse.

Dacryostenosis

Definition, Incidence, Etiology, and Pathophysiology. Dacryostenosis is defined as an obstruction of the nasolacrimal duct (Fig. 35-4). The condition usually presents either in the newborn period or in early infancy. Dacryostenosisis is a common abnormality, occurring in 1 of every 200 newborns.[24]

Dacryostenosis may result from the persistence of an embryonic fold of tissue located at the nasal terminus of the nasolacrimal duct or from a blockage of the duct by a mass of epithelial cells. The former etiology is unilateral, but the latter may be either unilateral or bilateral.[25] The older child may present with this problem as a result of trauma or chronic conjunctivitis.[46]

Clinical Manifestations and Diagnostic Studies. The first symptoms of this disorder are excessive

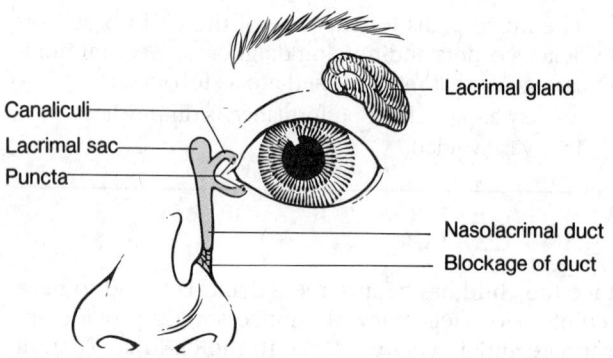

FIGURE 35-4
Dacryostenosis, obstruction of the nasolacrimal duct, is a common abnormality in newborns that can lead to infection if not treated.

tearing (called epiphora) and residual mucus on the eye lashes.[46] These symptoms may be notable in the newborn who ordinarily produces few tears. The infant normally develops the ability to shed tears by 3 weeks of age.[32] Other signs of an ongoing problem include a mucopurulent discharge that can be expressed with massage of the nasolacrimal duct and swelling in the area of the inner canthus of the eye.[25]

Persistence of dacryostenosis without appropriate management can lead to an infection of the nasolacrimal duct called dacryocystitis. Presence of this complication is indicated by erythema and edema over the lacrimal duct. It is also possible for conjunctivitis to occur along with dacryocystitis.[46]

There are no diagnostic tests for this disorder outside of a complete history and thorough physical examination. However, if dacryocystitis is suspected, a culture of the mucopurulent discharge can be obtained to confirm the diagnosis.

★ ASSESSMENT

Attention to the cardinal symptoms of excessive tearing, matting of the eyelashes, and punctal swelling are important to note when gathering the historic data. When examining the child, the nurse should gently massage the nasolacrimal duct to see if any mucous exudate can be expressed. The nurse also should look for signs of associated infection, such as purulent discharge or erythema of the conjunctiva. In the older child the nurse should ask when the symptoms first began to determine any temporal relationship to previous trauma or infection.

★ NURSING DIAGNOSES AND PLANNING

Based on assessment data discussed previously and in the preceding chapter, the following nursing diagnoses may apply to the family and child with dacryostenosis:

- High Risk for Infection related to an untreated dacryostenosis developing into a dacryocystitis.
- Body Image Disturbance related to excessive tearing and mucopurulent discharge from the eyes.

The nurse and child (or parents) together plan effective care based on the established nursing diagnoses. Several examples of expected outcomes follow:

- The parents demonstrate effective massage techniques.
- The parents exhibit correct use of antibiotic eye drops.
- The parents and child verbalize confidence in the resolution of the problem.

The nurse plans for the care of the child based on physician's orders and nursing diagnoses. Some general nursing care goals may be the following:

- The development of infection is avoided.
- Concerns about body image are diminished.

★ INTERVENTIONS: COLLABORATIVE AND INDEPENDENT

The most important instruction the nurse gives the parent of the child with dacryostenosis is how to massage the nasolacrimal duct to express mucous drainage. This maneuver is performed by gently stroking the area from the inner orbital rim (not over the nose or eye) to the inner canthus of the eye. Parents should be taught to massage the nasolacrimal duct three to four times a day. Massaging downward will help open the duct if no infection is present.

In the presence of an infectious process, massaging upward will help express purulent discharge. Frequent massage of the nasolacrimal duct and lacrimal sac can reduce the incidence of dacryocystitis.[46] The nurse should demonstrate this procedure and have the parent return and demonstrate it before terminating the visit.

The parents may be concerned about the infant's appearance with constant eye drainage. It is important for the nurse to explore the parents' feelings about the disorder and clarify the temporary nature of dacryostenosis with proper treatment. For the older child who acquires the disorder, emphasis may be placed on the fact that the drainage will resolve once aggressive treatment is begun. The nurse should also remind the child and/or parent that there are usually no long-term effects resulting from this condition.

Prophylactic antibiotic eye drops may be prescribed to decrease the chance of a secondary infection. In the case where a dacryocystitis has already occurred, the same antibiotic drops will be used to treat the infection. The nurse must teach the parents to instill these antibiotic eye drops correctly (see Chap. 25).

★ EVALUATION

Periodically the nurse and family evaluate the outcomes of care given. Examples of outcomes for the child and family with dacryostenosis were given under Nursing Diagnoses and Planning in this section.

On return visits the nurse evaluates the child for spontaneous resolution of the problem or any complications. The duct usually opens within 2 to 4 months.[32] By 12 months of age approximately 90% of these closed ducts have opened.[24] Ducts that do not open or cause chronic complications may need to be irrigated or probed by an ophthalmologist.[9] The nurse should inform the family of the child's progress with massage and prepare them in advance if further intervention will be needed.

Cataract

Definition and Incidence. A *cataract* is an opacity or cloudiness of the crystalline lens that consists of precipitated lens protein and results from physical or chemical changes within the lens.[17,32] Two distinct types of cataracts may occur—congenital and acquired. The majority of cataracts in children are congenital, with one of every 250 newborns (0.4%) having some form of a cataract. Between 10% and 38% of all blindness in children may be caused by congenital cataracts.[46] The remainder of cataracts in children are acquired through such causes as mechanical trauma, chemical exposures, radiation, toxic substances (such as long-term steroids and total parenteral nutrition), enzyme deficiencies, and diabetes.[9,32]

Etiology and Pathophysiology. Congenital cataracts may result from many viral, metabolic, hereditary, and even unknown causes.[32] Most of the infectious etiologies affect the fetus early in pregnancy when the lens is forming, specifically during the fifth to the eighth week of gestation. However, toxoplasmosis may detrimentally affect the fetus throughout the pregnancy.[25]

There are several classification systems for congenital cataracts. They may be typed most easily by their location and morphology. The polar kind is placed at the anterior or posterior pole of the lens and capsule and is associated with the prenatal vascular network surrounding the lens. The zonular type is an opacity of a lens layer or zone that leaves other parts, such as the embryonic nucleus and possibly the cortex, clear.[9]

With a total loss of transparency of the lens, the entire lens is opaque, but with membranous opacity, the lens is not only opaque but it also is thick and fibrotic.[46] Cataracts may be complete or incomplete (Fig. 35-5) and may be unilateral or bilateral. Failure to diagnose or treat cataracts may result in diminished visual acuity with possible long-term visual impairments for very young children who are still developing vision.

Clinical Manifestations. Two of the classic symptoms of cataracts in infancy are leukocoria and nystagmus. *Leukocoria* is a pupillary reflex that makes the pupil appear white due to the opacity of the lens (Fig. 35-6).

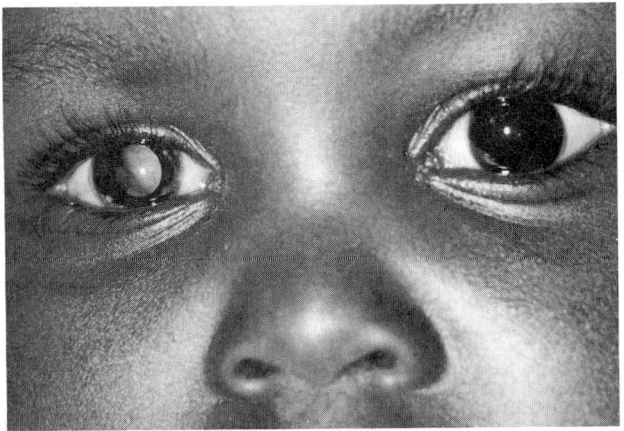

FIGURE 35-6
Leukocoria seen in a child with congenital cataracts (right eye). (Oski, F. A., et al. [1990]. *Principles and practice of pediatrics.* Philadelphia: J.B. Lippincott.)

Retrolental fibroplasia (RLF), retinoblastoma, and persistent hypoplastic primary vitreous also can cause leukocoria and must be excluded by diagnostic testing before the presence of a cataract is determined.[32] *Nystagmus* is an involuntary, oscillating movement of the eyeball. If nystagmus develops secondary to the cataract, it is usually present by 6 months of age in an infant born with congenital cataracts.

Cataracts often result in reduced visual acuity, depending on the location of the cataract. There is usually no pain associated with a cataract. Approximately 60% of children with congenital cataracts have additional ocular difficulties and the presence of cataracts is often linked with various other physical findings and congenital abnormalities.[32,46]

Diagnostic Studies. The ophthalmologist usually performs definitive tests for visual acuity if cataracts are suspected. Using the ophthalmoscope, the examiner can determine the presence of a red light reflex on the pupil. The absence of a red reflex (and especially the presence of a whitish pupil) should alert the practitioner to the possibility of a cataract. The presence of a cataract also can be determined with the use of a slit lamp, which provides binocular microscopic abilities in the examination.[32]

★ **ASSESSMENT**

The nurse who suspects a cataract from the child's clinical manifestations should obtain a thorough history concerning the pregnancy and neonatal course if the child is an infant and any predisposing factors if the child is older. The presence of other associated symptoms or syndromes also should be determined. On physical inspection the nurse needs to note the presence of any visible opacity of the lens or other ocular or systemic findings. Any abnormalities should be clearly and succinctly documented.

The nurse should screen for visual acuity to assist in the diagnosis of cataracts. The nurse also can note the presence of a white pupil or nystagmus. If there is an abnormality on visual screening coupled with symptoms of cataracts, referral to an ophthalmologist is indicated.

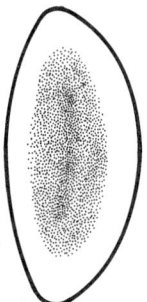
A Complete cataract

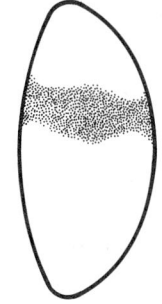
B Incomplete cataract

FIGURE 35-5
Cataracts are considered complete if the entire lens is affected (**A**) or incomplete if any part of the lens is opaque (**B**).

★ NURSING DIAGNOSES AND PLANNING

Based on assessment data discussed previously and in the preceding chapter, the following nursing diagnoses may apply to the family and child with a cataract:

- Altered Growth and Development related to sensory/perceptual deficit (visual).
- Anxiety regarding lack of knowledge about diagnosis, treatment, and prognosis.
- Altered Family Processes related to child's hospitalization for surgery.
- Body Image Disturbance related to diminished vision.
- High Risk for Injury related to decreased visual acuity.

The nurse and child (or parents) together plan effective care based on the established nursing diagnoses. Several examples of expected outcomes follow:

- The parents and child identify safety hazards.
- The parents discuss the benefits and risks of planned interventions.
- Family chooses aspect of child's care to provide.
- The child wears corrective lenses as instructed.
- The child demonstrates age-appropriate developmental behaviors.
- Parents and child identify safety hazards.

The nurse plans for the daily care of the child based on physician's orders and nursing diagnoses. Some general nursing care goals may be the following:

- Development is promoted.
- Parents and child understand information about cataracts.
- Injury is prevented.
- Parents become active members of the health team.

★ INTERVENTIONS: COLLABORATIVE AND INDEPENDENT

SURGICAL MANAGEMENT

The main form of treatment is surgical removal of the cataract, which in children generally means extracapsular cataract extraction or removal of all but the back part of the lens capsule. The anterior lens surface is aspirated through a small incision that is made at the edge of the cornea.[32]

The infant with a congenital cataract, especially when only one eye is affected, should have surgery performed within 3 weeks of birth to prevent deprivation amblyopia.[25] Children with a monocular congenital cataract develop this form of amblyopia due to greater visual stimulation in the unaffected eye. If either unilateral or bilateral congenital cataracts are untreated beyond 3 to 6 months of age, the prognosis for adequate vision is poor. Treatment for older children with acquired cataracts causing a visual disturbance is the same except that timing is not as crucial.[32]

Nursing interventions for the child diagnosed as having a cataract include teaching the family and child what a cataract is and how it alters vision. If surgical correction is indicated, the nurse provides the child and family with clear explanations about the events related to surgery. Preoperative nursing care includes administration of mydriatic eye drops to dilate the eyes before surgery.

Postoperatively, a pressure dressing is placed over the eye for 1 to 2 days and is removed by the surgeon. The child must be prevented from removing the eye patch during this time. Restraints or mitts worn on the hand may help prevent the child from tampering with the patch. After the patch is removed a bubble or shield is placed over the eye for up to 1 month for protection.

Often the child is allowed to go home the day of surgery and return to the surgeon's office for follow-up. Thus, clear discharge instructions must be given to the family as early as possible during the hospital course. The nurse should encourage quiet play for the child during the first postoperative days and discourage stooping and straining for the first few weeks after surgery.

MEDICATION THERAPY

Several types of eye drops, including ophthalmic antibiotics, steroids, and atropine, are given daily for several weeks postoperatively to prevent infection and curtail inflammation of the eye. The parents need to be taught how to administer these medications. The eye should be properly healed by 6 to 8 weeks after surgery.

VISUAL REHABILITATION

After surgery the child cannot focus well at close range because of the absence of the lens. Severe deprivation amblyopia is possible if the vision is not corrected. Contact lenses, either those that can be taken out or surgically implanted intraocular lenses, are preferred for visual rehabilitation of children after cataract surgery. The family needs to learn how to clean, insert, and remove the contact lens properly. With hard lenses, the parents must be taught to gradually increase the amount of time they are worn to prevent corneal damage. Glasses, preferably those with plastic lenses, are an alternative if contact lenses are not tolerated by the child.

PSYCHOSOCIAL SUPPORT

The nurse should spend time discussing the psychosocial implications of altered vision and cosmetic changes (due to the presence of the cataract or the use of glasses) with the family. Poor vision caused by a cataract or postoperative changes may greatly alter the child's ability to achieve normal developmental milestones. The nurse needs to work with the family to encourage the child's full developmental potential by demonstrating modifications (such as greater use of tactile and auditory stimuli) in the child's environment, which will enhance acquisition of developmental skills.

The nurse should explore the perceptions of the child and family related to cosmetic appearance and suggest alterations that may improve the child's external appearance and preserve his or her self-concept. Prompt surgical treatment of a large cataract or the use of attractive frames for glasses are two alternatives. In addition the nurse should provide anticipatory guidance on prevention of accidents that could occur because of the child's altered visual acuity.

★ EVALUATION

Periodically the nurse and family evaluate the outcomes of care given. Examples of outcomes for the child and family with a cataract were given under Nursing Diagnoses and Planning in this section.

Evaluation of nursing interventions should be an ongoing concern during each visit with the family to determine if the family correctly understands explanations given and is complying with the treatment regimen. Children who are being followed up and have not received surgical intervention must be monitored closely to determine if visual deficits have evolved. These families should be assessed frequently to ascertain if they are knowledgeable of symptoms that need prompt referral (i.e., worsening visual acuity, particularly unequal vision between the two eyes, nystagmus, and strabismus).

Glaucoma

Definition and Incidence. *Glaucoma* is the term used to describe an elevation of intraocular pressure. Glaucoma may occur in one or both eyes, and it may lead to optic nerve damage. Thus, untreated glaucoma in childhood may cause partial or complete blindness.

Developmental glaucoma is the general term for glaucoma that appears in childhood. Congenital and juvenile types of glaucoma have been described. Both eyes are affected in about 75% of children who have glaucoma.

Congenital glaucoma, the most common type of the developmental glaucomas, is responsible for 2% to 15% of blindness in schools for the blind. The presence of glaucoma at birth occurs in about 1 in every 10,000 children born with other developmental anomalies. The incidence of congenital glaucoma in children without other anomalies is approximately 1 in 30,000 live births.[52]

Juvenile glaucoma develops between the ages of 3 and 30. This form of glaucoma in children is similar to the open-angle type identified in adults. There are more boys than girls with juvenile glaucoma, and there is a history of the open-angle type of glaucoma in many of the families of affected children.

Etiology and Pathophysiology. Congenital glaucoma may be inherited through an autosomal recessive gene with weak penetration. About 60% of these children are diagnosed in the first 6 months of life.[46] Glaucoma is known to accompany other diseases or disorders such as neurofibromatosis, Marfan syndrome, or Sturge-Weber syndrome. Trauma, intraocular hemorrhage, inflammation (ureitis), and intraocular tumors also may contribute to the development of glaucoma. Glaucoma develops due to a blockage in the flow of the aqueous humor within the eye.[25] The aqueous fluid is secreted by the ciliary body and then circulates between the iris and lens, out into the anterior chamber, and ultimately to Schlemm's canal (see Chap. 33). Any obstruction to its flow along this passageway may lead to increased pressure within the globe (see Fig. 35-7).

Increased intraocular pressure initially may cause nonspecific symptoms, such as eye pain, tearing, and spasms of the lids. Further increased pressure within the eye eventually causes destruction of the ganglion cells of the retina, leading to ischemia and necrosis of the optic disc and nerve.[9] Necrosis of the optic disc causes blindness.

Clinical Manifestations. General symptoms that occur with glaucoma include photophobia, epiphora, blepharospasm (lid spasm), variable persistent pain, diminished vision with initial decrease in peripheral vision, and corneal edema accompanied by an enlarged eye with an increased corneal diameter and haziness (often called buphthalmos). Signs of progressive glaucoma may include a dilated pupil; thin, bluish sclera; enlarged globe

Narrow Angle Glaucoma

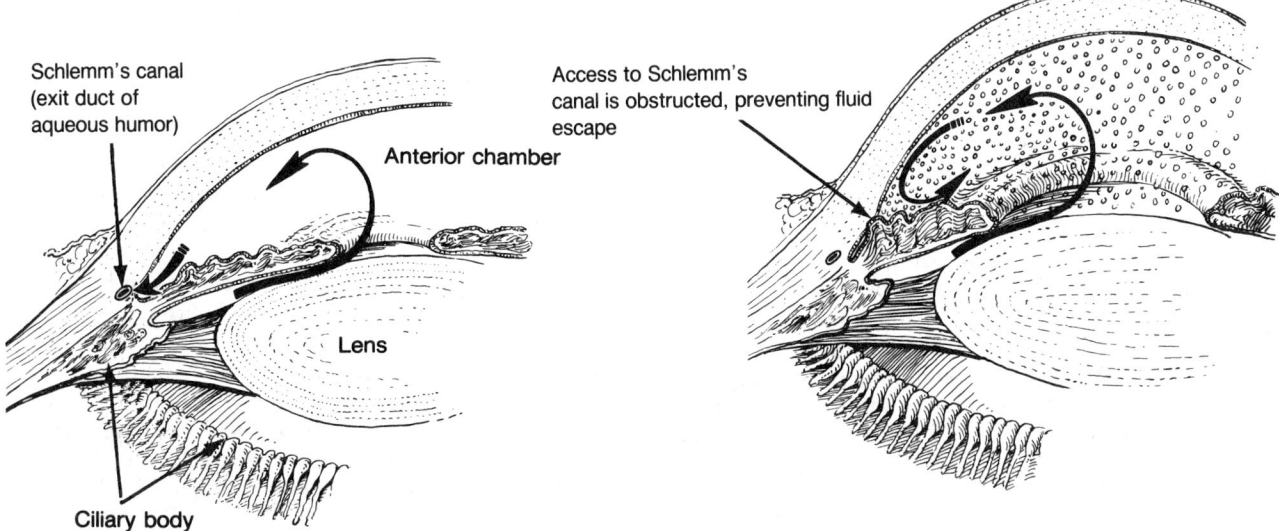

Schlemm's canal (exit duct of aqueous humor)

Anterior chamber

Access to Schlemm's canal is obstructed, preventing fluid escape

Lens

Ciliary body

Normal flow

Narrow-angle glaucoma

FIGURE 35-7

Glaucoma is caused by an obstruction to the flow of aqueous humor in the eye. (Lechliger, M., & Moya, F. *Introduction to the practice of anesthesia* [2nd ed.]. New York: Harper & Row.)

that feels firm to pressure; enlarged optic disc cup; and unusual behaviors due to the extreme sensory loss.[46]

Children with congenital glaucoma display most of these symptoms, depending on the severity of the disorder and how early it is diagnosed. Cardinal symptoms of congenital glaucoma are epiphora, photophobia, and enlargement of the anterior globe.[25] Juvenile glaucoma also is often accompanied by myopia and loss of peripheral vision. Pain, however, is rarely associated with this form, and these children do not have enlarged corneas.[32]

Diagnostic Studies. Initial evaluation of an acute attack of glaucoma may include gentle palpation of the child's eyeball, contrasting its tension to that of the examiner's eyeball.[32] This maneuver may distinguish glaucoma from conjunctivitis or iritis. Assessing visual acuity and visual fields as well as measuring the cornea vertically and horizontally offers additional information. Use of the ophthalmoscope to assess the optic disk is essential to determine if retinal changes have occurred.[25]

Tonometry is the means of directly measuring the intraocular pressure, with normal values ranging between 12 and 20 mmHg. Two different types of tonometers may be used, the Schiotz and the applanation. Both involve placing the instrument on the eyeball, and they may be difficult to use in a small child without anesthesia.[32] Gonioscopy also may be performed. This procedure allows a better view of the anterior portion of the eye through placement of contact lens instruments over the cornea and use of the slit lamp.[32]

★ ASSESSMENT

The astutely observant nurse working in a newborn nursery may identify an infant who demonstrates photophobia, one of the early signs of congenital glaucoma. Older infants who also have excessive tearing, an enlarged eyeball, a red eye, or blepharospasm also should be assessed for this disorder. If congenital glaucoma is suspected, the nurse should take a good history to determine if there is a family history of other syndromes or abnormalities that may accompany glaucoma. It is important for the nurse to be aware of such hereditary factors so that an accurate diagnosis can be obtained in the first year of life. If adequate treatment is begun early, visual loss can be prevented.

Older children who exhibit symptoms of glaucoma also should be screened to determine if any family members have glaucoma because glaucoma can result from an autosomal recessive inheritance pattern. Associated causes for the glaucoma, including syndromes, trauma, and inflammatory reactions, need to be considered. When obtaining such a history, the nurse should elicit a comprehensive description of the presenting symptoms, including how long they have been noticed and any treatments that have been helpful. This information is useful in determining which type of glaucoma the child may have.

★ NURSING DIAGNOSES AND PLANNING

Based on assessment data discussed previously and in the preceding chapter, the following nursing diagnoses may apply to the family and child with glaucoma:

- Pain related to increased intraocular pressure.
- High Risk for Injury related to increased ocular pressure following surgery for glaucoma.
- Anxiety related to knowledge deficit about the diagnosis, treatment, and prognosis.

The nurse and child (or parents) together plan effective care based on the established nursing diagnoses. Several examples of expected outcomes follow:

- The child and parents describe strategies used to maintain low intraocular pressure after surgery.
- The parents verbalize an understanding of treatment plans and prognosis.
- The parents verbalize an understanding of signs of complications that should be reported.
- The parents identify safety risks and measures taken to protect child.

The nurse plans for the daily care of the child based on physician's orders and nursing diagnoses. Some general nursing care goals may be the following:

- Pain is relieved.
- Injury is prevented.
- Anxiety is diminished.

★ INTERVENTIONS: COLLABORATIVE AND INDEPENDENT

MEDICATION THERAPY

Treatments for glaucoma may involve a trial of drugs aimed at decreasing the production or increasing the absorption of the aqueous humor. Such agents include cholinergic (e.g., pilocarpine) and adrenergic (e.g., timolol) agents, carbonic anhydrase inhibitors (e.g., acetazolamide), and hyperosmotic agents (e.g., glycerol).[25] Nurses should instruct the parents on how to administer these drugs, especially those instilled into the eye, and counsel parents on potential adverse effects.

SURGICAL MANAGEMENT

The most commonly used treatment, especially with congenital glaucoma, is surgery. The goniotomy, which requires cutting the membrane at the trabecular meshwork to allow outflow of aqueous humor, is the surgery of choice. This procedure may be repeated if it is unsuccessful the first time. Alternate procedures include trabeculectomy, peripheral iridectomy, and laser treatment.

The nurse should counsel the child preoperatively about the need for eye patches after surgery and even let the child try on the patches to become more familiar with their feel. The use of the eye medications and how they are instilled also should be discussed during preoperative teaching to reduce the child's anxiety about the postoperative course. Children experiencing pain and other symptoms before surgery should be reassured that most symptoms subside after surgery. Visual loss present at the time of surgery may or may not change postoperatively.

Postoperative nursing care of the child following a goniotomy usually involves the instillation of anti-inflammatory medications and covering the eye until the wound has healed. Discharge teaching for the parents includes a review of how to place an eye patch on the child and the best means of securing the patch. The parent also needs to be taught how to administer eye drops if the child is sent home with ophthalmologic medications.

TEACHING

Parents should be counseled preoperatively and postoperatively so that they are thoroughly informed about the child's diagnosis and prognosis. Parental anxiety about the glaucoma may be communicated to the child nonverbally and cause emotional problems for the child and parent. The parent also should be informed that the pain should subside with surgical intervention and that visual acuity may or may not change after surgery.

The child with poor visual acuity or blindness due to glaucoma requires the same interventions as any other child with very diminished vision (see "Blindness" in this chapter). The parents need to learn how to assist the child in dangerous situations to prevent secondary injury.

★ **EVALUATION**

Periodically the nurse and family evaluate the outcomes of care given. Examples of outcomes for the child and family with glaucoma were given under Nursing Diagnoses and Planning in this section. Have short-term goals been met? Are long-term goals still realistic?

LONG-TERM CARE

Children who are being treated for glaucoma using pharmacotherapy should be evaluated periodically to determine the effectiveness of the drugs. Those who have received surgical treatment also should be seen at intervals postoperatively to review their progress after surgery. Children showing worsening symptoms (i.e., photophobia, excessive tearing, an enlarged eyeball, red eye, blepharospasm) should be brought to the attention of the ophthalmologist for further evaluation. Some children require a change in their drug regimen or more than one surgery to arrest the process.

Strabismus

Definition and Incidence. *Strabismus* is the term used to indicate that the eyes are not straight or aligned bilaterally. Because the visual axis is not parallel, the eyes see two different images. Approximately 2% of all preschool children develop strabismus.[37] Several different definitions are listed in the accompanying display on terms used to describe strabismus.

Children with other congenital abnormalities have an increased incidence of strabismus. Approximately 50% of children who manifest strabismus do so by 1 year of age, and 80% develop symptoms by age 4.[32] Children who have a family history of strabismus should be carefully monitored for onset of symptoms because approximately half of all children who develop strabismus have a positive family history for this disorder.[11]

Etiology and Pathophysiology. The most common cause of strabismus is imbalance of the extraocular muscles. Other causes include cranial nerve palsies, poor vision, and strabismic syndromes.[37] The primary long-term effect of strabismus is the development of amblyopia due

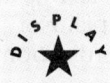

Terms Used to Describe Strabismus

Convergent (esotropia)—The eyes move nasally toward one another; often occurs with hyperopia as the eyes compensate for the refractive disorder by overconvergence of the eye muscles

Divergent (exotropia)—The eyes move away from one another; only a slight association with myopia but often occurs when the child is gazing at a distant object; may be present at birth

Monocular—Fixation with only one eye while the other eye deviates permanently; due to paralysis of the ocular muscles; child has a great likelihood of developing amblyopia due to this etiology

Alternating—Use of one eye at a time for fixation on a fluctuating basis; uses both eyes for vision and has a decreased chance of developing amblyopia

Nonparalytic—Constant deviation in all fields of gaze but not associated with eye muscle paralysis

Paralytic—Paralysis of certain extraocular muscles present but strabismus only apparent when the eye is moved in the direction of the affected muscle group

Accommodative—Divergence of the eyes (usually esotropia) in response to a large refractive error, most commonly a hyperopia or far-sightedness

Other terminology for describing this disorder are certain endings or words:

-tropia—Indicates continual presence of the strabismus

intermittent—Noncontinuous presence of the strabismus; added in front of the word that includes -tropia (i.e., intermittent esotropia)

-phoria—Strabismus seen only when the child is tested or during episodes of fatigue, illness, or stress; indicates a potential strabismus currently being controlled by the child (i.e., exophoria)

to suppression of the image of the deviating eye to avoid diplopia. Amblyopia may lead to permanent loss of vision in the affected eye in about half of children who have strabismus.[32]

Clinical Manifestations. Pseudostrabismus commonly occurs in infancy and does not represent a true strabismus or deviation of the eyes. With pseudostrabismus the eyes appear to turn inward bilaterally due to prominent epicanthal folds or a wide nasal bridge. As the nose grows and develops, this condition becomes less noticeable. Diagnostic tests are used to differentiate pseudostrabismus from true strabismus. Children with hypertelorism or facial asymmetry also may exhibit pseudostrabismus.[37]

Although the most apparent sign of this disorder is malalignment of the eyes, other symptoms may be present. The child may develop a compensatory squint, close one eye, or tilt the head to avoid seeing double.[37] With paralytic strabismus the child also may complain of a headache and show fine and gross motor incoordination.

Diagnostic Studies. The most common screening tests for strabismus can be easily performed by the nurse in any setting. The corneal light reflex or Hirschberg test is done by shining a light on the bridge of the nose and noting the relative position of the light reflection in each eye (Fig. 35-8). The child who does not have strabismus should reflect the light in corresponding parts of both corneas symmetrically. A positive test occurs when the light is centered in one eye but is off center in the opposite eye.[37]

The cover/uncover test requires that the child be asked to fixate on an object approximately 30 cm from his or her face and then cover one of the eyes with a cover card or hand. If the uncovered eye moves to fixate when the opposite eye is covered, then the uncovered eye most likely has strabismus. The examiner then quickly removes the cover and observes for any movement in the newly uncovered eye. Repeating the test on the other eye may determine if an alternating strabismus or amblyopia is also present. Other tests performed by the ophthalmologist include measuring the strabismus with prisms and fundoscopy, testing ductions and versions (types of eye movements), using the near point of convergence test and the Worth four dot test (performed by asking the child to recognize the colors of four dots or circles while wearing tinted glasses).

★ ASSESSMENT

When obtaining the history pertaining to strabismus, the nurse should ask the family whether they have noticed the child's eyes crossing or looking crooked and if so, at what age. The nurse needs to investigate if this anomaly was noticed in one or both eyes and if any treatment was instituted. If some form of treatment was given, it must be determined what type and for how long it was given.

Additional pertinent history includes any reports of blinking, rubbing, squinting, overreaching objects, and tripping.[11] Situational presence of strabismus (i.e., when the child is tired, sick, daydreaming, in bright lights, looking at a near or far object) may indicate a phoria. Obtaining an accurate family history, including any known strabismus, and a medical history for the child also is indicated.

On physical examination the nurse may perform the Hirschberg and cover tests to screen the child for strabismus. Visual acuity should be determined because half of all children with strabismus also have amblyopia. Other abnormal body movements, such tilting the head and squinting, should be noted, and an assessment of the child's extraocular movements should be obtained.

★ NURSING DIAGNOSES AND PLANNING

Based on assessment data discussed previously and in the preceding chapter, the following nursing diagnoses may apply to the family and child with strabismus:

- Altered Growth and Development related to sensory/perceptual deficit (visual).
- Anxiety (Parental) related to lack of knowledge about the treatments used for strabismus.

The nurse and child (or parents) together plan effective care based on the established nursing diagnoses. Two examples of expected outcomes follow:

- The child wears corrective lenses as instructed.
- The parents report diminished anxiety related to the child's strabismus and its treatment.

The nurse plans for the daily care of the child based on physician's orders and nursing diagnoses. Some general nursing care goals may be the following:

- Development is promoted.
- Parents understand information provided about strabismus.
- Acute symptoms are absent.

★ INTERVENTIONS: COLLABORATIVE AND INDEPENDENT

Once the nurse has assessed that the child has strabismus, an ophthalmology referral is indicated. The ophthalmologist may obtain additional information, but once the diagnosis is confirmed, treatment is instituted.

CONSERVATIVE MANAGEMENT

Conservative management includes occlusion therapy, eye exercises, corrective lenses, and medications. Patching the good eye to prevent amblyopia from developing is the most common form of occlusive therapy. Parents should be informed that therapeutic patching will not harm vision in the good eye, that patching alone will not straighten the eyes, that it is very important to limit patching to the time prescribed, that patches need to be worn

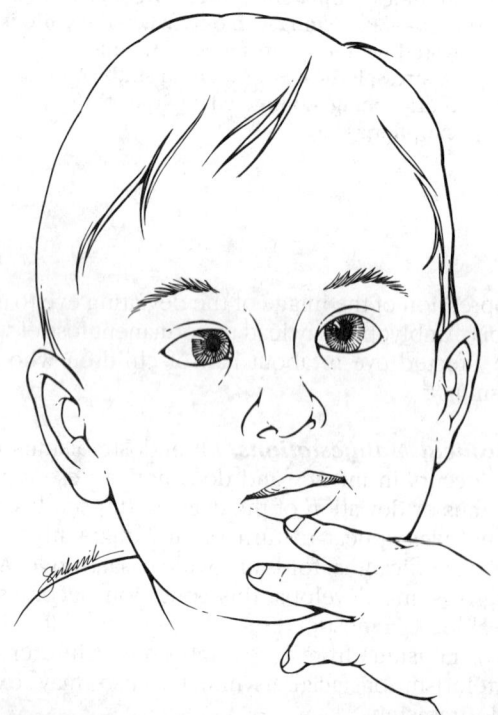

FIGURE 35-8
Example of strabismus during the Hirschberg test. Note asymmetry of the corneal light reflex.

on the face because patching over glasses is ineffective, and that returning for prescribed follow-up visits is essential.

Eye exercises may be helpful in a small number of children with limited-angle intermittent exotropia and double vision.[32] The exercises stress awareness of eye divergence and improving the use of both eyes to focus on a single image.

The use of glasses or bifocals for children with accommodative strabismus is a common form of treatment. Correction of the refractive error through glasses decreases the need for self-accommodation and therefore reduces the stimulus for excessive convergence (a means of achieving accommodation).

Anticholinesterase drugs that constrict the pupil and cause ciliary spasms occasionally are used to decrease the accommodative effort for children who have great difficulty wearing glasses.[37]

SURGICAL MANAGEMENT

Surgery may be indicated when glasses or other forms of conservative management cannot correct the child's strabismus. The three most common procedures are weakening procedures to decrease the effectiveness of an opposing muscle, strengthening procedures to increase the effectiveness of a synergistic muscle, and procedures to change the direction of the muscle action.[27] Parents should be told that the eyeball is not taken out in surgery, that the child may require more than one operation to straighten the eye, that it may be necessary to operate on both eyes to correct the deviation, that glasses often are prescribed after surgery to maintain the alignment, and that strabismus surgery will usually not change the child's reading ability or school performance.[28]

TEACHING

Helping the parents understand why a certain treatment has been prescribed and how to continue it at home is an important aspect of the nursing care for children with strabismus. If conservative management is indicated, the nurse must be sure the parents know how to position the patch or glasses on the child, how to conduct the exercises, and administer the prescribed drugs. For those who will undergo surgery preoperative teaching about what to expect after surgery and how to prepare the child is necessary.

Postoperatively the nurse may serve as the support person to the family and should provide appropriate discharge teaching concerning the use of dressings, eye drops, corrective lenses, and so forth. After discharge the nurse may serve as the continuing link between the family and the health care team.

★ EVALUATION

Periodically the nurse and family evaluate the outcomes of care given. Examples of outcomes for the child and family with strabismus were given under Nursing Diagnoses and Planning in this section. Have short-term goals been met? Are long-term goals still realistic? Planning for further nursing care takes into consideration complications.

Nursing evaluation of the child with strabismus should include the identification of any changes the child has experienced since the last medical visit. The nurse following a child for a phoria may need to take a thorough history and perform the Hirschberg and cover tests. The child who has been using any of the conservative types of management also should be reassessed for any progression in correction of the strabismus.

Amblyopia

Definition and Incidence. *Amblyopia*, or "lazy eye," is a loss of vision in one or both eyes unrelated to a specific organic problem. The child with amblyopia cannot see well due to poor visual stimulation, and the problem does not improve with the use of glasses.[28] This condition affects approximately 2% to 3% of the population and can be detected in the preschool years.[40] About 50% of children with amblyopia have strabismus. Conversely, 50% of children with strabismus also have amblyopia.[32]

Etiology and Pathophysiology. This problem has several etiologies, but the most common type in children is secondary to an untreated strabismus. Amblyopia arises from strabismus due to a suppression by the brain of the visual image in the deviating eye. The errant eye would otherwise cause double vision. This form also is referred to as strabismic amblyopia.[38]

Amblyopia also can result from a refractive error that is not the same in both eyes. This condition is referred to as refractive or passive suppression amblyopia or anisometropia in which the less affected eye is preferred for vision, and the eye with the greater refractive error becomes amblyopic. Deprivation amblyopia arises from organic eye problems, such as cataracts or ptosis, and occlusion amblyopia results from prolonged patching of the undeviated eye with strabismus.

Clinical Manifestations and Diagnostic Studies. Amblyopia by definition indicates a loss of vision in one or both eyes. If this condition results from diplopia or double vision associated with strabismus, the child may complain of headaches and difficulty focusing prior to the development of amblyopia.[32] A child may or may not complain of visual impairment with amblyopia but often will display other symptoms of visual impairment, such as overreaching or underreaching for an object.

A general rule of thumb is that a child who demonstrates a difference of two or more lines between eyes on the visual acuity chart should be referred to the ophthalmologist for evaluation of amblyopia.[9] Use of the cover/uncover test also may reveal a deviation of one eye or extreme irritability on the part of the child when the good eye is covered. An older child with amblyopia may experience a crowding phenomenon in which there is difficulty seeing figures on the Snellen chart when presented as a line but not when they are presented one at a time.[32]

★ ASSESSMENT

The nurse must assess the child at each well-child visit for deviation of the eyes for loss of visual acuity. Historic information from the parent concerning an occasional "wandering" eye or noticeable visual acuity problems may be extremely helpful in establishing this diagnosis. Performing screening tests, such as a visual acuity test appropriate for age and the cover/uncover test, are also important nursing assessments.

★ NURSING DIAGNOSES AND PLANNING

Based on assessment data discussed previously and in the preceding chapter, the following nursing diagnoses may apply to the family and child with amblyopia:

- Altered Growth and Development related to sensory/perceptual deficit.
- Anxiety related to parental knowledge deficit about the diagnosis and treatment of amblyopia.

The nurse and child (or parents) together plan effective care based on the established nursing diagnoses. Several examples of expected outcomes follow:

- The parents discuss the amblyopic condition and why it should be treated.
- The parents state that the reward system is helping the child cooperate with wearing the patch as prescribed.

The nurse plans for the daily care of the child based on physician's orders and nursing diagnoses. Some general nursing care goals may be the following:

- Development is promoted.
- Anxiety is diminished.

★ INTERVENTIONS: COLLABORATIVE AND INDEPENDENT

The nurse should provide counseling to the parents before referral and after diagnosis concerning what amblyopia is and why it should be treated. The parents should be informed about some of the causes contributing to the condition and potential visual problems if the condition is left untreated. Involving the parents in assuming the responsibility for adequate treatment ensures a better outcome for the child.

Correction of any refractive error through the use of glasses is the first line of treatment for amblyopia arising from a refractive disorder. Patching is the most common form of treatment for all types of amblyopia because occluding the vision in the better eye will stimulate the less used eye to see. This form of treatment is most effective in children younger than 6 years of age.[38] Other forms of treatment include pharmacologic occlusion, pleoptics (use of central fixation), prisms, and visual exercises.[32] Many of these treatments are discussed under "Strabismus" in this chapter.

Young children often do not like the patch and try to remove it. The nurse needs to work with the parent in establishing reward systems or special "treats" for wearing the patch appropriately. The patch may be prescribed for either intermittent or constant use throughout the day. The ophthalmologist should check the child's eyes at frequent intervals to rule out the development of occlusion amblyopia. Because this form of treatment may be continued for several months or even years, nursing support and continued contact with the parents is crucial in ensuring good compliance with the treatment regimen.

★ EVALUATION

Periodically the nurse and family evaluate the outcomes of care given. Examples of outcomes for the child and family with amblyopia were given under Nursing Diagnoses and Planning in this section.

The nurse should interview parents at each return visit concerning how they have implemented the patching routine and how the child responds to the patch. Tangible examples of how to implement a behavior modification program may assist the parents in enforcing the patching treatment.

Eye Infections

Definition and Incidence. Conditions causing edema and erythema of the eyelids as well as redness and tearing of the eye account for the majority of eye problems in children. Conjunctivitis is the most common of the conditions causing these symptoms. Orbital and periorbital cellulitis also account for a substantial number of these cases.

Conjunctivitis is an inflammation of the mucous membrane that overlays the eyeball. Infections account for most cases of conjunctivitis in children, but other causes, such as allergies, viral agents, systemic diseases, and environmental irritants, are possible. Periorbital cellulitis is an infection of the eyelid, while orbital cellulitis affects not only the eyelid, but also the globe.

Etiology and Pathophysiology. Conjunctivitis results from a variety of causative agents (Table 35-1). The most common bacterial agents include *Staphylococcus aureus, Haemophilus influenzae, Pseudomonas sp.*, and *Streptococcus sp.* The majority of these infections resolve spontaneously, but a small number of children, especially newborns, develop complications from an untreated infection. In addition, bacterial infections are very contagious.

Neisseria gonorrhoeae conjunctivitis, one type of ophthalmia neonatorum, can be spread to the newborn during passage through the birth canal. These bacteria can cause corneal ulceration, inflammation of other eye structures, and even septicemia. This condition occurs rarely in the United States because erythromycin or tetracycline is instilled into the eyes of all newborns prophylactically after birth.

Another type of infectious organism is the virus that may cause a bulbar (involving the covering of the eyeball up to the cornea) conjunctivitis commonly called "pinkeye" because of its characteristic appearance. Viral conjunctivitis usually clears without causing long-term effects but may be accompanied by upper respiratory symptoms. Because it can spread easily, the child should remain out of contact with other children for 10 to 14 days after symptoms first appear. Two more common types of viruses that cause conjunctivitis are adenovirus and herpes simplex.

Chlamydia conjunctivitis usually is manifested by an inclusion conjunctivitis (meaning that the virus causes large basophilic inclusion bodies within the cells of the conjunctiva). Chlamydia is a sexually transmitted disease

TABLE 35-1
Causative Agents of Conjunctivitis

Agent	Onset	Resolves	Comment
$AgNO_3$	Several hours after instillation	24–36 hours	$AgNO_3$ effective against gono-coccus but not *Chlamydia*
Bacterial gonococcus	2–4 days after birth	In days with treatment	Marked purulent discharge and edema
Chlamydia	5–12 days after birth	Days to a few weeks	Mild mucopurulent discharge, ba-sophilic intracytoplasmic inclusions in scrapings; may be associated with pneumonia (later onset)
Other bacteria	Any time	In days with treatment	Mild "sticky lids" to acute purulent inflammation, one or both eyes
Viral	Any time, initially in one eye	4 days to 2 weeks	May be associated with corneal changes
Herpes simplex	Any time, unilateral	About 1 week or may be recurrent	Often associated with skin lesions; steroids contraindicated
Allergic	In association with other symptoms; most common in spring	As allergies resolved— about 1 week	Itching followed by mild redness and tearing; "ropy" secretions; cobblestone papillae in vernal type

(Source: Avery, M. E., & Frist, L. R. [1989]. *Pediatric medicine*. Baltimore: Williams & Wilkins.)

and may be contracted by passing through the birth canal (ophthalmia neonatorum), by swimming in a contaminated pool, or by sexual transmission increasingly seen in adolescents.[32] One of the main complications of chlamydia conjunctivitis is scarring of the conjunctiva with corneal vascularization and opacification. This process develops after the acute infection.

Conjunctivitis also may appear as an allergic response to irritants (e.g., hair spray, cosmetics, and pollen) or may be part of a systemic allergic response. This response probably results from the release of histamine from sensitized immunoglobulin E (IgE) mast cells, and eosinophils are found on scrapings from the conjunctiva.[17] Other symptoms that may arise simultaneously with a systemic response include rhinitis, eczema, and asthma.

Cellulitis, a diffuse inflammatory process within solid tissues, is generally of bacterial origin in the eye tissues. Periorbital cellulitis may arise from infections due to trauma, insect bites, upper respiratory tract infections, and otitis media. Etiologies of orbital cellulitis may include infections of the sinuses, teeth, eyelids, and face. Orbital cellulitis should be treated promptly because an aggressive infection can invade the central nervous system.

Clinical Manifestations. The most common signs of conjunctivitis include hyperemia (redness of the conjunctiva), eye discharge, epiphora, and edema of the eyelids or of the conjunctiva (chemosis). These symptoms occur in different degrees depending on the causative organism. For instance, bacterial infections commonly cause a purulent or mucopurulent discharge; viral infections produce a watery exudate; and allergies and chlamydial infections provide a stringy type of discharge.[32] When the cornea also is involved, the condition is referred to as keratoconjunctivitis.

Cellulitis of the orbit shares some symptoms with conjunctivitis. Both conditions can cause swelling of the eyelid, although additional tenderness and warmth of the lid may occur with periorbital cellulitis. Children with orbital cellulitis present with malaise and fever, excessive swelling of the eyelid, proptosis (forward displacement of the eye with widening of the lids), chemosis, decreased vision, and painful and reduced movement of the eyeball.

Diagnostic Studies. Close inspection of the eye is the best means of initial diagnosis. Suspicion of conjunctivitis should be followed by culture or smear to determine the causative organism. Periorbital and orbital cellulitis also are diagnosed by inspection and culture. Both are easily recognized due to their characteristic and rather distinctive symptomatology. X-rays of the paranasal sinuses also are recommended because sinus infections often precede orbital cellulitis.[32]

★ **ASSESSMENT**

A thorough nursing assessment includes historic information concerning when the symptoms began and any predisposing factors. This assessment includes determining exposure to contagious diseases. Finding out when the symptoms began also may help in determining the length and severity of the infection. The nurse must also document descriptively any observations about the affected eye; a thorough description assists other health care providers with assessing the improvement of the eye during and after treatment. A referral to a pediatrician or an ophthalmologist may be warranted.

★ **NURSING DIAGNOSES AND PLANNING**

Based on assessment data discussed previously and in the preceding chapter, the following nursing diagnoses may apply to the family and child with eye infection:

- High Risk for Eye Injury related to an infection of the eye.

- Pain related to orbital conjunctivitis.

The nurse and child (or parents) together plan effective care based on the established nursing diagnoses. Several examples of expected outcomes follow:

- The parents demonstrate the correct method for instilling eye medication and applying compresses.
- The parents state precautions to inhibit spread of the infection.
- The child acknowledges improved comfort.

The nurse plans for the daily care of the child based on physician's orders and nursing diagnoses. Some general nursing care goals may be the following:

- Pain is relieved.
- Spread of infection is prevented.

★ INTERVENTIONS: COLLABORATIVE AND INDEPENDENT

Use of ophthalmic antibiotic preparations usually is recommended for the treatment of bacterial and chlamydial conjunctivitis. Oral antibiotics can be used for uncomplicated periorbital cellulitis, but orbital cellulitis requires prompt hospitalization and treatment with intravenous antibiotics.

Palliative treatment with cold compresses to the eyes several times a day is the treatment of choice for viral and allergic conjunctivitis. Discomfort may be relieved with acetaminophen. Bright lights hurt the eyes and should be avoided until discomfort abates.

An explanation to the parent about the child's eye disorder is another important part of the nursing role. Eye infections that are communicable (e.g., viral conjunctivitis) may require a period of isolation for the child, and the parent needs to understand the necessity for this precaution. It is extremely important for the parent to know what medications should be used for bacterial and chlamydial infections and how to administer either ophthalmic solutions or oral antibiotics or both.

The nurse should ensure prompt and appropriate referral for the child displaying symptoms of an eye infection. This referral includes written and verbal reporting of historic information and physical findings to an appropriate physician. Usually a pediatrician can adequately treat a simple conjunctivitis, but a cellulitis requires referral to an ophthalmologist.

★ EVALUATION

Periodically the nurse and family evaluate the outcomes of care given. Examples of outcomes for the child and family with an eye infection were given under Nursing Diagnoses and Planning in this section.

The nurse should keep in close contact with the child and family throughout treatment to promote compliance with the treatment regimen. Pertinent information concerning the disease and treatment course is essential to include in any discussion with the family. Follow-up contact with the family at routine well-child checkups is a good time to screen for progressive sequelae of the eye infection that may require an alternative treatment.

Eye Trauma

Definition and Incidence.   Injury to the eye may result from a blow or an inflicted wound. Trauma to the external and internal eye structures accounts for one third of all blindness in children younger than 10 years of age.[46] About 160,000 eye injuries per year occur in the age group between 5 and 17 years.[19]

Etiology and Pathophysiology.   Ocular trauma results from sports injuries, use of sharp toys or tools, abuse, explosives, or chemicals.[19] Injuries requiring prompt medical attention include lid lacerations, lacerations of the cornea and sclera, perforations of the globe, hyphemas (free blood in the anterior chamber), intraocular foreign bodies, orbital fractures, and burns. Corneal abrasions and subconjunctival hemorrhages, while not considered medical emergencies, often occur in children and should be evaluated by the primary health care provider.

Lacerations of the cornea or sclera and perforations of the globe may result in evulsion of uveal and vitreous material, damage of the lens tissue, hemorrhage, and even retinal detachment. Distortion of the pupil and absence of a red light reflex may be noted on ophthalmic examination. A hyphema often develops from blunt trauma to the eye. Damage to the root of the iris results in bleeding from the torn vessels and free blood entering the aqueous humor.

Foreign bodies may be of two types: irritants, such as dust or an eyelash causing tearing and photophobia, and those invading the globe. Penetrating intraocular foreign bodies may include such items as metallic foreign bodies, glass from broken windshields, sharp projectiles, and bullets. Orbital fractures usually occur from a blow to the eye and most often affect the floor of the bony orbit, called a blow-out fracture.

Caustic chemical burns are the most common cause of eye injury and are considered a true ocular emergency. Acid burns appear more severe, but alkali burns are more damaging because they may continue to erode the eye for days after the injury.[32]

Corneal abrasion is a common eye problem in children. Small abrasive foreign particles caught in the upper lid or scratches from a fingernail, sharp toy, or contact lens may cause this problem. Subconjunctival hemorrhages may occur as the newborn's face comes through the birth canal, and following Valsalva's actions such as coughing and sneezing. The small hemorrhages may be present upon waking in the morning without apparent cause.

Clinical Manifestations.   Injuries of the eyelid often result in periorbital ecchymosis (black eye) and edema. Blunt injury may cause a black eye or may lead to intraocular injuries that need further evaluation. Laceration of the eyelid is a more serious injury requiring prompt suturing to avoid difficulty with lid closure and further eye damage. A great deal of external bleeding may occur with a lid laceration. Evaluation for other ocular injuries should accompany inspection of a lid laceration.

Lacerations of the cornea or sclera often cause bleeding into the anterior chamber. The child also may complain of pain, photophobia, drowsiness, and poor vision. Depending on the location and extent of the injury, the child with a foreign body lodged in the eye may experience such symptoms as pain, impaired vision, irregular pupil, or extrusion of the vitreous humor through the wound.[32]

Common symptoms of an orbital fracture include initial lid emphysema (subcutaneous air under the lid tissue), protrusion of the globe, and diplopia. Limitation of eye movements is possible if one of the eye muscles has become entrapped. Enophthalmus, a sunken appearance of the globe, may appear after the lid swelling and redness disappear.[25] Injury to the globe occasionally results from an orbital fracture causing increased intraocular pressure, concussion sequelae, and tears of the intraocular structures.

Eye burns are classified by the degree of severity, in three stages, as follows: (1) hyperemia and inflammation, (2) vesicle and exudate formation, and (3) ischemia and necrosis. Symptoms of a chemical burn may not occur immediately, and their absence can be misleading when determining long-term implications.

A corneal abrasion may cause such symptoms as sudden pain, epiphora, light sensitivity, and diminished visual acuity. A subconjunctival hemorrhage is a small amount of bleeding in the conjunctiva and may be heralded only by the presence of bright red blood within the conjunctival sac. This hemorrhage is rarely associated with pain, and no other symptoms are usually present.

Diagnostic Studies. For the majority of these disorders, good nursing observation is the best diagnostic measure. Other methods used to diagnose certain eye injuries include use of fluorescein (a dye for the eye) and a slit lamp or ophthalmoscope to note a corneal abrasion. The slit lamp also may be used to determine the presence of a hyphema. X-rays, ultrasound, or CT scan often are used to ascertain the presence of a foreign body or orbital fracture.

★ ASSESSMENT

The nurse should first obtain an accurate history from the family concerning the circumstances surrounding the injury. Pertinent information includes the type of materials the child was playing with or around (e.g., sticks, sharp objects, BB guns), a description of how the accident occurred, and the initial appearance of the affected area (before a great deal of bleeding or edema developed). This information may assist in determining the type and extent of the injury. Eye burns are considered a medical emergency and should be treated with continuous irrigation before any other action is taken.

The nurse should closely inspect the eye structures for foreign bodies, swelling, discoloration, lacerations, and exudate. Presence of any of these signs or frank bleeding indicates that a referral is needed. Assessment of the child's visual acuity also is indicated to determine what structures have been affected and to serve as a baseline for comparison with the acuity present after treatment.

★ NURSING DIAGNOSES AND PLANNING

Based on assessment data discussed previously and in the preceding chapter, the following nursing diagnoses may apply to the family and child with eye trauma:

- High Risk for Injury (Permanent Visual Deficit) related to external trauma.
- Self-Esteem Disturbance related to disfiguration of the eye.
- Pain related to eye injury.
- Parental and Child Anxiety related to emergency care.

The nurse and child (or parents) together plan effective care based on the established nursing diagnoses. Several examples of expected outcomes follow:

- The child demonstrates feeling comforted by the presence of parents.
- The child and parents demonstrate decreased anxiety after procedures are explained.
- The child acknowledges diminished pain.
- The child and parents discuss openly their feelings about possible disfigurement.
- The child and parents discuss safety measures needed to protect the eyes from future injury.

The nurse plans for the care of the child based on physician's orders and nursing diagnoses. Some general nursing care goals may be the following:

- The eye is protected from further injury.
- Anxiety is diminished.
- Pain is relieved.

★ INTERVENTIONS: COLLABORATIVE AND INDEPENDENT

The types and duration of interventions for eye injuries depend on the nature of the problem. Simple periorbital ecchymosis involving injury to no other eye structures may be treated with cold compresses for the first day after the injury and with hot compresses thereafter. Lid lacerations are promptly sutured to prevent further eye damage. Lacerations of the cornea or sclera may require removal of the foreign body by an ophthalmologist, and the affected area may require suturing and proper placement of any underlying structures that may have been avulsed. Perforations of the globe require similar immediate referral to an ophthalmologist for excision of the foreign body and suturing.

Initial management of a hyphema is to gently cover the affected eye with a metal shield or the bottom of a Styrofoam cup until medical care can be obtained. Most children are hospitalized for several days until some of the bleeding has dissipated. Topical corticosteroids are occasionally used to reduce irritation in the eye.[39] Cycloplegic medications (i.e., atropine and cyclopentolate) that prevent ciliary muscle contraction may be used to allow the eye to rest and assist in the reabsorption of the blood. Continued patching is no longer believed necessary for adequate healing to occur.[39]

Removal of foreign bodies in the eye should be attempted only by an ophthalmologist because intraocular contents also may be removed. The eye should not be irrigated initially for the same reason. However, the nurse can carefully patch the eye to prevent further damage from rubbing or wiping after determining the child's visual acuity. Prompt referral to the ophthalmologist is then indicated. The most appropriate nursing care for a child with a suspected orbital fracture is prompt referral to an ophthalmologist for conclusive diagnosis and treatment. Antibiotics, oral decongestants, and cold compresses may be indicated before the decision for surgical repair of the bone is made.[32]

Corneal abrasions usually are treated with patching of the eyelid for 1 to 2 days postinjury to allow the epithelium to heal spontaneously. However, occlusion of one eye in preschool children may contribute to the development of esotropia (crossed eye). Therefore, patching should not be continued for more than 24 hours in very young children without close supervision by an ophthalmologist.[39]

Analgesics such as acetaminophen and cold compresses may ease the child's sensation of pain with a corneal abrasion. Prophylactic topical antibiotics may be prescribed, but steroids should be avoided lest the presence of infection be masked. A subconjunctival hemorrhage may be treated with cold compresses alone and usually resolves spontaneously within 1 to 2 weeks.[39]

EMERGENCY INTERVENTION IN BURNS

Burns, especially chemical burns, are a true ocular emergency. They require immediate and continuous irrigation of the eye with water or normal saline for at least 30 minutes after the injury or until medical supervision can be obtained. The stream should be directed from the inner canthus of the eye toward the outer canthus to avoid contamination of the other eye. The nurse may need assistance in keeping the child's eyes open during this procedure. The affected eye may be treated with one of several types of medications, and the child may even require hospitalization depending on the type and the extent of the burn.

COUNSELING AND TEACHING

Nursing care of the child with ocular trauma includes comfort measures to reduce the child's anxiety and perception of pain. Allowing the parents to be in close proximity to the child generally is the best comfort possible for very young children. The nurse should explain each procedure to the parents and child in advance to increase the child's compliance and decrease anxiety for the parents and child. Judicious use of pain medications when ordered is another nursing measure to reduce the child's perception of pain.

The nurse should explore with the child and parents their perception of the child's appearance. Facial disfigurement resulting from eye injuries may greatly affect the emotional status of the child and family. If wounds are expected to heal with little cosmetic damage, this information should be shared with the family as early in the treatment plan as possible. The surgeon can discuss possible surgical reconstruction with the family in cases where permanent scarring has occurred.

The nurse should discuss the treatment plan with the family to clarify any misconceptions they may have. The role of the nurse is also to serve as a contact person if questions arise. Furthermore, the nurse should actively participate in preventive care by teaching parents and older children how to avoid accidents that may cause eye injuries. This includes anticipatory guidance concerning proper use of chemistry sets and household chemicals, avoidance of sharp objects, and special care when using fireworks or power tools.

★ EVALUATION

Periodically the nurse and family evaluate the outcomes of care given. Examples of outcomes for the child and family with an eye injury were given under Nursing Diagnoses and Planning in this section.

If additional swelling, discharge, bleeding, or a fever develops, the nurse should immediately refer the child to the ophthalmologist for further evaluation. Likewise, diminishing visual acuity should be reported promptly.

Retrolental Fibroplasia (RLF)

Definition and Incidence. RLF, also called retinopathy of prematurity, is a disease incurred by premature infants exposed to supplemental oxygen for a long period of time. With RLF the retinal vasculature develops abnormal blood vessels with associated capillary constriction. Because the retinal circulation is not fully developed until 40 weeks' gestation, a preterm infant is most affected by adverse effects incurred within the retinal vasculature. Approximately 25% to 30% of preterm infants with a birthweight of 1700 g or less develop bilateral RLF.[9]

Etiology and Pathophysiology. Most sources espouse the concept that high concentrations of oxygen can cause vasoconstriction of vessels within the retina of a preterm infant causing irreversible capillary endothelial damage. However, at least one source proposes that hypoxia may be just as responsible for this process.[24]

Different staging systems exist for describing the development of the disorder, but basically the disease progresses from occlusion of some of the peripheral vessels, to neovascularization or proliferation of new vessels into the vitreous, then to possible leakage of the vessels and even scar formation. The development of scar tissue often causes detachment of the retina, which is seen as a white retrolental membrane.[9] Different infants may develop these symptoms to different degrees, and some with only early changes may have total regression of the disease.[32]

Clinical Manifestations. Retinal lesions indicative of RLF may be visualized using indirect ophthalmoscopy within several weeks after birth, even while the infant is still receiving oxygen. However, the retinal changes are more pronounced after oxygen therapy has been discontinued, usually between 4 and 8 weeks after birth.[4] Symptoms of the child with RLF are noticeable only as the child ages and demonstrates impaired visual acuity, strabismus, or blindness.[9]

Diagnostic Studies. Most neonatal units abide by the 1971 recommendations of the Committee on the Fetus and Newborn of the American Academy of Pediatrics, which state that all infants with a gestational age less than 36 weeks or a birthweight less than 2000 g who received supplemental oxygen should receive an ophthalmologic examination at the time of discharge from the nursery and again at 3 to 6 months of age. Examination require use of a dilating solution, the aid of a wire speculum to separate the lids, and inspection of the periphery of the retina using the indirect ophthalmoscope. If no active process is noted, the infant may be either discharged from the care of the ophthalmologist or rechecked again in 3 to 6 months. The infant with an active degenerative process needs close follow-up at 1- to 6-week intervals to determine the extent of the damage.

★ **ASSESSMENT**

The nurse working in the neonatal unit should be aware of the possibility of the development of RLF among preterm infants and should closely monitor the percentage of oxygen (PaO_2) and the length of time oxygen is administered to these children. The nurse also should assist in scheduling infants who fit the aforementioned parameters for eye examinations before nursery discharge and again after discharge. Any hint of poor vision, such as inability to fix or focus, in an infant who has reached 40 weeks of gestation should be reported to the appropriate physician to determine if a retinal examination should be performed.

★ **NURSING DIAGNOSES AND PLANNING**

Based on assessment data discussed previously and in the preceding chapter, the following nursing diagnoses may apply to the family and child with RLF:

- Altered Tissue Perfusion (Retinal) related to prolonged oxygen administration.
- Altered Growth and Development related to sensory/ perceptual deficit (vision).
- Altered Family Processes related to visually handicapped child.

The nurse and child (or parents) together plan effective care based on the established nursing diagnoses. Several examples of expected outcomes follow:

- The parents state that they understand the diagnosis, etiology, and prognosis.
- The parents use community resources to manage problems associated with having a visually handicapped child.
- The parents discuss activities planned to promote normal growth and development.

★ **INTERVENTIONS: COLLABORATIVE AND INDEPENDENT**

The nurse following these high-risk infants should determine which of them have developed RLF and need additional assistance. First the nurse should spend time with the family explaining the diagnosis and etiology of RLF. How altered tissue perfusion of the retina causes impaired vision also can be reviewed.

Further discussion with the family should center on the progressive nature of RLF even after hospital discharge and the importance of ongoing follow-up. Because the main reason for early diagnosis is early referral to a center for visually impaired children, the family must understand the importance of prompt intervention with the infant who has such a sensory loss. Finally, the nurse should assist the family in locating and using community resources to best care for their child.

★ **EVALUATION**

Periodically the nurse and family evaluate the outcomes of care given. Examples of outcomes for the child and family with RLF were given under Nursing Diagnoses and Planning in this section. Have short-term goals been met? Are long-term goals still realistic?

LONG-TERM CARE

On follow-up visits the nurse should evaluate the family's coping patterns and the progress of the child in achieving developmental tasks to determine whether the child is receiving optimum care.

Blindness

Definition and Incidence. Many of the visual disorders discussed previously in this chapter cause the child to be visually impaired. Low or poor vision is defined as central visual acuity between 20/60 and 20/200 in the better eye.[32] To be classed as legally blind the child must have a central visual acuity of 20/200 or less with correction in the better eye or a visual field of no greater than 20 degrees in the better eye.[9] The term *visual impairment* is used increasingly to describe children with poor eyesight.

Approximately 75% of children with visual impairment demonstrate symptomatology by 1 year of age, and half have a prenatal onset.[32] Approximately 5000 cases of legal blindness are diagnosed in children younger than 20 years of age each year.[19] Determining the child's visual acuity as early as possible is important to ascertain if the child may have a significant and debilitating visual impairment.

Etiology and Pathophysiology. Visual disturbances may occur from any of the disorders noted in previous sections, especially untreated refractive disorders, amblyopia, infection, glaucoma, cataracts, and trauma. Visual impairment in children and adolescents can be caused by many hereditary conditions; acquired problems, such as brain and primary eye tumors; and vascular disorders, such as diabetic and sickle cell retinopathy. Determining the etiology of the visual impairment helps in understanding the child's functional abilities and prognosis. The pathophysiology of the visual impairment depends on the etiology of the child's disorder. (Refer to other sections in this chapter for specific conditions.)

Clinical Manifestations. Because the perception and recognition of decreased visual acuity may differ at various ages, understanding normal vision in children is important in ascertaining abnormalities. Table 34-1 gives an overview of significant visual milestones at different ages. Any gross variance from these norms should be closely evaluated to determine whether the child has a visual impairment.

Children may not complain of poor vision and may have compensated for it at an early age. However, the child may display behaviors that signal to the observant parent or teacher that visual problems are present. These behaviors may include such actions as frequent rubbing of the eyes or blinking, a wandering or closed eye, facial distortions, preference for viewing objects either close up or at a distance, irritability, or a poor attention span.[32] The infant may be unable to achieve the normal visual milestones or may show developmental delays in reaching for objects and people or in social interaction. If other reasons for these behaviors cannot be determined, the possibility of visual impairment should be investigated.

Diagnostic Studies. The most important tests for visual acuity, as discussed under "Refractive Errors" in this chapter and in Chapter 34, are the Allen cards, the E chart, and the Snellen chart. These tests are used individually depending on the age of the child. The Hirschberg and cover tests are used to determine if the child has strabismus and may assist with the diagnosis of amblyopia. However, close observation of the child's behavior may provide information as valuable to the ophthalmologist as the results of these screening tests.

★ **ASSESSMENT**

The nurse should closely observe the child with questionable vision for variances from developmental or behavioral norms. Careful documentation of abnormalities is indicated. These behaviors should be monitored and, if they persist, may require referral.

Likewise, the child with suspected visual impairment should receive visual acuity testing and screening for strabismus and amblyopia if age appropriate. Abnormalities noted behaviorally or through visual screening should be reported promptly to the ophthalmologist for further testing and appropriate intervention.

The nurse needs to evaluate the impact of reduced vision on family functioning. Parents and siblings may overprotect the affected child or, conversely, may not provide enough safety measures. Altered family functioning also may occur in response to the child's diagnosis of impaired vision.

★ **NURSING DIAGNOSES AND PLANNING**

Based on assessment data discussed previously and in the preceding chapter, the following nursing diagnoses may apply to the family and child with blindness:

- High Risk for Injury related to inability to see.
- Altered Growth and Development related to sensory-perceptual alteration.
- Altered Family Processes related to care of the child with visual impairment.

The nurse and child (or parents) together plan effective care based on the established nursing diagnoses. Several examples of expected outcomes follow:

- The child maintains established norms for growth and development.
- The family discusses strategies to protect the child from injury.
- The family contacts support group and other available referrals.
- The parents use community resources for further visual care of the infant.
- The parents and child describe the meaning of the child's loss of vision to themselves.

The nurse plans for the care of the child based on physician's orders and nursing diagnoses. Some general nursing care goals may be the following:

- Safety precautions are instituted.
- Normal growth and development are promoted.
- Family members participate in caring for child.
- Grieving related to child's limitations.

★ **INTERVENTIONS: COLLABORATIVE AND INDEPENDENT**

GROWTH, DEVELOPMENT, AND SAFETY MEASURES

The child with limited or no vision needs every opportunity to develop the other senses to the maximum degree. Promoting this development should be the overall goal of the nurse working with such a child and family. The child also should be assisted in achieving maximum mobility, fine motor skills, social interaction, and language skills.

If the child requires certain adaptive equipment, such as glasses, magnifiers, large-print objects (e.g., books, phone dials, watches, calculators), or braille, the nurse should assist the family in obtaining this equipment. Aids such as storybook records or cassettes also may assist the young child in developing language skills. Other developmental tasks, such as crawling and walking, feeding, and toilet training should be encouraged at the same ages as sighted children but with modifications, such as ensuring an unobstructed environment for walking or helping guide the child's hands to the plate when eating. A home visit by a nurse may be helpful in determining if the home environment is conducive to learning and safe for the visually impaired child.

The nurse caring for the hospitalized child who is blind needs to provide the child with the same modifications and adaptive equipment used in the home setting. Rearrangement of the hospital room may be required to provide for the child's safety. If a family member cannot remain with the child during the hospitalization, the child should be accompanied by a hospital staff member whenever ambulation outside of the room is attempted. Obtaining a complete history from the family on the nursing admission assessment will provide the nurse with information concerning the modifications used by the child at home that need to be implemented during the hospital stay.

PSYCHOSOCIAL SUPPORT

The nurse working with the newly diagnosed child and family will need to offer support and guidance to them during this crisis period. Clarification of what the physician has told the family concerning the etiology of the visual impairment is essential. The family may deal with their grief in a variety of ways, and continued acceptance of them during this period will greatly enhance their eventual adjustment. Assisting the family to contact other families who have a child with a similar disability and informing the family about support groups such as the National Association for Parents of the Visually Impaired also may help the family accept and manage the impairment.

When the family is ready, the nurse should assist the family in locating appropriate resources. Many different programs are available for the visually impaired (such resources appear in a display at the beginning of the chapter), and the general goal of these programs is to assist the child in achieving independence. The nurse working with the family should find out what the child is learning and reinforce this knowledge with the family.

★ EVALUATION

Periodically the nurse and family evaluate the outcomes of care given. Examples of outcomes for the child and family with blindness were given under Nursing Diagnoses and Planning in this section. Have short-term goals been met? Are long-term goals still realistic?

LONG-TERM CARE

On follow-up visits the nurse should assess the parents' coping skills and ability to provide the child with appropriate stimulation. This assessment may be as informal as asking some leading questions or may be formalized into a standard questionnaire. Areas such as the child's ability to ambulate and feed independently, acquisition of language skills, and behavioral adjustment are most important to appraise.

The nurse also should discuss with the parents their perceptions of the center for the blind that the child is attending to see if this is a suitable placement. Determining if the school-age child is learning reading skills (either by braille or cassette players) is important to enhance further learning in school. Infants and small children not of appropriate age for these centers should be followed up closely; developmental screening tools such as the Denver developmental screening test can be used to determine whether the child is attaining developmental milestones appropriately.

The child with poor vision but without total blindness needs to be re-examined by the ophthalmologist periodically to document the degree of visual loss and make any adjustments to the use of poor-vision aids. These aids may include the use of glasses, contact lens, and magnifiers. Other adaptive equipment, such as rails in the bathtub and canes, also may be indicated.

Disorders of the Ears

Otitis Media

Early recognition, diagnosis, management, and parent and child education of otitis media are important for several reasons:

- Untreated middle ear infection can lead to variable conductive hearing loss that may impair a child's normal acquisition of speech and language.[16]
- Otitis media may predispose a child to chronic suppurative ear disease in later life.
- Middle ear infections account for one-third of all visits to the pediatrician's office, resulting in significant cost. About $2 billion is spent annually in the United States for the diagnosis and treatment of ear infections.[18]

Definition and Incidence.   *Otitis media* is defined as an inflammation of the mucosal lining of the middle ear. Inflammation of the middle ear is classified as otitis media without effusion, acute otitis media, or otitis media with effusion. The differentiations between these diseases are summarized in Table 35-2. Otitis media without effusion may be seen in the early stages of acute otitis media or during the resolution stage of acute otitis media.

Recognized as a disease continuum,[54] otitis media can fluctuate between acute suppurative otitis media and secretory otitis media. Inadequate treatment of acute suppurative otitis media may lead to otitis media with effusion (OME). Additionally, OME may follow an acute purulent otitis even after the infection has been treated with antibiotics, and the fluid in the middle ear is free of bacteria. In these cases the persistence of fluid in the middle ear provides a culture medium for bacteria or viruses that may be reintroduced from the nasopharynx or eustachian tube.

Otitis media occurs primarily in infants and young children. It is uncommon in adolescents. The initial episode of acute otitis media occurs most often at about 6 months of age. The age at the first episode is inversely related to the risk for future episodes of acute otitis media in the 12 months after the initial diagnosis. The reason for this association is not clear.

The incidence of otitis media is highest in the winter and early spring and lowest in the summer. This seasonal variation is attributed to the prevalence of the causative viral and bacterial organisms responsible for upper respiratory tract infections.

Children who are hospitalized in the pediatric intensive care unit (PICU) sometimes develop otitis media. Several variables, including immunosuppression, underlying disease state, length of stay in the unit, manipulation of the airway and the presence of indwelling tubes (endotracheal or gastric), may contribute to the increased occurence in this population.[14] The incidence of otitis media also has been documented as higher among children with congenital ear anomalies,[42] cleft palate, and Down syndrome.

Otitis media is almost twice as prevalent in white children as in urban African Americans, but native American, African and Australian aborigine, and Hispanic children have a higher incidence of middle ear infection than white American children. Other risk factors associated with otitis media include male sex, HIV infection, family history of otitis media, cigarette smoke exposure, and lower socioeconomic class.

Day care enrollment is associated with a higher incidence of otitis media. Children in group day care have many more episodes of otitis media than children in home

TABLE 35-2
Comparison of Types of Otitis Media*

Type and Synonyms	Definition	Appearance of Tympanic Membrane	Clinical Manifestations	Duration of Illness
Otitis media without effusion	Inflammation of the middle ear mucous membrane and tympanic membrane without evidence of a middle ear effusion	Erythema and opacification; mobility is normal; blebs or bullae may be present		
Acute otitis media (acute/suppurative, purulent, or bacterial otitis media)	Inflammation of the middle ear characterized by a rapid and short onset of clinical signs and symptoms	Full and bulging and opaque; may be erythematous; limited or no mobility of tympanic membrane	Acute onset of ear pain, fever, a purulent drainage through perforation of the tympanic membrane, pulling of the ear (in a young infant), irritability, anorexia, vomiting, diarrhea; hearing loss may be present	About 3 weeks
Otitis media with effusion (secretory, nonsuppurative, or serous otitis media)	Inflammation of the middle ear in which a collection of liquid is present in the middle ear space; noninfectious form of otitis media; tympanic membrane intact	Opacified; retracted or convex tympanic membrane; impaired mobility; full, bulging tympanic membrane; air-filled level, bubbles or both seen through a translucent tympanic membrane; effusion may be serous (thin, watery), mucoid (thick, viscid, mucous-like), purulent (pus-like liquid), or a combination of these	Asymptomatic; hearing loss may be present	Ranges from less than 3 weeks to more than 3 months: Acute: Duration of effusion is less than 3 weeks Subacute: Duration of effusion is from 3 weeks to 2–3 months Chronic: Duration of effusion is longer than 2–3 months

* Otitis media refers to inflammation of the middle ear without reference to etiology or pathogenesis. Three types are recognized.

day care.[47] Breast-feeding is associated with a significant decrease in the risk of recurrent acute otitis media in the first year of life.[8]

Etiology and Pathophysiology. To understand the pathophysiology of otitis media it is important to review the anatomy of the middle ear and adjacent structures shown in Figure 33-9 and understand their normal physiologic functions. Children are at higher risk for developing otitis media than adults because of the characteristics of the eustachian tube. In infants the eustachian tube lies horizontal or at an angle of 10 degrees in relation to the horizontal plane (compared to an angle of 45 degrees in an adult). Additionally, the infant's eustachian tube is shorter (18 mm in infants compared to 30 to 40 mm in adults) and is proportionately wider and less tortuous. The posterior third of the adult eustachian tube is osseous, and the anterior two-thirds is composed of membrane and cartilage. In contrast the infant's eustachian tube's osseous portion is longer and wider. The osseous portion of the normal eustachian tube remains open at all times, while the fibrocartilaginous portion is closed at rest and opens only during certain maneuvers. The mucous membrane lining that is continuous from the middle ear through the nose, nasopharynx, eustachian tube, and respiratory system spreads inflammation, infection, or obstruction from one area to another.

The normal eustachian tube serves several physiologic functions:

• It protects nasopharyngeal secretions from refluxing into the middle ear.
• It clears secretions produced within the middle ear into the nasopharynx.

• It ventilates the middle ear to allow for equilibration of pressure across both sides of the ear drum.

Middle ear infection can occur if any one of these three functions are disrupted.

If the eustachian tube is abnormally congested, blocked, or closed, a gradual absorption of oxygen and some of the nitrogen contained in the air becomes trapped in the middle ear space. The absorption of gas creates a buildup of negative pressure within the middle ear and results in transudation of serous fluid from the mucous membranes, thus inhibiting the normal drainage of fluid from the middle ear. Bacterial contamination of the fluid can occur because of reflux from the nasopharynx or from the capillaries of the middle ear's mucous membranes during an episode of bacteremia. If the fluid that refluxes into the middle ear is contaminated with bacteria, proliferation of the microbial pathogen will result in a suppurative, symptomatic otitis media.

The pathogenesis of otitis media results from conditions that block or impair aeration of the eustachian tubes, thus preventing the normal drainage of fluids from the middle ear. A variety of factors can lead to functional or mechanical obstruction. Functional obstruction results from obstruction or persistent collapse of the eustachian tube.

Mechanical obstruction of the eustachian tube can be intrinsic or extrinsic in origin. Intrinsic mechanical obstruction usually is secondary to mucosal inflammation related to upper respiratory infections or allergies. Inflammatory reactions result in obstruction of the eustachian tube mucosa or tympanic mucosal changes leading to persistence of middle ear effusion. Extrinsic mechanical obstruction usually is due to compression by tumor or adenoid tissue. These masses block the opening of the eustachian tube or obstruct eustachian tube lymphatics, resulting in transudation of fluid into the middle ear.

Nasal obstruction also may contribute to the pathogenesis of otitis media. Upper respiratory infection coupled with enlarged adenoids may increase the incidence of barotrauma during air flight.

The majority of otitis media cases are associated with a bacterial pathogenesis. The most prevalent bacterias isolated in infants and young children with otitis media are *Haemophilus influenzae* and *Streptococcus pneumoniae*. Recent studies have confirmed the role of viruses or a combined viral and bacterial infection in the etiology of acute otitis media.[3,12] The most common viruses identified in middle ear fluids are respiratory syncytial virus,[8] rhinovirus,[2] influenza virus, and enterovirus.[12]

Clinical Manifestations. Acute suppurative otitis media is characterized by rapid onset of signs and symptoms consistent with purulent effusion, fluid accumulation, and inflammation in the middle ear. Older children may complain of earache and hearing loss. Younger children may complain of ear pain or may pull on their ears or rub the affected side. Irritability, anorexia, lethargy, and general discomfort are the most common findings. Dizziness, unsteady gait, and tinnitus are less frequent complaints. Nasal congestion, often with purulent discharge from the same side as the earache, is also a common symptom. Younger children may experience vomiting or have loose stools. Fever is variable and often absent in one third or more of proven cases of bacterial otitis media.

If the tympanic membrane has ruptured, purulent discharge may be observed in the ear canal, and if the drainage has been present for several days, crusts and evidence of skin infection around the lobe and orifice of the external auditory canal may be observed. The child may complain of "clicking" or "popping" in the ear when swallowing. The child may describe a sensation of movement in the ear if air is present above the fluid level. Conductive or chronic hearing loss may occur in the affected ear.

Children with chronic suppurative otitis media may complain of a feeling of fullness in the ear and fluctuating hearing loss. A thin, straw-colored serous effusion is present as well as a mucoid effusion, which is cloudy or gray and has a glue-like consistency. Pain, fever, and discharge is usually absent. Otitis media with effusion is an asymptomatic disease except for possible hearing loss.

Diagnostic Studies. The basic components in diagnosis of otitis media include assessment of clinical signs and symptoms, examination of the external ear and its adjoining areas, otoscopic examination of the ear, and pneumatic otoscopy.[30] A thorough physical examination is performed to determine the presence of any concomitant upper respiratory tract infection or congenital defects. Head and neck examination includes assessment of the external ear, nose, oral cavity, nasopharynx, larynx, and neck for any masses, swelling, erythema, edema, tenderness, or discharge.

Examination of the tympanic membrane is performed by otoscopy, the most common diagnostic technique for

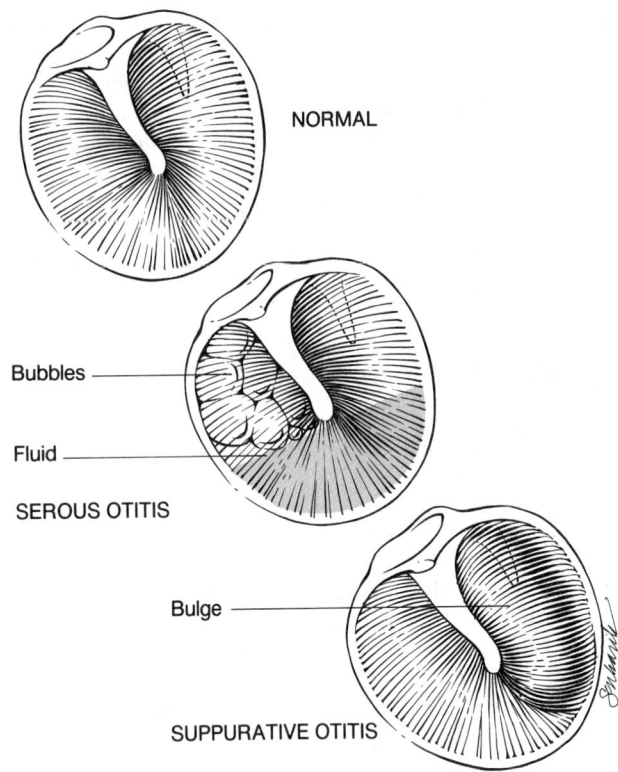

FIGURE 35-9
The tympanic membrane as visualized with the otoscope.

early detection of otitis media (Fig. 35-9). With acute suppurative otitis media a bulging bright red ear drum with decreased or absent light reflexes is observed. Bony landmarks may be absent or obscured due to opacification of the tympanic membrane. Children with secretory otitis media have a yellowish to orange discoloration of the drum due to the presence of purulent material behind the tympanic membrane. A fluid level may be visible behind the tympanic membrane, and perforation may be identified.

Pneumatic otoscopy is performed to assess the mobility of the tympanic membrane and to determine the presence of fluid or negative pressure in the middle ear (see Fig. 34-5B). Reduced mobility is conspicuous and diagnostic of middle ear fluid. The examiner determines if the tympanic membrane motion is bidirectional and brisk (normal), if mobility occurs in an outward direction only (negative middle ear pressure), or if mobility is sluggish or absent (fluid in the middle ear). The tympanic membrane has limited or absent mobility to pneumatic otoscopy with the presence of otitis media. The presence of fluid in the middle ear usually produces cloudiness and obscures the view of the middle ear structure. Air fluid levels or bubbles also may be observed.

Tympanometry in conjunction with pneumatic otoscopy can aid in confirming the diagnosis of otitis media. With middle ear effusion, pressure is reduced (i.e., more negative than -200 mm H_2O) and compliance is low. Tympanometry is accurate in detecting otitis media in children older than 7 months of age but may produce false negatives in younger infants.

An acoustic otoscope may be used in addition to a

pneumatic otoscopy in the diagnosis of otitis media.[26] The presence of fluid or thickening of the tympanic membrane increases sound reflection. Reflectivity is a function of the effective inelasticity of the tympanic membrane. The reflectivity is measured on a scale of 0 to 9 units. High reflectivity (5 to 9 units) suggests the presence of otitis media. Low reflectivity measures 0 to 5 units.

Tympanocentesis, a needle aspiration of middle ear contents, is not routinely performed because it is invasive and hazardous. For this reason the procedure should be performed only by a skilled pediatrician or an otolaryngologist. Tympanocentesis is indicated when one or more of the following is present[7,34]:

- Severe otalgia, serious illness, or appearance of toxicity.
- Unsatisfactory response to antimicrobial therapy.
- Onset of otitis media in a child who is receiving appropriate and adequate antimicrobial therapy.
- Presence of or potential for suppurative complications (if the benefits of obtaining additional information outweigh the risk of performing the procedure).
- Presence of otitis media in a newborn infant, a sick infant, or a child who is immunologically compromised in which an unusual organism is present.

★ ASSESSMENT

Nursing assessment includes obtaining a thorough history of previous ear infections, a recent history of upper respiratory infections, an allergy history, and a physical assessment. The physical assessment should determine the presence of tinnitus, ear pain, feelings of fullness in the ear, vertigo, or hearing loss. Young children may not be able to verbalize their pain, and the nurse must rely on cues, such as ear pulling, irritability, frequently putting fingers or foreign objects into the ear canal. Hearing loss should be determined using information from parents, siblings, and teachers to determine any abnormal hearing behaviors in the child. The accompanying display lists indications of abnormal hearing behaviors.

Mild to moderate conductive hearing loss is the most prevalent complication and cause of morbidity associated with otitis media. Accumulation of stagnant serous fluid can decrease sound transmission through the tympanic membrane and the bony ossicles of the middle ear. The hearing loss is usually reversible when the effusion is resolved. However, permanent conduction hearing loss can result in cases of recurrent acute or chronic otitis media.[8]

Nursing assessment also includes assessment of the level of knowledge the parent and child have regarding middle ear infections, including signs and symptoms, management, complications, and prevention of recurrent infection. Assessment also can determine the parents' compliance with the prescribed antibiotic treatment.

★ NURSING DIAGNOSES AND PLANNING

Based on assessment data discussed previously and in the preceding chapter, the following nursing diagnoses may apply to the family and child with otitis media:

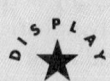

Nursing Assessment: Indications of Abnormal Hearing Behaviors

POOR HEARING AND UNDERSTANDING

- Fails to respond to speaker when addressed
- Does not respond to loud noises
- Does not turn head toward source of sound
- Does not respond to the telephone or doorbell
- Frequently asks speaker to repeat what was said
- Sit directly in front of the television with the volume turned up
- Abnormal speech, gestures used to communicate (pointing, grunting)

POOR BEHAVIOR AND POOR SOCIALIZATION HABITS

- Short attention span when watching television or during story telling
- Prefers to play alone rather than engage in group activities
- Is shy and withdrawn
- Talks loudly

POOR SCHOOL PERFORMANCE

- Not able to follow verbal instructions well; however, does well when observing others

- Anxiety related to knowledge deficit about condition and treatment.
- Pain related to inflammation and infection.
- Impaired Verbal Communication related to impaired hearing.
- High Risk for Injury (Falls) related to disturbance of balance and impaired ability to detect environmental hazards.
- Altered Growth and Development related to temporary conductive hearing loss.

The nurse and child (or parents) together plan effective care based on the established nursing diagnoses. Several examples of expected outcomes follow:

- The child sleeps without restlessness or waking.
- The child states that he or she feels relief from pain.
- The parents demonstrate correct method for cleaning the ear canal and inserting ear drops.
- The child's verbal skills are age-appropriate.

The nurse plans for the care of the child based on physician's orders and nursing diagnoses. Some general nursing care goals may be the following:

- Growth and development are promoted.
- Pain is relieved.
- Injury is prevented.

★ INTERVENTIONS: COLLABORATIVE AND INDEPENDENT

Children with otitis media usually are seen and treated as outpatients. Neonates suspected of otitis media, however, are admitted to the hospital for diagnosis and treatment because of the frequent association with sepsis, pneumonia, or meningitis. Parenteral antibiotics, parenteral fluid, and electrolyte therapy are usually necessary.

Nursing management of the child with otitis media includes promoting rest, relieving fever discomfort and pain, providing skin care, and teaching the parents or child regarding signs and symptoms, management, and prevention of otitis media.

MEDICATION THERAPY

Medical treatment is directed at eliminating or reducing any structural abnormalities contributing to blockage of the eustachian tubes and providing antibiotic therapy. Fifty percent of cases of acute suppurative otitis media resolve without sequelae in 3 to 4 weeks after appropriate antibiotic therapy. However, in 40% of cases the infection will persist for 4 weeks or more. In these children, antibiotics make the pus in the middle ear sterile but do not eliminate the fluid that has accumulated in the middle ear. The symptoms of otitis media are not eliminated. The remaining 10% of cases have persistent otitis media 90 days after the onset of the disease, even after appropriate antimicrobial therapy.

The choice of antibiotic initially should be based on the most likely causative organism until culture results provide more precise data. An appropriate choice would be amoxicillin 40 mg/kg in three doses or ampicillin 50 to 100 mg/kg in four doses. Amoxicillin is the preferred antibiotic because of fewer adverse reactions. Ampicillin must be administered 1 hour before or 2 hours after meals because absorption is significantly decreased when the drug is taken with food. Alternative antibiotics are used for specific organisms (Table 35-3).

Significant improvement usually is seen 48 to 72 hours after appropriate antimicrobial therapy is initiated.[7]

Parents should be instructed to contact the prescribing physician if otalgia (earache) or fever is not improved within 72 hours of therapy. Re-examination may reveal development of suppurative complications or development of a concurrent infection such as meningitis. If the child continues to have minimal signs of persistent infection (low-grade fever, failure to return to former activity), or if on otoscopic examination inflammation of the middle ear mucosa is still present, an additional 10-day course of antibiotics may be prescribed.

If severe earache or other toxic symptoms persist, then a tympanocentesis or myringotomy may be performed to provide immediate relief. Antibiotics may need to be re-evaluated based on culture results from the tympanocentesis.

Chemoprophylaxis or the use of antimicrobial agents for prolonged periods has been advocated[30,31] for children who have three episodes of acute otitis media in 6 months or four episodes in 12 months. Sulfisoxazole and amoxicillin in half their therapeutic doses are administered once a day for up to 6 months during winter and spring when respiratory infections are most frequent.

To relieve ear pain or discomfort analgesics such as acetaminophen (10 to 15 mg/kg per dose every 4 hours) may be useful initially until antibiotic therapy can eradicate the infection and decrease pain. Codeine (0.5 to 1.0 mg/kg per dose every 4 to 6 hours, not to exceed 3 mg/kg per day) may be prescribed with acetaminophen. Warm ear drops containing benzocaine may provide temporary relief if prescribed.

Decongestants, analgesics, and antipyretics may be used as adjunctive therapy. An oral decongestant, such as pseudoephedrine hydrochloride, may relieve rhinorrhea or nasal congestion. Antihistamines may be helpful for children with known or suspected nasal allergy. Steroids also have been used in the treatment of persistent OME with varying degrees of success.

TABLE 35-3
Antimicrobial Agents for Otitis Media

Drug	Recommended Dosage	Clinical Efficacy		
		Streptococcus pneumoniae	Haemophilus influenzae	Branhamella catarrhalis
Amoxicillin	40 mg/kg in three doses for 10 days	+	+	+
Ampicillin	50–100 mg/kg in four doses for 10 days	+	+	N/A
Amoxicillin-clavulanate	40 mg/kg in three doses	+	+	+
Cefaclor	40 mg/kg in three doses	+	+	+
Cefuroxime axetil	125 mg two times per day younger than 2 years	+	+	+
	250 mg two times per day older than 2 years			
Cefixime	8 mg/kg in one dose	+	+	+
Clindamycin	25 mg/kg in four doses	+	−	N/A
Erythromycin	40 mg/kg in four doses	+	−	+
Erythromycin-sulfasoxazole	40 mg/kg in four doses and 120 mg/kg in four doses	+	+	+
Trimethoprim-sulfamethoxazole	8 mg trimethoprim and 40 mg/kg sulfamethoxazole in three doses	+	+	+

Abbreviations: +, effective; −, not effective; N/A, not reported.
(Data from Bluestone, C. D., & Klein, J. O. [1990]. Otitis media, atelectasis, and eustachian tube dysfunction. In C. D. Bluestone & S. E. Stoll [Eds.]. *Pediatric otolaryngology*. Philadelphia: W.B. Saunders.)

TEACHING

If the ear drains by spontaneous rupture of the tympanic membrane, the nurse should teach the parent to clean the external ear canal several times daily with mild soap and water on cotton or gauze. Q-tips should be avoided because of potential hazards of pushing foreign matter further into the ear canal. When cleaning the ear canal of a young child, the parents should be taught to pull the ear lobe down and back to straighten the canal. In an older child the ear lobe should be pulled up and back. Positions are shown in Figure 25-11. The ear is dried after cleaning and a topical antibiotic applied if prescribed. Placing the child with the affected side down promotes drainage and clearance of the fluid.

If the child needs to take a trip by air, the parents should help their child swallow repeatedly, chew gum, or yawn during airplane ascent and descent to equilibrate atmospheric pressure and middle ear pressure. A small infant may be given a bottle. Older children could be taught to "pop" their ears by performing a modified Valsalva's maneuver. Air travel does not appear to adversely affect the course or sequelae of otitis media.[51]

Parents also should be taught the significance of nose blowing, sneezing, crying, or closed-nose swallowing in a child who has an open or abnormally patent eustachian tube. These activities may cause unwanted contaminated nasopharyngeal secretions to reflux into the middle ear. Parents also should be told that feeding in the reclining position and bottle propping can promote pooling of fluid in the pharyngeal cavity, increasing the chances of regurgitation and reflux of the feeding into the middle ear. An explanation of the anatomy of the eustachian tube helps the parents to appreciate the importance of compliance. The risk of aspiration secondary to propping the bottle also should be explained.

The nurse is responsible for determining the level of adherence to the prescribed medication routine. The most frequent drug-related factor in failure of antibiotic therapy is inadequate compliance.[8] Reasons for inadequate treatment usually are related to unpleasant taste of the drug, diarrhea, incorrect dosage schedules, and early termination. Parents need to know the importance of giving the full course of the antibiotic. Failure to give antibiotics as prescribed for acute otitis media may lead to persistence of the disease and complications, including exposure to additional antibiotics, hearing loss, and potential speech and language difficulties.

INFECTION PREVENTION

Therapeutic nursing modalities used to manage or prevent infection include control of allergies with food elimination and environmental control. Environmental control includes removing as much dust as possible from the home. Pillows, mattresses, stuffed furniture, rugs, stuffed toys, and animal hair are the main sources of dust. Even if the entire house cannot be environmentally controlled, the child's room should be. The room should be wet mopped and dusted from top to bottom including lights, window sills, shelves, closets, and molding. A disinfectant that prevents the growth of mold spores should be used. Smoking should not be allowed in the house.

SURGICAL MANAGEMENT

In cases of recurrent or persistent middle ear effusion that does not respond to antibiotic therapy, a myringotomy may be performed to provide immediate relief from pain and to promote drainage. Indications for a myringotomy with placement of ventilation tubes include persistence of fluid for 3 or more months per episode, presence of speech or language delay, presence of bilateral conductive hearing loss of 20 dB or more, the total number of episodes of otitis media, and a lack of response to suppressive antibiotic therapy.[23] Myringotomy is a surgical procedure in which an incision is made in the inferior portion of the tympanic membrane and the glue-like exudate is suctioned out to provide pressure equalization. Ventilatory tubes are then placed through the incision to facilitate the continuous drainage of fluid and encourage the equalization of pressure in the middle ear (Fig. 35-10). This procedure results in the drainage of the effusion, which enhances ventilation of the middle ear and helps to relieve any associated hearing loss. Children with severe symptoms, moderate to severe conductive hearing loss, delay in speech development, or learning problems attributable to hearing difficulties will benefit most from prompt insertion of ventilating tubes. Potential complications of myringotomy include hearing loss and infection.

PRESURGICAL AND POSTSURGICAL TEACHING

The desired outcomes of child and parent education include an understanding of home care to prevent complications of surgery. To reduce the anxiety associated with surgery the surgical procedure should be explained to the child and parents in easy terms. The expected length of surgery should be conveyed to the parents. Expected postoperative findings, including ear drainage, hearing loss, and pain, should be discussed prior to surgery with the child and parents. A small amount of reddish

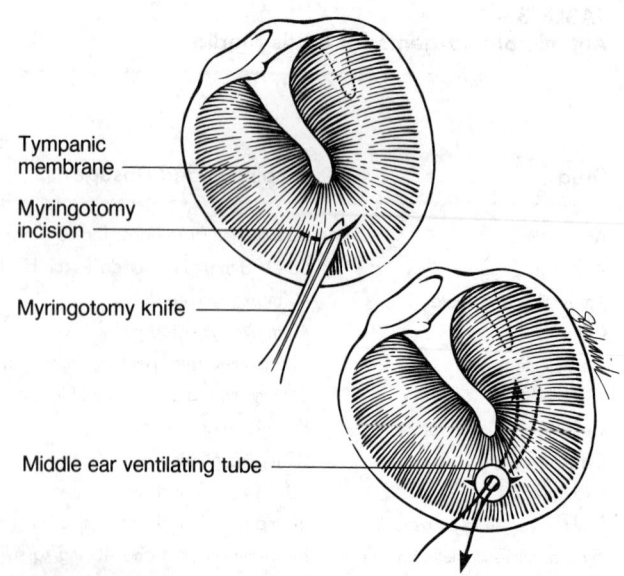

FIGURE 35-10

A myringotomy followed by placement of ventilating tubes is the treatment for recurrent or persistent middle ear effusion.

Tympanic membrane

Myringotomy incision

Myringotomy knife

Middle ear ventilating tube

drainage is normal during the first few days after surgery. Parents should be instructed to notify the surgeon if there is significant bleeding in the postoperative period or any bleeding after the third postoperative day. Frequent swallowing may be an early indication of hemorrhage and requires immediate medical attention. Vomiting of bright red blood, increased pain, persistent earache after the first 2 to 3 postoperative days, or a continuous elevated temperature may be signs of postoperative complications, including infection, hemorrhage, or edema.

Analgesics may be given to help control pain, and antipyretics may be given to help reduce fever. Ear pain or referred throat pain often occur during the first postoperative week and may be relieved with an ice collar applied to the child's neck for 10 to 15 minutes at a time. The child and parent also need to be taught that the ear must be kept dry. Earplugs may be used during swimming to prevent water from entering the ear. Diving is not allowed due to the risk of increasing middle ear pressure. Cotton covered with petroleum jelly is used to cover the external auditory meatus during bathing or washing of the hair to prevent contamination of the middle ear.

Parents should be told that the tympanostomy tube remains in place until it spontaneously falls out, about 6 to 12 months after insertion. The parents should inform the physician when this happens.

★ EVALUATION

Periodically the nurse and family evaluate the outcomes of care given. Examples of outcomes for the child and family with otitis media were given under Nursing Diagnoses and Planning in this section. Have short-term goals been met? Are long-term goals still realistic? Planning for further nursing care takes into consideration complications and long-term care.

COMPLICATIONS

Complications of otitis media, listed in the accompanying display, are either intratemporal or intracranial. The most dangerous complications of acute otitis media include mastoiditis, labyrinthitis, facial nerve paralysis, osteomyelitis, epidural abscess, otic hydrocephalus, meningitis, and brain abscess. Since the advent of antibiotics, the incidence of these complications is rare. Other complications associated with otitis media include perforation of the tympanic membrane, tympanosclerosis, fixation of the ossicles, cholesteatoma, chronic otitis media, and hearing loss.

The incidence of otitis media is highest during the first 3 years of life when acquisition of language occurs. A correlation between conductive hearing loss resulting from recurrent otitis media during the first 3 to 5 years of life and subsequent problems in the development of speech and acquisition of language and cognitive skills has been documented.[16] However, the long-term effects on language acquisition have been disputed.

Social and emotional development of the child also may be adversely affected, even with mild hearing loss of 15 to 25 dB in early childhood. A referral to speech therapy may be made if there is any concern of delayed or abnormal language development. Nursing responsi-

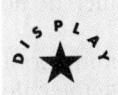

Possible Complications of Otitis Media

INTRATEMPORAL

Hearing loss
Chronic suppurative otitis media
Cholesteatoma
Tympanosclerosis
Ossicular fixation
Facial nerve paralysis
Tympanic membrane perforation
Mastoiditis
Labyrinthitis

INTRACRANIAL

Meningitis
Epidural abscess
Brain abscess
Otic hydrocephalus

---

bility includes educating the parents about these potential complications and the accompanying signs and symptoms that indicate complications.

LONG-TERM CARE

All infants and young children, particularly those at high risk for development or recurrence of otitis media, should be examined carefully during regular medical checkups. Gates and associates[20] recommend that hearing and middle ear screening should be done at least biannually in the first year of school and again 1 year later, preferably near the beginning and end of the school year when upper respiratory tract infections and chronic cases of otitis media tend to be the highest.

Children who are being treated for otitis media should be re-examined within 24 hours after the end of a course of antibiotic therapy to assess the response to the antibiotics and to determine the function and appearance of the eardrum. This appointment is important to determine if the infection has responded to therapy and to prevent development of OME.

Otitis Externa

Definition, Incidence, Etiology, and Pathophysiology. *Otitis externa*, commonly referred to as "swimmer's ear," is a localized or diffuse inflammation of the external auditory canal from the tympanic membrane to the external ear. This problem occurs predominantly during hot and humid weather (during the summer and autumn months).

Factors that predispose to acute and chronic otitis externa include frequent exposure to the water (e.g., swimming), trauma from foreign objects introduced into the ear (e.g., cotton-tipped applicators, bobby pins), use of ear plugs, hearing aid molds, use of ear drops,[22] or prolonged use of full-enclosure earphones (which do not allow for adequate ventilation of the ears).

Children swimming in chlorinated swimming pools are at risk for developing otitis externa because the chlorine helps break down the cerumen barrier coating the epithelium. In this state the epithelial lining can be easily invaded and infected by bacteria or fungi. Gram-negative organisms are the most common bacteria identified in otitis externa. Gram-negative organisms tend to be found in severe cases of otitis externa, while gram-positive organisms are found in the milder cases. Contaminated stagnant water in the external ear also may support bacterial growth.

Clinical Manifestations and Diagnostic Studies.

The first complaint of children with otitis externa is itching of the ear and having a feeling of a plugged ear. Inflammation of the external ear canal causes profound pain and swelling of the ear. Ear pain is experienced as early as 6 hours following epithelial damage to the ear canal. Any movement of the jaw or external ear aggravates the pain. The external canal is usually erythematous with preauricular and postauricular swelling. Fever may be present if the infection is severe. Conductive hearing loss and a feeling of "fullness" in the affected ear also may occur. A discharge is present if there is an infection. The ear canal is filled with a cheesy green-blue-gray discharge that is composed of bacteria, leukocytes, desquamated epithelial cells, and serous fluid. The discharge and edema may completely occlude the canal and contribute to vertigo.

Early recognition and diagnosis of otitis externa are important to prevent the spread of infection, which may progress to malignant otitis externa. Diagnosis usually is based on the typical clinical findings of a purulent and foul-smelling exudate and edema of the ear canal. Physical examination of the child will rule out other causes of ear pain, including parotiditis, periauricular adenitis, mastoiditis, dental abscesses, temporomandibular joint dysfunction, referred pharyngeal pain, acute purulent otitis media, and impacted foreign body.

Myringitis, inflammation of the tympanic membrane, may be identified on otoscopic examination. The eardrum will appear reddened, thick, and covered with flat vesicles. Epithelial damage often is visible in the ear canal.

★ ASSESSMENT

Nursing assessment includes obtaining a history of ear infections, exposure to water (during swimming or bathing), ear trauma or placement of objects into the external ear, and the use of earphones. The child should be asked about itching, pain, or discharge. Itching is the main symptom. Pain may occur when pressure is placed on the tragus, when the pinna of the ear is moved, or when chewing.

★ NURSING DIAGNOSES AND PLANNING

Based on assessment data discussed previously and in the preceding chapter, the following nursing diagnoses may apply to the family and child with otitis externa:

- Pain related to inflammation and infection.
- Altered Comfort (Itching) related to skin inflammation.
- Altered Health Maintenance related to knowledge deficit regarding condition, aural hygiene practices, complications, and prevention of future episodes of otitis externa.

The nurse and child (or parents) together plan effective care based on the established nursing diagnoses. Several examples of expected outcomes follow:

- The parents demonstrate correct actions for irrigating the ear.
- The parents describe measures that achieve comfort.
- The parents and the child who swims discuss recommended methods for ear care while swimming.

The nurse plans for the care of the child based on physician's orders and nursing diagnoses. Some general nursing care goals may be the following:

- Pain and itching are relieved.
- Effective ear care habits are established.
- Complications are prevented.

★ INTERVENTIONS: COLLABORATIVE AND INDEPENDENT

Medical management includes a thorough cleaning of the ear canal to remove all debris (including impacted cerumen) and treating the localized infection. Debris or exudate may be removed with gentle suction by the physician using a hypertonic saline solution, vinegar (5% acetic acid) diluted with an equal volume of water, or an acidified isopropyl alcohol solution. A soft rubber, silicon, or plastic catheter may be used to remove the cheesy exudate. Irrigation under pressure is not recommended because if a chronic draining otitis is the cause, material could be forced through a ruptured ear drum into the middle ear.

TEACHING

If indicated, the nurse should teach the parents how to irrigate their child's ear. Parents should be instructed to be sure to wash their hands prior to the procedure. A solution of half-strength hydrogen peroxide (mixed with equal parts of warm water) may be used. Parents are instructed about pulling the pinna to straighten the meatus. The irrigating tube is directed along the posterior wall of the canal. The water passes the wax or foreign object and rebounds off the drum to push the wax outward. The fluid is allowed to drain by gravity onto a clean towel or basin. This is painless. Any pain associated with syringing should be reported to the physician because it may indicate a perforation.

If the ear canal is swollen closed, ear drops containing polymyxin, neomycin, hydrocortisone, and propylene glycol will combat infection and decrease inflammation.[49] The nurse should instruct the parents about how to instill the drops. To instill the ear drops the child should be assisted to lie down with the affected ear upward. A cotton wick soaked with the drops is gently inserted into the external ear following instillation of the medication to facilitate contact of the medication with the skin. The child remains in this position for 5 minutes. Treatment is continued for 10 days if the infection extends beyond the skin of the ear canal as evidenced by fever, adenopathy, or cellulitis of the pinna.

Children who have severe infection may require parenteral therapy for 7 to 10 days with a combination of an aminoglycoside and an antipseudomonal penicillin, such as mezlocillin sodium (Mezlin) or piperacillin sodium (Pipracil). Systemic analgesics, such as acetaminophen and codeine, help relieve the pain. Use of a warm heating pad to provide intermittent dry heat also may help to relieve any pain or discomfort.

Parents and children are taught how to prevent future episodes of otitis externa. The child and parents are told that the goal is to keep the external ear canal clean and dry and to protect it from further trauma. Parents are taught not to use cotton-tipped applicators to clean the ears because this could push the cerumen or debris further into the ear canal.

Children on swim teams may be treated prophylactically with a few drops of a solution of equal parts of water and vinegar or vinegar and rubbing alcohol in each ear upon arising in the morning, after each swim, and at bedtime.[33] The solution must stay in the ear for at least 5 minutes. Limiting the stay in the water to less than 1 hour at a time may be beneficial. The ear should be dry for 1 to 2 hours before re-entering the pool. Water is drained from the ear by head shaking or by drying off with a towel. Custom molded ear plugs also may be used to prevent water from entering the external ear canal. Diving is avoided to prevent further increase in middle ear pressure. Parents and children are instructed on effective handwashing and daily cleansing of the ears. Baths or showers and shampoos may be allowed every other day if the child dries the ear canal immediately afterward.

★ EVALUATION

Periodically the nurse and family evaluate the outcomes of care given. Examples of outcomes for the child and family with otitis externa were given under Nursing Diagnoses and Planning in this section. Planning for further nursing care takes into consideration complications.

Children should return to the clinic or to the pediatrician's office 2 weeks after initiation of antibiotics to determine their effectiveness. Hearing loss should be assessed by an audiologist. The nurse should assess for resolution of signs and symptoms, reinforce earlier health care teaching, and assess knowledge and compliance to prevent future episodes of otitis externa.

COMPLICATIONS

Severe chronic otitis externa may result in deafness, adenopathy, fever, and severe pain. Malignant otitis externa is a severe form of the illness and usually occurs in children who are susceptible to infection, such as children with diabetes mellitus. If the infection extends to the middle and inner ear and to the central nervous system, severe sequelae can result including osteomyelitis of the base of the skull with involvement of cranial nerves VII and IX through XII.

Hearing Deficits and Language Disorders

Definition and Incidence. The sense of hearing is essential for formation of proper speech, language, and learning. The loss of hearing, regardless of degree, is considered a form of deafness and has especially detrimental implications for the developing child. Approximately 1 infant in every 1000 live births is born with a hearing deficit, and about 3 million children in the United States have a hearing impairment.[41]

Hearing loss is measured in decibels through the use of impedance audiometry and is categorized by the degree of loss as noted in Table 35-4. Any hearing loss greater than 20 dB in the frequency range for speech (500 to 200 Hz) may detrimentally affect the development of speech and learning.[46] Furthermore, when this deficit occurs in infants and children younger than 3 years of age, their language abilities may be permanently altered.[24] Testing infants and children suspected of having or at risk for developing a hearing impairment is therefore important. This testing can be done as early as 3 months of age.[46]

Speech and language disorders may manifest themselves as difficulty understanding speech, using language, or both. These are commonly referred to as either receptive, expressive, or mixed disorders, respectively. Because speech delays may result from hearing problems due to a receptive disorder, speech and hearing impairments are treated simultaneously.

Etiology and Pathophysiology. Another classification system for hearing loss is according to where the defect occurs in the auditory system. The two most frequent types of hearing loss are conductive and sensorineural. With a conductive loss there is some abnormality of the outer or middle ear involving such structures as the pinna, external auditory ear canal, tympanic membrane, ear ossicles, eustachian tube, and either the round or oval windows.[24] Usually this abnormality occurs from a mechanical defect in one of these structures. Common childhood problems contributing to conductive losses include acute otitis media, serous otitis media, cerumen plugs in the external ear canal, and defects of the ossicles.

A sensorineural hearing loss is caused by a defect in the inner ear or in the auditory pathway within the brain. This defect affects structures such as the semicircular ca-

TABLE 35-4
Hearing Impairment by Degree of Loss

Degree of Loss	Functional Impairment
0–14 dB	Normal hearing
15–30 dB	Mild hearing loss
31–50 dB	Moderate hearing loss
51–80 dB	Severe hearing loss
81–100 dB	Profound hearing loss

(Data from Weiss, C. E., & Lillywhite, H. S. [1981]. *Communicative disorders* (2nd ed.). St. Louis: C. V. Mosby.)

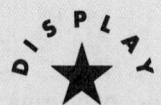

Etiology of Hearing Loss

CONGENITAL TYPES

- Perinatal infections (e.g., cytomegalovirus, rubella, herpes, toxoplasmosis, syphilis)
- Maternal ingestion of ototoxic drugs or exposure to radiation during pregnancy
- Chromosomal abnormalities (e.g., trisomy 13–15, trisomy 18)
- Genetic abnormalities (e.g., certain Y-linked and dominant forms)
- Atresia, stenosis, or other deformities of the ossicles arising from fetal maldevelopment
- Birth asphyxia
- Low birthweight (less than 2500 g)
- Erythroblastosis fetalis resulting from Rh incompatibility or extreme hyperbilirubinemia
- Family history of hearing impairment during childhood

ACQUIRED TYPES

- Childhood infections (e.g., measles, mumps, chickenpox, influenza, meningitis (especially *Haemophilus influenzae*), otitis media
- Childhood ingestion of ototoxic drugs (e.g., kanamycin, neomycin, or streptomycin), especially in infancy
- Structural disorders (e.g., chronic nasal obstruction and trauma)
- Neoplastic diseases and metabolic disorders (e.g., hypothyroidism)

(Data from Chow, M. P., Durand, B. A., Feldman, M. N., & Mills, M. A. [1984]. Handbook of pediatric primary care (2nd ed.). New York: Wiley; and Stone, C. [1990]. Clinical diagnosis and management of problems of the head, eyes, ear, nose and throat. In V. L. Millonig [Ed.]. The pediatric nurse practitioner certification review guide [pp. 131–132]. Potomac, MD: Health Leadership Associates, Inc.)

nals, the cochlea, and the auditory nerve. The condition may be congenital or acquired, as, for example, following certain infectious and metabolic disorders, use of ototoxic drugs, and trauma.

The two categories of etiologies are congenital and acquired. The accompanying display lists the more common disorders contributing to congenital and acquired hearing loss. Some common problems that may contribute to a delay in language acquisition include hearing loss (receptive disorder), orofacial changes such as unrepaired cleft palate, tongue thrust, malocclusion (expressive disorder), and neurologic disability or mental neurologic retardation (mixed disorder). Lack of appropriate environmental stimulation to develop speech also can contribute to a language delay. The three common areas of expressive speech impairments are articulation, fluency, and voice.

Clinical Manifestations. General indicators of hearing impairment in children are noted in Tables 35-5 and 35-6. In general, the child fails to demonstrate expected milestones in communication patterns and language acquisition skills. The child 0 to 3 years of age is most at risk for language disorders due to a hearing loss; therefore, this age group requires the closest observation for a potential problem.

Diagnostic Studies. Several types of diagnostic tests are available to assess the child's auditory ability. These are used if the child is at high risk for developing a hearing impairment or if there is reason to suspect a hearing problem. The brainstem auditory evoked potential (BAEP) is used especially for testing infants and children who are unable to respond volitionally (see Chap. 34).

Impedance audiometry can be used in children as young as 6 months of age. This diagnostic procedure is actually composed of three tests: static compliance (seldom used), tympanometry, and acoustic reflex testing.[35] Tympanometry assesses the compliance of the tympanic membrane as air pressure is changed within the external auditory canal. Acoustic reflex testing determines the response of the stapedial muscle in both ears to sound introduced in only one ear. Adequate stapedial muscle contraction indicates integrity of the reflex arc (VIII nerve, cerebellopontine angle, brainstem, VII nerve, stapedial muscle).

Behavioral assessment of the child, as noted in Table 35-5 and Chapter 34, is the initial means of screening for

TABLE 35-5
Nursing Assessment: Indicators of Hearing Impairment

Age	Hearing Impairments
0–3 months	Unable to respond appropriately to voice or noise
3–6 months	Does not make reflexive responses to loud and sudden noises (e.g., crying, body jerks, eye blinks)
7–12 months	Fails to demonstrate listening responses by turning the head, searching with the eyes, or quieting behavior in response to a sound or calling the child's name
1–2 years	Unable to say a variety of consonants and vowels with vocalizations, language not age appropriate
2+ years	Speech and language development clearly delayed, may have educational or behavioral problems

(Data from Chow, M. P., Durand, B. A., Feldman, M. N., & Mills, M. A. [1984]. *Handbook of pediatric primary care* [2nd ed.]. New York: Wiley; and Stone, C. [1990]. Clinical diagnosis and management of problems of the head, eyes, ear, nose and throat. In V. L. Millonig [Ed.]. *The pediatric nurse practitioner certification review guide* [p. 132]. Potomac, MD: Health Leadership Associates, Inc.)

TABLE 35-6
Nursing Assessment: Signs of Speech and Language Delay

Age	Speech Delays
6–9 months	Does not respond to sound heard behind or to the side
10–15 months	Fails to respond to his or her own name
15–18 months	Unable to understand or respond to "no-no," "bye-bye," and "bottle"
18–21 months	Unable to vocalize 10 different words
21–24 months	Cannot understand and respond correctly to simple commands (e.g., "sit down," "stand up")
24–30 months	Cannot point to body parts on request and has too much and inappropriate jargon or echoing
30–36 months	Speech unintelligible, even to family members; cannot demonstrate in, on, under, front, and back
36–42 months	Unable to say simple sentences and cannot ask simple questions; speech unintelligible to strangers
42–48 months	Fails to pronounce the final consonants of words
4–5 years	Cannot answer simple questions (e.g., "What do we sleep on?" "What is your name?" "What do you do when you are thirsty?"; unable to tell a boy from a girl or big from little; may stutter or show other signs of dysfluency
5–6 years	Unable to distinguish soft from hard and smooth from rough; cannot determine the use of common words (e.g., cook, stove, chair, house)

(Data from Weiss, C. E. & Lillywhite, H. S. [1981]. *Communicative disorders* [2nd ed.]. St. Louis: C. V. Mosby.)

auditory impairment. However, pure-tone audiometry is a tool often used in children 3 years of age and older. This test gives a visual image and numeric value to describe the child's hearing acuity. The normal hearing threshold ranges from 0 to 15 dB at between 250 and 8000 Hz. Table 35-4 describes abnormal hearing levels and their meaning.

Speech and language tests primarily identify problems with articulation, fluency, and voice. The child with speech problems is a candidate for more extensive speech and language testing. Several standardized tests are available to assess speech problems more definitively. These tests usually are administered by a professional speech pathologist.

★ ASSESSMENT

The nurse working with children of all ages is well situated to notice any auditory or vocal problems. Special attention should be given to pertinent historic information that may indicate a potential problem. Using the screening assessment included in Tables 35-5 and 35-6, the nurse should be able to determine potential or actual hearing and speech problems. If the nurse is unsure about the child's actual abilities, the parents or guardian should be questioned carefully concerning the child's responses to an auditory stimulus and speech production at home.

★ NURSING DIAGNOSES AND PLANNING

Based on assessment data discussed previously and in the preceding chapter, the following nursing diagnoses

may apply to the family and child with hearing deficits and language disorders:

- Impaired Verbal Communication related to poor speech production and language acquisition.
- Altered Growth and Development related to sensory-perceptual alterations (auditory).
- Altered Self-Concept related to auditory deficit.

The nurse and child (or parents) together plan effective care based on the established nursing diagnoses. Several examples of expected outcomes follow:

- The family states that they are using a reward system devised by the nurse and family.
- The family reports that they read to the child in an *en face* position.
- The parents state that the child participates in normal play with peers.
- The child discusses implications of hearing deficit with care providers.

The nurse plans for the daily care of the child based on physician's orders and nursing diagnoses. Some general nursing care goals may be the following:

- Skills or mechanical means for communication are learned.
- Normal growth and development continues.

★ INTERVENTIONS: COLLABORATIVE AND INDEPENDENT

Any child at risk of developing hearing problems or who shows early signs of developing them should be referred to the appropriate health care professional. The child's pediatrician should initially be alerted to the problem by the nurse or family member. The child may be referred on to an otolaryngologist who will determine if an audiologist is needed to analyze hearing difficulties or if a speech pathologist is needed to assess language problems using many of the diagnostic tools noted in the previous section.

Interventions for the hearing impaired child include hearing aids, auditory training (listening carefully to spoken language), lip reading, sign language, finger spelling, and speech training. These skills are usually taught in schools for the hearing impaired. Speech therapy to enhance the child's verbal skills is usually provided by a speech pathologist or speech therapist and may be offered through the school system, within hospital clinics, or in private practices.

PSYCHOSOCIAL SUPPORT

The nurse working with the child who uses a hearing aid may need to assist the family in developing a positive reward system to encourage the child to wear the device. This may take the form of a "star" or "sticker" chart, tokens, or points each time the hearing aid is worn. For every certain number of times the hearing aid is worn, the child earns a reward. Reading or speaking to small children while the hearing aid is being worn may be a positive reward in itself.

The nurse should encourage the family to take extra time each day to speak and read to the child in an *en face* position (face to face) and engage the child in conversation as much as possible. Engaging the child in normal activities for developmental age also should be suggested to the family. Outside play with peers, a school routine, and craft projects should be recommended. It is very important for the child to develop a good self-image and maximize his or her growth and development potential during the formative years. Engaging the child in various activities of daily living enhances the child's feeling of normalcy in spite of the hearing deficit.

Many of these same interventions apply to nursing care of the hospitalized child with a hearing loss. Nurses should determine from family members the most effective means of communicating with the child and clearly note this in the nursing plan of care for consistency throughout the hospital stay. If sign language or special communication boards are required, individuals who can use these techniques should care for the child. All hospital personnel who come into contact with the hearing impaired child should be informed of communication techniques unique to that child and use them when performing caregiving tasks.

The nurse may assist the family to provide optimum care for the speech and hearing impaired child by securing transportation, making appropriate referrals, and locating sources of funding for therapy. The compliance of the child and family in continuing the training program may be contingent on some of these factors. The family needs to realize that the earlier a speech and hearing impairment is diagnosed and treatment begun, the better the outcome for the child.

★ EVALUATION

Periodically the nurse and family evaluate the outcomes of care given. Examples of outcomes for the child and family with hearing deficits and language disorders were given under Nursing Diagnoses and Planning in this section. Have short-term goals been met? Are long-term goals still realistic?

LONG-TERM CARE

The nurse working with the family of a child with hearing or speech impairment should assess the progress of the child in therapy at intervals. Use of the guidelines noted in Tables 35-5 and 35-6 can assist the nurse to determine the age appropriateness of the child's responses. The nurse also should be a liaison with therapists and physicians providing the care to determine if the family is being supportive of the child or if there are any barriers to providing effective therapy. The nurse's role in follow-up is to offer support and assistance to the family in pursuing therapy for the child.

Disorders of the Nasal Region

Sinusitis

Definition and Incidence. *Sinusitis* refers to an inflammatory infection of the mucous membranes of the paranasal sinuses. The paranasal sinuses consist of the maxillary, ethmoid, frontal, and sphenoid sinuses (see Fig. 33-6). Sinuses are discussed in Chapter 33. The sinuses are lined with ciliated, mucus-secreting respiratory epithelium and are contiguous with the nasal mucosa of the respiratory tract. The appearance and size of the sinuses continually change and grow from infancy to adulthood.

As the child grows the maxillary sinus enlarges in width and height and eventually assumes a quadrilateral shape. It is the most common site of sinus infections in children older than 10 years.

The ethmoid sinus is present at birth, but it does not begin to develop until the fifth month and is not pneumatized until the second year. Ethmoid sinusitis is the most common form of sinusitis in childhood and is usually seen in infants and toddlers.

The sphenoid sinus is small at birth until it is pneumatized at age 3 or 4. Sphenoid sinusitis is less common because of its isolated position.

The frontal sinus does not appear until 5 or 6 years of age and does not become fully pneumatized until about age 8 or 9. Frontal sinusitis is uncommon in children until after the age of 10.

Sinusitis occurs most frequently in the fall, winter, and spring months when the incidence of upper respiratory tract infections also is at its highest. The actual incidence of sinusitis in children is not known.

Etiology and Pathophysiology. Retention of mucus in one or more of the paranasal sinuses may be due to obstruction of the ostia, reduction in the number of cilia, impaired function of the cilia, or overproduction or change in the viscosity of secretions.[48] The normal motility of the cilia usually protects the respiratory epithelium from bacterial invasion. However, some respiratory viruses may have a negative effect on the normal functioning cilia. Alterations in mucus, as in cystic fibrosis or asthma, also may impair ciliary activity.

Paranasal sinus mucosal swelling or mechanical obstruction may result in obstruction of the ostia and development of sinusitis. Acute sinusitis (lasting 1 to 3 weeks) usually results as a secondary complication of upper respiratory tract viral infections (following a common cold) or secondary to an allergic inflammation. There is also a strong association between sinus infections and other upper respiratory diseases, including reactive airway disease, otitis media, and immune deficiency.[44]

Mechanical obstruction of the sinuses is caused by septal deformities, intranasal or intrasinus neoplasms, and foreign bodies. Children who have choanal atresia, are nasally intubated, have a nasogastric tube in place, or have nasal packing in place are at greater risk for developing nosocomial bacterial sinusitis.

Chronic sinusitis (lasting more than 30 days) results when there is inadequate treatment of acute sinusitis. Chronic sinusitis results in a persistence of the infection, which may lead to permanent damage to the sinus mucosa.

Clinical Manifestations. Sinusitis is suspected if a recent upper respiratory tract infection (including the common cold) persists for greater than 10 days and symptoms are not improving. Children with sinusitis present with a persistent cough, purulent and copious nasal or postnasal discharge (signs similar to that of a common cold), and nasal obstruction. Fever, facial pain over the sinus areas, facial swelling, malaise, and halitosis are often reported by the parents. The presence of a cough or sore throat is usually secondary to a postnasal drip or to bronchial hyperactivity, which is usually worse at night or early in the morning. The cough may be dry or moist.

Children with maxillary sinusitis may complain of pain in the ear or in the teeth. With ethmoid sinusitis the lateral wall of the nose medial to the inner canthus of the eye may be tender. Children with sphenoid sinusitis will complain of a frontal, temporal, or retro-orbital headache that radiates to the occiput. In frontal sinusitis the child may complain of a headache or severe retro-orbital pain.

In the older child sinusitis is associated with complaints of dull persistent headaches (usually bilateral and frontomaxillary in location) and a sense of fullness or head congestion that clears poorly after an upper respiratory infection or typical cold. Periorbital swelling may be present and is most obvious in the early morning shortly after awakening. The swelling may decrease and actually disappear during the day but reappear the following morning. Fever may or may not be present.

Signs of chronic sinusitis include persistent nasal congestion, mild rhinorrhea, and a cough that persists for more than 30 days. A vague sinus headache may be present for a few hours after rising in the morning. Headaches are less severe with chronic sinusitis than with acute sinusitis. Postnasal drainage, sore throat, and throat clearing are common symptoms associated with chronic sinusitis. Change in voice quality may be evident if the nose and sinuses are closed off from the oral cavity, affecting the resonance of normal speech.

Diagnostic Studies. Simple upper respiratory tract infection and allergic inflammation, the most common risk factors for acute sinusitis, must be ruled out when making the diagnosis of sinusitis. Sinusitis is difficult to diagnose accurately from history alone or from external visual examination of the nose. Sinus transillumination, radiography, sinus aspiration, and nasal cytology are used in conjunction with clinical signs and symptoms to aid in diagnosis.

Sinus Transillumination. This technique is the most helpful and least expensive procedure available in the clinic setting for the diagnosis of maxillary or frontal sinusitis in an adolescent. Transillumination is performed in a darkened room with a penlight or with a transilluminator. To transilluminate the maxillary sinus the light is placed over the midpoint of the inferior orbital rim. The transmission of light through the hard palate is then assessed with the child's mouth open. To transilluminate the frontal sinus, the light is placed beneath the medial border of the supraorbital ridge. The bilateral symmetry of the glow is evaluated. If transillumination shows opacity or dullness, then infection is likely to be present. Differences in bone thickness, however, may give inaccurate results. Transillumination is not accurate in diagnosing

chronic sinusitis because changes indicating infection may be difficult to identify.

Radiography. Radiologic views for visualization of the maxillary and ethmoid sinuses may be taken to confirm the diagnosis. Figure 34-2 illustrates and explains the various views. If the radiograph reveals an air–fluid level, complete opacification of the sinuses, or mucosal thickening greater than 4 mm (measured from the lateral wall of the bone to the edge of the thickened mucosa inside the sinus), a presumptive diagnosis of sinusitis can be made. In children younger than 2 years of age x-rays may not be reliable, because the sinuses are not fully developed. Positive films have been seen in asymptomatic children. Similarly, films may be unremarkable in children with clinical indications of sinusitis. Therefore, diagnosis should not be based on radiographs alone.

Follow-up radiographs are indicated only in children who have long-standing or recurrent disease. If complications such as spread of infection or osteomyelitis are suspected, a CT scan may be obtained to provide more clarity of the sinuses. Cost and radiation exposure limit the routine use of this technology.

Sinus Aspiration. The most definitive way to diagnose sinusitis is to aspirate bacteria from the normally sterile sinus cavities. Aspiration of the sinus, however, should not be a routine procedure; it is indicated when the infection fails to respond to the usual medical therapy or when the child presents with intracranial or intraorbital complications of sinus infection. The maxillary sinus is the most accessible of the sinuses for needle aspiration. The puncture is performed under local anesthesia by the transnasal route with the needle directed beneath the inferior turbinate through the lateral nasal wall. If the child is apprehensive or too young to cooperate, a short-acting narcotic agent can be used for sedation. Sinus aspiration is usually not performed in children younger than 3 years of age because of the difficulty entering the small maxillary sinus and the possibility of damaging developing tooth buds.

Nasal Cytology. Nasal cytology may be useful in differentiating between an allergic or an infectious disease. The presence of a great number of eosinophils may suggest allergic rhinitis, whereas numerous polymorphonuclear cells may suggest an infection. However, nasal cytology lacks sensitivity and specificity, and results may be inconsistent with the child's history, physical examination, and x-ray findings. Culturing secretions of the nose, nasopharynx, or throat also is inadequate for identifying the organisms because contaminants from other sources are very likely.

★ **ASSESSMENT**

Nursing assessment should include obtaining a history of an upper respiratory infection, including a recent history of a cold. The duration and severity of respiratory signs and symptoms, the quality of nasal discharge, and the frequency and timing of cough should be obtained. The presence or absence of malodorous breath (despite good oral hygiene), morning headaches that subside during the day if the child is erect, puffiness around the eyes, dental discomfort, a history of allergies, and the use of cigarettes or passive smoking also should be determined.

The physical examination should include an assessment of the nasal mucosa, nasal septum, tonsillar and pharyngeal areas, cervical lymph nodes, and face for localized swelling. The examination may reveal purulent nasal discharge, swollen nasal turbinates, or even purulent secretions in the posterior pharynx. The nasal discharge may be thin or thick, clear, mucoid, or purulent. Any swelling or puffiness around the eyes should be determined.

★ NURSING DIAGNOSES AND PLANNING

Based on assessment data discussed previously and in the preceding chapter, the following nursing diagnoses may apply to the family and child with sinusitis:

- Pain related to inflammation and nasal discharge.
- Fluid Volume Deficit related to nasal drainage.
- Altered Health Maintenance related to knowledge deficit regarding condition, medications, and prevention of future infection.

The nurse and child (or parents) together plan effective care based on the established nursing diagnoses. Several examples of expected outcomes follow:

- The parents state that the child is consuming more liquids.
- The child's facial expressions indicate pain is relieved.
- The parents identify measures to use for comfort and fever reduction.
- The parents discuss adverse symptoms that will be reported.

The nurse plans for the care of the child based on physician's orders and nursing diagnoses. Some general nursing care goals may be the following:

- Pain relief is achieved.
- Fluid intake is improved.
- Complications are prevented.

★ INTERVENTIONS: COLLABORATIVE AND INDEPENDENT

The majority of children with sinusitis can be treated as outpatients unless there is severe illness with potential serious complications involving infection of the orbit, skull, meninges, or brain. The medical treatment of sinusitis is aimed at eradication of the bacterial pathogens and restoration of adequate sinus drainage.

MEDICATION THERAPY

Amoxicillin (40 mg/kg per day in three divided doses) is the therapy of choice. Ampicillin may be used, but it is associated with more side-effects such as diarrhea. Children with allergies to penicillin or cephalosporin are treated with trimethoprim (8 mg/kg per day) and sulfamethoxazole (40 mg/kg per day) given in two divided doses. The minimum length of treatment for acute sinusitis is 10 to 14 days.

Antihistamines may be used to decrease secretions, and decongestants may be used to shrink membranes and promote drainage. The effectiveness of antihistamines and decongestants is controversial. Parents and children should be warned against habitual use of decongestants because they may result in a chronically thickened nasal mucosa and worsening nasal congestion.

COMFORT MEASURES

Nursing care includes managing the fever and pain and promoting overall comfort of the child. Fever can be reduced by the use of antipyretics, and pain can be eased by the use of analgesics. Warm, moist packs over the sinus region also reduce the pain. The temperature of the warm packs should be carefully monitored to avoid accidental burning. To promote sinus drainage parents should be instructed to use a humidifier and to increase their child's fluid intake. Mucomyst or other mucolytic agents may be used to thin secretions.

SURGICAL MANAGEMENT

If several 3- to 4-week courses of medical therapy fail to alleviate the signs and symptoms, the child should be referred to an otorhinolaryngologist for possible irrigation and drainage of the sinuses. In children the usual surgical procedure is antral lavage, often with creation of antral windows by puncturing the bone between the inferior meatus and maxillary antrum to create a new accessory ostium. Purulent secretions or sometimes sterile glue-like material is washed out and a new opening for aeration and drainage is created. This procedure halts recurrent infections and alleviates chronic disease in some children. By relieving pressure in the sinus, oxygenation and blood flow improve, thus restoring compromised defense mechanisms. Drainage procedures usually are reserved for those who fail medical therapy with antibiotics or who have intracranial complications.

★ EVALUATION

Periodically the nurse and family evaluate the outcomes of care given. Examples of outcomes for the child and family with sinusitis were given under Nursing Diagnoses and Planning in this section. Planning for further nursing care takes into consideration complications.

COMPLICATIONS

Major complications result either from the contiguous spread or from the hematogenous dissemination of infection. Children who fail to respond to treatment within 24 to 48 hours or who present with neurologic findings are at risk for serious complications of sinusitis. Acute bacterial sinusitis may progress to osteomyelitis of the frontal bone, orbital cellulitis, retro-orbital abscess, cavernous sinus thrombophlebitis, meningitis, and brain abscess. The nurse should be alert for any signs that may indicate intracranial complications, including fever, chills, vomiting, headache, and blurred vision.

The parents also should be educated regarding these signs of sinusitis complication. If present, the primary physician should be notified as soon as possible. These complications may warrant referrals to neurosurgeons, ophthalmologists, and infectious disease experts. Hospitalization is required for the administration of intravenous antimicrobial therapy.

Disorders of the Mouth

Abnormal Dentition

Definition and Incidence. The common anomalies of developing teeth include abnormal number, size, shape, structure, and color. Dental caries are by far the most prevalent type of acquired tooth disorder in children. This problem affects about 75% of children by 5 years of age.[11]

Malocclusion of the teeth refers to malposition or malalignment of adjoining teeth. The incidence of malocclusion in school-age children and adolescents may be as high as 90%. However, only about 10% to 15% of these children experience difficulty from the malocclusion.[21]

Etiology and Pathophysiology. An especially detrimental condition in small children is bottle-mouth caries. This syndrome arises when children are consistently put to bed with a bottle containing a sweet or sugary fluid such as milk or juice. While sleeping, the liquid pools in the mouth, and the carbohydrates work in conjunction with bacteria to erode the erupting teeth. Children as young as 2 to 3 years of age can have severe dental decay resulting from this practice[11] (Fig. 35-11).

Problems with extra or missing teeth may arise due to hereditary patterns, problems during the initiation of tooth formation, and physical disruption of the dental lamina. Teeth that are too small or too large are thought to be due to vascular and neurogenic abnormalities. Abnormal shape of the teeth, which mostly affects the crowns and roots, occurs during the morphodifferentiation stage of tooth development and often results from autosomal dominant and polygenic patterns of inheritance.[15]

The three types of structural abnormalities most prevalent in erupting teeth are defects of enamel, dentin, and cementum development. These may arise during the histodifferentiation, apposition, or mineralization stages of tooth development and can cause weakness of the new teeth. Intrinsic anomalies of tooth color may result from etiologies such as blood-borne pigments (i.e., bile), drug administration, and hypoplastic-hypocalcified disease states.

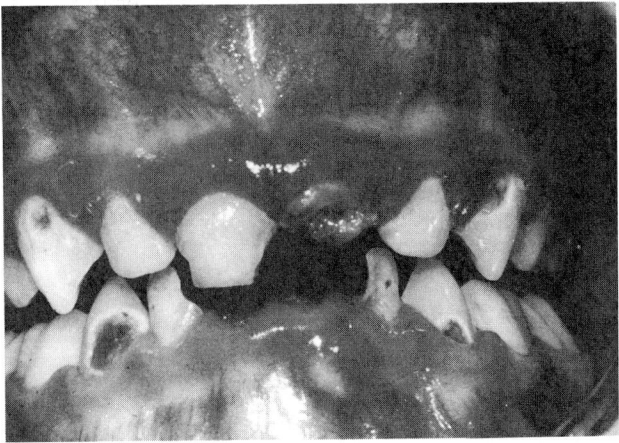

FIGURE 35-11
Bottle-mouth caries. (Oski, F. A., et al. [1990]. *Principles and practice of pediatrics.* Philadelphia: J.B. Lippincott.)

One of the most prevalent causes of tooth staining is from tetracycline antibiotics taken by a pregnant woman or administered to the child up to 8 years of age. Early tetracycline usage may result in permanent darkening of the teeth, especially the portion close to the gum line.[15] Use of tetracycline in young children at levels greater than 75 mg/kg usually causes enamel hyperplasia.[11]

Malocclusion of the teeth can cause difficulty chewing and therefore nutrition and digestive problems. Malocclusion also can lead to dental caries, speech impediments, and facial distortion. The majority of these problems arise from genetic skeletal deformities of the mandible and maxilla.

Periodontal disease usually arises due to inadequate nutrition and poor dental hygiene in children. An inflammation of the gums and supporting structures develops with bacterial colonization of the subgingival layer and eventual resorption of the bone or formation of root abscess. Because this condition can cause damage to the supporting structures of the teeth, the condition must be prevented if possible or quickly treated once it is diagnosed.

Clinical Manifestations. Abnormalities of tooth size, shape, number, structure, and color are usually self-evident on close inspection of the teeth. Cavities of the teeth present as discolorations on the tooth surface, between the teeth, or inside the chewing surfaces of the posterior teeth. In severe cases caries may appear at the juncture of the tooth and the gum and give the teeth a "moth-eaten" appearance.[11]

Malocclusions may be evident in various ways. Such irregularities as inappropriate jaw size for the developing teeth, hypertrophy or deviation of the mandible, asymmetry of the face, and too many or too few teeth may alter the structure of the mouth and cause difficulty in chewing. Any deviation from the normal occlusion pattern in which the top and bottom molars meet squarely together, and the top incisors slightly overlap and touch the bottom incisors should be suspected as a malocclusion.

Periodontal disease develops insidiously and may be difficult for parents to recognize until it is in its later stages. Some of the warning signs include gum bleeding with brushing, loose permanent teeth, a change in the bite pattern, halitosis, and pus that can be expressed between the teeth and gums.[36] It is rare for children to develop periodontal disease before puberty.[6]

Diagnostic Studies. Certain conditions, such as dental caries and malocclusion, may be diagnosed using x-rays of the teeth. These x-rays are usually ordered by the dentist or pedodontist after an initial examination. However, the majority of these disorders are primarily diagnosed by the dentist from keen inspection. A close examination of the oral cavity by the nurse cannot be overemphasized to determine the presence of abnormalities that need prompt intervention.

★ ASSESSMENT

Nurses working with children should carefully inspect the oral cavity as part of the routine assessment. Many parents do not have their child examined by a dentist at regular intervals. Therefore, many of the described abnormalities may progress unnoticed by the child and parents.

As part of a mouth inspection the nurse should note the number, position, shape, and color of the teeth. The total number of primary teeth after teething is completed is 20 (see Figs. 33-2 and 33-7). The number of permanent teeth varies depending on the child's age, but the total number possible when the child reaches maturity is 32. The position and shape of the teeth usually develop from central incisors to lateral cuspids to posterior molars. Tooth color varies but should be a uniform shade of white.

The nurse should observe for signs of dental caries by looking for discolorations of the teeth and should note the condition of the gums to rule out the presence of periodontal disease. Assessing the child's bite can help determine if malocclusion is a problem. The absence of teeth, wide spacing between teeth, and a crowded appearance of the teeth also indicate malocclusion.

★ NURSING DIAGNOSES AND PLANNING

Based on assessment data discussed previously and in the preceding chapter, the following nursing diagnoses may apply to the family and child with abnormal dentition:

- Altered Health Maintenance related to dental neglect.
- Altered Nutrition: Less Than Body Requirements related to difficulty chewing.
- Body Image Disturbance related to appearance of teeth.

The nurse and child (or parents) together plan effective care based on the established nursing diagnoses. Several examples of expected outcomes follow:

- The parents state that the child brushes his or her teeth twice daily.
- The parents identify the risks associated with placing the infant in bed with a bottle.
- The parents and child discuss possible orthodontic or other corrective procedures.
- The parents and child discuss nutritious eating habits.
- The child discusses feelings about appearance.

The nurse plans for the care of the child based on physician's orders and nursing diagnoses. Some general nursing care goals may be the following:

- Health maintenance practices are improved.
- Nutritional patterns improve.
- Acceptance of appearance.

★ INTERVENTIONS: COLLABORATIVE AND INDEPENDENT

The primary nursing intervention is to recognize dental problems needing referral to a dentist. These problems include obvious disorders as well as conditions that need close scrutiny and follow-up by the dentist. A good history concerning the child's dental development and tooth care assists the dentist in diagnosis.

COUNSELING AND TEACHING

The nurse should provide preventive counseling to parents concerning the need for twice-daily toothbrushing (preferably at bedtime and in the morning) beginning at the time of tooth eruption. Teaching should include instructions on wiping the gums of the infant with a soft wet cloth. Brushing with a tooth brush using toothpaste may be substituted for use of the cloth when the toddler is able to tolerate this procedure and can spit out the toothpaste. Flossing should be added when developmentally appropriate (approximately preschool age).

The nurse should provide preventive counseling to the parents of infants on the hazards of bottle-mouth caries. Parents should be encouraged to avoid putting the infant to bed with a bottle. The fluoride supply in the drinking water of the family's community also should be assessed by the nurse, and the family should be advised if the child needs supplemental fluoride (Table 35-7). Breast-fed infants who receive no fluoridated water in their diet should be given fluoride supplements. Parents also should be counseled not to give the child concentrated sweets for snacks because sugar may speed the development of dental caries.

Teaching parents about disorders diagnosed by a dentist also is indicated to clarify the problem for the child and parents and the reasons for the treatment prescribed. Examples would be the need for orthodontic work for malocclusions and invasive procedures for severe periodontal disease. Counseling also may increase the compliance of the family in following through on the treatment regimen.

The child who has poor nutritional intake due to an inability to chew well should be counseled about a soft or even liquid diet that will provide all necessary nutrients. Nurses can suggest foods in each of the designated food groups that can be eaten by the child (e.g., yogurt, pureed vegetables and meat, soft or mashed fruits). Use of a multivitamin supplement also may be indicated. Older children with body image problems resulting from

TABLE 35-7
Supplemental Fluoride Dosage Recommendations

Fluoride Content of Drinking Water	Dosage of Oral Fluoride		
	Age 0–2 Years	Age 2–3 Years	Age 3–14 Years
<0.3 ppm	0.25 mg/d	0.5 mg/d	1 mg/d
0.3–0.7 ppm	0	0.25 mg/d	0.5 mg/d

Approved by the American Academy of Pediatrics and the American Dental Association. Fluoride supplementation is unnecessary if the fluoride content of drinking water is over 0.7 ppm or if the patient is 15 years of age or older.
(Source: Belanger, G. K. & Casamassimo, P. S. [1987]. Teeth. In: Kempe, et al. [Eds.]. *Current pediatric diagnosis and treatment* [9th ed.]. Norwalk, CT: Appleton & Lange.)

poor dentition may be assisted by certain reconstructive or cosmetic dental procedures, such as crowns and partial dentures.

★ EVALUATION

Periodically the nurse and family evaluate the outcomes of care given. Examples of outcomes for the child and family with abnormal dentition were given under Nursing Diagnoses and Planning in this section. Have short-term goals been met? Are long-term goals still realistic?

LONG-TERM CARE

The nurse should evaluate the oral cavity at each visit with the child to observe for compliance with prophylactic and therapeutic dental treatments. Gradual resolution of previously noted problems as well as the development of new disorders needs to be thoroughly documented. The nurse serves as a vital link in helping the child to gain access to optimal dental care.

Cleft Lip and Cleft Palate

Definition, Incidence, Etiology, and Pathophysiology. Cleft lip and cleft palate are both congenital anomalies that are evident at birth. *Cleft lip*, previously referred to as a harelip, is displayed as a cleft or open space between the nasal cavity and the lip. The incidence of cleft lip, with or without cleft palate, is 1 in 1000 births.[10] *Cleft palate* involves absence of part or all of the structures making up the palate (i.e., the hard palate, soft palate, uvula, and maxillary teeth). The incidence of cleft palate is 1 in 2500 births.[10]

Cleft lip usually results from failure of the maxillary prominence to fuse with the medial nasal prominence and may occur unilaterally or bilaterally. The defect of cleft lip follows a multifactorial inheritance pattern and may occur along with cleft palate or other congenital anomalies. Cleft palate evolves from failure of the maxillary bone plate to close during embryonic life (see Chap. 33). Cleft palate also is believed to have a multifactorial or polygenic inheritance pattern, although specific environmental factors that predispose to cleft palate have not yet been identified.

Clinical Manifestations and Diagnostic Studies. Both of these disorders are apparent at birth. Even a small cleft palate should be easily noted on close visual inspection of the mouth area. As stated previously the disorders may present singly or in tandem and may be unilateral or bilateral (Fig. 35-12). The extent of the clefting, whether of the lip or palate, varies with each child.

Generally, the amount of oral and nasal involvement determines the extent of feeding and breathing problems the child may experience. The child with absence of both hard and soft palates often has difficulty sucking due to the loss of adequate suction in the oropharynx. Lack of oral suction may result in the pooling of secretions in the mouth. The child may swallow more air than usual due to the cleft palate and develop colic. Cleft lip occurring by itself tends to cause few feeding problems.[10]

Visual inspection is usually sufficient to assess func-

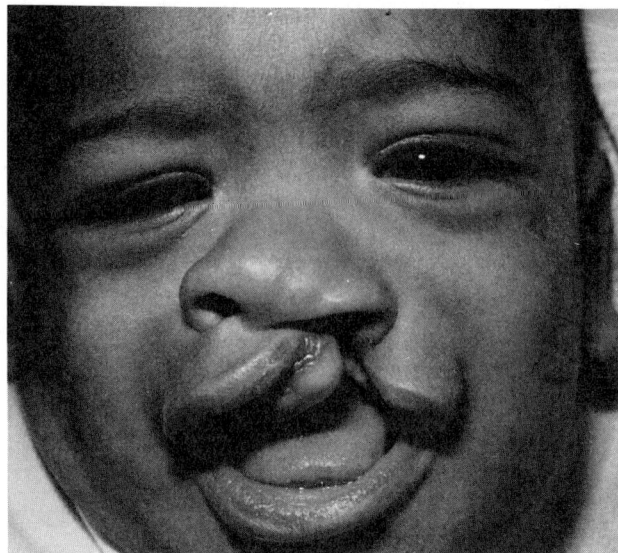

FIGURE 35-12
Unilateral cleft lip and palate. (Krause, C. J., et al. [1991] *Aesthetic facial surgery.* Philadelphia: J.B. Lippincott.)

tional deficiencies resulting from the anatomic defect. X-rays and possibly CT scan may be performed preoperatively to further assess the extent of the defect.

★ ASSESSMENT

The nurse examining the newborn with cleft lip or palate needs to describe clearly the location and extent of the defect. Documentation includes noting which anatomic structures are disrupted (i.e., lip, soft palate, or hard palate). The nurse also should delineate any functional problems the infant is having, such as respiratory and feeding irregularities. (The nurse should seek the guidance of the physician before introducing any fluids into the oral cavity of the newborn with cleft lip or palate.) Older children with cleft lip or palate should be closely monitored for hearing, speech, and dental difficulties.

★ NURSING DIAGNOSES AND PLANNING

Based on assessment data discussed previously and in the preceding chapter, the following nursing diagnoses may apply to the family and child with cleft lip or palate:

- Ineffective Airway Clearance related to pooling of secretions in the mouth.
- Sensory/Perceptual Alterations (Auditory) related to hearing loss secondary to chronic middle-ear effusion.
- Impaired Verbal Communication related to the anatomic defect.
- High Risk for Altered Parenting related to the birth of a child with a facial anomaly.
- Self-Esteem Disturbance related to the physical anomaly.
- Grieving (Parental) related to loss of the anticipated "perfect" child.

The nurse and child (or parents) together plan effective care based on the established nursing diagnoses. Several examples of expected outcomes follow:

- The parents demonstrate the ability to feed the infant successfully.
- The parents discuss the fact that there is no known cause for the cleft anomaly.
- The parents and child discuss their feelings about the anomaly.
- The parents and child demonstrate affection with physical closeness.

The nurse plans for the care of the child based on physician's orders and nursing diagnoses. Some general nursing care goals may be the following:

- Adequate air exchange is supported.
- The child, parents, and nurse develop effective communication skills.
- The child is incorporated into family activities.

★ INTERVENTIONS: COLLABORATIVE AND INDEPENDENT

PSYCHOSOCIAL SUPPORT

The nurse working with the family of the newborn with cleft lip or palate should be keenly aware of the psychological effects the birth of such a child may have on the family. The family may need to grieve the loss of the "perfect" child to accept a child with a defect. Due to its devastating cosmetic implications, cleft lip may be even harder for parents to cope with than cleft palate, which is structurally and functionally much more hazardous but not visible. When these children reach school-age, they too may need emotional support when dealing with such a cosmetic deficit. Explaining the defect to the family and clearly reinforcing the medical plan of care may help relieve the family's anxiety concerning the child's outcome.

Educating the family that no cause for clefting is known may relieve their guilt about having a child with this disorder. The nurse can explain to the parents that the initial cleft formation occurs by the 33rd to 35th day after conception, usually before the mother even realizes she is pregnant. The mother needs to be reassured that there was nothing that she could have done differently during her pregnancy to prevent the defect. Cleft lip or palate most frequently results from a multifactorial inheritance pattern, meaning that defects can recur in certain families throughout several generations. The parents may therefore want to question other family members about the incidence of these defects in past generations.

AIRWAY MAINTENANCE AND FEEDING MODIFICATIONS

The nurse must observe for and intervene if the newborn with cleft lip or palate displays symptoms of respiratory difficulties. Frequent oral suctioning may be indicated if the infant is unable to clear the airway. Most children born with these anomalies are able to feed by mouth but may need special soft nipples (premie nipples) or elongated nipples (lamb's nipples) to create an adequate seal for suction. Breast-feeding may be possible because the breast tissue occludes the palatal defect and allows enough suction in the oral cavity for the infant to swallow. A Brecht feeder (an Asepto syringe attached to a piece of rubber tubing) is useful for infants with very large cleft palates to allow the formula to pass directly to the pos-

terior oropharynx. The nurse should demonstrate any special feeding or suctioning instructions for the parents and assist them in performing these skills with the infant (Fig. 35-13).

SURGICAL MANAGEMENT

The first corrective surgery frequently is performed in the first few months of life. Cleft lip repairs are scheduled between birth and 3 months of age depending on the surgeon, while cleft palate repairs occur between 11 and 18 months of life, usually before speech begins. The cleft palate repair is generally accomplished by using tissue next to the cleft for flaps and moving these flaps to the midline to repair the cleft.

The nurse needs to prepare the family for the surgical procedure and postoperative course as early as possible. Realistic and concise information about the surgical interventions may assist acceptance by the parents concerning their child's condition. The nurse should also offer clarification about preoperative procedures, such as the orders regarding no oral feeding or medications. Postoperative needs, such as use of an intravenous (IV) line, humidification, and a clear liquid diet also should be reviewed.

Discharge instructions should include special care of the incision line. Incisional care includes a semisoft diet for approximately 21 days, no introduction of silverware or straws into the oral cavity, and avoidance of sucking and blowing actions. Parents should be instructed to rinse the child's mouth carefully after feedings with sterile water to remove all debris.

★ EVALUATION

Periodically the nurse and family evaluate the outcomes of care given. Examples of outcomes for the child and family with cleft lip or palate were given under Nursing Diagnoses and Planning in this section. Have short-term goals been met? Are long-term goals still realistic? Planning for further nursing care takes into consideration complications and long-term care.

COMPLICATIONS

Long-term problems, even after surgical repair, include speech and language, dental, and middle-ear difficulties.

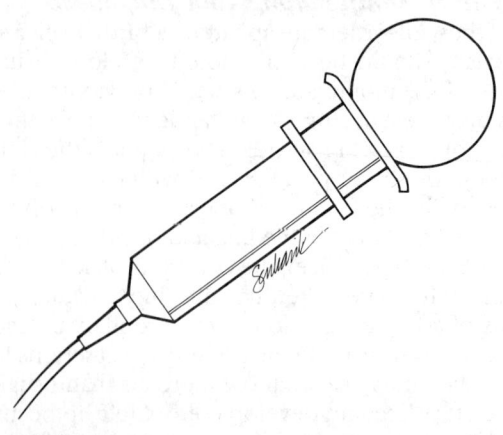

FIGURE 35-13
Brecht feeder.

Children with cleft palate may develop a hypernasal tone to their speech and have poor articulation of words. Dental deformities usually involve malocclusions of the upper anterior dental arch and result from both cleft lip and cleft palate. Children with cleft palate have frequent middle-ear effusions and infections resulting from eustachian tube dysfunction. These infections cause hearing loss and may further magnify the child's speech problems.

LONG-TERM CARE

On follow-up visits, the nurse should assess for resolution of existing physical problems and be alert for the development of new ones. Being astute to potential problems, such as speech and language difficulties, dental abnormalities, or middle-ear dysfunction, expedites the evaluation process. Exploring the feelings of the child and family helps the nurse to determine actual and potential coping difficulties and to evaluate the resolution of previous emotional problems.

When dealing with an older child with cleft lip or palate, the nurse should refer the child having speech and language, dental, or middle-ear problems to the appropriate health care provider for prompt intervention. The pediatrician or primary health care provider should closely monitor the frequency of ear infections and consult an otolaryngologist if the child develops a chronic condition or if hearing acuity is in question. Likewise, speech problems may be handled by a plastic surgeon or oral surgeon for organic etiologies and by a speech pathologist for functional disorders. The dentist or pedodontist needs to be consulted for jaw and tooth malalignments resulting from cleft lip or palate.

Disorders of the Throat

Nasopharyngitis

Definition and Incidence. *Nasopharyngitis* is more widely known as the common cold. Colds are highly communicable infections. The common cold accounts for nearly 3 million visits to the pediatrician's office annually. It is a frequent reason for absenteeism from school.

The risk of acquiring colds seems to be inversely related to age. Infants and preschool children have the highest incidence of colds: four to eight per year. Among preschoolers who have school-age siblings and who come from a large family, the occurrence of colds is higher. School-age children average three to five colds per year. Children who are enrolled in day care centers or nursery schools have more colds than children of similar ages who are cared for at home. The risk of spreading infection is higher in these environments. Spread of the common cold also can occur by person-to-person contact in public and private schools in an older child and adolescent.

Colds occur more frequently in the early spring, in the fall, several weeks after the start of school, and in the winter. The lowest incidence is in the summer.

Etiology and Pathophysiology. Viruses are the most common cause of colds. More than 200 viruses have been identified. Rhinovirus, however, is responsible for approximately one third of all colds. Other common viruses isolated are coronavirus, parainfluenza, respiratory syncytial, adenovirus, enterovirus, and influenza virus.

Bacteria are responsible for only 5% to 10% of all colds. Group A hemolytic streptococcus is the main bacterium identified. Other bacteria, including pneumococci and *Haemophilus influenzae*, can prolong the illness by causing a secondary infection.

Viruses are spread primarily in nasal secretions by inhalation or by close contact to an infected person by sneezing or coughing. Infection also can be spread by physical contact. Viruses are most commonly communicated from contaminated hands or from an inanimate object to a healthy individual. Viruses can live on surfaces for up to 72 hours. Once the child's hand is contaminated, self-inoculation onto mucosal surfaces can occur. Hand-to-nose or hand-to-eye contamination initiates viral proliferation on the epithelial surface of the nasopharynx.

After an incubation period of 2 to 4 days, during which time the virus replicates in the nasopharynx, cold symptoms will appear. Viral invasion results in local inflammation and submucosal edema with shedding and sloughing of the outermost layer of the nasopharynx mucous membrane. Edema and swelling of the mucous membranes follow with damage to the mucociliary clearance apparatus. Colds are self-limiting. The usual course is about 4 to 7 days, during which time the nasal epithelium regenerates. Symptoms generally subside within 2 weeks.

Clinical Manifestations and Diagnostic Studies. The earliest signs of a cold include mild nasal congestion; a thin, watery nasal discharge; and irritability. The nasal mucous membrane appears swollen and erythematous. By the second day sneezing, malaise, headache, runny eyes, anorexia, sore throat, and coughing usually accompany initial symptoms. Postnasal drip often contributes to nocturnal coughing. Fever may or may not be present. Infants younger than 2 to 3 years may have a fever with temperatures between 103° F and 104° F. Anorexia, vomiting, and diarrhea also may be present in young children with a common cold. Older child may have a low-grade fever or be normothermic.

As the cold progresses nasal congestion worsens with more purulent and serous nasal discharge. These symptoms continue for about a week, during which time the viruses are being shed from the nose. Although symptoms will usually subside within 1 week, the rhinitis and cough may persist for another 2 weeks while the epithelium is regenerating.

Nasopharyngitis is a localized infection; therefore, routine laboratory tests usually are not indicated. A throat culture may be performed to rule out beta-hemolytic streptococcal infection. A white blood cell count and differential will probably be normal or show a slight increase.

★ **ASSESSMENT**

Nursing assessment should include the child's recent exposure to an infected individual, crowds, or contaminated areas. The child's overall health status should be determined, including diet history, fluid intake, rest and play or work schedule, home environment, and any recent illnesses. A respiratory assessment should be performed to include rate, depth, ease, and rhythm of breathing. Nasal secretions should be assessed for volume, color, viscosity, and odor.

★ NURSING DIAGNOSES AND PLANNING

Based on assessment data discussed previously and in the preceding chapter, the following nursing diagnoses may apply to the family and child with nasopharyngitis:

- Altered Comfort related to malaise, headache, and fluctuating temperature.
- Altered Health Maintenance related to knowledge deficit regarding viral transmission and treatment of colds.

The nurse and child (or parents) together plan effective care based on the established nursing diagnoses. Several examples of expected outcomes follow:

- The child expresses relief from headache, stuffiness, and other symptoms.
- The parents identify factors to consider with use of medications.
- The parents and child identify means of preventing infection spread and remedies they plan to use at home to treat the cold.

The nurse plans for the care of the child based on physician's orders and nursing diagnoses. Some general nursing care goals may be the following:

- Cold symptoms are relieved.
- Spread of infection is prevented.

★ INTERVENTIONS: COLLABORATIVE AND INDEPENDENT

No remedy exists for the common cold. In young infants who are obligate nasal breathers, inflammatory edema of the nasal mucosa may create breathing difficulty. Suctioning to relieve the nasal obstruction is essential. Instilling several drops of normal saline in each nostril followed by bulb syringe suction may relieve nasal congestion. Humidifying the air or using a cool-mist water vaporizer may help to relieve nasal and pharyngeal discomfort. Elevating the head of the bed may be helpful to drain nasal secretions.

Treatment of the common cold is symptomatic in children. Acetaminophen may be given for pain or fever. Systemic and topical decongestants (oral phenylpropanolamine or pseudoephedrine) may be used to decrease nasal secretions and mucosal edema. Antihistamines and antihistamine–decongestant combinations are available as over-the-counter cold remedies. Parents should be cautioned that the antihistamine may cause lethargy, and the decongestant may cause jitteriness and irritability. Topical vasoconstrictors, nose drops, or nasal sprays may relieve nasal congestion but should not be used longer than 1 week because of the risk of nasal irritation and rebound congestion.

The parent should be told that adequate rest is needed to conserve the child's energy and minimize caloric expenditure. Optimal nutrition also is required for tissue repair. Fluid intake is essential to help keep fluid secretion thin. Hydration and throat lozenges help to relieve a dry, scratchy throat.

The child should be cared for at home during the first 2 to 3 days of the infection and not in day care, nursery school, or any school in which exposure to susceptible individuals can result in the spread of the infection. The nursing staff is responsible for teaching the family and child the proper handwashing technique. The use of disposable tissues helps to control droplets during sneezing or coughing. The desired outcome of parent education is to prevent the progression and spread of infection.

★ EVALUATION

The nurse and family evaluate the outcomes of care given. Examples of outcomes for the child and family with nasopharyngitis were given under Nursing Diagnoses and Planning in this section. Planning for further nursing care takes into consideration complications.

COMPLICATIONS

Symptoms generally last 5 to 8 days and then begin to subside. The most common complication of a bacterial nasopharyngitis is acute suppurative otitis media. Other complications include sinusitis (which may occur secondary to obstruction of the paranasal sinuses), adenitis, pneumonia, croup, and bronchitis. Signs of complications include a fever, worsening of symptoms, sore throat, or ear discomfort. Less significant complications include skin irritation due to wiping the nares, blowing the nose, or sneezing.

Pharyngotonsillitis

Definition and Incidence. *Tonsillitis* refers to an acute inflammation of the mucous membranes and structures of the throat, including the tonsils and their crypts. Acute tonsillitis and pharyngitis are usually concurrent infections. They can occur as a primary infection or as a complication of nasopharyngitis. Adenoiditis often accompanies tonsillitis in children. Acute tonsillitis may occur in all age groups. However, there is a higher incidence of the disease around 5 years of age.[35] Pharyngotonsillitis occurs more often in the winter and early spring months.

Etiology and Pathophysiology. Children with a decreased resistance to infectious disease and who have had previous episodes of viral pharyngitis or tonsillitis are more prone to develop pharyngotonsillitis. Overcrowding, poor nutrition, and lack of adequate ventilation have been associated with pharyngotonsillitis.

Pharyngotonsillitis can be of viral or bacterial origin. In one third of all cases of pharyngotonsillitis the causative agent is not known. In 14% of cases more than one agent is involved. The majority of these infections are viral in origin. A wide range of viruses may cause pharyngotonsillitis, including adenoviruses, Epstein-Barr virus, parainfluenza, coxsackievirus, influenza A, herpes simplex, enterovirus, *Mycoplasma pneumoniae*, *Candida albicans*, and respiratory syncytial viruses.

Bacteria account for only a small number of cases of pharyngotonsillitis. The primary cause of bacterial pharyngotonsillitis is hemolytic group A and β-hemolytic streptococcus.[43] Other bacteria isolated include *Streptococcus pyogenes, Neisseria gonorrhoeae, Corynebacterium diphtheriae, Haemophilus influenzae* type b, and *Staphylococcus aureus.*

Age is an important factor when predicting the causative agent. Viral tonsillitis is most common in children younger than 3 years of age, while hemolytic group A and B streptococcus tonsillitis is common in children older than 2 years of age and in early school-age children between 6 and 8 years of age. Hemolytic group A and B streptococcus is uncommon in children younger than 2 years of age; it occurs in only 3% to 4% of all cases of pharyngotonsillitis. Hemolytic group A and B streptococcus also is uncommon in neonates because of the transfer of maternal antibody *in utero.* Infection after adolescence also is uncommon probably because of the development of immunity to the more common varieties of streptococcal bacteria.

Viral and bacterial pharyngotonsillitis are highly communicable. The spread of infection (viral or bacterial) occurs by spreading salivary droplets or nasal discharges. Transmission is enhanced by close proximity. The respiratory particles can be transmitted through the air or by hands. The school and the home are the major localities where infection is spread.

Clinical Manifestations. Clinical manifestations follow an incubation period of 2 to 5 days. Viral and bacterial pharyngotonsillitis often display similar symptoms. A hemolytic group A and B streptococcus throat infection is characterized by a history of severe sore throat associated with muscular pain, high fever, chills, headache, sore throat, and malaise. Nausea, vomiting, and abdominal discomfort are early signs. The child complains of severe pain when swallowing. The pharynx is red, and the tonsils are embedded with whitish exudate. The anterior cervical lymph nodes are enlarged and tender. These systemic manifestations are the result of extracellular toxins released by the organism. Appearance of a rash may indicate manifestations of scarlet fever.

Viral pharyngotonsillitis typically is gradual in onset, often with nasal symptoms and low-grade fever. Adenoviruses can cause an exudative tonsillitis that is indistinguishable from streptococcal pharyngotonsillitis. Bacterial infection is associated with a high fever, nonpurulent conjunctivitis, and tenderness and edema of the cervical lymph nodes. Rhinitis and a cough are usually more often associated with viral tonsillitis.

Enteroviruses are manifested with a sudden onset of fever, sore throat, dysphagia, and vomiting. Small pale gray vesicles surrounded by erythema may appear on the soft palate, tonsils, and pharynx.

Children with chronic tonsillitis usually present with a recurrent sore throat. Their tonsils are enlarged and dusky red. The crypts are filled with purulent exudate. Enlarged and tender cervical lymph nodes are common. The posterior portion of the neck may be enlarged if both tonsils are involved. The child also may have malodorous breath.

If pharyngotonsillitis is associated with adenoiditis, the child has nasal obstruction with dry lips and oral mucous membranes secondary to mouth breathing. The voice may be muffled and nasal. A cough and malodorous breath are observed. The child also may have a decreased appetite because of impaired taste and smell secondary to nasal obstruction and mouth breathing.

Diagnostic Studies. Clinical findings alone are not diagnostic of a bacterial as opposed to viral pharyngotonsillitis. With viral pharyngotonsillitis the white blood cell count is usually normal. With a streptococcal infection the white blood cell count may be elevated (higher than 15,000 cells/mm³), indicating a bacterial infection. Also with a bacterial infection, leukocytosis with a shift to the left may be present, indicating the presence of new (immature) white cells to destroy pathogens.

Rapid viral antigen-detection tests and a rapid test for hemolytic group A and B streptococcal antigen have been proven to quickly identify the causative agent so that appropriate treatment can be initiated. These tests can be performed in the doctor's office or clinic and usually take no more than 10 minutes to 1 hour for the results to be obtained. Results, however, can produce a false-positive, particularly in children who are chronic carriers of streptococcal bacteria. In such cases a throat culture may be performed to identify significant bacterial pathogens.

★ ASSESSMENT

Early diagnosis of pharyngotonsillitis is important. Treatment should be initiated as soon as possible to prevent the spread of infection and to shorten the course of a bacterial illness so that the risk of complications can be minimized.

Baseline assessment should include a history of streptococcal infections, including the number of infections per year and a recent history of recurrent respiratory infections, sore throats, difficulty with swallowing, fever, and malaise. A family history of respiratory infection should be investigated.

Physical assessment should include examination of the tonsils and their crypts to determine the presence of edema and enlargement of tissues. Type of breathing should be determined (nasal versus mouth) as well as any malodorous breath. Energy level should be determined. A temperature should be taken to assess for the presence of fever. The physical assessment also should ascertain any ear pain, which might indicate an associated otitis media. Enlarged adenoids could block the eustachian tube, resulting in the accumulation of fluid in the ear and a buildup of negative pressure in the middle ear.

★ NURSING DIAGNOSES AND PLANNING

Based on assessment data discussed previously and in the preceding chapter, the following nursing diagnoses may apply to the family and child with pharyngotonsillitis:

- Pain related to inflammation of the pharynx.
- High Risk for Fluid Volume Deficit related to inadequate fluid intake.

- High Risk for Infection (Otitis Media) related to enlarged adenoids or tonsils.
- Altered Nutrition: Less Than Body Requirements related to impaired swallowing.
- Altered Health Maintenance related to knowledge deficit regarding the condition, treatment plan, signs and symptoms of complications, and prevention of future illnesses.
- Anxiety related to anticipated surgery.

The nurse and child (or parents) together plan effective care based on the established nursing diagnoses. A sample Nursing Care Plan for a 4-year-old boy undergoing a tonsillectomy is given here. Several examples of expected outcomes follow:

- The child expresses relief from sore throat and other discomforts.
- The parents state that the child is drinking more fluids and eating is improved.
- The parents and child discuss the benefits and risks of surgery.
- The parents describe appropriate precautions to use following surgery.

The nurse plans for the care of the child based on physician's orders and nursing diagnoses. Some general nursing care goals may be the following:

- Pain and other discomforts are relieved.
- Spread of infection to ears is prevented.
- Adequate nutrition and hydration are maintained.

★ INTERVENTIONS: COLLABORATIVE AND INDEPENDENT

For viral infections general supportive care with increased fluids, bedrest, analgesics, and antipyretics, such as acetaminophen, is recommended. Cool fluids may cause less pain when swallowing than warm or hot liquids or solid foods. Gargling with warm saline and using throat lozenges or sprays may be beneficial in relieving pain. The older child may use hard candy to assist in reducing the symptoms. Acute viral infections will usually resolve in 7 to 10 days.

MEDICATION THERAPY

Antibiotic therapy is prescribed if the infection is associated with a bacterial infection. Generally, antibiotic therapy is prescribed after rapid antigen screening or throat culture results have been obtained. Penicillin is the drug of choice for pharyngotonsillitis associated with group A streptococci infection. Oral penicillin 800,000 to 1.6 million IU daily for 10 days is usually prescribed. If penicillin G is prescribed, it must be given either before meals or 2 hours after meals. Phenoxymethyl penicillin may be given at any time. Dicloxacillin and ampicillin may be prescribed but are more expensive. The major disadvantage with oral therapy is noncompliance because the child usually appears to recover in 3 or 4 days. If oral therapy is prescribed, it is essential that the child completes the full course of therapy. If the parents appear unlikely to comply with the treatment plan, then a single intramuscular dose of benzathine penicillin G is indi-

cated. The dose is 600,000 IU for children weighing less than 60 lb, 900,000 IU for children weighing 60 to 90 lb, and 1.2 million IU for children weighing more than 90 lb.

Obtaining routine follow-up cultures after antimicrobial therapy is generally unnecessary. Relapse may occur in 20% of affected children, probably because of poor compliance with taking oral medications, reinfection from the household, or from contact with infected individuals.

SURGICAL MANAGEMENT

The efficacy of adenoidectomy and tonsillectomy is controversial. Indications for surgery include life-threatening conditions, including recurrent and persistent nasal or oral obstruction causing significant difficulty in swallowing, breathing, or speaking; hearing loss associated with large adenoids and tonsils; and cor pulmonale resulting from alveolar hypoventilation. Other reasonable indications for surgery include recurrent peritonsillary abscess, recurrent tonsillitis, suspected tonsilar tumor, persistent snoring or mouth breathing, and sleep apnea syndrome.[35]

Contraindications to surgery include tonsillitis in the acute phase, bleeding disease, and polio epidemics. Surgery is generally delayed for 2 to 3 weeks after an acute infection.

PREOPERATIVE CARE

The nurse's responsibility for the child who requires surgical intervention is to prepare the child and his or her parents for surgery. This includes explaining the need for surgery, the preoperative screening, the amount of time the procedure will take, the return from surgery, and what to expect after the surgery. The child is instructed not to eat or drink after midnight before the day of surgery. Prior to surgery a complete health history of the child is obtained, including recent colds, sore throats, bleeding tendencies, and allergies to drugs. A complete physical examination is performed.

POSTOPERATIVE CARE

After surgery the child is placed in a semiprone lateral position, which will facilitate drainage of fluid. As the child awakes, an upright position may be assumed. The nurse should observe for any signs of bleeding, emesis, or drainage and should note the color, amount, and frequency. Frequent swallowing may indicate drainage or bleeding. Suctioning is avoided to prevent trauma to the surgical area. Rapid heart rate, a weak pulse, and pallor could be signs of hemorrhage.

The nurse also should observe for signs of dehydration. Intake and output should be monitored. The child is encouraged to take small amounts of cool, clear liquids (e.g., jello, ice chips, popsicles), which will facilitate swallowing and help to relieve discomfort. IV fluids may be indicated for a young child to ensure adequate hydration. The diet may be advanced to soft foods (e.g., warm cereal or milk) the following day.

DISCHARGE PLANNING

Instructions for care of the child postoperatively should include when to call the doctor, mouth care, diet,

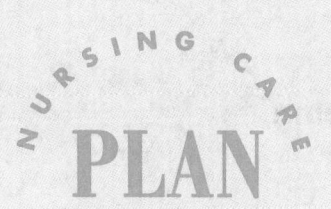

A 4-Year-Old Child Undergoing a Tonsillectomy

Assessment

Case Study Description

Tommy White, a 4-year-old, Caucasian male, has a history of chronic tonsillitis and adenoiditis that has recently contributed to pronounced mouth breathing and distortion of speech. He is scheduled for a tonsillectomy and adenoidectomy (T&A) on Friday and was seen in the preadmission clinic on Thursday for lab work and consultation with the anesthetist.

This is Tommy's first hospitalization. His clinic nurse assessed that Tommy was unaware of why he was having the operation and what body part would be affected. The nurse used dolls and pictures to teach Tommy about his impending hospitalization and operation. She also answered questions. On Friday, Tommy returned to the hospital for his surgery. He was admitted to the pediatric unit from the Recovery Room.

Assessment Data

On arrival to the pediatric unit: Awake, crying, and asking for his mother. Vital signs stable. No bleeding noted. Complains of sore throat. Refuses to drink. IV infusing in left hand.

Nursing Diagnosis	Intervention	Rationale
1. High risk for injury: bleeding related to surgery Supporting Data: • Immediately post-op T&A	Monitor for signs of bleeding: obvious blood from mouth, increased restlessness and swallowing.	Bleeding may occur from operative site in first 24 hours after surgery.
	Examine throat with flashlight every 4 hours and more often if indicated.	Good lighting helps to visualize throat well.
2. High risk for ineffective breathing pattern related to swelling of surgical site Supporting Data: • Immediately post-op T&A with potential swelling	Monitor respiratory status frequently for signs of distress: labored breathing, stridor, nasal flaring, cyanosis, tachypnea.	Symptoms of respiratory difficulty could indicate narrowing airway due to swelling.
	Maintain humidifier at bedside.	Loosens respiratory secretions.
	Elevate head of bed 30–45 degrees.	Facilitates drainage of secretions.
	Maintain ice pack around neck for 24 hours.	Decreases swelling.
	Monitor ability to swallow.	Increased difficulty could indicate narrowing airway.
3. Pain related to surgical procedure Supporting Data: • Post-op T&A • Complaints of sore throat • Crying • Refuses to drink	Assess level of pain and medicate accordingly.	Sore throats are expected after T&A; medicating every 3–4 hours as needed increases comfort and generally increases consumption of fluids.
	Encourage Tommy to drink cool liquids, no citrus juices.	Cool liquids are soothing to the throat, while citrus juices cause burning.
4. Impaired swallowing related to irritated nasopharyngeal cavity Supporting Data: • Refusal to drink • C/O sore throat	Evaluate relationship of refusal to drink to presence of pain; medicate if appropriate.	Children frequently refuse to swallow if their throat hurts or they think it will hurt.
	Encourage frequent sips of cool liquids.	Soothes throat.
	Maintain ice pack around neck for 24 hours.	Decreases swelling that can increase difficulty swallowing.

(Continued)

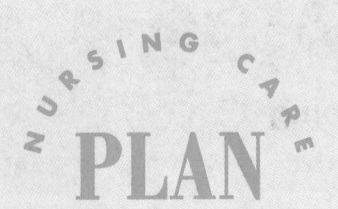

A 4-Year-Old Child Undergoing a Tonsillectomy (continued)

Nursing Diagnosis	*Intervention*	*Rationale*
5. High risk for fluid volume deficit related to increased fluid needs Supporting Data: • Refuses to drink • Potential for nausea and vomiting related to anesthesia	Maintain intravenous fluids as ordered until taking fluids by mouth well.	Children can become dehydrated quickly and need supplements when not taking fluids by mouth.
	Encourage frequent sips of cool clear liquids.	Child may tolerate small amounts frequently; large amounts quickly may cause vomiting; hot liquids increase blood supply at incision.
	Keep something at bedside for Tommy to drink.	He can drink whenever he wants to. Increases autonomy and control.
	Keep accurate intake and output.	An indicator of hydration status.
	Monitor for signs of dehydration: poor skin turgor, dry mucous membranes, elevated specific gravity.	Signs of dehydration indicate inadequate fluid intake: need to adjust IV rate after consult with physician; also encourage increased fluids by mouth.
	Measure and record amount and color of vomitus.	Vomiting is common after T&A, may be related to anesthesia or to pooling of blood in GI tract during surgery. Frequent vomiting could lead to dehydration; vomiting of new blood could indicate hemorrhage.
	Evaluate need for antiemetic and administer if needed as ordered.	Helps to decrease nausea and vomiting, which cause strain on sutures and discomfort.
6. High risk for infection related to traumatized tissue Supporting Data: • Post-op T&A • Raw surface with sutures	Monitor temperature every 4 hours; if elevated, every 2 hours.	Increasing temperature could be sign of infection.
	Notify physician if temperature above 101°F orally.	Treatment may need to be changed.
	Remove extra blankets.	Helps to reduce temperature.
	Dress lightly.	
	Sponge with tepid water.	
	Antibiotics as ordered.	Physicians frequently prescribe antibiotics prophylactically to prevent infection.
	Encourage fluids by mouth.	Good hydration decreases potential for infection.
7. Fear related to environment and procedures Supporting Data: • 4-year-old • First hospitalization • Crying	Encourage parents to be at bedside when Tommy arrives in his room.	Parents at bedside will give Tommy security and decrease some of the fear associated with the unknown.
	Show Tommy his room when he is fully awake.	Increases familiarity and decreases the unknown.
	Keep favorite toy at bedisde.	Familiar objects at bedside increase ability to cope with strange environment.
	Explain all procedures simply and carefully in terms of what he will see, feel, hear, taste, and smell.	Follows principles of preparing 4-year-old for procedures.

(Continued)

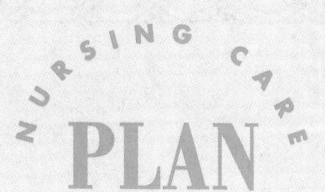

A 4-Year-Old Child Undergoing a Tonsillectomy (continued)

Nursing Diagnosis	*Intervention*	*Rationale*
	Tell Tommy how he can help during procedure and what his limits are.	Helps to minimize sense of loss of control.
	Provide dolls, puppets, and equipment for Tommy to play with.	Increases familiarity and allows for acting out of procedure and for ventilation of feelings.
8. Fear related to potential separation from family Supporting Data: • 4-year-old • Separation from family is a major threat to this age group	Encourage one parent to room-in with Tommy. If impossible, encourage frequent parental visitation and visitation of other close family and friends.	Separation from family is a major concern of this age group; having one parent stay decreases fear of separation and of hospitalization and facilitates coping.
9. Ineffective individual coping related to separation from family Supporting Data: • 4-year-old • First hospitalization	Encourage rooming-in. Allow Tommy choices when possible. Allow Tommy to visit playroom in the evening when fully awake and alert.	Decreases fear of separation, increases ability to cope with strange environment. Decreases sense of loss of control. The playroom is a fun, familiar, and secure place for children. Play also allows for ventilation of feelings.
10. Parental anxiety related to change in role functioning Supporting Data: • Tommy is an only child • First hospitalization for Tommy	Orient parents to hospital setting. Answer questions and provide explanations about all procedures. Allow parents to stay with Tommy and to participate in care.	Provides familiarity and decreases the unknown. Explanations allow for a better understanding of the situation and frequently will decrease anxiety about the child's condition. Allowing parents to stay with their child during the hospitalization increases their sense of control. By staying with the child they are constantly aware of the child's condition, which decreases anxiety associated with the unknown. Also gives parents the opportunity to watch how nurses interact and care for their child. Will reinforce feelings and practices of childrearing or help them change.

Evaluation

Tommy has no complications from surgery and is discharged on Saturday, the day after his surgery. He has a prescription for Amoxicillin three times a day for 10 days and for Tylenol with Codeine every 4 hours as needed for pain. Mrs. White has been given verbal discharge instructions by the physician, but states that she doesn't remember everything.

Expected Outcomes

• Tommy exhibits pain relief with nursing care.
• Tommy drinks juices and water periodically.
• Tommy expresses comfort with his parents at bedside.
• One parent remains at bedside around the clock.
• Mother discusses need for discharge teaching.

(This Nursing Care Plan was contributed by *Kay Jackson Cowen*, MSN, RNC, Lecturer, School of Nursing, The University of North Carolina at Greensboro, Greensboro, North Carolina.)

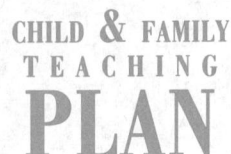

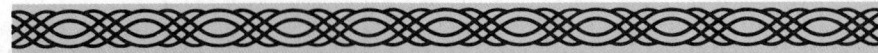

Home Care of the Child Following Tonsillectomy

Assessment

4-year-old Tommy is discharged from the hospital following an overnight stay after a T&A. He will return with his parents to their home in the country. Tommy attends pre-school full time. His father is a plumber and his mother is a part-time secretary, who has taken the next week off to care for Tommy. Both parents are high school graduates, and Mrs. White has taken several secretarial courses.

Because of his work schedule, Mr. White is not present at discharge. The focus of the nurse's teaching is Mrs. White, who has demonstrated basic understanding of her son's hospitalization and care, but difficulty remembering details.

Child and Family Objectives	Specific Content	Teaching Strategies
1. Describe signs of complications from surgery.	1. Explanation that Tommy is at risk for bleeding 5–8 days after surgery; symptoms include increased restlessness and increased swallowing in addition to obvious bleeding. Give Mrs. White phone numbers of physician and ER to contact immediately if child starts to bleed.	1. Use verbal explanation with a chance to ask questions. Have Mrs. White repeat signs and symptoms. Provide written list of signs of complications for Mrs. White to take with her.
	Possibility of Tommy's developing infection. Assess Mrs. White's ability to take a temperature. Advise her at what point she should call the physician.	If Mrs. White does not know how to take an oral temperature, demonstrate and allow for return demonstration.
2. Describe mouth care.	2. Rinse mouth frequently with warm water. May brush teeth as usual. Avoid astringent washes. No straws.	2. Discuss purpose of frequent rinsing: keeps mouth clean and promotes comfort.
		Explain that most mouth washes contain alcohol and would burn; are unnecessary. Demonstrate with straw how injury may occur.
3. Describe Tommy's dietary needs.	3. Advise to advance Tommy from liquids to soft foods as tolerated. No hard or spicy foods or citrus juices until appointment with physician.	3. Give verbal and written instructions with examples of soft foods that are acceptable.
4. Describe rest and activity requirements.	4. Advise quiet activities at home for 2 weeks.	4. Use verbal and written instructions with examples of quiet activities.
5. Discuss how to administer medications to Tommy.	5. Explain reason for and how to administer Amoxicillin (times, amounts).	5. Assess understanding of how to administer medications; if difficulty is noted, demonstrate and allow return demonstration.

(Continued)

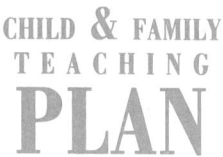

CHILD & FAMILY
TEACHING
PLAN

Home Care of the Child
Following Tonsillectomy (continued)

Child and Family Objectives	*Specific Content*	*Teaching Strategies*
6. State time for next appointment with physician.	6. Time and reason for follow-up.	6. Give appointment care.

Evaluation

- Mrs. White describes signs of complications to be reported.
- Mrs. White discusses proper mouth care for Tommy.
- Mrs. White identifies quiet activities she can use with Tommy.
- Mrs. White states importance of keeping next appointment with the physician.

(This Teaching Plan was contributed by **Kay Jackson Cowen, MSN, RNC,** Lecturer, School of Nursing, The Univrsity of North Carolina at Greensboro, Greensboro, North Carolina.)

activity, and expected healing. Parents are instructed to call the doctor if the child exhibits bleeding from the nose or throat or a fever greater than 101° F. Some bleeding may be normal for up to 10 days after surgery. The child is instructed to rinse his or her mouth frequently with warm water to keep the mouth clean and to minimize discomfort. The diet should consist of soft foods for the first 10 days after surgery. Acidic food, such as orange juice, grapefruit juice, and tomato juice, which can cause tissue irritation, is not to be taken. Straws are also not to be used to prevent accidental trauma to the surgical site. Aspirin is contraindicated to minimize bleeding tendency; acetaminophen is acceptable and may be beneficial to reduce earaches, which are not uncommon after surgery. The child should be told to avoid any strenuous activity until healing occurs. Rest is indicated for 2 weeks after surgery. See the sample Teaching Plan for further teaching ideas.

★ EVALUATION

Periodically the nurse and family evaluate the outcomes of care given. Examples of outcomes for the child and family with pharyngotonsillitis were given under Nursing Diagnoses and Planning in this section. Planning for further nursing care takes into consideration complications.

COMPLICATIONS

Inflammation of the tonsils and adjacent tissues results in erythema and development of exudate. The child is at risk for upper respiratory tract obstruction and otitis media because enlarged tonsils and adenoids impede normal drainage and ventilation of the eustachian tube. Complications of streptococcal pharyngotonsillitis include sinusitis, retropharyngeal abscess, cervical lymphadenitis,

otitis media, pneumonia, and peritonsillar abscess. Rheumatic fever and acute glomerulonephritis are late complications of streptococcal infections. The incidence of rheumatic fever has decreased significantly in recent years with an occurrence of less than 0.5% of streptococcal infections. Inflammation of the adenoids is often associated with tonsillitis; adenoidits could result in otitis media if the adenoids are large enough to block the eustachian tube.

Summary

Children with disorders of the head and neck predominately incur sensory deficits of vision, speech, or hearing. These maladies may result from a variety of etiologies, including congenital defects, infection, and trauma. The nurse plays a vital role in screening children for these problems, which are often of an insidious onset. Thus, recognition and referral are two of the most important roles the nurse plays in working with these children.

The nurse is an important member of the health care team in the diagnosis and early treatment stages by providing the family with support in accepting the diagnosis. Clarification of medical facts presented to the family is an equally important role. With the diagnosis of minor disorders as well as major abnormalities, the information and support the nurse provides may be an invaluable asset to the family.

Nurses also are essential in the intervention and follow-up stages of care for these children. With acute minor illnesses the nurse provides continuity if initial treatment plans did not work and may be the family's link to the physician for further care. The nurse's knowledge of available resources enhances the quality of care provided for the child and family.

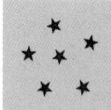

Ideas for Nursing Research

The care of a child with such sensory deficits as impaired vision, hearing, and speech is a challenging role for the nurse and inspires a variety of research possibilities. Nurses provide assistance in recognizing such disorders and often implement screening measures. During the diagnostic phase the nurse gives the family clarification and support. Nursing interventions and follow-up also are essential in helping the child and family stay compliant with the treatment regimen. The following areas need to be explored:

- Comparison of screening tools presently available for determination of hearing, language, and visual disorders
- Correlation of the results of standard developmental screening tests with screening tools for vision, speech, and hearing
- Evaluation of family coping styles and their impact on the child's ability to deal with the handicap
- Effects of different treatment modalities for the same disorder in assisting the child to function more optimally
- Effects of varying amounts of home interventions in supporting the treatment regimen for the same disorder
- Development of home-based therapy programs to more optimally integrate sensory-impaired children into society and school systems
- Evaluation of the impact that nurses have in recognizing and referring children with sensory deficits to appropriate management

References

1. Albin, R. E., Hendee, R. W., & O'Donnell, R. S. (1986). Craniofacial anomalies and their surgery. In R. J. Balkany & N. R. T. Pashley (Eds.). *Clinical pediatric otolaryngology*. St. Louis: C.V. Mosby.
2. American Academy of Pediatrics. Committee on Practice—Ambulatory Medicine. (1986). American Academy of Pediatrics Committee Statements: Vision, screening, and eye examination in children. *Pediatrics, 77*(6), 918–919.
3. Arola, M., Ziegler, R., Ruuskanen, O., et al. (1988). Rhinovirus in acute otitis media. *Journal of Pediatrics, 113*(4), 193.
4. Avery, M. E., & First, L. R. (1989). *Pediatric medicine*. Baltimore: Williams & Wilkins.
5. Behrman, R. E., & Kliegman, R. M. (1992). *Nelson textbook of pediatrics* (14th ed.). Philadelphia: W.B. Saunders.
6. Belanger, G. K., & Casamassimo, P. S. (1987). Teeth. In Kempe, C. H. et al. (Eds.). *Current pediatric diagnosis and treatment 1987* (9th ed.). Norwalk, CT: Appleton & Lange.
7. Bluestone, C. D. (1989). Modern management of otitis media. *Pediatric Clinics of North America, 33*(6), 1396.
8. Bluestone, C. D., & Klein, J.O. (1990). Otitis: Otitis media, atelectasis and eustachian tube dysfunction. In C. D. Bluestone & S. E. Stool (Eds.). *Pediatric otolaryngology*. Philadelphia: W.B. Saunders.
9. Boyd-Monk, H., & Steinmetz, C. G. (1987). *Nursing care of the eye*. Norwalk, CT: Appleton & Lange.
10. Byrne, W. J. (1990). The gastrointestinal tract. In R. E. Behrman & R. Kliegman (Eds.). *Nelson essentials of pediatrics* (pp. 377–410). Philadelphia: W.B. Saunders.
11. Chow, M. P., Durand, B. A., Feldman, M. N., & Mills, M. A. (1984). *Handbook of pediatric primary care* (2nd ed.). New York: Wiley.
12. Chonmaitree, T., Howie, V. M., Truant, A. L. (1986). Presence of respiratory viruses in middle ear fluids and nasal wash specimens from children with acute otitis media. *Pediatrics, 77*(5), 698.
13. Cohen, M. M. (Ed.). *Craniosynostosis: Diagnosis, evaluation, and management*. New York: Raven Press.
14. Derkay, C. S., Bluestone, C. D., Thompson, A. E., & Kardatske, D. (1989). Otitis media in the pediatric intensive care unit: A prospective study. *Otolaryngology—Head and Neck Surgery 100*(4), 292.
15. Dummett, C. O. (1988). Anomalies of the developing dentition. In J. R. Pinkham, P. S. Casamassimo, H. W. Fields, D. J. McTigue, A. J. Nowak (Eds.). *Pediatric dentistry—Infancy through adolescence*. Philadelphia: W.B. Saunders.
16. Eimas, P. D., & Kavanagh, J. F. (1986). Otitis media, hearing loss and child development: A NICHD conference summary. *Public Health Report, 101*(3), 289.
17. Ellis, P. P. (1987). Eye. In C. H. Kempe, H. K. Silver, D. O'Brien, & V. A. Fulginiti (Eds.). *Current pediatric diagnosis and treatment 1987* (9th ed.). Norwalk, CT: Appleton & Lange.
18. Frenkel, M. (1987). Acute otitis media—Does therapy alter its course? *Postgraduate Medicine, 82*(5), 84.
19. Garber, N. (1990). Health promotion and disease prevention in ophthalmology. *Journal of Ophthalmic Nursing and Technology, 9*(5), 186–192.
20. Gates, G. A., Northern, J. L., Ferrer, H. P., et al. (1989). Recent advances in otitis media. *Annals of Otology, Rhinology, and Laryngology, 98*(4), 39.
21. Grossman, L. K. (1987). Malocclusion. In R. A. Hoekelman et al. (Eds.). *Primary pediatric care*. St. Louis: C.V. Mosby.
22. Hawke, M., Wong, J., & Krajden, S. (1984). Clinical and microbiological features of otitis externa. *Journal of Otolaryngology, 13*, 289.
23. Heald, M. M., Matkin, N. D., & Meredith, K. (1990). Pressure-equalization (PE) tubes in treatment of otitis media: National survey of otolaryngologists. *Otolaryngology—Head and Neck Surgery, 102*(4), 334.
24. Hoekelman, R. A., Blatman, S., Friedman, S. B., Nelson, N. M., & Seidel, H. M. (1987). *Primary pediatric care*. St. Louis: C.V. Mosby.
25. Hollwich, F. (1985). *Ophthalmology—A short textbook* (2nd ed.). New York: Thieme-Stratton.
26. Jehle, D., & Cottington, E. (1989). Acoustic otoscopy in the diagnosis of otitis media. *Annals of Emergency Medicine, 18*(14), 396.
27. Kanski, J. J. (1990). *Synopsis of ophthalmology* (6th ed.). London: Butterworths.
28. Kaye, B. (1990). The cure for lazy eye. *Journal of Ophthalmic Nursing and Technology, 9*(3), 90–93.
29. Kershner, D. D., & Claussen, J. A. (1986). Craniofacial reconstruction: Perioperative care of the craniosynostosis patient. *AORN Journal, 44*, 554.
30. Klein, J. O. (1989). Otitis media. In J. E. Pennington (Ed.). *Respiratory infections: Diagnosis and management*. New York: Raven.
31. Klein, J. O., Tos, M., Hussl, B., et al. (1989). Recent advances in otitis media. *Annals of Otology, Rhinology, and Laryngology, 98*(4), 10.
32. Kovalesky, A. (1985). *Nurses' guide to children's eyes*. Orlando: Grune & Stratton.

33. Marcy, S. M. (1987). Swimmer's ear: Timely management tips. *Patient Care*, *21*(10), 28.

34. Medders, G., & Mattox, D. E. (1988). Update on otitis media: Pathogenesis and diagnosis. *Journal of Respiratory Diseases*, *9*(9), 37.

35. Myer, C. M., & Cotton, R. T. (1988). *A practical approach to pediatric otolaryngology.* Chicago: Year Book Medical Publishers.

36. Needleman, H. L., & Shusterman, S. (1989). Dentistry. In M. E. Avery & L. R. First (Ed.). *Pediatric medicine.* Baltimore: Williams & Wilkins.

37. Nelson, L. B. Disorders of ocular motility in childhood. *Journal of Ophthalmic Nursing and Technology*, *3*(6), 237–245.

38. Neumann, E., Friedman, Z., & Abel-Peleg, B. (1987). Prevention of strabismic amblyopia of early onset. *Journal of Ophthalmic Nursing and Technology*, *6*(6), 242–247.

39. Palmer, E. A. (1987). Periorbital and orbital edema. In R. A. Hoekelman et al. (Eds.). *Primary pediatric care.* St. Louis: C.V. Mosby.

40. Palmer, E. A. (1987). Visual disturbances. In R. A. Hoekelman, Blatman, S., Friedman, S. B., et al. (Eds.). *Primary pediatric care.* St. Louis: C.V. Mosby.

41. Riley, M. A. (1987). Hearing loss and other common auditory dysfunctions. Nursing care of the client with ear, nose, and throat disorders. New York: Springer.

42. Sando, I., & Takahashi, H. (1990). Otitis media in association with various congenital diseases. Preliminary study. *Annals of Otology, Rhinology, and Laryngology*, *99* (Suppl.), 23.

43. Schwartz, R. H., Hayden, G. F., & Wientzen, R. (1985). Children less than three-years-old with pharyngitis. *Clinical Pediatrics*, *25*, 4.

44. Shapiro, G. G. (1988). Sinusitis in children. *Journal of Allergy and Clinical Immunology*, *81*, 1025–1027.

45. Sims, N. H., & Roy, F. H. (1987). Vision screening. In R. A. Hoekelman et al. (Eds.). *Primary pediatric care.* St. Louis: C.V. Mosby.

46. Stone, C. (1990). Clinical diagnosis and management of problems of the head, eyes, ear, nose and throat. In V. L. Millong (Ed.). *The pediatric nurse practitioner certification review guide* (pp. 95 151). Potomac, MD: Health Leadership Associates.

47. Wald, E. R., Dashefsky, B., Byers, E., et al. (1988). Frequency and severity of infections in day care. *Journal of Pediatrics*, *112*, 540.

48. Wald, E. R. (1990). Rhinitis and acute and chronic sinusitis. In C. D. Bluestone & Stool, S. E. (Eds.). *Pediatric otolaryngology.* Philadelphia: W.B. Saunders.

49. Walike, J. W. (1979). Management of acute ear infections. *Otolaryngologic Clinics of North America*, *12*, 439.

50. Weiss, C. E., & Lillywhite, H. S. (1981). *Communicative disorders* (2nd ed.). St. Louis: C.V. Mosby.

51. Weiss, M. H., & Frost, J. O. (1987). May children with otitis media with effusion safely fly? *Clinical Pediatrics*, *26*, 567.

52. White, G. L., Liss, R. P., & Crandall, A. S. (1991). Congenital glaucoma. *Physician Assistant*, *15*(1), 45–46, 48–49.

53. Winston, K. R. (1985). Craniosynostosis. In R. H. Wilkins & S. S. Rengachary (Eds.). *Neurosurgery* (3rd ed.). New York: McGraw-Hill.

54. Yoon, T. H., Paparella, M. M., Schachern, P. A., & Lindgren, B. R. (1990). Morphometric studies of the continuum of otitis media. *Annals of Otology, Rhinology, and Laryngology*, *99*(Suppl.) 23.

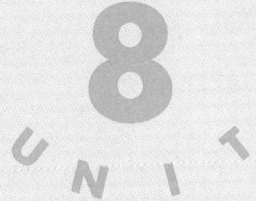

Nursing Care of Children With Altered Respiratory Function

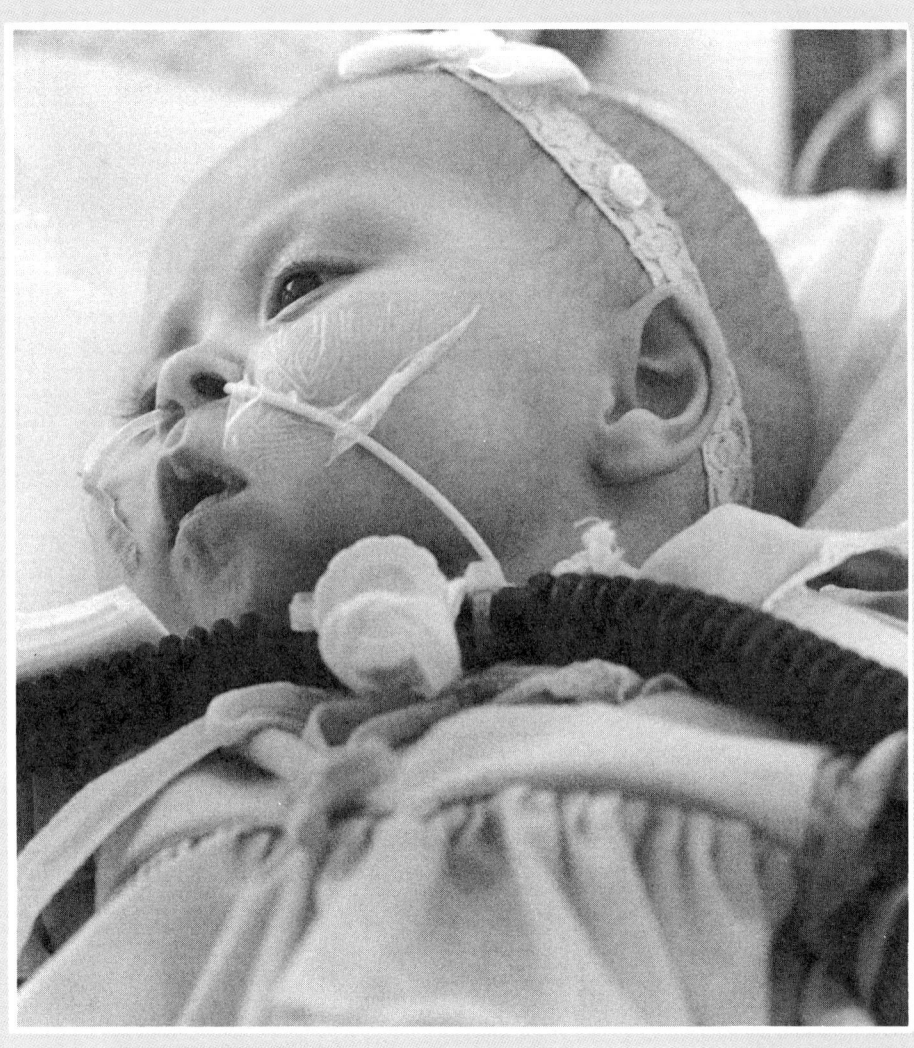

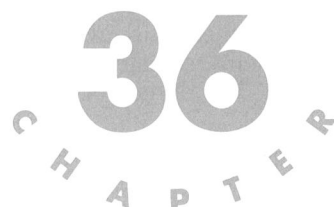 CHAPTER

Anatomy and Physiology of the Respiratory System

BEHAVIORAL OBJECTIVES

Describe fetal development of the
respiratory system.

Identify the anatomic structures of
the respiratory system.

Summarize the mechanics of
breathing.

Explain fetal preparation for the first
breath and the respiratory events that
occur at birth.

Describe the physiologic processes of
ventilation and perfusion.

Explain the respiratory system's role
in acid–base balance.

The respiratory system is responsible for transporting oxygen and carbon dioxide to and from the blood and for helping with the regulation of the body's acid–base balance. Because of the system's significance in indicating the general health status of children, it is one of the most routinely assessed systems in the body. Understanding dysfunctions of the respiratory system requires a fundamental grasp of the structure and function of the composite organs. This chapter reviews the anatomy and physiology of the respiratory system of the child, beginning with embryonic development and ending with developmental differences in infancy and childhood.

Embryonic Development

Three primary tissue layers constitute the primitive embryo. These are the endoderm or basal tissue layer, the mesoderm or middle layer, and the ectoderm. The developing respiratory system is derived principally from the endoderm. The lungs, airways, and the pleural cavity are structures rooted in endodermal tissue. However, support structures, such as the tracheal cartilage, respiratory muscles, pulmonary vessels, and pulmonary lymphatics, are generated from the mesodermal tissue.

Early Embryonic Period

Embryonic lung development occurs in five successive stages. The *early embryonic period* occurs 1 to 5 weeks after fertilization. The lungs initially appear as an outpouching (a diverticulum) on the ventral surface of the embryonic esophagus, or the foregut. This lung bud quickly divides into two bronchopulmonary pouches, giving rise eventually to the two mainstem bronchi. By the fifth week of gestation, the common tube from which the lung bud rises has differentiated into the esophagus and the laryngotracheal tube. Figure 36-1 shows early development of the lungs.

The early embryonic period is also a time of rapid pulmonary epithelial cell proliferation. These cells form the basic structure of the tissue complex of the respiratory tract. This period of rapid cell reproduction and growth is evidenced by the remarkable development and differentiation of the bronchopulmonary buds. The left bronchial bud gives rise to two secondary buds, the primitive upper and lower lung lobes. The right bronchus gives rise to three secondary buds, the rudimentary upper, middle, and lower, right lung lobes. At the end of 5 weeks, the gross rudimentary lung structures are present.

Pseudoglandular Period

The second stage of lung development, the *pseudoglandular period,* begins at the 6th week of gestation

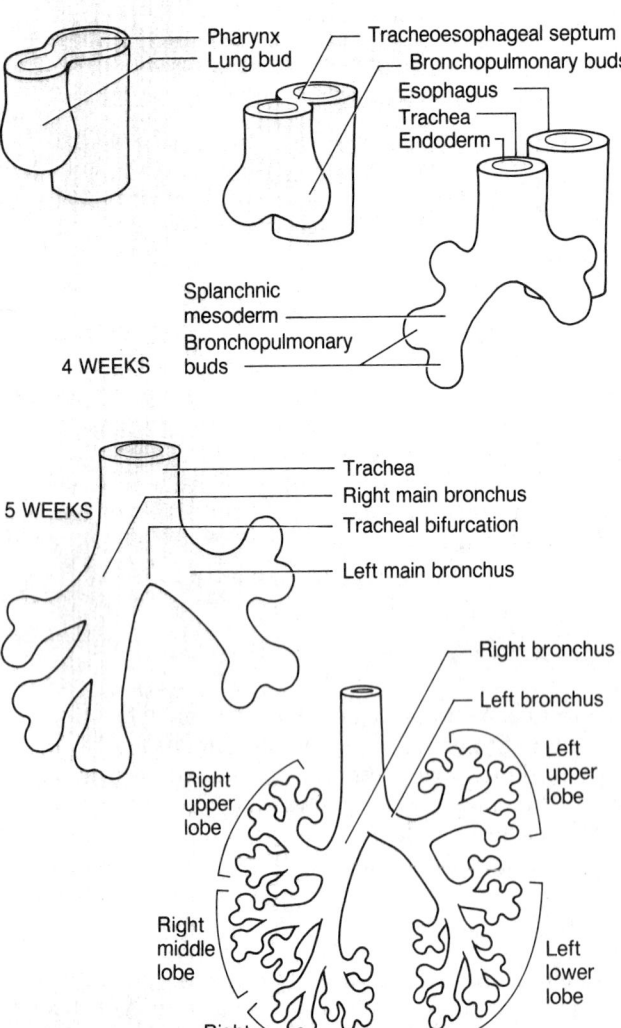

FIGURE 36-1
Early development of respiratory structures (4 through 6 weeks).

and continues through the 17th week. This stage is so named because the rudimentary lung has the appearance of a gland. The fundamental structures for air conduction, the entire tracheobronchial tree, are established. These include the mainstem bronchi, their secondary bronchi, and the bronchioles. In addition, 70% of the branching of the bronchi is complete.

During this period, the embryonic lung is rich in glycogen stores. This glycogen provides the nutrients needed for the rapid pulmonary cell development and differentiation occurring at this time. Toward the end of the pseudoglandular period, the bronchial arteries arise from the thoracic aorta and the intercostal arteries. Rudimentary veins also appear.

Canalicular Period

The *canalicular period* marks the third stage of embryonic lung development. This fetal stage, 13 to 25 weeks' gestation, is marked by the formation of alveolar ducts and alveolar cells that will eventually form alveoli. In addition, alveolar capillaries and the thoracic lymph system evolve and align closer to the alveolar ducts and primitive alveoli surfaces. The generation and multiplication of the alveolar capillaries are important steps necessary to facilitate oxygen and carbon dioxide transfer during extrauterine life.

Terminal Sac Period

The fourth stage of lung development is termed the *terminal sac period* and spans from 24 weeks' gestation through birth. Structurally, the bronchioles give rise to terminal sacs or primitive alveoli. Although the alveoli are present, they are thick-walled and narrow. In addition, the alveolar capillaries have not moved close enough to the alveoli sacs to lie directly on or next to them. Consequently, the diffusion gradient or the distance that oxygen and carbon dioxide must traverse between the alveoli and the capillaries is so great that oxygenation is inadequate. The implication of this anatomic arrangement is that while the biological equipment is present for extrauterine existence, development is insufficient to support life without artificial ventilatory support. Thus, infants born prior to 36 weeks' gestation typically develop acute respiratory problems such as hyaline membrane disease (also known as idiopathic respiratory distress syndrome) because of inadequate pulmonary structural development.

Biochemically, an important event occurs at the end of the canalicular period and during the terminal sac period that is essential for independent extrauterine existence. The alveolar epithelial cells lining the alveolar sacs differentiate into three special cell types: types I and II alveolar cells and the macrophage cells.

Type I alveolar cells primarily are involved with the formation of the interspace for gas exchange. Simply stated, these cells are responsible for the diffusion of oxygen from the alveoli into the pulmonary arterioles and carbon dioxide from the pulmonary capillary venules into the alveoli. Thus, for adequate oxygenation to occur in the extrauterine environment, the infant must have sufficient numbers of alveoli, mature type I alveolar cells, and alveolar capillaries within close approximation to the alveolar sac.

Type II alveolar cells are responsible for the storage and secretion of surfactant. Surfactant, a lipoprotein rich in cholesterol and phospholipids (including lecithin and sphingomyelin), is responsible for maintaining the spherical integrity of the alveoli. The presence of surfactant allows for equal distribution of air throughout the alveoli. Surfactant also prevents the alveoli from collapsing after expiration by trapping air inside, thereby maintaining functional residual capacity.

Alveolar sacs frequently have been compared to a cluster of grapes. In any cluster, the grapes vary in size; the alveolar sacs also vary in size. Because alveoli within a cluster have different radii, each alveolus requires a different pressure gradient for inflation, a phenomenon consistent with Laplace's rule. According to Laplace's rule, the surface tension within a sphere is inversely proportional to its radius. As the diameter of a sphere gets smaller, greater air pressure is required to inflate it. This concept is similar to taking two deflated balloons of varying sizes and inflating them. The balloon that is smaller requires greater air pressure for inflation than the larger-diameter balloon.

Similarly, following Laplace's rule, smaller alveoli would normally require greater pressure for inflation than larger ones. As air pressure flows to the area of least resistance, these smaller alveoli might not participate in the respiratory process because air would be shunted to the less resistant larger alveoli. The presence of surfactant lining each alveolus, however, reduces the surface tension of the alveolar wall, thus allowing all alveoli to be inflated under the same amount of pressure. Additionally, surfactant allows air to be trapped within the alveoli (functional residual capacity), so the walls of the alveoli do not fully collapse after each expiration. Subsequent inspiratory efforts are easily accomplished at a low pressure.

The production and storage of surfactant are not sufficient to support extrauterine life until the fetus has reached approximately 36 weeks' gestation. Prior to this time, low quantities and an immature form of surfactant make unassisted ventilation for the newborn infant difficult or impossible.

Surfactant is produced by a number of biochemical pathways. A predominant one in the developing fetus is the phosphytidylinositol (PI) pathway, which predominates until 32 weeks' gestation. The PI surfactant is very unstable and quickly used. Infants born prior to 32 weeks' gestation are thus more likely to suffer respiratory distress from hyaline membrane disease. The less stable PI surfactant is not as efficient in reducing the surface tension of the alveolar sacs. This deficit potentially interferes with alveolar stability by not allowing for consistent alveolar ventilation. Thus, smaller alveoli may become underinflated or overinflated, resulting in inadequate gas exchange and leading to hypoxemia and hypercarbia.

At about 32 to 34 weeks' gestation, a more stable form of surfactant is synthesized, phosphytidylglycerol (PG). PG surfactant is very stable and permits alveoli of differing sizes to inflate with equal amounts of pressure. It is possible to determine the presence of adequate levels of PG from analysis of amniotic fluid. PG surfactant is the form that persists for a lifetime. Thus, with the presence

of adequate amounts of PG, ventilation is such that oxygenation is optimal.

Surfactant maturity has in the past been estimated by measurement of lecithin and sphingomyelin (the L:S ratio). Ratio of these phospholipids is approximately equal until 35 weeks' gestation. With increasing age lecithin increases so that an L:S ratio of greater than 2:1 suggests surfactant maturity. However, levels of PG have been found to correlate better with surfactant maturity than the L:S ratio alone.[1] The trend is to use PG levels rather than L:S ratio for the purpose of estimating lung maturity.

A third type of alveolar cell is called a macrophage or scavenger cell, and it can be compared to a chimney sweep. These cells are responsible for the engulfment and digestion of foreign materials, primarily bacteria, that may find their way into the respiratory tract.

Alveolar Period

The final stage of lung development, termed the *alveolar period,* occurs from late fetal development through 8 years of life. At this time, the primary developmental activity is growth of the terminal sacs (alveoli), thinning of the alveolar tissue, and proliferation and approximation of the alveolar walls to the capillaries that will deliver fresh blood to the alveoli. The newborn infant has approximately 20,000,000 alveoli, and the number continues to increase until the eighth year of life when anatomic development is completed.[7]

Consequences of Abnormal Development

Many factors influence embryonic development of the lower respiratory tract. Either genetic or environmental conditions may interrupt or distort the development of structures in the growing embryo. Some of the consequences of abnormal embryonic development are described in Table 36-1.

Biochemical maturation of the respiratory system also can be affected during embryogenesis. Some preterm infants develop hyaline membrane disease (HMD), yet others do not. Preterm infants of heroin addicted mothers, for example, rarely develop HMD. Most mature infants have no respiratory problems at birth, but some mature

TABLE 36-1
Consequences of Abnormal Embryonic Development

Fetal Age (Weeks)	Structure	Anomalies at Birth
4–5	Trachea and esophagus	Failure of fusion of esophageal tube and tracheal tube into separate structures leads to tracheoesophageal fistula.
5–6	Lung lobes	Interrupted, delayed, or interference with development leads to hypoplasia of lung lobes.
8	Diaphragm	Failure of closure of diaphragmatic canals leads to diaphragmatic hernia with hypoplasia of the lung on the herniated side.

infants, such as those born to diabetic women, are at risk of developing HMD. Why are there such differing outcomes within similar patient populations?

The at-risk infants mentioned previously have one commonality: interference with biochemical development of surfactant. Fetuses exposed to chronic intrauterine stress are known to have accelerated biochemical lung maturation. Chronic fetal stress, such as intrauterine infection or persistent intrauterine malnutrition, induces accelerated fetal glucocorticoid synthesis and production. These glucocorticoids have been shown in fetal lamb studies to induce early production of mature surfactant (PG). In contrast, acute stress does not produce this effect. In fact, acute stress is typically a fetal hypoxic event that serves to temporarily "shut down" pulmonary biochemical activity.

The evidence that chronic stress enhances glucocorticoid production has provided the rationale for administration of the glucocorticosteroid betamethasone to pregnant women in preterm labor.[4] In an early experimental study of this treatment, neonates whose mothers had been given two doses of betamethasone before delivering preterm had a lower incidence of HMD compared to the infants of untreated women.[6] As a result of findings from this and other studies, women in preterm labor between 28 and 32 weeks' gestation have been given two doses of betamethasone to enhance the development of fetal surfactant.

Currently, betamethasone is used in conjunction with tocolytic drugs to prevent preterm labor and allow the infant to mature as much as possible *in utero*. For newborn infants at risk of developing HMD, doses of surfactant may be administered through the intratracheal route. Endotracheal surfactant was approved by the FDA in August of 1990 and is becoming widely used in level-two nurseries.[1]

Structure and Function

The respiratory system consists of the upper airway structures (nose, pharynx, larynx, and trachea) and the lower airway structures (bronchi, bronchioles, alveolar ducts, and alveoli). Air enters the upper airway and is warmed, moistened, and filtered, but no gas exchange occurs in this region. The nose and pharynx are discussed in Chapter 33, and the larynx and trachea are briefly discussed below. The primary focus of this chapter, however, is on the lower airway where gas transport is completed and exchange occurs (Fig. 36-2).

Larynx and Trachea

The larynx is formed by nine cartilages that vary in shape and size and by numerous folds of muscular tissue. It is positioned between the base of the tongue and the trachea. The laryngeal prominence, known as the Adam's apple, makes the position of the larynx easy to locate. The epiglottis is elastic and closes during swallowing to prevent the entry of oral contents into the airway. Vocal cords span either side of the opening into the larynx. The slit between the pair of vocal cords is known as the glottis.

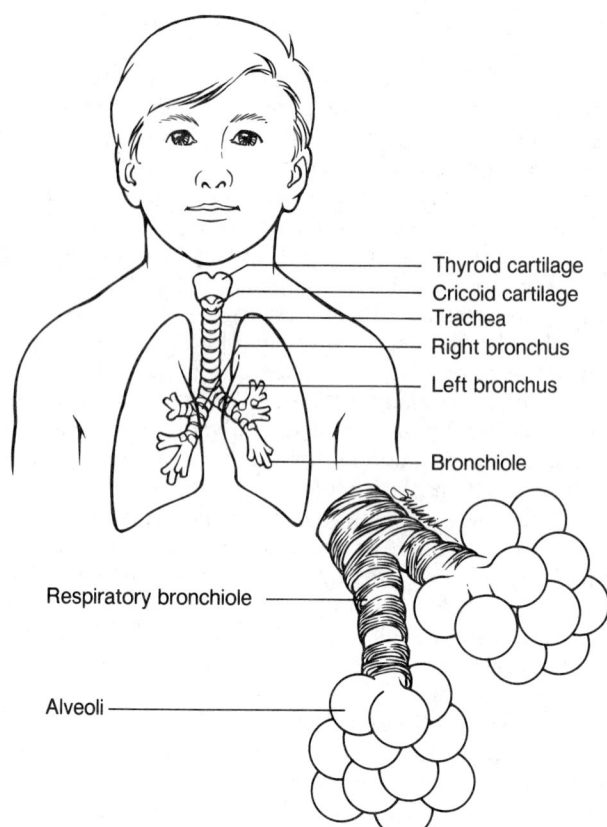

FIGURE 36-2
Structures of the lower respiratory system.

Two types of muscles are present in the larynx. Extrinsic muscles connect the larynx to nearby structures. Intrinsic muscles open and close the glottis and vary tension on the vocal cords. As air moves through the larynx, the vocal cords vibrate and can produce sound.

The larynx is lined with mucous membrane that is well supplied with mucus-secreting glands. Laryngeal mucosa is extremely sensitive and is readily stimulated by foreign particles. A protective cough reflex forcefully expels such materials. Inflammation of the mucous membrane reduces the size of the laryngeal opening and may interfere with air flow.

The trachea is a fibroelastic tube that connects the larynx to the bronchi. C-shaped cartilages situated along the length of the tube prevent its collapse. Large vessels entering and leaving the heart are located near the trachea and create a warm environment for the passage of air.

Mucous membranes similar to those in the larynx line the trachea. Cilia within the mucous membranes beat upward to carry mucus and contained materials toward the pharynx. Glands along the trachea keep the mucosa moist. Air that passes through the trachea is thereby moistened as well as warmed.

Thoracic Cavity and Mechanics of Breathing

The trachea, bronchi, and lung are housed in the thoracic cavity, a bony cage that is composed of 24 (12 pairs) of ribs and 12 thoracic vertebrae. The ribs are attached to the vertebrae posteriorly and the sternum anteriorly (Fig. 36-3). They are fixed in position by the intercostal muscles.

The thoracic cavity is divided into two pulmonary spaces containing the right and left lungs. The esophagus, trachea, heart, and large blood vessels lie between the lungs in the space known as the mediastinum. A two-layered membrane, the pleura, covers each lung and lines the thoracic cavity. The layer closest to the thoracic wall is termed the parietal layer; the other, closest to the lung surface, is called the visceral layer. The potential space between these two layers, the pleural space, contains a thin film of lubricating fluid that allows for the free, painless movement of the lungs during inspiration and expiration.

The apex of each lung extends 1.5 in above the clavicles, and the base of each reaches to the sixth rib anteriorly and the eighth rib posteriorly. The right lung is divided into upper, middle, and lower lobes, while the left lobe is divided into upper and lower lobes only. This anatomic difference in the number of lobes is necessary to accommodate the cardiac structures located within the mid and left thorax.

Inspiratory and expiratory actions of the thorax cause the ribs to flare and contract, with movement being at the points of attachment to the vertebrae and sternum. The diaphragm flattens and descends with inspiration and resumes its dome shape with expiration. The change in diaphragmatic shape alters intrathoracic pressure, allowing respiration to occur.

With inspiration, the intrathoracic pressure is decreased, and air is pulled into the lungs. The increased intrapulmonic pressure causes the ribs to expand or flare and the thoracic diameter to increase, giving the chest a barrel shape during inspiration.

The action of inspiration is analogous to stretching a rubber band to its limit. When the band is maximally stretched, contraction must occur. The thorax responds similarly; when inspiration has reached its limit, intrathoracic pressure exceeds extrathoracic pressure, the diaphragm relaxes, and the intercostal muscles begin to contract, causing the ribs to "collapse" around the lungs. The lungs also possess an elastic quality (compliance) so that at peak inspiration, excessive stretch of the tissue stimulates contraction, causing exhalation.

Lung elasticity, compliance, is an important feature in the work of breathing. Compliance enables the lung tissue to overcome resistance of the rigid structures of the airways (the bronchioles, bronchi, and trachea) and allow respiration. While compliance is a measure of lung elasticity, it is also a measure of surfactant production. Inadequate amounts of surfactant lower lung elasticity and make the work of breathing more difficult.

Accessory muscles are needed to assist the diaphragm with the mechanics of breathing. This group of muscles includes the sternocleidomastoids, the scapular elevators, scaleni, external intercostals, and the erectus muscles of the spine. The abdominals, internal intercostals, and the posterior inferior serrati are the muscle groups that aid in expiration. With inspiration, the diaphragm contracts, causing inward pulling of air. At the same time, the sternocleidomastoid, anterior serrati, and the scaleni muscles elevate the entire rib cage. When the lungs fully expand, the abdominal muscles contract and press the intrabdominal contents upward against the diaphragm to force air out. Simultaneously, the internal intercostals and the posterior serrati exert pressure, angling the ribs downward to facilitate exit of air.

Once breathing is established, continuous inspiration and expiration are the result of an interplay of the muscles of respiration, alterations in respiratory pressures, and the elasticity or compliance of the lung tissue and thoracic cavity.

Blood Supply

Blood to the pulmonary system is delivered through the pulmonary arteries that course along the bronchial tree and each of its branches to the terminal airways. The distal pulmonary arteries divide into alveolar capillaries and supply oxygenated blood to individual alveoli (Fig. 36-4). Following the exchange of oxygen for carbon dioxide, these capillaries empty into collecting venules, which drain into the bronchial veins. From these veins, the blood is transported to the pulmonary and azygos veins, which empty into the superior vena cava.

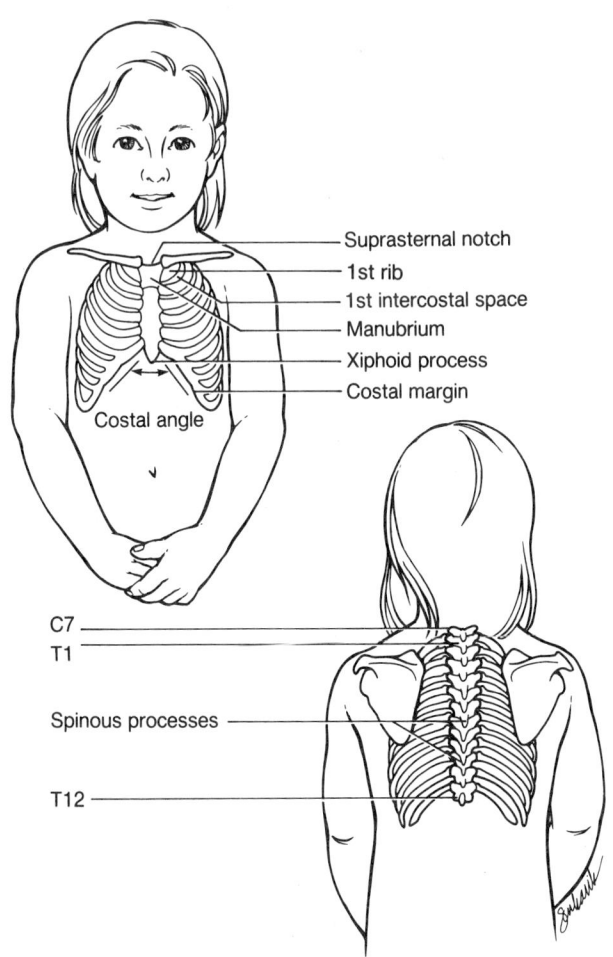

Suprasternal notch
1st rib
1st intercostal space
Manubrium
Xiphoid process
Costal margin
Costal angle

C7
T1

Spinous processes

T12

FIGURE 36-3
Bony landmarks of the anterior (**A**) and posterior (**B**) chest.

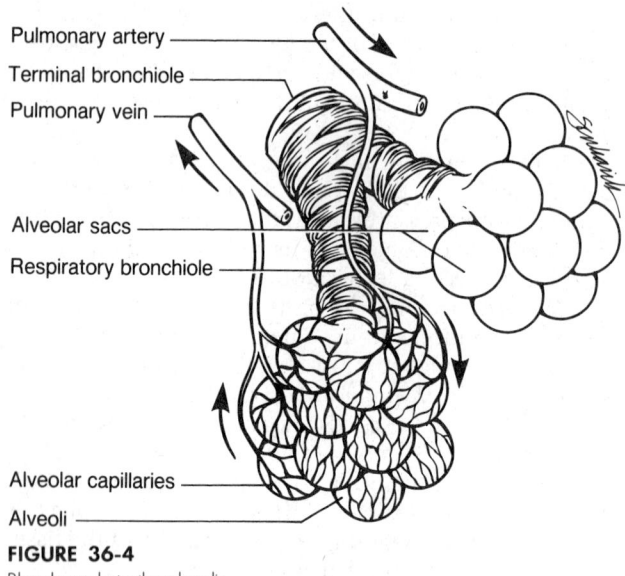

Pulmonary artery
Terminal bronchiole
Pulmonary vein

Alveolar sacs
Respiratory bronchiole

Alveolar capillaries
Alveoli

FIGURE 36-4
Blood supply to the alveoli.

Air Transport

Air transport to the lungs begins with the nose or mouth. Air transport for infants is primarily through the nose because they are obligatory nose breathers.[2] This phenomenon, which persists to 3 or 4 months of age, probably is due to the nose having a low airway resistance compared to higher air resistance created by the tongue falling back against the oropharynx with inspiration.[12] From the nose or mouth, air is transported through the larynx and into the trachea.

Beginning at the lower portion of the cricoid process, the most inferior of the cartilages forming the larynx, the trachea divides into the right and left mainstem bronchi. The bronchi differentiate further into smaller bronchi and bronchioles, the tubes that connect directly to the alveolar ducts.

The bronchi are specially configured to facilitate air transport to the alveoli and to protect the respiratory tract from foreign material. Dust particles that may be inhaled into the respiratory tract are propelled outward by mucous transport and ciliary action. The epithelial lining of the bronchi is composed of two mucous and one ciliary layer. Mucous glands and goblet cells in the bronchial epithelium produce mucus, which serves to entrap and float foreign particles. This mucus with the entrapped particles is swept upward along the respiratory tract by the ciliary lining of the bronchi. Through the action of coughing, foreign materials are expelled from the respiratory tract. While a cough reflex is present from infancy, children usually are unable to expectorate sputum with coughing until age 4 or after. This physiologic deficit is due to the underdevelopment of the ciliary lining of the bronchi until that time.

Developmental Differences

The primary differences in the respiratory system of a child compared to an adult are chest shape, lung ca-

pacity, respiratory rate, and pattern of breathing. The chest of the neonate is round, but it begins to change and become less barrel-shaped during the first year. By 10 years of age, the configuration is more elliptical, like an adult, with a flattened anterior–posterior diameter (Fig. 36-5).

Lung capacity is actually a reflection of the number and size of the alveoli. An infant has approximately 20,000,000 alveoli, compared to the 300,000,000 of an adult.[7] Logically, it is expected that the increased lung volume would correspond with growth of the child and subsequent lung tissue growth.

Structurally, the conducting airways (trachea, bronchi, and bronchioles) of the child up to age 8 are narrower and shorter than an older child and an adult. This makes children more prone to respiratory infections. The smaller airways and the inability to clear the airway with coughing in a very young child (up to age 4) potentiates problems with mucous obstruction more readily in this population than in older children and adults.

Infants' breathing is characterized by abdominal rather than chest movement because the accessory muscles of respiration are poorly developed and do not contribute much to the movement of the chest wall during inspiration. In infancy, the ribs articulate with the spine at a horizontal rather than an oblique slope that appears with later development. With inspiration and downward movement of the diaphragm, the abdomen becomes dome shaped, while the amount of thoracic flaring appears minimal. By age 3, the respiratory pattern demonstrates greater use of the chest muscles and less of the abdominal muscles.

A final developmental difference is the change in respiratory rates with age. Respiratory frequency decreases as body size increases. A newborn infant's respiratory rate fluctuates widely but becomes more stable within 1 to 2 days. The rate gradually slows through childhood (see Appendix).

System Physiology

The respiratory system's primary function is to transport oxygen to the alveoli in the lungs and to carry away carbon dioxide. Oxygen is absolutely necessary for normal cel-

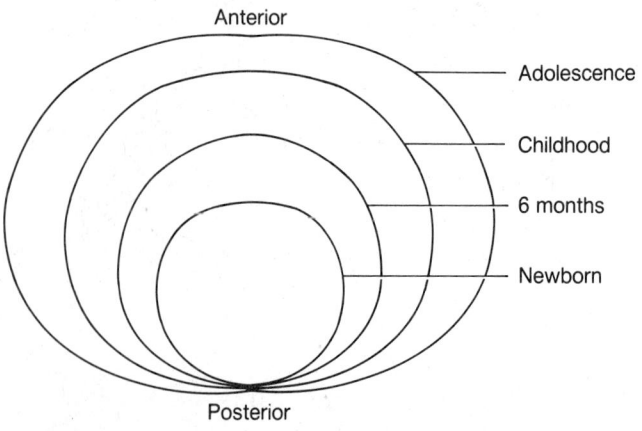

Anterior

Adolescence

Childhood

6 months

Newborn

Posterior

FIGURE 36-5
Age-related changes in chest configuration.

lular metabolic activity of the body. Oxygen deficit can have serious ramifications, affecting cell anabolism and tissue nourishment throughout the body. In addition to providing for air transport, the respiratory system is integral to the maintenance of the bicarbonate–carbonic acid balance necessary to maintain body pH.

The establishment of respiratory function is progressive from fetal preparation for the first breath until the the initial breath is taken. These processes are vital to permit ongoing ventilation, perfusion, and regulation of acid–base balance.

Fetal Preparation for the First Breath

Prior to birth, the process of gas exchange is managed by the placenta. In the circulatory system, the ductus arteriosus and the foramen ovale shunt blood away from the fetal lungs. Only 10% of the fetal cardiac output reaches the lungs. Enough oxygen-enriched blood is available to keep the pulmonic tissue vitalized but not enough to initiate respirations.

The low volume of blood flowing to the fetal lungs contributes to the maintenance of a high pulmonary vascular pressure (PVP). This high PVP creates a high resistance to blood through the pulmonary vascular channels, forcing more blood to be shunted away from the lungs. Low blood flow to the fetal lungs is essential to prevent the possibility of intrauterine respirations, which could lead to aspiration of amniotic fluid.

The fetal lungs are filled with approximately 50 ml of fetal lung liquid, a substance resembling plasma but with a lower protein content. The purpose of the fetal lung liquid is to provide for a slight distention of the alveoli, making the first breath at birth a little easier than if the alveolar walls were collapsed on themselves. The mechanics of this phenomenon may be compared to trying to inflate a wet balloon, which is very difficult because the walls of the balloon seem cemented to each other by the liquid. The alveoli would present a similar problem if they were not kept slightly open by the fetal lung liquid.

The fetal lung is moist, dark, and warm. This type of environment would normally provide an optimal medium for bacterial growth. However, the pH of the fetal lung liquid is slightly acidic. Pulmonary lung liquid thus inhibits bacteriostasis and reduces the potential for fetal pulmonary infection.

Preparation of the respiratory system for extrauterine functions is demonstrated by the occurrence of fetal breathing movements *in utero*. This phenomenon, noticed first by Vesalius, is the fetus "practicing" for extrauterine existence.[8] Vesalius noted that pregnant women displayed rhythmic movements of the abdominal wall over the uterus that were cyclic and predictable. Centuries later, Dawes also was intrigued by this phenomenon. He studied pregnant ewes by injecting radiopaque dye into the uterine cavity. On fluoroscopic examination he noted that the fetuses "breathed" the dye in and out of their upper airways. This dye never went below the larynx, but the accessory muscles of respiration were used.[3] Today,

the presence or absence of fetal breathing movements is used by perinatologists as one of the criteria in the biophysical profile of the fetus for determining fetal well-being.

The First Breath

The newborn baby's first breath is the result of an interplay of neurophysiologic and environmental stimuli. The neurophysiologic controls of respiration include the respiratory center (medulla), the central chemoreceptors (vagus and glossopharyngeal nerves), the peripheral chemoreceptors (aortic and carotid bodies), the cervical sympathetics, and reflex activity. Environmental factors also influence the first breath.

The process of birth is asphyxiating; the fetal blood PaO_2 (the partial pressure of oxygen in the arteries) falls to >20 mmHg, and a drop in blood pH indicates acidemia. The severe hypoxemia (PaO_2 >20 mmHg) acts as a direct stimulant to the central respiratory center (the medulla) and the central chemoreceptors, causing the infant to gasp. A low systemic pH also acts on peripheral chemoreceptors to stimulate respiration.

The PaO_2 sensors located in the aortic arch and the common carotid artery sinus are stimulated by hypoxemia. This action sends a message to the central chemoreceptors that the PaO_2 is low, stimulating the medulla to induce inspiration. A low systemic serum pH is also reflected in low cerebral spinal fluid pH. As the cerebral spinal fluid circulates from the ventricles through the foramina and into the spinal column, cranial nerves VII, IX, and X (facial, glossopharyngeal, and pharyngeal) are stimulated by the low pH. These cervical sympathetic nerves communicate with the peripheral chemoreceptors through the medulla or central receptor the information that acidemia due to hypoxia exists. Thus, respirations are stimulated by this pathway as well. What may appear to be a huge neuronal traffic jam is really an elaborate system of backups that ensures the possibility of respiration at birth.[2,4,8]

The passage of the infant through the vaginal canal during birth also facilitates the first respiration. The external pressure exerted on the descending infant's thorax increases the negative intrathoracic pressure. When the thorax is released from the vaginal passage, a recoil response occurs, causing a gasping intake of air into the lungs. The squeeze effect of vaginal delivery on the thorax is also instrumental in emptying the lung of about 25 ml of fetal lung liquid. This mechanism explains why the newborn infant typically requires gentle suctioning of the oral cavity to extract mucus and the lung liquid. The remaining lung liquid is absorbed by the pulmonary capillaries and lymphatics.

The vagus nerve also exerts control on respiration. Pulmonary stretch receptors located in the bronchioles stimulate the afferent pathways in the vagus nerve and stimulate expiration.

A reflex found only in the first weeks of life is Head's paradoxical reflex. This reflex may be an important force in the initiation of the first breath. When the trachea is inflated or distended with air, Head's reflex is stimulated, causing inflation of the alveoli. Neuronal transmission of this response is through the afferent paths of the vagus nerve. This reflex seems to lose its functional importance after infancy except during vigorous crying.[8]

Other reflex action helps to control respiratory rhythm by reacting to signals transmitted through the vagus nerve from stretch receptors located throughout the lungs in the walls of the bronchi and bronchioles.[5] When the lungs are inflated to maximal distention, the stretch receptors in the lungs are stimulated, activating exhalation. Conversely, a decrease in lung volume stimulates deeper inspiration. This automatic process is known as the *Hering-Breuer reflex,* and it is one of the body's protective mechanisms. Absence of this reflex, for example if the vagal nerve were severed, would produce slow, deep breathing, which may not be effective when more rapid respirations are needed, such as in the presence of increased metabolic or physical activity.

Finally, external environmental stimuli also activate respirations by stimulating the central nervous system generally. Noise, light, touch, and temperature in the delivery room are examples of stimuli that may positively affect the initiation of respirations.

While maturation of the respiratory system continues through the eighth year of life, the mechanics of air movement are established at the time of birth. Consequently, breathing is an almost unnoticeable function that becomes highly regarded when a pathologic condition exists. Without respiration, life obviously cannot be sustained.

Ventilation and Perfusion

At birth, it is estimated that the first breath requires 45 cm of water pressure for lung inflation to occur. Once the first breath is taken, the amount of pressure needed to effectuate respiration is only 5 cm of water pressure. The first respiration of the newborn infant inflates the pulmonary alveoli, dilates the pulmonary vessels, and establishes functional residual capacity (FRC, the amount of air left in the lung after expiration).

The first breath also leads to matching of ventilation to perfusion. Alveolar ventilation ($\dot{V}_A$) is the primary determinant of the rate at which oxygen is added and carbon dioxide is removed from the alveoli, the process of pulmonary gas distribution. Perfusion ($\dot{Q}$, capillary blood per minute) is the primary determinant of the rate at which oxygen is added to the pulmonary capillaries, the process of blood distribution in the lungs. Simply stated, ventilation and perfusion mean that for every 1 ml of air breathed in, 1 ml of blood is perfused with oxygen.

In reality, the structure of the lungs is such that $\dot{V}_A/\dot{Q}$ ratios vary between the apices and bases of the lungs. However, these variations are not pathologic. Clinically, situations may occur that significantly alter $\dot{V}_A/\dot{Q}$. Hyperventilation ($\uparrow\dot{V}_A$), for example, results in high PaO_2 and low $PaCO_2$. In hypoventilation, the opposite occurs.

High perfusion rates result in low PaO_2 and high $PaCO_2$. Rapid blood flow through the pulmonary vessels does not allow enough time for adequate diffusion of gases across the alveolar membrane to and from the alveolar capillaries. Conversely, low perfusion rates result in high PaO_2 and low $PaCO_2$.

Respiratory conditions that result in areas of pulmonary atelectasis can negatively affect $\dot{V}_A/\dot{Q}$. In this situation, areas of the lungs not being ventilated but still perfused will be reflected systemically as hypoxemia and hypercarbia ($PaO_2 \leq 50$ mmHg or $PaCO_2 \geq 45$ mmHg). In other conditions affecting perfusion but not ventilation, blood shunts from poorly perfused capillaries to normal ones. This condition, known as *intrapulmonary shunting,* also is reflected as hypoxemia and hypercarbia. More significantly, the amount of pulmonary dead space, areas not participating in gas exchange, increases. Thus alveoli that are ventilated but not perfused are dead spaces in the pulmonary system.

Regulation of Acid–Base Balance

Acid–base regulation is modulated through an interplay of the renal and respiratory systems. Cellular metabolism, enzyme reactions, and glycolysis, to name a few, are physiologic functions that are optimally performed in a somewhat alkaline medium with arterial *p*H ranging from 7.35 to 7.45. The renal system contributes to acid–base homeostasis through excretion or reabsorption of hydrogen (H^+) ions or bicarbonate (HCO_3^-) as needed.

By itself, the renal system is not an entirely efficient regulator of acid–base balance. The interaction of the respiratory system with the renal system is an important adjunct to acid–base homeostasis. Carbon dioxide (CO_2), when combined with HCO_3^- and H_2O, forms carbonic acid (H_2CO_3):

$$HCO_3^- + CO_2 + H_2O \rightarrow H_2CO_3 + HCO_3^-$$

The addition of the H_2CO_3 to the system can shift the balance of base to acid, making the system more acidic. This acid environment (*p*H <7.35) can impede physiologic function, especially at the cellular level.

The respiratory system regulates plasma CO_2 by way of alveolar ventilation. Hyperventilation in which CO_2 excretion is increased lowers $PaCO_2$, simultaneously reducing the number of CO_2 molecules available to combine with H_2O and HCO_3^- with a resultant increase in H_2CO_3. Alveolar excretion of CO_2 enhances renal excretion of H^+ and will reestablish a normal serum pH, thus acid–base balance.

Respiratory diseases or abnormalities negatively affect acid–base balance. Any condition in which alveolar ventilation is changed can result in acidosis or alkalosis. Therefore, the nurse needs to understand that asthma, croup, pulmonary atelectasis, aspirin poisoning, pneumonia, and the myriad of other conditions that directly or indirectly affect ventilation in children can manifest themselves in an acid–base disturbance.

Summary

Growth and development of the respiratory system begin soon after conception and continue into childhood. Prior to birth, the placenta manages the functions of ventilation and perfusion, but when respirations are established, these functions are assumed by the respiratory system. Understanding the development of the respiratory structures and the physiology of the respiratory system is essential for the accurate assessment of system functioning in the child.

References

1. Carlo, W. A., & Chatburn, R. L. (1988). *Neonatal respiratory care* (2nd ed.). Chicago: Year Book Medical Publishers.
2. Comroe, J. H. (1974). *Physiology of respiration* (2nd ed.). Chicago: Year Book Medical Publishers.
3. Dawes, G. S., Fox, H. E., Ledye, B. M., Liggins, G. C., & Richards, R. T. (1972). Respiratory movements and rapid eye movement sleep in the fetal lamb. *Journal of Physiology, 220,* 119–122.
4. Goodwin, J. W., Godden, J. O., & Chance, G. W. (1976). *Perinatal medicine: The basic science underlying clinical practice* (1st ed.). Baltimore: Williams & Wilkins.
5. Guyton, A. C. (1991). *Textbook of medical physiology* (8th ed.). Philadelphia: WB Saunders.
6. Liggins, G. C., & Howie, R. N. (1972). A controlled trial of an antepartum glucocorticoid treatment for prevention of the respiratory distress syndrome in premature infants. *Pediatrics, 50,* 515–518.
7. Moore, K. L. (1989). *Before we are born: Basic embryology and birth defects* (3rd ed.). Philadelphia: WB Saunders.
8. Slonin, N. B., & Hamilton, L. H. (1987). *Respiratory physiology* (5th ed.). St. Louis: CV Mosby.
9. Theibeault, D. W., & Gregory, G. A. (1986). *Neonatal pulmonary care* (4th ed.). Menlo Park, CA: Addison-Wesley.

Nursing Assessment and Diagnosis of Respiratory Function

BEHAVIORAL OBJECTIVES

Use functional health as a guideline for assessment of the child's respiratory system.

Describe the four components of the physical examination of the child's chest.

Identify deviations from normal findings of diagnostic tests of the respiratory system.

Describe the nursing responsibilities in caring for children who have procedures to diagnose or evaluate respiratory dysfunction.

Identify nursing diagnoses that are commonly used in the care of children with respiratory dysfunction.

Alterations of respiratory function are common problems in children from infancy through at least age 8 because development of the respiratory system is not complete until this age or thereafter. The respiratory system has an impact on other homeostatic mechanisms, including circulation, cellular metabolism, and gly-colysis; therefore, it is imperative that the nurse be adept at assessment of this system. No matter what the child's age, respiratory dysfunction can be reflected in other systemic manifestations, such as color (integumentary system), tachycardia or bradycardia (cardiac system), and level of consciousness (neurologic system).

Nursing Assessment

Because the child's respiratory compromise is the parents' primary concern, initial assessment begins with exploration of the reason for bringing the child to the health care provider or health care facility. The questions, "What?" "Where?" "When?" "Why?" and "How?" can be useful in obtaining medical information. For example, if the child's presenting problem is persistent cough, information may be obtained by asking questions similar to those presented in Table 37-1. Parents feel frustrated if initial questions focus on past events that may not seem relevant to the current problem.

Child and Family History

Nursing judgment is needed to determine when the broader base of historical information is best obtained. An exploration of the child's and family's response to aspects of the child's respiratory illness is, however, the basis for developing a plan of nursing care. The history may be organized around functional health.[8]

Health Perception and Health Management

The nurse interviewer begins with the mother's prenatal history and includes information that is known to have an impact on the developing fetus' respiratory system. Drugs taken by the mother in pregnancy, for example, can affect respiratory development. Infants whose mothers take heroin prenatally are at risk for having accelerated maturation of lung function, but they also may have arrested or delayed lung growth and subsequent retardation of height and weight due to insufficient oxygenation.

Important information about a woman's intrapartum course includes the infant's Apgar scores; whether resuscitation was required; presence of meconium in the amniotic fluid; and whether the infant was taken to the normal newborn nursery or to the neonatal intensive care unit. Problems that occur during the intrapartum period, which manifest as respiratory problems for the newborn, may have residual effects on the child later on.

The neonatal history focuses on any problems in the first 28 days of life that affected the respiratory system.

The newborn infant who had hyaline membrane disease complicated by chronic obstructive lung disease of the newborn (bronchopulmonary dysplasia) is prone to respiratory problems throughout childhood. This information is important in guiding the assessment of a child presenting with a respiratory disorder at a later date.

The history includes any medically managed or "home-remedy" managed respiratory problems prior to the onset of the current one. Questions focus on the usual course of the disease and the typical response to treatment. The nurse finds out if medications, prescribed or over-the-counter types, were taken or are being taken. Intervals between respiratory illnesses and whether hospitalization was required are important pieces of information. The nurse also inquires whether the child's immunizations are up-to-date because they offer protection against certain respiratory illnesses such as pertussis or diphtheria.

A complicated neonatal period will likely affect the parents' perception of their child's health in general. The parents of a child who had a respiratory problem at birth and recurrent respiratory illnesses during childhood may become overly protective of the child. Their perception might be that the child's lungs will never be "healthy." Therefore, they consider even minor upper respiratory infections a serious, life-threatening illness.

Nutrition and Metabolism

The assessment of the child's nutritional and metabolic status focuses on any food allergies or idiosyncrasies. Respiratory problems are sometimes associated with alterations in nutrition and allergies during childhood, because these frequently are precipitated by certain foods. If the child has an ongoing history of respiratory problems, its impact on the child's nutritional state is important information. For example, a disease such as cystic fibrosis affects both the respiratory and the gastrointestinal systems and thus has many manifestations of malnutrition. The child with severe asthma also may suffer nutritional deprivation due primarily to the stress of the respiratory compromise on the whole system.

Elimination

Children who suffer severe respiratory compromise due to illnesses affecting respiratory function often have elimination problems secondary to nutritional deficits. Frequently, upper respiratory infections are accompanied by gastritis. Has the child been vomiting? Does coughing stimulate vomiting? Gastrointestinal losses may further complicate respiratory disease-induced fluid and acid–base imbalances. The frequency, amount, consistency, and other unusual findings relative to defecation also must be questioned.

Activity and Exercise

Questioning the parents or, if appropriate, the child about normal exercise and activity patterns provides evidence of the effect of respiratory compromise on this function. Respiratory problems of a chronic nature, for example, can have a significant, negative impact on the

TABLE 37-1
Nursing Assessment: Questions for Assessing the Child When the Presenting Problem Is Persistent Cough

Areas of Assessment	Key Questions
What?	What is the nature of the cough? What makes it worse (activity, temperature, environment)? What makes it better (position change, humidity)? What does your child look like when coughing? What else happens during the coughing spell; is sputum produced; what color? Does blood or vomiting occur? What is your child like immediately afterward (tired, anxious, blue, gasping for air)? What does the cough sound like? What else accompanies the cough (fever, sweating)? What was your child's general state of health prior to the onset of the cough? What medicines is your child taking? What medicines do you usually give him or her when he or she is sick?
Where?	Where is your child most of the time when the coughing occurs (school, home)? Is the coughing painful, and where is the pain?
When?	When did the coughing start, and was it sudden in onset or gradual?
Why?	Why do you think your child has this cough?
How?	How do you think your child got this cough? How long has your child had this cough? How much does this cough interfere with your child's usual activities?

child's development, even causing developmental delays. A child with an acute respiratory disease, while not prone to developmental delay, may have interruption of normal activities of daily living. It is important to determine whether exercise is associated with respiratory distress. Should this child legitimately be excused from gym classes, for example, because the activities are too stressful to the respiratory system?

Sleep and Rest

The child with a racking cough at night eventually may suffer sleep deprivation syndrome if it is longstanding. This deficit may cause school-age children and adolescents to have difficulty concentrating in the classroom because they are perennially tired. The child's behavior may be construed by the teacher as apathy and inattentiveness. Rather than being understanding of the child's problem, the teacher may treat the child with disdain, which could negatively affect the child's self-esteem.

Cognition and Perception

Respiratory problems that cause decreased oxygenation can affect the child's behavioral or emotional state and may even affect cognitive and perceptual ability. Hypoxia or hypoxemia can cause irritability, drowsiness, and generalized fatigue. At times, emotional lability accompanies states of oxygen deprivation. It is important that the nurse ascertain the usual behavioral and emotional states of the child. This information will assist in determining the impact of the respiratory condition on the child's psychosocial integrity.

Oxygen deprivation of the brain, especially affecting the frontal areas (forebrain), can manifest itself in a short attention span or even confusion. This behavior may have a significant impact on the school-age child and adolescent child. The major activity of these age groups centers around school, where cognitive skills are imperative. Interruption of this ability can have far-reaching effects, such as feelings of inferiority or self-depreciation.

Self-Perception and Self-Concept

Assessment of the psychologic or behavioral domain often illuminates the child's self-perception. For the preschool and early school-age child, drawing pictures or playing with medical equipment generally aids in expressing ideas about the illness and its personal effect. The use of the Machover Draw-a-Person test can provide insight into the child's sense of body image and self-perception.

Determining what the child's developmental skills were before the illness and assessing what they are during the illness can assist the nurse in determining a child's self-concept. The use of pictures depicting health care delivery and asking the child to talk about them is useful in determining what the 10- to 13-year-old thinks about the illness. By adolescence, the child is usually able to respond to direct queries that are aimed at assessing self-perception. Does the child "see" himself or herself as a sick person or as a person with an illness that is only temporarily constraining?

Some children have personalities that make them more anxious than others. Respiratory compromise may exacerbate anxious feelings to the point of pathologic manifestations or worsening of the respiratory symptoms.

Role Relationship

Questioning regarding the child's social and personal history can clarify the effect of respiratory problems on role relations. Has the respiratory problem interfered with the child's social development or activity? Children with chronic respiratory conditions who have frequent hospitalizations or who miss many days of school are more likely to have delayed social development. The preadolescent in junior high and the adolescent in high-school are at the stage of development when social relations are being tested. Separation from peers and peer activities can have a devastating effect on social development that may be carried through to adulthood.

The nurse also assesses whether the child's respiratory illness has interfered with role relationships within the family. Do the parents believe that the other children in the family are being given less attention because of this ill child? Have usual family roles shifted due to the child's illness? How important are these changes? For example, has the mother had to quit working to care for this child, negatively affecting the family income and thus creating stress?

Sexuality and Reproduction

The sexuality and reproductive pattern of the child are assessed in general. For a more explicit delineation of this system, the reader is referred to Chapter 67. However, the nurse should be aware that certain diseases of the respiratory tract can negatively affect reproduction. Children with cystic fibrosis, for example, often are unable to have children due to infertility. This knowledge may be devastating to adolescents who foresee themselves as married and having a family later in life.

Coping and Stress Tolerance

Diseases of the respiratory system often can be exacerbated or ameliorated by how well the child copes with the stress of the illness. Anxiety provoked by the disease or its treatment may manifest itself in dyspnea, tachypnea, or episodes of hyperventilation beyond what is expected. Therefore, the nurse needs to gain insight into the child's typical responses to stress. Likewise, understanding the parents' strategies for handling problems associated with the child's illness is important.

Values and Beliefs

The nurse may explore the child's and parents' expectations for the child's future. What impact will the child's respiratory problems have on the ability to achieve those goals? Are spiritual values and beliefs or religious practices important in coping with the effects of the child's illness?

Other Information

The nurse obtains a family and genetic history as part of the information related to the history of this illness. The family history provides the nurse with information regarding communicable illnesses. Did a sibling develop chickenpox (varicella) within the last 7 days? Perhaps this child's respiratory symptoms are prodromal to the onset of the same disease. The nurse queries the parent regarding familial respiratory diseases, such as asthma. Did grandparents, the parents, siblings, or other significant family members have tuberculosis, pneumonia, or lung cancer? Have any other children in the family had respiratory problems, or did any of the children die due to a respiratory disease?

The family history includes questions regarding the environment of the home and neighborhood. Does anyone in the child's immediate family smoke? If this is an older child or adolescent, the nurse may determine if smoking has become a habit. Does the family live in a dense industrial area? Are toxic materials, such as furniture stripping or toxic cleaning solutions, frequently used in the home?

The genetic history determines the presence of any evidence of genetic faults or chromosomal abnormalities present in any generation beginning with the child's grandparents. Were any babies born in the family or past generations with conditions that could affect respiration? These conditions include diaphragmatic hernia, tracheoesophageal fistula, hypoplastic lungs, or neuromuscular diseases such as Duchenne's muscular dystropy.

Physical Examination

Before approaching the child for a physical examination, the parent or child is questioned about the effect of the respiratory condition on body systems. For example, questions regarding cardiac function and the effect

TABLE 37-2
Developmental Considerations in the Physical Examination of Respiratory Function

Technique	Infant	Child	Adolescent
Inspection	Chest round; Anteroposterior diameter = transverse diameter; Thoracic index (ratio of transverse diameter to anteroposterior diameter) is 1 at birth and 1.25 at 1 year of age; Smooth, rhythmic abdominal movements with breathing; Nose breathing expected.	Chest less round; anteroposterior diameter less than lateral diameter; Thoracic index 1.35 at 6 years of age; Abdominal movement with respirations common to about age 3, then more chest movement; By age 7, thoracic breathing dominant; Retractions and asymmetrical chest movements absent	Chest elliptical; lateral diameter two times greater than anteroposterior diameter; Chest and abdomen move in synchrony; bilateral symmetry of chest movement; Retractions and asymmetrical chest movements absent
Palpation	Depth of respirations: air felt on hand when placed near nose; Newborn—air felt at 2–3 in; older infant—air felt at 4–6 in; Respiratory excursions not palpated; Chest expands approximately 1.5 cm with inspiration; Tactile fremitus present if crying	Depth of respirations: Age 1–2—air felt at 5–6 in; Age 3–4—air felt at 8 in; age 5–6—air felt at 9 in; age 8–10—air felt at 10 in; Respiratory excursions equal on right and left sides; Tactile fremitus strongest over bronchi	Tenderness or masses absent; muscles firm, smooth, symmetrical; ribs aligned; Chest excursions equal bilaterally; Tactile fremitus strongest over bronchi
Percussion	Not done	Lungs slightly more resonant than in adolescents and adults	Resonance present; increased or decreased with respiratory dysfunction
Auscultation	Clear, loud bronchovesicular sounds; Fine rales common immediately after birth; May continue to be heard at the end of deep inspiration in normal newborns and older infants; As chest wall is thinner than adult, breath sounds are easily transmitted; Breath sounds may be difficult to hear unilaterally; Rarely are sounds absent; Sounds are diminished even with atelectases, effusion, empyema, and pneumothorax; Breath sounds may be diminished on the side of the chest opposite the direction in which the head is turned (positional); Wheezes are more common due to small airways	Breath sounds louder and harsher than in adults because stethoscope is closer to the origin of the sounds; Wheezes more common due to small airways	May differentiate vesicular, bronchial, and bronchovesicular sounds; Vocal fremitus—sounds loudest at upper and middle lobes along spinal column

of the respiratory illness on cardiac status are asked. "Do you feel like your heart is beating faster or wants to 'jump' out of your chest?" This might be an appropriate question to ask a 12-year-old. Changes in skin or lip color are questioned. Has the child had a fever with this illness? Has the child ever had a seizure either with this illness or with past respiratory problems?

A thorough history of the presenting problem, its effect on the child's function, a review of related information, and the impact of the illness on other systems of the body provides the foundation on which the actual physical examination is built. Information gleaned from these sources is beneficial to the nurse in guiding the examination and ultimately in correlating the physical findings with the historical information. No tool used in physical assessment can ever replace good skills acquired through the use of the nurse's senses. Thus, everything at the nurse's disposal is used and refined.

The examiner's sense of smell might identify an odor that is highly suspicious of certain diseases, such as the fruity, acetone breath of a diabetic. The eyes always should be roving and looking for the slightest deviation. A subtle elevation of the chest wall, a tinge of blue around the lips, a mouth partially open, or a slight but persistent flaring of the nares might suggest that there is some degree of respiratory compromise. Are there retractions with inspiration? Is the chest shape different from a well child's?

The nurse's ears should be sensitive to respiratory sounds that may be evident without the stethoscope. Do you hear the child wheezing? Are the respirations whistling? Are there unusual respiratory sounds with inspiration, expiration, or both?

The hands and fingers of the examiner need to develop sensitivity to vibrations transmitted through the chest wall. Touch also may reveal areas of tenderness on the chest or the presence of masses on the chest wall.

Ultimately the nurse uses all four techniques of examination: inspection, palpation, percussion, and auscultation. However, it is only in the last technique that any additional aid is used (the stethoscope) for data collection. Table 37-2 provides a summary of developmental considerations in examining the chest for respiratory function.

Prior to examination of the respiratory system, it is imperative that an environment that is not frightening or distressing to the child be established. Fear can significantly alter respirations and may inhibit an accurate assessment of the system. For a young child, it is sometimes helpful to let him or her explore the stethoscope, the nurse's "telephone," to ascertain that it will not cause pain. For any age patient, but especially the infant, warming the diaphragm of the stethoscope reduces the shock to the skin of a cold instrument. Babies typically do not like to be undressed and the cold stethoscope only serves to exacerbate their distress, altering respiratory rate and pattern and making precise assessment difficult. If an infant uses a pacifier for quieting behavior and if the respiratory distress is such that he or she can suck on one without respiratory difficulty, it is good to have such a device available. The nurse wants the child as quiet as possible when percussing and auscultating the lungs.

The school-age child and the adolescent have a greater need for privacy during a physical examination because the chest needs to be completely exposed. The pubescent girl with developing breasts will be concerned about modesty during the examination. The nurse provides an area that is free of interruption and in which care is given to respect the need for privacy in these age groups.

Examination of the respiratory system begins with assessing the child's vital signs. Because fever can directly affect respiratory rate, it is essential to determine if the child is normothermic, hyperthermic, or hypothermic. The heart rate is counted for a full minute. Aside from rate, the nurse ascertains the rhythm and quality of the heart rate. Are there rapid or skipped beats interspersed within the normal heart beats? Is this the result of oxygen deficit? What is the child's respiratory rate? Is there tachypnea, dyspnea, orthopnea, or irregular respirations? See inside front cover for normal respiratory rates.

Barness suggests that the depth of respirations be examined when the child is sitting and then again when the child is supine.[2] Decreased depth of respirations requires that the examiner's hand be closer than normal to the child's nose. In contrast, increased respiratory depth is evidenced by feeling air at a distance greater than normal.

Height and weight are assessed to determine if there has been any alteration in growth due to the respiratory illness. Children often lose weight with an acute respiratory disease such as croup. This loss typically reflects water lost through respiration and interruption of normal eating habits. Children with chronic respiratory conditions, however, may experience growth delays that are evidenced in the height and weight curves.

The blood pressure is measured. Variations around the norm of the blood pressure in children with a respiratory illness typically are due to problems of water loss (dehydration) that often accompany respiratory problems.

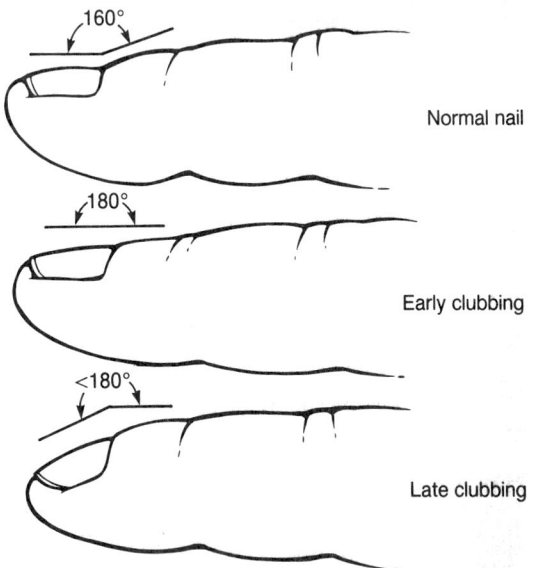

FIGURE 37-1

Clubbing of nails. Normal nail has approximately 160° angle between nail and nail base. In early clubbing, the angle between the nail and nail base is almost 180°. In late clubbing, the nail base is obviously swollen and the angle between nail and nail base is less than 180°.

TABLE 37-3
Abnormalities of Chest Contour

Abnormality	Description	
Barrel chest (normal in infancy)	The anteroposterior diameter is about equal; typically seen in chronic obstructive lung disease, such as severe asthma or cystic fibrosis	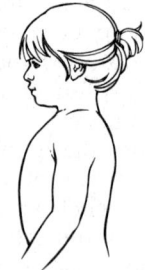
Pigeon chest (pectus carinatum)	The sternum juts anteriorly and the chest looks like that of a chicken	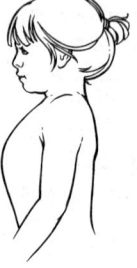
Funnel chest (pectus excavatum)	The sternum points posteriorly; may cause abnormal pressure on the heart, affecting function. In early infancy, funnel chest may result in midline sternal retractions.	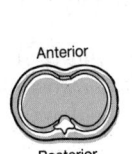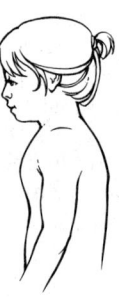
Lumbosacral deformities (kyphosis and scoliosis)	May cause limitation of lung capacity or expansion	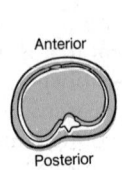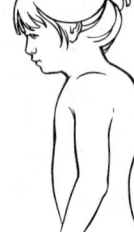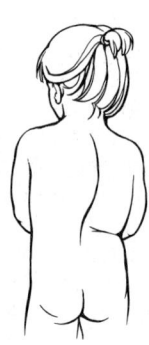
Enlargement of costochondral junctions (rachitic rosary)	Blunt, knobby, prominences that develop in the presence of long-term Vitamin D deficiency (rickets); beading of ribs may be visible and palpable; may be associated pigeon chest	

Table text adapted from Block, G., Nolan, J. (1986). Health assessment for professional nursing (2nd ed.). Norwalk, CT: Appleton-Century Crofts. Original art.

Inspection

In evaluating the respiratory system, the skin is inspected for any evidence of pallor or cyanosis. Infants and children may have a bluish, mottled appearance, which is more a reaction to environmental temperature than to oxygen deficit. To obtain a more accurate indication of central oxygenation, the oral mucosa should be inspected. A bluish tinge of the oral mucosa suggests an oxygen deficit. Cyanosis of the thoracic skin also may indicate severe hypoxia.

The nail beds are inspected for cyanosis or clubbing of the fingers and toes (Fig. 37-1). These signs typically are seen in children who have either a heart lesion, which causes cyanosis, or a long-standing respiratory problem. Pathophysiologic changes that occur in the fingers and toes as a result of chronic hypoxemia are described in Chapter 39.

The face is inspected for evidence of respiratory embarrassment. Flaring of the external nares typically is associated with respiratory distress. A drawn, tired appearance or at times a panicked look very often evidenced by raised eyebrows reflects the impact of respiratory compromise on the child's affectual well-being. Head movement and the position of the head and neck also are noted. Children in respiratory distress often will position themselves upright, with their jaw thrust forward. Noting whether the child is breathing through the nose or the mouth is important; nose breathing is typical. Mouth breathing is due to a variety of reasons, including nasal obstruction and swollen adenoids.

The thorax is inspected for configuration, contour, symmetry, and abnormalities.[7] Using the nipple line as a guide, the chest circumference is measured and recorded. The anterior–posterior diameter of the chest is compared to its lateral diameter. In the infant, these two measures are equal, a 1:1 ratio. By the time the child is 6 years old, the ratio of the anterior–posterior diameter to the lateral diameter is 1:2, the same as the adult's.[5] Changes in the ratio indicate pulmonary problems.

The chest is inspected for deformities. A prominent sternum that juts out anteriorly (pectus carinatum) or a sternum that is cavitated (pectus excavatum) may compromise lung expansion. Table 37-3 further explains abnormalities of chest contour.

Abnormal respiratory movements of the chest are noted. Are there retractions with inspiration, expiration, or both? Where are the retractions? Are they suprasternal, substernal, intercostal, subcostal, or supraclavicular (Fig. 37-2)? Retractions are due to the increased use of the accessory muscles of respiration. When airway obstruction is present, whether in the bronchi or alveolar ducts, the child uses the accessory muscles to assist with the normal respiratory mechanisms available. This is a compensatory measure used to exert greater force in inhaling, exhaling, or both. In young infants, slight head bobbing may be noted with each breath. This movement often indicates impending respiratory failure and is noticeable with the head supported on the caregiver's arm at the suboccipital area. This movement is caused by contraction of the scalene and sternocleidomastoid muscles, accessory muscles of respiration.

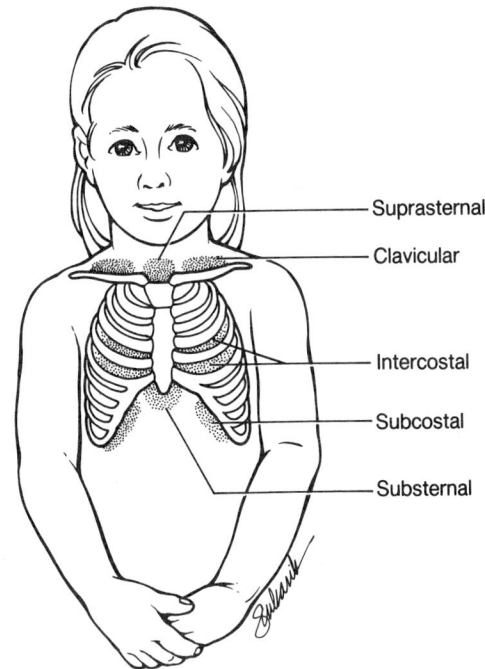

FIGURE 37-2
Areas where retractions are found in abnormal respiratory movements.

Finally, the overall movement of the chest is noted. Thoracic movement should be symmetrical bilaterally. Diminished or absent movement on one side may be evidence of respiratory obstruction, pneumonia, or a pneumothorax. Infants and children up to 7 years of age typically use the diaphragm for breathing, creating noticeable abdominal movement, rather than chest movement, with inspiration and expiration. Thus, with inspiration, the abdomen rises, and it falls with expiration. After 7 years of age, the abdomen and chest move together. Therefore, persistence of abdominal breathing in an older child may be due to a fractured rib or a respiratory illness.

The inspiratory time is evaluated in relation to expiratory time (I:E ratio) during a respiration cycle. The I:E ratio should be equal. However, in children with respiratory disorders, asthma for example, the expiratory phase is longer than the inspiratory phase. This compensatory mechanism is established to increase the length of time that inspired air remains in the alveoli. This facilitates both gas exchange and the functional residual capacity (FRC). Table 37-4 further identifies abnormal respiratory patterns.

Palpation

Palpation is performed with the palms and fingertips of the examiner's hands. To minimize discomfort for the child, the nurse should palpate with warm hands. The purpose of palpation is to detect any abnormalities of the chest, such as areas of swelling or tenderness, abnormal chest movements, and the presence or absence of vibrations (fremitus).[1]

Palpation for swelling or tenderness is performed with firm but light pressure. The examiner begins at the shoulders and moves the hands over all quadrants of

TABLE 37-4
Description of Abnormal Respiratory Patterns

Irregularities	Description
Tachypnea	Rapid superficial breathing rate is age dependent. In an infant or child of any age, respiratory rate of more than 60 signifies respiratory distress.
Bradypnea	Slow, deep breathing rate is age dependent. An infant or child who has been tachypneic but whose respiratory rate suddenly slows even to a rate normal for age should be evaluated for respiratory failure.
Apnea	Cessation of breathing in infants is of concern if it lasts longer than 20 seconds.
Hyperventilation	Fast, deep, and constant breathing: offsets O_2–CO_2 balance, causing dizziness, etc. Often it is a stress-related reaction.
Kussmaul's	Deeper than normal respiration; often seen in acidosis.
Cheyne-Stokes	Often in a critically ill patient; regular episodes of apnea occur within a regular breathing pattern.
Stertorous breathing	Rattly, snoring type of respiration; often heard in the terminal states.
Dyspnea	A subjective complaint of difficulty in breathing. In infants and children, frequently accompanied by retractions, nasal flaring, raised eyebrows, and head bobbing.
Orthopnea	A subjective complaint; air gets "stuffy" when child is sleeping, and he or she feels a need to sit up or sleep on extra pillows. Infants and young children may exhibit restlessness and irritability when placed in a horizontal position.

Adapted from Block, G., & Nolan, J. (1986). Health assessment for professional nursing (2nd ed.). Norwalk, CT: Appleton-Century Crofts.

the chest anteriorly, laterally, and posteriorly (Fig. 37-3). The hands remain in continuous contact with the chest, pausing at various points to apply firm, gentle pressure while noting the child's response. Palpation of areas of obvious swelling is done gently, noting the texture, temperature, and tenderness of the swelling. Tenderness along the ribs, the rib junctions (costochondral junctions), and the intercostal muscles is noted. A significant number of diseases can be manifested by thoracic tenderness. Leukemia, for example, often is associated with sternal tenderness.[1]

The intercostal spaces are palpated to determine whether the intercostal muscles are being used to assist breathing. If the movement of the rib interspaces feels excessive, the child may be having difficulty with air exchange. Decreased movement of the intercostal muscles causes suspicion of decreased respiratory activity or, in the worst case, paralysis of the intercostal muscles.

The nurse determines the equality of chest excursion by palpation. With the hands placed on either side of the spinal column at the 10th rib with thumbs touching in the midline, the child is instructed to take a slow, deep breath. With chest movement during inhalation, the examiner's hands should be displaced upward and away from the spinal column, causing slight separation of the thumbs. The nurse observes for equality of hand displacement. The movement of only one hand, for example,

indicates some respiratory compromise to the side not displaced.

Assessment of chest excursion is eliminated in the infant; however, the chest circumference may be measured at the level of the fourth intercostal space. In addition, the difference in chest circumference at inhalation and at exhalation may be used to ascertain if adequate excursion is taking place. Normally, there is approximately a 1.5 cm difference between the two measures.

With the palmar surfaces of the examiner's hand placed on the posterior chest, the presence or absence of vocal vibrations is noted. These vibrations, termed tactile fremitus, are palpated while the child repeats in a normal voice the number "99." This procedure is performed unilaterally; that is, the examiner's hand is placed at the top of the thorax to the right of the spinal column. When vibrations are felt, the hand is moved directly across to the left side. Using this zig-zag procedure, tactile fremitus is systematically evaluated from the top to the bottom of the posterior rib cage.

Tactile fremitus is normally strongest at the junction of the major bronchi and over the secondary bronchi but softer over the lower lung lobe segments. The presence or absence of tactile fremitus and the symmetry of intensity from side to side are noted. This procedure provides a gross examination for abnormality and is at least indicative of either fluid or consolidation in a lung segment. When palpating fremitus over fluid, the transmission of the vibration is decreased because fluid is a poor conductor. In contrast, tactile fremitus is increased over areas of consolidation. This examination can be performed in an infant if he or she is crying, but it is omitted in a quiet, nonvocalizing infant.

Percussion

The third phase of the chest examination is percussion. With the child either sitting or lying, the nurse places the long, middle finger of one hand firmly on the child's chest in an intercostal space; the palm and other fingers of the hand should be raised and not in contact with the chest. Using the middle or index finger of the other hand, the nurse uses the free hand to tap on the distal, interphalangeal joint of the finger that is in contact with the chest. The tapping hand is moved in a loose, striking fashion, keeping the wrist action fluid.

Chest percussion is performed to determine changes in tympany or resonance. If a lung segment is fluid filled or airless, the percussion sound is dull. Percussion over areas of consolidation or over a bony area such as the scapula elicits a flat sound (Table 37-5). Percussion notes on one side of the chest should be compared with sound produced in the same area on the opposite side.

Percussion of the posterior chest begins in the suprascapular area and extends to the 10th rib. Anteriorly, percussion starts at the infraclavicular space and extends midclavicularly to the 10th rib. Lateral percussion begins at the axillary line and extends to the eighth rib (see Fig. 37-3). This procedure generally is deferred from birth through 18 months of age because the information yielded at this age is not always reliable.

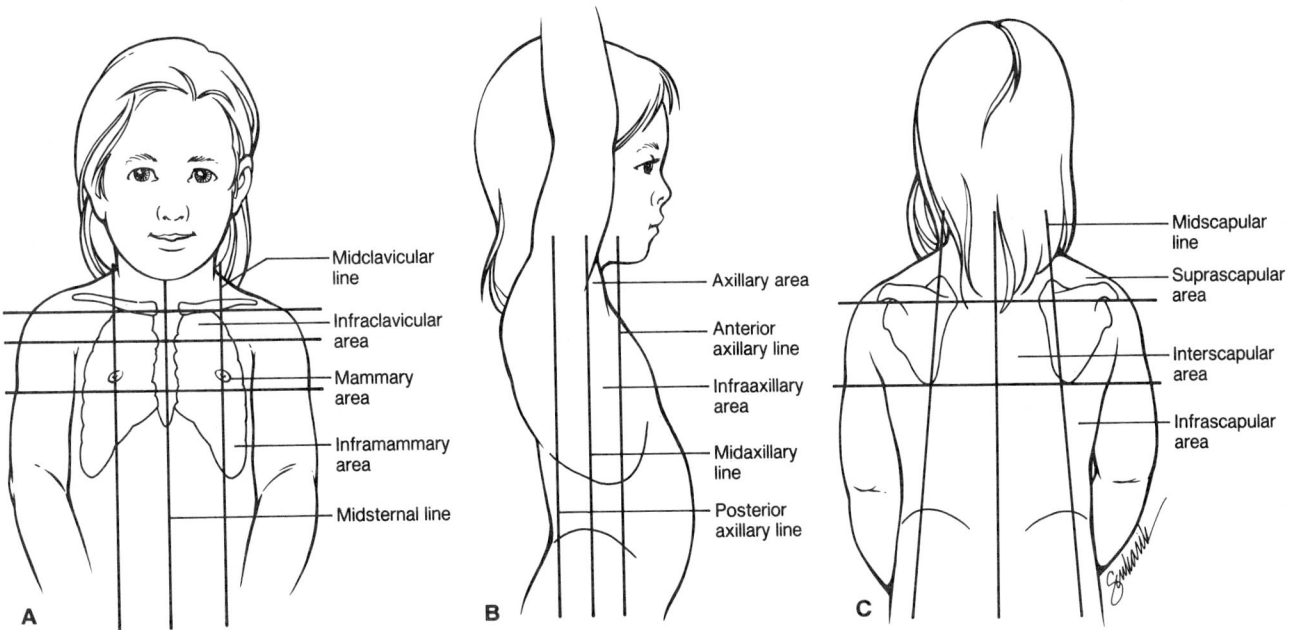

FIGURE 37-3
Areas of the chest used for percussion and auscultation. The examination is made anteriorly, laterally, and posteriorly.

Detection of a dull sound is expected when percussing over the left chest in the mammary area, from the midsternal line to the midclavicular line. This is because the examiner is tapping directly over the heart in a normal child. Likewise, dull sound is expected on the right chest wall in the midclavicular region from the 10th rib to the 8th rib because of the presence of the liver. Conversely, a noticeable resonant, tympanic sound may be elicited over the inframammary area in the left chest due to percussion over the empty stomach.

Auscultation

To eliminate any extraneous noise interference, the chest is auscultated without any clothing between the thoracic surface and the stethoscope. In the preschool-age child through adolescence, auscultation of the chest is best performed with the child in a sitting position, al-though supine is acceptable. During infancy, the nurse does well to auscultate the chest when the child is quiet; consideration of position is secondary. Placing the young child in a parent's arms often helps to quiet the child and allay anxiety while auscultating. Finally, the bell portion of the stethoscope head is used to isolate sound in an infant's chest, but the diaphragm of the stethoscope may be used for the child 18-months-old through adolescence. An infant stethoscope also may be used for infants younger than 18 months.

Information obtained from auscultation of the lungs is related to presence of normal, altered, or absent breath sounds. During normal respiration, the examiner should be able to distinguish among three types of breath sounds: bronchial, vesicular, and bronchovesicular. Table 37-6 describes and illustrates these breath sounds.

Breath sounds that are altered or added to normal sounds are called adventitious sounds, and these noises

TABLE 37-5
Percussion Notes and Their Characteristics

	Relative Intensity	Relative Pitch	Relative Duration	Example of Location
Flatness	Soft	High	Short	Thigh
Dullness	Medium	Medium	Medium	Liver
Resonance	Loud	Low	Long	Normal lung
Hyper-resonance	Very loud	Lower	Longer	Emphysematous lung
Tympany	Loud	High*	*	Gastric air bubble or puffed-out cheek

* Distinguished mainly by its musical timbre.
From Bates, B. (1991). A guide to physical examination (5th ed.). Philadelphia: JB Lippincott.

TABLE 37-6
Normal Breath Sounds

Sound	Relationship of Inspiration to Expiration	Diagram of Sound	Location	
			Normal	Abnormal
Vesicular	Inspiration > expiration	Inspiration Expiration	Throughout lung field	None
Bronchovesicular	Inspiration = expiration	Inspiration Expiration	First or second intercostal space, level of bifurcation of trachea	Peripheral lung
Bronchotubular	Inspiration < expiration	Inspiration Expiration	Over trachea	Lung area

Adapted from Fuller, J., & Schaller-Ayers, J. (1990). Health assessment. Philadelphia: JB Lippincott.

frequently are heard in a child with a respiratory problem. Adventitious sounds are described by the terms crackles, wheezes, rhonchi, and friction rub. Although these terms and others (including rales) have been used for many decades, their use is not standardized.[10,11] Novice practitioners may therefore need assistance in accurately describing what they hear on auscultation of the lungs. These sounds are described in Table 37-7. Neonates and infants also may make a "grunting" sound on expiration. This noise is made by air being forced against closed vocal cords and occurs in an attempt to keep small airways open.

When respiratory compromise is suspected, the nurse auscultates for vocal fremitus. The technique for this procedure is the same as that used for tactile fremitus except that a stethoscope is used. The child who is able to co-operate is instructed to say the number "99" or a word such as "Tennessee." Chest sounds are auscultated while the child speaks and should be loudest at the upper and middle lobes along the spinal column.

Bronchophony is an abnormal sound characterized by increased resonance. Thus, as the child repeats "99," the sound is very clear and intense. This finding in the presence of others, such as tactile fremitus and dull percussion, usually indicates a consolidation in the underlying area of the lung.

Another finding with consolidation is the presence of *egophony*. In this voice sound, the word that the patient repeats has a bleating quality to it. The examiner asks the child to repeat the word "Tennessee." When heard through the stethoscope the "EE" at the end of Tennessee will sound like a long "A."

TABLE 37-7
Adventitious Breath Sounds

Sound	Description	Cause
Discontinuous sounds (crackles)	Intermittent, nonmusical sounds	
Fine crackles	Soft, high-pitched, and very brief (5–10 msec)	Tiny explosions occur when small airways, deflated during expiration, pop open during inspiration
Coarse crackles	Somewhat louder, lower in pitch, and not quite so brief (20–30 msec)	Air bubbles flow through secretions or lightly closed airways during respiration.
Continuous sounds	Last notably longer than crackles (>250 msec) but do not necessarily persist throughout the respiratory cycle. Their musical quality distinguishes them from breath sounds.	
Wheezes	Relatively high-pitched with a hissing or shrill quality.	Wheezes and rhonchi are thought to occur when air flows rapidly through bronchi that are narrowed nearly to the point of closure. They often are audible at the mouth as well as through the chest wall.
Rhonchi	Relatively low-pitched with a snoring quality	
Pleural rub	Creaking, grating sounds that may be heard during both inspiration and expiration	When pleural surfaces become inflamed, they move jerkily as they are momentarily and repeatedly delayed by increased friction.
Stridor	A wheeze that is heard predominantly on inspiration; louder in the neck than over the chest wall	Indicates a partial obstruction of the airway in the neck (e.g., in the larynx or trachea).

Adapted from Bates, B. (1991). A guide to physical examination and history taking (5th ed.). Philadelphia: JB Lippincott.

The last test performed that always indicates consolidation is whispered *pectoriloquy*. The patient is asked to whisper "99." Because consolidated areas transmit noises better than fluid or air-filled areas, the sound heard by the examiner is very distinct, despite the patient's whispering.

The child's respiratory system can be affected by a variety of acute and chronic conditions. Viral infections such as chickenpox, genetic illnesses such as cystic fibrosis, and upper respiratory infections such as pneumonia can result in a wide range of dysfunction, from minor respiratory compromise to profound compromise. Skill in assessment of the respiratory system is needed to identify deviations from normal.

Diagnostic Tests

A number of diagnostic tests can be administered to confirm the presence or absence of a respiratory problem. Some of these are limited because of the age and ability of the child to follow directions and perform the test.

Laboratory Tests

Laboratory examination of blood specimens for *complete blood count* is appropriate when a child is admitted with a respiratory illness. Increases in hemoglobin and hematocrit in children with chronic respiratory diseases are common owing to a compensatory polycythemia. The body "thinks" that by increasing the number of red blood cells, more hemoglobin will be saturated with oxygen and oxygenation will improve. In contrast, low hemoglobin and hematocrit is diagnostic of anemia, which may affect respiratory function adversely by reducing the oxygen-carrying capacity of the blood. Leukocyte counts and white cell count differentials are routinely performed to ascertain the presence of an acute pulmonary infection. Children prone to allergies that manifest themselves as respiratory conditions are likely to have elevated eosinophils. Normal values of the blood components for children may be reviewed in Appendix A. The blood specimen also may be analyzed for *serum immunoglobulin levels*. Immunodeficiency diseases may cause recurrent respiratory infections and are diagnosed by analysis of serum immunoglobin levels (see Appendix A).

An analysis of *blood gases* often is needed in the presence of respiratory dysfunction to assess the child's oxygenation status and acid–base balance. This procedure and the required nursing care are described at the end of this section. Chapter 20 should be consulted for a review of normal values. Oxygenation status of the blood also may be monitored noninvasively using oximetry, which provides continuous measurement of hemoglobin saturation. Transcutaneous monitoring, which provides reliable information about trends of oxygen and carbon dioxide levels.

An order for *sputum collection* is common when a child has respiratory dysfunction. Obtaining the sputum specimen is not possible until the child is able to cough productively, about age 4. Unfortunately, an older child often refuses to expectorate sputum, and thus it may not be possible to carry out the order. For an infant or child suspected of having respiratory syncinctial virus, a *viral culture* may be performed with a specimen obtained from a nasopharyngeal swab or washing.

A *tuberculin skin test* may be required if the child has a history of contact with someone actively infected with the tubercle bacillus, but all children should be tested at 1 year of age and every 1 to 2 years thereafter. The procedure for tuberculosis testing is described in Chapter 9.

For a child suspected of having cystic fibrosis, a *sweat chloride test* may be performed.

Arterial Blood Sample

Description/Definition
Arterial blood sample is the most reliable index of ventilation and acid–base status.

Purpose
Arterial blood sample permits the analysis of actual oxygenation, carbon-dioxide retention, and loss of acid or base versus gain of acid or base by the blood buffer system. Such information provides the basis for making clinical decisions relative to administering (or not administering) oxygen, providing artificial ventilation, or administering (or not administering) bicarbonate.

Indications
- Respiratory embarrassment
- Respiratory obstruction
- Cyanosis
- Oxygen therapy
- Artificial ventilation
- Shock

Contraindications
None.

Preparation
A small infant should be positioned and held gently but firmly in an appropriate body alignment to obtain a sample from the temporal artery or the radial artery. In older infants and children, a local infiltration of 1% lidocaine over the brachial, radial, or femoral arteries is done to prevent unnecessary trauma to the puncture site. A heparinized syringe to prevent clotting of the blood should be used. A small basin of ice should be prepared to place the syringe with the blood sample. At least 2.5 ml of blood are needed to perform the analysis. The sample needs to be kept chilled to arrest metabolic reactions in the blood, including reactions that use oxygen. Therefore, the oxygen will remain stable, and the test results will accurately reflect the patient's ventilatory status and acid–base balance.

Developmental Considerations
None.

Nursing Implications
The nurse assists with drawing the arterial sample. Equipment should be ready and accessible to the phlebotomist. Care should be taken to avoid getting any air bubbles in the syringe after the sample is drawn because this can alter the test results. After the blood is drawn, the nurse applies firm pressure to the puncture site for 5 minutes to prevent hematoma or bleeding from the artery. Once it is assured that the puncture area is not bleeding a Band-Aid can be applied to the area. The nurse must keep in mind that handling blood products requires universal precautions to prevent any contamination to himself or herself or others.

Prior to drawing the blood sample, the nurse ascertains that the patient is quiet and not distressed. Allen's test needs to be performed and results documented if the radial artery is used. To perform the Allen's test, both the radial and ulnar arteries are compressed while the hand is elevated. Blanching of the hand will occur. Compression over the ulnar artery is released while pressure continues to be held on the radial artery. Hand color will return to normal if adequate collateral circulation is present.

Avoid any procedures that would tax the patient's respiratory system, such as postural drainage or suctioning, for at least 20 minutes prior to taking the arterial sample. Increased activity or stress can lower oxygenation and alter the outcome of the test. Finally, if changes in oxygen concentration delivered to the patient have been made, a sample of blood for gas analysis should not be drawn for at least 20 minutes.

Complications

- Hematoma of the sample site
- Oozing of blood from the sample site
- Anemia, especially in infants, from too frequent drawing of blood without replacement
- Infection of the sample site

Sweat Chloride Test

Description/Definition

The sweat chloride test is also known as the pilocarpine iontophoresis sweat test. The production of sweat is stimulated for chemical analysis of its chloride content. To conduct the procedure, an area on the forearm is washed with distilled water and dried. A small gauze square soaked with pilocarpine nitrate is laid on the untouched skin and an electrical lead (similar to an electrocardiogram lead) is placed over the gauze. A special, battery-operated machine delivers 2.5 amps of current onto the area, causing the pilocarpine to vibrate into the skin and begin simulating the production of sweat. After 5 minutes of stimulation, the electrode is removed and the reddened site is washed twice with distilled water. A piece of sterile filter paper or gauze (obtained from the laboratory) is removed immediately from the bottle with forceps and placed on the stimulated site. A square of plastic slightly larger than the gauze is fixed over the site with waterproof tape. The arm is then wrapped several times in plastic, and an elastic bandage holds everything in place. After 1 hour, the top dressings are removed, the gauze square next to the skin is quickly removed with forceps and carefully placed in the sterile bottle. The specimen is then taken to the laboratory for weight and analysis.

Purpose

This procedure is the best diagnostic test for cystic fibrosis, although other conditions may be associated with elevated concentrations of sweat electrolytes. However, most other conditions can be distinguished from cystic fibrosis by clinical manifestations of the disease. More than 60 mEq/L of chloride found in the sweat of children and adolescents is diagnostic of cystic fibrosis when one or more other criteria are present. However, values between 40 and 60 mEq/L are considered suggestive of the disease.[4]

Indications

- Chronic or productive cough
- Recurrent pneumonia or bronchiolitis
- Atelectasis
- Hemoptysis
- Infection with *Pseudomonas*
- *Staphylococcal pneumonia*

Contraindications

This test requires care and accuracy and is ideally done in a medical center in which the test is performed regularly by personnel familiar with the procedure.

Preparation

The procedure is explained to the parents and child in terms they understand. A nurse specialist or technician usually conducts the test without assistance, but the nurse's presence can be reassuring to the child and family. The skin of the test site cannot be touched while the procedure is being performed, because electrolytes inadvertently may be deposited on the site. The child's caregiver or nurse should have toys, books, or other articles ready so that the young child may be distracted during the short period of time that the site is being prepared. Older children may cooperate readily with age-appropriate explanations.

Developmental Considerations

The thigh may be used in very small infants to obtain enough sweat, but results may be unreliable because of their low production rates during the first few weeks of life.

Nursing Implications

The parents and child are assured that no pain is associated with the test, although the small test site may feel strange, as if the area has been "asleep" and is "waking up" while the current is flowing into the skin. Advocacy for the parent and child in obtaining adequate information about the test, its purpose, and the findings is essential. During the 1-hour wait for adequate sweat to form at the test site, the child should be dressed very warmly to encourage perspiration. A cap and sweater may be worn. Infants and young children may be wrapped in blankets and held closely by the caregivers to provide body heat. Older children may be encouraged to play outside in warm, humid weather. Fluids are encouraged to further enhance production of perspiration.

Complications

If more than 2.5 amps of electrical current are applied, a very small local skin burn may result. At least .1 g of sweat is needed for the test, but larger amounts are preferred to insure accuracy in the analysis. If inadequate amounts are produced, the test may need to be repeated, leaving the skin wrapped for several hours.

Sputum Collection/Tracheal Aspiration

Description/Definition

Sputum or tracheal aspirate is collected for laboratory analysis for the presence of bacteria or virus.

Purpose

Sputum can be used for a variety of tests, including cultures to diagnose bacterial infections, fungal diseases, presence of acid-fast bacilli, and anaerobic bacilli. When organisms are cultured, sensitivity to antibiotics may be determined. Sputum also can be used for cytologic studies to determine the presence or absence of malignant cells.

Indications

- Signs or symptoms of infectious processes, including elevated temperature, elevated white blood cell count, and signs and symptoms of respiratory distress.

Contraindications

None.

Preparation

Instruct the child and parents appropriately. In tracheal aspiration or when an uncooperative child requires suctioning to produce a specimen, restraints may be required to complete the procedure.

Developmental Considerations

Provide age-appropriate explanations. Older children's cooperation may be elicited.

Nursing Implications

Observe the child for increasing signs of respiratory distress if crying or protesting during the procedure. Also note the position of comfort for the child. If tracheal aspiration suctioning is required and respiratory distress is severe, the child may not tolerate the supine position.

Complications

None.

Procedures

Four types of diagnostic procedures may be used to evaluate respiratory problems in children: pulmonary function tests, radiologic examinations, endoscopies, and biopsies.

Pulmonary Function Tests

Description/Definition

Various types of lung function tests are performed to determine whether ventilation:perfusion ratios are normal, to assess lung volume, and to determine if airway obstruction exists. The more simple lung function tests include the following:

- Tidal volume—volume of air inhaled and exhaled during one normal respiratory cycle
- Vital capacity—maximum volume of air that can be forced from the lungs following maximum inspiration
- Functional residual capacity—volume of air remaining in the lungs following normal expiration
- Residual volume—volume of air remaining in the lungs following maximum exhalation
- Forced expiratory volume in 1 or 3 seconds—volume of air that can be forced from the lungs after maximum inspiration in 1 and 3 seconds

Purpose

Pulmonary lung function tests are done primarily to identify diseases that may cause a disturbance of lung function or that affect the mechanics of breathing.

Indications

- Hypoventilation
- Hypoxemia
- Hypercarbia
- Ventilator dependency

Contraindications

Unconscious patient.

Preparation

Instruct the child and parents appropriately. Some tests require that the nose be clamped; the child is assured that breathing will be possible despite this restriction. There are no restrictions relative to food intake; however, the pulmonary function tests should not be performed immediately after the child has eaten because vomiting may occur secondary to the coughing that the tests may stimulate.

Developmental Considerations

No developmental considerations exist relative to the actual performance of the test. However, older children can follow instructions.

Nursing Implications

It is important that the child be kept calm during the procedure because undue stress or anxiety may alter the test results.

Complications

None.

Radiologic Examinations

- Chest x-ray
- Fluoroscopy
- Bronchography

Description/Definition

Radiography (x-ray) enables visualization of the bony structures of the chest, lungs, major airways, and chest wall. Placing the child in various positions for x-rays enables the physician to see the shape of the airways.

Fluoroscopy produces radiographic images that can be seen on a television monitor, and it is used to evaluate regional ventilation and excursion of the diaphragm. Fluoroscopy also may be used during a barium swallow to diagnose the cause of choking, apnea, or color changes during feedings.

Bronchography is performed by instillation of a radiopaque material into the trachea and bronchi. The procedure is done under general anesthesia and is rarely indicated in children.

Purpose

X-ray with or without contrast material is useful for the diagnosis and location of obstruction or abnormality in the airway.

Indications

- Obstruction below an area that can be visualized by laryngoscope or bronchoscope

Contraindications

- Severe obstructive airway disease (fluoroscopy, bronchography)
- Allergy to iodine solutions (bronchography)

Preparation

No preparation is required for a simple chest x-ray or fluoroscopy except an explanation of the procedure. If a barium swallow is performed during the fluoroscopy, the child is fed or drinks the barium mixture.

The use of contrast media requires that the child be anesthetized. The same preparation for anesthesia for a respiratory procedure as delineated for bronchoscopy is applicable in this situation. Parental consent for the procedure should be obtained. The procedure should be explained to the parents and the child using age-appropriate methods.

Developmental Considerations

None.

Nursing Implications

Following the bronchography, the child should be monitored closely for any airway obstruction. The dye used for contrast is an aqueous solution of propyliodine, which is thick so that it will cling to the airway walls. Excess amounts of the solution can lead to respiratory distress. The use of anesthesia may inhibit the cough reflex, which may not return for some time after the procedure, necessitating suctioning and proper positioning of the child to prevent aspiration. Vital signs for a child recovering from anesthesia as described for bronchoscopy should be taken and recorded. Encouraging frequent oral intake of fluids when postanesthesia recovery is complete is important to maintain loose secretions that are easily expectorated or suctioned.

Complications

- Postprocedure aspiration
- Temporary suppression of cough and swallow reflex
- Allergic reaction to iodine-based contrast media

Endoscopies for Pulmonary Assessment

- Laryngoscopy
- Bronchoscopy

Description/Definition

Laryngoscopy is the visualization of the upper airway by means of a lighted laryngoscope.

Bronchoscopy is the visualization of the trachea, mainstem bronchi, and secondary bronchi by means of a lighted flexible scope.

Laryngoscopy is the least invasive of the two procedures and is done with relative ease even in small infants. It is an essential procedure when upper airway obstruction due to a foreign object is suspected. Laryngoscopy can be performed using a light sedative to quiet the child and a topical anesthetic if deemed necessary. The procedure is basically the same as that for insertion of an endotracheal tube.

Bronchoscopy is a more traumatic procedure physically and emotionally for a child. Following bronchoscopy, there is a tendency for airway mucous secretions to increase, which may add to any obstructive process already present. The use of atropine as a premedication aids in reducing mucous accumulation as well as serving to relax the smooth muscles of the bronchi. Bronchoscopy in children is done under general anesthesia and requires considerable skill.

Purpose

Laryngoscopy and bronchoscopy permit direct visualization of the upper ,airways which can aid in diagnosing the cause of obstruction. It is also useful for aspiration of thick, tenacious mucus; for harvesting of secretions for culture and histologic examination; and with bronchoscopy, for sampling of airway tissue for microscopic examination.[9]

Indications

- Foreign bodies or aspirates in upper airways
- Histologic studies

Contraindications

Bronchoscopy is best avoided in infants and young children.

Preparation

Obtain parental consent for procedures. Using age-appropriate techniques, the procedure should be explained to the child and the parents. The child should be not eat anything for a minimum of 6 hours before either procedure.

Developmental Considerations

- Infant—general anesthesia
- Child—same as infant
- Adolescent—sedated

Nursing Implications

In preparation for laryngoscopy, the child is supine with the head positioned in the "sniff" position to avoid overextension or underextension of the neck. Suction equipment is readied and in working order. A young child often requires restraints to avoid interfering with the procedure.

Bronchoscopy in pediatrics is routinely carried out under general anesthesia, and the child will require premedication for the procedure. Following the procedure, regular suctioning and postural drainage are required to handle the additional secretions that accumulate. As soon as the child is able, oral fluids should be offered frequently.

The nurse needs to monitor the child for any increasing respiratory distress, which may indicate swelling of the airway due to the trauma of the bronchoscope. Thus, respiratory rate and pulse rate should be monitored every 15 minutes for the first hour postprocedure, every 30 minutes for the next hour, and then as routinely ordered on the unit.

Complications

- Increased secretions, possibly leading to obstruction
- Infection
- Airway damage

Lung Biopsy

Definition/Description

Lung biopsy is performed to obtain a specimen of lung tissue through a closed-needle procedure or an open thoracotomy. The closed-needle procedure is performed with local anesthesia at the site of needle insertion through an intercostal space; this procedure usually is not performed on young children. The thoracotomy requires an incision to be made into the chest wall to expose lung tissue; the child receives general anesthesia.

Purpose

Tissue samples may be obtained for histology and culture through both methods of sampling. The open procedure also permits inspection of the exposed lung.

Indications

A lung biopsy is indicated when long-standing pulmonary dysfunction has not been diagnosed by other methods.

Contraindications

The condition of the child may not warrant this procedure, but even critically ill (hypoxic, anemic, thrombocytopenic, leukopenic) patients have withstood the procedure.

Preparation

For open thoracotomy, the child is prepared for surgery. The procedure should be explained and the operative permit signed. No physical preparation is required for the needle biopsy.

Developmental Considerations

Age-appropriate explanations are required.

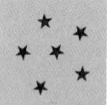

Ideas for Nursing Research

Repetitive assessment of children with respiratory dysfunction stimulates questions that need further investigations. The following topics are possible areas for nursing research:

- Coping differences between children of 10 and 12 years of age with chronic respiratory illnesses and children at the same ages with a chronic illness such as diabetes.
- The perceived body image of adolescents with chronic respiratory illnesses.
- Impact on siblings of a child with chronic respiratory illnesses.

TABLE 37-8
Selected Nursing Diagnoses Associated With Altered Respiratory Function

Data Analysis and Conclusions	Nursing Diagnoses
Health Perception and Health Management	
Parental verbalization regarding child's lack of growth	Altered Growth and Development related to effects of chronic respiratory illness
Growth measurements below 25th percentile on growth curve chart	
Sample statement by child: "The kids make fun of me at school and call me 'shrimp.'"	
Nutrition and Metabolism	
Child underweight, listless	Altered Nutrition: Less Than Body Requirements related to respiratory distress causing nausea, vomiting, and impaired gas exchange
Weight below 25th percentile of growth curve chart	
Eating accompanied by severe coughing spells typically resulting in vomiting	
Respiratory distress interferes with eating	
Elimination	
Reported problems of defecation, such as constipation or diarrhea	Altered Bowel Elimination related to poor nutrition
Abdominal distention	
Pain at defecation	
Need for oral or suppository agents to facilitate evacuation	
Bowel movements vary from q.o.d. to every third day	
Activity and Exercise: Sleep and Rest	
Tires easily with little activity	Activity Intolerance related to impaired gas exchange
Sleep frequently interrupted as a result of coughing spells	Sleep Pattern Disturbance related to persistence of cough
Mild exercise causes dyspnea	
Has difficulty concentrating for an extended length of time	
Oral cyanosis occurs with mild exercise	
Cognition and Perception	
Complains of frequent headaches	Altered Thought Processes related to impaired gas exchange and impact of respiratory illness on neurosensory function
Listless, lethargic	
Short attention span	
Academic level 1½ grades below age	
Irritable	
Self-Perception and Self-Concept	
Is afraid that "coughing will result in arrest of breathing"	Fear related to knowledge deficit regarding cough mechanism
Mother anxious that vomiting will cause aspiration	Maternal Anxiety related to lack of understanding regarding aspiration prevention
Child doesn't like school because "kids don't like me"	
Sexuality and Reproduction	
No evidence of secondary sex changes typical for age	Altered Sexuality Patterns related to impaired growth and development secondary to chronic respiratory condition
Child asks, "How come I don't have my period like the other girls?"	Anxiety related to lack of understanding of sexual maturation and factors affecting development
Mother concerned that chronic respiratory illness will cause sterility	
Coping and Stress Tolerance	
Child uses illness to manipulate parents.	Ineffective Family Coping related to fear of child's illness
Child's illness evokes great anxiety in parents.	Altered Family Processes related to lack of parenteral control
Parents are afraid to discipline child for fear of precipitating respiratory distress.	Ineffective Individual coping related to anger over illness
Child uses illness to manipulate peer relationships.	
Child has no special friends.	

Nursing Implications

Monitor vital signs postprocedurally. Observe for signs of bleeding, respiratory distress, and infection.

Complications

- With needle biopsy—pneumothorax
- With thoracotomy—postoperative hemorrhage or infection

Selected Nursing Diagnoses

After obtaining the history, performing the physical examination, reviewing results from the diagnostic tests, and tapping additional resources for information, the nurse carefully analyzes data obtained. Nursing diagnoses appropriate for the child with respiratory dysfunction become apparent and are used to develop a plan of care. Selected nursing diagnoses that may be appropriate for the child with respiratory dysfunction are presented by function in Table 37-8.

Summary

Accurate assessment of the respiratory system must be grounded in a thorough understanding of normal respiratory function. The respiratory system, which is responsible for oxygenation of the entire body, has an impact on other systems if it is compromised. The nurse needs to be able to correlate respiratory findings with other systemic responses to provide holistic care to the child. Inability to breathe without difficulty is very distressing to a child; this manifestation is equally distressing to the parents. Information obtained in the comprehensive data base help the nurse to diagnose dysfunction and to plan interventions that support the patient not only physiologically, but emotionally as well.

References

1. Athreya, B. H., & Silverman, B. K. (1986). *Pediatric physical diagnosis.* Norwalk, CT: Appleton-Century-Crofts.
2. Barness, L. A. (1991). *Manual of pediatric physical diagnosis* (6th ed.). St Louis: Mosby.
3. Bates, B. (1991). *A guide to physical examination and history taking* (5th ed.). Philadelphia: JB Lippincott.
4. Behrman, R., & Vaughan, V. (1992). *Nelson textbook of pediatrics* (14th ed.). Philadelphia: WB Saunders.
5. Block, G. J., & Nolan, J. (1986). *Health assessment for professional nursing: A developmental approach* (2nd ed.). Norwalk, CT: Appleton-Century-Crofts.
6. Carpenito, L. J. (1992). *Nursing diagnosis application to clinical practice* (4th ed.). Philadelphia: JB Lippincott.
7. Engel, J. (1989). *Pocket guide to pediatric assessment.* St. Louis: CV Mosby.
8. Gordon, M. (1991). *Manual of nursing diagnosis.* St. Louis: Mosby.
9. Hinshaw, H. C., & Murray, J. F. (1980). *Diseases of the chest,* (4th ed.). Philadelphia: WB Saunders.
10. Ward, J. (1989). Lung sounds: Easy to hear, hard to describe. *Respiratory Care, 34,* 17–19.
11. Wilkins, R., et al. (1989). Lung sound terminology used by respiratory care practitioners. *Respiratory Care 34,* 36–41, 1989.

38

CHAPTER

Nursing Planning, Intervention, and Evaluation for Altered Respiratory Function

BEHAVIORAL OBJECTIVES

List the most common disorders that affect the respiratory system in children.

Discuss the etiology, pathophysiology, clinical manifestations, and diagnostic procedures for infectious and noninfectious disorders of the respiratory system in children.

Apply nursing assessment to typical disorders of the respiratory system.

Describe the nursing interventions and medical and nursing management of children with respiratory system disorders.

Differentiate between the child and parent needs of the child with an acute versus a chronic disorder of the respiratory system.

Identify strategies to encourage child and parent adherence to treatment modalities.

The respiratory system plays an important role in the homeostasis of the entire body. Anatomy and physiology of the respiratory system are discussed in Chapter 36. Disorders of the respiratory system can involve the conducting airways or the gas exchange regions of the lungs. Conditions altering the normal function of the respiratory system can range from mildly unpleasant to life-threatening.

The larynx serves as the anatomic and functional transition point between the upper and lower airways. Chapter 35 includes a description of infectious and noninfectious conditions that affect the upper airway structures of the naso- and oropharynx. This chapter addresses respiratory disorders affecting the larynx and lower airways. For descriptive purposes, those disorders that include involvement of the larynx have been grouped as "upper airway" conditions, and those that occur beyond the larynx are grouped as "lower airway" conditions.

Disorders of the respiratory system may be divided into those that are infectious and those that are noninfectious. The most common respiratory tract infections in children include croup, bronchiolitis, and pneumonia, from a wide variety of viral and bacterial causative agents. Many infectious conditions are seasonal in nature and are rarely limited to a single anatomic region. Except for the first 3 to 6 months of life, when maternal antibodies offer acquired immunity, acute respiratory infections most commonly occur within the first 5 years of life. The incidence then declines due to growth and maturation of the lung, as well as the development of specific immunity. Severe respiratory infections can produce significant mortality in infants under the age of 5 years. Recurrent respiratory infections in childhood are particularly significant, because they may compromise the development of a mature, adult lung as it continues its growth throughout childhood.

The incidence and severity of respiratory disease are influenced by dynamic variables. Anatomic and genetic abnormalities; immunologic deficiencies; nutritional, environmental, social, and economic factors all play a role in the type and severity of respiratory illness. Several syndromes can occur at the same time or during the course of a single illness. One goal of nursing care is to return the child to optimal oxygenation and ventilation and to prevent further alterations in respiratory function. A second goal is to educate the child and the parents to behaviors that facilitate recovery from respiratory illness, and promote continued health and well-being. Resources and educational materials for families, teachers, and health care workers are given in the accompanying display.

Disorders of the Upper Airway

Upper airway disorders are the most commonly encountered respiratory conditions in ambulatory and hospitalized children. Presentation can range from mild to severe,

---

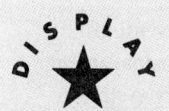

Resources for Families of Children With Altered Respiratory Function

American Lung Association
1740 Broadway
New York, NY 10019-4374

Cystic Fibrosis Foundation
6931 Arlington Road
Bethesda, MD 20814

American Association for Respiratory Care (AARC)
11030 Ables Lane
Dallas, TX 75229-2720

National Sudden Infant Death Syndrome Foundation
2 Metro Plaza
Suite 104
8200 Professional Place
Landover, MD 20785

National Sudden Infant Death Syndrome Clearinghouse
8201 Greensboro Drive
Suite 600
McLean, VA 22102

National Center for the Prevention of Sudden Infant Death Syndrome
330 N. Charles Street
Baltimore, MD 21201

Educational Materials

The American Lung Association (ALA) offers literature on asthma (e.g. "The Asthma Handbook," Home control of allergies, How to use your inhaler, and so forth), tuberculosis, smoking, and other topics (English and Spanish editions).

The ALA provides a school-based smoking cessation and prevention program entitled "Freedom from Smoking for Teens" designed for school professionals such as teachers, counselors, and nurses.

Many ALA chapters offer "CAMP SUPERSTUFF," a summer day camp for children with asthma. Contact the local ALA chapter for more information.

"An Introduction to Cystic Fibrosis for Parents and Children," written by James C. Cunningham, MD, and Lynn M. Taussig, MD (1988). This free, 95-page book, written for the lay person, is about the pathophysiology, diagnosis, and management of cystic fibrosis. Available from the Cystic Fibrosis Association.

Information on printed and audio-visual resources available concerning asthma, cystic fibrosis, respiratory care procedures, and so forth. Available from AARC.

"Asthma and You" coloring book, created by Children's Health Center, Phoenix, AZ, by Chris Mulligan, RN, MS, ANP, and Victoria Simpson, RN, PNP; cartoonist—Greg Pentkowski.
Also "Captain America: Return of the Asthma Monsters" Marvel Comic Books. Both available from Allen & Hanburys, A Division of Glaxo, Inc., 5 Moore Drive, Research Triangle Park, NC 27709.

"Super Cystic and Fabulous Fran Fibrosis" educational coloring book. Available from Organon, Inc., West Orange, NJ 07052 (Manufacturers of pancreatic enzymes).

Print and video educational resources for adolescents on such topics as AIDS awareness, sexually transmitted diseases, birth control, tobacco and drug use prevention, and other topics. Available from ETR Associates, P.O. Box 1830, Santa Cruz, CA 95061-1830.

and outcomes are directly correlated with early identification and appropriate intervention. Upper airway obstruction in children can be equated to acute cardiac emergencies in the adult. Therefore, rapid assessment of the child with upper airway obstruction is essential for the prevention of morbidity and mortality. The differential diagnosis of croup, epiglottitis, and foreign body aspiration is one of the most common and important in the care of children, because interventions for these conditions vary significantly. Table 38-1 lists the most common clinical findings associated with these three conditions.

Laryngotracheobronchitis

Definition and Incidence. Laryngotracheobronchitis (LTB), commonly referred to as croup, is an acute infection affecting the larynx, trachea, and bronchi. The parainfluenza viruses account for 85% of all cases of croup. It is an infection of the lower airway that is characterized by subglottic inflammation and edema, respiratory distress, and inspiratory stridor secondary to a variable degree of laryngeal obstruction. If signs and symptoms are recognized and appropriate treatment is initiated, the illness generally resolves in 3 to 7 days without associated morbidity or mortality. Foreign body obstruction or bacterial infection should be considered as a secondary contributing factor in children who fail to respond within this time period.

Although croup can be life-threatening, it is rarely fatal if promptly treated. However, the dramatic clinical appearance of the child during the acute phase can generate a great deal of distress and anxiety for the entire family. The nurse plays a valuable role in helping the child and family to cope with the acute episode by creating an environment of calmness and support.

In the United States, approximately 45,000 children are hospitalized annually with viral croup, with an average length of stay of 3 days.[99] Croup affects predominately infants and young children between the ages of 3 months and 3 years, with a peak in incidence in the second year of life. There is a higher incidence of viral croup in boys. More than 95% of children who suffer from classic acute croup have only one episode in their childhood. Spasmodic or allergic croup, different from and less common than acute croup, is related to a history of allergies, occurs predominantly at night in afebrile children, and may recur multiple times in childhood.[83]

The incidence of LTB is influenced by geographic location and season. Although viral croup can be seen throughout the year, it occurs most often during the cold weather seasons of late fall and winter. The seasonal variation is attributable to the virulence of the specific viral agent.

Etiology and Pathophysiology. Infants and young children are more susceptible to upper airway obstruction for three reasons: (1) their laryngeal airways are small in diameter and surface area; (2) their mucous membranes are vascular, and (3) the size of their glottic inlet and subglottic areas is small and can be rapidly obstructed by edema and spasm.

The virus often begins in the nasopharynx, ascending to the larynx, trachea, and bronchi. The airway mucosa becomes inflamed and edematous. Narrowing of the subglottic region secondary to the edema may significantly compromise airway diameter, leading to the characteristic inspiratory stridor associated with this condition. Increased mucus production and swelling of the vocal cords further compromise airway patency. Severe airway obstruction may necessitate endotracheal intubation.

Clinical Manifestations. The onset of viral croup is usually gradual, often preceded by a few days of upper respiratory infection with symptoms of rhinitis and cough. The earliest signs of viral croup include a harsh "barking" cough, inspiratory stridor, hoarse voice, and tachypnea (rapid and shallow breathing). These clinical findings occur secondary to narrowing of the diameter of the subglottic area of the trachea due to edema, spasm, and inflammation, all of which result in increased turbulence of air flow in the larynx and trachea. The child may complain of being tired and appear to be restless and irritable. The presence of a fever is variable. Within 24 hours, the signs and symptoms worsen with progressive respiratory deterioration.

Rales or rhonchi may be heard on chest auscultation in the child with severe croup, or breath sounds may be

TABLE 38-1
Differentiation of Clinical Manifestations of Three Upper Respiratory Diseases: Croup, Epiglottitis, and Foreign Body

	Croup	Epiglottitis	Foreign Body
Age	3 mo–3 y	2 y–5 y	6 mo–5 y
Onset	Gradual	Sudden	Usually sudden
Fever	Low-grade/moderate	High	None
Cough	Present/barking	Weak/absent	Sudden onset
Drooling	None	Present	None
Sore throat	Variable	Marked	None/variable
Voice	Hoarse	Muffled	Variable
Posturing	None	Upright	None
Choking	None	None	Before airway obstruction

diminished. Labored breathing with a prolonged expiration, and substernal, suprasternal, and intercostal retractions are also observed in severe cases. Stridor throughout the respiratory cycle may indicate only 1- to 2-mm airway patency at the level of the larynx. With significant obstruction, the child becomes cyanotic, pale, and lethargic. Symptoms can be variable throughout the day, increasing in severity at night. For most children with croup, the hallmark symptoms last for 3 to 4 days, although there may be persistence of upper respiratory symptoms.

Diagnostic Studies.   Diagnosis of croup is based on history, presenting signs and symptoms, and its clinical course. The differentiation of croup from epiglottitis is critical, because the management of these two conditions varies greatly. In cases where history and clinical presentation are ambiguous, the physician may need to confirm the diagnosis by gentle direct examination of the larynx or by obtaining an anterior–posterior and lateral x-ray of the neck. The radiograph of a child with croup usually demonstrates swelling and narrowing of the subglottic area, with a normal-sized epiglottis. Resuscitation equipment and personnel adept at intubation (ear, nose, and throat [ENT] specialists, anesthesiologists) should always be present when direct visualization of the upper airway is attempted, because the procedure may precipitate worsening airway obstruction, and necessitate immediate intubation.

★ ASSESSMENT

The nurse plays a major role in determining the severity of upper airway obstruction and the resulting impairment of gas exchange. Close observation of the child's respiratory status is essential. Assessment should be accomplished with minimal handling to prevent the worsening of airway obstruction and respiratory distress. The parents should be encouraged to stay with their child to minimize anxiety. Noxious and painful invasive procedures should be avoided if possible.

A complete history should be obtained on first encounter with the child. Important questions to ask include type of onset, prodrome of upper respiratory illness, fever, drooling, dysphagia, or cough? A child with croup presents with an upper respiratory prodrome of 1 to 3 days, fever is usually low grade, and a harsh, barking cough is present. Drooling, absence of cough, dysphagia, upright tripod posture, acute onset, and high fever are indicative of epiglottitis.

Respiratory assessment includes the identification and evaluation of stridor, retractions, respiratory rate, breath sounds, and color. Respiratory rate and use of accessory muscle are indicators of the adequacy of air exchange. Worsening airway obstruction increases resistance to air flow; therefore, nasal flaring, retractions, and increased respiratory effort are present. The intensity of stridor is not always helpful in determining the severity of subglottic obstruction; however, the absence of stridor with a concurrent increase in respiratory effort can be a harbinger of significant obstruction.

Consistent, repeated auscultation of breath sounds is necessary to determine air flow. The presence of decreasing breath sounds is indicative of progressive obstruction. Ideally, the same person should perform these repeated assessments to follow accurately the course of the disease. Changes in color are late signs of hypoxia; however, the absence of cyanosis does not preclude mild hypoxia. Alterations in level of consciousness can give an early indication of hypoxia. Anxiety is seen in children with air hunger, and hypoxia, lethargy, or obtundation indicate hypercapnia and respiratory failure.

Noninvasive monitoring of oxygen saturation by way of pulse oximetry (S_pO_2) and transcutaneous carbon dioxide monitoring (P_sCO_2) are invaluable in the assessment of severe respiratory illness. These devices allow the early identification of acute changes in arterial oxygenation and CO_2 without the need for invasive arterial blood gas (ABG) analysis. The clinical assessment of this objective data has been shown to aid in the determination of the severity of croup, and serves as a guide to the management of the child with severe croup.[40,108] A description of pulse oximetry and transcutaneous monitoring appears in the Noninvasive Monitoring section of this chapter.

Heart rate, rhythm, and blood pressure should be monitored. Tachycardia is a nonspecific indicator of hypoxia, because it is also present with fever and anxiety.

Although most children with croup present with only mild disease, a small percentage require aggressive intervention and hospitalization. Increased respiratory effort, significant changes in level of consciousness, or apnea requires the prompt notification of a physician.

★ NURSING DIAGNOSES AND PLANNING

Based on assessment data from above and Chapter 37, the following nursing diagnoses may apply to the family and child with LTB:

- Ineffective Breathing Pattern related to airway obstruction.
- Impaired Gas Exchange related to airway obstruction.
- Fluid Volume Deficit related to poor oral intake.
- Altered Nutrition: Less Than Body Requirements related to reduced appetite.
- Inability to Sustain Spontaneous Ventilation related to respiratory muscle fatigue.
- Anxiety related to airway obstruction, hospitalization, unfamiliar interventions, and separation from parents.
- Fear related to illness, home management, and when to seek medical help.

The nurse and child (or parents) together plan effective care based on the established nursing diagnoses. Several examples of expected outcomes follow:

- The parents provide comfort for the child.
- The parents participate in the child's care.
- The parents identify symptoms and appropriate care when attacks occur.

The nurse plans for the daily care of the child based on both physician's orders and nursing diagnoses. Some general nursing care goals may be the following:

- Symptoms of obstruction are relieved.
- Airway patency is maintained.
- Anxiety is diminished.

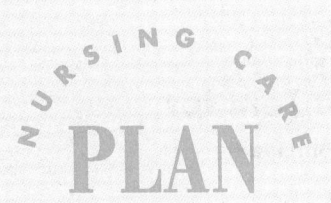

A 3-Year-Old Child in a Mist Tent for Laryngotracheobronchitis

Assessment

Case Study Description

Jonathan, age 3, accompanied by his parents, was admitted to the hospital with a diagnosis of acute viral laryngotracheobronchitis. He had been ill with a cold for about 3 days before the current respiratory illness. During the previous night, Jonathan had experienced several episodes of respiratory distress. His mother stated that Jonathan cries and resists when encouraged to drink, complaining that it hurts too much to swallow. Occasionally, when he does attempt to swallow fluids, his epiglottis spasms and he chokes. This reaction frightens Jonathan further and his refusal to drink has become adamant.

Now he is irritable, appearing tired and apprehensive. Jonathan is placed in a mist tent and immediately becomes fearful, crying and pushing at the tent sides, begging to be removed and held. His parents speak to him in reassuring, comforting tones, but appear to be reluctant to go too near the tent. Both parents appear tired from lack of sleep.

Jonathan's father works at night; his mother doesn't drive and needs to go home to care for two other children, ages 1 and 6, who are with a neighbor temporarily. When his parents leave, Jonathan cries and refuses the attempts of the nurse to comfort him.

Physician medication orders include aerosolized racemic epinephrine to be used as needed. A mist tent with oxygen also is ordered with instructions to monitor arterial saturation with pulse oximetry; oxygen concentration is to be regulated to insure arterial saturation greater than 95%. Fluids are begun intravenously.

Assessment Data

Vital signs on admission to the unit: T, 38.2°C; P, 150; R, 48. Examination reveals a barking cough, hoarseness, and obvious dyspnea with considerable inspiratory stridor and intercostal retractions. Skin appears pale and diaphoretic. Chest auscultation reveals rhonchi and rales. Skin turgor is poor. Analysis of blood gases revealed slight respiratory acidosis.

Nursing Diagnosis	Intervention	Rationale
1. Ineffective airway clearance related to respiratory tract inflammation, increased respiratory secretions, bronchospasms, and laryngeal edema.	Monitor vital signs, breath sounds, and signs of increasing respiratory distress q 30–60″ during acute distress and q 1–2′ otherwise.	Signs of increasing respiratory distress include tachypnea, head thrusting, retractions, stridor, nasal flaring, pallor, cyanosis, mouth breathing, labored and prolonged expiration, and diminishing breath sounds.
Supporting Data: • Dyspnea, barking cough, & hoarseness • Tachycardia & tachypnea • Rales, rhonchi, stridor, and retractions • Laryngeospasms • Restlessness & apprehension • Acute episodes of respiratory distress q 2–3 hrs	Place in position of comfort, usually semi or high Fowler's.	Upright position facilitates diaphragmatic movement and air intake, but child should not be *forced* to sit; will preferentially choose upright posture that will maximize diaphragmatic excursion. Nurse should work *with* Jonathan to maximize outcome.
	Keep in cool mist tent.	Moisture helps to thin respiratory secretions and open airways.
	Keep suctioning equipment and emergency intubation tray nearby.	If intubation is required, delay can be life-threatening.
	Administer medications as ordered.	Epinephrine causes vasoconstriction and reduces airway edema; effects are temporary.

(Continued)

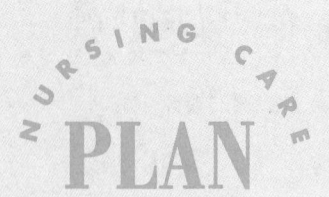

A 3-Year-Old Child in a Mist Tent for Laryngotracheobronchitis (continued)

Nursing Diagnosis	*Intervention*	*Rationale*
2. High risk for fluid volume deficit related to diaphoresis, difficulty swallowing, and increased metabolic rate. Supporting Data: • Fever • Diaphoresis • Refusal of oral fluids	Monitor intake and output, urine specific gravity, status of mucous membranes, and skin turgor. Offer clear liquids at room temperature as tolerated, but keep NPO during episodes of acute respiratory distress.	Urine output should be at least 2 ml/kg/hr and specific gravity between 1.003 and 1.020. Mucous membranes should be moist, and skin should rebound quickly when pinched. Dehydration should be avoided. Iced or hot liquids may stimulate laryngospasms. May aspirate with tachypnea.
3. Anxiety related to dyspnea and air hunger and separation from parents. Supporting Data: • Intermittent restlessness • Becomes highly agitated during acute episodes, then appears frightened and tense during aftermath • Unable to relax for 30–60″ following acute episodes of distress	Remain at bedside during acute episodes, maintaining a calm, reassuring approach. Encourage parents to remain with child as much as possible. Parent may go inside tent as desired to hold and comfort child; child may be removed from tent for consolation as status allows. Speak softly but firmly, encouraging him to take slow, deep breaths.	Crying and anxiety increase respiratory distress and hypoxia. Rapid changes during acute episodes require immediate intervention. Presence of parents and nurse is comforting and promotes rest. Parents need guidance on activities that will not jeopardize the child's respiratory status. Nurse sets tone for parent–child interactions and models desired behavior for parents.
4. Sleep pattern disturbance related to respiratory distress. Supporting Data: • Experiences more frequent episodes of acute respiratory distress at night; wakes q 2–3 hrs and remains awake 20–30″ following episodes	Administer sponge bath and fresh gown before bedtime. Place security objects from home inside tent. Play relaxing music.	Relaxation promotes rest, which is needed to conserve energy. Use familiar methods to comfort and promote sleep.
5. High risk for injury related to the use of combustible oxygen and electricity. Supporting Data: • Jonathan placed in mist tent with continuous oxygen	Post "NO SMOKING, OXYGEN IN USE" signs on the canopy and room door. Do not allow metal, friction, battery-operated, or electrical toys in tent when oxygen in use. Use only cotton blankets in tent. Place call light on outside of tent. Monitor tent equipment for electrical malfunction and safety hazards.	Oxygen is highly combustible. Precautions must be taken to prevent sparks.
6. High risk for hypothermia related to damp, cool interior of the mist tent. Supporting Data: • Mist tent supplies moist, cool air at temperature lower than room air	Monitor body temperature as needed, at least every 2–4 hours; keep tent temperature 18–20°C.	Cool temperatures are desired, but large body surface of small children increases risk of hypothermia. In children Jonathan's age, shivering increases oxygen consumption in order to produce heat.

(Continued)

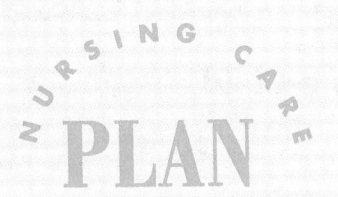

A 3-Year-Old Child in a Mist Tent for Laryngotracheobronchitis (continued)

Nursing Diagnosis	*Intervention*	*Rationale*
	Change gown and linens frequently; wipe sides of tent as needed.	Cool mist makes environment damp and encourages heat loss by evaporation from the skin. Hypothermia further compromises hypoxic child.
	Use hat, socks, and additional clothing if needed.	Core body temperature should remain 36–37.5°C.

Evaluation

- Adequate hydration is demonstrated by moist mucus membranes, good skin turgor, and drinking fluids when offered.
- Sleep is uninterrupted for at least 4-hour intervals.
- Personal injury and hypothermia are avoided.

Expected Outcomes

- Jonathan exhibits effective air exchange and absence of symptoms of acute respiratory distress.
- Jonathan responds to comfort measures by reduced crying, relaxed posture, and slower, deeper breathing.
- Parents remain at bedside as much as they can.

This Nursing Care Plan was prepared by Karen Wall, BScN.

★ INTERVENTIONS: COLLABORATIVE AND INDEPENDENT

Interventions are determined by the severity of disease. Most children can be managed at home, but up to 15% may require hospitalization, and 1% to 5% may require endotracheal intubation.[86,113] The Nursing Care Plan and Teaching Plan discuss the care of a preschooler with croup.

Children with severe respiratory symptoms or children who fail to respond to treatment may require further evaluation and hospitalization for treatment. Hospital management includes providing humidification, oxygen, fluids, racemic epinephrine, and possibly steroids. Children with mild cases of viral croup can be managed at home with cool mist, fluids, and appropriate education about observation for worsening airway obstruction. Guidelines for home treatment of croup are listed in the accompanying display.

HUMIDIFICATION AND OXYGEN THERAPY

Humidification and oxygen can be delivered by way of aerosol mask or face tent. The oxygen concentration is adjusted to maintain arterial saturation, as monitored by pulse oximetry, greater than 95%. The head of the bed should also be elevated slightly to minimize diaphragmatic compression of the lung and decrease the work of breathing (WOB). If a mist tent is used, the nurse should ensure safe operation of the tent, and that the mist is not so thick as to prevent adequate observation of the child. A further description of this care is given at the end of this chapter.

MEDICATION THERAPY

Racemic epinephrine by aerosol inhalation may be indicated for symptomatic obstruction that is refractory to mist alone. This pharmacologic intervention is felt to produce local vasoconstriction and reduce airway swelling, thereby decreasing airway obstruction. Aerosol administration by hand nebulizer (Fig. 38-1) is preferred over intermittent positive pressure breathing (IPPB). Nebulization is better tolerated and has fewer risks than IPPB. The beneficial effects of racemic epinephrine inhalation may last from 10 minutes to 2 hours. Treatment is given on a PRN basis and may be required every hour in severe cases. Any child receiving racemic epinephrine in the emergency room should be monitored for at least 2 hours after therapy before discharge, because the effects are transient and respiratory distress could recur. (Refer to the section in this chapter on Techniques and Technology in Pediatric Respiratory Care for a description of aerosol medication administration techniques.)

Antibiotics are not usually prescribed for viral croup unless there is suspicion of an underlying bacterial infection. Parenteral corticosteroids have been used to treat subglottic viral croup although their use remains contro-

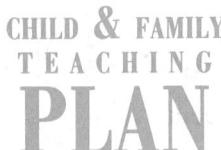

CHILD & FAMILY
T E A C H I N G
PLAN

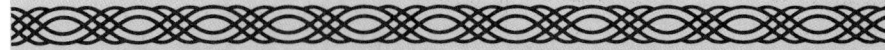

Helping Parents Cope With a Child With Laryngotracheobronchitis

Assessment

Three-year-old Jonathan has been hospitalized for 16 hours and the initial respiratory crisis has passed. His first night in the hospital was quite stressful. He woke every 2 hours in severe respiratory distress. When the episodes subsided, he remained tense, frightened, and restless until he fell back asleep after 20–30 minutes. In time, he responded better to the nurse's attempts to comfort but continued to ask for his mother.

Jonathan's parents return early the next morning, looking anxious and ill-at-ease. The father is overheard saying, "He must not be any better if he has to stay inside this tent all the time." Jonathan's mother remarks to the nurse, "I feel so helpless just standing here beside the crib watching him."

Neither parent finished high school, and none of the family has been hospitalized for illness. The parents seem overwhelmed by the activity and seriousness of Jonathan's illness. They listen intently when the nurse talks to them but have not asked questions.

Child and Family Objectives	*Specific Content*	*Teaching Strategies*
1. Discuss Jonathan's medical condition.	1. Laryngotracheobronchitis means "croup." Explain its cause and excellent prognosis.	1. Explain the term laryngotracheo-bronchitis. Use drawing or anatomical model of airway. Use familiar terminology, avoiding jargon and complex medical language.
2. Describe the benefits of therapeutic measures and the precautions that need to be taken.	2. Explain the use of the IV, medications, mist tent, and emergency equipment. Explain dangers of oxygen therapy matter-of-factly and the need for safety measures.	2. Point to each item as it is explained, making sure that parents see the specific area of discussion. Encourage questions by frequent pauses and asking the parents what else they would like to know.
3. Identify activities that will comfort and calm Jonathan.	3. Explain the effect of anxiety and crying on respiratory function. Suggest activities that other parents have used with their children.	3. Ask parents how they typically comfort Jonathan at home, what toys or other objects would soothe him. Encourage parents to hold and stroke their child.
4. Identify signs and symptoms of worsening respiratory distress and stressors that exacerbate condition.	4. Describe appearance and behaviors that need immediate attention and strategies that can be used at home for mild episodes, including use of a cool air vaporizer, a steamy bathroom, or taking the child outdoors into the cool night air.	4. Provide parents with a written list of symptoms that indicate an acute episode of respiratory distress and home treatment measures. Provide a written list of symptoms that should be reported to health care providers immediately. Provide phone numbers of physician and hospital for quick reference.

(Continued)

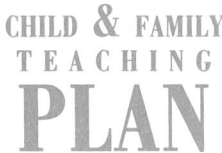

CHILD & FAMILY TEACHING PLAN

Helping Parents Cope With a Child With Laryngotracheobronchitis (continued)

Child and Family Objectives	*Specific Content*	*Teaching Strategies*
5. Express feelings related to the child's illness and his hospitalization.	5. Emergency situations in worsening conditions. Note that parents often experience feelings of guilt that treatment was delayed.	5. Inform parents that a child's illness can become worse quickly and that parents often have difficulty knowing what constitutes an emergency situation. Acknowledge that feelings of guilt and lack of confidence are common feelings. Praise parents appropriately for activities that provide comfort and demonstrate positive parenting skills.

Evaluation

- Parents accurately explain the cause, course, and prognosis for laryngotracheobronchitis.
- Parents explain the purpose of the treatment measures.
- Parents actively participate in assuring that safety measures are maintained.
- Parents actively participate in Jonathan's care when present.
- Parents provide comfort for him.
- Parents list appropriate measures they will take if Jonathan should develop croup again after discharge.
- Parents express satisfaction with the care the family received during the period of hospitalization.

This Teaching Plan was prepared by Karen Wall, BScN.

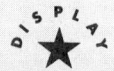

Parental Education: Guidelines for Home Treatment of Croup

- Stay calm to keep your child calm.
- Take your child into the bathroom, turn on the hot water, and close the door. Symptoms should begin to resolve in 5 minutes.
- Give the child clear fluids as tolerated.
- Avoid antihistamines. They can cause inspissation of secretions.
- Monitor respiratory rate.

Take your child to the doctor if the following conditions exist:

- Symptoms do not improve after being in the bathroom steam for 5 minutes.
- Breathing becomes more difficult or labored.
- Acute anxiety or restlessness develops.
- If drooling occurs, the child should be taken directly to the emergency room.

versial. Advocates believe that corticosteroid therapy reduces the severity and duration of respiratory symptoms. If prescribed, dexamethasone is usually the agent of choice.

FLUID THERAPY

Intravenous (IV) hydration at 1¼ to 1½ times the maintenance infusion rate compensates for the increased insensible water loss due to tachypnea and fever. The child with tachypnea and excessive WOB should not be allowed to have anything to eat or drink until the resolution of these symptoms.

PSYCHOSOCIAL SUPPORT

Anxiety can be diminished by allowing the parent to remain at the bedside, even when the child is in a mist tent. Separation of the child from the parent should not be forced just to place the child in a tent, and use of an aerosol mask or face tent allows the child to be held by the parents for extended periods outside the tent. Sedatives are not indicated because they cause respiratory depression and the inability to evaluate adequately a sedated child's level of consciousness (LOC). Rest should

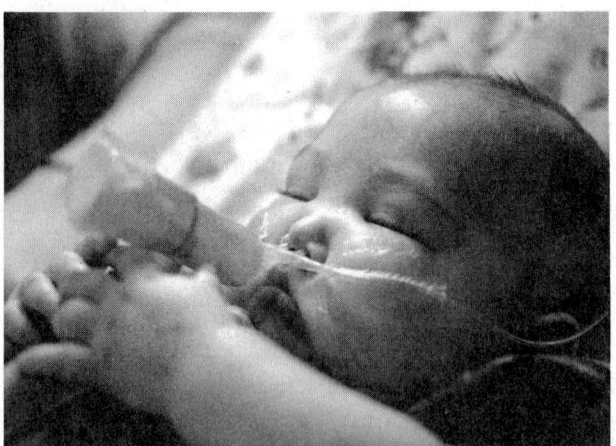

FIGURE 38-1
Infant with croup receiving an aerosol treatment by hand nebulizer.

be promoted to conserve energy. All procedures and treatments should be clearly explained to the parents and child, and invasive procedures such as ABGs should be avoided or kept to a minimum. Parents should be allowed to administer care as appropriate.

INTUBATION AND AIRWAY CARE

Endotracheal intubation may be indicated if the child is unresponsive to treatment, or demonstrates marked anxiety that changes to listlessness, increased respiratory effort, hypoxia, cyanosis, or decreased breath sounds. Occasionally, administration of a helium–oxygen gas mixture may serve as a temporizing measure until intubation personnel and site are ready.[89,104]

An endotracheal tube (ETT) one size smaller than usual is used because of the swelling, and to prevent complications associated with the presence of an artificial airway (e.g., subglottic stenosis). After intubation, the child receives continuous humidity by way of the ETT and, in some instances, may require continuous positive airway pressure (CPAP) to maintain adequate oxygenation. Mechanical ventilation is usually not required. Skilled nursing care ensures that the ETT does not become obstructed with secretions (vigilant suctioning) and that the child is not accidentally extubated. The child usually remains intubated about 5 days and is extubated when afebrile, clinically stable, and an air leak is present around the ETT. A tracheostomy is not recommended as an initial intervention, because the illness resolves in 4 to 5 days, at which time the artificial airway is no longer needed.[2,86]

TEACHING

Parental education remains a critical intervention, even in the hospitalized child. Health education is the cornerstone to the early identification and intervention of relapses or future episodes. Information includes counting respiratory rate and recognizing signs and symptoms of increased WOB and progressive respiratory distress. Discussion of the normal clinical presentation of croup enables parents to identify symptoms and intervene early. Any child with increased respiratory rate, restlessness, worsening retractions, and no relief of acute symptoms

after 5 minutes of humidification therapy should be brought to the hospital.

HOME MANAGEMENT

Home management includes providing an environment of high humidity or cool mist. Parents are instructed to position the child comfortably in the bathroom for 10 to 15 minutes with the shower running. A cool mist vaporizer may also be used and is preferred to warm mist vaporizers due to the risk of burns. Cool mist is felt to soothe the inflamed mucosa and decrease the amount of coughing.[113]

Home management also includes providing adequate hydration in the form of clear fluids. Encouraging the child to drink plenty of fluids will minimize dehydration, which tends to make respiratory secretions tenacious and difficult to expel. Antipyretics may be given to control fever.

★ EVALUATION

Periodically, the nurse and family evaluate the outcomes of care given. Examples of outcomes for the child and family with LTB were given under diagnoses and planning in this section. Have short-term goals been met? Are long-term goals still realistic? Planning for further nursing care takes into consideration complications and long-term care.

COMPLICATIONS

LTB usually is self-limiting and mild in presentation. Most children do not require hospitalization, and fewer still require an artificial airway. Inspiratory obstruction is maximal for the first 24 to 48 hours, although respiratory symptoms can last for a week. Morbidity is due to delayed identification and treatment of severe cases. Iatrogenic complications of endotracheal intubation include subglottic stenosis, tracheal or bronchial granulations, or pneumothorax. Acquired subglottic stenosis in LTB due to intubation is reported to range anywhere from 1% to 40%, with a mean of 5%.[86]

LONG-TERM CARE

Croup may recur in some children; therefore, appropriate parental education concerning early identification and intervention helps to minimize symptoms and prevent acute airway emergencies.

Epiglottitis

Definition and Incidence.   Epiglottitis is a disorder affecting the epiglottis, vallecula, and surrounding laryngeal tissue, characterized by acute onset, rapidly progressive inflammation, and swelling. Failure to diagnose this condition accurately and implement appropriate care in a timely manner may lead to fatal respiratory failure secondary to complete airway obstruction. Therapeutic interventions should occur promptly, avoiding any delays secondary to laboratory or radiologic assessment. The nurse's role requires monitoring the child for signs and symptoms of deterioration, preparing the child for emergency diagnostic and therapeutic procedures as quickly as possible, and supporting the child and parent through this life-threatening episode.

Epiglottitis most commonly occurs in children ages 2 to 5, with 70% of cases occurring in boys. This age range is in contrast to that seen with croup (3 months to 3 years), a condition that presents with some similar clinical characteristics but requires different interventions. Studies have shown that there is no consensus that epiglottitis has a seasonal variation.[65]

Etiology and Pathophysiology. *Hemophilus influenzae* type B is the organism responsible for approximately 85% of cases of epiglottitis. The infection is acquired most commonly through migration from the nasopharyngeal site, progressing down to the epiglottic area and the lower airways. The epiglottis and surrounding laryngeal tissues become acutely inflamed, with rapid swelling, leading to mechanical obstruction of the upper airway. The WOB increases and gas exchange is impaired, leading to respiratory failure with hypoxemia and hypercapnia. The clearance of lower airway secretions and inflammatory debris is also impaired due to the narrowed upper airway. Left untreated, the condition may rapidly deteriorate to asphyxia and respiratory arrest. Establishment of an artificial airway by way of endotracheal intubation or tracheostomy represents a primary, life-saving intervention in a large percentage of children who present with this condition.

Clinical Manifestations. Epiglottitis usually has an acute onset, with sore throat, hoarseness, and high temperature developing in a previously healthy child. Respiratory distress and increased WOB may manifest with tachypnea, dyspnea, and inspiratory stridor. Inspiratory retractions of the intercostal, supraclavicular, and suprasternal muscles are noticed. Breath sounds may be diminished, with expiratory rhonchi. The child appears highly anxious, sitting forward while gasping for air. Drooling and dysphagia are two characteristic signs of this condition. Direct visualization of the laryngeal tissues shows inflammation, with the epiglottis swollen, red, and stiff, and thick secretions coating the glottic area.

Diagnostic Studies. A diagnosis of epiglottitis is made based on history, signs, and symptoms, and is confirmed by direct visualization of the epiglottis and by lateral neck radiograph. Laryngoscopy for direct visualization of the airway must be performed in the operating room, in a controlled environment where appropriate anesthesia, intubation equipment, and personnel are available. The potential for total airway obstruction secondary to laryngospasm during visualization of the airway is extremely high, and unprepared personnel increase morbidity and mortality risks.

A lateral neck radiograph shows an enlarged epiglottis, distention of the hypopharynx, and a classic "thumb sign." A decision to transport the child to the radiology department must only be made after appropriate initial interventions have occurred based on the severity of the attack, and when a physician skilled in airway management is available to accompany the child during the diagnostic procedure.

★ **ASSESSMENT**

Frequent, thorough nursing assessment of the child with upper airway obstruction is crucial to the identification, management, and evaluation of epiglottitis. The clinical presentation of acute epiglottitis is classic; however, early manifestations of the disease can present diagnostic dilemmas to even the most experienced practitioner.

An accurate history lays the groundwork for further clinical evaluation. Objective data to be obtained include onset of illness, length of illness, fever, presence of dysphagia, absence of cough, stridor, complaints of sore throat, and the presence of drooling. The child with epiglottitis presents with a sudden onset of illness (6 to 10 hours) and marked temperature elevation (>39°C). The parents give a positive history for dysphagia, drooling, muffled voice, and sore throat.

Astute nursing observational skills provide invaluable information during the initial evaluation of the child. During the assessment of any child with upper airway obstruction, the parents must be present. Any intervention that facilitates the provision of a calm environment not only ensures the completion of an adequate database, but also diminishes the risk of acute airway obstruction precipitated by anxiety.

Respiratory assessment includes the evaluation of position of comfort, stridor, respiratory effort, and auscultation of breath sounds. The child with epiglottitis always assumes an upright or "tripod" posture, sitting forward leaning on the arms. The head is often held in the "sniffing" position with the jaw forward, mouth open, and the tongue protruding.[5,48] This position maximizes opening of the upper airway and helps to relieve airway obstruction (Fig. 38-2). These young patients resist any attempt to lay them supine, and, in fact, this maneuver is

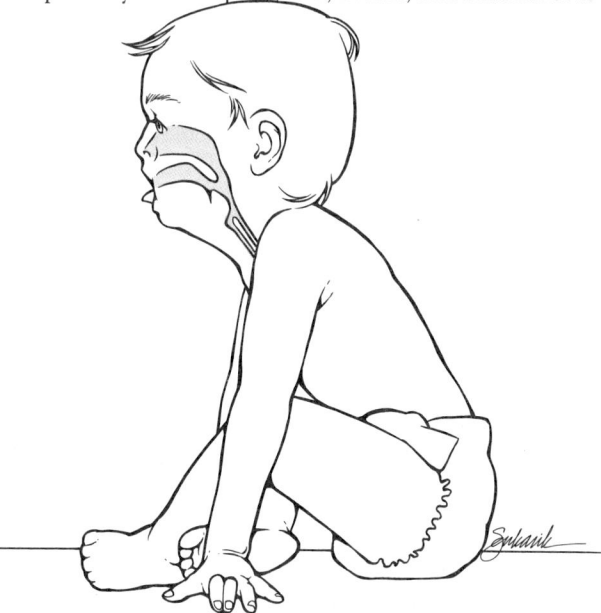

FIGURE 38-2

Characteristic posture of a child with acute epiglottitis. Sitting forward on hands, in the "tripod" position. Mouth open, tongue out, head forward and tilted up in the sniffing position, in an effort to relieve the acute airway obstruction secondary to the swollen epiglottis.

contraindicated because it can contribute to complete airway obstruction and respiratory arrest.

Inspiratory stridor can be present and is caused by turbulent air flow past the obstruction. As the obstruction worsens, the quality of the harsh sound intensifies; cessation of stridor indicates complete airway obstruction. Because stridor is not present in all cases of epiglottitis, the absence of this finding should not preclude the diagnosis of this condition.

Acute respiratory distress is always present and is abrupt in onset. Respiratory rate is increased, along with accessory muscle use and retractions of varying intensity. The need for continued respiratory assessment is critical to monitor for progressive deterioration, as well as to gauge therapeutic response to treatment. Auscultation is performed to determine the degree of air entry; the more significant the obstruction, the more diminished the breath sounds are. Rales and rhonchi may be present if there is concurrent pneumonia or pulmonary edema; however, these are not classic findings in acute epiglottitis. Cough is almost always absent, a finding that has been shown to be a sensitive indicator in differentiating epiglottitis from croup. Drooling is almost always present and is a classic clinical finding. Although the presence of drooling and the absence of cough are the most specific manifestations of epiglottitis, they may be absent in the child less than 18 months old, therefore making differential diagnosis problematic.[83] Complete blood count (CBC) and ABG evaluation are of little value and should be avoided until an artificial airway is secured. Pulse oximetry usually is well tolerated and is a useful monitor for alterations in oxygenation.

Assessment of the child's level of consciousness (LOC) is essential. An apprehensive, toxic child is a typical finding, whereas a depressed LOC is a late sign of significant hypoxia. Any disruption of the child can aggravate respiratory compromise; therefore, continued evaluation of the child's tolerance to the assessment process is of utmost importance. Any procedure that increases apprehension should be discontinued immediately.

Direct visualization of the larynx provides definitive diagnosis, but must not be attempted without the presence of a physician capable of difficult endotracheal intubations. Manipulation of the posterior pharynx or epiglottis can precipitate further swelling and induce laryngospasm, leading to complete airway obstruction. Routine examination of the oropharynx with any instrument should be avoided by unskilled personnel when epiglottitis is suspected.

Radiographic visualization of the soft tissues in the lateral neck can confirm the diagnosis. A thick epiglottic shadow that resembles an adult's thumb coupled with ballooning of the hypopharynx are radiographic characteristics of this condition.[70] Lateral neck films should be obtained only in the clinically stable child whose diagnosis is uncertain. Toxic, acutely distressed children *should not* be sent to radiology.

★ NURSING DIAGNOSES AND PLANNING

Based on assessment data from above and Chapter 37, the following nursing diagnoses may apply to the family and child with epiglottitis:

- Anxiety related to airway obstruction and hypoxia.
- Impaired Airway Clearance related to airway obstruction.
- Impaired Gas Exchange related to airway obstruction.
- Impaired Verbal Communication related to ETT.
- Fatigue related to acute illness and increased WOB.
- Ineffective Family Coping related to precipitate illness.

The nurse and child (or parents) together plan effective care based on the established nursing diagnoses. Several examples of expected outcomes follow:

- Effective breathing patterns are established.
- The parents provide emotional support for child.
- The parents exhibit understanding of the care and prognosis of the child.
- The parents establish a system for the child to communicate with them.

The nurse plans for the care of the child based on both physician's orders and nursing diagnoses. Some general nursing care goals may be the following:

- Increased air exchange is demonstrated.
- Anxiety is diminished.

★ INTERVENTIONS: COLLABORATIVE AND INDEPENDENT

The most important therapeutic interventions for the child with epiglottitis are the establishment of an artificial airway and antibiotic treatment of the causative organism. Other interventions are supportive to facilitate a return to previous activities of daily living.

ARTIFICIAL AIRWAY ESTABLISHMENT AND CARE

Once the diagnosis of epiglottitis is confirmed, the child should be monitored closely and never left unattended until the airway is secured. Endotracheal intubation is the preferred method, is as effective as tracheostomy, and is associated with fewer complications and shorter hospitalizations than tracheostomy.[5,48,65] Due to the swelling of the epiglottis, direct visualization of the vocal cords and glottic opening is virtually impossible. Therefore, the establishment of an endotracheal airway must always be accomplished by skilled physicians in a controlled environment. Usually, the child is intubated in the operating room under inhaled anesthesia by a pediatric anesthesiologist or ENT specialist. Endotracheal intubation is discussed further in the section of this chapter titled Care During Placement of the Endotracheal Tube.

When assisting with an intubation, the nurse should ensure that all the necessary equipment is available, not only for the immediate procedure, but for emergency resuscitation as well.

Once an airway has been established, IV access and all the necessary blood samples can be obtained. Any noxious procedures, such as blood samples, should be deferred until the child is intubated. The child is transferred to the pediatric intensive care unit (PICU) for further care.

Accidental extubation must be avoided. Iatrogenic complications due to intubation are prevented by vigilance and expert nursing care. Interventions aimed at the prevention of accidental extubation include soft wrist restraints, provision of diversional activities, IV sedatives, and parental education. The younger, anxious, uncooperative child may require more vigorous mechanical and pharmacologic restraints than older children. The use of these interventions should be made according to the individual child's needs, rather than to simplify nursing care.

Patency of the artificial airway is maintained through positioning, postural drainage, and endotracheal suctioning. Humidified gases are delivered to prevent drying of the airway and thickening of the secretions, in conjunction with sufficient oxygen to maintain arterial saturation >90%. This can be accomplished by way of T-piece or by CPAP. (See section on Care of the Child Requiring Mechanical Ventilation later in this chapter.) Rarely is mechanical ventilation required.

With appropriate antibiotic therapy, artificial airway support usually is required only for 48 hours. Extubation is accomplished after direct visualization of the epiglottis reveals a reduction in swelling, and there is presence of an air leak around the ETT, as evidenced by vocalization or with positive pressure hand ventilation using a bag-valve device. Postextubation stridor and cough usually respond to cool mist and nebulized racemic epinephrine. Continued observation in the PICU is necessary for 12 to 24 hours, until the potential need for reintubation is no longer a threat.

Some clinicians advocate the use of neuromuscular blocking agents to prevent accidental extubation.[65] However, others feel the risks of neuromuscular blockade outweigh the benefits.[3,48] All children receiving neuromuscular blockade require mechanical ventilation due to muscular paralysis, thereby creating greater risk if accidental extubation does occur. The sensation of paralysis is a frightening experience; therefore, all of these children require frequent IV sedation. The judicious use of sedatives in conjunction with age-appropriate diversions is as effective as neuromuscular blockade, without the potential adverse sequelae.

MEDICATION THERAPY

Empiric antibiotic therapy should be instituted based on knowledge of normal causative organisms. Antibiotic therapy should never be delayed until results from cultures and sensitivities are obtained. Once these values are known, adjustment of antibiotic coverage to more appropriate therapy can be accomplished. Initial therapy requires IV administration, with conversion to oral therapy when consecutive blood cultures are sterile, fever subsides, and the child is extubated and tolerating oral fluids. If *H. influenzae* is the etiologic agent, rifampin prophylaxis is recommended for household contacts with at least one child who is less than 48 months. Households in which all contacts are older than 48 months do not require rifampin.[1] Day care and nursery school prophylaxis is more complex, and the reader is referred to the American Academy of Pediatrics 1991 *Report of the Committee on Infectious Diseases* for guidelines.[1] Fever control is accomplished through the use of acetaminophen and tepid baths.

FLUID THERAPY

IV hydration is provided at maintenance rates appropriate for weight. Once oral fluids are tolerated, the IV can be heparin locked, and diet can be advanced as tolerated.

PSYCHOSOCIAL SUPPORT

Parental concerns center around issues of survival and the potential for handicap of their child. Prognosis can also influence the type and degree of parental concerns.[130] Providing accurate, timely, understandable information, and allowing for normal parenting to continue have been found to relieve parental stress in the PICU.[25]

Because the normal disease trajectory is short and full recovery is expected, every effort should be made to provide the parents with opportunities to care for their child. Unlimited visitation should be allowed for parents, siblings, and extended family while the child is in the PICU. The only constraints should be to maintain crowd control, while providing for patient safety.

Diversional and comfort activities can be developed in collaboration with child life specialists or physical therapists. As with any hospitalized child, developmental level must be taken into consideration when providing nursing care. Anticipatory preparation for procedures is essential, particularly in the stressful environment of the PICU. While the child is in the PICU, every effort must be made to control environmental stimuli and prevent sensory overload. Emotional responses to the hospitalization require continual evaluation to promote coping and to provide the parents with anticipatory guidance. It is not uncommon for children hospitalized in the PICU to experience night terrors and acute anxiety and to regress in developmental milestones. Anticipatory guidance around these issues helps parents understand their child's behavior after discharge from the hospital.

★ EVALUATION

Periodically, the nurse and family evaluate the outcomes of care given. Examples of outcomes for the child and family with epiglottitis were given under diagnoses and planning in this section.

Foreign Body Aspiration

Definition and Incidence. Foreign body aspiration is more common in infants and children than in adults. Smaller infant airways, incomplete food chewing due to the absence of molar teeth, a natural inquisitiveness about objects, and a certain level of carelessness on the part of adults all contribute to higher incidence in children. Eating while running also contributes to the incidence of foreign body aspiration. Recent data indicate that foreign body aspiration is the *number one* cause of accidental death in children under 1 year of age, and the fourth leading cause of death in children less than 4 years of age.[13]

Etiology and Pathophysiology. Although most objects aspirated into the respiratory tract are immediately expelled by coughing, objects may lodge in the larynx, trachea, or bronchi. The degree of symptomatology and seriousness depends on the size and location of the aspirated object. Food, such as peanuts and vegetables, is the most commonly aspirated item in children. The introduction of the Consumer Products Safety Act of 1979 set toy manufacturing standards and has led to a significant reduction in morbidity and mortality associated with aspiration of these objects.

Foreign body aspiration into the larynx and trachea that causes partial obstruction compromises air flow, leading to variable signs of respiratory distress. If unrecognized and untreated, the inflammatory reaction may further compromise the child, increasing morbidity and mortality. Complete airway obstruction represents an immediate life-threatening event, requiring emergency intervention such as the Heimlich maneuver, following American Heart Association standards.[58] (See Chap. 29.)

Aspiration of smaller objects may occur into a main stem or lobar bronchi, more often the right lung than the left. The degree of obstruction determines the associated pathology. An object that produces negligible obstruction may produce few symptoms and can remain in the airway for a prolonged time. Serious clinical signs and symptoms of respiratory distress can occur with significant bronchial obstruction, and pathologic changes may follow if not treated in a timely manner. Because airways naturally dilate during inspiration, a ball-valve type of obstruction may occur, in which gas passes by the obstruction on inspiration, but with airway narrowing on expiration the gas is trapped distal to the obstruction. This mechanism can lead to the development of obstructive emphysema or obstructive atelectasis, as well as chronic pulmonary suppuration.

Clinical Manifestations. Symptomatology depends on the site and degree of obstruction, and the stage at which the child presents. Partial obstruction in the trachea, larynx, or bronchi can produce cough, stridor, dyspnea, cyanosis, hemoptysis, and wheezing. Aphonia, hoarseness, and drooling are particularly characteristic of laryngeal obstruction. Significant bronchial obstruction may produce additional characteristic signs. Atelectasis distal to the obstruction may cause decreased breath sounds on the affected side, along with a dull percussion note. Conversely, the development of obstructive emphysema secondary to ball-valve obstruction produces a hyperresonant percussion note. Left undiagnosed and untreated, bronchial obstruction may lead to recurrent lobar pneumonia or recurrent episodes of what may be incorrectly diagnosed as asthmatic wheezing.

Diagnostic Studies. Because many of the signs and symptoms associated with foreign body aspiration also occur with croup, epiglottitis, and asthma, the history and physical examination are crucial to making the proper diagnosis and the subsequent initiation of appropriate treatment.

A blind finger sweep of the hypopharynx *is not* recommended in small children, because of the potential for increasing the obstruction by lodging the object even tighter and deeper in the larynx. Suspicion of laryngeal foreign body obstruction may be diagnosed by direct visualization of the hypopharynx and larynx. Chest radiographs may be used to make the diagnosis of foreign body aspiration in the trachea and bronchi but only if the object is radiopaque. More often, chest radiographs indirectly contribute to the diagnosis by demonstrating unilateral hyperinflation or atelectasis. Because bronchial obstruction is of greater magnitude during exhalation, both expiratory and inspiratory films should be obtained, if possible. Because infants are unable to cooperate with

techniques for obtaining inspiratory and expiratory films, a lateral decubitis film may be necessary. If chest radiograph results fail to confirm (or rule out) foreign body aspiration, but clinical signs persist, direct visualization of the lower airways by bronchoscopy may be required.

★ **ASSESSMENT**

Assessment of the child with suspected foreign body aspiration facilitates the differential diagnosis, helps determine the degree of airway obstruction, and aids in observing for worsening airway obstruction. The focus of this section is on solid object aspiration, such as peanuts, coins, and small toys. For further discussion on the aspiration of gastric contents, see section on Aspiration Pneumonia later in this chapter.

A careful history often reveals a sudden onset of choking and coughing. frequently, the event was witnessed by a parent or caregiver. However, in some situations, symptoms may subside, then reoccur at a later time. There is no previous history of fever or infectious prodrome.

Respiratory assessment determines the degree of obstruction, as well as the possible location of the aspirated object. Inspiratory stridor is common if the object has lodged in the supraglottic or glottic area. Expiratory stridor is present if the foreign body is below the cords. However, inspiratory and expiratory stridor may be present in situations where the foreign body is subglottic, fixed, and does not move with respiration.

Use of accessory muscles, presence of retractions, and chest expansion should be evaluated. Accessory muscle use and retractions indicate significant respiratory distress. Asymmetric chest expansion indicates obstruction of one bronchus, usually the right main stem.

The ability to talk and the quality of phonation must be assessed. The inability to talk indicates complete tracheal obstruction. A change in the voice usually indicates a laryngeal placement of the object. Normal phonation with a cough is usually indicative of a tracheal foreign body.[3] Auscultation may reveal wheezing or diminished or asymmetric breath sounds. The child should be continuously monitored for signs and symptoms of worsening obstruction and respiratory distress, including increased retractions and accessory muscle use, tachypnea, diminished breath sounds, tachycardia, dyspnea, and diminished LOC. Cyanosis is a late sign of hypoxia. Ongoing monitoring and evaluation are critical to the identification of progressive respiratory failure.

Chest radiographs may reveal the aspirated object, however organic material (e.g., peanuts, vegetables) will not be visible. Other nonspecific signs such as atelectasis, obstructive emphysema, or a mediastinal shift may be present.[3,131]

★ **NURSING DIAGNOSES AND PLANNING**

Based on assessment data from above and Chapter 37, the following nursing diagnoses may apply to the family and child with foreign body aspiration:

• Ineffective Breathing Pattern related to airway obstruction.

- Anxiety related to respiratory distress.
- Impaired Gas Exchange related to airway obstruction.
- Inability to Sustain Spontaneous Ventilation related to respiratory muscle fatigue.

The nurse and child (or parents) together plan effective care based on the established nursing diagnoses. Several examples of expected outcomes follow:

- The parents provide comfort and support for the child.
- The parents demonstrate knowledge and skill in emergency procedures for airway obstruction in a child.
- The child's normal patterns of daily activities are reestablished.

The nurse plans for the care of the child based on both physician's orders and nursing diagnoses. Some general nursing care goals may be the following:

- Effective breathing patterns are reestablished.
- Anxiety is diminished.

★ INTERVENTIONS: COLLABORATIVE AND INDEPENDENT

Interventions are aimed at support of respiratory function, relief of airway obstruction, and parental education.

CONTROL OF ANXIETY

The continual presence of the parents and a quiet, calm environment aid in the control of anxiety. Invasive, noxious procedures should be avoided to prevent further airway obstruction and worsening respiratory distress. Sedatives should not be given due to respiratory suppression and the limited ability to evaluate LOC in the sedated child.

Oxygen should be administered, even if the child is spontaneously breathing and stable. Noninvasive monitoring of oxygenation can be accomplished through the use of pulse oximetry. Emergency hand ventilation equipment should be kept close by.

Direct laryngoscopy and bronchoscopy, with direct visualization and removal of the object, is the definitive treatment. In the spontaneously breathing, stable child, the procedure may be performed in the operating room. The child with acute, complete tracheal obstruction requires emergency laryngoscopy for removal or tracheostomy/cricothyrotomy for emergency resuscitation.

Once the foreign body is removed, the nurse must continue to monitor the child's respiratory status. Airway edema may be present or may worsen; therefore, any indication of progressive airway obstruction should be reported to the physician. Humidified oxygen or air delivered by aerosol mask or face tent decreases secretion tenacity and facilitates mobilization of secretions. Deep breathing exercises, incentive spirometry, and coughing may aid in the resolution of atelectasis.

TEACHING

Most episodes of foreign body aspiration occur in children less than 5 years of age. The greatest risk is found in infants and toddlers. Therefore, anticipatory guidance and parental education are key interventions in the prevention of foreign body aspiration.

Normal growth and development should be reviewed. Early emphasis should be placed on infants' proclivity to place objects in their mouths. Small foods such as peanuts, hot dogs, jellybeans, and raw beans are to be avoided until 4 or 5 years of age. Toys with small removable objects should not be given to infants or toddlers. Pamphlets on child safety are helpful for parents to read, particularly after an acute episode of foreign body aspiration, because families only hear and retain a small percentage of any information given during stressful situations. Parents should also be encouraged to take a CPR class that includes the management of airway obstruction in infants and children.

★ EVALUATION

Periodically, the nurse and family evaluate the outcomes of care given. Examples of outcomes for the child and family with foreign body aspiration were given under diagnoses and planning in this section.

Tracheobronchomalacias

Stridor that appears at birth or within the first several weeks of life often leads to the diagnosis of laryngo-, broncho-, or tracheomalacia. These terms refer to congenital deformities of the laryngeal and supraglottic structures, or weakness of the cartilaginous tracheal and bronchial walls, all of which lead to airway collapse and obstruction. These congenital abnormalities are relatively rare. In the postnatal period, it is often difficult to distinguish this condition from trauma or aspiration at the laryngeal level.

In the case of tracheomalacia, there may be abnormally shaped tracheal rings, with protrusion of the posterior portion into the lumen of the trachea.

The structural abnormalities produce airway collapse on inspiration, and increases the WOB. In cases where major bronchi are involved, airway collapse may lead to secretion retention and obstructive atelectasis. Respiratory distress may become exaggerated with crying or with feeding, and may lead to poor oral intake, undernutrition, and lack of normal weight gain.

Symptoms associated with the malacias are directly related to the site and degree of abnormality. Breathing "noises" range from mild to loud crowing sounds with inspiration. The infant may exhibit inspiratory stridor, which often improves with placement of the child in the prone position with the neck hyperextended. Use of accessory muscles may be evident, along with sternal and substernal retractions in severe cases. Tachypnea and tachycardia may also be observed. Cyanosis is commonly not seen during normal breathing, but the child may exhibit transient episodes during feeding or crying.

The diagnosis of a malacia is made by direct visualization of the area in question. Laryngoscopy or bronchoscopy reveals alterations in the wall of the airway and narrowing of the airway lumen with respiration. Radiographs may reveal areas of narrowing of the larynx, trachea, or main stem bronchi, but are usually nonspecific with respect to cause.

★ NURSING IMPLICATIONS

Infants with tracheobronchomalacia vary in severity of symptomatology, which is directly related to the degree of collapsibility of the trachea or bronchus during respiration. The infant may exhibit tachypnea, wheezing, stridor, cough, and varying degrees of respiratory distress (signs and symptoms of acute respiratory distress are listed in a display in the Pneumonia section of this chapter), including chest retractions, hypoxia with cyanosis, nasal flaring, and anxiety related to acute hypoventilation with hypercapnia. Chest radiograph may reflect areas of hyperinflation related to interference with expiration. The symptoms often increase, sometimes dramatically, with episodes of forced expiration, as with crying. In mild cases of tracheobronchomalacia, the symptoms may become apparent only when the infant cries, whereas in more severe cases the infant may have complete collapse of the airway while crying, requiring emergency intervention such as hand ventilation and intubation. Symptoms often increase with respiratory infections because the unstable airway is further compromised by airway edema or increased mucus production and cough.[66]

Depending on the severity of the malacia, infants may become easily fatigued from the increased WOB. They may have a poor nutritional intake related to fatigue and have an increase in insensible fluid loss secondary to tachypnea and associated diaphoresis. Infants may be at risk for dehydration, and nurses must assess the infant for clinical signs of dehydration, and monitor intake and output accurately. Many nursing diagnoses are the same as those mentioned under previous upper airway disorders.

Tracheobronchomalacia may be treated medically or surgically depending on the severity and the length of the airway involvement. Medical treatment includes aerosolized bronchodilators to optimize the diameter of the airway lumen. Beta-2 bronchodilators such as albuterol or metaproterenol can be administered by hand nebulizer by way of mask or mouthpiece depending on the age of the child. This treatment may be done in conjunction with chest physiotherapy (CPT). (See section on Techniques and Technology in Pediatric Respiratory Care later in this chapter). Although CPT can assist with removal of accumulated secretions, it may be contraindicated in infants whose crying during the procedure leads to significant increases in airway collapse and respiratory distress.

In infants who have a short localized lesion, resection of the segment often is effective. Involvement of a long segment of airway may require various grafts such as rib and cartilage, which are used to stabilize the collapsing airway. These surgeries have had mixed results and are usually limited to severe cases.[30]

Infants and children with severe tracheobronchomalacia that extends through long segments of the airway often need a tracheostomy (see section on Care of the Child With a Tracheostomy later in this chapter) and the application of continuous positive airway pressure (CPAP). CPAP is a system by which positive pressure is applied throughout the respiratory cycle by way of the tracheostomy tube, with sufficient pressure to prevent airway collapse during expiration (Fig. 38-3). CPAP may be

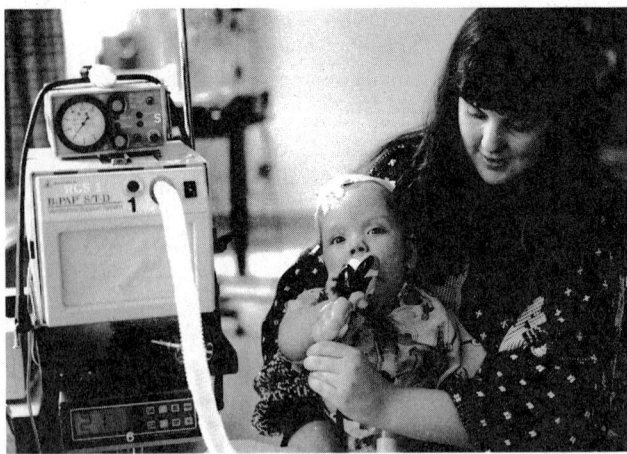

FIGURE 38-3
Infant with a tracheostomy on a CPAP/BIPAP system to support ventilation.

required for several months to stent the airway open, while allowing the child time to develop supporting structures and increase the airway lumen with maturation.

Parents need to be taught respiratory assessments, techniques for emergency bag/mask ventilation, and CPR. Because these children are often sent home with apnea monitors, parents require the skills necessary to set up and troubleshoot the equipment. Home oxygen equipment should be made available, and parents need to understand the indications for use, methods of application, and safety considerations in the home environment.

Because the CPAP system is large and has many connections, the apparatus poses restrictions on the infant and developmental delays may occur. Tracheostomies interfere with the infant's ability to vocalize and, therefore, inhibit the development of normal speech patterns. Nurses can teach parents alternative ways to stimulate the child as well as to make the system, and hence the infant, as portable as possible. Nurses and parents can work together to adjust the tracheostomy/CPAP system to work in the home if the parents can become experts in the system and develop a support network for respite care. Ensuring that the family has engaged a professional, supportive home respiratory care company to monitor the equipment routinely and respond to emergencies is an important aspect of home care. Families who are unable to take the infant home may experience failure in attachment with the child.

Bacterial Tracheitis

Bacterial tracheitis is a bacterial infection of the trachea and bronchi that is characterized by subglottic edema and the presence of copious amounts of thick, mucopurulent secretions in the trachea. This condition is an important cause of upper airway obstruction and can occur in children from several months old to early adolescence. Appearing with an acute onset or as a progressive disease, bacterial tracheitis is more common in the winter months.

An upper respiratory tract infection may contribute to bacterial invasion of the trachea. Whether viral infections play any role in the subsequent development of bacterial tracheitis is unclear.

Thick, stringy secretions adhere to the tracheal wall. The infection impedes mucociliary clearance, so that there is stasis of the secretions, leading to the formation of membranous webs and plaques. Areas of submucosal hemorrhage and granulation may be observed during the acute phase.

Bacterial tracheitis is often preceded by an upper respiratory infection followed by progressive deterioration of clinical status in 8 to 10 hours. Signs and symptoms of bacterial tracheitis are similar to those of viral croup or epiglottitis. However, drooling, usually seen with epiglottitis, is not present with bacterial tracheitis. The hallmark sign of bacterial tracheitis is the presence of large volumes of thick purulent secretions. As the illness progresses, a high fever with increased respiratory distress from progressive airway obstruction is seen.

Diagnosis is usually made after the child fails to respond to treatment for what is believed to be croup. Blood cultures are usually negative. The leukocyte count is elevated (usually higher than in viral croup) with a shift to the left indicating a bacterial infection. Bronchoscopy demonstrates thick mucus with disruption and sloughing of the tracheal mucosa. A lateral neck radiograph shows cloudiness of the tracheal air column with an irregularity or scalloping of the tracheal wall, and subglottic narrowing. A normal sized epiglottis rules out epiglottitis. Sloughed tracheal mucosa produces a vague density that may give a false impression of a foreign body. Chest radiograph may show the presence of pulmonary infiltrates. The diagnosis is confirmed by a culture of tracheal secretions.

★ NURSING IMPLICATIONS

Bacterial tracheitis shares many clinical features that are common to LTB and epiglottitis. Therefore, an accurate assessment is necessary to determine the interventions necessary to support the child. Obtaining an accurate history provides the foundation for further evaluation. Parents usually describe an initial prodrome of a febrile, mild upper respiratory infection, lasting 3 to 5 days. The child then develops a croupy cough, stridor, and difficulty in swallowing. Drooling usually is not present, and these children tolerate lying prone, in contradistinction to the child with epiglottitis.[33,60]

Further respiratory assessment reveals inspiratory and expiratory stridor, increased respiratory rate, and the use of accessory muscles. Cough and hoarseness progress as subglottic edema worsens and the volume of thick purulent tracheal secretions increases. A decrease in breath sounds indicates worsening obstruction.

Children with bacterial tracheitis usually are in significant respiratory distress and appear toxic. They do not usually improve when treated with bronchodilators, cool aerosol mist, or nebulized racemic epinephrine. Assessment and evaluation of all interventions are particularly important in this situation. Early identification of worsening respiratory distress or lack of response to interventions facilitates the institution of appropriate interventions.

If definitive diagnosis is questionable, examination of the oropharynx should be attempted, but only if the necessary equipment and personnel are available for endotracheal intubation. Bronchoscopy usually is performed in the operating room, revealing subglottic swelling, tracheal wall edema, and copious amounts of purulent secretions. Culture of tracheal secretions reveals the pathologic organism.[60,96]

Primary collaborative interventions are directed at maintaining airway patency, providing antibiotic therapy, and providing psychosocial support for the family and child.

Supportive interventions to maintain airway patency are determined by the severity and clinical progression of the disease. Children who have been ill for some time, those younger than 8 years of age, or those who demonstrate significant airway obstruction require debulking and suctioning of the purulent secretions under direct laryngoscopy, as well as endotracheal intubation.[33,96] Once endotracheal intubation is accomplished, the child is transferred to a PICU and placed on CPAP. (See section on Care of the Child Requiring Mechanical Ventilation later in this chapter.) Mechanical ventilation is rarely needed. Frequent endotracheal lavage with normal saline and suctioning are required to maintain patency of the ETT. Bronchoscopy may be used daily to clear tracheal secretions and to evaluate clinical progress. Extubation is performed once the fever has subsided, the amount and tenacity of secretions decrease, and there is an air leak around the ETT. Sedation and arm restraints may be necessary to prevent accidental extubation.

Children who are older or who present with milder disease can be managed by suctioning the trachea by way of direct laryngoscopy without intubation. This intervention may be necessary every day to remove the thick obstructive secretions.

IV broad-spectrum antibiotics are begun until culture and sensitivities are obtained. Antibiotic therapy is specified to cover the identified pathogen. Therapy should be continued for 10 to 14 days. Fever is controlled with antipyretics or tepid sponge baths.

Allowing parental participation in the care of the child is important to the support of family relationships. Ensuring the presence of the parents or a significant other also helps to decrease anxiety for the child. Parental education helps parents control their anxiety and achieve some mastery over a stressful situation. Education concerning the rationale for interventions and the expected hospital course is helpful.

Complications of bacterial tracheitis are primarily due to iatrogenic events or the virulence of the specific pathogen. Plugging of the ETT is a major concern because of the copious amounts of thick secretions produced. Respiratory failure due to ETT plugging, pneumothorax, or accidental extubation can occur.[33,34,60] Toxic shock syndrome has also been reported as a complication of bacterial tracheitis.[34,60]

Bacterial tracheitis has been implicated as a complication of endotracheal intubation, particularly in children with impaired immunologic defenses (e.g., children who use steroids, infants). Granulomas and ulceration can develop in the trachea due to mechanical damage from the ETT. Bacterial contamination by a virulent, resistant nosocomial organism can occur at the ETT site. A change in the color and consistency of secretions should alert the nurse to this possible complication.[41]

Bacterial tracheitis is capable of producing life-threatening airway obstruction. Delay in diagnosis and intervention significantly contributes to morbidity and mortality. Delay has been associated with cardiopulmonary arrest and death.[60,102] The usual hospital course is 14 days, endotracheal intubation (if necessary) is 2 to 4 days, and recurrences are uncommon.[102]

Acute Disorders of the Lower Airway

Bronchitis

Bronchitis is a nonspecific syndrome that seldom occurs as a primary disease in children but is usually secondary to respiratory conditions such as cystic fibrosis, asthma, or bronchiolitis. Bronchitis is an inflammatory process in the trachea and major bronchi; however, it may extend to the small bronchi and bronchioles. Bronchitis may be labeled as either acute or recurrent (chronic). The acute form usually resolves without therapy in 2 weeks, whereas the chronic form may persist for greater than 2 to 3 weeks. Chronic bronchitis is defined as 3 months or more of cough with expectoration for at least 2 years.[13] Bronchitis most often occurs in the winter months. It is more common in young children and is seen more commonly in boys than girls.

Bronchitis may be due to a viral or bacterial infection, or chemical or mechanical irritation of the bronchial epithelium. Rhinovirus, respiratory syncytial virus (RSV), influenza, and parainfluenza viruses have been isolated in children with bronchitis. Exposure to cigarette smoke during fetal development and postnatally has been shown to play a role in the development of bronchitis. Data also suggest that exposure to environmental pollutants such as ozone can contribute to chronic sputum production in childhood.[16]

Bronchitis causes inflammatory changes and edema of the airway mucosa. There is hyperplasia of the bronchial glands and hypersecretion of mucus into the lumen of the airways. In cases of what is termed "asthmatic bronchitis," there is a component of reversible airway obstruction secondary to constriction of bronchial smooth muscle.

The outstanding symptom of bronchitis is a cough. In the first 4 to 6 days of acute bronchitis, children have a dry, hacking, nonproductive cough. As the disease progresses, the cough becomes productive with purulent sputum. Fever, uncommon with bronchitis, is low grade if present. Diffuse expiratory rhonchi may be heard on chest auscultation. The presence of wheezing may indicate an underlying asthmatic component. The child may complain of chest pain, which is usually secondary to persistent coughing. Cough and mucus production often begin to subside by day 7 to 10 of the illness.

The chest radiograph may show increased bronchial markings or may be normal. The white blood cell (WBC) count is usually normal or may be elevated slightly. A sputum culture may be ordered to rule out other causes of the cough. Pulmonary function studies are not normally indicated.

★ NURSING IMPLICATIONS

Nursing assessment begins with a thorough history to determine the onset of illness, the severity of symptoms, and possible triggers. Usually, there is a prodrome of malaise and fever before the manifestation of respiratory symptoms. The assessment of respiratory function includes the determinations of respiratory rate, rhythm, depth, the presence and type of cough, and the amount of sputum produced. The presence of rales or wheezing should also be evaluated by chest auscultation.

Acute bronchitis usually presents with a dry harsh cough, upper respiratory congestion, and fever. Chronic bronchitis is characterized by cough and excessive mucus production for a minimum of 3 months. Respiratory tract irritants, such as air pollution and passive smoking, are often implicated in chronic bronchitis. A complete history and assessment of clinical symptoms help distinguish among acute bronchitis, chronic bronchitis, asthma, and sinusitis.[50] Many practitioners no longer use the diagnosis of chronic bronchitis in children, because it is nonspecific and can lead to the underdiagnosis of a primary disease such as asthma or gastroesophageal reflux.

Acute bronchitis is benign and self-limiting. Therapeutic intervention is symptomatic to control fever and cough. Antitussives, decongestants, and antihistamines can be given to control cough, congestion, and rhinorrhea. If vomiting occurs secondary to persistent coughing, fluid therapy may be indicated. Antibiotics are indicated only for secondary bacterial infection.

Therapy for chronic bronchitis should be directed toward the primary disease. Bronchodilators are indicated for asthma. Positioning techniques and altered feeding schedules should be instituted for gastroesophageal reflux. Parents should be taught that passive smoking aggravates lung disease and worsens the symptoms. Every effort should be made to encourage family members to stop smoking. Antimicrobial therapy is reserved for severe disease with secondary bacterial infection.[50]

The most common complications associated with bronchitis are secondary bacterial infection, pneumonia, and atelectasis. Outcomes with acute bronchitis are excellent; outcomes for chronic bronchitis vary with the underlying pathology.

Bronchiolitis

Definition and Incidence. Bronchiolitis refers to inflammation of the bronchioles. It occurs most commonly in children under the age of 2, with the highest incidence seen within the first 2 to 12 months of life. Bronchiolitis usually occurs in epidemics in the winter and early spring, in concurrence with the seasons for epidemics of RSV. Bronchiolitis outbreaks associated with the parainfluenza virus occur more often in the fall. RSV infections are so common that 100% of the population has been exposed by 2 years of age.[23] During RSV epidemics, infants are the most severely affected, with 80% of bronchiolitis hospitalizations occurring in infants 6 months old or younger. Morbidity and mortality are highest in this age group as well. Overall, 1% to 2% of all children who develop bronchiolitis require hospitalization.

Bronchiolitis affects boys more frequently than girls. Siblings in the home, a low socioeconomic status, and exposure to parental smoking (passive smoking) all increase the risk for developing bronchiolitis. Young children who attend day care are also at increased risk for contracting upper respiratory infections, which can progress to bronchiolitis.

Etiology and Pathophysiology. Bronchiolitis is caused most commonly by RSV, with two subtypes, A-subtype and B-subtype. A recent study suggests that knowledge of the RSV subtype might prove important in clinical management, because A-subtype was shown to be a more severe form in hospitalized children.[84] Approximately 90,000 children are hospitalized yearly with RSV bronchiolitis infections. Parainfluenza virus types I and III, adenovirus, enterovirus, influenza virus, and rhinovirus can also cause bronchiolitis. Some children may have more than one virus or may have a simultaneous bacterial infection.[123]

The spread of RSV bronchiolitis is by direct contact with respiratory secretions and is highly contagious. RSV is known to live for at least 30 minutes on clothing and up to 6 hours on surfaces such as a desk top. Introduced into a day care setting, RSV usually causes infection in all exposed children, who subsequently pass the infection on to their siblings at home. The incidence of nosocomial RSV infections also is high, with transmission occurring between health care workers contaminated with respiratory secretions.

Initially, the virus causes an infection of the upper respiratory tract. The virus spreads to the lower respiratory tract, involving the small bronchi and bronchioles. In the lower airways, the virus causes necrosis of the respiratory epithelium and destruction of the ciliated cells. Lymphocytes infiltrate the damaged areas resulting in submucosal edema and hemorrhage with increased production of a bronchiolar inflammatory exudate. Because of destruction of the ciliated cells, normal clearance of mucus from the tracheobronchial tree is impeded. (A month or more may be needed for cilia to regenerate.) Inflammatory cellular debris plugs the bronchioles, leading to increased airway resistance, decreased lung compliance, and impaired gas exchange. Areas of atelectasis and regional hyperinflation coexist, resulting in increased WOB, ventilation/perfusion ($\dot{V}_A/\dot{Q}$) mismatch, hypoxemia, and CO_2 retention, and respiratory acidosis in severe cases.

Clinical Manifestations. Bronchiolitis usually is preceded by a viral upper respiratory tract infection. The first indications of bronchiolitis may include rhinorrhea, cough, sneezing, and a low-grade fever. The child may also demonstrate irritability, a decreased appetite, and vomiting in the first few days of the illness. With the development of bronchiolitis, signs of increasing respiratory distress appear within 2 to 3 days after the initial onset of illness.

Characteristic clinical signs of bronchiolitis include inspiratory rales and expiratory wheezing on auscultation.

Other signs of respiratory distress observed in the child with bronchiolitis include tachypnea, nasal flaring, chest wall retractions (intercostal, subcostal, and suprasternal), tachycardia, and intermittent cyanosis. Hypoxemia and hypercarbia occur secondary to inadequate ventilation due to areas of overdistention and atelectasis. Shallow, rapid breathing represents the child's attempt to minimize the WOB due to air trapping and lung overdistention. Hyperinflation may be evidenced by a visible increase in the anteroposterior diameter of the infant's chest. A lack of appetite and increasing tachypnea make feeding difficult, and signs of dehydration may occur. Gastroesophageal reflux may develop secondary to compression of the stomach from lung hyperinflation.

Diagnostic Studies. The diagnosis of bronchiolitis usually is based on clinical signs and symptoms and the season of presentation. Other causes of airway obstruction including foreign body obstruction, lobar emphysema, and cystic fibrosis are ruled out. Signs and symptoms of bronchiolitis may mimic congestive heart failure, croup, or asthma. Chest radiograph may be normal or may show nonspecific changes including diffuse hyperinflation, increased bronchovascular markings, and patchy infiltration suggestive of pneumonia. ABGs show an increased $PaCO_2$ and decreased PaO_2. The white blood count usually is normal but, if increased, shows an increase in polymorphonuclear cells and bands (a shift to the left). Viral cultures may identify the causative viral agent.

Nasal washings and nasopharyngeal swabs are the preferred techniques for obtaining a specimen for analysis of the presence of the virus or its antigen. Derish et al[32] recently reported on the successful use of bronchoalveolar lavage in diagnosing RSV in four infants who had previously tested negative by nasopharyngeal swab. Rapid detection of RSV is possible by radioimmunoassays (RIA), by enzyme-linked immunosorbent assays (ELISA), or by direct fluorescent antibody assay.

★ ASSESSMENT

The nursing assessment of the child with bronchiolitis focuses on the severity of disease and the identification of etiologic factors. Viral bronchiolitis is a common childhood respiratory disease, and, in infancy, can become severe enough to require hospitalization for acute respiratory failure.[23,72] Bronchiolitis also is one of the most common causes of wheezing in infancy. Approximately 10% to 20% of infants with wheezing require hospitalization,[76] and 5% go on to acute respiratory failure.[72] Differential diagnosis may be problematic because the clinical syndrome of bronchiolitis is not entirely distinct from other lower respiratory diseases. Therefore, the nurse provides subjective and objective clinical data to support the identification and treatment of bronchiolitis.

The assessment process should begin with a complete history. Infants and small children with bronchiolitis present with a 1- to 3-day history of upper respiratory infection and low-grade fever.[14,23] The family should be questioned about the type, frequency, and severity of symptoms. How did the family treat the symptoms, and did this treatment work? Is anyone else in the family ill?

If so, what were the symptoms and how long did they last? A complete prenatal and neonatal history also should be obtained to assess for prematurity, low birthweight, congenital anomalies, and congenital heart disease.

Assessment of the home environment can support the differential diagnosis. Risk factors for bronchiolitis include family history of atopy or asthma, maternal smoking, no or limited breast-feeding, overcrowding, and low socioeconomic status.[23,85,114]

Pulmonary assessment includes the evaluation for tachypnea, retractions, use of accessory muscles, wheezing, and coryza. Auscultation determines the presence of wheezing, rales, rhonchi, and inspiratory stridor. Wheezing should be evaluated as to its quality and presence. A high-pitched wheeze usually indicates worsening airway obstruction. The disappearance of wheezing in combination with an increased WOB and respiratory distress indicates that air entry is absent or minimal ("silent lung"). The chest should be observed for symmetry of excursion and the use of accessory muscles. The presence of tachypnea, increased use of accessory muscles, and increased WOB are indicative of worsening airway obstruction. Cyanosis, apnea, and respiratory acidosis are late signs of respiratory failure, and they should precipitate rapid intervention and respiratory support.

Cardiovascular assessment requires the determination of heart rate and rhythm, blood pressure, and perfusion. Acutely ill infants who are tachypneic and feeding poorly are at risk for hypovolemia, which is manifested by tachycardia, cool extremities, increased capillary perfusion time (> 3 seconds), and diminished pulses. The presence of a normal blood pressure does not preclude the suspicion of hypovolemia and inadequate cardiac output due to compensatory mechanisms. Hypotension is a late and ominous sign, requiring rapid fluid administration and possibly pharmacologic intervention. Tachycardia or bradycardia can be seen with hypoxia.

Level of consciousness (LOC) is an important assessment parameter for any child with respiratory distress. Agitation can be an early sign of hypoxia. A decrease in LOC can indicate hypercarbia. All children should respond to pain, and infants older than 2 months should recognize their mother or primary caregiver.

★ NURSING DIAGNOSES AND PLANNING

Based on assessment data from above and Chapter 37, the following nursing diagnoses may apply to the family and child with bronchiolitis:

- Ineffective Breathing Pattern related to airway obstruction.
- Ineffective Airway Clearance related to airway obstruction.
- Impaired Gas Exchange related to increased secretions and ineffective airway clearance.
- Inability to Sustain Spontaneous Ventilation related to respiratory muscle fatigue.
- High Risk for Fluid Volume Deficit related to increased insensible loss and poor intake.
- Altered Nutrition: Less Than Body Requirements related to loss of appetite.
- Altered Parenting related to hospitalization.

The nurse and parents together plan effective care based on the established nursing diagnoses. Several examples of expected outcomes follow:

- The parents participate in the child's care.
- The parents discuss mode of spread of infection and isolation procedures.
- The parents demonstrate correct handwashing technique.
- The child's weight gain increases appropriately.

The nurse plans for the daily care of the child based on both physician's orders and nursing diagnoses. Some general nursing care goals may be the following:

- Effective breathing patterns are restored.
- Adequate hydration and oral intake are provided.
- Nosocomial infection is prevented.

★ INTERVENTIONS: COLLABORATIVE AND INDEPENDENT

MEDICATION THERAPY

The key to pharmacologic intervention is the aggressive use of nebulized β-adrenergic bronchodilators. However, in the emergency room setting, subcutaneous epinephrine or terbutaline may be used.[76,94] Often, distressed infants who present with wheezing respond to subcutaneous epinephrine, thereby preventing the need for hospitalization. Children less than 2 years old have a favorable response to subcutaneous adrenergic agents, as demonstrated by a decrease in respiratory rate and accessory muscle use. However, children younger than 18 months may require two to three doses before an appreciable improvement can be seen.[76]

Nebulized β-adrenergic agents include albuterol or metaproterenol, delivered by metered dose inhalers (MDI) with spacer, or by way of jet nebulizer, every 2 to 4 hours, or continuously if needed.[67,111] Albuterol promotes bronchodilation, decreases airway resistance, decreases WOB, and improves air exchange. Adverse effects include tachycardia and rhythm disturbances; however, these effects are seen less frequently due to selective β_2-adrenergic effects. During the administration of nebulized adrenergic agents, the nurse must continually evaluate heart rate and response to treatment. Children receiving continuous albuterol should be placed on a cardiorespiratory monitor and pulse oximeter. Theophylline also may be prescribed. The nurse should monitor for theophylline side-effects including vomiting, decreased appetite, restlessness, and irritability.

Ribavirin (Virazole), an antiviral drug, is approved by the U.S. Food and Drug Administration (FDA) for the treatment of RSV infections (bronchiolitis and pneumonia). Ribavirin is reported to decrease the duration of viral shedding and speed recovery from bronchiolitis. Studies indicate that early initiation of ribavirin may prevent serious sequelae of RSV infection and may shorten length of hospitalization.[49,87,116] Guidelines for the use of ribavirin in the treatment of RSV were issued by the American Academy of Pediatrics Committee of Infectious Diseases.[1] Ribavirin should be used for the following groups:

- Infants at high risk for severe RSV infection (congenital heart disease, bronchopulmonary dysplasia [BPD], other chronic lung conditions, certain premature infants, immunodeficiency states: transplants and chemotherapy).

- Infants hospitalized with severe RSV (PaO_2 less than 65 mmHg and elevated $PaCo_2$).
- Infants whose RSV disease state is not initially severe, but who may be at risk for a more complicated state by virtue of age (less that 6 weeks old), multiple congenital anomalies, and neurologic or metabolic disease.

Ribavirin is administered as an aerosol using a small particle aerosol generator (SPAG) unit, over a period of 12 to 20 hours/day, for 3 to 7 days. The SPAG unit delivers the aerosol medication to the child by way of oxyhood oxygen tent, mask, or ventilator. (See section on Techniques and Technology in Pediatric Respiratory Care later in this chapter for a detailed description of the use of ribavirin.)

Nurses should note that there is controversy concerning the safety of health care workers exposed to ribavirin.[52,56,82] The medication produces a residue that settles on all objects in the room, and environmental controls should be instituted to minimize exposure. The accompanying display lists caregiver precautions that are recommended to reduce exposure to ribavirin, and to screen staff who should avoid the care of an RSV-infected child receiving ribavirin.

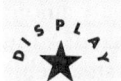

Precautions for Exposure of Health Care Workers to Ribavirin

- Pregnant women, and those pursuing conception within 6 weeks of potential exposure to ribavirin, should avoid contact with the drug.
- Health care workers should be screened for respiratory problems, reactive airways, or past skin/eye irritation from ribavirin exposure, and should avoid contact with the drug.
- Child should be placed in a private room, preferably with negative flow, or cohorted with other RSV children.
- The door should remain closed, and signs should be posted alerting staff and visitors to the presence of ribavirin.
- Gown, gloves, hair and shoe covers should be worn in the room. Handwashing before leaving the room is absolutely necessary.
- A surgical mask should be worn if environmental levels of the drug are at a minimum; otherwise, a respirator mask should be worn.
- Goggles should be worn by those with contact lenses.
- Whenever possible, SPAG unit should be turned off 3–5 minutes before breaking into delivery system to provide nursing care (suctioning and so forth).
- The drug may be administered on a schedule that includes nighttime.
- A scavenger system should be used when administering the drug to a nonintubated patient.

Antibiotic therapy is generally not indicated unless there is suspicion that there is a bacterial infection is superimposed.

OXYGEN THERAPY AND CHEST PHYSIOTHERAPY

Children who exhibit arterial desaturation require supplemental oxygen at levels necessary to maintain SaO_2 greater than 93% to 95%. Pulse oximetry should be used on any severely ill child receiving supplemental oxygen. Noninvasive monitoring permits the timely assessment of arterial oxygenation, without the need for invasive, painful ABG analysis. Oxygen can be administered by a variety of devices such as oxyhood, face tent, or nasal cannula, depending on the age of the child and the FiO_2 needs. (See section on Techniques and Technology in Pediatric Respiratory Care later in this chapter for a further discussion on oxygen delivery and pulse oximetry.)

Chest physiotherapy may be performed if the child tolerates the procedure and there is no increase in the WOB or desaturation during the procedure. The decision to institute chest physiotherapy should be based on an assessment that the child's normal mechanisms for secretion clearance are inadequate. Frequent suctioning may be necessary and regular repositioning promotes drainage of secretions.

MECHANICAL VENTILATION

Infants less than 2 months of age with RSV bronchiolitis are likely to require intubation.[87] However, mechanical ventilation is instituted in any child with severe respiratory failure who exhibits CO_2 retention, hypoxia, lethargy, or apnea. The length of mechanical ventilation required is usually anywhere from 48 to 96 hours. Once the child is extubated, supplemental oxygen should be continued. Many children demonstrate long-term oxygenation impairment after the clinical resolution of disease and may require oxygen therapy for several weeks. (See section on Care of the Child Requiring Mechanical Ventilation later in this chapter for further discussion of the nursing care of the intubated and ventilated child.)

HYDRATION AND NUTRITIONAL MANAGEMENT

Due to an increase in insensible water loss, and possible poor fluid intake, the child with bronchiolitis is at risk for dehydration. Fluid therapy should be given at maintenance rates. Blood glucose levels should be monitored, and hypoglycemia should be treated. The type of fluid therapy required is determined by serum electrolytes, osmolality, and serum glucose levels. Urine output should be monitored to evaluate fluid therapy and renal function. Urine output should be 0.5 to 1 ml/kg/h. Specific gravity (SG) also should be monitored. An elevated SG can indicate hypovolemia or renal dysfunction.

If the child is severely ill with an elevated respiratory rate, or requires mechanical ventilation, enteral nutrition should be instituted by way of a nasogastric tube. Reflux precautions should be taken in any child with significant respiratory distress requiring gavage feeding. Due to the increase in metabolic demands found with an increased WOB, caloric requirements may be as high as 150 to 200 calories/kg/day. An accurate calorie count must be done daily. Weekly plotting of weight gain on a growth chart is helpful in children who are hospitalized for prolonged periods.

PREVENTION OF NOSOCOMIAL INFECTION

The risk of nosocomial infection is linked to the length of stay, as well as to known risk factors such as cardiac disease and chronic lung disease. Secondary spread of RSV to hospitalized infants has occurred by way of contact with infected nursing, medical, and other hospital personnel. Transmission occurs by droplets through direct or close contact. The virus can live for one-half hour or more on the hands and for hours on environmental surfaces.[1,23] Thorough handwashing is the most effective way to prevent nosocomial spread. Masks and gowns have not been found to control the spread of RSV to other patients; however, goggles protect the provider when there is a splash risk. As with all patients, effective body substance isolation procedures should be followed. Surfaces must be decontaminated to prevent droplet spread. Contact isolation is recommended for infants or small children.[1] Children with BPD, cardiac disease, or lung disease and children who are immunosuppressed **should not** be housed with children who have positive RSV cultures.

TEACHING

Parents of children hospitalized with bronchiolitis should be allowed to participate in their child's care as much as possible. An open visiting policy must be maintained to support parental roles and the family unit. Screening of visitors is necessary if the child has RSV. The family should be taught about the mode of the spread of infection and the type of isolation procedures required. Family members should be educated about handwashing techniques, and they should be discouraged from handling other children. The nurse should be available to provide pertinent information on the child's daily progress, rationale for intervention, and the trajectory of illness.

★ EVALUATION

Periodically, the nurse and family evaluate the outcomes of care given. Examples of outcomes for the child and family with bronchiolitis were given under diagnoses and planning in this section. Have short-term goals been met? Are long-term goals still realistic? Planning for further nursing care takes into consideration complications and long-term care.

COMPLICATIONS

Most children with bronchiolitis do not require hospitalization. Only 5% progress to respiratory failure, and mortality is less than 1%.[1,72] The severity of illness is determined by underlying pathology and the etiologic organism. Children with congenital heart disease, BPD, chronic lung disease, prematurity, low weight, or young age are at greatest risk for severe disease.

Obliterative bronchiolitis is an infrequent consequence of acute lung injury. The pathogenesis includes intraluminal scarring and epithelial injury with subsequent sloughing and airway occlusion.[51] This complication should be suspected in the child who has persistent cough or wheezing, prolonged crackles, exercise intolerance after pulmonary injury, hyperinflation, hyperlucent lung syndrome, or respiratory symptoms in disproportion to radiographic findings.

LONG-TERM CARE

Most children who experience mild bronchiolitis recover normal lung function with no long-term sequelae. However, lung dysfunction may be present for years after severe bronchiolitis. Children who have a history of bronchiolitis have more symptoms of cough, wheezing, and reactive airways than normal controls.[35] Infants who have had RSV bronchiolitis have been shown to have subsequent symptoms of asthma; however, a direct correlation to the clinical diagnosis of asthma has not been found.[114] In some children, the sequelae of bronchiolitis decreases, with a reduction of wheezing and reactive airways. However, the presence of maternal smoking is directly correlated with long-term wheezing in children with a history of bronchiolitis.[85]

Pertussis

Definition and Incidence. Pertussis (whooping cough) is a highly communicable endemic and epidemic acute respiratory disease that affects children predominantly. Decreased access to immunization and a growing population of infants surviving congenital or neonatal illness have combined to produce a rise in the incidence of pertussis in the United States. The highest incidence of pertussis occurs in the first year of life, mostly among children who have not been properly immunized. A low level of family education, greater number of small children in the household, and crowded conditions are correlated with increased mortality. In the United States, the incidence is approximately equal in whites and nonwhites. The incidence in girls exceeds that in boys and is associated with increased severity and mortality.

Etiology and Pathophysiology. Pertussis is an infection of the upper respiratory tract caused by *Bordetella pertussis,* a gram-negative coccobacillus infectious only to humans. *B. parapertussis* and *B. bronchiseptica* have also been isolated from children with clinical whooping cough. Despite the high resistance of the adult population, resistance is poorly transmitted to the newborn. Transmission is by way of large aerosol droplets from the respiratory tract of symptomatic people, or by self-inoculation after touching a surface contaminated by a person with pertussis. The incubation period is usually 7 to 10 days with the bacteria residing in the respiratory tract.

B. pertussis is found attached to the superficial ciliated respiratory epithelium causing a marked endobronchial necrotizing inflammatory response. Shedding of cells into the lumen, inspissation of secretions, and paralysis of cilia can lead to areas of patchy atelectasis and pneumonia. Lobar and sublobular atelectasis, as well as bronchiectasis, are frequently seen. Interstitial or subcutaneous emphysema and pneumothorax may result from obstruction of large or small airways in severely affected infants.

Clinical Manifestations. The clinical manifestations of pertussis depend on the age and immunization status of the child, and the presence of complications (such as pneumonia and encephalopathy). The manifestations are denoted in specific stages: catarrhal, paroxysmal, and convalescent.

In the *catarrhal stage,* the onset is subtle, resembling a mild upper respiratory infection with rhinorrhea, low-grade fever, mild conjunctival infection, tearing, occasional sneezing, and a mild cough. This stage is the most infectious period and may last up to 14 days.

In the *paroxysmal stage,* the coughing progresses to become more forceful and appears as episodic paroxysms, occurring more frequently at night. At the height of the illness, the child may experience 10 to 20 episodes of paroxysms in a 24-hour period. There is little or no effective inspiratory effort between coughs. At the termination of the paroxysm, a long-drawn inspiratory effort is accompanied by a whoop, and the child frequently chokes or vomits. The cough is productive, and the vomitus is usually mucoid. After the episode, the child is exhausted and may have profuse sweating. In older children, a sense of fear or impending doom may precede the onset of paroxysm.

Apneic and cyanotic episodes lasting up to 60 seconds may occur during the paroxysm stage of pertussis, especially in early infancy. Most complications and deaths occur during the paroxysmal stage. Epistaxis and subconjunctival hemorrhage may also be present. The paroxysmal stage lasts 1 to 4 weeks or sometimes longer.

In the *convalescent stage,* the paroxysmal coughing gradually becomes less severe and less frequent. This stage can last from 1 to 6 months. During the convalescent stage, the child is usually free of the *B. pertussis* organism despite a persistent cough. Duration of illness in uncomplicated cases is usually 6 to 10 weeks. Weight loss or failure to gain weight may be observed in the young infant.

Diagnostic Studies. The diagnosis of pertussis is based on a characteristic history and physical examination. If a child presents with a history of paroxysmal cough for greater than 1 week associated with vomiting, whoops, or cyanosis, the child is suspected of having pertussis. Health care providers should consider the possibility of pertussis early and institute laboratory diagnostic procedures.

Lymphocytosis and an increase in total WBC count on a blood smear are usually present in classic pertussis. An increased WBC count greater than 15,000 with greater than 70% lymphocytes helps to confirm the diagnosis of pertussis. A WBC count greater than 50,000 is related to severe disease and a poor prognosis.

The best method for making the diagnosis of pertussis is to culture the organism from the nasopharynx. In obtaining the culture, a swab should be passed through the naris about 2 inches into the nasopharynx and left in place until coughing occurs.

★ ASSESSMENT

A thorough history is part of the initial assessment of the child with pertussis. A complete immunization history, as well as the investigation of any known exposures or ill household contacts is included. The nurse should determine from the parental interview the characteristic of their child's cough, presence of mucus during coughing, and presence of cyanotic episodes or periods when the child appears not to be breathing.

Assessment of the child's respiratory, fluid, and nutritional status is made. A complete respiratory assessment determines the stage of the disease process, the severity of illness, and the need for hospitalization.

The catarrhal stage mimics a mild upper respiratory infection, with mild coughing and rhinorrhea. The paroxysmal stage is manifested by the progression to severe paroxysms of coughing, often with a characteristic expiratory whoop, followed by vomiting. In infants less than 6 months, the whoop may be absent, with apnea being one of the most common manifestations.[1] Assessment of airway patency, air exchange on auscultation, and the use of accessory muscles determines if airway obstruction or atelectasis is present. Cyanosis is indicative of hypoxia and possible apneic episodes. Most children are afebrile.

Careful assessment of neurologic status is important, particularly after coughing paroxysms. Coughing spells often leave the child exhausted and lethargic. The determination of weight loss is important because paroxysms and exhaustion contribute to poor feeding and nutritional depletion.

★ NURSING DIAGNOSES AND PLANNING

Based on assessment data from above and Chapter 37, the following nursing diagnoses may apply to the family and child with pertussis:

- Fatigue related to coughing paroxysms.
- Ineffective Airway Clearance related to thick secretions.
- Anxiety related to frequent episodes of uncontrollable coughing paroxysms.
- Fluid Volume Deficit related to poor oral intake.
- Impaired Gas Exchange related to coughing and apneic episodes.
- Parental Anxiety related to lack of information about the disease, its treatment, and the child's prognosis.

The nurse and child (or parents) together plan effective care based on the established nursing diagnoses. Several examples of expected outcomes follow:

- The parents discuss decision regarding the child's immunizations.
- The parents maintain a calm, supportive environment for the child.
- The child eats small nutritious meals frequently.

The nurse plans for the daily care of the child based on both physician's orders and nursing diagnoses. A general nursing care goal may be the following:

- Incidence of paroxysms is reduced.
- Parents recognize symptoms that should be reported.
- Diversional activities keep child quiet.
- Transmission of pertussis is prevented.

★ INTERVENTIONS: COLLABORATIVE AND INDEPENDENT

Interventions for affected children are primarily supportive to manage apnea, cyanosis, feeding difficulties, and coughing paroxysms. Children less than 6 months of age should be hospitalized. Community intervention is directed at immunization and education.

The most effective method of preventing morbidity and mortality due to pertussis is through routine childhood immunization. The pertussis vaccine is a suspension of inactivated *B. pertussis* organisms combined with diphtheria and tetanus toxoid (DPT). Immunization also has been associated with milder disease forms in children who have not been completely vaccinated.

Information on immunization and the recommended schedule are given in Chapter 9. Parents should be educated regarding the reactions that may occur, and informed consent should be obtained before vaccines are administered.

Erythromycin is the most effective antimicrobial agent for treatment. When the drug is given in the catarrhal or paroxysmal stage, the organism is eradicated after 1 to 2 days. Treatment is continued for 14 days to prevent relapse. However, once paroxysms are present, antimicrobial therapy has no effect on the disease course. Corticosteroids and albuterol have shown some effect in diminishing the paroxysms of coughing.[1,64]

Rest is essential for the child with pertussis. Calming and comfort measures are implemented to prevent exhaustion. Diversional activity is an important part of the child's day and may help to decrease the number of paroxysmal coughing episodes. Family support centers around education and the continuation of normal parenting. The nurse's supportive, nonjudgmental attitude is critical because often these parents have chosen not to immunize their child; parental feelings of guilt are common. Therefore, the nurse should allow the parents to ventilate their feelings. The nurse is in a pivotal role to provide support and education about any concerns parents may have regarding immunization.

Nutrition is important to offset any weight loss. IV fluids may be necessary to maintain an adequate fluid balance. The child is encouraged to take frequent small feedings. Infants and children who become exhausted or congested may not feed well. Gavage or parenteral nutrition may be used.

Gentle nasopharyngeal suctioning may be required to clear the thick mucus. The procedure should be done carefully after a paroxysm because suctioning can precipitate a coughing episode; deep suctioning should be avoided. Humidified air and oxygen may be required in the presence of hypoxia. Pulse oximetry and transcutaneous O_2 and CO_2 monitoring are helpful in the ongoing evaluation of oxygenation and ventilation. Oxygen with hand ventilation bag and mask should always be at the bedside in the event of respiratory compromise.

Cardiorespiratory monitoring and close nursing supervision ensure early identification and intervention for apnea and bradycardia. Children should be isolated for 5 days after the initiation of antimicrobial therapy. If such therapy is contraindicated, the child must be isolated for 3 weeks after the onset of paroxysms.[1]

★ **EVALUATION**

The nurse and family evaluate the outcomes of care given. Examples of outcomes for the child and family with per-

tussis were given under diagnoses and planning in this section. Planning for further nursing care takes into consideration complications.

COMPLICATIONS

Complications from pertussis are seen most frequently in children less than 6 months of age and in children who have not been immunized. Complications from pertussis include pneumonia, atelectasis, subcutaneous emphysema, seizures, and encephalopathy. Mortality is increased in children who are under 1 year of age.

Central nervous system (CNS) disturbances occur most frequently during the paroxysmal stage and particularly in infants. The incidence of encephalopathy is approximately 1%. However the overall long-term prognosis for children with pertussis is favorable.

Prophylaxis for all close contacts is necessary regardless of age or immunization status. Erythromycin is the agent of choice, and therapy should last for 14 days. Pertussis immunization is recommended for all unimmunized contacts less than 7 years old.

Pneumonia

Pneumonia is an inflammation of the pulmonary parenchyma. Pneumonia occurs most often from infection, but also can be caused by aspiration of foreign substances into the lung or from inhalation of chemical irritants. Infectious pneumonias are discussed here, followed by aspiration pneumonia.

Infectious Pneumonias

Several epidemiologic factors play a role in the incidence of infectious pneumonia. These include age, gender, social environment, socioeconomic level, nutrition, underlying illness, and immunologic stability.

Viral Pneumonia. Viral pneumonia is the most common cause of lower respiratory tract infections in children age 4 and under. Several agents are responsible for pneumonia in this age group, including RSV, adenovirus, influenza and parainfluenza virus, cytomegalovirus, and rhinovirus. Children acquire a primary viral pneumonia secondary to an initial upper respiratory tract infection, with aspiration into the lower airways. Factors such as crowded living conditions, attendance at day care, and the presence of infected siblings all expose the majority of young children to viral organisms.

RSV is by far the most common and important cause of viral pneumonia. Peak seasons for RSV infections include the late fall and winter months, when cases reach epidemic proportions. Young children coming home from school with the newly acquired virus pass it on to their infant siblings. Whereas the older child may have only a mild viral upper respiratory infection, the infant sibling is often hospitalized with RSV pneumonia or bronchiolitis. RSV is so prevalent that almost all children have been exposed to the organism by 2 years of age.

The severity of illness correlates with the duration and level of viral shedding. The incubation period lasts 5 to 8 days, with viral shedding lasting anywhere from 3 days to 4 weeks. Pneumonia may be present with or without bronchiolitis. Fever and cough are consistent findings, with otitis media, rhinorrhea, pharyngitis, and conjunctivitis. Respiratory distress and impaired gas exchange can occur with severe RSV pneumonia, and intubation and mechanical ventilation may be necessary. Diagnosis of RSV pneumonia usually is made by culturing a swab of nasopharyngeal secretions.

Hospitalized infants suffering from an RSV infection are an important source of nosocomial infection. Nursing care should include effective aseptic techniques, keeping infected children separate from uninfected children, and minimizing the amount of cross-care that occurs between infected and noninfected patients.

Bacterial Pneumonia. Bacterial pneumonia is commonly caused by three major organisms: pneumococci, streptococci, and staphylococci. Bacterial pneumonia can occur anytime throughout the year, with no particular seasonal variation. Pneumonia in the newborn usually is a manifestation of an infection acquired from the mother just before or during delivery through the birth canal.

Pneumococcal pneumonia is the most common cause of lobar pneumonia. Occurrence is more common in the winter and early spring, and infection is transmitted by way of aerosol droplets. The organism gains access by aerosolization of nasopharyngeal contents into the lower airways, with proliferation in the lung parenchyma, where tissue necrosis can occur.

Streptococcal pneumonia may appear without evidence of illness or may follow a streptococcal upper airway infection. Streptococcal pneumonia is seen in the older child between the ages of 6 and 16. Hospitalization may be prolonged with this particular pneumonia due to an increased incidence of complications such as pleural effusion.

Staphylococcal pneumonia occurs most often in infants in the first year of life, often as a sequelae to a staphylococcal skin infection. It also is common to children with cystic fibrosis. Abrupt onset may occur, with the child presenting in a shocklike state, coupled with acute respiratory distress. Morbidity and mortality are highest with this type of bacterial pneumonia. Staphylococcal pneumonia is acquired by airborne and hematogenous routes. The airborne route is associated with an underlying viral respiratory tract infection. The hematogenous route is associated with soft tissue infection, although the exact mechanism of invasion is not fully understood.

Chlamydia Pneumonia. *Chlamydia trachomatis* is an intracellular microorganism with properties similar to that of gram-negative bacteria. It is the most common cause of newborn pneumonia, acquired from a maternal cervical infection. Organisms inoculate the eyes and nasopharynx during parturition, or by the ascending route in utero. Signs and symptoms include a persistent dry staccato cough, tachypnea, rhinorrhea, a history of conjunctivitis, and minimal or absent fever. The chest radiograph shows diffuse bilateral infiltrates.

Initiation of close follow-up care is important, especially in the first year of life of an infant who suffers a *Chlamydia* infection at birth, because recurrent wheezing, persistent abnormal chest radiograph, and altered pulmonary function have all been documented in these infants.[112]

Mycoplasma Pneumonia. *Mycoplasma* pneumonia is a common cause of pneumonia in children over the age of 4. *Mycoplasma* are small, free-living organisms classified separately from bacteria and viruses. The organism accounts for 75% of the pneumonias seen in children 5 to 15 years old.

Mycoplasma pneumonia is endemic, with epidemics occurring every few years; peak incidence is in the fall and early winter. Transmission is by exposure to aerosol droplets. The usual incubation period is 2 to 3 weeks. Asymptomatic people can carry the infective organism for several months after active infection. Signs and symptoms include rapid onset of fever, abdominal pain, headache, cough, sore throat, rales and rhonchi on auscultation, and loss of appetite. Transient joint pain and skin rashes are not uncommon. Chest radiograph findings are variable. Although most symptoms subside within 1 to 2 weeks, the cough may last for months.

Pneumocystis carinii Pneumonia. *Pneumocystis carinii* pneumonia occurs almost exclusively as an opportunistic infection in immunocompromised children. In the United States, it is restricted almost entirely to immunocompromised patients with deficient cell-mediated immunity, including those with congenital immunodeficiency and malignancy under treatment. *Pneumocystis carinii* is the primary pulmonary infection associated with individuals who have human immunodeficiency virus (HIV)-positive acquired immunodeficiency syndrome (AIDS). Children with lymphoma or leukemia are susceptible to developing pneumonia from this organism during remission.

Mode of direct transmission includes person-to-person transmission by the respiratory route and reactivation of latent infection as a result of immunosuppression. The period of incubation and communicability is unknown.

Clinical manifestations include a subacute, diffuse pneumonitis with dyspnea at rest, tachypnea, cough, and fever. Chest radiographs show bilateral interstitial infiltrate that can be more extensive than the clinical findings may suggest. ABGs show decreased PaO_2 and $PaCO_2$.

Incidence. Pneumonia is a common diagnosis in children, with the peak incidence occurring between 6 months and 5 years of age. Incidence declines after the age of 9. Boys are affected 25% more than girls. Poor socioeconomic status, large numbers of siblings, parental smoking, and preterm birth have all been associated with an increase in incidence of pneumonia in early childhood. Children living in urban areas are twice as likely to be diagnosed with pneumonia than children from rural areas.

Pathophysiology. Most organisms gain access by aerosolization of nasopharyngeal contents into the bronchi, with proliferation in the lung parenchyma, resulting in tissue necrosis. Pneumonias are categorized as lobar pneumonia, bronchopneumonia, or interstitial pneumonia, depending on the area of the lung affected. *Lobar pneumonia* refers to inflammation in all or a large segment of one or more pulmonary lobes. *Bronchopneumonia* originates in the terminal bronchioles, which become clogged with mucopurulent exudate and form consolidated patches in nearby lobules. *Interstitial pneumonia* refers to an inflammatory process confined within the alveolar walls (interstitium) and the peribronchial and interlobular tissues. Destruction of ciliated cells and bronchial mucous glands leads to sloughing of epithelium, resulting in edema of bronchial walls that become infiltrated with mononuclear cells and compromise tracheobronchial clearing.

Clinical Manifestations.   Clinical manifestations largely depend on the child's age and immune status, and the etiologic agent. The onset may be acute or insidious, with considerable variation in presentation. Symptoms may include mild to severe fever, rhinorrhea, cough, tachypnea, and malaise. Wheezing has been shown to occur more frequently with viral pneumonia than bacterial pneumonia.[124] Alterations in gas exchange secondary to the presence of secretions in the small airways may produce hypoxia. Dehydration may occur secondary to poor fluid intake and added loss of fluid from the respiratory system secondary to the increased minute ventilation.

In severe cases, respiratory muscle fatigue may lead to respiratory failure with impaired oxygenation, CO_2 retention, and respiratory acidosis. If respiratory failure develops, the child may require intubation and mechanical ventilation. Although overall mortality is extremely low in children who acquire a simple pneumonia, certain clinical situations may require immediate, aggressive therapy to avoid increased morbidity and mortality. At grave risk are young infants who acquire a bacterial pneumonia superimposed on a viral infection, children who are immunosuppressed, and children with chronic pulmonary conditions such as cystic fibrosis or BPD who acquire an acute pneumonia.

Diagnostic Studies.   Differentiating bacterial, viral, or other pneumonias based on clinical, laboratory, and radiologic findings is difficult. Clinical signs and symptoms include cough, respiratory distress, rhinorrhea, headaches, abdominal pain, anorexia, vomiting, fever, rales or wheezes on auscultation, and otitis media. These symptoms may be observed in either viral or bacterial pneumonia. The WBC count with differential, C-reactive protein, and chest radiograph do not help in a differential diagnosis of viral versus bacterial pneumonia.

In about half of childhood pneumonias, the causative pathogen is not identified. The limitations of current diagnostic techniques make proper identification of causative organisms and their appropriate antimicrobial treatment difficult. Several techniques are used in an attempt to identify the infecting organism in pneumonia. In children, the diagnosis of bacterial pneumonia can be made by isolating the infecting organism from sputum or pleural fluid. Although needle aspiration of the lung and culture of the aspirated pleural fluid is a more sensitive and specific diagnostic technique to identify the organism, the invasiveness of the procedure limits its use to only a few children with severe pneumonia.

In the young child, adequate sputum samples are rarely obtained for Gram's staining. Nasopharyngeal or throat cultures are of little value in diagnosing pneumonia, because multiple pathogens frequently reside in the upper airway, and there is a poor correlation between their presence in the pharynx and their responsibility for the pneumonia. In the older child, a sputum induction might be done using hypertonic saline (10% NaCl) aerosol or ultrasonic nebulizer using sterile water to induce cough and expectoration of a sputum sample.

★ ASSESSMENT

Nursing assessment of the child with pneumonia requires a thorough examination of the respiratory system because the number and severity of the clinical manifestations are highly variable. Depending on the child's age and the causative organism, the presenting manifestations may be as subtle as a low-grade fever with mild malaise, or so severe that the child is in acute respiratory distress, requiring intubation and mechanical ventilation.

Rate and quality of respirations compared with age norms are a priority at initial assessment. Quality of inspiration includes the presence of retractions, symmetry of chest movement, nasal flaring, and use of accessory muscles. Quality of expiration includes length of the expiratory phase, presence of audible wheezes, and accessory muscle effort.

Breath sounds on auscultation vary depending on lung field involvement and the stage of the disease. In the early stages, there may be scattered crackles, or breath sounds may be mildly decreased. An area of consolidation may produce tubular or bronchial breath sounds without other adventitious sounds. As the consolidation resolves, coarse crackles with rhonchi often are heard. The initial cough associated with pneumonia is usually hacking and nonproductive, progressing to wet and productive of clear or purulent sputum.

Systemic symptomatology includes fever, malaise, poor appetite, decreased oxygen saturation, cyanosis or pallor, complaints of generalized body ache, and chest pain. Young infants, especially under 2 months of age, may have a subnormal temperature, decreased food intake, and increased sleepiness or crankiness, without any signs of respiratory distress. They may present in the emergency room with signs of dehydration. Older children may complain of chest pain, productive cough with blood-tinged sputum, and chills. The nursing assessment display lists signs and symptoms of acute respiratory distress.

★ NURSING DIAGNOSES AND PLANNING

Based on assessment data from above and Chapter 37, the following nursing diagnoses may apply to the family and child with pneumonia:

- Activity Intolerance related to infectious process.
- Ineffective Airway Clearance related to infectious mucus production.
- Inability to Sustain Spontaneous Ventilation related to respiratory muscle fatigue.
- Anxiety related to air hunger.
- Altered Family Processes related to the child's illness/hospitalization.

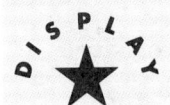

Nursing Assessment: Signs and Symptoms of Acute Respiratory Distress in Otherwise Healthy Children

Mild

- Increased respiratory rate
- Tachycardia
- Minimal or absent diaphoresis
- Mild substernal retractions in younger child, no retractions in older child
- May be restless/irritable but consolable; interested in play with low frustration tolerance; moving about
- Able to suck with rests; diminished interest in food
- Stable oxygen saturation in high 90s
- Breath sounds may have scattered wheezes, rales, rhonchi, mild diminishment, or may be clear
- Blood gases have stable pH/oxygen and carbon dioxide may be altered or normal
- Face, finger, toe color remains pale pink

Moderate

- Tachypnea
- Tachycardia
- Diaphoresis
- Nasal flaring, grunting
- Substernal, intercostal, and supraclavicular retractions; use of accessory muscles
- Prolonged expiratory phase of respiration
- Too fatigued to suck or eat, poor appetite
- Pallor or mild cyanosis (''duskiness'')
- Irritable, cries easily but not long due to shortness of breath, lies down and is not interested in environment.

- Older child has increased anxiety and complains about shortness of breath; calls for primary caregiver
- Oxygen saturation decreased
- Blood gases have decreased oxygen and/or increased carbon dioxide; pH may be normal or borderline acidosis
- Breath sounds significantly diminished, wheezes, rales

Severe

- Tachypnea or bradypnea
- Tachycardia or bradycardia
- Hypertension or hypotension
- Diaphoresis
- Severe retractions or minimal chest movement
- Prolonged expiratory phase of respiration with expiratory grunt
- May be in stupor, unconscious
- No crying, may have generalized hypotonia
- Peripheral and/or central cyanosis or severe pallor
- Breath sounds are diminished (minimal air movement audible)
- Significantly decreased oxygen saturation
- Blood gases have low oxygen, high carbon dioxide, and acidotic pH

- High Risk for Fluid Volume Deficit related to decreased nutritional intake and increased losses.
- Hyperthermia related to infectious process.
- Anxiety (Caregiver) related to lack of information about disease process, contagiousness, treatment regimen, and prevention of complications.
- Altered Nutrition: Less Than Body Requirements related to poor appetite and persistent cough.
- Sleep Pattern Disturbance related to persistent cough.

The nurse and child (or parents) together plan effective care based on the established nursing diagnoses. Several examples of expected outcomes follow:

- Factors that aggravate activity intolerance are identified.
- The parents demonstrate accurate assessment skills to identify and avoid complications.
- The parents demonstrate comfort and calming skills.
- The child sleeps for uninterrupted periods of time.
- The parents and child use effective coping skills to diminish anxiety.
- The parents state they have sought professional counseling regarding sexually transmitted diseases.

The nurse plans for the daily care of the child based on both physician's orders and nursing diagnoses. Some general nursing care goals may be the following:

- Normal breathing and eating patterns are restored.
- Cross-contamination to other family members is avoided.

★ INTERVENTIONS: COLLABORATIVE AND INDEPENDENT

Care of the child with infective pneumonia includes the administration of antimicrobial drugs, other pharmacologic support, oxygen, bronchial hygiene, fluids, and education. Nurses need to understand the causative organism and treatment regimen of the child's illness to establish necessary isolation techniques and continuous physical assessment with realistic expectations for the results of therapy. Ongoing assessment is necessary to identify respiratory deterioration and promote recovery.

MEDICATION THERAPY

Although there are many antibiotics available to treat bacterial pneumonias, effective antiviral agents are limited.

Viruses render children more susceptible to secondary bacterial complications. Hence, children with viral pneumonia may be treated prophylactically with antibiotic therapy, depending on culture results, the practitioner's clinical assessment, and other susceptibility criteria, such as age.

Drugs of choice for treatment of *Pneumocystis carinii* pneumonia are trimethoprim-sulfamethoxazole (TMP-SMZ) or pentamidine. Major side-effects of TMP-SMZ include bone marrow suppression, fever, and rash, all of which may complicate the clinical picture of the underlying immunosuppressive disorder. Pentamidine is an alternative, administered IV or intramuscularly (IM) therapeutically, and by IV or aerosol inhalation prophylactically. Because IM administration of pentamidine is associated with abscesses at the injection site, the IV route is preferred in the immunosuppressed child.[53]

The administration of aerosolized pentamidine requires the use of specialized equipment and techniques. Figure 38-4 shows a child receiving an aerosol pentamidine treatment. Some states have created guidelines for proper, safe administration of aerosolized pentamidine in an effort to control the health care worker's environmental exposure to the medication. Precautions for pentamidine administration by nursing or respiratory care personnel are highlighted in the accompanying display. The child should be sequestered in a private room, if possible, during administration, with the door closed, and caregivers should wear a mask during the actual administration of the medication to the child. These protective behaviors have an added importance because there have been reports of an increasing incidence of resistant strains of tuberculosis present in HIV-positive AIDS patients who develop *Pneumocystis carinii* pneumonia and may require aerosol pentamidine therapy.[18,90]

Children who exhibit wheezes on auscultation may be treated with bronchodilator medication. These medications may be given orally or by aerosol inhalation by way of hand nebulizer or metered dose inhaler (MDI) (see section on Techniques and Technology in Pediatric Respiratory Care later in this chapter). Bronchodilators relax bronchial smooth muscle to increase lumen size,

Precautions for Safe Administration of Aerosolized Pentamidine

- Patient should be in a private room, preferably with negative flow, with the door closed.
- A special nebulizer should be used, with filters to trap exhaled aerosol particles.
- Staff should be screened before exposure to pentamidine. Those who have a history of diabetes, reactive airways, eye irritation to previous exposure, or those who are pregnant should be exempt from administering the drug.
- A mask and gloves should be worn by the therapist during medication administration.
- The flow to the nebulizer should be turned off whenever the child removes the mouthpiece to cough, rest, and so forth.

which facilitates improved ventilation and gas exchange, and enhances the opportunity for coughing and expectoration of mucus and detritus from the infected airways.

OXYGENATION

Oxygen is administered to optimize oxygenation. The use of a cool aerosol by way of mask, face tent, or hood helps add humidity to the airways, facilitating mobilization of secretions. Pulse oximetry can be used to monitor oxygen saturation, to evaluate the response to oxygen therapy, and to alert the nurse to changes in the clinical condition. (See section on Techniques and Technology in Pediatric Respiratory Care later in this chapter.)

FLUID THERAPY

Children with infections and respiratory distress have a greater insensible loss of fluids through diaphoresis and tachypnea. They may have a significant decrease in fluid intake from loss of appetite and fatigue from respiratory distress, rendering them unable to eat. Nasal congestion may interfere with the infant's ability to suck. IV fluids may be necessary to avoid dehydration, especially in the infant.

BRONCHIAL HYGIENE THERAPY

Chest physiotherapy techniques including postural drainage and percussion can assist with the drainage of mucus and cellular debris from the affected lobe(s). Although the rhythmic clapping on the chest may be soothing to some children, many cry during the procedure, which represents a form of deep breathing in the child too young to do so on request. Hence, crying is not necessarily a reason to avoid this treatment. Techniques and illustrations are found in Chapter 25.

The benefits of CPT may be enhanced when administered in conjunction with aerosolized bronchodilators in children receiving both therapies. Nurses should coordinate their schedule with respiratory care staff when necessary to optimize the effectiveness of these two in-

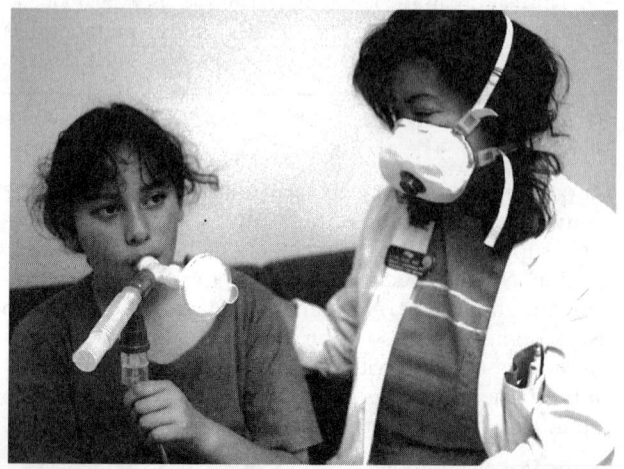

FIGURE 38-4
Eight-year-old child receiving aerosolized pentamidine treatment. Note that the respiratory therapist is wearing a protective mask.

terventions. Nasopharyngeal or oral suctioning may be required in the child with copious amounts of secretions.

TEACHING AND COUNSELING

Most children with pneumonia are treated as outpatients; therefore, parents must leave the primary care setting of the emergency room with knowledge and skills to enhance the child's care and promote compliance with treatment. Nurses must teach families the basic concepts of cross-contamination and methods of protecting other family members. Parents need to be taught assessment skills to identify complications of pneumonia and to promote early treatment in future pulmonary infections. Parents need to acquire the skills to administer aerosol treatments and oral antibiotics. When parents seem unable to comprehend the outpatient care, a public health nurse consultation is indicated, or inpatient care should be considered. A medical interpreter should be arranged for parents with language differences that could diminish the effectiveness of communication.

Family counseling may be indicated when a newborn acquires a pneumonia from an infected mother. Infants who have *Chlamydia* pneumonia are frequently born to young, socioeconomically deprived mothers whose medical histories reflect an increased risk for sexually transmitted diseases. In caring for the family unit, the nurse should counsel the mother to be treated, and suggest prenatal screening for subsequent pregnancies. Safe sex guidelines and their rationale should be discussed, with printed materials to support the discussion.

★ EVALUATION

The nurse and family evaluate the outcomes of care given. Examples of outcomes for the child and family with infectious pneumonia were given under diagnoses and planning in this section.

Aspiration Pneumonia

Definition and Incidence. Aspiration pneumonia or pneumonitis is an inflammatory response in the lung resulting from the aspiration of foreign substances. This response may be triggered by a variety of causes, including aspiration of gastric contents after vomiting, smoke inhalation, accidental aspiration of hydrocarbon-based household cleaning products, or aspiration of a foreign body. This type of pneumonia is often seen in infants who have gastroesophageal reflux or tracheoesophageal fistula.

Pathophysiology. The extent and type of pathologic features differ depending on the causative agent, although there are similarities. Irritation to the airway mucosa and lung parenchyma leads to mucosal edema, ciliary stasis, and inspissation of secretions and aspirated substances, leading to impaired airway clearance. Airway irritant receptors are often stimulated, producing a cough that is usually nonproductive and, in some cases, bronchospasm. Atelectasis can develop, leading to ventilation/perfusion (V/Q) mismatch and hypoxemia. Alveolar epithelium may be damaged, producing alveolar-capillary membrane leak and pulmonary edema, further compro-

mising gas exchange. Toxicity associated with the aspiration of certain chemicals may extend beyond the pulmonary system, leading to CNS depression, renal toxicity, cardiomyopathy, and hepatosplenomegaly.

Clinical Manifestations. History and physical presentation play a key role in the diagnosis of aspiration pneumonitis. Sick children found in the presence of open bottles of household liquids should immediately receive emergency care.

The child with aspiration pneumonia may exhibit tachypnea, tachycardia, nonproductive cough, and rhonchi on auscultation. Diffuse wheezing may be present secondary to airway edema, or may be localized from foreign body aspiration. Cyanosis, retractions, and lethargy may be present. The aspiration of certain household substances may leave a characteristic odor on the breath. Fever may occur shortly after the event or may develop within 24 to 48 hours, depending on the causative agent. CNS depression may be present on admission or may progressively develop over the initial 12 to 24 hours.

Diagnostic Studies. In instances of impaired gas exchange, pulse oximetry readings reflect a low S_pO_2. Pulse oximetry is an unreliable tool for assessing oxygenation in the child suspected of smoke inhalation, because pulse oximeters overestimate actual S_pO_2 in the presence of carbon monoxide inhalation, leading to a false reassurance about oxygenation. Children with potential lung injury from smoke inhalation require an ABG with oximetry to assess levels of oxyhemoglobin (HbO_2) and carboxyhemoglobin (COHb) directly. Radiographic findings in fluid or vomitus aspiration usually show variable areas of patchy density with air trapping. Laboratory tests are of little value in the diagnosis of aspiration pneumonia, other than to confirm the specific substance that might have been ingested.

★ ASSESSMENT

Assessment of the child with aspiration pneumonia includes obtaining a complete history and physical examination. Respiratory alterations depend on the volume and type of substance aspirated, and the location of the aspiration within the lungs. The child may exhibit tachypnea, tachycardia, and a decrease in oxygenation by pulse oximetry. Auscultation reveals wheezes or rales, which may be localized or diffuse.

Infants with gastroesophageal reflux or tracheoesophageal fistula are susceptible to developing aspiration pneumonia. Gastroesophageal reflux is a relaxation or incompetence of the esophageal sphincter muscle, which allows stomach contents to return up the esophagus, and be aspirated down the trachea. The disorder is commonly seen in early infancy due to immaturity of sphincter control, and it usually resolves over time. Reflux is also seen in neurologically impaired children, such as those with cerebral palsy, probably due to altered nerve innervation of the sphincter muscle.

Tracheoesophageal fistula is a congenital malformation in which the trachea and esophagus are joined, allowing ingested food to pass into the lungs (see section on Tracheoesophageal Abnormalities in Chap. 59). Soon after birth, the infant usually presents with respiratory symptoms, including cough, choking, and cyanosis.

★ NURSING DIAGNOSES AND PLANNING

Based on assessment data from above and Chapter 37, the following nursing diagnoses may apply to the family and child with aspiration pneumonia:

- Impaired Gas Exchange related to airway obstruction and inflammation.
- Ineffective Breathing Pattern related to airway obstruction.

The nurse and child (or parents) together plan effective care based on the established nursing diagnoses. Several examples of expected outcomes follow:

- The parents demonstrate correct positioning of child.
- The parents demonstrate respiratory assessment skills.
- The parents discuss handwashing, smoke-free environment, and sibling care.

The nurse plans for the daily care of the child based on both physician's orders and nursing diagnoses. Some general nursing care goals may be the following:

- Upper airway is kept clear.
- Adequate gas exchange is achieved.
- Further incidence of aspiration is avoided.

★ INTERVENTIONS: COLLABORATIVE AND INDEPENDENT

Interventions are aimed at supporting gas exchange, bronchial hygiene, pharmacologic therapy, positioning and feedings, and parental education. Severe, diffuse aspiration may require intubation and mechanical ventilation. Aspiration pneumonia caused by congenital abnormalities such as tracheoesophageal fistula invariably require surgical correction.

The child may require oxygen therapy in conjunction with cool aerosol mist to help mobilize aspirated contents. Pulse oximetry can be used to monitor oxygenation. Other measures to facilitate optimal gas exchange include placing the head of the bed at a 30- to 45-degree elevation for children with tracheoesophageal fistula. In the child with gastroesophageal reflux, the mattress should be raised at the head with the child harnessed or supported in the prone position at all times.

The child with tracheoesophageal fistula should be made NPO, and a suction catheter should be placed in the upper esophageal pouch for drainage of excessive mucus and drool. Feedings should be done slowly, and the infant should be in an upright position afterwards, avoiding bouncing and increased abdominal pressure.

Nasopharyngeal suctioning may be necessary to keep the upper airway clear of any gastric contents that might otherwise be aspirated. Chest physiotherapy with postural drainage is sometimes necessary to help mobilize secretions from the affected lung segments. However, in gastroesophageal reflux, CPT should only be done while the stomach is empty, immediately before feedings, to avoid reflux. Postural drainage is contraindicated in a child with an unrepaired tracheoesophageal fistula.

Antibiotics are indicated to treat any infection that occurs secondary to aspiration of gastric contents, or as a consequence of an acute inflammatory response in the lung. If the child exhibits wheezing, aerosolized bronchodilators may also be administered as needed.

Parents should be taught positioning measures and other methods to avoid aspiration. Regular assessment of any relationship observed between regurgitation and cough in the infant should also be reviewed.

Nurses should teach parents respiratory assessment skills to promote early care for the child who remains prone to complications or recurrence. Parents are also taught skills such as the indications for and methods of administering oral or aerosol medications at home. The importance of follow-up care must be emphasized, and parameters for seeking immediate medical care must be discussed in detail. Information about home contagion control, such as handwashing and sick sibling awareness, is given. Facts about children living within a smoking environment and the increased incidence of respiratory problems are discussed with parents as a prophylactic measure for avoiding future pulmonary illness.

★ EVALUATION

The nurse and family evaluate the outcomes of care given. Examples of outcomes for the child and family with aspiration pneumonia were given under diagnoses and planning in this section.

Depending on the causative factors and severity of an aspiration pneumonia, some infants may continue wheezing episodes and remain susceptible to other pulmonary infections long after resolution of the aspiration pneumonia. Some scarring and fibrotic changes may be seen on chest radiograph, which may resolve only after months or years have passed. Infants with congenital heart disease or chronic lung disease, such as BPD, are not only more susceptible to aspiration pneumonia but to long-term sequelae as well.

Tuberculosis

Definition and Incidence. Tuberculosis (TB) is an infectious disease caused by *Mycobacterium tuberculosis*. TB is characterized by stages of inflammatory infiltrations, formation of tubercles, caseation, necrosis, abscesses, fibrosis, and calcification. Primary TB refers to the initial infection, which progresses through a series of stages terminating in dormant calcified lesions. Secondary TB usually implies a reactivation from a healed primary lesion. The respiratory system is the most common site of a primary TB infection.

It is estimated that 1 billion people worldwide are infected with TB, with 1 to 3 million deaths occurring annually from TB.[57] The U.S. Department of Health and Human Services, Centers for Disease Control reported 25,701 cases of active TB in 1990 in the United States, an increase of 15.8% since 1985.[18] Risk factors for developing TB include diabetes, particularly poorly controlled insulin-dependent diabetes, corticosteroid or immunosuppressive therapy, primary or secondary malnutrition, acquired or congenital immunodeficiency disease, and children with malignancies of lymphoid tissue.

There are some areas in the United States in which the incidence of TB is higher, such as large metropolitan areas where the problems of homelessness, overcrowding, and the lack of access to medical services favor the transmission of TB. Additionally, the incidence of TB has risen in metropolitan areas with a higher density of HIV-infected patients, where it is manifesting with increasing frequency as a secondary infection. Urban areas are also populated with new immigrants from developing countries that are associated with a higher incidence of TB.

Etiology and Pathophysiology. Children usually acquire the infection from contact with an infected adult, usually in the immediate household. Children rarely infect other children. Children with primary TB infection are the reservoir from which future cases emerge. Therefore, it is important to identify infected children early so treatment and education can be initiated. Unidentified disease is largely responsible for new infections.

Transmission most often occurs by way of infected aerosol droplets that become airborne when the actively infected person coughs, sneezes, or laughs. For the infection to be transmitted, the bacilli must be inhaled and implanted on lung tissue. The particle size must be 5 mm or smaller for the bacilli to travel to the lower airways; larger particles are effectively filtered out by the upper respiratory tract. Poor ventilation can also increase the risk of transmission.

In primary TB, infection with *Mycobacterium tuberculosis* results in a localized pneumonitis at the alveolar site. The inflammatory response in the alveolar tissue triggers polymorphonuclear cells, which phagocytize but do not kill the bacilli. Sensitization to the tuberculin antigen and development of a tubercle lesion at the site of infection follows in the next 2 to 4 weeks after exposure. The lesion undergoes stages of necrosis, encapsulation with scar tissue, and calcification. Most often, the disease arrests at this stage. If the disease progresses at the time of primary infection, erosion into a central airway can cause dissemination throughout the lung. Involvement of a blood vessel can lead to hematogenic distribution of the organism throughout the body.

Miliary TB refers to small lesions resulting from systemic dissemination, involving a variety of organs such as the brain, liver, kidney, or bones. Reactivation of a dormant primary lesion produces what is termed secondary TB. Although the reactivation may be localized, necrotic cavitation of lung tissue can be extensive and can lead to clinical signs and symptoms of respiratory impairment.

Clinical Manifestations. Clinical presentation varies from asymptomatic with only a positive skin test to extensive pulmonary and systemic involvement. In most cases, the child with primary TB does not have any specific recognizable clinical signs and symptoms other than a positive skin test and calcified lesions on chest radiograph. A child with secondary TB infection may demonstrate a fever and a mild cough, with weight loss and night sweats as the disease progresses. Young infants may be characterized as "failing to thrive." Although pulmonary symptoms are limited, wheezing or decreased breath sounds and tachypnea may be present if there is bronchial obstruction.

Diagnostic Studies. Diagnosis of TB is based on the tuberculin skin test, clinical signs and symptoms, bacteriologic tests, and chest x-ray.

Tuberculin Skin Test. The tuberculin skin test is the most valuable test for the control of TB. The screening of children for TB is based on three premises: TB is curable; TB is a progressive disease; and the progression from infection to disease is preventable with medications.

The American Academy of Pediatrics (AAP) recommends annual tuberculin skin testing in children from high-prevalence settings including those living in families with a case of positive TB, American Indian children, and children of parents who have recently immigrated from Asia, Africa, the Middle East, Central and South America, or the Caribbean.[1] All HIV-infected children should have purified protein derivative (PPD) status determined regularly, although absence of a skin reaction does not rule out infection. In children who are considered at low risk, the AAP recommends routine testing at 12 to 15 months of age, before entering school, and in adolescence unless local epidemiologic circumstances dictate differently.[1] The tuberculin test is discussed in Chapter 9.

The interpretation of skin tests in children can be complicated by other vaccines to which the child has been exposed. Additional factors can also lead to false-positive and false-negative tuberculin test results. The accompanying display lists several factors that can influence the accuracy of TB skin testing, a discussion of which is beyond the scope of this textbook.

Bacteriologic Tests. Gastric contents or aspirated bronchopulmonary secretions usually are requested by the physician to isolate the tubercle bacilli in infants. Extrapulmonary specimens are analyzed by staining, culturing, and determining histologic appearance. The pulmonary specimen undergoes fluorescent and nonfluorescent testing to determine the presence of the tubercle bacilli. Performance of an induced sputum may be done on older children to determine the presence of the acid-fast bacilli.

Chest Radiograph. An anteroposterior and lateral chest radiograph is obtained on every child with a positive skin test. Asymptomatic children may show no abnormalities other than calcified lesions, whereas symptomatic children may have some pulmonary abnormality including parenchymal inflammation or localized, nonspecific infiltrates. Lymph node involvement is a characteristic finding in childhood TB and is seen on radiograph as progressive hilar lymph node enlargement. Compression from the enlarged lymph node can result in bronchial obstruction, destruction of the bronchus, and formation of thick caseum in the lumen that may occlude the bronchus. Pleural effusions, calcifications, and miliary lesions may occur with childhood TB. Cavitation is usually not seen earlier than adolescence.

★ **ASSESSMENT**

The nursing history and assessment for a child with a positive skin test for TB should include questions re-

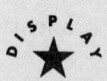

Factors Influencing TB Skin Test Results

False-Positive Skin Tests

- Reactions caused by nontuberculosis myco-bacteria
- Children previously vaccinated with bacille Cal-mette-Guérin (BCG)
- Errors in interpreting the reaction seen at the in-jection site

False-Negative Skin Tests

- Use of bad tuberculin products
- Administration errors during the injection
- Errors in interpreting the reaction seen at the in-jection site
- Physiologic factors in the child, to include:
- Febrile infection that causes temporary anergy
- Recent vaccination with a live virus (e.g., mea-sles, mumps, and so forth)
- Metabolic or nutritional imbalances
- Certain diseases affecting the lymphoid organs
- Children currently on corticosteroids or immu-nosuppressive drugs

garding the presence of general malaise, fatigue, exercise intolerance, anorexia, weight loss, cough, fever, and night sweats. Although cough is usually mild, the sputum may be blood-streaked or mucopurulent. Chest assessment should include respiratory rate, rhythm, excursion, symmetry of movement, inspiratory-to-expiratory (I:E) ratio, and use of accessory muscles. Chest auscultation should be done to determine the presence of rhonchi or wheezes, or diminished breath sounds. The degree of respiratory distress is determined from the symptomatology noted (see display on Nursing Assessment: Signs and Symptoms of Acute Respiratory Distress in Otherwise Healthy Children earlier in this chapter). However, many children with a positive skin test for TB may be asymptomatic.

Temperature should be obtained to determine the presence of fever, and lymph nodes should be inspected and palpated for inflammation and tenderness. Lymph node inflammation usually occurs in the cervical and supraclavicular areas.

A search for the infected person must be completed to find and treat the source of the child's infection. Therefore, a nursing history should include questions regarding all people living in the household, including other close contacts such as babysitter and the people in the babysitter's home. The same physical symptom history should be obtained from all contacts, including history of positive TB skin tests and recent travel. All contacts should have a TB skin test and, if positive, a chest radiograph. A chest radiograph is also warranted in the presence of a negative skin test if physical symptoms are present. Siblings should be evaluated and tested because of their similar contact pattern and close proximity to each other.

★ NURSING DIAGNOSES AND PLANNING

Based on assessment data from above and Chapter 37, the following nursing diagnoses may apply to the family and child with TB:

- Ineffective Breathing Pattern related to decrease in total lung capacity.
- Anxiety related to lack of knowledge about illness, management, reinfection, and transmission prevention.
- High Risk for Infection Transmission related to noncompliance with medical and nursing regimens.
- Altered Nutrition: Less Than Body Requirements related to anorexia from chemotherapy.

The nurse and child (or parents) together plan effective care based on the established nursing diagnoses. Several examples of expected outcomes follow:

- The parents discuss infectious aspects and prognosis of tuberculosis.
- The child reports consumption of small and frequent nutritional feedings.
- The parents state symptoms to report in the child or other family members that should be reported.
- The parents demonstrate good hygiene techniques.
- The child covers mouth while coughing and sneezing, followed by handwashing.

The nurse plans for the daily care of the child based on both physician's orders and nursing diagnoses. A general nursing care goal may be the following:

- The family understands the need for long-term care
- Infection to others is avoided.

★ INTERVENTIONS: COLLABORATIVE AND INDEPENDENT

Historically, TB has caused much suffering and death. However, since the advent of chemotherapy, TB has been curable with relatively little morbidity. Parents need to understand this new prognosis to diminish their fears and perhaps encourage compliance regarding the chemotherapy and other preventive measures.

Isolation is rarely necessary because most children with pulmonary TB are noninfectious. In fact, most children are successfully treated on an outpatient basis.

CHEMOTHERAPY

Chemotherapy is the most important treatment for TB. The primary antituberculosis drugs are isoniazid (INH), rifampin (RMP), pyrazinamide, ethambutol hydrochloride, and streptomycin sulfate. The most common combination of drugs used in the treatment of children is INH and RMP; the others may be used if an INH/RMP combination is not tolerated or, less frequently, if the strain of TB is drug resistant. Treatment with a combination of INH and RMP for 9 months is recommended for pulmonary disease, whereas the same treatment is extended to 12 to 18 months for extrapulmonary disease. Treatment for 9 months with INH and RMP cures 98% of the cases when given once daily for the first 1 to 2 months, then either once daily or twice per week for the remaining months.[118] Treatment with INH and/or RMP may be given prophylactically to children who have been exposed with (class 2) or without (class 1) a positive skin test (Table 38-2).

SURGICAL MANAGEMENT

Surgery is necessary when tissues that are the source of the infection are not accessible to drug therapy. This may include surgery for pulmonary lobe resection or rigid bronchoscopy for polyp removal in a bronchus.

ACTIVITY PROMOTION AND NUTRITIONAL MANAGEMENT

Nursing management supports rest, meaning the child may do activities that do not cause fatigue and may increase activity as tolerance increases. Nutrition is often difficult to promote in the anorexic child, yet is important for adequate healing and resistance to further infection. Small, frequent meals of desired foods can often increase nutritional intake.

TEACHING

Parents must be educated about the drug regimen and the importance of full treatment with prophylaxis. Parents should be instructed to report symptoms of liver toxicity of the chemotherapeutic drugs, such as nausea, vomiting, jaundice, malaise, right upper-quadrant abdominal pain, fever, and anorexia.

Prevention of the disease is the major goal of parent education. Parents must be able to recognize the symptoms of the disease in other family members and contacts so they can be directed toward treatment. They must be taught good hygiene, especially good handwashing, and avoidance of contact with sputum with proper disposal of contaminated material. Children must be taught to use tissues to cover their mouths when they cough and sneeze, with proper handwashing afterward.

PUBLIC HEALTH INVOLVEMENT

The public health department should be notified regarding all cases of TB and suspected sources of the infection. A public health nurse visit to the home can assist the parents with methods to decrease contagiousness and support chemotherapy compliance. Hospitalized children may be visited by family members who may also be infected; nurses should therefore screen each visitor to avoid spread in the hospital setting. Asymptomatic children may be sent to school and lead a relatively unrestricted life. Older children with active TB should be restricted from contact sports and protected from fatigue and stress.

★ **EVALUATION**

Periodically, the nurse and family evaluate the outcomes of care given. Examples of outcomes for the child and family with TB were given under diagnoses and planning in this section.

Atelectasis

Atelectasis is characterized by a loss of lung volume, leading to alveolar collapse. Collapse can occur in a small portion of one lung segment, an entire lobe, or through-

TABLE 38-2
Classification of Persons Exposed to or Infected With *Mycobacterium tuberculosis*

Class	Exposure History	Infection (Skin Test)	X-Ray Result	Culture Result	Clinical Signs	Plan of Care
0 No tuberculosis exposure, not infected	Neg	Neg	Not done	Not done	None	
1 Tuberculosis exposure, no evidence of infection	Pos	Neg	Not done	Not done	None	If exposure is within 3 months consider preventative therapy.
2 Tuberculosis infection, no disease	Pos	Pos	Neg	Neg	None	Preventative chemotherapy may be indicated
3 Tuberculosis: clinically active	Pos	Pos/neg	Pos/neg	Pos/neg	Pos	Chemotherapy
4 Tuberculosis: not clinically active	Pos	Hx of pos	Pos (but stable)	Neg	None	
5 Tuberculosis suspect (diagnosis pending)	Pos	Results pending	Results pending	Results pending		(Patients to remain in this class no longer than 3 months) Reclassify once results obtained

Source: American Thoracic Society and the Centers for Disease Control (1990). Diagnostic Standards and Classification of Tuberculosis. *American Review of Respiratory Diseases, 142,* 725.

out both lungs. Airway obstruction from secretions or mucous plug, tumor, or an aspirated foreign body can produce atelectasis. External compression of lung tissue from conditions such as pneumothorax or pleural effusion may also contribute to a loss of lung volume. A variety of postoperative factors can also predispose the child to the development of atelectasis. These include the use of anesthetics or narcotics that suppress coughing and deep breathing, pain and immobility. The common feature is a failure on the part of the child to take periodic deep breaths and cough.

Pathophysiologic changes and clinical manifestations depend on the extent of the atelectasis. Localized atelectasis may lead to mild tachypnea, with decreased breath sounds in the affected area. If the cause is foreign body aspiration, localized wheezing may be heard on auscultation. Flexible fiberoptic bronchoscopy may be used diagnostically to confirm the presence of a foreign body and may be used therapeutically to extricate the foreign body.

Involvement of an entire lobe may lead to impairment of gas exchange and hypoxemia. Diffuse atelectasis secondary to postoperative factors can contribute to mild hypoxemia, tachypnea, and increased WOB. Breath sounds may be distant or absent in the lower lobes, with a dull percussion note. If the child is encouraged to take several deep breaths and cough, crackles may subsequently be heard. A fever may develop 24 to 48 hours postoperatively. Chest radiograph findings may show decreased lung volumes.

If secretion retention is the cause of localized atelectasis, measures to enhance mobilization of secretions may be indicated. These include adequate systemic hydration, aerosol therapy, CPT, positive expiratory pressure (PEP) mask therapy, and, in some instances, bronchodilators in patients with a history of chronic reactive airways disease.

Incentive spirometry is useful in the older, cooperative child. A number of units are available; some can be entertaining for the child and family. One bedside unit has a clown whose nose illuminates when a preset volume is achieved. Other disposable units use colored balls or water that moves when the appropriate volume is achieved (Fig. 38-5). The technique must be explained to the child and family before it is attempted. Demonstrations can be incorporated into the preoperative teaching program. Alternative maneuvers for smaller children include blowing bubbles or paper objects across a flat surface. This therapy must not exhaust the child; six maneuvers every 2 hours while awake is usually sufficient. Deep breathing exercises can be attempted in older children, although measuring results is difficult because many children self-limit inspiratory volume. The goal of any deep breathing maneuver is to increase the child's tidal volume to twice normal or greater if tolerated.

Mechanically ventilated children can develop atelectasis secondary to ineffective cough, pulmonary disease, or inappropriate ventilator settings. These children usually respond to the application of positive end-expiratory pressure (PEEP; see section on Care of the Child Requiring Mechanical Ventilation later in this chapter) and hyperinflation with endotracheal suctioning. Frequent turning or positioning in a chair is important. Severe persistent atelectasis, such as seen in right middle lobe syndrome, may require bronchoscopy and lavage to clear mucous plugs.

Atelectasis usually resolves over time, particularly with good nursing care. Continued assessment of breath sounds and daily chest radiographs help monitor therapeutic response. Many children can leave the hospital postoperatively with atelectasis and suffer no significant alteration in gas exchange.

★ NURSING IMPLICATIONS

Atelectasis is primarily a complication of surgery, endotracheal intubation, foreign body aspiration, or airway compression. The first step toward the assessment of atelectasis is the identification of those children who are at risk for the development of this complication.

Respiratory signs include decreased breath sounds or a change in the pitch of breath sounds over the atelectatic lung. Changes often are difficult to hear in the small child or infant due to transmission of breath sounds throughout the lung fields. Chest expansion may be asymmetric or decreased on the involved side. WOB can be significantly increased if the atelectasis is severe or widespread. Chest radiography reveals intrapulmonary opacification and a shift of the intrathoracic structures toward the area of atelectasis. Any child with atelectasis requires frequent auscultation to determine response to therapeutic interventions.

Early mobility, ambulation, and frequent position changes are the primary interventions to prevent and treat atelectasis. Deep breathing maneuvers are also helpful in the resolution of atelectasis. Positioning with the head of the bed up and maximal inspiration reverse the microatelectasis associated with hypoventilation.[42]

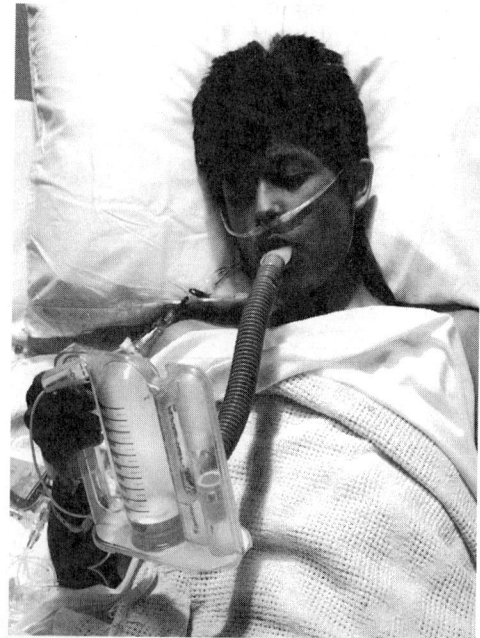

FIGURE 38-5

Twelve-year-old boy performing incentive spirometry after cardiac surgery.

Pleural Conditions

Pleural Effusion

Definition and Incidence. A pleural effusion is a collection of fluid in the pleural space. Pleural effusion fluid may represent a transudate, exudate, blood, or chyle (lymph fluid). A *hydrothorax* is a collection of noninfectious serous fluid in the pleural space. A pleural effusion caused by blood is called a *hemothorax*. A *chylothorax* occurs when lymph fluid finds its way into the pleural space. *Empyema* refers to the presence of pus in the pleural cavity.

The incidence of pleural effusion in the pediatric population is low. Many of the conditions that predispose to the development of a pleural effusion (congestive heart failure, liver failure, lung abscess, and so forth) are not commonly seen in children. The most common causes of pleural effusion in the pediatric patient are chest trauma, necrotizing pneumonia, and malignancy.

Etiology and Pathophysiology. Pleural effusion develops when the movement of fluid into the pleural space exceeds its rate of removal. The fluid may represent an exudate (protein content greater than 3.0 g/ml) or transudate (protein content less than 3.0 g/ml).[13] Several mechanisms are responsible for the accumulation of fluid in the pleural space. These include (1) increased capillary permeability, (2) either increased capillary hydrostatic pressure or decreased colloid osmotic pressure in the vascular bed perfusing the thoracic structures, (3) increased negative intrapleural pressure, and (4) alterations in pleural space lymphatic drainage.

Exudative pleural effusions develop in conditions in which capillary permeability is increased, such as pulmonary infections or infarctions, malignancies, lupus, or rheumatoid arthritis. Empyema may develop secondary to infection, either primary or secondary to trauma, or from rupture of a lung abscess. Hemothorax results from chest wall trauma, thoracic surgery, or a vascular rupture. Injury or infection involving thoracic duct outflow can lead to the development of a chylothorax. Congestive heart failure, liver or renal impairment, or malignancy can produce a hydrothorax.

Accumulation of fluid in the pleural cavity leads to compression of the adjacent lung tissue, producing atelectasis. Depending on the extent of the pleural effusion, gas exchange may be impaired and WOB increased as the child attempts to reexpand the collapsed lung tissue. Additionally, significant extravasation of vascular volume into the pleural space can deplete vascular volume, leading to hemodynamic compromise.

Although small amounts of pleural fluid can be reabsorbed into the vascular and lymph system, the evacuation of the pleural space by way of thoracentesis may be necessary to avoid complications. Failure to remove large volumes of fluid can lead to the development of a fibrothorax. In this situation, the pleural surfaces fuse to form a fibrous, calcified tissue, which can lead to a chronic restrictive lung condition. A decision to perform thoracentesis is based on clinical presentation and pleural fluid type and volume.

Clinical Manifestations. The clinical presentation varies depending on type and cause, volume of fluid, and underlying conditions. In mild pleural effusion, the child may exhibit tachypnea, decreased breath sounds, and a dull/flat percussion note on the affected side. Pleuritic pain most often occurs in association with an inflammatory condition. With a moderate to large pleural effusion, positional dyspnea may be present, with hypoxia and respiratory failure.

Diagnostic Studies. Chest radiograph confirmation requires that the pleural effusion occupy at least 15% to 20% of the pleural space. An upright posteroanterior film may show a hazy consolidation at the lateral base of the lung, with obliteration of the costophrenic angle. Thoracentesis may also be performed for diagnostic purposes.

Analysis of the pleural fluid determines if it is an exudative or transudative process. Exudates are milky (chylothorax), bloody, or turbid. Transudates are clear or straw-colored and odorless. Pleural fluid should be sent for cell count, culture and sensitivity, specific gravity, glucose and protein analysis.[73] Aspiration of a sample of pleural fluid allows for the analysis of protein content and other markers that help identify the cause of the pleural effusion and guide its management.

★ ASSESSMENT

Accumulation of pleural fluid can be small and asymptomatic or large, producing significant respiratory distress. Respiratory signs and symptoms include tachypnea, increased respiratory effort, retractions, decreased breath sounds or a change in the pitch of breath sounds, and pleuritic pain. Fever may or may not be present, depending on the underlying etiology. Chest radiographs demonstrate the effusion, with large effusions producing a contralateral shift of the mediastinal structures. Often, small accumulations of pleural fluid are noted incidentally on routine chest radiographs.

Knowledge of risk factors and those conditions that are associated with pleural effusions helps the nurse to anticipate those children who may develop this condition. Congestive heart failure, postoperative cardiac surgery, postcardiotomy syndrome, pneumonia, trauma, and malignancies are all associated with effusions.

★ NURSING DIAGNOSES AND PLANNING

Based on assessment data from above and Chapter 37, the following nursing diagnoses may apply to the family and child with pleural effusion:

- Impaired Gas Exchange secondary to fluid accumulation.
- Altered Breathing Pattern secondary to decreased lung volume.

★ INTERVENTIONS: COLLABORATIVE AND INDEPENDENT

Interventions are determined by the severity of the effusion, the amount of respiratory distress that it causes, and the underlying etiology. Small effusions, particularly those caused by congestive heart failure, can be treated with diuretics. Treatment may not be necessary if the effusion is well tolerated. Often, daily monitoring by chest radiograph and careful assessment of the child are all that is required while the effusion is spontaneously reabsorbing.

Moderate or large effusions require thoracentesis or chest tube insertion (see Table 38-3). The child with chylothorax is placed on a medium-chain triglyceride diet to decrease thoracic lymphatic flow and to help in the resolution of the chylothorax. Once the chylothorax resolves, the child may start a regular diet.

★ EVALUATION

Continued assessment after therapeutic intervention is necessary to evaluate the response to therapy. Chest auscultation and evaluation of the WOB determine the efficacy of treatment and help in the identification of a reaccumulation of pleural fluid.

Adequate chest tube function and the insertion site must be assessed frequently. Adverse effects are usually due to inappropriate insertion technique, inadvertent clamping of the chest tube, accidental disconnection of the chest tube, and inappropriate set-up of the drainage unit. Complications include liver, diaphragm, or spleen injury from the thoracentesis. Pleural infection and empyema can occur secondary to poor technique.

Pneumothorax

Definition and Incidence. Pneumothorax is a condition in which air accumulates in the pleural space, resulting in partial or complete collapse of the adjacent lung. A *spontaneous pneumothorax* occurs when an alveolar structure ruptures and air leaks into the pleural space. Penetrating injury to the chest wall, lung, or internal mediastinal structures can also produce pneumothorax. A *tension pneumothorax* is a life-threatening condition in which the air in the pleural space is trapped under increasing positive pressure. The overall incidence of pneumothorax is extremely low in the general pediatric population.

Etiology and Pathophysiology. Pneumothorax occurs most commonly from iatrogenic reasons, such as positive pressure ventilation, or with perforation of the lung from thoracentesis, biopsy, central line insertions, or tracheostomy.[13] Other causes include trauma to the chest wall, and pneumonias. Children with asthma and cystic fibrosis may suffer recurrent spontaneous pneumothorax due to the chronic hyperinflation and coughing associated with these conditions.

Pneumothorax occurs secondary to movement of air into the pleural space. Spontaneous pneumothorax results from rupture of an alveolar bleb or cyst, allowing air to leak into the pleural space. Blunt objects can penetrate the chest wall and introduce air into the pleural space. Contact with the alveolar surface from fractured ribs or foreign body injury, or from various diagnostic or therapeutic interventions, can cause an alveolar tear, leading to an air leak into the pleural space. Injury or disease of the trachea, esophagus, or large bronchi can also lead to air leak and pneumothorax. Positive pressure mechanical ventilation can also produce lung rupture and pneumothorax.

These conditions lead to the accumulation of air in the pleural space on the affected side. Compression of the adjacent lung tissue can produce atelectasis and impaired gas exchange, depending on the size of the pneumothorax. A tension pneumothorax is particularly dangerous and requires immediate measures to evacuate the trapped air from the pleural space.

Clinical Manifestations. The signs and symptoms associated with pneumothorax depend on its size and the degree of underlying lung disease. In an otherwise healthy child, a small pneumothorax may produce mild pleuritic pain on the affected side, accompanied by tachycardia, tachypnea, and dyspnea. In a child with compromised pulmonary function, or on mechanical ventilation, even a small pneumothorax can lead to respiratory failure with hypoxemia and hypercapnia.

A large pneumothorax can produce all of the above signs and symptoms. Additionally, asymmetric movement of the chest wall may be noted on inspiration, with the affected side lagging behind. The percussion note on the affected side will be hyperresonant, and the breath sounds may be diminished. There may be a shift of the mediastinum to the affected side, as evidenced by a shift in the point of maximal impulse, or by palpating the trachea at the sternal notch. Jugular vein distention is sometimes visible, and subcutaneous emphysema may be palpable at the apex of the lung or neck. A tension pneumothorax secondary to positive pressure ventilation causes a shift of the mediastinum to the unaffected side, as the lung tissue is compressed. Hypoxemia, hypercapnia, and cardiovascular collapse ensue if untreated.

Diagnostic Studies. The diagnosis of pneumothorax is based on history and clinical presentation and is confirmed by chest radiograph. An end-expiration upright chest film is of most diagnostic value, especially in questionable cases. The outline of the visceral pleura and the opaque lung on the affected side can be seen with hyperlucent (dark) intrapleural air seen between the lung and the chest. A shift of the mediastinum may also be visible. Subcutaneous air may be visible in the soft tissues of the neck and chest. In the newborn, transillumination of the chest on the suspected side with a special light can demonstrate *translucency,* which is indicative of air in the pleural space.

★ ASSESSMENT

Pneumothoraces can be small and well tolerated, or, conversely, they can be large, producing significant respiratory distress. Respiratory assessment includes auscultation of breath sounds to determine absence or a change in pitch. Physical examination reveals dyspnea and increase in the WOB. The child may indicate pleural pain when a moderate or large pneumothorax is present.

A tension pneumothorax presents emergently with acute respiratory and cardiovascular decompensation. Sudden deterioration manifests with acute cyanosis, hypoxia, arterial desaturation, hypotension, and bradycardia. This condition is an emergency and requires the immediate notification of the physician. Additionally, the child on the ventilator should immediately be given 100% oxygen.

★ NURSING DIAGNOSES AND PLANNING

Based on assessment data from above and Chapter 37, the following nursing diagnoses may apply to the family and child with pneumothorax:

- Impaired Gas Exchange related to lung collapse.
- Pain related to the chest tube.
- Impaired Mobility related to chest tube.

The nurse and child (or parents) together plan effective care based on the established nursing diagnoses. Several examples of expected outcomes follow:

- The parents discuss the need for chest tube.
- The child ambulates with parental support.

The nurse plans for the daily care of the child based on both physician's orders and nursing diagnoses. Some general nursing care goals may be the following:

- Gas exchange is improved.
- Comfort is improved.

★ INTERVENTIONS: COLLABORATIVE AND INDEPENDENT

A small pneumothorax may require only close monitoring until it is reabsorbed. Symptomatic pneumothorax requires chest tube insertion connected to water seal and possibly suction. Emergent tension pneumothorax requires immediate needle aspiration of the accumulated air, followed by chest tube insertion. Interventions for chest tubes are listed in Table 38-3.

Monitoring includes ongoing respiratory assessment, pulse oximetry, and blood gas analysis if warranted. Care must be taken to ensure the proper maintenance of the chest tube and collection chamber. Daily chest radiographs may be necessary to monitor for the resolution of the air accumulation. Once the chest tube is discontinued, care must be taken to monitor the child closely to assess for possible reaccumulation.

★ EVALUATION

Most pneumothoraces resolve over time. The length of time for reabsorption depends on the underlying etiology. Iatrogenic complications can occur secondary to improper chest tube insertion technique. Adverse sequelae from iatrogenic causes include liver laceration, damage to the diaphragm, and lung injury. Pleural infection is also possible.

Chronic Respiratory Disorders

Asthma

Definition and Incidence. Asthma is the most common chronic pulmonary condition in childhood, and its incidence appears to be on the rise. It is estimated that over 10 million Americans suffer from asthma, and

that 10% to 12% of children exhibit signs and symptoms compatible with a diagnosis of asthma. The onset of childhood asthma occurs by the age of 2 in more than 50% of cases, and by the age of 5 in 80% of afflicted children.[46] A major educational effort was initiated by the National Heart, Lung and Blood Institute (NHLBI) in the late 1980s. In 1991, the National Institutes of Health (NIH) published the National Asthma Education Program report, entitled "Guidelines for the Diagnosis and Management of Asthma."[93] The report is aimed at reversing the rising morbidity and mortality statistics by the year 2000.

The prevalence of childhood asthma varies according to a number of demographic variables including age, sex, geographic location, and race. Although death from asthma in children is uncommon, there is a growing concern regarding the rise in frequency, severity, and mortality. Certain age-specific characteristics and mechanisms of hyperresponsiveness produce a significant problem with underdiagnosis of asthma in children. Unfortunately, the adage "all that wheezes is not asthma" has led clinicians to seek other diagnoses for the child who presents with wheezing.

Asthma is a disease characterized by hyperreactivity of airways, encompassing airway hyperresponsiveness to various stimuli, reversible airway obstruction, and airway inflammation. The "twitchiness" of the airways is dynamic and variable, with components of bronchospasm, edema, inflammation, and increased sputum production. Changes in the severity of airway obstruction can occur spontaneously or with therapeutic interventions, and the child may be symptom-free with normal pulmonary function between acute asthma attacks.

Etiology and Pathophysiology. The primary characteristic of asthma is airway hyperresponsiveness. A variety of immunologic and nonimmunologic stimuli can initiate the cascade of events that leads to the development and manifestations of asthma. Multiple immunologic stimuli can trigger bronchial hyperreactivity, producing airway smooth muscle contraction, inflammation, and chemotaxis. Sensitivities to aspirin, monosodium glutamate (MSG), sulfites, and other substances are included. Nonimmunologic factors include multiple physical and chemical stimuli (dusts, molds, pollens, and so forth), gastroesophageal reflux, and viral infections.

The terms *extrinsic* and *intrinsic* are also used to categorize two types of asthma. Extrinsic or allergic asthma is commonly associated with specific allergens, has onset in childhood and is associated with a positive family history for asthma. Intrinsic asthma has more nonspecific causative factors and is usually adult-onset.[100] A combination of intrinsic and extrinsic factors contributes to the age of onset, type, and severity of asthma.

A complex interaction of events occurs during an asthma attack. In response to stimuli, the airways of an asthmatic child undergo cell activation, leading to the release of inflammatory mediators from mast cells, macrophages, and epithelial cells. Secondary biochemical activations produce changes in airway smooth muscle tone, mucociliary function, and epithelial permeability.

Response to these changes determines the severity of an asthma attack. Airway narrowing from edema, bron-

TABLE 38-3
Nursing Intervention: Care of the Child With a Chest Tube

Nursing Action:	Rationale
Setting up System	
1. Set up. Obtain required equipment: Sterile gloves, mask, hat Antiseptic solution Local anesthetic Sterile drapes Syringes Needles No. 15 scalpel Suture, needle holder Chest tube Collection chamber Thoracostomy tray	1. All equipment must be sterile to prevent complications. Assembly of all equipment ensures a smooth procedure.
2. Set up collection system. Fill water seal chamber with sterile H_2O to 2-cm mark. If suction is ordered, fill suction chamber with sterile H_2O to appropriate level. Connect to suction source; water should bubble gently in suction chamber.	2. Sterile H_2O must be used to prevent contamination of the system and infecting the patient. Water seal chamber must be filled to maintain negative intrapleural pressure and prevent lung collapse. The level of the H_2O in the suction chamber determines the amount of suction, not the degree of bubbling.
3. Explain procedure to patient and family.	3. Patient/family preparation helps control anxiety.
4. Premedicate with analgesic or sedative.	4. To control anxiety and pain, the physician also should administer a local anesthetic to the proposed insertion site.
Insertion	
1. Continually monitor respiratory and cardiovascular function during insertion procedure.	1. Continuous monitoring of respiratory function alerts the nurse to possible complication or ineffective analgesia/anesthesia.
2. Connect collection chamber and place sterile, occlusive dressing over insertion site once chest tube (CT) is inserted.	2. Sterile and occlusive dressing prevent infection.
3. Obtain chest radiograph.	3. Assess proper placement of CT and determine adequate function.
Monitoring Collection System	
1. Document amount and color of drainage.	1. Evaluation of type and severity of effusion and need for possible fluid replacement.
2. Maintain tube patency by gently milking the tube as needed. *Never strip chest tubes.*	2. Prevents occlusion of CT. Stripping can produce excessively negative pressures, producing lung contusion, and can worsen bleeding.
3. Change collection chamber if it fills completely.	3. Ensures continuous drainage.
4. Check water seal level daily. Keep at 2-cm level. Observe for fluctuation of the water level.	4. Must maintain fluid level to maintain negative intrapleural pressure. Fluctuation occurs during respiration; normal is 2 to 6 cm. Fluctuation is due to changes in the intrathoracic pressure. In spontaneously breathing children, the water level rises with inspiration and falls on expiration; this is reversed in mechanically ventilated children.
5. Observe for bubbling in the water seal chamber.	5. Bubbling in the water seal chamber indicates a patient or system air leak. A patient air leak is noted if the bubbling stops when the CT is momentarily clamped near the insertion site. A patient air leak requires notification of the physician. If the bubbling persists while the tube is clamped, there is a system air leak. Make sure all connections are tight and that there are no holes in the system.
6. Maintain water level and bubbling in suction chamber at prescribed level.	6. Ensures the proper amount of suction generated. Absence of bubbling in suction chamber indicates kink in suction tubing.
7. Keep tube loops and collection chamber lower than patient.	7. Promotes drainage.
Patient Monitoring	
1. Assess child's respiratory status and breath sounds. Observe for fine crackling under the skin.	1. Monitor for complications and effectiveness of CT. Subcutaneous emphysema indicates the proximal fenestration of the CT is not in the pleural space.
2. Change dressing according to hospital policy. Assess site for exudate, erythema.	2. Prevent infection.

(Continued)

TABLE 38-3
(Continued)

Nursing Action:	Rationale
3. Monitor child's temperature, assess for signs and symptoms of infection.	3. Alert caregivers to possible infection.
4. Allow child to get out of bed, ambulate, or to be held by parent. *Never clamp chest tube for prolonged periods.*	4. Normalize experience as much as possible. Promote return to activities of daily living.
Removing Chest Tube	
1. Explain procedure to child and family and pre-medicate patient.	1. Decreases anxiety; controls pain.
2. Remove chest tube rapidly during inspiration; must be done by experienced personnel.	2. Rapid removal during inspiration helps prevent lung collapse.
3. Cover insertion site with sterile petroleum jelly dressing.	3. Prevents infection and leakage of air into pleural space.
4. Obtain chest radiograph.	4. Determines if effusion/pneumothorax has reaccumulated after CT is removed.
5. Document.	5. Aids communication among health professionals.

chospasm, and hypersecretion of mucus leads to air being trapped behind obstructed airways. Functional residual capacity (FRC) rises toward total lung capacity, helping to tether the airways open, but also increasing WOB. Accessory muscles are used to maintain ventilation in the presence of the acute hyperinflation. Hypoxemia occurs secondary to V/Q mismatch in severe attacks. Cardiovascular changes include increased pulmonary vascular resistance (PVR) and systemic vascular resistance (SVR) secondary to the hypoxemia and hyperinflation.

Clinical Manifestations. The clinical presentation of a child with asthma varies depending on the severity of the attack. The onset, duration, and frequency of signs and symptoms vary from person to person. In mild asthma, signs or symptoms of airway obstruction may be absent, and routine pulmonary function tests may be normal. With increasing severity, however, manifestations of airway obstruction are more evident. The child may exhibit tachypnea and tachycardia, increased WOB, and use of accessory muscles. Expiratory wheezes may be heard on auscultation, or by the naked ear in severe cases, and the expiratory phase is markedly prolonged. Cough is often present, with limited production of thin clear sputum. Changes in clinical appearance may be gradual or may progress rapidly to acute distress and respiratory failure. A condition known as "status asthmaticus" may develop, in which the child fails to respond to maximum therapeutic interventions. These children require admission to critical care units for aggressive intervention, which, in many cases, may include intubation and mechanical ventilation for respiratory failure.

Diagnostic Studies. The diagnosis of asthma is based on a combination of history, physical assessment, and laboratory and pulmonary function tests. Laboratory studies include CBC and sputum analysis for eosinophilia, or elevated serum IgE. Unfortunately, the absence of positive findings does not rule out asthma. Skin testing for specific IgE antibodies to common allergens can also contribute to the diagnosis of asthma. A recently developed multiantigen radioallergosorbent test (RAST) for children, the Phadiatop Paediatric, has shown excellent correlation with clinical diagnosis in screening children 7 years of age or younger for atopic disease.[129]

Pulmonary function tests, including peak expiratory flow rate (PEFR) and basic spirometry (FEV1.0, FVC, % FEV1.0/FVC) will be abnormal. ABGs reveal mild hypoxemia and hypocapnia with the onset of the attack. In the child with known asthma, the clinical presentation in the emergency department guides the clinician in selecting therapy and deciding whether there is a need for hospitalization. History, physical examination findings, pulmonary function, and response to therapy all play a role in determining the severity of an asthma attack and the need for hospitalization. SaO2 and PEFR or FEV1.0,[45,63] degree of dyspnea,[63] and duration of symptoms[79] have all been postulated as valuable indices for predicting the need for hospitalization. The degree of pulsus paradoxus has also been advocated as an index of the severity of an asthma attack.

★ **ASSESSMENT**

An adequate assessment of the asthmatic child is critical to determine the severity of disease, necessary interventions, and therapeutic response. Inadequate assessment has been implicated in the undertreatment of acute asthma with a resulting increase in morbidity.[63]

Obtaining a detailed history is the first step in the assessment process. Familial history of atopic disease (e.g., allergic rhinitis, atopic dermatitis, asthma) is commonly found in asthmatic children. About 40% of children with severe asthma have one parent similarly affected.[93] If both parents are asthmatic, the incidence rises to 80%.[59] Other pertinent subjective data to be obtained include onset of symptoms, type of onset, history of cough, change in behavior, a history of an upper respiratory infection, history of bronchospasm or wheezing, exposure to known allergens, and use of bronchodilator and steroids to control symptoms and outcomes of previous attacks.[12]

Often, the parents or the child can identify known triggers that precipitate acute attacks. The stimuli include environmental inhalants such as dust, molds, pollens, smoke, paint fumes, and air pollution.[93] There is a significant association between acute asthmatic attacks and elevated ambient sulfur dioxide levels, with an estimated 9% of all asthmatics sensitive to elevated concentrations of sulfate.[55,75] Other known triggers include exertion, temperature changes, and emotional upsets. Documentation of significant historical findings, in conjunction with a complete physical assessment, helps in the differential diagnosis, as well as in determining appropriate therapeutic intervention.

It is unnecessary and inappropriate to separate the child from the parents during the objective evaluation. The separation can precipitate undue anxiety, exacerbate clinical symptomatology, and impede clinical assessment. The severity of acute attacks can be assessed and documented through physical examination and laboratory data.[78]

The first step is to observe the child in a position of comfort (e.g., held by parents, sitting upright). Evaluation of respiratory effort, respiratory rate, retractions, use of accessory muscles, dyspnea, grunting, and diaphragmatic movement is best facilitated when the child is not agitated. The degree of respiratory effort is an important determinant of airway obstruction. The use of accessory muscles correlates most closely with lung function in the child.[63] The presence of paradoxical diaphragmatic movement or apnea indicates respiratory muscle fatigue and should precipitate emergent supportive care.

Auscultation of the chest is performed to determine alterations in air flow and the presence of air trapping. Wheezing signifies obstruction and should be documented according to its presence in the respiratory cycle. Wheezing can occur at end expiration, throughout expiration, or during the entire respiratory cycle. However, the degree of wheezing proves to be a weaker correlate of disease severity than the use of accessory muscles. Therefore, the presence or absence of wheezing *alone* should not be used as a single assessment parameter.[63] Decreased breath sounds or the absence of wheezing found in the presence of significant WOB indicates severe asthma, often labeled as the "silent chest" due to almost complete airway obstruction.[78,121] The presence of wheezes reassures the nurse that at least some air exchange is occurring!

Cardiovascular assessment includes evaluation of heart rate, blood pressure, systemic perfusion, and pulsus paradoxus. Tachycardia is a frequent finding in acute episodes and may also be secondary to the administration of theophylline or β-agonists; blood pressure should be normal. Pulsus paradoxus is assessed by obtaining a blood pressure during inspiration and again during expiration. During inspiration, a reduction of systolic blood pressure of greater than 15 mmHg is abnormal. This effect is secondary to the large negative intrapleural pressures (i.e., minus 100 mmHg) that are generated during inspiration

in acute asthma. This alteration increases systemic afterload, thus decreasing cardiac output (CO). A pulsus paradoxus of more than 20 mmHg is indicative of severe airway obstruction.[78] Another indicator of decreased cardiac output is peripheral perfusion. An increase in capillary filling time (i.e., >3 seconds), cool skin, decreased pulses, and pale, mottled extremities can indicate compromised cardiac output. Cyanosis indicates significant hypoxia and severe impairment of gas exchange.

LOC should be evaluated in all children with respiratory distress. Restlessness, confusion, and agitation are important although nonspecific signs of hypoxia. Lethargy or obtundation (mental dullness) is found more frequently with hypercapnia.

★ NURSING DIAGNOSES AND PLANNING

Based on assessment data from above and Chapter 37, the following nursing diagnoses may apply to the family and child with asthma:

- Activity Intolerance related to reactive airways.
- Ineffective Airway Clearance related to reactive airways.
- Decreased Cardiac Output related to changes in intrapleural pressure.
- Impaired Gas Exchange related to reactive airways.
- Inability to Sustain Spontaneous Ventilation related to respiratory muscle fatigue.
- Fluid Volume Deficit related to poor oral intake.
- Anxiety related to lack of information about the disease, treatment, and long-term outcomes.
- Ineffective Family Coping: Compromised related to chronic illness.

The nurse and child (or parents) together plan effective care based on the established nursing diagnoses. Several examples of expected outcomes follow:

- The child participates in planning self-care management.
- Stimuli known to precipitate acute attacks are avoided when possible.
- Parents demonstrate skill in caring for child during acute episodes.
- Parents discuss symptoms that indicate need for interventions by health care personnel.
- The child participates in routine exercise as tolerated.

The nurse plans for the care of the child based on both physician's orders and nursing diagnoses. Some general nursing care goals may be the following:

- Hypoxic episodes are minimized.
- Comfort measures are effective in limiting acute episodes.
- Fluid and electrolyte balance is maintained.
- Parents participate effectively in child's care.

★ INTERVENTIONS: COLLABORATIVE AND INDEPENDENT

The nurse may care for the asthmatic child in a variety of settings and in acute or chronic conditions. The following interventions begin with care of the child in an acute episode. The section ends with discharge planning and long-term care interventions.

In emergency care, the priority is ongoing monitoring of respiratory function while providing life-saving functions. Figure 38-6 is a flowchart of actions to take in the emergency room and possible outcomes.

OXYGENATION

Children with severe asthma are hypoxic secondary to V/Q mismatch. Increasing the fraction of inspired oxygen (FiO_2) to the lung helps diminish systemic hypoxia. The concentration of oxygen should be sufficient enough to maintain S_pO_2 >90%. The availability of pulse oximeters can help in titrating oxygen delivery to meet established therapeutic goals, avoiding the need for invasive, painful ABGs. Oxygen therapy should be initiated at 2 L/min by nasal cannula or 40% O_2 by face mask. Some children require higher concentrations to maintain adequate oxygenation. Oxygen flow rates for nasal cannulas should not exceed 6 L/min. Various oxygen masks or face tents are capable of delivering higher concentrations of O_2. Mist tents are to be avoided because the heavy mist can aggravate bronchospasm, and visibility of the child is impaired. (See section on Techniques and Technology in Pediatric Respiratory Care later in this chapter for an explanation of oxygen delivery systems.)

MEDICATION THERAPY

The aim of pharmacologic intervention is to promote bronchodilation and to inhibit inflammation. Bronchodilators are the cornerstone of interventions for the asthmatic child. The most frequently administered agents include nebulized β-agonists agents (albuterol, terbutaline, or metaproterenol), anticholinergic drugs (atropine or Atrovent), methylxanthines (theophylline, aminophylline), steroids, and IV isoproterenol (Table 38-4). Antihistamines and cough suppressants may be detrimental in the treatment of asthma and are not indicated.[122]

Aerosolized second- and third-generation β-agonists are preferred due to minimal cardiac side-effects as compared to older agents such as epinephrine. These drugs promote direct bronchodilation by stimulating the β_2 receptors in bronchial smooth muscle, enhance mucociliary clearance, improve respiratory muscle contractility, and inhibit mast cell degranulation. Administration during acute episodes is facilitated by way of a jet nebulizer through a mask or mouthpiece (Fig. 38-7A). Nebulizers require only tidal volume breathing and, therefore, are preferred over MDI in acutely ill, uncooperative, or uncoordinated children. However, once the child is stable, an MDI may be substituted. Figure 38-7B shows a 7-year-old asthmatic child using an MDI with spacer and mask for a bronchodilator treatment. IPPB is contraindicated in children with obstructive airway disease.[77]

Bronchodilators such as albuterol and metaproterenol are β_2-selective and possess few cardiac side-effects such as tachycardia, vasodilation, and dysrhythmias. Peak onset of action is usually 30 to 60 minutes, and duration is 4 to 6 hours. However, for the child with severe bronchospasm, frequency of administration can be increased to every 30 minutes, or continuously if needed. Albuterol has been found to have minimal side-effects, to promote decreased use of accessory muscles, and to improve max-

imal expiratory flow when used on a continuous basis.[7,67] Figure 38-8 shows a 3-year-old girl with asthma performing a maneuver to measure PEFR to assess response to inhaled bronchodilators.

The actions of aminophylline include CNS stimulation, improved respiratory muscle contractility, bronchodilation, vasodilation, and diuresis. Although this agent has been used for years, many pediatric pulmonologists reserve the use of this agent for severe asthma that is nonresponsive to the β_2 agents.[122] Any child receiving continuous IV administration of aminophylline requires hospitalization and close monitoring. Initiation of therapy requires a loading dose administered over 20 minutes, then the institution of a continuous infusion.[78] Careful monitoring for signs and symptoms of toxicity, including nausea, vomiting, restlessness, delirium, tachycardia, dysrhythmias, and convulsions is required. Children with seizures secondary to theophylline toxicity are often refractory to anticonvulsant therapy and have a poor outcome.[91] Blood levels should be monitored 1 hour after the bolus, at 12 hours to determine steady state, then every 24 hours thereafter. Therapeutic levels are 10 to 20 mg/dL, and toxicity is associated with levels higher than 20 mg/dL.[6,78]

Atropine is not routinely used to treat asthmatics; However, it is useful in some children who are refractory to or who do not tolerate more conventional pharmacologic interventions with β_2 therapy. Atropine is administered by nebulizer and has a longer action than the nebulized β_2 agents. Administration frequency is every 4 hours. Side-effects include tachycardia, dry mouth, urinary retention, and restlessness. An alternative drug is Atrovent, a congener of atropine, supplied as an MDI in the United States. It is usually administered at two to four puffs per dose interval and can be given in conjunction with β_2 aerosol medications by administering the Atrovent MDI after the β_2 treatment.

Isoproterenol requires continuous infusion, cardiorespiratory monitoring, placement of an arterial line, and admission to an intensive care unit (ICU). This agent is a nonselective β-agonist and is reserved for the child in acute respiratory failure with carbon dioxide retention. Serious side-effects include increases in myocardial O_2 consumption, tachycardia, dysrhythmias, and vasodilation. Concomitant administration of aerosolized β-agents is usually discontinued to help minimize cardiovascular side-effects. Weaning of isoproterenol occurs when ABGs have normalized and clinical improvement is demonstrated. Once the continuous infusion is discontinued, aerosolized β_2 treatments are resumed.[78]

An attractive alternative to isoproterenol is continuous nebulized albuterol. This therapeutic intervention possesses fewer side-effects than isoproterenol. Use of either IV isoproterenol or continuous nebulized albuterol may help prevent the need for mechanical ventilation in severely ill asthmatic children.[20,78]

Corticosteroids should be administered to all severe asthmatics requiring hospitalization. These agents are used for their antiinflammatory effects, as well as their synergism with β_2 agonists, thus improving bronchodilation. A 5- to 7-day course is usually instituted and has not been found to result in adrenal suppression. Concurrent administration of an H_1 receptor agonist is rec-

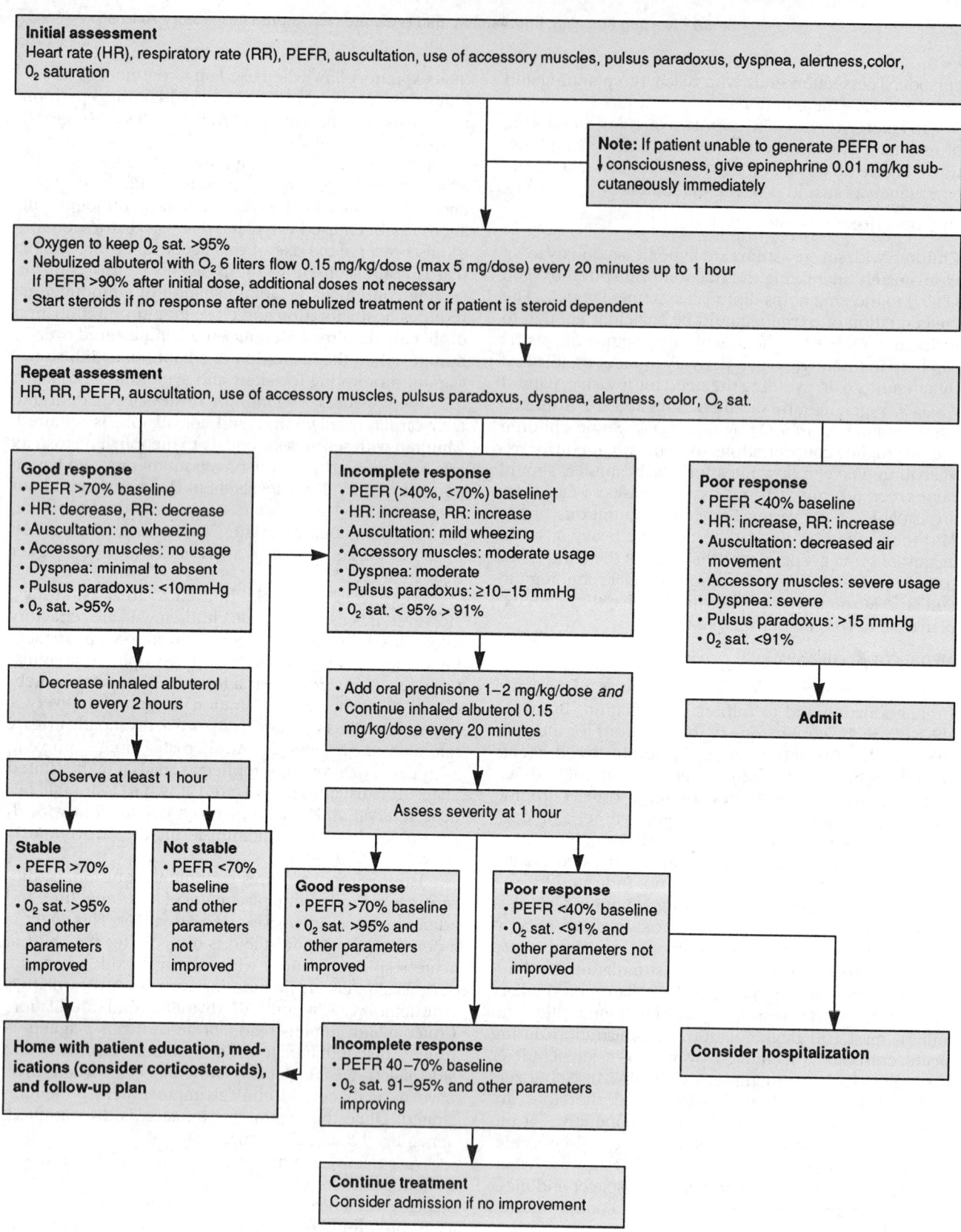

Initial assessment
Heart rate (HR), respiratory rate (RR), PEFR, auscultation, use of accessory muscles, pulsus paradoxus, dyspnea, alertness, color, O_2 saturation

Note: If patient unable to generate PEFR or has ↓ consciousness, give epinephrine 0.01 mg/kg subcutaneously immediately

- Oxygen to keep O_2 sat. >95%
- Nebulized albuterol with O_2 6 liters flow 0.15 mg/kg/dose (max 5 mg/dose) every 20 minutes up to 1 hour
  If PEFR >90% after initial dose, additional doses not necessary
- Start steroids if no response after one nebulized treatment or if patient is steroid dependent

Repeat assessment
HR, RR, PEFR, auscultation, use of accessory muscles, pulsus paradoxus, dyspnea, alertness, color, O_2 sat.

Good response
- PEFR >70% baseline
- HR: decrease, RR: decrease
- Auscultation: no wheezing
- Accessory muscles: no usage
- Dyspnea: minimal to absent
- Pulsus paradoxus: <10mmHg
- O_2 sat. >95%

Incomplete response
- PEFR (>40%, <70%) baseline†
- HR: increase, RR: increase
- Auscultation: mild wheezing
- Accessory muscles: moderate usage
- Dyspnea: moderate
- Pulsus paradoxus: ≥10–15 mmHg
- O_2 sat. < 95% > 91%

Poor response
- PEFR <40% baseline
- HR: increase, RR: increase
- Auscultation: decreased air movement
- Accessory muscles: severe usage
- Dyspnea: severe
- Pulsus paradoxus: >15 mmHg
- O_2 sat. <91%

Decrease inhaled albuterol to every 2 hours

- Add oral prednisone 1–2 mg/kg/dose *and*
- Continue inhaled albuterol 0.15 mg/kg/dose every 20 minutes

Admit

Observe at least 1 hour

Assess severity at 1 hour

Stable
- PEFR >70% baseline
- O_2 sat. >95% and other parameters improved

Not stable
- PEFR <70% baseline and other parameters not improved

Good response
- PEFR >70% baseline
- O_2 sat. >95% and other parameters improved

Poor response
- PEFR <40% baseline
- O_2 sat. <91% and other parameters not improved

Home with patient education, medications (consider corticosteroids), and follow-up plan

Incomplete response
- PEFR 40–70% baseline
- O_2 sat. 91–95% and other parameters improving

Consider hospitalization

Continue treatment
Consider admission if no improvement

* Therapies are often available in a physician's office. However, most acutely severe exacerbations of asthma require a complete course of therapy in an Emergency Department.

† PEFR % baseline refers to the norm for the individual, established by the clinician. This may be % predicted based on standardized norms or patient's personal best.

FIGURE 38-6

Emergency department management of children with acute exacerbation of asthma. Therapies are often available in a physician's office. However, most acutely severe exacerbations require a complete course of therapy in an emergency department.

TABLE 38-4
Drug Dosages in Acute Exacerbation of Asthma in Children

Drug	Available Form	Dosage	Comment
Inhaled β_2-Agonist			
Albuterol			
Metered-dose inhaler	90 μg/puff	2 inhalations every 5 min for total of 12 puffs, with monitoring of PEFR or FEV to document response	If not improved, switch to nebulizer. If improved, decrease to 4 puffs every hour.
Nebulizer solution	0.5% (5 mg/ml)	0.1–0.15 mg/kg/dose up to 5 mg every 20 min for 1–2 h (minimum dose 1.25 mg/dose) 0.5 mg/kg/h by continuous nebulization (maximum 15 mg/h)	If improved, decrease to 1–2 h. If not improved, use by continuous inhalation.
Metaproterenol			
Metered-dose inhaler	650 μg/puff	2 inhalations	Frequent high-dose administration has not been evaluated. Metaproterenol is not interchangeable with beta$_2$-agonists albuterol and terbutaline.
Nebulizer solution	5% (50 mg/ml)	0.1–0.3 ml (5–15 mg). Do not exceed 15 mg.	
	0.6% unit dose vial of 2.5 ml (15 mg)	As above 5–15 mg. Do not exceed 15 mg.	
Terbutaline			
Metered-dose inhaler	200 μg/puff	2 inhalations every 5 min for a total of 12 puffs	
Injectable solution used in nebulizer	0.1% (1 mg/ml) solution in 0.9% NaCl solution for injection Not FDA approved for inhalation.		Not recommended because not available as nebulizer solution. Offers no advantage over albuterol, which is available as nebulizer solution.
Systemic β-Agonist			
Epinephrine HCl	1:1000 (1 mg/ml)	0.01 mg/kg up to 0.3 mg subcutaneously every 20 min for three doses.	Inhaled β_2-agonist preferred.
Terbutaline	(0.1%) 1 mg/ml solution for injection in 0.9% NaCl.	Subcutaneous 0.01 mg/kg up to 0.3 mg every 2–6 h as needed. Intravenous 10 μg/kg over 10 min loading dose. Maintenance: 0.4 μg/kg/min. Increase as necessary by 0.2 μg/kg/min and expect to use 3–6 μg/kg/min.	Inhaled β_2-agonist preferred.
Methylxanthines			
Theophylline	Aminophylline (80% anhydrous theophylline)	Loading dose:* If theophylline concentration known: every 1 mg/kg aminophylline will give 2 μg/ml increase in concentration. Loading dose:* If theophylline concentration is unknown: —No previous theophylline: 6 mg/kg aminophylline —Previous theophylline: 3 mg/kg aminophylline Constant infusion rates:* Infusion rates to obtain a mean steady-state concentration of 15 μg/ml: Age 1–6 mo 6 mo–1 y	 0.5 mg/kg/h aminophylline 1.0 mg/kg/h aminophylline

(Continued)

TABLE 38-4
(Continued)

Drug	Available Form	Dosage	Comment
		1–9 y	1.5 mg/kg/h aminophylline
		10–16 y	1.2 mg/kg/h aminophylline
Corticosteroids			
Outpatients:	Oral prednisone, predniso- lone, or methylprednisolone	1–2 mg/kg/day in single or di- vided doses	Reassess at 3 days. Only a short burst may be needed. No need to taper dose.
Emergency Department or hospitalized patients:	Methylprednisolone IV or PO	1–2 mg/kg/dose every 6 h for 24 h then 1–2 mg/kg/day in di- vided doses q 8–12 h	Length depends on re- sponse. May only need a few days.

* Check serum concentration at approximately 1, 12, and 24 hours after starting the infusion.
From National Asthma Education Program Expert Panel Report (1991). ''Guidelines for the diagnosis and management of Asthma.'' Bethesda, MD: NIH/NHLBI publication no. 91-3042.

ommended during steroid therapy to alkalinize gastric pH and prevent gastric ulcer formation.[77,122]

HYDRATION

Adequate hydration is essential to decrease mucus vis- cosity and improve mucociliary airway clearance. In- creased insensible water loss can occur secondary to hy- perventilation. Dehydration can also occur due to decreased fluid intake and the diuretic effect of theoph- ylline. Correction of dehydration and provision of maintenance fluids are critical. Monitoring of electrolytes, serum osmolality, and urine specific gravity is necessary to prevent overhydration.

The increased negative intrapleural pressure that oc- curs during asthmatic attacks facilitates interstitial edema around the bronchioles. This effect, in combination with excessive fluid therapy, can precipitate pulmonary edema. Therefore, normal water balance should be maintained according to the individual child.[19,77]

MECHANICAL VENTILATION

In spite of aggressive therapy, a small number of children develop progressive respiratory failure and require en- dotracheal intubation and mechanical ventilation. This intervention should be instituted in an ICU by experi- enced personnel. Certain pharmacologic agents, includ- ing morphine, meperidine, tubocurarine, and atracurium, can induce bronchospasm and should be avoided for in- duction and intubation of the asthmatic child.

Mechanical ventilation is instituted to facilitate a long expiratory phase while maintaining normal minute ven- tilation. Bronchodilator and corticosteroid therapy is continued. ABG monitoring is used to evaluate response to therapy. Manipulation of suctioning of the ETT can precipitate bronchospasm and, therefore, should be kept to a minimum. Intratracheal administration of lidocaine can help blunt this reflexive response.

These children are extremely difficult to ventilate due to their severe bronchospasm and are at high risk for iat-

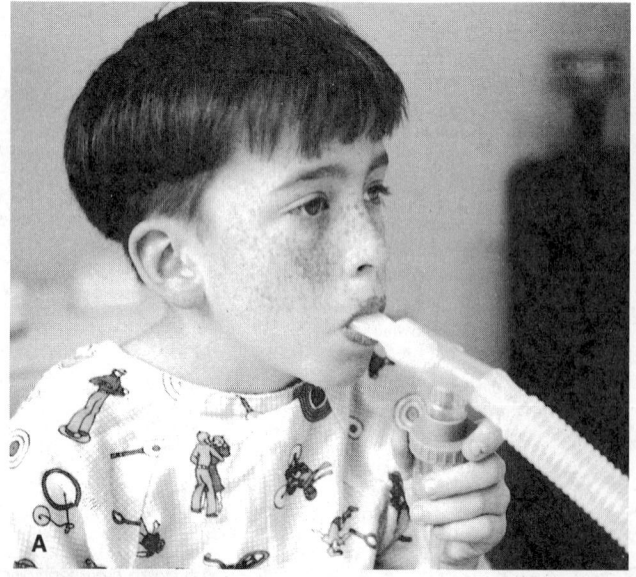
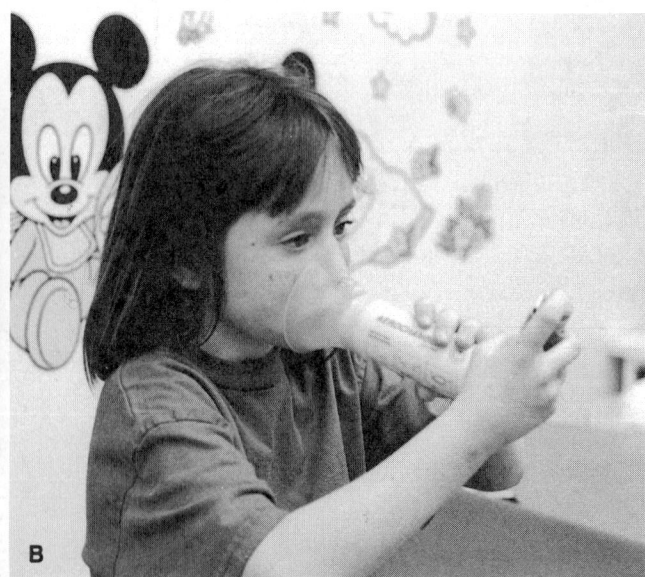

FIGURE 38-7
Aerosolized medications. (**A**) Nine-year-old child taking an aerosol medication treatment by hand nebulizer. (**B**) Seven-year- old girl self-administering a metered dose inhaler (MDI) bronchodilator with a spacer device.

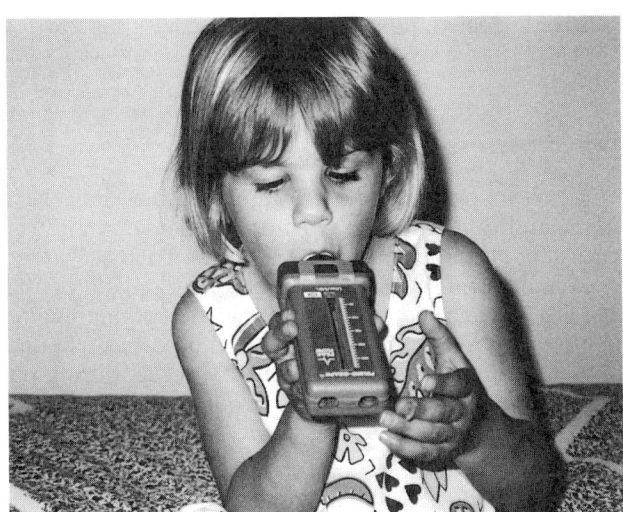

FIGURE 38-8
Three-year-old asthmatic child using her peak flowmeter to measure PEFR after a bronchodilator treatment.

rogenic complications such as pneumothorax. Vigilant attention to ventilator settings and monitoring data, coupled with the judicious use of sedatives or paralyzing agents where indicated, can reduce morbidity and mortality risks. Weaning is determined by individual patient progress. Once extubation is achieved, continuous oxygen therapy is necessary as determined by arterial saturation and blood gas analysis. (For further discussion on interventions for the mechanically ventilated child, see section on Care of the Child Requiring Mechanical Ventilation later in this chapter.)

PSYCHOSOCIAL SUPPORT

Children suffering from an acute asthmatic attack experience acute anxiety, panic, and a fear of impending death. Hypoxia can potentiate the anxiety. Frequently, parental anxiety compounds the child's feelings. Parental anxiety increases in direct correlation with disease severity.[12A]

The nurse is in a pivotal position to provide emotional support for the family and child. Provision of a calm, quiet atmosphere is essential. Allowing as much parent/child control of therapeutic interventions as possible can be beneficial. The use of breathing maneuvers that allow slow exhalation (about 1.5 to 3 times inspiratory time) or pursed-lip breathing is helpful during acute episodes of wheezing.[122] Patient and family education is critical during all interventions. Improving knowledge base and understanding the rationale for therapy promote mastery of needed skills and help relieve anxiety. Participatory management is useful, particularly in children who have a long history of acute asthma.

Use of sedatives in the nonintubated child should be avoided because of the risks of respiratory depression. However, in severely agitated children, chloral hydrate is useful due to its minimal respiratory depressant effects. Careful monitoring of respiratory effort and S_pO_2 is necessary if these pharmacologic agents are used. All children on mechanical ventilation require IV sedation to diminish anxiety and promote synchronization of breathing with the ventilator.

ACTIVITY MANAGEMENT

Regular exercise is recommended, particularly swimming, gymnastics, and cycling. Asthma does not preclude participation in other competitive sports if the child tolerates them. Routine exercise improves pulmonary function, as well as self-esteem, and is an important factor in facilitating socialization.

For those children with exercise-induced asthma (EIA), treatment with cromolyn or albuterol 15 minutes before exercising is effective.[10] Minimizing airway moisture loss can be accomplished by covering the nose and mouth with the hand during exercise, or by nasal rather than mouth breathing. Adequate hydration with oral fluids also maintains airway moisture. Communication with coaches and physical education teachers regarding the need for bronchodilators, and the importance of self-pacing for the child prevents misunderstanding. Collaborative evaluation of the exercise regimen is important to a self-managed program. Life experiences can become normalized for the growing child once EIA is controlled.

DISCHARGE PLANNING

The family and child should be involved in the multidisciplinary approach to developing a therapeutic plan. Self-management and techniques to cope with acute episodes are critical to compliance and outcomes.

Patient education can be facilitated through various community programs and literature from organizations such as the American Lung Association (see resource list at beginning of this chapter). Topics to be discussed include the pathology of asthma, actions and side-effects of the drugs, and the normal trajectory of illness. Environmental stimuli that trigger acute attacks should be avoided or minimized. However, strict control is usually unnecessary. Parental smoking around the asthmatic child should be discouraged[93] (see also section on Long-Term Care below).

Therapeutic respiratory maneuvers for acute attack should be taught to the child and family. Effective technique in the administration of inhaled medications is also essential. Key points for the effective use of inhalers include:

- The inhaler must be shaken before every activation
- A slow, deep inspiration is required, with the inhaler activated at the beginning of inspiration
- The inhaler is activated once for each inspiration
- Holding the breath for 5 to 10 seconds at the completion of inspiration improves drug deposition.

A spacer is used for young children who cannot properly use a metered dose inhaler (MDI).

One important aspect of care is the incorporation of the treatment program into the family lifestyle. Normal growth and development must be facilitated. Children who experience frequent attacks or hospitalizations may develop delays in normal development task attainment. The long-term illness trajectory must be discussed with parents and child. Counseling may be required to help deal with anxiety, behavioral problems, or overprotection.

Evaluation of the impact on the family determines if coping mechanisms are appropriate. In the child with frequent exacerbations, school absenteeism can become a problem. Evaluation of school performance is required, and a collaborative plan must be developed with the family, school nurse, and teachers.

Noncompliance becomes a key issue with the adolescent who already is struggling with issues of self-esteem and peer pressures. The adolescent may try to hide the illness from peers, and the normal parent–child struggles that occur during adolescence can be aggravated by asthma. With support and education provided by the health team, parents can learn to "let go" while the adolescent becomes more responsible for his or her own care.

Among care teaching issues is establishment of guidelines for the family in case of an acute episode. Such guidelines are suggested in the accompanying display.

★ EVALUATION

Periodically, the nurse and family evaluate the outcomes of care given. Examples of outcomes for the child and family with asthma were given under diagnoses and planning in this section. Have short-term goals been met? Are long-term goals still realistic? Planning for further nursing care takes into consideration complications and long-term care.

COMPLICATIONS

Undertreatment and underrecognition of asthma have been implicated in increased morbidity and mortality statistics for children in the past 10 years. To avoid undertreatment, asthma must be treated on an ongoing basis, not just during acute episodes. Evaluation of ongoing responses to therapy ensures improved outcome.[46] Remission of clinical symptoms frequently occurs during puberty, and a few children actually outgrow their asthma. If asthma is severe by 14 years of age, the condition usually continues into adulthood.

In a small percentage of children, asthma becomes life-threatening. Risk factors for the development of life-threatening asthma include:

*   Early onset of less than 1 year of age
*   Frequent hospitalizations to control exacerbation
*   Noncompliance with prescribed regimen

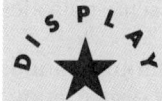

Patient Teaching: Guidelines for Family Management of a Child's Asthma Episode

Steps to Manage an Asthma Episode at Home

*   Know your child's early warning signs so you can begin treatment early.
*   Give the prescribed amount of medicine at the times or intervals the doctor has indicated. If your treatment plan includes increased dosage or a second medicine to be used during episodes, give it as instructed. If you need to give more medicine than prescribed, notify your clinician.
*   Remove, if possible, an allergen or irritant if it triggered the child's episode. Treatment is less effective if there is continued exposure to a trigger.
*   Keep yourself and your child calm and relaxed.
*   Have your child rest while you observe the progress of therapy.
*   To monitor your child's condition, note change in body signs like posture, difficulty breathing, wheeze, and cough. If you have a peak flowmeter, test the child's peak flow rate 5–10 min after each treatment to see if air flow is returning to normal.
*   Call a family member, friend, or neighbor to help you if needed.
*   Call the clinic, doctor's office, or hospital for help if needed.

Signs to Seek Medical Care

Not all asthma episodes require a visit to the doctor. There are several signs that parents can use to decide if a trip to the doctor or emergency department is needed. If any one of these signs is present, seek emergency treatment for your child.

*   Wheeze, cough, or shortness of breath gets progressively worse, even after the medicine has been given and had time to work. Most inhaled bronchodilator medications produce a noticeable and significant effect within 5–10 min. Discuss with your doctor the time your child's medications take to work.
*   Peak flow rate declines or stays the same after treatment with bronchodilators or drops to 50% or less of the child's normal baseline level (personal best or predicted, as determined by the clinician). Discuss this peak flow level with your doctor.
*   Child has a hard time breathing. Signs of this are:
    —Child's chest and neck are pulled or sucked in with each breath.
    —Child is hunched over.
    —Child is struggling to breathe.
*   Child has trouble walking or talking.
*   Child stops playing and cannot start any activity again.
*   Child's lips or fingernails are grey or blue. If this happens, take your child to the doctor or emergency room IMMEDIATELY!

From National Asthma Education Program Expert Panel Report. (1991). "Guidelines for the diagnosis and management of asthma." Bethesda, MD: NIH/NHLBI publication no. 91-3042.

- Asthma that produces unexpected rapid deterioration of pulmonary function
- Dependence on steroids.[93]

Some children with severe, persistent asthma can be predisposed to the development of chronic obstruction pulmonary disease as adults. However, a direct causal relationship has not been found. Atelectasis, pneumothorax, thoracic deformity, decreased bone density, psychological problems, and respiratory failure are complications seen more frequently in children who suffer from asthma.[46]

LONG-TERM CARE

Long-term management is aimed at maintaining respiratory function, minimizing symptoms and acute episodes, and supporting normal lifestyle.

Nebulized β-agonists are the preferred drug for ongoing treatment. Albuterol or metaproterenol are administered by way of MDI with or without a spacer. Maintenance treatment is every 4 to 6 hours. Children with infrequent episodes may use inhalers for the duration of asthmatic symptoms. Recently, capsules filled with powdered β-agonists have become available (Rotacaps) for use as an alternative to MDI; however, their application in the pediatric population has not been well-documented. For children who are refractory to inhaled treatment, oral β-agonist agents are also available either as a tablet or syrup. However, these oral agents have more systemic side-effects and can contribute to restlessness and irritability. Aminophylline is used to treat children who are less responsive to β-agonists. Long-term side-effects of aminophylline include alterations in behavior. Serum levels should be monitored, and families need to be informed of the drugs and conditions that alter theophylline clearance.

Cromolyn sodium is used to prevent bronchospasm but is ineffective for the treatment of acute attacks. Cromolyn is administered by way of MDI or hand nebulizer and has few side-effects, other than occasional cough and bronchospasm. These side-effects can be prevented by the administration of a bronchodilator before or with cromolyn inhalation.

Systemic steroids are infrequently used for prolonged periods. Aggressive therapy with the previously mentioned agents should be instituted before steroids. Administration of oral steroids should be every other day to prevent adrenal suppression, and withdrawal should be achieved as soon as possible.

Inhaled steroids are recommended for children older than 5 years of age with chronic moderate or acute asthma. Therapy is usually begun after there has been a trial of cromolyn sodium. Once the child has been stabilized on inhaled steroids, the cromolyn sodium may be discontinued.[93] If the child is receiving aerosolized bronchodilators, either by nebulizer treatment or MDI, the inhaled steroids should be taken *after* the bronchodilators to maximize topical deposition in the lower airways.

Cystic Fibrosis

Although there is no cure for cystic fibrosis (CF), and the disease is ultimately fatal, the nurse can play a valuable role in supporting the child and family members, providing family education, and fostering adherence to respiratory and nutritional interventions. These efforts can relieve symptoms, minimize exacerbations, and even slow the insidious progression of the disease. Current management regimens, including respiratory therapy, antibiotics, and nutritional support, have contributed to extending the median life expectancy to the age of 27, a significant improvement over 20 years ago.[43,70]

Definition and Incidence. Cystic fibrosis is a hereditary disorder of the exocrine glands, affecting a variety of body systems including the airways, pancreas, intestinal tract, and sweat glands.

The incidence of CF is approximately 1 in every 2000 births, with a lower prevalence in African Americans and Asian Americans. It continues to rank as the leading fatal genetic disease in whites. CF is an autosomal recessive disorder, with an estimated 1 in 20 whites (5%) in the United States being carriers of the gene. According to theoretical genetic probabilities, when both parents carry the CF gene, 25% of children will have CF, 50% will carry the gene but not have CF, and 25% will neither have CF nor carry the gene. In 1989, the gene (CFTR) responsible for CF was cloned, opening new horizons for advances in prediction, diagnosis, and treatment of this disease in the future.

Etiology and Pathophysiology. The respiratory system involvement is the most significant aspect of CF, ultimately responsible for the morbidity and 90% of the mortality. Large volumes of thick, dry secretions are produced by the bronchial mucous glands. This problem coupled with abnormalities in ciliary motility leads to chronic secretion retention, producing diffuse airway obstruction, increasing airway resistance and contributing to areas of atelectasis. A large percentage of children with CF also have a component of airway hyperreactivity, further increasing airway resistance. Airway obstruction leads to V/Q mismatch, altering effective gas exchange and affecting oxygenation.

Secretion retention leads to chronic colonization and recurrent infection with gram-positive and gram-negative organisms such as *Staphylococcus aureus, Pseudomonas aeruginosa,* and *Pseudomonas cepacia.* As many as one third of acute pulmonary exacerbations may occur secondary to nonbacterial infections such as influenza, and can be severe.[101] The presence of secretions in the airways can contribute to the development of bronchiectasis, as well as trapping gas behind the immobile secretions. This process leads to an increase in Functional Residual Capacity (FRC) and Total Lung Capacity (TLC), a classic "barrel chest" appearance, and obstructive pulmonary disease. Chronic hypoxemia leads to increased Pulmonary Vascular Resistance (PVR), pulmonary hypertension, and, ultimately, cor pulmonale.

Nutritional abnormalities occur secondary to dysfunction of the pancreas and intestine. Pancreatic enzymes are abnormally thick, and obstruction of their secretory tubes leads to inadequate breakdown of dietary fats and proteins. Malabsorption of nutrients in the intestinal tract contributes to poor growth and development. Chronic undernourishment adversely affects respiratory muscle strength and function, particularly significant in people with CF, because their resting energy expenditure (REE) requirements have been shown to be greater than for the normal population.[8] Respiratory muscle dysfunction contributes to increased O_2 consumption and CO_2 production, increased energy expenditure and WOB, and ineffective gas exchange and secretion clearance. There is a close link between nutritional status and pulmonary function, which together influence the progression of the condition.

The pathophysiologic changes that occur with CF vary in onset and intensity. In some children, primary involvement of the respiratory system occurs shortly after birth, with fatality in the first year of life. In others, CF may not manifest until early childhood, adolescence, or, rarely, early adulthood. Girls are particularly susceptible to an increase in respiratory dysfunction as they enter puberty. Although the exact reason for this gender difference is unknown, changes in hormonal activity are thought to play a role.

Clinical Manifestations. The clinical manifestations of CF depend on the age of the child and the intensity of signs and symptoms. At birth, approximately 10% to 20% of infants born with CF exhibit meconium ileus. Parents may notice loose, frequent, foul-smelling stools. Infants born with rectal prolapse should be evaluated for CF, because this condition is rarely found in other infants.

In childhood, frequent respiratory infections, chronic cough, and poor growth may be seen. The cough is usually productive, with purulent, foul-smelling sputum during periods of acute infection. Chest auscultation reveals rhonchi, with tachypnea, a prolonged expiratory phase, and wheezes during acute exacerbations. As the disease progresses, airway obstruction leads to pulmonary hyperinflation with an increased anteroposterior chest diameter (barrel chest). Spontaneous pneumothorax may occur with coughing, due to the rupture of cystic areas of the lung. Hemoptysis occurs in some children who have advanced disease.

Gas exchange abnormalities produce chronic hypoxemia and eventually CO_2 retention. The chronic hypoxemia may produce digital clubbing (see Chapter 37), increased PVR, and cor pulmonale. Cyanosis may be seen during acute exacerbations, or continuously in severe cases.

Children with CF often require repeated hospitalizations for acute exacerbations, at which time they receive IV antibiotics and fluids, intensive respiratory care, and nutritional support. Eventually, the person develops respiratory failure, with severe hypoxemia and hypercapnia. The decision is ultimately made either to intubate and mechanically ventilate the child, or to provide comfort measures and support the family through the impending death.

More people with CF are reaching adulthood and facing issues involving abnormal reproductive function. Most males with CF are sterile, due to obstruction of the epididymis and vas deferens, preventing adequate sperm counts. In the female, thickened vaginal secretions alter sperm motility and viability, which, coupled with irregular menses, makes conception difficult. Although puberty is delayed and the aforementioned abnormalities exist, pregnancy is still possible. Unfortunately, the added stress of pregnancy can exacerbate CF and speed its progression.

Diagnostic Studies. Cystic fibrosis may be diagnosed at birth or it may be unrecognized until early adulthood, depending on the clinical manifestations and severity of the disease. A family history of CF, coupled with signs and symptoms as described earlier, contribute to a diagnosis. Definitive diagnosis of CF is made by performing a sweat chloride test. The pilocarpine iontophoresis sweat test is recommended by the Cystic Fibrosis Foundation. A sweat test is positive if the chloride level is greater than 60 mEq/L in children or 80 mEq/L in adults (see Chapter 37).

Pulmonary function studies serve to quantify the degree of impairment, assess response to therapeutic interventions, and provide serial information on the progression of the disease. Chest radiographs demonstrate the degree of hyperinflation, bronchiectasis, and cardiomegaly, and are used during acute exacerbations to identify pneumonia infiltrates. Sputum cultures aid in identifying specific pathogens responsible for acute exacerbations. ABGs are used to establish the adequacy of oxygenation and ventilation during acute exacerbations, and serial ABGs contribute to evaluation the progression of the disease. Pulse oximetry also can be used in lieu of ABGs to monitor adequacy of oxygenation.

★ ASSESSMENT

During the first postpartum days, when the neonate with CF has not yet developed pulmonary symptoms, bilious vomiting, distended "doughy" colon on palpation, and dry, tan-colored rectal meconium may indicate a meconium ileus. Because up to .20% of infants with CF are born with a meconium ileus, early diagnosis, intervention, and parental teaching can be initiated. A nursing history obtained from parents of older children includes stools that are foul-smelling, greasy, loose, and frequent, and a failure to thrive. The child's health history includes serious pulmonary infections and symptoms of respiratory compromise.

Because the diagnosis of CF may be delayed until childhood, a child may present in the emergency room in mild to severe acute respiratory distress (see display on Nursing Assessment: Signs and Symptoms of Acute Respiratory Distress in Otherwise Healthy Children earlier in this chapter). A diligent health history with physical examination may raise questions that go beyond the acute presenting symptoms. The physical signs may include a stature that is small for age, barreled chest, prominent development of chest accessory muscles and abdomen indicating increased chronic respiratory work, and some degree of nailbed clubbing from chronic hypoxemia. Cough is usually present, and breath sounds reveal rhonchi on expiration. The skin may taste salty, and serum electrolytes may reflect hyponatremia or hypochloremia. Although a chest radiograph may indicate acute changes responsible for respiratory distress, it may also reflect chronic changes such as cystic areas, hyperinflation, fibrotic changes, and cor pulmonale.

The child with established CF needs ongoing nursing assessment. Daily health habits, such as exercise, diet, and stress management, can indicate areas that need change, education, and compliance. Specific measures to maintain pulmonary toilet and to avoid infection may change frequently; hence, child/parent education is an ongoing process. Flare-up or worsening of pulmonary status is indicated by an increased cough or wheeze, increased sputum production, decrease in exercise tolerance, increased feelings of fatigue, decrease in lung function by pulmonary function tests (PFTs), weight loss and poor appetite, and fever.[24]

★ NURSING DIAGNOSES AND PLANNING

Based on assessment data from above and Chapter 37, the following nursing diagnoses may apply to the family and child with cystic fibrosis:

- Ineffective Airway Clearance related to thick, sticky mucus production.
- Ineffective Breathing Pattern related to acute respiratory distress or chronic respiratory failure.
- High Risk for Infection related to thick mucus production with ineffective clearance.
- Altered Nutrition: Less Than Body Requirements related to intestinal malabsorption.
- Altered Health Maintenance related to multidimensional disease.
- High Risk for Activity Intolerance related to chronic pulmonary disease.
- Altered Growth and Development related to multiple hospitalizations.
- High Risk for Caregiver Role Strain related to inexperience with caregiving.
- Anxiety related to lack of knowledge concerning disease process, bronchial hygiene, home total parenteral nutrition (TPN), and other care procedures.

The nurse and child (or parents) together plan effective care based on the established nursing diagnoses. Several examples of expected outcomes follow:

- The parents demonstrate adequate skill in chest physiotherapy.
- The parents construct a schedule to include treatment in family activities of daily living.
- The child demonstrates ability to self-administer PEP therapy.
- The child participates in a regular exercise program as tolerated.
- The parents identify high-calorie, high nutritional needs of child.
- The parents discuss the financial and time demands the child's care places on their lives.
- The parents express a desire to provide protective measures for their child's environment.

The nurse plans for the daily care of the child based on both physician's orders and nursing diagnoses. General nursing care goals may include the following:

- Symptoms of pulmonary disease are minimized.
- Optimum growth and development are promoted.

★ INTERVENTIONS: COLLABORATIVE AND INDEPENDENT

Chest physiotherapy (CPT), bronchodilators (aerosol and oral), and antibiotics are used for the treatment and prevention of pulmonary infection. Oxygen may be needed to treat hypoxemia. Pancreatic enzymes and other nutritional approaches are used to enhance physical growth and development. Exercise is encouraged not only to promote pulmonary toilet and pulmonary function, but also to enhance emotional and social development of the chronically ill child.

BRONCHIAL HYGIENE

Various techniques may be employed to facilitate removal of the large volumes of sputum produced with CF. These measures include CPT, PEP mask therapy, and autogenic drainage (AD). CPT includes percussion, vibration, postural drainage, and coughing to move thick tenacious mucus from small airways to larger airways. Percussion is done with a cupped hand, plastic percussor, or mechanical (electrical) percussor on the chest over the area to be drained (Fig. 38-9). Vibration is a technique by which the chest wall is vibrated on exhalation to encourage secretion movement. These two methods are enhanced with postural drainage, a method using gravity to assist mucus movement by positioning the child such that the lobe to be drained is higher than the main stem bronchi. (See Figs. 25-17 and 25-18.) An effective cough can remove the secretions from the larger airways.

CPT should be completed before meals to avoid emesis from coughing and positioning, but *after* a bron-

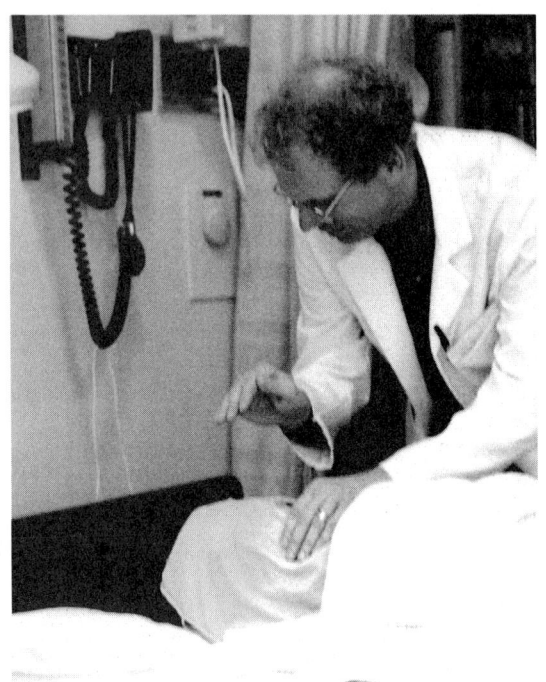

FIGURE 38-9
A child with cystic fibrosis receiving percussion therapy while in a postural drainage position.

chodilator treatment to increase the effectiveness of the treatment. CPT must become a regular part of home care for the child with CF. Parents are taught to increase CPT when the signs of pulmonary infection occur. Nurses work with parents to resolve problems regarding schedule of treatments and medications, while considering realities such as the need for day care when both parents work. Other family members and friends can be taught effective CPT methods to maintain compliance and give parents respite.

Positive Expiratory Pressure (PEP) therapy is an alternative technique for mobilizing pulmonary secretions in the child with cystic fibrosis.[81] Figure 38-10 shows a child performing PEP mask treatment and lists the steps involved. Children as young as 5 years of age can be taught PEP therapy. PEP can be performed by mask or mouthpiece, and can be done in conjunction with a nebulizer or MDI treatment. There is a potential for improved compliance with PEP because the therapy can be self-performed, and it usually raises equivalent amounts of sputum as with CPT, in one-half to one-third the treatment time. Self-administered PEP therapy by inpatients has significant cost-saving potential, because it does not require respiratory therapists, physical therapists, or nursing personnel to assist with CPT sessions.

Autogenic drainage (AD) is another technique for mobilizing secretions. The technique requires a series of controlled breaths at three variable lung volumes, in conjunction with huff coughing. As with PEP therapy, the child sits up in a chair and performs the therapy without the assistance of another person. Due to the controlled breathing required to perform AD, the procedure is usually not taught to children under the age of 12.

A study by Davidson[27] has shown both AD and PEP to be as effective as CPT in mobilizing secretions in adult patients with CF. Further research is needed to establish the role of these two techniques in children. However, because both PEP and AD can be self-performed while sitting up, they offer several advantages over conventional CPT in terms of convenience, comfort, and potential in-hospital cost savings. Because children with CF chronically produce large volumes of sputum, the ultimate goal of the health care provider is to facilitate the use of whichever secretion clearance technique best meets the lifestyle and preference of the person.

ACTIVITY PROMOTION

A regular exercise program within the limits of symptoms has been shown to benefit the pulmonary system. Activities such as swimming facilitate mucociliary clearance, improve muscle performance, reduce oxygen consumption, and enhance psychological well-being. Children with CF should be encouraged to engage in exercise and sports activities as a regular part of their lifestyle, with appropriate education and monitoring to minimize symptoms.

MEDICATION THERAPY

IV antibiotics for 14 to 21 days or more often are required for improvement of the clinical signs of pulmonary infection. Frequent and long hospitalizations are stressful for the child as well as disruptive to the whole family system. Home IV therapy can be a cost-containing and therapeutically effective option in some cases while allowing children to remain in their own environment and on their established schedule. A supportive and experienced home health care team can increase the success of home IV therapy. Home IV therapy often requires an indwelling catheter. Parents should know the basic assessment and care of the IV catheter to enhance safety, even when a home health care team is involved.

Aerosolized antibiotics may be administered by hand nebulizer during hospitalization or in the home. Aminoglycosides such as tobramycin or gentamicin, or a broad spectrum penicillin may be topically delivered to the infected airways, enhancing the treatment of gram-negative pulmonary infections.[43] Because these medications may produce cough or bronchospasm, bronchodilators are usually ordered by MDI or nebulizer in conjunction with aerosolized antibiotics. The MDI bronchodilator should be taken before the antibiotic treatment. Nebulized bronchodilators can be taken in a separate treatment before the nebulized antibiotic, or both medications may be mixed together in the nebulizer for a single treatment, which represents a savings of time and cost. Drugs such as albuterol and tobramycin are chemically compatible for up to 7 days if refrigerated, enhancing the ease of outpatient aerosol antibiotic therapy in the home setting.[47]

Bronchodilators may be indicated in those children with CF who have hyperreactive airways and wheezing, with a component of reversible airway obstruction. Beta$_2$-agonists may be administered by hand nebulizer, MDI, or orally. Children may be taught to take their MDI at an early age, using a spacer device with the mask to enhance lung deposition. Assessment of response to inhaled bronchodilators by measurements such as PEFR is recommended to quantify improvement. A study by Eggleston et al[38] indicated that long-term use of inhaled bronchodilators in children with CF who had bronchial

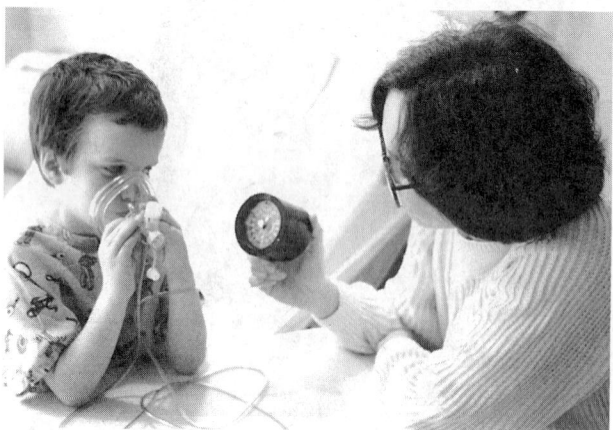

FIGURE 38-10

PEP mask therapy. 1. Child sits comfortably with elbows on table. 2. Child places mask over mouth and nose and creates a tight but comfortable seal. 3. Child takes a deep breath in, using his diaphragm, and holds inspiration for 3 seconds. 4. Child actively but not forcefully exhales, producing a pressure between 10 and 20 cmH$_2$O. 5. Child repeats steps 3 and 4 for 10 to 15 breaths. 6. Child removes mask and performs two to three huff coughs to raise secretions. 7. Child repeats steps 3 to 6 two to four times per session.

hyperreactivity produced sustained improvement in lung function.

A few children with CF respond well to inhaled or oral mucokinetic agents. The mycolytic drug Mucomyst may be given by hand nebulizer to promote the mobilization of pulmonary secretions. Although less commonly used in recent years, Mucomyst can be administered orally to treat mucoid intestinal obstruction. Organidin or guaifenesin also have been used orally to enhance pulmonary mucokinesis.

Several other pharmacologic agents recently have been to be evaluated in the treatment of cystic fibrosis. Intravenous immune globulin (IVIG) therapy may be indicated in selected children with advanced CF who manifest hypogammaglobulinemia and specific antibody deficiencies. Recombinant human deoxyribonuclease 1 (rhDNase) has been administered to children with CF by aerosol inhalation. The medication cleaves DNA in the purulent sputum, reducing viscosity and enhancing secretion clearance. The nonsteroidal antiinflammatory drug ibuprofen is also being studied.[71]

NUTRITIONAL MANAGEMENT

The goal of nutritional therapy is to promote adequate growth and development. Because the child with CF has increased metabolic demands with decreased absorption, this goal is often difficult to achieve. Many children need as much as 200 kcal/kg/day to maintain growth similar to their peers. The diet consists of high protein and low or moderate fat with pancreatic enzymes, adequate hydration, and supplemental vitamins. Diet consultation from a qualified nutritionist can assist with individualizing a palatable diet for the child as well as supporting and educating the family with the changing dietary needs of the growing child. Nurses must assist parents to understand the need for pancreatic enzyme therapy so that their children absorb the ingested nutrients. Nasogastric tube feedings may be needed to give extra calories throughout the nighttime to supplement regular meals and snacks during the daytime. Tube feedings may prevent or delay the necessity of TPN. Parents must be taught proper tube placement techniques, care, and assessment skills to avoid aspiration into lungs that are already compromised.

SURGICAL MANAGEMENT

A variety of surgical interventions may be pursued in certain cases of advanced pulmonary disease. One possible procedure is a lung resection for chronic segmental or lobar collapse, or occasionally for massive pulmonary hemorrhage. More dramatic surgery is organ transplantation of one or both lungs, or heart–lung transplantation. Although mortality is high with these procedures, future advancements in patient selection, surgical techniques, and postoperative management probably will increase the value of these interventions.[43,120]

GENETIC TESTING AND COUNSELING

Nurses must understand the basic genetic possibilities for the family and direct them to a genetic counselor. Genetic testing can identify a person who carries the CF gene; the parents' siblings and their future mates may find this information helpful. Genetic testing also can identify the fetus affected by CF. After the options are discussed with the parents, a nonjudgmental atmosphere can encourage them to explore their values and beliefs in view of the information. Because children with CF are living to be adults, they too need genetic counseling to make informed decisions regarding reproduction.

PSYCHOSOCIAL SUPPORT

Psychosocial assessments are needed for the family of a child with CF. Parental ability to comply with the increasing demands of the child with CF is crucial to the preventive care and well-being of the child. Financial demands, such as medical costs and underemployment due to time constraints, can stress the whole family unit. Frequent hospitalizations can place a parent in the stressful position of having to leave the sick child or lose the job. The progressive chronicity of the disease with increasing illnesses and general demise of a loved child is emotionally upsetting and depressing to most parents, siblings, and other caregivers. Some of these stressors may be relieved by state, county, or federal assistance. Social workers may be able to coordinate the benefits for the family unit, as well as psychotherapeutic assistance and referrals. Home health care nurses can assist parents with the coordination of home care needs. All members of the health care team need to provide empathy and therapeutic listening. Subjects to discuss with children and their families are listed in the accompanying display.

Parents need to be aware of protective measures regarding their child's pulmonary status. Chemicals, dust,

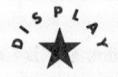

Patient Teaching: Educational Needs of a Family of a Child With Cystic Fibrosis

- Signs and symptoms of respiratory distress
- Signs and symptoms of pulmonary infection
- Chest physical therapy, postural drainage and schedules
- Supplemental oxygen administration—assessment of need and method
- Administration of aerosolized medications and schedule
- Oral medication administration (enzymes, supplement, antibiotics)
- Aseptic technique for central or peripheral IV medication administration
- TPN set-up, administration, insertion, and problem management
- Nasogastric tube placement and assessment for correct placement
- Feeding pump set-up and problem management
- Weight, height, and plot on growth chart
- Assessment of stools; assessment for bowel obstruction
- Protecting the child from airborne hazards (smoke, dust, chemicals)
- Emergency care and CPR
- Support group and CF Foundation contacts
- Importance of follow-up care

sawdust, and other airborne hazards of everyday life should be discussed with parents. A passive smoking environment is harmful for all children and especially for the child with CF. Parents must protect the child with CF from siblings and friends who have infections, because an upper respiratory infection may have extremely detrimental effects on the child.

★ **EVALUATION**

Periodically, the nurse and family evaluate the outcomes of care given. Examples of outcomes for the child and family with CF were given under diagnoses and planning in this section. Have short-term goals been met? Are long-term goals still realistic? Planning for further nursing care takes into consideration complications and long-term care.

COMPLICATIONS

Children with CF have repeated hospitalizations for recurrent pulmonary infection, chronic nutrient malabsorption, and other complications. Table 38-5 lists complications and their causes with possible interventions. As the child grows older, his or her physical condition deteriorates and the child becomes more technology-dependent. Although the lifespan of children with CF has increased remarkably, most die as teenagers or young adults.

Pulmonary complications are the cause of most hospitalizations and of death. Upper airway complications such as sinusitis and nasal polyps can be painful but usually do not cause major problems. However, bronchiec-

tasis and cor pulmonale are complications of CF that can be life-threatening, and treatment is sought to diminish the signs and symptoms, because these cannot be reversed. Pneumothorax and pulmonary hemorrhage can occur from the rupture of tissues weakened by chronic inflammation in the lung. These complications need emergency care and can often be reversed.

Because of malabsorption of nutrients in the gastrointestinal system, the child often fails to thrive. Occasionally, thick mucus and abnormal stools cause a bowel obstruction, usually treatable by mucolytic agents and enemas, and rarely needing surgery. Less common but serious complications include diabetes mellitus, cirrhosis of the liver, and gallstones.

LONG-TERM CARE

The follow-up care of a person with CF is best accomplished by a multidisciplinary team, consisting of various physician specialists, nursing specialists, nutritionists, respiratory therapists, physical therapists, social workers, and genetic counselors. The team goal is to provide preventive as well as interventional care for the changing needs and status of the child with CF. Care is often provided at a medical center that operates a specialized CF center with a trained multidisciplinary staff.

Bronchopulmonary Dysplasia

Definition and Incidence. Bronchopulmonary dysplasia (BPD) is a chronic lung disease that develops in infants secondary to treatment at birth for other respi-

TABLE 38-5
Complications of Cystic Fibrosis With Causes and Interventions

Complication	Cause	Interventions
Sinusitis	Thick, sticky mucus in sinuses	Antihistamines, decongestants, antibiotics
		If severe, sinus flushing
Polyps	Unknown	Nothing
	Mucous gland problem	If severe, surgical removal
Clubbing of fingers/toes	Sign of chronic tissue hypoxemia	Nothing
Bronchiectasis	Inflamed and damaged airways become stretched and floppy	CPT, cough, postural drainage, PEP
Hemoptysis	Inflamed airway lining	If mild, nothing
Pulmonary hemorrhage	Inflammation and erosion of tissue	Depends on degree of bleeding
	Artery rupture	Emergency care or observation
Pneumothorax	Inflamed tissue erodes	Depends on degree of pneumothorax; may need chest tube
	Air leaks into pleural space	Emergency care or observation
Cor pulmonale	Heart failure related to high resistance of pulmonary vasculature	Diuretics, oxygen
Bowel obstruction	Thick mucus	Mucolytic agents, enemas
	Dry, sticky stool	If severe, surgical removal
Cirrhosis of the liver	Bile duct obstruction with mucus	Nothing
Diabetes mellitus	Unknown	See Diabetes Mellitus.
	Possible pancreatic scarring	
Gallstones	Unclear. Possible alteration in fat and bile acid metabolism.	Surgical removal if symptomatic.

ratory conditions such as respiratory distress syndrome (hyaline membrane disease). Factors that predispose to the development of BPD include prematurity and low birthweight, coupled with exposure to positive pressure mechanical ventilation with high concentrations of oxygen for extended periods of time. As many as 40% of preterm low birthweight infants treated with mechanical ventilation for hyaline membrane disease are estimated to develop BPD, although the precise overall incidence remains unknown because the definition and reporting of BPD differ among institutions.[70] Advances in obstetrics, neonatology, and newborn respiratory care have contributed to increased survival of low birthweight infants, which has led to a rise in the incidence of BPD over the past 10 years.

Etiology and Pathophysiology. The exact etiology of BPD is unclear, although there are several contributory factors, most of which are iatrogenic. In the preterm, low birthweight infant born with immature lungs, decreased lung compliance with edema, increased airway reactivity, and mucus plugging frequently requires the use of positive pressure ventilation and high inspired oxygen concentration to prevent hypoxia and hypercarbia. Although necessary, the use of oxygen >60% is associated with direct damage to lung tissue, causing an inflammatory response that increases airway edema and resistance. The use of positive pressure damages fragile lung tissue, causing hyperinflation and disruption of alveolar structure. Mechanical ventilation, pulmonary infections, poor nutrition, barotrauma, and patent ductus arteriosus (PDA) add to the likelihood that BPD will develop. The resultant injury includes coexistent areas of alveolar fibrosis, atelectasis, and cystic overdistention, all poorly involved in gas exchange.

After recovery from ventilatory support, carbon dioxide retention and hypoxemia remain, and oxygen is required to maintain an adequate PaO_2. Airways exhibit chronic inflammation, edema, and hyperreactivity, with bronchospasm, increased secretions, and decreased mucociliary clearance. Hydration therapy may lead to pulmonary edema due to leaking pulmonary capillary beds from alveolar epithelial lung injury. Pulmonary hypertension is commonly present, and cor pulmonale may develop in advanced cases.

Mortality for BPD is reported as 10% to 30%, with a high incidence within the first year of life in severe cases.[17] For those infants who survive their hospitalization and move into childhood, pulmonary function abnormalities are common for the first few years. Obstructive lung disease with hyperreactive airways may persist into the school years; however, the majority of children recover normal lung function by the age of 7 to 10, as their lungs mature and heal.[9] In preterm infants who developed chronic lung disease, neurodevelopment and academic performance at age 8 have been shown to be compromised.[103] However, these deficits have not been a universal finding, and further research is needed.

Clinical Manifestations. The clinical presentation of infants with BPD varies widely based on a continuum of the disease process. Most infants show signs of chronic respiratory distress with tachypnea, substernal retractions, rales, wheezes, copious secretions, cyanosis on room air, and activity intolerance. ABGs and noninvasive monitoring data demonstrate hypoxemia and hypercapnia.

Signs of right heart failure may be present. Edema may be difficult to assess in the older infant but can be noted most easily around the eyes. The liver may be enlarged, and jugular vein distention may be observed. Pulmonary edema may occur with normal fluid administration.

The infant with BPD is usually thin with weight and height in the bottom 50th percentile. Increased WOB can consume much of the caloric intake or can adversely affect adequate feeding and fluid intake, contributing to growth failure.

Diagnostic Studies. The diagnosis of BPD is usually made based on history, clinical presentation, pulmonary function tests (PFTs), and chest radiograph. PFTs can be invaluable in measuring lung function but are difficult to obtain in the infant. Common findings include increased airway resistance, decreased compliance (increased lung stiffness), and increased functional residual capacity (FRC). Chest radiograph reveals characteristic streakiness with concomitant areas of hyperinflation and atelectasis, and a flattened diaphragm and enlarged heart in more severe cases. Electrocardiography and echocardiography may show evidence of right heart hypertrophy secondary to increased pulmonary vascular resistance in severe cases.

★ **ASSESSMENT**

Assessment of the child with BPD should begin with a thorough history to evaluate the age of onset and severity of disease. Severity may range from mild respiratory alterations requiring bronchodilators and diuretics, to severe respiratory dysfunction requiring tracheostomy and mechanical ventilation. The clinical presentation of BPD is directly related to these conditions.[4,17] Other data to obtain from the family include feeding problems, oxygen requirements, pharmacologic support, activity tolerance, growth and development issues, previous illnesses, and hospitalizations. Parents are usually sensitive to nonspecific changes in their child's status, and any parental concerns or "gut feelings" should be acknowledged and investigated.

Respiratory assessment of the child with BPD should include examination of respiratory rate, use of accessory muscles, presence of retractions, color, activity tolerance, and auscultation. An elevated respiratory rate, a prolonged expiratory phase, retractions, and the use of accessory muscles indicate a worsening respiratory status. A child with significant reactive airways may present with wheezing. Fluid overload and pulmonary edema are manifested by the presence of rales, wheezing, and increased WOB. Activity intolerance and poor feeding can be nonspecific signs of worsening hypoxia and increased oxygen demands. Although cyanosis usually is a late sign of hypoxia, a baseline assessment, either objectively or from the history should be made to determine if the presence of cyanosis is a significant finding, because many of these children are normally slightly cyanotic. Clubbing is secondary to chronic hypoxia. An assessment of oxygen saturation by way of pulse oximetry should be made on a routine basis. Chest radiographs and PFTs may be obtained. As with any child who has chronic respiratory disease, positive respiratory findings should be compared to baseline or historical data to determine their significance.

The cardiac assessment should include not only the assessment of normal cardiovascular function, but also should evaluate the cardiorespiratory interaction. Heart rate and blood pressure evaluation should be obtained while the child is at rest and not agitated. The child may be tachycardic when awake and active, but the heart rate may return to normal when asleep. A heart rate appropriate for age during sleep can be a sign of normal well-being for the child with BPD. Perfusion should be appraised by determining capillary filling time, pulses, and skin temperature, and observing for the presence of mottling. Peripheral edema and hepatomegaly are found with worsening right-sided heart failure secondary to hypoxic pulmonary vasoconstriction.

When awake, the child's ability to interact with the environment should be evaluated. The child should be playful (especially in personal–social areas of development) and able to interact with others. Decreased interaction with surroundings may be an early sign of illness. Activity intolerance usually is noted in compromised children with BPD secondary to the inability to meet the increased oxygen demands required for active play. The child may rest more frequently and not play as long, or may seem more passive than other children the same age. A decreased tolerance (less than baseline) for activity may indicate progressive illness or deterioration.

It is important to note subtle changes in the child's feeding patterns. Does the child take longer to feed? Does the child take as much formula? Is cyanosis noted with feeding? Does the child vomit some of the feeding? What is the child's activity level after feeding? Feeding difficulties are frequent findings in the child with BPD. Assessment of nutritional status is imperative because adequate caloric intake is critical for the growth and development of these fragile children.

★ NURSING DIAGNOSES AND PLANNING

Based on assessment data from above and Chapter 37, the following nursing diagnoses may apply to the family and child with BPD:

- Ineffective Airway Clearance related to reactive airways and poor cough.
- Activity Intolerance related to chronic hypoxia.
- Impaired Gas Exchange related to reactive airways and airway inflammation.
- Inability to Sustain Spontaneous Ventilation related to respiratory muscle fatigue.
- Altered Growth and Development related to chronic hypoxia and decreased nutrition.
- Anxiety (Parental) related to knowledge deficit of home oxygen therapy, bronchodilator administration, and diuretics.
- Altered Nutrition: Less Than Body Requirements related to decreased oral intake.

- Ineffective, Family Coping related to chronic illness.
- Social Isolation (Family) related to time spent in child's care.
- Dysfunctional Ventilatory Weaning Response related to inability to cooperate.

The nurse and parents together plan effective care based on the established nursing diagnoses. Several examples of expected outcomes follow:

- The parents participate in infant stimulation programs.
- The parents cuddle infant as much as possible.
- The infant rests between periods of routine care.
- The parents discuss home care options and community services.
- The parents construct a schedule in which they spend time with their other children and alone as a couple.
- The parents identify safety rules concerning oxygen use in the home.

The nurse plans for the daily care of the child based on both physician's orders and nursing diagnoses. Some general nursing care goals may include the following:

- Effective respiratory rate and gas exchange are achieved.
- Developmental milestones are facilitated.
- Adequate nutrition is supported.

★ INTERVENTIONS: COLLABORATIVE AND INDEPENDENT

The child with BPD frequently spends several months in the hospital depending on the severity of the disease process and the ability of the family to care for the infant on oxygen at home. General management interventions of the child with BPD are given in Table 38-6.

MECHANICAL VENTILATION

Most infants who develop BPD are born prematurely and require mechanical ventilation within the first week of life for a minimum of 3 days.[22] Once BPD has developed, these infants often require positive pressure ventilation and oxygen therapy during the neonatal period for prolonged periods of time. Occasionally, an infant requires a tracheotomy for long-term mechanical ventilation. This intervention usually is performed at 2 to 4 months of age in those infants who are not demonstrating clinical improvement.[98] Many infants who require prolonged mechanical ventilation and are clinically stable, and who have supportive home environments, may be cared for at home.

Because children with BPD are at increased risk for serious respiratory infections from normal respiratory pathogens, they frequently require hospitalization during acute respiratory illness. A small number of these children require mechanical ventilation to support respiratory function until resolution of the acute insult. Usual indications for mechanical ventilation in these children include worsening hypoxia and arterial desaturation in spite of increased oxygen administration, increased WOB, alterations in the level of consciousness, and hypercapnia relative to the child's baseline.

OXYGENATION

The severity of lung disease determines the need for supplemental oxygen therapy. Because most infants with BPD

TABLE 38-6
General Management of the Child
With Bronchopulmonary Dysplasia

Pathophysiologic Manifestations	Interventions
Right heart failure/cor pulmonale	Diuretics
Reactive airways/bronchospasm	Bronchodilators
	Diuretics
	Steroids
Hypoxia/pulmonary hypertension	Oxygen therapy/pulse oximetry
Increased CO_2/respiratory failure	Mechanical ventilation if appropriate
Alveolar fibrosis/emphysema	Steroids
Copious secretions/loss of ciliary function	Chest physiotherapy
Poor growth	High-calorie formula
	Serial monitoring of height, weight, and head circumference
Electrolyte alterations	Potassium chloride replacement
	Arginine chloride
	Calcium replacement
Activity intolerance	Planned rest periods
	Increase oxygen delivery

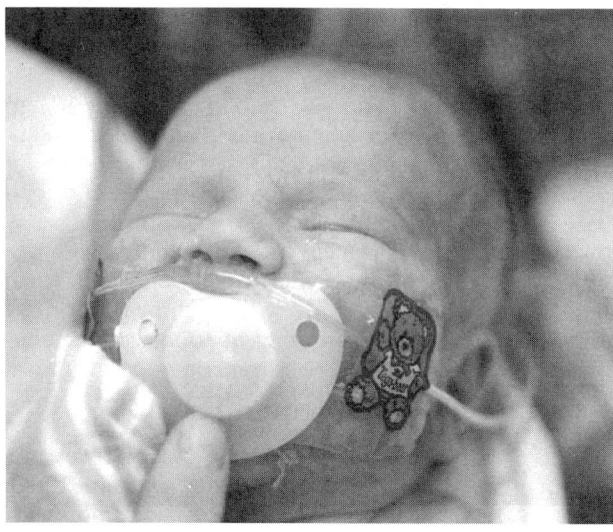

FIGURE 38-11
An infant with BPD receiving oxygen by way of nasal cannula. Protective skin barrier is applied to the skin, over which the cannula is held in place with an adhesive product such as Tegaderm.

have marked hypoxemia, supplemental oxygen is required to maintain PaO_2 greater than 50 mmHg. The duration of oxygen therapy and FiO_2 requirements gradually decrease as lung function improves. Most infants who require oxygen therapy after discharge from the hospital are clinically stable receiving from 1/16th to 2 L/min.

Oxygen is commonly delivered by way of nasal cannula to infants with BPD. The flow should be set to maintain blood oxygen saturation greater than 90% during all activities. This level of oxygenation helps to prevent episodes of pulmonary hypertension due to hypoxic pulmonary vasoconstriction. Oxygen saturation can be monitored by pulse oximetry continuously or intermittently during a variety of infant activities. Weaning the child with BPD off oxygen is much slower than in children with other acute pulmonary diseases. Weaning should be attempted gradually, as determined by clinical response, activity level, feeding, weight gain, and arterial saturation. The process may take some children months to years to achieve.[22] Oxygen saturation should be checked more frequently after weaning occurs, because hypoxia can occur several hours to even days later.

Several methods have been developed to hold the oxygen cannula in place. Many children tolerate small pieces of tape directly on the face. However, infants and children with sensitive skin may require a small piece of skin barrier placed on the skin to prevent maceration and ulceration from the cannula and tape (Fig. 38-11). In some older children, the cannula may be secured to a hat.

CHEST PHYSIOTHERAPY

Many children with BPD produce copious amounts of tenacious secretions. These children often require secretion clearance maneuvers to facilitate drainage and clearance. Chest percussion, vibration, and postural drainage

are effective in those children who have a large volume of sputum production. However, this technique should be used cautiously in children with reactive airways disease. A complete evaluation of the child, the need for therapy, and the response to therapy is important, particularly because chest physiotherapy can increase oxygen consumption, worsen hypoxemia, induce agitation, and worsen V/Q mismatch.[36,42] Other secretion clearance techniques, such as PEP mask therapy, may be more efficacious in BPD children with copious secretions.

MEDICATION THERAPY

Pharmacologic intervention is aimed at the promotion of bronchodilation, control of the pulmonary inflammatory changes, and the control of cor pulmonale. Inhaled bronchodilators commonly used in BPD include albuterol, Alupent, and isoetharine. Commonly used oral medications include the methylxanthines, albuterol, and metaproterenol. These agents promote pulmonary smooth muscle relaxation, decrease wheezing, and improve respiratory function. Frequently, bronchodilators are required for acute respiratory illness and not for long-term therapeutic management.[22,28]

Systemic steroids may be used to reverse the inflammatory process found with BPD. Dexamethasone facilitates weaning from oxygen and mechanical ventilation in some infants who are refractory to conventional treatment. Therapy should not exceed 5 days if clinical effect is not apparent.[28] A short course of systemic steroids may also be indicated during acute respiratory illness in some children.[22]

Children with BPD are more susceptible to severe respiratory infection than their peers, with almost half of these children rehospitalized for acute respiratory illness during their first year of life. Therefore, pharmacologic intervention often is required in these children. Antimicrobial therapy is determined by the etiologic organism. RSV is a major pathogen in these children, necessitating the use of ribavirin therapy.

Diuretic therapy is a mainstay of pharmacologic intervention for the management of congestive heart failure (CHF) and cor pulmonale in children with BPD.[28] Furosemide or the thiazides are used to reduce pulmonary edema and improve lung compliance. Side-effects include volume depletion, chloride deficiency, hypokalemia, and metabolic alkalosis. Fluid balance, electrolytes, and acid–base balance must be monitored. Potassium chloride replacement therapy is usually needed. Children with persistent, severe hypochloremic metabolic alkalosis may require replacement therapy with arginine chloride to prevent further potassium wasting. Spironolactone is often added to promote diuresis while sparing potassium.

FLUID AND NUTRITIONAL MANAGEMENT

Children with BPD poorly tolerate excessive or even normal amounts of fluid intake. Intolerance is manifested by a marked tendency to accumulate excessive amounts of fluid in the lungs. Therefore, fluid restriction is instituted to reduce pulmonary edema. As discussed above, these children also require chronic diuretic therapy to control lung fluid.

Sensitivity to fluid administration makes nutritional management problematic. The risks and benefits of supporting nutritional requirements with fluid restriction must be evaluated. Caloric requirements in children with BPD are higher than in their peers, up to 150 to 200 kcal/kg/day. Total parenteral nutrition (TPN; hyperalimentation) may be necessary early in the course of illness, and high-calorie formulas are necessary long-term to promote nutritional intake while meeting necessary fluid restrictions. Often, these infants are poor feeders, exhibit food aversion, and have delayed oral motor skills. Therefore, they may require supplemental gavage or gastrostomy feedings.

SUPPORT OF GROWTH AND DEVELOPMENT

Chronic hospitalization, sequelae of preterm birth, and intensity of illness can contribute to developmental delay. Delays in gross motor and fine motor skills are most noticeable; cognitive and personal–social skills can be preserved. Height, weight, head circumference, and developmental screening should be corrected for gestational age. Early intervention and developmentally sensitive infant stimulation programs are critical to the identification and support of growth and development.

ACTIVITY MANAGEMENT

Activity intolerance must be evaluated so that the plan of care can be adjusted to the child's individual needs. The child should be allowed rest periods during routine care and feedings. Care activities should be carefully scheduled so that rest periods are uninterrupted. Increasing the child's oxygen liter flow during activities may be necessary to support the increase in oxygen requirements.

FAMILY SUPPORT

The birth of a child normally is a joyful experience; however, the birth of a preterm infant who develops BPD is met with grief. The parents must let go of their vision of a perfect baby and begin to deal with reality. Chronic sorrow is a normal reaction that may last a lifetime, particularly when parents are faced with the multiple stressors that are associated with chronic illness. Identification of family and community supports requires a multidisciplinary approach, using the social worker, primary medical provider, nursing services, and others who are sensitive to cultural and religious needs.

Social isolation can occur secondary to the amount of time and expense the care of a chronically ill child requires. The family should be informed of community services, respite agencies, and home care options. Coping and adaptation are supported through parental education, positive reinforcement of parenting tasks, the provision of respite care, and the empowerment of families with chronically ill children. Every effort should be made to normalize the child's and family's experience. Siblings should be allowed special time with their parents, to prevent feelings of abandonment and isolation, and parents should be encouraged to spend time together to enhance the maintenance of a strong couple relationship.

HOME MANAGEMENT

Caring for the child with BPD at home is less expensive and provides the child with a supportive environment in which to grow and develop. The family can be together again, incorporating the child with BPD into the family lifestyle. Home health nurses can provide parental support, problem solving, and ongoing assessment. A home health nurse also can provide care for the child during the night and respite periods.

Equipment in the home provides optimal mobility for the child and parent. Extension tubing from the main oxygen source in the home can allow the child increased freedom of movement and activity. Oxygen provided in small, lightweight liquid oxygen systems allows the parent to transport the child more conveniently. Because oxygen supports combustion, parents and other caregivers must be educated about necessary safety precautions. Smoke alarms and fire extinguishers should be installed. The appropriate monitors, such as pulse oximetry, apnea monitors, or ventilator disconnect monitors, with functioning alarms are necessary to alert caregivers to possible complications. (See Chapter 21 for a discussion of home care for the chronically ill child.)

Expected outcomes of family teaching are listed in the accompanying display.

★ EVALUATION

Periodically, the nurse and family evaluate the outcomes of care given. Examples of outcomes for the child and family with BPD were given under diagnoses and planning in this section. Have short-term goals been met? Are long-term goals still realistic? Planning for further nursing care takes into consideration complications and long-term care.

COMPLICATIONS

Outcomes and survival of children with BPD continue to improve with the advancement of technology and the understanding of the etiology and pathophysiology of BPD. Complications include frequent respiratory infections requiring hospitalization, pulmonary hypertension, right-sided heart failure, and cor pulmonale. Morbidity is secondary to preterm birth and the severity of disease. Mental

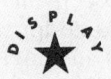

Patient Teaching: Expected Outcomes of Family Teaching for the Child With Bronchopulmonary Dysplasia

- Explain the purpose of oxygen in the human body
- Describe signs of respiratory distress and appropriate interventions
- List symptoms of respiratory infection
- Demonstrate ability to administer medications correctly
- Demonstrate effective chest physiotherapy technique
- Demonstrate use of nasal cannula and care of affected skin
- Demonstrate use of oxygen tank, home oximeter, and/or apnea monitor
- Describe appropriate changes in family/child lifestyle and routine related to child's care
- Describe appropriate safety measures needed with oxygen therapy
- Demonstrate effective infant CPR
- Identify primary health care provider and the plan for follow-up medical care
- Discuss the nutritional plan of care and fluid restriction
- Identify changes in child's fluid status
- Identify potential stressors in home care
- Name available family/community supports

retardation, developmental delays, cerebral palsy, and learning disabilities can occur.

Mortality is between 10% and 25%, with most deaths occurring in the first year of life secondary to acute respiratory infections.[22] Pulmonary dysfunction has been found in adolescents and young adults with a history of BPD. Although most of these individuals were asymptomatic, the long-term impact of the findings on later adulthood can only be postulated.[95] The major respiratory sequelae include airway obstruction, reactive airways, and hyperinflation.

LONG-TERM CARE

The identification of a primary health care provider is of critical importance for children with BPD, so that continuity of care can be maintained. Standard immunizations are recommended for all children at the normal intervals. Routine screening is necessary for the early identification of vision and hearing deficits. Follow-up visits should include the assessment of pulmonary function, cardiac function, growth and development, nutritional balance, fluid and electrolyte status, and response to interventions.

The family's ability to cope with the child on oxygen at home should be assessed. Is the family getting enough sleep? Has the cost of equipment and nursing care not covered by insurance placed a heavy financial burden on the family? Has the relationship between the parents changed? How are the siblings coping? These issues are

extremely important because they can affect family stability and the quality of the care that the child receives.

Apnea Disorders

Definition and Incidence. Apnea is the absence of air flow to the lower airways. Three specific classifications of apnea may be applied to the pediatric population: apnea of prematurity, apnea of infancy, and obstructive sleep apnea. Apnea may be *central* in origin, related to cessation of respiratory activity; *obstructive,* which refers to ineffective respiratory efforts due to upper airway obstruction; or *mixed.*

Central apnea of less than 15 seconds without any associated signs or symptoms is considered normal in the infant. Apneic episodes are considered abnormal if they last 20 seconds or longer, or if they are associated with cyanosis, bradycardia, pallor, or hypotonia, regardless of length. Apnea in the infant should be distinguished from periodic breathing, which is a normal breathing pattern during sleep. With periodic breathing, the infant exhibits apneic episodes of 3 to 5 seconds, followed by progressively faster respirations. Periodic breathing in excess of 4% of sleep time is considered abnormal.

Apnea of prematurity occurs in more than 50% of infants born at less than 32 weeks of gestation and can occur during sleep, feeding, or urination. Clinical interventions depend on the frequency, severity, and duration of the apneic episodes. *Apnea of infancy* occurs in term and postterm infants, may last up to 20 seconds or greater, and can be associated with significant clinical deterioration. This frightening, unexplained event requires close assessment and monitoring because up to 50% of infants have repeated episodes. *Obstructive* sleep apnea occurs in a small percentage of infants and children and is caused by a variety of age-specific congenital or pathologic conditions.

Etiology and Pathophysiology. The cause of *apnea of prematurity* is not known but is believed to be associated with immaturity of the respiratory control center within the brainstem. Central apnea is most commonly seen, with total absence of respiratory effort, and the infant exhibits bradycardia, cyanosis, pallor, and flaccidity. The infant has variable respiratory responses to hypoxia and hypercapnia and may be unable to respond by initiating a breath to correct the problem. Other causes of apnea of prematurity include sepsis, hypothermia, gastroesophageal reflux, seizures, meningitis, intraventricular hemorrhage, hypoxia, hypoglycemia, and anemia. Clinical interventions depend on the frequency, duration, and severity of episodes.

Apnea of infancy occurs in term and postterm newborns, infants, and children. The NIH consensus statement describes infant apnea of 15 seconds or less as normal, versus apneic episodes of 20 seconds or greater (or shorter) and associated with cyanosis or pallor, bradycardia, and marked hypotonia, as abnormal.[21] The infant may exhibit choking or gagging activity before the apnea, and observers become startled by what appears to be a life-threatening event requiring CPR. Although brainstem or upper airway dysfunction may be identified as a causative factor in some infants, no underlying disease or condition can be identified in as many as 50% of cases. Accurate diagnosis of the underlying cause helps guide the clinician in developing a specific care plan. It is important to identify not only the duration of infantile apneic periods, but also the physiologic responses (desaturation, bradycardia, no changes, and so forth) to determine how best to monitor the infant and to implement necessary interventions when warranted. Infants who suffer apnea have an increased incidence of SIDS. These life-threatening events are sometimes referred to as "near-miss SIDS."[70]

Obstructive sleep apnea occurs secondary to partial or complete closure of some portion of the upper airway during inspiration. Findings may include snoring, repeated episodes of apnea, hypoventilation, hypoxemia, and an abnormal sleep pattern. The child may sleep restlessly and assume unusual positions in bed (sometimes sitting) to breathe easier. Enuresis and morning headaches may be common. Growth and development may be delayed. Anatomic abnormalities that produce obstructive sleep apnea manifest within the first 6 months of life. In the preschool or school-age child, enlarged tonsils and adenoids are the most common cause of obstructive sleep apnea. Occasionally, children who are extremely obese may suffer from obstructive sleep apnea and alveolar hypoventilation, the classic Pickwickian syndrome. Chronic obstructive sleep apnea with associated hypoventilation, hypoxemia, and hypercapnia may lead to polycythemia, pulmonary hypertension, and right ventricular hypertrophy.

Therapeutic interventions for obstructive sleep apnea depend on the seriousness of the condition. Apneic episodes associated with an oxygen saturation drop of more than 5%, a P_sO_2 drop of 8 mmHg or greater, or a rise in end-tidal CO_2 of 2% or greater may indicate the need for specific treatment.[70]

Clinical Manifestations. Apnea is usually noted by the parents caring for the infant at home. The parent brings the child to the emergency room because of apnea, cyanosis, pallor, and limpness that has led the family to initiate some form of resuscitative efforts including vigorous stimulation or mouth-to-mouth resuscitation. By the time the family arrives at the hospital, though, the infant frequently is breathing and appears normal. Previously, these events were called "near-miss SIDS" or "aborted SIDS" but have recently been renamed "apparent life-threatening events" (ALTE), because the diagnosis of SIDS is made postmortem. Infants who experience apneic episodes as inpatients may exhibit changes in monitoring data. Pulse oximetry readings may deteriorate, and PaO_2 values drop, whereas P_sCO_2 levels rise.

Diagnostic Studies. Diagnostic studies should be done to identify or rule out known causes of apnea of infancy. General tests that should be completed when the clinical presentation is nonspecific include CBC, electrolytes, calcium, glucose, chest radiograph, electroencephalogram (EEG), electrocardiogram (ECG), esophageal pH monitoring, barium swallow, and upper gastrointestinal study. Additional tests such as a sleep study (polysomnography), septic work-up, nuclear mag-

netic resonance imaging (MRI), and bronchoscopy may be done if a specific condition is suspected. Home apnea monitoring serves as an early warning sign of an apneic event and as a mechanism for documenting the frequency of apneic events.

Apnea of Infancy

★ **ASSESSMENT**

Infants hospitalized and monitored for apneic episodes are assessed for the particular features of the episode. Initially, after the apnea alarm sounds, the nurse quickly determines whether the episode is truly an apneic episode or a mechanical problem with the monitor. During an apneic episode, the nurse monitors the infant for heart rate, color, pulse oximetry S_pO_2, muscle tone, and movement. Seizure activity, if any, is assessed for duration, body movement, eye deviation, and presence of respiratory effort. If possible, determination of the order of the events can be helpful diagnostically, that is, whether the apnea was preceded by or occurred after any seizure activity.

Events and timing of the episode are important elements of assessment. Whether the child was sleeping, feeding, or crying is important to note. Emesis in the mouth or on linens can reflect apnea related to gastrointestinal reflux. Postapneic episode efforts to breath and cough, level of consciousness, and amount of intervention required to resume normal breathing patterns are necessary to report for safety measures and are also diagnostically helpful.

Because many conditions and illnesses may have apnea as part of their symptomatology, a general and thorough physical assessment must be included. Clues to other illnesses, such as fever as it relates to infective disease, jaundice secondary to hyperbilirubinemia, and neurologic irritability as it relates to intercranial hemorrhage or encephalopathy, must be included in the general assessment of the infant.

The nurse needs to assess the parents' knowledge level regarding apnea monitoring equipment and resuscitation techniques, and their ability to cope with their infant's apneic episodes. Having them speak about the episode(s) is not only therapeutic for the parents but also can assist the nurse in identifying knowledge, skill, and support needs.

★ **NURSING DIAGNOSES AND PLANNING**

Based on assessment data from above and Chapter 37, the following nursing diagnoses may apply to the family and child with apnea of infancy:

- Ineffective Breathing Pattern related to periods of apnea.
- Anxiety (Parental) related to knowledge deficit regarding apnea monitoring and apnea treatment.
- Compromised Family Coping related to stress of infant's condition.

The nurse and parents together plan effective care based on the established nursing diagnoses. Several examples of expected outcomes follow:

- The parents discuss their concerns regarding the infant's condition and treatment.

- The parents demonstrate accurate operation of apnea monitoring and troubleshooting the monitoring equipment.
- The parents demonstrate techniques to stimulate the infant to breathe.
- The parents participate in CPR training.

The nurse plans for the daily care of the child based on both physician's orders and nursing diagnoses. A general nursing care goal may include the following:

- Apneic episodes will be recognized and treated promptly.
- Parents will gain confidence in their assessment and intervention skills.

★ INTERVENTIONS: COLLABORATIVE AND INDEPENDENT

Management of apnea in infancy primarily involves the use of drugs and home monitoring. Methylxanthines such as theophylline and caffeine work well in infants with apnea related to the central nervous system (CNS), due to their stimulant effects. Although theophylline may have side-effects including fussiness, irritability, and hyperactivity, it is readily used because it is available as an elixir preparation and therapeutic serum blood levels are easily monitored. A general guideline for the discontinuation of the medication in infants with apnea is when they have had few numbers of alarms or apneic episodes that did not require any intervention for 2 to 3 months.[21]

TEACHING

Apnea in infancy is similar to chronic illness because it persists over time, has an uncertain prognosis, and is manageable but not curable. Sensitive health care practitioners acknowledge parents' concerns regarding their infant's condition and apnea treatment. Teaching is ideally done individually rather than in a group setting. In this manner, the nurse can teach specifically to the family's needs including sophistication level, specific clinical manifestations of the infant, and specific fears and skills of the parents. Written materials are needed to reiterate instructions, and return demonstrations by parents are an effective way to practice newly acquired skills.

Parents must learn the proper method of applying an apnea monitor to their infant, including correct placement of leads and connections, and a systematic approach to troubleshooting the monitor. They must learn to assess quickly the status of their infant once the alarm has sounded and to intervene effectively and safely. Nurses are able to teach parents about the practical aspects of apnea monitoring, differentiating mechanical problems from true apnea. Nurses teach parents to assess systematically their infant's status and to intervene beginning with mild stimulation, proceeding all the way to full CPR if necessary. Parents are taught safety issues, such as avoidance of vigorous shaking during the episode.

★ EVALUATION

Periodically, the nurse and family evaluate the outcomes of care given. Examples of outcomes for the child and family with apnea of infancy were given under diagnoses and planning in this section. Have short-term goals been met? Are long-term goals still realistic?

LONG-TERM CARE

Ongoing follow-up care is done by the primary health care practitioner, subspecialist, such as pediatric pulmonologist or apnea team, and the vendor for the apnea monitor. The family is monitored for adherence to the treatment plan, and the infant is followed up for the pattern of apneic episodes. Assessment of family stress is made as an ongoing process, and a referral to a family counselor is made if necessary. Discontinuation of medications and, eventually, the apnea monitor can be a stressful separation process, and each family needs to be individually assessed and supported according to individual needs.

Obstructive Sleep Apnea

★ ASSESSMENT

Obstructive sleep apnea can occur in children of all ages and requires careful observation of the child during sleep, because it can usually be detected by simple observation and auscultation over the mouth and nose. Inspiratory efforts usually do not cease during obstructive apnea; therefore, careful observation and recording of intensity and frequency of these efforts along with sleep state, presence of snore, position, and frequency of arousal are useful for diagnostic purposes. Monitoring of oxygen saturation, carbon dioxide levels, and heart rate during these episodes is useful for determination of severity and safety. Duration of apnea, reaction of the child, and degree of intervention necessary to resume effective breathing should be noted.

Associated symptoms identified from a nursing history and physical examination are important to note. Parents often describe their child's sleep as restless, and the child may assume unusual positions to breathe more effectively. Mood, responsiveness, and development may be impaired from sleep deprivation, because these children sometimes wake with headaches and may be somnolent or irritable throughout the day. Parents are frequently sleep-deprived; they may wake frequently with concern for their child or because of their child's snoring or restlessness. Ability to cope with stress and the parent–child relationship may be impaired related to sleep deprivation.

On physical examination, the nurse observes for craniofacial abnormalities, such as micrognathia or macroglossia. Abnormalities during feeding, such as frequent sighs, breathlessness with suck, nasal regurgitation of food, and difficulty in swallowing, can indicate mouth and throat abnormalities that otherwise may not be apparent. Therefore, habits and characteristics are important to note for safety measures and diagnostic purposes.

★ NURSING DIAGNOSES AND PLANNING

Based on assessment data from above and Chapter 37, the following nursing diagnoses may apply to the family and child with obstructive sleep apnea:

- Impaired Gas Exchange related to apneic episodes.
- High Risk for Activity Intolerance related to sleep deprivation.
- Altered Family Processes related to sleep deprivation.
- Fatigue related to interrupted sleep.
- Altered Growth and Development related to sleep deprivation.
- Anxiety (Parental) related to cause of obstructive disorder, techniques and technology for intervention, and emergency measures.
- High Risk for Altered Parenting related to fear of apneic episodes, sleep deprivation, and coping with stress.
- Sleep Pattern Disturbance related to apnea.
- High Risk for Suffocation related to anatomic or physiologic obstruction causing apnea.

The nurse and child (or parents) together plan effective care based on the established nursing diagnoses. Expected outcomes may be similar to those listed for apnea of infancy.

The nurse plans for the daily care of the child based on both physician's orders and nursing diagnoses. Some general nursing care goals may include the following:

- Apneic episodes will be recognized and treated promptly.
- Age-appropriate developmental patterns will be established.
- Coping mechanisms will be used to manage anxiety.

★ INTERVENTIONS: COLLABORATIVE AND INDEPENDENT

The goal of treatment is to maintain a patent airway to avoid the morbidity and mortality associated with prolonged tissue anoxia. Interventions are directly related to the cause of the obstruction. In older children, the treatment often is surgical. If the obstruction is caused by enlargement of the tonsils and adenoids, a tonsilloadenoidectomy is performed. Obstruction caused by craniofacial abnormalities may be corrected by reconstructive surgery, or, if reconstruction is not possible, a tracheostomy is done as a palliative procedure (see section on Care of the Child With a Tracheostomy later in this chapter).

The use of methylxanthine medications may be effective in reducing obstructive apnea in premature infants (see section on Apnea of Infancy earlier in this chapter). Another nonsurgical technique in infants and older children involves the use of continuous positive airway pressure (CPAP, BiPAP), applied to the nasopharynx by way of a nasal mask in the spontaneously breathing child. This technique uses positive pressure to splint the airway open, preventing total airway collapse during the respiratory cycle.

A child with obstructive apnea may be discharged from the hospital with an apnea monitor. Parent education regarding the home use of an apnea monitor is similar to that described under apnea of infancy. Parents must also learn effective interventions ranging from mild stimulation to CPR. Specific techniques for establishing a patent airway may need to be taught, based on the reason for the obstruction in their child. Nurse–parent teaching is best conducted in a one-on-one situation to adapt to the specific needs of the child. Nurses should acknowledge and be sensitive to the anxiety produced in parents by the apneic problem, home apnea monitor, and use of resuscitation techniques on their child. Telephone follow-up by the primary health care practitioner and specialists can support the family and enhance coping.

★ EVALUATION

Periodically, the nurse and family evaluate the outcomes of care given. Examples of outcomes for the child and family with obstructive sleep apnea were given under diagnoses and planning in this section.

Sudden Infant Death Syndrome

Sudden infant death syndrome (SIDS), also known as crib death, is the sudden and unexpected death of an apparently normal infant, which remains unexplained after autopsy. SIDS is the leading cause of death in infants age 1 to 12 months, with an incidence of approximately 2 cases per 1000 live births.[70] The incidence of SIDS in preterm infants, infants having apneic episodes, infants with prenatal drug exposure, and siblings of SIDS victims is higher than in the general population. A variety of factors associated with an increased risk of SIDS are listed in the accompanying display. There may be as high as a 10% morbidity in near-SIDS infants who require mouth-to-mouth or cardiac resuscitation.

There are no pathologic, histologic, or clinical data to explain why SIDS occurs. The only common finding in SIDS is the apparent observation that cessation of respiration (apnea) preceded death. Abnormal function of the respiratory control systems in the brain appears to be the most obvious explanation for SIDS. However, no consistent abnormalities in respiratory control have been identified in normal infants or infants with apparent life threatening events that would serve to predict SIDS.

The typical scenario for SIDS is that the parents wake to find that the infant has died while asleep. The infant may have mucus on the outside of the nose and mouth but otherwise looks undisturbed. Parents report not hearing any crying or struggling throughout the night.

Family Support

When an infant dies of SIDS, the parents are overwhelmed with grief and feelings of guilt and remorse. Denial and anger, particularly at the health care team or each other, are often present. The nurse becomes an active listener, support person, and resource for the parents. Active listening skills are important so that the nurse can allow parents to express their feelings.

The amount of time and resources needed to come to terms with their grief varies according to family coping strategies and support systems. Another, although often overlooked, important aspect of intervention is the inclusion of babysitters, family friends, siblings, and extended family into the grief counseling.

Counseling should begin with the sharing of recent findings on the causes and known facts about SIDS. Parents often review in their minds, or out loud, the weeks

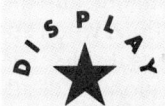

Factors Associated With an Increased Incidence of SIDS

Maternal Characteristics	*Infant Characteristics*
Lower socioeconomic status	Male
Less than 20 years of age	Prematurity or Small for Gestational Age
Nonwhite	Low APGAR scores
Previous fetal death	Previous need for resuscitation
Cigarette smoking	(history of ALTE)
Substance abuse	Multiple births
Poor prenatal care	Previous SIDS sibling
Illness during pregnancy	Poor feeder
	History of upper respiratory infection before SIDS event

Data from Koff, P. B., Eitzman, D. V., & Neu, J. (1988). Neonatal and pediatric respiratory care. *St. Louis: Mosby.*

immediately preceding the event, in search of a reason for the death of their infant. This review occurs secondary to a need to identify cause and effect, making the event easier to understand. However, caution must be exercised in this situation, particularly when friends and family members may have old-fashioned ideas as to the reasons for SIDS, influencing the parents' perception of the event. Siblings often fabricate in their minds reasons for the infant's death. Parents must be alerted to the possibility of misinterpretation on the sibling's part; a satisfactory explanation allays intense adverse reactions.

Parental support groups are helpful. These groups provide a network of social supports, composed of families who have suffered from a similar event. Often, social workers are group facilitators, providing additional resources and support. Organizations available for information on SIDS are listed at the beginning of this chapter.

Other community resources can be found by contacting the state health department for information. Many children's hospitals and public health departments offer support groups, literature, and home visits. Books and pamphlets are helpful to reinforce information and counseling given by health care members.

A postmortem examination is essential to identify the cause of death. Postmortem results should be communicated as quickly as possible to the parents.

Although subsequent siblings of a SIDS infant demonstrate a less than 2% recurrent risk for SIDS, many siblings of SIDS victims are monitored at home for apnea to relieve parental anxiety.[29] Unfortunately, the efficacy of this intervention remains unproven.

Evaluation of coping is an ongoing process, and follow-up by the primary health care provider is important. The resolution of grief and the posttraumatic adjustment require time. One must be aware of the fact that these families never "get over" this event, and chronic grief is a normal adaptation to SIDS. Anticipatory guidance should focus on the typical feelings and responses of other parents. Validation of feelings, listening, and reflection are important counseling skills the nurse can use when helping a family cope with SIDS.

Apparent Life-Threatening Events (ALTE) or Near-Miss SIDS

ALTE are episodes of apnea, color change, changes of muscle tone, and sometimes choking or gagging. Vigorous stimulation or resuscitation is needed to revive the infant.[29] A careful history is necessary to establish if there has been any previous upper respiratory infection, feeding problems, sleeping problems, prenatal risk factors (e.g., maternal drug ingestion), prematurity, birth trauma, seizures, history of apnea, or medication ingestion. Physical examination includes a complete neurologic examination, developmental testing, and evaluation of cardiac and pulmonary function. The nurse also should obtain an accurate description from the caregiver as to the events preceding the episode, how the infant looked, and the amount and type of resuscitation required.

Management decisions are based on the severity of the episode. Infants are often admitted to the hospital for a complete work-up, including cardiorespiratory monitoring, EEG, ECG, and a sleep study. Infants demonstrating apnea and bradycardia are treated with methylxanthines (aminophylline or caffeine).[29] Infants who continue to demonstrate apnea or who have an abnormal pneumogram are sent home on an apnea monitoring program. Parents must also be taught infant CPR before discharge. Appropriate referrals to public health nurses, vendor supports, and community services are important. The primary caregiver must be informed of all interventions to enable appropriate follow-up.

Techniques and Technology in Pediatric Respiratory Care

The majority of conditions that adversely affect a child's pulmonary system require some level of intervention aimed at treating or supporting the child's respiratory function during the illness. These interventions include oxygen and humidity therapy, aerosol medication administration, chest physiotherapy and other secretion clearance maneuvers, incentive spirometry, continuous positive airway pressure, and mechanical ventilation. As more institutions consolidate care in this era of cost-containment, nurses are assuming greater responsibility for the direct administration of respiratory care. The nurse is expected to understand the basic rationale for respiratory interventions and their specific goals. Additionally, a knowledge of the equipment and techniques allows the nurse to safely and optimally monitor normal and adverse response to therapy.

Noninvasive Monitoring

Several technologies are available for continuous, noninvasive monitoring of respiratory status. These include pulse oximetry (S_pO_2), transcutaneous monitoring of PO_2 (P_sO_2) and PCO_2 (P_sCO_2), and capnometry, which measures end-tidal carbon dioxide ($ETCO_2$) in respiratory gases. These devices give the nurse immediate access to information regarding oxygenation and ventilation that would otherwise require an invasive, painful ABG to obtain. The nurse, however, should *always* act based on physical assessment findings (vital signs, cyanosis, LOC, and so forth), irrespective of how reassuring the numbers displayed on these noninvasive monitors may be.

Pulse Oximetry

Pulse oximetry uses the principles of light absorption and plethysmography to measure the amount of oxyhemoglobin in arterial blood. A probe is applied to an arterial vascular site, such as the finger or toe of the child. Two light-emitting diodes (LEDs) pass light through the digit, and a photodetector on the opposite side of the digit measures the amount of transmitted light, based on the amount of "red" blood (hemoglobin bound with oxygen) present in the arteries. The measurement is converted to an S_pO_2 reading, along with a display of pulse rate, computed from the pulsatile movement of arterial blood at the probe site (Fig. 38-12).

A knowledge of the oxyhemoglobin desaturation curve is important to understand how the S_pO_2 correlates with PaO_2. Several physiologic and environmental factors can influence the accuracy of the pulse oximeter, and the nurse should be aware of these considerations when applying the pulse oximeter and interpreting its results. The pulse oximeter can serve as an excellent monitor of adequacy of oxygenation, as well as a device for weaning oxygen therapy and assessing response to interventions such as bronchodilator therapy, suctioning, and CPT.

Transcutaneous Monitors

Transcutaneous monitors measure skin surface PO_2 and PCO_2. A heated probe is applied to the surface of the skin, most commonly the abdomen, inner thigh, or upper arm of the infant. The probe "arterializes" capillary blood, so that O_2 and CO_2 at the skin surface correlate more closely with arterial O_2 and CO_2. Special electrodes within the heated probe measure the skin surface O_2 and CO_2. These measurements are assumed to correlate to the values in arterial blood. As with the pulse oximeter, multiple physiologic and environmental factors influence the validity of the device. The transcutaneous monitor is used most often to recognize blood gas trends in the newborn intensive care nursery (ICN), or with the infant in PICU, often in conjunction with the pulse oximeter (Fig. 38-13).

Capnometers

Capnometers measure the amount of CO_2 in respiratory gases and are mostly limited to use with mechanically ventilated children in the PICU. An adaptor is placed at the point where the endotracheal tube connects to the ventilator circuit. Infrared light passes through the adaptor continuously, where it is exposed to gases the child inhales and exhales. The amount of exhaled CO_2 gas is measured, and that signal is converted to an end-tidal CO_2 reading. This value correlates indirectly with the arterial CO_2 ($PaCO_2$). As with the transcutaneous monitor, this device is used primarily to note trends in CO_2 levels based on changes in clinical status or response to interventions, such as ventilator parameter changes. Endotracheal CO_2 monitoring can be particularly useful in weaning a child from mechanical ventilation, decreasing the

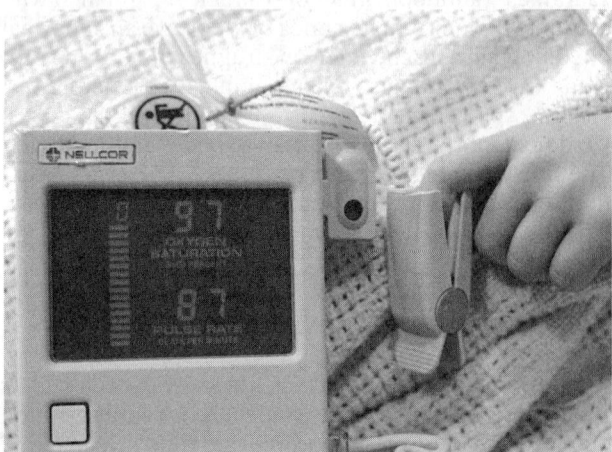

FIGURE 38-12
An example of a pulse oximeter used to measure arterial oxygen saturation (SpO_2).

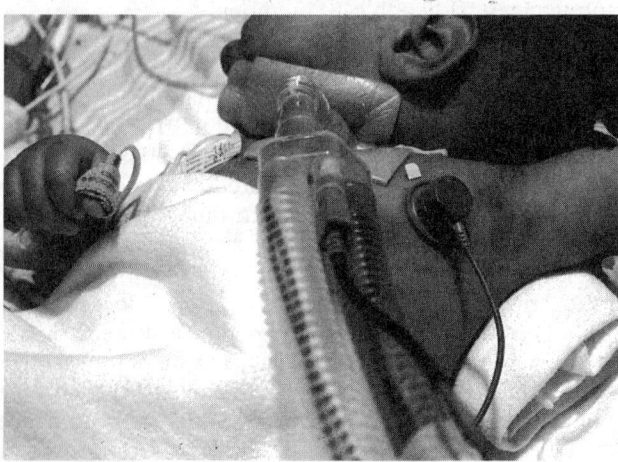

FIGURE 38-13
An infant on mechanical ventilation, on a noninvasive pulse oximeter (right thumb), and transcutaneous CO_2 monitor (upper chest).

need for repeated ABGs with every ventilator change. The accuracy of these devices is also subject to physiologic and environmental factors.[26]

Oxygen and Humidity Therapy

Oxygen

A variety of devices are used to administer oxygen. These devices and their advantages and disadvantages and effectiveness and risks are outlined in Chapter 25. The common goal of this equipment is to raise the child's PaO_2. In the presence of a low PaO_2 as determined by ABGs, or low pulse oximetry S_pO_2 or transcutaneous P_sO_2, oxygen may be ordered. Orders should include type of device and desired liter flow. Specific outcome criteria are also advisable in children. (For example, the goal may be to titrate liter flow to maintain $S_pO_2 > 95\%$).

Common oxygen delivery devices include nasal cannula, blow-by cannula, nasal catheter, face mask, oxygen hood, Isolette, and mist tent (croupette). (Information on this equipment is given in Chapter 25. Figure 25-16 illustrates some of this equipment.) Oxygen delivery devices operate at clinician-set oxygen flow rates measured in liters per minute. Actual FiO_2 is variable, depending on a variety of factors such as breathing pattern, age of the child, and fit. A humidifier may be used with these devices to add moisture to the dry gas delivered by way of the flowmeter from the hospital's wall oxygen delivery system.

A particularly important use of the nasal cannula is in the management of infants with BPD. Oxygen-dependent infants may require small but critical levels of oxygen to maintain adequate S_pO_2 and to reduce pulmonary hypertension. Oxygen flowmeters with calibrations as low as 1/16th L/min may be required to deliver low levels of oxygen to the infant. Correct application of the nasal cannula in the nares of these infants ensures consistent delivery and avoids pressure necrosis, particularly when the child is discharged home on O_2 (see section on Interventions: Collaborative and Independent for bronchopulmonary dysplasia earlier in this chapter).

Humidity

The primary goals of humidity therapy are to (1) aid in bronchial hygiene, and (2) humidify gases breathed through an artificial airway. In many acute and chronic respiratory conditions, there is an abundance of secretions that may be difficult to mobilize and expectorate. Children with pneumonia, croup, or CF may benefit from the use of an aerosol to add humidity to the airway. Aerosols are particulate water and are commonly administered by way of a large volume nebulizer (500 ml) filled with sterile water. Large-bore tubing is connected to the nebulizer, and the aerosol is delivered from the distal end of the tubing to the child by way of mask, face tent (Fig. 38-14), or tracheotomy collar. The nebulizer usually is connected to an oxygen flowmeter for its gas supply, and adjustment of the nebulizer collar allows for entrainment of air to adjust FiO_2 delivery.

Newborns and small infants may receive aerosol by way of a hood (Fig. 25-16C), which allows for control of

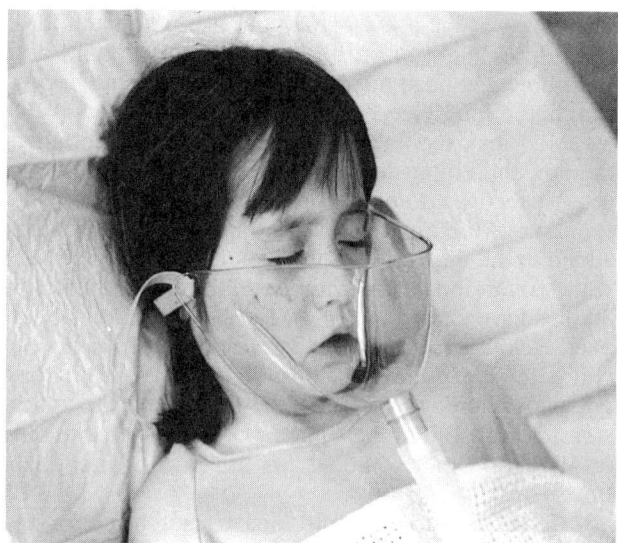

FIGURE 38-14
A child receiving humidity and oxygen by way of an aerosol face tent.

FiO_2, humidity, and temperature. Adjustment of liter flow should be sufficient to flush out exhaled CO_2 (>7 L/min), but not so high that the cool gas blowing over the infant's head causes hypothermia. An oxygen analyzer should be placed inside the hood, on the mattress at the level of the infant's face, for continuous monitoring of FiO_2.[107]

Although less commonly used than in the past, aerosol tents may still be used in the treatment of children with croup (Fig. 25-16D). "Croup tent" therapy controls four environmental factors: FiO_2, humidity, temperature, and filtered gas. Cool mist by way of tent can be soothing to the irritated, swollen airway mucosa of the infant with croup. When delivering oxygen by way of tent, any toys or equipment that might cause a spark should be avoided.

In the child with a tracheostomy, the normal upper airway humidification system is bypassed, requiring the use of added humidity. Although the use of a nebulizer with a tracheotomy collar is common, more therapists are using heated wick-type humidifiers to supply the added moisture needed to avoid secretion stasis. Use of this type system reduces the infection risks associated with nebulizers and may represent a cost-saving because less frequent equipment changes are required.

Aerosol Medication Administration

A variety of pharmacologic agents may be administered by inhalation to the child with pulmonary disease. These include bronchodilators, steroids, antiasthma drugs (cromolyn sodium), and antimicrobials. Two basic techniques for aerosol medication delivery exist: hand nebulizers and metered dose inhalers (MDI). Most of the bronchodilator medications lack specific dose recommendations for children age 8 or younger; nurses should consult the respiratory care department or the pharmacy at their hospital for specific dosing guidelines. Typically, a dose less than the standard adult dose (some references suggest 0.02 mg/kg body weight) is mixed with 1 to 3 ml normal saline and administered using a hand nebulizer, by way of mask or mouthpiece. Older children should be taught to breath in slow and deep and hold their breath at peak inspiration to enhance drug deposition in the lung (see Fig. 38-6A).

MDI may serve as an alternative to hand nebulizer therapy, thereby saving considerable time and cost. Because effective use of MDI requires coordination of inspiration with canister activation, spacer devices are often added to the delivery system. Even infants may use MDI with spacer and mask, without compromising efficacy. Studies have shown that a MDI with spacer may be just as efficacious as a hand nebulizer in acutely ill infants and children.[115] An additional consideration in teaching parents and children the use of MDI is that most of the topical steroids available in the United States are available only in MDI form, not solutions for use in hand nebulizer treatments.

Certain pulmonary conditions warrant the use of specific medications by inhalation. Racemic epinephrine is often given in the treatment of croup, or for postextubation stridor. Tobramycin or gentamicin may be ordered for the topical treatment of pulmonary infection in the child with CF admitted with acute exacerbation. Pentamidine may be administered prophylactically in immunosuppressed children at risk for an opportunistic infection with *Pneumocystis carinii* (see section on Pneumonia earlier in this chapter). Cromolyn sodium, a prophylactic antiasthma drug used to reduce the incidence of asthma attacks, can be taken either by hand nebulizer or MDI. Cromolyn sodium is chemically compatible for mixing with most bronchodilators for administration as a single nebulizer treatment (see section on Interventions: Collaborative and Independent for asthma earlier in this chapter).

Ribavirin Administration

Ribavirin (Virazole) is a synthetic antiviral agent approved by the FDA for the treatment of RSV. The drug is supplied as a 6-g vial of crystalline powder that is reconstituted with 300 ml sterile water, for a dose of 20 mg/ml. Delivery of the full dose requires administration for 10 to 20 h/day, over a course of 3 to 5 days. A recent study by Eglund et al[39] examined higher doses (60 mg/ml) for shorter duration with favorable results.

A Small Aerosol Particle Generator (SAPG) unit aerosolizes the medication for delivery by way of oxyhood, aerosol mask or face tent, or by "croup tent". Although the manufacturer cautions against its use in conjunction with mechanical ventilation due to the risks of ET tube obstruction from residue build-up, reports have supported its use in this manner.[31,97,116]

Concerns exist regarding environmental exposure to ribavirin by health care workers (see section on Interventions: Collaborative and Independent for bronchiolitis earlier in this chapter). Although studies in baboons and rats have shown teratogenic and mutagenic properties, no data exist demonstrating these risks in humans. Nevertheless, guidelines such as suggested in the display "Precautions for Exposure of Health Care Workers to Ribavirin" in this chapter should be considered. Nurses working in hospitals where ribavirin is administered are encouraged to collaborate with their institution's environmental health and safety officers to ensure that the ribavirin delivery system minimizes exposure.

Secretion Clearance Techniques

Certain pulmonary conditions predispose to increased volumes of secretions that require mobilization and expectoration. Traditional techniques for bronchial hygiene include coughing and deep breathing, and chest physiotherapy (CPT).

CPT includes postural drainage, which uses gravity to drain different lung segments, coupled with percussion or vibration on the chest wall over the segments being drained. These three techniques are discussed in Chapter 25, and Figs. 25-17 and 25-18 illustrate the various drainage positions for infants and children. Effective CPT requires a minimum of 3 to 5 minutes in each drainage position and should be used only in conditions characterized by large volume sputum production. Infants with BPD and children with CF represent two specific pulmonary conditions where CPT has been shown beneficial.

Recently, alternatives to CPT have been used at selected institutions. These include autogenic drainage (AD) and positive expiratory pressure (PEP) mask therapy (see section on Interventions: Collaborative and Independent for cystic fibrosis earlier in this chapter). Both techniques have considerable potential as secretion clearance techniques that may supplement or replace traditional CPT. AD and PEP hold the potential for having considerable impact on hospital and outpatient costs and compliance, because both techniques are self-performed by the child while sitting up. Figure 38-15 shows a 9-year-old girl receiving PEP treatment by mouthpiece.

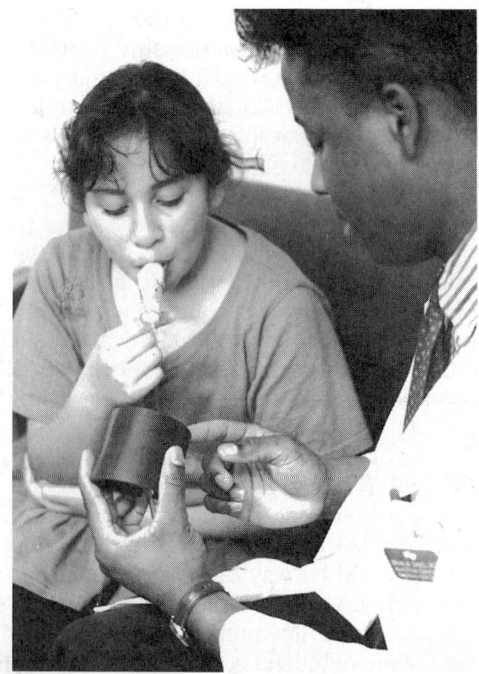

FIGURE 38-15
A child receiving PEP treatment by mouthpiece, an alternative to mask PEP for the older child.

The ThAIRapy vibrating vest also represents a relatively new secretion clearance technique. ThAIRapy uses a vest connected to hoses through which pneumatic vibrations of air are applied to the chest wall to move the secretions up the airways. Vests are available for use in children as young as 7 years old. Limited research is available to identify the long-term clinical role that this device will play in the treatment of children with conditions such as CF.[127]

Incentive Spirometry

Atelectasis may develop in certain medical conditions but most often is associated with postoperative abdominal or thoracic surgery. The most effective way to reexpand collapsed lungs is through deep, spontaneous inspirations. Incentive spirometry (ICS) can serve as a valuable therapy for visually stimulating deep inspiration in the child. Various devices have been developed, all of which act to assist the child in taking deep breaths (see Fig. 38-5). Instructions for children receiving ICS should include taking a deep, sustained inspiration, followed by a 3-second breath hold, then exhalation. For optimal use in the postoperative treatment or prophylaxis of atelectasis, ICS should be done each waking hour times ten breaths.

Continuous Positive Airway Pressure

Continuous positive airway pressure (CPAP) is a technique for applying positive pressure to the airway in a child who is spontaneously breathing, either by way of the natural airway or through an endotracheal or tracheostomy tube. The child receives a flow of gas to supply inspiratory needs, then exhales through a resistor, which provides continuous positive pressure to the airways. CPAP can be applied by way of mechanical ventilator set in the CPAP mode, or less expensively using a "homemade" CPAP system or commercially available CPAP device such as the Respironics SleepEasy or BiPAP. These latter devices are compact and can be effectively used in the home setting. BiPAP was developed to apply CPAP and low-level pressure support to people by way of a tight-fitting nasal mask or nasal prongs.

Indications for the use of CPAP include the treatment of central or obstructive sleep apnea, or in conditions where there are problems with oxygenation but not hypercapnia. CPAP is also frequently used as a final step before extubation when infants and children are being weaned from mechanical ventilation.

The nurse should be familiar with the CPAP system and associated alarms to provide safe, timely interventions should the system malfunction. Home care companies can serve as excellent resources for bridging the information gap for parents who are faced with taking their child home from the hospital on CPAP.

Mechanical Ventilation

Positive pressure mechanical ventilators are generally of two varieties, either volume-cycled or time-cycled.

Volume-cycled machines deliver a preset volume of gas at selected time intervals and are usually used in older infants and children. The ventilator delivers breaths at preset time intervals (control mode) or in conjunction with spontaneous inspiratory efforts of the patient (assist-control [A/C] or synchronized intermittent mandatory ventilation [SIMV]). The clinician also sets the other parameters such as FiO_2 and PEEP to maximize ventilator performance and gas exchange, and a variety of alarms to alert the caregivers to alterations in ventilator operation.

Time-cycled ventilators deliver a breath for a preset inspiratory time, up to a preset pressure limit. The machine can operate in the control, A/C, or IMV/SIMV mode. As with volume ventilators, these machines allow for setting FiO_2, PEEP, and other parameters. Time-cycled ventilators are used in the ICN or on infants in the PICU. The nurse must possess special assessment skills and be able to apply specific nursing interventions to ensure that the child continues to receive appropriate, safe ventilatory support. A knowledge of the basic operation of the ventilator and appropriate interventions should equipment fail is critical to the continued well-being of the child receiving mechanical ventilation.

Care of the Child Requiring Mechanical Ventilation

Intubation and mechanical ventilation become necessary when the child is unable to sustain adequate gas exchange with spontaneous ventilation. Intubation should be performed by skilled clinicians in an environment where oxygen and hand ventilation are available for use. In children younger than 8 years, an uncuffed ETT is used to maximize lumen size and to minimize trauma to the small, fragile trachea. Guidelines for selection of ET tube size based on age and weight are shown in the accompanying display. After placement of the ET tube, the nurse assumes a primary role in maintaining its stability and patency.

Children in Respiratory Failure

Acute Respiratory Failure

Acute respiratory failure (ARF) can occur as a sequelae to a variety of pulmonary, cardiac, neurologic, and metabolic conditions. The common factor associated with ARF is the inability of the pulmonary system to maintain gas exchange sufficient to meet metabolic demands. Hypoxemia and hypercapnia are present, with respiratory acidosis. Management of ARF often requires intubation and mechanical ventilation in a critical care setting.

Adult respiratory distress syndrome (ARDS) is a particular type of acute lung injury that can lead to ARF in children. ARDS is a clinical syndrome that occurs as a complication of illness or injury. Sepsis and septic shock, and gastric aspiration represent the two most common conditions that predispose to the development of ARDS. Nurses caring for critically ill children should acquire an understanding of the predisposing factors and clinical manifestations of ARDS.

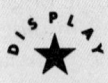

Pediatric Endotracheal Tube and Suction Catheter Size Guidelines

Age	Internal Diameter	Suction Catheter French Size
1–6 mo	3.0	6
6–12 mo	3.5	6–8
12–18 mo	4.0	8
18–36 mo	4.5	8–10
3–4 y	5.0	10
5–6 y	5.5	10–12
6–7 y	6.0	12
8–9 y	6.0–6.5	12
10–11 y	6.5–7.0	12–14
12–14 y	7.5	14

Endotracheal Tubes

ETT Size
  • For children > 1 year of age

$$ETT\ (in\ mm) = \frac{Age\ (in\ years)}{4} + 4$$

• Diameter of tip of the child's little finger approximates the ETT external diameter.

Most children 8 years and younger do not require cuffed ETTs.

Intubation for upper airway obstruction (as in croup, epiglottitis): use ETT 1 or more sizes smaller than usual because airway is already narrowed.

Although the pathophysiology associated with ARF is predominantly dependent on the primary condition, a common clinical manifestation includes a decrease in PaO_2, even on supplemental oxygen, and an increase in $PaCO_2$. This imbalance occurs secondary to some combination of increasing shunt, V/Q mismatch, and increased deadspace/tidal volume (Vd:Vt) ratio. The child may exhibit tachypnea, dyspnea, increased WOB, cyanosis, retractions, and use of accessory muscles. Neurologic alterations correlate with the degree of ventilatory fatigue and hypercapnia. The pH is acidotic, secondary to the acute retention of carbon dioxide. Other clinical findings relate to the specific etiologic condition.

The diagnosis of ARF is made based on clinical findings and ABGs. Chest radiograph or other imaging findings may help explain the cause (pneumonia, foreign body aspiration, and so forth) of ARF. Pulmonary function studies are not diagnostic but help support the clinical findings and quantify the seriousness of the condition, such as in cases of myasthenia gravis or Guillain-Barré. Laboratory studies such as CBC and body fluid cultures assist in identifying the need to treat primary or secondary infectious causes of ARF.

Chronic Respiratory Failure

Due to advances in medical care and technology, an increasing number of children are surviving acute illness and are left with long-term disability. Disease processes that produce chronic respiratory failure (CRF) can be divided into three major categories: chronic lung disease/BPD, neurologic/neuromuscular dysfunction, and congenital defects. In children with CRF, the disability may require prolonged dependence on oxygen therapy and mechanical ventilation.

Clinical manifestations of CRF include the continued need for mechanical ventilation, secondary to elevated CO_2 levels or the inability to maintain adequate ventilation. The child either tolerates slow weaning from the ventilator or may not tolerate ventilator weaning at all. Tracheostomy tubes are required to maintain long-term airway support, and gastrostomy tubes may be needed to maintain adequate nutrition.

Placement alternatives for the ventilator-dependent child are limited. Many children remain in the ICU for extended periods of time, sometimes years. Special units have been developed at some institutions to care for the ventilator-dependent child outside of the ICU. These units provide a less stressful setting for parents to learn to care for their child, using a developmental/wellness approach. Because the number of long-term facilities that permanently care for a ventilator-dependent child is limited, some families care for their child on a ventilator at home. This decision is made only after the family and health care team consider family readiness, financial feasibility, home capability, and other factors that affect home care.

★ ASSESSMENT

The presence of an artificial airway and mechanical ventilator does not ensure appropriate ventilatory support. An essential aspect of the assessment of the mechanically ventilated child is the ongoing evaluation of the efficacy and adequacy of ventilatory support. Methods of assessment include physical examination, ABG analysis, chest radiograph, and vital sign parameters. The nurse's subjective assessment of whether the child "looks good" or "looks bad" is often much more telling and more important than objective data.

Assessment of heart rate, blood pressure, color, and perfusion is necessary to determine the adequacy of ventilatory support. Bradyrhythmias, hypotension, cyanosis, and decreased perfusion may indicate hypoxia and respiratory insufficiency. Chest excursion should be symmetric with normal chest wall movement on inspiration. Auscultation of the chest determines if breath sounds are present, equal, or abnormal. If breath sounds over the right chest are louder than the left, right mainstem intubation should be suspected. The absence of breath sounds, in combination with abdominal distention and arterial desaturation, indicates esophageal intubation. The absence of breath sounds on one side in the presence of acute clinical deterioration may indicate pneumothorax.

The quality of the breath sounds should be assessed to determine if atelectasis, bronchospasm, secretions, or effusions are present.

Invasive and noninvasive monitors may be used. ABGs, pulse oximetry, transcutaneous monitors, and end-tidal CO_2 monitors are invaluable when assessing the adequacy of ventilatory support.

Assessment is made of the level of consciousness and how well the child tolerates mechanical ventilation. Ventilator/patient asynchrony (the child is "fighting" the ventilator) is manifested by frequent coughing, agitation, frequent "high pressure" alarming of the ventilator, and changes in vital signs. Agitation can indicate hypoxia, whereas lethargy may indicate hypercapnia. Ongoing assessment of child and family coping, behavioral responses, and efficacy of all interventions is needed.

★ NURSING DIAGNOSES AND PLANNING

Based on assessment data from above and Chapter 37, the following nursing diagnoses may apply to the family and child using mechanical ventilation:

- Ineffective Airway Clearance related to ETT obstruction and diminished or absent cough.
- Impaired Gas Exchange related to ineffective ventilatory support.
- Ineffective Breathing Pattern related to ventilator asynchrony.
- Altered Growth and Development related to disruption of normal activities of daily living.
- Impaired Verbal Communication related to endotracheal intubation.
- Altered Parenting related to the intensive care environment.
- Anxiety related to the intensive care environment.
- Altered Nutrition: Less Than Body Requirements related to inadequate intake.
- Sleep Pattern Disturbance related to sensory overload.
- Dysfunctional Ventilatory Weaning Response related to inability to cooperate.

The nurse and parents together plan effective care based on the established nursing diagnoses. Several examples of expected outcomes follow:

- The child exhibits comfort from swaddling, positioning, and diversional activities.
- The child exhibits pain relief and sedation from medications.
- The parents maintain regular interactions with the child.
- The child rests between care procedures.
- The parents perform a return demonstration of range of motion exercises and suctioning.
- The parents participate in care of the child.
- The parents use alternative methods of communication with the child.
- The parents construct a schedule allowing for normal activities and school.
- The parents discuss their concerns about the child's condition and the outcome.
- The parents state their interpretation of what they have been told concerning the child's condition.
- The parents state they have made environmental adaptations for the child's home care.

- The parents describe their understanding of available community resources.

The nurse plans for the care of the child based on both physician's orders and nursing diagnoses. Some general nursing care goals may include the following:

- Adequate airway clearance and gas exchange are maintained.
- Behaviors appropriate to age group are increased.
- Adequate nutrition is achieved.

★ INTERVENTIONS: COLLABORATIVE AND INDEPENDENT

The nurse has a primary role in the stabilization and assessment of adequate placement and patency of the ETT. Endotracheal intubation should be an elective procedure to prevent anticipated respiratory failure. However, emergency intubations are occasionally needed, and the nursing staff should be familiar with specific procedures to allow for controlled intubation in any situation. If a skilled practitioner is not immediately available, the child usually can be supported with 100% oxygen and bag-valve mask manual ventilation until expert help arrives.

CARE DURING PLACEMENT OF THE ENDOTRACHEAL TUBE

Nursing actions for care during the endotracheal intubation procedure and the care and monitoring afterwards are given in Table 38-7. The nurse ensures that the appropriate equipment and monitors are at the bedside and in working order.

During the procedure, the nurse monitors the heart rate and arterial saturation continuously. Bradycardia and arterial desaturation indicate profound vagal stimulation or hypoxia, and the practitioner performing the intubation should be alerted immediately. The intubation may need to be aborted momentarily, and the child may need to be briefly manually ventilated with bag-mask and 100% oxygen until clinically stable.

Once the child has been successfully intubated, the lungs must be auscultated to evaluate tube placement. Symmetric chest excursion, equal breath sounds, normal heart rate, and appropriate arterial saturation should be present. If right mainstem or esophageal placement is suspected, the child should be extubated and reintubated. Absolute confirmation of ETT placement is established with chest radiograph; the tip of the ETT should be 2 to 3 cm above the carina. Care should also be taken when moving or turning the child, because the position of the ETT in the trachea changes when the head and neck are moved. Flexion of the neck moves the ETT toward the carina, whereas extension moves the ETT away from the carina and toward the larynx. Accidental extubation can occur secondary to extension of the neck in infants due to their anatomically short trachea.

Stabilization of the ETT can be accomplished in various ways. Taping of the ETT should be performed by two people to prevent slippage of the tube and accidental extubation. The skin is usually prepped with benzoin, and a skin barrier may be applied to prevent skin maceration under the tape. The taping configuration varies and is usually determined by unit or institutional pref-

TABLE 38-7
Nursing Intervention: Care of the Child With an Endotracheal Tube

Nursing Action: Care During Procedure	Rationale

1. Gather supplies:
  Cardiac monitor
  Pulse oximeter
  Bag, mask, 100% oxygen
  Suction source
  Laryngoscope handle and blade with functioning bulb
  Stylet
  Tape, benzoin, skin barrier to stabilize endotracheal tube (ETT)
  Gloves, protective eyewear
  NG tube if not already present
  Necessary medications as ordered
  Appropriate sized ETT
	1. Gathering all supplies prior to procedure facilitates a smooth intubation.
	
	Appropriate blade sizes:
	  Premature infant—0 straight
	  Term infant—1 straight
	  Small child—1 straight
	  Child—2 straight
	  Large child—2–3 straight or curved
	  Adolescent/Adult—3 straight or curved

2. Use uncuffed ETT in child under 8 y. If cuffed tube is used, note cuff pressure. (Cuff pressure should not exceed 25 cm H_2O.)	2. Excessive cuff pressure can contribute to ischemic damage of the tracheal wall, contributing to subglottic stenosis. Use only cuffed ETT with high-volume, low-pressure cuffs.
3. Place child on monitors, check that suction is properly set up and functioning, and ensure that bag and mask are correctly assembled and connected to 100% oxygen.	3. These actions provide safety measures for prompt intubation and care.
4. Monitor child and equipment during procedure.	4. Practitioner must be alerted immediately if a problem arises so the procedure can be aborted.
5. Securely tape ETT above lip, using protective skin barrier for long-term intubation.	5. ETT must be securely taped to prevent tube movement or dislodgement. One of the most common causes of accidental extubation is loose tape.
6. Hand ventilate while auscultating the mouth or neck, to determine if an air leak around the ETT is audible. An air leak should be audible around 25 cm H_2O.	6. In children, the narrowest portion of the airway is the cricoid, not the cords. The use of the properly sized ETT is critical to the support of adequate ventilation and the prevention of subglottic edema.

Nursing Action: Suctioning	Rationale
1. Place a tape measure on the side of the bed, indicating the length of the ETT. Measure the suction catheter before insertion into the ETT.	1. Only the ETT is suctioned to clear secretions. Turning the head will not introduce the catheter into the contralateral mainstem bronchus.
2. Suction the ETT only. Do not force or insert until resistance is met.	2. Insertion of the catheter into the airway until resistance is met causes tracheal wall damage and possible granuloma formation.
3. Oxygenate and hyperventilate before suctioning.	3. These actions help to prevent hypoxia, arterial desaturation, and hypercarbia associated with suctioning.
4. Provide analgesia or sedation if necessary. Apply soft wrist restraints on small children who are unable to cooperate.	4. Control of anxiety and chemical or mechanical restraints can help prevent accidental extubation. Use only as needed, as determined by individual patient response.
5. Supply continuous suction, appropriate sized suction catheter, and tonsillar suction at bedside.	5. Suction equipment must be available at all times in case the child requires ETT or oral suctioning.
6. Suction the ETT, using two glove sterile technique. Suction only when the patient needs it.	6. This maneuver maintains patency of the ETT. Sterile technique is necessary to prevent acquired infection. Two gloves protect the nurse. Excessive suctioning can contribute to tracheal wall damage and may not be tolerated by the patient.
7. Assess the patient's response to suctioning (heart rate, perfusion, arterial saturation).	7. Response to therapeutic intervention requires continual evaluation to determine efficacy of treatment and possible adverse sequelae.
8. Oxygenate and hyperventilate after suctioning.	8. These actions help prevent hypoxia, arterial desaturation, and hypercarbia associated with suctioning.

Nursing Action: Monitoring and Continuous Care	Rationale
1. Provide continuous cardiorespiratory, arterial saturation, and end-tidal CO_2 monitoring.	1. Monitoring allows the timely identification of complications. Tachycardia or bradycardia, arterial desaturation, or CO_2 retention can be seen with ETT obstruction and hypoxia. Monitoring also allows for the timely assessment of response to therapeutic intervention.
2. Provide manual ventilation bag connected to O_2 source, appropriately-sized face mask, and extra ETT at bedside.	2. Equipment must be at bedside in case of accidental extubation or emergency reintubation.
3. Assess breath sounds and chest excursions every hour.	3. Such assessments determine proper placement of ETT. Absent or decreased breath sounds can indicate esophageal intubation or ETT obstruction. Breath sounds heard only on the right indicate right mainstem intubation. Respiratory assessment helps in the early identification of atelectasis or pneumothorax.
4. Turn/reposition every 2 h as tolerated.	4. Frequent position changes can help prevent atelectasis and pressure sores.
5. Provide passive range of motion (ROM) exercises.	5. Passive ROM helps prevent contractures.
6. Provide age-appropriate diversional activities as tolerated.	6. Diversional activities help normalize the environment and support normal growth and development.
7. Provide age-appropriate methods of nonverbal communication (e.g., magic slate, pen and paper, sign language).	7. Children who are intubated are unable to speak and need a means of communication for normal growth and development.
8. Allow parents to participate actively in child's care.	8. Normalize the environment and support the parental role.

erence. Figure 38-16 illustrates one possible taping configuration. Once the ETT is secured, the breath sounds should be auscultated to ensure proper tube placement.

SUCTIONING

Ensuring ETT patency is a primary nursing function when caring for the intubated child and is accomplished by periodic suctioning of the ETT. The frequency of ETT suctioning is determined by the child's condition, amount and consistency of secretions, size of the ETT, and the child's tolerance of the procedure. Children with copious secretions and small ETTs may require suctioning more frequently (e.g., every 1 to 2 hours). Children who do not produce large amounts of secretions and who do not tolerate the procedure, or who have underlying pathology that is adversely affected by ETT suctioning (for example, pulmonary or intracranial hypertension) should be suctioned less frequently (e.g., every 6 hours).[80,131]

The procedure must be performed in a sterile manner, using two gloves and an appropriately sized suction catheter (see display on Pediatric Endotracheal Tube and Suction Catheter Size Guidelines earlier in this chapter and Table 38-7). If necessary, nonbacteriostatic normal saline lavage may be used in those children with tenacious secretions; however, lavage should not be required routinely because the appropriate use of humidified, warm air should prevent the formation of thick secretions. Hyperventilation and preoxygenation must be used before suctioning to prevent profound arterial desaturation, hypercapnia, and bradycardia; a second person uses a manual ventilation bag and oxygen source. The amount of preoxygenation requirements varies from 10% greater than what the child is receiving up to 100% oxygen. The amount of positive pressure generated during manual ventilation should be measured by a manometer directly in line with the ventilation bag. Care should be taken to avoid excessive peak pressures during hand ventilation; usually peak pressures equal to those produced by the mechanical ventilator are sufficient. Hyperventilation and preoxygenation should be administered for five to ten breaths before and after each suction pass. The child should be continually monitored to assess for adverse effects and tolerance.

Before suctioning, the length of the ETT should be determined, and a measuring tape should be placed on the side of the bed to indicate ETT length. The suction catheter should be passed to the end of the ETT only. Excessive, forceful insertion of the catheter until resistance is met (at the carina) is contraindicated and can result in tracheal mucosa damage. Suctioning should be performed to clear the ETT of secretions only. It is not possible to suction selectively the right or left mainstem bronchus by turning the head and therefore should not be attempted. Routine turning of the head can produce excessive movement of the ETT, resulting in tracheal damage. Careful evaluation is necessary to determine the risks and benefits of routine suctioning in each child.

MEDICATION THERAPY

The goals of pharmacologic intervention are to facilitate a smooth intubation, control pain, and provide sedation if needed. The agents used may vary according to physician preference. For sedation during intubation, short-acting benzodiazapine, sodium pentothal, or ketamine is often used. A short-acting neuromuscular blocking agent is used for short-term paralysis (e.g., vecuronium, succinylcholine). However, long-term pharmacologic support should be individualized according to underlying pathology and needs of the child.

Pain should be controlled by an analgesic. Often, in the critical care setting, continuous infusions are used, with periodic bolus administration according to need. Frequently used agents for pain control include morphine sulfate and fentanyl. Side-effects include respiratory depression and transient hypotension. Respiratory depression is not an issue in those children who are supported by mechanical ventilation, so this is not a sufficient criterion to withhold analgesia. However, analgesic administration must be reevaluated in those children who are being weaned from mechanical ventilation, in whom spontaneous ventilation is desired.

Sedation often is required in agitated children who

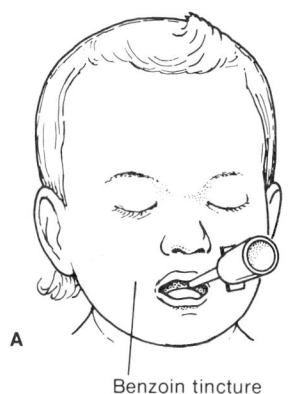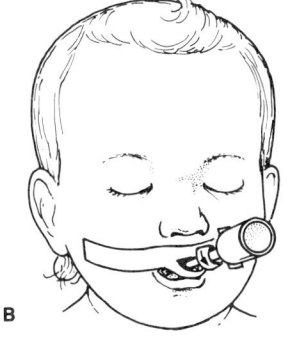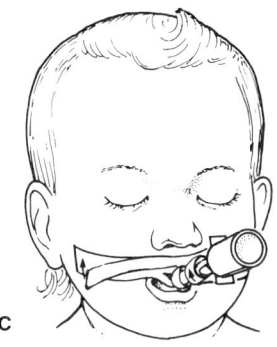

Benzoin tincture

FIGURE 38-16
One method for taping the endotracheal tube. (**A**) The area is prepared and painted with tincture of benzoin, and hypoactive squares are placed on each cheek. (**B**) The unsplit end of the tape is fixed to the square on the cheek. The upper end of the split tail is carried over the upper lip onto the opposite cheek and fastened securely. The lower split tail is brought under the tube and wrapped around in a spiral fashion. (**C**) A second split tail is applied in a similar fashion to the other cheek.

have no underlying physiologic reason for agitation (e.g., hypoxia), are preverbal, not comforted by normal measures (e.g., swaddling, positioning, diversional activities), or are asynchronous with the ventilator. Frequently used agents are chloral hydrate, midazolam, or Valium. Assessment as to the need for and efficacy of sedation is necessary. The routine administration of sedatives to simplify nursing care is inappropriate and should be avoided.

Neuromuscular paralysis is occasionally required in those children who remain asynchronous with the mechanical ventilator, in spite of sedation. Pharmacologic paralysis is *not equated* with sedation. Full cognitive awareness can be maintained while paralyzed with these agents; therefore, the concurrent use of sedatives is *required* in all children who are pharmacologically paralyzed. A common indication of inadequate sedation is tachycardia and blood pressure elevation. The use of paralytic agents must be individually adjusted to specific need, rather than routinely used.

Children who are pharmacologically paralyzed require vigilant monitoring and nursing care. These children are at greater risk if accidental extubation occurs due to their inability to generate spontaneous ventilation. Frequent turning and strict attention to appropriate body alignment are also important. Prevention of contractures, pressure sores, joint hyperextension, and dislocation are critical nursing functions. Normalization of the critical care experience should continue through parental participation in care and auditory diversions. Parental teaching helps allay anxiety and educates regarding the rationale for intervention. Parents and nursing staff should continue to explain procedures and talk to the child as normal, always assuming the presence of cognitive function.

MANAGEMENT OF OXYGEN DEMAND

Children requiring intubation and mechanical ventilation often are unable to meet excessive oxygen demands. The nurse is in a position to intervene and minimize oxygen demands.

Fever, pain, shivering, and agitation should be controlled because they all can increase oxygen consumption.[37,88,106] Infants should be cared for in a neutral thermal environment or under a radiant warmer, to prevent nonshivering thermogenesis and brown fat metabolism. WOB can increase oxygen consumption by 40% or more.[128] Anemia must be avoided and may require correction with red cell infusion. The maintenance of hemoglobin at 12 to 15 g% improves arterial oxygen content and supports oxygen delivery to the tissues.[131]

Many routine nursing procedures can adversely affect oxygen delivery and consumption. The nurse must be aware of individual tolerance of normal nursing procedures and schedule care accordingly. Procedures such as bed baths, weighing, suctioning, turning, and physical therapy can increase oxygen consumption. The adverse effects of these interventions are manifested by arrhythmias, hypotension, arterial desaturation, and agitation.

NUTRITIONAL MANAGEMENT

The mechanically ventilated child is at risk for nutritional depletion as well as fluid overload. Therefore, the provision of adequate calories can become problematic. Often, fluid therapy is at one half to three quarters of maintenance level during the acute period of illness. Fluids can be increased gradually as the child improves and as determined by underlying pathology. Nutritional support should be instituted as soon as possible, usually within 3 days of intubation. The enteral route is preferred; however, parenteral nutrition should be started if needed.

Enteral feedings can be given by either nasogastric tube or gastrostomy tube. Gastrostomy is usually reserved for children requiring long-term nutritional or mechanical ventilatory support. Feedings can be advanced as tolerated, until the appropriate caloric requirements are met, taking into consideration any excessive nutritional demands or existing depletion. The child exhibiting gastroesophageal reflux can be positioned prone, placed in an infant seat, or placed with the head of the bed up. Tube feeding can be provided in children receiving pharmacologic paralysis because these agents do not interfere with smooth muscle motility. The diet should be balanced to avoid large carbohydrate loads because the respiratory quotient (the amount of CO_2 produced through metabolism) of carbohydrates is high, resulting in an increase in CO_2 production. Hypercarbia can be problematic for the child in respiratory failure.[110]

Inadvertent starvation of the mechanically ventilated child results in muscle wasting and difficulty in weaning from mechanical ventilation. Many children who have been critically ill, without appropriate nutritional support, require parenteral or enteral feeding before successful weaning can be accomplished.[11,125]

PSYCHOSOCIAL SUPPORT OF THE CHILD

The PICU environment is designed to meet the complex needs of the critically ill child through the provision of round-the-clock nursing and medical care, technological support, and new, often invasive therapeutic interventions. Consequently, the critical care milieu is noisy, bright, foreign, and threatening to parents and child. The adverse effects of this environment include sleep disturbances, behavior changes, night terrors, hallucinations, and changes in circadian and biologic rhythms.

During the acute stages of illness, the focus of care is often on physiologic support. However, nursing care cannot be limited to short-term goals. The nurse must continue to support the long-term, dynamic needs of growth and development. An environment must be created that allows for the continuation of normal parent–child interactions, ensuring the continued development of the child's social and cognitive skills. Additional variables that affect the ventilator-dependent child's perception and adaptation to the environment include the use of sedatives, neuromuscular paralysis, and the ETT that precludes normal vocalization.

Frequent painful invasive procedures, frequent handling, and sensory overload all contribute to sleep deprivation. The use of sedatives that reduce rapid eye movement sleep phases also contributes to overall sleep disturbances.[126] Rest periods must be built into the care plan. Clustering of daily procedures can permit longer periods of either free play or sleep. Care must be taken never to perform painful procedures on a sleeping child.

Preparation for all procedures is important—even infants should be awakened before painful interventions.

Emotional needs of the child can be met by allowing for normal parenting to occur and minimizing the periods of separation from family and friends. Unlimited visiting and active participation by the parents in the child's care should be encouraged. The parents can bring in diversional activities, such as tapes of the child's favorite music, favorite movies, games, or video or cassette tapes made of the family, to be used when the parents cannot be present. Provision of alternative methods of communication for intubated children re-enhances their sense of control and mastery over a threatening situation. Strategies include the use of a small grease board for those who can write or the use of simple sign language techniques. Toddlers frequently respond to pictures of different facial expressions to indicate feelings. Siblings of any age can be allowed to visit most patients after a simple screening for communicable diseases and evaluation of coping styles and relationships. Care must be taken, however, to prepare siblings for the sights and sounds of the PICU before visiting. A postvisit debriefing helps clarify misconceptions or questions the sibling may have.[74]

Normal growth and development can be facilitated by the provision of age-appropriate toys and activities. The child life specialist and physical therapist are invaluable resources to the nurse who cares for the ventilator-dependent child. A collaborative plan should be developed that incorporates normal activities of play or school into the plan of care. Timing is of critical importance, however, especially in the child who has suffered a protracted illness. Ongoing assessment is vital to determine the child's readiness, as well as response to developmental interventions. Signs of adverse response, or overstimulation, include agitation, inability to self-comfort, and withdrawal. For age-appropriate developmental interventions, see Table 38-8. General nursing interventions for various ages during painful procedures are given in Table 25-9.

PSYCHOSOCIAL SUPPORT OF THE PARENTS

Parental stress in the PICU is multifaceted and complex. Common stressors include loss of parental role, lack of access to their child, lack of knowledge about their child's condition, and concerns about their child's survival and long-term prognosis. Reduction of parental stress facilitates parental adaptation to the PICU, enabling parents to become active, informed participants in their child's care.

Youngblut and Jay[130] found that parents were most concerned about outcome (e.g., physical handicap, brain damage) and survival after emergent admission to the PICU. Parents' concerns were not lessened by a good prognosis, indicating that staff perceptions about outcome may be different than parents'. Carter et al[15] found that change in the parental role was the most stressful area for parents. Financial considerations do not seem to surface until some days later during the hospitalization.[15,130]

Strategies to decrease parental stress are aimed at parental education, development of trust and respect, and the promotion of role attainment. Clear, concrete information must be provided in an environment that is free from excessive stimulation. Explanations need to be re-

peated, and the nurse encourages for questions and the clarification of issues.

Nursing interventions that allow for parental participation in their child's care are effective in decreasing parental stress. However, collaborative interventions should never be forced on the family. Parents can be taught to bathe, hold, read to, diaper, do range of motion exercises with, and suction their child. However, the nurse should not expect parents to manage their child's care completely at all times. Parents need permission to leave their child for breaks, for meals, or to go home. Nurses should be nonjudgmental of the frequency and type of care parents wish to provide.

WEANING AND EXTUBATION

Weaning from ventilatory support can be rapid and simple, or it can be slow and complex. Weaning should begin when:

- Resolution of underlying pathology has occurred
- Cardiovascular stability is achieved
- ABGs are within expected normal range for the child
- Muscle strength is sufficient to support spontaneous respiratory function
- A leak around the ETT is apparent

The method chosen for weaning should be determined by the child's condition and underlying pathology. Common methods used to wean mechanical ventilation include CPAP, T-piece, and pressure support.

Before extubation, the nurse should ensure that emergency intubation equipment is readily available, should the child fail the extubation attempt and require reintubation. Oral feedings are withheld for a few hours before and after extubation. Once the child is extubated, he or she is placed in humidified oxygen at a level necessary to maintain adequate arterial saturation. The nurse is responsible for the frequent assessment of respiratory function for at least 24 hours after extubation. The presence of inspiratory stridor, accessory muscle use, and increased WOB indicates postextubation subglottic edema. This condition usually responds to aerosolized racemic epinephrine.

A chest radiograph should be obtained 4 hours after extubation to determine the presence of a pneumothorax or atelectasis. The child should be encouraged to cough or use deep breathing maneuvers to facilitate secretion clearance if warranted. Chest physiotherapy and nasopharyngeal suctioning should be avoided immediately after extubation, because these maneuvers can trigger laryngospasm and upper airway obstruction.

DISCHARGE PLANNING FOR HOME VENTILATION

Parents of a child requiring chronic ventilatory support have the option of taking the child home. Ventilatory support can be variable, ranging from simple CPAP, to ventilation during sleep only, to complete mechanical support. The advantages of home ventilation programs include cost-effectiveness, reestablishment of the family unit, and the facilitation of the child's normal growth and development.[44,54,109]

Discharge planning for the ventilator-dependent child usually begins 2 to 3 months before discharge. An interdisciplinary approach is used. After a thorough as-

TABLE 38-8
Nursing Interventions: Age-Appropriate Developmental Interventions for Ventilator-Dependent Children

Age	Gross Motor/Fine Motor	Personal/Social	Cognitive/Language
1–2 months	Place in prone position with toys in line of vision Pick up and hold several times a day Move arms/legs together/up and down during diapering/vital signs Remove restraints Position with hands together	Provide face-to-face action Use exaggerated faces and speech Stroke gently during baths/diaper changes Warn infant before procedure by calling name and stroking cheek. Comfort infant when finished Swaddle Maintain eye contact and let suck on pacifier during feeding	Talk to quietly during vital signs and diaper changes Play music Hang a mobile over bed Record parents reading books/stories and play when parent is absent Provide cuddly toy
3–4 months	Place in prone position Sit up for chest physiotherapy, feeding Put in infant seat with hip and shoulder rolls Offer bright rings/rattles Bathe in tub of water, tickle feet, exercise legs and arms Position with hands/knees together Loosen clothing and let move around	Use en face positions Smile and talk to infant Hold and cuddle during feeding and after procedures Stimulate laugh by light tickling Put mirrors in cribs	Talk to or sing to during baths and diapering Provide bright colored toys and change often Hang mobile Tie bells to crib Call name, speak directly to infant Keep regular nap and bedtime rituals
5–8 months	Support sitting, roll on beach ball to stand Put on floor or playpen with toys Sit in corner chair, put easily grasped objects within reach Give toys to bang/squeak Play pat-a-cake Put on side with rolls, help roll over	Practice different facial expressions Play peek-a-boo Smile during feedings, frown during painful procedures, comfort afterward Introduce foods, let play with food, smear on hands and help get to mouth Keep nap and bedtime rituals	Read stories, and play tapes of parents reading at bedtime and naps While bathing, name body parts, play peek-a-boo with toys, and name movements such as splashing and washing While diapering, talk about sensations, hot/cold, wet/dry, say up/down, explain all acting movements Provide activity board Put parents' pictures inside bed and call by name
8–12 months	Encourage floor play, roll on beach ball to stand Pull to sitting with hands Encourage hand–hand transferring Give different textures to play with: yarn/tape/dressing packages/bright paper	Continue introducing foods. Put in lap/infant seat/high chair to feed Let experiment with food Let feed self regardless of mess. Protect tracheostomy with towel Play games, pat-a-cake, peek-a-boo Put in playpen near door, have different people talk and play Keep nap and bedtime rituals Introduce cup Praise *all* achievements Assess need for security blanket Put mirrors at bedside, point to child and call name	Play hide and seek with toys Name sounds (hear the phone/TV/water running) and sights (toys, equipment, people), body parts Read picture books, let child turn pages Echo any sounds made above ventilator Give stacking toys/boxes/bags Teach "no" Start sign language: help/hi/bye Encourage memory by giving simple commands—give me the _____
12–24 months	Continue standing, and walking exercises Give push/pull/riding toys Help dance to music Let turn pages of books, finger paint, put rings on stick	Encourage self-feeding Ignore temper tantrums, watch for respiratory distress only, speak calmly afterward Maintain nap and bedtime rituals Let sleep during night Take outside with portable ventilator Assess toilet training	Give stackable toys, container toys, crayons, finger paints, blocks, big jigsaw puzzles Name body parts Help with dressing by pulling off socks and shoes Read books, name objects Name colors and have child point Give simple commands—hand me _____, open the box

(Continued)

TABLE 38-8
(Continued)

Age	Gross Motor/Fine Motor	Personal/Social	Cognitive/Language
			Teach repositioning on/in/under
24–36 months	Give room to walk	Use spoon and cup to eat	Name pictures
	Help string large beads, use scissors, color with crayons or paint	Maintain feeding rituals	Give simple directions—where is _____, give me _____
		Let play with other children	Teach no/yes, prepositions
	Give play dough	Maintain nap and bedtime rituals	Read books
			Let help in dressing self
36–48 months	Encourage walking/hopping/ stairs	Secure toilet training	Teach relationships, big/bigger
	Give push/pull toys	Get around other children	Expand sign language
	Ball play	Play pretend games	Encourage to mimic adult behavior
	Have child imitate circle/cross when drawing	Help get undressed and dressed	Teach colors, read books
School age		Encourage child to participate in own care and promote independence as much as possible	Provide honest explanations
		When appropriate, accept child's need to direct procedures	Promote reading to increase knowledge of words and their meaning
		Identify strengths and provide opportunity to develop them	Encourage and provide environment for intellectual curiosity, as well as allow time for fum
		Promote involvement with peer groups, encourage friendships	Promote hospital school attendance
		Apply consistent, firm, and reasonable discipline when needed	
Adolescence		Allow as much independence as possible	Vocational rehabilitation service referral if appropriate
		Develop skills for self-care	Collaborate with school personnel
		Respect need for privacy	
		Encourage opportunities to encounter opinions, values, and beliefs that may differ from their own	
		Acknowledge feelings, facilitate family sharing feelings	

sessment of family readiness, motivation, and financial support, a home evaluation is made. The home environment must be outfitted with electrical outlets, fire safety equipment, and possibly wheelchair ramps.

Emergency planning includes notification of utility companies that a ventilator-dependent child is living in the home, so that emergency power back-up is made a priority. Emergency back-up equipment such as a generator, portable suction, and resuscitation bag must be available. A disaster plan must be developed with local community resources and the Red Cross in the case of natural disaster or fire.[119]

Parental education centers around the total care of the child, including tracheostomy care, suctioning, hand ventilation, special feeding, care of the ventilator, and CPR. The accompanying display lists objectives to be accomplished. The family should be connected with community resources that supply home care, respite care, educational mainstreaming, and support.

★ EVALUATION

The nurse and family constantly evaluate the outcomes of care given. Examples of outcomes for the child and family using mechanical ventilation were given under diagnoses and planning in this section. Planning for further nursing care takes into consideration complications.

COMPLICATIONS

Complications secondary to mechanical ventilation include pneumothorax, pneumonia, oxygen toxicity, and barotrauma. Iatrogenic effects of endotracheal intubation include subglottic stenosis, bacterial tracheitis, and airway mucosal damage. Outcomes for the child requiring mechanical ventilation are determined by the cause of respiratory failure.

Care of the Child With a Tracheostomy

A tracheostomy is a alternative airway created by surgical intervention. An incision is made on the neck and into the trachea below the vocal cords, and a plastic (sometimes metal) tube is placed into the trachea and comes out to the skin. The tube is secured with ties around the

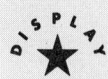

Patient Teaching: Expected Outcomes of Family Teaching for a Child on Home Ventilation

- Verbalize why the child is on the ventilator/CPAP
- Discuss purpose of the ventilator/CPAP
- Verbalize concerns or fears regarding home ventilation
- Demonstrate appropriate care of the artificial airway
- Demonstrate how to use the ventilator/CPAP
- Demonstrate the setting up and operation of ventilator/CPAP
- Demonstrate troubleshooting ability for ventilator/CPAP
- Demonstrate change of tubing circuits
- Verbalize cleaning procedure for tubing, humidifier, and other circuit pieces
- Demonstrate appropriate use of monitors
- Verbalize appropriate equipment placement in the home
- Identify vendor resources for maintenance of equipment
- Identify resources for emergencies or disasters
- Identify emergency backup plans in case of ventilator breakdown, power failure, or natural disasters
- Verbalize modifications in family/child lifestyle and routine related to child's care needs
- Identify resources for home nursing and respite care

neck to hold it in place. A new tracheostomy has sutures through the trachea, which are brought outside and secured to the skin so that the trachea can be held open in the event of accidental decannulation. These sutures are removed once the ostomy site has healed and the opening to the trachea is formed.

A tracheostomy is created to bypass an anatomic or physiologic obstruction of the airway. These obstructions may occur from a congenital problem, such as severe tracheobronchomalacia, subglottic stenosis, and various craniofacial anomalies. Acquired obstructions include hemangiomas and neoplasms of the throat and airway. The need for tracheostomy may be related to acute infectious disease causing obstruction, such as epiglottitis or croup. Neurologic problems causing vocal cord paralysis, such as trauma to the skull base and neck or conditions such as an Arnold-Chiari malformation, may warrant the creation of a tracheostomy.

The need for long-term mechanical ventilation also necessitates the creation of a tracheostomy, because long-term oral and nasal intubations traumatize nasal, oral, supra- and subglottic tissues. Children with neuromuscular diseases or those requiring long-term ventilation as a result of chronic respiratory disease or multisystem failure are included.

★ NURSING DIAGNOSES AND PLANNING

Many nursing diagnoses that can be used with the child who has altered respiratory function were discussed throughout this chapter. The following nursing diagnoses may also apply to the family and child with a tracheostomy:

- Anxiety related to knowledge deficit regarding tracheostomy procedures and care.
- Body Image Disturbance related to artificial breathing orifice.
- Impaired Verbal Communication related to tracheostomy tube.
- Altered Family Processes related to long-term hospitalization.
- Altered Growth and Development related to lack of vocalization and impedance of movement.
- High Risk for Infection related to tracheostomy incision.
- High Risk for Tube Obstruction related to ineffective humidification or ineffective secretion clearance.
- High Risk for Injury (Choking) related to aspiration of food, emesis, or foreign body.
- High Risk for Altered Parenting related to stress surrounding home tracheostomy care.
- Impaired Physical Mobility related to need for CPAP, ventilation, or humidity.
- Self-Care Deficit (Feeding and Bathing) related to possible food and water deposits into tracheostomy tube.

The nurse and child (or parents) together plan effective care based on the established nursing diagnoses. Several examples of expected outcomes follow:

- The parents discuss anatomy and physiology of throat and altered breathing techniques.
- The child's skin integrity is maintained.
- The child participates in speech therapy.
- The parents demonstrate effective use of bedside equipment.
- The parents demonstrate troubleshooting skills.
- The parents identify telephone numbers of emergency care and support persons or groups.

The nurse plans for the care of the child based on both physician's orders and nursing diagnoses. Some general nursing care goals may include the following:

- Airway patency is maintained.
- Satisfactory family processes are established.
- The child achieves normal developmental milestones.

★ INTERVENTIONS: COLLABORATIVE AND INDEPENDENT

CARE OF THE SURGICAL SITE

As with any incision, the site is inspected for drainage and increasing erythema. However, tracheostomy incisions are left open without approximating edges. Because the tracheostomy tube partially blocks the view of the incision, the area behind the tracheostomy tube must be inspected carefully to visualize tears, necrosis, and pressure points and rashes. Some serosanguineous discharge is expected from the site for the first 2 to 3 days, whereas

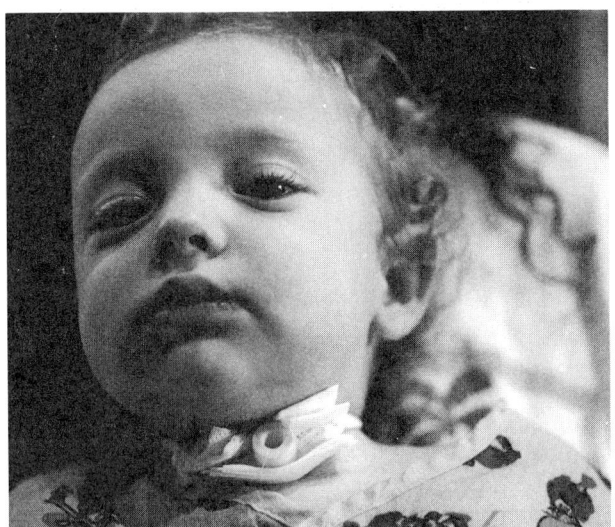

FIGURE 38-17
A child with the tracheostomy tube in place with the dressing.

purulent drainage is not. When purulent drainage is noted, careful inspection is important to determine whether the drainage originates from the surgical site or from the lumen of the tube representing pulmonary secretions.

The site is cleansed with half-strength hydrogen peroxide followed by a normal saline rinse and dried at least twice daily until healed. A dressing made of nonshredding material is placed under the tube flanges and around the base (two by two with slit is convenient to use) to soak up discharge from the surgical site (Fig. 38-17). The dressing may be omitted after the surgical site has healed or may be continued to protect the skin in children with secretions. Once the site is healed, tracheotomy care is performed once daily and as necessary to inspect and clean the underlying skin.

A new tracheostomy site is painful not only because it is a newly created incision, but because a relatively rigid tube is placed through the incision, potentially causing friction on a highly sensitive site. Frequent neck moves, especially in crying infants, increase the potential friction. Appropriate pain control methods should be considered for the child's comfort.

CARE OF THE TRACHEOSTOMY TIES

The tracheostomy tube is held in place by nonfrayable, durable ties that are changed daily because they become saturated with secretions. Infants with short necks and many skin folds are prone to skin breakdown, especially in the first weeks after the tracheostomy is performed. Careful inspection around the perimeter of the neck is necessary to observe for skin breakdown and rashes. Protective covering for skin and foam padding on tracheostomy ties may be indicated to prevent or treat skin breakdown as well as promote comfort.

Changing the tracheostomy ties must be done safely to avoid accidental decannulation. If the child is unable to cooperate, is fearful or crying, an extra person is necessary to hold and console the child. New ties are looped through the flanges of the tube and tied in a double square knot **before** the old ties are removed. One continuous tie is threaded through both flanges such that only one knot site is needed, thereby decreasing the odds of loosening knots (Fig. 38-18). The ties should be tight enough to allow only one small adult finger between the neck and the tie.

In infants with short necks and many skin folds, it may be important to have a tracheostomy extender over the tracheostomy to protect the lumen from being occluded by the infant's abundant chins. This apparatus may be a piece of plastic snuggly fitting over the tracheostomy tube, protecting the lumen by supporting the skin while the neck is flexed. Infants with constant oxygen or humidity needs may have sufficient protection from the mist collar.

SUCTIONING

Suctioning is performed regularly to assist the child with secretion removal and to avoid tracheostomy tube plug-

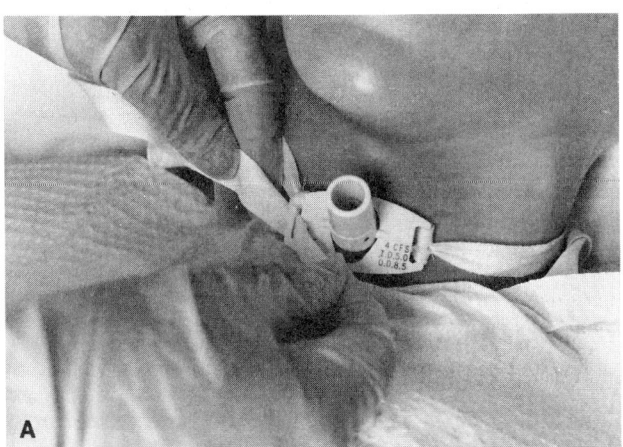
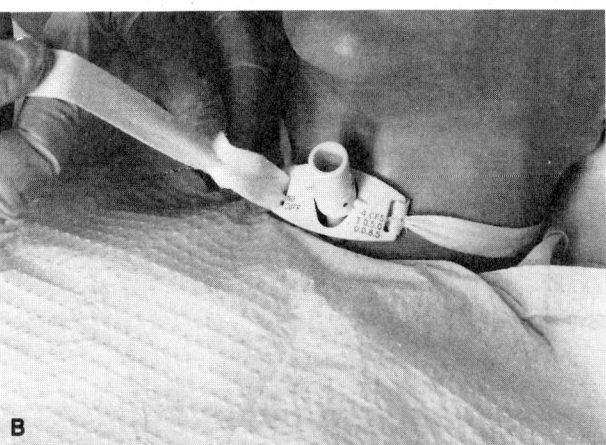

FIGURE 38-18
Ties secured to the faceplate of the tracheostomy. (**A**) The slit end of one clean tie is threaded through the one eyelet of the faceplate and held with a finger through the loop. (**B**) The other end of the tie is threaded through the slit and pulled taut against the faceplate.

ging. Therefore, the child should be suctioned when mucus is draining from the tube, when the child seems anxious, when the chest seems congested, and with any other sign of respiratory distress. Table 38-9 gives nursing actions for suctioning.

Suctioning is done with sterile technique while the child is hospitalized. If the child has a good cough, suctioning beyond the end of the tube is not necessary because this may cause tracheal inflammation leading to the formation of granulation tissue. Therefore, deep suction is defined as 0.5 cm beyond the end of the tracheostomy tube. Placement of a marked catheter or measuring tape near the bedside indicating the maximum depth of suctioning is a useful reference for nurses and parents.

Suction catheters are available in various sizes and styles. The size chosen should be half the size of the tracheostomy tube lumen; otherwise, the catheter may obstruct the whole airway. Vacuum pressure applied is between 80 and 100 mmHg. Another consoling person who can restrain the anxious child may be necessary. Oxygenating the child with 100% oxygen by bag-valve hand ventilation before and after each suction pass may be necessary for the oxygen-dependent child, or the child in distress, to prevent hypoxia. Instillation of sterile saline drops is sometimes necessary to loosen thick secretions for successful aspiration. The catheter is inserted into the tracheostomy tube without applying suction. Once the catheter has been inserted to the maximal safe distance, suction is applied by occluding the side port of the catheter with the thumb, and the catheter is withdrawn using a circular motion over 3 to 4 seconds. The child is allowed to rest between each aspiration, while the nurse reassesses the child's respiratory status. This process is repeated until the trachea is clear.

HUMIDIFICATION

Normally, air entry to lungs is humidified by nasal and oropharynx mucosa. The child with a tracheostomy has this natural humidification bypassed. A humidification system is applied to avoid thickening of secretion and occlusion of the tracheostomy tube lumen. Depending on the child's needs, humidification may be required constantly or at nighttime and naps only. Children requiring supplemental oxygen need constant humidification to avoid the drying effects of oxygen. Humidification and warmth promote growth of bacteria and, therefore, equipment requires daily cleaning and frequent changes to avoid infective complications. Adequate oral intake is also helpful for the maintenance of thin secretions.

CHANGING THE TRACHEOSTOMY TUBE

Tracheostomy tubes require routine changes to avoid obstruction from encrusted secretions and to avoid infections. Frequency of tube changes is dictated by the child's need and usually done every 1 to 2 weeks. Nursing actions in tube changes are given in Table 38-10.

The procedure requires two caregivers, one to position, hold, and console the child and the other to change the tube. Emergency equipment, such as oxygen, a hand ventilation system with tracheostomy adapter, mask, and smaller tracheostomy tube, should be available and operational. Suctioning is performed to decrease secretions before the procedure. The new tracheostomy tube is prepared with sterile technique, with obturator and ties in place. The child is positioned with head slightly extended. Old ties are cut, and the old tube is removed. The new tube is inserted with a smooth forward and downward motion, the obturator is removed, and the respiratory status is assessed. Ties are secured around the neck once the patency of the airway is ensured.

MANAGEMENT OF TRACHEOSTOMY TUBE COMPLICATIONS

Thick secretions can be avoided in a child who is well-hydrated and uses a mist collar. The amount of time that a child uses a mist collar is assessed by need. All children requiring oxygen need constant humidification due to the drying effects of oxygen. Children who have thick secretions should be suctioned after instilling sterile normal saline drops to lubricate and loosen thick and crusted secretions. Prophylactic suctioning of the tube in the child with thick secretions is done every 2 to 4 hours, even if

---

TABLE 38-9
Nursing Intervention: Suctioning the Child With a Tracheostomy

Nursing Action	Rationale
1. Select size of catheter.	1. The catheter should be half the size of the tube diameter to avoid occlusion.
2. Turn on vacuum source.	2. Vacuum pressure should be 80–100 mmHg to avoid hypoxia and atelectasis during procedure.
3. Position child on back and ask for help to hold the child if necessary.	3. Another person helps to avoid strain, promote comfort, and avoid decannulation.
4. Instill drops of sterile normal saline in tracheostomy tube.	4. Normal saline helps to loosen thick and crusted secretions in tube.
5. Insert catheter without suction to 0.5 cm beyond end of tube.	5. This action clears tube without irritating mucosa.
6. Apply suction and withdraw catheter from tube in a twisting motion over 3–4 s.	6. This action cleans secretion in all of tube without causing hypoxia and anxiety
7. Allow child to rest 30–60 s before repeating suction.	7. In addition to providing some rest for the child, this period gives the nurse time to assess need for more suction and avoid hypoxia and to check oxygen saturations.

TABLE 38-10
Nursing Intervention: Changing a Tracheostomy Tube

Nursing Action	Rationale
1. Prepare new tracheostomy tube with obturator and ties in place.	1. With this action, the tube can be tied into place quickly and safely. The child will be without tube for minimal time.
2. Recruit assistance to hold and console child.	2. The tube has to be replaced quickly; the child may protest or move. A second person facilitates tube placement.
3. Place pillow or roll under shoulders.	3. The roll slightly extends the head and optimizes position of trachea for recannulation.
4. Cut old ties and remove old tube quickly.	4. Quick (but safe) movements aid in replacing old tube with new.
5. Slide new tube in place.	5. Tube slides into place with a forward/downward movement.
6. Remove obturator and check respiration.	6. Placement of tube is checked by noting air passage through tube.
7. Tie snuggly around neck as soon as assessment is complete.	7. This action avoids decannulation and maintains airway.

the tracheostomy sounds clear, to avoid plugging of the tube.

Skin breakdown and rashes occur around the tracheostomy stoma and along the perimeter of the neck where the ties create pressure. Dampness from a mist collar and moistness in skin folds can promote skin breakdown and infection. All areas are inspected thoroughly at least once daily. Treatment of the skin breakdown depends on the cause and area. Pressure sores on the neck from ties require frequent cleansing and padding of the ties. Ties cannot be loosened because of the risk of accidental decannulation. Skin and incision site breakdown at the ostomy site requires increased cleansing with hydrogen peroxide and normal saline and frequent split gauze changes under the flanges of the tube. Depending on the extent of the infection, systemic antibiotics may be indicated. Antifungal and antibiotic ointments are often applied. All areas of skin irritation and breakdown need frequent evaluation and documentation regarding the progress of healing.

Two extra tracheostomy tubes, one of the same size and the other one size smaller, always are present at the bedside for emergency tube changes. Scissors are near the bedside to cut the tracheostomy ties. A child with a partial or complete occlusion of the tracheostomy tube often appears anxious, has chest retractions, and becomes cyanotic with decreasing oxygen saturation occurring suddenly or over a short period of time. The child is not able to clear the occlusion with a cough.

When obstruction is noted, the first nursing action is to call for help while preparing to suction the tracheostomy. Because the child is anxious, extra hands are necessary to hold the combative child. Normal saline drops are instilled, and a suction catheter is passed into the tube, trying to regain patency and clear the tube. When patency cannot be regained after one effort, tracheostomy ties are cut and the tracheostomy tube is removed and replaced. If the child has had an accidental decannulation, the tube is replaced as soon as possible. Depending on the child's pathology, the child may or may not be able to breathe without a tracheostomy tube. A new tube, the same size, is replaced in the method mentioned in Table

38-10. If using the same size is not possible, a size smaller is inserted, and, if this is not possible, oral intubation should be performed.

PROMOTION OF GROWTH AND DEVELOPMENT

Tracheostomy set-ups, with all their connections and tubing, can interfere with a child's freedom to move and, hence, interfere with growth and development. Specific measures to stimulate motor learning are done by nurses and taught to parents. Elongation of tubing to allow for improved mobility may be accomplished. Creeping on the floor is possible with careful observation, and stimulation to walk should be promoted. If possible, the child is taken off the mist collar during these activities and special attention is given to avoid foreign body occlusion of the tracheostomy tube.

Speech is inhibited by the tracheostomy tube, because air does not pass through the vocal cords. A Passey-Muir valve, applied to the end of the tracheostomy tube, directs air through the vocal cords assisting the child to create sound and learn to speak. However, not all children can tolerate the increased resistance to air flow through the tracheostomy tube. Older children with tracheostomies, with the assistance of a speech therapist, can be taught to speak by covering the tracheostomy tube. After decannulation, a child may need speech therapy to gain the speech skills delayed by tracheostomy intervention. The accompanying display summarizes the home care education requirements for parents caring for a child with a tracheostomy.

★ **EVALUATION**

The nurse and family evaluate the outcomes of care given. Examples of outcomes for the child and family with a tracheostomy were given under diagnoses and planning in this section.

Summary

Respiratory disease is the most common cause of acute and critical illness in children. Many of the diseases are

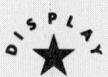

Patient Teaching: Educational Needs of a Family Providing Home Care of a Child With a Tracheostomy

Basic anatomy and physiology of the throat and alteration in breathing with a tracheostomy

Equipment needed at bedside for all care and emergencies

Respiratory assessments and signs and symptoms of distress

Skin assessments, signs and symptoms of breakdown, and interventions

Routine skin care of the tracheostomy including skin assessment and care, ostomy site care, and tie changes

Assessment for secretion thickness and infection. Importance of good hydration

Assessment for need of suctioning and methods

Application and troubleshooting of apnea monitors during sleep

Assessment of tube occlusion and method of changing during an emergency and routine

Cardiopulmonary resuscitation adapted to the child with a tracheostomy

System of emergency care and phone numbers in the home

Telephone numbers of suppliers and method of restocking supplies

Another person who is able to learn all of the above to provide respite and support to parents

Telephone numbers of support groups or another person with a child who has a tracheostomy

Ideas for Nursing Research

Children with chronic respiratory conditions may be seen in the health care system repeatedly throughout childhood. Recurrent contact with these families provides an excellent opportunity for long-term nursing investigations. Likewise, the frequent appearance of many children with acute respiratory conditions in the health care provider's office presents a large population available for inclusion in an empirical study. Areas of investigation that nurses might consider include the following topics:

- Effective strategies for preparing the family for home care of the child with a chronic respiratory condition.
- Creative methods that encourage a child's cooperation with respiratory toileting measures.
- Techniques that would motivate children to take prescribed medication by mouth or aerosol.
- Methods of reducing stress for children whose respiratory conditions are exacerbated by intense emotions.
- Clarification of the nurse's role on the multidisciplinary health team that provides care to children with chronic respiratory conditions.
- Confirmation of the defining characteristics of nursing diagnoses typically used with children who have altered respiratory function.

mild and self-limiting; however, severe respiratory disease can produce significant morbidity and mortality, especially in infants and small children. Early intervention, ongoing evaluation of the response to therapy, and the incorporation of primary nursing and family-centered care all contribute to improved outcomes.

New respiratory interventions and techniques are being used or are under clinical trials in children. Artificial exogenous surfactant (for example, Exosurf or Survanta) is being used to treat preterm infants with respiratory distress syndrome. This intervention reduces the severity of respiratory failure and speeds recovery and weaning from mechanical ventilation. Therefore, this intervention may be expected to decrease the frequency of chronic lung disease in the newborn and also may be useful in the child who is suffering from respiratory failure secondary to surfactant washout (that is, ARDS).

Extracorporeal membrane oxygenation (ECMO) is an artificial blood pump/oxygenator that is used to bypass the lungs and heart in severe pulmonary disease. It is effective in the treatment of neonatal meconium aspiration and persistent pulmonary hypertension, with severe respiratory failure. This technological intervention facilitates improved recovery without the iatrogenic effects of mechanical ventilation (e.g., pneumothorax, oxygen toxicity, chronic lung changes). ECMO also is undergoing

clinical trials for the support of newborns with diaphragmatic hernia and hypoplastic lungs.

High-frequency ventilation (HFV) is an alternative to conventional ventilation that uses breathing rates of 400 to 2400 with low tidal volumes. HFV has been found to be useful in patients with bronchopleural fistulas and severe air leak syndromes. Clinical trials are underway evaluating the efficacy of high-frequency ventilation in children with ARDS.

The care of the child with pulmonary disease requires an interdisciplinary team approach to problem identification and support. In spite of the technological and scientific advances, the health care team must not lose sight of the fact that the patient is still a child. Normalization of the hospital environment is important. Every effort must be made to promote the child's developmental level and coping strategies. Support of the family unit is of primary importance, because they will continue to nurture and care for young children long after recovery and discharge.

References

1. American Academy of Pediatrics. (1991). *Report of the Committee on Infectious Diseases.* Elk Grove Village, IL: Author.
2. Anas, N. G., & Goodman, G. (1990). Croup. In D. L. Levin & F. C. Morris (Eds.), *Essentials of pediatric intensive care.* St. Louis: Quality Medical.
3. Backofen, J. E., & Rogers, M. C. (1987). Upper airway disease.

In M. C. Rogers (Ed.), *Textbook of pediatric intensive care.* Baltimore: Williams & Wilkins.

4. Bancalari, E., & Gerhardt, T. (1986). Bronchopulmonary dysplasia. *Pediatric Clinics of North America, 33,* 1.

5. Battaglia, J. D. (1986). Severe croup: The child with fever and upper airway obstruction. *Pediatrics in Review, 7,* 227.

6. Benitz, W. E., & Tatro, D. S. (1988). *The pediatric drug handbook* (2nd ed.). Chicago: Year Book Medical.

7. Bentur, L., et al. (1992). Controlled trial of nebulized albuterol in children younger than two years of age with acute asthma. *Pediatrics, 89,* 133.

8. Berquist, W. E. (1991). *Metabolic assessment: Value for the CF patient.* Symposium conducted at the Cystic Fibrosis Western Regional Caregivers Conference, San Francisco, CA.

9. Blayney, M., Kerem, E., Whyte, H., & O'Brodovich, H. (1991). Bronchopulmonary dysplasia: Improvement in lung function between 7 and 10 years of age. *Journal of Pediatrics, 118,* 201.

10. Blue, C.L. (1988). Exercise induced asthma: The "silent asthma." *Journal of Pediatric Health Care, 2,* 167.

11. Boegner, E. (1990). Modes of ventilatory support and weaning parameters in children. *AACN—Clinical Issues in Critical Care Nursing, 1,* 378.

12. Boynton, R. W., Dunn, E. S., & Stephens, G. R. (1988). *Manual of ambulatory pediatrics* (2nd ed.). Boston: Scott, Foresman.

12A. Brook, V., Weitzman, A., & Wigal, J. K. (1991). Parental anxiety associated with a child's bronchial asthma. *Pediatric Asthma, Allergy, and Immunology, 5,* 15.

13. Burton, G. G., Hodgkin, J. E., & Ward, J. J. (1991). *Respiratory care: A guide to clinical practice* (3rd ed.). Philadelphia: Lippincott.

14. Carlsen K. H., Larsen, S., Bjerve, O., & Leegaard, J. (1987). Acute bronchiolitis: Predisposing factors and characterization of infants at risk. *Pediatric Pulmonology, 3,* 153.

15. Carter, M. C., Miles, M. S., Buford, T. H., & Hassanein, R. S. (1985). Parental environmental stress in pediatric intensive care units. *Dimensions in Critical Care Nursing, 4,* 180.

16. Castillejos, M., et al. (1992). Effects of ambient ozone on respiratory function and symptoms in Mexico City schoolchildren. *American Review of Respiratory Disease, 145,* 276.

17. Cavender, B. S. (1990). Nursing diagnoses and interventions in bronchopulmonary dysplasia: A case study. *AACN—Clinical Issues in Critical Care Nursing, 1,* 331.

18. Centers for Disease Control. (1991). Tuberculosis morbidity in the United States: Final data, 1990. Atlanta: *MMWR, 40.* 5-3, 23.

19. Chantarojanasiri, T., Nichols, D. G., & Rogers, M. C. (1987). Lower airway disease: Bronchiolitis and asthma. In M. C. Rogers (Ed.), *Textbook of pediatric intensive care.* Baltimore: Williams & Wilkins.

20. Chipps, B. (1989, November 16). Aerosol therapy for continuous bronchodilation. Pulmonary Medicine Seminars lecture presented at Updates in Cardio-Pulmonary Medicine, Sacramento, CA.

21. Consensus statement. (1987). NIH consensus development conference on infantile apnea and home monitoring. *Pediatrics, 79,* 292.

22. Conte, V. H. (1992). Bronchopulmonary dysplasia. In P. L. Jackson & J. A. Vessey (Eds.), *Primary care of the child with a chronic condition.* St. Louis: Mosby Year-Book.

23. Corey, M. A., & Clore, E. R. (1991). Management of the infant with respiratory syncytial virus. *Journal of Pediatric Nursing, 6,* 93.

24. Cunningham, J. C., & Taussig, L. M. (1991). An introduction to cystic fibrosis for the patient and family. Cystic Fibrosis Foundation. Bethesda, MD.

25. Curley, M. A. Q. (1988). Effects on the nursing mutual participation model of care on parental stress in the pediatric intensive care unit. *Heart and Lung, 17,* 82.

26. Curley, M. A. Q., & Thompson, J. E. (1990). End-tidal CO_2 monitoring in critically ill infants and children. *Pediatric Nursing, 16,* 397.

27. Davidson, A. G. F., McIlwaine, P. M., Wong, L. T. K., Pirie, G. E., & Nakielna, E. M. (1988). Comparison of positive expiratory pressure and autogenic drainage with conventional percussion and drainage techniques (abstract). *Pediatric Pulmonology, 137*(Suppl 2).

28. Davis, J. M., Sinkin, R. A., & Aranda, J. V. (1990). Drug therapy for bronchopulmonary dysplasia. *Pediatric Pulmonology, 8,* 117.

29. Davis, N., & Sweeney, L. (1989). Infantile apnea monitoring and SIDS. *Journal of Pediatric Health Care, 3,* 67.

30. deLormier, A., Harrison, M., Hardy, K., Howell, L., & Adzick, S. (1990). Tracheobronchial obstructions in infants and children. *Annals of Surgery, 212*(3), 277–289.

31. Demers, R. R., Parker, J., Frankel, L. R., & Smith, D. W. (1986). Administration of ribavirin to neonatal and pediatric patients during mechanical ventilation. *Respiratory Care, 31,* 1188.

32. Derish, M. T., Kulhanjan, J. A., Frankel, L. R., & Smith, D. W. (1991). Value of bronchoalveolar lavage in diagnosis of severe respiratory syncytial virus in infants. *Journal of Pediatrics, 119,* 761.

33. Donaldson, J. D., & Matltby, C. C. (1989). Bacterial tracheitis in children. *Journal of Otolaryngology, 18,* 101.

34. Dudin, A. A., Thalji, A., & Rambaud-Cousson, A. (1990). Bacterial tracheitis among children hospitalized for severe obstructive dyspnea. *Pediatric Infectious Disease Journal, 9,* 293.

35. Duiverman, E. J., Neijens, H. J., van Strik, R., Affourtit, M. J., & Kerrebijn, K. F. (1987). Lung function and bronchial responsiveness in children who had infantile bronchiolitis. *Pediatric Pulmonology, 3,* 38.

36. Dulock, H. L. (1991). Chest physiotherapy in neonates: A review. *AACN—Clinical Issues in Critical Care Nursing, 2,* 446.

37. Earp, K. J. (1989). Thermal gradients and shivering following open heart surgery. *Dimensions in Critical Care Nursing, 8,* 266.

38. Eggleston, P. A., Rosenstein, B. J., Stackhouse, C. M., Mellits, E. D., & Baumgardner, R. A. (1991). A controlled trial of long-term bronchodilator therapy in cystic fibrosis. *Chest, 99,* 1088.

39. Eglund, J. A., et al. (1990). High-dose, short-duration ribavirin aerosol therapy in children with suspected respiratory syncytial virus infection. *Journal of Pediatrics, 117,* 313.

40. Fanconi, S., et al. (1990). Transcutaneous carbon dioxide pressure for monitoring patients with severe croup. *Journal of Pediatrics, 117,* 710.

41. Farber, H. J., & Berg, R. A. (1991). Bacterial tracheitis as a complication of endotracheal intubation. *Pediatric Pulmonology, 11,* 87.

42. Fedorovich, C., & Littleton, M. T. (1990). Chest physiotherapy, evaluating the effectiveness. *Dimensions of Critical Care Nursing, 9,* 68.

43. Fick, R. B., & Stillwell, P. C. (1989). Controversies in the management of pulmonary disease due to cystic fibrosis. *Chest, 95,* 1319.

44. Field, A. L., Coble, D. H., Pollack, M. M., & Kaufman, J. (1991). Outcome of home care for technology-dependent children: Success of an independent, community-based case management model. *Pediatric Pulmonology, 11,* 310.

45. Geelhoed, G. C., Landau, L. I., LeSouef, P. N. (1990). Oximetry and peak expiratory flow in assessment of acute childhood asthma. *Journal of Pediatrics, 117,* 907.

46. Goldenhersh, M. J., & Rachelefsky, G. S. (1989). Childhood asthma: Overview. *Pediatrics in Review, 10,* 227.

47. Gooch, M. D. (1991). Stability of albuterol and tobramycin when mixed for aerosol administration. *Respiratory Care, 36,* 1387.

48. Goodman, G., Anas, N. G., & Siegel, J. D. (1990). Epiglottitis. In D. L. Levin & F. C. Morriss (Eds.), *Essentials of pediatric intensive care.* St. Louis: Quality Medical.

49. Groothuis, J. R., et al. (1990). Early ribavirin treatment of respiratory syncytial viral infection in high risk children. *Journal of Pediatrics, 117,* 792.

50. Guerra, I. C., & Shearer, W. T. (1990). Acute and chronic bronchitis. In F. A. Oski (Ed.), *Principles and practice of pediatrics.* Philadelphia: Lippincott.

51. Hardy, K. A., Schidlow, D. V., & Zaeri, N. (1988). Obliterative bronchiolitis in children. *Chest, 93,* 460.

52. Harrison, R., & Bellows, J. (1988). Health care worker exposure to ribavirin aerosol. *Field Investigation FI-86-009.* Berkeley, CA: California Department of Health Services.

53. Hauger, S. (1991). Approach to the pediatric patient with HIV infection and pulmonary symptoms. *Journal of Pediatrics, 119(1),* part 2, s25–s33.

54. Hazlett, D. E. (1989). A study of pediatric home ventilator management: Medical, psychosocial and financial aspects. *Journal of Pediatric Nursing, 4,* 284.

55. Henry, R. L., et al. (1991). Asthma in the vicinity of power stations: II. Outdoor air quality and symptoms. *Pediatric Pulmonary, 11,* 134.

56. HESIS Hazard Alert. (1990, December). Ribavirin. *Hazard Evaluation System and Information Service,* Department of Industrial Relations, State of California.

57. International Union Against Tuberculosis/World Health Organization Study Group. (1982). Tuberculosis control: Report of a Joint IUAT/WHO Study Group. Geneva: World Health Organization.

58. JAMA–AHA Standards and guidelines for cardiopulmonary resuscitation and emergency cardiac care. (1986). *JAMA, 255,* 2841.

59. Kadlec, J. V., & Bellanti, J. A. (1985). The immune system. In A. R. Colon & M. Ziai (Eds.), *Pediatric pathophysiology.* Boston: Little, Brown.

60. Kasian, G. F., et al. (1989). Bacterial tracheitis in children. *Canadian Medical Association Journal, 140,* 46.

61. Kaufman, J., & Hardy-Ribakow, D. (1988). What parents need to know about trach care. *RN, 51,* 99.

62. Kennelly, C. (1987, July/August). Tracheostomy care: Parents as learners. *Maternal-Child Nursing, 12,* 264.

63. Kerem, E., et al. (1991). Clinical-physiologic correlations in acute asthma of childhood. *Pediatrics, 87,* 481.

64. Kerfoot, F. E. (1989). The perils of pertussis. *Journal of Pediatric Nursing, 4,* 277.

65. Kimmons, H. C., & Peterson, B. M. (1986). Management of acute epiglottitis in pediatric patients. *Critical Care Medicine, 14,* 278.

66. Kitterman, J. (1987). Tracheal lesions. In A. Rudolf & J. Hoffman (Eds.), *Pediatrics* (p. 1371). Los Altos, CA: Appleton & Lange.

67. Klassen, T. P., et al. (1991). Randomized trial of salbuterol in acute bronchiolitis. *Journal of Pediatrics, 118,* 807.

68. Kline, M. W., & Shearer, W. T. (1991). A national survey on the care of infants and children with human immunodeficiency virus infection. *Journal of Pediatrics, 118(5),* 817–821.

69. Knowles, M. R., et al. (1990). A pilot study of aerosolized amiloride for the treatment of lung disease in cystic fibrosis. *New England Journal of Medicine, 322,* 1189.

70. Koff, P. B., Eitzman, D. V., & Neu, J. (1988). *Neonatal and pediatric respiratory care.* St. Louis: Mosby.

71. Konstan, M. W., Hoppel, C. L., Chai, B., & Davis, P. B. (1991, June). Ibuprofen in children with cystic fibrosis: Pharmacokinetics and adverse effects. *Journal of Pediatrics, 118(6),* 956–964.

72. Lebel, M. H., Gauthier, M., Lacroix, J., Rousseau, E., & Buithieu, M. (1989). Respiratory failure and mechanical ventilation in severe bronchiolitis. *Archives of Disease in Childhood, 64,* 1431.

73. Leonard, S. R., & Nikaidoh, H. (1990). Thoracentesis and chest tube insertion. In D. L. Levin & F. C. Morriss (Eds.), *Essentials of pediatric intensive care.* St. Louis: Quality Medical.

74. Lewandowski, L. A. (1992). Psychosocial aspects of pediatric

75. Litovitz, T. L. (1985). Ecology of childhood. In A. R. Colon & M. Ziai (Eds.), *Pediatric pathophysiology.* Boston: Little, Brown.

76. Lowell, D. I., Lister, G., Von Koss, H., & McCarthy, P. (1987). Wheezing in infants: The response to epinephrine. *Pediatrics, 79,* 939.

77. Lubinsky, P., & Anas, N. G. (1990). Inhaled medications. In D. L. Levin & F. C. Morriss (Eds.), *Essentials of pediatric intensive care.* St. Louis: Quality Medical.

78. Lubinksy, P., Anas, N. G., & Davis, S. L. (1990). Acute severe asthma. In D. L. Levin & F. C. Morriss (Eds.), *Essentials of pediatric intensive care.* St. Louis: Quality Medical.

79. Lulla, S., & Newcomb, R. W. (1980). Emergency management of asthma in children. *Journal of Pediatrics, 97,* 346.

80. Lulu, J. A., & Myer, M. L. (1991). Mechanical ventilation considerations in complex congenital heart disease. *Critical Care Nursing Clinics of North America, 3,* 609.

81. Mahlmeister, M. J., Fink, J. B., Hoffman, G. L., & Fifer, L. F. (1991). Positive-expiratory-pressure mask therapy: Theoretical and practical considerations and a review of the literature. *Respiratory Care, 36,* 1218.

82. Mahlmeister, M. J., Guglielmo, B. J., & Harrison, R. (1988). We are concerned about ribavirin exposure (Letter to the editor). *Respiratory Care, 33,* 809.

83. Mauro, R. D., & Poole, S. R. (1988). Is it croup? A guide to diagnosis and treatment. *Contemporary Pediatrics, 5,* 51.

84. McConnochie, K. M., Hall, C. B., Walsh, E. E., & Roghmann, K. J. (1990). Variation in severity of respiratory syncytial virus infections with subtype. *Journal of Pediatrics, 117,* 52.

85. McConnochie, K. M., & Roghmann, K. J. (1989). Wheezing at 8 and 13 years: Changing importance of bronchiolitis and passive smoking. *Pediatric Pulmonology, 6,* 138.

86. McEniery, J., Gillis, J., Kilham, H., & Benjamin, B. (1991). Review of intubation in severe laryngotracheobronchitis. *Pediatrics, 87,* 847.

87. McMillan, J. A., et al. (1988). Prediction of the duration of hospitalization in patients with respiratory syncytial virus infection: Use of clinical parameters. *Pediatrics, 81,* 22.

88. Mims, B. C. (1989). Physiologic rational of S_vO_2 monitoring. *Critical Care Nursing Clinics of North America, 1,* 619.

89. Mizrahi, S., Yaari, Y., Lugassy, G., & Cotev, S. (1989). Major airway obstruction relieved by helium/oxygen breathing. *Critical Care Medicine, 14,* 986.

90. Montgomery, A. B., et al. (1990). Occupational exposure to aerosolized pentamidine. *Chest, 98,* 387.

91. Morriss, F. C. (1990). Methylxanthine poisoning. In D. L. Levin & F. C. Morriss (Eds.), *Essentials of pediatric intensive care.* St. Louis: Quality Medical.

92. Nassos, P. S., Yajko, D. M., Sanders, C. A., & Hadley, W. K. (1991). Prevalence of *Mycobacterium avium* complex in respiratory specimens from AIDS and non-AIDS patients in a San Francisco hospital. *ARRD, 143,* 66.

93. National Institutes of Health–National Asthma Education Program. (1991). *Guidelines for the diagnosis and management of asthma.* National Heart, Lung, and Blood Institute, US Department of Health and Human Services. Publication No. 91-3042.

94. Newcomb, R. W. (1989). Use of adrenergic bronchodilators by pediatric allergists and pulmonologists. *American Journal of Diseases in Children, 143,* 481.

95. Northway, W. H., et al. (1990). Late pulmonary sequela of bronchopulmonary dysplasia. *New England Journal of Medicine, 323,* 1793.

96. Orenstein, J. B., Thomsen, J. R., & Baker, S. B. (1991). Pneumococcal bacterial tracheitis. *American Journal of Emergency Medicine, 9,* 243.

97. Outwater, K. M., Meissner, C., & Peterson, M. B. (1988). Ri-

bavirin administration to infants receiving mechanical ventilation. *American Journal of Diseases in Children, 142,* 512.

98. Overstreet, D. W., Jackson, J. C., van Belle, G., & Truog, W. E. (1991). Estimation of mortality risk in chronically ventilated infants with bronchopulmonary dysplasia. *Pediatrics, 88,* 1153.

99. Paskerkamp, H., & Chernick, V. (1989). Acute upper airway infection. In R. M. Chernick (Ed.), *Current therapy of respiratory disease-3.* Philadelphia: Decker.

100. Porth, C. M. (1990). *Pathophysiology: Concepts of altered health states* (3rd ed.). Philadelphia: Lippincott.

101. Pribble, C. G., Black, P. G., Bosso, J. A., & Turner, R. B. (1990). Clinical manifestations of exacerbations of cystic fibrosis associated with nonbacterial infections. *Journal of Pediatrics, 117,* 200.

102. Rabie, I., McShane, D., & Warde, D. (1989). Bacterial tracheitis. *Journal of Laryngology and Otology, 103,* 1059.

103. Robertson, C. M. T., Etches, P. C., Goldson, E., & Kyle, J. M. (1992). Eight-year school performance, neurodevelopment, and growth outcome of neonates with bronchopulmonary dysplasia: A comparative study. *Pediatrics, 8,* 365.

104. Rogers, M. (1989). Upper airway diseases. In *Handbook of Pediatric Intensive Care.* (pp 25–40). Baltimore: Williams & Wilkins.

105. Ronczy, N., & Beddome, M. A. (1990). Preparing the family for home tracheostomy care. *AACN—Clinical Issues in Critical Care Nursing, 1*(2), 367.

106. Rutherford, K. A. (1989). Advances in the treatment of oxygenation disturbances. *Critical Care Nursing Clinics of North America, 1,* 659.

107. Sayler, J. W., & Chatburn, R. L. (1990). Patterns of practice in neonatal and pediatric respiratory care. *Respiratory Care, 35,* 879.

108. Sayler, J. W., & Lewis, D. D. (1990). Pulse oximetry: Application in the pediatric and neonatal critical care unit. *Clinical Issues in Critical Care Nursing, 1,* 339.

109. Scharer, K., & Dixon, D. M. (1989). Managing chronic illness: Parents with a ventilator dependent child. *Journal of Pediatric Nursing, 4,* 236.

110. Schlichtig, R., & Sargent, S. C. (1990). Nutritional support of the mechanically ventilated patient. *Critical Care Clinics, 6,* 767.

111. Schuh, S., et al. (1990). Nebulized albuterol in acute bronchiolitis. *Journal of Pediatrics, 117,* 633.

112. Sheahan, S. L., & Seabolt, J. P. (1989). *Chlamydia trachomatis* infections: A health problem of infants. *Journal of Pediatric Health Care, 3,* 144–149.

113. Skolnik, N. S. (1989). Treatment of croup. *American Journal of Diseases in Children, 143,* 1045.

114. Sly, P. D., & Hibbert, M. E. (1989). Childhood asthma following hospitalization with acute viral bronchiolitis is infancy. *Pediatric Pulmonology, 7,* 153.

115. Sly, R. M. (1991). Aerosol therapy in children. In The American Association for Respiratory Care aerosol consensus statement—1991. *Respiratory Care, 36,* 994.

116. Smith, D. W., et al. (1991). A controlled trial of aerosolized ribavirin in infants receiving mechanical ventilation for severe respiratory syncytial virus infection. *New England Journal of Medicine, 325,* 24.

117. Southall, D. P., Thomas, M.G., & Lambert, H. P. (1988). Severe hypoxaemia in pertussis. *Archives of Diseases in Childhood, 63,* 598.

118. Starke, J. R., & Taylor-Watts, K. T. (1989). Tuberculosis in the pediatric population of Houston Texas. *Pediatrics, 84,* 28–35.

119. Steele, N. F., & Morgan, J. (1989). Emergency planning for technology-assisted children. *Journal of Pediatric Nursing, 4,* 81.

120. Theodore, J., & Lewiston, N. (1990). Lung transplantation comes of age. *New England Journal of Medicine, 322,* 772.

121. Traver, G. A., & Martinez, M. (1988). Asthma update, part I. Mechanisms, pathology and diagnosis. *Journal of Pediatric Health Care, 2,* 221.

122. Traver, G. A., & Martinez, M. (1988). Asthma update, part II. Treatment. *Journal of Pediatric Health Care, 2,* 227.

123. Tristram, D. A., Miller, R. W., McMillan, J. A., & Weiner, L. B. (1988). Simultaneous infection with respiratory syncytial virus and other respiratory pathogens. *American Journal of Diseases in Children, 142,* 834.

124. Turner, R. B., Lande, A. E., Chase, P., Hilton, N., & Weinber, D. (1987). Pneumonia in pediatric outpatients: Cause and clinical manifestations. *Journal of Pediatrics, 111,* 194.

125. Uauy, R., & Mize, C. E. (1990). Starvation in the PICU. In D. L. Levin & F. C. Morriss (Eds.), *Essentials of pediatric intensive care.* St. Louis: Quality Medical.

126. Warner, J., & Norwood, S. (1991). Psychosocial concerns of the ventilator dependent child in the pediatric intensive care unit. *AACN—Clinical Issues in Critical Care Nursing, 2,* 432.

127. Warwick, W. J., & Hansen, L. G. (1991). The long-term effect of high-frequency chest compression therapy on pulmonary complications of cystic fibrosis. *Pediatric Pulmonology, 11,* 265.

128. White, K. M., Winslow, E. H., Clark, A. P., & Tyler, D. O. (1990). The physiologic basis for continuous mixed venous oxygen saturation monitoring. *Heart and Lung, 19,* 548.

129. Wood, R. A., Schuberth, K. C., & Sampson, H. A. Value of a multiantigen radioallergosorbent test in diagnosing atopic disease in young children. *Journal of Pediatrics, 117,* 882.

130. Youngblut, J. M., & Jay S. S. (1991). Emergent admission to the pediatric intensive care unit: Parental concerns. *AACN—Clinical Issues in Critical Care Nursing, 2,* 329.

131. Zander, J., & Hazinski, M. F. (1992). Pulmonary disorders. In M. F. Hazinksi (Ed.), *Nursing care of the critically ill child* (2nd ed.). St. Louis: Mosby.

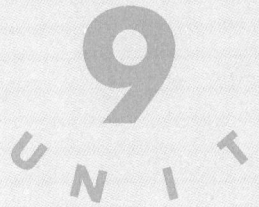

UNIT 9

Nursing Care of Children With Altered Cardiovascular Function

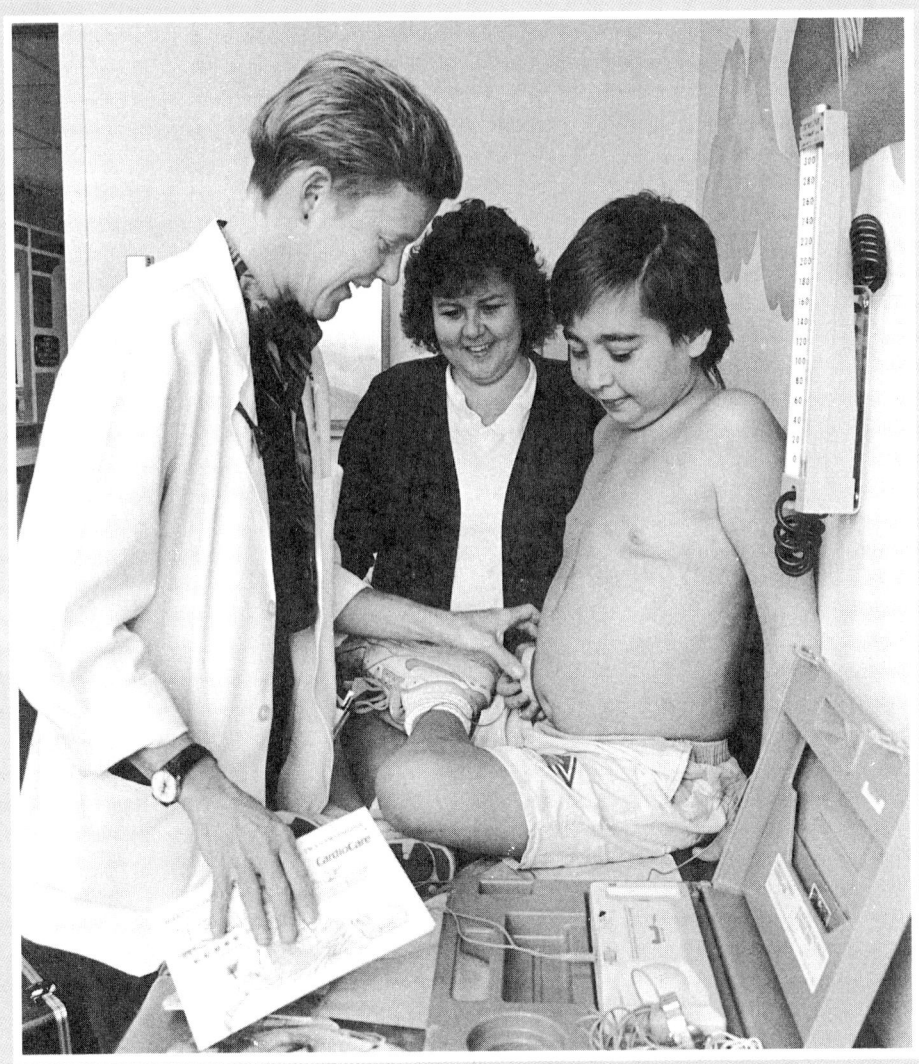

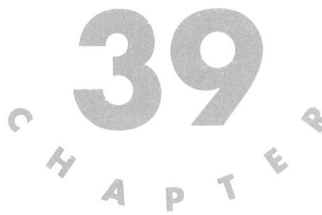
Anatomy and Physiology of the Cardiovascular System

BEHAVIORAL OBJECTIVES

Discuss the embryonic development of major cardiac structures.

Identify anatomic structures in the mature cardiovascular system and their function.

Diagram the electrical conduction pathway in the heart.

Describe neural and hormonal regulation of the cardiovascular system.

Explain the cardiac cycle and its relation to cardiac function.

Differentiate between fetal and postnatal circulation.

The cardiovascular system delivers oxygenated blood and nutrients to all body cells and removes deoxygenated blood and metabolic waste products. The cardiovascular system has specialized structures consisting of a *pumping unit* (the heart), a *circuit* (arteries, veins, and capillaries) that transports blood throughout the body, and numerous *valves* that regulate blood flow through the heart and vessels. The heart also has its own electrical system to maintain its rate and rhythm, but neural and hormonal systems complement the heart's intrinsic regulatory mechanism.

From conception throughout the postnatal period and childhood, the heart undergoes changes in size, structure, and function. A basic understanding of fetal cardiogenesis and later development establishes a foundation for understanding normal cardiac findings as well as abnormal development. This chapter is an introduction to the cardiovascular system, its embryogenesis, anatomy, and physiology.

Embryonic Development

Development of the cardiovascular system begins early in fetal life with cardiac structures forming during the third to eighth weeks of gestation. By the end of the eighth week, the heart beats and is one of the first organ systems to function in utero. This early development permits the fetus to provide for nutritional, respiratory, and excretory needs of developing cells and tissues. The embryonic design of the cardiovascular system, however, also must anticipate the shift that will occur later

981

in the centers of metabolic activity. Functions managed by the placenta prenatally are transferred to the respiratory, digestive, and renal systems after birth. The following section highlights the major events of embryogenesis of the cardiovascular system. Although the development of each of the major structures is discussed separately, all are developing simultaneously.

Cardiac Tube

Early in pregnancy, the embryo relies on diffusion as a means of nutrient and waste exchange, but, as the embryo grows, it requires its own transport system for servicing the developing structures. Long before the heart is recognizable as a tubular structure, cells with heart-forming capacity are localized in the mesoderm. During the first 3 weeks of gestation, the mesoderm thickens and splits into two layers, the somatic and the splanchnic mesoderm. Whereas the somatic mesoderm evolves into other structures, the splanchnic mesoderm differentiates into a variety of cardiac structures within a fluid-filled space that becomes the pericardial cavity.

The splanchnic mesoderm initially forms a pair of tubes that soon fuse into a single endocardial tube. This primitive heart tube ultimately forms the endocardium, the inside lining of the heart. It is enveloped by a single fold of tissue that is formed by the rudiments of the myocardium, the muscular middle layer of the heart.

As the heart tube matures, sequential dilated areas appear to suggest the future structures of the heart. These regions are the sinoatrium (the sinus venosus joined with the common atrium), ventricle, bulbus cordis, and truncus arteriosus (Fig. 39-1). In the mature heart, they become, respectively, the atria, the left ventricle, the right ventricle, and the aorta and pulmonary artery.[1,2,7,11,21] Blood enters at the sinoatrium and leaves through the truncus arteriosus.

Rapidly elongating within the pericardial cavity, the heart tube is forced into a complex pattern of bends that enhances the formation of the cardiac chambers. Factors regulating the direction of the looping are poorly understood but thought to be related to the velocity and pressure of blood flowing through the cardiac tube. Nevertheless, the bending heart tube finally achieves the familiar cardiac contour. Approximately 28 days after conception, the ebb and flow of blood cells through the heart begin.

Right and Left Atria

In the developing heart tube, endocardial cells proliferate and give rise to bulges of tissue within the canal; these thick pads are known as endocardial cushions. Other tissue located at the top of the atrium, called the septum primum, grows down and fuses with the endocardial cushions. Likewise, tissue known as the septum secundum grows from the superior and posterior wall of the atrium. As the partition develops, the septum secundum forms the flapped opening known as the foramen ovale. By 5 weeks' gestation, the septation of the atria is complete and blood flows from the right to the left sides through the foramen ovale, which closes after birth.[2,7,11,23]

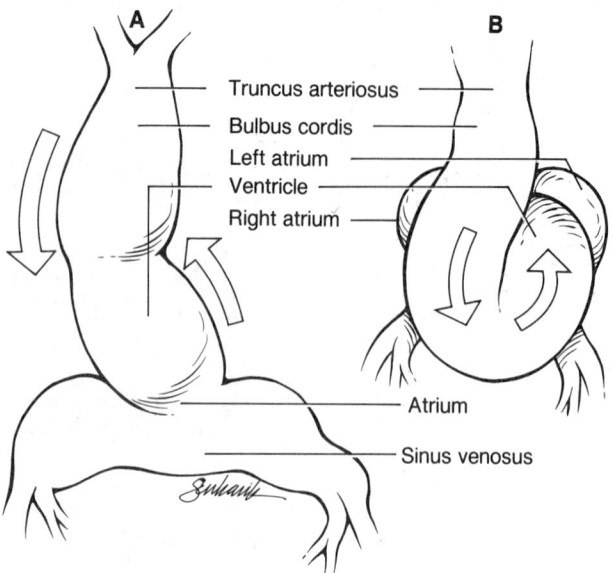

FIGURE 39-1
Changes in the cardiac tube during the fourth week of gestation. A single tube elongates and bends upon itself (**A**) to achieve the familiar cardiac contour (**B**).

Right and Left Ventricles

Early in fetal development, the heart tube elongates and bends to bring the ventricle gradually to a position posterior to the atrium. Continued growth of the cardiac tube also stimulates the absorption of the proximal end of the bulbus cordis into the right side of the common ventricle. About the same time, the ventral surface of the ventricle shows a distinct, median, longitudinal groove, which begins to divide the one ventricle into two chambers.

Between the fourth and eighth week of fetal life, the muscular interventricular septum grows toward the endocardial cushions. Extension of the endocardial cushions and swellings of other tissue fuse and form the membranous ventricular septum. This tissue merges with the muscular interventricular septum to complete the ventricular septum.[2,11,23] For a while, an interventricular foramen exists, but, unlike the foramen ovale between the atria, the communication between the ventricles is rapidly obliterated. By 8 weeks' gestation, there is little trace of the foramen's existence.

Atrioventricular Valves

In the primitive heart, the atrioventricular (AV) communication is a single opening; the sinoatrium empties into a common ventricle. With the division of the atrium and ventricle into left and right sides, however, openings between the chambers require new structures to help regulate the flow of blood. Flaps of tissue arise from localized proliferations of endocardial tissue on the walls of the atrioventricular canal.

Each flap differentiates as a mass of fibrous tissue and becomes connected to special muscles of the ventricle (papillary muscles) by cords of connective tissue (chor-

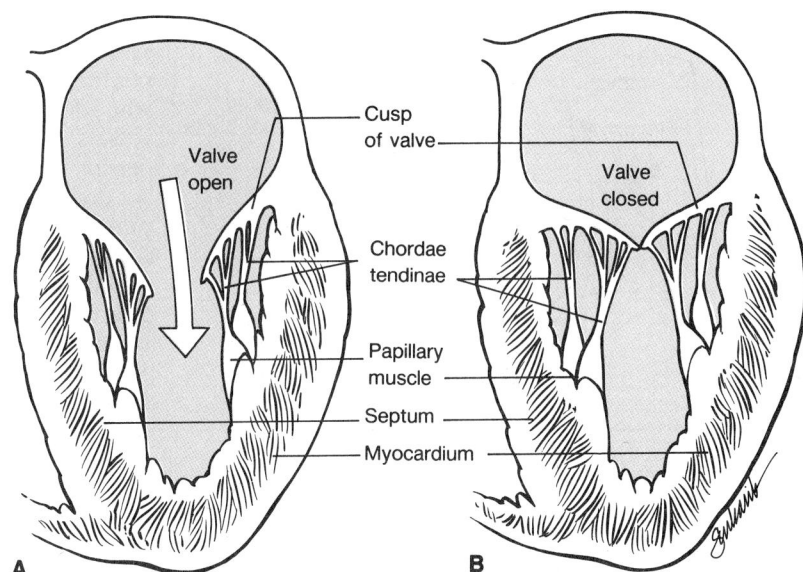

FIGURE 39-2

Detail of the atrioventricular valve action. (A) To open, the papillary muscles contract and the chordae tendineae pull the valve open, allowing blood to fill the ventricles. (B) When the ventricles are full, the valve closes to prevent backflow of blood into the atria.

dae tendineae; Fig. 39-2). Three flaps or valvular cusps are formed around the right atrioventricular canal, creating the tricuspid valve. The two flaps of tissue on the left side create the mitral (bicuspid) valve. These valves control blood flow from the upper chambers (atria) into the lower chambers (ventricles).

Aorta and Pulmonary Artery

As mentioned previously, the proximal portion of the bulbus cordis is incorporated into the wall of the right ventricle. During the fifth week of gestation, the remainder of the bulbus cordis is divided into two channels by a spiral septum that appears as ridges of tissue. Similar ridges are found in the truncus arteriosus and are directly continuous with those of the bulbus cordis. The ridges enlarge and fuse to form the aorticopulmonary septum, creating a pulmonary trunk and a systemic trunk. These two trunks ultimately twist around one another and become the pulmonary artery and the ascending aorta, respectively (Fig. 39-3). The semilunar valves (pulmonary and aortic valves) form inside the two vessels when truncal septation is almost completed and function to maintain blood flow in one direction, away from the heart.[11,23]

Aortic Arch

The aortic arch pattern is laid within the first 4 weeks of gestation, but it is transformed into the familiar arrangements of arteries around 7 weeks. This structure begins as six pairs of aortic arches that proliferate from the distal truncus arteriosus. The arch pairs I, II, and V undergo regression and involution. By the fourth week, they disappear without leaving any permanent structures. Arch pair III forms the connection of the carotid arteries. The right arch IV forms the right subclavian artery, and, with contributions from the divided truncus and bulbus, the left IV arch becomes the ascending arch of the aorta. The proximal segment of arch pair VI forms branches of

the pulmonary artery, but the distal segment persists as the ductus arteriosus. The ductus arteriosus permits blood flow to be shunted directly from the aorta to the pulmonary artery because little blood is needed in the lungs in utero.[7]

Pulmonary Veins

The pulmonary veins begin to develop early in the third week of gestation. The primitive pulmonary vein arises as a sprout of endothelium out of the left atrium and joins the pulmonary capillary plexus on the lung buds. This pulmonary vein, as well as the sinus venosus and the bases of the right and left pulmonary veins, are all absorbed into the dorsal wall of the left atrium. Consequently, four separate pulmonary venous orifices are formed in the left atrium (Fig. 39-4). The pulmonary veins allow blood from the lungs to enter into the left heart and be pumped to the body.

Consequences of Abnormal Development

The complexity of the events leading to the formation of the four-chambered heart and vascular pathways presents many opportunities for malformations to occur. Most congenital heart defects are caused by abnormal division or faulty separations of the heart tube, and failure of specific vessels or tissues to grow during the time frame of normal development. For examples of specific anomalies that occur as a result of disturbances in the formation of the heart and blood vessels, refer to Table 39-1. These defects are explained in detail in Chapter 41.

Structure and Function

Without a mechanism to circulate the blood, it cannot perform its many roles. The basic structures of the car-

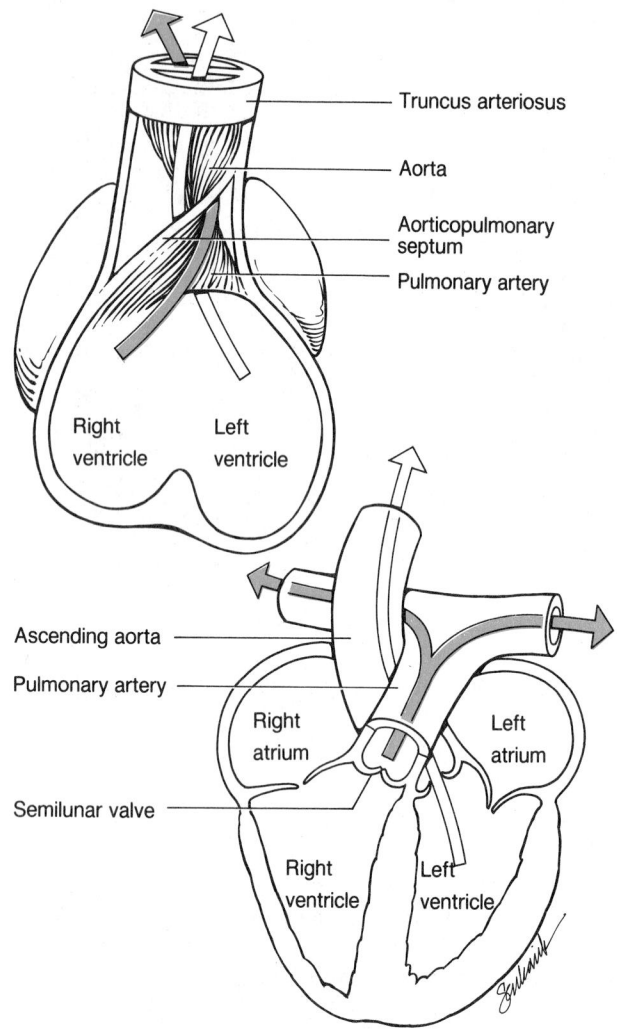

FIGURE 39-3

Formation of the aorta and pulmonary artery. (**A**) The aorticopulmonary septum separates the truncus arteriosus and begins to spiral. (**B**) The aorta and pulmonary artery become distinct, and semilunar valves form.

diovascular system are the heart, which pumps the blood, and the blood vessels, which distribute and collect it. A variety of valves lie within the heart and vessels to regulate the direction of blood flow.

Heart

Location, Position, and Appearance

The heart is located in the anterior thoracic cavity between the lungs. It lies in the mediastinum, with approximately one third to the right of the median plane and two thirds to the left (Fig. 39-5). The lower border of the heart forms a blunt point known as the apex, which lies on the diaphragm, pointing to the left. The upper border of the heart lies just below the second rib. The great vessels that enter and leave the heart in the superior region help secure its position.

On the outside, the heart is encased by a loose-fitting sac called the pericardium, which is composed of a fibrous portion and a serous portion. The sac is made of the tough, white fibrous tissue, which attaches to the large blood vessels emerging from the base of the heart. The fibrous portion of the pericardium fits loosely around the heart but does not adhere to it. The serous portion of the pericardium is further distinguished into two layers: the parietal layer, which lines the fibrous pericardium, and the visceral layer, which lies on the heart. Between the visceral and parietal layer is a potential space that contains a small amount of pericardial fluid, which lubricates and protects the heart by reducing friction during cardiac contraction.

Layers of Heart Wall

The visceral layer of the pericardium is composed of connective tissue. It adheres to the outside of the heart and is called the *epicardium*. This layer contains adipose tissue, the cardiac blood vessels, and nerves.

The *myocardium* is the thick middle layer of the heart. It consists of specialized, striated muscle fibers that are interlaced together in bundles. Similar to skeletal muscle, the cardiac muscle cells are composed of sarcomeres, the basic contractile units that contain thick filaments composed of myocin and thin filaments of actin. The thick and thin filaments overlap each other but are not connected. During contraction, the filaments slide together in a serial fashion to shorten the muscle.

Cardiac muscle cells, however, are different from skeletal muscles in their ability to contract as a unit. All cardiac muscle cells contain intercalated disks, dense structures at the ends of the fibers that form a strong bond and maintain cell-to-cell cohesion. When a wave of electrical current is generated, the stimulus is transmitted from one muscle cell to another. Excitation arising anywhere in the atria or ventricles is able to spread out over all the fibers until the last cell is activated. This property explains the "all or none" response of heart muscle; when stimulated, the heart either responds with excitation of all its fibers or gives no response at all.

Another difference between myocardial muscle and skeletal muscles is the abundance of energy units (called

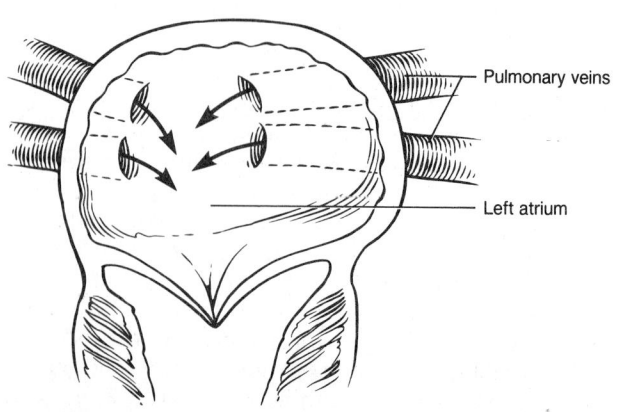

FIGURE 39-4

Four pulmonary veins open into the left atrium.

TABLE 39-1
Consequences of Abnormal Embryonic Development

Fetal Age (Weeks)	Structure	Anomalies at Birth
3	Pulmonary veins	Total anomalous pulmonary venous return (TAPVR)—four types: • Supracardiac • Cardiac • Infradiaphragmatic • Mixed
4–6	Atrial septum	Atrial septal defects (ASD)—three types: • Secundum ASD (center) • Primum ASD (lower) • Sinus venosus ASD (high)
4–8	Ventricular septum	Ventricular septal defects (VSD)–five types: • Infracristal VSD • Supracristal VSD • Endocardial cushion defect • Muscular VSD • Membranous VSD
4–8	Endocardial cushion region	Endocardial cushion defect—two major types: • Partial AV canal • Complete AV canal Ventricular septal defects Atrial septal defects
5–7	Pulmonary artery and aorta	Persistent truncus arteriosus tetralogy of Fallot (TOF)—four defects: • Ventricular septal defect • Pulmonary stenosis • Displacement of aorta • Right ventricular hypertrophy Pulmonary stenosis (PS) Transposition of the great vessels (TGA) Pulmonary atresia (PA)
5–7	Aortic arch	Coarctation of the aorta (COTA) Interrupted aortic arch Aortic atresia Patent ductus arteriosus Vascular rings

mitochondria) within the cells. Myocardial cells require high-energy compounds to contract repetitively over a lifetime. Because the heart muscle never rests, the large number of mitochondria provides the necessary elements, such as adenosine triphosphate (ATP), to avoid accumulation of an oxygen debt from anaerobic metabolism. In contrast, skeletal muscles have relatively short repetitive and sustained contractions and, therefore, require fewer mitochondria.

Cardiac muscle cells also have a protective period of time during which the heart muscle cannot respond to stimulation and produce another contraction. This absolute refractory period prevents tetanic contractions like those that may occur in excessive stimulation of skeletal muscle. Refractoriness and other physical properties of myocardial tissue are described in the accompanying display.

On its inner surface, parts of the myocardium have raised, ridgelike projections called papillary muscles. These structures attach to thin but strong fibrous cords that connect to the valves that are located between the atria and the ventricles. Contraction and relaxation of the papillary muscles control the opening and closure of the mitral and tricuspid valves.

A third, delicate layer lines the interior of the myocardial wall and is known as the *endocardium*. The endocardial connective tissue is thin and transparent over the interior ventricular walls but thicker in the atria.

Chambers

The heart is primarily a muscular organ that consists of four chambers, two *atria* above and two *ventricles* below. The atria serve as collecting or intake chambers. Because blood flows readily into the lower chambers, needing little assistance from atrial contraction, the atria have thin muscular walls. The ventricles are much thicker than the atria because they require greater strength for pumping. The right ventricle pumps blood primarily to the low-resistance pulmonary circuit and, therefore, is only about 3 mm thick. The left ventricle, however, is responsible for high-pressure pumping of blood to the entire systemic circulation; its muscle mass is 10 to 13 mm thick. The

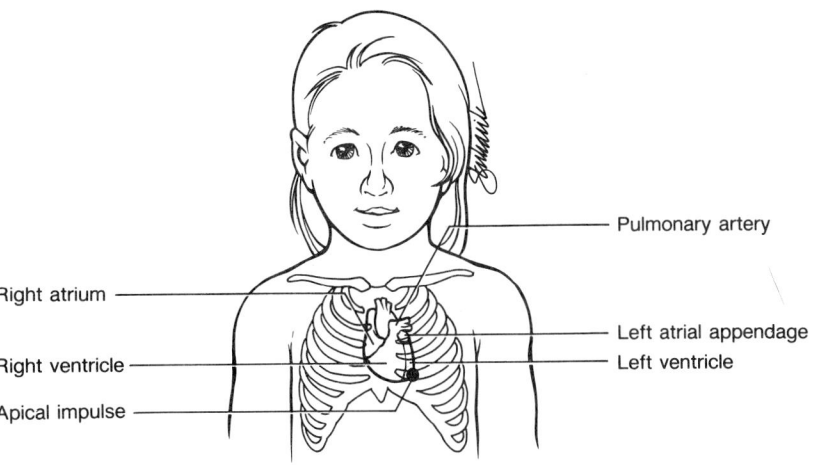

FIGURE 39-5
Diagram representing actual orientation of heart structures in relation to the chest wall, showing the atria behind the ventricles, which project toward the anterior chest wall.

Right atrium

Right ventricle

Apical impulse

Pulmonary artery

Left atrial appendage

Left ventricle

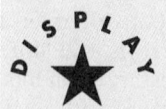

Properties of Myocardial Tissue

Automaticity—Ability of the heart to spontaneously initiate and maintain its own impulse rate without extrinsic neurohormonal control. Intrinsic control centers of the heart are called "pacemaker cells." Fluid and electrolyte balance rather than the nervous system is believed responsible for the property of automaticity.

Conductivity—Ability of cardiac muscle cells to transmit an electrical impulse to adjacent cells.

Contractility—Ability of heart muscle fibers to shorten in response to electrical stimuli.

Excitability—Ability of cardiac muscles to respond to an electrical stimulus. When stimulated, the heart muscle responds with the strongest possible contraction (the "all or nothing" principle). Excitability is influenced by neural and hormonal factors, oxygen availability, and numerous other conditions.

Extensibility—Ability of heart muscle to stretch as the chambers fill with blood between contractions.

Rhythmicity—The regular pattern of the initiation and conduction of electrical impulses in the heart. The electrical charge generated in the pacemaker cells causes a four-phased response: stimulation, transmission, contraction, and relaxation.

Refractoriness—Time during which heart muscle is responding to a stimulus and will not respond to another. During the absolute refractory period, the heart does not respond to any stimulus no matter how strong. During the relative refractory period, the heart slowly regains excitability and could respond to a strong stimulus.

---

right ventricle is located in the anterior chest, and the left ventricle is posterior to it. Structures of the heart are diagrammed in Figure 39-6.

Valves

Blood flows through the upper and lower chambers of the heart in only one direction because of the presence of atrioventricular (AV) valves, which are thin fibrous leaflets or cusps. The tricuspid valve, which has three cusps, is between the right atrium and right ventricle. The mitral valve has two cusps and is between the left atrium and the left ventricle.

Semilunar valves (pulmonary and aortic) prevent backflow of blood from the pulmonary artery to the right ventricle and from the aorta to the left ventricle. These one-way valves open with a forward pressure gradient of blood, and they close with a backward pressure gradient. The AV valves require almost no backflow to cause closure, whereas the semilunar valves require a strong backflow. The semilunar valves must withstand higher pressures and velocities of blood ejection and, therefore, are thicker and stronger than the AV valves.

Blood Supply

Although the heart chambers are filled with blood, cardiac tissue requires its own blood supply. This is provided from the right and left coronary arteries that branch off the aorta and feed into the myocardium. The right

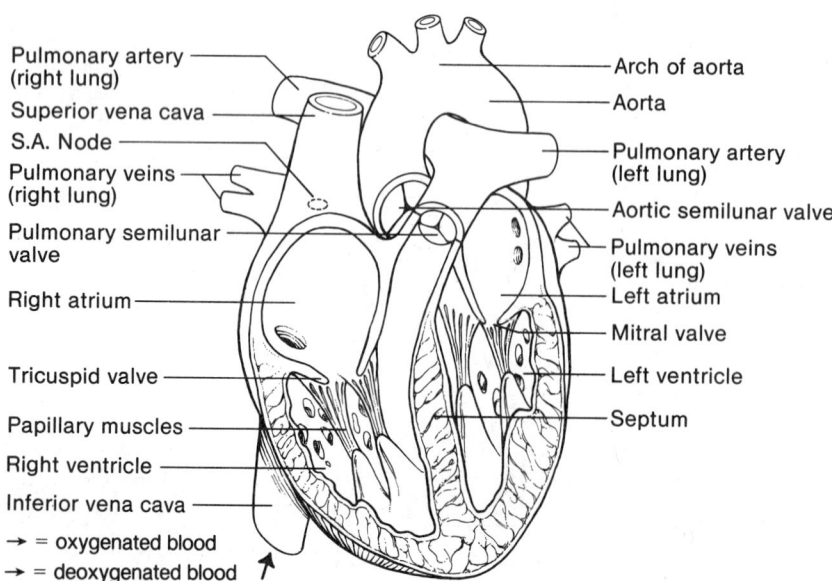

FIGURE 39-6
Structures of the heart with normal blood flow. Colored arrows indicate flow of oxygenated blood; black arrows indicate flow of deoxygenated blood. (Fuller, J., & Shaller-Ayers, J. [1990]. *Health assessment: A nursing approach.* Philadelphia: Lippincott.)

coronary artery mainly supplies the right ventricle. The left coronary artery is larger and branches further to supply blood to the remainder of the heart. A rich capillary blood supply provides oxygen needed for metabolism within the cardiac muscle cells. The ratio of about one capillary per every myocardial fiber enhances the diffusion of oxygen, carbon dioxide, and other substances in a short, rapid pathway. Venous drainage is similar: coronary veins collect the blood from heart tissues and converge to form a single large vein that empties into the right atrium.

Electrical Conduction

The cardiac conduction system is the heart's intrinsic electrical activity that is responsible for generating electrical impulses and conducting the impulses throughout the heart to stimulate myocardial contraction. The conduction pathway follows a clearly defined route through the heart (Fig. 39-7).

The origin of the cardiac impulse is the *sinoatrial (SA) node* that is embedded in the wall of the right atrium near the orifice of the superior vena cava. Known as the heart's pacemaker, the SA node sends the electrical impulse through the atria along three internodal tracts: anterior, middle, and posterior. Impulses are transmitted along internodal tracts that extend to the *atrioventricular (AV) node,* which is located in the lower part of the interatrial septum.

The AV node consists of transitional cells that conduct the electrical impulse at a slower rate than the SA node, thereby permitting atrial contraction before ventricular activity. The AV node connects to junctional tissue, a complicated network of fibers that form the *bundle of His* (AV bundle). The AV bundle extends through the AV valve and crosses the muscular interventricular septum,

where it divides into the right and left bundle branches. Both branches further subdivide into subendothelial *Purkinje fibers,* which are embedded into their respective ventricles. As the electrical impulse is transmitted, it passes through the AV bundle into the right and left branches to the Purkinje fibers; the ventricular myocardium receives the electrical transmission that causes the ventricles to contract.

On a cellular level, the electrical properties of the myocardium and pacemaker cells go through phases known as polarization, depolarization, and repolarization. Polarization occurs when the cardiac cell has negative ions inside the cell and positive charges outside the cell and is ready for electrical stimulation. Depolarization transforms the cell from a resting state to an electrically active state. Repolarization is the return of the cardiac cell to its resting state, waiting for stimulation.

The electrical impulses are created by the exchange of electrolytes such as sodium and potassium across cell walls. Shifts of electrolytes change the electrical charge within and outside the cell. These changes affect the electrical composition of the cell and allow for the electrical impulse to be transmitted from one cell to another.

The electrical activity of the heart is conducted to the external surface of the body where it can be recorded by means of an electrocardiogram (ECG). The electrocardiograph consists of several electrodes that are placed at strategic points on the body and connected to a galvanometer. On graph paper, the electrocardiograph machine records the waves of electrical activity, and these are arbitrarily labeled by the letters P, Q, R, S, and T. The accompanying display explains the association between the cardiac cycle and the ECG tracing. The normal ECG pattern is illustrated in Figure 39-7.

Abnormal cardiac rhythm or rates place the person

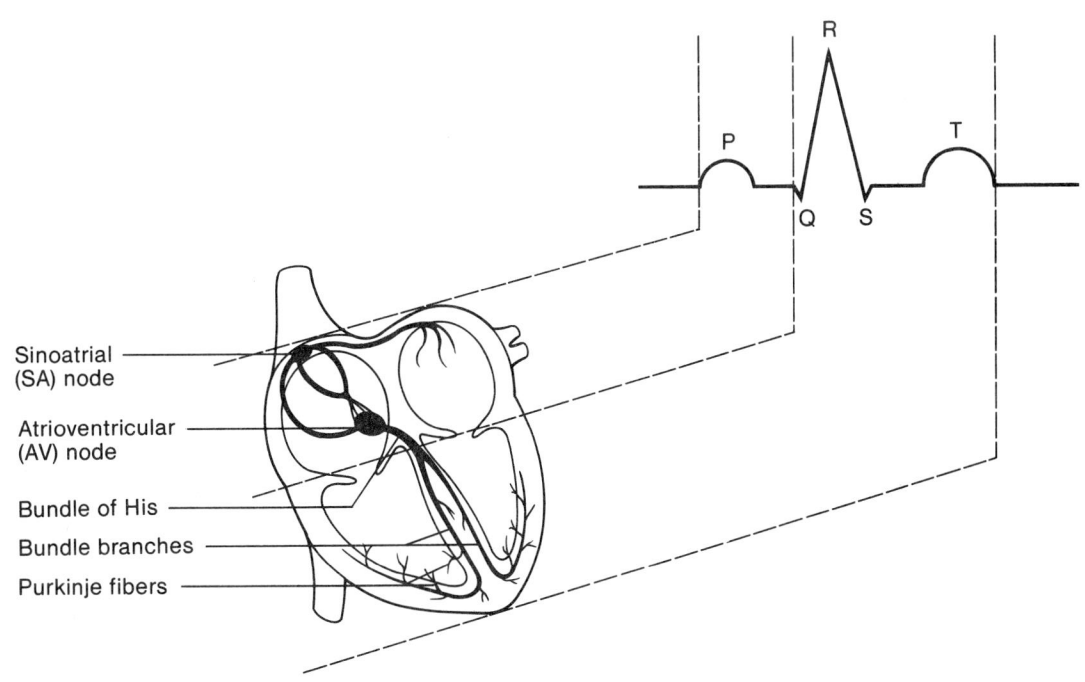

FIGURE 39-7
The cardiac conduction system in relation to the electrocardiogram. (Fuller, J., & Shaller-Ayers, J. [1990]. *Health assessment: A nursing approach.* Philadelphia: Lippincott.)

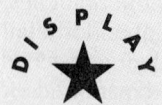

Association Between Cardiac Cycle and the ECG Tracing

P wave—Reflects the electrical excitation of the left and right atria. The P wave should precede each QRS complex.

P-Q interval—Indicates a pause during which the electrical impulse proceeds from the atria to the ventricles; the time elapsed from the onset of atrial excitation to the onset of ventricular excitation.

P-R interval—Indicates the time between sinus node depolarization and ventricular depolarization.

QRS complex—Evidence of ventricular excitation; duration indicates the time of ventricular conduction.

S-T interval—Indicates the delay between depolarization and repolarization.

Q-T interval—Represents the time from the onset of ventricular depolarization to the end of ventricular repolarization; interval shortens as heart rate increases.

T wave—Reflects recovery from excitation in the ventricles.

---

at risk. Extremely rapid or slowed heart rate can contribute to cardiac failure, which subsequently results in inadequate delivery of oxygen to cells throughout the body. Cardiac failure (congestive heart failure or shock) can be a serious outcome of a faulty conduction system.

Cardiac Performance

Cardiac performance depends on cardiac output (CO) and the peripheral vascular resistance. *Cardiac output* is the volume of blood pumped by the ventricles per minute (measured in liters per minute). Cardiac output is calculated by multiplying *stroke volume* (the volume of blood a ventricle ejects during systole) by the *heart rate* (heart beats per minute). This action may be expressed by the formula $CO = SV \times HR$. A heart rate (HR) of 70 beats/min with a stroke volume (SV) of about 60 ml/beat would generate cardiac output of 4.2 L/min.[8,9,22]

Cardiac output increases when there is an increase in heart rate or stroke volume. Heart rate is affected by numerous factors including exercise, emotions, and illness. Stroke volume depends on many factors including preload, afterload, and contractility. *Preload* is the volume of blood in the ventricles at the end of diastole, immediately before the onset of ventricular contraction. *Afterload* is the resistance against which the ventricles must pump. *Contractility* is the force of contractions generated by the myocardium under given loading conditions.

Neural and Hormonal Control

Although intrinsic mechanisms are essential to its functioning, regulation of the cardiovascular system is also influenced by complex interactions of the nervous and endocrine systems. Both the sympathetic and parasympathetic components of the autonomic nervous system contribute to the regulation of heart rate and contractility. Likewise, epinephrine and norepinephrine exert regulatory influence on the heart's performance.

Parasympathetic fibers originate in the medulla of the brain and send messages by way of the vagus nerve to the conduction center (SA and AV nodes). Stimulation of the vagus nerve causes the heart rate to slow (sinus bradycardia), and it also has a depressant effect on myocardial contractility.

Sympathetic fibers originate in the cervical and thoracic portion of the spinal column and enter the chain of paravertebral ganglion that travel to the heart. Norepinephrine, a natural neurotransmitter, is secreted during sympathetic stimulation and is stored in sympathetic nerve fibers. It is released when there is depolarization of the sympathetic neurons. These neurons innervate tissue that have α- and β-adrenergic receptors and cause the "fight or flight" response of increased heart rate, increased contractility, and peripheral vasoconstriction. Alpha receptors in the blood vessels are responsible for vasoconstriction, whereas beta receptors found in the specialized conducting cells mediate heart rate and contractility. Beta$_2$ receptors are found in the coronary arteries and cause vasodilation.

Baroreceptors (stretch receptors) are located in the aortic arch and the carotid sinuses, and they are also important in regulating the cardiovascular system. These pressure receptors respond to changes in arterial blood pressure by transmitting signals to the vasomotor and vagal centers of the brain. A rise in arterial blood pressure causes the baroreceptors to inhibit the sympathetic nervous system and stimulate the parasympathetic nervous system, resulting in a decreased arterial blood pressure. A drop in arterial blood pressure subsequently causes baroreceptors to be inhibited; sympathetic stimulation increases and results in a rise in heart rate, in contractility, and a rise in arterial blood pressure.

Epinephrine and norepinephrine, mentioned above, influence the cardiovascular system in an opposite manner. Norepinephrine is a generalized vasoconstrictor, but epinephrine typically dilates the vascular bed.

Vessels

Types

There are three types of blood vessels: arteries, veins, and capillaries. An *artery* carries blood away from the heart and, with the exception of the pulmonary artery and its branches, carries oxygenated blood.

Arterial lumens are large, and their walls are thick. They are made of elastic tissue that propels the flow of blood forward and accommodates the high pressures created as blood is expelled from the left ventricle. The arteries are constructed of three layers: the intima or smooth inner lining; the media or elastic middle layer, which allows pulsatile flow; and the adventitia or outer arterial layer, which is the supportive structure.

Arterioles are microscopic arteries. They are responsible for blood flow distribution, and they are the major site of resistance to blood flow. The arteriolar walls are made of smooth muscle that adjusts blood flow according to organ and tissue demands. Arterioles further subdivide into multiple *capillaries,* single-cell vessels that branch into all tissues. Precapillary sphincters regulate blood flow into the capillary beds in a slow and steady rate without pulsation. The capillaries carry out their functions of oxygen and nutrient delivery and the exchange of waste products between the blood and the interstitial fluid of the body.

Blood is removed from the capillary bed by microscopic vessels called *venules,* structures that transport the blood to larger vessels. *Veins* carry deoxygenated blood (except the pulmonary veins) toward the heart and, ultimately, empty into either the superior or inferior vena cava. These two vessels empty into the right atria of the heart.

Great Vessels of the Heart

The two great vessels of the heart are the pulmonary artery and the aorta. The *pulmonary artery* is located anterior to the aorta and at its base is a semilunar valve that has three cusps. This valve prevents backflow of blood during cardiac contractions. The pulmonary artery bifurcates into the right and left pulmonary artery and enters into the right and left lungs, allowing deoxygenated blood to be delivered from the heart to the lungs.

The *aorta* is a thick-walled vessel that supplies blood to the systemic circulation. At the base of aorta, a semilunar valve constructed of three cusps controls the directional flow of blood. As the aorta leaves the heart, it forms an arch that branches into smaller arteries that serve the head, neck, and upper body. The aorta descends through the thorax and abdomen, branching as needed to provide blood to the rest of the body.

Developmental Changes

Previous discussion has indicated the remarkable changes that occur in the cardiac structures in the embryo and fetus, but physical characteristics of the cardiovascular structures continue to change after birth. In infancy, the ratio of heart size to total body size is larger, and the heart requires a larger space within the thoracic cavity. Growth and development of the child result in a reduction of that ratio. Yet during the first year, the weight of the heart doubles; by 5 years, it quadruples; and by 9 years, the heart weighs six times as much as at birth.

At birth, the size of the ventricular walls are approximately equal, but, with the demands of peripheral circulation after birth (see below), the left ventricular wall becomes thicker than the right. The position of the heart

also changes. At birth, it assumes a horizontal position, but, as the heart grows, it shifts to lie lower and more obliquely.

As the child's body lengthens, the heart increases in size to meet the growing demands of the circulatory system. Likewise, the walls of blood vessels become thicker to manage the increasing blood pressure. Systolic blood pressure quickly rises during the first 6 weeks after birth but then slows until puberty, when it rises to adult levels.

System Physiology

Circulation

Fetal Circulation

Fetal circulation is well-developed in utero to meet the demands of the growing fetus. Because the lungs are essentially nonfunctional and the liver is only partially functional, most of the blood flows to the placenta and the brain. After birth, the prenatal functions of the placenta are delegated to other systems. Fetal structures not needed after birth are the placenta, umbilical vessels, foramen ovale, ductus arteriosus, and ductus venosus (Fig. 39-8).

In the fetus, oxygenated blood from the placenta travels by way of the *ductus venosus* and connects the umbilical vein to the inferior vena cava, bypassing the liver. The blood that enters the inferior vena cava is shunted from the right atrium to the left atrium through the *foramen ovale.* Blood enters the left ventricle and is

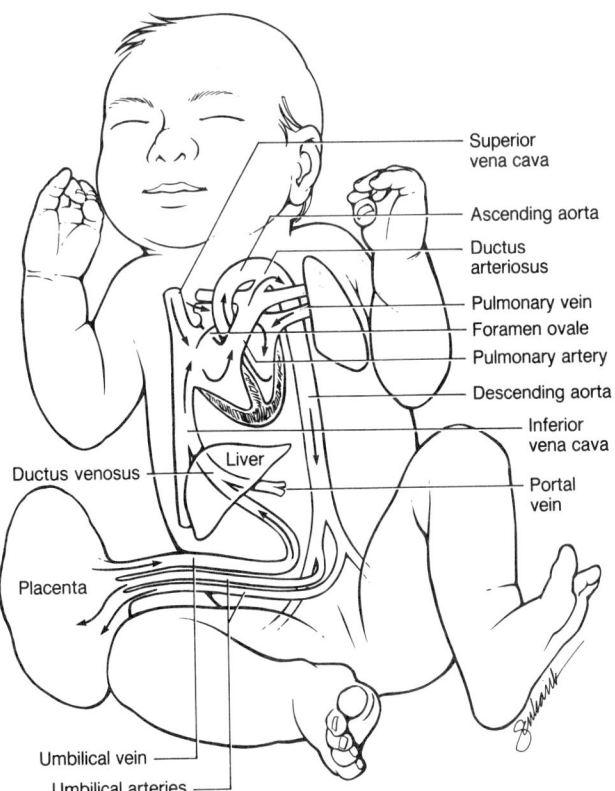

FIGURE 39-8
Fetal circulation.

preferentially routed toward the brain and upper extremities. After circulating, blood from the head and upper body drains to the superior vena cava, and blood from the lower extremities empties into the inferior vena cava. Both vessels empty into the right atrium. Blood flows from the right atrium through the pulmonary artery and directly to aorta by way of the *ductus arteriosus.* The shunt prevents most blood from entering the nonfunctional lungs. Blood flow continues by way of the aorta into the lower extremities and limbs. The aorta branches to the umbilical arteries, and blood is returned to the placenta.

Postnatal Circulation

When the infant is born, two significant events immediately effect the change from fetal to neonatal circulation. The first event is the infant's initial breath of air, and the second is the infant's separation from the placenta. After these events, the baby must rely on its own lungs for oxygen.

When placental circulation is replaced by the pulmonary circulation, the following changes occur to the structure and function of the cardiovascular system:

1. *Pulmonary vascular resistance (PVR) decreases* and pulmonary blood flow increases; therefore, pulmonary artery pressure decreases.
2. *Foramen ovale functionally closes* as a result of pressure changes in the right and left atria.
3. *Ductus arteriosus closes* as a result of increased oxygen tension in arterial blood.
4. *Ductus venosus closes* as a result of the loss of blood flow from the placenta.
5. *Systemic vascular resistance increases* as a result of removal of the low-resistance placenta.[1,14]

With the lungs expanded and the increase of alveolar oxygen (20 to 50 mmHg), the pulmonary vascular resistance (PVR) is lowered. Within a few hours after birth, there is marked increase in pulmonary blood flow. The PVR continues to diminish slowly in the next 6 to 8 weeks, and the smooth muscle of the pulmonary arterioles begins to thin.[14] The PVR continues to decrease until the child is 2 years old. The role of the PVR is an important determinant in the outcome of many congenital heart defects; it can also help protect the pulmonary circulation from volume overload.[15]

Functional closure of the foramen ovale occurs with pressure changes within the atrium. When PVR drops, the right atrial pressure is lowered; when the pulmonary venous return increases, left atrial pressure increases. The pressure causes the flapped opening between the atria (foramen ovale) to close. Although functional closure occurs soon after birth, anatomic closure may take several weeks.

The closure of the ductus arteriosus occurs within 15 to 20 hours after birth, primarily as a result of a constricting effect of the oxygen tension of the arterial blood. The smooth muscle of the ductus arteriosus responds to the oxygen, thus functionally closing the ductus arteriosus (Fig. 39-9).

The ductus venosus constricts as blood flow is stopped with the loss of the placenta. The umbilical ar-

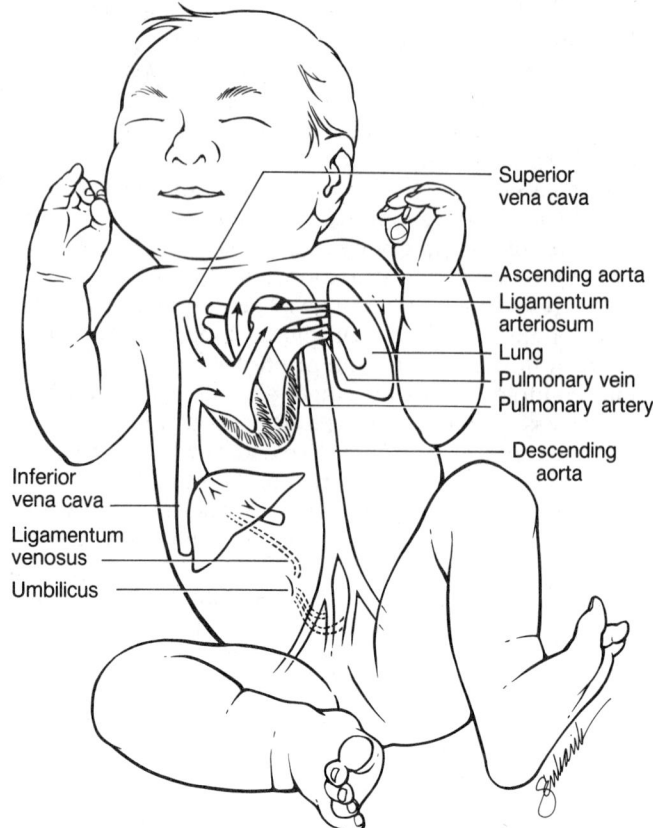

FIGURE 39-9
Postnatal circulation.

teries, veins, and ductus venosus constrict within 3 to 7 days and undergo fibrous infiltration.[11,18,19]

Cardiac Cycle

A cardiac cycle is a complete heartbeat consisting of a contraction phase (systole) and a relaxation phase (diastole) of both the atria and the ventricles. At the beginning of one cycle, the two atria contract simultaneously; as they relax, the two ventricles contract and relax. This sequence of action creates a kind of "milking" action to the movements of the heart. Each cardiac cycle requires approximately 0.8 second, producing a heart rate of 75 beats/min. As the heart rate increases, the contraction and relaxation phases shorten.[22]

The events of the cardiac cycle can be broken into four periods: ventricular filling, atrial contraction, isovolumetric contractions, and ventricular rapid ejection.

Rapid Ventricular Filling. During mid to late diastole, deoxygenated blood returns from body tissues by way of the superior and inferior vena cava into the right atrium. Simultaneously, oxygenated blood arrives from the lungs by way of the pulmonary veins and empties into the left atrium. Pressure within the empty ventricles is low, but pressure within the atria increases with continuing inflow of blood. Rapid filling of the ventricles occurs because the AV valves are open to allow passage of blood from the upper to lower chambers.

Atrial Contraction.   About 80% of the deoxygenated venous blood flow enters the atria and goes directly into the ventricle before atrial contraction begins. At the end of diastole, the SA node discharges, the atria depolarizes, and atrial contraction occurs. This action is sometimes called the "atrial kick," and it forces additional atrial blood to enter the ventricles.

Isovolumetric Contraction.   At the start of systole, pressure within the ventricles begins to build. The AV valves close so that no blood can flow backwards into the atria, and the semilunar valves remain closed because of the higher pressure in the arterial circuit. Therefore, the volume of blood within the ventricles remains constant during the initial ventricular contraction despite increased pressure within the chambers.

Ventricular Ejection.   When pressure within the ventricles exceeds aortic and pulmonary arterial pressure, the semilunar valves open. Deoxygenated blood from the right ventricle is pumped to the pulmonary circulation, and oxygenated blood from the left ventricle is pumped out to the systemic circulation. The blood ejected during ventricular systole occurs in the first third of this phase.

After ventricular ejection, diastole begins, and as pressure in the ventricles falls below that in the aorta and pulmonary artery, the semilunar valves close to prevent backflow of blood into the ventricles. The vena cava and the pulmonary veins fill the atria with blood. Because pressure in the atria is greater than that in the ventricles, the AV valves open to permit blood flow into the ventricles. One cardiac cycle, a single heart beat, is thereby completed, and the sequence begins anew.[3,5]

Pulmonary Circulation

Output of the right ventricle equals that of the left ventricle; therefore, the flow of blood through the pulmonary and systemic circuits is the same. Pulmonary circulation is, however, a low-pressure and low-resistance system in comparison to the systemic circulation. Therefore, the pulmonary vessels are thinner and larger in diameter than the systemic vessels. The pulmonary artery pressure is normally 25/10 mmHg, and a large stroke volume is well-accommodated in the pulmonary vascular bed. The pulmonary circuit carries the deoxygenated venous blood away from the heart by way of the pulmonary artery which bifurcates into the right and left main branches. The right and left pulmonary arteries supply blood to their respective lungs. Blood travels to the pulmonary capillary bed in the alveoli where oxygen and carbon dioxide exchange occurs. After oxygenation, the pulmonary venous blood returns to the left atrium by way of four pulmonary veins. The four pulmonary veins differ from the systemic veins in that they carry highly oxygenated blood.

Systemic Circulation

Systemic circulation is the flow of blood in the remainder of the body, exclusive of the lungs. Numerous vessels connect the heart to all body tissues, providing especially well for vital organs. Blood first enters an arterial system made up of the aorta, arteries, arterioles, and capillaries. Arteries branch off the aorta to deliver oxygen to the capillaries in the tissues.

After leaving the capillaries, the deoxygenated blood and waste products travel back to the heart by way of the venous circulation. The smaller venules coalesce to form larger veins; and wall thickness increases as lumen size increases. Blood flow through these vessels increases as it reaches the superior and inferior vena cava and returns to the heart. Smooth muscle within the vein walls regulates the amount of blood by contracting and relaxing to adapt to the body's needs.

Summary

The cardiovascular system is a complex transport system that is well-organized and efficient. It delivers oxygen, nutrients, and other substances to every body cell and tissue in the amounts required without interruption. From a complicated embryonic phase to major changes in the circulatory route after birth, the developing cardiovascular system presents many opportunities for anomalies to occur. Knowledge of the anatomy and physiology of the cardiovascular system is essential to performing a comprehensive assessment of this dynamic transport system.

Acknowledgements

The Departments of Pediatric Cardiology and Nursing Education, Children's Hospital, Oakland.

Dedicated In Memory Of

Stanley M. Higashino, M.D.
Chief of Cardiology
Children's Hospital, Oakland
1930–1991

References

1. Adams, F. H., & Emmanouilides, G. C. (1989). *Moss' heart disease in infants, children and adolescents* (4th ed.). Baltimore: Williams & Wilkins.
2. Amplatz, K., Moller, J., & Castaneda-Zuñiga, W. R. (1986). *Radiology of congenital heart disease.* New York: Thieme Medical.
3. Berne, R. M., & Levy, M. N. (1992). *Cardiovascular physiology* (6th ed.). St. Louis: Mosby.
4. Clare, M. D. (1985). Care of infants and children with cardiac disease. *Heart and Lung, 14*(3), 218–222.
5. Cohn, P. (1985). *Clinical cardiovascular physiology.* Philadelphia: Saunders.
6. Curley, M. A. Q. (1985). *Pediatric cardiac dysrhythmias.* Bowie, MD: Brady Communications.
7. Fink, B. W. (1991). *Congenital heart disease: A deductive approach to its diagnosis* (3rd ed.). St. Louis: Mosby.
8. Ford, R. D. (Ed.). (1986). *Cardiovascular care handbook.* Springhouse, PA: Springhouse.
9. Goerke, J. (1988). *Cardiovascular physiology.* New York: Raven Press.
10. Guzzeta, C. E., & Dossey, B. M. (1992). *Cardiovascular nursing.* St. Louis: Mosby.

11. Hazinski, M. F. (1992). *Nursing care of the critically ill child* (2nd ed.). St. Louis: Mosby.
12. Lamb, J., & Carlson, V. (1986). *Handbook of cardiovascular nursing.* Philadelphia: Lippincott.
13. Park, M. K. (1988). *Pediatric cardiology for the practitioner* (2nd ed.). St. Louis: Mosby.
14. Perloff, J. K. (1987). *The clinical recognition of congenital heart disease* (3rd ed.). Philadelphia: Saunders.
15. Ream, A., Fogdall, R., et al. (1982). *Acute cardiovascular management, anesthesia and intensive care.* Philadelphia: Lippincott.
16. Rogers, M. C. (1987). *Textbook of pediatric intensive care.* Baltimore: Williams & Wilkins.
17. Rosendorff, C. (1983). *Clinical cardiovascular and pulmonary physiology.* New York: Raven Press.
18. Row, R. D., Freedom, M. R., & Mehrizi, A. (1987). *The neonate with congenital heart disease.* Philadelphia: Saunders.
19. Tarhan, S. (1988). *Cardiovascular anesthesia and postoperative care* (2nd ed.). St. Louis: Mosby.
20. Underhill, S. (1989). *Cardiac nursing* (2nd ed.). Philadelphia: Lippincott.
21. Vander, A. J., Sherman, J. H., & Luciano, D. S. (1990). *Human physiology: The mechanisms of body function* (5th ed.). New York: McGraw-Hill.
22. Vincent, R. N., & Collins, G. F. (1986). Cardiac embryology and fetal cardiovascular physiology. *Critical Care Quarterly, 9*(2), 1–5.
23. Wenger, N., Hurst, J. W., & McIntyre, M. C. (1980). *Cardiology for nurses.* New York: McGraw-Hill.

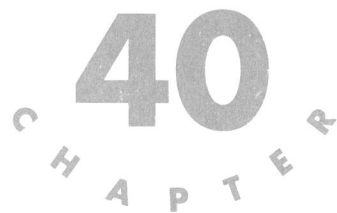

40

CHAPTER

Nursing Assessment and Diagnosis of Cardiovascular Function

BEHAVIORAL OBJECTIVES

Use functional health as a guideline for assessment of the child's cardiovascular function.

Describe the components of a physical examination of an infant or child with an alteration in cardiovascular function.

Describe diagnostic tests used in the cardiovascular assessment of the child and the nursing care required.

Identify nursing diagnoses commonly used in the care of children with cardioovascular dysfunction.

Nursing assessment of the cardiovascular system begins with a thorough health history. The assessment focuses on the child's health patterns, and, as the baseline data are collected, actual or potential cardiovascular problems are revealed. The child's and family's concerns must be elicited and reported in an organized, objective, and systematic fashion that accounts for developmental and age-appropriate behaviors.

Attention is given first to primary concerns, because the child and family give them priority. The parents, for example, may be most worried about their child's size; they may be less concerned about the child's blue skin tone (cyanosis), rapid respirations, feeding difficulties, and easy fatigability. Responding first to the family's primary concerns builds trust between the nurse and the family and can result in a more collaborative relationship in meeting the child's health care needs.

Once the primary concerns are addressed and rapport has been established, the nurse proceeds by obtaining a history from the child and family. Physical examination, diagnostic laboratory tests, and cardiovascular procedures also contribute significantly to the comprehensive database. Critical analysis of assessment data determines the nursing diagnoses to be used in planning care for the child.

994   Nursing Care of Children With Altered Cardiovascular Function

Nursing Assessment

Child and Family History

Children who present with suspected or known cardiovascular dysfunction need to be assessed comprehensively with focus on the effects of the disorder. The following section explains how the health history can be obtained using functional health as a format for nursing assessment and diagnosis with sample questions and observations of behavior.

Health-Perception and Health-Management

Assessment of health-perception and health-management may begin with a focus on historic data about prenatal and postnatal events. This information may be useful in establishing a diagnosis of congenital heart disease during infancy. The mother may be asked to describe the pregnancy, labor, and birth. Did the mother have any infections or chronic diseases during pregnancy? Did she smoke or use drugs? Is there a history of heart problems in the family? Have there been early infant deaths in the family? How has the child's growth and development compared with other children of the same age? How often does the child have acute illnesses like colds or other respiratory infections?

The family's and child's perception and management of the child's cardiovascular health are assessed. Questions may be asked about modes of treatment, compliance to therapy, and views on outcomes and expectations of therapy. What is your understanding of the heart problems? Is the child on any medication? What things do you do to take care of the cardiovascular condition? What are your concerns about your child's health? What worries your child?

Nutrition and Metabolism

The overall nutritional status of the child is a significant indicator of the child's cardiovascular status. Observations should focus on general growth and weight gain; both may be delayed in children with congestive heart failure and cyanotic heart disease.[17] A child with cardiovascular dysfunction usually shows a more significant weight loss than height deficit. The child's feeding patterns are also key data in assessing cardiovascular dysfunction, because respiratory problems and fatigue often develop while feeding. What is child's respiratory pattern at rest? What changes occur in respiratory pattern with feeding? How long after a meal does the respiratory pattern return to normal? Does the child's color change with activity?

Questions relevant to nutrition and metabolic patterns of the cardiovascular child include: What is the child's diet (i.e., 24-hour recall)? Is the child breast- or bottle-fed? What is the child's usual feeding schedule? How much is taken? How long does each feeding take? Does the child turn blue during feedings? Does child breathe faster or harder during feedings? Does child grunt? What is the strength of the infant's sucking reflex?

Have there been significant weight gains or losses? Have you noticed a decrease in child's ability to feed (e.g., fatigue, less intake, longer to feed)?

Elimination

The patterns of excretory function may indicate problems of congestive heart failure. The assessment focuses on the renal, bowel, and integumentary systems. Relevant questions are: What is the child's usual bowel and urinary elimination pattern? Has the pattern changed recently? Does the child seem to be retaining fluid (puffy face, hands, and feet)? Is the abdomen distended? Does the child become cyanotic when defecating? Does the child have excessive perspiration? What causes the child to perspire? How often are clothes changed due to wetness?

Activity and Exercise

The child's activity and exercise are best assessed with an understanding of age-appropriate activities and developmental norms. A child who is inactive, easily fatigued, and intolerant of exercise may be displaying symptoms of cardiovascular dysfunction. Questions may include: What is the child's typical day? How many hours are spent in the crib, being held, and playing? What types of activity does the child enjoy (e.g., sports, recreational games)? What changes have you noticed in the child's activity? Are there decreases in the child's activity level? Does the child keep up with other children? How far can the child walk or run? How many flights of stairs can the child walk up (with or without becoming tired)? Does the child participate in self-care activities?

Sleep and Rest

Children who develop congestive heart failure or cyanotic heart disease may have altered sleep–rest patterns. They may require upright positioning to enhance respiratory comfort, may awaken easily, and may be restless and irritable sleepers. The quality and quantity of sleep and rest, the position for sleep (upright, prone side, supine), and expression of restfulness are included in the assessment. Sample questions include the following: How many hours does the child sleep per night? Does the child awaken during the night? Does the child take naps? How often? Length? In what position does the child sleep? Is the child restless or bothered by nightmares? Where does the child sleep (with parents or alone)?

Cognition and Perception

Cognition and perception are assessed to evaluate the child's and family's ability to understand and manage the cardiovascular problem. This also helps to determine if cardiovascular dysfunction may be contributing to alterations in the child's cognitive or perceptual abilities. The assessment of cognition and perception is enhanced by closely observing the child and family during the interview process. Observations include attention span, language communication skills, memory, learning styles, and decision-making skills. The nurse should observe the child's and the parents' ability to hear, see, talk, and concentrate on the conversation. Does the child or family have any sensory deficits? Is the child in pain or discomfort (describe duration, onset, frequency)? Do the child or parents have fears or concerns? What is child's and parents' perception of the child's cardiovascular status? What questions do the child or parents have? How would they best learn new information about the child's condition or therapy (e.g., demonstration, video, or reading)?

Self-Perception and Self-Concept

The child with a cardiovascular disorder may experience physical limitations, developmental delays, psychological stress, and emotional changes. These changes may have a negative influence on the child's self-concept. During the interview process, the nurse observes for nonverbal cues such as body posture and movement, eye contact, voice patterns, and gestures; these may give clues about the child's self-concept and self-esteem. Questions for children include the following: How do you describe yourself? How you feel about yourself? How does your appearance or activity compare with other children your age? Do you feel sad, depressed, angry, or fearful? Why? When? Parents may be asked about behavioral problems, progress in school, and the child's involvement in social activities.

Role Relationships

Cardiovascular disorders can be disruptive to family interrelationships, causing problems such as sibling jealousy, parental disagreement, and increased involvement of extended family members. Children with cardiovascular problems are often overprotected and overindulged by their families. Families may enforce little discipline, and the role relationships may not be clearly defined. Observations of the child–caregiver interaction are noted. Are the parents and other family members supportive, nurturing, and loving to the child? Does the child manipulate the parent? Questions for the family may include: What is the family structure? Who are the primary caregivers? How do the family members feel about the child's cardiovascular problem? Do the siblings understand the child's problems? How is the child disciplined? Are expectations for this child's behavior similar to those of the siblings?

Relationships of the child and parents with others outside the family may also be assessed. How does the child relate to peers? How does the child do in school? Does the child have any close friends? Are there adults other than the parents who relate well with the child? Sometimes a teacher or coach is able to provide encouragement, motivation, and direction not accepted from family members.

Sexuality and Reproduction

Disturbances in cardiovascular function may influence the child's sexuality and feelings of masculinity or femininity. Age and developmentally appropriate questions should be asked about sexuality and reproduction: How do you feel about being a boy or girl, or becoming a man or woman? How do your sexual characteristics compare with others your age? Have medications changed aspects of sexuality such as libido or menses? Are there concerns about becoming a parent in the future?

Coping and Stress Tolerance

The child's cardiovascular problem is typically a major stressor on the family's lifestyle and presents alterations in the family system. The family may react to the information with fear, guilt, mourning, and loss of a "perfect child." The family's and child's response to the stress is defined as the *coping pattern;* therefore, questions focus on the child's and family's ability to manage problems. Sample questions include: How did the family cope with learning about the heart problem? How has the child's cardiovascular problem caused the family to change behavior? Who are the child's and family's sources of support or help? How does the child and family solve or handle problems? Give an example of a stressful situation and how it was handled.

Values and Beliefs

Cardiovascular dysfunction has multiple implications for the child's and family's value-belief system. Often preexisting values and cultural beliefs can influence the family's perceptions of the disorder and compliance with treatment plans. The nurse needs to explore general areas related to culture and religious beliefs, including symbolism regarding the heart. Questions may include: Has the child's cardiovascular problem interfered with usual cultural or religious practices? How does the heart problem affect goals for the child or family? Have they had to reevaluate individual or family beliefs or priorities because of the heart problem? Are there cultural or religious practices that they feel are not accepted in the health care system? Are there cultural or religious practices that they think may help the child?

Physical Examination

The physical examination may confirm or rule out a suspected cardiovascular problem. For example, if the health history reveals an infant is a poor feeder, sleeps excessively, breathes fast, and perspires easily, the nurse may suspect congestive heart failure and focus the examination on related physical findings. A comprehensive history provides invaluable guidance in performing the physical examination for the child with heart problems.

The examination is conducted in a well-lit room with the child in a sitting position. The examination can also be performed while the infant or young child is in the parent's lap to promote an atmosphere that is quiet and nonthreatening.

A typical approach to the examination is in the order of inspection, palpation, auscultation, and percussion; this sequence works with the cooperative child. However, with a sleeping child, the nurse may try to inspect and auscultate before palpating and percussing to prevent waking a sleeping child who may subsequently become uncooperative. Inspection, palpation, and auscultation are the three most beneficial methods in the cardiovascular examination. Percussion is a less useful method for contributing data; however, it can be an important method in determining heart and liver size and placement.

General Information

When approaching the cardiovascular examination, general information is first obtained, followed by in-depth and specific investigation. The examination usually begins with general physical assessments, which include appearance, vital signs, size measurements, color, muscular tone, skeletal development, and activity level.

General appearance and the overall nutritional status of the child are first observed. Are there any obvious abnormalities with the child? Does the child look unusual? The astute nurse notes any obvious problems that may suggest specific congenital heart disease. For example, many chromosomal abnormalities that are manifest in obvious physical features are associated with congenital heart problems. Does the child appear too thin or overweight? Thinness may indicate inadequate nutrition related to the heart problem, whereas overweight may be associated with cardiovascular conditions that cause fluid retention and edema.

Vital signs, including temperature, pulse, respirations, and blood pressure, are measured carefully in the cardiovascular assessment (Fig. 40-1). A child suspected of an acquired cardiovascular problem should have a temperature taken using an age-appropriate route (oral, rectal, axillary, tympanic). Significant fever may be caused by viral or bacterial infections, dehydration, or toxins. Any of these causes have implications for the cardiovascular system. For example, fever as seen in acute rheumatic fever and Kawasaki disease has significant cardiovascular sequelae.[19]

The pulse is carefully measured and noted for its rate, regularity, rhythm, and quality. Normal pulse rates for children are given in the front of the book. Abnormal findings related to pulse are described in Table 40-1. Pulses can be palpated and auscultated in several areas, as discussed in Chapter 25. Pulses should be compared in the right and left arm and then the arm and leg for quality and rate. In the absence of dysfunction, pulses are usually equal in rate and rhythm in all sites. A comparison of the radial and femoral pulse is extremely important in the cardiovascular examination, especially when coarctation of the aorta is suspected. If there are bounding, full pulses in the upper extremities and weak, absent pulses in the lower extremities, coarctation of the aorta can be highly suspected.[19]

Respiratory rate, rhythm, and quality are evaluated by inspection, palpation, and auscultation. Respiratory rate is counted for a full minute while the child is at rest; an elevated respiratory rate is often an early sign of congestive heart failure. Is the breathing comfortable or distressed? Does the child exhibit retractions, deep respirations, or grunting sounds? Is the child able to breathe better in the upright position? Abnormal breath sounds such as rales may be indicative of congestive heart fail-

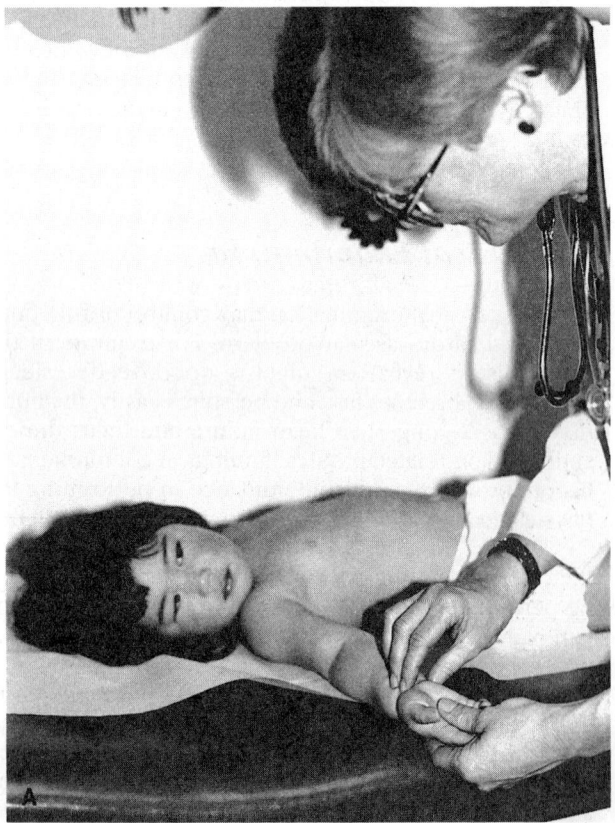
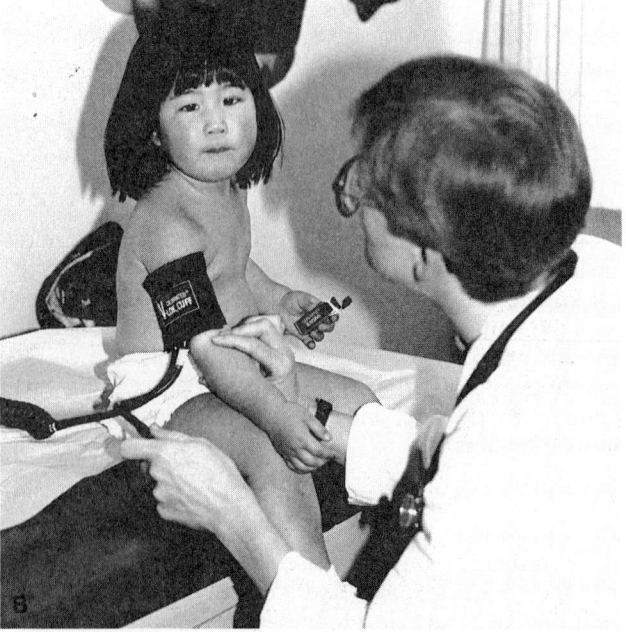

FIGURE 40-1
Vital signs are important in a cardiovascular assessment. The nurse takes the radial pulse (**A**) and the blood pressure (**B**).

TABLE 40-1
Abnormal Findings Related to Pulse

Finding	Definition/Meaning
Pulse alterans	One strong beat, next weak beat; pulses alternate in amplitude from beat to beat; occurs with severe heart strain, left-sided failure
Bounding pulse	Pulse pressure increased, pulse is strong; accompanied by increased stroke volume, decreased peripheral vascular resistance; occurs with patent ductus arteriosus
Brisk pulse	Widened pulse pressure
Diminished femoral pulses	Decreased pulse pressure in lower body; occurs with coarctation of the aorta
Decreased, thready peripheral pulse	Low or decreased cardiac output; occurs in circulatory shock; pulse is weak and small
Bradycardia	Decreased pulse rate; occurs with congenital heart block or a degree of heart block, and digitalis toxicity
Tachycardia	Increased pulse rate; occurs with excitement, fever, congestive heart failure, and dysrhythmia
Pulses paradoxus	Pulse diminished perceptibly in amplitude on inspiration; can occur in pericardial tamponade

ure.[19] Chapter 37 gives more detail about comprehensive assessment of the respiratory system.

Blood pressure is a basic and important measurement in cardiovascular assessment. The use of proper equipment and technique (as discussed in Chap. 25) is essential. Normal blood pressure values for children are listed at the front of this book. The child should be quiet and still when obtaining the blood pressure; an excited, agitated child may cause an inaccurate blood pressure reading. The normal range of blood pressure differs with the child's age.

The child's measurements (height, weight, head circumference) are entered on standard growth charts. The percentile is noted, and growth patterns are evaluated for a progressive upward trend compared with the standardized growth curve at each visit. A child with cardiac dysfunction may demonstrate retarded growth patterns, especially with slow weight gain.

Inspection

The skin is evaluated for color, because cyanosis or paleness is a strong manifestation of cardiac dysfunction. A grayish cast to the skin, mucous membranes, lips, nailbeds, and sclera indicates cyanosis; this assessment is especially important for dark-complexioned children whose skin color may not reveal cyanotic symptoms at first glance. The cyanosis may become noticeable or increase during exercise or activities such as feeding, defecation, and movement. Cyanosis of the extremities (acrocyanosis) in neonates is a common and normal finding that decreases when the newborn is warm and active. In all cases, the degree and distribution of any form of cyanosis require thorough investigation. Pallor may be seen in infants due to vasoconstriction that results from congestive heart failure or severe anemia.

Sweat on the forehead is often seen in infants with congestive heart failure. It usually occurs during activity such as feeding or crying. This symptom is a compensatory reaction of the sympathetic nervous system in an attempt to increase cardiac output.[19]

The fingernails are inspected for clubbing. *Clubbing* is a widening and thickening of the end of the fingers and is usually a late sign of a severe, long-standing hypoxia. Chapter 37 provides more information on assessing the degree of clubbing. Cyanosis of the nailbeds should also be noted in the fingers and toes.

The musculoskeletal system is inspected for muscular tone, posture, and size. Cardiovascular dysfunction can manifest as poor posture, loss of muscle tone, and size. The nurse should observe the child's gait, posture, and movements. The child is asked to perform simple age-appropriate motor skills (e.g., stand on one foot, climb flight of stairs, and so forth). Children with cyanotic heart disease may assume a knee-chest or squatting position to help improve arterial oxygen saturation. This position increases systemic vascular resistance, thereby reducing right to left shunting in the heart.

The activity level of a child must also be carefully observed and investigated. Assessment of activity intolerance is noted by behaviors such as poor feeding, need for prolonged rest periods after play, decreased ability to keep up with peers, periods of restlessness, increased sleep, and the need for upright positions while sleeping. Children with congestive heart failure exhibit signs of easy fatigability, poor feeding abilities, loss of muscular tone, and increased respiratory effort.

The chest wall is inspected for obvious deformities, which may result from cardiac enlargement. The anterior chest is inspected from left to right sides; both sides should be symmetric. A precordial bulge may be seen if the heart has been enlarged for a prolonged period; acute dilation of the heart does not cause a pericardial bulge.[17]

Palpation

The skin is palpated for temperature, which is directly correlated to adequate circulation. With low cardiac output states, the peripheral blood supply is shunted to vital organs; peripheral organs such as skin lose nutrient supply and warmth. Therefore, coolness of the extremities may indicate a low cardiac output.

Assessment for edema is appropriate when congestive heart failure is suspected, although edema is a late sign because of the increased vascular and hepatic capacitance in young children. Periorbital edema, scrotal edema, and generalized body puffiness are all important indicators. Edema is assessed by gently pressing on an area for up to 5 seconds. A depression of the skin remains with pitting edema.[9]

Palpation specific to the cardiovascular system includes the apical and peripheral pulses, thrills, and heaves. Apical and peripheral pulses have already been described as part of the general information obtained at the beginning of the examination. Thrills are of diagnostic significance and are best felt with the palm of the examiner's hand and not with the fingertips[19] (Fig. 40-2). *Thrills* are low-frequency vibrations caused by the blood flowing from one chamber of the heart to another through a narrow valvular opening or an abnormal septal defect. They occur with loud murmurs (grade 3 or higher) and

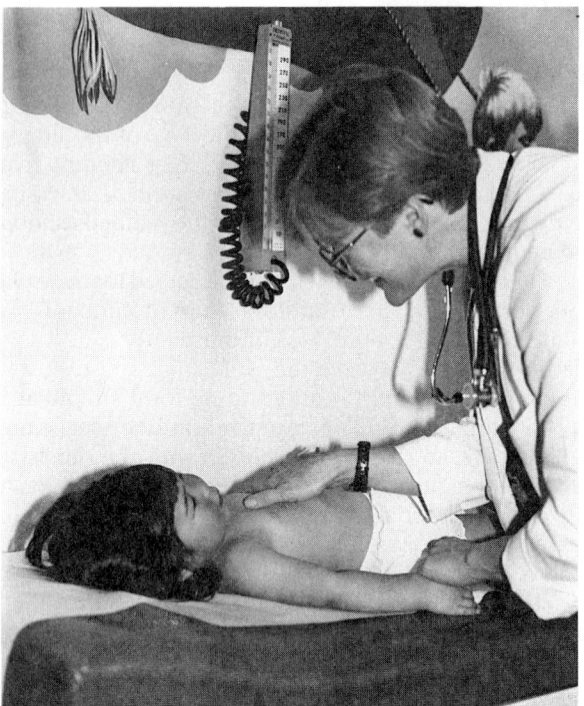

FIGURE 40-2
The nurse palpates for cardiovascular thrills with the palm of her hand.

are found in the same area as the murmur. Thrills also may occur over the carotid artery and the suprasternal notch, but thrills in this area are felt by fingertip palpation. These thrills are suggestive of aortic or pulmonary valve problems or possibly a carotid bruit.

Heaves are associated with fluid volume overload problems. A heaving pulsation can be felt at the lower left sternal border and may be characteristic of right ventricular hypertrophy. A thrusting impulse or heave is felt at the apex of the heart, which is displaced outward and downward.

Auscultation

Auscultation of the heart is one of the most valuable methods of cardiovascular examination for determining normal versus abnormal cardiac findings. Technical skill acquired through repetitive practice in a quiet setting is imperative to obtain accurate information. The new nurse should seek out expert advice from a skilled practitioner. A stethoscope with a bell and diaphragm is needed. Low-frequency sounds such as murmurs are best heard with the bell, and high-frequency sounds such as rubs are heard with the diaphragm. Stethoscopes should be carefully selected to match the size of the child (see Chap. 25).

The auscultatory cardiovascular assessment should include heart rate, rhythm and regularity, intensity and quality of heart sounds, diastolic and systolic sounds, and the presence of abnormal sounds. Auscultation the aortic, pulmonic, tricuspid, and mitral areas (Fig. 40-3A). The respiratory system is included with assessment of the cardiovascular system because abnormal breath sounds may

be indicative of pulmonary edema and congestive heart failure (see Chap. 37).

The nurse should auscultate while the child is first in an upright, sitting position (see Fig. 40-3B) and then in a reclining, supine position (see Fig. 40-3C). If further examination is needed, the child may be asked to stand and lean forward or to lie on the left side to identify or clarify abnormal sounds. The diaphragm of the stethoscope is used first to identify high-pitched sounds (S_1 and S_2); the bell is used to identify lower-pitched sounds (S_3 and S_4). Table 40-2 summarizes normal and abnormal heart sounds. The transmission of sound is usually easier when there is less muscle and fat content; therefore, auscultation of heart sounds is usually easier in a child than in an adult.

The heart rate should be compared with the peripheral pulse rate, which was obtained earlier. Normal heart sounds are identified. The first heart sound (S_1) is the closure of the mitral and tricuspid valves, the beginning of systole, and is best heard at the lower left sternal border, the apex of the heart. A splitting of S_1, the almost imperceptible pause between the closure of one valve and then the other, is normal in children.

The second heart sound, the beginning of diastole, is the closure of aortic and pulmonic valves. S_2 is best heard in the upper left sternal border or pulmonic area. Normal splitting of S_2 may be heard on inspiration; the first component is aortic closure, and the second is pulmonic closure. S_2 splitting during expiration is considered abnormal.

A third heart sound (S_3) is commonly heard in young children. S_3 occurs early in diastole and is due to blood passing through the mitral valve and entering the empty left ventricle.

The fourth sound (S_4) is rarely heard and is always abnormal; it is the atrial contraction during the end of diastole.

The last auscultatory step is to determine the presence of murmurs or other sounds. A *heart murmur* is defined as a sound lasting longer than other heart sounds and described as vibrations within the heart chambers or in the vessels. Murmurs are caused by turbulent blood flow that is obstructed or abnormal. A common heart murmur results from abnormal blood flow between two chambers or two vessels; regurgitation of blood between valves, septal defects, or vessels; constricted blood flow between a valve or vessel; and increased blood flow through valves and vessels. Each murmur is evaluated in terms of intensity, timing (systole or diastole), location, transmission, pitch, and quality (musical, vibratory, blowing). Table 40-3 provides information to be used in describing auscultatory findings of the heart.

Innocent murmurs, also called functional murmurs, arise from cardiovascular structures without anatomic abnormality. The sounds are caused by blood passing through a normal heart or vessel and are not related to pathology. Over 80% of children have an innocent murmur during childhood.[19] Innocent murmurs are most common beginning at age 3 to 4 years and are always associated with normal ECG and x-ray findings.

Murmurs may be difficult to distinguish from pericardial friction rubs. A friction rub is grating, high-pitched, scratchy, and is heard throughout systole and diastole.

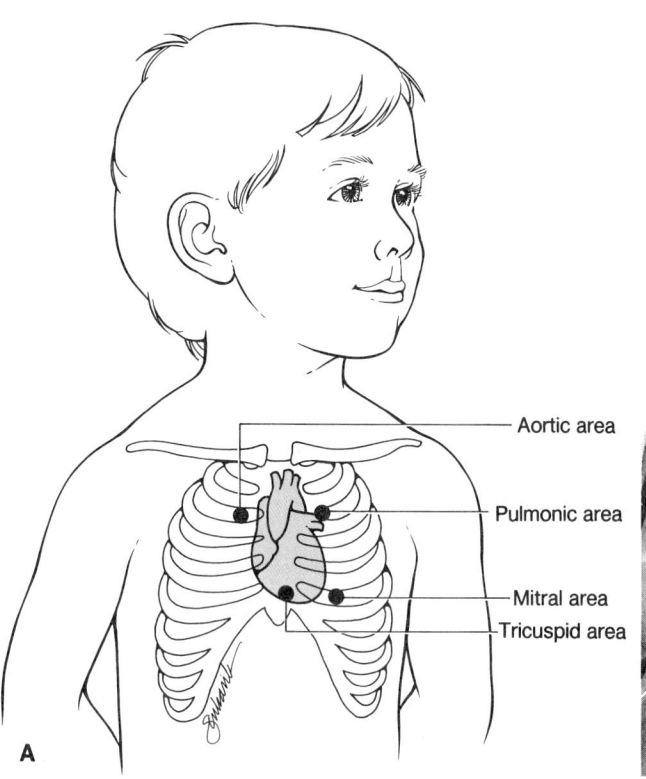

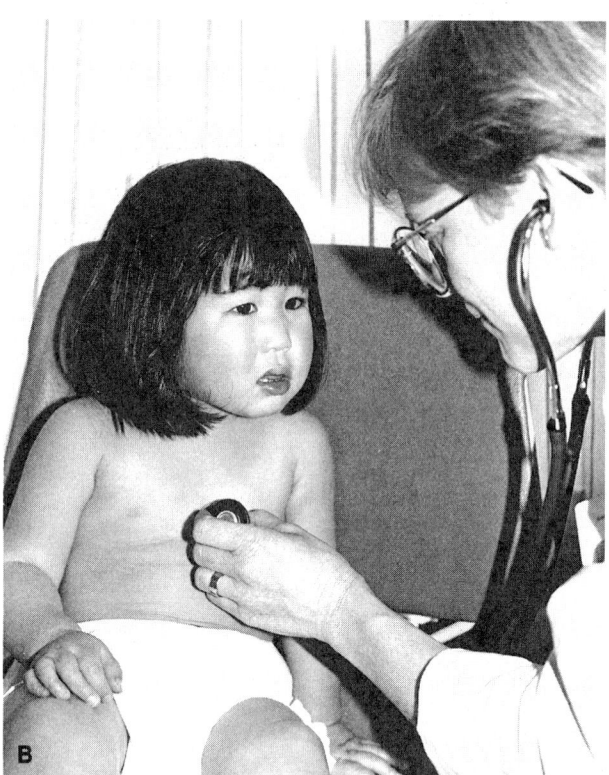

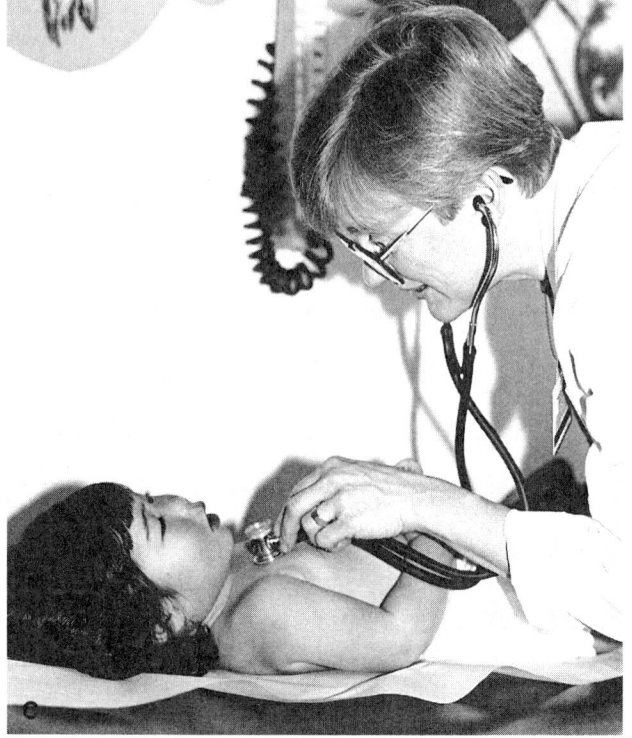

FIGURE 40-3

One of the most valuable methods of cardiovascular examination is auscultation of the heart. (**A**) Areas of auscultation in a child. (**B**) Auscultation in an upright position. (**C**) Auscultation in a supine position.

These sounds are caused by inflammation of the layers of the pericardium and are considered abnormal. Friction rubs are usually best heard in the third interspace to the left of the sternum.

Diagnostic Tests

Specialized tests are performed on children suspected of having a cardiovascular problem. During these tests, the child and family may be fearful and anxious. The nurse's responsibilities include carefully and sensitively explaining the purposes and procedures of the tests, familiarizing the child and family with the equipment to be used, providing psychosocial support, assisting with the test, and providing follow-up care and information. Details of common laboratory studies and diagnostic procedures for children with suspected cardiovascular dysfunction are described below.

TABLE 40-2
Summary of Normal and Abnormal Heart Sounds

Heart Sound	Ausculatory Site and Location	Characteristics
S_1 (Closure of mitral and tricuspid valves simultaneously)	Mitral (apical) area	Heard best/loudest at apex
	<2 years: 4th left interspace lateral to the left midclavicular line	Heard best with diaphragm of stethoscope (low-frequency sound)
	>2 years: 5th left interspace medial to midclavicular line	May be split
S_2 (Closure of aortic and pulmonic valves)	Aortic area: 2nd right interspace close to sternum	S_2 is louder than S_1
	Pulmonic area: 2nd interspace, just to left of sternum	Split S_2 is physiologically normal (increased split with inspiration)
		Heard best with diaphragm of stethoscope
S_3 (Rapid filling of ventricle)	Apical area	May be normal or pathologic
	<2 years: 4th left interspace lateral to left midclavicular line	Described as a "gallop"
		Sounds like "Ken-tuc-ky"
	>2 years: 5th left interspace medial to midclavicular line	Heard as a faint, low-pitched sound with bell of stethoscope
S_4 (Atrial contraction)	Mitral area	Pathologic, atrial gallop
	<2 years: 4th left interspace lateral to left midclavicular line	Decreased ventricular compliance
		Heard as soft, brief sound
	>2 years: 5th left interspace medial to midclavicular line	Sounds like "Ten-nes-see"
		Louder on inspiration
		Best heard with bell of stethoscope
Pericardial friction rub (Movement of the heart against the pericardium)	Extracardiac sound	High-pitched, scratchy sound
	3rd interspace to left of sternum	Heard throughout systole and diastole
		Usually indicates inflammation of pericardial sac
Continuous murmur (May indicate patent ductus arteriosus)	Pulmonic area	Begins in systole and continues without interruption through S_2 into diastole
	2nd left interspace; radiates to 1st interspace below left clavicle	
Innocent (functional) murmur	Mid lower sternal border or lower left sternal edge and apex	Grade 3 or less
		Always systolic
		Does not radiate
		Louder in supine than sitting position
		Normal chest x-ray and ECG
		No other cardiac pathology
Carotid bruit (Turbulence in the brachycephalic or carotid arteries)	Right/left supraclavicular area over the carotid arteries	Early systolic ejection murmur
		Thrill felt over carotid
		An innocent murmur
Venous hum (Turbulence in the jugular venous system)	Right/left infra-supra-clavicular area	Continuous murmur
		Diastolic sound louder than systolic
		Heard in upright position

Laboratory Tests

A variety of laboratory tests are performed on children suspected of having a cardiovascular problem. A *complete blood count* is often performed to evaluate the cardiac status. Normal values are in Table 40-4. The *hematocrit* (HCT) measures the percentage, by volume, of packed red blood cells (PRBC) in a whole blood sample. The purpose of a hematocrit is to aid the diagnosis of abnormal states of hydration, polycythemia, and anemia.

Total hemoglobin measures the grams of hemoglobin (Hgb) found in 1 dL (100 ml) of whole blood. Hgb concentration correlates closely with RBC count. The he-

moglobin test measures the severity of anemia or polycythemia.

Hemoglobin and hematocrit values are increased in cyanotic heart disease and may be lowered in congestive heart disease. Polycythemia, an increase in red blood cells, is a compensatory reaction of the body to aid in the circulation of the unoxygenated blood caused by cyanotic heart disease. Polycythemia can cause clotting disorders because it increases viscosity of blood. Conversely, polycythemia decreases platelet aggregation, thus predisposing a severely cyanotic child to bleeding disorders.[19]

Erythrocyte sedimentation rate (ESR) measures the time required for erythrocytes in a sample of whole blood

TABLE 40-3
Description of Heart Murmurs

Finding	Description
Timing	
Systolic	Heard with first heart sound (S₁)
	Early, mid, or late systolic murmur
Throughout systole	Pansystolic or holosystolic murmur
Diastolic	Heard with second heart sound (S₂)
	Early, mid, or late diastolic murmur
Late diastolic	Called presystolic
Location of maximum intensity	Described in terms of intercostal interspace and relation to sternum (right, upper mid, or lower sternal border, midclavicular, or axillary line)
Radiation or transmission from point of maximum intensity	Other areas where murmur is heard from the point of maximum intensity
Intensity	
Grade 1	Very faint; usually normal but may be abnormal
Grade 2	Quiet but audible with stethoscope; normal or abnormal
Grade 3	Moderately loud, usually abnormal
Grade 4	Loud; associated with a thrill; abnormal
Grade 5	Very loud, may be heard with stethoscope barely on chest; associated with thrill; abnormal
Grade 6	May be heard with stethoscope off chest; associated with thrill; abnormal
Pitch	High, medium, or low sounds
Quality	Blowing, rumbling, harsh, or musical sounds

to settle to the bottom in a vertical tube. ESR is a sensitive nonspecific test that is frequently the earliest indicator of disease. It is used to monitor inflammatory or malignant disease and to aid in the detection of myocarditis, endocarditis, rheumatoid heart disease, and Kawasaki disease.[19] For any suspected infectious process of the cardiovascular system, *blood cultures* are usually obtained.

Hemostasis is the process in which the body protects the circulatory system from blood loss. If hemostasis is altered, blood tests such as bleeding time, platelet count, clotting time, and prothrombin time (protime) are ordered to assess the body's ability to clot and produce blood cells. (See Unit 10 for more information on hematologic function.)

Arterial Blood Gases. Analysis of blood gases (ABGs) are performed on a sample of blood drawn from a percutaneous arterial puncture or from an arterial line. Blood pH and the partial pressures of oxygen (PaO_2) and carbon dioxide ($PaCO_2$) are measured. ABGs demonstrate the efficiency of pulmonary gas exchange, determine the acid–base level of blood, assist in monitoring for cardiac disorders and the efficiency of the cardiac pump, and, if mechanical respiratory control systems are in use, assess the ventilatory setting.

PaO_2 values indicate how much oxygen the lungs are delivering to the blood; $PaCO_2$ values indicate how effi-

ciently the lungs eliminate carbon dioxide; and pH indicates the acid–base level of the blood. Table 40-5 gives normal values for blood gases in children. In children with cyanotic congenital heart disease (CHD) an increase in FiO_2 (delivered oxygen) does not significantly increase the child's PaO_2.

Procedures

The diagnostic procedures used to evaluate cardiovascular system problems in children include the chest x-ray, electrocardiogram, echocardiogram, cardiac catheterization, and magnetic resonance imaging.

Chest Roentgenogram (Chest X-Ray)

Description/Definition

Radiographic test used for evaluating cardiovascular problems and pulmonary vasculature. In a routine chest x-ray, posterior–anterior view and left lateral views are obtained. The chest x-ray provides images of the thorax, mediastinum, heart, and lungs.

Purpose

To provide information regarding (1) cardiac size, shape, and position; (2) enlargement of cardiac chambers; (3) pulmonary blood flow and pulmonary vascular markings; (4) status of lung parenchyma and presence of vascular or bony abnormalities; (5) position of catheters and pacemaker wires.

Indications

Suspected cardiac problems.

Contraindications

First trimester of pregnancy.

(Protective lead shields or apron should be worn by health personnel to decrease exposure to radiation.)

Preparation

Nurse should explain procedure to child and family, including purpose, how it is performed, and why the results are important. The nurse should allay fears about radiation exposure and familiarize the child with equipment. Explanations that there is no physical pain or discomfort during administration of test and that the child must be still are beneficial.

Developmental Considerations

- Infant: Positioning and soft restraints may be necessary.
- Child: Positioning for comfort; positive reinforcement.
- Adolescent: As for child; may use in-depth, clear explanations.

Nursing Care

Supportive care to child and family.

Complications

None.

Electrocardiography

Description/Definition

Electrocardiogram (ECG) is a recording of the electrical forces of the heart. The ECG records the conduction, magnitude, and duration of the electrical activities of the heart (see Chap. 39).

TABLE 40-4
Blood Indices of Cardiovascular Function

Test		Normal Range*		Deviation	Clinical Importance
		%	(Mean −2 SD)		
Hematocrit (ml/100 ml)	*Infant:*			High	Neontal heart failure
	1 day	51	(42)		Cyanotic heart disease
	1 mo	44	†(33)		
	6 mo–2 y	36	†(33)		Polycythemia
	Child:				
	2–6 y	37	(34)	Low	Anemia
	6–12 y	40	(35)		Heart failure
	Adolescent:				
	12–18 y				
	Male	43	(36)		
	Female	41	(37)		
Hemoglobin (g/100 ml)	*Infant:*	16.5	(13.5)	High	Cyanotic heart disease
	1 day	13.9	(10.7)		
	1 mo	12.0	(10.5)		Polycythemia
	6 mo–2 y				
	Child:			Low	Bacterial endocarditis
	2–6 y	12.5	(11.5)		
	6–12 y	13.5	(11.5)		
	Adolescent:				
	12–18 y				
	Male	14.5	(13.0)		
	Female	14.0	(11.5)		
Erythrocyte sedimentation rate (mm/h)	*Newborn:*			Increased	Acute rheumatic fever
	Child:	0–4			Acute myocardial infection
	Adolescent:	4–20			Transplant rejection
	Male:	0–10			
	Female:	0–20		Decreased	Congestive heart failure
					Polycythemia
					Renal failure with heart failure

* Norms taken from Groono, M. G. (1991). *The Harriet Lane handbook* (12th ed.). St Louis: Mosby.

Different types of ECG include exercise ECG and ambulatory (Holter) electrocardiograms. Exercise ECGs measure cardiovascular effects of controlled physical stress (treadmill walking or stationary bike riding). Ambulatory ECGs record the events of the heart's electrical activity for 24 hours or longer while the child performs usual activities and experiences.

Purpose

To provide information regarding (1) heart rate; (2) abnormal rhythms (dysrhythmias); (3) chamber size, myocardial strain; (4) the relative position of the heart; (5) indications of myocardial ischemia; (6) evaluations of artificial pacemaker and cardiotonic drugs.

Indications

Suspected cardiovascular problems with rate or rhythm abnormalities, enlarged cardiac size or displacement, myocardial ischemia, or evaluation of therapies.

Contraindications

None.

Preparation

Explain to child and family that the ECG test is conducted by either a trained technician or a registered nurse. ECGs are painless and easy to administer. Explain that electrodes with jelly are placed on child's skin; jelly may feel sticky. The electrodes transmit electrical impulses of the heart to the ECG machine, and the test takes 5 to 10 minutes. Preparation of the child should focus on decreasing fears and promoting cooperation.

Developmental Considerations

- Infant: Parent may be allowed to hold child quietly.
- Child: Generally cooperate with instruction to sit still.
- Adolescent: Privacy needs to be assured.

Nursing Care

Educational and emotional care.

Complications

None.

TABLE 40-5
Arterial Blood Gases in Children

Finding	Normal Range*	Deviation	Clinical Interpretation
pH	Neonate: 7.32–7.42	Low	Acidosis due to congestive heart failure or shock respiratory failure
	Child: 7.35–7.45	High	Alkalosis
pCO₂	Infant: 30–40 mmHg	Low	Metabolic acidosis (compensated) or respiratory alkalosis
	Child: 35-45 mmHg	High	Metabolic alkalosis (compensated) or respiratory acidosis
HCO₃	Infant: 20–26 mEq/L	Low	Metabolic acidosis or respiratory alkalosis (compensated)
	Child: 22–28 mEq/L	High	Metabolic alkalosis or respiratory acidosis (compensated)
pO₂	Infant: 60–80 mmHg	Low	Hypoxemia
	Child: 80–100 mmHg	High	O₂ therapy

* Values taken from Hazinski, M. F. (1992). *Nursing care of the critically ill child* (2nd ed.). St. Louis: Mosby.

Echocardiography

Description/Definition

Echocardiography is a noninvasive diagnostic test that provides data on cardiovascular structures and functions. Echocardiograms are the reflection of ultra-high frequency sound waves that are passed through the chest wall and heart. The sound waves are either reflected from tissue or absorbed and passed through to different layers in the chest cavity. The ultrasonic impulses are sent to a recorder and visualized on a video screen; permanent videotapes may be obtained.

The most common techniques are motion-mode (M-mode) and two-dimensional (cross-section). M-mode is a graphic recording of motion of the cardiac structure along with the ECG. A single ultrasound beam strikes the heart, producing a vertical view of cardiac structures. This M-mode provides important information on the chamber dimensions, wall thickness, and left ventricular function parameters. Information on valve motion and the detection of pericardial effusions may also be recorded.

In two-dimensional echocardiography (2DE), the ultrasound beam rapidly sweeps a spatial orientation of the great veins, atria, ventricles, valve, and great arteries. It provides a cross-sectional or fan-shaped view of cardiac structures.

Three monitor leads are placed on the child's chest (as if child was having an ECG). A water-soluble gel is applied to the end of the transducer and to the child's skin and chest area. The small transducer is passed smoothly back and forth over the chest wall and angled in various planes to record the patterns made by tissue and fluid in the chest.[17]

Purpose

To diagnose and evaluate congenital heart defects; to measure the chambers of the heart; to diagnose hypertrophic cardiomyopathies; to detect tumors, thrombi, and vegetations; to evaluate cardiac function; to detect pericardial effusions.

Indications

Child suspected of cardiovascular dysfunction.

Contraindications

None.

Preparation

Explain to the child and family the purpose of the test. Explain that the test takes 30 to 60 minutes and that the room may be darkened slightly to aid visualization. Reassure the child that it is safe and painless and that lying still is essential. Explain that the child may feel a slight vibrating sensation or "tickle" as the transducer is moved along the chest and that the child will be able to watch heart beat on television screen.

Developmental Considerations

Same as for chest x-ray and ECG.

Nursing Care

- Educational and emotional care.
- Sedation is only necessary for children who are unable to hold still. The child is positioned in a supine or left side-lying position in bed or on a stretcher.
- The child may be asked to sit up.

Complications

None.

Cardiac Catheterization

Description/Definition

Despite the tremendous advances in noninvasive diagnostic tests for congenital heart defects, cardiac catheterization and angiography remain important diagnostic tools to obtain certain detailed information about a cardiac defect and its hemodynamics. Electrophysiologic data also may be obtained in some cases. Interventional catheterization is used for treating selected defects that otherwise would need surgical intervention (see Chapter 44 for Interventional Catheterization discussion).

Cardiac catheterization refers to the insertion of a radiopaque catheter through an artery or vein into the heart. Fluoroscopy is used to monitor the location and movement of the catheter. Catheterization provides pressure measurements within the heart chambers and great vessels. Altered pressure measurements often indicate conditions that involve obstruction to blood flow to certain areas of the heart or great vessels. Oxygen saturations help identify the presence and proportion of shunting within the heart or in the vascular systems. Other measurements such as cardiac output also are obtained.

Angiocardiography is included in the cardiac catheterization procedure. This process involves injecting contrast material into the heart through the catheter to view the anatomy of the heart and surrounding vessels. The pictures obtained are known as cineangiograms (cine). Digital subtraction angiography is a more recent, sophisticated technique in which part of the cine can be subtracted from the entire picture to better visualize one specific part.

Cardiac catheterization is performed in a catheterization laboratory in which specialized radiographic equipment is located. In addition, monitors, oxygen, neonatal thermoregulating equipment, and other emergency supplies are available.

In the infant and neonate, catheterization is performed via the right or left femoral artery and vein; umbilical vessels may be used in the neonate. In the older child, the antecubital fossa sometimes is used as an alternative to the femoral access. Percutaneous puncture or cutdown is used to access the vein or artery.

Prior to catheterization, the access site is cleansed and draped. Following the administration of local anesthesia, a catheter is inserted into the vessel and passed to the heart; the catheter enters the right

TABLE 40-6
Selected Nursing Diagnoses Associated With Altered Cardiovascular Function

Data Analysis and Conclusion	Nursing Diagnosis
Health Perception and Health Management	
Below growth curve for height, weight, head circumference; loss of weight, failure to thrive; inability to suck or feed well; increased emesis; medications that decrease appetite; decreased interpersonal contacts due to hospitalization; no stimulation from primary caregiver because of long hospitalization	Altered Growth and Development related to cardiovascular condition, lack of nutrition, medication, knowledge deficit of primary caregiver, hospitalization, or separation from primary caregiver
Nutrition and Metabolism	
Report of increased sweating, edema, increased respirations; increased weight; diuretic therapy; abnormal electrolyte panel	Fluid Volume Excess related to congestive heart failure, electrolyte imbalance, or decreased cardiac output
Activity and Exercise	
Abnormal/irregular heart rate; poor peripheral pulses; poor capillary filling time; signs of pulmonary edema (tachypnea, dyspnea, tachycardia, increased temperature, extreme irritability, color mottled, pale); fatigue and restlessness; parent reports child ''is tired, not able to keep up with others, takes long naps, turns blue with activity''	Decreased Cardiac Output related to poor cardiac function, dysrhythmias, increased or decreased fluid volume
Rapid respirations, dyspnea, tachypnea; retractions; nasal flaring; cyanosis (mucous membranes, sclera, central, circumoral); abnormal ABGs; clubbing of fingers; abnormal breath sounds	Impaired Gas Exchange related to decreased tissue perfusion secondary to pulmonary edema or cyanotic heart disease
Sleep and Rest	
Wakes frequently through night; sleeps upright or at 45-degree angle; reports of nightmares, insomnia; unable to stay awake at school; stress due to hospitalization and need for cardiac diagnostic procedures	Sleep Pattern Disturbance related to fear and anxiety, interrupted sleep, respiratory discomfort, or hospitalization
Self-Perception and Self-Concept	
Reports of obsessive, compulsive behaviors; aggressive behavior with caregivers; increased pulse, BP, palpitations	Fear related to loss of body function, invasive cardiac procedure (catheterization), or surgery
	Altered body image related to decreased size and decreased activity
Role Relationship	
Child born with congenital heart defect; parent expresses concerns about role; prolonged hospitalization of infant; parent expresses concern about care of other children at home	High Risk for Altered Parenting related to birth of child with CHD, home care of other children, role changes

heart from a venous access and the left heart (via aorta) from an arterial access. Usually the vein is entered first; the catheter enters the right heart from the inferior vena cava and passes consecutively into the right atrium, the right ventricle, and the pulmonary artery.

After the right-sided structures are evaluated, the catheter can be pulled back into the right atrium and passed across a septal defect or the patent foramen ovale into the left atrium. The foramen ovale remains probe patent in 25% of the adolescent population. The catheter also may enter the left atrium from the right heart by means of a septal puncture. From the left atrium, the catheter may be passed into the left ventricle and then, if necessary, into the aorta. If passage across the septal wall is not possible, the artery may be cannulated and the left side of the heart entered from the aorta.

Intravenous heparin may be administered to prevent clotting and embolic phenomenon. At the end of the procedure, protamine often is given to reverse the anticoagulant effects of heparin.

When the cardiologist has completed these measurements, the angiograms are taken. These help identify any anatomical defects or shunting of blood as a result of the specific heart defect. The radiopaque contrast material used for obtaining angiograms has been associated with several side effects such as hot flushes, dysrhythmias, headache, restlessness, nausea, and other allergic reactions (Lloyd-

Jones, 1986). These symptoms are rarely life-threatening and are usually transient. New solutions with fewer side effects have been developed recently and are being used.

An electrophysiologic study may be performed as part of a catheterization to evaluate a child's conduction system. This type of study is particularly useful in children with dysrhythmias. Catheters with tiny electrodes are used to record directly the heart's electrical impulses and to stimulate the conduction system.

When the catheter is removed, direct pressure is applied to the site for at least 10 minutes to prevent bleeding. The test usually takes from 1 to 3 hours to perform, depending on the ease of venous/arterial access and the amount of information that needs to be gathered. Abdominal and chest x-rays often are taken after the procedure to demonstrate renal anatomy and rule out other lesions or detect any perforation of the vessels entered during the catheterization.

Purpose

To provide information regarding one or more the following areas:

- Pressure, flows, and resistance in the systemic and pulmonic circulations.

- Oxygen content, saturation, and tension.
- Structure defects (e.g., septal and valvular abnormalities, shunts).
- Coronary arteries and great vessels.
- Myocardial function.
- Electrophysiology.

Indications

Suspected cardiovascular problems.

Contraindications

- Coagulopathy
- Poor renal function

Preparation

After determining what the patient/family already knows about the catheterization, the nurse should explain the purpose of the test, using age-appropriate teaching methods for the child. Both emotional and physical care are described. It is important to allow time for the child and his family to discuss the information provided and to ask questions. The nurse must be aware of the child's and parents' anxiety resulting from the condition and anticipated catheterization. Frequently the parents are not sure of the diagnosis or treatment plan until after the catheterization. These uncertainties increase their anxiety.

Development Considerations

- Infant:
  - Precatheterization teaching focuses on parents.
- Toddler:
  - Alleviation of separation anxiety.
  - Favorite toy to cath lab.
  - Support, comfort measures.
- Preschool:
  - Coloring book with pictures of procedure.
  - Play therapy—IV equipment, dolls.
  - Tour of lab.
  - Favorite toy to lab.
  - Distraction techniques during procedure if awake.
- School-age:
  - Give simple, clear explanations with pictures of procedure.
  - Play therapy (for young school-age children).
  - Tour of lab.
  - Distraction techniques during procedure if awake.
- Adolescent:
  - Clear, thorough explanations.
  - Tour of lab.
  - Ensure privacy.
  - Headphones/music during procedure.

Precatheterization Nursing Care

- NPO—usually 4 hours prior to procedure (length of time may vary with age of patient).
- Nursing assessment; documentation of precatheterization vital signs and hypersensitivities, height, and weight.
- Surgical prep (shave and scrub) as needed.
- Signed consent.
- Play therapy with nurse or child life specialist to mimic selected aspects of catheterization procedure (e.g., administration of sedation, IV insertion).
- Tour of catheterization laboratory.
- Sedation administration.
- Positioning patient (i.e., supine, restraints as needed).
- EKG monitoring.
- IV insertion as needed.

Additional Precatheterization Care

- Medical history and physical.
- Pre-anesthesia visit (optional).
- CXR, EKG, echocardiogram if not performed recently.

- CBC and urinalysis if not performed recently; type and cross-match may be needed for infants.
- Discontinuation of anticoagulant therapy.

Postcatheterization Nursing Care

- Postcath care is based on the possible complications of cardiac catheterization. Monitor vital signs q 15 minutes × 1 hr then q 1 hr (avoid measuring blood pressure on affected extremity). Position affected extremity straight to decrease risk of bleeding.
- Observe pressure dressing covering site of catheter insertion for blood loss/hematoma; if bleeding occurs, apply direct continuous pressure to the site.
- Check quality of pulses distal to the catheterization site (compare left and right side for symmetry).
- Record color, perfusion, capillary filling, warmth of affected extremity.
- Ensure adequate urine output.
- Resume oral intake gradually; encourage fluids when child is able to take fluids successfully.
- Remove pressure bandage as ordered and replace with BandAid.
- Provide age appropriate diversional activity for child that is awake.
- Give discharge instructions.
- The child is discharged when fully recovered from the procedure. The child should be eating a regular diet, maintaining adequate intake and output, and able to ambulate. It is also important that the family understand postcatheterization care. Written and verbal instructions are given to the family:
  - Resume regular activity.
  - Report fever over 100°F oral/101°F rectal.
  - Report increased redness, swelling, drainage from site.
  - Change BandAid at groin as necessary for infants with soiled diapers.
- The family and child must have a clear understanding of the findings of the catheterization, the treatment options, and the recommendations for further intervention (i.e., surgery, medication)

Complications

- Thrombophlebitis
- Pulmonary embolism
- Vagal nerve response
- Bleeding, hematoma, hemorrhage
- Arterial embolus/obstruction
- Dye reaction
- Infection
- Cardiac tamponade
- Dysrhythmias
- Cerebrovascular accident
- Cardiac perforation
- Hypoxemia
- Altered renal perfusion (due to metabolism of contrast media)

Magnetic Resonance Imaging

Description/Definition

Magnetic resonance imaging (MRI) is a diagnostic modality that uses two forms of energy: radio and magnetism. MRI is based on magnetic fields and a computer that produces images. A magnetic field surrounds the child and causes hydrogen ions in the body to line up in a certain fashion. When the ions move back to their original position, a signal is released and processed by the computer. MRI is a noninvasive procedure and has tremendous potential for evaluation of the cardiovascular system. MRI can identify the heart and vessels in sharp contrast and can identify the anatomic aberrations of many congenital heart defects.[15]

Purpose

To provide information regarding (1) cardiovascular anatomy; (2) diagnostic information on many congenital heart defects; (3) tumors, postoperative evaluation, blood clots, cardiomyopathies, infections.

Indications

Suspected cardiovascular problems.

Contraindications

None.

Preparation

Nurse should explain MRI and reassure child that there is no discomfort or pain but that the child must be completely still during the test. Infants and small children require sedation to ensure stillness and are restricted to clear liquids for 4 hours before the examination. Children are encouraged to go to the toilet before the test starts. Most physicians routinely sedate young children with oral medications to ensure that the child lies still throughout the procedure.

Techniques for monitoring the child during the examination must be altered because normal monitoring equipment cannot be used if it contains metal. The metal can interfere, alter, or distort the magnetic field and decrease the quality of the image. Blood pressure cuffs are replaced with plastic connectors, and ECG tracings can be obtained with nonferrous electrodes. Respirations are monitored with a pneumatic tube. As MRI technology advances, other monitoring devices will be developed.

Developmental Considerations

- Infant:
  - Safety restraints.
  - Clear liquid 4 hours before test.
  - Sedation.
- Toddler:
  - Sedation as needed.
  - Safety precautions.
- Child:
  - Thorough explanation.
  - Play therapy.
- Adolescent:
  - Clear explanation.

Nursing Care

Teaching and emotional support.

Complications

None.

Selected Nursing Diagnoses

Once the history is taken and the physical examination is complete, the nurse critically studies the information that was obtained. Analysis of the comprehensive database yields nursing diagnoses, statements that describe the child's response to the cardiovascular problem.[5,7] Nursing diagnoses appropriate for the child with cardiovascular dysfunction are used to develop a plan of care. Selected nursing diagnoses that may be appropriate for the child with cardiovascular dysfunction are presented by function in Table 40-6.

Summary

The assessment of a child's cardiovascular status is an important part of the nurse's role. Nurses must be sen-

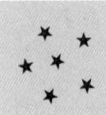

Ideas for Nursing Research

In the assessment and diagnosis of cardiovascular function, the nurse is faced with opportunities to improve the delivery and quality of nursing care. Nursing research is one way to investigate identified problems formally. The following areas need to be explored:

- Design for a pediatric cardiovascular assessment tool for nurses to use in practice.
- Development of standardized nursing diagnoses for the pediatric cardiovascular patient.
- Strategies to decrease child/parental fears related to cardiovascular procedures.
- Preoperative teaching for cardiac procedures/ surgeries in an institution.
- Appropriate teaching materials relevant to the care of the cardiovascular patient (e.g., pacemaker care, feeding issues, CPR).

sitive, understanding, and objective in conducting the interview and in performing the physical examination. Nurses are also responsible for assisting with cardiovascular diagnostic tests, particularly in providing the child and family with accurate information and physical and emotional preparation. Once the assessment is complete, the nurse must analyze the accumulated data and formulate nursing diagnoses. This process demands a sound knowledge base of physiologic and developmental norms in children.

Acknowledgements

Sarah Higgins, R.N., Ph.D.
Cardiology Clinical Nurse Specialist
Department of Pediatric Cardiology
Children's Hospital, Oakland

Elizabeth Cook, R.N., M.S.
Cardiology Clinical Nurse Specialist
Department of Pediatric Cardiology
Children's Hospital, Oakland

The Departments of Pediatric Cardiology and Nursing Education, Children's Hospital, Oakland.

Dedicated In Memory Of

Stanley M. Higashino, M.D. (1930–1991)
Chief of Cardiology
Children's Hospital, Oakland

References

1. Agamalian, B. (1986). Pediatric cardiac catheterization. *Journal of Pediatric Nursing, 1*(2), 73–79.
2. Arciniegas, E. (1985). *Pediatric cardiac surgery*. Chicago: Yearbook Medical.

3. Bates, B. (1991). *A guide to physical examination and history taking,* (5th ed.). Philadelphia: Lippincott.

4. Bavin, R. (1983). Pediatric cardiac preoperative teaching: A family centered approach. *Focus on Critical Care, 10*(3), 36–43.

5. Ulrich, S. P., Canale, S. W., & Wendell, S. A. (1990). *Nursing care planning guides* (2nd ed.). Philadelphia: Saunders.

6. *Cardiovascular care handbook.* (1986). Springhouse, PA: Springhouse.

7. Carpenito, L. J. (1992). *Handbook of nursing diagnoses* (4th ed.). Philadelphia: Lippincott.

8. Doenges, M. E. (1991). *Nurse's pocket guide: Nursing diagnoses with interventions* (3rd ed.). Philadelphia: FA Davis.

9. Fuller, J., & Schaller-Ayers, J. M. (1990). *Health assessment: A nursing approach.* Philadelphia: Lippincott.

10. Gordon, M. (1991). *Manual of nursing diagnosis.* St. Louis: Mosby.

11. Greene, M. G. (1991). *The Harriet Lane handbook* (12th ed.). St. Louis: Mosby.

12. Hazinski, M. F. (1992). *Nursing care of the critically ill child,* (2nd ed.). St Louis: Mosby.

13. Higgins, S. S., & Kashani, I. A. (1984). Congestive heart failure: Parent support and teaching. *Critical Care Nurse,* July/August (4), 21–24.

14. Higgins, S. S., & Kashani, I. A. (1986). The cyanotic child: Heart defects and parental learning needs. *MCN: American Journal of Maternal Child Nursing, 11*(4), 259–262.

15. Higgins, C. B., & Riscak, H. (1987). *Magnetic resonance imaging of the body.* New York: Raven.

16. Kashani, I. A., & Higgins, S. S. (1986). Counseling strategies for families of children with heart disease. *Pediatric Nursing, 12*(1), 38–40.

17. Ludomirsky, A., & Huhta, J. (1987). *Color Doppler of congenital heart disease in the child and adult.* New York: Futuro.

18. Malasanos, L., Barkauskas, V., & Stoltenberg-Allen, K. (1990). *Health assessment* (4th ed.). St. Louis: Mosby.

19. Park, M. K. (1988). *Pediatric cardiology for practitioners* (2nd ed.). Chicago: Yearbook Medical.

20. Perloff, J. K. (1987). *The clinical recognition of congenital heart disease.* Philadelphia: Saunders.

21. Rehm, R. S. (1983). Teaching cardiopulmonary resuscitation to parents. *MCN: American Journal of Maternal Child Nursing, 8,* 414–441.

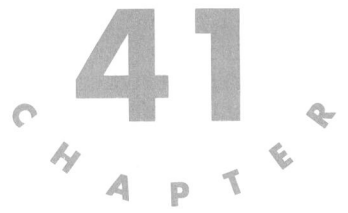

Nursing Planning, Intervention, and Evaluation for Altered Cardiovascular Function

BEHAVIORAL OBJECTIVES

Explain the etiology, pathophysiology, and clinical manifestations of congestive heart failure.

Describe nursing assessments, diagnoses, and interventions typically appropriate for the child with congestive heart failure.

Diagram the flow of blood in the hearts of children who have common congenital heart lesions.

Highlight important components of general nursing care for the child who undergoes interventional cardiac catheterization or open-heart surgery.

Compare the psychosocial needs of the family with a child who has corrective cardiac surgery to those of the family with a child undergoing heart transplantation.

The inherent symbolism of the heart makes the diagnosis of heart disease in children particularly difficult for families. The heart is seen not only as a pump but also as the center of life, love, and feelings. Even a relatively simple, asymptomatic problem may stimulate greater fear and concern than a more life-threatening problem in another part of the body.

Caring for a child with a serious heart condition creates a high level of stress for a family. The threat of death, feelings of guilt or inadequacy, and the treatment regimen can profoundly affect parenting styles and family life. The physical, emotional, social, and financial costs may be enormous for parents and siblings, as well as for the affected child. Nurses who care for children with disorders of the heart are, therefore, challenged to provide not only expert technical care, but also sensitive and effective psychosocial care for the child and family.

1009

The majority of children with heart disease have congenital heart disease (CHD), anatomic abnormalities of the heart structure that occur during fetal development and are present at birth. A number of acquired cardiac conditions also are seen in children. Both congenital and acquired conditions are discussed in this chapter. Because many of the conditions have the potential to cause congestive heart failure (CHF), the chapter opens with a full discussion of this serious complication. Likewise, the chapter includes the care of the child undergoing interventional cardiac catheterization and corrective cardiac surgery because many of the conditions may be treated successfully by these interventions. The chapter closes with a discussion of the care of a child undergoing heart transplantation.

Congestive Heart Failure

Definition and Incidence. CHF is a symptom related to an underlying cardiac etiology; it should not be considered a disease. CHF is characterized by myocardial dysfunction and decreased cardiac output (CO). The heart is unable to sustain a sufficient CO to meet the metabolic demands of the body.[91]

CHF usually develops within the first 3 or 4 months of life in children who have certain congenital heart defects. The incidence of CHF decreases markedly in late infancy. CHF may occur later in childhood following surgical repair of CHD.

Etiology and Pathophysiology. CHF is usually due to an excessive workload placed on a normal myocardium. In the first year of life, CHF is commonly due to congenital heart defects,[91] which commonly result in either a volume or pressure overload on the heart. Volume overload (high preload) occurs when there is an abnormal connection between the systemic and pulmonary circulations. This connection results in a left-to-right shunt and increases pulmonary blood flow. The shunt and increase in pulmonary blood flow cause overcirculation, which makes the heart work harder. Pressure overload (high afterload) occurs when there is an obstruction to pulmonary or systemic blood flow. The result, again, may be overcirculation or an increase in myocardial function to exceed the pressure transmitted by the obstruction.

CHF also may develop in the child with nonstructural conditions that impair cardiac contractility such as myocarditis, ischemia, and endocrine or metabolic disorders. Tachydysrhythmias resulting from drugs, electrolyte imbalances, or any number of causes also can impair cardiac contractility. Other conditions such as anemia, sepsis, obstructive lung disease, and endocrine disorders place high output demands on the heart and are, therefore, possible causes of CHF in children. Finally, CHF may be attributed to surgical correction of a congenital heart lesion due to intraoperative myocardial damage.

CHF may be classified as right-sided or left-sided failure.[5] In right-sided heart failure, the right ventricle functions poorly, causing increased central venous pressure and venous engorgement throughout the body. Increased systemic venous hypertension contributes to enlargement of the liver and peripheral edema. In left-sided

heart failure, function of the left ventricle is suboptimal and contributes to increased pressure in the left atrium and the pulmonary veins. Increased pulmonary pressure occurs and results in pulmonary edema. Infants and young children usually present with biventricular (both right- and left-sided) CHF. Consequently, signs of both systemic and pulmonary venous engorgement are typically observed.

The time of onset of symptoms of CHF may provide a clue to the etiology of the heart anomaly.[91] In infants with congenital heart defects, the onset of symptoms may be related to alterations in hemodynamics as the infant's circulation pattern makes the transition from fetal to mature circulation (see Chap. 39 for a comparison). Cardiac conditions that may be associated with the timing of manifestations of heart failure are presented in Table 41-1.

As CO diminishes, the cardiac muscle hypertrophies and dilates with the additional effort to meet body demands for oxygen. Simultaneously, the inadequate CO, followed by reduced arterial blood pressure, stimulates vascular stretch receptors and baroreceptors in the aorta and carotid arteries, triggering the sympathetic nervous system. Release of catecholamines and stimulation of β-receptors increase the rate and force of myocardial con-

TABLE 41-1
Common Causes of Congestive Heart Failure in Children and the Ages at Which They Generally Occur

Age	Cardiac Anomaly or Condition
Premature infant	Patent ductus arteriosus
Birth to 1 week	Hypoplastic left heart syndrome
	Severe coarctation of the aorta
	Interrupted aortic arch
	Patent ductus arteriosus
	Myocarditis
	Transposition of the great arteries
1 week to 3 months	Ventricular septal defect
	Endocardial cushion defect
	Coarctation of the aorta
	Truncus arteriosus
	Supraventricular tachycardia
	Critical aortic stenosis
	Total anomalous pulmonary venous return
	Anomalous left coronary artery from pulmonary artery
3 months to 1 year	Tricuspid atresia
	Endocardial cushion defect
	Single ventricle
	Large ventricular septal defect
	Large patent ductus arteriosus
	Total anomalous pulmonary venous return
Over 1 year	Endocarditis
	Myocarditis
	Rheumatic fever
	Cardiomyopathy

(Adapted from Park, M. K. (1988). *Pediatric cardiology for practitioners* (2nd ed., p. 310). Chicago: Year Book Publishers.)

traction. Catecholamines also increase venous tone, thereby facilitating return of the blood to the heart. Circulation to the skin, extremities, splenic bed, and kidneys is diminished in an attempt to improve blood flow to the vital organs (heart, lungs, and brain). Decreased renal blood flow stimulates the release of renin, angiotensin, and aldosterone, causing retention of water and sodium and contributing to the development of hypervolemia. Increased blood volume contributes to increased left and right ventricular end-diastolic pressure, resulting in pulmonary and systemic venous engorgement. Sympathetic cholinergic receptors in the skin also may be stimulated.

This complex network of cardiac reserve mechanisms compensates as long as possible to maintain a sufficient CO. Consequently, signs of poor systemic perfusion do not occur until the compensatory mechanisms have been exhausted. The clinical manifestations of CHF are directly linked to the pathophysiologic processes (Fig. 41-1).

Clinical Manifestations. Infants and children with CHF typically appear ill, but signs and symptoms depend on the degree of cardiac reserve available to meet the body's needs.[12 (p.1019)] As compensatory mechanisms fail, hemodynamic changes become evident. Decreased myocardial function, pulmonary congestion, and systemic venous congestion produce classic signs of CHF. The range of possible clinical manifestations exhibited by the body systems is presented in Table 41-2. However, the clinical presentation of individual children may vary, producing clusters of the signs and symptoms.

Initially, decreased CO produces sympathetic nervous system response, which results in preservation of blood flow to vital organs (heart, lungs, and brain) and decreased perfusion to the nonvital organs. Early symptoms of decreased perfusion may be subtle because the compensatory mechanisms are effective initially. Eventually, if CO is severely decreased, a significant reduction in perfusion to all organs occurs.

Generally, tachycardia is an early sign of decreased CO and is an adaptive mechanism to attempt to provide oxygen to poorly perfused tissues.[91 (p.897)] Eventually, when the heart muscle receives reduced flow, ischemic changes occur and contractility is accelerated. Ineffective ejection from the left ventricle results in pulmonary congestion that causes tachypnea, thoracic retractions, nasal flaring, wheezing, crackling sounds upon auscultation, and a chronic, hacking cough. Respiratory effort that is rapid and labored is the most common overt clinical sign of CHF. Infants may have difficulty feeding because of difficulty breathing.

Ineffective ejection from the right ventricle produces systemic congestion. Clinical manifestations of systemic edema are less common in infants and children than adults with severe CHF.[6] In older children, as pulmonary edema increases, arterial oxygen saturation declines, and cyanosis becomes evident. The most consistent symptom

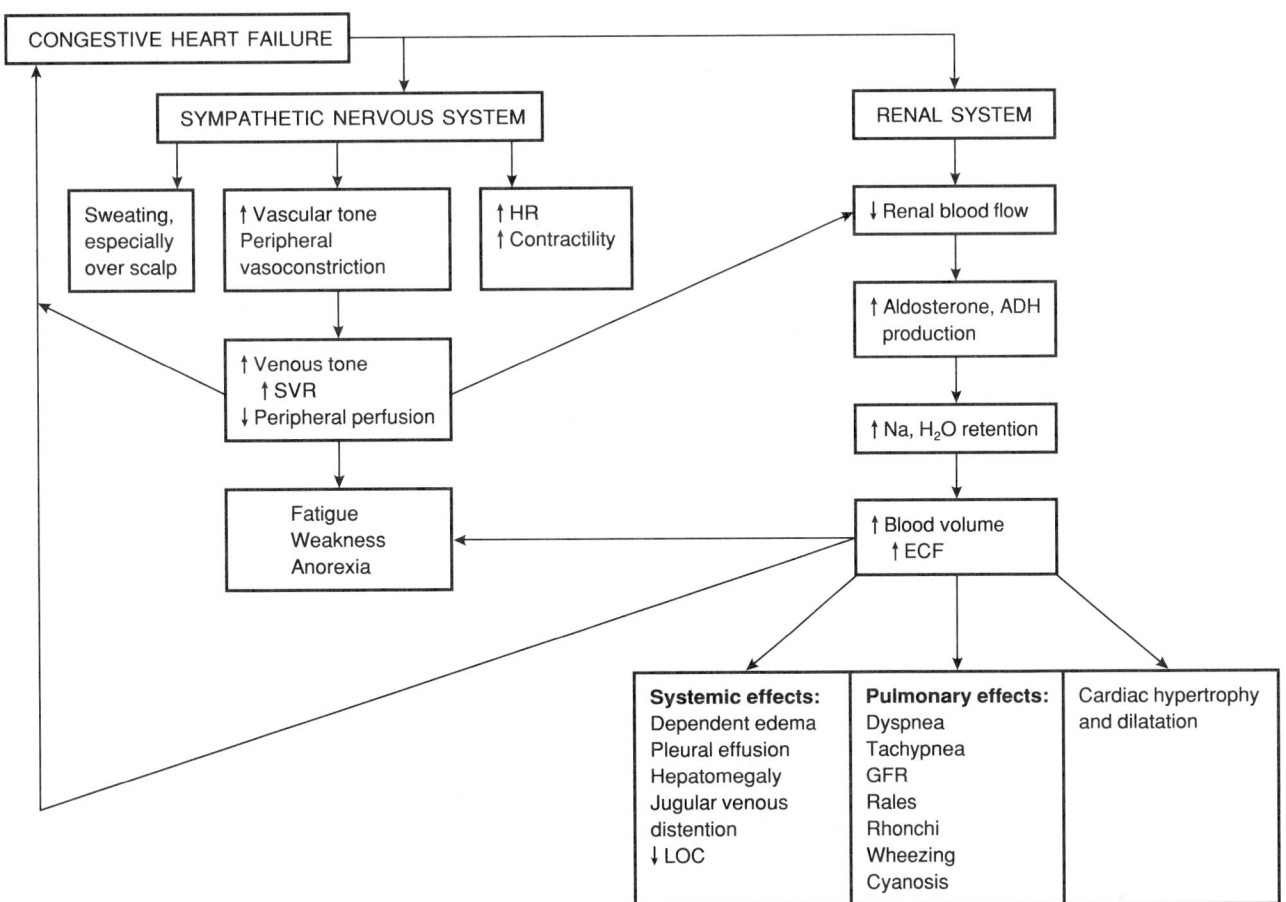

FIGURE 41-1
Pathophysiology of congestive heart failure. (Courtesy of Eleanor Hedenkamp, 1989.)

TABLE 41-2
Clinical Manifestations of Congestive Heart Failure

Body System With Findings	Explanation
Cardiovascular System	
Tachycardia	Compensatory sympathetic nervous system effect causing increased release of adrenal catecholamines in response to decreased cardiac output and diminished lung compliance
Hyperactive precordium and precordial bulge	Associated with forceful myocardial contraction and cardiac enlargement
Thready pulses, narrow pulse pressure	Due to impaired myocardial contractility
Edema (periorbital, rarely have sacral) or ascites	Right ventricular hypertrophy and right-sided failure
Gallop rhythm (extra heart sounds S_3 and S_4)	Due to ventricular dilation and excess preload
Hepatomegaly and splenomegaly	Ventricular hypertrophy and right-sided failure
Respiratory System	
Tachypnea	Pulmonary congestion secondary to increased pulmonary blood flow leading to atelectasis and decreased oxygenation
Intercostal, supra/subcostal retractions, nasal flaring, grunting, and dyspnea	Decreased compliance of the lungs requires greater exertion for ventilation
Rales, cough	Pulmonary edema in the alveolar spaces
Orthopnea	Allows blood to pool in lower extremities; decreases venous return; reduces pressure of abdominal organs on diaphragm
Peripheral Vasculature System	
Pale, cool, mottled skin	Sympathetic vasoconstriction of peripheral vessels creating redistribution of blood flow to major organs such as the brain and heart
Diaphoresis, especially on the scalp	Stimulation of cholinergic fibers; fatigue and poor tolerance for exertion
Gastrointestinal (GI) System	
Slow and poor feedings, poor suck, falls asleep during feedings, tolerates only small amounts of formula	Increased energy consumption during simultaneous eating and breathing
Poor weight gain/growth failure	Decreased caloric consumption, augmenting imbalance between energy requirements and caloric consumption
Formula intolerance, vomiting	Reduced GI perfusion due to preferential distribution of blood to major organs
Abdominal distention	Due to air swallowed with rapid breathing
Central Nervous System	
Lethargy, irritability	Insufficient cardiac output to maintain optimal cerebral blood flow
Decreased muscle tone	Diminished blood flow to musculature and lack of movement
Renal System	
Reduced urine output	Decreased blood flow to the kidneys and reduced glomerular filtration rate
Abnormal weight gain	Related to sodium and water reabsorption or fluid retention (edema)

of systemic congestion is enlargement of the liver.[91] (p.898) Other manifestations include neck vein distention in the older child, periorbital or peripheral dependent edema, and ascites.

Other body systems produce symptomatology that is directly related to the state of decreased perfusion.[88] Cerebral perfusion is maintained at normal levels by compensatory mechanisms during the early stage of decreased CO. Later, the child exhibits restlessness, agitation, and anxiety, and this behavior progresses to confusion and combativeness. Severely decreased cerebral perfusion eventually results in the loss of consciousness. Decreased renal perfusion results in activation of the renin–angiotensin mechanism, which produces sodium and water retention, decreased urinary output with in-

creased urine specific gravity, and, if untreated, anuria and acute tubular necrosis. Decreased gastrointestinal (GI) perfusion causes nausea and vomiting, decreased bowel sounds and activity, and potentially paralytic ileus or necrotizing enterocolitis. Decreased perfusion to the skin results in pallor or cyanosis, mottling, diaphoresis, decreased temperature and pulses, and, eventually, necrotic changes. Decreased perfusion to the hepatic system causes decreased hepatic metabolic function. Decreased perfusion to the musculoskeletal system produces weakness and fatigue.

Diagnostic Studies. There is no single diagnostic test for CHF.[54] (p.8) A chest x-ray that demonstrates cardiomegaly may be indicative of CHF. The location and configuration of the heart and pulmonary vasculature also may be evaluated with the chest x-ray. Ventricular hypertrophy and conduction anomalies may be diagnosed through an electrocardiogram (ECG). An echocardiogram may show chamber enlargement, valve competency, and impaired myocardial functioning. Blood studies may be desired to assess electrolytes, glucose, blood gases, and counts of the blood components. Cardiac catheterization may be used to define the specific defect and its hemodynamic effect. In most cases, however, the diagnosis of CHF is made on the basis of the history and observation of the clinical manifestations.

★ ASSESSMENT

Obtaining a detailed history of the child and family is essential, and it should include observations indicative of long-standing cardiac problems including delay of growth, feeding difficulties, and the presence of frequent respiratory infections. A complete cardiac assessment of the child should include auscultation of the child's chest, pulses, blood pressure in both upper and lower extremities, and other general cardiovascular assessments (described in Chap. 40). Because CHF eventually compromises ventricular output and affects both pulmonary and systemic perfusion, an effective approach for examining the child is to focus on the perfusion parameters (e.g., tachycardia) outlined in Clinical Manifestations. Astute inspection, palpation, and auscultation are essential during this process.

Observation of the child's general appearance is important for recognition of physical changes as well as differences in behavior and mental status. General body size, weight, and development are compared to expected norms for age. The child's response to activity is noted. Cutaneous findings that may be observed include color, diaphoresis, and the presence of edema in the face or extremities. Further inspection may reveal distention of neck veins, respiratory distress, the presence of a hyperactive or bulging precordium, and abdominal distention associated with ascites. Restlessness or lethargy, air hunger, and anxiety should be noted. A checklist for characteristics of mental status may be useful and may reveal subtle changes over time.

Vital signs should be carefully assessed. Arterial blood pressure is maintained in *early* cardiac failure; sympathetic neural stimulation of the vasomotor center increases vasomotor tone and heart rate. Assessment of the child in *late* CHF, however, reveals bradycardia, hypotension, and dysrhythmia. As systemic venous engorgement progresses, the central venous blood pressure rises. Peripheral pulses are palpated simultaneously with the apical pulse to detect pulse deficits, and peripheral pulses are palpated simultaneously in the upper and lower extremities to determine any variation in intensity. Peripheral pulses may be bounding or thready depending on the cardiac defect. CO is assessed indirectly by determining skin temperature and capillary refill. The skin is cool and clammy, and the capillary refill time is lengthened in CHF.

The physical examination of the child with CHF is focused on the cardiovascular, respiratory, renal, and GI systems. Auscultation of the heart, chest, and abdomen may reveal subtle or pronounced symptoms, depending on the level of cardiac failure. Palpation of the abdomen may reveal enlargement of the liver. In severe CHF, percussion of the abdomen reveals shifting dullness, and a fluid wave may be elicited if two examiners are present to perform the technique (see Chap. 46). Increase in abdominal girth due to ascites may be tracked accurately by using inked landmarks for the placement of the tape measure. Urinary output and specific gravity should be measured.

Assessment of the emotional and psychosocial status of the child and family is essential if holistic, family-centered nursing care is to be provided. The nurse observes child and family interactions with the health team and with each other. Because many affected children are infants, nursing assessment should focus on parent–infant attachment and family functioning. Parents are at times reluctant to invest too much emotional involvement with a newborn who has a congenital defect as a protective psychological defense against possible loss of the child. Reactions of the older child to the physical manifestations of CHF should also be noted because many are fearful and anxious. The child and family undoubtedly have needs for information and education that should be assessed with sensitivity and care. Adjustment to school should be evaluated. Nurses also need to assess other family stressors such as the care of other children, the need for housing and meals during the child's hospitalization, and financial concerns.

★ NURSING DIAGNOSES AND PLANNING

Based on assessment data from above and Chapter 40, the following nursing diagnoses may apply to the family and child with CHF:

- Activity Intolerance related to tachycardia, tachypnea, dyspnea, and other signs of CHF.
- Anxiety related to dyspnea, tachycardia, discomfort due to CHF, and knowledge deficit about condition, diagnostic studies, and treatment plan.
- High Risk for Ineffective Family Coping related to diagnosis of CHF, hospitalization, and knowledge deficit.
- Fatigue related to tachycardia, tachypnea, dyspnea, feeding problems, and other signs of CHF.
- High Risk for Impaired Skin Integrity related to vulnerability of skin secondary to edema and poor tissue perfusion.
- High Risk for Altered Growth and Development related to growth failure, poor muscle tone, poor feeding, and other signs of CHF.
- High Risk for Infection related to reduced body defenses, debilitated state, and other signs of CHF.
- High Risk for Altered Nutrition: Less Than Body Requirements related to poor feeding, poor growth patterns, poor suck, formula intolerance, fatigue, and other signs of CHF.
- High Risk for Altered Parenting related to poor feeding, poor weight gain, poor muscle tone, and other signs of CHF.
- High Risk for Social Isolation of Parents related to sick infant requiring complex care, frequent hospitalizations, feeding problems, and other problems related to CHF.

The nurse and parents together plan effective care based on the established nursing diagnoses. Several examples of expected outcomes follow:

- The child demonstrates sufficient energy and strength to perform required activities.
- The parents and child use effective coping mechanisms in managing anxiety.
- The parents demonstrate nurturing behavior toward the child.
- The child demonstrates behaviors appropriate to age group.

The nurse plans for the daily care of the child based on both physician's orders and nursing diagnoses. Some general nursing care goals may be the following:

- Corrective surgery is performed successfully.
- Adequate cardiac function is attained and maintained.

★ **INTERVENTIONS: COLLABORATIVE AND INDEPENDENT**

The major goals of therapy for the care of the child with CHF include improving cardiac contractility, decreasing oxygen demands of the body, and removing excess intravascular fluid. The therapy for CHF includes medication therapy, fluid therapy, and comfort measures and thermoregulation.

MEDICATION THERAPY

Digitalization. Due to its rapid onset and decreased risk of toxicity, digoxin is the drug of choice for the treatment of CHF in children. Digoxin increases cardiac contractility and slows the conduction through the atrioventricular (AV) node. The major effect of digoxin is to slow the heart rate while improving the contractility of the heart.

When digoxin is initiated in a child, several doses must be administered over a 24-hour period initially to provide a therapeutic serum digoxin level. A total digitalizing dose is given initially, but this dose is usually administered intravenously in divided doses that are separated by 8 hours.[54] The first dose is typically one half of the digitalizing dose, and the second and third doses are usually one quarter of the dose. When the digitalizing doses are completed, a maintenance dose of digoxin is provided. The maintenance dose is typically one fourth of the total dose used to achieve digitalization, divided equally and given twice a day.

Careful calculation of the dosage of digoxin is vital because toxic levels are possible. Two health professionals should calculate the dose separately, and it should be written in micrograms as well as in the volume of the preparation to be given. For example, 30 μg or 0.6 ml of Lanoxin elixir may be calculated and prepared from supplies that are available as 0.05 mg/ml or 50 μg/ml. General guidelines regarding dosages for children of different ages are provided in Table 41-3.

The child is most often hospitalized during the digitalization process so the heart rhythm can be monitored for therapeutic effects of the medication. Digitalization at home is possible with competent caregivers and medical care close by. Side-effects of digoxin include bradycardia, heart block, premature ventricular contractions,

TABLE 41-3
Usual Digitalizing and Maintenance Dosages With Normal Renal Function Based on Lean Body Weight

Age	Digitalizing Dose* (mcg/kg)		Daily Maintenance Dose (mcg/kg)
	Oral	IV	
Premature	20–30	15–25	20%–30% of the loading dose†
Full term	25–35	20–30	
1–24 months	35–60	30–50	
2–5 years	30–40	25–35	25%–35% of the loading dose†
5–10 years	20–35	15–30	
Over 10 years	10–15	8–12	

* IV digitalizing doses are 80% of oral digitalizing doses.

† Projected or actual digitalizing dose providing desired clinical response.

Gradual digitalization is accomplished by beginning an appropriate maintenance dose. The range of percentages provided above can be used in calculating this dose. Dosage guidelines provided are based upon average patient response; substantial individual variation can be expected.

Infants and children: Individualize dosage. Divided daily dosing is recommended for infants and young children under 10 years of age. Children over 10 require adult dosages in proportion to their body weight. Drug Facts and Comparison, 1992 edition. Facts and Comparisons, Inc., St. Louis, p. 568.

anorexia, nausea, vomiting, and diarrhea. When digitalis toxicity is questioned, a serum digoxin level may be obtained. Nontoxic serum digoxin levels vary from hospital to hospital but typically are in the range of 1.1 to 2.2 ng/dl. Digoxin levels are inaccurate in neonates.

The presence of clinical symptoms of toxicity may be more accurate than the digoxin level in some situations. The incidence of toxicity is more common in preterm infants, because they have a longer serum half-life of digoxin than older children. Hypokalemia, hypercalcemia, and a low serum magnesium level predispose a child to digoxin toxicity.

Assessment of the child's heart rate and potassium level should be performed before digoxin administration, and any irregularity of heart rhythm, rate, or hypokalemia should be reported. Digibind, a specific antidote for digoxin toxicity is available and is recommended for life-threatening toxicity; however, little research is available on this antidote.

Discharge teaching related to digoxin administration should include review of the side-effects, actions, accurate dosage, as well as guidelines for administration of the medication (see the accompanying display). If one dose is forgotten or vomited, the dose should not be repeated. The parent should contact the physician if two consecutive doses of the medication are missed. The family is also instructed to watch for signs of toxicity and to keep the medication out of the reach of children.

The family should always plan ahead and refill the prescription before the digoxin bottle is empty. Teaching the family how to count the child's heart rate is generally unnecessary, but nurses should confirm that parents' knowledge is accurate. The family should never increase or decrease the digoxin dose unless the cardiologist has

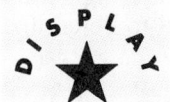

Patient/Parent Teaching: Guidelines for Digoxin Administration

Concept/Problem	What to do	Comments
Missed dose	Give next dose at regular time. Do not make up for missed dose. (If the missed A.M. dose is remembered before 12 noon or the missed P.M. dose is remembered before 12 midnight, it can be given and the regular digoxin schedule resumed.)	If two or more doses are missed in a row, notify your physician.
Vomited dose	Give next dose at regular time. Do not make up for vomited dose.	If two or more doses are vomited in a row, notify your physician.
Overdose or accidental ingestion	Take child immediately to the *nearest* emergency room. Bring the digoxin bottle with remaining medicine with you.	Don't waste time at home trying to make the child vomit. An overdose can be fatal. Digoxin should be stored out of reach of children.

Signs of:
  Anorexia
  Diarrhea
  Vomiting
  Lethargy
  Fever
  Difficulty breathing
	Contact your physician.	These symptoms can be signs of digoxin toxicity or a normal childhood illness that could affect digoxin's effect on the heart. It is important to have the child evaluated to determine the proper course of treatment.

1. Give the medicine at the same time each day, preferably 1 hour before or 2 hours after meals. _____ A.M. _____ P.M.
2. Give the digoxin directly and not mixed with food because the entire dose may not be ingested.
3. Your child's cardiologist is: _____
   Phone: _____

   Pediatric clinical
   nurse specialist: _____
   Phone: _____

The top half of the display is reprinted from Joffe, M. (1987). Pediatric digoxin administration. Dimensions of Critical Care Nursing, 6(3), 143. *Copyright 1987 Hall Johnson Communications, Inc. Reproduced with permission. For further use contact the publisher at 9737 West Ohio Avenue, Lakewood, CO 80226.*

recommended this change. The dose of digoxin is increased as the child continues to grow.

Diuretic therapy. Although digoxin usually improves cardiac contractility and CO sufficiently, diuretic therapy is typically needed to enhance removal of excess intravascular fluid volume. The use of diuretics in children, however, must be considered carefully, and electrolyte values must be assessed closely. An adequate serum concentration of chloride is required for sodium excretion. When the child's serum chloride and potassium levels are low, the excretion of sodium is limited. In turn, there is an increase in renal excretion of hydrogen ions that results in metabolic alkalosis. Consequently, diuretic administration is contraindicated when a child has metabolic alkalosis and low serum chloride or potassium levels. Diuretics should also be avoided or used with caution in a child with hypovolemia and hypotension.

When a diuretic is needed for acute, severe CHF in the ill child, intravenous furosemide (Lasix) is the drug of choice. This diuretic has a rapid onset and encourages the excretion of sodium, chloride, and water. However,

other diuretics such as ethacrynic acid, chlorothiazide, or spironolactone may be given. These medications, their use, and side-effects are summarized in Table 41-4.

The nurse is responsible for documenting the administration of the diuretic and should include time, dosage, and route. When a diuretic is given, accurate measurement of intake and output is necessary to determine effectiveness of the medication; any decrease in urinary response must be reported to the physician.

Serum electrolytes must be determined routinely. Foods high in potassium such as bananas, oranges, and legumes may be encouraged to balance the child's electrolyte status. However, when a high-potassium diet is ineffective, electrolyte replacements such as elixir of potassium chloride may be administered to correct the imbalance. Oral potassium chloride supplements of 1 to 2 mEq/kg/day may be necessary to maintain a normal serum potassium level. The potassium chloride elixir can be mixed in punch or juice to disguise its bitter taste and to avoid the GI irritation that occurs with the medication.

Discharge teaching should include the correct dosage

TABLE 41-4
Diuretics Used for Congestive Heart Failure

Medication and Use	Side-Effects
Furosemide (Lasix)	Electrolyte depletion, especially potassium
IV: To reduce edema rapidly when due to cardiac, hepatic, or renal dysfunction; especially effective for acute congestive heart failure (CHF) and pulmonary edema	Watch for rapidly occurring diuresis that may lead to hypotension and hypovolemia
	May precipitate digoxin toxicity (potassium depleting)
	Transient deafness, tinnitus, vertigo, dizziness
PO: Appropriate for long-term management of hypertension (HTN)	Possible increased ototoxicity with aminoglycosides
Hydrochlorothiazide (Diuril, Esidrix, Hydrodiuril)—carbonic anhydrase inhibitors	Hypokalemia
	Hyperuricemia
CHF and HTN	Hyperglycemia
Spironolactone (Aldactone)—potassium-sparing diuretic	Hyperkalemia
Often used as adjunct to potassium-losing diuretics for edema and HTN	GI upset (anorexia, nausea, vomiting, diarrhea), CNS effects (headache, drowsiness, ataxia, confusion)
	Used with caution in children with renal impairment
Ethacrynic acid (Edecrin)	May cause hypokalemia, cause dehydration, reduced blood volume, tetany and metabolic alkalosis
Renders urine more acidic; diuresis and electrolyte loss more pronounced than with other diuretics. Often effective in patients refractory to other diuretics.	Observe for excessive diuresis
	May need potassium supplement

and administration of the diuretics as well as the side-effects and actions of the medications. Parents should be instructed to call the physician if the child develops any side-effects or if the child has vomiting or diarrhea for an extended period of time. Diuretic therapy may be discontinued during the illness to avoid dehydration, but the family should not discontinue any medication unless they have contacted the physician.

FLUID BALANCE MONITORING

Management of appropriate fluid balance in the child with CHF is an important component of therapy. Strict and accurate measurement and documentation of all the child's intake and output help maintain assessment of fluid status. All diapers or pads exposed to urine must be weighed to calculate urine output accurately. The normal urine output in children is 1.0 to 2.0 ml/kg/h.

All fluid intake must also be calculated and documented on the child's flow record. Intravenous fluids, including flushes or other incidental fluids, must be considered in the total fluid intake. Fluid restriction is not typically required in the infant with CHF, because fluid restriction leads to calorie restriction and the fluid status is typically managed with diuretics. In the older child, CHF is treated with fluid restriction. However, limiting fluid intake in children is difficult. Using small cups or other containers and filling them completely gives the child the illusion of receiving more volume.

Precise measurement of the child's weight at the same time on the same scale each day should be per-

formed to evaluate any weight loss or gain. A significant weight gain or loss must be investigated to determine fluid retention or fluid loss.

NUTRITIONAL MANAGEMENT

Assessment of the child's nutritional status is important; adequate caloric and protein intake is needed to promote growth. Infants with CHF may have difficulty coordinating breathing, sucking, and swallowing. Small, frequent feedings may be tolerated, but nasogastric feedings may be necessary if the child is tachypneic and requires an hour or more to feed 1 to 2 ounces of formula. In severe cases, continuous NG or GT feedings may be given at night and feedings by mouth during waking hours to enhance caloric intake.

Concentrated formula preparations may be necessary when the infant tolerates only small feedings. These formula additives provide adequate calories while permitting the infant to take less fluid/formula. The use of Polycose, Sumacal, MCT (medium chain triglyceride) oil, corn oil, and other supplements in the feeding are beneficial in the long-term care and growth of the infant with moderate to severe CHF and allows the child to gain weight before open-heart surgery.

Feeding the infant with CHF is frustrating for the family and medical team. Vomiting, formula intolerance, slow feeding, and the infant's poor suck intensify the stress of having a child with CHF. The use of a soft nipple, upright feeding position, and frequent rest periods help the infant with CHF tolerate feedings. In addition, small frequent feedings allow the infant rest periods and prevent abdominal distention and vomiting.

Providing education, advice, and support is an important role of the health team when working with parents of children with CHF. Allowing a mother time away from the ill child is important and allows the mother time to do things for herself and enhances coping mechanisms. A teaching pamphlet related to feeding the infant with CHF is also available from the American Heart Association. The intervention of a clinical nurse specialist, lactation consultant (for breast-feeding mothers), or other health team member to assist families with feeding issues can be beneficial.

COMFORT MEASURES

The infant with CHF is typically more comfortable in a semi-Fowler's position, because diaphragmatic movement and lung expansion are improved. The infant breathes much easier, and respiratory distress is relieved. The use of an infant seat helps to support the child and prevents sliding down or off to the side. The use of a therapeutic mattress on the bed and frequent position changes helps to prevent skin breakdown that can occur with poor tissue perfusion and edema accompanying CHF.

The use of cool mist or humidified oxygen may be necessary for the infant in moderate to severe CHF to improve oxygen delivery to the tissues. Oxygen is best administered by way of a noninvasive route such as a tent or oxygen hood. Suctioning of the nasopharynx may be needed to maintain a patent airway.

Morphine sulfate may be administered to some children with severe CHF for its sedative effect and its action in improving pulmonary edema. This narcotic must be used cautiously, however, because it can cause respiratory depression. Chloral hydrate may be used, because it causes little respiratory depression and few side effects.

Organization of the child's care is critical to reduce stress that could potentiate the effects of CHF. Careful planning of procedures to allow frequent rest periods and uninterrupted sleep diminishes strain on the heart, which is already decompensated. However, developmentally appropriate stimulation and planned diversional play activities are crucial for children with CHF.

A neutral thermal environment prevents excessive oxygen consumption and stress in the compromised child. The child's temperature should be maintained around 37° C to prevent excessive oxygen consumption. An external heating device may be needed, and environmental precautions (such as avoiding drafts or placement near cold windows) are needed to prevent heat loss.

PSYCHOSOCIAL SUPPORT

To the family or child, the term congestive heart failure may mean that "the heart is failing or stopping," and their anxiety is heightened. Explaining the diagnosis and treatment plan in clearly understood terms is essential. The anxiety of the family can be minimized by the nurse whose presence and concern are visible to the child and family. Nurses can provide the information about services available in the agency and encourage communication between the family and other members of the health team. A referral to a social worker may be needed to investigate avenues of financial or other assistance for which the family may be eligible. At times, simple considerations such as making provisions for showering or for meals to be served in the child's room can do much to comfort the family and win their trust.

TEACHING

Education regarding CHF including its etiology, pathophysiology, and medical management is important to diminish the family's anxiety and to help them cope with the multiple stressors that affect their lives while the child is ill. If surgical intervention is planned, the family needs information about the procedure and what to expect preoperatively and postoperatively, as well as a clear description of the surgical procedure. A Teaching Plan later in this chapter outlines preoperative teaching. Prognosis and expected long-term outcomes should be discussed. Although the physician is responsible for providing much of this information initially, the nurse has a responsibility to ensure that the family understands it. Most families want to participate in making decisions about the child's care, but they need adequate information and time to provide informed consent. The nurse may need to review information more than once and use different teaching strategies before the family comprehends fully what they need to know.

MONITORING OF SIGNS AND SYMPTOMS

The care of the child with moderate to severe CHF is complex and requires a true team approach. The child must be monitored continually for symptoms of an exacerbated condition including continued tachycardia, diminished urinary output, poor peripheral pulses, tach-

ypnea, respiratory distress, and an enlarging liver. Changes in eating patterns and changes in mentation such as lethargy or irritability should be noted. Laboratory studies for glucose, electrolytes, and pH should be analyzed carefully for subtle changes; blood gases should be obtained when metabolic or respiratory status is questionable. Careful documentation of the child's clinical status is required to ensure that medical treatment and nursing care plans are formed on accurate information.

★ EVALUATION

Fortunately, CHF usually resolves after corrective surgery of the underlying congenital heart lesion. Children with inoperable cardiac lesions continue to have worsening heart failure that becomes intractable to medical management. These children may become candidates for cardiac transplantation when their failure can no longer be treated medically.

Congenital Heart Disease

Definition and Incidence. Congenital heart disease (CHD) refers to structural or functional heart anomalies that are present at birth, although symptoms may not be detected until much later.[37] There are more than 40 recognized individual heart defects, and these can occur in innumerable combinations. Several congenital defects that occur in children are described in detail in this chapter.

The specific incidence of CHD is variously reported as between 4 to 10 in every 1000 live births.[37] The wide range of reported incidence can be explained partly by methodology and the lack of consistency in anomalies included in some surveys. Also, some conditions that are common in preterm infants and other conditions that become apparent later in life are not included in the lower rates; the addition of these figures would increase the total incidence. Furthermore, the number of aborted or stillborn infants with CHD is thought to be significant, and, if estimates of occurrence in this population were included, the reported incidence of CHD would be even greater.

Etiology and Pathophysiology. Few specific causes of CHD have been identified.[71] Environmental factors including radiation, pollution, chemicals, viruses such as rubella, and certain drugs have been implicated. Maternal factors thought to affect the fetus include age over 40, insulin-dependent diabetes, alcoholism, and drug use. Heredity does not appear to be a significant contributing factor. However, the incidence may increase slightly if a parent has a diagnosis of CHD or has another child with a heart anomaly. CHD is closely associated with a number of syndromes including Down, Turner, and others. The vast majority of cases, however, are attributed to multifactorial (genetic–environmental interaction) causes, not to any single influence,[71] and other congenital defects are likely to be present.

Blood normally flows from one area of the body to another as a result of the pumping action of the heart and pressure differentiation, following the path of least resistance from high to low pressure (see Chap. 39). Defects that allow blood to flow from the high pressure in the left side of the heart to the low pressure in the right side result in increased pulmonary blood flow and CHF. Other defects cause decreased pulmonary blood flow and result in cyanosis. Some defects are indefinite or complex, presenting wide variation in the degree of cyanosis and amount of pulmonary blood flow.

Congenital cardiac anomalies may be classified in various ways. The traditional method is to group conditions on the presence or absence of cyanosis.[11] (p.32) Although these categories are useful, they imply that the clinical manifestations of the anomalies are distinct. It should be noted, however, that children with acyanotic defects may eventually develop cyanosis, and children who have what are known as cyanotic defects at times have normal skin coloring. This variation in clinical manifestations is a result of the complexity of some defects and individual physiologic response to the problems.

To provide additional description, congenital cardiac anomalies are further categorized into hemodynamic characteristics describing the flow of blood to the lungs: either increased or decreased pulmonary blood flow. Variations in the pattern of pulmonary blood flow occur when blood is shunted through abnormal openings in the heart walls or between the major vessels, or when the normal flow of blood is obstructed.

Clinical Manifestations. Clinical manifestations of the anomalies vary greatly depending on the hemodynamic effects of the lesion. Signs and symptoms commonly associated with each of the major congenital heart anomalies are described below. In general, the two major clinical findings in the infant with CHD are cyanosis and CHF.[54]

The cyanosis associated with CHD is caused by hypoxia and, if not treated, can lead to acidosis and death. Blueness of the mucous membranes, nailbeds, and skin is indicative of systemic hypoxia. Clinical cyanosis is hardly visible until arterial saturation is around 85% and then only if the hematocrit is high. If the hematocrit is low, arterial saturation may be even lower before cyanosis is clearly visible.[6]

Interventions. Fortunately, the options and opportunities available for children diagnosed with CHD are dramatically changing. Little more than 30 years ago, a diagnosis of CHD was a death sentence for most children, because heart disease can affect every other body system adversely. Medical management with medication and palliative procedures and treatments, then as now, offered only a chance at stabilization and extended life. There were few surgical options, and they were seen as major and technically challenging procedures. Advances in closed-heart surgery began and continued in the third and fourth decades of this century, but the 1950s were highlighted by the development and successful use of a cardiopulmonary bypass (CPB) machine. Each following decade has seen dramatic progress and hope offered in the repair of increasingly complex lesions, culminating with the advent of heart and heart–lung transplantation in children. Of children hospitalized for CHD during infancy, over half require surgery before the end of their

first year.[6] The nursing care required for children with cardiac surgery is presented after a discussion of the various defects. A sample Nursing Care Plan is outlined under the section on Ventricular Septal Defect.

Acyanotic Congenital Heart Defects With Normal or Decreased Pulmonary Blood Flow

The defects placed in this category are known as obstructive lesions because they cause some degree of impairment to the flow of blood either within the heart or within the great vessels. This group of anomalies includes those that fail to cause cyanosis even in the presence of decreased pulmonary blood flow, because no desaturated blood is in the systemic circuit. However, when the anomaly is severe and compensatory mechanisms fail, cyanosis may eventually develop.

In this group of cardiac lesions, blood follows the normal circulatory pathway, unless another defect is also present. The most common obstructive lesions are pulmonary stenosis, aortic stenosis, and coarctation of the aorta (COA). After a general discussion of etiology and pathophysiology, the definition, the incidence, clinical manifestations, and general interventions are described for each defect.

Stenosis is the narrowing of a particular heart structure or blood vessel that impairs the flow of blood. As the heart is developing in utero with the stenosis, normal blood flow is usually reduced proportionate to the degree of narrowing. Those structures that receive diminished blood supply are often hypoplastic (underdeveloped) at birth. Restoring normal blood flow in the heart with surgery can stimulate growth, often to near-normal size.

The hemodynamic effects depend on the severity of the lesion, and the degree of obstruction is described as mild, moderate, or severe. In mild cases, few hemodynamic effects are noticed. When the affected areas are completely occluded or missing (atresia), structures proximal to the defect become overworked and dysfunctional. Distal structures are often dilated secondary to the jetstreaming of blood through the stenotic area. As CO decreases, perfusion beyond the stenosis is significantly reduced. Severe stenosis is a life-threatening condition in the newborn, and immediate intervention is needed.

Pulmonary Stenosis

Definition and Incidence. Pulmonary stenosis is a narrowing of the right ventricular outflow tract. The narrowing may occur in the infundibulum (the widened space leading to the pulmonary artery), below the pulmonary valve, in the valve, or in the main or branch pulmonary arteries. The most common lesion is valvular stenosis in which the cusps of the pulmonary valve are thick and form a domelike obstruction during systole,[12] as shown in Figure 41-2. Pulmonary stenosis occurs in 5% to 8% of all congenital heart defects, and many have associated cardiac lesions.[8] (p.79)

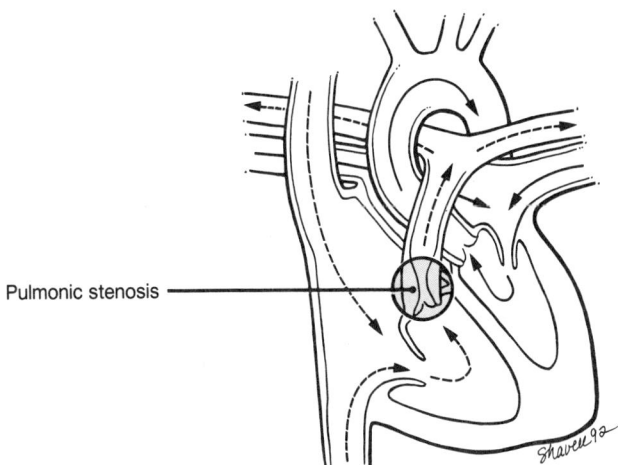

FIGURE 41-2
In pulmonary stenosis, the right ventricular outflow tract narrows.

Clinical Manifestations.   The signs and symptoms of pulmonary stenosis vary greatly depending on the severity of the narrowing. A systolic murmur is typically heard over the pulmonic area at the upper left sternal border, and a thrill is present if the stenosis is severe. When present at birth, a severe pulmonary stenosis may cause no symptoms as long as the ductus arteriosus remains patent and allows blood flow to the lungs. Once the ductus arteriosus begins to close, the lungs do not receive an adequate flow of blood. The neonate becomes severely hypoxemic and begins to exhibit respiratory distress, cyanosis, and other signs of developing CHF with systemic venous engorgement. In marked contrast, an older child with mild pulmonary stenosis may be asymptomatic, and the pulmonary stenosis is detected only by accident. Children with moderate defects may experience fatigue and dyspnea with exercise or other exertion, because blood flow to the lungs is insufficient to meet increased needs for oxygen.

Diagnostic Studies.   A chest x-ray of the infant or child with pulmonary stenosis demonstrates decreased pulmonary vascular markings, dilation of the main pulmonary artery, and, possibly, right-sided cardiomegaly. The ECG can also be used to document right ventricular hypertrophy. Further evaluation with an echocardiogram can confirm the presence of right atrial and right ventricular hypertrophy and thick pulmonary valve leaflets with decreased mobility. Right ventricular hypertension may be diagnosed with cardiac catheterization.

Interventions.   For infants with severe PS, an infusion of prostaglandin E_1 may be necessary to maintain patency of the ductus arteriosus until further treatment is possible. The prognosis for children with pulmonary stenosis has been greatly improved with the use of balloon angioplasty. In this procedure, a cardiac catheterization is performed (see Chap. 40), and a balloon on the end of the catheter is inflated in the stenosed region. As the pulmonary valve or artery is opened, normal blood flow from the right ventricle is possible.

For more serious defects, a closed pulmonary valvotomy may be performed to open the leaflets of the pulmonary valve. After a sternotomy is performed to expose the heart, the vessels are clamped momentarily to prevent blood from entering the heart. A small incision is made in the pulmonary artery, the fused leaflets are quickly incised, and the arterial incision is closed.

When severe stenosis is present, more complex surgical procedures are possible. The right ventricular outflow tract may be revised, the pulmonary valve may be removed, or a shunt may be created between systemic blood flow and the pulmonary artery. The use of CPB is needed for these intricate surgical procedures inside the heart. Children who have successful repair of pulmonary stenosis have an excellent prognosis and can expect excellent health in adulthood.[31]

Aortic Stenosis

Definition and Incidence.   Aortic stenosis is a narrowing or obstruction in the path of systemic blood flow leaving the left ventricle (Fig. 41-3). The defect can occur above the aortic valve (supravalvular), below the valve (subvalvular), or at the valve annulus (valvular). Valvular stenosis is the most common defect and often results from the presence of only two cusps rather than the normal tricuspid (3 cusps) valve. However, the stenotic aortic valve may be tricuspid, or rarely, unicuspid. In valvular stenosis, the leaflets are thickened and the commissures between them are fused to varying degrees.

Aortic stenosis comprises 5% of all congenital heart defects.[77 (p.80)] Boys are four times as likely as girls to have aortic stenosis.

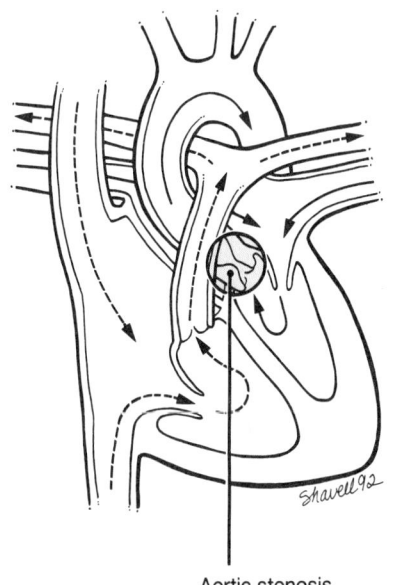

Aortic stenosis

FIGURE 41-3
Normally, blood flows through the right side of the heart and through the lungs. However, in aortic stenosis, the path of systemic blood flow leaving the left ventricle narrows or is obstructed (shown in the circle). When the aortic valve, which separates the left ventricle from the aorta, does not open properly, the pressure in the left ventricle rises.

Clinical Manifestations.   The infant born with severe or critical aortic stenosis may be asymptomatic until the ductus arteriosus begins to close. In this instance, ductal blood flow is needed to provide systemic blood flow because the left ventricular outflow tract is obstructed. Once the ductus arteriosus closes, however, blood flow through the aorta is markedly diminished. The infant may die suddenly in cardiovascular collapse.

The infant born with severe or critical aortic stenosis presents with cardiomegaly, left ventricular hypertrophy, severe CHF, poor peripheral perfusion, and acidosis. In contrast, children with mild or moderate disease often are asymptomatic and have normal growth and development. They may display only mild symptoms of dyspnea or exercise intolerance. Peripheral pulses are normal or decreased. Angina is rare and difficult to recognize as such. A systolic murmur is heard at the right upper sternal border (possibly also at the left sternal border in infants) and radiates to the carotids and jugular fossa. Thrills may be palpable at the second right intercostal space and jugular fossa. When aortic insufficiency is present, a diastolic murmur of aortic regurgitation is heard.

Diagnostic Studies.   When aortic stenosis is present, a chest x-ray shows a normal-size cardiac silhouette despite left ventricular hypertrophy. The ECG, however, can reveal the ventricular hypertrophy. Signs of left ventricular strain may develop, including flattening or inversion of the T wave and depression of the ST segment. The echocardiogram reveals the level of the obstruction, left ventricular wall thickness, and an estimated pressure gradient across the obstruction. A cardiac catheterization confirms the presence of left ventricular hypertension and reveals the gradient (pressure difference) from the left ventricle to the aorta.

Interventions.   The neonate who presents with critical aortic stenosis requires immediate medical intervention to reestablish ductal blood flow and to reverse any respiratory or metabolic acidosis that is present. Once the neonate is stabilized, the current therapy is a cardiac catheterization to attempt balloon dilation of the aortic valve. Before the advent of interventional catheterization, these neonates required an open valvulotomy. This mode of treatment required the use of CPB and was considered very high risk because of the ventricular dysfunction typically associated with aortic stenosis.

The infant or older child who presents with a mild or moderate aortic stenosis usually requires little medical management other than monitoring the degree of stenosis. Aortic stenosis is known to be a progressive disorder that usually requires surgical intervention at some point. During serial evaluations, the defect is monitored for its effect on heart size, left ventricular function, left ventricular wall thickness, and the pressure gradient across the obstruction. Surgical intervention is usually recommended when the pressure gradient is greater than 50 mmHg. The procedure depends on the type of defect. With supravalvular or subaortic stenosis, a membrane is present and requires resection. When valvular aortic stenosis is diagnosed, an open aortic valvulotomy is done. Children with aortic stenosis may require further surgery depending on the success of the first operation. In

the cases of supravalvular and subvalvular aortic stenosis, the tissue membrane may grow back or the membrane may attach to the aortic valve; removing the tissue also could damage one of the valve leaflets. Therefore, another valvulotomy may be required, with or without replacement of the valve. Valve replacement is delayed until adulthood whenever possible to allow the child to finish growing and negate the need for subsequent valve replacements.

When a young child does require valve replacement, a choice is made between a tissue valve (homograft) or a mechanical valve. The placement of a mechanical valve in the heart requires a lifetime of anticoagulant therapy. Postoperative complications following surgery for aortic stenosis are persistent stenosis, restenosis of the aortic lumen, and acquired aortic insufficiency.

The child with aortic stenosis should abstain from competitive athletic participation and should refrain from sustained activities that provide no opportunity for rest. Anaerobic activities such as weight-lifting are not recommended.

The long-term prognosis of aortic stenosis depends on the amount of left ventricular dysfunction. Aortic stenosis that has caused enlargement of the left ventricle with thickening of the ventricular wall produces more risks. A 25% mortality rate is associated with surgical intervention in these cases. Although the quality of life into adulthood has been reported as good, some people may develop residual problems in their middle adult years.[31]

Coarctation of the Aorta

Definition and Incidence.   Coarctation of the aorta (COA) is an abnormal, discrete narrowing of the aorta that causes an obstruction to blood flow on the left side of the heart. Blood flow through the aorta is reduced and causes decreased perfusion beyond the narrowing. Coarctations are located in the region of the embryologic ductus arteriosus. They are classified by their location in relation to the ductus, that is, preductal, juxtaductal, and postductal (Fig. 41-4). COA is the cause of about 8% of the cases of known CHD, and it occurs more frequently in males.[77 (p.03)] Nearly one third of all children with Turner's syndrome have COA.

Clinical Manifestations.   When the obstruction is mild, the child is usually asymptomatic, and the coarctation may not be detected until later years. Older children are usually diagnosed during a routine physical examination when systemic hypertension is noticed. Blood pressure in the upper extremities is typically higher than that in the lower extremities. Femoral pulses may also be diminished. A systolic murmur may be heard over the left chest anteriorly and between the scapulae posteriorly. In older children whose bodies have compensated for the aortic defect by establishing collateral circulation, a continuous murmur can be heard radiating over the back.

The newborn with severe obstruction is critically ill, exhibiting severe signs of CHF that are precipitated by the extreme resistance against which the left side of the heart must pump. Within the first week of life, these infants exhibit symptoms of low CO and CHF. Respiratory distress and acidosis may be expected. If blood flow be-

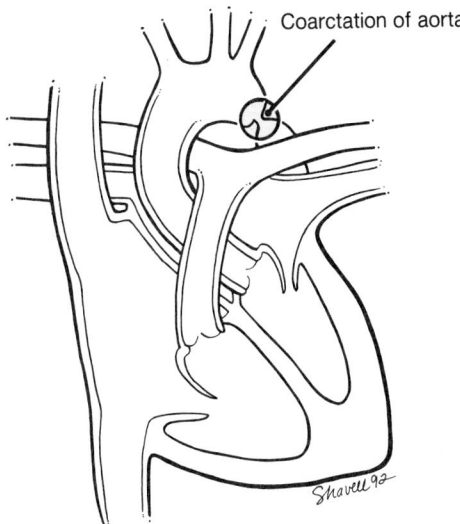

FIGURE 41-4

In coarctation of the aorta, there is an abnormal narrowing (shown in the circle) of the aorta that causes an obstruction to the blood flow on the left side of the heart. Because of this narrowing, the pressure in the aorta and left ventricle increases. To help carry blood through the narrowing, blood vessels around it enlarge.

yond the coarctation is significantly reduced by the obstruction, peripheral perfusion is severely compromised and results in weak peripheral pulses, cold and pale skin, and prolonged capillary refill time (CRT greater than 2 seconds).

Diagnostic Studies. The chest x-ray of a symptomatic infant shows cardiomegaly and pulmonary venous congestion. The x-ray of an older, asymptomatic child may show a heart of normal size. At times, the narrowing of the aorta produces a silhouette that looks like the letter "E" or the number "3." In children over 5 years of age, the dilated intercostal arteries that provide collateral circulation may erode the interior surface of the ribs and cause a notched appearance of the ribs that is seen on x-ray.

An ECG further evaluates the coarctation and may reveal mild, left ventricular hypertrophy in the older child. However, a young infant less than 3 months of age will have evidence of biventricular hypertrophy. An echocardiogram documents the presence and location of the coarctation as well as other anomalies that may be present. Cardiac catheterization is used to determine the exact location of the coarctation and other aortic arch anomalies, and to evaluate collateral circulation or associated defects.

Interventions. Once stabilized with endotracheal intubation and mechanical ventilation, severely symptomatic infants require medical management with a prostaglandin E_1 infusion to reestablish blood flow through the ductus arteriosus. A less severely ill infant presenting with early symptoms of CHF may be treated effectively with digoxin and diuretics. These infants are followed closely until elective repair is appropriate. Surgical intervention is usually recommended when the child develops irretractable CHF or systemic hypertension.

Repair of the coarctation is accomplished through a left lateral thoracotomy incision; CPB is generally unnecessary. However, the aorta is cross-clamped during the repair, and, if there is concern about blood flow distal to the aorta, the CPB is used. Two different methods are used to repair the COA. The first procedure is a left subclavian arterioplasty, and it may be used in infancy and early childhood. The child's left subclavian artery is ligated distally, opened, and extended down the aorta as a patch. This method, known as the subclavian flap, is preferred because it allows maximal postoperative aortic growth and has minimal risk of restenosis. In older children, coarctation repair is usually accomplished by the second method: an end-to-end anastomosis with removal of the narrowed segment of the aorta. Should restenosis occur, balloon angioplasty via cardiac catheterization is often used to dilate the recoarcted area, avoiding the need for further surgery.

After coarctation repair, most older children have significant postoperative hypertension that is managed with antihypertensives. As a rule, the hypertension gradually subsides, but residual murmurs are common. Rarely, postoperative mesenteric vasculitis or arteritis occurs in the immediate postoperative period and can produce abdominal pain or distention that can lead to GI bleeding and bowel necrosis if untreated. Paralysis after coarctation repair is also rare but is thought to result from diminished circulation to the spinal artery during surgery.

Acyanotic Congenital Heart Defects With Increased Pulmonary Blood Flow

Acyanotic congenital heart lesions with increased pulmonary blood flow are those that permit blood to pass between the systemic and pulmonary circulation through an abnormal opening. These lesions allow minimal mixing of desaturated venous blood with saturated arterial blood in the systemic circulation; blood is shunted left-to-right through the defect in the heart or great arteries. Pulmonary blood flow is increased, thereby producing pulmonary congestion and respiratory distress. Cyanosis usually is not seen, because all systemic blood flow is oxygenated. In severe cases, systemic blood flow may be diminished due to poor cardiac function from CHF. The most common acyanotic defects with increased pulmonary blood flow are patent ductus arteriosus (PDA), ventricular septal defect (VSD), atrial septal defect (ASD), and atrioventricular septal defect (AVSD).

Patent Ductus Arteriosus

Definition and Incidence. Patent ductus arteriosus (PDA) occurs when the normal muscular fetal structure connecting the pulmonary artery and aorta fails to close completely after birth (Fig. 41-5). A persistent PDA occurs more frequently in females and accounts for 5% to 10% of the total number of congenital cardiac lesions, excluding preterm infants.[77] [(p.73)] PDA presents more frequently in children living in high altitudes. Incidence also increases in the children of mothers reporting rubella

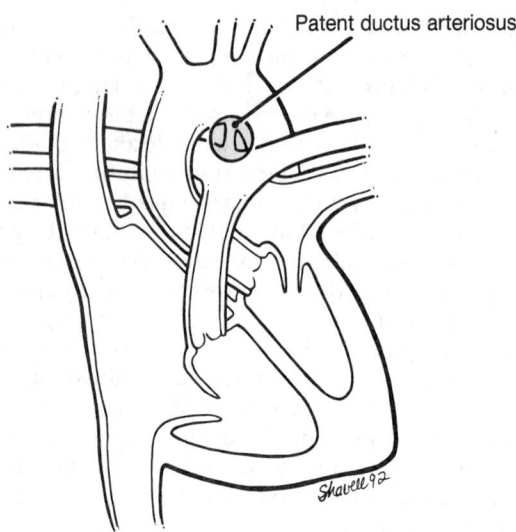

Patent ductus arteriosus

FIGURE 41-5

In patent ductus arteriosus, a connection (shown in the circle) exists between the aorta and pulmonary artery. Pressure is higher in the aorta than the pulmonary artery, and blood flows from the aorta through the patent ductus arteriosus into the pulmonary artery. This means there is an excess volume of blood flowing through the lungs.

exposure during the first trimester of pregnancy. PDA frequently occurs alone but also is associated with other cardiac defects such as COA and VSD.

Etiology and Pathophysiology.   The ductus arteriosus is a structure 1 cm in length and diameter that forms during the fifth to seventh week of gestation and links the pulmonary artery to the aorta. Blood is shunted directly from the heart into the systemic circulation, thereby bypassing the lungs during fetal development. When the infant takes the first breath, the pulmonary vessels dilate, paO_2 increases, and the pulmonary vascular resistance falls. As the oxygen content in the blood increases, the ductal tissue contracts and eventually becomes fibrotic. If these processes do not occur, a ductus remains patent. Closure typically begins within 12 days but the ductus may not be completely closed until 21 days after delivery. Although the ductus can spontaneously close at any time, it is unlikely to close independently after 1 year of age. Prematurity, hypoxia, and scarring of the ductus during a fetal rubella infection increase the incidence of PDA.

The hemodynamics of PDA depend on the size of the ductus and the pulmonary vascular resistance. For example, a small PDA creates high resistance to blood flow through the ductus. Limited blood is shunted through the PDA. A large PDA creates a different situation: after birth, the resistance in the pulmonary and systemic system is almost equal and little or no shunting occurs through the ductus. As the pulmonary resistance falls during the next 4 to 6 weeks, a pressure gradient is created between the aorta and the pulmonary artery. Thereafter, the pressure in the aorta is higher than the pressure in the pulmonary artery, and blood is shunted continuously from the aorta across the patent ductus to the pulmonary artery and the lungs. This altered circulation leads to an increased volume load on the left side of the heart and

increased pulmonary vascular congestion. Over time, the hemodynamic effects of a large PDA could lead to an increased pulmonary resistance and, potentially, increased right ventricular pressure and hypertrophy.

Clinical Manifestations.   Clinical manifestations of the defect vary in direct proportion to the amount of shunting from the aorta to the pulmonary artery. Children with a small PDA are asymptomatic. PDA is typically identified during a routine physical examination with symptoms of bounding peripheral pulses and widened pulse pressure. Frequent respiratory infections, poor growth, and fatigue upon exertion are seen in children with a larger PDA. If pulmonary vascular obstruction develops, cyanosis of the lower extremities may develop.

In contrast, the premature infant with PDA may present with CHF and may require immediate intervention. The infant often appears gravely ill, experiencing tachypnea, retractions, and hypoxemia. Oxygen requirements consistently increase.

The classic sign of PDA is a loud, continuous "machinery" type heart murmur that is initially heard only in systole. Over time, the harsh and uneven sound becomes continuous as the blood shunts throughout systole and diastole. The murmur is best auscultated along the second left intercostal space and under the left clavicle. The murmur may be associated with a thrill over the suprasternal notch or along the upper left sternal border.

Diagnostic Studies.   The appearance of the heart on x-ray depends on the degree of left-to-right shunting through the PDA. The heart may appear normal in the asymptomatic child. However, the x-ray usually displays a large left ventricle and left atrium, dilated pulmonary artery and aorta, and increased pulmonary vascularity. The child's ECG may be normal, or it can display left ventricular or biventricular hypertrophy. An echocardiogram may document a large left atrium and ventricle, the presence of the ductus arteriosus, and the size of the shunt. A cardiac catheterization is not necessary to diagnose a classic PDA but may be performed if other cardiac anomalies are suspected or if the child presents in an atypical manner.

For the infant with some of the complex cyanotic congenital heart lesions, the presence of PDA is essential and beneficial. The infant with a ductal-dependent cyanotic lesion may develop cyanosis when the ductus begins to constrict or close. Prostaglandin E_1 (PGE_1) is a potent ductal dilator and is used to maintain ductal patency in these particular cases. Specific lesions for which PGE_1 is indicated are identified throughout the chapter.

★ **ASSESSMENT**

Most infants and children with PDA remain asymptomatic until early childhood; therefore, ongoing assessment of the child's growth and development is an important component of well-child care. A detailed history of feeding patterns, activity tolerance, and respiratory infections may assist in the diagnosis of an acyanotic congenital heart lesion. A complete cardiac assessment of this child during the well-child examination (i.e., auscultation of the chest, evaluation of peripheral pulses, and measurement of blood pressure) assists in the identification of high-risk children.

The premature neonate in the neonatal intensive care unit is most seriously affected by PDA. Therefore, close assessment of this high-risk neonate to identify symptoms of tachypnea, retractions, and an increasing need for oxygen is an important component of the nursing assessment.

Interventions. Most children with PDA remain asymptomatic and undergo elective surgical closure of the ductus arteriosus in early childhood. All PDAs should be closed in childhood because of the risk of bacterial endocarditis from the turbulent blood flow around and through the ductus. The only exception to elective PDA closure is the child with pulmonary vascular disease, who should be evaluated carefully to determine the risks associated with surgical closure.

The medical management of the symptomatic premature neonate with PDA is much more intense and complex than for the older child. The use of diuretics and fluid restrictions is recommended during the early stage of treatment to reduce the manifestations of CHF. When infants do not respond to 48 hours of conservative medical management, pharmacologic interventions may be instituted. Digoxin may be added to the medical regimen. However, this medication must be used cautiously due to the high risk of digoxin toxicity in the premature neonate. Indomethacin, a prostaglandin inhibitor, may be given to the neonate during the first 14 days of life to promote the closure of the ductus arteriosus, but it is contraindicated in the presence of hyperbilirubinemia, necrotizing enterocolitis, bleeding dyscrasias, and renal or GI disease. Medical management of the high-risk neonate is successful in more than 60% of the cases. Surgical closure of the ductus arteriosus is indicated when indomethacin fails.

Most cardiac centers recommend closure of PDAs regardless of their size and degree of shunting, because of the potential for endocarditis. Closure of the PDA is usually accomplished through a left lateral thoracotomy incision during closed-heart surgery. The ductus is divided, and the severed ends of the ductus are closed with suture.

During the past few years, cardiologists have developed an "umbrellalike" occlusion device to be used during a cardiac catheterization to close the PDA. This device is introduced from the aorta into the ductus and into the pulmonary artery where it is permanently inserted to block the flow of blood through the ductus. Perhaps in the next decade this cardiac catheterization intervention may become the treatment of choice for children with PDA to avoid the surgical risk. This catheter occlusion procedure is being used in some cardiac centers for elective closure of the PDA. However, the long-term results remain unknown.

Children undergoing PDA closure have an excellent prognosis. The elective closure of the PDA causes less than a 1% mortality risk. Postoperative complications after PDA closure are uncommon but may include injury to the recurrent laryngeal nerve and result in hoarseness, or the left phrenic nerve may be injured and lead to paralysis of the left hemidiaphragm. The ductus arteriosus is occasionally tied with suture and not divided (partic-

ularly in the high-risk neonate), and this procedure may lead to reopening of the ductus. As a result, most cardiac surgeons ligate and divide the ductus arteriosus.

Atrial Septal Defect

Definition and Incidence. An atrial septal defect (ASD) is an abnormal communication between the right and left atria that permits blood to be shunted from left to right through the atrial septum (Fig. 41-6). The size of the ASD varies from a pinhole to the absence of the entire septum, resulting in a common or single atrium. The ASD can be located anywhere along the septum and is classified as ostium primum, ostium secundum, or sinus venosus according to its position.

The ostium secundum type of ASD is located in the region of the foramen ovale and is the most common. An ostium primum defect is located near the lower portion of the atrial septum and may be associated with a mitral valve abnormality. The sinus venosus defect is located near the junction of the superior vena cava and the right atrium and may be associated with pulmonary vein abnormalities. The ASD more frequently occurs in females and accounts for 5% to 10% of all CHD.[77] (p.69)

Etiology and Pathophysiology. The atrial septum develops during the fourth to sixth week of gestation. In normal fetal circulation, the foramen ovale, an opening in the atrial septum, permits blood to bypass the lungs during fetal development. After birth, as the left atrial pressures increase, the foramen ovale normally closes. When the atrial septal layers of the fetus fail to fuse completely, an ASD develops.

The hemodynamic impact of the ASD occurs as the infant grows and the pulmonary circulation develops less resistance than the systemic circulation. A higher pressure thus exists in the left atrium than the right atrium, shunting the blood through the ASD from the left to right. Increased compliance of the right atrium and ventricle leads to an

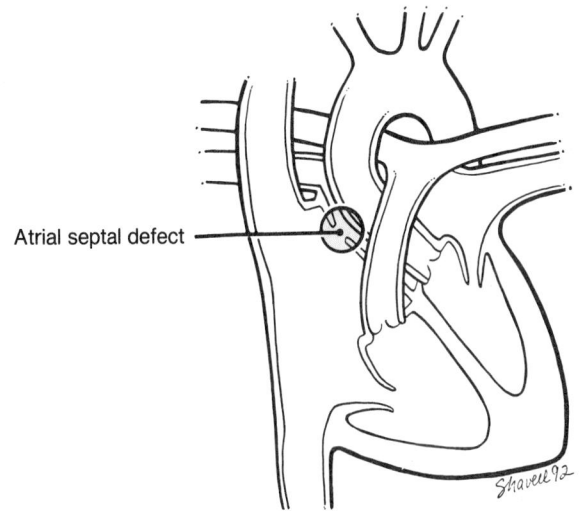

Atrial septal defect

FIGURE 41-6

In an atrial septal defect, there is an abnormal communication between the right atrium and left atrium, allowing blood to be shunted from left to right through the atrial septum.

increase in the pulmonary blood flow. The flow to the lungs may be two to four times greater than normal.

Clinical Manifestations. Children with ASDs are generally asymptomatic until late childhood or adolescence. A child with a small ASD typically displays normal patterns of growth and development and has normal tolerance of exercise. A moderate to large ASD may restrict the child's exercise capacity, and the child may be smaller than his peers. Other clinical signs of ASD are based on the size of the shunt and may include a history of more frequent respiratory infections and dyspnea after extreme exertion. If the ASD is large, the child may develop CHF later in childhood.

Most children with ASD are diagnosed during a well-child examination when the characteristic systolic ejection murmur is noted. Heart sounds are heard best at the upper left sternal border; the S_1 sound is normal, but the S_2 is fixed and widely split. The murmur is the sound of increased blood flow across a normal pulmonary valve.

Diagnostic Studies. The chest x-ray of the child with an ASD may demonstrate pulmonary artery, right atrium, and right ventricle enlargement. Increased pulmonary vascularity due to the increased pulmonary blood flow may be noted. The ECG may be normal or indicate right atrial and ventricular enlargement. An echocardiogram is used to identify the size and location of the defect and to provide an estimate of the size and direction of the shunt. Cardiac catheterization may be unnecessary if the other diagnostic studies are adequate, but it may be used to confirm the diagnosis and to quantify the volume of the shunt.

Interventions. Children with a significant shunt through the ASD are treated medically with digoxin and diuretics if signs of CHF are present. The use of a high-caloric formula is indicated to enhance weight gain in the infant with significant CHF. Although spontaneous closure of the ASD has been reported during the first 2 years of life and some defects may decrease in size over time, most children with an ASD require surgical intervention.

Elective surgical closure of the ASD usually is performed in the preschool or early school-age years. Surgical closure is indicated earlier for the rare child who experiences significant CHF and failure to thrive because of an ASD.

Closing the ASD requires open-heart surgery and is performed through a median sternotomy with the use of CPB. Some cardiac surgeons may still use a right anterolateral thoracotomy incision below the breast for better cosmetic results in the female patient; however, this approach has been associated with an increased risk of air embolism. Hypothermia may be used for the infant undergoing this surgery. Depending on the size of the defect, the lesion is closed by direct suture, or by inserting a patch made of the child's own (or bovine) pericardium or woven prosthetic material.

After an ASD closure, children have an excellent prognosis. The elective closure of the ASD has a mortality rate of less than 1%.[76] (p.111) Possible postoperative complications include heart block, atrial arrhythmias, a resid-

ual ASD, or CHF due to a noncompliant left ventricle. The heart size may remain abnormally large but returns to normal within 2 years postoperatively. Children whose large shunts have been repaired demonstrate enhanced physical development soon after surgery.

Major strides continue to occur in the field of interventional catheterization. Closure of small or moderate ASDs has been accomplished using an umbrella patch inserted through a catheter onto the atrial septum during cardiac catheterization. These children require close medical follow-up, and the procedure remains investigational in most cardiac centers. However, during the next decade, catheter closure of the simple ASD may become the preferred approach.

Ventricular Septal Defect

Definition and Incidence. A ventricular septal defect (VSD) is an abnormal communication between the right and left ventricle that permits blood to shunt from the left ventricle into the right ventricle (Fig. 41-7). The size of the VSD varies from a pinhole to a defect so large that the entire septum is absent, resulting in a common or single ventricle. The VSD can be located in different areas of the septum, and the membranous type is most common. VSDs in the muscular portion of the septum or in other locations are less likely.

VSDs are the most common congenital cardiac lesion in all groups and account for 20% to 25% of the total number of cardiac lesions.[77] A VSD is frequently associated with other cardiac defects such as transposition of the great vessels, COA, and PDA. In complex defects, such as truncus arteriosus and tetralogy of Fallot (TOF), the VSD is an important component of the defect that allows for an exit of blood from the ventricles or provides mixing of desaturated and oxygenated blood. VSD occurs

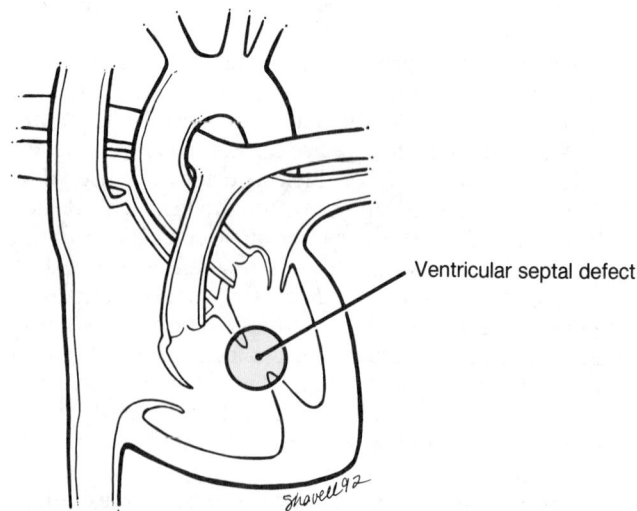

FIGURE 41-7

In a ventricular septal defect, there is a hole in the wall of the septum that separates the left ventricle from the right ventricle. Normally, the oxygen-poor blood flows through the superior vena cava and inferior vena cava into the right atrium, the right ventricle, and the pulmonary artery. In a ventricular septal defect some of the oxygen-rich blood from the left ventricle flows through the defect and recirculates through the lungs.

more frequently in males and in children with Down syndrome.

Etiology and Pathophysiology. The ventricular septum is comprised of membranous and muscular tissue and develops during the fourth to eighth week of gestation. When this tissue development is inadequate, an abnormal communication between the right and left ventricle occurs.

The hemodynamic significance of the VSD is related to its size and location, as well as to the reactivity of the child's pulmonary vasculature. At birth, the right ventricular pressure normally equals the left ventricular pressure. As the infant grows, the pulmonary circulation develops less resistance than the systemic circulation, resulting in higher pressure in the left ventricle than the right. In the infant with a VSD, blood begins to shunt from the left to right ventricle around 6 to 8 weeks after birth, and pulmonary blood flow is increased.

Initially, the right side of the heart may handle the increased pulmonary blood flow from the VSD, but the overload eventually leads to an increased right ventricular and right atrial workload, resulting in CHF. The increased right ventricular pressure from the left-to-right shunting of blood through the VSD causes the heart muscle to hypertrophy. The hypertrophy with increased pulmonary blood flow and right heart workload leads to increased pulmonary vascular resistance.

With a large, untreated VSD, the increased resistance may cause right-to-left shunting of blood through the VSD. Cyanotic heart disease and advanced pulmonary vascular obstructive disease (Eisenmenger syndrome) may develop. Once the flow of shunted blood is reversed, the pulmonary vascular disease is irreversible. Development of this serious heart disease is rare.

Approximately 75% of children with a small muscular VSD experience spontaneous closure of the defect by the age of 6 years due to growth of the muscular cardiac tissue. About 50% of small membranous defects close spontaneously within 10 years of life. Other membranous defects and the moderate to large muscular type of defect almost always require surgical intervention.

Clinical Manifestations. The clinical symptoms are directly related to the size of the VSD and the amount of shunting that occurs through the defect. Children with small VSDs typically have no clinical symptoms and display normal patterns of growth and development; the cardiac lesion is usually found during routine physical examination. The VSD causes a loud, harsh pansystolic murmur that is best auscultated at the left lower sternal border and may transmit throughout the chest. The intensity of the murmur may not always be indicative of the size of the VSD, because sounds from a small VSD may be louder than those from a moderate or large defect.

The child with a moderate-size VSD may experience only exercise intolerance and increased susceptibility to upper respiratory infections. However, the child with a large, untreated VSD is typically thin, diaphoretic, tachycardic, and tachypneic. Affected children are often irritable, difficult to feed, lethargic, and difficult to manage medically. Therefore, children with large VSDs may present with failure to thrive and CHF early in infancy. Cyanosis is absent, and peripheral pulses are normal unless the heart has begun to fail.

Diagnostic Studies. The chest x-ray of the child with a VSD typically reveals enlargement of the right atrium, right ventricle, and pulmonary artery, as well as increased pulmonary vascularity due to the increased pulmonary blood flow. The ECG may demonstrate left ventricular hypertrophy and cardiomegaly. Echocardiographic findings indicate the presence of shunting and cardiomegaly. Cardiac catheterization may be performed to evaluate the pulmonary vasculature and the amount of shunting into the pulmonary vessels.

Interventions. A child who has a small VSD and is asymptomatic is followed regularly in the outpatient cardiology department to assess for spontaneous closure or change in the status of the lesion. Every child with a VSD should receive prophylactic antibiotic coverage during elective procedures (such as dental, upper respiratory, or urologic procedures) and at other times when there is an increased risk of bacteremia (see section on Endocarditis later in this chapter). The small VSD may require surgical closure on an elective basis before school entry if it fails to close spontaneously before that time.

If a child has a moderate-size VSD, cardiac catheterization is performed to assess pulmonary vascular resistance. Surgery is performed to close the defect if this resistance is increasing. However, a child who remains asymptomatic with a normal pulmonary vascular resistance should be followed medically to allow the VSD a chance to close spontaneously. When the VSD remains unchanged, the child typically undergoes elective surgical closure of the lesion before entry in school.

Children with large VSDs are the most difficult to manage medically, because they frequently develop CHF, pulmonary infections, and elevated pulmonary vascular resistance early in life. The large VSD is typically in the membranous portion of the heart and does not close spontaneously. The infant develops CHF early and requires digitalization and diuretic therapy. The use of high-caloric formulas to enhance weight gain also may be initiated at this time. The infant is maintained on medical treatment for as long as possible, allowing the child a chance to gain weight before surgery. This child is at a significant risk for the development of endocarditis, and thus aggressive prophylactic antibiotic therapy is indicated. Surgical therapy is necessary when the infant has CHF that fails to respond to the medical therapy. It also is indicated for any child developing high pulmonary vascular resistance and failure to thrive. Such a situation is addressed in the sample Nursing Care Plan and Teaching Plan for an infant with VSD that has progressed to CHF.

Closure of the VSD requires open-heart surgery. This corrective procedure is performed through a median sternotomy with the use of CPB and hypothermia. Depending on the size of the defect, the lesion is closed by direct suturing or the use of a woven prosthetic patch. Postoperative complications include CHF, heart block, and a residual VSD. Heart block may be transient or permanent, requiring a pacemaker due to damage to the conduction system.

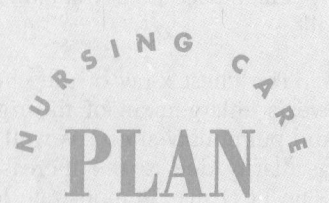

An Infant Requiring Surgery for Ventricular Septal Defect and Congestive Heart Failure

Assessment

Case Study Description

Julio Rodriquez is 6 months old. When he was age 2 months, an echocardiogram revealed a large membranous ventricular septal defect (VSD), and he has taken Digoxin, Lasix, and Aldactone since the first hospitalization. His formula is 24 cal/oz, and he takes 2 to 3 oz over 30 to 60 minutes about 7 times per day. His parents are young, Spanish-speaking, Mexican immigrants. There are two older siblings at home; grandparents have come from Mexico to help care for older children. The parents are very concerned about the baby's condition and frightened of this hospitalization and potential plans for surgery.

Mr. Rodriquez takes responsibility for answering questions through Spanish-speaking health aide; Mrs. Rodriquez nods and occasionally murmurs additional information. The history is difficult to follow, and the family knows only that Julio's "heart has a hole in it." They seem unsure what to expect during this hospitalization. When asked, the parents state that they have been praying for Julio and lighting candles for him; religion seems an important part of their lives.

Treatment involves planned hospitalization for cardiac catheterization and possible surgery.

Assessment Data

Thin and pale; weighs 6.0 kg: has fallen from the 50th to 5th percentile on the growth chart in the past 4 months. His heart rate is 140, respiratory rate is 50 to 60 with mild nasal flaring and inter- and subcostal retractions. He is irritable and diaphoretic during examination. His mother states that he becomes diaphoretic during feeding.

Auscultation: a grade 3–4/6 systolic murmur is heard over the left sternal border, and it is loudest along lower left region.

On examination, the liver is palpable about 3 cm below the right costal margin. ECG indicated biventricular hypertrophy; cardiomegaly and pulmonary overcirculation are confirmed by chest x-ray; echocardiogram reveals enlarged VSD.

Nursing Diagnosis	Intervention	Rationale
PREOPERATIVE		
1. Possible complication: decreased cardiac output related to congestive heart failure (CHF)	Monitor for deterioration of status: • Vital signs (BP, P, R) may be placed on electronic monitors	Tachycardia and tachypnea due to sympathetic nervous system response caused by a decreased cardiac output; low blood pressure is a late sign of diminished cardiac output (CO).
Supporting Data: • Thin and small for age; pale • Diaphoretic with modest effort • Tachycardia (P = 140) • Tachypneic (R = 50 to 60) with nasal flaring and retractions • Irritable and difficult to feed • Hepatomegaly • ECG, chest x-ray, and echocardiogram confirm diagnosis	• Pulmonary perfusion (respiratory rate, presence and degree of retractions, nasal flaring, grunting)	Overcirculation to lungs results in pulmonary engorgement leading to respiratory distress.
	• Peripheral perfusion (presence and quality of pulses in extremities, temperature of skin, color of skin, diaphoresis, capillary refill time)	Decreased CO results in poor pulses, cool, pale skin, with prolonged capillary refill time (i.e., greater than 2 s) and diaphoresis.
	• Daily weight (on same scale, at same time, prior to feeds, and dressed in same clothing)	A weight gain of over 50 g over a 24-h period for infants less than 1 year old may indicate fluid retention, as a result of CHF.

(Continued)

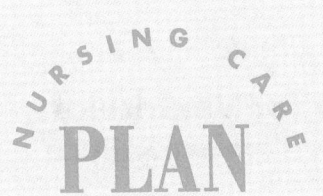

An Infant Requiring Surgery for Ventricular Septal Defect and Congestive Heart Failure

Nursing Diagnosis	*Intervention*	*Rationale*
	Administer medications as ordered (i.e., Digoxin, Lasix, and Aldactone).	Digoxin increases the contractility of the heart; Lasix and Aldactone help remove excessive fluid volume and improve CO by reducing congestion.
	Monitor electrolytes, especially potassium (hypokalemia manifested by arrhythmias, nausea, vomiting, diarrhea).	Lasix depletes potassium, resulting in hypokalemia, which may precipitate arrhythmias and digoxin toxicity. Aldactone may offset hypokalemia as it is potassium sparing.
	Monitor digoxin serum level.	Digoxin toxicity chiefly manifested by arrhythmia in infants. Need to maintain therapeutic levels.
	Monitor intake and output.	Precise calculations and documentation needed to ensure accurate fluid replacement.
2. Altered nutrition: less than body requirements related to poor feeding secondary to CHF Supporting Data: • In 5th percentile weight for age norms • Takes only 2–3 oz formula in 30–60 min. • Increased diaphoresis when feeding	Monitor caloric intake, daily weight, intake and output, feeding behaviors. Discuss findings with physician and adjust formula mix or feeding method (nipple or gavage) as needed. Promote quiet environment during feeding; keep child's head elevated during and after feeding; place child on side or prone after feeding.	CHF results in poor perfusion of the GI tract along with increased work of the heart during feeding; children in CHF require significantly greater caloric intake (up to 150–170 kcal/kg/day) due to increased caloric needs. Position promotes intake and digestion, reduces the incidence of vomiting during and after feeding.
3. Discomfort related to effects of CHF Supporting Data: • Irritability • Diaphoresis with exertion	Provide comfort measures: • Position for comfort; maybe semi-Fowler's or prone • Use soothing talk and touch during procedures • Avoid thermal stress • Use oxygen hood as ordered	Minimizing caloric expenditure reduces degree of hypoxia; provides more energy to optimize cardiac contractility and improve CO. Supplemental oxygen to correct hypoxia and improve poor tissue perfusion.
4. Anxiety related to air hunger. Supporting Data: • Strained expression and crying when approached • Fussy and irritable • Does not sleep well	Promote/continue home routines as much as possible; approach in calm manner; comfort by rocking, placing child's favorite blanket or music box nearby; encourage mother to be present as much as possible. Avoid unnecessary handling and disturbing when asleep.	Infants respond to sensorimotor activities such as touch, motion, and sound. Approach preserves unnecessary energy expenditure for crying efforts. Diminished anxiety improves air intake, decreases energy expenditure, and enhances emotional comfort. Unnecessary handling increases oxygen consumption and anxiety.
5. Altered growth and development related to poor growth associated with chronic heart disease. Supporting Data: • No social smile • Inactive with no attempt to reach out or mobilize self	Prepare teaching plan for parents explaining expected behaviors, effect of chronic illness on growth and development, and anticipatory needs for stimulation when condition improves.	Failure of parents to understand long-term effects of chronic heart disease may contribute to anxiety; knowledge can contribute to informed decision making about Julio's treatment. Parents need knowledge to help stimulate Julio so he can reach his fullest potential for growth and development.

(Continued)

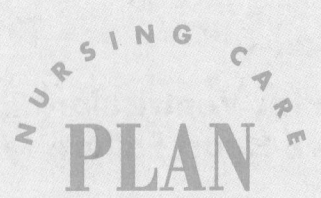

An Infant Requiring Surgery for Ventricular Septal Defect and Congestive Heart Failure

Nursing Diagnosis	*Intervention*	*Rationale*
• Parents observe that he doesn't behave as older siblings did at 6 months		
6. Parental anxiety related to lack of understanding of Julio's illness, plan for care, and prognosis	Establish rapport with family by spending time in room and attending to their comfort needs (comfortable chairs, pillows, meals in room, linens for freshening up in unit facilities).	Family responds to demonstrations of caring and concern and are more receptive to teaching strategies.
Supporting Data:		
• Gave confusing history through Spanish-speaking health aide. Were not sure why physicians wanted Julio hospitalized.	Permit liberal visitation from other family members as possible.	Family solidarity and support especially important in Latino culture.
• Parents cry frequently and express great concern when nurse is in the room.	Develop teaching plan to incorporate basic information about the VSD, how it will be treated, and the long-term prognosis.	Information helps calm fears and allows parents to become active participants in the decisions made about Julio's care.

Evaluation

Diagnostic tests confirm the severity of the VSD but no other cardiac defects, the presence of CHF, and Julio's deteriorating status. He has remained lethargic but relatively comfortable when undisturbed. Feedings have been given primarily by nasogastric tube; Julio's weight and electrolytes have stabilized.

After 2 days of hospitalization in which extensive teaching has been done, Mr. and Mrs. Rodriquez give permission for Julio to have a surgical repair of the VSD with use of cardiopulmonary bypass. They understand that the procedure is expected to repair the congenital cardiac defect, and that Julio's outlook for normal growth and development is excellent.

Julio's grandparents and older siblings have visited, and all remain visibly concerned by his condition. The primary nurse has established a good relationship with the family, and they readily call for help when needed and verbalize their gratitude for the nurse's kindness.

A palliative surgery for the treatment of a VSD is known as a pulmonary artery banding. This closed-heart surgery is performed through a lateral thoracotomy. Prosthetic material is placed around the main pulmonary artery to restrict pulmonary blood flow. The symptoms of CHF and pulmonary vascular disease are thereby reduced. The procedure is typically reserved for the infant who would be at high risk for open-heart closure of the VSD. However, because of success rates with corrective surgery, the use of palliative pulmonary artery banding has been abandoned unless additional cardiac lesions make the complete repair difficult or impossible.

Interventional cardiac catheterization procedures are being perfected to permit closure of the VSD in the catheterization laboratory. A prosthetic patch that can be released through the end of a catheter and attached to the ventricular septum is being investigated at this time and may be used routinely for small to moderate lesions in the near future. Successful repair of VSD in childhood generally enables children to grow into adulthood without cardiac problems.[31]

Atrioventricular Septal Defect

Definition and Incidence. The atrioventricular septal defect (AVSD) is one of the endocardial cushion defects and occurs as an abnormality of the atrial septum, ventricular septum, and AV valves. This defect may occur in a partial or complete form. A partial form of AVSD exists when the defect is in the lower part of the atrial septum near the AV valves, and clefts of the mitral and/or tricuspid valve are present; the ventricular septum remains intact. A complete AVSD is complex and may include deficient septal tissue in either the atrium, the ventricle, or both structures, and a large AV valve that is common to both sides of the heart.

AVSD accounts for approximately 2% of all congenital heart defects, and it is the most common cardiac anomaly

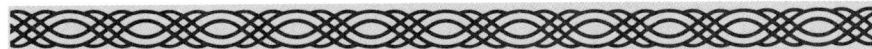

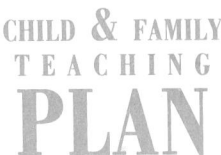

CHILD & FAMILY
T E A C H I N G
PLAN

Preparation for Open Heart Surgery for Congestive Heart Failure

Assessment

Julio has been hospitalized with congestive heart failure due to a large VSD (see accompanying Nursing Care Plan). The parents are intelligent, and both have finished grade school. They ask many questions of their Spanish-speaking nurse. They know little about Julio's condition or what is proposed for this hospitalization. The pediatric cardiologist has indicated that Julio's condition will not improve without surgery. The pediatric surgeon has spoken with the parents and encouraged them to give permission for surgery. After consultation with the surgeon to validate the proposed plans, the nurse uses information obtained in observation of and interaction with the Rodriquez parents to formulate the following teaching plan.

Child and Family Objectives	Specific Content	Teaching Strategies
1. Describe the heart defect, its general effect on blood flow, and its relationship to Julio's symptoms.	1. Describe the heart with four sections and blood that flows into the lungs from one side and into the body system from the other. Explain that too much blood goes to lungs, causing increased workload on Julio's heart. Symptoms are due to pulmonary engorgement and congestive heart failure.	1. Teaching should be done by a Spanish-speaking nurse or other health care provider who has an accurate understanding of the cardiac defect and is able to speak in terms familiar to the parents. Use a model of the heart or simple illustration to point out the specific problem area. Explain the clinical manifestations in simple terms. For example, "When Julio doesn't get enough air, he has to work hard when he sucks on the bottle. He gets tired before he gets enough to eat. We have put this tube in Julio's stomach so that he can rest and still get enough to eat." In deference to Latino customs, Mr. Rodriquez is given the opportunity to take leadership in asking questions, but Mrs. Rodriquez also should be acknowledged individually.
2. Describe the surgical plan and its expected benefits.	2. Explain in simple terms how the VSD will be closed and how blood flow will be forced to take the preferred route through the heart and body. The effect of the repair on Julio's symptoms can be attributed to the improved flow of blood out to the body and reduced amount of blood to the lungs, enabling the heart to beat more effectively.	2. Use the same model or diagram to make a direct comparison with changes that will occur as a result of surgery. Speak slowly, pointing to the illustration or his/her own body for emphasis and clarity. Care should be taken to avoid a patronizing tone; rather, the parents should be treated as important members of Julio's interdisciplinary health team.

(Continued)

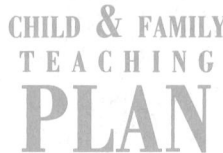

CHILD & FAMILY
T E A C H I N G
PLAN

Preparation for Open Heart Surgery for Congestive Heart Failure (continued)

Child and Family Objectives	*Specific Content*	*Teaching Strategies*
3. Return demonstrate comforting interaction with Julio and aspects of care.	3. Parents are usually eager to know what they can do to contribute to the child's comfort. They may be able to touch, hold, and talk to him, depending on symptoms.	3. Demonstrate what the parents can do, thus diminishing their fears about hurting Julio. Give appropriate praise when they interact. Parents feel valued when their skills are recognized and interactions are encouraged.
4. Verbalize activities to promote Julio's growth and development after the surgery.	4. The effects of chronic illness on Julio's growth and development are explained, as is the benefit of surgery. Julio will benefit from social interactions with family members when his physical condition improves.	4. Supply a written description of expected behaviors of the 6-month-old infant for future reference. Spanish pamphlets on child development may be obtained. Reassure parents that Julio's failure to thrive is due to physical illness, not to any known mental defect or other problem.
5. Verbalize fears and concerns related to Julio's condition.	5. The seriousness of Julio's condition preoperatively should be acknowledged. However, the parents can be reassured that most children who have Julio's problem recover well from surgery. Normal growth and development may be expected in the future.	5. Be available and present continuously and win the parents' confidence. State that most parents are terribly worried about their ill children. Introduce other parents whose children have successfully recovered from similar surgery; they will give encouragement.

Evaluation

- Julio's parents cried less.
- Julio's parents spoke optimistically about the surgery and its benefit on Julio's health.

A Spanish-speaking nurse was assigned to Julio's care on the day shift, and the parents eagerly engaged in conversation, asking questions and admitting their concerns. They looked at "before and after" pictures of a child who had similar surgery and beamed in anticipation that their Julio would do as well in a few months.

The parents gave permission for the surgery, and the nurse revised the teaching plan to provide new information about Julio's transfer to the operating room and his admission to the pediatric intensive care unit.

---

found in children who have Down syndrome.[77 (p.75)] AVSD may also occur in combination with other complex forms of CHD.

Etiology and Pathophysiology. The AV valves are comprised of endocardial cushions that begin to develop during the fourth week of gestation. In early embryonic development, the endocardial cushions are filled with cardiac jelly, but the tissue later develops into leaflets whose edges begin to approximate each other and even-

tually fuse to form the stem of the atrioventricular canal. When tissue development is interrupted or inadequate, abnormal communications between the atria or ventricles may persist, or the AV valve may be incompletely formed. The defects are thereby formed by the end of the fifth week of gestation.

Hemodynamic impact of the AVSD is related to the extent of the defect, whether it is partial or complete. Immediately after birth, the pulmonary vascular resistance is high, and, although the AVSD is present, minimal shunting of blood occurs. However, the infant's pulmonary vascular resistance normally falls during the first 3 months of life, and a left-to-right intracardiac shunt develops through the AVSD, causing an increase in pulmonary blood flow.

In children with a partial AVSD, the cleft in the mitral valve produces a degree of mitral insufficiency, but this regurgitation is hemodynamically insignificant. The left-to-right shunt through the ASD produces an increase in right ventricular volume. The development of pulmonary vascular disease is uncommon in the partial AVSD.

In the complete AVSD, the pulmonary vascular resistance decreases. The degree of shunting depends on the size of the defect and the pressure in the pulmonary vascular bed. Shunts at the atrial level produce right atrial enlargement and increase in right ventricular volume. Shunts at the ventricular level result in increased pulmonary blood flow. When pulmonary blood flow is increased, pulmonary venous return to the left heart is increased, causing left atrial enlargement. Increased volume and high pressure flow to the pulmonary bed and severe mitral insufficiency produce marked pulmonary congestion and marked signs of CHF. Pulmonary vascular disease may be expected to develop during the first year of life in the infant with complete AVSD.

Clinical Manifestations. Clinical manifestations of AVSD are directly related to the type of defect (partial or complete), the amount of left-to-right shunt, the level of pulmonary vascular resistance, and the degree of AV valve insufficiency. A child with the partial form of AVSD may remain asymptomatic or present signs and symptoms similar to children who have ASDs. However, a systolic murmur is heard as blood regurgitates through the defective mitral valve.

Infants with a complete AVSD are often irritable and difficult to feed, and readily fatigue with effort. Failure to thrive, recurrent respiratory infections, and signs of CHF, with or without pulmonary hypertension, usually appear in infancy. Auscultation of the heart reveals a systolic murmur and fixed splitting into the second heart sound. When mitral insufficiency is present, a systolic murmur is heard at the apex of the heart.

Diagnostic Studies. A chest x-ray of the child with a partial form of AVSD reveals slight enlargement of the heart. The effect of right ventricular overload is noted with slightly increased pulmonary vascular markings. In the child with a complete AVSD, the chest x-ray detects pronounced cardiomegaly and vascular markings. The heart of a child who has severely increased pulmonary vascular resistance may be less enlarged, but the central pulmonary arteries are enlarged, and the lung fields are clear.

An ECG usually indicates marked right ventricular hypertrophy and also may show left ventricular hypertrophy. The PR interval may be prolonged. An ECG is valuable to assess the degree of AV valve incompetence and can confirm the presence of shunting and the characteristic deformity of the left ventricular outflow tract. A cardiac catheterization may be used to define the direction and magnitude of shunting in both pulmonary and systemic circulation. The cardiac catheterization also is used to obtain important data about the degree of pulmonary hypertension and the amount of resistance within the pulmonary vascular bed.

Interventions. Because children with partial AVSD are typically asymptomatic, no medical intervention is required before elective repair of the defect after it is discovered. The repair is elective and done when the child reaches school age. Surgery may be completed earlier in children who present with symptoms or severe mitral regurgitation. The corrective procedure is performed through a median sternotomy with the use of CPB.

The ASD is generally repaired with a pericardial or prosthetic patch. A tricuspid or mitral valvuloplasty may be performed to decrease the amount of AV valve insufficiency. Clefts in the valve leaflets are usually closed with sutures. Total repair of the AV valve is difficult, and a degree of AV valve insufficiency usually exists postoperatively. A small percentage of children may require further surgical intervention, but most children recover well without the need for further interventions.

Corrective open-heart surgery is recommended for children with a complete AVSD. An incision is made through the right atrium, and the common AV valve leaflets are divided and separated from any attachments. The atrial defect may be closed with one or two separate patches. The AV valve tissue is mounted to the septal defect patch, and a valvuloplasty is performed to make the AV valve as competent as possible. The left-sided AV valve may be left with three rather than two leaflets.

Operative risks are highest in symptomatic infants and those children with preoperative symptoms such as left ventricular hypoplasia, pulmonary hypertension, and severe mitral regurgitation. Postoperative complications after repair of the AVSD include low CO, dysrhythmias (heart block), hemorrhage, respiratory failure, and persistent CHF. Occasionally, hemolysis or coagulopathy occurs when a degree of mitral valve regurgitation is present and may be related to a dehiscence in the valve repair. Mechanical ventilation is expected postoperatively to control pulmonary hypertension through hyperventilation, and weaning from the ventilatory support system is accomplished gradually and cautiously. Pharmacologic paralysis and sedation are common to reduce cardiac effort during the first few days postoperatively.

After repair for AVSD, most children lead active and normal lives. Follow-up with a pediatric cardiologist is needed for monitoring the function of the mitral valve. Prophylaxis against endocarditis is recommended. A small group of children may experience residual, continuing pulmonary hypertension and may need additional treatment.

Cyanotic Congenital Heart Defects With Normal or Decreased Pulmonary Blood Flow

Cyanotic congenital cardiac defects with decreased pulmonary blood flow result in a condition known as hypoxemia. Hypoxemia occurs when desaturated, unoxygenated blood from the systemic venous system enters the systemic arterial system through a shunt from the right to left side of the heart. Cyanosis becomes apparent when mucous membranes, nailbeds, and skin become hypoxic. The various lesions permit some or all of the systemic venous blood to bypass the lungs. Cardiac anomalies included in this group are tetralogy of Fallot (TOF), tricuspid atresia (TA), and pulmonary atresia (PA).

Tetralogy of Fallot

Definition and Incidence. Tetralogy of Fallot (TOF) received its name from a French physician who identified four specific cardiac abnormalities that occur simultaneously. The four component anomalies of TOF are: (1) a large VSD, (2) right ventricular outflow tract obstruction (sometimes called pulmonary stenosis), (3) displacement of the aorta toward the right side (overriding of the aorta), and (4) right ventricular hypertrophy (Fig. 41-8). TOF may also occur in conjunction with other defects such as pulmonary atresia, absent pulmonary valve, and AVSD. TOF is the most frequent cardiac anomaly that is recognized beyond infancy, and it accounts for about 10% of all congenital heart defects.[77 (p.148)] The following discussion refers to TOF as a single defect and not as part of a larger, more complex cardiac anomaly.

Etiology and Pathophysiology. TOF occurs as a result of abnormal fetal development, although the precise embryonic events are not clear.[82] Inadequate development in the region where the pulmonary artery should emerge prevents outflow of blood from the heart; collateral circulation from the aorta may supply the lungs with blood.[12 (p.964)] A malalignment of embryonic tissues causes a large VSD that displaces the aorta so that it lies directly over the ventricular septum. Right ventricular hypertrophy develops in response to the increased workload that occurs with obstructed pulmonary blood flow.

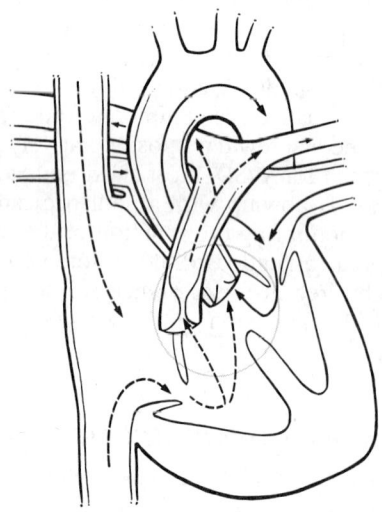

FIGURE 41-8

In tetralogy of Fallot, four specific anomalies occur simultaneously. They are (1) a large ventricular septal defect (also shown in Fig. 41-7); (2) right ventricular outflow tract obstruction (sometimes called pulmonary stenosis; also shown in Fig. 41-2); (3) displacement of the aorta toward the right side; and (4) right ventricular hypertrophy.

The severity of obstructed pulmonary blood flow determines the hemodynamic changes expected with TOF. When obstruction is mild, the right ventricular pressure is only slightly elevated, and there is minimal shunting of blood through the VSD. The resistance to pulmonary blood flow is approximately equal to the systemic blood flow, creating what is known as a "balanced defect," with mild or absent hypoxemia. When pulmonary blood is severely obstructed, a large amount of venous blood is shunted through the VSD from the right ventricle into the aorta, producing arterial oxygen desaturation. The more severe the obstruction, the greater the right-to-left shunt through the VSD. Unoxygenated blood bypasses the lungs and enters the aorta directly. Thus, oxygenated blood is mixed with unoxygenated blood, and hypoxemia is significant.

Clinical Manifestations. The most apparent clinical manifestation of TOF is cyanosis, but it is directly proportional to the degree of right ventricular outflow tract obstruction. A newborn with PDA may have minimal cyanosis until the ductus begins to close. As the infant grows and becomes more active, the right ventricular outflow tract obstruction becomes more severe. Right-to-left shunting may at first occur only during periods of exertion, such as when the infant cries. Periodic episodes of hypoxemia cause hypercyanosis, commonly referred to as "tet spells." Children become extremely anxious during these episodes and may lose consciousness.

As the severity of the pulmonic stenosis increases, the child with TOF exhibits exercise intolerance and dyspnea, as well as delayed motor development. A squatting position may be assumed by children old enough to walk because it improves pulmonary blood flow by increasing the resistance in the systemic circuit and reducing the right-to-left shunt. The tips of the fingers and toes become clubbed from the effects of hypoxemia. With time and increased obstruction to pulmonary blood flow, cyanosis eventually occurs even when the child is at rest. Polycythemia eventually ensues, and the untreated child is at risk for associated problems such as cerebral vascular accidents, brain abscesses, and coagulopathies associated with increased platelet number or function.

A systolic ejection murmur, caused by blood trying to flow across the stenotic pulmonary outflow tract, is heard at the second intercostal space at the upper left sternal border. A thrill may be present over the same area. Bruits may be heard over the child's back if collateral circulation to the lungs has developed. A raised sternum (sternal lift) indicates the presence of right ventricular hypertrophy.

Diagnostic Studies. Chest x-rays reveal a narrow mediastinum with a cardiac contour in the shape of a boot. The apex of the heart appears elevated due to right ventricular hypertrophy. Pulmonary vascular markings are usually decreased unless collateral vessels to the lungs are present. ECG demonstrates right ventricular hypertrophy. The echocardiogram confirms the presence of the four component defects of TOF. Size of the pulmonary arteries may be assessed with a two-dimensional echocardiogram. Cardiac catheterization is used to establish the exact nature of the defects, to measure the existing pressure gradients in the heart, and to determine the degree of desaturation.

Interventions. The child with mild right ventricular outflow tract obstruction is monitored closely until surgical repair is performed, as early as 3 to 4 months of age. The determination of age at surgical repair depends totally on the extent of the cardiac defect and its clinical manifestations. Infants who present with severe cyanosis within the first two days of life have a severe form of TOF. Prior to surgery, they may require prostaglandin E_1 to maintain ductal patency and pulmonary blood flow until cardiac catheterization and surgery can be done. For infants and children who develop hypercyanotic spells, oxygen and a weight-appropriate dose of morphine sulfate should be available. During a spell, the nurse should place the child in the knee-to-chest position and notify the physician. When circumstances are not favorable for a complete repair, a palliative surgical procedure such as the modified Blalock-Taussig anastomosis may be performed. Complete repair of the TOF requires a median sternotomy and CPB to close the VSD and to repair the right ventricular outflow tract.

After repair of the TOF, children may develop postoperative complications including CHF, dysrhythmias, low cardiac output, and neurologic symptoms. Right bundle branch block may develop as a result of either a right ventriculotomy or closure of the VSD. Poor postoperative results usually are related to severity of the original defect.[82 (p.96)] However, children with early surgical correction of the TOF usually demonstrate excellent cardiovascular function for years after surgery (see section on Endocarditis for prophylactic antibiotic coverage to prevent bacterial endocarditis).

Tricuspid Atresia

Definition and Incidence. Tricuspid atresia (TA) is the absence of the tricuspid valve or the presence of an inperforated tricuspid valve, which is located on the right side of the heart (Fig. 41-9). The resulting absence of blood flow to the right ventricle causes it to become hypoplastic, and the pulmonary artery serving the lungs atrophies. A VSD is usually present and permits blood flow to the lungs from the left ventricle. TA accounts for 1% to 2% of all congenital heart defects in infancy.[77 (p.101)]

Etiology and Pathophysiology. The tricuspid valve is formed during the fifth week of gestation as a result of the blending of endocardial cushion tissue and a portion of the ventricular septum. The embryologic events that lead to the development of TA is unclear, but the defect may be due to an abnormal development of the AV canal, an abnormality in the endocardial cushions on the right side of the heart, or an early fusion of the tricuspid leaflets.[82 (p.99)] Children with TA may have associated cardiac defects in addition to or rather than the VSD, including transposition of the great arteries, patency of the ductus arteriosus, and collateral circulation to the lungs.

Tricuspid atresia results in an obligatory shunt from the right atrium to the left atrium through a patent foramen ovale or an atrial septal defect. This shunt results in a

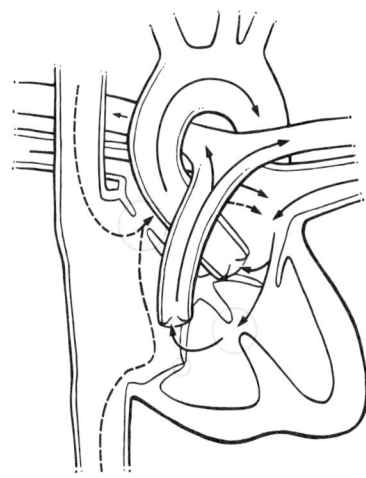

FIGURE 41-9

In tricuspid atresia, the tricuspid valve is completely closed (shown in the circle), resulting in absence of blood flow to the right ventricle, causing it to become hypoplastic and atrophying the pulmonary artery to the lung.

mixing of desaturated systemic venous blood and fully saturated pulmonary venous blood. This desaturated blood is then pumped by the left ventricle. A large percentage of the blood flows out of the aorta, but a small portion may flow through the ventricular septal defect into the right ventricle. This volume is small, however, due to the right ventricular pressure relative to a small chamber size and the associated stenosis of the pulmonic valve and hypoplastic pulmonary vessels. Blood also reaches the pulmonary artery through the ductus arteriosus. When pulmonary blood flow is restricted significantly, hypoxia and acidosis result. Without surgical treatment, many infants die within the first 6 months of life.[82 (p.102)]

Clinical Manifestations. Clinical manifestations vary depending on the extent of pathology in the heart. In most cases, TA causes significant obstruction to pulmonary blood flow. Infants present with cyanosis and rapidly develop respiratory distress and acidosis as the ductus arteriosus closes. Immediate intervention is needed.

In contrast, if a large VSD is present, the infant exhibits signs of CHF from increased pulmonary blood flow. This complication occurs most often between 4 and 12 weeks of age. Characteristic behavior of the infant includes irritability and difficulty feeding. A harsh systolic murmur along the left sternal border, loudest at the left lower sternal border, accompanies a VSD. Often, however, no murmur is heard when a VSD is not present.

Diagnostic Studies. In the child with TA, a chest x-ray reveals a normal cardiac size, but diminished pulmonary blood flow. An ECG confirms the presence of hypertrophy in both atria and left ventricle. Echocardiography reveals the absence of the tricuspid valve as well as the relationship of the major cardiac arteries. Diagnosis of the TA may be confirmed with cardiac catheterization, which reveals right-to-left shunt at the atrial level. Samples of systemic arterial blood reveal low oxygen saturation.

Interventions. When severe cyanosis is present, prostaglandins E_1 may be initiated to maintain ductal patency. The Rashkind procedure, a balloon atrial septostomy may be performed during cardiac catheterization.[77] (p.102) This procedure allows blood to exit freely from the right atrium. While several palliative procedures are available, many institutions are repairing the main defect in very young infants. The choice of the exact surgical procedure depends on factors such as the infant's size, the size of the vessels to be used, and the surgeon's preference.[82] (p.102) Surgical correction is typically accomplished with a modification of the Fontan procedure, that is, a right atrium-to-pulmonary artery anastomosis. Postoperatively, right-sided pressures are high and systemic venous engorgement leads to pleural effusions. Hypoalbuminemia also occurs from protein loss. Chylothorax may develop and is treated with chest tube therapy and a fat-modified diet. Long-term results of surgical repairs for children with TA are being evaluated.[12] (p.970)

Pulmonary Atresia

Definition and Incidence. Pulmonary atresia (PA) is the complete closure of the pulmonary valve annulus (Fig. 41-10). This defect is often accompanied by a small, hypoplastic, thick-walled right ventricle and a small, malformed tricuspid valve. The main pulmonary artery also is often hypoplastic due to the absence of blood flow in utero. To maintain life, there must be some type of communication with the pulmonary circuit such as a PDA or patent foramen ovale. PA is diagnosed in less than 1% of all children with CHD.[8] (p.102)

Etiology and Pathophysiology. Two types of PA are recognized. In the first, the PA occurs with a VSD, an enlarged right ventricle, and an insufficient tricuspid valve. In this type, the pulmonary valve does not exist. Unoxygenated venous blood from systemic circulation enters the right ventricle, passes through the VSD into the left ventricle, and into the aorta. The second type of PA occurs in the presence of an intact ventricular septum, a small right ventricle, and a small, stenotic tricuspid valve orifice. With the second type, unoxygenated systemic blood enters the right atrium and passes into the left atrium across an atrial defect or patent foramen ovale, enters the left ventricle, and exits through the aorta. Blood that enters the right ventricle regurgitates into the right atrium through a variably incompetent tricuspid valve. In many infants, right-sided heart failure occurs due to tricuspid regurgitation and increased right atrial pressure.

Clinical Manifestations. Most of the infants with PA develop obvious cyanosis soon after birth. The hypoxia progresses as the ductus arteriosus constricts, and CHF develops. A heart murmur is not present unless PDA exists. However, without rapid medical management, the prognosis is poor.[8] (p.103)

Diagnostic Studies. Chest x-ray and ECG may reveal the enlarged chambers of the heart. An echocardiogram usually gives evidence of the atretic pulmonary valve and hypoplasia of the right ventricle and tricuspid valve. The atrial communication can be visualized, and its size can be estimated. Cardiac catheterization reveals an atrial right-to-left shunt and desaturation of systemic arterial circulation.

Interventions. Medical management of PA is initiated with the administration of prostaglandin E_1 into the ductus arteriosus through an umbilical catheter to prevent closure of the PDA.[82] (p.99) A balloon atrial septostomy may be performed during the cardiac catheterization to improve the right-to-left atrial shunt. Open-heart surgery to repair the PA is usually done when the child is between 4 and 6 years of age.[36] (p.260) Repair may be accomplished by either the modified Fontan procedure (see Tricuspid Atresia), or the Rastelli procedure, during which a conduit with a valve is placed between the right ventricle and pulmonary artery. Postoperative complications include CHF, low CO, hemorrhage, rhythm abnormalities, and neurologic insults. The long-term outlook for children who have repair of the PA depends on the extent of the cardiac defect and the type of repair. Many children have residual anomalies that influence cardiac function adversely.[31]

Cyanotic Congenital Heart Defects With Increased Pulmonary Blood Flow

Cyanotic cardiac lesions with increased pulmonary blood flow are lesions in which the blood from the pulmonary and systemic circulation mix. The mixing of unoxygenated blood from the venous system and the oxygenated blood in the arterial system produces cyanosis. In the neonate, excessive pulmonary blood flow generally does not develop until the pulmonary vascular resistance begins to fall. When the pulmonary vascular resistance decreases, these neonates develop signs of CHF. Four

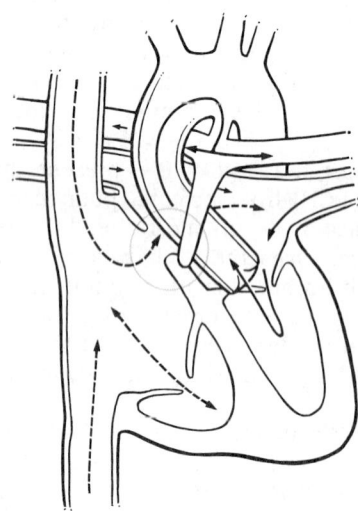

FIGURE 41-10

Pulmonary atresia is the complete closure of the pulmonary valve annulus, resulting in no blood flow to the lungs. Note the atrial septal defect, which allows blood to flow from the right atrium into the left atrium, left ventricle, and aorta; the closed pulmonic valve from the right ventricle to the pulmonary artery; and, thus, the hypoplastic pulmonary artery and its branches.

common lesions placed in this category are included in this chapter: anomalous pulmonary venous return, truncus arteriosus, transposition of the great arteries (TGA), and hypoplastic left heart syndrome (HLHS).

Total Anomalous Pulmonary Venous Return

Definition and Incidence. Anomalous pulmonary venous return occurs when one or more of the pulmonary veins drains oxygenated blood from the lungs into the right atrium rather than into the left atrium. Blood may enter the right atrium either directly or indirectly through the vessels in the systemic venous system that ultimately drain into the right atrium. When all of the pulmonary veins are misplaced, the condition is known as total anomalous pulmonary venous return (TAPVR). Partial anomalous pulmonary return exists when only some of the pulmonary veins fail to drain into the left atrium. This section confines discussion to TAPVR.

TAPVR occurs most often as an isolated defect and accounts for 1% of congenital cardiac lesions and is four times as likely to affect males as females.[77] In TAPVR, the pulmonary veins from the lungs join to form a confluence behind the left atrium. The confluence does not connect to the left atrium but empties into the left innominate vein, the right superior vena cava, the inferior vena cava, the portal vein, or the coronary sinus (Fig. 41-11). TAPVR has been classified into four types depending on the level at which the confluence drains: supracardiac, cardiac, infracardiac, and mixed.

Etiology and Pathophysiology. TAPVR occurs during the third week of gestation when the common

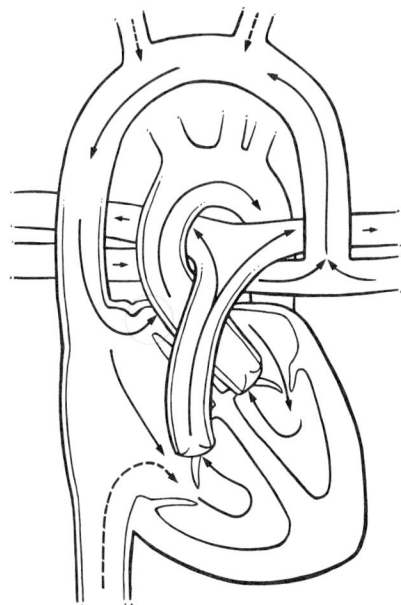

FIGURE 41-11
In total anomalous pulmonary venous return, pulmonary veins from the lungs join to form a confluence behind the left atrium. Blood enters the right atrium rather than the left atrium through the vessels in the systemic venous system. This illustration shows the possible drainage routes: left innominate vein; right superior vena cava; coronary sinus; inferior vena cava; and portal vein.

pulmonary vein fails to connect into the left atrium. An interatrial opening such as an ASD is essential for survival. Pulmonary venous return reaches the right atrium, causing systemic venous blood and pulmonary venous blood to mix before it is shunted to the left atrium through the ASD. Systemic arterial oxygen is proportional to the amount of pulmonary blood flow. In the supracardiac and cardiac types of TAPVR, there is no obstruction, pulmonary venous return is large, and systemic arterial blood is only minimally desaturated. However, the right atrium, right ventricle, and pulmonary artery enlarge to compensate for the increased blood volume. An obstruction to pulmonary venous return occurs in the infracardiac type of TAPVR, however. Pulmonary venous return is diminished, and systemic arterial blood is poorly saturated. The right atrium maintains a normal size, but the left atrium and ventricle are small.

Clinical Manifestations. Children with TAPVR present clinical symptoms that depend on the anatomy of the defect and the hemodynamic alterations. The more severe the obstruction to pulmonary venous return, the more severe the clinical course. Within the first few days of life, newborns with severe obstruction present with marked cyanosis, CHF, and respiratory distress. Cardiac findings may reveal a loud and single S_2, a gallop rhythm, but no heart murmur.

When TAPVR occurs without pulmonary obstruction, the child usually presents with growth retardation, mild cyanosis, and early signs of CHF. Repeated pneumonia is a common finding. The physical examination reveals a hyperdynamic cardiac impulse with dysrhythmia. A widely split and fixed S_2 is heard with a systolic ejection murmur at the upper left sternal border.

Diagnostic Studies. When a pulmonary venous obstruction is present, the ECG demonstrates right axis deviation with right ventricular hypertrophy. The chest x-ray shows a normal heart size with increased pulmonary vascular markings. The echocardiogram reveals enlargement of the right heart structures, presence of an interatrial communication, and discontinuity of the pulmonary veins and left atrium. Cardiac catheterization is used to confirm the diagnosis and locate the anomalous pulmonary venous connection. Pressure measurements obtained at the time of catheterization document the presence of pulmonary hypertension. These children cannot be expected to live more than a few weeks without surgery.[8 (p.100)]

When TAPVR presents without obstruction in the pulmonary venous blood flow, the ECG demonstrates right axis deviation with right atrial and right ventricular hypertrophy. The chest x-ray shows cardiomegaly with increased pulmonary vascular markings. An abnormal ("snowman") configuration of the heart may be visible. The echocardiogram reveals enlargement of the right heart structures, presence of an interatrial communication, and discontinuity between the pulmonary veins and left atrium. Cardiac catheterization is performed to confirm the diagnosis and to locate precisely the anomalous pulmonary venous connection. Pressure measurements obtained at the time of catheterization document the presence of pulmonary hypertension.[4]

Interventions.   The infant who presents with obstructed TAPVR requires aggressive management for CHF and pulmonary edema. Medical management is aimed at stabilizing the respiratory and cardiovascular status until surgery is performed. The infant with unobstructed TAPVR is assessed for the degree of CHF and pulmonary hypertension. Surgical intervention may not be needed immediately for survival; however, it usually is planned as soon as the diagnosis is confirmed.

Surgical repair of TAPVR is done through a median sternotomy with the use of CPB and profound hypothermia. The repair consists of eliminating the anomalous pulmonary venous connection, anastomosing the pulmonary veins to the left atrium, closing the interatrial communication, and ligating the patent ductus, if present. Specific surgical procedures depend on the nature of the defect. The degree of pulmonary venous obstruction before surgery determines the degree of risk for postoperative complications. Postoperative complications include pulmonary venous obstruction, pulmonary hypertension, low CO, dysrhythmias, and pulmonary edema. There is a 10% to 25% mortality rate for infants undergoing surgical repair for TAPVR.

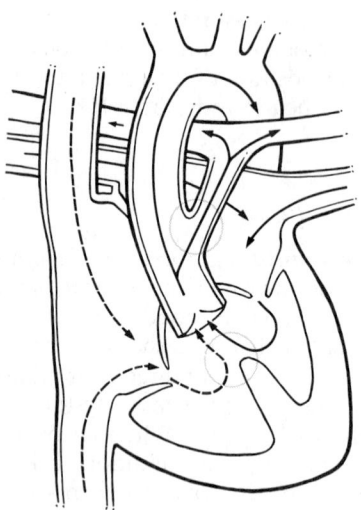

FIGURE 41-12

In truncus arteriosus, only one blood vessel rather than two leaves the heart, providing a common route for blood leaving both the right ventricle and left ventricle. This illustration shows type I truncus arteriosus.

Truncus Arteriosus

Definition and Incidence.   Persistent truncus arteriosus is a congenital cardiac lesion in which only one blood vessel (rather than the usual two) leaves the heart to provide systemic, pulmonary, and coronary circulation. A VSD is usually present. Truncus arteriosus rarely occurs and accounts for less than 1% of all congenital cardiac lesions.[77 (p.105)] Truncus arteriosus may be classified into four categories according to the origin of the pulmonary arteries. At times, terminology such as pseudotruncus and hemitruncus have been used to classify truncus arteriosus. However, these terms are confusing and are no longer appropriate.

Etiology and Pathophysiology.   During the 21st to 28th day of gestation, the common truncus arteriosus normally divides to form the aorta and pulmonary artery. When this division or separation does not occur, the common truncus arteriosus persists as the only vessel arising from the heart to provide both pulmonary and systemic circulation. With this defect, formation of the ventricular septum also is usually incomplete and a VSD is present.

Truncus arteriosus provides a common route for blood to leave both the right and left ventricles of the heart (Fig. 41-12). As the pulmonary vascular resistance decreases during the newborn period, the pulmonary blood flow becomes excessive. The large VSD allows equalization of left and right ventricular pressures and mixing of saturated and desaturated blood.

Clinical Manifestations.   A majority of children with truncus arteriosus present early in life with signs of CHF. The clinical course is determined by the amount of blood flow to the lungs, which, in turn, depends on the pulmonary vascular resistance and size of the pulmonary arteries.

Children with truncus arteriosus usually do not present with cyanosis because there is excessive pulmonary blood flow. However, they typically present with the usual signs of CHF: tachypnea, poor feeding, and diaphoresis. Truncal valve insufficiency also is common and further compounds the CHF. The natural history of this disease is such that 65% of children die within the first 6 months and 75% within the first year.[4]

A harsh systolic ejection murmur at the left sternal border is characteristic of the VSD associated with truncus arteriosus. A thrill may be present. A click follows the first heart sound and arises from the truncal valve. The second heart sound, single or split, can be loudly heard over the second intercostal space at the right sternal border. Truncal valve insufficiency produces a blowing diastolic murmur at the lower left sternal border. A diastolic rumble is heard at the apex of the heart when pulmonary blood flow is excessive.

Diagnostic Studies.   The ECG reveals a normal sinus rhythm with biventricular hypertrophy. The chest x-ray reveals cardiomegaly, increased pulmonary vascular markings, and absence of the main pulmonary artery segment. Echocardiography is helpful in diagnosing truncus arteriosus, because the VSD and the origin of the pulmonary arteries from the main trunk can be visualized.

Cardiac catheterization is used for definitive diagnosis before surgical repair. This invasive study is done to determine pulmonary artery anatomy, pressures in the pulmonary arteries (to determine pulmonary vascular resistance), function of the truncal valve, and coronary artery anatomy.[29]

Interventions.   Symptomatic infants with truncus arteriosus are treated medically to reduce the symptoms of CHF. The effects of this type of treatment for CHF are not long-lasting. At one time, temporary, palliative surgery was recommended but was associated with high mortality. Persistent excessive pulmonary blood flow can lead to pulmonary vascular disease; therefore, complete surgical repair is recommended in symptomatic infants early in life.

Surgical repair of truncus arteriosus is done through a median sternotomy using CPB. At times, profound hypothermia also is used during surgery. One or both pulmonary arteries are detached from the main trunk, and the aorta is repaired with suture. The VSD is closed with prosthetic material, the pulmonary arteries are divided from the truncus, and continuity is established between the right ventricle and the pulmonary arteries. Postoperative complications are similar to those of other repairs. The long-term outlook for truncus arteriosus depends on two factors: the function of the truncal valve and the longevity of the extracardiac conduit. The conduit must be replaced later at least once to accommodate the child's growth and physical development.[12 (p.977)]

Transposition of the Great Arteries

Definition and Incidence. Transposition of the great arteries (TGA) occurs when the aorta arises from the right ventricle and the pulmonary artery arises from the left ventricle (Fig. 41-13). TGA is the second most common heart defect, comprising about 5% of all children with congenital heart defects and occurring more frequently in males.[8 (p.87)]

Etiology and Pathophysiology. Between the third and fourth week of gestation, the common trunk (truncus arteriosus) normally divides into the aorta and pulmonary artery. Incomplete growth of the spiral ridge of tissue from which the two vessels arise results in the abnormal placement of the two vessels. TGA can be associated with or without a VSD.

The neonate with TGA and no VSD essentially has two separate paths of circulation. In the first, venous blood from the inferior and superior vena cavae enters the right atrium, goes to the right ventricle, and flows out the aorta to the systemic circulation without ever being oxygenated.

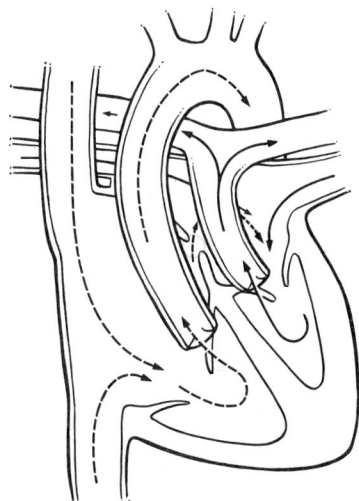

FIGURE 41-13
In transposition of the great arteries, the major blood vessels leaving the heart originate from the opposite ventricles than normal: the aorta arises from the right ventricle, and the pulmonary artery arises from the left ventricle.

In the second path, oxygenated blood from the pulmonary veins enters the left atrium, goes into the left ventricle, and flows out the pulmonary artery to the lungs without going into the systemic circulation.

For survival, the infant with TGA must have an anatomic communication between the pulmonary and systemic circulation. Mixing of blood from these two separate circulations occurs through the foramen ovale and ductus arteriosus. The foramen ovale shunts blood from the left atrium to the right atrium, allowing oxygenated blood from the pulmonary circulation to mix with unoxygenated blood in the systemic circulation. The ductus arteriosus connects the aorta and pulmonary artery and allows blood from the systemic circulation to enter the pulmonary circulation.

The neonate with TGA and a VSD has communication between the two paths of circulation that permits mixing of desaturated and saturated blood. The pattern of blood flow through the heart is similar to TGA without VSD, with the exception that blood from the right ventricle flows to the left ventricle by way of the VSD. This blood flow pattern occurs because the pressure in the pulmonary circulation is lower than that in the systemic circulation. Shunting begins as the neonate's pulmonary vascular resistance falls. As blood is shunted to the pulmonary circulation, the left atrial pressure rises from an increase in blood volume, causing a left-to-right shunt through the foramen ovale.

Clinical Manifestations. Clinical manifestations of an infant with TGA depend on the amount of mixing of blood between the systemic and pulmonary circulations. Infants whose mixing depends on a small patent foramen ovale and patent ductus become cyanotic as the structures close through normal physiologic events. Infants become markedly cyanotic and develop signs of CHF within the first 24 hours of life and are ill. Infants with an atrial or ventricular opening have better mixing and are less cyanotic; however, the infant with a VSD may be more prone to CHF. Pulmonary vascular obstructive disease sometimes develops within the first year of life despite a normal amount of blood going to the lungs.

On cardiac examination, the neonate who has TGA without VSD may not have a murmur, but S_2 may be louder than normal. The neonate with TGA and a VSD has a loud S_2, a holosystolic murmur best heard at the fourth intercostal space left of the sternum, and a thrill may be present.

Diagnostic Studies. An ECG typically reveals right ventricular hypertrophy. The chest x-ray shows cardiomegaly and a narrow mediastinum with increased pulmonary vascular markings. The cardiac silhouette may be "egg-shaped."[76] An echocardiogram confirms the diagnosis of TGA and demonstrates the arterial–ventricular discordance. The presence of a VSD or other anomalies also is documented. Cardiac catheterization is performed to document the presence of coexisting defects, the relationship of the great vessels, and the origins of the coronary arteries.

Interventions. During a cardiac catheterization, a balloon septostomy is done to provide the neonate with a larger pulmonary-to-systemic shunt. An IV infusion of prostaglandin E_1 (PGE_1) is begun to lower systemic and pulmonary vascular resistance and to maintain the patency of the ductus arteriosus. Pulmonary blood flow subsequently improves and raises oxygen saturation. When the neonate has an associated VSD, lowering the pulmonary vascular resistance may cause CHF.

Neonates with TGA undergo surgical repair soon after diagnosis. Palliative procedures are available when the neonate's cardiac anatomy makes early repair unsuitable. If pulmonary stenosis or atresia is associated with the TGA, surgical repair through the Rastelli procedure is the usual option. Definitive repair consists of switching the right- and left-sided structures either at the atrial level, at the ventricular level, or at the greater artery level. The latter is called a Jatene procedure (arterial switch), and it is believed to have improved long-term results in comparison to other corrective procedures performed in the past (Mustard and Senning procedures). Complications associated with the Mustard and Senning procedures are systemic venous obstruction, superior vena cava syndrome (edema of face and head, pleural effusion, and chylothorax), pulmonary venous obstruction, and dysrhythmia. A potential complication of the arterial switch is stenosis at the site of the pulmonary, aortic, or coronary artery anastomoses.

Hypoplastic Left Heart Syndrome

Definition and Incidence. Hypoplastic left heart syndrome (HLHS) consists of underdevelopment of the left-sided heart structures (Fig. 41-14). The problems that can occur alone or in combination include a hypoplastic left ventricle, aortic and/or mitral valve atresia, and hypoplasia of the aortic arch. HLHS comprises 2% of all the congenital heart defects. Without early medical and surgical intervention, HLHS is fatal.

Etiology and Pathophysiology. The semilunar valves develop in the fifth week of gestation; incomplete

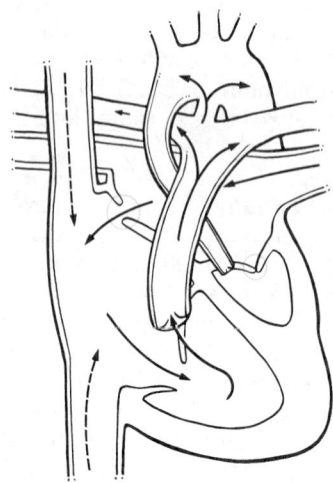

FIGURE 41-14

In hypoplastic left heart syndrome, left-sided structures of the heart are underdeveloped. Problems include hypoplastic left ventricle, aortic or mitral valve atresia, and hypoplasia of the aortic arch.

development results in a narrow or closed aortic valve. In the presence of stenosis or atresia of the aortic valve, other left heart structures, such as the left ventricle, ascending aorta, and transverse aortic arch also fail to develop normally. Growth of these heart structures depends proportionally on the antegrade blood flow from the ductus arteriosus.

Hypoplasia of the left heart structures does not permit adequate systemic blood circulation. Neonates with this condition depend on blood flow from the pulmonary artery to the aorta through the ductus arteriosus. The ductus arteriosus routes blood to the aorta. Unoxygenated blood is thereby delivered to the systemic and coronary circulations. When severe obstruction of the mitral aortic valve is present, the pressure in the left atrium rises to allow left-to-right shunting of blood through the foramen ovale.

Clinical Manifestations. Neonates with HLHS, as with other neonates with congenital heart defects whose systemic blood flow depends on the ductus arteriosus, present as healthy newborns. In a few hours or days, the ductus arteriosus begins to close, and the infant becomes symptomatic. Tachypnea, cyanosis, and other signs of diminished systemic circulation develop, and the condition of the infant rapidly deteriorates. Peripheral pulses, initially normal, diminish when the systemic perfusion is compromised. A specific murmur usually is not associated with this defect.

Diagnostic Studies. The ECG shows a right ventricular hypertrophy with decreased left ventricular forces. The chest x-ray reveals cardiomegaly and increased pulmonary vascular markings. Underdevelopment of the left heart structures is demonstrated on the echocardiogram. Cardiac catheterization is performed to assess the presence of tricuspid valve regurgitation or COA.

Interventions. Until recently, HLHS was felt to be a lethal defect with no viable treatments available. Neonates affected with HLHS did not receive medical or surgical intervention and usually died within the first few weeks of life. Now, at least two options are available: surgical repair that is accomplished in multiple stages or heart transplantation. The success of surgical repair (the Norwood procedure) depends on the infant's medical condition and the complexity of the existing cardiac anomalies.

Neonates with HLHS can be managed medically on a PGE_1 infusion until the physicians and family decide which approach they prefer. The PGE_1 reopens the ductus arteriosus. Before surgical intervention, every attempt is made to normalize blood gases and to maintain a stable respiratory status. The use of mechanical ventilation and oxygen is avoided, if possible, to avoid decreasing pulmonary vascular resistance and causing a greater flow of blood to the lungs.

If transplantation is desired, infants with HLHS remain hospitalized while waiting for a donor heart to become available. The first stage of surgical repair may be needed to permit survival.

Regardless of the severity of a congenital heart defect, the effect upon the child and family has long-term implications. The outlook for children with CHD is constantly improving as new techniques, procedures, and medications are developed. As adolescents who underwent surgery in infancy or childhood reach adulthood, long-term results of their physical and psychosocial well-being will become available. While corrective surgery is generally preferred, children with complex defects may become candidates for cardiac transplantation.

Acquired Heart Disease

Acute Rheumatic Fever

Definition and Incidence. Rheumatic fever (RF) is an inflammatory disease that follows untreated group A β-hemolytic streptococcal pharyngitis. Although the most serious manifestation of acute RF is carditis, other parts of the body may be affected in the inflammatory process, including the joints, the brain, and the skin.[7 (p.692)] Treatment of the pharyngitis with antibiotics almost totally reduces the risk of RF.

RF is considered the most common cause of acquired heart disease in children worldwide, but the incidence has declined sharply during this century in the United States and in western European countries.[7] However, recent studies suggest that the incidence of RF is increasing in the United States.[51] The incidence is greater for children in underdeveloped countries, in crowded, inadequate housing, and in poor living conditions with poor hygiene and poor nutrition.

RF usually occurs in children between 6 and 15 years of age with a peak incidence at 8 years of age.[77 (p.131)] Seasonal variation in incidence in the United States is expected, with more frequent outbreaks in the late winter and early spring when streptococcal infections are most common.[56 (p.539)] Approximately 3% of children who have not previously experienced RF develop this complication after an untreated streptococcal pharyngitis.[7]

Etiology and Pathophysiology. The onset of symptoms of acute RF typically occurs approximately 3 weeks after an upper respiratory tract infection with group A β-hemolytic streptococcus. Many researchers believe that genetic susceptibility to RF is associated with a state of immune hyperreactivity to the streptococcal antigens.[7 (p.694)] Autoimmune processes have likewise been suggested as the cause of acute RF.[56] However, pathogenesis of the disorder remains unclear.

During the acute phase of RF, the streptococci present in the upper respiratory system release a large number of toxins and enzymes that diffuse out from the site of infection. An inflammatory reaction in the connective tissue of the heart, joints, and skin leads to edema and a cellular infiltration of the lymphocytes. The heart may dilate, and the joints swell.

The acute phase of RF lasts 2 to 3 weeks and is followed by a proliferative phase that is limited to the heart. Large aggregates of cells form around an avascular center of fibrinoid and are called Aschoff bodies. These vegetations may be present in any area of the myocardium but often localize in the mitral valve area. They result in fi-

brotic scarring that may lead to permanent cardiac damage.[56]

Clinical Manifestations. Variation in clinical findings is common and depends on the site of involvement, the severity of the attack, and the stage at which the child is first examined. The principal manifestations of RF, however, are noted in the heart, joints, skin, and central nervous system (CNS). They are discussed in order of occurrence in this section.

Polyarthritis is the most common presenting complaint; it occurs in approximately 75% of the cases.[56] Swelling, tenderness, redness, warmth, pain, and limitation of motion in the joint tissue are typical manifestations. The knees, ankles, elbows, and wrists are affected most often. Typically a migratory polyarthritis, more than one joint may be involved either simultaneously or in succession. The polyarthritis lasts approximately 3 weeks and leaves no permanent damage. Arthralgia differs from polyarthritis and is a minor manifestation of RF. It is characterized by pain in one or more joints *without* evidence of inflammation, tenderness, or limitation of motion.

Carditis occurs in over 50% of all children with RF and is the most serious clinical symptom. Carditis can be fatal during the acute stage or can lead to permanent valve damage. Scarred areas, especially along the mitral and aortic valves, interfere with cardiac function. The presence of a tachycardia out of proportion for the degree of fever and a new organic murmur are distinctive signals of rheumatic carditis. The murmur is typically a high-pitched, blowing holosystolic murmur but also may include a low-pitched, mid-diastolic murmur along the left sternal border. Carditis can eventually lead to significant CHF, pericarditis, pericardial effusions, precordial pain, pericardial friction rubs, cardiomegaly, and aortic and/or mitral regurgitation. Mild carditis may disappear within a few weeks, but severe carditis may last 2 to 6 months.

CNS involvement is manifested by chorea (also called Sydenham chorea or St. Vitus dance) in approximately 10% of children with RF, particularly in prepubertal girls. It may occur alone or with the other manifestations of the disease. Chorea is involuntary, purposeless movements, which are usually preceded by poor coordination and deterioration in school work. These rapid and random involuntary movements particularly affect the muscle groups of the face and arms. The movements are usually aggravated by emotional stress. Emotional lability and personality changes are common. Chorea is self-limiting and subsides within a few weeks or months.

Subcutaneous nodules are round, hard, freely movable painless swellings, which usually surround the bony prominences of the wrists, elbows, knees, and ankles. They occur in 10% of the cases and have a significant association with carditis. Generally, they appear several weeks after the onset of RF.

Erythema marginatum is the classic skin rash of RF, but it is present in less than 5% of affected children. The rash begins as a slightly red, raised, nonpruritic macule. It extends outward to form rings with definite margins. The rash commonly appears over the trunk and inner areas of the arms and legs but may fade and reappear for several months. The rash tends to disappear after exposure to cold and reappear after a hot shower.

Other symptoms of RF include abdominal pain, weakness, fatigue, pallor, weight loss, unexplained epistaxis, and a low-grade fever that peaks during the midafternoon.

Diagnostic Studies. No single laboratory test can confirm a diagnosis of acute RF. Consequently, a set of findings known as the revised Jones' criteria have been recommended by the American Heart Association to be used in confirming the diagnosis of RF in children.[23] These criteria consist of three groups of clinical and laboratory findings. The criteria listed in the accompanying display include presence of the major and minor manifestations of RF, laboratory findings, and supportive findings. Diagnosis of acute RF is probable when:

- Two major criteria are present or
- One major criterion plus two minor criteria are present
- Positive evidence of a preceding streptococcal infection is present (absence of this element makes the diagnosis doubtful).

A positive throat culture for group A streptococci and an elevated or rising antistreptolysin-O (ASO) titer are reliable tests for evidence of a prior streptococcal infection. The ASO titer measures the concentration of antibodies formed in the blood against streptolysin-O, a streptococcal extracellular product that causes red blood cell lysis. The ASO titer rises 5 to 7 days after the infection and reaches peak levels in 3 to 4 weeks after the streptococcal infection.[7 (p.699)]

Other laboratory data that may be obtained include an erythrocyte sedimentation rate (ESR) and C-reactive protein test. The ESR confirms the presence of an inflammatory process, but it is nonspecific. The C-reactive protein is another sensitive indicator of inflammation.

Inaccurate diagnosis of RF is generally due to misinterpretation of physical and laboratory findings. Cautious use of the Jones' criteria and streptococcal antibody tests should help prevent diagnostic errors.

Interventions. The goals and objectives of the health care team include treatment of the streptococci infection, prevention of permanent cardiac damage, palliation of the other symptoms, prevention of recurrences of the disease, and emotional support for the child and family.

When the child is admitted with symptoms of RF, the nurse's assistance in the collection of the appropriate laboratory studies is an essential part of the child's care. When RF is suspected, a complete blood count (CBC), ESR, C-reactive protein, throat culture, ASO titer, chest x-ray, and ECG should be obtained. The child receives 0.6 to 1.2 million units of benzathine penicillin G intramuscularly to eradicate the streptococcus.[7] Although penicillin is the antibiotic of choice, erythromycin may be used as a substitute in children sensitive to penicillin.

The child is placed on bedrest during the inflammatory process if carditis is diagnosed. The ESR is a helpful guide in determining the amount of time bedrest is needed, the usual period being a few days to 1 to 2 weeks.[77 (p.134)] Physical exercise and activity are avoided until the child's baseline heart rate returns to its normal range. Gradual resumption of activities is recommended.

When the diagnosis of acute RF has been confirmed, treatment with anti-inflammatory agents such as aspirin is initiated for mild cases of carditis and arthritis. Aspirin also helps reduce the child's fever and discomfort. It is

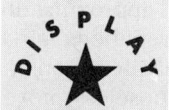

Jones' Criteria (Revised) for Guidance in the Diagnosis of Rheumatic Fever*

Major Manifestations

Carditis
Polyarthritis
Chorea
Erythema marginatum
Subcutaneous nodules

Minor Manifestations

Clinical:
   Fever
   Arthralgia
   History of previous rheumatic fever or rheumatic heart disease
Laboratory:
   Acute phase reactants (↑ Erythrocyte sedimentation rate, C-reactive protein, leukocytosis)
ECG: Prolonged PR interval

PLUS

Supporting Evidence of Streptococcal Infection

Increased ASO or other streptococcal antibodies
Positive throat culture for Group A streptococcus
Recent scarlet fever

* *The presence of two major criteria, or of one major and two minor criteria, indicates a high probability of acute rheumatic fever. The evidence of a preceding streptococcal infection greatly strengthens the possibility of rheumatic fever.*

given in a dose of 60 to 100 mg/kg/day, and blood salicylate levels are maintained between 20 and 25 mg/100 ml. Prednisone is reserved for cases of moderate to severe carditis. It typically is given for 3 to 5 weeks, and then doses are gradually withdrawn. Aspirin is not given to children receiving prednisone until the last week of treatment.

Prophylactic treatment against recurrences is begun with the first dose of antibiotic given during the acute phase. When the acute phase has ended, the child must receive either monthly intramuscular injections of 1.2 million units of benzathine penicillin G or 200,000 units of penicillin orally twice a day for at least 5 years after the acute attack.[7 (p.702)] Because the risk of recurrent RF is greatest in this time span, effective family teaching for follow-up care is essential. In addition to the routine doses, affected children also are given additional prophylactic antibiotics before dental, upper respiratory, or urologic procedures.

Treatment of CHF may include bedrest, restriction of fluids and salt, digoxin, diuretics, and oxygen. Symptoms of chorea are treated by reducing the physical and mental stress for the older child and by using appropriate measures for protection in the environment. Children with severe chorea may need anticonvulsant to help control random movement.

Children who have rheumatic arthritis without carditis are treated only with salicylates. Children initially are given aspirin, 50 to 75 mg/kg/day, divided into four doses.[7 (p.702)] Some dosage adjustment may be needed to achieve therapeutic results, but salicylate therapy usually is continued for 2 weeks and gradually withdrawn over the following 2 to 3 weeks.

Prognosis. The presence or absence of permanent cardiac damage in the child with RF determines the long-term follow-up and prognosis. Typically, the severity of the heart involvement at the time of the initial assessment is directly proportional to the severity of the residual heart disease.[56] Because each recurrence of RF increases the severity of the cardiac valve involvement, the need for prophylactic treatment cannot be overemphasized. When there is no evidence of carditis, complete physical recovery is typical.

Cardiomyopathies

Definition and Incidence. A cardiomyopathy is a disease of the myocardium and may be considered either primary or secondary. Primary cardiomyopathy is not associated with other cardiovascular or systemic diseases; the cause is often speculative or unknown. In secondary cardiomyopathy, however, the condition is thought to be related to another disease such as Duchenne's muscular dystrophy, Kawasaki disease, collagen diseases, thyroid dysfunction, drug toxicity, and hemochromatosis. The discussion of cardiomyopathies in this chapter is limited to primary conditions that affect infants and children. The incidence of a cardiomyopathy is approximately 1% of all cardiac disease in children, but it is responsible for at least 5% to 8% of the cardiac deaths in this population.

Etiology and Pathophysiology. Primary cardiomyopathies are classified according to anatomic and functional features: congestive (dilated), hypertrophic, and restrictive (Fig. 41-15). The course of heart disease in the child depends on the type of cardiomyopathy present. Therefore, each type is discussed separately.

Congestive or dilated cardiomyopathy is most prevalent in children and is sometimes associated with a history of viral infection. The condition is characterized by massive cardiomegaly due to enlargement of all four chambers. Weak systolic contractions permit stasis of blood in the heart and establish high risk for the development of thrombi. This type cardiomyopathy is characterized by gradual deterioration of left ventricular function resulting in low CO and the development of CHF.

Hypertrophic cardiomyopathy is known by many other names including asymmetric hypertrophic cardiomyopathy and idiopathic hypertrophic subaortic stenosis (IHSS). This condition generally is diagnosed in adolescents and young adults and is thought to be transmitted

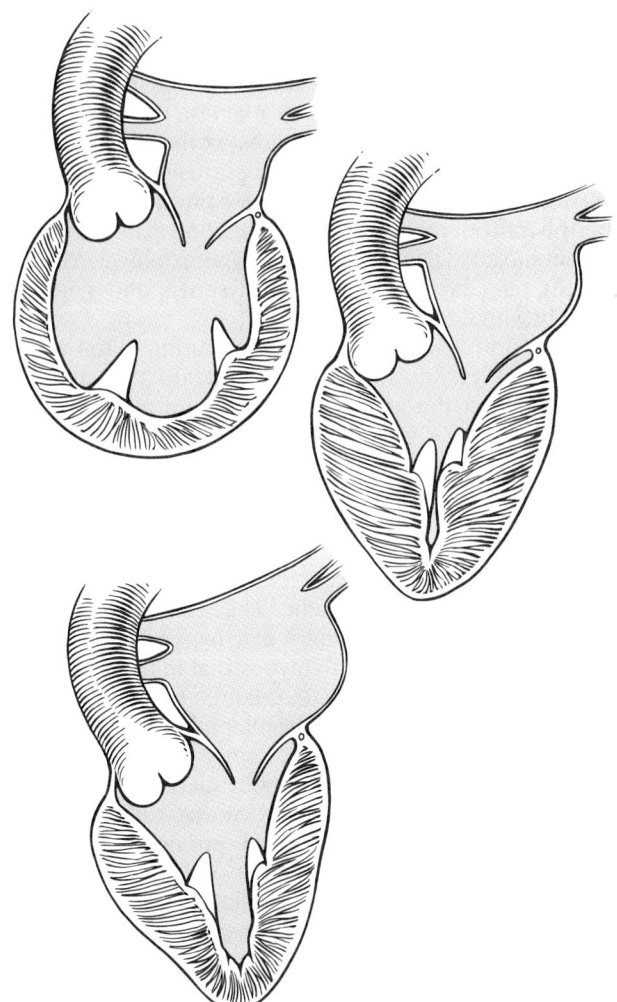

FIGURE 41-15
Primary cardiomyopathies occurring in children and adolescents. Congestive cardiomyopathy is most prevalent in children and may be associated with a history of viral infection. Hypertrophic cardiomyopathy generally occurs in adolescents and young adults and may be the result of genetic transmission. Restrictive cardiomyopathy is the least common of the three types.

genetically. The disease leads to progressive and asymmetric thickening of the myocardium, particularly along the ventricular septal region. The thickened tissue invades the ventricular chambers, leading to a reduced cavity size and obstruction of the aorta and pulmonary arteries (right and left ventricular outflow obstruction). It is a progressive disease that may lead to sudden death, particularly during exercise. The disease is familial in one-third of the cases.

The restrictive type of cardiomyopathy has features that resemble many aspects of the dilated type. It is the least common of the three cardiomyopathies and is characterized by stiff ventricular walls that lead to restricted ventricular filling during diastole.

Endocardial fibroelastosis (EFE) is a form of restrictive cardiomyopathy seen in infants. Although its cause is usually unknown, EFE may be related to a prenatal viral infection. EFE often results in marked and diffuse thickening of the endocardium and may lead to severe regurgitation. Over a period of time, the chambers of the heart become dilated as the endocardium thickens.

Clinical Manifestations. Depending on the type of cardiomyopathy, the child may be asymptomatic with only mild evidence of cardiac dysfunction. Typically, when the child becomes symptomatic, significant cardiac involvement has occurred. The child may present with weakness, dyspnea, palpitations, exercise intolerance, and signs of CHF. As the illness progresses, the child has signs of low CO, decreased peripheral perfusion, cardiac dysrhythmias, and chest pain. Progression of CHF leads to peripheral edema, ascites, cough, cool, pale skin, and hepatomegaly. The child with a hypertrophic cardiomyopathy may experience angina, dyspnea, and syncope, usually with exercise.

A systolic ejection murmur, indicating mitral regurgitation or left ventricular outflow obstruction, is often auscultated at the apex of the heart and along the left sternal border. A gallop rhythm also may be noted. An active apical impulse and a left ventricular heave may be present in cardiomegaly.

Diagnostic Studies. The chest x-ray reveals cardiomegaly, with predominant left ventricular enlargement and pulmonary engorgement. The ECG is normal or shows evidence of left ventricular hypertrophy and ST segment changes related to myocardial injury. Atrial and ventricular arrhythmias are noted often on the ECG. The echocardiogram displays ventricular hypertrophy and dilation with poor contractility. It may also demonstrate ventricular septal thickening, or obstruction of the left or right ventricular outflow tracts. A cardiac catheterization is performed to rule out structural cardiac disease, evaluate the degree of left ventricular outflow obstruction, evaluate other hemodynamics including pulmonary vascular disease, or obtain an endomyocardial biopsy.

Interventions. Initial treatment of the child with a cardiomyopathy is directed at correcting any reversible or treatable cause of the disease. Unfortunately, most children presenting with cardiomyopathies do not have reversible disease. Care is directed toward alleviating symptoms of CHF as described earlier in the chapter.

The goal of treatment for congestive cardiomyopathy is to decrease the work of the heart. Hydralazine, Minipress, and Nipride may be used to cause arterial dilation and arteriolar relaxation, thereby decreasing resistance against which the heart must pump. Anticoagulants such as Coumadin occasionally are used to decrease the development of thromboemboli caused by the sluggish blood flow through the congested heart. All these treatments for the congestive cardiomyopathy are palliative, and the prognosis is poor.

The goals in the treatment of hypertrophic cardiomyopathy are to decrease the outflow obstruction and increase the blood volume in the left ventricle. Beta-blocking agents such as propranolol (Inderal) are used effectively to decrease the rate and contractile force of the heart. This action allows an increased filling time during diastole. Calcium channel blocking agents also have been used to decrease the contractile force of the heart and increase filling time. Drugs that have opposing effects on the heart must be avoided in the child with this type of cardiomyopathy. The prognosis of hypertrophic cardiomyopathy is unpredictable, especially in children who are asymptomatic.

The goals for treatment of restrictive and congestive cardiomyopathy are similar. The treatment includes lowering the resistance against which the heart pumps and controlling arrhythmias. The treatment for restrictive cardiomyopathies is essentially palliative.

Sudden death due to a fatal arrhythmia may occur in any form of cardiomyopathy. Careful monitoring and management of the arrhythmia are crucial through frequent Holter (24-hour) monitoring of the ECG. Progressive restriction of the child's physical activity may be required. Competitive sports and strenuous physical activity are discouraged. Creative diversional interventions need to be planned when the child's activity must be limited.

Some cardiac surgeons in medical centers may attempt surgical intervention with these children. Damaged valves may be repaired or replaced, or a portion of the enlarged ventricular septum may be excised. However, these procedures have a relatively high mortality rate.

The most viable option for children with end-stage cardiomyopathy is heart transplantation. Many advancements have occurred with pediatric heart transplantation, and the survival rate has improved significantly. However, children with restrictive cardiomyopathy are not ideal candidates for heart transplantation due to underlying systemic pathology. (See Heart Transplantation in this chapter for more details.)

Endocarditis

Definition and Incidence. Endocarditis is an inflammatory process caused by an infection of a valve or inner lining of the heart. Previously referred to as bacterial endocarditis, the condition is now known by a more comprehensive term: infective endocarditis (IE). This term refers to infective processes that are amenable to medical and surgical treatment.[44 (p.719)]

The incidence of IE has increased in children. Almost half of children with IE are 10 years of age or older, but, occasionally, IE is found in infants and very young children.[44 (p.719)]

Etiology and Pathophysiology. Endocarditis is usually caused by bacteria or fungi that enter the bloodstream and lodge somewhere inside the heart or great vessels. Microorganisms are more likely to settle, grow, and vegetate in areas where there is blood turbulence created by stenotic structures or other cardiac defects. *Streptococcus viridans* is the most common causative organism, but staphylococci may also be responsible.

Microorganisms can enter the bloodstream at various sites. A localized infection, a traumatized area, surgery, or even an invasive procedure may enable the normal flora to enter the sterile bloodstream. For example, dental procedures that cause bleeding of the gums may result in the introduction of α-hemolytic (viridans) streptococci. Procedures or surgery involving the nonsterile GI or genitourinary (GU) tracts may cause bacteremia.

Although endocarditis can occur in the absence of underlying heart problems, it generally occurs in children who have CHD. Certain congenital heart defects such as TOF, VSD, left-sided valvular disease, and systemic-pulmonary arterial communications are associated with a higher incidence of endocarditis.[31] Children with prosthetic heart valves and prosthetic grafts also have an increased risk for developing IE.[77 (p.124)]

Untreated endocarditis results in severe complications. Thrombi from the vegetations can become dislodged and travel to other organs, including the brain, lungs, and kidneys, causing occlusion of affected vessels. Embolic events in ophthalmic vessels can produce sudden blindness. Symptoms of confusion and delirium may develop as a result of the embolic events and encephalopathy.

CHF may result from the direct or indirect effects of IE on the cardiac structure. Vegetation may directly damage the structure on which it has lodged, or it may indirectly alter the function of the heart through the disease process. This type of CHF is difficult to treat, particularly when the infective process is still active. Causative agents also may affect the conductive system of the heart, causing serious arrhythmias. CHF may produce pulmonary edema and mask the presence of endocarditis.

Clinical Manifestations. IE simulates many diseases and may be difficult to recognize, especially if the child has no history of cardiac abnormalities. Two types of endocarditis have been described: subacute and acute. Subacute endocarditis is characterized by a slow onset, and an unexplained, intermittent low-grade fever. The child may have experienced weight loss, may be anorectic, and may complain of headache, malaise, myalgia, or other nonspecific symptoms. A review of the history may reveal dental work, urinary tract manipulation, or other procedures done weeks or even months before the onset of symptoms. The physical examination may reveal a low-intensity heart murmur, as well as splinter hemorrhages (small splinter-appearing hemorrhages below the fingernail). Janeway lesions (small, painless hemorrhages on the palms and soles) and Osler's nodes (tender red nodes at the ends of the fingers) are relatively rare in children.[44 (p.723)]

In contrast, acute endocarditis is characterized by a high fever associated with body stiffness and rigidity. A new, significant heart murmur develops, and petechiae appear on the skin, conjunctiva, and oral mucosa. Sometimes occurring within hours, the onset of symptoms is much more sudden than in subacute endocarditis.

Diagnostic Studies. The presence of IE usually is substantiated with a positive blood culture, indicating the causative microorganism. Other abnormal laboratory findings include leukocytosis anemia, elevated ESR, and microscopic hematuria. The chest x-ray may show signs of cardiomegaly. Echocardiography may confirm the diagnosis of IE by revealing the presence of vegetations; however, the diagnosis is not ruled out if no vegetation is recognized.[44 (p.724)]

Interventions. When IE is suspected, antibiotics known to be effective in treating staphylococcal and streptococcal infections are started intravenously immediately after blood is drawn for blood cultures. If necessary, changes are made in the antibiotic orders after the culture results are available. Serum antibiotic levels are monitored to ensure therapeutic levels, and blood cultures are drawn regularly to evaluate the effectiveness of the medications. The length of antibiotic treatment is determined by the causative organism and the child's response to therapy, but generally lasts 4 to 6 weeks. Emboli from vegetations can become dislodged and travel to the brain, lungs, kidney, bowel, or spleen causing occlusion of affected vessels. CNS symptoms of headache, confusion, and delirium may occur. Special interventions are needed to prevent depression as a result of extended hospitalization and repeated venipunctures.

Surgical intervention is sometimes recommended for the treatment of endocarditis, particularly when a prosthetic material is present. Removal of the prosthetic material (a patch, valve, or shunt) is indicated for the following conditions: persistent bacteremia, repeated embolic events, malfunctioning of a valve or graft, and bacteriologic relapse after therapy.

The most effective way to treat IE continues to be prevention. Children with certain congenital heart defects need to follow a prophylactic regimen that involves meticulous oral and dental care. Antibiotics should be administered routinely prior to all dental procedures that may lead to bleeding of the gums, any surgical procedure, or procedures that involve mucosal surfaces or contaminated tissue such as the GI or GU tracts. The American Heart Association has developed guidelines for prophylactic antibiotic coverage to prevent bacterial endocarditis. An example of the guidelines is shown in the accompanying display.

Prognosis. Over the years, the prognosis for IE has dramatically improved due to an increased awareness of the disease, early diagnosis, and prompt treatment. However, mortality remains high, ranging from 10% to 30%. Mortality seems to be associated with neurologic complications (such as a cerebrovascular accident), that is manifested by lethargy, confusion, and/or paresthesia or paralysis. Those children experiencing recurrent infections also have a higher mortality. Thus, prevention remains the primary goal in treating IE.

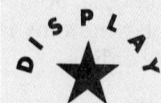

Prevention of Bacterial Endocarditis

Who requires SBE prophylaxis?

1. All unoperated congenital cardiac defects except an uncomplicated atrial septal defect
2. Rheumatic and other acquired valvular abnormalities
3. All postoperative cardiac patients *except* those with no residua 6 months after pacemaker implantation, heart transplantation, or repair of atrial septal defect, ventricular septal defect, or patent ductus arteriosus
4. Any patient with a previous episode of endocarditis even in the absence of underlying heart disease
5. Hypertrophic cardiomyopathy
6. Mitral valve prolapse

What procedures are indications for SBE prophylaxis?

1. All dental procedures likely to involve bleeding (extraction, cleaning, drilling). *Note:* Shedding of primary teeth and adjustment of orthodontic appliances do not require prophylaxis.
2. Tonsillectomy, adenoidectomy, bronchoscopy (using rigid bronchoscope), or any surgical procedure involving respiratory mucosa. *Note:* Not necessary for endotracheal intubation or myringotomy with tube insertion.
3. Incision and drainage of infected tissue
4. Any surgical or invasive procedure involving the gastrointestinal or genitourinary system. *Note:* Not necessary for endoscopy without biopsy, urethral catheterization in the absence of infection, hernia repair, circumcision, lacerations not requiring sutures.

Regimen for Procedures Involving Dental, Oral, or Upper Respiratory Tract Procedures:

Initial dose: 1 h before procedure orally, or 30 min before IM or IV. Follow-up dose: ½ initial dose 6 h later.

1. *Standard* Initial Dosages (Any of the following are acceptable)

	Route	<30 kg (66 lb)	>30 kg (66 lb)
Amoxicillin	Oral	50 mg/kg	3.0 g
Pen VK	Oral	50 mg/kg	2.0 g
Ampicillin	IV or IM	50 mg/kg	2.0 g
Aqueous penicillin G	IV or IM	50,000 units/kg	2 million units

2. *Penicillin allergy* or patients on *daily rheumatic fever prophylaxis*:

	Route	<30 kg (66 lb)	>30 kg (66 lb)
Erythromycin ethylsuccinate	Oral (2 h before)	20 mg/kg	800 mg
Erythromycin stearate	Oral (2 h before)	20 mg/kg	1.0 g
Clindamycin	Oral or IV	10 mg/kg	300 mg

Regimen for High-Risk Patients (prosthetic valve or previous SBE) or for Gastrointestinal/Genitourinary Procedures:

1. *Standard*
   Initial Dose: Ampicillin 50 mg/kg (max. 2.0 g) plus gentamicin 2 mg/kg (max. 80 mg) IM or IV
   Follow-up Dose: Amoxicillin 25 mg/kg (max. 1.5 g) orally 6 h later or repeat parenteral dose 8 h later.
2. Patients with *penicillin allergy*
   Initial Dose: Vancomycin 20 mg/kg (max. 1.0 g) IV *over* 1 h starting 1 h before plus gentamicin as above.
   Follow-up Dose: Not necessary for vancomycin; gentamicin same dose 8 h later.

(Courtesy of Children's Hospital of Pittsburgh. Modified from recommendations by the American Heart Association. (1990). JAMA *264:2919–2922. © American Medical Association.)*

Kawasaki Disease

Definition and Incidence. Kawasaki disease was first described in Japan in 1967 by the physician for whom the condition is named. Also known as mucocutaneous lymph node syndrome (MLNS), Kawasaki disease is a generalized febrile illness accompanied by significant disease of the heart, especially vasculitis of the coronary arteries with the formation of aneurysms.[77] (p.129)

Although Kawasaki disease remains prevalent in Asian children, particularly Japanese and Korean, it has been identified throughout the world. Of the affected children, 80% are under 5 years of age, and males are more susceptible than females.[90] (p.640) The disease occurs more frequently in late winter and in early spring, and recurrent epidemics have been noted in some regions. However, no evidence of person-to-person transmission has been confirmed.[10] (p.529)

Etiology and Pathophysiology. The etiology of Kawasaki disease has not been identified. Investigations have focused on microorganisms including rickettsiae, propionibacteria, streptococci, and house dust mites. However, nonorganic agents such as mercury and carpet shampoo have also been studied.[90] (p.641) Interest also has been expressed in the theory of a retrovirus as the causative agent, but the virus has yet to be identified. The syndrome is believed to represent an immunologic response of a child to an external agent: infectious, antigenic, or toxic.[67] (p.887)

Kawasaki disease is an acute inflammatory condition that is characterized by generalized, systemic microvasculitis. When the disease was first described, the condition was considered severe but self-limiting because all affected children recovered. However, some deaths do occur and are almost always attributed to cardiovascular involvement.[67] Almost all of the deaths occur suddenly about 3 to 7 weeks after the onset of illness, but death occasionally occurs years after apparent recovery from Kawasaki disease.

Early in the disease process, there is extensive inflammation of the small cardiac vessels that serve the myocardium. Cardiac pathology may continue with the development of necrotizing coronary arteritis with dilation of the vessels and the possible formation of aneurysms. In some children, the large number of platelets in the coronary vessels may gradually occlude the lumen and lead to myocardial infarction with sudden death. In other children, cardiac involvement results in pericardial effusion, serious dysrhythmias, and malfunctioning of the mitral valve, and CHF.

Although only 20% of children who have Kawasaki disease develop coronary artery aneurysms, it is thought that there is some type of coronary vessel involvement in *all* patients. Of those aneurysms that do develop, usually during the fourth week of the illness, up to two thirds regress without any treatment.

The generalized vasculitis can affect all body systems. Some children with Kawasaki disease develop aseptic meningitis. GI symptoms may include abdominal pain or diarrhea and, occasionally, vomiting. A few children may have hepatic or gallbladder enlargement. Arthritis or arthralgia may also occur.

Clinical Manifestations. Six major clinical features of Kawasaki disease have been described: fever, conjunctival congestion, changes in the oral mucosa, changes in the extremities, skin changes, and lymphadenopathy,[67] as shown in the accompanying display. In general, three phases of the illness are apparent. The acute phase lasts about 10 days and is followed by the subacute phase, which persists 12 to 25 days. The convalescent phase ends 6 to 8 weeks after the onset of the illness, but laboratory values may not normalize until much later.

An abrupt onset of *fever* may herald the illness with spiking to 104° F or more several times throughout the acute phase. An elevated temperature usually persists for about 10 days but may last 3 weeks or longer. *Conjunctival congestion* appears within 24 to 48 hours after the onset of fever. Although the eyes are "bloodshot," no exudate or other abnormality is present. *Changes in the oral mucosa* also appear with 24 to 48 hours after the onset of fever. Erythema of the entire oral mucosa is apparent. Enlargement of the lingual papillae results in the development of "strawberry tongue." The lips become dry and fissured, making intake of food and fluids difficult. Oral symptoms may persist until the 9th day but generally subside by the 12th day.

Changes in the extremities are distinctive. Erythema of the soles and palms appears 3 to 5 days after the onset of illness. Edema of the hands and feet is indurative, feeling hard to the touch. Children appear to be in constant pain and discomfort and may resist movement of the extremities. However, the changes in the extremities subside about 10 days after their appearance and are followed by desquamation of the fingertips and toes, palms, and soles. The skin peels in an unusual manner as a complete, thick layer. Transverse furrows (Bow's lines) may appear across the middle of the nails during the convalescent phase, about 2 months after the onset of illness.

Criteria Used to Diagnose Kawasaki Disease (Must meet 5 of the 6)

Fever for more than 5 days
Conjunctival infection
Oral changes
- Erythema, fissuring, or crusting of lips
- Diffuse oropharyngeal erythema
- "Strawberry" tongue

Extremity changes
- Generalized purple-red discoloration appears on palms and soles
- Indurative, firm edema of hands and feet
- Desquamation of tips of fingers and toes about 2 weeks from onset of illness
- Transverse grooves across fingernails 2 to 3 months after onset of illness

Erythematous rash
Enlarged lymph node mass

(Data from Neches, W. H. (1990). Kawasaki disease. In J. H. Moller & W. A. Neal (Eds.), Fetal, neonatal, and infant cardiac disease. Norwalk, CT: Appleton & Lange.)

The most pronounced *skin change* is the appearance of an erythematous rash a few days after the onset of the fever. The rash is generalized and resembles rubeola. Pruritus is expected. This symptom usually lasts about 5 to 7 days.

Lymphadenopathy also appears shortly after the onset of symptoms and typically lasts until the 10th day. Lymph node enlargement is pronounced in the cervical region, but it is not tender and rarely shows redness.

Each phase of Kawasaki disease has particular features related to the heart. Severe tachycardia and a gallop rhythm occur most often during the acute phase. However, more serious problems arise during the subacute phase. The child may present with signs of CHF, pericardial effusions, serious arrhythmias, and malfunctioning of the mitral valve.

Diagnostic Studies. The diagnosis of Kawasaki disease is confirmed if it follows the clinical course previously described. During the acute phase, the white blood cell (WBC) count and the ESR rise. During the subacute phase, the platelet count is elevated. Between 15 and 25 days into the course of illness, the platelets peak at 600,000 to 1.8 million. When the child's ESR returns to normal, the convalescent phase of the disease is over.

Electrocardiography and echocardiography are used to monitor the child's cardiac status. Echocardiography is useful in diagnosing aneurysms of the coronary arteries and monitoring overall function of the heart. Cardiac catheterization sometimes is needed to confirm aneurysms through angiography.

Interventions. Supportive care is the main objective for the treatment of Kawasaki disease because a cure is not yet available. Some type of anti-inflammatory medication is needed to reduce the generalized, multisystem inflammatory process. Aspirin usually is the drug of choice, and it is given in doses up to 100 mg/kg/day during the acute phase.[77] [(p.131)] Serum salicylate levels must be monitored to maintain therapeutic levels. After the fever subsides, the dose is reduced for 2 weeks to 30 mg/kg/day, and then to 10 mg/kg/day. Low doses are continued for about 3 months and sometimes up to 1 year. Aspirin should be given for a longer period if coronary artery aneurysms are present. Gamma globulin also has been found helpful in preventing severe dilatations of the coronary arteries.

It is generally recommended that the child with Kawasaki disease be hospitalized during the acute phase. Thereafter, children are seen frequently as outpatients to detect any developing complications. If CHF develops, it is treated cautiously with digitalization and diuretics.

Coronary artery bypass surgery has been performed in a few children who have developed anginalike symptoms as a result of the cardiac damage of Kawasaki disease.[90] Use of a variety of vein grafts has yielded varying results. Internal mammary artery grafts are favored.

Children in the acute and subacute phase often feel miserable. They experience discomfort from the severe edema, fever, and joint pains. Irritability and refusal of food and water are common. Mobility frequently is restricted because of the effects of the illness. The nurse should provide as many comfort measures as possible including pain medication, gentle passive range of motion exercises, and a quiet, soothing environment. If the child's oral intake is inadequate, a calorie count and dietary supplements may be necessary. Lip balm and anesthetic mouthwashes may provide temporary relief.

The nurse, along with the recreational therapist, provides the child with age-appropriate diversions within the prescribed physical restrictions. Activities using fine motor skills are difficult for children with involvement of the extremities and are not recommended.

Prognosis. The long-term prognosis of children with Kawasaki disease is not known.[67] Recovery is usually complete in children who do not develop coronary vasculitis.[12]

Cardiac Dysrhythmias

Definition and Incidence. Disturbances in the heart's rhythm are called dysrhythmias. Basic terms used to describe dysrhythmias include the following: *tachycardia* is a heart rate elevated above the upper limit of normal for a given age group; *bradycardia* is heart rate below the lower normal limits; and *arrhythmia* is an alteration in either time or force of the heart beat. The frequency and clinical significance of dysrhythmias differ between the adult and child.

Dysrhythmias recently have been observed more frequently in infants and children than in previous years. Approximately 1% of all newborns are thought to experience abnormal heart rhythm, but most infants outgrow the disturbance in early infancy. The increase in the incidence of dysrhythmias in children is related to improvements in diagnostic techniques and the fact that children who survive repair of congenital heart defects are prone to rhythm disturbances.[12] Some dysrhythmias are commonly found in children who have no evidence of heart disease.

Etiology and Pathophysiology. Childhood dysrhythmias may be caused by an intrinsic cardiac mechanism that is unaccompanied by other cardiac anomalies. However, children with congenital heart defects are prone to disturbances in the cardiac conduction system that often lead to a dysrhythmia. Other children experience dysrhythmias immediately after corrective cardiac surgery due to transient injury of the conduction system and surgically induced hemodynamic changes.

Extrinsic mechanisms also are known to precipitate dysrhythmias in children. Metabolic abnormalities and electrolyte or acid–base imbalances, for example, may produce conduction disturbances. Diseases of the heart such as myocarditis also may lead to alterations of the rhythm, rate, and conduction pathways of the cardiac system. Invasive procedures such as cardiac catheterization, intubation, suctioning, and insertion of hemodynamic monitoring lines can precipitate a dysrhythmia. Finally, systemic infections, medications, and collagen vascular disease may increase the incidence of dysrhythmias in children.

The heart's conduction system and the cardiac cycle are discussed in Chapter 39. Common dysrhythmias, grouped according to their origin in the heart, are discussed briefly below. Several tracings are given as examples. However, a text on interpretation of ECGs can provide a more detailed discussion of dysrhythmias.

Sinus Node Rhythms. *Sinus tachycardia* is a heart rate that is persistently higher than the upper limit of normal for age. This condition is typically noted as a heart rate of more than 200 beats/min in the infant and more than 140 to 160 beats/min in the child. Sinus tachycardia is caused by anxiety, fever, shock, and anemia.

Sinus bradycardia is a heart rate that is below the lower limit of normal for age. A heart rate of less than 100 beats/min in the infant and less than 80 beats/min in the young child usually is considered abnormal. Sinus bradycardia is caused by hypoxia, respiratory acidosis, increased intracranial pressure, or vagal stimulation.

Sinus arrhythmia is a phasic variation in the heart rate, increasing during inspiration and decreasing during expiration. This arrhythmia is considered a variation of a normal pattern.

Atrial Rhythms. In atrial rhythms, the impulse originates somewhere in the atria outside the sinus node. A *premature atrial contraction* (PAC) is an early P wave due to origin outside of the sinoatrial (SA) node. This rhythm is seen in healthy children.

Atrial flutter and atrial fibrillation are rapid atrial rates of over 300 beats/min due to structural heart disease or myocarditis.

Atrial tachycardia or supraventricular tachycardia (SVT) is a dysrhythmia that originates from the atrium or AV node and causes a rapid, regular heart rate of 200 to 300 beats/min. A heart rate this rapid leads to decreased ventricular filling and CO. Over half the cases are idiopathic in a normal child, but known causes include infection, fever, and CHD. The problem occurs more frequently in infants under 3 months of age, particularly in males. Both the onset and end of tachycardia may be spontaneous and abrupt. The dysrhythmia may last from a few minutes to several hours.

Nodal Rhythm. Nodal rhythm, also called junctional rhythm, is characterized by the AV node functioning as the main pacemaker of the heart resulting in a slower than normal rate and the absence of P waves. The rhythm may be caused by cardiac surgery or digoxin toxicity.

Ventricular Rhythms. A *premature ventricular contraction* (PVC) is a bizarre, wide QRS complex that occurs abnormally early in the cardiac cycle. PVCs may be a result of myocarditis, CHD, or digoxin. However, PVCs also may occur in an otherwise healthy child. It is treated if it occurs frequently and causes hemodynamic instability.

Ventricular tachycardia (VT) is a series of PVCs that usually signifies serious cardiac dysfunction (Fig. 41-16). This tachycardia leads to extremely low CO or ventricular fibrillation.

Ventricular fibrillation is characterized by bizarre QRS complexes of varying sizes with a rapid and irregular heart rate. Severe hypoxia, severe electrolyte disturbances, and myocarditis may cause fibrillation. Immediate intervention is crucial because the rapid rhythm does not allow for effective contractions or sufficient time for ventricular filling; inadequate CO ensues.

AV Conduction Blocks. AV conduction blocks are a disturbance between the normal sinus impulse and the ventricular response. One example of this dysrhythmia is complete heart block—absolute failure of the atrial impulse to conduct to the ventricle (Fig. 41-17). The ventricles and atrium contract at different rates. A slower heart rate and lower CO result.

Wolff-Parkinson-White Syndrome. Wolff-Parkinson-White (WPW) syndrome is a tachydysrhythmia that results from an abnormal conduction pathway between the atrium and the ventricle that bypasses the normal delay of conduction in the AV node (Fig. 41-18). The abnormal pathway may be detected on the ECG by a delta wave.

Clinical Manifestations. The child presenting with a dysrhythmia may not exhibit any clinical symptoms if the rhythm has not affected CO. Problems are often identified during hospitalization for another condition or during a well-child examination. Infants with symptomatic dysrhythmias may present with the clinical manifestations of CHF discussed earlier in the chapter. Older children may present with syncope, palpitation, or chest pain.

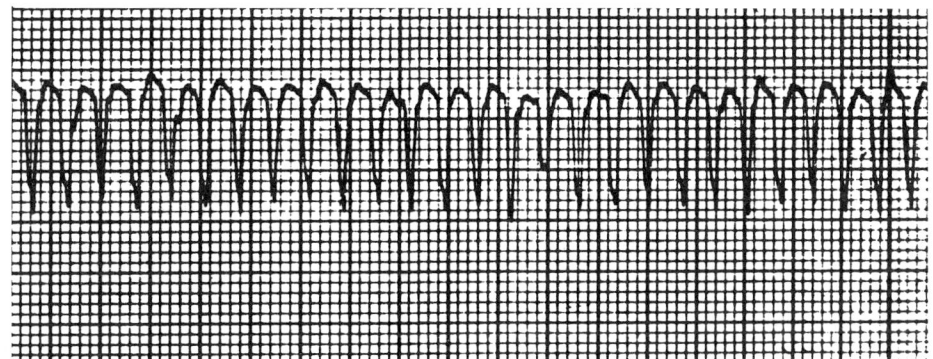

FIGURE 41-16
Ventricular tachycardia in an infant. The ventricular rate is 500 per minute, and the QRS duration is only 0.045 second. This may be mistaken for supraventricular tachycardia. However, the notched morphology of the QRS complexes, as well as the discordance between the QRS complexes and the T waves (QRS pointing upward and T waves pointing downward), is extremely suggestive of ventricular tachycardia, even though the QRS duration is normal. In sinus rhythm, this infant had a QRS duration of 0.025 millisecond with a completely different QRS morphology. (Oski, F. A., DeAngelis, C. D., Feigin, R. D., & Warshaw, J. B. (Eds.). (1990). *Principles and practice of pediatrics.* Philadelphia: Lippincott.)

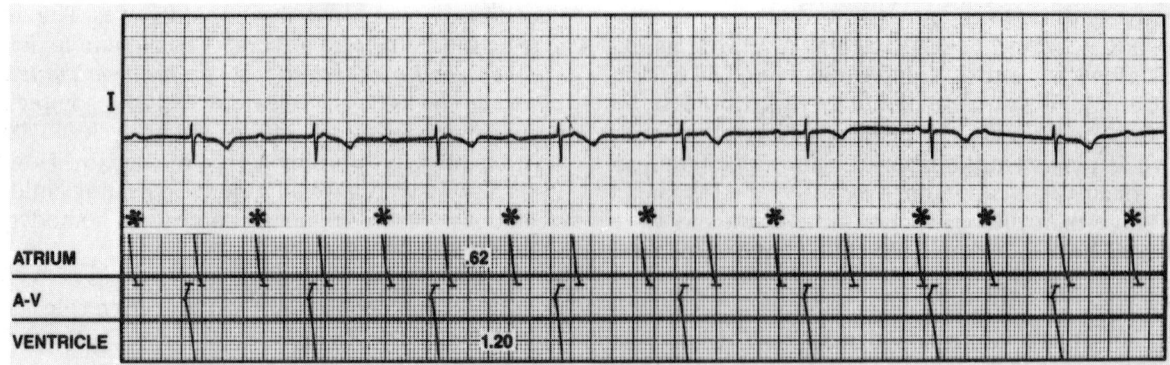

FIGURE 41-17

Complete AV block in a 1-month-old child. The atrial rate is 97/min (cycle length of 0.62 second), and the ventricles are controlled by a junctional, narrow QRS rhythm at a rate of 50/min (cycle length 1.20 seconds). The P waves with asterisks should conduct to the ventricles, (i.e., they occur beyond the end of the preceding T wave and they do not change the ventricular rate). There is complete AV dissociation, with no relationship of the P waves to the QRS complexes. (Oski, F. A., DeAngelis, C. D., Feigin, R. D., & Warshaw, J. B. (Eds.). (1990). *Principles and practice of pediatrics*. Philadelphia: Lippincott.)

Diagnostic Studies. Technologic advances in the detection of dysrhythmias have improved the care of these children significantly. An ECG is usually the first diagnostic study obtained when the child has a dysrhythmia. However, a transient dysrhythmia may best be obtained from a rhythm strip produced by a bedside cardiac monitor.

Cardiac monitoring equipment must be carefully examined to ensure its accurate function. Abnormal ECG patterns due to conditions outside the heart are called artifacts. Dry or loose electrodes, damaged cables, or interference from other equipment are common causes of artifacts and must be ruled out before determining whether the child has a dysrhythmia.[40]

A Holter monitor may be used to provide documentation of dysrhythmia activity during a 24-hour period. The ECG leads are attached to the body and worn continuously until removed by the technician. The unit is operated from a battery pack that is strapped to the waist.

Transtelephonic ECG monitoring permits the identification of dysrhythmias to occur at any time. The family is given a battery-powered transmitter and instructions on its use. When the child begins to experience cardiac symptoms, the transmitter is placed on the child's chest, and the other end of the monitor is placed over the mouthpiece of a telephone receiver. The abnormal rhythm is transmitted to a central ECG receiving center for analysis.

Exercise stress testing may also be done to observe the effect of exertion on the heart. Chest pain, palpitations, and dysrhythmias may be initiated by the accelerated demands for oxygen during exercise. An echocardiogram (described in Chap. 40) may be performed to rule out any structural or functional cardiac disease.

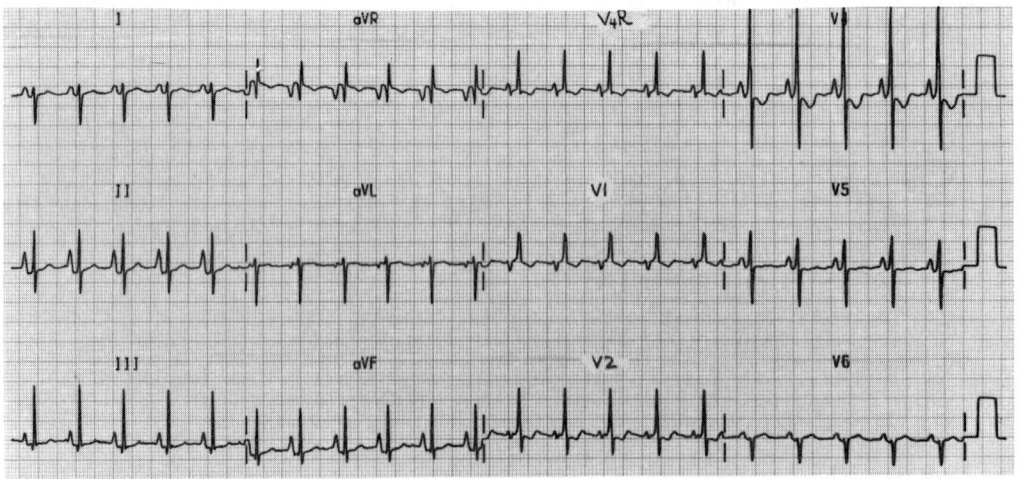

FIGURE 41-18

Wolff-Parkinson-White syndrome in a baby. In the limb leads, no delta wave is apparent. In lead V$_4$, the short PR interval (0.075 second), the delta wave, and the bizarre QRS morphology are seen most easily. Note that the P waves are tall and broad, indicating atrial enlargement. This patient had just undergone conversion from supraventricular tachycardia to sinus rhythm. Frequently, the P waves show atrial enlargement immediately after conversion. (Oski, F. A., DeAngelis, C. D., Feigin, R. D., & Warshaw, J. B. (Eds.). (1990). *Principles and practice of pediatrics*. Philadelphia: Lippincott.)

The relatively recent use of invasive procedures for analyzing dysrhythmias in children has resulted in a more precise diagnosis of the conduction system disturbance. One invasive procedure, an electrophysiologic study, is performed during a cardiac catheterization by introducing electrode catheters into the right ventricle. Dysrhythmias are induced by electrically stimulating selective regions of the heart. Various medications are administered during the procedure to determine which medication can best treat the dysrhythmia.

Transesophageal recording is another invasive procedure performed to stimulate dysrhythmias. When an electrode catheter is inserted into the lower esophagus, dysrhythmias may be induced indirectly.

★ INTERVENTIONS: COLLABORATIVE AND INDEPENDENT

Precise diagnosis of the dysrhythmia is necessary for establishing a logical plan of medical intervention.[13] Interventions are aimed at treating the cause, and individualized management of each child is required.

MEDICATION THERAPY

A variety of drugs has been used to treat children with dysrhythmias, and pediatric cardiologists are typically involved in the management of children placed on antiarrhythmic drugs. For many years, digitalis derivatives were used for the treatment of tachycardia, but current recommendations discourage its use.[13] Still, digoxin is the drug of choice for the initial pharmacologic treatment of SVT, as it not only slows the heart rate through the vagal effect on the SA node but also shows AV conduction. Tachycardia may be effectively terminated with the use of intravenous verapamil, a "slow channel" blocking drug. Verapamil should not be instituted if digoxin has been used, however. Adenosine and ATP may also be used for some children. Procainamide (Pronestyl), propranolol (Inderal), and quinidine are other useful medications for the treatment of some tachycardias.

In the treatment of bradycardia, atropine, an anticholinergic, may be given to increase the SA node discharge. Isoproterenol (Isuprel), a sympathomimetic drug, also may be given to increase the child's heart rate. Lidocaine is the drug of choice in the treatment of ventricular dysrhythmias.

VAGAL STIMULATION

Neonates and infants with some tachycardias may respond to interventions other than medication. For example, measures may be initiated to stimulate vagal tone, thereby slowing the heart rate.[13] One approach requires the application of an ice bag to the infant's face for no more than 15 seconds. In another technique, the face is immersed in very cold water for 6 to 7 seconds.

CARDIOVERSION

Cardioversion may be initiated when the cause of tachycardia is unknown or when the neonate or infant is critically ill.[13] It may be initiated when the child exhibits signs of cardiovascular decompensation. Cardioversion uses external electrical current to the heart to interrupt the dysrhythmia. The current depolarizes the heart fibers to promote the return of normal sinus rhythm. The child is typically sedated before the procedure and the defibrillator delivers 1 to 2 watt-seconds/kg. Antiarrhythmic drugs may be used in conjunction with cardioversion.

PACEMAKER THERAPY

The use of a permanent pacemaker for dysrhythmias is usually avoided, because it treats only symptoms, not the cause. Furthermore, the implantation technique can be difficult.[13] Although the indications for pacemaker therapy are not agreed upon, it has been used in the treatment of both bradycardia and tachycardia, generally to provide relief until surgical intervention is possible. The development of new pacemakers that control heart rate according to activity, CO, and respirations has increased the flexibility of their use. Some models provide overdrive pacing or cardioversion functions when heart rates exceed the limits programmed into the pacemaker's computer.

The child who has a pacemaker implanted will require continuous ECG monitoring to assess pacemaker function during the initial postoperative period. The nurse will need to know the programmed rate and possible variations with the particular type of pacemaker used. As the child recovers, the nurse begins special discharge teaching and should refer to the manufacturer's guidelines as discharge teaching is planned. The family must receive complete instructions about the pacemaker. Wound care, heart rate checks, and transtelephonic monitoring of the pacemaker are also included in discharge teaching. The importance of carrying a pacer identification card and using a Medic Alert badge is emphasized. For the child with a life-threatening dysrhythmia, parents may need to learn cardiopulmonary resuscitation.

SURGICAL MANAGEMENT

Surgical obliteration of abnormal pathways is performed when the dysrhythmia is producing significant cardiac decompensation and no other treatment is effective. This therapy requires the use of CPB and open-heart surgery. The conduction system is identified by mapping, and the abnormal pathways are divided to render them inoperative. Because many of these procedures are relatively new, the long-term effects of such surgery are unknown.

Prognosis. Infants and children with isolated dysrhythmias have an excellent prognosis. These children usually remain on medication for at least a year and have no activity restrictions. However, children with chronic dysrhythmias that are resistant to antiarrhythmic therapy have a more serious prognosis. Experimentation with various drug regimens and frequent hospitalizations often are necessary in the treatment of these children.

Hypertension

Definition and Incidence. Hypertension refers to a consistent state of elevated blood pressure in which the systolic and/or diastolic blood pressure is above the 95th percentile for age and sex on at least three different occasions.[40 (p.1020)] Blood pressure refers to the force exerted by blood against the wall of a vessel, namely an artery. When the lumen of the artery or the amount of fluid within the artery changes, blood pressure also changes. Thus, the term *hypertension* indicates that either the volume of blood has increased or the size of the lumen of the arteries has become smaller. *Primary (essential) hypertension* refers to the chronic elevation of blood pressure not attributable to underlying disease. *Secondary hypertension* results from another condition or structural anomaly of the cardiovascular system and is more common than primary hypertension in infants and children.[79]

In the United States, the incidence of hypertension in children 3 to 18 years of age is estimated to be 1% to 2.5%. More males than females develop hypertension. The same incidence of hypertension occurs in both white and African-American children until puberty, but at this age, African-American children are at a higher risk than white children. Thus, in the pediatric population, the person at highest risk for developing hypertension is the African-American male adolescent.

Etiology and Pathophysiology. The exact cause of primary hypertension is not yet known. Heredity, race, and gender have been investigated as likely causes.[94] Salt and calcium intake, stress, and obesity are also thought to influence the development of essential hypertension.[40] Evidence is accumulating that precursors of primary hypertension (epidemiologic or biochemical markers) are present in young children, although symptoms are not manifest.[40 (p.1023)] The future confirmation of these predictors will simplify diagnosis and intervention.

Over 90% of secondary hypertension results from renal parenchymal or renal artery disease and COA.[77 (p.183)] Various endocrine and neurologic conditions are also known to cause hypertension. Medications such as oral contraceptives and steroids used for long-term therapy also may be implicated.

The effects of persistent hypertension may be recognized throughout the child's body. The heart progressively hypertrophies, and coronary artery disease develops. Vascular changes in the eyes include linear hemorrhages and papilledema. Smaller retinal blood vessels narrow, and larger arteries become wide, tortuous, and irregular. Vascular degeneration also may occur in the brain and may result in large or small cerebral hemorrhages. Renal damage is also due to vascular changes and may include narrowing of some arteries, leading to loss of kidney tissue, and, ultimately, renal failure.

Clinical Manifestations. Hypertension has been called the "silent killer" because patients with hypertension are frequently asymptomatic. Hypertension may be recognized during a routine examination, but overt signs and symptoms may not be recognized until the disease is well advanced and its effects are irreversible. Blurred vision, severe headaches, seizures, marked irritability, and, occasionally, severe back or abdominal pains are definite warning signs. Hypertensive encephalopathy may be recognized by the presence of fever, vomiting, ataxia, stupor, and seizures.[79 (p.1029)] Untreated chronic hypertension eventually leads to clinical manifestations of heart failure, coronary artery thrombosis, cerebrovascular accident, or kidney failure.

Diagnostic Studies. It may be possible to prevent the devastating effects of hypertension with early diagnosis and intervention. The main diagnostic tool is accurate blood pressure measurement. (See Chapter 25 for assessment guidelines and techniques.) Blood pressure should be routinely assessed in children over 3 years of age. However, when there is some reason to suspect hypertension in a younger child, even an infant, the blood pressure should be measured. If a child's blood pressure is in the 90th to 95th percentile for age, follow-up in a physician's office or clinic is essential. Possible causes of secondary hypertension are explored by taking in-depth family history and performing blood studies, x-rays, and other diagnostic tests.

★ **INTERVENTIONS: COLLABORATIVE AND INDEPENDENT**

Nonpharmacologic interventions for primary hypertension are rarely effective when used alone to treat primary hypertension. However, some reduction of blood pressure may be achieved through weight loss, a low-salt diet, physical fitness, and avoidance of those factors known to elevate blood pressure. Biofeedback techniques may also be used.[79]

Several types of medications are available for emergency and long-term use, although the use of some drugs in infants and children has been poorly investigated.[40 (p.1025)] The blood pressure may be reduced rapidly with the intravenous administration of a vasodilator such as hydralazine, diazoxide, nitroprusside, or minoxidil. The underlying pathophysiology helps direct the choice of drugs for long-term use, but diuretics, adrenergic blockers, and renin–angiotension agents are commonly used and administered orally. Diuretics such as hydrochlorothiazide, furosemide, and spironolactone reduce the excess body fluid and exhibit direct antihypertensive actions (Table 41-5). They are used for mild hypertension or as an adjunct to other drug therapy.[40] Medications that act in the CNS include β-, central, and α-adrenergic antagonists. Beta-blockers reduce blood pressure by reducing heart rate and decreasing the force of contraction; alpha-blockers promote peripheral vasodilation to produce a fall in blood pressure. Vasodilators tend to be short acting and may cause sodium and water retention. However, they are potent drugs that may be used in severe hypertension.[40] Renin-angiotension inhibitors also are sometimes used for severe hypertension. When the underlying pathophysiology is poorly understood, sympatholytic agents such as reserpine, methyldopa, or clonidine may be needed[79] (see Table 41-5).

Children being treated with antihypertensive medications require consistent monitoring of blood pressure and evaluation of possible side-effects of the drug(s). Blood tests for drug levels, electrolytes, BUN, and creatinine often are necessary. Adjustments in dosage or types of medicines are not uncommon, especially considering that systemic hypertension is a lifelong disease.

Because the child probably has been asymptomatic, it is often difficult for the patient and family to understand the importance of compliance with diet, exercise, and medication regimens. The family and child, if old enough,

TABLE 41-5
Medications Used for Systemic Hypertension

Medication and Use	Side-Effects
Beta-Adrenergic Antagonists	
Metoprolol (Lopressor) Selectively inhibits beta receptors; used for hypertension	Fewer adverse reactions than nonselective adrenergic blockers for children with pulmonary disease Contraindicated for children with CHF, asthma, chronic lung disease, but fewer adverse effects to lungs due to selective beta actions
Propranolol (Inderal) Treatment of ventricular and supraventricular dysrhythmia	Antagonizes effects of bronchodilators (e.g., Isuprel) Oral dose may cause GI distress Lightheadedness and other CNS changes may occur Decreased respiratory function Dysrhythmias (sinus bradycardia, atrioventricular block) Worsening of CHF Hypotension Peripheral neuropathy
Central-Adrenergic Inhibitors	
Methyldopa (Aldomet) Moderate to severe hypertension; often used in conjunction with diuretics	Hemolytic anemia Positive direct Coombs' test Postural hypotension Heart block CHF Bronchospasm, hypoglycemia Parasympathetic overactivity (diarrhea, allergy, bradycardia, increased risk of peptic ulcer) Cold extremities CNS effects (fatigue and drowsiness) GI effects (nausea and constipation)
Clonidine (Catapres) Same as Aldomet	Same as Aldomet Dryness of mouth, nose, and eyes Gynecomastia in males Abrupt withdrawal may cause rapid rise in systolic and diastolic blood pressures
Alpha$_1$-Adrenergic Antagonists	
Prazosin hydrochloride (Minipress) Same as Aldomet	Same as Aldomet May also cause loss of consciousness (related to dose and sodium depletion)
Vasodilators	
Hydralazine (Apresoline) Potent hypotensive agent PO: Chronic forms of hypertension IV: Hypertensive emergencies May be given in combination with other antihypertensives or diuretics	*Common:* Headaches, tachycardia, palpitations, nausea, vomiting, diarrhea, anorexia, angina *Others:* nasal congestion, flushing, dyspnea, lacrimation, edema, dizziness, tremors, muscle cramping, depression, psychotic reactions, allergic reactions, GI bleeding, blood abnormalities ("lupuslike" syndrome seen with prolonged therapy)
Minoxidil (Loniten) For severe, symptomatic hypertension not manageable with other drugs	Pericardial effusion with tamponade Hypertrichosis ECG changes (magnitude and direction of T wave) Edema Shortness of breath Faintness Angina May exacerbate CHF, pulmonary hypertension, and renal impairment

(Continued)

**TABLE 41-5
(Continued)**

Medication and Use	Side-Effects
Angiotensin-Converting Enzyme Inhibitor	
Captopril (Captopen)	Serious nephrotoxicity, especially with preexisting renal disease
Treatment for hypertension, refractory CHF	Tendency toward producing hyperkalemia
	Impaired immune response (neutropenia, agranulocytosis), pancytopenia, skin rash, photosensitivity, taste alterations, and excessive hypotension

need to be aware of the later consequences of uncontrolled hypertension. That hypertension can be controlled for a normal, productive life must also be stressed. Contact with other children who have hypertension through personal introduction at the clinic or through a support group may encourage compliance with the recommended elements of self-care.

The Child Undergoing Therapeutic Cardiac Catheterization

Cardiac catheterization is widely used in the diagnosis of CHD and other cardiac problems. Precise details of anatomy are revealed, or pressure in the chambers is accurately measured in preparation for cardiac surgery. Chapter 40 contains basic information about the diagnostic procedure.

In recent years, cardiac catheterization has been used not only for diagnostic purposes, but also as a route for therapeutic interventions. This section describes some of the interventions that can be accomplished by cardiac catheterization. The display on cardiac catheterization in Chapter 40 should be consulted for a review of nursing care that should be provided for children and their families. In general, older children and their parents benefit from preparation using different media that contain descriptions of the procedure and the sensations the child will experience.[21]

Types of Procedures

Septostomy. Balloon septostomy is a lifesaving procedure that is used in infants with congenital heart defects in which blood must traverse an intraatrial communication to return to active circulation.[64 (p.160)] Defects such as TGA, TAPVR, and other complex defects associated with hypoplastic right or left ventricles require an opening in the atrial septum.

Both the Rashkind and Edwards-Miller catheters are fitted with balloons; the cardiologist makes a selection based on the size of the infant. Access to the venous system is achieved through the umbilical or femoral vein (Fig. 41-19). With the balloon deflated, the catheter tip is passed through the right atrium, through the foramen ovale, and into the left atrium. The balloon is inflated and quickly but smoothly pulled across the atrial septum into the right atrium. To ensure that the enlarged opening is

patent, the balloon is deflated, advanced back into the right atrium, inflated, and the movement is repeated two to four times until no resistance to the inflated balloon is encountered. After the successful septostomy, the pressures in the right and left atria should be essentially equal, and the infant's hemodynamic status should be greatly improved.

In the older infant or child whose atrial septum has begun to thicken, the initial septostomy may be accomplished with a catheter that is fitted with a blade instead of a balloon.[49 (p.329)] Using essentially the same procedure described above, the atrium is cut initially with the Park blade catheter. The opening is enlarged with a balloon catheter.

Valve Dilations. Balloon valvotomy is used primarily for pulmonary valve stenosis, but it has also been used for aortic valve stenosis, and in rheumatic mitral valve stenosis.[49 (p.330)] The procedure is used on patients of all ages from newborn through adulthood.[63 (p.161)] After the catheter reaches the heart, a guidewire is advanced to avoid the catheter's occlusion of the small opening. The deflated balloon is advanced along the guidewires to the correct position in the narrowed valve. The balloon is promptly inflated and deflated (Fig. 41-20). The procedure is repeated with a larger balloon until the valve is dilated.

Angioplasty. The most common vascular problem that might need dilation in neonates and infants is COA.[49] Although surgery is often needed later to provide per-

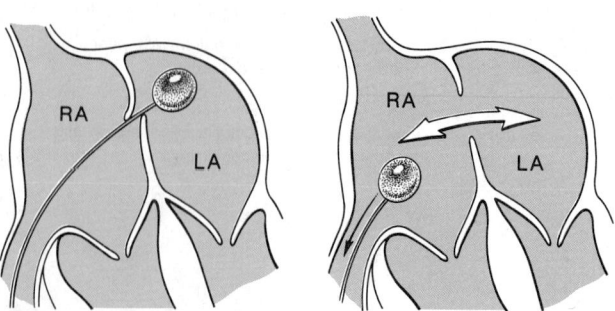

FIGURE 41-19

In balloon septostomy (Rashkind procedure), a catheter is advanced through the inferior vena cava (**A**) into the left atrium (LA). After the balloon is inflated, it is rapidly pulled back into the right atrium (RA) (**B**). This activity creates an opening in the wall between the atria.

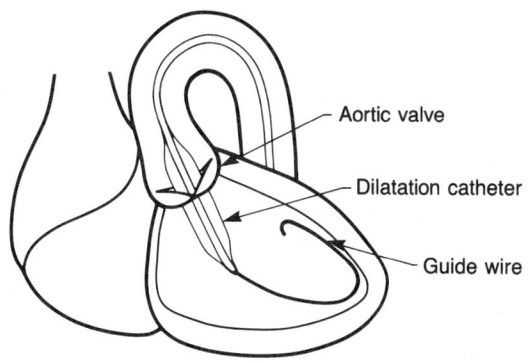

FIGURE 41-20
Balloon valvotomy. Cross-sectional view of heart illustrating guidewire and dilatation catheter positions across the aortic valve. The guidewire is curved to prevent ventricular dysrhythmias or puncture. (Hudak, C. M., Gallo, B. M., & Benz, J. J. (1990). *Critical care nursing: A holistic approach* (5th ed.). Philadelphia: Lippincott.)

manent correction of the defect, temporary relief may be provided by angioplasty. In this procedure, vascular access is achieved through either the umbilical or femoral vein. As with valve dilation, the catheter is passed over a guidewire and across the area of stenosis and is inflated (Fig. 41-21). The area of stenosis is stretched. Clinical studies indicate that the angioplasty accomplishes the dilation by tearing the intimal and medial layers of the vessel, thereby increasing the risk of aneurysms. Follow-up of children who have angioplasty is therefore essential.

Vessel Embolization and Intracardiac Occlusion. Cardiac catheterization procedures may be used to close PDA and ASDs.[49] In this technique, a cardiac catheter is positioned at the defect and a small device made of fabric and wire or polyurethane is deposited. The device occludes the defective opening, and permanent sealing is achieved by the natural formation of a thrombus and growth of tissue into the fabric of the device.

The Child Undergoing Cardiac Surgery

Cardiac surgery remains a common intervention for various types of congenital heart defects. The surgery may be either palliative or corrective. Palliative surgery usually bridges the gap between the need for immediate intervention and corrective surgery, particularly in those children who are in poor condition. At times, depending on the severity of the condition, palliation is the only treatment for the defect.

Parents who have been aware of the eventual need for surgery for their child may experience anxiety long before surgery is scheduled. Their anxiety often escalates as the time for surgery approaches. Parents realize that what they have dreaded is about to happen and that their worst fears may be realized. Providing proficient and sensitive nursing care to families through this period of acute stress is a significant nursing challenge. Sample Nursing

Care and Teaching Plans for a child with CHF requiring surgery are given earlier in this chapter.

The age of the child influences the amount of anxiety or stress that is experienced. Because many of the children undergoing cardiac surgery are infants, more psychosocial support may be appropriate for the parents than the child. However, the nurse's awareness of psychosocial development in young children is essential to the provision of appropriate interventions.

Preoperative Phase

★ **ASSESSMENT**

When the child is admitted for cardiac surgery, the nurse obtains a comprehensive history through a logical, organized approach such as the use of functional health patterns as described in Chapter 40. Understanding the effects of the child's congenital heart defect helps the nurse to anticipate findings from the physical examination. After admission, measures of the blood pressure, heart and respiratory rate, and weight are obtained. The child's color, skin temperature, quality of peripheral pulses, and capillary refill time in extremities are assessed. Heart and lung sounds are auscultated, and tissue perfusion is evaluated, as described in "Congestive Heart Failure" in this chapter.

Accurate assessment of the child's and family's level of understanding of the procedures to be done, as well as their current level of anxiety, provides additional information for development of the nursing care plan. Questions the nurse could investigate include: What previous, if any, experiences has this child had related to hospitalization? What new experiences will this child and family encounter during this hospitalization? What does the family know about the child's heart condition and the

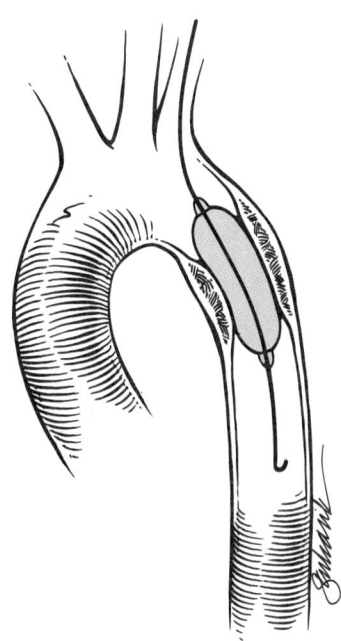

FIGURE 41-21
Angioplasty.

proposed surgical procedure? What outcome does the family expect?

The fear of the unknown produces great anxiety for the child and family. Fears of surgical risks or even of death may be expected. The impact of these emotions on the behavior and coping abilities of the child and family cannot be overestimated. To provide effective interventions, the nurse needs to explore cultural and religious beliefs and understand the practices that the family finds helpful during times of stress.

★ NURSING DIAGNOSES AND PLANNING

Based on assessment data from above and Chapter 40, nursing diagnoses may relate to both physical and psychosocial problems. The following nursing diagnoses focus on psychosocial issues and may apply to the family and child who is hospitalized for cardiac surgery:

- Fear related to inadequate information or distorted perceptions about the cardiac surgery.
- High Risk for Ineffective Family Coping related to inadequate psychological resources, unsatisfactory support system, or sensory overload.
- Fatigue related to extreme stress and lack of sleep or rest.

Together, the nurse and parents plan effective care based on the established nursing diagnoses. Several examples of expected outcomes follow:

- The parents and child use effective coping mechanisms in managing anxiety.
- The child demonstrates behaviors appropriate for age group.
- The child expresses individual fears.

The nurse plans for the care of the child based on the physician's orders and nursing diagnoses. Some general nursing goals may include the following:

- Palliative or corrective surgery is performed successfully.
- Adequate cardiac function is attained and maintained.

★ INTERVENTIONS: COLLABORATIVE AND INDEPENDENT

PARENT AND PATIENT TEACHING

When surgical intervention is planned, preoperative teaching usually is begun by the cardiologist, cardiothoracic surgeon, and office or clinic nurses. General concepts are presented to the parents and child concerning types of repair, general postoperative course, and prognosis.

Before hospitalization, parents often want to help in preparing their child for surgery. Children may want to know what to expect during the hospitalization. Offering simple, honest answers to the child's questions helps relieve anxiety and makes admission to the hospital less stressful. Preadmission visits to the hospital and pediatric unit may be offered to the parents and child. Books are also available to assist parents in preparing their child for hospitalization.

Recommendations for telling children about the plans for hospitalization are related to age. Because of their developmental inability to conceptualize, toddlers and preschoolers should be told about coming to the hospital only 2 to 5 days before the admission. The length of preparation time should increase as the child gets older. Older school-age children and adolescents, therefore, would be told as soon as the admission was planned.

While some children may be admitted to the hospital on the day before surgery, the trend is toward hospital admission on the same day as the surgery in order to defray costs. In such cases, the majority of the preparation occurs the week before the surgery on an outpatient basis. Diagnostic procedures such as blood work, chest x-ray, ECG, and echocardiogram should be discussed. The nurse must ensure that the child and the parents have a basic understanding of cardiac function and pathophysiology.

Additional teaching is needed to prepare the child and family with more specific information about the surgery. The toddler probably does not understand anything more complex than "Dr. Jones is going to fix your heart." For older children, the surgical procedure is explained and preoperative and postoperative expectations are described.

In some institutions, the anesthesiologist, intensive care nurse, surgeon, and the cardiologist meet with the child and parents the day before surgery. All members of the team explain their roles in caring for the child. The child and family should learn what type of surgery is planned, who will administer anesthesia, what type of preoperative medications will be given, and what restrictions on food, fluid, or activities are required.

The intensive care nurse or clinical nurse specialist may prepare the child and parents for the immediate postoperative period. The nurse may describe how the child will appear, what equipment will be used, and the basic purposes of invasive tubes and lines. The discussion should include chest tubes, endotracheal tube, central lines, nasogastric tubes, and Foley catheters. Parents are given a description of procedures and activities expected in the intensive care unit (ICU), particularly within the first 6 to 12 hours postoperatively. Information about the ICU visitation policy is also provided.

The child may be told about the noisy ICU environment, the need for monitoring physical status, the inability to talk while intubated, and the availability of pain medication. The need for postoperative chest physiotherapy is discussed, because the child's active participation is required when the endotracheal tube has been removed. Older children may be interested in eating and can understand that feeding will begin once bowel sounds resume and the child is extubated. Children who require long-term intubation may be started on nasogastric feedings to provide postoperative caloric needs.

Parents and adolescents may appreciate a tour of the ICU, but some may decline the offer. If so, their choice of not touring should be respected. However, the reluctance of parents to view the ICU should be remembered during their first visit to the ICU. Adequate explanations of the physical surroundings need to be provided for the family.

PSYCHOSOCIAL SUPPORT

Although infants cannot understand verbal explanations, they certainly respond to comforting for anxiety associated with an unfamiliar environment. Separation from parents is a significant cause of anxiety for the older infant. During the preoperative phase, therefore, the primary caregiver should be encouraged to stay with the infant through the night. However, parents should not be shamed when they need to spend time with their other children at home. Rather, the nurse can help the family by reassuring that the child will receive attention and care. Favorite blankets or stuffed animals may be brought into the hospital to promote the child's sense of security.

Young children benefit from preoperative play therapy. Puppets, dolls, or even painting may be used to help explain certain postoperative procedures. Practicing certain techniques such as chest physiotheraphy also may be helpful.

Particular age-specific fears need to be kept in mind. Recognition of these fears is important because they may promote further anxiety. The nurse needs to acknowledge these fears as being real for the child and must clarify any misperceptions. Reinforcing the indications for surgery may be helpful. However, providing reassurance, understanding, and comfort is an important strategy for the nurse to use in calming the fearful child.

Parents and families find that the care and encouragement of staff members are helpful during this time of stress. As needed, the clinical nurse can act as the liaison between other members of the health team and the parents. Allied health members who may be helpful include the social worker, clergy, family therapy, or psychological services. Furthermore, the nurse can anticipate basic needs such as a cot, linens, meals, access to a telephone, and other basic considerations. The family should be allowed to accompany the child to the door of the surgical suite. In some institutions, parents may be allowed to remain with their child through induction of anesthesia. Such practical interventions are long remembered and appreciated by frightened and concerned parents.

PHYSIOLOGIC MONITORING

Although little physical care may be needed preoperatively, the child's intake and output should be recorded. The temperature is monitored at least every 4 hours, and any elevation is reported to the cardiologist immediately. Preoperatively, an elevated temperature may indicate a viral or bacterial process and may necessitate postponement of the surgery.

Intraoperative Phase

★ INTERVENTIONS: COLLABORATIVE AND INDEPENDENT

PSYCHOSOCIAL SUPPORT

During the surgery, the family needs to be directed to an area where they can wait in comfort. The nurse can ensure that the surgical personnel know the family's location and can contact them readily. Interim reports can encourage families who wait for an extended time. Attention to anxiety of the family members and attention to physical needs for nutrition, exercise, and elimination may be provided by the waiting room volunteer or by the nurse,

depending on the institution's facilities. The family may appreciate a visit from a clergy member or members of the health team with whom they have established rapport.

SURGICAL MANAGEMENT

Cardiac surgery can either be closed-heart or open-heart. Common surgical procedures are described in the accompanying display. With closed-heart surgery, the heart is not opened, and CPB is not needed; the surgical repair takes place outside of the main heart structure. For example, if the PDA needs to be ligated, the heart does not have to be entered because the ductus is positioned outside the heart between the aorta and pulmonary artery. Closed-heart surgery usually is performed through a lateral thoracotomy incision that extends from the midaxillary line to the scapula.

In contrast, open-heart surgery is accomplished through a median sternotomy in which the sternum is separated and requires the use of CPB to maintain a relatively bloodless field during repair. The heart–lung machine is primed with heparin to prevent clotting of blood in the CPB circuit. During the bypass, blood from the inferior and superior vena cavae drains into the heart–lung machine instead of the right atrium. A special oxygenator and filtration system provide the same basic functions as the lungs: to provide blood with oxygen and to remove carbon dioxide. Blood exits the machine and enters the systemic system through the aorta, oxygenated and filtered. The heart–lung machine controls how fast the blood flows through the body; a low flow rate reduces the child's metabolic needs during surgery. The steps in CPB are diagrammed in Figure 41-22.

Hypothermia may be used with open-heart surgery, particularly if a child weighs less than 10 kg and the repair is complex. Techniques that keep the child's body colder than normal (18° C to 32° C) drastically reduce the amount of oxygen needed for cellular metabolism.[24] In general, the more extensive the surgery, the greater the reduction needed in body temperature. Hypothermia allows the surgeon to discontinue the heart–lung machine for a brief period (around 40 minutes).

Cardioplegia also is used for extensive open-heart surgeries. An instillation of an electrolyte solution stops all activity of the heart and preserves the heart muscle. These procedures permit the surgeon to work on a motionless heart.

MONITORING FOR POTENTIAL COMPLICATIONS

The use of CPB, hypothermia, and cardioplegia has implications for the postoperative period. Use of the CPB significantly increases operative time and the number of suture lines in the heart and vessels. Function of the myocardium may therefore be diminished, and the risk of postoperative bleeding may be increased. Blood cells may be traumatized as they flow though the heart–lung machine and contribute to the formation of thrombi. Furthermore, use of the CPB can destroy coagulation factors and result in significant coagulopathy.

Hypothermia also increases risks during the postoperative period. As the hypothermic child is warmed, oxygen usage is increased to maintain the body's normal oxygen demands. Additional oxygen is needed to respond to the body's metabolism rate that increases in an attempt

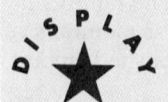

Surgical Procedures Used to Repair Congenital Heart Defects

Blalock-Hanlon Septectomy

Removes atrial septum surgically to promote better mixing of oxygenated and venous blood; used particularly for transposition of the great arteries.

Blalock-Taussig (B-T) Shunt

Creates a communication between the right or left subclavian artery and the right or left pulmonary artery. Some of the blood from the aorta enters the pulmonary system, establishing pulmonary blood flow. Pulses in corresponding upper extremity will not be palpable.

Modified B-T Shunt

Implies that a prosthetic shunt was used between the subclavian and pulmonary arteries as opposed to directly anastomosing the subclavian to the pulmonary artery.

Central Shunt

Creates a communication between the aorta and the pulmonary artery; functions on the same principle as Waterston-Cooley and B-T shunts. Principal difficulty is sizing hole to promote optimum pulmonary blood flow yet not overperfuse lungs to point of causing CHF or pulmonary hypertension. Chief advantage is that procedure permits bilateral pulmonary artery growth.

Fontan Procedure

Routes systemic venous blood flow directly from the right atrium into the pulmonary arteries or by a hypoplastic right ventricle. Procedure has been modified since introduction in 1971.

Glenn Anastomosis

Creates a communication between the superior vena cava (SVC) and the pulmonary artery (PA), thus bypassing SVC venous return from the right atrium; generally done using right SVC to right PA; may also be done on the left. Creates an increased amount of pulmonary blood flow under low pressure. Used mostly for tricuspid atresia; recently used as 1st stage of a two-stage Fontan procedure (referred to as a "Bidirectional Glenn"). Unique complication is the SVC syndrome.

Jatene Procedure

Transposes the great arteries above the semilunar valves. Also called an "arterial switch" operation. Coronary arteries are removed from the aorta before the switch and then transplanted into the aorta at its new location. Used primarily in correction of the transposition of the great arteries.

Mustard or Senning Procedure

Reverses blood flow pattern at the atrial level. Also called an "atrial switch" operation. An intra-atrial baffle diverts systemic venous blood to the lungs by way of the mitral valve and left ventricle. Pulmonary venous blood crosses over to the tricuspid valve, right ventricle, and aorta. Used for transposition of the great arteries.

Pott's Anastomosis

Creates a communication between the descending aorta and the left pulmonary artery; based on the same principles used in the central shunt, Waterston-Cooley, and B-T shunt. Initially difficult to control size of shunt; may cause CHF. Later, difficult to close.

Pulmonary Outflow Tract Enlargement With Patch

Places a prosthetic or pericardial patch across the pulmonary outflow tract, possibly across pulmonary valve annulus, and into the main pulmonary artery. Depending on technique, cardiopulmonary bypass may or may not be needed, although bypass more often used. Smaller than normal pulmonary arteries expected to grow due to increased amount of blood flow.

Rastelli Procedure

Closes the ventricular septal defect (VSD) with a baffle that directs blood from the left ventricle, through the VSD, and into the aorta. The pulmonic valve is closed, and a conduit is placed from the right ventricle to the pulmonary artery. Used for transposition of the great arteries when a VSD and severe pulmonary stenosis are also present. Requires replacement of conduits as child grows.

Waterston-Cooley Anastomosis

Creates a direct communication between the back of the ascending aorta and the front of the right pulmonary artery where they overlap. An opening is made between the back of aorta and front of right pulmonary artery, and the two are sewn together. Works on same principle as B-T shunt. Opening may be too large, increasing pulmonary blood flow too much, resulting in CHF and pulmonary hypertension. Distorts the right pulmonary artery and may necessitate reconstruction later.

1. Patient's deoxygenated blood enters the bypass circuit from the venous cannulas in the superior and inferior vena cavae.
2. Blood is temporarily held in the reservoir.
3. The oxygenator adds oxygen and removes carbon dioxide from the patient's blood.
4. The heat exchanger initially cools, then rewarms the patient's blood.
5. Roller pumps pump the blood through the circuit and back to the patient.
6. Oxygenated blood is returned to the ascending aorta by way of the aortic cannula.

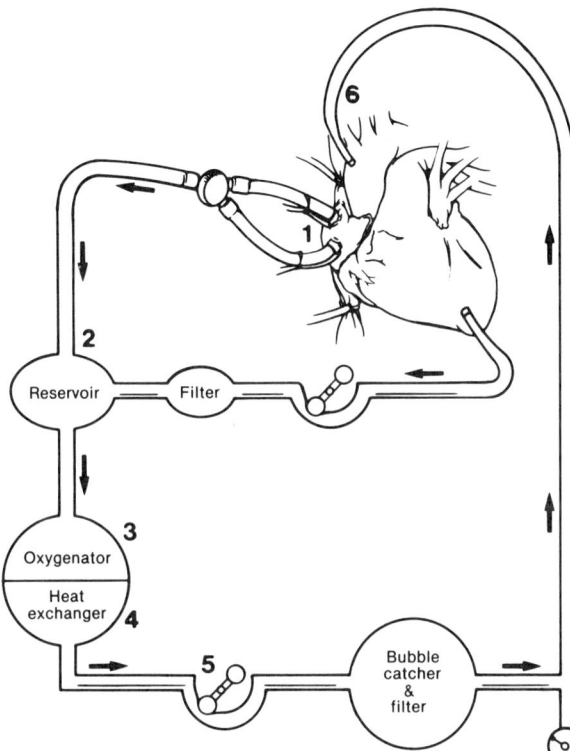

FIGURE 41-22

Flow of blood through the cardiopulmonary bypass circuit. (Hudak, C. M., Gallo, B. M., & Benz, J. J. (1990). *Critical care nursing: A holistic approach* (5th ed.). Philadelphia: Lippincott. Adapted from Calkins JM: Pumps, primes, and perfusion techniques. In Conahan, T. J. (1982). *Cardiac anesthesia.* Stoneham, MA: Butterworths.)

to raise the core body temperature. The body may not recognize when the normal temperature of 37° C has been reached. Therefore, the child may develop a fever, often up to 38° C to 40° C rectally.

The state of cardioplegia induced in the operative phase predisposes the heart's muscle to poor contractility in the early postoperative phase. Cardioplegia solution is a mixture of electrolytes. Until the myocardial depressant effects of cardioplegic solutions have worn off, the heart is not able to pump efficiently, and CO may be compromised.

The respiratory system also is adversely affected by cardiac surgery. Whether open- or closed-heart surgery is performed, the child is intubated and anesthetized, and spontaneous respirations cease. With mechanical ventilation, the respiratory muscles are not actively used, and alveoli have a greater tendency to collapse. Respiratory

distress may follow. The longer the surgery, the greater the anesthesia's negative impact on the respiratory system.

If a surgical procedure necessitates the use of CPB, the lungs do not receive any blood flow. It is thought that the lungs are tolerant of this deprivation because of hypothermia and the time-limited use of the bypass machine. However, lung function in the immediate postoperative period may be adversely affected.

The last major intraoperative factor that affects the child's postoperative course is the hemodynamic and anatomic results of the operative procedure. Depending on the child's age, preoperative circulation may have been different from the circuit established with surgery. Before surgery, the heart and body may have adapted to the hemodynamics of the heart defect. Postoperatively, the repair may contribute to compromise of CO. For example, complete heart block may develop from a VSD repair because of intraoperative damage to the conductive system. A less than adequate heart rate may decrease CO enough to produce symptoms. Likewise, children with preoperative polycythemia and coagulopathies are at a greater risk for postoperative bleeding.

Postoperative Phase

★ ASSESSMENT

In the immediate postoperative period, the child is placed in an ICU. The nurse needs to be especially alert to the physiologic changes, which, if unrecognized, could result in morbidity or mortality for the child. Assessment of both pulmonary and systemic perfusion is necessary to determine the adequacy of the CO. If the child's CO is adequate, pulses are easily palpable, capillary refill time is about 2 seconds, and the temperature of the skin is warm or cool, depending on the child's body temperature. Arterial blood gases do not indicate an acidosis. Oxygen saturation measures are within an acceptable, predetermined range, depending on the child's defect and repair. If the child is extubated, no respiratory distress is noted; respiratory rate is within normal limits, and no retractions are visible. Neurological status of the child is intact. Urine output is considered adequate if the infant produces at least 1 cc/kg/h and the older child produces 1 to 2 ml/kg/h.[24] The child's body temperature is closely monitored to avoid hyperthermia.

After the child has been transferred out of the ICU, general principles of assessment remain essentially the same as in the ICU. CO is monitored through manifestations of organ functioning and tissue perfusion. Respiratory status is monitored closely. Body temperature also is assessed frequently to detect the possible development of infection.

When the child begins taking a regular diet, assessment of nutritional intake is needed because children often have poor appetites postoperatively. Children who are at risk for systemic venous engorgement from long-term, high right-sided pressures tend to be intolerant of food because of engorgement of the liver; this condition usually resolves with time.

★ NURSING DIAGNOSES AND PLANNING

Based on the assessment data from above and Chapter 40, the following nursing diagnoses may apply to the child undergoing cardiac surgery:

- Anxiety of Parents related to appearance and behavior of child.
- Altered Comfort related to surgical procedure.
- Body Image Disturbance related to the appearance of the surgical incision.
- Altered Family Processes related to hospitalization of the child and loss of parental role.
- Altered Nutrition: Less Than Body Requirements related to loss of appetite after surgery.
- High Risk for Fluid Volume Deficit related to postoperative bleeding.
- Potential Complication: Cardiac/Vascular related to surgical repair.
- Potential Complication: Respiratory related to inadequate tissue perfusion.
- Potential Complication: Metabolic related to infection.
- Potential Complication: Renal/Urinary related to inadequate urinary output.

The nurse and child (or parents) together plan effective care based on the established nursing diagnoses. Examples of expected outcomes include the following:

- Parents relate less anxiety after teaching.
- The child relates relief after the administration of an effective comfort measure.
- The child shares feelings about how the self is viewed.
- The parents participate in the care of the child.
- The child increases oral intake to levels appropriate for size.

★ INTERVENTIONS: COLLABORATIVE AND INDEPENDENT

PHYSIOLOGIC MONITORING

When the child first arrives in the ICU, the nurse carefully monitors the child's airway, temperature, blood pressure, heart rate and rhythm. Because many factors depress myocardial contractility and decrease CO, the nurse must be prepared to administer medications to improve contractility of the heart muscle. These medications, referred to as inotropes, may include dopamine, dobutamine, and digoxin.

Capillary membrane permeability is reduced because of the effects of CPB, hypothermia, and cardioplegia. The reduction in permeability causes fluid imbalances that may further reduce CO. As the child's body temperature returns to normal after being hypothermic, the vessels dilate, causing a hypovolemic state. Insufficient fluid volume intravascularly results in decreased blood pressure. Careful monitoring of the blood pressure, heart rate, central venous pressure, temperature, urine output, and other signs of tissue perfusion are required continuously to prevent sudden effects of fluid imbalances. Fluid replacement should be given, usually in boluses of 5 to 10 cc/kg over 20 to 60 minutes; this fluid may be infused immediately if severe signs of decompensation occur. Either crystalloid or colloid fluids may be used.

Urine output may be excessive immediately postoperatively because diuretics often are used when discontinuing CPB. These medications promote diuresis and help reduce the amount of "third spacing," that is, fluid accumulating in the extravascular space (edema) due to altered cell membrane permeability.

Fever alters hemodynamics in children of all ages. The neonate is particularly sensitive to any changes in thermoregulation. Hyperthermia causes the events previously described, but in small infants, the events occur in a more dramatic fashion. Hypothermia also results in significant hemodynamic changes. The neonate cannot shiver to increase body temperature; thus, brown fat stores are broken down to provide heat, and the use of oxygen increases. In particular, neonates should be kept in a strict neutral thermal environment, maintaining body temperature near 37° C to keep oxygen requirements at a minimum.[85] Heat is provided by using overhead lamps or radiant warmers.

Blood gases or noninvasive techniques of monitoring respiratory status (pulse oximetry or transcutaneous monitoring) should be performed regularly. Changes of ventilator settings should be made to meet the demands of the patient's metabolism. That is, if a child develops a fever, the body's metabolic rate significantly increases to maintain adequate CO, blood pressure, and organ perfusion. This acute demand for oxygen needs to be provided by the ventilator because the child cannot compensate because of anesthesia and sedation. Thus, the nurse must continuously observe the child for signs of inadequate oxygenation that may result in hypoxia and acidosis. Hypoxia may be recognized by presence of altered blood gases; pale, cold, clammy skin; bradycardia; tachypnea with possible retractions or nasal flaring in the extubated child; decreased neurologic sensorium; or increased irritability. Unless the child is hypotensive, the head of the bed should be elevated to a 30-degree angle to facilitate diaphragmatic expansion and to promote drainage of fluid from the chest cavity.[85]

When children begin to wake up, they may exhibit agitation by thrashing about and pulling at the lines. Agitated children, especially infants, often become unstable physiologically. Heart rate and blood pressure increase, ventilation becomes more difficult, and hypoxemia and bradycardia often develop. In these instances, infants and children are sedated again and may be pharmacologically paralyzed until they are stable and ready to become less technology-dependent. Less agitation is typical after the care providers and surroundings are more familiar. The child is greatly comforted by the presence of a parent or other family member in the room.

When extubated, the child needs to be monitored for further signs of respiratory decompensation, which may necessitate re-intubation. The extubated child often does not take deep breaths due to the effects of anesthesia, narcotics, or pain. To avoid respiratory acidosis, the child needs to be reminded to breathe deeply. Analgesia and sedation should be used with discretion because each may further depress respiratory drive and make the child more acidotic. Vigorous pulmonary toilet with coughing and deep breathing is done every 1 to 2 hours. When awake, younger and less cooperative children may prefer blowing bubbles or blowing up balloons as deep breathing techniques. Pulmonary toilet is more effective when the child is pain free and can avoid splinting, shallow breathing, and weak coughing. Therefore, pain medication is administered as often as necessary. Pain assessment tools and scales are helpful in determining the child's level of pain (see Chap. 28 concerning children with pain). Continuous monitoring, perhaps with pulse oximetry, is useful.

PREVENTION OF COMPLICATIONS

The diagnosis of *hemorrhage* is usually determined when chest tube drainage is greater than 3 cc/kg/h.[85] Immediate correction of the bleeding is imperative. Protamine sulfate may be administered if bleeding is caused by a heparin-induced coagulopathy. More often, however, blood products with coagulation factors such as platelets, cryoprecipitate, fresh frozen plasma, or whole blood are given to reverse the coagulopathic effects of the CPB. If bleeding cannot be controlled with blood products or medications, the child is taken back to the operating room for exploratory surgery.

If chest tube patency is not maintained, fluid may accumulate around the heart and prevent it from emptying. This phenomenon is known as *cardiac tamponade.* Chest tube patency is maintained by milking or stripping the chest tubes every 20 minutes immediately postoperatively. When drainage has decreased, the procedure is done less frequently. Stripping and back stripping should be performed by knowledgeable and experienced caregivers, because these techniques may produce tension pneumothorax.

When working with chest tubes, the nurse must not only ensure that they are draining adequately but also that there is no *air leak* in the system. If there is an air leak, the specific area of leakage should be determined, and the child should be closely monitored for signs or respiratory distress. Air leaks may eventually lead to pneumothoraces.

Cardiac tamponade can occur later in the immediate postoperative course. A decrease in systolic blood pressure, increase in heart rate, increase in central venous pressure, a narrowing pulse pressure (difference between systolic and diastolic pressures), and muffled heart tones are signs of tamponade. Chest x-ray or echocardiogram is used to confirm fluid in the pericardial space, if time permits.

The tamponade developing immediately postoperatively is treated by returning the child to the operating room for evacuation of the blood. Sometimes, when a tamponade occurs later in the postoperative course and does not create significant symptoms, a pericardial tap may be performed. In this procedure, a needle is inserted into the pericardial space and the fluid is aspirated with a syringe.

Dysrhythmias are not uncommon postoperatively and are associated particularly with certain surgical procedures. Any surgical repair that is performed near the conduction system may cause a dysrhythmia. The dysrhythmia may be temporary due to inflammation in the area or permanent due to direct injury to the conductive fibers. The most common dysrhythmias observed after cardiac surgery are supraventricular tachycardia, various degrees of heart block, and right bundle-branch block.[85]

When dysrhythmias occur, the child must be assessed immediately for evidence of compromised CO. In children, atrial dysrhythmia tends to be more common than ventricular dysrhythmia. Atrial dysrhythmias usually do not disturb CO as much as those that are ventricular in origin. Antidysrhythmics should be readily available and are given when symptoms result from the abnormal heart beat. Lidocaine is usually given for ventricular arrhythmias, but digoxin and quinidine more often are used for supraventricular tachycardia. Isuprel and atropine are commonly used for slow heart rates. Cardioversion, a procedure in which a synchronized electrical impulse is passed through the heart to resume the normal sequence of conduction (sinus rhythm), may be used for those tachydysrhythmias that cause sudden decompensation or do not respond to pharmacologic management.

If the child had preoperative *pulmonary hypertension,* there is a greater risk after surgery for an inadequate CO due to failure of the right ventricle from pumping against high resistance in the lungs. Depending on the degree of vascular changes, the blood pressure in the lungs may return to normal over days, months, or years. However, the child may be unstable immediately postoperatively due to unpredictable reactions of the lungs to the newly established blood flow. This problem may be especially severe in infants.

In older children with preoperative pulmonary hypertension, conditions that trigger pulmonary hypertensive episodes need to be avoided in the postoperative phase. Examples of such conditions include inadequate oxygenation, acidosis, hypothermia, poor ventilation, low glucose levels, and low calcium levels.

Pulmonary hypertension also can adversely affect gas exchange. Several other conditions such as poor chest tube functioning, atelectasis, pleural effusion, anesthesia, pain, and poor ventilation all can result in reduced gas exchange. When monitoring infants' oxygen saturation levels, the nurse should remember that neonates can tolerate much lower oxygen saturations because their fetal saturations were only about 25%.

Metabolic acidosis often occurs immediately postoperatively due to hypovolemia. Often, once fluid has been replaced, the acidosis corrects itself. If it does not, sodium bicarbonate may be given to reverse the acidosis.

Respiratory acidosis occurring immediately postoperatively is usually a result of inadequate ventilation. If the child is on a ventilator, adjustments should be made to increase the amount of minute volume (the amount of air entering the lungs per minute). In infants and younger children, the mean inspiratory pressure or respiratory rate is adjusted; in an older child or adolescent, the tidal volume is adjusted instead of the inspiratory pressure due to different types of ventilators used. Unless the child is hypotensive, the head of the bed should be raised to a 30-degree angle to facilitate expansion of the diaphragm and to promote drainage of fluid from the chest cavity by way of the chest tubes.[85]

Infection is another possible complication of surgery. When cardiac surgery is performed, multiple invasive lines and catheters are inserted with a sterile technique. Contamination greatly increases the risk of postoperative infection. Therefore, it is imperative that the nurse practice strict sterile technique with all invasive procedures, including dressing changes, Foley care, and changing intravenous tubing.

Many precautions are taken to reduce the spread of infection, but handwashing is the most effective intervention. Antibiotics may be ordered prophylactically preoperatively and usually for 2 to 3 days postoperatively. Lines and catheters are removed as soon as possible. Should a temperature develop within the first 2 days after surgery, pulmonary atelectasis is suspected and treated with vigorous pulmonary toilet, acetaminophen, and an analgesic. The fever usually resolves within hours after this treatment has been started.

The nurse watches for subtle signs of infection: temperature instability, poor feeding, fatigue, pale or mottled appearance. Incisions and intravenous sites need to be assessed closely for signs of infection such as inflammation and drainage, especially if it is purulent in character. An infection should be suspected if a fever develops or persists after 72 hours postoperatively.[92]

Children with pain are discussed in Chapter 28 with pharmacologic and nonpharmacologic methods of alleviating pain.

PSYCHOSOCIAL SUPPORT

Despite preoperative teaching, parents find seeing their child in the ICU a traumatic experience. The first visit postoperatively often is the most difficult. The child has numerous tubes and is edematous, restrained, and almost naked in a noisy room.

Parents' responses vary. Some parents are open in expressing their fears and anxieties; others may be closed and uncommunicative; still others may exhibit feelings in more overt behaviors and may be considered "difficult." The nurse should assist the family by comforting them, offering additional information, and providing reassurance about the child's condition. Asking how the parents are coping and how the staff can help them is important. The nurse also encourages parents to touch and talk to their child.

As the child's condition becomes more stable, parents are encouraged to spend time with their child and to become involved in physical care as much as possible or as much as they desire. For example, family members may want to assist in helping the child to ambulate or to perform pulmonary toileting. Such involvement may lessen parents' feelings of role alteration.

When intensive care is no longer needed, the child is transferred to the general pediatric unit. This transition is usually an adjustment for both the patient and family. The intensive unit offered continuous nursing care, and the nurse was available immediately. However, the child and family may feel that inadequate care is being delivered on the general unit. The cardiologist, clinical nurse specialist, and staff nurse need to help the child and family understand that such intense observation is no longer needed. This part of the hospitalization is primarily intended to help the patient and family prepare for home. The child, if old enough, and the family should become actively involved in the care. Diversional activities, often organized by Child Life Specialists, encourage the child to engage in play, both medical and nonmedical. Trips to the playroom often become the highlight of the child's day.

CONTINUING CARE

After open-heart surgery, a child occasionally develops a persistent low-grade temperature about a week postoperatively.[92] The child may complain of chest pain. Pleural and pericardial effusions may develop; a pericardial friction rub may be auscultated. A chest x-ray shows enlargement of the heart, and ECG changes are evident. The ESR may be elevated. This group of manifestations is known as the "postcardiotomy syndrome." The cause remains unclear, although it is thought to be part of an autoimmune process. If this syndrome develops, aspirin therapy is started to reduce the pericardial inflammation and may be continued for several months. Steroids also may be used for their anti-inflammatory effects. Bedrest is recommended until all symptoms of pericarditis subside. Close outpatient monitoring is planned to evaluate for pleural effusions, respiratory distress, or any other problems. Families are instructed to notify the cardiologist of any chest pain, fever, or difficulty breathing.

Postoperatively, the child has a high caloric need of approximately 100 to 110 calories/kg/day. A poor appetite may make it difficult for the child to consume this amount. Antacids, given to relieve GI distress, often are not effective. The child's weight is monitored at least daily. If significant weight loss occurs, supplemental additives or formulas are given to achieve the daily caloric goal. Consultation with the nutritionist may be beneficial.

DISCHARGE PLANNING

Discharge planning begins in the early postoperative period. For example, the child and parents can begin to learn about the prescribed medications and their indications. Later, when discharge is imminent, the child and parents need to know the dosage, method of administration, and side-effects of each medication. They should be expected to administer the medications safely before discharge. A written schedule of dosages and administration times is helpful to ensure that the child receives the medication properly at home.

The family needs to know what symptoms should be reported to the cardiologist. Fever, nausea, vomiting, diarrhea, irritability, and difficulty with feedings may indicate an infection or the development of CHF.

Activity limitations should be specific to each child. Limitations usually are imposed for several weeks after discharge to promote healing of the sternum. Younger children tend to pace themselves adequately, but the activity of older children and adolescents may be more difficult to control. If the older child ignores the limitations, the reasons for the restrictions should be emphasized. Sometimes children feel a strong desire for control and independence, yet they also need the security of knowing that a loved-one is there as a caretaker.

In preparing the child and family for discharge, the nurse should be sensitive about the anxieties associated with going home. For example, the family may have nonspecific fears or they may worry about postoperative complications developing at home, the child's future, and quality of life. Information is given about resources available to both the child and the family. Phone numbers may be provided for a variety of people including the cardiologist, clinical nurse specialist, visiting or public health nurse, psychiatrist, or family therapist. Emphasis is placed on treating the child as normally as possible to help reduce the risk of future behavior problems.

After returning home, children, particularly infants, toddlers, and preschoolers, may show signs of regression. For example, an older infant who drinks from a cup may begin using a bottle again postoperatively. Similarly, a toddler or preschooler who is toilet-trained may have "accidents" during and after hospitalization. Sleep disturbances are not uncommon. The nurse should alert parents to such responses after hospitalization. Given time, the child eventually returns to prehospitalization behavior.

The child's school nurse is notified of any restrictions or any medications the child may need during school hours. Children usually are encouraged to participate in physical education postoperatively, as soon as it is recommended by the cardiologist or surgeon.

★ EVALUATION

Periodically, the nurse and family evaluate the outcomes of care given. Examples of outcomes for the child undergoing cardiac surgery were given under Planning in this section. Have short-term goals been met? Are long-term goals still realistic?

Heart Transplantation

Orthotopic heart transplantation refers to the removal of a recipient's heart and the implantation of a donor heart in the same place. This type of surgery offers life and hope to those children with heart muscle disorders or complex cardiac pathology that cannot be treated effectively with conventional surgery. Although infants were among early transplant recipients in the late 1960s, it was not until adult transplantation became more successful a decade later that children began being considered seriously as candidates. Relatively few transplants have occurred in children, and most have been within the past 5 years; therefore long-term results are unknown.[17 (p.973)] Ethical considerations of heart transplantation in children continue to be debated. Religious and cultural beliefs of families are considered.

Older children were the first pediatric recipients of transplanted hearts because their size made it easier to find suitable donor organs. In addition, they could participate in the treatment decision. In the 1980s, with increased experience and success with both adults and older children, physicians began to offer infants and younger children the benefits of this technology. Limited donor organ availability, however, is a significant deterrent to transplantation in infants and young children.

Transplantation is not a cure for heart disease or dysfunction. Rather, it is an exchange of one chronic condition for another. The procedure requires lifelong compliance with medication, follow-up tests, and treatments, as well as acceptance of an uncertain future. Children who are potential transplantation candidates have no other medical or surgical options available to them and are not expected to survive more than a few months without surgery. Transplants are most frequently performed in

cases of cardiomyopathies, followed by complex congenital heart defects. Specific criteria to determine candidates for heart transplantation are listed in the accompanying display.[1 (p.974)]

Diagnostic Studies. Preparation for heart transplantation requires that the cardiac diagnosis is confirmed and that the use of other therapy is ruled out. A cardiac catheterization is usually performed. This diagnostic test is particularly important for those children who are suspected of having high pulmonary vascular resistance. During the catheterization, the resistance is measured precisely. Children with exceptionally high resistance have a greater risk for developing right ventricular failure after heart transplantation. Therefore, a heart–lung transplantation may be recommended.

If a child has a cardiomyopathy, an endomyocardial biopsy is obtained to verify the type of cardiomyopathy. In addition, potential recipients are carefully evaluated to diagnose other chronic illnesses that would limit survival after transplantation. End-stage renal or liver disease and unresolved malignancy are examples of conditions that would prevent a child from being accepted as a candidate for heart transplantation.

Blood tests are done to determine the child's blood type and past exposure to infectious diseases. The blood type is essential in matching a donor heart. Compatible blood types and weight range are the two critical criteria in successful donor–recipient matching. Differing serology histories between the donor and recipient create potential problems that need to be prevented. For example, if a recipient tests negative for cytomegalovirus (CMV) but receives a heart from a donor who tests positive, the child may develop the CMV infection, which has proven to be devastating to immunosuppressed patients. If a mismatch is documented, antiviral medications are given to the recipient postoperatively to prevent the infection. The limited preservation time of the donor heart prohibits prospective tissue typing in most cases (see also Chaps. 42 and 43).

Diagnostic studies are also performed on the donor's heart to certify that it is a suitable organ. An echocardiogram is used to validate the heart's structural integrity.

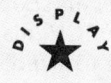

Indications for Heart Transplantation in Children

End-stage acquired cardiomyopathy
Endocardial fibroelastosis
Untreatable congenital heart disease
Unresectable cardiac tumor
Premature ischemic heart disease
Failed cardiac transplant graft

(Data from Cameron, D. E., & Reitz, B. A. (1989). Heart and heart-lung transplantation. In F. H. Adams, G. C. Emmanouilides, & T. A. Riemenschneider (Eds.), Moss' heart disease in infants, children, and adolescents (p. 974). Baltimore: Williams & Wilkins.)

Additional assessments are made to rule out ischemic damage.

★ ASSESSMENT

After being accepted as a candidate for a heart transplantation procedure, the child and the family begin a difficult waiting period. The wait may be only a few hours, or it may extend to many weeks or months. Some children die of their disease before a donor heart can be found. Guilt about waiting for another child to die is common. The nurse who has contact with families who are waiting may ask open-ended or leading questions that would encourage parents and children to reveal their feelings. For example, the nurse may say, "Waiting is difficult for most families, and many feel strange about waiting for a donor heart. What kinds of ideas keep coming to your mind?" Another question may be, "How is waiting for the procedure affecting your lives?"

The nurse also can assess the completeness and accuracy of the parents' and child's knowledge base. Some families may have done intense investigation about the procedure and need clarification or confirmation of their knowledge. Other families have only rudimentary understanding of the child's cardiac problem and the transplantation process. Teaching should not be initiated before the nurse has assessed what the child and family know, what they want to know, and the learning styles of the family members.

★ NURSING DIAGNOSES AND PLANNING

Many of the nursing diagnoses discussed earlier in the section on the child having cardiac surgery are applicable to the child having cardiac transplantation.

★ INTERVENTIONS: COLLABORATIVE
    AND INDEPENDENT

Preparation of the child and family for surgery is difficult because no one knows exactly when or if the procedure will take place. Overpreparation is a real risk and may lead to heightened anxiety or depression. Becoming familiar with hospital equipment that may be used posttransplant may be helpful for young children. Books about hospital experiences are useful for all ages. Details about the immediate postoperative period in the ICU may be too much information for young children to handle far in advance; older children may appreciate and need this information as soon as the candidacy has been determined.

When a donor heart is found, the child is admitted to the hospital and the usual preoperative routines are begun. There may be little time for preparation. Immunosuppression therapy is started preoperatively. The child is taken to the operating room, and the removal of the heart is timed to coincide with the removal and examination of the donor heart in another room, or its arrival at the hospital after distal procurement.

The operative period is an emotional and difficult time for parents. Meeting the ICU staff, being informed about progress in the operating room, and having a chance

to talk to other families and health care team members can be helpful during this trying time.

Cardiac transplantation requires the use of CPB (see Fig. 41-22). The recipient's aorta is divided just above the aortic valve, and the pulmonary artery is divided just above the pulmonary valve. The right and left atria are excised at the atrioventricular junction, leaving a posterior shell of the atria. The left and right atrial walls of the graft are anastomosed to the remaining portion of the recipient's heart. The pulmonary artery and the aorta are anastomosed. This surgery is illustrated in Figure 41-23.

The transplantation surgery results in two unique phenomena. First, the denervation of the autonomic nervous system occurs because of the atrial suture line of the surgical repair. Second, the recipient has two P waves: one from his own SA node and one from the donor's SA node. The recipient's SA node impulse does not cross the suture line and, therefore, does not initiate contraction. The donor's SA node initiates the QRS complex and contraction. The suture lines electrically isolate the two sets of P waves.

POSTOPERATIVE CARE

Postoperative care is similar to recovery from other heart surgery, with additional emphasis on protective isolation

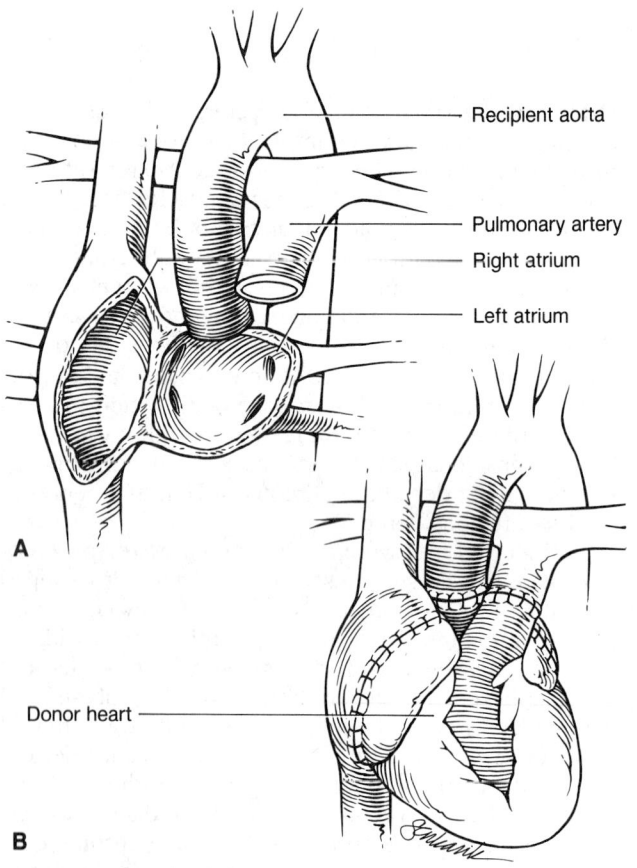

FIGURE 41-23.
Heart transplantation. **A,** The recipient's aorta is divided just above the aortic valve, and the pulmonary artery is divided just above the pulmonary valve. The right and left atria are excised at the atrioventricular junction, leaving a posterior shell of the atria. **B,** The right and left atrial walls of the graft are anastomosed to the remaining portion of the recipient's heart, and the pulmonary artery and aorta are anastomosed.

and on prevention of rejection. Infection and rejection are the leading causes of death in the post-transplant period. In the first 3 weeks postoperatively, infections are usually bacterial; later, infections are usually viral. The child who has an infection is febrile, tachycardiac, and exhibits signs of poor peripheral perfusion.

The presence of rejection may be manifested by complaints of fever, tachycardia, weakness, nausea, and flulike symptoms. If the rejection is severe, CO is compromised and is manifested by dysrhythmias, ventricular gallop, low blood pressure, poor peripheral perfusion, and neurologic sequelae ranging from lethargy or irritability to loss of consciousness. The confirmation of rejection may be sought with an ECG or with an echocardiogram. However, an endomyocardial biopsy, performed through a cardiac catheterization procedure, is the only reliable method of surveying for rejection. Toddlers and older children undergo biopsies frequently in the first few months after transplantation, and these procedures are done every 6 months as the rejection is controlled.

Approximately 90% of children experience rejection within the first 3 months after transplantation; virtually every child experiences at least one episode of rejection.[17] As time from the surgery increases, rejection becomes less frequent, and it is uncommon after the first year. One rejection episode per patient per year is expected.[17] Long-term survival may be limited by problems with coronary artery disease caused by chronic rejection.

High-dose immunosuppression is especially needed immediately after surgery because this is the period of greatest risk for rejection. Immunosuppressants must be taken for life. Blood levels of these medications are monitored closely to maintain maximum effectiveness. Immunosuppression dosages are augmented if rejection episodes occur. Lymphoma or renal dysfunction are potential long-term complications caused by immunosuppressive therapy.

DISCHARGE PLANNING

Attention should be given to discharge planning early in the post-transplant period. Nurses should encourage as much independence and autonomy as possible for the child and the family. Older children or parents begin learning about medications quickly, and within a few days may be responsible for their administration. Because hypertension is a common sequela of the immunosuppressive medicines and hypotension is a hallmark of rejection, a blood pressure cuff of the correct size is obtained and the parents are taught how to measure the blood pressure. Other teaching includes a diet restricted in cholesterol and saturated fat, and the signs of complications that must be reported.

Although the child has a chronic condition, emphasis is placed on seeing and treating the child as healthy. The family may need support and help in allowing the healthier child to do more and changing their lifestyles appropriately. Care needs to be taken in long-term follow-up to assess the child's peer relationships and dependence on parents. Often transplant recipients are seen as being different by their peers and becoming part of the peer group is difficult. In addition, the child may have a problem achieving age-appropriate independence if parents

Ideas for Nursing Research

Nurses who care for children with cardiovascular disorders have many opportunities to explore issues related to their clinical specialty. Possible topics for empirical investigation, include:

- Effects of crying in the child with chronic hypoxia.
- Limits of exercise tolerance in children with cyanotic heart defects or stenotic lesions.
- School performance of children with cyanotic heart disease.
- Child and family adjustments to the child with chronic cyanosis.
- Quality of life after repair of heart defects or cardiac transplantation.
- Accurate assessment technique for postoperative pain.
- Effective feeding techniques for infants with congestive heart failure.

are overprotective. Vulnerable child syndrome is discussed in Chapter 20 and illustrated in Figure 20-1.

★ **EVALUATION**

With a healthy donor heart, children often recover quickly after transplantation surgery; this is especially true for children who have become sick suddenly, as with some of the cardiomyopathies. Those who have been sick for many months or years are cachectic and debilitated, and, unfortunately, slower recoveries and higher morbidity and mortality after transplantation are expected. Survival statistics for children after heart transplantation surgery are constantly improving as new techniques, procedures, and medications are developed.

Summary

The child who has heart disease is often critically ill and in need of urgent intervention. The nurse who understands the etiology, pathophysiology, and course of the cardiac diseases can offer accurate information to the family and can develop an appropriate and comprehensive plan of care. Many children have congenital heart defects that can be effectively corrected with surgery. A few children may be candidates for heart transplantation. Knowledge of medical and surgical interventions enables nurses to provide complex physical care with confidence. Yet, patient teaching and sensitive psychosocial support are necessary to make the hospitalization experience less traumatic for children and their families. The role of nurses who care for children with alterations in cardiac function is therefore demanding, but the opportunities to provide comprehensive, family-centered nursing that makes a difference in patient outcomes are frequent and satisfying.

References

1. Adams, F. H., Emmanouilides, G. C., & Riemenschneider, T. A. (Eds.). (1989). *Moss' heart disease in infants, children, and adolescents* (4th ed.). Baltimore: Williams & Wilkins.

2. Addonizio, L. J., Hue, D. T., Fuzesi, L., Smith C. R., & Rose, E. A. (1989). Optimal timing of pediatric heart transplantation. *Circulation, 80*(5), 84–89.

3. Anderson, T. M. (1990). Indications and candidacy for heart transplantation in children. In J. M. Dunn & R. M. Donner (Eds.), *Heart transplantation in children.* Mt. Kisco, NY: Futura.

4. Arciniegas, E. (1985). *Pediatric cardiac surgery.* Chicago: Year Book Medical.

5. Artman, M., Parrish, M. D., & Graham, T. P. (1983). Congestive heart failure in childhood and adolescence: Recognition and management. *American Heart Journal, 105*(3), 471–480.

6. Avery, M. E., & First, L. R. (Eds.). (1989). *Pediatric medicine.* Baltimore: Williams & Wilkins.

7. Ayoub, E. M. (1989). Acute rheumatic fever. In F. H. Adams, G. C. Emmanouilides, & T. A. Riemenschneider (Eds.), *Moss' heart disease in infants, children, and adolescents* (4th ed.). Baltimore: Williams & Wilkins.

8. Bailey, N. A., Lay, P., & Loma Linda University Infant Heart Transplant Group. (1989). New horizons: Infant cardiac transplantation. *Heart and Lung, 18*(2), 172–178.

9. Bardy, G. H., Ivey, T. D., Coltorti, F., Stewart, R. B., Johnson, G., & Greene, H. L. (1988). Developments, complications and limitations of catheter-mediated electrical ablation of posterior accessory atrioventricular pathways. *American Journal of Cardiology, 61*(4), 309–316.

10. Baum, M. F., Cutler, D. C., Fricker, F. J., & Trimm, R. F. (1991). Physiologic and psychological growth and development in pediatric heart transplant recipients. *Journal of Heart and Lung Transplantation, 10*(5), 848–855.

11. Bayne, E. J. (1988). Etiology, diagnosis, and management of congenital cardiac disorders. *Comprehensive Therapy, 14*(8), 31–40.

12. Behrman, R. E., & Vaughan, V. C. (1992). *Nelson textbook of pediatrics* (14th ed.). Philadelphia: Saunders.

13. Benson, D. W., & Dunnigan, A. Disturbances of cardiac rhythm. (1990). In J. H. Moller & W. A. Neal (Eds.), *Fetal, neonatal, and infant cardiac disease.* Norwalk, CT: Appleton & Lange.

14. Betocchi, S., et al. (1987). Effects of verapamil administration on left ventricular diastolic function in systemic hypertension. *American Journal of Cardiology, 59*(6): 624–629.

15. Bradlyn, A. S., Christoff, K., Sekora, T., O'Dell, S. L., & Harris, C. V. (1986). The effects of a videotape preparation package in reducing children's arousal and increasing cooperation during cardiac catheterization. *Behaviour Research and Therapy, 24*(4), 453–459.

16. Bull, C. (1986). Interventional catheterisation in infants and children. *British Heart Journal, 56*(3), 197–200.

17. Cameron, D. E., & Reitz, B. A. (1989). Heart and heart–lung transplantation. In F. H. Adams, G. C. Emmanouilides, & T. A. Riemenschneider (Eds.), *Moss' heart disease in infants, children, and adolescents.* Baltimore: Williams & Wilkins.

18. Castanada, A. R., Mayer, J. E., Jonas, R. A., Lock, J. E., Wessel, D. L., & Hickey, P. R. (1989). The neonate with critical congenital heart disease: Repair—A surgical challenge. *Journal of Thoracic and Cardiovascular Surgery, 98*(5), 869–875.

19. Clark, E. B. (1989). Congenital cardiovascular defects in infants with Down syndrome. *Pediatrics in Review, 11*(4), 99–100.

20. Click, L. A. (1985). Cardiac arrhythmias in infants and children. *Critical Care Quarterly, 8*(3), 9–18.

21. Cohen, J. A., & Hasler, M. E. (1987). Sensory preparation for patients undergoing cardiac catheterization. *Critical Care Nursing, 7*(3), 68–73.

22. Cohn, H. E., Freed, M. D., Hellenbrand, W. F., & Fyler, D. C.

(1985). Complications and mortality associated with cardiac catheterization in infants under one year: A prospective study. *Pediatric Cardiology, 6*(3), 123–131.

23. Committee on Rheumatic Fever and Bacterial Endocarditis (1982), American Heart Association. (1984). Jones criteria (revised) for guidance in the diagnosis of rheumatic fever. *Circulation, 69*(11), 204A–208A.

24. Drinkwater, D. C., & Laks, H. (1989). Principles of pediatric heart surgery. In F. H. Adams, G. C. Emmanouilides, & T. A. Riemenschneider (Eds.), *Moss' heart disease in infants, children, and adolescents.* Baltimore: Williams & Wilkins.

25. Duszynski, S. (1989). Pediatric ECG interpretation—A self study text. Milwaukee: Maxishare.

26. Ector, H., Holvoet, G., Witters, E., Ferdinande, P., & DeGeest, H. (1985). Catheter technique for electrical ablation of the atrioventricular conduction system. *Chest, 88*(5), 676–679.

27. Edmunds, L. H., & Wagner, H. R. (1985). Congenital anomalies of the mitral valve. In Arciniegas, E. (Ed.), *Pediatric cardiac surgery.* Chicago: Year Book Medical.

28. Ettedgui, J. A. (1991). Balloon angioplasty and valvotomy. In Neches, W. H., Park, S. C., & Zuberbuhler, J. R. (Eds.), *Perspectives in pediatric cardiology: Pediatric cardiac catheterization* (vol. 3). Mt. Kisco, NY: Futura.

29. Fink, B. W. (1985). *Congenital heart disease—A deductive approach to its diagnosis.* Chicago: Year Book Medical.

30. Fricker, F. J., et al. (1990). Experience with heart transplantation at the University of Pittsburgh and Children's Hospital. In J. M. Dunn & R. M. Donner (Eds.), *Heart transplantation in children.* Mt. Kisco, NY: Futura.

31. Gersony, W. M. (1989). Long-term follow-up of operated congenital heart disease. *Cardiology Clinics, 7*(4), 915–923.

32. Guindi, M. M., & Waley, V. M. (1987). Coronary sinus thrombosis: A potential complication of right heart catheterization. *The Canadian Journal of Surgery, 30*(1), 66–67.

33. Harjula, A. L. J., Heikkila, L. J., Nieminen, M. S., Kupari, M., Keta, P., & Matilla, S. P. (1988). Heart transplantation in repaired transposition of the great arteries. *Annals of Thoracic Surgery, 46*(6), 611–614.

34. Hazinski, M. F. (Ed.). (1992). *Nursing care of the critically ill child.* St. Louis: Mosby.

35. Hellenbrand, W. E., & Mullins, C. E. (1989). Catheter closure of congenital cardiac defects. *Cardiology Clinics, 7*(2), 351–368.

36. Higgins, S. S., & Kashani, I. A. (1986). The cyanotic child: Heart defects and parental learning needs. *MCN, 11*(4), 259–262.

37. Hoffman, J. I. (1990). Congenital heart disease; Incidence and inheritance. *Pediatric Clinics of North America, 37*(1), 25–43.

38. Huhta, J. C., et al. (1987). Surgery without catheterization for congenital heart defects: Management of 100 patients. *Journal of the American College of Cardiology, 9*(4), 823–829.

39. Hutchings, S. M., & Monett, Z. (1989). Caring for the cardiac transplant patient. *Critical Care Nursing Clinics of North America, 1*(2), 245–261.

40. Ingelfinger, J. R. (1989). Systemic hypertension. In F. H. Adams, G. C. Emmanouilides, & T. A. Riemenschneider (Eds.), *Moss' heart disease in infants, children, and adolescents* (4th ed.). Baltimore: Williams & Wilkins.

41. Joffe, M. (1987). Pediatric digoxin administration. *Dimensions in Critical Care Nursing, 6*(3), 136–146.

42. Kanakriyeh, M. S., Mulins, C. E., Parisi, F., Petry, E. L., & Bailey, L. L. (1989). Late hemodynamic results after orthotopic heart transplantation in early infancy. *Catheterization and Cardiovascular Diagnosis, 18*(4), 232–236.

43. Kaplan, E. L. (1987). The startling comeback of rheumatic fever. *Contemporary Pediatrics, 4*(11), 20–34.

44. Kaplan, E. L., & Shulman, S. T. (1989). Endocarditis. In F. H. Adams, G. C. Emmanouilides, & T. A. Riemenschneider (Eds.), *Moss' heart disease in infants, children, and adolescents* (4th ed.). Baltimore: Williams & Wilkins.

45. Krabil, K. A., et al. (1987). Echocardiography vs. cardiac catheterization diagnosis of infants with congenital heart disease requiring cardiac surgery. *American Journal of Cardiology, 60*(4), 351–354.

46. LaMontagne, L. L. (1987). Children's preoperative coping: Replication and extension. *Nursing Research, 36*(3), 163–167.

47. Lau, K. C., Leung, M. P., & Lo, R. N. S. (1986). Retrograde transfemoral catheterization of the left ventricle in children with aortic valve stenosis. *Pediatric Cardiology, 7*(2), 79–82.

48. Lawrence, P. A., & Wieczorek, B. H. (1987). Congenital valvular heart disease. *Journal of Cardiovascular Nursing, 1*(3), 18–25.

49. Lock, J. E. (1990). Cardiac catheterization. In J. H. Moller & W. A. Neal (Eds.), *Fetal, neonatal, and infant cardiac disease.* Norwalk, CT: Appleton & Lange.

50. Lock, J. E., Cockerham, J. T., Keane, J. F., Finley, J. P., Wakely, P. E., & Fellows, K. E. (1987). Transcatheter umbrella closure of congenital heart defects. *Circulation, 75*(3), 593–604.

51. Lock, J. E., Keane, J. F., & Fellows, K. E. (1986). The use of catheter intervention procedures for congenital heart disease. *Journal of the American College of Cardiology, 7*(6), 1420–1423.

52. Lundquist, C. B., Osson, S. B., & Varnauskas, E. (1986). Transseptal left heart catheterization: A review of 278 studies. *Clinical Cardiology, 9*(1), 21–26.

53. Malinowski, L. M., & Doyle, J. E. (1985). Cardiac catheterization of the neonate. *American Journal of Nursing, 85*(1), 60–62.

54. Malinowski, P., & Yablonski, C. (1986). Congenital heart disease in infants: Nursing assessment. *Critical Care Quarterly, 9*(2), 6–23.

55. Malinverni, R., Francioli, P. B., Glauser, M. P. (1987). Comparison of single and multiple doses of prophylactic antibiotics in experimental streptococcal endocarditis. *Circulation, 76*(2), 376–382.

56. Markowitz, M. (1992). Rheumatic fever. In R. E. Behrman & V. C. Vaughan (Eds.), *Nelson textbook of pediatrics* (14th ed.). Philadelphia: Saunders.

57. Martin-Duran, R., et al. (1986). Comparison of Doppler-determined elevated pulmonary pressure with pressure measured at cardiac catheterization. *American Journal of Cardiology, 57,* 859–863.

58. Mavroudis, C., et al. (1988). Infant orthotopic cardiac transplantation. *Journal of Thoracic and Cardiovascular Surgery, 96,* 912–924.

59. Medelin, G. J., et al. (1989). Interventional catheterization in congenital heart disease. *Radiologic Clinics of North America, 27*(6), 1223–1240.

60. Medicus, L. (1987). Kawasaki disease: What is this puzzling childhood illness? *Heart & Lung, 16*(1), 55–60.

61. Mersch, J. (1985). End-stage cardiac disease: Cardiomyopathy. In M. K. Douglas & J. A. Shinn (Eds.), *Advances in cardiovascular nursing.* Rockville, MD: Aspen.

62. Miller, G. A. H. (1985). Balloon valvuloplasty and angioplasty in congenital heart disease. *British Heart Journal, 54*(3), 285–289.

63. Mullins, C. E. (1989). Pediatric and congenital therapeutic cardiac catheterization. *Circulation, 79*(6), 1153–1159.

64. Mullins, C. E. (1989). Therapeutic cardiac catheterization. In F. H. Adams, G. C. Emmanouilides, & T. A. Riemenschneider (Eds.), *Moss' heart disease in infants, children, and adolescents* (4th ed.). Baltimore: Williams & Wilkins.

65. Murphy, C. (1989). Educating people with congenital heart disease. *Journal of the Medical Association of Georgia, 78*(5), 286–290.

66. National Heart, Lung, & Blood Institutes Task Force on Blood Pressure Control in Children. (1987). *Report of the Second Task Force on Blood Pressure Control in Children—1987* (pp. 1–33). Bethesda, MD: U. S. Department of Health and Human Services, Public Health Service, National Institutes of Health.

67. Neches, W. H. (1990). Kawasaki disease. In J. H. Moler & W. A. Neal (Eds.), *Fetal, neonatal, and infant cardiac disease.* Norwalk, CT: Appleton & Lange.

68. Neches, W. H. (1991). Transcatheter occlusion. In W. H. Neches, S. C. Park, & J. R. Zuberbuhler (Eds.), *Perspectives in pediatric cardiology: Pediatric cardiac catheterization* (Vol. 3). Mt. Kisco, NY: Futura.

69. Netz, H., Madu, B., & Röhner, G. (1987). Heparinization during cardiac catheterization in children. *Pediatric Cardiology, 8*(3), 167–168.

70. Ng, L., & Mickols, O. J. (1986). Nursing management of the postoperative cardiac surgical patient in the critical care unit. In C. E. Rackley (Ed.), *Advances in critical care cardiology* (pp. 211–233). Philadelphia: F. A. Davis.

71. Nora, J. J. (1989). Etiologic aspects of heart diseases. In F. H. Adams, G. C. Emmanouilides, & T. A. Riemenschneider (Eds.), *Moss' heart disease in infants, children, & adolescents.* Baltimore: Williams & Wilkins.

72. Ogborn, M. R., & Crocker, J. F. S. (1987). Investigation of pediatric hypertension. *American Journal of Diseases in Children, 141*(11), 1205–1209.

73. Page, G. G. (1985). Patent ductus arteriosus in the premature neonate. *Heart & Lung, 14*(2), 156–163.

74. Palacios, I., et al. (1987). Percutaneous balloon valvotomy for patients with severe mitral stenosis. *Circulation, 75*(4), 778–784.

75. Pankey, G. A. (1986). Infective endocarditis: Changing concepts. *Hospital Practice, 21*(3), 103–110.

76. Park, M. K. (1988). *Pediatric cardiology for practitioners* (2nd ed.). Chicago: Year Book Medical.

77. Park, M. K. (1991). *The pediatric cardiology handbook.* St. Louis: Mosby–Year Book.

78. Phillips, J. M., & Raviele, A. A. (1985). Diagnostic and therapeutic techniques in pediatric cardiology: Past, present, and future. *Critical Care Quarterly, 8*(3), 1–7.

79. Pruitt, A. W. (1992). Systemic hypertension. In R. E. Behrman & V. C. Vaughan (Eds.), *Nelson textbook of pediatrics* (14th ed.). Philadelphia: Saunders.

80. Rao, P. S. (1989). Balloon dilatation in infants and children with cardiac defects. *Catheterization and Cardiovascular Diagnosis, 18*(3), 136–149.

81. Rashkind, J. (1985). Interventional cardiac catheterization in congenital heart disease. *International Journal of Cardiology, 7*(1), 1–11.

82. Rees, A. H., Solinger, R. E., & Elbl, F. (1987). *Handbook of pediatric cardiology.* St. Louis: Green.

83. Roberts, W. C. (1987). Frequency of systemic hypertension in various cardiovascular diseases. *American Journal of Cardiology, 60*(9), 1E–8E.

84. Rocchini, A. P., Katch, V. L., Grekin, R., Moorhead, C., & Anderson, J. (1986). Role for aldosterone in blood pressure regulation of obese adolescents. *American Journal of Cardiology, 57*(8), 613–618.

85. Rotondi, P. (1986). Intensive care unit management of the postoperative cardiac surgery patient. *Critical Care Quarterly, 9*(2), 49–63.

86. Shear, C. L., Burke, G. L., Freedman, D. S., & Berenson, G. S. (1986). Value of childhood blood pressure measurements and family history in predicting future blood pressure status: Results from 8 years of follow-up in the Bogalusa heart study. *Pediatrics, 77*(6), 862–869.

87. Shuman, S. T., et al. (1984). Prevention of bacterial endocarditis: A statement for health professionals by the Committee on Rheumatic Fever and Infective Endocarditis of the Council on Cardiovascular Disease in the Young. *Circulation, 70*(6), 1123A–1127A.

88. Slota, M. C. (1987). Assessment of systemic perfusion in the child. *Critical Care Nurse, 7*(4), 68–73.

89. Smallwood, S. B. (1988). Preparing children for surgery: Learn-

ing through play. *Association of Operating Room Nurses' Journal,* *47*(1), 177–186.

90. Takahaski, M., & Lurie, P. R. (1989). Abnormalities and diseases of the coronary vessels. In F. H. Adams, G. C. Emmanouilides, & T. A. Riemenschneider (Eds.), *Moss' heart disease in infants, children, and adolescents* (4th ed.). Baltimore: Williams & Wilkins.

91. Talner, N. S. (1989). Heart failure. In F. H. Adams, G. C. Emmanouilides, & T. A. Riemenschneider (Eds.), *Moss' heart disease in infants, children, and adolescents* (4th ed.). Baltimore: Williams & Wilkins.

92. Talner N. S., & Lister, G. (1989). Perioperative care of the infant with congenital heart disease. *Cardiology Clinics, 7*(2), 419–438.

93. Tanaka, M., et al. (1987). Quantitative analysis of narrowings of intramyocardial small arteries in normal hearts, hypertensive hearts, and hearts with hypertrophic cardiomyopathy. *Circulation, 75*(6), 1130–1139.

94. Thomas, S. P., & Groer, M. W. (1986). Relationship of demographic, life-style, and stress variables to blood pressure in adolescents. *Nursing Research, 35*(3), 169–172.

95. Trento, A., Griffith, B. P., Fricker, F. J., Kormos, R. L., Armitage, J., & Hardesty, R. L. (1989). Lessons learned in pediatric heart transplantation. *Annals of Thoracic Surgery, 48*(5), 617–622.

96. Watkins, L. O., Weaver, L., Odegaard, V. (1986). Preparation for cardiac catheterization: Tailoring the content of instruction of coping style. *Heart & Lung, 15*(4), 382–389.

97. Weinhaus, L., & Lababidi, Z. (1987). Catheter rupture during balloon valvuloplasty. *American Heart Journal, 113*(4), 1035–1036.

98. Wesolowski, C. A. (1988). Self contracts for chronically ill children. *MCN, 13*(1), 20–23.

99. Zellers, T. M., Driscoll, D. J., Humes, R. A., Feldt, R. H., Puga, F. J., & Danieson, G. K. (1989). Glenn shunt: Effect on pleural drainage after modified Fontan operation. *Journal of Thoracic and Cardiovascular Surgery, 98*(5), 725–729.

10
UNIT

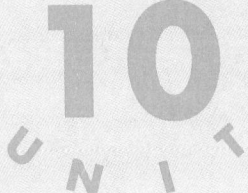

Nursing Care of Children With Altered Hematologic Function

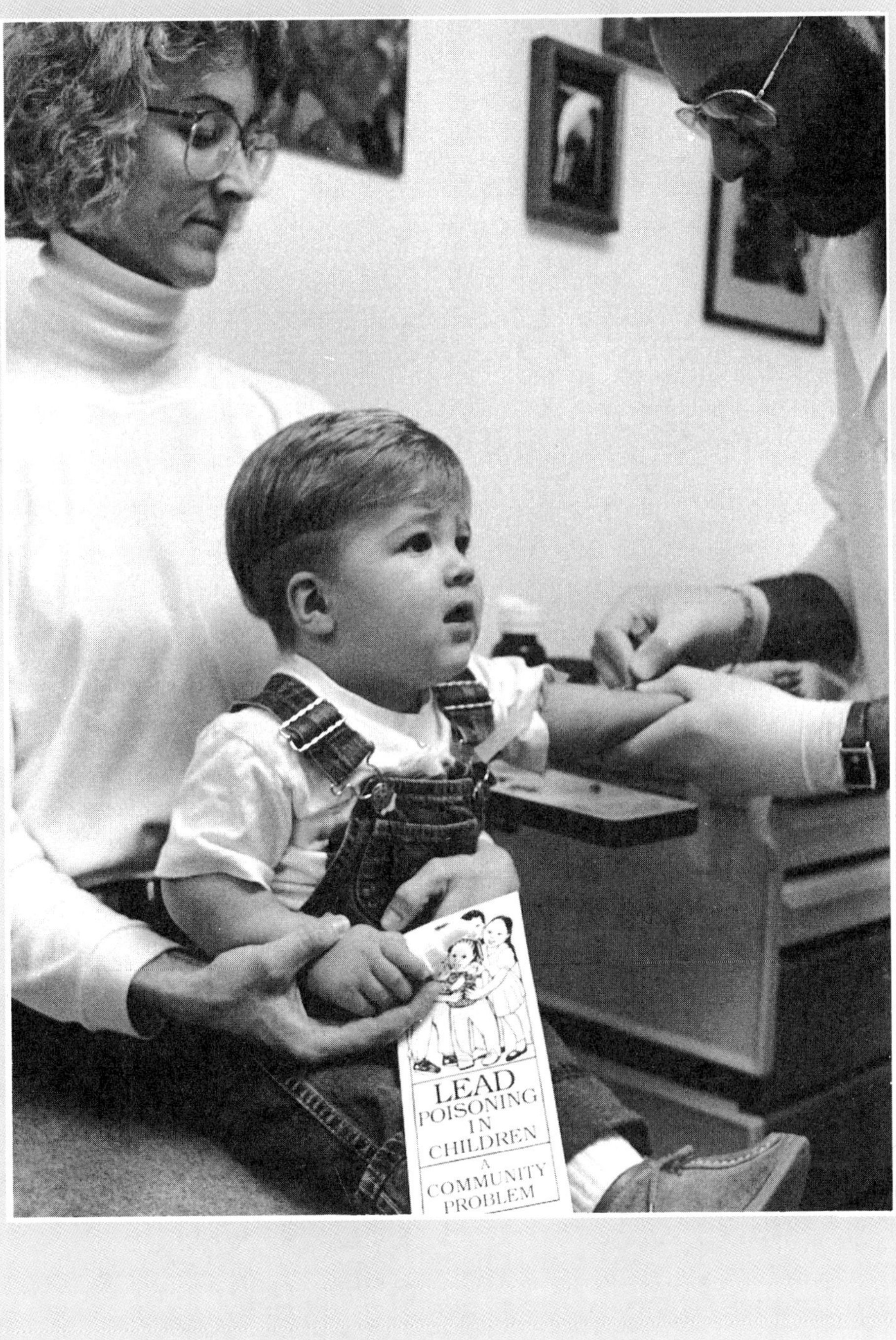

LEAD
POISONING
IN
CHILDREN
A
COMMUNITY
PROBLEM

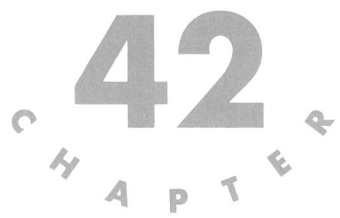

Anatomy and Physiology of the Hematologic System

BEHAVIORAL OBJECTIVES

Discuss embryonic development of blood formation.

List various categories of blood cells and explain their functions.

Discuss normal values of blood cell counts at various ages.

Describe hematopoiesis and its regulation.

Blood is considered to be a form of connective tissue, with an intercellular substance made up of the blood plasma and the cellular component consisting of erythrocytes (red blood cells; RBCs), leukocytes (white blood cells; WBCs), and thrombocytes (platelets). Hematopoiesis is the formation of the various blood cells, from *hemo* meaning blood and *poiesis* meaning production.[12] This chapter describes hematologic function by examining the functions of the various formed elements of the blood: transport of oxygen and carbon dioxide between the lungs and the rest of the body, phagocytosis and other defense mechanisms, and hemostasis.

Embryonic Development

Blood formation begins early in human embryonic life in specialized centers called blood islands. Hematopoiesis begins in these blood islands of the yolk sac in the second week of life from stem cells called hemocytoblasts, which were formerly undifferentiated mesenchyme cells.[4] Hemopoietic cells are transferred from the yolk sac to the embryo proper by the sixth week of embryonic life. Initially, the liver is established as the major hemopoietic center (at about 1 month of intrauterine life); at this time, production of RBCs dominates, with moderate production of platelets and macrophages, and only minor production of WBCs. The spleen also functions as an erythropoietic organ from the third to fifth fetal months. In the last half of gestation, there is a shift in hematopoiesis to the bone marrow, and, by birth, most blood formation takes place in the bone marrow.[11] In human beings, the bone marrow produces all the erythrocytes, granulocytes, monocytes, and platelets and supplies either precursors of lymphocytes or actual lymphocytes to the spleen, lymph nodes, and other lymphatic tissues. Although the liver is hematopoietically inactive in humans after birth, it reserves its potential for hematopoiesis, which can be resumed in cases of bone marrow failure.[7]

After birth, there is further change in the sites of hematopoiesis. In infancy, most of the medullary spaces in bones are filled with red marrow, the term given to actively hemopoietic bone marrow. Gradually, during childhood, fatty tissue or yellow marrow replaces the red marrow of long bones. In older children and adults, active blood formation occurs in the marrow of selected bones; ribs, sternum, vertebrae, pelvis, skull, clavicles, and scapulae. In circumstances of severe hematologic stress (e.g., after hemorrhage), the yellow marrow of the long bones of the extremities can resume active hematopoiesis.

Consequences of Abnormal Development

Abnormal development in the embryo leads to death, arrested development, or congenital problems, as indicated in Table 42-1. Also, a number of genetically linked blood disorders may lead to hematologic dysfunction in newborns and children. For example, sickle cell anemia, glucose-6-phosphate dehydrogenase deficiency (G-6-PD), pyruvate kinase deficiency, hereditary spherocytosis, Wiskott-Aldrich syndrome, hemophilia, and thalassemia syndrome are genetically linked or transmitted. More information on each of these disorders is found in Chapter 44.

Structure and Function

There are a variety of ways to categorize blood cells, depending on whether the focus is on the cell of origin in the blood-forming marrow or on the functional capabilities of the cell. Generally, blood cells are considered to be one of three groups: RBCs or erythrocytes, WBCs or leukocytes, and platelets or thrombocytes. Each of these is considered here. Whereas erythrocytes and thrombocytes each make up a complete category, leukocytes are further subdivided into eosinophils, neutrophils, basophils, monocytes, and lymphocytes, each of which has

TABLE 42-1
Consequences of Abnormal Embryonic Development

Fetal Age	Structure	Anomalies at Birth
2 weeks	Blood islands of the yolk sac, hematopoiesis.	Termination of growth
6 weeks	Hemopoietic cells are transferred to the embryo from the yolk sac; liver is major hemopoietic center.	Development arrested
3–5 months	Spleen also functions as an erythropoietic organ.	
6–9 months	Shift of hematopoiesis to the bone marrow.	Congenital aplastic anemia, Fanconi's anemia, Blackfan-Diamond syndrome

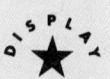

Categories of Blood Cells

Erythrocytes—Red blood cells (RBCs)
Leukocytes—White blood cells (WBCs)
   Granular leukocytes (granulocytes)
      Eosinophils
      Neutrophils
      Basophils
   Agranular leukocytes
      Monocytes
      Lymphocytes
Thrombocytes—Platelets

specific functions. Eosinophils, neutrophils, and basophils are termed granular leukocytes (or granulocytes) because of the appearance of granules in their cytoplasm when stained in vitro. Monocytes and lymphocytes are agranular leukocytes.

When considering the process of hemopoiesis, the blood cells may be categorized according to the precursor cell line from which each originates. Although there is not complete agreement as to theories of hemopoiesis, a commonly held belief is that pluripotent stem cells exist in bone marrow. From this cell or cells come all of the populations of blood cells found in a blood smear, through a series of maturational stages that take place in the bone marrow. This theory is the monophyletic theory. It differs from the polyphyletic theory, which states that there are specific stem cells for each of the classes of blood cells or that there are at least two stem cells, one of which develops into granulocytes, lymphocytes, and monocytes and the other into erythrocytes and megakaryocytes (which produce thrombocytes). In any case, there is direct evidence for the existence of stem cells at early stages of the development of any of these cell lines; severe but sublethal irradiation of bone marrow cells has been shown to induce chromosomal damage in subsequent clones of cells of the various hematopoietic cell lines as seen by the same distinctive karyotype. Stem cells in the fetus occur in both fetal liver and bone marrow, but later (in the adult) are found in bone marrow, the major site of hemopoiesis in adults.

Two other terms are used to describe categories of blood cells, and these also refer to the developmental sites. Cells that both originate in bone marrow and essentially complete all stages of development there are termed *myeloid cells*. These cells are considered to have come from myeloid stem cells, which take several forms as they differentiate. For example, myeloid stem cells may differentiate into granulocyte/monocyte progenitors (precursor cells), erythroid progenitors, or megakaryocyte progenitors. A separate stem cell, termed the *lymphoid stem cell,* differentiates into two classes of lymphocytes, at least one which completes its maturation outside of the bone marrow. Each category of cells is discussed in detail.

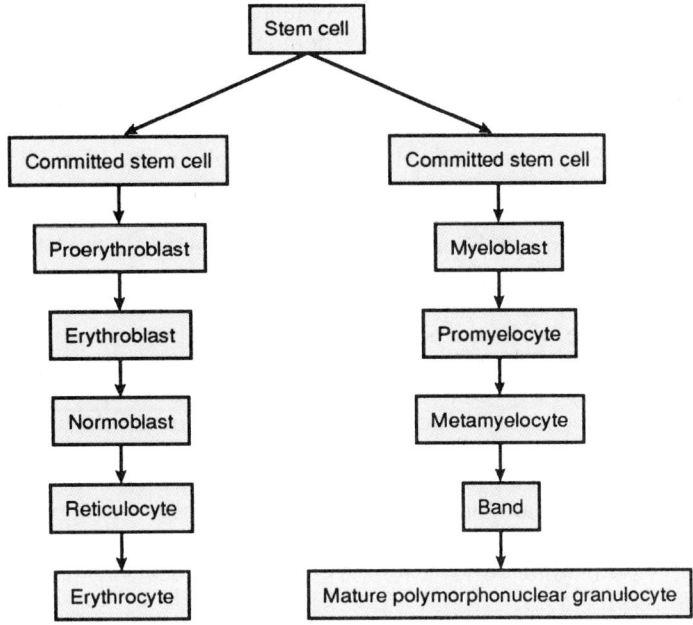

FIGURE 42-1
Stages of development of erythrocytes and leukocytes.

Erythrocytes

The RBC, called the erythrocyte, develops from erythroblasts, precursor cells in the bone marrow, which differentiate through a series of changes that result in the biconcave non-nucleated mature erythrocyte. The stages of development are: proerythroblast, erythroblast, normoblast, reticulocyte, and erythrocyte (Fig. 42-1). Although the early precursor cells are nucleated, as cellular differentiation occurs there is condensation and finally extrusion of the nucleus and production of hemoglobin. Although loss of the nucleus makes the red cell a better carrier of oxygen, it imposes a finite life span because the nucleus is needed to direct the replacement of vital enzymatic proteins necessary to cell reproduction.[11] As the cell matures into an erythrocyte, it loses the ability to make any more hemoglobin and it assumes its characteristic biconcave disk shape (Fig. 42-2). The whole process of differentiation is stimulated by the action of erythropoietin, whose own synthesis and secretion from the kidney are stimulated by decreases in tissue oxygenation.

Because the major purpose of the RBC is to transport oxygen and carbon dioxide between the lungs and tissues, the control of RBC production necessarily involves the recognition of hypoxia. Although in the adult male, the erythrocyte count is 4.5 to 5.9 million/mm³, the reticulocyte count is only 1.0% to 2.0% of the total RBCs. In the newborn and infant, laboratory figures are different, in that larger percentages of reticulocytes are present, reflecting the active erythropoiesis that occurs in the developing fetus. The greater the amount of erythropoiesis that is occurring, the greater the numbers of immature erythrocytes that are released into the circulation. The reticulocytes survive as such for approximately 24 hours before maturing into RBCs. In the 3-month-old fetus, blood samples contain about 90% reticulocytes; the 6-

month fetus' blood sample contains from 15% to 30% reticulocytes, and the newborn has only 4% to 6% reticulocyte count. A gradual reduction in the numbers of immature cells occurs, and, by the third month, blood samples of the normal infant show reticulocyte levels approximately the same as adults (1% to 2%). Age-relevant changes in the erythrocytes are also seen, from 4.0 to 6.6 million/mm³ in a 1-day-old child, followed by a gradual decrease to a nadir at 2 months of age of 2.7 to 4.9 million RBCs/mm³. There is a gradual increase until, by age 12, levels almost as high as levels (4.7 to 6.1 million/mm³)

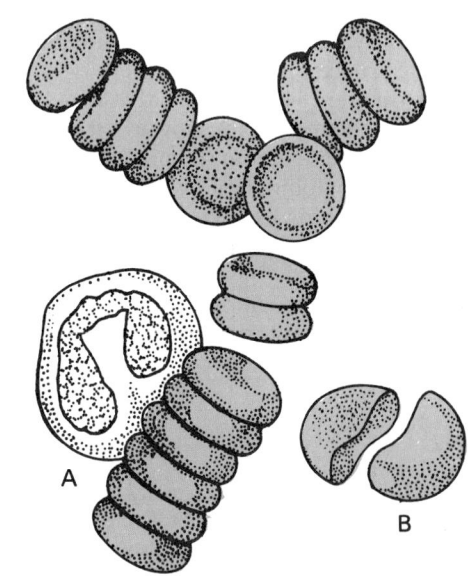

FIGURE 42-2
Grouped red blood cells. (**A**) One white blood cell is shown. (**B**) Red cell split to show its biconcave shape. (From Rosdahl, C. B. [1991]. *Textbook of basic nursing* [5th ed.]. Philadelphia: Lippincott.)

of erythrocytes are reached. The normal range of laboratory values is given in the Appendix.

Antigens and Major Blood Groups

Red blood cells contain genetically determined antigens on the cell membrane that result in recognition of four major blood groups: A, B, AB, and O. These antigens react with antibodies present in the plasma of incompatible people to cause agglutination (clumping) of the blood. A person with type A blood has the A antigen and the anti-B antibody; a person with type B blood has the B antigen and the anti-A antibody. The AB blood group has both antigens and neither antibody, so it is compatible with any other blood group as the recipient of blood. People with type O blood have both antibodies but neither antigen, so their blood is considered a universal donor type (Table 42-2). The Rh factor is an additional antigen contained in the membrane of the erythrocytes of some people (85% of Caucasians); people with the Rh factor are termed Rh-positive. People who lack the Rh factor are said to be Rh-negative and will synthesize antibodies to the factor if exposed to the Rh factor.[5]

Hemoglobin and Transportation of Gases

The main function of RBCs is the transport of oxygen from the lungs to the tissues in oxygenated blood and the transport of carbon dioxide (a by-product of normal metabolism) from tissues to the lungs. Circulation is illustrated in Figure 39-9. *Hemoglobin,* a major component of the erythrocyte, is responsible for the red cell's ability to transport gases. Hemoglobin is a substance consisting of a protein, globin, attached to iron-containing pigments called heme groups. Heme gives hemoglobin its unique ability to bind with oxygen and carbon dioxide for easily reversible transport. A hemoglobin molecule is made up of two pairs of polypeptide chains, with each chain having a heme group attached to it. Various hemoglobins are found in the embryo, the fetus, and the adult, depending on the chemical makeup of the polypeptide chains in each. The six different hemoglobins that may be found are the embryonic hemoglobins Gower 1, Gower 2, and Portland; the fetal hemoglobin, hemoglobin F; and the adult forms of hemoglobin, hemoglobins A and A_2. The embryonic hemoglobins completely disappear by the third month of gestation as the fetal hemoglobin becomes more dominant.

This fetal form of hemoglobin reaches a peak of about 90% of the hemoglobin produced at about the sixth month

of fetal life, and then begins to decrease. The newborn's hemoglobin consists of 40% to 70% fetal hemoglobin, which decreases by the end of infancy to about 1% to 2% of the total hemoglobin, with the adult forms making up the rest. Fetal hemoglobin in small amounts may be present throughout the lifetime of a person. The apparent purpose of the presence of fetal hemoglobin during the gestational period is to facilitate the uptake of oxygen at lower oxygen tensions, which exist in fetal circulation, and also the greater discharge of carbon dioxide. The presence of fetal hemoglobins in larger than normal amounts may be seen in disease states (thalassemia), particularly those accompanied by hematologic stress.[5]

Methemoglobin is the form of hemoglobin continuously being formed in normal red cells, in which iron has been oxidized and is no longer capable of carrying oxygen. Methemoglobin does not normally accumulate in the blood because it is reduced to regular hemoglobin by an enzymatic reaction that converts the iron from a ferric to a ferrous state.[8] However, if RBCs are exposed to excess oxidant drugs or toxins, methemoglobinemia may develop and cause problems in the release of normal amounts of oxygen to the tissues.

Levels of hemoglobin vary depending on the age of the fetus and infant. From a concentration of 15 to 22 g/dL in the newborn, the level normally drops to its lowest point at around 3 to 6 months of age (less than 10 g/dL), representing the body's rapid rate of growth and creating a state of physiologic anemia. Physiologic anemia results in part from the shortened survival of the fetal red cell, sizable expansion of blood volume that accompanies growth during the first 3 months of life, and the marked decrease in erythropoiesis that occurs with onset of respiration and the rise at that time of arterial oxygen saturation from 45% to 95%. The decrease in erythropoiesis is secondary to a massive drop in erythropoietin that accompanies the high arterial oxygen saturation of blood reaching the kidneys. These events are part of a physiologic adaptation to extrauterine life.

The physiologic anemia seen in normal infants is even more marked in the premature infant. The hemoglobin level may fall to 7 to 9 g/dL by 3 to 6 weeks of age. To confound the problem, premature infants are born with a small reserve of vitamin E, which has an important role in red cell stability.[1]

Phagocytosis

When the RBC has lived out its normal life span, (approximately 120 days), it is destroyed by the process of phagocytosis by cells in the spleen, liver, and the bone marrow. The spleen particularly plays a role in destruction of normally senescent RBCs. Iron is salvaged from the used hemoglobin and recycled to the bone marrow for use in the production of new hemoglobin. Part of the used hemoglobin is degraded to bilirubin, a pigment that stains the body tissues, skin, and sclera if present in increased amounts. This tinge of color in tissues caused by hyperbilirubinemia is referred to as jaundice. Normal bilirubin is 0.2 to 1.4 mg/100 ml of blood. An increase in the indirect type or unconjugated portion of bilirubin, which rises as a result of destruction of hemoglobin, is seen in hemolytic anemias, but jaundice is not necessarily

TABLE 42-2
ABO Blood Group System

Blood Group	Antigen	Antibody
A	A	Anti-B
B	B	Anti-A
AB (Universal recipient)	A and B	No antibodies
O (Universal donor)	No antigens	Anti-A and Anti-B

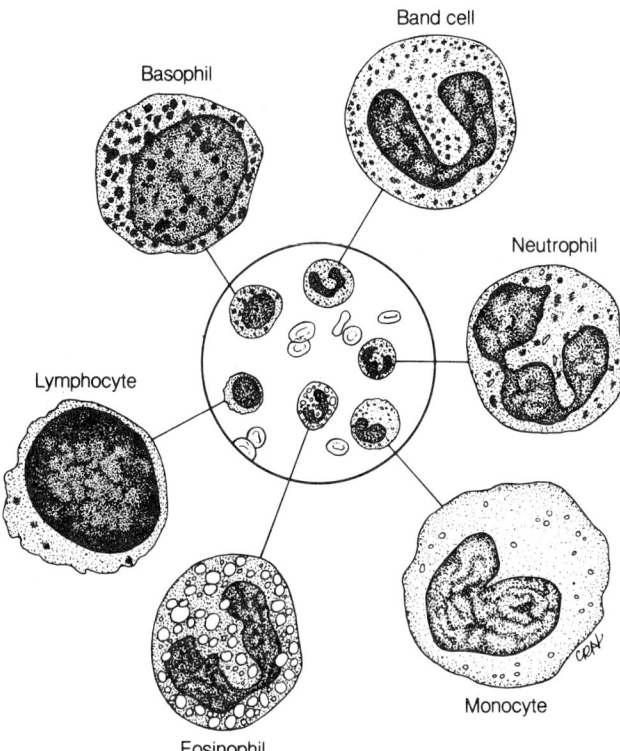

FIGURE 42-3

Types of white blood cells (leukocytes). Note comparison to red blood cells (the smaller cells) in the circle. Band cells are immature granulocytes.

seen if hepatic function is normal. The normally functioning liver can excrete the excess heme pigments in the feces, which is reflected by measurements of fecal urobilinogen.

Leukocytes

Leukocytes or WBCs are actually five different kinds of cells, each having distinct functions and particular characteristics (Fig. 42-3). The five classes of WBCs in the circulation are: the neutrophils, eosinophils, and basophils (which make up the granular leukocytes) and the monocytes/macrophages and lymphocytes (which make up the agranular leukocytes). As a group, these cells have important functions concerned with resistance to infection and disposal of products of cellular breakdown. Awareness of normal values is important because characteristic changes in the WBC and differential counts occur in many diseases. Some aspects of the process of leukopoiesis were discussed earlier; each cell line proceeds through multiple steps of maturation until the mature form of the cell is found in the blood. Immature precursors of white cells are sometimes found in the circulation and have diagnostic significance. The number of circulating WBCs at birth is high, ranging from 9,000 to 38,000 cells/mm³ of blood. The mean level falls to about 12,000 cells/mm³ by the end of the first week and continues to decrease to 5,000 to 10,000 cells/mm³ by the end of the first year of life.

Granular Leukocytes

The granular leukocytes go through the following stages of development: committed stem cell, myeloblast, promyelocyte, metamyelocyte, band, and mature polymorphonuclear granulocyte (see Fig. 42-1). A "shift to the left" is the term describing an increase in the number of band (or other immature) forms of granulocytes (see Fig. 42-3). A shift to the left occurs when the bone marrow is being stimulated to increase production of the granulocytes, such as during an infectious process. The granular leukocytes have in common the appearance of granules in their cytoplasm and a multisegmented nucleus.

The *neutrophil* is the predominating type of granulocyte, representing 54% to 62% of the total number of WBCs (see Fig. 42-3). Band neutrophils account for about 3% to 5% of the total WBCs. The granules are called *lysosomes* and contain digestive enzymes, which can act on bacteria or other particles ingested by neutrophils. The neutrophils are found in several compartments within the body. The mitotic compartment consists of the most immature forms, which are found in the bone marrow. The maturation compartment consists of the more mature forms of precursor cells, the metamyelocytes and band forms; these are no longer capable of dividing (so can only differentiate and mature) but still reside in the bone marrow. There is a marrow storage compartment consisting of a reserve of mature neutrophils, which can be rapidly mobilized.

It takes approximately 6 to 11 days for a cell to develop from a myeloblast to a mature neutrophil capable of functioning in the peripheral blood. Once in the circulation, neutrophils exist in two compartments, which can readily exchange cells. The circulating granulocytic compartment and the marginal compartment are of approximately equal size. The latter contains neutrophils sequestered in small blood vessels, which can quickly be mobilized into the circulating compartment if needed. Neutrophils do not exist in the circulation for long, perhaps 6 to 9 hours, after which they enter the tissue pool, where their primary function of phagocytosis is carried out. They are attracted to areas of inflammation and bacterial proliferation. Neutrophils are capable of random locomotion as well as directed locomotion (chemotaxis), probably in response to substances released by bacteria or damaged tissues.

The major function of neutrophils is phagocytosis, the engulfing and digesting of particles and cells that may be harmful to the body. Neutrophils are attracted to areas of bacterial proliferation and inflammation by responding to substances secreted by lymphocytes in the area of tissue that is infected or inflamed.

Abnormalities of neutrophil count can be of two types: neutrophilia or neutropenia. *Neutrophilia,* or an increase above normal in numbers of neutrophils, is seen in infection. The increase is seen as cells in the marginating pool are shifted to the circulating compartment cells. In addition, cells from the marrow storage compartment are released into circulation and the bone marrow is stimulated to increase production of neutrophils. There is a normal ratio between myeloid and erythroid elements (the M/E ratio) of bone marrow, which can be seen on bone marrow examination. This M/E ratio is normally 2:

1 to 4:1. When there is hypertrophy of the neutrophilic series (the major portion of the myeloid series), this M/E ratio may be increased to 5:1 to 10:1. *Neutropenia* is seen when counts are below 2500 cells/mm³. As neutrophil counts fall, increasing risk of infection is seen, including opportunistic infections.

Basophils are granulocytic leukocytes that contain large amounts of heparin and histamine in the large blue coarse granules that fill the cytoplasm (see Fig. 42-3). Basophils account for under 1% of the circulating leukocytes and are not obviously phagocytic. Their high content of heparin and histamine makes them similar to the mast cells that are located in tissues, and basophils may be precursors of the mast cells. Basophils play an important role in systemic allergic reactions such as anaphylaxis, during which they degranulate and release heparin and histamine into the bloodstream. They increase during asthma attacks and in inflammatory conditions. Basophils are thought to be vital for the prevention of clot formation and may counteract the coagulant effect that inflammation has on the RBCs. Normal levels in the blood are low or nonexistent, certainly less than 1% of the total WBCs.

Eosinophils are also present in low amounts in the circulating blood, comprising less than 5% of total WBCs (see Fig. 42-3). They are only weakly phagocytic. Because their number increases during allergic attacks, their function is thought to be a detoxification of foreign proteins. They are present in large numbers in the mucosa of the gastrointestinal tract and in the lung. Their increase is most pronounced during invasion of the tissues by parasites. Eosinophilia also occurs in drug reactions, such as codeine or penicillin sensitivity.

Agranular Leukocytes

Monocytes are a form of agranular leukocyte, with a large lobulated nucleus and only fine granules in the cytoplasm (see Fig. 42-3). They account for 1% to 5% of the total WBCs and are increased in such diseases as protozoan infection, bacterial endocarditis, and tuberculosis. Monocytes are immature cells that spend about 8 hours in the circulation before migrating into tissues where they assume their mature stage as macrophages. Macrophages are especially dense in organs such as the liver, spleen, lung, and lymph nodes where they provide a protective mechanism against invasion of microbes. Both monocytes and macrophages are efficient phagocytes for bacteria, extraneous matter, and dead neutrophils. Monocytes are sensitive to corticosteroids, showing decreased movement, chemotaxis, and bactericidal activity after exposure to even low levels of corticosteroids. Monocytopenia is seen in chronic infections and during recovery from infections.

Lymphocytes are categorized as an agranular leukocyte (see Fig. 42-3). Lymphocytes make up 25% to 33% of the WBCs. Lymphocytes originate in the bone marrow but differentiate in lymphoid structures such as the thymus, lymph nodes, spleen, liver, and intestines. The two large categories of lymphocytes (T cells and B cells) both have important functions in defense mechanisms in the body. Their function is the recognition of and response to eliminate foreign organisms or materials in the body.

The lymphocytes originate from a stem cell called a lymphoblast and develop through a sequence similar to other blood cells with an intermediate stage of prolymphocyte and then to one of two forms of mature lymphocyte. The mature lymphocyte differentiates in the influence of either the bone marrow or the thymus gland and subsequently becomes part of a pool of B-lymphocytes or T-lymphocytes.

The *thymus-dependent lymphocyte,* or *T cell,* expresses cell-mediated immune responses. There are a number of subpopulations of T cells identified, the most familiar being the T-helper cells, which are the prime target of the human immunodeficiency virus (HIV). The normal cellular immune response involves the release of cytotoxic agents and the synthesis of lymphokines by activated T cells. The lymphokines help activate other cells such as macrophages, B-lymphocytes, and cytotoxic T cells, to name a few.

The *B cell,* thought to complete its differentiation in the bone marrow, is responsible for humoral immunity. B cells are transformed into plasma cells, which secrete immunoglobulins (antibodies) into the bloodstream. Antigen–antibody reactions frequently activate a complex of serum proteins called the complement system, which, acting together, lead to lysis of the antigen-bearing cell. The antigen–antibody complement system also markedly increases the phagocytic function of the macrophages that act in the nonspecific portion of the immune response. The role of the lymphocytes in immune responses is a critical one, sometimes most clearly revealed by the genetic or acquired lack of one or more of the lymphocyte populations.

The infant is born with an immature immune system, which is not effective in providing immunity to infection. However, the fetus receives preformed antibodies from its mother, reflecting her experience with infectious agents, and thus receives passive immunity to otherwise dangerous infections. These antibodies, which crossed the placenta, have a finite life span, so the concentration in the infant's serum falls rapidly within the first few months of life. The lowest levels of immunoglobulins are between the second and fourth months, during which time the infant is not yet able to mount an adequate immune response of his own. This period of physiologic hypogammaglobulinemia is short-lived as the infant's own immune system begins to respond to antigens in the environment in increasing amounts during the first year of life.

Additional protection against infection is afforded the infant who is breast-fed. Breast-fed infants have lower mortality and morbidity than do infants who are formula-fed.[2] Human milk has been found to contain an antibody, immunoglobulin A,[10] polymorphonuclear leukocytes, and lymphocytes that are active against a number of bacteria.[6]

Platelets and Coagulation

The smallest of the blood's formed elements are the platelets, or thrombocytes. The platelets function in homeostasis, have a role in phagocytosis, and an integral role in the process of coagulation. Platelets are actually non-nucleated fragments of the megakaryocytes, the precursors of thrombocytes in the bone marrow. The normal range of platelets in the newborn is from 150,000 to 350,000 cells/mm³; after a week, the count can be expected to be the same as in an adult, 150,000 to 400,000 cells/mm³. Normal intravascular clot formation continually consumes about 15% of the circulating platelets.[5] Circulating platelets have a life span of up to about 10 days, so are being replenished constantly to maintain a normal count in the bloodstream.[11] Little is known about the source of thrombopoietin, a hormone presumed to stimulate the production of platelets from megakaryocytes in the bone marrow. The kidney may be the source of thrombopoietin, and other colony-stimulating factors (CSF) such as interleukin-3 may help modulate platelet production.[3]

If the integrity of a vessel wall is destroyed, platelets adhere to the inner surface of the vessel. They form a plug, which slows and stops the flow of blood. As the platelets are degraded, a platelet factor is released that interacts with other substances in the blood plasma to form a fibrous clot. Platelets release serotonin, which acts as a vasoconstrictor and further contributes to the slowing of the blood flow.[11] The total process of coagulation is much more complex than this description of platelet function would suggest and involves at least 13 factors that must interact in a carefully synchronized cascade to effect hemostasis. Clotting factors are listed in Table 42-

TABLE 42-3
Clotting Factors

Official Number	Synonym	Contemporary Version
I	Fibrinogen	I (Fibrinogen)
II	Prothrombin	II (Prothrombin)
III	Tissue thromboplastin	III (Tissue factor)
IV	Calcium	IV (Calcium)
V	Labile	V (Labile factor)
		VI PF₃ (platelet coagulant activities)
		VI PF₄
VII	Stable factor	VII (Stable factor)
VIII	Antihemophilic factor	VIII AHF (antihemophilic factor)
		VIII VWF (von Willebrand factor)
		VIII RAg (related antigen)
IX	Christmas factor	IX (Christmas factor)
X	Stuart-Prower factor	X (Stuart-Prower factor)
XI	Plasma thromboplastin (antecedent)	XI (Plasma thromboplastin antecedent)
XII	Hageman factor	XII HF (Hageman factor)
		XII PK (Prekallikrein Fletcher)
		XII HMWK (High-molecular-weight kininogen)
XIII	Fibrin-stabilizing factor	XIII Fibrin-stabilizing factor

The Roman numerals and synonyms designating each clotting factor accepted by the International Committee on Blood Clotting Factors are located in the left-hand columns. Note the absence of factor VI. The version in the right-hand column incorporates more recently recognized clotting factors but is not officially recognized.
(Green, D. [1978]. General considerations of coagulation proteins. *Annals of Clinical and Laboratory Science*, 8[2], 95–105.)

3 and discussed further in Chapter 44. Coagulation cascades may be extrinsic or intrinsic. The mechanism is illustrated in Figure 42-4. Coagulation cascades are important in understanding disorders of platelets. Cascade is discussed further in Chapter 44.

Platelets control both the development and lysis of clots. When the platelet count is under 25,000 to 50,000 cells/mm³, thrombocytopenia is said to occur. Spontaneous bleeding can occur when the level of platelets is below 25,000 cells/mm³.

System Physiology

Hematopoiesis Regulation

Regulation of hematopoiesis is necessary both to ensure an adequate number of functional circulating blood cells and to prevent overproduction of cells. For example, the production of RBCs is regulated by a protein hormone synthesized by juxtaglomerular cells in the kidney. The hormone, erythropoietin, may be produced by other tissues as well. Erythropoietin is produced during hypoxia and stimulates cells in the bone marrow to differentiate into erythroblasts, the precursors to mature erythrocytes.

It has been presumed for some time that leukopoietic hormones also exist; the prompt response of the bone marrow with production of WBCs in appropriate circumstances such as infection suggests that there is careful regulation of the process of leukopoiesis. Studies of a group of factors labeled colony-stimulating factors (CSF) demonstrate that these factors control various steps in the complex process of WBC development. CSF are a group of glycoproteins that stimulate WBC production, maturation, and function. Their name stems from the observation that, in tissue-culture systems, these factors stimulate the growth of colonies of maturing WBCs from their hematopoietic precursors. Under normal conditions, CSF are synthesized continuously by a large number of cells in the body, such as lymphocytes, macrophages, endothelial cells, and others. Some of the specific CSF are: interleukin-3, which stimulates a wide variety of cells to differentiate; granulocyte-macrophage-CSF, which stimulates the production of granulocytes and macrophages; granulocyte-CSF, which stimulates granulocyte production and enhances neutrophil function; and interleukin-5, which stimulates production of eosinophils specifically. Although much is not known about the normal mechanisms of leukopoiesis, there is great interest in the role of these leukopoietic factors in normal physiology as well as the potential for clinical application in disease such as cancer and aplastic anemias.[3,9]

Summary

Hematologic functions are constantly being effected by the cells described above, carried throughout the body in the liquid portion (plasma) of the fluid connective tissue called blood. Using the erythrocytes, leukocytes, and platelets, the blood is one of the major homeostatic forces of the body, maintaining the integrity of the body.

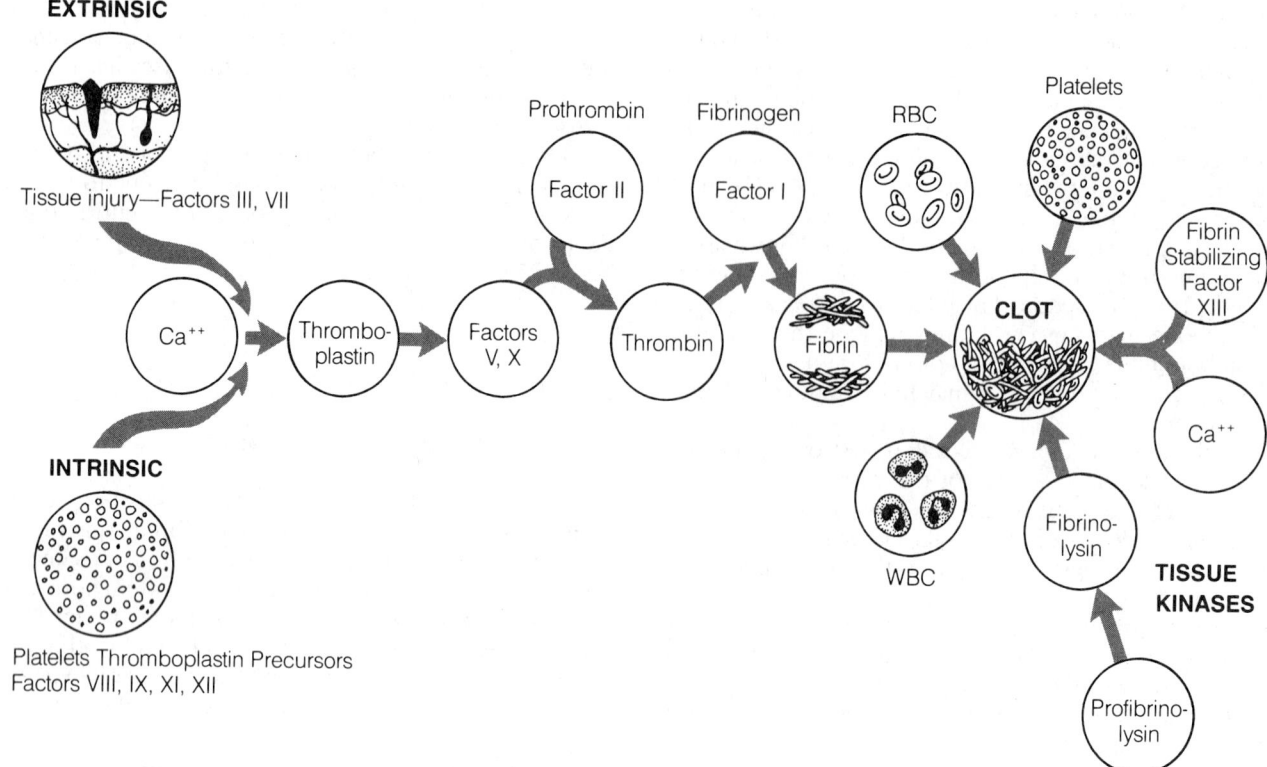

FIGURE 42-4

Coagulation cascades—the blood-clotting mechanism. The schematic drawing represents the factors essential to change blood into a solid gel. The entire chain reaction in which fibrinogen (a plasma protein) is converted to fibrin (the clot) takes place at the site of vessel damage. (Adapted from Feller, I., & Archambeault, C. *Nursing the burn patient*. Ann Arbor: The Institute for Burn Medicine. From Smeltzer, S. C. & Bare, B. G. [1992] *Brunner & Suddarth's textbook of medical-surgical nursing* [7th ed.]. Philadelphia: Lippincott.)

Blood carries respiratory gases, nutrients, and wastes; it contains the cellular and humoral agents that fight and control infections. Complicated processes regulate the maintenance of adequate numbers of blood cells to carry out the important functions of blood. Because abnormalities in the quantity or quality of blood cells are seen so commonly in disease states of infants and children, diagnostic procedures related to blood cells are a mainstay of medical practice. As nurses increase their skills in recognizing the characteristics of abnormal blood parameters, they become more astute in instituting measures of care directed at addressing the common problems associated with such abnormalities.

References

1. Behrman, R. E., & Vaughan, V. C. (1992). *Nelson textbook of pediatrics* (14th ed.). Philadelphia: Saunders.
2. Cunningham, A. S. (1977). Morbidity in breast-fed and artificially fed infants. *Journal of Pediatrics, 90*, 726–729.
3. Dexter, T. M., Garland, J. M., & Testa, N. G. (1990). *Colony-stimulating factors: Molecular and cellular biology*. New York: Marcel Dekker.
4. Gilchrist, F. G. (1968). *A survey of embryology*. New York: McGraw-Hill.
5. Griffin, J. P. (1986). *Hematology and immunology: Concepts for nursing*. Norwalk, CT: Appleton-Century-Crofts.
6. Parmely, M. I., Beer, A. E., & Billingham, R. E. (1976). In vitro studies on the T-lymphocyte population of human milk. *Journal of Experimental Medicine, 144*, 358.
7. Patten, B. M. (1968). *Human embryology* (3rd ed.). New York: McGraw-Hill.
8. Rapaport, S. E. (1971). *Introduction to hematology*. New York: Harper & Row.
9. Robinson, W. A. (1988). Clinical use of colony-stimulating factors. *Mediguide to Oncology, 8*(3), 1–4.
10. Tomasi, R. B. (1972). Secretory immunoglobulins. *New England Journal of Medicine, 287*, 500.
11. Weiss, L. (1977). *The blood cells and hematopoietic tissues*. New York: McGraw-Hill.
12. Wintrobe, M. M. (1980). *Blood, pure and eloquent: A story of discovery, of people, and of ideas*. New York: McGraw-Hill.

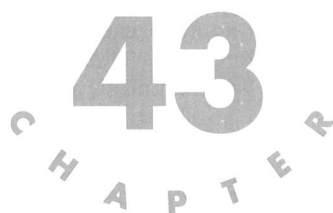

Nursing Assessment and Diagnosis of Hematologic Function

BEHAVIORAL OBJECTIVES

Use functional health as a guideline for assessment of the child's hematologic function.

Describe developmental considerations in the physical examination of a child with possible hematologic dysfunction.

Describe the laboratory tests used to diagnose hematologic dysfunction.

Describe tests and findings pertinent to the three divisions of disorders.

Identify nursing diagnoses commonly used in the care of children with hematologic dysfunction.

B lood is a significant fluid of the body in conveying information about a child's health. Hematologic disorders are organized into three areas: disorders of red cell function, disorders of white cell function, and disorders of platelet and coagulation function. These are further subdivided in Chapter 44 into production, maturation, and destruction.

This chapter discusses how to assess the child with a hematologic disorder. Descriptions of pertinent history and physical assessment findings unique to each disorder (red, white, and platelet and coagulation) are followed by a discussion of the diagnostic studies used to determine specific hematologic disorders in children.

Nursing Assessment

Child and Family History

A child diagnosed with a disorder in hematologic function requires a complete nursing history before physical assessment. The purpose of the history is to gather information needed to assess the severity of the disease state and causative factors. The nursing history should also assess the child and family responses to stress and usual coping styles. The type and extent of history vary depending on whether this is a newly diagnosed disorder or the child has a chronic illness (i.e., sickle cell anemia or hemophilia). A newly diagnosed child requires a complete nursing history.

1077

The child seen for follow-up care requires an ongoing assessment that focuses on specific problems since the last visit.

A complete nursing history of the patient establishes the database for the nurse, providing a guide for continued evaluation. This database changes and expands as the child develops. Nursing considerations should include hereditary implications, past medical history, current health perception, activity, and perceptual and coping patterns of the patient and family.

A careful family history of the child who has a hematologic disorder is important. Many of the hemolytic anemias and bleeding disorders are inherited. Examples include sickle cell anemia, β-thalassemia, glucose-6-phosphate dehydrogenase (G6PD) deficiency, von Willebrand's disease, and hemophilia.

Health Perception and Health Management

A general overall health assessment is required for the child with a disorder in hematologic function. This assessment should include a family history of hematologic disorders, birth history, past medical history, and psychosocial history of the child and family.

A child with a possible diagnosis of iron deficiency anemia often has no significant symptoms of anemia, therefore the nursing database provides vital information regarding the disease severity. Children with chronic forms of anemia, such as sickle cell anemia or β-thalassemia, require a complete history of previous hospitalizations and blood transfusion therapy. Baseline laboratory data are important to assess because these children have hemoglobin levels at which they function normally. A decreased hemoglobin level can be an in-

dication of a number of serious disorders, and the laboratory data is used to classify childhood anemias. If the child has had multiple transfusions, documentation of periodic ferritin levels should be noted because these children often require iron chelation therapy. If the child is on chelation therapy, use of desferoxamine should be noted (Fig. 43-1).

The patient with a diagnosis of sickle cell anemia has the potential for multiple problems. Nursing history and physical examination of the patient with sickle cell anemia are complex. This patient requires an in-depth review of past family history of sickle cell disease or trait, past medical history of the patient, and a complete review of systems. A nursing history should include a social history of the family and how knowledgeable the family is about sickle cell disease.

Children with impaired white blood cell function are at great risk for the acquisition of infections including unusual infections caused by fungal, protozoal, or viral agents. Infections must be treated aggressively and without delay. The history should include questions regarding exposure to infectious diseases, especially varicella zoster (chickenpox), immunizations received, and descriptions of recent illnesses or fever. Children with impaired white cell function must be assessed for signs and symptoms of infections during each health care encounter. Unfortunately, the usual signs and symptoms of infection may be altered due to decreased white cell function.

Patients with suspected aplastic anemia should have a nursing history that includes family history of the disease. Documentation of the presence of prenatal and congenital malformations is important because of a high incidence of aplastic anemia in children with multiple congenital anomalies. The history should include exposure to drugs, household chemicals, irradiation, and in-

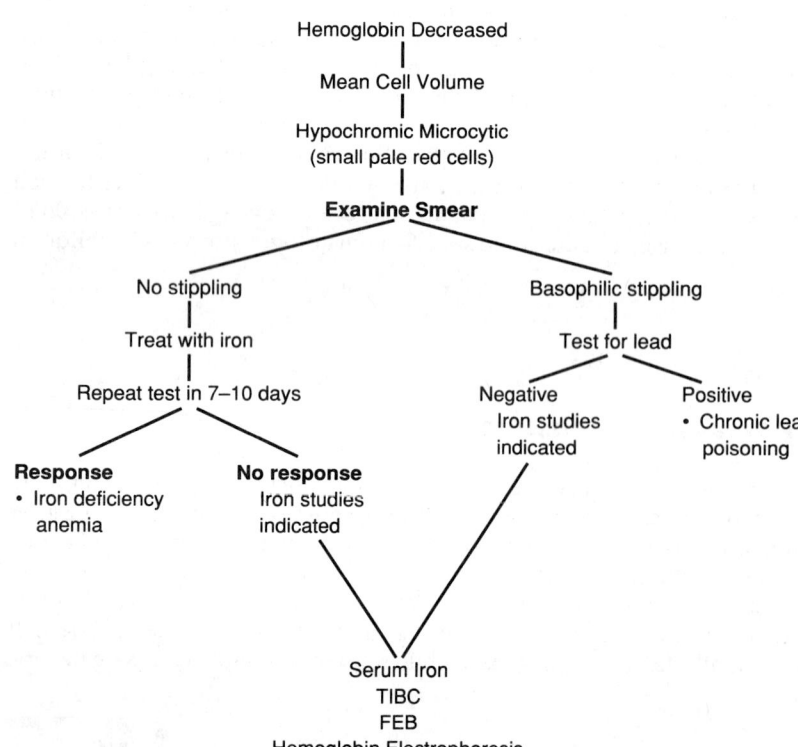

FIGURE 43-1

Iron deficiency anemia may be indicated when hypochromic microcytic cells are found. If the child does not respond to therapy, further studies are indicated. (From: Patterson, K.L. [1985]. The childhood anemias. Pediatrics: Nursing update. Volume 1, lesson 4. Princeton, NJ: Continuing Professional Education Center, 2:8.)

fections (e.g., hepatitis and mononucleosis). The history of the patient with aplastic anemia is more extensive than the physical assessment. Patients may show signs of anemia or a bleeding disorder, but the diagnosis is usually based on laboratory findings (Fig. 43-2).

An initial history of a patient with suspected hematologic malignancy should begin with a history of presenting symptoms. The child may complain of bone pain, lethargy, frequent infections, epistaxis, bruising, and enlarged lymph nodes. Nursing history should state all symptoms first and then incorporate the past medical history of the child. The past medical history should be aimed at past childhood illness, difficulty with bleeding, and immunization history.

The history of a patient with a potential bleeding disorder should include a review of the patient's medical history and family history with a focus on bleeding disorders. A general review of systems should follow. The patient with a diagnosis of von Willebrand's disease can be either male or female. In some instances, the clinical manifestations of the disease may not become apparent until later in life. The history given by family members may be a diagnostic clue as to the type of bleeding disorder suspected in the patient. A history of bleeding disorders in all family members, including grandparents, parents, aunts, uncles, cousins, and siblings, should be ascertained. Females with disorders in platelet and coagulation must have a thorough menstrual history, paying particular attention to menorrhagia.

Assessment of patients at high risk for bleeding dis-

orders (family history of hemophilia) should begin before birth. It should be noted, however, that approximately 30% of new cases diagnosed with hemophilia have no family history of the disorder. Data to be collected include the mother's carrier status, complete history of all family members with the disease, past medical history of the patient to include hepatitis and HIV status, and current health status of the patient. To determine the patient's level of function, the history should include a review of knowledge pertaining to the disease, self-perception (e.g., body image, sexuality, coping techniques), number of bleeds per month the patient experiences (both treated and untreated), home infusion programs, and activity level (school/home/play/work). Finally, questions aimed at establishing the impact of chronic illness on the patient and family should be asked.

The chronicity of the majority of the hematologic diseases mandate a comprehensive financial assessment. This assessment should include questions related to family finances and health insurance coverage. Often referral to social services early in the diagnostic period will assist the nurse in this assessment and planning for the individual child and family.

Nutrition and Metabolism

A careful nutritional assessment for any child is imperative. However, for the child with a hematologic disorder, the nutritional assessment may diagnose a specific disorder such as iron deficiency anemia. A child suspected

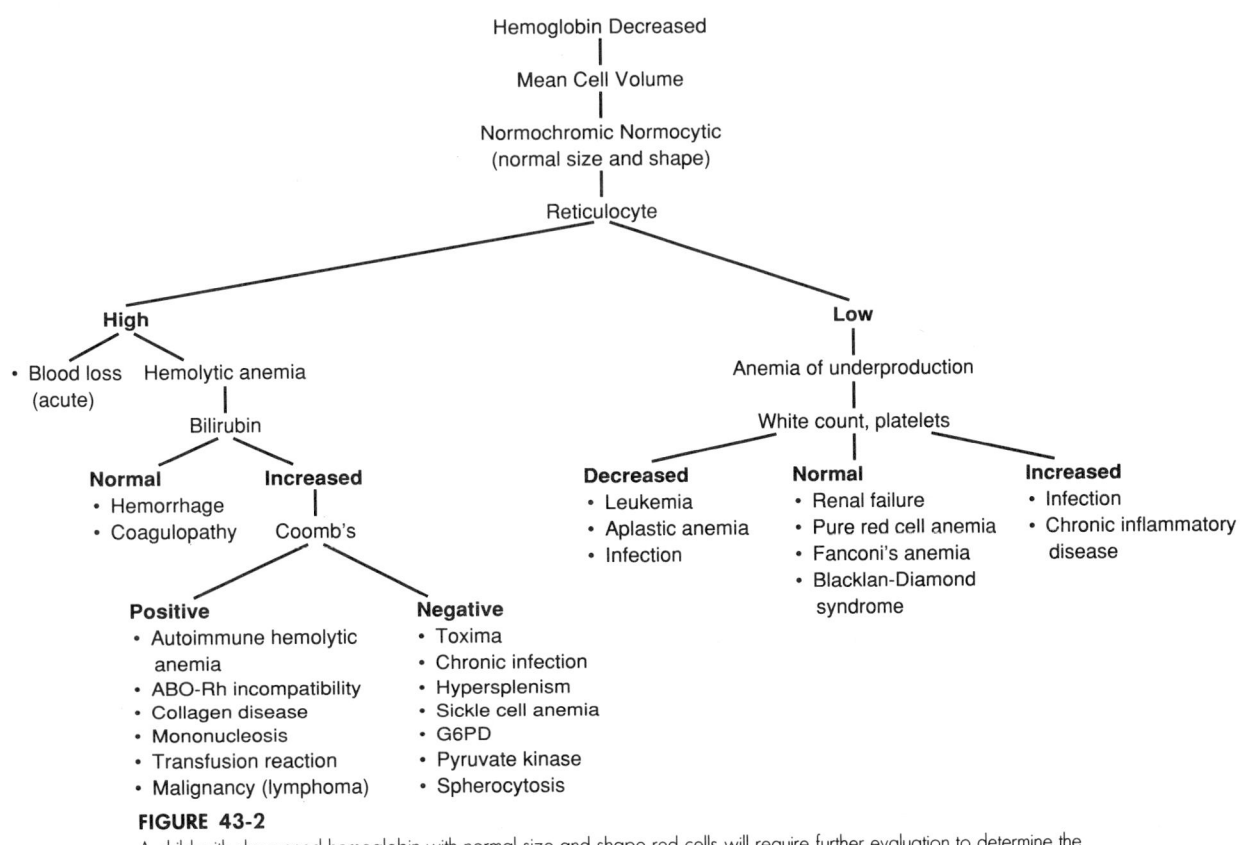

FIGURE 43-2

A child with decreased hemoglobin with normal size and shape red cells will require further evaluation to determine the etiology of the anemia. (*From:* Patterson, K.L. [1985]. The childhood anemias. *Pediatrics: Nursing update.* Volume 1, lesson 4. Princeton, NJ: Continuing Professional Education Center, 2:8.)

of having iron deficiency should have a careful food intake assessment, with particular attention to iron-rich foods. Milk intake in the young infant should be carefully documented. Often infants who ingest cow's milk throughout the day and have no other dietary source of iron are at high risk for the development of iron deficiency anemia. In addition, a history of pica points to possible iron deficiency.

The child with sickle cell anemia should have an assessment of usual daily fluid intake. These patients must increase their fluid intake during periods of sickling crisis. Parental understanding of the methods to prevent sickling crisis by increasing fluid intake should be ascertained.

Children with G6PD deficiency enter a hemolytic crisis if they ingest certain foods, medications, or chemicals (e.g., analgesics, antipyretics, antimalarials, and sulfonamides). Careful assessment of the ingestion of these items aids in determining complications of this disease.

Children with disorders of white cell function have altered healing ability. Therefore, a careful assessment of previous wound healing should be undertaken. Children with sickle cell anemia have altered healing secondary to repeated sickling infarction episodes similar to diabetic patients.

A history of pallor or paleness in a child with a possible diagnosis of anemia should be noted to include any color changes in the mucous membranes or conjunctiva. Increased bruising or petechiae may point to a decrease in the platelet count or another bleeding disorder.

Patients with hemophilia and similar bleeding disorders must pay careful attention to their dental care. A careful dental assessment would include: How often does the child see the dentist? How many times a day does the child brush his or her teeth? Do the child's gums bleed with brushing? How are mouth bleeds normally treated?

Elimination

Children with disorders in coagulation and platelet function must have any history of bleeding from the rectum noted. Also, changes in stool characteristics that indicate bleeding should be noted (e.g., black, tarry stools). Children who are taking iron replacements have stools that are tarry and green. Diarrhea or constipation may be a side-effect of iron replacement therapy. This change is normal and should be expected.

Parents of children with sickle cell anemia often report enuresis into the late childhood years and when the child is in the hospital for hydration treatment for crisis. This phenomenon is due to hyposthenuria. When the kidneys are subjected to repeated sickling episodes, damage to the renal tubules cause loss of the ability to concentrate the urine. Parents and children should be taught that hyposthenuria is a normal complication of sickle cell anemia.

Activity and Exercise

It is essential to determine the child's activity level because it may need to be modified for safety reasons. Children with anemia often report fatigue. Children with sickle cell anemia should avoid strenuous aerobic exercise because of the increased possibility of sickling with lowered oxygen concentration in the blood. The activity level of these children must be documented, and appropriate anticipatory guidance must be given.

Children with hemophilia or other disorders in platelet or coagulation function may not be able to perform those activities that are typical of their age group, due to the risk of bleeding.

Sleep and Rest

Children with chronic anemia adjust to the lowered oxygen-carrying capacity and often do not report fatigue unless the hemoglobin level falls below 7.0 g/dL. Children who have an acute fall in hemoglobin level should be assessed for fatigue. These children need frequent rest periods.

Children under assessment for bleeding disorders must limit their activity or maintain complete bedrest until treatment corrects the bleeding tendencies.

Cognition and Perception

Patients with iron deficiency anemia may have central nervous system changes, such as irritability, or behavioral changes that require careful assessment. Children with chronic diseases such as sickle cell anemia and hemophilia have repeated painful episodes during crisis and bleeding episodes. The pain related to these diseases must be carefully assessed so that appropriate interventions can be evaluated. Children require developmentally appropriate pain assessment techniques as described in Chapter 28. These assessments include descriptions of the child's response to previous analgesic administration as well as assessment of how the child copes with painful medical procedures.

Self-Perception and Self-Concept

Evaluation of the patient with a disorder in hematologic function regarding self-concept, body image, and sexuality must be appropriate for the patient's developmental level. Open-ended questions, both verbal and written; interview techniques; and observation of family members contribute to a comprehensive assessment.

Role Relationship

The child with a disorder in hematologic function deals with many psychosocial issues. The child with a chronic blood disorder such as hemophilia, sickle cell anemia, or leukemia has frequent clinic visits and hospitalizations, which may lead to prolonged school absences. The child may not be able to participate in contact sports and thus may be excluded from some peer groups. Some patients with hemophilia actually become the daredevil of the group, perhaps showing their ability to perform difficult tasks.

Chronic illness in a child has an impact on the entire family. Overall assessment of family relationships and family functioning should be ongoing throughout the

TABLE 43-1
Developmental Considerations in the Physical Examination of Hematopoietic Function

Organ/System	Infant	Child	Adolescent
Skin	May be mottled if cold	Bruising may be normal if on legs and arms	Bruising may be normal if on legs and arms
Lymph	Small movable nontender nodes may be present	Small movable nontender nodes may be present	
Liver	Palpable 0–3 cm below costal margin	Palpable 1–2 cm below costal margin	Non-palpable
Spleen	May be palpable under ribs	May be palpable under ribs	Non-palpable

treatment process. Assessment of how parents usually discipline their children is important as disorders of platelet and coagulation function may require parents to substitute alternative approaches to disciplining their child. In addition, the child with a chronic illness needs to assume responsibility for his care as he matures. Ongoing assessment in this area is necessary to provide guidance for the transfer of care from parents to the mature child.

Sexuality and Reproduction

Issues in sexuality and reproduction are important for the child with an inherited hematologic disorder such as sickle cell anemia, β-thalassemia, or hemophilia. The parents and child should he assessed as to their understanding of the genetic inheritance of the specific disorder so that informed choices can be made about future reproduction.

The child who must receive multiple blood product transfusions in treatment of the specific illness must be assessed as to his or her understanding of the transmission of bloodborne illnesses, especially HIV infection. Assessment of the understanding of the need for and practice of precautions for sexual intercourse that must be taken to protect both partner and patient should be ongoing in these high-risk patients.

The development of secondary sexual characteristics is often delayed in children with sickle cell anemia. Tanner staging should begin in preadolescence and continue throughout maturity.

Coping and Stress Tolerance

The child with a disorder in hematologic function may present to the office or the emergency room with sudden onset of anemia, infection, bleeding, bruising, or the appearance of petechiae. The parents of the child are often extremely frightened because the child is ill, and a hematologic malignancy is often one of the possible reasons given for the abnormalities in the child. Obtaining a complete history may be difficult for the nurse in the initial encounter. The complete history may need to be taken in parts, beginning with the most important areas first (e.g., history of the present illness, drug and food allergies, and usual patterns of coping, like favored toys).

The complete nursing database can be completed later when parent and child stress levels are lower.

Other chronic hematologic illnesses have acute exacerbations of the illness, like sickle cell crisis. During these episodes, the family is under stress. The nurse must assess for changes in usual patterns of coping that might alert the nurse to concurrent problems in the family. In addition, the families of children with chronic illnesses should have periodic updates of the nursing history because significant changes in the family may have occurred that may impact the child and family's ability to cope (e.g., divorce or death of a parent or close family member).

TABLE 43-2
Abnormal Findings on the Physical Examination of the Hematopoietic System

Body Part	Abnormal Findings
Head	Sunken fontanelle, decreased head circumference, prominent forehead, protruding maxilla
Eyes	Sunken eyes, papilledema, sclera yellow, petechial lesions
Ears	Membranes not intact or showing scarring, bleeding
Nose	Bleeding, petechial lesions, decreased secretions, tenderness, nasal flaring, thick discharge
Throat	Swelling, redness, petechiae, bleeding, pale, mucosal breakdown, oozing gums, abscess formation
Neck	Tenderness on palpation; masses; nodules that are hard, firm, spongy, non-movable, and tender on palpation
Heart	Murmurs; tachycardia; gallop rhythm; prominent active heaving or thrusting precordium
Lungs	Tachypnea, decreased breath sounds, dullness over lung fields, decreased chest expansion, rales, rhonchi
Abdomen	Palpable liver > 2 cm below costal margin, palpable spleen, palpable mass, no bowel sounds present, enlarged inguinal nodes, distention after voiding
Genitourinary system	Palpable masses, abnormal bleeding patterns, mucosal breakdown
Skin	Pallor, temperature, dry texture, decreased turgor, rashes, erythema, jaundice, bleeding, petechiae, bruising, swelling, cyanosis, abscess formation
Extremities	Swelling, tenderness, decreased range of motion, warm to touch, decreased peripheral pulses, concave nailbeds, pallor

Values and Beliefs

The child and family should be assessed for their understanding of the inheritance of a particular hematologic disorder. Often the child and family have conflicting feelings regarding this issue. Careful assessment in this area is important so that referral to a mental health specialist can be made to assist the family in resolving these issues.

Parents of children with hematologic disorders often have to face subjecting their child to a blood transfusion. Since the discovery of HIV, people are reluctant to receive blood product transfusions. Education and support are necessary to increase the family's and child's understanding of the need for and risks involved in receiving human blood products. In addition, parents may have religious reasons to refuse a blood transfusion for their child (e.g., Jehovah's Witnesses).

Physical Examination

The physical assessment of the child with a disorder in hematologic function focuses on all organ systems. Disorders related to the hemopoietic system are observed through symptoms documented in the history and signs observed on physical examination. Table 43-1 outlines developmental considerations in the physical exam; Table 43-2 outlines abnormal findings on the physical examination of the child's hematopoietic system.

Diagnostic Tests

The diagnostic tests used in treatment of hematologic function include a simple blood test and bone marrow aspiration. These tests are described here. Abnormalities in other routine laboratory studies, such as the urinalysis and chemistry profile, are listed in Table 43-3 as to how they relate specifically to disorders in hematologic function.

Laboratory Tests

Various analyses can be made with a blood specimen. Common hematologic laboratory tests are summarized in the tables of this chapter. The procedures for collecting blood are discussed in Chapter 25. The nurse should be familiar with the common normal blood values so deviations can be recognized. Normal values are given in the Appendix.

In addition to the normal variants of hemoglobin that exist at various stages of human development (see Chap. 42), there are several indices of normal function of erythrocytes (Tables 43-4 and 43-5). Among these are hematocrit values, the mean corpuscular volume (MCV), the mean corpuscular hemoglobin (MCH), and mean corpuscular hemoglobin concentration (MCHC). Hematocrit is the percentage of RBCs in the total blood volume; normal values for adults are: male, 41 to 53, and female, 36 to 46. By comparison, the hematocrit for a day-old neonate is 48 to 69, with a drop by the age of 2 months to 28 to

TABLE 43-3
Hematologic Dysfunction Found in Routine Laboratory Studies

Test	Abnormalities in Specific Hematologic Diseases
Urinalysis	
Specific gravity	May be low in sickle cell anemia secondary to hyposthenuria; not reliable indication of hydration status in these patients
pH	No specific findings
Albumin	No specific findings
Bile	May be present in hemolytic anemia
Blood	May be present in patients with thrombocytopenia secondary to bleeding in kidney, bladder
Ketones	No specific findings
Chemistry Profile	
Total bilirubin Direct bilirubin	Elevated in hemolytic anemia secondary to lysis of blood cell
Total protein Albumin	May be decreased in childhood chronic illnesses as a measure of nutritional status
Serum glutamic-oxaloacetic transaminase (SGOT) Serum glutamate pyruvate transaminase (SGPT)	May be elevated in patients on chemotherapy with associated liver toxicities or leukemic infiltrates in liver, or in children who have had repeated blood product transfusions secondary to hepatitis
Lactate dehydrogenase (LDH)	May be elevated in hematologic malignancies as an indication of cell destruction
Alkaline phosphatase (Alk Phos)	May be elevated during sickle cell crisis
Blood urea nitrogen (BUN)	Elevated with bleeding in the gastrointestinal tract
Uric acid	Elevated in acute lymphocytic leukemia during induction therapy secondary to cell lysis; also elevated in children with sickle cell anemia

TABLE 43-4
Age-Related Changes in Hemoglobin (Hb) and Mean Corpuscular Volume (MCV) in Newborns to 6 Months of Age

Age	Hb	MCV
Birth (cord values)	13.6–19.6	106
1 day	21.2	106
1 week	19.6	101
2 weeks	18.0	96
3 weeks	16.6	93
4 weeks	15.6	91
2 months	13.3	85
3 months	12.5	84
4 months	12.4	79
6 months	12.3	78

(With permission from: Patterson, K. L. [1985]. The childhood anemias. *Pediatrics: Nursing update*, Volume 1, Lesson 4. Princeton, NJ: Continuing Professional Educational Center, 2:8.)

42. By adolescent years, hematocrit levels rise to near adult levels: 37 to 49 for males and 36 to 46 for females.

MCV is a measure of the average volume or size of a red blood cell and is determined by dividing the hematocrit by the total number of RBCs. An elevated MCV occurs when the red blood cells are abnormally large, as in megaloblastic anemias. A decreased MCV is seen in iron deficiency anemia or thalassemia, when the RBC is microcytic. Levels are higher in the neonate than in the infant and young child, and there is a gradual increase from a level of 70 to 86 cuμ in the infant to the adult levels of 80 to 100 cuμ.

MCH is computed by dividing the hemoglobin concentration by the number of RBCs. It represents the average amount of hemoglobin in a red blood cell. The causes for abnormal values closely resemble those for MCV. Newborn levels are 32 to 24 pg/cell, compared to normal adult levels of 27 to 31 pg/cell.

MCHC represents the average concentration or percentage of hemoglobin in a single red blood cell. It is derived by dividing the hemoglobin by the hematocrit. If the cell has a deficiency of hemoglobin or is hypochromic as in iron deficiency, the MCHC is decreased. Normal levels at birth are 30% to 36% Hgb/cell; in infancy, 30% to 36% Hgb/cell; and for the normal adult, 31% to 37% Hgb/cell.

Red Cell Dysfunction. The laboratory assessment of the child with a disorder in red cell function is usually simple. A complete blood count with reticulocyte count is often all that is required initially. From the results of these tests, others are prescribed by the physician or the nurse practitioner.

Anemia is generally defined as a reduction in the red cell mass or the blood hemoglobin concentration.

Based on normal hemoglobin measures, anemia would be defined as any hemoglobin level less than the lower range for age. However, these values are only guidelines. A patient whose usual hemoglobin concentration falls toward the upper limits of normal may be anemic if the present hemoglobin level is at the lower limits of normal.

Anemias may be classified by one of two approaches: morphologic and physiologic. Anemias may be classified morphologically according to red cell size, shape, and color. With this type of classification, anemias are divided into three categories: hypochromic microcytic anemias, macrocytic anemias, and normochromic normocytic anemias.

The morphologic approach to classifying anemias is based on the red cell's appearance as reported by the red blood cell indices. Hypochromic microcytic anemia is characterized by small, pale red blood cells. MCV and MCH are below normal. Macrocytic anemias are characterized by large red cells as indicated by an increased MCV and MCH. Normochromic normocytic anemias have normal values for MCV and MCH.

Morphologic classification of anemias is the method most widely used by nurse practitioners and physicians. It provides a classification system based on laboratory results. In addition, this system provides a more orderly method for ruling out certain diagnoses when trying to establish the cause for a particular anemia.

The physiologic approach includes three categories: (1) disorders of red blood cell production in which the rate of red cell production is less than would be expected for the degree of anemia, (2) disorders of red cell maturation, and (3) disorders of red cell destruction or hemolytic anemias.

The physiologic classification of anemias provides a basis to plan and implement nursing care for anemic pa-

TABLE 43-5
Age-Related Changes in Hb and MCV by Age and Sex From 1 Year to Adult

Sex	Age (yr)	Hb (g/dL)*	MCV (ccμ)
Males and females	1–2	12.3 (10.7–13.8)	79 (67–88)
	3–5	12.5 (10.9–14.4)	81 (73–91)
	6–8	12.8 (11.0–14.3)	82 (74–92)
	9–11	13.2 (11.4–14.8)	84 (76–94)
Males	12–14	14.0 (12.0–16.0)	85 (77–94)
	15–17	14.8 (12.3–16.6)	87 (79–95)
	18–44	15.3 (13.2 17.3)	89 (80–99)
	45–64	15.2 (13.1–17.2)	90 (81–101)
	65–74	14.9 (12.6–17.4)	91 (81–103)
Females	12–14	13.4 (11.5–15.0)	86 (73–95)
	15–17	13.5 (11.7–15.3)	88 (78–98)
	18–44	13.5 (11.7–15.5)	90 (81–100)
	45–64	13.7 (11.7–16.0)	90 (81–101)
	65–74	13.8 (11.7–16.1)	90 (81–102)

* Median values and 95% confidence intervals.
(With permission from: Patterson, K. L. [1985]. The childhood anemias. *Pediatrics: Nursing update*, Volume 1, Lesson 4. Princeton, NJ: Continuing Professional Educational Center, 2:8.)

TABLE 43-6
Laboratory Tests Commonly Used in Diagnosing Anemia in Children

Test	Description
Complete Blood Count	
Hb	Hemoglobin is an iron-containing protein that is the basic component of red cells and is the vehicle of O_2 and CO_2 transport. Normal values vary with age.
Hct	Percentage of the volume of a blood sample occupied by red blood cells. Rough measure of erythrocyte concentration. Not as sensitive as Hb for anemia screening.
RBC	Cells that carry Hb. Is not used to evaluate anemia but is used in determining indices.
WBC and differential	Number and type of infection-fighting cells. Not used in diagnosing anemia except in cases of malignancy. Leukemia and hypersegmented neutrophils accompany the megaloblastic anemia of pernicious anemia.
MCV	Mean corpuscular volume, one of the red cell indices. Average volume of each RBC. Undergoes same changes as MCV in iron deficiency anemia.
MCH	Mean corpuscular hemoglobin, one of the red cell indices. Average weight of hemoglobin in the RBC. Undergoes same changes as MCV in iron deficiency anemia.
Peripheral smear	Identifies variations in RBC size, shape, structure, Hb, and staining properties that identify certain properties of red cells in anemia.

Basophilic stippling: (aggregated ribosomes)	Thalassemia Lead poisoning Iron deficiency
Howell-Jolly bodies: (nuclear remnants)	Asplenia, hyposplenia Pernicious anemia Dyserythropoietic anemias Severe iron deficiency anemia
Heinz bodies: (denatured or aggregated hemoglobin)	Thalassemia Unstable hemoglobins Asplenia Chronic liver disease
Spherocytes:	Hereditary spherocytosis Acquired hemolytic anemia
Schistocytes:	Hemolytic-uremic syndrome DIC Vasculitis Prostheses (heart valves)
Target cells:	Hemoglobins S, C, D, and E Thalassemias Lead poisoning
Sickle cells:	Sickle cell anemia

Test	Description
Iron Studies	
Serum iron	Concentration of iron bound to transferrin.
Transferrin saturation	Percentage of serum iron divided by TIBC. Widely used as a confirmatory test to diagnose iron deficiency anemia.
Serum ferritin	Ferritin is a storage form of iron in liver, reticuloendothelial cells, and bone marrow. Not predictable in diagnosing iron deficiency in infants.
TIBC	Capacity of plasma for binding iron, which is limited by the transferrin content. Normally, transferrin is approximately one third saturated with iron; so, if the plasma iron is 100 mg, TIBC would be 300 mg.
Free erythrocyte protoporphyrin (FEP)	Binds with iron to form heme. Low levels of iron do not allow normal amounts of heme construction, so FEP accumulates. Lead also blocks the conversion of iron and FEP to heme, so lead toxicity also causes elevated FEP levels.
Miscellaneous	
Reticulocyte count	An immature RBC released by the bone marrow that matures within 2 days of release. An increased count means the bone marrow is responding to an anemia by making RBCs faster than normal.
Indirect bilirubin	The fraction of total bilirubin that reflects Hb breakdown from RBCs. Increased levels with hemolysis.
Coomb's	A measure of antibody formation in cases of hemolytic anemia. If positive, antibodies are present; if negative, no antibodies are present. Useful in distinguishing congenital hemolytic syndromes from antibody-mediated hemolysis.
Hgb electrophoresis	Method of determining percentages of certain types of hemoglobins. Used in diagnosis of sickle cell anemia, thalassemia, and other hemoglobinopathies
Bone marrow aspiration	Cellular changes in marrow are diagnostic of many abnormalities. Used only to diagnose anemias that cannot be ascertained by laboratory work alone.
Stool for occult blood	Used to identify bleeding from the GI tract.

(With permission from: Patterson, K. L. [1985]. The childhood anemias. *Pediatrics: Nursing update*, Volume 1, Lesson 4. Princeton, NJ: Continuing Professional Education Center, 2:8.)

TABLE 43-7
Normal White Blood Cell Counts From Birth to 6 Years

Age	Leukocytes	Neutrophils (%)	Lymphocytes (%)
Birth	9.0–30.0	61	31
1 month	5.0–19.5	35	56
2 years	6.0–17.0	33	60
4 years	5.5–15.5	42	50
6 years	5.0–14.5	51	42

tients. For example, if RBC maturation is impaired, the nursing goal is to provide interventions that promote erythropoiesis, such as increasing dietary iron intake. If the anemia results from red blood cell destruction, the nursing goal might include blood replacement as well as interruption or prevention of the destructive cycle.

The common tests used in the diagnosis of childhood anemias are described in Table 43-6.

White Cell Dysfunction. The white blood cell count (WBC) and differential are useful guides in the diagnosis, treatment, and prognosis of various childhood illnesses. Normal granulocyte counts and lymphocyte counts vary during childhood (Table 43-7). In addition, African-American children generally have lower white counts than white children, primarily due to decreased numbers of neutrophils.

Lymphocytes are involved in cell-mediated immunity (see Chap. 27). These types of white cells are involved

TABLE 43-8
Laboratory Assessment of White Cell Function

Test	Description	Clinical Implications
White blood count	Number of WBC/mm³ of blood	Increased in infection. May be increased or decreased in presence of leukemia. Some viral infections may decrease WBC. Chemotherapy will decrease total WBC. Normal values vary according to age (see Table 43-7).
Differential	Quantification of WBC types in blood	
Neutrophils:		
Segs (polys)	Primary defense in bacterial and fungal infections, can phagocytize and kill bacteria	Will be elevated in infections. Chemotherapy will decrease total number of segs and bands.
Bands (stab)	Immature neutrophil, increased in number during infections, can also phagocytize and kill bacteria	Will be markedly elevated in bacterial infection (>segs), called a left shift.
Lymphocytes	Involved in development of antibody and delayed hypersensitivity reactions, elevated in viral infections	Will be elevated in viral infections. A lymphocytosis is normal in toddlers. May be elevated in the early stages of acute lymphocytic leukemia.
Monocytes	Large phagocytic cells involved in early phase of inflammatory response	Markedly elevated numbers indicate bone marrow recovery from effects of chemotherapy.
Eosinophils	Increased in allergic disorders, parasitic diseases	Children with asthma or allergic disorders will have markedly elevated eosinophilic count.
Basophils	Contain histamine; function unknown	
Immunoglobulin levels	Level of circulating immunoglobulin is measure of body's ability to form antibodies against infections	Children with low levels of immunoglobulins are at great risk for infections. Actual levels vary with age.
IgG	Bacterial protection	
IgA	Viral protection	
IgM	Bacterial protection	
Skin test reactivity	Tests of immune function, especially T-cell function	Usually the child is tested with antigens that he should react against as control. Absence of any reactivity is a poor prognostic sign. Antigens are given by intradermal injection or by a multi-test device. Careful documentation of the location of each antigen is critical in test interpretation.
Bone marrow aspiration	Determines marrow cellularity and morphology, presence or absence of neutrophils and precursors, neutrophil maturation	Abnormalities of cell lines determine disease state.

TABLE 43-9
Bone Marrow Classification of Acute Leukemia in Children

	Acute Lymphoblastic Leukemia	Acute Nonlymphoblastic Leukemia
Special Stains		
Sudan black	−	+
Peroxidase	−	+
Auer rods	−	+
Morphology		
FAB	+	−
Immunology		
T-cell marker	+	−
B-cell marker	+	−
CALLA	+	−
Cytogenetics		
Philadelphia chromosome	+/−	−

also in fighting viral infections. The neutrophils are the most important phagocytic cells defending the body against bacterial and fungal infections. They are formed in the bone marrow and are called to sites of infections by the processes described in Chapter 27.

Leukopenia exists when the white blood cell count is below normal for age. Usually, this is a WBC count of less than 4000. If the absolute granulocyte count is less than 1500, the child is considered neutropenic. The absolute neutrophil count is calculated by the following formula. If the lab results are: WBC 3200 Seg^{20} Band^5 Lymph^{60} Mono^{10} Eos^5, then WBC × (% seg + bands) = ANS (3200 × 0.25) = 700. The absolute neutrophil count is used primarily in the treatment of a child with cancer. This count is important in determining when a child has sufficiently recovered enough from previous therapy to start chemotherapy again. In addition, this count is used to determine when a child is at great risk for infection. Any child with a fever (T > 101°F or 38°C) and an ANC < 1000 is considered to have a life-threatening illness until proven otherwise.

Neutropenia can result from underproduction in the bone marrow, increased destruction in the circulation, or sequestration of white blood cells from the circulating pool. The average life span of a white blood cell is 6 to 8 hours. The primary laboratory evaluation of white blood cell and immune function includes the tests listed in Table 43-8.

Aplastic anemia and childhood leukemia are diseases in which combinations of hematologic dysfunction are characteristic. Aplastic anemia may be idiopathic or secondary to ingestion of certain drugs, chemicals, or infections, commonly viral infections such as hepatitis. Laboratory findings would include pancytopenia, with decreased reticulocyte count. Examination of the bone marrow shows marked decreased or absence of hematopoietic cells and replacement by fatty tissue containing reticulum cells, lymphocytes, plasma cells, and tissue mast cells. Many times, a bone marrow biopsy is needed to exclude the possibility of poor sampling technique.

A child suspected of having acute lymphocytic leukemia shows changes in the blood count, which may include a decreased hemoglobin, a decreased platelet count, and a decreased or increased white count. The marrow is usually replaced by leukemic blasts, with a resultant decrease in other hematopoietic cells. Once the leukemia has been destroyed, the bone marrow returns to normal function. Thereafter, bone marrow suppression is caused by the antineoplastic drugs used to treat the leukemia. Table 43-9 lists the bone marrow classification studies used to diagnose childhood leukemias.

Platelet and Coagulation Dysfunction. Idiopathic thrombocytopenia purpura (ITP) is the most common cause of thrombocytopenia that occurs in childhood. ITP is characterized by an increased destruction of platelets, usually caused by an immune-mediated process. This disorder is diagnosed based on pertinent history data and a drop in platelet count. Tests are employed to rule out other disorders in which thrombocytopenia is a manifestation (Table 43-10). The use of bone marrow examination to rule out aplastic anemia or a malignancy is controversial. Many clinicians feel that, if steroids are to be used to treat ITP, one must determine that some other, more serious, disorder of the bone marrow is not present. Tests have been developed to determine platelet surface-bound antibodies. These tests are usually available only

TABLE 43-10
Diagnostic Tests Used in Idiopathic Thrombocytopenia Purpura (ITP)

Test	Result	Clinical Implications
Platelet count	<100,000	Determine severity of bleeding potential, response to therapy
Bone marrow aspiration	Normal erythroid and myeloid cells, increased megakaryocytes	Rule out aplastic anemia, leukemia
Antinuclear antibody	Positive	May indicate systemic lupus erythematosus, Evans' syndrome, or other autoimmune disorders
Coombs	Positive	
Serum complement	Decreased	
Antiplatelet antibody	Present	Determine presence of surface antibodies, and predict response to steroid or gamma globulin treatment

in tertiary care centers. The antiplatelet antibody tests are useful in predicting response to steroids or gamma globulin treatment, especially in recurrent or chronic forms of ITP.[6]

Disorders in coagulation are diagnosed by actual measurement of the specific coagulation factor suspected to be involved. Usually the problem is noted by routine clotting studies such as the prothrombin time (PT) and the partial thromboplastin time (PTT). Table 43-11 describes the common tests used in the diagnosis of disorders in platelet and coagulation function.

Procedures

Most disorders in hematologic function are identified by simple laboratory tests. The bone marrow aspiration or biopsy is used to determine specific hematologic function. Although this test is not indicated in all patients with disorders of hematologic function, it is employed in the diagnostic evaluation of many diseases in this area.

There is uniformity of aspirates taken from multiple sites of hematopoietic tissue, so a marrow aspirate taken from one site is a good reflection of overall hematopoietic

TABLE 43-11
Laboratory Evaluation of Platelets, Platelet Function, and Blood Coagulation

Test	Normal Range	Deviations	Clinical Implications
Platelet count	150,000–450,000	Count <100,000 indicates thrombocytopenia	Child must avoid activities that could cause injury
			Count < 25,000 could result in spontaneous bleeding
			Will see increased bruising or petechiae
			Normal life span of platelet 8–10 days
			⅔ of the body's platelets are in the circulating pool and ⅓ are in the splenic pool.
Examination of the blood smear	Normal size/number of platelets present	A disproportionate number of large platelets may indicate an increased platelet turnover, suggesting peripheral platelet destruction rather than impaired platelet production.	Common in idiopathic thrombocytopenia purpura
Platelet aggregation	Platelets will aggregate/cluster together when exposed to the agents epinephrine, thrombin, ADP, ristocetin	Absence or decreased aggregation curves	Primarily used for von Willebrand's disease
Antiplatelet antibodies	Absent	Present	Indicates peripheral destruction of platelets
			Present in idiopathic thrombocytopenia purpura or patient who has had multiple platelet transfusions
Blood Coagulation			
Prothrombin time (PT)	Child/Adult: 13 s	>14 s	Detects deficiencies in extrinsic pathway, mainly factor VII
Partial thromboplastin time (PTT)	Child/Adult: 30–45 s	>45 s	Detects factor deficiencies in intrinsic pathway VIII, IX (XI, XII)
If both PT and PTT are prolonged			Common pathway (XI, thrombin, fibrinogen)
Fibrinogen	200–400 mg/dL	<200	Indicates combined platelet and clotting disorders, decreased in disseminated intravascular coagulation syndrome
Bleeding time	<9 min	>9 min	Associated with any bleeding disorder
			Child must be as calm as possible during the test or bleeding time will be prolonged
Clotting factors	Measured by activity level and antigen level	Measured by decreased or absent levels	Factor VIII deficiency (hemophilia A)
			Factor IX deficiency accounts for 15% of all patients with hemophilia B
			von Willebrand's disease will have low but not absent levels of factor VIII activity and antigen

activity. A study of the bone marrow can give valuable information for evaluating normal and diseased states. In the infant, the best sites for bone marrow aspiration are the proximal tibia and posterior iliac crest. The posterior iliac crest is the preferred site in older children (Fig. 43-3).

Bone Marrow Aspiration/Biopsy

Description/Definition

Insertion of a special aspirate or biopsy needle in the space and aspiration of a sample. Bone marrow plug removal for close examination of the hematologic system and a wide variety of hematologic diseases. Several sites can be used: posterior or anterior iliac crest (posterior is most common), anterior tibia (primarily in newborns and young infants), vertebral bodies, and the sternum.

Purpose

The study provides an evaluation of marrow cellularity, specific types of cells present, including any cells foreign to the marrow (e.g., malignancy), and maturation of the blood cell lines.

Indications

- Confirmation of a severe or complicated hematologic disorder.
- Rule out malignant metastasis to the bone marrow.

The biopsy usually is obtained if an aspirate sample is inadequate to diagnose the disorder.

Contraindications

- Diagnosis can be made by blood tests alone.

Special precautions must be taken when a bone marrow aspirate or biopsy must be done on a child with a disorder of platelet function. The puncture site should be watched carefully for bleeding. Immediately after the procedure, pressure should be applied for 5 to 10 minutes. A pressure bandage should be applied, and the site should be observed hourly for 4 to 8 hours. The medical and nursing staff should be prepared to give platelet support if bleeding occurs in spite of the above measures.

Preparation

The parent and child should be given specific information about the indications for and steps of the procedure. In addition, the child should be provided with strategies to cope with the pain involved with this procedure.[13] See Chapter 28 for additional coping strategies to help children undergoing painful medical procedures.

Usually, the child is given sedative medications; medications vary with the practice standards of each institution. The current trend is to provide conscious sedation for children undergoing this procedure. If the child is to receive heavily sedating agents, he or she should be NPO at least 4 to 6 hours before the procedure to prevent the risk of aspiration. Emergency equipment should be available, and a person should be identified to be responsible solely to assess the child's respiratory status during the procedure.

The patient is positioned based on the site to be used. For the posterior iliac crest site, the child is placed on the stomach, with a small pillow or support under the hips (see Fig. 43-1). The skin is cleansed with a disinfectant and sterilely draped. The skin, subcutaneous tissue, and periosteum are infiltrated with a local anesthetic. For the aspiration, a large-gauge needle is placed into the bone. A twisting motion is used. The patient reports this to feel like a hard pressure. The stylet is removed, and a small amount of fluid (0.2 to 1.0 ml) is aspirated. This aspiration causes a severe, sharp pain, which subsides immediately after stopping the aspiration. The needle is removed, and pressure is applied to the puncture site for a few minutes. Usually, a small pressure bandage is placed over the site.

If a biopsy is to be obtained, a different needle is used. This needle has a tapered edge and a stylet that extends beyond the needle. The needle is placed into the marrow space according to the procedure described above, but, instead of aspirating, the special needle is twisted and rocked back and forth several times to "core out" a small piece of the bone marrow. Both procedures usually take 10 to 15 minutes.

Developmental Considerations

Tibial site is commonly used in neonates and young infants.

- Infants: May need sedative medications to ensure the child remains still during procedure.
- Toddlers: In addition to sedative medications, have parents or a comforting surrogate present during procedure.
- Preschool and School-Age: Therapeutic medical play as preparation; parental presence encouraged.

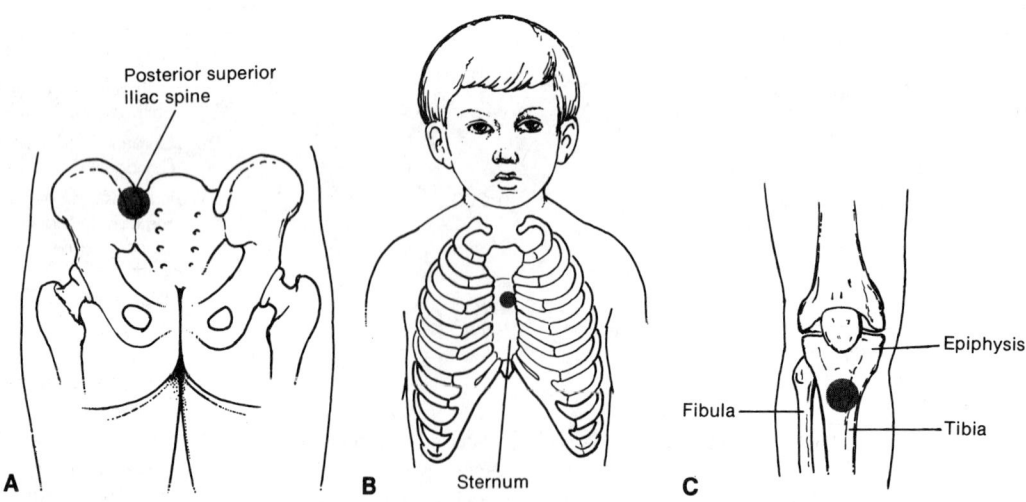

FIGURE 43-3
Preferred sites for bone marrow aspiration. (**A**) Anterior or posterior iliac crest is used at any age. (**B**) The sternum is used for children over 6 years of age. (**C**) The tibia is used in infants and children through 2 years of age. (Skale, N. [1992]. *Manual of pediatric nursing procedures.* Philadelphia: J. B. Lippincott.)

TABLE 43-12
Selected Nursing Diagnoses Associated With Altered Hematologic Function

Data Analysis and Conclusions	Nursing Diagnosis
Health Perception and Health Management	
Mother of patient newly diagnosed with acute lymphocytic leukemia asks for any reading material about leukemia treatment. School-age child with hemophilia asks to learn to give his own factor.	Altered Health Maintenance related to knowledge deficit regarding treatment regimen, dietary, prescription, observation and reporting of symptoms, follow-up care of disease, health promotion activities.
Child with acute lymphocytic leukemia and absolute neutrophil count of 250 asks to go to school. Child newly diagnosed with acute lymphocytic leukemia has temperature of 102°F. Child with acute lymphocytic leukemia is exposed to varicella at school. Child asks why he must take Bactrim if he is not sick.	High Risk for Infection related to immunosuppression from chemotherapy
Child with idiopathic thrombocytopenia purpura wants to ride his bike. Child with acute lymphocytic leukemia and platelet count of 30,000 is playing catch with a baseball. Child with hemophilia wants to play football. Child with acute lymphocytic leukemia needs intramuscular injection.	High Risk for Injury related to low platelet count
Nutrition and Metabolism	
Child with sickle cell anemia wants to go to zoo on hot summer day. Child with sickle cell anemia has flu and starts to complain of back pain 3 days later.	High Risk for Fluid Volume Deficit related to extreme heat
Elimination	
Child with sickle cell anemia has problem with bedwetting. Specific gravity of urine of child with sickle cell anemia is 1005, but child appears to be mildly dehydrated. Child newly diagnosed with T-cell acute lymphocytic leukemia has drop in urine output 8 h after initiation of chemotherapy.	Altered Urinary Elimination related to renal damage from disease or therapy
Activity and Exercise	
Child with aplastic anemia and Hb of 7.5 complains of headache and dizziness when standing up quickly. Child newly diagnosed with acute lymphocytic leukemia returns from school early.	Activity Intolerance related to anemia
Child with hemophilia has right knee contracture.	Impaired Physical Mobility related to damage from repeated bleeding into the joint
Cognition and Perception	
Child newly diagnosed with acute lymphocytic leukemia is preparing for discharge, and mother asks what to do if child gets a fever at home. Father of child with hemophilia calls nurse when he is unable to get IV in to give factor VIII. Mother of child with sickle cell anemia wonders whether her other children have the disease.	Knowledge Deficit related to diagnosis, treatment plan, side-effects of treatment, management of side-effects, genetic counseling
Mother of child with relapsed acute lymphocytic leukemia wonders whether bone marrow transplant is too hard a treatment for her son. Family of child with relapsed acute lymphocytic leukemia wants further therapy, but insurance plan does not cover experimental drugs.	Decisional Conflict related to treatment of child
Adolescent with hemophilia learns he is HIV positive.	Ineffective Individual Coping related to acquistion of a life-threatening disease secondary to treatment of primary chronic illness
Mother of child with sickle cell anemia wonders whether she should have more children. Mother of child with thalassemia major asks about in utero testing for the disease.	Decisional Conflict related to genetic counseling regarding inherited diseases
Self-Perception and Self-Conflict	
Toddler with acute lymphocytic leukemia cries when nurse takes him into treatment room. Child with hemophilia denies that his arm hurts.	Fear related to medical procedures
Family of child going for bone marrow transplant asks to speak to psychologist.	Anxiety related to life-threatening illness
Child with acute lymphocytic leukemia says he will not go to school if his hair falls out. Adolescent with non-Hodgkins fears vomiting with chemotherapy	Anxiety related to side-effects of treatment

TABLE 43-12
(Continued)

Data Analysis and Conclusions	Nursing Diagnosis
Adolescent with aplastic anemia in laminar airflow unit for bone marrow transplant refuses to care for Hickman. Child with acute lymphocytic leukemia refuses to eat. Child with sickle cell refuses to go to school. Adolescent with non-Hodgkins lymphoma, hospitalized now for 2 months, refuses to talk to any staff member.	Powerlessness related to illness-related regimen
Adolescent with hemophilia, recently diagnosed with AIDS, contemplates suicide. Adolesent with acute lymphocytic leukemia insists that mother cannot leave the hospital.	Hopelessness related to deteriorating physiologic condition
Adolescent with non-Hodgkins lymphoma cries when she combs her hair and handfuls fall out, says, "I'm not going back to school until my hair comes back."	Body Image Disturbance related to side effects of treatment
Sexuality and Reproduction	
Adolescent with hemophilia, recently found to be HIV positive, asks about sex.	Altered sexuality patterns related to concern of spreading disease

- Adolescents: Might benefit from using a Walkman during procedure to assist in coping.

Nursing Care

The nurse is responsible for preparation of the child and family. This may take the form of verbal descriptions, books, videotape of the procedure, or referral to a child-life specialist or psychologist to provide specific cognitive or behavioral coping techniques.

If the child is to receive sedative medication, the nurse is to monitor the child's vital signs and respiratory status during and after the procedure until the child is fully awake.

After the procedure, the nurse should observe the puncture site for signs of bleeding or infection. If the child's platelet count is below 100,000, the nurse should be ready for the possibility of increased bleeding from the puncture site.

The dressing over the puncture site should remain in place for 24 hours to help prevent infection in the site.

Complications

- Infection or bleeding at the puncture site.
- Mild to moderate pain at the site can occur up to 1 to 2 days after the procedure and should be treated with an analgesic.

Selected Nursing Diagnoses

After obtaining the history, performing the physical examination, reviewing results from the diagnostic tests, and tapping additional resources for information, the nurse carefully analyzes data obtained. Nursing diagnoses appropriate for the child with a hematologic dysfunction become apparent and are used to develop a plan of care. Selected nursing diagnoses that may be appropriate for the child with hematologic dysfunction are presented by function in Table 43-12. Chronic illness and pain are discussed in Chapters 21 and 28, respectively.

Summary

Blood is a significant fluid in assessing a child's health. The history and types of tests may be divided into an etiologic organization of disorders: red cell, white cell, and platelet and coagulation dysfunction. The child and family history helps to establish information used in as-

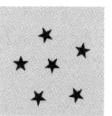

Ideas for Nursing Research

There is much controversy in the literature regarding sedation versus cognitive/behavioral preparation for bone marrow aspiration. Usually, the child is given sedative medications to help relax the child during the procedure. Medications used vary with the practice standards of each institution. The trend is to provide conscious sedation for children undergoing this procedure. Children who will require repeated bone marrow aspirates (e.g., children with hematologic malignancies) need to be assessed as to whether repeated conscious sedation or cognitive/behavioral techniques should be employed with each procedure. Little research has been done to document the long-term effects on the child of either approach. Research has focused solely on alleviating pain and behavioral distress involved with the procedure. The following areas need to be explored:

- Long-term effects of sedation during bone marrow aspiration/biopsy at different developmental levels.
- Long-term effects of cognitive/behavioral preparation for bone marrow aspiration/biopsy.
- Pain control practices in sickle cell crisis and hemarthrosis.
- Infection control practices for the neutropenic patient.
- Patient/family education for chronic illness such as sickle cell anemia or hemophilia.
- Management of fatigue in the anemic patient.
- Computerization of a comprehensive nursing database for the child with a chronic illness.

sessing the severity of the disease state and causative factors.

Diagnostic tests in hematologic function include a simple blood test and bone marrow aspiration. Initially, a complete blood count with reticulocyte count is sufficient. The results of this test determine if further testing needed. Bone marrow aspiration or biopsy is used to determine specific hematologic function.

References

1. Alexander, M., & Brown, M. (1979). *Pediatric history taking and physical diagnosis for nurses* (2nd ed.). McGraw-Hill.
2. Bates, B. (1991). *A guide to physical examination and history taking.* (5th ed.). Philadelphia: J. B. Lippincott.
3. Buchanan, G. R. (1980). Hemophilia. *Pediatric Clinics of North America, 27*(2), 309–326.
4. Charache, S. (1986). Advances in the understanding of sickle cell anemia. *Hospital Practice, 21*(2), 173–190.
5. Chow, M., Durand, B. A., Feldman, M. N., & Mills, M. A. (1984). *Handbook of pediatric primary care* (2nd ed.). New York: John Wiley & Sons.
6. Droske, S. C., & Francis, S. A. (1981). *Pediatric diagnostic procedures.* New York: John Wiley & Sons.
7. Emami, A., et al. (1987). Idiopathic thrombocytopenia purpura in children: New therapeutic considerations. *Kansas Medicine, 88*(11), 317–319.
8. Klopovich, P. M. (Ed.). (1983). Blood disorders in children [Special issue]. *Issues in Comprehensive Pediatric Nursing, 6.*
9. Lanzkowsky, P. (1980). *Pediatric hematology/oncology.* New York: McGraw-Hill.
10. Nathan, D. G., & Oski, F. A. (Eds.). (1992). *Hematology of infancy and childhood* (4th ed.). Philadelphia: W. B. Saunders.
11. Oheve-Frempong, K., & Schwartz, E. (1980). Clinical features of thalassemia. *Pediatric Clinics of North America, 27,* 403–420.
12. Oski, F. A. (1985). Iron deficiency: Facts and fallacies. *Pediatric Clinics of North America, 32*(2), 493–497.
13. Patterson, K. L., & Ware, L. L. (1988). Coping skills for children undergoing painful medical procedures. *Issues in Comprehensive Pediatric Nursing, 11*(2–3), 113–143.
14. Walker, R. W., & Walker, W. (1984). Idiopathic thrombocytopenia, initial illness and long-term follow-up. *Archives of Disease in Childhood, 59,* 316–322.
15. Wallach, J. (1983). *Interpretation of pediatric tests: A handbook synopsis of pediatric, fetal and obstetric laboratory medicine.* Boston: Little, Brown.
16. Walters, I., Baysinger, M., Buchanan, J., et al. (1983). Complications of sickle cell disease. *Nursing Clinics of North America, 18*(1), 139–229.
17. Yip, R., Johnson, C., & Dallman, P. R. (1984). Age-related changes in laboratory values used in the diagnosis of anemia and iron deficiency. *American Journal of Clinical Nutrition, 39,* 427–436.

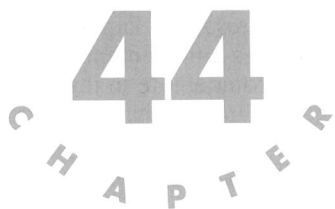

44

CHAPTER

Nursing Planning, Intervention, and Evaluation for Altered Hematologic Function

BEHAVIORAL OBJECTIVES

Explain how hematologic diseases can be grouped by etiologic factors (hematologic trio).

Discuss the basic pathology of disorders of red blood cells, white blood cells, and platelets.

State several nursing diagnoses common to pediatric patients with altered hematologic function and their families.

Discuss basic nursing interventions for children with hematologic disorders.

Describe guidelines for administration of blood and blood products.

The simplest organization of hematologic disease entities is grouping them by etiologic factors occurring in the three blood cells. This hematologic trio of red blood cells (RBCs), white blood cells (WBCs), and platelets can each be further subdivided into categories of production, maturation, and destruction. Such a subdivision creates a manageable framework of categories for organization by the nurse.

Thinking critically within this framework encourages the nurse to identify common interventions for the diseases within a particular subdivision. Implementation of these common interventions enables the nurse to move the ill child significantly toward the overall goal of restored hematologic function.

This framework is used for the organization of this chapter. General nursing implications for hematologic dysfunction are discussed at the beginning of each section. Disorders of RBC production, maturation, and destruction, WBC production and maturation, platelet production and maturation, and coagulation are discussed along with specific disorders.

1093

Disorders of Red Blood Cells

RBCs are the oxygen transport system of the body. RBCs are biconcave discs (see Fig. 42-2). Formed in the bone marrow, RBCs are released into the body's circulation and destroyed at the end of their normal life span of 120 days. If either the shape or the hemoglobin is altered, the ability of the RBC to function is hampered.

Problems of the RBC can be divided into three categories: disorders of production, maturation, and destruction. Problems can arise because the bone marrow does not produce enough RBCs. Perhaps the bone marrow is functioning appropriately, but the RBCs do not mature correctly. The materials available to the bone marrow may be inferior or scanty. Or the problem may be inappropriate destruction of the RBC. Knowing the etiology of the disorder is helpful in establishing appropriate nursing goals and interventions. Therefore, the disorders of the RBC in this section are divided among production, maturation, and destruction categories.

Disorders of RBC Production

Nursing Interventions for Disorders of RBC Production

Nursing interventions for the child affected with a disorder of RBC production are fourfold: oxygenation, teaching, restoration of RBC production, and psychosocial support. Table 44-1 details these nursing interventions.

Oxygenation. Adequate oxygenation to the tissues is the initial goal. Hemoglobin and hematocrit values provide indicators of oxygenation. Comparison of a series of values offers information about positive or negative changes in tissue oxygenation. If the hemoglobin value drops below 6 g/dL, transfusion with packed RBCs would increase the body's ability to transport sufficient oxygen. Packed RBCs are usually the blood product of choice because increasing the number of RBCs, not increasing the fluid volume, is the means to achieving improved oxygenation of the tissues. A hemoglobin of 11 g/dL is usually the targeted value, indicating sufficient hemoglobin to oxygenate the tissues adequately.

The caregiver can also monitor the child's activity level as an indicator of adequate oxygenation. This monitoring is an excellent opportunity for nurses to involve parents in the care of their child because parents know the usual behaviors of their child better than anyone else. They are essential allies in determining whether the child is limiting strenuous activity to conserve energy or whether the child is participating in normal activities at a normal intensity. If the parents are not available for assistance in this monitoring, the nurse depends on knowledge of normal childhood development in conjunction with knowledge of the particular child from personal observation or shared knowledge from other colleagues.

In many instances, the disorders of RBC production include scenarios of prolonged anemia: hemoglobin values of less than 6 g/dL for greater than 6 months. If prolonged anemia occurs, the heart achieves adequate oxygenation by working harder, by pumping the available RBCs more often to achieve adequate tissue oxygenation. The increased pumping rate results in an enlarged cardiac muscle, just as lifting arm weights results in larger bicep muscles. This compensation causes enlargement of the heart. If the heart is required to compensate in this way for extended periods (i.e., years), cardiac damage occurs. To provide opportunity to prevent such cardiac damage, serial chest x-rays offer information regarding any changes in the heart size.

Teaching. A second goal is an informed caretaker. Each of the disorders of RBC production has a specific etiology and pathophysiology. The nurse must determine how to convey appropriate information about the disorder to the caretaker. In particular, the nurse conveys the necessity for serial hematocrit and hemoglobin evaluations. Knowledge about adequate tissue oxygenation is essential for the successful management of the disorder. Caretakers should receive the parameters for normal values (e.g., a hemoglobin of 11 g/dL). Compliance with the prescribed schedule of serial hemoglobin and hematocrit checks is an indicator of successful integration of information taught. Noncompliance requires careful ascertainment as to the reasons for noncompliance. Sometimes the reasons are as straightforward as inadequate transportation to the laboratory. However, other times the reasons for noncompliance are complex, including differing cultural values of health and philosophies of life. The caretaker should also be prepared for the required actions if the values are below normal (e.g., a hemoglobin of 6 g/dL would initiate measures for a transfusion). An accompanying display lists guidelines for the administration of blood products.

Some of the disorders of RBC production require prolonged transfusion treatment. When this is the case, chelation therapy is instituted to prevent iron overload or hemosiderosis. Caretakers need to be informed of this possibility at the initiation of transfusion therapy. When chelation therapy is necessary, the caretaker and, if appropriate, the child need instruction about the method of chelation. Most institutions use portable infusion pumps to deliver the chelating agent subcutaneously; however, the chelating agent can also be administered intravenously. The subcutaneous infusion usually requires 6 to 8 hours for 6 days each week. This can be scheduled to coincide with the child's sleep. The caretaker needs instruction about using the particular infusion pump as well as information about inserting a subcutaneous needle. If intravenous infusion is preferred, it can be accomplished simultaneously with the transfusion.

Restoration of RBC Production. Another goal of nursing intervention is the restoration of RBC production. This should be monitored by serial reticulocyte counts, hemoglobin, and hematocrit levels, laboratory values that indicate bone marrow activity. A rising reticulocyte count is an early indication that RBCs are being prepared to be released into circulation. Once a stable RBC volume has been achieved, the reticulocyte count also remains stable. The hemoglobin and hematocrit levels are indicators of the circulating RBCs.

The nurse is also involved in the administration of

TABLE 44-1
Nursing Interventions: General Care of Children With Disorders of RBC Production

Goal	Intervention	Evaluation
Provide adequate oxygenation to tissues	*Oxygenation:*	
	Check serial hematocrit and hemoglobin	Hematocrit and hemoglobin are in normal limits (Hgb 11 g/dL)
	Transfuse if hemoglobin < 6 g/dL	
	Monitor child's activities for change in intensity of activity	Activities are within normal limits
	Take serial chest x-ray to evaluate heart size if anemia is prolonged (Hgb < 6 g/dL for 6 months)	Heart is not enlarged
Keep caretaker informed	*Teaching:*	
	Teach regarding disease process	Appropriate questions are asked and answered
	Teach regarding need for serial Hct and Hgb checks	Caretaker complies with schedule
	Teach regarding parameters for transfusion	
	Teach regarding need for possible chelation therapy; if transfusion therapy	
Restore RBC production	*Restoration of production:*	
	Take serial reticulocyte count and check hemoglobin and hematocrit	
	Administer medication:	
	ATG	
	• Have emergency equipment on hand	
	• Give test dose	
	• Monitor vital signs every 20 min for an hour, then every hour	
	• Monitor IV site to avoid extravasation	
	If extravasation occurs,	
	• Stop infusion	
	• Notify physician	
	• Administer subcutaneous Benadryl at site	
	• Apply ice	
	• Elevate	
	• Evaluate site for burnlike wound	
	• Avoid infection of wound with cleansing, antibiotic application, and sterile dressing	
	Bone marrow transplantation (see Chap. 31)	
	Androgens	
	• Prepare child and family for physical and psychological impact of masculinization (i.e., secondary sexual changes, deepening voice, facial and pubic hair, enlargement of penis or clitoris, muscle development)	
Provide a healthy psychosocial environment	*Psychosocial support:*	
	Discuss disease prognosis with child (fears, anger, guilt)	Age-appropriate openness occurs between child and caretakers regarding disease, therapy, and prognosis
	Discuss prognosis with caretakers	
	Incorporate age-appropriate play into regimen (use of puppets if > 24 mo)	

medications that stimulate RBC production. Antithymocyte globulin (ATG) is one such medication. The precautions for its administration are listed in Table 44-1. Androgens are another medication that can be employed in the stimulation of RBC production. This class of medications is not more difficult to administer than are other medications. However, the physical changes wrought by these preparations do create a definite psychological impact. Caretakers and the children need to be prepared for the masculinization that is a side-effect of these drugs. The length of time before the evidence of masculinization varies depending on the dosage, specific preparation, and route of administration. The changes include deepening voice, facial and pubic hair growth, enlargement of the penis or clitoris, and muscle development. Discussion of these impending changes between the health care team and the caretaker is essential for continued compliance with the androgen treatment regimen. Bone marrow transplantation is discussed in Chapter 31.

Psychosocial Support. A healthy psychosocial environment is another goal of the nurse. A myriad of items constitute a healthy psychosocial environment for the well child. When an illness complicates the equation, the health care team is valuable in offering suggestions for dealing with the stress of illness. Initially, the caretaker should receive information about the prognosis of the disease in an atmosphere that is relaxed and allows the caretaker to ask questions freely. After the information is shared, emotional responses such as fear, anger, and guilt should be addressed.

After this discussion of emotional issues, the caretaker and health care team need to formulate a method for talking with the child about these same issues. Knowledge of normal growth and development plus particular information about the child are crucial at this point. Some school-age and teenage children are able to discuss these factors, whereas younger and less verbal children need to use puppets, drawings, imaginary friends, role play, stuffed animals, and dolls. The goal of a healthy psychosocial environment is greatly aided by a sense of openness between the child and the caretakers concerning the disease, its treatment, and the prognosis. As with a healthy child, the development of a healthy psychosocial environment in an ill child is a series of interactions that do not produce results as predictably as immunizations. The nurse must be vigilant in the continual evaluation of the child's psychosocial environment and in the implementation of strategies to achieve such a goal.

Aplastic Anemia

Definition and Incidence. Aplastic anemia is an unusual blood disorder in which the bone marrow fails to produce RBCs, WBCs, and platelets. In other words, it is a complete failure of the marrow to produce hematologic elements. The failure of the bone marrow to function can be either acquired or congenital.

The incidence of aplastic anemia is approximately 1 per 100,000, and the prognosis is poor with mortality of over 70%. Of those affected, 50% die within 6 months to 1 year.

Etiology and Pathophysiology. Congenital aplastic anemia is idiopathic and is usually described in conjunction with Fanconi's anemia. *Fanconi's anemia* is a syndrome in which the affected child may have a combination of the following characteristics: short stature, congenitally absent radii and thumbs, malformed kidneys and abnormal heart, microcephaly (abnormally small skull), microphthalmos (abnormally small eyes), dark pigmentation with café-au-lait spots, and *pancytopenia* (reduction in all cellular components of the blood). Fanconi's anemia is transmitted as an autosomal recessive trait.

Acquired aplastic anemia usually results from exposure to a chemical or from an illness causing hematopoiesis to stop. Several exposures or conditions are known to cause acquired aplastic anemia. They are (1) irradiation, (2) compounds containing benzene such as petroleum products, paint, shellacs, and dyes, (3) chemotherapeutic agents and antibiotics such as chloramphenicol, (4) severe infections such as hepatitis or sepsis, (5) conditions that cause replacement of the marrow such as leukemia or lymphoma, and (6) idiopathic causes. The exact pathophysiology of aplastic anemia is unknown.

Clinical Manifestations. The clinical manifestations of aplastic anemia, whether congenital or acquired, are directly related to the bone marrow failure. When all three components are severely decreased, as in aplastic anemia, the tasks of the components are not completed and cause specific, distinct problems. However, because the symptoms of pancytopenia are subtle, the clinical manifestations of aplastic anemia are usually insidious. The lack of functioning RBCs means that anemia is present. When the hemoglobin and hematocrit are sufficiently decreased, the practitioner can observe pallor, lethargy, and shortness of breath with excursion. However, these signs of anemia are evident in children only when the hemoglobin falls below 5 to 6 g.

The lack of WBCs, *neutropenia*, results in a susceptible host, which leaves the child open for a multitude of infections. The child often has recurring infections, because he cannot defend himself from opportunistic organisms.

A low platelet count, *thrombocytopenia*, causes increased potential for bleeding, because the coagulation system is missing a vital component for its successful function. The child presents with petechiae on mucosal surfaces initially and on other body surfaces later. There may be blood in the urine and stool, or there may be spontaneous bleeding.

Diagnostic Studies. Aplastic anemia is definitively diagnosed with a bone marrow aspiration. The marrow is examined for the presence of precursors of all hematologic lines: erythroid elements, myeloid elements, and platelets/megakaryocytes. In aplastic anemia, the marrow is replaced with a fatty substance instead of precursors for mature hematologic elements.

★ **ASSESSMENT**

The nursing assessment for a child suspected of having aplastic anemia was discussed in Chapter 43. The assessment includes obtaining information about:

- Exposure to chemicals containing benzene, such as petroleum products, insecticides, paints, and dyes.
- Recent infections and their resolution.
- Use of antibiotics, particularly chloramphenicol.
- Activity level and any change.
- Bleeding episodes.
- Color of urine and stool.

★ NURSING DIAGNOSES AND PLANNING

Based on the assessment data from above and Chapter 43, the following nursing diagnoses may apply to the child with aplastic anemia:

- High Risk for Injury related to spontaneous bleeding.
- High Risk for Injury related to complications of blood transfusion.
- High Risk for Infection related to inadequate primary defenses.
- Activity Intolerance related to weakness caused by anemia.
- Social Isolation related to priorities of life-saving procedures.
- Knowledge Deficit regarding the disease and its treatment and complications.

The nurse, child, and parents together plan effective care based on the established nursing diagnoses. Several examples of expected outcomes follow:

- The child participates in quiet activities in bed.
- The family visits child whenever procedures are not being performed.
- The family describes complications and how they should respond.

The nurse plans for the daily care of the child based on both doctor's orders and nursing diagnoses. Some general nursing care goals may be the following:

- Blood products are administered safely.
- Infection is prevented.

★ INTERVENTIONS: COLLABORATIVE AND INDEPENDENT

The goal in management of a child with aplastic anemia is the restoration of hematologic function of the bone marrow. There are two medical approaches to accomplishing this goal: (1) immunosuppressive therapy to remove the presumed immunologic functions that prolong aplasia and (2) replacement of the bone marrow through transplantation. The nursing goals are to administer the drugs and blood safely, prevent infection, and educate the family regarding possible complications (see Table 44-1).

Bone marrow transplantation is the treatment of choice if a compatible donor and funding are available. Because bone marrow transplantation is a highly specialized procedure, the child should be transferred to an institution that specializes in the preparation, procedure, and recovery. Bone marrow transplantation is discussed in Chapter 31.

MEDICATION THERAPY

If bone marrow transplantation is unavailable, drug treatment is employed. Drugs used in treating aplastic anemia include antithymocyte globulin (ATG) or antilymphocyte globulin (ALG), which are drugs produced by injecting lymphocytes obtained from surgical patients other than the child into research animals. After the animals have produced the desired globulin, it is harvested and injected into the child. The mechanism of action is unclear, but in some cases the drug stimulates the bone marrow to produce erythroid and myeloid elements as well as platelets. Some researchers believe that the aplasia is caused by some mechanism of autoimmunity. Employed to stimulate erythropoiesis, ATG is administered intravenously over 12 to 16 hours, but the optimum interval for therapy is under investigation. ATG should be administered with caution because of the risk of anaphylactic reactions. The child should receive a test dose of the medication with emergency equipment at hand. After initial safety has been determined, the full dose can be given. However, emergency equipment should remain at hand because reactions can occur at any time. Subsequent administration of ATG depends on the response seen in the hematologic function of the child. Parents and child should be prepared for a gradual response, if any, of 3 to 6 months.

Before the availability of ATG and ALG, androgens were the treatment of choice for aplastic anemia. Testosterone causes the fatty marrow to become hyperplastic with erythroid precursors, but the exact mechanism is unknown. The testosterone can be administered either orally (oxymetholone and fluoxymesterone) or intramuscularly (nandrolone decanoate and testosterone enanthate) on a daily or weekly schedule, respectively. Sometimes corticosteroids are used in conjunction with testosterone therapy as an enhancer. The child and parents must be prepared for the masculinizing side-effects of this androgen therapy.

PREVENTION OF BLEEDING

The thrombocytopenic child also has periodic platelet counts to determine the need for platelet transfusions and precautions. Prevention of bleeding is the major nursing concern. The child must be protected from environmental hazards as well as activities that would cause bleeding. Spontaneous bleeding rarely occurs unless the platelet count is less than 20,000. Caretaker and parental education should also include information about the signs and symptoms of internal bleeding (i.e., dizziness, fainting, headaches, blood in the urine or stool, hemoptysis, blurred vision, and altered sensorium). Complete education materials should provide information regarding the appropriate way to contact the primary health care provider should these symptoms occur, as well as techniques to stop external bleeding (pressure at the appropriate point).

ADMINISTRATION OF BLOOD PRODUCTS

Nursing interventions hinge around pancytopenia and the side-effects of the therapies. Because a child with pancytopenia has few or no red or WBCs or platelets, he must be protected from the symptoms of anemia, neutropenia, and thrombocytopenia. Because this triad of symptoms is the classic presentation of one with leukemia, the nursing intervention is similar to leukemia. The child should receive transfusions as needed to provide adequate oxygenation of the tissues. Periodic hemoglobin and hematocrit evaluation provides the necessary data for determining the transfusion schedule. Administration of blood products is more fully detailed in the accompanying display, Nursing Interventions: Guidelines for the Ad-

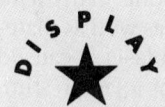

Nursing Interventions: Guidelines for the Administration of Blood Products

I. Review of basics when giving blood products
  A. Identify recipient before beginning infusion.
  B. Do not vent plastic blood containers.
  C. Use clot filter in administration set.
  D. Do not add any medications or solutions to blood product, except isotonic NaCl or ordered plasma expanders.
  E. Mix components thoroughly before use.
  F. Check unit for hemolysis; supernate should be clear; if suspicious, return to blood bank for reevaluation.
  G. Obtain baseline patient assessment including vital signs.

II. Whole Blood
  A. Contains all the cellular and plasma components of donor blood.
  B. Indicated only for those patients with symptomatic deficit in oxygen-carrying capacity combined with hypovolemic shock.
  C. Acts as a source of RBCs to carry oxygen to tissues and as a blood volume expander with proteins and coagulation properties.
  D. Contraindications: (1) any anemia that can be pharmacologically treated, (2) if other volume expanders can be used, (3) coagulation deficiencies.
  E. Side-effects and hazards:
    1. Hemolytic transfusion reactions may be caused by undetected serologic incompatibilities but more often are caused by some clerical or identification error. Signs and symptoms: shock, chills, fever, dyspnea, chest/back pain, headache, hemoglobinuria, and bilirubinuria. Nursing interventions: (1) discontinue transfusion; (2) notify physician to manage shock; (3) judiciously administer fluids and diuretics. Delayed hemolytic reactions may mimic autoimmune hemolytic anemia, but usually the course is benign and requires no treatment.
    2. Transmission of infectious diseases continues to be a risk despite improved screening of donors and collected blood. Viral hepatitis may be transmitted 10% of the time. Other diseases include malaria, syphilis, brucellosis, CMV, Epstein-Barr, and AIDS.
    3. Alloimmunization of recipient is not life-threatening, but may require selective administration of subsequent transfusions.
    4. Febrile reactions, with or without chills, occur in 0.5% to 1.0% of transfusions.
    5. Allergic reactions such as urticaria occur in 3% of transfusions. Urticaria may be decreased by premedication with antihistamine.
    6. Circulatory overload reactions such as pulmonary edema occur when excessive volume is given. Particular risk is present in chronic severe anemia because of decreased RBC mass and increased plasma volume.
    7. Bacterial contamination is extremely rare since the introduction of disposable equipment. But if gram-negative bacilli are present, aggressive measures to combat toxic shock are essential.
    8. Air embolism: Signs and symptoms: chest pain, cough, dyspnea, and shock. Nursing Interventions: (1) patient on left side with head down. This traps the air in the right atrium; (2) notify physician.
    9. Iron overload with resultant hemosiderosis happens in patients given repeated transfusions over long periods of time. This iron overload can be prevented with chelation therapy.
    10. Metabolic complications can occur when massive amounts of blood (>patient's blood volume in a few hours) are rapidly infused. Complications: citrate toxicity, acidosis, hypothermia, and microaggregates.
  F. Dosage and administration depend on clinical situation. Do not give slower than over 4 h.

III. Red Blood Cells
  A. Collected from plasma by either centrifugal or gravitational force.
  B. Provide source of RBCs for oxygen-carrying capacity and mass for volume replacement.
  C. Indicated in patients with a symptomatic deficit in oxygen-carrying capacity. RBCs are preferred to whole blood in patients with cardiac disease, chronic anemia, liver or kidney disease. RBCs must be compatible but not ABO identical.
  D. Contraindications: (1) with pharmacologically correctable anemia; (2) with coagulation deficiencies; (3) with ABO incompatibility. RBCs must be ABO compatible.
  E. Side-effects and hazards: same as whole blood except removal of plasma reduces amount of metabolites and antibodies and lessens risk of circulatory overload.
  F. Dosage and administration: 1 ml/kg will raise hematocrit 1%. Must use clot filter and can be warmed. Infuse in approximately 4 h.
  G. RBCs leukocytes removed. This blood component is modified by the addition of sedimenting agents to remove leukocytes. At least 70% of leukocytes must be removed and 70% of the original RBCs must remain. RBCs leukocytes removed is indicated for patients with febrile reactions due to leukocyte antibodies. They may also be combined with irradiation to prevent graft versus host disease.

(Continued)

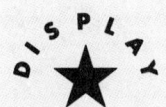

Nursing Interventions: Guidelines for the Administration of Blood Products (continued)

H. Washed RBCs. Removes 85% of leukocytes and 99% of plasma. Retains > 80% of original RBCs.

I. Frozen RBCs or deglycerolized. RBCs can be preserved by adding glycerol, an endocellular cryoprotective agent. The component may be stored for 3 years. When thawed, 70% of original RBCs are retained. Thawing and washing remove glycerol before administration. Age is based on days before freezing. Frozen cells are phenotyped before freezing.

J. Rejuvenated RBCs. Addition of rejuvenation solution allows freezing and subsequent deglycerolization. Causes increased ATP levels and gives cells characteristics of only several storage days.

IV. Plasma
   A. Anticoagulated clear liquid portion of whole blood separated from whole blood.
   B. Actions are volume expansion with plasma proteins and as a source of nonlabile clotting factors.
   C. Indications: (1) blood volume replacement in hypovolemia; (2) patients with severe hypoproteinemia; (3) source of factor IX.
   D. Not used for replacement of labile coagulation factors.
   E. Side-effects: chills, fever, hemolytic and allergic reactions, circulatory overload.
   F. Dosage and administration: 1 unit of plasma (180–275 ml) has approximately 200 units of factor IX. Use clot filter at a rate of 10 ml/min.

V. Fresh Frozen Plasma
   A. Anticoagulated clear liquid portion of whole blood that is separated and frozen within a few hours.
   B. Action includes: source of coagulation factors (V, VIII, XI) and can provide plasma proteins for vascular volume expansion.
   C. Indications: control of bleeding in patients who require labile coagulation factors that are not available.
   D. Do not use if specific concentrates are available.
   E. Dosage and administration: contains 400 mg fibrinogen and 200 units factor VIII. Infuse at approximately 10 ml/min.

VI. Plasma Platelet Rich
   A. Contains plasma and platelets.
   B. Acts to provide platelets for thrombocytopenic patients and proteins for vascular volume expansion.
   C. Needed only when need for platelets is coupled with hypovolemia.
   D. Not used if hypovolemia is not a problem.

VII. Cryoprecipitated AHF (antihemophilic factor)
   A. Preparation containing factor VIII of plasma from whole blood.

B. Acts as a source of coagulation factors VIII, XIII, and fibrinogen.

C. Indications: hemophilia A, factor VIII deficiency, von Willebrand's disease.

D. Used only with a specific coagulation defect.

E. Side-effects and hazards; viral hepatitis, febrile and allergic reactions, and AIDS. ABO-compatible is preferred.

F. Dosage and administration: level of factor VIII varies with each clinical situation. Each unit contains 80 units AHF plus 150 mg of fibrinogen. Usually give a loading dose, then a maintainance dose 12 h later. (Desired factor VIII level % × patient's plasma volume in ml/100 × average units factor VIII per cryo (80) = #bags of cryo AHF.) Infuse at approximately 10 ml/min.

VIII. Platelets
   A. Concentrate of megakaryocyte cytoplasmic fragments from one unit of whole blood and suspended in a small amount of original plasma. (May contain large number of lymphocytes.)
   B. Acts to correct a hemostatic deficit in thrombocytopenic patients.
   C. Indications: treatment of bleeding due to thrombocytopenia or functionally abnormal platelets.
   D. Not used if bleeding is not related to abnormal or low platelets.
   E. Side-effects: chills, fever, allergic reaction, viral hepatitis, AIDS. Repeated transfusions may lead to alloimmunization of HLA antigens. Refractory state may develop where only HLA-matched platelets will help. ABO-compatibility can be a problem if the component is grossly contaminated with RBCs.
   F. Dosage and administration: Usual unit contains 5.5×10^{10} platelets suspended in 20–30 ml plasma. Use clot filter. 1 unit/m² will raise platelet count approximately 10,000. Infuse one unit every 10 min. (Platelets from pheresis process should be infused more slowly.)

IX. Platelet Pheresis
   A. Collected from single donor during 2–3 hour cell separation.
   B. Volume is usually 200–500 ml plasma with 35×10^{10} platelets.
   C. Use only when random donor concentrates are not effective.

X. Granulocytes
   A. Prepared from whole blood by various buffy coat extractions and sedimentation techniques. Concentration varies from $0.5–2 \times 10^9$ granulocytes.
   B. Provide granulocytes, which can ingest and kill bacteria.

(Continued)

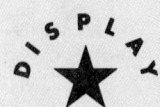

C. Used for patients with neutropenia and infection not responsive to antibiotics or other treatment modalities.
D. Not used until antibiotics have been tried. If no bone marrow recovery is expected, then granulocytes are not helpful. The components must be ABO-compatible
E. Side-effects: chills, fever, allergic reactions,

viral hepatitis, CMV, graft versus host disease. The side-effects may be diminished by premedication with Benadryl and Demerol.
F. Granulocyte pheresis achieves much higher levels of harvest—5–30 × 10⁹ granulocytes.
G. Administered over 2–4 h with close observation for reactions.

(Adapted from: *American Red Cross*. [1991]. Circular of information for the use of human blood and blood components. *Washington, D.C.: American Red Cross publication* no. 1751.)

---

ministration of Blood Products. Activity level should be determined by the child.

INFECTION CONTROL

If the child is hospitalized, the nurse must protect the neutropenic child from exposure to infections. Scheduled WBC counts determine the risk of infection and signal recovery. Depending on the hospital policy, reverse isolation may be employed. The child must be protected from infectious visitors as well as hospital employees. The nurse should be instrumental in the appropriate use of play and activity to avert the psychological isolation and depression that can occur. If the child is at home, the nurse should teach the caretaker about appropriate precautions. Family members do not usually need to use protective garments or special techniques when interacting with the child because he has some immunity to the family's illnesses.

PSYCHOSOCIAL SUPPORT

The psychosocial interventions required in aplastic anemia revolve around the issue of a child with a catastrophic disease. Because most laypeople are not familiar with aplastic anemia, there is fear of contagion and misunderstanding. The nurse should equip the family with accurate information and printed material so that they can answer the questions and concerns that friends may have. Preparing the family for the possibility of social isolation is necessary. Usually, education is the key to overcoming this problem. The family members may experience depression related to the severity of the disease and the poor prognosis. Talking about these issues before their occurrence can be extremely helpful when family members are assured that such feelings are normal and expected. The parents should know that psychological counseling is available if they wish to seek such help.

Family members often overlooked in situations like aplastic anemia are the siblings. In the turmoil revolving around their brother or sister, the siblings can easily feel neglected. Sometimes siblings experience guilt for wishing something bad on the affected sibling. As a result of this guilt, the family may see conciliatory behavior, retreating, or anger. Other siblings feel bitterness toward

the affected sibling because he seems to be getting all the parental attention. Nurses can and should prepare families for these possibilities. Often, awareness of the potential for unintentional negligence of a sibling is enough to assist the family in preventing its occurrence.

The child with aplastic anemia is the center of countless procedures, conversations, and evaluations. It is crucial for the nurse to remember that, once the imminent danger of the disease has abated, this child needs social interaction with his or her family and friends if possible. If the social interaction is omitted, the child is abandoned to deal alone with fears and imaginings. The key to dealing with any disease is creating an environment that is as normal as possible, including play, praise, discipline, friends, family, and rest.

DISCHARGE PLANNING

The discharge planning from the initial hospitalization should include arrangements for the next clinic visit or blood count at the local health unit; information about the side-effects of the procedures or medications; limitations, if any, on activity; foreknowledge regarding typical psychological reactions of the child and family; and appropriate telephone numbers should an emergency occur.

RESOURCES

An evaluation of the family situation with particular attention to transportation arrangements should be made. The nurse may be able to help the caretaker arrange for the required blood counts and subsequent transfusions by using community agencies and resources. For example, there may be transportation services available through a local service organization or financial support for lodging at a Ronald McDonald House. Because many families have both parents working outside the home or are single-parent families, this evaluation of needs can be crucial in securing the appropriate health care for the child.

Because aplastic anemia is a rare disorder, local support groups for this specific disease are unusual. However, parents may find other support groups helpful. For example, parents of children with other blood disorders may be available in the area and may fulfill the parents' need to talk with someone else. The Aplastic Anemia

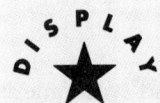

Resources for Children and Families

National Association for Sickle Cell Disease, Inc.
4221 Wilshire Boulevard
Los Angeles, CA 90010

Howard University
Center for Sickle Cell Disease
2121 Georgia Avenue, NW
Washington, DC 20059

National Sickle Cell Disease Program
National Heart, Lung, and Blood Institute
7550 Wisconsin Avenue, Room 504
Bethesda, MD 20205

Aplastic Anemia Foundation of America
P.O. Box 22689
Baltimore, MD 21203

National Hemophilia Foundation
19th West 34th Street
New York, NY 10011

Foundation of America (AAFA) supports research and distributes informational brochures. The brochures are free and prepared for nurses, social workers, physicians, patients, and the general public. The accompanying display lists resources for children and families.

★ EVALUATION

Periodically, the nurse and family evaluate the outcomes of care given. Example of outcomes for the child and family with aplastic anemia were given under planning in this section. Have short-term goals been met? Are long-term goals still realistic? Planning for further nursing care also takes into consideration complications and long-term care.

COMPLICATIONS

Complications of aplastic anemia relate to the pancytopenic nature of the disease and the adverse effects of treatment. The complications of anemia (decreased RBCs) are insufficient oxygen to the tissues and enlargement of the heart due to overwork. Neutropenia (decreased WBCs) results in the risk of demise from an overwhelming opportunistic infection. Hemorrhage is the complication of thrombocytopenia (decreased platelets). Because treatment involves the administration of blood products, complications include hemosiderosis (iron overload), AIDS, hepatitis, and production of antibodies to platelets. The complications of bone marrow transplantation are discussed in Chapter 31. The use of ATG can result in anaphylactic reaction and death.

Blackfan-Diamond Syndrome

Definition and Incidence. Pure red cell aplasia or Blackfan-Diamond syndrome is a rare, congenital condition in which the bone marrow fails to produce RBCs. The bone marrow contains normal elements for the myeloid line of cells and for the platelets, but does not produce the appropriate precursors for erythrocytes.

Blackfan-Diamond syndrome is most commonly evident in infants and affects males and females equally.

Etiology and Pathophysiology. The transmission of the syndrome is unclear; however, there are cases in which a familial transmission is strongly implicated. The prognosis depends on the success of corticosteroid therapy. If the child does not respond to corticosteroid therapy, life depends on blood transfusions. Children receiving multiple transfusions are at risk for hemosiderosis and hemochromatosis (varying degrees of iron overload) with death typically occurring in the second decade. The terminal event might be congestive heart failure due to siderotic (iron toxicity) myocardial disease and ischemia, steroid-associated infections, or transfusion-associated liver disease.

Clinical Manifestations. The affected infant displays the effects of anemia between the second and sixth month of life (i.e., pallor, listlessness, increased sleeping, and fatigue with activity). All these symptoms are extremely difficult to ascertain in the infant. This typical timetable of 2 to 6 months of age at diagnosis indicates that the intrauterine hematopoiesis was normal and the symptoms listed subsequently appear gradually. Although there are some inconclusive arguments supporting a biochemical deficiency as the basis of the syndrome, the reason for the cessation of normal erythropoiesis is unclear. Some children experience such a profound anemia that immediate transfusion is required to prevent heart failure and death.

Diagnostic Studies. Blackfan-Diamond syndrome is diagnosed by the examination of a bone marrow aspirate. Microscopic evaluation of the marrow reveals normal marrow with the exception of few or absent RBC precursors. The levels of erythropoietin are usually normal, but there is lack of erythropoietic activity in the marrow and blood. The peripheral blood smear demonstrates a normochromic, macrocytic anemia without biochemical or morphologic abnormalities. The reticulocyte count is low despite the normal to high levels of erythropoietin.

★ ASSESSMENT

Initially, the nurse is instrumental in the preparation of the child and family for the diagnostic tests. Because the child is too young for explanations, he or she benefits greatly from the comfort found in the parent's arms. Because a young child is attuned to the stress and anxiety experienced by the parents, the nurse may be helpful in comforting the child as well. The parents must be informed about the tests to be performed. In addition, they probably have questions, even if unspoken, regarding the nature of the illness their child is facing. Because Blackfan-Diamond syndrome has a guarded prognosis, the nurse must be honest but hopeful in the information given to the parents.

The nurse should elicit pertinent data regarding the family history. Because Blackfan-Diamond syndrome has been demonstrated to be familial in some cases, it is helpful to know if this particular family has knowledge of such a condition in the past. If there is evidence of a familial trait, the child's parents may be referred for genetic counseling after the initial trauma of diagnosis is completed.

★ NURSING DIAGNOSES AND PLANNING

Based on the assessment data from above and Chapter 43, the following nursing diagnoses may apply to the child with Blackfan-Diamond syndrome:

- High Risk for Injury related to administration of treatments.
- High Risk for Injury related to complications of blood transfusion.
- Anxiety related to change in family's health status.
- Fear related to possibility of child's death.
- Anticipatory Grieving related to possibility of death.
- Ineffective Individual Coping (Child) related to psychosocial vulnerability to required treatments.
- Knowledge Deficit regarding side-effects of corticosteroid therapy.

The nurse, child, and parents together plan effective care based on the established nursing diagnoses. Several examples of expected outcomes follow:

- The parents express emotions regarding child's illness and prognosis.
- The parents discuss treatment regimen, complications, and prognosis.
- The child verbalizes concerns regarding treatment.
- The parents exhibit comfort in discussing the disorder with the child.

The nurse plans for the daily care of the child based on both doctor's orders and nursing diagnoses. Some general nursing care goals may be the following:

- Blood products are administered safely.
- Erythropoietic function is restored.
- Erythropoietic function is stabilized.

★ INTERVENTIONS: COLLABORATIVE AND INDEPENDENT

The goal of therapy for Blackfan-Diamond syndrome is the restoration of erythropoietic function. Nursing care is directed toward safe administration of treatments and healthy adaptation of the child and family to a chronic illness. Nursing interventions include:

- Preparation of the child for diagnostic tests.
- Eliciting pertinent family history.
- Referral for genetic counseling if appropriate.
- Discussion of fears and anxieties with the parents.
- Instruction about corticosteroid therapy, timing and side-effects.
- Administration of safe transfusions.
- Instruction for home chelation therapy.

Blackfan-Diamond syndrome is treated with corticosteroids and/or transfusions. Some children spontaneously resume erythropoietic function, whereas others depend on treatment for their lifetime.

MEDICATION THERAPY

Corticosteroid therapy, which stimulates the marrow to produce RBCs, is initiated immediately in large doses (2 to 4 mg/kg/day of prednisone or its equivalent). Usually within 1 to 3 weeks, there is evidence of red cell precursors in the bone marrow followed by a reticulocytosis, and, in 4 to 6 weeks, the hemoglobin returns to normal. At this time, the corticosteroid dose is gradually decreased to determine the lowest possible dose at which erythropoiesis will continue. The dose may be as low as 2.5 mg/day of prednisone. Some children respond well to alternate-day regimens or 4 days a week regimens. Because some children with Blackfan-Diamond syndrome outgrow the condition, the corticosteroid therapy should be periodically discontinued to determine if the child has outgrown the need for the therapy. Because the normal life span of an RBC is 120 days, the child must be able to produce more than one cycle of RBCs. Production of healthy RBCs that maintain normal levels of hemoglobin is evidence of cure.

When the nurse begins teaching the caretaker about the corticosteroid therapy, it is imperative that the caretaker understand that the therapy must be given. To discontinue the therapy, particularly in the early stages of the regimen, can be lethal. The side-effects of corticosteroid therapy include: masking of infections, weight gain, rapid mood swings, and delayed or retarded growth. Many children do not experience these side-effects once the dose is decreased.

ADMINISTRATION OF BLOOD PRODUCTS AND IRON CHELATION

While waiting for the resumption of erythropoietic function, the child must be supported with transfusions. Washed packed RBCs are the transfusion of choice because the washed RBCs have less potential for causing an incompatibility reaction in the child (see the display on guidelines for administration of blood products).

Approximately 25% of children with Blackfan-

Diamond syndrome do not respond to corticosteroid therapy and must be supported indefinitely with transfusion therapy. Because the child is expected to receive multiple transfusions (as often as every 3 weeks) to maintain a hemoglobin of approximately 10 g/dL, an iron chelation program must be started concurrently. The chelation program minimizes the deleterious effects of hemosiderosis and hemochromatosis (iron toxicity). The iron chelation agent (usually Desferal) is administered intravenously or subcutaneously. Often the child receives subcutaneous Desferal by way of a portable infusion pump during sleep for 6 days a week and intravenous Desferal concurrently with the transfusion.

PSYCHOSOCIAL SUPPORT

The psychosocial interventions initially focus on the parents. The parents must be offered an opportunity to express their fear, anger, and grief about their child's disease. Counsel that encourages expression of these emotions is helpful.

Once the children are old enough to know that they are different from peers (around 15 to 18 months of age), the nurse should encourage the caretaker to talk with the child about the need for therapy. For example, the child may indicate verbally or behaviorally that he knows other children, perhaps siblings, do not require the same therapy. The caretaker could respond that the treatments help the child be healthy and strong. As the child's understanding increases, more details should be provided. The subject should be dealt with in a matter-of-fact manner. The child's questions should be answered honestly, yet at an age-appropriate level. Parents are often nervous about the child's questions, but, if they have discussed the possibilities with the nurse, they are much better prepared to handle the inquiries.

★ EVALUATION

COMPLICATIONS

The major complications of Blackfan-Diamond syndrome are related to the transfusion therapy, which risks incompatibility reactions, infection from contaminated blood, and iron overload. Incompatibility reaction and infection have a relatively low incidence due to the improved and scrupulous methods of blood preparation available. Iron overload (hemosiderosis and hemochromatosis) can be minimized with the institution of an iron chelation program in which the chelating agent (Desferal) is administered subcutaneously over 8 to 10 hours by way of a portable infusion pump for 6 days a week. When the child receives a transfusion, a concurrent infusion of intravenous Desferal can be used. This combination of subcutaneous and intravenous chelation greatly reduces the incidence of iron overload and the long-term detrimental effects of hemosiderosis.

LONG-TERM CARE

The long-term management of Blackfan-Diamond syndrome involves numerous clinic visits to evaluate the progression of corticosteroid and/or transfusion therapy. During the clinic visits, nurses should determine whether the child is receiving the appropriate medication on the prescribed schedule. After this ascertainment, the nurse should ask questions related to any untoward side-effects of the therapy as well as questions related to the child's growth and development. The caretaker may also experience some renewed anxiety, fear, or grief later in the course of treatment.

Blackfan-Diamond syndrome is most often managed in the home environment. The nurse is instrumental in helping the parents foresee problems and troubleshoot those problems, whether they be physical care problems or emotional stress problems. Hospitalization is not the routine management of this syndrome. However, if hospitalization is necessary, the child and parents need the emotional support that every family needs at a nonelective admission to the hospital. In addition, the family will likely experience renewed fear and anxiety regarding the overall prognosis of the disease. Sensitivity to these emotions by the nursing staff can enhance the quality of care to the child and the family.

Because Blackfan-Diamond syndrome is rare, the likelihood of a support group or community resources specifically designated for this syndrome is negligible. However, there may be assistance and support available with other families receiving care through the hematology/oncology department of the nearby children's hospital. Several phone calls by the nurse can ascertain the availability of services in a given area.

Transient Erythroblastosis of Childhood (TEC)

Transient erythroblastosis of childhood (TEC) is an illness in which the bone marrow fails to produce adequate numbers of RBCs. The etiology is unknown. This severe anemia is typically diagnosed in children between the ages of 8 months and 5 years. The child demonstrates severe anemia, reticulocytopenia, and decreased red cell precursors in the bone marrow. The child presents a clinical picture of severe anemia. Remission occurs spontaneously but without a recognized timetable. The anemia requires supportive therapy with transfusions of RBCs until spontaneous remission occurs. The condition does not recur.

TEC is a particularly frightening disease for parents because the health care team is not able to answer the questions about etiology or length of illness. Yet, the team usually conveys the seriousness of the disease by insisting on immediate treatment with blood transfusions and hospitalization for observation. The nursing care of a child receiving transfusions is discussed in the display on administration of blood products. The emotional care for the child and family is like that for any hospitalization with appropriate emotional support for the family members and age-appropriate activities for the child.

Anemias Secondary to Malignancies of Childhood

Anemias complicating other diseases are common. Some examples of such diseases are malignancies treated with bone marrow depressing agents, bronchiectasis, osteomyelitis, rheumatic fever, rheumatoid arthritis, ulcerative colitis, and advanced renal disease. Although the pathophysiology of the primary disease is different, the secondary anemias are similar. The secondary anemias are usually normochromic, normocytic with normal to low reticulocyte counts. The RBC life span is moderately decreased because of increased RBC destruction by a hyperactive reticuloendothelial system. The anemia is typically caused by depressed bone marrow activity and depressed erythropoietin production. This secondary anemia is differentiated from other anemias by the presence of normal total iron-binding capacity (TIBC), low serum iron, and iron saturation. The bone marrow demonstrates normal cellularity with adequate red cell precursors.

The treatment and nursing care should focus on the primary disease. Usually adequate treatment of the pri-

mary disease results in satisfactory management of the secondary anemia.

Disorders of RBC Maturation

Nursing Interventions for Disorders of RBC Maturation

Nursing interventions for the child affected with a disorder of RBC maturation are threefold: oxygenation, teaching, and restoration of RBC maturation. Table 44-2 details these nursing interventions.

Oxygenation.   Adequate oxygenation of tissues is the initial goal. As discussed in the section titled "Nursing Interventions for Disorders of RBC Production," serial

TABLE 44-2
Nursing Interventions: General Care of Children With Disorders of RBC Maturation

Goal	Intervention	Evaluation
Provide adequate oxygenation of tissues	Oxygenation:	
	Check serial hematocrit and hemoglobin	Hct and Hgb are in normal limits (Hgb 11 g/dL)
	Transfuse if hemoglobin < 6 g/dL	
	Monitor child's activities for change in intensity of activity	Activities are within normal limits
	Take serial chest x-ray to evaluate heart size if anemia is prolonged (Hgb < 6 g/dL for >6 months)	Heart is not enlarged
Keep caretaker informed	Teaching:	
	Teach regarding disease process	Appropriate questions are asked and answered
	Teach regarding need for therapy and scheduled regimen	Caretaker complies with regimen
	Teach regarding implications if therapy is not initiated and continued	
Restore normal RBC maturation	Restoration of Production:	
	Make serial microscopic evaluations of peripheral smears	RBC indices [MCV, MCH, MCHC] are normal
	Make serial evaluations:	
	• Erythrocyte protoporphyrin	
	• Transferrin saturation	Transferrin > 16%
	• Ferritin	
	• Zinc protoporphyrin	
	• Blood lead levels	
	If iron deficiency	
	• Provide supplemental iron source (vitamin supplement and dietary sources)	Compliance with treatment regimen
	• Teach regarding side-effects: teeth staining, darker/green stools, constipation	
	• Teach regarding enhancement of absorption before meals, avoid milk, eat foods rich in vitamin C	
	If lead poisoning	
	• Remove offending source of lead	Child is not exposed to lead
	• Chelation therapy if blood lead levels ≥ 45 µg/dL	Blood lead levels return to normal
	• Evaluate changes in symptoms (i.e., abdominal pain, anorexia, vomiting, constipation, irritability, increased sleeping time, loss of developmental milestones, seizures, or ataxia)	No symptoms

hemoglobin and hematocrit values are indicators of available oxygen transport mechanisms. The child's activity level is also a gross indicator of adequate oxygenation. Transfusion with packed RBCs would be initiated if the hemoglobin value was less than 6 mg/dL. The targeted hemoglobin level is 11 g/dL. When hemoglobin levels remain less than 6 g/dL for longer than 6 months, the child's heart size should be evaluated by way of chest x-ray. Serial x-rays assist the health care team in the avoidance of heart enlargement.

Teaching. A second goal of the nurse in the management of the child with a disorder of RBC maturation is an informed caretaker. The caretaker needs factual information about the child's disorder, which can be provided through an oral exchange, review of printed material, referral to parental or child support groups, and viewing of videos or other media that would be appropriate to the situation. Once the disorder has been discussed and appropriate questions have been asked and answered, discussion of the need for therapy and the scheduled regimen should follow. All the factual information about the disorder is presented to inform the caretaker about the treatment and subsequent schedule. Realizing that not all caretakers share the nurse's philos-

ophy about health, the nurse should present information about the need for therapy and its implications in a neutral manner. The nurse is striving to inform the caretaker so that the caretaker has the knowledge and tools to make an intelligent decision about therapy. This neutral presentation of information can be the most difficult task of nursing.

Restoration of RBC Maturation. The third goal in the management of disorders of RBC maturation is the restoration of normal RBC maturation. Normal maturation is achieved by the removal of an offending element such as lead in lead poisoning, or by the addition of missing elements such as iron supplementation in iron deficiency anemia. Laboratory values do not restore normal maturation; however, evaluation of appropriate values provides information about the circulating RBCs. The nurse can participate in the serial microscopic evaluations of peripheral blood smears. The RBC indices (mean corpuscular volume [MCV], mean corpuscular hemoglobin [MCH], and mean corpuscular hemoglobin concentration [MCHC]) are within normal ranges when the RBCs are maturing correctly. These indices measure the RBC volume, hemoglobin, and hemoglobin concentration. Other elements that are helpful in determining normal RBC

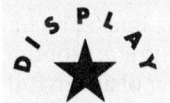

Myths or Misconceptions About Iron Deficiency

Fallacy: Iron deficiency is rarely observed in populations cared for by pediatricians in private practice. "While it must be acknowledged that the prevalence of iron deficiency anemia is much higher among infants in the lower socioeconomic groups, with as many as 30% being anemic and an additional 25% being iron deficient, iron deficiency, with or without anemia, does occur in the population of infants and children served by pediatricians in private practice. Iron deficiency anemia also occurs in affluent adolescents. A survey of Yale University undergraduates found that 17.9% of the females had a hemoglobin of less than 12.0 g/dL in association with an MCV of less than 80 fl and were presumed to be iron deficient."

Fallacy: Infants are born iron deficient. "Throughout gestation the fetus tends to maintain a constant iron content of about 75 mg/kg. Unless extreme, the presence of maternal iron deficiency does not appear to compromise the iron endowment of the fetus. The hemoglobin concentration in the cord blood of infants born to anemic, iron-deficient mothers does not differ from that of infants born to iron-sufficient mothers until maternal hemoglobin values fall below 6.0 g/dL."

Fallacy: Exclusively breast-fed infants require iron supplementation by 6 months of age. "The iron of human milk has a much greater bioavailability than has been observed with any other form of food. Studies employing radioisotopes have shown that approximately

50% of the iron in human milk is absorbed when fed to healthy 6-month-old infants. When 6-month-old infants who are breast-fed are contrasted with infants receiving an iron-fortified formula, the rate of iron accumulation, the serum iron, transferrin saturation, and hemoglobin values are found to be identical. It appears safe to conclude from the available data that the exclusively breast-fed infant does not require any form of iron supplementation for at least the first 6 months of life and probably for the first 9 months of life. The introduction of solid foods may compromise the unique bioavailability of iron from human milk. It would seem prudent, when solid foods are introduced, to choose foods that are a good source of iron to compensate for this reduction in iron bioavailability. Iron-fortified infant cereal appears to be a logical first food."

Fallacy: Iron deficiency is not associated with systemic manifestations. "There is mounting evidence that iron deficiency, even in the absence of anemia, can produce behavioral alterations. Studies using the Mental Development Index (MDI) of the Bayley Scales of Infant Development have been tested in numerous situations by various researchers and all concluded that iron therapy positively influenced the children's performance. Iron deficiency can affect the behavior and intellectual attainment of infants."

(From: *Oski, F. A.* [1985]. *Iron deficiency facts and fallacies.* Pediatric Clinics of North America, 32[2], 493–497.)

maturation are erythrocyte protoporphyrin, transferrin, ferritin, zinc protoporphyrin, and blood lead.

Iron Deficiency Anemia

Definition and Incidence. Iron deficiency anemia is the most prevalent nutritional disorder in the United States. This anemia is prominent in the age groups that are experiencing rates of rapid growth (i.e., toddlers, adolescents, pregnant and lactating women). The September 1986 issue of *MMWR (Morbidity and Mortality Weekly Report)* reported that the prevalence of iron deficiency anemia in children has declined in the United States from 7.8% to 2.9% over a 10-year span.[49] This decline in the incidence can be attributed to two factors. First, improvement in nutrition of infants and children has been the key. Government-supported programs like WIC have successfully decreased the incidence of iron deficiency anemia. In addition, the increased availability of fortifying iron, level of fortification, and consumer label information in infant formulas and cereals have allowed the consumer to purchase products that are more useful in preventing iron deficiency anemia than products were in the past. The mechanisms for reporting iron deficiency anemia have also been improved.

The primary cause of iron deficiency anemia in the United States is an inadequate dietary supply of iron. Of course, anything that causes a decrease in the supply of iron, its absorption, or synthesis can cause iron deficiency anemia.

Etiology and Pathophysiology. Iron deficiency occurs in three stages. In the initial stages of iron depletion, the ferritin and hemosiderin iron stores are depleted. In the second stage of iron-deficient erythropoiesis, the serum iron levels fall and the iron-binding capacity rises. In the third and final stage, or clinically obvious iron deficiency anemia, the hemoglobin falls and anemia develops as the iron deficiency affects heme synthesis.[2]

Authors have debated the bioavailability of iron in various foods, but the issues are unresolved. Rees, Monsen, and Merrill[36] documented positive improvement in the commercial availability of iron-fortified products over the past 10 years.

In contrast, Fomon[17] has concluded that the routine use of elemental iron powders to fortify foods is not satisfactory because these powders are not absorbed and are inferior to ferrous sulfate. The debate is certain to continue; however, the decline in incidence of iron deficiency anemia is certainly encouraging.

Clinical Manifestations. As in any anemia, clinical manifestations of the disorder are directly related to the effects of decreased hemoglobin and the resultant decreased oxygen-carrying capacity. The insidious onset of iron deficiency anemia usually results in only "soft" clinical signs. Many times the children are thin because they suffer not only from iron deficiency, but also from general nutritional deficiency. Other anemic children are chubby. They are frequently dubbed "milk babies" because their diets have included large quantities of whole milk to the exclusion of other foods. Because cow's milk has been identified as a gastrointestinal (GI) irritant causing mi-

croscopic, chronic blood loss from the GI tract, these "milk babies" are chubby but anemic. The microscopic blood loss in the infant is caused by the incomplete digestion of cow's milk and the subsequent irritation of the GI tract. It is necessary to point out that this microscopic loss is not sufficient to cause any problem other than anemia.

Diagnostic Studies. No one laboratory test confirms or rejects the diagnosis of iron deficiency anemia. Only when the practitioner uses several tests in conjunction can the diagnosis be confirmed. The tests listed in Table 44-3 are considered the important studies in determining the cause of anemia.[33]

★ ASSESSMENT

The interview of a potentially anemic child can produce valuable information. However, the nurse interviewing a child and parents must be astute in the history-taking process. The age of the child is extremely important because the peak incidence of iron deficiency anemia is 10 to 18 months. The other times during which rapid growth is occurring should also signal the nurse to be on the alert for this type of anemia, because these rapid growth periods create a higher demand for iron when the usual diet does not contain any additional sources of iron. Other factors that are important to note during the history are race, neonatal history, dietary habits, drug intake, recent infection, and family history of blood disorders. Routine screening for anemia should occur at 1 year of age in full-term infants and at 6 to 9 months of age in preterm infants. Screening also should occur between 2 and 3 years, at 5 years, and in adolescence.

TABLE 44-3
Laboratory Studies Used to Determine Cause of Anemia

Tests	Description
Hemoglobin level	Normal level depends on the age of the patient. However, if the anemia is hypochromic microcytic in nature, as an iron deficiency anemia, then a decrease in the hemoglobin concentration precedes any change in the hematocrit.
Mean corpuscular volume	All the RBC indices (MCV, MCHC, and MCH) parallel the decrease in hemoglobin concentration.
Serum iron and total iron binding capacity	These tests are used together to determine the iron supply to the bone marrow (serum iron/TIBC × 100 = TSI [transferrin saturation index]). If either of these values is used singly, accuracy of findings is hampered. Both can be influenced by infections, and serum iron also is subject to wide diurnal variations
Free erythrocyte porphyrin	Functional index of the adequacy of iron delivery to the erythroid marrow. The porphyrin ring, necessary to the development of hemoglobin, is formed before the insertion of iron to form heme. Therefore, in iron deficiency anemia, there would be a build-up of porphyrin.
Serum ferritin	Serum ferritin concentration is directly related to macrophage iron stores, and it parallels the changes of iron stores.

★ NURSING DIAGNOSES AND PLANNING

Based on the assessment data from above and Chapter 43, the following nursing diagnoses may apply to the child with iron deficiency anemia:

- Altered Nutrition: Less Than Body Requirements related to insufficient or imbalanced diet.
- Altered Nutrition: More Than Body Requirements related to large quantities of whole milk in diet.
- High Risk for Activity Intolerance related to lower iron stores.
- High Risk for Altered Parenting related to lack of knowledge regarding adequate diet.
- Knowledge Deficit related to iron supplementation.

The nurse, child, and parents together plan effective care based on the established nursing diagnoses. Several examples of expected outcomes follow:

- The caretaker identifies foods rich in iron and how to adapt them to family's diet.
- The caretaker complies with iron supplementation regimen.
- The child expresses desire to become healthier by eating well-balanced diet.
- The child identifies need for iron supplementation.

The nurse plans for the daily care of the child based on both doctor's orders and nursing diagnoses. A general nursing care goal may be the following:

- Hemoglobin reaches the desired level.

★ INTERVENTIONS: COLLABORATIVE AND INDEPENDENT

IRON SUPPLEMENTATION

Treatment consists of oral ferrous sulfate in a dose of 5 or 6 mg/kg/day. It is important to realize that higher doses of ferrous sulfate do not replenish the depleted iron stores any more rapidly than the recommended dosage. This dosage of iron should be administered before meals. It is helpful to remind parents that milk and eggs are inhibitors of iron absorption and that vitamin C is an enhancer of iron absorption. Thus, the nurse can suggest that each dose be given with 4 oz of orange juice or other vitamin C-enriched drink before a meal. Permanent staining of teeth can be minimized if the liquid is administered through a straw, thus avoiding contact between the teeth and the liquid.

Often the most difficult part of nursing management is achieving compliance with the prescribed regimen. Iron therapy is no exception. The side-effects include nausea, GI disturbance (including diarrhea or constipation), green/black stools, anorexia, and staining of teeth if the liquid form is used. In addition, the restoration of iron stores requires treatment for at least 2 to 3 months. Although follow-up hemoglobin levels need to be checked, there is great diversity in the recommendations for the spacing of these follow-up visits. Pochedly and May[33] recommend weekly hemoglobin levels and reticulocyte counts until the hemoglobin reaches the desired level. After this achievement, the iron supplementation should continue for an additional 2 months.

Patterson[30] recommends rechecking the reticulocyte count 10 days after the therapy is initiated. If there is a response to the therapy, further follow-up of hemoglobin and reticulocyte count should be obtained at 1-month intervals. If there has been no response, the practitioner must investigate noncompliance as well as other possible diagnoses. Specifics regarding follow-up can be determined by the population served, the practicality in any situation (time and expense), and the existing policies within an institution.

DIET THERAPY

Initial counseling with the parents or caretakers should include information regarding dietary sources of iron. Information should be tailored to the age of the child as well as to the educational level of the parents.

Iron-fortified infant formulas and iron-fortified infant cereals are important sources of iron for infants and toddlers. Good sources of iron include lean meat, fish, and poultry; cooked dried peas, beans, and lentils; dark green leafy vegetables; dried fruit; potatoes; whole-grain and enriched bread; fortified cereals; and nuts and nut butters. The iron content of whole-grain products, enriched cereals, and legumes is particularly important for vegetarians and people who must limit purchases of more costly sources of iron, such as meat.[15] Including foods that are sources of ascorbic acid increases the absorption of iron in a meal.

PREVENTION

The American Academy of Pediatrics recommends ways nurses can be influential in the prevention and early detection of anemias. The recommendations for nurses are found in the accompanying display.

★ EVALUATION

Periodically, the nurse and family evaluate the outcomes of care given. Example of outcomes for the child with iron deficiency anemia were given under planning in this section. Have short-term goals been met? Are long-term goals still realistic?

Lead Poisoning

Definition and Incidence. Lead poisoning is an acquired condition in which the blood levels of lead are above normal. It can cause severe mental, emotional, and physical impairment. The normal level of lead in the body is less than 9 μg per 100 ml of whole blood. Lead levels above 10 μg per 100 ml of whole blood are categorized into four classes of increasing risk of lead toxicity, as listed in Table 44-4. Implications of lead poisoning are discussed in Chapter 53.

Lead poisoning is usually seen between the ages of 1 and 6 years in children living in old, deteriorating housing. Because the primary source of lead for lead poisoning is leaded paints, young children playing in these homes exhibit pica (the consumption of non-food stuffs) and from the consumption of the leaded paint dust or chips become poisoned. The ingested lead accumulates in the blood and tissues of the body. The incidence of lead poisoning has declined since the introduction of lead-free

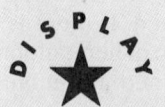

Prevention and Early Detection of Anemias by Nurses

- Iron supplementation from one or more sources should start no later than 6 months of age in full-term infants and no later than 2 months of age in preterm infants.
- In formula-fed infants, the most convenient and best sources of supplemental iron are iron-fortified formulas and two servings per day of iron-fortified cereal.
- The intake of supplemental iron should not exceed 1 mg/kg/day for a full-term infant and 2 mg/kg/day for preterm infants, to a maximum intake of 15 mg/day.
- The maintenance of breast-feeding for 6 months or more should protect against the development of iron deficiency anemia in full-term infants.

- Commercially available infant formulas are preferable to fresh milk during the first 6–12 months of age.
- If an infant receives fresh cow's milk after 6 months of age, his total daily milk intake should not exceed 3 cups or 24 oz. Infants who continue to receive formula after 6 months of age should receive no more than 1 qt of formula per day to encourage the introduction of iron-rich foods and establish the pattern for a more varied diet.
- No more than a 1-month supply of iron preparation should be kept in the home to prevent accidental poisoning.

(Based on recommendations of: *The American Academy of Pediatrics, Committee on Nutrition. [1985]. Pediatric nutrition handbook [2nd ed.]. Elk Grove Village, IL: The Academy.*)

paint in the United States in the 1940s. Another common source of lead is improperly glazed glassware. Lead toxicity has neurologic effects: learning disorders, mental retardation, seizure disorders, and encephalopathy; therefore, the effective prevention of lead poisoning by screening programs is a goal of health care.

Etiology and Pathophysiology. The etiology of lead poisoning, also known as plumbism, is directly related to environmental exposure to lead, which is absorbed through the respiratory and GI tracts. Food, air, and water all contain lead. However, only those people who are exposed to unusual, repeated, or concentrated sources of lead are at risk for lead poisoning.

Lead poisoning occurs when abnormally high levels of lead are introduced into the body, disrupting heme synthesis. The lead inhibits several enzymatic reactions in the production of heme. The levels of lead are directly related to the amount of bone marrow depression seen.

TABLE 44-4
Classes of Lead Poisoning Risk

Class	Blood Level Concentration (μg/dL)
CLASS I (low risk)	Lead < 9
CLASS IIA (rescreen)	Lead 10–14
CLASS IIB (moderate risk)	Lead 15–19
CLASS III (high risk)	Lead 20–44
CLASS IV (urgent risk)	Lead 45–69
CLASS V (urgent risk)	Lead ≥70

(Source: Centers for Disease Control. [1991]. Preventing lead poisoning in young children. Washington, D.C.: U.S. Department of Health and Human Services, Public Health Service, Centers for Disease Control, p. 46.)

The production of erythrocytes in the bone marrow is slowed, or the erythrocytes produced are abnormal. As a result of the enzymatic inhibition, the erythrocytes do not have enough heme to produce healthy hemoglobin and are, therefore, microcytic and hypochromic. Morphologically, these microcytic, hypochromic erythrocytes are indistinguishable from those found in the anemia of iron deficiency.

Adults absorb only 5% to 10% of the lead available in the air and diet, whereas children absorb as much as 40% to 50% of the available metal. The child absorbs more airborne lead than adults because of the proportionately greater lung space to body weight in the child. With these differences in absorption, it is obvious that children are at much greater risk of lead poisoning than adults in the same environment. Lead is also absorbed more readily in hosts whose diets are high in fat and deficient in iron, calcium, magnesium, zinc, and copper. Fat-rich diets provide a suitable medium for lead storage in the body, whereas deficiencies in iron, calcium, magnesium, zinc, and copper are enhancers of lead storage.

Recent research has found serious central nervous system problems related to blood lead levels as low as 10 μg/dL.[10A] The blood levels used for screening and treating lead poisoning have been lowered as more effective screening tests have been developed. Growth, hearing, and IQ are found to be decreased with blood levels ≤10 μ/dL.[10A]

Clinical Manifestations. Children with mild lead poisoning present a subtle clinical picture including vomiting, abdominal pain, headaches, hyperirritability, anorexia, and decreased play activity. The child with more severe lead poisoning presents a much more alarming picture with the onset of acute encephalopathy. Usually, parents of children with severe lead poisoning can, in retrospect, identify the vague symptoms of mild lead poisoning 4 to 6 weeks before the onset of acute encephalopathy. Persistent vomiting, ataxia, altered consciousness, seizures, and signs of increased intracranial pressure are the signs of severe lead poisoning (see Table 44-4).

Diagnostic Studies. Careful physical examination of the child with mild lead poisoning usually reveals little, if any, information. Laboratory results are more helpful. Microscopic evaluation of the peripheral blood smear demonstrates microcytic, hypochromic erythrocytes as well as basophilic stippling. X-rays of long bones, if obtained, show "lead lines." Free erythrocyte protoporphyrin (FEP) is another laboratory test. FEP levels, which would be normal if the heme production were normal, are elevated because the lead inhibits heme production resulting in excess FEP. However, FEP is not a sensitive test for identifying children with blood levels below about 25 μg/dL. Electrochemical techniques, usually anodic stripping voltrametry (ASV), and atomic absorption spectroscopy (AAS) are used to assess levels < 25 μg/dL.

★ ASSESSMENT

The goal for nursing assessment is to ascertain which children are at risk for exposure to lead, which children have elevated levels of lead, and which children have dietary habits increasing their susceptibility to lead poisoning. Questions related to these issues should be included in every visit to the health care facility. The accompanying display lists priority groups for screening for lead poisoning.

Especially susceptible to lead poisoning are infants and toddlers living in old housing where lead paint may have been used or where renovations may be creating lead flaking; living near lead smelting plants or with people working in lead smelting industry; living near busy traffic areas where exhaust fumes are high; and practicing pica regularly.[3]

An erythrocyte protoporphyrin (EP) level, which determines metabolic effects of lead, should be given initially at 9 to 15 months of age. Screening is continued at 3- to 6-month intervals.[3]

★ NURSING DIAGNOSES AND PLANNING

Based on the assessment data from above and Chapter 43, the following nursing diagnoses may apply to the child with lead poisoning:

- High Risk for Injury (Mental, Physical, or Psychosocial) related to ingestion of lead.
- Diversional Activity Deficit related to lack of stimulation by caretaker.
- Altered Growth and Development related to results of lead in body.
- Ineffective Individual Coping related to knowledge deficit of lead poisoning.
- High Risk for Altered Parenting related to perceived threat to personal integrity.
- Altered Nutrition: Less Than Body Requirements related to inadequate diet.

The nurse, child, and parents together plan effective care based on the established nursing diagnoses. Several examples of expected outcomes follow:

- The family identifies hazards of lead in the environment.
- The family participates in removing lead from environment.
- The child consumes a diet low in fat and high in iron.
- The family seeks special instruction for child who has learning deficits because of the lead poisoning.

The nurse plans for the daily care of the child based on both doctor's orders and nursing diagnoses. Some general nursing care goals may be the following:

- Lead is removed from body.
- Source of lead is removed from environment.
- Further lead poisoning is prevented.

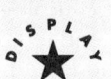

Priority Groups for Screening for Lead Poisoning

Children ages 6 months to 6 years

- who live in or are frequent visitors to deteriorated housing built before 1960
- who live in housing built before 1960 with recent, on-going, or planned renovation or remodeling
- who are siblings, housemates, or playmates of children with known lead poisoning
- whose parents or other household members participate in a lead-related occupation or hobby
- who live near active lead smelters, battery recycling plants, or other industries likely to result in atmospheric lead release

(From: *Centers for Disease Control, U.S. Department of Health and Human Services.* [*1991*]. Preventing lead poisoning in young children [p. 40]. Washington, D.C.: U.S. Department of Health and Human Services.)

★ INTERVENTIONS: COLLABORATIVE AND INDEPENDENT

The goal of treatment is threefold if the child's lead levels are elevated: (1) removal of the source of lead from the child's environment, (2) implementation of diet low in fat and high in iron, and (3) removal of lead from the body by chelation (if lead level is $\geq$45 μg/dL).

LEAD REMOVAL

The nurse can guide the family in finding the source of the poisoning. If the cause is the paint in the house, it has to be removed. The nurse can advise the parents on how to remove the paint. Children must be removed from the house while this is done, because lead in the air from the flaking of paint can be damaging. The house should be washed completely after the paint removal. New paint should be applied to surfaces.

If the family is financially unable to remedy the situation, this removal may prove difficult when the source is paint chips. Social workers are a valuable resource in this type of situation; political involvement may also be necessary. Personal approaches to the city council, the school board, or the public health department may achieve action that not only benefits the identified child but also protects other children in similar situations.

NUTRITIONAL MANAGEMENT

The family needs diet advice on how to help rebuild the child's nutritional status. Institution of a low-fat diet with adequate supplies of calcium, magnesium, zinc, iron, and copper should accompany the removal of the offending lead source. The low-fat diet prevents any more lead from being bound and stored in the fat tissues of the body.

IRON CHELATION

If the blood lead level is greater than or equal to 70 μg/dL, chelation must be instituted. Blood lead values between 30 and 69 μg/dL may also result in chelation. The nurse should refer to specific institution protocols for instruction. Whenever chelation is begun, calcium disodium edetate CaNa$_2$EDTA is given intramuscularly at dosages ranging from 1 g/m^2/d to 1.5 g/m^2/d at intervals of every 4 to 12 hours for 5 to 7 days. CaNa$_2$EDTA is contraindicated in children with impaired renal function. Dimercaprol (British anti-lewisite; BAL) is used when CaNa$_2$EDTA is contraindicated, or it is used in combination with CaNa$_2$EDTA when the blood lead levels are extremely high (>70 μg/dL). Following the typical course of intramuscular chelation with resultant decreasing blood lead levels, an oral chelating agent is begun. The oral agents (e.g., D-penicillamine, succimer) also cause renal toxicities; attention to renal function is necessary.

If encephalopathy is present, BAL is added to the regimen. Additionally, fluid and electrolyte management is crucial because CaNa$_2$EDTA is a nonmetabolizable drug excreted solely by the kidneys. Management of seizures and other problems of encephalopathy is critical but routine.

Children should be prepared for the intramuscular injections, which are painful. The injection site must be rotated also. Management of problems of encephalopathy, especially of seizures, is critical but routine.

TEACHING

The major patient and family teaching is related to the prevention of lead exposure or prevention of further exposure. Some families may need assistance in identifying hazards and in improving the environment in which their children live and play. The caretaker needs guidance in finding activities for the toddler so that thumbsucking and the practice of pica are defeated by other outlets. Instruction must also include appropriate diets to diminish the effects of the lead in the system. If the child has learning deficits, the nurse can direct the parents to appropriate local agencies and institutions where the child can be trained.

EMERGENCY INTERVENTION

When lead poisoning causes an emergency situation, nursing interventions include the management of seizures, establishment of adequate renal output, and restoration of normal cardiac rhythm. Adequate renal func-

tion and subsequent urinary output of at least 0.5 to 1 ml/kg/h must be achieved so that the chelation agents can be excreted. However, fluids and electrolytes must be balanced with the need to minimize increased intracranial pressure. Once adequate renal function has been established and the seizures are controlled acutely, chelation of the circulating lead is begun. BAL is used initially, followed by CaEDTA. When the patient becomes asymptomatic, the BAL is usually discontinued and CaEDTA is administered alone. If symptoms continue, the treatment with BAL and CaEDTA can be cautiously extended.

★ EVALUATION

Periodically, the nurse and family evaluate the outcomes of care given. Examples of outcomes for the child with lead poisoning were given under planning in this section. Have short-term goals been met? Are long-term goals still realistic?

Thalassemia Syndromes

Definition and Incidence. Thalassemia is an autosomal recessive condition in which inappropriate synthesis of some of the polypeptide chains of hemoglobin causes a deficiency in normal hemoglobin. The resultant erythrocytes are hypochromic.

Thalassemia, meaning blood disorder in the people by the sea, is associated with those living in Mediterranean areas. Research has indicated that thalassemia is the result of mutations in mRNA protecting the host from malaria. Typically, people with thalassemia syndromes have ancestors from areas affected by malaria.

Etiology and Pathophysiology. The β-thalassemia trait (the most common form) is found in 3% to 10% of Americans with Italian or Greek ancestors and in 0.5% of African-Americans. Other ethnic groups are also affected but to a much lesser extent. The actual genetic etiology of the thalassemia syndromes has not been identified. It is unlike other hemoglobinopathies in that there are no chemical abnormalities in the hemoglobin present in the host.

The body normally produces several types of polypeptide chains of hemoglobin classified as alpha, beta, delta, and gamma, all of which are produced in proportion to the body's need for certain types of hemoglobin. For example, during fetal development, the body needs hemoglobin F, which is composed of beta and delta polypeptide chains. But in later development, the need for hemoglobin F decreases with a corresponding decline in beta and delta polypeptide chains production. Hemoglobin F is replaced by more hemoglobin A, which is composed of alpha and beta polypeptide chains.

In thalassemia syndromes, the proportion of different polypeptide chains is abnormal. When the available polypeptide chains combine, they form variations of hemoglobin with varying abilities to carry oxygen, resulting in erythrocytes with decreased life spans. The proportion of normal hemoglobin available to the host determines the severity of the syndrome and the clinical manifestations.

The nomenclature used with thalassemia syndromes can be confusing. The terms alpha, beta, major, and minor are all used to describe thalassemia syndromes. The designation of β-thalassemia signifies that the host has an inability to produce normal amounts of the beta polypeptide chain of hemoglobin. α-Thalassemia means the host cannot produce enough alpha polypeptide chains. The designation of thalassemia major or minor denotes heterozygous or homozygous transmission of the disease, respectively. With heterozygous transmission of the syndrome, the clinical manifestations are usually milder than those seen with the homozygous form.

Clinical Manifestations. Clinically, the presentation of thalassemia depends on the severity of the syndrome in the particular child (Fig. 44-1). In β-thalassemia minor, the symptoms are a hypochromic, microcytic anemia. The MCV is decreased as is the MCH. The symptomatology is vague and nonspecific. Many times β-thalassemia minor is confused with iron deficiency anemia. However, when it does not respond to the therapeutic trial of iron supplementation, further investigation should reveal the thalassemia syndrome. One way to lessen the confusion with iron deficiency anemia is the Mentzer formula, which divides the MCV by the RBC count (MCV/RBC count). If the value is >13.5, iron deficiency is suggested. If the value is <11.5, β-thalassemia trait is suggested.

The clinical picture of β-thalassemia major (Cooley's anemia) usually begins in the second 6 months of life, when the child has a severe hemolytic anemia, requiring transfusion to sustain life. Because the child is not producing adequate normal hemoglobin, the body accelerates erythropoiesis, which is accomplished by hypertrophy of bone marrow sites, particularly in the head region. This reactivation or acceleration of erythropoiesis in the head region is the basis for the classic facies of thalassemia. The child has frontal bossing (protuberance) and an exaggerated overbite because of the bone marrow hypertrophy in the frontal bone and the maxillary bones.

Hypertrophy in other bone marrow sites can cause thinning of the long bones with resultant fractures. The child who has β-thalassemia major also demonstrates enlargement of the spleen and liver. The complexion has a greenish-brown tint because of hemosiderosis (deposition of iron from destroyed red cells into the tissues). Frequently, these children also have growth delay because there are concurrent endocrine disorders. Diabetes may occur as a result of pancreatic hemosiderosis.

Diagnostic Studies. In the child with thalassemia syndromes, the physical symptoms are vague in mild cases and also in severe cases if evaluated early in the course of the disease. The diagnosis is based on laboratory data, which show a decrease in hemoglobin, MCV, and MCH. The RBC value is usually normal to increased, and the MCHC is normal or decreased. It is important to note that the decrease in MCV is usually striking and disproportionate to the decrease in hemoglobin and hematocrit. Microscopic evaluation reveals a hypochromic, microcytic anemia with some target cells, which look exactly like their name—a target. The target cells are not diagnostic alone, but in conjunction with other data are useful in the determination of diagnosis. Depending on the severity of the syndrome, the microscopic evaluation may also demonstrate other abnormalities such as poikilocytosis, ovalocytosis, and nucleated red cells. Poikilocytes are large, irregular, malformed RBCs; ovalocytes are elliptical RBCs; and nucleated red cells contain a nucleus. In children with severe thalassemia, a skull x-ray demonstrates the classic "raised hair" picture.

Once a tentative diagnosis has been reached, the hemoglobin can be analyzed to determine which polypeptide chain is deficient. This specific information is helpful in discussion of prognosis and treatment with the parents.

⭐ **ASSESSMENT**

The child with a thalassemia syndrome may present at the health care facility with vague symptomatology or, if

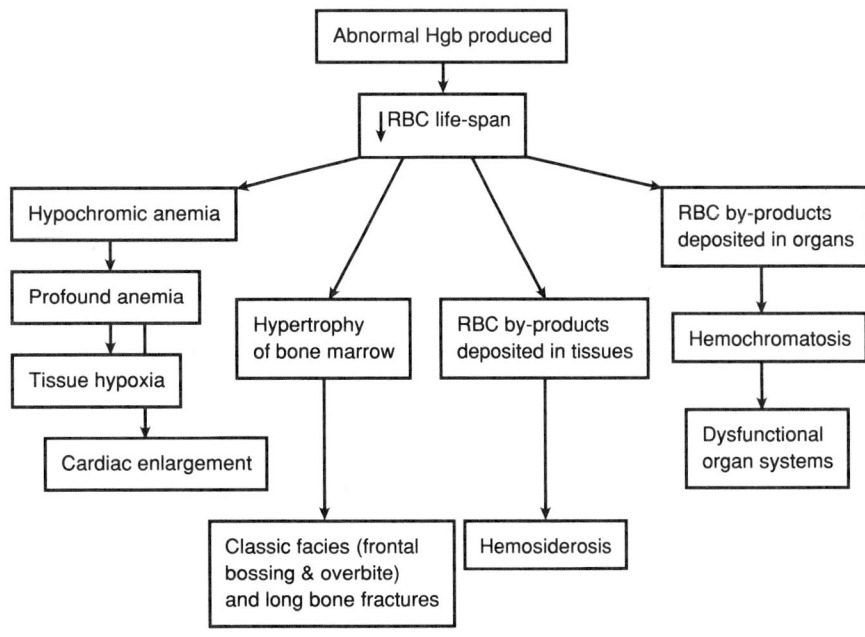

FIGURE 44-1
Summary of thalassemia syndromes.

the syndrome has gone undetected for a long period of time, the presentation may be dramatic. Factors of which the nurse must be cognizant include children with ancestors in areas affected with malaria and children with hypochromic, microcytic anemia not responding to iron supplementation. If parents remember a relative who had some sort of blood problem, this type of knowledge can be a clue for the nurse obtaining the history.

★ NURSING DIAGNOSES AND PLANNING

Based on the assessment data from above and Chapter 43, the following nursing diagnoses may apply to the child with thalassemia:

- High Risk for Injury related to blood transfusion.
- Altered Family Processes related to chronic illness and treatment.
- Ineffective Individual Coping related to situational crises.
- Activity Intolerance related to generalized weakness from anemia.
- Social Isolation related to periodic treatment protocol.

The nurse, child, and parents together plan effective care based on the established nursing diagnoses. Several examples of expected outcomes follow:

- The parents discuss their concerns about caring for a child with chronic illness.
- The child verbalizes emotions centered on chronic illness, transfusion therapy, and iron chelation.
- The child maintains social contacts with close friends.

The nurse plans for the daily care of the child based on both doctor's orders and nursing diagnoses. A general nursing care goal may be the following:

- Safety is maintained during blood transfusion.

★ INTERVENTIONS: COLLABORATIVE AND INDEPENDENT

There is no cure for thalassemia, so treatment is used to keep the condition under control. The medical management goal is to maintain normal hemoglobin levels through the use of blood transfusions. Nursing care involves assisting with transfusions and iron chelation; assisting the patient and family to cope with a chronic illness; and helping the child develop social relationships in school and with friends.

ADMINISTRATION OF BLOOD PRODUCTS AND IRON CHELATION

Most transfusion regimens attempt to maintain the child's hemoglobin between 9 and 10 g/dL. Depending on the severity of the syndrome, the use of transfusion therapy allows the child to maintain an age-appropriate activity level, grow at the usual rate, avoid hypertrophy of the bone marrow tissue and the resulting facial deformities, and avoid splenomegaly due to extramedullary erythropoiesis. The schedule for transfusion is usually every 4 to 6 weeks.

As with any transfusion regimen, the side-effects must be minimized. Transfusions carry the risk of transmitting infectious disease, including AIDS. The most problematic side-effect of transfusion therapy is iron overload. Because each transfusion delivers 200 mg of iron that cannot be excreted physiologically, hemosiderosis can quickly become a serious problem. Early institution of iron chelation therapy minimizes the demise of the child from myocardial siderosis, a common terminal event for children with thalassemia before the widespread use of iron chelation therapy. Iron chelation therapy using subcutaneous, or intramuscular deferoxamine slows hemosiderosis considerably. Infusions of deferoxamine (20 to 40 mg/kg/day) for 10 to 12 hours promote urinary excretion of 15 to 60 mg Fe/day. This level of urinary excretion is usually sufficient to create a negative iron balance. Chelation-induced iron unloading can be enhanced by ascorbate supplements.

Teaching the parents or caretaker and child about the technique is essential to accurate and effective use. For the school-aged child, the nurse should address the issue of stigma and isolation from other children. Preparation for the child's resumption of normal activities should include discussion of peers' possible reactions to the affected child. Depending on the situation, the nurse may offer to talk with the child's teachers and classmates, an interaction beneficial for all involved. Fears are addressed and allayed; children are exposed to health care workers; curiosity is quelled; and valuable communication is established between the child, the school, the health care facility, and classmates.

★ EVALUATION

Periodically, the nurse and family evaluate the outcomes of care given. Examples of outcomes for the child with thalassemia were given under planning in this section. Have short-term goals been met? Are long-term goals still realistic? Planning for further nursing care also takes into consideration long-term care and complications.

Disorders of RBC Destruction

Nursing Interventions for Disorders of RBC Destruction

Like disorders of RBC production and maturation, nursing interventions for disorders of RBC destruction include actions to ensure adequate tissue oxygenation and informed caretakers. Additionally, the nurse takes actions to help restore normal RBC life span. Table 44-5 details the nursing care for disorders of RBC destruction.

Oxygenation. To ensure adequate oxygenation of the body's tissues, the nurse is initially involved in making certain that the body has enough transport mechanisms for the needed oxygen. This can be accomplished through the evaluation of serial hemoglobin and hematocrit levels, transfusion when values are less than 6 g/dL, and institution of chelation therapy.

Teaching. Informing the caretaker is the second goal in the nursing management of disorders of RBC destruction. The caretaker needs information about the dis-

TABLE 44-5
Nursing Interventions: General Care of Children With Disorders of RBC Destruction

Goal	Intervention	Evaluation
Provide adequate oxygenation of tissues	*Oxygenation:*	
	Check serial hematocrit and hemoglobin	Hematocrit and hemoglobin are normal (Hgb 11 g/dL)
	Transfuse if hemoglobin < 6 g/dL	
	Monitor child's activities for change in intensity	Activities are within normal limits
	Take serial chest x-rays to evaluate heart size if anemia is prolonged (Hgb < 6 g/dL for 6 months)	Heart is not enlarged
Keep caretaker informed	*Teaching:*	
	Teach regarding disease process	Appropriate questions are asked and answered
	Teach regarding need for serial Hct and Hgb and electrophoresis evaluations	Caretaker complies with treatment regimen
	Teach regarding parameters for transfusion	Caretaker complies with transfusion schedule
	Teach regarding need for chelation therapy	Caretaker complies with chelation program
	Teach regarding situations precipitating RBC destruction (i.e., altitude, decreased oxygen, increased stress, dietary factors)	Caretaker avoids situations predisposing to RBC destruction
	If splenectomized, teach regarding need for pneumococcal prophylactis	Pneumococcal pneumonia is avoided
Restore normal RBC life span	*Restore RBC life span:* If SS anemia,	
	• Suppress HgbS production with hypertransfusion therapy • Serial Hgb electrophoresis • Chelation therapy if transfusion therapy is prolonged • Teach caretaker regarding symptoms of SS crisis and appropriate solicitation of health care	HgbS < 40% Chelation therapy is appropriately instituted Caretaker recognizes symptoms and seeks health care
	If G6PD or pyruvate kinase deficiency,	
	• Avoid offending dietary sources	Child avoids specific dietary offenders

order, the prescribed treatment plan, and the implications of compliance or noncompliance. The caretaker also needs information concerning the situations that precipitate RBC destruction. With glucose-6-phosphate dehydrogenase (G6PD) deficiency, particular foods or chemicals in foods are the stimuli precipitating RBC destruction. Substances with oxidant properties are the ones to be avoided. Some more commonly used drugs that have oxidant properties are the antipyretics, sulfonamides, antimalarials, and naphthaquinolones. The fava bean is a food that also has oxidant properties. Although the fava bean is not a staple in the United States, it is a dietary staple of people from Middle Eastern countries. With sickle cell anemia, decreasing amounts of available oxygen cause the RBCs to sickle. Strenuous activities at high altitudes, such as mountain climbing and rappelling,

would be contraindicated in people with sickle cell anemia. Air travel in unpressurized cabins would also be contraindicated.

The caretaker also requires information regarding the risk of pneumococcal sepsis. Children under the age of 5 are rarely splenectomized because of the overwhelming risk of sepsis. The use of prophylactic antibiotics and immunizations against pneumococcal, meningococcal, and *Hemophilus influenzae* sepsis are effective strategies to combat overwhelming sepsis.

Restoration of Normal RBC Life Span. The ultimate goal with the disorders of RBC destruction is achievement of normal RBC life span. This can be accomplished by the avoidance of situations that precipitate RBC destruction (see Table 44-5). The avoidance of ox-

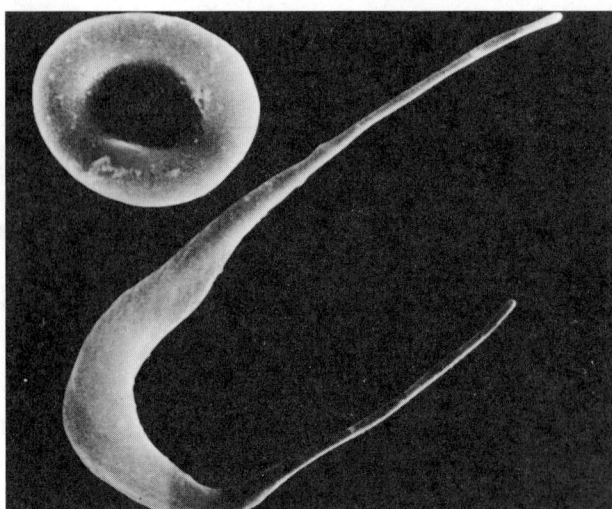

FIGURE 44-2
A normal and a sickled red blood cell.

idant compounds for those affected with G6PD deficiency results in normal RBC life span.

Sickle Cell Anemia

Definition and Incidence. Sickle cell anemia is one of several hemoglobinopathies, which are characterized by a hemoglobin variant replacing the normal adult hemoglobin.The erythrocytes have less than a normal life span of 120 days. Sickle cell anemia is a homozygous condition in which the hemoglobin in the erythrocyte forms the characteristic "sickled" shape when oxygen concentrations are less than normal. Figure 44-2 shows the difference between a normal RBC and a sickled cell.

Sickle cell *trait* is the related heterozygous condition; it occurs in approximately 8% of the African-American population in the United States. Sickle cell anemia may occur in 25% of children when both parents have the sickle cell trait. This easy transmission of the trait and the condition means that genetic counseling is in order for those people identified as having the sickle cell trait. Recent advances in prenatal diagnosis allow the identification of sickle cell trait or anemia before birth.

Etiology and Pathophysiology. The gene responsible for sickle cell anemia causes a single substitution of valine at one point on the beta polypeptide chain of hemoglobin. This one substitution results in the linear, sickle-shaped crystals of hemoglobin in conditions with less than normal concentrations of oxygen. The RBCs containing the sickle hemoglobin do not have the ability to travel through the smaller blood vessels, thus occluding the vessel. Oxygen is deprived from tissues distal to the occlusion so the distal tissues experience a "stroke."

Clinical Manifestations. The clinical manifestations for the child with sickle cell anemia are varied. However, the presentation is usually the result of persistent vaso-occlusive crises and hemolytic anemia. The spleen is often enlarged even though its function is di-

minished, resulting in hyposplenism. The spleen is not able to accomplish its phagocytic or reticuloendothelial functions. Because the spleen cannot function properly, these children are at increased risk for pneumococcal sepsis or meningitis. The body is unable to contain this infection, because of the hyposplenic state: an overwhelming sepsis occurs, requiring immediate intervention to prevent demise. Mortality can be as high as 25% in children who contract pneumococcal meningitis or sepsis.

The presenting factor usually involves a sickle cell crisis associated with these crises: vaso-occlusive, sequestration, or aplastic, as illustrated in Figure 44-3.

Vaso-occlusive Crises. Sickle cell anemia may present in infancy with a typical symmetric swelling of hands and feet, the result of infarctions in the small blood vessels of the hands and feet. The presentation of "hand and foot syndrome" is a classic clue to sickle cell disease because it is an early manifestation of the vaso-occlusive crises seen in sickle cell disease (see Fig. 44-3). The erythrocytes sickle in relation to stress: an infection, a virus, or decreased concentrations of oxygen. The stress alters the surface tension of the erythrocyte; the hemoglobin crystallizes in long chains; and the characteristic biconcave shape of the RBC becomes a sickled cell.

This sickled cell occludes the blood vessel.

Depending on the site and size of the occlusion, the clinical manifestations vary. If the site of the occlusion is the small, distal bones of the hands and feet, then hand and foot syndrome is seen. If the site is the liver, altera-

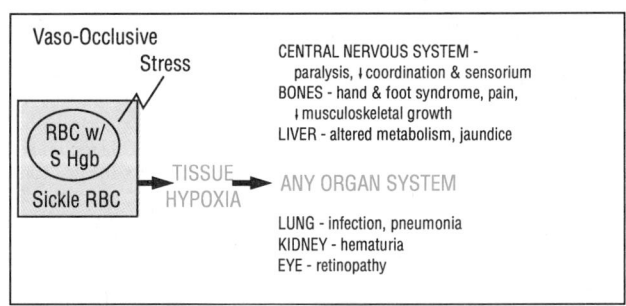

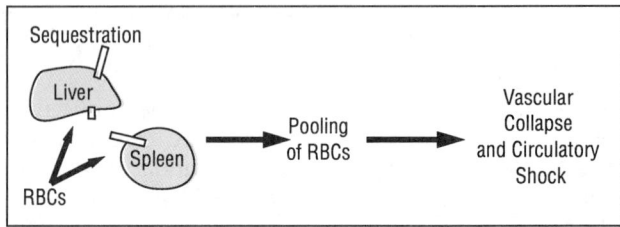

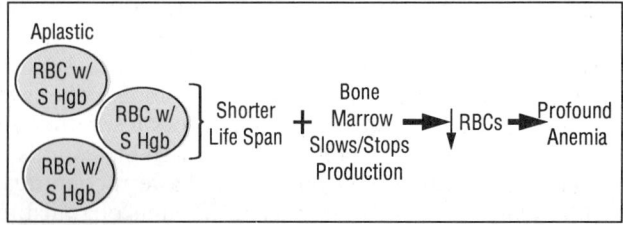

FIGURE 44-3
Sickle cell crises and their effects.

tions in metabolism are evident, such as jaundice. If the site is the central nervous system, alterations in sensorium, or coordination may be evident. There may also be evidence of paralysis if the central nervous system occlusion is large enough.

Sequestration Crises. Children with sickle cell anemia may also experience sequestration crises, which are the result of pooling of large amounts of blood in the spleen and liver (see Fig. 44-3). The reason for the pooling is unknown. Because a major portion of the circulating blood is pooled in the spleen and liver, the child rapidly develops circulatory shock. The child in sequestration crisis must be supported with transfusion therapy and adequate hydration. Transfusion and hydration therapy usually promote remobilization of the pooled blood.

Aplastic Crises. Aplastic crises in sickle cell anemia result due to the shortened life span of the erythrocyte with sickle hemoglobin (see Fig. 44-3). In the aplastic crisis, bone marrow cannot produce enough normal erythrocytes to maintain adequate levels of oxygen to the tissues. The erythrocytes with hemoglobin S carry oxygen, but, because they are destroyed before they can deliver oxygen to all the tissues, the bone marrow cannot keep up with the hemolysis. A profound anemia results. The child must be supported with transfusions until a balance is achieved between normal new cells and those destroyed.

Diagnostic Studies. The diagnosis can be made as early as 3 months of age, but may be missed until the child is a preschooler. However, sickle cell anemia can only be definitively diagnosed after 6 months of age. A sickle cell prep can be used as a screening test. The definitive test in determining sickle cell anemia is a hemoglobin electrophoresis establishing the presence and percentage of hemoglobin S. The amount of fetal hemoglobin in the newborn obscures the detection of hemoglobin S. As the fetal hemoglobin decreases, the hemoglobin S increases. Usually by 6 months of age the concentration of hemoglobin S is large enough for detection with the sickle cell prep.

Often, affected children are evaluated not because of any symptoms, but because of their parents' family history and suspicion that the child might have sickle cell anemia. As technology improves, early detection of sickle cell anemia will become more common.

The peripheral blood smear of the child with sickle cell anemia also yields valuable information even though it is not definitive information. The smear demonstrates irreversibly sickled cells, target cells, Howell-Jolly bodies, poikilocytes, nucleated red cells, and hypochromia. The hemoglobin is usually between 6 and 8 g/dL.

★ ASSESSMENT

Nurses play an integral role in the detection of sickle cell anemia. Screening tests on all susceptible children greatly decrease the long-term complications of undetected disease. Susceptible children include those with a positive family history and black children. In addition, screening for sickle cell trait is also important. Those people carrying the sickle cell trait need to be informed of the implications for their offspring. When both parents carry the

sickle trait, they need to know that there is a 25% chance that every offspring will have sickle cell anemia and a 50% chance that every offspring will have sickle cell trait (Fig. 44-4). Genetic counseling can be helpful for those affected with the sickle trait or with sickle cell anemia.

The symptoms of a child in sickle cell crisis are related to either vaso-occlusive crises or hemolytic anemia. The vaso-occlusive crises present with symptoms of pain and possible swelling at the affected site. If the site of the crisis is the central nervous system, the child may experience a change in sensorium, altered consciousness, or paralysis. Symptoms of a hemolytic anemia include weakness, fatigue, dyspnea with exertion, pallor, and tachycardia. The child in sequestration crisis would show signs of circulatory shock because a large volume of blood is pooled in the splenic area. This pooling or sequestration reduces the available volume of circulating blood, resulting in circulatory shock.

★ NURSING DIAGNOSES AND PLANNING

Based on the assessment data from above and Chapter 43, the following nursing diagnoses may apply to the child with sickle cell anemia:

- High Risk for Injury (Bleeding) related to physical activity.
- Pain related to tissue anoxia.
- Activity Intolerance related to possible crises.
- Diversional Activity Deficit related to curtailment of physical activity.
- Altered Family Processes related to situational transition.
- Hopelessness related to chronic nature of condition.
- Knowledge Deficit regarding cause and treatment of disease.

The nurse, child, and parents together plan effective care based on the established nursing diagnoses. Several examples of expected outcomes follow:

- The child and parents describe hemophilia, its cause, its course, and chronic nature.
- The child verbalizes relief of pain from vaso-occlusive crises.

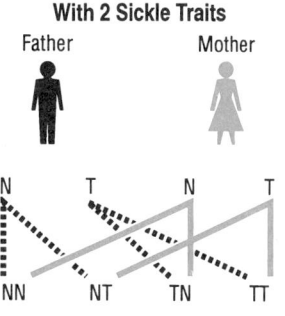

With 2 Sickle Traits

Therefore with each pregnancy, 25% chance of sickle cell anemia 50% chance of sickle cell trait 25% chance of normal hemoglobin

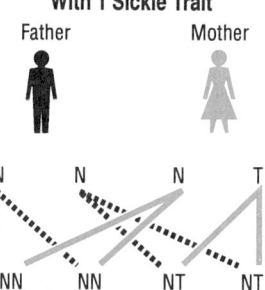

With 1 Sickle Trait

Therefore with each pregnancy, 50% chance of sickle cell trait 50% chance of normal hemoglobin

N = *normal hemoglobin*   T = *sickle cell trait*

FIGURE 44-4

Genetic transmission of sickle cell trait.

- The child and family identify activities that should be avoided.
- The child participates in normal social activities.
- The family uses appropriate emotions to discuss the transitions it must make because of the disease in the family.
- The family participates in genetic counseling.

The nurse plans for the daily care of the child based on both doctor's orders and nursing diagnoses. Some general nursing care goals may be the following:

- Sickling is prevented.
- Hydration is provided.
- Adverse effects of crises are minimized.

★ INTERVENTIONS: COLLABORATIVE AND INDEPENDENT

Although there is no cure for sickle cell anemia, the management is twofold: (1) prevention of the sickling phenomenon by promotion of adequate oxygenation and hydration, and (2) treatment of the medical emergency of sickle cell crisis. Table 44-1 presents some of these interventions.

The goal of management of sickle cell anemia is to prevent or minimize the adverse effects of vaso-occlusive, sequestration, and aplastic crises. To prevent the crises, the hemoglobin S concentration must not exceed 40%. In addition, certain situations such as flying in unpressurized aircraft, undue stress due to illness, and activity at high elevations, such as mountain climbing, should be avoided. These situations increase the likelihood of sickling of the erythrocytes.

MEDICATION THERAPY

The ideal drug or combination of drugs is one that would inhibit the sickling (polymerization) of the abnormal hemoglobin, while having little effect on the oxygen affinity of the hemoglobin molecule. Most drugs available seem to increase the oxygen affinity, which increases hemoglobin and hematocrit and, thus, the viscosity of the blood. This increased viscosity should be avoided, because it increases the risk of vaso-occlusive crises. The lower hemoglobin and hematocrit are, in fact, protective in the child with sickle cell anemia.[47]

SYMPTOM MANAGEMENT

Sickle cell anemia crises are not always so easy to predict but can be minimized with hypertransfusion programs. The intent is to suppress hemoglobin S concentration to less than 40% by supplying normal hemoglobin by way of transfusions. Serial hemoglobin electrophoresis provides detailed information about the differing concentrations of hemoglobin. As discussed earlier, a regimen of extended transfusions requires chelation to prevent iron overload or hemosiderosis.

When crises do occur, the symptoms of the particular crisis must be managed. For example, if the crisis is a vaso-occlusive event affecting the lower limbs, management would include pain relief, hydration, rest, and correction of any acidosis. While the crisis is managed, there must also be a simultaneous lowering of the concentration of hemoglobin S, which can be effectively lowered by transfusion with normal hemoglobin A blood or by dilution of the patient's blood with other expanders. Hemoglobin electrophoresis can determine the exact concentration of all hemoglobin present. The need for additional transfusion therapy can be determined.

Some children with sickle cell anemia have frequent vaso-occlusive crises. These children are in pain and quickly learn that narcotics are extremely effective in the relief of their pain. When used knowledgeably, narcotics are extremely effective and are not addictive. The nurse must be extremely careful in the assessment of pain in these children, because too much narcotic for too little pain leads to addiction, but not enough narcotic for existing pain is ineffective as well as incompassionate. The dilemma is clear. The interpretation of clinical situations is not.

TEACHING

Patient and family teaching is essential to combat adequately the problems of sickle cell anemia. The need for genetic information and counseling has already been discussed. Other issues requiring instruction are:

- Unrestricted activity when not in crisis.
- Avoidance of situations precipitating a crisis.
- Compliance with routine health checks.
- Symptoms of crises.
- Access to health care when crisis occurs.

The nurse can instruct the family members on the most expedient way to achieve emergency health care in their particular community.

Nurses providing education through the school systems and local health departments can have a significant impact on the health of this susceptible population.

PSYCHOSOCIAL SUPPORT

For psychological reasons, the nurse needs to address the issue of differentness with the child older than 4 or 5 years. Parents of the child with sickle cell anemia need to have the opportunity to express their feelings about having a child with sickle cell anemia and the burden it may impose. It does not matter to the parent whether they knew there was a risk of sickle cell anemia or not; whenever parents learn that their child is not normal, there can be feelings of guilt, anger, frustration, confusion, or helplessness. Discussion of these possibilities is an important role of the nurse.

EMERGENCY INTERVENTION

When there is a sequestration crisis, the nurse assists with the administration of oxygen by way of mask, cannula, or endotracheal tube, the establishment of an intravenous line, insertion of a urinary catheter, obtaining baseline weight, monitoring vital signs, securing samples for laboratory measures such as blood gases, and the safe administration of ordered medications. The nurse should also elevate the child's legs to prevent any further pooling of blood in the extremities and to enhance the blood return to the heart. Volume expanders are effective in both sequestration and vaso-occlusive crises because they effectively decrease the viscosity of the blood and subsequently decrease the percentage of circulating hemoglobin S.

Emergency situations also require a special attentiveness to the parents of the ill child. A nurse staying with the parents as a comforter and liaison for information would be ideal. When circumstances are not ideal, the nurse specialist should provide parents with periodic updates of the measures taken and their child's response to them.

★ EVALUATION

Periodically, the nurse and family evaluate the outcomes of care given. Examples of outcomes for the child and family with sickle cell anemia were given under planning in this section. Have short-term goals been met? Are long-term goals still realistic? Planning for further nursing care also takes into consideration complications and long-term care.

COMPLICATIONS

The complications of sickle cell anemia are those occurring as a result of a crisis. The specifics of the complication are directly related to the organ system or systems affected. For example, if the central nervous system is affected during a vaso-occlusive crisis, the child may experience a stroke with residual motor and mental deficits. The management of the stroke in a child with sickle cell anemia is like that of an adult with a stroke except for the developmental issues that coexist. In working with the child, the nurse must remain aware of the normal cognitive, emotional, and physical development of the child.

Depending on the severity of the complications, such as stroke, there are also financial and emotional challenges with which the parents and family must deal. The nurse should be instrumental in assessing the family's need and readiness for discussion. Sometimes the nurse is the appropriate one for the parents to talk with, but in other circumstances a referral to the social work, pastoral, or financial aid department is more appropriate. The nurse's assessment of need is crucial to effective intervention with the child and the family.

LONG-TERM CARE

Long-term management of the child with sickle cell anemia involves periodic evaluations of the amount of hemoglobin S in the child's blood in conjunction with appropriate developmental screening and preventive health care. The frequency of the evaluations is determined by the severity of the child's condition and the family's access to the health care facility.

Those affected with sickle cell anemia have an unusually high susceptibility to pneumococcal sepsis. Mortality of up to 25% merits particular attention. The preventive measure most often employed for children less than 2 years old is daily prophylactic doses of penicillin, which usually affords the child protection from this devastating complication. Children older than 2 years can successfully receive the pneumococcal polysaccharide vaccine for protection against systemic pneumococcal infections.

Families with children affected with sickle cell anemia should be informed of any local and national support groups. Information and support are available through the organizations listed in the display near the beginning of the chapter.

Glucose-6-Phosphate Dehydrogenase Deficiency (G6PD)

Definition, Incidence, and Pathophysiology. G6PD deficiency is a rare condition causing hemolytic anemia that is transmitted on the X chromosome. G6PD, an enzyme necessary for RBC survival, functions to oxidize compounds that would otherwise destroy the RBC. One such normally produced compound is hydrogen peroxide. The affected person with G6PD deficiency does not produce enough of this enzyme to oxidize the hydrogen peroxide. The unoxidized hydrogen peroxide causes the hemoglobin to denature and to precipitate into the RBC where it is captured into inclusions called Heinz bodies. RBCs with precipitated hemoglobin cannot transport oxygen to the tissues in the required efficient manner. Therefore, all RBCs with Heinz bodies are quickly destroyed by the spleen because of their inefficiency.

G6PD deficiency has a wide range of clinical manifestations based on the severity of the defect. If the child is affected with a severe G6PD deficiency, hemolysis of RBCs on a massive level ensues. On the other hand, if the condition is only mild, the hemolytic anemia will also be mild.

In many cases of G6PD deficiency, hemolysis is triggered by the ingestion of oxidant compounds, a condition usually occurring within 48 to 96 hours after ingestion of the oxidant drug. Examples of such oxidant compounds are antimalarials, sulfonamides, nitrofurans, antipyretics, and analgesics. There are some oxidant compounds not in listed classifications that also cause hemolytic anemia in children affected with G6PD deficiency. They include probenicid, chloramphenicol, vitamin K, and naphthalene. If these drugs are needed for treatment of an illness, it is necessary to question the child or family of any knowledge of G6PD deficiency in their family history.

Members of ethnic groups who have a higher susceptibility (from 5% to 40%) to the deficiency are Italians, Greeks, Mediterraneans, Middle Easterns, Africans, and Orientals. In the United States, 13% of African-American males and 2% of African-American females are affected with G6PD deficiency.

Clinically, the affected newborn with G6PD deficiency may have hyperbilirubinemia, kernicterus, and jaundice. In older children with a mild form of the condition, nurses may only see a compensated hemolytic process.

G6PD deficiency is diagnosed by the actual evaluation of G6PD activity in the RBC. Levels of activity must be less than 10% of normal to be diagnostic for G6PD deficiency. The severity of the condition depends on the decrease in the enzyme activity. New RBCs have higher enzyme activity than do older cells. Therefore, after recovery from a hemolytic episode has begun, the G6PD level may be within normal limits. Several weeks may need to elapse before a diagnostic value can be obtained.

Nursing Implications. The major role for the nurse in dealing with children affected with G6PD deficiency is the prevention of hemolytic episodes. Instruction about avoidance of oxidant compounds is the major thrust. In addition, the nurse can be instrumental in the screening of high-risk people. Should a hemolytic episode occur, the goal of treatment is restoration of normal hemoglobin levels and tissue oxygenation. Transfusions may be necessary, but the hemolytic episodes are usually self-limiting (see Table 44-1).

Pyruvate Kinase Deficiency

Pyruvate kinase deficiency causes the RBC to have a shortened life span. As a result, the affected child experiences a hemolytic anemia. Pyruvate kinase deficiency is caused by the homozygous expression of an autosomal recessive gene. This particular gene inhibits the production of the enzyme pyruvate kinase. The deficiency of the enzyme pyruvate kinase results in a decreased amount of adenosine triphosphate (ATP). This decreased energy source for the RBC causes potassium to leak from the RBC, thereby causing the early destruction of the RBC.

In the mild form of the deficiency, no clinical symptoms are evident. Only a compensated hemolytic process is accidentally found during an investigation of some other problem. In the more severely affected, clinical manifestations include hyperbilirubinemia, jaundice, anemia, and kernicterus. Appearance of symptoms is directly dependent on the severity of the enzyme deficiency.

Pyruvate kinase deficiency is diagnosed through the actual measurement of the RBC enzyme. If the level of enzyme activity is less than 10% of normal, a diagnosis of pyruvate kinase deficiency is made.

The treatment goal is the maintenance of normal levels of hemoglobin, RBCs, and tissue oxygenation (see Table 44-1). In some affected people, transfusion therapy may be needed during severe anemia or aplastic episodes. Splenectomy may be considered if the affected child has substantial transfusion requirements. The splenectomy should not be considered before 5 years of age because of the risk of pneumococcal sepsis.

Hereditary Spherocytosis

Hereditary spherocytosis is the most common hemolytic anemia resulting from a structural defect in the RBC. The condition is transmitted as an autosomal dominant trait. Although hereditary spherocytosis has been documented in all ethnic groups, there seems to be a predilection for people with a northern European ancestry.

The etiology of hereditary spherocytosis is a defect in the proteins or lipoproteins of the RBC membrane. The defective RBC membrane, unusually permeable in hereditary spherocytosis, allows the intracellular concentration of sodium to increase through the cation pump. Along with the increased intracellular sodium, the use of ATP also increases. The RBC is destroyed because of metabolic overload from the increased intracellular sodium and use of ATP as well as from loss of the cell membrane.

The RBC membrane defect also results in the characteristic spheric shape of the cell. The different properties of the normal biconcave disk RBC as opposed to the abnormal spherically shaped RBC should be noted. The normal RBC can increase its volume in relation to its surface area and it can more easily negotiate smaller blood vessels because of its flexibility. The abnormal spherocyte cannot increase its volume because it has already reached its capacity for that surface area. Its spheric shape is also rigid, and, therefore, it cannot negotiate the smaller blood vessels as easily as can its normal counterpart.

As these spherocytes circulate through the body, they must traverse the splenic circulation, a process that involves tiny apertures in the splenic cords. Because the abnormally rigid spherocyte has extreme difficulty negotiating these channels, it becomes stuck and lysis follows. The spleen effectively removes the abnormal cells from circulation, which causes a hemolytic anemia in the host.

The severity of hereditary spherocytosis varies among people but is usually similar within families. In newborns, the manifestations include anemia and hyperbilirubinemia. In older children, the anemia and hyperbilirubinemia are accompanied by slight jaundice, reticulocytosis, splenomegaly, and moderate marrow expansion. The school-aged child and adolescent may present with pigmentary gallstones.

The definitive tests for diagnosis of hereditary spherocytosis are the osmotic fragility and autohemolysis tests. Because of their inability to increase their volume to surface area, spherocytes rupture much more easily than do normal cells. The spherocytes are much more fragile. The autohemolysis test for normal cells results in the lysis of less than 5% of the cells stored for 48 hours. With hereditary spherocytosis, lysis of cells is greatly increased (15% to 45%). In conjunction with the clinical symptoms of anemia, reticulocytosis, and hyperbilirubinemia, these two tests are definitive for the diagnosis of hereditary spherocytosis.

Nursing Implications. There is no cure for the RBC membrane defect. However, the hemolytic symptoms can be relieved by a splenectomy, which should be cautiously considered in young children because of the risk of overwhelming sepsis after the procedure. Splenectomy is only offered to those children with uncompensated hemolytic anemia who are older than 5 years of age.

When the affected child is unable to maintain a compensated hemolytic state, as in an aplastic crisis or infection, the goal of treatment is supportive. The aplastic crisis or infection is usually self-limiting, and, therefore, the compensated hemolytic state resumes.

Disorders of White Blood Cells

WBCs are the body's defense system. As a group, they circulate through the body patrolling for foreign organisms and materials. When such organisms and materials are located, WBCs activate a complicated and effective system to conquer and destroy the invaders. The majority of the WBCs' work is defense against infection and neutralization of cellular breakdown.

WBC × Neutrophil % = Real Number of Functioning Neutrophils

EXAMPLE:
3 YR-OLD BOY
WBC = 11000 (11.0 × 10³)
% NEUTROPHIL = 47%
ABSOLUTE NEUTROPHIL COUNT = 5170

FIGURE 44-5
Determination of absolute neutrophil count.

Diseases of the WBCs typically are manifested through the breakdown of the body's defense against infections. Sometimes the weakened resistance to infection is related to decreased numbers of WBCs. Determination of the absolute neutrophil count can be helpful at this point (Fig. 44-5). In other instances, the increased susceptibility to infection is related to defective WBC function. Like the diseases of the RBC, the diseases of the WBC can be divided into categories of etiology.

The most important WBC disorder is the category of leukemias. This category of diseases and their treatment are discussed in relation to neoplastic disease in Chapter 31. The other WBC diseases are much less common. Even so, knowledge of all disorders of WBCs is critical for the nurse.

Nursing Interventions for Disorders of WBC Function

The nursing interventions for disorders of the WBC can be divided into four goals: caretaker knowledge, prevention of viral and bacterial illnesses, prompt intervention when illness occurs, and restored normal WBC function. These goals are discussed in Table 44-6.

Teaching. The initial goal is a caretaker who is knowledgeable about the signs and symptoms of the disorder. Information about the specific disorder can be conveyed by the nurse through oral or written media. It

TABLE 44-6
Nursing Interventions: General Care of Children With Disorders of WBC Production, Maturation, and Destruction

Goal	Intervention	Evaluation
Keep caretaker informed	*Teaching:* Teach regarding disease process Teach regarding altered signs of illness Teach regarding appropriate channels of health care if ill	Caretaker asks appropriate questions and expresses understanding about disease and signs of illness Caretaker identifies plans to seek consultation when illness is present
Prevent bacterial and viral illnesses	*Prevention of Illnesses:* Prophylactic antibiotics, if appropriate	Caretaker complies with prophylactic antibiotic regimen by drug levels
	Protective isolation if absolute neutrophil count is < 2000	Child complies with isolation plan
	Avoid others with known illnesses if neutrophils < 5000	Child actively avoids people with known illness
	Teach child regarding personal hygiene	Good hygiene practices are evidenced
Intervene promptly if illness occurs	*Intervention:* Obtain cultures to determine organism causing illness	Caretaker contacts health care provider to assess signs of illness
	Begin antibiotics at therapeutic dose	Antibiotics are delivered on schedule
	Evaluate antibiotic choice based on culture and sensitivity results	Signs of illness are diminished
		Cultures are made of blood, urine, skin lesion
	Teach regarding appropriate channels of health care when ill	
Restore normal WBC function	Serial WBC with differential	Normal WBC for age
	If leukemia, • Normal remission by bone marrow aspirate evaluation	Cellularity of bone marrow is normal
	If neutropenia, • Removal of source or cause	Quantity and function of neutrophils are normal
	If chronic granulomatous disease, • Symptomatic relief	

is critical for the caretaker to understand that the disease causes masking of the usual signs of illness—fever, swelling, redness—because of the underlying WBC abnormality. Individual children respond differently to illness. Caretakers and health care staff should determine over time the usual response of the child. In some children, a fever of 100°F or flushed cheeks are indicative of a serious infection. In others, a nonspecific lethargy or fatigue is the only clue the caretaker notices. The initial stages of such an exercise in discernment can be harrowing for the parents. The health care team needs to be supportive of questions, able to reassure caretakers by examination of the child, and compassionate about their anxiety.

Many of the children with disorders of WBCs are managed through a specific outpatient clinic that has an "on call" system, which channels questions to a rotating member of the health care team. Teaching the caretakers how to access this system is vital to their comfort after discharge from the hospital. The caretaker's questions, expression of understanding, and identification of plans to seek consultation when illness is suspected are measures of the caretaker's knowledge.

Prevention of Bacterial and Viral Illnesses. Prevention of bacterial and viral illnesses is another goal for the children affected with disorders of WBCs. Prophylactic antibiotics can be used if the child is particularly susceptible to certain illnesses. For instance, children with leukemia frequently receive Bactrim as a prophylaxis against pneumocystis. Figure 44-5 details the method to determine absolute neutrophil count. Periodically, the caretaker needs to know the child's absolute neutrophil count so that appropriate protective measures can be begun. If the value is less than 5000, the child needs to avoid people who are known to be ill. If the value is less than 2000, the child needs to be placed in protective isolation. Protective isolation means that all those coming in contact with the child should wear masks and gloves to prevent the transmission of airborne germs and contact fomites. Instruction of the child regarding personal hygiene is also a valuable method to prevent illnesses. Handwashing is of utmost importance.

Prompt Intervention. Once an illness is detected, the nurse should assist in the collection of culture specimens. These children need antibiotics at therapeutic doses immediately. The choice of antibiotics can be evaluated and changed, if necessary, based on the results of the culture and sensitivity reports. Timely delivery of medications is a central part of the nurse's role. The symptoms of illness, however slight, diminish and the subsequent cultures clear once the appropriate antibiotic is delivered.

Resumption of Normal Function. The ultimate goal for these disorders is the resumption of normal WBC function. Serial evaluation of WBC differentials provides information about the circulating WBCs. Normal cellularity of the bone marrow provides additional information about the body's response, whether decreased, normal, or accelerated. The laboratory can also perform specialized tests that evaluate the function of neutrophils. The

nurse assists in the collection of the necessary specimens. When neutropenia is the disorder and an offending material or compound can be identified, removal of the substance is the way to restore normal WBC function. The suppurative lesions seen with Chronic Granulomatous Disease (CGD) require drainage and appropriate skin care. The location of the lesion dictates the type and frequency of dressing. Pain control for these lesions depends on the extent and location of the lesion. Leukemia treatment and nursing interventions are discussed in Chapter 31.

Disorders of WBC Production

Neutrophilia

Neutrophilia or increases in WBCs occur for two reasons: (1) There can be an increase in the circulation of WBCs or (2) there can be an increase in the production of WBCs.

In the healthy body, there are circulating WBCs, which are referred to as the circulating granulocytic compartment. In addition, there are WBCs called the marginal compartment, which are held in reserve in the small blood vessels for situations or conditions that require rapid mobilization of additional WBCs.

Neutrophilia occurs as a healthy response to generalized or localized infections when the body recognizes the threat and responds with increased WBCs. The neutrophils increase, as do all other types of WBCs, eosinophils, basophils, lymphocytes, and monocytes. Many times, the peripheral blood contains more immature WBCs, such as metamyelocytes, than usual. This increase in immature cells is sometimes referred to as a "shift to the left." This phrase refers to the manner in which WBCs are usually divided in counting procedures. The more immature cells are typically recorded on the left.

Young children demonstrate a more dramatic neutrophilia than do adults. Because of this dramatic increase in neutrophils, the WBC count can resemble that of chronic myelogenous leukemia. Differentiation between the neutrophilia of infection (leukemoid reaction) and that of chronic myelogenous leukemia can be achieved by noting the activity of alkaline phosphatase and bone marrow changes. In chronic myelogenous leukemia, the alkaline phosphatase is decreased and there are bone marrow changes. With neutrophilia from infection, alkaline phosphatase activity is increased; the entire line of neutrophils is hyperactive and there are no changes in the bone marrow.

Neutropenia

Neutropenia is a substantial reduction in the number of circulating WBCs. This reduction of neutrophils, whether from a congenital or acquired cause, results in a host that is at increased risk of infection. The host is at particular risk from infections of the skin, lungs, and the mucosa of the buccal and rectal regions.

Chronic neutropenia is a condition of mild neutropenia in young children. The etiology of the decreased WBCs is unknown. Clinically, the child has recurrent skin and lung infections as well as oral and rectal ulcerations. The usual signs of infections (redness, swelling, and fever) are either decreased or absent because the child does not have enough neutrophils to mount these reactions; therefore, caretakers need to be sensitive to subtle signs and symptoms in the child. Treatment of neutropenia is the institution of appropriate antibiotic therapy. There are some reported cases in which the child outgrows this chronic neutropenia and assumes a normal WBC count. The transmission of the condition is uncertain because there have been documented cases of both autosomal recessive and dominant transmission.

Acquired neutropenia is a condition of reduced neutrophils as a result of viral illnesses. Roseola, rubella, influenza, autoimmune disorders, and copper deficiency have each been documented as precipitants of neutropenia. The neutropenia associated with viral illnesses is usually transient. However, in some instances of severe viral illness, the overwhelming nature of the disease is signaled by the degree of neutropenia. With autoimmune disorders such as rheumatoid arthritis and lupus erythematosus, associated neutropenia can be alleviated with corticosteroid therapy. In the limited number of cases of neutropenia associated with copper deficiency, the neutropenia is relieved with the replenishment of necessary copper. It is also important to note that acquired neutropenia occurs in diseases with bone marrow insufficiency, such as leukemia. The treatment for bone marrow deficiency diseases frequently involves medications whose side-effects include severe neutropenia. Some examples of these drugs are methotrexate, nitrogen mustard, ionizing radiation, and benzene compounds.

Drug-induced neutropenia associated with a systemic infection is a condition of substantially reduced neutrophils in the peripheral blood and bone marrow. The most common offenders are drugs from the aminopyrine, thiourea, sulfonamide, and semisynthetic penicillin families. If a profound neutropenia occurs concurrent with the administration of any of these compounds, the possible offending drug should be discontinued immediately. The infection should be treated with appropriate antibiotics determined from the culture and sensitivity procedures. In most cases, drug-induced neutropenia is self-limiting once the offending agent is removed; the bone marrow responds quickly to produce the entire granulocytic line of cells. Once bone marrow recovery begins, there is peripheral evidence of recovery within 4 to 5 days.

Transient neutropenia of the newborn can occur in conjunction with severe infections such as cytomegalic inclusion disease, toxoplasmosis, or bacterial sepsis. Antibiotic therapy should be instituted after diagnosis of the infection. This neutropenia usually lasts between 4 and 6 weeks even with antibiotic treatment.

Disorders of WBC Maturation

Chronic Granulomatous Disease

Chronic granulomatous disease is an X-linked recessive condition in which the host is unable to kill invading bacteria and viruses despite normal numbers of circulating neutrophils. The WBCs have a defect in the intracellular mechanism that normally destroys such invading organisms. The WBC phagocytizes the offending organism but is unable to destroy the offender.

Clinically, the host manifests recurrent suppurative skin lesions, enlarged regional lymph nodes, frequent respiratory infections, hepatomegaly, and splenomegaly. Treatment is the prompt institution of appropriate antibiotics for the offending organism. Frequently, these children develop abscesses, which should be drained promptly. The demise of the child with chronic granulomatous disease usually results from an overwhelming sepsis. Careful observation for infections by caretakers followed by quick attention from the health care team minimizes the complications of the disease (see Table 44-6).

Disorders of Platelets and Coagulation

Blood within the human body must achieve a delicate balance. On one hand, blood must be fluid so that it can flow freely through all the vessels, delivering nutrients and gathering wastes. On the other hand, blood must be able to repair damaged vessels so that the fluid blood does not escape from the circulation. This delicate balance within the blood is achieved by the interaction of the vessels, the platelets, and the host of enzymes known as the coagulation cascade.

The normal interaction of this triad successfully balances the body's need for freely flowing blood and its need to repair damaged vessels through coagulation. The blood vessels must maintain a smooth intimal surface so that the blood can flow freely through its channels. The small blood vessels must also be able to handle interruption of its integrity with vasoconstriction and local tissue pressure control. Second in the triad maintaining hemostasis are the platelets, which are responsible for adhering to damaged vessel walls, aggregating to form platelet plugs, serving as templates for coagulation reactions, and maintaining vascular integrity.[8] Finally, the coagulation cascade, a series of enzymatic reactions, converts a dozen or so factors into a clot (see Fig. 42-4).

Diseases and disorders of the platelets and coagulation can be divided according to etiology: disorders of platelet production, disorders of platelet maturation, and disorders of coagulation.

Nursing Interventions for Disorders of Platelet Production

Nursing interventions for disorders of platelet production are fourfold and are detailed in Table 44-7. They are caretaker knowledge, restoration and maintenance of normal platelet count, intervention in viral and bacterial infections, and management of bleeding.

Teaching. The caretakers and child need factual information regarding the disease process, the planned therapy, and how to access the health care system as needed. When this information is assimilated successfully, the caretaker understands the disease, complies with the

TABLE 44-7
Nursing Interventions: General Care of Children With Disorders of Platelet Production

Goal	Intervention	Evaluation
Keep child and caretaker informed	*Teaching:*	
	Teach child/caretaker regarding disease process	Child and caretaker give evidence of understanding of presented material
	Teach child/caretaker regarding therapy plan	Child complies with therapy regimen
	Teach child/caretaker regarding activity restrictions	Child complies with activity restrictions and has limited number of bleeding episodes
	Teach child/caretaker regarding access to health care	Appropriate access to health care is used as needed
Restore normal platelet count and Maintain adequate platelets	*Platelet Restoration:*	
	Make serial platelet counts	Platelet counts are WNL for age
	Transfuse with platelets	Bleeding ceases
Manage bleeding effectively	*Bleeding Management:*	
	Treat cause of bleeding (i.e., viral and bacterial infections)	Host is free of infections

therapy plan (or makes an informed decision to be non-compliant), and appropriately accesses the health care system when necessary. Information particular to the platelet disorders is related to activity restrictions. Parameters for restricted activity need to be defined for the child and the caretaker.

The physician sets the specific value at which contact activity should be eliminated. In some cases, the value is 20,000 platelets/mm³. In others, it is 50,000. Whatever the actual value, the activities that should be eliminated are those that might result in contact injuries and bleeding. For example, basketball and football are sports in which contact injuries frequently occur. Although roller skating and jumping on the bed do not necessarily involve contact with other people, these activities might result in a fall or a blow to some body part with resultant bleeding. Any activities that possess the potential for a bleeding injury should be eliminated within the set parameters. Compliance with these instructions is evidenced by appropriate restrictions and a limited number of bleeding episodes.

Restoration and Maintenance of Normal Platelet Count. Restoration and maintenance of normal platelet counts is the central issue in the management of these disorders. Serial platelet counts confirm treatment successes and failures. The targeted goal for platelet counts is set by combining the normal for age value with the child's clinical condition. It is important that the child, as opposed to the laboratory value, be treated. When the clinical condition and the laboratory value indicate that a platelet transfusion is necessary, the guidelines for administration of platelets listed in the display on Administration of Blood Products should be employed. One unit of platelets usually raises the child's platelet count by 200/kg or 12 × 1000/m³, assuming there are no destructive processes or antiplatelet antibodies present.

Intervention in Viral and Bacterial Infections. If the cause of bleeding is something other than trauma, such as viral or bacterial infections, the offending agent should be eliminated. The nurse assists with the collection of specimens for cultures and administers the ordered antibacterial or antiviral medications correctly. Cessation of bleeding and negative second cultures show that the treatment has been successful.

Management of Bleeding. Sometimes bleeding occurs spontaneously or without an identifiable cause. When this is the case, the bleeding should be contained as quickly as possible. Usually, the containment is achieved with a platelet transfusion. The most dangerous site for spontaneous bleeding is intracranially. Caretakers need to know that signs and symptoms of intracranial bleeding include headache, neurologic signs, altered consciousness, and seizures. If the hemorrhage occurs in a joint, swelling and pain are the major indicators; if within the lung, coughing up blood and dyspnea; if within the GI or urinary tracts, obviously bloody stools or pink-red urine. Examination by the health care team is essential for the well-being of the child.

Disorders of Platelet Production

Idiopathic Thrombocytopenic Purpura

Definition and Incidence. Idiopathic thrombocytopenic purpura (ITP), a bleeding disorder, is characterized by the sudden onset of petechiae, purpura, and bleeding in an otherwise healthy child. Often, there is a history of a recent viral illness. The peripheral platelet count is low (less than 20,000/mm³), whereas there are normal to increased numbers of megakaryocytes. There is no associated anemia or leukopenia.

This usually benign bleeding disorder occurs most often in children younger than 10 years of age. Most cases occur between the ages of 2 and 5 years. The incidence seems to be more common in white children, with both sexes affected equally. This increased incidence in fair-skinned children may be related to the difficulty of diagnosing purpura in dark-skinned children. ITP happens suddenly and presents a dramatic clinical picture. However, 90% of children affected have a complete spontaneous recovery within 6 months without receiving any treatment. The other 10% develop chronic ITP requiring treatment to sustain adequate platelet counts.

Etiology and Pathophysiology. The etiology of ITP is unclear. In the 1980s, research demonstrated an immune basis for the bleeding disorder, but the specific mechanism of disease has not been pinpointed. The current idea of etiology is one of an antigen–antibody complex that alters the platelet membrane, resulting in removal of defective platelets from the peripheral circulation. Because the researchers have narrowed the cause to an immune one, some of the recent literature refers to idiopathic thrombocytopenic purpura as immune thrombocytopenic purpura.

The characteristic bleeding of ITP is caused by some undefined mechanism that suddenly destroys the circulating platelets by sequestration within the reticuloendothelial system, usually the spleen. Current technology has demonstrated the presence of platelet-associated IgG (PAIgG) in children with ITP. Although the specific site and character of the platelet-associated IgG are undetermined, it is recognized that the PAIgG level correlates with the degree of thrombocytopenia (i.e., the greater the level of PAIgG, the greater the thrombocytopenia). Although the incidence of intracranial hemorrhage is only 1% of those affected with ITP, this rare complication merits rigorous observation of the affected child.

Clinical Manifestations. The child with idiopathic thrombocytopenia purpura presents with petechiae, purpura, and bleeding. The complete blood count (CBC) demonstrates abnormally low platelets ($<20,000/mm^3$) but normal red cell and white cell indices. The child does not act ill, but the extensive nature of the petechiae, purpura, and bleeding causes alarm for all who see the child. The history usually reveals a recent viral illness.

Diagnostic Studies. It is necessary to define the level of risk for intracranial bleeding in the child suspected of having ITP. An initial CBC with platelet count provides information about all the hematologic lines. A platelet count less than $20,000/mm^3$ merits restriction of activity associated with potential trauma and elimination of all drugs that affect platelet function (e.g., aspirin and aspirin products coated to protect the GI tract).

With newer techniques, one is able to obtain platelet indices that can differentiate ITP from acute leukemia and aplastic anemia. Table 44-8 lists these differentiations. The mean platelet volume (MPV) is like the mean corpuscular volume used for red cells. The MPV rises when there are increased numbers of young platelets in the circulation, as is the case in ITP. The platelet distribution width (PDW) denotes the variability of platelet size. A

TABLE 44-8
Platelet Indices Differentiating Idiopathic Thrombocytopenic Purpura (ITP)

	Acute Leukemia	Aplastic Anemia	ITP
Platelet count	Decreased	Decreased	Decreased
Mean platelet volume (MPV)	Normal	Normal	Increased
Platelet distribution width (PDW)	Normal	Normal	Increased

wide variation of sizes causes the PDW to increase, whereas a population of uniformly sized platelets would cause the PDW to decrease. One would see an increase of the PDW in ITP because of the wide variety in sizes of platelets released into the circulation. The platelet indices provide confirmation of a clinical diagnosis of ITP and do not constitute diagnostic information in and of themselves.

Examination of a bone marrow aspirate is necessary to rule out the possibility of leukemia, neuroblastoma, or lymphoma, conditions that can be confused with ITP. In the adolescent with ITP, it is necessary to rule out the possibility of systemic lupus erythematosus. It is necessary to have the information from the bone marrow aspirate before beginning any steroid therapy.

★ **ASSESSMENT**

Initially, the nurse determines if the bleeding is massive enough to constitute an emergency. If so, appropriate emergency action should be taken. If the bleeding does not constitute an emergency, the nurse can assess the child at a more leisurely pace. The nursing assessment should include historic information, with particular attention to recent illnesses and family history of immune disorders.

★ **NURSING DIAGNOSES AND PLANNING**

Based on the assessment data from above and Chapter 43, the following nursing diagnoses may apply to the child with ITP:

- Fear related to medical procedures and side-effects.
- Anxiety related to life-threatening condition.
- High Risk for Injury (Bleeding) related to low platelet count.
- Activity Intolerance related to need for bedrest.
- Body Image Disturbance related to side-effects of medication.
- Knowledge Deficit regarding disease process, thrombocytopenia risks, and precautions.

The nurse, child, and parents together plan effective care based on the established nursing diagnoses. Several examples of expected outcomes follow:

- The child plays with medical equipment involved in procedures.
- The child and parents verbalize concerns related to possibility of death.

- The child resumes some activities as platelet count rises.
- The adolescent discusses side-effects of drugs that are not permanent.
- The child and family describe thrombocytopenia precautions and rationale.

The nurse plans for the daily care of the child based on both doctor's orders and nursing diagnoses. A general nursing care goal may be the following:

- Serious injury is prevented.

★ INTERVENTIONS: COLLABORATIVE AND INDEPENDENT

The treatment goal of ITP is the restoration of normal platelet counts so that bleeding does not occur. This is accomplished pharmacologically with corticosteroids. If the ITP is resistant, IV IgG can be used, as well as splenectomy. The major concerns for the family are protection of their child from trauma and further bleeding and the adjustment of all involved with an acute illness. The sample Nursing Care Plan presents care of a child with ITP.

TEACHING

Parents are usually upset because of the dramatic and sudden nature of ITP. Therefore, they should be given as much information as possible. Although a diagnosis of ITP cannot be established immediately, when the health care team is reasonably certain of the diagnosis, the parents need to know the usual benign course of this bleeding disorder.

Because the most serious complication of ITP is intracranial hemorrhage, the child and parents should receive instruction regarding the symptoms signaling such an event. Of particular importance are headache, neurologic signs, altered consciousness, and seizure, any of which should be investigated by the health care team for underlying cause. Also affected with the bleeding of ITP can be other organ systems such as pulmonary, GI, and genitourinary (GU). The nurse should teach parents to recognize signs of bleeding from these systems (e.g., coughing up blood, bloody urine and stools).

MEDICATION THERAPY

There is controversy in the health literature about the efficacy of steroid therapy in ITP. Prednisone at doses of 1 to 2 mg/kg/day for 2 to 3 weeks causes a rise in the platelet count, but the risks of prednisone therapy in young children are certainly a deterrent. Literature on ITP suggests that the increased platelet count induced with prednisone does not lessen the risk of intracranial hemorrhage nor does the prednisone shorten the course of the disorder. Prednisone therapy, however, does allow the child to engage in activities that would be prohibited if the platelet count remained below 20,000/mm³. Eighty to ninety percent of children with ITP experience thrombocytopenia for 3 weeks. Those children who remain thrombocytopenic after 6 months from diagnosis are among the 10% who have chronic ITP.

The children with chronic ITP pose a therapeutic challenge. They must have adequate platelet counts, yet the risks of prolonged prednisone therapy (or resistance to previous courses of prednisone) and the postsplenec-

tomy risk of overwhelming sepsis are prohibitive in young children. The viable option to this therapeutic dilemma is the use of intravenous gammaglobulin (IgG), which achieves a significant rise in the platelet count similar to that seen with prednisone. Effective in those children who have become resistant to the corticosteroid therapy, intravenous IgG is so costly that it is usually reserved for those children who have become resistant to steroids. The intravenous IgG is administered usually in doses of 400 mg/kg for 5 consecutive days. Most often, the child's platelet count rises substantially within 3 to 8 days. Should the child's platelet count fall or an episode of bleeding occur, subsequent doses can be given. This therapy with intravenous IgG can be continued until remission is achieved or splenectomy can be safely performed. If splenectomy is required, the bleeding of ITP is resolved.

It is necessary to emphasize that, although the child with ITP needs serial platelet counts, the clinical condition of the child is more important in determining therapy than are the laboratory values. Children who maintain platelet values greater than 50,000/mm³ without bleeding usually do not need any treatment.

★ EVALUATION

Periodically, the nurse and family evaluate the outcomes of care given. Examples of outcomes for the child and family with ITP were given under planning in this section. Have short-term goals been met? Are long-term goals still realistic?

Wiskott-Aldrich Syndrome

Wiskott-Aldrich syndrome is an X-linked, recessively transmitted bleeding disorder characterized by thrombocytopenia, eczema, and heightened susceptibility to infection. The specific underlying etiology is unclear; however, there is a structural defect in the circulating platelets and a decrease in the function of the T and B cells. Examination of the bone marrow reveals normal to increased numbers of megakaryocytes. However, the platelets released into circulation are defective and have a decreased life span. But, donor platelets transfused into the affected person have a normal life span, a phenomenon that suggests a platelet defect.

The children affected with Wiskott-Aldrich syndrome usually present during infancy with bloody diarrhea or hemorrhage. The immunologic studies reveal markedly elevated serum levels of IgA and IgE, but decreased serum levels of IgM. The function of T and B cells is reduced, but not as dramatically as seen in combined immunodeficiency disease. The affected child is unable to produce appropriate antibodies, and the function of T and B cells deteriorates over time.

Treatment with transfer factor has been encouraging because it raises the platelet count. Transfer factor, a factor present in lymphocytes and sensitized to particular antigens, can be administered to unsensitized people. There are a few cases in which bone marrow transplantation has been successful. Steroids and splenectomy have no beneficial effect on the syndrome. Children affected with Wiskott-Aldrich syndrome usually die before the age of 10. Most often, the terminal event is either a hemorrhage or an overwhelming infection.

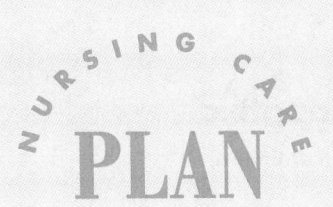

A 4-Year-Old Child With Idiopathic Thrombocytopenic Purpura

Assessment

Case Study Description

Michelle, a white female, is 4 years of age. She lives with both parents and three siblings, ages 5, 9, 12. Both her mother and father work, so Michelle goes to a day care center. All other siblings are in school.

Her growth and development have been normal, and she has achieved all developmental milestones. According to her pediatrician's records, all her immunizations are up to date. She has no known allergies and has never been hospitalized. Michelle has had frequent ear infections but has not had one in over a year. About a week ago, she had an upper respiratory infection.

This morning, Michelle woke up, ate breakfast, and dressed herself. Dad dropped her off at the day care center at 7:30 AM. Around 10:00 AM, her teacher noticed Michelle had several bruises. She asked her if she had fallen or if someone had pushed her. Michelle had no idea where she got the bruises and stated she felt fine. Michelle's teacher decided to call her mother and tell her about the situation. Her mother was concerned and told the teacher to keep an eye on her.

As the day went on, Michelle developed more bruises and had some pinpoint purplish spots all over her body. At 1:30 PM, Michelle's teacher called her mother and told her she should come and pick her up. Michelle's mother brought her to the emergency room at the hospital.

Assessment Data

Four-year-old white female with multiple bruises. Mother states she was fine this morning and has no history of trauma. Michelle has not taken any medications and has no known allergies.

Gen: Active child in no apparent distress. Multiple bruises, petechiae, and crusted blood at both nares.

Vital signs: Temperature 37.6 p.o. Heart rate 116. Respirations 18. Blood pressure not done. Physical examination is normal except for purpuric lesions ranging from pinpoint to large ecchymoses over the entire body.

Laboratory data:

CBC–WBC 6.5   S70
    Hb 13.3   B1
    Hct 38.5   M2
    Plt ct 2000   L20

Bone Marrow Aspiration: Increased number of megakarocytes. Consistent with idiopathic thrombocytopenia purpura.

Nursing Diagnosis	Intervention	Rationale
1. Fear and anxiety related to medical procedures, potentially life-threatening condition, side-effects of treatment	Explain disease process and relate information regarding planned treatment.	Family fears and anxieties can be decreased when explanation of disease, its treatment, and outcomes are given.
Supporting Data: • Rapid progression of condition • Parents alarm at bleeding • Family indicates its lack of knowledge of ITP	Describe all procedures, allow child to play with medical equipment.	Explanation of all procedures before performing them helps decrease anxiety related to unfamiliar procedures. Therapeutic play can allow the child to express fears and potential misconceptions regarding medical procedures.
	Allow time for patient and family to discuss their fears. Encourage open and	

(Continued)

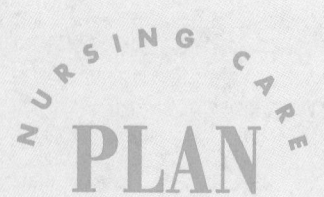

A 4-Year-Old Child With Idiopathic Thrombocytopenic Purpura (continued)

Nursing Diagnosis	Intervention	Rationale
	honest communication within the family.	Use of active listening and supportive counseling enables parents and child to express fears and concerns, thereby helping them to resolve conflicts.
2. High risk for injury related to low platelet count Supporting Data: • Platelet count—2000 • Multiple bruises • Petechiae	Monitor vital signs, heme test urine/stool/emesis. Hold pressure over puncture sites for 5 min.	Assessment for internal bleeding
	Do not use rectal temps or blood pressure cuffs.	Rectal temps may cause mucosal bleeding. Blood pressure cuffs may cause soft tissue injuries.
	Administer medications as prescribed.	Medications administered on time help decrease disease process.
	Pad child's bed rails, arm/leg joints.	Protection from injury decreases bleeding episodes.
3. Activity intolerance related to need for bedrest Supporting Data: • Platelet count—2000	Child must be placed on bedrest until platelet count > 10,000.	Limiting patient's activity lessens risk of spontaneous bleeds.
	Minimal activity with platelet count > 20,000–100,000.	Child up for short distances will foster independence.
	No IM medications with platelet count < 50,000.	Prohibiting IM medications decreases bleeding into the muscle.
	No strenuous exercise until disease state has resolved.	The less activity the less chance for potential injury.
4. Body image disturbance related to bruises and side-effects of medications	Educate child/adolescent that disease usually subsides within a few months. Side-effects from drugs are not permanent.	Adolescents especially are often concerned with alteration in body appearance.
5. Knowledge deficit regarding disease process and thrombocytopenia risks and precautions.	Provide written and verbal communication regarding ITP and recommended treatment.	Parents and children often are too anxious to absorb initial verbal communication.
	Provide written and verbal communication regarding thrombocytopenia precautions to be used at home.	Parents need security of knowing how to reach medical team if necessary.

Evaluation

- The child and family express normal emotions concerning the disease, treatment, and side-effects.
- The child exhibits no further signs of serious injury.
- The child verbalizes understanding of the temporary condition of bruising.
- The child and family describe thrombocytopenia precautions and rationale for each.
- The child resumes normal activities after recovery from disease.

Nursing Implications. The nursing role with children with Wiskott-Aldrich syndrome is one of support for a catastrophic disease. The episodic nature of the syndrome means that the child and caretakers are well acquainted with the working of the health care system. In addition, the cyclic process of the syndrome can create an emotional and spiritual roller coaster for all involved. Assistance with the emotional and spiritual issues can be coordinated by the nurse. Identification of the family's needs combined with referral to specific resources in the hospital and community enhances the manner in which the family copes with this catastrophic disease. The emotional and spiritual care of the child and the family is of utmost importance. The nurse's interventions for emotional and spiritual issues should be tailored to the developmental stage of the child as well as the functional level of the family.

Disorders of Platelet Maturation

Schönlein-Henoch Syndrome (Anaphylactoid Purpura)

Schönlein-Henoch syndrome is a nonthrombocytopenic purpura characterized by vasculitis of the small vessels in the skin causing a distinctive rash and involvement of the renal and GI systems and joints. Although the etiology of the syndrome is unknown, it is not rare. It is seen more often in children between the ages of 2 and 8 years and affects boys twice as often as girls. The prognosis is excellent for those with a mild case consisting of purpuric rash and arthritis. The usual duration is only a few days. Children with more severe cases may be ill for 4 to 6 weeks, and those with extreme cases may have smoldering symptoms for up to a year.

Clinically, the child with Schönlein-Henoch syndrome may present with a distinctive rash. This nonpuritic rash has a centrifugal distribution primarily on the legs and sometimes the buttocks. Many times the rash is a purpura and matures, as do ecchymoses (red to purple to rust, then fading to normal skin color). Two thirds of the children with the syndrome have arthritis in the large joints. The swelling, tenderness, and pain with motion usually resolve spontaneously within a few days of the syndrome's onset, but some children experience recurrent joint pain during the course of the syndrome. Renal involvement demonstrates a mild azotemia (increased urea in the blood) and hypertension. The potential for chronic renal disease is the most serious complication of Schönlein-Henoch syndrome. Sometimes the purpuric rash can be confused with that of septicemia or early meningococcemia. Blood cultures using blood expressed from the lesions differentiate the two. Schönlein-Henoch syndrome has a negative blood culture.

Nursing Implications. Because treatment for Schönlein-Henoch syndrome is symptomatic, comfort measures for swelling, tenderness, and pain of the joints are the symptomatic interventions for the nurse. Monitoring for signs of hypertension and collection of blood specimens for azotemia are additional tasks for the nurse. The nurse should be instrumental in teaching the family how to comfort the child most effectively. Offering instruction and example in the techniques of distraction, massage, imagery, and relaxation can be helpful for the family and child. The nurse should also provide the family with appropriate telephone numbers so that the family can contact the health care team with any questions or concerns.

Disorders of Coagulation

Nursing Interventions for Disorders of Coagulation

Nursing interventions for disorders of coagulation are detailed in Table 44-9. They are caretaker information, minimalization of bleeding episodes, management of bleeding, and psychosocial support.

Teaching. As stated in nursing interventions for disorders of platelet production in Table 44-7, the information that the child and caretaker should receive about the disorders of coagulation are related to the disease process, the therapy plan, access to health care, and activity restrictions.

Prevention of Bleeding Episodes. Minimization of bleeding episodes is another nursing goal. This can be accomplished by teaching the child and caretaker to recognize and avoid situations that invite trauma or accidents. Standard precautions such as use of seat belts and car safety seats should always be taken. Use of protective helmets when bicycling and body shields or pads when playing noncontact sports is essential. Education of caretakers to think critically about activities and their potential for injury can occur through example, role play, written materials, or videos. Talking with other caretakers of children similarly affected provides emotional support as well as information about safety.

Once a deficient coagulation factor is identified, the laboratory can determine the level at which bleeding occurs in each person. Maintaining a factor level greater than the identified bleeding level prevents hemorrhage. Periodic evaluation of the factor level is required in the treatment plan. In some disorders, platelet transfusion is needed to restore hemostasis. In DIC, the paradoxical situation of bleeding and clotting may require both the platelet transfusion to stop bleeding and a simultaneous infusion of heparin to prevent clotting. Each unit of platelets raises the platelet count by $12 \times 1000/m^3$ or 200/kg.

Management of Bleeding. Nursing interventions also involve the effective management of bleeding episodes. If the bleeding episode is an emergency situation (e.g., circulatory shock), the nurse assists in the establishment of an effective airway, insertion of an intravenous line, obtaining ongoing vital signs, insertion of a urinary catheter, collection of needed specimens for ordered laboratory tests, and the administration of ordered medications. The hemorrhage is usually stopped with the replacement of the deficient coagulation factor or by a transfusion of platelets. Success of the interventions is the cessation of bleeding and laboratory values indicating

TABLE 44-9
Nursing Interventions: General Care of Children With Disorders of Coagulation

Goal	Intervention	Evaluation
Inform child and caretaker	*Teaching:*	
	Teach child/caretaker regarding disease process	Appropriate questions are asked and understanding of presented information is evidenced
	Teach child/caretaker regarding therapy plan	
	Teach child/caretaker regarding activity restrictions	
	Teach child/caretaker regarding access to health care	
Minimize bleeding episodes	*Minimize Bleeding:*	
	Teach child/caretaker to recognize and avoid situations inviting trauma or accidents	Number of bleeding episodes are limited Family appropriately accesses health care
	Maintain sufficient levels of deficient coagulation factor	Factor levels > level for bleeding by periodic lab evaluations
	Transfuse with platelets (may need simultaneous infusion of heparin)	Platelet count is normal
Manage bleeding effectively	Stop bleeding by replacing deficient coagulation factor	No further bleeding occurs Factor levels are normal by lab evaluation
	Monitor site of bleeding for resolution (cranium, joint, muscle, abdomen)	Pain and swelling decrease; neurologic exam is stable and normal; vital signs are stable
Provide healthy psychological development	*Psychosocial Support:*	
	Provide age-appropriate developmental experiences	Appropriate developmental milestones are achieved
	Discuss chronic nature of condition and social implications with caretakers and child	Fears, doubts, anger, sadness are expressed normally for situation
	Advise concerning genetic counseling	Appropriate questions are asked of health care personnel.

normal factor levels or platelet counts. The signs and symptoms of bleeding depend on the site of hemorrhage. Equally so are the evidences of bleeding resolution. Hemorrhage within the cranium produces neurologic signs; in the joints and muscles, signs of pain and swelling; and in the abdomen, signs associated with the kidney, urinary, and GI tracts.

Psychological Support. Fostering healthy psychological development is another nursing goal in the care of the child affected with a coagulation disorder. Because of its chronic nature, this is of more importance with hemophilia than with the acute nature of DIC or von Willebrand's disease. Chronic disease requires the family and the child to make adaptations for not only the issues of disease process and treatment, but also for financial, social, emotional, and spiritual issues. The emotions of fear, doubt, anger, and sadness should be addressed. These myriad issues cannot be dealt with in one discussion with the nurse but require ongoing dialogue with the entire health care team. Once particular areas of concern or need are identified, appropriate referrals can be initiated. For example, a teenager may be asking questions about reproductive capacity and the effects of hemophilia on any offspring. Genetic counseling might be helpful in an-

swering these questions. Coordination of these issues and the needed services is a vital role of the nurse. One of the guidelines for assessment of a healthy psychological environment is the achievement of appropriate developmental milestones. Hopefully, the child with a coagulation disorder can accomplish many, if not all, of the normal developmental milestones.

Hemophilias

Definition and Incidence. The hemophilias are X-linked, recessively transmitted bleeding disorders with congenital decreased activity or absence of a coagulation factor in the coagulation cascade. In hemophilia A, the affected factor is factor VIII; in hemophilia B, factor IX is affected. Clinically, hemophilia A and B cannot be differentiated; diagnosticians must rely on laboratory tests specific for factor activity for differentiation. The most common type of hemophilia is hemophilia A; it is also called factor VIII deficiency. The second most common type is hemophilia B, also called factor IX deficiency or Christmas disease. Eighty percent of hemophilias are hemophilia A; 15% are hemophilia B. The designation of Christmas disease resulted from the disease's first docu-

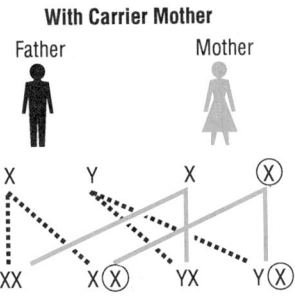

With Carrier Mother

Father   Mother

XX   X(X)   YX   Y(X)

Therefore with each pregnancy,
50% chance of normal coagulation
25% chance of carrier state
25% chance of hemophilia

With Hemophiliac Father

Father   Mother

(X)X   (X)X   YX   YX

Therefore with each pregnancy,
50% chance of normal coagulation
50% chance of carrier state

(X) = *hemophilia gene*

FIGURE 44-6
Genetic transmission of hemophilia.

TABLE 44-10
Classification of Severity of Hemophilia

Severity	Description
Severe form of hemophilia	Factor level less than 1% of normal
Moderate form of hemophilia	Factor level between 1% and 5% of normal
Mild form of hemophilia	Factor level between 5% and 25% of normal
Subclinical form of hemophilia	Factor level between 25% and 50% of normal

mentation in the literature at Christmas 1952, and one of the patients described had the surname of Christmas.

Because hemophilia is an X-linked disorder, it is almost always seen in males. The exceptions would be either the female offspring of a hemophiliac father and carrier mother or a naturally occurring mutation. Figure 44-6 presents a genogram of transmission of hemophilia. The incidence of hemophilia is approximately one case in every 10,000 people.

Pathophysiology.   For adequate coagulation to occur in the body, the levels of factors VIII and IX must be above 50%. Factor levels less than 50% of normal result in changes in the body's ability to stop bleeding. Because there can be varying deficiencies in hemophilia, there is a severity classification system that is based on the factor levels (Table 44-10). Although hemophilia is recognized as a genetic disorder, there is no known cause for hemophilia. It is simply a congenital deficiency. Understanding the coagulation cascade is crucial to understanding the bleeding seen in hemophilia (see Fig. 42-4).

Clinical Manifestations.   Hemophilia A and B are clinically undistinguishable from one another and are discussed together. All clinical manifestations of hemophilia are related to the prolonged bleeding so well known in hemophiliacs. The bleeding may be from an obvious injury, a spontaneous bleeding episode within a joint, or an internal or external bleeding episode that may result in circulatory shock.

The first clinical manifestation of severe hemophilia is bleeding in the neonate, usually from the umbilical cord stump or from a circumcision. In the milder cases, bleeding may not be noticed until the child becomes mobile. At that time, the child exhibits unusual bruises and prolonged bleeding from small injuries or spontaneously from soft tissue.

The most common sites of bleeding in hemophiliacs are the joints. Hemarthroses are painful when they occur. Swelling and pain are present as well as the common consequence of chronic damage to the joint. Bleeding may occur at any other site in the body: soft tissue, intra-

muscular bleeding, intracranial hemorrhage, visceral bleeding, and so forth. The clinical manifestations of the bleeding are dictated somewhat by the location of the bleeding. Hematuria is common.

Diagnostic Studies.   Hemophilia is definitively diagnosed through a specific assay for either factor VIII or factor IX. Before doing the specific assays, several laboratory tests can be helpful in the determination of the diagnosis. The partial thromboplastin time (PTT), which is greatly prolonged in those affected with hemophilia, evaluates the time required for the clotting of plasma, which has been activated when calcium and platelets are added. The normal value is 25 to 40 seconds. Prolongation of the PTT demonstrates a deficiency in any of factors XII, XI, IX, and VIII. The factors are listed according to placement in the coagulation cascade (see Fig. 42-4).

The prothrombin consumption time determines the amount of prothrombin consumed in the coagulation cascade. Normally, the amount of prothrombin in the serum is decreased when compared to plasma. Prothrombin is decreased in serum because it is used during the first part of the coagulation cascade involving factors XII, XI, IX, and VIII. If there is an abnormality in the first part of the coagulation cascade, the prothrombin in the serum is not used and is similar to that contained in the plasma.

In the thromboplastin generation test blood is titrated to determine the specific factor deficiency. The actual test, using a mixture of plasma, serum, and platelets, estimates the time required to form thromboplastin at regular intervals.

If the PTT, the prothrombin consumption time, and thromboplastin generation time are abnormal, a distinction must be made between deficiency of factor VIII and IX. The specific deficiencies can be differentiated by the correction of the abnormal tests. For example, if tests can be corrected with normal plasma adsorbed with barium sulfate, but not with serum, factor VIII is deficient. If the tests can be corrected with serum, but not with plasma, factor IX is deficient. Knowing that normal plasma absorbed with barium sulfate retains factors VIII and XI, whereas normal serum contains factors XI and IX is helpful. Therefore, how the abnormal tests are corrected is crucial information in the determination of specific factor deficiencies. In addition to these tests, the laboratory can determine the activity levels of individual factors with specific assays.

★ **ASSESSMENT**

In almost all cases of hemophilia, there is a history of prolonged bleeding and easy bruisability. As well, there may be a family history of hemophilia or other bleeding disorder. The nurse's careful and complete questions illuminate important information. Depending on the severity of the bleeding, the nurse examines the child and makes an assessment about the critical nature of the situation. If the situation is not critical, time can be spent in the examination of the child and answering the caretakers' questions and concerns.

The diagnostic evaluation for hemophilia involves a battery of blood tests, for which the nurse must prepare the child and family. The nurse must consider the critical nature of the situation, the developmental level of the child, and the anxiety and knowledge levels of the parents.

★ **NURSING DIAGNOSES AND PLANNING**

Based on the assessment data from above and Chapter 43, the following nursing diagnoses may apply to the child with hemophilia:

- Anxiety related to threat to health status.
- Pain related to bleeding episodes.
- Activity Intolerance related to possible bleeding episodes.
- Powerlessness related to bleeding episodes.
- Hopelessness related to chronic nature of disease.
- Social Isolation related to inability to engage in physical activity.
- Fear related to probable financial burden.
- Knowledge Deficit regarding cause and treatment of disease and signs of bleeding episodes.

The nurse, child, and parents together plan effective care based on the established nursing diagnoses. Several examples of expected outcomes follow:

- The caretaker identifies prevention of and signs of bleeding episodes with appropriate steps to be taken.
- The child and parents express their feelings of powerlessness and hopelessness.
- The child participates in quiet activities with siblings and friends.
- The child verbalizes relief during painful episode.
- The family contacts a local hemophilia organization for support.

The nurse plans for the daily care of the child based on both doctor's orders and nursing diagnoses. Some general nursing care goals may be the following:

- Number of bleeding episodes reduced.
- Blood factors are delivered safely.

★ **INTERVENTIONS: COLLABORATIVE AND INDEPENDENT**

There is no method to correct the underlying congenital deficiency of hemophilia. The goal of treatment for hemophilia is the minimization of bleeding episodes and of residual effects by appropriate action when the bleeding episodes do occur.

ADMINISTRATION OF BLOOD PRODUCTS

Administration of the deficient factor from a variety of sources is the medical treatment of choice. Although the treatment of choice has been the administration of purified factor concentrates, in the mid-1980s the incidence of AIDS in hemophiliac patients was traced to factor concentrates, which are commercially prepared by extracting the specific factor from large volumes of human plasma (2000 to 25,000 donors). Because the severely affected hemophiliac could require two doses of the deficient factor each week, it is possible that the hemophiliac could be exposed to as many as 300,000 donors each year.[12] The risk of contacting AIDS and hepatitis became greatly increased because of the increased exposure.

Because of improved quality assurance programs and more stringent laboratory controls, since 1986 the factor concentrates have been free of HIV, the virus causing AIDS. However, this heat-treated concentrate still can infect the recipient with hepatitis. A newer, more expensive (four times) product is reported to be free of the risk of hepatitis. Other treatment options are fresh plasma, fresh-frozen plasma, cryoprecipitate, and cryoprecipitate concentrates. Arginine desmopressin (DDAVP) is also a therapeutic option for mild bleeding. With the new techniques of recombinant DNA, the production of specific factors at affordable prices will be possiblle in the near future. Each of the sources of coagulation factor has varying concentrations of the desired factor. The dosage depends on the severity of the bleeding and the chosen source. Table 44-11 lists the activity of the factor required to stop the bleeding at various sites.[28] The nursing interventions for the specific factor therapy are detailed in the earlier display related to Administration of Blood Products.

PSYCHOSOCIAL SUPPORT

The child and family affected with hemophilia need the attention that all children and families need when faced with the reality of a chronic illness. There are financial, emotional, physical, spiritual, and intellectual burdens that must be borne. The nurse's assessment of the family's needs and receptiveness is crucial in initiation of appropriate instruction as well as in referrals to financial aid, social work, school, marriage and family counselors, and pastoral care.

TABLE 44-11
Factor Level Required to Stop Bleeding

Site	Factor Level	Treatment Duration
Joints	10%–20%	2 days
Muscle or tissue	10%–20%	2–3 days
Iliopsoas muscle, calf, or under-arm musculature	30%	3–5 days
Mouth, tooth extraction, minor surgery	30%	5 days
Intracranial, intrathoracic and GI, fractures	30%–50%	4–14 days
Major operations	>50%	2–3 weeks

Often the child with hemophilia feels isolated because of the illness and may, in fact, be isolated. The necessary limitation of activities associated with trauma and the days missed from school because of hemarthoses and clinic visits all contribute to actual isolation for the child. The isolation can result in poor performance in school, immature attitudes toward peers, hopelessness, and despair. An awareness of these common events can be helpful in minimizing their deleterious effects. The nurse must also recognize the stress with which the other people in the family are dealing. Depending on the individual nurse's expertise, the nurse can be helpful in working through some of these challenging areas. In other instances, it is more appropriate to initiate referrals for the family. The National Hemophilia Foundation offers a variety of services and information for the child and the family. The nurse should strongly encourage the family to contact this organization as a source of information and support. The address was given earlier in this chapter.

TEACHING

After the diagnosis has been confirmed, the nurse plays an important role in educating the family about hemophilia and its effects on their lives. Initially, the teaching should be focused on the physical care of the child. The caretaker must know the signs of bleeding and the appropriate action to initiate should bleeding occur. Administration of the deficient factor can always be accomplished at the hospital/hemophilia clinic. However, because some of the affected children do not live close to the facility, home administration is another means to accomplish treatment. Home administration of medication means that the caregiver and later the affected child must know the safe procedures for reconstitution and intravenous administration of the deficient coagulation factor. Effective instruction regarding the procedure, as well as discussion of channels of communication for the family, are crucial for the success of home treatment. Concerns of the family and child with hemophilia are addressed in the accompanying Teaching Plan.

★ EVALUATION

Periodically, the nurse and family evaluate the outcomes of care given. Examples of outcomes for the child and family with hemophilia were given under planning in this section. Have short-term goals been met? Are long-term goals still realistic? Planning for further nursing care takes into consideration complications.

COMPLICATIONS

The complications of hemophilia are related either to bleeding episodes or to the chronic nature of the disease. The most common physical complication is a result of hemarthoses, which causes irreversible damage to the structures allowing mobility. The ideal management is prevention of hemarthroses. The second choice is to minimize the extent of bleeding. And, finally, if mobility is sufficiently impaired, surgical correction in the damaged joint is a last resort. The risk of intracranial hemorrhage is small, but the morbidity is high. All caretakers must be informed of the signs and symptoms of such an event.

Another physical complication of hemophilia is a direct result of the therapy—infectious diseases transmitted through the therapy. Limited to human donors, the sources of coagulation factors have become contaminated with the viruses causing hepatitis and AIDS. Because there has been a major offensive in the laboratories processing donated blood and those preparing factor concentrates to eliminate the risk of transmitting infectious diseases, the blood and its by-products are much safer today. This is of little comfort for those already exposed to the life-threatening diseases. As research continues, safer and more effective sources of coagulation factors will be available to those in need.

Von Willebrand's Disease

Von Willebrand's disease is a dominantly transmitted bleeding disorder characterized by decreased adhesiveness of platelets. Children affected with von Willebrand's disease usually are concurrently affected with immune disorders. The incidence is uncertain, but estimates are that there is approximately one case of von Willebrand's disease to every two or three cases of hemophilia A and B combined.

The etiology of von Willebrand's disease is complex because the affected child has decreased factor VIII (sometimes factor IX) but does not have the classic bleeding of hemophilia. The cause of this discrepancy between von Willebrand's disease and hemophilia is the structure of the factor VIII molecule, which is composed of two major parts. The low-molecular-weight component contains the coagulating properties. The high-molecular-weight component contains three subgroups: (1) the factor VIII antigen, (2) the von Willebrand factor, and (3) the ristocetin cofactor. In von Willebrand's disease, the von Willebrand factor is missing or decreased. The von Willebrand factor, responsible for causing the platelets to adhere to the small vessel walls maintaining hemostasis, acts as an intercellular glue, attaching platelets to the exposed subendothelium of the small vessels.[8] The platelets are normal, but they are restricted in their function. In some cases of von Willebrand's disease, there are deficiencies in all three subgroups of the high-molecular-weight component of factor VIII.

The child with von Willebrand's disease usually presents early in childhood with a bleeding episode from the skin or mucous membranes. The child may also have bleeding from the GI tract or the nose, after dental work, or from minor surgery. The disease's intensity lessens with age.

The partial thromboplastin time is prolonged in this condition as in hemophilia. The bleeding time is elevated in von Willebrand's disease but is normal in hemophilia. Other specific and highly specialized laboratory tests to evaluate the levels of the various parts of the factor VIII molecule can be helpful in strengthening the diagnosis, but the PTT and bleeding time can provide almost definitive results.

Nursing Implications. The goal of therapy in von Willebrand's disease is the restoration of normal platelet function by replacement of the deficient component of the factor VIII molecule. Any blood fraction containing

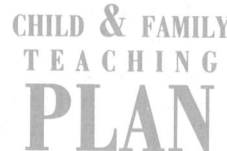

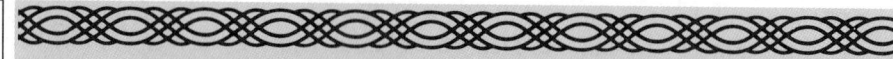

Concerns Related to Hemophilia

Assessment

Peter, a 5-year-old boy, has been diagnosed with mild hemophilia A after a lingering bruise to the left shoulder.

This is the only child for these parents. Family live near paternal grandparents in a modest, suburban, three-bedroom home. Insurance through father's employer will cover the majority of the inpatient expenses and a small part of the medications and outpatient expenses. Both parents completed high school. The mother is the primary caretaker, but had begun to share after-school care of the boy with the nearby paternal grandparents. The father is interested, but works 15 hours a day and is not readily available on weekdays.

Parents identified that they do not know anyone with hemophilia and are not sure what will happen to Peter. The nursing diagnosis, Health maintenance, altered, related to a knowledge deficit regarding hemophilia, was made.

Child and Family Objectives	Specific Content	Teaching Strategies
1. Identify the reason for bleeding in hemophilia.	1. Explain the network of coagulation factors that produce hemostasis and the effect of the deficient factor on bleeding.	1. Use diagrams, charts, or figures of the coagulation cascade.
2. Exhibit an understanding of the treatment plan for hemophilia.	2. Explain the levels of factor availability. Describe the serial collection of blood samples to verify factor concentration. Discuss the sequence of the collections. Describe the procedures that will be used in the treatment. Answer all questions about disease and treatment. Describe and explain all these issues with Peter on an age-appropriate level. Enlist Peter's cooperation.	2. Use chart of factor levels. Show specific tubes used for collection. If interested, show lab where assays are performed. Encourage questions and allow enough quiet time with parents so that they are able to ask questions comfortably. The school-age child needs factual information about the disease and its treatment so that he can cooperate.
3. Identify activities that would be hazardous if factor level is low.	3. Situations that could pose a bleeding threat. Discuss parameters set by physician for activity restrictions.	3. Encourage child and caretakers to think about their neighborhood, home, and play areas. Role play how the child will react to imposed restrictions.
4. Prepare for bleeding episode.	4. Management of bleeding episode. Signs and symptoms of bleeding. Signs of emergency bleeding. Change in sensorium, blurred vision, racing pulse or heart, seizures.	4. Use list of community telephone numbers. Role play situations at school, home, and neighbors' homes. Chart of signs and symptoms handout. Use check-list.

(Continued)

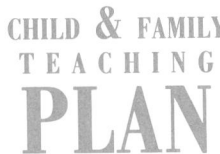

CHILD & FAMILY TEACHING PLAN

Concerns Related to Hemophilia (continued)

Child and Family Objectives	Specific Content	Teaching Strategies
5. Verbalize feelings related to chronic nature of hemophilia.	5. Caretakers discuss feelings of disappointment, fear, stigma, anger, sadness.	5. Encourage openness.
	Child discusses similar feelings.	Use separate sessions. May employ puppets, drawings, or clay.

Evaluation

- The child and caretakers identify the reason for bleeding in hemophilia and describe the disease process.
- The child and caretakers discuss the treatment plan for hemophilia.
- The child and caretakers explain activity restrictions based on factor level parameters set by physician.
- The child and caretakers identify situations with high potential for trauma and accidents.
- The child and caretakers formulate a plan for avoiding situations that place child at risk for injury.
- The child and caretakers verbalize plan and actions in the event of a bleeding episode.

---

the needed component can be used in treating von Willebrand's disease. The options include fresh-frozen plasma, cryoprecipitate, and some factor VIII concentrates (the highly purified forms are not helpful). These options are useful, but the risks of transmitting bloodborne diseases and of inducing immunologic abnormalities must be considered. The increased commercial availability of heat-treated blood fractions has reduced the risk of transmission of diseases.

Another treatment option for these children is 1-desamino-8-D-arginine vasopressin, more commonly known as desmopressin or DDAVP. DDAVP can temporarily correct the bleeding defect by causing the release of endogenous procoagulant factor VIII and von Willebrand factor. This treatment option should be used as the treatment of choice because of its effectiveness and its lack of risk in transmitting other diseases.

Disseminated Intravascular Coagulation (DIC)

Disseminated intravascular coagulation (DIC) is a complex disorder involving thrombosis and bleeding. DIC occurs as a result of endothelial injury, which can be caused by any noxious stimuli. Some of the more common causes in children are anoxia, hypotension, endotoxins, antigen–antibody complexes, tumor by-products, and viruses.

DIC is usually an acute complication of another pathologic condition. Several conditions that predispose a patient to DIC are shock, sepsis, obstetric complications, acute leukemia, acute nonlymphocytic leukemia, disseminated malignancies, massive trauma, and giant hemangiomas.

The pathophysiology of disseminated intravascular coagulation begins with the endothelial injury by the noxious stimuli (Fig. 44-7). The endothelial injury results in the release of tissue factor and the subsequent activation of the extrinsic coagulation cascade (see Fig. 42-4). The endothelial injury also exposes the collagen of the vessel with the subsequent activation of the intrinsic coagulation cascade. These two events occur in such rapid succession that there is a depletion of the coagulation factors as well as depletion of platelets. In addition to the activation of the intrinsic and extrinsic coagulation cascades, the endothelial injury causes plasminogen activator release resulting in fibrinolysis. DIC is sometimes confusing because the endothelial injury causes clotting (through the activation of both coagulation cascades) as well as bleeding (through the process of fibrinolysis).

As the coagulation cascades are activated, fibrin is generated and deposited in the small vessels. The deposition of the fibrin in the small vessels can cause thrombosis and jeopardize tissue viability distal to the thrombos. The rapid utilization of coagulation factors and platelets creates a situation in which the patient is prone to bleeding. In addition, the deposition of fibrin activates the normal fibrinolytic response, which exacerbates the hemorrhagic process.

Disseminated intravascular coagulation is sometimes

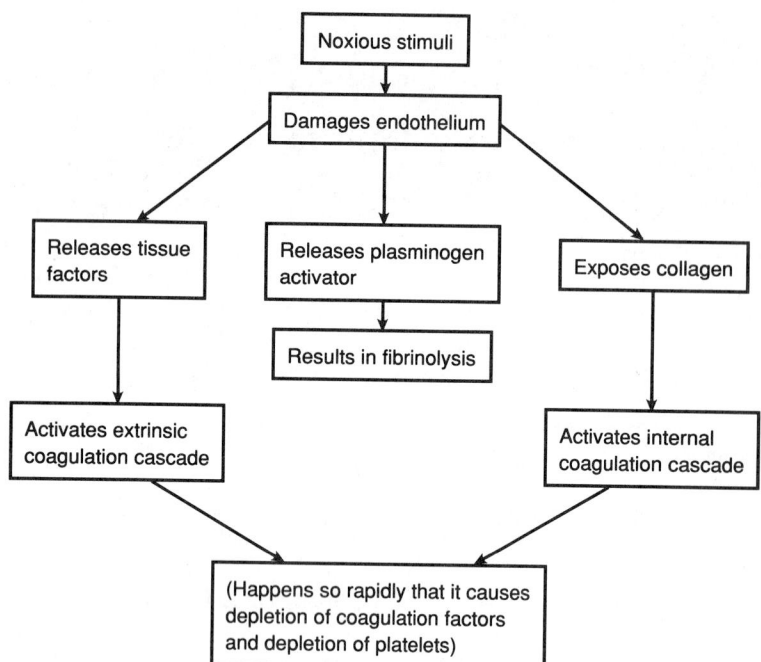

FIGURE 44-7

Summary of pathologic track of disseminated intravascular coagulation. The endothelial injury causes both clotting (through coagulation cascades) and bleeding (through fibrinolysis).

evident because of the multiple thromboses; in other patients, it is evident because of overwhelming bleeding. The manifestations are varied in intensity. However, the cardinal signs of DIC are coagulation factor depletion, thrombocytopenia, and fibrinolysis.

The laboratory values in DIC are congruent with depletion of coagulation factors and platelets. The prothrombin time is prolonged. The platelets are reduced. The fibrinogen is reduced usually to less than 100 mg/dL, and the fibrin degradation products are markedly elevated.

Nursing Implications. The goal of treatment in disseminated intravascular coagulation is the maintenance of intravascular volume and tissue oxygenation. RBCs are required for tissue oxygenation, and volume replacement is frequently required to maintain volume. Although the goal of maintaining volume and oxygenation is readily accepted, there is much controversy over the administration of coagulation products and anticoagulants. Each patient must be evaluated individually, and the benefits and risks of either therapy must be weighed carefully.

The generation of thrombin with its resulting coagulation factor and platelet depletion must be halted. In addition, the depleted coagulation factors need to be restored. If the source of bleeding cannot be quickly identified or requires time for resolution, such as in the patient with nonlymphocytic leukemia, the treatment of choice is as follows. The patient should receive full therapeutic doses of heparin and subsequent transfusions of platelets and fresh-frozen plasma. The heparin stops the continuing thrombosis and intravascular coagulation and the platelets and plasma restore clot-promoting materials for normal hemostasis.

Because DIC is a complex and often frightening disorder, the parents and child are typically alarmed. The nurse should be instrumental in calming all involved with appropriate information. Because DIC is usually a com-

plication of another pathology, the family may need help in separating the two processes. There are many physical tasks for the nurse to perform and monitor in DIC, but there are the important emotional and psychological issues as well. An efficient nurse sets priorities, allowing the safe delivery of treatments and medications as well as the compassionate interaction with the child and the family.

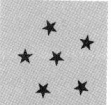

Ideas for Nursing Research

Blood cell changes are seen in many diseases and conditions in children. Nurses need to have an understanding of how such changes affect the care required. Also, some dysfunctions are genetically related. Nursing care of children with hematologic dysfunction can be improved by research. The following areas need to be explored:

- Effects of antibiotics and other medications on normal blood cell counts.
- Common synergistic effect of iron deficiency on permanent changes seen in lead poisoning.
- Effect of teaching programs at diagnosis of sickle cell disease and on social adjustment and prevention of complications.
- Use of intravenous IgG in chronic ITP.
- Development of a prenatal diagnosis for hemophilia.
- Effectiveness of teaching safety measures to parents of children with conditions of decreased platelet counts.
- Side-effects of administration of colony-stimulating factors.

Summary

Grouping disease entities by etiologic factors can simplify and successfully organize hematologic dysfunction. The hematologic trio of RBCs, WBCs, and platelets can further be divided into etiologic categories of production, maturation, and destruction. Such a division is helpful for the nurse and creates a framework for organization of understanding and care. Within this framework, the nurse can identify common interventions for the diseases within a particular subdivision. General nursing interventions for most hematologic diseases are the following: oxygenation; teaching, psychosocial support; restoration of blood cell production, maturation, and life span; prevention of or intervention in bacterial and viral illnesses; and prevention and management of bleeding episodes. Each disease entity has specific medical care and nursing interventions.

References

1. Accardo, P., Whitman, B., Caul, J., & Rolfe, U. (1988, January). Autism and plumbism: A possible association. *Clinical Pediatrics, 27*(1), 41–44.
2. Aldouri, M. A., Wonke, B., Hoffbrand, A. V., et al. (1987). Iron state and hepatic disease in patients with thalassemia major, treated with long term subcutaneous desferrioxamine. *Journal of Clinical Pathology, 40,* 1353–1359.
3. American Academy of Pediatrics, Committee on Environmental Hazards and Committee on Accident and Poison Prevention. (1987). Statement on childhood lead poisoning. *Pediatrics, 79*(3), 457–465.
4. Berkman, S. A., Lee, M. L., & Gale, R. P. (1988, April). Clinical uses of intravenous immunoglobulins. *Seminars in Hematology, 25*(2), 140–152.
5. Bhambhani, K., Inoue, S., & Sarnaik, S. A. (1988, February). Seasonal clustering of transient erythroblastopenia of childhood. *American Journal of Diseases of Children, 142*(2), 175–177.
6. Bickis, U. (1988, January). Lead-induced neuropathy. *American Journal of Public Health, 78*(1), 95.
7. Biller, J. A., & Yeager, A. M. (Eds.). (1981). *The Harriet Lane handbook.* Chicago: Year Book Medical.
8. Burns, E. R. (1987). *Clinical management of bleeding and thrombosis.* Boston: Blackwell Scientific.
9. Bussel, J. B., et al. (1988, January–February). Combined plasma exchange and intravenous gammaglobulin in the treatment of patients with refractory immune thrombocytopenic purpura. *Transfusion, 28*(1), 38–41.
10. Camitta, B. M. (1988, February 6). Criteria for severe aplastic anaemia. *Lancet,* (8580), 3.
10a. Centers for Disease Control (1991). Preventing lead poisoning in young children. Washington, D.C.: U.S. Department of Health and Human Services.
11. Clark, M., Royal, J. & Seeler, R. (1988, February). Interaction of iron deficiency and lead and the hematologic findings in children with severe lead poisoning. *Pediatrics, 81*(2), 247–254.
12. Dugdale, M. (1988, February). Current problems in hemophilia: Consequences of successful therapy. *Journal of the Tennessee Medical Association, 81*(2), 97–100.
13. Dunston, T. (1988, January 9). The problems of diagnosing iron deficiency. *South African Medical Journal, 73*(1), 3–4.
14. Emami, A., et al. (1987, November). Idiopathic thrombocytopenic purpura in children: New therapeutic considerations. *Kansas Medicine, 88*(11), 317–319.
15. Eschleman, M. M. (1983). Introductory nutrition and diet therapy (2nd ed.). Philadelphia: J. B. Lippincott.
16. Finan, A. C., et al. (1988, February). Nutritional factors and growth in children with sickle cell disease. *American Journal of Diseases in Children, 142*(2), 237–240.
17. Fomon, S. J. (1987). Bioavailability of supplemental iron in commercially prepared dry infant cereals. *Journal of Pediatrics 110*(4), 660–661.
18. Hertrampf, E., et al. (1986). Bioavailability of iron in soy-based formula and its effect on iron nutriture in infancy. *Pediatrics, 78*(4), 640–645.
19. Imholz, B., et al. (1988, February). Intravenous immunoglobulin (i.v. IgG) for previously treated acute or for chronic idiopathic thrombocytopenic purpura (ITP) in childhood: A prospective multicenter study. *Blut, 56*(2), 63–68.
20. Jandl, J. H. (1987). *Blood: Textbook of hematology.* Boston: Little, Brown.
21. Junghans, R. P., & Sacher, R. A. (1987). Iron metabolism and hypochromic anemias. In D. H. Pittiglio & R. A. Sacher (Eds.), *Clinical hematology and fundamentals of hemostasis.* Philadelphia: Davis.
22. Kelting, S., & Johnson, C. (1987). Erythropoiesis and neonatal blood transfusions. *MCN: American Journal of Maternal Child Nursing, 12*(3), 172–177.
23. Kuross, S. A., Rank, B. H., & Hebbel, R. P. (1988, April). Excess heme in sickle erythrocyte inside-out membranes: Possible role in thiol oxidation. *Blood, 71*(4), 876–882.
24. Lang, J. M., Amaral, D., Audhuy, B., Barats, J. C., Boilletot, A., & Oberling, F. (1987). High dose intravenous IgG followed by splenectomy versus splenectomy alone in idiopathic thrombocytopenic purpura refractory to steroids. *Nouvell Revue Francaise d'Hematologie, 29*(5), 285–287.
25. Lenarsky, C., Weinberg, K., Guinan, E., et al. (1988, January). Bone marrow transplantation for constitutional pure red cell aplasia. *Blood, 71*(1), 226–229.
26. Mallouh, A. A., & Asha, M. (1988, February). Beneficial effect of blood transfusion in children with sickle cell chest syndrome. *American Journal of Diseases in Children, 142*(2), 178–182.
27. Marty, J. (1987). Aplastic anemia including pure red cell aplasia and congenital dyserythropoietic anemia. In D. H. Pittiglio & R. A. Sacher (Eds.), *Clinical hematology and fundamentals of hemostasis.* Philadelphia: Davis.
28. Matthias, F. R. (1987). Blood coagulation disorders: Hemorrhagic diatheses and thromboembolic diseases. New York: Springer-Verlag.
29. O'Neil-Cutting, M. A., & Crosby, W. H. (1987). Blocking of iron absorption by a preliminary oral dose of iron. *Archives of Internal Medicine, 147,* 489–491.
30. Patterson, K. L. (1985). The childhood anemias. *Pediatrics: Nursing Update, 1*(4), 2–8.
31. Pittiglio, D. H., & Sacher, R. A. (1987). *Clinical hematology and fundamentals of hemostasis,* pp. 52–54. Philadelphia: Davis.
32. Pizarro, F., Amar, M., & Stekel, A. (1987). Determination of iron in stools as a method to monitor consumption of iron fortified products in infants. *American Journal of Clinical Nutrition, 45,* 484–487.
33. Pochedly, C., & May, S. L. (1987). Iron deficiency anemia in children. *American Family Physician, 35*(5), 195–200.
34. Pootrakul, P., Joesphson, B., Huebers, H. A., & Finch, C. A. (1988, April). Quantitation of ferritin iron in plasma, an explanation for nontransferrin iron. *Blood, 71*(4), 1120–1123.
35. Reding, D., & Amare, M. (1988, February). High-dose intravenous gamma globulin therapy for immune thrombocytopenia. *Wisconsin Medical Journal, 87*(2), 11–13.
36. Rees, J. M., Monsen, R. S., & Merrill, R. K. (1985). Iron fortification of infant foods: A decade of change. *Clinical Pediatrics, 24*(12), 707–710.
37. Ricerca, B. M., & Storti, S. (1987). Differentiation of iron defi-

ciency from thalassaemia trait: A new approach. *Haematologica, 72,* 409–413.

38. Rock, G., Tittley, P., & Taylor, J. R. (1988, March). Abnormal platelet von Willebrand factor interaction in patients with TTP. *American Journal of Hematology, 27*(3), 179–183.

39. Rodeghiero, F., Castaman, G., DiBona, E., Ruggeri, M., Lombardi, R. & Mannucci, P. M. (1988, February). Hyperresponsiveness to DDAVP for patients with type I von Willebrand's disease and normal intra-platelet von Willebrand factor. *European Journal of Haematology, 40*(2), 163–167.

40. Rodgers, G. P., Roy, M. S., Noguchi, C. T., & Schechter, A. N. (1988, March). Is there a role for selective vasodilation in the management of sickle cell disease? *Blood, 71*(3), 597–602.

41. Sabio, H., McKie, V. C., & Davis, P. C., Jr. (1987, November). Idiopathic thrombocytopenic purpura in childhood: A current perspective. *Journal of Medical Association of Georgia, 76,* 771–773.

42. Stehr-Green, J. K., Holman, R. C., Jason, J. M. & Evatt, B. L. (1988, April). Hemophilia-associated AIDS in the United States, 1981 to September 1987. *American Journal of Public Health, 78*(4), 439–442.

43. Stekel, A., Olivares, M., Cayazzo, M., Chadud, P., Llaguno, S., & Pizarro, B. F. (1988). Prevention of iron deficiency by milk for-tification. II. A field trial with a full-fat acidified milk. *American Journal of Clinical Nutrition, 47,* 265–269.

44. Takahashi, H., Tatewaki, W., Nagayama, R., et al. (1987). Heat-treated factor VIII/von Willebrand factor concentrate in platelet-type von Willebrand's disease. *Haemostasis, 17*(6), 353–360.

45. Vaughan, V. C., McKay, R. J., & Behrman, R. E. (1979). Nelson textbook of pediatrics (11th ed.). Philadelphia: W. B. Saunders.

46. Wallmark, A., Ljung, R., & Nilsson, I. M. (1987, December). Determination of factor IX allotypes for carrier identification in haemophilia B. *British Journal of Haematology, 67*(4), 427–432.

47. Zeringer, H., & Pittiglio, D. H. (1987). Hemolytic anemias: Intracorpuscular defects; III. The hemoglobinopathies. In D. H. Pittiglio & R. A. Sacher (Eds.), *Clinical hematology and fundamentals of hemostasis.* Philadelphia: Davis.

48. Zipursky, A., Brown, E. J., Watts, J., et al. (1987). Oral vitamin E supplementation for the prevention of anemia in premature infants: A controlled trial. *Pediatrics, 79*(1), 61–68.

49. Declining anemia prevalence among children enrolled in public nutrition and health programs in selected states, 1975–1985. (1986). *Morbidity & Mortality Weekly Report, 35,* 36.

50. Zipursky, A., et al. (1987, January 17). Iron deficiency—Time for a community campaign? *Lancet,* (8525), 141–142.

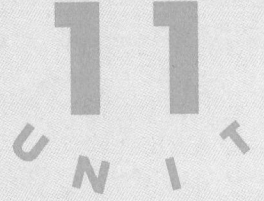

Nursing Care of Children With Altered Renal Function

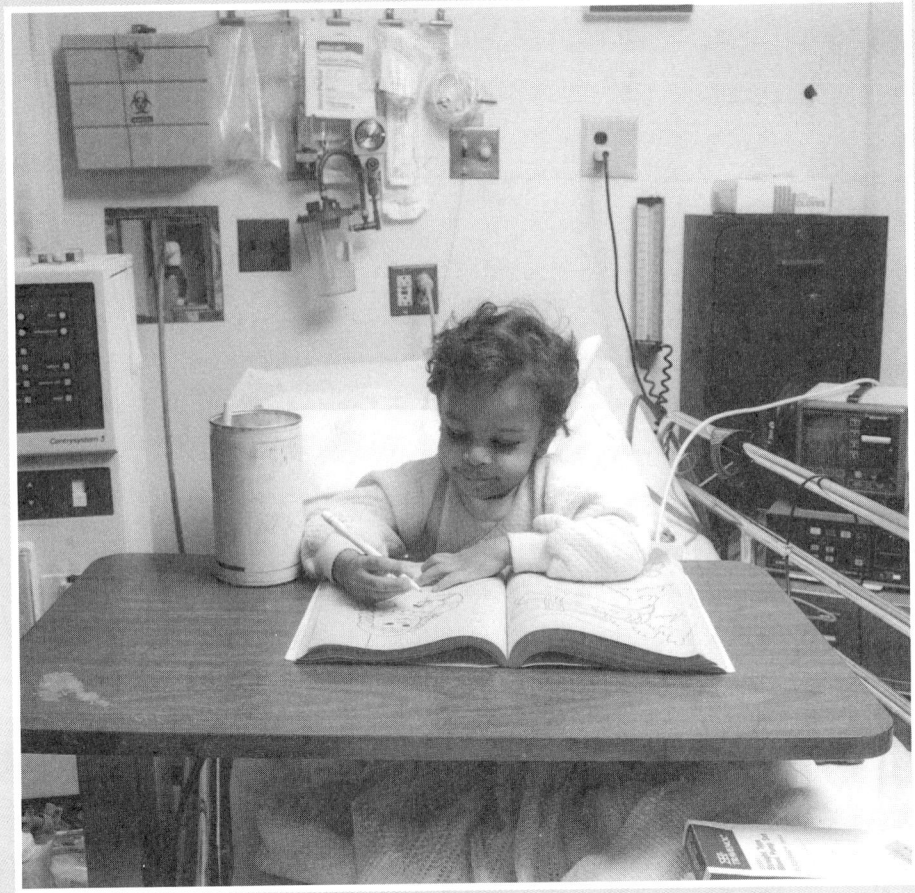

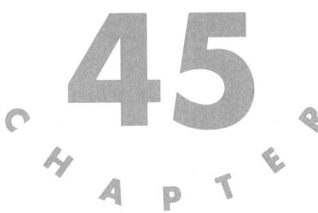

45

C H A P T E R

Anatomy and Physiology of the Renal System

BEHAVIORAL OBJECTIVES

Identify the major anatomic structures of the renal system.

Discuss the three stages of embryonic development of the kidney.

Describe the components of the nephron.

Trace the blood supply through the kidney.

Discuss the kidney's role in maintaining fluid and electrolyte balance.

Identify the metabolic wastes removed by the renal system.

Explain the kidney's role in regulating acid–base balance.

List the major hormones controlled by the renal system.

The kidneys are the major organs of the renal system. These specialized, paired organs are positioned retroperitoneally and are located in front of and to the sides of the vertebral column. They lie between the 12th thoracic and the 3rd lumbar vertebrae. The right kidney is positioned beneath the liver and is usually 1 to 2 cm lower than the left kidney (Fig. 45-1). The size of the kidneys increases with the growth of the child. At full growth, they measure 5 to 7 cm wide, 11 to 13 cm long, and 2.5 cm thick. Each kidney comprises 0.5% of the body's weight at birth and 0.2% at maturity.[8,10–12]

If the surface of the kidneys could be visualized in the newborn, they would appear lobulated. The lobules decrease in number with maturity and vary from one person to another.[8] The kidneys are covered with a strong fibrous capsule composed of connective tissue that becomes the outer covering for the adjacent structures that collect urine.[11] The kidneys are often embedded in a mass of adipose tissue that helps hold them in place.

The hilus of the kidney is the concave fissure along the medial border. From this region, the renal artery and renal vein connect with the abdominal aorta and the inferior vena cava, respectively. The renal pelvis, which funnels urine to the ureter, also connects at the hilus. Likewise, nerves and lymphatics enter and exit the kidney at this site.

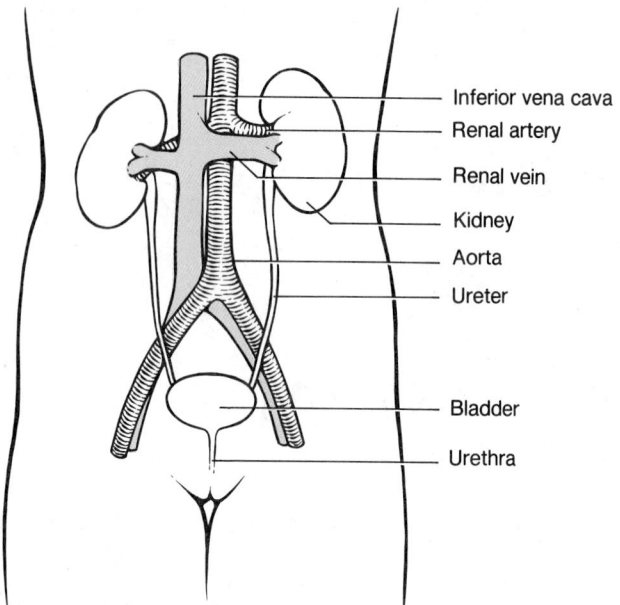

FIGURE 45-1
Organs and accessory structures of the renal system.

Despite this deceptively simple exterior, the renal system is complex. It is responsible for the control and regulation of fluids and waste products. The renal system also plays an important role in electrolyte and acid–base balance, as well as in the production and control of several hormones. The overall functioning of the renal system is critical for maintaining physiologic homeostasis from fetal growth through adult life. By understanding how the renal system functions, the nurse has a clearer understanding of the nursing needs of children with renal disorders.

Embryonic Development

The kidneys develop from the mesoderm, which is a primary germ layer of the embryo. Embryonic development of the renal system occurs sequentially in three overlapping stages: the pronephros, mesonephros, and metanephros. These stages may be considered as progressive differentiation of tissues along a continuum of development (Fig. 45-2).

Pronephros Stage

The pronephros stage begins at the third week of gestation with the appearance of the first renal tubules. Approximately seven pairs of pronephric tubules develop, but as new tubules develop in the posterior region, older tubules in the anterior region degenerate. The pronephric duct evolves from the nephrogenic tissue and eventually becomes the functional excretory duct of the mesonephros.[7,8,10]

Mesonephros Stage

The mesonephros stage begins during the third to fourth week of gestation. Mesonephric tubules arise from

the tissue bed, and each connects laterally to what was originally the pronephric duct but which is called the mesonephric or Wolffian duct. These new ducts empty into the cloaca, which eventually becomes the bladder and rectum.

The earliest nephrons are formed with a primitive Bowman's capsule distinguished at the proximal ends. Along with the development of a complete glomerulus, some of the convoluted tubules can be differentiated during this period. By the 11th to 12th week, the mesonephros regresses and the metanephros development begins.[7,10]

Metanephros Stage

The metanephros stage marks the development of the permanent kidney in humans. From the fifth week of gestation, the ureteral bud grows and divides dorsally. By the 13th week to 14th week, lobular collecting systems are distinguishable in the kidney as they develop from ureteral bud branches.[7,10]

The kidney of a human fetus is able to form urine at 10 to 12 weeks of gestation.[1] Fetal urine is a protein- and sugar-free filtrate of fetal plasma. During the latter stages of pregnancy, fetal urine provides a major source of am-

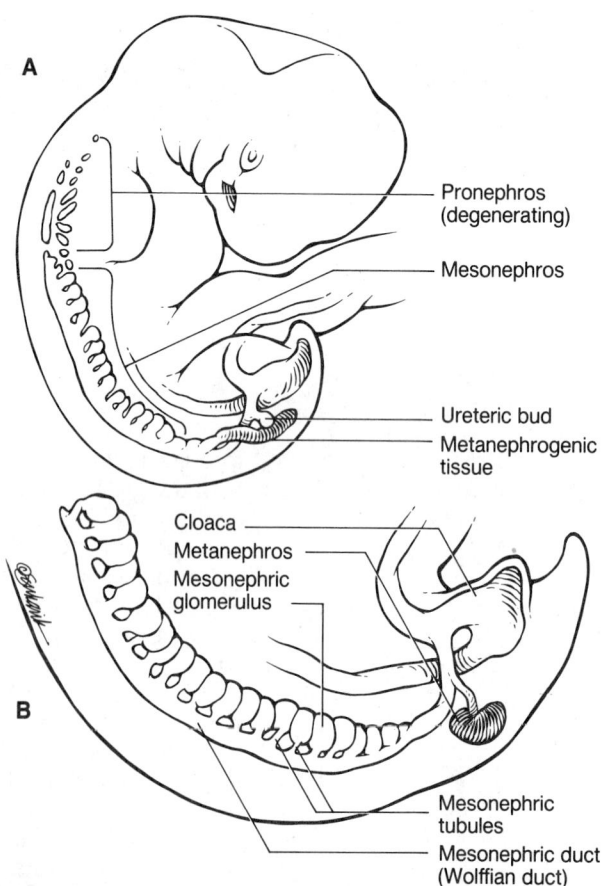

FIGURE 45-2
Embryonic development of the renal system. **(A)** Progressive degeneration of the pronephros and development of the mesonephros and early metanephros stages. **(B)** Enlarged detail shows progression to the later metanephros stage.

TABLE 45-1
Consequences of Abnormal Embryonic Development

Fetal Age Weeks	Structure Formed	Anomalies at Birth
3–4	Pronephros	Renal agenesis
	Mesonephros	Potter's syndrome
5	Beginning of metanephros	Renal agenesis
8–9	Pelvis and ureter developing	Posterior urethral valves
		Multicystic kidneys
	Some functioning nephrons	Dysplastic kidneys
20–22	Clearly demarcated medulla and cortex	Renal hypoplasia
		Polycystic disease
	One third of nephrons formed	Medullary cystic disease

factors including: a decrease in renal vascular resistance, an increase in systemic blood pressure, effective filtration pressure, and an increase in glomerular permeability.[4] The periods when structural and functional maturity occur are addressed in their corresponding sections of this chapter.

Consequences of Abnormal Development

It is difficult to pinpoint precisely abnormal renal development with a specific stage of development because there is much overlapping of these stages. The time frames in Table 45-1 have been speculated by experts in an attempt to determine when suspected teratogenic agents may impair development.[7,12]

Structure and Function

A longitudinal cross section of the kidney reveals three distinct areas of renal structure: the cortex, the medulla, and the pelvis. Anatomic features in these regions are diagrammed in Figure 45-3 and discussed below.

Kidney

Cortex

The outer section of the kidney is known as the cortex; it is approximately 1 cm wide in the mature kidney. The cortex contains 85% of all nephrons and their surrounding blood supply.

niotic fluid. Continuous equilibrium of amniotic fluid is maintained as it is swallowed and reabsorbed by the fetus.

During the 12th to 16th weeks of gestation, the kidney establishes its full number of lobes. By the 14th or 15th weeks, well-developed vascular patterns are established. At 16 weeks, it is possible to distinguish the cortex and medulla of the kidney as a result of the development of the arterial patterns.[6] The last period of renal development begins at 32 to 36 weeks. During the last trimester of pregnancy, the kidney triples in size as a result of glomerular, interstitial, and tubular growth.

During gestation, one of the many functions of the placenta is to serve as a hemodialyzer for the fetus. At birth, after clamping of the umbilical cord, a marked increase in renal functioning occurs. The rapid maturation of renal function is thought to be the result of several

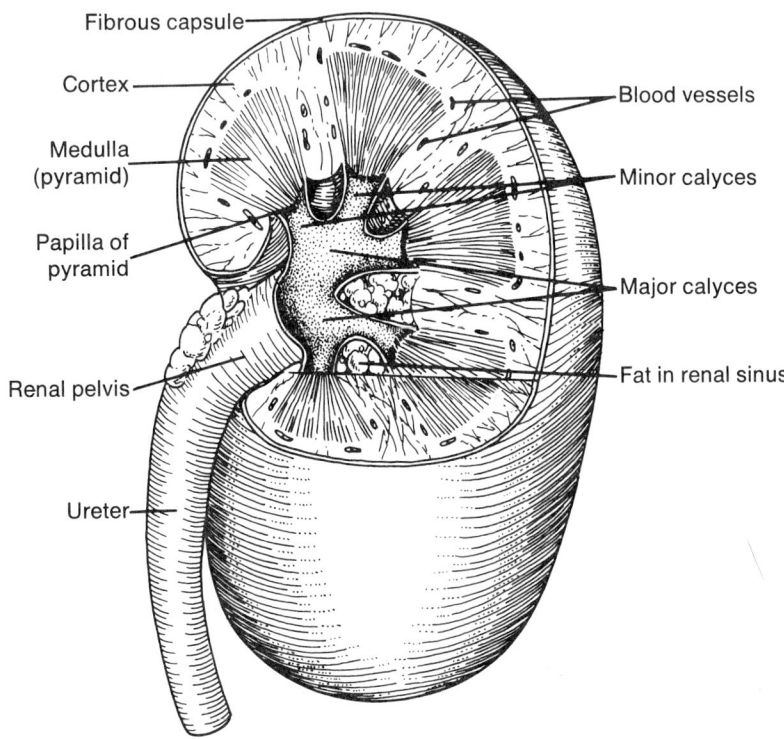

FIGURE 45-3
Cross section of the kidney with blood supply.

Medulla

The medulla is the inner portion of the kidney. It is approximately 5 cm wide in the mature kidney and contains portions of the collecting system and renal pyramids. Each pyramid in the medulla forms a single lobe. Between pyramids are the columns of Bertin, composed of cortical tissue.[2] The medulla also contains the juxtamedullary nephrons and their surrounding blood vessels.

Pelvis

The structures of the renal pelvis are responsible for the collection and transport of urine from the kidney. Urine formed in the nephron passes through the renal papilla at the base of the pyramids. It flows through the minor calices, which enclose the papilla. Several minor calices join to form the major calices, which converge to constitute the renal pelvis. Urine passes through the ureteropelvic junction and into the ureter.

Nephron Structures

Each kidney contains about 1 million nephrons, the microscopic functional units of the kidney. Of these nephrons, 85% originate in the outer region of the cortex,

and the remaining 15% arise out of the cortical area immediately adjacent to the medulla. The latter are known as juxtamedullary nephrons. Although all of the nephrons are responsible for producing urine, the juxtamedullary nephrons regulate urine osmolality to a greater extent than the cortical nephrons[11] (Fig. 45-4).

Glomerulus

Nephrons consist of a glomerulus and a tubule. Glomeruli are clusters of capillaries that originate in afferent arterioles, divide into capillary networks, and merge to form the efferent arterioles. Each glomerulus is surrounded by a balloonlike sac known as Bowman's capsule. The capsule consists of two layers: the visceral layer closely applied to the glomerulus, and the outer parietal layer. Bowman's capsule opens into the proximal convoluted tubule.

Tubules

Fluid filtered in the glomeruli enters the proximal convoluted tubule, the second longest portion of the nephron. It is composed of columnar cells containing mitochondria that facilitate the active transport of solutes.[9]

As the proximal convoluted tubule straightens and narrows, it becomes the loop of Henle. Short loops of

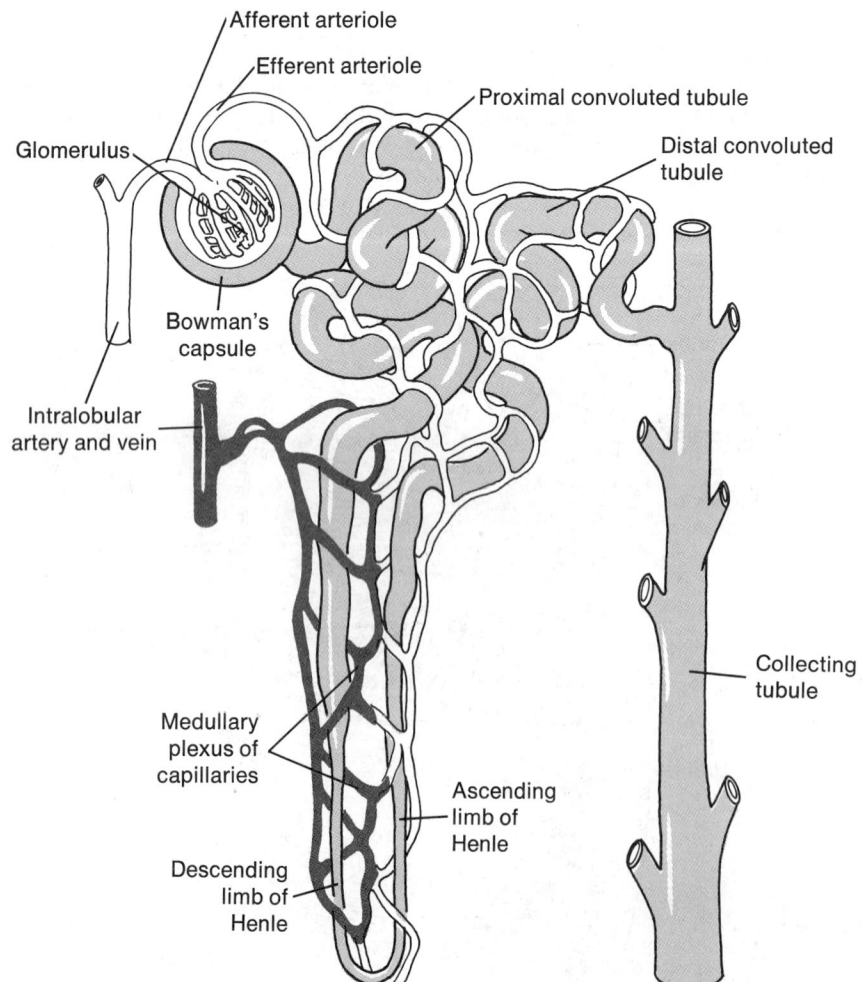

FIGURE 45-4

Detailed structure of a single nephron with blood supply.

Henle are found in cortical nephrons whereas long loops are found in juxtamedullary nephrons. The loop of Henle ascends and widens, then becomes the distal convoluted tubule. Multiple distal tubules empty into a single collecting duct, the longest portion of the nephron. After urine travels through the papillary collecting ducts and enters into the calyx, it is in its final composition and concentration, ready for excretion.[12]

The juxtaglomerular apparatus is located near the distal convoluted tubule and the glomerulus (Fig. 45-5). This is the portion of the kidney where renin is formed (see section entitled "Hormonal Control").

The cell structure of nephrons varies from one segment to another, but the entire nephron is lined with a continuous layer of cells known as the basement membrane. This basement membrane supports the structural integrity of the nephron, and it permits the rapid passage of filtrates to the collecting ducts.[11]

Nephrons of the newborn differ from those of the adult in their dimension and characteristics. Relative to its glomerulus, the proximal tubule is underdeveloped.[7] However, by 6 months of age, the anatomic glomerular tubular relationships are near adult levels.[1]

Another characteristic of the newborn kidney is the variation in size among individual nephrons. Nephrons increase in size as they mature. The increase in renal size during maturation and growth parallels the development of renal function.[7]

Blood Supply

As the kidneys develop, their blood supply is obtained by way of several arteries branching from the aorta.

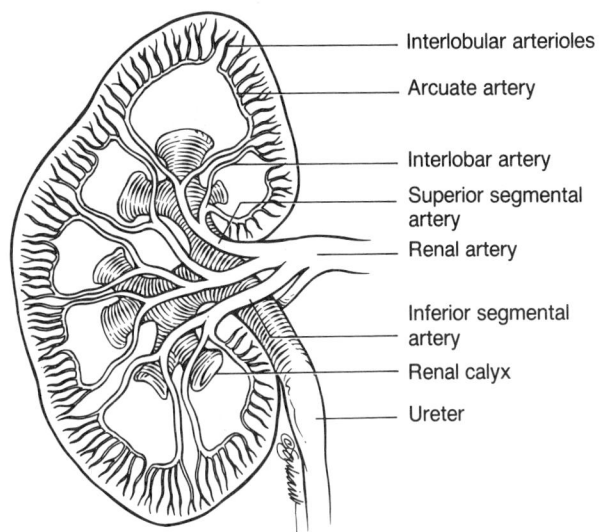

FIGURE 45-6
Arterial blood supply to the kidney.

There is degeneration or coalescence of these multiple branches as the kidneys grow until a single pair of renal arteries remains. The renal veins develop in a similar pattern.[6]

The renal artery enters the hilus of the kidney and branches into segmental arteries that extend to the anterior and posterior sections of the kidney. These segmental arteries supply the interlobal arteries that enclose the renal pyramids. As the interlobar arteries reach the base of the pyramids, bordering the medulla and cortex, they become the arcuate arteries (Fig. 45-6).[6,8,11] Interlobular arteries branch from the arcuate arteries and progress through the cortex to the periphery of the kidney.

The afferent arterioles emerge from the interlobular arteries to supply blood to the glomeruli. One afferent arteriole enters each glomerulus. Blood supply leaves the glomerulus by way of an efferent arteriole. The efferent arteriole branches into the peritubular and vasa recta capillaries (Fig. 45-7).[3]

Peritubular capillaries supply the proximal and distal tubules and are found mainly in the cortex. The vasa recta capillaries supply the loop of Henle and are located primarily in the medulla where blood flow is slower. These capillaries drain into venules.[11]

The venous system of the kidney is patterned in a similar manner as the arterial system. The capillaries form venules, which flow into interlobular veins, to arcuate veins, to interlobar veins, to the renal vein, which exits the hilum of the kidney to the inferior vena cava.

The following are important aspects regarding the kidneys' blood supply: (1) Renal circulation requires 20% to 30% of the total cardiac output. (2) When a renal artery is occluded, the area it supplies becomes infarcted. Arteries of renal circulation are end arteries and do not anastomose with other branches. (3) The renal cortex receives 75% of the blood supply to the kidneys. This rich perfusion accounts for the fact that blood flows through the cortex at a faster rate than it flows through the medulla.[6]

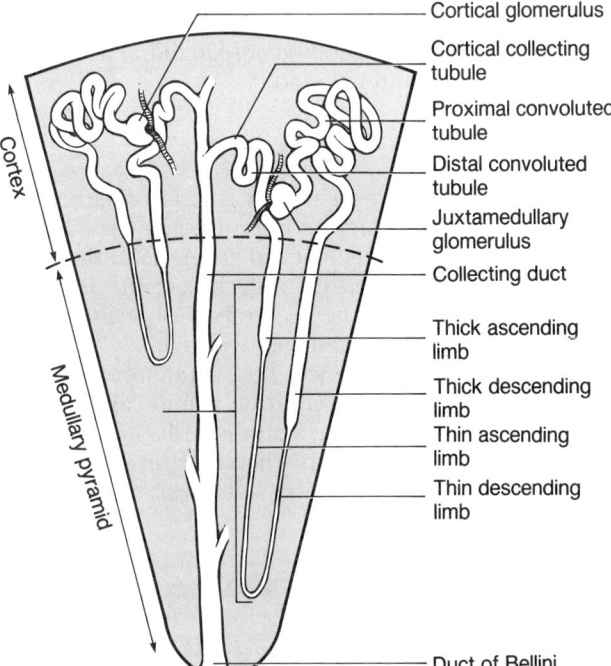

FIGURE 45-5
Cortical and juxtamedullary nephrons.

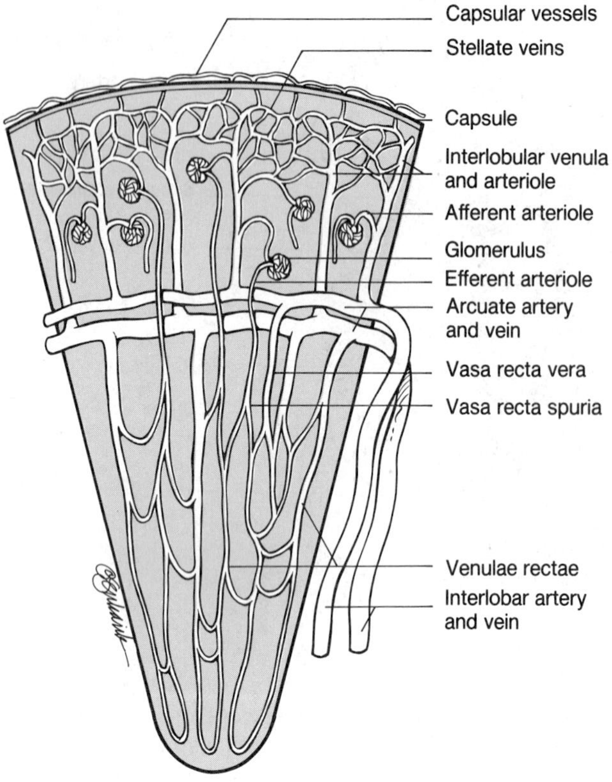
Capsular vessels
Stellate veins
Capsule
Interlobular venula and arteriole
Afferent arteriole
Glomerulus
Efferent arteriole
Arcuate artery and vein
Vasa recta vera
Vasa recta spuria
Venulae rectae
Interlobar artery and vein

FIGURE 45-7
Blood supply to the nephrons.

Nephron Functions

Each segment of the nephron has distinct roles, including filtration, reabsorption, and secretion. The functions of the glomerulus, proximal tubule, loop of Henle, distal tubule, and collecting duct are addressed separately in the following section.

Glomerulus

The production of urine begins with the glomerulus. The main function of the glomerulus is to filter fluid, known as glomerular filtrate, from the blood into Bowman's capsules. To aid in accomplishing this task, the glomerular membrane is 100 to 500 times as permeable as the usual capillary. It is, however, selective, denying passage of protein and other cellular elements of the blood. The glomerular filtrate is equivalent to an isotonic ultrafiltrate of plasma.[2,5]

Because the renal artery branches directly from the aorta, blood perfuses the glomerulus at a high pressure. Each minute the renal blood flow to both kidneys is approximately 1200 ml. Of this volume, approximately 650 ml are plasma. The glomeruli filter about 125 ml/min of the plasma as a result of filtration pressure. In a 24-hour period, over twice the body weight is filtered through the glomeruli. The tubules reabsorb 99% of the filtrate.[2,5]

The rate of glomerular filtration is affected by several variables. Developmentally, the newborn and infant have a lower glomerular filtration rate than the adult as a result of: (1) lower glomerular membrane permeability, (2) lower perfusion pressure, and (3) a smaller surface area available for filtration.[1,6] Generally, the glomerular filtration decreases with hypotension, localized renal ischemia, exercise, pain, and dehydration. An increase in glomerular filtration may occur with hypertension.[2]

Proximal Tubule

The primary urine that emerges from the glomeruli may be considered ultrafiltrate because it contains none of the corpuscular elements of the blood and is nearly protein-free. All the soluble substances in the filtrate are present in a concentration about equal to plasma concentration. The proximal tubule reabsorbs 60% to 70% of the glomerular filtrate. Along with the filtrate, there is rapid reabsorption of sodium, chloride, potassium, and calcium, and a slower reabsorption of magnesium and uric acid. Nearly all nutritionally important components of the ultrafiltrate are also reabsorbed, including glucose, amino acids, and ascorbic acid. The proximal tubule secretes and buffers hydrogen and ammonium ions, and it alone secretes weak organic acids and bases.[2,8]

Loop of Henle

The loop of Henle reabsorbs approximately 25% of the filtered ions. Chloride is actively reabsorbed and produces an electrochemical gradient to allow passive reabsorption of sodium. By reabsorbing chloride and sodium, the high osmolality of the medullary interstitium is maintained. Reabsorption of these ions creates a hypotonic filtrate. Most of the filtered magnesium is also reabsorbed in the loop of Henle.[11]

Distal Tubule

The distal tubule begins the process of the final adjustment of urine composition. It is in this segment that sodium and chloride are reabsorbed due to the action of aldosterone. Calcium is also reabsorbed in the distal tubule. Magnesium is reabsorbed or secreted, and hydrogen ions are secreted and buffered.[11]

Collecting Duct

In the collecting duct, urea is reabsorbed and secreted until equilibrium between the tubular fluid and the renal interstitium is reached. There is further reabsorption of sodium and chloride based on the body's needs. Potassium may be reabsorbed or secreted, and hydrogen ions are secreted and buffered.

The presence or absence of the antidiuretic hormone (ADH) determines the final urine volume and concentration. With ADH present, water is reabsorbed and the urine is more concentrated. When ADH is absent, urine is dilute and produced in large volumes.[8,11]

System Physiology

Fluid Balance

The kidneys are the body's most important organs for fluid regulation. They not only regulate water excretion but they do so in a manner that meets the specific needs of the body. Depending on the fluid requirements of the body, the kidney can produce dilute or concentrated urine.

As previously described, the glomerulus filters a large volume of fluid each day, although by the time this filtered fluid travels through the entire nephron, only a fraction of the glomerular filtrate is left to become urine.

Glomerular filtrate passes through the highly permeable proximal tubule and the descending loop of Henle where most of it is reabsorbed. It enters the ascending loop of Henle and the distal tubule where a small amount of reabsorption occurs. The volume of fluid reabsorbed in the collecting tubule and collecting duct depends on the presence or absence of ADH. The kidney has the unique ability to excrete either large amounts of water with minimal solutes or a greater quantity of solutes with minimal water loss.[8,11]

Most infants are not able to concentrate urine to their full ability until after 1 year of age. This delay is a result of an immature loop of Henle and a decreased response of the collecting tubules to ADH.[1]

Electrolyte Balance

The kidneys are the principal organs in the regulation and maintenance of electrolyte balance. As is true with water balance, the kidneys are able to regulate precisely the amount of each electrolyte excreted.

A fraction of the sodium filtered through the glomerulus is excreted in the urine. The proximal tubule reabsorbs 65%, the loop of Henle 25%, the distal tubule 6%, and the collecting duct 2% to 4%.

Sodium reabsorption is enhanced by a decreased glomerular filtration rate and by aldosterone secretion. Aldosterone, a mineralocorticoid secreted by the adrenal cortex, increases the reabsorption of the sodium and water. Excretion of sodium is enhanced by an increased glomerular filtration rate and by a decreased production of aldosterone.[9]

Chloride is reabsorbed with sodium in the tubules at approximately the same percentages. Acidosis enhances chloride excretion whereas alkalosis enhances its reabsorption.[9,11]

Potassium is also largely reabsorbed by the tubules. Whereas nearly 100% may be reabsorbed in the proximal tubule, it is actively and passively secreted in the distal tubule. The renal excretion of potassium is enhanced by an elevated serum potassium, alkalosis, aldosterone secretion and an increased tubular flow rate.[9,11]

Calcium is reabsorbed in the proximal tubule at 65%, the loop of Henle at 20% to 25%, and the distal tubule at 10%. Reabsorption of calcium is enhanced by a decreased glomerular filtration rate, the excretion of parathyroid hormone, and a reduction in plasma calcium.[9]

Phosphate is reabsorbed in the proximal tubule. Reabsorption is enhanced by a decreased glomerular filtration rate and the presence of sodium. Excretion is enhanced by an increased glomerular filtration rate and the parathyroid hormone.[9]

Newborn kidneys have some limitations in their ability to maintain electrolyte balance. If given an increased sodium intake, their excretion ability is limited. The liability in electrolyte balance may be due to the neonate's inability to increase the glomerular filtration adequately and to the limited ability of the distal tubule to reabsorb sodium. By 1 year of age, their full ability to excrete a sodium load is achieved.[1]

Excretion of Metabolic Wastes

One of the best known functions of the kidneys is their ability to excrete metabolic waste products. Urea is a nitrogenous waste product of protein metabolism. Nearly all of the urea produced is filtered by the glomeruli. The tubules reabsorb approximately half of the filtered urea, and the remainder is excreted in the urine.

Several factors influence the production and excretion of urea including the glomerular filtration rate, the presence of fever or infection, and the body's hydration status. Because the production and excretion of urea is affected by nonrenal factors, the level of serum urea or BUN alone is not an accurate indicator of renal function.

Creatinine, another important waste product, is the end result of muscle cell metabolism. Creatinine is produced at a constant rate proportional to the body's muscle mass. It is filtered at the glomerulus, but it is not reabsorbed or secreted in the tubules. Because creatinine is produced at a steady rate and its excretion is regulated by glomerular filtration, a serum creatinine level is a reliable indicator of renal function.[9,11]

Acid–Base Balance

Another function of the renal system is to maintain an acid–base balance. The kidneys participate in this process along with the blood buffers and the lungs. The renal role begins within approximately 24 hours after a change in pH occurs and may continue for several days.[11]

The renal system's main contribution in acid–base balance is to regulate the plasma bicarbonate. Regulation is accomplished by: (1) reabsorbing bicarbonate in the tubules, (2) excreting excess bicarbonate, and (3) replenishing depleted bicarbonate stores. Bicarbonate levels are replenished by combining carbon dioxide (CO_2) with water (H_2O) to form carbonic acid (H_2CO_3) and excreting the excess hydrogen ion (H^+) leaving bicarbonate (HCO_3).[11,12]

The nephron is able to adjust urine pH from 4.5 to 8 depending on the needs of the body. The kidney responds to acidosis by stimulating the reabsorption of bicarbonate in the proximal tubule and the secretion of hydrogen ions in the distal tubule, resulting in excretion of an acid urine with urine pH as low as 4.5. In response to alkalosis, the tubules reabsorb less bicarbonate and secrete less hydrogen, causing an increased excretion of bicarbonate in the urine. Urinary pH may increase to 8 depending on the level of correction required.[9,11]

Hormonal Control

The renal system participates in the production and control of several hormones, including activated vitamin

D, renin, erythropoietin, and prostaglandins. The origin and function of each are reviewed in this section.

Vitamin D exists in an inactive state in the liver. It is activated in the cortex of the kidney. Stimulation to activate vitamin D is provided by the secretion of parathyroid hormone. Because the active version of vitamin D (1,25-dehydroxy vitamin D_3) is made in the body, it is considered a hormone and not a vitamin.[11,12]

The major role of activated vitamin D is to stimulate calcium and phosphate absorption in the intestine. If there is a deficiency in this hormone, the intestine decreases its absorption of calcium and, consequently, plasma calcium decreases. Failure to calcify the newly forming bones of infants and children normally results in rickets. Children with renal disease are unable to activate vitamin D and require oral supplements to improve calcium absorption.[12]

Renin is neither a real hormone nor does it work alone to increase vascular pressure. It is, however, responsible for initiating an important cycle to aid in blood pressure control. Renin is actually an enzyme that is secreted into the blood by the juxtaglomerular apparatus of the kidney. Once it is in the bloodstream, renin acts as a catalyst to split angiotensin I from the plasma protein, angiotensinogen. The liver is responsible for producing and secreting angiotensinogen, and it is always present in high concentrations in the plasma. Angiotensin I is converted to angiotensin II by another enzyme as blood flows through the lungs. Angiotensin II is the active hormone that enters the kidney and other organs by way of arterial circulation.

Renin is released when there is a decreased perfusion pressure, especially in the afferent arterioles. It promotes the production of angiotensin II, which causes vasoconstriction, stimulates thirst, and promotes the release of aldosterone. Aldosterone enhances sodium reabsorption in the renal tubules and causes an increase in plasma sodium. The actions of angiotensin II and aldosterone work to increase perfusion pressure, which, in turn, decreases renin secretion.[8,11,12]

Erythropoietin is an important hormone secreted by the kidneys. The action of erythropoietin is to stimulate the bone marrow to produce erythrocytes. This hormone is released when there is a decrease in oxygen to the kidneys, as in anemia or poor renal blood flow. Children with chronic or end-stage renal disease have a decreased ability to produce erythropoietin and are subsequently often anemic.[12]

The kidneys are also responsible for producing the prostaglandin hormones. Prostaglandins are found primarily in the papilla of the kidneys. They are also found in other areas of the body, including the prostate gland from which they received their name. Although there are several types of prostaglandins, most act as vasodilators. They also weaken the kidney's response to the renin–angiotensin system and promote the excretion of sodium and water.[8,11]

Summary

From the period of embryonic development, the renal system evolves as a structure critical to the maintenance of life. Although fully functioning at birth, the renal system continues to mature during childhood. The kidneys, specifically the nephrons, assume responsibility for removing metabolic wastes from the blood and for maintaining fluid, electrolyte, and acid–base balance, resulting in a precisely controlled urine output. The renal system is also responsible for production and control of certain hormones. With its own intricate roles, the renal system works with other systems of the body to maintain overall homeostasis.

References

1. Avery, G. B. (1987). *Neonatology, pathophysiology and management of the newborn* (3rd ed.). Philadelphia: Lippincott.
2. Brundage, D. J. (1980). *Nursing management of renal problems* (2nd ed.). St. Louis: Mosby.
3. Edelmann, C. M. (1978). *Pediatric kidney disease,* Vol. I. Boston: Little, Brown.
4. Fine, R. (1982, August). Symposium on pediatric nephrology. *Pediatric Clinics of North America, 29*(4).
5. Guyton, A. C. (1991). *Textbook of medical physiology* (8th ed.). Philadelphia: Saunders.
6. Hollerman, C. E. (1979). *Pediatric nephrology.* Medical Outline Series. Garden City: Medical Examination Publishing.
7. Holliday, M. A., et al. (1987). Pediatric nephrology (2nd ed.). Baltimore: Williams & Wilkins.
8. Knox, F. G. (1978). *Textbook of renal pathophysiology.* Hagerstown: Harper and Row.
9. Lancaster, L. E. (1991). *Core curriculum for nephrology nursing* (2nd ed.) Pitman: Jannetti.
10. Netter, F. H. (1983). *The CIBA collection of medical illustration.* Vol. 6: *Kidneys, ureters, and urinary bladder.* West Caldwell, NJ: CIBA.
11. Richard, C. J. (1986). *Comprehensive nephrology nursing.* Boston: Little, Brown.
12. Vander, A. J. (1991). *Renal physiology* (4th ed.). New York: McGraw-Hill.

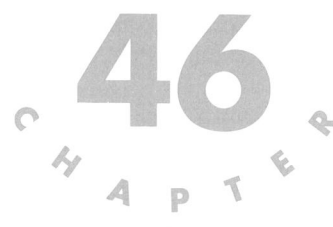

46

C H A P T E R

Nursing Assessment and Diagnosis of Renal Function

BEHAVIORAL OBJECTIVES

Use functional health as a guideline for assessment of the child's renal function.

Describe the components of a complete physical examination of the child's renal function.

List the common blood and urine indices tested to determine renal diseases.

Describe the noninvasive and invasive tests used to diagnose renal dysfunction.

Identify nursing diagnoses commonly used in the care of children with renal dysfunction.

Comprehensive assessment of renal function includes information collected by several members of the health care team. The nurse may be responsible for interviewing the child and family to obtain a health history and for performing a physical examination. Additional information is usually gathered from reports of diagnostic tests that are ordered by the physician, and from others who assist in caring for the child. This chapter provides guidance in performing the interview and examinations and interpreting findings from diagnostic tests. Examples of nursing diagnoses that are commonly associated with children who have renal dysfunction are also provided.

Nursing Assessment

Nursing assessment of the child with renal disease is built on a foundation of background data that have led to the suspicion or medical diagnosis of impairment in renal function. Although the assessment is ongoing, extensive information may be obtained in the initial contacts with the child and family. Thereafter, care should be taken to avoid repetitious questioning; available records may be studied for historic information. The nursing assessment for the current problem begins with a history in which functional health patterns are reviewed.

Child and Family History

When the child is known to have renal impairment, the nursing history emphasizes the impact that the condition has had on the child and the family's patterns of functioning.[9] Nursing judgment should be used in determining when the interview should be conducted with the child and family jointly or separately.

Health-Perception and Health-Management

Assessment of health-perception and health-management begins by asking the child and parents to describe their perceptions of the child's health status. Many parents have the misconception that renal insufficiency or end-stage renal disease is reversible. They often act on this belief by seeking a "cure" through prayer or folk medicine and may refuse to have their child begin dialysis. The parents may be asked why they sought medical care; many are able to articulate their concerns and perceptions regarding their child's health status when this question is asked.

Adherence to the medical plan needs to be assessed. What medications or medical regimen has been prescribed? Does the child have difficulty taking the medications or completing the regimen? The family may be asked matter-of-factly how often treatments or medications go undone. If the child and family feels accepted and comfortable with the nurse, they are more inclined to reveal their inability to perform required medical care.

The family's ability to obtain follow-up medical care needs to be explored. Does the family own a car, or is public transportation readily available to them? If transportation is available, does the family have the income for frequent trips to the clinic or dialysis center?

Inquiry should be made about health practices that the family employs. Does the family seek medical assistance for ongoing health needs as well as when a medical crisis occurs? Are routine health maintenance needs such as immunizations being provided along with treatment for the child's renal condition?

Nutrition and Metabolism

Assessment of nutrition and metabolism is crucial for children with renal disease because they may have altered metabolic states related to their illness. They may require complex renal diets and fluid restrictions. The nurse must carefully explore past and present nutritional practices to ensure comprehensive understanding of this health pattern.

Can the family accurately describe the renal diet and fluid restrictions? Who is responsible for the child's diet? Does the school-age child carry bag lunches to school or eat at the cafeteria? Are the child's meals prepared separately, or is an attempt made to serve similar foods to the entire family?

The child's current nutritional status may be assessed by obtaining a 3-day diet history to determine typical caloric intake and types of foods consumed. Because a recall of the past three days may be unreliable, instructions may be given to obtain information in the near future, with the child or parents recording all types and amounts of food eaten in a given time frame. The nurse should be aware that there may be inconsistencies between what the parent perceives the child to eat and what the child actually eats.

Evaluation of the child's and family's ability to adhere to the prescribed renal diet is of great importance. The ill child's stage of development may affect ability to follow the special diet. Does the infant refuse to eat, spit out the nipple, arch its back, turn its head, or vomit when fed formula? Does the toddler refuse to eat required foods? Is mealtime a battle with the toddler? Does the toddler exhibit manipulative behaviors related to food? Does the school-age child sneak restricted foods while at school? Is the adolescent's choice of food affected negatively by peer pressure?

The child with renal insufficiency or end-stage renal disease is usually anorectic secondary to uremia. Often the family gives anything the child would like to eat, even if the food is not on the prescribed diet, because of their child's lack of interest in food. Does the family perceive the child's diet as medically important or useless? The child may be asked why the renal diet has been ordered. Children may believe that they are being punished for their illness with the renal diet and fluid restrictions.

The child's rate of growth also needs to be ascertained. What did the child weigh at birth? Did the child follow a normal growth curve before presenting with kidney disease? Has the child's linear growth slowed or stopped? Has the child gained more than 2 to 3 lb in a period of 1 week? A height and weight chart is used to plot the growth on all children with kidney disease.

Elimination

Assessment of elimination is of obvious importance for any child with suspected renal problems because the information could possibly reveal early indicators of renal disease. Certain renal conditions such as nephrosis or renal insufficiency significantly decrease the child's number of urinary voidings in a 24-hour period. Other factors also influence the frequency of a child's urination, such as the child's age or the amount of fluid consumed. Newborns and infants usually urinate 12 to 20 times every 24 hours, toddlers urinate 6 to 10 times in a 24-hour period, and school-age through adolescent children urinate only 4 to 6 times in a 24-hour period. These norms must be considered when evaluating how often the child urinates.

An assessment of not only frequency and pattern of urination but also changes in the color or in the odor of the urine is important. Normal urine is straw-colored or a clear to light medium yellow, due to the presence of the pigment urochrome. Normal urine should have little odor. If the child complains of a strong foul odor, the odor may be due to a kidney or urinary tract infection. Does the child have burning or pain on urination? If the child being assessed is unable to articulate pain, the family should be asked if the child cries, grunts, or pulls his legs up to his abdomen when voiding. These are all classic signs of a kidney or urinary tract infection.

Whether the child has difficulties with wetting the bed at night needs to be determined. Bedwetting (enuresis) should be considered a normal event during the first 5 to 6 years of life but thereafter should be considered dysfunctional. The cause of enuresis may be either emotional or physiologic. Some children have a renal tubular concentrating defect that causes the kidneys to produce exceptionally large volumes of urine. This volume, in turn, leaves the child vulnerable to bedwetting. How often does the child wet the bed? How long has this been a problem for the child? Has the child ever experienced a dry night? Does the child drink large volumes of fluid before bedtime? The child with a concentrating defect drinks large amounts of liquid to replace the fluid lost. Does the family view bedwetting as a problem? What methods does the family use for coping with the bedwetting?

If the child is on dialysis, the nurse should assess the effectiveness of the particular therapy used by the child. Assessment of the child on hemodialysis would include asking the child or family if they are able to palpate the arteriovenous shunt for a thrill. Does the child or family palpate the shunt regularly? Does the child complain of edema during the first 24 hours after hemodialysis? The child on hemodialysis should not have any signs of fluid overload during the initial hours after dialysis.

Assessment of the child on home peritoneal dialysis would include first a review of the fluid exchanges, then a review of symptoms. How often does the child perform dialysis? Is at least 75% of the dialysate infused into the peritoneum drained off? This amount must be removed from the peritoneum to ensure adequate ultrafiltration of the waste products and electrolytes. Does the child complain of edema? Has the child ever had a weight gain of 2 or more pounds in a day? Does the child ever complain of shortness of breath? All of these symptoms would indicate ineffective peritoneal dialysis.

Activity and Exercise

Renal disease can be a draining and emotional illness. The child may experience feelings of lethargy from the uremic condition and, therefore, be unable to perform age-appropriate activities. Has the infant met its developmental milestones? Does the school-age child attend school? Is the adolescent able to attend social functions?

Assessment of the child's self-care abilities provides insight into activity and exercise patterns. Taking prescribed medications, measuring blood pressure, and performing peritoneal dialysis (if over the age of 12) are examples of self care activities. Are the medications stored at a level that the child can reach? Are the medications labeled so that the child can easily read them? Does the child have an automated or manual blood pressure cuff? Is the dialysis equipment at a level they can reach? Are medications premixed in the dialysate container? Is a clean, quiet area provided for the child to complete dialysis?

Sleep and Rest

Assessment of the child's sleep and rest may reveal problems related to the child's renal disease or required medications. Certain renal problems may cause the child to have difficulties sleeping, whereas others may predispose the child to lethargy.

Any recent changes in the child's sleep and rest habits are questioned. A child with renal insufficiency may become tired and lethargic during a normal day's activity when their disease approaches end stage. Does the toddler take more naps than usual? Does the school-age child take a nap after school instead of playing with friends? Does the adolescent stay home on weekends to go to bed early? Is the child difficult to get up in the morning?

The child with nephrotic syndrome or a renal transplant is usually on medications that may cause hyperactivity. Often families with a child on these medications have difficulty attempting to get their child to rest or sleep quietly throughout the night. Has the family noticed a change in the child's rest habits since the initiation of these medications? What methods have been tried to promote rest and sleep? Are the medications given in the morning instead of the evening to allow for a more restful night's sleep?

The child with enuresis generally experiences frequent interruptions during the night due to a wet bed. How many times a night is the child typically disrupted due to this enuresis? Is the child able to return to sleep after waking up with a wet bed? How long is the child awake? Have the parents noticed that the child is overly tired during a day's activities?

Cognition and Perception

The child's and family's cognition and perception are assessed in relation to the child's kidney disease. Does the family understand the basic functions of the kidneys? To what degree does the family understand the child's disease and mode of therapy? What is the child's perception of the renal disease? The family's depth of knowledge about renal disease should be explored thoroughly to plan nursing interventions.

Information regarding how the child and parents best learn content and skills is crucial when developing a teaching plan related to the renal condition. At what level do the child and family read? Does the child or parent have a visual or hearing problem? Does the child or parent prefer learning new information by written, oral, or visual aids?

Pain is an unfortunate accompaniment to renal disease. How much pain does the child experience? Where is the pain, and what does it feel like? How does the child respond to the pain? Does the child perceive pain as punishment? How does the family view pain? What do they believe about the appropriate expression of pain?

Self-Perception and Self-Concept

Renal disease often has an effect on a child's sense of body image and self-concept. The child may be asked to explain feelings about personal elimination patterns, edema, or other physical side-effects the kidney disease has caused. A toddler or school-age child may have difficulty verbalizing these feelings but might be able to draw a self-portrait that could be analyzed at a later time. The older child is normally reluctant to express the feelings of self-doubt or self-worth that are frequently experienced. These children should be asked leading questions that direct their answers. The nurse may say, for example, "Some children who have the same condition have told me that they feel different from other children. Tell me how you feel about yourself." This type of dialogue may be more productive if conducted with the child alone and not in the family's presence.

Some forms of renal disease eventually lead to kidney failure. In these situations, the child's level of depression or fear about the potential loss of kidney function and the possibility of dialysis or transplantation needs to be assessed. The child may express feelings of sadness, hopelessness, anger, or anxiety about this loss. Is the child having difficulty going to school and interacting with peers? Is all attention and energy focused on the renal condition? Many children with renal failure live in constant fear of death but are afraid to bring the issue up because of concern about hurting their parents and other loved ones.

Assessment for personal identity confusion is especially appropriate when the child has received a kidney transplant. Older school-age children and adolescents sometimes believe that they will take on the characteristics of the person who donated their kidney. For example, the girl with a male's kidney may fear becoming masculine. Does the child ever fantasize about the person who donated the kidney? Has the child written a letter of thanks for the donation of a kidney? This act often finalizes the transfer of organs for the child.

Role Relationships

The effect of the child's renal disease on the social roles of family members and on the family structure should be explored. Has the child's illness alienated siblings? Do the siblings resent the ill child for the parent's extra time and attention? Sometimes the siblings of ill children feel left out and wish that they too could become ill.

Alterations in effective parenting secondary to the child's illness may also be explored. Parents of ill children often become overly permissive because they are afraid of scolding a child that is so medically fragile. In comparison to other children in the home, how is the ill child disciplined? Do family rules apply to this child as well as the siblings?

The child's social interaction with peers also needs to be assessed. Does having kidney disease keep the child from attending typical childhood activities such as sleep-overs? Do frequent clinic appointments and hospitalizations keep the child from interacting with his peers and siblings? Are there signs of social isolation? Asking the child how the medical therapies and appointments could be adjusted to allow for more social interaction may provide areas for further exploration and adjustment.

Sexuality and Reproduction

Renal disease can have a great impact on a child's sexuality. Younger children should be assessed for feelings of maleness and femaleness as they compare themselves to same-sex peers. Does the child have friendships with others of the same or opposite sex? Is the adolescent sexually active? Is there concern about the normalcy of the sexual feelings experienced? Does the presence of catheters, fistulas, or multiple scars affect the child's self-image, and, in turn, feelings of sexuality?

The nurse may also assess the family's feelings in regards to their child's sexuality. Does the family view the child as a sexual being? How does the family support the child's sexual maturation? Are topics related to sexuality open for discussion between the ill child and parents?

Children also need to be assessed for signs of sexual abuse because these children often present with multiple kidney problems. Does the child have frequent kidney and urinary tract infections? Is the child timid and reserved when questioned about sexuality and relationships? Is the child's language and interest in sexual matters appropriate for the age?

Coping and Stress Tolerance

The child's and family's ability to adapt and cope with the symptoms, treatment, and impact of renal disease needs to be explored in the history. Changes in family routine should be noted. What resources do the child and family use for support during crisis? Has the family ever had a "breakdown" due to crisis? Previous patterns of ineffective coping may be recognized if the child and family are asked to describe how they managed one specific stressful situation in the past.

Values and Beliefs

The assessment of function is completed with an examination of the family's value and belief pattern. The child and family may be asked about the occurrence of spiritual crisis that is often associated with an illness, change in body image, or loss of an organ. What are the family's religious beliefs regarding the child's illness? Does the family believe in performing blood transfusions or other medical therapies? Are there conflicts in values between the child and the family?

Physical Examination

Developmental considerations in the physical examination of the child's urinary system are discussed in Table 49-1.

The child is carefully observed during the interview, because the general appearance of the child may reveal more than subtle physical findings.[1] The child's general height, weight, and posture are evaluated in a developmental perspective. Grooming and cleanliness are noted. Is there an odor to the child? Severe uremia produces a foul body odor emitted by way of the skin pores in most children. The face should tell whether the child feels well or is in acute distress, is chronically ill, lethargic, or responsive.

The nurse generally begins the physical examination by taking anthropometric measurements. These measurements include: height or length, head circumference (in infants), weight, triceps skin folds, and arm muscle area. The evaluation of the triceps skin folds or arm muscle area may be based on chronologic age, height age, or bone age. Calculations may be plotted on a growth chart.

Vital signs are also taken. Blood pressure is measured using an age-appropriate sized cuff. If hypertension is detected, the blood pressure should be taken in both arms in the supine, standing, and sitting positions. Temperature is measured to assess for a possible infection.

General Approach

The child's skin is examined for color, integrity, and markings. Paleness may be present if the child has anemia or uremia, but the skin may also have a brownish color caused by uremia. An inspection of the skin for hydration and dryness is important. Skin turgor is tested by lifting a small amount of skin from the back of the hand of the older child or the abdomen of the infant. If the child is well hydrated, the skin should snap back quickly, but a delay in return usually occurs with dehydration. Scratch marks may indicate the pruritus of uremia. Ecchymosis related to abnormal platelet function may be found throughout the body. White bands and ridges in the nails may indicate significant protein malnutrition from nephrosis.

The nurse observes for periorbital edema, puffiness around the eyes. Dependent edema of the extremities is diagnosed by depressing two fingers into the tissue surrounding the ankle. If an impression in the skin remains for several seconds, pitting edema is present.

Next, the child's hair is examined for amount, color, and texture. Thinning of the hair may occur due to antihypertensives, immunosuppressants, or protein malnutrition. Hirsutism may also be secondary to some antihypertensives or immunosuppressants. The hair may be brittle from hypoparathyroidism.

Another important observation is the position of the child's ears. Some genetic renal disorders are characterized by low-set ears. The upper portion of the pinna should measure equal with or above the outer canthus of the eye. Nerve deafness is associated with some cases of renal tubular acidosis and with some forms of nephrosis and hypoparathyroidism. Deafness may suggest the possibility of heredity nephropathy or, if renal function is impaired, previous aminoglycoside therapy.[11]

The internal eye is examined for changes. Examination of the fundus may reveal the ravages of hypertension with arterial narrowing, hemorrhages, exudates, and papilledema. Scleral calcification may be a consequence of hypercalcemia or uncontrolled hypherphosphatemia. A beam of light from a penlight directed across the cornea reveals its degree of smoothness and clarity. Cloudiness over the cornea may indicate cataracts, a possible side-effect of prednisone therapy, which is commonly used for treatment of renal disease.

Lips, buccal mucosa, and gums are examined for hydration and color. Dry buccal mucosa and dry chapped lips may indicate failing renal function. Pale lips and buccal mucosa may be a sign of anemia. The child's dentition should be examined for hygiene and appearance. Chronic hypocalcemia may cause the child's teeth to become darkened and brittle.

Inspection of the head is followed by an examination of the cardiovascular and respiratory systems. The child is first placed in a supine position to examine the pulses for rate, rhythm, and volume. The femoral pulses should always be palpated for coarctation due to renal failure or hypertension. The point of maximal impulse (PMI), or apex of the heart, is assessed and should be visible at the fifth intercostal in the midclavicular line after the age of 7. Before this age, the apex is normally felt at the fourth intercostal, just to the left of the midclavicular line. The PMI should be easily palpated in children over the age of 2. A weak PMI may indicate a pericardial effusion or heart failure secondary to medications or failing kidneys. A shift to the left of the PMI might reveal left ventricular heart failure possibly caused by renal failure. The child's heart rate and character are assessed for any abnormalities or changes. Murmurs may indicate a high cardiac output from chronic anemia. A friction rub may indicate pericarditis secondary to severe uremia.[2]

Examination of Chest

With the child in a sitting position and the shirt removed, the chest is observed for the character and rate of respirations. The rate of respiration varies from 30 to 50 breaths a minute at birth, to 16 to 20 at 6 years of age, and to 14 to 16 at puberty. Hyperventilation suggests metabolic acidosis secondary to renal disease. A rapid respiratory rate with increased respiratory effort points to pulmonary edema.[2] Dyspnea may also be observed in the child with severe anemia as the child struggles to obtain enough oxygen for metabolic needs.

With the child still sitting, breath sounds are auscultated. Breath sounds should be clear. Presence of rales and rhonchi may indicate an opportunistic infection caused by the child's immunosuppressant therapy. Diffuse, fine crepitations at both lung bases suggest pulmonary edema.

Examination of Abdomen

As the assessment moves to the abdomen, the child puts the shirt on to prevent the possibility of becoming chilled. The child is placed in a supine position, and assessment is begun with inspection. The location of scars that may indicate previous renal surgeries such as nephrostomy tubes, dialysis catheters, or transplantations are noted. Location of the nipples is also important, because low-set nipples are often an indicator of genetic renal disorders. Abdominal distention may be present as a consequence of ascites, or enlargement of the kidneys due to hydronephrosis, a tumor, or retention of urine in the bladder.[2]

The tone or musculature of the abdomen is observed for its presence and character. Absence of abdominal wall musculature is characteristic of prune belly syndrome, a genetic kidney disease, and is obvious in infancy. The abdomen lacks complete musculature, the bowels lay freely inside the skin on either side of the child, and peristaltic waves are easily visualized throughout. The absence of abdominal musculature caused by prune belly

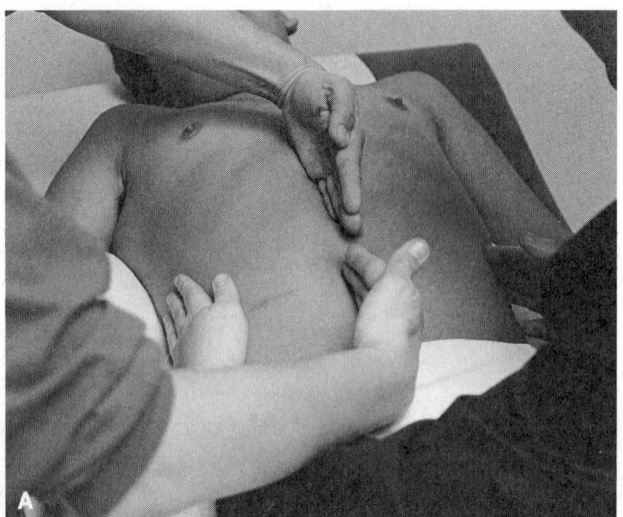

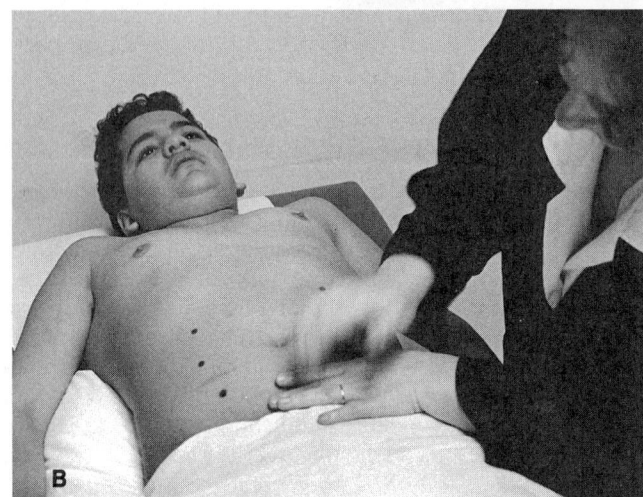

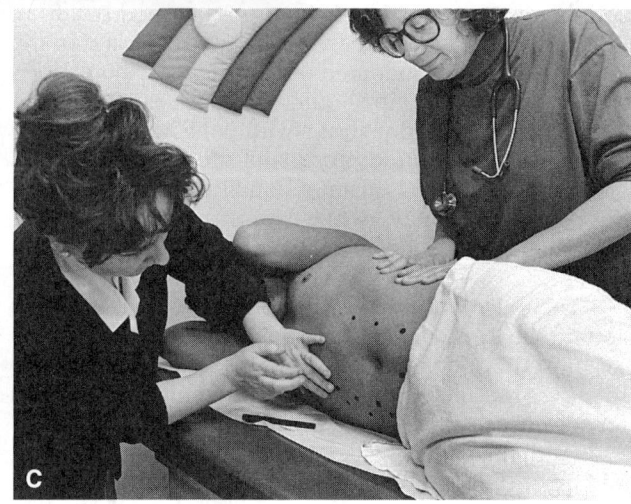

FIGURE 46-1

Two tests are used to determine presence of ascites, common with chronic kidney disease. (**A**) Fluid wave test. The edge of the nurse's hands are placed along the midline of the child's abdomen while the examiner strikes on flank. The opposite flank is felt for wave of fluid transmitted during the strike. An easily palpated wave suggests ascites. (**B**) Test for shifting dullness. *Left:* Examiner percusses abdomen for areas of dullness. These areas are marked. *Right:* Patient is turned to a second position and the same areas are percussed. Considerable shifts of dullness indicate ascites. (Photos by Kathy Sloane, courtesy of Children's Hospital, Oakland, CA.)

syndrome is less obvious in the older child, and it may be revealed only when the recumbent child is asked to fold his arms above his chest and to raise his shoulders off the bed. This motion causes an upward movement of the umbilicus.

The assessment of the abdomen continues with auscultation. Renal vascular sounds are auscultated over the kidneys posteriorly with the bell side of the stethoscope in the child with hypertension. A murmur in this area may suggest constriction of one of the renal arteries. Bowel sounds are auscultated in all four quadrants but may be diminished in the child with peritoneal dialysis as a result of the fluid surrounding the bowel in the peritoneum.

After auscultation of the abdomen, the nurse percusses the abdomen. A distended abdomen with bulging flanks and little tympany suggests fluid or solid masses. Two tests can be easily performed to determine the presence of ascites: the fluid wave test and the test for shifting dullness (Fig. 46-1). The fluid wave test is performed with the child in the supine position. An assistant is asked to place the edge of the hand firmly along the midline of the child's abdomen. One flank is struck sharply as the opposite flank is felt for a wave of fluid transmitted from the strike. An easily palpated wave suggests ascites.[3] The test for shifting dullness is easily obtained by percussing for areas of dullness with the child in one position. The borders of dullness are first marked; the child shifts positions and the examiner percusses again. Considerable shift of the areas of dullness indicates free abdominal fluid, or ascites, common with chronic kidney disease.

After the child sits upright, the costovertebral angle is percussed for tenderness. Percussion is accomplished by placing the palm side of the left hand over the costovertebral angle and striking the hand with the ulnar side of the right hand. The presence of pain or tenderness may indicate a kidney infection or disease.

After careful inspection, auscultation, and percussion, the abdomen is palpated to explore further for signs of kidney disease. The child returns to the supine position. To palpate the right kidney, the left hand is placed under the child's right loin, between the rib cage and iliac crest. The examiner's right hand is placed below the right costal margin with fingers pointing left. The hands are pressed firmly together as the child is asked to take a deep breath. The lower pole of the right kidney may or may not be palpable. To palpate the left kidney, the same technique is used but with the examiner standing on the child's right side. The left loin is supported with the left hand, and palpation is done with the right hand.[3] Palpation of the left kidney is more difficult, and it is usually not located because of its higher position. Both kidneys are normally difficult to palpate in the older child but are easily palpated in the neonate.

The transplanted kidney is palpated for tenderness or warmth. Transplanted kidneys are placed retroperitoneally and can be palpated easily with the child in the supine position. Superficial palpation is used to outline the kidney. The presence of pain or warmth is characteristic of rejection.

Examination of Musculoskeletal System

After examination of the abdomen, the musculoskeletal system is assessed. Knee and wrist joints are observed for bony, painless swelling, the classic sign of renal rickets.[1] The presence of rickets may be a consequence of the early osteomalacic phase of uremia, osteodystrophy, or renal tubular disease. Any skeletal disproportion caused by uremic osteodystrophy should also be noted. Arm span and leg length are compared, as well as the child's sitting and standing height. Muscle mass also needs to be assessed. Hemihypertrophy of the legs is occasionally associated with a neuroblastoma or with medullary sponge disease.[2] Another common finding in the child with osteodystrophy is knock-knee, a condition that is identified by having the child walk across the room while observing the gait. Measurements of the intermalleolar distance are obtained to determine severity. The neonate is examined for congenital dislocation of the hips, a common finding in infants with congenital renal disease.

Deformities of the spine may indicate renal disease. The sacral area is examined for a patch of pigmentation or a tuft of hair, subtle signs that may point to an underlying spinal deformity, which may be responsible for a neuropathic bladder.[2]

Diagnostic Tests

Laboratory Tests

Urinalysis. Urine and blood tests are the most common studies performed to assess renal function. A routine urinalysis is the simplest and often the most fruitful screening test for renal dysfunction. The nurse plays an important role in obtaining an accurate urinalysis and is usually the person who either obtains or instructs the child and family on how to collect the specimen properly. An error in the collection technique could result in a costly false reading.

When collecting a routine urine sample, the first voided specimen of the day is preferred because it has the highest acidity and concentration. The routine urine sample may be voided into a bedpan or urinal, but preferably into a clean urine container. The analysis must be performed within 30 minutes of collection because some casts degenerate rapidly in a voided urine, and phosphates and urates may precipitate on standing. Table 46-1 gives urinary indices.

Clean Catch Urine. Clean catch urine samples are required when a culture and sensitivity are desired, providing a clean but not sterile sample. Obtaining this sample requires meticulous cleaning of the perineal area or penis. The nurse should assist the child 10 years and under and provide careful teaching for the older child. For the infant or toddler not yet toilet-trained, a sterile urinary bag needs to be applied to the perineum to collect the urine. Sometimes a catheter may be required to obtain a clean catch urine on a child not yet toilet-trained. Preparation and methods for collecting urine specimens are discussed in Chapter 25.

24-Hour Urine. Twenty-four hour urine specimens are obtained to determine various urine indices that cannot be determined with a spot urine test, such as creatinine clearance. Refer to the accompanying display for the steps in collecting a 24-hour urine.

Blood Tests. The blood tests most frequently ordered to evaluate renal function are blood urea nitrogen (BUN) and creatinine. These tests are frequently referred to as "renal function tests." Urea is formed in the liver as a by-product of protein catabolism and is excreted by the kidneys. The blood concentration of urea is therefore related to the excretory function of the kidneys and serves as an index of function. BUN, however, is sometimes more reflective of protein ingestion rather than true renal function.

Creatinine, like BUN, is excreted entirely by the kidneys and is therefore directly proportional to renal function. Creatinine is a catabolic product of creatine, which is used in skeletal muscle contraction. The daily production of creatinine depends on muscle mass, which fluctuates little; therefore, the creatinine level fluctuates little. This makes creatinine the most accurate of the two values to measure renal function.

The normal BUN/creatinine ratio is about 20:1. When the BUN level rises out of proportion to the creatinine, dehydration, gastrointestinal (GI) bleeding, or malnutrition are suspected. When the levels rise together, kidney disease or failure are indicated. Refer to Table 46-2 for blood indices of renal function.

Creatinine Clearance Test. The creatinine clearance test is the most accurate method for measuring renal function, more accurate than simple blood tests such as BUN and creatinine, or urine tests. The creatinine clearance study is preferred because it is not affected by outside factors, and it shows less normal variability.

Creatinine clearance is a measure of the glomerular filtration rate (GFR), that is, the number of milliliters of filtrate made by the kidneys per minute. This test can be stressful for the child because it requires a blood speci-

TABLE 46-1
Urine Indices of Renal Function

Test	Appropriate Ranges	Deviations	Clinical Implications
Color	Clear yellow-gold	Cloudy	Presence of bacteria
		Hematuria	Trauma
			Glomerular nephritis
			Systemic lupus erythematosus
		Light	Dilute
		Dark	Concentrated
Specific gravity	Newborn: 1.001–1.020	High	Dehydration
	Older infants and children: 1.001–1.030		Presence of protein or glucose
		Low	Excessive fluid intake
			Decreased antidiuretic hormone
			Dehydration
pH	Newborn: 5.0–7.0	>7	Nephritis
	Older infants and children: 4.7–7.8	>8	Polycystic kidney disease
			Tuberculosis
			Kidney calculi
			Kidney trauma
Red blood cells (RBC)	None	Microscopic hematuria	Lower urinary tract infection
			Lupus erythematosus
			Malignant hypertension
			Glomerulonephritis
			Trauma
			Calculi
White blood cells (WBC)	1–2	>2	Urinary tract infection
			Pyelonephritis
Granular casts	None	>1	Glomerulonephritis
			Pyelonephritis
			Proteinuria
Crystals	None	>1	Calculi
			Hyperparathyroidism
Creatinine clearance	1–8 days: 17–60 ml/min/1.73 m²	Diminished	Renal impairment
	1–4 weeks: 26–68 ml/min/1.73 m²		
	1–6 months: 39–114 ml/min/1.73 m²		
	6–12 months: 49–157 ml/min/1.73 m²		
	12–18 months: 62–191 ml/min/1.73 m²		
	2–12 years: 89–165 ml/min/1.73 m²		

men and a 24-hour urine sample. Young children who must wear a urine collection device for this length of time often find the process frustrating. Creatinine clearance is determined by the formula indicated in the accompanying display about creatinine clearance test. The value determined for the creatinine clearance test may be individualized to the child by using the corrected creatine clearance formula. The laboratory needs the child's height and weight to determine body surface area using a standard nomogram.

Procedures

Laboratory tests are often not sufficient in diagnosing renal disease; more direct evaluation of the system is re-

quired. X-ray films and invasive diagnostic tests may be ordered. The major noninvasive and invasive tests are discussed in the following section.

Scout Film (KUB)

Description/Definition

X-ray of the abdomen, often called a kidney-ureter-bladder (KUB) film.

Purpose

KUB offers a one-dimensional view of the entire renal system, useful in evaluating the size of the kidneys, which can aid in early diagnosis of

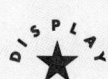

Guidelines for a 24-Hour Urine Collection

1. Explain the procedure to the child and family.
2. Instruct the family to keep the urine on ice or in the refrigerator.
3. Discard the urine from the first void.
4. Indicate the starting time on the container.
5. Collect all urine voided during the 24-hour period. If one specimen is discarded, the 24-hour urine must start again.
6. Remind the child to void before defecating so that the urine is not contaminated by feces.
7. Collect the last sample as close as possible to the end of the 24-hour period.

chronic disease process, obstructive uropathy, or cystic disease. It is also useful in identifying renal calculi.

Indications
- Unexplained renal symptoms
- Rising BUN or creatinine
- Difficulties voiding

Contraindications
- None

Preparation
The child and family should have the study explained to them by the physician or nurse. Prepare as for routine x-ray film.

Developmental Considerations
None

Nursing Care
The child is placed in a supine position for the film. The nurse should have the child lay still without breathing while the film is taken. The

TABLE 46-2
Blood Indices of Renal Function

Test	Appropriate Range	Deviations	Clinical Implications
Sodium	Infant: 139–146 mEq/L Child: 138–145 mEq/L Adolescent: 135–151 mEq/L	Hypernatremia Hyponatremia	Renal disease secondary to decreased output Dehydration Severe nephritis Edema Chlorothiazide diuretics Decreased blood flow to kidneys secondary to decreased cardiac output
Potassium	<10 days of age: 3.5–6.0 mEq/L >10 days–adolescent: 3.5–5.0 mEq/L	Hyperkalemia Hypokalemia	Inadequate excretion due to renal failure Acidosis Acute renal failure with oliguria or anuria Renal tubular acidosis Chlorothiazide diuretics Nephritis
Chloride	Infant: 95–110 mEq/L Child: 101–108 mEq/L Adolescent: 98–108 mEq/L	Hyperchloremia Hypochloremia	Dehydration Anemia Chlorothiazide diuretics
Calcium	Infant: 7.0–12.0 mg/dl Child: 8.0–10.5 mg/dl Adolescent: 8.5–10.5 mg/dl	Hypercalcemia Hypocalcemia	Kidney disease secondary to inadequate elimination Prolonged use of diuretics Hyperparathyroidism secondary to renal insufficiency
Phosphorus	Infant and child: 4.0–7.0 mg/dl Adolescent: 3.0–4.5 mg/dl	Hyperphosphatemia	Renal insufficiency and severe nephritis accompanied by elevated BUN and creatinine
Blood urea nitrogen	Infant: 5–15 mg/dl Child–Adolescent: 10–20 mg/dl	Increased Increased	Kidney failure (acute or chronic) Urinary obstruction Dehydration Excessive protein intake Hemorrhage
Creatinine	Infant: 0.2–0.4 mg/dl Child: 0.3–0.7 mg/dl Adolescent: 0.5–1.0 mg/dl	Increased	Kidney failure (acute or chronic) Obstruction of urinary tract

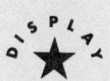

Creatinine Clearance Test

Creatinine clearance = UV/P

U = Number of mg/dl of creatinine excreted in the urine over 24 hours.

V = Volume of urine, in ml/min.

P = Serum creatinine in mg/dl

To individualize the CrCl test to the child, nomograms are used to find the body surface area (expressed in square meters, m²).

Corrected Creatinine Clearance

Corrected CrCl

$$= \frac{\text{Measured CrCl (see above formula)} \times 1.73}{\text{Body Surface Area (in m}^2\text{)}}$$

KUB may be performed on the clinical unit with the child in bed or in the radiology department.

Complications

None

Renal Ultrasound

Description/Definition

An ultrasound probe is moved back and forth over the renal area; ultrasonic waves from the probe reflect from the renal structures to the probe and produce an image on the ultrasound computer.

Purpose

The renal ultrasound is an accurate, noninvasive procedure used to determine kidney size and shape. Ultrasound easily identifies thinning of the renal cortex, edema, masses, cysts, and obstructive uropathy.

Indications

- Hydronephrosis
- Chronic parenchymal disease
- Kidney transplantation rejection
- Cystic kidney disease
- Neurogenic bladder

Contraindications

None

Preparation

The child and parents should have the test explained to them by the physician, and the nurse should reinforce the information. Ideally, the child should be NPO for 6 to 12 hours before the study to eliminate bowel gas. Sedation may be required for some children.

Developmental Considerations

Infant: If the child is agitated, prepare with rectal chloral hydrate, 8 mg/kg.

Child: If the child is agitated, prepare with oral chloral hydrate, 8 mg/kg.

Adolescent: No sedation required.

Nursing Care

Chloral hydrate sedation is administered before the study. Once in ultrasound, the child is instructed to lay supine.

Complications

None

Intravenous Pyelography (IVP)

Description/Definition

Iodinated radiographic contrast medium is administered intravenously; the medium is secreted and concentrated by the renal tubules. X-ray films are taken at 30 seconds, then every 5 minutes for up to 30 minutes. If the patient has poor renal function, delayed films may be obtained at 1 hour, 8, 12, or 24 hours.

Purpose

IVP outlines complete renal anatomy quite well. Retroperitoneal masses may be identified because they shift the ureters. Cysts, tumors, calculi, and obstructions can be easily observed.

Indications

- Difficulty voiding
- To obtain complete picture of renal anatomy
- Possible kidney stones
- Possible tumors or malignancy

Contraindications

- Iodine allergy
- Sickle cell anemia

Preparation

Assess the child for past allergic reactions to iodinated radiographic contrast mediums, iodine, or seafood. The child should receive cathartics or an enema the evening before the study. The nurse warns the child and family about hot flushing and a salty taste in the mouth that may occur when the dye is administered.

Developmental Considerations

Infant: Not useful in neonates due to their renal concentrating deficit. Children less than 2 years of age should be NPO after midnight. Eight ounces of fluid are allowed in the morning before the study. The test should be scheduled early to prevent dehydration.

Child: Children more than 2 years of age sometimes are given a cathartic the night before the procedure; they are NPO after midnight. A Fleet enema is given in the morning before the procedure.

Adolescent: Same as child.

Nursing Care

Intravenous access is established and the iodinated radiographic contrast material is administered in a bolus push. During the study, the child should be observed closely for a reaction to the contrast material. After the study, the child is encouraged to drink extra fluids.

Complications

1. Allergic reaction to contrast material
2. Sickling and infarction of renal tissue in child with sickle cell anemia
3. Congestive heart failure

Renal Scan (Radiorenography)

Description/Definition

A radioactive isotope (e.g., I^{131}, technetium, hippuran) is administered intravenously and excreted by the kidney. External radiation detector probes are placed over the kidneys to determine blood flow by noting the appearance and disappearance of the radioactive material in the

TABLE 46-3
Selected Nursing Diagnoses Associated With Altered Renal Function

Data Analysis and Conclusion	Nursing Diagnosis
Health Perception and Health Management	
Uncontrolled BP. Sudden change in lab values. Examples: BUN, creatinine, calcium, phosphorus. Fluid overload. Repeated relapses in condition. Misses scheduled appointments. Verbalizes hopelessness or confusion about therapy.	Altered health maintenance related to knowledge deficit, frustration, or hopelessness.
Nutrition and Metabolism	
Poor appetite. Weight loss. Decreased muscle mass. Low serum protein. Proteinuria. High BUN for creatinine ratio.	Altered nutrition (less than body requirements) related to strict renal diet, anorexia, CAPD protein loss, loss of taste, loss of vitamins, loss of protein in urine.
Increased appetite. Weight gain. Steroid-induced diabetes mellitus. Hypertension. Sedentary activities.	Altered nutrition (more than body requirements) related to increased caloric intake from steroid therapy or altered metabolism of nutrients.
Areas of redness. Skin breakdown. Poor skin turgor. Poor wound healing.	Impaired skin integrity related to altered nutritional/metabolic processes, edema, poor wound healing due to steroids.
Fever. Oral candidiasis. UTI (urinary tract infection) burning on urination, frequency. Backache. Wounds/pus. Increased WBC. Abdominal pain. Upper respiratory infection.	High risk for infection related to impaired immune system from uremia or side-effects of medications, altered skin integrity, peritonitis from peritoneal dialysis or poor wound healing.
Activity and Exercise	
Fatigue. Dyspnea. Increased pulse rate. Unable to attend school. Decrease in physical activities.	Activity intolerance related to uremia and anemia.
Shortness of breath. Rales, wheezing. Dyspnea. Orthopnea. Hyperventilation.	Ineffective breathing pattern related to fluid retention/overload leading to congestive heart failure or pulmonary edema, metabolic acidosis, or abdominal distention during peritoneal dialysis.
Change in BP, pulse, CVP; EKG changes (arrhythmias, tall T waves). Restlessness. Massive diuresis. Early transplant rejection.	Decreased cardiac output related to arrhythmias from potassium retention (hypertension) or volume deficit following renal transplantation.
Decreased strength. Low stamina. Bone pain. Changes in bone density noted on x-rays. Fractures. Low serum calcium.	High risk for injury related to muscle weakness or bone changes from demineralization.
Preoccupation with drinking. Sneaking excess fluid. Refusing to eat with others.	Diversional activity deficit related to fluid restrictions.
Pallor. Dyspnea. Fatigue. Hct <30%. EKG changes (arrhythmias and tall T waves). K$^+$ >5.5 mEq. Edema.	Altered tissue perfusion related to anemia, arrhythmia or edema.
Unable to attend school. Unable to attend family functions. Hypertension. Weight gain >2 lb/week. Failure to seek proper medical support. Missing appointments. Altered electrolytes. Elevated BUN and creatinine.	Impaired health maintenance related to stress, financial strain or decreased family support associated with chronic renal diseases and their treatment (dialysis, transplant).
Elimination	
Frequency. Urgency. Hesitancy. Painful voiding. Decreased or absent voiding.	Altered urinary elimination pattern related to nocturia, dysuria, or renal failure.
Straining at stools. Hard stools. Infrequent passage. Abdominal distention. Anorexia or nausea. Headache.	Constipation related to lack of exercise, decreased fluid intake, decreased fiber in diet, decreased peristalsis and abdominal distention associated with peritoneal dialysis, phosphate binding medications (antacids), or bedrest.
Decreased urine output. Decreased weight, BP, CVP. Increased pulse rate. Dizziness. Sweating. Decreased skin turgor. Thirst. Increased hematocrit.	High risk for fluid volume deficit related to dialysis or diuretic therapy.
Decreased urine output. Increased weight, BP, CVP and pulse rate. Edema (face, periorbital, hands, sacrum, ankles). Dyspnea. Congestive heart failure. Pulmonary edema. Increased BUN and creatinine. Decreased hematocrit.	Fluid volume excess related to acute or chronic renal failure, nephrotic syndrome or excess dietary sodium.
Cognition and Perception	
Verbal report of pain. Facial grimacing. Guarding. Self-focusing. Changes in BP, P, R. Sweating. Restlessness. Refusing procedures. Crying on urination. Holding urine.	Pain related to diagnostic procedures, therapeutic procedures, or urinary tract infections.
Confusion. Poor concentration. Poor memory. Lethargy. Apathy. Decline in school grades.	Altered thought processes related to uremic buildup of toxic waste products or depression over chronic illness.
Not following prescribed regimen. Multiple questions. Anxiety. Refusal of treatment. Does not trust medical team.	Anxiety related to lack of knowledge about renal disease, diagnostic and therapeutic procedures, or medications.
Self-Perception and Self-Concept	
Restlessness. Insomnia. Withdrawn. Questioning. Trembling. Sweating.	Anxiety/Fear of the unknown related to knowledge deficit or lack of experience with disease, procedures, or treatment options.
Refusal to look at, touch, or care for catheters or scars. Changes in socialization patterns. Verbalizes negative feelings about body. Fear of negative reaction by others. Refusal to attend school or interact with peers. Obsession with appearance. Adolescent refuses to have relationships with opposite sex.	Body image disturbance related to catheters, surgical scars, short stature, medication side-effects (Cushing's syndrome, "moon face," acne, weight gain, excessive hair growth on face, arms, or back).
Awareness of kidney transplant as "foreign body." Guilt feelings over cadaver donor's death. Overidentifies with the cadaver donor: feels that they will take on some of their personality. Feelings that they should have died instead.	Personal identity disturbance related to transplanted kidney.

(Continued)

TABLE 46-3
(Continued)

Data Analysis and Conclusion	Nursing Diagnosis
Role-Relationship Disturbances	
Expression of grief. Hopelessness. Withdrawal. Depression. Dependency.	Grieving related to loss of function of a major body part and lifestyle changes.
Verbalizes fear and concern. Reluctance to visit. Unrealistic goals. Blames self. Expresses resentment. Inappropriate questions or behavior. Delays treatment.	Altered parenting related to anxiety over child's illness.
Withdrawal. Depression. Anger. Regression.	Social isolation related to separation from family and friends due to hospitalization or home-bound education, appearance (fear of rejection by peers), decreased financial resources (may create lifestyle changes for the family).
Sexuality and Reproduction	
Verbalizes concerns. Questioning. Inappropriate sexual behavior. Change in relationships. Amenorrhea. Impotence.	Sexual dysfunction related to uremia resulting in decreased sexual drive and infertility.
Coping and Stress Tolerance	
Anger and hostility. Depression. Withdrawal. Regression. Sleep disturbances.	Ineffective individual coping related to hospitalization (forced separation), body image changes, or powerlessness over chronic condition.
Grief. Guilt. Anger and hostility. Depression. Withdrawal. Abuse/neglect. Misses appointments.	Ineffective family coping related to diagnosis and prognosis, disruption of lifestyle, financial worries, or guilt.

kidneys. The time of uptake and excretion of the radioactive material is calculated.

Purpose

Visualizes renal vascularization and function of the kidneys. Useful in determining perfusion and function of a transplanted kidney.

Indications

- Identifying direct primary renal disease (i.e., glomerulonephritis, acute tubular necrosis, and so forth)
- Transplantation rejection
- Renal infarction
- May be used in place of IVP for children with allergies to the contrast material

Contraindications

None; only a tracer dose of radioactive material is used.

Preparation

The child and family should have the test explained to them by the physician. Assurance is given that the child is exposed to low doses of radiation and that no side-effects are expected. No special preparation is required other than placement of a heparin lock or intravenous line. The nurse reinforces that the child should not experience any pain or discomfort once the intravenous line is established.

Developmental Considerations

Infant: The young child requires restraint on a papoose board.
Child: None
Adolescent: None

Nursing Care

Intravenous access is established, and the radiologist or radiologic technologist administers the radioactive isotope. The child is placed in the supine position. The nurse needs to encourage the child to remain still during the procedure.

Complications

None

Renal Biopsy

Description/Definition

A small amount of renal tissue is removed by open or percutaneous technique either in the operating room or radiology department. A closed biopsy using a percutaneous needle is much more common than open biopsy. With closed biopsy, the kidney is identified by ultrasound, a biopsy needle is inserted, and a small piece of cortical tissue is removed. Open biopsy requires a surgical incision to expose the kidney and obtain a specimen.

Purpose

Renal biopsy permits the study of renal histology at any point during the course of the disease. Useful for diagnosing unexplained hematuria, steroid-resistant nephrosis, persistent glomerulonephritis, and unexplained hypertension. The biopsy identifies early rejection versus immunosuppressant toxicity in transplantation.

Indications

- Transplantation rejection
- Possible cyclosporine toxicity of transplanted kidney
- Hematuria
- Nephritis unresponsive to therapy

Contraindications

- PT, PTT, or bleeding times elevated

Preparation

The physician and nurse should explain to the child why the procedure is being done and what the experience will be like. The child to receive local anesthesia needs to be taught how to take deep breaths and hold them on cue.

Developmental Considerations

Infant: Children younger than 10 years of age are usually biopsied under general anesthesia
Child: Same as infant
Adolescent: Children older than 10 years of age are sedated and biopsied under ultrasound

Nursing Care

Intravenous access must be established for both the closed and open biopsy. The child younger than 10 years must be prepped for surgery

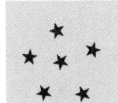

Ideas for Nursing Research

The complexity of renal disorders often makes nursing assessment and diagnosis a lengthy process that is tiring to the child and family. Nurses have an opportunity to investigate ways to make data collection more effective and efficient. The following areas need to be explored:

- The methods of interviewing that are most effective in different ages of children with renal dysfunction.
- Determine the method to do the most accurate nutritional assessment on the child with renal disease.
- Best teaching methods for promoting understanding of renal diagnostic procedures in young children.
- How to avoid repetition of assessment data collection when a child with a chronic renal condition has repeated hospitalizations.

---

per physician's order. All children should receive sedation before going for the procedure. The child is placed in the prone position with a pillow or sand bag used to elevate the mid body area. The nurse should instruct the child older than 10 years receiving local anesthesia to take deep breaths during the procedure and to hold a deep breath when the needle is inserted. Immediately after the procedure, a pressure dressing and sand bag should be applied. The child remains in the prone position for 30 to 60 minutes and on bedrest for 24 hours. The biopsy dressing should be checked for bleeding and vital signs checked every 10 minutes the first hour and, based on findings, progressively decreased to once every hour. All urine should be checked for hematuria, and intake and output need to be monitored for 24 hours. The nurse should encourage the child to drink large amounts of fluid to prevent clot formation or urine retention. The nurse must monitor for flank pain, sudden weakness, fainting, and rapid pulse.

Complications

- Hemorrhage
- Infection
- Hematoma

Selected Nursing Diagnoses

After obtaining the history, performing the physical examination, reviewing results from the diagnostic tests, and tapping additional resources for information, the nurse carefully analyzes data obtained. Nursing diagnoses appropriate for the child with renal dysfunction become apparent and are used to develop a plan of care. Selected nursing diagnoses that may be appropriate for the child with renal dysfunction are presented by function in Table 46-3.

Summary

The comprehensive assessment of the child with renal disease necessitates a focused history using functional health and a thorough physical examination involving all body systems. Laboratory data as well as noninvasive and invasive diagnostic studies are crucial in diagnosing renal disease. Nursing diagnoses are determined according to the functional health pattern and help the nurse to provide appropriate physiologic, psychological, and sociologic care. All of this information is compiled in a nursing care plan that directs nursing care for the child with symptoms associated with a renal disease.

References

1. Barness, L. A. (1992). *Manual of pediatric physical diagnosis* (6th ed.). St. Louis: Mosby.
2. Barratt, T. M., & Chantler, C. (1987). Clinical evaluation. In T. M. Barratt, M. A. Holliday, & R. L. Vernier (Eds.), *Pediatric nephrology* (5th ed.). Baltimore: Williams & Wilkins.
3. Bates, B. (Ed.). (1991). *A guide to physical examination* (5th ed.). Philadelphia: Lippincott.
4. Dracopoulos, D. T., & Weatherly, J. B. (1983). Chronic renal failure: The effects on the entire family. *Issues in Comprehensive Pediatric Nursing, 6.*
5. Edelmann, C. (1978). *Pediatric kidney disease.* Boston: Little Brown.
6. Fine, R. N., & Gruskin, A. B. (1984). *End stage renal disease in children.* Philadelphia: Saunders.
7. Flannery, L. (1978). Adaptation to chronic renal failure. *Psychosomatics, 19,* 784.
8. Giovannelli, G. G., New, M. I., & Gorini, S. (1981). *Hypertension in children and adolescents.* New York: Raven Press.
9. Gordon, M. (1991). *Manual of nursing diagnosis.* St. Louis: Mosby.
10. Lancaster, L. E. (1984). *The patient with end stage renal disease* (2nd ed.). New York: Wiley.
11. Levine, D. Z. (1991). *Care of the renal patient* (2nd ed.). Philadelphia: Saunders.
12. Lum, G. M., & Todd, J. K. (1991). Kidney and urinary tract. In W. E. Hathaway, et al. (Eds.), *Current pediatric diagnosis and treatment.* Norwalk, CT: Appleton & Lange.
13. Neff, E. J. (1987). Nursing the child undergoing dialysis. *Issues in Comprehensive Pediatric Nursing, 10,* 3.
14. Polise, K. (1985). The renal system. In L. L. Hayman, & E. M. Sporing (Eds.), *Handbook of pediatric nursing.* New York: Wiley.
15. Sachs, B. L. (1977). *Renal transplantation: A nursing perspective.* Flushing, NY: Medical Examination Publishing.
16. Seidel, H. M., & Chantler, C. (1975). Clinical evaluation. In T. M. Barratt, M. A. Holliday, & R. L. Vernier (Eds.), *Pediatric nephrology.* Baltimore: Williams & Wilkins.
17. Southby, J., & Moore, J. (1983). Nursing diagnosis for a child with end stage renal disease. *Journal of the American Association of Nephrology Nurses and Technicians, 10,* 23–27.
18. Ulrich, B. (1989). *Nephrology nursing concepts and strategies.* Norwalk, CT: Appleton & Lange.

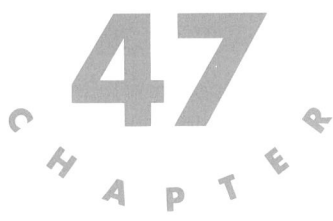

47

CHAPTER

Nursing Planning, Intervention, and Evaluation for Altered Renal Function

BEHAVIORAL OBJECTIVES

Distinguish between the clinical manifestations of acute and chronic renal failure.

Differentiate between acquired and congenital renal disorders.

Discuss important nursing assessments and interventions critical to detecting and monitoring physiologic complications in the child with altered renal function.

List nursing diagnoses that are commonly applicable to the child with altered renal function.

Discuss the medical therapy and treatment modalities commonly prescribed for children with altered renal function.

Compare advantages and disadvantages of peritoneal dialysis and hemodialysis for the child and family.

Outline the nursing care typically needed for the family and child who has a kidney transplantation.

Discuss the potential effects of chronic renal failure and end-stage renal disease on the growth and development of the child.

Describe the psychosocial impact of chronic renal failure and end-stage renal disease on the child and family.

The kidneys have a critical function in maintaining homeostasis. Damage or disease of the kidneys, therefore, has the potential to affect all other body systems and contribute to acute or chronic conditions. Nursing care for children with altered renal function demands comprehensive assessment and continuous monitoring of physiologic status. Providing psychosocial support for the child and family at various stages of illness and treatment is equally important. The nurse plays a critical role in teaching the child and family about renal disease, its treatment, and home care regimens. Ongoing evaluation of the impact of chronic renal insufficiency on the child's growth and development cannot be overemphasized.

Renal dysfunction occurs in children as a result of inherited, congenital, or acquired conditions. Because many renal disorders have the potential to cause acute renal failure (ARF), progress to chronic renal failure (CRF) and end-stage renal disease (ESRD), this chapter begins with those problems. Specific inherited or acquired conditions that result in renal dysfunction follow. The collaborative and independent nursing interventions needed to maintain and improve the child's health and well-being are emphasized.

Acute Renal Failure

Definition and Incidence. Acute renal failure (ARF) is the sudden deterioration of the kidney's ability to manage regulatory and excretory functions. This condition may also be called acute tubular necrosis or acute tubular insufficiency. Few children develop ARF, but it is a life-threatening event when it occurs.

ARF results in the accumulation of metabolic waste products in the blood, decreased urine output, and altered fluid and electrolyte balance. When nitrogenous waste products accumulate in the blood, a condition known as *azotemia* exists; if the waste products generate toxic symptoms, the condition is called *uremia*. ARF is said to be present when either blood urea nitrogen (BUN) is in excess of 100 mg/dL or oliguria (less than 300 cc/m^2/day or <1 cc/kg/h) is present.[23]

ARF can be either reversible or irreversible. Children with reversible ARF can expect to have complete recovery in approximately 6 months. Those who have irreversible renal failure develop uremia and require dialysis and/or transplantation.

Etiology and Pathophysiology. In ARF, there is tissue injury causing a severe reduction of renal function to such an extent that maintenance of body homeostasis is impossible. Three general classifications based on cause have been established: prerenal, renal, and postrenal failure. The conditions that contribute to these causes are listed in Table 47-1.

Prerenal failure occurs when blood flow to the kidneys is markedly diminished. The kidneys have no preexisting anatomic or physiologic defect; they simply receive inadequate circulatory perfusion. The most common prerenal cause of ARF is hypovolemia associated with blood loss, trauma, or gastrointestinal (GI) losses. GI losses include vomiting and diarrhea, which can result in severe dehydration, causing hypovolemia, and resulting in diminished perfusion of the kidneys and, ultimately, ARF. Recovery from prerenal causes is typical.

Renal causes of ARF, in contrast, result when the kidney tissue is insulted or damaged primarily by the presence of disease or toxins. In this situation, the glomerular capillaries and tubules are unable to function. Glomerulonephritis, for example, may damage the glomeruli, whereas toxic agents may destroy renal tubules. Recovery of kidney function is unusual with renal causes of ARF.[3]

Postrenal causes of ARF result when there is an anatomic or functional barrier in the flow of urine from the kidneys to the urethral meatus. These obstructions may be temporary and result in little damage if corrective surgery is performed. If a congenital anomaly is involved, the problem may go unnoticed until permanent renal damage occurs, or only temporary relief may be obtained with corrective surgery. These children may develop a chronic renal condition.[44]

In all types of ARF, there is a critical reduction in the glomerular filtration rate (GFR) thus preventing formation of urine in the customary volume and composition. The BUN level quickly rises, and tubular reabsorption of sodium from the proximal tubules is prevented. As a result, sodium concentration increases in the distal tubules and

TABLE 47-1
Causes of Acute Renal Failure in Children

Prerenal	Renal	Postrenal
Hypovolemia:	Glomerulonephritis	Urinary calculi
Gastroenteritis	Nephrotic syndrome	Blood clots
Hemorrhage	Interstitial nephritis	Tumors:
Burns	Hemolytic uremic syndrome	Wilms' tumor
Hypotension:	Malignant hypertension	Neuroblastoma
Sepsis	Periarteritisnodosa	Congenital structural anomalies
Hypothermia	Intravascular coagulopathy	Foreign body
Shock	Nephrotoxins:	Trauma
Heart failure	Accidental ingestion of drugs or poison	
Hypoxia:	Heavy metals (mercury, gold, lead, arsenic)	
Respiratory distress syndrome	Antineoplastics	
Pneumonia	Anesthetics	
Renal vascular obstruction	Antimicrotics	
	Anti-inflammatories	
	Contrast media	
	Snakebite	
	Pesticides	
	Fungicides	

stimulates the renin mechanism explained in Chapter 45. Angiotensin is released and stimulates local vasoconstriction of the afferent arterioles and more retention of sodium. Sodium retention expands the extracellular volume and blood volume, which increases blood pressure and decreases urine volume. Figure 47-1 diagrams the complex effects of renal failure.

Damage to the kidneys from acute failure varies depending on the underlying cause. Necrosis of the renal cortex may be complete or incomplete, and the extent of damage determines whether some function is likely to return. Likewise, the amount of necrosis of the renal tubules varies with underlying causes and duration of ARF. The body is unable to regenerate an entire nephron if the basement membrane has been destroyed, but it may regenerate individual tubular cells.[44] The prognosis of ARF, therefore, depends on the cause, the extent of the renal damage, the effectiveness of treatment, and the development of complications.

Clinical Manifestations. Frequently, ARF may be due to more than one factor, and the presenting symptoms may vary. The most common complaint is the sudden decrease in urine output, although in some types of ARF the urine volume may be close to normal.[3] The child is generally lethargic and may appear pale and edematous. Nausea and vomiting are not unusual. Hypertension is common and may cause central nervous system irritability

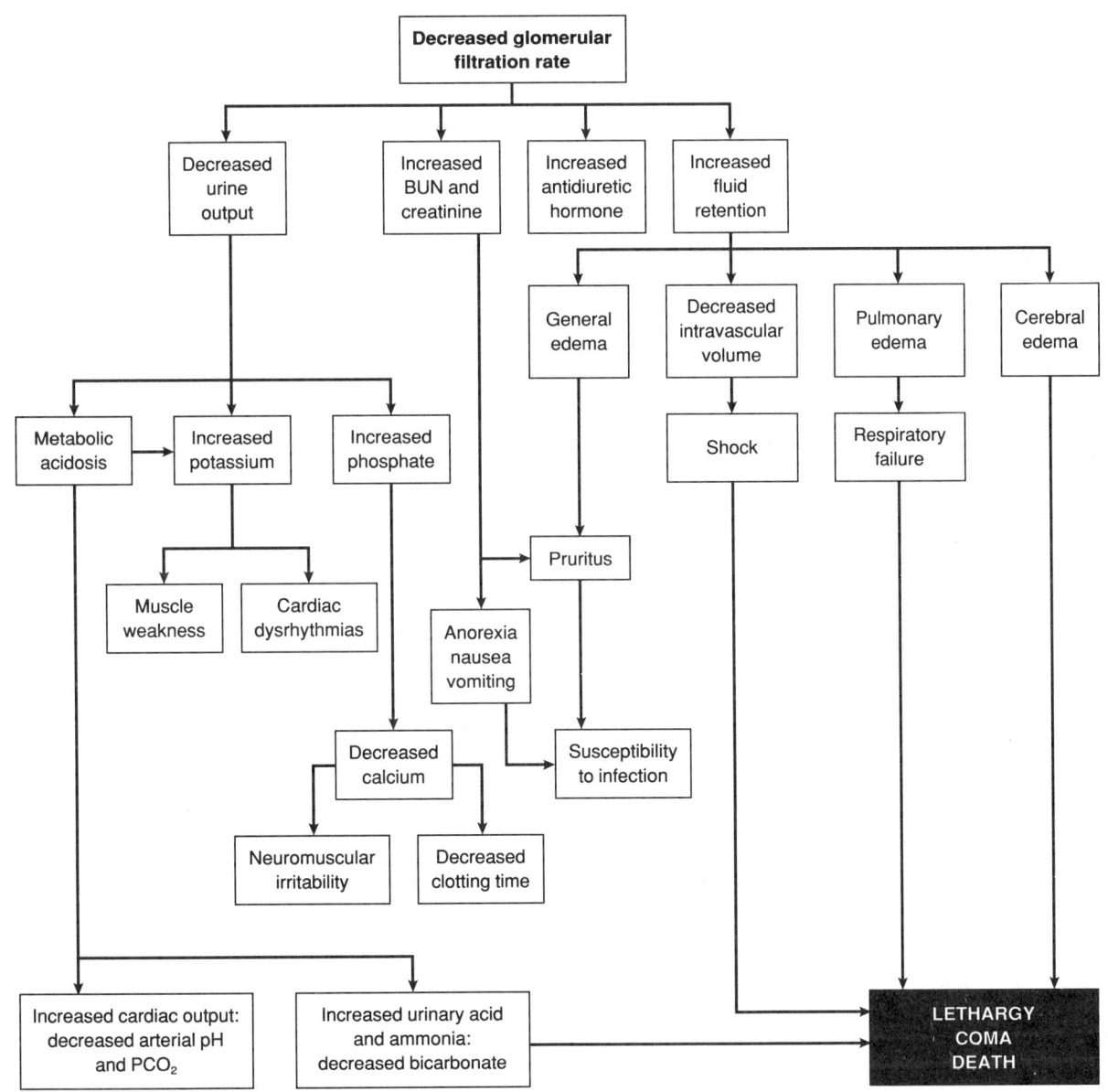

FIGURE 47-1
Complex effects of renal failure. The life-threatening progress of kidney failure results primarily from the decrease in the glomerules filtration rate as shown on the flowchart. Two other effects heighten the complications caused by the impaired filtration. Increased secretion of the enzyme renin sets up a chain of events that exacerbates fluid retention. Decreased levels of the hormone erythropoietin inhibit red blood cell production in the bone marrow and thus contributes to anemia. (Coleman, E. [1986]. When the kidneys fail. *RN, 49,* 28–34.)

and, eventually, seizures. As fluid overload progresses, pulmonary edema and congestive heart failure are possible.[40]

The child with a prerenal cause related to hypovolemia frequently presents with clinical signs of dehydration: hypotension, tachycardia, poor perfusion, sunken eyes, dry mucous membranes, and poor skin turgor. With careful volume replacement, there can be rapid improvement in kidney perfusion and kidney function. In reversible ARF, the changes in the kidney progress through the following three phases:[23]

- *Initiation phase*—A sequence of events is set in motion that injures the tubular epithelial cells by ischemia or by a toxin.
- *Maintenance phase*— The GFR remains relatively low for several days or weeks depending on the severity of the initiating insult.
- *Recovery phase*—Improvement in renal function is characterized by gradual and progressive restoration of GFR and tubule function. During this phase, there is frequently an abrupt diuresis with high urine output.

Although most children with ARF recover, some etiologic factors such as chronic obstruction lead to permanent renal impairment. In time, these children develop CRF and, ultimately, ESRD.

Diagnostic Studies. Previously healthy children with ARF typically seek medical care for unmistakable symptoms. A comprehensive assessment usually suggests the diagnosis and underlying causes. Common findings of blood work may reveal anemia, hyponatremia, hyperkalemia, hypocalcemia, metabolic acidosis, and elevated BUN, creatinine, uric acid, and phosphate. Urinalysis shows diminished output, and, if the ARF is a result of hypovolemia, specific gravity and pH are elevated; casts, crystals, and red blood cells (RBC) may be present if ARF is due to renal causes. Chest x-ray may reveal cardiomegaly and pulmonary congestion if renal failure is advanced. Obstructions may be evaluated with abdominal x-ray, renal ultrasound, and a renal scan. Renal biopsy may be required to determine the exact cause of renal failure. Detailed information regarding renal diagnostic procedures can be found in Chapter 46.

★ ASSESSMENT

A complete history and thorough physical assessment are extremely important to help determine etiology and develop the plan of care. The history explores when the parents first noticed that the child was ill. A recent history of a GI or upper respiratory infection is not uncommon. Changes in the child's urinary output and the presence of blood in the urine are important to note, as well as the child's ability to take and retain fluids.

As ARF develops, fluid accumulates in the tissues and pallor is evident. Urine output diminishes and is dark in color. If the renal failure is advanced, signs of congestive heart failure, hepatosplenomegaly, and increasing pressure in the central nervous system may be exhibited. Physical examination, including vital signs and weight, with particular attention to fluid status, is imperative. A

guide to nursing assessment by systems is described in Table 47-2.[34]

★ NURSING DIAGNOSES AND PLANNING

Children with ARF have unique needs. However, based on the assessment data from above and Chapter 46, the following nursing diagnoses may apply:

- Fluid Volume Excess related to decreased urine output, sodium retention, or fluid intake above amount allowed.
- Altered Nutrition: Less Than Body Requirements related to anorexia, nausea, vomiting, dietary restrictions, or altered taste sensation.
- Activity Intolerance related to anemia and/or congestive heart failure.
- Anxiety/Fear (child) related to unfamiliar environment and painful procedures.
- Anxiety/Fear (parental) related to knowledge deficit regarding normal kidney function, acute renal failure, treatment plan, and hospitalization.

The nurse and child (or parents) work together to plan effective care based on the established nursing diagnoses. Several examples of expected outcomes follow:

- The child participates in age-appropriate activities.
- The family describes potential complications and actions to take for each.
- The child is free of infection.
- The child demonstrates that his or her nutritional needs are met.
- The child and family return to normal activities of daily living.

The nurse's plans for the daily care of the child are based on both physician's orders and nursing diagnoses. Some general nursing care goals for restoring renal function may be the following:

- The child's chemical and laboratory findings are within the normal limits (urinalysis, complete blood count [CBC], serum BUN, and creatinine).
- The child's blood pressure is within normal limits for age and sex.

★ INTERVENTIONS: COLLABORATIVE AND INDEPENDENT

When the risks are known and ARF is impending, the condition sometimes may be prevented by prompt initiation of fluid therapy and other measures. With the onset of symptoms of renal failure, however, the primary plan is supportive until the kidneys recover. (ARF that persists to CRF is discussed in the following section of the chapter.) General management includes control of fluids and electrolytes, maintenance of normal blood pressure, and treatment of the underlying causes and resulting complications. Nurses have both collaborative and independent responsibilities in providing care.

FLUID THERAPY

When prerenal causes of ARF are found, the need for volume replacement is readily apparent. With hypovolemia, intravascular volume is expanded by the intravenous (IV) administration of isotonic saline. After this in-

TABLE 47-2
Nursing Assessment of Acute Renal Failure: A Systems Approach

Body System	Clinical Manifestation	Assessment
Urinary system	Urine output: Decrease in initial phase, gradually increases during maintenance phase, and progresses to normal during recovery phase Urinary tract infection	Monitor intake and output accurately Monitor blood and urine electrolytes Serum BUN and creatinine Monitor vital signs Perform cultures of urine and blood
Gastrointestinal system	Nausea and vomiting Anorexia Altered taste sensation Diarrhea or constipation Stomatitis Gastrointestinal bleeding Weight loss Muscle wasting	Monitor diet intake (usually need increased caloric intake and decreased Na^+, K^+, and protein in diet) Observe for hematemesis and melena Monitor serum BUN and K^+ (usually elevated)
Cardiovascular system	Arrhythmias due to hyperkalemia and hypocalcemia Pericarditis Initial phase (especially prerenal) hypotension, but hypertension common Volume overload Congestive heart failure	Monitor BP, pulse, and heart sounds Observe for hypovolemia (poor skin turgor, poor perfusion, tachycardia, sunken eyes, dry mucous membranes) Signs of overload (cardiac gallop rhythm, edema of feet and hands, puffy face, neck veins distended, and hepatomegaly)
Respiratory system	Acidosis Hyperventilation Upper respiratory infection Pneumonia Pulmonary edema	Monitor respirations and blood gases Chest x-ray Breath sounds: pulmonary rales start at base of lungs then generalize
Neurologic system	Weakness Myoclonus Disorientation Headache	Determine level of consciousness, irritability versus lethargy Observe for seizure activity
Integumentary system	Rashes Itching/dryness Purpura	Monitor for bruises, skin integrity Monitor CBC, especially platelet count
Hematopoietic system	Anemia Frequently WBC increased Platelet count decreased	Observe for pallor Monitor hemoglobin and hematocrit—signs of bleeding, coagulation studies

fusion, a child who is dehydrated generally voids within 2 hours.[3] Failure to void requires reassessment to determine whether the kidneys are functioning. If laboratory and clinical evaluations confirm that the child is adequately hydrated, diuretic therapy may be considered.[44] Fluid restriction is essential for children who fail to produce adequate urine output (>1 cc/kg/h) after volume expansion or the use of diuretics.

During the maintenance (oliguric) phase, the fluid therapy plan is designed to replace all losses including insensible loss (increased with fever), any drainage (nasogastric [NG], chest, diarrhea), and urine output. The nurse needs to monitor all intake closely, including intravenous (maintenance plus that used for medication administration), oral (food and fluids), and mist from humidified air.

The adequacy of fluid therapy is best determined by changes in weight, which the nurse measures on the same scale at the same time of day or every 12 hours. Weight is expected to stabilize or increase slightly until the kidneys regain function. As kidney function returns, urine output increases and may become voluminous, causing a rapid decline in body weight. This diuresis is characteristic of the recovery phase.

The nurse is responsible for titrating the IV fluids and monitoring the child's response by ongoing assessment. Fluid volume must be watched carefully to avoid hypervolemia during the oliguric state and resulting hypertension. Conversely, during the diuretic stage of the disease, hypovolemia must be avoided to prevent further renal damage.

ELECTROLYTE THERAPY

Hyperkalemia is life-threatening because it causes cardiac toxicity; it must be treated aggressively and promptly. Children with ARF should receive low potassium-containing fluid, foods, or medications until renal function is re-established. The body's excess potassium must be depleted. Kayexalate, a sodium polystyrene sulfonate resin, is often administered at a dose of 1 g/kg body weight by mouth or by rectum. It may be repeated every 2 to 4 hours in an emergency situation and every 6 hours for temporary maintenance. Kayexalate actually removes potassium by exchanging sodium ions for potassium ions. Kayexalate should be mixed with sorbitol, which promotes an osmotic diarrhea to ensure adequate GI loss and prevents constipation or fecal impaction.[12,52]

If the serum potassium continues to rise, emergency measures may include the IV administration of calcium gluconate, sodium bicarbonate, or a combination of glucose with regular insulin. The effects of these measures, however, are short-term. IV calcium gluconate protects the heart from the effects of hyperkalemia but does not decrease serum potassium. When a child with renal failure is acidotic, sodium bicarbonate causes the potassium to enter the cells, temporarily lowering the serum potassium level. The combination of glucose and insulin causes glucose to go into the cells and take potassium with it. In a life-threatening crisis, the emergency measures already mentioned may be used or dialysis may be initiated.[12,23]

If serum potassium is 6.0 mEq/L or higher, the child should be placed on continuous cardiac monitoring. The appearance of tall, peaked T waves is the earliest sign of hyperkalemia and demands rapid notification of the physician. As the child's condition becomes worse, the ST segment is depressed, the P–R component is prolonged, and the QRS interval becomes wider (see Chap. 39 for discussion of the normal electrocardiogram). If unchecked, ventricle fibrillation and cardiac arrest ensue.

CARDIOVASCULAR CONTROL

Hypertension may be present and should be treated by decreasing the fluid and sodium load and by using antihypertensive drugs. In children with hypertensive encephalopathy, irritability, headache, or convulsions may be present. These signs are usually associated with an acute, rapid rise in blood pressure rather than chronic hypertension. Diazoxide or hydralazine may be administered by IV push, or sodium nitroprusside by continuous IV drip. Nifedipine, propranolol, captopril, or Minipress may be given orally.[23] After administration of the antihypertensive, a fall in blood pressure may be seen in 15 to 20 minutes. However, additional doses may be required.

DIET THERAPY

Maintaining good nutrition is extremely important due to the fact that severe catabolism occurs with ARF. Healing of the kidneys and prevention of complications requires adequate calories to maximize energy metabolism. For the child who has been healthy previously, the diet should be as unrestrictive as possible—usually low in sodium, potassium, and protein but high in carbohydrates, fats, and vitamins. Use of dietary supplements such as Ensure or Sustacal may be needed to meet the nutritional and caloric requirements.

The renal dietitian is a valuable member of the health team for these acutely ill children. Nurses may need to assume responsibility for obtaining the dietitian's assistance and facilitating the contacts made with the child and family. Reinforcement of teaching done by the dietitian is also an important nursing responsibility.

If renal failure persists beyond a week, the nutritional plan is altered, depending on the child's ability to maintain adequate intake. Tube feedings or the use of parenteral alimentation (central or peripheral) is sometimes necessary. The IV use of high glucose and essential amino acids results in a positive nitrogen balance, a decrease in BUN, and improved healing.[10,23]

RENAL REPLACEMENT THERAPY

The patient's overall clinical condition and the progression of renal failure determine the need for dialysis. No one index or laboratory value can be used arbitrarily to make a decision to proceed with dialysis; each child is evaluated individually for development of life-threatening symptoms of renal failure. Indications for dialysis include congestive heart failure, hypertension, pulmonary edema, hyperkalemia, arrhythmias, pericarditis, encephalopathy, or seizures.[23] When dialysis is used, the child's diet can be liberalized and IV nutritional support can be increased. Both hemodialysis and peritoneal dialysis are discussed in detail at the end of this chapter.

If fluid overload is the primary concern manifested by congestive heart failure, pulmonary edema, or hypertension, continuous fluid removal may be indicated. A new therapeutic regimen, continuous arteriovenous hemofiltration (CAVH) is available.[23] Figure 47-2 illustrates the components of the CAVH system. With CAVH, it is possible to adjust the amount of fluid removed from the body, a feature that is advantageous when increases in fluid intake are needed for nutritional maintenance. CAVH may continue as long as needed.

The CAVH procedure is performed in the intensive care unit and requires one-to-one monitoring. Placement of venous and arterial lines is necessary for the procedure to begin. Blood is pumped from the child's artery through a filter (membrane), which primarily removes fluid. Blood is returned through the venous access.

INFECTION CONTROL

Children with ARF are at increased risk for infection due to (1) a decrease in the ability of the immune system to function, (2) altered nutritional status, and (3) the necessity for invasive procedures. Infection with subsequent electrolyte imbalance may cause death in a small percentage of children with ARF; therefore, prevention of these complications is a priority. All members of the health team should practice good medical asepsis, with special attention to handwashing. Nurses may be advocates in protecting children from unnecessary exposure to pathogens through screening of visitors for communicable infections and in promoting cleanliness of the environment. Frequent assessment for symptoms of infection, prompt reporting of changes to the physician, and accurate and prompt execution of orders (i.e., obtaining cultures, administration of antibiotics) are mandatory.[44]

SURGICAL MANAGEMENT

Along with medical treatment of the effects of ARF, surgical interventions may be required in postrenal condi-

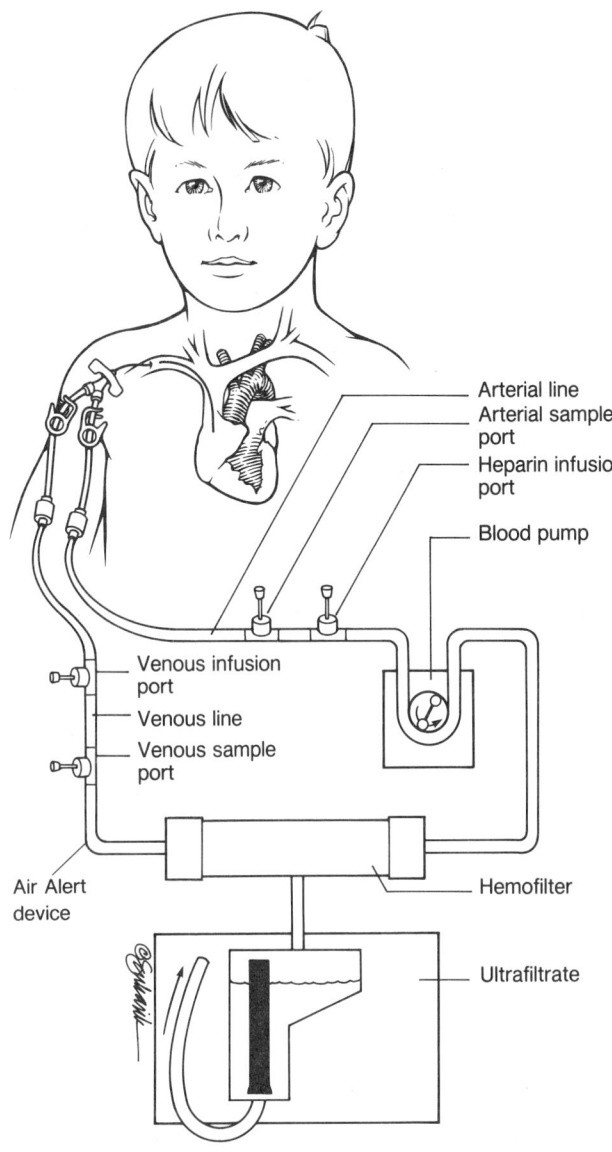

FIGURE 47-2
Components of a continuous arteriovenous hemofiltration (CAVH) system.

When surgery is required, preoperative teaching is needed and must be appropriate for the age and development of the child. Families are extremely anxious, and many have difficulty processing new information. The learning plan should include frequent assessment of their level of understanding and a review of information as needed. Encouraging the child and family to ask questions and to express fears and concerns facilitates this process.

Education may also be provided to emphasize the risks of infection and the need for preventive measures. The most common sources of infection are from the respiratory or urinary system. Content of the teaching plan to prevent infections is presented in the display. Scrupulous handwashing by professionals on the health care team in the family's presence can reinforce this aspect of teaching.

Teaching of child and family about the dietary plan is also important. For this plan to be effective, the cooperation of the entire family is necessary. Education and understanding contribute to the success of the plan.

Children who have altered nutrition (less than body requirements) related to anorexia, altered taste sensation, nausea, vomiting, diarrhea, and dislike of dietary restrictions need special consideration. The nursing goal is to have the child consume an adequate amount of calories to maintain a positive nitrogen balance, as evidenced by maintaining body weight, and good skin integrity. The following suggestions may be beneficial in improving nutritional intake:

- Include the child's food "likes" as much as possible.
- Encourage family to bring foods that have been calculated in the dietary plan from home.
- Provide small, frequent feedings to help increase caloric intake.
- Consult a dietitian for use of dietary supplements.

COOPERATION ENCOURAGEMENT

Nursing interventions may also be directed toward the child's cooperation with therapeutic regimens. This experience with renal failure may be frustrating for a child, the family, and the care providers. Often, the child be-

---

tions. The obstruction (a stone, blood clot, or tumor) may be removed. The goal is to restore the normal manufacture and flow of urine. Surgical procedures may also be required for the placement of access sites for dialysis, or for the insertion of a central venous catheter for nutritional support. Postoperative complications and nursing care are the same as for any child undergoing surgery. However, these children are at higher risk for bleeding and infection.

TEACHING

The child and family undoubtedly have a knowledge deficit related to hospitalization, renal failure, diagnostic procedures, and treatment plan. Many times, parents feel responsible for their child's illness, and the nurse can provide understanding and education to help them manage their guilt feelings. It is the responsibility of the nurse to assess the learning needs and to develop an individualized learning plan.

Methods to Reduce Risk of Infection

- Use good handwashing.
- Provide good oral hygiene.
- Give daily bath with special attention to skin care.
- Perform careful assessment for any breaks in skin.
- Monitor for signs and symptoms of infection.
- Report complaints of dysuria, cough, or any other symptoms.
- Use meticulous aseptic technique for procedures.
- Provide a restful environment to prevent fatigue.

comes preoccupied with the constant thought (psychological desire) of drinking, in addition to experiencing physiologic thirst. The fluid limit should be explained in terms the child can understand, and the child should be encouraged to verbalize frustrations and concerns regarding the fluid limit.

The nurse's creativity is needed in developing a plan of care to manage successfully the problems associated with limited fluid intake. The plan should involve the child, thereby giving some control and independence in making decisions. For the school-age child, tickets can be made to equal the total of the 24-hour oral intake. At the beginning of each shift, the child is given tickets for the time frame and is allowed to decide what fluid is purchased and when to drink it. The nurse may need to help the child plan for meals and medication time. High caloric liquids rather than water are encouraged.

The use of diversional activities to distract the child from constantly thinking about "drinks" may involve family members and games. Prizes for winning games may include simple rewards such as a sticker or being read a story—whatever seems desirable from the child's point of view. Positive reinforcement for complying with the fluid restriction is important in the motivation for the child to continue to comply.

Other interventions may be considered. For example, IV fluids may be decreased to a minimum to permit the child to drink as much of the 24-hour intake as possible. Low-sodium foods can be encouraged to decrease thirst. Frozen fluids such as popsicles may be used; they last longer and sometimes are more satisfying. Likewise, chewing gum, sour balls, and ice cubes may be preferred.

For the toddler and preschooler, all cups and water or fluid sources need to be controlled. Children can be creative in obtaining liquids from toilets, sinks, other children, and parents. A sign on the *child* as well as on the bed stating "ask nurse about restricted fluids" is necessary. Food trays should be carefully observed for "hidden" fluids such as the juice in a dish of canned fruit.

PSYCHOSOCIAL SUPPORT

Because ARF often happens suddenly, the child and family may not have time to develop effective coping mechanisms. The nurse's role is to be supportive, reassuring, and understanding while the child and family endure this traumatic experience. For example, the nurse may give parents time to talk with health care providers away from the child. Similarly, the ill child may be given a chance to talk to the nurse in private.

Parents generally benefit from the nurse's presence, because this indicates caring and concern for the child. The nurses' brief visits to the child's room when no procedures or treatments are planned can be reassuring. Parents often feel reluctant to leave the hospital but become fatigued from the constant strain of attending their ill child. Parents who feel rested and well nourished are more likely to provide the type of emotional support and care that their child needs. Nurses can give parents opportunities to acknowledge their feelings of fear or guilt about leaving the child and confirm that these feelings are not unusual. Nevertheless, parents can be encouraged to take time away from the child to care for themselves.

Parents and the child should be given information regarding the pathologic condition, treatments, and expected outcomes. A positive attitude maintained by the nursing staff also can give the family encouragement. Parents may be reassured that most children with ARF respond well to treatment and fully recover.

The nurse is the key in helping the family and child through the normal fears and concerns that may be exaggerated due to hospitalization, the acuteness of renal failure, the diagnostic procedures, and treatments. Families may need help getting their questions answered; nurses may make arrangements for those on the health care team who can provide information to talk with the family.

DISCHARGE PLANNING

Most children who recover from ARF do not require any special drugs, diet, or therapy. After improvement of the renal condition, the best treatment is healthful living: a balanced, nutritious diet; plenty of fluids; adequate rest; and exercise as tolerated.[44]

Occasionally, a child may need to be discharged on antihypertensive medication. If so, discharge planning includes teaching regarding the procedure for taking a blood pressure, and signs and symptoms of hypotension and hypertension. The side-effects of all medications as well as appropriate time and dosage are explained.

While reviewing medications and diet, special attention focuses on financial and cultural issues surrounding the family's ability to follow the prescribed plan. Ideally, the family is referred to a renal dietitian with expertise in including ethnic foods within the dietary restrictions. The medical social worker should be contacted to assist with referrals for financial assistance.

★ EVALUATION

Periodically, the nurse and family evaluate the outcomes of care given. Examples of outcome criteria for ARF were given under Planning in this section. Have short-term goals been met? Are long-term goals still realistic? Planning for further nursing care also takes into consideration long-term care.

LONG-TERM CARE

Follow-up care is usually done in nephrology clinics where weight, blood pressure, urinalysis, and serum chemistries are monitored. The duration of continuing care depends on individual needs, which are related to the underlying cause of the ARF. Throughout the course of follow-up, the nurse needs to reassess continuously the child's or family's learning needs. Prevention of infection (decreased exposure to those who are ill, good handwashing, and so forth), immunizations, and routine dental care are part of well-child care that should be included.

Chronic Renal Failure and End-Stage Renal Disease

Definition and Incidence. Chronic renal failure (CRF) is a progressive reduction of renal function. With CRF, there is a destruction of nephrons to the point that the kidneys are unable to meet the excretory and metabolic needs of the body. The progression of CRF varies depending on etiology. Children with congenital lesions usually experience a slow, downhill course over a period of years. Those children with acquired renal disease, however, may have a rapid decline in kidney function over a period of months or a prolonged course of renal disease followed by a rapid decline.

The GFR is the indicator used to determine severity of CRF. The lower the GFR, the greater the loss of renal function.[52] CRF in children is relatively rare.[33,34]

CRF progresses from decreased renal reserve to renal insufficiency, and finally, to end stage renal disease (ESRD). ESRD occurs when the kidneys can no longer maintain fluid and electrolyte balance, and the signs and symptoms of uremia appear in spite of treatment with diet, medication, and transfusions. By the time ESRD develops, 90% of the nephrons are usually destroyed, and the GFR is diminished to 10% or less than normal.[34]

The incidence of ESRD in children is relatively low compared with that of the adult population. Depending on the criteria used for accumulating the incidence data, the number of children presenting yearly with ESRD varies from less than 1 to 3.5 children per million people.[33] The discrepancy in numbers is attributed to the variation in the ages of patients and demographic data used to calculate rates.

The progression to ESRD depends on the initial cause of renal dysfunction, the effectiveness of medical interventions, the child's ability to adhere to the prescribed plan of care, and the child's ability to remain free of secondary illnesses and injury. Children and parents alike need to understand the irreversible nature of the disease and recognize that the end stage requires decisions regarding the treatment plan for renal replacement therapy.

Etiology and Pathophysiology. A correlation exists between the age of the child when renal failure is first diagnosed and the cause of CRF. In children under the age of 5 years, CRF is often the result of anatomic abnormalities. In the child over 5, CRF caused by acquired glomerular disease or by hereditary disorders is common.[3] Examples of these categories of disorders are listed in Table 47-3.

Early in the course of renal disease, the child is usually asymptomatic and gives evidence of only minimal biochemical changes. CRF may go undetected until the condition is advanced.

The progression of CRF is remarkably similar no matter what initiates the process. When damage occurs to a nephron, other nephrons assume the work load to meet the metabolic and nutritional needs of the body. Hypertrophy and hyperplasia of the remaining nephrons occur in the attempt to maintain the solute clearance function. Eventually, the overload causes a decrease in the nephron's ability to excrete effectively and results in azotemia and clinical uremia.[33]

The stages of CRF are recognized primarily by the development of symptoms. Laboratory values are not definitive, and children present individualized responses to alterations. The three stages of CRF may be recognized by the following patterns:

TABLE 47-3
Causes of Chronic Renal Failure and End-Stage Renal Disease in Children

Congenital	Acquired
Renal malformations:	Chronic glomerulonephritis
Renal hypoplasia	Rapidly progressive glomerulonephritis
Renal dysplasia	
Severe vesicoureteral reflex	Membranoproliferative glomerulonephritis
Obstructive uropathy	
Hereditary disorders:	Focal glomerulosclerosis
Alport syndrome—hereditary nephritis	Chronic pyelonephritis
Congenital nephrotic syndrome	Henoch-Schönlein purpura—anaphylactoid
Polycystic kidney disease	
Cystinosis	Goodpasture's syndrome
Bartter's syndrome	Hemolytic uremic syndrome
Oxalosis	Nephrotic syndrome
	Sickle cell nephritis
	Lupus erythematosus nephritis
	Hypertension
	Vascular thrombosis
	Cortical necrosis
	Bilateral Wilms' tumor

- *Diminished renal reserve*—reduced renal function without the accumulation of metabolic wastes in the blood.
- *Renal insufficiency*—metabolic waste begins to accumulate in the blood resulting in elevated BUN, serum creatinine, uric acid, and phosphorus levels.
- *Uremia*—excess amounts of nitrogenous waste accumulate in the blood because the kidneys can no longer maintain homeostasis.[33,47]

Clinical Manifestations. The onset of CRF is usually insidious. Symptoms vary from child to child and develop in no particular order. Fatigue, pallor, and the loss of appetite are frequently the first signs parents observe. The active, alert, healthy-looking child begins to sleep more than usual and takes on a pale and sickly appearance.[53] Complaints of headaches are common. The child becomes disinterested in school and is unable to keep up with peers.

One of the most devastating consequences of chronic renal disease in children is the development of bone deformities related to calcium and phosphorus disturbances (described below) and poor nutrition. The resulting skeletal deformities may prevent adequate ambulation and impair growth. Sexual maturation also is delayed or inhibited in children with CRF because the pathophysiology of the condition may create imbalances in the gonadal hormone levels. Both of these side-effects have a profound influence on psychosocial development of the child.[33]

Besides the appearance and behavior of the child, renal failure contributes to specific clinical manifestations discussed below.

Azotemia/uremia—the accumulation of nitrogenous waste products in the blood leading, ultimately, to toxic symptoms such as anorexia, nausea, vomiting, diarrhea, headache, drowsiness, mental slowness, stupor, coma, muscle twitching, and seizures. An elevated BUN and serum creatinine give evidence that glomerular filtration is severely impaired. Deposits of urea crystals may appear on the skin (''uremic frost'') and cause dryness and itching. An unpleasant breath odor may become apparent.

Metabolic acidosis—derangement of acid–base balance. In the normally functioning kidney, the kidneys excrete acid and conserve bicarbonate. As glomerular filtration fails in CFR, serum bicarbonate falls as it is wasted by the kidneys, and metabolic acidosis results.

Electrolyte imbalance—disturbed serum levels of sodium, potassium, calcium, and phosphates. Most children with CFR are able to maintain normal *sodium* levels if dietary intake is adequate. Some causes of CFR (e.g., anatomic anomalies) may promote sodium wastage, whereas other children who have hypertension, edema, or congestive heart failure may retain too much sodium. *Potassium* levels usually are maintained until renal function seriously deteriorates. Hyperkalemia occurs as a result of impaired glomerular filtration and possibly from excessive intake of potassium. *Phosphates* are retained as the GFR diminishes, and plasma *calcium* levels fall correspondingly.

The failing kidneys are unable to excrete phosphorus, and there is a decrease in the absorption of calcium due to abnormal metabolism of vitamin D. In response to the low serum calcium level, the parathyroid glands release parathyroid hormone, which, in turn, stimulates the release of calcium from the bones to provide adequate amounts to maintain electrolyte balance. Secondary hyperparathyroidism leads to the development of osteitis fibrosa and renal osteodystrophy, a condition once called ''renal rickets'' that ultimately leads to growth retardation.[3]

Anemia—low levels of RBC. Several variables contribute to this common finding in children with CRF. The major factor is the kidneys' diminished production or activation of erythropoietin, which stimulates bone marrow to produce RBC. Other contributions to anemia include the fact that the life span of erythrocytes is shortened as the presence of uremic toxins increases. Inadequate dietary intake of iron and folic acid may also contribute to the development of anemia.

Hypertension—elevated arterial pressure. Renal ischemia activates the renin–angiotensin mechanism and causes hypertension in many children who have CRF. The difficulties in regulating fluid volume further aggravate hypertension.

The clinical picture of children with ESRD can be disconcerting. The child may have congestive heart failure as a result of hypervolemia and uncontrolled hypertension. The neurologic status of the child may also deteriorate, and seizures may occur in the presence of hypertension. At times, bleeding occurs due to a decreased platelet count and abnormalities of platelet function. Blood and urine indices reveal serious deterioration in the child's condition. Hyponatremia, hyperkalemia, and hypocalcemia may be present. The child gives evidence of metabolic acidosis, and BUN and serum creatinine levels are markedly elevated.

Diagnostic Studies. A variety of studies is needed to confirm the diagnosis, determine the extent of renal damage, and monitor the progression of renal impairment. Blood studies are essential and are expected to show low hemoglobin and hematocrit as well as leukopenia. The derangement of electrolytes is evident in findings of hyponatremia, hypocalcemia, hyperkalemia, and hyperphosphatemia. The BUN, uric acid, and serum creatinine are increasingly elevated as renal function declines. Hormone levels (estrogen and progesterone in girls and testosterone in boys) may also show lower than normal values.

Urine studies show a low specific gravity and diminished GFR. Chest x-ray and echocardiography may be needed to determine the status of the heart, and bone films may be used to evaluate bone deterioration. Investigations of the kidneys may include angiography, ultrasound, isotope scan, and biopsy. All of these procedures are discussed in Chapter 46.

★ **ASSESSMENT**

CRF pervades all body systems and affects the emotional, social, and psychological well-being of the child and family. The care of children with CRF is complex and demands a wide range of understanding of the child's response to the illness as well as the family's. A comprehensive assessment of functional health is invaluable in establishing a broad database (see Chap. 46). The physical assessment should focus on detecting signs or symptoms of complications related to fluid–electrolyte and acid–base imbalance, anemia, infection, bone disease, and growth retardation. The nurse should assess for edema (most frequently seen in face, feet, and legs), pallor, and bruising. Vital signs are particularly important in assessment of fluid status. The development of hypertension, a gallop heart rhythm, and dyspnea suggest the onset of congestive heart failure; these signs may be accompanied by fatigue, activity intolerance, anorexia, orthopnea, and cough.

★ **NURSING DIAGNOSES AND PLANNING**

The complexity of CRF and its ability to disturb all other body systems makes the identification of nursing diagnoses essential to plan care in an organized, goal-directed manner. Based on the assessment data from above and Chapter 46, the following nursing diagnoses may apply:

- Fluid Volume Excess related to renal failure.
- Altered Nutrition: Less Than Body Requirements related to anorexia, diet restrictions, nausea, and vomiting.
- High Risk for Infection related to decrease in immune system functioning.
- High Risk for Injury related to bone changes, neuropathy, and muscle weakness.
- Grieving related to loss of renal function and changes in lifestyle.
- Fear/Anxiety related to hospitalization, separation from family and friends, painful procedures, and lack of knowledge about disease, diagnostic procedures, hospitalization, and treatment plan.
- Altered Comfort (pruritus) related to uremia.
- Self-Esteem Disturbance related to body image, changes secondary to growth retardation.
- High Risk for Noncompliance related to complex med-

ical therapy (i.e., diet and fluid restrictions, medications, and dialysis treatment).

- Ineffective Individual and Family Coping related to life-long chronic illness.

The nurse and child (or parents) work together to plan effective care based on the established nursing diagnoses. Several examples of expected outcomes follow:

- The child maintains school work at an appropriate level.
- The child and family demonstrate understanding of medication and its purpose and side-effects.
- The child and family discuss renal replacement therapy with a child undergoing such therapy.
- The family participates in support groups.

The nurse develops plans for the daily care of the child based on both physician's orders and nursing diagnoses. Some general nursing care goals in CRF and ESRD may be the following:

- Complications are prevented.
- Adequate calories and proteins are maintained.
- Blood levels are maintained.

Most children with chronic renal disease progress gradually over time to ESRD. These children are followed through pediatric nephrology clinics for years; therefore, they have time to adjust to diet restrictions and medications associated with renal disease.

The child and family are the most important members of the care team and should be included in all aspects of care[18,28] (Fig. 47-3). The family must be motivated to participate fully in the plan if success is to be ensured. If families are motivated to care for their child, they can overcome obstacles that may seem insurmountable to the health care team.

★ INTERVENTIONS: COLLABORATIVE AND INDEPENDENT

The medical plan is supportive and aimed at preventing complications. The treatment of chronic renal disease can

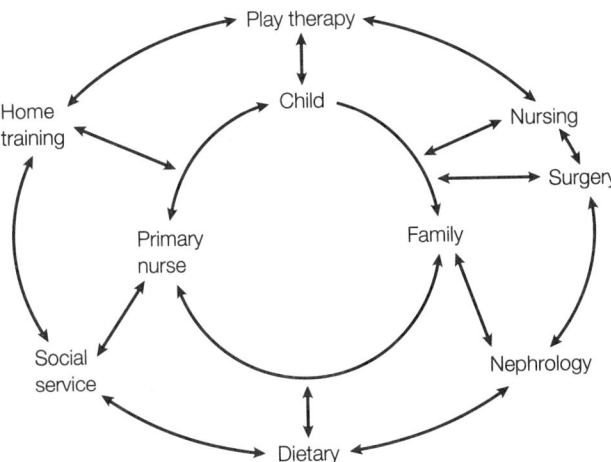

FIGURE 47-3
Model shows the central place of the child and family within the health care team. (Fine, R. A. & Grusken, A. B. [1984]. *End stage renal disease in children.* Philadelphia: Saunders.)

be categorized into (1) treatment directed toward either reversing the primary disease process or preventing deterioration of kidney, (2) treatment directed toward the secondary medical consequences of CRF, and (3) treatment directed toward supporting or replacing the kidney function once ESRD has developed.[33]

Nursing interventions required for the child with CRF are tailored to individual needs. General interventions, however, are related to diet, medications, activity, teaching, and psychosocial support. Each of these responsibilities is discussed below.

DIET THERAPY

Dietary management of renal disease is extremely important in CRF and as the child approaches the end stage. The nutritional goal is to maintain adequate calories and protein for growth while limiting the excretory demands on the kidney. Specific diet modifications depend on the underlying disease process, how much residual kidney function the child has, laboratory studies, and the development of complications. Some of the common dietary considerations are sodium and fluid restrictions to prevent hypertension and congestive heart failure; and potassium restriction to prevent hyperkalemia and cardiac arrhythmias. Restriction of phosphorus intake and the addition of phosphate binders, vitamin D, and calcium can prevent or treat bone disease.[46]

Children with CRF are often anorectic and usually fail to take in adequate calories to meet the energy demands of their bodies. Caloric intake can be improved by adding unrestricted amounts of carbohydrates and fats to the diet. Sugar, jam, and honey are examples of foodstuffs that may be encouraged. Protein intake is often restricted to limit uremic symptomatology and should, therefore, be of high biologic quality with the essential amino acids.[46] Eggs and milk have excellent biologic value, as do meat, fish, and fowl. Vitamin supplements may also be considered.

Experimental evidence has shown that hyperphosphatemia and elevated calcium/phosphorus products lead to the renal deposition of calcium phosphate, which contributes to a decline in kidney function. Therefore, dietary counseling resulting in lower serum phosphorus levels may prolong the decline in kidney function.[46]

Constipation is a major problem for children with CRF and ESRD, especially for those on dialysis. Primary causes of constipation include restrictions of fresh fruits and vegetables to prevent elevated potassium levels, fluid restrictions, phosphorus binders in the form of calcium carbonate, and lack of exercise due to fatigue caused by anemia. Constipation may be reduced by the increase of bulk in the diet, as for example, in popcorn. Stool softeners may also be prescribed. A highly competent, sympathetic dietitian is required to formulate a palatable diet that takes into consideration the child's food preferences, ethnic background, and social situation.[33]

BLOOD REPLACEMENT

Because anemia is a major complication of chronic and ESRD, blood replacement and protection from unnecessary loss are important interventions. Blood transfusions of packed red blood cells are generally the prescribed treatment.[21,47,52] Blood transfusions immediately raise hemoglobin and hematocrit, improving the child's energy level, but these effects are temporary. The risk of transmitting viral infections like hepatitis B and raising serum ferritin levels must be weighed against the potential risks of anemia.

Immunization or prophylaxis against hepatitis B virus is being used in many dialysis centers.[47] Children must be monitored monthly for hepatitis to prevent the spread of this infection. These children should be considered infectious and precautions should be observed, especially in handling blood and peritoneal fluid.

Iron overload from repeated blood transfusions may be treated with an iron chelating agent such as desferrioxamine (Desferal). This agent binds the iron, which is eventually removed during the dialysis treatment.[47]

MEDICATION THERAPY

Various therapeutic regimens, including utilization of immunosuppressive drugs, have been employed to fore-stall the progression of various glomerular diseases.[33] See Table 47-4 for medications used for children with CRF. Because many drugs are excreted by the kidneys, dosage must be monitored carefully to achieve maximum effectiveness and minimum risk of toxicity. The nurse assists the child to take medications as prescribed and alerts the family to side-effects or precautions.

A new therapy for the anemia associated with CRF and ESRD is the medication Epoetin alfa (Epogen), which was recently approved by the Food and Drug Administration. This drug is a glycoprotein manufactured by recombinant DNA technology, and it has the same biologic effects as endogenous erythropoietin normally produced by the kidneys. Epogen stimulates the bone marrow to manufacture RBC, thereby raising levels of hemoglobin and hematocrit. The use of Epogen has been shown to decrease the need for transfusions and to improve the child's sense of well-being.

Epoetin alfa is used primarily for children receiving hemodialysis or peritoneal dialysis. Patients are started on a schedule of three times per week with doses of 50 to 150 units per kilogram of body weight. Children on hemodialysis receive the medication at the end of their treatment by IV push. Children on peritoneal dialysis are given the medication subcutaneously three times per week.

Side-effects of Epoetin alfa include hypertension, headache, seizures, tachycardia, nausea and vomiting, clotting in the vascular access, hyperkalemia, diarrhea, and shortness of breath. Children on the drug need to be monitored carefully with special attention to blood pressure and hematocrit. Monitoring of the child's serum ferritin level, total iron binding capacity (TIBC), and percentage of saturation also is necessary to ensure that there is adequate iron for red cell formation. Iron supplements in the form of IV iron dextron (Imferon) or oral iron may be necessary. Dosage and frequency of the drug are adjusted as needed. Each renal center has adapted manufacturer recommendations to meet the needs of their patient population.

ACTIVITY PROMOTION

The approach to children with chronic renal disease is to encourage normal activities for age and ability. School attendance is essential to support development of age-appropriate socialization.[52] However, due to bone disease and growth failure, many children develop an aversion to school because they are frequently awkward and unable to keep up with peers. These children require support and encouragement to manage these disabilities.[33]

Physical activities should be encouraged both at school and at home. With the support of the health care team, the educational personnel can make a plan to help mainstream the child into the school system.[52] The nurse is the key person to facilitate education of the teachers, school nurse, and other children. The child and family may need additional psychosocial support from a professional counselor to enhance adaptation and prevent maladjustive behavior.[30]

TEACHING

Knowledge provides the child and family with the power to make intelligent choices about the treatment plan. Ed-

TABLE 47-4
Medications Used for Chronic Renal Failure

Medication	Use/Action
Immunosuppressive Drugs	Prevent progression of glomerular closure
Prednisone	
Cyclophosphamide (Cytoxan)	
Antihypertensive Drugs	Control hypertension
Captopril (Capoten)	
Prazosin hydrochloride (Minipress)	
Nifedipine (Procardia)	
Hydralazine hydrochloride (Apresoline)	
Diuretics	Control hypertension
Chlorothiazide (Diuril)	
Furosemide (Lasix)	
Metolazone (Zaroxolyn)	
Vitamin D Analogues	Treat and prevent renal bone disease
Dihydrotachysterol (DHT)	
Calcitriol (Rocaltrol)	
Calcium Supplements	Treat and prevent renal bone disease
Calcium gluconate	
Calcium carbonate	
Os-Cal	
Antacids With Aluminum—used for short term only—can become aluminum toxic:	Treat and prevent renal bone disease
Basaljel	Treat elevated serum phosphorus
Dialume	
Amphojel	
Antibiotics	Treat or prevent urinary tract infection
Ampicillin	
Furadantin	
Co-trimoxazole (Septra, Bactrim)	
Folic Acid and Vitamin Supplements	Supplement dietary restrictions
Nephrovite	

ucation is a team effort with the nurse being the primary educator and coordinator. The child and family need to know about all medications prescribed, including dosage, frequency, purpose, and side-effects. The family is instructed in the technique of blood pressure monitoring and signs and symptoms of hypertension and hypotension. The nurse also supports the dietitian by assessing knowledge of diet and referring the family for follow-up when necessary.

Ideally, education starts early because there is a tremendous amount of information to process. Information should be given in a style and manner that the child and family can understand. Translation of information into understandable language, both verbally and in writing, is imperative.

Because the outcome of CRF is irreversible, the child and family require assistance in anticipating future needs such as renal replacement therapy (dialysis or transplantation). The nurse has an important role in the family's understanding of needs and facilitating the transition to more complex medical management. By organizing and planning each visit, the nurse can review previous information, answer questions, and introduce new information. The nurse should schedule a tour of the dialysis unit and encourage the child and family to talk with others undergoing similar treatments.

As renal function diminishes, surgery is scheduled to create the access for dialysis. The elective scheduling of this event provides the child and family with opportunities for optimal care and decreases the stresses that emergency surgery would stimulate. During the healing process, the child and family can learn to care for the access site and begin to cope with the reality that dialysis is imminent.

ADVOCACY

With long-term care needed by children with CRF, the role of the nurse as a patient advocate is continuously used. The child and family need to be able to make informed decisions, and the alert, caring nurse ensures they have accurate and comprehensive information. The child also can be protected from unnecessary examinations or procedures that might result from the large number of care providers involved in the treatment plan. When considering the number of laboratory tests ordered, for example, the timing of these tests and the trauma to the child may be overlooked. As an advocate, the nurse may question the necessity of repeated tests in short time frames. Issues of cost are also important to consider, and the nurse advocate can find ways to minimize waste and unnecessary expense.

Obtaining appropriate resources for the family is another aspect of advocacy. Social workers, for example, are valuable to these families for many reasons. One of the most important is in helping families to maintain access to the health care system. The financial burdens of CRF and ESRD are overwhelming; families often need guidance to obtain eligibility for services and benefits. The social worker can keep them informed of federal, state, and local funding available for these children and assist the families to use available resources. The nurse can facilitate the communication between the social worker and the family.

PSYCHOSOCIAL SUPPORT

Encouraging the child to participate in normal age-appropriate activities helps progression through normal developmental stages and gives the child a sense of control and ability to cope with the chronic renal condition. The health team, including family members, can facilitate the child's development of self-respect and a positive self-concept by also encouraging participation in self-care. This process requires planning *with* the child in setting goals. The plan must be established to provide measurable and achievable goals in a step-by-step process. Positive reinforcement is obtained not only by reaching the goal, but also by the verbal praise and acknowledgement of the health care team. Behavior modification techniques appropriate for age may include charts with stars for daily accomplishments and toys for reaching larger goals.[18,30]

Adolescents can be difficult to motivate; a mutually agreed upon contract can be useful. These children are struggling for psychosocial independence while managing a disease process that typically requires dependence on machines, medications, and others for support. Helping the adolescent to set realistic goals for school or vocational training is a challenge.[18,30]

Children have the best potential for physical rehabilitation when the family has strong support systems and effective communication patterns. Children from supportive, secure family backgrounds are better able to cope psychosocially with illness if they have developed a basic sense of trust, security, competence, and self-confidence. Children from deprived backgrounds and less supportive families may be overwhelmed by fear and depression.[18,30,33] Therefore, they may need referral for outside resources, more education, and more encouragement to express their concerns and fears.

Families need to be encouraged to ventilate their frustrations in dealing with renal disease and their chronically ill child. Negative feelings that mount from daily long-term caregiving can stress the family to the point that coping is difficult.[30] Support from other families experiencing the same concerns and frustration is often beneficial. Organized support groups can be a source of encouragement and a place to share information, but families often find that they have inadequate energy and time to devote to these groups. Instead, families frequently develop supportive relationships with one another while waiting for clinic appointments or during dialysis treatments. Nurses may facilitate these relationships by introducing people and encouraging exchange of information.

One troublesome aspect of ESRD is the uncertainty concerning course and prognosis. Uncertainty creates confusion and anxiety for the child and family, as well as for the health care team. The care plan requires frequent reassessment and modification of interventions. The child and family need to be flexible because diet orders and medication schedules may change frequently. There are often unplanned events, such as infections, reactions to medication, clinic visits, or surgery related to the site of dialysis access.

★ EVALUATION

Periodically the nurse and family evaluate the outcomes of care given. Examples of outcome criteria for CRF and

ESRD were given under Planning in this section. Have short-term goals been met? Are long-term goals still realistic? Planning for further nursing also takes into consideration long-term care.

LONG-TERM CARE

A tertiary clinical facility is necessary for the management of children with CRF and/or ESRD. Furthermore, an interdisciplinary team of health professionals must provide comprehensive, individualized, quality care to these children and their families and assistance in resolving the complex problems that arise.[33] The coordinator of the team is usually a pediatric nephrologist who is assisted by other physicians including pediatric surgeons and pediatric urologists. Other essential members of the team are (1) a renal dietitian who is knowledgeable and sympathetic toward the needs of the child with renal disease, (2) a medical social worker with a strong background in pediatric chronic illness, a working knowledge of Medicare benefits and regulations, as well as an ability to use available resources effectively, and (3) technically competent nurses with specialized psychosocial skills and training in caring for chronically ill children.

As ESRD develops, the child and family have two primary options: conservative treatment or active renal replacement therapy. Conservative therapy consists of the treatment of secondary problems and the reduction of pain and suffering. Parents may elect to use only conservative management, particularly if there are other existing debilitating conditions such as severe mental retardation when the child would not comprehend the procedures and would adapt poorly.[21] Because conservative treatment ultimately leads to death, it is important that the family be given maximum psychosocial support in implementing their decision.[33] Renal replacement therapy is discussed later in this chapter.

Acquired Conditions Causing Renal Dysfunction

Nephrotic Syndrome

Definition and Incidence. Nephrotic syndrome is a renal disorder that encompasses many forms of glomerular disease. These include differences in clinical course, response to treatment, and prognosis. Nephrotic syndrome is actually a functional state, defined by the presence of the following clinical findings: massive proteinuria, hypoalbuminemia, hyperlipidemia, and edema.[27,29,37]

Nephrotic syndrome is classified as primary or secondary (Table 47-5). Primary nephrotic syndrome occurs from disease localized in the glomeruli of the kidneys. Secondary nephrotic syndrome results from systemic diseases that have a destructive effect on the glomeruli.

The most common type of primary nephrotic syndrome is minimal change nephrotic syndrome (MCNS). In approximately 85% of children with nephrotic syndrome, the condition results from minimal change or "nil" disease of the kidneys and is responsive to steroid therapy. Other terms such as idiopathic nephrotic syndrome, lipoid nephrosis, steroid-responsive nephrotic

TABLE 47-5
Causes of Nephrotic Syndrome

Primary Nephrotic Syndrome	Secondary Nephrotic Syndrome
Minimal change nephrotic syndrome	Infections
Congenital nephrotic syndrome (Finnish type)	Bacterial
	Poststreptococcal glomerulonephritis
Chronic glomerulonephritis	Infective endocarditis
Focal glomerulosclerosis	Ventriculoatrial shunt infections
Membranous glomerulopathy	Syphilis
Membranoproliferative glomerulonephritis	Viral
Mesangial proliferative glomerulonephritis (Berger's disease)	Hepatitis B
	Cytomegalovirus
	Acquired immunodeficiency syndrome
	Varicella
	Protozoal
	Malaria
	Neoplasms
	Wilms' tumor
	Lymphomas
	Multisystem disease
	Systemic lupus erythematosus
	Connective tissue disease
	Henoch-Schönlein purpura
	Diabetes mellitus
	Heredity disorders
	Sickle cell disease
	Alport's syndrome
	Toxins and drugs
	Bee stings
	Poison ivy and poison oak
	Penicillamine
	Heavy metals
	Mercury
	Vaccines
	Tridione
	Captopril
	Heroin
	Other
	Renal arterial stenosis
	Hemolytic uremic syndrome
	Chronic inflammatory disease (amyloidosis)

syndrome, and foot process disease have been used to identify this condition. MCNS affects 1.6 out of every 100,000 children under 16 years of age; the typical age is from 18 months to 6 years. Males are affected more than females by a 2:1 ratio. Although MCNS is not inherited, familial occurrence is estimated in 2% to 3% of cases.[27]

Congenital nephrotic syndrome is an inherited type of primary nephrotic syndrome, which is transmitted through autosomal recessive genes. It is most commonly reported in children of Finnish extraction.[29] This rare disorder comprises only 1.5% of all cases of nephrotic syndrome in children. It occurs during the first year of life, and most of these children are born preterm. Males and females are equally affected. Congenital nephrotic syndrome presents like nephrotic syndrome in the older child; however, it is characterized by a progressive loss of renal function, and the prognosis is poor. Death usually ensues, but dialysis and renal transplantation have been successful with some of these children.

Primary nephrotic syndrome is also associated with several types of chronic glomerulonephritis. Of these, focal glomerulosclerosis is the most common, and it constitutes 6% to 12% of all nephrotic syndrome during childhood.[29] In contrast to children with MCNS, these children are less responsive to steroid therapy, and 30% to 40% have renal insufficiency.[29] The renal biopsy is abnormal, with evidence of sclerosis in some of the glomeruli.

The classification of secondary nephrotic syndrome refers to renal involvement occurring as a result of some other systemic disease or evident cause. Secondary nephrotic syndrome accounts for 15% to 20% of nephrotic syndrome in childhood. The most common causes of secondary nephrotic syndrome occur in systemic lupus erythematosus and Schönlein-Henoch purpura.[29] Nephrotic syndrome has also been reported in patients with acquired immunodeficiency syndrome (AIDS). Because of the diverse causes of secondary nephrotic syndrome, glomerular tissue injury may be of minimal change or show morphologic features of various forms of chronic glomerulonephritis. Glomerulonephritis is discussed more fully later in this chapter.

Etiology and Pathophysiology. MCNS is the most common type of nephrotic syndrome occurring in childhood. Unless otherwise stated, the following discussion refers to children with MCNS.

Nephrotic syndrome is a disease of unknown etiology, but it has been associated with immunologic causes. Abnormal immunoglobulins have been found in children presenting with nephrotic syndrome.[37] The onset of nephrotic syndrome has been linked to the occurrence of respiratory tract infections, and some of these children have an increased incidence of allergic disorders such as asthma, hay fever, and urticaria. Circulating immune complexes have been reported in children and adults with nephrotic syndrome, but their role in the disease process remains poorly understood.[29]

Another view about the pathogenesis of nephrotic syndrome suggests that two underlying defects are present: (1) there is an abnormal persistence and proliferation of a subclass of T cells, and (2) the increased glomerular permeability in nephrotic syndrome results from a circulating lymphocyte product that injures the glomerular basement membrane.[29] Although the exact role of the immune system and its relationship to the development of nephrotic syndrome is not fully understood, the successful treatment of nephrotic syndrome with steroids and other immunosuppressive agents lends strong support to the theory that nephrotic syndrome has an immunologic origin.

The primary abnormality in nephrotic syndrome is heavy proteinuria due to a change in the permeability of the glomerular basement membrane. The glomerular capillary barrier, normally impermeable to albumin and other large proteins, allows proteins to leak and pass through to the urine. In addition to excessive urinary loss of protein, a significantly increased portion of circulating albumin is catabolized by the kidney. A decreased serum protein (hypoalbuminemia) develops.

Changes in oncotic pressure cause fluid to shift from the intravascular space to the interstitial space causing edema. A decrease in the intravascular volume activates antidiuretic hormone secretion and the renin–angiotensin system. This process leads to an increased retention of salt and water, which further aggravates the edema (Fig. 47-4).

Over the last 60 years, the prognosis for children with nephrotic syndrome has dramatically improved. The availability of steroids and the treatment of infections with antibiotics have reduced the complications of this disease and the incidence of mortality in children with nephrotic syndrome. In general, one out of six children requires only one course of steroids.[37] The majority may continue to relapse until they reach adolescence. Of these children, 66% to 75% reach remission. The others continue to relapse into adulthood.[37]

Although the overall prognosis for children with MCNS is favorable, the outcome for children with other forms of nephrotic syndrome is less certain. Response to steroids is less predictable for children with chronic glomerulonephritis. For children with focal glomerulosclerosis, ESRD may occur in 20% to 50% of patients after 5

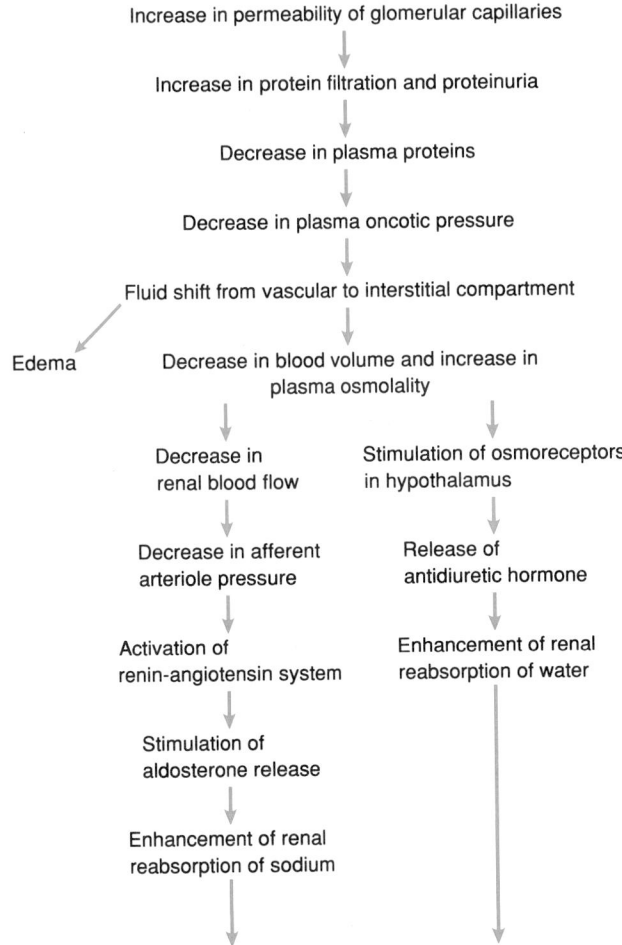

FIGURE 47-4

Pathophysiologic mechanisms that lead to edema formation in the nephrotic syndrome. (Richard, C. J. [Ed.]. [1986]. *Comprehensive nephrology nursing* [p. 139]. Boston: Little, Brown.)

to 10 years of follow-up.[29] Children that progress to ESRD may be candidates for renal transplantation. There is a risk of reoccurrence of nephrotic syndrome even after transplantation.[29]

Clinical Manifestations.   Edema is the cardinal sign of nephrotic syndrome, and it often first appears in the periorbital region. Edema may also be noted in dependent areas of the body such as the hands, ankles, feet, and genitalia.[29] Body weight increases as edema progresses, and ascites and pleural effusion may also be present in children with untreated or long-standing disease. Pallor, fatigue, and lethargy accompany the edema.

The presence of massive proteinuria and marked hypoalbuminemia establishes the diagnosis of nephrotic syndrome in a child with edema.[29] Hypercholesterolemia and generalized hyperlipidemia are also seen in nephrotic syndrome. The severity of hyperlipidemia is generally related to the severity of the nephrotic syndrome. Other factors that may affect the degree of hyperlipidemia in nephrotic syndrome are the patient's age, diet, presence of renal failure, and use of corticosteroids. There is evidence to suggest that the elevated serum lipid levels are a result of increased hepatic synthesis and decreased catabolism.[29]

The frequency with which hematuria, hypertension, and reduced GFR occur in children with nephrotic syndrome depends on the nature of the underlying glomerular disease. GFR is normal in most children. Decreased levels of renal function are often transient and reflect poor renal perfusion and hypovolemia.[3] Gross hematuria is rare, but microscopic hematuria is reported in 10% to 20% of children.[27] Urine output may be decreased, and the color may be concentrated. Blood pressure is usually normal or may be slightly elevated. As a group, children with chronic glomerulonephritis present with several distinct clinical and laboratory findings that differentiate them from children with MCNS.

Diagnostic Studies.   Diagnostic evaluation includes a comprehensive *urinalysis,* which typically shows a 3+ to 4+ protein spill and elevated specific gravity. Microscopic hematuria may be found. Although most renal function tests are normal, a decreased creatinine clearance has been reported in approximately 30% of children with nephrotic syndrome.[29]

Specimen collection for quantified protein is often difficult because of the age group of these children. However, the diagnosis of nephrotic syndrome is confirmed with 100 mg/kg/day or greater than 1 g/m²/24 h of urinary protein excretion.[29] The serum albumin is less than 2.5 g/dL and, because an inverse relationship exists between the serum albumin and cholesterol level, cholesterol level is greater than 200 mg/dL. Total serum proteins are always decreased.

Other *blood studies* are generally ordered and include CBC, electrolytes, BUN, creatinine, calcium, and pH. The hematocrit and hemoglobin may be increased or decreased secondary to hemoconcentration or hemodilution. The serum sodium may be decreased because of trapping in the interstitial space. Calcium may be low due to the loss of vitamin D metabolites in the urine. The BUN and creatinine are usually normal.

A *renal biopsy* is not routinely done on all patients with nephrotic syndrome unless the child is unresponsive to the initial therapeutic regimens, or if MCNS is unlikely.[29] It is estimated that if renal biopsies were carried out on all children with nephrotic syndrome, 80% would have MCNS, which is responsive to steroids, and the biopsy would have been unnecessary.[27] The pathologic hallmark of MCNS is the absence of any significant glomerular or interstitial inflammation noted on renal biopsy. Hematuria, casts, and abnormal renal function are unusual for MCNS and are almost always indicative of more serious disease.[29]

★   ASSESSMENT

The admission history should include questions as to when the parents first noted that the child was ill. Were there any events that seemed to precipitate or precede the onset of edema? Have there been any recent immunizations or allergic episodes? Can recent infections or upper respiratory tract infections be recalled? Has the child experienced flulike symptoms including fever, diarrhea, or vomiting? Have the parents noticed a change in urinary patterns? When and where did the edema first appear? Have they noticed any behavioral changes in the child such as irritability or loss of appetite? Has anyone in the family been ill recently? Does anyone in the family have kidney disease?

Although the suggested questions may elicit strong evidence of the onset of the nephrotic syndrome, not all children display obvious symptoms of illness. Many cases of nephrotic syndrome have an insidious onset and may go unnoticed until the condition is advanced.

The physical examination should include baseline vital signs including temperature, pulse, respirations, and blood pressure. The general appearance of the child should be noted. Does the child appear ill? How would the comfort level and behavior of the child be described? Breath sounds should be auscultated for the presence of adventitious sounds and air exchange. The presence and extent of fluid retention/edema should be evaluated. Special areas to assess for edema include the periorbital region, upper and lower extremities, abdomen, and genitalia (scrotum and labia).

Skin breakdown, which can occur as a result of edema, should be assessed. Signs and symptoms of infection should be noted. Peripheral perfusion should be assessed by checking the circulation to extremities: peripheral pulses, color, temperature, capillary refill, and sensation. Because a child who is edematous may also have a depleted intravascular volume, signs of hypovolemia and shock should also be assessed.

★   NURSING DIAGNOSES AND PLANNING

Based on the assessment from above and Chapter 46, the following nursing diagnoses may apply:

- Fluid Volume Excess related to edema, or movement of interstitial fluid into the intravascular space during treatment.
- High Risk for Fluid Volume Deficit related to hypovolemia secondary to loss of fluid from the intravascular space.

- Pain related to edema, and Pain secondary to inflammation from peritonitis.
- High Risk for Impaired Skin Integrity related to frequent, loose stools and edema.
- Activity Intolerance related to edematous extremities and decreased lung expansion secondary to ascites.
- Diversional Activity Deficit related to the need for bed rest or hospitalization.
- Fear related to the inability to open eyes secondary to severe periorbital edema.
- Altered Nutrition: Less Than Body Requirements related to anorexia and protein loss.
- Altered Nutrition: More Than Body Requirements related to an increased appetite secondary to steroid therapy.
- High Risk for Infection related to suppressed immunity secondary to steroid therapy and the disease.
- Body Image Disturbance related to an edematous appearance and side-effects of steroid therapy.
- Social Isolation related to edematous appearance.
- Ineffective Individual or Family Coping related to changes in usual roles, frequent hospitalizations, and chronic kidney disease.
- Anxiety related to knowledge deficit regarding disease process and treatment, home care instructions.

The nurse and child (or parents) work together to plan effective care based on the established nursing diagnoses. Several examples of expected outcomes follow:

- The child is infection free.
- The child demonstrates appropriate growth and development for age.
- The child and family resume normal activities of living.
- The family preserves normal family functioning.

The nurse develops plans for the daily care of the child based on both physician's orders and nursing diagnoses. Some general nursing care goals for restoring renal function may be the following:

- Urine is protein free.
- Blood pressure is within normal limits for age.
- Edema is resolved.
- Fluid and electrolyte balance is restored.
- Body weight is stabilized and weight gain is appropriate for age.
- Nutritional needs are met, including a return to a state of positive nitrogen balance.
- Side-effects of steroids are minimal, and growth retardation is prevented.

★ INTERVENTIONS: COLLABORATIVE
   AND INDEPENDENT

Children with nephrotic syndrome present a challenge to the nurse, who must continually assess the child for the development of serious complications. These complications include altered fluid and electrolyte balance, infection, and adverse reactions to steroid therapy. Nursing care of a child with nephrotic syndrome is discussed in the Nursing Care Plan. Prompt reporting of clinical findings and referral to the physician for treatment are essential. In addition to collaborative problems, there are many independent interventions the nurse may initiate, including strategies to increase comfort, improve nutritional status, and prepare for home care.

MEDICATION THERAPY

During the 1950s, *corticosteroids* began to be used to treat nephrotic syndrome, and they remain as the primary treatment modality today. Prednisone is the most common form of corticosteroid used in this country. The goal of steroid therapy is to induce a remission of proteinuria and to maintain this remission.[29]

The dose and schedules of prednisone administration may vary. However, initial therapy usually includes the daily administration of prednisone at 2 mg/kg/day until the urine is protein free. A response is usually seen in 2 to 4 weeks. After the initial therapy, the child is placed on a maintenance regimen of prednisone every other day for 4 weeks. The dose and schedule of prednisone are tapered until it is discontinued.

The response of children to treatment with steroids depends largely on the underlying renal histology. Most children with MCNS go into remission after treatment with steroids.[29] One out of 6 children requires one course of prednisone only; the majority relapse until adolescence. At that time, 66% to 75% reach remission.[37]

Treatment with corticosteroids is the primary treatment in inducing a remission in children with nephrotic syndrome. It is imperative that these children receive *all* doses of medication ordered at the scheduled time. This may be difficult when toddlers or preschool-age children refuse to take the prednisone. The nurse must work with the family in determining a consistent method of giving the medication that the child will accept. Because prednisone is bitter and tastes terrible, crushing and mixing it with applesauce, cherry syrup, or other food or fluids may help the child to take the medication. Effective interventions should be on the nursing care plan so that all nurses are aware of how the child prefers to take the medication.

Including the parents in the administration of prednisone while the child is hospitalized assists in compliance at home. If it is a struggle to give each dose of prednisone to the child while in the hospital, it is unlikely that compliance at home will be maintained. This omission could severely affect the child's recovery, and the nurse must stress the critical nature of drug administration with the parents. The nurse should also acknowledge to parents that medication administration to toddlers is not an easy task, even for nurses!

Diuretic therapy is usually not indicated unless there is severe fluid retention and edema causing the child to be extremely uncomfortable.[29] Furosemide (Lasix) at a dose of 1 to 2 mg/kg given once or twice daily may be of some benefit. Zaroxolyn is used in combination with furosemide.

The use of salt-poor *albumin* should be restricted to children who have persistent edema, vascular insufficiency, or oligoanuria of several days' duration.[37] The dose of albumin is 1 g/kg/24 h, followed by a dose of Lasix given IV. The child needs to be monitored carefully during the albumisol infusion for signs of circulatory overload and hypertension caused by the shift of subcutaneous fluid into the intravascular space.

(text continued on page 1182)

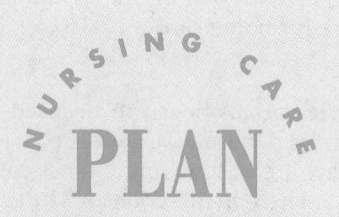

A Child With Possible Nephrotic Syndrome

Assessment

Case Study Description

Ricardo is a 3-year-old Hispanic child admitted to the hospital for ruling out nephrotic syndrome. This is his first hospital admission. Ricardo is the youngest of five children. Father is the decision maker for the family. Mother is the primary caretaker of the children. Parents moved from Mexico 2 years ago. They speak very little English.

Assessment Data

Subjective:

Parents report that Ricardo hasn't been his usual self the last couple of weeks. He is less active and wants to lie down a lot. He seems to breathe harder, and he gets out of breath quickly. His clothes are tight, and his shoes don't fit. Father thought he was just growing until Ricardo woke up yesterday morning with his eyes swollen shut. That's when father decided to bring Ricardo to the hospital. Mother reports that Ricardo seems to be urinating less often. He hasn't gone to the bathroom since yesterday around dinner time. Mother reports that Ricardo has always been very healthy. He is "normal" like the other children. Ricardo is potty trained. Father states Ricardo is their favorite child. Mother nods her head and agrees.

Objective:

Ricardo is fussy and irritable. Cries when approached and clings to mother. Uncooperative with physical examination and procedures. Afebrile. Tachypneic with respiratory rate of 40. Apical pulse is rapid at 130. Blood pressure is slightly elevated at 120/80. Ricardo has generalized edema, with marked periorbital edema such that the eyes are swollen shut. Scrotal edema is noted. Ricardo's abdomen is moderately distended. Bowel sounds are present.

Laboratory findings reveal 2+ proteinuria, decreased serum albumin of 2.3 g/dL, and elevated serum cholesterol of 240 mg/dL.

Growth and development are normal for age.

Nursing Diagnosis	Intervention	Rationale
1. Fluid volume excess related to altered renal function secondary to extracellular shift from serum protein loss Supporting data: • Edema • Abdominal distention • Proteinuria • Tachypnea/tachycardia • Decreased urine output	Monitor vital signs closely. Use appropriate size BP cuff. Label cuff with child's name to be used consistently for measurement.	Close observation of vital signs is necessary for early detection of fluid balance complications and circulatory overload/shock.
	Obtain daily weights before breakfast. Weigh on same scale with same amount of clothing.	Accurate, precise measurements are necessary for indication of renal function, fluid balance, and response to treatment.
	Monitor respiratory and cardiovascular status.	
	Auscultate breath sounds and for the presence of adventitious sounds.	
	Observe closely during Albumisol infusions if prescribed.	Child may develop circulatory overload and hypertension caused by the shift of fluid subcutaneously into the intravascular space.
	Accurate recording of intake and output with 8-hour totals.	
	Dipstick urine for protein.	
	Obtain urine specific gravity.	
	Monitor progression of edema	
	Measure abdominal girth over umbilicus daily.	

(*Continued*)

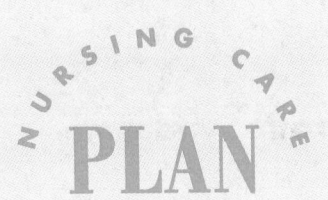

A Child With Possible Nephrotic Syndrome
(continued)

Nursing Diagnosis	*Intervention*	*Rationale*
	Administer diuretics as ordered; monitor response and for signs and symptoms of hypokalemia.	A drop in serum K^+ can occur with diuretic therapy.
	Limit salty foods; No added salt (NAS) diet preferred, but must be palatable to the child to provide adequate nutritional intake.	Excessive salt in diet can aggravate edema.
	Elevate head of bed.	Position assists with lung expansion. Ascites may cause upward displacement of the diaphragm and cause respiratory distress.
2. High risk for fluid volume deficit related to hypovolemia secondary to the shift of fluid from the intravascular space. Supporting data: • Child with nephrotic syndrome may have marked edema, but have a decreased blood volume.	Monitor peripheral perfusion. Monitor respiratory rate and heart rate; report upward trends to the physician. Monitor BP/hypotension; report downward trends to the physician.	These are important indicators of intravascular volume depletion. Identifying subtle signs may prevent the child from progressing to shock.
3. Altered Nutrition: less than body requirements related to anorexia and protein loss Supporting data: • Parental report of poor appetite and decreased intake of a few week's duration • Proteinuria • Hypoalbuminemia • Hospitalization and salt restriction may aggravate the situation • Toddler/preschool children may be "picky" eaters	Initiate calorie count. Consult dietitian regarding high-protein, low-salt diet that is palatable to the child. Assess food preferences and allow the child to choose foods. Provide small frequent feedings and nutritious snacks. Encourage parental participation. Establish meal time routines. Allow child to eat in playroom and to go to cafeteria with family as condition improves. Discuss family's bringing in food from home or restaurant. Provide positive reinforcement to child. Assist child with eating while eyes are swollen shut.	Diet of high biologic protein value improves nitrogen balance and prevents malnutrition. Involving parents, making the eating experience fun, pleasant, and similar to home routines are effective strategies to encourage nutrition in the toddler and preschool age groups
4. High risk for infection related to altered immune response secondary to the disease process and steroid therapy Supporting data: • Although not fully understood, children with nephrotic syndrome are at risk for infection secondary to altered immune responses • Child began course of prednisone	Monitor temperature Assess for signs and symptoms of infection, especially sepsis and peritonitis Notify physician for fever, vomiting, diarrhea, abdominal pain, redness or rash over abdomen Place patient with noninfectious roommate	Infection can be a life-threatening complication in the child with nephrotic syndrome Indicators of peritonitis. Prompt treatment with antibiotics is necessary Decrease child's exposure to infected persons

(*Continued*)

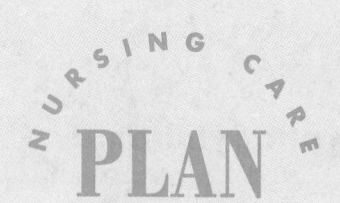

A Child With Possible Nephrotic Syndrome
(continued)

Nursing Diagnosis	Intervention	Rationale
	Screen visitors and inform family that visitors who are ill or exposed to contagious disease such as chickenpox should not visit	
	Administer antibiotics as ordered and monitor patient for side-effects and adverse reactions (e.g., ampicillin rash)	
	Use scrupulous handwashing and aseptic technique	
	Observe family hygiene habits, and instruct as necessary	Family needs to continue infection control techniques when child is discharged
5. High risk for impaired skin integrity related to edema, diarrhea, and decreased activity Supporting data: • Generalized edema of extremities • Periorbital edema • Scrotal edema • Frequent, loose stools • Bedrest	Monitor skin for breakdown or infection Monitor circulation to extremities Separate skin folds and gently wash and thoroughly dry	Pressure from edema impedes circulation and may lead to skin breakdown Edema is a source of discomfort for the child Prevention of skin breakdown is essential to decrease the risk of infection
	Separate skin folds with cotton gauze Apply loose, nonrestrictive clothing (diapers included) Avoid the use of tourniquets; if necessary, protect skin with cloth or 4 × 4. Avoid the use of tape when possible. Tape on extremities with IVs should be checked frequently so tape doesn't become too tight Change patient position at least q2h Apply egg crate mattress or sheep skin Elevate extremities with pillows Apply scrotal support Inspect buttocks for breakdown	
	Gently cleanse buttocks with mild soap and water after each stooling Expose buttocks to air Obtain order for protective ointment, (e.g., Desitin) if buttocks are reddened	Frequent, loose stools and prolonged contact with the skin can lead to breakdown and infection
	Elevate the head of the bed Cleanse eyes with warm saline Consolidate venipunctures whenever possible	
6. Fear (child) related to unfamiliar environment, decreased vision secondary to swollen eyelids Supporting data:	Allow and encourage family to stay with child and participate in care Provide consistency of caretakers	Interventions support coping in the preschool-age hospitalized child

(Continued)

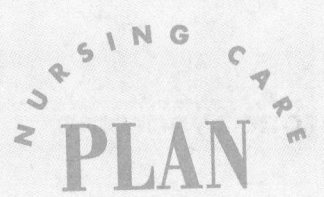

A Child With Possible Nephrotic Syndrome
(continued)

Nursing Diagnosis	*Intervention*	*Rationale*
• Excessive crying • Clinging to mother • Uncooperative and "fights" procedures • Separation from family • Eyelids swollen shut • Preschool age • First hospitalization	Assign Spanish-speaking nurses if possible Encourage parents to bring in favorite toys or objects from home—stuffed animal, blanket, and so forth While eyes are swollen, provide diversional activities that entertain and don't frustrate the child—read stories, sing songs, play music As edema subsides offer other age-appropriate activities as tolerated—coloring books, simple puzzles, cars and trucks Consult child life specialist to assist with bedside activities and therapeutic play Send child to playroom as tolerated Prepare child for procedures using strategies appropriate for the preschool child: parental presence, equipment play, doll play, stories about hospitalized children	
7. Altered family processes related to sudden illness and hospitalization. Supporting data: • Youngest and favorite child • Disrupted family routine • Financial burden of hospitalization • Nephrotic syndrome can lead to long-term chronic renal failure	Use Spanish interpreters whenever possible Assign primary nurse to coordinate nursing care Allow family to express concerns and feelings Reinforce and clarify treatment and medical plan When appropriate, point out indicators that the child is improving	Communicating with the family in their native language decreases anxiety and fear Strategies to promote coping in parents of hospitalized children
8. Anxiety (parental) related to knowledge deficit about disease process, treatment plan, home care regimen Supporting data: • Child's first admission to the hospital • Newly diagnosed • Family will need to learn procedures to be done at home to prevent infection and relapse (steroid administration, urine dipstick for protein, special diet, signs of infection and relapse)	Explain disease process and treatment in terms the family can understand Provide verbal and written information in Spanish as much as possible—use hospital interpreter Develop a teaching plan for discharge that is "phased in" throughout the child's hospitalization (refer to teaching plan for child with nephrotic syndrome in this chapter)	Successful treatment of nephrotic syndrome depends on parental understanding and follow-through with the treatment plan to prevent relapse and complications

(Continued)

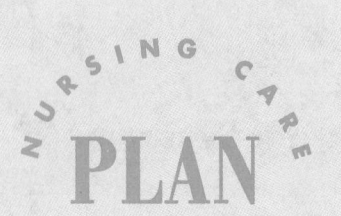

NURSING CARE
PLAN

A Child With Possible Nephrotic Syndrome
(continued)

Evaluation

- Vital signs normal for age
- Appropriate urine output for age
- Return to most recent weight
- Edema resolves
- Urine is free of protein

Expected Outcomes

- Child eats 50% of meals
- Child's skin is free from breakdown
- Child is free of infection
- Child and family experience decreased fear and anxiety
- Family discusses disease and rationale for treatment
- Family complies with home care regimen
- Child regains/maintains normal fluid and electrolyte balance.

Cytoxic agents such as Cytoxan, chlorambucil, and nitrogen mustard may be prescribed for children who do not improve with steroids, who relapse promptly after steroids are stopped, or who show significant toxic effects to steroids such as growth failure, hypertension, or a cushingoid appearance. A renal biopsy is always indicated before the use of these agents, and they should be used with extreme caution.[37] Short-term side-effects of cytoxan include bone marrow suppression, transient alopecia, and the risk of hemorrhagic cystitis. Long-term effects of these drugs may include sterility and the risk of carcinogenesis.

DIET THERAPY

The child's nutritional status should be evaluated. An early, accurate recording of nutritional intake is important. A calorie count should be initiated as needed. For some children, food intake is calculated by the number of bites eaten. Because appetite is often poor, the child's likes and dislikes need careful consideration. This information should be recorded on the nursing care plan. Small, frequent feedings may also be helpful.

The prescribed diet is generally liberal. "No added salt diets" are generally recommended to avoid aggravating the edema that is secondary to salt and water retention. Salty foods such as pizza and potato chips, or adding the salt from a shaker to foods should be avoided. Excessive protein intake is unnecessary, but the protein in the diet should be of high biologic value. Fluids are generally provided as desired by the child, unless there is refractory anasarca (generalized edema).

If the child does not eat food prepared in the hospital, parents may bring food prepared at home. Parents should be instructed not to add salt to the food. Seasoning substitutes for salt should be discussed with the family. The assistance of a dietitian is extremely helpful in planning a diet that is nutritious, reasonable in salt content, and

yet palatable to the child. Dietary planning is particularly important in cultures where highly seasoned foods are preferred.

MONITORING FOR COMPLICATIONS

All patients with nephrotic syndrome should be placed on strict *intake and output*. It is imperative that the nurse keep an accurate record. Parents and the child (if old enough) should be instructed to save all urine or stool and to notify the nurse of any emesis. Careful weighing of diapers including urine and stool is important. Parents should be instructed to notify the nurse of any foods or fluids that are ingested by the child. Parents may not know that foods such as gelatin and ice cream need to be counted as fluid intake.

All *urine should be checked with a dipstick for protein* and recorded. Because parents need to dipstick the urine at home, teaching should begin while the child is hospitalized. Urine also should be inspected for gross hematuria. Intermittent checking of urine specific gravity may be ordered.

Caregivers need to obtain *daily weight* to monitor retention of fluid. The child should be weighed at least once daily, at the same time of day and on the same scale. Diapers should be removed from infants, and older children should be weighed with a minimum amount of clothing. All nurses need to be consistent with the procedure. Because the weight of the child on admission is used, the initial weight should be validated by another nurse. Weight also should be rechecked any time there is a large discrepancy from a previously recorded weight. Weight always should be obtained and recorded in kilograms to facilitate the calculation of appropriate medication dosages.

Close observation of the extent of edema is necessary. The abdominal girth may be measured once a day to determine the extent of ascites. The measurement should always be taken at the same position. It is helpful to mark the area around the umbilicus with indelible ink so that the tape measure is always positioned in the same area and consistent measurements are obtained.

After admission, *vital signs* should be obtained to establish a baseline and should be taken at least every 4 hours. Vital signs may be done more often if the child is hypertensive or has signs or symptoms of hypovolemia. An extremely edematous child may be hypotensive and have decreased circulating blood volume. It is imperative that the nurse reassess the circulatory and cardiovascular status whenever vital signs are obtained.

Blood pressure (BP) measurement should be obtained using the same cuff that all other nurses are using. The cuff may need to be labeled with the child's name. Differences in cuff size may affect the readings obtained. The bladder of the BP cuff should completely wrap around the circumference of the child's arm and the width of the cuff should cover 2/3 of the child's upper arm. A cuff that is too small may make a normotensive child appear hypertensive.

The nurse must continually monitor the child's *fluid and electrolyte status*. Response to diuretic therapy, including the development of hypokalemia, is of vital importance. Frequent vital signs and close observations of respiratory distress or circulatory overload should be performed during Albumisol infusions.

Attention needs to be given to *skin inspection and care* because skin breakdown may occur as a result of edema. Skin should be gently washed with soap and water and thoroughly dried. Skin folds formed wherever body surfaces touch may be separated with cotton gauze. Extremities may be elevated with pillows to decrease edema and venous congestion.

Circulatory checks to extremities should be done routinely. The use of tourniquets should be avoided when possible because they are extremely painful to a child with swollen extremities and also can contribute to skin irritation. If necessary, a 4 × 4 gauze or cloth can be placed under the tourniquet when blood is drawn or IV therapy is initiated. Taping of extremities being used for IV therapy should be checked frequently so that the tape has not become too tight secondary to increased swelling from the extremity being in a dependent position. Clothing should be nonrestrictive.

The perineal area should be inspected for the extent of labial or scrotal edema. These areas also should be gently cleansed and thoroughly dried. Scrotal support may increase the child's comfort. Because diarrhea may occur as a result of infection or an edematous GI mucosa, the buttocks should be protected against skin breakdown. Diapers should be changed frequently, and the buttocks should be gently washed with mild soap and water. Desitin or other ointments may be helpful in protecting and healing the affected area.

Because children with nephrotic syndrome have an increased risk and incidence of infection, they should be protected by the use of good *medical asepsis*. Scrupulous handwashing and personal hygiene are essential. Children should not be roommates of other children with known or suspected infections that are contagious. The nurse should alert the physician whenever infection is even remotely suspected. It is important to remember that steroid therapy may suppress signs and symptoms of infection in these children. Temperatures elevated even slightly above normal should be monitored closely and reported to the physician. Abdominal distention, rigidity, pain and tenderness, absent bowel sounds, and a red rash over the abdomen indicate peritonitis, a serious complication in these children.

POSITIONING

If the ascites is severe enough to push up on the diaphragm so that lung expansion is difficult and causes discomfort for the child, the head of the bed should be kept elevated. The use of an egg crate or air flow mattress may increase the child's comfort and prevent pressure to body parts. For the child who is afraid or unable to move because of generalized edema, the nurse should assist with repositioning the child in bed as needed to increase comfort and prevent skin breakdown.

ACTIVITY PROMOTION

Because the child's activity is generally not restricted unless edema is severe, the nurse needs to determine the activity level best tolerated by the child. Activity level may change over the course of the hospitalization as edema resolves. The child should be encouraged to resume as many normal daily activities as possible. If ambulation is difficult, a wheelchair or wagon for younger children is appropriate. The leg extensions on the wheelchair should be up if edema in the lower extremities is severe. Playroom or schoolroom activities appropriate for the child's age should be encouraged.

PSYCHOSOCIAL SUPPORT

Because many of these children are long-term patients and repeated hospitalizations are possible, the nurse must take measures to reduce the stress of hospitalization and foster the child's normal progression through the stages of growth and development. Psychosocial support to the child and family is continuous, and their ability to cope effectively is re-evaluated with each readmission to the hospital or return to the outpatient setting.

Because fear of the hospital and procedures is so great for toddlers and preschool-age children, the nurse needs to incorporate individualized preprocedural strategies in the nursing care plan, especially for procedures the child finds most frightening. School-age children may be particularly sensitive about an edematous appearance and looking "funny." These feelings should be acknowledged by the nurse. It is important for the nurse to tell the child when an improvement in edema is observed. Appropriate reassurance that the swelling will abate is often comforting to the child and parent. Children should be encouraged to socialize with peers when they are ready. A roommate may be helpful until the child is ready to be around other children in a group, as in going to the playroom.

When periorbital edema is severe enough that the eyes are swollen shut, the child may be particularly fearful. Whenever possible, the same nurse should care for the child. It is extremely important that all health professionals let the child know what they are going to do before they touch the child. Because the child's normal ability to engage in activities is limited, the nurse and family can provide audio activities such as reading stories to the child, singing, or playing records or tapes. Familiar objects from home such as special blankets or stuffed animals should be kept close to the child because hugging these objects helps the child feel secure. Parents should be encouraged to hold and stay close to the child. The child and family should be assured that the periorbital edema will subside and that the child will be able to see soon. The nurse should also explain to the parents that keeping the head of the bed elevated or placing pillows under the child's head while up in the wagon helps the edema resolve.

DISCHARGE PLANNING

Discharge planning is extremely important and includes not only a teaching plan, but ensuring that the family returns for follow-up. A teaching plan is provided here for the mother of Ricardo, the child discussed in this chapter's Nursing Care Plan. Generally, the family should be comfortable with dipsticking the urine for protein and administering the prednisone, and should feel knowledgeable about the prescribed diet. Side-effects of prednisone should be discussed with the family. The family and child (if old enough) should be assured that many side-effects of prednisone will resolve when the drug is stopped. However, they should also be reminded regularly that prednisone must be taken consistently to treat this disease effectively.

Parents should also be aware of signs and symptoms of relapse and when they should call the physician. Suspected infections should be immediately reported to the physician. Infection control techniques should also be discussed with the family. The need for yearly tuberculin skin tests is reinforced; corticosteroids suppress the protective inflammatory response and may permit the establishment of a tuberculosis infection.

The family should clearly understand when the child should come back for follow-up care; the importance of ongoing evaluation needs heavy emphasis. Finally, the family should know how to reach the physician at any hour of the day or night.

★ EVALUATION

Periodically the nurse and family evaluate the outcomes of care given. Examples of outcome criteria for nephrotic syndrome were given under Planning in this section. Have short-term goals been met? Are long-term goals still realistic? Planning for further nursing care also takes into consideration complications and long-term care.

COMPLICATIONS

Several complications may occur in the child with nephrotic syndrome. Infection is a serious problem and is a cause of mortality in these patients. Cellulitis, bacteremia, and peritonitis may occur. *Streptococcus pneumoniae* is the organism most commonly seen as the cause of infections. Other gram-negative organisms such as *Escherichia coli* and *Hemophilus influenzae* may also be seen.[29] Altered immune systems in patients with nephrotic syndrome and treatment with steroids appear to be re-

sponsible for the increased risk of infection in these patients. Early detection of infections is of primary concern. Peritonitis or other life-threatening infections are treated with ampicillin and an aminoglycoside such as gentamicin.

Other complications of nephrotic syndrome include an increased risk of vascular thrombosis secondary to a hypercoagulable state. Mild transient renal impairment is also well known in severe cases of nephrotic syndrome. Malnutrition may occur as a result of negative nitrogen balance secondary to abnormal protein loss through the urine and increased protein catabolism.

Relapse, defined as the return of edema and proteinuria, is a concern in the management of nephrotic syndrome. Two thirds of children have one or more relapses. Each relapse is treated with a course of steroids. Growth retardation is a well-known side-effect of prolonged administration of steroids. However, studies show that "catch-up" growth can occur after steroids are discontinued.[29]

CRF may develop in children whose responses to treatment include: frequent relapses, steroid toxicity, steroid resistance, and unresponsiveness to cytoxic agents. It is estimated that 10% of children are resistant to all forms of therapy and go on to develop CRF.[6]

LONG-TERM CARE

Clinic visits should include obtaining the child's weight, checking for edema, and performing a urinalysis or urine dipstick for protein. Serum chemistries are needed to evaluate renal function. Blood pressure should also be measured. Toxicity from steroid therapy is evaluated. There should be opportunity to discuss concerns such as absence from school and relationships with friends for the school-age child. Side-effects from prednisone such as moon-face and weight gain may affect the child's social relationships and school attendance. The initiation of social services for interventions may be appropriate.

Clinic visits may also include a nutrition evaluation. Dietary management of excessive weight gain and an increased appetite caused by the prednisone should be discussed. It may be necessary to limit caloric intake and provide the child and family with sample menus for the day. Follow-up teaching by a dietitian may be indicated.

Home visits are generally not necessary, unless the nurse feels that follow-up reinforcement of teaching regarding dipsticking of urine and prednisone administration is necessary. When compliance with the treatment plan is in doubt, or return for follow-up is a concern, a home visit is essential.

Support for the child in school may be needed, and tutoring should be arranged when possible. If a child feels sensitive about physical appearance and it is affecting attendance at school, the school nurse may volunteer to speak to the child's classmates.

Repeated hospitalizations for relapse, the development of complications, and the progression of renal failure can be frightening and discouraging for the child and family. Consistent caregivers are needed, and referral to the social service department is appropriate. If the child does progress to CRF, nursing interventions appropriate for these children should be initiated.

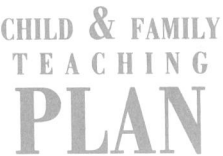

CHILD & FAMILY TEACHING PLAN

Parental Care of a Child With Nephrotic Syndrome

Assessment

Ricardo is a 3-year-old Hispanic child who was admitted to the hospital to rule out nephrotic syndrome. The diagnosis was confirmed. Ricardo's condition has stabilized. He will be discharged soon.

Ricardo's family moved to the United States from Mexico 2 years ago. He is the youngest of five children, ranging in age from 3 years to 14 years. The family lives in a small apartment along with the maternal grandmother. Mother is the primary caretaker of the children, and says that she will be the one coming in for teaching. Mother speaks very little English. She brings the eldest daughter who is 14 with her to translate. Her daughter understands English fairly well. Ricardo's father is very interested and supportive, but only visits occasionally because of working two jobs. He also speaks very little English.

The family's finances are limited. They use public transportation. They are a very close-knit and loving family, deeply concerned about Ricardo, their "baby." Mother has expressed fear about the need for Ricardo to take steroids. She has heard that they are very "bad."

Child and Family Objectives	Specific Content	Teaching Strategies
1. Learn importance of and steps in medication regimen.	1. Review purpose and side-effects of prednisone and Lasix. *Prednisone*—Prednisone is the major treatment of nephrotic syndrome. It *must* be taken every day. It is necessary that the medication be tapered by the physician and not stopped abruptly. Side-effects: increased appetite; fluid retention and wt gain; hyperactivity; dry skin; striae; flushing of cheeks; bruising; GI bleeding; risk of infection; moon face; growth retardation. Not all children experience all side-effects or to the same degree. *Most* side-effects disappear when the drug is stopped. *Lasix*—"water pill." Side-effects: dehydration, potassium loss. Prednisone and Lasix administration. (time, dose, technique)	1. Contact Spanish interpreter to assist with verbal and written instructions. Review and reinforce information in several teaching sessions. Primary nurse to instruct family for consistency of information given. Be open to mother's concerns about steroids. Correct misconceptions as necessary. Keep physician informed of mother's feelings. Reassess mother's ability to assess serious complication (infection, GI bleeding, dehydration). Reassure mother child's response to steroids will be closely monitored. Have mother come in to administer PM doses of medication. Assign Spanish-speaking nurse if possible. Use daughter for translation when necessary, or call hospital translator.

(Continued)

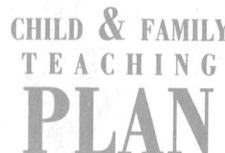

CHILD & FAMILY
TEACHING
PLAN

Parental Care of a Child With Nephrotic Syndrome (continued)

Child and Family Objectives	Specific Content	Teaching Strategies
		Demonstrate crushing medications in small amount of applesauce.
		Plan for at least three return demonstrations.
2. Demonstrate accurate dipstick urine procedure with reporting of results.	2. Explain purpose and importance of urine dipstick for protein.	2. Have mother observe urine dipstick procedure.
	Reinforce that the doctor will use the daily diary to see how the child is responding to treatment. It will be necessary to continue this at home.	Plan for at least three return demonstrations.
		Develop daily record for mother to record results at home. Begin practicing recording results.
		Arrange for family to have urine dipstick supplies before discharge.
		Assess need for community health nurse follow-up.
	Explain the meaning of relapse.	Assess verbal understanding by discussing relapse several times before discharge.
	Review signs and symptoms of relapse: 2+ protein spill, 1–2 lb weight gain, increase in puffiness and swelling such that clothes are tight and shoes won't fit.	Discuss in Spanish.
		Plan to be present when physician speaks with mother whenever possible. Reinforce and clarify information discussed.
3. State *when* and *how* to call physician.	3. Physician should be notified for signs and symptoms of relapse, fever, vomiting or diarrhea, exposure to communicable diseases such as chickenpox.	3. Provide simple written instructions in Spanish.
	Stress the importance of notifying the physician immediately for any of the above reasons.	Give mother a list of names and phone numbers of how to get medical assistance at any hour of day or night.
4. Verbalize understanding of infection.	4. Review general signs and symptoms of infection.	4. Schedule several sessions with mother to discuss.
	Review signs and symptoms of peritonitis: vomiting, abdominal pain, diarrhea.	Ask mother to repeat signs and symptoms.
	Review oral and axillary routes of taking temperature.	Give mother written information before discharge.
	Reinforce fever as an important sign of infection.	Determine method and temperature-taking device to be used at home.
		Schedule a minimum of three return demonstrations.

(Continued)

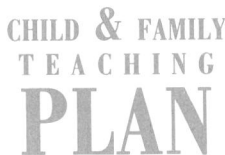

CHILD & FAMILY
T E A C H I N G
PLAN

Parental Care of a Child With Nephrotic Syndrome (continued)

Child and Family Objectives	*Specific Content*	*Teaching Strategies*
	Reinforce that use of thermometer is most accurate method of determining fever, and to check child's temperature when he is flushed, feels hot, and is irritable.	Ensure that mother has temperature-taking supplies before discharge.
	Instruct parent to notify physician for temperature >38° C.	
	Infection control measures: good handwashing, avoidance of large crowds, and avoidance of exposure to infectious person when possible.	Assess hygiene measures and health habits at home, and instruct as needed. Role model good handwashing technique. Give praise for good hygiene habits observed in the hospital.
5. Discuss prescribed diet and concerns related to it.	5. Well-balanced, nutritious diet and avoidance of excessive salt intake.	5. Allow mother time to express concerns of avoiding salty foods in family lifestyle. Assess home nutrition habits. Contact dietitian to discuss prescribed diet and alternative ways to season food instead of salt. Provide mother with pictures of "do" and "don't" foods. Have mother plan sample menu for the day. Ensure that diet is palatable to the child so that adequate intake of nutrients is not jeopardized.

Evaluation

- Mother states purpose and side-effects of medications.
- Mother identifies serious side-effects from medications that warrant notification of the physician.
- Mother demonstrates correct medication administration.
- Mother correctly demonstrates dipstick procedure with accurate recording of results in daily diary.
- Mother states signs and symptoms of relapse.
- Mother describes signs and symptoms of infection.
- Mother identifies measures to decrease risk of infection.
- Mother provides appropriate foods for Ricardo.

Hemolytic Uremic Syndrome

Definition and Incidence.   Hemolytic uremic syndrome (HUS) is one of the most common causes of ARF in childhood.[3] Classic or primary HUS generally occurs in children under 6 years of age, but it is most common in infancy and early childhood. However, it may also occur in the school-age child. There is an increased frequency of the occurrence of HUS in families, and genetic linkage has been suggested, but patterns of inheritance have not yet been found.[49]

Like nephrotic syndrome, HUS is characterized by a group of clinical manifestations. The triad of symptoms usually presented is thrombocytopenia, hemolytic anemia, and ARF (uremia). HUS was first described in 1955 when five children who died were found to have illnesses that were characterized by this triad. Over 1200 cases have been reported since HUS was originally recognized.[19]

Etiology and Pathophysiology.   The cause of HUS is not known, but increasing evidence suggests that HUS is caused by bacterial toxins. In some children, HUS has been preceded by gastroenteric infections caused by *E. coli, Salmonella, Shigella,* and other less common organisms. HUS may also follow an upper respiratory infection or other viral conditions.

In HUS, the primary injury is to the endothelial cells that line the blood vessels in the kidneys (Fig. 47-5). The endothelial cells that form the basement membrane of the glomeruli swell and detach. This injury is thought to activate protective local clotting mechanisms. Subsequently, platelets and fibrin are deposited in the lumina of the glomeruli, arterioles, and small arteries. Clotting and the formation of thrombi lead to obstruction of blood flow in the kidney. Renal insufficiency develops, causing hematuria and proteinuria, and progresses to ARF with oliguria and azotemia.[49]

Anemia develops as a result of the shortened life span of the erythrocytes that are damaged as they try to traverse the occluded renal vessels. Likewise, platelets are also destroyed, and thrombocytopenia results. The liver and spleen remove the damaged erythrocytes and platelets from circulation and therefore may become enlarged (hepatosplenomegaly).

Clinical Manifestations.   Children with HUS usually present with a recent history of gastroenteritis or an upper respiratory infection or viral illness. They may have been ill with vomiting and diarrhea of blood-streaked stools. The family may report that the child has recently become unusually pale, has no appetite, and has not been up to normal activity levels. Parents may also report that the child has been irritable and seems to be urinating less frequently, sometimes with mild hematuria.

Physical examination reveals a child with pallor due to anemia. The presence of bruising and petechiae depend on the extent of thrombocytopenia. Signs and symptoms of ARF ranging from mild dysfunction to complete renal shutdown are present. Decreased urine output, the presence of edema, and an elevated blood pressure may be expected. Pulmonary edema and congestive heart failure are late manifestations secondary to fluid overload. Hypoxia may result secondary to anemia, and approximately 50% of children with HUS have transient episodes of hypertension that must be treated.[49]

Significant involvement of the central nervous system is indicated by the presence of tremors, seizures, and stupor. Generalized seizures occur in up to 40% of children diagnosed with HUS.[49] Patients with hyponatremia and severe azotemia are particularly at risk, but cerebral infarcts may also contribute to seizures in some children.[49]

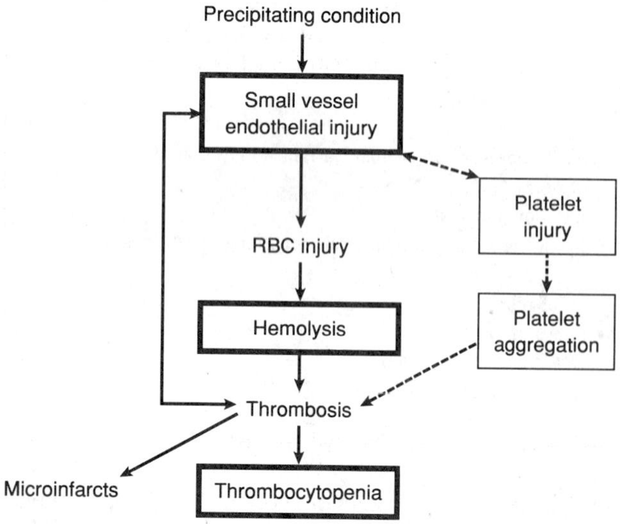

Diagnostic Studies.   The child's recent history and current clinical picture suggest the diagnosis of HUS, but blood and urine studies provide necessary confirmation. Hemoglobin may be in the range of 5 to 9 g/dL and, with an elevated reticulocyte count, provide evidence of hemolytic anemia. The platelet count typically is low (20,000 to 100,000/mm³), and WBC are elevated to 30,000/mm³.[3] Coagulation studies are generally normal.

Other findings are consistent with those seen in children with ARF. The degree of fluid and electrolyte imbalance varies with the extent of renal failure, but BUN and serum creatinine levels are elevated, and hyperkalemia, hypocalcemia, and hyperphosphatemia may be present. The urine may be positive for blood and protein, and specific gravity is low.

Renal biopsy is not indicated unless renal failure persists more than 2 weeks or if laboratory findings do not provide adequate confirmation. Thrombocytopenia is a contraindication for performing renal biopsy.

★   **ASSESSMENT**

The nursing history must include the same information discussed when assessing a child with ARF. In addition, specific questions regarding the onset of flulike symptoms, blood-streaked diarrhea, pallor, bruising, and irritability or seizures are essential.

Physical examination includes assessment of the degree of pallor, including inspection of the lips and nailbeds. The skin should be inspected for bruises, petechiae, and the presence of edema. The child's hydration status should be assessed; the child may be dehydrated as a result of diarrhea and vomiting even though edematous. These children are also assessed for signs and symptoms of congestive heart failure and fluid overload. Heart sounds and breath sounds are auscultated for the presence of a gallop rhythm and adventitious sounds. The nurse also assesses for changes in neurologic functioning such as irritability, lethargy, and seizure activity.

FIGURE 47-5

Pathogenic mechanisms in hemolytic uremic syndrome. (Adapted from Eknoyan, G., & Riggs, S. [1989]. Thrombotic thrombocytopenic purpura and hemolytic uremic syndrome. In S. Massry & R. Glassock [Eds.], *Textbook of nephrology* [Vol. I; p. 733]. Baltimore: Williams & Wilkins.

★ NURSING DIAGNOSES AND PLANNING

Nursing diagnoses for the child with HUS include those applicable for the child in ARF. Based on the assessment data from above and Chapter 46, the following nursing diagnoses may also apply:

- High Risk for Injury related to a low platelet count and seizures.
- High Risk for Impaired Skin Integrity related to frequent loose stools and edema.
- Fluid Volume Deficit related to vomiting and diarrhea.
- Fatigue related to anemia.

Planning and sample goals and expected outcomes are discussed in the section on ARF.

★ INTERVENTIONS: COLLABORATIVE AND INDEPENDENT

Children with HUS are acutely ill and demand aggressive medical management and intensive nursing care. More than 90% of the children diagnosed with HUS survive the acute phase, and most of them recover normal renal function.[3] The remainder are left with residual renal failure, and a child may occasionally require long-term dialysis treatment. As with acute renal failure from other causes, immediate attention must be given to fluid and electrolyte balance. Other interventions include blood replacement and medications. Nursing interventions also include diet modification, monitoring for complications, teaching, and emotional support. Dialysis may be required for severe renal impairment, especially if congestive heart failure is present.

FLUID AND ELECTROLYTE THERAPY

Children who are dehydrated from vomiting and diarrhea require fluid therapy, but care must be taken not to further impair renal functioning. Fluids are usually restricted to 350 to 400 ml/m^2/24 h plus the replacement of urinary and GI losses. Hyperkalemia is treated with the administration of a cation exchange resin such as Kayexalate; dialysis may be indicated.

Maintaining the child's fluid restriction is an extremely important nursing intervention. Because the majority of these children are so young, they do not understand why the fluid restrictions are necessary; the cooperation of parents must be enlisted. Individualized strategies regarding fluid restriction should be added to the nursing care plan. Approaches for management of fluid restriction are discussed in the acute renal failure section.

BLOOD REPLACEMENT

Blood transfusions of packed red blood cells are ordered to improve severe anemia, but platelet infusions are generally not indicated unless the child is actively bleeding. If the platelet count is less than 50,000/mm^3 and the child must undergo an invasive procedure such as vascular access for the initiation of dialysis, platelet infusions are indicated.[49]

Investigations into the use of other therapies including heparin, plasma infusions, and fibrinolytic agents such as urokinase have been attempted. Vitamin E therapy and IV immunoglobin G (IgG) infusions have also been used. Most recently, plasmapheresis and exchange transfusions have been tried. So far, none of these specific therapies has been proven to be advantageous over general supportive therapy in the treatment of these children.[49]

MEDICATIONS

Antihypertensives such as nifedipine and hydralazine are used to control elevations in blood pressure.[49] Children may also be treated prophylactically with anticonvulsants for seizures if they exhibit any signs of neuromuscular irritability such as muscle twitching. The dosage of all drugs is evaluated in light of current renal function.

DIET THERAPY

The child's nutritional needs must be met, yet the child with HUS is often anorectic. Nursing strategies that improve the child's nutritional intake are essential. Dietary management includes a high-calorie, high-carbohydrate diet that is limited in sodium, potassium, protein, and phosphorus. Small frequent feedings of a prescribed diet that is still palatable to the child are important. The child's food preferences and dislikes are recorded on the nursing care plan.

Consultation with a dietitian should be initiated to assess the child's nutritional needs and assist the child and family to understand the need for the prescribed diet. The dietitian fits the child's normal dietary habits into the prescribed diet whenever possible, and this accommodation can do much to improve the child's oral intake and nutritional status.

If diarrhea is persistent and severe, or bowel ischemia is present, the child may need to remain NPO. Total parenteral nutrition (TPN), appropriately modified for the child with renal impairment, is indicated to maintain positive nitrogen balance.

ACTIVITY PROMOTION

The nurse should observe the child's level of fatigue and activity intolerance related to anemia. Appropriate activities should be planned. This may mean quiet play and providing diversional activities at the bedside. Activities can be increased as the child's condition improves.

MONITORING FOR COMPLICATIONS

Accurate measurement of intake and output is essential, including stool and vomitus whenever possible. Stool and urine are measured separately, but this is sometimes difficult in the infant and toddler age groups. Assessment of fluid balance includes hydration status and evaluation for hypovolemia and shock. The child receiving IV fluids or blood should be observed closely for hypertension and fluid overload secondary to increased intravascular volume.

It is imperative that the child be monitored closely for signs and symptoms of deteriorating renal function. Interventions for the child in various phases of ARF are applicable here, including the initiation of dialysis.

Accurate measurement of blood pressure is extremely important, and upward trends should be reported to the physician. Irritability and complaints of headache or dizziness are symptoms that can alert the nurse to a hypertensive episode.

The child should be assessed for alterations in neurologic function, and any muscle twitching should be reported to the physician immediately. Seizure precautions should be initiated.

The nurse should monitor the child for bleeding. All output, including emesis, urine, and stool should be inspected for gross blood and tested for occult blood. Tissue injury should be prevented by avoiding IM injections and rectal temperatures. After venipuncture, pressure should be applied to the site.

Skin assessments are made regularly to avoid breakdown. Frequent, loose stools may cause excoriation of the skin on the buttocks; therefore, diapers should be changed frequently, and the perineal area should be gently washed and dried after each soiling. Ointments such as Desitin may assist in healing the affected area.

TEACHING

The nurse must continually assess the family's understanding of the medical plan and treatments. Because one third or more of the children with HUS require dialysis, families of those children need an orientation to the dialysis unit and information about what will happen. Close collaboration with the dialysis nurses is essential.

This is a fearful time for families. To have a healthy child become acutely ill so quickly and require kidney dialysis is frightening news. The family may fear that the child will not survive. The nurse can create an environment that allows the family to ventilate their concerns and fears freely. It is reassuring to families to know that most children with HUS do extremely well and regain normal kidney function.

PSYCHOSOCIAL SUPPORT

The nurse can initiate strategies to decrease the stress of hospitalization for the infant and young child. Children should be prepared for all procedures in a manner appropriate for their level of growth and development. The assistance of a child life specialist may be beneficial in providing activities for the child at the bedside and to assist with therapeutic play, perhaps with a doll (Fig. 47-6). Above all, the family should be encouraged to visit and to participate in the child's care.

Because it is likely that the child will require one or more blood transfusions, the parents may be fearful of AIDS. The family should be encouraged to discuss their fears with the physician. Nurses can reassure the family that the blood supply is carefully tested for AIDS. The possibility of donor-directed blood should be an option discussed with the family.

The chapter section on ARF should be reviewed for more discussion of emotional support.

DISCHARGE PLANNING

The complexity of discharge planning and the degree of long-term care required depend on the extent of residual renal dysfunction. Home care instructions for all children with HUS should include clarification of medications, diet, and fluid plan. Follow-up appointments need to be stressed and reinforced with the family. Generally, visiting nurse referrals are not needed unless the family is unlikely to return for follow-up or if noncompliance with medications such as antihypertensives is a concern. The family

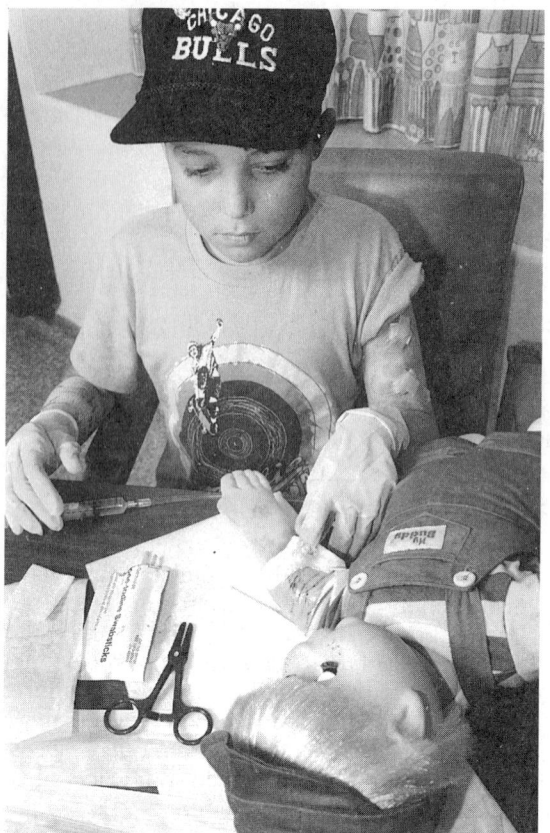

FIGURE 47-6
School-age boy in therapeutic play with doll. Children are encouraged to perform procedures they have experienced on the dolls.

should be instructed to call the physician for fever, weight gain, and return of edema, decreased urination, flulike symptoms, and the inability to take prescribed medications.

For the few numbers of children who require continued treatment with dialysis, a much more extensive discharge plan needs to be developed. Discharge planning guidelines and long-term management would follow those for the child requiring ongoing hemodialysis or peritoneal dialysis.

★ EVALUATION

Evaluation criteria given earlier in this chapter for the child with ARF may be used for the child with hemolytic uremic syndrome.

Acute Poststreptococcal Glomerulonephritis

Definition and Incidence Glomerulonephritis is an inflammation of the glomeruli in the kidneys. It may be a primary condition or occur secondary to a host of systemic diseases. The symptoms range from mild to severe, and the clinical course varies from acute to rapidly progressive, or it may become chronic. Table 47-6 provides a comparison of these three major forms of glomerulonephritis. Glomerulonephritis is also classified by

TABLE 47-6
Glomerulonephritis: Comparison of Three Major Clinical Forms

	Acute	Rapidly Progressive	Chronic
Occurrence of glomerular changes	Days to weeks	Weeks to months	Months to years
Renal dysfunction	Usually reversible and self-limiting	Aggressive, *rapid* progression to end-stage renal disease	Irreversible chronic renal failure to end-stage renal disease
Causative factors	*Infection.* Group A beta hemolytic strep*	Acute glomerulonephritis	Persistent underlying disease process
	Strep viridens—infective bacterial endocarditis	Drugs	Membranoproliferative glomerulonephritis*
	Staph bacteremia and staph epidermis—ventricular atrial shunt infections	Toxic agents	
		Idiopathic causes	
	Viral diseases	Goodpasture's syndrome	
	Parasitic diseases		
	Fungal diseases		
	Systemic diseases: Systemic lupus erythematosus		
	Henoch-Schönlein purpura		

* Most common cause.
Source: Glassock, R. (1989). Glomerular diseases, Part 1: Syndromes of glomerular diseases. In S. Massry & R. Glassock (Eds.), *Textbook of Nephrology* (2nd ed.). Baltimore: Williams & Wilkins.

the extent of renal injury, as shown in the display on classification of glomerular tissue injury.

Although several types of glomerulonephritis have been identified, acute poststreptococcal glomerulonephritis (APSGN) is the most common type in children, and it occurs as a result of a previous infection by group A beta-hemolytic strep.[51] APSGN is most prevalent in school-age children with the average age of onset being 6 to 7 years of age; less than 5% of affected children are under 2 years. Males are usually affected more than females by a 2:1 ratio.[4] Cases of APSGN can occur sporadically in populations, but outbreaks of epidemic proportions have also occurred. Analysis of the children affected during epidemics has revealed a 1:1 male-to-female ratio. Because of the prevalence of upper respiratory infections in the winter, the incidence of APSGN is higher during these months.

Etiology and Pathophysiology Streptococcal infections of the upper respiratory tract and skin are known to precipitate the onset of APSGN. Pharyngitis and impetigo are often the sites of initial infection, although the latter is less common.[51] A latent period of 1 to 2 weeks exists between the onset of the initial infection and the onset of nephritis.

APSGN is known as an immune complex disease, but the exact pathogenic mechanism is not well understood. It is suggested that antibodies are produced by the body in response to a streptococcal infection and that these antibodies are directed against "self" antigens in the kidney. Antigen–antibody complexes are deposited on the epithelium of the glomerular basement membrane, causing the kidney to become enlarged and edematous. Inflammation and obstruction lead to tissue injury. Glomerular filtration is impaired, resulting in ARF with varying degrees of severity.

The prognosis for children with APSGN is generally favorable. Resolution of the disease and return of normal renal function occur in a few weeks. Second attacks of APSGN are known but are unusual. Recurrent bouts of nephritis may be suggestive of underlying chronic renal disease.

Clinical Manifestations. Children presenting with APSGN have classic signs and symptoms after an antecedent streptococcal infection. The onset of APSGN is generally abrupt, although the severity of symptoms can range from asymptomatic microscopic hematuria with normal function to ARF. Parents usually bring the child to the physician because of hematuria and edema. Gross hematuria, described as cola- or tea-colored urine, is

Classification of Glomerular Tissue Injury in Glomerulonephritis

Diffuse: all glomeruli are affected
Focal: some glomerular involvement
Segmental: portions of individual glomeruli are involved
Membranous: the glomerular capillary wall thickens
Proliferative: the number of glomerular cells increase
Crescent formation: proliferation of epithelial cells; glomerular cell death and cessation of function
Sclerosis: scar tissue within the glomeruli

present in the majority of patients. Their urine is a dark, concentrated, reddish-brown color. Even if overt hematuria is absent, all children with APSGN have microscopic hematuria as well as red cell casts. Oliguria and proteinuria are expected, and urine specific gravity is high.

Initially, mild periorbital edema is a common finding, but generalized edema may also occur in varying degrees of severity in affected people. Causes of edema include a decreased GFR, resulting in the retention of sodium and water. The degree of proteinuria may also affect the extent of edema.

Hypertension ranging from mild to moderate is a common finding in children with APSGN. Occasionally, severe hypertension is present and can precipitate the onset of encephalopathy with seizures.

Diagnostic Studies The criteria for diagnosis of APSGN is based on (1) the presence of glomerular injury (i.e., hematuria, proteinuria, and red cell casts), and (2) confirmation of previous infection with group A beta-hemolytic strep. Laboratory tests are similar to those for children who develop ARF due to other causes.

Confirmation of a poststreptococcal infection is achieved by positive skin or throat cultures and an elevated antistreptolysin (ASO) titer. However, the severity of APSGN is not indicated by the level of elevation in the ASO titer. In addition, depression of hemolytic complement activity and serum C3 levels are typically seen.

Chest x-ray findings consistently reveal cardiomegaly (usually mild); pulmonary edema and pleural effusions are also common. Renal biopsies are usually not indicated but may be obtained when there is an atypical presentation of APSGN, to identify a specific type of glomerular lesion, or for persistent symptomatology.

★ ASSESSMENT

Nursing assessment of children with APSGN is similar to any child presenting with ARF. The degree of hematuria and amount of urine output should be assessed. Weight gain and the extent of edema are important indicators. The family's knowledge of a recent streptococcal infection is ascertained, and the ill child is assessed for signs and symptoms of current infection. Family screening for streptococcal infection is also important to help prevent recurrence.

★ NURSING DIAGNOSES AND PLANNING

Nursing diagnoses and planning for the child with APSGN are essentially the same as those suggested for ARF.

★ INTERVENTIONS: COLLABORATIVE AND INDEPENDENT

Medical therapy is generally supportive to manage symptoms and generally follows that already discussed for ARF. Antibiotic therapy is generally not indicated unless positive cultures are present.[4,51] Hypertension and edema are managed with antihypertensive medications, diuretic therapy, and dietary sodium restrictions. Protein restrictions are initiated if the child has marked azotemia. Fluid retention in APSGN is managed by fluid restriction and diuretics, such as furosemide, if necessary.

ACTIVITY PROMOTION

Bedrest is generally recommended for the child with severe hypertension and significant edema. In the absence of these findings, the child should be allowed activity as tolerated. Studies have shown no direct beneficial effect of imposed strict bedrest on the outcome of APSGN.[4,51] However, if bedrest is ordered, the nurse can provide diversional activities at the bedside. Many of the children with APSGN are of school age, and activities appropriate for this age group should be provided. Clarifying and liberalizing activity should be discussed with the physician as the child's condition improves. Prolonged imposition of strict bedrest on a school-age child that is normally physically active and socializing with peers may contribute to the stress of hospitalization and affect the child's ability to cope.

MONITORING

Constant monitoring of the child's fluid and electrolyte status and early recognition of complications are important. Maintaining fluid limits is essential and includes developing strategies that cause the least frustration and distress for the child.

TEACHING

Child and family teaching should include explanations of treatment and procedures including fluid limits, frequent monitoring of vital signs (especially blood pressure), daily weight, and laboratory tests. Preprocedural strategies should be initiated as appropriate for the child's level of growth and development (i.e., most often for the school-age child). In addition, the importance of compliance with fluid limits, dietary requirements, and the saving of urine for measurement should be reinforced and cannot be overemphasized.

DISCHARGE PLANNING

Discharge instructions to the family include clarification of diet and medications, signs and symptoms of renal dysfunction, and when to notify the physician. Instructions for subsequent appointments should be clarified, stressing the necessity of follow-up care. The nurse may need to instruct the family on how to take the blood pressure and dipstick the urine at home. Home health agency referrals are usually not necessary unless the family is unlikely to return for follow-up.

★ EVALUATION

Outcome criteria for the child with ARF may be applied also to the child with APSGN.

COMPLICATIONS

Common complications of APSGN include circulatory overload and congestive heart failure, severe hypertensive episodes with or without hypertensive encephalopathy and seizures, and fluid and electrolyte imbalances typically recognized in children with ARF. Severe, persistent oliguria with azotemia or total anuria is rare in APSGN.

Hemodialysis or peritoneal dialysis may be indicated to manage ARF in these patients.

LONG-TERM CARE

Long-term care of the child with APSGN includes follow-up return visits to the clinic or physician's office for assessment of renal function. The frequency of visits depends on the individual child and the severity of the disease. Microscopic hematuria and proteinuria may persist for several months. Follow-up visits include blood pressure measurement and examination of the urine for red cells and protein. Penicillin prophylaxis against subsequent infections with nephrotogenic strains of group A beta-hemolytic strep is not routinely recommended.

Lupus Nephritis

Systemic lupus erythematosus (SLE) is an autoimmune disease characterized by fever, weight loss, rash, arthritis, and an assortment of other symptoms (see Chap. 28). The majority of children with SLE develop renal involvement that varies from mild asymptomatic disease to rapidly progressive glomerulonephritis and renal failure. As in acute poststreptococcal glomerulonephritis, immune complexes are deposited in the glomeruli. As the disease advances, more glomeruli are injured, resulting in inflammation and the formation of thrombi.[45]

Effective treatment of lupus nephritis is primarily drug therapy with the steroid prednisone. Immunosuppressive agents such as cyclophosphamide are indicated for more severe forms of nephritis. Cyclosporine is being investigated in the treatment of membranous lupus nephropathy.[2]

Plasmapheresis has also been tried on a limited basis for exacerbations of lupus. The aim of plasmapheresis is to remove antigens, antibodies, and immune complexes through plasma exchange. However, no significant benefits of plasmapheresis over conventional therapy with prednisone and oral cyclophosphamide have been demonstrated.[2]

Although children with SLE generally respond well to drug therapy, the condition is only controlled, not cured. The risk of relapse with severe nephritis endures. Continued treatment by an interdisciplinary health team is mandatory.[3]

Henoch-Schönlein Purpura Nephritis

Henoch-Schönlein purpura (HSP) is one of the common systemic diseases of childhood that results in glomerular injury. Peak incidence occurs around 4 years of age. The disease is thought to be an immune-complex disease, but its exact cause is unclear. Nearly all children with HSP have some histologic evidence of renal involvement.[11]

Children with HSP may be asymptomatic, or they may develop mild hematuria. Other symptoms may include a rash on the buttocks and lower extremities, arthritis, and abdominal pain. Renal involvement is usually detected within 1 month of the onset of HSP, but may appear later.[3]

Varying degrees of nephritis including proteinuria, hypertension, and reduced GFR appear, and nephrotic syndrome is common in affected children. Treatment for HSP nephritis is generally supportive, and the prognosis is excellent. A small percentage of children, however, develop ESRD.[11]

Goodpasture's Syndrome

This disorder was first identified in 1919 by Ernest Goodpasture during a flu epidemic. A patient who had hemorrhagic pneumonitis died, and glomerulonephritis was discovered on autopsy. Goodpasture's syndrome is a disorder with a distinct triad of clinical manifestations: pulmonary hemorrhage, glomerulonephritis, and the presence of circulating antiglomerular basement membrane (anti-GBM) antibodies in the plasma.[25,45] Young adult males are most often affected by this disease, but it does occur in older children and adolescents.

The etiology of Goodpasture's syndrome is unknown. Anti-GBM antibodies are produced in response to glomerular, tubular, or alveolar basement antigens. The stimulus for the production of anti-GBM antibodies remains unclear. Mini-epidemics of Goodpasture's syndrome and seasonal peaks during the spring months suggest an infectious etiology. Influenza A has been documented in some cases. Environmental exposure to hydrocarbons has also been suggested as a possible cause.[45]

The clinical presentation of Goodpasture's syndrome may vary. Signs and symptoms include flulike complaints, hematuria, hemoptysis, and anemia. Clinical manifestations depend on the degree of glomerular and pulmonary injury.[45] The disease can be fatal due to rapidly progressive glomerulonephritis and life-threatening pulmonary hemorrhage with respiratory failure.

Treatment of Goodpasture's syndrome is directed at trying to control the underlying pathology. Medical management includes suppressing the inflammatory response and removing the number of circulating antibodies.[25,45] Plasmapheresis, steroids, and immunosuppressive agents such as cyclophosphamide may improve both renal and pulmonary signs and symptoms. Dialysis may be required for treatment of ARF. Some children progress to ESRD and are candidates for renal transplantation.

Congenital and Inherited Conditions Causing Renal Dysfunction

Alport's Syndrome

Alport's syndrome is the most common type of hereditary nephritis, and it is transmitted as an autosomal dominant disorder. The nature of this inherited defect is unclear, but the syndrome has a more severe clinical course in males. Some families have no history of renal disease, suggesting that there is a high spontaneous mutation rate for the abnormal gene. Besides renal involvement, children with Alport's syndrome may also develop hearing loss and cataracts.[3,40]

Few renal changes may be identified in children less than 10 years of age. Then, glomeruli begin to thicken and sclerose. Tubular atrophy follows with further degeneration of the nephrons.

Affected children present with a wide variation of symptoms. Some have only microscopic hematuria, but others have recurrent episodes of gross hematuria and manifestations similar to chronic glomerulonephritis. If the child has few symptoms, the presence of proteinuria indicates the need for renal biopsy and confirmation of the diagnosis.

The medical and nursing plans are symptomatic and supportive. Males with Alport's syndrome frequently develop CRF that progresses to ESRD during the second to third decade of life. These children are good candidates for dialysis and renal transplantation. Females usually live a normal life with minimal hearing impairment. Genetic counseling should be included as part of the care plan.[3,40]

Bartter's Syndrome

Bartter's syndrome is a rare congenital disorder that affects the renal tubules. The condition is of an autosomal recessive origin and is more common in African Americans.[11] Physical features characteristic of Bartter's syndrome include a large head, down-turned mouth, and protruding pinnae of the ears.

Bartter's syndrome may be identified in early infancy; some children are born preterm. Presenting signs and symptoms include growth failure, poor feeding, dehydration, vomiting, constipation, polyuria, and excessive thirst.[42] Affected children crave salt and experience muscle weakness.

The exact underlying pathology of this defect is still not fully understood, but there is an inability of the kidney tubules to reabsorb chloride ions. Renal biopsy findings include hyperplasia of the cells adjoining the glomerululi (juxtaglomerululi apparatus). The basic defect triggers the appearance of hypokalemia, metabolic alkalosis, hypochloremia, and hyperaldosteronism. Excess production of prostaglandins is thought to encourage the secretion of renin; however, these children are not hypertensive. Overproduction of prostaglandins is thought to contribute to the other clinical findings of this disorder.[3]

Medical treatment of children with Bartter's syndrome is symptomatic and directed at restoring sodium and fluid volume. Potassium chloride supplements may be required in amounts up to 10 mEq/kg/day to prevent muscle weakness and cardiac arrhythmias.[13] Prostaglandin inhibitors such as aspirin and indomethacin are prescribed to alleviate manifestations of this disease.[3,43]

Children with Bartter's syndrome require monitoring for development of renal toxicity. Glomerulonephritis develops in some children and may progress to ESRD.[42]

Cystinosis

Cystinosis is inherited as an autosomal recessive trait, and affected children have distinctive physical features

including blond hair, fair complexion, and bone deformities from rickets. They may also experience photophobia and hypothyroidism. Cystinosis is an accumulation of cystine in the kidneys that causes progressive renal damage and usually results in CRF within the first decade of life.[3,17,42] The condition may appear in infancy or in childhood.

Infants with nephropathic cystinosis present to the health care system with failure to thrive, polyuria, polydipsia, and episodes of dehydration. The juvenile form of cystinosis appears after the age of 3 and has the same but less severe clinical manifestations. Early treatment requires meticulous attention to fluid and electrolyte balance. Children with cystinosis tolerate dialysis and transplantation as well as any other child with ESRD.

Nephrogenic Diabetes Insipidus

Nephrogenic diabetes insipidus (NDI) is a rare, X-linked recessive disease, clinically characterized by polyuria, polydipsia, and impairment in urine-concentrating ability. These symptoms occur because of complete (in males) or partial (in females) tubular unresponsiveness to the action of vasopressin (antidiuretic hormone). Differential diagnosis is needed between NDI and pituitary diabetes insipidus.

During infancy, affected males may experience dehydration caused by hypernatremia, and repeated episodes have been associated with seizures. Mental retardation may follow. Other clinical features are malnutrition and short stature.

Primary treatment plans include providing nutrition (calories) and maintaining hydration.[17,36,42] NDI is a chronic condition, but the prognosis is good if hypernatremic dehydration can be avoided.[3]

Renal Tubular Acidosis

Renal tubular acidosis (RTA) is a disorder of the renal tubules characterized by a sustained metabolic acidosis, urine pH >5.4, and hyperchloremia.[1] Principal forms of the condition are distal RTA (type I; classic) and proximal RTA (type II). Both distal and proximal RTA occur as a result of primary or secondary causes, which are listed in Table 47-7.

In distal RTA, the distal tubules of the nephrons are defective and unable to establish an adequate gradient of pH between blood and urine in the distal tubules.[1] Inability of the distal tubule to secrete hydrogen ion reduces the formation of acids and carbon dioxide in the tubular lumen. Urine pH cannot be reduced below 5.8 despite severe systemic acidosis.[3] Sodium bicarbonate is lost and results in hyperchloremia and hypokalemia, but the hypokalemia is less severe than that found in proximal RTA. Distal RTA may be complicated by excessive loss of calcium in the urine that leads to bone demineralization, retarded bone age, and the precipitation of calcium phosphate in the tubules (nephrocalcinosis).[3,42] The deposition of calcium in the kidneys may accentuate tubular dysfunction.[42]

TABLE 47-7
Classification of Renal Tubular Acidosis

Proximal	Distal
Isolated	Isolated
Sporadic	Sporadic
Hereditary	Hereditary
Fanconi's syndrome	Secondary
Primary	Interstitial nephritis
Secondary	Obstructive
Inherited	Pyelonephritis
Cystinosis	Transplant rejection
Lowe's syndrome	Sickle cell nephropathy
Galactosemia	Lupus nephritis
Hereditary fructose intolerance	Ehlers-Danlos syndrome
Tyrosinemia	Nephrocalcinosis
Wilson's disease	Hepatic cirrhosis
Medullary cystic disease	Elliptocytosis
Acquired	Medullary sponge kidney
Heavy metals	Toxins
Outdated tetracycline	Amphotericin B
Proteinuria	Lithium
Interstitial nephritis	Toluene
Hyperparathyroidism	
Vitamin D deficiency rickets	

Adapted from Behrman, R. E., & Vaughan, V. C. (1992) *Nelson Textbook of Pediatrics.* Philadelphia: Saunders.

In proximal RTA, the proximal tubules of the nephrons are defective in reabsorbing bicarbonate. Excessive bicarbonate is lost in the urine, and plasma bicarbonate levels decrease. Sodium and potassium are lost along with bicarbonate, resulting in depletion of fluid volume and hypokalemia.

In children who have substantial systemic acidosis, a urine pH <5.5 supports the diagnosis of proximal RTA.[3] With urinary bicarbonate loss, the serum bicarbonate level falls until it reaches a threshold at which bicarbonate wasting ceases. At this level (15 to 18 mEq/L), the quantity of filtered bicarbonate is reduced to an amount that can be totally reabsorbed by the tubules. The urine becomes acidified because the distal tubules are intact.[3]

Children with RTA present with growth retardation and symptoms related to metabolic acidosis.[43] If acidemia is severe, anorexia, vomiting, hyperventilation, and vascular collapse may occur.

Children with proximal RTA require therapy with sodium bicarbonate 10 mEq/kg/day to correct acidosis. Lower maintenance doses of sodium bicarbonate at 2 to 3 mEq/kg/day are usually required to treat distal RTA sufficiently.

Children with RTA usually grow normally once the acidosis is corrected. Alkaline therapy in most cases is lifelong, and potassium may be needed to correct deficits. Preservation of renal function with distal RTA is excellent if therapy is initiated before severe nephrocalcinosis develops.[42]

Sickle Cell Nephropathy

Sickle cell anemia is an autosomal dominant inherited disease usually seen in African Americans, although it can affect Caucasians of Mediterranean descent. Most children with sickle cell disease eventually experience renal involvement that is characterized by hematuria, urinary concentrating defect, enuresis, proteinuria, and nephrotic syndrome. Medical management is directed at supportive and symptomatic treatment, which includes prevention of dehydration and blood transfusions to correct anemia. Sickle cell neuropathy is reversible in some children. Others, however, progress to ESRD and are candidates for dialysis and transplantation.[3,53]

Renal Replacement Therapy

Renal replacement therapy consists of dialysis and/or renal transplantation. Although dialysis may be used for an extended period of time to control symptoms of renal failure, it offers no cure of the underlying problem. Generally, the ultimate goal of treatment for ESRD is successful kidney transplantation.

Dialysis

Simply stated, dialysis is the passage of a solute and fluid through a semipermeable membrane. During the dialysis treatment, waste products and excess fluids are removed from the blood by way of osmosis, diffusion, and ultrafiltration. Two types of dialysis are available: hemodialysis and peritoneal dialysis. A comparison of these two modalities is presented in Table 47-8.

Until recently, hemodialysis was the standard treatment for long-term management of children with renal failure. The development of new peritoneal dialysis techniques, however, has revolutionized the approach to long-term care and make it the preferred method for many children. Hemodialysis remains the treatment of choice for ARF that may result from poisoning or drug toxicity. Decisions about the type of dialysis also depend on variables such as the size of child, available family support systems, living arrangements, distance from hospital or dialysis center, and psychosocial functioning of the child and family.

Peritoneal Dialysis

Peritoneal dialysis is the ideal treatment for most children because it allows them the opportunity to be at home and to participate in normal childhood activities such as school and extracurricular commitments. Because this procedure is performed every day, it requires fewer diet and fluid restrictions and often fewer medications than hemodialysis. Some studies suggest that children treated with peritoneal dialysis have an improved nutritional status and grow better due to the absorption of dextrose in the fluid used for exchange.[20]

Peritoneal dialysis is a procedure that uses the peritoneal membrane for the removal of solutes and excess water. A patent catheter surgically placed in the peritoneal cavity is essential for effective treatment. Most of the time, the child is taken to the operating room for catheter insertion; however, some pediatric dialysis centers perform this procedure at the bedside.

A variety of styles and sizes of catheters are available. After the catheter is placed in the peritoneal cavity, it is

TABLE 47-8
Comparison of Peritoneal Dialysis and Hemodialysis

Peritoneal Dialysis	Hemodialysis
Independent lifestyle	Dependent on dialysis staff
Child/family responsibility to perform every day	Transportation to dialysis center three times a week
Child has control but constantly reminded of illness	Child can deny disease between treatments
Can attend school every day	Misses some time at school; decreased peer involvement
Potential for growth may be greater due to increased calories from dialysate	Potential for growth is questionable
External peritoneal catheter	Vascular access usually internal, requires needle insertion for each treatment
Hypertension rare	Hypertension frequently related to fluid overload
Chemistry clearance stable because treatment performed daily	Wide fluctuations in chemistries (44–64 h between treatments)
Fewer diet and fluid restrictions	Diet and fluid restriction: low-sodium, low-potassium, low-phosphorus diet
Infrequent blood transfusions	Blood transfusion common
''Burn out'' for child or family common because of constant care required	Health care team responsible for performing treatment; travel and vacation easier for child and family
Peritonitis is primary complication	Access complications (infection, clotting) most common
Need to store at least 1 month's supplies and equipment for machine	No storage space required
Flexibility in schedule is possible	Care of siblings and family schedule planned around dialysis schedule

tunneled out the subcutaneous tissue to exit through the skin on the abdomen (Fig. 47-7). A watertight seal at the site where the catheter enters into the peritoneal cavity is of utmost importance.[48] This seal prevents leaking that could result in peritonitis, the primary complication of peritoneal dialysis.

Peritoneal dialysis uses a simple technique that can be safely performed at home even on small children. A warm solution of fluid and solutes called dialysate is instilled through the catheter into the peritoneal cavity, allowed to dwell for a specified time, and then to drain.

The volume of dialysate needed for the exchange is calculated by the child's size and weight, with 30 to 50 cc/kg used as general rule.[47]

Dialysate is commercially available in dextrose concentrations of 1.5%, 2.5%, and 4.25% and contains sodium, calcium, and potassium. The higher the concentration of solutes, the greater the osmolarity and the more fluid that will be removed from the body. The concentration of dextrose used is determined by the amount of fluid that needs to be removed to maintain normal body weight.

Because the abdominal catheter provides direct ac-

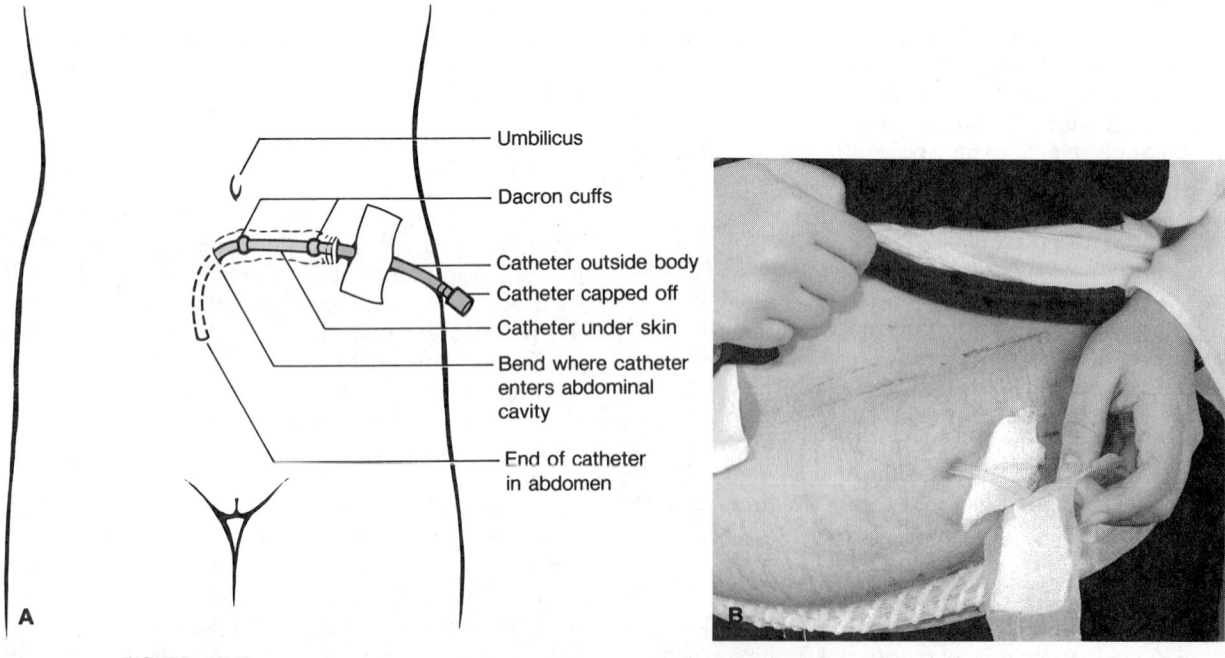

FIGURE 47-7
Peritoneal dialysis procedure. (**A**) Placement of peritoneal dialysis catheter. Approximately two-thirds of the catheter is under the skin or in the child's abdomen. (Redrawn from Gabriel, R. [1987]. *A patient's guide to dialysis and transplantation.* Boston: MTP Press.) (**B**) Peritoneal catheter exit site in an adolescent girl.

cess to the peritoneal cavity, the connection and disconnection procedure must be performed with strict aseptic technique to reduce the risk of infection. Bacteria introduced into a high-dextrose, warm, dark environment, through a break in the system or technique, can readily result in peritonitis.

Types of Peritoneal Dialysis. Over the last 12 years, peritoneal dialysis techniques and equipment for children have improved. In the beginning, the technique of *intermittent peritoneal dialysis* (IPD) was used. This treatment used a machine to deliver the dialysate but took 10 to 12 hours, 3 to 4 days per week. This treatment may still be used as an interim plan while a catheter site is healing or home training is completed. Now, however, continuous ambulatory peritoneal dialysis (CAPD) or continuous cycling peritoneal dialysis (CCPD) are preferred to maintain the child in the best metabolic balance.

CAPD and CCPD are performed every day at home by the child or the family. Home training requires approximately a 2- to 3-week commitment to learn the principles of aseptic technique, technical aspects of the plan, accurate assessment of the child, troubleshooting, and treatment of complications. The health care team is available by telephone for consultation and support.[21]

Continuous ambulatory peritoneal dialysis (CAPD) is performed four to five times a day in a clean, quiet environment. Individual bags of dialysate are warmed with a heating pad or K-pad. The warm dialysate is instilled in the prescribed volume. Once the solution has infused, the tubing is clamped, rolled up with the bag, and placed in a pocket or secured to the body. The child goes about normal daily activities.

In approximately 4 hours, the tubing and bag are positioned lower than the abdomen to drain the used dialysate, which contains the waste products and fluid that have crossed the peritoneal membrane. Used dialysate is assessed for volume, clarity, presence of fibrin, or blood. The child's fluid status is assessed using measures of weight, blood pressure, pulse, and sense of well-being. These findings help in the selection of the concentration of dextrose that will achieve the desired body weight.

The next bag of dialysate is prepared, and the transfer of the "spike" from one bag to another is done aseptically. Everyone in the room is required to wear a mask; doors and windows are closed, and activity in the room is kept to a minimum (Fig. 47-8). After the connection is secure, the fresh dialysate is infused by gravity, and the tubing and bag are placed in the pocket. This process takes approximately 30 minutes, depending on volume being used and adequacy of inflow and outflow. Keeping dialysis ongoing throughout the day and night permits the BUN and creatinine to be maintained at stable levels.

Another form of peritoneal dialysis is *continuous cycling peritoneal dialysis* (CCPD). This treatment is performed every night while the child sleeps. It requires a cycling machine that automatically opens and closes the tubing for inflow and outflow of the dialysate (Fig. 47-9). The physician prescribes the type and volume of fluid and frequency of the exchanges. At bedtime, the child or parent sets up the machine with the appropriate dialysate to achieve an optimal body weight. The connecting procedure is simple and is accomplished in approximately 15 minutes. The treatment generally takes 10 hours per night with 6 to 10 exchanges occurring during that time. As the child sleeps, warm dialysate infuses into the peritoneal cavity, dwells for a predetermined time, and drains. In the morning, the disconnect procedure is performed, allowing the child to be free of interruptions during normal daily activities.

Two positive features of CCPD are a decrease in frequency of opening the system and an increase in freedom during the day. Disadvantages, however, include the decreased mobility required during the treatment time and the time and knowledge required to correct problems

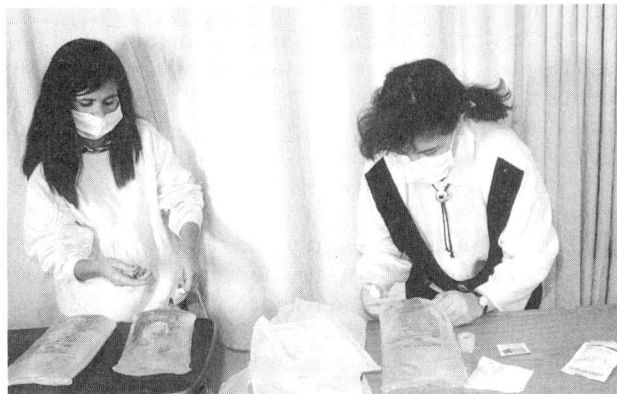

FIGURE 47-8
Two adolescent girls in different stages of a continuous ambulatory peritoneal dialysis (CAPD) exchange.

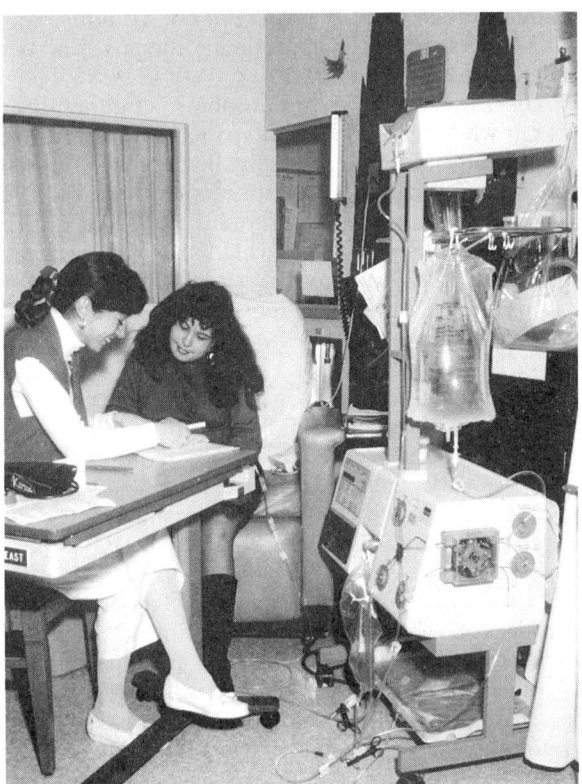

FIGURE 47-9
Adolescent girl in training for home peritoneal dialysis using a cycling machine.

when the machine alarms.[21,47] Both CAPD and CCPD require storage of at least 1 month's supplies in the home. Cost of both methods are similar.

Complications. Although CAPD and CCPD are the optimal form of chronic dialysis for most children, the procedures are not without risk. Possible complications that are related directly to the dialysis procedure include fluid overload, dehydration, abdominal or muscle cramps, and dizziness. These problems can usually be corrected by altering the amount, flow rate, and temperature of the dialysate. Technical complications related to the catheter include obstruction by fibrin or blood, occlusion or obstruction of the catheter by the omentum, or a kink in the catheter.

Peritonitis is the most common complication and results from entry of bacteria during the frequent opening of the dialysis system. The child with peritonitis frequently has abdominal pain, nausea, and vomiting. The dialysate appears cloudy, and the child may have fever. Treatment is usually started at home by flushing the peritoneal cavity with three rapid exchanges of dialysate and, in the last bag, a predetermined antibiotic is injected (usually cephalosporin).[47]

After the family calls the dialysis center, the child and the *first* bag of dialysate that was drained from the peritoneal cavity in the exchange are brought to the hospital. Culture, cell count, and Gram's stain are performed on a sample of this dialysate to determine the causative organism. *Staphylococcus epidermidis* and *Staphylococcus aureus* are commonly found, but *Pseudomonas,* other gram-negative organisms, and fungi also can cause peritonitis.[47] Antibiotics are usually continued for 2 weeks, and during this time the cell count and cultures are repeated to ensure that appropriate therapy has been implemented.

This treatment plan for peritonitis is frequently carried out with the child as an outpatient. However, occasionally, the child is so clinically ill with fever, dehydration, and pain that hospitalization is required for a few days. Frequent episodes of peritonitis can lead to scarring of the peritoneal membrane, which may result in loss of the membrane's ability to dialyze sufficiently. Some infections (especially fungal) require removal of the peritoneal catheter to allow the membrane to heal. Hemodialysis is then required for 4 to 6 weeks.

Localized infection at the exit site of the catheter may also complicate the child's condition. With "tunnel infection," edema, tenderness, and warmth are noted along the subcutaneous catheter route, and purulent drainage may be seen on the old dressing. Culture and sensitivity of the exudate are required, but infections in these sites typically respond well to antibiotic therapy.

"Burnout" for the child and family is another serious complication. These children are chronically ill and frequently wait years for a kidney transplantation. Performing peritoneal dialysis daily with responsibility for assessment, planning, and performing the care can lead to stress and unrelieved fatigue of caregivers. Nurses may be able to help the family to devise a plan for respite care.

Despite the many advantages of peritoneal dialysis, there are situations when hemodialysis remains the treatment of choice. Some families are unable to assume the

responsibility for daily treatments because of crisis within the family, living arrangements (e.g., not enough room for supplies and the machine or unable to maintain asepsis), as well as medical or psychosocial concerns.

Hemodialysis

Hemodialysis is a procedure that uses an "artificial kidney" (dialyzer) when the child's own kidneys can no longer function effectively. After access to the child's vascular system is established, blood flows from the access, through a dialyzer, and by the process of diffusion, osmosis, and filtration, fluid and metabolic waste products are removed. The "clean" blood returns to the child's circulation through the vascular access. This procedure is usually performed three times a week for periods of 3 to 5 hours for each treatment. Most children receive hemodialysis treatments in pediatric dialysis units. Some families, if highly motivated, may perform this treatment at home after completing a specialized training program.

Types of Vascular Access. Two basic types of vascular access are used for hemodialysis: external devices and internal fistulas (Figs. 47-10 and 47-11). *External devices* are typically used for the acute or unplanned event and include the subclavian catheter, the femoral catheter, and the Scribner shunt. These devices are generally placed while the child is under anesthesia in the operating room, and as soon as the child is recovered, the access may be used for the dialysis procedure.

The most common external device is the subclavian catheter (see Fig. 47-10A). When placed, the catheter is tunneled under the skin into the superior vena cava. It is threaded into the right atrium of the heart to ensure adequate blood flow to perform the dialysis procedure. The catheter may exit anywhere on the chest wall, but it is typically positioned near the clavicle (see Fig. 47-10B). Placement of the femoral catheter is less difficult, and if the child is too unstable to go to the operating room, the procedure may be performed at the bedside.

There are many sizes and styles of catheters used for hemodialysis; preference is given to the largest size catheter that the child's blood vessels can accommodate. A single-lumen catheter is typically used in small children or infants. However, a large, double-lumen catheter can be used in most children and is preferred to achieve optimal blood flow through the dialysis system.

Insertion of a Scribner shunt requires a surgical procedure that is usually performed in the operating room. In this procedure, two cannulas are inserted, one into an artery, and one into a vein (see Fig. 47-11C). The Silastic tubing is tunneled under the skin to the surface, and the two pieces of tubing are joined by a straight Teflon connector. Blood is able to circulate from the artery, through the shunt tubing, and return to the vein.

The size of the child and the veins available dictate the location of the Scribner shunt.[41,48] Ideally, the shunt is located in the most distal site possible so that more proximal sites are available in the future if the shunt needs to be moved. Typically, Scribner shunts are located in the forearm, but they occasionally are placed in the legs. The smallness of distal vessels in young children, however, often necessitates the location of Scribner shunts

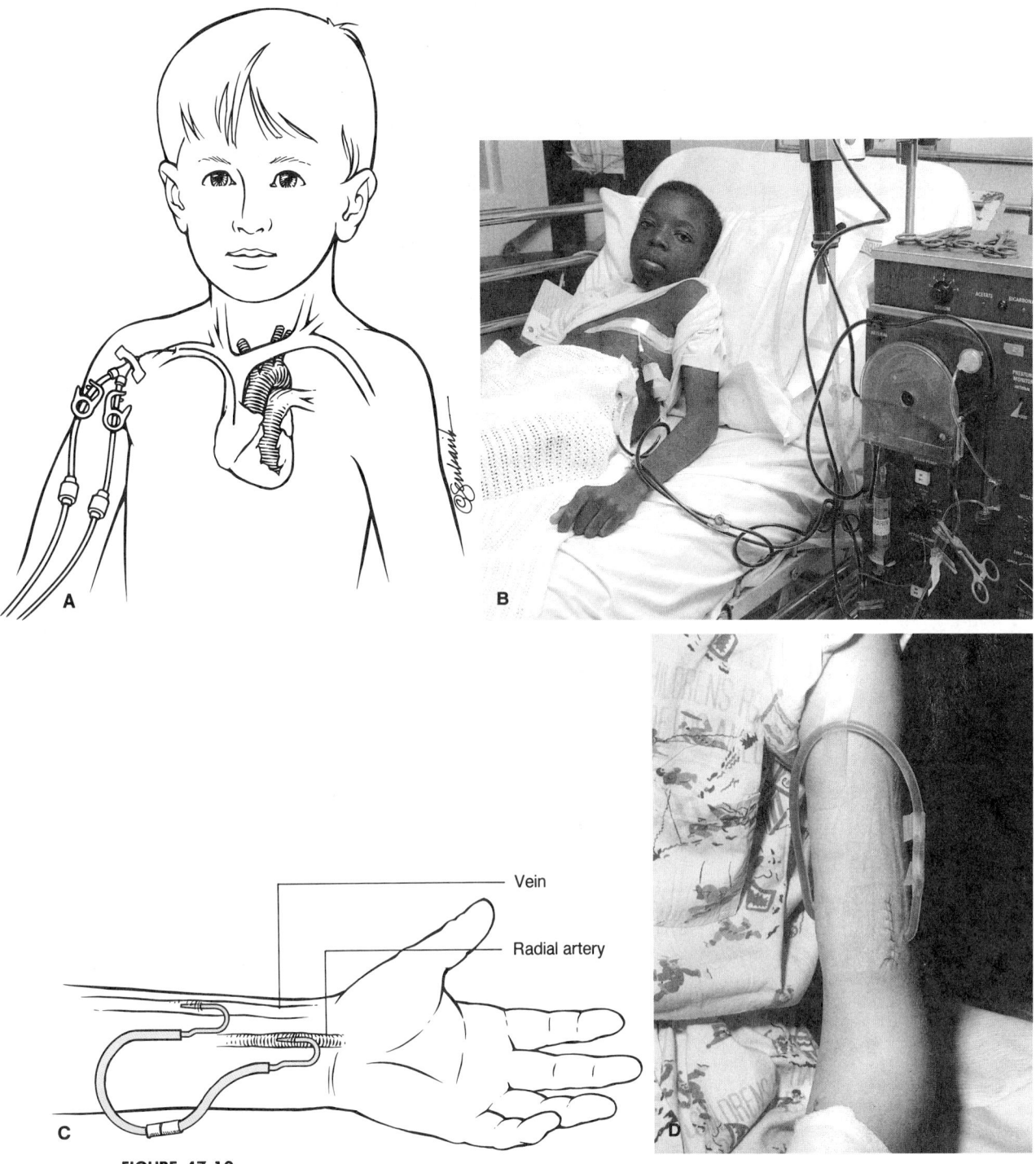

FIGURE 47-10
External devices for vascular access in hemodialysis. (**A & B**) Subclavian catheter. (**A**) Placement of subclavian catheter. (**B**) Adolescent boy undergoing hemodialysis treatment using a subclavian catheter. (**C & D**) Scribner shunt. (**C**) Scribner shunt consists of a Silastic tubing with one tip inserted into an artery and the other tip inserted into a vein. (**D**) Adolescent girl with a Scribner shunt in the upper arm. Ends can be connected while the patient is not on dialysis.

in the upper arm or lower leg, near the ankle (see Fig. 47-10*D*).

The external devices are generally viewed as a short-term solution to the need for vascular access, but they have been used for extended periods of time in many children, up to 2 years or more. This type of access is ideal for small children who find medical treatments traumatic, because the dialysis treatment requires no in-

vasive, painful procedures once the device is in place. Young children in the developmental stage when fears of body mutilation are heightened are good candidates for use of one of these external devices.

Two types of *internal fistulas* may be used to establish vascular access for hemodialysis: the "graft fistula" and the Cimino-Brescia fistula. For long-term hemodialysis, the most common vascular access used in the school-age

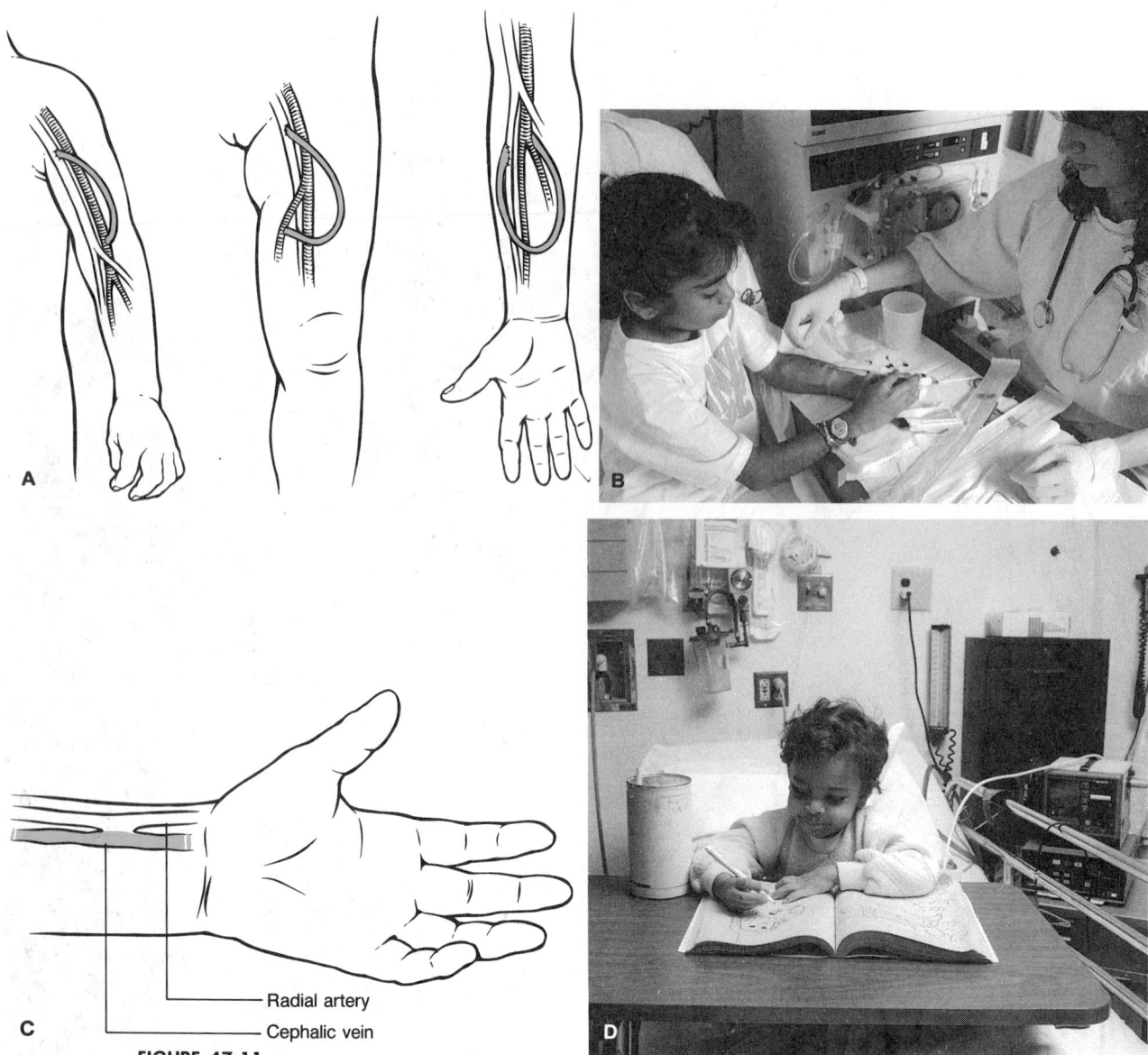

FIGURE 47-11

Internal fistulas for vascular access in hemodialysis. (**A**) Anatomic sites for placement of internal graft fistulas. (**B**) A school-age girl involved in self-care is injecting xylocaine intradermally before the insertion of the dialysis needle into her fistula. (**C**) Creation of an arteriovenous fistula requires the side-by-side anastomosis of an artery and a vein that are readily accessible. (**D**) A young boy plays while he is having hemodialysis.

child and adolescent is the graft fistula, also known as a vascular prosthesis. The fistula is created by tunneling a segment of polytetrafluoroethylene (PTFE), commonly available as Gortex or Impra, under the skin to establish a connection between an artery and a vein of the leg or arm (see Fig. 47-11A). The graft remains under the skin and is accessible only by insertion of a needle through the skin. A local anesthetic is typically injected before the use of the graft fistula for the hemodialysis procedure (see Fig. 47-11B).

After the graft fistula is created, postoperative edema may persist for a few weeks. Although the graft may be used as early as 10 days, there is less potential for complications such as bleeding, infection, and clotting if the graft is allowed to mature and heal completely for 2 to 6 weeks.[41]

The Cimino-Brescia fistula is theoretically the best type of vascular access because it does not require implantation of a foreign body. Creating the fistula requires a simple surgical procedure to create a side-to-side or end-to-side anastomosis of an artery and a vein (see Fig. 47-11C). Larger children, especially adolescent males, are ideal candidates for this type of vascular access because their blood vessels are larger than those found in smaller children. Use of the fistula requires the insertion of either two large (16 to 17 gauge) needles or one needle (usually 14 gauge) with a Y connecter each time hemodialysis is performed.

Like the external devices, the internal fistulas are placed at the most distal site permitted by the age and size of the child. Consideration is also given to the handedness of the child so that placement in the dominant side is avoided. Careful planning of the access site is necessary to permit freedom of movement during the dialysis procedure. Children often play, color, or write while hemodialysis is in progress if the vascular access does not interfere (see Fig. 47-11D).

Preoperative and Postoperative Nursing. Because surgical procedures are required to create all vascular accesses for dialysis, preoperative preparation is mandatory and must be appropriate for the child's level of growth and development. Communication between the child's nurse and the operating room staff during the procedure is necessary to keep the family informed of progress. Allowing the family the choice of going up to the operating room preoperatively and also seeing their child postoperatively in the recovery room are options that are offered at many pediatric facilities. Parental presence can help to decrease anxiety caused by separation and fear of the unknown.

Postoperative assessment of vital signs, pain, bleeding, and patency of the access and maintaining asepsis of the site are important nursing functions. Nursing care of the access is vital because it is the child's "lifeline" to dialysis. If a catheter is used, it needs to be assessed carefully for signs of bleeding or infection. Symptoms of infection should be reported immediately to ensure prompt treatment with antibiotics and the prevention of sepsis. Assessment for patency of the catheter is usually done by dialysis nursing staff at the time of treatment; it is flushed with a heparin solution to prevent clotting between treatments.

Assessment of blood flow in the Scribner shunt requires visual assessment of the color of blood flowing through the Silastic tubing. The blood should be a bright red cranberry color. If it appears dark or if the plasma and cells separate, blood flow is inadequate and clotting of the shunt is imminent. The tubing should be warm to touch, and when pinched, the tubing should refill with blood quickly.

The flow of blood through surgically created fistulas is assessed by listening with a stethoscope and hearing the "bruit," the swishing sound of the flow of blood from an artery through the graft. The flow of blood also can be felt by palpating the fistula; this sensation is called a "thrill." Any changes found through the assessment should be reported immediately to the physician to ensure prompt treatment to attempt to save the access and prevent further complications. General precautions regarding care of the child with an access are presented in the accompanying display.

Dialyzer. Once vascular access has been established, a dialyzer or "artificial kidney" must be selected. Factors considered in making the selection of the dialyzer for the individual child include the following:

- Efficiency of chemistry clearance—how well electrolyte balance is restored and toxins removed.
- Ultrafiltration rate—the capacity of the membrane to let fluid move through its pores.
- Blood volume required—the percentage of child's blood needed in the dialyzer at one time during dialysis.

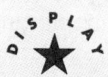

General Precautions for Children With Vascular Access

- The access is the child's "*lifeline*" to the dialysis machine and it must be guarded.
- The access should not be used for routine laboratory tests or medications.
- *Only* personnel experienced in the technical aspects of its use should handle it.
- The access should be protected from injury; external tubing should be secured to body.
- Tight, restrictive clothing should be avoided on extremity with the access.
- Blood pressures and venipunctures are discouraged in the vascular access extremity.
- The signs and symptoms of infections must be reported immediately.
- Patients with external access must *always* carry clamps with them.
- Any break in the dialysis system has the potential for infection.
- Any bleeding at the site of access should be controlled by direct pressure.

- Surface area of the dialyzer—the amount of blood needed to circulate in the machine for efficient functioning.

The hemodialysis procedure requires that the dialyzer and tubing be primed with fluid before the procedure begins. Inflowing blood is treated with small amounts of heparin to prevent formation of clots. The blood and the dialysate are pumped through the dialyzer in opposite directions. Hemodialysis treatments are efficient, and the dialyzer is able to remove adequately the excess fluid and metabolic wastes that have accumulated over 44 to 68 hours in about 4 hours.

Complications. Because hemodialysis is so efficient, it is likely to result in problems related to rapid changes in blood volume and chemistry. Children may experience nausea or vomiting, headaches, muscle cramps, and dizziness or lightheadedness. Occasionally, the acutely ill or uremic child experiences severe symptoms associated with what is called *disequilibrium*. This is a complex group of symptoms that includes changes in blood pressure, headache, mental confusion, restlessness, irritability, twitching, jerking, and sometimes seizures, which, if untreated, can progress to coma and death. Prevention is the best plan and requires starting with a less efficient dialyzer, slower blood flow, and shorter treatment times. Drugs such as mannitol or phenobarbital may be administered to prevent cerebral edema and to raise the central nervous system's threshold for seizures. Other complications associated with the hemodialysis treatment are clotting, hemorrhage, or infection of the vascular access, sepsis, severe hypotension, or severe hypertension.

Over the last 20 years, there have been great technological improvements in hemodialysis equipment;

however, accidents may still occur. There may be technical or human error resulting in air embolism, clotting of the dialyzer, rupture of the dialyzer, hemolysis due to the dialysate being hypotonic or hypertonic, or pyrogenic reactions from contamination of the system. Numerous references and handbooks on the intricacies of hemodialysis are available and should be consulted for more detailed information.

Interventions: Collaborative and Independent

Whether the child is hospitalized or is receiving outpatient dialysis, the nurse is in an ideal position to support the medical plan and provide informed and concerned care. As the primary caregiver, nurses provide ongoing assessment, recognize health problems, and initiate actions to correct them. The general responsibilities of the dialysis nurse are summarized in the accompanying display.

Nurses have an important responsibility to the child and family as the primary patient advocate. The nurse is the key link for the child and family to the health care system and the resource person to triage questions and concerns to appropriate health care members.

Teaching.   Finally, the nurse must assume the role of educator. Listed below are some of the topics to be included in a teaching plan.

- Normal kidney function
- What is kidney disease?

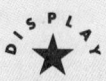

General Nursing Interventions for Children Receiving Dialysis

- Educate the child and family about the dialysis program (i.e., health care team, dialysis unit, and procedures).
- Monitor fluid and electrolyte status by accurate intake and output, weights, vital signs, and recognizing changes in health status.
- Help the child incorporate food preferences into the dietary plan to improve intake and nutrition while maintaining limitations.
- Administer medications as prescribed and monitor for their effectiveness as well as side-effects.
- Infuse blood or blood products as needed for the correction of anemia.
- Use aseptic technique when performing procedures.
- Recognize signs and symptoms of infection, promptly reporting them to the physician and administering antibiotics as ordered.
- Report any concerns of the child and family to appropriate health team members, such as physician, dietitian, social worker.
- Perform prescribed treatments (i.e., dialysis) following hospital procedures and reporting complications.

- How dialysis works
- What is peritoneal dialysis?
- What is hemodialysis?
- Dialysis access care
- Medications
- Participation in dialysis treatment
- Age-appropriate self-care
- Emergency procedures
- Preparation for kidney transplantation

The individualized needs of the child and family dictate the priorities of teaching.

Transplantation

All children who have ESRD and are undergoing dialysis, are usually considered for renal transplantation. Dialysis is generally viewed as an interim mode of therapy for the child until a donor kidney is available. Recently, some dialysis centers have started placing children on the waiting list for renal transplantation before starting dialysis. This trend may be ideal because the child and family ultimately may be spared the trauma and stress of long-term dialysis.

Preparation for kidney transplantation includes determining whether the kidney will be obtained from a living relative or from a cadaver. Of living relatives who are candidates to donate a kidney, an identical twin is the best match, followed by siblings and parents. Compatibility of recipient and donor tissue is determined by laboratory tests performed before transplantation. These tests include ABO blood typing, white cell cross-match, mixed lymphocyte culture (MLC), and HLA typing. (HLA stands for histocompatability-linked antigen and is the primary determinant of rejection of transplanted tissue.)

Kidney transplantations from cadavers are less successful than those from living relatives. Children who are to receive a cadaver kidney are placed on a waiting list. Many families are forced to wait a long time for the transplantation because of the shortage of available and suitable kidneys.

Many ethical questions arise out of this shortage of donor organs. How are decisions made regarding who will be the recipients? What criteria are used in the decision-making process? For a more complete discussion of ethical issues, readers should consult texts on professional ethics.

In addition to determining the histocompatibility of the donor and recipient, many other parameters are assessed before transplantation. These variables include not only the physical condition of the child, but emotional and psychosocial readiness of the child and family. Many kidney transplantation centers use pretransplantation checklists or protocols to ensure that all potential recipients and donors receive consistent and thorough evaluation and preparation.

★   ASSESSMENT

In addition to monitoring the effects of ongoing renal impairment, the child undergoing renal transplantation requires the routine assessments for anyone undergoing surgery. However, critical attention needs to be given to assessing the child for signs and symptoms of infection before surgery. Symptoms including fever, cough, and runny nose must be reported to the physician immediately, even if only subtle signs are noted.

The nurse should also assess the child's and family's knowledge and understanding of the transplantation procedure and treatment protocols. Their level of anxiety and fears related to surgery, rejection, and the child's prognosis should be assessed. How do the child and family feel about receiving a donor organ? If the donor is a family member, how does the donor feel about giving up a kidney and the potential effect its loss has on the donor's health and well-being? How certain is the family that they will be able to comply with a lifelong medication regimen to prevent rejection? Are they fully aware of the side-effects of immunosuppressive drugs, including changes in physical appearance?

After renal transplantation, the nurse must constantly assess the child's fluid and electrolyte balance and the functioning of the transplanted kidney. Observing the child for signs and symptoms of rejection and infection is critical. In addition, the nurse needs to assess the child for general complications after surgery such as atelectases, ileus, and pain.

★ NURSING DIAGNOSES AND PLANNING

Nursing diagnoses for any child experiencing general surgery are applicable to the child undergoing renal transplantation. However, the following nursing diagnoses may also be applicable preoperatively:

- Anxiety (Child and Family) related to surgery and knowledge deficit about the transplantation procedure and treatment plan.
- Fear (Child and Family) related to rejection of the new kidney or of complications that would cause the child to lose the kidney and return to dialysis.
- High Risk for Decisional Conflict related to risk/benefits of dialysis versus transplantation.

Additional postoperative nursing diagnoses may be the following:

- High Risk for Infection related to altered immunity secondary to immunosuppressive medications.
- Altered Nutrition: More Than Body Requirements related to increased appetite and oral intake secondary to steroids.
- Body Image Disturbance related to receiving a donated kidney and the side-effects of steroids and other immunosuppressive agents.
- Anxiety regarding home care and follow-up.
- High Risk for Noncompliance With Medical Therapy at Home related to lifelong need to follow through (i.e., daily doses of immunosuppressive medications and altered physical appearance from side-effects of the medications).

Expected outcomes for children who have undergone renal transplantation may include the following:

- The child is free of infection.
- The child continues to progress through normal stages of growth and development.

- The child engages in age-appropriate behaviors and activities including healthy peer and social relationships.
- The child and family demonstrate understanding of the lifelong treatment regimen.
- The child and family describe healthy coping mechanisms they have developed to manage the ongoing threat of loss of the transplanted kidney.
- The child and family resume activities of daily family living.

Some general nursing care goals for restoring function after transplantation may be the following:

- Maximal functioning of the transplanted kidney is evidenced by adequate urine output, normal serum chemistries.
- Episodes of rejection are minimized and effectively treated so that renal function is restored.
- Side-effects of immunosuppressive therapy are minimized.

★ INTERVENTIONS: COLLABORATIVE AND INDEPENDENT

PREOPERATIVE CARE

Nursing care of the child undergoing renal transplantation includes assisting the child to be in an optimal physiologic and mental state before transplantation. Achieving this goal requires the approach of a multidisciplinary health team. Children receiving a kidney from a living relative are fortunate to have time for preparation at a reasonable pace. A child receiving a cadaver may be called at any time, day or night.

Potential sources of infection, such as dental caries or chronic sinusitis, should be treated before transplantation.[32] Preoperative nursing care involves ensuring that all pretransplantation procedures are completed before surgery. Transplantation centers generally have a protocol with which all team members should be familiar. Close collaboration and communication among all members of the health care team, especially between the dialysis nurse and the child's unit nurse, are essential to ensure that all items on the preoperative transplantation checklist are completed.

Admission procedures should be completed in a timely manner so that the child can be taken to the operating room without delay. Laboratory work includes final cross-matching (which may take a few hours), electrolytes levels, CBC, and coagulation studies. Radiologic procedures, such as chest x-ray, may be ordered.

In addition to standard preoperative checklist procedures, the transplantation recipient needs preoperative doses of prophylactic antibiotics and immunosuppressive agents. The child needs to be dialyzed just before surgery and may receive a blood transfusion.

Initial doses of immunosuppressive agents are given intravenously just before surgery and include drugs such as Solu-Medrol, azathioprine (Imuran), and cyclosporine. Protocols for immunosuppressive therapy vary at different transplantation centers.

The child and family should be informed that the child will be in the intensive care unit after surgery for close observation and monitoring. A tour of the intensive care unit should be presented as an option. Teaching includes what to expect postoperatively, such as the monitoring equipment used in the intensive care unit, the presence of IV and central venous pressure (CVP) lines, the need for Foley catheter, and frequent vital signs.

The child and family should be told that the urine may look bloody at first, that this discoloration is normal and will gradually clear. They should know that the amount of urine produced after the transplantation is different for each recipient and varies depending on how soon the new kidney starts working to full capacity. The nurse in the intensive care unit checks the amount of urine at least every hour and keeps the physician informed.

An explanation of where the kidney will be placed, what the incision will look like, and the type and location of the incisional dressing should be included. The use of a doll, body diagram, and printed materials are helpful to prepare for the surgery. Samples are shown in the accompanying display of educational materials.

Preparation routinely done for any child anticipating surgery is necessary and includes teaching about the need for NPO status before surgery. Anticipatory guidance is given about the gradual progression of diet, pulmonary care, and activity in the postoperative period. The child is reassured that medication will be given for pain and that it will be given through the IV line, not by intramuscular injections.

Although psychological preparation for the transplantation begins as soon as the decision is made in favor of transplantation, support for the child and family to ex-

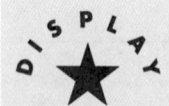

Educational Materials for Children With Renal Disease

Me and My Kidneys (coloring book)
by Carol Hayes and Tamara Stephenson, 1989
St. Joseph's Hospital and Medical Center, Phoenix, AZ
May purchase from:
    Renal Services
    St. Joseph's Hospital and Medical Center
    P. O. Box 2071
    Phoenix, AZ 85001

A Kid and a Kidney
by Pamela W. Graham, MSW, and Paula L. Mandel, BS
illustrated by Paula L. Mandel, BS
May purchase from:
    Paramedical Trust Funds
    Department of Nursing Education
    1755 N. W. 12th Avenue
    Miami, FL 33136

My Kidney Transplant
by Dianne Kegg, RN
For information, write to:
    Indiana University Hospitals
    1100 W. Michigan Street
    Indianapolis, IN 46223

Special Care for Special Needs
by Susan Saver, et al.,
University of Minnesota,
Department of Pediatric Nephrology

Helping Children Cope—Anatomically Correct "Zaadi Dolls"
For information, write to:
    The Zaadi Company
    836 Chelmsford Street
    Lowell, MA 01851

Kelly Kidney Teaching Doll
Designed and created by:
Janice McCormick
Tulane University Medical Center
New Orleans, LA 70112

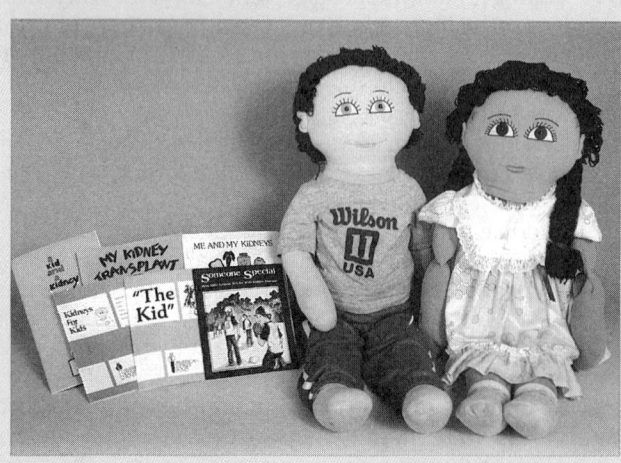

Samples of dolls and printed materials available for teaching the child and family.

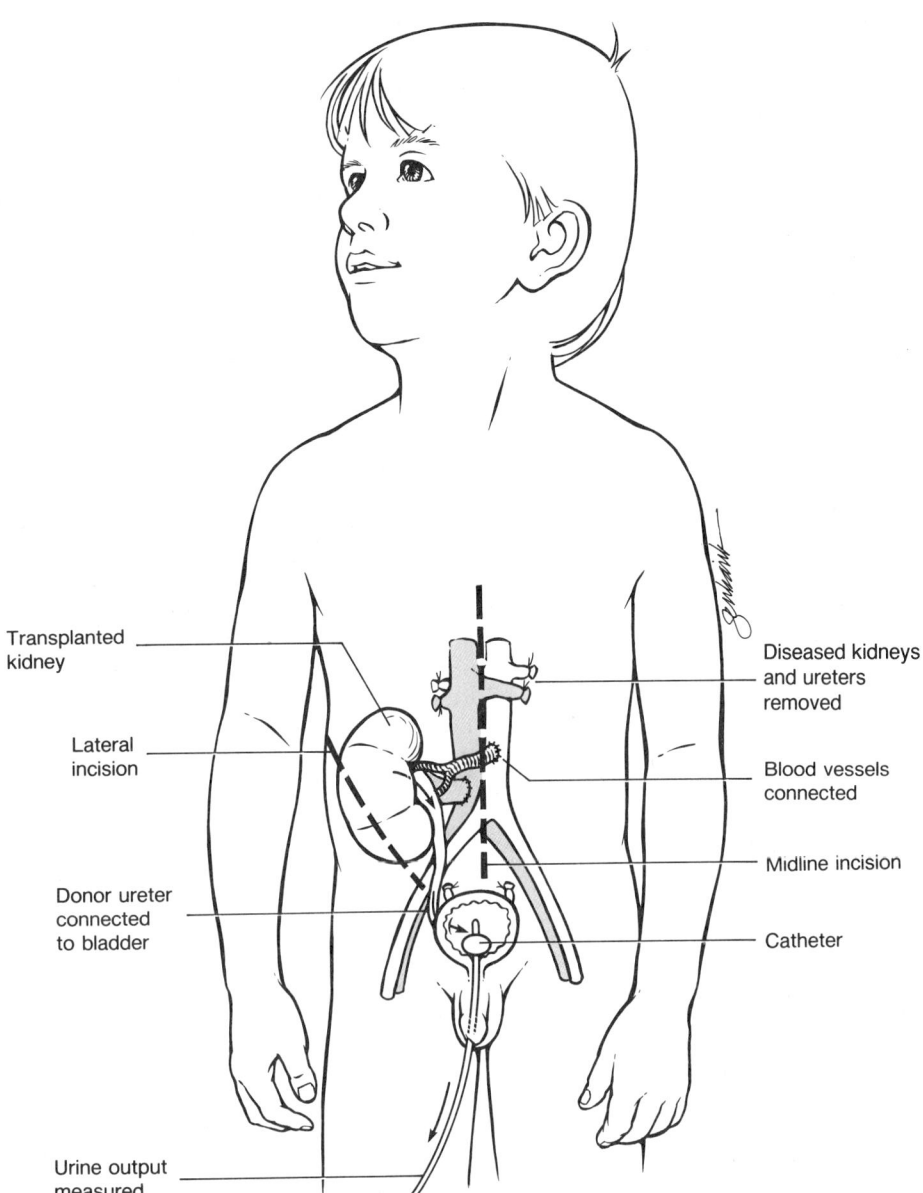

Transplanted kidney

Lateral incision

Donor ureter connected to bladder

Diseased kidneys and ureters removed

Blood vessels connected

Midline incision

Catheter

Urine output measured

FIGURE 47-12

Anatomic representation of a kidney transplant in children. Diseased kidneys have been removed.

press their feelings should be encouraged to continue at the actual time of transplantation. Visits from the social worker before surgery can be helpful to the family. Although this is an exciting and hopeful time, it is not without concern and fear.

OPERATIVE CARE

During renal transplantation, the child receives general anesthesia. The child's own kidneys are generally not removed unless they are an ongoing source of infection or uncontrolled hypertension.[39] Surgical placement of the transplanted kidney into a child is similar to placement in an adult. In the child over 20 kg, the donor renal artery is anastomosed to the common iliac artery of the recipient. The renal vein is anastomosed to the common or external iliac vein.[39] In the child under 20 kg, the kidney is generally transplanted intraabdominally. The donor artery is anastomosed to the recipient aorta, and the donor vein is anastomosed to the recipient vena cava. Small pediatric

kidneys may be placed in the extraperitoneal position.[39] Donor ureters are transplanted into the recipient's bladder (Fig. 47-12).

During the surgical procedure, care is directed at (1) keeping the child warm, (2) maintaining hemostasis, and (3) ensuring cardiovascular stability and acid–base balance. It is essential that an adequate circulating fluid volume be maintained. Before revascularization of the kidney, Lasix and mannitol may be given to promote diuresis and stimulate the flow of urine.[39] Before surgical closure, the open wound is irrigated with an antibacterial solution to prevent sepsis.

POSTOPERATIVE CARE

Children who receive renal transplantations are generally admitted to the intensive care unit after surgery. The care of the child includes fluid and electrolyte management and close observation for the functioning of the transplanted kidney. The functional status of the kidney varies among individuals after transplantation. There may be immediate function with a return to normal BUN and serum creatinine levels within several hours or days after surgery. Other children experience anuria, oliguria, or massive diuresis. In some children, the kidney permanently fails due to technical complications or rejection.[32]

During the immediate postoperative period, medical therapy includes supporting the child to maintain fluid and electrolyte balance so that there is an adequate cardiac output to perfuse the kidney. The goal of fluid management is to maintain optimal hydration.[39] Maintenance fluids are given, and urine volume is replaced hourly cc/cc with dextrose/saline solutions.[38] If the child is anuric and experiencing volume overload, fluids are restricted.[39] Serum electrolytes are closely monitored.

Urine output is measured every hour, and the physician should be notified promptly if the urine output decreases below parameters set for the child, or if the urine output drops 50% from the previous hour. It is critical that the flow of urine not be impeded by blood clots; the patency of the Foley catheter must be maintained through irrigation if necessary.

Postoperatively, the child needs close attention regarding pain management. These children require IV morphine postoperatively, and it should be given as frequently as necessary to keep the child comfortable. Parents usually assist the nurse in assessing the child's pain.

Postoperative nursing care includes psychosocial support given to the transplantation donor as well as the recipient. How does the donor feel about having lost a kidney? Many times recipient and donor would like to be united as soon as possible after surgery because they are close relatives. Concern for each other's well-being is often strong. The nurse should be receptive to these needs and should support communication efforts.

MONITORING FOR COMPLICATIONS

Postoperative complications of renal transplantation include the appearance of acute tubular necrosis (ATN), infection, rejection, cardiac arrhythmias secondary to electrolyte imbalances, bleeding, hyperglycemia, technical complications that obstruct the flow of urine, and pulmonary complications secondary to general anesthesia and surgery.

A primary goal of treatment is to suppress the child's immune response to the transplanted kidney. Rejection episodes can occur at various times after transplantation, and they are classified as hyperacute, acute, or chronic.

Hyperacute rejection occurs on the operating room table or within hours of the transplantation. This immediate rejection is a humoral immune response and occurs when the transplantation recipient possesses preformed antibodies to antigens in the donor kidney. Hyperacute rejection rarely occurs because of the advances in cross-matching techniques.[31]

Acute rejection is seen frequently in the postoperative period and up until the end of the first year. Symptoms of acute rejection include a decreased urine output, fever, swelling, and tenderness over the transplanted kidney, weight gain and edema, malaise, hypertension, and rising BUN and creatinine levels. Acute rejection episodes are treated with high doses of IV Solu-Medrol over a 3-day

period. Approximately 80% of rejection episodes can be reversed by increased doses of prednisone or Solu-Medrol.[31]

Chronic rejection occurs several months to several years after transplantation. There is a progressive loss of renal function. Chronic rejection may be asymptomatic and insidious, eventually leading to loss of the transplanted kidney and a return to dialysis.[8]

Protocols for immunosuppressive therapy vary among transplantation centers. Prednisone is used in combination with azathioprine (Imuran) or cyclosporine A. Cyclosporine, approved for use in 1983, has replaced Imuran as the drug of choice in many transplantation centers. Cyclosporine selectively inhibits cell lymphocyte activity, while being minimally toxic to other hematopoietic cells.[31] In other words, cyclosporine prevents tissue rejection, but leaves the transplantation recipient enough immunity to fight infection.[16]

Unfortunately, a major side-effect of cyclosporine is nephrotoxicity. Concern about the potential of early acute nephrotoxicity has led to changes in immunosuppressive treatment protocols, which may delay initiating cyclosporine until several days after transplantation, or until serum creatinine decreases to a specific level.[38] The nurse must ensure that serum trough levels of cyclosporine are drawn at the appropriate time (i.e., 30 minutes before administration) and that, if the level is within an acceptable range, the drug is given on time. Trough levels of 175 to 250 are acceptable for the first 90 days posttransplantation.[38] Prednisone is often tapered after surgery to decrease side-effects. Before administrating Imuran, the nurse must always check the white blood cell count. If the WBC is less than 4000, the dose may need to be withheld.[9]

Other immunosuppressive agents are also used in the treatment of acute rejection episodes. These include antilymphocyte preparations such as ATG, and more recently, Orthoclone OKT3. OKT3 is a monoclonal antibody highly specific, affecting only T lymphocytes, which are the primary cells involved in acute rejection.[19] Children being treated with IV infusions of OKT3 require close monitoring and observation. Adverse reactions include anaphylaxis, fever, chills, dyspnea, wheezing, and general flulike symptoms. Adverse reactions are minimized with pretreatment medications such as Solu-Cortef, acetaminophen, and Benadryl. Symptoms may also subside with subsequent doses of OKT3.[8,20]

Regardless of the immunosuppressive agent prescribed, the nurse must ensure that the child receives all doses of medication ordered. Double checking the physician's order sheet against the child's medication record is recommended before giving the next dose of medication. It is essential that the nurse clarify any discrepancies or questions before administering the drug. Accuracy of the measured dose should be checked by another nurse before it is given to the child.

Infection is a major cause of death after renal transplantation. In addition to common bacterial and viral infections, these immunosuppressed children are at increased risk for life-threatening infections caused by viruses (*Varicella* and cytomegalovirus), fungi (*Cryptococcus* and *Aspergillus*), and parasites (*Pneumocystis carinii*).[14]

Monitoring for development of infection includes frequent checks of the surgical incision. Infection control measures such as scrupulous handwashing and strict aseptic technique during procedures need continued reinforcement. Preventing postsurgical pneumonia through aggressive pulmonary care and encouraging ambulation is especially important in these children.

Children with renal transplantations should be assessed for signs and symptoms of *ARF* and ATN. Nursing assessment and interventions discussed in the section in this chapter on ARF would apply to children undergoing transplantation as well.

The child's condition usually stabilizes a few days after surgery, and transfer to the general pediatric unit is possible. Monitoring for complications continues to be a crucial role of the nurse.

DISCHARGE PLANNING

The long-term success of a kidney transplantation largely depends on the child's and family's willingness and ability to perform the self-care activities necessary to minimize the risks of rejection and infection.[9] Each child and family should receive a structured teaching plan. Most renal transplantation centers use a transplantation coordinator to ensure that all teaching is completed before discharge. A nephrology clinical nurse specialist is often designated to fulfill this role.

In addition to formalized teaching sessions with the family, the clinical nurse specialist coordinates the teaching done by other health team members such as the primary nurse and dietitian. Although all children and families receive standardized home care instructions, teaching must allow for individualized needs as well. Factors to consider include how well the child is doing after the transplantation, culture and language, previous transplantations, and the ability of the child and family to learn what they absolutely need to know before going home. The clinical nurse specialist and primary nurse must communicate regularly to ensure that the child and family's individualized needs are being incorporated into the discharge plan.

Nurses play a critical role in preparing the child and family for discharge. Failure of the family to comply with the prescribed medical regimen can lead to serious, life-threatening complications and loss of the kidney. Side-effects from immunosuppressive medication that cause visible physical changes may be reason enough for the child to stop taking the medications. This is especially true for older school-age children and adolescents. Essential discharge teaching strategies include verbal and written instructions of the critical components of home care needs. Teaching should be in the family's native language whenever possible. Additional teaching materials include videotapes, booklets, and pamphlets for renal transplantation recipients. Critical components of discharge teaching include:

MEDICATION

The family is taught about the administration of immunosuppressive agents such as prednisone and cyclosporine. Ample opportunities should be provided for the child and family to practice administration of these drugs so that they are comfortable before discharge. Cyclosporine administration includes the need to take the medication in a glass cup with milk, chocolate milk, or orange juice. Side-effects of these immunosuppressive agents should also be discussed. The importance of taking these medications each day cannot be overemphasized with the family. The physician should be notified immediately if the child is unable to take prescribed doses of immunosuppressive agents for any reason.

DIET THERAPY

The renal dietitian primarily instructs the child and family on the prescribed diet that they need to follow at home. A nutritious diet that is low in calories is needed to prevent weight gain from steroid therapy. Sodium restriction is often prescribed to control weight gain caused by fluid retention. The prescribed diet is individualized and depends on the degree of functioning of the new kidney. In any case, the dietitian and nurse must work with the child and family to make sure that the prescribed diet is palatable and incorporated into the family's usual dietary patterns, with regard to cultural preferences whenever possible. In contrast to the diet and fluid restrictions that are necessary for management of ESRD, the prescribed diet after renal transplantation is often much more liberal and a welcome change to the child and family.

ACTIVITY PROMOTION

After renal transplantation, children are encouraged to get adequate exercise. Activity is needed to help control weight gain from steroids, but it also allows the child to engage in age-appropriate activities that are so important to psychosocial well-being. Contact sports such as football are restricted to avoid injury to the transplanted kidney.

INFECTION CONTROL TECHNIQUES

Infection is a major cause of morbidity and mortality in transplantation recipients. The child and family should be taught measures they can take to decrease the risk of developing an infection. These include good handwashing, personal hygiene, and limiting exposure to infectious illness by avoiding ill children and large crowds. Suspected exposure to contagious diseases such as chickenpox should be reported to the physician immediately.

WHEN TO NOTIFY THE PHYSICIAN

The child and family should be encouraged to call the physician or other members of the transplantation team whenever questions or concerns arise. Problems may be of either a physical or a psychological nature. In addition, the child and family should be aware that they must notify the physician of any signs and symptoms of infection, rejection, or side-effects of immunosuppressive agents, because these circumstances may lead to life-threatening illness or loss of the transplanted kidney. Signs of "kidney trouble" include: fever; urine output less than usual; pain and tenderness over the transplanted kidney; aches and pains in arms and legs; swelling or puffiness around face, hands, or ankles; inability to take prescribed immunosuppressive; general symptoms of a cold or the "flu"; exposure to infectious illness.[7] The family must be provided with a list of phone numbers readily available that they can call any time, day or night. The importance of not waiting too long to call for assistance must be continually reinforced with the family. Time can make a difference in preventing serious complications and saving the transplanted kidney.

OUTPATIENT FOLLOW-UP

The family should be introduced to the outpatient nephrology staff before discharge. The importance of follow-up visits is emphasized with the child and family. Clinic visits are essential to monitor kidney functioning, toxicity, and side-effects of immunosuppressive drugs, and to obtain general psychosocial support for the child and family. Children undergoing renal transplantations require the ongoing physical, psychosocial, and financial assistance that can be provided by caregivers in renal transplantation centers. They have the resources and expertise available to support the child and family. National organizations such as the Kidney Foundation provide support to these families as well. A list of these resources is given in the accompanying display.

★ EVALUATION

The nurse and family evaluate the outcomes of care given. Examples of outcome criteria for transplantation were given under Planning in this section.

COMPLICATIONS

Common complications experienced by the child who has received a kidney transplantation have been discussed above. In the long-term, other possible complications may include hepatic dysfunction, hypertension, growth retardation, steroid-induced diabetes, cataracts, bone demineralization, aseptic necrosis, recurrent kidney disease,

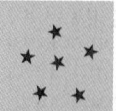

Ideas for Nursing Research

The complex nature of renal dysfunction ensures a never-ending quest for knowledge that will improve nursing care for these children. Some questions that may be investigated include:

- What is the relationship of selected teaching variables such as timing of information, the number of educators, and type of patient education materials to compliance?
- What are factors that identify the child as "high-risk" for ineffective coping with chronic renal disease?
- What factors are related to coping with the ongoing fear of rejection after transplantation?
- Does the number of previous rejection episodes, previous transplants, and time after transplantation affect coping?
- Of the following factors, which one contributes to the most absences from school in the child with chronic renal disease?
  1. Outpatient treatment schedules
  2. Complications of the illness resulting in readmissions to the hospital
  3. Lack of support at school
  4. Disturbances in body image and self-esteem

atherosclerotic heart disease, malignancies, and chronic allograft rejection.[20,40]

LONG-TERM CARE

Initially, even children that are doing well after the transplantation need to come back to clinic several times a week. It may be difficult for the child and family to come back for all scheduled visits to the clinic. The family may have to travel long distances at inconvenient times. The health care team must be sensitive to the family's needs and provide support or assistance with transportation and flexible appointment scheduling whenever possible.

Summary

Children with alterations in renal function present many challenges to the pediatric nurse due to the acute and chronic nature of this complex body system. Many children present with life-threatening acute illness but recover and resume a normal life with normal renal function having been restored. Other children progress through the stages of CRF to ESRD. These children encounter many of the stressors of other chronic conditions.

There are many frustrations for the child, family, and health care team. Emotional reactions of the child and family are predictable, and the nurse who understands the responses and anticipates them is better prepared to provide assistance. Renal disease is often unpredictable, requiring frequent changes in the treatment plan. To be able to maintain a delicate balance between "ideal" health

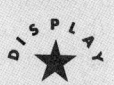

Resources for Children and Families

American Kidney Fund
7315 Wisconsin Avenue, 203E
Bethesda, MD 20014

National Kidney Patients Association
1024 Cottman Avenue, Suite 3
Philadelphia, PA 19111

National Kidney Foundation
2 Park Avenue
New York, NY 10006
(investigate local branches of this foundation)

Magazine "For Patients Only"
20335 Ventura Blvd., Suite 400
Woodland Hills, CA 91364

American Association of Kidney Patients
1 Davis Boulevard
Suite LL-1
Tampa, FL 33606

care and ensuring quality of life is a constant struggle. Awareness of and sensitivity to the family's culture, values, and beliefs give the health care team insight into their acceptance of the treatment plan.

There are many rewards in providing care to these children and their families. These include developing ongoing relationships with families, supporting the family through times of despair, and seeing the family once again take control over their lives through knowledge and support given by the health care team. Perhaps the ultimate reward is sharing in the joy of a new kidney and knowing that it affords the child and family an opportunity for a restoration of health and a return to a near normal life.

References

1. Avery, M., et al. (1989). Nephrology. In M. Avery & L. First (Eds.), *Pediatric medicine.* Baltimore: Williams & Wilkins.
2. Balow, J., & Austin, H. (1989). Renal involvement in multisystem disease and heredofamilial diseases, Part 1. Lupus nephritis. In S. Massry & R. Glassock (Eds.), *Textbook of nephrology* (2nd ed.). Baltimore: Williams & Wilkins.
3. Behrman, R., Vaughan, V., & Nelson, W. (Eds.). (1992). The urinary system. In *Nelson textbook of pediatrics.* Philadelphia: Saunders.
4. Boineau, F., & Lewy, J. (1989). Glomerular diseases, Part 3A, Poststreptococcal glomerulonephritis. In S. Massry & R. Glassock (Eds.), *Textbook of nephrology* (2nd ed.). Baltimore: Williams & Wilkins.
5. Bressler, R. (1987). The child undergoing renal transplantation. In C. S. Greenberg (Ed.), *Nursing care planning guides for children.* Baltimore: Williams & Wilkins.
6. Bressler, R. (1987). The child with nephrotic syndrome. In C. S. Greenberg (Ed.), *Nursing care planning guides for children.* Baltimore: Williams & Wilkins.
7. Bressler, R. (1989). *Home care instructions for kidney transplant patients.* Unpublished paper, Division of Nephrology, Children's Hospital Los Angeles.
8. Bressler, R. (1989). *OKT3 infusion instructions for nurses.* Unpublished paper, Division of Nephrology, Children's Hospital Los Angeles.
9. Bressler, R. (1989). *Renal transplantation.* Unpublished paper, Division of Nephrology, Children's Hospital Los Angeles.
10. Brown, R. O. (1988). Nutritional support in acute renal failure. *American Association of Nephrology Nurses and Technicians Journal* (1983) 25–29.
11. Cameron, J. (1989). Renal involvement in multisystem disease and heredofamilial disease, Part 5: Henoch-Schönlein purpura nephritis. In S. Massry & R. Glassock (Eds.), *Textbook of nephrology* (2nd ed.). Baltimore: Williams & Wilkins.
12. Carbone, V., & Bonato, J. (1985). Nursing implications in the care of the chronic hemodialysis patient in the critical care setting. *Heart & Lung, 14*(6), 570–578.
13. Chesney, R., & Novello, A. (1989). Defects of renal tubular transport. In S. Massry & R. Glassock (Eds.), *Textbook of nephrology* (2nd ed.). Baltimore: Williams & Wilkins.
14. Chmielewski, C. (1987). Early recognition of infection after renal transplantation. *American Nephrology Nurses' Association Journal, 14*(6), 389–391.
15. Coleman E (1986). When the kidneys fail, *RN 49,* 28–34.
16. Cook, C. V., & Harwood, C. H. (1985). Cyclosporine in transplantation. *Heart and Lung, 14*(6), 529–540.
17. DeFronzo, R. A., & O Thier, S. (1986). Inherited disorders of renal tubule function. In B. Brenner & F. Rictor (Eds.), *The kidney.* Philadelphia: Saunders.
18. Diamond, R. P. (1986). Psychosocial care of the child with ESRD.

In A. Nissenson & R. Fine (Eds.), *Dialysis therapy.* Philadelphia: Hanley & Belfus.
19. Eknoyan, G., & Riggs, S. (1989). Renal involvement in multisystem diseases and heredofamilial diseases, Part 9: Thrombotic thrombocytopenic purpura and hemolytic uremic syndrome. In S. Massry & R. Glassock (Eds.), *Textbook of nephrology* (2nd ed.). Baltimore: Williams & Wilkins.
20. Farrel, M. (1987). Orthoclone OKT3: A treatment for acute renal allograft rejection. *American Nephrology Nurses' Association Journal, 14*(6), pp. 373–376.
21. Fine, R., Salusky, I., & Ettenger, R. (1987). The therapeutic approach to the infant child and adolescent with end-stage renal disease. *Pediatric Clinics of North America, 34*(3), 789–801.
22. Gabriel, R. (1980). *A patient's guide to dialysis and transplantation.* Boston: MTP Press.
23. Gaudio, K. M., & Siegel, N. J. (1987). Pathogenesis and treatment of acute renal failure. *Pediatric Clinics of North America, 34*(3), 771–787.
24. Glassock, R. (1989). Glomerular diseases, Part 1: Syndromes of glomerular diseases. In S. Massry & R. Glassock (Eds.), *Textbook of nephrology* (2nd ed.). Baltimore: Williams & Wilkins.
25. Glassock, R. (1989). Renal involvement in multisystem diseases and heredofamilial diseases, Part 6: Goodpasture's syndrome. In S. Massry & R. Glassock (Eds.), *Textbook of nephrology* (2nd ed.). Baltimore: Williams & Wilkins.
26. Gradus, D., & Ettenger, R. (1982). Renal transplantation in children. *Pediatric Clinics of North America, 29*(4), 1013–1038.
27. Grupe, W. E. (1986). Management of primary nephrotic syndrome. In R. J. Postlewiate (Ed.), *Clinical paediatric nephrology.* Bristol, England: Wright.
28. Johnson, R. S. (1984). The role of the social worker in the management of the child with ESRD. In R. Fine, & A. Grushkin (Eds.), *End-stage renal disease in children.* Philadelphia: Saunders.
29. Kher, K., Sweet, M., & Makker, S. P. (1988). Nephrotic syndrome in children. *Current Problems in Pediatrics, 18*(4), 197–251.
30. Klingenstein, J. A. (1986). Successful rehabilitation of the renal client. In C. Richard (Ed.), *Comprehensive nephrology nursing.* Boston: Little, Brown.
31. Kottra-Buck, C. (1986). Renal transplantation. In C. Richard (Ed.), *Comprehensive nephrology nursing.* Boston: Little, Brown.
32. Kottra-Buck, C., & Ruse, L. A. (1986). Complications following renal transplantation. In C. Richard (Ed.), *Comprehensive nephrology nursing.* Boston: Little, Brown.
33. Korsch, B., & Fine, R. (1985). Chronic kidney diseases. In N. Hobbs & J. Perrin (Eds.), *Issues in the care of children with chronic illness.* San Francisco: Jossey Bass.
34. Lancaster, L. (1982). Renal failure: Pathological physiology, assessment and intervention. *Critical Care Nurse, 2*(1), 40–54, 59–63.
35. La Valle, S. (1986). Infectious and obstructive diseases of the kidney. In C. Richard (Ed.), *Comprehensive nephrology nursing.* Boston: Little, Brown.
36. Lieberman, E. (1976). *Clinical pediatric nephrology.* Philadelphia: Lippincott.
37. Lieberman, E. (1987). *Idiopathic nephrotic syndrome.* Unpublished paper. Division of Nephrology, Children's Hospital Los Angeles.
38. Lieberman, E. (1988). *Renal transplant protocol.* Unpublished paper. Division of Nephrology, Children's Hospital Los Angeles.
39. Lum, C. T., Wassner, S. J., & Martin, D. E. (1985). Current thinking in transplantation of infants and children. *Pediatric Clinics of North America, 32*(5), 1203–1232.
40. Lux, L. L., & Roper, K. E. (1987). Alteration in child health: Biophysical emphasis [renal function]. In M. J. Smith, T. Goodman, & N. Ramsey (Eds.), *Child and family concepts of nursing practice.* New York: McGraw-Hill.

41. Matsumoto, T., Simonian, S., Kholussy, A. M. (1987). *Manual of vascular access procedures.* Norwalk, CT: Appleton-Lange.

42. Opas, L., & Lieberman, E. (1989). Fluid and electrolyte disorders in infants and children. In S. Massry & R. Glassock (Eds.), *Textbook of nephrology* (2nd ed.). Baltimore: Williams & Wilkins.

43. Postlewaite, R. J. (1986). Renal tubular disorders. In R. J. Postlewaite (Ed.), *Clinical paediatric nephrology,* Bristol, England: Wright.

44. Richard, C. (1986). Acute renal failure. In C. Richard (Ed.), *Comprehensive nephrology nursing.* Boston: Little, Brown.

45. Richard, C. (1986). The kidney and systemic disease: Nephrotic syndrome and renal vascular disorders. In C. Richard (Ed.), *Comprehensive nephrology nursing.* Boston: Little, Brown.

46. Roberts, C. E. (1984). Dietary treatment in early stages of chronic renal failure. *Contemporary Dialysis, 5*(7), 47–53.

47. Sauer, S. N., & Nolander, M. E. (1989). The pediatric renal patient. In B. T. Ulrich (Ed.), *Nephrology nursing: Concepts and strategies.* Norwalk, CT: Appleton & Lange.

48. Sherman, N. J. (1986). Acute and chronic access in pediatric patients. In A. Nissenson & R. Fine (Eds.), *Dialysis therapy.* Philadelphia: Hanley & Belfus.

49. Siegler, R. L. (1988). Management of hemolytic-uremic syndrome. *Journal of Pediatrics, 112*(6), 1014–1020.

50. Strauss, J., Zilleruelo, G., Freundlich, M., & Abitol, C. (1987). Less commonly recognized features of childhood nephrotic syndrome. *Pediatric Clinics of North America, 34*(3), 591–605.

51. Sweet, M., & Travis, L. (1986). Acute nephritic syndrome. In R. J. Postlethwaite (Ed.), *Clinical pediatric nephrology.* Bristol, England: Wright.

52. Weiss, R. (1988). Management of chronic renal failure. *Pediatric Annals, 17*(9), 584–589.

53. Weiss, R., & Spitzer, A. (1983). Renal failure in childhood. *Comprehensive Therapy, 9*(12), 31–40.

Consultants

Jane Dzinovic, BSN, RN, Nurse Manager of Dialysis, Children's Hospital, Los Angeles

Gary Lerner, MD, Medical Director, Hemodialysis Unit, Children's Hospital, Los Angeles

Ellin Lieberman, MD, Head, Division of Nephrology, Children's Hospital, Los Angeles

Debbie Litwin, MN, RN, Clinical Nurse Specialist Nephrology. Transplant Coordinator, Children's Hospital, Los Angeles

Karen Van Wert, MSN, RN, NP, Division of Nephrology, Children's Hospital, Los Angeles

UNIT 12

Nursing Care of Children With Altered Urinary Function

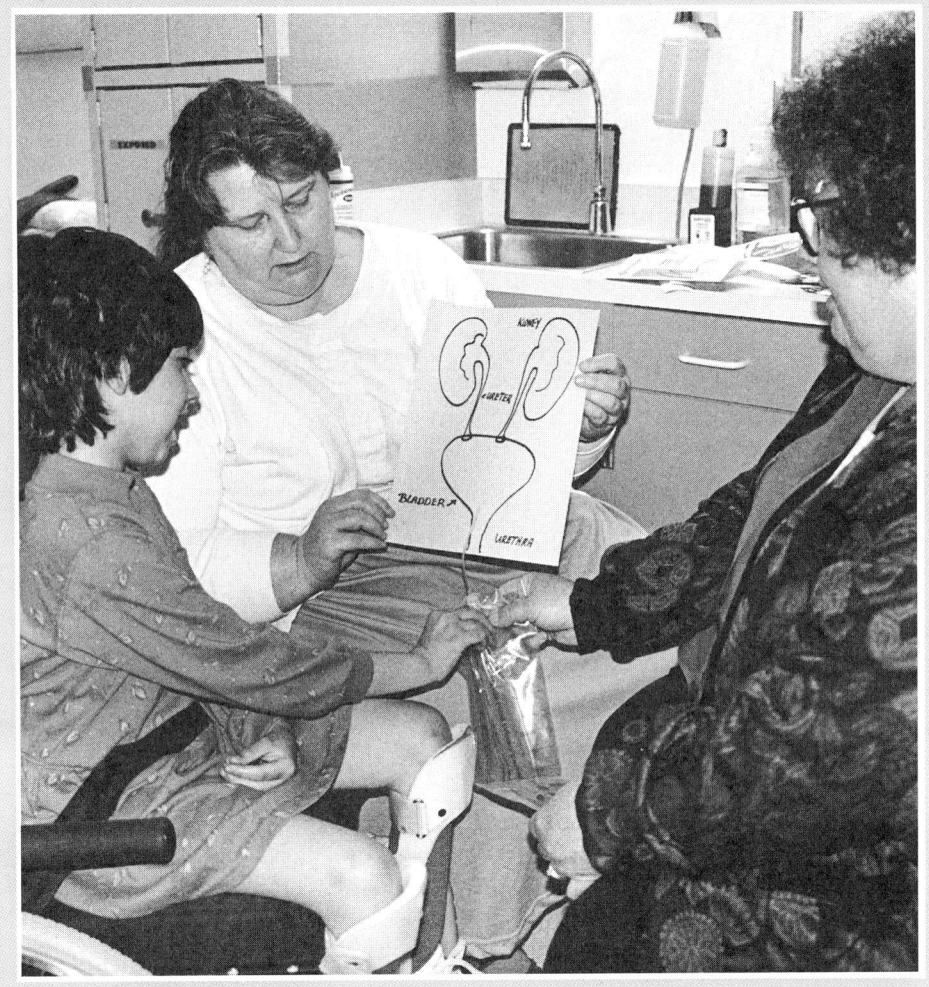

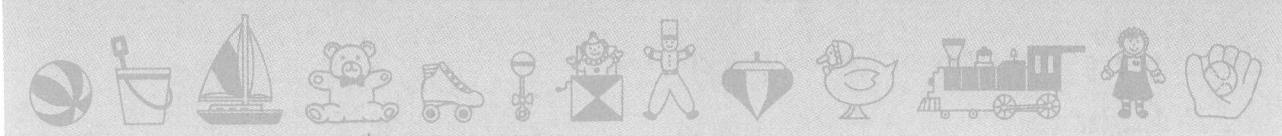

48
C H A P T E R

Anatomy and Physiology of the Urinary System

FEATURE OF THIS CHAPTER

Consequences of Abnormal Embryonic Development, Table 48-1

BEHAVIORAL OBJECTIVES

Describe the embryonic structures that differentiate into the organs of the urinary system.

Identify the components of the ureterovesical unit.

Explain the neural innervation of the detrusor muscle and components of the sphincter mechanism.

Describe the functions of the urethrovesical unit during urination.

List the stages a child progresses through in the attainment of urinary continence.

The anatomy and physiology of the renal system was discussed in Chapter 45. This chapter continues the discussion of urine formation, transportation, and elimination.

The purpose of this chapter is to discuss urinary tract anatomy and physiology, to provide a basis for assessing urinary system function, and to enhance the reader's understanding of the impact of urologic dysfunction on the health and development of the affected infant, child, or adolescent.

Embryonic Development

Kidney and Ureter

Primitive renal function in the growing fetus begins in the second to fourth week of development (see Chap. 45 and Fig. 45-2). Pronephrons arise from intermediate mesoderm during the second week of development and give rise to 6 to 10 tubules found at the ventral borders of the primitive spinal column. These are the wolffian bodies that connect the wolffian duct and cloaca. They function as primordial kidneys until the fourth week of gestation. After the first month, the wolffian bodies cease to function and disappear.[35,40]

As the pronephrons cease to act as primitive kidneys, the mesonephrons assume the tasks of renal function in the developing fetus. The mesonephrons develop around the fourth week of gestation shortly before the pronephrons degenerate, arising from the intermediate mesoderm just caudal to the tissue that gave rise to the wolffian bodies. These structures are more highly developed than the pronephrons and possess a structure analogous to Bowman's capsule. As the mesonephrons grow, they move toward the primary nephric duct as it migrates caudally toward the cloaca to form the mesonephric duct. After connecting with the primary nephric duct, the mesonephric tubules assume an S shape and elongate to enhance their ability to filter blood from adjacent capillaries. The mesonephrons degenerate around the eighth week of life and form a vestigial structure that no longer possesses renal function but contributes to development of male sexual organs.[40]

The metanephrons are the final phase of renal development in the fetus. This nephric system develops from both the intermediate mesoderm and the mesonephric duct. The metanephrons appear as an outgrowth of the mesonephric duct as it moves toward the cloaca. They produce a ureteral bud that grows cephalad as the metanephric cap continues to enlarge. This metanephric cap continues to differentiate while the ureteral buds develop into the renal pelves and collecting ducts. The metanephrons continue to develop into mature nephrons as the kidneys slowly ascend to their normal retroperitoneal position by moving cephalad and rotating to a 90-degree angle from the spinal column.[35]

Bladder and Urethra

As the fetus reaches a size of 4 mm (a 4-week-old embryo), the primitive gut forms a blind sac whose end resembles a tail. An ectodermal depression develops under the root of this tail and sinks in toward the hindgut until only a thin membrane separates the primitive digestive tract and outside body. This depression is called the proctodeum, and the membrane forms part of the cloaca. The cloaca develops into two portions, the posterior urorectal and anterior urogenital sinus. This division occurs because of progressive, caudal extension of the urorectal

fold, which, along with a dense layer of mesenchyme, disrupts the cloacal membrane and replaces it with a dense fibrous sheath separating the primordial rectum from the urogenital sinus. The urogenital sinus develops into the urinary bladder (Fig. 48-1).[35,40]

The urogenital sinus originates as a tubular structure continuous with the allantois. It is further divided into two segments, a superior urinary portion and inferior genital portion formed by fusion of the müllerian ducts and müllerian tubercle at approximately the ninth week of gestation. The superior or urinary portion of the urogenital sinus forms the bladder, the proximal urethra in the male and entire urethra in the female. The distal segment develops into the distal urethra in the male and lower portion of the vagina in the female.[40,41]

The development of the urethra in the male and female is not completely understood. It arises from the urogenital sinus but is profoundly influenced by factors that govern the development of the genitalia. The development of the sexual organs and external genitalia is discussed in Chapter 66.

Consequences of Abnormal Development

Abnormal growth of the embryonic urinary system causes congenital anomalies that are significant to the nursing care of patients with altered urinary function (Table 48-1). Failure of the metanephrons to ascend or rotate; failure of ureteral bud development; abnormal development of the metanephrons, principally affect the production of urine and are discussed in Chapter 50. Abnormal development of the ureteral bud may result in a number of congenital anomalies that exert varying effects on urinary tract function.

Ureterocele is caused by persistence of epithelium at the ureteric bud/mesonephric junction when the fetus is approximately 10 mm in size. Ureterocele causes narrowing of the ureter on the affected side and often causes obstruction of that portion of the kidney it drains. Significant obstruction of the lower ureteral segment may arise from ureterovesicle abnormalities that interfere with

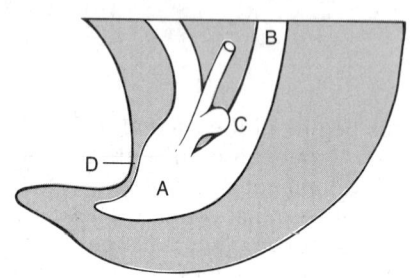
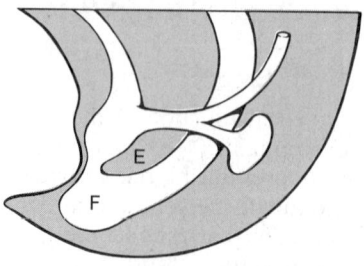
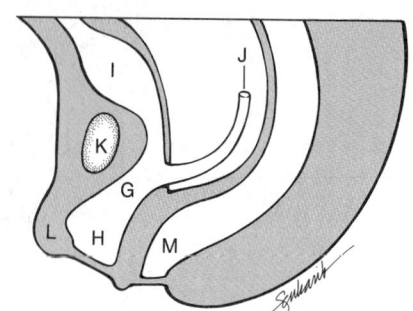

FIGURE 48-1

Embryology of lower urinary tract. *Left,* Structures of lower urinary tract including cloaca and primitive gut at approximately 6 weeks' gestation: cloaca (**A**), midgut (**B**), hindgut (**C**), and cloacal membrane (**D**). *Middle,* Movement of cloaca caudal (toward the tail) and separation of urogenital sinus (**E**) from rectum (**F**); approximately 7 weeks' gestation. *Right,* At approximately 8 weeks' gestation, there is further differentiation of urogenital sinus into pelvic region (**G**), genital region (**H**), and urinary region (**I**) that will mature as urinary bladder. Also shown are wolffian duct (**J**), primitive symphysis pubis (**K**), genital tubercle (**L**), and rectum (**M**).

TABLE 48-1
Consequences of Abnormal Embryonic Development

Fetal Age in Weeks	Structure Formed	Anomalies at Birth
4	Mesenchymal cells migrate between surface ectoderm and urogenital sinus	Exstrophy of the bladder
5–8	Ureteral bud	Ureteral duplication
		Ureterocele
		Megaureter
		Vesicoureteral reflux
6	Division of the cloaca	Rectovesicle, rectourethral, or rectovestibular fistula with imperforate anus
	Descent of the bladder	Urinary fistula
		Urachal cyst
		Urachal diverticulum
	Proximal urethra	Epispadias

alignment of the ureter and trigone or from extrinsic compression. Embryonic abnormalities also may affect the renal pelvis. The most commonly affected area is the ureteropelvic junction (UPJ). Anomalies of the bladder and urethra may profoundly alter urinary transport, storage, and elimination functions. Incomplete knowledge of the embryonic development of the urethra hampers an understanding of certain urethral congenital anomalies. Failure of fusion of various urethral folds may contribute to various states of hypospadias, but the etiology of this defect remains unclear.[40] The embryonic origins of other known congenital anomalies of the urethra such as posterior valves also remain poorly elucidated.[22]

Structure and Function

Kidney

The kidneys are a pair of reddish brown, oval organs that lie on either side of the thoracolumbar spinal column in the retroperitoneal area (see Fig. 45-1). In the neonate, the kidneys have a lobular surface and comprise approximately 1/80 of body weight compared to 1/240 in the adult.[34] An adult woman's kidneys are only slightly smaller than an adult man's. The left kidney is positioned slightly higher than the right because of the liver.[45]

Each kidney is composed of two regions: (1) renal pelvis and calices and (2) renal parenchyma. Urine formed in the renal parenchyma is collected within pyramids that drain into papillae and combine to form a minor calix. Each kidney contains 8 to 18 renal pyramids that drain into 3 to 13 minor calices which, in turn, combine to form 2 to 3 major calices and drain into the renal pelvis for transport to the urinary bladder[45] (see Chap. 45 and Fig. 45-3).

The kidneys are bounded by a dense, fibrous capsule that is loosely adherent to the cortex. Each kidney is supported by perirenal fascia and perinephric fat. They are further surrounded by Gerota's fascia along with the adrenal glands.[45]

The blood supply of the kidneys arises directly from the aorta. One or multiple renal arteries branch off the abdominal aorta at a nearly 90-degree angle and enter each kidney near the hilus. After entering the renal parenchyma, the renal arteries continue to branch off at approximate right angles, causing rapid decrease in blood flow needed for efficient urine formation. The veins that drain the kidneys are approximately parallel to the renal arteries. The renal veins empty directly into the inferior vena cava. In the normal person, the number of renal veins mirror the number of renal arteries. Lymphatic drainage of the kidneys is by way of para-aortic and paravenacaval nodes. The kidneys are under autonomic neural control.[45]

The principal function of the kidneys is the *formation of urine*. A detailed discussion of renal function related to urine formation, regulation of acid–base balance, maintenance of blood pressure, and production of erythropoietin is provided in Chapter 45. A gross description of the urinary transport function of the kidneys is provided to give a greater understanding of the potential for altered renal function associated with abnormalities of urine transport, storage, and elimination.

Renal Pelvis and Ureter

Each renal pelvis and ureter is a continuous muscular tube that arises at the hilum of the kidney and terminates at the bladder. The kidneys, renal pelves, and ureters comprise the upper urinary tracts. The renal pelvis is a cone-shaped structure that receives urine from the major calices for transport to the ureter. The ureter is a long muscular tube that connects the renal pelvis and bladder. It is gently curved but not as tortuous as the small bowel. After narrowing at the ureteropelvic junction, the ureters course over the psoas muscle, past the sacroiliac joints, and terminate in a detubularized segment called the trigone at the bladder base.[44]

The internal diameter of the ureter varies along its length. Three areas of narrowing particularly significant for the child with altered urine transport function due to urinary calculi are the ureteropelvic junction, the area adjacent to the iliac arteries, and the ureterovesical junction[44] (Fig. 48-2).

The microscopic structure of the ureters is composed of three histologic layers. An inner mucosal layer is bounded by a layer of smooth muscle bundles and outer adventitia. The ureteral mucosa consists of transitional cell epithelium similar to that found in the bladder. The muscular layer of the ureteral wall is significant because it causes the peristaltic waves that transport urine from kidney to bladder. The smooth muscle of the ureteral wall is a single layer of helical patterned bundles that branch in multiple directions. It normally contracts in response to mechanical stretch without the need for neural stimulation even though peristalsis can be influenced by neural and hormonal factors.

The neural innervation of the ureters arises from the celiac, mesenteric, and hypogastric plexus, providing the ureters with a rich supply of adrenergic and cholinergic receptors that modulate ureteral peristalsis. The blood supply of the renal pelves and ureters varies among people. Arterial blood enters the ureters by way of an arterial plexus found in the adventitia. The upper ureters and renal pelves typically are supplied by branches of the renal, adrenal, or gonadal arteries. The lower ureters typically receive arterial blood from branches of the common iliacs, obturator or external iliacs. Other lower ureters are supplied by the deferential artery of the male or uterine artery of the female. A venous plexus in the ureteral submucosa drains deoxygenated blood from the ureters. The venous drainage system typically mirrors the arterial supply.[10]

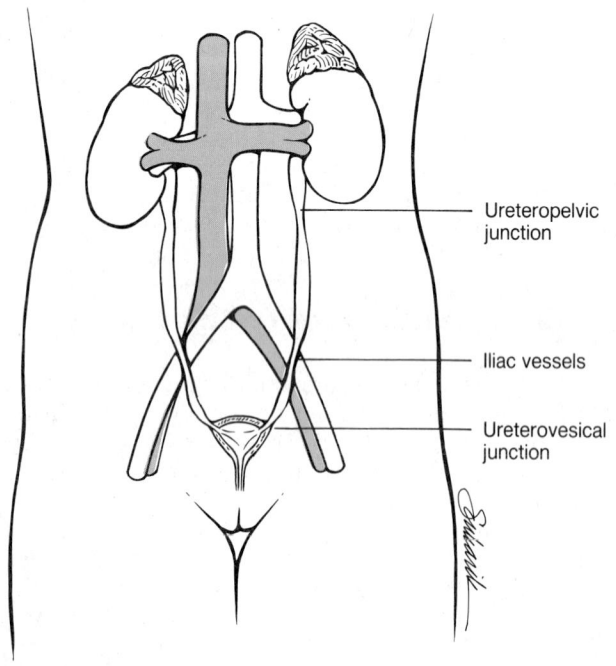

FIGURE 48-2
Ureters. Three areas of narrowing of ureteral course: ureteropelvic junction, the area where the ureter crosses the iliac arteries, and ureterovesical junction.

The lymphatic drainage of the ureters also varies among people. The upper ureters and renal pelves are commonly drained by the para-aortic or renal nodes. Lower ureteral segments are typically drained by common or external iliac nodes.[10]

The principal function of the ureters is the *transportation of urine from kidney to bladder*. The smooth muscle bundles of the ureteral wall are well-suited for this task. Like the smooth muscle of the bowel wall, ureteral smooth muscle contracts in response to mechanical stimuli such as stretch caused by urine entering the renal pelvis. When a sufficient volume of urine collects in the renal pelvis, intrinsic pacemakers located near or in the renal pelvis stimulate a peristaltic wave that pushes a bolus of urine through the ureter and into the bladder. The urine travels only one direction, from kidneys toward the bladder. Flow of urine in the normal direction is termed *efflux*.

A single peristaltic wave empties only a portion of the contents of the renal pelvis but is soon followed by subsequent waves that cause efficient transport of urine from renal collecting system to lower urinary tract.[41] An increase in urine output by the kidneys causes more rapid filling of the renal pelvis and more vigorous peristalsis of the ureters, whereas decreased urinary output results in ureteral peristaltic waves that are less frequent and of less magnitude.

Ureteral peristalsis is further modulated by neural stimulation. Sympathetic stimulation of alpha-adrenergic receptors in the ureteral wall increases peristalsis. In contrast, stimulation of beta-adrenergic receptors in the ureteral wall decreases peristalsis. The influence of parasympathetic stimulation on ureteral peristalsis is not known. Stimulation of the parasympathetic nervous system may increase ureteral peristalsis by activating cholinergic receptors or by releasing catecholamines that indirectly stimulate ureteral smooth muscle bundles.[43,44]

Ureterovesical Unit

The ureterovesical unit or junction is functionally distinct from the ureter or bladder. It is the place where the ureter tunnels through the bladder wall into the trigone (Fig. 48-3). The junction is located near the base of the bladder at the outer aspect of the trigone and consists of three components: a segment of intravesical ureter, trigone, and adjacent bladder wall.

The intravesical ureter tunnels into the bladder wall at its posterolateral aspect for approximately 2.0 to 2.5 cm before terminating at an orifice in the lateral trigone. The intravesical ureter is divided into intramural and submucosal segments. The intramural ureter is approximately 1.5 cm long and surrounded by detrusor muscle bundles. The submucosal ureter lies directly under the bladder mucosa and is approximately 0.8 cm in length.

Ureteral smooth muscle bundles near the ureterovesical unit as well as those of the intravesical ureter are oriented differently than bundles in the upper ureters. These bundles are arranged in a longitudinal rather than helical pattern and continue from ureter to adjacent trigone in the bladder base. This arrangement promotes closure of the intravesical ureter and helps prevent *reflux*

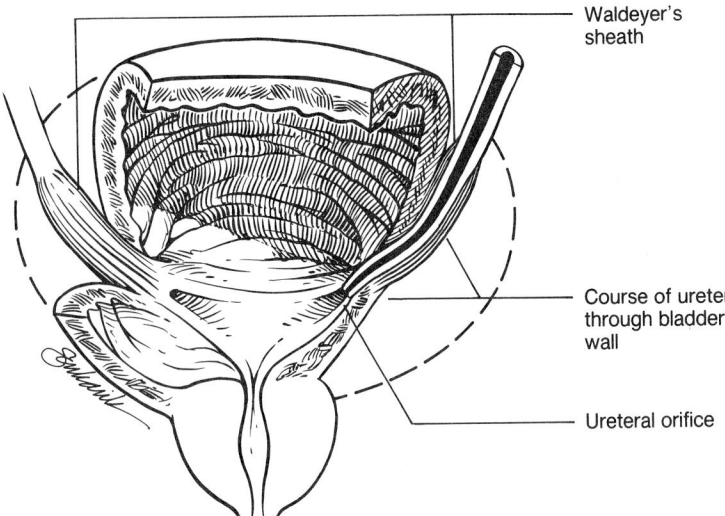

FIGURE 48-3
Ureterovesical junction. (**A**) The course of the ureter through the bladder wall, (**B**) the location of the ureteral orifices, and (**C**) presence of Waldeyer's sheath.

or the backward travel of urine from bladder to upper urinary tract.[41]

The ureteral segments immediately adjacent to the bladder and the intravesical ureter are surrounded by Waldeyer's sheath, a fibromuscular structure that helps anchor upper and lower urinary tracts. Waldeyer's sheath originates from the ureteral wall just above the bladder and surrounds the intramural ureter before fusing with the trigone and fixing the distal ureter to the bladder wall.[41,42]

The trigone muscle also forms a component of the ureterovesical unit. The trigone is a triangular muscle located in the bladder base with its apex extending into the proximal urethra. It is a detubularized extension of the ureter that assists in the prevention of urinary reflux and further anchors the lower and upper urinary tracts. The superficial trigone consists of longitudinally oriented smooth muscle bundles that originate in the intravesical ureter, fan out from the ureteral orifice, and terminate near the external urethral meatus of the female or verumontanum of the male. The deep trigone originates from smooth muscle bundles of Waldeyer's sheath to form a base for the muscle. It terminates at the meatus where urethra meets bladder in a dense fibromuscular structure.

The bladder wall adjacent to the intravesical ureter and trigone is the final component of the ureterovesical unit. As the intravesical ureter and Waldeyer's sheath enter the bladder, they are surrounded by detrusor muscle bundles. This arrangement helps anchor the ureters to the bladder while allowing some flexibility for the ureter to slide in and out of the vesicle wall.[41]

The principal function of the ureterovesical unit is to *allow efflux of urine from kidneys to bladder while preventing reflux of urine from bladder to kidneys.* During bladder filling, the intravesical ureter remains closed between ureteral peristaltic waves due to active and passive factors. The longitudinally arranged smooth muscle bundles, assisted by the trigone, actively promote closure of the intravesical ureter. In addition, a number of passive factors also contribute to closure of the ureterovesical junction, including the oblique angle at which the intravesical ureter enters the bladder wall, the length of the intravesical ureter, the ratio of intramural ureter to sub-

mucosal ureter, and the support of the adjacent bladder wall.[31,39]

As the bladder fills, the ureterovesical junction maintains a relatively low closure pressure. Nonetheless, because of the interaction between ureter and bladder, this flap valve remains closed even during precipitous rises in intravesical pressure so that reflux of urine from bladder to upper urinary tracts is prevented. However, as a bolus of urine travels from the upper ureters due to a peristaltic wave, the relatively low closure pressure maintained during normal vesicle filling is temporarily overwhelmed and urine enters the bladder. As filling progresses, closing pressure rises slightly as the bladder wall becomes progressively distended, and increasingly vigorous contractions are needed to fill the distended bladder.

During voiding, the ureterovesical junction is subjected to a sustained increased pressure (30 to 60 cm H_2O) as the bladder wall contracts. The prevention of reflux during micturition is assisted by active contraction of the trigone and intravesical ureter that begins several seconds before the corresponding detrusor contraction and lasts for a brief period after the bladder is emptied. During this period, no efflux or reflux of urine between ureter and bladder occurs.[14]

Urethrovesical Unit

Like the ureterovesical unit, the urethrovesical unit is defined by way of functional as well as anatomic characteristics. The urethrovesical unit, also known as the lower urinary tract, consists of the bladder, bladder neck, urethra, adjacent pelvic floor muscles, and supportive structures (Figs. 48-4 and 48-5).

Bladder

The bladder is a hollow, muscular organ. During infancy, the bladder is an abdominopelvic organ; its neck lies above the symphysis pubis, and the dome of the filled bladder may be palpated just under the umbilicus. As the child matures, the bladder assumes its place in the true pelvis just before puberty. In the adolescent and adult,

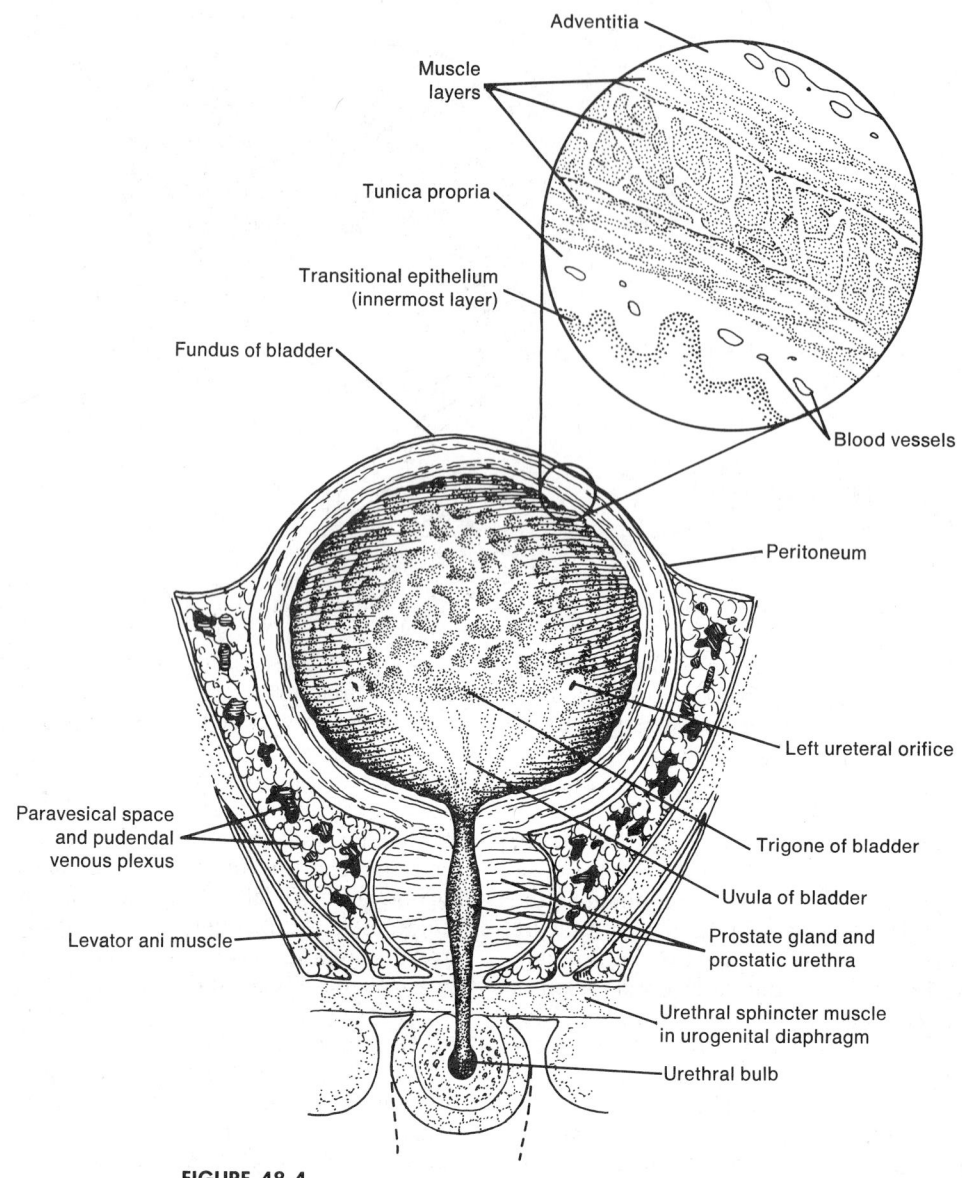

FIGURE 48-4

Cross section of male urinary bladder with microscopic inset of bladder wall.

the empty bladder lies entirely within the pelvis and the bladder neck lies posterior to the symphysis pubis.[11,37]

The size and shape of the bladder vary according to the amount of urine it contains. The empty bladder assumes the shape of a tetrahedron. As it fills, the bladder becomes more spherical and may be observable as a bulge in the lower abdomen when it contains 500 cc or more.[14]

The bladder is characterized by two inlets (the ureteral orifices) and a single outlet. The organ may be divided into three regions: the body of the bladder, often referred to as the detrusor; the base of the bladder that contains the ureteral orifices and trigone; and the bladder neck that marks the origin of the urethra.

The body of the bladder contains an apical surface and superior, right, and left inferolateral aspects. The wall of the bladder body contains four distinct histologic layers. The vesicle of the bladder is lined by a transitional cell epithelium often called the *urothelium*. This cellular lining is four to six cells deep in the empty bladder. As

the bladder fills, the urothelium accommodates increased volumes by smoothing of gross and microscopic folds and by stretching of intracellular structures designed to maximize surface area per milliliter of volume. The urothelium of the bladder is specialized for the needs of urinary storage; it forms a particularly tight physiologic membrane that is impermeable to reabsorption of urine components.[33]

The lamina propria lies adjacent and is loosely adherent to the urothelium. It is found throughout the body of the bladder and contains many elastin fibers that allow it to accommodate vesicle filling as well as blood vessels that provide nutrition for the urothelium and smooth muscle of the bladder wall.[28]

The smooth muscle of the bladder wall is termed the *tunica muscularis or detrusor muscle*. It contains smooth muscle bundles supported by a collagenous framework.[28] The muscle bundles of the detrusor are arranged in a complex meshwork of circular and longitudinally ori-

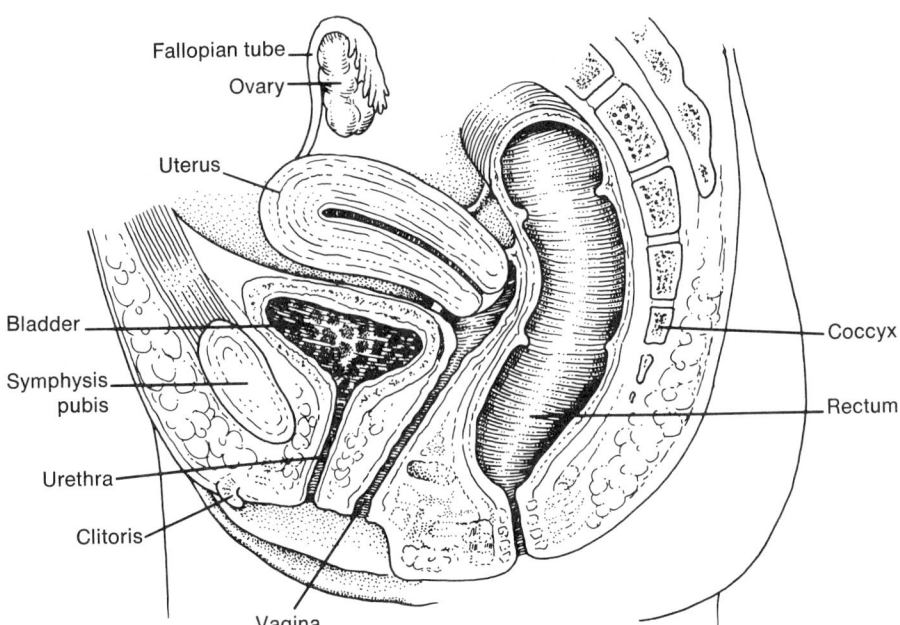

FIGURE 48-5
Cross section of female pelvis.

ented cells; the existence of discreet layers remains un-proven.[13,41] From a physiologic perspective, the variably oriented bundles are best conceptualized as a single muscular unit.[13] The outermost histologic layer of the bladder wall is the adventitia. It is composed of fibroelas-tic tissue and is loosely connected to the peritoneal fascia which help maintain the bladder in its appropriate ana-tomic position.[28]

The base of the bladder is triangular and contains the trigone and ureteral orifices described previously. It lies superior to the seminal vesicles and adjacent to the rectum in the male and adjacent to the anterior vaginal wall in the female.[37]

The bladder neck contains the urethral orifice and is located adjacent to the bladder base. Like the body of the bladder, it contains a urothelium, lamina propria, smooth muscle tunic, and adventitia. Unlike the body of the blad-der, however, the smooth muscle of the vesicle neck is histologically and physiologically distinct.[25] In the male, the bladder neck is characterized by a collar of circular smooth muscle bundles that extend into the proximal urethra to the level of the superior prostatic border.[13] It is often referred to as the internal sphincter, although its importance as an active continence mechanism remains unestablished.[19] In the female, the bladder is character-ized by longitudinally or obliquely arranged smooth muscle bundles that promote bladder neck closure during bladder filling but contributes little to active closure of the urethral sphincter mechanism.[13]

The urinary bladder is under autonomic control, which is modulated by the brain, brainstem, and spinal cord. Parasympathetic innervation of the bladder arises from the pelvic plexus, which originates at sacral spinal roots 2 to 4. Sympathetic innervation is provided by the hypogastric plexus, which arises from spinal segments T10 or T12 to L2.

Arterial blood reaches the bladder by way of the ves-ical arteries, which are branches of the internal iliac, hy-pogastric, obturator, and inferior gluteal arteries. In the female, branches of the uterine and vaginal arteries also reach the bladder. Venous drainage does not typically mirror arterial supply as it does in the kidneys and ureters. Venous blood typically exits the bladder by way of the plexus of Santorini and a paravesicle neurovascular sheath before emptying into the inferior hypogastric vein. The lymphatic channels of the bladder drain from the uro-thelium to vesicle, external iliac, hypogastric, and com-mon iliac nodes.[41]

Urethra

The urethra is a hollow, collapsible tube that serves as a conduit for urinary evacuation and barrier to passive urinary leakage during bladder filling. Because of signif-icant differences in gross anatomy, the male and female urethras are discussed separately.

Male. The male urethra originates at the bladder neck and terminates at the distal portion of the glans penis (see Fig. 48-4). In the adult male, the urethra is approx-imately 23 cm long and is divided into two segments. The proximal urethra is closest to the bladder. The blad-der neck and preprostatic urethra are characterized by a circular band of smooth muscle tissue that forms an in-ternal sphincter. The prostatic urethra tunnels approxi-mately 3 cm through the prostate and terminates at the gland's apex. It lies near the anterior surface of the gland and is characterized by a raised posterior aspect that con-tains the verumontanum and prostatic secretory ducts. The membranous urethra lies immediately distal to the prostatic urethra, is approximately 2 to 2.5 cm long, and forms the least distensible portion of the urethra. The membranous urethra contains specialized slow twitch skeletal muscle fibers that form the rhabdosphincter.

The conduit or distal urethra tunnels through the penis and terminates at the external meatus, is approxi-mately 15 cm in length, and serves as a conduit for the expulsion of urine or semen. The bulbous and pendulous portions of the distal urethra begin at the termination of the membranous segment and tunnel through the corpus spongiosum of the penis to the glands before expanding into the fossa navicularis. The fossa navicularis is a widened area in the urethral course approximately 2.5 cm in length; it terminates at the ellipsoid external meatus.[45]

The microscopic anatomy of the male urethra is marked by three distinct histologic layers. The lumen of the urethra is lined by columnar epithelium near the bladder that changes to a squamous epithelium as it extends to the fossa navicularis. Mucus-secreting glands are scattered throughout the epithelial lining of the male urethra.[28]

Beneath the urethral epithelium is a submucosal layer that contains a rich vascular network and numerous arteriovenous communications. The muscular layer of the male urethra begins at the level of the bladder neck and is most abundant in the membranous segment. Smooth muscle bundles are arranged in a circular orientation at the bladder neck and short preprostatic urethra. Within the membranous urethral segment, an outer layer of smooth muscle bundles are bounded by the slow twitch, C-shaped skeletal muscle fibers of the rhabdosphincter.[13]

The blood supply of the male urethra arises from the urethral artery, which is a branch of the internal pudendal artery. Venous blood is drained by way of the pudendal plexus and deep vein of the penis. Innervation of the urethra is provided by branches of the pudendal nerve, and lymphatic channels are drained by deep subinguinal nodes.[41]

Female. The female urethra is conceptualized as a single functional segment comparable to the proximal urethra in the male (see Fig. 48-5). In the female, the urethra exits the bladder neck at a 16-degree angle relative to the meatus, tunnels anterior and inferior to the symphysis pubis, and terminates just above the vaginal vestibule. It is approximately 3.5 to 5.0 cm in length. The final portion of the female urethra is anatomically fused with the vaginal wall.[13,41]

The microscopic anatomy of the female urethra is characterized by three histologic elements. The epithelial lining of the urethra begins as columnar cells that flatten to squamous epithelium near the meatus. Mucus-secreting glands are particularly abundant in the female urethra. Beneath the epithelium lies a submucosal vascular cushion that contains a complex network of arteries, veins, and arteriovenous communications. The muscular layer of the urethral wall is marked by smooth muscle bundles. In the middle segment of the urethra, an inner layer of slow twitch skeletal muscle fibers are found, which comprise the female rhabdosphincter.[13]

The innervation of the female urethra arises from branches of the internal pudendal nerve. The female urethra receives arterial blood from branches of the vesical arteries. Venous blood is drained by way of the vesical veins and clitoral plexus. Lymphatic channels are drained by way of the inguinal, hypogastric, and obturator nodes.[45]

Pelvic Floor

The pelvic floor is comprised of skeletal muscle fibers, fascia, and ligaments. The pelvic floor contains three principal muscles: the levator ani, coccygeus, and pubococcygeus. Each muscle extends from the pelvic bone to the pubis, symphysis, perineal body, prostate, or rectum. The muscles of the pelvic floor act as a single functional sling that maintains the pelvic viscera in its proper position. They also surround the membranous urethra and contribute to its sphincter mechanism. This muscular unit may be referred to as the pelvic diaphragm.[13]

The pelvic floor also contains the pubourethral ligaments in the female and puboprostatic ligaments in the male, which assist in maintaining the urethrovesical unit in its proper anatomic position. In addition, the perineal body, a fibrous, fat-laden plug that lies between the membranous urethra in the male and the vaginal wall and anorectal junction in the female, contributes to support of the urethra and bladder.[13] Indirect support is supplied by reflections of the endopelvic fascia, which act as "false ligaments."[14]

System Physiology: Function of the Urethrovesical Unit

Micturition

The principal functions of the urethrovesical unit are *storage and evacuation of urine produced by the kidneys.* Gaining voluntary control of urethrovesical function represents a developmental milestone for the child known as *continence.*

Three principal physiologic mechanisms govern the maintenance of continence in the human being. They are a bladder wall capable of both passive filling and active contraction, an intact nervous system that allows voluntary control of the micturition reflex within a complex social and cultural framework, and a competent sphincter mechanism.

Bladder Wall Capability

Normal urinary control relies on the bladder wall to perform two dramatically different functions. During a prolonged filling period, the bladder must remain in a relaxed state and act as a passive filling and storage compartment. In contrast, the bladder wall must mount a contraction of sufficient magnitude and duration to empty itself completely within a brief period of less than 2 minutes during micturition.

Filling. To act as a filling and storage compartment, the bladder wall relies on active and passive components to accommodate volumes of 500 cc or more. The active component of the bladder wall is the detrusor muscle, which, under neural modulation, remains in a relaxed state until an appropriate time for voiding occurs. Noncontractile or passive components also contribute to the bladder's distensibility. They are the collagenous framework of the detrusor, elastic and connective tissue of the lamina propria, and the expansive properties of the urothelium.

During filling, the detrusor muscle and noncontractile components of the bladder are so distensible that the pressure exerted against urine stored in the bladder remains relatively low and constant despite volumes that vary between 5 cc and 500 cc or more. Mathematically, this relationship is described by Laplace's law (Pdet = FpiR^2, where Pdet = the pressure of the detrusor or bladder wall, F = force, and R = radius of the bladder wall), which states that as the force exerted against the wall of a spherical object such as the bladder increases with filling, so does the radius. Because these two factors tend to cancel one another, the pressure exerted by the bladder wall against the intravesical contents (urine) tends to remain less than 15 cm H$_2$O even though volume varies significantly.

Active or passive factors may significantly alter the bladder's ability to act as an efficient filling and storage compartment. A hyperactive or *unstable* contraction of the detrusor muscle may curtail normal bladder filling and cause uncontrolled bladder emptying. A sustained detrusor pressure rise during bladder filling, termed *poor compliance,* also may compromise its ability to act as a storage compartment. Poor compliance occurs in response to detrusor hypertonicity noted as a sustained increase in the resting tone of the smooth muscle of the bladder wall. More commonly, poor compliance occurs in the presence of abnormality of the bladder's passive vesicoelastic properties caused by an increase in the amount of collagen in the detrusor or replacement of muscle and collagen with fibrotic tissue in response to obstruction, infection, inflammation, or denervation.[16]

Emptying. Bladder emptying requires contraction of smooth muscle contained within the vesical wall in coordination with relaxation of muscular components of the urethral sphincter mechanism. The normal detrusor contraction begins with neurologic stimulation. As a result, intravesical pressure rises, which, coupled with a simultaneous reduction of urethral resistance, allows the bladder to completely evacuate itself of urine.

The efficiency of a contraction is affected by the magnitude of urethral resistance, vesicoelastic and contractile properties of the bladder wall, and by the ability of the nervous system to activate the detrusor muscle for a sufficiently long period to empty itself completely. Obstruction of the bladder outlet, poor compliance of the bladder wall, or inefficient neural modulation of the detrusor muscle may interfere with the bladder's ability to contract efficiently.

Neural Control of the Micturition Reflex

Urinary continence requires the smooth muscle of the bladder wall to function in a significantly different manner than smooth muscle of the bowel or ureters. Bladder filling and emptying are controlled by a neurogenic modulatory system that extends from the vesicle wall to the brain. This complex modulatory system forms the cornerstone of social continence by allowing the child to master the ability to *initiate a voluntary bladder contraction* or *stable bladder* and to postpone micturition until an appropriate opportunity occurs.

Brain. The net effect of the brain's contribution to bladder function is the inhibition of detrusor contractions

until the person wishes to urinate. Although the interactions that allow the brain to accomplish this task are not completely understood, the principal structures that contribute to bladder stability have been identified.

A detrusor motor area exists in each hemisphere of the prefrontal lobes that is thought to contribute to prevention of bladder contractions in the continent person (Fig. 48-6). Abnormality of this area results in a loss of bladder stability.[7]

The thalamus also contributes to the modulation of bladder function. The thalamus is a collection of nuclei that relay input from lower brain areas to higher structures. These nuclei process input from sensory, somatic, and autonomic pathways including those that govern the urethrovesical unit.[6] Abnormality of the thalamus results in a loss of bladder stability possibly caused by functionally separating the bladder from the inhibitory influence of the detrusor motor area.

The limbic system influences both somatic and visceral functions including those of the urethrovesical unit. In experimental animals, stimulation of the limbic system is associated with modulation of the detrusor reflex.[12] Any role the limbic system may play in the brain's modulation of bladder function in humans remains unknown.

The hypothalamus affects behavior patterns associated with sexual function and voiding habits. Unfortunately, its influence on bladder and urethral function in the human remains unclear.[7]

The basal ganglia are a set of nuclei that constitute a portion of the extrapyramidal tracts. The nuclei of the basal ganglia assist the body in achieving fluid voluntary and involuntary movements by modulating muscle tone

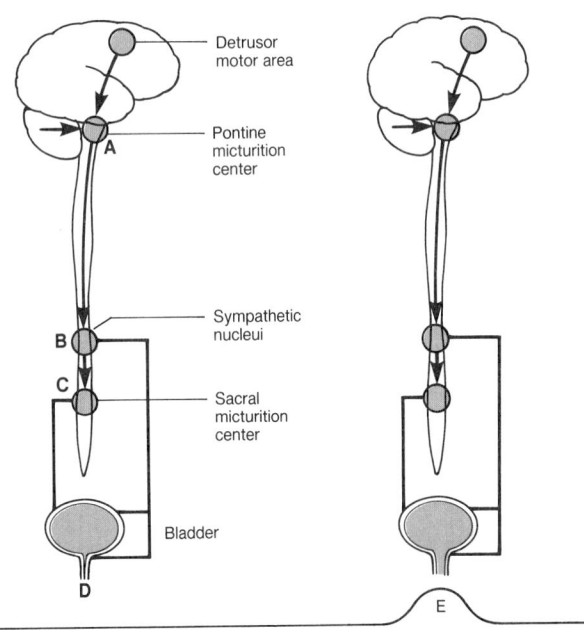

CMG pressure

FIGURE 48-6

Neural modulation of lower urinary tract. The lower urinary tract receives input from multiple centers in the brain and brainstem (pontine micturition center) to control micturition (**A**). The spinal cord modulates lower urinary tract function by way of the sacral micturition center (**B**) and sympathetic nuclei in thoracolumbar segments T10-L2 (**C**). Cystometrogram (CMG) represents bladder filling (**D**) and voiding (**E**).

including detrusor reflex activity.[18,36] Dysfunction of the basal ganglia, such as that noted in parkinsonism, results in loss of the brain's inhibitory influence over the bladder with resulting detrusor instability.[32]

The cerebellum also contributes to the extrapyramidal system in the human. In addition to regulating the force and rate of volitional movements, it contributes to the body's ability to maintain its position in space.[18] Like the basal ganglia, abnormality of the cerebellum results in loss of bladder stability and may cause dysfunction of the ability to relax the pelvic floor muscles in preparation to initiate micturition.[27]

Brainstem. The dorsal aspect of the pons exerts a significant modulatory role on urethrovesical function.[1,16,21] Two regions modulate detrusor and sphincter function. An "m region" is responsible for the initiation of the detrusor reflex (bladder contraction). An adjacent "l region" coordinates detrusor reflex activity and pelvic floor muscle activity necessary for the maintenance of sphincter closure during bladder filling and storage and sphincter relaxation needed for efficient bladder emptying.[17,21]

Spinal Cord and Peripheral Nerves. The spinal cord is the pathway for communication between end organs such as the bladder and brain (see Fig. 48-6). Communication between bladder wall and cerebrocortical centers is mediated by reticulospinal pathways located in the lateral columns.

Two spinal centers have particular significance for bladder function. Sympathetic outflow from the thoracolumbar cord (T12-L2) travels to the bladder wall and bladder neck by way of the hypogastric plexus. Sympathetic innervation promotes bladder filling and storage by way of relaxation of smooth muscle bundles in the detrusor and excitation of the circular smooth muscle of the vesicle neck. Abnormality of the thoracolumbar center may result in dyssynergia of the circular smooth muscle of the vesicle neck and obstruction of the bladder outlet.[20]

The sacral micturition center is the location of the parasympathetic outflow to the bladder as well as the nuclei that innervate skeletal muscles of the pelvic diaphragm. Parasympathetic innervation travels to the bladder by way of the pelvic plexus. Stimulation of the sacral micturition center is necessary for the detrusor to mount a contraction needed for efficient evacuation of urine. Abnormality of the sacral micturition center results in urinary retention due to impaired or absent detrusor contractility.[20]

Bladder Wall. The neural control of smooth muscle in the bladder wall arises from neuromuscular junctions located throughout the detrusor. The neuromuscular junctions of the bladder innervate smooth muscles cells on a nearly 1:1 basis under control of the autonomic nervous system. Because these junctions receive direction from multiple modulatory centers in the brain and spinal cord, the bladder (unlike smooth muscle organs located in the intestinal or upper urinary tract) is under voluntary control although ephaptic transmission probably occurs under certain circumstances.

Many neuromuscular junctions in the bladder wall release acetylcholine under parasympathetic control causing detrusor contraction and micturition. Other junctions contain adrenergic vesicles under sympathetic control. Excitation of these neural junctions promote relaxation of the detrusor.[5]

Detrusor muscle bundles also respond to noncholinergic, nonadrenergic neurotransmitters. Adenosine triphosphate (ATP) is a purinergic neurotransmitter that may contribute to detrusor muscle contraction. It is not known whether ATP acts as a cotransmitter released only in conjunction with acetylcholine or whether it acts independently of cholinergic release.[9] Other potential neurotransmitter substances also have been identified in *in vitro* studies of bladder muscle strips including vasoactive intestinal polypeptide, substance P, and others.[8,30] Their role in bladder motor activity or sensation perception remains unclear.

Paracrine and endocrine substances also influence detrusor contractility. The bladder synthesizes prostaglandins E_1, E_2, and $F_{2\alpha}$. Prostaglandin E_2 enhances detrusor contractility while inhibiting urethral smooth muscle tone and is predominate in lower urinary tract function.[24] Estrogens indirectly affect detrusor contractility by stimulating the synthesis of prostaglandins.[4,29]

Urethral Sphincter Mechanism

Urinary continence is not explained solely by the innervation of the urinary bladder, which renders the detrusor under voluntary control. The urethrovesical unit also must rely on the competence of the urethral sphincter mechanism to prevent urinary leakage due to the physical stresses that the bladder frequently experiences during activities of daily living.

The urethral sphincter mechanism is the combination of a number of passive and active factors that combine to ensure urethral closure during bladder filling and storage (Fig. 48-7). This conceptualization of the urethral sphincter mechanism is complementary to the traditional concepts of an internal mechanism located at the bladder neck and external mechanism located at the middle third of the female urethra and membranous urethra in the male.

The softness of the urethral epithelium contributes to sphincter closure because of its impressive ability to mold or deform itself in response to extrinsic compression. The urethral epithelium's ability to conform to varying configurations is best demonstrated when a catheter is passed into the bladder. Continence is maintained in spite of the potentially disruptive presence of a relatively stiff tube in the urethral lumen because the epithelium deforms its shape to fill in the potential space caused by the catheter's presence.[46]

The ability of the urethral epithelium to form a watertight seal is further enhanced by the mucosal secretions produced by the urethra. Mucosal secretions lower surface resistance and further fill microscopic gaps needed to produce a seal impermeable to urine.[38,46]

The vascular cushion of the urethral wall also contributes to the sphincter mechanism. This rich arteriovenous network enhances urethral wall pliability and may

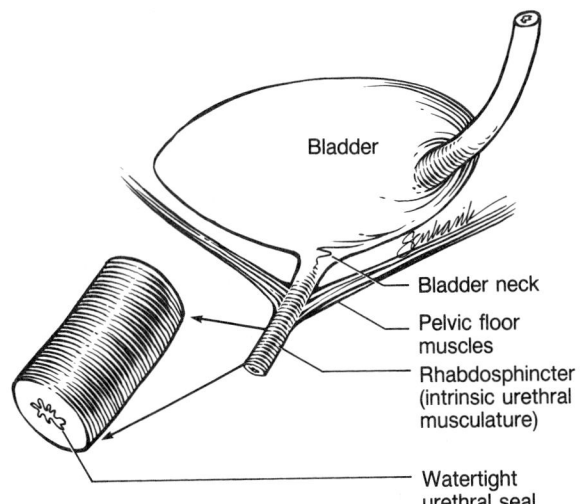

FIGURE 48-7
Urethral sphincter mechanism. The watertight urethral seal depends on the (1) plasticity of the urethral mucosa, (2) presence of mucus, and (3) vascular cushion. Tension that maintains urethral closure in the presence of physical stress relies on smooth muscle within the urethra located near the bladder neck, the rhabdosphincter, and the pelvic floor muscles. The pelvic floor muscles and pelvic ligaments also assist in sphincter function by providing support maintaining the urethra in its proper anatomic position.

contribute to the closure pressure needed to maintain a leakproof seal during periods of physical stress.[38]

Skeletal and smooth muscle within the urethral wall provide active tension needed to maintain sphincter closure in response to variable intravesical pressures produced by physical stress. The rhabdosphincter is the principal structure that provides active tension needed to maintain urethral closure during bladder filling and storage. The slow twitch fibers are ideally suited for the prolonged tension needed for consistent continence under the stresses of physical movement. The smooth muscle bundles in the bladder neck and urethra contribute to sphincter tension by supplementing the considerable active closure pressure provided by the rhabdosphincter.[19,38]

The periurethral muscles that form the pelvic diaphragm contribute to urethral closure during periods of intense physical stress. These fibers are anatomically and functionally distinct from the rhabdosphincter. They are characterized by a mixture of fast and slow twitch muscle cells that reflexively or volitionally respond to particularly intense stressors such as coughing, sneezing, or lifting a heavy object.[41]

The skeletal muscles of the pelvic floor are modulated by the pyramidal tracts originating in the cerebral cortex. A periurethral muscle motor area is located in the sensorimotor cortex adjacent to the central sulcus. Motor impulses from the brain travel to the pelvic floor muscles by way of the pudendal nerve, which receives its impulses from the corticospinal tracts of the spinal cord. This volitional tract interacts with reflex loops between the pons and pudendal nerve to provide coordination between pelvic floor and bladder muscles.[2]

The structures of the pelvic floor, including muscles, ligaments, and fascial coverings, also contribute to the

urethral sphincter mechanism by way of their passive, supportive properties. By maintaining the urethrovesical unit in its proper position, the muscular elements of the urethra function at optimal length and orientation, and the urethral wall remains under the influence of abdominal pressure variations needed to maintain continence during periods of intensive physical stress.[15]

Attaining Continence— A Developmental Perspective

The attainment of continence is a developmental task for the growing child that can be divided into phases comparable to other maturational milestones such as mastery of language or fine motor skills. A complete understanding of the development of continence recognizes that the equipment needed for urinary control represent a combination of social and cognitive skills as well as maturation of the physiologic apparatus necessary for bladder stability and volitional control of the sphincter mechanism.

Infancy. During the first year of life, continence is not an issue. Bladder filling is a passive, reflexive event that proceeds until stretch receptors in the bladder wall trigger the pontine micturition center. When stimulated, the dorsal pons initiates a detrusor contraction mediated by the parasympathetic nervous system. At the same time, the pontine sphincter coordination center causes relaxation of the sphincter mechanism allowing the bladder to empty its contents.

Age 1 to 2. Between the first and second year of life, the infant develops proprioceptive bladder sensations and an awareness of bladder fullness.[26] The bladder probably remains unstable or independent of volitional control; the child may use this newly acquired awareness of sensation and increasing control over the pelvic diaphragm muscles to postpone urinary leakage temporarily until a toilet is reached. The child is likely to exhibit short periods of diurnal continence but reverts to incontinence while asleep.

Age 3 to 5. Somewhere between 2 and 4 years, diurnal control becomes well established and nocturnal enuresis begins to subside.[26] In 1955, Klackenberg[23] studied 315 children between ages 1 and 5 and discovered that the development of urinary control was not well correlated with "toilet training" efforts by caretakers. The poor correlation between parental training regimens and the development of continence is best explained by remembering that urinary control is difficult or impossible before the brain centers that govern bladder stability are mature. As this maturational process occurs, diurnal urinary control is completed and nocturnal enuresis disappears. The key difference between the child with a stable versus unstable bladder is the ability to *initiate a volitional contraction and to postpone bladder contractions.* Before bladder stability is attained, the child is forced to rush to the toilet with little or no warning because the perception of bladder fullness is quickly followed by an unstable or uncontrolled contraction that begins the process of urination. After the development of stability, the child retains the perceptions of urinary urgency but gains the ability to *postpone* any contraction until he reaches the toilet and to *voluntarily initiate* a contraction.

Age 5. Blomfield and Douglas observed that by the age of 4 1/2 years 88% of their subjects had acquired complete diurnal and nocturnal urinary continence.[3] Adequate bladder control is demonstrated by a diurnal voiding pattern of every 2 hours or less often, absence of nocturnal urinary leakage, and nocturia 0 to 1 time per night. The continent child should be able to postpone urination and initiate micturition even if an intense desire to void is not perceived. Stress urinary incontinence is never normal and should be treated as a dysfunctional voiding state regardless of the child's age.

Summary

The principal functions of the urinary tract are the formation, transportation, and elimination of urine. Urine is formed in the kidneys and transported by the ureters to the bladder in a flow called efflux. Smooth muscles promote closure of the ureter to prevent reflux or the backing movement of urine from the bladder to the upper urinary tract. This promotion of efflux and prevention of reflux are the function of the ureterovesical unit. The urethrovesical unit, the lower urinary tract includes the bladder, bladder neck, urethra, and adjacent pelvic floor muscles and supportive structure. The bladder fills, stores, and empties the urine through micturition. This is accomplished through neural control of the bladder through messages from the brain. The urethral sphincter mechanism is a combination of passive and active factors that ensure urethral closure during bladder filling, storage, and opening for emptying. Attaining continence is a developmental task that requires mature physiologic apparatus with social and cognitive skills.

References

1. Barrington, F. J. F. (1925). The effect of lesion on hind- and mid-brain on micturition in the cat. *Journal of Experimental Physiology, 15,* 81–102.
2. Bhatia, N. N., & Bradley, W. E. (1983). Neuro-anatomy and physiology: Innervation of the lower urinary tract. In S. Raz (Ed.), *Female urology.* Philadelphia: Saunders.
3. Blomfield, J. M., & Douglas, J. W. B. (1956). Bedwetting: Prevalence among children aged 4–7 years. *Lancet, 1,* 850.
4. Borda, E., Chaud, M., Gutinsky, N., Ortiz, C., Gimeno, M. F., & Gimeno, A. L. (1983). Relationships between prostaglandins and estrogens on the motility of isolated rings from the rat urinary bladder. *Journal Of Urology, 129,* 1250–1253.
5. Brading, A. (1987). Physiology of bladder smooth muscle. In M. Torrens & J. F. B. Morrison (Eds.), *Physiology of the lower urinary tract.* London: Springer-Verlag.
6. Bradley, W. E. (1986). Physiology of the urinary bladder. In P. C. Walsh, R. F. Gittes, A. D. Perlmutter, & T. A. Stamey (Eds.), *Campbell's urology* (5th ed.). Philadelphia: Saunders.
7. Bradley, W. E., & Scott, F. B. (1978). Physiology of the urinary bladder. In J. Harrison, P. C. Walsh, A. D. Perlmutter, R. F. Gittes, & T. A. Stamey (Eds.), *Campbell's urology* (4th ed.). Philadelphia: Saunders.
8. Burnstock, G. (1985). Nervous control of smooth muscle by transmitters, cotransmitters and modulators. *Experientia, 41,* 869–874.
9. Burnstock, G., Dumsday, B., & Smythe, A. (1972). Atropine resistant excitation of the urinary bladder: The possibility of transmission via nerves releasing a purine nucleotide. *British Journal of Pharmacology, 44,* 457–61.
10. Davis, J. E., Hagerdoorn, J. P., & Bergmann, L. L. (1981). Anatomy and ultrastructure of the ureter. In H. Bergmann (Ed.), *The ureter.* New York: Springer-Verlag.
11. Duckett, J. W., & Caldamone, A. A. (1992) Bladder and urachus. In P. P. Kelalis, L. R. King, & A. B. Belman (Eds.), *Clinical pediatric urology* (3rd ed.). Philadelphia: Saunders.
12. Evarsden, P., & Ursin, T. (1968). Nervous control of urinary bladder in cats: I. The collecting phase. *Acta Physiologica Scandinavica, 72,* 157.
13. Gosling, J. A., & Chilton, C. P. (1984). The anatomy of the bladder urethra and pelvic floor. In A. R. Mundy, T. P. Stephenson, & A. J. Wein (Eds.), *Urodynamics: Principles, practice and application.* London: Churchill-Livingstone.
14. Gray, M. L., & Broadwell, D. C. (1989). Genitourinary system. In J. Thompson, G. McFarland, J. Hirsh, S. Tucker, & A. Bowers (Eds.) *Mosby's manual of clinical nursing* (2nd ed.). St. Louis: Mosby.
15. Gray, M. L., & Dougherty, M. C. (1987). Urinary incontinence—pathophysiology and treatment. *Journal of Enterostomal Therapy, 14,* 152–162.
16. Griffiths, D. J. (1984). Hydrodynamics and mechanics of the bladder and urethra. In A. R. Mundy, T. P. Stephenson, & A. J. Wein (Eds.), *Urodynamics: Principles, practice and application.* London: Churchill-Livingstone.
17. Griffiths, D. J., Holstege, G., Dalm, E., & DeWall, H. (1990). Control and coordination of bladder and urethral function in the brainstem. *Neurourology and Urodynamics, 9,* 63–82.
18. Guyton, A. C. (1991). *Textbook of medical physiology* (8th ed.). Philadelphia: Saunders.
19. Hadley, H. R., Zimmern, P. E., & Raz, S. (1986). The treatment of male urinary incontinence. In P. C. Walsh, R. F. Gittes, A. D. Perlmutter, & T. A. Stamey (Eds.), *Campbell's urology* (5th ed.). Philadelphia: Saunders.
20. Hald, T., & Bradley, W. E. (1982). *The urinary bladder: Neurology and dynamics.* Baltimore: Williams & Wilkins.
21. Holstege, G., Griffiths, D. J., De Wall, H., and Dalm, E. (1986). Anatomical and physiological observations on supraspinal control of bladder and urethral sphincter muscles in the cat. *Journal of Comparative Neurology, 250,* 449–461.
22. King L. R. (1992). Posterior urethra. In P. P. Kelalis, L. R. King, & A. B. Belman (Eds.), *Clinical pediatric urology* (3rd ed.). Philadelphia: Saunders.
23. Klackenberg, G. (1955). Primary enuresis: When is a child dry at night? *Acta Pediatrica Scandinavica, 44,* 513.
24. Klarskov, P., Gerstenberg, T., Ramirez, D., Christensen, P., & Hald, T. (1983). Prostaglandin Type E activity predominates in urinary tract smooth muscle in vitro. *Journal of Urology, 129,* 1071–1074.
25. Kluck, P. (1980). The autonomic innervation of the human urinary bladder, bladder neck and urethra: A histochemical study. *Anatomical Record, 198,* 439–447.
26. Kramer, S. A. (1992). Surgical treatment of urinary incontinence. In P. P. Kelalis, L. R. King, & A. B. Belman (Eds.), *Clinical pediatric urology* (3rd ed.). Philadelphia: Saunders.
27. Leach. G. E. (1982). Urodynamic manifestations of cerebellar ataxia. *Journal of Urology, 128,* 348.
28. Leeson, C. R., & Leeson, T. S. (1985). *Textbook of histology* (5th ed.). Philadelphia: Saunders.
29. Levin, B. M., Frances-Schofer, M., & Wein, A. J. (1980). Estrogen induces alteration of autonomic distribution in the rabbit urinary bladder. *Federal Proceedings, 39,* 296.
30. Levin, R. (1990). *New transmitters and receptor mechanisms—implications for drug therapy.* Second Urology Research Con-

ference: Physiology of the Lower Urinary Tract. Houston, July 1990.

31. Levitt, S. B., & Weiss, R. A. (1992). Vesicoureteral reflux: Natural history classification and reflux nephropathy. In P. P. Kelalis, L. R. King, & A. B. Belman (Eds.), *Clinical pediatric urology* (3rd ed.). Philadelphia: Saunders.

32. Lewin, R. J., Dillard, G. W., & Porter, R. W. (1967). Extrapyramidal inhibition of the urinary bladder. *Brain Research, 4,* 301.

33. Lewis, S. (1990). *Bladder epithelial permeability.* Second Urology Research Conference: Physiology of the Lower Urinary Tract. Houston, July 1990.

34. Olsson, C. (1992). Anatomy of the upper urinary tract. In P. C. Walsh, R. F. Gittes, A. D. Perlmutter, & T. A. Stamey (Eds.), *Campbell's urology* (6th ed.). Philadelphia: Saunders.

35. Pinck, B. D. (1981). Embryology of the upper urinary tract. In S. 1-Askari, M. Golimbu, & P. Morales (Eds.), *Essentials of basic sciences in urology.* New York: Grune & Stratton.

36. Porter, R. W. (1967). A pallidal response to detrusor contraction. *Brain Research, 4,* 381.

37. Sarma, K. P. (1969). *Tumors of the urinary bladder.* New York: Appleton-Century-Crofts.

38. Staskin, D. R., Zimmern, P. E., Hadley, H. R., & Raz, S. (1985). Pathophysiology of stress incontinence. *Clinics in Obstetrics and Gynecology, 12,* 357–368.

39. Stephens, F. D., & Lenaghan, D. (1962). Anatomical basis and dynamics of vesicoureteral reflux. *Journal of Urology, 87,* 669.

40. Tanagho, E. A. (1981). Embryology of the genitourinary system. In D. R. Smith (Ed.), *General urology.* Los Altos, CA: Lang.

41. Tanagho, E. A. (1986). Anatomy and surgical approach to the urogenital tract. In P. C. Walsh, R. F. Gittes, A. D. Perlmutter, & T. A. Stamey (Eds.), *Campbell's urology.* Philadelphia: Saunders.

42. Waldeyer, W. (1891). Uber die insel des Gehirns der anthropoiden. *Korrespondenzblatt der Deutschen Gessellschaft fur Antropologie, Ethnologie and Urgeschichte, 22,* 110.

43. Weiss, R. M. (1981). Effects of drugs on the ureter. In H. Bergmann (Ed.), *The ureter.* New York: Springer-Verlag.

44. Weiss, R. M. (1992). Physiology and pharmacology of the renal pelvis and ureters. In P. C. Walsh, R. F. Gittes, A. D. Perlmutter, & T. A. Stamey (Eds.), *Campbell's urology* (6th ed.). Philadelphia: Saunders.

45. Williams, P., & Warwick, R. (1980). *Gray's anatomy.* Philadelphia: Saunders.

46. Zinner, N. R., Sterling, A. M., & Ritter, R. C. (1980). Role of inner urethral softness in urinary incontinence. *Urology, 16,* 115.

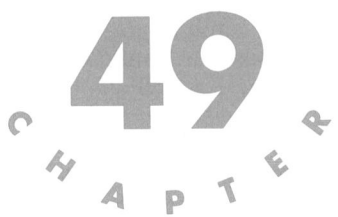

49

C H A P T E R

Nursing Assessment and Diagnosis of Urinary Function

BEHAVIORAL OBJECTIVES

Use functional health as a guideline for assessment of the child's urinary function.

Describe the components of a complete physical examination of the school-age child's urinary system.

Identify four physical findings that indicate a potential urologic emergency in the neonate.

Describe noninvasive and invasive tests used to diagnose urinary dysfunction.

Identify nursing diagnoses that are commonly used in the care of children with urinary dysfunction.

Assessment of the child with altered urinary function identifies abnormalities of urine formation, transport, storage, and elimination. The nursing assessment also focuses on the interactions between urologic disease and normal functional health. Assessment is an ongoing process that requires synthesis and evaluation of data obtained from historical review obtained from the patient and family, findings from physical examination, and information gathered from diagnostic tests of urinary structure and function.

Nursing Assessment

Child and Family History

Health Perception and Health Management

The family's response to a urologic abnormality and expectations concerning potential nursing or medical management programs can be assessed by asking a series of questions. Gather information of the mother's pregnancy, labor, and delivery. Were urologic abnormalities detected or suspected because of prenatal ultrasonography? Was the pregnancy or labor and delivery marked by complications? Identify the ages and health history of the child's siblings, and explore any familial history of urologic abnormalities, including multicystic or polycystic kidney disease, vesicoureteral reflux, urinary calculi, urinary tumors, hypertension, or congenital defects.

The health perception and health management assessment includes asking the parents to describe their perceptions of the affected child's health status since birth. Ask the parents to differentiate between a disease and handicap, or disease and dysfunctional condition. Many parents fail to distinguish a handicap such as spina bifida or dysfunctional state such as enuresis from a disease state. They often act on this perception by seeking a "cure" for the child's condition and may refuse to accept caring measures such as intermittent catheterization or behavioral modification routines because they perceive that these measures fail to cure the problem.

Strategies used by the family to manage acute health care problems such as urinary tract infection or fever due to unknown cause can be evaluated by asking the child and family to identify symptoms they feel justify a visit to a health care professional. Their knowledge of the symptoms of common acute urologic conditions such as lower or upper urinary tract infection or acute obstruction are assessed by direct questions.

Inquire about preventive measures the family employs to avoid problems associated with abnormal urinary function. Can they identify the importance of adequate fluid intake in the prevention of urinary tract infection? Do they use urinary containment devices or behavioral modification strategies to manage urinary leakage? Or do they ignore the condition or treat urinary leakage as misbehavior deserving punishment?

When appropriate, ask the child what his or her perceptions of urologic problems are and what goals, if any, provide evidence of improvement. Does he or she wish to graduate to "big boy" or "big girl" pants, or is the child content to remain in diapers? Assess the child's perceptions of urologic abnormality by using unambiguous and open-ended questions or directions. Ask the child to complete the sentence, "Leaking urine is like . . . ." Listen carefully to the language and key terms the child uses to answer these questions, and evaluate the key words and concepts used to describe experiences with impaired urinary function. Does the child perceive urinary leakage as a medical condition or as misbehavior? Does the child believe that punishment is proper treatment for bedwetting or soiling clothing?

Nutrition and Metabolism

Assessment of the child and family's nutrition and metabolism explores patterns of fluid and nutritional intake and their impact on urine formation, transport, and elimination. Ask the family to list the type, volume, and timing of beverages the child consumes. Are fluids consumed with meals only? Does the child sip beverages between meals? What percentage of the fluids consumed in a 24-hour period consists of water or clear juices, and what percentage consists of carbonated or caffeine-containing beverages? Does the child with nocturnal urinary leakage problems refrain from consuming liquids for a brief period before bedtime? If so, how long? Follow

this assessment with a voiding diary (Fig. 49-1) to supplement the historical report with more objective data concerning voiding patterns whenever feasible.

Evaluation of the child and family's general nutritional habits is completed to assess the impact of renal or urologic abnormality on physical growth patterns. A height-weight chart is used as a screening instrument, and more detailed assessment is indicated when potential abnormalities in growth patterns are suspected. This information is crucial when caring for the child who forms urinary calculi in the presence of a metabolic disorder that may respond to dietary manipulation. The information is also valuable when caring for a patient with retarded growth due to impaired renal function.

Elimination

Assessment of the urinary and fecal elimination is crucial for the nursing care of any child with a urologic abnormality. Evaluate the patient's urinary and fecal elimination patterns within a developmental framework (see Chap. 48). A checklist is used to define the child's voiding history; related urologic, neurologic, and general medical conditions; surgical history; and current medications. A sample of a voiding history assessment checklist is given in the accompanying display. The accuracy of this checklist is then verified with a voiding diary, physical examination, and review of diagnostic data.

The voiding dysfunction assessment checklist begins with the child's bladder management program and spontaneous voiding pattern. Many children will be managed with diapers. Assess the appropriateness of diaper use from a developmental perspective. Is the child too young for toilet training, or are diapers used for urine containment because of persistent incontinence or as a method of punishment?

Other children with voiding abnormalities are managed by intermittent cathetherization. Determine the catheterization schedule employed and ask whether leakage occurs between catheterizations. Establish whether the child is able to catheterize himself or herself and which family members or caretakers can help with the procedure as needed. Assess how the child contains any urinary leakage experienced between catheterizations.

Certain children with profound voiding abnormalities manage their bladders via an indwelling catheter. Determine how long the catheter has been in place and how often a new catheter is inserted. Ask the family to describe how they care for the catheter and what types of urinary collection devices are used when the child is awake and asleep. Does the child leak urine around the catheter? If so, ask what type of urinary containment device is used to contain incontinence and determine what measures have been taken to correct the problem.

Children who void spontaneously also may experience altered urinary elimination patterns. The nurse first assesses diurnal and nocturnal voiding patterns. Many children will have difficulty quantifying their voiding patterns, and a voiding diary may help. Ask the child and family if the child can sit through a movie without urinating or determine the child's schedule at school and how often he or she must urinate during a typical day. Assess the child's nocturnal voiding pattern and differ-

Instructions:

1. Measure all amounts of urine using the plastic cup provided or another measuring container marked with "cc's" or "ounces".
2. Record the amount you urinated under the column marked "Amount Voided".
3. Record the amount you obtain with catheterization under the column marked "Cath Volume".
4. Record the amount you drink under the column marked "Amount Drank".
5. If you experienced a leakage place a check beside the approximate time it occurred. Do not try to estimate amounts.

TIME	AMOUNT VOIDED	LEAKAGE	AMOUNT DRANK	CATH VOLUME

FIGURE 49-1

Simple Voiding Diary. The simple voiding diary provides information concerning patterns of urinary elimination, incontinence, and fluid intake. The information sought is tailored for each patient. A graduated container is required when the voided volume is recorded. (Courtesy of the Shepherd Spinal Center, Atlanta, GA 30309.)

entiate between nocturia, nocturia with subsequent incontinence, and enuresis. A child experiences nocturia if awakened during the night by a desire to void. Nocturia with incontinence occurs when the child is awakened by a desire to void but fails to reach the toilet before urinating. Nocturnal enuresis occurs when a child urinates before awakening. Using a voiding diary, evaluate the type of incontinence the affected child is experiencing. The symptom of stress incontinence occurs when the child or family observes urinary leakage associated with physical exertion, such as position changes or abdominal straining. Urge incontinence occurs when the child notes urinary leakage related to a pronounced desire to void. The child typically states he or she cannot reach the toilet in time. Parents or caretakers may note that the child rushes to reach the toilet and may squat in an attempt to prevent incontinence. Reflex incontinence occurs when the child empties his or her bladder in an uncontrolled manner in the absence of any sensations of urgency. Children with continuous or "total" incontinence are never dry. They may experience extraurethral incontinence due to congenital anomaly or a surgically created stoma (uri-

nary conduit) with failure to store urine, or they may note a continuous dribble from an ectopic structure or small fistula superimposed on an otherwise normal voiding pattern.

Determine the family's impressions of the child's urinary flow pattern. A normal or explosive flow pattern is marked by urination with a good-caliber stream and without interruption of hesitancy greater than 15 to 30 seconds. The child with a normal or explosive pattern may void with urgency that may be accompanied by urge incontinence. An intermittent voiding pattern is often accompanied by hesitancy initiating a urinary stream and straining to enhance bladder emptying. The child is often completely unaware of this behavior. A poor-dribbling voiding pattern also may be associated with hesitancy to void and straining or compressing the bladder in an attempt to enhance the urinary stream.

Assess the child's sensations of filling whenever feasible. The normal child should experience a mild sensation of urgency centered at the urethral meatus or glans penis approximately 1 hour before urinating. This sensation is initially suppressed but will recur and become

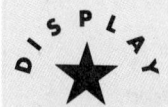

Voiding History Assessment Checklist

Instructions: Check, circle, or fill in the blank for each section of this checklist to provide a thorough assessment of voiding function of the infant, child, or adolescent.

Voiding History

Was the child ever successfully toilet trained? No _____ Yes _____
At what age? _____

Date of onset of current symptoms: _____
Bladder management program:
Diapers _____
Pads/incontinent briefs _____
Credé every _____ hours
Intermittent catheterization every _____ hours.
Indwelling catheter for _____ (days/months/years)
Spontaneous voider:
Diurnal frequency every _____
Nocturia _____ times per night
Incontinence: Stress _____ Urge _____ Reflex _____ Continuous _____
Enuresis _____
Quality of urinary stream:
Explosive _____ Normal _____ Intermittent _____ Poor/Dribbling _____
Strains to void? Yes _____ No _____
Hesitancy initiating stream? Yes _____ No _____
Sensations of bladder filling: Hypersensitive _____ Normal _____ Diminished or Absent _____

Urinary retention: Acute _____ Chronic _____ Feelings of incomplete emptying _____

Related Urologic Conditions

Urinary tract infection:
Symptoms of infection: Yes _____ No _____
Documented infections: Current _____ Chronic _____ Recurrent Infections _____
Urinary tract infections associated with fever: Yes _____ No _____
Vesicoureteral reflux: No _____
Yes: Left _____ Right _____ Bilateral _____
Grade: _____
Urinary calculi: No _____
Yes: _____ Type: _____
Urologic anomalies: _____
Urologic tumor: _____

Related Neurologic Conditions

Spinal cord abnormalities:
Myelomeningocele _____
Meningocele _____
Spina Bifida Occulta _____
Sacral Dysraphism _____
Sacral Agenesis _____
Sacral Tumor _____
Traumatic Injury (Level: _____)
Developmental delay _____
Closed head injury _____
Cerebral palsy _____
Central nervous system tumor: _____
Other: _____

(Continued)

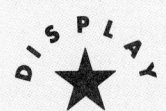

Voiding History Assessment Checklist (continued)

Related Medical History

Medical Conditions

Diabetes _____
Tumor of the _____
Renal disease: Renal insufficiency _____ Renal failure _____
Imperforate anus? Yes _____ No _____
Bowel habits: every _____
           Constipation: Yes _____ No _____
           Fecal incontinence: Yes _____ No _____
Other: _____

Surgical History

Current Medications

more persistent as the child postpones urination. Ultimately, the child will cope with this sensation by voiding, which gives a feeling of relief and sensation of complete bladder emptying. Children with urge incontinence often report pain associated with the occurrence of unstable bladder contractions. Other children will experience absent sensations of feeling or rely on sensations of abdominopelvic distention to determine bladder fullness.

Urinary retention occurs when the child is unable to complete emptying the bladder by voiding. The child with acute urinary retention experiences a sudden cessation of micturition, requiring indwelling or intermittent catheter drainage. Other children may experience chronic retention requiring prolonged catheterization or manual bladder compression (Credé's maneuver) to empty their bladders. Determine whether the child feels he or she completely empties the bladder. Even children who void spontaneously may experience feelings of incomplete emptying often associated with objectively demonstrable urinary retention.

Explore other urologic conditions that affect the child's urinary function. Urinary tract infection alters lower tract function and elimination patterns. Determine whether the child experiences symptoms of lower urinary tract infection (urinary frequency greater than every 2 hours, pain or burning with urination, and change in appearance or odor of urine). Does the patient have a history of documented urinary tract infections? Do they recur, or does the infection persist despite appropriate antibiotic therapy? A history of urinary tract infections associated with fever is suggestive of upper urinary tract infection and potential vesicoureteral reflux. Determine whether the child has a known occurrence of vesicoureteral reflux and the extent and severity (grade) of the condition.

Urinary function also is affected by the presence of tumors or congenital anomalies of the genitourinary tract. Determine whether these conditions exist and what treatments have been used to restore normal urinary function.

Because of the close relationship between lower urinary tract function and central nervous system function, an assessment of the child's urinary function includes a detailed review of neurologic function. Determine any known neurologic conditions that affect the brain, spinal cord, or peripheral nerves. Evaluate whether the child is affected by a developmental delay due to neurologic deficit or other factors.

Other medical conditions may affect urinary function. Diabetes is a common childhood disorder that impacts on renal and lower urinary tract function. Tumors of the abdomen, pelvis, or structures adjacent to the brain or spinal cord may affect urinary tract function. Subtle, neuropathic voiding abnormalities often cause fecal as well as urine elimination disorders. Determine the child's bowel habits (frequency and consistency of stool) and whether fecal incontinence persists past the third year of life.

Explore the child's surgical history, and evaluate whether any operative procedures may affect urinary function. Surgical procedures of the abdomen, pelvis, brain or spinal cord, spinal column, or cranium may directly affect urinary structures or indirectly compromise urinary function by affecting the neurologic status of the lower urinary tract.

Review the child's current medications, and identify any drugs that are likely to affect urinary function. Commonly implicated agents include diuretics, cold preparations containing a decongestant, anticholinergics, psychotropic drugs, antianxiety agents, antihypertensives, antiasthmatics, and narcotics.

Activity and Exercise

The child should be assessed with particular attention to activities that affect the child's ability to accomplish the tasks necessary to void or empty the bladder via catheterization. Observe the child in a variety of activities and over time. Does the child have sufficient dexterity, mental awareness, and mobility to move to the toilet and empty his or her bladder? Assess environmental influences that enhance or impede the ability to transfer onto the toilet. These include the physical distance to a toilet; physical barriers that may impede mobility, such as heavy doors or height of the commode; and availability of handicap aids, if needed. Determine the child's dexterity in removing clothing, such as lowering undergarments and britches, unfastening buttons, and manipulating zippers.

Sleep and Rest

Assess the child and family's sleep and rest patterns and define the extent that they are affected by altered urinary elimination. Determine whether an intermittent catheterization schedule necessitates arising at night or whether an enuretic child is awakened at night to empty his or her bladder. Evaluate the number of times a child with nocturia is wakened during the night by the desire to void and whether other family members arise with the child.

Cognition and Perception

The child's cognitive awareness of bladder elimination, including perceptions of bladder filling and need to eliminate urine in a socially appropriate manner, is assessed by asking specific questions. Can the child identify when the bladder is full? Did the child have time to get to bathroom from the time of the sensation to voiding? Where is the bathroom?

Self-Perception and Self-Concept

Ideally, the child is interviewed away from the presence of parents and siblings as well as with family members present. Ask the child to describe his or her experiences with voiding dysfunction or urologic disease within the home and while at school or to draw and describe a picture of his or her body. Question the child concerning beliefs related to urinary elimination. Determine whether the child and family view urinary elimination as a sinful or dirty act or whether elimination is discussed under any circumstances. Particularly note the language that the child and family use to describe acts related to urinary elimination, and incorporate this language into patient teaching and care.

Many urologic conditions provoke profound feelings of guilt, humiliation, and shame in the affected child and other family members. The affected child is usually hesitant to discuss these feelings. Younger children are often better able to express their feelings through play or drawing. Ask the older child or adolescent a leading question, such as "Leaking urine makes me feel like . . . ?" Allow the child to express feelings of self-perception and relationships with others in the child's own context of meaning. Following assessment of the child's perceptions of self-concept and relationships with others, query the parent's perceptions of the child's self-concept and ability to relate to family members, peers, and other adults.

Role Relationships

The family relationships are observed primarily in the health center environment. Home assessments are encouraged when feasible. Questions addressing the various role relationships should be discussed with the entire family as well as with parents, siblings, and the "sick" child separately. The use of drawings can be effective in identifying underlying strengths and concerns in the family.[14]

Sexuality and Reproduction

Assessment for younger children focuses on how they perceive their maleness or femaleness and how they compare themselves to age-matched peers, older or younger siblings, or friends and adults. Assessment of the adolescent also focuses on sexual and reproductive behaviors and the patient's assessment of his or her desirability as a sexual partner.

Coping and Stress Tolerance

Explore how the child and parents handle stressors related to urologic abnormality. Identify the strategies the child uses to cope with urinary symptoms, and allow the child to vocalize frustrations. Provide the parents opportunities to identify and vocalize their feelings and frustrations concerning the child's urologic condition. Evaluate the family's responses to the stresses related to health problems in the home setting, clinic, or hospital whenever possible.

Values and Beliefs

Ask patients to describe their goals in life related to career relationships and lifestyle whenever feasible. Explore parental expectations relevant to these issues, and evaluate the consistency of perceptions between the affected child and other family members. Ask the child and parents to share their perceptions of how a urologic abnormality may impact on these goals and whether they believe these problems can be overcome.

Physical Examination

General Approach

Physical examination of the urologic system in the infant, child, or adolescent is completed within the context of a complete nursing assessment. Inspect the general body habitus of the patient for general state of health and any signs of apparent distress. Observe the patient's height, weight, and posture within a developmental perspective. Note the grooming and dress, facial expression, presence of body odors, and interactions within the immediate environment. Observe the integument, eyes, and mucous membranes for the state of hydration and evidence of failing renal function. Measure the patient's vital signs, including blood pressure, in the supine, standing, and sitting positions to assess for hypertension associated with abnormal renal function. Measure the patient's temperature to assess for signs of systemic infection, including upper urinary tract infection.[4,9]

Examine the patient for costovertebral angle tenderness prior to abdominal examination if infection is suspected to determine the presence of upper urinary tract infection and degree of tenderness. Place a hand just below the angle formed by the intersection of the costal margin at the lower aspect of the rib cage and vertebral column, make a fist with the opposite hand, and *gently* tap over the hand to determine presence of tenderness.

Have the patient empty his or her bladder and obtain a urine specimen for urinalysis, microscopic examination, and culture if feasible. Place the patient in a supine position and examine the abdomen. Begin the examination by observing for the general size and shape of the abdomen, pelvis, and genitalia. Observe the skin for signs of surgical or other scars, rashes, or lesions. Inspect the umbilicus for evidence of displacement, inflammation, or hernia. Assess the abdomen for signs of bulging, masses, or asymmetry.[1] Inspect the suprapubic area of the pelvis from the patient's side for signs of bulging or mass. Note whether any mass reaches beyond the true pelvis to the umbilicus or further.

Percuss the abdomen to gain a general orientation to significant landmarks, including the liver, spleen, bowel, and bladder. Percuss the bladder by working down from a position superior to the umbilicus. Choose a point where percussion reveals a hollow, resonant sound like that heard over loops of bowel. Percuss downward from the midline toward the symphysis pubis until the sound changes to dull, indicating urine in the bladder. Follow percussion by light palpation of abdominal organs to determine muscular resistance, marked abdominal tenderness, and superficial masses.[1]

Deep palpation of the abdomen is used to detect the presence of subtle or deep abdominal masses. The kidneys are easily palpable only in the infant. Palpate the right kidney by placing one hand behind the patient's lower rib and iliac crest. Place the other hand over the overlying abdomen, below the costal margin. Gently but firmly press the hands together when the abdomen is maximally relaxed prior to inspiration. The lower pole of the kidney is then palpable. The left kidney is palpated by using the same maneuver from the opposite side of the patient.[1]

Follow examination of the abdomen by inspection of the external genitalia, including the penis, scrotum, and scrotal contents in the male, and labia, vagina, and urethral meatus in the female. Techniques of examination are discussed in Chapter 9.

Physical examination of the urinary system in the infant, child, or adolescent is completed by observation of the urinary stream whenever feasible. In the infant, urination is typically elicited by exposing the genital area to air or by gently stroking the pubic skin or inner aspects of the thigh. The stream is then observed for caliber, force, and interruption. In the male infant the urinary stream should arch above the penile meatus and travel several inches or more away from the body. Its caliber should approximately that of a pencil lead and should continue, without interruption, until the bladder is emptied. The female infant also produces a stream that clears the labia to form an arch that typically terminates between the legs. Straining or grunting during urination should not occur as the infant empties the bladder.

In the older child or adolescent, observation of the voided urinary stream is completed by hydrating the patient and asking him or her to void into a toilet or electronic urinary flowmeter. The nurse provides the child or adolescent with a quiet and private environment. Assume a position behind and at an oblique angle from the toilet to observe micturition away from the patient's direct line of vision. The patient is then asked to void and the stream is assessed for caliber, force, interruption, and associated straining. The patient should be able to produce an uninterrupted urinary stream approximately the size of a large pencil lead that does not spray between the legs or wet the shoes. The child should complete micturition within 10 to 30 seconds after the stream begins and the adolescent within 60 seconds. It is not unusual for the child to enhance micturition with abdominal straining, but the straining should not be marked or associated with an intermittent stream. Boys may milk the urethra several times after micturition is completed to empty the distal portion of the urethra but should not experience a persistent post-void dribble. The older child or adolescent should report a feeling of complete bladder emptying after voiding is terminated. Table 49-1 summarizes the developmental considerations in the physical examination of the genitourinary system.

Examination of the Neonate

Physical examination of the neonate focuses on delineation of urinary structures and the exclusion of a number of findings that may indicate an urgent or emergent urologic condition. Detection of any of these conditions warrants immediate referral to a physician for detailed evaluation and intervention.

Inspection of the abdomen, pelvis, and genitalia may reveal obvious congenital anomalies that require rapid

TABLE 49-1
Developmental Considerations in the Physical Examination of Genitourinary Function

	Infant	Child	Adolescent
Abdomen			
Inspection	Protuberant (upright and supine position)	Protuberant (upright position only) Concave (supine position)	Concave (upright and supine position)
	Absent scars, rashes, lesions	Absent scars, rashes, lesions	Absent scars, rashes, lesions
	Superficial venous pattern	Superficial venous pattern	Absent venous pattern
	Umbilical cord remnant for first 2 weeks of life	Cutaneous remnant of umbilicus may protrude or remain flush with skin	Cutaneous umbilical remnant may protrude or remain flush with skin
	Absent hernia	Absent hernia	Absent hernia
Percussion	Full bladder percussible above umbilicus	Full bladder percussible near umbilicus	Bladder with 150 ml percussible at suprapubic area
			Bladder with >500 ml percussible at umbilicus
Palpation	Easily palpable	May not be palpable	Rarely palpable
	Absent masses, tenderness	Absent masses, tenderness	Absent masses, tenderness
	Lobulated surface	Smooth surface	
Costovertebral Angle		Absent tenderness	Absent tenderness

care. Exstrophy of the bladder or cloacal exstrophy typically causes great anxiety among parents and may indicate multiple organ system abnormalities that require care. Imperforate anus (absence of anal sphincter tone with prolapse of the rectum) often is associated with urinary system abnormalities, such as rectovaginal fistula, and potentially compromised bladder function. The presence of ambiguous genitalia requires postponement of assignment of a name or other indicators of a phenotypic sex until a genotypic or "assigned" sex is determined (see Unit 18).

Examination of the abdomen in the infant may reveal the presence of an abdominal mass. Approximately one half of abdominal masses in neonates arise from the kidneys, and most are traced to abnormalities of the urinary tract, retroperitoneal area, or genital tract. The most common finding is hydronephrosis due to multicystic or polycystic kidney.[15] Determination of an abdominal mass warrants immediate referral to a physician for detailed evaluation.

Abnormalities found during urine examination or of observation of the infant's urinary elimination patterns also may constitute a urologic emergency. The discovery of gross or microscopic hematuria in the infant's urine may indicate obstruction of the urinary tract, thrombosis of the renal vein or polycystic kidney, tumor, or other abnormality. Each of these conditions requires rapid evaluation and intervention when encountered in the infant.[15]

Observation of an abnormal voided stream or urine elimination pattern also may indicate a urologic condition requiring rapid evaluation and intervention. Micturition should occur within the first 12 to 24 hours in the newborn.[13] Absent urination may indicate a serious abnormality of urine formation, transport, or elimination. The presence of a poor urinary stream associated with straining and distention of the pelvis often indicates bladder outlet

obstruction due to presence of urethral valves, tumor, polyp, or neuropathic bladder.[11,15]

Examination of the Infant and Child

Physical assessment of the infant or child focuses on delineation of physical findings related to a specific complaint and as a screening examination to detect potentially serious conditions that may remain asymptomatic.[4]

General assessment focuses on a determination of renal status and presence of systemic infection or illness. Retarded or slowed growth patterns may indicate insufficient renal function. Infection of the upper urinary tract typically causes the patient to appear acutely distressed with marked fever (101° F or greater) and may be associated with systemic infection or sepsis.

Examination of the abdomen and pelvis may reveal the presence of a mass. Unlike the neonate, an abdominal mass in the child raises the suspicion of malignancy (Wilms' tumor is most common), in addition to the possibility of renal hydronephrosis due to obstructive uropathy or multicystic or polycystic kidney. The presence of a pelvic mass may indicate presence of a full or overdistended bladder relieved by micturition. Persistent mass may indicate the presence of solid tumor such as rhabdomyosarcoma.

Examination of the Adolescent

Examination of the adolescent also centers on detection of physical findings related to a specific complaint and exclusion of findings that indicate potentially serious, undetected conditions. In addition to abnormalities of urine formation, transport, and elimination, adolescents carry a higher risk than younger children for certain urologic abnormalities commonly found among adult populations, such as urinary calculi and sexually transmitted disease.

Because of developmental issues related to privacy and independence, the adolescent may be examined away from the parents. Particular attention is paid even to vague symptoms. The determination of urinary elimination patterns and observation of the voided urinary stream are particularly important when abnormalities are suspected. Thorough examination of the abdomen and pelvis is completed using warm hands and a slow, deliberate approach to relieve anxiety.

Physical examination of the adolescent requires particularly careful evaluation of the genital system as well as the abdomen and pelvis. This evaluation includes assessment of sexual development, determination of sexual behaviors, and detection of signs of sexually transmitted infections. Refer to Chapter 67 for discussion of the examination of the male and female genital tract.

Diagnostic Tests

Laboratory Tests

Laboratory indices of urinary function may be found in Chapter 46, Tables 46-1 and 46-2.

Procedures

Commonly used diagnostic procedures in assessing the urinary system are found in the following section. Procedures have been divided into five major categories, including radiographic studies, ultrasonographic studies, radionuclide studies, cystoscopic examinations, and urodynamic testing. Intravenous pyelogram is described in Chapter 46.

Radiographic Studies

LINEAR TOMOGRAPHY

Description

A series of x-rays that provides a single view of differing linear planes of the kidney. Tomography is typically performed as a part of the intravenous pyelogram (IVP).

Purpose

Linear tomography allows a more detailed anatomic description of the kidney compared with plain-film intravenous pyelography, which gives a summative view of multiple planes of tissue.

Indications

Urinary calculi: The IVP allows assessment of kidney size and position and detection of the size and ratio of renal parenchyma to caliceal collecting system. It also provides data on the size and contour of renal pelves and ureters and gross appearance of the urinary bladder.

Contraindications

All patients who are having IVPs are questioned concerning allergy to iodine-bound contrast media. A history of allergy to shellfish also may provide a clue to potential allergy to contrast material. Significant dehydration or renal insufficiency may contraindicate testing.[7]

Preparation

Informed consent may be required. Bowel preparation for the IVP is begun the night before examination. The patient is typically not allowed to eat solid foods for 6 to 12 hours prior to study.

Developmental Considerations

Infants 12 months of age or less concentrate contrast material poorly. They typically require a greater dosage per kilogram body weight than do older children. Rapid rehydration following evaluation by IVP is indicated to avoid complications.

Nursing Interventions

Explain the procedure to the child and family before testing is begun. Adequate fluid hydration prior to and following test is maintained.

Complications

Related to the IVP portion of the examination:

- Hypersensitivity to contrast material.
- Acute renal insufficiency.

CYSTOURETHROGRAPHY (CYSTOGRAM, VOIDING CYSTOURETHROGRAM)

Description

Serial x-rays of the bladder and urethra following intravesical infusion of an iodine-bound contrast material. The cystogram consists of filling the bladder via a catheter while taking radiographic pictures of the pelvis and abdomen; the voiding cystourethrogram also allows radiographic assessment of the bladder and urethra during micturition.

Purpose

The cystogram provides a detailed anatomic picture of the urinary bladder. Vesicoureteral reflux is detected by the retrograde movement of contrast from the bladder to the ureters or renal pelvis. Inspection of the contour of the ureter and renal pelvis allows grading of reflux (see Chap. 50). Voiding cystourethrography also allows assessment of the urethra during micturition. Anatomic obstruction or disruptions of the urethra may be detected by voiding cystourethrography.

Indications

- Bladder or urethral anomalies.
- Vesicoureteral reflux.
- Voiding dysfunction.
- Recurrent urinary tract infections.
- Febrile urinary tract infection.

Contraindications

Contact allergy to iodine-bound substances.

Preparations

Food and fluids may be consumed prior to voiding cystourethrogram.

Developmental Considerations

None.

Nursing Interventions

Patient must be catheterized for examination unless an indwelling urethral catheter is in place. The need for catheterization and feelings experienced during the procedure are carefully explained to the child prior to testing. Inform the family that catheterization requires preparation of the genital area with a cool liquid soap followed by insertion of lubrication directly into the urethra in selected cases. Insertion of the catheter will cause a temporary sensation of pressure and urethral irritation that should subside when the catheter is in place. Removal of the catheter should cause minimal or no discomfort.

Complications

During the first 24 hours following catheterization, the child may experience magnified sensations of urgency to urinate. Adequate hydration and soaking in a warm bath will relieve this discomfort. Dysuria that persists beyond this period may indicate urinary tract infection and warrants contacting the physician for urine culture and appropriate treatment. Antibiotic prophylaxis following catheterization for cystourethrography is used in select cases at the physician's discretion.

RADIOGRAPHIC EVALUATION OF DIVERSIONS AND URINARY RESERVOIRS

Description

Iodine-bound contrast material may be infused to any surgically created urinary reservoir or conduit (i.e., ileoconduit, Indiana pouch, Koch pouch, ileocecal reservoir, etc.) and serial x-rays taken.

Purpose

Radiographic assessment of a surgically created urinary conduit or reservoir is used to detect reflux from the diversion to the kidneys and provides an assessment of the size and configuration of the diversion. Cinefluoroscopy using provocative maneuvers such as filling with contrast or physical exertion may be used to test the competence of a continent reservoir.

Indications

- Detect morphology of conduit or reservoir.
- Incontinence of continent reservoir.
- Detect and grade reflux in nonrefluxing reservoir.

Contraindications

Contact hypersensitivity to iodine-bound substances.

Preparation

None.

Developmental Considerations

None.

Nursing Interventions

See Cystourethrography. Catheterization of the urinary reservoir is required for infusion of contrast materials, but discomfort is rarely associated with this procedure. Assist the radiologic staff with catheterizations as indicated.

Complications

- Hypersensitivity to contrast material.
- Rupture of reservoir or conduit.

RETROGRADE URETHROGRAM

Description

A series of x-rays of the urethra produced by gentle retrograde injection of contrast material infused via a catheter or syringe placed at the urethral meatus.

Purpose

The retrograde urethrogram is typically limited to male patients. It provides a detailed description of urethral anatomy.

Indications

Used to detect a stricture or diverticulum or diagnose disruption of the urethral prior to catheterization when urinary trauma is suspected.

Contraindications

Contact hypersensitivity to iodine-bound substances.

Preparation

None.

Developmental Considerations

None.

Nursing Interventions

Explain to the child and family that the catheter or catheter-tipped syringe will be placed into the distal urethral meatus. Emphasize that placing the syringe is not analogous to injection of the penis or urethra with a needle or catheterization of the bladder.

RETROGRADE PYELOGRAPHY

Description

X-rays of the ureter and renal pelvis obtained by infusion of iodine-bound contrast material injected directly into the ureters via a retrograde fashion. Access to the ureter is attained by cystoscopic examination with identification and catheterization of the ureteral orifice.

Purpose

Provides a detailed anatomic views of the renal pelvis and ureter. The retrograde pyelogram is currently used less often than more noninvasive procedures such as intravenous pyelography.

Indications

Structural abnormality not completely evaluated by IVP.

Contraindications

Contact hypersensitivity to iodine-bound materials.

Preparation

See Cystoscopy.

Developmental Considerations

See Cystoscopy.

Nursing Interventions

See Cystoscopy. Assess the patient for flank pain, fever, and chills for 48 hours following testing. Obtain urine and blood cultures in consultation with the physician if symptoms occur.

Complications

Pyelonephritis or acute ureteral overdistension of the pelvis and ureter are potential complications of the retrograde pyelogram.

COMPUTED TOMOGRAPHY OF THE URINARY SYSTEM (ABDOMINOPELVIC CT)

Description

A series of transverse tomographic views of specific planes throughout the abdomen, including the urinary system. A computer is used to measure densities of various structures imaged that allows clinicians to distinguish whether structures consist of air, fluid, bone, or solid tissue.

Purpose

CT is used to assess the size and extent of spread of renal and retroperitoneal masses.

Indications

Abdominopelvic CT also is used to evaluate cystic renal disease, inflammatory lesions, or marked hydronephrosis.[5]

Contraindications

Allergies to intravenous injection of contrast material. Certain procedures require intravenous administration of iodine bound contrast materials. When a contrast-enhanced CT is ordered, all patients are questioned concerning allergy to iodine-bound contrast media. A history of allergy to shellfish also may provide a clue to potential allergy to contrast material. Significant dehydration or renal insufficiency may contraindicate testing.[7]

Preparation

For contrast-enhanced CT, informed consent may be required, and bowel preparation is begun the night before examination; otherwise none.

Developmental Considerations

Sedation may be required for the younger child or infant because examination requires the child to lie quietly in a supine position for a prolonged period.

Nursing Interventions

Explain the procedure to the child and family before testing is begun. The procedure is noninvasive unless contrast is injected. Vital signs are monitored during and for the first 1 to 2 hours following use of sedation.

Ultrasonographic Studies

RENAL AND BLADDER ULTRASOUND

Description

Nonradiographic, noninvasive examination of urinary studies using sonographic techniques.

Purpose

Allows examination of the anatomy of the kidneys, ureters, and bladder. Dilated ureters also may be detected. Ultrasound allows assessment of renal parenchyma and caliceal system.

Indications

Assessment of renal size, hydronephrosis, renal tumors, and urinary calculi. It allows approximation of bladder volume before and following micturition and assessment of bladder wall thickness or presence of tumors.

Contraindications

None.

Preparation

None.

Developmental Considerations

None.

Nursing Interventions

Explain the procedure to the child and family, emphasizing that the examination will not hurt and does not require radiation exposure.

Complications

None.

Radionuclide Studies

DTPA SCAN

Description

Serial analog (visual) images and digital data gathered from the kidneys, ureters, and bladder following intravenous injection of a technetium 99m DTPA radionuclide preparation. The substances are rapidly concentrated in the kidneys, reflecting renal perfusion. The kidneys will rapidly clear the material by filtration without significant excretion or tubular retention. Thus, the test allows assessment of renal function reflected by the glomerular filtration rate.[8] A DTPA scan also allows visualization of the ureters and bladder.

Purpose

The DTPA scan produces both analog images of the urinary system and digital data concerning renal perfusion and filtration of the radionuclide. Visual images allow qualitative assessment of kidney size, renal parenchymal mass, and signs of obstruction of the renal pelvis or ureters. Digital readings allow semiquantitative or quantitative assessment of renal vascular perfusion and comparative renal function

(i.e., right kidney function vs. left kidney). Urinary obstruction is assessed by giving furosemide and comparing digital curves of renal washout in response to this potent diuretic. The normal kidney is expected to filter and excrete the radionuclide rapidly, whereas an obstructed kidney continues to collect and concentrate the tracer.

Indications

Urinary obstruction, assessment of right versus left parenchymal function, and glomerular filtration rate may be calculated from the scan.

Contraindications

None.

Preparation

An intravenous infusion may be started either 30 minutes prior to examination to insure adequate hydration before examination or immediately prior to testing to allow injection of the radionuclide material. Intravenous access is maintained during the study to provide access for furosemide administration. A urinary catheter may be inserted for every child who undergoes examination or selectively when vesicoureteral reflux or ureteropelvic obstruction is suspected.

Developmental Considerations

None.

Nursing Interventions

Explain the procedure to the child and family before testing is begun. Adequate oral hydration is maintained during and following examination.

Complications

Infiltration of intravenous infusion site may cause discomfort.

DMSA SCAN

Description

A series of analog images and digital data gathered from the kidneys following intravenous injection of a technetium 99m DMSA preparation. The material is tightly bound to cells of the renal cortex and allows detailed assessment of cortical function.

Purpose

The DMSA scan allows the best assessment of the renal parenchyma and differential kidney function. It is also useful for assessment of renal scarring following upper urinary tract infection. It does not allow visualization of the ureters or bladder.

Indications

- Calculation of differential renal function (most accurate of radionuclide techniques).
- Detection of renal scars.

Contraindications

None.

Preparation

Testing requires intravenous administration of a single bolus of radionuclide material followed by serial images of the kidneys. Catheter placement, prolonged intravenous hydration, or injection of furosemide are not typically used as a part of the DMSA scan.

Developmental Considerations

None.

Nursing Interventions

Explain the procedure to child and family prior to testing.

Complications

Infiltration of intravenous infusion site may produce discomfort.

RADIONUCLIDE CYSTOGRAPHY (NUCLEAR CYSTOGRAM)

Description

Serial images of the bladder and ureters following intravesical infusion of a radionuclide preparation. The most commonly used substance is technetium 99m DTPA.

Purpose

Radionuclide cystourethrography exposes the child to only a fraction of the radiation that a voiding cystogram does. Nonetheless, the anatomic detail of the study is not as detailed as that provided by cystourethrography, and the urethra is not visualized.

Indications

The study is used to detect vesicoureteral reflux but does not allow accurate determination of the extent (grade) of the condition.

Contraindications

None.

Preparation

The child is catheterized, then an infusion of saline into which the radionuclide material is injected follows. Prophylactic antibiotic prophylaxis may be used in selected patients (see Cystourethrography.)

Developmental Considerations

None.

Nursing Interventions

Explain the procedure to the child and family before testing is begun.

Complications

Urinary tract infection.

Cystoscopic Examination

Description

Evaluation of the urethra, bladder wall, trigone, bladder neck, and ureteral orifices using direct visualization via a metal or flexible sheath and fiberoptic technology. Catheterization and injection of the ureters (retrograde pyelogram) may be combined with cystoscopy when indicated.

Purpose

Cystoscopy allows detailed examination of the structures visible within the lower urinary tract, including the proximal urethra, bladder neck, trigone, ureteral orifices, and bladder wall. Its use is weighed against its expense and invasive nature.

Indications

Cystoscopy is used in selected cases of recurrent urinary tract infections, hematuria, vesicoureteral reflux, or when bladder calculi, tumor, congenital anomalies, or foreign bodies are suspected. Its role in children with neuropathic or idiopathic bladder dysfunction remains unclear.[6]

Contraindications

Current urinary tract infection.

Preparation

The child typically can take nothing by mouth for the night preceding testing. Examination is completed in the operating suite or in an adjacent cystoscopic suite. The patient is placed in a lithotomy position, draped in a sterile fashion, and prepared with a povidone-iodine solution. A metal or flexible sheath is gently inserted into the bladder through the urethra. Fluid is infused throughout the procedure, and the bladder is regularly drained as it fills.

Developmental Considerations

The infant or child is typically examined under general anesthesia or with spinal anesthesia and systemic sedation.

Nursing Interventions

Fully explain the procedure before testing is begun. Following examination, the child may experience mild dysuria that is relieved by repeated urination and adequate hydration. Transient, mild hematuria often occurs but should cease after the first 24 to 48 hours following assessment.[3]

The patient is monitored for fever and chills, which indicate potential upper urinary tract infection. Blood or urine cultures are obtained if symptoms occur.

Complications

Febrile urinary tract infection.

Urodynamic Testing

SIMPLE URODYNAMIC ASSESSMENT: VOIDING DIARY

Description

The voiding diary is a paper-and-pencil tool used to determine urine elimination patterns.

Purpose

The voiding diary is used to assess patterns of urinary elimination and incontinence. It gives a more accurate assessment of functional capacity than does complex urodynamic testing.

Indications

The voiding diary is used to establish a working diagnosis of instability, stress, overflow, or continuous incontinence.

Contraindications

None.

Preparation

None.

Developmental Considerations

Parents must be recruited to maintain diary for younger children or toddlers.

Nursing Interventions

The voiding diary is completed by the child, parent, or nursing staff. Different tools are used that give varying amounts and kinds of information. Evaluate the goals of assessment, the environment that data will be gathered in, and the motivation of the person(s) who will gather and record these data.[10] Choose an appropriate form based on this assessment. A simple take-home diary may include the volume of fluid consumed and the volume and time voiding occurs (see Fig. 49-1). Incontinence is typically indicated by a check mark. Fully explain the procedure and gain the child and family's cooperation before beginning assessment. Provide the patient's family with multiple copies of the diary, a graduated container to collect and measure voided or catheterized urine volumes, and a simple instruction sheet for using the diary. Instruct the patient to maintain the diary for a 2- to 4-day period, including a week day and weekend day whenever feasible. If data are collected within the hospital or inpatient environment, use nursing staff to supervise data collection. A more complex form may be chosen based on the goals of assessment and availability of professional staff to assist in data collection (Figs. 49-2 and 49-3).

Complications

None.

DATE	INI	TREATMENT	TIME		DATE		DATE		DATE		DATE		DATE	
						in.		in.		in.		in.		in.
ord.		Bladder Program		I.C.										
				Reflex										
				Foley/Void										
d.c.				I.C.										
				Reflex										
				Foley/Void										
ord.				I.C.										
				Reflex										
				Foley/Void										
d.c.				I.C.										
				Reflex										
				Foley/Void										
				I.C.										
				Reflex										
				Foley/Void										
				I.C.										
				Reflex										
				Foley/Void										

FIGURE 49-2
Bladder Program Flowsheet. This voiding diary compares indwelling catheter, intermittent catheterization (IC) program, voided, and reflex voiding volumes. This diary is used for spinal cord–injured subjects, and data are compiled by the nursing staff. It is particularly useful for comparing volumes generated via reflex or spontaneous voiding versus volumes generated from catheterized residuals. (Courtesy of the Shepherd Spinal Center, Atlanta, GA 30309.)

COMPLEX URODYNAMIC TESTING

Description

Urodynamics is a set of tests used to measure lower urinary tract function during bladder filling and micturition. Urodynamic testing typically consists of a cystometrogram, which assesses bladder pressure as a function of volume during bladder filling and voiding; an electromyogram of the pelvic floor muscles; and urinary flow study. Urodynamic assessment may be combined with simultaneous radiographic assessment of the bladder and urethra (see Cystourethrography). Urethral pressure also may be assessed. Drugs are occasionally given to assess their effect on bladder function.

Purpose

Urodynamics offers a quantitative and semiquantitative of lower urinary tract function. Bladder filling is assessed via the cystometrogram combined with an electromyogram. This combination of tests allows assessment of functional bladder capacity, proprioceptive sensations of bladder filling, and compliance of the bladder wall in response to passive filling and stability of the detrusor. The electromyogram offers clues to the sphincter response to bladder filling. Further information regarding urethral closure pressure during filling is obtained when the cystometrogram-electromyogram is combined with continuous urethral pressure measurement. A screening assessment of micturition is obtained by measuring the urinary flow. A more complete assessment is obtained by combining urinary flow measurement with bladder contraction pressures and electromyogram.

Indications

Complex urodynamics is indicated in cases of neuropathic bladder dysfunction, dysfunctional voiding states due to unknown causes, and urinary retention due to obstruction or deficient detrusor function.

Contraindications

- Current urinary tract infection.
- Acute pain rendering patient immobile.

Preparation

The child is asked to arrive for assessment with a full bladder if feasible. An initial urinary flow study is then completed prior to any catheterization procedure. The child will be catheterized for a cystometrogram, which will be uncomfortable (see Cystourethrography). A tube may be placed in the rectum. Advise the patient that placement of the rectal tube will not hurt but may give a feeling of passing gas. The tube is not expected to produce a bowel movement. The electromyogram of the pelvic floor muscles is done via patch electrodes or needle or hooked-wire electrodes. Patch electrodes are noninvasive but less accurate than needle or hooked-wire electrodes, which require one or two needle sticks for proper placement. The urethral pressure study requires a second catheterization. Prophylactic antibiotics are often given following testing.

Developmental Considerations

Urodynamics can be performed on all age groups when sufficient nursing and technical expertise is available.

Nursing Interventions

Fully explain the testing procedure to the child and family before assessment is begun.

Complications

Urinary tract infection.

Selected Nursing Diagnoses

Nursing diagnoses are based on findings from the nursing assessment, physical examination, and diagnostic studies. The defining characteristics assist in identifying the nursing diagnoses. Selected nursing diagnoses associated with

(text continued on page 1242)

Program: _____

Fluid Restrictions: _____

Comments (ie, urgency, cognition): _____

_____

_____

_____

_____

_____

Date: _____

INTAKE graph (vertical axis: 600, 550, 500, 450, 400, 350, 300, 250, 200, 150, 100, 50, 0)

TIME: 2300, 2400, 0100, 0200, 0300, 0400, 0500, 0600, 0700, 0800, 0900, 1000, 1100, 1200, 1300, 1400, 1500, 1600, 1700, 1800, 1900, 2000, 2100, 2200, 24-HOUR TOTAL

TOTAL

INSTRUCTIONS:

1. Graph volume of fluid intake and urinary output using the following code:
2. Code: INTAKE = black dots
   - OUTPUT = void = black dots
   - v = spont
   - s = stim when both obtained
   - CATH = black x's
   - PVR's to be graphed on the same time coordinate as spont void or incontinent
   - INCONT = "+" or "0" in designated block at base of output graph
   - + = large 0 = small
3. Approximate time to closest hour
4. Approximate amount to closest cc

OUTPUT graph (vertical axis: 700, 650, 600, 550, 500, 450, 400, 350, 300, 250, 200, 150, 100, 50, 0)

INCONT

TIME: 2300, 2400, 0100, 0200, 0300, 0400, 0500, 0600, 0700, 0800, 0900, 1000, 1100, 1200, 1300, 1400, 1500, 1600, 1700, 1800, 1900, 2000, 2100, 2200, 24-HOUR TOTAL

TOTAL

FIGURE 49-3

Rehabilitation Bladder Program Record. A more complex voiding diary compares voided volume, catheterized volume, and fluid intake in a chart format. It is useful for determining urine elimination patterns following catheterization during acute illness or a neurologic insult. (Courtesy of Emory University Hospital, Atlanta, GA.)

TABLE 49-2
Selected Nursing Diagnoses Associated With Altered Urinary Function

Data Analysis and Conclusion	Nursing Diagnosis
Health Perception and Health Management	
Change in laboratory values; relapse in condition; poor hygiene habits; lack of adaptive behaviors; lack of financial resources	Altered Health Maintenance, related to knowledge deficit regarding physiologic condition
Nutrition and Metabolism	
Weight loss; poor appetite; low serum protein; pale conjunctival and mucous membranes; poor muscle tone; loss of hair; proteinuria	Altered Nutrition: Less Than Body Requirements, related to inability to absorb nutrients due to physiologic factor
Elimination	
Urinary frequency; urgency; nocturia	Altered Urinary Elimination, related to abnormal pattern of urinary elimination
Urinary incontinence; sensory deficit; dexterity deficit; inadequate privacy; inadequate lighting	Functional Incontinence, related to involuntary or uncontrolled leakage of urine influenced by environmental and functional factors
Urinary incontinence, absent sensations of bladder filling; detrusor instability; absent urge to void	Reflex Incontinence, related to uncontrolled leakage of urine associated with neurologic lesions above the sacral micturition center but caudal to the pontine micturition center
Urinary incontinence associated with physical exertion; urinary urgency; urinary frequency	Stress Incontinence, related to physical exertion such as coughing or exercise
Continuous urinary leakage not associated with urgency or physical exertion leakage of urine; unsuccessful bladder control training; nocturia; unawareness of incontinence	Total Incontinence, related to extraurethral leakage of urine from a fistulous opening in the urinary system
Urgency; urinary frequency; nocturia; urinary incontinence; detrusor instability; preservation of detrusor-sphincter coordination	Urge Incontinence, related to uncontrolled leakage of urine associated with a marked desire to urinate caused by detrusor instability
Poor force of urinary stream; hesitancy when initiating stream; urinary frequency; nocturia; dribbling incontinence; urinary residual (>100 ml or 20% of total bladder volume)	Urinary Retention related to incomplete bladder emptying after micturition caused by deficient detrusor function
Activity and Exercise	
Decreased strength; inability to get to toilet; severe pain; inability to undress; inability to carry out proper toileting hygiene	Toileting Self-Care Deficit, related neuromuscular impairment
Fatigue; dyspnea; increased pulse rate; inability to attend school; inability to walk far; decrease in physical activities	Activity Intolerance, related to physiologic defect
Sleep and Rest	
Nocturia; verbal complaint of lack of sleep; verbal complaint of interrupted sleep; increasing lethargy and listlessness; yawning; lack of concentration	Sleep Pattern Disturbance, related to voiding urgency at night
Self-Perception and Self-Concept	
Refusal to look at or touch part of body with defect; verbalization of negative feelings about self; refusal to attend school; refusal to socialize with peers	Body Image Disturbance, related to physiologic defect
Verbalization of lack of control over situation and future; depression over condition; non-compliance in monitoring progress; alienation from others; anger	Powerlessness, related to chronic condition
Roles and Relationships	
Verbalizes concerns about other family members; anger; fear; anxiety; alienation from professional care givers	Parental Role Conflict, related to interruption of family life caused by child's hospitalization
Inability to attend school; confined to hospital room; withdrawal; no eye contact; depression; regression; infrequency of family visits	Social Isolation, related to hospitalization
Sexuality and Reproduction	
(Adolescent) verbalizes problems; physical defect prohibits sexual intercourse; value conflicts; friend of opposite sex does not visit; seeks confirmation of desirability	Sexual Dysfunction, related to biopsychosocial alteration of sex
Coping and Stress Tolerance	
Anger taken out on health care workers; withdrawal; inability to meet basic needs; inability to problem solve; inappropriate use of defense mechanisms; regression	Ineffective Individual Coping, related to lack of maturity in handling situation
Neglect of child; infrequent visits; arrives late for visits; does not keep promises; inability to accept medical diagnosis; agitation; hostility	Disabling Individual Family Coping, related to parent's inability adequately to express personal concerns

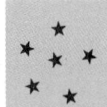

Ideas for Nursing Research

Under the current nursing diagnosis framework, dysfunctional voiding states are described by the general label of Altered Urinary Elimination or by more specific labels such as Stress or Reflex Incontinence. This system often makes establishing a proper diagnosis difficult in the clinical setting. Altered Urinary Elimination fails to define any specifics of an abnormal condition and is useful only as a preliminary diagnosis until further assessment is completed. Nursing research can help identify a simpler, clearer diagnostic taxonomy for dysfunctional or abnormal voiding states that derives its conclusions from data gathered by nursing assessment strategies. Such a taxonomy will assist nurses to identify, refine, and evaluate interventions designed to relieve patients who suffer adverse effects of altered urinary function. Ideas for nursing research related to assessment of urinary system function include the following:

- The role of the voiding diary in the assessment of urinary incontinence.
- The accuracy (sensitivity and specificity) of the voiding diary in detecting an unstable bladder (urge or reflex incontinence) versus complex urodynamics.
- The role of complex urodynamic testing in the prediction of upper urinary system distress or compromised function.
- The role of observation of voided stream versus assessment of the uroflow tracing.
- The implications of urinary incontinence and enuresis in the school-age child and adolescent.

altered genitourinary function are presented by function in Table 49-2.

Summary

The assessment of the child with altered urinary function is derived from historical information from the child and family, physical examination, and data from laboratory and diagnostic testing. Determining appropriate nursing diagnoses requires ongoing synthesis and evaluation of assessment data that are reflected in a nursing care plan that addresses symptoms arising form a urologic abnormality and the impact exerted by this condition on the patient's overall biophysical and psychosocial health.

References

1. Bates, B. (Ed.). (1991). *A guide to physical examination* (5th ed.). Philadelphia: Lippincott.
2. Gordon, M. (1991). *Manual of nursing diagnosis.* St. Louis: Mosby.
3. Gray, M. L., & Broadwell, D. C. (1989). Genitourinary system. In J. M. Thompson, G. K. McFarland, J. E. Hirsch, S. M. Tucker, & A. C. Bowers (Eds.) *Mosby's manual of clinical nursing* (2nd ed.). St. Louis: Mosby.
4. Hoekelman, R. A. (1991). The pediatric physical examination. In B. Bates (Ed.), *A guide to physical examination* (5th ed.). Philadelphia: Lippincott.
5. Hoffman, A. D. (1992). Uroradiology: Procedures and anatomy. In P. Kelalis, L. King, & A. Belman (Eds.), *Clinical pediatric urology* (3rd ed.). Philadelphia: Saunders.
6. Kroovand, R. L. (1992). Cystoscopy. In P. Kelalis, L. King, & A. Belman (Eds.), *Clinical pediatric urology* (3rd ed.). Philadelphia: Saunders.
7. Lerner, J., & Khan, Z. (1982). *Manual of urologic nursing.* St. Louis: Mosby.
8. Majd, M. (1992). Nuclear medicine. In P. Kelalis, L. King, & A. Belman (Eds.), *Clinical pediatric urology* (3rd ed.). Philadelphia: Saunders.
9. Malasanos, L., Barkhaus, V., Moss, M., & Stoltenberg-Allen, K. (1990). *Health assessment* (4th ed.). St. Louis: Mosby.
10. Norton, C. (1986). *Nursing for continence.* Beaconsfield, England: Beaconsfield.
11. Parrott, T. S., & Woodard, J. R. (1976). Urologic surgery in the neonate. *Journal of Urology, 116,* 506–508.
12. Seidel, H. M., Ball, J. B., Dains, J. E., & Benedict, W. E. (1991). *Mosby's guide to physical examination* (2nd ed.). St. Louis: Mosby.
13. Sherry, S. N., & Kramer, I. (1955). The time of passage of first stool and urine by the newborn infant. *Journal of Pediatrics, 46,* 158.
14. Spinetta, J., & Deasy-Spinetta, P. (1981) *Living with childhood cancer.* St. Louis: Mosby.
15. Woodard, J. R. (1992). Neonatal and perinatal emergencies. In P. C. Walsch, R. F. Gittes, A. D. Perlmutter, & T. A. Stamey (Eds.), *Campbell's urology* (6th ed.). Philadelphia: Saunders.

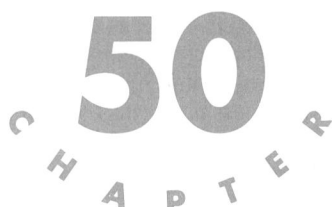

Nursing Planning, Intervention, and Evaluation for Altered Urinary Function

50
CHAPTER

BEHAVIORAL OBJECTIVES

Identify three anomalies of the upper urinary tract.

List the most common urologic disorders associated with the prune belly syndrome.

List the discharge teaching issues related to the care of the infant with spinal bifida and neuropathic bladder following neurosurgical closure of the myelodysplastic defect.

Apply knowledge of the pathophysiology of urinary obstruction to the care of the child with retention due to ureteropelvic junction obstruction.

Describe three management options for enuresis in a school-age child.

Describe the postoperative nursing care of the toddler who undergoes ureteroneocystostomy for vesico-ureteral reflux.

Differentiate between the signs and symptoms of lower and upper urinary tract infections.

Describe the medical and surgical treatment options for a Wilms' tumor.

Abnormal urinary function in the infant, child, or adolescent occurs as a result of tumor, obstruction, or infection of the urinary system or as a response to congenital anomaly. Medical management of children with altered urinary system function attempts to alleviate or ablate the factors causing distress to urinary function. The nursing management of these children centers on physical and psychosocial care during periods of illness caused by urologic abnormality and on strategies that enable the affected child and family to moderate their behavior and environment to maximize overall health and minimize the adverse effects of a dysfunctional urologic condition.

Congenital Anomalies

Anomalies of the Kidneys

Definition and Incidence. A congenital anomaly of the kidney occurs when adverse conditions influence renal embryogenesis. Anomalies of number exist when a child has one or more than two kidneys. *Renal agenesis* exists when no trace of kidney tissue can be identified. Unilateral agenesis is the absence of a single kidney. Its absolute incidence is unknown. Bilateral renal agenesis is the absence of any kidney tissue and is incompatible with life. It most commonly occurs as a feature of Potter's syndrome. *Supernumerary kidneys* exist when more than two anatomically complete kidneys develop. They are the rarest of all the renal congenital anomalies.[30]

Anomalies of position exist when the kidneys fail to ascend and rotate into their normal retroperitoneal location. A *malrotated kidney* is typically turned along its vertical axis from its normal position of 90 degrees relative to the spinal column (Fig. 50-1). It occasionally results in compromised urinary system function due to obstruction. The *pelvic or sacral ectopic kidney* is located in the true pelvis or the space created by the pelvic bone. In certain instances the pelvic kidney does not interfere with urinary function and may remain undetected. A pelvic kidney is clinically significant when it is accompanied by structural abnormalities that interfere with urine formation and transportation. The absolute incidence of clinically significant pelvic kidneys is unknown. An *intrathoracic kidney* is even rarer than a pelvic kidney. It rarely causes significant urologic abnormality.

Anomalies of *renal fusion* exist when the kidneys share a common plane of tissue. A horseshoe kidney, or fusion of two kidneys joined by an isthmus of tissue that crosses the midline, is the most common form. It is associated with abnormal renal function only when accompanied by structural defects of the pelvis or ureteral course. In certain instances, a kidney will cross over the spine to the contralateral side. In many instances, the congenitally crossed kidney will fuse with its partner, forming a condition called *crossed fusion ectopia*.[30]

Etiology and Pathophysiology. The etiology of renal agenesis remains unclear. The development of the kidney was discussed in Chapter 48. Congenital agenesis of the kidney occurs when the process is arrested or never begins. It is unclear whether absence of the ureteric bud or an intrinsic defect in the metanephric tissue is primarily responsible.[30]

The pathophysiology of unilateral renal agenesis arises from abnormalities of the remaining kidney, which also may be affected by the pathologic process that caused the contralateral kidney to fail to develop. A solitary kidney in a child with renal agenesis may be malrotated or ectopic. The remaining kidney will undergo compensatory hypertrophy or enhanced growth in an attempt to overcome the reduced mass of nephrons available to filter the blood. Urinary function is significantly compromised when structural abnormalities cause obstruction, hydronephrosis, and abnormalities of the remaining kidney. Renal agenesis also may be associated with nonurologic anomalies of the genitalia, gastrointestinal tract, and skeletal and cardiovascular systems. It is a well-recognized feature of certain multisystem syndromes.[30]

The etiology of the malrotated or ectopic kidney is unknown. Abnormalities of ascent and rotation may occur because of ureteral bud or metanephric pathology as well as genetic, vascular, or teratogenic factors. Most commonly, however, anomalies of renal position are associated with abnormal development of the vertebral bodies.[51]

The pathophysiology of ectopia and malrotation anomalies arises from structural abnormalities that affect the upper urinary tract. Rotation of the kidney on its vertical axis may result in obstruction and hydronephrosis. These factors place the kidney at increased risk for urinary stasis, infection, and compromised parenchymal function.[30]

Malrotated, ectopic kidneys also are at increased risk of vesicoureteral reflux and associated nephropathies. Up to 50% of all pelvic or sacral ectopic kidneys are difficult to detect with intravenous pyelography (IVP) because of compromised renal function.[30]

The pathophysiologic process that produces an anomaly of one kidney's position also may affect the contralateral side. The ureter of the contralateral, normally positioned kidney is more likely to enter the renal pelvis at an abnormally high position, causing poor drainage of calices with chronic urinary stasis and hydronephrosis. In addition, the contralateral kidney is at greater risk for multicystic defect with compromised renal function.

The intrathoracic kidney is most commonly found among males on the left side. The rare instances of intrathoracic kidneys have not been associated with the high incidence of structural abnormalities characteristic of pelvic ectopia.[30]

The etiology of renal fusion anomalies also remains unclear. The pathologic process that leads to fusion probably occurs during early embryonic development. Pathophysiologic changes in urinary function arise when fusion is associated with structural or vascular abnormalities. The most common form of fusion, horseshoe kidney,

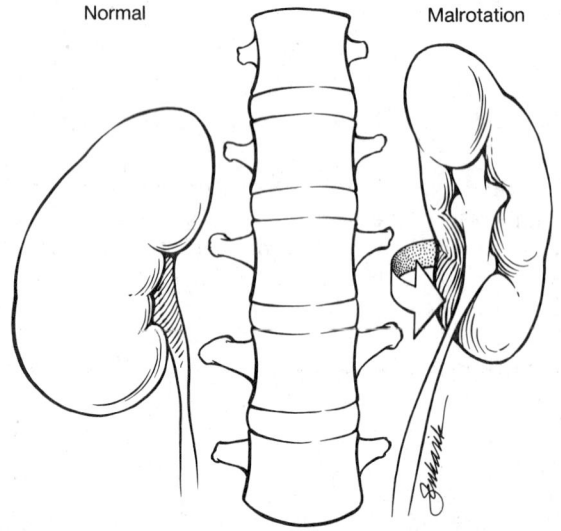

FIGURE 50-1
Malrotation of the kidney.

is always associated with malrotation of the kidneys and may be associated with ectopia. Horseshoe kidney may be noted as a feature of a multisystem syndrome or genetic defects. Affected infants often die, although the renal anomaly is rarely fatal. Other children may have completely normal renal function and a horseshoe kidney that remains undetected except as an incidental finding. Between one third and two thirds of all children with horseshoe kidneys have associated genitourinary anomalies. Ureteral duplication, cryptorchidism, and anomalies of the urethra are most common. Congenital anomalies of the cardiovascular, skeletal, and gastrointestinal systems also may accompany horseshoe kidneys but are typically milder than those associated with renal ectopia.[30] Horseshoe kidneys also are at increased risk for development of Wilms' tumor.[48]

Clinical Manifestations. Renal anomalies are detected when obstructive uropathy or symptoms of compromised renal function produce clinically apparent infection, pain, or signs of end-stage kidney disease. Bilateral renal agenesis is noted in a neonate with multiple congenital anomalies that rapidly lead to death. Anuria and abnormal genitalia are common findings, although death typically occurs due to respiratory failure. Unilateral renal agenesis is most commonly detected during assessment of a febrile urinary tract infection characterized by flank pain, fever, nausea, vomiting, and dysuria that occurs during the first 5 years of life. A child with significantly compromised renal function due to an abnormal remaining kidney may present with failure to thrive or other signs of renal failure.[30] Multiple congenital anomalies also provide a clue to the possibility of renal agenesis.

An ectopic or pelvic kidney also becomes clinically apparent when structural abnormalities compromise urinary function. Hydronephrosis is a common finding and may be detected as a lower abdominal mass on physical examination or by urinary tract imaging studies when obstructive uropathy is suspected. An ectopic kidney also may be detected during evaluation of urinary tract infection. Many pelvic kidneys are detected during routine urinary tract assessment in the presence of multiple congenital anomalies. In other instances, deteriorating renal function and failure to thrive may lead to detection of renal ectopia.

The horseshoe kidney typically presents with one of two scenarios. It may be associated with multiple congenital anomalies requiring evaluation of the urinary system. In other instances, structural or vascular abnormalities may cause infection and pain due to obstruction or hypertension due to vascular abnormalities or poor renal function.[30]

Renal anomalies are most commonly identified by radiographic imaging studies performed for evaluation of urinary tract infections.

Diagnostic Evaluation. Renal anomalies are most commonly identified by radiographic imaging studies performed for evaluation of urinary tract infections. Diagnostic evaluation for renal agenesis includes the following examinations and tests. Physical examination will reveal an abdominal mass with hydronephrosis or Potter's

facies noted with bilateral agenesis. Other congenital anomalies may be present. Laboratory findings include a normal or elevated serum blood urea nitrogen (BUN) and creatinine if bilateral agenesis is present. Imaging studies are helpful in the diagnosis: kidney, ureter, and bladder (KUB) radiographic examination reveals an absence of renal shadow on the affected side; IVP reveals an absence of concentration and secretion of fluid on affected side, compensatory hypertrophy (symmetric enlargement without hydronephrosis), of the contralateral kidney, *or* hydronephrosis of the contralateral kidney with or without evidence of poor function (delayed concentration of contrast material). In the DTPA radionuclide scan, there is absent function on the affected side, normal function of the contralateral kidney, or evidence of obstruction when challenged by furosemide (Lasix) injection. In the renal ultrasonography, there is an absent renal image on the affected side, enlarged pole-to-pole measurement of contralateral kidney (compensatory hypertrophy), or hydronephrosis. Vascular supply is absent on the affected side in renal arteriography.

In ectopic kidney, the physical examination may reveal an abdominal mass with hydronephrosis. Genital or other congenital anomalies may be present. Serum BUN and creatinine are normal unless both kidneys are dysplastic. In imaging studies, KUB reveals an absent renal shadow in the retroperitoneal space of the affected side; the shadow may be detected in the intrathoracic space or true pelvis. On the IVP, the location of the affected kidney is aberrant (pelvis or lower thoracic space) with evidence of poor function in 50% of pelvic kidneys; rotation of kidney on vertical axis is common. If there is a contralateral kidney, normal function or hydronephrosis and evidence of poor function is present. A short, straight ureter appears on the affected side or is dilated, with evidence of upper urinary tract obstruction. Renal ultrasonography reveals absence of renal image in peritoneal space of affected side; renal shadow may be undetectable because of bony pelvis or overlying ribs. An asymmetric hemitrigone appears on the affected side during cystoscopic examination.

Physical examination is unremarkable or reveals presence of other congenital anomalies when the client has a horseshoe kidney. Laboratory findings include normal or elevated serum BUN and creatinine with renal dysplasia. In the KUB, there is a renal isthmus shadow crossing the midline. IVP reveals malrotation of the renal axis bilaterally, with lower poles in closer proximity than upper poles, and either normal concentration of contrast material or varying degrees of renal atrophy with poor concentrating ability on the affected side. Atypical ureteral course is anterior to the kidney. Hydronephrosis may be detected. A voiding cystourethrogram is normal or marked by vesicoureteral reflux. A renal ultrasonography reveals presence of isthmus. Hydronephrosis may be detected. Computerized tomography (CT) scan also shows the presence of the isthmus. On the arteriography, an abnormal vascular supply appears on the affected side.

★ ASSESSMENT

The nurse combines knowledge of anatomic and functional studies of the urinary tract with assessment of the child's bladder elimination function, past history of potential or documented urinary tract infections, and general health to evaluate the severity of the anomaly on the child's function and general well-being.

The nurse obtains a careful history of any past urinary tract infections and of febrile episodes due to unclear causes. This information may implicate a prior history of compromised urinary function with infection. The parents are asked to identify what signs and symptoms they believe indicate potential urinary tract infection; the nurse assesses the accuracy of their responses. The child's voiding habits are explored and compared with developmental norms. A child who experiences altered urinary elimination patterns for his or her age group is further assessed by use of a voiding diary to elucidate potential neuropathic or functional bladder disorders that may influence urologic function in the presence of a renal anomaly.

The child's general health and growth and development are evaluated. Significantly compromised renal function causes generally poor nutritional intake and compromised growth. In contrast, acute renal insufficiency in the presence of obstruction and an anomalous urinary system will produce rapid weight loss with nausea, vomiting, and potential fluid volume abnormalities, often in conjunction with a febrile urinary tract infection.

The child is assessed for coexisting congenital anomalies of the genital, skeletal, and gastrointestinal systems. The nurse is particularly sensitive to abnormalities of the reproductive system remembering that genital anomalies (urethral duplication with abnormal voiding, undescended testis, rudimentary or abnormal uterus and vagina) are found in many children with unilateral renal agenesis, ectopic or pelvic kidneys, or horseshoe kidney.

★ NURSING DIAGNOSES AND PLANNING

Based on the assessment data from above and the preceding chapter, the following nursing diagnoses may apply:

- High Risk for Infection, related to chronic disease.
- High Risk for Fluid Volume Deficit related to deviations affecting absorption of fluids.
- Fluid Volume Excess related to compromised regulatory mechanisms.
- Altered Nutrition: Less Than Body Requirements related to inability to absorb nutrients.
- Altered Growth and Development related to effects of physical disability.
- Altered Urinary Elimination related to urinary obstruction.

Other functionally related nursing diagnoses are given in Table 49-2 in Chapter 49.

The nurse and child (or parents) work together to plan effective care based on the established nursing diagnoses. Several examples of expected outcomes are as follows:

- The child participates in safe sports activities.
- The child maintains adequate fluid intake.
- The family consults a nutritionist for an appropriate diet.
- The family states the signs of urinary tract infection.

The nurse plans for the daily care of the child based on both physician's orders and nursing diagnoses. Some

general nursing care goals for restoring renal function may be the following:

- Adequate protein intake is maintained.
- Renal function is preserved.
- Urinary drainage is restored.
- Infection is prevented or eliminated.

★ INTERVENTIONS: COLLABORATIVE AND INDEPENDENT

Management of a renal anomaly is determined by the extent to which it compromises urinary function. In many instances, the anomaly is associated with a normal contralateral system and remains asymptomatic. The nurse explains to the child and family that a person with a single kidney is expected to live a normal life. The family is advised that adequate protein intake necessary for normal growth and development should be provided despite advice in the popular literature promoting limited protein intake for persons with a single kidney. The family also is advised that evidence exists that *excessive* protein intake should be avoided because it may compromise renal function over a prolonged period.[7] Refer the family to a nutritionist as indicated for advice concerning an appropriate diet.

Consult the physician concerning the advisability of participating in contact sports. Football, rugby, wrestling, and other contact sports are typically avoided because of the potential of trauma to a solitary or ectopic kidney. Remind the child and family that adequate exercise is, nonetheless, encouraged and that sports such as track, swimming, and baseball carry less risk of injury and fulfill needs for exercise, recreation, and competition.

In other instances, urinary system function is compromised from the time the child presents for care. In this case the principal goal of management is the restoration of urinary drainage and transport and preservation of renal function. These children typically present with a febrile urinary tract infection and may have urosepsis. Immediate care is aimed at eradicating infection, reducing the fever, and reversing associated dehydration and electrolyte and nutritional deficits. Intravenous fluids containing dextrose and appropriate electrolytes are begun. Broad-spectrum, parenteral antibiotic therapy is instituted in accordance with medical orders, and urine is collected for culture and sensitivity reports.

An appropriate antipyretic is given to reduce fever, which may exceed 102° F. Vital signs are monitored every 2 to 4 hours, and the child is closely assessed for signs of septic shock (hypotension with cool, clammy skin and disorientation) until the fever subsides. Following report of the urine culture and sensitivity and reduction of fever, the child is placed on a single, oral antibiotic agent. Intravenous fluid therapy is discontinued in consultation with the physician and when the child is able to tolerate food.

Following immediate care for the presenting urinary tract infection, the urinary system is assessed for structural defects. Urinary obstruction causes stasis of urine that predisposes the child to infection, and compromised renal function and vesicoureteral reflux cause reverse peristalsis of infected urine from bladder to kidney, which may cause pyelonephritis. Surgical interventions may be used to repair a structural anomaly of the upper urinary tract, or a severely defective kidney may be removed, particularly if it is associated with hypertension or infection or contributes less than 15% of total renal function. (Refer to "Obstructive Uropathies" in this chapter for discussion of nursing care related to upper urinary tract obstruction.)

In other instances, structural urologic abnormalities may not require surgical reconstruction, and conservative measures are used to prevent and treat infection. The nurse teaches the parents measures to prevent infection, including adequate fluid intake, and to recognize the signs of lower and upper urinary tract infection, should they occur. These include painful urination, change in the odor of urine, change in urine color and consistency, and presence of fever or abdominal or pelvic discomfort. The family is taught to seek medical care for urine culture if infection is suspected and to alert nurses and physicians of the potential for urinary tract infection if their child is evaluated by clinicians unfamiliar with the child's history.

Children with a solitary kidney and otherwise normal function are taught to monitor themselves for signs and symptoms of urinary tract infection. They are advised to have annual blood pressure checks and assessment of the upper urinary tracts if suboptimal function of the remaining kidney or structural abnormality is found on initial evaluation.

★ EVALUATION

The nurse and family periodically evaluate the outcomes and criteria. Examples of expected outcomes for kidney anomalies were given under "Nursing Diagnoses and Planning" in this section. Have short-term goals been met? Are long-term goals still realistic? Planning for further nursing care also takes into consideration complications and long-term care.

COMPLICATIONS

Urinary tract infection is often the first clinically apparent complication of a renal anomaly. The infection is typically severe and involves the upper urinary tract, causing fever. Advanced cases of upper urinary tract infection may be complicated by systemic bacterial infection, which rapidly leads to septic shock and death if not promptly treated.

Compromised renal function also may complicate a renal anomaly. The kidney may be congenitally dysplastic and contain immature, nonfunctioning renal tissue or develop parenchymal scars from infection. Once a certain mass of renal tissue is damaged, the kidney begins predictable course of steadily declining function and failure.[8]

LONG-TERM CARE

The long-term management of children with a renal anomaly focuses on maintaining the long-term health of functioning renal tissue. The family of a child with recurrent urinary tract infections also must learn to recognize and act when signs of cystitis occur. They are followed by annual evaluation of the upper urinary tracts and serum creatinine test. Their growth and development is assessed annually, and their diets may be monitored on an ongoing basis by a clinical nutritionist in consultation with a nephrologist.

Children who present with irreversibly compromised kidney function are referred to a nephrologist for ongoing care related to end-stage renal disease.

Anomalies of the Renal Pelvis and Ureter

Definition and Incidence. Anomalies of the renal pelvis and ureter arise when the development and migration of the ureteric bud is arrested or prevented (Fig. 50-2). A *bifid renal pelvis* is the division of the renal pelvis into two compartments that fuse at the ureteropelvic junction (UPJ; see Fig. 50-2*A*). It occurs in as many as 1 in 10 live births and does not compromise urinary function.

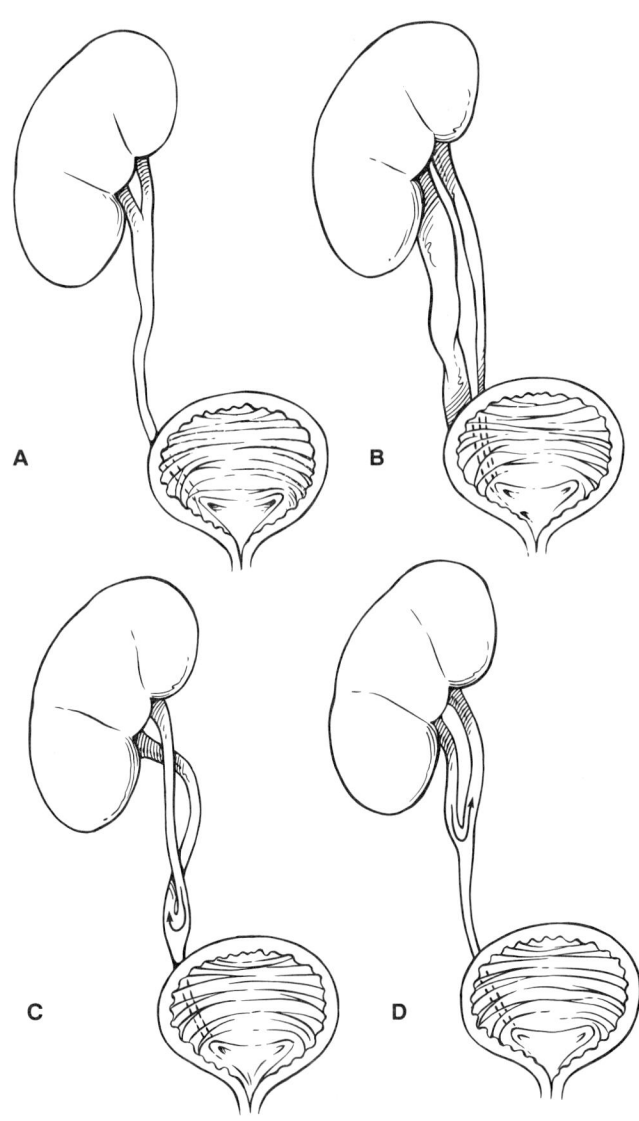

FIGURE 50-2

Several anomalies of the ureteral pelvis and ureter. (**A**) Bifid renal pelvis. (**B**) Complete ureteral duplication. (**C & D**) Incomplete ureteral duplication: (**C**) V-shaped duplication. (**D**) Y-shaped duplication with yo-yo peristalsis.

Ureteral duplication is divided into two forms: complete and incomplete. *Complete ureteral duplication* is the existence of two ureters that originate from a single kidney and terminate into the bladder via distinct orifices (see Fig. 50-2*B*). Each ureter has its own pelvis and drains a separate pole of the kidney. *Incomplete ureteral duplication* exists when a ureter with a single orifice bifurcates into two branches somewhere along its course from kidney to bladder. Bifurcation of the lower third of the ureter is most common. It is called a "V" shaped ureter, whereas division of the upper ureteral segment forms a "Y" shaped ureter[31] (see Figs. 50-2*C* and *D*).

Incomplete or complete ureteral duplications are the most common of all urologic anomalies. Duplication anomalies are more commonly found in girls, and bilateral duplication anomalies are not uncommon.[31]

Ureteral ectopia occurs when the ureter terminates into a structure other than the trigone.[31] Ectopic ureters may terminate into the bladder neck, prostatic urethra, seminal vesicle, or ejaculatory duct in males and bladder neck, distal urethra, or vestibule in females. They rarely open into the rectum. Ectopic ureters are more common in females, and approximately 70% are associated with duplication anomalies, with the upper ureteral segment at greater risk.

A *ureterocele* occurs when the ureter ends in a cystic dilation that protrudes into the bladder vesicle. Two forms of ureterocele, simple and ectopic, occur. A *simple ureterocele* may represent a congenital anomaly or acquired condition. The orifice lies in a normal position within the lateral aspect of the trigone. An ectopic ureterocele also arises from the terminal portion of the ureter to protrude into the bladder lumen (Fig. 50-3). It is "ectopic" because it arises from a ureter whose orifice does not terminate

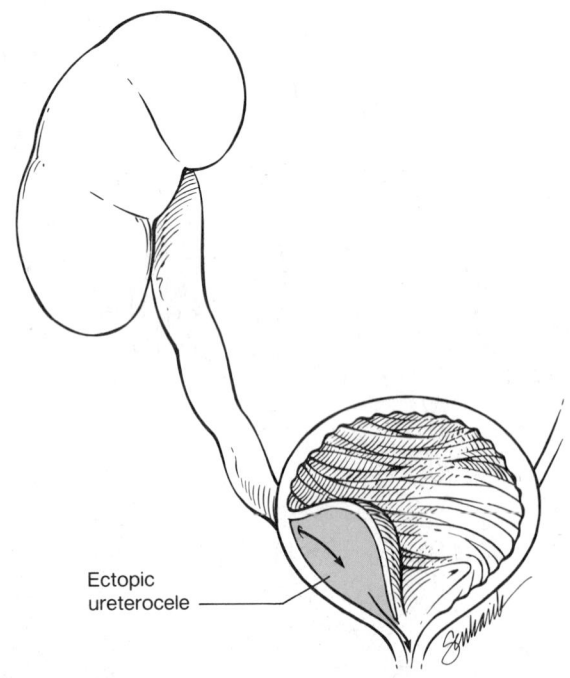

FIGURE 50-3
An ectopic ureterocele is one in which the ureter terminates and protrudes into the bladder lumen.

into the trigone. The incidence of ureterocele is not known.

Etiology and Pathophysiology. The etiology of the bifid renal pelvis is unknown. The condition occurs when division of the caliceal system of the developing kidney extends into the renal pelvis.

The etiology of ureteral duplication anomalies also remains incompletely elucidated. An autosomal dominant gene may place certain persons at increased risk for duplication anomalies.[31]

Many duplicated ureters pose no threat to the urinary system and are treated as a variant of normal. Duplicate ureters are clinically significant when they obstruct the drainage of the upper urinary tracts or are associated with vesicoureteral reflux and infection. Ureteral duplication anomalies are sometimes associated with obstruction, particularly when complicated by a ureterocele.

More commonly, complete duplication anomalies are complicated by vesicoureteral reflux. The lower segment is particularly susceptible to reflux because it is laterally placed in relation to the ectopic ureter and often enters the bladder wall via a straight rather than oblique course. Reflux rarely involves both ureters.

Incomplete ureteral duplication arises when a single ureteric bud divides during development, creating an aberrant branch. It can occur at any time during ureteral development. Affected children are at increased risk of upper urinary tract infection because of stasis and reverse peristalsis. Flank pain may be produced by rapid fluid ingestion with resulting intermittent obstruction and overdistention of the renal pelvis.[31]

Ureteral ectopia arises from an abnormality in the embryonic development of the terminal portion of the wolffian duct. During normal development, the ureter forms a convex loop that tilts toward and fuses with the urogenital sinus. In contrast, the ectopic ureter arises from a point more cephalad along the metanephric tissue, causing it to cling to the duct longer than normal. The ectopic ureter becomes transposed to the normally placed ureter and is carried more toward the bladder neck or developing reproductive system and genitalia. An ectopic ureter is often associated with ectopic ureterocele and complete duplication anomaly.[51]

Pathophysiologic effects on urinary function are influenced by the location of the ureteral orifice and the presence of associated ureterocele. Infection also is associated with ectopic ureterocele. If the ureteral orifice inserts into the proximal urethra, continence is maintained but the ureter is obstructed, placing the urinary tract at increased risk of stasis and infection. In boys the ureter may open into the membranous or, more commonly, into the prostatic urethra, also causing obstruction. The ectopic ureter is typically dilated and refluxes because it does not tunnel through the bladder wall.[51]

The etiology of simple and ectopic ureteroceles remain unclear. Simple or "adult" ureterocele was once thought to be an acquired condition. More recently, evidence has been introduced that supports the theory that simple ureterocele is, indeed, a congenital anomaly.[63]

Infection and obstruction may accompany simple ureterocele and compromise urinary function. The ureterocele is rarely large enough to obstruct the bladder outlet, but ureteropelvic obstruction as well as reflux and associated urinary tract infection are sometimes noted.[13]

An ectopic ureterocele may be associated with infection, obstruction, and renal dysplasia. Urinary tract infection is particularly severe in young infants; high fever and renal failure are often presenting symptoms. Among older children, hematuria and signs of lower urinary tract infection are more likely.[31] Obstruction and renal dysplasia also are associated with ectopic ureterocele.

Clinical Manifestations.   Congenital anomalies of the renal pelvis and ureter are noted when complications occur. The bifid renal pelvis may remain undetected throughout a person's life or present as an incidental finding during urologic evaluation for unrelated pathology.

Incomplete or complete ureteral duplications also may remain undetected or may present only as an incidental finding during urologic investigation for unrelated pathology. Clinically significant duplex ureteral systems most commonly present as urinary tract infection. Signs and symptoms of obstruction (flank pain, fever, vomiting) also may occur.

Ectopic ureters may present as incontinence or infection. The urinary leakage is typically continuous and dribbling in nature and superimposed on an otherwise normal voiding pattern. Girls with ureteral ectopia may experience a continuous, watery vaginal discharge if the ureteral orifice is located in the vestibule. Ectopic ureters that are located within the sphincter mechanism may present with signs and symptoms of obstruction.

A simple ureterocele or small ectopic ureterocele may not produce any significant disturbance in urinary function and remain silent throughout childhood or be detected only as an incidental finding. Urinary tract infection is the most common presenting complaint of clinically significant ureteroceles. The infection may be severe and associated with fever and hematuria. Infants may present with signs of acute renal insufficiency (vomiting, fever, failure to thrive). The urinary frequency, urgency, and urge incontinence sometimes associated with ureterocele often arises from associated cystitis rather than structural defects of the sphincter mechanism or neuropathic instability incontinence, although sphincter incompetence may be noted. Urinary retention and difficulty emptying the bladder may associated with ectopic ureteroceles.[31]

Diagnostic Evaluation.   A bifid renal pelvis may remain undetected because the physical examination is unremarkable and laboratory findings are normal. An IVP shows duplication of the renal pelvis and absent obstruction.

The diagnosis of a ureteral duplication usually is made during urologic investigation for infection or multiple congenital anomalies. Physical examination is unremarkable and laboratory findings are normal in incomplete ureteral duplication. The IVP may show an accessory ureteral branch that branches from a single orifice in the bladder, "Y" anomaly of ureter (aberrant branch at proximal one third of ureter) or "V" anomaly (aberrant ure-

teral branch near ureterovesical junction). Ultrasound shows ureteral dilation on the affected side, and cystoscopic examination reveals a single ureteral orifice on the affected side.

In complete ureteral duplication, there is an unremarkable physical examination or signs of urinary tract infection. Serum creatinine and BUN are normal or elevated if renal function is compromised because of dysplasia or infection. IVP shows complete duplication of the ureter from the vesical orifice to the renal pelvis of the affected kidney. The superiorly placed ureteral branch will drain the lower pole of the kidney, and an inferiorly placed pole will drain the upper pole. Lower pole ureterohydronephrosis and upper pole reflux are commonly observed. A voiding cystourethrogram reveals reflux into the lower pole. Ectopic ureterocele may be noted. Dilation of the collecting system of the lower pole is shown in ultrasound. DTPA radionuclide scan shows poor drainage of the lower pole of the affected kidney following furosemide challenge if UPJ or lower ureteral obstruction is present. Cystoscopic examination reveals duplication of ureteral orifices on the affected side. Ectopic ureterocele is commonly associated, and reflux is often noted.

In ectopic ureter, the physical examination is unremarkable, or there may be signs of urinary tract infection with fever and obstruction. Laboratory findings are normal. IVP reveals a ureter that opens into a structure other than the bladder base (trigone). There is dilation and obstruction of the affected system if the ureter terminates at prostatic or membranous urethra. Cystoscopic examination identifies the ureteral orifice at the bladder neck with proximal urethra, or the orifice may be absent from bladder or urethra.

Physical examination in a simple ureterocele is unremarkable, or there may be signs of urinary tract infection. IVP is unremarkable for obstruction. Cystogram reveals cystic dilation of the lower ureteral segment with a spherical filling defect at the bladder base. Cystoscopic examination reveals cystic dilation of the terminal ureteral segment with the ureteral orifice located in bladder base.

Ectopic ureter and ureterocele are typically present in the context of a urinary tract infection, often associated with signs of obstruction. Diagnosis of ectopia and ureterocele are made by radiographic imaging study. The physical examination is unremarkable or there may be a cystic swelling near the urethral meatus or anterior vaginal wall. A normal or elevated serum BUN and creatinine with compromised renal function are shown as a laboratory finding. In IVP, a complete ureteral duplication anomaly is revealed. Hydronephrosis and ureteral dilation are common, and poor function with renal dysplasia may occur. In a voiding cystourethrogram, there is a larger cystic dilation at the bladder base than that associated with simple ureterocele; reflux into the ureter draining lower pole is common. Ultrasound reveals dilation of the lower pole on the affected side, with small pole-to-pole renal size noted with dysplasia. DTPA radionuclide scan indicates an obstruction of the upper pole with ectopia of the lower ureter on the affected side. DMSA radionuclide scan reveals a compromised or scarred renal parenchyma of the upper pole resulting from infection or obstruction. Cystoscopic examination reveals cystic dilation of the terminal ureteral segment. The ureteral orifice is ectopic in location (bladder neck).

★ ASSESSMENT

Nursing assessment of the infant or child with ureteral duplication involves evaluation of the severity of the anomaly and its probable influence on urinary function. This evaluation is completed in consultation with the physician and is based on data collected from radiographic and functional studies of the upper urinary tracts. Three urologic problems are associated with ureteral duplication anomalies: (1) reflux, which is most common in the lower pole ureter of a complete duplication anomaly; (2) obstruction of the upper pole ureter if it opens in the bladder neck or proximal urethra; or (3) incontinence if the upper pole ureter opens distal to the urethral sphincter mechanism. Assessment of these problems is discussed in "Obstructive Uropathy," "Altered Urinary Elimination: Voiding Dysfunction," and "Vesicoureteral Reflux" later in this chapter.

Nursing assessment of the child with a simple ureterocele requires evaluation of its effects on urinary function. The urologic problems associated with simple ureterocele are reflux on the affected side and obstruction of the bladder neck. The nursing assessment of these conditions is discussed in "Obstructive Uropathies" and "Vesicoureteral Reflux" later in this chapter.

Nursing assessment of patients with ectopic ureter or ureterocele focuses on identification of altered urinary function in the presence of a congenital anomaly and evaluation of its effects on the child's growth and development.

★ NURSING DIAGNOSES AND PLANNING

Based on the assessment from the previous section and the preceding chapter, the following nursing diagnoses may apply:

- Anxiety related to surgery and results.
- High Risk for Infection related to reflux.
- Pain related to surgical procedures.
- Altered Urinary Elimination related to surgery.
- Urinary Retention related to obstruction.

Other functionally related nursing diagnoses are discussed in Table 49-2 in Chapter 49.

The nurse and child (or parents) work together to plan effective care based on the established nursing diagnoses. Several examples of expected outcomes are as follows:

- The child and family discuss goals of surgery and results.
- The child expresses comfort from pain relief therapy.

The nurse plans for the daily care of the child based on both physician's orders and nursing diagnoses. Some general nursing care goals for restoring urinary function may be the following:

- Postoperative urine will be pink or light red.
- Adequate hydration and nutrition are supported postoperatively.
- Renal function is preserved.

★ INTERVENTIONS: COLLABORATIVE AND INDEPENDENT

The nurse reassures the family that a bifid renal pelvis is a variant of normal and will not produce altered urinary function. Further counsel the family that altered urinary function present when bifid renal pelvis is detected is due to anomalies other than the bifid pelvis.

Management of the child with incomplete ureteral duplication focuses on treatment of associated conditions of reflux, urinary tract infection, and obstruction. The nursing care of these patients is discussed in "Urinary Tract Infection," "Obstructive Uropathy," and "Vesicoureteral Reflux" later in this chapter.

Management of the patient with ectopic ureter and ureterocele is complex because these anomalies typically coexist and are usually accompanied by a complete duplication anomaly. Because the affected renal pole and collecting system are significantly abnormal, surgery is usually required to restore acceptably normal urinary function. The surgical approach to these children is not straightforward. The affected upper renal pole is typically dysplastic and often a source of infection. It rarely contributes significantly to total renal function, and removal is often justified. In addition, the associated ureterocele contributes to obstruction of the bladder outlet as well as dysplasia of the affected upper renal pole. Reflux of the affected or adjacent ureter also may occur.[31]

Surgical options include heminephrectomy (removal of the affected renal pole and ureter), with excision of a portion of the associated ureterocele if the upper renal pole is not salvageable, or ureteropyelostomy (surgically joining the upper pole collecting system into the lower pole renal pelvis with removal of the lower pole ureter near the bladder) when the upper pole parenchyma is salvageable. Surgical reconstruction also extends to the lower urinary tract. In certain instances, decompression of a ureterocele with heminephrectomy of the upper pole and partial ureterectomy may be sufficient to cause spontaneous diminution of the ureterocele and spontaneous correction of associated reflux over a period of months. In other instances, open surgical excision of the ureterocele with reimplantation of refluxing ureters is required, particularly when the ureterocele is large and the associated reflux severe.[53]

If the child is acutely ill due to febrile urinary tract infection and compromised renal function, the ureterocele may be simply "unroofed" or incised and allowed to drain using a transurethral approach. Unroofing a ureterocele offers the advantage of avoiding surgery for the child already compromised by infection and renal insufficiency but fails definitively to correct the structural abnormalities that originally led to urologic disease. The effect of unroofing a ureterocele is to reverse urinary stasis and infection caused by obstruction at the bladder base. Unfortunately, reflux of the unroofed ureter almost inevitably occurs, which itself may lead to further infection and renal damage.[53]

PREOPERATIVE CARE IN RECONSTRUCTION OF THE UPPER URINARY TRACT

Prior to surgery of the upper urinary tract, the family and child are given a simple explanation of goals of surgery.

The nurse emphasizes that surgery is expected to maximize function of the child's viable urinary system by removing the most severely affected, anomalous tissue. Reassure the toddler or preschool boy experiencing castration anxiety that the surgery will not harm his penis. Advise the family that the surgical incision will be located at the affected flank or abdomen. Older children and adolescents may require shaving from nipples to the midthigh of the affected side.

POSTOPERATIVE CARE

Following surgery, the child will return to the nursing unit with a flank or abdominal dressing, urethral catheter, and intravenous fluid line. A Penrose or other wound drain also may be present in the wound. The nurse routinely assesses the incisional dressing for signs of excessive bleeding, urine output, or infection. Because the pelvocaliceal system of the diseased pole is separate from the lower pole, the wound should not produce copious urine output, although frequent dressing changes may be needed to protect the wound from irritation due to serosanguineous drainage. Inform the physician of the presence of copious urinary drainage from the wound because this finding may indicate loss of integrity of the surgically repaired kidney.

The nurse monitors urine output on an hourly basis during the first 12 to 24 hours following surgery and every 4 to 8 hours until the Foley catheter is removed. Hematuria is expected during the initial postoperative period, and the color of the urine will be pink or light red. The physician is promptly contacted if excessive bleeding with bright-red output and clots is noted. Markedly decreased or absent urine output may indicate obstruction of the Foley catheter. Consult the physician concerning gentle irrigation of the catheter with saline if these signs occur.

Intravenous fluids are administered during the initial postoperative period to maintain adequate hydration and for nutritional support. Bowel sounds may be absent or reduced for a brief period following nephrectomy because of irritation to the retroperitoneum. Assess the child for return of normal bowel sounds, and offer oral fluids in consultation with the physician. Intravenous fluids are discontinued after the child is able to tolerate oral fluids and solid foods.

The nurse assesses the child for evidence of postoperative pain and determines the source of the pain. The nurse is alert for nonverbal indications of pain in a child or infant and uses an assessment tool specifically designed for eliciting information about pain. Intermittent cramping pain located in the suprapubic area is typically caused by bladder spasm. The nurse checks for catheter patency and consults the physician concerning administration of medications.

Gastrointestinal pain presents as intermittent, cramping discomfort throughout the abdomen. Oral fluid and food intake are avoided until bowel irritation subsides. Occasionally, a nasogastric tube is used to relieve marked pain.

Incisional pain presents as a dull, aching discomfort. The nurse restricts excessive movement and uses proper positioning to relieve incisional pain. Analgesics are administered as indicated in consultation with the physician.

Assist the child regularly to cough, turn, and deep breathe to avoid potential pulmonary complications following heminephrectomy, especially if a flank incision is used. The nurse auscultates the child's chest daily following surgery and promptly notifies the physician if congestion and fever or purulent sputum from the respiratory passages are noted.

Following removal of the catheter, the child is monitored for reinstitution of normal voiding habits. The nurse encourages the child to drink an adequate volume of fluid and maintains a record of voided volumes and fluid intake.

PREOPERATIVE CARE IN RECONSTRUCTION OF THE LOWER URINARY TRACT

Reconstruction of the lower urinary tract may require simple unroofing of the ureterocele or open surgery and ureteroneocystostomy (reimplantation of the ureters). Refer to "Vesicoureteral Reflux" later in this chapter for a discussion of nursing interventions for the child undergoing reimplantation of the ureter.

The child and family are given a brief explanation of the surgical procedure and its goals. The nurse reinforces the concept that the unroofing procedure is not a definitive cure but a temporizing measure designed to decompress the ureterocele and prevent further damage to the urinary system until definitive surgical correction can be completed. The family is reminded that unroofing a ureterocele is expected to cause the affected ureter to reflux and that prophylactic antibiotics and routine follow-up assessment are essential. The male preschooler or toddler is reassured that the surgery will not harm his penis.

POSTOPERATIVE CARE

Nursing management following unroofing of a ureterocele centers on the control of hematuria, prevention of infection, and preservation of renal function. The surgical procedure is typically performed in a cystoscopic suite. The child is placed under general anesthesia, and a sheath (metal catheter used to introduce telescopes and other cystoscopic instruments into the bladder) is inserted into the bladder through the urethra. The ureterocele is visualized, and its protuberant wall is trimmed until it is flush with the bladder wall.

The child returns to the nursing unit with a Foley catheter in place; an intravenous line may or may not be present. The child should experience minimal discomfort following unroofing of a ureterocele associated with bladder wall irritability and instability (uncontrolled detrusor contractions). The urine output is monitored from the catheter for evidence of hematuria. The urinary output should be pink or light red to yellow. Bright-red blood and clots are not expected and warrant consultation with the physician. Intravenous fluids are discontinued after the child is able to tolerate oral liquids, typically the same day as the surgical procedure. The child may be discharged the following day unless urinary tract infection or compromised renal function justifies further in-hospital therapy.

★ **EVALUATION**

Periodically, the nurse and family evaluate the outcomes and criteria. Examples of outcome criteria for anomalies of the renal pelvis and ureter were given under "Nursing

Diagnoses and Planning" in this section. Have short-term goals been met? Are long-term goals still realistic? Planning for further nursing care also takes into consideration complications and long-term care.

COMPLICATIONS

The principal complications associated with ureteral anomalies are urinary tract infection, obstruction, and diminished renal function. The management of these complications is discussed above.

LONG-TERM MANAGEMENT

The long-term nursing management of children with ureteral anomalies center on the prevention and management of associated vesicoureteral reflux, infection, and compromised renal function. Refer to "Obstructive Uropathy," "Urinary Tract Infection," and "Vesicoureteral Reflux" in this chapter and Chapter 47 "Nursing Interventions of Children with Alterations in Renal Function" for discussion of nursing care related to these conditions.

Anomalies of the Bladder: Exstrophy and Epispadias

Definition and Incidence.   Exstrophy is a spectrum of anomalies that affect the urinary tract, genitalia, and bony pelvis. Among the forms of exstrophic anomalies, 30% are epispadial with anomalous opening of the urethra, 10% are cloacal exstrophies with externalization of

the bladder and portions of the gastrointestinal tracts, and 60% are classic exstrophy anomalies, characterized by externalization of the posterior bladder wall in the present of an epispadial urethra. Classic exstrophy is a rare anomaly, occurring in approximately 1 in 30,000 live births. It occurs in boys three times more often than in girls and is associated with a variety of other anomalies.[66]

Etiology and Pathophysiology.   The etiology of bladder exstrophy remains unclear. During the third week of gestation, the cloacal membrane is bordered by primitive genital tubercles. By the fourth week, the anterior portion of the cloacal membrane retracts from the umbilical cord, allowing development of the anterior abdominal wall caudal to the umbilicus.[10] Failure of separation of the cloacal membrane causes the genital tubercles to complete an anomalous coalescence with an externalized bladder or epispadial or open urethra and diastasis, or abnormal separation, of the symphysis pubis.

Separation of an abnormally large cloacal membrane prior to partitioning of the cloacal pouch by the urorectal septum will produce cloacal exstrophy, causing the cloaca to remain externalized in conjunction with an exstrophic, bifid bladder separated by ileocecal bowel.[15]

Epispadias without externalization of the bladder, a milder form of exstrophy, occurs when the overdeveloped or persistent cloaca causes splaying of the bladder neck and urethra. Although any portion of the urethra may be affected by the anomaly, the most common form of epispadias is "complete," characterized by sphincter incompetence and continuous urinary leakage.

Clinical Manifestations.   In *classic exstrophy*, the exstrophied bladder appears as a grossly obvious mass of red tissue of the suprapubic area leaking urine through an open urethra. The symphysis is separated; the severity of the diastasis correlates with the size of the exstrophied bladder.[15] Associated congenital anomalies are common.

In cases of *complete epispadias* without exstrophy, the bladder remains an internal organ, although the urethra is laid open (Fig. 50-4). When epispadias involves the glandular urethra, the glans penis is split dorsally and the meatus is located in an abnormally proximal location at the coronal sulcus. If the penile urethra is involved, the splayed dorsal groove extends to the urethral meatus located between the symphysis pubis and coronal sulcus. In other cases, the entire penile urethra is affected and the splayed dorsal groove extends over the penile course with an obviously incompetent meatus located at the pubopenile junction.[27]

Diagnostic Evaluation.   Exstrophy and epispadias are evident on physical examination. There is a red bulging mass in the midline of the suprapubic area. The urethra is detubularized (splayed open) to the bladder neck, and there is diastasis of the symphysis pubis. Laboratory findings are normal. An IVP is normal or reveals ureterohydronephrosis if the exstrophy is not closed during infancy.

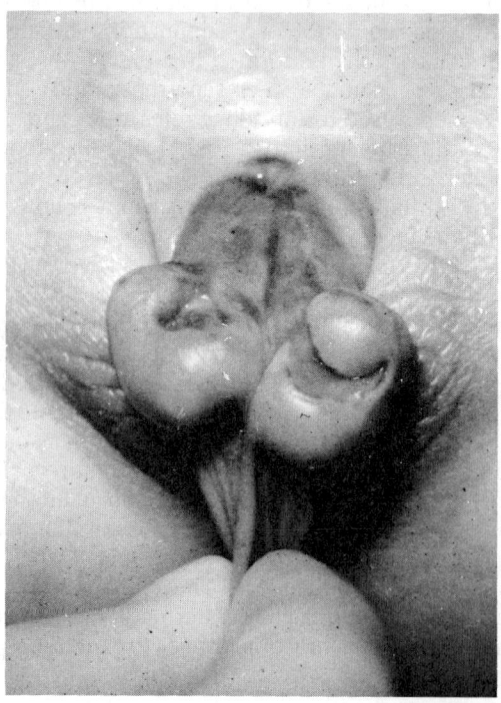

FIGURE 50-4

Isolated epispadias without exstrophy. The bladder neck is intact in this child, and urinary continence is good but not excellent. Note also the incomplete duplication of glans. (From Avery, G. B. [1987]. *Neonatology: Pathophysiology and management of the newborn* [3rd ed.]. Philadelphia: Lippincott.)

★ ASSESSMENT

Nursing assessment of exstrophy focuses on the severity of the anomaly and the extent to which urinary function is compromised. The most profound dysfunction caused by exstrophy is a complete loss of the bladder's ability to store urine due to both externalization of the posterior wall and deformities of the urethral sphincter mechanism. Assessment of the child's urine elimination patterns will reveal continuous leakage due to outlet incompetence and loss of vesicle integrity. The nurse also assesses the exposed bladder mucosa for evidence of thickening or irritation and consults with the physician to gain understanding of upper urinary tract function.

The nurse assesses the family's response to the presence of a disfiguring congenital anomaly. They are questioned regarding their knowledge of medical plans and their perceptions of their infant. The nurse reassures the family that, with corrective surgery, restoration of a relatively normal appearance of the genitalia is expected. Explore their plans for care of the infant during the prolonged period during which repair occurs, and ask them to identify support in their extended family or social network.

★ NURSING DIAGNOSES AND PLANNING

Based on the assessment data from above and the preceding chapter, the following nursing diagnoses may apply:

- Preoperative
  - Family Coping: Potential for Growth related to disfiguring anomaly.
  - Altered Mucous Membrane related to exposed bladder epithelium.
  - High Risk for Infection related to inadequate primary defenses.
  - Altered Urinary Elimination related to the anomaly.
- Postoperative
  - Altered Urinary Elimination related to upper tract deterioration.
  - Urinary Retention related to obstruction.
  - High Risk for Infection (urinary tract) related to surgical trauma.
  - Body Image Disturbance related to urinary incontinence.
  - High Risk for Impaired Skin Integrity related to urinary incontinence.
  - Pain related to initial postsurgical voiding.

Other functionally related nursing diagnoses are discussed in Table 49-2 in Chapter 49.

The nurse and child (or parents) work together to plan effective care based on the established nursing diagnoses. Several examples of expected outcomes are as follows:

- The parents discuss their reaction to disfiguring anomaly.
- The parents demonstrate aptitude in cleansing area and drying the skin with hair dryer on warm.
- The child obtains urinary continence.

The nurse plans for the daily care of the child based on both physician's orders and nursing diagnoses. Some general nursing care goals may be the following:

- The exposed bladder mucosa is protected from contamination and trauma.
- Urinary output reflects preoperative level.
- Continuous incontinence is resolved or reduced.

★ INTERVENTIONS: COLLABORATIVE AND INDEPENDENT

PARENTAL SUPPORT

Initial nursing interventions center on assisting the family to cope with the realities of a child with a disfiguring congenital anomaly. The affected family members often have feelings of alarm and revulsion toward the child's disfigurement, which is likely to generate feelings of guilt and shame. The nurse assists the family to cope with this crisis by reassuring the family that their anxiety and revulsion are a response to the child's anomaly rather than the child as a human being.

The nurse explains that the anomalies are repairable with a staged surgical approach, immediate consultation with a pediatric urologist will occur, and reconstructive surgery is expected to produce an aesthetically acceptable appearance and to restore acceptable bladder and reproductive function.

The family is assisted in identifying sources of support within the medical community, their extended family, and social network as they learn to cope. The parents are helped to identify a counselor to deal with feelings of anxiety, guilt, or shame if the crises associated with the birth of a baby with bladder exstrophy compromises or disables normal coping mechanisms.

Educate the family that exstrophy is not a genetic defect. Advise the affected family that the chances of producing another child with exstrophy are low as are the chances that this child will produce a baby with exstrophy.[57]

PREVENTION OF TRAUMA

Nursing care of the affected infant focuses on protecting the exposed bladder mucosa prior to initial surgical closure. The mucosa is susceptible to contamination with environmental pathogens and trauma from shearing and pressure. The nurse places the child in a temperature-regulated Isolette without clothing to reduce friction against the bladder mucosa. The affected area is covered by a piece of Silastic or plastic wrap to reduce trauma produced by movement against Isolette linen.[15]

Because the exstrophic bladder continuously leaks urine, the nurse protects the adjacent skin with daily cleansing and thorough drying of the skin, using a dryer on its lowest setting, and by applying a moisture barrier such a Desitin ointment or a skin sealant such as Bard Protective Barrier Film, United Skin Prep, Hollister Skin Gel, or a benzoin preparation.[22]

PREVENTION OF INFECTION

Because the child is susceptible to urinary tract infection, the nurse routinely assesses the child for signs of urinary tract infection, change in urine odor, or unexplained fever. The physician is consulted promptly to obtain a urine culture if symptoms appear.

SURGICAL MANAGEMENT

Three management plans may be used for the child with bladder exstrophy. The anomaly may be left unrepaired and the child treated with a urinary containment system. Associated complications such as infection and trauma to the exposed bladder mucosa are managed as they arise. Unfortunately, this approach has a number of distinct disadvantages that render it unacceptable: a disfiguring anomaly that significantly compromises the child's self-esteem and body image; lifelong continuous urinary incontinence; and compromised sexuality and sexual function. Nonsurgical management also carries a significant risk of urinary tract infection and ongoing trauma to the exposed bladder mucosa that will ultimately undergo squamous metaplasia and a significant risk of adenocarcinoma during the second or third decades of life.[10]

Two surgical options exist for the repair of bladder exstrophy: urinary diversion or primary repair closure. Urinary diversion offers the advantage of allowing closure or removal of the anomalous bladder and preserves the upper urinary tracts for a number of years. However, with refinements in staged surgical repair of exstrophy, urinary diversion has become undesirable because of persistent incontinence, and greater risk of upper urinary tract deterioration over time.[10]

The most attractive alternative remains the staged surgical repair of the defect because it restores more nearly normal urinary and genital anatomy and function, promoting optimal growth and development. The goals of primary surgical closure of the exstrophied bladder are to internalize the exposed mucosa and reapproximate the symphysis pubis followed by repair of the epispadias designed to render the sphincter competent and the child continent.[10]

The initial surgical repair ideally occurs during the first week of life but may be postponed as long as 6 months in certain instances. The exstrophied bladder is closed, but the epispadias and incompetent bladder neck are left untouched to preserve upper urinary tract function until more extensive lower tract reconstruction is feasible. In addition, attention is directed to the closure of the abdominal wall and approximation of the symphysis pubis.[10]

PREOPERATIVE CARE IN INITIAL SURGERY

Prior to surgery, the nurse reviews the goals of the procedure with the family. The parents are advised that the procedure will include complete reapproximation of the urethra in girls and urethral reconstruction and penile lengthening in boys. They are further advised that the procedure is *not* expected to produce continence and that the infant will continue to experience continuous urinary leakage per urethra due to sphincteric incompetence.

The nurse informs the parents that the child will return from the surgical suite with a suture line where the exstrophied bladder was located, a suprapubic catheter, and intravenous fluid line in a peripheral venous site. The older infant who undergoes iliac osteotomies will have an apparatus for immobilization of the pelvic bone.

POSTOPERATIVE CARE

The upper urinary tracts are drained via ureteral catheters placed during surgery that empty into the bladder, which is, in turn, drained via a suprapubic tube. The suprapubic tube provides temporary drainage for the newly closed bladder and protects the reconstructed urethra from trauma. The nurse monitors the urine output for excessive bleeding and volume. The urine will be yellow or pink and should not contain bright-red blood or clots. Gross hematuria is reported promptly to the pediatric urologist because the neonate or infant cannot tolerate prolonged blood loss as well as the older child or adult.

The urinary output from the newly closed bladder should reflect preoperative levels. A decline in urine output may indicate blockage of a ureteral catheter with obstruction of the upper urinary tracts or blockage of the suprapubic tube. The nurse routinely assesses the patient for signs of urinary obstruction (flank or abdominal tenderness or mass, vomiting, and decreasing urinary output) and reports findings promptly to the physician.

The surgical wound will be closed by sutures and may contain a drain. The wound may produce serosanguineous fluid but should not drain excessive amount of urine. The wound and drain are monitored by the nurse for signs of infection (edema, erythema, purulent discharge) and for excessive urine output. The dressing is changed as needed, and a skin barrier or protective skin sealant is applied to prevent irritation from wound exudate.

The older infant who undergoes osteotomies with primary bladder closure will have a pelvic demobilization device in place; mobility is limited but not obliterated by use of the device. The nurse assists the parents in positioning and holding their child as appropriate. The nurse provides care appropriate to the device used. The infant is assessed for pain, and the nurse determines the location and cause of the pain. Intermittent, unstable contractions of the bladder (spontaneous, uncontrolled detrusor contractions often referred to as "bladder spasms") may produce a sudden cramping pain that is intense but of short duration. Nonverbal indications of pain (crying, changes in body posture and expressions) are likely to be associated with leakage of urine around the catheter. Unstable contractions are produced by bladder irritability or overdistention.

The nurse helps the child reduce pain by reducing excessive movement and environmental stimuli and consults the physician concerning analgesics and antispasmodics for bladder spasms.

Intravenous fluids are administered during the initial postoperative period. Small amounts of clear liquids are offered; intravenous therapy is discontinued when the child is able to tolerate oral fluids.

CARE BETWEEN FIRST- AND SECOND-STAGE REPAIR

During the period between primary closure of the exstrophied bladder and repair of the bladder neck, the child experiences continuous urinary leakage from the epispadic urethra. The nurse teaches the parents to monitor the child for signs and symptoms of urinary tract infection and to intervene promptly if infection occurs. Refer to "Urinary Tract Infection" in this chapter for nursing care of the child with predisposition for infection.

The nurse assists the parents in prevention of skin breakdown caused by urinary incontinence. Advise the parents that their child is particularly prone to altered integrity of the pelvic skin because of constant urinary exposure. Assist them to develop a program for daily cleansing of affected skin areas with complete drying using a dryer at lowest heat setting and for application of a skin sealant or moisture barrier as indicated. Advise the family to seek care if a rash develops in the perineal area that does not respond to their care regimen within 3 to 5 days.

SECOND-STAGE SURGICAL REPAIR

Bladder neck reconstruction compromises the second-stage surgical reconstruction for the child with exstrophy and the primary reconstruction for the child with classic epispadias. Because the care is markedly similar, both are discussed in this section.

Bladder neck reconstruction for the epispadic child is typically undertaken during the third to fifth year of life. This delay serves several useful purposes: it allows the bladder to gain a capacity of 60 to 90 ml and allows the parents to adjust to the concept of intermittent catheterization, should it be necessary.

The Young-Dees-Leadbetter procedure is commonly used for second-stage exstrophy or primary epispadias repair.[10] The bladder base is rolled into a tubularized structure that forms the new urethra. The resulting urethra measures approximately 3 to 3.5 cm in length with a diameter of 1.5 to 2 cm. This procedure is often combined with augmentation of the bladder and almost always is accompanied by reimplantation of the refluxing ureters that commonly accompany the exstrophy-epispadias anomaly.

PREOPERATIVE CARE IN SECOND-STAGE SURGERY

Prior to surgery, the goals of the procedure are explained to the parents. The surgery is expected to resolve or greatly reduce the continuous incontinence associated with outlet incompetence by constructing a sphincter mechanism from the bladder base. The surgery is not expected to produce hydronephrosis of the upper urinary tracts, but close assessment during the months following surgery is essential. Advise the parents that reimplantation of the ureters is designed to resolved reflux and will render the child less susceptible to urinary tract infection.

POSTOPERATIVE CARE

Bladder augmentation, when performed, is designed to enhance bladder capacity but will not improve detrusor contractility. The nursing care related to augmentation and intermittent catheterization is discussed in "Altered Urinary Elimination: Voiding Dysfunction" in this chapter.

The parents have been prepared for the child's return from the surgical suite with a suprapubic catheter, urethral stent, and intravenous fluid line. The nurse monitors the suprapubic catheter for amount and character of output. The urine will be lightly blood tinged but should not be bright red or have excessive clots. The nurse reports the presence of excessive bleeding promptly to the physician.

The nurse restricts the child's mobility and reinforces the tape and dressings used to secure the urethral stent and suprapubic catheter as needed. Should the urethral stent be accidentally removed from the urethra, the child is placed on strict bedrest and the physician contacted promptly. The nurse should not attempt to recatheterize the urethra.

The urethral stent is typically removed 10 to 14 days postoperatively. Clamp the suprapubic tube for a voiding trial in consultation with the physician after stent removal. Advise the child and family that complete urinary control rarely occurs until several months following surgery. Advise the child that voiding may cause some discomfort during the first several days but that this feeling will subside as the bladder is repeatedly emptied.

Observe the child's urinary stream during these initial voiding trials for force, caliber, and constancy. The urinary stream should be relatively continuous and of the caliber of a pencil lead. Consult the physician to obtain complex uroflowmetry if an abnormal voiding pattern is suspected. Children with urinary incontinence and epispadias may need coaching concerning proper voiding habits. The discomfort experienced during initial voiding attempts may cause the child to develop sphincter dyssynergia caused by fear of discomfort with micturition. Teach the child who inappropriately contracts the sphincter to isolate, contract, and then relax his or her pelvic floor muscles, first in isolation of and then in conjunction with micturition.

Maintain a voiding diary during initial voiding trials, and assess the child for potential urinary retention. Measure the postvoid residual volume at least three times during the postoperative period in consultation with the physician and begin an intermittent catheterization schedule if necessary.

★ EVALUATION

Periodically the nurse and family evaluate the outcomes and criteria. Examples of outcome criteria for exstrophy and epispadias were given under "Nursing Diagnoses and Planning" in this section. Have short-term goals been met? Are long-term goals still realistic? Planning for further nursing care also takes into consideration complications and long-term care.

COMPLICATIONS

Urinary tract infection, upper urinary tract deterioration, loss of perineal skin integrity, and trauma to the bladder mucosa are the principal complications related to the period before primary closure of the exstrophied bladder. Potential loss of skin integrity due to continuous urinary leakage in the perineal area and urinary tract infection are the principal complications associated with the period between primary bladder closure and bladder neck reconstruction. Urinary retention, hydronephrosis, and persistent urinary leakage may complicate the period following bladder neck reconstruction. The management of these complications is discussed in the previous section.

LONG-TERM MANAGEMENT

Following repair of the bladder neck, the child with epispadias and exstrophy is likely to continue to experience difficulties with urinary leakage. Continuous urinary leakage is typically reduced to stress urinary incontinence, and urinary retention may occur. Routine follow-up visits are mandatory to manage altered urinary elimination and assess the status of the upper urinary tracts.

The nurse shows the family how to complete a voiding diary during a 2- to 3-day period prior to follow up appointments; the results are discussed with the child and family during the visit. Persistent stress urinary incontinence is initially managed by pelvic floor exercises. The nurse teaches the child to isolate and contract the periurethral muscles using both endurance and resistive exercises. Have the child contract the pelvic floor muscles as vigorously as possible for 10 consecutive 10-second intervals with up to 50 repetitions daily or every other day.[24] Integrate these exercises into a game, and encourage the parents to participate with the child to promote maximum compliance.

The child and family are reassured that complete urinary control may take months or several years to develop. The parents are advised that continence often improves with increasing age and peer pressure to have "dry pants." In addition, prostatic growth associated with puberty may provide extra dryness for boys.[10]

Anomalies of the Urethra: Hypospadias

Definition and Incidence.　Hypospadias is a congenital defect of the penis characterized by malformation of the anterior urethra distal to the sphincter mechanism. The hypospadias defect is described by the position of the aberrant urethral meatus, which varies from penile-scrotal junction to distal shaft and its association with chordee or penile curvature (Fig. 50-5).

The incidence of clinically significant hypospadias is approximately 1 in 300 male children, although mild forms of the defect may occur more often. The incidence is greatest in the presence of a family history of hypospadias.

Etiology and Pathophysiology.　Although a precise description of the etiology of hypospadias has not been elucidated, it is thought to arise from a multifactorial genetic defect. This hypothesis accounts for its familial and racial predispositions.

Others have theorized that hypospadias represents a mild intersex state.[14] Although hypospadias and ambiguous genital defects may be associated in certain instances, it seems unlikely that a true intersex state exists since hypospadias often occurs in a genotypic-normal male with descended testes.

The embryology of urethral development was discussed in Chapter 48. Failure of fusion between the genital folds with incomplete union of the ventral aspects of the preputial tissues results in hypospadias. Hypospadias is typically accompanied by some degree of lateral curvature of the penis termed *chordee.* The pathophysiologic mechanisms that cause the formation of a chordee also remain unclear.

Clinical Manifestations.　The effects of the abnormal embryologic processes that produce hypospadias and chordee are immediately obvious on inspection of the genitalia. The urethral meatus is located proximal and ventrally to its usual site, and the penis is often displaced caudally with varying degrees of lateral curvature due to presence of a chordee. The meatus may be circular in shape or markedly elongated with significant stenosis. It is occasionally covered with delicate skin and may be located so near the penile-scrotal junction that the defect is labeled a "vaginal hypospadias."

The penile skin also is altered by the hypospadias defect. The skin distal to the hypospadias is marked by a "V" shaped defect and absent frenulum. Two lateral raphes of tissue extend from this "V" shaped defect to the penile dorsum, creating an anomaly that resembles the eyes of a cobra or the cowl of a monk's hood.[14] The corpora cavernosa may remain unaffected or may be rendered hypoplastic in the presence of a chordee. The corpora spongiosum distal to the hypospadias defect is abnormal or absent.[14]

A number of other congenital anomalies may be found in cases of hypospadias. The most common are undescended testis (cryptorchidism) and inguinal hernia. Anomalies of the upper urinary tracts also may be present, particularly when the hypospadias defect is severe. Defects involving other organ systems are uncommon.[42]

Diagnostic Evaluation.　Hypospadias is obvious on physical examination. The urethral meatus is ventrally located (distal shaft to penoscrotal junction). There is caudal location of the penis (displaced toward rectum) and lateral curvature of the penile shaft. The frenulum is absent. A cobra's eye or monk's cowl defect of genitalia is present. Undescended testis occurs in 9% to 10% of cases and inguinal hernia in 9% of cases. An invasive physical examination called *infusion cavernosometry* discloses a normal penis (straight, bilateral erection) or

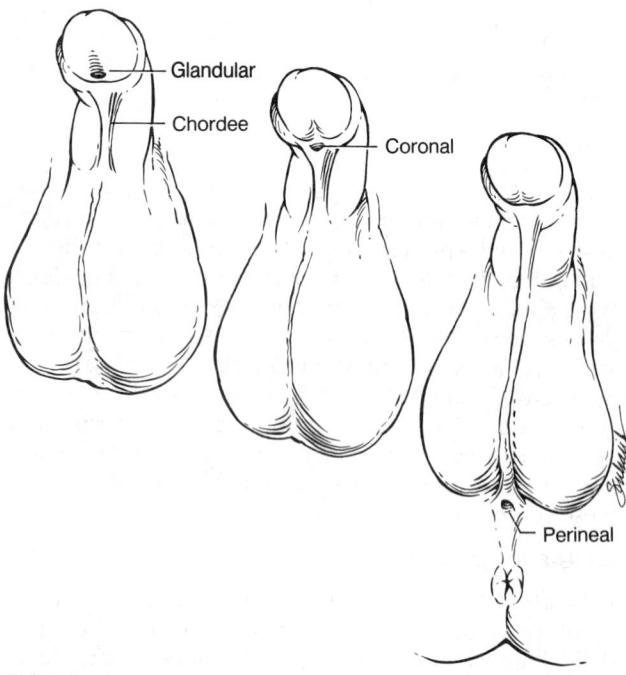

FIGURE 50-5
Typical hypospadias. The defect is described by anatomic location of the aberrant urethral meatus and its association with the chordee.

curvature of the penis. Imaging studies include the IVP, which is normal or shows the presence of obstructive uropathy; renal ultrasound, which is normal or shows evidence of obstructive uropathy; and voiding cystourethrography, which is normal or shows the presence of vesicoureteral reflux.

★ ASSESSMENT

The nursing assessment of the patient with hypospadias focuses on the extent to which the defect compromises urinary system function and self-concept. Physical assessment of the male infant with hypospadias centers on inspection of the genitalia. The urethral meatus is located by visual inspection, and its location is confirmed by observation of voiding. The meatus also is assessed for its shape, size, and flexibility, and the penile skin is inspected for presence of lateral tissue raphes and presence of a frenulum. The glans and distal shaft are assessed for their size and shape. The location of the penis relative to other perineal structures (particularly rectum and scrotum) is determined. The penis is examined in both flaccid and erect states to determine the presence and degree of curvature related to chordee.

The infant also is assessed for presence of associated congenital defects, particularly undescended testis, inguinal hernia, or ambiguous genitalia. Results of imaging studies are reviewed for evidence of associated upper urinary tract anomalies, including renal agenesis, ureteropelvic obstruction, or vesicoureteral reflux.

Ongoing nursing assessment also focuses on the extent to which hypospadias affects body image, particularly as it relates to sexual and urinary function. This evaluation begins with assessment of the family's response to the presence of a genital defect at birth, followed by examination of the child's response to hypospadias before, during, and after surgical repair.

The nurse determines how the parents plan to care for the child during the stage prior to consideration of surgical repair and their perceptions of how the hypospadias defect will ultimately affect the urinary and sexual function.

Assessment of the child's response to hypospadias begins during the toddler or early childhood period. The nurse assesses the child's responses to his genitalia by observation followed by more structured evaluation when feasible. The nurse encourages the younger child to draw a picture of his body just after a bath (naked, including genitalia) and ask the child to tell a story about the picture. A child psychologist or other developmental expert is consulted to evaluate the content of this story for perceptions of self-concept related to his genitalia and problems or frustrations with the appearance or function of these structures. The nurse provides opportunities for older children or adolescents verbally to express feelings concerning the appearance and function of the genitalia and encourages them to draw and describe their appearance whenever feasible. The responses of peers will profoundly affect the adolescent's response to his appearance.

The nursing assessment following hypospadias repair also focuses on physical assessment of the residual defect (if any) and cosmetic appearance of the penis, observation of micturition, and evaluation of emotional impact on the child and family.

★ NURSING DIAGNOSES AND PLANNING

Based on the assessment data from above and the preceding chapter, the following preoperative and postoperative nursing diagnoses may apply:

- Knowledge Deficit regarding management of hypospadias.
- High Risk for Altered Parenting related to expectations of perfect infant.
- Body Image Disturbance related to perception of anomaly.
- Anxiety related to results of surgical repair.
- Constipation related to inactivity.
- Pain related to surgical procedure.
- Impaired Physical Mobility related to restraint.
- High Risk for Impaired Skin Integrity related to immobility.
- Impaired Social Interaction related to immobility.

Other functionally related nursing diagnoses are discussed in Table 49-2 in Chapter 49.

The nurse and child (or parents) together plan effective care based on the established nursing diagnoses. Several examples of expected outcomes are as follows:

- The parents verbalize their relief that defects can be repaired.
- The child interacts with other children despite immobility during the postoperative period.
- The child maintains normal bowel movements postoperatively.

The nurse plans for the daily care of the child based on both physician's orders and nursing diagnoses. Some general nursing care goals for restoring penis and urethra function may be the following:

- Integrity of skin is monitored.
- A normal-appearing and functioning penis is established.

★ INTERVENTIONS: COLLABORATIVE AND INDEPENDENT

PARENTAL SUPPORT

Following diagnosis, the nurse begins teaching the family about management of the child with hypospadias. The nurse advises the parents that the hypospadias defect is confined to the distal portion of the urethra and is not expected to cause permanently altered urinary elimination function. Surgical intervention is commonly undertaken to repair a hypospadias defect. The repair is typically completed in a one- or two-stage operative procedure, and the consulting surgeon will review the details of these procedures prior to definitive repair. The family is reassured that surgery is expected to establish a normal-appearing and functioning penis and their child is expected to have normal voiding and sexual function.

The nurse advises the family that the appropriate age for surgical repair of hypospadias is determined in consultation with the pediatric urologist and that repair is typically completed prior to school age. No ideal age for repair exists because of individual differences; the child's psychosocial and emotional needs primarily determine the timing of surgery.[4]

SURGICAL REPAIR

More than 200 variations of surgical repair for hypospadias have been described[4,14]; a number of the more commonly used techniques are listed in Table 50-1. Although each of the repairs contains unique elements, all share the following elements. Meatoplasty and glanuloplasty require the construction of an elliptic-shaped meatus exiting from the distal portion of a normally shaped glans penis. Orthoplasty, the resection or removal of associated chordee with restoration of a straight penile shaft, accompanies these maneuvers. Urethroplasty also is completed, which requires tubularization of the affected urethral segment, allowing micturition and passage of semen through the urethra and out the meatus. Repair of the penile shaft is then undertaken. It requires covering the entire structure with skin followed by scrotoplasty to insure a normal cosmetic appearance of the adjacent genital area.[14]

A two-stage surgical repair has been used to treat hypospadias since the late nineteenth century. A one-stage repair was introduced in 1900 and revised extensively beginning in the 1940s. The feasibility of a one-stage procedure with its obvious advantages is now well established, although two-stage procedures remain in use among boys with more extensive defects.[14] The nursing management of the patient following hypospadias repair is influenced by the type of procedure used and the age of the patient.

PREOPERATIVE CARE

Prior to surgical repair, the family is given an explanation of the elements of the procedure and its goals. The rationale for a one-stage versus two-stage procedure is provided by the surgeon, and an ideal age for repair is determined.

Surgical repair at a relatively early age (3 to 9 months) is often undertaken and offers the psychosocial advantage of repairing the defect prior to or in the early stages of genital awareness (6 to 18 months). However, technical considerations may require the administration of testosterone to stimulate sufficient penile growth for repair.

The nurse teaches the parent to rub a 5% testosterone cream on the child's skin daily for a period of 3 weeks. A small amount is worked completely into the skin and the family is taught to apply the cream using gloves or careful and thorough handwashing immediately following application. Alternately, intramuscular testosterone may be administered by the nurse deep into the lateral aspect of the thigh muscles (vastus lateralis) weekly for 3 weeks. If injection is used, the parents are taught to monitor for side effects.

POSTOPERATIVE CARE

Immediately following surgery, the child will return to the nursing unit with a relatively large perineal dressing that serves to secure a suprapubic tube, compress the wound to prevent excessive bleeding, and protect the repair from environmental contamination. The penis is typically wrapped in gauze surrounded by a self-adhering elastic tape.

The dressing and suprapubic catheter are left in place and protected from inadvertent removal. The younger child is restrained to prevent unintentional contact with the surgical site and the sheets are tented in a semicircular frame to prevent adherence to the penis or dressing. Urinary or bloody drainage from the wound is reported promptly to the physician. Inadvertent or spontaneous removal of the suprapubic tube also is reported to the physician, and *no* efforts are made to replace the tube without direct physician consultation.

ACTIVITY PROMOTION

Mobility is severely limited for the first 48 to 72 hours following surgery, and moderate restrictions are maintained for 7 to 10 days until the suprapubic tube and larger dressing are removed.[21] During the first 2 to 3 postoperative days, the child is confined to the bed and required to remain in a supine position. Following this period, activity is increased, but the child may remain bedridden for an additional 7 to 10 days.

The nurse prepares the family for this period of limited mobility and encourages them to obtain multiple diversionary activities that the child may engage in, such

TABLE 50-1
Common Hypospadias Repairs

Procedure	Stages Required	Description
Chordee release (Spence-Allen)	Requires subsequent urethroplasty	Release of chordee with skin repair
Staged urethroplasty (Byar's, Browne, Durham-Smith, others)	First-stage chordee release required	Tubularization of defective urethral segment
MAGPI (meatal advancement glanuloplasty) (Duckett)	One-stage repair	Chordee repair with urethroplasty and meatal advancement with glans repair; used for smaller, distal defects
Flip-flap (Mathieu, Devine-Horton)	One-stage repair	Similar to MAGPI with skin flap for urethroplasty; for distal defects
Preputial free graft (Devine-Horton)	One-stage repair	Extensive chordee repair with urethroplasty requiring skin graft or island graft used for proximal defects
Preputial island flap (Duckett)		
Adjacent island flap (Hinderer, Desprez, Broadbent)		

as story books, tapes, or toys that can be manipulated while the child is supine. Restrain the child only when indicated, and administer sedatives as needed in consultation with the attending physician. Offer the child repeated assurances that his immobility is only temporary and in no way is an act of punishment. Encourage social interactions with siblings, other patients, or volunteer hospital staff.

The nurse assists the child's family to reduce frustrations associated with temporary immobility in a typically active child by encouraging a rotation of caretakers and shorter visits by one caretaker rather than prolonged contact by a single significant other. Encourage the parents to use friends, extended family members, hospital volunteer staff or other social support networks to allow time away from the child as needed.

Careful assessment and rapid interventions designed to reduce pain also assist the child to cope with immobility following hypospadias repair. Assess the child's pain for its character, duration, and likely etiology. Bladder spasms may occur and typically cause short bursts of cramping or stabbing pain centered in the bladder area. Administer anticholinergic medications if bladder spasms occur. Postoperative wound discomfort is typically of prolonged duration and may be aggravated by movement of the pelvic muscles. Administer analgesic or narcotic medications if wound pain occurs.

Immobility also increases the potential for altering bowel elimination and skin integrity. Prophylactic stool softeners may be used to prevent constipation and straining for a bowel movement during the immediate postoperative period. The nurse evaluates the child's postoperative bowel function according to the baseline habits taken in the history. Adequate fluid intake and fiber-rich foods are encouraged. The immobile child is daily assessed for altered skin integrity. Pillows or other supports are used to afford maximal mobility. The sedated or neurologically impaired child's positions are regularly changed to avoid pressure sores.

TEACHING

The family is taught to bathe and monitor the child's skin for altered integrity. The child participates in self-care activities whenever appropriate. The nurse reassures the child that he will be able to return to his former level of self-care following removal of dressings and tubes.

The child and family are typically quite anxious concerning surgical outcomes and are easily frightened if all aspects of medical and nursing care plans are not fully comprehended. The nurse reassures the family that the initial appearance of the penis following dressing removal will be significantly improved following a prolonged healing process. The nurse also emphasizes that urinary and sexual function are expected to be reach normality following repair.

★ EVALUATION

The nurse and family evaluate the outcomes and criteria. Examples of outcome criteria for were given in "Nursing Diagnoses and Planning" in this section. Have short-term goals been met? Are long-term goals still realistic? Plan-

ning for further nursing care also takes into consideration complications and long-term care.

COMPLICATIONS

The principal complications following hypospadias repair are persistent chordee, meatal stenosis, urethral stricture or stenosis, urethral diverticula, and fistula.[4] The likelihood of persistent chordee depends on surgical repair and extent of the initial defect. Curvature of the penis may require further surgical repair and repeated evaluation.

Meatal stenosis (narrowing) will cause a reduction on the force of the urinary stream that is often accompanied by spraying or splitting. Stenosis represents a frustrating complication for the affected patient; it is corrected by meatoplasty or by simple dilation. Urethral stenosis or stricture also presents as a reduction in the force of a urinary stream. It is usually treated by urethral dilation but occasionally requires urethroplasty (open surgical repair of the urethra).

Urethral diverticula are herniations of the urethral mucosa from its normal tubular configuration caused by postoperative infections or urethral stenosis.[4] Urethral fistulas are abnormal tracts between the urethral lumen and skin. They cause urine to exit the urethra at an abnormal location during micturition. Surgical repair is indicated if urethral diverticula interfere with voiding or when fistulas do not spontaneously close.

LONG-TERM MANAGEMENT

Patients are routinely assessed 2 to 4 weeks following discharge from the hospital and again at 6 months to 1 year following repair. Parents and patients are taught to monitor for complications and to seek follow-up care if urinary or sexual function is compromised.

Certain patients who have undergone unsuccessful attempts to repair hypospadias defects require much more extensive long-term follow-up care. The nurse reassures these patients that surgical advances have been achieved within the past several decades and that subsequent surgery offers a realistic chance of improving their repair. Additional surgical repair is undertaken when sexual or urinary function is compromised or when the cosmetic appearance of a repair is unacceptable to the affected male. Evaluation of the long-term psychosocial effects of hypospadias are completed by the nurse, and referral to an appropriate counselor is indicated when unresolved issues related to self-concept and body image remain despite surgical repair.

Urologic Manifestations of Multisystem Congenital Anomalies

Prune Belly Syndrome

Definition and Incidence. Prune belly syndrome is a congenital defect characterized by deficient abdominal musculature, enlarged ureters and bladder, and undescended (cryptorchid) testes (Fig. 50-6). Other terms for the disorder are *triad syndrome,* referring to the three principal anomalies (enlarged mid and lower urinary tract, abdominal wall defect, and cryptorchidism) or

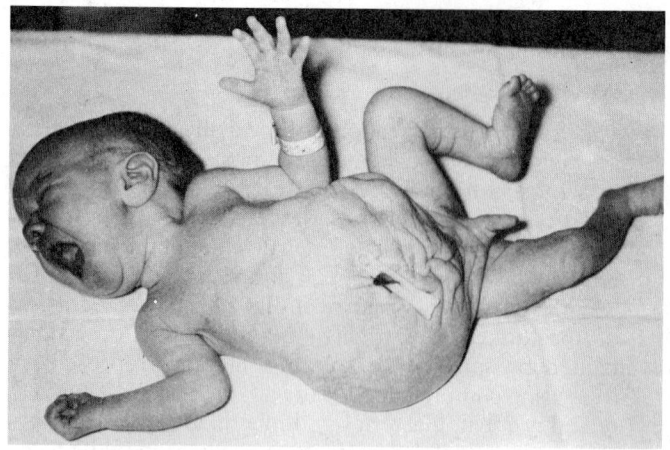

FIGURE 50-6
Typical congenital deficiency of the abdominal musculature found in prune belly. Note the undescended testes. (From Avery, G. B. [1987]. *Neonatology: Pathophysiology and management of the newborn* [3rd ed.]. Philadelphia: Lippincott.)

Eagle-Barrett syndrome.[77] Nonetheless, because of its descriptive nature and wide use, the term *prune belly syndrome* is used in this discussion.

The syndrome typically affects boys rather than girls; the simultaneous occurrence of urinary and abdominal wall defects in a female infant is extraordinarily rare.[77]

Etiology and Pathophysiology. The etiology of prune belly syndrome remains elusive; four explanations predominate. Bruton[9] and Wigger and Blanc[72] postulate that prune belly syndrome arises from a mesenchymal tissue defect that affects the migration of thoracic somite buds. Unfortunately, this theory does not fully explain the association of deficient abdominal musculature with urologic and testicular abnormalities.[59]

An intrinsic defect of the urinary tract also has been blamed for the development of prune belly syndrome. The defect may be an intrinsic abnormality of smooth muscle development or the aftermath of obstruction of the prostatic urethra. The nature of the intrinsic defect and exact mechanisms remain unclear.[59]

A defect in yolk sac development also has been attributed to the development of prune belly syndrome.[61] Because the yolk sac plays a crucial role in the formation of the chorionic cavity, a defect in this process may result in some of the abnormalities often seen in prune belly syndrome. Unfortunately, this explanation does not completely account for the cryptorchid testes and urinary tract disorders that complete the most common defects that define the syndrome.

The pathophysiology of prune belly syndrome lies in its deleterious effects on the abdomen and urinary and reproductive systems.

Abdominal Defects. The abdominal wall defect is characterized by a patchy, asymmetric or virtually absent mass of somatic muscle. The abdominal wall musculature is typically absent in the lower and mid-abdominal region with deficient, abnormal muscle predominant in the upper and lateral abdominal regions. The flanks often bulge, and the thorax is typically flared at the intercostal margin due to deficient support from the abdomen.[77]

Urinary Defects. The urinary system is adversely affected from the kidney to proximal urethra (Fig. 50-7). The kidneys often demonstrate some degree of dysplasia and hydronephrosis. The extent of renal dysplasia varies

significantly both among affected children and within the urinary system of a single child.

The ureters of the child with prune belly syndrome are grossly dilated and tortuous. On radiographic examination they resemble small bowel segments rather than the thin, delicate ureters seen in unaffected children. The contractility of the affected ureter is compromised by deficient innervation and replacement of smooth muscle bundles with fibrous tissue.

The prune belly bladder is enlarged with deficient (hypotonic) detrusor contractility. The bladder wall is thickened (though not trabeculated) and irregular in shape, often having an hourglass configuration. The dome of the bladder may be enlarged, forming a pseudodiverticulum. The trigone is also markedly large with an unusually wide space between the ureteral orifices. The bladder neck is widened and may be hard to demonstrate clearly by cystography.[77]

The proximal urethra is widened, and the prostatic urethra assumes a triangular configuration. Although these

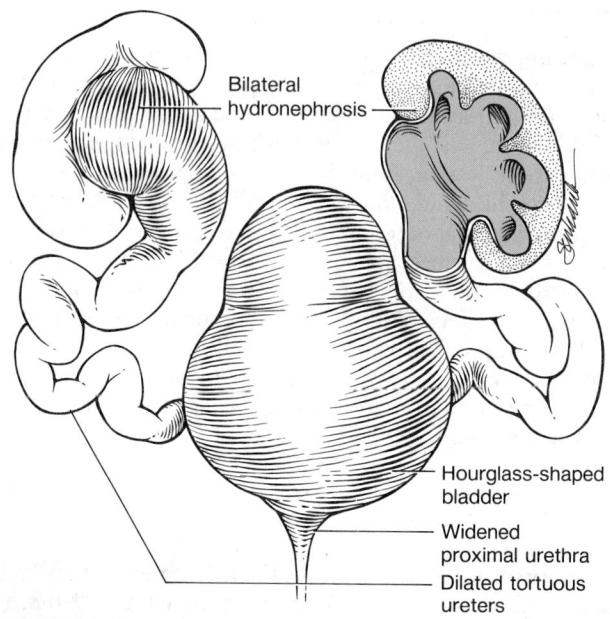

Bilateral hydronephrosis

Hourglass-shaped bladder

Widened proximal urethra

Dilated tortuous ureters

FIGURE 50-7
Urinary system defects in prune belly.

findings are reminiscent of obstruction, evidence of anatomic or functional obstruction is uncommon.[77]

The urinary defects of prune belly syndrome adversely affect virtually every child with the syndrome. The severity of renal dysplasia exerts a profound influence on urine formation function and the child's ultimate prognosis.[77] The large, tortuous ureters that characterize prune belly syndrome compromise urine transport from kidney to bladder because of insufficient smooth muscle contractility, obstruction, and retrograde movement (reflux) The enlarged bladder typically carries a large residual due to deficient detrusor contractility. As a result, urinary transport and elimination functions are further compromised and the effects of urinary stasis are magnified. Some children experience improved ureteral and bladder function as they mature, whereas others experience deteriorating function.

Reproductive Defects. Failure of testicular descent into the scrotum also occurs. The defect is typically bilateral, and the testes lie high in the abdomen as opposed to the inguinal canal or scrotal outlet. In addition to cryptorchidism, the vas deferens also may be affected by prune belly syndrome.[59]

Data concerning the long-term effects of prune belly syndrome on male reproductive function are scant because of the relatively poor prognosis associated with the condition until the last decade. No cases of fertility have been documented in the medical literature.

Other Defects. Although characteristic defects associated with prune belly syndrome involve only the abdominal wall and urinary and reproductive systems, other congenital anomalies also may be noted. *Respiratory function* is compromised because of deficient abdominal wall musculature and residual effects of in utero oligohydramnios. Oligohydramnios causes pulmonary hypoplasia, whereas the effect of deficient abdominal wall musculature leads to insufficient aeration of all pulmonary lobes, with increased susceptibility to pneumonitis.[77]

The effect of prune belly syndrome on pulmonary function arises from the degree and severity of hypoplasia and abdominal muscle deficiency. Hypoplasia often leads to pneumomediastinum or pneumothorax. The affected child is particularly prone to death from respiratory failure during the neonatal period. Fortunately, infants who survive this period are likely to overcome hypoplasia and regain a more optimistic prognosis.

Lobar atelectasis and pneumonia also compromise respiratory function because the abdominal muscles needed for forceful inspiration are absent or deficient. This deficiency is particularly pronounced when the affected child must cough effectively to remove excess pulmonary secretions produced as a response to anesthesia or sedation.

Orthopedic anomalies are sometimes associated with prune belly syndrome and are thought to occur as a result of compression defects caused by in utero oligohydramnios. The severity of orthopedic defects vary from mild dimpling of the elbows and knees to club foot (talipes equinovarus), congenital hip dislocation, dysplasia of the hips, absence of a limb, or polydactylism.[59]

Malrotation of the gut is the most common *gastrointestinal anomaly*, although imperforate anus also may occur. Constipation accompanies the syndrome but is usually attributed to deficient abdominal musculature rather than intrinsic colorectal defects.[77]

The most common *cardiac defects* are ventriculoseptal defect, atrioseptal defect, and tetralogy of Fallot.

Clinical Manifestations. The presence of prune belly syndrome is immediately obvious on physical inspection. The abdomen of the neonate assumes a flaccid, wrinkled appearance, leading to the descriptive term "prune belly." In contrast, inspection of an older child or adult will reveal a more subtle pot-bellied defect with absent wrinkles, even on assumption of a supine position.[59,77] The thorax will flare near the intercostal margin, and the flanks will bulge due to muscular deficiency.[77]

The limbs will be normally developed or may show affects of orthopedic anomalies. The child's respirations will appear normal at rest but effective coughing is absent.[77]

Diagnostic Evaluation. A definitive diagnosis of prune belly syndrome is made soon after birth. Physical examination reveals flaring of thorax; poor respiratory excursion with poor use of accessory muscles with maximal inspiration; decreased breath sounds over dependent pulmonary lobes with atelectasis; and normal heart sounds or murmur consistent with congenital defect. Kidneys are palpable and mildly to markedly enlarged; bladder is palpable and enlarged (above the umbilicus); and testes are above the scrotum and impalpable. Body limbs are normal, or dimples appear at knees and elbows. Dislocated hips, club foot, or an absent limb may be noted. In the neonate or infant, there is marked absence of abdominal musculature with wrinkled, protruding contour. In the older child or adolescent, there is a protuberant abdomen with absent wrinkles. Serum BUN and creatinine are normal, or elevated with significant, bilateral renal dysplasia. Imaging studies are helpful in making the diagnosis. An IVP reveals bilateral hydronephrosis; dilated, tortuous ureters; enlarged bladder; and poor concentration of dye during neonatal period or if dysplasia present. Voiding cystourethrography reveals an enlarged bladder with thickened wall, trabeculation rarely, and bladder neck often open during filling. Vesicoureteral reflux is commonly diagnosed. Voiding urethrogram shows enlarged prostatic urethra and may demonstrate stenotic or atretic membranous portion. For ultrasound, refer to IVP. In the DTPA radionuclide scan, there is an enlarged pelvocaliceal system with delayed excretion of radionuclide; it is often difficult to distinguish obstruction and deficient muscle contractility, and poor concentration of radionuclide is noted if dysplasia present. DMSA radionuclide scan reveals accurate evaluation of differential renal function when dysplasia suspected or confirmed. The Whitaker test shows differentiated obstruction of the upper urinary tract from delayed excretion of dye due to weak ureteral muscle function. Cystoscopic examination reveals a widened prostatic urethra. The membranous urethra may be narrowed. The trigone is markedly enlarged, ureteral orifices are laterally placed, and reflux is commonly noted. The bladder wall is enlarged and thickened, but trabeculation is absent. A urodynamic assessment reveals a large capacity with urinary residual due to deficient detrusor function; occasionally, the residual is caused by obstruction of the bladder outlet.

★ ASSESSMENT

The nursing assessment of the child with prune belly syndrome focuses on identification of significant defects that characterize the syndrome for that child and determination of the adverse effects of these on urinary, pulmonary, and reproductive function. The nurse completes a physical examination of the child, including the thorax and abdomen. The thoracic examination includes evaluation of pulmonary function, including general state of oxygenation, respiratory excursion, and ability to cough. Evaluation of the effects of prune belly syndrome on thoracic structures also includes auscultation of the heart to determine murmurs or other signs of congenital cardiac anomalies. Detailed discussions of the principles of assessment of respiratory and cardiac function are presented in Chapters 37 and 40.

Evaluation of the urinary system begins with assessment of the abdomen and its contents. The abdominal wall is inspected for size, shape, and contour, followed by auscultation of bowel sounds. The kidneys and bladder are easily palpable because of abdominal weakness. They often are enlarged because of megacystis and hydronephrosis, respectively. The infant's voiding habits are assessed by maintenance of a voiding diary and by observation of voided stream. The infant with prune belly syndrome should urinate within the first 12 to 24 hours following birth. The stream may be normal or intermittent to poor in character due to insufficient detrusor contractility or obstruction.

The nurse also reviews laboratory and radiographic or other diagnostic tests to determine the extent to which congenital anomalies caused by prune belly defect will compromise urinary, pulmonary, and reproductive function. These include laboratory findings relevant to renal function and radiographic, radionuclide, and ultrasonic evaluation of the urinary tract.

Assessment of the older child or adolescent with prune belly syndrome also centers on evaluation of the effects of the syndrome on urinary, pulmonary, and sexual function whenever appropriate.

★ NURSING DIAGNOSES AND PLANNING

Based on the assessment data from above and the preceding chapter, the following nursing diagnoses may apply to the neonate or infant with prune belly syndrome:

- Altered Urinary Elimination related to anatomic obstruction.
- Urinary Retention related to anatomic obstruction.
- Altered Tissue Perfusion: Renal related to interruption of flow.
- Altered Growth and Development related to effects of physical disability.
- High Risk for Infection (Urinary Tract) related to urinary stasis.
- Ineffective Breathing Pattern related to deficient abdominal musculature.

- Ineffective Airway Clearance related to obstruction.

Nursing diagnoses related to childhood and adolescent development include the first five above and the following:

- Body Image Disturbance related to psychosocial experiences.
- Sexual Dysfunction related to retrograde ejaculation.

Nursing diagnoses related to surgical procedures have been discussed in other sections. Other functionally related nursing diagnoses are discussed in Table 49-2 in Chapter 49.

The nurse and child (or parents) together plan effective care based on the established nursing diagnoses. Several examples of expected outcomes are as follows:

- The parents demonstrate ability to monitor the infant for signs of compromised renal function.
- The adolescent discusses concerns about sexuality.

The nurse plans for the daily care of the child based on both physician's orders and nursing diagnoses. Some general nursing care goals in restoring renal function may be the following:

- Adequate urinary drainage is maintained.
- Urinary stasis is prevented.
- Infection is prevented.
- Renal function is maintained.
- Trauma to underlying viscera is prevented.

★ INTERVENTIONS: COLLABORATIVE AND INDEPENDENT

The family often feels shocked and fearful in the presence of a physically disfiguring defect. The nurse offers the family a realistic overview of the most common findings associated with prune belly syndrome while reassuring them that, with treatment, the prognosis is typically quite good.

The neonate is placed on an apnea monitor until initial assessment of the respiratory function is completed. A detailed discussion of the care of the infant at risk for pulmonary complications related to ineffective breathing patterns or hypoplasia is presented in Chapter 38, "Nursing Interventions for Alterations in Respiratory Function."

The nurse begins anticipatory monitoring of the child for evidence of micturition. Unless voiding is absent after the first 24 hours or some other atypical finding is detected, medical urologic assessment is postponed for the first days of life. Following assessment of the urologic manifestations of prune belly syndrome, an initial bladder management program is established. This often consists of allowing the child to void spontaneously in the diapers or may require teaching the parents to perform clean intermittent catheterization if significant urinary retention is detected.

The nurse evaluates the success of this bladder management with a voiding diary that includes volume of oral intake and urinary output. The voided volume is approximated by weighing diapers.

CONSERVATIVE VERSUS SURGICAL MANAGEMENT

Considerable controversy exists among urologic surgeons whether the infant with prune belly syndrome is best managed by conservative (nonsurgical) means or by reconstructive surgery of the urinary tract.[59,74,77] Conservative management is clearly favored among patients with milder forms of the syndrome. These infants are allowed to void spontaneously and are managed in diapers. Although they are carefully monitored for urinary tract infections, prophylactic antibiotic therapy or intermittent catheterization is used only when recurrent infections occur.

When conservative (nonsurgical) management of prune belly uropathies is used, the nurse assists the family to institute an appropriate bladder management program according to the needs of their child and prescribed medical recommendations. The nurse teaches the affected family to monitor their child for signs of urinary tract infection, including foul-smelling urine, dysuria and hematuria, or fever. They are also taught to maintain a voiding diary as needed and to monitor the child for signs of compromised renal function such as vomiting, poor appetite, and failure to thrive.

Many children with more severe forms of prune belly syndrome require surgical intervention to attain an acceptable level of urinary system function. The goals of surgery are to promote adequate urinary drainage, maximize the smooth muscle potential of the ureters and bladder, and prevent urinary stasis, infection, and declining renal function.[74]

Surgical intervention may begin quite early in life. The most common initial procedure is some form of temporary urinary diversion designed to promote optimal urinary drainage. A cutaneous vesicostomy is often performed. This procedure offers the advantage of bypassing the need for extensive manipulation of the bowel and allows the child to be managed in diapers similar to unaffected children. The procedure requires a small transverse incision halfway between umbilicus and symphysis pubis where the bladder is brought to the skin and a small opening (stoma) is left to provide continuous urinary drainage.

PREOPERATIVE CARE

The nursing management of the child undergoing cutaneous vesicostomy begins prior to surgery. The nurse emphasizes the goals of surgery as a form of *temporary* urinary diversion designed to prevent urinary retention and its complications while allowing the parents to manage their child's urine output in the diaper rather than a pouch. The parents are advised that creation and subsequent closure of the vesicostomy are relatively simple procedures and that closure will occur after the child grows enough to allow more definitive urinary tract repair.

POSTOPERATIVE CARE

Following creation of the vesicostomy, the child returns to the nursing unit with a suprapubic tube in the vesicostomy site and an intravenous fluid line. The nurse monitors urine output for volume and character. The urine may be yellow or lightly blood tinged. Bright-red urine or clots are not expected and are reported promptly to the physician.

The intravenous fluid line is discontinued as soon as the child tolerates oral fluids, usually the same day. The child may experience discomfort following vesicostomy surgery caused by painful bladder spasms. The nurse assesses the pain for its character, duration, and location. Bladder spasm are often alleviated simply by ensuring that the suprapubic tube is draining adequately. Consult the physician concerning the use of anticholinergic or antispasmodic medications if spasms persist.

TEACHING

Advise the parents that the vesicostomy site will drain urine almost continuously. Urinary leakage is contained in a diaper similar to unaffected children, but the nurse should warn the parents that the skin adjacent to the vesicostomy stoma will be exposed to constant moisture and must be adequately protected to prevent loss of integrity. Teach the parents to change the diapers on a routine basis (approximately every 2 hours) and as needed in accordance with defecation schedules. Have the parents apply a moisture barrier with diaper changes and to clean and dry the skin daily. Teach the family to use a hair dryer on low setting to promote maximal drying of the skin adjacent to the stoma during daily cleansing. Instruct the parents regularly to monitor the peristomal skin for rashes and to report changes to their primary health care professional as indicated.

TEMPORARY DIVERSION OF UPPER URINARY TRACT

If a specific obstruction of the urinary tract lies above the level of an enlarged, hypotonic bladder, temporary diversion of the upper rather than lower urinary tract is indicated.[74] A cutaneous pyelostomy is performed by creating an opening between the renal pelvis and overlying skin. Like the vesicostomy, the stoma is viewed as temporary. Postoperatively, the child is managed in diapers rather than an external pouch, and the peristomal skin is monitored routinely.

RECONSTRUCTIVE SURGERY

Definitive surgical reconstruction of the severely affected urinary tract, which typically consists of ureteral and bladder repair, is performed in a nonstaged procedure. Surgery is performed through a single transperitoneal incision. Reconstruction of the ureters consists of reimplantation of refluxing ureters into a more medial aspect of the trigone in an antirefluxing manner, with resection of redundant ureteral length and infolding or tapering of the dilated ureter as indicated. Reconstruction of the bladder consists of reduction cystoplasty or the resection of the enlarged bladder dome and reapproximation of the remaining bladder borders in a watertight fashion.[74]

The nursing care of the child following open surgery of the bladder and ureteral reimplantation is discussed in "Altered Urinary Elimination: Voiding Dysfunction" and "Vesicoureteral Reflux" in this chapter.

Occasionally, obstruction of the bladder outlet will require internal urethrotomy. The procedure is performed transurethrally using an Otis urethrotome or under direct visualization using a resectoscope. The nursing care of the patient undergoing transurethral resection of obstructive tissue is presented in "Obstructive Uropathy" in this chapter.

MANAGEMENT OF ABDOMINAL WALL DEFECT

The deficient abdominal wall musculature associated with prune belly syndrome also is addressed by nonsurgical or surgical management. The nursing management of this aspect of care focuses on prevention of trauma to the underlying viscera and recognition of body image issues produced by the defect.

The infant is managed initially without any type of protective device. The nurse advises the parents to avoid tight-fitting clothing, diapers, or restrictive devices that might constrict blood flow to abdominal contents. In addition, they are advised to avoid trauma to the child's abdomen such as that caused by a walker or car seat that restrains the child with a lap rather than chest belt.

As the child begins to ambulate, a support or corset device is chosen. The device should offer support and protection to the abdomen and give a cosmetically normal appearance when worn underneath clothing. The device should be constructed of an elasticized material that "breathes" freely to prevent excessive perspiration or discomfort. An ideal corset extends from shoulders to mid-thigh and contains a properly sized opening for the genitalia and anus.

Surgical placation of the abdominal wall offers the advantage of providing a more cosmetically acceptable appearance of the abdomen but little or no improvement of bladder or respiratory function.[77] The procedure is typically deferred until the child reaches a sufficient age to give consent for this elective procedure.

CARE RELATED TO UNDESCENDED (CRYPTORCHID) TESTES

Even though the fertility potential of the child with prune belly syndrome is significantly compromised, the testes are brought to their normal scrotal position whenever possible. Restoration of the testes from an intra-abdominal to scrotal position is done via some form of orchiopexy procedure. The goals of surgery are to maximize androgenic and potential spermiogenic function of the affected testes and to prevent potential complications of leaving an undescended testis in the abdomen. The care of the patient undergoing orchiopexy is discussed in Chapter 69.

★ EVALUATION

Periodically the nurse and family evaluate the expected outcomes. Examples of outcome for prune belly syndrome were given in "Nursing Diagnoses and Planning" in this section. Have short-term goals been met? Are long-term goals still realistic? Planning for further nursing care also takes into consideration complications and long-term care.

COMPLICATIONS

The principal complications related to prune belly syndrome result from compromised pulmonary, urinary, and renal function. Potential pulmonary complications include respiratory failure due to hypoplasia of the lungs.

The complication is seen in the neonatal period; it is often severe and may cause early death but subsides after the first months of life. Those patients who do not experience hypoplasia or who survive the neonatal period also may experience a predisposition toward pulmonary complications, including atelectasis and pneumonia caused by ineffective coughing and poor maximal inspiration due to abdominal wall muscle deficiency.

The principal urinary system complications are deficient renal function and urinary tract infection. Renal insufficiency arises from dysplasia present from birth or as a complication of reflux, urinary stasis, and infection caused by obstruction or deficient smooth muscle function. Urinary tract infections arise from urinary stasis, and retention and may be complicated by the presence of vesicoureteral reflux allowing bacteria to ascend from the lower to upper urinary tracts.

LONG-TERM MANAGEMENT

The long-term management of the child with prune belly syndrome includes ongoing assessment and prevention of pulmonary and urinary complications as well as persistent issues of body image, self-concept, and sexual function faced by the older child and adolescent.

As the older child with prune belly syndrome grows, he or she becomes increasingly aware of the cosmetic defect created by abdominal wall muscle deficiency. The child may feel overweight or weak because of the lax abdominal configuration. In addition, the older child or adolescent may feel inadequate or frustrated when unable to participate in contact sports due to the considerable risk of injury to underlying organs.

The nurse assesses the affected patient's body image by observation of behaviors and through direct questioning or use of a self-portrait as indicated. The child or adolescent is provided with rationale for all restrictions in activity and assisted in exploring alternate diversional activities and athletic according to his or her interests. The child is encouraged to attain adequate exercise by activities such as running, swimming, or other sports that do not require physical contact or place undue risk of abdominal injury.

The nurse explores issues of sexual activity and fertility with the male adolescent or adult with prune belly syndrome. Provide factual information that fertility has not yet been documented among males with the prune belly syndrome but that erections and the sensations of orgasm are expected. The nurse assists the patient to identify experts in reproductive function as needed to discuss realistic alternatives for family planning.

Imperforate Anus

Definition and Incidence. Imperforate anus is a broad term that applies to a number of anorectal defects caused by abnormal cloacal development.[1] Several systems of classification of imperforate anus exist. One of the most commonly used was proposed by Ladd and Gross,[37] who identified four principal variants of imperforate anus based on physical examination and surgical implications. Since then, the International Classification

System for anorectal anomalies has been formulated that classifies imperforate anus according to the level of the defect relative to the pelvic floor musculature.[55] Within this system, imperforate anus is the result of a low (translevator), intermediate (infralevator), or high (supralevator) lesion or miscellaneous (early) lesion resulting in cloacal exstrophies or persistent urogenital sinus.

The incidence of imperforate anus lesions is approximately 1 in 5000 births. Its occurrence is important in any discussion of altered urinary system function because of the association between imperforate anus and urologic defects.

Etiology and Pathophysiology. Although the etiology of imperforate anus remains unclear, it is known that the defect arises from abnormal development and separation of the cloacal membrane. Imperforate anus lesions lie along a spectrum of cloacal anomalies. The most severe form occurs as early as the fourth week of fetal development, resulting in cloacal, renal, spinal, and lower extremity anomalies, and is incompatible with life. Imperforate anus states represent a milder form of this defect. Nonetheless, the anorectal defect is viewed as the presenting sign of a more extensive congenital anomaly rather than an isolated finding.[1]

The level of lesion causing an imperforate anus state corresponds with the level of arrested descent of the urorectal septum. Particularly high and early lesions result in the persistent cloacal anomaly noted in females. Arrest at a slightly lower level causes the high or supralevator imperforate anus state. This lesion is characterized by communication between the posterior cloaca (primitive rectum) and anterior cloaca (urogenital sinus) that is noted as rectourethral fistula in males or a rectovaginal fistula in females.[4]

Low imperforate anus lesions occur even later in fetal development, after the urorectal septum has completed its descent. These lesions present as more isolated gastrointestinal defects rather than multiorgan system abnormalities noted in higher lesions.[4]

Urologic Manifestations. Structural urologic defects associated with imperforate anus are usually confined to higher (infralevator or supralevator) lesions. Children with a supralevator imperforate anus lesion have a 30% chance of associated urologic defects. The most common anomalies include renal agenesis, renal dysplasia, UPJ obstruction, ureteral duplication anomalies, malrotated or ectopic kidney, and lower urinary tract anomalies. In contrast, only 10% of patients with infralevator lesions have urinary system anomalies.[5]

Children with imperforate anus lesions are at increased risk for lower urinary tract anomalies, including voiding dysfunction and vesicoureteral reflux. Neuropathic bladder dysfunction is identified in as many as 10% of children with intermediate or high imperforate anus lesions,[22] and vesicoureteral reflux may be found in as many as 47% of patients with higher lesions or 19% of patients with imperforate anus at any level.[45]

The significance of voiding dysfunction and vesicoureteral reflux is highlighted by the association of imperforate anus states with lumbosacral spine abnormalities. Lower spine abnormalities are reported in as many as 38% of patients with supralevator lesions.[12] These defects cause a neuropathic bladder in affected children. In addition, the effects of extensive abdominopelvic surgery required to perform pull-through procedures for repair of the anorectal defect exert an as yet unmeasured effect on bladder and sphincter function. Unfortunately, no study reviewed adequately screens the incidence of dysfunctional states among a large group of children with imperforate anus, although some reports suggest that urinary incontinence may resolve by puberty.[46]

Clinical Manifestations. Inspection of the rectum and buttocks at birth may reveal the presence of imperforate anus. The anus may be located in its normal position or may be caudally displaced in association with an anal dimple. The opening is stenotic or absent and may be covered by a thin strip of epithelium bulging from meconium in the bowel. The epithelium adjacent to the anal opening is abnormal in appearance. Presence of a fistula to the urethra or vagina may be detectable by gentle rectal probing (unless rectal agenesis has occurred) or endoscopic examination.

The urologic manifestations of imperforate anus are more subtle. Presence of a rectovesical or rectourethral fistula is made by direct inspection or may be detected as a result of urinary tract infection or bladder overdistention. Urinary obstruction may be detected by the presence of an abdominal mass, whereas agenesis of a kidney remains silent unless contralateral renal dysplasia is present.

Diagnostic Evaluation. Physical examination in imperforate anus reveals stenosis of the anal canal, absence of the anus, or aberrant placement with stenosis; presence of a rectovaginal fistula with meconium in the vagina; abdominal distention with retention of meconium; rectovesical fistula with bladder distention; aberrant appearance of buttocks or lower extremity with lumbosacral spine or other orthopedic anomalies; and evidence of cardiac anomalies (poor development, blue or dusky skin color with inadequate oxygenation of peripheral tissues). Laboratory findings show that serum BUN and creatinine are normal or elevated with significant dysplasia and contralateral renal agenesis. Imaging studies reveal the following: KUB is normal or shows presence of lumbosacral anomaly, and IVP reveals normal or absence of kidney (agenesis), malrotation of kidneys along the vertical axis, ureteral dilation with reflux, trabeculation of the bladder with neuropathic dysfunction, or poor concentration of contrast material due to renal dysplasia. A renal bladder ultrasound shows normal or absent kidney, ureteral dilation, and thickened bladder wall. The cystogram/voiding cystourethrogram (VCUG) is normal or shows presence of vesicoureteral reflux. Urodynamic studies are normal, or there is evidence of urinary retention due to deficient detrusor function or obstruction of the bladder outlet with sacral spinal anomalies associated with deficient detrusor contractility, and sphincter incompetence. Endoscopic studies reveal the presence of a rectourethral, rectovaginal, or rectourethral fistula; aberrant ureterotrigonal orifices with vesicoureteral reflux; trabeculation of the bladder wall; or sphincter incompetence with neuropathic bladder dysfunction.

★ **ASSESSMENT**

The nurse regularly assesses the child for evidence of spontaneous voiding within 12 to 24 hours after birth. A voiding diary that includes approximate urinary output (via weighing diapers) and a record of fluid intake is completed to assess urinary elimination patterns. The voided urinary stream is assessed for force, caliber, and presence of intermittency. The postvoid residual is assessed in consultation with the physician using catheterization or ultrasonic assessment of the bladder immediately after micturition occurs. The nurse also reviews the results of imaging and endoscopic examination of the urinary system to determine the presence of structural urinary tract defects.

Repeated assessment of urine elimination patterns is undertaken any time the child or family perceive a change in voiding patterns or following reconstructive surgery of the rectal area. This assessment includes a voiding diary kept for a period of 2 to 3 days, documentation of postvoid residual, and provocative testing for presence of stress urinary incontinence. The nurse consults the physician concerning complex urodynamic testing or performance of upper urinary tract imaging studies when urinary elimination patterns change.

★ **NURSING DIAGNOSES AND PLANNING**

Based on the assessment data from above and the preceding chapter, the following nursing diagnoses may apply:

- Altered Urinary Elimination related to anatomic obstruction.
- Urinary Retention related to anatomic obstruction.
- Stress Incontinence related to incompetent bladder outlet.
- High Risk for Infection (Urinary Tract) related to urinary retention, vesicoureteral reflux.
- Sexual Dysfunction related to altered body structures.

Other functionally related nursing diagnoses are discussed in Table 49-2 in Chapter 49.

The nurse plans for the daily care of the child based on both physician's orders and nursing diagnoses.

★ **INTERVENTIONS: COLLABORATIVE AND INDEPENDENT**

The nursing management of urologic manifestations of imperforate anus is guided by identification of specific structural or functional abnormality. Detailed discussion of the most common urologic defects associated with imperforate anus are contained throughout this chapter.

Spina Bifida Defects

Definition and Incidence. Spina bifida, or spinal dysraphism, is a congenital anomaly characterized by failure of closure of the vertebral column. Spinal bifida is further defined by the degree of herniation or protrusion of neural tube contents through this opening. *Spina bifida occulta* is the mildest form of the anomaly and

refers to the abnormal opening of the posterior vertebral laminae in conjunction with noticeable bony defects such as absence of the spinous processes or hemivertebrae. The overlying skin may be normal in appearance or may show a tuft of hair or subcutaneous lipoma.

Spina bifida with meningocele is characterized by abnormal fusion of the posterior vertebral laminae and protrusion of the meninges through the skin causing a cyst on the back. *Spina bifida with myelomeningocele* is the most severe form of the anomaly. It is similar in appearance to meningocele except for the herniation of elements of the spinal cord in addition to meninges and spinal fluid into the protruding cyst.

Spina bifida defects occur in approximately 1 in 1000 live births in the United States. When spina bifida occurs in one child, the risk for future siblings rises.

Spina bifida defects are most frequently noted in the lumbosacral region of the spine, although any portion of the cord may be affected. The significance of spina bifida defects is important to any discussion of urologic nursing because of its association with neuropathic bladder dysfunction.

Etiology and Pathophysiology.

Voiding Dysfunction.   Normal bladder function relies on the input of multiple modulatory centers of the central nervous system. When a spina bifida defect causes abnormal nervous system function, neuropathic bladder function results. In the case of spina bifida occulta, the defect is often subtle; voiding and bowel dysfunction may occur, but obvious motor defects are uncommon. At the opposite extreme, spina bifida with myelomeningocele causes profound motor deficit of the lower extremities as well as severe bowel and bladder dysfunction.

Spina bifida defects affect multiple levels of the nervous system, and neurologic function may be further altered by bony growth and development. Thus, a variety of dysfunctional voiding states will be found that are affected by maturation as well as the location and extent of the original defect.

Because of the variable neurologic defects associated with myelodysplasia, it is impossible to define a typical or classic dysfunctional voiding pattern caused by spina bifida. Nonetheless, certain general characteristics can be identified, based on the child's age and general location of the spinal and neural defect.

During the neonatal period, spina bifida defects typically cause one of several dysfunctional voiding patterns. A defect that causes complete failure of sacral spinal function results in absence of detrusor reflex contractions (detrusor areflexia) with or without loss of bladder wall compliance. The sphincter mechanism is typically incompetent, and denervation of the rhabdosphincter and periurethral musculature may produce a stiff, noncompliant urethral wall with obstruction superimposed on a pattern of stress incontinence.

As a result, urine elimination is characterized by poor, dribbling urinary leakage produced when filling of the noncompliant bladder exceeds urethral closure pressure or when sudden physical exertion causes stress urinary incontinence. The urinary tract is at high risk for infection and compromised renal function.

When the neurologic defect caused by a spina bifida defect is centered above the sacral micturition center, hyperreflexic detrusor contractions occur that produce a voiding pattern similar to the normal infant. These contractions are typically accompanied by uncoordinated or dyssynergic sphincter response caused by the spinal defect.

Other infants with spina bifida defect have preservation of detrusor reflex contractions and synergic sphincter response to micturition. Their voiding patterns mimic normal infants. As a result, they are unlikely to develop infections or upper urinary tract distress during the first year of life *unless* their neurologic status changes, causing alteration of urinary tract function.

As the child grows, the dysfunctional voiding pattern of infancy changes. The bladder wall often becomes poorly compliant, and the detrusor muscle may change from hyperreflexic to areflexic or hyporeflexic. The dyssynergic sphincter mechanism typically becomes incompetent and noncompliant, causing passive obstruction of the outlet. As a result, the urinary elimination pattern is characterized by overflow type leakage. Although these children may experience relatively little urinary leakage if placed on an intermittent catheterization program, recurrent urinary tract infections and compromised renal function often occur because of chronically elevated pressures generated by the poorly compliant, obstructed lower urinary tracts.

In other children, the detrusor becomes hypotonic or areflexic but the bladder wall remains relatively compliant (distensible). In these children, the sphincter mechanism is likely to be incompetent, but the urethral wall typically remains compliant and urethral leak pressures remain less than 40 cm H_2O. These children have absent or significantly diminished sensations of bladder filling and marked urinary stress incontinence. They are less likely to suffer compromised renal function and infection.[41]

Still other children experience persistent detrusor hyperreflexia with sphincter dyssynergia. Their voiding patterns are characterized by brief dry periods followed by uncontrolled micturition with intermittent stream and persistent residuals. They are unlikely to experience stress urinary incontinence, but they also are at high risk for compromised renal function and infection.

Vesicoureteral Reflux. Because children with spina bifida have neuropathic bladders, they are particularly prone to the development of secondary vesicoureteral reflux. Those children at greatest risk have lower urinary tracts that are exposed to chronically high pressures. Refer to "Vesicoureteral Reflux" in this chapter for a detailed discussion of the pathophysiology and related nursing care.

Renal Dysfunction. Neuropathic bladder function, if left untreated, ultimately compromises a child's survival because of its deleterious effects on renal function. Although most infants with spina bifida defects are born with adequate renal function, some develop renal failure due to abnormal lower urinary tract function. The etiology of compromised renal function among children with spina bifida arises from certain dynamic characteristics of the neuropathic bladder. Gallaway and associates[19] have identified five urodynamic parameters that differentiate a "hostile" versus "nonhostile" neuropathic bladder. They are outlet resistance, sphincter behavior, bladder wall compliance, detrusor hyperreflexia, and reflux.

Clinical Manifestations. The presentation of the spina bifida defect depends on the severity of the associated neural tube defect. Spina bifida occulta often remains undetected unless bowel and bladder dysfunction warrant investigation of the neurologic system. In contrast, spina bifida with meningocele or myelomeningocele is readily apparent with birth or with prenatal ultrasonic assessment.

The back deformity of spina bifida is characterized by a midline cyst causing a skin defect. The lower extremities may be misshapen and have grossly apparent muscle atrophy. In addition, the cranium may show signs of hydrocephalus because of Arnold-Chiari defect. The anal sphincter is patulous, and dribbling urinary leakage may be observed during physical exertion such as crying.

Diagnostic Evaluation. The following is observed on physical examination: cyst-like deformity of back near midline *or* lipoma or hair-bearing tuft over defect; and lower extremities with normal or reduced movement. Laboratory findings reveal normal or elevated serum creatinine and BUN with markedly compromised renal function. IVP is normal or shows evidence of hydronephrosis due to neuropathic bladder function. Cystogram or voiding cystourethrogram shows passive funneling of bladder neck with sphincter incompetence, trabeculated bladder with detrusor hyperreflexia, or poorly compliant bladder wall; reflux is noted in certain cases and may be high grade and bilateral. DTPA radionuclide scan is normal, or there is evidence of poor upper urinary tract drainage relieved by placement of indwelling catheter and continuous drainage of the lower urinary tract. DMSA radionuclide scan is normal, or there is evidence of renal scarring and compromised renal function due to reflux with infection. Nuclear cystogram is normal, or shows evidence of vesicoureteral reflux that may be high grade. For results of a urodynamic examination, refer to the previous discussion. In the endoscopic examination, there is passive funneling of bladder neck with sphincter incompetence and trabeculation with certain dysfunctional voiding states. Reflux may be noted.

★ ASSESSMENT

The assessment of the child with spina bifida defects focuses on several issues. Altered urinary elimination may cause urinary tract infection and renal damage in the infant, toddler, child, or adolescent. In the child and adolescent, dysfunctional voiding carries the added burden of incontinence. Bladder and bowel incontinence and marked physical handicaps adversely affect the child or adolescent's physical and psychosocial development, particularly in issues related to self-esteem, body image, toileting, and hygiene.

During the first year of life, the goal of nursing management is the identification of dysfunctional voiding states that pose an undue risk of urinary tract infection and compromised renal function. Newborns with meningocele or myelomeningocele are closely observed for the onset of voiding. Diapers are weighed to determine urine output volume, and the physician is informed if spontaneous voiding is not noted within the first 12 to 24 hours after delivery.

Most infants with spina bifida and myelomeningocele undergo neurosurgical repair of their defect during the first hours or days of life. In addition, most experience placement of a ventroperitoneal shunt for hydrocephalus during the first month of life. Because each procedures may affect voiding function, voiding patterns are reassessed following both surgeries. This assessment includes voiding diary and observation of the urinary stream. Stress incontinence is assessed by observation of dribbling leakage during gentle compression of the pelvis or crying. Urinary retention is assessed by catheterization or ultrasound of the bladder following micturition.

Baseline renal function is assessed by use of appropriate imaging studies and review of laboratory creatinine and BUN values. These studies are repeated as appropriate to determine progressive changes in urinary function throughout the first year of life.

Definitive assessment of bladder function among infants is determined by complex urodynamic assessment. Testing is completed during the first 4 to 6 weeks of life, and the results are used to determine the potential that a dysfunctional voiding state will compromise the function of the upper urinary tract or lead to infection.

Assessment of urine elimination patterns continues as the infant matures into a toddler and young child. In addition to assessment of the lower urinary tract function in relation to renal function, assessment also focuses on the establishment of a bladder management program that establishes an acceptable level of continence.

The nurse continues an assessment of upper urinary tract function and urinary tract infection through evaluation of urine cultures and review of data from appropriate imaging studies.

In addition to issues related to urinary system function, the nurse assesses psychosocial issues related to altered urine elimination patterns during early childhood. Although all children are managed in diapers during infancy, children with spina bifida are typically managed in diapers up to the period immediately preceding school. As they continue to grow and mature, issues related to bladder and bowel control may cause social isolation, depression, and disturbances in body image and self-esteem. The nurse refers the affected child to an appropriate counselor when these issues interfere with mental or physical well-being.

Assessment of urine elimination patterns and incontinence continues into adolescence. In addition to these issues, the adolescent must cope with even greater emphasis on issues of body image, self-esteem, and mastery of self-care skills needed for a maximally independent adult life. The nurse continues to assess the adolescent's response to these issues as he or she moves toward a goal of living as an adult free of complete dependence on family members.

★ **NURSING DIAGNOSES AND PLANNING**

Based on the assessment data from above and the preceding chapter, the following nursing diagnoses may apply to children of all ages and adolescents:

- Altered Urinary Elimination related to neurological impairment.
- Urinary Retention related to bladder outlet obstruction and/or deficient contractility.
- Stress Incontinence related to sensory motor impairment.
- Reflex Incontinence related to neuropathic condition.
- High Risk for Infection (urinary tract) related to bladder weakness.
- High Risk for Impaired Skin Integrity related to altered sensation.
- Altered Tissue Perfusion: Renal related to integrity of arterial flow.
- Stress Incontinence related to neuropathic urethral function.
- Body Image Disturbance related to urinary incontinence.
- Self-care Deficit: Toileting, Bathing, and Hygiene related to neuromuscular impairment.

Additional nursing diagnoses for the adolescent may include the following:

- Chronic Low Self-Esteem related to perception of physical defects.
- Social Isolation related to delay in accomplishing developmental tasks.
- Sexual Dysfunction related to biopsychosocial alterations of sexuality.
- Altered Sexuality Patterns related to impaired relationships with significant others.

Other functionally related nursing diagnoses are discussed in Table 49-2 in Chapter 49.

The nurse and child (or parents) together plan effective care based on the established nursing diagnoses. Several examples of expected outcomes are as follows:

- The parents list methods to monitor the child for urinary tract infections.
- The child exhibits proficiency in self-catheterization.
- The adolescent participates in a rehabilitation program for independent living.

The nurse plans for the daily care of the child based on both physician's orders and nursing diagnoses. Some general nursing care goals may be the following:

- Incontinence is reduced.
- Tests reveal bladder's potential for infection and renal compromise.
- Individualized management plans evolve.
- Infection is prevented.

★ **INTERVENTIONS: COLLABORATIVE AND INDEPENDENT**

INFANT CARE AND PARENTAL SUPPORT

Parents of the child with spina bifida are reassured that the physical defect is treatable and that the prognosis for their baby is quite good with proper care. In contrast, the nurse avoids predictions concerning the magnitude of physical handicaps or associated loss of bowel and bladder function. Rather, the parents are advised that each child is unique and that it is necessary to adopt a "wait and see" philosophy concerning the nature and extent of physical handicaps.

The nurse also reassures the parents that their feelings of fear and anger are normal. They also are warned that they may face a greater than normal risk of bearing other children with spina bifida defects and are counseled to seek consultation with an appropriate physician before planning further pregnancies.

FOCUSED ASSESSMENTS

An initial bladder management program typically consists of diaper management with or without intermittent catheterization program or Credé maneuver program. The nurse reinforces the particulars of this program and teaches the family to monitor the child for urinary tract infection. They are advised to monitor the child regularly for a change in urine odor or voiding patterns and to seek medical care promptly should symptoms of infection occur.

The nurse begins assessment of the neonate's urinary elimination pattern during the first hours of life. Spontaneous voiding should occur within the first 12 to 24 hours after birth. The nurse checks all diapers for evidence of micturition and assesses the lower abdomen for evidence of bladder distention. A catheter is inserted if bladder distention or other signs of urinary retention occur.

Following neurosurgical repair of myelomeningocele or meningocele, the nurse reassesses bladder elimination patterns. Certain infants experience a brief period of spinal shock possibly produced by surgical manipulation. This condition causes detrusor areflexia or absence of bladder contractions and urinary retention. Retention is managed by intermittent or indwelling catheter until spontaneous contractions return. Infants who do not experience urinary retention are managed in diapers.

Urodynamic assessment is completed within the first month of life. The timing of this examination varies among individual children; typically it occurs after spontaneous voiding has returned following neurosurgical repair.

INFECTION PREVENTION

Children with spontaneous bladder contractions and appropriate (coordinated) sphincter response are assessed as relatively low risk for upper tract distress and infection. They are managed by diapers alone. Follow-up upper tract imaging studies and repeat urinalysis and urine culture are obtained as indicated or per established protocol (Table 50-2). Urodynamic studies are repeated if the voiding pattern or findings on upper tract imaging studies change or if urinary tract infections occur.

In contrast, infants with spontaneous contractions and dyssynergic (uncoordinated) sphincter response are assessed as high risk for upper urinary tract distress and may be placed on an intermittent catheterization program in addition to diaper management. The nurse teaches the parent to perform catheterization using clean technique. The catheterization schedule is determined in conjunction with the pediatric urologist. Antispasmodic or anticholinergic medications are added if voiding pressures are elevated; upper tract imaging studies and urine cultures are performed on a frequent basis.

Infants with hyporeflexic or areflexic detrusor contractions and urinary retention also may be managed by an intermittent catheterization program or Credé voiding if vesicoureteral reflux is not present.

If the bladder proves to be high risk for upper urinary tract distress and evidence of compromised renal drainage is present on initial evaluation, the child may undergo temporary urinary diversion to prevent further deterioration. The most common surgical procedure is vesicostomy. The nursing care related to this procedure is discussed earlier in this chapter.

CARE OF THE CHILD

Ongoing assessments of urinary tract infection are performed throughout the toddler and childhood period. As the child approaches school age, the nurse consults the parents and pediatric urologist concerning institution of a bladder management program designed to free the child from dependence on diapers.

Repeat urodynamic testing begins the process of designing such a program. For the child with detrusor hyperreflexia and adequate bladder wall compliance, an anticholinergic or antispasmodic medication is added to the intermittent catheterization program to promote dryness between catheterizations. An α-sympathomimetic (such as pseudoephedrine) may be used to improve sphincter function when stress incontinence is found.

Around age 4 to 6 years the child is taught to self-catheterize. The nurse schedules a specific appointment for instruction. A teaching plan for intermittent catheterization is shown in the display. Catheterization is further discussed under "Interventions" in the "Altered Urinary Elimination: Voiding Dysfunction" section later in this chapter. The principles of catheterization, that is, clean, dry hands and a clean, dry catheter, are emphasized. An appropriate position for catheterization is determined; sitting in the wheel chair or standing before a toilet is preferred when feasible. After demonstrating appropriate handwashing technique, the child is allowed to manipulate the catheter and to locate the urethral meatus. Consistent adherence to a scheduled regimen is emphasized. The child is encouraged to begin catheterization under parental supervision and to continue catheterization in a relatively independent manner at school under the school nurse's supervision and in cooperation with her or his teacher. The nurse emphasizes the accomplishment of this skill as a sign of "growing up" and praises the child when self-catheterization is mastered. The mastery of this skill assists the child in gaining self-esteem and a feeling of control over bodily functions that will assist her or him in beginning school.

Pharmacologic agents often assist in reducing the magnitude of incontinence without completely resolving leakage. The nurse encourages the family to remove diapers from the child and use an appropriate pad or incontinent brief system whenever feasible. This simple strategy assists the child in growing "beyond" diapers, gaining self-esteem associated with beginning school. The nurse uses voiding diaries and repeated clinic visits to evaluate the success of the child's bladder management program.

The child who experiences marked leakage due to deficient detrusor function and pronounced sphincter incompetence with low leak pressure also may be managed by intermittent catheterization and α-sympathomimetic medications. Unfortunately, this regimen often fails to

TABLE 50-2
Long-term Assessment and Management of the Child With Spina Bifida and Neuropathic Bladder

Assessment	Nursing Management Goals
Infancy (0–1 yr)	
Month 1	Prevent infection and compromised renal function.
Urinalysis	Contain urinary leakage.
Urine culture	
Upper tract imaging study	
Urodynamics	
Voiding cystourethrogram*	
Month 3	
Upper tract imaging study†	
Urinalysis and urine culture‡	
Month 6	
Upper tract imaging study†	
Urinalysis and urine culture	
Month 9	
Upper tract imaging study†	
Urinalysis and urine culture	
Year 1	
Upper tract imaging study	
Urinalysis and urine culture	
Toddler/Childhood	
Year 2–4	
Annual upper tract imaging study†	Prevent infection and compromised renal function.
Urinalysis and urine culture, annual or when needed.	Establish bladder management program to maintain child free of diapers and maximally dry between catheterizations.
Repeat urodynamics with voiding cystourethrography, annual with high-risk bladder	
Year 5	
Urinalysis and urine culture	Teach child to manage bladder program with minimal parental supervision.
Upper tract imaging study	
Urodynamics, with or without voiding cystourethrography	
Year 6–12	
Urinalysis and urine culture, annual and when needed	
Upper tract imaging study, annual and when needed	
Adolescence	
Year 13–18	
Urinalysis and urine culture, annual and when needed	Prevent infection and compromised renal function.
Upper tract imaging study, every other year†	Establish bladder management program that frees adolescent from diapers and establishes maximal dryness between catheterization.
Urodynamics with or without voiding cystourethrogram, when needed	Contain urinary leakage using appropriate pad or incontinent brief system.

* Voiding cystourethrography is performed more frequently if vesicoureteral reflux is present.
† Upper urinary tract imaging studies are performed more frequently for the high-risk bladder.
‡ Urinalysis and urine culture are performed when signs or symptoms of urinary tract infection occur.
Adapted from Bauer, S. B. (1985): Urodynamic evaluation and neuromuscular dysfunction. In P. P. Kelalis, L. R. King, & A. B. Belman (Eds.), *Clinical pediatric urodynamics* (pp. 283–310). Philadelphia: Saunders.

resolve urinary leakage. Surgical reconstruction of the lower urinary tract in the form of pubovaginal sling for girls or artificial urinary sphincter for girls or boys may be required to overcome sphincter incompetence. A newer technique, the transurethral or periurethral injection of a collagen substance, is under investigation for its potential to correct stress incontinence caused by sphincter incompetence.

The child with detrusor hyporeflexia or areflexia, poor bladder wall compliance, and an elevated leak pressure also may be managed by intermittent catheterization program and antispasmodic or anticholinergic medications.

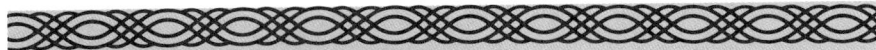

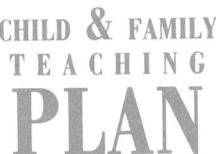

CHILD & FAMILY TEACHING PLAN

Intermittent Catheterization

Assessment

Steve is a 12-year-old black child diagnosed with spina bifida and myelomeningocele at birth. He is status postrepair of spina bifida defect and ventroperitoneal shunt. Steve has a history of five urinary tract infections over the past year; the last infection was associated with fever. Urodynamic testing reveals poorly compliant bladder wall and absent vesicoureteral reflux. Upper tract imaging study (IVP) reveals moderate left hydronephrosis, which represents a change from previous studies.

Steve undergoes augmentation cystoplasty and will manage his bladder by intermittent catheterization program postoperatively. He is of normal intelligence and motivated to "stay dry."

The family consists of mother who has high school education. Estranged father does not visit. The child and his mother reside with the maternal grandmother in a rural area.

Both the child and mother have good eyesight and manual dexterity. The grandmother also has good vision corrected by glasses and adequate dexterity despite mild arthritis.

Mother, child, and grandmother state that they have "heard of" intermittent catheterization but do not know how to perform the procedure.

Child and Family Objectives	Specific Content	Teaching Strategies
1. Identify rationale for performing catheterization and learn principles of catheter program.	1. Goals of catheterization: regular and complete bladder emptying to prevent overdistension, infection, and incontinence. Hands are clean and dry. Lubrication is used for easy insertion. Emphasize that sterile technique is not required for catheterization at home.	1. Use appropriate language (aimed at person with fifth-grade education) to explain goals. Supplement explanation with anatomic drawings as feasible. Use simple explanation. Compare catheter to care of eating utensils. Provide with written instruction sheet of step-by-step procedure. See display (Patient Teaching for Self-Care: Technique for Performing Intermittent Catheterization) later in this chapter.
2. Practice catheterization technique until it is learned correctly.	2. Demonstrate technique several times during hospital stay following augmentation procedure. Allow parent, grandmother, and child to assume the task one step at a time. Begin by allowing them to gather supplies and wash hands. Advance to allowing them to hold catheter and identify meatus. Follow by allowing them to insert catheter, first with assistance, then under observation only. Reinforce skill for each member of the family to relieve excessive reliance on any one person. Materials for catheterization: clean, dry catheter (size determined in	2. The written steps provided to family should be followed each time. Encourage the child and family to participate.

(Continued)

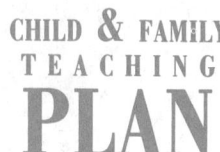

Intermittent Catheterization (continued)

Child and Family Objectives	Specific Content	Teaching Strategies
	consultation with physician); water-soluble lubricant (large tube acceptable if family taught to recap between uses); soap and water for washing hands (moist towelettes acceptable *only* when soap and water not available).	
3. Establish appropriate catheterization schedule.	3. Consult physician concerning schedule for catheterizations (i.e., every _____ hours). Discuss with family to tailor catheterization schedule around usual family routines.	3. Use simple explanations of importance of maintaining the schedule of regular, complete bladder emptying. Provide family with written schedule (clock face, time sheet, etc.) to reinforce verbal instructions.
4. Identify strategies to cope with potential complications.	4. Teach family: • To recognize signs and symptoms of urinary tract infection. • To observe urine for presence of blood. • To contact doctor if blood noted in urine or at urethral meatus. • To discontinue catheterization prior to notification of physician. • To contact local physician for urine culture if signs of infection occur. • To identify a resource person for family to call with questions.	4. Use simple explanations and written instructions to reinforce content provided. Resource person such as urologic nurse clinician can reinforce initial instructions and assist family to cope with unforeseen situations as they learn to manage bladder via catheterization program.

Evaluation

- Family and child identify rationale for catheterization program.
- Family and child verbalize the three principles of clean catheterization technique: clean, dry hands; clean, dry catheter; and lubrication for easy insertion.
- Mother, child, and grandmother demonstrate proper technique for catheterization, including assembly of materials; preparation of catheter, including lubrication; and washing and storage of catheter.
- Child and family verbalize a schedule for catheterization that takes family routines into account.
- Family identifies potential complications and strategies to manage these situations.

Unfortunately, this program often offers only a temporary answer because hostile bladder function (bladder conditions discussed earlier that threaten renal function) typically necessitates surgical reconstruction of the lower urinary tract to prevent recurrent infections and deterioration of renal function.[41]

CARE OF THE ADOLESCENT

The adolescent initially manages incontinence by a combination of intermittent catheterization and pharmaco-

logic agents. When these measures fail, the adolescent is advised to consult a urologist concerning surgical options designed to promote optimal continence.

In addition to these problems, the adolescent faces issues of independence in self-care and self-determination frustrated by physical handicap and bowel and bladder dysfunction. Left unresolved, these issues cause significant depression and loss of self-esteem. The nurse remains continuously aware of these issues and assists the adolescent to adopt an aggressive philosophy that urinary and bowel incontinence are unacceptable. The patient is provided with multiple opportunities to discuss issues of body image, self-esteem, sexuality, and the need for a productive and satisfying adult life. The adolescent is referred to a local or regional rehabilitation program designed to teach independent living and care skills whenever feasible.

SURGICAL MANAGEMENT

The child or adolescent with poor bladder wall compliance and high urethral leak pressure (40 cm H_2O or greater) often requires surgical reconstruction of the urinary tract to prevent persistent infections and deteriorating renal function. Urinary diversion, such as vesicostomy, is appropriate for the toddler or very young child, but augmentation enterocystoplasty is preferred for the older child or adolescent.

This surgical procedure requires isolation of a segment of bowel from the fecal stream by cutting a segment of small or large bowel and reanastomosing the remaining ends to reseal the intestinal tract. It is detubularized (reshaped into a dome-like structure) and placed on the bladder. The surgeon may use large or small bowel.[29] The augmentation procedure may be combined with reimplantation of refluxing ureters and a reconstruction of an incompetent sphincter mechanism via sling procedure, implantation of an artificial sphincter, or injection of collagen.

A newer procedure, the gastrocystoplasty, has been used for reconstruction of the hostile neuropathic bladder. The gastrocystoplasty is created in a manner similar to the enterocystoplasty using a segment of the fundus of the stomach. Two potential advantages, acidic secretions that exert a bacteriostatic effect in the urine and reduced secretion of mucus, make the gastrocystoplasty a viable alternative to augmentation procedures using bowel for certain patients.

PREOPERATIVE CARE

Intermittent catheterization is taught as a prerequisite to surgery. During the days before surgery, the nurse reviews the explanation of the procedure with the family. Because the procedure often involves more than one operation, special emphasis is placed on the goals of the current procedure.

A urine culture is obtained prior to hospital admission, and bacteriuria is eradicated using sensitivity-determined antibiotic therapy. The child is admitted to the hospital prior to the day of surgery and a bowel prep (consisting of liquid diet with cleansing enemas) is completed. The nurse explains the purpose of the bowel prep to the child and family. Oral fluids are used to prevent dehydration until the preoperative night, and intravenous fluids are used if necessary to prevent excessive fluid volume and electrolyte loss. Preoperative anti-infective agents are administered to reduce the chances of infection.[29]

POSTOPERATIVE CARE

The child returns from the operative suite with an intravenous fluid line and nasogastric, urethral, and suprapubic tubes. The nurse regularly assesses all drainage tubes for patency, character, and volume of output.

The nasogastric tube is used to allow the bowel to rest and heal following surgical manipulation. It is removed following the return of normal bowel sounds indicating adequate peristalsis. The intravenous line is used to provide carbohydrates, fluid volume, and needed electrolytes while the bowel is healing. It is removed also after bowel sounds return and the patient is able to tolerate oral fluids and food.

The urethral and suprapubic tubes are placed to allow adequate drainage of the augmented bladder and to prevent overdistention.[29] Two catheters are used to allow a back-up system should one become occluded by mucus or other debris. The nurse assesses each drainage tube for patency every 2 hours and maintains a regular record of the patient's urinary and gastrointestinal tube output. The urinary output is assessed for color and presence of blood, clots, and mucus. The urine may be lightly pink tinged or yellow and cloudy; blood clots or bright-red blood are not expected in the urinary output. Mucous strands will be noted. The physician is consulted if either tube becomes occluded; gentle irrigation with sterile saline may be used to restore patency.

In addition, catheter patency is promoted by the maintenance of adequate fluid intake by intravenous or oral routes. Advise the child and family that these mucous strands will persist for several months in the newly augmented bladder but are expected to subside over the first postoperative year. Adequate fluid intake and cranberry juice are given to reduce the viscosity and obstructive potential of mucous strands.

The nurse regularly assesses the child for pain following surgery using an appropriate assessment tool. The location and duration of the pain is determined to assist in proper management. Sharp, stabbing, or cramping pain of short duration located in the lower abdomen or suprapubic area is typically caused by contraction of the augmented bladder. Check the bladder catheters for patency, and administer antispasmodic or Lomotil (see following discussion) to relieve discomfort caused by bladder spasms.

Dull, chronic discomfort of the lower abdomen or pelvic area is typically caused by incisional pain. Proper positioning and limiting movement in combination with analgesics prescribed by the physician will relieve incisional pain.

TEACHING

Following removal of surgical tubes, the significance of intermittent catheterization and adequate fluid intake are re-emphasized. The principles and technique of catheterization are reviewed and reinforced, and the patient and family are given opportunities to demonstrate proper technique before discharge.

The nurse teaches the child and family the potential complications associated with augmentation enterocystoplasty. These include recurrence of urinary tract infection or leakage or rupture of the vesicle. Urinary tract infection is managed as it was prior to surgical reconstruction. The child and family are advised to watch for a change in urinary status and symptoms of discomfort similar to those associated with infection prior to augmentation. They also are advised that infection may cause increased contractility of their augmented bladder, producing feelings of abdominal cramping and leakage.

Urinary leakage not associated with infection is dramatically reduced following augmentation cystoplasty. Patients with high leak pressures or dyssynergic sphincter function prior to augmentation may remain completely dry between catheterizations, and patients with lower leak pressures may report feeling completely dry even though mild stress urinary leakage is noted on urodynamic testing.

Persistent urinary leakage is typically caused by two factors: contraction of the augmented bladder or sphincter incompetence. Leakage is assessed by a voiding diary and urodynamic assessment. The nurse provides the child with a voiding diary (see Chap. 49) to assess functional capacity and factors associated with leakage.

MEDICATION MANAGEMENT

Incontinence due to contractions of the augmented bladder is managed by antispasmodic or anticholinergic medications or by Lomotil. The nurse teaches an appropriate schedule for administration of these medications and advises the family of potential side effects. Expected side effects of antispasmodic or anticholinergic medications are dry mouth and constipation. The family is advised to maintain the child's bowel program and adequate intake of fluid and dietary fiber to prevent constipation. More serious side effects include blurred vision and hallucinations. The family is advised to contact the physician promptly and discontinue the medication should these symptoms occur.

Lomotil, a mixture of a synthetic narcotic (diphenoxylate) and atropine, may be even more effective in controlling unwanted contractions of an augmented bladder than a pure antispasmodic preparation. In addition to the side effects associated with an anticholinergic, the narcotic agent may exacerbate constipation and produce drowsiness.

Urinary leakage due to sphincter incompetence may be managed by an oral α-adrenergic agonist such as pseudoephedrine. More often, this condition requires additional surgery such as artificial urinary sphincter or other bladder neck–tightening procedure.[29]

★ **EVALUATION**

The nurse and family evaluate the outcomes and criteria. Examples of outcome criteria for the child with spina bifida were given in "Nursing Diagnoses and Planning" in this section. Have short-term goals been met? Are long-term goals still realistic? Planning for further nursing care also takes into consideration complications and long-term care.

COMPLICATIONS

The three principal complications associated with altered urinary system function due to spina bifida are urinary tract infection, incontinence, and compromised renal function. The key to successful prevention of these complications lies in ongoing, routine surveillance of urinary system function. A protocol for surveillance is provided in Table 50-2.

Obstructive Uropathy

Definition and Incidence. An obstructive uropathy occurs when a structural abnormality or dysfunctional condition causes urinary stasis, infection, and/or compromised urinary and renal function. The most common sites of obstruction of the developing urinary system are the UPJ, ureteral course, ureterovesical junction, bladder outlet, and proximal or sphincteric urethra.

Etiology and Pathophysiology.

Obstructive Lesions. An understanding of the pathophysiology of an obstructive uropathy arises from appreciation of the nature of obstruction and its effects on the urinary system. An obstruction occurs when mechanical or physical factors restrict flow within a system. As a result, the system must produce greater energy to maintain a flow rate equal to that produced before obstruction occurred. Mathematically, the relationships between flow, pressure and resistance within a system are expressed by a form of Bernoulli's equation:

$$\text{Resistance} = \frac{\text{Pressure}}{\text{Flow}}$$

In this equation, *pressure* denotes the amount of energy a system, such as the urinary tract, must produce to complete its work (the transport of urine from kidneys to outside the body), and the term *flow* represents the result of that work. The term *resistance* denotes a number of factors, including turbulence and the variable widths of the passages urine must travel through, that influence the smooth outflow of urine.

In the normal urinary tract, an acceptable balance among pressure, resistance, and flow exists so that the person is able efficiently to transport and evacuate urine at a relatively low pressure. When obstruction exists, however, the resistance to flow rises and the flow of urine decreases. The urinary tract responds by attempting to restore a normal flow rate by increasing pressure. It is the deleterious results of this process that cause the obstructive uropathies commonly found in patients with altered urinary system function.

A urologic obstruction is defined by its location within the urinary tract and the nature of the obstructive lesion. An obstruction can occur virtually anywhere in the urinary tract, from calix to distal urethra. Depending on its severity, an obstruction will affect the entire portion of the tract that lies proximal to the constriction.[69]

Obstruction of the urinary tract is further defined according to the nature of the lesion. Intrinsic obstruction occurs when the lumen of a urinary structure is blocked because of an anatomic or functional abnormality. In contrast, an extrinsic obstruction occurs when elements outside the urinary system cause compression of the outflow path. These lesion may be congenital or acquired.[69] Common obstructive lesions affecting children are listed in Table 50-3.

Obstructive Uropathy and the Upper Urinary Tract. The result of an obstructive condition is noted primarily within that portion of the urinary system proximal (upstream) of the lesion. The effects of obstruction on the upper urinary tract are influenced by the severity

TABLE 50-3
Causes of Obstructive Lesions of the Urinary System

Site of Obstruction	Cause

Calix	Intrinsic obstruction
	  Infundibular stenosis
	  Infundibular inflammation
	  Tumor
	  Trauma
	Extrinsic obstruction
	  Vascular compression
	  Compression from tumor

Ureteropelvic junction	Intrinsic obstruction
	  Narrowed acontractile segment
	  High insertion into pelvis
	  Obstructing calculi
	Extrinsic obstruction
	  Aberrant vessels
	  Adhesions or fibrous bands

Ureteral course	Intrinsic obstruction
	  Stricture
	  Inflammation
	  Obstructing calculi
	Extrinsic obstruction
	  Retrocaval ureter
	  Aberrant vessels

Ureterovesical junction	Intrinsic obstruction
	  Narrowed acontractile segment
	  Obstructing calculi
	Extrinsic obstruction
	  Thick, noncompliant bladder wall

Bladder outlet and proximal urethra	Intrinsic obstruction
	  Bladder neck hypertrophy
	  Bladder neck contracture
	  Urethral polyp
	  Posterior urethral valves
	  Stricture
	  Dyssynergic or nonrelaxing sphincter mechanism
	Extrinsic obstruction
	  Bladder diverticula
	  Tumor

Adapted from Kelalis, P. P. (1985). Anomalies of the urinary tract: Renal pelvis and ureter. In P. P. Kelalis, L. R. King, & A. B. Belman (Eds.), *Clinical pediatric urology* (pp. 672–725). Philadelphia: Saunders; King, L. R. & Levitt, S. B. (1986). Vesicoureteral reflux, magaureter, and ureteral reimplantation. In P. C. Walsh, R. F. Gittes, A. D. Perlmutter, & T. A. Stamey (Eds.), *Campbell's urology* (pp. 542–578). Philadelphia: Saunders; and Walker, R. D. III. (1987). Vesicoureteral reflux. In J. Y. Gillenwater, J. T. Grayhack, S. S. Howards, & J. W. Duckett (Eds.), *Adult and pediatric urology* (pp. 1676–1706). Chicago: Year Book.

and duration of the lesion. Ureteral dilation and hydronephrosis (enlargement of the renal pelvis and collecting system) are commonly noted.[20]

Following obstruction, the ureteral segments that lie above the obstructive site are subjected to increased resistance to flow. They attempt to compensate by increasing the number (frequency) and strength (amplitude) of peristaltic contractions. As a result, ureteral and renal pelvic pressures rise and the ureter begins to enlarge (dilate). During an acute phase, within minutes or hours of a partial or complete obstruction, this produces discomfort as pain receptors in the ureteral wall are stretched. If the obstruction persists, pressure will fall as a result of permanent damage to the ureteral wall.[20]

Obstruction of a ureter also affects the kidney it drains. During the first few weeks following ureteral occlusion, the kidney will become enlarged due to urinary stasis and dilation of the collecting system. This enlargement is accompanied by damage to the renal parenchyma over time.[20]

The process that causes progressive renal damage in the presence of obstruction was elucidated in an animal model. During the first hours following complete renal obstruction, the papillae of the kidney flatten and the distal portion of the nephrons dilate. This causes dilation of the proximal portion of the nephron. By the end of the first week, the urine collecting tube begins to show signs of atrophy and necrosis. During the second week following obstruction, progressive dilation of the collecting and distal tubules of the nephron continues and atrophy of the proximal tubules begins. By the fourth week following obstruction, there is a 50% loss of functioning parenchymal mass, and by the eighth week only a 1-cm shell of nonfunctioning parenchyma remains.[20]

Although bilateral renal damage inexorably leads to renal failure, the human body is able to compensate for unilateral renal damage by compensatory growth of the contralateral kidney. Although the biochemical factors that initiate this change are not known, research into certain renotropic factors that incite renal hypertrophy presents exciting potential for academic growth and clinical practice.

Obstructive Uropathy and the Lower Urinary Tract. The effects of obstruction on the lower urinary tract also are influenced by the condition's severity and duration. The principal effects of obstruction on the bladder and urethra are the restriction of urinary outflow and decompensation of smooth muscle bundles of the bladder wall.

Obstruction of the lower urinary tract causes a loss of diameter at the bladder outlet (neck) or urethral lumen. This constricts the ability of the bladder to empty itself by reducing the volume of urine able to exit the urethra within a given period. As a result, residual urine in the bladder persists despite what was previously an adequately strong contraction. The lower urinary tract attempts to compensate for urinary residual by increasing both the amplitude and duration of a bladder contraction.[21] Unfortunately, this forces the detrusor muscle to hypertrophy, causing an increase in the ratio of collagen to smooth muscle bundles in the bladder wall.[67]

Ultimately, the process of bladder outlet obstruction causes loss of bladder wall compliance. As a result, the chronically elevated pressures compromise ureteral function by forcing them to operate at a higher pressure to transport urine past the thickened, hypertrophied bladder wall. Ureteral dilation, in turn, initiates the process of hydronephrosis and compromised renal function, completing the deleterious cycle of events that characterize obstructive uropathy.

Clinical Manifestations. Because of increased sophistication in ultrasound techniques, obstructive uropathy may be detected prior to birth. More commonly, however, severe cases are detected during the neonatal period, and more subtle cases of obstructive uropathy are detected when infection or discomfort complicate the already compromised urinary system.

Acute urinary obstruction presents as pain, commonly complicated by urinary tract infection. The pain associated with acute urinary obstruction is typically intense and may be centered in the flank or lower back. It often radiates to the groin and testes in boys and to the labia majora in girls.[58]

Urinary tract infection associated with obstruction is common. The infection often involves the upper urinary tract, causing fever, nausea, and vomiting. Irritative voiding symptoms consisting of painful urination (dysuria), urinary frequency, urgency, and hematuria are common.

Chronic obstruction of the urinary tract is not often associated with pain. The obstructive uropathy may be detected during urologic evaluation for recurrent urinary tract infections or for altered growth and development when renal function is compromised. In many instances, the presence of congenital anomalies such as prune belly syndrome or imperforate anus associated with urinary system abnormality may lead to diagnosis of obstructive uropathy.

Diagnostic Evaluation. During physical examination, an abdominal mass is noted in the infant or child with hydronephrosis; findings may be obscured by abdominal muscle guarding in older children or adolescents. Laboratory findings are normal unless bilateral compromised renal function is present. An IVP shows an enlarged renal collecting system (hydronephrosis) with normal or thin rim of renal parenchyma. The ureters are dilated proximal to the obstructive lesion. The cystogram/VCUG is normal or shows a trabeculated bladder with thickened wall if obstruction exists at the vesicle outlet or urethra. A renal and bladder ultrasound reveals hydronephrosis of kidney, normal or enlarged ureters, and thickened bladder wall if obstruction is at the bladder outlet or urethral course. The DTPA radionuclide scan shows increased concentration of radionuclide on affected side with incomplete washout of DTPA substance when challenged by furosemide. DMSA radionuclide scan shows normal or reduced differential function of the affected kidney. On endoscopic examination, there is a normal urethrogram or a narrowed urethral segment is revealed. The bladder wall is trabeculated if the obstruction is located in the lower urinary tract; ureteroscopy will reveal ureteral enlargement proximal to the obstructive lesion. A urodynamic examination shows a poor or intermittent flow pattern with increased contraction pressure and increased calculated resistance value during the pressure-flow study if a lower urinary tract obstruction is present. The Whitaker test shows obstruction between renal pelvis and the ureterovesical junction.

⭐ **NURSING IMPLICATIONS**

The nursing care of patients with obstructive uropathy is determined by the location, etiology, and severity of the lesion. Within the context of this discussion, three obstructive lesions commonly encountered when caring for children with altered urinary function are discussed in subsequent sections. They are UPJ obstruction, ureteral obstruction, and posterior urethral valves causing bladder outlet obstruction.

COMPLICATIONS

The complications of obstructive uropathy are urinary stasis, compromised renal function, and infection. Urinary stasis occurs when urine transport and evacuation are compromised despite attempts to overcome resistance by increased pressure. Left uncorrected, this process becomes more pronounced as the affected urinary structures dilate and hypertrophy.

The association of urinary tract infection with obstructive uropathy is influenced by the location and etiology of the obstruction. The nursing care of the child with an infected urinary tract is presented in "Urinary Tract Infection" in this chapter.

Ureteropelvic Junction Obstruction

Definition and Incidence. UPJ obstruction exists when intrinsic or extrinsic factors compromise urine transport from the renal pelvis to proximal ureter (Fig. 50-8). The most common intrinsic factors leading to UPJ obstruction are abnormal development or acquired disease of the smooth muscle bundles at the junction causing replacement of muscle with fibrous tissue or abnormally high insertion of the ureter into the renal pelvis.[31]

Extrinsic factors also may obstruct the UPJ. Kinks, bands or adhesions may form around the UPJ causing dysfunctional angulation, high ureteral insertion or compression of the junctional lumen. Aberrant blood vessels also cause or exacerbate obstruction of the UPJ.[31]

Etiology and Pathophysiology. See "Obstructive Uropathy" introductory discussion.

Clinical Manifestations. The most common presenting symptom of UPJ obstruction among infants is abdominal mass produced by a hydronephrotic kidney. Signs of compromised renal function, including fever, nausea, vomiting, and failure to thrive, also may be found.[31]

Among older children, UPJ obstruction presents as vague, poorly localized abdominal pain often mistaken for gastrointestinal disorders. The child typically complains of paraumbilical pain associated with nausea and vomiting that mimics symptoms of irritable colon or gastroenteritis. In other instances, the pain is localized to the flank and is colicky in nature. Discomfort caused by UPJ obstruction is exacerbated by copious fluid intake. This finding often serves as a valuable clue to the presence of the condition.[31]

Gross hematuria also may indicate the presence of UPJ obstruction, but urinary tract infection is not a common initial finding.[31] The rare incidence of infection is explained by the high location of the obstruction in relation to the lower urinary tract. As expected, the association of UPJ obstruction and infection is common when the condition is complicated by vesicoureteral reflux.

Diagnostic Evaluation. Physical examination reveals an abdominal mass in infants or younger children. Laboratory findings comprise an elevated serum BUN and creatinine when renal function is compromised bilater-

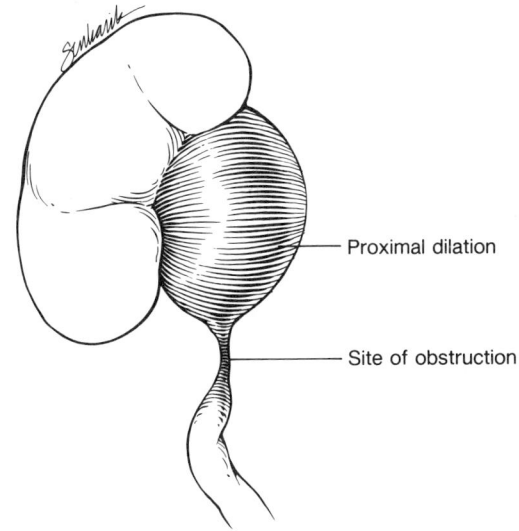

- Proximal dilation

- Site of obstruction

FIGURE 50-8
Ureteropelvic junction obstruction.

ally. Imaging studies include the following findings. On the IVP, a hydronephrosis of affected kidney(s) is revealed; there is a dilated renal pelvis but normal ureter distal to UPJ. Cystogram/VGUG is normal or shows presence of vesicoureteral reflux. Renal and bladder ultrasound also shows hydronephrosis of the affected kidney with absent ureteral dilation. Arteriography reveals presence of aberrant vessels. DTPA radionuclide scan reveals increased concentration of radionuclide of affected kidney(s) with delayed or absent washout in response to furosemide challenge. On the urodynamic examination, an increased pressure gradient between renal pelvis and UPJ is evident on the affected side.

★ ASSESSMENT

The nursing assessment of the child with UPJ obstruction centers on assessment of renal and urinary function compromise. In the infant, the nurse questions the parents for any signs of potential abdominal pain indicating potential obstruction, including bouts of crying following feeding or other episodes of increased fluid intake. The parents are questioned concerning previous bouts of unexplained fever or episodes of known urinary tract infection. A growth and height assessment is made, and the child's current status is compared with previous records to assess potential altered growth due to renal insufficiency. The nurse also obtains a history of periods of poor appetite and nausea and vomiting.

The nurse assesses the older child for the onset, location, character, and duration of flank or abdominal pain. The child and family are asked if these episodes correlate with increased fluid intake. Obtain a history of gastrointestinal troubles such as irritable colon or gastroenteritis that may represent previously undetected clues to obstructive uropathy. Growth and development is assessed, and comparison is made between current levels and previous patterns. The nurse questions the child and family concerning the color and character of urine output. They are asked specifically if the urine has ever been bright

red (indicating fresh blood in the urine) or dark red or amber (indicating old blood in the urine).[58] The child and family are also questioned concerning irritative voiding symptoms (urinary frequency, urgency) that may indicate a history of urinary tract infection.

★ NURSING DIAGNOSES AND PLANNING

Based on the assessment data from above and the preceding chapter, the following nursing diagnoses may apply:

- Altered Tissue Perfusion: Renal related to integrity of blood vessels.
- Altered Urinary Elimination related to anatomic obstruction.
- Altered Growth and Development related to anatomic obstruction.
- High Risk for Infection (Urinary Tract) related to inadequate primary defenses.
- Pain related to surgical procedure.
- Ineffective Airway Clearance related to limited movement.

Other functionally related nursing diagnoses are discussed in Table 49-2 in Chapter 49.

The nurse and child (or parents) together plan effective care based on the established nursing diagnoses. Several examples of expected outcomes are as follows:

- The child and parents discuss concerns related to growth and developmental tasks.
- The child participates in coughing and deep breathing exercises.
- The child remains infection free.

The nurse plans for the daily care of the child based on both physician's orders and nursing diagnoses. Some general nursing care goals may be the following:

- Postoperative urine is pink or yellow.
- Obstruction is relieved.
- Optimal renal and urinary function are restored.
- Infection is prevented.

★ INTERVENTIONS: COLLABORATIVE AND INDEPENDENT

SURGICAL RECONSTRUCTION

Surgical correction is the most common means of medical treatment for clinically significant obstruction. The goal of corrective surgery is to relieve obstruction and restore optimal renal and urinary function. In certain instances, however, nephrectomy is required when renal function is severely compromised, posing a threat to the child's current or future health.[31]

Corrective surgery for UPJ obstruction is preferred when the kidney contributes 20% or more to urinary function and when it is producing hypertension. Pyeloplasty is the definitive corrective surgery for obstruction. The goal of surgery is to identify and remove the dysfunctional ureteral segment causing obstruction or reinsert the ureter into the renal pelvis in a manner that improves optimal urinary drainage. Various operative techniques are used (Table 50-4).

TABLE 50-4
Techniques of Pyeloplasty

Procedure and Indication	Description
Y–V Intrinsic obstruction	Reconstruction of UPJ without resection of aberrant tissue; requires minimal manipulation of kidney and vascular supply.
Spiral flap Markedly long segment of fibrous ureter	Creation of a broad flap of enlarged pelvis dissected and used to reconstruct UPJ; contraindicated with high ureteral insertion.
Dismembered Shorter aberrant ureteral segment	Resection of aberrant ureteral segment with spatulation and reanastomosis of healthy renal pelvis with ureter; contraindicated when tension must be used to join pelvis and ureter.

Pyeloplasty may be accompanied by surgical manipulation of aberrant blood vessels in certain instances. In this case, the goal of surgery is both to establish normal drainage of the urinary tract and to avoid creating local ischemia and systemic hypertension by indiscriminate ligation of aberrant blood vessels that supply the kidneys.[56]

PREOPERATIVE CARE

The goals and purpose of the surgical procedure are reviewed with the child and family. A urine culture is obtained in consultation with the physician, and bacteriuria is eradicated prior to surgical manipulation of the kidney using anti-infective chemotherapy. The urologic surgeon may place a ureteral or percutaneous stent in the severely affected kidney to promote decompression of the renal pelvis 3 to 6 days prior to surgery. The nurse monitors the urine output from this tube for volume, color, and character. The affected kidney may diurese on decompression, causing increased urinary output and relief from pain. The nurse re-emphasizes that this relief represents the effects of a temporary diversion method and that surgery is still indicated for permanent correction of obstruction.

POSTOPERATIVE CARE

The child will return from the operating suite with a flank incision, intravenous fluid line, and percutaneous or ureteral stent. The nurse monitors all drains for volume, character, and color of urinary output. The urine will be pink or yellow; the presence of bright-red blood or clots in the urine is promptly reported to the physician. During the first postoperative day, urinary stents are monitored as often as hourly for patency, and occlusion is reported promptly to the physician.

The child is carefully monitored for signs of pain and discomfort. Assess the child's pain for location, duration, and intensity using an assessment tool for the pediatric patient whenever feasible. It is often difficult to distinguish postoperative wound pain from pain produced by obstruction. Postoperative wound pain in the child who has undergone pyeloplasty is particularly pronounced because of the necessity of a flank incision in many cases. Flank incision pain is relatively continuous and aggravated by certain positions and activity, especially coughing or deep breathing. In contrast, pain due to unexpected postoperative obstruction typically crescendos as the obstruction worsens. It is unrelieved by position changes and unaffected by coughing or deep breathing.

After assessing the source of the pain, the nurse assists the patient to relieve discomfort via adequate urinary drainage or positional changes as indicated. Analgesic or narcotic medications are administered to relieve persistent pain as directed.

Scrupulous aseptic technique is used when caring for percutaneous tubes to prevent inadvertent kidney infection. The tube is securely attached to the patient's flank by dressings that are monitored for exudate or urine output. Prophylactic antibiotic medications are administered to prevent infection as directed.

The nurse takes special care to prevent respiratory complications associated with ineffective airway clearance due to limited movement and pain. Appropriate pain medications are administered prior to routine "turn, encourage cough and deep breathing" exercises, and the patient is monitored routinely for signs of respiratory infection.

The ureteral or percutaneous stent is typically removed by the seventh postoperative day. Following stent removal, the nurse assesses the patient for signs of obstruction, including flank or abdominal pain. The family is advised of signs of obstruction; they are taught to seek medical help promptly should these symptoms occur.

MANAGEMENT OF THE FAILED, OBSTRUCTED KIDNEY

Nephrectomy rather than pyeloplasty becomes the procedure of choice when obstruction of the UPJ is of sufficient duration and severity to irreparably damage the affected kidney. In this instance, the goal of surgery is to prevent systemic renovascular hypertension associated with allowing a nonfunctioning kidney to remain in an otherwise healthy child. The nursing care related to nephrectomy is discussed in "Urinary System Tumors" in this chapter.

★ **EVALUATION**

The nurse and family evaluate the outcomes and criteria. Examples of outcome criteria were given in "Nursing Diagnoses and Planning" in this section. Have short-term goals been met? Are long-term goals still realistic? Planning for further nursing care also takes into consideration complications and long-term care.

COMPLICATIONS

See "Obstructive Uropathy" introductory discussion.

LONG-TERM MANAGEMENT

The results of pyeloplasty are evaluated 3 to 6 months after surgery by repeat IVP, ultrasonography, and/or radionuclide studies. The nurse reassures the parents that although the physical appearance of the urinary tract assessed by ultrasound or IVP may not show marked improvement, evaluation is based on functional rather than morphologic improvement. Therefore, DTPA radionuclide scans produce definitive results, and radiographic procedures or ultrasound are best conceptualized as adjunctive tests.

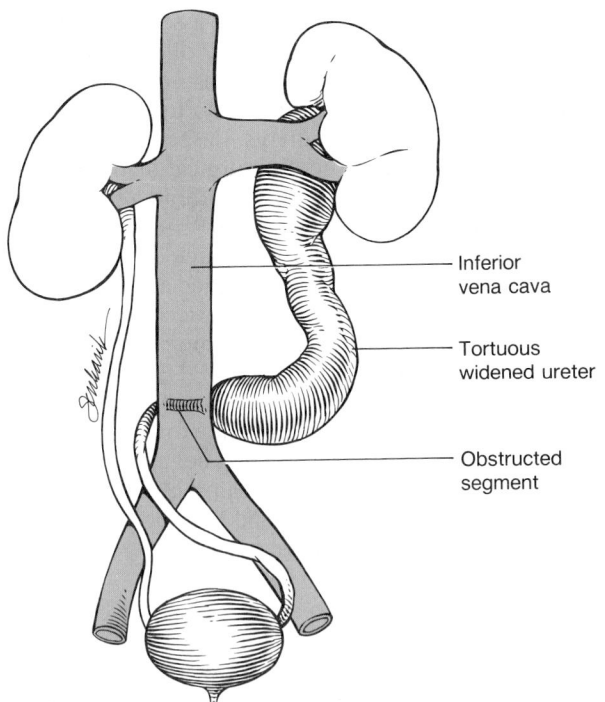

FIGURE 50-9
Retrocaval ureter. An aberrant blood vessel produces extrinsic obstruction.

Labels on figure:
Inferior vena cava
Tortuous widened ureter
Obstructed segment

Long-term management of the child with UPJ obstruction also requires prospective monitoring for renal failure that may progress over months or years in spite of technically successful reconstruction. Advise the parents that their child should undergo annual assessment of height and weight, serum creatinine and BUN, and blood pressure. Emphasize to the parents that the child must be fully informed of the risk for prolonged complications related to abnormal renal function, including annual blood pressure assessment, throughout his or her adult life.

Ureteral Obstruction

Definition and Incidence. Ureteral obstruction occurs when the ureteral course is constricted due to mechanical or anatomic factors. Intrinsic factors that contribute to ureteral obstruction include stricture, valves, diverticula, or atresia. The ureteral course also may be obstructed by a polyp, tumor, or obstructing calculi.[32] Extrinsic factors causing ureteral stricture include retrocaval ureter or aberrant blood vessels (Fig. 50-9). Obstruction of the ureterovesical junction by congenital defects, acquired disease states, or iatrogenic causes also may obstruct the ureter and is often described by the terms *megaureter* or *megaloureter* (Fig. 50-10A).

Etiology and Pathophysiology. See the "Obstructive Uropathy" introductory discussion.

Clinical Manifestations. The presenting signs of ureteral obstruction are typically pain produced by acute blockage or infection presenting as a complication of chronic ureteral obstruction. In certain instances, an obstructed ureter is detected during evaluation of the urinary system for related congenital anomalies such as exstrophy or epispadias defect, prune belly syndrome, or imperforate anus.

Diagnostic Evaluation. If hydronephrosis is present in an infant or young child, an abdominal mass is felt on physical examination. A normal or elevated serum BUN and creatinine appear if renal function is compromised. Imaging studies include an IVP, which reveals an enlarged, tortuous ureter(s) with hydronephrosis of affected kidney(s); and the cystogram/VCUG, which is normal. A renal and bladder ultrasound reveals an enlarged ureter(s) and hydronephrosis. DTPA radionuclide scan shows increased concentration of radionuclide material in the affected kidney with poor or equivocal response to furosemide challenge (response is affected by

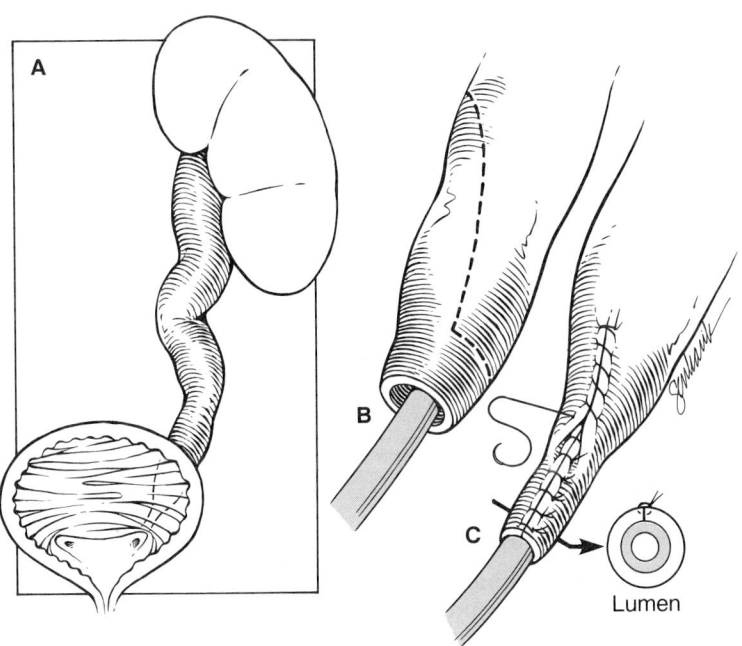

FIGURE 50-10
Ureteral tapering procedure. (**A**) Congenital megaureter. (**B**) Ureteral wall is incised and extra tissue removed. (**C**) Ureter is reconstructed with narrower lumen.

Labels on figure: A, B, C, Lumen

size of the ureter and location of the lesion). Urodynamic examination reveals a high-pressure gradient between the renal pelvis and UPJ regardless of size or location of the obstructive lesion.

★ ASSESSMENT

Nursing assessment of the obstructed ureter centers on identifying the source of obstruction and its effects on urinary and renal function. The nurse obtains a history of signs and symptoms of urinary tract infection and abdominal discomfort. Urinary elimination patterns are assessed with the use of a voiding diary and observation of voided stream to rule out the possibility of a dysfunctional voiding state. These results are used with the findings of the physical examination and imaging and laboratory study results to determine the extent of compromise to urinary system function caused by obstruction.

Renal function is assessed by determining current height and weight compared with previous findings. In addition, any history of weight loss, nausea and vomiting, or failure to thrive is assessed to determine the extent to which renal function is compromised.

★ NURSING DIAGNOSES AND PLANNING

Based on the assessment date from above and the preceding chapter, the following nursing diagnoses may apply:

- Altered Tissue Perfusion: Renal related to obstruction.
- Altered Urinary Elimination related to anatomic obstruction.
- Altered Growth and Development related to effects of physical anomaly.
- High Risk for Infection (Urinary Tract) related to inadequate primary defenses.
- Pain related to surgical procedure.

Other functionally related nursing diagnoses are discussed in Table 49-2 in Chapter 49.

The nurse and child (or parents) together plan effective care based on the established nursing diagnoses. Several examples of expected outcomes are as follows:

- The child changes positions regularly to relieve incisional pain.
- The parents describe symptoms of urinary tract infection to report.
- The child remains infection free.

The nurse plans for the daily care of the child based on both physician's orders and nursing diagnoses. Some general nursing care goals may be the following:

- Bladder spasms are minimized.
- Optimal drainage is improved.

★ INTERVENTIONS: COLLABORATIVE AND INDEPENDENT

URETERAL RECONSTRUCTION

Surgical reconstruction of the affected segment is indicated when intrinsic ureteral obstruction exists. The method of reconstruction is determined by the location and type of lesion and the degree of associated uropathy. Ureteral stricture may be treated by dilation or surgical reconstruction. Transureteroureterostomy is performed by resecting the aberrant ureteral portion and reanastomosing the remaining segments. Cases of extrinsic ureteral obstruction are treated by surgical manipulation of the offending structure with or without resection and reanastomosis of the affected ureter.[32]

Surgical correction of an obstructed ureter is even more difficult in the markedly enlarged and tortuous ureter or megaureter. In these cases, resection of an aperistaltic obstructive segment is supplemented by in-folding or tapering of the wide ureter. Ureteral tapering requires creation of a transverse suprapubic incision through which the ureter is freed from its connection to the bladder wall (see Fig. 50-10B). The obstructing segment is resected along with a portion of the remaining ureteral wall to narrow the remaining lumen (see Fig. 50-10C). The goal is to improve optimal drainage and to enhance reimplantation of ureteral orifice into bladder wall.

Ureteral in-folding is an alternative surgical approach to tapering (Fig. 50-11). The megaureter is exposed and the obstructing segment resected. Ureteral narrowing is then accomplished by folding the ureter so that an optimal width is obtained. The principal advantage to this approach is the limited need to dissect and reanastomose the ureter with the associated risk of vascular damage.

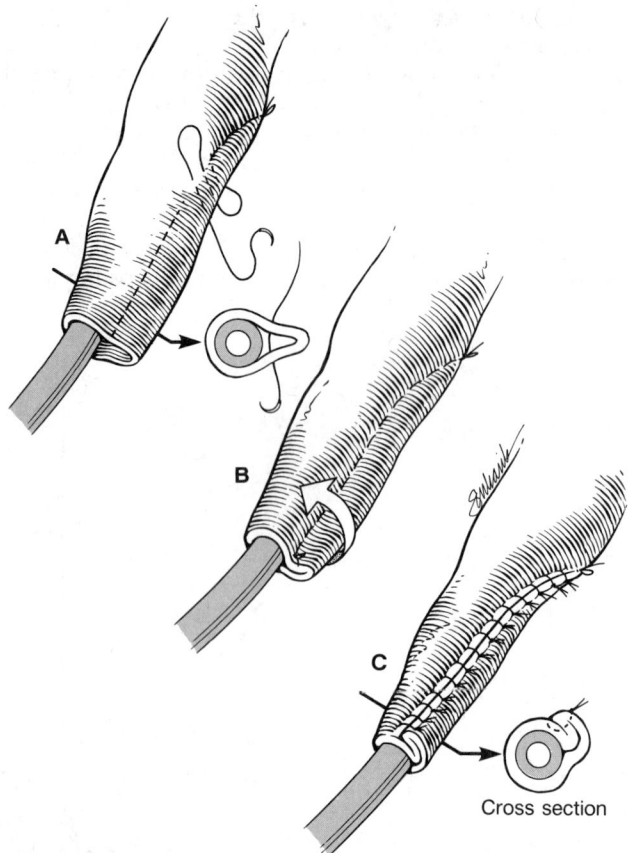

Cross section

FIGURE 50-11

Ureteral infolding procedure narrows lumen without incising ureteral wall. (A) Megaureter in Fig. 50-10A is resected. (B) Ureter is infolded to reduce caliber. (C) Sutures are left in place without incising and reconstructing ureteral wall.

PREOPERATIVE CARE

The nurse reviews the goals and purpose of the procedure. Urine culture is obtained prior to surgery in consultation with the physician, and sensitivities are used to render the child's urinary tract infection free.

POSTOPERATIVE CARE

The child returns from the surgical suite with an intravenous fluid line, ureteral stent and Foley catheter, and suprapubic or abdominal incision. The nurse monitors output from the Foley catheter for volume, color, and signs of hematuria. The urine is expected to be pink or yellow; the presence of bright red blood or clots is promptly reported to the physician.

The child may experience pain from the surgical site, from unexpected ureteral obstruction, or from painful bladder spasm. The nurse determines the location, intensity, character, and duration of pain to determine appropriate management strategies. Bladder spasms cause an intermittent, cramping pain centered in the suprapubic area. Urine often leaks from around the catheter in response to bladder spasm. Management focuses on insuring adequate Foley catheter drainage and observing that the patient's bladder is not overdistended. Excessive activity also may be limited to reduce irritation produced by traction of the catheter balloon against the bladder neck. Anticholinergic medications are administered to reduce the occurrence of spasms in consultation with the physician.

In contrast to bladder spasm, discomfort from the surgical wound presents as a more constant, aching pain, also located in the suprapubic or abdominal area. It is exacerbated by movement and relieved by proper positioning and splinting during deep-breathing or coughing exercises. Incisional pain is managed by proper positioning of the patient, limitation of excessive activity as indicated, and administration of analgesic medications as directed.

Pain due to unexpected obstruction of the ureter presents as discomfort in the abdomen or flank that rapidly crescendos into intense pain not relieved by positional changes or restriction of activity. Obstruction may be accompanied by reduced urinary output or excessive blood clots or debris in the urine. Pain from obstruction is managed by rapid notification of the physician.

Removal of the ureteral stents and Foley catheter is accomplished by the physician approximately 7 days after surgery. Following stent removal the patient is monitored for signs of obstruction discussed earlier. Patterns of urinary elimination are monitored by a voiding diary, which is kept until bladder micturition habits return to preoperative norms.

The patient and family are taught the signs of acute ureteral obstruction and are advised to seek care promptly should symptoms occur. In addition, they are advised to monitor the child carefully for signs of urinary tract infection and to seek care should it occur.

★ EVALUATION

COMPLICATIONS

See "Obstructive Uropathy" introductory discussion.

LONG-TERM MANAGEMENT

The success of ureteral reconstruction is assessed approximately 3 to 6 months after surgery by repeat IVP, ultrasound, and/or functional radionuclide scan. The nurse reassures the family that the gross appearance of the urinary system may or may not appear dramatically different. Instead, the family is prepared to rely on the results produced by functional assessment of the urinary tract, such as that obtained by DTPA scan or Whitaker assessment.

The family is advised that urinary tract infection, recurrent obstruction, and compromised renal function may occur as late-onset complications of ureteral obstruction with surgical reconstruction. They are taught signs to observe. They are assisted in arranging annual check-ups, including assessment of growth and development patterns, serum creatinine and BUN, and blood pressure. The parents are advised to teach their child that complications of abnormal renal function may occur many years after technically successful ureteral reconstruction and require annual blood pressure screening throughout adult life.

Urethral Valves

Definition and Incidence.   Urethral valves are embryologic leaflets that block urinary outflow in the male's posterior urethra, producing obstructive uropathy. Four types of valves are described as follows:

Type I valves are formed from posterior mucosal folds distal to the verumontanum. They represent an abnormal fusion of the caudal end of the cisternae of the normal urethra.

Type II valves are tissue folds that originate in the verumontanum and terminate near the bladder neck.

Type III valves are formed by a marked fusion of the anterior folds of the verumontanum or a congenital urethral membrane.

Type IV valves are formed by a deep infolding of the anterior and anterolateral walls of the membranous urethra. They are often associated with prune belly syndrome.[16,61]

Once considered exceedingly rare, the incidence of urethral valves has been determined to be more common than expected since the advent of voiding cystourethrography. The absolute incidence of the condition remains unknown.[32]

Etiology and Pathophysiology.   See the "Obstructive Uropathy" introductory discussion.

Clinical Manifestations.   Because of increased sophistication associated with antenatal ultrasonography, the obstructive uropathy associated with total or nearly total bladder outlet obstruction may be detected before birth. In other instances, valves are detected during routine assessment of the neonate's urine elimination patterns. Affected boys often void with a poor or intermittent stream and strain or grunt to enhance bladder emptying. Nonetheless, a strong urinary stream does not preclude the possibility of valves.

Neonatal examination of boys with urethral valves usually reveals bilateral abdominal masses due to hydronephrosis, with a pelvic or lower abdominal mass representing the overdistended bladder. Voiding is often accompanied by straining and poor force of stream.[74]

Other children present with signs of renal insufficiency, such as nausea, vomiting and metabolic acidosis, that may be confused with respiratory distress syndrome. In certain instances, the urinary tract is compromised by infection and sepsis, even during the first days of life.[44]

Approximately half of the children born with valves are not detected during the neonatal period. Later clinical manifestations present as signs of obstructive uropathy, including pain, dysuria with infection, and abdominal or flank mass detected on physical examination.[16]

Diagnostic Evaluation. Physical examination reveals a bilateral abdominal or flank mass due to hydronephrosis or a lower abdominal mass or pelvic mass due to bladder distention. Abdominal or flank pain in the older child is due to obstruction. There are normal or elevated serum BUN and creatinine levels with compromised renal function. IVP reveals hydronephrosis of both kidneys; ureters are enlarged and tortuous; and the bladder wall is thickened and trabeculated. In certain cases, hydronephrosis with moderately enlarged ureters and trabeculation, large bladder diverticula may be present. Cystogram/VCUG show trabeculated, thickened bladder wall or moderate trabeculation with large diverticula; vesicoureteral reflux may be present. Renal and bladder ultrasound shows bilateral hydronephrosis with enlarged ureters and thickened bladder wall. Because the cusps or leaflets of urethral valves collapse during retrograde irrigation or instrumentation, they are often not noted during routine cystoscopic examination. Urethral valves are best seen when the endoscopic telescope is placed distal to the verumontanum and the irrigation valve is left open, allowing antegrade bladder emptying. A pressure-flow study demonstrates poor flow pattern with high voiding pressures consistent with outlet obstruction. Filling cystometrogram may demonstrate reduced functional capacity and poor compliance due to marked trabeculation.

★ ASSESSMENT

Much of the nursing assessment of urethral valves relies on evaluation of urinary elimination patterns. The nurse assesses micturition patterns in the child with suspected valves with the use of a voiding diary and observation of the voided stream. The voiding diary typically reveals frequent episodes of micturition with small functional capacity and large residual urine assessed by ultrasound or catheterization. Observation of the voided stream typically reveals a poor or intermittent stream and straining in an attempt to maximize bladder evacuation.

The nurse also assesses the extent of the associated obstructive uropathy through data from physical examination, evaluation of growth and development patterns, and laboratory and imaging studies. A history of fevers of uncertain origin or changes in urine color and odor may indicate a poorly documented history of urinary tract infection.

★ NURSING DIAGNOSES AND PLANNING

Based on the assessment data from above and the preceding chapter, the following nursing diagnoses may apply:

* Altered Tissue Perfusion: Renal related to obstruction.
* Altered Urinary Elimination related to anatomic obstruction.
* Altered Growth and Development related to effects of physical anomaly.
* High Risk for Infection (Urinary Tract) related to inadequate primary defenses.
* Urinary Retention related to blockage.

Nursing diagnoses related to transurethral resection may be the following:

* Altered Urinary Elimination related to catheterization.
* Altered Tissue Perfusion: Peripheral Ureteral related to surgical trauma.
* High Risk for Infection (Urinary Tract) related to inadequate primary defense.
* Pain related to surgical procedure.

Other functionally related nursing diagnoses are discussed in Table 49-2 in Chapter 49.

The nurse and child (or parents) together plan effective care based on the established nursing diagnoses. Several examples of expected outcomes are as follows:

* The parents demonstrate ability to monitor the child for bleeding postoperatively.
* The parents verbalize understanding of toilet training for the boy with valve disease.

The nurse plans for the daily care of the child based on both physician's orders and nursing diagnoses. A general nursing care goal may be the following:

* Optimal urinary flow is improved.

★ INTERVENTIONS: COLLABORATIVE AND INDEPENDENT

TEMPORARY URINARY DIVERSION

The initial management of urethral valves in the neonate remains controversial. In many instances, acute medical illness and uncertainty related to eventual bladder function justify the use of a temporary urinary diversion. The most commonly used procedure is the vesicostomy, which effectively bypasses the obstructing valves while allowing management with diapers rather than a pouch-type device. The nursing care related to vesicostomy diversion is discussed in ''Prune Belly Syndrome.''

DEFINITIVE VALVE REPAIR

Definitive repair of urethral valves requires surgical resection of the valve cusps with or without reconstruction of refluxing ureterovesical valves and dilated ureters. Resection of urethral valves is performed via transurethral resection using a resectoscope to ablate the valve cusps and Bugbee electrode to fulgurate the remaining mucosa. The goal of ablation is to remove completely all obstructing leaflets, leaving a smooth urethral course for optimal urinary flow.[16]

POSTOPERATIVE CARE

The patient will return from the operating or cystoscopic suite with a urethral catheter in place. The nurse monitors output from the catheter for volume and consistency. The urine may be pink tinged but should not be bright red or contain clots. If excessive hematuria is detected, gentle traction is placed against the catheter after checking to see that the balloon is inflated to provide hemostasis and the physician is notified promptly. The urethral catheter is removed after allowing time for the urethral mucosa to heal, usually within the first 1 to 3 postoperative days.

Pain and discomfort following resection of valves are assessed for duration, location, and character. Bladder spasms are characterized by brief, cramping pain in the suprapubic area. Urethral irritation is noted as prolonged burning centered in the penis. The nurse manages discomfort by limiting excessive movement prior to catheter removal to minimize irritation from the catheter balloon. A urinary antispasmodic, such as oxybutynin (Ditropan), combined with a urinary analgesic such as phenazopyridine (Pyridium) is administered to relieve discomfort as directed. Following catheter removal, residual irritation from resection is alleviated by warm sitz baths and adequate hydration.

Following catheter removal, the patient is assessed for urine elimination patterns and for residual hematuria. The family is advised that the child may pass some dark-red "scabs" and pink-tinged urine within 7 to 10 days following catheter removal. They are reassured that the presence of these scabs are expected and indicate healing at the surgical site. The nurse teaches the parents to monitor their child for the presence of excessive bleeding (bright-red blood or multiple clots) and promptly to seek care if symptoms occur.

In many instances, simple ablation of the urethral valves is not sufficient to reverse the obstructive uropathy caused by bladder outlet obstruction. Detailed discussions of the nursing care related to ureteral reconstruction and vesicoureteral reflux are presented in "Ureteral Obstruction" and "Vesicoureteral Reflux," respectively.

★ **EVALUATION**

The nurse and family evaluate the outcomes and criteria. Examples of outcomes for the child with urethral valve disease were given in "Nursing Diagnoses and Planning" in this section. Have short-term goals been met? Are long-term goals still realistic? Planning for further nursing care also takes into consideration complications and long-term care.

COMPLICATIONS

In addition to the complications associated with obstructive uropathy, the child with urethral valves also faces potential complications related to surgical resection. Residual valve tissue due to incomplete resection may cause persistent obstruction and exacerbate the original obstructive uropathy. In contrast, overzealous resection may result in sphincter damage and lead to stress urinary incontinence. The nursing care related to the child with stress incontinence is presented in "Altered Urine Elimination: Voiding Dysfunction" in this chapter.

LONG-TERM MANAGEMENT

The long-term management of urethral valves is determined by the severity of associated obstructive uropathy. Lower urinary tract function may return to a relatively normal state following relief from obstruction, but trabeculation and compromised detrusor contractility may persist. The nurse advises the family of the boy with a history of valve disease to proceed with toilet training at a normal age but cautions the parents that potential problems gaining control may occur.

Prolonged voiding dysfunction in the infant is assessed by its effects on urinary and renal function as well as its effects on the child's social and emotional development. If problems with urinary control are associated only with wet diapers, then the family may be encouraged to allow toilet training to wait while the child grows and obtains greater bladder size and functional capacity. In contrast, voiding dysfunction associated with repeated urinary tract infections or signs of upper urinary tract distress, such as development of secondary vesicoureteral reflux or febrile infections, must be managed by more aggressive measures, such as an intermittent catheterization program or surgical reconstruction of the poorly compliant bladder.

The nurse completes a screening assessment of bladder function with a careful history of urine elimination patterns and a voiding diary. Definitive assessment also relies on complex urodynamic assessment as well as repeated imaging studies of upper urinary tract function.

Ongoing assessment of renal function also is necessary for managing the child with urethral valve disease. Annual measurement of serum creatinine and BUN, growth patterns, and blood pressure are indicated and should extend throughout the adult years.

Urinary System Tumors

Upper Tract Tumors

Definition and Incidence. The most common malignancy of the upper urinary tract in children is the *Wilms' tumor,* also called *renal embryoma* or *nephroblastoma.* Wilms' tumor is an embryonal malignancy of the kidney with mixed histopathology. It accounts for 95% of all cancers found in the entire urinary system prior to age 16 years.[36] It occurs in approximately 7.8 in 1 million children between the ages of 1 and 14, accounting for 6.2% of cancers in white children and 7.9% of all malignancies in black children in the United States.[3] Other tumors affecting the upper urinary tracts are renal cell carcinoma and transitional cell carcinomas of the renal pelvis and ureters. Because of its marked prevalence, discussion in this section is limited to the Wilms' tumor. Wilms' tumor is also discussed in Chapter 31.

Wilms' tumors are further defined by staging systems. Currently, the system proposed by the National Wilms' Tumor Study Group (NWTS-3) is widely accepted and is used in this discussion.[17] The staging system is explained in Table 50-5.

Etiology and Pathophysiology. The etiology of Wilms' tumor remains unclear. It is thought to arise from

TABLE 50-5
Staging System for Wilms' Tumor

Stage	Description
I	Tumor contained in one kidney; excised surgically without extension beyond margins of resection.
II	Tumor extends beyond kidney; completely excised surgically.
III	Tumors have residual nonhematogenous tumor cells confined to abdomen.
IV	Tumor characterized by distant metastases involving lung, liver, bone, or brain.
V	Tumor involves both kidneys, severely limiting surgical resection as an option.

abnormal proliferation of the metanephric blastema interfering with differentiation of metanephric ducts into mature tubules and glomeruli.[11] Chromosomal factors also are postulated to influence the likelihood of developing a Wilms' tumor during infancy or childhood.[3]

A propensity for development of Wilms' Tumor is noted among children with Beckwith-Weidemann syndrome. The syndrome is characterized by visceromegaly of the kidney, liver, pancreas, adrenal cortex, and testis. Omphalocele, microcephaly, mental retardation, and macroglossia (enlargement of the tongue) also may occur.

Hemihypertrophy, an uncommon congenital defect characterized by asymmetry of the body that may represent a mild form of the Beckwith-Wiedemann syndrome, is associated with development of Wilms' tumor. Genitourinary anomalies, including hypoplasia, fusion anomalies, and ectopic kidneys, also may place a child at risk for development of renal embryoma.

Wilms' tumor presents with a variety of histopathologic characteristics. Although a detailed description of the pathology or renal embryoma is beyond the scope of this discussion, it is important to note the general pathologic findings associated with a favorable or unfavorable prognosis.

Three histopathologic characteristics are considered unfavorable when attempting to eradicate Wilms' tumor because their presence accounts for 60% of related deaths while comprising only 10% of all new malignancies. *Anaplasia* is a variance in nuclear size of malignant cells associated with marked hyperchromatism and abnormal mitotic figures. It typically occurs in older children and is more ominous when found throughout the tumor rather than confined to a focal area. A *rhabdoid* tumor is characterized by uniformly large cells with prominent, large nucleoli. Rhabdoid neoplasms exhibit a marked tendency to metastasize to the brain and lung. They occur more commonly in infants and may be associated with primary central nervous system tumors of different etiology. *Clear cell* tumors also indicate an unfavorable outcome. Clear cells are characterized by scanty cytoplasm and faint nuclei. They occur more frequently in males and place the child at greater risk for bony metastasis.[11]

Favorable histopathologic variants of Wilms' tumors include multilocular cysts, congenital mesoblastic nephroma, and rhabdomyosarcoma. They are considered "favorable" because they are less likely to metastasize

and, in certain instances, may undergo some degree of spontaneous regression.[11]

Malignancy of the urinary system causes subtle, then severe compromise of urologic and distant organ system function leading to illness and death unless treatment successfully eradicates cancer cells without unduly harming adjacent normal tissue structures.

Local invasion by a Wilms' tumor leads to distortion of the urinary collecting system and may extend into the renal pelvis, causing obstruction and hematuria. The progressing tumor crowds normal renal parenchyma, eventually replacing it with malignant cells. Tumor cells may invade adjacent structures, including renal and extrarenal blood vessels. Hypertension may arise due to local invasion of the renal artery or may occur as a result of renin secretion from the tumor itself. Hematogenous and lymphatogenous metastasis involve distant sites, including liver, bone, lung, and brain as well as hilar, periaortic, or distant lymphatic chains.[11]

The principal prognostic factors are the stage of tumor at the time of diagnosis and its size and histologic characteristics. Minor predictors of prognosis include the patient's age (younger children are more likely to have more favorable histologic characteristics), presence of tumor spillage during surgery, and the presence of local extension patterns.[11] Fortunately, improvements in therapeutic modalities have strengthened the prognosis of affected children who must deal with the physical and psychosocial impact of a childhood malignancy.

Clinical Manifestations.   Wilms' tumor is typically diagnosed in a well-appearing child noted to have an abdominal mass or enlarging abdomen on routine physical examination (Fig. 50-12). The mass is generally confined to one side of the abdomen; vague pain is associated in approximately one third of affected children.[11] Gross hematuria is noted in 10% to 12% of children at the time of diagnosis; urinalysis reveals that an even larger number will have microscopic hematuria. Approximately 63% will experience hypertension; weight loss, fever, and malaise are more uncommon and may indicate the presence of metastatic disease.[75]

Diagnostic Evaluation.   Physical examination of the child with Wilms' tumor reveals a smooth abdominal mass. Hypertension is present in 63% of cases. Laboratory findings include urinalysis, which only rarely shows hematuria; urine culture to rule out bacteriuria; serum creatinine and BUN, which are normal or elevated if renal function is compromised; normal urinary catecholamine levels (excludes possibility of neuroblastoma); and hematocrit and hemoglobin, which may be acutely depressed after surgical manipulation. The IVP confirms two kidneys, the affected kidney with distortion of renal shadow and caliceal drainage system due to tumor invasion, radiolucent area in tumor with hemorrhage or necrosis; calcification of central tumor elements is rare, and egg-shell appearance may be seen at the periphery.[11] Renal ultrasound reveals distortion of renal parenchyma and caliceal collecting system due to mass effect. Arteriography visualizes a vascular pattern of poorly visualized, malignant kidney. CT scan of the abdomen shows the presence of a mass with distortion of renal architecture

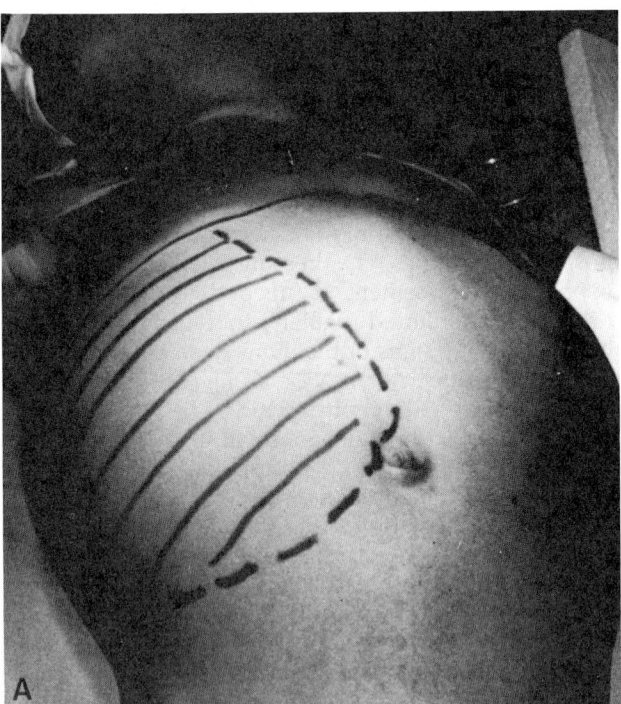

FIGURE 50-12
Enlarged abdomen of a 7-year-old boy with Wilms' tumor. (From Pizzo, P. A., & Poplack, D. G. [1989]. *Principles and practice of pediatric oncology.* Philadelphia: Lippincott.)

and metastasis to abdominal viscera or lymph nodes detectable on chest x-ray; the presence of pulmonary metastasis is seen.

★ ASSESSMENT

The nursing assessment of the child with Wilms' tumor centers on evaluation of the extent that the mass has affected urinary and other organ system function and evaluation of the psychosocial impact this unexpected finding exerts on the affected child and family.

Assessment of the immediate psychosocial impact of the diagnosis of a malignancy also is undertaken when the diagnosis is established. Adult family members typically feel anxiety, fear, and dread. Even the very young affected child will detect these emotions in the parent's behavior and react with marked anxiety. Both child and parents are provided opportunity to express feelings related to the diagnosis of a malignant tumor. The nurse uses this time to begin to explore coping opportunities needed to face the immediate crisis and the issues related to definitive treatment of Wilms' tumor.

★ NURSING DIAGNOSES AND PLANNING

Based on the assessment data from above and the preceding chapter, the following nursing diagnoses may apply:

- Initial Diagnoses
  - Altered Tissue Perfusion: Renal related to integrity of blood vessels.
  - Anxiety related to situational crises.

- Family Coping: Potential for Growth related to adaptive tasks.
- Ineffective Family Coping related to discrepancy of coping styles regarding disability.
- Ineffective Denial related to displacement of fear of impact of condition.
- Defensive Coping related to difficulty in reality-testing perceptions.
- Ineffective Individual Coping related to situational crises.
- Tumor Resection
  - Altered Tissue Perfusion: Peripheral related to surgical procedure.
  - Decreased Cardiac Output related to surgical procedure.
  - Ineffective Airway Clearance related to surgical procedure.
  - High Risk for Infection (Respiratory) related to inadequate primary defenses.
  - Pain related to surgical incision.
- Radiotherapy
  - Diarrhea related to radiotherapy.
  - Altered Nutrition: Less Than Body Requirements related to loss of appetite.
  - High Risk for Impaired Skin Integrity related to radiation effects.
  - Altered Growth and Development related to multiple caretakers.
  - Altered Tissue Perfusion: Hepatic related to obstruction caused by tumor invasion.
- Chemotherapy
  - Diarrhea related to chemotherapy.
  - Altered Nutrition: Less Than Body Requirements related to nausea and vomiting.
  - High Risk for Impaired Skin Integrity related to chemotherapy.
  - Body Image Disturbance related to weight loss and alopecia.
  - Altered Oral Mucous Membrane related to chemotherapy.
  - Pain related to nausea and vomiting.
  - Altered Tissue Perfusion related to removal of one kidney.

Other functionally related nursing diagnoses are discussed in Table 49-2 in Chapter 49.

The nurse and child (or parents) together plan effective care based on the established nursing diagnoses. Several examples of expected outcomes are as follows:

- The family discusses their anxieties about the child's condition.
- The child expresses feelings of anger related to cancer.
- The child exhibits proper splinting during postoperative coughing.
- The child eats frequent, small meals postoperatively.

The nurse plans for the daily care of the child based on both physician's orders and nursing diagnoses. Some general nursing care goals may be the following:

- Healthy kidney maintains support of urinary system.
- Optimal nutrition is maintained.
- Fluid intake and output balance is maintained.
- Optimal urinary flow is improved.

★ INTERVENTIONS: COLLABORATIVE AND INDEPENDENT

SUPPORT FOLLOWING INITIAL DIAGNOSIS

Because the diagnosis of Wilms' tumor is typically established in an otherwise healthy appearing child, the family faces a significant crisis as they struggle to redefine the affected member as having cancer. Feelings of anxiety, fear, and dread are experienced by adult caretakers, which are reflected in even the very young child. The affected child also experiences intense anxiety and confusion as he or she attempts to cope with news that they have a serious illness even though they do not "feel bad."

Immediately following diagnosis and explanation of the immediate medical care regimen, the nurse provides the family with a reasonably private environment to allow expressions of grieving or fear. The nurse assists the family to identify resource persons and make short-term plans related to immediate medical care plans. Long-term prognosis is avoided; the nurse emphasizes that appropriate medical treatment offers realistic hope for cure and encourages the family to face their crisis by attempting to cope with immediate tasks, or "one step at a time."

The child also is forced to cope with the realities of cancer, and he or she draws from very limited life experience. The child often reacts with denial or prolonged anger. This anger is often aimed at parents or nurses with whom they feel most able to express their anxiety. Although nurses, parents, and other caretakers may feel uncomfortable when confronted with these feelings, they know they are a portion of the child's coping mechanisms.

The nurse assists the child to cope with anxieties by continuing to show acceptance of feelings of anger and fear while placing realistic and prudent limits on inappropriate (self-destructive or potentially harmful) behaviors. Children are provided ample opportunities to express their frustrations with aspects of care but are given repeated explanations of why uncomfortable tests or therapeutic modalities are necessary. The nurse encourages the child and family to participate in support groups or to seek individual or family psychological counseling as indicated.

SURGICAL MANAGEMENT

Surgical resection of the tumor is undertaken routinely to reduce the tumor mass unless cancer affects both kidneys. The tumor is approached via a transverse transperitoneal or thoracoabdominal incision, with the patient in an oblique position and the affected kidney facing upward. The entire tumor is resected or removed, taking care not to disrupt its contents and seed the exposed surgical area. The entire kidney, perinephric fat, and Gerota's fascia, is often taken, but the adrenal gland, included in a classic radical nephrectomy, may be spared in certain instances.[11]

PREOPERATIVE CARE

The nurse offers a simple explanation of the purpose and goals of the surgery. The parents and child are reassured that the remaining kidney will be able to carry out the work of both kidneys.

POSTOPERATIVE CARE

The child will return from the operative suite with a thoracoabdominal or flank dressing, intravenous fluid line, nasogastric tube, and Foley catheter. The nurse monitors the child for signs of blood loss during the immediate postoperative period. The vital signs are obtained at least every 4 hours around the clock, and a hematocrit and hemoglobin are typically obtained the first and second postoperative nights. The dressing is left undisturbed except for reinforcement as needed. Nonetheless, the dressing is monitored regularly for signs of exudate or blood loss. Any signs of bleeding, such as pallor; rapid, weak pulse with tachypnea; or falling blood pressure are rapidly reported to the physician.

The nurse also maintains rigorous pulmonary toilet throughout the immediate postoperative period to prevent potential complications. The child is taught to cough and deep breathe prior to surgery, and these maneuvers are repeated on a regular basis during the postoperative period. Because the child has a relatively large thoracoabdominal or transperitoneal incision, normal deep breathing and coughing are compromised by discomfort. The nurse plans for these difficulties by using proper splinting and positioning and by arranging the pulmonary toilet schedule around pain medication administration. Routine assessment of breath sounds by auscultation and monitoring of temperature for fever are used to evaluate the effectiveness of pulmonary toileting procedures following tumor resection.

The child is regularly assessed for pain following surgery using a pediatric assessment tool. The nurse assesses pain for its location, character, duration, and likely etiology. Incisional pain is typically located over the abdomen or flank; it is characterized as dull and of long duration. Wound pain is relieved by analgesics administered in consultation with the physician and by proper positioning and restriction of excessive movement. Abdominal pain produced by irritation from extensive tumor resection also is localized in the abdomen. In contrast to incisional pain, it is characterized by sharp, cramping pain of limited duration that is likely to recur. It is relieved by adequate drainage from the nasogastric tube, analgesics as needed, and time.

Following return of normal bowel sounds, the nasogastric tube is removed and the child is allowed to drink oral fluids with slow progression to solid foods. The intravenous fluid line is discontinued when the patient tolerates oral fluids.

The Foley catheter is routinely assessed for patency, volume, and character of urinary output. The urine is expected to be yellow or light pink during the first postoperative day. The Foley catheter is typically discontinued 72 hours after surgery.

CARE RELATED TO RADIATION THERAPY

Radiotherapy is used in both preoperative and postoperative care of the Wilms' tumor. During the preoperative period, the goal of therapy is to "debulk" or reduce the size of the tumor in an attempt to make surgical intervention more efficacious. Preoperative radiotherapy also serves to lessen the likelihood of rupture of the tumor during surgical manipulation. Postoperative radiation is designed to increase long-term survival rates.

The nursing management of the child receiving radiotherapy for Wilms' tumor begins before treatment is initiated. The nurse reviews the goals of treatment, emphasizing that the process of radiotherapy is not painful. The patient and family are warned that radiotherapy of the abdominal area may produce diarrhea, nausea, and loss of appetite. Diarrhea is typically transient and is managed by changing the diet to clear liquids, including juices and beverages rich with calories and electrolytes, especially sodium and potassium. The child is then advanced to solid foods as the diarrhea subsides; small meals and avoidance of fried foods are encouraged.

Loss of appetite and nausea also are treated by dietary manipulation. The child is fed in multiple, small meals with flexibility in the variety of foods offered given with consideration of the child's likes and dislikes. The parents are advised that meals are often consumed slowly and that reheating the meal is preferable to forcing the child to eat at one sitting. The child often requires a rest period following a meal to lessen nausea and vomiting. In addition, nonfatty and nonspicy foods are often better tolerated and beverages containing calories from complex carbohydrates and essential electrolytes are encouraged. Oral antiemetics may be required to control nausea and vomiting resulting in nutritional and fluid volume deficits.

Teach the family to monitor the child for altered skin integrity due to radiation effects and to report any problems to the nurse or physician. Baby oil or lanolin is used on affected areas in consultation with the radiotherapist. Itching is relieved by use of cornstarch, A and D, or hydrocortisone ointments.

The family is advised to monitor the child for more serious toxic effects of radiotherapy, including anemia with impaired gas exchange and increased susceptibility to infection due to neutropenia. The nurse teaches the family to recognize signs of anemia such as fatigue, intolerance of normal activities, and pallor of the skin. The family is advised that the child should avoid large crowds and activities requiring excessive exertion. In addition, the nurse counsels the family to promptly report fever and signs of respiratory or urinary tract infection to the physician.

CARE RELATED TO CHEMOTHERAPY

Chemotherapy is principally used to improve survival rates following surgical resection. Vincristine and doxorubicin are used in combination for many Wilms' tumors. In addition, actinomycin-D and vincristine are used for stage I tumors with favorable histologic characteristics. Investigations into the usefulness of chemotherapy in eradication of Wilms' tumor will focus on the use of further protocols requiring multiple chemotherapeutic agents and comparative studies of chemotherapy versus radiotherapy.[11]

The nursing care of the child undergoing chemotherapy for Wilms' tumor begins prior to the initiation of treatment. The goals of treatment are explained and the particulars of a given regimen are discussed in consultation with the physician. The family is taught to monitor the child for potential side effects, including altered nutritional intake related to nausea and vomiting and altered bowel elimination patterns due to diarrhea. The nursing actions designed to alleviate these adverse effects are similar to those discussed under "Care Related to Radiation Therapy."

The nurse also teaches the family and child to care for loss of oral mucous membrane integrity due to effects of chemotherapy or infection. The child is encouraged to maintain a routine of oral hygiene and to avoid hot beverages or particularly spicy foods. Popsicles or cold beverages may offer temporary relief from cracked, sore membranes. Topical numbing agents such as viscous lidocaine also may be used according to medical direction if indicated. Candidal infection also may impair oral tissue integrity. Fungal infection is treated by nystatin suspension or suppository in consultation with the physician.

Renal and urinary system function also may be affected by chemotherapy, particularly following surgical removal of one kidney. The nurse encourages the patient to maintain adequate fluid intake. Beverages should be chilled whenever feasible and consumed in small amounts throughout the day. Fluids rich in complex carbohydrates and containing needed electrolytes, such as Gatorade, serve a dual purpose. They assist the kidneys in excreting renal clearance of chemotherapeutic end products and reduce impaired nutrition caused by diarrhea and nausea and vomiting.

Patients undergoing chemotherapy for Wilms' therapy also are at risk for body image disturbance related to weight loss and alopecia. These effects are important for the child at any age but are particularly devastating for the adolescent. The nurse counsels the child concerning these effects *before* the initiation of treatment and reassures them that changes in appearance are temporary and reversible.

The nurse assists the child and family to obtain an appropriate wig before hair loss occurs. Consult the physician or oncology nurse specialist concerning use of ice cap or tourniquet device, remembering the controversy concerning the effectiveness of these modalities.[17] The adolescent is reassured that hair will grow back after chemotherapy is discontinued. Female patients are advised that their hair may have additional curl. Male adolescents may fear loss of weight loss, muscle mass, and physical ability as much as they fear loss of hair. They also are reassured of the temporary effects of chemotherapy and reminded of the necessity of therapy despite its unpleasant effects.

★ **EVALUATION**

The nurse and family evaluate the outcomes and criteria periodically. Example of outcomes for the child with Wilms' tumor were given in "Nursing Diagnoses and Planning" in this section. Have short-term goals been met? Are long-term goals still realistic? Planning for further nursing care also takes into consideration complications and long-term care.

COMPLICATIONS

The complications of Wilms' tumor arise from its propensity to recur and those related to treatment modalities.

Recurrence of Wilms' tumor typically is noted as appearance of distant metastasis. Once considered incurable, these children now can look forward to a 43% rate of cure, if the tumor has a favorable histology, due to advances in chemotherapy and radiotherapy. The survival rate decreases for children with unfavorable histology characteristics.[11]

The acute complications related to surgery are hemorrhage leading to shock and death unless promptly reversed. The risk of hemorrhage is increased by the nature of the surgical procedure. Patients may experience internal bleeding only indirectly detectable by changes in serum hematocrit and hemoglobin, followed by alterations in vital signs and mental status. A significant risk of pulmonary complications also exists because of the wound location and thoracic discomfort.

The acute complications of chemotherapy and radiotherapy occur because these treatment modalities attack all rapidly proliferating body cells, malignant or normal. Bone marrow and hepatic toxicities represent serious complications of chemotherapy or radiotherapy and justify suspension of treatment until untoward effects are reversed.[11]

The long-term effects of chemotherapy and radiotherapy include renal failure and bowel obstruction. Altered growth and development also occurs as a result of radiation therapy on the developing musculoskeletal system.[11] Long-term follow-up management is needed to identify and treat these complications.

LONG-TERM MANAGEMENT

Repetition of imaging studies to rule out recurrent tumor is undertaken for at least 5 years following termination of successful therapy. In addition, measurement of height and weight are obtained annually to evaluate the potential effect of treatment on musculoskeletal growth and development.

Lower Tract Tumors

Definition and Incidence. Malignant tumors of the lower urinary tract are rare in childhood. The most common tumor is the *rhabdomyosarcoma*. The tumor arises from the primitive mesenchyme and resembles muscle tissue noted in developing fetuses. It originates in the submucosa of the bladder neck, trigone, or dome. Occasionally, the tumor may arise from adjacent structures such as the prostate, soft tissue of the pelvis, uterus and vagina, or paratesticular structures.[58] The disease affects white children approximately twice as often as black children. It typically affects persons under 4 years of age but may occur at any time throughout childhood including adolescence. This tumor is also discussed in Chapter 31.

Other tumors of the lower urinary tract system include transitional cell carcinomas of the bladder, leiomyosarcomas of the bladder, and various malignant tumors involving the urachus.[58] Because rhabdomyosarcoma is by far the most common lower tract malignancy, the present discussion is limited to this tumor.

Rhabdomyosarcoma is further defined by its stage. Many staging systems have been proposed. Perhaps the most commonly used system was proposed by the Intergroup Rhabdomyosarcoma Study,[18] as shown in Table 50-6.

Etiology and Pathophysiology. The etiology of rhabdomyosarcoma remains unclear. The tumor is some-

TABLE 50-6
Staging System for Rhabdomyosarcoma

Stage	Description
I	Tumors localized; completely resected by surgery.
II	Divided into three subtypes as follows: IIa: Tumors visible only locally; regional nodes grossly normal even though microscopic evidence exists despite surgical resection. IIb: Tumors exhibit regional nodal disease; amenable to surgical resection with no evidence of microscopic residual. IIc: Tumors exhibit evidence of nodal involvement with evidence of microscopic disease after surgical resection.
III	Tumors have extensive local invasion; not amenable to complete surgical resection.
IV	Tumors have distant metastases at time of diagnosis.

what unique because it arises from visceral smooth muscle yet resembles developing striated muscle tissue. It originates from the submucosa of the bladder wall and moves toward the ureteral and urethral orifices. The tumor reduces the size of the bladder vesicle with polypoid projections that may extend out the urethral meatus and into the vagina of girls.[58]

Like any malignancy, the pathophysiology of rhabdomyosarcoma arises from the tumor's propensity for uncontrolled growth causing invasion of local structures and metastasis to distant sites. The ultimate result is disruption of genitourinary function followed by compromise of distant organ system function, which leads to death of the affected child or adolescent.

Lymphatic node metastasis and hematogenous metastasis occur as the disease advances; children with primary tumors of the prostate are particularly prone to distant lesions. The principal sites for metastasis are lungs, bone, and liver.

Clinical Manifestations. The most common presenting feature is altered urinary elimination patterns arising from obstruction. Acute urinary retention and difficulty expressing the urinary stream arise as the tumor occludes the bladder outlet.[58] This leads to frequency, urgency, and urge incontinence. Urinary retention, stasis, and infection eventually result. Gross hematuria, palpable mass, anemia, and signs of compromised renal function also are noted in certain cases.

Diagnostic Evaluation. Physical examination reveals a palpable mass of the suprapubic area from bladder distention and tumor. A normal or elevated serum creatinine and BUN are present with obstructive uropathy. There may be a normal or depressed hematocrit and hemoglobin due to blood loss from the tumor. IVP reveals ureterohydronephrosis due to obstruction and a filling defect of the lower aspect of the bladder vesicle caused by tumor presence. Cystogram/VCUG reveals a filling defect of the lower aspect of the bladder. Cystoscopic examination indicates presence of lobulated, white extensions of the tumor.

★ ASSESSMENT

Nursing assessment centers on the determination of the extent that the tumor has invaded local structures and metastasized to distant sites, causing compromise of organ system function, and the severity of psychosocial distress produced by the diagnosis of cancer.

The nurse assesses the child or adolescent for patterns of altered urinary elimination. A voiding diary is rarely maintained because an initial diagnosis of tumor is typically made by physical examination. The nurse reviews the results of laboratory, radiographic, and cystoscopic findings to determine the extent of disease and its effects on general health.

The nurse also begins assessment of the family and child's responses to a diagnosis of cancer. This assessment includes identification of supportive resources among family and friends (see "Assessment" in the "Upper Tract Tumors" section).

★ NURSING DIAGNOSES AND PLANNING

Nursing diagnoses and planning in lower urinary tract tumors are similar to nursing diagnoses and planning for upper tract tumors.

★ INTERVENTIONS: COLLABORATIVE AND INDEPENDENT

PARENTAL SUPPORT

Following initial diagnosis of rhabdomyosarcoma, the family and child or adolescent must rapidly readjust their lives to cope with the demands required to combat a malignant tumor. Often the family feels alarmed, anxious, and frustrated as they begin to accept the realities associated with a malignant tumor. In addition, the child must begin to accept the reality of a potentially life-threatening cancer as well as the adjustments associated with surgical resection that disturbs body image. The younger child is particularly susceptible to ineffective coping mechanisms such as chronic defensive or denial reactions that may hinder her or his ability to cope with immediate medical care regimes. The nurse is aware of this danger and continues to offer support and reassurance to the child.

The nurse assists the parents to manage their child without guilt, reassuring them that the tumor is not a product of their behaviors or abilities as caretakers. The parents are advised that their child or adolescent must face extremely difficult issues related to mortality, body image, and self-concept with limited life experiences to draw on. They are particularly warned that the child may choose inappropriately to blame them or involved health care professionals. The nurse advises parents to remind the child continuously of the goals and necessity of each step in the health care regimen. The nurse also assesses the family on an ongoing basis for signs of dysfunctional coping mechanisms and refers them to counselors or other professionals as indicated.

CATHETERIZATION

The immediate goal of physical care of the child with rhabdomyosarcoma is the relief of urinary obstruction.

The placement of a suprapubic or urethral Foley catheter is used to palliate obstruction until adequate staging and related diagnostic work-up can be completed and a definitive plan of care decided on.

The nurse maintains this urinary drainage by monitoring urinary output for volume and character. The urine may be clear yellow, or it may be red with gross hematuria. The nurse assists the child or adolescent to maintain adequate fluid intake and monitors the urine for signs of excessive bleeding, which is reported promptly to the physician. The tube is maintained in place and secured as needed to prevent inadvertent withdrawal and to minimize risk of infection. The patient is reassured that the catheter is temporary.

Following appropriate diagnostic work-up and initial staging, a definitive plan of care is undertaken. Historically, radical surgery alone has proven to be inadequate, resulting in an unacceptable low survival rate. The addition of radiotherapy has also proved to be disappointing.

CURRENT TREATMENT

Currently, treatment consists of a regimen of radical surgery, followed by postoperative radiotherapy and 2 years of adjunctive chemotherapy, which has significantly improved the survival rate of 64% to 86%. The regimen typically consists of tumor resection; cystoprostatectomy is typically but not always required. Postoperative radiotherapy is then used on all except stage I patients. The regimen consists of 3500 rads given over a 4-week period if microscopic residual is noted and 4000 to 4500 rads for grossly evident residual disease.[64]

Chemotherapy consists of a combination of vincristine, actinomycin-D, and cyclophosphamide given at 4-week intervals. The chemotherapy is typically given prior to surgical resection in an attempt to reduce the tumor, whereas radiation is used at the operative site to control local invasion.[58]

The nurse informs the family and child that surgery is planned in accordance to the response to chemotherapy and that resection is delayed purposely to enhance the child's response to therapy rather than to suit scheduling conveniences. Typically, chemotherapy is begun and a 50% reduction in tumor size is expected after the completion of the second course of drugs. If this occurs as predicted, surgical resection or radiotherapy is planned.

CARE RELATED TO PARTIAL CYSTECTOMY

Limited resection (subtotal cystectomy with or without radical prostatectomy) is undertaken whenever possible. The extent of resection relies on intraoperative findings. If, after 16 weeks and additional chemotherapy, residual disease remains, more complete resection or radiotherapy is again considered.[58]

The nursing care of the patient undergoing partial cystectomy begins prior to surgery. The goals of surgery are explained to the family. The older patient undergoes a preoperative shave from umbilicus to mid-thigh.

The patient returns from the operative suite with a urethral catheter, intravenous fluid line, and lower abdominal incision. The nurse meticulously maintains an open, patent drainage system to prevent rupture of the newly reconstructed bladder wall. Urinary output is assessed for volume character and color. The urine is lightly pink or red tinged for the first several days following surgery. Bright-red blood or clots are not expected and should be reported promptly to the physician.

The indwelling catheter is removed as soon as the urine returns to a clear, yellow consistency to minimize the risk of postoperative infection. The nurse closely monitors the patient for spontaneous voiding following catheter removal. The adolescent or child is reassured that initial stinging on urination is relieved by multiple episodes of voiding. The patient is assisted to receive adequate fluid intake, and a warm bath may be used to provide relief from discomfort associated with urethral irritation following catheter removal. The patient who is unable to void spontaneously must be recatheterized after a reasonable trial to avoid overdistention of the newly reconstructed bladder wall.

The nurse also monitors the surgical wound and dressing. The dressing may exude a moderate amount of serosanguineous drainage requiring frequent changes. Urinary output from the wound will be absent or minimal because the goal of surgery is a watertight seal at the bladder. Purulent or bloody drainage indicates rupture of the operative site or infection. These events are not expected and warrant rapid consultation with the physician.

The intravenous fluid line is maintained only until the child is able to tolerate oral fluids, usually during the first postoperative night. Gastrointestinal irritation is minimal or absent following partial cystectomy because the procedure requires little or no bowel manipulation.

The nurse evaluates the patient for pain following partial cystectomy on an ongoing basis using a pediatric assessment tool. The pain is evaluated for its duration, location, and character. Painful bladder spasms may occur because of resection of the detrusor muscle. Pain from bladder spasms is short in duration, centered in the suprapubic area, and sharp and stabbing in nature. It is managed by insuring adequate bladder drainage, avoiding excessive movement that may produce traction by the inflated catheter against the vesicle outlet, and administering anticholinergic medications as indicated. Incisional pain also is centered in the suprapubic area but of longer duration and is characterized by a dull, boring sensation. It is treated by limiting excessive movement and analgesics as indicated.

TOTAL CYSTECTOMY WITH INCONTINENT URINARY DIVERSION

Total, or radical, cystectomy is undertaken when a tumor is too locally invasive to allow partial resection of the bladder wall. The bladder is removed along with the prostate and seminal vesicles in the male and bladder urethra, lower ureters and anterior vagina in the female. It is always followed by creation of a new urinary reservoir (incontinent diversion) or urinary conduit (urostomy) to provide adequate urinary elimination (Fig. 50-13).

Creation of a urinary conduit requires isolation of a relatively short segment (15 to 20 cm) of small bowel caudal to the jejunum. Commonly, a segment of ileum is chosen that lies close to the ileocecal valve. It is isolated from the fecal stream and brought to the lower abdominal quadrant and everted through the skin in a budded fashion. The opposite end is closed, and the ureters are im-

planted in the conduit. The conduit is constructed in a peristaltic manner so that urine flows in the same direction as normal ileal peristalsis, promoting urinary elimination. The conduit is not a storage area; urine is expected to flow from the urostomy in a continuous manner, requiring a pouching system for containment.[22]

PREOPERATIVE CARE

The patient is admitted to the hospital several days prior to surgery for adequate bowel preparation, including oral agents to promote bowel evacuation and enemas that will continue to the morning of surgery. The nurse administers the prep according to medical orders while insuring that the child does not experience excessive fluid and electrolyte depletion through administration of intravenous replacement fluids. The patient is placed on a low-residue diet prior to surgery and is switched to clear liquids approximately 72 hours prior to the procedure. The child or adolescent is encouraged to consume adequate fluids; beverages rich in electrolytes such as Gatorade are particularly encouraged. Intravenous fluids are used for the child who is unable to retain oral fluids during the bowel prep.

The nurse also helps prepare the bowel by administration of appropriate anti-infective agents as directed prior to surgery. The child is closely monitored for intolerance to these agents, and the physician is informed if the child is unable to tolerate the agent or shows signs of allergic reaction.

The nurse assists the child or adolescent to begin the difficult transition required by altering the anatomy of the urinary system. An enterostomal therapy (ET) nurse is consulted to begin the process of acclimating the patient to the demands of caring for an ostomy. This nurse also assists the patient to begin the emotional process needed to cope with disturbed body image produced by creation of a conduit for urine elimination.

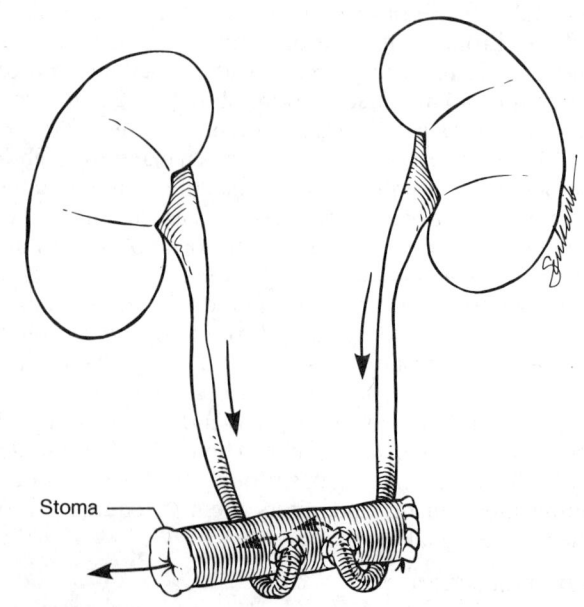

FIGURE 50-13
Bricker ileal conduit (incontinent diversion).

The nurse reassures the patient that he or she will be able to participate in all activities engaged in prior to creation of the diversion except contact sports and weight lifting. The child or adolescent is encouraged to express fears related to a changed body image and another adolescent with an ostomy is allowed to visit the patient whenever feasible. The nurse maintains ongoing consultation with the ET nurse concerning the emotional progress of the child and obtains psychiatric assistance when indicated.

POSTOPERATIVE CARE

Following surgery the child returns to an intensive care unit with an intravenous fluid line, nasogastric tube, abdominal incision with dressing, incisional drain, and urethral catheter used to evacuate fluid from the surgical site at the bladder. The nurse monitors all drains for character and volume of output. The stoma is pouched with a clear device with an antireflux pouch and spout, allowing continuous drainage into a bedside bag and regular inspection of the budded ostomy. The stoma will be large and edematous; it is inspected regularly for signs of viability and continuity with the abdomen. A dark reddish or black color or signs of separation of the stoma from abdominal skin are reported promptly to the physician. The nurse also monitors this drainage system for urinary output. The output is usually blood tinged but should not have excessive bright-red blood or clots. A decreased output in the pouching system may indicate ileal ureteral leak or compromised renal function. The nurse first assesses drainage from all other sources, such as incisional drain, urethral catheter, and so forth, to determine if a disruption of ureteral ileal anastomosis is likely. The physician is then consulted.[58]

The incisional wound is routinely assessed for output and characteristics of exudate. Urinary output should be minimal or absent, as should bloody discharge. The nurse also monitors drainage from the incisional drain and regularly assesses vital signs and hematocrit and hemoglobin values if excessive bleeding is suspected.

Rigorous pulmonary toilet is essential following cystectomy with creation of a urostomy to prevent nosocomial respiratory infection. The nurse assists the patient to turn, cough, and deep breathe to counteract the effects of stasis of secretions and ineffective airway clearance patterns. Auscultation of the chest for evidence of atelectasis or stasis of secretions is undertaken every 48 hours following surgery until the patient is able to ambulate. Administration of analgesics is coordinated with pulmonary toilet regimens to encourage adequate mobilization of respiratory secretions.

The nasogastric tube also is monitored for volume and character of output. Greenish-brown output is expected from the tube; the presence of bloody drainage is reported promptly to the physician because this may indicate gastrointestinal hemorrhage. The tube is routinely irrigated with saline as ordered, usually every 2 hours. If output from the tube ceases, the suction device is checked and the tube is first irrigated with saline. If this does not produce results, consult the physician concerning repositioning or replacing the tube as indicated. Because extensive manipulation of the bowel is required

for surgery, the tube is left in place until adequate bowel sounds return.

The patient's intravenous fluid line is left in place until she or he is able to tolerate oral fluids. During this period, the nurse maintains careful records of all fluid intake and output from drains and monitors the patient for evidence of fluid or electrolyte imbalance. Any changes are reported promptly to the physician.

The nurse also assesses the child for pain on an ongoing basis using a pediatric assessment tool (see Chap. 28). The pain is evaluated for its duration, location, and character. Incisional pain is characterized by long-lasting abdominal discomfort that has a dull, boring character. It is treated by proper positioning and analgesics in consultation with the physician. Gastrointestinal discomfort is shorter in duration and produces a "cramping" discomfort. It is treated by insurance of adequate nasogastric tube drainage and removal of the tube when adequate peristalsis returns. Nasal discomfort created by the presence of the nasogastric tube is alleviated by the use of petroleum jelly.

The nurse also assesses the patient for altered skin integrity associated with tubes, drains, dressings, or the pouching system. Regular inspection of all affected skin areas is completed with dressing, tube, or drainage manipulations, and ongoing consultation with the ET nurse is maintained whenever skin problems arise.

Following the acute postoperative period, the nurse begins evaluation and care aimed at assisting the adolescent or child to cope with disturbed body image produced by the surgery. The ET nurse will proceed with instruction of pouch and pouching changes at whatever pace the patient is able to tolerate. The nurse maintains regular consultation with the ET nurse and assists with ostomy care as needed. The patient is provided ample opportunity to discuss issues related to the urostomy. The nurse assesses the child and family's acceptance of the ostomy by evaluating their ability to participate in pouch changes or observe the procedure or look at the pouch as others perform these functions. The child is reassured that the stoma will shrink to approximately the size of a quarter or smaller as the edema resolves. Issues concerning sexuality and self-concept typically are not resolved by the time of hospital discharge, but continued nursing and medical care are provided as the family and child resolve these issues at their own pace.

CARE RELATED TO CONTINENT URINARY DIVERSION

Advances in surgical technique have led to the development of a number of techniques for creating a continent urinary diversion. The indications for continent diversion in the child with rhabdomyosarcoma are identical to those for incontinent diversion, with the exception that consideration is given to the greatly increased amount of bowel required for the procedure.

The continent ileal urinary reservoir or Koch pouch was the first widely used continent diversion (Fig. 50-14A). It requires to isolation of 60 to 70 cm of ileum with intact mesentery and vascular supply. The middle portion of this segment is detubularized and opened to form a urinary reservoir, and the entrance and exits to the reservoir have nipple valves created by intussusception, or telescoping the ileum back through its own lumen. The

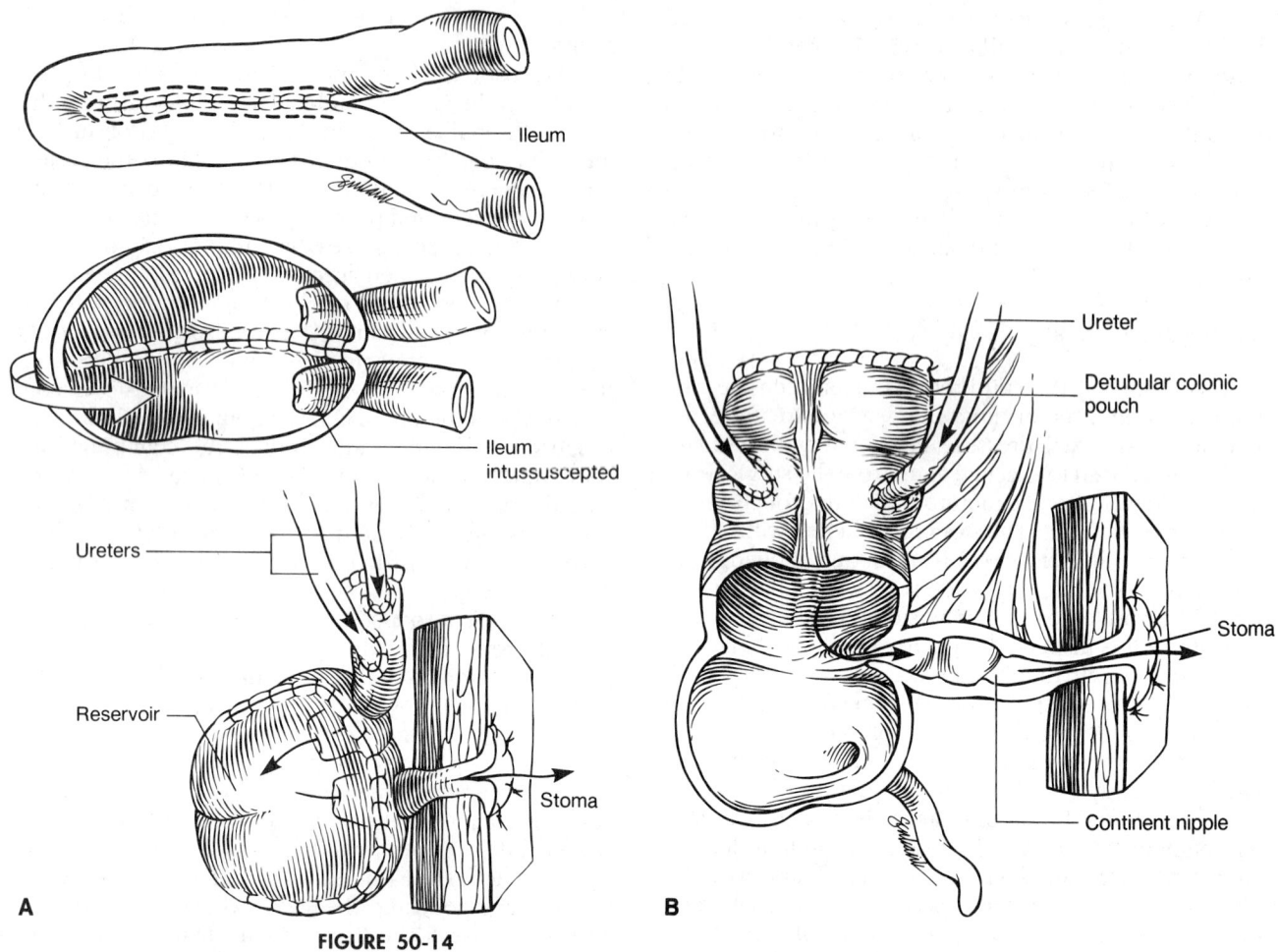

Ileum

Ileum
intussuscepted

Ureters

Reservoir

Stoma

A

Ureter

Detubular colonic
pouch

Stoma

Continent nipple

B

FIGURE 50-14
Two types of continent diversions. (**A**) Koch pouch. (**B**) Indiana (ileocecal) reservoir.

ureters are reimplanted into the proximal nipple, and the distal valve is used as a stoma that is continent of urine. The stoma is drained regularly by a red rubber catheter, and clean gauze is used to protect the stoma from trauma.[43]

Because of the association of the Koch pouch with mechanical and metabolic complications, other alternate techniques have been devised. These techniques use large bowel segments to create urinary reservoirs less prone to the metabolic complications associated with the Koch pouch.[34] For example, the ileocecal reservoir uses a portion of the distal ileum along with segments of the cecum and ascending colon to create a urinary reservoir (Fig. 50-14*B*). The ureters are anastomosed to the ascending colon in an antirefluxing manner, and the ileum is fashioned into a continent mechanism via an abdominal stoma. The patient cares for the device with catheterization in a manner similar to the Koch pouch.[23]

CARE RELATED TO RADIOTHERAPY AND CHEMOTHERAPY

Refer to "Upper Tract Tumors" earlier in this chapter.

★ EVALUATION

The nurse and family evaluate the outcomes and criteria periodically. Have short-term goals been met? Are long-term goals still realistic? Planning for further nursing care also takes into consideration complications and long-term care.

COMPLICATIONS

The principal complications related to tumors of the lower urinary tract are those produced by the propensity of a malignant tumor to invade local structures and metastasize to distant sites and those produced by medical interventions designed to eradicate the tumor.

The complications associated with partial cystectomy are rupture of the reconstructed bladder and tumor recurrence due to residual disease or tumor spillage. The risk of rupture is minimized by the maintenance of adequate bladder drainage during the immediate postoperative period. Tumor spillage is minimized by careful surgical technique, including lavage of the bladder prior to bladder incision and isolation of the bladder from the surgical wound with packs. Tumor proliferation associated with surgical manipulation is further alleviated by careful timing of the procedure following adequate chemotherapy to reduce tumor size and postoperative radiotherapy to prevent excessive local spread.

The complications associated with chemotherapy and radiotherapy are discussed in "Upper Tract Tumors" earlier in this chapter.

LONG-TERM MANAGEMENT

Long-term follow-up care for the prevention of tumor recurrence is absolutely essential for patient survival. Routine imaging studies and blood studies are typically undertaken for 5 years following the termination of treatment. In addition, a urinary diversion requires ongoing care, including ET nurse follow-up, to insure that the patient maintains an acceptable pouching system with intact peristomal skin and absent urinary leakage. Any diversion, continent or conduit, requires ongoing imaging of the upper tracts to insure that the reconstructed urinary system does not compromise renal function.

Altered Urinary Elimination: Voiding Dysfunction

Definition and Incidence. A dysfunctional voiding state exists when a child experiences uncontrolled or involuntary loss of urine or inability to empty the bladder after reaching the age of social continence. A dysfunctional voiding state is clinically significant when it produces a social or hygienic problem perceived by the child, family, or social group or when urinary or renal function is compromised.

Voiding dysfunction is further defined by the use of classification systems that allow differentiation between the various symptoms and causes that lead to the nursing diagnosis of altered urinary elimination. Three classification schemes used by nurses are outlined in Table 50-7.

Dysfunctional voiding states can be divided into four categories: stress urinary incontinence, instability incontinence, urinary retention associated with overflow (paradoxical incontinence), and extraurethral or constant incontinence.[22-24] Stress urinary incontinence occurs when urine loss is produced by physical exertion. Instability incontinence occurs when bladder contractions occur involuntarily. The concept of bladder stability and instability presupposes that a person has reached an age where physiologic maturity and cultural expectations should insure control of bladder function. Urinary retention is the inability to empty the bladder completely. It is typically associated with paradoxical, or overflow, urinary incontinence. Extraurethral incontinence exists when the urethral sphincter mechanism is bypassed, causing continuous or constant incontinence. The principal strength of this system is its clearly stated defining characteristics for identifying types of incontinence. A potential weakness is the lack of a broad label for describing voiding dysfunction before a more specific diagnosis is determined.

Other systems of classifying dysfunctional states also are used by nurses. The North American Nursing Diagnosis Association uses a classification scheme for incontinence based on one broad label and six more specific diagnoses. Within this system, altered urinary elimination describes any condition that results in a disturbance in urine elimination. The more specific diagnoses are (1) stress incontinence, which implies a loss of urine of less than 50 ml, occurring with increased abdominal pressure; (2) total incontinence, which implies a continuous and unpredictable loss of urine; (3) urge incontinence, which occurs soon after a strong sense of urgency to void, happens at somewhat predictable intervals when a specific volume is reached; and (4) functional incontinence, which is the condition that exists when there is an involuntary, unpredictable passage of urine. The strength of this system is its identification of a broad working diagnosis for urinary incontinence and recognition of the impact of environmental and functional factors on urinary function. A potential weakness is the vagueness of differentiating characteristics of the more specific diagnoses.

A functional classification system also has been advocated to describe altered urine elimination patterns.[2] This system contains two broad categories: "failure to store urine" and "failure to empty urine." Beneath these broader descriptive titles are two further titles: "because of the bladder" and "because of the outlet." The functional classification is easily correlated with the two phases of bladder function, filling and emptying, so that failure to store is seen as a filling deficit and failure as a evacuating deficit. The phrase "because of the bladder" implies dysfunction of the detrusor muscle, so that "failure to store because of the bladder" implies instability and "failure to empty" implies deficient detrusor contractility. The phrase "because of the outlet" implies either incompetence of the outlet or the opposite state, obstruction. Thus, "failure to fill because of the outlet" implies stress urinary incontinence, whereas "failure to empty because of the outlet" implies obstruction. The principal strength of this system is labels that are easy to comprehend. A potential weakness is the failure of a label for extraureteral leakage and functional incontinence.

The incidence of voiding dysfunction among children is difficult to identify because sociocultural as well as physiologic factors define continence.

TABLE 50-7
Classification Schemes for Voiding Dysfunction: Altered Urine Elimination*

Gray and Dougherty	Functional	NANDA
Stress incontinence	Failure to store, because of the outlet	Stress incontinence
		Total incontinence
Instability incontinence	Failure to store, because of the detrusor	Urge incontinence
		Reflex incontinence
		Functional incontinence
Urinary retention (overflow incontinence)	Failure to empty, because of the detrusor	Urinary retention
	Failure to empty, because of the outlet	
Extraurethral incontinence (constant incontinence)		Total incontinence

* The nursing diagnosis Altered Urine Elimination applies to any dysfunctional voiding state. NANDA = North American Nursing Diagnosis Association.

Adapted from Gray, M. L. & Dougherty, M. C. (1987). Urinary incontinence: Pathophysiology and treatment. *Journal of Enterostomal Therapy 14*, 152–162. Kim, M. J., McFarlan, G. K., & McLane (1987). *Handbook of nursing diagnosis* (Eds.). St. Louis: Mosby; Barrett, D. M. & Wein, A. J. (1991) Voiding dysfunction: Diagnosis, Classification, and Management. In J. Y. Gillenwater, J. T. Grayhack, S. S. Howards & J. W. Duckett (eds.). Adult and pediatric urology. (2nd ed.). Chicago: Mosby Year Book; and Wheatley, J. K. (1983). Causes and Treatment of bladder incontinence. *Comprehensive Therapy*, 9, 27.

Etiology and Pathophysiology. Although multiple classification schemes for voiding dysfunction have been proposed, the taxonomy proposed by Wheatley[71] and modified by Gray and Dougherty[22,24] is used for this discussion.

Stress incontinence occurs when the sphincter mechanism allows urinary leakage during physical exertion. The causes of stress incontinence among children are structural abnormality of the sphincter mechanism, acquired sphincter damage, or congenital or acquired abnormality of the neurologic mechanisms that modulate sphincter activity.

Acquired stress urinary incontinence is relatively rare among children. The condition occurs when the child is subjected to trauma of the pelvic floor or urethra, or it can be due to iatrogenic damage from transurethral resection of bladder, internal urethrotomy for bladder neck stenosis, or "Y-V" plasty.[35]

Stress urinary incontinence also may result from acquired or congenital abnormality of the neural modulators of the sphincter and pelvic floor. Spina bifida defects or sacral agenesis are associated with sacral cord or cauda equina damage, whereas trauma or disease of the lower spinal segments may denervate the urethral sphincter.

Instability incontinence presents as two conditions affecting children. *Urge incontinence* occurs when the child is unable to suppress bladder contractions in response to social norms despite having exceeded the age of 4 years, when bladder control should be mastered. No detectable abnormality is found for many children who suffer from diurnal instability incontinence. Some investigators postulate that these children have an immature bladder or suffer from a maturational lag of the supraspinal control of detrusor function,[44] whereas others theorize that subtle forms of neuropathy cause obvious voiding dysfunction without obvious motor or sensory deficits detectable by traditional neurologic examination.[19] *Reflex incontinence* is the leakage of urine caused by uncontrolled bladder contractions in the absence of sensations of urgency. It is caused by spinal lesions on injury that interrupts sensory and motor pathways between the brain and bladder.

Nocturnal enuresis is the occurrence of instability incontinence during sleep. Night-time control also should be completed by the age of 4 years, although the clinical significance of enuresis without simultaneous occurrence of diurnal leakage is guided by the magnitude of the social and hygienic problems it creates rather than by any threat to urinary function.

The etiology of enuresis also remains unclear. Perhaps the most widely accepted explanation for enuresis is a maturational lag. This hypothesis presupposes that affected children lack complete development of the cortical modulation of bladder control. The result is a failure of detrusor inhibition during sleep.[50]

Enuresis has also been associated with sleep disorders. Dysfunctional circadian rhythms of antidiuretic hormone secretion are postulated to lead to abnormal diuresis that peaks during the first several hours of somnolence and overloads functional bladder capacity, causing enuresis during deeper sleep stages.[54]

Psychosocial factors are also postulated to exert an influence on the occurrence of enuresis. Clinical observations support the existence of "secondary enuresis," or a new onset of bedwetting, in response to psychosocial stress such as birth of a new sibling or divorce. Nonetheless, no persuasive evidence exists to support hypotheses that enuresis occurs because of psychopathology.[50]

Genetic factors also have been associated with enuresis. The occurrence of enuresis is greater among siblings and the offspring of enuretic parents.

Urinary retention is caused by two conditions: deficient detrusor function and bladder outlet obstruction. *Deficient detrusor function* or *bladder muscle weakness* occur because of congenital or acquired conditions. Detrusor weakness may arise because of congenital neuropathic abnormalities of the lower spinal cord, such as lumbosacral spina bifida defects, sacral agenesis, or sacral teratoma. Acquired conditions, such as spinal cord injury of the lumbosacral segments, osteomyelitis of the vertebral bodies, or extensive surgical procedures of the lower spine or abdominopelvic contents, also may contribute to detrusor weakness with urinary retention.[35]

Obstruction of the bladder outlet also causes urinary retention. Structural congenital anomalies such as meatal stenosis, urethral valves, polyps, or diverticula may produce urinary retention and obstruction, even prior to birth. Acquired conditions, including bladder neck contracture, tumor, foreign body, or abscess, also may obstruct the vesicle outlet and cause urinary retention.[35] Functional obstruction of the bladder outlet also exists when the sphincter fails to relax during detrusor contraction. This condition arises as an neurogenic response among children with spinal cord abnormalities or as a learned response among certain children with diurnal instability incontinence.

Extraurethral leakage is particularly common among children. The constant urinary leakage produced by bypassing the sphincter mechanism may be caused by congenital (ectopia) or acquired conditions (fistula) or by design (surgically created stoma). Urinary ectopia resulting in continuous incontinence occurs when the sphincter mechanism is bypassed. Ureteral ectopia distal to the sphincter mechanism or in the vaginal vestibule is the most common form of the condition.[24] Other congenital defects causing extraurethral leakage include accessory or duplication of the urethra.[35]

Urinary fistula is a condition that exists when an abnormal tract exists between the lower urinary tract and adjacent structure, resulting in constant urinary leakage. Fistulas in children are caused by penetrating pelvic trauma, as a complication of malignant lesions, or as a surgical complication.

Surgically created stomas may be used temporarily or permanently to divert urine flow from the ureters, bladder, or urethra. The most common forms of urinary diversion among children are pyelostomy (creation of an incontinent stoma between renal pelvis and skin), ureterostomy (creation of a stoma between ureter and skin), and vesicostomy (creation of a stoma between bladder vesicle and skin). An ileal conduit is created when malignant tumor or other conditions necessitate cystectomy or permanent defunctionalization of the bladder.

Clinical Manifestations. Voiding dysfunction presents as altered urinary elimination patterns commonly accompanied by some form of uncontrolled urinary leakage. Stress urinary incontinence presents as uncontrolled urine loss accompanied by physical exertion. If the associated sphincter incompetence is mild, then leakage is noted only with vigorous exercise or with marked abdominal pressure increase caused by coughing or sneezing. When the sphincter is markedly incompetent, leakage is noted even with minimal physical exertion such as changing positions.

Diurnal instability incontinence is characterized by urinary frequency, sensations of urgency to void, and leakage when the sensation of urgency is perceived. Affected children often assume a characteristic squatting position with the heel pressed into the perineum to obstruct the urethra and prevent wetting. Nocturnal enuresis may be associated with diurnal instability incontinence or occur as a distinct entity.

Urinary retention also presents as frequent voiding episodes. Enuresis or nocturia (awakening from sleep to void) often accompany diurnal frequency. Overflow or paradoxical incontinence, leakage despite the inability to empty the bladder completely, also is noted in association with urinary retention. Frequently, patients are completely unaware of their inability to empty the bladder and retention is detected only on examination of the urinary system for related conditions such as infection or incontinence of unknown etiology.

Extraurethral urinary leakage may be easily detectable, particularly if it is the result of surgical intent or a large fistula. The resulting leakage is voluminous and not related to urgency or physical exertion. In contrast, extraurethral leakage due to ureteral ectopia is more subtle and presents as a continuous dribble superimposed on an otherwise normal voiding pattern.

Diagnostic Evaluation. Physical examination reveals the following signs of voiding dysfunction: *stress incontinence* is associated with signs of pelvic floor denervation, such as patulous rectum; *instability incontinence* is associated with normal findings or signs of central nervous system abnormality; *urinary retention* is associated with bladder distention, normal abdominal examination, or signs of mass with hydronephrosis; and *extraurethral leakage* is associated with abnormal perineum with epispadias or exstrophy anomaly *or* single orifice in female with cloacal anomaly *or* fistula or surgically created stoma, and altered perineal skin integrity due to continuous exposure to urine.

Laboratory tests include normal serum BUN and creatinine or elevated values with compromised renal function.

Imaging studies may be normal or may show evidence of problems. An IVP is normal or shows evidence of hydronephrosis and ureteral enlargement due to obstructive uropathy. An ectopic ureter is noted with ectopia and dribbling incontinence. Cystogram/VCUG shows leakage with coughing with *stress incontinence;* trabeculation of bladder wall due to *instability incontinence* (particularly when complicated by obstruction); extravesicle leakage of contrast material with fistula; and presence of an accessory or duplicate urethra. Renal and bladder ultrasound are normal or show evidence of obstructive uropathy.

Urodynamic examination reveals the following: *stress incontinence* shows a normal cystometrogram or large bladder capacity due to denervation, quiet pattern and absent bulbocavernosus response due to pelvic floor denervation on sphincter electromyogram, and low or abnormally high maximum closure pressure and evidence of leakage in response to coughing demonstrated on urethral pressure study; *instability incontinence* shows occurrence of bladder contractions during filling cystometrogram; *urinary retention* produces a pressure-flow analysis consistent with weak detrusor (poor or intermittent flow and low-pressure contraction) or obstruction (poor or intermittent flow with high-pressure contraction), and dyssynergia of pelvic floor muscles may be noted; and *extraurethral leakage* may have normal findings.

Further diagnosis is made by cystoscopic examination, which reveals the following: *stress incontinence* shows abnormal funneling of proximal urethra and bladder neck noted with sphincter incompetence; *instability incontinence* shows normal findings or presence of trabeculation; *urinary retention* shows abnormally large bladder capacity with smooth wall due to detrusor weakness or evidence of obstructive uropathy due to obstruction; and *extraurethral leakage* shows the presence of a fistula or ectopic urinary structure.

★ ASSESSMENT

Nursing assessment centers on determining the type of incontinence and the extent to which it compromises urinary tract function. The nurse questions the child and family concerning patterns of urine elimination and strategies used to contain leakage. The family is asked if there is any known history of urinary tract infections or symptoms of infection, including changes in urine odor and dysuria. The nurse elicits any known history of neurologic history and determines bowel habits as well as achievement of developmental milestones and general physical ability.

The neurologic system is examined for evidence of subtle neuropathy, such as differences in size of lower extremities or feet. The pelvis is investigated for evidence of altered sensorium; the nurse determines whether sensations of bladder filling are present and centered in the penis or clitoral area as opposed to the abdomen.

Observation of micturition and a voiding diary form an essential component for any assessment of dysfunction. The voiding diary is used to document objectively and verify historical information provided about voiding habits. The diary also provides information about functional bladder capacity and may assist in determining functional aspects of voiding, particularly related to sensory, motor, or cognitive deficits. Observation of the voided stream is most useful for attempting to determine potential urinary retention manifested by poor or intermittent urinary stream. Assessment of residual by use of catheterization or ultrasonic evaluation done in consultation with the physician is necessary for complete assessment of potential urinary retention.

The nurse also assesses the psychosocial implications of a dysfunctional voiding state on the child and family using a structured interview. Open-ended questions are used to ascertain the meaning of incontinence as perceived by the parents, siblings, and affected child. Asking the family to complete the statement, "Leaking urine is like . . ." is a particularly useful technique when interviewing the family affected by incontinence.

★ NURSING DIAGNOSES AND PLANNING

Based on the assessment data from above and the preceding chapter, the following nursing diagnoses may apply to the initial diagnoses:

- Altered Urinary Elimination related to multiple causality.
- Stress Incontinence related to incompetent bladder outlet.
- Urge Incontinence related to unstable (hyperactive) bladder contractions.
- Reflex Incontinence related to neurologic impairment.
- Functional Incontinence related to sensory impairment.
- Total Incontinence related to neurologic dysfunction.
- Urinary Retention related to bladder outlet obstruction.
- High Risk for Infection (Urinary Tract) related to inadequate primary defenses.
- Dysreflexia related to bladder distention.
- Self-Esteem Disturbance related to embarrassing accidents.
- Sexual Dysfunction related to altered body function.
- Altered Sexuality Patterns related to altered body functions.
- High Risk for Impaired Skin Integrity related to excretions.

Other functionally related nursing diagnoses are discussed in Table 49-2 in Chapter 49.

The nurse and child (or parents) together plan effective care based on the established nursing diagnoses. Several examples of expected outcomes are as follows:

- The parents demonstrate accurate methods of care.
- The parents demonstrate ability to maintain a timed voiding schedule.
- The parents and/or child demonstrate adequate handwashing in preparation for catheterization.
- The child discusses methods of avoiding embarrassing situations.

The nurse plans for the daily care of the child based on both physician's orders and nursing diagnoses. Some general nursing care goals may be the following:

- A suitable containment system is found and used.
- Continence is improved.

★ INTERVENTIONS: COLLABORATIVE AND INDEPENDENT

Management of the incontinent child includes nonpharmacologic strategies in addition to traditionally recognized medical or surgical interventions.

PROVISION OF A CONTAINMENT SYSTEM

The most immediate need for the child with urinary leakage is to assist the family to identify an adequate urinary containment system. This system must consider the volume of urine leaked, the coexistence of fecal soiling, and

the child's age and developmental status. An adequate system to contain urinary leakage should prevent soiling of garments, minimize or abate odor, and fit under the child's clothing without creating excessive bulk or noise with movement. Ideally, the urine containment system also helps prevent altered perineal skin integrity by minimizing the volume of urine that remains in contact with the skin.

A child up to the second or third year of life is managed in diapers because they provide an adequate and socially acceptable containment device, even in the presence of extraurethral leakage. They are capable of absorbing large amounts of urine and minimize associated odor. Although they appear bulky and may rustle under clothing, diapers are a cultural norm for infants, and detection of their presence does not produce loss of self-esteem. In addition, many diapers are manufactured in a manner that minimizes urine exposure to the skin, helping to prevent loss of skin integrity.

Among school-age children or adolescents, however, a diaper is less acceptable. Finding commercially available diapers is difficult because few children require them as compared with infants. Although the diaper adequately contains a large amount of leakage that can be expressed at once or over time, its bulkiness is a problem for the affected child who must endure the humiliation of being labeled a "baby." As an alternative, the family of the school-age child is encouraged to consider a pad if urinary leakage is relatively mild and if the volume of leakage at a single episode is small.

The older child or adolescent with more marked leakage or the child with instability incontinence who may leak 200 to 300 ml in a single episode may require more protection than a pad offers. These children should investigate incontinent briefs. An incontinent brief system combines cloth underwear or pants with a disposable pad system that fits into the cloth pants (Fig. 50-15). These systems offer several distinct advantages over diapers.

Among selected boys, a condom drainage system may be preferable to a pads or incontinent briefs (Fig. 50-16). The condom offers the advantage of limiting the skin exposed to urine. The disadvantages are the difficulty fitting many boys with an appropriately sized condom, the potential for penile skin breakdown, and the need for leg bag drainage. The condom should fit snugly around the flaccid penis and offer sufficient distensibility to allow for an erection. The condom may be coated with an adhesive, may have an adhesive strip or may utilize an inflatable cuff to contain urine. The condom must be watertight and adhere to the penis for at least one day. The end of the condom that fits over the penile shaft must be stiff enough to prevent twisting of the condom and obstruction of urine flow into the collection bag.

The leg bag should have non-rubber elastic straps. The straps must fit to the bag tightly and resist extensive movement and stress. The leg bag also must be backed by a breathable, non-rubberized surface to prevent irritation to the underlying skin. Certain bags may be placed in a cloth sack resembling a sock and attached to the leg. The tubing that connects the bag and condom should be adjustable and fit securely. The valve used to empty the leg bag should be easy to manipulate, preferably with a single hand.

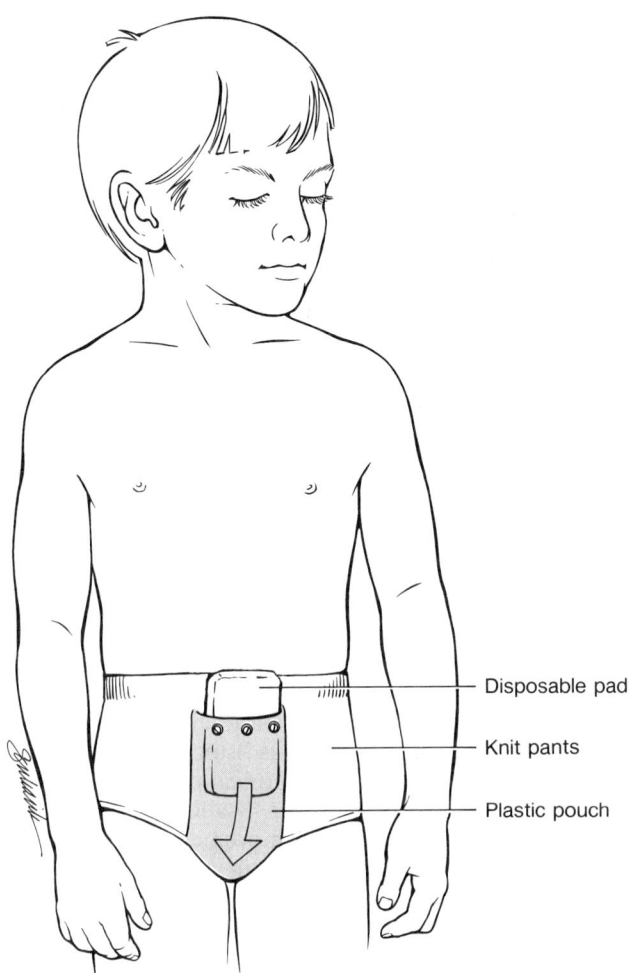

FIGURE 50-15
Incontinent brief system. A disposable pad is inserted into a plastic pouch in the front of the cloth briefs. The waistband and legs are elasticized for better fit.

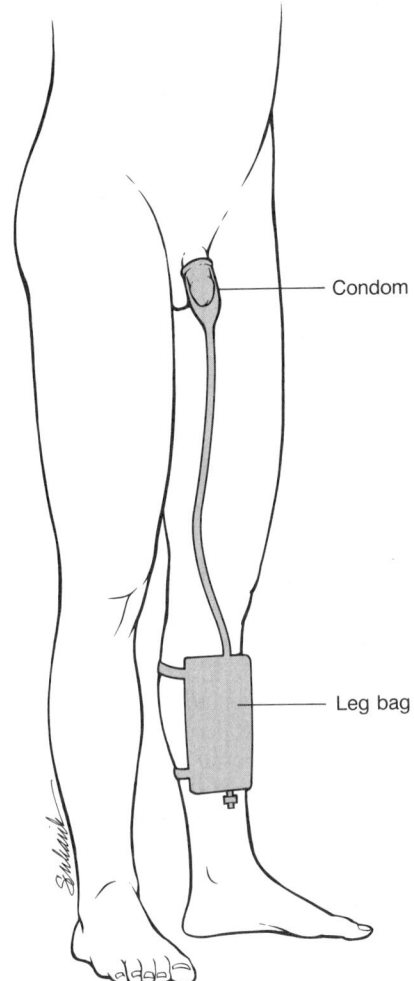

FIGURE 50-16
Condom catheter with leg bag.

MANAGEMENT OF STRESS INCONTINENCE

Stress incontinence may be managed by exercise regimens, pharmacologic manipulation, or surgical intervention. Pelvic floor exercise has limited usefulness in children as compared with adults, since children more often experience severe sphincter deficiencies rather than pelvic descent. Specific indications for pelvic floor muscle exercises are discussed throughout this chapter.

Pharmacologic manipulation also may be used to treat mild to moderate stress incontinence. α-Sympathomimetics are available in several over-the-counter preparations that may be administered to children in consultation with the physician (Table 50-8). These agents work by increasing the efficiency of the smooth muscle and vascular components of the urethral sphincter mechanism. Pseudoephedrine (Sudafed) or ephedrine is used. The medications should not be given in a preparation containing antihistamine, which can cause drowsiness, or caffeine, which may cause anxiety or hyperactivity. Occasionally, imipramine (Tofranil) is given because it exerts an α-sympathomimetic and antispasmodic effect.

The nurse advises the family and child that the goal of therapy is to improve continence but that the drug may not completely cure the condition. The family is assisted in arriving at a suitable schedule for administration of the drug based on the child's daily activities. The child needs the drug while he or she is awake and active and not asleep.

TABLE 50-8
Drugs* Used to Alter Bladder Function

Drugs Used to Reduce Bladder Instability	
Propantheline	(Pro-Banthine)
Methantheline	(Banthine)
Oxybutynin	(Ditropan)
Flavoxate	(Urispas)
Dicyclomine	(Antispas, Bentyl)
Terodoline	(Terolin)
Drugs Used to Increase Bladder Contractility	
Bethanechol chloride	(Urecholine, Duvoid)
Drugs Used to Reduce Sphincter Incompetence	
Ephedrine	(Various OTC products)
Pseudoephedrine	(Various OTC products)
Phenylpropanolamine	(Various OTC products)

* Generic drug names are provided, followed by trade name(s) in parentheses.
OTC = over the counter.

The child is monitored for potential side effects, and the family is taught to do the same. The child's blood pressure is monitored after beginning these agents, and the child is assessed for hyperactivity or signs of hypersensitivity to the drug.

Because of the severity of leakage associated with sphincter damage, many children with stress incontinence must undergo surgery to alleviate their situation. A number of procedures may be used. Urethral suspension is similar to techniques that are sometimes used when sphincter incompetence is mild to moderate. Fascia, bladder flaps, or muscle flaps have been used to fashion slings that are wrapped around the urethra to increase bladder outlet resistance. Periurethral or transurethral injection of a collagen substance is under investigation and may offer a valuable treatment modality for stress incontinence caused by sphincter incompetence. The artificial urinary sphincter offers another treatment modality for these patients.

PREOPERATIVE CARE IN ARTIFICIAL URINARY SPHINCTER SURGERY

The purpose and goals of artificial urinary sphincter surgery are explained to the child and family. They are advised that the device is expected to reduce urinary leakage markedly but that it may not completely cure urinary leakage. A successful outcome is defined as reducing urinary leakage to one pad per day for boys and two pads per day for girls. The child will return from surgery with a *deactivated* device and is expected to experience continuous urinary leakage via the urethra until the device is activated. The child and family are shown a model of the device and taught to activate and deflate the pump (Fig. 50-17). This opportunity is used to assess the child for manual dexterity in manipulating the pump device.

A urine culture is obtained, and bacteria are eradicated from the urinary tract using sensitivity-guided antibiotic therapy. Even if the culture is negative, pro-

phylactic antibiotics, usually a cephalosporin, are administered prior to surgery.[2]

POSTOPERATIVE CARE IN ARTIFICIAL URINARY SPHINCTER SURGERY

The child will return from the surgical suite with an intravenous fluid line, perineal dressing, and closed-system retropubic drain. The child is allowed to drain urine via the urethra; an indwelling Foley catheter is not typically used because of the risk of infection.[2]

An adequate urinary containment system is established, and the surgical drain is assessed for volume and characteristic of drainage. The surgical dressing also is evaluated for exudate and signs of infection. Prophylactic intravenous antibiotics are continued for 4 days postoperatively, followed by oral medications for an additional 14 days.[2]

The child is assessed for pain using an appropriate pediatric assessment tool whenever appropriate. The character, duration, and location of the pain are determined as well as factors that aggravate or alleviate it. A sharp, intermittent suprapubic pain is probably caused by bladder spasm due to postoperative irritability. Administer antispasmodic or anticholinergic medications to alleviate painful bladder spasm as listed in Table 50-8.

A persistent, dull, aching perineal pain is caused by operative wound pain. The pain is alleviate by proper positioning and restriction of movement as indicated. Analgesics are administered for pain as indicated.

The child is discharged from the hospital on the sixth or seventh postoperative day unless complications occur. The nurse teaches the family to apply gentle downward traction to the deflation pump to insure that it remains in an accessible location in the scrotum or labia. They are warned *not* to attempt to manipulate or activate the pump before instructed.

The child will be readmitted to the inpatient unit for a 2- to 3-day period for pump activation. Urine culture is obtained and sterile urine is ensured by use of therapeutic or prophylactic antibiotics administered prior to activation. An x-ray of the abdomen and pelvis is obtained to confirm the location and integrity of the implant. The pump is mechanically manipulated under anesthesia to the activated or "on" position, which closes the urethral cuff, placing closure pressure against the urethral lumen. The child returns to the nursing unit with an indwelling catheter in place.[2]

The indwelling catheter is removed soon after the child recovers from anesthesia. After the catheter is removed, the child and family are retaught to deflate the pump (now placed in the labia or scrotum) every 3 hours until voiding with the artificial device becomes a reality (see Fig. 50-17). If indicated, the child resumes a clean intermittent catheterization program.

Prior to discharge, the parents are taught to monitor for potential long-term complications related to artificial sphincter implantation. They are pump erosion, mechanical failure, and infection. Pump erosion presents as fever with lower abdominal pain or as an unexplained recurrence of severe stress incontinence. The family is taught to seek medical care immediately should these symptoms occur.

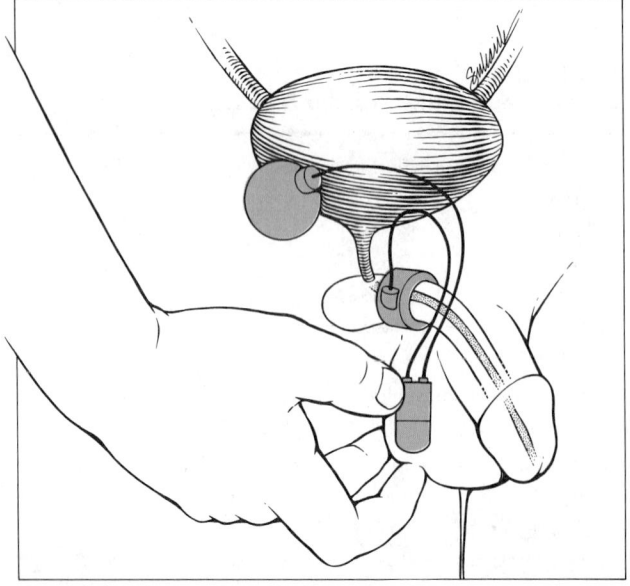

FIGURE 50-17
Artificial urinary sphincter in a boy.

Mechanical failure may cause the cuff to remain in a closed or open position. Although both results are anxiety provoking for the affected child and family, failure of cuff opening presents a medical emergency because the child is rendered in a state of acute urinary retention. Teach the family to seek medical care promptly should mechanical failure occur and to ensure that the physician providing emergency care is aware of the presence of an artificial sphincter device and is familiar with its use.

The risk of infection by the artificial device is lessened by meticulous intraoperative sterile procedure and judicious use of prophylactic antibiotics prior to the invasive urologic instrumentation. Teach the family to monitor the child for signs of implant infection (lower abdominal pain and fever) and to seek their urologist's advise concerning the use of a first-generation cephalosporin prophylaxis prior to subsequent invasive procedures.

MANAGEMENT OF DIURNAL AND NOCTURNAL INSTABILITY AND INCONTINENCE

The treatment of diurnal and nocturnal instability incontinence is influenced by the underlying etiology and its likelihood to produce upper urinary tract distress. For the purposes of this discussion, emphasis is placed on incontinence due to idiopathic or subtle neuropathy in the otherwise health child. A detailed discussion of neuropathic instability incontinence is presented in "Spina Bifida Defects" in this chapter.

Instability incontinence may respond to a variety of treatment modalities. When the diagnosis is established, the nurse teaches the family to begin a timed voiding schedule with fluid control. Timed voiding consists of requiring the patient to void at 2-hour intervals during waking hours. The patient is required to refrain from voiding except at these 2-hour intervals.

The timed voiding schedule is designed to accomplish two goals. An unstable bladder contraction is triggered by provocative maneuvers such as filling. Often, the child who has never gained bladder control either tries to void at the first sign of urgency or simply gives in and resigns herself or himself to a state of wet clothes. Instituting a timed voiding schedule encourages the child to regain some amount of control over urine elimination in a constructive, nonpunitive manner. In instances of relatively mild bladder instability, instituting a timed voiding schedule may greatly alleviate or resolve a problem with incontinence. A bladder drill is a behavior modification technique that encourages progressive gains in functional bladder capacity. By postponing micturition, in spite of the occurrence of unstable contractions, the child slowly builds the bladder's functional capacity and a more acceptable of urine elimination is established.[28]

Fluid control is combined with timed voiding bladder therapy. Many parents and some health care professionals cling to the axiom that incontinence is relieved by simply restricting fluids. Although this strategy may temporarily reduce the symptom, it offers no permanent solution and may adversely affect urinary and other organ system function. The goals of fluid control therapy are to ensure adequate intake while avoiding periods of excessive drinking.

The success of such a program requires a motivated child, motivated parents, and careful coordination with teachers and other caretakers (such as day care personnel). The nurse assists the child and family in identifying the persons who must participate in this timed voiding, fluid control management plan.

Communicate the rules of the regimen as well as its goals and purpose to these persons by letter or telephone conversation as indicated.

If the program is unsuccessful, the physician is consulted concerning the addition of anticholinergic or antispasmodic medications (see Table 50-8). Oxybutynin (Ditropan) or propantheline (Pro-Banthine) are commonly used agents. A medication is begun at a relatively small dose and gradually increased as the child is able to tolerate it. The child and family are taught to monitor for side effects and to distinguish "nuisance effects" from potentially harmful side effects.

A dry mouth is expected when an antispasmodic or anticholinergic medication is used. The child is warned to expect to experience more thirst, but fluid control regimens are not altered. Constipation also may occur as a side effect. As well as ensuring adequate fluid intake, the addition of apple or prune juice to fluid choices and foods high in fiber typically reverses altered bowel elimination.

Potentially harmful side effects of anticholinergic and antispasmodic medications include flushing and intolerance to heat, blurred vision, or hallucinations. Flushing and heat intolerance are relatively common side effects and may cause the child to experience fevers following vigorous exertion. The nurse teaches the parents to monitor the child for redness of the face, chest, and arms following play. They are advised to take an axillary temperature if color changes are noted. Flushing, which is particularly prominent during hot summer months, is typically managed by dosage reduction. Many children must be removed from antispasmodic medication therapy during hot summer months.

Blurred vision and hallucinations indicate potential toxicity related to anticholinergic use. The nurse advises the parents to discontinue the drug and promptly contact their physician should these symptoms occur.

Occasionally, anticholinergic and antispasmodic medications are used pharmacologically to paralyze the bladder and an intermittent catheterization program is instituted. The goal of therapy in this instance is to convert the bladder to a storage vesicle, allowing it to be emptied only by catheterization. The disadvantages of the procedure are the increased likelihood of significant side effects produced by larger doses of antispasmodic medications and the need to substitute catheterization for spontaneous micturition.

Pelvic floor stimulation provides an alternate, nonpharmacologic therapy for diurnal instability incontinence. Therapy relies on the use of transcutaneous, transrectal, or surgically implanted pudendal nerve stimulation. Pelvic floor stimulation exploits the physiologic relationship between the pelvic plexus and pudendal nerve. By stimulating the pudendal nerve, the pelvic plexus is reflexively inhibited,[6] which prevents unstable bladder contractions. Because the pudendal nerve enervates the entire pelvic floor musculature, stimulation may be applied transcutaneously, intravaginally, or intrarectally. The amount of stimulus required to stimulate the pudendal nerve does not produce pain. Stimulation is a passive exercise; the child and family are taught to use a take-home probe device daily for 15-minute periods or by a radio device that activates the surgically implanted stimulator.

Surgical or cystoscopic procedures are rarely used for otherwise normal children with diurnal and nocturnal instability incontinence.

MANAGEMENT OF ENURESIS

The management of enuresis remains controversial. Because it typically resolves spontaneously with maturation and rarely poses a threat to renal function, anticipatory management is often encouraged, particularly among children prior to school age. The nurse reassures the parents and recommends rubber-coated undersheets and absorptive pads when aggressive treatment is postponed. Aggressive management consisting of pharmacologic or conditioning therapy is instituted when enuresis poses a significant social and hygienic problem perceived by the affected patient and family.

One of the most popular forms of management of enuresis is conditioning therapy using an alarm system (Fig. 50-18). The goal of therapy is to condition the child to arise at night in response to a desire to void rather than wetting the bed. The child uses an alarm device. As soon as the child begins wetting, a buzzer alarms and arouses the child from sleep. The system is used continuously for a 2-week period.

Alarm therapy is reportedly effective 70% of the time, but relapse rates are as high as 30%. Relapses are commonly treated by repeated conditioning.[50]

Pharmacologic therapy is aimed at preventing either unstable bladder contractions or excessive diuresis during sleep. Imipramine may be given 2 hours prior to sleep. The success rate is approximately 40%, with an additional 10% to 20% of children who are significantly improved. The recurrence rate is significant, and side effects of insomnia, nervousness, and gastrointestinal disturbances may occur.[50]

The use of antidiuretics for enuresis has been advocated by Danish investigators.[54] Their conclusions are based on observations of diurnal variance of circadian serum levels of antidiuretic hormone in enuretic and normal children. This therapy has recently enjoyed widespread use in the United States. DDAVP (desmopressin acetate) is administrated as nasal drops prior to sleep.

MANAGEMENT OF URINARY RETENTION

Nursing care is instituted to relieve the symptoms of retention and to remove the cause of the condition. The resolution of urinary retention relies on decompression of the urinary system at regular intervals. The two most commonly used alternatives are indwelling or intermittent catheterization.

Indwelling catheterization is preferred when bladder drainage is temporary due to obstruction or reversible detrusor insufficiency. Intermittent catheterization is preferred when drainage is likely to be required over a prolonged period.

Intermittent catheterization is taught by the nurse. Success requires a motivated nurse, patient, and family. Prior to teaching, the nurse confers with the attending physician and an appropriate schedule is decided on. The nurse then confers with the family to discern the child and family's daily routines and evaluates the resources available for accomplishing a routine catheterization program.

When catheterization is taught in an inpatient unit, the goal of instruction is gradually to increase the family's independence in performing the procedure while decreasing the nurse's role in catheterization to that of observer. The procedure is explained with emphasis on underlying principles of clean, dry hands; a clean, dry catheter; and adequate water-soluble lubricant (see display on patient teaching).

The parents and child wash their hands while the nurse evaluates their technique. After adequate cleaning is assured, the child is taught to handle the catheter with confidence and to coat the catheter with a water-soluble lubricant. The child is taught to place the catheter at the urethral meatus and to insert gently until urine returns from the tube. Several strategies are emphasized to insure complete bladder emptying, such as straining and gently repositioning the catheter after urine flow ceases. Following adequate emptying, the nurse teaches the child to pinch the catheter to avoid inadvertent spillage and then to remove the catheter.

The family is taught to rinse the catheter with cool water following each use and to clean the tube thoroughly with warm water and soap prior to repeated use. Emphasize the importance of washing and drying prior to repeated use. Warn the child and family to *never* store a catheter in any solution prior to use. Refer to the detailed teaching plan concerning intermittent catheterization earlier in this chapter.

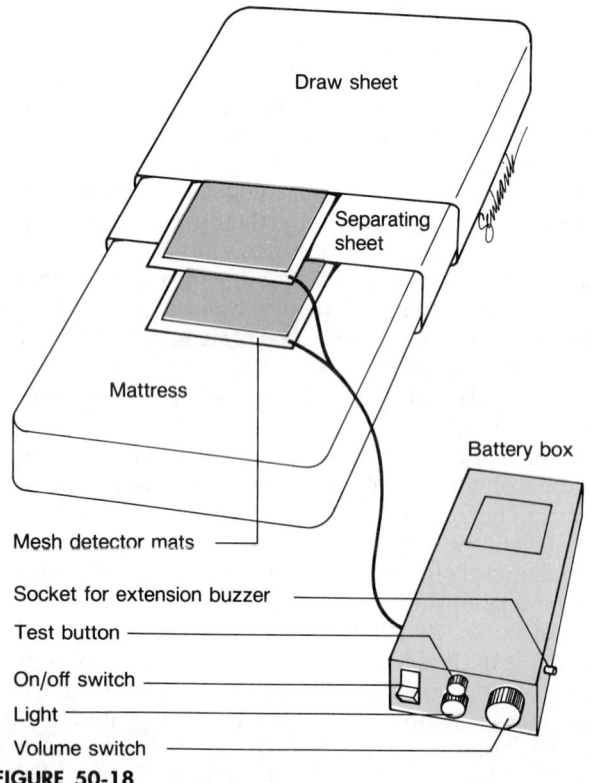

FIGURE 50-18
Alarm system for enuresis.

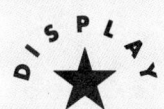

Patient Teaching for Self-Care

Technique for Performing Intermittent Self-Catheterization

1. Wash hands thoroughly, rinse, and dry.
2. Lubricate catheter using water-soluble jelly; placing lubricant in paper towel and applying thin layer to catheter end is acceptable.
3. Wash urethral meatus prior to insertion using soapy wash cloth or towlette if soap and water are not available.
4. Gently insert catheter until urine flows.
5. When urine ceases flowing, gently advance tube first further in the bladder then out to ensure complete evacuation. Gentle manual compression of the suprapubic area is acceptable.
6. The urine can be collected in toilet or urinal-type container as feasible.
7. Withdraw catheter slowly after pinching tube to prevent spillage of urine from the tube.
8. Wash the catheter in warm, soapy water and run water through lumen to ensure patency.
9. Rinse catheter with cool tap water and store in dry container. The catheter should be stored for reuse in a DRY place. Never store the catheter in any type of solution.
10. Wash hands.

Treatment of the factors that underlie urinary retention may require pharmacologic manipulation or surgical reconstruction. Deficient detrusor function occasionally may present as a symptom of a changing neurologic lesion amenable to surgical manipulation. More commonly, it is caused by irreversible neurologic deficits such as myelomeningocele or sacral agenesis so that intermittent catheterization on a permanent basis remains the most viable solution. Rarely, a new onset of urinary retention may be treated with pharmacologic manipulation.

Urinary retention caused by bladder outlet obstruction, in contrast to deficient detrusor function, is typically managed by surgical manipulation. Refer to "Obstructive Uropathy" in this chapter for discussion of surgical options and related nursing care.

MANAGEMENT OF EXTRAURETHRAL INCONTINENCE

Extraurethral incontinence due to surgically created urinary stomas is managed by a pouching system or diapers. Extraurethral incontinence due to urinary fistula or ectopia is managed by a urinary containment system (discussed previously).

★ EVALUATION

The nurse and family evaluate the outcomes and criteria periodically. Example of outcomes for the incontinent child were given in "Nursing Diagnoses and Planning" in this section. Have short-term goals been met? Are long-term goals still realistic? Planning for further nursing care also takes into consideration complications and long-term care. An example of nursing care of a child with voiding dysfunction is given in the nursing care plan display.

COMPLICATIONS

The principal complications of dysfunctional voiding states are urinary tract infection, recurrent or refractory leakage, and compromised renal function.

Urinary tract infection is a common complication of incontinence, particularly when associated with retention. The nursing management of urinary tract infections focuses on treatment of existing infection and prevention of recurrence. Current infection is treated by obtaining urine culture and using laboratory sensitivities to guide appropriate antibiotic therapy. Detailed discussion of the management of infection is presented in "Urinary Tract Infection" in this chapter.

When urinary retention is the principal component of the dysfunctional voiding state, intermittent catheterization or temporary indwelling Foley drainage is instituted. In contrast, when urinary retention is not the principal difficulty, other measures may be used to relieve the situation.

The nurse manages the complication of dyssynergia with instability incontinence by biofeedback training. The child is taught to isolate and contract and relax the pelvic floor muscles using a hand-held device or urodynamic mainframe connected to patch electrodes placed over the external anal sphincter. Following mastery of pelvic muscle contraction and relaxation, the child is taught to maintain a relaxed state during micturation to promote complete bladder emptying.

Persistent urinary leakage or recurrent leakage after a dry period is particularly frustrating for the child experiencing a voiding dysfunction. When a child who has gained a reasonable level of dryness experiences recurrence of leakage, the nurse first evaluates the possibility of urinary tract infection, which may exacerbate leakage. A urine culture is obtained. If the culture is negative, a voiding diary is begun and the characteristics of persistent or recurrent leakage are identified.

Compromised renal function is a serious complication of voiding dysfunction. In every patient with incontinence, assessment of renal function with laboratory analysis and/or imaging studies is undertaken. In addition, complex urodynamic evaluation may be indicated

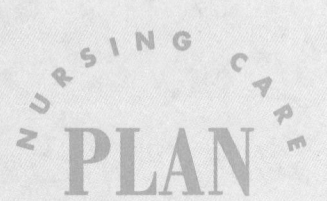

A Child With Voiding Dysfunction

Assessment

Case Study Description

A 9-year-old girl presents with complaints of urinary urgency, frequency (every 1 hour), diurnal incontinence associated with urgency and enuresis. History of four documented urinary tract infections over past year; none associated with fever.

Past history of never gaining full bladder control. Urinary stream assessed as intermittent. Neurologic examination assessed per referring physician as normal.

Assessment Data

Voiding diary.

Functional capacity of 100–180 ml with frequency of ½ to 1 hour during day hours. Incontinent episodes correlate with sensations of urgency and with episodes of increased fluid intake. Enuresis 3 of 3 days assessed.

Inspection of external genitalia

Within normal limits.

Complex urodynamic testing, results: Instability incontinence with reduced functional capacity. Pressure-flow analysis demonstrates intermittent stream with dyssynergic sphincter response. Moderate postvoid residuum (30% of total bladder volume).

Neurologic examination.

Within normal limits.

Nursing Diagnosis	Intervention	Rationale
1. Altered urinary elimination Supporting Data: • History of urinary frequency, urgency, diurnal leakage, and enuresis • Voiding diary consistent with historical report • Functional capacity found to be 100–180 ml of urine • Urodynamic testing shows bladder instability	Assist child to identify proper urinary containment device (pad for undergarments).	A proper incontinence containment system is used to protect clothing and to avoid excessive loss of esteem associated with "wet britches." The pad also assists in reduction of associated odor and reduces likelihood of loss of skin integrity.
	Begin timed voiding regimen: 1. Begin child on every 1½ hour protocol during waking hours. 2. Set goal of every 3 hours during daytime hours.	Timed voiding schedule with bladder drill is used to increase functional capacity in attempt to reduce frequency and diurnal leakage.
	Begin fluid control regimen. 1. Begin with reduction of fluids with meals to 8 oz and 3–4 oz/hr awake. Ensure minimum adequate intake based on age and body weight.	Fluid control helps child avoid excessive intake resulting in greater likelihood of incontinent episodes and frequency.
2. High risk for infection (urinary tract) Supporting Data: • Four documented episodes over past year	Begin biofeedback training control of pelvic floor muscles. 1. Using electromyographic recorder and perineal patches, teach child to contract pelvic floor muscles.	Intermittent stream and dyssynergic stream promote larger than normal residual urine volume and turbulence, allowing milking of distal urethral flora into bladder. Relaxation of pelvic floor muscles promotes good bladder evacuation and lessens risk of infection.

(Continued)

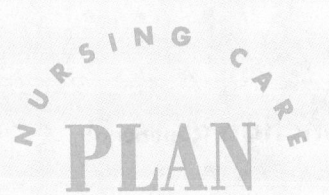

NURSING CARE PLAN

A Child With Voiding Dysfunction (continued)

Nursing Diagnosis	Intervention	Rationale
• Urodynamic evidence of intermittent stream with dyssynergic sphincter and moderate postvoid residual	2. Teach child to contract and relax these muscles (Kegel exercises). 3. Combine the contraction technique prior to micturition followed by relaxation and voiding. 4. Evaluate results using uroflowmetry.	

Evaluation

On reassessment at 4 weeks, the child was found to have slightly improved diurnal frequency but persistent episodes of incontinence. The urinary stream remained normal pattern with absent postvoid residual. Urinalysis showed no evidence of infection.

Nursing Diagnosis	Intervention	Rationale
1. Altered urinary elimination	Consult physician concerning anticholinergic or antispasmodic medication to be added to initial regimen. Continue bladder drill regimen. Teach family and child about the medication, including schedule, side effects (constipation, flushing with heat intolerance, and blurred vision). Reassure the child and family that dry mouth is to be expected and is not harmful.	Pharmacologic agent assists child to gain functional capacity and reduce likelihood of diurnal incontinence. Pharmacologic manipulation used as adjunct to bladder training program.
2. High risk for infection	Continue to reinforce importance of pelvic floor relaxation technique with micturition.	Relaxation of sphincter during voiding encourages complete bladder emptying and reduces risk of infection.

Evaluation

On follow-up 4 weeks later, the child was found to have success at holding urine for 1 and ½ hour periods during the day. Incontinent episodes less than one per 10 days.

Nursing Diagnosis	Intervention	Rationale
1. Altered urinary elimination (persistent diurnal frequency and occasional leakage) Supporting Data: • Diurnal frequency remains every 1½ hours • Occasional incontinent episodes persist	Increased timed voiding regimen to every 2 hours, use telephone conversation to increase by ½ hour to goal of every 3 hours via recheck every 2 weeks.	Diurnal frequency is reduced, and diurnal leakage is dramatically reduced using pharmacologic agent and timed voiding routine. Nonetheless, the goal is to establish normal voiding habits with no leakage.
2. Altered urinary elimination (enuresis)	Obtain alarm system. Use alarm system for 2-week trial period *after* diurnal voiding patterns reach acceptable level.	Enuresis is managed by establishing a pattern of nocturia (awakening to void) rather than leakage while asleep.

(Continued)

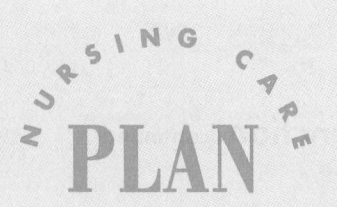

A Child With Voiding Dysfunction (continued)

Nursing Diagnosis	Intervention	Rationale
	Choose device that is sewn in child's undergarments to decrease interval between beginning of voiding and alarm activation.	An alarm system modifies the child's behavior to recognize urge to void and awaken to urinate.
	Teach parents and child proper use of the alarm using manufacturer's insert and principles of diurnal bladder management program.	
Evaluation	Follow-up evaluation 6 months after child has used enuretic device and timed voiding regimen with pharmacologic manipulation reveals diurnal frequency of 3 hours during waking hours and nocturia twice per night with enuretic episodes less than one per month. No reports of diurnal incontinence in past 4 weeks.	

to assess the potential threat that the bladder poses to renal function. When urodynamic evaluation reveals that the bladder fills and/or empties at higher than normal pressures, aggressive means are used to preserve renal function. The nurse assists the family to prevent deterioration of renal function by emphasizing the importance of repeat imaging studies of the upper urinary tracts and adherence to catheterization and medication regimens.

LONG-TERM MANAGEMENT

Successful management of dysfunctional voiding states requires ongoing evaluation and flexibility in treatment regimens. Because of the social stigma associated with incontinence, families are likely to seek treatment only as a last resort. They often have unrealistic expectations of virtually instant results with the institution of medication or a surgical procedure. They are frustrated when results are less than perfect and may interpret vague plans for follow-up care and repeat evaluation as a subtle indication that their child's problem is unimportant or a behavioral rather than actual dysfunctional health problem.

The nurse prevents the development and propagation of these destructive attitudes by outlining a definite schedule for follow-up care in consultation with the physician. The complex and chronic nature of urinary incontinence is explained to the child and family, and realistic goals are set during initial assessment. Although follow-up care must be individualized for each child, repeat clinic visits are indicated after a new bladder management program is initiated, following a change in medication regimen, or when leakage recurs. Routine follow-up care also occurs on an annual or semiannual basis until the voiding dysfunction is resolved. Routine follow-up assessment includes repeat voiding diaries as indicated, evaluation of voided urinary stream, and assessment of residual. Renal function analysis with ultrasound of the

kidneys and serum BUN and creatinine complete the evaluation.

Urinary Tract Infection

Definition and Incidence. A urinary tract infection occurs when pathogens invade and colonize the kidneys, ureters, bladder, or urethra. An infection of the urinary tract is defined according to its location. Urethritis refers to infection of the urethra, cystitis implies bladder infection, and pyelonephritis indicates pathogenic colonization of the upper urinary tracts. This system for defining infection is particularly applicable in the clinical setting because it provides valuable clues concerning presentation and appropriate clinical management.

Urinary tract infections also are defined according to their natural history and response to antibiotic therapy. Stamey[60] described urinary tract infections according to four categories: (1) first time infection; (2) recurrent infection; (3) persistent infection; and (4) unresolved bacteriuria. This category is particularly useful when examining the likely etiology of an infection and when considering long-term management.

The incidence of urinary tract infections varies with age and the presence of predisposing factors such as obstructive uropathy or voiding dysfunction. The incidence of the first episode of symptomatic bacteriuria among girls is greatest during the first year of life. The incidence then steadily decreases through the adolescent years. Among boys, the first year of life also carries the greatest risk of symptomatic bacteriuria, presumably due to detection of clinically significant congenital anomalies affecting urinary system function. In contrast to girls, though, the incidence drops dramatically and remains low through the adolescent years.[73]

Etiology and Pathophysiology. The pathophysiology of urinary tract infections is defined by the virulence of the invading organism (pathogen) and the susceptibility of the host. The body uses two defense mechanisms against colonization of the urinary tract. The first mechanism is urinary constituents in combination with the mechanical action of flow from upper to lower tract to outside the body. Normal urine maintains a *p*H of 6.0 or less and an osmolality that is bacteriostatic to common urinary pathogens. More importantly, the mechanical action of urinary flow continuously washes bacteria downstream in preparation for expulsion from the bladder.[49]

The second line of defense is the walls of the urinary tract. This is demonstrated by experiments requiring instillation of the bladder with bacteria. Following inoculation, the bladder wall responds rapidly to bacterial invasion. Within 30 minutes, polymorphonuclear leukocytes are noted in the bladder wall. Within 2 hours, the entire wall contains plentiful white blood cells, and within 24 hours, clumps of white blood cells are detectable in the urine.[29]

The most common route of bacterial entry into the urinary tract is ascending from the urethra. Blood-borne or lymphatic-spread bacteria also may cause infection but are rarely seen in the clinical setting. Urinary stasis due to obstruction or deficient muscle contractility compromises these defense mechanisms and increases host susceptibility to infection. Vesicoureteral reflux also compromises host-defense mechanisms by promoting the retrograde movement of bacteria from lower to upper urinary tract. Second-line defense mechanisms also are compromised due to disease states that interfere with hematogenous and lymphatic immune mechanisms.[49]

The virulence of the bacterial pathogen also exerts a profound influence on the likelihood of urinary tract infection. *Pathogenic virulence* refers to the pathogen's ability to bypass or overwhelm host-defense mechanisms and establish an infection.[49] For example, certain strains of *Escherichia coli* are known to adhere to the walls of the urinary tract, thus defeating its principal mechanical defense against infection. Extensive investigation of the virulence of various bacterial strains has been sparked by these observations of virulence among particular strains of *E. coli.* Although a consensus has not been reached, current investigational efforts have identified biochemical markers that are associated with a particular virulence for lower and upper urinary tract infection. Further investigations may offer valuable insights to the pathogenesis of urinary tract infection.

The most common pathogenic organism noted in first infection is *E. coli*, followed by strains of *Klebsiella, Proteus, Enterobacter,* and *Pseudomonas.* These pathogens comprise the normal flora of the gut and enter the urinary tract by way of an ascending urethral route. Among older children, gram-positive bacteria, including *Enterococcus* and *Staphylococcus* species, have been associated with clinically significant infection, although they are not predominant pathogens among infants.[49]

In addition, a number of pathogens noted among adolescents or children who are victims of sexual abuse probably represent sexually transmitted urinary tract infections. These include *Chlamydia trachomatis, Ureaplasma urealyticum,* and *Neisseria gonorrhoeae.* They are typically associated with urethritis among boys and silent infection among girls.[49]

Clinical Manifestations. The clinical manifestations of urinary tract infection are influenced by the location of the infection. Infections occur in upper urinary tract (involving the kidneys, renal pelvis, and ureters), lower urinary tract (bladder and trigone), and urethra.

Urethritis. The most common presenting complaint among boys with demonstrable urethritis is dysuria or burning associated with urination and bloody or clear urethral discharge. Sexually transmitted urethritis is suspected when the discharge is purulent, regardless of the age of the child. Urethritis is relatively uncommon among girls. Chemical urethritis due to exposure to bubble bath solutions or chlorinated water may present as dysuria and bloody discharge noted in undergarments.[49]

Cystitis. Lower urinary tract infection among boys and girls causes urinary frequency, urgency, and abdominal or lower back pain. Cystitis rarely causes true bladder instability among normal children but is likely to exacerbate leakage among children with pre-existing incontinence. Fever is *not* typically associated with lower urinary tract infection. When fever does occur, it does not exceed 100° F.

In certain instances, bacteriuria may exist even when the child is asymptomatic. This presentation is particularly common for the child with neurologic and altered pelvic sensations. In this instance, a change in urinary odor or subtle changes in the energy level of the affected child may be the only symptoms of infection.

Pyelonephritis. In contrast to lower urinary tract infections, upper urinary tract infection is associated with fever greater than 100° F. The child typically presents with abdominal and flank pain in addition to dysuria and urinary frequency; nausea, vomiting, and poor appetite also may occur. Among infants, upper urinary tract infection often presents as failure to thrive with dehydration and vomiting, although variations in body temperature may not be as marked as those seen in older children.

Diagnostic Evaluation. The physical examination reveals an inflamed urethral meatus in urethritis and costovertebral angle tenderness in upper urinary tract infection. Laboratory findings in urethritis include a negative urinalysis and urine culture and a urethral swab culture positive for specific pathogens or negative if *C. trachomatis* or viral pathogens are present. In cystitis, the urinalysis is positive for white blood cells (pyuria) and bacteria (bacteriuria) and the urine culture is positive (bacterial colony count >10^5). The blood culture is negative for systemic infection. In pyelonephritis, the urinalysis is positive for bacteriuria and pyuria with a positive urine culture (bacterial colony count >10^5) and a blood culture positive for systemic infection. The IVP is normal for urethritis; renal scarring may be present if infections are complicated by reflux; unsuspected structural anomalies or obstructive uropathy may be noted. The cystogram/VCUG is normal for urethritis. Reflux may be noted, particularly if upper urinary tract infections are known or suspected. DMSA radionuclide scan is normal or has evidence of renal scarring due to vesicoureteral reflux with recurrent pyelonephritis. DTPA radionuclide scan is normal, or unsuspected obstruction of upper urinary tract may be revealed. A cystoscopic examination in urethritis reveals inflammation of the urethra with hemorrhagic patches, particularly predominant in the bulbar urethra in boys. In cystitis, there is inflammation of the bladder wall and trigone; cystic lesions may be noted. Urodynamic examination is normal, or there may be evidence of a voiding dysfunction consistent with urinary retention or functional outlet obstruction, such as vesicosphincter dyssynergia or poor bladder wall compliance.

★ ASSESSMENT

The nursing assessment of the child with symptoms of urinary tract infection focuses on localization of the infection to the upper or lower urinary tract or urethra. The nurse also assesses the likelihood that the infection represents a first or recurrent infection or unresolved bacteriuria. The family is also questioned concerning potential contributing factors such as dysfunctional voiding state or history of vesicoureteral reflux.

The nurse begins to determine the location of the infection by investigating the possibility of urethral discharge. A bloody urethral discharge may represent nonspecific urethritis, whereas a purulent discharge raises the possibility of high-risk sexual behavior (intercourse without barrier protection) in the adolescent or sexual abuse in the younger child.

When urethral discharge is absent, the nurse attempts further to localize the infection to the bladder or upper urinary tract. The nurse asks the child and family if infection is associated with fever. If so, are they aware of the temperature in degrees? High fever raises a suspicion of upper urinary tract infection, whereas low-grade or absent fever indicate probable lower tract infection. Upper versus lower urinary tract infection is further differentiated by exploring other symptoms associated with infection. A child who is nauseated and vomiting and exhibits signs of systemic illness is more likely to be experiencing upper urinary tract infection in contrast to the child's whose symptoms are restricted to lower urinary tract irritability.

A urethral swab is collected if discharge is present by *gently* inserting a sterile swab into the distal urethra. The child experiences marked discomfort when the procedure is performed and is restrained *before* insertion of the swab to avoid unintentional urethral laceration. A urine specimen is obtained whenever urinary tract infection is suspected. A voided specimen may be acceptable, but a catheterized sample is often indicated. The nurse chooses a small catheter, which is introduced after a water-soluble lubricant is inserted into the distal urethra. A 2% lidocaine jelly preparation may be used prior to catheter insertion to reduce urethral discomfort. The preparation is inserted into the urethra approximately 3 to 5 minutes prior to instrumentation, and the urethra is occluded to optimize the medication's effect. The procedure is contraindicated if the patient has an allergy to lidocaine.

Assessment is completed when review of laboratory findings, imaging studies, and cystoscopic examination is combined with historical data and physical examination to determine the location of infection and its classification as first, unresolved, persistent, or recurrent episode.

★ NURSING DIAGNOSES AND PLANNING

Based on the assessment data from above and the preceding chapter, the following nursing diagnoses may apply:

- Related to Urethritis
  - Pain related to urination.
  - Altered Urinary Elimination related to urinary tract infection.
  - High Risk for Infection (Recurrent Urethritis) related to increased exposure.
- Related to Cystitis
  - Pain related to urinary tract infection.
  - Altered Urinary Elimination related to urinary tract infection.
  - High Risk for Infection (Urinary Tract) related to inadequate host defense mechanisms.
- Related to Pyelonephritis
  - Pain related to urinary tract infection.
  - Hyperthermia related to urinary tract infection.
  - Altered Urinary Elimination related to urinary tract infection.
  - Altered Nutrition: Less Than Body Requirements related to poor appetite.
  - Fluid Volume Deficit related to urinary frequency.
  - Altered Tissue Perfusion related to urinary frequency.

Other functionally related nursing diagnoses are discussed in Table 49-2 in Chapter 49.

The nurse plans for the daily care of the child based on both physician's orders and nursing diagnoses. Some general goals for the child with urinary tract infection may be the following:

- Fluid and electrolyte balance is maintained.
- Infection is eliminated.

The nurse and child (or parents) together plan effective care based on the established nursing diagnoses. Several examples of expected outcomes are as follows:

- The child and/or parents describe the medication regimen, including schedule and side effects.
- The child uses comfort measures for pain.

★ INTERVENTIONS: COLLABORATIVE AND INDEPENDENT

MANAGEMENT OF URETHRITIS

After a diagnosis of urethritis is established, the nurse institutes comfort measures to alleviate pain. The child is encouraged to sit in a tub of warm water at least twice daily to relieve pelvic floor muscle tension and irritative symptoms. Adequate fluid intake is maintained to prevent dehydration, and analgesics are used if indicated following consultation with the physician.

If specific urethritis is diagnosed, an antibiotic agent is prescribed. Intramuscular penicillin is commonly used for *N. gonorrhoeae* infection, and an oral tetracycline is used when *C. trachomatis* is documented or suspected. Referral to an appropriate counselor is essential for the sexually active adolescent to prevent recurrence of sexually transmitted disease, and referral to family and protective social services is required for the younger child found to be the victim of sexual abuse.

MANAGEMENT OF CYSTITIS

Following diagnosis of cystitis, the child is placed on an appropriate antibiotic based on laboratory sensitivity reports. The nurse institutes comfort measures, including warm baths and reassurance that irritative symptoms are transient. A urinary analgesic such as phenazopyridine is administered in consultation with the physician. Bladder drill regimens are temporarily suspended in the child with instability incontinence, and reassurance is given to the child with recurrent incontinence.

All children with cystitis are encouraged to drink liberal amounts of fluids. The nurse dispels myths concerning the advantages of cranberry or citrus juices and urine pH.[26] Rather, the child is encouraged to drink adequate amounts of a variety of juices and large amounts of water. Carbonated or caffeinated beverages are generally avoided because of their reportedly irritative effect on the bladder mucosa in certain children.

The nurse assists the child and family to determine an appropriate schedule for taking a prescribed medication and to monitor for common side effects. A variety of antibiotic agents are used for urinary tract infections. A trimethoprim-sulfamethoxazole preparation (Bactrim or Septra) is often prescribed. The dosage schedule is twice daily, preferably in the morning and before bedtime. The family is instructed to give the medication with a glass or bottle of juice or water and taught to monitor the child for rashes indicating a hypersensitive reaction and for diarrhea.

Nitrofurantoin (Macrodantin) is administered four times daily. The drug is given with meals or a snack and a glass of juice or water. The family is warned to monitor the child for rashes indicating a hypersensitive response to the drug or gastrointestinal upset (nausea and vomiting).

Other commonly used antibiotic agents include the cephalosporins, penicillins, and fluoroquinolines. The nurse uses recognized reference books and package inserts to review administration regimens and potential side effects prior to patient administration in the hospital or clinic setting.

MANAGEMENT OF PYELONEPHRITIS

Treatment of febrile urinary tract infections in the infant or acutely ill older child often requires hospitalization. The nursing management of these children begins prior to results of urine culture. Dehydration and nutritional deficits are palliated by administration of intravenous fluids. The intravenous line also is used for administration of parenteral antibiotics until urine cultures are obtained. The child is commonly placed on a parenteral penicillin or ampicillin to treat potential gram-positive organisms and an aminoglycoside to treat potential gram-negative organisms. Elevated fever is treated with antipyretic agents as indicated.

Following results from urine and blood cultures, a more specific antibiotic is chosen based on laboratory sensitivity report. As the fever begins to subside and symptoms of nausea and vomiting cease, the intravenous line and parenteral medications are discontinued and the child is switched to an oral antibiotic. The nurse encourages the child to drink liberal amounts of fluid and monitors the vital signs closely for evidence of recurrent fever. Discharge from the hospital occurs after the child is tolerating oral fluids and solid food and when sings of systemic illness have subsided.

★ EVALUATION

The nurse and family evaluate the outcomes and criteria periodically. Example of outcomes for the child with urinary tract infection were given in "Nursing Diagnoses and Planning" in this section. Have short-term goals been met? Are long-term goals still realistic? Planning for further nursing care also takes into consideration complications and long-term care.

COMPLICATIONS

The principal complications of urinary tract infection are recurrence and persistence of bacteria despite antibiotic therapy. The goal of recurrence prevention in urinary tract infection is the enhancement of host-defense mechanisms and judicious use of prophylactic or suppressive anti-infective agents. The family is warned of the potential for recurrence. The family is instructed to ensure adequate fluid intake every day to optimize movement of pathogens out of the urinary tract. The child is advised to avoid bubble baths that may irritate the urethra. The nurse emphasizes proper hygiene during diaper changes or following urination or defecation.

Persistent or frequent recurrence of urinary tract infections often indicates undetected structural anomalies of the urinary tract or potential presence of associated conditions such as vesicoureteral reflux or obstruction. Urologic evaluation is completed when infection persists despite appropriate antibiotic therapy. Referral to a pediatric urologist is necessary.

Unresolved bacteriuria may indicate incorrect choice of antibiotic in the absence of a laboratory sensitivity report or inadvertently incorrect choice due to contamination of the urine specimen. The nurse obtains a urine culture in consultation with the physician, and therapy is redirected based on laboratory findings.

LONG-TERM MANAGEMENT

The long-term management of patients with urinary tract infections centers on identification of the factors that contribute to recurrence in an attempt to break this cycle. Urologic anomalies are treated, and contributing factors are eliminated or suppressed. Host-defense mechanisms may be strengthened by the use of prophylactic anti-infective agents. Adequate oral fluid intake is established to optimize urinary flow, and a catheterization program is begun if retention prevents adequate elimination of urine regularly.

Follow-up care is also indicated when the recurrent infections occur despite suppressive or preventive management. The nurse assists the family to identify a strategy to obtain a urine specimen for culture and sensitivity report. The specimen is ideally obtained without requiring excessive and expensive office visits, and appropriate medications are often prescribed by telephone conversation with a pharmacist under the direction of a physician.

When the symptoms of recurrent urinary tract infection include high-grade fever with or without vomiting and dehydration, the family is taught to seek medical care immediately.

Hematuria

Definition and Incidence. Hematuria is defined as the presence of red blood cells in the urine. *Gross hematuria* is noted when blood is visible to the naked eye; *microscopic hematuria* is when red blood cells are visible only on microscopic examination. Among children, nephritis is the most common cause of gross hematuria.[42]

Etiology and Pathophysiology. Multiple sources of urinary tract bleeding may account for hematuria. Glomerular sources of hematuria commonly noted in children include poststreptococcal glomerulonephritis or glomerulonephritis caused by another species of bacteria. Familial nephritis (Alport's syndrome), is characterized by progressive nephritis and ocular deafness due to neural causes and transmitted by an autosomal-dominant gene. Other sources, including benign familial hematuria and sporadic hematuria, also can be traced to glomerulopathy. Systemic diseases, including hemolytic uremic syndrome, systemic lupus erythematosus, subacute bacterial endocarditis, and shunt nephritis, also may cause hematuria that is traceable to a glomerulopathy.[62]

Hematuria from renal origin affects the parenchyma or vascular supply of the kidney(s). Malignant tumor of the renal parenchyma may produce hematuria, alerting the clinician to a serious underlying disease. Renal vein or renal artery thrombosis, arteriovenous malformation, or renal cortical necrosis also may cause hematuria.[42]

Obstruction of the urinary system may produce intermittent hematuria. UPJ obstruction or obstructing calculi may produce gross or microscopic bleeding. Other sources of hematuria arise from the urinary tract. When urinary tract infection is present and both hematuria and proteinuria (presence of protein in the urine) are noted, suspicion of a coexisting glomerulonephropathy is raised.[42]

Trauma to the urinary system due to blunt or penetrating trauma, including blunt trauma to the flank affecting the kidneys, may produce hematuria. The introduction of a foreign object into the urinary system via urethra also may produce bleeding noted in the urine.

Certain drugs (piperacillin, anticoagulants, and cyclophosphamide) may also produce hematuria as a side effect.

Clinical Manifestations. Gross hematuria presents as discolored urine. A bright-red color indicates recent bleeding, and darkly colored (often described as "tea" or "cola") colored urine indicates older blood. It is important to remember that other factors than blood may cause discoloration of the urine and that hematuria is established after urinalysis, including microscopic examination. Hematuria may present in the presence or absence of other suggestive findings. Hematuria that coexists with irritative voiding symptoms and dysuria raises the suspicion of urinary tract infection. Hematuria in the presence of intense flank or pelvic pain raises a suspicion of calculi. Hematuria in the presence of proteinuria indicates the possibility of underlying glomerulonephropathy, whereas hematuria in the presence of hypertension suggests the potential of associated renal vascular abnormality.[42]

Diagnostic Evaluation. Physical examination in hematuria reveals bruising of the abdomen or pelvis with renal or bladder trauma; an abdominal or pelvic mass with tumor or obstructive hydronephrosis; and costovertebral tenderness with pyelonephritis. Several laboratory findings will indicate hematuria. The serum BUN and creatinine will be elevated with compromised renal function. The serum streptococcal antibody titer is elevated, or there is depressed total hemolytic complement level (C3) with acute poststreptococcal glomerulonephritis. Urinalysis is significant for (1) red blood cells on gross or microscopic examination; (2) white blood cells and bacteriuria with cystitis; (3) white blood cells and parasites in urine with schistosomiasis; or (4) red blood cells and proteinuria with renal involvement. The KUB shows presence of urinary calculi. The IVP has delayed excretion if renal function is compromised or shows hydronephrosis when an obstruction is present; evidence of urinary calculi may be present. There is evidence of extravasation of contrast in the presence of trauma. DTPA radionuclide scan shows compromised function or evidence of obstruction. The DMSA radionuclide study also shows compromised renal function. A renal arteriogram reveals evidence of renal artery thrombosis or arteriovenous malformation or of extravasation with penetrating trauma of the artery. The renal venogram shows evidence of thrombosis or arteriovenous malformation or of extravasation with penetrating trauma. The voiding cystourethrogram shows evidence of lower urinary tract trauma (extravasation) and a filling defect with presence of a lower urinary tract tumor. The retrograde urethrogram shows abnormal urethral course with trauma. Cystoscopic examination reveals inflammatory lesions of the bladder wall and a tumor of bladder wall or urethra.

⭐ **ASSESSMENT**

The evaluation of gross or microscopic hematuria in a child requires a particularly thorough history and physical examination. Hematuria is a symptom, not a disease, and definitive management is based on detection of the underlying cause. Initially, the patient is tested for presence of urinary tract infection. If the history reveals recent residence in or travel to Africa, evaluation of infection with *Shistosoma haematobium* is undertaken.[42]

Once urinary system infection is excluded as the cause of hematuria, investigation of renal disease is begun. The coexistence of proteinuria and hematuria is suggestive of glomerulopathy. Poststreptococcal or postbacterial glomerulonephritis is evaluated by blood tests for antibody titers or hemolytic complement level changes. Other renal causes of hematuria are evaluated in the context of a consultation with a pediatric nephrologist. Renal biopsy and investigation of systemic disease are sometimes indicated.

★ **NURSING DIAGNOSES AND PLANNING**

Based on the assessment data from above and the preceding chapter, the following nursing diagnoses may apply:

- Altered Urinary Elimination related to anatomic obstruction.
- Altered Tissue Perfusion related to trauma.

Other functionally related nursing diagnoses are discussed in Table 49-2 in Chapter 49.

The nurse and child (or parents) together plan effective care based on the established nursing diagnoses. Several examples of expected outcomes are as follows:

- The parents consult their physician regarding underlying cause.

The nurse plans for the daily care of the child based on both physician's orders and nursing diagnoses. A general nursing care goal may be the following:

- Adequate hydration is maintained.

★ **INTERVENTIONS: COLLABORATIVE AND INDEPENDENT**

Because hematuria is a symptom, its management is related to the underlying cause. The nurse advises the family to consult their physician for evaluation of the symptom. Because hematuria can be intermittent, the family is advised to consult the physician soon after detectable (gross) hematuria is noted.

Hematuria associated with infection is managed by copious hydration, sensitivity-guided anti-infective therapy, and evaluation of the underlying cause when appropriate. Hematuria associated with abdominal or pelvic trauma is managed by bedrest and hydration or by surgical repair when renal or lower urinary tract injury is severe. The nurse assists the parents to arrange diversionary activities for the child limited to bedrest following blunt renal trauma. Adequate hydration with clear liquids and juices is maintained, and the child's urine is regularly evaluated for presence of blood. Urinalysis is used to monitor resolving hematuria when gross bleeding is no longer evident.

The management of hematuria associated with renal disease is discussed in Chapter 47.

★ **EVALUATION**

The nurse and family evaluate the outcomes and criteria periodically. Planning for further nursing care also takes into consideration complications and long-term care.

COMPLICATIONS

The complications of hematuria are influenced by the underlying pathologic process that produces blood in the urine. The principal immediate complication of significant hematuria related to obstruction, calculi, or bacteriuria is systemic spread of infection leading to sepsis or shock.

LONG-TERM MANAGEMENT

The long-term management of the child who experiences hematuria is determined by the underlying cause. The long-term management of renal disorders is discussed in Chapter 47.

Vesicoureteral Reflux

Definition and Incidence. Vesicoureteral reflux is the backward movement of urine from the lower to upper urinary tract. Reflux is of clinical significance in children because of its adverse affects on renal function and propensity to place the urinary tract at risk of infection.[38,52]

Vesicoureteral reflux is further defined by its grade. Although a number of grading systems have been proposed, the system promulgated by the International Reflux Study Committee is used in this discussion.[68] In this system, five grades of reflux are described (Table 50-9). Reflux is graded by noting the severity of regurgitated contrast material infused into the bladder via cystography or cystourethrography. In grade I reflux, contrast material is noted only in the affected ureter, which is not dilated. Grade II reflux is characterized by contrast reaching the renal pelvis without dilation of the upper tracts. Grade III reflux is characterized by contrast material up to the renal pelvis and mild dilatation of the renal collecting system and ureter. Grades IV and V reflux are characterized by progressive dilation and tortuosity of the ureters with clubbing of the calices.

The incidence of vesicoureteral reflux among healthy children remains unclear because of ethical contraindi-

TABLE 50-9
Grading System for Vesicoureteral Reflux

Grade and Description

I
Reflux noted only in affected ureter that is not dilated.

II
Reflux reaches renal pelvis without dilation of upper tracts.

III
Reflux ascends to renal pelvis and mild dilation of renal collecting system and ureter.

IV
Reflux with marked distention of renal pelvis, calices, and ureter.

V
Reflux characterized by progressive dilation and tortuosity of ureters without clubbing of calices.

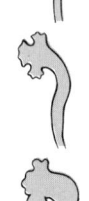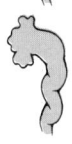

cations related to performing invasive radiographic studies on healthy children; it is thought to be less than 1%.[38] The association of reflux with symptomatic urinary tract infections is particularly strong in infants and very young children who are likely to have shorter submucosal ureteral tunnels and ureterovesical junction incompetence.[33]

The incidence of reflux is greater among offspring and siblings of individuals with known vesicoureteral reflux. Although the cause of this familial disposition remains unclear, studies have found a relationship between the presence of histocompatibility agents detectable on the lymphocytes that further implicate a genetic predisposition toward the condition.[38]

Etiology and Pathophysiology.   Two pathophysiological processes, dysfunction of the UPJ and voiding dysfunction, contribute to a child's risk of reflux. The presence of ureterovesical junction incompetence due to functional and structural factors is called *primary reflux. Secondary reflux* refers to the development of reflux in a previously competent ureterovesical junction because of a dysfunctional voiding state.

The three structural features most important to normal ureterovesical junction function are the angle of entry into the bladder wall, length of the submucosal ureteral segment, and the support of adjacent detrusor muscle bundles in the bladder wall (see Chap. 48). Of these factors, the length of the submucosal ureteral segment is the most significant in the prevention of reflux. Among infants and very young children, the submucosal ureteral segment tends to be shorter than among older children. This developmental characteristic places them at higher risk for experiencing reflux. Primary reflux may represent a congenital characteristic of the ureterovesical junction that may correct itself with maturation or may reflect a more serious structural defect that is unlikely to resolve spontaneously.[38]

Secondary reflux is the result of a dysfunctional voiding state that places stress on the competence of the ureterovesical junction. A dysfunctional voiding state may be the sole cause of reflux, or it may exacerbate reflux in a marginal or mildly impaired junction.

Bladder wall compliance also affects the likelihood of reflux. Gray and Walther[25] found a correlation between poor bladder wall compliance and unsuspected reflux in adults, and a relationship between bladder wall compliance and upper tract deterioration, including vesicoureteral reflux, among myelodysplastic children has been observed.

Often children experience a combination of factors.

Reflux and Infection.   The association of reflux and upper urinary tract infection is well established and represents the most common complication of the condition.[33] Because reflux allows urine to regurgitate from the lower urinary tract (bladder) to the upper urinary tract (ureters and kidney), simple urinary tract infections that begin in the bladder via an ascending urethral route are transmitted to the upper urinary tracts and kidneys. As a result, fever and systemic illness occur. Following invasion of the kidney, bacteria enters the blood stream, and sepsis and shock may occur if the infection is not promptly treated. Renal function also may be acutely compromised, particularly when infection occurs among infants or younger children.

Reflux and Renal Function.   Because the process of reflux begins in the lower urinary tract, it first affects distal tubular function while sparing the glomerulus. These early changes in renal function are subtle and reversible. Later changes affect the glomeruli, causing more obvious compromise in renal function, size, and growth.[68]

Reflux, whether or not it is associated with infection, has the propensity to produce scars of the renal parenchyma. A renal scar is an area of dysmorphic tissue that causes asymmetry of the kidney's shape. The result is a loss of functioning nephrons and some degree of compromised function.

Reflux also affects the kidney's growth and development. This retardation of growth is exacerbated in the presence of higher grades of reflux or when reflux is complicated by recurrent infections. It is alleviated when antibiotics or surgical intervention effectively prevent recurrences.[68]

Reflux also affects general growth and development. Wettlaufer,[70] a nurse researcher, found that children experienced significant gains in height and weight above that accounted for by normal growth patterns following surgical correction of their reflux.

Clinical Manifestations.   The most common presenting symptoms of vesicoureteral reflux are caused by urinary tract infection. Urinary tract infection causes altered patterns of urine elimination, including frequency, urgency, and dysuria. Nocturia may be noted among older children, and nocturnal enuresis is seen in younger children. The urine often assumes a strong odor and may appear cloudy and concentrated. Infection involving the upper urinary tracts is characterized by fever, nausea, vomiting, and poor appetite. The infant may be severely dehydrated and present with failure to thrive due to vomiting with infection and acute renal insufficiency, whereas the older child may present with hypertension and symptoms of infection, particularly if the kidneys are scarred.[68]

Flank pain also may present a clue to the presence of reflux. Among infants, reflux may be associated with a colicky discomfort that can be confused with gastroenteritis. Older children usually are able to localize their pain to the flank area during micturition or when the bladder is very full.[68]

Diagnostic Evaluation.   A physical examination shows signs of systemic infection, including fever and mild to severe dehydration. The blood pressure is normal or elevated if renal scarring is significant. Urinalysis may be normal, or bacteriuria or pyuria may be evident. The urine culture also may be normal, or bacterial colony forming units (CFU) $>10^5$ may be present. Serum creatinine and BUN are normal or elevated in renal failure. In a cystogram/VCUG, there is presence of contrast material in the affected ureter and renal pelvis. The IVP may be normal or show evidence of ureteral tortuosity, blunting, or calices if reflux is high grade. Failure to concentrate contrast material occurs if renal function is compromised or failed. DTPA radionuclide scan is normal, or there is evidence of compromised renal function. DMSA radionuclide scan shows evidence of renal scarring; this is the best definitive determinant of differential renal function in cases of unilateral reflux nephropathy. Radionuclide cystogram indicates the presence of reflux; it *does not* allow determination of grade. Cystoscopic examination reveals normal ureteral orifices or lateral displacement with abnormal anatomic presentations. This examination allows assessment of the urethra and the adjacent bladder wall. In the urodynamic examination, the results are normal or there is evidence of a dysfunctional voiding state.

★ ASSESSMENT

The nursing assessment of the child with known or suspected vesicoureteral reflux centers on the determination of current or recurrent urinary tract infections and renal function and its effects on general health and development. Because the child with reflux often presents with acute infection, the initial evaluation centers on the identification of urinary tract infection and evaluation of systemic complications. Urine is obtained for culture and sensitivities, and blood cultures are obtained. The child is assessed for signs of altered nutritional status and fluid volume deficit.

A history of previous urinary tract infections is elicited from the family. If infection has never been documented by culture, the nurse asks the parents to recall episodes when the child may have exhibited signs of infection, including foul-smelling, cloudy urine lasting for several days or periods of dysuria or urinary frequency that were not evaluated by urinalysis and culture. The parents are asked if the child has had previous episodes of unexplained fevers or febrile illness diagnosed as gastroenteritis that may provide clues to previously undiagnosed urinary tract infections.

Following control of the initial acute episode, reflux is evaluated by voiding cystourethrography or radionuclide cystography to determine the presence and grade of reflux. Potential dysfunctional voiding states are evaluated by use of a voiding diary and observation of the voided stream as well as historical review of the child's voiding habits.

In addition, the child's height and weight are determined and plotted on a standardized chart for comparison to national standards and previous values to determine the potential effect on general growth and development.

Because of the increased risk of reflux among siblings, the family is advised to consult a pediatric urologist concerning screening tests for reflux.

★ NURSING DIAGNOSES AND PLANNING

Based on the assessment data from above and the preceding chapter, the following nursing diagnoses may apply:

- Altered Urinary Elimination related to urinary tract infection.
- Hyperthermia related to urinary tract infection.
- Pain related to urinary tract infection.
- Fluid Volume Deficit related to vomiting.

- Altered Nutrition: Less Than Body Requirements related to vomiting and poor appetite.
- Altered Renal Tissue Perfusion related to scarring.
- High Risk for Infection (Urinary Tract) related to traumatized tissue.
- Altered Urinary Elimination related to scarring.
- Altered Tissue Perfusion: Renal related to inadequate blood supply.
- Altered Growth and Development related to compromised renal function.

Other functionally related nursing diagnoses are discussed in Table 49-2 in Chapter 49.

The nurse and child (or parents) together plan effective care based on the established nursing diagnoses. Several examples of expected outcomes are as follows:

- The family describes side effects of antibiotic medications to be administered.
- The family demonstrates appropriate methods of monitoring the child for recurrent urinary tract infection.
- The child voids within 6 to 8 hours of catheter removal.
- The parents comply with prescribed antibiotic medication regimen.

The nurse plans for the daily care of the child based on both physician's orders and nursing diagnoses. Some general nursing care goals may be the following:

- Condition is resolved.
- Further infection is prevented.
- Normal urinary pattern is established.

★ INTERVENTIONS: COLLABORATIVE AND INDEPENDENT

Two basic therapeutic options exist for the management of vesicoureteral reflux. Pharmacologic prophylaxis may be provided while waiting for the condition to resolve spontaneously. Surgical management requires temporary prophylaxis with antibiotic agents followed by definitive resolution of the refluxing ureter(s) by reimplantation into the bladder base.

MEDICATION THERAPY

Following diagnosis of reflux in a child, each is placed on prophylactic antibiotics to prevent the occurrence or recurrence of infection.

The ideal medication for prophylaxis should be inexpensive, effective on a variety of common urinary pathogens, and produce no adverse side effects.

No medication completely fulfills all requirements, although several agents offer satisfactory results.[76] Nitrofurantoin is effective against most common urinary tract pathogens, including *E. coli* and *Klebsiella*. It exerts virtually no effect on the flora of the distal colon and rectum because it is absorbed or excreted before reaching this point, but it is associated with rare but significant side effects. Trimethoprim-sulfamethoxazole in combination also is effective against common urinary pathogens but affects the normal flora of the distal colon and rectum and can cause the development of bacterial strains resistant to oral medications in rare instances.

The cephalosporins also may be used for antibiotic

prophylaxis. Cephalexin (Keflex) achieves acceptable therapeutic concentrations in the urine and exerts antimicrobial activity against a wide spectrum of common urogenital pathogens. It exerts relatively minimal effect on rectal flora; side effects or allergic reactions are rare but may occur.

TEACHING

The nursing role in medical management is primarily educational. The family is taught when to administer the medication and to monitor for potential side effects.

The nurse obtains a voiding diary when urinary output patterns are not clear.

The nurse teaches the family how to prepare and properly administer the medication as indicated. Table 50-10 lists administration and storage guidelines and possible side effects. Proper positioning and gentle restraint of the head are taught to prevent aspiration. Other medications are available in a powder form, which may be mixed with small amounts of beverages or with food. The family is taught to give these medications by mixing with a relatively small amount of food to insure administration of the entire dose. The nurse teaches the family to mix bitter or unpleasant agents with iced beverages to disguise the taste as needed.

The family is taught to store and date medications for maximum therapeutic effect (see Table 50-10). Oral

TABLE 50-10
Patient Teaching: Preparation and Administration of Common Prophylactic Antibiotic Agents

Drug*	Administration	Storage	Side Effects
Nitrofurantoin (Macrodantin)	Powder is reconstituted with sterile water without preservatives or may be mixed with milk, water, fruit juice, or formula. Capsules given to older child with meals or snack.	Powder form or capsules maintained in cool, dry place.	Nausea, vomiting common; drug is administered with milk or meals to minimize gastric irritation.
			Staining of teeth may occur if powdered form of drug is crushed prior to administration; administer with juice, milk, formula, or water followed by additional beverage to avoid prolonged contact with teeth.
			Hypersensitivity reactions: skin eruptions, urticaria, drug fever, arthralgia; teach family to discontinue drug and contact physician promptly should reaction occur. Hypersensitivity also may present altered pulmonary function (rare among children) such as allergic pneumonitis or exacerbation of asthma noted within first 2 weeks of therapy; teach family to discontinue drug and contact physician promptly should pulmonary reaction occur.
			Subacute pulmonary sensitivity may occur after first 2 weeks of therapy, noted as increasing malaise, cough, dyspnea; teach family to contact physician and discontinue drug should symptoms occur.
			Drug may cause or exacerbate peripheral neuropathies (uncommon); teach family to monitor for increasing numbness or motor activity of extremities, discontinue drug, and notify physician should symptoms occur.
			Drug may color urine brown.
Trimethoprim-Sulfamethoxazole (Septra, Bactrim)	Oral suspension available in grape or cherry flavors, given with adequate fluid to lessen potential adverse effect on renal function; administration with food may delay absorption.	Oral suspension; tablets stored in cool, dry place (refrigeration not required); store in light-minimizing container, avoid excessive exposure to light.	Hypersensitivity response; rash, nausea and vomiting, fever; teach family to discontinue drug and contact physician at first sign of rash or skin eruption.
			Hypersensitivity response may progress to Stevens-Johnson syndrome in rare cases, manifested by erythema multiforme lesions, high fever, headache, marked stomatitis, rhinitis, urticaria, balanitis; teach family to contact physician promptly and discontinue use of drug should symptoms occur.
			Repeat kidney function studies (serum creatinine and BUN) recommended for prolonged use; consult physician to establish proper schedule for assessment.
			Excessive exposure to sunlight may cause photosensitive response, lessened by reduced dosage; teach family to monitor for symptoms and restrict exposure if indicated.
Cephalexin (Keflex)	Given as oral suspension or tablets; administration with meals will delay but not reduce proportion of drug absorbed.	Store oral suspension in refrigerator, shake well before each use; discard unused portion after 14 days; tablets stored in cool, dry place (<86°F).	Hypersensitivity reactions, including anaphylactic response, occur rarely; teach family to monitor for allergic response, discontinue medication, and contact physician promptly should rash, urticaria, or respiratory symptoms (wheezing, etc.) occur.
			Diarrhea also may occur; teach family to give yogurt or buttermilk to re-establish normal intestinal flora; teach family to contact physician if diarrhea persists.

* Trade name shown in parentheses.

suspensions may require storage in a refrigerator, and tablets or capsules typically require storage away from heat above 86° F. The family is taught to check drugs for manufacturer's label concerning expiration of potency and to discard any medication once the expiration date is reached.

The nurse also teaches the family to monitor the child for recurrence of urinary tract infection and to seek medical care aggressively should symptoms of infection occur. Parents are taught to ask their primary care provider to assess a voided urine specimen any time their child experiences fever or symptoms suggestive of urinary tract infection. Urine cultures are obtained whenever microscopic examination reveals bacteriuria and pyuria.

Parents of a younger child or infant who presents with fever and inability to tolerate feedings are advised to seek immediate care through a hospital emergency or immediate care department.

SURGICAL MANAGEMENT

The discovery that lower grades of reflux (I to III) may subside spontaneously with use of prolonged suppressive antibiotic therapy has obviated the need for surgical intervention among many children. Nonetheless, so many other children with reflux greatly benefit by surgery that it remains a viable part of a treatment program.[76]

The principal indications for surgery are higher grades of reflux (IV, V) and poor control through antibiotic therapy. Surgery is indicated among children with higher grades of vesicoureteral reflux because longitudinal studies have demonstrated that they have only a 50% rate of spontaneous resolution of the condition due to maturation even after several years and run the risk of additional renal function compromise if the condition remains uncorrected. In addition, surgery may be contemplated among children with grade III vesicoureteral reflux who have cystoscopic evidence of structural anomaly of the vesicoureteral junction despite an adequate period of conservative management. In any instance, when surgery is potentially indicated, careful consideration also is given to the child's risks when on prolonged antibiotic use versus undergoing a surgical procedure.[76]

Other patients are considered surgical candidates even though they have lower grades of vesicoureteral reflux when febrile infections recur despite prolonged prophylactic antibiotic therapy. Unreliable compliance with prescribed antibiotic regimens is the most common cause of failed medical therapy in lower grade reflux, although some patients may be prone to breakthrough infections due to unknown factors despite appropriate therapy.[76]

The question of surgical versus medication management also arises in the child or adolescent with newly diagnosed, persistent vesicoureteral reflux despite several years of appropriate therapy. Because this patient has little chance of spontaneous resolution[68] compared with the infant or young child, the decision to perform surgery relies on its potential to prevent further compromise of renal function due to scarring. Although surgical intervention does lower the incidence of pyelonephritis, it does not arrest the progression of pre-existing scars or the onset of renal insufficiency in the already compromised patient.[39]

Regardless of the indications for surgery, the goal remains the prevention of vesicoureteral reflux by the establishment of a reasonably long submucosal tunnel located at the bladder base in the trigone. This goal is realized by any one of a number of procedures that lengthen the intramural portion of the ureter, often in combination with placement of the ureter in a more physiologically advantageous location near the medial aspect of the trigone.[31]

The surgery is typically performed via a Pfannenstiel's incision; the bladder is opened; and the ureters are mobilized and reimplanted into the bladder in a "nonrefluxing" manner.[31]

Subureteric injection of Teflon paste has been reported as an alternative to open surgical correction of vesicoureteral reflux. Use of this procedure remains controversial.[40] A newer technique of injection of glutaraldehyde cross-linked collagen is under investigation.

PREOPERATIVE CARE

Prior to surgery, the procedure is explained to the family and child using appropriate language and extensive visual aids as indicated by the child's age and cognitive level. The nurse obtains a urine culture and consults with the physician concerning treatment of infection prior to surgery if bacteriuria is detected.

POSTOPERATIVE CARE

The child returns from the surgical suite with a suprapubic tube or urethral catheter in place. The nurse monitors the urinary output for volume and evidence of catheter patency. Loss of patency and bladder overdistention are prevented by careful assessment of output volume and by regular inspection of the drainage system. The physician is contacted promptly should the catheter become occluded. The nurse refrains from disconnecting the system to avoid infection, particularly if ureteral stents are incorporated into the bedside drainage system. The urine should be pink or light red; gross bleeding and clots are not expected, and the physician is contacted promptly should they occur.

Indwelling ureteral stents are sometimes used after ureteroneocystostomy to prevent obstruction of the ureterovesical junction. The stents are typically positioned in such a way that they extend through the catheter via two holes created by the surgeon and into the closed urinary drainage system. This allows the catheters to be easily removed with the urethral catheter. Tape and proper positioning of the exposed catheter and bedside collection bag are used to prevent inadvertent loss of adequate urinary drainage.

The nurse monitors the child for presence of pain using a specific assessment tool for pediatric patients whenever feasible. This assessment includes determination of the location, duration, and character of the pain. Sharp, cramping pain is attributable to bladder spasm from the indwelling catheter. The nurse assesses the catheter tubing to ensure patency and lightly percusses the bladder to rule out overdistention. Movement is restricted to minimize the occurrence of spasms and an anticholinergic-antispasmodic agent such as oxybutynin or propantheline is administered as directed. Dull, prolonged pain may occur because of the incision and is treated by repositioning and restricted movement and by analgesics or narcotics in consultation with the physician.

The catheter is typically removed by the second or third postoperative day[31] to lessen the risk of nosocomial infection and prolonged hospital stay. The nurse closely monitors the child to ensure the ability to void following catheter removal. The child is told that voiding may sting or burn at first but is encouraged to drink fluids and to void repeatedly to lessen this discomfort. The physician is contacted concerning recatheterization if the child is not able to void within 6 to 8 hours after catheter removal or despite palpable bladder distention and desire to urinate. Urination is encouraged by allowance of adequate privacy, provision of adequate fluids, and placing the child in a warm tub as needed.

An imaging study is typically obtained prior to hospital discharge. An IVP or DTPA radionuclide scan is commonly chosen. The nurse explains to the child and family that this examination is designed to insure that significant obstruction does not exist following surgery. They are also informed that this procedure *does not* ensure that the reflux has been resolved and that further assessment is essential to ensure that definitive resolution.

★ EVALUATION

The nurse and family evaluate the outcomes and criteria periodically. Example of outcomes for the child with ves-

icoureteral reflex were given in "Nursing Diagnoses and Planning" in this section. Have short-term goals been met? Are long-term goals still realistic? Planning for further nursing care also takes into consideration complications and long-term care.

COMPLICATIONS

The complications related to medical or conservative management are untoward effects of antibiotic medications and the danger of breakthrough infection. Common side effects of the certain medications used for anti-infective prophylaxis are listed in Table 50-10. Although serious complications related to antibiotic therapy are rare and easily overlooked, they are, nonetheless, significant or even fatal unless promptly reversed.

The potential for breakthrough infection also is significant because there is a strong correlation between the formation of scars and suboptimal or insufficient renal function in childhood and adulthood.[65] Recurrent pyelonephritis places the kidney at higher risk for formation or scars or further compromise of renal function. Complications related to surgical intervention are persistent or recurrent reflux and obstruction. Obstruction is assessed by imaging studies of the upper urinary tracts. Obstruction may, itself, cause flank pain and infection that may be misconstrued as recurrence of reflux prior to more detailed assessment. Minimal degrees of obstruction may be noted after surgery that regress as healing continues

---

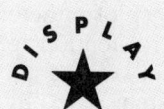

Follow-Up Assessment of the Child With Reflux

Medical Management

Following Diagnosis of First Infection

Month 1:   Urine culture,* baseline height and weight, baseline blood pressure, baseline BUN and serum creatinine, voiding diary; urodynamics if voiding diary or history suggestive

Month 2:   Urine culture

Month 3:   Urine culture

Month 6:   Urine culture (unless infection occurs in interim)

Month 9:   Urine culture

Year 1:   Urine culture, height and weight, blood pressure, serum creatinine and BUN

Following Spontaneous Resolution of Reflux

Annual: Height and weight, serum creatinine and BUN, blood pressure

Surgical Management

Following hospital discharge:	Therapeutic dosage of antibiotic for 2 weeks followed by resumption of daily prophylaxis until absence of reflux shown by imaging study
4–8 weeks following discharge:	Renal ultrasound to rule out obstruction
8–16 weeks following discharge:	Voiding cystourethrogram or radionuclide cystogram to assess absence of vesicoureteral reflux

Repeat upper urinary tract imaging study (IVP, radionuclide scan, ultrasonography) used when significant renal scars exist.

Repeat voiding cystourethrography or radionuclide cystography if urinary tract infection recurs.

* *Urine cultures obtained more frequently if recurrent infections occur or when microscopic examination of suspicious urine reveals bacteriuria and/or pyuria.*

Data from Levitt, S. B., & Weiss, R. A. (1985). Vesicoureteral reflux: Natural history, classification, and reflux nephropathy. In P. P. Kelalis, L. R. King, & A. B. Belman (Eds.), Clinical pediatric urology (pp. 355–380). Philadelphia: Saunders.

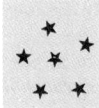

Ideas for Nursing Research

Many potential areas for nursing research exist. Perhaps the most important caveat for the new researcher interested in nursing aspects of altered urinary system function is to remember to allow the situation to determine the approach to research rather than attempting to "fit" a research tool or methodology to a convenient clinical problem. Children and adolescents with altered urinary system function suffer physical and emotional pain as they attempt to cope with their disease, tumor, or dysfunctional condition. Research that addresses the cause and solutions to these problems will alleviate immeasurable suffering for the person at the bedside as well as many others who face similar problems. Ideas for nursing research related to planning and intervention of altered urinary system function include the following:

- The natural history of the silent condition known as compromised renal/urinary function.
- Exercises that benefit children in rehabilitation of sphincter muscle control and learning continence.
- The nonsurgical and nonpharmacologic methods that increase continence among children with physical handicaps and neuropathic bladder and bowel.
- The role for electrostimulation in children with instability incontinence.
- Whether children with reflux should be routinely screened by noninvasive urodynamic testing to exclude voiding dysfunction.
- What is appropriate screening test(s) for siblings of children with reflux.

and edema lessens. Surgical intervention is indicated only when obstruction is persistent or progressive.[31]

Persistent or recurrent reflux may occur because of surgical technique or because of a dysfunctional voiding state placing the ureterovesical junction at high risk for incompetence. Complex urodynamic investigation is indicated whenever voiding dysfunction is suspected as the underlying cause of reflux. The success of subsequent procedures will rely on resolution of the dysfunctional voiding state prior to repeat reimplantation.

The long-term complications of reflux are hypertension and renal failure. Hypertension typically develops in young adults who have experienced vesicoureteral reflux as children, particularly when they have significant residual scarring of one or both kidneys. The etiology of their hypertension probably represents the result of increased renin production by the affected kidney(s) caused by segmental parenchymal ischemia.

Renal failure occurs in many of these children. The associated risk factors are recurrent febrile urinary tract infection, renal scarring, and hypertension. The etiology of renal failure remains obscure, although a glomerulo-

pathy or result of chronic pyelonephritis has been implicated.[68]

LONG-TERM MANAGEMENT

The long-term management of reflux is crucial for successful resolution and preservation of optimal renal function. The nurse emphasizes the critical importance of long-term follow-up at every stage of management. Data base systems and protocols for follow-up are often useful for the nurse in the clinic or office setting, particularly if large numbers of patients are being cared for at any given time. A summary of routine follow-up assessment for the child with vesicoureteral reflux is shown in the accompanying display.

Summary

The nursing management of children with altered urinary system function addresses both the immediate complaint and its impact on general health, well-being, and function. The nurse synthesizes knowledge of the interrelationships between upper and lower urinary tract function to preserve optimal renal function and effective urinary transport, storage, and elimination.

Nursing care ranges from preoperative and postoperative care to emotional support of the parents and child with disfiguring anomalies. The child's self-concept is addressed, and sexual dysfunction is considered. Because parents provide much of the care at home, discharge planning and teaching are important nursing responsibilities.

References

1. Agatstein, E. H., & Ehrlich, R. M. (1986). Imperforate anus, persistent cloaca and urogenital sinus outlet obstruction. In P. C. Walsh, R. F. Gittes, A. D. Perlmutter, & T. A. Stamey (Eds.), *Campbell's urology*. Philadelphia: Saunders. pp. 1922–1933.
2. Barrett, D. M., & Wein, A. J. (1991). Voiding dysfunction: Diagnosis, classification and management. In J. Y. Gillenwater, J. T. Grayhack, S. S. Howards, & J. W. Duckett (Eds.), *Adult and pediatric urology*. pp. 1001–1100. Chicago: Year Book.
3. Belasco, J. B., Chatten, J., & D'Angio, G. J. (1984). Wilms' tumor. In W. Sutow, D. Fernbach, & T. Vetti (Eds.), *Clinical pediatric oncology*. St. Louis: Mosby. pp. 793–804.
4. Belman, A. B. (1985). Urinary problems associated with imperforate anus. In P. P. Kelalsi, L. R. King, & A. B. Belman (Eds.), *Clinical pediatric urology*. Philadelphia: Saunders.
5. Belman, A. B., & King, L. R. (1972). Urinary tract anomalies associated with imperforate anus. *Journal of Urology, 108,* 823.
6. Bradley, W. E. (1986). Physiology of the urinary bladder. In P. C. Walsh, R. F. Gittes, A. D. Perlmutter, & T. A. Stamey (Eds.), *Campbell's urology* (pp. 129–185). Philadelphia: Saunders.
7. Brenner, B. M., Meyer, T. W., & Hostetter, T. H. (1982). Dietary protein intake and the nature of progressive renal disease: The role of hemodynamically mediated injury in the pathogenesis of progressive glomerulosclerosis in aging, renal ablation and intrinsic renal disease. *New England Journal of Medicine, 307,* 652.
8. Brundage, D. (1986). Renal system. In J. M. Thompson, G. K. McFarland, J. E. Hirsch, S. M. Tucker, & A. C. Bowers (Eds.), *Clinical nursing*. St. Louis: Mosby. pp. 1031–1104.
9. Bruton, O. C. (1951). Agenesis of abdominal musculature with

genitourinary and gastrointestinal tract anomalies. *Journal of Urology, 66,* 607.

10. Caldamone, A. A. (1991). Anomalies of the bladder and cloaca. In J. Y. Gillenwater, J. T. Grayhack, S. S. Howards, & J. W. Duckett (Eds.), *Adult and pediatric urology.* (2nd ed.) Chicago: Year Book. pp. 2023–2054.

11. D'Angio, G. J., Duckett, J. W., & Belasco, J. B. (1985). Tumors: Upper urinary tract. In P. P. Kelalis, L. R. King, & A. B. Belman (Eds.), *Clinical pediatric urology.* Philadelphia: Saunders. pp. 1157–1188.

12. Denton, J. R. (1982). The association of congenital spinal anomalies with imperforate anus. *Clinical Orthopaedics and Related Research, 162,* 91.

13. Diard, F., Eklof, O., Lebowitz, R., & Mauoseth, K. (1981). Urethral obstruction in boys caused by prolapse of simple ureterocele. *Pediatric Radiology, 11,* 139.

14. Duckett, J. W. (1987). Hypospadias. In J. Y. Gillenwater, J. T. Grayhack, S. S. Howards, & J. W. Duckett (Eds.), *Adult and pediatric urology* (pp. 1880–1915). Chicago: Year Book.

15. Duckett, J. W., & Caldamone, A. A. (1985). Congenital disorders of the bladder. In W. F. Hendry & H. N. Whitfield (Eds.), *Textbook of genitourinary surgery* (pp. 178–202). London: Churchill-Livingstone.

16. Duckett, J. W., & Snow, B. W. (1986). Disorders of the urethra and penis. In P. C. Walsh, R. F. Gittes, A. D. Perlmutter, & T. A. Stamey (Eds.), *Campbell's urology.* Philadelphia: Saunders. pp. 2000–2030.

17. Farewell, V. T., D'Angio, G. J., Breslow, N., & Norkool, P. (1981). Retrospective validation of a new staging for Wilms' tumor. *Cancer Clinical Trials, 4,* 167–171.

18. Gaiger, A. M., Soule, E. H., & Newtown, W. A., Jr. (1981). Pathology of the rhabdomyosarcoma study: Experience of the intergroup rhabdomyosarcoma study. *National Cancer Institute Monograph, 56,* 19–27.

19. Gallaway, N. T. M., Mekras, J. A., & Webster, G. D. (1989, May). *A Score to predict upper tract deterioration in myelodysplasia.* Presented at the American Urological Association Annual Meeting, Dallas, Texas (Abstract No. 633).

20. Gillenwater, J. Y. (1986). Pathophysiology of urinary obstruction. In P. C. Walsh, R. F. Gittes, A. D. Perlmutter, & T. A. Stamey (Eds.), *Campbell's urology* (pp. 542–578). Philadelphia: Saunders.

21. Gosling, J. A., & Dixon, J. S. (1983). Detrusor morphology in relation to bladder outflow obstruction. In F. Hinman, Jr. (Ed.), *Benign prostatic hypertrophy.* New York: Springer-Verlag. pp. 666–671.

22. Gray, M. L., & Broadwell, D. C. (1986). Genitourinary system. In J. M. Thompson, G. K. McFarland, S. M. Tucker, J. E. Hirsch, & A. C. Bowers (Eds.), *Clinical nursing.* St. Louis: Mosby. pp. 1203–1364.

23. Gray, M. L., & Dobkin, K. (1989). Genitorurinary system. In J. M. Thompson, G. K. McFarland, S. M. Tucker, J. E. Hirsch, & A. C. Bowers (Eds.), *Clinical nursing.* St. Louis: Mosby. pp. 1806–1153.

24. Gray, M. L., & Dougherty, M. C. (1987). Urinary incontinence: Pathophysiology and treatment. *Journal of Enterostomal Therapy, 14,* 152–162.

25. Gray, M. L., & Walther, M. M. (1987, March). *Incidental finding of reflux on urodynamics.* Presented at the Southeastern Section, American Urological Association, Boca Raton, Florida.

26. Howe, S. H., & Bates, P. (1987). The cranberry juice cure: Fact or fiction? *AUAA Journal (Urologic Nursing), 8* (1), 13–16.

27. Jeffs, R. D., & Lepor, H. (1986). Management of the exstrophy-epispadias complex. In P. C. Walsh, R. F. Gittes, A. D. Perlmutter, & T. A. Stamey (Eds.), *Campbell's urology.* Philadelphia: Saunders. pp. 1882–1927.

28. Jeter, K. (1990). Treating and managing incontinence. In K. Jeter, N. Faller, & C. Norton (Eds.). *Nursing for continence.* Philadelphia: Saunders. pp. 65–90.

29. Kay, R., & Straffon, R. (1986). Augmentation cystoplasty. *Urologic Clinics of North America, 13,* 295–306.

30. Kelalis, P. P. (1985a). Anomalies of the urinary tract: The kidney. In P. P. Kelalis, L. R. King, & A. B. Belman (Eds.), *Clinical pediatric urology* (pp. 643–671). Philadelphia: Saunders.

31. Kelalis, P. P. (1985b). Anomalies of the urinary tract: Renal pelvis and ureter. In P. P. Kelalis, L. R. King, & A. B. Belman (Eds.), *Clinical pediatric urology* (pp. 672–725). Philadelphia: Saunders.

32. King, L. R. (1985). Obstructive uropathy: Ureter and uretero-vesical junction. In P. P. Kelalis, L. R. King, & A. B. Belman (Eds.), *Clinical pediatric urology* (pp 486–512). Philadelphia: Saunders.

33. King, L. R., & Levitt, S. B. (1986). Vesicoureteral reflux mega-ureter, and ureteral reimplantation. In P. C. Walsh, R. F. Gittes, A. D. Perlmutter, & T. A. Stamey (Eds.), *Campbell's urology* (pp. 542–578). Philadelphia: Saunders.

34. Kosko, J. W., Kursh, E. D., & Resnick, M. I. (1986). Metabolic complications of urologic intestinal substitutes. *Urologic Clinics of North America, 13,* 193–200.

35. Kramer, S. A. (1985). Surgical treatment of urinary incontinence. In P. P. Kelalis, L. R. King, & A. B. Belman (Eds.), *Clinical pediatric urology* (pp. 326–344). Philadelphia: Saunders.

36. Kramer, S. A., & Kelalis, P. P. (1991). Pediatric urologic oncology. In J. Y. Gillenwater, J. T. Grayhack, S. S. Howards, & J. W. Duckett (Eds.), *Adult and pediatric urology.* (2nd ed.) Chicago: Year Book. pp. 2245–2288.

37. Ladd, W. E., & Gross, R. E. (1934). Congenital malformations of anus and rectum: Report of 162 cases. *American Journal of Surgery, 23,* 167.

38. Levitt, S. B., & Weiss, R. A. (1985). Vesicoureteral reflux: Natural history, classification, and reflux nephropathy. In P. P. Kelalis, L. R. King, & A. B. Belman (Eds.), *Clinical pediatric urology* (pp. 355–380). Philadelphia: Saunders.

39. Malek, R. S., Svensson, J. P., & Torres, V. E. (1983). Vesicoureteral reflux in the adult: Factors in pathogenesis. *Journal of Urology, 130,* 37–40.

40. Malizia, A. A., & Woodard, J. R. (Personal Communication). Potential for granuloma formulation following injection of polytef in experimental animal.

41. McGuire, E. J., Woodside, J. R., & Borden, T. A. (1981). Prognostic value of urodynamic testing in myelodysplastic patients. *Journal of Urology, 126,* 205.

42. Moel, D. I. (1985). Urinalysis investigation of hematuria and renal biopsy. In P. P. Kelalis, L. R. King, & A. B. Belman (Eds.), *Clinical pediatric urology* (pp. 76–92). Philadelphia: Saunders.

43. Monte, J. E., MacGregor, P. S., Fazio, V. M., & Lavery, I. (1986). Continent ileal urinary reservoir (Koch pouch). *Urologic Clinics of North America, 13,* 251–260.

44. Mundy, A. R. (1985). The unstable bladder. *Clinics in Obstetrics and Gynecology, 12,* 15.

45. Narasmiharo, K. L., Prasad, G. R., Mukhopadhyay, B., Katariya, S., Mitra, S. K., & Pathak, I. C. (1983). Vesicoureteral reflux in neonates with anorectal anomalies. *British Journal of Urology, 55,* 268.

46. Nixon, H. H., & Puri, P. (1977). The results of treatment of anorectal anomalies: A thirteen to twenty year follow up. *Journal of Pediatric Surgery, 12,* 27.

47. North American Diagnosis Association. (1990). Taxonomy I: Revised 1990. St. Louis: Author.

48. Pappis, C. H., Moussatos, G. H., Constantinides, C. G., & Karis, M. (1979). Bilateral nephroblastoma in a horseshoe kidney. *Journal of Pediatric Surgery, 14,* 483.

49. Parrott, T. S. (1989). Cystitis and urethritis. *Pediatrics in Review, 10,* 217–222.

50. Parrott, T. S., & Woodard, J. R. (1979). The importance of cystourethrography in neonates with imperforate anus. *Urology, 13,* 607.

51. Perlmutter, A. D. (1985). Enuresis. In P. P. Kelalis, L. R. King,

& A. B. Belman (Eds.), *Clinical pediatric urology*. Philadelphia: Saunders. pp. 311–325.

52. Polk, H. C., Jr. (1965). Notes on Galenic urology. *Urological Survey, 15*, 2.

53. Retik, A. B. (1986). Ectopic ureter and ureterocele. In P. C. Walsh, R. F. Gittes, A. D. Perlmutter, & T. A. Stamey (Eds.), *Campbell's urology* (pp. 2089–2115). Philadelphia: Saunders.

54. Rittig, S., Noorgard, J. P., Pedersen, E. B., & Djurhuus, J. B. (1987, May). *Nocturnal diuresis and urinary osmolality in enuretics*. Presented at the American Urological Association Annual Meeting, Anaheim, California.

55. Santulli, T. V., Keisewetter, W. B., & Bill, A. H., Jr. (1970). Anorectal anomalies: A suggested international classification. *Journal of Pediatric Surgery, 5*, 281.

56. Shaeffer, A. J., & Grayhack, J. T. (1986). Surgical management of ureteropelvic junction obstruction. In P. C. Walsh, R. F. Gittes, A. D. Perlmutter, & T. A. Stamey (Eds.), *Campbell's urology* (pp. 2505–2533). Philadelphia: Saunders.

57. Shapiro, E., Lepor, H., & Jeffs, R. D. (1984). The inheritance of the exstrophy-epispadias complex. *Journal of Urology, 132*, 308.

58. Smithson, W. A., & Benson, R. C., Jr. (1985). Tumors: Lower genitourinary tract. In P. P. Kelalis, L. R. King, & A. B. Belman (Eds.), *Clinical pediatric urology* (pp. 1189–1201). Philadelphia: Saunders.

59. Snow, B. W., & Duckett, J. W. (1991). Prune belly syndrome. In J. Y. Gillenwater, J. T. Grayhack, S. S. Howards, & J. W. Duckett Eds.), *Adult and pediatric urology*. Chicago: Year Book. pp. 1921–1938.

60. Stamey, T. A. (1980). *Pathogenesis and treatment of urinary tract infections*. Baltimore: Williams & Wilkins.

61. Stephens, F. D. (1983). *Congenital malformations of the urinary tract*. New York: Praeger.

62. Strickler, G. B. (1985). Renal parenchymal disease. In P. P. Kelalis, L. R. King, & A. B. Belman (Eds.), *Clinical pediatric urology* (pp. 972–990). Philadelphia: Saunders.

63. Tanagho, E. A. (1981). Anatomy of the genitourinary tract. . In D. R. Smith (Ed.), *General urology*. Los Altos, California: Lange. pp. 311–325.

64. Tefft, M. (1981). Radiation of rhabdomyosarcoma in children: Local control in patients enrolled into the intergroup rhabdomyosarcoma study. *National Cancer Institute Monographs, 56*, 75.

65. Torres, V. E., Malek, R. S., & Svensson, J. P. (1983). Vesicoureteral reflux in the adult: II. Nephropathy, hypertension and stones. *Journal of Urology, 130*, 41–44.

66. Turner, W. R., Ransley, P. G., & Williams, D. I. (1980). Variants of the exstrophic complex. *Urology Clinics of North America, 7*, 493.

67. Turner-Warwick, R. T. (1984). Bladder outflow obstruction in the male. In A. R. Mundy, T. P. Stephenson, & A. J. Wein. Urodynamics: Principles, practice, and application, pp. 183–204.

68. Walker, R. D., III (1987). Vesicoureteral reflux. In J. Y. Gillenwater, J. T. Grayhack, S. S. Howards, & J. W. Duckett (Eds.), *Adult and pediatric urology* (pp. 1676–1706). Chicago: Year Book.

69. Weiss, R. M. (1986). Physiology and pharmacology of the renal pelvis and ureter. In P. C. Walsh, R. F. Gittes, A. D. Perlmutter, & T. A. Stamey (Eds.), *Campbell's urology*. Philadelphia: Saunders.

70. Wettlaufer, J. (1989, May). *Growth patterns following surgical repair of vesicoureteral reflux*. Presented at the American Urological Association Allied, Inc. Annual Assembly, Dallas.

71. Wheatley, J. K. (1983). Causes and treatment of bladder incontinence. *Comprehensive Therapy, 9*, 27.

72. Wigger, H. J., & Blanc, W. A. (1977). The prune belly syndrome. *Pathology Annual, 12*, 17.

73. Winberg, J. (1986). Urinary tract infections in infants and children. In P. C. Walsh, R. F. Gittes, A. D. Perlmutter, & T. A. Stamey (Eds.), *Campbell's urology*. Philadelphia: Saunders. pp. 831–867.

74. Woodard, J. R. (1986). Neonatal and perinatal emergencies. In P. C. Walsh, R. F. Gittes, A. D. Perlmutter, & T. A. Stamey (Eds.), *Campbell's urology*. Philadelphia: Saunders. pp. 2217–2243.

75. Woodard, J. R. (1986). Wilms' tumor. In S. D. Graham (Ed.), *Urologic oncology*. New York: Raven Press. pp. 403–422.

76. Woodard, J. R., & Rushton, G. (1987). Reflux uropathy. *Pediatrics Clinics of North America, 34*(5), 1349–1364.

77. Woodard, J. R., & Trulock, T. S. (1986). Prune belly syndrome. In P. A. Walsh, R. F. Gittes, A. D. Perlmutter, & T. A. Stamey (Eds.), *Campbell's urology* (pp. 2159–2167). Philadelphia: Saunders.

Nursing Care of Children With Altered Neurologic Function

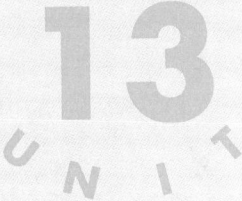

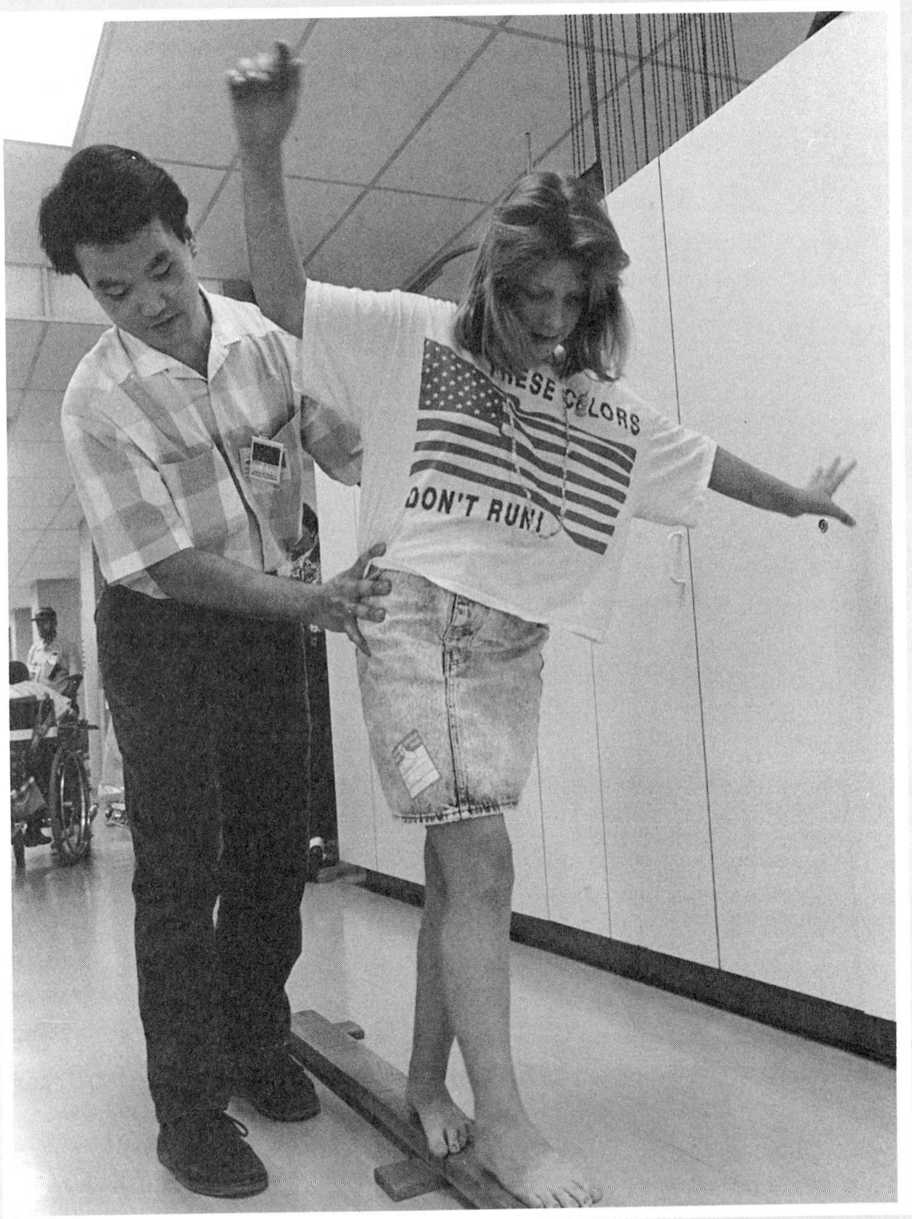

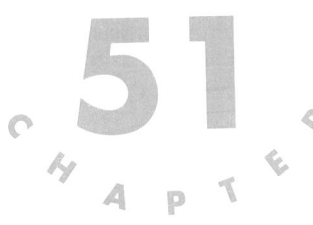

Anatomy and Physiology of the Nervous System

BEHAVIORAL OBJECTIVES

Describe the embryologic development of the nervous system.

Identify the structures and organs that comprise the nervous system.

Identify the physiologic function of the structures and organs that comprise the nervous system.

Describe the normal anatomy and physiology of the neurologic system.

Impulses travel throughout the body through a complex network of nerve pathways. Neurons receive afferent (sensory) impulses from the peripheral nerves or sensory receptors and transmit efferent (motor) impulses to effector organs (muscles and glands). Neuroglia support, protect, and supply nutrients to nerves of the central nervous system.

The basic components of the nervous system are nerve cells (*neurons*) and supporting cells (*neuroglia*). Dendrites carry impulses to nerve cells; each dendrite has a receptor that receives stimuli and initiates sensory impulses. Axons carry impulses from the nerve cells. Axons of the white matter in the brain, spinal cord, and nerve trunks are covered with a myelin sheath; unmyelinated axons are found in the gray matter. Synapses permit the transmission of impulses between axons and dendrites or cell bodies. Neurotransmitters, primarily acetylcholine and norepinephrine, are involved in the transmission of nerve impulses across the synapses.

The nervous system has two major divisions: the central nervous system and the peripheral nervous system. The central nervous system is composed of the brain and spinal cord. The peripheral nervous system has two functional divisions: the somatic nervous system, which regulates bodily responses to the external environment, and the autonomic nervous system, which regulates visceral response to the internal environment.

The central nervous system is protected by the skeletal structures of the skull and vertebrae. It is bathed in cerebrospinal fluid and covered by the meninges. The spinal cord, an extension of the medulla, carries ascending and descending tracts of nerve fibers and is divided into cervical, thoracic, lumbar, and sacral segments.

The peripheral nervous system consists of 31 pairs of spinal nerves and 12 pairs of cranial nerves that are associated with the brainstem. Peripheral nerves carry sensory impulses to or efferent impulses from the central nervous system. Input can be voluntary or involuntary. The somatic division of the peripheral nervous system is composed of two types of fibers. *Afferent* (sensory) fibers carry information, such as temperature, pain, and input from the special senses (vision, hearing, taste, and smell). Somatic *efferent* (motor) fibers regulate voluntary control of skeletal muscles.

The autonomic nervous system controls involuntary functions. It has sympathetic and parasympathetic divisions. In the autonomic nervous system afferent impulses from visceral organs are carried to the brain, while efferent fibers innervate visceral smooth muscles, glands, and cardiac muscle. The sympathetic division prepares the body for the "fight or flight" response. The parasympathetic division maintains homeostasis of body function.

Embryologic Development

The development of the nervous system is complex. Any factor that interrupts this normal process may cause malformations of the central nervous system and conditions incompatible with extrauterine life. Any alteration in normal development of the nervous system or injury to a normally developing system may appear as abnormal development of the infant or child. Not all abnormalities in development manifest themselves immediately at birth. For example recognition of an alteration may be delayed until that part of the nervous system becomes fully functional (e.g., cerebral palsy may not be recognized until the child attempts to walk).

Neural Tube and Crest

The neural tube forms the brain and spinal cord. At approximately 3 weeks' gestation the dorsal ectoderm of the embryo is transformed into specialized neural tissue, the neural plate.[18] This process is called *induction*. This plate invaginates into a neural groove with neuroepithelial cells forming the wall of the groove, the *neural folds* (Fig. 51-1). The walls of the midportion of the neural groove then begin to close progressively (Fig. 51-2) caudally and rostrally. The rostral portion of the neural tube forms the brain, while the caudal portion forms the spinal cord. The tube closes by the 4th week following conception and forms a neural canal.[18] The ventricles of the brain and the spinal cord form from the neural canal.

During the process of neural tube formation some lateral cells separate from the walls of the groove forming the neural crest. Peripheral nervous system structures,

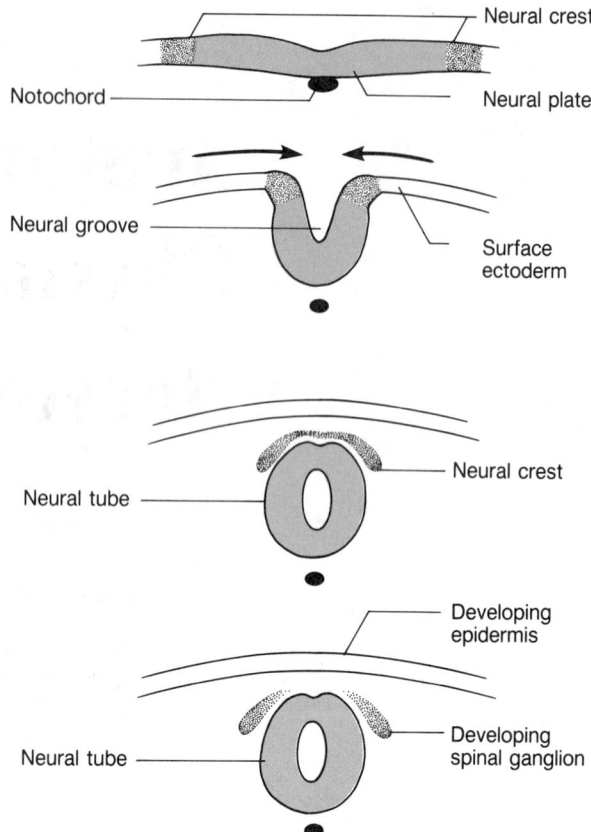

FIGURE 51-1

Formation of the neural tube, groove, and crest. (After Moore, K. L. [1988]. *The developing human: Clinically oriented embryology* [4th ed.]. Philadelphia: W. B. Saunders, reprinted by permission.)

the adrenal medulla, and melanoblasts are formed from the neural crest. Body ectoderm then covers the neural tube and crest.

Major Subdivisions of the Brain

Before the neural tube completely closes, the rostral end forms the forebrain (prosencephalon), the midbrain (mesencephalon), and the hindbrain (rhombencephalon).

The forebrain differentiates into the telencephalon and the diencephalon. Telencephalic vesicles give rise to the cerebral hemispheres and lateral ventricles. The thalamus, hypothalamus, optic nerve and retina, posterior pituitary, pineal body, and third ventricle arise from the diencephalon. The choroid plexus is formed by ependymal cells and vascular mesenchyma on the roof of this and other ventricles in the brain.

The walls of the mesencephalon thicken as nerve fibers connecting higher and lower centers of the nervous system continue to grow. As the central canal narrows and thickens, the aqueduct of Sylvius forms. The midbrain also gives rise to cranial nerve nuclei, the red nucleus, substantia nigra, tectum, and cerebral peduncles.

The hindbrain differentiates into metencephalon and myelencephalon. The cerebellum and pons arise from the metencephalon. The medulla oblongata, the fourth

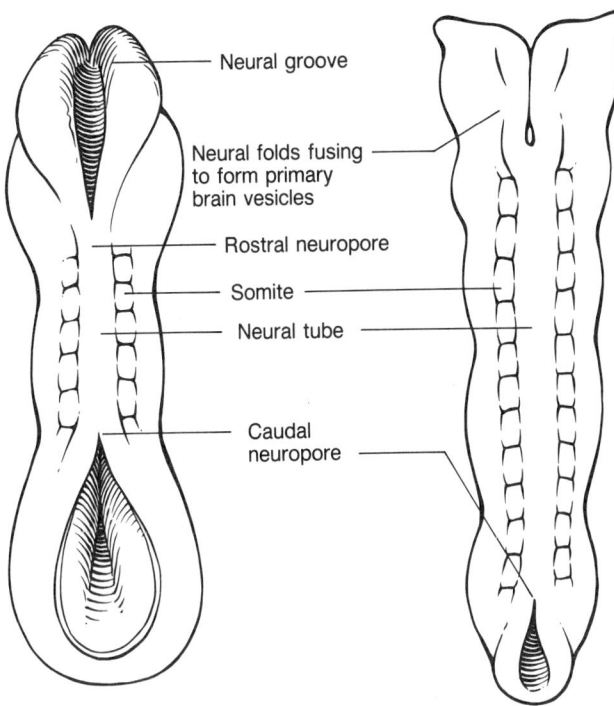

FIGURE 51-2
Closure of the neural tube begins at the central portion and proceeds anteriorly and posteriorly. (After Moore, K. L. [1988]. *The developing human: Clinically oriented embryology* [4th ed.]. Philadelphia: W. B. Saunders, reprinted by permission.)

ventricle, and the choroid plexus form from the myelencephalon.

In the embryo the spinal cord fills the vertebral canal. However, the vertebral column and dura mater grow faster than the spinal cord. Therefore, as the fetus matures the cord no longer extends the entire length of the canal. At approximately 6 months the cord reaches the first sacral vertebra; at 40 weeks' gestation the spinal cord extends to the second or third lumbar vertebra. In an adult the spinal cord extends to the level of the first lumbar vertebra.[18]

Brain and Spinal Nerves

Brain differentiation has occurred and development of cranial nerves has begun by 5 to 6 weeks postconception.[18] At approximately 12 weeks' gestation the gross structures of the brain and spinal cord are complete.[22]

The brain continues to grow and develop after birth, with most brain growth taking place during the first year of life. At birth the brain reaches 25% of its adult weight; by 6 months it reaches 50%; by 1 year it reaches 70%; and by 3 years it is 90% of adult size.[23] The brain grows by hyperplasia during the prenatal period, by hyperplasia and hypertrophy from birth to 6 months, and by hypertrophy until puberty.[4] Genetic, environmental, and nutritional factors are major influences on development of the central nervous system.[4]

Myelination

In the late fetal period formation of myelin sheaths in the spinal cord begins, and most nerve tracts are not fully functioning until myelinization occurs.[18] This process continues throughout childhood and possibly into adulthood.[11] Complete myelinization of fiber tracts is associated with full function of those tracts.

At birth myelinization of the peripheral nervous system, optic pathways, and bulbar structures accounts for crying, sucking, and primitive reflexes in the newborn. Myelinization occurs in a cephalocaudal direction. As a result children are able to sit before standing and stand before walking. This is followed by the ability to control bowel and bladder function. When there is a delay or impairment in myelinization, attainment of developmental milestones at anticipated intervals may be negatively affected.

Reflexes

By the time the fetus reaches 28 weeks the nervous system is able to control some of the body functions, and some weak reflexes are present. This has implications for assessment of gestational age and viability of preterm infants. At 40 weeks' gestation the newborn possesses numerous vital reflexes. Adaptation to extrauterine life depends on reflex function. As the central nervous system matures some of these primitive reflexes disappear, and actions become intentional.

Consequences of Abnormal Development

A number of central nervous system defects are associated with an abnormality in neural tube closure (Table 51-1). A defect in closure with the rostral or cranial end of the neural tube can inhibit development of the brain. When cerebral tissue is missing and remaining brain tissue is exposed due to lack of a cranium, the condition is termed *anencephaly*.

If there is a defect in the spinal column, the meninges or meninges and spinal cord may protrude through the vertebral opening exposing neural tissue. This condition is called *spina bifida occulta, meningocele,* or *myelomeningocele* depending on the severity of involvement.

Hydrocephalus is caused by an abnormal accumulation of cerebrospinal fluid. The normal structure and function of the cerebrospinal fluid pathway can be affected by the following:

- An obstruction of flow in the ventricles, often in the aqueducts,

TABLE 51-1
Consequences of Abnormal Embryonic Development

Fetal Age in Weeks	Structure Formed	Anomalies at Birth
4	Closure of caudal neuropore	Spina bifida, meningocele, meningomyelocele
	Closure of rostral neuropore	Cranial meningocele, anencephaly

- An obstruction or impaired absorption of cerebrospinal fluid outside the ventricular system, or
- Excessive production of cerebrospinal fluid due to a tumor of villi similar to the choroid plexuses.

Arnold-Chiari malformation is a congenital herniation of the cerebellum and medulla through the foramen magnum into the vertebral column. This herniation causes an obstruction in the flow of cerebrospinal fluid through the fourth ventricle.

Microcephalus occurs when the brain is small and underdeveloped. In this condition the forebrain is most affected. Due to genetic or environmental causes the cranium remains small and the head circumference falls below average because the growth of the cranium is partially caused by the pressure of the growing brain.

Structure and Function

Central Nervous System

Brain

The brain is a mass of gray and white nerve tissue comprising the two hemispheres of the cerebrum, the cerebellum, and the brainstem (Fig. 51-3). It is encased by the cranium and protected by the meninges. Brain growth is related to cranial growth, although deviations in head circumference may be caused by a growth disorder not involving the brain.

At birth the bones of the skull are not completely ossified. Two midline fontanels also are present. The diamond-shaped, anterior fontanel at the juncture of the frontal and coronal sutures remains open until 12 to 18 months of age. The triangular, posterior fontanel at the juncture of the lambdoidal and sagittal sutures closes by

2 months of age. These flexible suture lines allow the brain room to grow. Head circumference should be plotted on a graph to determine whether growth is proceeding as anticipated (see the head circumference chart in Chap. 9).

Cerebral Hemispheres. The two cerebral hemispheres serve as the "control center" for the nervous system. They are composed of convoluted gray matter positioned above a core that contains primarily white matter, as well as basal nuclei (gray matter) and the lateral ventricles. The left and right hemispheres are connected by the corpus callosum, a band of fibers that permits the transmission of impulses from the lobes of one hemisphere to corresponding sections of the opposite hemisphere. A deep, longitudinal fissure partially separates the two hemispheres above the level of the corpus callosum.

The cerebral cortex, the outer layer of the cerebral hemispheres, receives, processes, analyzes, and integrates impulses and stores information in the form of memory. The cerebral cortex integrates mental processes and controls body function, movement, and behavior.

The convoluted surface of the cerebral cortex has fissures, gyri (elevated portions), and sulci (depressions) that increase the surface area of the brain. The central sulcus separates the frontal and parietal lobes of each hemisphere, and the lateral sulcus separates the frontal and parietal lobes from the temporal lobe.

The inner core of white matter forms tracts or commissures that permit the interaction between the cortical areas and other parts of the nervous system. The white matter contains three types of myelinated fibers with specialized function:

- Projection, afferent, and efferent fibers carry impulses between the cortex and distant areas of the central nervous system.
- Short- and long-association fibers carry impulses within each individual hemisphere.
- Commissural fibers carry impulses between the two hemispheres.

The basal ganglia, two collections of gray matter, are positioned in the central portion of each hemisphere. Each basal ganglion is formed by a caudate nucleus, the putamen, the globus pallidus, and the amygdaloid nuclear complex. The basal ganglia receive input from the cerebral cortex by means of the projection fibers, the primary motor area, and sensory areas. Efferent (output) fibers from the globus pallidus go to the thalamus and are relayed to other parts of the central nervous system.

The basal ganglia control and integrate motor activities in conjunction with the cerebral cortex and cerebellum. These structures and the reticular formation form the extrapyramidal motor system. The extrapyramidal system regulates patterns of automatic movements, muscle tone, and posture needed for locomotion, whereas the pyramidal tracts (corticospinal tracts) regulate both voluntary and motor activities. Pyramidal tracts are formed by fibers that pass from the primary motor area of the cerebral cortex through the medulla where they decussate (cross over) and descend to the spinal cord.

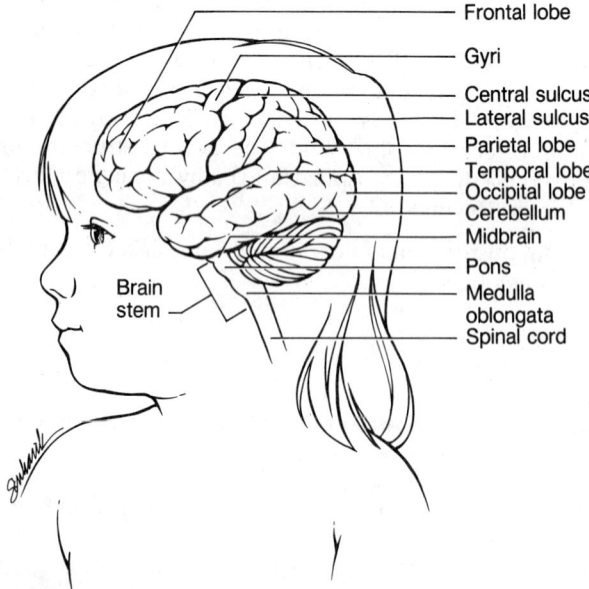

Frontal lobe
Gyri
Central sulcus
Lateral sulcus
Parietal lobe
Temporal lobe
Occipital lobe
Cerebellum
Midbrain
Pons
Medulla oblongata
Spinal cord

Brain stem

FIGURE 51-3

External surface of the brain showing major lobes of the cerebrum, the cerebellum, and divisions of the brainstem.

Lobes. Each cerebral hemisphere is divided into four major anatomical lobes: frontal, temporal, parietal, and occipital (see Fig. 51-3). These lobes are named for the cranial bones that encase them.

The frontal lobe includes two major areas, the primary motor area and Broca's speech area. The primary motor area regulates body movements. Impulses transmitted through fibers from the right hemisphere govern the left side of the body and vice versa. Broca's speech area in the left frontal lobe is the portion related to the motor aspects of speech formation. The left hemisphere usually is dominant and controls language, math, and analytic function in right-handed individuals, but the converse is not always true. The left hemisphere usually is considered dominant for speech regardless of hand dominance.[5]

The parietal lobe is the primary somatesthetic (sensory) area. Each lobe receives and interprets tactile and kinesthetic sensory impulses from the opposite side of the body. Differences in distances, sizes, and shapes of objects and the intensity of the stimuli in contact with the skin are identified. Sensory impulses from the right side of the body are received by the left somatesthetic area; afferent impulses from the left side of the body are received by the right somatesthetic area.

The temporal lobes contain the primary auditory centers, which permit understanding of language. The occipital lobes contain the primary visual cortex. The visual cortex in each hemisphere is associated with perception from the opposite half of the visual field.

Each hemisphere of the brain also contains the insula and part of the limbic lobe. Little is known about the insula, which lies deep in the lateral sulcus. The limbic lobe surrounds the brainstem, is composed of parts of each of the four major lobes, and is associated with expression of emotions and the effects of emotion on autonomic function.

Brainstem. The brainstem, composed of the medulla oblongata, pons, and midbrain, connects the higher brain centers with the cerebrospinal cord (see Fig. 51-3). Ascending and descending tracts pass through the brainstem, which serves as a relay and reflex center. Each section of the brainstem is associated with specific cranial nerves.

The medulla is located just above the foramen magnum and serves as a connection between the brainstem and the spinal cord. Ascending sensory tracts carry pressure and vibratory sensations, two-point tactile discrimination, and conscious muscle proprioception. Descending motor fibers from the motor cortex of the cerebral hemisphere pass through the pyramids on the anterior surface of the medulla and cross over (decussate) to the other side of the brainstem. As a result the right hemisphere controls the left side of the body, while the upper part of the cortex controls muscles found in the lower portion of the body.

The glossopharyngeal (IX), vagus (X), accessory (XI), and hypoglossal (XII) nerves arise from this area (Table 51-2). The medulla contains cardiac, vasomotor, respiratory, coughing, sneezing, swallowing, salivary, and vomiting reflex centers.

The pons connects the midbrain with the medulla and links the cerebellum with other structures of the nervous system. Through cerebellar peduncles on each side

TABLE 51-2
Cranial Nerves: Origin and Function

Cranial Nerve	Composition	Origin	Function
Olfactory (I)	Sensory	Nasal mucosa	Smell
Optic (II)	Sensory	Retina	Vision
Oculomotor (III)	Motor	Midbrain	Eye movement, pupil constriction
Trochlear (IV)	Motor	Midbrain	Eye movement (down, in)
Trigeminal (V)	Motor	Pons	Jaw movement
	Sensory	Face/head	Skin (face, anterior scalp), mucosa (eyes, nose, mouth), tongue/teeth
Abducens (VI)	Motor	Pons	Eye movement (lateral)
Facial (VII)	Motor	Pons	Facial movement, tears, salivation
	Sensory	Tongue	Taste (anterior two thirds of tongue—sweet, sour, salt)
Vestibulocochlear (VIII)	Sensory	Pons, vestibular branch, cochlear branch	Balance, hearing
Glossopharyngeal (IX)	Motor	Medulla	Swallow/gag reflex, abdominal viscera
	Sensory	Tongue/pharynx	Taste (posterior tongue—bitter)
Vagus (X)	Motor	Medulla	Swallow/gag reflex, abdominal viscera
	Sensory	Viscera	Thoracic/abdominal viscera
Accessory (XI)	Motor	Medulla	Head movement, shoulder movement
Hypoglossal (XII)	Motor	Medulla	Tongue

of the pons, descending fibers leave the cerebral hemisphere, decussate, and enter the opposite cerebellum. Cranial nerves associated with this area include the trigeminal (V), abducens (VI), facial (VII), and vestibulocochlear (VIII).

The midbrain is the upper portion of the brainstem and contains the substantia nigra and the red nucleus. The substantia nigra is a nuclear mass containing dopamine and additional neurotransmitters. The red nucleus plays a part in postural and righting reflexes. The oculomotor nerves (III) and trochlear nerves (IV) arise from this area.

The reticular formation is composed of gray matter within the brainstem, contains motor and sensory nerves, and receives impulses from somatic and visceral systems. The reticular activating system alerts or arouses and coordinates reflexes and voluntary movement.

Diencephalon. The diencephalon is a mass of gray matter located between the midbrain and the cerebral hemispheres. It contains the epithalamus, including the pineal gland, one pair of thalami, usually referred to as the thalamus, connected by an intermediate mass, and the hypothalamus.

The thalamus routes and relays sensory impulses (vision, hearing, taste, touch) to specific areas of the cerebral cortex. It also aids in interpretation of sensations such as pain, pressure, and temperature. The nuclei of the thalamus are involved in maintaining wakefulness, regulating autonomic responses, and integrating motor functions.

The hypothalamus is located below the thalamus and controls the sympathetic and parasympathetic divisions of the autonomic nervous system. This organ performs the following functions:

- Regulates temperature
- Maintains water balance
- Controls activities of the endocrine system
- Controls appetite
- Plays a part in sleep and wake states
- Influences emotional expression and sexual behavior.

Cerebellum. The cerebellum is located in the posterior cranial cavity behind the medulla and pons and below the posterior portion of the cerebral hemispheres (see Fig. 51-3). The cerebellum integrates and coordinates voluntary muscle activity and maintains balance, muscle tone, and equilibrium. It is covered by the tentorium, which separates it from the posterior aspect of the cerebrum. The cerebellum is composed of three parts—an outer cortex of gray matter, an inner body of white matter, and four pairs of nuclei.

The cerebellum is connected to the brainstem by three pairs of peduncles (fibrous bands). Through these peduncles, afferent and efferent impulses are transmitted between peripheral and cortical areas and the cerebellum.

Ventricles. The four ventricles of the brain are cavities connected by channels called *foramina.* The ventricles, which contain cerebrospinal fluid, serve a protective function for the brain and spinal cord (Fig. 51-4). These ventricles are lined with ependyma and contain the choroid plexuses, which are vascular extensions of the pia mater, the innermost meningeal layer. Most of

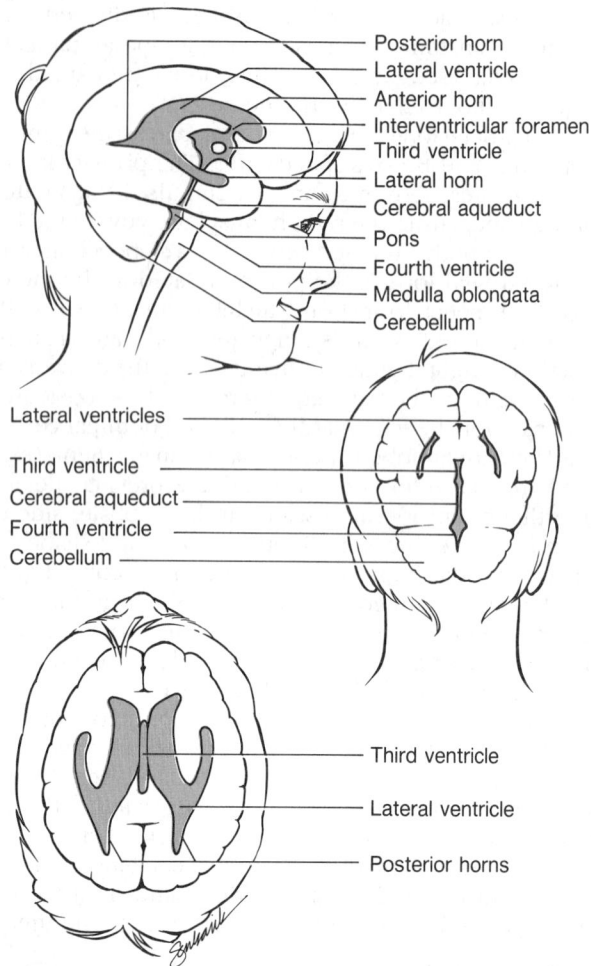

FIGURE 51-4
Ventricles of the brain: lateral view (**top**), posterior view (**middle**), and superior view (**bottom**).

the cerebrospinal fluid is continually secreted by the choroid plexuses found in all the ventricles.

Each cerebral hemisphere has one lateral ventricle (the right and left make up the first and second ventricles). Cerebrospinal fluid flows from the lateral ventricles, by way of the paired foramen of Monro, to the third ventricle in the diencephalon; through the aqueduct of Sylvius to the fourth ventricle in the medulla; through the foramen of Luschka and foramen of Magendie to the cisterna magna; to the subarachnoid spaces of the brain and spinal cord (see Fig. 51-4).

Hydrostatic pressure and motion of the choroid plexuses move the fluid downward through the ventricles to the subarachnoid spaces of the brain and spinal cord. The fluid is then absorbed by the arachnoid villi and enters the venous circulation.

Spinal Cord

The spinal cord is a cylindrical structure lying within the vertebral canal (Fig. 51-5). In older infants and adults, the spinal cord extends from the medulla to approximately the first or second lumbar vertebra. The 31 pairs of spinal nerves originate in the spinal cord. (See Peripheral Nervous System in this chapter.)

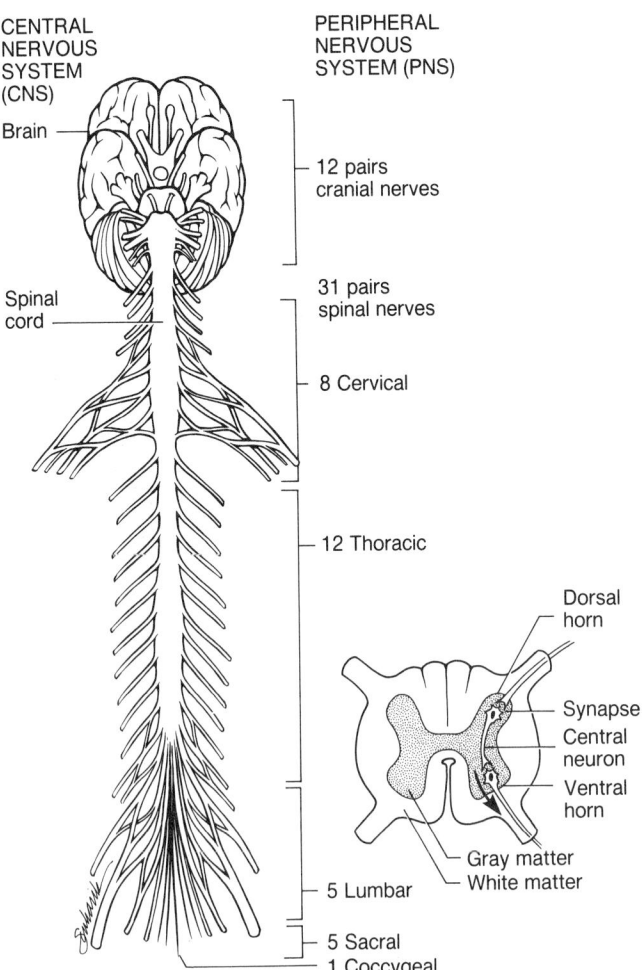

CENTRAL
NERVOUS
SYSTEM
(CNS)

Brain

Spinal
cord

PERIPHERAL
NERVOUS
SYSTEM (PNS)

12 pairs
cranial nerves

31 pairs
spinal nerves

8 Cervical

12 Thoracic

Dorsal
horn

Synapse
Central
neuron
Ventral
horn

Gray matter
White matter

5 Lumbar

5 Sacral
1 Coccygeal

FIGURE 51-5

The spinal cord and vertebral column showing location of spinal nerves and vertebrae. Enlarged vertebrae showing gray and white matter and horns. (After Memmler, R. L., Cohen, B. J., & Wood, D. L. [1992]. *Structure and function of the human body* [5th ed.]. Philadelphia: J. B. Lippincott, reprinted by permission.)

The spinal cord is divided into segments containing ascending, descending, or associative bundles of fibers called tracts. Ascending tracts in the white matter allow sensory impulses to reach the brain, and descending tracts allow motor impulses to exit the brain to the spinal nerves. The spinal cord has two enlarged areas: the cervical enlargement contains the spinal nerves supplying the upper extremities and the lumbar enlargement contains nerves supplying the lower extremities.

The cord is composed of an internal H-shaped core of gray (unmyelinated) matter surrounded by white (myelinated) matter (see Fig. 51-5). The gray matter, composed of nerve cell bodies and fibers reaching into the white matter, contains internuncial neurons that transmit impulses between neurons contained in the brain and spinal cord. These neurons integrate spinal cord reflexes and motor movements.

The reflex arc, in simple form, is composed of a sensory neuron and a motor neuron connected by one or more internuncial neurons. A peripheral receptor receives a stimulus. The sensory neuron generates an impulse that travels from the neuron to the central nervous system and onward to the effector organ. This mechanism permits a reflex response to occur that is independent of the higher brain centers. Reflexes are associated with one or more segmental levels of the spinal cord and may be described as superficial, deep, or visceral. Superficial reflexes, also called cutaneous reflexes, occur when the skin surface is stimulated. Deep reflexes occur in response to stimulation of muscles and tendons, such as the knee-jerk reflex. Visceral reflexes occur when visceral nerves are stimulated. Reflexes also may be described as normal and abnormal or pathologic.

The gray matter of the spinal cord is divided into two anterior or ventral horns and two posterior or dorsal horns. The transverse gray commissure connects the left and right portions. The anterior horns contain anterior motor neurons through which impulses travel from the cord to the skeletal muscles to permit movement. Sensory fibers arise from the dorsal horn.

The white matter is divided into the left and right posterior funiculi, positioned between the dorsal horns. Two anterior funiculi are located between the two ventral horns. A lateral funiculus is found on the sides of the gray matter.

Cerebrospinal Fluid. The cerebrospinal fluid that surrounds the brain and spinal cord is a clear, colorless fluid secreted by the choroid plexuses. It contains protein, glucose, electrolytes, oxygen, and carbon dioxide. The cerebrospinal fluid normally contains no or few cells. Substances found in the cerebrospinal fluid usually are equal to or less than the concentration of the same substances found in blood plasma.

Cerebrospinal fluid cushions the central nervous system from injury, regulates intracranial pressure, carries nutrients to the cells, and removes waste products. The normal spinal fluid pressure is a function of the rate of fluid production and reabsorption. An abnormally high production, obstructed flow, or decreased absorption of cerebrospinal fluid increases intracranial pressure.

Meninges. The brain and spinal cord are completely covered and protected by three membranes: the dura mater, arachnoid membrane, and pia mater (Fig. 51-6). The meninges cover and protect the brain and spinal cord.

The dura mater is the tough, outermost membrane formed by dense connective tissue. The dura mater extends from the foramen magnum to the level of the second sacral vertebra where it terminates as a fibrous cord—the coccygeal ligament. The dura has two layers: the periosteal layer, which adheres to the inner surface of the cranium and is rich in blood vessels and nerves, and the inner meningeal layer. Occasionally, these layers separate and form large venous sinuses that permit drainage of cerebrospinal fluid and cerebral blood. The dura extends into and forms partitions in the brain. These extensions are called the falx cerebri, which separate the cerebral hemispheres; the falx cerebelli, which divide the cerebellar hemispheres; and the tentorium cerebelli, which separate the cerebellum from the occipital lobe of the cerebrum.

The subdural space lies between the dura and the arachnoid. This space contains tiny blood vessels and a

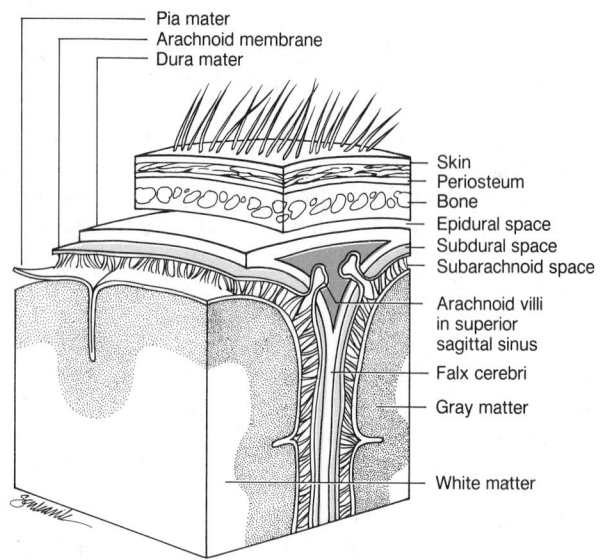

FIGURE 51-6
The meningeal layers of the brain.

The entire spinal cord receives its blood supply from one anterior spinal artery and one pair of posterior spinal arteries and their branches. Both the anterior and posterior spinal arteries are branches of the vertebral artery. The venous system of the brain and spinal cord is continuous.

Blood–Brain Barrier. The blood–brain barrier is an anatomic and physiologic mechanism that separates the parenchyma of the brain and the cerebrospinal fluid from direct contact with arterial blood. The cerebral endothelial cells of capillaries, joined by tight junctions, and neuroglial cells slow or prohibit the movement of certain substances that could pass through capillary walls located in other parts of the body.[12] This mechanism controls the transport of various chemicals, disease-producing organisms, and other substances and protects the brain from harm.

The Peripheral Nervous System

The peripheral nervous system is composed of 12 pairs of cranial nerves and 31 pairs of spinal nerves. Roman numerals are used to identify each of the cranial nerves, most of which emerge from the brainstem (see Table 51-2). Each of the spinal nerves is named for the segment of the spinal cord from which it emerges. There are 8 cervical (C), 12 thoracic (T), 5 lumbar (L), 5 sacral (S), and 1 coccygeal spinal nerves.

The dorsal (posterior) sensory root and ventral (anterior) motor root are the sites for attachment of the spinal nerves to the cord. All spinal nerves contain a combination of dorsal and ventral roots. These roots unite, leaving the spinal column through the intervertebral foramina as a single spinal nerve. This single spinal nerve trunk and the autonomic fibers become a peripheral nerve containing visceral and somatic fibers.

Some peripheral nerves contain only sensory fibers and some only motor fibers. However, the majority of peripheral nerves are mixed, containing sensory and motor fibers. When visceral organs and skin surface follow a single spinal nerve pathway, injury to an internal organ can cause referred pain in another part of the body.

After each spinal nerve leaves the cord it separates into anterior (ventral) or posterior (dorsal) branches. Ventral rami innervate the muscles and skin of the front and sides of the body, including the extremities (Fig. 51-7). The dorsal rami innervate the muscles of the back and segments of the skin overlying them. These individual areas of skin are called *dermatomes*. While each nerve innervates a specific corresponding dermatome, there is some overlap of neighboring spinal nerves innervating these dermatomes.

Underlying muscle areas served by these motor roots are called *myotomes*. Divisions of the ventral rami include the cervical, brachial, and lumbosacral plexuses. These plexuses, networks of spinal nerves and blood vessels, are the source of major peripheral nerves to the extremities.

The microscopic peripheral sensory receptors may be classified as general sense receptors or special sense receptors. General sense receptors, found in the skin and

small amount of cerebrospinal fluid that prevent the membranes from adhering to one another. The arachnoid membrane, a thin, delicate, avascular membrane, encases the subarachnoid space. The subarachnoid space between the arachnoid and the pia mater also contains cerebrospinal fluid.

Cisterns are cavities in the subarachnoid space formed by separations of the pia and arachnoid membranes. Into the largest of these, the cisterna magna, the foramina of the fourth ventricle open. The lumbar cistern, the site for a spinal tap, is located at L4.

The pia mater is a delicate, vascular membrane that adheres to the spinal cord and the surface contours of the brain, following its folds (gyri) and furrows (sulci). The pia mater is composed of two layers: the intima pia, the innermost membrane, and the epipial layer, which carries blood vessels to the spinal cord.

Associated Structures and Functions

Vascular Supply to the Brain and Spinal Cord. The common carotid artery divides into the internal and external carotid arteries. The internal carotid or its branches, such as the anterior cerebral artery and middle cerebral artery, supply the cortex, dura, and deep structures of the brain. The left and right subclavian arteries form one pair of vertebral arteries. These vessels enter the skull through the foramen magnum, unite as the basilar artery, and branch into the posterior cerebral arteries. The vertebral arteries and branches supply blood to the posterior part of the brain.

The circle of Willis, at the base of the brain, is formed by the juncture of the internal carotid, anterior and posterior communicating arteries, and anterior and posterior cerebral arteries. The circle of Willis provides a mechanism for the interchange of blood between the arterial systems (internal carotid and basilar arteries).

The dural sinuses permit the venous blood to leave the brain. These sinuses empty into the internal jugular vein and reenter the general circulation.

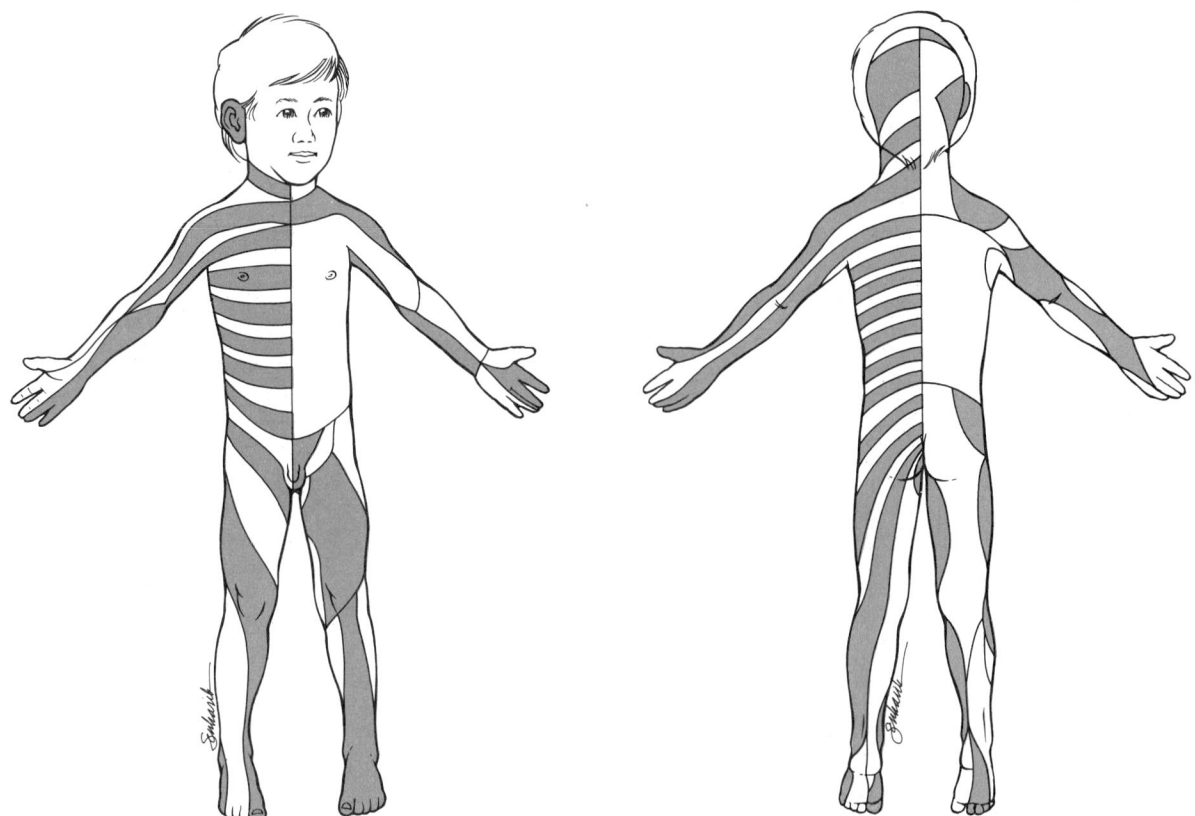

FIGURE 51-7
Innervation of dermatomes: anterior and posterior. (Evans, O. B. [1987]. *Manual of child neurology*. New York: Churchill Livingstone, reprinted by permission.)

body wall, permit the recognition of temperature, touch, pain, and location and position of the body parts. Spinal nerves carry general sense impulses to the spinal cord. Special sense impulses, such as vision, hearing, taste, and smell, are carried to the brain by the associated cranial nerves.

Sensory receptors are termed exteroceptors, proprioceptors, and interoceptors. *Exteroceptors*, located in the skin, permit recognition of pain, pressure, temperature, and touch. *Proprioceptors*, located in the body wall, permit recognition of location and position of body parts. *Interoceptors*, located in the visceral organs, receive sensory information related to visceral activities and are part of the autonomic nervous system.

Information is carried to and from the central nervous system by the peripheral nerves. The dorsal root fibers carry afferent impulses from the peripheral nerves into the cord through the spinal pathways. The ventral root carries efferent impulses to the periphery. The afferent component of the cranial nerves relays sensory input (vision, taste, smell, hearing) to the brain, while the efferent component of cranial nerves controls movements of the face, eyes, tongue, and neck (see Table 51-2).[6,9,10,20,21]

Autonomic Nervous System

The autonomic nervous system (ANS) is an involuntary system that controls the activities of the visceral organs and regulates respiratory, digestive, circulatory, excretory, and sexual functions (Fig. 51-8). ANS has both afferent and efferent fibers. While the autonomic nervous system and somatic pathways use the same peripheral nerve pathways, the efferent pathways of these systems are unique.

In the autonomic nervous system the motor pathways involve two neurons and a synapse. These neurons are referred to as preganglionic or postganglionic motor neurons. The preganglionic motor neuron extends from the central nervous system to a ganglion and synapse. The postganglionic fiber extends from the ganglion and synapse to the effector organ. This distinguishes the autonomic system from the voluntary nervous system, which has no synapses. Rather, in the peripheral nervous system after exiting the central nervous system, somatic motor neurons extend axons from the gray matter of the spinal cord directly to the effector organs. No synapses are involved.

The brainstem, hypothalamus, and spinal cord receive sensory impulses and transmit reflex responses to visceral effectors (smooth muscles, cardiac muscle, and glands). Sensory information is transmitted by way of the cranial nerves in the brainstem so reflex activities can occur or by peripheral nerves to the spinal cord and higher brain centers. Afferent impulses from nerves in the internal organs do not reach the higher brain centers. For this reason sensation from the viscera often is vague and difficult to localize.

Sympathetic and Parasympathetic Divisions. The

autonomic nervous system is divided into the sympathetic (thoracolumbar division) and parasympathetic (cranio-

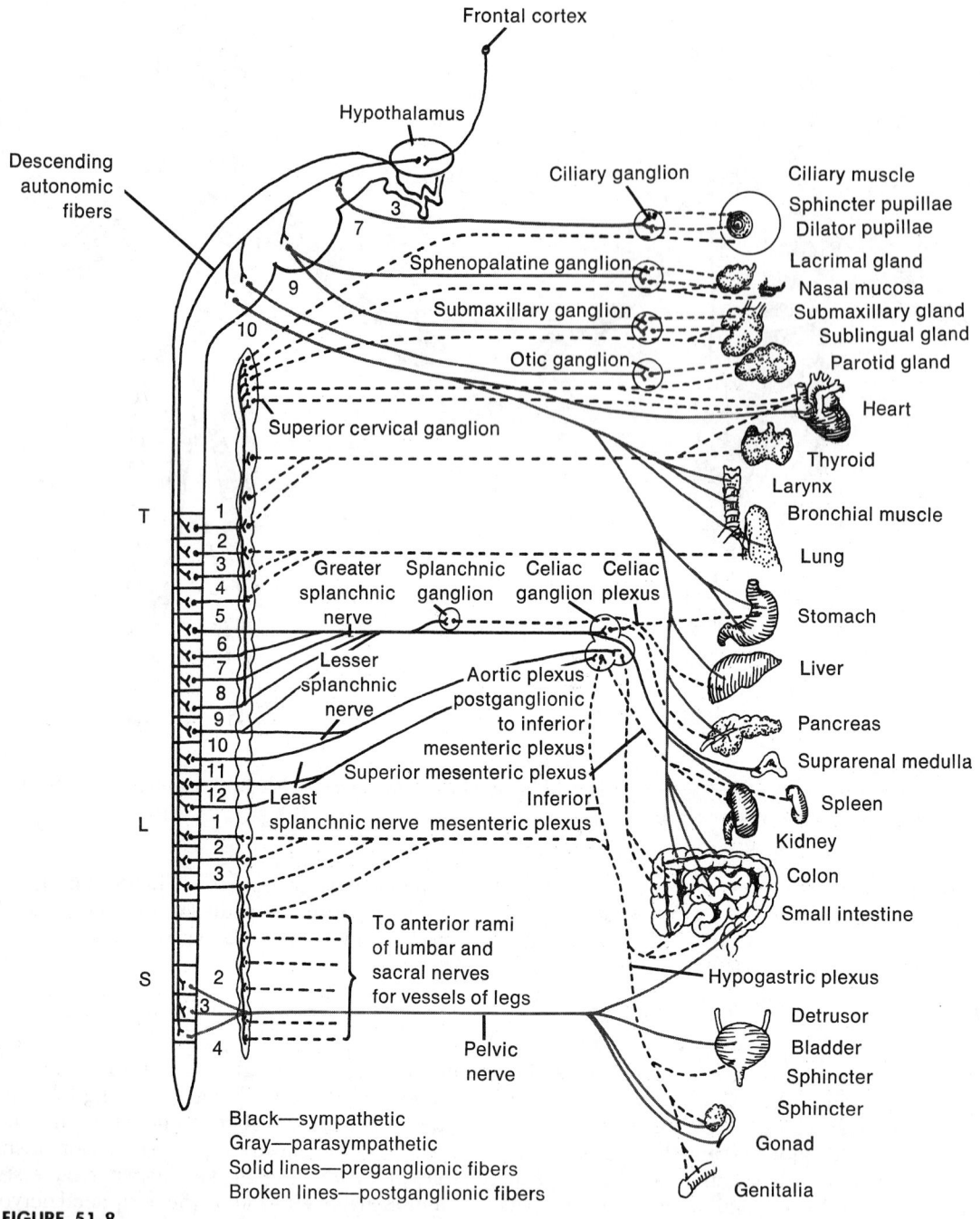

Frontal cortex

Hypothalamus

Descending autonomic fibers

Ciliary ganglion — Ciliary muscle
Sphincter pupillae
Dilator pupillae

Sphenopalatine ganglion — Lacrimal gland
Nasal mucosa

Submaxillary ganglion — Submaxillary gland
Sublingual gland

Otic ganglion — Parotid gland

Superior cervical ganglion — Heart

Thyroid
Larynx
Bronchial muscle
Lung

Greater splanchnic nerve Splanchnic ganglion Celiac ganglion Celiac plexus — Stomach

Liver

Lesser splanchnic nerve

Aortic plexus postganglionic to inferior mesenteric plexus — Pancreas

Superior mesenteric plexus — Suprarenal medulla

Least splanchnic nerve — Spleen

Inferior mesenteric plexus — Kidney

Colon
Small intestine

To anterior rami of lumbar and sacral nerves for vessels of legs

Hypogastric plexus

Pelvic nerve

Detrusor
Bladder
Sphincter
Sphincter

Gonad

Genitalia

Black—sympathetic
Gray—parasympathetic
Solid lines—preganglionic fibers
Broken lines—postganglionic fibers

FIGURE 51-8

Parasympathetic fibers of the autonomic nervous system are shown in black. Sympathetic fibers are shown in color.

sacral division) components. In the sympathetic division two cord-like chains of paravertebral ganglia, extending from the level of the base of the skull to the coccyx on either side of the spinal cord, form sympathetic trunks. Preganglionic fibers of the sympathetic division follow the path of a thoracic or lumbar spinal nerve to the sympathetic trunk. The sympathetic nerve trunk and common spinal nerve trunk are united by the gray and white components of the rami. The white ramus innervates blood vessels, sweat glands, and muscles of hair follicles, and the gray ramus innervates the viscera.

Lateral ganglia in the sympathetic trunk contain sympathetic neurons that release norepinephrine and send

fibers to the viscera. The sympathetic division sends fibers to glands and involuntary muscle. The sympathetic trunks also contain unmyelinated preganglionic fibers, primarily unmyelinated postganglionic fibers, and both myelinated and unmyelinated afferent fibers. Branches of postganglionic fibers reach the autonomic plexuses, cranial and spinal nerves, and organs.

The parasympathetic division includes some sacral and cranial nerve fibers, such as the motor fibers of the vagus nerve. Parasympathetic preganglionic fibers originate in the brain, hypothalamus, and spinal cord and leave the craniosacral areas of the cord following the route of a visceral nerve. They synapse with autonomic ganglia in or near the walls of effector organs. Autonomic nerve endings release neurotransmitters. The type of neurotransmitter released, acetylcholine or norepinephrine, depends on whether the neuron is sympathetic or parasympathetic; each produces a specific effect on the visceral organs. The effects of secretion of acetylcholine are called cholinergic or parasympathetic. Effects of norepinephrine are called adrenergic or sympathetic.

Most body organs receive stimuli from both the sympathetic and parasympathetic nervous systems, as shown in Table 51-3. The sympathetic component stimulates the organs and prepares the body for stressful physical and emotional situations, initiating the fight or flight response. The sympathetic division also inhibits organs, such as those in the urinary and digestive systems, that are not involved in the response to stress. The parasympathetic nervous system inhibits visceral organ activities and restores equilibrium after a stress response.

Special Senses

Special sense organs include receptors for vision, hearing, taste, and smell. These are distinguished from the general senses of pain, pressure, touch, temperature, and position.

The external structures of the eye—the cornea, aqueous humor, lens, and vitreous body—receive light waves. These waves are refracted, received by receptors in the retina, and transmitted to the occipital lobe cortex where they are interpreted. The optic nerve (II) carries

visual impulses from rods and cones in the retina, while the ophthalmic branch of the trigeminal nerve (V) transmits somatesthetic impulses from the eye to the brain. Extrinsic muscles move the eyeballs. Intrinsic muscles are responsible for control of pupil size and shape of the lens. Oculomotor (III), trochlear (IV), and abducens (VI) nerves regulate muscles that move the eyeballs. The pupils of the newborn respond to light. Because newborns are hyperopic, they see best about 8 to 12 inches from the face. As early as 2 to 3 years of age visual acuity may reach 20/20 to 20/30.[2]

The ear has a role in hearing and equilibrium. Sound waves pass through the external ear to the tympanic membranes. Vibrations of the membrane, carried by the malleus, incus, and stapes in the middle ear, are transmitted to the perilymph and endolymph fluid in the inner ear. Movement of the endolymph causes receptors to transmit impulses to the temporal lobe of the cortex. The vestibulocochlear nerves (VIII) are involved in the transmission of these impulses. The vestibule and three semicircular canals of the middle ear have receptors for equilibrium. Infants are especially responsive to the human voice. Hearing acuity affects the child's ability to imitate and learn sounds and thus influences the development of language.

Receptors for salty, sweet, sour, and bitter sensations are located in the taste buds of the tongue. The facial (VII) and glossopharyngeal (IX) nerves transmit these sensations to the brain. The sense of taste is present at birth. The acuity of this sense is affected when the sense of smell is impaired, as with a cold.

Receptors for smell are found in the mucosal lining the upper portion of the nasal cavity. Sense impulses are carried to the olfactory centers of the brain through the olfactory nerve (I). The sense of smell is present at birth. For example, newborns are able to sense the odor of breast milk. Odors are recognized quickly, but when odors persist the olfactory receptors rapidly adapt and become desensitized to that odor.

System Physiology

The brain is the center of consciousness, thought, personality, creativity, memory, reason, judgment, and emotion. Different parts of the brain regulate and coordinate body processes and functions. An intact central nervous system is required for normal growth, development, and function.

The spinal cord serves as a connection between the peripheral nerves of the body and the brain. The major functions of the cord include transmission of sensory impulses to the brain through the ascending tracts, transmission of motor impulses from the brain to the nerves that supply muscles or glands through the descending tracts, and regulation of reflex activities.

The sensory organs, vision, hearing, taste, and smell, are regulated by the cranial nerves. The way in which an infant perceives the world and responds to the world is governed by and through the interactive processes of the neurologic system. The importance of understanding the relationships between the ability to perceive stimuli and respond appropriately is learned. The neonate is born

TABLE 51-3
Effects of the Sympathetic and Parasympathetic Systems on Selected Organs

Effector	Sympathetic System	Parasympathetic System
Pupils of eye	Dilation	Constriction
Sweat glands	Stimulation	None
Digestive glands	Inhibition	Stimulation
Heart	Increased rate and strength of beat	Decreased rate and strength of beat
Bronchi of lungs	Dilation	Constriction
Muscles of digestive system	Decreased contraction (peristalsis)	Increased contraction
Kidneys	Decreased activity	None
Urinary bladder	Relaxation	Contraction and emptying
Liver	Increased release of glucose	None
Penis	Ejaculation	Erection
Adrenal medulla	Stimulation	None
Blood vessels to		
Skeletal muscles	Dilation	Constriction
Skin	Constriction	None
Respiratory system	Dilation	Constriction
Digestive organs	Constriction	Dilation

(Memmler, R. L., Cohen, B. J., & Wood, D. L. [1992]. *Structure and function of the human body* [5th ed.]. Philadelphia: J. B. Lippincott.)

with certain reflexes to assist in the adjustment to extra-uterine life. These reflexes ultimately are replaced with other reflexes as the infant grows and develops. Interruptions in the development of the brain and spinal column have significant implications for the infant.

Summary

The nervous system regulates voluntary and involuntary responses and permits the body to adjust to the internal and external environment. The system is highly integrated. No one component functions independently of other components. The next two chapters further develop the assessment of the nervous system. It is important to understand the underlying anatomy of the nervous system and the relationship of the transmission of stimuli from the internal and external environment to relate alterations of this system to observed changes in infants and children.

References

1. Beck, F., Moffat, D. B. & Davies, D. P. (1985). *Human embryology* (2nd ed.). Boston: Blackwell Scientific Publications.
2. Behrman, R. E., Kliegman, R. M., Nelson, W. E. & Vaughan, V. C. (1992). *Nelson textbook of pediatrics* (14th ed.). Philadelphia: W.B. Saunders.
3. Bellack, J. P., & Bamford, P. A. (1984). *Nursing assessment: A multidimensional approach.* Monterey, CA: Wadsworth Health Sciences Division.
4. Bobak, I. M., & Jensen, M. D. (1987). *Essentials of maternity nursing: The nurse and the childbearing family.* St. Louis: C.V. Mosby.
5. Carpenter, M. B., & Sutin, J. (1983). *Human neuroanatomy* (8th ed.). Baltimore: Williams and Wilkins.
6. Chaffee, E. E., & Lytle, I. M. (1980). *Basic anatomy and physiology* (4th ed.). Philadelphia: J.B. Lippincott.
7. Chusid, J. G. (1985). *Correlative neuroanatomy and functional neurology* (19th ed.). Los Altos, CA: Lange Medical Publications.
8. Clemente, C. D. (1985). *Anatomy of the Human Body* (by Henry Gray) (30th American ed.). Philadelphia: Lea and Febiger.
9. Crouch, J. E. (1985). *Functional human anatomy* (4th ed.). Philadelphia: Lea and Febiger.
10. Davis, B. O., Holtz, N. & Davis, J. C. (1985). *Conceptual human physiology.* Columbus: Charles E. Merrill.
11. Evans, O. B. (1987). *Manual of child neurology.* New York: Churchill Livingstone.
12. Guyton, A. C. (1991). *Textbook of medical physiology* (8th ed.). Philadelphia: W.B. Saunders.
13. Hall-Craggs, E. C. B. (1985). *Anatomy as a basis for clinical medicine.* Baltimore: Urban and Schwarzenberg.
14. Heimer, L. (1983). *The human brain and spinal cord: Functional neuroanatomy and dissection guide.* New York: Springer-Verlag.
15. Lewis, M. (1990). *Clinical aspects of child and adolescent development* (3rd ed.). Philadelphia: Lea & Febiger.
16. Memmler, R. L., Cohen, B. J., & Wood, D. L. (1992). *Structure and function of the human body* (5th ed.). Philadelphia: J.B. Lippincott.
17. Moore, K. L. (1989). *Before we are born: Basic embryology and birth defects* (3rd ed.). Philadelphia: W.B. Saunders.
18. Moore, K. L. (1988). *The developing human: Clinically oriented embryology* (4th ed.). Philadelphia: W.B. Saunders.
19. Nauta, W. J. H., & Feirtag, M. (1986). *Fundamental neuroanatomy.* New York: W.H. Freeman and Company.
20. Pallett, P. J., & O'Brien, M. T. (1985). *Textbook of neurological nursing.* Boston: Little, Brown and Co.
21. Price, S. A., & Wilson, L. M. (1992). *Pathophysiology: Clinical concepts of disease processes* (4th ed.). St. Louis: Mosby.
22. Porth, C. M. (1990). *Pathophysiology: Concepts of altered health states* (3rd ed.). Philadelphia: J.B. Lippincott.
23. Reeder, S. J., & Martin, L. L. (1992). *Maternity nursing: Family, newborn and women's health care* (17th ed.). Philadelphia: J.B. Lippincott.
24. Romero, R., Pilu, G., Jeanty, P., & Hobbins, J. C. (1988). *Prenatal diagnosis of congenital anomalies.* Norwalk, CT: Appleton and Lange.
25. Stern, J. T. (1988). *Essentials of gross anatomy.* Philadelphia: F.A. Davis.
26. Williams, P. L., Warwick, R., Dyson, M. & Bannister, L. H. (1989). *Gray's anatomy.* (37th ed.) New York: Churchill Livingstone.

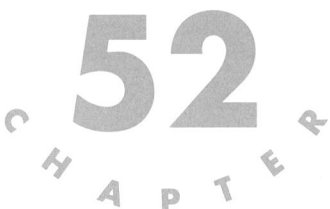

Nursing Assessment and Diagnosis of Neurologic Function

BEHAVIORAL OBJECTIVES

Describe the components of a complete history and physical examination of the child's neurologic function.

Differentiate between the assessment procedures for infants, children, and adolescents.

Identify the appropriate equipment for a comprehensive neurologic assessment.

Describe the preparation of infants, children, and adolescents for selected neurologic diagnostic procedures.

Identify nursing diagnoses that are commonly used in the care of children with neurologic dysfunction.

Nursing assessment of an infant, child, or adolescent and family usually falls into one of three categories: screening examination as a portion of a routine assessment, an in-depth examination specific to a child's complaint or human response noted by the nurse, or continuous evaluation of a patient's status to detect improvement or deterioration. The screening examination should include at least one or two items from each section of the complete neurologic examination. The complete neurologic examination is performed only when there is reason to believe the child has an unidentified neurologic problem or deficit. The complete neurologic assessment is lengthy, detailed, and time consuming. Continuous evaluation of the patient's status occurs most frequently in acute care settings. Abbreviated assessment forms for a neurologically impaired infant and for a neurologically impaired child can be conducted in 5 minutes. The most accurate neurologic diagnoses are based on detailed descriptions in the history and physical examination. Most neurologic disorders are hereditary, so a detailed family history is crucial.

Nursing Assessment

Establishing rapport and earning the child's trust early by discussing items of interest to the child make assessment easier. Play and other forms of interactive assessment are therefore critical to the neurologic portion of a history and physical examination. A game can be made out of "closing your eyes and touching your nose" or of standing with eyes closed and imagining something good. The neurologic test tasks are easily developed into games.

School-age children should be assessed for neurologic "soft signs" when the history or physical examination suggests neurologic deficits. *Soft signs* are a group of ambiguous or minor neurologic aspects of gross and fine motor control, coordination, balance, and sensation. The relationship between these features and the function or dysfunction of the central nervous system is uncertain. Soft signs are of particular value in assessing children who have reported "school problems." Many of these soft signs can be detected through observation of the child and family during the interview for the history. The accompanying display lists neurologic soft signs.

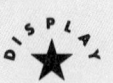

Neurologic Soft Signs

Easily distracted
Short attention span
Labile emotions
Impulsiveness
Deficits of perception—space, time, form, movement
Learning problems—reading, writing, and arithmetic
Articulation and language problems
Hypoactivity
Mild flaccidity or rigidity
Asymmetrical deep tendon reflexes
Hyperactivity—excessive, sustained, and purposeless movements
Poor coordination—poor quality of execution of movements
Poor sense of position
Unusual body movements
No established handedness

Child and Family History

The interview may begin by talking about everyday events with the parents to establish rapport and indicate the nurse's interest and concern. The child and family should be observed for grooming, color, posture, overall behavior, and appearance. Clues to their values, likes, and dislikes may be discovered through conversation with the parents. Whenever possible ask questions and talk directly with the child. Talking only to the parents suggests that the child is not expected to know much or to participate, and this may interfere with the development of rapport and trust between the child and the examiner.

Health Perception and Health Management

Note the general appearance of the child and caregiver (e.g., type and condition of attire, cleanliness, nutrition, and grooming). Assess for congruence between appearance, affect, and answers given by the child and parent. Lack of congruence suggests a problem (e.g., lack of trust, lack of understanding of the level of language, a need to be approved of by the interviewer, or emotional problems not yet expressed). The following questions should be asked: How has the family's general health been during the last few years? Has the child missed school; has the caregiver missed work? How often do family members have cold or flu symptoms? What are the current health problems of the child, each sibling, and parent(s)? What is the occupation of each parent?

Assess age of the child and the age of the caregivers. What grade is the child in, and what is the educational history of each parent? Does the child seem to be developing normally for his or her age? Does the caregiver believe the child is developing at about the same rate as other children of the same age? Is the child developing

faster, slower, or at about the same rate as the parents and siblings at that age? Obtain a complete developmental history of the family.

Assess the definition of health and its value to the child and caregivers, their financial status, and their pattern of seeking health care. What kind of health problems are most common in this family, and how have they dealt with them (e.g., folk remedies, surgery)? How easy has it been to follow a physician's or nurse's suggestions? Assess the family history of accidents. Does the child seem "accident prone"? What does the child or the caregiver believe must be done to maintain health; that is, what steps are taken to maintain or promote health (e.g., use of seat belts, visits to the physician and dentist, amount of sleep, administration of vitamins, amount of exercise)? What is the child's and family's immunization history. How has the child's current illness affected the family?

If appropriate, ask what the perceived cause of this illness is and what actions were taken when the symptoms were perceived. Determine the results of this action.

If appropriate, ask what things are most important to the child and caregiver while they are at the physician's office and how the nurse could be most helpful.

Nutrition and Metabolism

What was the child's birth weight and growth percentile? What was the child's weight at 6 and 12 months of age? Does the child or the parents think the child's weight is appropriate for height?

Determine the typical daily food and fluid intake for the child and caregiver. Compare this with the calculation of fluid maintenance requirements for weight. Ask about the child's appetite and food preferences. At what time of day does the child seem to have the biggest appetite? How many and what kind (if any) of vitamin supplements does the child take? Does the child's daily diet include grains, milk, vegetables, meat, and fruit? How much cheese and milk does the child consume daily? What are the favorite family snack foods, drinks, and so forth? Are there routine family meal times, or does everyone eat on their own schedule?

Is there a history of vomiting? If so, when does the vomiting occur (before or after meals)? Does the child complain of nausea?

Does the child have any food allergies? Have there been any skin problems (e.g., dryness, cracking, peeling, new moles, lesions)? Do cuts and bruises heal quickly? Is there a history of dental caries or gingivitis?

Elimination

When was the child toilet trained? Were there any difficulties with the toilet training? Determine the child's elimination pattern—frequency, consistency, color, odor, discomfort. How frequently does the child have diarrhea or constipation? When is the child most likely to have diarrhea? How does the caregiver handle constipation? What are the child's words for urination and defecation? Does the child perspire, and if so, is it often and to excess?

Determine the child's urinary elimination habits, including color, odor, amount, frequency, and history of toilet training. Does the child wet the bed at night? Is there a history of urinary tract infections?

Are there household pets in the family? How is elimination of their wastes handled? What are the child's feelings about and play activities with the household pets?

Activity and Exercise

Ask about the exercise pattern of the child and family (type, regularity, tolerance). How does the child respond to exercise? What type of play activities does the child enjoy the most?

Describe the child's play pattern: frequency, playmates, active or passive, variety, stimulation, energy level, stamina. How often and what kind of interactive play does the caregiver or each parent initiate with the child?

Is the child able to feed, bathe, dress, and groom himself or herself? What activities must be performed by the caregiver and how often? Who is responsible for housekeeping, transportation, and so forth? Does the child seem clumsy or less coordinated than other children of the same age? Does the child have full range of motion in all joints? Are the muscles firm? Is the child more or less strong than other children of the same age?

Sleep and Rest

Determine the child's sleep pattern and nap routine. How many hours of sleep does the child get each 24 hours? Does the child seem to be rested and ready for the day upon awakening? Does the child have difficulty getting to sleep? How long does is take for the child to fall asleep after going to bed? Does the child make a strong effort to delay bedtime? What kind of help does the child need to go to sleep (e.g., bedtime story, teddy bear, snack, night light, music)? Describe the child's normal bedtime routine. Does the child have nightmares? If

so, what kind and how often? What helps the child recover from them? How often does child awaken during the night? Does the child sleepwalk or sleep excessively? Describe the parents' sleep patterns.

Has the child or any family member had seizures, muscle twitching dizziness, muscle weakness, or paralysis? Have there been any fainting spells? Has the child had periods of being shaky or unsteady on his or her feet?

Cognition and Perception

Does the child or family have any difficulty with hearing or vision? When were these last checked? Does the child seem to be having trouble remembering things? Has the child been having rapid mood changes? What kind of grades does the child earn in school (if appropriate)?

Has the child or the family had any numbness, tingling, or decreased sensation? Has the child complained of headaches? If so, how often, in what location on the head, and how was the pain described? How does the child usually describe pain? Does the child generally have a low or high tolerance to pain? Do any family members have frequent headaches? If so, what kinds? How is pain managed in the family? What kinds of medications are used? Is there a history of drug, alcohol, or cigarette use? Is there any mental retardation in the family tree? Is there a history of head trauma? Has the child ever lost consciousness? Has anyone else in the family ever lost consciousness? Has the child or anyone in the family ever had a convulsion?

Does the caregiver describe providing care for the child as easy, average, or difficult? Would the caregiver describe the child as high strung or easygoing?

Has anyone in the family had an early death, nervous breakdown, degenerative illness, or mental illness? How much do the child and the parents know about the child's current illness and its treatment? What is their understanding about what will happen to the child? How has this illness affected them? What is their understanding of the medications, diet, activity restrictions, and caregiving requirements?

Self-Perception and Self-Concept

What is the general mood of the family and the child? Does the child generally feel good about himself or herself? Is the child often depressed, anxious, happy, sad, moody, annoyed, fearful, or out of control? What helps the child and family improve their moods? How does the family describe its status in the community?

How does the child describe himself or herself? Does the child ever lose hope? Do the parents ever lose hope? What helps when this happens? On a scale of one to five Do the parents rate the child nervous (five) or relaxed (one), assertive (five) or passive (one)? How does the child rate himself or herself on the same scale? Does the child spend a great deal of time dressing and grooming? Is the child concerned about appearance?

Role Relationship

Describe a typical school day for the child. Describe the child's best friends. Does the child serve as a leader or a member of his or her group? What role does the child assume in the family? How has the illness affected his or her family role? Describe the family structure and the way decisions are made in the family. Does the child have much support in the family? Does the child feel good about relations with the family? How involved is the family in community activities? Are there supportive extended family members in the community? Does the child feel lonely? If so, how frequently? How does the family describe their stress level? To which member of the family does the child feel the closest?

How does the child respond to separation from parents? How dependent or independent is the child? Does the child have temper tantrums? If so, how are they handled? Does the child have discipline problems or school adjustment problems? How does the child relate to peers?

Sexuality and Reproduction

How does the child relate to the parent of the opposite sex? Has the child developed secondary sex characteristics? How does the child or adolescent feel about sexuality? Would the child and family describe the child as more feminine or masculine? Is child satisfied with his or her sexual identity? What kind of questions has the child asked regarding sexuality? How did the parents respond?

Is the adolescent sexually active and satisfied with sexual activity? Does the adolescent anticipate any problems? Would the adolescent like to make any changes? When did menstruation start?

Does the adolescent have any difficulty during menstruation? Does the adolescent use any contraceptives? If so, are there problems with the contraceptive? If a child seems precocious, the previous questions may be addressed to him or her.

Coping and Stress Tolerance

How does the child handle problems, stress, anger, and frustration? Does the child need help to handle these emotions or is he or she self-regulated and coping well? How do the family and parents handle problems? Who decides how problems are handled? What are favorite strategies for handling problems (e.g., ignore or discuss them)? Describe support systems of the family and patient. To whom does the patient turn most often for support? What life stressors and family stressors is the family experiencing?

Values and Beliefs

What does the child consider the most important things in life? If the child could change any part of life, what would be changed? What plans does the child or adolescent have for the future? What plans does the family have for the child's future? How might these plans be affected by the child's illness? How important is religion? Does religion help when difficulties arise? Are there any family "rules" that everyone thinks are important? Is the family generally getting what it wants out of life?

TABLE 52-1
Equipment Needed for Neurologic Assessment

Equipment Needed	Function
Percussion hammer	Evaluate reflexes
Sterile needles (two)	Test responses to pain
Coin or tongue depressor	Evaluate sensory discrimination and sensation
Cotton balls	Evaluate sensory discrimination and sensation
Cotton-tipped applicator	Evaluate superficial sensation and corneal reflexes
Two test tubes (one filled with hot water, one cold)	Evaluate hot and cold sensation
Penlight	Assess pupillary response
Transillumination collar with flashlight (newborn only)	Illuminate skull or brain to assess brain growth
Tongue depressor millimeter pupil gauge (see Fig. 52-1)	Assess pupil size
Ophthalmoscope (advanced)	Evaluate optic disc
Tuning fork	Assess hearing/vibration
Ticking watch	Evaluate hearing
Small samples of sugar, salt, peanut butter, orange or banana extract	Evaluate taste and smell
Plastic tape measure (centimeters)	Measure size/symmetry
Stethoscope	Assess bruits/vital signs
Sphygmomanometer	Assess blood and pulse pressure
Red ball or yarn	Assess visual fields and eye movements
Eye charts (Snellen "E" or animal picture)	Assess visual acuity
Denver II	Assess development of children younger than 6 years

Physical Assessment

The equipment needed for a complete neurologic examination is listed in Table 52-1. The equipment should be within reach before the examination is begun. A neurologic assessment should be approached systematically. The same format should be followed whenever possible so that parts of the examination are not forgotten. The examination can be divided into five parts: general, mental, or emotional; head and neck; cranial nerves; motor and sensory responses; and reflexes. Knowledge of the child's developmental and cognitive stage is essential. The examination must be geared to the child's level of understanding because cooperation is essential to ensure accurate data. A checklist for a physical examination for infants, children, and adolescents is presented in Table 52-2. An explanation of some of the testing procedures follows.

The neurologic examination for newborns and infants is different than that for older children and adults. The newborn examination includes eliciting infant reflexes as a means of evaluating central nervous system integrity. The newborn examination often is performed within the first 24 hours of life; however, an evaluation of the newborn's neurologic system is most accurate when per-

TABLE 52-2
Developmental Considerations in the Physical Examination of Neurologic Function

Check ✓ if normal, NE if not examined, − if abnormal. Describe abnormal findings.

Infant	Child	Adolescent
General: Head/Neck	**General: Head/Neck**	**General: Head/Neck**

Infant	Child	Adolescent
_____ Head symmetry/normal cephalic	_____ Head symmetry/normal cephalic	_____ Normocephalic, symmetrical
_____ Head circumference in centimeters (2 cm>chest)	_____ Head circumference (5 to 7 cm<chest)	_____ No lumps or tenderness
_____ Lateral anterior fontanel measurements (up to 16 mo)	_____ Good muscle tone; no hypotonia or hypertonia	_____ Normal hair distribution
_____ Vertical anterior fontanel measurements (up to 16 mo)	_____ Well-coordinated movements	_____ No lesions
_____ Less than 1 cm transillumination in frontal area of skull; none at occipital base (up to 12 mo)	_____ No bruits over skull	_____ Eyes, brows, and lids: good alignment, symmetrical
_____ No swelling or nodes palpated on skull	_____ Full range of motion in neck	_____ Lids: no lag
_____ No bulging of fontanels	_____ Eyes, brows, lids: good alignment, symmetrical, no lag	_____ PERRLA
_____ No marked pulsations in fontanels	_____ Normal hair distribution	_____ Full range of motion in neck
_____ No dilatation of scalp veins	_____ No lesions	_____ Good posture, muscle tone
_____ No bruits heard over skull	_____ No lumps or tenderness	_____ Well-coordinated movements
_____ No sutures palpable for past 6 months	_____ PERRLA	
_____ Describe head position when resting	_____ No abnormality of pattern of papillae or coating of tongue	
_____ No head lag (past 3 months)	_____ Color of tongue: _____	
_____ Raises head when prone (infant)	_____ Tongue not enlarged or protruding	
_____ Holds head erect when sitting	_____ No impairment in movement of tongue	
_____ Pinna of ears on horizontal plane with outer canthus of eye and occipital protruberance	_____ No shortening of frenulum (child can elevate tip of tongue to produce _t, d, n, l_ sounds)	
_____ Size of lower jaw proportional to rest of head	_____ No profuse or decreased salivation	
_____ No bulging or "bossing" of frontal area of skull	_____ No discoloration of gums	
_____ No tenderness or pain over scalp, occiput	_____ Number of teeth present: _____	
_____ Eyes, brows, and lids: good alignment, symmetrical	_____ Teeth present appropriate for age	

Cranial Nerves	Cranial Nerves	Cranial Nerves
_____ N.I.: Not checked in child younger than age 2 (have child older than age 2 close eyes and identify peanut butter or chocolate)	_____ N.I.: Identifies peanut butter, orange, or peppermint smell with eyes closed	_____ N.I.: Correctly identifies odors
_____ N.II.: Age: Birth Test: Hold bright object in front of eyes to attract attention, then move from side to midline. Response: Elementary fixation—can follow to the midline.	_____ N.II.: Age: 3 to 5 years Test A: Pediatric eye chart or Denver II Test B: Test color discrimination with color blocks. Test C: Test peripheral vision by having child look straight ahead as you wiggle your finger in each of the four fields approaching a 90-degree angle from behind Response: 20/30 visual acuity	_____ N.II.: Normal visual fields Visual acuity corrected OD _____ / _____ OS _____ / _____
_____ N.II.: Age: 1 to 3 months Test: Move bright colored object in front of eyes to attract attention, then move it through a full 180-degree range. Response: Binocular fixation, follows moving object through 180 degrees.		_____ Fund:
		_____ Optic disks: Flat, yellow, margins clear
_____ Age: 3 to 5 months Test: Same—also observe for fixation on distant objects. Response: Can fixate on objects beyond 3 ft		_____ Physiologic cup flat
		_____ Arteries, veins: normal ratio
		_____ No AV nicking, hemorrhage, or exudate

(Continued)

TABLE 52-2
(Continued)

Check ✓ if normal, NE if not examined, − if abnormal. Describe abnormal findings.

Infant	Child	Adolescent
Cranial Nerves	**Cranial Nerves**	**Cranial Nerves**

Infant	Child	Adolescent
_____ Age: 5 to 7 months Test: Hold the four different colored Denver II test blocks in palm before child Response: Prefers red and yellow		_____ N.III.: PERRLA
_____ Age 7 to 12 months Test A: Attract attention to raisin held in your palm near infant Test B: Begin screening amblyopia by covering each eye alternately as child observes raisin or other object Response: Fixates on raisin and will try to pick it up		_____ Intact fields of gaze
_____ N.II.: Age: 12 to 18 months Test A: Show pictures Test B: Give pencil and paper Response: Stares at pictures, scribbles on paper		_____ No ptosis or lid lag
_____ Age: 18 months to 3 years Test: Use Denver II Eye Screening chart Response: 20/40 visual acuity		_____ N.IV.: Downward medial movement of eyes intact
_____ N.III. N.IV.: Same as adolescent	_____ N.III.: PERRLA	_____ N.V.: Sensory perception of pain, light touch, and temperature are intact in the ophthalmic, maxillary, and mandibular divisions
_____ N.V.: Same except blowing lightly on eyes will elicit corneal reflex in infants and children Response: Blinks in response to blowing on eyes	_____ Intact fields of gaze	
	_____ No ptosis or lid lag	_____ Motor function strong with clenched teeth
	N. IV, V, VI, VII, VIII, IX, X, XI, XII same as adolescent	_____ Corneal reflexes present
_____ N.VI.: Nystagmus is normal up to 4 months		_____ N.VI.: Lateral deviation of eye intact
_____ N.VII.: Have child mimic facial expressions, such as frown, smile, nose wrinkled, eyes squinting Response: Symmetrical movements		_____ No nystagmus
		_____ *N.VII.: Facial muscles strong and symmetrical
_____ N.VIII.: Age: Birth to 4 months Suspend infant at 30-degree angle and rotate each direction in a complete circle, observing eye response Response: Eyes will oscillate (nystagmus) in the direction of rotation		_____ Taste present on anterior tongue
		_____ *N.VIII.: Auditory acuity normal to ticking watch or whisper
_____ Age: 4 to 18 months Test: Attract attention to silent toy on one side, then use bell on opposite side outside of peripheral vision—orienting response-to-noise test; note response and repeat on opposite side Response: 4 to 5 months—eyes widen, turns head slightly in direction of sound, seems to listen 6 to 7 months—head turns toward sound 8 months—eyes determine source of sound		_____ Air conduction greater than bone conduction (Rinne)
		_____ No lateralization (Weber)
		_____ N.IX., N.X.: Normal gag reflex
		_____ Soft palate and uvula symmetrical with upward movement
		_____ Taste present on posterior tongue
_____ N.IX.: Same as adolescent		_____ N.XI.: Sternocleidomastoids and trapezii muscles strong, symmetrical
_____ N.X.: Same as adolescent		
_____ N.XI.: Infant—observe head control 18 months—have child imitate shrugging or lifting of shoulders		_____ N.XII.: Tongue symmetrical, no deviation, atrophy, or fasciculation
_____ N.XII.: Pinch nostrils Response: Opens mouth and raises tip of tongue		

(Continued)

TABLE 52-2
(Continued)

Check ✓ if normal, NE if not examined, − if abnormal. Describe abnormal findings.

Infant	Child	Adolescent
Motor	**Motor**	**Motor**
(For children between ages of 1 month and 5 years give Denver Developmental Screening Test.) Observe:	Observe:	Observe:
_____ Activity level	_____ Activity level	_____ *Normal gait, heel-to-toe, deep knee bends, walking on heels and toes
_____ Mobility (Walking? Crawling? Scooting?)	_____ Posture symmetrical	_____ *Romberg negative
_____ Coordination of spontaneous and induced movements	_____ Normal gait, heel-to-toe, deep knee bends	_____ Good coordination: Finger-to-nose, patting leg, heel-to-shin
_____ Eye–hand coordination	_____ *Romberg negative	_____ Grip strong, no tremor or drift of arms
_____ Hand position	_____ Good coordination: Finger-to-nose, patting leg, heel-to-shin	_____ Muscles—no atrophy, asymmetry, fasciculations, involuntary movements, or abnormal positions
_____ Neat pincer grasp (9 months and older)	_____ Grip strong, no tremor or drift of arms	_____ Muscles firm, strong; symmetrical strength
_____ Good grasp	_____ Muscles—no atrophy, asymmetry, fasciculations, involuntary movements, or abnormal positions	
_____ Resting position	_____ Muscles firm, strong; symmetrical strength	
_____ Range of motion for each major joint to check muscle tone		
_____ Coordination while rising from supine to standing position		
Motor Sensory	**Motor Sensory**	**Motor Sensory**
_____ Withdrawal of extremity following painful stimulus	_____ *Pain perception intact	_____ *Pain perception intact
_____ Change in facial expression following painful stimuli	_____ Perception of light touch, temperature, and vibration intact	_____ Perception of light touch, temperature, and vibration intact
_____ Movement or withdrawal of extremity stimulated by stroking	_____ Normal position sense and point discrimination	_____ Normal position sense and point discrimination
_____ Vertical suspension positioning	_____ Normal stereognosis and number identification	_____ Normal stereognosis and number identification
Mental Status and Speech	**Mental Status and Speech**	**Mental Status and Speech**
_____ Alertness	_____ *Orientation to person, place, time	_____ *Orientation to person, place, time
_____ Quality of cry	_____ Alert, conscious	_____ Alert, conscious
	_____ Recent and remote memory good	_____ Recent and remote memory good
	_____ Recites nursery rhyme	_____ Recites nursery rhyme
	_____ Dress and behavior appropriate	_____ Serial sevens, threes normal
	_____ Mood: _____	_____ Able to abstract
		_____ Dress and behavior appropriate
		_____ Mood: _____
Reflexes	**Reflexes**	**Reflexes**
(Use semiflexed finger instead of reflex hammer)	(0 to 4 scale; normal is 2+)	(0 to 4 scale; normal is 2+)
_____ Rooting reflex (up to 4 months)	_____ *Biceps (C5, C6)	_____ *Biceps (C5, C6)
_____ Moro reflex (up to 6 months)	_____ *Triceps (C7, C8)	_____ *Triceps (C7, C8)
_____ Brudzinski's sign	_____ *Brachioradialis (C5, C6)	_____ *Brachioradialis (C5, C6)
_____ Kernig's sign	_____ Abdominal (T8, T9, T10; T10, T11, T12)	_____ Abdominal (T8, T9, T10; T10, T11, T12)
_____ Sucking reflex	_____ Cremasteric (L1, L2)	_____ Cremasteric (L1, L2)
_____ Tonic neck reflex (up to 6 months)	_____ *Knee jerk (L2, L3, L4)	_____ *Knee jerk (L2, L3, L4)
_____ Grasp reflex (up to 4 months)	_____ *Ankle (S1, S2)	_____ *Ankle (S1, S2)
_____ Landau (up to 24 months)	_____ Plantar (L4, L5, S1, S2)	_____ Plantar (L4, L5, S1, S2)
_____ Parachute (from 9 months)	_____ Brudzinski's sign	_____ Brudzinski's sign
_____ Babinski's (up to 18 months)	_____ Kernig's sign	_____ Kernig's sign

Key: PERRLA, pupils equal reaction response to light and accomodation; N.I, olfactory nerve; N.II, optic nerve; AV, atriovenous nerve; N.III, oculomotor nerve; N.IV, trochlear nerve; N.V, trigeminal nerve; N.VI, abducens nerve; N.VII, facial nerve; N.VIII, vestibulochlear nerve; N.IX, glossopharyngeal nerve; N.X, vagus nerve; N.XI, accessory nerve; N.XII, hypoglossal nerve.

formed on or after day 10. Evaluation before 10 days may not yield the infant's best performance because much energy is expended in adapting to extrauterine life.

Infant examination

The infant must be *dry, comfortable, rested,* and *fed* to elicit the best performance. An optimal time for a neurologic evaluation is 2 to 2.5 hours after a feeding.

General. Observe the infant's position. Are the extremities flexed or extended? Is the infant sleeping? Is the infant moving in sleep or still? Are respirations regular or irregular? As the examination progresses, note how the infant responds to stimuli, such as crying, symmetrical grimacing, eyes focusing, irritability, and changes in skin color. Is the infant attempting to respond and interact with the environment or the examiner, or is the infant shutting out the environment? This assessment will provide a good indication of the infant's neurologic competence. Note the quality of the cry; it should not be shrill or high pitched.

Head and Neck. Observe the infant systematically for asymmetry, areas of swelling, discolorations, alignment and symmetry of eyes, eyebrows, and eyelids. Draw an imaginary horizontal line from the eye to the ear as in Figure 52-1. The findings are abnormal if the pinna of the ear falls below that line or if the ear is rotated toward the occiput more than 10 degrees.

Measure the anterior fontanel in centimeters using a tape measure. The bones, sutures, and fontanels are shown in Figure 33-5. Measure the lateral distance between the junction of the sagittal and coronal sutures from the left apex to the right apex. It helps to hold the tape down with one finger while stretching it from one apex to the other. A lateral or anterior–posterior measurement of the anterior fontanel should not exceed approximately 3 cm. If the actual fontanel measurement exceeds 3 cm, a mean fontanel size (L + W/2) should be calculated. Take the sum of the apex-to-apex measurement for the lateral (width) and the anterior–posterior measurements (length) and divide by two. The range for mean anterior fontanel size in the newborn is 1 to 3.5 cm. Mean fontanel

diameters greater than 3.5 cm indicate skeletal disorders, chromosomal disorders, or conditions such as malnutrition, rubella, progeria, or hypothyroidism. Larger anterior fontanels often are associated with hydrocephalus. The posterior fontanel should measure approximately 0.5 cm.

Flex the head on the chest to check for resistance or nuchal rigidity. Turn the head from side to side to check for full range of motion. Check the grasp reflex by helping the infant curl its fingers around your index finger and gently pull the infant to a sitting position. Note how far the head lags behind as you pull the infant to a sitting position. Often the infant can bring the head upright for a few seconds. After 3 months of age the infant's head should not lag behind the shoulders as he or she is pulled to a sitting position. Head lag is a good indicator of overall tone and development. It also is useful in evaluation of cranial nerve XI. Palpate the skull for tenderness, swelling, and bulging.

Cranial Nerves. Holding the infant almost upright and shielding the eyes from overhead lights encourages him or her to open the eyes. Check the eyes for a corneal reflex blink by directing a puff of air onto the eyes while open. You will need assistance to hold the eyes open when checking to determine the size and whether the pupils are equally responsive, react to light, and accommodate equally (PERRLA). Some neonates can mimic adult facial expressions if given time to study them. Make a face, such as a frown or wrinkled nose, or stick out your tongue and determine whether the infant has symmetrical movements when trying to mimic your face.

Motor and Sensory. Use red yarn or a red ball to attract the infant's attention. Note motor activity coordination as the infant attempts to grasp it. Administer the Denver II (see the Appendix) to children between the ages of 1 month and 5 years, and observe for the items on the checklist. Infants younger than 1 month of age should be tested with the Brazelton Newborn Assessment Scale (NBAS) described in Chapter 11. Premature infant development may be assessed with a refinement of the NBAS called the Assessment of Premature Infant Behavior, which also is described in Chapter 11. Development is a critical factor in assessing neurologic integrity. To test

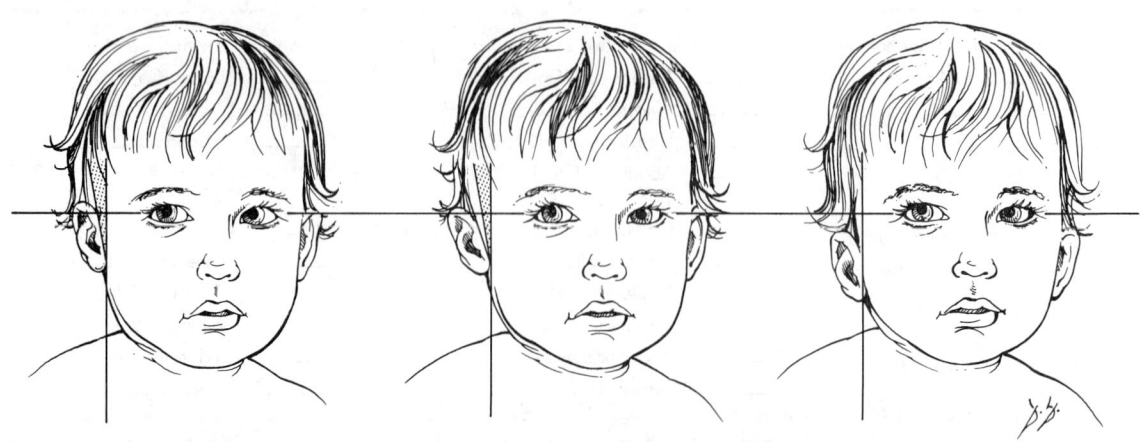

FIGURE 52-1
Alignment of ears with eye plane. (**Left,** normal ears; **center,** abnormally angled ear; **right,** low-set ears.)

the infant's sensory abilities flick the sole of the infant's foot with your fingers. Note the facial expression, total body response, and extremity response. Stroke an extremity and determine whether the infant attempts to move or withdraw the stroked extremity.

Reflexes. Refer to Chapter 11 for a description of the methods of eliciting neonatal reflexes. Superficial and deep-tendon reflexes in infants may yield highly variable results because of the immaturity of the system and minimal nerve myelination. Asymmetry or absence of the plantar grasp is abnormal and suggests a lower spinal column defect. The tonic neck reflex (TNR) appears at 2 or 3 months and disappears by 6 months. It is elicited by laying the infant supine and turning the head to one side (see Fig. 11-3). The infant will assume a typical "fencer's" position, extending the arm and leg on the side to which the head was turned, while flexing the other arm and leg. A persistent TNR suggests a neurologic defect. Moro's reflex should disappear by 6 months. It is sometimes called the startle reflex, which is confusing because the startle reflex is never lost. The classic "C" positioning of the fingers and adduction of the arms to the midline, shown in Figure 52-2, distinguish Moro's reflex from the startle reflex. Throwing the arms to the side when startled

is a reflex that a healthy person never loses. A persistent Moro's reflex indicates a serious neurologic deficit.

The Landau reflex appears between 4 and 6 months of age and disappears at approximately 24 months of age. In the Landau reflex the infant extends the head, trunk, and hips when held in a horizontal prone position across the examiner's hands (see Fig. 11-2). The parachute reflex appears at 9 months and persists throughout life. Hold the infant in a prone position and rapidly lower him or her toward the examining table. This stimulates the parachute reflex and causes the infant to extend the arms, hands, and fingers to break the fall. Babinski's reflex is positive from birth until after the infant has been walking for some time but disappears by 18 months. Babinski's reflex consists of the infant flaring the toes and extending the big toe when the sole of the foot is stroked on the lateral aspect. The absence of a Landau, Parachute, or Babinski's reflex in an infant when it should be present is a significant indicator of a central nervous system defect, possibly cerebral palsy.

Child and Adolescent Examination

The neurologic responsiveness of a child older than 2 years is similar to that of adults, because 75% of cortical development is complete by 2 years of age.[1] For this reason a child and adolescent are discussed together. The approach to the child will be more playful, whereas the adolescent should be approached as an adult.

General. Observe the child to determine whether his or her activity and behavior seem appropriate for age and development. If not, adjust language to the appropriate level. Begin talking about things in which you have observed the child to be interested, such as Sesame Street characters, dolls or puppets in the room, or pets that were discussed while taking the history. Take cues for approaching the adolescent from the attire and personal items visible. Once the child appears to relax, begin with nonpainful, nonthreatening assessment items. Begin with quiet activities and progress to the gross motor assessments and reflexes. Model the desired behavior for the child.

Head and Neck. Demonstrate the full range of motion of the neck and ask the child to copy. Playing a game of "monkey see, monkey do," in which the child must imitate exactly what the examiner does, is an excellent way to test cranial nerves and motor and sensory function. Listen to the skull with a stethoscope to determine bruits, and allow the child to listen to yours.

Cranial Nerves. The olfactory nerve (I) is checked by asking the child to identify an odor on a piece of cotton with the eyes closed. Eye charts, the pediatric "E" or the Snellen depending on age, are used to evaluate the visual acuity of the optic nerve (II). The oculomotor, trochlear, and abducens nerves (III, IV, and VI) usually are tested as a unit. Ask the child or adolescent to follow an object or the examiner's fingers as they move in all directions. If the oculomotor nerve is involved, the child will have difficulty looking up, down, or toward the nose. Check for ptosis of the eyelid. The trochlear nerve (IV) is in-

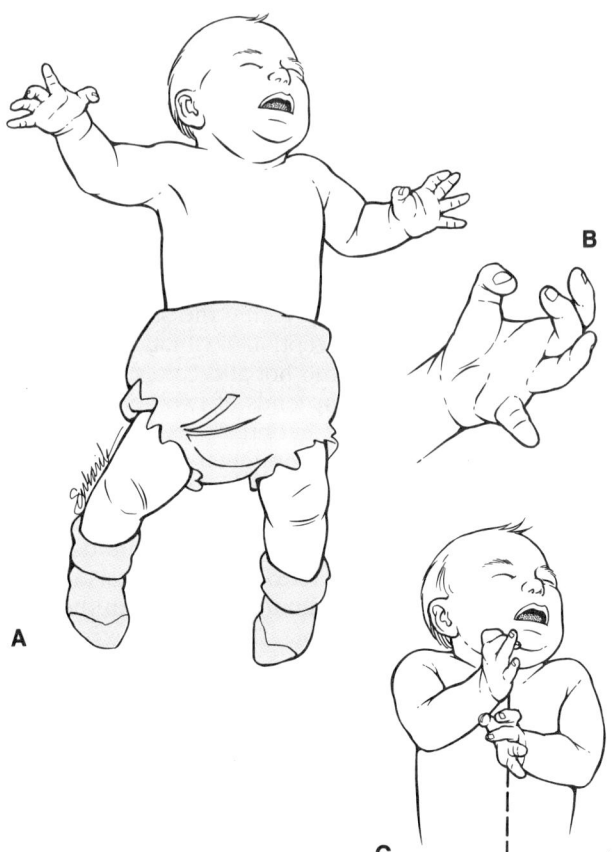

FIGURE 52-2

(A) Neonate in the startle reflex (Moro reflex) with arms thrown out. (B) In the Moro reflex the child's hand goes into a classic "C" position. This is seen only in the first 6 months of life. (C) In the actual startle reflex the infant's arms come back toward the body in midline position. The startle reflex is never lost; the Moro reflex, with the hand in a "C" position is an indication of a serious neurologic defect in an older child.

volved when the child has difficulty looking downward and to the outside. If the abducens nerve (VI) is affected, the child will not be able to look laterally (to the side). Note whether the child's eyes move smoothly or with constant involuntary cyclical movements (nystagmus). When checking the pupils for PERRLA (also oculomotor [III]), darken the room. Ask the child to look at a specific point. Note the size and shape of the pupil. A tongue depressor pupil gauge made from taping a paper millimeter pupil chart to a tongue depressor may be held beside the child's head to get a more accurate measurement of pupil size[2] (Fig. 52-3A). Note whether the pupils are equal in size. Ask the child to focus on a specific object on the other side of the room, and then ask the child to look at something you are holding in your hand. The pupil size should decrease (constrict) as the child looks from the distant object to the close object. This is called accommodation. Shine a pen light briefly into each eye, and note how quickly, smoothly, and equally the pupils constrict to the light.

The trigeminal nerve (V) is first tested by lightly touching the child's cheek, forehead, and jaw with a wisp of cotton (see Fig. 52-3B). A difference in response on opposite sides should be noted, and this indicates a decreased or increased sensitivity to light touch. Test for sensitivity to warm and cold objects in the same manner. The corneal reflex is tested by lightly touching the cornea from the side (so the child does not see it) with a wisp of cotton. Be sure to touch the cornea and not just the sclera. Ask the child to open the mouth; look for symmetry or deviation of the jaw. Ask the child to copy you, and clench the jaw while you palpate the temporal and masseter muscles for strength.

Look for symmetry as you ask the child to imitate a grimace (see Fig. 52-3C), wrinkled forehead, frown, smile, and raised eyebrows. Ask the child to keep eyelids closed as you attempt to open them. These tests are used to evaluate the facial nerve (VII). Only the cochlear portion of the acoustic nerve (VIII) is normally tested because special equipment is needed to test the vestibular portion. Hold a ticking watch away from the children's ear and ask them to tell you when they can hear it as you move it toward the ear. Repeat the procedure moving the watch away from the ear. Be sure to test both ears. A whispering sound also can be used to test hearing. Use a tuning fork to test air and bone conduction of sound. Strike the tuning fork against your palm, and place the point on the top of the child's head. Ask whether the sound is heard in the middle or more to one side or the other (*lateralization* test). The sound should be heard in the center. Strike the tuning fork again, and place the point (base) on the mastoid process behind the child's ear. Ask the child to let you know when the sound is no longer heard. Next, strike the fork and hold the vibrating portion next to the ear, and have the child tell you when it can no longer be heard. In general the child's air conduction should be better than bone conduction.

The glossopharyngeal nerve (IX) and vagus nerve (X) are tested together. If the child can swallow and speak clearly without hoarseness and if soft palate movement is symmetrical when the child says "ah," the vagus is considered to be intact. Touch each side of the back of the throat with a tongue depressor to check the gag reflex.

The accessory nerve (XI) can be tested by palpating the sternocleidomastoid and trapezius muscles for strength as the child shrugs his or her shoulders against resistance and turns the head. The hypoglossal nerve (XII) is tested by asking the child to stick out the tongue. Note any tremors or deviations of the tongue.

Motor and Sensory. The motor and cerebellar systems can be checked at the same time. Muscles are checked for strength against resistance and size, and the smoothness or fluidity of motion, coordination, and balance of those muscles indicates cerebellar function. While the child is sitting use "monkey see, monkey do" to have the child pat the legs simultaneously, alternating the hand between supination and pronation positions (see Fig. 52-3D); place the heel to the shin, and move it up to the knee on each side; touch the finger to the nose with eyes open and then closed (see Fig. 52-3E); and touch the finger to the examiner's finger with eyes open (see Fig. 52-3F). Check the grip in both hands for strength and equality, and then have the child push down and then up against resistance from the examiner's hands. Test both arms and legs against resistance with the knee and elbow flexed. Check muscles for atrophy, asymmetry, fasciculation, involuntary movements, or abnormal positions. Watch the child walk normally back and forth across the room, while checking for gait and heel-to-toe walking (see Fig. 52-3G). Check balance with deep knee bends, walking on heels, and walking on toes. Have child stand with both feet together and arms raised straight out in front for several seconds. Note any drift in arms or tendency to "list" to one side. Repeat this procedure for several seconds with the child's eyes closed for the Romberg test (see Fig. 52-3H).

To test the sensory system check for perception of sensation (temperature, touch, and vibration) on corresponding sides of the body and extremities. Pain perception is checked by lightly pricking the skin with a pin. Use the tuning fork for perception of vibration, the cotton ball for light touch, and the hot and cold test tubes for temperature. Use the sharp ends of two applicators for two-point discrimination. Check the proximal, distal, and each side of each extremity for light touch, temperature, vibration, and pain. Ask the child to identify a nickel (if older than 5 years) and several other familiar objects placed in the child's hand one at a time (stereognosis). The eyes should be closed for both stereognosis and graphesthesia (recognizing a number written on the hand with the end of an applicator). Compare sides.

Mental Status and Speech. Ask children to tell you their name, address, and telephone number if they are preschool age or older. Children older than age 8 also should be able to tell you the day and time. Ask them to tell you about what happened the first day they went to school and the last time they were at school to determine recent and remote memory. Ask children to recite a nursery rhyme, and then ask them to tell you what it means (ability to abstract). Children aged 7 or older may be asked to repeat up to seven-digit numbers, while younger children do well to remember and repeat one less digit than their age (i.e., children age 5 can repeat four-digit numbers). Children can point to a face on a "happy face"

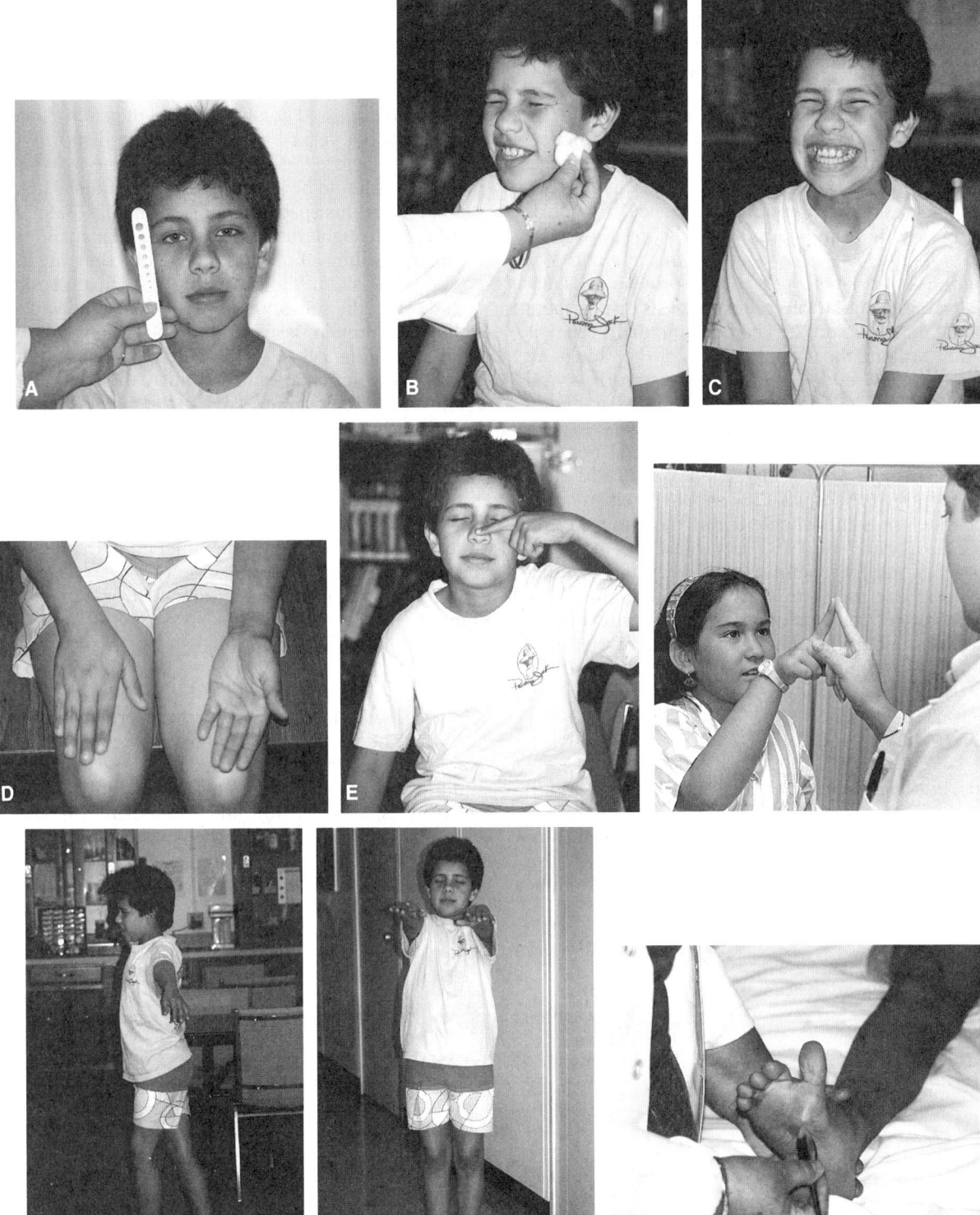

FIGURE 52-3

Neurologic examination of a child. (**A**) A tongue depressor is prepared to gauge the size of the pupil. (**B**) Trigeminal nerve is tested with a piece of cotton. (**C**) The child grimaces to indicate control of the facial nerve. (**D**) Alternate pronation-supination of palms. (**E**) The child moves finger to nose with eyes closed. (**F**) With eyes open the child extends finger to examiner's finger. (**G**) Heel-to-toe walking with arms extended out to sides. (**H**) Romberg test. (**I**) positive Babinski. (All but F are courtesy of Dr. Donna Deanne, Wright State University, Dayton, OH.)

chart to indicate their mood or how they feel. You may question them about their friends, activities, and favorite school subjects to give an idea of their general affect concerning these activities or relationships.

Reflexes. Deep-tendon reflexes are elicited by tapping briskly with a reflex hammer on a bony prominence, such as the radial styloid process or a tendon. This test is shown in Figure 9-12. This action stretches the muscles slightly and results in a contraction (reflex), which is graded on a scale from one to four. A score of two is a normal response; one is slow, and both three and four are abnormally brisk responses. An abnormal biceps tendon reflex or brachioradialis reflex suggests involvement of cervical nerves V and VI. The brachioradialis reflex is elicited by striking the styloid process of the radius. An abnormal triceps tendon reflex suggests that cervical nerves VI, VII, and VIII are involved. The patellar tendon reflects the function of lumbar nerves II, III, and IV. The Achilles tendon reflects the function of sacral nerves I and II. The presence of Babinski's reflex in a child older than 18 months is abnormal. Care should be taken not to use too much pressure when eliciting the Babinski's reflex, because it can cause a voluntary withdrawal in normal children that may be confused with the pathologic Babinski's response. Stroke the ball of the foot lightly from the lateral aspect to the medial aspect. Extension or dorsiflexion of the big toe along with fanning of the other toes suggests pyramidal tract disease (see Fig. 52-3*I*).

Diagnostic Tests

Specific diagnostic tests to investigate abnormal findings in the history and physical examination may be ordered by the physician. Noninvasive diagnostic tests usually are ordered before proceeding to the more invasive and often painful procedures. Children with alterations in neurologic functioning may be performing at a cognitive level well below their chronologic age; therefore, it is important to assess the child's level of perception prior to the explanation of the diagnostic tests.

The timing of preparation for diagnostic tests depends on the age and coping ability of the child. Children younger than 4 years usually are prepared shortly (5 to 10 minutes) before the test is to be performed. No painful procedures should be performed in the patient's hospital room, so that this space remains essentially "safe" from painful and frightening procedures. Explanations for younger children should begin before they are transported to the site of the procedure. Explanations should include all of the sensory experiences the child will have: sight, smell, touch, taste (if appropriate), and hearing. Relating experiences to child's everyday sensations helps him or her to anticipate and assimilate the experience in a nonthreatening manner. Trust in the nurse is improved when the child experiences no "surprises" associated with a planned procedure.

Older children who have good coping skills and a good sense of time may be prepared several hours before the procedure or as soon as the nurse knows it has been ordered. This time enables the older child to prepare for the procedure and allay unnecessary anxiety. Again, tell children what they will experience from all of their senses.

Laboratory Tests

A variety of laboratory tests is performed on a child suspected of having a neurologic problem. These tests may include a complete blood count, blood glucose, creatinine phosphokinase, phenylalanine, urea nitrogen, electrolytes, liver function, and tests for toxic substances, such as lead or drugs. Indices for blood and cerebrospinal fluid (CSF) in neurologic function are given in Tables 52-3 and 52-4, respectively.

TABLE 52-3
Blood Indices of Neurologic Function

Test	Appropriate Ranges	Deviations	Clinical Implications
Creatinine phosphokinase	Neonate: 10 to 300 IU/L Child: Male 0 to 20 IU/L Female 0 to 50 IU/L	Increase	Convulsions Cerebral infarction Subarachnoid hemorrhage Central nervous system trauma
Glucose Fasting Blood sugar	Premature: 20 to 60 mg/dl Neonate: 30 to 80 mg/dl Child: 60 to 100 mg/dl Adolescent: 70 to 110 ml	Increase	Brain trauma
Phenylalanine	L4 mg/100 ml	Increase >15 mg/100 ml	Phenylketonuria
Uric acid		Increase	Level poisoning

TABLE 52-4
Cerebrospinal Fluid Indices of Neurologic Function

Test	Appropriate Ranges	Deviations	Clinical Implications
Bilirubin White blood cell count (WBC)	Negative Premature: <18 Neonate: <15 leuko-cytes/mm^3 Child: 0 to 5 cells/mm^3	Increase	Aseptic meningitis (WBC 1000 to 2000/mm^3 or higher—mostly polymorphonuclear leukocytes)
Color	Crystal clear, colorless	Turbid, cloudy	Meningitis Cryptococcal infection
		Yellow	Bilirubinemias
		Pink	Cerebral hemorrhage Subrachnoid hemorrhage
Glucose	Neonatal: 20 to 40 mg/dl Child: 20 to 40 mg/dl Adolescent: 50 to 80 mg/dl	Decrease	Bacterial meningitis (<40 mg to 40% blood glucose) Primary brain tumor Viral meningoencephalitis
		Increase	Brain tumors with increased intercranial pressure Mumps
Pressure	50 to 180 mm H$_2$O (varies with size)	Increased	Space-occupying lesions such as intercranial tumors, intracerebral bleeding Meningitis Encephalitis Neurosyphilis Hydrocephalus Hydrocephalus with large pool cerebrospinal fluid
Protein	Neonate: 60 to 120 mg/dl Child: 15 to 45 mg/100 ml (lumbar) 5 to 15 mg/100 ml (ventricular)	Increase	Aseptic meningitis Bacterial meningitis (100 to 500 mg/100 ml) Brain abscess Brain tumors Guilain-Barré syndrome Subarachnoid hemorrhage Syphilis
Total cell count	0.8 mm^3	Increase	Infection
Total cell count		Decrease of abnormal cells	Brain tumors, cranial infarct Encephalitis (subacute viral) Meningitis Surgical trauma, central nervous system

Procedures

Diagnostic studies are considered noninvasive and invasive. Noninvasive procedures are the following: x-rays of the skull and spinal columns; echoencephalography; electroencephalography; computerized axial tomography; visual, auditory, and sensory evoked responses; brain electrical activity map; transillumination; and nuclear magnetic resonance. The following are invasive procedures: transcephalic impedance; cerebral angiography; brain scans; pneumoencephalography or ventriculography; electroneurography; electromyography; lumbar tap; and ventricular or subdural tap.

X-Rays of Skull and Spinal Column

Description/Definition

Radiographic "pictures" of the patient's head or spinal column.

Purpose

Skull and spinal column radiography allows detection of traumatic fractures and bony changes associated with space-occupying lesions, increased intracranial pressure, and congenital malformations.

Indications

- Trauma of the skull or spinal column.
- Persistent headaches.

- Signs associated with increased intracranial pressure.
- Suspicion of congenital malformation.

Contraindications

None.

Preparation

The machinery is large, cold, and often frightening to the child. Preschoolers and older children may benefit from seeing the equipment or pictures of the equipment ahead of time. Particular attention should be paid to explaining that the table may feel cool or cold and that the machine may make a whirring sound similar to an electric can opener followed by a click while it is taking the "picture." Children also should be told that they may have to remove their clothes and wear a gown that opens down the back.

Developmental Considerations

None.

Complications

None.

Echoencephalography

Description/Definitions

Ultrasound waves are pulsed through the open fontanels through paddles to discern a displacement of brain structures. It is used regularly in the neonatal intensive care units for early detection of intraventricular hemorrhage in neonates.

Purpose

Ultrasonography allows detection of inflammation, intracranial hemorrhage, hydrocephalus, and malformations of the brain or spinal column in infants and neonates.

Indications

- Suspicion of spinal or brain anomalies or malformations.
- Screening for intracranial bleeding.
- Suspicion of hydrocephalus.
- Inflammation.

Contraindications

None.

Preparation

No preparation or follow-up care is needed.

Developmental Considerations

None.

Complications

None.

Electroencephalography (EEG)

Description/Definition

Amplified brain electrical activity from several different points is recorded on a graph.

Purpose

EEG is used to analyze focal or generalized abnormalities of brain function.

Indications

- Pinpointing the location of structural lesions.
- Diagnosis and localization of seizure foci.
- Study of normal and abnormal sleep.
- Diagnosis of brain death.

Contraindications

- Child who is restless.
- Child who is unable to lie quietly or sleep during procedure.

Preparation

The procedure takes approximately 45 minutes and involves the attachment of electrodes to several points on the scalp. The hair must be washed before and after the procedure. Washing before the procedure removes hair oils and debris that might interfere with the accuracy of the signals. Washing the hair after the procedure removes the excess conduction jelly from the hair.

Developmental Considerations

Young children may benefit from seeing a picture of a child receiving an EEG and feeling an electrode before undergoing for the procedure. This prepares them for the sensations they will feel and reduces the fear of pain associated with the procedure.

Complications

None.

Computerized Axial Tomography

Description/Definition

A combination of x-ray and computer technology is used to obtain a series of pictures of different tissue densities of intracranial structures. The child is placed supine on a horizontal table that moves inside a large circular structure. The machine is similar to being inside a large donut that completely encircles the child's head. The procedure may last for a full hour, and the child must be still throughout the procedure.

Purpose

Computerized axial tomography (CAT) is useful for detecting vascular irregularities, hemorrhage, lesions, tumors or masses, and ventricular size. The slightest changes in density of tissues is detected, facilitating early diagnosis of lesions.

Indications

- Neurologic trauma.
- Loss of consciousness.
- Hydrocephalus.
- Vascular anomalies, lesions, or tumors.

Contraindications

None.

Preparation

The child and parents must be informed about the procedure and that the physician may decide to use an intravenous contrast medium to enhance the pictures. Infants and young children probably will be sedated because of the need to remain still throughout the procedure.

Developmental Considerations

Young infants may need sedation to remain still for 1 hour. An infant optimally should be fed approximately 30 minutes before examination, so that he or she is likely to sleep during the majority of procedure. Sedation may still be advisable, depending on how soundly the infant sleeps.

Nursing Implications

Describe the process and equipment completely, so the child will know what to expect. Hair ornaments must be removed.

The child is usually restricted from fluids (NPO) prior to the study. An infant should be fed before the study to enhance relaxation. Allow the child to express feelings following the procedure.

Complications

Observe the injection site for thrombi when a contrast medium is used.

Visual, Auditory, and Sensory Evoked Potentials

Description/Definition

These studies are similar to an EEG; however, they yield specific information about conduction pathways to specific areas of the brain. They consist of applying an appropriate stimulus to the skin, eyes, or ears, while recording the intensity of the stimulus and the time required for the response to be reflected by the electrodes placed over the corresponding area of the cerebrum.

Purpose

Evoked potentials (EPs) are used to assess the function of primary sensory pathways, such as vision, sensation, and hearing. The brain and sensory pathways are assessed for sensory function.

Indications

- Cortical dysfunction.
- Brainstem dysfunction.
- Spinal and peripheral nerve disorders.
- Degenerative disorders.

Contraindications

None.

Preparation

The procedure is painless, and other than an explanation of the procedure, no special nursing care is required.

Developmental Considerations

Young children may need sedation to remain still throughout the procedure.

Infants should be fed 30 minutes before the procedure to enhance their likelihood of sleeping throughout the procedure. Sedation may still be ordered to help the infant remain still.

Complications

Mild skin discomfort may be experienced where electrodes were placed.

Brain Electrical Activity Map

Description/Definition

This procedure is a computerized topographical map using EEG and EP data. These maps provide concise spatiotemporal summaries of electrical activity from the scalp electrodes of the EEG and EP. A numerical matrix is used to generate the image in the computer and can be stored for later reference and statistical manipulation.[3]

Purpose

The brain electircal activity map (BEAM) is used to identify the areas of the brain that are being used in association with specific activities and states.

Indications

- Assessing hearing problems, school problems, and speech problems.[1]
- Predicting developmental delays in infants but limited by the difficulty in keeping the infant still and quiet.

Contraindications

None.

Preparation

This procedure requires the same preparation as an EEG. The child must be still throughout, unless patterns of movement are being studied. Hair must be washed before and after the procedure.

Development Considerations

Infants must be very still throughout the procedure. If the infant has been fed approximately 30 minutes to 1 hour before the procedure begins, he or she is more likely to sleep through the procedure.

Complications

None.

Transillumination

Description/Definition

A light source, such as a Chun gun or a flashlight (with a dark rubber collar surrounding the lighted end), is used to illuminate the skull. The infant is carried into a dark room, and the end of the light source is placed flush against the head. The distance from the light source to the outer limit of the illuminated area is measured on each side of the head over each lobe.

Purpose

This procedure is used to detect anencephaly or asymmetrical development of cerebral lobes.

Indications

- Hydrocephalus.
- Anencephaly.

Contraindications

None.

Preparation

No special preparation is needed.

Developmental Considerations

None.

Complications

None.

Nuclear Magnetic Resonance

Description/Definition

This procedure directs radiowaves through the skull to the nuclei of the structure to be evaluated. Radiowave energy is absorbed and moves or resonates, thereby emitting a pulse that the nuclear magnetic resonance converts into a proton map. A picture is developed that distinguishes between structures. Solid tumors are darker than the surrounding structure and are sharply outlined. No radiation is involved, and small structures are clearly depicted.

Purpose

Magnetic resonance images are used to evaluate the soft tissues of the brain and spinal column for trauma or congenital abnormalities.

Indications

- Tumors or space-occupying lesions.
- Hemorrhage, edema, or ischemia.
- Vascular disorders.
- Congenital malformations.
- Degenerative disorders.

Contraindications

None.

Preparation

Children and parents need complete explanations. The child may need to rehearse the procedure, which also helps in assessing the need for sedation. All metal objects must be removed because they interfere with the radiowaves.

Developmental Considerations

Sedation may be required for young children and infants to help them remain still throughout the procedure.

Complications

None.

Transcephalic Impedance

Description/Definition

Transcephalic impedance (TCZ) is measured by placing two needle electrodes 2.5 cm apart just inside the anterior hairline and two more electrodes at the inion (external occipital protuberances), which are also 2.5 cm apart. A TCZ meter powered by a 9-V battery is activated, and a digital reading is recorded. This procedure may be performed weekly or as desired. Infants without an increase in TCZ during the first 5 or more weeks of life tend to have abnormal intelligence as measured by the Bayley Mental Scales at 1 year of age.[4]

Purpose

TCZ is used to predict developmental and neurologic outcome for neonates at 1 year of age. In healthy preterm infants TCZ should increase weekly at an average of 1.36 Ohm/wk as the brain develops and matures.[5] TCZ is used to assess function of the brain in the neonate.

Indications

- Severe asphyxia.
- Intraventricular hemorrhage.
- Lethargic or very ill preterm infants.
- Hypotonic infants or spasticity.

Contraindications

The needles occasionally are disturbing to infants; therefore, this may cause agitation.

Preparation

Cleanse the forehead well. Explain the procedure to the parents.

Developmental Considerations

None.

Nursing Implications

Nursing preparation may include cleaning the needle sites with antiseptic solution and explaining the procedure to the parents.

Complications

Potential for inflammation or infection of needle sites, but this incidence is very rare.

Cerebral Angiography

Description/Definition

A radiopaque substance is injected into the femoral, brachial, or carotid arteries, and radiograph skull films are taken sequentially as the substance moves through intracranial and extracranial blood vessels.

Purpose

The procedure detects displacement of blood vessels by space-occupying lesions (subdural hematoma, tumor, or hydrocephalus); changes in flow patterns (malformations or thrombosis); and structural abnormalities (aneurysms, vascular malformations).

Indications

- Vascular anomalies.
- Cerebral lesions.

- Cerebral hemorrhage.
- Tumors.

Contraindications

Allergies to the radiopaque die or acute cerebral hemorrhage during the labile period are contraindications for angiography.

Preparation

Parents and children should understand that the procedure may take several hours and will involve administration of medication to cause relaxation; the head will be immobilized during the procedure; and the child may experience a burning sensation when the radiopaque material is injected.

Developmental Considerations

Age-appropriate comfort measures should be used. Young children should be given an opportunity to engage in therapeutic play that enables them to resolve unexpressed feelings about the procedure.

Nursing Implications

Nursing care following the procedure requires careful monitoring of the injection site for potential thrombus formation, arterial spasms, petechiae, hematoma, and bleeding. A pressure dressing is maintained over the site, and ice packs may be applied to reduce bleeding. The arm or leg involved is kept immobile, and the skin temperature, color, and distal pulses are checked every half hour for the first 4 hours and then every 2 hours for the next 6 hours. Neurologic and vital signs must be checked every hour for the first 4 hours and every 2 hours for the next 6 hours to detect allergic reactions to the contrast medium or cerebral vascular accident secondary to the procedure. The child should be watched for seizure development, increased intracranial pressure, and consciousness.

Complications

Allergic reactions to the contrast medium, cerebral vascular accidents, seizures, loss of consciousness or changes in levels of consciousness, and increased intracranial pressure are potential complications.

Brain Scans

Description/Definition

A radioisotope substance consisting of molecules too large for diffusion across the blood–brain barrier is injected intravenously. The brain is then scanned for the radioactive substance, which should be found in the venous sinuses.

Purpose

A lesion that interferes with the blood–brain barrier will show up on the scan because the lesion allows the radioactive indicator substance to diffuse in the diseased brain tissue.

Indications

- Detecting brain tumors.

Contraindications

None.

Developmental Considerations

None.

Nursing Implications

Nursing preparation involves explaining what the child should expect and describing the equipment and location of the injection site. No follow-up care is required other than observing the injection site for bleeding or hematoma.

Complications

None.

Pneumoencephalography or Ventriculography

Description/Definition

These procedures are rarely performed on children because they cause great discomfort and involve complications, and the information can be gathered from a CAT scan. Air of a contrast medium is injected into the subarachnoid space and ventricular system. X-rays are then taken to localize a brain tumor, assess patency of the ventricles, and identify cerebral anomalies. The air or contrast medium is injected through the fontanels in infants, but a burr hole must be drilled into the skull of older children to allow the injection needle to be inserted into the ventricles.

Purpose

Rarely used for diagnostic purposes.

Indications

- Localize brain tumors.
- Assess patency of ventricles.
- Identify cerebral anomalies.

Contraindications

Increased intracranial pressure or dehydration may be contraindications.

Preparation

Preparation for the procedure involves explanations to the parents and child, shaving and cleansing the scalp where the burr hole will be placed, NPO if general anesthesia will be given, and explanation of the effects of any preoperative medication.

Developmental Considerations

The procedure is much less involved when the fontanels are open because no burr hole is required. The child, infant, and adolescent *must* be kept flat after the procedure to prevent subdural hemorrhage and incapacitating headaches.

Nursing Implications

The child may be NPO for 6 to 8 hours before the test. Postoperatively the child is observed for signs of bleeding, shock, hemorrhage, increasing intracranial pressure, and infection. Vital signs should be monitored every 30 minutes for the first 2 hours and then every 4 hours for the rest of the day. Headaches may occur and are particularly uncomfortable for children undergoing pneumoencephalogram. Analgesia may be required for the headache, which may be aggravated by movement. The child with a pneumoencephalogram is kept *flat*, while the child having a ventriculogram may elevate the head approximately 10 degrees. Position following both procedures should be changed every 2 hours.

Complications

Increased intracranial pressure, vomiting, fever, and meningitis are potential complications.

Electroneurography (Nerve Conduction Studies)

Description/Definition

An electrical stimulus is applied to peripheral nerves while an oscilloscope records the sensory nerve action potential and the compound muscle action potential. Sensory and recording electrodes are placed along the nerve pathway to measure responses. The distance the impulse traveled is then divided by the conduction time, and the result is reported as the conduction velocity of the nerve under study.

Purpose

Serial studies may be used to trace degeneration with time or increase in conduction velocity.

Indications

- Sensory deficits or injuries.

Contraindications

None.

Preparation

The child and family should be told about the nature and purpose of the test and the procedure should be explained. The child should be allowed to feel the electrodes and should be told that there will be a tingling sensation much like when the "funny bone" is hit. The child must remain still throughout the recording.

Developmental Considerations

Infants may need sedation to remain still.

Complications

None.

Electromyography

Description/Definition

Needle electrodes are inserted into the muscle to be tested. An oscilloscope measures and records muscle action potentials induced by muscle movement.

Purpose

This test is used to differentiate among central nervous system, neurogenic, and neuromuscular transmission disorders.

Indications

- Determine the type of myopathy in children with muscle weakness or sensory disorders.

Preparation

The child and family should be told the nature and purpose of the test and how it is conducted.

Developmental Considerations

The older child should know that it will feel like "mosquito bites" or at least tingle when the electrodes are activated. The younger child should at least know that there is some discomfort associated with the needle electrodes. Some children may need sedation.

Complications

None.

Lumbar Tap

Description/Definition

A needle is introduced into the subaranchoid space between the third and fourth lumbar vertebrae below the level of the spinal cord (Fig. 52-4A). Sterile technique is used, and the child must remain absolutely still with the back bowed (see Fig. 52-4B). A manometer is attached to the end of the spinal needle to determine cerebral spinal fluid (CSF) pressure, a Queckenstedt test is performed (compression of neck veins to determine effect on CSF pressure), and CSF is collected in sequential tubes. It is essential that the tubes be accurately numbered in sequence.

Purpose

To examine CSF for cell count, invading organisms, sensitivity, protein, sugar, and pressure; or to introduce medications.

Indications

- Increased intracranial pressure
- Meningitis or encephalitis
- Central nervous system hemorrhage

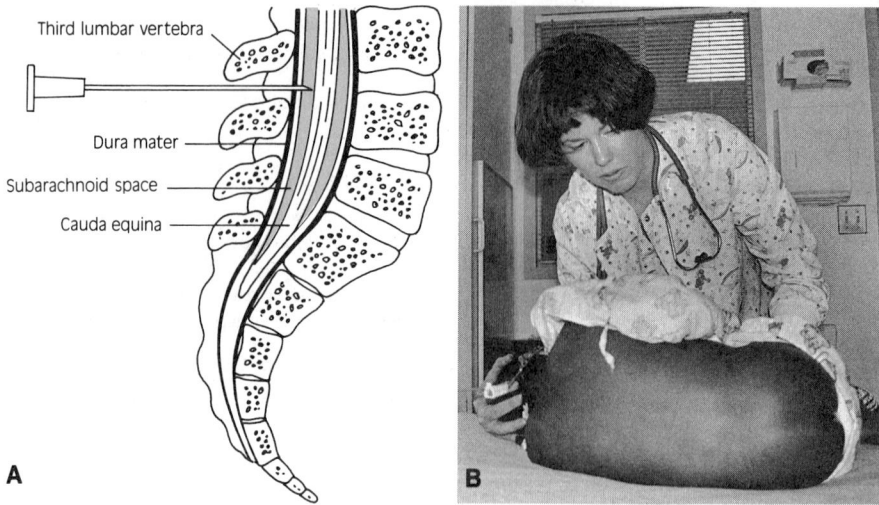

FIGURE 52-4

Lumbar puncture test. (**A**) The lumbar puncture needle is inserted between the third and fourth lumbar vertebrae. (**B**) Positioning of the child for a lumbar puncture. (Photo by Kathy Sloane. Courtesy of Children's Hospital, Oakland, CA.)

Contraindications

Contraindicated with severely increased intracranial pressure.

Preparation

Children and parents should have the procedure explained at their level of understanding. The child, toddler, or infant is placed in a side-lying position with both the knees and head flexed, and the head touching the chest. This position causes the back to bow out (see Fig. 52-4C) and opens the lumbar vertebral spaces. The child should be given constant verbal reassurance and support.

Developmental Considerations

Infants or neonates may be held in a sitting position on the examining table or a parent's lap.

Nursing Care

Some pain may be experienced when the needle is inserted. The nurse is responsible for positioning the child with the head and knees flexed towards the chest while lying on one side. While facing the child, grasp the back of the child's head with one hand and encircle the knees from behind with the other arm so that the child is held securely with the back in a bowed position. Observe for tolerance of the procedure and provide constant verbal support. Label and number the CSF tubes in the order they were collected.

Following the procedure keep the child flat. Loss of CSF associated with the procedure puts pressure on the cerebral veins should the child's head be lifted. This elevation of the head can cause a subdural hematoma and at the very least a severe headache. Encourage fluids to replace lost CSF, and provide for therapeutic play. A lumbar punction can be a traumatic procedure for a child.

Complications

Subdural hemorrhage, meningitis, and headaches are potential complications.

Ventricular or Subdural Tap

Description/Definition

A needle is inserted through the infant's anterior fontanelle into the subdural space (subdural tap) or through the brain tissue to the lateral ventrical. If the fontanelle is closed, a craniotomy is necessary. CSF pressure is measured, and samples of CSF are removed as in the lumbar tap for microscopic examination.

Purpose

Ventricular taps usually are performed to remove CSF from the ventricles for microscopic examination (see Lumbar Tap in this chapter) or to relieve and measure intracranial pressure. Subdural taps are used to remove fluid accumulations from subdural hematomas or effusions.

Indications

*   Increased intracranial pressure.
*   Meningitis or encephalitis.
*   Central nervous system hemorrhage.
*   Subdural hematoma or subdural effusion.

Contraindications

Extremely agitated infants may need to be sedated.

Preparation

Obtain consent to shave the hair over the fontanelle. During the procedure the infant is positioned supine with the top of the head facing the physician. The nurse may wrap a larger infant in a mummy restraint. The head must be held firmly throughout the procedure to prevent movement.

Developmental Considerations

Infants should have been fed more than 30 minutes prior to the procedure to enhance sleepiness if the infant can tolerate oral feedings. A pacifier may be helpful in calming some infants, but some infants may be too distressed to draw comfort from the pacifier.

Nursing Care

It is imperative that the infant be kept perfectly still while the needle is inside the skull. Care must be taken to label and number CSF collection tubes sequentially. Following the procedure a pressure bandage is applied to the site, and the infant should rest in an infant seat or in a semiupright position to reduce leakage from the tap site. Observe for leakage of CSF from the site of the puncture. Observe closely for signs of fever, headache, or increased intracranial pressure (described in detail in Chap. 53). Older children may benefit from therapeutic play following the procedure.

TABLE 52-5
Selected Nursing Diagnoses Associated With Altered Neurologic Function

Data Analysis and Conclusion	Nursing Diagnosis
Health Perception and Health Management	
Mental retardation	
Developmental lag; demonstrated lack of understanding of personal hygiene; observed inability to take responsibilities	Altered Health Maintenance related to lack of ability to make deliberate and thoughtful judgments
Frequent seizures	High Risk for Injury related to episodic seizures
Unsuccessful medication regimen	
Socially and physically active child; unrealistic view of risk	
Nutrition and Metabolism	
Comatose	Altered Nutrition: Less Than Body Requirements related to inability to ingest food
Poor muscle tone	
Spinal injury; immobility	
Areas of redness; skin breakdown, poor skin turgor	Impaired Skin Integrity related to physical immobility
Elimination	
Paralysis; abdominal distention; hard stools; infrequent passage; headache; appetite impairment	Constipation related to immobility
Spinal injury; incontinence; no urge to void or feelings of bladder fullness	Reflex Incontinence related to neurologic impairment
Mental retardation; incontinence; nocturia; no toilet training	Altered Urinary Elimination related to mental disabilities
Activity and Exercise	
Decreased strength; inability to get to toilet; severe pain; inability to undress; inability to carry out proper toileting hygiene	Toileting Self-Care Deficit related to neuromuscular impairment
Inability to move on the bed; inability to transfer and ambulate; limited range of motion; imposed restrictions of movement	Impaired Physical Mobility related to neuromuscular impairment
Fatigue; dyspnea; increased pulse rate; inability to attend school; inability to walk far; decreased physical activities	Activity Intolerance related to physiologic defect
Sleep and Rest	
Agitation; frequent awakenings during night; lack of sleep; verbal complaint of interrupted sleep; nightmares; increasing lethargy and listlessness; yawning; lack of concentration	Sleep Pattern Disturbance related to interrupted sleep
Cognition and Perception	
Verbal report of pain; facial grimacing; guarding; self-focusing; sweating; restlessness; crying	Pain related to injury
Inappropriate or absent speech response; decreased auditory comprehension; confusion; inattention to noises; slurring speech	Impaired Verbal Communication related to change in level of consciousness
Memory deficit; inaccurate interpretation of environment; distractability	Altered Thought Processes related to change in level of consciousness
Disorientation; inaccurate interpretation of environmental stimuli; hallucinations; impaired communication; lethargy; comatose; altered behavior	Sensory/Perceptual Alterations related to changes in level of consciousness
Verbalized uncertainty about choices; verbalization of undesired alternative actions; delayed decision making; distress	Decisional Conflict related to care of child with microcephaly
Self-Perception and Self-Concept	
Facial expression of fear; verbal expression of fear; child withdraws and becomes quiet; crying or whimpering	Fear related to frequent tests and treatment
Periodic trips to hospital for treatment; restlessness; apprehension; facial tension; clinging to parents; crying and whining	Anxiety related to separation from parents
Verbalization of lack of control of situation and future; depression about condition; noncompliance in monitoring progress; alienation from others; anger	Powerlessness related to chronic condition
Spinal cord injury; verbal expression of impairment; withdrawal from family and friends; negative feelings about body; preoccupation with injury; verbal expression of hopelessness	Body Image Disturbance related to neuromuscular impairment

(Continued)

TABLE 52-5
(Continued)

Data Analysis and Conclusions	Nursing Diagnosis
Roles and Relationships	
Verbalizes concerns about other family members; anger; fear; anxiety; alienation from professional caregivers	Parental Role Conflict related to interruption of family life caused by child's hospitalization
Inability to attend school; confined to hospital room; withdrawal; no eye contact; depression; regression; infrequency of family visits	Social Isolation related to hospitalization
Sexuality and Reproduction	
Spinal cord injury; verbal expression of concerns; knowledge deficits about alternatives; impaired social relationships	Altered Sexuality Patterns related to neuromuscular disabilities
Coping and Stress Tolerance	
Anger taken out on health care workers; withdrawal; inability to meet basic needs; inability to problem solve; inappropriate use of defense mechanisms; regression	Ineffective Individual Coping related to lack of maturity in handling situation
Denial of change of health status; inability to become involved in problem solving and goal setting; anger; lack of effort to move toward independence	Impaired Adjustment related to disability requiring change in lifestyle

Complications

Cerebral tissue injury or meningeal lacerations may result from movement of the needle during the tap. Keeping the infant still is essential. Meningitis or encephalitis is rare but possible.

Selected Nursing Diagnoses

After obtaining the history, performing the physical examination, reviewing results from the diagnostic tests, and tapping additional resources for information, the nurse carefully analyzes data obtained.[6] Selected nursing diagnoses that may be appropriate for the child with neurologic dysfunction are presented by function in Table 52-5.

Summary

A complete neurologic examination is performed only when there is reason to believe that a child has an unidentified neurologic problem. It is a lengthy, detailed, and time-consuming assessment. Most neurologic disorders are hereditary, so a detailed family history is crucial. Neurologic test tasks can be developed into games and play. Soft signs are a group of minor neurologic aspects of both gross and fine motor control, coordination, behavior, and sensation. Soft signs are of particular value in assessing children with school problems. A systematic neurologic assessment should be used for general or mental and emotional health, head and neck, cranial nerves, motor and sensory responses, and reflexes.

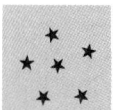

Ideas for Nursing Research

Much work is needed to standardize nursing diagnoses most commonly used in neurologic nursing. Research is needed to correlate neurologic soft signs with school problems. Nursing needs to develop more sensitive assessment tools for detecting subtle signs of neurologic difficulty, such as those displayed by children who were very premature. This could be helpful in primary intervention for subtle developmental or learning problems. The following areas need to be explored:

- Short standardized neurologic screening examinations related to nursing diagnoses.
- Standardized essential history information for nursing diagnoses in neurologic dysfunction
- Relationship between subtle signs of neurologic difficulty in premature infants and later learning disability.
- Impact/interaction of drugs on normal and impaired neurologic function.

References

1. Slota, M. C. (1983). Pediatric neurological assessment. *Critical Care Nursing, 3*(6), 106–112.
2. Lord-Feroli, K., & Maguire-McGinty, M. (1985). Toward a more objective approach to pupil assessment. *Journal of Neurosurgical Nursing, 17*(5), 309–312.
3. Borg, E., Spens, K., Tonnquist, I., & Rosen, S. (1987). Brain map: New possibilities in diagnosis of central auditory disorders? *Acta Oto-Laryngologica (Stockholm), 103,* 612 617.
4. Ellison, P., Heimler, R., & Franklin, S. (1987). The relationship of transcephalic impedance, head growth and caloric intake to outcome in preterm infants. *Acta Paediatrica Scandinavica, 73,* 820.
5. Ellison, P., & Evers, J. (1981). Trancephalic impedance in the neonate: An indicator of intracranial hemorrhage, asphyxia and delayed maturation. *Journal of Pediatrics, 98,* 968–971.
6. Standards Committee of the American Association of Neuroscience Nurses. (1984). *Journal of Neurosurgical Nursing, 16*(2), 117–120.

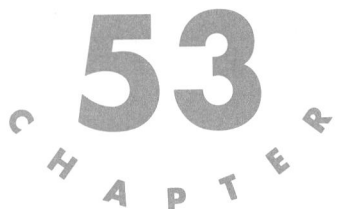

53

C H A P T E R

Nursing Planning, Intervention, and Evaluation for Altered Neurologic Function

BEHAVIORAL OBJECTIVES

Describe the major congenital anomalies affecting the central nervous system.

Discuss the impact of central nervous system injuries.

Discuss increased intracranial pressure in relationship to various types of head injuries.

Discuss nursing implications for spinal cord injuries.

Describe nursing implications for common neurologic infections.

Describe care provided for children with seizure disorders.

Discuss nursing implications for common functional disabilities of the central nervous system.

List nursing diagnoses commonly applied to children with neurologic dysfunction.

Nursing care for disorders of neurologic function is among the most exacting and taxing of all forms of nursing care. Precise assessment and monitoring of all systems is required because even minute changes may signal catastrophic deterioration of the child's condition.

Parents are fearful for their child's life and are concerned about possible permanent disabilities. Parents of children with visible physical alterations in neurologic function will be concerned about the social stigma of having a child with a visible imperfection. Often parents must deal with guilt feelings that they should have been able to prevent this condition for their child, and they are anxious about the child's welfare.

Parents' emotional distress is communicated to the child and may cause an increase in the child's anxiety. This anxiety consumes energy that might otherwise be devoted to healing and may prolong or exacerbate the child's condition. Therefore, it is critical for the nurse to be aware of parents' distress and intervene to allay

1353

anxiety, guilt, and despair. The parents' perception of the child's condition and potential outcome has a direct impact on the progress of the child's recovery.

The family of a child with a neurologic dysfunction may need support from an organization specific to the child's needs. One of the responsibilities of the nurse is to guide the family to such an organization. Resources for children and families with altered neurologic function are listed in the accompanying display.

Congenital Anomalies of the Central Nervous System

Faulty closure of the bony prominences or neural tube of the central nervous system (CNS) can result in mild defects, such as spina bifida occulta, or severe defects, such as anencephaly, which is incompatible with life. During the third and fourth week of prenatal development the critical formation of the neural tube takes place.

The overall incidence of neural tube defects is 1 per 1000 live births in the United States, but the estimates vary geographically.[21] When a woman gives birth to a child with a neural tube defect, the risk of occurrence in subsequent pregnancies increases to 2% to 5%. For families with two affected children the recurrence risk is 6% to 10%.[7] Therefore, genetic counseling may be helpful to the family if more children are desired.

Many neural tube alterations are apparent at birth or shortly thereafter. These include anencephaly, microcephaly, hydrocephalus, encephalocele, and spina bifida. The etiology for the majority of these alterations is thought to be genetic predisposition accompanied or triggered by environmental factors, such as maternal infections or drug ingestion.

Congenital anomalies or abnormalities of the CNS usually are obvious at birth or shortly thereafter. Intelligence and "normal" appearance are highly valued attributes in American society, so the birth of a child at risk for these features increases the parents' grief reaction to the loss of their imagined "perfect child." Mental retardation accompanies some congenital abnormalities, and parents often worry about their child's intelligence potential. Early recognition of congenital anomalies enables early intervention to maximize the child's potential development. Parents need reassurance immediately and frequently about their child's prognosis and the possibility of mental retardation.

Parents of children with anomalies will experience all phases of grief for their loss of the "perfect" child they had anticipated. Their first response to the diagnosis may be "Why me?" or "What did I do to deserve this?" They may also experience anticipatory grieving for the death of their child. This grieving is discussed in Chapters 20 and 21. Grieving in death is discussed in Chapter 32.

Anencephaly and Microcephaly

Anencephaly is the absence of the entire brain or at least both cerebral hemispheres. The cause of anencephaly is unknown, and the incidence varies from 1 to 5 per 1000 live births. The malformation occurs more frequently in girls than in boys and is more common in white children. The true incidence may be difficult to determine because of the high rate of spontaneous abortions of affected fetuses in early pregnancy. Complete anencephaly is incompatible with life; however, some infants may survive for a few days if enough brainstem tissue is present to support extrauterine life. The brain tissue that is present is frequently exposed because the skull is also defective.[18]

Microcephaly (a small head) is a rare condition that is characterized by a small skull, mental retardation, and inadequate or interrupted brain growth. Microcephaly is diagnosed in infants whose head circumference is at least 1 cm less than the chest circumference 3 days after birth. The head circumference at 6 months of age is 33 cm or less. Microcephaly may result from recessive genetic disorders, uterine infections such as rubella or cytomegalic inclusion disease, maternal phenylketonuria, or maternal alcoholism.[18]

Children with microcephaly have a long, narrow, receding forehead; a small cranium; and a flat occiput. The fontanels are either small or closed. Because brain growth is subnormal, the head is disproportionately small when compared to the rest of the body. The degree of neurologic abnormality and mental retardation varies from mild to severe. There is no known treatment for microcephaly.

Diagnostic Studies. Neural tube defects can be detected prenatally by examining the mother's blood serum between the 16th and 20th weeks of pregnancy. If the serum level of alpha-fetoprotein (AFP) is elevated, an amniocentesis should be performed to confirm the diagnosis. An amniocentesis can detect anencephaly with 90% certainty. Closed defects (spina bifida occulta) are covered by skin. Because this type of lesion has no opening to allow communication with amniotic fluid, the AFP level does not rise. Ultrasound examination *in utero* also is helpful for detecting neural tube disorders. Once the diagnosis of a neural tube defect is confirmed, the parents must decide whether they wish to have an abortion or carry the infant to term.

★ **NURSING INTERVENTIONS: COLLABORATIVE AND INDEPENDENT**

Because there is no medical treatment associated with anencephaly and microcephaly, both of which usually are apparent at birth, nursing management primarily consists of parental support for the parents' disappointment, grief, and loss. Seeing the baby frequently helps parents come to terms with reality and facilitates coping. The primary nursing diagnoses follow:

- High Risk for Infection related to exposed brain tissue.
- Dysfunctional Grieving related to the loss of the anticipated "perfect child."
- Anticipatory Grieving related to probable death of the infant.

The major objective of care is to promote the highest level of development possible for the microcephalic child. The degree of mental retardation or neurologic abnormalities is not known at birth, and these infants re-

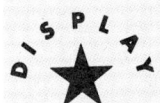

Resources for Children and Families With Altered Neurologic Function

Family Support

Epilepsy Foundation of America
4351 Garden City Drive
Landover, MD 20785

The Exceptional Parent (magazine for parents of
   children with disabilities)
605 Commonwealth Avenue
Boston, MA 02215

Guillain-Barré Syndrome Support Group
P.O. Box 262
Wynnewood, PA 19096

March of Dimes Birth Defects Foundation
1275 Mamaroneck Avenue
White Plains, NY 10605

National Association of Mothers of Special Children
9079 Arrowhead Court
Cincinnati, OH 45231

National Easter Seal Society
70 East Lake Street
Chicago, IL 60601

National Head Injury Foundation
333 Turnpike Road
Southboro, MA 01772

The National Tay-Sachs & Allied Diseases Association
385 Elliott Street
Newton, MA 02164

Spina Bifida Association of America
1700 Rockville Pike, Suite 540
Rockville, MD 20852

United Cerebral Palsy Association, Inc.
66 East 34th Street
New York, NY 10016

Pediatric Rehabilitation

National Head Injury Foundation
333 Turnpike Road
Southboro, MA 01771

National Spinal Cord Injury Association
149 California Street
Newton, MA 02158

National Spinal Cord Injury Hotline
National Study Center for Emergency Medical Service
22 South Greene Street
Baltimore, MD 21201

American Spinal Injury Association
250 East Superior Street, Room 619
Chicago, IL 60611

National Rehabilitation Information Center
Catholic University of America
447 Eighth Street, NE
Washington, DC 20017

National Information & Referral Service
P.O. Box 4008
Austin, TX 78765

Children's Defense Fund
1520 New Hampshire Avenue, NW
Washington, DC 20036

National Center for Law and the Handicapped
P.O. Box 477
University of Notre Dame
Notre Dame, IN 46556

National Information Center for Handicapped Children
   and Youth
P.O. Box 1492
Washington, DC 20013

National Institute for Handicapped Research
Mail Stop 2305
Office of Special Education and Rehabilitation Services
Washington, DC 20202

National Institute of Neurological and Communicative
   Disorders and Stroke
Building 31, Room 8A 06
National Institutes of Health
Bethesda, MD 20205

Commission on Accreditation of Rehabilitation Facilities
2500 North Pantano Road
Tucson, AR 85715

Special Olympics
1701 K Street, NW
Suite 203
Washington, DC 20202

National Rehabilitation Association
633 South Washington Street
Alexandria, VA 22314

American Physical Therapy Association
1156 15th Street, NW
Suite 500
Washington, DC 2005

American Occupational Therapy Association
1383 Piccard Drive
Rockville, MD 20850

Nursing Organizations

American Trauma Society
Trauma Coordinators Subcommittee
1400 Mercantile Lane, Suite 188
Landover, MD 20785

Society of Trauma Nurses
Suite 1000
888 17th Street, NW
Washington, DC 20006

Association of Rehabilitation Nurses
2506 Gross Point Road
Evanston, IL 60201

quire frequent assessment and follow-up. Parents will need emotional support as they grieve for the loss of their anticipated "perfect child" and develop a positive attitude toward their infant. In all other respects the newborn infant should receive the standard nursing care. A multidisciplinary approach with continued family support regarding the child's care and education is important.

Hydrocephalus

Definition and Incidence. *Hydrocephalus* is an abnormal accumulation of cerebrospinal fluid (CSF) in the brain resulting from an obstruction of circulation of CSF through the ventricles, interference with the absorption of the CSF from the subarachnoid space, and occasionally excessive production of fluid by the choroic plexus. Although the word hydrocephalus (Greek) literally means water on the brain, increased intracranial pressure (ICP) also must be present for the condition to be pathologic. Congenital hydrocephalus is estimated to occur in 3 or 4 of every 1000 births.[14]

Etiology and Pathophysiology. Congenital hydrocephalus can result from intrauterine infections, including rubella, cytomegaloviruses, toxoplasmosis, and syphilis. Hydrocephalus may be classified as either communicating or noncommunicating, depending on whether CSF circulates or communicates from the lateral ventricles in the center of the brain where it is made to the outside of the brain (subarachnoid space) where it is absorbed. The circled areas in Figure 53-1 represent small passages that can easily become obstructed: foramen of Monroe (interventricular), aqueduct of Sylvius, foramen of Luschka and foramen of Magendie, and the arachnoid villi.

Noncommunicating hydrocephalus (obstructive or internal) is due to a blockage that prevents CSF flow to the subarachnoid space where it can be absorbed. See the accompanying display on types of noncommunicating hydrocephalus.

Communicating hydrocephalus results from an excessive production of CSF flowing to the subarachnoid space or an inability of the villi to absorb it. The obstruction to the villi's absorption of CSF occurs more often as a complication of CNS infections or head injuries than as a congenital anomaly. This form of hydrocephalus may be secondary to fibrous tissue formation in the arachnoid villi caused by hemorrhage or infection.

Acquired hydrocephalus is most commonly caused by infections of the CNS, such as bacterial meningitis. Other causes include tumors, ruptured aneurysms, cranial arteriovenous malformations, cerebral trauma, and systemic bleeding disorders, which produce an inflammatory response and eventual fibrosis of the subarachnoid villi. Intracranial hemorrhage in a preterm infant frequently results in the development of hydrocephalus.

The pathophysiology consists of continued production of CSF that either cannot flow out of the ventricles or cannot be reabsorbed at a rate to keep pace with production. (Enough CSF is normally produced to replace the entire volume three times every 24 hours.) Obstruction causes the CSF to accumulate, ICP to increase, brain

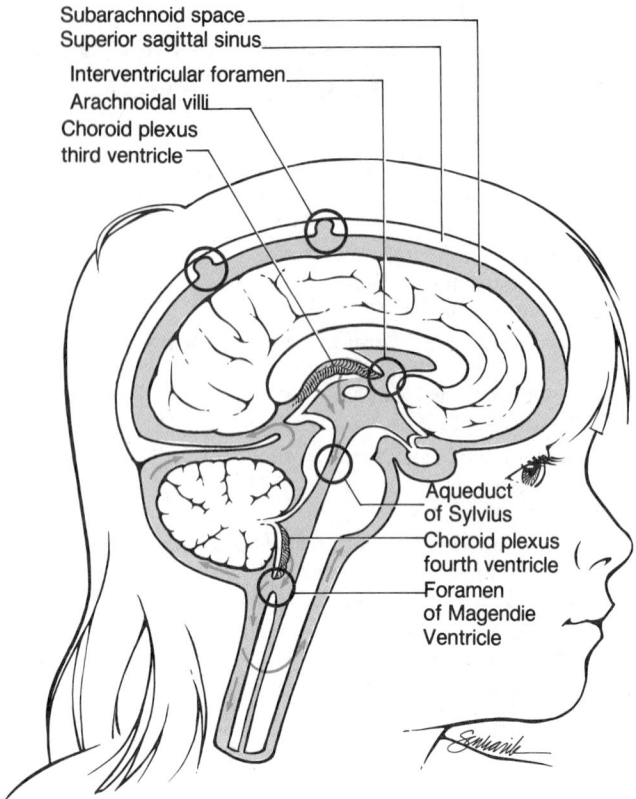

FIGURE 53-1
Circulation of cerebrospinal fluid and potential obstruction sites.

tissue to be displaced, and ultimately brain tissue to be destroyed (see Increased Intracranial Pressure section later in this chapter).

Clinical Manifestations. The most prominent sign of hydrocephalus in infancy is the enlargement of the head before the cranial sutures have fused. In older infants and children neurologic signs frequently are the result of increased ICP. Increased ICP and subsequent dilation of the ventricles produce similar findings in all children with hydrocephalus independent of the primary cause.

Rapidly progressing hydrocephalus produces symptoms very early as ventricular dilation occurs. Nonspecific symptoms include headaches that vary in intensity, location, and duration; lethargy; drowsiness; nausea; vomiting; loss of appetite; and diplopia. Changes in vital signs include bradycardia, hypertension, and altered respiratory patterns and rates. These nonspecific symptoms are most frequently the result of increased ICP and are discussed in more detail in a later section in this chapter.

Significant dilation of the ventricles must take place before abnormal enlargement of the head is evident. In young infants an abnormal frontal skull contour may develop. This is called frontal bossing and is characterized by a prominent forehead. The scalp veins become dilated and prominent. Upward gaze may be impaired due to midbrain pressure. The sclerae above the irises frequently are visible; this is a diagnostic sign called the *setting sun*, as shown in Figure 53-2*A*. Bulging fontanels may be present without noticeable head enlargement. Lower-extremity spasticity may develop as fibers from the cortical motor areas are stretched.

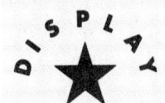

Types of Noncommunicating Hydrocephalus

Arnold-Chiari Malformation: Congenital malformation of the brainstem, cerebellum, and fourth ventricle that is displaced into the foramen magnum or upper cervical canal. If the cerebrospinal fluid (CSF) flow from the fourth ventricle is not obstructed by this displacement, it is classified as communicating rather than noncommunicating hydrocephalus.

Chiara II Malformation: Congenital malformation of the medulla oblongata, cerebellum, and fourth ventricle that causes obstruction of the foramen of Magendie and foramen of Luschka. Often associated with myelomeningocele.[12]

Dandy-Walker Malformation: Congenital atresia of the foramen of the fourth ventricle (Luschka and Magendie), resulting in an enlarged ventricle.

Stenosis of the Aqueduct of Sylvius: Congenital malformation creating blind forks (deadened passages) or acquired narrowing of the passage connecting the third and fourth ventricles. Hemorrhage associated with trauma or inflammation of the narrow passage associated with infection may lead to adhesions or gliosis.

Tumors or hematomas may obstruct the flow of CSF out of the foramina of Luschka and Magendie.

If hydrocephalus progresses, development of lower brainstem functions may be disrupted. Difficulties in sucking and feeding become evident along with the presence of a shrill, high-pitched cry. If untreated, the skull continues to enlarge because of the increased pressure; the cortex is destroyed, and mental retardation may result.

Diagnostic Studies. During infancy increases in head circumference faster than the normal rate indicate a need for further diagnostic evaluation. Routine daily head circumference should be monitored in infants with suspected hydrocephalus, myelomeningocele, and intracranial infections.

Abnormal transillumination may be observed in children younger than 2 years if the cranium is thin and the ventricles are moderately enlarged. Transillumination consists of wrapping the end of a flashlight with soft, black rubber. The infant is taken into a completely dark room and the flashlight is placed against the infant's skull (see Fig. 53-2B). The width of the red illumination from the edge of the flashlight collar to the edge of the red illumination is measured on each side of the occiput, the parietal bones, and the frontal bone. The occipital measurements should be the smallest, and the frontal should be the largest. Frontal bone transillumination in the newborn averages 1 cm or less, and there should be minimal or no transillumination in the occipital area. Asymmetrical transillumination suggests brain anomalies.[10]

Computerized tomography (CT) permits visualization of specific brain tissue and CSF-filled spaces and greatly facilitates evaluation. Examination of CSF should be considered to rule out occult infections that may be responsible for the development of hydrocephalus. CSF circulation and obstructions can sometimes be visualized

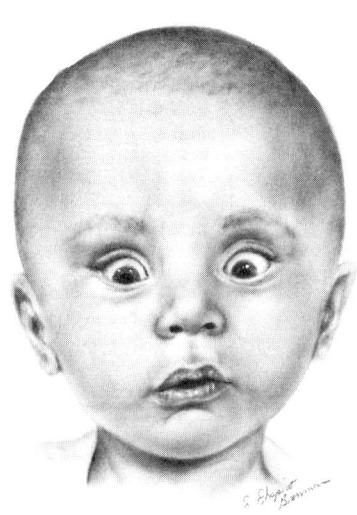

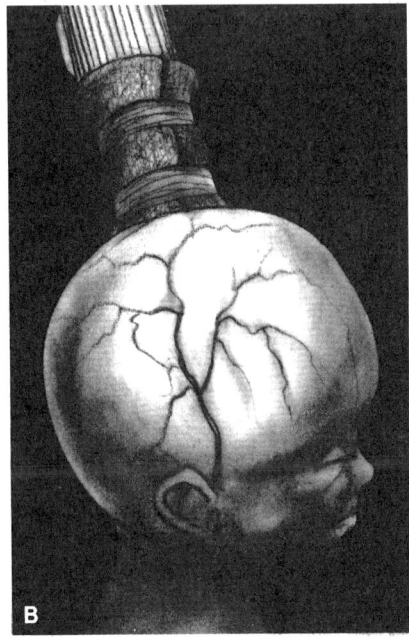

FIGURE 53-2
Hydrocephaly. (**A**) The eyes are deviated downward, revealing the upper scleras and creating the "setting sun" sign. (Redrawn from Paine, R. S. [1960]. Neurological examination of infants and children. *Pediatric Clinics of North America, 7,* 476.) (**B**) Transillumination of the skull in advanced cases of hydrocephaly produces a glow of light over the entire cranium. (Source: Bates, B. [1991]. *A guide to physical examination and history taking.* [5th ed.]. Philadelphia: J. B. Lippincott.)

A

B

by injecting dye into the lumbar subarachnoid space and obtaining serial CT scans to measure the flow of CSF. Other studies, such as angiography, radioisotope scanning, air encephalography, and echoencephalography, may be needed to diagnose hydrocephalus.

★ ASSESSMENT

Although hydrocephaly may be present at birth, generally it becomes apparent in the first few weeks of life. An infant with diagnosed or suspected hydrocephalus must be carefully observed for signs of increasing ICP (see Intracranial Pressure in this chapter). The infant's head is measured daily at the point of largest measurement—the occipitofrontal circumference. If possible, this measurement should be taken by the same individual to reduce the chance of discrepancies. Head circumference normally increases 2 cm each month for the first 3 months of life and 1 cm each month from 3 to 6 months. Increases in head circumference from 6 to 12 months of age average 1 cm/mo. Therefore, in full-term infants head growth should not exceed 0.5 cm/wk for the first 3 months. Head growth in critically ill premature infants may not exceed 0.25 cm/wk.[24]

Fontanels and suture lines should be gently palpated for size, tenseness, and separation. Suture lines with a separation greater than 5 mm suggest hydrocephalus. An infant whose anterior fontanel measures more than 5 cm laterally or anterior to posterior should be watched carefully for hydrocephalus. Vital signs and levels of consciousness need to be carefully and routinely assessed to detect changes reflecting deterioration. Difficulty feeding, irritability, and shrill, high-pitched crying should be noted and reported.

★ NURSING DIAGNOSES AND PLANNING

Based on the assessment data discussed previously and in the preceding chapter, the following nursing diagnoses may apply to the child with hydrocephalus:

- Dysfunctional Grieving related to the loss of the "perfect child."
- Pain related to pressure in the head.
- Visual Sensory/Perceptual Alterations related to sensitivity to stimuli.
- Altered Nutrition: Less Than Body Requirements related to feeding difficulties.
- High Risk for Injury related to shunt or incision.
- Anxiety related to knowledge deficit about hydrocephalus, its cause, and its treatment.

The nurse and parents together plan effective care based on the established nursing diagnoses. Several examples of expected outcomes follow:

- The parents discuss their disappointments with a less-than-perfect child.
- The parents state that they have contacted a support group.
- The parents demonstrate ease in handling the infant with enlarged head or shunt.
- The parents describe the medical reasons for regular follow-up.

The nurse plans for the daily care of the child based on physician's orders and nursing diagnoses. Some general nursing care goals may include the following:

- Irritability is kept to a minimum.
- Infant tolerates feeding.
- Infant remains infection free.
- Shunt operates as planned.

★ NURSING INTERVENTIONS: COLLABORATIVE AND INDEPENDENT

MEDICAL MANAGEMENT

Medical therapy designed to decrease CSF production has been used for infants and children who have slowly progressing hydrocephalus with few signs and symptoms. A pharmaceutical approach also has been used when the condition prohibits surgery. Pharmacologic agents that can be used to reduce the production of CSF include acetazolamide, digoxin, furosemide, and glycerol.[14,44] These agents usually are successful for relatively short periods of time and have not been as effective as surgical therapy.

SURGICAL MANAGEMENT

Surgical therapy is the most effective means of treating hydrocephalus. Several types of surgical intervention commonly are used. If there is a direct obstruction of CSF flow, such as a neoplasm, cyst, or hematoma, surgical therapy is aimed at removing the obstruction and restoring CSF flow. If CSF production is excessive, fluid production may be reduced by endoscopic choroid plexus extirpation (removal of a portion of the choroid plexus tissue). Plastic surgery ventriculostomy of the third or fourth ventricle may be performed to establish communication between the ventricle and the cisterna interpeduncularis.

The most widely used procedure and the treatment of choice for communicating hydrocephalus and infantile noncommunicating hydrocephalus is placement of a mechanical shunt system to circumvent the normal CSF pathways. A catheter is surgically placed into one of the lateral ventricles, usually the right, and is connected to a one-way valve system (Holter valve, Pudenz-Heyer-Schulte valve) that opens when the pressure in the ventricle exceeds a certain baseline value. As fluid drains from the ventricles and lowers the pressure, the valve closes and remains shut until the pressure rises again. The valve often is placed beneath the scalp in the postauricular area. The distal end of the valve is connected to a catheter that is placed in the right atrium of the heart (ventriculoatrial) or into the peritoneal cavity (ventriculoperitoneal). The latter is shown in Figure 53-3. Therefore, the fluid flows directly from the lateral ventricles back into the system circulation, bypassing the site of mechanical or functional obstruction in CSF absorption. If the shunt system becomes obstructed, kinked, or disconnected, symptoms will recur if the hydrocephalus is still active. Both types of shunts might require periodic revision as the child grows. Surgically placed shunt systems are not curative, but they do effectively treat the symptoms and stop progression of the ventricular dilation.[28]

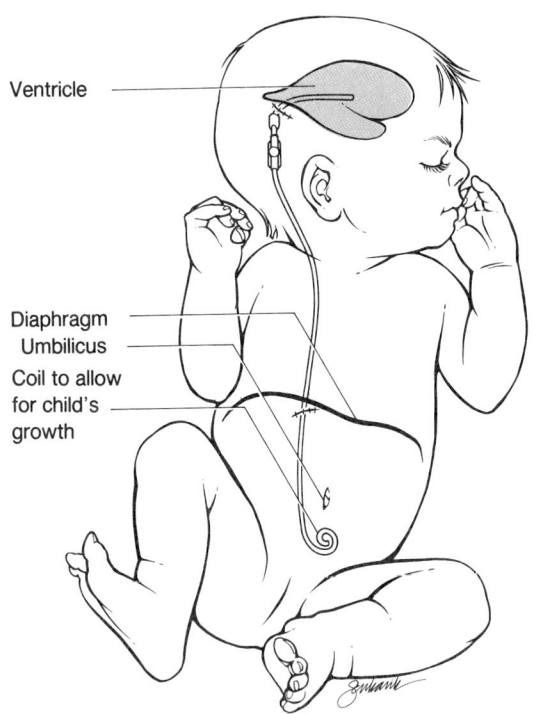

Ventricle

Diaphragm
Umbilicus

Coil to allow
for child's
growth

FIGURE 53-3
The most widely used treatment for hydrocephalus is a mechanical shunt. The ventriculoperitoneal shunt is illustrated here, but a ventriculoatrial shunt is used also.

PREOPERATIVE CARE

Preoperative nursing care of the child with hydrocephalus is supportive and assessment oriented. The child must be monitored for neurologic changes that may be indicate an increasing ICP (see Increased Intracranial Pressure in this chapter). Daily measuring and recording of the occipitofrontal circumference is mandatory because it indicates a worsening condition. The anterior fontanel must be palpated at least once each shift for size, tension, or bulging and the results recorded in the nurses' notes.

Frequently these children are irritable and lethargic and exhibit seizure activity. Pain and pressure in the head makes them extremely sensitive to stimuli. Noise and bright light should be kept to a minimum. Vital signs should be monitored frequently for widening pulse pressure and decreasing heart rate. Some physicians prefer the head of the bed to be elevated 30 degrees to assist with venous return and decrease ICP; others want it elevated no more than 15 degrees; some want the bed kept flat.

The infant may have difficulty tolerating feedings. Increased ICP may be accompanied by vomiting that is not associated with nausea. The infant may feel hungry and suck rapidly, only to vomit shortly thereafter. Small frequent feedings and frequent burping may help prevent vomiting and the subsequent dehydration. Placing the infant in a right side-lying position and elevating the head slightly after feeding also may decrease the incidence of vomiting. Care must be taken to support the large head and to prevent neck strain. Frequent rest periods between feedings and procedures must be provided. Stimulation should be kept to a minimum.

POSTOPERATIVE CARE

The primary concern of postoperative care is observation for the development of increased ICP (indicating that the shunt is not functioning properly) or too rapid drainage of CSF (a depressed fontanel), which may result in a subdural hematoma or brain herniation.

The infant or child should be positioned on the inoperative side to prevent pressure on the shunt valve. The head of the bed should be kept flat to help prevent rapid reduction of the intracranial fluid and subsequent subdural hemorrhage. Sedation should be avoided because it may mask important changes in the level of consciousness (LOC).

Nursing management also includes observing the child for possible shunt or incisional infection. Signs of local inflammation at the operative sites along with an elevated temperature, elevated white blood cell count, and behavioral changes, such as poor feeding and lethargy, should be recorded and reported immediately to the physician.

The family needs to understand the shunting procedure and requires education in preparation for discharge. Support groups can be extremely helpful in helping educate and prepare families for discharge. Commonly parents are afraid to handle these children because of the fear that they might harm or displace the shunt. The nurse must reassure them that normal activity and handling will not interfere with the shunt function.

Parents also need to understand the need for routine medical follow-up to determine shunt effectiveness. Furthermore, they need to be educated about signs and symptoms that require immediate medical evaluation. Family members are taught to observe the child for lethargy, headache, vomiting, fever, stiff neck, seizures, pupil changes, weakness, visual disturbances, and behavioral changes that need to be reported to the child's health care provider.

PARENTAL SUPPORT

Nursing care includes helping the parents accept the diagnosis and explaining the surgical procedure to them. If the child's head is markedly enlarged or the child displays neurologic deficits and symptoms of increased ICP, parents more readily accept the fact that something is wrong with the child. Because hydrocephalus is commonly diagnosed at birth, the grief and pain most parents face can make this an extremely difficult time. The nurse must identify sources of support for these parents and help them talk about their feelings and expectations.

★ EVALUATION

Periodically the nurse and family evaluate the outcomes of care. Examples of outcomes for the child and family with hydrocephalus were given under Nursing Diagnoses and Planning in this section. Have short-term goals been met? Are long-term goals still realistic? Planning for further nursing care takes into consideration complications.

COMPLICATIONS

Immediately following surgery, a rapid decrease in ICP can result in the cerebrum separating from the dura, rupturing small blood vessels, and causing a subdural hematoma. In an infant a markedly sunken fontanel, restlessness, or agitation may indicate too rapid decompression. Subdural hematomas more frequently occur in older children whose fontanels are closed and ventricles are greatly enlarged.

Shunt infections are relatively common and at times are accompanied by the development of ventriculitis. In case of infection, massive doses of antibiotics are administered intravenously or directly into the ventricles. If the infection cannot be eradicated by antibiotic therapy, the shunt will need to be surgically replaced. CSF can be withdrawn through the shunt reservoir to diagnose an infection.

LONG-TERM CARE

Hydrocephalus will arrest spontaneously in approximately 40% of children who exhibit near-normal intelligence. Untreated, hydrocephalus is associated with a 50% to 60% mortality rate. Even with surgical treatment, only about 33% are considered neurologically and intellectually normal.[4] The majority of children with treated hydrocephalus exhibit physical and developmental handicaps, such as ataxia, spastic diplegia, poor motor coordination, mental retardation, and perceptual disturbances.

Encephalocele

Definition and Incidence. An *encephalocele* is a herniation of brain tissue, the meninges, or both through a defect in the skull that produces a sac-like structure (Fig. 53-4). The most common site of this cranial cleft is the occipital area (about 75%), but they can occur anywhere. This malformation has an estimated incidence of 1 to 3 per 100,000 live births and therefore occurs less frequently than other neural tube defects.

Etiology and Pathophysiology. The exact cause of encephalocele formation is not known, although recessive inheritance factors and environmental influences may be implicated in some instances. If a simple hole exists in the cranium without protrusion of brain tissue, the defect is referred to as cranium bifidum occultum. The size of the encephalocele may range from a small protrusion to a large sac containing meninges and brain tissue. Encephaloceles rarely occur as a solitary malformation and frequently are associated with abnormalities of the cerebral hemispheres, cerebellum, and midbrain.[2]

Clinical Manifestations. The clinical findings are variable and depend in part on whether there are associated cerebral malformations, including hydrocephalus, and how much of the brain is displaced into the protruding sac. Lesions that are composed only of meninges have a good prognosis, and the infant may develop normally without motor or mental deficits. When the meninges, brain tissue, and CSF are involved, as in encephalomeningocele, brain damage is inevitable, and hydrocephalus, seizures, and mental retardation commonly occur. Other disabilities associated with this malformation include ataxia, spasticity, blindness, and impairment of eye

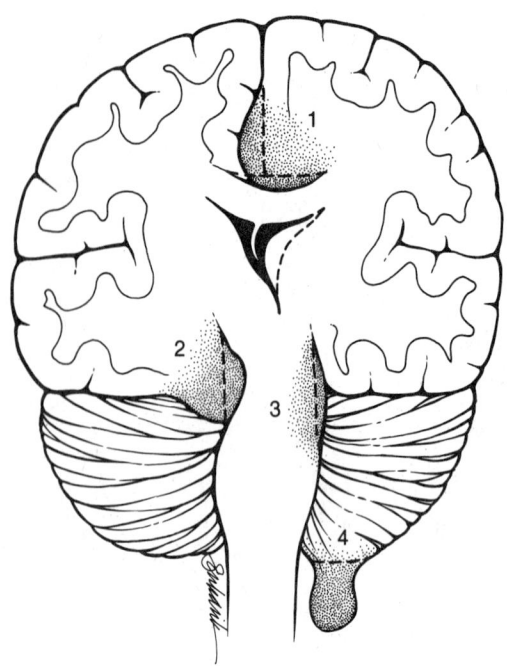

FIGURE 53-4
Brain herniation is a complication of primary head injuries. **1,** cingulate or across the falx; **2,** uncal (lateral transtentorial) herniation involves displacement of the medial portion of the temporal lobe across the tentorium into the posterior fossa; **3,** central (transtentorial) herniation involves downward displacement of the cerebral ventricles; and **4,** In Cerebellar herniation, the cerebellar tonsils move downward through the foramen magnum and compress the medulla.

movement. In severe cases of encephaloceles death before 1 year of age is not uncommon.

Diagnostic Studies. The diagnosis usually is apparent at birth. A CT scan is reasonably accurate in determining the contents of an encephalocele. Palpatation and transillumination may aid in the differential diagnosis.

★ ASSESSMENT

Nursing assessment data can aid in the diagnosis of encephalocele and are useful in determining the plan of care. Observation and notation of motor behaviors the infant demonstrates may be useful in determining the degree of neurologic involvement. Normal and abnormal reflexes need to be recorded as well as information concerning feeding difficulties. Because hydrocephalus and seizure activity commonly occur with this malformation, the nurse needs to be aware of the associated signs and symptoms and routinely assess the infant for these complications.

★ NURSING DIAGNOSES AND PLANNING

Nursing diagnoses depend, to some extent, on the degree of neurologic impairment. Based on assessment data discussed previously and in the preceding chapter, the following nursing diagnoses may apply to the family and child with an encephalocele:

- Impaired Skin Integrity related to surgical repair.

- High Risk for Infection related to possible rupture of herniated sac.
- Altered Nutrition: Less Than Body Requirements related to feeding difficulties.
- High Risk for Injury related to seizures.
- Dysfunctional Grieving related to the loss of the "perfect child."
- Anticipatory Grieving related to possible death of the infant.
- Altered Family Processes related to guilt or blame regarding origin of disability.
- Anxiety related to knowledge deficit about diagnosis, prognosis, surgical intervention, and home care.

The nurse and parents together plan effective care based on the established nursing diagnoses. Several examples of expected outcomes follow:

- The parents discuss their disappointments with a less-than-perfect child.
- The parents discuss their concern about the possibility of death of the infant.
- The parents communicate with each other their feelings concerning the infant.
- The parents describe the condition of the child and its ramifications for their family life.

The nurse plans for the daily care of the child based on physician's orders and nursing diagnoses. Some general nursing care goals may be the following:

- Skin care is maintained.
- Positioning prevents pressure on encephalocele.
- Nutrition is maintained.
- Assessments are made to prevent seizure complications.

★ NURSING INTERVENTIONS: COLLABORATIVE AND INDEPENDENT

SURGICAL MANAGEMENT

Treatment consists of surgical removal of the sac and closure of the defect depending on the severity of the defect. In the case of a severe defect with multiple associated complications, the decision may be made not to repair the encephalocele surgically. A decision not to close the defect is made if the infant has severe nerve and brain involvement with decreased chances of survival or if the parents decide not to have the defect repaired for financial reasons. Early closure is especially important if the sac does not have a good skin covering because of the increased likelihood of infection. A cranioplasty may need to be performed to repair a large cranial defect. If hydrocephalus is present or develops, a shunt may need to be inserted.

PREOPERATIVE CARE

Before surgery infants should be carefully positioned to prevent pressure being placed on the encephalocele. Such pressure can lead to rupture of the sac and subsequent decompression of the CSF (with resulting herniation of brain tissue) and possibly to infection. Pressure also may force CSF from the sac into the intracranial compartment causing an increased ICP. Vital signs, serial head circumference measurements, wound characteristics, signs of increased ICP, and motor responses need to be recorded, and abnormalities should be reported to the physician. Feeding problems commonly are present due to difficulty holding and positioning the child and an increased ICP (lethargy and poor sucking reflex). The optimum position for feeding is cradled in the nurse's arms with the meningocele protected. However, if this position is not feasible, the child may be fed in a side-lying position in the isolette. The head should be elevated slightly.

POSTOPERATIVE CARE

After surgery positioning is again important until the incision is healed. The child must be observed frequently for signs of increased ICP, vital signs, neurologic changes, pupillary changes, and behavior changes such as irritability and lethargy. Maintenance of bodily functions and meticulous skin care are primary nursing concerns. Prevention of infection is crucial.

★ EVALUATION

Periodically the nurse and family evaluate the outcomes of care. Examples of outcomes for the child and family with encephalocele were given under Nursing Diagnoses and Planning in this section.

Myelodysplasia

Definition and Incidence. The term *myelodysplasia* refers to a group of CNS disorders that occur during embryonic development and are characterized by malformations of the neural tube. Failure of the neural plate to close as it forms the neural tube during the first trimester of gestation results in spinal defects known as spina bifida occulta, meningocele, and myelomeningocele. *Spina bifida occulta* is a defect that results from incomplete closure of the vertebral laminae in which the meninges or neural tissue are not exposed at the skin surface (Fig. 53-5). *Meningocele* is a defect in which the meninges and CSF protrude through the vertebral defect forming a sac-like cyst. *Myelomeningocele* involves protrusion of the spinal cord nerve roots, meninges, and CSF through the vertebral defect. Most children diagnosed with meningoceles also have Arnold-Chiari malformations and hydrocephalus.[11]

The incidence of these malformations ranges from 1 to 5 per 1000 live births and is more common in girls. Women who have had one child born with such a defect have a 2% to 5% greater chance of having a subsequent child with a similar malformation. Two affected children in the same family increase the risk to between 10% and 15%.[39] Affected mothers have a 3% chance of having a child with a similar defect. The incidence varies with ethnic population and geographic sites, but the highest number of myelodysplasia cases are found in Great Britain.[21]

Pathophysiology. Spina bifida occulta must be present before meningocele and myelomeningocele lesions can occur. Spina bifida occulta most frequently occurs at the fifth lumbar or first sacral level but may be present at any point along the spinal canal. A meningocele

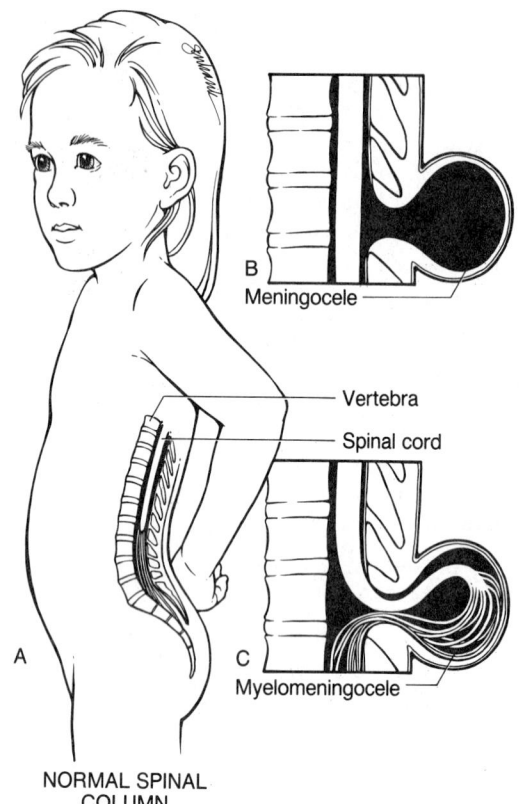

B
Meningocele

Vertebra

Spinal cord

A   C
Myelomeningocele

NORMAL SPINAL
COLUMN

FIGURE 53-5

Cross-section of a normal spine compared to a meningocele and myelomeningocele.

is a soft, cyst-like mass containing meninges and CSF; it is apparent at birth, most frequently in the lumbosacral or sacral area. The spinal nerve roots may be misplaced, but their function remains intact. When a myelomeningocele is present and spinal cord segments are involved in the cystic mass, the most prominent clinical manifestation is flaccid paralysis of the lower extremities. Because the lower motor and sensory neurons are damaged at and below the level of the defect, varying degrees of motor, sensory, reflex, and sphincter dysfunction are present.

Clinical Manifestations. Some cases of spina bifida occulta may go undetected throughout life. The condition frequently is benign and asymptomatic. External skin abnormalities, such as an overlying dimple, tuft of hair, or small nevus or hemangioma may be present.

Meningoceles can be as large as an orange or as small as a dime. They generally occur in the lumbar region and are soft, fluid-filled sacs covered with abnormal skin or meninges. Because no nervous tissue is involved, they frequently transilluminate (a light can be shone through them) clearly. Spinal nerve roots may be displaced; however, normal nerve function remains intact. Surgical repair is required to prevent infection. Hydrocephalus may be associated with or develop as a result of this condition.

A myelomeningocele is more severe than a meningocele because the spinal cord and nerve roots may stop at the level of the lesion. The sac may be as large as a grapefruit, and CSF frequently leaks through the thin membrane that covers it. Paralysis, sensory loss, and in-

continence of the bladder and bowel are common and are determined by the level of the lesion. The majority of children with a lumbar or lumbosacral myelomeningocele develop hydrocephalus, and 70% to 80% require treatment for the hydrocephalus.[11] The hydrocephalus results from embryonic malformations of the CSF circulation in the brain, most notably of the lower brainstem and cerebellum (Arnold-Chiari malformation). Functional motor disability is greatest with lesions at L3 and above.

Diagnostic Studies. A meningocele or myelomeningocele is obvious at birth. The degree of motor-sensory function can be assessed through a complete neurologic examination and careful observation. X-rays of the skull and entire spinal column frequently are used to rule out lesions or malformations not evident from the physical examination. Magnetic resonance imaging and ultrasound are useful in determining the presence and extent of hydrocephalus. Daily head circumference measurements and palpation of the fontanels also aid in monitoring the development of hydrocephalus. Cultures of spinal fluid and blood may be performed to monitor the development of infection.

★ ASSESSMENT

Myelodysplasia lesions other than spina bifida occulta have a sac-like protrusion that may contain meninges, CSF, a portion of the spinal cord, and nerve roots. It is important to assess whether the sac is leaking fluid. Motor and sensory functions need to be carefully assessed. With myelomeningocele little or no movement may be seen in the legs, hips, and feet. There also may be dribbling of urine and feces. Hydrocephalus also may be apparent. The degree and extent of neurologic deficit depends on the level of the myelomeningocele: The higher the lesion, the greater the deficit. Children with high lumbar or thoracic lesions frequently die before 10 years of age from infections.

★ NURSING DIAGNOSES AND PLANNING

Based on assessment data discussed previously and in the preceding chapter, the following nursing diagnoses may apply to the family and child with a myelodysplasia:

- High Risk for Infection related to exposed tissue.
- Bowel Incontinence related to neurologic impairment.
- Functional Urinary Incontinence related to neurologic impairment.
- High Risk for Impaired Skin Integrity related to incontinence.
- High Risk for Peripheral Neurovascular Dysfunction related to malformation.
- Impaired Physical Mobility related to limited position changes.
- Altered Health Maintenance related to lack of knowledge regarding care of child.
- Altered Role Performance related to an ill child.

Other parental diagnoses (Anticipatory Grieving, Dysfunctional Grieving, and Altered Family Processes) were discussed earlier in the chapter along with expected outcomes.

The nurse and child (or parents) together plan effective care based on the established nursing diagnoses. Several examples of expected outcomes follow:

- The parents perform range-of-motion exercises with child.
- The parents talk to the child while performing care.
- The parents provide tapes of family voices and sounds.

The nurse plans for the daily care of the child based on physician's orders and nursing diagnoses. Some general nursing care goals may be the following:

- Infant remains infection free.
- Bowel routine is established.
- Skin is kept clean and dry.

★ NURSING INTERVENTIONS: COLLABORATIVE AND INDEPENDENT

The goals of orthopedic management include promoting the child's mobility and preventing musculoskeletal deformity. The areas most often involved in treatment include the feet, knees, hips, and spine. Management techniques include the use of exercise, casts, braces, and surgical procedures on soft tissue and bone. Maintenance of good anatomic alignment is essential to provide functional posture and support. Ambulation is possible with the use of braces, walkers, and crutches.

Nursing care of the child with myelodysplasia involves acute care following birth and care during later hospitalizations. Lifelong health care frequently is required and is best achieved by a multidisciplinary team that consists of nurses, physicians, rehabilitation therapists, social workers, and psychologists. The child with myelodysplasia requires intensive nursing care both preoperatively and postoperatively.

MEDICAL MANAGEMENT

Careful monitoring and evaluation of the child's urinary tract and renal function are essential. Urologic evaluation is performed early with the goal of treatment to prevent urinary retention, infection, and renal damage. Periodic contrast radiography is essential to evaluate the status of the urinary tract because a normal urinary collecting system at an early age does not exclude the possibility of later deterioration. Periodic urine cultures also are required. Intermittent catheterization and medications can promote complete emptying of the bladder. Cholinergic agents may be used to treat a hypotonic bladder, while a hypertonic bladder may be treated with antispasmodics. Occasionally surgical diversion of the urinary tract (ureteroileostomy or ileal conduit) may be necessary when other measures fail to prevent urologic complications.

SURGICAL MANAGEMENT

Meningocele commonly is treated by surgical closure of the defect within 24 hours of birth. Early closure reduces the incidence of infection and damage to the spinal cord and nerve roots. Early closure also may enhance bonding because the infant will be easier to hold and care for after surgery. The child must be carefully observed for complications such as meningitis, hydrocephalus, and spinal cord dysfunction following surgery.

Surgical management of the child with myelomeningocele is more complex. Treatment begins at birth and continues throughout the child's life. Physicians may disagree about the most appropriate care for a child born with myelomeningocele. Frequently these children suffer from other severe defects along with infection and hydrocephalus. Some physicians recommend no surgical intervention, while others advocate repair of every defect. This decision-making process is extremely difficult for parents. Giving them as much information as possible and providing emotional support may help them make these difficult decisions.

Early closure of the myelomeningocele (within 48 hours) is advocated by most physicians, especially when the lesion is leaking fluid. This early treatment reduces the risk of infection and might prevent further neurologic impairment. However, some physicians advocate a late closure (between 1 week and 10 months) when the child is larger to reduce the risk of further nerve damage or to determine whether the child will survive the inevitable infections.

Skin grafting and multiple surgical procedures often are necessary to completely repair the defect. The presence of infection, hydrocephalus, and hemorrhage may require treatment prior to surgery. Antibiotics are administered before, during, and after surgery. The operative site must be protected from contamination and pressure; therefore, positioning of the child is important. Hydrocephalus may be present before surgical repair of the myelomeningocele, or it may develop postsurgically. A surgically placed ventricular shunt may be indicated to divert CSF and reduce ICP.

PREOPERATIVE CARE

Preoperative care of the meningeal sac is of utmost importance. The covering over the defect usually is very thin and fragile; therefore, the surface must be kept clean and protected. Topical antibiotics and moist saline dressing may be prescribed. If the sac is open, sterile dressings must be maintained. The infant should be kept prone with the head turned to the side to protect the sac. The use of a Bradford frame or small rolls and sandbags may facilitate proper positioning. The infant's hips should remain abducted with a pad to prevent dislocation, and the feet are kept in a neutral position with a small roll under the ankles. Bowel dysfunction in the toddler and older child can be managed by dietary measures and a regular, timed bowel routine. Softeners and suppositories often are effective in such bowel programs.

Neurologic assessment includes observation of sensorimotor function (spontaneous movement, response to stimulation) and any changes that indicate neurologic deterioration. Elevated or subnormal temperature, irritability, pallor, vomiting, or nuchal rigidity (stiff neck) may be early signs of a meningeal infection. Because hydrocephalus is common, head circumference should be monitored at least daily, if not every 8 hours. Fontanels should be observed and palpated for size, tenseness, or bulging every 4 hours. Other signs of increased ICP are discussed under Clinical Manifestations.

Meticulous skin care also should be provided. Incontinence of urine and feces is common and represents a major threat of brain infection through the sac or incision. Diapers and clothing are not used, but pads are placed under the infant and changed frequently. The skin should be kept clean and dry, and the position should be changed every 1 or 2 hours. When the infant is positioned prone, the chin, cheeks, and tip of the nose should be assessed frequently for development of pressure sores. Side-lying positions, when permissible, place the hips in flexion and reduce arm use. A rolled blanket must be used to support the back in side-lying positions, and the lesion must be protected at all times.

Feeding may be routine depending on the plans for surgery. The infant should be held for feedings because this provides for needed position changes, facilitates feeding and burping, and provides the sensory stimulation and cuddling necessary for psychosocial development. Intake should be recorded accurately, and daily weight should be obtained.

POSTOPERATIVE CARE

Following surgery, the nurse should observe the infant's vital signs, neurologic signs, and elimination. The nurse also should look for the development of hydrocephalus and infection in the surgical area. Head circumference, fontanel presentation, and behavioral changes should be recorded and reported to the physician.

The prone position also is the most common position used following surgery. Again, diapers and clothing should not be used until the incision is well healed. Range-of-motion exercises should be instituted when permissible. Parents may be taught these exercises and included in the plan of care to enhance their feeling of active involvement in their child's care.

SENSORY STIMULATION

Visual and auditory stimulation are required to maintain the child's development level. Brightly colored objects and pictures should be placed within the child's visual field. These should be changed frequently so that they continue to provide stimulation. Talking to the infant while providing care, music boxes, recordings of family voices, and radios are useful forms of auditory stimulation.

PSYCHOSOCIAL SUPPORT

The nurse can promote bonding between parents and child. Parents should be encouraged to stroke and speak to their child. A sitting position near the baby's head will help encourage eye contact. Participation in the child's care should be encouraged when possible. The parents should be taught how to feed, exercise, hold, and comfort the baby whenever the infant's condition permits.

DISCHARGE PLANNING

Before discharge the family will need information regarding skin care, range-of-motion exercises, bowel and bladder programs, shunt function if one was placed, signs of hydrocephalus, and general methods of care. Because this information can be overwhelming, parents need to be assured of their ability to care for their child. They also need to know where to get assistance when needed. Community health nurses, the myelodysplasia team or clinic, community support groups, and the Spina Bifida Association of America can provide resources, educational materials, and emotional support to families.

Anticipatory guidance regarding future hospitalizations for shunt revisions and orthopedic care needs to be provided. The need for periodic clinic or physician contact should be stressed and an explanation of routine tests provided.

★ EVALUATION

Periodically the nurse and family evaluate the outcomes of care. Examples of outcomes for the child and family with myelodysplasia were given under Nursing Diagnoses and Planning in this section.

LONG-TERM CARE

As the child grows mobility training becomes important. Routine bowel and bladder programs need to be initiated by age 2. Parents will continue to require assistance and support as they guide their child toward a more independent lifestyle. Each developmental level presents specific issues or problems for the child and parents; however, continued nursing interventions will aid these families in the achievement of realistic goals.

Injuries Affecting the Central Nervous System

Accidents are the primary cause of CNS injuries (see Chap. 30). Both parents and child may experience guilt feelings concerning the accident. They may believe they could have prevented the injury. Children may recall admonitions against climbing the tree, skate boarding without a helmet, and so forth. They may overreact by becoming fearful of disobeying. The young child may believe the injury is punishment for wrongdoing. Children may be relieved to learn that these feelings are normal and that no one is blaming them. Unfortunately, some parents may blame the child or blame the other parent for not preventing the accident in an attempt to relieve or deny their own sense of guilt. In terms of long-range outcomes for the child, the nurse's treatment of the parents' and child's guilt feelings is as important as the critical life-saving interventions.

Central Nervous System (Head) Injuries

Damage to CNS tissue may range from concussion (transient loss of cerebral function or consciousness) to brain death. Blood, air, and pus are substances that are extremely caustic to brain tissue. Brain cells with direct exposure to any one these substances are destroyed. Children have a fat layer between their scalp and skull bones that cushions the impact of a blow and reduces the potential injury. The increased fragility of tissue and higher cerebral blood volume increase the risk of brain damage and hemorrhage.

Falls, accounting for 50% of head injuries in children, frequently occur when the child is playing; climbing trees, fences, furniture, and play equipment; and riding bicycles or tricycles. Motor vehicle accidents cause 25% of head injuries, with the child being injured as a passenger or struck by a vehicle as a pedestrian. The remaining 25% of head injuries occur from a variety of sources, including child abuse and battering; being struck on the head by an object such as a baseball or baseball bat; or running into a stationary object such as a car, wall, or door. As in all childhood accidents head injury occurs almost twice as often in boys compared to girls. The highest incidence of head injury occurs between the ages of 8 and 9 years with a secondary peak incidence in boys at 12 to 13 years.

When a head injury occurs the brain is subjected to acceleration, deceleration, or a combination of the two known as contrecoup injuries (Fig. 53-6). *Acceleration* injuries occur when the head remains stationary and is hit by a moving object. *Deceleration* injuries occur if the child's head is moving and hits a stationary object. In *contrecoup* injuries the side of the brain that was struck or the site of impact (*coup*) may not be the site of the greatest cerebral injury because the brain on the opposite side of the head is thrown against the skull and tends to rebound (contrecoup). This movement occurs because the brain floats freely in CSF, while the brainstem is stable. As the brain strikes the inner rough surface of the cranial vault, blood vessels, nerve tracts, brain tissue, and other structures are bruised and torn. Thus, a blow to the frontal

region can cause severe injury to the occipital area as a result of contrecoup injury (see Fig. 53-6). The vector of the force moving the brain within the skull causes shearing stresses along the interface between structures of different density. Gray matter of cell bodies may rapidly accelerate, while the white matter or axons tend to lag behind. The most serious effects of shearing forces frequently are in the area of the brainstem.

Increased Intracranial Pressure

Increased ICP is a clinical manifestation of head injuries that requires the most astute nursing observations for early detection and prevention of additional tissue damage.

Definition. *Increased ICP* can be defined as increased pressure exerted within the cranium. Normal ICP values vary between 0 and 10 mmHg, but the generally accepted measure of normal ICP is a value less than 15 mmHg. Normal ICP is a result of the balance between the fixed volume of the cranium and the volume of brain tissue, blood, and CSF (i.e., cranial volume = brain tissue + blood + CSF). Brain tissue accounts for approximately 80%, interstitial fluid approximately 10%, and blood approximately 10%. According to the Monro-Kellie doctrine, when the volume of brain tissue, blood, or CSF changes, the brain uses autoregulatory mechanisms to maintain homeostasis and keep ICP within normal range. When the balance of intracranial contents is disrupted or compensatory mechanisms are insufficient, increased ICP is the result.

Etiology and Pathophysiology. Causes of increased ICP differ according to the age of the child. The most common causes include trauma, tumors, hemorrhage, and CNS infections. Table 53-1 provides a summary of the common causes of ICP according to age.

The skull is considered a semiclosed container with a fixed volume. The intracranial volume includes brain tissue, CSF, and blood. For the ICP to remain constant, an increase in the volume of any of the intracranial contents must be accompanied by a decrease in the volume of the other contents. For example, in a patient with hy-

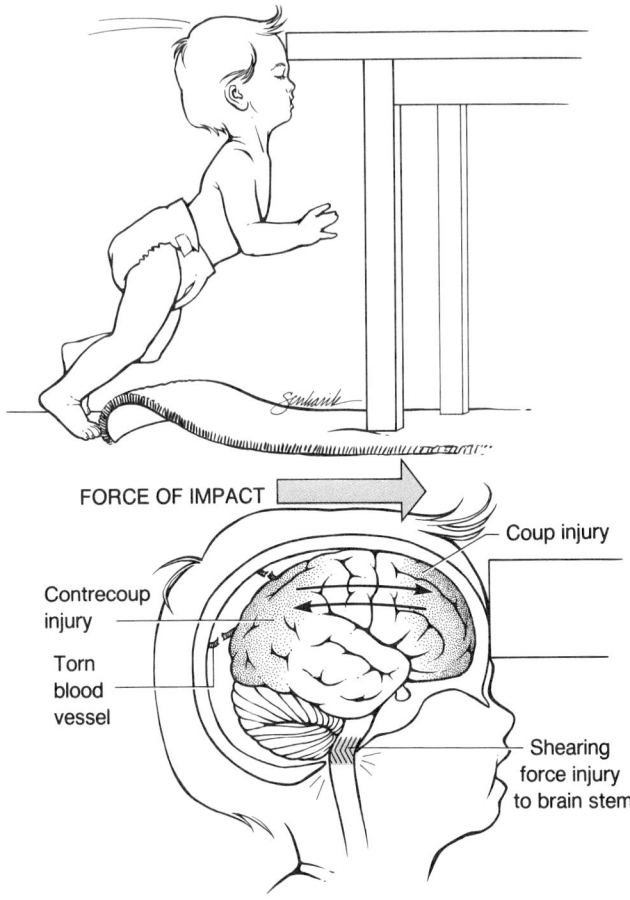

FIGURE 53-6
Example of a deceleration injury such as head striking windshield. (**A**) Original impact. (**B**) Shift in brain following impact that causes (**C**) rupture of veins supporting brain. (**D**) Illustration of shearing force. (**E**) Damage caused by movement of brain over rough bony skull prominences.

TABLE 53-1
Age-Related Causes of Increased Intracranial Pressure

Newborn	Infant and Preschooler	Older Child and Adolescent
Birth trauma	Brain tumors	Brain tumors
Hemorrhage	Central nervous system infections	Diabetic ketoacidosis
Hydrocephalus	Diabetic ketoacidosis	Guillain-Barré syndrome
Perinatal asphyxia	Head trauma	Head trauma
	Hydrocephalus	Vascular disorders
	Hypercapnia	
	Hypoxia	
	Reye's syndrome	

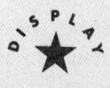

Common Volume Changes Associated With Increased Intracranial Pressure

Increased extracerebral volume
  Blood (epidural and subdural hematomas)
  Cerebrospinal fluid (CSF) (hydrocephalus)
  Effusion (subdural)
  Inflammatory exudate (empyema, purulent meningitis)
Increased intracerebral volume
  Blood: intravascular (increased cerebral perfusion), extravascular (hemorrhage)
  Edema: intracellular (cytotoxins), extracellular (vasogenic)
  Mass lesion (abscess, neoplasm, vascular malformation)
Increased intraventricular volume
  Blood (intraventricular hemorrhage)
  CSF (obstruction of flow, inflammatory exudate, or mass)

drocephalus, the excess CSF triggers compensatory mechanisms that decrease cerebral blood flow and further compromise brain tissue volume. As CSF continues to accumulate and changes in the cerebral blood flow and brain tissue volume are maximized, an increase in the ICP is inevitable. The open fontanels and sutures of an infant younger than 18 to 24 months provide some measure of protection. However, they can expand only so much, and as pressure increases so does the compression of vital structures of the brain.

The pathophysiology of increased ICP, regardless of the cause, is a result of an increase in volume within the skull with subsequent inability to compensate. The pathologic changes in volume are most commonly a result of increased extracerebral volume, increased intracerebral volume, and increased intraventricular volume. Examples of these are provided in the display on common volume changes associated with increased intracranial pressure.

Clinical Manifestations. The signs and symptoms of increased ICP vary depending on the rate (acute or chronic) at which the pressure increases, the cause of the disorder, and the age of the child. Early symptoms of increased ICP include irritability, restlessness, difficulty sucking, anorexia, headache, and nausea. Changes initially are subtle and may occur for hours. Children generally are poor reporters of headache; therefore, the first symptoms of increased ICP are irritability and restlessness. An infants may rub his or her head and turn it from side to side to indicate the presence of a headache.

Intermediate symptoms of increased ICP indicate worsening pressures and include projectile vomiting, tense or elevated fontanel in children younger than 18 months, severe headaches, sluggishness, unequal response of pupils to light, diplopia (double vision), visual field defects (loss of central of peripheral vision), blurred vision, papilledema (edema of the optic disc), decreased

pulse, increased systolic pressure, and seizures. Vital sign changes are important indicators of the condition.

As the ICP continues to increase the signs and symptoms of late stages are more severe. Late symptoms include decreased LOC, decreased reflexes, decreased respiratory rate or change in pattern (Cheyne-Stokes, inspiratory spasm, acute apnea), elevated temperature, herniation of the optic disc, dilated pupils, sunset eyes, decorticate or decerebrate posturing, and eventually death. Early, intermediate, and late symptoms are summarized in Table 53-2.

Rapidly increasing ICP or values in excess of 15 mmHg are considered a medical emergency. Displacement of brain tissue (herniation) into an adjacent space is a severe complication of increased ICP. *Tentorial herniation* (displacement of cerebral tissue inferiorly across the barrier between the cerebrum and brainstem) results in damage to cerebral and brainstem structures, compression of blood vessels, and CSF flow obstruction. Tentorial herniation can rapidly bring about permanent brain damage and even death; therefore, the nurse must be aware of the signs and symptoms. These include ipsilateral (same side as the lesion) dilatation of the pupil due to pressure on the oculomotor nerve; Cheyne-Stokes respirations, which may progress to hyperventilation and eventually to cessation of respirations; and a positive Babinski's reflex.

Herniation of the brainstem through the foramen magnum (the sole outlet of the cranium after fontanel closure) located at the base of the skull where the spinal cord and brainstem meet is another lethal complication

TABLE 53-2
Early, Intermediate, and Late Symptoms of Increased Intercranial Pressure

	Early Symptoms	Intermediate Symptoms	Late Symptoms
General	Irritability Restlessness Lethargy	Decrease in pulse and increase in systolic blood pressure Seizures Sluggish, unequal pupillary response Papilledema Projectile vomiting	Decreased level of consciousness Decreased reflexes Decreased respiration or change in pattern Elevated temperature Herniation of optic disc Dilated pupils Decorticate and decerebrate posturing
Infant	Poor feeding Increased pitch of cry Full scalp veins Tense fontanel Rubbing head	Tense, bulging fontanel in child younger than 18 months Shrill cry Increased head circumference	Prominent scalp veins Enlarged head (prominent frontal portion over the eyes) Sunset eyes
Child	Headache Anorexia Nausea or vomiting Unsteady gait	Severe headache Blurred vision Diplopia	See general

of increased ICP. If the pressure of the CSF surrounding the spinal cord decreases suddenly (i.e., a spinal tap or lumbar puncture), the brainstem can be sucked down through the foramen magnum. Death is almost instantaneous.

Diagnostic Studies. Diagnosis of increased ICP is based on the history and the presenting behaviors. Computerized axial tomography (CAT) is useful in diagnosing mass lesions, cerebral edema, and select causes of increased ICP.

ICPs can be monitored with both noninvasive and invasive sensors. An external noninvasive sensor when applied to the anterior fontanel is a useful indicator of ICP. The applanation principle applied with these types of devices is based on the fact that the fontanels elevate or bulge as ICP increases. This movement of the fontanel (either up or down) expresses ICP values. One such noninvasive monitor is the Ladd monitor (Ladd Research Industries, Inc., Burlington, VT), which uses a pneumatic tube and bellows with a fiber optic sensor. Caution should be used in the application of the sensor because application force of the sensor can affect the accuracy of the measurements.

ICPs also can be monitored with three types of invasive devices: the intraventricular catheter, subarachnoid screw, or epidural probe (Fig. 53-7). The intraventricular catheter is threaded into the lateral ventricle (see Fig. 53-7A), filled with saliva, and attached to a transducer and monitor that provide constant measurement of the ICP. Advantages of the intraventricular catheter include the following: is the most accurate form of ICP measurement; allows drainage of CSF to decrease pressure; and provides a route for intraventricular medications. Disadvantages are that the intraventricular catheter is difficult to place and may traumatize cerebral tissue during insertion, excessive CSF drainage could precipitate subdural hematoma formation due to tears of cortical veins, and the risks of infection are increased.

The subarachnoid screw requires a burr hole through the skull to insert a screw or stopcock into the subarach-

noid space (see Fig. 53-7B). A monitor and transducer can then be connected to the screw through the pressure tubing. Advantages of the subarachnoid screw include the following: is less invasive, which lowers the risk of infection, and provides accurate ICP readings in people whose ventricles are too small for the intraventricular catheter. Disadvantages include the following: The screw cannot be used to drain CSF; there is a risk of brain herniation through the drill hole; and there is a risk of CSF leakage through the dura mater.

The epidural probe is the least invasive monitoring device. A tiny fiber optic sensor is inserted through a burr hole into the epidural space (see Fig. 53-7C). Advantages include the following: Infection risk is lowered, and the transducer does not need to be repositioned with patient movement. Disadvantages include the inability to drain CSF and the inability of some epidural probes to be recalibrated after insertion.

ICP monitoring also can be used to estimate cerebral perfusion pressure (CPP). CPP is a helpful guide to estimate the adequacy of cerebral circulation. Normal CPP ranges from 70 to 100 mmHg. Measures of CPP less than 50 mmHg are associated with brain ischemia and lead to further cerebral damage. CPP can be calculated by subtracting the ICP from the mean arterial pressure (i.e., CPP = mean arterial pressure − ICP).

⭐ **ASSESSMENT**

Because increased ICP can have serious complications, including death, nurses must become familiar with and able to recognize its signs and symptoms. The Glasgow Coma Scale (GCS) is a universally accepted standardized screening tool nurses can use to assess neurologic status (see Chap. 30). Although the GCS is useful, it cannot replace a complete neurologic assessment. The typical ongoing bedside assessment should focus on the patient's LOC, vital signs, pupillary response, motor function, and motor responses.

LEVEL OF CONSCIOUSNESS

LOC may serve as the most valuable estimate of neurologic function and indicate increased ICP. LOC may be divided into five categories: alert, lethargic, stuporous, unconscious, and comatose. The alert patient is awake, oriented to person and place, and responsive to stimuli appropriate for developmental level. If the patient is alert, it is important to assess alterations in actions and mental status. For instance, a high pitched cry, hyperirritability, hypertonicity, fatigue, and drowsiness may be initial indicators of increasing ICP. The lethargic patient appears drowsy but easily awakens and responds to minimal stimulation. The stuporous child is difficult to arouse, confused, and irritable; statements may be incomprehensible. The unconscious child responds only to painful stimuli, and the comatose patient is totally unresponsive.

VITAL SIGNS

Vital sign changes can be good indicators of increasing ICP. Alterations in respirations can be specific indicators of increasing ICP. Respirations should be observed for 1 full minute with careful examination of the pattern. As increasing ICP gets closer to the center of the brain's vital

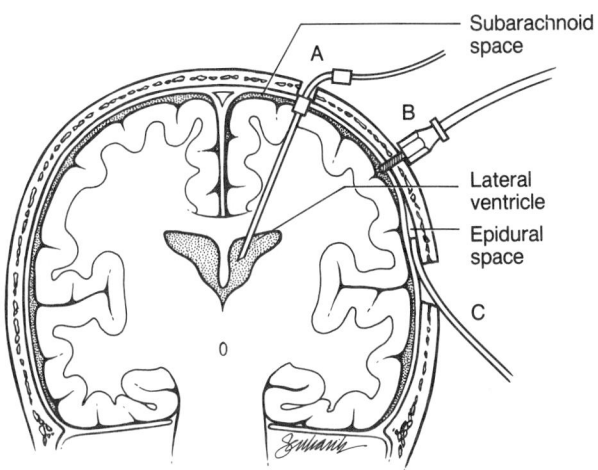

FIGURE 53-7

Three invasive devices to monitor intracranial pressure. (**A**) Intraventricular catheter into lateral ventricle. (**B**) Subarachnoid screw into subarachnoid space. (**C**) Epidural fiber optic sensor into epidural space.

Subarachnoid space

Lateral ventricle

Epidural space

centers, the respiratory patterns will change. Cheyne-Stokes breathing is associated with disturbances in the cerebral hemispheres and the basal ganglia. Respirations gradually increase in rate and volume until they reach a climax, then gradually subside and cease entirely for approximately 5 to 50 seconds when they begin again. Central neurogenic hyperventilation is associated with disturbances in the brainstem's lower midbrain to middle pons area; it also follows transtentorial herniation. Respirations are rapid (usually greater than 24/min), continual, regular, and deep. Apneusis (prolonged inspiration with a 2- to 3-second peak followed by an expiratory pause) is associated with disturbances in the middle to lower pons area and with brainstem damage, such as an infarct of the pons. Cluster breathing is associated with disturbances involving the upper medulla area. Respirations consist of irregular spurts of breathing followed by periods of apnea. Ataxia (or Biot's) breathing is associated with disturbances in the medulla. Respirations are irregular, unpredictable, and consist of deep and shallow random breaths and pauses. Abnormal breathing patterns associated with increased ICP are listed in the accompanying display.

Changes in systolic blood pressure and pulse also can indicate an increasing ICP. Normal systolic blood pressure is greater than ICP. When the ICP equals or exceeds the systolic pressure, the cerebral arteries become compressed, decreasing the blood supply to the brain and causing ischemia. Brain ischemia triggers an increased systolic blood pressure to compensate for the increased ICP, attempting to restore blood supply to the brain. The heart further responds by pumping more forcefully and slowly (40 to 60 beats per minute). When possible, blood pressure should be determined consistently on the same arm and with the child in the same position for reliable interpretation.

Abnormal temperatures may result from increased ICP when the pressure affects the hypothalamus. Rectal temperatures should be taken every 2 to 4 hours. If the temperature increases or if treatment to decrease the temperature has been instituted, it may be necessary to check every 30 minutes to 1 hour.

PUPILLARY RESPONSE

Abnormal pupil response and eye movement can indicate increased ICP, especially if the midbrain and upper pons of the brainstem are involved. Normally, pupils are equal in size (2 to 6 mm in diameter) and react readily to light.

An intracranial hemorrhage may cause the pupil on the affected side to be dilated and possibly fixed (the pupil no longer constricts to a beam of light). However, a condition known as anisocoria causes one pupil to be up to 2 mm larger than the other and is normal in 17% of all people. Consider different pupil sizes an indication of increased ICP unless you can document anisocoria, especially if subsequent assessments indicate that the pupil continues to increase in size.

To determine pupil response, shine a penlight directly at the pupil. A brisk contraction of the pupil is the normal response. A sluggish response—or no response—indicates a disturbance on the same side of the brain as the abnormal pupil (ipsilateral response). If the child's pupil or pupils suddenly become fixed and fully dilated, this signals a neurosurgical emergency that demands immediate attention.

Assessment of eye movement also may provide information regarding the ICP. If the conscious child can follow the nurse's fingers up, down, sideways, and obliquely, returning to the center point with each movement, then cranial nerves III, IV, and VI are not affected by an increased ICP. The eyes should always move as a pair, which is a phenomenon known as *conjugate eye movement*. Disconjugate eye movement occurs when the eyes move independently of one another, indicating pressure in cranial nerves III, IV, or VI.

In an unconscious child if the eyes are pointing in different directions, they are disconjugate. If the eyes are pointing in the same direction but frequently gaze to the left or right, an infarct in the cerebral cortex (the eyes will look *toward* the damaged hemisphere) or an abscess (the eyes will look *away* from the damaged hemisphere) may exist.

The "doll's eye" (the oculocephalic reflex) test should not be performed on children for whom fractures of the cervical vertebrae have not been ruled out. More than 50% of children with severe head injury have multiple injuries. This test involves moving the head briskly from side to side with the eyelids open. If the eyes move in the *opposite* direction than the way the head is turned, this is a normal response and the patient is said to have "positive doll's eyes." If one or both eyes remain fixed, the child has "negative doll's eyes," which probably results from pressure on the midbrain and upper pons of the brainstem.

MOTOR FUNCTION AND MOTOR RESPONSE

Motor function and motor response may be assessed simultaneously. Careful observation may elicit needed information. First, the nurse should observe for normal spontaneous movement of all extremities. The infant may be enticed to reach for a brightly colored object or a favorite toy to assess motor response and function. Older children can be assessed by their ability to follow simple commands, such as raising their arms or sticking out their tongue. Finger grasp alone is not a good indication of the ability to follow commands because some children do this as a motor reflex. Instead, the child should be asked to repeatedly grasp and release the nurse's fingers. This assesses motor response, and a relative weakness when comparing the right to the left may indicate motor function disturbances. If the child follows simple com-

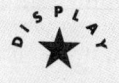

Abnormal Breathing Patterns Associated With an Increased Intracranial Pressure

Cheyne-Stokes breathing
Central neurogenic hyperventilation
Apneusis
Cluster breathing
Ataxia breathing

mands, test the motor strength of their flexors and extensors. Use your hand to create a resistance for them to pull against or push away. Also test for arm drift by having the child close their eyes and extend their arms, palms up. A weak arm will drift down and the hand will pronate. By comparing the right side to the left, any difference in strength will be noted.

If the child is unconscious or does not respond to spoken commands, motor function and response may be tested by resorting to a painful stimulus. When applying a painful stimulus, remember that the unconscious patient still feels pain. The pain itself can trigger a sympathetic response and cause the ICP to increase. Therefore, apply the painful stimulus only for the time needed to elicit a response. For a peripheral nerve pain stimulus, press your thumbnail against the child's nail bed. For a central nerve pain stimulus, apply pressure to the supraorbital ridge above the eye. Avoid using sternal rubs because they cause trauma and ecchymosis. An appropriate response is the child pushing away or withdrawing from the source of pain. An inappropriate response is decorticate posturing (flexor rigidity; flexion of upper extremities) or decerebrate posturing (extensor rigidity; pronation of forearms and hands). Figure 53-8 illustrates examples of decorticate and decerebrate posturing. These postures reflect brainstem dysfunction.

Increasing restlessness or exaggeration of any sign or symptom may occur suddenly or be slow in onset. Early recognition of changes and immediate treatment of the child's condition is essential.

★ NURSING DIAGNOSES AND PLANNING

Based on assessment data discussed previously and in the preceding chapter, the following nursing diagnoses may apply to the family and child with increased ICP:

- High Risk for Fluid Volume Deficit related to treatment.
- Fluid Volume Excess related to treatment.

- Ineffective Breathing Pattern related to increased ICP.
- High Risk for Impaired Skin Integrity related to immobility.
- Altered Nutrition: Less Than Body Requirements related to altered LOC.
- Sensory-Perceptual Alterations related to increased ICP.
- High Risk for Injury related to seizure activity.
- High Risk for Peripheral Neurovascular Dysfunction related to ICP.
- Impaired Physical Mobility related to altered LOC.
- Fear related to treatment.
- Anxiety related to change in environment.

The nurse and child (or parents) together plan effective care based on the established nursing diagnoses. Several examples of expected outcomes follow:

- The child's skin remains free of signs of skin breakdown.
- The child rests between nursing activities.
- The parents remain with the child, conditions permitting.
- The parents exhibit a feeling of calm when dealing with the child.

The nurse plans for the daily care of the child based on physician's orders and nursing diagnoses. Some general nursing care goals may be the following:

- Child's LOC and motor and sensory function improve.
- Blood gases and vital signs remain within normal limits.
- Child's breath sounds remain clear.
- Child's cornea remains free of lacerations.

★ NURSING INTERVENTIONS: COLLABORATIVE AND INDEPENDENT

Treatment depends on the cause and severity of the increased ICP. Surgery may be indicated for an increased ICP that results from a tumor, obstruction of CSF, or hem-

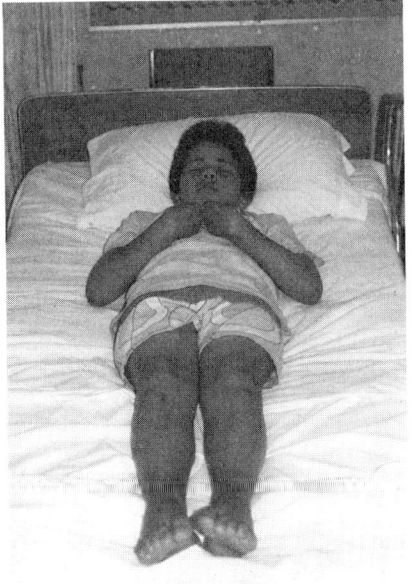
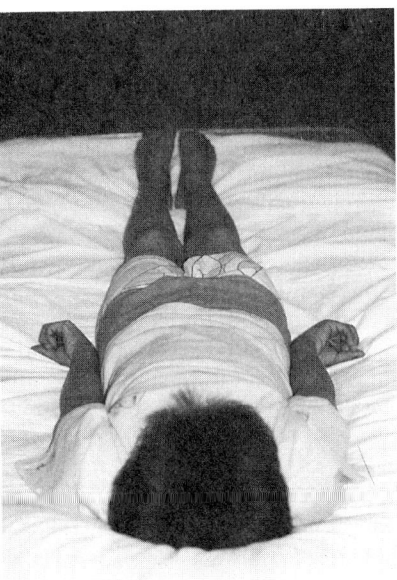

FIGURE 53-8

Postures reflecting brainstem dysfunction. (**A**) Decorticate posturing; (**B**) decerebrate posturing.

A

B

orrhage. If cerebral edema is the cause, treatment is directed at reducing the edema. Whatever the cause, medical and nursing therapy is primarily supportive. Once increased ICP is suspected or documented, treatment must be prompt to prevent further cerebral ischemia.

MEDICAL MANAGEMENT

The major medical treatments for an increased ICP are hyperventilation, fluid restriction, osmotic diuresis, removal of CSF, blood pressure control, corticosteroids, and high-dose barbiturate therapy. Acute subdural and epidural hematomas require surgical treatment.

Induced hyperventilation usually is the most rapid and effective method of reducing ICP. In some children a decrease of maintenance fluids to two thirds or one half of normal levels may be all that is required to decrease ICP. Adequate intravascular volume must be maintained to prevent hypotension; however, excessive free water administration can cause a reduced serum osmolarity and increased cerebral edema. Normal (0.9%) saline with an osmolarity of 310 mOsm/L is probably the best intravenous fluid to administer.

Mannitol (20% to 25%) has become the most frequently used osmotic agent. It is relatively impermeable to the blood–brain barrier, thereby drawing fluid from the brain into the plasma.

Diuretics differ from osmotic agents by removing sodium and water and by decreasing CSF formation, which also can decrease ICP. Furosemide and other renal loop diuretics have shown an ability to reduce ICP. Diuretics directly reduce serum-brain water, which decreases CSF formation. Combinations of osmotic agents and diuretics are frequently used when one method alone is inadequate to lower ICP.

Removal of CSF through a ventricular catheter or a subarachnoid screw rapidly reduces ICP. CSF drainage is most useful for brief periods to reduce ICP during plateau waves. A closed CSF drainage system is necessary to reduce the risks of infection. CSF for examination may be obtained easily with drainage systems.

Control of blood pressure is of great importance because hypotension can result in further brain ischemia. Conversely, even moderate hypertension can exaggerate cerebral edema. In each child there is a point at which blood pressure decreases without a parallel reduction in ICP. When this occurs volume expansion, control of arrhythmias, and sympathomimetic drug therapy should be initiated to keep the systolic blood pressure above 100 mmHg and the mean CPP above 50 mmHg at all times. Somewhat lower levels can be tolerated in neonates (mean blood pressure usually is less than 50 mmHg), but the precise safe limits are not known.

Corticosteroids are used to reduce ICP; however, the benefits of steroid usage remain controversial. The mechanism by which steroids reduce cerebral edema is not known.

If the increased ICP fails to be controlled by the medical therapies already described, high-dose barbiturate therapy may be initiated. Barbiturates decrease cerebral blood flow and metabolism, which subsequently results in a prompt reduction in cerebral blood volume and ICP.

MONITORING

Data collection and around-the-clock observation with periodic assessments are the primary tasks of nursing when a child has ICP. To individualize care and monitor changes, the nurse must be aware of the child's admitting condition and the possible cause of the elevated ICP, vital signs, and LOC. The parents can provide much valuable information and should be included in the child's care as much as possible.

LOC should be assessed hourly or more frequently if necessary. Pupillary responses should be monitored and recorded, noting reaction to light, size, and equality. Vital signs should be assessed at least every 2 hours or as ordered by the physician. Even subtle changes in these signs should be reported to the physician.

An accurate intake and output should be monitored hourly. When fluids are restricted the total amounts should be divided so that the majority of oral intake can be during waking hours, days, and evenings. When an osmotic or diuretic agent is used urinary output must be monitored carefully to detect urinary retention. Indwelling catheters will provide the most accurate record of output. The nurse must also observe for signs of circulatory overload and pulmonary edema, as well as dehydration and circulatory collapse.

If an ICP monitoring system is used, the nurse must be aware of specific nursing policies and procedures regarding its care. Some general guidelines include monitoring the child for signs of infection; frequent calibration of the transducer and monitor to ensure accurate readings; and checking the catheter, screw, or probe patency frequently. If these structures become occluded with blood or brain tissue, the physician should be notified immediately. Any sudden changes in ICP should be reported to the physician. If stopcocks are present in the system, they should be positioned to prevent excessive CSF drainage or leakage.

POSITIONING

In most cases nursing management includes elevating the head of the bed 30 degrees to promote venous return. Increases in ICP can be avoided when changing the child's position by avoiding neck flexion, neck extension, and rotation of the head. Sandbags sometimes are required to maintain the head in a neutral position. Side-lying or supine positions can be used, but prone positions should be avoided due to neck vein obstruction.

Care to prevent the child from injury is also the responsibility of the nurse. Restraints should be avoided if at all possible because pulling at the restraints increases ICP. Having someone stay with the child can decrease the chance of self-injury. Proper positioning, using sheepskin, keeping the side rails up, and frequent massaging over bony prominences reduce the chances of pressure ulcers and flexion contracture formation.

REST PROMOTION

Nursing and medical care should be planned carefully to avoid overstimulation. Nursing measures should be kept to a minimum because general hygiene measures (oral, body, and catheter cleaning routines) and position changes produce transient increases in ICP. Because endotracheal tube suctioning increases ICP, the nurse should allow at least 15-minute uninterrupted rest periods following suctioning episodes. Avoid, for example, taking vital signs, giving a bed bath, changing linens, and repositioning the child all at the same time. Constant stimulation tends to increase the ICP.

Situations involving increased ICP are frightening to the parents and the child. Anxiety and fear increase the blood pressure and the ICP. Therefore, prior to touching the child, it is necessary for the nurse to explain every procedure to the child and what will be done. For the child with an altered state of consciousness, speaking in a calm and soothing tone of voice along with gentle touch may decrease the child's anxiety, blood pressure, and ICP.

GENERAL CARE

Hyperthermia increases the chances of febrile seizures and hypoxia and increases the cerebral metabolic rate. If fever is present, antipyretics and cooling devices should be used. The nurse also can maintain a cool room temperature, keep the child uncovered, and if necessary, gently sponge the child with cool water. If shivering occurs, any or all measures should be discontinued.

Frequently the child will have an endotracheal or tracheostomy tube to ensure a patent airway and to provide means to hyperventilate the child. The nurse is responsible for respiratory care, including suctioning, to maintain clear respiratory passages. In most cases chest percussion and postural drainage are contraindicated because they cause an increase in the ICP.

Occasionally the child's corneal reflexes might be impaired, resulting in incomplete eye closure. Subsequent drying of the eye and corneal ulceration may occur. If drying is a problem, the nurse should obtain orders to instill artificial tears routinely to provide necessary lubrication.

NUTRITIONAL MANAGEMENT

Nutritional needs can be provided in the form of enteral nutrition (nasogastric or gastrostomy tube feedings) or parenteral nutrition (hyperalimentation). Regardless of the type, amount, and method of tube feeding, the nurse must assess the child's ability to tolerate feedings and prevent possible aspiration. At 2- to 4-hour intervals the nurse can assess the amount of tube feeding residual by aspirating fluid from the feeding tube. Residuals should be recorded to indicate trends, and if greater than 100 ml, the physician should be notified. The head of the bed should be elevated, and tube feedings are frequently colored (avoid red because it may imitate blood) to indicate aspiration during respiratory suctioning. If hyperalimentation is the choice for nutritional support, the nurse must ensure that catheter dressings are occlusive and maintain sterility at the insertion site. Hyperalimentation lines should not be used for intravenous piggyback drug administration or intravenous push medications due to possible drug interactions and contamination of the line.

PARENTAL SUPPORT

Support of the parents is an essential nursing function. Because parents may have difficulty understanding and accepting procedures such as the insertion of intraventricular catheters or subarachnoid screws, the nurse must carefully explain brain anatomy and assure them that the catheter or screw does not injure brain tissue.

Nurses should encourage parents to remain with their child when conditions permit. The nurse must, however, be aware that parental anxiety can indirectly affect the child. The parents' questions and concerns should be answered directly and honestly. The nurse can provide some anticipatory guidance to lessen parental fear of the unknown.

★ EVALUATION

Periodically the nurse and family evaluate the outcomes of care given. Examples of outcomes for the child and family with increased ICP were given under Nursing Diagnoses and Planning in this section.

Intracranial Hemorrhage

The major varieties of intracranial hemorrhage are a result of perinatal trauma (subarachnoid and intraventricular hemorrhage [IVH]) or cranial trauma (epidural and subdural hematomas). Perinatal trauma refers to adverse effects on the fetus during labor and delivery or in the neonatal period. The pathogenesis of neonatal subarachnoid or IVHs is not entirely known, but the majority of hemorrhages appear to relate to birth trauma involving the cranium or hypoxic events (especially with perinatal asphyxia). Trauma is the dominant contributing factor in epidural and subdural hemorrhage, usually as a result of a blow to the head.

Intraventricular and Subarachnoid Hemorrhage

Definition and Incidence. IVH can be defined as the presence of blood or bleeding into the intraventricular space. It occurs primarily in premature infants as the major cause of brain injury during infancy. The incidence of IVH has decreased from a high of 49% reported in the late 1970s and 1980s to less than 29% in infants weighing less than 2000 g.[34] The incidence of IVH is directly correlated with the degree of prematurity. Premature infants with weights less than 1500 g (3½ lb) are at the greatest risk for IVH. Fortunately, survival rates for all infants, especially those less than 1000 g birthweight, are increasing.[47]

Subarachnoid hemorrhage is the presence of blood or bleeding into the subarachnoid space. Subarachnoid hemorrhage occurs in both premature and full-term infants as a result of birth trauma or anoxia. The exact incidence of this complication is not known.

Etiology and Pathophysiology. Although the exact predisposing factors associated with perinatal IVH and subarachnoid hemorrhages are not known, the following factors have been implicated through research: birth trauma, hypoxic–ischemic insults, intracranial hypertension, capillary vulnerability between 23 and 36 weeks' gestation, platelet and coagulation disturbances, and impaired cerebral blood flow.[47] Subarachnoid bleeding most commonly originates from the fragile subarachnoid and subpial venous plexus.[39] In IVH the site of bleeding is the subependymal germinal matrix, which is ventrolateral to the lateral ventricles. Hemorrhage from the choroid plexus occurs in approximately 50% of infants with IVH and germinal matrix hemorrhage.[47] Both types of hemorrhage are associated with the development of hydrocephalus as a result of subarachnoid adhesions or intraventricular disruption of CSF drainage.

Clinical Manifestations. Preterm infants with a small subarachnoid hemorrhage rarely demonstrate clinical symptoms, but a lumbar puncture will reveal bloody CSF. A CAT scan usually confirms the presence of hemorrhage without indicating the site of origin. Term infants with small subarachnoid hemorrhages frequently demonstrate seizure activity on the second day of life. Again, lumbar puncture will reveal bloody CSF (200 to 4000 red blood cells/mm). These infants with small arachnoid hemorrhages usually recover with minimal evidence of hemorrhage. However, infants with larger subarachnoid collections of blood may show severe obtundation, seizures, and a unilaterally dilated pupil.

Three clinical states are commonly associated with IVH. Some infants with IVH demonstrate no clinical symptoms. Some infants deteriorate in a catastrophic manner soon after the onset of bleeding. These children demonstrate apnea and bradycardia. They also commonly exhibit decerebrate rigidity with clonic movements. Their eyes may converge or conjugately deviate, and the pupils become fixed. These infants frequently become flaccid and die within minutes or hours. Saltatory deterioration, which is less dramatic, may occur for several days. Respiratory difficulties of varying severity occur during the first week of life. Neurologic signs such as a decrease in tone occur with other subtle changes. Fontanel bulging may occur but usually only after several weeks.

The prognosis in severe hemorrhage regardless of the site is extremely poor; death may result in these cases (approximately 10% to 50% mortality). Although most infants recover from less severe bleeding episodes, complications such as hydrocephalus, cerebral palsy (CP), seizures, and impaired mental capacities may occur.

Diagnostic Studies. The most frequently used tests to confirm the diagnosis of a subarachnoid hemorrhage or IVH include a CT scan and lumbar puncture. The CT scan permits visualization of blood dispersed within brain tissue, while the lumbar puncture reveals the presence of blood in the CSF. Other diagnostic tests may include electroencephalogram (EEG), ultrasonography, and subdural taps.

★ **ASSESSMENT**

An IVH or subarachnoid hemorrhage can precipitate an increased ICP. Therefore, the nurse should assess the child closely for signs that ICP is rising. Abnormalities in vital signs (bradycardia, hypotension, widening pulse pressure) could be present.

Seizures, which may occur on the second day of life (sometimes they occur earlier or later), would indicate the possibility of a subarachnoid hemorrhage. Seizures may not only be caused by neurologic damage; severe metabolic disturbances and withdrawal in the narcotic-addicted infant also can precipitate seizure activity. Neonatal seizures differ from the typical tonic–clonic seizures associated with adults and older children. Neonatal seizures typically involve intermittent periods of hypertonia with jerking of one or more extremities and deviation of the eyes. On rare occasions the only symptoms of seizures might be rapid eye blinking, repetitive mouthing, apnea, and circumoral cyanosis.

The neurologic damage associated with subarachnoid hemorrhages and IVH frequently causes weak, asymmetric, or hypoactive reflexes. Muscle tone is affected and becomes either hypotonic or hypertonic. Hemiparesis is a common finding; therefore, the nurse should make a careful notation and exploration of one-sided weakness.

Because hydrocephalus is a major complication associated with subarachnoid hemorrhage and IVH, daily head circumference should be performed on all infants. Because bulging or full fontanels also is a sign of increased ICP and hydrocephalus, they should also be assessed regularly.

★ **NURSING DIAGNOSES AND PLANNING**

Based on assessment data discussed previously and in the preceding chapter, the following nursing diagnoses may apply to the family and child with an IVH or subarachnoid hemorrhage:

- High Risk for Injury related to seizure activity.
- Impaired Physical Mobility related to neuromuscular impairment.
- High Risk for Peripheral Neurovascular Dysfunction related to cephalic complications.
- Sensory-Perceptual Alterations related to seizure activity.
- Powerlessness related to long-term prognosis of child's illness.

Other diagnoses (Altered Family Processes and Anticipatory and Dysfunctional Grieving) were discussed earlier in this chapter.

The nurse and child (or parents) together plan effective care based on the established nursing diagnoses. Several examples of expected outcomes follow:

- The family progresses through recognized stages of grieving.
- The family demonstrates effective communication within the family unit.
- The family participates actively in decision making.
- The family verbalizes confidence in its ability to cope with the child's neurologic dysfunctions.
- The family seeks help from appropriate referral agencies.

The nurse plans for the daily care of the child based on physician's orders and nursing diagnoses. Some general nursing care goals may be the following:

- Vital signs are maintained.
- Body processes are maintained.

★ NURSING INTERVENTIONS: COLLABORATIVE AND INDEPENDENT

MEDICAL MANAGEMENT

The treatment of catastrophic bleeding is primarily providing cardiorespiratory support. Some physicians use lumbar puncture to relieve acute pressure. Others routinely perform lumbar punctures for the first 2 days following hemorrhage to remove fluid to minimize the amount of blood remaining in the ventricles and subarachnoid villi. Osmotic agents frequently are administered to cause diuresis and decrease CSF secretion. If coagulation deficiencies are present, they are treated as necessary. Because seizures are common, anticonvulsive agents such as phenytoin and phenobarbital are prescribed. Even in the absence of seizures prophylactic therapy is routinely initiated. Medical treatment is primarily supportive for infants with IVH and subarachnoid hemorrhage. Individual signs and symptoms are treated as they occur.

NURSING MANAGEMENT

Nursing management in the acute phase includes physical care of the infant and emotional support for the family. Physical care interventions are supportive and include maintenance of essential bodily processes, rest, warmth, minimal handling, elevation of the head, and sedation as prescribed.

Because hypoxia, hypotension, and bradycardia are common in this infant population, cardiac, apnea, and oxygen saturation monitors can assist in close observation of vital signs. Oxygen should be administered as ordered.

Neonatal seizures also should be treated on a prophylactic or routine basis. As noted previously neonates do not exhibit the typical tonic–clonic seizures, so the nurse must be an astute observer to monitor the infant for seizure activity. Phenobarbital frequently is the drug of choice, and blood levels should be maintained around 20 mg/ml.

Other interventions should be aimed at preventing neurologic handicaps. All infants with intracranial hemorrhage require range-of-motion exercises and therapeutic positioning to treat abnormalities of movement, weakness, tone, and paralysis. Interventions should always be clustered during waking periods to allow the infants an opportunity to rest.

PARENTAL SUPPORT

Parents require emotional support. Even if the child does well initially, complications such as hydrocephalus, seizure activity, mental retardation, and cerebral palsy may occur weeks or even years later. Parents need support in dealing with this uncertainty.

The nurse encourages ventilation of feelings of anxiety, guilt, and despair. The family should be made to understand that these feelings are normal. The nurse assists the family in forming realistic expectations regarding the child's condition and behavior as well as expectations for themselves. Realistic goals reduce family frustration, and achieving goals increases the child's sense of competence.

The impact of the illness on all family members should be considered. Siblings (or spouses) may feel jealous of the time the parent(s) spend at the hospital with the ill child. Siblings may "act out" or display inappropriate attention-getting behaviors. The nurse helps the family learn to view problems from one another's point of view. Family members are encouraged to accept the feelings of others as valid and to express their own feelings and needs.

The nurse and family explore available choices or options and the probable outcome of each option. The nurse assesses the family's support systems and refers the family to appropriate community support groups. Others who have experienced similar situations can share how they handled issues of control and feelings of helplessness. The nurse should be alert to concerns regarding the financial burden of the child's illness. The nurse refers the family to social services.

The family is urged to take time for themselves and to continue with outside interests. Family members need periodic relief from constant attendance at the bedside. A break can replenish energy and perspective. The family can go for a walk or for a meal together while their child is receiving nursing care.

★ EVALUATION

Periodically the nurse and family evaluate the outcomes of care given. Examples of outcomes for the child and family with intraventricular and subarachnoid hemorrhage were given under Nursing Diagnoses and Planning in this section. Planning for further nursing care takes into consideration complications.

COMPLICATIONS

If the child survives the initial insult, complications such as hydrocephalus, neurologic disabilities, mental retardation, seizure disorders, and CP may develop. These disabilities are treated as they develop; they might resolve prior to hospital discharge, continue for several months, or last throughout the infant's life span.

Epidural and Subdural Hematomas

Definition and Incidence. An *epidural hematoma* is bleeding into the space between the dura and the skull, usually as a result of severe head trauma (Fig. 53-9). Epidural hematomas frequently are unilateral and are more common in children older than 2 years. Epidural hemorrhage is rare in the newborn and accounts for only about 2% of observed neonatal intracranial hemorrhage.[39]

Subdural hematomas are at least five to 10 times more frequent than epidural hematomas in infants and toddlers (see Fig. 53-9). A subdural hematoma is venous bleeding into the space between the dura and arachnoid membrane. This bleeding usually occurs with head trauma, and 75% are bilateral.[11]

Etiology and Pathophysiology. Subdural hematomas in the neonate frequently are the result of excessive molding of the skull during birth. Subdural hematomas also may be the result of ventricular shunting, hyperna-

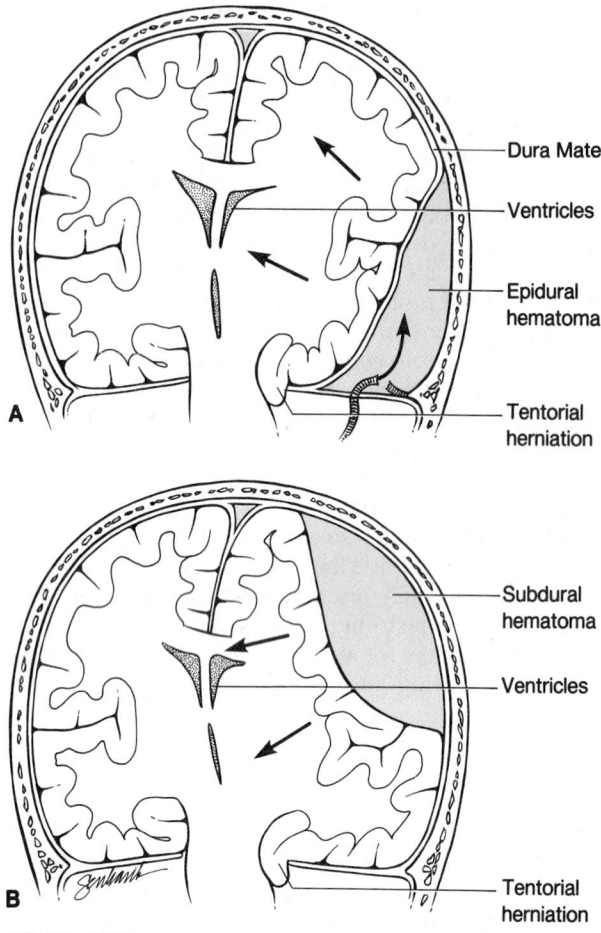

FIGURE 53-9
Epidural and subdural hematomas. (**A**) Epidural hematoma. Note the broken blood vessel and the shift in the midline structures of the brain. (**B**) Subdural hematoma.

tremic dehydration, hemodialysis, coagulation deficiencies, anticoagulant therapy, meningitis, neoplastic infiltration of the meninges, and violent shaking of infants and children. A subdural hematoma frequently is the result of a tear in the arachnoid that allows blood from the small bridging veins between dura and pia mater to collect in the subdural space. Subdural hematomas are classified as acute, subacute, or chronic depending on the severity of the venous bleed.

Epidural hematomas frequently are arterial in origin as a result of a tear in the middle meningeal artery (see Fig. 53-6). Because the bleeding is arterial, rapid compression of the brain occurs. Occasionally, epidural hematomas may be the result of a venous bleed that originates with a laceration of the sagittal or transverse dural sinus. Epidural hematomas are more common in children because the dura is not so firmly attached to the skull surface as it is in older people.

Clinical Manifestations. Typically the child with an epidural hematoma presents the following picture: a history of head injury, a brief period of unconsciousness, and after regaining consciousness a period of apparent well-being for minutes or hours. The lucid period is not always present in children as it is in adults. Then signs of cortical compression, such as vomiting, headache, loss

of consciousness, convulsions, or hemiparesis (epidural hemorrhage is commonly unilateral) develop. Anemia from a substantial blood loss is a prominent sign. This type of hemorrhage constitutes a neurologic emergency. The bleeding needs to be stopped, and the clot needs to be evacuated immediately. This type of injury raises ICP and is potentially fatal if not treated promptly.

As mentioned previously subdural hematomas are classified as acute, subacute, or chronic. Acute subdural hematomas occur within 3 days of the initial injury and carry a high mortality (more than 50%) because of secondary injuries related to edema and increased ICP. The clinical picture is similar to that of an epidural hematoma except that there is definitely no lucid interval. In subacute hematomas symptoms develop between 3 days and 3 weeks following injury. There may be a period of improvement in the LOC and neurologic symptoms, but this is followed by deterioration if the hematoma is not removed. Symptoms of chronic subdural hematoma may occur 3 weeks to up to 6 months following injury. Occasionally the child and parents may not even remember the initial head injury. Seepage of blood into the subdural space occurs very slowly. Because blood in the subdural space is not absorbed, fibroblastic activity encapsulates the hematoma. Even if further bleeding does not occur, this encapsulated hematoma creates an osmotic gradient (due to cell lysis) that pulls fluid from the subarachnoid space into the area. This encapsulated mass increases in size and exerts pressure on the cranial contents. Subtle mood changes, irritability, drowsiness, confusion, apathy, seizures, and decreasing consciousness for days or months are signs of a subdural hematoma.

Diagnostic Studies. A CT scan is the most commonly used diagnostic test because it can differentiate between subdural and epidural hematomas. Skull x-rays are indicated when palpable skull defects or significant scalp swelling is present.

Lumbar puncture is not a good choice for diagnostic study with head injury due to the danger of brainstem herniation. Subdural taps occasionally are useful for diagnosis but usually are reserved for children who cannot be transported for CT scanning safely or rapidly enough.

★ ASSESSMENT

The most important indication of head injury is the LOC of the child immediately following the injury and during the following hours, days, or weeks. Orientation, short-term memory, and state of alertness need to be assessed at regular intervals. Confusion, amnesia of the incident, headache, and drowsiness are common in most children, as is vomiting once or twice following the injury. With rapidly developing unconsciousness, focal signs are related to the area of the brain involved. These symptoms can include ipsilateral (same side) pupil dilation and contralateral (opposite side) hemiparesis.

An accurate history of the head injury event should be obtained from eyewitnesses if possible. The areas of the head involved in the injury, how long the child was unconscious, whether the child regained consciousness, and behaviors that occurred after the event can provide useful information in the diagnosis and treatment of head injury.

Other signs and symptoms that need to be assessed include facial asymmetry, pupil size, equality and reaction of pupils to light, cranial lumps or bruises, clear drainage from the nose or ears and whether that drainage tests positive for glucose (CFS has high glucose levels, whereas secretions do not), blurred or double vision, slurred or incoherent speech, sleepiness or difficulty in awakening, attention span, and seizures. Common presentations in younger children include pallor, anemia, poor feeding, irritability, poor motor response, hyperreflexia, and increased muscle tone. Late signs in younger children include increasing head circumference, full and tense anterior fontanel, and delayed development. Other late signs observable in all children include fever higher than 101° F (not associated with infection), decreased pulse rate, widening pulse pressure, stiff neck, muscle weakness, paralysis, Battle's sign (bruising behind the ears), and racoon eyes (bruising around the eyes). The two latter signs indicate a basal skull fracture.

Because both epidural and subdural hematomas have the potential to increase ICP, these children need to be assessed according to the criteria discussed earlier in this chapter in the section Increased Intracranial Pressure. Careful, ongoing bedside assessment must be routinely performed so that life-threatening events may be avoided.

★ **NURSING DIAGNOSES AND PLANNING**

Based on assessment data discussed previously and in the preceding chapter, the following nursing diagnoses may apply to the family and child with an epidural or subdural hematoma:

- Altered Family Processes related to an ill child.
- Altered Thought Processes related to neurologic impairment.
- Impaired Verbal Communication related to neurologic impairment.
- Anxiety related to threat in interactional patterns.
- Pain related to ICP.

Other common nursing diagnoses and expected outcomes have been discussed in previous sections on CNS injuries in this chapter.

★ **NURSING INTERVENTIONS: COLLABORATIVE AND INDEPENDENT**

Appropriate nursing interventions also have been discussed under Increased Intracranial Pressure and Intraventricular and Subarachnoid Hemorrhage in this chapter. An estimated 80% of children with head injuries have excellent to good recovery, depending on the prompt initiation of medical care. Children who appear to have had a mild injury with no loss of consciousness or a temporary loss of consciousness without other neurologic behaviors, such as concussion or contusion, will be discussed later in this chapter.

Children with more severe head injuries, such as those who have lost consciousness for more than a few minutes, and those with other focal or diffuse neurologic signs must be hospitalized until their condition stabilizes

and neurologic signs disappear. Treatment of the more seriously injured child is observational and supportive.

The child can be maintained on clear liquids if able to take fluids by mouth and if vomiting is not a concern. Fluids usually are limited to 75% of normal daily intake because of cerebral edema. Cerebral edema and increased ICP must be observed for and treated. Osmotic agents and diuretics may be used. Cerebral edema also is treated with corticosteroids and hyperventilation through controlled ventilation. Blood gases should be monitored closely if a ventilator is used. ICP monitoring also can be beneficial.

If fluid draining from the nose, ears, or both is positive for glucose, the draining fluid is probably CSF. The head of the child should be elevated to reduce drainage, and antibiotics should be given to reduce the risk of meningitis because the CSF draining from the ear represents a direct opening between the skull and ear canal.

SURGICAL MANAGEMENT

As a rule the closer to the time of the injury that symptoms of compression occur, the more extreme is the amount of blood loss. Surgical treatment consists of two options: burr holes to relieve the pressure; and/or craniotomy for evacuation of the hematoma, to cauterize or ligate the torn artery or vein, and to repair dural lacerations.

Subdural punctures through the lateral aspect of a patent anterior fontanel sometimes are useful in the treatment of subdural hematomas. A needle is inserted through the fontanel into the subdural space and the collected blood is aspirated with a syringe. Subdural punctures can be repeated daily to empty the subdural space. If after 2 weeks of daily subdural punctures, bleeding has not ceased, surgery is generally necessary to halt bleeding.

MONITORING FOR COMPLICATIONS

The key to successful nursing management of the child with a head injury is a careful, thorough assessment and observation of subtle changes in the child's LOC. Frequently the decision concerning surgical intervention is partially based on nursing observations. Therefore, it is imperative that nurses document their assessments clearly, accurately, and completely. Pupillary responses and vital signs often are checked at least every 15 minutes until the child improves; the frequency of the pupillary and vital sign checks can then be decreased.

Daily weights are useful in the maintenance of an accurate intake and output. Because these children frequently are fluid restricted or treated with osmotic agents and diuretics to control cerebral edema, fluid balance needs to be carefully monitored.

REST PROMOTION

All efforts that might increase ICP should be avoided. Nursing care is clustered to provide uninterrupted periods of rest. However, the nurse should record the child's heart rate, blood pressure, ICP, and oxygenation level before, during, and after caregiving as a basis for evaluating how the child tolerated the interventions. The environment should be kept as quiet as possible. Needs should be anticipated to decrease the amount of crying. Position changes should be made slowly. Stool softeners frequently are given to avoid straining on defecation. The head of the bed also should be elevated to decrease pressure.

Restlessness can be managed with diphenhydramine or chloral hydrate, and headaches can be treated with acetaminophen. Narcotics should be avoided whenever possible because of their neurologic effect, which can hamper further assessments. Anticonvulsants can be administered either prophylactically or following seizure activity.

CARE OF THE UNCONSCIOUS CHILD OR CHILD WITH A CRANIOTOMY

A child who is unconscious requires meticulous nursing care. Hyperventilation and a clear airway must be maintained. The child should be turned and suctioned every 2 hours or as necessary. The child's response to turning and suctioning should be evaluated to determine the relative merit and need for continuing these interventions. Proper positioning to promote venous drainage is mandatory. Controversy exists concerning whether the head should be elevated, and if it is elevated, whether it should be elevated 15 or 30 degrees. Elevating the head 15 degrees increases venous drainage without requiring as much increase in blood pressure compensation for gravity as an elevation of 30 degrees.

If the child has had a craniotomy, the nurse should observe carefully for any signs of hemorrhage, and the dressing should be inspected frequently for large amounts of blood or other drainage. If Jackson-Pratt drains are present following surgery, they should be kept depressed, and the amount, consistency, and color of drainage should be noted.

PARENTAL SUPPORT

Parents of children who have suffered a serious head injury need substantial informational and emotional support. Nurses need to keep the parents informed about the child's condition, about procedures and treatments, and about the nursing care. Nurses should encourage parents to stay with their child and participate in the child's care as much as possible when conditions permit.

★ EVALUATION

Periodically the nurse and family evaluate the outcomes of care given. Examples of outcomes for the child and family with an epidural or subdural hematoma were given under Nursing Diagnoses and Planning in this section. Planning for further nursing care takes into consideration complications.

COMPLICATIONS

In approximately 5% of children with head injuries, generalized seizures can occur immediately following the injury to up to 4 years after the injury. Late seizures frequently are the result of brain tissue scarring. Anticonvulsant medications are prescribed until the child has been free of seizures for 2 years; the medication is then gradually tapered.

Mental retardation, loss of motor function, and hydrocephalus also may occur following head trauma and intracranial hemorrhage. Growth and developmental delays are not uncommon following a severe head injury.

Cerebral Concussions and Contusions

Definition and Incidence. A *concussion* is the most frequent type of closed head injury. Concussion is defined as a transient loss of consciousness that persists for seconds or up to hours with amnesia immediately following the event. Concussion is common in contact sports such as football.

Cerebral contusion is a more severe type of injury, causing hemorrhagic lesions (bruising) in brain tissue. Contusion produces a loss of consciousness along with a neurologic deficit; this differentiates contusions from concussions. Contusions are less common in infants and children when compared to adults, and contrecoup injuries are relatively rare in infants.

Etiology and Pathophysiology. Concussion and contusion frequently are the result of a coup injury (injury to the brain at site of impact) or a contrecoup injury (injury to the brain opposite the site of impact; see Fig. 53-6). The original impact accelerates the brain, which decelerates when it strikes the opposite cranial wall. The risk of concussion or contusion is great in falls, motor vehicle accidents, and contact sports.

The blunt force causing a concussion generally is less than that which could produce a fracture. The temporary loss of consciousness is believed to be the result of stretching or shearing strain on the brainstem. Recovery usually is complete within 48 to 72 hours.

Contusions represent petechial hemorrhages along the superficial aspect of the brain. There may be multiple sites of brain injury (coup and contrecoup). Contusions are a result of the brain striking the inner rough, irregular surface of the skull and are more likely to occur in the occipital area than in the frontal lobes.

Clinical Manifestations. Concussions result in no morphologic abnormality of the brain or neurologic deficits. Loss of consciousness, usually for a brief period, occurs. The typical signs and symptoms associated with concussion include lethargy, vomiting, and irritability. Three types of amnesia commonly are associated with concussion. *Temporary anterograde amnesia* refers to memory loss of events following the injury. This amnesia frequently lasts only several hours and gradually improves. *Temporary retrograde amnesia* is a memory loss of events prior to the injury. Events that occurred years earlier are sometimes forgotten. Memory may gradually improve with time. *Permanent retrograde amnesia* is a memory loss for the seconds or minutes prior to the injury, which will not improve.

Contusions are accompanied by a loss of consciousness that may exceed 24 hours. Symptoms may include lethargy, confusion, coma, blood pressure and heart rate disturbances (as a result of cerebral edema and increased ICP), vomiting, urinary incontinence, and focal neurologic signs such as weakness, sensation disturbances, and visual impairment. Contusion to the brainstem can produce abnormal respirations from Cheyne-Stokes respirations to apnea. Depending on the site and extent of the hemorrhagic focal lesion, signs may vary from a mild transient weakness to prolonged unconsciousness and paralysis.

Diagnostic Studies. The diagnosis of concussion is determined by the presenting signs and symptoms and the history of the injury or event. Because no morphologic neurologic damage occurs with concussion, no diagnostic tests aid in this diagnosis.

A CT scan can assist in the diagnosis of contusion by allowing visualization and by pinpointing the location of the petechial hemorrhagic brain lesions. A CT scan is an important diagnostic procedure to differentiate contusions from the early stages of more severe intracranial hemorrhages (epidural and subdural hematomas). Skull x-rays are useful in determining whether a fracture exists.

★ ASSESSMENT

The signs and symptoms of head injuries are similar to those of differing diagnoses, so the nursing assessment must be carefully and thoroughly administered to assist in pinpointing the exact neurologic dysfunction. A head-to-toe assessment should be completed on each infant and child with emphasis on the LOC, pupillary response, vital signs, and motor response and function. After a careful initial assessment, repeated assessments must be performed at routine intervals, depending on the severity of the child's state, to determine whether the condition is improving or deteriorating.

A history of the event that precipitated the injury should be obtained from eyewitnesses or from the child if possible. If the child suffered a loss of consciousness, determining how long he or she was unconscious and the effect of arousal can be useful.

Careful observation for signs of cerebral edema, intracranial hemorrhage, and increased ICP should be incorporated into the assessment of any child who has suffered even minor head trauma. Even a child who appears well without apparent neurologic damage at the moment may be suffering from a catastrophic life-threatening event.

★ NURSING DIAGNOSES AND PLANNING

Based on assessment data discussed previously and in the preceding chapter, the following nursing diagnoses may apply to the family and child with a cerebral concussion or contusion:

- Altered Thought Processes related to temporary amnesia.
- Pain related to brain injury.
- High Risk for Injury related to seizure activity.
- Fear related to injuries.
- Anxiety related to threat to interaction patterns.
- Sensory/Perceptual Alterations related to altered sensory transmissions.

Other common nursing diagnoses and expected outcomes have been discussed in previous sections on CNS injuries in this chapter.

The nurse and child (or parents) together plan effective care based on the established nursing diagnoses. Several examples of expected outcomes follow:

- The child maintains a fluid balance.
- The parents list symptoms to observe and report.

- The child discusses the injury and circumstances leading up to it.
- The parents discuss their concerns about the outcome of the injury.

The nurse plans for the daily care of the child based on physician's orders and nursing diagnoses. Some general nursing care goals may be the following:

- Vital signs are maintained.
- Major neurologic impairment symptoms are absent.
- Motor and sensory function are maintained.
- Any symptoms of further impairment are reported to the physician immediately.
- Pain is kept to a minimum.

★ NURSING INTERVENTIONS: COLLABORATIVE AND INDEPENDENT

Careful observation is necessary so more severe head injuries can be recognized if they develop. Other nursing care of the child with a concussion or contusion is primarily supportive and educational. The child should be monitored frequently for changes in LOC, motor function, and sensory function. Maintaining adequate fluid intake or monitoring intravenous fluid therapy, observing for side or toxic effects of drug therapy (diuretics, corticosteroids, or anticonvulsants), maintenance of an adequate airway, enforcement of strict bedrest, observing for CSF leaks, and monitoring vital signs are nursing responsibilities. Management of a child with a suspected contusion is supportive and observational. Hospitalization is routine. Frequent neurologic checks are necessary to monitor the presence or absence of neurologic symptoms. Cerebral edema and an increased ICP are possible complications. Steroids are commonly given to limit cerebral edema and increase the child's resistance to stress. In the hospital environment the nursing staff is responsible for assessing the same conditions as those about which the parents were instructed when taking the child home. Observed changes need to be reported to the physician because they can indicate a greater problem, such as an intracranial bleed.

TEACHING

Educating the child and family regarding the child's condition, medications, plan of care, and care following discharge are important. The family should be alerted to observe for signs of decreasing LOC in case the child develops a subdural hematoma.

Children who appear to have had a mild head injury with no loss of consciousness or a brief loss of consciousness followed by alertness without neurologic deficits can be observed by parents at home. However, the injury may cause some minor symptoms, such as headache, drowsiness, and vomiting. These symptoms commonly disappear after a short time. Parents should be instructed to observe the child at 1- to 2-hour intervals and report any of the following if they occur: clear fluid or blood draining from the ears or nose; prolonged periods of sleep that differ from the child's normal pattern; difficulty or listlessness in awakening the child; frequent forceful vomiting; behavioral changes in temperament; seizures or uncoordinated jerking movements; and weakness or lack of arm or leg movement. If the child is admitted to the hospital following a mild concussion, careful observation for a period of 24 to 36 hours usually is all that is required.

★ EVALUATION

Periodically the nurse and family evaluate the outcomes of care given. Examples of outcomes for the child and family with a cerebral concussion or contusion were given under Nursing Diagnoses and Planning in this section. Planning for further nursing care takes into consideration complications.

COMPLICATIONS

Some children develop what is known as post-traumatic or postconcussion syndrome. This condition consists of severe headaches, dizziness, tinnitus, double vision, difficulty focusing, personality changes, poor coordination, learning difficulties, and depression. The syndrome is self-limiting and resolves spontaneously within 1 year.

Approximately 5% of children who experience head injuries develop post-traumatic seizures. These generalized seizures may develop immediately following the injury or up to 4 years later, but most occur within 1 to 3 months. Anticonvulsant medications are administered until the child has been seizure free for 2 years; the medication is then gradually withdrawn.

Spinal Cord Injuries

Definition and Incidence. Spinal cord injuries can be defined as damage to the vertebral column (vertebrae and intraventricular articulations), the spinal cord itself, or the spinal cord nerve roots. About 10,000 new patients per year in the United States are rendered paraplegic or quadriplegic as a result of spinal cord injuries, but trauma to the vertebrae and spinal cord account for less than 5% of childhood injuries. Spinal cord injury is more common in boys (82%) than in girls (18%). Approximately 50% of spinal cord injuries occur between the ages of 15 and 25 years.[11] Also, 5% to 20% of spinal cord injuries are associated with acute head injuries.

Etiology and Pathophysiology. During infancy birth injury is the most common cause of spinal cord trauma. It is most likely to occur with spinal hyperextension due to a forceful breech extraction. The majority of these injuries result in cord transection in the midcervical region to the upper thoracic region.

In older children trauma to the spinal cord is most commonly caused by automobile accidents, falls, and sports injuries in which the spine is either hyperextended or flexed beyond its normal range. Crushing injuries to the spine and its contents are rare but are most often the result of impact from falling from a considerable height or diving into shallow water. The pathologic manifestations of spinal cord injury vary from complete severance to contusion and compression.

Trauma to the spinal cord may result from internal or external stressors. Internal stressors, the most common, consist of damage to the spinal cord in which no entry into the spinal cord has occurred. Examples of such injury include fractures, dislocation injuries of the vertebral column, or violent agitation that injures the cord. Severe acceleration–deceleration injuries, such as whiplash, cause squeezing or shearing damage to the cord. An external stressor, such as a knife or bullet, causes a direct entry wound into the spinal cord from the outside. The incidence of teenagers who receive external injuries to the spinal cord as a result of being shot or stabbed is increasing.

Damage to the spinal cord frequently is due to a sudden narrowing of the spinal canal, in which the cord is caught between the lamina of the lower vertebrae and the body of the upper vertebrae, which causes cellular damage to the cord tissue. Secondary causes of damage include ischemic tissue necrosis as a result of hemorrhage (most commonly the anterior spinal artery and vertebral artery), hematoma formation, edema, structural changes of white and gray matter, and a local biochemical response to trauma.

The most common sites of injury in children are at levels T12, L1, C5 and C6, and C1 and C2 (Fig. 53-10). The terms transected and severed are frequently used; however, it is rare for the cord to be completely severed or transected. More appropriate classification of spinal cord injury may be complete versus incomplete. A *complete lesion* is one in which there are no clinical signs of any cord function below the level of the injury. *Incomplete lesions* have some preservation of sensory or motor functions below the level of injury. A lesion that presents

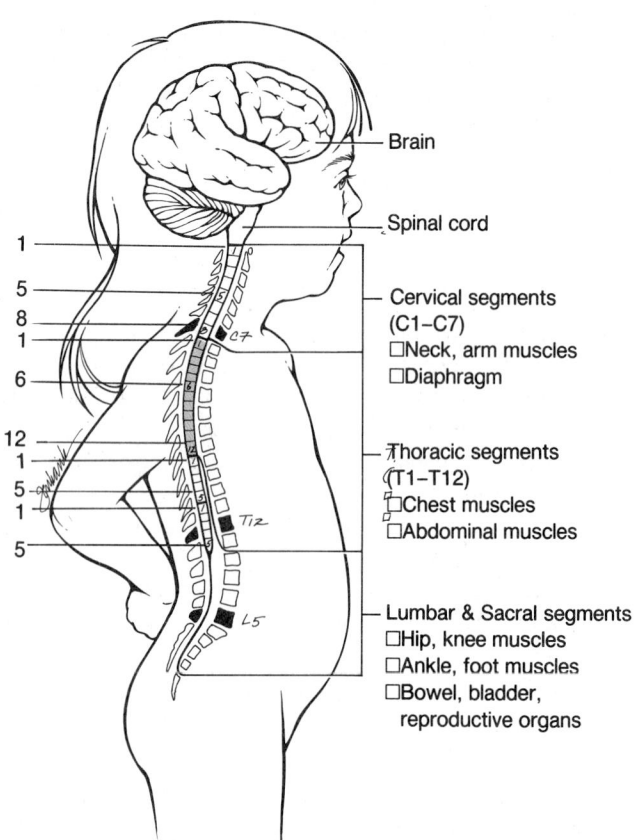

FIGURE 53-10

The level of a spinal cord injury determines the degree of function that can ultimately be regained.

as complete and remains so over the following 24 to 72 hours has a poor prognosis regarding return of function. An incomplete lesion has at least the possibility of partial return of function. However, there is no clinical way to differentiate between a complete spinal cord injury and someone who is in severe spinal shock. In other words all lesions have the possibility of being incomplete and should be treated as such.

Clinical Manifestations. The clinical signs and symptoms of spinal cord injuries usually are divided into three distinct phases. Useful predictions concerning the return of basic bodily functions cannot be made at the time of accident. An improvement in neurologic function may not be evident for weeks or months until the child has progressed through the first two phases of recovery.

First Recovery Phase. Immediately after the injury the child manifests symptoms of spinal shock syndrome or diaschisis. Spinal shock results in a suppression of reflexes below the level of injury due to disruption of central and autonomic pathways. The local effects of cord edema and ischemia produce a physiologic presentation of complete spinal cord injury even in the absence of an anatomic severance. These cause a loss of sensory and motor functions, reflex activity, and flaccid paralysis below the level of injury. The exact signs and symptoms depend on the location and severity of the cord damage. However, most children with a spinal cord injury experience some spinal shock with the following signs and symptoms:

- Loss of reflexes, and sensory and motor functions at or below the level of damage
- Loss of temperature and vasomotor control (including the ability to sweat)
- Loss of bowel or bladder function
- Flaccid paralysis of affected muscles.

An injury at C1 to C2 is incompatible with life. Lower cervical fractures produce paralysis of all four extremities (quadriplegia) with some involvement of respiratory muscles. Lower thoracic level injuries and lumbar level injuries often are accompanied by varying degrees of flaccid paralysis involving the lower extremities (paraplegia), bladder, and rectum.

The problems related to this first phase usually are the result of prolonged inactivity: atrophy of paralyzed and noninvolved muscles, negative nitrogen balance as a result of depression and loss of appetite, calcium loss from bone with resultant urinary calculi, atonic bladder and urinary retention, respiratory difficulty with higher lesions, great risk of pressure sores, reduced cardiac output and plasma volume, and inability to regulate body temperature with higher lesions.

Spinal shock typically lasts from 1 day to 6 weeks with much autonomic reflex cord function returning in about 3 weeks. Usually the shorter the period of spinal shock, the greater the degree of recovery.

Second Recovery Phase. During the second phase of recovery flaccid paralysis is replaced by spinal reflex activity, which results in spastic paralysis. Frequently parents and children misinterpret these sudden spastic movements that occur in paralyzed limbs as normal movement. Minor stimuli, such as stroking the leg or spontaneous crying, sometimes are sufficient to stimulate spastic tremors that contract muscles.

Spasticity creates different problems compared to those associated with flaccid paralysis. Spasticity predisposes the child to contractures, especially the hip adductor, knee flexor, and heel tendons. Hypertonicity of the bladder and bowel occur, causing forceful emptying instead of dribbling associated with the first phase.

The return of spinal reflexes can lead to autonomic dysreflexia, an emergency situation. Autonomic dysreflexia results from an increase in sympathetic activity that causes the systolic blood pressure to rise over 200 mmHg. The child frequently experiences a severe occipital headache, sweating on the forehead, pupillary constriction, bradycardia and flushing of the face and upper extremities, tachycardia or cardiac arrhythmias, and piloerection. Seizures and retinal or cerebral hemorrhages may result from the increased blood pressure.

The usual causes of autonomic dysreflexia are an overdistended bladder, bowel, or stomach. Treatment consists of immediate removal of the cause. The bladder should be emptied gradually to reduce the risk of decompression-induced hypotension. Digital dilatation or glycerin suppositories usually are sufficient to stimulate a bowel movement to reduce overdistention. Enemas should be avoided because large volumes only distend the bowel further. Other suggestions for treatment include elevation of the child's head to reduce ICP and administration of an antihypertensive agent if ordered. The best treatment is prevention by immediate investigation of early signs of distress. The child and nurse must be alert for the development of this complication. Reflex activity in a child with high-cord injury reaches its maximum in about 2 years and then diminishes.

Third Recovery Phase. In the final stage of cord injury neurologic signs are stabilized regarding loss and recovery of sensory and motor functions. For instance if compression of the spinal cord was only from edema, which is relieved, no permanent disability occurs. However, young children and infants with cervical or high thoracic injuries are prone to develop curvature of the spine because of muscle tension and spasticity. The major emphasis of the third recovery phase is rehabilitation, which will be discussed later.

Diagnostic Studies. Diagnosis requires a clinical history of the injury, neurologic examination, and x-rays. Spinal cord injury should be suspected whenever a child has sustained a trauma that had any degree of force. Spinal radiographs usually are normal in children with spinal cord injuries, although fracture or dislocation may be detected. Radiographs must be taken carefully and with sufficient lifting help to prevent further cord damage. If a spinal tap is performed, CSF usually is bloody and has a decreased protein count. CT scans are useful to rule out intracranial injuries.

★ **ASSESSMENT**

A history of the injury event is a vital part of all nursing assessments. The nature of the injury can provide valuable clues regarding the type and degree of suspected damage. A complete neurologic examination should be performed on any child suspected of having spinal cord injury. The neurologic examination can determine if damage occurred, and if so, the extent and level of cord damage with resultant impairments can be examined. To rule out spinal cord injury, it must be determined that reflex arcs are functioning, sensory tracts are intact when each dermatome is examined, and voluntary motor response is present by assessing the ability to move an extremity or body part against gravity. Guidelines are given in Table 53-3.

The nurse's assessment of reflexes with motor and sensory functioning are detailed in Chapter 52. It is important to test reflexes specific to the child's age. Also, the nurse must remember that the child in spinal shock may not demonstrate any reflexes or motor or sensory function below the lesion. The loss of reflexes and motor or sensory function may not be permanent.

★ NURSING DIAGNOSES AND PLANNING

Based on assessment data discussed previously and in the preceding chapter, the following nursing diagnoses may apply to the family and child with a spinal cord injury:

- Inability to Sustain Spontaneous Ventilation related to trauma to chest or spinal cord.
- Ineffective Breathing Patterns related to neurologic impairment.
- High Risk for Aspiration related to paralyzed functions.
- High Risk for Altered Body Temperature related to trauma affecting temperature regulators.
- Altered Skin Integrity related to immobilization.
- Altered Nutrition: Less Than Body Requirements related to increased nutritional needs.

- High Risk for Fluid Volume Deficit related to failure of regulator mechanisms.
- Diversional Activity Deficit related to long-term immobilization.
- Reflex Incontinence related to neurologic impairment.
- Urinary Retention related to neurologic impairment.
- Constipation related to decreased activity.
- High Risk for Disuse Syndrome related to paralysis.
- Self-Care Deficit related to paralysis.
- Anxiety related to change in health status.

Many other nursing diagnoses are applicable to the child who is paralyzed. The previous list is only a few of the common diagnoses.

Just as there are many nursing diagnoses applicable to a child with a spinal cord injury, the expected outcomes are numerous. The following are only a few based on plans made by the nurse and parents together.

- The child participates in breathing exercises and assisted coughing.
- The child's skin remains intact.
- The child maintains a good nutritional diet.
- The child participates in diversional activities.
- The child participates in self-care to the best of his or her ability.
- The child expresses a normal range of emotions regarding the injury and outcome.

The nurse plans for the daily care of the child based on physician's orders and nursing diagnoses. Some general nursing care goals may be the following:

- Normal alignment is restored.
- Spinal area is stabilized.

TABLE 53-3
Nursing Assessment: Guidelines for Assessing Level of Spinal Cord Lesion

Cord Level Associated With Motion	Cord Level Associated With Sensation	Observe Movement and Test Sensation of Body Part	Ask the Child to . . .
C3 to C5	C4	Shoulders, chest, abdomen	Shrug shoulders, take a deep breath (assess diaphragm movement)
C5	C6	Elbow (radial side)	Bend elbow
	T1	Ulnar side	
C6	C6	Wrist	Bend wrist
C8 to T1	C6	Thumb	Make a fist, oppose thumb to each fingertip
	C1	First two digits	
	T1	Little finger	
T5 to T12		Abdomen	Tighten abdomen
	T4	Nipple line	
	T10	Navel	
	L1	Pubis	
L1 to L3	L2	Hip	Flex hip
L2 to L4	L3	Knee	Straighten leg
L5, S1, and S2	L5	Toes	Wiggle toes
S2 to S4	S5	Perineum	Tighten sphincter muscle around your finger

- Compromised neurologic areas are decompressed.
- Early rehabilitation begins.

★ NURSING INTERVENTIONS: COLLABORATIVE AND INDEPENDENT

Nurses are one of several participants in the interdisciplinary team responsible for this child. This team should be composed of physicians from various specialties, occupational and physical therapists, teachers, social workers, psychologists, and vocational counselors with expertise and experience in children with spinal cord injuries. Frequently this interdisciplinary team can be involved in the care of these children for years after discharge from the institution.

The nursing care of the paraplegic or quadriplegic child is complex and is concerned primarily with prevention of complications and maintenance of functions.

The four goals of treatment for any spinal cord injury include:

- Restoration of normal alignment of the spine and its structures
- Early assurance of complete stability of the injured spinal area
- Decompression of compromised neurologic structures
- Early rehabilitation to a productive life.

EMERGENCY INTERVENTION

Initial care of a child with a spinal cord injury begins at the scene of the accident. Rescue personnel have been educated and trained in stabilization and transfer techniques to reduce the possibility of further injury. The use of cervical immobilization devices, such as the Philadelphia collar and back boards, can assist in stabilization of the spine and its structures. If conscious, the child should be calmed, reassured, and advised not to move. As soon as safely possible the child should be transferred to a medical center with personnel specially trained in the care of children with spinal cord injuries.

INITIAL MANAGEMENT

Management during the first phase is supportive with treatment aimed at preventing further neurologic damage, preventing complications, and maintaining vital functions.

Intravenous fluids, corticosteroids, oxygen, maintenance of blood pressure, prophylactic heparin, urethral catheterization, and nasogastric suction often are useful in the initial management phase. A potent diuretic frequently is used for approximately 10 days to decrease spinal cord edema, which could further compromise blood supply to sensitive cord tissue. To prevent aspiration the child should not be given anything by mouth or any drugs that would mask neurologic changes.

CARE IN THE SECOND PHASE

The focus of medical treatment during the second phase is primarily rehabilitative and is aimed at returning the child to his or her home. Drug therapy may include nitrofurantoin to prevent bladder infection; large doses of vitamin C to enhance protein use and to acidify the urine; diazepam, baclofen, or dantrolene sodium to relieve skeletal muscle spasms; and analgesics to relieve pain

caused by the tissue trauma and paresthesias above the level of the spinal cord injury.

SURGICAL MANAGEMENT

Operative intervention is infrequent but may be necessary to remove dangerously placed bone fragments. Surgery is performed only if one of the following conditions exists:

- There is an opening in the dura.
- Abdominal wounds are communicating with the spinal cord.
- Bone is impinging directly on the cord or nerve root.
- Despite aggressive medical treatment, there is an increasing, neurologic deficit.

During surgery the doctor may fuse the spine (with bone chips from the iliac crest or rib strut) or use wires and rods to support the bones as they heal. Postoperative external bracing may continue for 3 months for cervical injuries or up to 9 months for thoracolumbar injuries.

RESPIRATORY CARE

The child with a cervical injury above C_4 will require continuous respiratory assistance. The child may receive oral or nasotracheal intubation initially; however, a tracheostomy tube eventually will be placed to prevent tissue sloughing, facilitate clearing of secretions, and provide access for long-term ventilator dependence. Even if respiratory personnel are responsible for establishing and maintaining ventilatory equipment, the nurse should be knowledgeable about how the equipment works and should routinely assess the prescribed rate and volume to assure proper functioning. A phrenic nerve pacemaker (stimulator) device may be implanted in some children to stimulate diaphragmatic contractions and initiate respirations. Again, nurses must understand its function and operation.

Children with lesions below C_4 rarely are ventilator dependent but usually are unable to cough and deep breathe effectively. Decreased vital capacity, oxygen distribution, and respiratory reserves all contribute to respiratory difficulty, resulting in susceptibility to respiratory tract infections. A variety of breathing exercises and assistive devices may be used to stimulate deep breathing and to increase the elastic qualities of the lung, which will facilitate a productive cough. Incentive spirometry, intermittent positive-pressure breathing devices, nebulized oxygen, chest physiotherapy, assisted coughing, and suctioning as necessary may be performed routinely throughout the day.

TEMPERATURE CONTROL

With autonomic dysfunction, temperature regulation can create problems. The child is unable to sweat and will become hyperthermic if too warmly covered; conversely, dilated capillaries lose a great deal of heat to the environment if the child is not covered enough. A child with an elevated temperature that cannot be corrected by environmental changes should be evaluated for respiratory or urinary tract infection.

IMMOBILIZATION

Children frequently are immobilized for long periods with a variety of cervical traction devices. Crutchfield and

Gardner-Well tongs may be inserted into the skull (Fig. 53-11). This procedure is very frightening to children and parents and should be explained thoroughly prior to the procedure. Halo traction also is frequently used (see Fig. 53-11*C*). With traction devices a child should be turned approximately every 2 hours to prevent skin breakdown. (Always be sure to log-roll.)

Bed or frame devices with or without the use of traction also may be used to help immobilize the child. The stryker frame securely wedges the child between two frames that pivot, allowing frequent turning between prone and supine positions without disturbing spinal alignment. Kinetic beds (such as the Restcue) gently rock the patient side to side in a cradlelike motion that helps combat the complications of immobility (such as deep-vein thrombosis, orthostatic hypotension, stasis of pulmonary secretions, and decubitus ulcers) while maintaining the patient's position.

MAINTENANCE OF SKIN INTEGRITY

Children with spinal cord injuries are at increased risk for pressure sores because they lack sensation and vasomotor control, cannot change their position without assistance, and have decreased peripheral circulation. Normal pressure from body weight can cause tissue ischemia in as little as 30 minutes. Initially the child should be turned (with a log-roll technique) at least every 2 hours around the clock. Alternating pressure mattresses, egg carton mattresses, and sheepskins is helpful in preventing pressure sores. The areas most prone to breakdown include the sacrum, scapulae, heels, and occiput when in a supine position; the trochanters and the lateral aspect of the ankles, heels, and knees when in a side-lying position; and the ischial tuberosities when in a sitting position. Foam elbow, heel, and sacrum protectors and gentle massage can be helpful. Skin must be kept clean and dry, especially for children who are incontinent.

The common type of pressure lesion begins in deeper tissues and is not visible until a later stage. Areas that feel firm, warm, or irregular or appear to be only slightly reddened require immediate careful examination. Maintaining intact skin requires much less nursing care than caring for a pressure ulcer.

NUTRITIONAL MANAGEMENT

The child with a spinal cord injury has increased nutritional needs, which include a diet high in protein, calories, and vitamins. If edema is not a problem, fluids should be maintained at 1500 to 2000 ml/d. Inactivity results in muscle wasting and calcium loss from bone, which can predispose the child to renal calculi. Ascorbic acid can be used to acidify the urine, thereby reducing the likelihood of stone formation. Monitoring the child's weight is a useful measure of fluid balance and caloric requirements.

BLADDER TRAINING

Every child with a spinal cord injury needs to be evaluated urologically because bladder function may not always be predictable. When the bladder is denervated, as in lower motor neuron damage or the acute stage of spinal shock, the bladder wall is flaccid, and overdistention can occur. Usually an indwelling catheter is used during the acute treatment phase, but intermittent catheterization also is acceptable. When the bladder is emptied only periodically, as with intermittent catheterization, dribbling is likely to occur due to lack of sphincter tone. If dribbling is a problem, external collection devices should be used for boys and diapers or incontinent pants for girls to reduce the likelihood of skin breakdown.

Bladder training can be achieved through methods such as intermittent catheterization and triggering mechanisms such as bladder pressure (Credé's maneuver). Even if reflex activity returns and spontaneous bladder

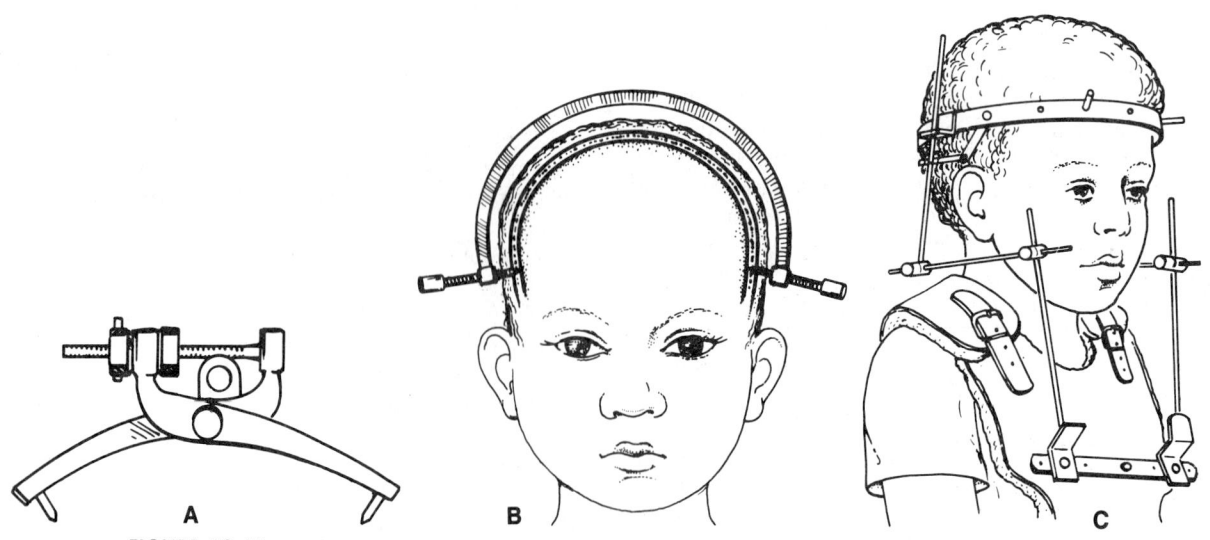

FIGURE 53-11
Long-term immobilization may be accomplished with Crutchfield tongs (**A**) or Gardner-Wells tongs (**B**) placed through burr holes in the skull or with a halo body vest (**C**). (Source: **A** and **C**, Skale, N. [1992]. *Manual of pediatric nursing procedures.* Philadelphia: J. B. Lippincott. **B**, Smeltzer, S. C., & Bare, B. G. [1992]. *Brunner and Suddarth's textbook of medical-surgical nursing.* [7th Ed.]. Philadelphia: J. B. Lippincott.)

emptying occurs, complete emptying is prevented. The older paraplegic child can be taught to express urine manually and to perform self catheterization, but the quadriplegic or younger child must rely on a parent or significant other to perform these procedures. Because renal problems and failure due to repeated infections are the most common causes of death in the postacute phase of spinal cord injury, bladder management is extremely important. Periodic urine cultures and oral antimicrobials frequently are ordered prophylactically (see Chap. 50).

BOWEL TRAINING

Successful bowel training usually is easier to manage than bladder training. A high-roughage diet is important to provide bulk. Bowel movements may be regulated by insertion of a glycerin or bisacodyl (Dulcolax) suppository once each day at the same time to establish a defecation pattern. Stool softeners, such as Colace, can be administered if the stool appears hard. Digital stimulation may be all that is required in some children to initiate evacuation. This may be accomplished by inserting a gloved finger gently into the child's rectum.

REMOBILIZATION

One of the major problems after spinal cord injury is retraining the child's body to adjust to vertical positions after having been maintained supine for long periods. Blood tends to pool in dilated vessels below the level of injury when these children are placed in a vertical position. Hypotension, light-headedness, dizziness, and fainting sometimes occur. Children must be reacclimated to an upright position to prevent vascular pooling. This must be accomplished gradually by elevation of the head to approximately a 30-degree angle twice a day for 20 to 30 minutes. As the child adjusts to this change in position the amount of time and angle can slowly be increased until the child is ready to begin using a wheelchair. This process may require several weeks.

ACTIVITY PROMOTION

Maintaining good body alignment and prevention of pressure areas reflects good nursing care, but children with spinal cord injuries also require movement. Supportive devices frequently are necessary to prevent complications such as footdrop. High-top gym shoes routinely applied can help maintain the feet in a correct position. Range-of-motion exercises, both passive and active, should be planned with the guidance of the child's physical therapist. If the child suffers from spastic paralysis, administration of antispasmodics such as diazepam are helpful. It is important to maintain and increase the strength of the child's intact musculature. The exercise plan should be coordinated among the nursing, physical therapy, and occupational therapy teams to be most effective.

Figure 53-12*A* illustrates an example of a play activity that can be used with an immobilized child. The child can throw bean bags with strings attached at various targets and retrieve them using the attached string. Other children can become involved in the game, making it competitive for older children. Nurses must use their imaginations to improvise games that provide active movement for an immobilized child.

PSYCHOSOCIAL SUPPORT

Unexpected injuries and hospitalization accompanied by immobilization are traumatic to children and their families. Psychological care of the child and family is difficult,

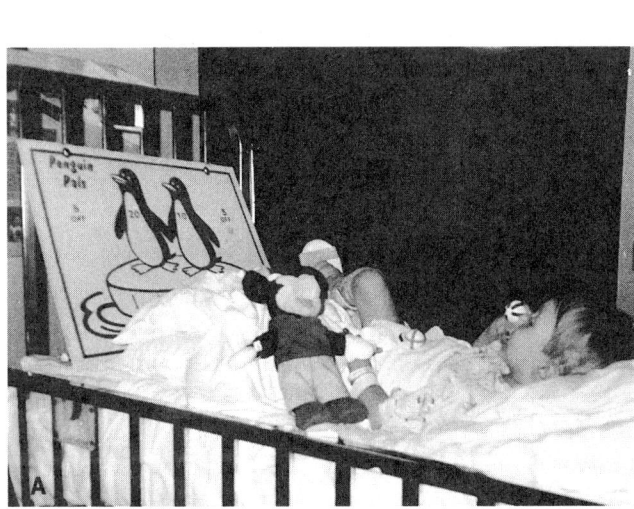
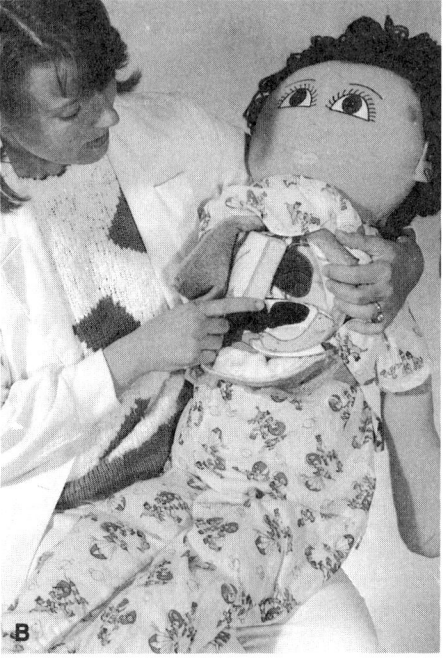

FIGURE 53-12
Play activities serve many purposes. (**A**) Play activity planned for the child in bed allows optimal movement and distraction.
(**B**) Specially equipped dolls can help children comprehend injury to internal organs. (Illustrations provided by Ellen Reynolds, Children's Hospital of Pittsburgh.)

but it is just as important as physical care. Spinal cord injury and its effects disrupt developmental goals and lifelong plans of the child and parents. During the acute phase shock, disbelief and denial are common. The child experiences an increased dependency, and a loss of control over body functions creates changes in self-concept and body image.

After the initial acute phase, children and parents experience anger, anxiety, and depression. The child frequently is confronted with issues of mobility and self-care and is faced with learning new skills. The parents are confronted with financial problems and long-term rehabilitation needs. Support groups of other parents who have experienced similar difficulties are an invaluable resource both emotionally and materially in helping parents cope with hospitalization and home care of their injured child.

Young children may benefit from explanations using specially equipped dolls that illustrate the internal organs and structures (see Fig. 53-12*B*). Play therapy with a therapeutic play kit enables these children to express their feelings of anger through play. In addition these children need opportunities for active play to express their pent up aggressions associated with immobilization. These children normally would be actively running and engaging in activities to express and release their aggressive feelings; when they are immobilized this normal means of expression is denied them at the very time they need to express their anger about the painful procedures they must endure.

Due to the emotional and physical changes that occur, these children commonly fluctuate between emotional states. Appropriate communication, mutual trust, professional respect, and sincere interest in the child and family should emphasize hopeful signs without giving false reassurance.

REHABILITATION

Parents may need assistance in selecting rehabilitation programs and rehabilitation facilities. Guidelines are presented in the accompanying displays on selecting pediatric rehabilitation programs and what to look for when visiting a spinal cord injury facility. Referrals should be made as indicated for home health assistance and support groups. The nurse should discuss with the parents the services available from resource agencies and support groups. The parents may be given a list of resource agencies similar to the list in the display at the beginning of this chapter.

★ EVALUATION

Periodically the nurse and family evaluate the outcomes of care given. Examples of outcomes for the child and family with a spinal cord injury were given under Nursing Diagnoses and Planning in this section. Planning for further nursing care takes into consideration complications.

COMPLICATIONS

Children who suffer spinal cord injuries require meticulous care. Contractures, pressure sores, respiratory infections, and urinary tract infections can be repeated lifelong problems depending on the quality of care these children receive. Most frequently the child with spinal cord injuries faces complications associated with immobility. Heterotrophic ossification is one such example. Heterotrophic ossification is ectopic bone growth between denervated muscle layers near major joints. This process occurs below the level of the lesion immediately after the injury and may continue for years. Children who have developed such heterotrophic bone growth should not be forced to exercise the involved extremity. Heterotrophic ossification occurs most frequently in the elbows and hips and can be differentiated from contractures by x-ray. Spontaneous regression of heterotrophic bone is the rule, but surgical excision occasionally is required to restore joint function.

Lead Poisoning

Lead poisoning is discussed on a cellular level in Chapter 44.

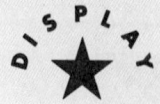

Guidelines for Selection of Pediatric Rehabilitation Programs

- Early intervention (i.e., coma stimulation, therapeutic positioning, and range of motion)
- Developmental model (rehabilitation professionals with pediatric training)
- Interdisciplinary model (regular team and family meeting)
- Family-centered care (therapeutic leaves or weekend passes)
- Individualized care programs (individual treatment plans)
- Prevention and anticipation (written criteria and procedures for back transfers and acute emergencies)
- Established links to special education programs
- Defined goals of reintegration and independence
- Focus on abilities and enhancement of strengths and functional abilities (adaptive equipment for communication and mobility)
- Commission on Accreditation of Rehabilitation Facilities accreditation or criteria incorporated into program

(Developed by C. J. Wright, MSN, RN, Trauma Rehabilitation Coordinator, Children's National Medical Center, 1990.)

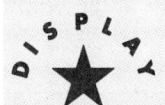

Pediatric Rehabilitation: What to Look for When Visiting a Spinal Cord Injury Facility

General Information

- How many patients are at the facility?
- How many patients have injuries similar to your child's?
- How many patients are in a similar age group as your child?
- Are the patients with similar injuries treated on the same unit?
- Does the facility offer a specific program for spinal cord-injured children?
- What are the visiting rules and family participation policies?
- What are the rules regarding leaves of absence for therapeutic home visits (i.e., weekend pass)?
- What accreditation does the center have: Commission on Accreditation of Rehabilitation Facilities (CARF), American Spinal Cord Injury Association (ASIA), Joint Commission on Accreditation of Healthcare Organizations (JCAHO)?
- When families visit, is there parking and overnight accommodations?
- How long is your child expected to be there?
- Are there model apartments where the patient and family can spend time together before the patient is discharged?
- Who helps plan for discharge, equipment, and adaptations to home transportation?

Staffing

- Who will be your child's primary physician, and what is their specialty?
- Is there a doctor at the facility at all times?
- How far will the patient be from an acute care hospital in case of changes in health?
- How often will the family see the doctor?
- Are there educational classes for patients and families on special needs, such as skin care, bowel and bladder care, sexual counseling?
- How often will the patient be receiving therapy, and what types of therapy are available?
- Are there special education teachers?
- What special psychological services are provided for the spinal cord-injured child and family?
- How often does the interdisciplinary team meet? How often are family conferences held?

- The *rehabilitation team* should include

  Physical medicine
  Psychiatry
  Occupational therapy
  Rehabilitation nursing
  Speech therapy
  Nutrition
  Psychology
  Physical therapy
  Neuropsychology
  Special education
  Child life
  Social services
- *Available specialties*: Pediatrics; pediatric surgery; pulmonary; urology; gastroenterology; plastic surgery; ear, nose, and throat; neurology; neurosurgery

Follow-Up Care

- Does the center have its own outpatient department?
- Is someone responsible for making sure that patients receive follow-up care?
- Can your child have follow-up care close to home?
- Will his or her records from rehabilitation be sent to the acute care hospital for follow-up?
- Who will identify community resources for health care, equipment, recreation?
- Where does your child's equipment get repair or routine maintenance?
- Will the doctors at the acute care hospital get reports on your child's progress?

Environment

- At lunch time are the children eating in their rooms or in a lunch room with the other patients?
- Ask for a planned schedule of activities.
- Look around to see in the morning/afternoon whether the patients are in their beds or involved in an activity (e.g., physical therapy, group activities, orientation activities).
- Is there access to a pool for aquatic therapy?
- Examine the facility for accessibility by wheelchair on and off the rehabilitation unit.
- Look at school and play rooms for age-appropriate signs, toys, and activities.

(Adapted from C. J. Wright, MSN, RN, Trauma Rehabilitation Coordinator, National Spinal Cord Injury Hotline, 1986.)

Definition and Incidence. Lead poisoning (plumbism) poses a serious health hazard to children younger than age 6. The Centers for Disease Control (CDC)[5A] report that adverse effects from lead exposure may occur at blood lead levels as low as 10 µg/dL. Lead poisoning usually is a result of ingestion of nonfood substances (pica). Lead can be found in improperly fired lead-glaze pottery, water from lead pipes, lead-sealed containers, and batteries. In 1973 federal legislation banned the use of lead paint in homes; however, layers of lead paint and leaded plaster are common in older inner-city dwellings. Some recent studies also indicate that soil in areas surrounded by inner-city highways have elevated levels of lead attributed to automobile exhaust. Approximately 4% of American children younger than age 6 have elevated blood lead levels.

Etiology and Pathophysiology. Lead poisoning most commonly results from the ingestion of paint or plaster chips containing lead. Research studies have indicated an increased risk of lead poisoning associated with respiratory exposure to lead dust.[5A] Ingested lead is excreted slowly through the kidneys, the intestines, and to some extent the sweat glands. Repeated ingestion of lead will exceed the rate of excretion, causing attachment of lead to the erythrocytes in the circulatory system and deposition of excess lead in the tissues. Damage occurs in three major systems of the body: the hematologic, renal, and neurologic systems. The effect of lead on body systems is due to disruption of cellular transport mechanisms. Usually bone marrow is affected first and microcytic anemia results. Hemoglobin formation is prevented or retarded because lead interferes with the biosynthesis of heme. Hemoglobin precursors, especially erythrocyte protoporphyrin (EP), increase when the blood lead concentration in the body exceeds 5 to 10 μg/dl. Coproporphyrin and δ-aminolevulinic acid are increased in the urine when the blood lead concentration in the body reaches 80 μg/dl of whole blood. Lead also is toxic to the cells in the proximal renal tubules, causing abnormal secretion of protein, glucose, amino acids, and phosphates. Calcium function also may be impaired. Although lead damages bone marrow and the cells of the renal tubules, its effect on these tissues is reversible.

The effects of lead on the CNS are the most significant, however, because they are not believed to be reversible. In the CNS lead causes an increase in membrane permeability, which causes a fluid shift into brain tissue, producing increased ICP, ischemia, and cellular destruction. Acute encephalopathy manifested by hypertension, intellectual deficits, seizures, cerebral edema, coma, and even death may result.

Clinical Manifestations. Symptoms of chronic lead ingestion may not appear for months depending on the amount ingested. Common early symptoms include anorexia, abdominal pain, anemia, constipation, nausea, vomiting, clumsiness, irritability, apathy, lethargy, and underachievement in school.[41,45] If lead ingestion continues or larger blood levels are present, common symptoms include hepatosplenomegaly, ataxia, seizures, increased ICP, fever, and coma. In addition the child has hypochromic, microcytic anemia and basophilic stippling. The CSF may have increased protein level, and "lead lines" (areas of increased density) may be evident near the epiphyseal line of long bones on x-ray examination.

Diagnostic Studies. Screening procedures for lead poisoning are based on the lead level in the blood. In high risk communities routine screening is done by a fingerstick specimen. Elevated blood lead levels are followed by a venous sampling. Erythrocyte protoporphyrin (EP) tests are not sensitive to lead levels between 10 and 25 μg/dL and therefore are not recommended for routine screening.[5A] See also Table 44-4 for classification of lead poisoning risks.

When the blood lead level exceeds 10 mg/100 ml, further studies are indicated. Other signs of lead poisoning include lead in the urine and hair, increased protein and sources of lead in the CSF, a blue lead line in the gums, and increased density in long bones at the epiphyseal line.

⭐ **ASSESSMENT**

Some children are brought to the health care facility because parents have observed them eating paint chips, chewing on window sills, or teething on other painted items. Paint tastes sweet, and ingestion of paint chips off the floor or walls may occur repeatedly. All children who live in homes built before 1940 should be screened annually for lead poisoning due to the accumulation of lead-based paints. When older apartments and homes are remodeled or old paint is scraped prior to painting, parents need to be informed of the risks of lead poisoning. Children are exposed to lead when adults in the home have jobs or hobbies where there is exposure to lead (furniture refinishing, making stained glass, plumbing, motor vehicle parts).

The health history is the most important portion of a nursing assessment of children with potential lead poisoning. If the child has a known history of eating paint chips, the nurse may want to begin the history by determining whether the child has other hand-mouth habits, such as thumb or finger sucking, biting fingernails, or putting everything into the mouth. Eating habits should be explored, especially those that may cause inadequate nutrition, such as calcium, iron, or zinc deficiencies. Determine whether the child has a compulsion to eat specific inedible items repeatedly (pica), such as ashes, clay, starch, or plaster. Assessment of maternal–infant interaction during questioning for the history may indicate maternal deprivation or inadequate parental care, which may be associated with the development of pica. Developmental milestones should be evaluated to determine developmental delays. The nurse should determine if there is a history of change in behavior or behavioral problems, such as excessive irritability or aggressive behavior, impulsiveness, hyperactivity, lethargy, decreased interest in play, and learning difficulties.

The history should include a careful assessment of the child's living conditions. Does the environment include old housing, crowded urban address, poverty, or a lead smelter in the neighborhood? Do household members have hobbies (artist paint) or occupations that include the use of lead? Have any folk remedies been used to treat the child that might contain lead? What kind of pottery is used in the home? Some older Mexican pottery contains lead, as does lead crystal.

The only symptom that can be noticed on a routine physical examination is the presence of a blue lead line along the child's gums. This bluish black line usually appears on the gums about 1 mm from the gum margin around each tooth. The blue lead gum line does not appear where teeth are missing. Therefore, nurses need to routinely examine children's gums for the presence of this blue line. Also, the parents should be questioned concerning whether the child has ever been observed chewing on window sills or eating paint chips off the walls or floor, whether recent remodeling of the house has occurred, and whether parental jobs and hobbies involve lead.

★ NURSING DIAGNOSES AND PLANNING

Based on assessment data discussed previously and from the preceding chapter, the following nursing diagnoses may apply to the family and child with lead poisoning:

- High Risk for Injury related to lead exposure.
- Pain related to chelation injections.
- Fear related to injection therapy.
- Altered Thought Processes related to lead ingestion.
- Diversional Activity Deficit related to lack of diversional activity in environment.

The nurse and child (or parents) together plan effective care based on the established nursing diagnoses. Several examples of expected outcomes follow:

- The parents describe the reason for concern related to lead ingestion.
- The child maintains balanced urinary output.
- The child expresses normal emotions through play activities.
- The child demonstrates interest in play activities.
- The parents verbalize an understanding of planning and preparing regular, well-balanced meals.

The nurse plans for the daily care of the child based on physician's orders and nursing diagnoses. Some general nursing care goals may be the following:

- The source of lead is removed from environment.
- Lead is removed from body.
- Seizures are prevented.
- Increased ICP is prevented.
- Mental retardation is prevented.

★ NURSING INTERVENTIONS: COLLABORATIVE AND INDEPENDENT

Treatment of lead poisoning is based on the following:

- Detection of the source of lead and its removal from the environment, if possible.
- Administration of chelating agents to remove lead from the body.
- Maintenance of adequate urine output.
- Prevention of complications, such as seizures and an increased ICP.
- Careful follow-up and routine screenings.

PREVENTION

First-level nursing management should focus on prevention of lead poisoning by identifying and screening children at risk. The mortality rate can be as high as 25% following acute encephalopathy. Even treated children of prolonged exposure may show residual effects, such as mental retardation, seizures, and behavioral disturbances (see Chap. 44).

MEDICATION THERAPY

High blood lead levels require immediate treatment with chelating agents. Chelating agents combine with lead in the blood and enhance its excretion in the urine. Calcium disodium edentate (CaEDTA) removes lead from soft tissue and bone (but not red blood cells). It is administered either intravenously or intramuscularly for 5 days, stopped for 2 days, and then restarted for another 5 days as necessary. Adequacy of urine output must be determined before the first dose of CaEDTA is given.

When CaEDTA or dimercaprol (BAL) are administered intramuscularly, as many as 12 injections a day may be required for up to 5 days. Injections must be rotated carefully and recorded in the nurses' notes. The child will need careful preparation for the injection because they are very painful. Therapeutic play with needle play may assist the child in coping with repeated painful injections and can provide a means of expressing anger, frustration, and feelings of powerlessness. Injections should be administered in the treatment room or any area other than the child's room so that the child maintains a sense of safety from pain in his or her own room. Careful records of intake and output are necessary, because CaEDTA and lead are toxic substances to kidney cells. Chelation is also discussed in Chapter 44.

BAL also can be given intramuscularly into a large muscle mass, but it should not be injected into the same site that is used to give CaEDTA. BAL injections are so painful they are usually given with procaine. Both drugs remove calcium from the body, so serum calcium levels need to be monitored periodically. Penicillamine is an oral chelating agent used for children who do not tolerate CaEDTA or BAL. It enhances urinary secretion of lead and may be given for 3 to 6 months. Children receiving penicillamine must be monitored carefully for side-effects, such as rash, enuresis, abdominal pain, and decreased platelets or white blood cells.[42]

MONITORING FOR COMPLICATIONS

Nursing care also includes periodic neurologic assessment and measurement of intake and output. Due to cerebral edema, seizure precautions are necessary. All aspects of nursing care described for a child with an increased ICP may be appropriate for a child with acute encephalopathy as a result of lead poisoning.

COUNSELING AND TEACHING

Needle play and aggressive play, such as throwing bean bags or pounding peg boards or clay, provide needed outlets to express frustration and anger.

Nursing care includes helping parents find day care if necessary, learn how to stimulate their children, and organize play groups to keep children interested in activities other than pica. Parents may need assistance in planning menus to treat nutritional deficiencies. Consistent meal times may reduce the need for pica activity, especially if the child is only allowed to eat at mealtimes. Parents need support and assistance in understanding the multiple aspects of the child's condition. Appropriate referrals may assist parents in relocating or deleading the home and in finding financial support for day care.

★ EVALUATION

Periodically the nurse and family evaluate the outcomes of care given. Examples of outcomes for the child and family with lead poisoning were given under Nursing Diagnoses and Planning in this section.

Neurologic Infections

Neurologic infections are dangerous because of potential loss of life or function, and because of this they are particularly frightening to parents. Parental anxiety can be communicated to the child, thereby increasing the child's anxiety and energy demands. Providing emotional support for the parents while providing the child with attentive nursing care promotes rest and healing for the child. Successful nursing management requires vigilant attention to changes in the child's condition. Initial assessment must be as thorough as the child's energy reserves and condition allow to provide an adequate baseline for assessing minute deleterious changes. Altered LOC, decreased responsiveness, increased ICP, blood pressure changes, abnormal posturing, and increased tension or bulging of the fontanel in the infant signal critical changes in condition.

Meningitis

Definition and Incidence. Meningitis is an acute inflammation of the meninges (the three membranes that envelop the brain and spinal cord). Meningitis encompasses two major diagnostic groups: bacterial meningitis and viral (aseptic) meningitis.

The incidence of bacterial meningitis in the first 5 years of life ranges between 35 to 50 per 100,000. The greatest occurrence of cases (90%) are diagnosed between the ages of 1 month and 5 years, but the greatest risk of developing meningitis occurs between 6 and 12 months.

Etiology and Pathophysiology. Bacterial meningitis most commonly results from the dissemination of microorganisms from a distant site of infection. Bacteremia allows these pathogens to invade the CNS, stimulating an inflammatory response in the meningeal tissues. The most common pathogenic agents in approximately 95% of bacterial meningitis cases are *Haemophilus influenzae*, *Streptococcus pneumonia*, and *Neisseria meningitides*. These bacteria are thought to invade the CSF by way of the choroid plexus of the cerebral ventricles. Meningitis also may be caused or may result from direct inoculation into the subarachnoid space through dural defects or traumatic injuries.

The choroid plexuses, ependyma, and pia mater respond to the infection by becoming more permeable to serum protein, which increases protein levels in the CSF. During the infectious stage, less glucose travels across the inflamed choroid plexus, resulting in lower glucose levels of the CSF. As the bacteria invade the meninges, purulent material develops over the base and surface of the brain; it may appear in the ventricles and finally cause obstruction of CSF flow. As a defense mechanism white blood cells invade the CSF.

Aseptic meningitis is an obsolete term used to describe all the types of meningitis that are not caused by bacteria. Aseptic meningitis has been defined as an acute illness with meningeal signs and symptoms, absence of bacteria, and a relatively short benign course. With current better culture methods the exact organisms causing aseptic meningitis can be isolated. Approximately 97% of the cases referred to as aseptic meningitis actually are viral meningitis. Viral meningitis is an inflammation of the meninges resulting from a virus (herpes group, adenovirus, enteroviruses, influenza, or rubella). Viral meningitis is most common in July, August, and September. Numerous causes result in the other 3% of aseptic meningitis and include such pathogens as *Mycobacterium tuberculosis*, rickettsia, fungi, and cysticercosis.

In viral or aseptic meningitis the pathogen usually enters the system by oral ingestion and is absorbed into the bloodstream. The pathogen then crosses the blood-brain barrier from the blood into the CSF. The amount of inflammation generally is minimal, causing the child to have a headache, some photophobia, nausea, and sometimes fever. Usually the inflammation is not severe enough to result in a stiff neck or positive Brudzinski's or Kernig's sign.

Clinical Manifestations. The early diagnosis of meningitis in infants younger than 6 months of age may be difficult because signs of meningeal irritation are not prominent. Table 53-4 lists the clinical manifestations of meningitis for neonates, infants, and children by age group. In young infants, particularly in infants 2 or 3 months or younger, nuchal rigidity often is absent, and the only specific indicator of meningitis may be increased tension or bulging of the anterior fontanel due to increased ICP. Because early recognition of meningitis in

TABLE 53-4
Clinical Manifestations of Meningitis

Age Group	Symptoms
Neonates (younger than 1 month of age)	Poor feeding
	Poor acceptance
	Hypothermia or hyperthermia
	Irritability
	Decreased activity
	Tense or bulging anterior fontanel
	Tachycardia or bradycardia
Infants	Fever (low or high grade)
	Anorexia
	Vomiting
	Seizures
	Grimacing, lethargy
	High-pitched cry
	Crying with position changes
	Nuchal rigidity
Children	Photophobia
	Fever
	Chills
	Diplopia
	Delirium, irritability, stupor, coma
	Projectile vomiting
	Kernig's and Brudzinski's signs
	Rash (petechial and purpuric with meningoccoci)

the young infant is difficult, spinal fluid usually is examined in all young infants with unexplained fever and unusual symptoms of illness.

The clinical features of meningitis can be categorized into four main divisions: (1) infection, (2) meningeal inflammation, (3) changes in behavior and LOC, and (4) neurologic abnormalities. The signs and symptoms of infection may be characterized by a sudden or gradual onset of low- or high-grade fever. Other symptoms include a cold or minor illness that increases in severity, chills, malaise, poor feeding, lethargy, rash, and tachycardia (due to temperature elevation).

Meningeal inflammation results in classic features associated with meningitis. When headaches, pain or stiffness in the back and neck (nuchal rigidity), vomiting, and Kernig's and Brudzinski's signs are present, meningitis should be suspected.

Changes in behavior and LOC may be difficult to evaluate in young infants, but parental observations may provide useful information. The sensorium frequently is clear at onset, except for transient delirium. Irritability is a common finding and a high-pitched cry occurs when position is altered in young infants. Lethargy and decreased responsiveness may progress to stupor and coma if the ICP increases. Anorexia also is common in children of all ages.

Neurologic abnormalities may include photophobia, impairments in cranial nerves, losses in motor or sensory function, changes in reflexes, and other ophthalmic problems. Generalized seizures accompany meningitis in infants, but convulsions are possible at any age. Observation for the signs and symptoms of increased ICP is critical. Papilledema, bradycardia, and abnormal breathing patterns frequently accompany an increased ICP.

Diagnostic Studies. The diagnosis of meningitis is confirmed based on the history, clinical presentation examination of CSF, and blood work. In bacterial meningitis the CSF usually is cloudy, has a high white blood cell count, has increased protein levels, and has decreased glucose level. The CSF should be cultured to identify the causative organism so that specific antibiotic therapy may be instituted.

Blood tests frequently yield an elevated complete blood count, an increased proportion of polymorphonuclear granulocytes, and decreased serum sodium. Cultures of the blood, urine, and nasopharynx also may be taken to identify a causative organism. A chest x-ray also should be performed to determine the presence of pneumonia.

The symptoms preceding viral (aseptic) meningitis depend on the etiologic agent. The parotid swelling of mumps, respiratory or gastrointestinal symptoms, and skin manifestations such as measles or chickenpox are common presenting symptoms.

★ ASSESSMENT

A complete history should be obtained to gather data that may indicate behavioral changes. Subjective symptoms should be investigated, such as a severe, throbbing headache; muscle pains; backache; stiff neck; and chills. Hyperthermia, hypothermia, bradycardia, and tachycardia

may be presenting symptoms. The child's LOC needs to be carefully assessed. Reflex changes, resistance to neck flexion, and positive Kernig's and Brudzinski's signs are classic findings in meningitis. An infant's fontanels require careful inspection and palpation. Skin lesions preceded by a rash are common in meningococci meningitis. Pneumonia or otitis media frequently precedes pneumococcal and *Haemophilus* meningitis.

★ NURSING DIAGNOSES AND PLANNING

Based on assessment data discussed previously and in the preceding chapter, the following nursing diagnoses may apply to the family and child with meningitis:

- High Risk for Injury related to seizure activity.
- Pain related to neurologic involvement.
- Sensory/Perceptual Alterations related to isolation.
- Altered Nutrition: Less Than Body Requirements related to anorexia.
- High Risk for Impaired Skin Integrity related to drug therapy.
- Altered Family Processes related to situation crises.
- Anxiety related to spread of contagious disease.

The nurse and child (or parents) together plan effective care based on the established nursing diagnoses. Several examples of expected outcomes follow:

- The parents stay by child's side as much as possible.
- The child exhibits that he or she is comfortable.
- The child maintains balanced urinary output.

The nurse plans for the daily care of the child based on physician's orders and nursing diagnoses. Some general nursing care goals may be the following:

- Vital signs are stabilized.
- Complications are recognized early.
- A quiet, restful environment is maintained.

★ NURSING INTERVENTIONS: COLLABORATIVE AND INDEPENDENT

The principles of treatment generally include support of the patient, including ventilation and circulation as needed; prompt identification of the infecting organism; early intravenous antimicrobial therapy; and early recognition and therapy of complications such as cerebral edema and hyponatremia.

ISOLATION

The child with meningitis should be placed in isolation until the causative organism is identified. For bacterial meningitis respiratory isolation should be maintained for 24 hours after the initiation of antimicrobial therapy. Viral meningitis requires excretion precautions for the duration of hospitalization.

MONITORING FOR COMPLICATIONS

Nursing management of the child with meningitis requires careful observation and assessment skills. Changes can occur rapidly in 24 to 48 hours. The nurse needs to observe and record changes in behavior, LOC, increased

ICP, increased number or severity of seizure activity, and posturing.

Vital signs should be monitored every 15 minutes to 1 hour initially until stable. Cardiac and apnea monitors frequently are helpful. Head circumference should be measured and fontanels inspected at least every 8 hours.

MEDICATION THERAPY

Drug therapy usually is a combination of chloramphenicol and penicillin until culture and Gram's stain results are known. However, infants younger than 2 months of age generally receive gentamycin (or tobramycin) and ampicillin. Large doses of the penicillin are given because of its relatively low toxicity and poor diffusion into spinal fluid across the blood–brain barrier. Chloramphenicol is discontinued if the infectious agent proves to be susceptible to penicillin. If the child is allergic to penicillin or the infectious strain (*H. influenzae*) has become resistant to penicillin, chloramphenicol is the drug of choice. Chloramphenicol may be given orally, whereas penicillin requires intravenous routes due to the large dosages. All patients with meningitis are treated with antimicrobial agents for 10 to 14 days or longer if the patient remains febrile or exhibits even mild symptoms. Corticosteroids and mannitol occasionally are used to treat cerebral edema. Diazepam, dilantin, or phenobarbital may be used to treat seizure activity.

Maintaining intravenous lines for the administration of antibiotics is extremely important. Restraints are sometimes required to prevent interruption of intravenous therapy. When restraints are used they must be applied carefully and released periodically to provide range-of-joint motion and promote circulation. Also, because large doses of antibiotics are given, careful inspection of the site is necessary so that infiltration, redness, or swelling can be recognized before more serious problems occur. Accurate records of intake and output need to be maintained. Urine output and specific gravity may indicate development of inappropriate antidiuretic syndrome, a complication of meningitis. Daily weights also provide useful information regarding input and output. The child generally is observed for 24 hours after the last dosage of antibiotics and then discharged without need for further medication.

NUTRITIONAL MANAGEMENT

Feedings may need to be slow, small, and frequent due to the anorexia most of these children experience. Parenteral fluid may be necessary to supplement oral intake. If vomiting is a problem or the child is unable to handle oral feedings, tube feedings may be required.

STRESS MANAGEMENT

During the acute stage the child should be kept quiet in a darkened room. Sudden loud noises may increase neurologic irritation and discomfort. Nursing care should be organized so that extended periods of rest are provided. Large numbers of visitors should be discouraged, but when possible, parents are encouraged to stay with the child to provide a sense of security for the child.

PROPHYLAXIS AND PREVENTION

Household contacts as well as those exposed at day care or school are at risk of developing secondary cases of meningitis within the first week after exposure. The drug of choice for prophylaxis frequently is rifampin. Doses of 20 mg/kg per day for 4 days are recommended for children, while adults receive 600 mg/day for 4 days. Children younger than age 5 should receive the *H. influenzae* vaccine. The HiB vaccine is given at 2, 4, 6, and 15 months of age. This measure will greatly reduce the incidence of secondary cases of meningitis.

Because meningitis frequently occurs after a primary infection, its prevention should be emphasized by nurses. Parents should understand the need to complete the prescribed antibiotic therapy used in the treatment of children with sinus, ear, and respiratory infections. Furthermore, the need for prophylactic therapy must be emphasized during periods of meningitis outbreaks.

PARENTAL SUPPORT

Parents may feel guilty for not recognizing how ill the child was and not seeking medical attention earlier. Nurses should reassure the parents that these feelings are normal, and they should explore whether they could have sought medical attention earlier. Emotional support and education are therefore important.

★ EVALUATION

Periodically the nurse and family evaluate the outcomes of care given. Examples of outcomes for the child and family with meningitis were given under Nursing Diagnoses and Planning in this section. Planning for further nursing care takes into consideration complications.

COMPLICATIONS

The major factors that influence the outcome of meningitis are the age of the child and the infecting organism. The younger the child, the greater the risk for complications due to the immaturity of the child's brain. Residual effects occur in approximately 35% of children who have *H. influenzae* meningitis.

Common complications include subdural effusions, hydrocephalus, developmental delays, and visual and hearing deficits. It has been estimated that 10% of these children develop hearing impairments; 15% to 34% develop language disorders or delays; 2% to 4% have visual impairment; 3% to 7% suffer motor impairments; 2% to 8% continue with seizure activity; and 10% can be classified as mentally retarded.

Subdural Effusion

Subdural effusions are an accumulation of fluid from the bloodstream that has been drawn into the subdural space between the dura mater and the intermediate meningeal layer. Protein enters the subdural space from dural blood vessels, which are abnormally permeable to meningitis. The protein in the subdural space causes fluid to follow by osmotic action. Subdural effusions are most frequently seen in cases of *H. influenzae* meningitis, especially in cases in which treatment has been delayed.

Usually a few days after the onset of *Haemophilus* encephalitis, approximately 50% of children develop a subdural effusion. When a subdural effusion is present, fever generally persists and deep tendon reflexes are hyperactive or asymmetric.

Once a subdural effusion is diagnosed by CT scan or subdural tap, treatment frequently consists of close observation. Once the meningitis treatment is initiated, protein leakage will stop, and the effusion will be absorbed. See nursing interventions under Meningitis in this chapter.

Encephalitis

Definition and Incidence.   *Encephalitis* is an acute and severe inflammation of the brain parenchyma. Acute viral encephalitis often is a result of arbovirus and herpes simplex infections. Chronic encephalitis usually is a result of postviral diseases, such as measles, mumps, and chickenpox, which may result in a CNS infection.

Etiology and Pathophysiology.   Arbovirus encephalitis results from a tick- or mosquito-borne virus that directly invades the CNS. After a mosquito or tick bite, the virus rapidly localizes in the CNS and produces congestion, edema, and small hemorrhages in the brain. Neuroviral lesions with nerve cell necrosis, destruction, and foci of intracellular infiltration are widespread through the brain and spinal cord.

Herpes simplex encephalitis is the most common form of encephalitis. The diagnosis of herpes simplex encephalitis may be difficult because symptoms are similar to acute functional psychosis, subarachnoid hemorrhage, meningitis, tumor, or abscess. This form of encephalitis usually causes extensive neural damage mostly to gray matter. The frontal and temporal lobes are the most frequently involved sites. A serious complication of herpes simplex encephalitis can be a residual syndrome in which fluent dysphasia and an inability to process new information intellectually are a chronic problem.

Encephalitis resulting from rubeola and mumps is thought to be an autoimmune reaction occurring in the neural tissues. These communicable disease forms are preventable by immunization.

Clinical Manifestations.   Disease onset can be acute or insidious, with fever, headache, seizures, hemiparesis, nuchal rigidity, ataxia, dysphasia, altered mental status, difficulty chewing or swallowing, blurred vision, diplopia, and facial muscle weakness. If untreated, lethargy or restlessness may progress to stupor and coma.

After an acute phase the child may remain comatose for days, weeks, or longer (sleeping sickness). Most children generally recover, although the mortality rate is high with herpes simplex encephalitis. Residual effects, such as headache, fatigue, personality changes, behavior disturbances, mental deterioration, impaired motor function, seizures, or irritability, may persist in 60% of the cases. The usual course of the disease is 2 to 3 weeks, with symptoms subsiding in about 7 to 10 days.

Diagnostic Studies.   The diagnosis depends on clinical signs and isolation of the causative organism from the blood or spinal fluid. Spinal tap results will reveal an increased CSF pressure and an increased white blood cell count. Isolation of the virus from either blood or CSF may take weeks.

★ ASSESSMENT

Observation is the key to accurate assessment of the child with encephalitis. A baseline neurologic examination should be completed and recorded for later comparison. The child should be closely monitored for signs of meningeal irritation and symptoms of increasing ICP (vomiting, headache, convulsions, pupillary changes, and LOC changes). Vital signs recorded at routine intervals and changes in temperature, heart rate, and blood pressure need to be reported immediately. Signs of cranial nerve involvement (diplopia, blurred vision, and dysphagia), abnormal sleep patterns, and behavioral changes also should be noted.

★ NURSING DIAGNOSES AND PLANNING

Based on assessment data discussed previously and in the preceding chapter, the following nursing diagnoses may apply to the family and child with encephalitis:

- High Risk for Injury related to seizure activity.
- Pain related to fever.
- High Risk for Infection Transmission related to environmental factors.
- Altered Nutrition: Less Than Body Requirements related to LOC.
- Activity Intolerance related to need for prolonged rest.
- Altered Thought Processes related to LOC.

The nurse and child (or parents) together plan effective care based on the established nursing diagnoses. Several examples of expected outcomes follow:

- The child resumes normal sleep patterns.
- The child increases activity level each day.
- The child verbalizes that he or she is comfortable.

The nurse plans for the daily care of the child based on physician's orders and nursing diagnoses. Some general nursing care goals may be the following:

- Seizure activities are controlled.
- Fever is reduced.
- Vital signs are stabilized.
- A quiet, restful environment is maintained.

★ NURSING INTERVENTIONS: COLLABORATIVE AND INDEPENDENT

Treatment is supportive and palliative in nature. Isolation of the child during the acute infectious stage is sometimes necessary, depending on the causative organism.

MEDICATION THERAPY

Cerebral edema is treated with intravenous administration of hypertonic solutions, steroids, and diuretic therapy. Anticonvulsants are given to control seizure activity. Acetaminophen, cool sponge baths, and hypothermia may be initiated to reduce fever. Sedatives are sometimes indicated to control restlessness and sleep disorders. Antibiotics are not frequently given due to the viral syndrome of encephalitis. Steroids should not be used in the case of herpes simplex encephalitis because they are thought to increase the spread of herpes virus through nervous tissue. Adenine arabinoside frequently is given intravenously with herpes encephalitis.

GENERAL CARE

Nursing management of children with encephalitis is similar to care of children with meningitis and unconscious children. Routine assessments should focus on neurologic and vital sign changes. Meticulous skin care and position changes should be instituted early to prevent skin breakdown. Care should be clustered to provide prolonged periods of rest. Frequently children with encephalitis experience reversal of sleep patterns and tend to sleep during the day and remain wakeful and restless at night. Maintenance of nutrition and hygiene are important aspects of care. Physical therapy and graduated exercises should be continued until spontaneous activity has resumed.

The family should be supported during all phases of the child's illness. Because it is difficult to predict the outcome of the illness, parental anxiety may be high. If long-term rehabilitation is necessary, the nurse may help the family prepare for a prolonged hospitalization.

TEACHING

Nurses also must help educate parents concerning the necessity of immunization against rubeola and mumps. Furthermore, parents can be taught measures that reduce the likelihood of transmission of mosquito-borne infections. The public health department should become involved in epidemic encephalitis outbreaks.

★ EVALUATION

Periodically the nurse and family evaluate the outcomes of care given. Examples of outcomes for the child and family with encephalitis were given under Nursing Diagnoses and Planning in this section.

Brain Abscess

Definition and Incidence. A *brain abscess* is a collection of exudate (pus, microorganisms, and serum) that most commonly forms in the cerebrum, the subdural space, or the epidural space. Boys are more likely to develop a brain abscess than girls. Brain abscesses are rare in infants younger than 1 year of age, but the incidence escalates rapidly as age increases. Approximately one third of all reported brain abscesses occur in children. The overall estimated incidence of brain abscesses is 2 to 3 per 10,000 general hospital admissions.[39]

Etiology and Pathophysiology. Although brain abscesses are not common in children, early recognition and treatment can possibly prevent fulminating meningitis. The cause of brain abscesses may be any of the organisms that cause meningitis, as described previously. Forty percent of brain abscesses are caused by mastoid and middle-ear infections. Approximately 10% are the result of sinus infections. Metastatic abscesses are the most common (approximately 50%) and result from lung infections or abscesses, skin infections, or acute bacterial endocarditis.

The infected site may be either a pocketed mass of exudate outside the dura resulting from infection of the overlying bone or a localized collection trapped in the subdural space. Bacteria enter the brain from another source of infection as discussed previously. The bacteria cause a localized inflammatory reaction characterized by edema, hyperemia, leukocyte infection, and parenchymal softening. Several days after infiltration, liquefaction and necrosis of brain tissue results in a cystic mass of exudate. This mass may be enclosed by an abscess wall from migration of fibroblasts.

Clinical Manifestations. The signs and symptoms vary with the location of the abscess. However, acute clinical manifestations of brain abscesses may include headache, malaise, anorexia, chills, fever, and neurologic signs, such as motor or sensory impairment, speech disorders, and seizure activity. These clinical manifestations frequently are the result of a mass lesion within the skull and subsequent signs of increased ICP.

Diagnostic Studies. The diagnosis of brain abscesses depends on the history of an infection and localizing signs found on neurologic examination. Skull films, CAT scan, arteriograms, EEG, ventriculography, and transfontanel cannulation may be helpful in localizing brain abscesses. Cultures from the suspected site of primary infection may assist in identification of the causative organism.

★ ASSESSMENT

Assessment criteria for brain abscesses are similar to those for meningitis and encephalitis. A thorough health history should be obtained with emphasis on whether the child has recently had a viral, ear, or sinus infection. A physical examination of the child may reveal signs of infection and those commonly associated with increased ICP. Focal signs may be present, which will help determine the brain abscess location.

★ NURSING DIAGNOSES AND PLANNING

Nursing diagnoses that may apply to the child with a brain abscess are similar to those discussed under Meningitis and Encephalitis in this chapter.

★ NURSING INTERVENTIONS: COLLABORATIVE AND INDEPENDENT

Treatment of a brain abscess includes the administration of antibiotics, attempts to reduce brain swelling, and surgical evacuation of the lesion. Surgical excision is only possible if the abscess is well encapsulated. When possible, the abscess may be cannulated and drained. The sac may then be injected with antibiotics. Mortality from all forms of treatment may range between 30% and 45%.[39]

Nursing care of a child with a brain abscess is similar to the care described for a child with meningitis or encephalitis. Antibiotics should be administered as ordered.

Phenytoin and phenobarbital also may be required to treat seizure activity. Cerebral edema and an increased ICP frequently are treated with osmotic diuretics (mannitol and urea) and glucocorticoids (dexamethasone).

If a surgical procedure has been performed to remove or drain the abscess, frequent neurologic assessments and vital signs are still important. The nurse should continue to watch for signs of meningitis (nuchal rigidity, headache, chills, and fever). The dressing should be changed frequently using aseptic technique, and the color, amount, and consistency of drainage should be recorded.

Meticulous skin care, caloric intake, careful positioning, and ambulation should be instituted as soon as possible to prevent secondary complications. Parents should understand the need for prompt medical attention if the child develops otitis media, mastoiditis, or upper respiratory and sinus infections.

★ EVALUATION

Periodically the nurse and family evaluate the outcomes of care given. Examples of outcomes for the child and family with brain abscess are similar to those given under Nursing Diagnoses and Planning for Meningitis and Encephalitis in this chapter.

Depending on the initiation and success of the treatment for a brain abscess, future complications may include recurrence of the infectious process, epilepsy, or mental retardation.

Reye's Syndrome

Definition and Incidence. *Reye's syndrome* is a disorder of acute onset, usually occurring 3 to 7 days after a viral infection, such as measles, chickenpox, influenza, or an upper respiratory infection. The syndrome is characterized by severe noninflammatory encephalopathy with edema of the brain, fatty infiltration and degeneration of the liver, high blood levels of ammonia, and hypoglycemia.

Late winter and early spring are peak seasons for Reye's syndrome, which affects children between birth and 19 years, with peaks at ages 6 and 11. White children are more often affected; however, African American infants younger than 1 year of age from lower socioeconomic urban areas are affected more than white infants. Reye's syndrome is a worldwide problem that affects both sexes. Mortality rates differ, but nationally rates vary between 40% and 50%.[17] Increased awareness, early detection, and prompt treatment have reduced the mortality rate to about 5% in recent years.

Etiology and Pathophysiology. Although the etiology and pathogenesis of Reye's syndrome remain speculative, it usually is associated with a previous viral syndrome. The encephalopathy that develops is a result of hepatic dysfunction, which causes hypoglycemia and increased blood and brain levels of ammonia and lactic acid.

In children with Reye's syndrome there appears to be fatty infiltration of the liver with no evidence of inflammatory changes. There also appears to be fatty de-

generation of the kidneys, heart, lungs, skeletal muscle, and pancreas. Mitochondria within the liver cells swell, which is believed to interfere with the detoxification of waste products. This inability to detoxify waste products is believed to be responsible for the increased levels of ammonia and lactic acid. Glycogen also is decreased or absent from the liver hepatocytes. Increased ammonia levels and resulting hypoglycemia contribute to the encephalopathy.

Retrospective studies between 1980 and 1985 indicate that children who received salicylates (aspirin) during the preceding viral infection were more likely to develop Reye's syndrome.[17] It is therefore recommended that children with influenza or varicella illnesses not receive salicylates. Some studies also suggest that the use of phenothiazine during a prodromal illness may induce the occurrence of Reye's syndrome. Other theories of causation include the possibility of a hereditary enzyme deficiency or exposure to environmental toxins. Investigations are continuing into possible causes of Reye's syndrome.

Clinical Manifestations. Most occurrences of Reye's syndrome are apparent 3 to 7 days after a systemic viral illness. The child frequently appears to be recovering when recurrent vomiting occurs. Vomiting persists and is associated with nausea, anorexia, and listlessness. The clinical manifestations of Reye's syndrome are divided into five stages of increasing severity, as listed in Table 53-5. Patients with a milder form of Reye's syndrome (stage I) proceed from the vomiting phase to a neurologic phase. Subtle cognitive and behavioral changes may progress to somnolence, but often these children progress into a delirious phase (stage II). Excessive stimulation of the sympathetic nervous system during stage II may be manifested; visual hallucinations are not uncommon. These symptoms may progress to a light coma. If the child continues to deteriorate into a deeper coma and decorticate posturing (stage III), mortality rates are significantly higher. Occasionally children who do not respond to treatment plummet beyond deep coma and lose

TABLE 53-5
Stages of Reye's Syndrome

Stage	Description
I	Vomiting, confusion, lethargy, and drowsiness. Responds to verbal commands, and pupillary reactions are normal. Mother may detect subtle cognitive and behavioral changes and apathy.
II	Irritability, disorientation progressing to delirium, hyperventilation, restlessness, combativeness, hyperactive reflexes, and sluggish pupillary reaction but appropriate responses to painful stimuli. Tachypnea, tachycardia, fever, and diaphoresis may indicate excessive sympathetic stimulation.
III	Obtundation progressing to coma, decorticate rigidity, hyperventilation, and sluggish pupillary reaction.
IV	Decerebrate rigidity, deepening coma, pupils fixed and dilated, apneic spells, and loss of doll's eye reflex and corneal reflexes. Eventual loss of brainstem function.
V	Flaccidity, loss of deep tendon reflexes, seizures, and respiratory arrest.

brainstem function (stage IV). Recovery from stage IV is unlikely. Stage V is characterized by seizures and respiratory arrest.

Coagulation abnormalities also can be severe in Reye's syndrome. A prolonged prothrombin time is common. Disseminated intravascular coagulopathy develops in some instances.

Diagnostic Studies. Biochemical evidence of hepatic dysfunction is recognized as one of the most important diagnostic studies confirming Reye's syndrome. Serum glutamic-oxaloacetic transaminase and serum glutamate pyruvate transaminase (SGPT) are elevated to twice normal levels. Bilirubin levels remain normal or only slightly elevated. A liver biopsy that reveals fatty droplets uniformly distributed throughout cells may be performed.

The white blood cell count often is elevated, commonly to more than 20,000/μl. Acetone is present in the urine, and dehydration may be reflected by elevated blood urea nitrogen and creatine levels. Hypoglycemia, hyperammonia, hypothrombinemia, prolonged prothrombin time, elevated serum amino acid and free fatty acids, and respiratory alkalosis with a metabolic acidosis are common findings.

★ ASSESSMENT

A thorough health history should be obtained from the child's parents. The parents should be questioned specifically as to whether the child had a recent upper respiratory infection, chickenpox, measles, or influenza. It is important to determine whether the child received aspirin during this recent illness.

Because nursing and medical interventions depend on the stage of Reye's syndrome, assessment criteria should be directed to determining whether the child exhibits behaviors associated with stage I, II, III, IV, or V (see Table 53-5). A history of the child's behavior and progression of illness can be solicited from the parents. Further information can be collected during the physical examination and through continuing observation.

A thorough nursing assessment should yield information that permits easy classification of the child's stage of illness. LOC needs to be recorded for baseline data. Is the child lethargic, restless, combative, or comatose? The child's posture also is important. Does the child exhibit hyperactive reflexes, flexor posturing, extension posturing, or rigidity? Are signs and symptoms of an increased ICP present? (Refer to Increased Intracranial Pressure in this chapter.) Vital signs may reveal evidence of sympathetic overstimulation (tachycardia, tachypnea, fever, diaphoresis, and pupillary dilatation).

★ NURSING DIAGNOSES AND PLANNING

Based on assessment data discussed previously and in the preceding chapter, the following nursing diagnoses may apply to the family and child with Reye's syndrome:

- Fluid Volume Deficit related to vomiting.
- Fluid Volume Excess related to cerebral edema.

- Altered Cerebral Tissue Perfusion related to rapid brain swelling.
- Anxiety related to changes in conscious environment.
- Pain related to cerebral edema.
- Decreased Cardiac Output related to rapid, deteriorating progress of disease.
- Altered Family Processes related to guilt.

If the child's condition progresses, some of the diagnoses and interventions listed under Increased Intracranial Pressure are appropriate.

The nurse and child (or parents) together plan effective care based on the established nursing diagnoses. Several examples of expected outcomes follow:

- The child's body is maintained in the proper position.
- The child verbalizes understanding of his or her surroundings.
- The child verbalizes that he or she is comfortable.
- The parents remain with the child as much as allowed.
- The parents exhibit normal emotions concerning the child's illness.

The nurse plans for the daily care of the child based on physician's orders and nursing diagnoses. Some general nursing care goals may be the following:

- Fluid and electrolyte balance is maintained.
- Diuretic therapy is successful.
- Vital signs are stabilized.

★ NURSING INTERVENTIONS: COLLABORATIVE AND INDEPENDENT

All children with suspected Reye's syndrome should be admitted to an intensive care unit. Upon admission the diagnosis should be confirmed and the disease stage and neurologic symptoms recorded as a baseline. Because progression through the stages can occur in a matter of hours, close observation is mandatory.

The outcome and prognosis usually are good. The best indicator of outcome is the child's neurologic stage at the time of admission. Children in stage I frequently recover in 24 to 72 hours, while children in stage III frequently die (40%) or recover with residual neurologic deficits (10%). Prognostic indicators of a poor outcome for the child include clinical manifestations greater than stage II on admission, cerebral perfusion pressure less than 50 mmHg, ammonia levels greater than 300 mg/100 ml, hyperosmolality greater than 350 mOsm/L, and severe hypocapnia.

The method and aggressiveness of treatment for Reye's syndrome are determined by the condition or stage classification of the child when first seen. A child may progress from stage I to stage V in as few as 24 to 48 hours.

FLUID AND ELECTROLYTE THERAPY

The child mildly affected with Reye's syndrome who exhibits vomiting and lethargy requires immediate correction of fluid and electrolyte imbalances. Hypoglycemia should be corrected immediately and a dextrose solution should be maintained as high as 300 mg/100 ml using solutions containing 25% dextrose. Hemorrhagic complications generally are controlled with vitamin K or fresh frozen plasma. Hyperthrombia should be treated (without antipynetics) to prevent increased cerebral metabolic requirements. Furthermore, some degree of fluid restriction is necessary to forestall or prevent the occurrence of cerebral edema. Oral intake should be limited and frequently is discontinued. Oral neomycin may be used to inhibit absorption of ammonia from the gut. Monitoring blood glucose, serum ammonia, and plasma osmolality routinely is required.

The more seriously ill child who exhibits delirium or coma, posturing, sympathetic overstimulation, and pupillary changes will deteriorate rapidly without aggressive management. Peritoneal dialysis and exchange transfusions have been used to eliminate toxic materials from the vascular department (the result of hepatic failure).

Rapid, progressive, massive brain swelling with compromise of cerebral arterial perfusion is thought to be the major cause of death in children with Reye's syndrome. Therefore, vigorous diuretic therapy is instituted when the illness appears to be progressing beyond stage I. Fluids should be restricted to 50% of maintenance requirements. Mannitol is given in intermittent doses to reduce cerebral edema. ICP monitoring and Swan-Ganz catheter placement frequently are used to monitor anti-edema therapy. The head of the bed may be elevated to facilitate venous drainage from the head. Elective intubation may be necessary to control hypoxia and hypercapnia. Mechanical ventilation is used to maintain $PaCO_2$ levels in the range of 20 to 25 mmHg and PaO_2 levels 80 to 100 mmHg. Dexamethasone and hypothermia also may be used to decrease cerebral edema or ICP.

When these measures are unsuccessful in controlling ICP, barbiturate coma may be induced, and CSF may be drained from the ventricles. For further information on treatment of an increased ICP, see Increased Intracranial Pressure in this chapter.

GENERAL CARE

Nursing care of the child with Reye's syndrome is similar to that for the child with increased ICP. The nurse should routinely observe for the clinical signs and symptoms of increasing ICP. Cardiac, pulmonary, and intracranial monitoring are routine. Aseptic care of these various devices is a must.

Complications of prolonged bedrest can be prevented by supportive care. Proper positioning, use of egg crate mattresses, and meticulous skin care should be provided to prevent skin breakdown. Tactile stimulation, bright lights, and loud noises should be limited as much as possible due to their effects on the child's irritability and ICP. Hyperthermia should be corrected to normal or sometimes subnormal levels to decrease cerebral metabolism. Cooling blankets, cool room temperature, and sponge baths may be instituted rather than antipyretic therapy.

PSYCHOSOCIAL SUPPORT

Because children with Reye's syndrome are disoriented or comatose, as their condition improves the hospital environment is frightening. Reorientation and a careful explanation of nursing activities may help reduce some of the anxiety. Parents should be encouraged to stay and participate in the child's care when possible.

Parents require a great deal of support. Because the prognosis is uncertain, parents need to be updated and receive as much information as possible. As with other neurologic infections, parents may feel guilty about not seeking medical attention sooner. Also, nurses need to practice primary prevention by teaching parents to avoid aspirin-containing products when treating childhood illnesses.

★ EVALUATION

Periodically the nurse and family evaluate the outcomes of care given. Examples of outcomes for the child and family with Reye's syndrome were given under Nursing Diagnoses and Planning in this section. Planning for further nursing care takes into consideration complications.

COMPLICATIONS

Herniation of the brainstem due to an increased ICP is the most severe complication of Reye's syndrome. Other complications include respiratory and renal failure, pancreatitis, cardiac arrythmias, and diabetes insipidus. Residual neurologic abnormalities may be present in approximately 10% of children who recover.

Guillain-Barré Syndrome

Definition and Incidence. *Guillain-Barré syndrome* (also known as Landry's paralysis, acute febrile polyneuritis, infectious polyneuritis, acute segmental demyelinating polyradiculoneuropathy, and inflammatory polyradiculoneuropathy) is a rapidly developing, reversible disorder that involves loss of the myelin sheath of peripheral nerves. The anterior and posterior roots at spinal segmental levels also are involved, and they demyelinate and degenerate. The incidence appears to be increasing in children, with the greatest susceptibility reported in children between the ages of 4 and 10 years. However, the syndrome also has been reported in infants younger than 1 year of age. Boys and girls are equally susceptible.[4]

Etiology and Pathophysiology. Although the exact cause of this demyelination remains unknown, Guillain-Barré syndrome often follows a viral infection of the upper respiratory tract or gastrointestinal tract. Other theories suggest that Guillain-Barré syndrome is an autoimmune disorder, possibly occurring in response to an infection.

Regardless of the etiology, Guillain-Barré syndrome causes degenerative changes in the spinal nerve roots and peripheral muscles. In the early stage of this disorder inflammation and edema occur around the axon. With time patchy demyelination of the sheath around the axon occurs, which results in slowed or aborted nerve impulse transmission. An ascending paralysis, which may be partial or complete, follows.

Clinical Manifestations. The first symptoms of this infectious disorder frequently include weakness or paresthesia (tingling, numbness, or heightened sensitivity) of the lower extremities. Sensory symptoms usually are milder than the motor impairments. An ascending paralysis rapidly progresses; this may stop at any spinal level or result in total paralysis, including respiratory paralysis. (Up to 30% require mechanical ventilation.) Although most children are only moderately impaired by the disorder, deaths during the acute phase afflict approximately 5%; 10% to 20% incur significant residual neurologic disability; and 5% to 10% may experience a relapse.[39,37]

The child may present with diffuse weakness and sluggish or absent tendon reflexes. Shallow respirations and a weak cough are the early signs of intercostal muscle involvement. Autonomic instability and signs of meningeal irritation, such as nuchal rigidity and back stiffness, may be present. Muscle wasting usually is not a problem due to the rapid progression of the paralysis. Tenderness or deep pain may be present with pressure or movement of muscle tissue. Cranial nerves may become involved, and the facial cranial nerve is most often affected. Urinary retention, postural hypotension, loss or increase in sweating, hypertension, tachycardia, and inverted "T" waves on electrocardiogram may be present.

Motor function returns in a descending pattern, which means the arms regain function before the legs. Remyelinization occurs at a rate of approximately 1 mm/d, so recovery can take up to 6 months depending on the amount of myelin sheath degeneration. Recovery usually begins within 3 to 4 weeks. The ability to walk is one of the last motor functions to be regained.

Diagnostic Studies. No conclusive diagnostic tests can confirm Guillain-Barré syndrome. The diagnosis frequently is made by ruling out other disease processes, such as heavy metal intoxication, porphyric or diphtheric polyneuropathy, infectious mononucleosis or acute hepatitis related polyneuritis, and other toxins such as tri-o-cresyl phosphate. Nerve conduction velocity usually is depressed, although it may be normal during the early stage. Electromyography can distinguish between the demyelination present in Guillain-Barré and other diseases. CSF analysis may reveal elevated protein levels and elevated pressures. The cell count of the spinal fluid usually is less than 10 cells/mm.[21]

★ ASSESSMENT

A thorough health history may reveal a recent viral illness and an ascending pattern of muscle weakness. Because the signs and symptoms of Guillain-Barré range from minor (slight loss of muscle strength) to severe (respiratory muscle paralysis), routine complete neurologic examinations are required to measure increasing weakness and muscle involvement. The child must always be monitored closely for the development of respiratory distress resulting from a reduction in tidal volume and vital capacity due to muscle paralysis. Increasingly shallow respirations and a weak cough are early signs of involvement of the intercostal respiratory muscles.

★ NURSING DIAGNOSES AND PLANNING

Based on assessment data discussed previously and in the preceding chapter, the following nursing diagnoses may apply to the family and child with Guillain-Barré syndrome:

- Ineffective Airway Clearance related to decreased energy.
- Impaired Gas Exchange related to decreased energy.
- Pain related to pressures and movement.
- Urinary Retention related to general muscle weakness.
- Functional Incontinence related to general muscle weakness.
- Impaired Verbal Communication related to intubation.
- Self-Care Deficit related to paralysis.
- Activity Intolerance related to fatigue.
- Diversional Activity Deficit related to boredom with same environment.
- Social Isolation related to altered state of wellness.

The nurse and child (or parents) together plan effective care based on the established nursing diagnoses. Several examples of expected outcomes follow:

- The child demonstrates comfort in communicating by assistive devices.
- The child exhibits pleasure with being read to.
- The child verbalizes that he or she is comfortable.
- The child participates in range-of-motion exercises as paralysis decreases.

The nurse plans for the daily care of the child based on physician's orders and nursing diagnoses. Some general nursing care goals may be the following:

- Vital signs are stabilized.
- Progress of clinical manifestations is monitored on a flow chart.
- Proper body alignment is maintained.
- Range-of-motion exercises are performed.

★ NURSING INTERVENTIONS: COLLABORATIVE AND INDEPENDENT

Medical management basically is supportive because no specific treatment exists. There seems to be a lot of controversy about the use of corticosteroids with Guillain-Barré patients. Some studies have shown that corticosteroids improve recovery time, and others indicate that they do not alter the course of the disease.[37] If corticosteroids are to be administered, they need to be started early in the illness.

Supportive management includes treatment for hypotension or hypertension, intubation and mechanical ventilation if respiratory musculature is involved, tracheotomy if mechanical ventilation is required for several weeks, and use of a kinetic bed to manage problems associated with prolonged bedrest (respiratory, autonomic, and musculoskeletal problems).

Plasmapheresis (plasma exchange) has been used experimentally for those with Guillain-Barré syndrome. The rationale is that if the syndrome is an autoimmune disorder, plasma exchange can remove the myelin-destroying antibodies and ultimately improve recovery time. Plasmapheresis has shown significant improvement in at least 60% of experimental cases.[37]

NURSING MANAGEMENT

Nursing care will determine the clinical course and the recovery time. Because care is mostly supportive, frequent observations of neurologic status are necessary to monitor the ascent and degree of paralysis. The strength of leg, trunk, and arm muscles should be compared to previous assessments. Keeping a flow chart is useful to monitor the progress of clinical manifestations.

Respiratory involvement evidenced by use of accessory muscles, decreasing tidal volumes, and vital capacities should be the focus of routine assessments. Respiratory insufficiency may be demonstrated by signs of confusion, increased pulse, sweating, and restlessness. Materials for selective intubation should be kept at the bedside to prevent complications associated with respiratory distress.

SUPPORT OF COMMUNICATION

If the child is intubated or unable to speak due to paralysis, some form for communication needs to be arranged. Questions that may be answered yes or no can be accomplished with head nods. Communications boards with the alphabet or pictures also may help.

Because the child cannot call for help easily, special devices may be used to assist in calling for the nurse. One such device is placed on the pillow so that by rolling their head to either side, a nurse call is initiated. Other creative devices may be designed by the multidisciplinary team. Even with a device for summoning the nurse, frequent checks by nursing staff are important to reassure the child.

ACTIVITY PROMOTION

Divisional activity is important, and parents can participate. Reading to the child, sitting at the bedside, and talking will help to stimulate the child while in the hospital. Once paralysis begins to improve, occupational, physical, and play therapy may be instituted according to the child's capacity.

Other aspects important to the child's care include elevating the head 30 degrees and providing proper body alignment, meticulous skin care, passive and active range-of-motion exercises, proper nutrition to aid healing and prevent muscle wasting, and maintenance of a clean airway.

PSYCHOSOCIAL SUPPORT

Guillain-Barré syndrome is frightening to the child and parents. Careful explanations concerning the course of the disease and recovery may alleviate some of this anxiety. Parents should be encouraged to spend as much time as possible at the bedside.

DISCHARGE PLANNING

Once recovery begins discharge plans need to be completed. Arrangements for assistive devices and tutorial services for a school-age child should be planned for in-home care. Parents need to be educated and prepared for situations that may arise at home. In most instances recovery is complete but slow.

Acquired Immunodeficiency Syndrome

Care of the patient with acquired immunodeficiency syndrome (AIDS) probably is the greatest health care challenge of this decade.

Definition and Incidence. The Centers for Disease Control (CDC) lists AIDS as a "reliably diagnosed disease that is at least moderately indicative of an underlying cause of reduced resistance reported to be associated with that disease."[22] New cases of pediatric AIDS identified between 1982 and 1989 number 1000 nationwide.[50] Estimated incidence for AIDS in children for 1991 range from 3200 cases[38] to 10,000 cases.[31] Approximately 40% of all patients with AIDS are reported to demonstrate neurologic symptoms.

AIDS represents the ninth leading cause of death among children between 1 and 4 years of age and the seventh leading cause of death in children between 15 and 24 years of age.[30]

Etiology and Pathophysiology. AIDS is believed to be caused by the human immunodeficiency virus (HIV), which is an RNA group virus that causes persistent cellular infection. The virus selectively infects and destroys T-helper lymphocytes, resulting in impaired cell-mediated immunity. Cell-mediated immunity protects an individual from infections (viral, fungal, and bacterial) as well as from some forms of cancer. Therefore, children with AIDS have an increased susceptibility to infection, many of which are life-threatening.

Infection with HIV does not necessarily mean that the child will develop AIDS. To fully develop the disease three conditions must be present: infection with the virus, impaired immunity, and life-threatening neoplasms or infections. The spectrum of this illness includes AIDS-related complex (ARC). People with ARC have been infected with AIDS but do not demonstrate characteristics of the disease in the full sense. Approximately 6% to 20% of these ARC individuals develop AIDS within 2 years.

Transmission of AIDS occurs primarily by sexual contact or blood transfusion. AIDS cannot be transmitted by casual contact. The virus must have direct contact with the bloodstream by injection or through cracks in the mucous membranes. The virus is very fragile when outside the human body. Furthermore, it is believed that the AIDS virus is cell specific; it must encounter T4 lymphocytes, certain B lymphocytes, or cells of the CNS to multiply.[35]

A wide range of incubation periods have been reported, with the mean incubation period being approximately 4.5 years. Incubation times as short as 3 weeks and as long as 7 years are not uncommon. Children who develop AIDS most frequently are infected during birth from an HIV-positive mother or have received contaminated blood products.

Clinical Manifestations. Neurologic involvement occurs in 40% to 73% of all patients with AIDS. Neurologic symptoms frequently are a direct result of infiltration of the CNS by specific organisms, encephalopathy secondary to metabolic disturbances, or symptomatic peripheral neuropathy.

Viral CNS opportunistic infections seen in AIDS patients include aseptic meningitis. Symptoms include an acute febrile response, headache, and meningeal signs. The course usually is self-limiting and nonprogressive. Patients with aseptic meningitis frequently have fifth, seventh, and eight cranial nerve deficits.

Herpes group CNS infections also are common in AIDS patients. Fever, seizures, aphasia, focal neurologic deficits, and an increased white blood cell count in the CSF are common.

Nonviral CNS infections common in the AIDS population include cerebral toxoplasmosis, one of the most common infections in animals and humans. Toxoplasmosis causes chronic and inflammatory abscesses scattered throughout the cerebral hemispheres. Fever, altered mental status, and focal deficits commonly are seen depending on the location of the infection. The mortality rate associated with toxoplasmosis is approximately 70%.

Progressive multifocal leukoencephalopathy (PML), a degenerative disorder, also is common in AIDS patients. It is caused by reactivation of parvoviruses that lie dormant in approximately 90% of the population when the immune system is normal. In the AIDS population PML causes focal neurologic signs, such as aphasia, hemiparesis, blindness, and ataxia. Symptoms usually progress to death in a matter of months.

The most often cited clinical neurologic presentation is progressive dementia. The syndrome has been referred to as subacute encephalitis, subacute encephalopathy, and more recently AIDS dementia complex (ADC). Early findings associated with ADC in children include developmental delays, loss of reflexes, lack of coordination, irritability, visual disturbances, difficulty concentrating, recent memory loss, and an inability to perform school work or complex activities. Assessment later in this stage reveals severe confusion, little spontaneous or verbal behavior, and a vacant stare. Motor impairments occur late and include weakness, spasticity, seizures, ataxia, and incontinence.

Diagnostic Studies. Blood tests and tissue samples are taken to determine the presence of HIV or HIV antibodies. A number of disorders mimic AIDS, so a major portion of diagnosis is ruling out other probable causes, such as Wiskott-Aldrich syndrome or severe combined immunodeficiency disease. Specific criteria for the diagnosis of AIDS in children younger than 13 years of age include one of the following: confirmed HIV in tissues or blood, symptoms meeting CDC case definition, or HIV antibody. Infants younger than 13 months of age must display one of the following: symptoms meeting CDC case definition, confirmed HIV in tissues or blood, or HIV antibody and evidence of both cellular and humoral deficiency and symptoms.

★ ASSESSMENT

The primary targets of AIDS in children are the neurologic, respiratory, and gastrointestinal systems. A careful history and physical assessment may reveal developmental delays, loss of reflexes, lack of coordination, irritability, visual disturbances, difficulty concentrating, recent memory loss, and an inability to perform school work or complex activities.

★ NURSING DIAGNOSES AND PLANNING

Based on assessment data discussed previously and in the preceding chapter, the following nursing diagnoses may apply to the family and child with AIDS:

- High Risk for Infection related to immune system weakness.
- High Risk for Infection Transmission related to highly infectious virus.
- Pain related to progression of disease.
- Altered Thought Processes related to neurologic involvement.
- Ineffective Individual Coping related to personal vulnerability.
- Altered Growth and Development related to effects of physical disability.
- Social Isolation related to altered mental status.
- Situational Low Self-Esteem related to social prejudices.
- Caregiver Role Strain related to prognosis of the condition.

The nurse and child (or parents) together plan effective care based on the established nursing diagnoses. Several examples of expected outcomes follow:

- The child remains free from opportunistic infections.
- The child discusses normal range of feelings caused by the disease.
- The child continues his or her schooling.
- The family seeks help from a support group.
- The family states symptoms of disease advancement for which they should contact their health care worker.

The nurse plans for the daily care of the child based on physician's orders and nursing diagnoses. A general nursing care goal may be the following:

- Spread of infection is prevented.

★ NURSING INTERVENTIONS: COLLABORATIVE AND INDEPENDENT

No specific therapy exists for AIDS; the majority of therapy is aimed at prevention of infection. Research also is promising new approaches to correct immune system defects with bone marrow transplants, lymphokine, interferon, and interleukin-2.

Specific treatments for the neurologic symptoms associated with AIDS include zidovudine to control disease progression, intravenous gamma globulin to reduce episodes of bacterial infections, treatment of secondary herpes encephalitis with acyclovir, and treatment of specific symptoms as they manifest.

Care for the child with AIDS includes nutritional support, consistent personal and oral hygiene, aggressive pulmonary toileting, developmentally appropriate diversional activities, education of the child and family, psychosocial counseling for the child and family, and support for reintegration into the community. AIDS is a chronic disease, and as such it requires frequent readmission and continuing strain on family resources. See Chapter 21 for additional information on care of the child with a chronic illness and Chapter 27 for a further discussion on AIDS.

INFECTION CONTROL

The nurse must identify actual and potential problems that the AIDS child may develop to plan successful nursing care. The single most important aspect of care is to prevent infection, either acquired or opportunistic. Therefore, the child and family need to be educated concerning rapid evaluation of any fever or possible infection, proper nutrition, skin and mouth care, and the establishment of good hygiene practices.

The nurse caring for a hospitalized child with AIDS must strictly adhere to appropriate infection control measures to protect the child and the nurse as identified in hospital policy. Proper cleansing of surfaces contaminated with body fluids is essential in the hospital and at home. It should be emphasized that there are no documented instances of AIDS transmission from casual contact. However, some nurses continue to remain reluctant to care for AIDS patients. In hospitals in which nurses may choose their primary patients, the child with AIDS has a good chance of getting a nurse who wants to care for him or her.

PSYCHOSOCIAL SUPPORT

AIDS is a deadly disease, and its victims confront issues of death and dying, social isolation, moral prejudice, and overwhelming psychological needs.

The child and family need continuing psychological and physical support from significant others. Parents need to express feelings in a safe environment and have relief periodically to provide effective care for their child. Support groups across the country have been established to help children and families deal with these issues.

★ EVALUATION

Periodically the nurse and family evaluate the outcomes of care given. Examples of outcomes for the child and family with AIDS were given under Nursing Diagnoses and Planning in this section. Planning for further nursing care takes into consideration complications (see Chap. 27).

Seizure Disorders

Epilepsy, a term first used by Hippocrates, is derived from the Greek verb meaning "to seize upon" or "take hold of." However, the term epilepsy has a negative connotation that dates back to the thought that evil spirits caused people to have "fits." The current terminology for this condition is *seizure,* which is the English translation for the Hippocratic term epilepsy.

The definitions and usage of the terms epilepsy and seizure remain controversial. Some clinicians use the term seizure to describe a nonrecurrent, nonchronic event, while the term epilepsy describes chronic and recurrent seizure disorders. Others describe both seizures and epilepsy as convulsive disorders. In this chapter the term seizure refers to both acute and recurrent disorders.

Definition and Incidence. A seizure is defined as a sudden electrical discharge of a group of neurons in the brain that results in a transient impairment of consciousness, movement, sensation, or memory. A seizure is a symptom of an underlying disorder. Most commonly, seizure activity is classified according to etiology, clinical manifestation, and site of origin and specific electroencephalographic patterns. At least 50 conditions that may cause seizures are known.

Approximately 2 to 4 million people in the United States are afflicted with some type of seizure disorder. Seizure disorders are among the most commonly observed neurologic dysfunction in children, although the exact incidence is unknown. The incidence for epileptic seizures during the first decade of life is estimated at 60 per 100,000 children. However, rates of childhood seizure activity have been as low as 3 per 1000 and as high as 20 per 1000. The variability in estimates reflects differences in definitions of epilepsy, populations studied, and differences in epidemiologic methods. Approximately 6% of all children experience a febrile condition once, and 50% of this group may have a subsequent seizure that may not be associated with an elevated temperature.[39]

Etiology and Pathophysiology. Seizure disorders have numerous and varied causes based on primary and secondary factors. Also, seizure disorders are caused by different problems in various age groups.

Primary seizures (also called idiopathic, essential, genuine, or genetic seizures) are the result of an unidentified cause. A predisposition to this type of seizure tends to occur in some families who are believed to inherit a lower neuronal threshold that results in vulnerability to abnormal neuronal discharges.

Secondary seizures (also known as acquired, symptomatic, or organic) result from identifiable causes. Secondary seizures frequently are the result of pathologic processes, toxic exogenous or endogenous substances, disturbances in metabolism, or fever. Pathologic processes include congenital abnormalities, such as the arteriovenous malformation porencephalia; infectious problems, such as meningitis and encephalitis; space-occupying lesions, such as tumors (benign or malignant, primary or metastic), cystic masses, abscesses, and hematomas; head trauma; actual neuron damage from deficient states, such as hypoxia, anoxia, and hypoglycemia; hemorrhages in the cranial cavity; acute cerebral edema; digestive disorders, such as the leukodystrophies; and cerebrovascular accidents.

Toxic exogenous and endogenous substances also may result in seizure activity. Some of the substances include pentylenetetrazol (Metrozol), alcohol intoxication or its abrupt withdrawal, lead encephalopathy, and shigella or salmonella ingestion. Metabolic disturbances that result in interferences in essential requirements, such as oxygen, calcium, sodium, glucose, and magnesium, may precipitate seizures. Other metabolic states that have been associated with seizure activity include alkalosis, uremia, hyperbilirubinemia, and disorders of amino acid metabolism. Finally, fever is another factor that may precipitate a seizure in some children.[26,39,40]

The child's age at first seizure may provide a clue to the cause of the disorder. In the neonatal group frequent causes of seizures include birth injuries (oxygen deficiencies and traumatic hemorrhages) and congenital anomalies of the brain. Other common causes of seizure disorders in this age group are metabolic disorders (hypoglycemia and hyperbilirubinemia), neonatal tetanus, narcotic withdrawal in infants born to addicted mothers, and meningitis.

Idiopathic seizures usually are seen for the first time in children 1 month to 3 years of age; tuberous sclerosis is a frequent cause of seizures at this time. Electrolyte imbalances, ingestion of foreign toxic substances, hypoglycemic episodes, and subdural hematomas are other causative factors in this age group.

In children older than 3 years of age seizures that result from acute infections are less common. However, residual neuronal damage from former injuries may precipitate seizures at this time. Disease states that may increase the likelihood of seizure disorders in this population include renal disorders (uremia and hypertension), degenerative disorders, space-occupying lesions, metabolic disorders, and the hormonal and metabolic changes associated with adolescence.

Regardless of the cause and type of seizure, a seizure can occur whenever the threshold on nerve cells is lowered, resulting in an excessive discharge of electrical impulses. These excessive electrical impulses may arise from a central area of the brain that immediately affects consciousness; localized areas of the cerebral cortex, producing manifestations limited to that particular anatomic focus; and localized areas of the cortex that spread to other portions of the brain.

The group of hyperexcitable cells responsible for seizure activity are referred to as the epileptogenic focus. These epileptogenic discharges can be identified on EEG tracings, which assist determination of their location. Normally these hyperexcitable cells are restrained from spreading their electrical discharge to surrounding cells by normal inhibitory mechanisms. However, in response to a variety of physiologic stimuli, such as hypoglycemia, electrolyte imbalances, dehydration, overhydration, emotional stress, and endocrine chances, the normal inhibiting mechanisms are weakened. This permits the epileptogenic focus to spread to surrounding synaptically related cells.

Although the pathophysiology of seizures is not clear, several conditions have been identified that may precipitate excessive discharges. Some experts believe seizure activity is the result of alterations in the cellular-sodium potassium pump, a change in the cells' permeability to sodium, or an excess of excitatory neurotransmitters. Whatever the cause, seizures occur as a result of excessive excitatory influences or insufficient inhibititory influences.

Clinical Manifestations. Clinical manifestations may be broken down into various categories based on phases of a seizure, classifications of seizures, and unclassified seizures.

Phases of a Seizure. Seizure activity occurs in several phases: prodromal, ictal, and postictal.

Prodromal Phase. In the prodromal phase the child may undergo mood or behavioral changes called prodromes (warning symptoms). Prodromes may precede a seizure by hours or days and include an aura. The aura is a peculiar sensation experienced by some people just before the onset of a seizure and may be explained as a flash of light, metallic flash, or an unusual sound or smell. An aura serves two useful purposes: It provides a warning so that safety measures may be taken, and it may provide a reliable clue to the origin of the discharge. For instance visual hallucinations implicate the occipital or temporal lobe; verbal phenomena originate in the dominant hemisphere; unusual tastes, odors, visceral sensations, or dream-like cloudiness have a temporal lobe origin.

Ictal Phase. As seizure activity begins so does the ictal phase. Muscle contraction during a seizure can be either clonic, tonic, or jacksonian. Clonic contractions produce rhythmic motions due to opposing muscles alternately contracting and relaxing. Tonic contractions cause the child to become rigid because all of the involved muscles are maintained in contraction for a period of time. Jacksonian contractions begin with muscle twitching or tremors that spread from one area to another. Furthermore, seizure activity may involve the entire body, one side, or one or more body parts. Eye movements also are obvious during seizure activity. Bilateral discharges cause the eyes to move upward, and unilateral discharges cause the eyes to deviate to the opposite side. Loss of consciousness commonly accompanies a seizure and indicates a generalized cortical involvement.

Postictal Phase. In the postictal phase immediately following a seizure behavior may be varied. The child may be drowsy, confused, uncoordinated, and display some motor or sensory impairment. Behavioral changes, weakness, or the inability to move part of the body may be an indication of the epileptogenic focus area.

Classification of Seizures. The International Classification of Epileptic Seizure developed by the International League Against Epilepsy developed a uniform system of classifying seizures.[8] This system of classification recognized that seizures can be separated into two fundamental types: those of focal or partial origin and those that are generalized from the onset. Seizures that do not fall into the focal or generalized categories are considered unclassified.

Focal (Partial) Seizures. Focal (partial) seizures are caused by abnormal electric discharges from epileptogenic foci from a specific region of the cerebral cortex. The focus of the seizure usually is secondary to an underlying condition that causes damage to brain tissue. Focal lesions include scar tissue from trauma or surgery, atrophy, malformations, or space-occupying lesions. The frontal, temporal, and parietal lobes are most often involved in focal seizure activity. Focal seizures are of three types: psychomotor (complex), motor, or sensory-motor (Table 53-6).

Psychomotor seizures often are observed in children from 3 years of age through adolescence and are more

TABLE 53-6
Characteristics of Focal (Partial) Seizures

Psychomotor	Motor	Sensory-Motor
Cognitive disruption	Clonic activity of any muscle group but mostly hand and face	Tingling or numbness of a body part
Automatism		
Visual, auditory, olfactory hallucinations	Jacksonian seizure	Visual, auditory, taste, or olfactory sensations
No recall of behavior	Autonomic symptoms: diapluresis, tachycardia, flushing	
Postictal state		Odd posturing
Age 3 years or older		Age 8 years or older
	No postictal state	

common in adults. Complex seizures are sometimes referred to as temporal lobe seizures because temporal lobe foci are the most common. This seizure type can alter behavior and produce automatisms (performed unconsciously), such as lip smacking, chewing, drooling, swallowing, grimacing, and picking hand movements. Many different sensory experiences can precede automatisms. The most frequent is a strange abdominal discomfort accompanied by odd or unpleasant tastes or odors, complex auditory or visual hallucinations, and a wild-eyed appearance and jumbled repetitive phrases.

A wide variety of motor behavior may be observed during a psychomotor attack. However, the attacks frequently are stereotypic and occur in a similar manner each time. The primary features of psychomotor seizures in children are confusion and purposeless, repetitive activity (automatism), most often followed by postictal sleep or confusion. Psychomotor seizures typically last from 30 seconds to several minutes.

Motor seizures originate in the frontal lobe; they begin in the head or face. The most common form is referred to as an aversive seizure, in which the eyes or hands turn away from the affected side. Another common form is the sylvian seizure, which most commonly occurs during sleep. This type involves tonic–clonic movements of the face, increased salivation, and arrested speech. Rarely, jacksonian motor seizures occur. Jacksonian seizures involve adjacent areas of the motor cortex and therefore affect a greater body area. For example a seizure may begin in the fingers, spread to the arm, and then move to the entire side of the body. Focal motor seizures most often are clonic, begin slow and intensify, and last from 5 seconds to several minutes.

Sensory-motor seizures are uncommon in children younger than 8 years. These seizures are characterized by visual sensations, tingling, numbness, pain, prickling, or paresthesias. Tonic–clonic movements or odd posturing may follow these sensations.

Generalized Seizures. Generalized seizures involve abnormal electric charges that occur bilaterally within the brain. There are basically four types: absence seizures, tonic–clonic seizures, myoclonic seizures, and atonic seizures (Table 53-7).

Absence (petit mal) seizures commonly occur in children 5 to 12 years of age. They frequently are discovered when the child begins school. Teachers may complain that the child has a tendency to daydream and appears unable to concentrate on subjects at hand. On close inspection the child has staring or blinking spells accompanied by a loss of consciousness that may last a few seconds. Absence seizures may number in the hundreds each day and interfere with normal functioning.

In this type of seizure the abnormal electric discharge rapidly spreads from the epileptogenic focus to the entire cerebral cortex. This rapid electric discharge results in only brief losses of consciousness. Absence seizures commonly last for 2 years; approximately 50% of children no longer experience seizures after this time. However, in adolescents absence seizures can progress to become tonic–clonic seizures.

Tonic–clonic (grand mal) seizures are the most common type of seizure and are associated with convulsions. These seizures may occur at any time, often are preceded by a warning (aura), and are characterized by the tonic or stiffening phase followed by the clonic or jerking phase. After a seizure the child will experience a postictal period.

Tonic–clonic seizures commonly occur shortly after the warning aura. Some children know to seek help and lie down, while others may seek privacy due to embar-

TABLE 53-7
Characteristics of Generalized Seizures

Absence	Tonic–Clonic	Myoclonic	Atonic
Petit mal seizures	Grand mal seizures	Brief, rapid contractions of upper extremities	Akinetic seizures (drop seizures)
5 to 12 y	Most common type	Lasts 1 to 2 s	3 to 12 y
Daydreaming, vacant staring, blinking followed by loss of consciousness for a few seconds	Preceded by aura	No loss of consciousness	Transient loss of trunk and muscle tone
	Tonic (rigidity) phase lasts a few seconds followed by clonic (twitching): convulsions, incontinence, inability to manage saliva, tongue biting, loss of consciousness	No postictal period	Associated with myoclonic jerks
		One of least severe forms	Frequent falls
May occur 100 times a day		*Infantile spasms* (head drop seizure 3 to 12 mo)	No loss of consciousness
Frequently resolved in 2 y	Lasts up to 5 min	Flexion/extension of head, trunk, and extremities	Functional impairment
	Postictal period of several hours	May occur 100 times a day	May occur 100 times a day
	Headache upon awakening	No loss of consciousness	
		Disappear but progress to focal, psychomotor, or generalized seizures	
		Develop severe retardation	
		High mortality rate	

assment. If the child is not sitting or lying when the seizure activity begins, they will fall. The child undergoing a seizure may become cyanotic due to hypoxia. The eyes often roll up, and the pupils become dilated. An overall rigidity is noted as muscles clamp down. It is not uncommon for the tongue to become lacerated as the jaws contract. The tonic period may last only a few seconds followed by the clonic stage in which the muscles twitch. This twitching results in uncontrolled movements of some or all body parts; thus, the term convulsions evolved. During this clonic stage incontinence of urine and feces and the inability to handle saliva, which may appear as foaming at the mouth, may be observed. Tonic–clonic seizures usually last 5 minutes or less and are followed by a postictal period of deep sleep or confusion for several hours. A headache is common when the child awakens.

Myoclonic seizures may be present in children with metabolic encephalopathies, degenerative disorders, and infectious processes. Children who experience myoclonic seizure exhibit brief, rapid contractions of the upper extremities. Usually this is a single jerk of one or more muscle groups, lasting only 1 to 2 seconds. The trunk and lower extremities are rarely involved. This forceful contraction may cause the child to throw or drop an object being held. No loss of consciousness occurs.

Myoclonic seizures occur most often on awakening and are common in retarded children with nonprogressive static encephalopathies due to a variety of causes. Myoclonic seizures respond well to treatment and are considered one of the least severe forms of seizure disorders.

Infantile spasms also termed salaam or head-drop seizures are a form of myoclonic seizure. Affected infants are usually 3 to 12 months of age. During this episode the head, trunk, and limbs may be flexed or extended symmetrically, or the trunk and head may quickly extend while the limbs remain flexed. Hundreds of these rapid seizures may occur per day. No loss of consciousness or postictal period is evident with infantile spasms. Clinically these infants seem colicky and jittery, and they may manifest spells of laughing and smiling. Normal activity and attention to the environment are constantly interrupted by these spells, especially when the child is stimulated.

Infantile spams gradually resolve, even in the absence of treatment. Fifty percent of children become free of spasms by age 2; persistent spasms beyond age 5 are rare. Unfortunately, cessation of spasms is accompanied by severe retardation and focal, psychomotor, or generalized seizures in approximately two thirds of surviving children. Only approximately 10% of children who develop infantile spasms will have normal intelligence. Mortality rates have been reported to be as high as 15% to 20%.

Atonic seizures sometimes are called drop attacks. They are most common in children between the ages of 3 and 12 years. Atonic seizures consist of a transient loss of trunk and muscle tone, which causes the child to fall. Atonic seizures may be associated with myoclonic jerks.

Patients often describe the child as clumsy and uncoordinated due to the frequent falls. Because no loss of consciousness occurs, diagnosis may be hampered by a delay in seeking medical attention. Like absence seizures, hundreds of drop attacks may occur each day.

A variety of functional impairments, including intelligence, perceptual, motor, and mental deficiencies frequently are associated with atonic seizures. It is believed the abnormal electric discharge begins in the centrencephalon and extends to the brainstem and peripheral muscles.

Unclassified Seizures. There are seizures (not included in the International Classification of Seizures) that either clinically or electrographically do not meet the established criteria. Pseudoseizures, febrile seizures, and status epilepticus are unclassified seizures.

Pseudoseizures. Pseudoseizures closely resemble seizure activity, which makes diagnosis difficult. They most often occur in children and adolescents; girls are affected twice as often as boys. Electrographic studies indicate that no abnormal electric discharge occurs within the brain with pseudoseizures. Most experts conclude that pseudoseizures are psychologically determined. Clinical manifestations of pseudoseizures differ from true seizure activity. A witness is almost always present, and pseudoseizures last longer than most epileptic seizures. The child may obey commands and demonstrate eye focusing during these episodes. Abnormal motor activity is present; however, protective mechanisms remain intact (such as breaking a fall or protecting the head from hitting the ground). No tongue biting, incontinence, or dilatation of the pupils occurs. Postictal confusion does not occur. Pseudoseizures require psychotherapeutic treatment or hypnosis.

Febrile Seizures. Febrile seizures usually are transient in children and occur in association with a fever. Febrile seizures are among the most common neurologic disorders of childhood, occurring in 2% to 4% of children younger than 5 years of age. Because of a lowered seizure threshold, children between the ages of 6 months and 6 years are susceptible to seizures when their temperature rises above 38.8° C (101.8° F). Febrile seizures occur with increased frequency in children younger than 18 months of age. Twice as many boys as girls experience febrile seizures, and there appears to be an increased susceptibility in families, indicating a possible genetic disposition.

The cause of febrile seizures is uncertain. The majority of febrile seizures occur within the first 24 hours of an illness, often as the temperature is rapidly increasing. In some children the first indication of an illness may be the seizure. Febrile seizures commonly accompany an upper respiratory or gastrointestinal infection, and 25% of these children may suffer recurrent seizures with subsequent infections. As the number of febrile seizures increases, the severity of the seizures also increases.

The degree of the fever is not the precipitating factor in the seizure. Once the fever has fallen and rises a second time during an illness, some children will not seize again, even though the previous precipitating temperature elevation has been reached or exceeded. The speed with which the fever escalates is more important in some children than the degree of increase in temperature.

A febrile seizure can be diagnosed only after other causes that may precipitate this activity have been excluded. CNS infections and inflammation, acute metabolic disorders, aberrations in water and electrolyte balance, and structural lesions must be ruled out.

The recurrence rate for febrile seizures has been reported to be between 25% and 50%. Approximately 33% of recurrences take place within 1 year of the first seizure. Also, children who exhibit febrile seizures have an increased risk for developing a chronic seizure disorder.

Status Epilepticus.   Status epilepticus is defined by the international classification as repeated seizures occurring so frequently as "to produce a fixed and enduring epileptic condition." Consciousness is not regained between seizures. Approximately 5% to 10% of the pediatric seizure population will have a status epilepticus attack at some time. Approximately 50% of children with this condition are younger than 2 years of age. The mortality rate has been reported to be as high as 50%. Death often is caused by cardiac or respiratory arrest from the seizure activity alone or in combination with medications used to stop the convulsions. Sepsis, meningitis, encephalitis, trauma, or toxic or metabolic encephalopathies may result in status epilepticus and must be evaluated rapidly and early in the child who is having recurrent seizures.

Status epilepticus represents a medical emergency not only because of an underlying treatable cause, but also because 15% to 20% of children suffer permanent neurologic damage. Frequent causes of status epilepticus in a child with a known seizure disorder include noncompliance with anticonvulsive therapy and subtherapeutic levels of the anticonvulsant. Children without a history of seizure activity who experience an attack of status epilepticus frequently have suffered a head trauma that results in a subarachnoid or intracerebral hemorrhage, encephalitis or meningitis, hypoglycemia or hyponatremia, or an acute drug or alcohol withdrawal syndrome.

Status epilepticus may involve any type of focal or generalized seizure; however, tonic–clonic activity is the most common and poses the greatest threat due to risk of anoxia, cardiac dysrhythmias, and systemic lactic acidosis. Focal status epilepticus usually involves a repetitive clonic-type movement of the face or arms. An absence status may exist, in which clinically no muscle activity is seen, but confusion and inattention are present.

Diagnostic Studies.   The process of diagnosis in a child with a seizure disorder includes determining the type of seizure the child has experienced and determining the underlying cause of the seizure. A detailed history should be obtained from a reliable source with emphasis on a description of the seizure, parts of the body involved, length of attack, behavior following the seizure, age at onset, precipating factors (fever, infection, falls, anxiety, fatigue, sensory stimulation), and previous medical record.

Laboratory studies that may prove to be of value include blood chemistries (blood urea nitrogen, electrolyte levels, liver function tests, calcium and phoshorous levels, studies for toxic substances); a complete blood cell count (to rule out lead poisoning); and a white cell count for signs of infection. Blood and urine amino acid levels may help in diagnosing a metabolic etiology for the seizures.

A lumbar puncture usually is part of the diagnostic workup for seizures. Spinal fluid is analyzed for cell count, glucose, protein levels, and serology. An elevated opening pressure may indicate a space-occupying lesion (e.g., hemorrhage or tumor).

The EEG is the most useful tool for evaluating seizure disorders in children. This is a physiologic recording and does not determine the underlying cause; that is, a tumor may not be distinguished from a blood clot. An EEG is useful in localizing the focus of onset of a seizure, determining the various seizure types (high-voltage spikes are seen in grand mal seizures; wave patterns are observed in petit mal seizures), and recording the activity for future comparisons. There are various manipulation procedures that may be used during an EEG to stimulate a seizure: sleep or sleep deprivation prior to the EEG, hyperventilation, flashing lights, and loud noises.

Skull x-rays and CAT scans also are useful. Skull films may reveal cranial growth asymmetry or intracranial calcifications. A CT scan allows visualization of anatomic structures inside the skull (tumors, infarctions, edema, hemorrhage, congenital lesions, vascular abnormalities), which may aid in the diagnosis of underlying causes.

★ **ASSESSMENT**

Because the onset, characteristics, and progression of seizure activity may help determine the type and location of a seizure, the nurse begins an assessment by taking a complete and detailed history. Accurate descriptions of the seizure's onset and pattern may help pinpoint its cause. Possible precipitating factors, such as menses, drugs, lack of sleep, stress, head trauma, encephalitis, meningitis, diabetes, hypertension, and febrile seizures, should be investigated. Also, a complete medication history (noncompliance with medication regimens may contribute to seizure activity) and family history of neurologic disorders should be obtained. When possible the child should be questioned about the presence of an aura or other prodromal symptoms (mood or behavioral changes, unusual sound or smell, nausea, metallic taste, flash of light). However, if the child is seizing, the physical assessment should be limited to direct observation and recording of specific behaviors. Historic information can be obtained later.

★ **NURSING DIAGNOSES AND PLANNING**

Based on assessment data discussed previously and in the preceding chapter, the following nursing diagnoses may apply to the family and child with seizures:

- Sensory/Perceptual Alterations related to altered sensory integration.
- High Risk for Injury related to seizure activity.
- Ineffective Airway Clearance related to seizure activity.
- Altered Oral Mucous Membranes related to medication.
- Body Image Disturbance related to seizure activity.
- Ineffective Individual Coping related to seizure activity.
- Situational Low Self-Esteem related to seizure activity.
- Anxiety related to threat to self-concept.
- Fear related to subsequent seizure activity.
- Ineffective Management of Therapeutic Regimen related to developmental age.

The nurse and child (or parents) together plan effective care based on the established nursing diagnoses. Several examples of expected outcomes follow:

- The family demonstrates a knowledge of protection methods during seizures.
- The child describes precautions to take when there is a warning of seizure activity.
- The child and family describe medications and possible side-effects.
- The child participates in school activities as directed by health care workers.

The nurse plans for the daily care of the child based on physician's orders and nursing diagnoses. Some general nursing care goals may be the following:

- Protection is provided during seizure activity.
- Medication provides relief with no or few side-effects.
- Diet therapy is maintained by family.

★ NURSING INTERVENTIONS: COLLABORATIVE AND INDEPENDENT

Management of seizure activity falls into four categories:

- Use of anticonvulsant medications
- Removal of causative and precipitating factors
- Protection of the child during seizure activity
- Education of the child and family regarding seizure activity.

MEDICATION THERAPY

The drugs used to control seizures are outlined in Table 53-8. Approximately 70% to 80% of children who experience seizures benefit from anticonvulsants. Anticonvulsants raise the seizure threshold or prevent the spread of abnormal electric discharges by desensitizing normal neurons to the barrage of stimulation from the seizure focus. The choice of anticonvulsant drugs is based on the type of seizure disorder being treated, the dosage required to achieve therapeutic levels, the side-effects produced, and the availability of alternative drugs in case the first drug fails. Generally one drug is chosen to treat the seizure disorder and is given in increasingly higher doses until a therapeutic blood level is reached. If the child continues to seize, a second drug may be started and given until it reaches a therapeutic blood level. Because children absorb, metabolize, and excrete anticonvulsant drugs at different rates, an individualized dosage regimen is necessary.

Periodic drug therapy re-evaluation is important to assess the continued effectiveness during rapid growth and physical or emotional stress and when the child has been seizure free for more than 2 years. If the child has remained seizure free for 2 years, he or she may be slowly weaned from anticonvulsant therapy. However, some children require lifelong therapy. All follow-up examinations should include frequent blood cell counts, liver studies, urinalysis, and measurements of anticonvulsant blood serum levels.

When a decision has been made to terminate anticonvulsant therapy, medication should be gradually reduced for a period of weeks. Sudden withdrawal of these drugs can precipitate an increase in the number and severity of seizures.

NUTRITIONAL MANAGEMENT

In some cases fasting has been effective in reducing seizures. A diet that restricts proteins and carbohydrates stimulates ketosis and acidosis. It is generally believed that ketone has a tranquilizing effect and raises the seizure threshold. Approximately 80% of caloric requirements should be supplied by fats. Fluid restriction creating a negative fluid balance also increases the ketogenic effect.

Although anticonvulsant therapy remains the most successful treatment for seizures, a ketogenic diet may be beneficial for children who respond poorly to anticonvulsant treatment. The diet is most effective in children between the ages of 2 and 5 years.

SURGICAL MANAGEMENT

When seizure activity is thought to be caused by a tumor, hematoma, progressive cerebral lesion, or other operable condition, surgical treatment is initiated. However, when anticonvulsant therapy has proven unsuccessful and a distinct epileptogenic focus is believed to be responsible for seizures, a surgical excision may be considered. The goal is to remove the epileptogenic focus with as little neurologic deficit as possible. Sometimes the seizure focus is in a part of the brain that is not accessible, and too much brain damage would occur when attempting to reach it. Occasionally the scar tissue from the operation may be a future site for seizure activity; therefore, the child may continue to have seizures even after surgery. Surgical excision does not eliminate the need for anticonvulsant therapy until the child is free of seizures for at least 4 years.

MONITORING AND PROTECTION DURING SEIZURE ACTIVITY

During a seizure, protecting the child and observing seizure activity are of the utmost importance. Care directives are based on the phase and severity of the seizure.

Someone should stay with the child during the seizure. The child should be placed face down or on the side to keep the airway clear, especially to keep the tongue from sliding back in the throat. Nothing should be placed in the child's mouth. Protect the child from injuries caused by thrashing of the body. Do not confine the child's movements but move objects out of the way. If the child stops breathing, this is part of the seizure; normally the child will begin to breathe again on his or her own.

If the child is hospitalized, one of the nurse's responsibilities is to observe and make notes on the seizure. It is important to note the time of onset and behavioral characteristics immediately prior to the attack. Frequently the child will fall or emit a cry just prior to the seizure. Observe the parts of the body involved and the order and character of the movements. Did muscle twitching originate in the face, arms, or legs? How did it progress? Check the direction of the eyes for nystagmus and note changes in pupillary size. Record any bladder or bowel incontinence, lip or tongue biting, apnea, cyanosis, increased salivation, or head deviation that accompanies the seizure. Because hypoxia occurs during some seizures, observe changes in respiratory patterns, and assess airway status.

TABLE 53-8
Common Anticonvulsant Drugs

Medication	Indications	Usual Dosage	Therapeutic Serum Level	Side-Effects or Adverse Reactions
Barbiturates				
Phenobarbital (Luminal or Mebaral)	All seizure states. Safest overall drug. May be given in combination with other drugs	1 to 5 mg/kg per day in children. Long half-life; may be taken once a day	20 to 40 mg/ml	Drowsiness, dizziness, fever, depression, irritability, rash, ataxia, megaloblastic anemia, osteomalacia, nystagmus, hyperactivity. Decreases warfarin absorption, potentiates valproic acid and phenothiazine. Tolerance may develop
Primidone	Generalized tonic–clonic seizures. May be the drug of choice for partial and complex partial seizures	10 to 20 mg/kg per day	7 to 15 mg/ml	Contains phenobarbital so it has similar side-effects. Drowsiness, nausea, ataxia, nystagmus, rash, anemia, diplopia. Potentiated by isoniazid
Hydantoin				
Phenytoin (Dilantin)	Tonic–clonic seizures, complex and other partial seizures, psychomotor for seizures, status epilepticus	5 to 10 mg/kg per day. Half-life is 24 hours; may be taken once a day	9 to 20 mg/ml	Gastrointestinal upset, ataxia, nystagmus, diplopia, acne, hirsutism, dermatitis, hypocalcemia, osteomalacia, agranulocytosis, megaloblastic anemia, leukopenia, increased cholesterol, lupus-like syndrome, insulin suppression, gingival hyperplasia. Causes discoloration of urine (red, pink, brown). Increases metabolism of digitalis and warfarin
Miscellaneous				
Carbamazepine, complex and other (Tegretol)	Tonic–clonic seizures, partial seizures, psychomotor seizures	7 to 20 mg/kg per day. Half-life is short, so must be taken every 8 hours	4 to 10 mg/ml	Dry mouth, nausea, vomiting, drowsiness, ataxia, dizziness, jaundice, edema, rash, skin eruptions, leukopenia, aplastic anemia, pancytopenia. Decreased phenytoin levels may cause inappropriate secretions of ADH in toxic levels and low urine output
Ethosuximide (Zarontin)	Absence attacks, minor motor seizures	20 to 30 mg/kg per day	40 to 90 mg/ml	Gastrointestinal upset, drowsiness, dizziness, headache, hiccups, loss of appetite, euphoria, irritability, urinary frequency, swelling of tongue, leukopenia, abnormal liver function
Valproic acid (Depakene)	Partial, simple, and complex absences initially, multiple seizures	10 mg/kg per day. 40 mg/kg per day maximum	50 to 100 mg/ml	Nausea, vomiting, drowsiness, ataxia, transient hair loss, diarrhea and stomach cramps when toxic levels are reached, altered bleeding times, liver toxicity
Benzodiazepines				
Diazepam (Valium)	States epilepticus, severe tonic–clonic seizures	2 to 10 mg/dose given IV to stop a seizure. Half-life is short; give in conjunction with an anticonvulsant		Sedation, respiratory arrest, fatigue, ataxia
Clonazepam (Clonopin)	Myoclonic and akinetic seizures, minor motor, absence attacks, and complex partial attacks	0.1 to 0.2 mg/kg per day	20 to 50 mg/ml	Lethargy, drowsiness, dizziness, thick speech, hypotonia, hyperactivity, anorexia, rash, thrombocytopenia, hypersalivation, behavior changes

Vital signs should be recorded after the seizure activity has ceased.

During the postictal stage the nurse reassures an adequate airway and checks for apparent injury (tongue lacerations, results of a fall, or tonic–clonic activity). Also, the child's neurologic status should be described, noting behavioral changes, confusion, lethargy, transient local paralysis, expressive or receptive aphasia, weakness, headache, and sleep patterns after the seizure.

Assessment of the child's immediate environment also is the responsibility of the nurse. Objects that could cause harm should be removed from the vicinity. Side rails should always be in the upright position to prevent falls; some institutions pad bed rails to prevent injury during seizure activity.

TEACHING AND COUNSELING

The child and family members need teaching and counseling regarding the disease and its prognosis. Anxieties are high, and everyone needs to be reassured that (in most cases) the child can lead a fairly normal life once the seizures are controlled. Parents must learn how to manage seizure activity to avoid being overprotective.

The parents and child must learn the importance of taking the anticonvulsant medication regularly. The medication may need to be taken for many years. Once the initial diagnosis has been made and the seizures are controlled by medications, the child is able to return to school and a lead normal life. Certain precautions must be taken, at least temporarily. For instance, some children may need to wear protective helmets. Bicycle riding and some activities should be curtailed until the child is seizure free for at least 6 months. It is advisable for the child to wear a Medic Alert bracelet if the child still has seizures or is in an environment where his or her companions may not know the diagnosis. Adolescents may want to learn to drive; regulations regarding driving vary from state to state.

In addition to learning about the disease and its prognosis, the parents will need to know how to care for the child during seizure activity. The nurse can share the same information he or she needs to know (given in the previous section). The parents should also be taught to observe activities prior to the seizure that may indicate an aura or a cause for the seizure.

Parents and children need in-depth education regarding dosage and side-effects of anticonvulsants (see Table 53-8). Further subjects to be discussed with the family are presented in the accompanying Teaching Plan.

★ EVALUATION

Periodically the nurse and family evaluate the outcomes of care given. Examples of outcomes for the child and family with seizures were given under Nursing Diagnoses and Planning in this section.

Degenerative Disorders

Alterations in neurologic function classified as degenerative are among the most difficult for the child, family, and nurse. These alterations are progressive and render the child increasingly dependent and incapacitated with the knowledge that the condition usually is terminal. The comfort of the child and family are high priorities. Care is provided to assist the child in remaining as independent as possible for as long as possible. Self-care procedures are simplified to make life more bearable for the child and family and to provide emotional support while preventing complications. Eventually the child loses all intellectual and voluntary motor functions, becoming totally helpless and unresponsive. Nursing management for children with degenerative neurologic disorders is presented here and in Table 53-9. Nursing assessment and

diagnoses relative to the specific disorder are presented after a discussion of that disorder.

Nursing Management of Children With Degenerative Neurologic Disorders

Major elements of caring for children and families of children with degenerative neurologic disorders include prevention of injury, prevention of infection, precise and meticulous monitoring of vital signs and intake and output, provision of adequate nutrition, maintenance of skin integrity, maintenance of mobility, prevention of contractures for as long as possible, and emotional support of child and family.

Prevention of Injury

Loss of motor coordination, sensory input, and cognitive function contribute to the risk for accidental injury in children with neurodegenerative disorders. Protective helmets may be helpful when falls, seizures, or severe lack of motor coordination are present. Creating a safe environment by padding sharp corners of furniture is helpful with small children. Assistive devices such as walkers, canes, and crutches to provide mobility and safety may be helpful. Safety restraints on wheelchairs and other equipment should always be used. Chest restraints, shoulder straps, bolster pads, and other devices for head support protect children from injury in wheelchairs and automobiles. When the child is too large for a conventional car seat but too unstable for a conventional seat belt, special harnesses, adapted car seats, and travel chairs with retractable wheels that may also double as wheelchairs may be the answer to providing safety.

Weakness of the neck and trunk can lead to injury or airway obstruction if the child slumps sideways or forward in a chair and cannot regain an upright position. Appropriate positioning and postural support maintain the child's functional body alignment and protect the child from potential injury.

Prevention of Infection

Limited mobility, loss of motor coordination, and immunologic deficits add to the risk of infection in children with neurodegenerative disorders. Children with the highest risk may be placed on prophylactic antibiotics. Respiratory and urinary infections are common, and the child should be protected from contact with people who have respiratory or other infections.

Provision of Adequate Nutrition

Children experiencing loss of motor coordination, loss of sensory feedback and integration, and progressive loss of consciousness require intervention to maintain adequate nutrition. Initially children may need eating implements to be altered, such as padding the handles of knives, forks, and spoons, to help feed themselves. Soft nipples or syringe feeders may be needed. The type

TABLE 53-9
Nursing Diagnoses and Interventions for the Child With a Degenerative Neurologic Disorder

Nursing Diagnosis	Nursing Interventions	Rationale
Anxiety related to knowledge deficit regarding diagnosis, treatment, and prognosis	Teach child and family what they do not already know about the diagnosis, treatment, and prognosis for the child.	An individualized teaching plan enhances its effectiveness and coping.
Sensory perceptual alterations related to impaired sensation, loss of consciousness, and decreasing cerebral function	Protect child from injury; sensations of heat, pain, or body position may be lost.	Prevention of pain and injury allows child to use resources for maintenance.
	Provide orienting stimuli, such as television, clock, or calendar.	Disorientation increases anxiety and consumes energy that could be used for healing and maintenance.
	Encourage parents to touch and talk to child to enhance orientation.	
	Note and post signs regarding perceptual deficits to alert all caregivers (e.g., double vision, no sensation left side, child cannot talk).	Alerting other professionals to sensory deficits improves quality of care.
	Check neurologic signs and sensation on a regular basis and report increasing sensory deficits.	Early recognition of increasing sensory deficits facilitates caregiving and decreases accidents.
Altered thought processes related to loss of cerebral function and increased intracranial pressure	Establish communication, either verbal, written, eyeblinks, or hand squeezes to signify yes or no.	Communication decreases anxiety and enhances cooperation.
	Eliminate distractions, such as television or radio, and establish eye contact with child before speaking. Speak slowly, distinctly, and loud enough to be heard. Use simple language and short sentences.	Attention span and powers of concentration may be limited. These techniques enhance concentration.
	Repeat important information and reinforce as necessary.	Repetition enhances retention, which may be difficult with memory losses.
Impaired physical mobility related to loss of function, increased intracranial pressure, and loss of consciousness	Provide passive range-of-motion, stretching, and elongation exercises.	Stretching, elongation, and range-of-motion exercises maintain existing joint motion.
	Seek consultation of physical and occupational therapists regarding best position for child and most appropriate exercises.	
	Use mobilizing devices to increase locomotion and independence.	Mobilizing devices provide support and increase independence.
High risk for injury related to seizures or loss of nerve function	Provide a safe environment: • Side rails up • Padded side rails if indicated • Durable toys appropriate to developmental level and manipulative ability • Protective helmet for children prone to falls when walking • Restraints while in wheelchair or vehicles • Seizure precautions for children who also have seizure disorder.	Routine safety precautions prevent injuries from seizures and from uncontrolled or uncoordinated movements.
	Provide sufficient rest before exercise and during the day.	Fatigue may increase accidental injuries and precipitate seizures.
	Teach the family how to provide safety at home (when appropriate).	These precautions increase the child's safety while at home.
	Supervise child during bathing, swimming, or climbing. Pad sharp edges of tables and other furniture. Carpet stairs. Supervise use of stove, sharp toys, or utensils. Children who fall frequently should wear a protective helmet.	
Pain	Administer pain medication as ordered without allowing pain to build to a severe level before medication is given.	Administering pain medication before pain becomes severe enhances comfort and decreases amount of medication needed to relieve pain.
	Use distraction and relaxation techniques to assist in reduction of pain.	These techniques reduce perception of pain.

(Continued)

TABLE 53-9
(Continued)

Nursing Diagnosis	Nursing Interventions	Rationale
Fear and anxiety related to progressive loss of previous abilities and approaching death	Encourage child and family to express feelings of fear and anxiety.	Expressing feelings enhances coping.
	Provide child with drawing materials or crayons, and ask child to draw a picture of a person or family.	Children's drawings are nonverbal representations of themselves and their feelings, and they enhance coping.
	Allow child's favorite diversional activities and incorporate them into care plan.	Diversional activities take the child's mind off of health status and enhance coping.
	Allow child to discuss feelings about death. Answer child's questions honestly.	Discussion of impending death allows child to allay fear and prepare for separation from family.
Impaired verbal communication	Establish a communication system for child based on family input (hand gestures, communication board, eye blinks to indicate yes or no).	Communication is essential for establishing rapport, gaining cooperation, and providing child with a sense of security.
	Provide child with means of summoning the nurse in an emergency if use of the call button is not possible.	Provision for summoning emergency assistance enhances sense of security and safety.
Body image disturbance; chronic low self-esteem; personal identity disturbance; altered role performance	Assist child to express feelings about loss of body function and loss of independence.	Expression of feelings assists understanding and enhances coping.
	Provide child and family with choices about activities, and provide opportunities for as much self-direction and independence as condition permits.	Choices and self-direction allow a sense of control and achievement, which enhance self-esteem.
Altered nutrition: less than body requirements related to loss of motor control	Provide assistance with feeding if motor deficits are present and tube feed when appropriate (see Chap. 59 for care of child requiring tube feeding).	Assistance with feeding increases consumption and decreases potential for aspiration.
	Ensure adequate fluid intake, especially cranberry juice, between tube feedings.	Increased fluids soften stools and flush kidneys to prevent stone formation.
High risk for impaired skin integrity	Turn and position every 1 to 2 hours on a special mattress (egg crate foam, water bed, or other types of special mattresses that alternate pressure points).	Turning and repositioning help to prevent pressure sores and improve circulation to muscles.
	Inspect skin for pressure areas, and provide frequent skin care.	Areas of friction or pressure can cause skin breakdown.
Impaired gas exchange and ineffective airway clearance	Turn, cough, and deep breathe every 2 hours.	Immobility leads to pooling of secretions; mobilizing secretions reduces potential for static pneumonia.
	Suction and perform chest physiotherapy as necessary to remove pooled secretions.	
	Elevate head of bed 15 to 30 degrees.	Elevation of head reduces gravitational pressure on diaphragm during breathing.
	Position child on side if unresponsive and not intubated.	Side-lying position maintains patent airway.
Ineffective breathing patterns	Monitor skin color, respiratory rate, pattern, tidal volume, and blood gases frequently to determine respiratory efficiency.	Early detection of ineffective breathing patterns prevents complications, cyanosis, and death.
	Provide oxygen therapy as directed.	Supplementary oxygen enhances diffusion.
High risk for infection	Use aseptic technique when performing intrusive procedures.	Stress of illness increases cortisol levels and leads to immunosuppression and increased susceptibility to infection.
	Keep open wounds clean, dry, and free from urine or feces.	

of food or its consistency may need to be altered to allow the child as much independence as possible when eating. Impaired control of oral muscles may result in difficulty swallowing, sucking, closing lips, chewing, or moving food in the mouth. Abnormal reflex patterns, such as tongue thrust or jaw clamping; loss of gag and swallowing reflexes; and gastroesophageal reflux may increase the risk of airway obstruction or aspiration. Gavage feeding or gastrotomy tubes eventually are necessary to augment oral feedings and maintain nutrition when oral feedings are no longer possible. Consultation with an occupational therapist may be helpful in designing individualized feeding techniques.

Prevention of Impaired Skin Integrity

Impaired movement and sensation added to the increased risk of injury create the risk for skin breakdown. Decreased sensitivity to pain and poor coordination or the presence of orthopedic appliances that do not fit properly leave the child susceptible to pressure sores. Special bed mattresses, such as gel, flotation, water beds, alternating pressure or high-density foam, and wheelchair pads, prevent pressure sores over bony prominences. Using sheepskin pads and keeping the bed linen free of wrinkles reduces friction, which predisposes the child to pressure sores. Daily inspection of the child's skin for injured or reddened areas and daily massages are recommended.

Maintenance of Mobility

Impaired mobility problems range from difficulties with fine motor coordination to total body paralysis. Adaptations must be made in clothes, tools to assist with dressing (such as hooks to assist with buttons and shoes), bedrooms to promote ease of rising and usefulness, and bathrooms for wheelchairs, walkers, bath chairs, and grab bars. Use of scooter boards, carts, wheelchairs, and crutches or canes can help the child to gain and maintain mobility for as long as possible.

Range-of-motion exercises every 4 hours are essential to prevent contractures and maintain flexibility in joints. Once the child becomes bedridden, all of the problems of immobility must be anticipated and prevented as much as possible. As long as the child has mental and fine motor function, toys may be adapted to provide diversional activity and exercise.

Promotion of Family Coping

Ineffective family coping patterns are common among families of children with degenerative neurologic disorders, and one of the major nursing responsibilities is to prevent maladaptive coping.[23] Nursing strategies that enhance adaptation include listening to concerns and feelings and providing positive reinforcement for parenting and for efforts toward participation in the care of the child; listening to fears and allaying anxiety when possible; explaining that parents of children with this disorder often feel guilty for bearing the child, for leaving the child's side, or for failing to prevent the disorder. Encourage parents to take time together away from the child so that the time with the child is more helpful and less emotionally draining. Parents need to plan special times to spend with their other children. The attention required by the child with a degenerative disorder is excessive and detracts from the time available for other siblings, who resent the loss of attention and the excessive demands of the ill child. Family counseling is critical for maintenance of family integrity; divorce frequently accompanies a diagnosis of a degenerative neurologic disorder.

Psychosocial Support

Every child with a degenerative neurologic disorder is at risk for low self-concept related to poor body image and loss of coordination. Role playing difficult situations is an important means of enabling the child to prepare for and cope with situations that could be detrimental to his or her self esteem. Nurses are in a prime position to assess factors that inhibit positive self-image and work with both the child and family to understand and intervene in self-concept issues. Planned activities consistent with the child's abilities, maintenance of independence, and contact with peers for as long as possible are essential. Meeting and socializing with other children with similar disorders may be helpful. Referral for special counseling, group counseling, and occupational therapy can improve self-esteem and self-concept.

Tay-Sachs Disease

Definition, Incidence, Etiology, and Clinical Manifestations. *Tay-Sachs disease* is an autosomal recessive disorder that results in neurologic deterioration. The allele or gene responsible for production of the enzyme hexosaminidase A does not function properly. Hexosaminidase is important in the metabolism of gangliosides, a class of glycosphingolipids that is specific to nerve and brain tissue. Lack of the hexosaminidase A enzyme causes the accumulation of sphingolipids in all cells of the body, but functional disorders are manifested primarily in the CNS. A characteristic feature of Tay-Sachs is a cherry red spot on the macula surrounded by a grayish white rim. It is caused by the accumulation of lipids in the retinal ganglion cells in the foveal region of the eye.

The clinical picture of the disorder is characteristic. One of the earliest signs of the disorder is an exaggerated startle response to noise (hyperacusis). Between 2 and 6 months of age an infant with Tay-Sachs begins to display apathy and loss of interest in the environment. Interaction with parents is decreased and finally is absent. Mental retardation occurs, along with a progressive loss of vision, motor function, and control. Progressive spasticity and hyperreflexia; tonic, myoclonic, or grand mal seizures; and decerebrate posturing may occur in the late stages of the disorder, along with feeding difficulties, emaciation, and progressive abnormal enlargement of the head. Most children with Tay-Sachs die between 3 and 6 years of age.

Tay-Sachs is inherited by children of parents who both carry a deleterious recessive allele. Each parent is normal in appearance and health but carries the mutant gene in a recessive pattern. The chances of a couple having a child with Tay-Sachs when both parents are carriers is one in four. The incidence of Tay-Sachs among the average population is 1 in 300, and in the Ashkenazi (Eastern European Jewish) population it is 1 in 25. The incidence in the New York City Jewish community is estimated to be 1 in 16 according to Merz.[25]

Diagnostic Studies. The basic defect in Tay-Sachs is the absence of the enzyme hexosaminidase A in all body tissues. The diagnostic procedure most commonly used is measurement of the enzyme in amniotic fluid cells through amniocentesis early in the pregnancy. After delivery the enzyme can be measured in serum or white cells for diagnosis.

★ **ASSESSMENT**

Assessment for hyperreflexia and exaggerated startle reflex in response to noise (hyperacusis) should be performed on infants (particularly Jewish infants) who present with apathy or progressive loss of motor function during the first 6 months following a normal birth and neonatal period. Affected infants will develop progressive hypotonia and blindness along with increasing feeding difficulties. They may develop spasticity, seizures, and decerebrate posturing. Developmental milestones will be delayed or not achieved, and death usually occurs in the preschool years.

★ **NURSING DIAGNOSES AND PLANNING**

Based on assessment data discussed previously and in the preceding chapter, the following nursing diagnoses may apply to the family and child with Tay-Sachs:

- Self-Care Deficit related to progressive loss of mental and motor function.
- Sensory/Perceptual Alterations related to progressive loss of vision and mental retardation.
- Anticipatory Grieving related to prognosis of progressive degeneration/death.
- Altered Family Processes related to terminally ill child.
- Anxiety related to knowledge deficit regarding disease management and complications.

The nurse and child (or parents) together plan effective care based on the established nursing diagnoses. Several examples of expected outcomes follow:

- The family demonstrates an understanding of the disease and steps for protection of the child.
- The child performs at an optimal level for the stage of disease.
- The parents make an appointment for genetic follow-up.

The nurse plans for the daily care of the child based on physician's orders and nursing diagnoses. Some general nursing care goals may be the following:

- The family learns to manage the physical care of the child.
- The parents plan for the progression of their child's illness.

★ **NURSING INTERVENTIONS: COLLABORATIVE AND INDEPENDENT**

There is no cure for the disorder, so interventions for Tay-Sachs disease are palliative. The central foci for nursing management are maintaining the child at optimal developmental level, supporting the parents in their grief, teaching the parents how to feed the child to prevent aspiration and how to provide comfort measures for the child, and referring the parents for genetic counseling regarding future family planning.

PREVENTION

The only way to treat Tay-Sachs is to prevent it, which is very difficult. Ultra-Orthodox Jewish law proscribes abortion, and contraception is permitted only under strict conditions. Most Ultra-Orthodox Jews opt not to take the simple blood test that identifies carriers of the recessive disorder. Identification as a carrier can result in psychological difficulties, because the backgrounds of both boys and girls are examined along with medical histories before a marital match is consummated. Families in which a member has been designated a carrier may be labeled as having a "tainted bloodline," thereby affecting the marriageability of the entire kindred.

Chevra Dor Yeshorim (Association of an Upright Generation) is a program proposed by a New York rabbi that provides confidential screening for the Tay-Sachs allele. It has been so effective that it is now available in most large cities in the United States. All individuals taking the blood test are assigned a number, and test results are filed at the screening centers by number alone. Names are not recorded, so there is no possibility of stigmatization. Carriers learn their status as carriers only if they are matched with another carrier. Families are thus allowed to report that the match has failed for any number of reasons and to look for new matches.

★ **EVALUATION**

Periodically the nurse and family evaluate the outcomes of care given. Examples of outcomes for the child and family with Tay-Sachs were given under Nursing Diagnoses and Planning in this section. The reader is referred to Chapter 32 for a discussion on terminally ill children and nursing interventions for the child and family.

Subacute Sclerosing Panencephalitis

Definition and Incidence. *Subacute sclerosing panencephalitis* (SSPE) is a rare complication following infection with measles virus, which appears 5 to 6 years after the acute disease. It also may follow immunization with live measles vaccine virus. It is included under degenerative disorders because of its chronic course and the absence of clinical manifestations of infection.

The estimated incidence of SSPE is 1 per 100,000 cases of natural measles and 1 per 1 to 2 million doses of attenuated measles vaccine. The incidence has declined as the use of measles vaccine has increased in different geographic areas, but the overall incidence in the population is still estimated to be between 1 and 4 per 1 million population depending on the geographic location.[4,1] The frequency of SSPE is higher in developing countries and rural populations. Children who are intensely exposed to measles from extended contact with an ill sibling or who contract measles at an early age are at greater risk for SSPE. Boys are three to four times more likely to acquire the disorder than girls. Because cerebral degeneration usually appears 7 years after the primary infection, the peak incidence is between 8 and 14 years of age. However, cases have been reported in children younger than 2 years of age and in adults older than 21.

Etiology and Pathophysiology. SSPE is a progressive cerebral degenerative disease that usually is fatal within 2 years of onset. The exact pathophysiology is unknown. Changes in the brain include perivascular lymphocytic infiltrates, intranuclear inclusion bodies in neurons and glial cells, proliferation of astrocytes and microglial cells, perivascular cuffing, and diffuse mononuclear infiltration of the cerebrum along with demyelinization. The widespread loss of cortical neurons is responsible for the first clinical manifestations of the disorder.

Clinical Manifestations. The first clinical manifestations of the disorder are insidious changes in behavior, personality, and intellect. School failure and emotional lability are more readily detected by the parent than the subtle personality changes, which initially may be attributed to normal developmental changes. Disruptive behavior in school and declining grades in a child who has previously been successful often are the presenting symptoms. Emotional outbreaks may be especially difficult for the parents and frightening for the child, who may feel out of control. As the disorder progresses myoclonic jerks or dystonic movements interfere with ambulation. Grand mal seizures may occur. Finally the child slips into a coma and develops decorticate rigidity followed by death within 2 years of the onset of the disorder.

Diagnostic Studies. Definitive diagnosis of SSPE is based on isolation of a measles-like virus in the brain, high titers (1:128) of measles virus antibody in the CSF, elevated gamma globulin, and a characteristic EEG pattern consisting of regularly repeated bursts of generalized high-voltage slow-wave complexes.

★ **ASSESSMENT**

A careful history is the most important aspect of assessment for SSPE. Previously normal children presenting with emotional lability, disruptive school behavior, and declining grades require thorough documentation of contact with measles virus and immunization records. Check for recent life disruptions in the family or major life stressors, such as a recent move, new school, or death in the family to rule out an emotional disorder. The nurse should attempt to obtain an accurate picture of the child's personality, behavior, grades, and gait before the onset of symptoms. Particular attention should be given to the history related to achievement of developmental milestones. A review of previous Denver II results in children younger than age 6 may give a more definitive picture of the loss of motor function.

The child's motor function should be closely observed and compared with muscle strength and symmetry for each side of the body. The child's level of involvement in sports and school activities should be assessed. The child's description of his or her disorder may be helpful in planning for each individual perspective.

★ **NURSING DIAGNOSES AND PLANNING**

Based on assessment data discussed previously and in the preceding chapter, the following nursing diagnoses may apply to the family and child with SSPE:

- High Risk for Injury related to myoclonic movements.
- Sensory/Perceptual Alterations related to decreasing cerebral function and demyelinization.
- Altered Thought Processes related to loss of cerebral function.
- Impaired Physical Mobility related to demyelinization.
- Altered Family Processes related to progressive factor of illness.
- Powerlessness related to progressive deterioration.
- Knowledge Deficit regarding illness, treatment, and prognosis.

Many other nursing diagnoses may evolve. Some of these are discussed in Table 53-9.

The nurse and child (or parents) together plan effective care based on the established nursing diagnoses. Several examples of expected outcomes follow:

- The family demonstrates understanding of the disease.
- The family states methods it is using for accident prevention for the child.
- The parents relate the importance of the care they are giving the child.

The nurse plans for the daily care of the child based on physician's orders and nursing diagnoses. Some general nursing care goals may be the following:

- Injury is prevented.
- Parents and child discuss the illness and the prognosis together.

★ **NURSING INTERVENTIONS: COLLABORATIVE AND INDEPENDENT**

Treatment is palliative and is designed to keep the child as comfortable as possible. There is no cure. Nursing management is supportive and protective (see Table 53-9). If the child is cared for prior to loss of consciousness, safety and prevention of potential injury due to loss of muscular coordination and myoclonic movements are principal concerns. Emotional support for the child and parents is central because of the terminal nature of the disorder and because of the anguish associated with the loss of previously normal function. It is important for parents to feel that they are actively "doing something" for their child. They feel frustration with the inexorable progressive deterioration and lack of hope for a cure. Ultimately, powerlessness may become the prominent nursing diagnosis for the family, along with grief and guilt.

★ EVALUATION

Periodically the nurse and family evaluate the outcomes of care given. Examples of outcomes for the child and family with SSPE were given under Nursing Diagnoses and Planning in this section.

Ataxias

Degenerative disorders specific to the spinocerebellar pathways or basal ganglia usually are genetically determined (autosomal recessive transmission) with an unknown etiology. Some are detectable in early infancy, while others are not manifested until late childhood or adolescence. Children and parents are subjected to the psychological trauma and social stigma attached to progressive visible distortions of movement and coordination.

Friedreich's Ataxia

Definition and Incidence. Friedreich's ataxia is actually a group of heterogeneous metabolic disorders that involve progressive cerebellar and spinal cord dysfunction. As underlying metabolic disturbances are clarified, the dominant inheritance disorders will be classified differently than the autosomal recessive inheritance disorders. The onset varies but usually occurs in late childhood or adolescence.

Etiology and Pathophysiology. Degenerative changes related to unclear metabolic disturbances are found in the spinocerebellar, posterior column, and corticospinal tracts. Degeneration and necrosis of cardiac muscle fibers also may be present. Death usually is due to myocardial failure. Peripheral neuropathy may be present and may lead to the development of a positive Babinski's reflex.

Clinical Manifestations. Progressive loss of coordination in the arms and gait disturbances are usually the presenting symptoms. Characteristic pes cavus (very high arches in the feet), hammer toes, and scoliosis often accompany this disorder. Loss of tendon reflexes, a positive Babinski's reflex, muscle weakness (usually distal) and muscle atrophy, intention tremors, dysarthria, and occasionally nystagmus are present. Progressive loss of sensation occurs, especially in the feet, along with loss of position and vibration senses. Cardiomegaly, cardiac failure, and arrhythmias are sometimes the symptoms that cause the parents to seek help.

Diagnostic Studies. The diagnosis is based almost exclusively on the clinical manifestations. Electrocardiograph changes indicating cardiomyopathy and nerve conduction studies that show peripheral neuropathic slowing of nerve conduction velocity may support the diagnosis, but there are no definitive laboratory examinations on which to base the diagnosis. Clinical manifestations, which are often considered to be pathognomonic, include absent ankle jerks, positive Babinski's reflex, and ataxia.

★ ASSESSMENT

Children presenting with cardiac complaints who also display gait disturbances and a positive Babinski's sign should have a comprehensive review of their history. A history that shows progressive gait disturbances, perhaps a history of falling, poor coordination, loss of ability in sports, or history of difficulty in physical education activities is suspicious and should be referred for nerve conduction studies. If the child has Friedreich's ataxia, a loss of coordination in the arms usually follows the initial gait problems. Areflexia (lack of reflexes) or hyperreflexia and spasticity may be present, along with the pathognomonic ataxia, positive Babinski's reflex, and lack of or hyperreflexive ankle jerks. Inability to walk is present by early adulthood.

The home should be assessed for safety precautions. The need for mechanical support devices to aid the child and family in performing activities of daily living and level of family functioning should be determined. At some point family counseling and therapy may become necessary to cope with the emotional strains associated with caring for a child diagnosed with a progressive degenerative and ultimately terminal neurologic disorder.

Older children should be assessed for disturbances in self-concept related to loss of independence, loss of coordination, change in appearance, and inability to communicate with peers.

★ NURSING DIAGNOSES AND PLANNING

Based on assessment data discussed previously and in the preceding chapter, the following nursing diagnoses may apply to the family and child with Friedreich's ataxia:

- High Risk for Injury related to gait difficulties and loss of coordination.
- Impaired Physical Mobility related to progressive loss of coordination.
- Decreased Cardiac Output related to cardiac failure.
- Ineffective Airway Clearance related to cardiac failure.
- Fluid Volume Excess related to cardiac failure.
- Altered Tissue Perfusion related to cardiac failure.

The nurse and child (or parents) together plan effective care based on the established nursing diagnoses. Several examples of expected outcomes follow:

- The family states the methods it is using to protect the child.
- The parents state the importance of promoting rest for their child.

Many other nursing diagnoses may evolve. Some of these are discussed in Table 53-9.

The nurse plans for the daily care of the child based on physician's orders and nursing diagnoses. Some general nursing care goals may be the following:

- The child is protected from injury.

- The child is able to use mechanical support devices to assist in activities of daily living.

★ NURSING INTERVENTIONS: COLLABORATIVE AND INDEPENDENT

There is no cure and no effective treatment for this disorder. Genetic counseling may be appropriate, but medical interventions are largely palliative. Some physicians recommend orthopedic surgery for the pes cavus and scoliosis, but most physicians avoid procedures requiring immobilization for recovery. Prolonged immobilization speeds the already relentless progressive loss of muscular coordination.

Nursing management is supportive and is directed toward assisting parents to deal with their grief, guilt over bearing a child with a genetic impairment, emotional burden of caring for a child suffering progressive degeneration, and increased specialized care requirements associated with loss of mobility, coordination, and sensation. See the display in this chapter on nursing management for the family of the child with an alteration in neurologic functioning. Care of the child is directed toward symptomatic care of sensory, motor, and systemic impairments. The problems of loss of independence and mobility, seizures, impaired vision and hearing, cardiac and respiratory difficulties, and feeding problems require nursing attention. Nursing care for children who present with cardiac failure is directed toward reducing the cardiac workload and enhancing cardiac output. Nursing interventions include promoting rest, monitoring activity, meticulous recording of intake and output and daily weights, measuring abdominal girth, and changing the child's position frequently. Administering prescribed cardiac medications, such as digoxin and diuretics, and noting their effect on the child are important. Nursing care for children with cardiomegaly and cardiac failure is covered in Chapter 41. General nursing care for Friedreich's ataxia is discussed in Table 53-9.

★ EVALUATION

Periodically the nurse and family evaluate the outcomes of care given. Examples of outcomes for the child and family with Friedreich's ataxia were given under Nursing Diagnoses and Planning in this section.

Ataxia-Telangiectasia

Definition and Incidence. *Ataxia-telangiectasia* is another autosomal recessive disorder that results in a specific immunologic dysfunction associated with progressive cerebellar degeneration. The telangiectasia portion of the name comes from the vascular lesions formed by dilated small blood vessels on the bulbar conjunctiva, the external ears, the nasolabial folds, and the flexor creases of the extremities. Contrary to Friedreich's ataxia, neurologic manifestations of ataxia-telangiectasia usually appear during infancy. The incidence of malignancies such as lymphomas and brain tumors is increased in children with ataxia-telangiectasia, which is presumed to be related to the immunologic dysfunction.

Etiology and Pathophysiology. This disorder is complex, and the etiology is not totally understood. Degeneration is limited to the spinocerebellar tracts and the cerebellum. It is not clear how the cerebellar degeneration and the immunologic disorder are related. Affected infants have immunologic deficits and associated thymic dysfunction, but the etiology is unclear. The immunologic disorder renders the infant susceptible to frequent sinopulmonary infections. The etiology of the telangiectasia is also unknown. Death occurs as a result of infection, malignancy, or pulmonary failure.

Clinical Manifestations. The earliest manifestations are neurologic and begin in infancy. Infants walk late with a characteristic ataxic gait. Tendon reflexes are diminished or absent. Eye movements are characteristics of the disorder. Involuntary eye movements are retained, but voluntary movements on command are difficult or impossible. Later in childhood nystagmus, intention tremor, choreoathetosis, and progressive dysarthria occur. The telangiectatic skin changes appear by 5 years of age.

Manifestations of immunologic deficiency are variable. Some children rarely experience sinopulmonary infections, while others have frequent recurrent sinopulmonary infections. There are usually no palpable lymph nodes, and tonsillar tissue is diminished or absent. Scoliosis may appear in late childhood, and by early adolescence independent ambulation is difficult to impossible. Mild dementia may occur in the late states of the disorder, and death occurs by adolescence or early adulthood.

Diagnostic Studies. Five laboratory tests are used to discriminate ataxia-telangiectasia from CP or Friedreich's ataxia: (1) Serum immunoglobulin (Ig) levels show a decrease or absence of IgA and IgE. (2) Blood counts show a decrease in the number of circulating small lymphocytes. (3) Delayed hypersensitivity reactions to intradermal injections of *Candida* or mumps antigens are decreased or absent. (4) Skin sensitization reactions to dinitrochlorobenzene are usually absent. (5) Serum levels of AFP are often increased.

★ ASSESSMENT

Ataxic CP and Friedreich's ataxia have similar presenting symptoms. In infancy the task is often to discriminate ataxia-telangiectasia from CP. The absence of a positive Babinski's sign and the presence of the characteristic eye movements along with the late onset of Friedreich's ataxia make it relatively easy to distinguish telangiectasia. However, distinguishing CP from telangiectasia is based on the differential laboratory studies. Infants with ataxic gaits, involuntary eye movements, and delayed motor development or coordination should all be referred for laboratory studies to rule out CP.

The Denver II may be used to establish the child's functional level of activities of daily living and motor achievement, as well as language and social development. The home environment must be assessed for environmental safety precautions and sources for infection. Home care will depend on the child's functional level; once that is assessed attention is given to determining the need for mechanical supports to assist in child care and the emotional condition of the family. Family functioning should be assessed to determine the need for family counseling.

★ NURSING DIAGNOSES AND PLANNING

Based on assessment data discussed previously and in the preceding chapter, the following nursing diagnoses may apply to the family and child with ataxia-telangiectasia:

- High Risk for Injury related to gait difficulties and loss of coordination.
- Impaired Physical Mobility related to progressive loss of coordination.
- High Risk for Infection related to immonologic deficiencies.
- High Risk for Peripheral Neurovascular Dysfunction related to cerebellar degeneration.
- Ineffective Individual Coping related to personal vulnerability.
- Ineffective/Disabling Family Coping related to unexpressed feelings of guilt and anxiety.

Many other nursing diagnoses may evolve. Some of these are discussed in Table 53-9.

The nurse and child (or parents) together plan effective care based on the established nursing diagnoses. Several examples of expected outcomes follow:

- The family states methods it is using for environmental protection of the child.
- The parents state the importance of protecting the child from infections.
- The parents demonstrate normal emotional ranges for guilt and anxiety.

The nurse plans for the daily care of the child based on physician's orders and nursing diagnoses. Some general nursing care goals may be the following:

- The child remains infection free.
- The child participates in activities of daily living with assistance.

★ NURSING INTERVENTIONS: COLLABORATIVE AND INDEPENDENT

There is no cure for ataxia-telangiectasia. Gamma globulin replacement therapy has not been successful. Prompt treatment of infections is the treatment of choice. Malignancies may be surgically removed if their location permits and the parents agree. Pulmonary complications are treated palliatively.

Nursing management of the infant or child with ataxia-telangiectasia is directed toward preventing infections, assessing and planning for maintenance of as much mobility as possible, providing supportive care for the child and family, preventing injuries, and enhancing acceptance of diminishing competency. Nursing care for children who present with lymphomas and other oncologic problems is covered in Chapters 31 and 44. Nursing care for children experiencing respiratory failure is covered in detail in Chapter 38.

★ EVALUATION

Periodically the nurse and family evaluate the outcomes of care given. Examples of outcomes for the child and family with ataxia-telangectasia were given under Nursing Diagnoses and Planning in this section.

Myasthenia Gravis

Definition and Incidence. *Myasthenia gravis* is a disorder of the neuromuscular junction, specifically of the postsynaptic junction. There is a deactivation of the acetylcholine receptor sites, which impairs normal impulse transmission to the muscle. Myasthenia gravis is thought to be autoimmune in nature.

Children with myasthenia gravis are categorized into three groups: those with congenital myasthenia gravis, those with neonatal myasthenia gravis, and a those referred to as juvenile, who may develop myasthenia gravis any time after birth. The initial signs and symptoms develop before age 20 in approximately 20% of patients. Girls are affected approximately three times more frequently than boys. Also, the incidence is higher in African American women. The incidence is 2 to 10 people per 100,000.

Etiology and Pathophysiology. The exact cause of myasthenia gravis and its origin remain controversial. Some theories suggest that myasthenia gravis results from insufficient receptor protein production, while others believe that abnormal receptor sites cause this disorder. The most widely accepted theory postulates that an autoimmune disorder blocks, deactivates, or destroys acetylcholine receptor sites. Several autoimmune antibodies are suspected, such as IgG antibodies, thyroglobulin, rheumatoid factor, and complement components 3 and 9.

Regardless of the cause, the basic physiologic defect in myasthenia gravis is that compound action potentials are limited and may not pass onto the muscle at the neuromuscular junction. Muscle contraction is thereby inhibited, and increasing weakness occurs with increased activity.

Congenital myasthenia gravis occurs at birth and persists. Neonatal myasthenia gravis develops within 72 hours of birth in approximately 12% of infants born to mothers with myasthenia. Children with neonatal myasthenia gravis experience transitory symptoms that subside by 12 weeks of age and are subsequently normal. Juvenile myasthenia gravis is identical to adult forms and usually has an onset after age 10 and a higher incidence in girls.

Clinical Manifestations. The most important clinical sign of myasthenia gravis is skeletal muscle weakness, which can be relieved by rest and worsened by exercise. The muscles supplied by the cranial nerves are most often affected. Therefore, muscles involved in swallowing, coughing, and gagging may lose their power to protect the airway. Loss of facial expression, ptosis, and diplopia are common. As the disease progresses proximal muscles of the arms and legs may be affected. Respiratory muscles can become too weak to function, leading to acute respiratory distress. Bulbar involvement also may be present, causing dysarthria, dysphagia, and difficulty chewing.

Children with neonatal myasthenia gravis exhibit poor sucking, choking, weak cry, expressionless face, floppy and weak limbs, obscene or Moro's reflexes, periods of apnea, and other respiratory problems following birth. Children with congenital myasthenia gravis characteristically exhibit ocular muscle weakness initially. Other muscle groups eventually become involved and may progress to sudden respiratory death. The most common symptoms of juvenile myasthenia gravis are paralysis of the ocular, bulbar, and skeletal muscles. Symptoms are usually more pronounced in the late afternoon and evening. Exercise and excitement may proliferate symptoms, and rest may relieve them.

Diagnostic Studies. Myasthenia gravis should be suspected in children exhibiting any evidence of cranial muscle weakness and progressive muscle fatigue after exertion. Because myasthenia gravis may be associated with a variety of other autoimmune disorders (systemic lupus erythematosus, thyroiditis, rheumatoid arthritis), thyroid tests, serum creatinine phosphokinase, sedimentation rate, and antinuclear antibody levels usually are performed. A CAT scan of the thymus also may be performed.

Most commonly the diagnosis of myasthenia gravis is confirmed by observing the child's response to an anticholinesterase drug. Tensilon (edrophonium) or Prostigmin (neostigmine) can be administered in small doses intravenously (IV). This IV administration of an anticholinesterase in children with myasthenia gravis causes a dramatic revival of exhausted muscles in approximately 1 minute. Improvement lasts approximately 5 minutes. Edrophonium usually is used to test the ocular and oropharyngeal muscles, while neostigmine is preferred when evaluating limb strength.

Edrophonium also may be used to determine if a patient needs more anticholinesterase (myasthenic crisis) or whether they have too much (cholinergic crisis). Edrophonium will improve symptoms of myasthenic crisis and excaberate symptoms of cholinergic crisis. Atropine, a cholinergic reactivator, can be given in cholinergic crisis.

★ ASSESSMENT

A careful history of children suspected of having juvenile myasthenia gravis may reveal a variable and unpredictable course, characterized by remissions and exacerbations. Congenital and neonatal forms of myasthenia gravis usually are recognized by behavioral and physical symptoms shortly after birth.

When assessing a child with myasthenia gravis, the degree of muscular paralysis should be determined. Careful attention must be paid to the degree of ocular and oropharyngeal weakness. The child also should be observed for ptosis, diplopia, weak facial movements, and inability to swallow, cough, or gag. It is also important to assess respiratory muscle involvement. Is dyspnea or apnea present? Despite muscle weakness, muscles rarely atrophy. Respiratory effort should be observed to determine whether intercostal and diaphragm muscles are

compromised. In older children there is a tendency for the head to fall forward, and children may hold their jaw closed with their hands. The extent of upper and lower extremity weakness also must be determined.

★ NURSING DIAGNOSES AND PLANNING

Based on assessment data discussed previously and in the preceding chapter, the following nursing diagnoses may apply to the family and child with myasthenia gravis:

- High Risk for Injury related to muscle weakness.
- Impaired Verbal Communication related to oropharyngeal weakness.
- Altered Nutrition: Less Than Body Requirements related to inability to swallow.
- Fatigue related to increased energy required to perform activities of daily living.
- Activity Intolerance related to generalized weakness.
- Self-Care Deficit related to generalized weakness.
- Ineffective Airway Clearance related to inability to cough.
- Anxiety related to knowledge deficit regarding medication therapy.

Many other nursing diagnoses may evolve. Some of these are discussed in Table 53-9.

The nurse and child (or parents) together plan effective care based on the established nursing diagnoses. Several examples of expected outcomes follow:

- The parents demonstrate understanding of medication regimen, adverse side-effects, and medication interactions.
- The family states the importance of providing rest periods for the child.
- The child and family learn the importance of avoiding emotional and physical stress.

The nurse plans for the daily care of the child based on physician's orders and nursing diagnoses. Some general nursing care goals may be the following:

- Muscle strength is maintained for as long as possible.
- The child is protected from injury.

★ NURSING INTERVENTIONS:
 COLLABORATIVE AND INDEPENDENT

Children with both congenital and juvenile myasthenia gravis will require lifelong medical and nursing supervision. Successful nursing management and education can lessen the stress and anxiety experienced by the child and family. The parents and child (if older) should be educated about the importance of proper medication dosage and routine and the side-effects. The symptoms of both myasthenic and cholinergic crisis should be reviewed.

Emphasis should be placed on planning the child's activities to avoid severe fatigue. Frequent rest periods throughout the day may be required. Strenuous activities should be discouraged. Energy-saving devices such as wheelchairs can lessen fatigue.

Because respiratory distress or failure is possible in children with myasthenia gravis, patients and occasionally siblings should become certified in basic life support. The family and child should also receive teaching about prevention of aspiration, infection, and emotional stress. Emotional and physical stress can precipitate a myasthenic crisis, which requires immediate medical attention.

MEDICATION THERAPY

Treatment for myasthenia gravis involves the administration of anticholinesterase. Anticholinesterase is useful because it inhibits the hydrolysis of acetylcholine by acetylcholinesterase at the neuromuscular junction. This allows acetylcholine to accumulate at synapses, thus increasing stimulation of the existing receptor sites. Improved nerve impulse transmission results in improved muscle strength.

Pyridostigmine (Mestinon) is frequently the drug of choice due to its long action, fewer side-effects, and stable blood level. The initial dosage is approximately 30 mg every 4 hours in older children and approximately 5 mg every 4 hours in infants. Dosages are gradually increased until a satisfactory response is obtained. During this time the child must be closely observed for cholinergic crisis (overmedication with anticholinesterase). Symptoms of overmedication include excessive lacrimation and salivation, sweating, abdominal cramps, diarrhea, vomiting, bradycardia, and respiratory muscle weakness.

Thymectomy (surgical excision of the thymus gland) may be performed. This procedure removes a source of antigen production and reduces the immune response. Corticosteroids also may be used in children with a poor response to anticholinesterase. Steroids can reduce the immune response by reducing the amount of antibodies. Plasmaphoresis and immunosuppressive drugs (Imuran) can be helpful in reducing the circulating antiaceytylcholine receptor antibodies in the plasma, thereby reducing the symptoms for a limited time in some patients.

Drugs that should be avoided in children with myasthenia gravis include diuretics that induce hypokalemia (increase muscular weakness), sedatives, narcotics, curare, antiarrhythmic drugs such as procainamide and quididine, magnesium sulfate, aminoglycosides, polymyxin antibiotics, and quinine.

★ EVALUATION

Periodically the nurse and family evaluate the outcomes of care given. Examples of outcomes for the child and family with myasthenia gravis were given under Nursing Diagnoses and Planning in this section.

Functional Neurodisabilities

Neurologic functional disabilities fall into four broad categories: neuromuscular manifestations such as CP, attention-deficit manifestations with or without hyperactivity, sensory integration deficit manifestations, and learning disabilities. Each category refers to a group of disabilities that is thought to result from injury or insult to the brain during the perinatal period or early infancy. Insults or injuries may be the result of a single event, such as a

hypoxic period during delivery or an IVH resulting from trauma or stress during the neonatal period. Cumulative episodes of hyoxemia or hyperoxemia or multiple small IVHs also are implicated.

CP refers to a select group of permanent disabilities manifested in neuromuscular disorders. Attention deficit disorders (ADD) are a group of neurologic soft signs associated with a short attention span but no accompanying hyperactivity. Hyperactivity along with a short attention span is classified as an ADD with hyperactivity. Sensory integration deficits or dysfunctions refer to difficulty integrating the myriad of sensory stimulations bombarding the neurologic system. These children have difficulty organizing and interpreting sensations and planning appropriate activity. Sensory input is received but may not be correctly perceived. The manner in which the child's brain processes the information it receives may be dysfunctional. Learning disabilities may be related to delayed development of the eye musculature and coordination rather than to visual acuity or mental aptitude.

CP and mental retardation were the first identified diagnostic categories because their clinical manifestations were so obvious. Minimal brain dysfunction and dyslexia were the next categories identified to explain reading difficulties and qualitative developmental problems that did not fit into other categories. Advances in analysis of brain function, understanding of mental data processing, and precision in assessment tools have enhanced the diagnosis of functional disabilities. Help is now available for development delayed by neurologic dysfunction: Developmental optometrists now provide specialized evaluation of visual development and therapy in addition to visual acuity screening to enhance motor and perceptual skills related to visual learning problems. Occupational therapists use sensory integration exercises to overcome neurologic deficits resulting from early brain trauma. Support groups provide self-help and emotional outlets for both parents and children afflicted with neurologic dysfunctions.

Cerebral Palsy

Definition and Incidence. *Cerebral palsy* refers to an alteration in motor function resulting from a hypoxic or anoxic injury to the motor cortex, cerebellum, or basal ganglia. CP is the most common permanent physical disability found in children. Estimated incidence is 1.5 to 5 per 1000 live births or approximately 25,000 new cases per year. Cerebral palsy can be classified as athetoid, ataxic, rigid, or spastic, as listed in Table 53-10, depending on the location of the trauma and the type of neuromuscular movements manifested by the child.

Etiology and Pathophysiology. The principal cause of CP is damage associated with ischemia, hypoxia, or asphyxia in low birth weight, preterm infants (Table 53-11). The next most common cause is perinatal asphyxia followed by birth trauma. Congenital infections, metabolic conditions, and intrauterine ischemic events are rare causes of CP.[33] Etiologic factors associated with CP occurring in the prenatal, perinatal, or postnatal period may contribute either singly or cumulatively to the develop-

TABLE 53-10
Classifications of Cerebral Palsy

Classification	Pathophysiology and Movement Characteristics
Athetoid (dyskinetic) (kernicterus, hemolytic disease)	Damage to basal ganglia results in uncontrolled and involuntary movements that are intensified by stress or emotional tension. Movements tend to disappear during sleep.
Ataxic (least common) (cerebral hypoplasia hypoglycemia)	Damage to cerebellum manifests in loss of balance (equilibrium), coordination, and kinesthetic sense. Gait is staggering or unsteady. May be unilateral with falling toward one side only.
Rigid (cortical trauma)	Damage to cerebral cortex anterior horn cells causes loss of inhibiting function to flexor and extensor muscles. Muscles remain in a constant state of tension and resistance.
Spastic (periventricular hemorrhage, ischemia, infarction, hemiplegia, quadriplegia)	Damage to anterior horn cells in cerebral cortex results in exaggerated muscle responses in selected muscle groups.

ment of CP. Isolated hypoxic events have long been associated with CP. New evidence suggests that cumulative effects of repeated hypoxemic episodes may make the neonate more vulnerable to IVH, resulting in CP.[13]

No characteristic pathophysiologic pattern is evident. Neurologic lesions such as atrophy, loss of neurons, laminar degeneration associated with wider sulci or narrower gyri, or gross malformations may be present. Damage occurs in the anterior horn cells of the cortex, the cerebellum, or the basal ganglia. Table 53-10 lists the etiologic factors and pathophysiology associated with each major classification of CP. Multiple handicaps frequently are present in children with CP because of the nature of the etiologic factors. Asphyxia and trauma are pervasive injuries. Convulsive disorders are common, along with nearsightedness, strabismus, hearing deficits, and speech disorders. More than 50% of children with CP also have mental retardation.

Clinical Manifestations. The most common form of CP is the spastic diplegia of prematurity caused by hypoxic infarction or hemorrhage in the area adjacent to the lateral ventricles. The reflex arc usually is intact and the characteristic physical manifestations are increased muscle tone, increased stretch reflexes, and frequently weakness. Hypotonia or decreased muscle tone lasting a few weeks or months to a year are the earliest clinical signs. Very tense muscles are the most obvious clinical manifestation. Affected children tend to walk on their toes because of a tight heel cord. They often have strabismus, speech difficulties, and feeding difficulties.

Athetoid or dyskinetic CP is caused by kernicterus or hemolytic diseases that damage the basal ganglia. The result is uncontrolled and involuntary worm-like movements that are aggravated or intensified by emotional tension or stress. Continuous uncontrollable movement maintains joint mobility and prevents deformities. All extremities, the neck, trunk, tongue, and facial muscles usually are involved. Eyes tend to converge toward the midline and are displaced upward, yielding a conjugate upward gaze. High frequency hearing losses and deafness

are common. Drooling and imperfect speech articulation (dysarthria) combined with the hearing losses make it difficult to communicate with the child.

Ataxic CP is less common and is caused by hypoglycemia or cerebral hypoplastic damage to the cerebellum. Ataxia CP is manifested by a loss of balance, coordination, and kinesthetic sense. The typical gait is wide based and staggering or unsteady and may be one sided. Rapid repetitive movements are difficult. Reaching for objects may be accompanied by disintegration of upper extremity movements. Ocular or visual problems are common, and both position and touch are affected. Development is very slow during the first 3 to 5 years of life, but cerebellar coordination tends to improve as the child grows.

Rigid CP is uncommon. Rigid CP is caused by trauma to the anterior horn cells of the cortex and causes a loss of inhibition function in both the flexor and extensor muscles. Muscle tone is continuously high in both tension and resistance, which results in deformities and a lack of active movement.

Traumatic postnatal head injuries sometimes result in a mixed type of CP manifested by a combination of spastic and athetoid movements. These children are severely disabled physically and possibly mentally.

Diagnostic Studies. The primary diagnostic tools are the medical developmental history and the neurologic examination. Definitive diagnosis of CP rarely occurs prior to 18 months or 2 years of age. The first clue may be failure to achieve developmental milestones. Infants at high risk for CP, such as infants with low birth weight (less than 2500 g), or very low birth weight (less than 1500 g) usually are followed in developmental clinics until school performance is satisfactory. Early detection allows early developmental intervention, which is thought to prevent or reduce residual deficits.

Harris[16] reports significant neuromotor predictors of CP using the movement assessment of infants instrument[6] at the 4-month chronologic age developmental follow-up visit. The instrument is a valid, reliable, 65-item neuromotor assessment of muscle tone, primitive reflexes, automatic reactions, and volitional movement.

Additional diagnostic tests such as electroencepha-

TABLE 53-11
Etiology of Cerebral Palsy

Prenatal	Perinatal	Postnatal
Intrauterine ischemic events	Low birth weight	Intraventricular hemorrhage
Rubella in the first trimester	Premature birth	Cerebral vascular accident
Congenital brain anomalies	Asphyxia	Infections
RH/ABO incompatibility	Intrauterine ischemic events	Encephalitis
	Infections	Meningitis
	Birth trauma	Trauma/ischemic events
	Hypoglycemia	Hypoglycemia
	Overdose of maternal medications	Hyperbilirubinemia
		Hyperosmolarity
		Poisonings

lography or tomography may be needed, and screening for metabolic defects and serum electrolytes help rule out brain tumors and progressive degenerative diseases. Supplemental developmental assessments from developmental optometrists, physical therapists, and occupational therapists may be helpful in documenting the precise disabilities and formulating a plan of therapy. An interdisciplinary approach is the most beneficial.

★ ASSESSMENT

Early detection of infants with CP enables early intervention programs, which can prevent some disabilities and mediate the long-term effects of others. The newborn with evidence of asymmetric strength or movement of an extremity, a tendency to keep legs extended, scissoring leg movements, rigidity when held, and difficulties with sucking and swallowing should be given a thorough neurologic examination and referred for developmental follow-up. Infants with low birth weight or low 5-minute Apgar scores or infants who have sustained head trauma, hypoxia, metabolic insults, and perinatal infections should also receive developmental testing in follow-up visits.

Often the first evidence of CP is a delay in the attainment of developmental milestones. Nurses detecting developmental delays should refer these infants for precise developmental testing by physical therapists trained to evaluate motor function. Definite diagnoses of CP cannot be made before 6 months of age and often not until 2 or 3 years of age, but physical therapy interventions for specific motor problems can be instituted as soon as a problem is identified. Caution should be used in predicting outcomes or labeling deficits such as CP because of preconceived public notions about CP and the attendant anxiety and social stigma. Often parents have a more positive attitude when specific problems are identified and approached without the label of CP.

★ NURSING DIAGNOSES AND PLANNING

Based on assessment data discussed previously and in the preceding chapter, the following nursing diagnoses may apply to the family and child with CP:

- High Risk for Injury related to uncoordinated movements.
- Impaired Physical Mobility related to uncoordinated movements.
- Self-Care Deficit related to uncoordinated movements.
- Impaired Skin Integrity related to immobility.
- Altered Nutrition: Less Than Body Requirements related to feeding difficulties.
- High Risk for Activity Intolerance related to fatigue and perceptual and cognitive impairment.
- Impaired Verbal Communication related to neuromuscular impairment.
- Altered Family Processes related to child's dysfunction.
- High Risk for Caregiver Role Strain related to amount of caregiving tasks.

These nursing diagnoses and others are discussed in the Nursing Care Plan for a 9-year-old child with cerebral palsy.

The nurse and child (or parents) together plan effective care based on the established nursing diagnoses. Several examples of expected outcomes follow:

- The family demonstrates an ability to feed the child properly.
- The family demonstrates knowledge of proper positioning.
- The child performs activities of daily living to the best of his or her ability.
- The family demonstrates a method of skin assessment for possible breakdown.
- The child participates in an adaptive communication method.
- The family states that it is seeking further counseling regarding coping with the dysfunction.
- The child participates in activities with other children.

The nurse plans for the daily care of the child based on physician's orders and nursing diagnoses. Some general nursing care goals may be the following:

- Injury is prevented.
- A means of communication is provided.

★ NURSING INTERVENTIONS: COLLABORATIVE AND INDEPENDENT

Dramatic achievements in human factors engineering, ergonomics, and bioelectric engineering have resulted in energy-efficient braces and new mobilization devices that help prevent and reduce deformities associated with CP. Antique mobilizing devices such as crutches and wheelchairs are being replaced by energy-efficient, creative, wheeled scooter boards and wheeled go-carts that provide mobility without restricting upper or lower extremity function. Computer technology coupled with knowledge advances in engineering have enabled children with spastic quadriplegia CP to become independently mobile, exercise some control over their environment, and communicate with assistive devices. Unfortunately, most of this equipment is very expensive. Few individuals are able to acquire the necessary funding. Long-term benefits from this equipment remain to be established.[27]

Therapeutic management of the child with CP is designed to assist children to achieve their maximum potential as productive independent members of society. Toward this end, program goals include:

- Early detection and intervention to correct deformities and prevent associated problems.
- Locomotion, self-help, and communication as soon as possible.
- Optimum appearance and integration of motor functions.
- Equipment and education adapted to individual child's needs.
- Active involvement of parents in rehabilitation program.
- Positive approach to problems and enhancement of child's self-esteem.

A team approach is the most effective form of intervention. Nurses, orthopedic surgeons, physical and oc-

(text continued on page 1423)

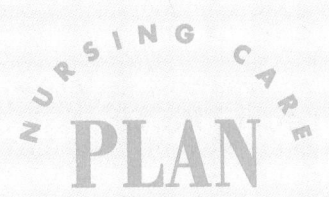

A 9-Year-Old Child With Cerebral Palsy

Assessment

Case Study Description

Leon is a 9-year-old African American boy with cerebral palsy and sensory motor deficits (quadriplegia) secondary to trauma during birth. He has a tracheostomy and receives tube feedings through a gastric feeding tube. Leon has been admitted to the hospital two to three times a year for the past 9 years for various procedures and illnesses. The most common admitting diagnosis for Leon has been bronchitis or aspiration pneumonia associated with gastric reflux.

Leon's medical diagnoses for this admission are food intolerance, abdominal pain, and reflux. He is scheduled for surgery to revise the fundoplication he had 4 years ago and to reduce the reflux of his gastric contents into the esophagus.

Leon's mother has expressed concern that her husband's salary as an electrician and his private health insurance are inadequate for Leon's health care expenses. Nursing care is provided 8 hours a day for 6 days each week by a home health agency. Leon's mother can call her own mother for help when she needs to get away from the house, but she has expressed feelings of being "tied down." She has been neglecting her own health needs to save time and money for Leon's care.

Leon has difficulty communicating verbally, but he seems to have average or above average intelligence. He is in special education classes and will soon be acquiring a computer, which he can use with a stick in his mouth.

Nursing Diagnosis	Intervention	Rationale
1. Impaired verbal communication	Observe and question parents regarding most effective means of communicating with Leon. Establish a communication system for Leon based on family input (hand gestures, communication board, sign language, computer, or voice synthesizer).	Communication is essential for establishing rapport and gaining cooperation for the implementation of nursing care.
	Use Leon's preferred means of communicating: eye signals, blinking, and minimal use of communication board.	Effective communication devices provide comfort and security for Leon.
	Provide a special extension to the nurse call button that can be activated by contact with Leon's head so that he can summon a nurse in an emergency.	Providing for summoning emergency assistance enhances Leon's sense of security and safety.
2. Alteration in comfort: pain	Administer pain medication as ordered without allowing pain to build to a severe level before medication is given.	Administering pain medication before pain becomes severe enhances comfort and decreases amount of medication needed to relieve pain.
	Provide cimetidine or ranitidine as ordered.	These drugs neutralize gastric acid and reduce hydrochloric acid production.
	Use distraction and relaxation techniques to assist in reduction of pain.	These techniques reduce perception of pain.

(Continued)

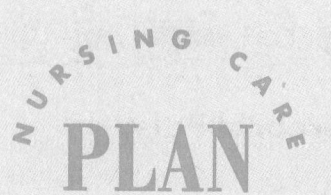

A 9-Year-Old Child With Cerebral Palsy
(continued)

Nursing Diagnosis	*Intervention*	*Rationale*
3. High risk for infection related to surgical wound and high risk for aspiration of gastric reflux	Wound care: keep incision clean and dry, and prevent contamination (see Nursing Management of Child With Surgical Interventions in this chapter).	Keeping the wound clean and dry reduces chances of acquiring infection.
	Turn, cough, and deep breathe every 2 hours after surgery.	Leon is susceptible to respiratory infections, and mobilizing his secretions reduces potential for static pneumonia.
4. Impaired physical mobility	Provide passive range-of-motion, stretching, and elongation exercises.	Stretching, elongation, and range-of-motion exercises maintain existing joint motion and reduce tension and spasticity in muscles.
	Seek consultation of physical and occupational therapists regarding best position for Leon and most appropriate exercises.	
	Use mobilizing devices to increase locomotion and independence. Leon has a special wheelchair that he operates with his mouth.	Mobilizing devices provide support, increase independence, and reduce deformity.
5. High risk for injury related to uncontrolled, uncoordinated movements	Provide a safe environment: • Side rails up • Padded side rails if indicated • Durable toys appropriate to developmental level and manipulative ability • Protective helmet for children prone to falls when walking • Restraints while in wheelchair or vehicles • Seizure precautions for children who also have seizure disorder	Routine safety precautions prevent injuries from uncontrolled or uncoordinated movements.
	Provide sufficient rest before exercise and during the day.	Tense/spastic muscles require a great deal of energy, and fatigue may increase accidental injuries.
	Teach the family how to provide safety at home (when appropriate—not applicable for Leon). Supervise child during bathing, swimming, or climbing. Pad sharp edges of tables and other furniture. Carpet stairs. Supervise use of stove, sharp toys, or utensils. Children who fall frequently should wear a protective helmet.	These precautions increase the child's safety while at home.
6. High risk for knowledge deficit related to treatment and prognosis	Assess family knowledge about fundoplication procedure, and prepare Leon and his parents for the surgical fundoplication (see Nursing Care Plan for Child Experiencing Orthopedic Surgery, Chap. 62).	Assessment of learning needs before implementing the teaching plan enhances its effectiveness.

(Continued)

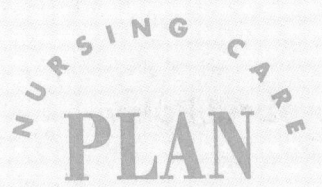

A 9-Year-Old Child With Cerebral Palsy
(continued)

Nursing Diagnosis	*Intervention*	*Rationale*
7. Self-care deficit: feeding, dressing/ grooming, toileting, and bathing/ hygiene	Provide complete care for Leon, including all activities of daily living, but provide him with choices about food, clothing, timing of care, and options for care. Allow Leon's mother to assist with care if she desires.	Leon is unable to care for himself, and his mother has the constant care of him at home and may benefit from a respite.
8. High risk for disturbance in self-concept: body image, self-esteem, personal identity, and role performance	Using eye signals, assist Leon to express his feelings about his care and being in the hospital or having surgery again.	Expression of feelings assists understanding and enhances coping.
	Provide Leon with choices about activities, and provide him with an opportunity to be self-directing and develop new skills. (A computer that can be operated by a stick in Leon's mouth has been ordered for him.)	Choices and self-direction allow Leon a sense of control and achievement, which enhance self-esteem.
9. High risk for diversional activity deficit	Assess Leon's favorite diversional activities and incorporate them into his care. He enjoys physical contact and having his father tussle with him in the bed.	Diversional activity enhances rapport, provides an outlet for tension and anxiety, and promotes rest.
10. High risk for social isolation related to Leon's communication/ interaction difficulties	Explore opportunities for Leon to communicate with other children using his computer when it arrives, and suggest program resources to his parents.	Communication with other children is the first step toward establishing and developing relationships that can sustain children through the difficulties inherent in living.
	Provide opportunities and assist other children to learn how to interact with Leon.	
11. High risk for ineffective individual coping	Assist Leon to anticipate potentially stressful situations. Assist Leon to role play difficult situations at school, and teach him how to handle the reactions of others to his efforts to establish communication and interaction.	Role playing provides the child with an opportunity to experiment with various coping strategies for stressful situations in a nonstressful environment.
12. High risk for alteration in family process related to Leon's need for constant physical care and financial burden of repeated hospitalizations	Explore potential sources of financial assistance to decrease need for Leon's father to work overtime and weekends. Explore potential for additional caregiving support or day care facility to allow Leon's mother some respite from constant caregiving demands.	Financial assistance will decrease burden of Leon's health care costs and decrease guilt for Leon and his family.
	Refer parents to social services for additional suggestions for decreasing financial burdens and acquiring respite from pressure of Leon's constant caregiving needs. Community fund raisers may be conducted by newspapers or appropriate support groups.	Additional assistance with Leon's physical caregiving will enable his mother and father to meet more of their own needs.

(Continued)

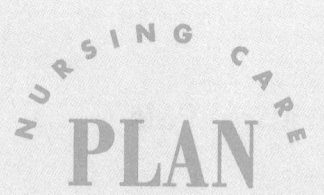

A 9-Year-Old Child With Cerebral Palsy
(continued)

Nursing Diagnosis	*Intervention*	*Rationale*
13. High risk for alteration in nutrition: less than body requirements related to feeding difficulties and increased energy requirements related to sustained increased muscle tension	Provide all caregiving before feeding so Leon can rest without interruptions for at least 1 hour following feeding.	Interruptions facilitate reflux and decrease speed of absorption.
	Position Leon in a sitting position for his tube feeding with good alignment of his extremities.	Gravity facilitates the passage of food.
	Instill warmed tube feeding (some children prefer room temperature, but Leon likes his warm) using force of gravity.*	Feeding should flow in slowly for approximately 30 minutes to simulate normal time for food consumption.
	Instill 30 to 60 ml of sterile water following tube feeding and cap end of tubing or cover with gauze.	Water rinses tubing to maintain patency. Covering tube opening prevents accidental ingestion of inedibles.
	Open cap over gastric tube as needed, elevate end, and massage or knead abdomen to relieve gas.	Gas associated with tube feedings is painful and may be relieved by elevating tube and massage.
	Ensure adequate fluid intake, especially cranberry juice, between tube feedings.	Increased fluids soften stools and flush kidneys to prevent stone formation.
	* See Nursing Care Plan for Child With Alteration in Nutrition Chapter 59 for more detail on tube feeding.	
14. High risk for activity intolerance related to fatigue and perceptual or cognitive impairment	Leon fatigues quickly, so his activity and caregiving should be limited to 30 minutes or less at a time.	Fatigue decreases coping and increases sensations of pain.
15. High risk for impaired skin integrity	Turn and position Leon every 1 to 2 hours on a special mattress (egg crate foam, water bed, or other types of special mattresses that alternate pressure points).	Turning and repositioning prevent pressure sores and improve circulation to muscles.
	Inspect skin for pressure areas and provide frequent skin care. Check braces, scooters, and other ambulation devices for pressure or friction areas.	Areas of friction or pressure can cause skin breakdown.

Evaluation

- Leon demonstrates as much independent mobility as his condition permits.
- Leon cares for self as much as condition permits.
- Leon is free of injury and pressure sores.
- Leon communicates his needs to caregivers using a bell attached to a mouthpiece.
- Leon's family participates in planning and providing care.
- Leon's family sets realistic expectations and allows Leon some independence. (They encouraged him to get the computer and will support his learning to use it.)
- Leon's family participates in community support group and has substantial support from grandparents.
- Leon and his family demonstrate effective coping and problem solving.
- Leon's mother calls her mother for help and is now seeking financial help for Leon's health care expenses.

cupational therapists, language specialists, education specialists, psychologists, social workers, and behavior technologists may all be involved in the care of one child.

MEDICAL MANAGEMENT

Medical management of the child with CP consists of surgical and pharmacologic treatment of spasticity and pharmacologic treatment of infections with antibiotics. Treatment with diazepam (Valium) and other medications for spasticity has questionable usefulness for improving muscle tone. Sedating side-effects of the medications used to produce muscle relaxation must be balanced with improved muscle function.

SURGICAL MANAGEMENT

Common surgical procedures include tenotomy of adductors along with obturator neurectomies (hamstring release and lengthening the tendons) to improve mobility, even though spasticity may not be corrected. A few medical centers are performing dorsal rhizotomies (severing the spinal cord roots that produce abnormal muscle contractions) or ventrolateral thalamotomies (destroying small portions of the basal ganglia) to improve the child's ability to walk.[32,19] Gastrostomy tubes may have to be inserted surgically to supplement or replace oral feeding for children who have severe oropharyngeal involvement or recurrent aspirations. Nissen fundoplication is a surgical procedure frequently required by children with severely debilitating CP who are fed through a gastrostomy tube. This procedure involves surgically tightening the esophageal fundus into the stomach to decrease reflux of gastric contents into the esophagus.

INDIVIDUALIZED CARE

Many people think children with CP are automatically mentally retarded, but that is not always the case. Some children have normal intelligence that has not been developed because no one thought they could do anything. Refer to Chapter 20 for the care of the mentally retarded child. Unless it is known that the child is mentally retarded, the child should be approached with a positive attitude and normal expectations. Nursing care is highly individualized, but all children need to feel accepted by the nurse and approached with dignity and the expectation that they can achieve what is required of them. Expectations should be based on the degree of pathologic involvement and the child's functional level.

Children with CP usually are treated at home unless they have a severe infection or require surgery. Care of the child hospitalized for orthopedic procedures is no different than that for any other child experiencing orthopedic surgery; however, activities of daily living may require adaptations that challenge the nurse.

Major elements of nursing care for families and children with CP include provision of adequate nutrition, prevention of injury and infection, maintenance or promotion of mobility, prevention of interrupted skin integrity, promotion of adequate communication, and psychosocial support of the family and child.

NUTRITION MANAGEMENT

A high calorie diet and increased fluid intake are required because of increased caloric needs from muscle tension and spasticity. Increased fluids are necessary to replace increased insensible losses associated with the constant motion and to decrease chances of urinary infections.

Feeding difficulties result from a weak or absent suck reflex, muscular spasms during swallowing, inability to coordinate chewing activity, difficulty controlling tongue or lips, persistence of infantile reflexes such as tongue thrust or hyperactive bite or gag reflex, and inability to fully close lips or jaw. Consultation and collaboration with an occupational therapist or physical therapist with specialized training in feeding difficulties is the most effective method of developing feeding efficiency for the child. Nursing interventions may include the following:

- Provide soft and semisoft foods.
- Use Teflon-coated utensils to minimize trauma from hyperactive bite reflex.
- Place food on center of tongue and press down gently with the spoon while avoiding contact with the lips. This helps the child avoid or minimize the tongue thrust reflex.
- Facilitate swallowing with upward stroking of the neck.
- Place middle finger under child's chin to assist with closing the jaw.

Proper positioning of the child for feeding is essential. Specially adapted chairs provide trunk and head support for the child in the upright position. The arms should be well supported in a position to assist with feeding as much as the child is capable. Feet should be supported firmly. The head may be slightly flexed, but it should face forward as much as possible. Prevent hyperextension of the neck.

PREVENTION OF INJURY

Loss of motor coordination, sensory input, and cognitive function contribute to the risk for accidental injury in children with neurodegenerative disorders. Protective helmets may be helpful when falls, seizures, or severe lack of motor coordination are present. Creating a safe environment by padding sharp corners of furniture is helpful with small children. Assistive devices, such as walkers, canes, and crutches, provide mobility and safety. Safety restraints on wheelchairs and other equipment should always be used. Chest restraints, shoulder straps, bolster pads, and other devices for head support protect children from injury in wheelchairs and automobiles. When the child is too large for a conventional car seat but too unstable for a conventional seat belt, special harnesses, adapted car seats, and travel chairs with retractable wheels that may double as wheelchairs may provide the necessary safety protection.

Weakness of the neck and trunk can lead to injury or airway obstruction if the child slumps sideways or forward in a chair and cannot regain an upright position. Appropriate positioning and postural support maintain the child's functional body alignment and protect the child from potential injury.

ADAPTATION OF MOBILITY

Impaired mobility problems range from difficulties with fine motor coordination to total body paralysis. Adaptations must be made in clothes, tools to assist with dressing (such as hooks to assist with buttons and shoes), bedrooms to promote ease of rising and usefulness, and bathrooms for wheelchairs, walkers, bath chairs, and grab bars. Use of scooter boards, carts, wheelchairs, and crutches or canes can assist the child to gain and maintain mobility.

Range-of-motion exercises every 4 hours are essential to prevent contractures and maintain flexibility in joints. Children who are bedridden have all of the problems of immobility that must be anticipated and prevented as much as possible. As long as the child has mental and fine motor function, toys may be adapted to provide diversional activity and exercise.

PREVENTION OF SKIN BREAKDOWN

Impaired movement and sensation increase the risk of skin breakdown. Decreased sensitivity to pain and poor coordination or orthopedic appliances that do not fit properly leave the child susceptible to pressure sores. Braces, splints, and casts must be inspected to detect worn pads or poor alignment. Special bed mattresses such as gel, flotation, water beds, alternating pressure or high-density foam, and wheelchair pads prevent pressure sores over bony prominences. Using sheepskin pads and keeping the bed linen free of wrinkles reduces friction, which predisposes the child to pressure sores. Daily inspection of the child's skin for injured or reddened areas and daily massages are recommended.

COMMUNICATION MANAGEMENT

When children with CP have severe involvement of the oropharyngeal muscles or larynx resulting in poor speech, the nurse must determine from the parents how the child communicates. If there is no effective communication system, then the nurse can assist in developing one that facilitates interaction so that the child's needs are known. This reduces the child's, the family's, and the staff's frustration. Gestures, sign language, typewriters, communication boards, voice synthesizers, or simple systems such as looking up for no and down for yes may be devised.

PSYCHOSOCIAL SUPPORT

Maladaptive family coping patterns are common among families of children with CP, and one of the major nursing responsibilities is to prevent maladaptive coping.[23] Nursing strategies that enhance adaptation include listening to concerns and feelings and providing positive reinforcement for parenting and for participating in the care of the child; listening to fears and allaying anxiety when possible; and explaining that parents of children with this disorder often feel guilty for bearing the child, for leaving the child's side, or for failing to prevent the disorder. Encourage parents to seek counseling, to take time together away from the child so the time with the child is more helpful and less emotionally draining, and to spend time with their other children. The attention required by the child with CP is excessive and detracts from the time available for other siblings, who resent the loss of attention and the excessive demands of the ill child. Family counseling is critical for maintenance of family integrity.

The family is the most important influence on the child's self-concept. Emotional support of the family and suggestions for ways they can promote the child's self-esteem are the best ways to support the child. CP is accompanied by physical evidence of the disability. This often is accompanied by social stigma with which both the child and the family must cope. The social stigma and physical disabilities increase the risk for low self-concept and poor body image. It is important for children to talk about their disability and how it affects them. Nurses are in a prime position to assess factors that inhibit positive self-image and work with the child and family to understand and intervene in self-concept issues. Planned activities consistent with the child's abilities, maintenance of independence, and contact with peers are essential. Meeting and socializing with other children with similar disorders may be helpful. Referral for special counseling, group counseling, and occupational therapy can improve self-esteem and self-concept.

★ EVALUATION

Periodically the nurse and family evaluate the outcomes of care given. Examples of outcomes for the child and family with CP were given under Nursing Diagnoses and Planning in this section.

Attention Deficit Disorders

ADDs are the most common neurobehavioral problems of the pediatric age group. Two categories of ADD were identified in the Revised Diagnostic and Statistical Manual of Mental Disorders, third edition (DSM-IIIR)[2]: ADD with hyperactivity and ADD without hyperactivity. Symptoms were divided into separate criteria for inattention, impulsivity, and hyperactivity. The DSM-IIIR[3] lists 14 symptoms and states that the presence of eight of these symptoms is required for the diagnosis of attention deficit hyperactivity disorder (ADHD).

Definition and Incidence. ADDs are described by the American Psychiatric Association[3] as a disease of infancy characterized by developmentally inappropriate impulsivity, inattention, and hyperactivity. These children have difficulty persisting with tasks and problems and have difficulty organizing and completing their work. The incidence is estimated at between 1% and 20% in North America for those with ADHD and between 7% and 41% for learning disabilities or ADD without hyperactivity.[20] The wide variation in estimates of prevalence of ADD results from sampling problems in the research studies. Some investigators limit the sample to children younger than 6 and others sample children through adolescence.[43] It is one of the most frequently diagnosed childhood disorders in North America.

Etiology and Pathophysiology. ADDs were once classified as minimal brain disorders, which is inaccurate because there is no evidence of true brain damage.[5] The myth that ADD is caused by brain injury has little substantiation in the literature. Evidence now indicates that genetic factors are largely responsible for ADD, and it tends to run in families.[48] ADD is 10 times more common in boys than in girls, and there is an increased risk if the mother or both parents had ADD.[43]

Clinical manifestations include sloppy schoolwork that is performed impulsively and contains many omissions, insertions, oversights, and misrepresentations of easy items. Children appear not to listen or not to hear instructions. Hyperactive ADD children have difficulty sitting still and exhibit excessive running, climbing, and rapid physical movement from one area to another. Activity tends to be haphazard rather than goal directed, and it is poorly organized. Symptoms vary, but the onset usually occurs before 3 years of age, and the hyperactivity seems to decline by adolescence. Other symptoms are present throughout childhood, and teenagers may exhibit depressive symptoms or aggressive behavior.[46]

Learning difficulties, frustration, low self-esteem, and poor or altered peer relationships ensue and may be the precursors to personality disorders sometimes seen in these individuals as adults.[3] Enuresis and encopresis without physical bases also may be associated with ADD.

Diagnostic Studies. Diagnostic evaluation for ADD or ADHD is based on a thorough history from the parents and the school, physical and neurologic examinations, a special neuromaturational examination, intelligence and achievement tests, and lead, thyroid, and chromosome laboratory studies. CAT scans and EEGs may be performed to rule out other disorders. Hearing tests may be conducted to rule out hearing deficits, and psychological testing may be performed by a licensed psychologist specializing in neuropsychology to determine the magnitude of learning and attention difficulties and attendant emotional disorders.

Definitive diagnosis is based on the absence of organic problems and the presence of eight symptoms from the list of 14 presented in the DSM-III.[3] The symptoms are listed in descending order of discriminatory power (see Chap. 18).

★ ASSESSMENT

Nursing assessment of ADHD involves an accurate history from school personnel and parents. Children have diffi-

culty following instructions, sitting still in class, and organizing and completing their work. They may interrupt parental conversations, are impulsive, and are easily distracted. Children have difficulty following the rules in games, which does not endear them to other children. Documentation of history and observed behavior is then sent with a referral to the physician for diagnosis.

★ NURSING DIAGNOSES AND PLANNING

Based on assessment data discussed previously and in the preceding chapter, the following nursing diagnoses may apply to the family and child with ADD:

- High Risk for Injury related to hyperactivity.
- Self-Esteem Disturbance related to inability to organize work.
- Impaired Social Interaction related to disregard of social proprieties.
- Ineffective Management of Therapeutic Regimen related to inability to sustain interest.
- Caregiver Role Strain related to bizarre behavior.
- Compromised Ineffective Family Coping related to developmental disability of child.

The nurse and child (or parents) together plan effective care based on the established nursing diagnoses. Several examples of expected outcomes follow:

- The parents demonstrate correct use of pharmacotherapy.
- The family participates in family counseling.
- The family uses an effective reward system.

The nurse plans for the daily care of the child based on physician's orders and nursing diagnoses. Some general nursing care goals may be the following:

- A structured environment is created in the school.
- The child and family discuss effective coping strategies.

★ INTERVENTIONS: COLLABORATIVE AND INDEPENDENT

Medical management consists of a behavior modification regimen accompanied by pharmacotherapy with stimulants to reduce the hyperactivity (Table 53-12). Reactions

TABLE 53-12
Psychostimulants for Children With Attention Deficit Hyperactivity Disorder*

Medication	Usual Dosage	Frequency	Maximum Daily Dosage
Methylphenidate	0.3 mg/kg to 0.6 mg/kg	b.i.d.	0.8 mg/kg b.i.d. or 60 mg/d
Pemoline (Child older than 6 y)	2.25 mg/kg 56.25 to 75 mg	Daily Daily	112 mg/d
Dextroamphetamine	0.15 to 0.3 mg/kg	Early AM, noon, and sometimes 4:00 PM	40 mg/d

* Table developed from data reported in Munoz-Millan, R., & Casteel, C. (1989). Attention-deficit hyperactivity disorder: Recent literature. *Hospital and Community Psychiatry, 40*(7), 699–707.

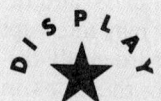

Management of Attention Deficit Hyperactivity Disorders

BEHAVIORAL MANAGEMENT

- Structured, small-classroom environment
- Removal from disturbing or distracting influences
- Curriculum modifications/remediation for specific learning disability and provision for optimal timing of activity sequences
- Self-contained classrooms versus open classrooms or mainstreaming (learning disability classroom or behavioral disabiity classroom)
- Behavior modification with *immediate rewards* in conjunction with pharmacologic therapy
- Special summer camps, group activities

DIETARY MANAGEMENT

- Elimination of food coloring from diet rarely effective
- Low and excess blood sugar may influence behavior of some children

PARENTAL TRAINING

- Instruction in effective parenting techniques including strict discipline with *immediate rewards* to child for appropriate behavior
- Family therapy to deal with intrapsychic conflict and sibling conflict related to increased attention and immediate rewards for Attention Deficit Hyperactivity Disorder child

COGNITIVE-BEHAVIOR THERAPY

- Modeling
- Positive reinforcement
- Time out

PSYCHOPHARMACOLOGY

- Individual psychotherapy for child in addition to family therapy
- Psychostimulants

of the child to food colorings may be assessed to determine related behavioral alterations, but this is rarely the stimulant. An interdisciplinary team is the most effective means of managing children with ADD because modifications of the educational environment are necessary, counseling for the child and family is helpful, parents need to be trained in effective parenting techniques, and the pharmacotherapy may need supervision.

The accompanying display summarizes the management of ADDs. Successful nursing management and education can lessen the stress and anxiety experienced by the child and family. The parents and child (if older) should be educated about the importance of proper medication dosage and routine as well as the side-effects. Management of the behavior problems is important and requires immediate attention. Parental effectiveness training and family counseling are essential. Immediate rewards are necessary for ADD children because they have such short attention spans that delayed rewards have no meaning or are counterproductive. Siblings tend to resent the extra attention and immediate rewards given ADD children. Family counseling is helpful in dealing with these issues. Individual psychotherapy is an important component of therapy to provide support for the emotional lability, immaturity, and disturbed interpersonal relationships that often accompany this disorder.

★ **EVALUATION**

Periodically the nurse and family evaluate the outcomes of care given. Examples of outcomes for the family and

child with ADD were given under Nursing Diagnoses and Planning in this section.

Summary

Precise assessment and monitoring of all systems are essential in care of the child with altered neurologic function. Even minute changes signal catastrophic deterioration in the child's condition. Parents are fearful for the child's life and about possible permanent disabilities. If the child has visible physical alterations, the anxieties of the parents are compounded by concerns about social stigma.

Congenital anomalies of the CNS usually are obvious at birth or shortly thereafter. Anticipatory grieving may be part of the parents' reaction to such a child. Accidents are the primary cause of CNS injuries, and parents and children may feel guilty about the accident.

Increased ICP is a clinical manifestation of head injuries that requires the most astute nursing observations for early detection and prevention of additional damage. Neurologic infections are dangerous because of the risk of loss of life or function. Initial assessments must be as thorough as the child's energy level will allow. Seizure disorders are among the most commonly observed neurologic dysfunction in children.

Degenerative disorders are difficult because a once alert and seemingly normal child progressively becomes dependent and incapacitated. Functional neurodisabilities fall into four broad categories: neuromuscular, attention deficit, sensory integration deficit manifestations, and learning disabilities.

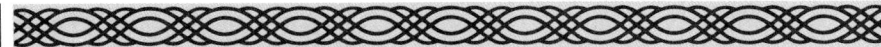

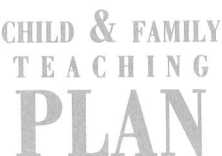
CHILD & FAMILY
T E A C H I N G
PLAN

Care of the Child Experiencing Seizures

Assessment

Ruth S. is an 8-year-old African American who recently was diagnosed with seizure disorder. She has been started on anticonvulsants and has noted a decrease in seizure activity. Ruth describes an aura of a flash of light prior to the seizure. Ruth and her parents are frightened by the seizures and want to know what they should do to protect Ruth. The nursing diagnosis Anxiety related to knowledge deficit was formulated, and the nursing intervention included the development of this teaching plan.

Child and Family Objectives	Specific Content	Teaching Strategies
1. Describe diagnosis, prognosis, and general care for seizures.	1. Etiology of seizures, prognosis, and record keeping. Factors for which a physician should be called for emergency assistance.	1. Provide handouts. Show brain activity on a drawing of the brain. Provide examples of normal and abnormal electroencephalograms; discuss and provide time for questions and answers.
2. Describe methods of protecting the child generally and during seizures.	2. Routine safety precautions help prevent injuries during seizures. Supervise child during bathing, swimming, and climbing.	2. Provide list of safety guidelines for parents.
	Pad sharp edges of tables and other furniture, and carpet stairs. Children who frequently fall should wear helmet.	Tour home with parents to decide environmental changes to make in home.
	Provide the following care during a seizure: Turn child or child's head to side. Open airway by extending neck. Clear surrounding area of objects that might cause injury. Place pad or coat under child's head. *Do not* restrict child's movement. *Do not* place anything in the child's mouth.	Provide a written list of guidelines for care during and following a seizure.
	Keep a record of seizures, noting frequency, time, origin, progression of seizure activity, and child's behavior following seizure.	Provide a checklist for parents to complete after each seizure.
	Reorient child to environment following the seizure.	Provide objects of orientation: clock, calendar. Discuss with parents that loving and touching help speed orientation.
3. Describe medication therapy and side-effects to observe for.	3. Anticonvulsant medications prevent or diminish seizure activity. Administer anticonvulsants as ordered (accurately and consistently).	3. Provide written description of medication, including possible side-effects. Discuss what to do if side-effects occur.

(Continued)

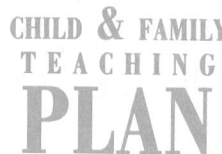

CHILD & FAMILY
TEACHING
PLAN

Care of the Child Experiencing Seizures
(continued)

Child and Family Objectives	Specific Content	Teaching Strategies
	Administration of medications: what, how, and when. Do not give other medications unless first cleared by physician treating seizures. Adverse side-effects should be discussed.	Stress importance of taking medication exactly as directed.
4. Demonstrate measures of psychosocial coping.	4. Encourage child to express anger, fear, sense of rejection, loss of control.	4. Role play, play with dolls, discussion.
	Encourage child to participate in decision making whenever possible.	
	Children need activities that will not precipitate seizure activity.	Demonstrate "quiet" activities: bean bags, paper basketballs.
	Knowledge assists child to take precautions to prevent seizures or protect self.	Help child find causative factors. Discuss importance of aura and what child should do when aura occurs.
	Counseling helps child understand self, feelings, and means of expressing self.	Refer family to support groups or counseling.
	Assist child to anticipate potential stressful situations.	Role play seizure at school and how to handle reactions of peers; dating; getting a job; obtaining a driver's license; peer pressure to take drugs or alcohol.
5. Maintain good oral health habits.	5. Discuss the importance of good oral hygiene, because anticonvulsant medications may cause hypertrophy of the gums.	5. Arrange a meeting with a hygienist; provide soft toothbrush, dental floss, gum massager. Demonstrate correct use of these items with return demonstration. Teach how to use electric toothbrush if dentist recommends.

Evaluation

- Ruth and family demonstrate knowledge of seizures, precautions, medications, and adverse side-effects.
- Ruth and family report that home environment provides protection from injury during seizures.
- Ruth and family express feelings appropriately.
- Ruth demonstrates effective coping and growing self-esteem.
- Ruth and family discuss use of support groups and community resources.
- Ruth practices good oral hygiene.

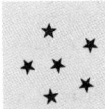

Ideas for Nursing Research

The nurse who is working with children with neurologic problems has a unique opportunity to explore methods for improving the immedicate response to treatment and level of rehabilitation. Neurologic disorders range from congenital birth anomalies to traumatic injuries and the implications for nursing care are quite diverse. Some ideas for nursing research include the following:

- Effects of head elevations of 0, 15, and 30 degrees on the intracranial pressure (ICP) of children with head injuries
- Effects of position changes on heart rate and ICP for children with head injuries
- Effect of 4 to 6 hours of undisturbed rest each night on the length of hospital stay
- Caregiving procedures that increase ICP and how long it takes the child to return to preprocedure ICP, blood pressure, and heart rate levels
- Comparison of various types of mattresses on the incidence of pressure sores in comatose children
- Effectiveness of various stress reduction strategies in reducing stress associated with neurologic treatments for children

References

1. Aaby, P., Bukh, J., Lisse, I., et al. (1984). Risk factors in subacute sclerosing panencephalitis: Age and sex-dependent host reactions or intensive exposure? *Review of Infectious Diseases, 6,* 239–250.
2. American Psychiatric Association Committee on Nomenclature and Statistics. (1980). *Diagnostic and statistical manual of mental disorders* (3rd ed.). Washington, DC: American Psychiatric Association.
3. American Psychiatric Association Committee on Nomenclature and Statistics. (1987). *Diagnostic and statistical manual of mental disorders, revised* (3rd ed.). Washington, DC: American Psychiatric Association.
4. Behrman, R., & Vaughn, V. C. (1987). *Nelson's textbook of pediatrics.* Philadelphia: W.B. Saunders.
5. Cantwell, D., & Baker, L. (1987). Attention-deficit disorder in children: The role of the nurse practitioner. *Nurse Practitioner, 12*(7), 37–54.
5A. Centers for Disease Control. (1991) Preventing lead poisoning in young children. Bethesda, MD: U.S. Department of Health and Human Services, Public Health Service.
6. Chandler, L., Andrews, A., & Swanson, M. (1980). *The movement assessment of infants: A manual.* Rolling Bay, WA: Author.
7. Cohen, F. L. (1987). Neural tube defects: Epidemiology, detection and prevention. *Journal of Obstetrical, Gynecological and Neonatal Nursing, 16*(2), 105–115.
8. Commission on Classification and Terminology of the International League Against Epilepsy. (1981). Proposal for revised clinical and electroencephalographic classification of epileptic seizures. *Epilepsia, 22,* 489–501.
9. Davis, D. M. (1988). Reye's syndrome—1986. *Journal of Emergency Nursing, 14*(2), 110–111.
10. Evans, J. C. (1981). Newborn assessment. In J Fox (Ed.). *Primary health care of the young.* New York: McGraw Hill, 94–136.
11. Foo, D. (1985). Spinal cord injury and spinal shock. *Emergency Care Nursing, 1*(2), 77–82.
12. Gabriel, R. S., & McComb, J. G. (1985). Malformations of the central nervous system. In J. H. Menkes (Ed.). *Textbook of child neurology* (3rd ed.) (pp. 189–270) Lea & Febiger.
13. Gorski, P., Huntington, L., & Lewkowics, D. (1987). Handling preterm infants in hospitals: Stimulating controversy about timing stimulation. In N. Gunzenhauser (Ed.). *Infant stimulation.* Skillman, NJ: Johnson & Johnson Baby Products Company Pediatric Round Table Series *13,* 43–50.
14. Grant, L. (1984). Hydrocephalus: An overview and update. *Journal of Neurosurgical Nursing 16*(6), 313–318.
15. Hanley, D. F. (1988). When to suspect viral encephalitis. *Patient Care 22*(13), 77–91.
16. Harris, S. (1987). Early neuromotor predictors of cerebral palsy in low birthweight infants. *Developmental Medicine and Child Neurology, 29,* 508–519.
17. Hurwitz, E. S., et al. (1985). Public health service study on Reye's syndrome and medications. *New England Journal of Medicine, 313*(14), 849–857.
18. Huttenlocher, P. (1987). The nervous system. In R. Behrman & V. Vaughn (Eds.). *Nelson's textbook of pediatrics* (13th ed.) (pp. 1274–1330) Philadelphia: W.B. Saunders.
19. Laitinen, L., Nilsson, S., & Fugl Meyer, A. (1983). Selective posterior rhizotomy for treatment of spasticity. *Journal of Neurosurgery, 58,* 895–899.
20. Lambert, N. & Sandoval, J. (1980). The prevalence of learning disabilities in a sample of children considered hyperactive, *Journal of Abnormal Child Psychology, 8,* 33–50.
21. Lemire, R. (1988). Neural tube defects. *Journal of Child Neurology, 3*(2), 2, 46.
22. Levy, R., et al. (1985). Neurological manifestations of the acquired immunodeficiency syndrome: Experience as UCSF and review of the literature. *Journal of Neurosurgery, 62,* 475–479.
23. Macedo, A., & Posel, L. (1987). Nursing the family after the birth of a child with spina bifida. *Issues in Comprehensive Nursing, 10*(1), 55–65.
24. McMillan, J. A., Neiburg, P. I., & Oski, F. A. (1977). *The whole pediatrician catalog.* Philadelphia: W.B. Saunders.
25. Merz, B. (1984). Matchmaking scheme solves Tay-Sachs problem. *Journal of the American Medical Association, 248*(19), 2636–2637.
26. Mitchell, M. (1989). *Neuroscience nursing: A nursing diagnosis approach.* Baltimore: Williams & Wilkins.
27. Molnar, G. (1985). Cerebral palsy. In G. Molnar (Ed.). *Pediatric rehabilitation* (pp. 420–467). Baltimore: Williams & Wilkins.
28. Nellhaus, G., Stumpf, D., & Moe, P. (1987). Neurologic and muscular disorders. In H. Kemp, et al. (Eds.). *Current pediatric diagnosis and treatment* (9th ed.) (pp. 645–729) Norwalk, CT: Appleton & Lange.
29. Nikas, D. L. (1987). Critical aspects of head trauma. *Critical Care Nursing, 10*(1): 19–44.
30. Novello, A., et al. (1989). Final report of the U.S. Dept of Health and Human Services secretary's work group on pediatric human immunodeficiency virus infection and disease: Content and implications. *Pediatrics, 84*(3), 547–555.
31. Oleske, J., Connor, E., & Boland, M. (1988). A perspective on pediatric AIDS. *Pediatric Annals, 17*(5), 319–321.
32. Palmer, F. B., et al. (1988). The effects of physical therapy on cerebral palsy: A controlled trial in infants with spastic diplegia. *New England Journal of Medicine, 318*(13), 803–808.
33. Paneth, N. (1986). Etiologic factors in cerebral palsy. *Pediatric Annals, 15,* 191, 194–201.
34. Perlman, J. M., & Volpe, J. J. (1987). Prevention of neonatal intraventricular hemorrhage. *Clinics in Neuropharmacology, 10*(2), 126–142.

35. Perlstein, L. M., & Ake, J. M. (1987). AIDS: An overview for the neuroscience nurse. *Journal of Neuroscience, 29*(6), 296–299.

36. Pollack-Latham, C. L. (1987). Intracranial pressure monitoring: Patient care. *Critical Care Nursing, 7*(6), 53–73.

37. Provenzale, J. M. (1987). Treatment modalities in Guillain-Barré syndrome. *Hospital Practice, 22*(3), 93–104.

38. Rogers, M. (1988). Pediatric HIV transmission: Epidemiology, etiopathogenesis, and transmission. *Pediatric Annals, 17*(5), 324–331.

39. Rudolph, A. M. (1987). *Pediatrics* (18th ed.). Norwalk, CT: Appleton & Lange.

40. Santilli, N., & Sierzant, T. L. (1987). Advances in the treatment of epilepsy. *Journal of Neuroscience Nursing, 19*(3), 141–157.

41. Schwartz, J., Angle, C., & Pitcher, H. (1986). Relationship between childhood blood lead levels and stature. *Pediatrics, 77*(3), 281–288.

42. Shannon, M., Graef, J., & Lovejoy, F. (1988). Efficacy and toxicity of b-penicillamine in low-level lead poisoning. *Journal of Pediatrics, 112*(5), 799–804.

43. Shaywitz, S., & Shaywitz, B. (1984). Diagnosis and management of attention deficit disorder: A pediatric perspective. *Pediatric Clinics of North America, 31*(2), 429–458.

44. Shinnar, S., et al. (1985). Management of hydrocephaly in infancy: Use of acetazolamide and furosemide to avoid CNS shunts. *Journal of Pediatrics, 107*(1), 31–37.

45. Shukla, R., et al. (1989). Fetal and infant lead exposure: Effects on growth in stature. *Pediatrics, 84*(4), 604–612.

46. Silver, L., & Brunstetter, R. (1986). Attention deficit disorder in adolescents. *Hospital Community Psychiatry, 37*(6), 596–607.

47. Volpe, J. J. (1989). Intraventriculr hemorrhage and brain injury in the premature infant: Neuropathology and pathogenesis. *Clinics in Perinatology, 16*(2), 387–411.

48. Wendorf, B. (1987). Attention deficit disorder: Addressing the biological issues in behavioral disorders. *Family Systems Medicine, 5*(3), 293–303.

49. Whieldon, D. (1987). Emergency: Pediatric head trauma. *Patient Care, 21*(11), 192–204.

50. Williams, A. (1989). Nursing management of the child with AIDS. *Pediatric Nursing, 15*(3), 259–261.

14

UNIT

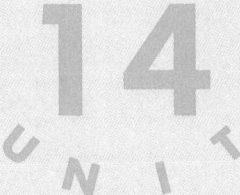

Nursing Care of Children With Altered Endocrine Function

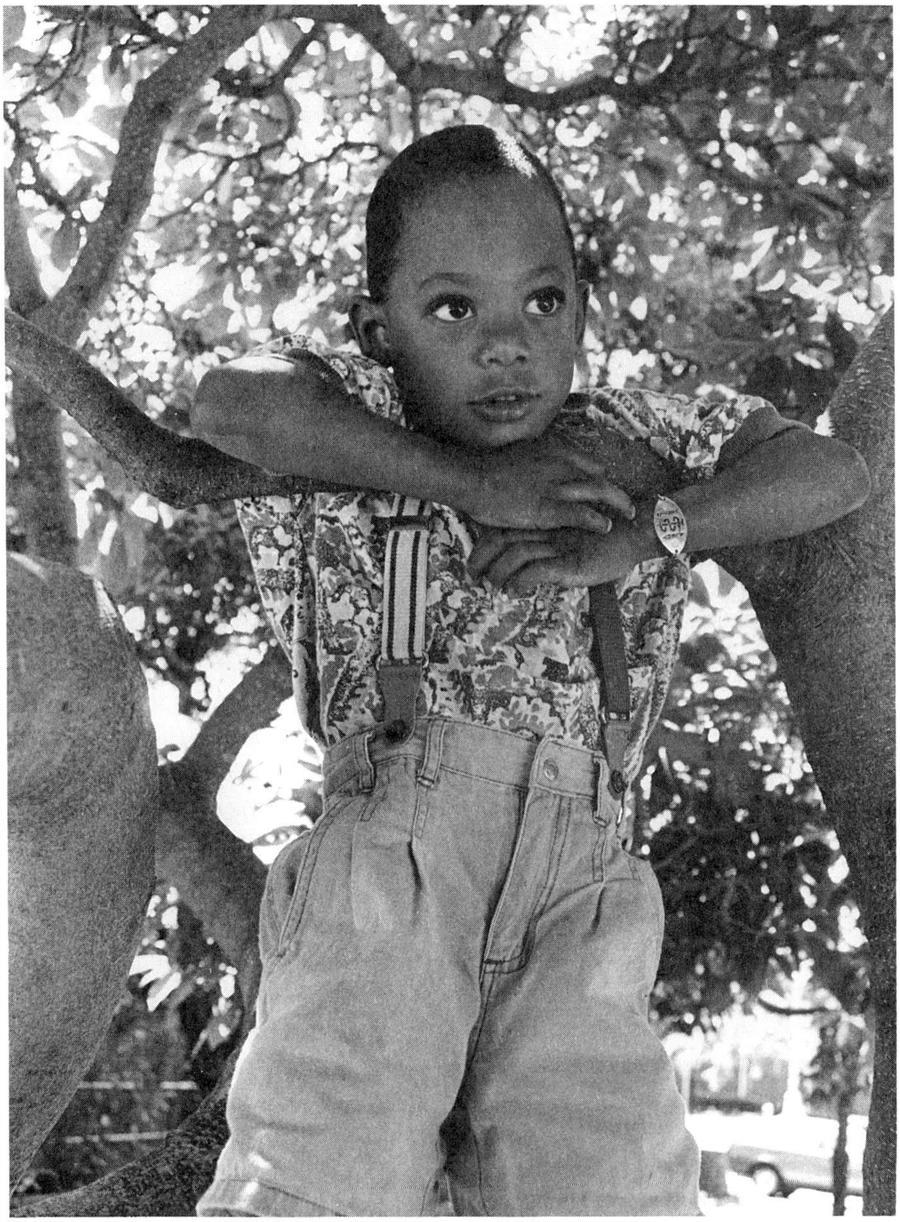

54

Anatomy and Physiology of the Endocrine System

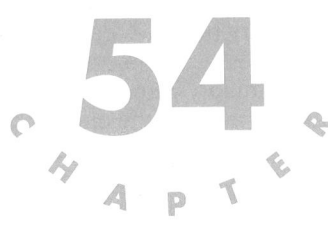

BEHAVIORAL OBJECTIVES

Describe the general embryonic development of the endocrine system.

Identify the consequences of abnormal embryonic development of the endocrine glands.

Describe the structure and function of the major endocrine glands.

Explain the role of the endocrine glands and their hormones in maintaining homeostasis.

Explain the mechanisms of hormone regulation and action during childhood.

Endocrinology is the study of communication and control within a living organism through chemical messengers that are synthesized and secreted by that organism. The body's cells and tissues are highly developed, and the endocrine system provides a communication network capable of regulating and integrating their functions. Growth, maturation, metabolic function, and reproduction are controlled by the endocrine system through hormones produced and secreted by specialized glands. The glands of the endocrine system include the hypothalamus, pituitary, thyroid, parathyroid, adrenal, endocrine pancreas, ovary, and testes. Their locations are shown in Figure 54-1.

A *gland* is a group of specialized cells that can synthesize and secrete chemical messengers called hormones in response to specific signals. There are two types of glands: endocrine and exocrine. *Endocrine glands* secrete their hormones directly into the bloodstream and act on remote tissues sensitive to their action (target tissues). Endocrine glands are the focus of this chapter. *Exocrine glands* secrete substances that usually are released into ducts and carried to an internal or external body surface. Examples of exocrine glands include the salivary, sebaceous, and sweat glands.

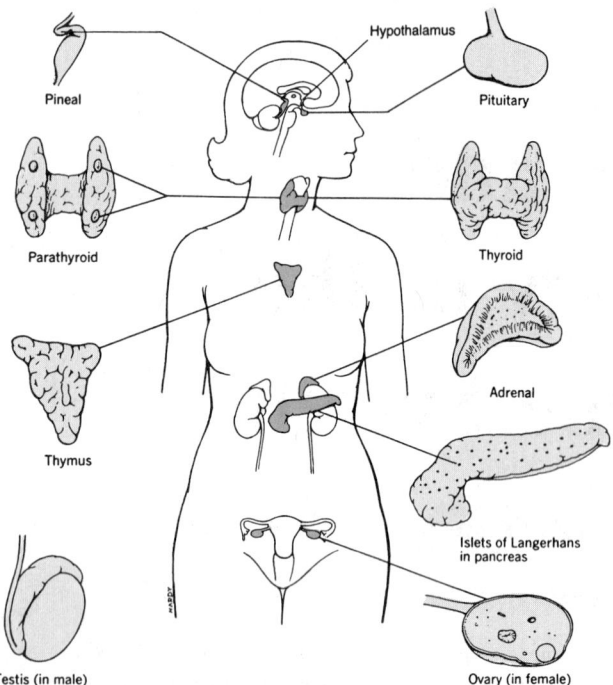

FIGURE 54-1

Location of the major endocrine glands in the body.

This chapter provides the information necessary to help nurses achieve a basic understanding of the endocrine system: its embryologic roots, its glands, the hormones produced by the glands, and the actions and interplay of the hormones as they work to maintain homeostasis.

Embryonic Development

The embryonic origins of the endocrine glands differ not only in their cell types, but also in their relationship to the hypothalamus. The hypothalamus is an integral part of the central nervous system that is derived from neural ectoderm of the diencephalon area. Early in embryonic development the anterior midline projection of the hypothalamus moves forward and meets with the developing Rathke's pouch to form the pituitary stalk and posterior pituitary gland.[40] Other projections of the hypothalamus are connected to the autonomic nervous system, the limbic system, and other parts of the developing nervous system. Hypothalamic-releasing hormones are detectable in the fetus by 11 weeks' gestation.

Near the end of the embryonic period, the main organ systems are established. During the fourth to fifth week of embryonic development a distinct pattern of cartilaginous structures, called the branchial arches, are formed from the fusion of two hollow ectodermal processes. Outpouches of the foregut lining, called pharyngeal pouches, develop between the arches. Rathke's pouch, a single, medial outpouching that grows from the primitive oral cavity, gives rise to the anterior lobe of the pituitary gland. A second outpouching of the neural ectoderm develops into the pituitary's posterior lobe, which remains connected to the hypothalamus by the pituitary stalk or

infundibulum. The connection between the posterior lobe of the pituitary and the brain persists, but the lumen of Rathke's pouch disappears.[40] The infundibulum becomes elongated, and the pituitary becomes embedded in the sella turcica.[21]

The gross features of the pituitary gland are recognizable, and secretory granules appear by the end of the third month of fetal life.[3,22] Derived from a common stem cell, the major secretory cells of the pituitary synthesize, process, and release various secretory granules. Upon entering the interstitial fluid these granules dissolve to become soluble hormones that enter the bloodstream of the fetus. The pituitary gland seems to synthesize growth hormone (GH) and adrenocorticotropin hormone (ACTH) first, and these are followed by thyroid-stimulating hormone (TSH), follicle-stimulating hormone (FSH), luteinizing hormone (LH), and finally prolactin (PRL) at approximately 20 weeks' gestation.[11] The stage of fetal development when pituitary hormone secretion is initiated and maintained has not been definitely established.

The thyroid gland appears during the fourth week of fetal development from a single medial outpouch in the floor of the second pharyngeal pouch. This outpouching undergoes elongation, and the medial portion of the thyroid gland arises as a bilobate shape at the base of the tongue.[26,40] The thyroid gland descends to its position in front of the trachea by the seventh week. The thyroglossal duct then undergoes dissolution and fragmentation, leaving a small dimple at the posterior third of the tongue by the eighth week of fetal life.[26] During the eighth week of gestation thyroglobulin is synthesized by the follicular cells of the thyroid. Trapping of iodine is followed by iodination of tyrosine near the 10th week.[16] These are the new materials of thyroid hormone synthesis. The fetal pituitary–thyroid axis functions independently of the mother by midgestation.

The lateral portion of the thyroid gland arises from the neural crest. The lateral portion, where C cells are formed, fuses with the medial portion of thyroid tissue in its upper lateral aspects. C cells produce calcitonin and have been found in many other tissues in the body. It is thought, however, that the C cells located in other tissues arise embryologically from a different source.[26]

The parathyroid glands are formed during the fifth week of fetal development. The dorsal wings of the third and fourth pharyngeal pouches differentiate into parathyroid tissue. They migrate inferiorly to rest on the upper and lower poles of the thyroid gland.[1,40]

The adrenal cortex and medulla are formed from separate embryologic tissues. Primitive sympathetic cells derived from the neuroectoderm migrate ventrally to form the neural crest. Some of these cells remain in close association with the developing sympathetic nervous system and give rise to the extra-adrenal chromaffin cells and chromaffin cell bodies. Other pheochromoblasts invade the developing adrenal cortex to form the primitive adrenal medulla. Extra-adrenal cells mature before the 11th week of gestation. Postnatally most extra-adrenal chromaffin cells degenerate, while those of the adrenal medulla mature.[23,40]

The adrenal cortex arises from the coelomic mesoderm medial to the wolffian ridge penetrated by cells arising from the nervous system. By eight weeks of fetal life the cortex has formed two distinct zones. A central, larger fetal zone and a thin rim of definitive cortex later form the adult adrenal cortex. Between the second and third month of gestation the adrenal glands are much larger than the kidneys. Fetal production of some adrenal hormones begins around midtrimester in response to ACTH and PRL stimulation.[4,36] The inner zone involutes shortly before birth and disappears between 3 and 12 months of age. During this time the permanent cortex starts to differentiate into three zones that are well established by 3 years of age.

The pancreas houses the islets of Langerhans cells, the endocrine tissue of the pancreas. The islets of Langerhans cells arise from the ends of the parenchymatous pancreatic tissue during the third month of fetal life and are scattered throughout the gland. Originally islet cells are seen as single cells among the exocrine cells of the terminal pancreatic tubules and then as clusters of cells within the exocrine basement membrane. These clusters of cells lose their connection with the exocrine tissue to form islets.[39,43] The individual islet cells increase in size and replicate. Insulin secretion begins during the fifth month of gestation. The fetus and young child have the greatest relative volume of islet cell mass.[5] Basal insulin levels in the fetus are similar to the mother's insulin level.

Current beliefs regarding sexual differentiation state that male and female embryos possess bipotential gonads that develop into ovaries unless testes-organizing factors actively interfere. The development of the undifferentiated gonads into normal ovaries or testes is initially determined by the sex chromosomes.[41,42] The gonads appear during the fourth week of development as a pair of ridges that differentiate from the mesodermal cells as the gonads develop. Ovaries are distinguishable from testes by 6 weeks' gestation. Pituitary gonadotropin levels, which are higher in girls, are detectable by 11 weeks' gestation. By 12 weeks' gestation the fetal ovary begins estrogen secretion. Follicles develop as granulosa cells form spheres around oocytes following stimulation by fetal gonadotropins.[19,40] At birth ovarian follicle development is complete.[19]

The descent of the testes appears to be in response to hormonal and mechanical control. In the first 3 months of fetal life the testes are stimulated by placental chorionic gonadotropins. At 11 weeks' gestation LH produced by the fetal pituitary gland stimulates testosterone synthesis in the fetal testes.[24] The fetal testes secrete two hormones necessary for normal internal and external male sexual differentiation. The Leydig's cells produce testosterone, which stimulates paired wolffian ducts to differentiate into vas deferens, seminal vesicles, and epididymis. Antimüllerian factor inhibits the formation of female organs. Testosterone is critical to male external genital development and to the synthesis of androgens, which are essential for the development of the glans penis, penile urethra, and scrotum.[28] After 12 weeks' gestation testosterone production is gonadotropin dependent.

The regulation of the fetal endocrine system is not totally independent but uses the precursor hormones secreted by the placenta and others obtained from the mother.

Consequences of Abnormal Development

The consequences of abnormal development of the hypothalamus are closely linked with defects in brain formation and differentiation.[38] These defects carry a high risk for mortality in the fetal and neonatal period.[8] Consequences of abnormal embryonic development of the hypothalamus and other endocrine glands are summarized in Table 54-1.

Structure and Function

The endocrine glands are located throughout the body (see Fig. 54-1) and are primarily involved with governing the body processes of growth, maturation, metabolic functions, and reproduction through the action of their hormones. In fact the Greek meaning of the word hormone is to arouse to activity. Hormones are produced and released into the bloodstream when their action is needed and inhibited when their effect is achieved. The following sections describe the locations of the endocrine glands, the hormones they produce, and the actions of the hormones.

Hypothalamus

The hypothalamus lies below the third ventricle of the brain and is surrounded by the optic chiasm anteriorly, the sulci formed by the temporal lobes laterally, and the mamillary bodies posteriorly. The pituitary stalk descends from its central region, the median eminence.[39] Composed of numerous nuclei (collections of nerve cells of similar structure and function), the hypothalamus is concerned with regulation of body processes, temperature, thirst, hunger, satiety, and adaptive and sexual behaviors. The cell projections (axons) of the supraoptic and paraventricular nuclei form the posterior pituitary gland. These projections release their hormones directly into the blood vessels of the posterior pituitary. Other nuclei of the hypothalamus located near the median eminence synthesize and secrete hormones into the hypothalamic–hypophyseal portal system.[8] The hypothalamic-hypophyseal portal system carries hypothalamic-releasing and -inhibiting hormones (known chemical structures) or factors (unknown chemical structures) to the anterior lobe of the pituitary gland.

The hypothalamus and the anterior pituitary are components of an integrated functional unit, an information relay system (Fig. 54-2). Specialized neuronal cells of the hypothalamus are responsive to changes in the internal and external environments.[43] The hypothalamus is crucial for the regulation of growth, reproduction, adrenal function, thyroid function, and water balance. The pituitary gland's ability to synthesize and secrete hormones can be inhibited or stimulated by hypothalamic hormones.[32] Hypothalamic hormones include gonadotropin-releasing hormone (GnRH), growth hormone-releasing hormone (GHRH),

TABLE 54-1
Consequences of Abnormal Embryonic Development

Embryonic Event	Consequence
Anencephaly Holoprosencephalic syndromes	• Poor chance of fetal survival • Absent hypothalamus • Absent or hypoplastic pituitary gland • Maldevelopment of the target organs
Partial form of holoprosencephalic syndrome (Kallmann's syndrome)	• Anosmia secondary to agenesis of olfactory lobes • Hypogonadotropic hypogonadism secondary to lack of hypothalamic gonadotropin-releasing hormone production
Absence or hypoplasia of anterior pituitary	• Extremely uncommon • Absence usually incompatible with life • Hypoplasia may be mild or severe • Severe hypopituitarism (hypoglycemia and adrenal failure that leads to shock)
Agenesis of the thyroid gland	• Congenital hypothyroidism
Nondescent of the thyroid gland (lingual thyroid)	• Thyroid tissue may remain along the pathway of the thyroglossal duct, including the trachea, larynx, and posterior pharynx, all of which would be susceptible to all thyroid disease processes
Elongated descent of the thyroid gland	• May lead to substernal, preaortic, or pericardial thyroid
Failure of the thyroglossal duct to atrophy	• Cystic, dilated, or infections of the thyroglossal duct may occur as the child ages
Agenesis or dysgenesis of the parathyroid glands	• Partial or absence of C cells • Occasional abnormalities or absence of parathyroid glands (DiGeorge syndrome)
Gonadal dysgenesis male and female	• Lack of secondary sexual characteristics, sexual infantilism
Agenesis or hypoplasia of Leydig's cells	• Minimal masculinization to hypoplastic male genitalia (male pseudohermaphroditism)
Germinal cell aplasia	• Usually normal male genitalia; sterile (Sertoli's cell only syndrome, DelCastillo syndrome)
Atrophy of fetal testes after 16 weeks' gestation	• Normal male external genitalia with anorchia (absent testes) (vanishing testis syndrome)
Agonadia (testicular regression syndrome)	• Gonads are absent, external genitalia abnormal, all but rudimentary müllerian or wolffian derivatives absent

thyrotropin-releasing hormone (TRH), corticotropin-releasing hormone (CRH), somatostatin (also known as growth hormone-inhibiting hormone), and prolactin-inhibiting factor. The functions of hypothalamic hormones are summarized in Table 54-2.

GHRH has a specific action on the GH cells of the anterior pituitary. It releases GH stored in the pituitary and serves as a raw material necessary for the synthesis of GH.[8,32] Somatostatin inhibits GH secretion and thyrotropin-releasing hormone (TRH). The release of other pituitary hormones is not inhibited.[21]

TRH is the stimulus for TSH and PRL release. Specific areas of the hypothalamus synthesize and release TRH into the pituitary portal system. TRH is released episodically with the greatest secretion just before the onset of sleep. There is evidence that TRH is involved in the stress response and is sensitive to changes in environmental temperature. Increased production of TSH in response to cold has been demonstrated only in infants and young children during surgical hypothermia.[26,43]

CRH is the principle stimulus for pituitary ACTH. Glucocorticoids provide feedback inhibition of CRH release, thereby inhibiting gonadotropin secretions. Some studies have shown that CRH causes a general arousal and suggest that it also may have an integrative role in the response to stress. The stress response includes biologic responses as well as modification of behavior appropriate to the stress.[43] Negative feedback control is exerted by adrenal cortisol.

GnRH neurons secrete autonomously. Hormones are released in cyclical patterns that repeat every 60 to 90 minutes. The sex steroids and other hormones alter the frequency and amplitude of GnRH pulses. GnRH binds to specific receptors in the anterior pituitary. It regulates the release of stored gonadotropins and the synthesis of gonadotropins. As the central nervous system matures, GnRH secretion is inhibited.[8] During puberty the normal pulsatile pattern for adults is established.

The hypothalamus is the origin of the neuron cell bodies that terminate in the posterior lobe of the pituitary gland. In the posterior lobe the terminals are organized into a secretory mechanism that discharges directly into the blood. Both vasopressin and oxytocin (not significant in childhood) are synthesized in the hypothalamic nuclei and transported along the neurohypophyseal tract to the posterior pituitary, which stores and releases these hormones under central control.[3,8]

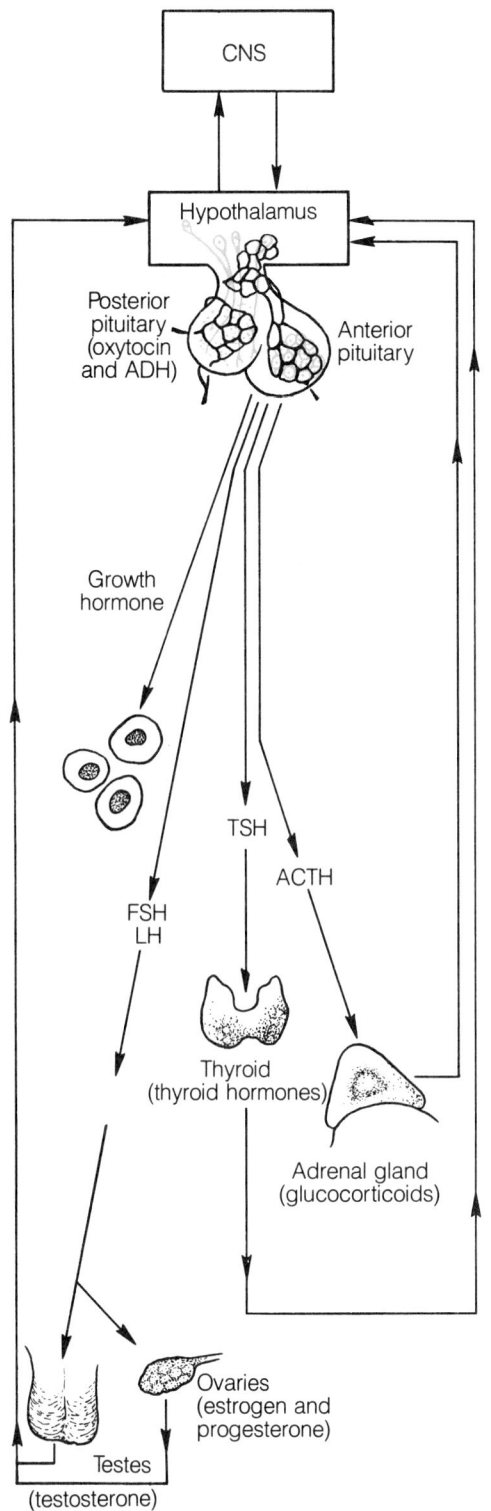

FIGURE 54-2
Control of hormone production by hypothalamic-pituitary-target cell feedback mechanism. Hormone levels from the target glands regulate the release of hormones from the anterior pituitary by means of a negative feedback system. (Source: Porth, C. M. [1990]. *Pathophysiology: Concepts of altered health states* [3rd ed.]. Philadelphia, J. B. Lippincott.)

TABLE 54-2
Major Actions of Hypothalamic Hormones

Hormones	Actions
Growth hormone-releasing hormone (GHRH)	• Stimulates secretion of growth hormone (GH) from the anterior of the pituitary
Somatostatin (growth hormone inhibiting hormone, GHIH)	• Inhibits GH secretion • Inhibits thyrotropin-releasing hormone (TRH) • Inhibits insulin and glucagon secretion • Decreases secretion of thyroid-stimulating hormone (TSH), parathyroid hormone (PTH) • May inhibit prolactin and adrenocorticotropin hormone (ACTH)
Thyrotropin-releasing hormone (TRH)	• Stimulates TSH and prolactin secretion from the anterior pituitary
Corticotropin-releasing hormone	• Stimulates the release of ACTH
Prolactin-releasing factor (PRF)	• Stimulates prolactin release from the anterior pituitary gland
Prolactin-inhibiting factor (PIF)	• Inhibits release of prolactin
Gonadotropin-releasing hormone (GnRH)	• Stimulates the secretion of luteinizing hormone (LH) and follicle stimulating hormone (FSH) from the anterior pituitary

(Data from Cooper, P. E., Martin, J. B. [1990]. Physiology and pathophysiology of the endocrine brain and hypothalamus. In K. L. Becker (Ed.). *Principles and practice of endocrinology and metabolism.* Philadelphia: J. B. Lippincott; Gray, D. P. [1990]. Mechanisms of hormonal regulation. In K. L. McCance & S. E. Huether (Eds.). *Pathophysiology: The biologic basis for disease in adults and children.* St. Louis: C.V. Mosby.)

Pituitary Gland

The pituitary gland (also called the hypophysis) consists of an anterior (adenohypophysis) and posterior (neurohypophysis) lobe. It lies in the sella turcica at the base of the brain in the sphenoid bone. It weighs approximately 0.5 g, and 75% of its weight is the larger anterior lobe. The diameter of the gland is approximately 1 cm.[11]

The blood supply to the anterior pituitary is provided by the hypophyseal artery, a branch of the internal carotid artery, and by the hypothalamic–hypophyseal portal system. The cells of the pituitary extract hypothalamic hormones and other raw materials from the blood to produce new hormones.[6] The blood supply to the posterior lobe of the pituitary is largely separate from the anterior lobe and is provided by the inferior hypophyseal arteries.

Anterior Lobe

The anterior lobe of the pituitary gland consists of three major types of cells: the acidophils (alpha cells), which secrete GH; basophils (beta and delta cells), which secrete LH, FSH, TSH, and ACTH; and chromophobes (gamma cells), which secrete PRL. These cells are arranged in groups surrounding blood sinuses.

The anterior lobe of the pituitary gland secretes hormones that regulate the other major endocrine glands of the body. The six hormones produced by the anterior lobe are GH, ACTH, TSH, LH, FSH, and PRL. With the exception of GH each of the hormones has a direct action on a target organ (Table 54-3).

Growth Hormone. GH stimulates somatic growth, thereby increasing the size of almost all the tissues of the body. Generally GH enhances the use of proteins, conserves glucose, and uses fat stores. GH release is controlled by the hypothalamus (GHRH) and regulated by negative feedback and neural control mechanisms. GH secretion can be stimulated or inhibited by neurogenic, metabolic, or hormonal influences. Exercise, fasting, sleep, hypoglycemia, and stress are examples of GH stimulants. Psychosocial factors and chronic illnesses can inhibit or suppress GH in some children.[2]

Adrenocorticotropin Hormone. ACTH directly influences the adrenal cortex to produce steroids. The production of ACTH is under control of the hypothalamus, and rising blood levels of cortisol provide feedback inhibition. ACTH secretion is stimulated in response to physical and psychological stressors and by the redistribution of body nutrients.[11,43]

Thyroid-Stimulating Hormone. TSH has a direct effect on the size and vascularity of the thyroid gland. As TSH levels increase the thyroid gland enlarges due to an increase in iodine transport and synthesis of triiodothyronine (T_3) and thyroxine (T_4). TSH secretion is inhibited when T_3 and T_4 levels increase, but when blood concentrations of T_3 and T_4 levels fall, the pituitary gland receives a message to secrete more TSH and increase production of T_3 and T_4.[11,26] The thyroid hormones maintain metabolic rate, help with adaptation to cold temperatures, and are vital to central nervous system development, particularly in children younger than 3 years of age.[43]

Gonadotropins: Luteinizing Hormone and Follicle-Stimulating Hormone. LH and FSH are secreted from the anterior pituitary gland in response to hormone signals from the hypothalamus and the gonads (see Fig. 54-3). LH and FSH communicate information obtained from the central nervous system and the environment to the reproductive system. LH and FSH stimulate cell growth and maintenance in both the testes and ovaries.[6]

LH and FSH levels are regulated by GnRH, and they reach peak secretion at approximately 24 weeks of fetal life. GnRH, LH, and FSH secretion then falls to low levels that persist from late gestation until shortly before the onset of puberty, around the age of 10. As this time approaches levels begin to rise after and during the onset of a nighttime sleep cycle. As puberty progresses LH levels continue to increase in the frequency and amplitude of pulses until a mature adult pattern is established. It is thought that puberty results when the hypothalamus begins releasing GnRH with increasing frequency and amplitude.[6,25] Secretion of LH and FSH from the anterior lobe of the pituitary gland leads to subsequent secretion of gonadal hormones evidenced by increased growth velocity and the appearance of secondary sexual characteristics.

LH stimulates steroidogenesis in both sexes, particularly testosterone synthesis from Leydig's cells in the

boy and from theca cells in the girl. FSH binds to the Sertoli's cells and spermatogonic membranes in the testes to stimulate spermatogenesis in the male. Although FSH is necessary in the initial maturation of spermatogenesis during puberty, adult men can maintain normal sperm production in spite of low FSH levels.[6] In girls granulosa cells are responsive to FSH, which stimulates follicular development and estradiol production.[7] LH also induces ovulation from the mature follicle in girls and exerts a partially stimulatory effect on spermatogenesis in boys, probably due to increases in intracellular levels of testosterone.[39]

Prolactin. PRL is another hormone secreted by the anterior pituitary gland. The highest PRL levels are found during fetal development. PRL levels fall rapidly after birth and stabilize to normal prepubertal levels. Boys maintain the prepubertal levels well into adulthood, while girls demonstrate increasing levels during puberty that are maintained as they mature.[11,43] PRL secretion may be influenced by several hormones, including estrogens and thyroid hormones. In the menstrual cycle PRL may increase prior to the preovulatory LH surge. PRL levels increase during sleep cycles and fall abruptly upon awakening. Exercise and stress have been found to increase the secretion of PRL.

PRL's role in stimulating breast growth is questionable, but its role in the initiation and maintenance of lactation is recognized. The secretion of milk proteins, fats, sugars, and the electrolyte content of breast milk is controlled by PRL.[11,43] The mechanism by which suckling releases PRL is not completely understood.

Posterior Lobe

The posterior lobe of the pituitary is connected to the hypothalamus by the pituitary stalk (infundibulum).[8] The posterior lobe consists of nerve-like cells known as pituicytes that originate in the hypothalamus. The hormones of the posterior pituitary, vasopressin, and oxytocin are formed in the hypothalamic nuclei and are transported down the nerve fibers. The hormones are then stored in terminal dilations for later use. The process by which these hormones are packed in granules and transported to the pituitary has not been well explained.[9,37]

Vasopressin. Vasopressin (antidiuretic hormone or ADH) plays an important role in water conservation and maintenance of body fluid osmolality, blood volume, and blood pressure.[43] Vasopressin acts on the collecting ducts and distal tubules of the kidneys to increase their permeability to water, thereby decreasing the formation of urine. Although blood volume and pressure influence the secretion of vasopressin, the most important regulator of vasopressin release is the osmotic pressure of plasma, which is mediated by specialized neurons called osmoreceptors that are located mainly in the hypothalamus.[33] The sensitivity of the osmoregulatory system varies during normal aging and can be affected by posture, pregnancy, and menses. Osmoreceptors seem to have a set point below which vasopressin release is suppressed and above which vasopressin is stimulated.[37] Therefore, concentrated body fluids stimulate vasopressin secretion and in-

TABLE 54-3
Major Actions of Endocrine Hormones

Pituitary Gland			Cortisol	Mobilizes amino acids from proteins in plasma and muscle
Anterior Lobe				Promotes fat mobilization
Growth hormone (GH) or somatotropin (SH)	Stimulates growth of cells, bones, and tissues			Antagonizes the action of insulin
	Increases protein synthesis			Influences the immune system, plasma volume, maintenance of blood pressure, and cardiac output
	Decreases rate of carbohydrate use and resistance to insulin			Acts as an anti-inflammatory
	Increases mobilization and use of fats for energy			Necessary for life
	Necessary for normal growth and development		Androgens ‡	Produces many secondary sexual characteristics in boys and girls (e.g. growth of sexual hair)
Thyroid-stimulating hormone (TSH)	Promotes growth and secretory activity of the thyroid gland			Maintains secondary sexual characteristics
	Necessary for normal growth and development		*Medulla*	
Adrenocorticotropin hormone (ACTH)	Influences the secretory output of the adrenal cortex (cortisol and adrenal androgens)		Catecholamines Norepinephrine	Acts as an alpha-receptor stimulator whose action is excitatory (vasoconstriction, increased blood pressure, intestinal relaxation)
Follicle-stimulating hormone (FSH)	Stimulates gametogenesis in boys and girls			Regulates basic metabolic processes, including glycogenolysis, lipolysis, inhibition of insulin release, and electrolyte transport
Luteinizing hormone (LH)				
Prolactin (PRL)	Acts directly on the mammary gland and is responsible for initiation and maintenance of lactation		Epinephrine	Acts as an alpha- and beta-receptor stimulator for which actions are primarily inhibitory and metabolic (increases contractility and excitability of the heart muscle, causing increased cardiac output)
Posterior Lobe				
Antidiuretic hormone (ADH) or vasopressin	Regulates osmolarity and body water volume			
	Increases permeability of the collecting ducts in the kidneys, thereby decreasing urine formation by increased water reabsorption			Increases blood flow to muscles, brain, and viscera
Oxytocin	Stimulates uterine contractions at parturition			Increases the basal metabolic rate
	Stimulates release and flow of breast milk			Enhances blood glucose
Thyroid Gland				Inhibits smooth muscle contractions
Thyroxine (T_4)	Regulates the metabolic and oxidative rates in tissue cells		**Pancreas**	
Triiodothyronine (T_3)	Stimulates growth and development of various tissues at critical periods, including the central nervous system and skeleton		Insulin	Regulates glucose, protein, and lipid metabolism
				Promotes the transfer of glucose across the cell membrane
	Influences rate of metabolism of lipids, proteins, carbohydrates, water, vitamins, and minerals			Inhibits the release of glucose from the liver, promoting hepatic glucose storage
	Maintains cardiac rate, force, and output			Potentiates the action of growth hormone
	Necessary for muscle tone and function		Glucagon	Acts as a counter-regulatory hormone to insulin with epinephrine, GH, and the glucocorticoids
Calcitonin	Lowers serum calcium by opposing bone-reabsorbing effects of PTH, prostaglandins, and calciferols by inhibiting osteoclastic activity			Increases blood glucose
	Lowers serum phosphate levels			Promotes amino acid transport from the muscle
Parathyroid Glands				Decreases protein synthesis
Parathyroid hormone (PTH)	Maintains normal calcium levels in the blood			Decreases lipolysis and ketone formation
	Regulates phosphorous metabolism and increases the rate of calcium reabsorption in the renal tubules		**Gonads**	
			Ovaries	
	Enhances the rate of calcium reabsorption from bone		Estrogen	Develops and maintains the development of secondary sexual characteristics
	Influences the rate of calcium for the gastrointestinal tract			Promotes proliferation of specific cells in the body, leading to maturation of the reproductive organs
Adrenal Glands				Prepares the endometrium for implantation of the fertilized ovum
Cortex				
Mineralocorticoids	Influences electrolyte concentrations and fluid volume		Progesterone	Prepares uterus for pregnancy
Aldosterone*	Stimulates renal tubules to reabsorb sodium and excrete potassium			Prepares breasts for lactation
	Necessary for life		*Testes*	
Glucocorticoids†	Promotes the conversion of protein to carbohydrate (gluconeogenesis and the storage of carbohydrate as glycogen)		Testosterone	Develops and maintains primary and secondary sexual characteristics in boys
Cortisol				Ensures normal sperm production

* Aldosterone is the major mineralocorticoid; others include 11-deoxycorticosterone and 18-hydroxy-11-deoxycorticosterone.

† The principal glucocorticoid is cortisol; others include cortisone and corticosterone.

‡ The primary androgens secreted during adrenarche are dehydroepiandrosterone and androstenedione.

crease reabsorption of water in the kidney. In contrast dilute body fluids suppress vasopressin and decrease reabsorption of water from the kidneys.[33]

Oxytocin. This hormone stimulates the smooth muscle of the pregnant uterus at term. High levels of oxytocin have been found in the fetus at the time of delivery, raising questions about the role of the fetus in determining the onset of labor.[3] However, oxytocin does not appear to be essential for the initiation of labor. The role of oxytocin in lactation is better understood. Suckling of the infant at the breast stimulates the release of oxytocin, which then causes the release of stored milk from the mammary alveoli and ducts.

Thyroid Gland

The thyroid gland is a two-lobed gland located at the interior aspect of the neck. The lobes are arranged on each side of the trachea below the larynx. They are connected by an isthmus that lies on the upper part of the trachea. The gland is well vascularized and composed of follicular and parafollicular cells. Follicular cells are irregular in size and shape. They contain a colloid or jelly-like substance called thyroglobulin that is secreted by the columnar epithelial cells that line the follicle.[26] Iodides trapped from ingested foods are transported into the thyroid, are oxidized, and are combined with the amino acid tyrosine to form hormonally inactive iodotyrosines and coupling of iodotyrosines to form hormonally active T_3 and T_4. These hormones are stored in thyroglobulin and released into the bloodstream as needed.[16,20] T_3 is more active, but its action is short-lived.

The action of the thyroid gland is closely regulated by the anterior lobe of the pituitary and the hypothalamus under feedback control. The stimulation of the hypothalamus may be modulated by higher centers in the brain. The thyroid hormones are essential for normal physical growth, maturation, and mental development. They regulate the metabolic and oxidative rates in body cells. Metabolism of proteins, carbohydrates, lipids, vitamins, and minerals is controlled by the thyroid hormones.[20]

The parafollicular cells (C cells) are derived from the neural crest. Calcitonin is produced by the C cells of the thyroid gland and acts as an anti-parathormone (PTH) hormone, thereby serving to maintain calcium and phosphorous homeostasis.[28] At the bone site calcitonin decreases the amount of calcium and phosphorus released from bone as it increases the amounts of calcium and phosphorus excreted in the urine. Calcitonin seems to work only when acute changes in serum calcium levels occur. The importance of calcitonin in the regulation of mineral metabolism is unclear.[1]

Parathyroid Glands

The parathyroid glands, usually four, are independent of the thyroid gland in structure and function. The parathyroids are small reddish glands located on the upper and lower poles of the thyroid. The glands are composed of closely packed epithelial cells richly supplied with capillaries[1] (see Table 54-3).

Mineral homeostasis is achieved through the maintenance of calcium concentrations in the blood, and the parathyroid glands regulate this activity. The target organs of PTH are the bones and kidneys. In bones PTH requires vitamin D to increase osteoclastic activity and decrease osteoblastic activity. In the kidneys PTH causes increased reabsorption of calcium and excretion of phosphorus by decreasing the absorption of renal tubular phosphate.[12,28] The combined effect of PTH on bones, kidneys, and the intestine is to raise the serum level of calcium.

Adrenal Glands

The adrenal glands are small pyramidal shaped glands that rest on the upper pole of each kidney. The blood supply to the adrenal glands is provided from numerous arterial twigs that form a sinusoidal circulation in the adrenal cortex and medulla. A single vein drains each adrenal gland. The adrenal gland consists of two sections: the cortex or outer layer and the medulla or inner layer.[29,31] The functions of the adrenal cortex and medulla are outlined in Table 54-3 and are discussed below.

Adrenal Cortex

The adrenal cortex is divided into three zones: the zona glomerulosa or outer zone, zona fasciculata, and the zona reticularis. In general these zones are not very well defined but have specific functions. The zona glomerulosa is mainly concerned with biosynthesis of mineralocorticoids, of which aldosterone is the most active. The zona fasciculata and the zona reticularis, which are controlled by pituitary ACTH, produce glucocorticoids and androgens.[31] Cortisol is the major glucocorticoid secreted. Although there are other hormones secreted by the adrenal cortex, only the major ones are addressed in this chapter.[4,29]

Aldosterone, a mineralocorticoid, is essential for life. Aldosterone's major action is on the excretion of electrolytes by the kidneys. It stimulates the absorption of sodium, which then attracts chloride and causes its reabsorption into the blood. In this way the sodium and chloride content of the extracellular fluids is maintained, as is the circulating fluid volume, because water is reabsorbed with the sodium. The reabsorption of potassium is suppressed, and the sodium and potassium balance is maintained. Other stimulants of aldosterone secretion include an increase in extracellular potassium, a decrease in extracellular sodium, and an increase in angiotensin levels.[4,29,43] The rate of aldosterone synthesis is modulated by angiotensin II and potassium. Angiotensin II is responsible for the regulation of blood pressure and salt and water homeostasis by the renin–angiotensin system.[29]

Most glucocorticoid effects are a result of the action of cortisol in response to pituitary ACTH. Glucocorticoids affect the metabolism of glucose, protein, and fat. They also have an effect on inflammation, immunity, wound healing, muscle, and myocardial activity. Elevated levels of cortisol cause negative feedback to the pituitary and the suppression of ACTH. Physical and psychological stress lead to immediate increases in ACTH production and cortisol secretion.[4,30]

Androgens, sex steroids secreted by the adrenal gland, are considered weak compared to the action of testosterone and estrogen from the gonads. However, androgens are the primary stimulus for the onset of adrenarche (appearance of sexual hair). Adrenarche is the maturational increase in production of adrenal androgens in response to changes in the pattern of ACTH secretion by the anterior pituitary gland. Adrenarche, which precedes the onset of puberty by about 2 years, promotes increased stimulation of the ovaries in girls and the testes in boys that continues throughout puberty.[43] Adrenal androgens also are necessary for maintenance of secondary sexual characteristics in adulthood.

Adrenal Medulla

The adrenal medulla forms the central portion of each of the adrenal glands. The chromaffin cells of the adrenal medulla are innervated by preganglionic sympathetic nerve fibers from the splanchnic nerves. The chromaffin cells have chromaffin granules that are similar to the storage and secretory granules of other glands. These granules are highly specialized and consist of an outside membrane and its soluble contents. When an adrenomedullary cell mobilizes chromaffin granules toward the cell surface, they discharge their contents into the pericellular fluid in response to stimulation by the sympathetic nervous system.[43]

The hormones secreted by the adrenal medulla are referred to as catecholamines. The sympathetic nervous system operates through neurochemical transducers (catecholamines) that convert neuronal activity into physiologic responses. The sympathoadrenal system is under the direct control of the central nervous system and regulates the functions that enable the body to adapt to emergency situations.[43,44]

The primary medullary catecholamines are epinephrine and norepinephrine, and their functions are described in Table 54-3. The action of the sympathetic nervous system and that of hormones secreted by the adrenal medulla are similar. Although epinephrine and norepinephrine cause similar responses from target sites in the body, they are not identical. Epinephrine acts on both alpha and beta receptors in the body, and its effects are mainly inhibitory (dilation and relaxation). Norepinephrine acts only on alpha receptors, and its effects are mainly excitatory (constriction and contraction).[23,44] Therefore, epinephrine has more impact on cardiac activity than norepinephrine and can increase cardiac output. In contrast norepinephrine is much more effective in causing constriction of blood vessels and is effective in elevating blood pressure.

The activity of the adrenal medulla changes constantly to meet the metabolic needs of many tissues and to maintain the constancy of the internal environment (homeostasis). Some stressors that stimulate the sympathoadrenal system include fear, anger, psychological and physical stress, pain, blood loss, hypoglycemia, and bodily injury. The physiologic effects of catecholamines decrease rapidly.[44]

Pancreas

The pancreas is an exocrine and an endocrine gland that lies retroperitoneally behind the stomach, with its head and neck near the curve of the duodenum. Its main body extends across the posterior abdominal wall with its tail touching the spleen. It is composed of two types of tissues: the acini, which secrete digestive juices into the duodenum (exocrine), and the islets of Langerhans, which secrete insulin and glucagon directly into the bloodstream. The islets contain alpha (glucagon) and beta (insulin) cells (see Table 54-3). These cells function independently of the pancreatic system of ducts and are highly vascularized. There are more than one million islet cells that secrete hormones into the bloodstream. Glucose is the major stimulus for the release of insulin, although protein ingestion also serves as a stimulant. Catecholamines secreted by the adrenal medulla inhibit the action of insulin.[13,43]

Insulin affects every cell of the body, but its main effects occur in the liver and muscle. It facilitates the passage of glucose from the intravascular to the intracellular space by activating insulin receptors that promote glucose transport. Glucose can then be used as a direct energy source, converted to glycogen for storage, or converted into the lipid synthesis pathway to promote lipid accumulation in the cell. Release of glucose from the liver is inhibited by insulin, thereby increasing hepatic storage of glucose. Synthesis of fatty acids and glycerol is increased as lipid mobilization from adipose tissue stores is inhibited.[13,17] Insulin potentiates the action of GH, secreted by the pituitary gland, by stimulating amino acid uptake into cells and promoting cell growth and multiplication.[13,43]

Glucagon, which is produced by the alpha cells of the pancreas, releases glycogen from the liver. This action increases blood glucose levels. Insulin, epinephrine, GH, and cortisol work together to maintain homeostasis when a person is in a fasting state.[13]

Gonads

The gonads include the ovaries in girls and the testes in boys. The many changes that occur during puberty are part of a series of events that begin *in utero* and reach completion during adulthood. Hypothalamic control mechanisms (GnRH) that are suppressed during childhood are reactivated at the time of puberty, possibly due to the maturation of the central nervous system and the decreased sensitivity of the hypothalamus to the negative feedback system of gonadal sex steroids. During puberty these events lead to the stimulation of the ovaries in girls and the testes in boys.[41] This period is also called gonadarche. Functions of the gonadal hormones are summarized in Table 54-3.

Ovaries

The ovaries are almond shaped organs that produce feminizing hormones. They consist of two layers: the cortex and the medulla. The outer cortical portion of the ovary is concerned with the development of the ova and secretion of ovarian hormones. Theca and granulosa cells in the cortex produce estrogen and progesterone. Under the influence of the anterior pituitary hormones LH and FSH, the follicles begin to mature.[7] Thecal cells surround the growing follicle and produce estrogens, which are released into the bloodstream. The ruptured follicle (ovulation) leads to the development of the corpus luteum. The corpus luteum and the granulosa cells of the late follicular and midcycle phase secrete progesterone.[34,39] The ovarian medulla houses connective tissues that contain blood vessels and smooth muscle fibers.

Testes

The testes are composed of glandular tissue covered by fibrous tissue. In addition to producing sperm the testes function as an endocrine gland. Testosterone is produced by Leydig's cells that are located in the interstices between seminiferous tubules (see Table 54-3). It is responsible for the distinguishing characteristics of the masculine body.[41]

Testosterone levels are extremely high at birth but fall off rapidly in the early neonatal period. Little testosterone is produced during childhood until the onset of puberty. Testosterone secretion after puberty causes the penis, scrotum, and testes to enlarge until the completion of pubertal development at approximately 20 years of age. At the onset of puberty testosterone stimulates the growth of hair in a male pattern, hypertrophy of the laryngeal mucosa, enlargement of the larynx, increased skin thickness, initial increased secretion of sebaceous glands, increased muscle development, and nitrogen retention.[18,43]

The number and amplitude of hypothalamic GnRH pulses increase as boys advance through puberty. Pituitary LH stimulates the Leydig's cells to secrete testosterone, which works as the negative feedback to inhibit LH secretion. FSH has little effect in boys until the onset of maturation of spermatozoa when Sertoli's cells are stimulated. Later in puberty the levels of LH and FSH remain constant throughout the day, as does the level of testosterone.[18]

System Physiology

Hormones are synthesized by glands from chemical substances or raw materials found in the blood. Some glands produce more hormone than the body needs and have the ability to store the excess hormone in the gland itself. Secretion of hormones into the bloodstream occurs in response to a chemical or nervous stimuli. Hormonally responsive cells exist in a complex and continually changing environment of fuels and ions, and the changes that occur in them are the result of both the nonhormonal and hormonal matrix in which they are bathed.[43] The following sections describe how the endocrine system interacts with its surrounding environment, the body.

Response of Target Cells

Hormones are chemical messengers recognized by discriminators on or in sensitive cells and, by elaborate

means, transduced into a response. Often the response generated by the hormone involves acceleration of some biochemical processes and concurrent inhibition of others.[43] A target cell is any cell in which the hormone binds to its receptor. The response of a target cell is determined by the differentiated state of the cell. A cell can exhibit several responses to a single hormone.

The hormone receptors have two functions: (1) a recognition domain that binds the hormone, and (2) a domain that signals the recognition of the hormone into an intracellular function.[17] Hormone action seems to be dependent on the presence within the target cell of a chemical reaction. The rate of this reaction can be influenced by the hormone. As a target cell uses a hormone its chemical structure is altered, thereby making it inactive. Target cells have receptors inside the cell or on their surface that can bind the hormone and trigger a response in the cell (Fig. 54-3). Hormones do not act on cells without specific receptors for that hormone. Because of the repetitive production, use, and inactivation of hormones, they must be continually secreted by the glands. They cannot be reused or recirculated in the body.[19]

Hormone Transport

When hormones are released into the circulatory system by the endocrine glands, they are distributed throughout the body. There are two main groups of hor-

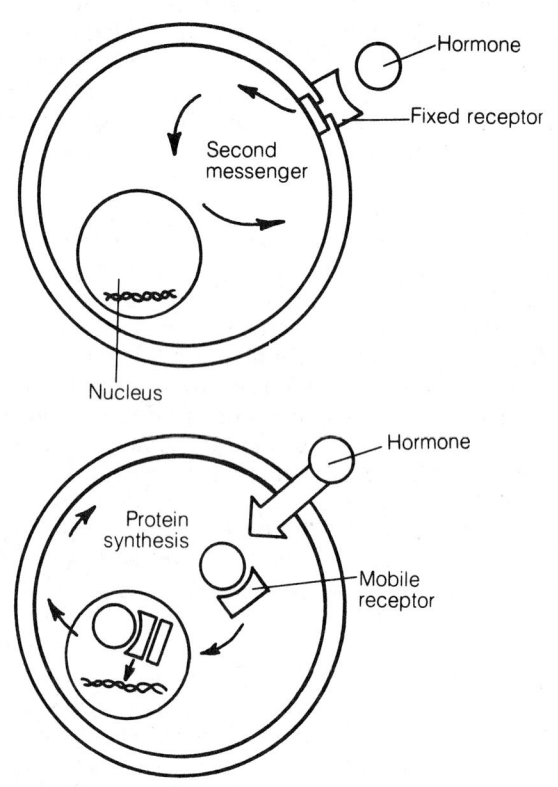

FIGURE 54-3
The two types of hormone-receptor interactions: the fixed membrane receptor, (**top**), and the intracellular mobile receptor, (**bottom**). (Source: Porth, C. M. [1990] *Pathophysiology: Concepts of altered health states* [3rd ed.]. Philadelphia, J. B. Lippincott.)

mones: peptide hormones, sometimes known as water-soluble hormones, and steroid and thyroid hormones, also known as lipid-soluble hormones.[6]

Generally the steroid and thyroid hormones are lipid soluble and circulate bound to carrier proteins. The amount of bound hormone usually is determined by the amount of available binding proteins.[17] Examples of known binding proteins include corticosteroid-binding globulin and thyroid-binding globulin. There is evidence that specific plasma membrane receptors exist and that they serve a transport function for their respective hormones. After secretion steroid and thyroid hormones associate with carrier proteins. These hormones then cross the plasma membrane and encounter receptors either in the cytosol or the nucleus of the target cell.[43]

Receptors for most peptide hormones are located in the plasma membranes of cells. These hormones are called first messengers. The peptide hormones include pituitary hormones, hypothalamic hormones, parathyroid hormones, and insulin. Peptide hormones interact with outwardly facing plasma membrane-limiting receptors, and they do not have to be internalized to elicit their effects. Hormone receptor interaction results in a highly coordinated biologic response that may involve many individual cellular components, some of them at a distance from the plasma membrane.[17,19]

Hormones classified as peptides regulate intracellular metabolic processes through intermediary molecules called *second messengers*. They are called second messengers because the hormone itself is the first messenger.[17,43] The second messenger increases intracellular cyclic AMP (cAMP), which mediates the metabolic effects of the hormones. The receptors for the peptide hormones act first to recognize the hormone on the plasma membrane and then bind with the hormone. Once recognition and binding have occurred, the hormone-receptor complex initiates the transmission of an intracellular signal by way of a second messenger.[17] Some hormones use cAMP, and others use calcium or phosphatidylinositol metabolites as their intracellular signal. cAMP is the intracellular signal for hormones such as ACTH, ADH, CRH, somatostatin, calcitonin, LH, FSH, PTH, and glucagon. It is possible that other mediators are involved in this process.[43]

The receptors on the plasma membranes are continuously synthesized and degraded so that changes in receptor concentration may occur within hours. Both receptor affinity and concentration are regulated by intracellular and extracellular mechanisms that include physiochemical environment (*p*H, temperature, sodium, and calcium levels), urea concentration (levels of cAMP), lipid matrix of the plasma membrane (cholesterol concentration), hormone levels, stage of growth and development, diet, exercise, and drugs.[17,43]

Rhythm of Hormonal Secretions

Rhythmicity is a basic property of biologic processes. It appears that many of the hormones secreted by endocrine glands demonstrate a circadian rhythm, that is a rhythm that has a cycle length of approximately 24 hours. GH and ACTH have diurnal variations linked with the

sleep–wake cycle.[30] Other hormones like LH and FSH are secreted in complex patterns that are set by internal clocks that function over many time scales: the lifetime of the individual from the embryonic period onward through childhood, puberty, maturation and reproduction, and senescence.

The pineal gland is an endocrine organ derived from the neuroectoderm of the embryo from an outgrowth of the diencephalon. In the adult it is located near the posterodorsal aspect of the diencephalon. One hormone secreted by the pineal is called melatonin, which appears to be closely linked to the light-dark environment. The nocturnal secretion of melatonin does not appear to be related to sleep stage. Additionally, melatonin secretion is highest early in life and decreases dramatically near the time of the hormonal activation of puberty through adulthood. The consequences of altered melatonin levels are unknown.[35] It is possible that the pineal and its hormones have a major role in the rhythmicity of endocrine hormones.

Feedback Control

There are different methods by which the rate and quantity of hormone secretion are controlled. Regulation of hormone secretion is achieved by the use of feedback systems that provide precise monitoring and control of the cellular environment (see Fig. 54-3).

One mechanism for the regulation of hormone levels is negative feedback. Every gland has a tendency to oversecrete the hormone it produces. Once the desired physiologic effect is achieved, information is sent back to the producing gland to halt further secretion. Likewise, as the gland undersecretes and the physiologic effect of the hormone lessens, feedback to the producing gland causes it to increase hormone production. Negative feedback is seen in the relationships among the hypothalamus, the anterior pituitary gland, and the peripheral endocrine glands controlled by the pituitary hormones.[10,17] The hypothalamus secretes hormones that stimulate or inhibit the release of specific anterior pituitary hormones, which then stimulate a peripheral gland to secrete hormone and, with sufficient stimulation, to grow. This feedback system allows for the secretion of hormones in response to the body's need for them.[10]

Another feedback mechanism is positive feedback, which occurs when hormone secretion continues to trigger additional hormone secretion. This mechanism is uncommon within the endocrine system.[17] Feedback mechanisms also can be described in terms of short, ultrashort, and long feedback loops. These terms are used to describe regulation of the hormone secretion by the hormones themselves.[17]

Summary

The endocrine system serves as a communication network that coordinates the responses necessary to maintain homeostasis and preserve the survival of the organism. Endocrine hormones affect target cells with appropriate receptors that are able to initiate specific cell functions or activities. The receptors for hormones reside on the plasma membrane or in the intracellular compartment of a target cell. Water-soluble (peptide) hormones circulate throughout the body in an unbound form. Lipid-soluble (steroid) hormones bound to carrier proteins circulate throughout the body. All hormones are produced in the amounts required to maintain homeostasis. They are shed from the body by processes of metabolic inactivation or excretion. Therefore, a constant basal production of hormones is maintained. The endocrine glands release their hormones under the influence of other glandular-based releasing factors, neural influences, or both. Most hormone levels are regulated by negative feedback mechanisms.

Hormones are not secreted at uniform rates. Some hormones are regulated by intrinsic controls, for example the adrenal steroid hormones that are released in a diurnal (daily) pattern or gonadotropin and female sex hormones that maintain a cyclic rhythm. Extrinsic factors of hormone regulation include external stimuli, such as stress, pain, and injury, which can override the existing normal feedback mechanisms. Understanding the origins of the endocrine system, its structure and function, and its importance in regulating metabolic processes is vital to the nurse's ability to assess a child who has an endocrine disorder.

References

1. Aurbach, G. D., Marx, S. J., & Spiegel, A. M. (1985). Parathyroid hormone, calcitonin, and the calciferols. In J. D. Wilson & D. W. Foster (Eds.). *Williams textbook of endocrinology* (7th ed.) (pp. 1137–1217). Philadelphia: W.B. Saunders.

2. Bercu, B. B. (1990). Disorder of growth hormone neurosecretion. In F. Lifshitz (Ed.). *Pediatric endocrinology* (2nd ed.) (pp. 43–60). New York: Marcel Dekker.

3. Bode, H. H. (1990). Disorders of the posterior pituitary. In S. A. Kaplan (Ed.). *Clinical pediatric endocrinology*. (pp. 63–86). Philadelphia: W.B. Saunders.

4. Bondy, P. K. (1985). Disorders of the adrenal cortex. In J. D. Wilson & D. W. Foster (Eds.). *Williams textbook of endocrinology* (7th ed.) (pp. 822–839). Philadelphia: W.B. Saunders.

5. Bonner-Weir, S. (1990). Morphology of endocrine pancreas. In K. L. Becker (Ed.). *Principles and practice of endocrinology and metabolism* (pp. 1064–1068). Philadelphia: J.B. Lippincott.

6. Bremner, W. J. (1990). Pituitary gonadotropins and their disorders. In K. L. Becker (Ed.). *Principles and practice of endocrinology and metabolism* (pp. 152–156). Philadelphia: J.B. Lippincott.

7. Bronson, R. A. (1990). Poly-cystic ovaries. In F. Lifshitz (Ed.). *Pediatric endocrinology* (2nd ed.) (pp. 294–306). New York: Marcel Dekker.

8. Cooper, P. E., & Martin, J. B. (1990). Physiology and pathophysiology of the endocrine brain and hypothalamus. In K. L. Becker (Ed.). *Principles and practice of endocrinology and metabolism* (pp. 98–104). Philadelphia: J.B. Lippincott.

9. Culpepper, R. M., Herbert, S. C., & Andreoli, T. E. (1985). The posterior pituitary and water metabolism. In J. D. Wilson & D. W. Foster (Eds.). *Williams textbook of endocrinology* (7th ed.) (pp. 614–652). Philadelphia: W.B. Saunders.

10. Darlington, D. N., & Dallman, M. F. (1990). Feedback control in endocrine systems. In K. L. Becker (Ed.). *Principles and practice of endocrinology and metabolism* (pp. 38–45). Philadelphia: J.B. Lippincott.

11. Daughaday, W. H. (1985). The anterior pituitary. In J. D. Wilson & D. W. Foster (Eds.). *Williams Textbook of Endocrinology* (7th ed.) (pp. 492–567). Philadelphia: W.B. Saunders.

12. Downs, R. W. Jr. (1990). Hypoparathyroidism and other causes of Hypocalcemia. In K. L. Becker (Ed.). *Principles and practice of endocrinology and metabolism* (pp. 447–457). Philadelphia: J.B. Lippincott.

13. Drash, A. L. (1990). Management of the child with diabetes mellitus: Clinical course, therapeutic strategies and monitoring techniques. In F. Lifshitz (Ed.). *Pediatric endocrinology* (2nd ed.) (pp. 681–700). New York: Marcel Dekker.

14. Erickson, G. F., & Schreiber, J. R. (1990). Morphology and physiology of the ovary. In K. L. Becker (Ed.). *Principles and practice of endocrinology and metabolism* (pp. 776–788). Philadelphia: J.B. Lippincott.

15. Fort, P. (1990). Thyroid disorders in infancy. In F. Lifshitz (Ed.). *Pediatric endocrinology* (2nd ed.) (pp. 437–456). New York: Marcel Dekker.

16. Granner, D. K. (1990). Hormonal action: In K. L. Becker (Ed.). *Principles and practice of endocrinology and metabolism* (pp. 25–38). Philadelphia: J.B. Lippincott.

17. Gray, D. P. (1990). Mechanisms of hormonal regulation. In K. L. McCance & S. E. Huether (Eds.). *Pathophysiology: The biologic basis for disease in adults and children* (pp. 564–593). St. Louis: C.V. Mosby.

18. Griffin, J. E., & Wilson, J. D. (1985). Disorders of the testes and male reproductive tract. In J. D. Wilson & D. W. Foster (Eds.). *Williams textbook of endocrinology* (7th ed.) (pp. 259–311). Philadelphia: W.B. Saunders.

19. Guyton, A. C. (1992). *Human physiology and mechanisms of disease* (3rd ed.). Philadelphia: W.B. Saunders.

20. Ingbar, S. H. (1985). The thyroid gland. In J. D. Wilson & D. W. Foster (Eds.). *Williams textbook of endocrinology* (7th ed.) (pp. 682–815). Philadelphia: W.B. Saunders.

21. Kaplan, S. A. (1990). Growth and growth hormone: Disorders at anterior pituitary. In S. A. Kaplan (Ed.). *Clinical pediatric endocrinology* (pp. 1–62). Philadelphia: W.B. Saunders.

22. Kovacs, K., & Horvath, E. (1990). Morphology of the pituitary in health and disease. In K. L. Becker (Ed.). *Principles and practice of endocrinology and metabolism* (pp. 109–124). Philadelphia: J.B. Lippincott.

23. Landsberg, L., & Young, J. B. (1985). Catecholamines and the adrenal medulla. In J. D. Wilson & D. W. Foster (Eds.). *Williams textbook of endocrinology* (7th ed.) (pp. 891–966). Philadelphia: W.B. Saunders.

24. Lanes, R. (1990). Ambiguous genitalia, micropenis, and cryptorchidism. In F. Lifshitz (Ed.). *Pediatric endocrinology* (2nd ed.) (pp. 353–376). New York: Marcel Dekker.

25. Lee, P. (1990). Physiology of puberty. In F. Lifshitz (Ed.). *Pediatric endocrinology* (2nd ed.) (pp. 217–248). New York: Marcel Dekker.

26. LiVolsi, V. A. (1990). Morphology of the thyroid gland. In K. L. Becker (Ed.). *Principles and practice of endocrinology and metabolism* (pp. 267–271). Philadelphia: J.B. Lippincott.

27. MacGillivray, M. H., & MacGillivray, B. (1990). Hypogonadism and chromosome disorders. In F. Lifshitz (Ed.). *Pediatric endocrinology* (2nd ed.) (pp. 377–412). New York: Marcel Dekker.

28. Mimouni, F., & Tsang, R. C. (1990). Parathyroid and vitamin D-related disorders. In S. A. Kaplan (Ed.). *Clinical pediatric endocrinology* (pp. 427–453). Philadelphia: W.B. Saunders.

29. New, M. I., Del Balzo, P., Crawford, C., & Speiser, P. W. (1990). The adrenal cortex. In S. A. Kaplan (Ed.). *Clinical pediatric endocrinology* (pp. 181–234). Philadelphia: W.B. Saunders.

30. Pang, S., & Riddick, L. (1990). Hirsuitism. In F. Lifshitz (Ed.). *Pediatric endocrinology* (2nd ed.) (pp. 259–292). New York: Marcel Dekker.

31. Pescovitz, O. H., Cutler, G. B. Jr, & Loriaux, D. L. (1990). Synthesis and secretion of corticosteroids. In K. L. Becker (Ed.). *Principles and practice of endocrinology and metabolism* (pp. 579–591). Philadelphia: J.B. Lippincott.

32. Pugliese, M. T. (1990). Neuroendocrine disorders. In F. Lifshitz (Ed.). *Pediatric endocrinology* (2nd ed.) (pp. 877–892). New York: Marcel Dekker.

33. Raiti, S. (1990). Diabetes insipidus. In F. Lifshitz (Ed.). *Pediatric endocrinology* (2nd ed.) (pp. 863–876). New York: Marcel Dekker.

34. Rebar, R. W., Kenigsberg, D., & Hodgen, G. D. (1990). The normal menstrual cycle and the control of ovulation. In K. L. Becker (Ed.). *Principles and practice of endocrinology and metabolism* (pp. 788–798). Philadelphia: J.B. Lippincott.

35. Reiter, R. J. (1990). The pineal gland. In K. L. Becker (Ed.). *Principles and practice of endocrinology and metabolism* (pp. 104–109). Philadelphia: J.B. Lippincott.

36. Rittmaster, R. S., & Cutler, G. B. Jr. (1990). Morphology of the adrenal cortex and medulla. In K. L. Becker (Ed.). *Principles and practice of endocrinology and metabolism* (pp. 572–578). Philadelphia: J.B. Lippincott.

37. Robertson, G. L. (1990). Physiology of vasopressin, oxytocin, and thirst. In K. L. Becker (Ed.). *Principles and practice of endocrinology and metabolism* (pp. 222–230). Philadelphia: J.B. Lippincott.

38. Rogol, A. D. (1990). Hypothalamic and pituitary disorders in infancy and childhood. In K. L. Becker (Ed.). *Principles and Practice of Endocrinology and Metabolism* (pp. 171–183). Philadelphia: J.B. Lippincott.

39. Rosenfield, R. L. (1990). The ovary and female sexual maturation. In S. A. Kaplan (Ed.). *Clinical pediatric endocrinology* (pp. 259–324). Philadelphia: W.B. Saunders.

40. Sadler, T. W. (1985). *Langman's medical embryology*. Baltimore: Williams & Wilkins.

41. Simpson, J. L., & Rebar, R. W. (1990). Normal and abnormal sexual differentiation and development. In K. L. Becker (Ed.). *Principles and practice of endocrinology and metabolism* (pp. 714–740). Philadelphia: J.B. Lippincott.

42. Styne, D. M. (1990). The testes: Disorders of sexual differentiation and puberty. In S. A. Kaplan (Ed.). *Clinical pediatric endocrinology* (pp. 367–426). Philadelphia: W.B. Saunders.

43. Tepperman, J., & Tepperman, H. M. (1987). *Metabolic and endocrine physiology* (5th ed.). Chicago: Year Book Medical Publishers.

44. Voorhees, M. L. (1990). Disorders of the adrenal medulla and multiple endocrine adenomatosis syndrome. In S. A. Kaplan (Ed.). *Clinical pediatric endocrinology* (pp. 235–258). Philadelphia: W.B. Saunders.

Nursing Assessment and Diagnosis of Endocrine Function

BEHAVIORAL OBJECTIVES

Use functional health as a guideline
for assessment of the child's
endocrine function.

Describe the components
of a complete physical examination
for a child's endocrine function.

Explain nursing responsibilities
in preparing children and families
for diagnostic tests associated
with endocrine disorders.

Identify nursing diagnoses that are
commonly used in the care of
children with endocrine dysfunction.

Many endocrine disorders are insidious and do not become clinically apparent for a long time. Using the benefit of hindsight, it is not unusual to determine that a child has had an endocrine condition for years, often dating back to the newborn period. Using the framework of functional health to obtain the clinical history, the nurse can elicit important information that frequently is overlooked or deemed unimportant to the child's family because of its prolonged evolution.

Endocrine conditions often require significant adjustment on the part of the child and the family, and a comprehensive database helps the nurse and other members of the health care team to provide effective, holistic care. This chapter provides general guidelines for the nurse to follow in eliciting pertinent history, performing the physical examination, and understanding the laboratory evaluation in the clinical assessment of a child with an endocrine disorder. Nursing diagnoses commonly used with children who have endocrine disorders also are identified.

Nursing Assessment

Child and Family History

Useful data include past growth measurements (obtainable from the family doctor, the "baby book," or school records), heights and weights of family members, and medical information concerning the health of close relatives. Time may be needed for distant family members to be contacted for pertinent information.

1447

Health Perception and Health Management

The family's perception of the child's health significantly colors the conduct of the nursing assessment and must be ascertained early in the history-taking process. Appraisal of health perceptions includes those held by the historian(s), most commonly the parents, and the child. The nurse must establish a setting in which the family and child can talk openly. Feelings associated with endocrine conditions that present precipitously may be very different from those associated with endocrine problems that emerge over a long period of time. Parents may feel guilty when their child is being evaluated for a chronic illness. These feelings may arise from a perception that medical care was not sought soon enough or from a sense of responsibility for the child's condition. Denial on the part of one or both parents, the child, or other significant family members or friends is an important perception and may feed into feelings of guilt. A knowledge of these issues will enable the nurse to collect data in an effective, nonthreatening way.[1,8]

To assess the family's understanding of the child's health status, the nurse notes the chief concern. The child and parents express in a few words the reason the child is having the evaluation. The nurse also should ask about the decision-making process that led the family to seek medical care. Who is concerned? The endocrine evaluation may have been scheduled at the urging of the child, the child's physician, relatives, or parents. The family may not recognize the need for medical evaluation.[8]

The child's perception of the illness may range from a sense of feeling "different" from peers, to a surprisingly accurate understanding of the problem. It is important to recognize misconceptions about the condition early in the history-taking process. Teasing, difficulty with socialization, changing academic or physical performance, and other variables affect the child's understanding of the problem.

Children's perception of their health problems varies depending on their stage of psychosocial development. Young children are concerned about separation or loss, while older children tend to worry more about body integrity and socialization issues. Unless specifically asked, children are unlikely to volunteer this sensitive information. Familiarity with the principles of child development (see Chap. 8) enables the nurse to ask the right questions depending on the specific clinical situation.

The child's perception of the impact of the endocrine condition on his or her lifestyle needs to be assessed to plan appropriate teaching. Much of this assessment occurs after the condition is diagnosed and treatment is proposed, but valuable information and insight into how the child might manage a health problem can be obtained as part of the initial history. To learn about the child's understanding of the presenting problem, the nurse can ask if anyone else with the same problem is known. The child's knowledge of the impact of the endocrine condition on that person's daily activities influences personal application of the information.

While children's health concerns tend to revolve more around socialization issues and short-term consequences, parents typically are more concerned about morbidity and long-term consequences. The parents' understanding of the illness and their fears surrounding it have an effect on the initial gathering of information. Taking the parents aside and offering them an opportunity to express concerns privately and to ask questions will eventually benefit the child.

As with the child, it is important to assess the parents' background regarding the chief complaint. The mother of a newly diagnosed diabetic child whose sister died prematurely from complications of diabetes, for example, will have a different perception of her child's illness than a mother who has not been touched by this disease. Many families are ill-served by misinformation disseminated by the media and shared by well-meaning relatives and acquaintances. Endocrinology is such a rapidly evolving field of medicine that is not uncommon for patients to receive erroneous and outdated information, even from the physician who makes the referral.

Assessment of the family's previous experience with health management is important. The nurse should ask about the child's previous routine care, whether any medications (including vitamins) are taken, and the degree of compliance with previously prescribed treatment regimens. It is useful to know the family's response to the health problems of other family members because they are likely to respond similarly to the present situation. This information will be useful as future treatment plans are formulated.

The nurse should assess the patient's socioeconomic status, at least in a cursory manner. Financial pressures may influence initial fact gathering and future plans. The diagnosis and treatment of endocrine conditions can be very expensive. The nurse may be aware of avenues of financial aid and can share this general information at the time of the interview. This assistance may alleviate major concerns and set the stage for more effective fact gathering.

Nutrition and Metabolism

To enjoy normal growth and development, children need an adequate diet, normal assimilation of ingested calories, and normal metabolism.[3] Endocrine disease can affect any of these processes. Adequacy of diet is assessed with specific questions concerning the timing and content of typical meals and snacks, food preferences, and aversions. Recent changes in appetite or eating habits are noted. Assimilation is assessed with questions regarding digestion (vomiting, bloating, food intolerance) and elimination. The nurse asks about a history of constipation, diarrhea, or abnormal stool patterns. Cellular metabolism is difficult to assess historically but may be suggested by a change in weight, either recently or by long-term patterns.

Graphic representation of a child's growth data is a cornerstone of the nursing assessment of a child with an endocrine disorder.[6,9] Plotting measurements on a growth chart defines the child's growth pattern and reveals deviations from a previously established pattern. To optimize the value of the growth chart, the nurse gathers as many past measurements as possible. The parents' records (e.g., baby book), pediatrician, school nurse, and physical education teacher are potential sources of height and weight measurements.

Significant disease of any organ system can affect a child's growth pattern.[6,8,9] Most endocrine conditions that compromise growth are associated with growth failure. However, some cause accelerated growth. The relationship between height and weight also is revealing and may provide diagnostic clues.

Elimination

The history of elimination patterns includes a description by the child or parent of established patterns and noted changes. The timing of deviations from established patterns is important. If the child has experienced a change in elimination pattern, the nurse determines when the change occurred and whether it occurred suddenly or gradually. Some abnormal elimination patterns may have existed from birth. Many years of an unusual elimination pattern, such as one stool per week or chronically liquid stools, may seem normal to the child and family. The nurse should ask specific questions regarding characteristics of the stool (frequency, color, consistency, smell, floating, blood, mucus, pain, straining) and urine (frequency, concentration, blood, color, pain, straining).

Activity and Exercise

Assessment of physical activity as related to the child's age includes questions regarding types of exercise, frequency, and stamina during participation in activities. Any changes, especially in the child's strength or stamina, should lead the nurse to ask additional questions about the nature, timing, and character of the changes. Many endocrine disorders have an insidious onset. Subtle changes in a child's activity level may suggest a diagnosis.

Sleep and Rest

Because a wide variation in normal sleeping patterns exists among children, the nurse needs to ascertain the child's particular pattern. The child's normal bed time, ease of falling asleep, and usual length of uninterrupted sleep are noted. Incidence of insomnia, frequency and length of naps, inappropriate sleep patterns, or difficulties arising in the morning are assessed and recorded.

The nurse inquires about the restfulness of the child's sleep. Children with a thyroid disorder, for example, may not sleep soundly and may toss all over the bed, leaving their bedding in disarray the following morning. Questions about snoring, bed wetting, nightmares, and sleepwalking are important. The nurse should ask about the sleeping patterns of other members of the household. It may be learned, for example, that an older brother's rock band practices at the house between 8:00 PM and midnight on weekdays, explaining the patient's lack of adequate sleep!

Cognition and Perception

The nurse asks about the child's motor, personal and social, and language milestones. School performance should be assessed, determining whether there have been recent changes in performance. Some endocrine disorders are manifest in behaviors such as sluggishness, lethargy, and disinterest; others cause increased aggressiveness or difficulty in concentration.

Hearing and vision should be explored historically, with questions pertaining to hearing acuity, tinnitus, and balance. Vision is assessed by asking questions relevant to visual acuity ("Can you see the blackboard from the back of the room?"), and to peripheral vision ("Can you see out of the corner of your eye?"). Sensory deficits sometimes are associated with endocrine disorders.

Self-Perception and Self-Concept

Because most endocrine diseases are chronic, they can be expected to have a significant impact on a child's feeling of self-worth. Assessment of the child's self-perception is helpful when it is time to tailor future intervention strategies. Exploration of these psychosocial areas also may have diagnostic significance. Some endocrine problems, such as thyroid disease, may be manifested as a personality change and reflected in altered self-esteem.

The child's self-esteem is assessed by determining how the child "fits" in a variety of social settings. The number of friends at school, participation in extracurricular activities, and general preferences reveal much about a child's feelings of self-worth and self-acceptance. School performance and any change in a previous pattern should be explored with the child and parents.

Children presenting for an endocrine evaluation may be motivated by a concern with body image. The child who is shorter or heavier than the rest of the peer group may have low self-esteem. The child's verbalization of concerns and feelings illuminates issues to be addressed in the nursing care plan.

Role Relationship

Socialization issues may have diagnostic significance and need to be considered when formulating the care plan. In the evaluation of the child with an endocrine problem, attention is directed to areas that can be affected when a child is significantly different from the peer group or other members of the family. Areas to which attention should be directed include relative stature, timing of puberty, and age appropriateness of attitudes and activities.

The nurse determines who lives with the child and the child's relationships with the rest of the family. Questions should include the child's sibling order, noting inappropriate rivalry. The marital status of the parents (e.g., step-parents, stepsiblings) is recorded.

To adequately assess the child's adaptation in the family, the nurse may need to interview the child and parents separately. Some questions concerning marital discord are better asked apart from the child. The child's role relationships outside the family also are explored. Children with short stature often are relegated to a subordinate role in peer relationships. To evaluate peer relationships, the nurse asks about the child's friends. A good way to do this is by asking the best friend's name. Adolescents should be asked about interest in the opposite sex and dating relationships.

Sexuality and Reproduction

Many endocrine conditions affect sexual development. In some conditions sexual development is accelerated, while in others it is retarded. The nurse should assess gently whether the patient feels "normal," keeping in mind that most adolescents have limited knowledge about normal pubertal development. The timing of physical milestones and the cadence of sexual development are explored (see Tables 66-3 and 66-4 and Figs. 66-6 through 66-9). Children with delayed puberty may experience a long time between sexual milestones, while children with early puberty usually pass through them quickly (see Chap. 66).[4,5,10] Questions regarding the timing of milestones in the parents and siblings are important because these characteristically are similar within families. Information about the pubertal development of parents and siblings may be useful in establishing a diagnosis and assessing the impact of a pubertal disorder on the child and family.[1]

Menstruation is affected by a number of endocrine conditions.[7] The timing of the first menstrual period (menarche) should be recorded, along with the frequency and character (duration, amount of bleeding, presence or absence of cramping) of the menstrual periods. The date of the last normal menstrual period is noted.

Coping and Stress Tolerance

The ability of the child and family to adapt to stress has a significant impact on the child's long-term prognosis.[1] Key areas of concern are the acceptance of a chronic illness and the ability to adapt current lifestyles to necessary treatments. Some endocrine disorders require the family to be prepared for episodes of acute instability. By gathering information about experiences that required coping skills, the nurse can design the care plan to prepare the family for the future. The nurse asks about instances of successful coping as well as failures. Stress tolerance (physical response) may be impaired in some endocrine conditions.

Values and Beliefs

The perceived impact of the diagnosis on the family's and child's goals affects their acceptance and compliance with treatment. Questions should address religious and cultural beliefs, noting areas of concern. Consequences of certain endocrine conditions may have a more significant impact on some families than others. For example, the prospect of infertility is likely to be troubling to families whose religion or culture emphasizes childbearing. Understanding the family's values and beliefs concerning sexual topics is very important when gathering information or helping shape treatment plans for endocrine conditions that affect genitalia or sexual function. Religious restrictions should be known. For example, patients who practice religious avoidance of pork should not be prescribed pork-derived insulin.

Physical Examination

The physical examination focuses on detecting aberrations seen in children with endocrine disorders. Spe-

TABLE 55-1
Developmental Considerations in the Physical Examination of Endocrine Function

System	Infant	Child	Adolescent
Head and neck	Patency and size of fontanel; symmetry of head, eyes, and ears Dentition appropriate for age Absence of cleft lip/palate Absence of goiter	Symmetry of head, eyes, ears Dentition appropriate for age Absence of goiter	Symmetry of head, eyes, and ears Dentition appropriate for age Absence of goiter
Chest	Symmetry, absence of breast development Normally spaced nipples	Breast development (Tanner stage)	Breast development (Tanner stage) Gynecomastia in boys
Abdomen	Absence of umbilical hernia, symmetry	Fat distribution	Fat distribution
Genitourinary	Absence of genital ambiguity, absence of hair, absence of odor and/or discharge	Absence of hair or pubertal changes Testicular descent in boys Sexual development (Tanner stage) Absence of odor or discharge	Sexual development appropriate for age (Tanner stage) Absence of odor or discharge
Musculoskeletal	Absence of disproportionality, muscle tone (hypotonic versus normal versus spastic)	Absence of disproportionality Absence of short metacarpals Absence of muscle weakness	Absence of disproportionality Absence of short metacarpals Absence of muscle weakness
Neurologic	Absence of hypotonia Absence of tremor	Absence of tremor Absence of hyporeflexia or hyperreflexia Absence of gait disturbance Normal stance	Absence of tremor Absence of hyporeflexia or hyperreflexia Absence of gait disturbance Normal stance
Integument	Absence of abnormal texture or coloring (hyperpigmentation or vitiligo) Absence of excessive nevi	Absence of abnormal texture or coloring (hyperpigmentation or vitiligo) Absence of excessive nevi	Absence of abnormal texture or coloring (hyperpigmentation or vitiligo) Absence of excessive nevi

cific areas to which the nurse should direct attention are outlined below. A summary of developmental considerations is presented in Table 55-1.

Measurements

Physical measurements and evaluation of growth are critically important in the assessment of the child with a suspected endocrine condition.[2,6] Calculated growth based on previous measurements must be interpreted cautiously if the accuracy of the data cannot be ascertained. This caution is particularly true if the time span between measurements is less than 1 year. Because growth rates normally are expressed as growth per 12 months, errors in measurement taken over shorter time intervals may be exaggerated and an inaccurate indicator of growth. Conversely, measurements taken over a long period of time are valuable because the significance of the error is minimized.

The accuracy of the nurse's measurements can be assured if the equipment is properly calibrated and the child is measured using a standardized technique (see the accompanying display on guidelines for accurate height measurements). Height, weight, heart rate, and blood pressure should be measured for every child. Head circumference is measured on all children younger than 36 months. Depending on the circumstance, other physical parameters, such as arm span, upper to lower segment ratios, and sitting heights, are measured.[2]

Growth Patterns

Height, weight, and head circumference are plotted on standard, sex-specific growth charts. Growth charts produced by the National Center for Health Statistics commonly are used. There are two sets of standard charts: birth to 36 months and 2 to 18 years, each for boys and girls. These are presented in the appendix. It is important to measure children correctly when using the standard growth charts. The examiner should note that the infant growth charts for boys and girls are graphic records of supine length, weight, and head circumference. The charts for older children track standing heights and weights. Growth data for children between the ages of 2 and 3 years may be plotted on either of the charts. Length is plotted on the infant chart (birth to 36 months), and height is plotted on the older children's charts (2 to 18 years).

The growth charts define normal growth patterns. After the third year, height measurements typically follow the standard percentile curves. Deviations from the norm (crossing percentiles) are readily apparent.

Head and Neck

Because some endocrine conditions are associated with facial anomalies, the head and neck are inspected for obvious dysmorphology, such as cleft lip or palate, asymmetry, or other unusual appearance.[2] The eyes should be inspected carefully. The nurse notes the child's

---

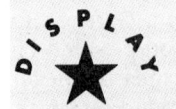

Nursing Assessment: Guidelines for Accurate Height Measurements in Infants, Children, and Adolescents

LENGTH MEASUREMENT: INFANT OR CHILD YOUNGER THAN 3 YEARS OF AGE

- Infants are measured in the supine position on a horizontal stadiometer or a flat firm surface with a head stop and foot board.
- *Supine* measurements are plotted on the infant (birth to 36 months) sex-specific NCHS growth chart.
- *Standing* measurements are plotted on the older child (2 to 18 years) sex-specific NCHS growth chart.

PROCEDURE FOR SUPINE MEASUREMENT

1. Lay the child in the supine position, with head gently held against a stationary right angle.
2. Hold the knees straight and the feet flexed to 90 degrees.
3. Gently press a rigid right angle against the baby's feet.
4. Record the measurement to the nearest 3 mm (⅛ in).

HEIGHT MEASUREMENT: CHILD AND ADOLESCENT

- *Standing heights* are obtained for children older than 3 years using a stadiometer or a rigid wall-mounted measuring tape with a rigid right angle. (The sliding arm device on physicians' scales is considered inaccurate.)

PROCEDURE FOR STANDING MEASUREMENT

1. Position the child with feet together; heels, buttocks, shoulders, and back of head are all touching the wall. Ensure that the knees are not bent.
2. Gently support the child's mastoid processes, center the child's head, and ensure that the child's line of sight is parallel to the floor.
3. Lower a rigid right angle down the stadiometer or measuring tape until it gently touches the child's head.
4. Record the measurement to the nearest 3 mm (⅛ in).

position of gaze (conjugate or not), pupil symmetry, and any obvious abnormalities. Visual acuity can be assessed grossly. The mouth is inspected for deviations from normal (high arched or cleft palate). The dentition is inspected, noting either early or retarded dental development. A single upper central incisor is sometimes seen with growth hormone deficiency. Multiple caries or abnormal enamel may indicate a calcium or phosphorus problem. The neck is inspected and palpated for the presence of thyroid enlargement or masses.

Chest

The chest is inspected for symmetry, deformities (shield chest, pectus carinatum, pectus excavatum), and breast development. The presence or absence of hypertrophied costochondral junctions ("rachitic rosary") is noted. Breast development in boys and girls is noted and assigned a Tanner stage (see Tables 66-3 and 66-4). A large percentage of boys in midpuberty will normally have a small degree of gynecomastia (breast development), which usually spontaneously regresses.[9]

Abdomen

The abdomen is inspected, and fat distribution is noted. Children with adrenal disorders may have "central obesity" with thin arms and legs, and others with growth hormone deficiency may have persistence of ripply "baby fat." The abdomen is palpated for the presence of organomegaly or masses.[2,9]

Pelvic Region

Some endocrine disorders manifest themselves by changes in the genitalia, which are inspected. Any abnormalities in anatomy or development for age are noted. Girls are inspected for enlarged clitoris, labial fusion, and vaginal estrogen effect. The presence of estrinized vaginal mucosa (pink) in a young girl is evidence of early puberty. Vaginal discharge or odor and the presence of masses in the inguinal canals are considered abnormal. Boys are inspected for phallic size, position of the urethral opening, testicular descent and size, scrotal development, and other abnormalities. The amount and distribution of pubic hair is noted and recorded by assigning a Tanner stage for both sexes[2,6,9] (see Tables 66-3 and 66-4 and Figs. 66-7 and 66-9).

Musculoskeletal System

Some endocrine conditions, for example hypothyroidism, are associated with disproportional growth, while others affect growth but not proportions (e.g., growth hormone deficiency). The nurse notes unusual body habitus or disproportionality. Unusually long or short extremities are noted. Arm span and sitting heights are measured if abnormal proportions are suspected. The hands and feet are inspected for unusual features (short metacarpals, bowlegs (genu varum), or knock-knees (genu valgum). Gait is observed and abnormalities noted. The muscles are palpated and gross strength, symmetry, and consistency are noted.[2,9]

Neurologic Signs

The nurse notes the presence or absence of a tremor, which may signal thyroid disease, and assesses the child's gait, stance, and deep tendon reflexes. Absence of the sense of smell is associated with isolated gonadotropin (luteinizing hormone [LH] and follicle-stimulating hormone [FSH]) deficiency causing pubertal delay. Endocrine conditions may affect a child's mental status. Signs of lethargy, hyperactivity, or unusual nervousness should be noted.[2,9]

Integument

The skin is inspected for hair distribution, texture (rough, soft, moist, dry, oily), acne, hyperpigmentation, depigmentation (vitiligo), cafe-au-lait spots, and nevi. The skin is affected by a number of endocrine conditions.[2,9]

Diagnostic Tests

Laboratory Tests

Because the role of the endocrine system is achieved through blood-borne hormones, blood tests play a major role in the evaluation of the child with a suspected endocrine disease. Hormones may be measured directly in the blood, or the metabolites of the hormones may be measured in the urine. Some endocrine tests can be performed with one blood sample. In many cases, however, the evaluation of hormonal concentrations in the blood is more complicated.

Hormonal concentrations may be extremely variable, depending on age, sex, stage of sexual development, time of day, nutritional status, and other factors. Some hormones are secreted in a periodic fashion. Cortisol, for example, is produced by the adrenal cortex with a circadian (daily) rhythm. Cortisol levels are measurable any time during the day, but levels vary depending on the time. Other hormones, such as growth hormone, normally are not detectable at certain times of the day. Insulin levels vary depending on the timing of meals. A child suspected of a hyperinsulin condition (for example an insulin-secreting tumor) usually needs to fast for the diagnosis to be made. LH and FSH (the gonadotropins) concentrations are high before birth, low in childhood, and gradually rise during puberty. The frequency of pituitary secretion of these hormones varies depending on the age and sexual stage of the child.[2,9]

To evaluate the endocrine system, specialized testing often is required. The process may entail serial sampling of blood or manipulation of the endocrine system with medications that either stimulate or suppress hormone production. These specialized tests usually are performed using an indwelling catheter (heparin lock) for repeated blood sampling. Blood indices of endocrine evaluation are listed in Table 55-2.

A routine urinalysis often is included in an endocrine evaluation. Other urine tests aimed at answering specific concerns relating to certain parts of the endocrine system may be obtained. As with blood tests some tests may be conducted on one sample of urine. Other tests may require serial urine collections. Timed urine collections

TABLE 55-2
Blood Indices of Endocrine Function

Test	Appropriate Range*	Deviations	Clinical Implications
Growth hormone	>10 ng/ml after pharmacologic stimulation	<10 ng/ml	Growth hormone deficiency
Somatomedin C or IGF-I	Normals specific for laboratory and child age	Low	Growth hormone deficiency Malnutrition
17 hydroxyprogesterone	Less than 200 ng/dl	Elevated	Adrenal hyperplasia, in poor control
Karyotype	46 xy (male) 46 xx (female)	Abnormal karyotype associated with many syndromes	45 xo Turner's syndrome, 47 xxy Klinefelter's syndrome, 15 q Prader-Willi syndrome
Luteinizing hormone and follicle-stimulating hormone	Prepubertal: <10 mIU/ml After puberty: 10 to 25 mIU/ml	Elevated with precocious puberty Low Very high	Primary gonadal failure, precocious puberty Hypogonadotrophic Hypogonadism Primary gonadal failure
Total T₄	4.5 to 12.5 µg/dL	Elevated Low	Hyperthyroidism Increased thyroid-binding globulin (TBG) Hypothyroidism Decreased TBG
T₃ resin uptake	33% to 50%	Elevated Low	Hyperthyroidism Decreased TBG Hypothyroidism Increased TBG
Thyroid-stimulating hormone (TSH)	0.3 to 5.0 mIU/ml	Elevated Low	Primary hypothyroidism Hyperthyroidism TSH deficiency Normal
Calcium	Premature 6 to 10 mg % Full term <1 wk 7 to 12 Child 8 to 10.5 Adult 8.5 to 10.5	Low Elevated	Hypocalcemia due to rickets, hypoparathyroidism Hyperparathyroidism
Phosphorus	<1 y 4.2 to 9.0 mg % 1 y 3.8 to 6.2 2–5 y 3.5 to 6.8 Adult 3.0 to 4.5	Low Elevated	Rickets, renal phosphate loss (X-linked rickets), hyperparathyroid Renal disease, hypoparathyroid, neonatal tetany

Alkaline phosphatase	<2 y 150 to 400 U/L
	2 to 10 y 100 to 300
	11–18 y
	  Male: 50 to 375
	  Female: 30 to 300
	Adult: 30 to 100
		Low
		
		Elevated
			Hypoparathyroid
			Hypophosphatasia
			
			Rickets, hyperparathyroid, familial

* Normal ranges vary between laboratories. Compare patient values to normals for the laboratory performing the tests.

are useful because the endocrine system is dynamic and many hormone levels fluctuate during the day. Timed urine collections for assay of hormones or their metabolites reflect the body's total production of the substance with time. Urine indices of endocrine evaluation are listed in Table 55-3.

Procedures

Radiographic tests or other imaging techniques frequently are part of the endocrine evaluation. As with blood and urine tests, specific testing is ordered depending on the suspected diagnosis. One of the most frequently ordered radiographic tests is an evaluation of

skeletal maturation, or "bone age." The patient's radiograph (usually of the hand and wrist) is compared with standards for age. Some endocrine conditions are associated with retarded skeletal maturation (hypothyroidism, growth hormone deficiency, constitutional delay), while others cause an accelerated bone age (precocious puberty, hyperthyroidism). More sophisticated imaging techniques are useful when specifically required. These include ultrasound, magnetic resonance imaging, computed tomography scans, and nuclear medicine studies.[2,9]

Stimulation tests frequently are part of an endocrine evaluation. The procedure used to accomplish this testing is presented here with examples of stimulation tests in Table 55-4.

TABLE 55-3
Urine Indices of Endocrine Function

Test	Appropriate Range*		Deviations	Clinical Implications
Microalbumin	<25 mg/24 hours		Elevated	Diabetic nephropathy
Vanillylmandelic acid	Age	mg/g/creatine	Elevated	Excess production of catecholamines: Pheochromocytoma Neuroblastoma
	<1 y	3 to 17		
	1 to 2 y	4 to 12		
	2 to 15 y	2 to 11		
	Adults	1.5 to 7.0		
Pregnanetriol	Age	mg/24 h	Elevated	Excess production of 17 hydroxyprogesterone (17 OHP)
	Infants	≤0.2		
	Children	≤1.0		Adrenal hyperplasia in poor control
	Adults	≤2.0		
Free cortisol	Age	mg/g/creatine	Elevated	Cushing syndrome
	prepubertal	7 to 25		
	Adult man	7 to 45		
	Adult woman	9 to 32		

* Normal ranges vary between laboratories. Compare patient values to normals for the laboratory performing the tests.

Provocative Blood Testing to Evaluate the Endocrine System

Description/Definition

Hormone production or release is stimulated or suppressed to evaluate function of the endocrine system.

Purpose

Stimulation tests frequently are part of an endocrine evaluation. Random hormone levels may not reflect endocrine function accurately. Often it is necessary to stimulate or suppress legs of the hypothalamic–pituitary–end-organ axes to evaluate the integrity of the system as a whole. Examples include evaluation of the growth

hormones–somatomedin-c, hypothalamic–pituitary–thyroid, hypothalamic–pituitary–adrenal, and hypothalamic–pituitary–gonadal axes.

Indications

Suspected endocrine conditions in which random hormone determinations are inadequate (e.g., growth hormone deficiency, borderline hyperthyroidism, adrenal insufficiency).

Contraindications

None.

Preparation

Explain the procedure to the child and family, assuring that the child is properly prepared for the test. (For example, prior to a glucose

TABLE 55-4
Examples of Stimulation Tests Used to Diagnose Endocrine Disorders

Test	Purpose	Stimulant	Nursing Observations
Growth hormone (GH) stimulation	Diagnose GH deficiency	Insulin	Hypoglycemia
		L-dopa	Nausea
		Clonidine	Hypotension
		Arginine	
		Glucagon	Nausea
Thyroid-releasing hormone (TRH) stimulation	Assess axis: hypothalamic–pituitary–thyroid Diagnose thyroid disease: hypothyroidism, hyperthyroidism	TRH	Transient blood pressure, pulse alterations, flushing, urge to urinate
Luteinizing hormone-releasing hormone (LHRH) stimulation	Assess axis: hypothalamic–pituitary–gonadal Diagnosis of pubertal disorders	Gonadotropin-releasing hormone	None
Adrenocorticotrophic stimulation	Assess axis: hypothalamic–pituitary–adrenal	ACTH	None
Glucose tolerance test	Assess glucose tolerance Evaluation of acromegaly	Glucose	Nausea

TABLE 55-5
Selected Nursing Diagnoses Associated With Altered Endocrine Function

Data Analysis and Conclusions	Nursing Diagnosis
Health Perception and Health Management	
Repeated admissions for minor illnesses; nausea, vomiting, and diarrhea; appears very ill.	Altered health maintenance related to knowledge deficit about sick day management and inadequate child care arrangements
Parents given information on adjusting medication in times of stress; instructions not followed.	
Parents recently divorced; lives with each parent on alternate weeks.	
Frequently left alone in mornings when parent leaves for work; illness not recognized early.	
Nutrition and Metabolism	
Child very excitable and cries easily; tremor in fingers.	Altered nutrition: less than body requirements related to high caloric demands resulting from increased metabolic rate
Skin flushed with heat intolerance; wearing sleeveless blouse without sweater or coat in winter.	
Weight in lowest fifth percentile for height on growth chart.	
Elimination	
Reports hard, formed stool two times a week; pain and difficulty with defecation.	Constipation related to decreased metabolic rate
Dislikes raw fruits and vegetables.	
Fluid intake about 1500 ml/day.	
Physically inactive; no afterschool play outdoors.	
Activity and Exercise	
Parents report child has athletic potential, but child acts exhausted with minimal exercise.	Activity intolerance related to effects of excessive metabolic rate
Frequent outbursts and episodes of disruptive behavior in school.	
Tachycardia and tachypnea noted on examination.	
Sleep and Rest	
Parents report that child is in constant motion; acts exhausted but cannot sleep when put to bed. Has not slept through the night in several weeks. Sleeplessness gradually becoming more pronounced.	Sleep pattern disturbance related to impaired metabolism
Self-Perception and Self-Concept	
Child expresses difficulty participating in sports events with peers. Reports teasing by peers and feelings of inadequacy.	Self-esteem disturbance related to altered growth and development
Growth failure; in lowest fifth percentile of growth chart.	
Mother reports difficulty finding age-appropriate clothing in stores.	
Role Relationship	
Parents express despair and guilt over child's illness.	Altered family processes related to the presence of chronic illness in child
Parental reluctance to administer injections with statements such as "I can't bear to hurt him," and "When I approach him with the medication, his screaming tears me apart."	
Parents acknowledge lack of family, social, and spiritual support systems; child is never left with an alternate caregiver.	
Sexuality and Reproduction	
Peers (age 15) experienced puberty 2 to 3 years ago.	Self-esteem disturbance related to delayed development of secondary sex characteristics
Has child-like body characteristics.	
No breast buds or pubic hair.	
Stated that "Everyone treats me like I'm a child. No one believes me when I tell my age."	

(Continued)

TABLE 55-5
(Continued)

Data Analysis and Conclusions	Nursing Diagnosis
Feet don't touch floor when sitting in standard sized desk or chair.	
Coping and Stress Tolerance	
Separated from family and peers during hospitalization at medical center; home 50 miles away. Has missed 1 week of classes at high school.	Grieving related to perceived effects of chronic disease on lifestyle and goals
Diagnosed with insulin-dependent diabetes mellitus 3 days ago. Withdrawn and refuses to leave room or engage in conversation with staff.	
Refuses to look at educational materials or participate in self-care.	
Values and Beliefs	
Parents and child verbalize uncertainty as to need for treatment.	Decisional conflict related to lack of information regarding side-effects of medication and long-term result of noncompliance
Unable to state benefits or risks of medication accurately.	
Local college track star recently admitted use of steroids. Media publicity on effects of steroid use.	
Parents report fear for their child's long-term health.	

tolerance test, the patient should be loaded with carbohydrates. Many tests require the patient to be fasting.) Prepare the necessary supplies and obtain informed consent, if required.

Developmental Considerations

- Infant: Encourage parent to bring favorite toys or security blanket.
- Child: Encourage child to bring a quiet game, book, or favorite toy. Explain the procedure in age-appropriate terms.
- Adolescent: Encourage patient to bring a book or diversional activity. Explain the procedure in age-appropriate terms. Invite the child to ask questions or voice concerns.

Nursing Implications

- Establish venous access with an indwelling catheter (heparin lock or intravenous saline).
- Obtain baseline vital signs.
- Obtain baseline blood sample in correct collection tube.
- Administer indicated medication for the test.
- Obtain and handle blood samples properly at prescribed times.

Selected Nursing Diagnoses

After obtaining the history, performing the physical examination, and reviewing results from the diagnostic tests, the nurse carefully analyzes the data obtained. Nursing diagnoses appropriate for the child with endocrine dysfunction become apparent and are used to develop a plan of care. Selected nursing diagnoses that may be appropriate for the child with endocrine dysfunction are presented by functional health in Table 55-5.

Summary

Children with endocrine disorders often present with a perplexing array of physical signs and symptoms. The assessment requires a good knowledge base, patience, sensitivity, and a willingness to adapt the process to each encounter. A comprehensive database includes a thorough history obtained from the child and family, a thorough physical examination, and analysis of the findings of diagnostic tests. From this composite of information the nurse is able to begin establishing nursing diagnoses that are used to develop a plan of care. Refinement of the

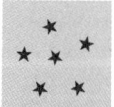

Ideas for Nursing Research

Nurses who are employed in office or clinic settings in which children are evaluated for endocrine disorders have many opportunities to participate in investigations related to assessment and diagnosis. While some research may be initiated by the physician or other members of the medical team, other ideas can be developed by nurses. The following areas need to be explored:

- Evaluate the frequency and accuracy with which heights and weights are obtained by the primary caregiver.
- Determine the frequency and accuracy of methods used to interpret growth measurements that are obtained.
- Investigate the factors that most successfully contribute to the construction of a comprehensive database, including setting, personal characteristics, and behaviors of the interviewer and data collection tools.
- Examine the effectiveness of methods used to assess the child's perception of self as it relates to the endocrine disorder.

nursing care plan depends on the specific endocrine disorder and the individual needs or problems of the child and family.

References

1. Gordon, M., Crouthamel, C., Post, E. M., & Richman, R. A. (1982). Psychosocial aspects of constitutional short stature: Social competence, behavior problems, self-esteem, and family functioning. *Journal of Pediatrics, 101*, 3. pp. 477–480.
2. Kaplan, S. A. (1990). Growth and growth hormone: Disorders of the anterior pituitary. In S. A. Kaplan (Ed.). *Clinical pediatric endocrinology* (pp. 1–62). Philadelphia: W.B. Saunders.
3. Lowery, G. H. (1986). *Growth and development of children* (8th ed.). Chicago: Year Book Medical Publisher.
4. Marshall, W. A., & Tanner, J. M. (1969). Variations in the pattern of pubertal changes in girls. *Archives of Diseases in Childhood, 44.* pp. 291–300.
5. Marshall, W. A., & Tanner, J. M. (1970). Variations in the pattern of pubertal changes in boys. *Archives of Diseases in Childhood, 45.* pp. 13–23.
6. Rieser, P., & Underwood, L. E. (1989). *Growing children: A parents' guide* (2nd ed.). Chapel Hill: University of North Carolina.
7. Rosenfeld, R. L. (1990). The ovary and female sexual maturation. In S. L. Kaplan (Ed.). *Clinical Pediatric endocrinology* (pp. 259–323). Philadelphia: W.B. Saunders.
8. Solomon, S. B. (1986). Children with short stature. *Journal of Pediatric Nursing, I*, 2. pp. 80–89.
9. Stanhope, R., & Brook, C. G. D. (1989). Disorders of puberty. In C. G. D. Brook (Ed.). *Clinical paediatric endocrinology* (2nd ed.) (pp. 189–212). Blackwell Scientific Publications.
10. Styne, D. M. (1990). The testes: Disorders of sexual differentiation and puberty. In S. L. Kaplan (Ed.). *Clinical pediatric endocrinology* (pp. 367–425). Philadelphia: W.B. Saunders.

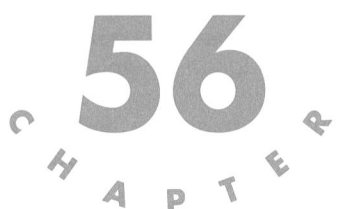
Nursing Planning, Intervention, and Evaluation for Altered Endocrine Function

BEHAVIORAL OBJECTIVES

Describe symptoms commonly observed in children with altered function of each of the endocrine glands.

Discuss the medical therapy and treatments usually prescribed for children with selected endocrine dysfunctions.

Discuss the nursing assessments and interventions typically needed for children with selected endocrine dysfunctions.

Distinguish between normal and abnormal patterns of linear growth and weight gain.

Outline the adaptations needed in the lifestyle of the child newly diagnosed with diabetes mellitus and the family.

Describe the psychosocial implications of common endocrine alterations.

Children with endocrine disorders often have no visible signs of their health problems; they may not appear ill in any physical way. Yet, some children with endocrine disorders cannot eat the foods that other children enjoy, or they may need to adhere to schedules that other children do not understand. Some endocrine disorders change only the rate of growth, and the child otherwise has a completely normal appearance. Expectations related to children's size create problems for them with adults and peers. For example, children who are small for their age may not be included in peer activities. In contrast, fast-growing children are often treated as if they are older than their years, and they may seem "dumb" to similar-sized but older children. Children with endocrine alterations sometimes experience psychosocial distress more than adverse physical effects of their condition.

Children with endocrine disorders do not endure their condition alone. These children have parents and other loved ones who are reminded frequently of the sometimes precarious health of their children. The family, therefore, is inextricably linked to the child's health care, and nursing care is vital not only for the child with the disorder but for the family as well. The accompanying display provides a sampling of support agencies for families with endocrine dysfunction to use as resources.

Endocrinopathy

Endocrine disorders can arise from problems at three different levels within the system. *Primary problems* are the result of malfunction of an endocrine gland. The pancreas, for example, may shut down the production of insulin. *Secondary problems* occur when a healthy endocrine gland fails to be stimulated to function by the master gland (the pituitary gland). Glands that depend on pituitary stimulation are the thyroid, adrenal cortex, and gonads. *Tertiary endocrinopathies* occur as a result of problems within the hypothalamus, the central nervous system control center of the endocrine system that stimulates the pituitary gland. The interrelationships among these three levels of endocrine function have been explained in Chapter 54. Whether the problems arise at the primary, secondary, or tertiary level, the end result is the same: insufficient production or overproduction of the necessary hormones. Most endocrine problems in children result from the production of too little hormone.

Other pathologic processes present in the child's body can complicate the diagnosis and treatment of endocrine problems. For example, essential organs, such as the liver or kidneys, must be healthy in order to use hormones affecting their function. A condition in which the target organs fail to respond to stimulation from the endocrine system is called *end-organ failure.* Another pathologic condition occurs when tumors arise and secrete hormones independently of the endocrine gland. Endocrinopathy can also occur as a result of external factors that damage the healthy endocrine system; these problems are known as *iatrogenic conditions.* For example, children receiving immunosuppressive therapy for treatment of asthma, allergic rhinitis, or juvenile arthritis may experience shutdown of the adrenocortical-pituitary-hypothalamic feedback system. When the external source of hormone is removed, the endocrine gland is unable to respond.

Some groups of children experience an increased risk for endocrine alterations and must be assessed carefully for early signs of hormone imbalances. For example, children who have had radiation treatment, especially to the cranium, and children with damage to the central nervous system are at risk to develop endocrine disorders. The increased life span of children who formerly succumbed quickly to brain tumors and other life-threatening conditions suggests that these children will continue to be seen in the health care system in increasing numbers. Other children at risk for endocrine alterations include infants born to mothers who have hyperthyroidism and the children of a parent who has a genetically-linked endocrinopathy. Early identification of endocrine disorders in these high-risk populations increases the likelihood that treatment can be successfully instituted.

In this chapter, the alterations of the endocrine system are organized around the levels of endocrine function. First, disorders of endocrine glands that are under pituitary control are presented. Basic understanding of the thyroid gland, adrenal cortex, and gonads is necessary to understand the pituitary problems that are discussed in the following sections. The chapter concludes with alterations that occur in endocrine glands not under pituitary control.

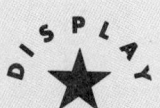

Resources for Families With Altered Endocrine Function

Association for Glycogen Storage Disease, PO Box 896, Durant, IA 52747.

The Association for Children with Russell-Silver Syndrome, Inc., 22 Hoyt Street, Madison, NJ 07940.

Congenital Adrenal Hyperplasia Support Association, Inc., 10 County Highway, #4, Wrenshall, MN 55797.

Human Growth Foundation, 7777 Leesburg Pike, PO Box 3090, Falls Church, VA 22043.

Little People of America, PO Box 126, Owatonna, MN 55060.

Magic Foundation, 770 Alexandria Drive, Naperville IL 60565. (growth disorders support group)

Pediatric Endocrinology Nursing Society, 3648 Deerfield Place, Ann Arbor, MI 48103.

Prader-Willi Syndrome Association, 5515 Malibu Drive, Median, MN 55436.

Turner Syndrome Society of the U.S., 15500 Wayzata Boulevard, Wayzata, MN 55391.

U.S. Department of Health and Human Services, Public Health Service, National Institutes of Health: Facts About Precocious Puberty.

Diabetes Mellitus

American Diabetes Association, Inc., 1660 Duke Street, Alexandria, VA 22314.

Canadian Diabetes Association, 123 Edward Street, Suite 601, Toronto, Ontario, Canada M56 1E2.

Juvenile Diabetes Foundation International, 23 East 26th Street, New York, NY 10010.

Juvenile Diabetes Foundation International—Canada, 4632 Yonge Street, Suite 201, Willowdale, Ontario, Canada M2N 5M1.

National Diabetes Information Clearinghouse, Box NDIC, Bethesda, MD 20205.

Altered Thyroid Gland Function

The thyroid gland produces hormones that control the metabolic rate of the entire body and are essential for life. The thyroid gland is under the direction of the hypothalamic-pituitary system through which the hypothalamus produces thyrotropin-releasing hormone (TRH), which stimulates the production of thyroid-stimulating hormone (TSH) from the pituitary. TSH initiates the release of the hormones triiododthyronine (T_3) and thyroxine (T_4) from the thyroid gland. Because the functions of the two hormones are essentially the same, the term *thyroid hormone* is typically used (see Fig. 54-3.)

Hypofunction of the thyroid gland is far more common in childhood than is hyperfunction. Although an alteration in thyroid function can be caused by dysfunction at the pituitary level (secondary hypothyroidism), primary hypothyroidism is the most common thyroid alteration in children. Goiter, an enlargement of the thyroid gland, is another alteration of thyroid structure that may appear in the presence or absence of other thyroid gland disorders.

Primary Hypothyroidism

Definition and Incidence. A low concentration of circulating thyroid hormone (T_3 and T_4) results in slowed metabolism, affecting all body systems. Thyroid hormone is essential to linear growth, and during prenatal life, infancy, and to age 2 years. It also is essential for normal brain development. Without thyroid hormone, an infant fails to develop physically and mentally, but its absence in older children does not affect intellectual potential.

Primary hypothyroidism may be present at birth (congenital), or it may develop at any time in a person's life (acquired). *Congenital hypothyroidism* is the most common cause of primary hypothyroidism; it occurs in 1 in 2500 live births.[6] Acquired hypothyroidism may be attributed to a variety of conditions, but it is often due to thyroiditis. Thyroiditis is any inflammation of the thyroid gland that results in injury or damage to thyroid tissue. Different types of thyroiditis may occur, but chronic autoimmune thyroiditis is the usual cause of acquired hypothyroidism; its incidence may be as high as 1% in school-age children. Both congenital and acquired hypothyroidism occur more frequently in females than males.

Etiology and Pathophysiology. *Congenital hypothyroidism* may result from a variety of conditions. Sometimes, familial tendencies for thyroid disorders can be identified, and, rarely, the mother has a history of treatment early in pregnancy for thyroid disease. Enzymatic defects of thyroid hormone synthesis may occur. In many instances, the cause of congenital hypothyroidism is undetermined.

Congenital hypothyroidism most often appears as the result of defects in the embryonic development of the thyroid gland (thyroid dysgenesis). Thyroid tissue may be completely absent (aplasia) or partially present (hypoplasia), and the tissue may be located in the normal position or anywhere between the neck and tongue (an ectopic location). When a remnant of the gland is present, enough thyroid hormone may have been produced that severe symptoms of deficiency are not evident at birth, but symptoms develop as growth and developmental demands for the hormone increase. If hypothyroidism is unrecognized and untreated at birth, infants fail to grow at a normal pace, and profound mental retardation develops.

A low concentration of circulating thyroid hormone is common in sick premature infants, occurring in as many as 25% of these newborns.[18] However, this finding, sometimes called *sick euthyroidism,* represents an appropriate physiologic response to the critical nature of the infant's condition; the lower metabolic rate conserves essential energy. Treatment is not necessary because the condition is self-correcting.

Acquired hypothyroidism (juvenile hypothyroidism) is recognized after the age of 2 years and may be attributed to a wide variety of defects. The condition may be considered iatrogenic, as when neck radiation or surgery damages the gland and diminishes its function. In other children, dietary deficiency of iodine, essential for the synthesis of thyroid hormone, results in hypothyroidism. This condition is almost unheard of today, as the typical American diet is rich in iodine.

Thyroiditis is another cause of acquired hypothyroidism, and it occurs in several forms. Diseases such as tuberculosis, mumps, and other acute inflammatory conditions may contribute to the development of thyroiditis. The usual cause of thyroiditis is an autoimmune process called Hashimoto thyroiditis[12] (also known as autoimmune thyroiditis or lymphocytic thyroiditis). This autoimmune condition often is associated with chromosomal abnormalities, such as Down syndrome, Turner syndrome, and Klinefelter syndrome, as well as with other diseases with autoimmune components (e.g., diabetes mellitus and rheumatoid arthritis). Hashimoto thyroiditis is more prevalent in adolescents than in younger children.

In Hashimoto thyroiditis, the thyroid gland is infiltrated with lymphocytes, and antithyroid antibodies may be identified in the circulation. Knowledge of the basic immunologic defect is limited and the mechanism of thyroid gland destruction is poorly understood. Faulty synthesis of thyroid hormone stimulates release of TSH, which causes the thyroid gland to become hyperactive and enlarged. The loss of thyroid function and subsequent appearance of clinical symptoms occur gradually as the gland is destroyed slowly.

Some children have a low concentration of thyroid-binding globulin (TBG), the vehicle for carrying thyroid hormone in the bloodstream. Children with low TBG, however, have normal amounts of unbound T_4, and hypothyroidism is not present. TBG deficiency is a benign genetic disorder; treatment is not indicated.

Clinical Manifestations. Newborns with *congenital hypothyroidism* seldom exhibit any physical signs of the condition. Without routine screening, only 10% to 15% of infants with this disorder would be diagnosed by 3 months of age.[18] A newborn with congenital hypothyroidism might have a markedly open posterior fontanel, an umbilical hernia, or prolonged physiologic jaundice, but classic signs of congenital hypothyroidism may not be noted until later in life.

Affected infants often display feeding difficulties, primarily because of a lack of interest and general sluggishness. They cry little, sleep more than usual, and often have a subnormal pulse rate and body temperature. The skin may be mottled and cold to touch. Because these symptoms appear gradually, diagnosis may be delayed.

By 6 months of age, untreated infants exhibit the classic hypothyroid symptoms: arrest of growth; a large, protruding tongue; hypotonia; hoarse cry; coarse facial features; poor feeding; and constipation. Unfortunately, the manifestations of hypothyroidism generally indicate that significant intellectual potential has already been lost. Infants who are untreated until 6 months of age will be profoundly and irreversibly mentally retarded. If the condition is recognized and treated by the age of 3 months, these infants can achieve a mean IQ of 89.[18]

The clinical manifestations of *acquired hypothyroidism* depend on the age of the child at onset and on the extent of the dysfunction. Typically, the older the child is at onset, the less effect on growth and development. With the onset of acquired hypothyroidism, all metabolic processes become depressed, and growth arrest is the most notable feature. A sample chart is given in Figure 56-1. The heart rate slows, the pulse and blood pressure decrease, pulse pressure narrows, generalized puffiness develops, and weight gain ensues. With progression of the condition, the hair stops growing and becomes coarse. Facial features also coarsen, and children experience cold intolerance and dry skin. The thyroid gland may hypertrophy in an attempt to produce adequate hormones, forming a goiter.

In accordance with the reduced metabolic rate, children with hypothyroidism become physically inactive, further decreasing their caloric consumption. Children

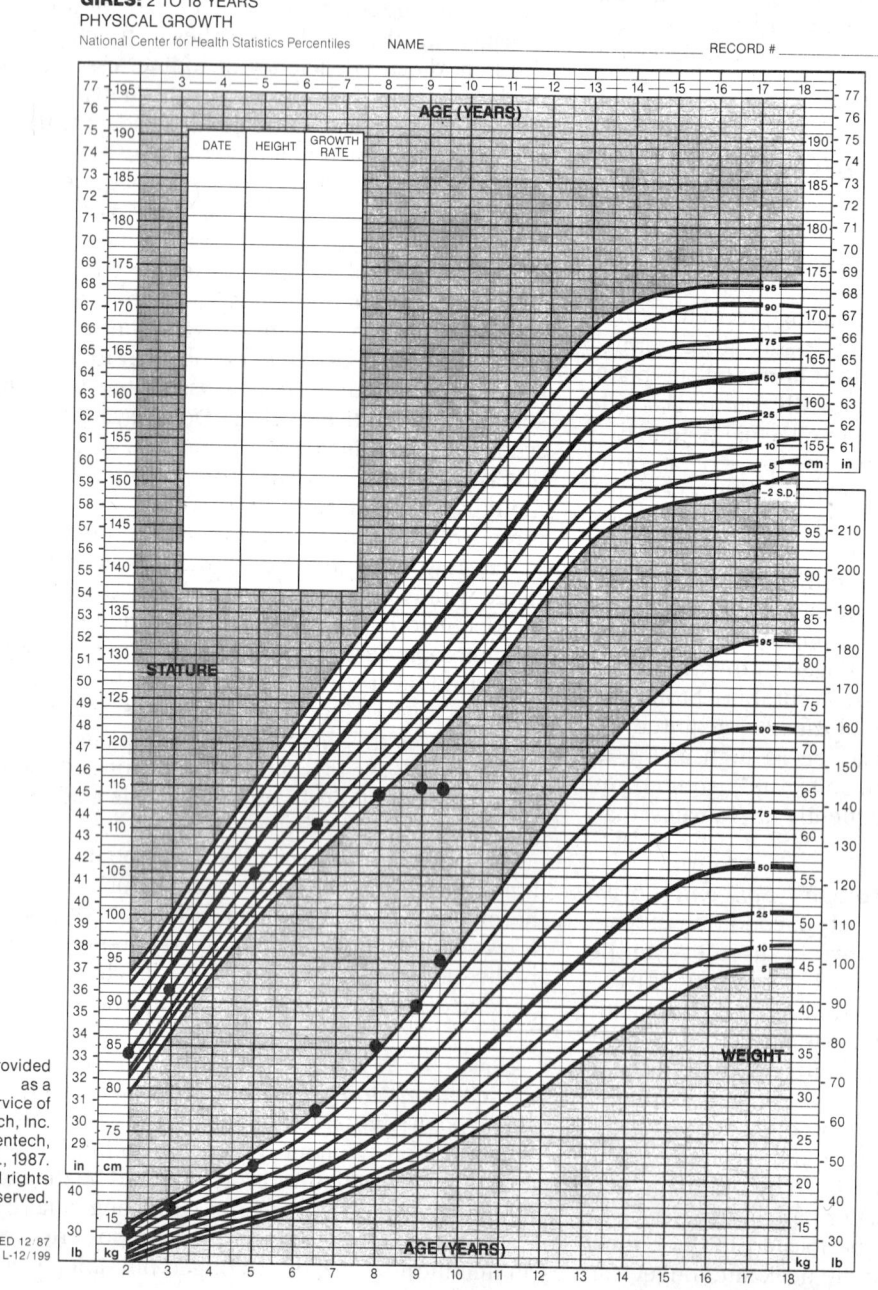

GIRLS: 2 TO 18 YEARS
PHYSICAL GROWTH
National Center for Health Statistics Percentiles

FIGURE 56-1

Growth chart of a girl with onset of acquired hypothyroidism before age 6. There are already abnormalities on her growth chart with a subtle weight gain at age 6 and a change in height percentiles from the 25th to the 10th percentile. By age 8 her weight gain and growth speed are clearly abnormal, although the child is not yet "short." She was not diagnosed until age 9½ when she was seen for her "obesity."

often perform well in school and are pleasant playmates. However, they do their school work slowly and may go to bed quite early because they feel so tired.

Diagnostic Studies. The devastating effects of untreated congenital hypothyroidism have prompted many countries to mandate neonatal screening programs.[18] Within a few days of birth, a blood sample, obtained from a puncture of the heel or toe, is tested for a variety of metabolic disorders, including hypothyroidism. For those infants whose T_4 concentration is outside the normal range, the serum concentrations of TSH and T_4 are subsequently obtained via venipuncture. Infants with congenital hypothyroidism have a low concentration of T_4 and a high concentration of TSH. TSH concentration increases in an attempt to stimulate the absent or inadequate thyroid gland.

A nuclear scan may be performed prior to the initiation of therapy to determine the presence and location of thyroid tissue. Early treatment is of utmost concern and should not be delayed significantly if the scan cannot be obtained promptly.

Blood studies are required for older children suspected of having acquired hypothyroidism. Serum concentrations of TSH, T_4, and thyroid antibodies help determine whether the deficiency is primary (thyroid gland dysfunction—low T_4, high TSH) or secondary (pituitary gland dysfunction—low T_4, low or normal TSH). In Hashimoto thyroiditis, high concentration of antibodies are identified. In children with no symptoms of hypothyroidism and a low T_4, an assessment of free T_4 and TBG concentration is obtained. In cases of TBG deficiency, the TBG level is low, but the free T_4 level remains normal.

Bone age x-rays may be used to evaluate the degree and duration of the hypothyroid condition. The more severe or prolonged the hypothyroid condition, the greater the delay in bone age to be expected. Therefore, the greatest delay in bone age would be expected in infants born with thyroid agenesis and the least delay in older children with recently acquired hypothyroidism.

★ **ASSESSMENT**

Any infant in the newborn nursery with a pronounced open posterior fontanel should be evaluated for congenital hypothyroidism. In addition to the state screening program requiring heel-stick blood samples, venous blood is obtained for T_4 and TSH concentration and is sent immediately to the hospital laboratory. These samples can be analyzed (within 2–3 days), prior to obtaining the screening results from the state laboratory.

An assessment of infants who have failed the state screening program includes obtaining a behavioral history of sleeping, eating, and bowel patterns and levels of alertness. Physical examination may reveal subtle signs of hypothyroidism, but most often is normal. Growth parameters are obtained, including length, nude weight, and head circumference.

The range of normal thyroid hormone concentration in the blood is higher in infants and children than in adults (see Chap. 55). When evaluating laboratory values, the nurse must be aware of the age-specific ranges for the laboratory used. If the nurse relies on the printed adult range, signs of hypothyroidism may be overlooked.

Routine health assessment of all children requires that a growth chart be used to plot their linear growth and weight gain. Study of this chart can be useful in identifying the onset and progress of the disease. Further, a series of school pictures may be used to document the progression of facial changes that accompanies acquired hypothyroidism.

★ **NURSING DIAGNOSES AND PLANNING**

Based on the assessment data discussed in the previous section and in the preceding chapter, the following nursing diagnoses may apply to the family and children with hypothyroidism:

- Altered Family Processes related to grief over loss of perfect baby.
- Altered Growth and Development related to effects of hypothyroidism.
- Anxiety related to lack of knowledge about hypothyroidism and its treatment.

The nurse and child (or parents) together plan effective care based on the established nursing diagnoses. Several examples of expected outcomes are as follows:

- The parents discuss the side-effects of the initial medication.
- The parents verbalize feelings about the child's condition to the nurse and each other.
- The parents discuss plans to provide age-appropriate stimulation for development.
- The parents administer the medication appropriately.

The nurse plans for the daily care of the child based on both the physician's orders and nursing diagnoses. Some general nursing care goals may include the following:

- The child achieves full potential for physical and mental growth and development.
- The family understands the need to continue a life-long regimen of medication and monitoring.

★ **INTERVENTIONS: COLLABORATIVE AND INDEPENDENT**

MEDICATION THERAPY

The goal of treatment is to achieve and maintain the child's thyroid hormone concentration within a normal range for age (euthyroid state). This state is accomplished by daily replacement of thyroid hormone using oral tablets of synthetic T_4. Because T_3 is converted to T_4 for use within the body, its replacement is unnecessary. Synthetic T_4 (L-thyroxine) is easily obtained in tasteless, inexpensive tablets that can be chewed, crushed, or swallowed whole. This medication is taken daily.

When an infant is strongly suspected of having congenital hypothyroidism, thyroid replacement may begin after obtaining venous blood samples but prior to obtaining results of the diagnostic tests. If the suspected diagnosis is ruled out, several days of unneeded thyroid replacement will cause the infant no harm and is preferred to withholding a treatment that is so critical to neurologic development. Full replacement doses of L-thyroxine (10

μg/kg) are given daily, and the dose is gradually lowered to about 2 to 3 μg/kg by adolescence.[6] The decreased dosage follows the normal decline of the basal metabolic rate as the child ages. In infants with partial thyroid function, treatment may be given until the child is 3 years of age and past the critical time of brain growth. The child then is re-evaluated after treatment is discontinued for a determination of future thyroid replacement needs.

Children with acquired hypothyroidism may have had the condition for many years. These children need a gradual institution of treatment with L-thyroxine to avoid initiating symptoms of hyperthyroidism, although temporary behavior changes are to be expected. Irritability, jumpiness, and insomnia may occur as the body adjusts to the increased amounts of T_4, and these symptoms may persist for several weeks. The dose for children aged 5 to 10 years is begun at a low level and is gradually increased to 3 to 5 μg/kg daily. This dose is lowered to 2 to 3 μg/kg daily as the child ages.[6]

TEACHING

With the current trends for early discharge from the newborn nursery and home birth, the possibility of delay or omission in screening infants for hypothyroidism is increased. Because congenital hypothyroidism often is not evident at birth, the importance of neonatal screening cannot be overstressed to parents. Obtaining these blood samples must be a priority for nurses, because prompt diagnosis and treatment are essential to correct the condition and to prevent permanent brain damage.

Unless profoundly hypothyroid, affected infants are given full replacement doses of L-thyroxine immediately, not gradually as in older children. The onset of side-effects may be dramatic. Parents should be told to expect the infant to experience sleep disturbances and increased crying for at least several days. These unpleasant behaviors can be a significant stressor in the lives of new parents, who may already be exhausted.

In older children in whom hypothyroidism may have been undiagnosed for some time, families need to be prepared for the changes in behavior that will occur as a result of treatment. Children will become more active and animated. The nurse describes the more active behavior as a positive and healthy change.

Families need to be educated about the lifetime need for thyroid replacement in their children. Taking the medication daily may be difficult, because hypothyroidism may remain a hidden disorder. Children who skip doses often explain that they do not feel "better" when they do take it. L-thyroxine has a long half-life, and there are no obvious reactions from taking the drug sporadically. Nevertheless, better control is achieved with constant blood concentration of T_4. The nurse works with the child and family to make taking the medication a daily habit. Sticker charts may be helpful to younger children, and medication boxes marked with the days of the week can be helpful to older children. Most importantly, annual re-education about the purpose and need for this medication is necessary.

Parents should be told that generic L-thyroxine is not suitable for children, because these preparations lack the consistency that growing children require.[18] Several brand-name products (e.g., Synthroid, Levothyroid) are available at slightly higher cost. Parents also need to be aware of the potential dangers of accidental overdose and take appropriate safety measures for all the children in their home. If the medication is missed one day, the dose should be made up the next day. The tablets may be crushed and mixed with a small amount of water or formula. However, parents should be cautioned to avoid mixing an infant's medication in a full bottle because of the potential of partial dosing if the bottle is not finished.

★ EVALUATION

The nurse and family periodically evaluate the outcomes of care given. Examples of outcomes for the child and family with hypothyroidism were provided under "Nursing Diagnoses and Planning" in this section. Have the short-term goals been met? Are the long-term goals still realistic? Planning for further nursing care takes into consideration the development of complications and long-term care.

COMPLICATIONS

Without treatment, infants with hypothyroidism remain small and mentally deficient. Treatment begun within 45 days of life is associated with a normal IQ at 5 to 7 years of age. The degree of intellectual impairment, if any, is linked to the length of time infants remain in a hypothyroid state.

For unknown reasons, children with acquired hypothyroidism may never reach their full genetic potential for height, although they may exhibit marked catch-up growth after onset of treatment.[12] The intellectual capacity of these children is unimpaired.

LONG-TERM CARE

Periodic assessment is needed to evaluate the growth and the adequacy of thyroid replacement. Once treatment is initiated, infants with congenital hypothyroidism typically experience a phase of rapid catch-up growth. Infants who were overweight and puffy due to poor circulation from the slowed metabolism of hypothyroidism may not gain weight during these weeks, but they grow steadily after this settling phase. Any infant who does not gain weight and grow needs to be evaluated for undertreatment.

Children with acquired hypothyroidism often have a period of rapid statural growth after treatment has begun, but they may experience weight loss as their metabolism is stimulated by L-thyroxine. Once these children are in a euthyroid state, they grow and gain weight at a normal rate. Slowing of growth rate, change in height percentile, or gain in weight may signal undertreatment.

Children with hypothyroidism require monitoring of their blood concentration of TSH and T_4 to ensure that an adequate amount of replacement hormone is being given. If an inadequate dosage of L-thyroxine is taken, the TSH concentration increases in an attempt to stimulate production of thyroid hormone. TSH concentration that is higher than the normal range indicates the need to have a higher level of circulating thyroxine, regardless of the level of T_4 measured in the blood. Undertreatment may occur when only T_4 values are obtained. In infancy, after the desired dosage has been established, TSH and

T_4 concentrations are checked two to four times each year, but throughout childhood and adolescence, the concentration is checked less frequently (once or twice a year).

Adolescent girls with hypothyroidism require future-oriented counseling that stresses the importance of adequate thyroid replacement during pregnancy. Ideally, women should have excellent control (euthyroid state) prior to conception.

Hyperthyroidism

Definition and Incidence. Hyperthyroidism is a condition in which a high concentration of thyroid hormone stimulates increased metabolic function throughout the body. Table 56-1 compares the clinical manifestations of hypo- and hyperthyroidism. Hyperfunction of the thyroid gland is rare in infants and young children. Almost all hyperthyroidism in children is due to Graves disease. Most cases occur during adolescence, and it is seen three to six times more often in girls than in boys.[6]

Etiology and Pathophysiology. Hyperthyroidism is most often caused by an autoimmune process within the thyroid gland that stimulates excessive secretion of thyroid hormone. Graves disease is the most common cause of hyperthyroidism in children.[10]

Both immunologic and genetic factors are recognized as etiologic factors in Graves disease. It is thought that the condition produces an immunoglobulin that binds to the receptors for TSH in the thyroid gland. The binding stimulates the thyroid to produce its hormone; hyperthyroidism results. There is a high familial incidence of Graves disease, and it sometimes accompanies other conditions, such as Down syndrome, diabetes mellitus, hypoadrenalism, and collagen disease.

Neonatal Graves disease is a rare condition associated with maternal Graves disease. Infants receive thyroid-stimulating immunoglobulins across the placenta from the mother. This disorder is an emergency condition, because the hypermetabolic state it causes in the infant can result in severe brain damage. The mortality rate is 20% unless these infants receive prompt treatment at birth.[20]

Clinical Manifestations. In older children, the onset of symptoms from Graves disease is often gradual. Symptoms range from mild irritability and sleep disturbances to tachycardia and weight loss, despite a voracious appetite. Children may become excitable, cry easily, and develop a tremor of the fingers. Skin flushing, fever, heat intolerance, and sweating are not uncommon. A staring expression is often noted, although severe exophthalmos (bulging eyes) is uncommon in children. There is often enlargement of the thyroid gland (goiter). Some adolescents have significant school problems because of their hyperactivity; occasionally, a psychiatric disorder is blamed for the behavior patterns. Affected children are generally normal in height but are underweight. Typical growth changes for an adolescent with Graves disease are seen in the chart in Figure 56-2.

The onset of neonatal hyperthyroidism occurs in utero, and the symptoms are present at birth. These infants have tachycardia, restlessness, flushed skin, fever, and staring eyes. They may have goiter, jaundice, and failure to thrive, although their appetite is voracious.[11] The condition may be transient or occur as a classic form of Graves disease.

Diagnostic Studies. Serum blood concentrations of TSH, T_4, and thyroid antibodies are obtained. In the presence of Graves disease, these tests reveal normal or low TSH levels with high concentrations of T_4 and antibodies to the gland. The antibodies are the result of the autoimmune process that is destroying the thyroid tissue. High concentrations of maternal thyroid stimulating antibody during pregnancy predicts the risk of graves disease in the neonate. Excessive TSH production is a rare finding that would prompt a pituitary evaluation, including a computed tomography (CT) scan of the head.

Children with a goiter or an unusual thyroid gland (with asymmetry or nodules) require additional evaluation. An ultrasound may be performed to identify the size and placement of thyroid tissue. A radionuclide scan may also be needed and often shows a rapid and diffuse concentration of the radioactive material in the enlarged thyroid gland.

★ **ASSESSMENT**

The initial concerns of health care providers are the level of toxicity and the symptoms present in the child. An extensive history from older children generally reveals the onset of this disorder and subsequent development of symptoms. Physical examination includes temperature, heart rate, blood pressure, height, and weight. Typical findings are described in Table 56-1. Notation is made of any difficulty that the child has with swallowing due to enlargement of the thyroid gland. The thyroid gland is gently palpated and measured. Linear growth and weight gain patterns are determined and plotted on a growth chart.

TABLE 56-1
Comparison of Possible Clinical Manifestations of Hypothyroidism and Hyperthyroidism

Hypothyroidism	Hyperthyroidism
Growth arrest	Irritability; nervousness
Weight gain	Weight loss; ↑ appetite
Bradycardia; narrow pulse pressure	Tachycardia; wide pulse pressure
Hypotension	Hypertension
Constipation	Increased gastric motility
Coarse, dry skin	Smooth, silky skin
Cold intolerance	Heat intolerance
"Marble statue" quiet	Restlessness; tremor
Fatigue	Sleeplessness
Delayed relaxation of deep tendon reflexes	Brisk deep tendon reflexes
Delayed dental development	Proptosis

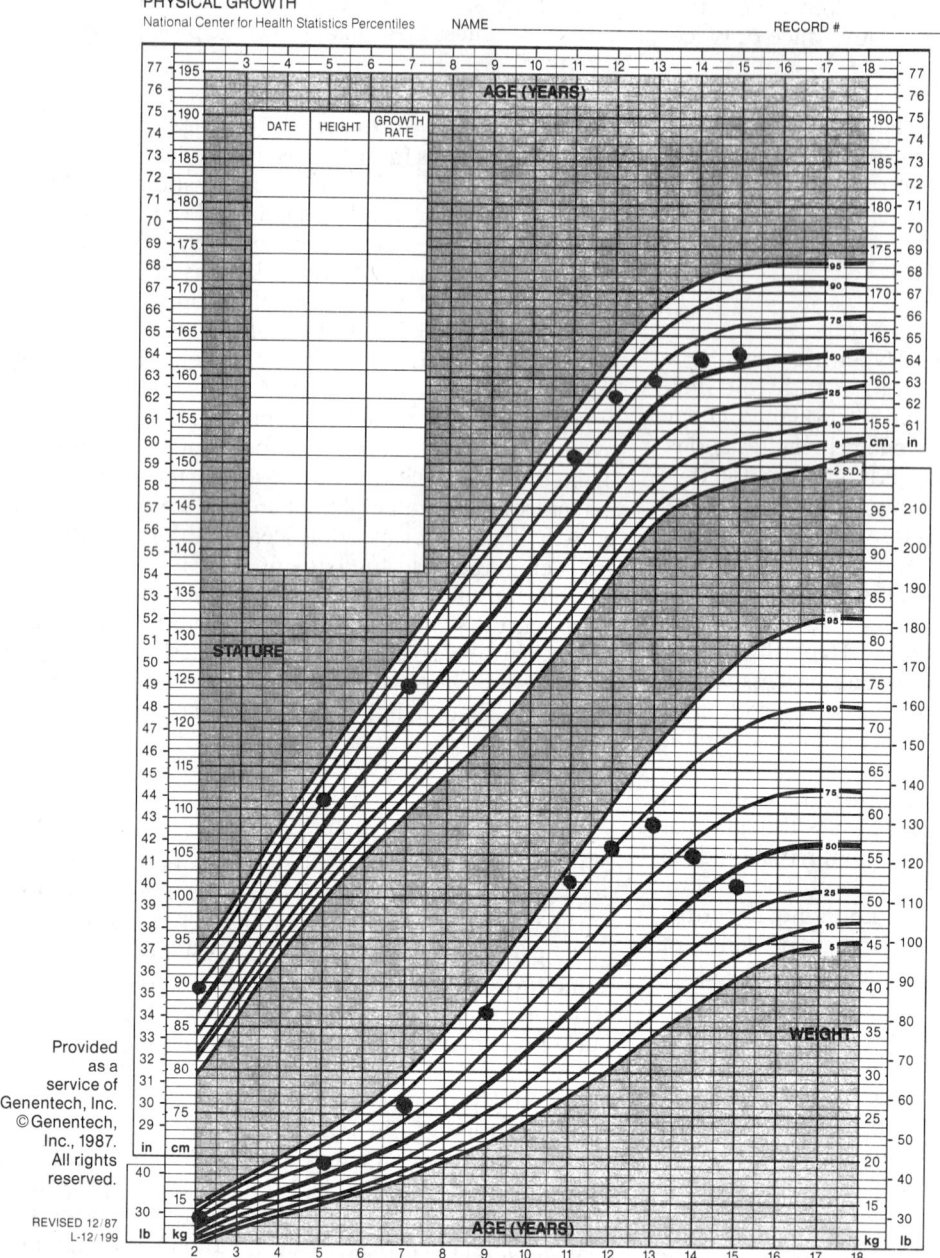

GIRLS: 2 TO 18 YEARS
PHYSICAL GROWTH
National Center for Health Statistics Percentiles   NAME _____   RECORD # _____

FIGURE 56-2

Typical growth changes for an adolescent girl with Graves disease. Note the weight loss after age 13; she had already achieved her final height. Her weight loss was not due to dieting or exercise, but to the excessive metabolic rate prompted by her high blood concentration of T_4.

Nurses working in the antepartum, labor and birth, and postpartum areas need to obtain a thyroid disease history on every mother. Although mothers with a history of altered thyroid function may have no active symptoms and consider their disease cured, their infants are at high risk.

★ **NURSING DIAGNOSES AND PLANNING**

Based on the assessment data discussed in the previous section and the preceding chapter, the following nursing diagnoses may apply to the family and children with hyperthyroidism:

- High Risk for Activity Intolerance related to effects of excessive metabolic rate.
- Anxiety related to a knowledge deficit about effects of hypothyroidism.

- Altered Nutrition: Less Than Body Requirements related to high caloric demand resulting from high metabolic rate.
- Sleep Pattern Disturbance related to impaired metabolism.
- Impaired Swallowing related to thyroid gland enlargement.
- Altered Growth and Development related to weight loss or inappropriate weight for height.

The nurse and child (or parents) together plan effective care based on the established nursing diagnoses. Several examples of expected outcomes are as follows:

- The parents state the child has curtailed activities following diagnosis.
- The parents and child describe the dose and routine for medication therapy accurately.

- The parents discuss the benefits and risks of surgery or radiation therapy.
- The parents describe strategies used to meet child's nutritional needs.

The nurse plans for the daily care of the child based on both the physician's orders and nursing diagnoses. Some general nursing care goals may include the following:

- The child and family understand the need to continue with a lifelong regimen of medication and monitoring.
- The child gains to optimum weight for height.
- The child develops improved relationships with family and peers.

★ INTERVENTIONS: COLLABORATIVE
   AND INDEPENDENT

Treatment of children with hyperthyroidism is aimed at reducing the overactivity of the thyroid gland. Affected children initially must curtail their activities and avoid physical and emotional stress to avoid additional stress of the body systems.[6] If symptoms are severe and not well-controlled at home, the child might require hospitalization. The cause of hyperthyroidism determines the medical and surgical intervention and influences nursing care.

MEDICATION THERAPY

The initial treatment for Graves disease is to administer oral propylthiouracil (PTU) or another of the thioneamides, such as methimazole (Tapazole). These drugs are accumulated in the thyroid gland and prevent the production of excessive thyroid hormone. When administered to children several times daily, these antithyroid drugs may induce a permanent remission.

PTU is usually the drug of choice because of the speed with which it produces results. Initially, PTU, 300 mg, is given daily, usually 100 mg every 8 hours; dosage may vary with the size of the child and extent of symptoms. If larger daily doses are required, the frequency of administration is increased rather than the amount of each dose.

Clinical improvement generally occurs with the first 2 weeks of administration of PTU and a normal metabolic state is achieved in about 6 weeks. As the thyroid hormone concentration decreases, the dose of PTU is reduced gradually until the child is placed on a maintenance dose of 50 mg every 8 hours. Typically, therapy is continued for at least 1 year; if the thyroid gland is then of normal size and is functioning well, treatment is discontinued.

PTU treatment can cause temporary side-effects, including skin rash, itching, and arthritis, but these reactions are generally mild. Transient leukopenia is not uncommon, and it is typically asymptomatic. Rarely, the drug causes agranulocytosis (severe leukopenia), usually early in the course of treatment, and this reaction often is accompanied by fever and sore throat. In these instances, the PTU is discontinued immediately, and treatment of the infection is begun.

Adrenergic antagonists, such as propranolol (Inderal), may be used as an adjunct to PTU to alleviate severe symptoms that sometimes result from hyperthy-roidism. When beta-blocker agents are required, they are discontinued as soon as a euthyroid state is achieved.

When children are treated with medication, clear directions are given about the nature of the drug and its administration. Side-effects are described, and directions are given about notifying the physician if any of the effects are experienced. Parents are warned that thyrotoxicosis (severe symptoms of hyperthyroidism) may be precipitated by sudden discontinuation of an antithyroid drug. Any barriers to obtaining the necessary medication are identified, and solutions to the problems are explored. A referral to social service agencies may be appropriate.

Nursing care also includes discussions about the long-term management of hyperthyroidism and its prognosis. The nurse's comprehensive understanding of the condition and its medical treatment is invaluable in providing parents with additional information or in reinforcing the physician's explanation.

SURGICAL MANAGEMENT

When drug therapy does not induce a permanent remission, two long-term treatment choices remain: The gland can be surgically removed (thyroidectomy) or the child can ingest oral radioactive iodine to obliterate the gland. This choice is difficult for most families. Surgery may involve a total or partial excision of the thyroid gland. Total removal of the gland results in permanent hypothyroidism. Partial resection may allow for the eventual return of the disease or onset of hypothyroidism. The surgeon decides what amount of thyroid tissue to remove.

Prior to thyroidectomy, the child is treated with antithyroid drugs until a euthyroid state is achieved. About 2 weeks before surgery, Lugol's solution (an iodine preparation) is given in small amounts (5 drops twice a day) to reduce the vascularity and function of the thyroid gland. This medication is bitter and should be diluted in juice or another liquid.

During the surgical procedure, great care is taken to leave the parathyroid glands intact. If the glands are inadvertently removed, profound hypoparathyroidism and hypocalcemia result. Surgical complications are rare when the procedure is performed by highly skilled surgeons, but laryngeal nerve damage and anesthesia mishaps are possible.

Postoperative nursing care focuses on the detection of thyroidtoxicosis ("thyroid storm") the sudden release of excessive thyroid hormone into the bloodstream during surgery.[53] Symptoms include fever, tachycardia, diaphoresis, shock, and death, if untreated. This crisis can occur any time within the first postoperative day, but it is most likely to occur during the surgical procedure.

Postoperative nursing observations also include the recognition of hypocalcemia in the event that the parathyroid glands were accidentally damaged or removed during surgery. Symptoms of irritability to external stimuli, gastrointestinal disturbance (vomiting, abdominal cramping, and diarrhea), convulsions, and tetany should be reported immediately, because the condition can be fatal.

RADIATION THERAPY

Radioactive iodine (I^{131}) is used to obliterate the thyroid gland when medical treatment is not feasible or effective and surgery is contraindicated or refused. This treatment is seldom selected, however, because of concerns about exposure to radiation that could result in complications, including thyroid carcinoma, leukemia, thyroid nodules, and genetic mutations. With this form of treatment, however, the actual exposure to radiation is extremely low, and long-term risks are negligible.[6] The radiation option eventually results in permanent hypothyroidism, requiring lifelong administration of synthetic thyroid hormone tablets to maintain a euthyroid state.

PSYCHOSOCIAL SUPPORT

Children with hyperthyroidism and their families benefit from nursing interventions related to the management of symptoms while waiting for the selected method of treatment to take effect. Because these children are overactive and susceptible to fatigue, they need a quiet environment in which rest can be encouraged. Their sensitivity to warmth may necessitate dressing in layers that can be discarded if room temperature cannot be adequately controlled. Physical activity is restricted to conserve energy. School-age children may be able to continue their classroom work, but active play needs to be minimized until symptoms improve.

Disruptive behaviors related to hyperthyroidism should be explained to teachers. Affected children often experience emotional outbursts that they are unable to control; these episodes may embarrass the child and interfere with peer relationships. Decreased environmental stress and promotion of relaxation strategies help children remain in better control of their behavior.

DIET THERAPY

Children's increased metabolic rate increases their daily nutritional needs. Foods of good nutritional value are preferred to those that provide only calories, and vitamin supplements may be needed. Appetites of children with

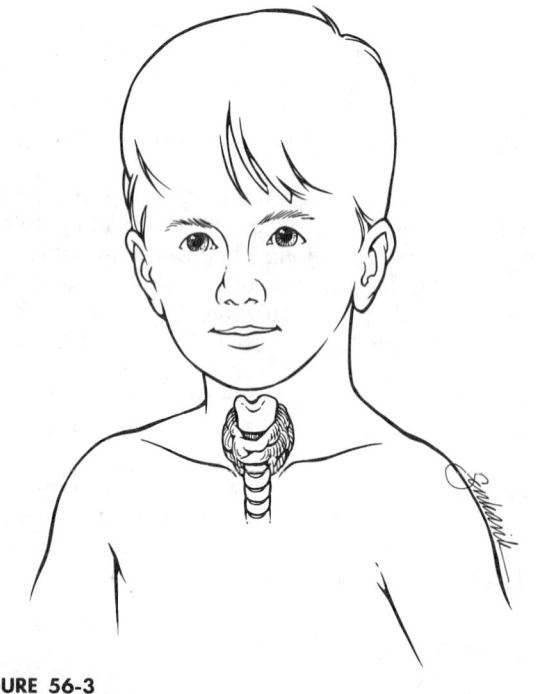

FIGURE 56-3
Simple goiter.

hyperthyroidism typically are better satisfied with smaller, more frequent meals during the day and evening. Fears about gaining weight are allayed with explanations about the impact of the increased metabolic rate. Referral to a nutritional counselor may be helpful to parents in managing this aspect of their child's condition.

★ EVALUATION

The nurse and family periodically evaluate the outcomes of care given. Examples of outcomes for the child and family with hyperthyroidism were given under planning in this section. Have short-term goals been met? Are long-term goals still realistic?

LONG-TERM CARE

Follow-up care for children with hyperthyroidism is needed to monitor the effectiveness of treatment. Surveillance of serum concentration of T_4 and TSH are essential, as is alertness to side-effects of medications. If remission is achieved with medical intervention alone, the possibility of relapse is explained to children and their parents.

Children whose thyroid gland has been surgically removed or obliterated by radioactive iodine need lifelong replacement of thyroid hormone. Adequate replacement can be ascertained only with regular evaluation by health care providers. The child's and family's familiarity with symptoms of inadequate or excessive thyroid replacement needs to be assured.

Goiter

A goiter is an enlargement of the thyroid gland, and it may occur as the result of either hypothyroidism or hyperthyroidism. The condition also has been noted in people who have normal function of the thyroid gland. When thyroid enlargement occurs in a euthyroid person and does not result from inflammation or neoplastic disease, it is called a *simple* or *colloid goiter* (Fig. 56-3). Incidence of this condition is highest in girls before and during pubertal years.

In most children who have simple goiters, no extrinsic cause of the condition is discovered, and iodine deficiency is rarely identified. Therefore, simple goiters are believed to result from some intrinsic, possibly inborn, abnormality.

Simple goiters are evaluated with thyroid antibody titers and radionuclide iodine studies. Children generally have no symptoms other than the enlarged thyroid gland, which is palpated during the physical examination. Some children with simple goiters are treated with L-thyroxine to prevent the development of nodules. Other children are not treated, but the size and progression of the goiter is monitored.

In cases of goiter from thyroiditis, L-thyroxine may be given to reduce the thyromegaly. This treatment is instituted even when the enlarged thyroid gland produces enough thyroxine, because an external supply of thyroxine reduces the demands of TSH on the thyroid gland and allows the gland to rest and eventually return to its normal size.

Altered Adrenal Gland Function

The adrenal gland produces an array of hormones, some of which are also synthesized elsewhere in the body (see Chap. 54). Cortisol and aldosterone are essential to life. Under the action of the adrenocorticotropic hormone (ACTH) produced by the pituitary gland, the adrenal cortex releases cortisol continuously, but increases production in times of physical or emotional stress. Disorders that prevent the production or release of these hormones present some of the most devastating and dangerous endocrine problems seen in children. Specific adrenal conditions are numerous, and only a few seen in children have been selected for discussion in this chapter.

Primary Adrenal Insufficiency: Addison Disease

Definition and Incidence. Primary adrenal insufficiency (also called *primary adrenocortical insufficiency*) results when the adrenal gland is damaged or absent. This condition exists in numerous forms, and a review of medical literature reveals that no consistent presentation of the disorders exists. One way to consider adrenocortical insufficiency, however, is to compare the chronic with the acute form. The term *Addison disease* is used to denote the chronic condition that develops gradually as the adrenal cortex is destroyed and cannot produce sufficient amounts of the glucocorticoid cortisol and the mineralocorticoid aldosterone. Acute adrenocortical insufficiency results with destruction of adrenal tissue.

Etiology and Pathophysiology. *Chronic primary adrenal insufficiency* (Addison disease) may result from a variety of conditions, the most common of which is idiopathic atrophy of the adrenal gland. This condition is thought to result from an autoimmune process in which the body, for some unknown reason, develops antibodies against adrenal tissue. Under the direction of the immune system, the adrenal cortex is slowly destroyed. Addison disease sometimes appears in conjunction with other autoimmune conditions, such as insulin-dependent diabetes mellitus (IDDM), Hashimoto thyroiditis, and acquired immune deficiency syndrome (AIDS).

Infectious diseases also constitute an important etiology of Addison disease. Tuberculosis once was a relatively common cause of adrenocortical destruction. Systemic fungal infections also are known to contribute to gradual degeneration of the adrenal cortex.

Acute adrenocortical insufficiency may be attributed to trauma, such as adrenal hemorrhage in the newborn following prolonged labor and the difficult delivery of a large infant.[55] Fulminating infections may also cause acute symptoms. For example, meningococcemia may lead to adrenal hemorrhage with secondary cardiovascular shock (Waterhouse-Friderichsen syndrome). In other instances, metastatic disease or its treatment with radiation therapy leads to rapid destruction of the adrenal gland. The adrenal gland also may be absent or hypoplastic at birth.

Because 90% of adrenocortical function can be lost before symptoms become apparent, children with adrenal dysfunction may not appear ill; however, they are at great risk for severe complications when they are sick. The marginally adequate adrenal reserves suddenly become inadequate to meet the rising demand for cortisol during times of stress.

Diminished amounts of aldosterone from the adrenal cortex result in fluid and electrolyte imbalance because the distal tubules of the nephrons are unable to conserve sodium. Sodium, therefore, is lost in increasing amounts through the kidneys. As the volume of extracellular fluid is depleted, blood volume diminishes and blood pressure decreases. Serum concentration of sodium decreases (hyponatremia), and potassium concentration increases (hyperkalemia) because the cation exchange in the distal tubules can no longer take place at a normal rate. Decreased amounts of cortisol from the adrenal cortex result in a decline in hepatic gluconeogenesis and an increase in tissue glucose uptake. Hypoglycemia results and gives rise to clinical symptoms that are described in the following paragraphs. The presence of hypoglycemia in a child with symptoms of shock suggests the diagnosis of acute adrenal hyposecretion, because blood sugar is increased by the "stress hormones" in persons with normally functioning adrenal glands.

As the concentration of circulating adrenal hormones decreases, the intrinsic feedback mechanism stimulates secretion of ACTH and melanocyte-stimulating hormone (MSH) from the pituitary gland.

Clinical Manifestations. The onset of symptoms of Addison disease may be so gradual that they are unrecognized until the affected child is seen in the pediatrician's office for a discussion of signs that may be vague. Other children will be diagnosed with acute adrenocortical hypofunction when they become gravely ill following a minor illness or trauma. Infants born without adrenal glands are gravely ill immediately or soon after birth.

Chronic deficiency of the adrenocortical hormones results in weakness, anorexia, and weight loss due to altered carbohydrate metabolism and electrolyte imbalances. Although anorexia is common, affected children may crave salty foods because of the sodium deficit. If hypoadrenalism is untreated, gastrointestinal symptoms, including nausea, vomiting, and diarrhea, develop. Dehydration (flushed skin, elevated temperature, and dry mucous membranes) may ensue.

Children with chronic adrenocortical insufficiency often appear to have a suntan with no bathing suit lines because of the elevated MSH. Pigmentation may be apparent first on the face and hands and especially noticeable on the areolae and genitalia. Increased pigmentation may also be seen on the gums, in the palmar creases, and at pressure points, such as the elbow and the knee. Chronically low cortisol and aldosterone production also causes hypotension and a diminished heart rate. Children may appear fatigued and listless because of their altered stress response ability.

Some children with Addison disease have a history of recent emotional problems and may be in counseling for behavior disturbances. Depression has been reported as the psychiatric symptom seen most often in association with adrenal failure. Moodiness and withdrawal may be early signs. These problems are a result of pathophysiologic changes, not all of which are well understood.

Children with acute adrenal insufficiency may present in a condition that quickly becomes life-threatening. An adrenal crisis occurs when there is severe depletion of cortisol due to either an increased need for cortisol or a decreased availability of cortisol. A child with a severe injury that destroys both adrenal glands also experiences an adrenal crisis. Some children may have an acute adrenal injury, leading to an adrenal crisis that resolves and never becomes a chronic condition. This circumstance is typically seen in the intensive care setting with children who have had extensive abdominal surgery or trauma.

Adrenal crisis precipitates gastrointestinal symptoms such as nausea, vomiting, and diarrhea that may be accompanied by signs of central nervous system involvement (convulsions, stupor, and coma). As the child's condition deteriorates, the pulse becomes rapid and weak, blood pressure declines, respirations become shallow, and the skin becomes cold, clammy, and cyanotic. These signs herald circulatory collapse, which is fatal when the condition is untreated.

Newborns with acute primary adrenal insufficiency are gravely ill shortly after birth and are in danger of seizures, shock due to hypoglycemia, and electrolyte imbalance. Symptoms such as tachycardia, tachypnea, hyperpyrexia (fever), cyanosis, cold and clammy skin, and hypotension are obvious signs of the critical nature of the problem. These infants do not have the hyperpigmentation seen in older children with long-standing adrenal hypofunction.

Diagnostic Studies. When adrenal failure is suspected, measurements of serum cortisol, glucose, and electrolyte levels are obtained immediately, because these children are at risk for shock and vascular collapse. If the child is already in shock, the diagnosis may be made using clinical manifestations alone, and treatment with replacement fluid and hormones begins immediately. Laboratory values are not consistent, but hypoglycemia, hyponatremia, and hyperkalemia often are evident in primary adrenocortical insufficiency. The plasma concentration of cortisol is low in an early-morning specimen or when the child is stressed. Urinary free cortisol may be subnormal.[55]

Antibody testing shows a high antibody titer to the adrenal gland in children with Addison's disease. Serum antibodies for other endocrine glands at risk for autoimmune destruction, such as the thyroid, gonad, and pancreas, are checked.

Further blood testing may be performed to assess the integrity of the hypothalamic-pituitary-adrenal axis. An intravenous injection of synthetic ACTH causes a healthy adrenal gland to increase secretion of cortisol within 30 to 60 minutes. When ACTH is given to a child with a damaged adrenal gland, the cortisol concentration remains unchanged.

Abdominal x-rays, ultrasonography, and CT scans may be helpful in diagnosing adrenal disease or damage. An electrocardiogram may reflect the changes associated with hyperkalemia. An electroencephalogram may show changes in brain wave patterns.

★ ASSESSMENT

The nurse's primary concern for children with Addison disease is the potential for circulatory collapse and shock. Admission to the hospital is expected for infants or children with severe illness at the time of diagnosis. Securing intravenous access is the first priority, but blood studies are obtained rapidly to determine the extent of the existing fluid and electrolyte imbalances. Other diagnostic tests may be performed depending on the seriousness of the presenting signs and symptoms.

The nursing history should include the diet profile of the child, especially exploring the symptom of salt craving. This investigation may help ascertain the onset and duration of the disorder. Any concerns about the child's recent school performance and behavior are included in the history. A history of linear growth and weight gain is obtained and plotted on a growth chart. A recent history of weight loss is not uncommon, and growth may have been inhibited. Chronic exhaustion and an increased desire for sleep are noted. A review of body systems may elicit information about the gastrointestinal symptoms mentioned previously.

Physical examination includes recumbent and sitting blood pressure measurement to assess for postural hypotension, determination of the heart rate, and examination of the skin for areas of increased pigmentation. Height and weight measurements are compared with previous observations to determine growth patterns. Abdominal tenderness may be present in children who have gastrointestinal complaints.

Because androgens are produced by the adrenal cortex as well as by the gonads, sexual development of the child is noted. Preadolescent and adolescent girls may have less pubic and axillary hair development than is expected for their age and degree of breast development. The ovaries contribute androgens and stimulates some sexual hair development, but many girls will never have much sexual hair as a result of the loss of adrenal function. Testicular androgens in boys overwhelm their adrenal androgens, and they generally do not experience altered sexual development.

★ NURSING DIAGNOSES AND PLANNING

Based on assessment data discussed in the previous section and the preceding chapter, the following nursing diagnoses may apply to the family and children with primary adrenal insufficiency:

- Anxiety (Child and Parents) related to insufficient knowledge about illness and its treatment.
- Fluid Volume Deficit related to abnormal fluid loss.
- Altered Nutrition: Less Than Body Requirements related to anorexia.
- Activity Intolerance related to fatigue and generalized weakness.

The nurse and child (or parents) together plan effective care based on the established nursing diagnoses. Several examples of expected outcomes are as follows:

- The parents describe the plan for drug therapy at home and side effects of the drugs administered.
- The parents demonstrate competence in injection techniques.
- The parents discuss strategies to be used to improve fluid and dietary intake to desired levels.
- The parents express diminished anxiety as the child's condition stabilizes.

The nurse plans for the daily care of the child based on both the physician's orders and nursing diagnoses. Some general nursing care goals may include the following:

- Medications are taken as prescribed.
- The child's height and weight patterns indicate steady growth.
- The child's normal activity patterns are resumed.

★ INTERVENTIONS: COLLABORATIVE AND INDEPENDENT

Many children with adrenocortical insufficiency begin treatment as outpatients. Children with severe electrolyte imbalances or dangerous hypotension, however, need hospitalization to correct their electrolyte concentrations. All children with this disorder require the specialized expertise of a pediatric endocrinologist. Nursing care of the hospitalized child focuses on adequate replacement of hormones, fluid, and electrolytes, as well as close monitoring of clinical symptoms and serum electrolytes. Education of the child and parents is essential to relieving their anxiety and promoting adherance to the medical regimen.

FLUID AND ELECTROLYTE REPLACEMENT

Treatment for acute adrenal insufficiency must be immediate and intense to restore balance of electrolytes, fluids, and hormones. An intravenous solution of 0.9% saline solution in 5% glucose is used to correct hypoglycemia and sodium loss. During the first hour of therapy, the child should receive 20 ml/kg of the fluid, but the rate is adjusted to provide 60 mg/kg over the following 24 hours.[55] A gradual resumption of oral fluid intake diminishes the risk of nausea and vomiting, which would lead to further dehydration.

HORMONE REPLACEMENT

In acute adrenocortical insufficiency, a high concentration of blood cortisol is achieved with a water-soluble preparation of hydrocortisone given with intravenous fluids. Large doses can be used safely; infants may receive as much as 25 mg at 6-hour intervals, and older children may receive 75 mg at 6-hour intervals during the first 24 hours. The dose may be reduced during the next 24 hours if the child's condition improves. After 48 hours, intravenous fluids may be discontinued and oral preparations of cortisol and aldosterone administered.

With chronic adrenal insufficiency, both glucocorticoids (cortisol) and mineralcorticoids (aldosterone) must be replaced. Cortisol is replaced with hydrocortisone tablets (Cortef), given three to four times a day or cortisone acetate given twice or three times daily. Prednisone, which needs to be given only twice daily, is avoided during the growing years because it is much more growth suppressive than hydrocortisone. Physiologic production of cortisol is 15 to 20 mg/m² (body surface area) per day, but adequate replacement doses vary among individual children. Gastric irritation may accompany administration of cortisone but may be minimized by ingestion with food or the use of an antacid.

Aldosterone is replaced once or twice daily with fludrocortisone acetate (Florinef Acetate) tablets, at a dose of 0.05 to 0.2 mg daily. This medication does not need to be increased during times of stress or illness. All these medications are well tolerated by children.

Although the adrenal cortex produces androgens, these hormones also are supplied by the gonads; supplemental dosages are unnecessary for boys or girls with primary adrenal insufficiency.

MONITORING PHYSICAL SIGNS

When the child is hospitalized, the nurse monitors the blood pressure and intake and output closely.[55] Accurate and frequent blood pressure measurement is important because hypotension indicates inadequate hormone replacement and electrolyte imbalance. In contrast, hypertension may signal excessive replacement. Hydration is assessed by carefully recording intake and output and by observation of skin turgor. Level of consciousness should be assessed regularly while the child is acutely ill.

DIET THERAPY

Children must have free access to salt and salty foods. Despite fludrocortisone coverage, they may continue to lose sodium and experience salt craving. Parents should be told that an increase in the desire for salt may be a sign of hormone imbalance. This symptom should prompt parents to call the physician, who may increase the child's medication doses and ask them to go to a laboratory to obtain electrolyte studies.

TEACHING

Once the child has been stabilized, the emphasis of nursing care shifts to education about the long-term implications of adrenocortical insufficiency. For children who have experienced a severe illness, the need for daily medication is clear. Children with minimal symptoms, however, may not believe the need is great, and they may tire quickly of taking the multiple doses of medication that are required daily.

Parents need to understand the function of the adrenal gland so they can appropriately substitute for its function. In times of stress, the normal adrenal gland increases its production of cortisol, and this response must be mimicked in the child with adrenal insufficiency. A rule-of-thumb approach is that when a child has a minor illness, the cortisol dose should be doubled at each administration until the child is well. A more serious illness that keeps the child home from school requires a tripling of the dose.

Vomiting, accidents, severe fatigue, surgery, and other highly stressful situations produce immediate and intense needs that can best be met with an injection of hydrocortisone. Parents must be educated in the administration of intramuscular injections. They are instructed to give the injection immediately when the need is recognized, before they call the physician or go to the emergency department.

Most parents are reluctant to give their child intramuscular injections even when they have been taught the technique. By hesitating to provide this injection to their child, the child becomes more ill and in risk of shock and death. Parents who witness the miraculous recovery of an almost comatose child after an injection of cortisol will never hesitate again. Giving an unnecessary dose of cortisol has little impact on the health of a child, but failing to give a needed dose may lead to a fatal outcome. All children must wear medical alert tags that explain their dependency on cortisol (Fig. 56-4). These tags are not safe for infants to wear but can be secured to their car seats.

Many parents have fears about the use of steroids for their children. They may have heard about the side-effects of prednisone, such as acne, hirsutism, buffalo hump, and obesity. These parents need to be taught about the difference between replacement of missing hormones and use (or abuse) of steroids for other purposes. They also need to be aware that chronic overdosage with the prescribed replacement hormones leads to weight gain and

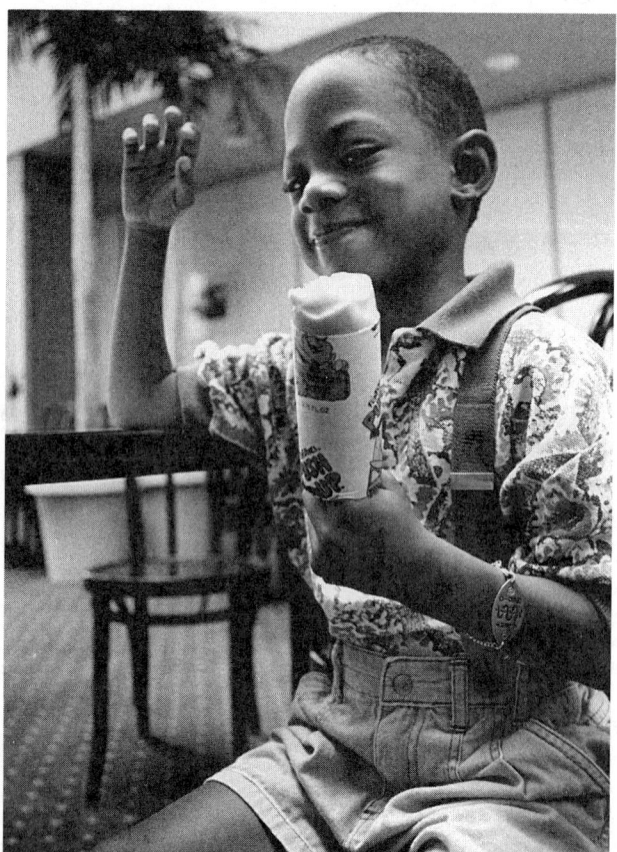

FIGURE 56-4
Medic Alert tags may be worn for a variety of conditions that require specific care in case of injury or emergencies. (Photo by Kathy Sloane.)

poor growth and that follow-up visits are vital to monitoring these patterns.

PSYCHOSOCIAL SUPPORT

Parents of infants or children who experience adrenal crisis need much emotional support. As with any critically ill child, parents needs information about the nature of the child's condition and regular progress reports about the child's response to treatment. Because the child's physiologic response to drug therapy is generally rapid and dramatic, each sign of improvement is encouraging to frightened parents.

Emotional lability is sometimes seen in Addison disease, despite excellent control. The cause of this disturbance is unknown. Families may benefit from counseling, and if the nurse is unable to provide adequate assistance, a referral should be made to a mental health professional who is knowledgeable about the impact of chronic illness on children and their families.

★ **EVALUATION**

The nurse and family periodically evaluate the outcomes of care given. Examples of outcomes for the child and family with primary adrenal insufficiency were given under planning in this section. Have the short-term goals been met? Are the long-term goals still realistic? Planning for further nursing care takes complications and long-term care into consideration.

COMPLICATIONS

Children with Addison disease are at risk for other autoimmune endocrine deficiencies as well. These conditions generally occur later in the adolescent or adult years. Regular physical examinations will screen for these problems. Serum antibodies to the gonads, thyroid, and pancreas are obtained when there are concerns about disease in these glands.

LONG-TERM CARE

Children with primary adrenal insufficiency need to be seen several times each year in the pediatric endocrinologist's office or clinic to monitor their physical condition, including blood pressure, heart rate, weight and height gains, and degree of skin pigmentation. Serum electrolytes are obtained, and testing may include urine sodium concentration to measure the adequacy of the fludrocortisone dose.

Children with well-controlled primary adrenal failure should grow and develop normally. During times of illness, they require additional doses of cortisol, and they may need daily electrolyte determinations at an outpatient clinic for the duration of the stressful period. They are not at risk for more illnesses than are their siblings, but they require more care when they are ill.

Over-production of melanin may continue to cause a slightly tanned appearance, even in children with well-controlled Addison's disease. There is no health risk associated with this finding. A change in pigmentation, however, may be associated with high levels of ACTH and is indicative of poor cortisol coverage. This development should prompt a re-evaluation.

Congenital Adrenal Hyperplasia

Definition and Incidence. Congenital adrenal hyperplasia (CAH) is a group of conditions that can cause adrenocortical insufficiency. Each condition results from a deficiency of one of the enzymes needed for normal synthesis of hormones by the adrenal cortex. In its classic form, CAH is a life-threatening condition that occurs in 1 in 12,000 births in the United States.[69] Infants generally are diagnosed at birth or shortly thereafter. CAH is also known as *adrenogenital syndrome* or *congenital virilizing adrenogenital syndrome* because of the effect the adrenal hormones can have on the genitals of the newborn child.

Late-onset CAH (also called cryptic CAH) is a condition recognized relatively recently that occurs primarily in girls and women. These individuals present later in childhood with symptoms of excessive androgen production. They seldom have severe cortisol deficiency but experience hirsutism and menstrual irregularities.

Etiology and Pathophysiology. In CAH the adrenal glands are intact, but one of the enzymes needed to synthesize cortisol (and sometimes aldosterone) is absent. The common type of CAH (90%) is an autosomal recessive disorder that causes deficiency of 21-hydroxylase, an enzyme that is essential to form both cortisol and aldosterone. This deficiency results in the severest form of the disorder. Another type of CAH is due to 11-β-hydroxylase deficiency, which blocks the production of cortisol, but not aldosterone. Other rare enzyme deficiencies may occur as well.

At 3 months' gestation, the fetus already produces its own supply of cortisol.[69] Lack of cortical response stimulates (through the negative feedback loop to the pituitary) an excessive ACTH response. This continual ACTH message to the adrenal glands results in hyperplasia of adrenal tissue, and because the adrenal pathway to androgen production is not blocked, excessive androgen production is stimulated. High concentrations of testosterone during the 12th to the 20th weeks of fetal development stimulate excessive growth and development of the external genitalia of female infants, a process known as *virilization*. The genitalia of male infants with CAH may be unaffected or somewhat enlarged.

Clinical Manifestations. CAH is generally diagnosed at birth or within a few weeks. Fetal genital development is under the direction of circulating hormones, regardless of the child's karyotypes.[55] Some girls may be so fully masculinized at birth that immediate determination of the baby's gender is impossible or that male gender is mistakenly assigned (pseudohermaphroditism). In mild cases, female infants have only a slightly enlarged clitoris, but in severely affected infants, the clitoris has a distinct penile shape, including urethral displacement onto the shaft of the clitoris. The labia may be rugated and fused, appearing scrotal. The vagina may be incomplete, ending in a blind pouch. In spite of the external appearance, the uterus and ovaries are normal, because their development is directed by the female chromosome pattern.

Male infants with CAH often escape detection at birth. They can have somewhat large genitals for age and increased pigmentation of the scrotum, but these characteristics may be considered normal by the examiner. However, at 5 to 10 days of age, they may develop a severe electrolyte imbalance with symptoms of adrenal crisis, including dehydration, vomiting, wasting, and shock. This presentation is a medical emergency, described earlier as acute adrenocortical insufficiency.[67] CAH occurs with varying amounts of salt wasting, depending on which enzymes are missing from the complex process of steroid production.[69]

Children with partial enzyme absence may be diagnosed with CAH during childhood. Sufficient cortisol and aldosterone may be produced to meet daily needs, but a severe illness results in collapse. Undiagnosed children with this condition grow quickly due to the effects of excessive androgens and are very tall for their age. Girls may have clitoromegaly; boys often have an enlarged penis, scrotum, and prostate. Both sexes develop pubic and axillary hair; acne is common. If these children are not treated, the adrenal androgens may mature the hypothalamic-pituitary axis and initiate true precocious puberty. They may have rapid advancement of bone maturation, leading to premature closure of the epiphyses and significantly short adult stature.

Diagnostic Studies. When children present with signs of adrenal crisis, serum electrolyte levels are obtained immediately to determine the extent of sodium depletion. Serum concentration of adrenal steroids are obtained using RIA. In fact, routine screening for CAH in newborns has been proposed to facilitate earlier diagnosis and treatment.[69] The implementation of this program has begun in several states. If the ACTH stimulation test is performed, serum concentration of 17-hydroxyprogesterone (17-OHP) are elevated in classic CAH. Unstimulated 17-OHP is elevated, as well.

Chromosome studies are needed in children with any degree of sexual ambiguity so that genetic gender can be established. Ultrasound studies are done to assess development of the vaginal vault and uterus in girls with CAH. Procedures for prenatal diagnosis of CAH with genetic analysis of amniotic fluid or chorionic villus biopsy have been developed in recent years.[69]

★ **ASSESSMENT**

Newborns with CAH are often critically ill and may be sent to a tertiary care center after their electrolyte levels have been stabilized. Care for children with adrenal crisis is described in the section on primary adrenal insufficiency.

All somatic measures are obtained and accurately recorded. Children diagnosed in later childhood need a growth chart developed to visualize previous patterns of growth. The genitalia should be carefully examined and described in the record. Notation is made of any intercurrent illnesses and the need to increase cortisol either orally or by injection. Patterns of salt craving are noted. Psychosocial assessment includes information about gender identity, school performance, and behavior.

Developing a genogram with the parents helps reveal

previous infant deaths, stillbirths, or sudden, unexplained deaths. Notation is made of any relatives who matured quickly or who were exceptionally short adults. These findings may have been the result of undetected CAH and cortisol deficiency.

★ NURSING DIAGNOSES AND PLANNING

Based on assessment data discussed in the previous section and the preceding chapter, the following nursing diagnoses may apply to the family and child with congenital adrenal hyperplasia:

- Fluid Volume Deficit related to abnormal fluid loss.
- Anxiety related to lack of knowledge about the newborn's chronic illness and/or sexual ambiguity.
- Body Image Disturbance related to sexual ambiguity.
- Altered Growth and Development related to hormone imbalance and failure to follow expected growth and maturation patterns.
- Sexual Dysfunction in females related to virilization of the genitalia.

The nurse and child (or parents) together plan effective care based on the established nursing diagnoses. Several examples of expected outcomes are as follows:

- The mother discusses the benefits of breast feeding.
- The parents describe their feelings about the gender decision.
- The child demonstrates comfort with the gender identity.
- The child exhibits behavior appropriate to age group.

The nurse plans for the daily care of the child based on both the physician's orders and nursing diagnoses. Some general nursing care goals may include the following:

- Parents understand the implications of their decisions regarding gender.
- Therapeutic levels of hormones are maintained.
- Fluid and electrolyte balance is maintained.

★ INTERVENTIONS: COLLABORATIVE AND INDEPENDENT

The priorities of care for children with CAH depend on clinical manifestations of the condition. Children in adrenal crisis need intense care, as described earlier. The birth of an infant with ambiguous genitalia who is not critically ill may require only the care generally given to any newborn. However, the parents' need for education and psychosocial support is obvious.

HORMONE REPLACEMENT

Treatment for the child with CAH is aimed at two related goals. The first is to supply the essential hormones that will stabilize electrolytes and fluid balance, and the second is to decrease the production of ACTH and to prevent further stimulation of androgen (testosterone) production. ACTH is released when the body has insufficient cortisol, so achieving the first goal also resolves the second. Achievement of these goals is a difficult task. Cortisol needs are not smooth and predictable, especially in infancy. Undertreatment with cortisol leads to increased ACTH production (excessive androgens) and risk of adrenal crisis with vascular collapse. Overtreatment leads to excessive weight gain and growth failure. The pattern of oral cortisol replacement supplies a child's daily needs and suppresses the normal early-morning secretion of ACTH. This goal can be achieved by supplying the largest dose of cortisol at bedtime. The other doses are scheduled throughout the day, generally on awakening and in the early afternoon.

DIET THERAPY

In the newborn, a diagnosis of CAH is a good reason to promote and support breast-feeding. Children who are breast-fed are less likely to vomit, and breast milk, with its increased sodium content, is the ideal food for the salt-wasting infant.[13] If additional sodium is needed, parents are given a prescription or directions for preparing saline supplements. Older children with adrenal insufficiency require free access to table salt and foods rich in sodium. This freedom can be an adjustment for health-conscious parents who have limited the use of these foods and do not use table salt. Additional salt usually is required during hot weather and for sustained physical exertion due to increased sodium loss through the skin. Parents are instructed to observe their child's eating habits pertaining to the need for salt. A pattern of increased desire for salty foods might signal that the child is receiving insufficient medication.

PSYCHOSOCIAL SUPPORT

The birth of a child with CAH is a crisis for the family.[13] This is especially true when the newborn has ambiguous genitals and the parents are unable to announce the gender to family and friends. There can be no fast answers, because the laboratory studies required for diagnosis may take several days (see section on ambiguous genitalia in Chap. 68).

The nurse plays a major role in listening to the parents' concerns and in encouraging them to express their feelings. Of great importance is the nurse's role in affirming the gender of the child once it has been established. After this time, the nurse and all staff should refer to the newborn as "she" or "he," never "it" or "the baby." Privacy during diaper changes is important. Attempts to use the virilized girl for teaching purposes with medical or nursing students should be done with great sensitivity for the parents' and child's feelings.

SURGICAL MANAGEMENT

Female infants whose CAH is recognized early often require reconstructive surgery to feminize the appearance of the external genital area. Surgical procedures to decrease the size of the clitoris may be initiated during infancy. Later, surgery may be necessary to create a vaginal outlet for menstrual flow. Some surgeons wait to begin vaginal reconstruction until the girl is old enough to participate in the necessary dilatation of the vagina. Without dilatation, adhesions form. Young women who use tampons or who are having regular sexual intercourse maintain a patent vagina without mechanical dilatation.

These procedures may take place over the course of many years and are intrusive and potentially painful. The nurse assists in preparing the child for surgery with age-appropriate explanations. Although the same procedure may be repeated many times, the child is continually growing and developing new cognitive skills and must be re-educated at each step.

TEACHING

Education of the parents with regard to administering hormone medication, monitoring for signs of deficiency, and providing supplementary injections has already been discussed.

Parents who have a child with ambiguous genitalia or pseudohermaphroditism have many questions about the cause of the condition, the options available for treating the child, and the long-term prognosis. The nurse needs a sound knowledge base about the condition and an ability to explain the complex endocrine anomaly in terminology parents can understand. If surgery is planned, diagrams and pictures of the procedures are extremely useful. An open, unhurried approach to the parents and child encourages them to ask questions until they receive all the information they need. Parents generally need time to reflect on the information they have received and often benefit from the nurse's follow-up. Explanations may need to be repeated, or new information may be desired.

When parents understand that their child's anomaly is a result of an inherited genetic trait, they may experience feelings of guilt. The nurse can acknowledge these feelings and provide reassurance that the condition was not the result of oversight or negligence on their part. Referral to a spiritual advisor, social worker, or psychologist may be helpful.

GENETIC COUNSELING

Because the parents of a child with CAH are both carriers of the autosomal recessive gene, they need to be advised that future pregnancies incur a 25% risk that the child will have CAH. Some physicians prescribe high doses of cortisol for these mothers early in a future pregnancy to decrease ACTH production and virilization in the fetus. Amniocentesis is performed in the second trimester to determine the sex of the child and the need for continued treatment. If the fetus is female, the mother will continue cortisol therapy to decrease virilization of the fetus. Treatment usually begins before 12 weeks of pregnancy, but it is currently unclear how effective this regimen can be. All parents should be referred to an endocrine specialist for management of future pregnancies.

★ EVALUATION

The nurse and family periodically evaluate the outcomes of care given. Examples of outcomes for the child and family with congenital adrenal hyperplasia were given under planning in this section. Have the short-term goals been met? Are the long-term goals still realistic? Planning for further nursing care takes complications and long-term care into consideration.

COMPLICATIONS

Girls with poorly controlled CAH may have excessive virilization, including hirsutism (male patterns of body hair), clitoromegaly, and menstrual irregularities.[69] Overtreatment leads to excessive weight gain and poor growth.[55]

Frequent blood tests and 24-hour urine collections are required to monitor hormone and electrolyte balance. Testicular tumors may occur in boys with poorly suppressed ACTH production.[6]

LONG-TERM CARE

Children with CAH need to be followed closely in the pediatric endocrinology ambulatory care setting. Infants are seen every 2 to 3 months, and older children return at least three times each year. They may grow unusually fast and be taller than their peers, or they may grow poorly and be quite small. If ACTH production is not well suppressed, excessive androgens promote true precocious puberty and closure of the growth plates. These children have a significantly short stature in adulthood.

Adrenal Insufficiency Due to Exogenous Suppression

Definition and Incidence. When children are given cortisol over extended periods to treat illness, the function of their own adrenal glands is suppressed. The high serum concentration of cortisol maintained by medication prevents the normal feedback loop to the hypothalamus or pituitary gland from operating. When the external source of cortisol is withdrawn, the temporary absence of ACTH stimulation to the adrenal gland results in diminished endogenous cortisol production. This condition is termed "adrenal insufficiency due to exogenous suppression." The increasing use of corticosteroids for a variety of childhood illnesses has led to an increasing incidence of this condition.

Etiology and Pathophysiology. With exogenous adrenal suppression, the adrenal glands are healthy, but do not receive ACTH stimulation to produce the essential glucocorticoid, cortisol. Instead, adequate or even excessive circulating levels of cortisol are obtained from an external source. The lack of stimulation produces secondary adrenal cortex atrophy.[55] When the external source of cortisol is removed, the adrenal cortex is unable to respond adequately.

Children may have exogenous adrenal suppression from the use of steroids in the treatment of conditions such as asthma, purpura, and inflammatory bowel disease. Steroid treatment needs to be withdrawn gradually over several weeks to allow the ACTH-adrenal system to recover. Although 90% of children will have a fully functioning ACTH-adrenal system within 6 months of ending treatment, they should be considered at risk for adrenal suppression during illness for as long as 18 months.[55]

Although corticosteroids have been available primarily through prescription in the past, cortisone creams are now available over the counter. These products can make a rash disappear almost overnight. They are believed to be of no harm when used in small amounts but have great potential for innocent abuse. For example, cortisone cream may be used by parents for diaper rash. Even if a thin layer of cortisone cream is applied, the large surface area treated provides a remarkably large dose. This effect is greatly magnified by the waterproof diaper. Occasional use is unlikely to cause adrenal suppression; however, long-term use may contribute to breakdown of the skin, further increasing the absorption rate of the cortisone cream and leading to adrenal suppression.

Clinical Manifestations. Children with exogenous adrenal suppression may present with weight gain and failure to grow, but have no other symptoms. The innocuous signs may progress to profound symptoms when the child becomes ill or is stressed. The symptoms of primary adrenal insufficiency are described in the preceding paragraphs. Excessive long-term cortisol supplementation eventually results in the development of Cushing syndrome.

Diagnostic Studies. When exogenous adrenal suppression is suspected, measurements of serum cortisol and electrolytes are obtained immediately, because these children are at risk for vascular collapse and shock. An ACTH stimulation test is done to determine the adrenal gland's ability to respond to ACTH. After giving an intravenous or intramuscular dose of ACTH, the child with a normal response has a peak serum cortisol level higher than 20 μg/dl or an increase of 10 μg/dl from baseline. If the blood concentration of cortisol remains unchanged, primary rather than secondary insufficiency is suspected.

★ **ASSESSMENT**

When a child presents with symptoms of acute adrenal insufficiency, the primary concern is the potential for collapse and shock. The history should include specific questions about the use of prescribed steroids for existing chronic illness. Asking about the use of diaper rash ointment for infants is important.

★ **NURSING DIAGNOSES AND PLANNING**

In addition to the nursing diagnoses that were described previously in the section on primary adrenal insufficiency, the following may also be applicable:

- Impaired Skin Integrity related to prolonged use of cortisone cream.
- Anxiety related to outcome of acute illness.
- Altered Health Maintenance related to insufficient knowledge about the effects of long-term steroid use.

The nurse and child (or parents) together plan effective care based on the established nursing diagnoses. Several examples of expected outcomes are as follows:

- The parents state they have discontinued using cortisone cream.
- The parents describe the potential effects of long-term steroid use and withdrawal.

The nurse plans for the daily care of the child based on both the physician's orders and nursing diagnoses. Some general nursing care goals may include the following:

- Diminished anxiety as knowledge increases.
- Height and weight gain return to normal for age.

★ **NURSING INTERVENTIONS: COLLABORATIVE AND INDEPENDENT**

Dosages for therapeutic steroids given to children must be carefully tapered over 2 to 4 weeks.[6] The process of weaning children from exogenous steroids may be complicated by the underlying disease, as well as by symptoms of steroid withdrawal such as nausea, vomiting, lethargy, and myalgia. Those children receiving inadvertent cortisol should have the source removed (e.g., the cortisone diaper cream).

★ **EVALUATION**

The nurse and family periodically evaluate the outcomes of care given. Examples of outcomes for the child and family with adrenal insufficiency due to exogenous suppression were given under planning in this section.

The child who has had a temporary suppression of the adrenal gland should have ACTH testing of adrenal responsiveness to determine a return to normal function. Catch-up growth and weight gain may continue for several months. These children may need injections of cortisol before surgical procedures for as long as 12 months following the cessation of their cortisol treatment.[6]

Adrenocorticotropic Hormone Deficiency

Insufficient production of ACTH by the pituitary gland or the cortical releasing factor by the hypothalamus results in an inadequate secretion of the adrenocortical hormones. These conditions may be attributed to hypopituitarism, cranial radiation, or trauma. These children do not produce sufficient cortisol, but their aldosterone levels are within normal limits.

Hyperfunction of the Adrenal Cortex: Cushing Syndrome

Definition and Incidence. *Cushing syndrome* refers to a constellation of clinical findings that results from sustained tissue exposure to excessive cortisol. When excessive ACTH is produced by the pituitary gland and stimulates the adrenal gland to release excessive amounts of hormones, the condition is called *Cushing disease*. These conditions are uncommon in children. However, the incidence of hypercortisolism has increased concomitant with the use of exogenous steroids to treat a host of medical disorders in children.

Etiology and Pathophysiology. During infancy and early childhood (to about the age of 7 years), Cushing syndrome most often results from a malignant adrenal tumor, usually an adenoma or carcinoma.[6,55] Thereafter, tumors of the pituitary gland (basophilic adenomas) are more likely, and they cause secondary adrenal hyperplasia (Cushing disease). Adrenal tumors are rare in childhood, but when they occur, they are exceptionally virulent and have a poor prognosis for long-term survival.

Cushing syndrome also occurs as a side-effect of steroid therapy; this condition may be referred to as a *cushingoid syndrome*. Iatrogenic Cushing syndrome can occur in children receiving cortisol therapy with oral medication or other preparations, such as eye drops and skin creams. Long-term use of these preparations eventually leads to the loss of the ACTH-adrenal feedback loop. Children develop the features of excessive cortisol exposure from an external supply, but their adrenal gland is unable to respond to additional body requirements during times of illness or stress (see earlier section on adrenocortical insufficiency.)

Increased adrenal secretion of cortisol results in an exaggeration of the physiologic actions of cortisol. Cortisol influences metabolism by increasing gluconeogenesis, which results in protein catabolism and fat accumulation.[55] Cortisol also plays a major role in the body's coping defenses against internal and external stressors (see Chap. 54). All these actions are exaggerated in the child with Cushing syndrome.

Clinical Manifestations. Typical signs of excessive cortisol production include gradual but profound growth arrest, with height often below the third percentile on the growth chart. Weight gain, the development of a round face with prominent, flushed cheeks ("moon facies"), and a large pad of fat located on the posterior neck ("buffalo hump") are expected. Obesity is common, but the extremities are thin, and strength is diminished because of muscular wasting. Thinning of the skin and development of purplish striae ("stretch marks") on the hips, abdomen, and thighs are thought due to the loss of collagen. Bruises and petechiae may result from capillary fragility related to protein loss.

Demineralization of the bones, especially the spine, is common and can contribute to bone fractures.[55] Emotional lability or mental disturbances can result from excess cortisol, which influences brain metabolism. Hypertension is not a consistent finding, but it may occur secondary to the salt-retaining activity of cortisol and the resulting increase in blood volume.[55]

If an adrenal tumor also secretes androgens, there may be development of pubic hair and acne, deepening of the voice, and enlargement of the clitoris in girls.[6] These children generally have normal or accelerated growth patterns. However, pubertal development may be delayed, and girls beyond menarche may experience amenorrhea.

Cushing syndrome is sometimes suspected in children who have gained weight rapidly and become obese. A key distinction between Cushing syndrome and exogenous obesity, however, is the linear growth rate. Children who are obese from exogenous causes usually have an excellent rate of growth. Excessive cortisol is growth-suppressive, and children with Cushing syndrome usually fall below expected growth rate norms for their age.

Diagnostic Studies. Blood studies are ordered to determine cortisol and electrolyte concentration. With hyperadrenalism, serum cortisol is increased, but the normal fluctuations that occur in healthy children may make an analysis of the laboratory findings difficult.[6] Serum electrolytes are measured to determine sodium concentration, but they are typically within normal limits. A differential blood cell count may show decreased lymphocytes and eosinophils with increased polymorphonuclear neutrophils and erythrocytes.[55]

Additional studies, such as the synthetic ACTH stimulation test, may be ordered. The ACTH stimulation test can be used to differentiate primary adrenal tumors from other causes of Cushing syndrome. A 6-hour intravenous infusion of ACTH further raises the levels of plasma cortisol in children with adrenal hyperplasia and in some children with adenoma. However, no response is expected in children with adrenal carcinoma or iatrogenic Cushing disease.[55]

Diagnostic urine tests may include a 24-hour collection to measure excretion of cortisol and androgens. Most children with Cushing syndrome have an elevated urinary cortisol level, but androgens may be within normal limits. Ultrasound or scanning with magnetic resonance imaging (MRI) or CT is used to identify tumors in the hypothalamic-pituitary region or in the abdominal area. X-rays may be used to determine bone age.

★ ASSESSMENT

The interview with the child and family includes a discussion to determine the onset of symptoms. Changes in the child's appearance and behavior are reviewed, and the parents' concerns are elicited. Also included in the interview are questions pertaining to possible external cortisol exposure in the form of creams or drops and oral medications for medical disorders. The nurse also asks about other family members taking cortisone preparations. All of the child's current medications should be examined to be certain the child is not receiving cortisol in error.

During the physical examination, the skin is inspected for the characteristic purple striae often seen in areas of weight gain, such as the abdomen and thighs. Rapid weight gain that produces red striae is not due to cortisol excess. The presence of bruises or petechiae is noted, as are the patterns of fat deposits in the body and muscle wasting in the extremities. Vital signs are assessed to determine the presence of hypertension.

★ NURSING DIAGNOSES AND PLANNING

Based on assessment data discussed in the previous section and the preceding chapter, the following nursing diagnoses may apply to the family and child with Cushing syndrome:

- High Risk for Injury related to demineralization of the bones and muscle weakness.
- Decreased Activity Tolerance related to weakness and fatigue.
- Body Image Disturbance related to physical and behavioral changes.
- Altered Health Maintenance related to insufficient knowledge of Cushing syndrome, its causes, symptoms, and treatment.

The nurse and child (or parents) together plan effective care based on the established nursing diagnoses. Several examples of expected outcomes are as follows:

- The child exhibits increased energy and resumes age-appropriate activities.
- The child who has had surgical removal of the adrenal glands or the pituitary gland states he or she is taking replacement hormones as prescribed.
- The child or parents describe the disease process, causes, factors contributing to symptoms, and the procedures for cure or symptom control.

The nurse plans for the daily care of the child based on both the physician's orders and nursing diagnoses. Some general nursing care goals may include the following:

- The child exhibits catch-up growth and reversal of changes in physical appearance.
- Injury is avoided.

★ INTERVENTIONS: COLLABORATIVE AND INDEPENDENT

Nursing care of the child with Cushing syndrome depends on the cause. Tumors of the adrenal or pituitary glands usually require surgical removal of the gland. The loss of the adrenal glands ensures a sudden withdrawal of circulating cortisol. Symptoms of adrenal crisis, discussed earlier, are prevented with carefully prescribed replacement therapy. The surgical removal of the pituitary gland results in panhypopituitarism, the absence of all the hormones normally produced by pituitary tissue. Teaching related to the administration of replacement hormones and to the recognition of danger signs is needed.

Cushing syndrome due to use of steroid preparations or drugs requires a different approach. If the supply of cortisol is from accidental sources, the drug is withdrawn. If the child has been receiving excessive doses of prescribed medication, the dosage is reduced to reverse the symptoms.

★ EVALUATION

The nurse and family periodically evaluate the outcomes of care given. Examples of outcomes for the child and family with Cushing syndrome were given under planning in this section.

Hyperfunction of the Adrenal Medulla: Pheochromocytoma

The adrenal medulla and sympathetic nerve endings produce epinephrine, norepinephrine, and other catecholamines. These hormones protect the child from hypoglycemia by mobilizing energy stores. This mechanism is activated by nutritional needs and in times of stress. The principal disorder of the adrenal medulla is pheochromocytoma.

Definition, Incidence, Etiology, and Pathophysiology. Pheochromocytoma is a tumor of that arises from chromaffin cells, usually in the adrenal medulla. Fewer than 5% of these tumors are reported in children, but when they do occur, more than 50% have multiple tumors. Although most of the tumors are located on the adrenal gland, they may appear at other sites in the abdomen,

chest, or pelvis. The incidence of pheochromocytoma is greater in boys, and the peak age of occurrence is between 9 and 12 years.

Often inherited as an autosomal dominant genetic trait, pheochromocytoma is associated with other syndromes or tumors, but it is generally benign. The overproduction of catecholamines (epinephrine, norepinephrine, and dopamine) by the tumor produces the clinical manifestations of the disorder.

Clinical Manifestations and Diagnostic Studies. The clinical manifestation of pheochromocytoma varies with quantitative variations in tumor secretions, but hypertension is almost always present. Hypertension may be sustained, or it may occur intermittently. Acute hypertensive episodes cause headache, tachycardia, sweating, pallor, and vomiting. Seizures are possible if the hypertension is untreated. Children typically display good appetites, but hypermetabolism prevents weight gain; in fact, growth failure may be pronounced. Symptoms such as polyuria and polydipsia and abdominal or chest pain are also possible, as are orthostatic hypotension, heat intolerance, and diaphoresis. The intermittent occurrence of symptoms in some children may mistakenly suggest a psychological rather than organic cause. Environmental or personal stress may augment symptoms.

A 24-hour urine specimen collected when the child is symptomatic may reveal a concentration of catecholamines and metabolites in excess of 300 μg. Plasma catecholamines may also be measured and reveal high levels. An abdominal MRI or CT scan can detect tumors as small as 1 cm.[44]

★ NURSING IMPLICATIONS

The nursing history should investigate the incidence of similar symptoms in other family members. A description of the onset of symptoms is helpful in determining the organic basis of the disease. The comprehensive physical examination includes careful measurement of the somatic parameters and the blood pressure.

Several nursing diagnoses may apply to the child with pheochromocytoma, depending on the duration of the illness. Two commonly used diagnoses are the following:

- Anxiety related to the acute onset of uncontrollable symptoms.
- Altered Growth and Development related to sustained hypermetabolic state.

The treatment of choice with pheochromocytoma is surgical removal of the tumor. To prevent intraoperative and postoperative complications, children must be placed on medication to achieve pharmacologic control of their symptoms 2 to 3 weeks before surgery is scheduled. An alpha-adrenergic blocking agent, such as phenoxybenzamine (Dibenzyline), is given orally twice a day. Side-effects of these drugs include nasal congestion, gastrointestinal irritation, and hypotension.[44] Propranolol is given as an adjunct.

Preoperative teaching about the effects of the medication and its administration is accompanied by information about the surgical procedure to be performed. The vital signs are monitored frequently, with alertness to degeneration of vascular status and signs of congestive heart failure. Stress reduction measures, such as quiet and rest, are encouraged.

Unilateral or bilateral adrenalectomy is typically performed, depending on the location of the pheochromocytoma. Manipulation of the adrenal gland can precipitate the release of adrenal hormones into the circulation, stimulating an extreme rise in blood pressure. However, a precipitous decrease in blood pressure from the sudden withdrawal of catecholamines places the child at grave risk for shock during surgery and until 48 hours later. If bilateral adrenalectomy is performed, the child is treated for chronic adrenocortical insufficiency with intraoperative hydrocortisone and lifelong oral steroid replacement.

If all existing tumor has been removed, symptoms should abate in the early postoperative period. Long-term follow-up is needed, however, because recurrence of the tumor is possible in later years. Outcome criteria are similar to those described for chronic adrenocortical insufficiency.

Altered Gonadal Function

During puberty many hormonally-mediated changes take place that alter the physical appearance, emotions, behavior, and interests of a child. Distinguishing between what is considered "normal" and "abnormal" may be difficult. Issues pertaining to sexual development and maturation are especially stressful.

A great deal of variation is possible in the timing and pace of normal sexual maturation in children, and the transformation can begin at either end of the normal age range. Likewise, puberty can be completed relatively quickly, or it can continue into young adulthood. Early or late development can be a source of great anxiety for the adolescent and parents. Puberty and maturation of secondary sexual characteristics are discussed in Chapter 66.

Causes for altered timing of puberty may be familial in nature, related to environmental factors, or the result of an underlying disease process. Whatever the cause, the child and family face uncertainty and fear related to the child's future development; these emotions are compounded by the sensitive nature of issues related to sexuality. Children who are obviously different from their peers because of premature or delayed development have many psychosocial needs.

Similar to other endocrine disorders, altered sexual development may be the result of a primary, secondary, or tertiary cause. *Primary causes* are those involving an abnormality or absence of the gonads (testes or ovaries). There may be a lack of stimulation from the pituitary gland (secondary) or the hypothalamus (tertiary). Pituitary and hypothalamic hypofunctions generate conditions that are clinically identical, because both result in inadequate pulsatile release of luteinizing hormone (LH) and follicle-stimulating hormone (FSH), that stimulate the gonads to mature. A comprehensive discussion of the disorders may be found in the medical pediatric endocrinology literature; more common alterations in gonadal function of children have been selected for inclusion in this text.

Delayed Sexual Development

Definition and Incidence. Delayed puberty is defined as the lack of breast development in girls by age 13 to 13.5 years or the lack of testicular enlargement in boys by age 13.5 to 14 years. The failure to progress in puberty to menarche (girls) or to adult genital development (boys) is also defined as delayed sexual development. Although the condition occurs in both genders, boys are more likely to seek evaluation for this problem because of teasing from their peers and an inability to compete successfully in athletic events. All children with the problem, however, require a thorough evaluation.

Etiology and Pathophysiology. Constitutional delay of adolescence represents one end of the spectrum of normal variation in the timing and pace of puberty. It is the most frequent cause of delayed puberty. In many instances, there is a family history of relatives who entered puberty later than did their peers. This variant is considered a normal pattern and requires no treatment. These children eventually achieve full sexual maturity, although often not until age 20 or older.

Delayed puberty can be related to deficiency of gonadotropin-releasing hormone (GnRH) produced in the hypothalamus or gonadotropins (LH and FSH) produced in the pituitary gland. A wide variety of conditions, which are summarized in the accompanying display on causes of delayed development, may affect the production of these hormones that are necessary for the initiation of sexual maturation. These disorders require medical treatment.

Other causes of delayed sexual development include congenital or acquired disorders of the testes or ovaries, known as *hypogonadism*. Likewise, children treated previously for cancer with chemotherapy or abdominal radiation may have primary gonadal dysfunction.

Genetic disorders also can cause delayed sexual development. For example, Klinefelter syndrome, a cause of primary hypogonadism in boys, results from two or more X chromosomes; this condition occurs in approximately 1 in 750 males. The diagnosis may not be evident until the testes fail to enlarge at adolescence (see discussion on Klinefelter syndrome in Chap. 68). Turner syndrome, a chromosomal anomaly found in girls, results in incomplete or absent ovarian development. This condition is described in the following section.

Other disorders of the endocrine system can be responsible for delayed puberty. Untreated hypothyroidism, for example, may lead to delayed puberty.[46] Excess glucocorticoids due to medication prescribed or endogenous secretion also can be associated with pubertal delay.[46]

Finally, sexual development may be delayed secondary to another condition in the child. Systemic illness may lead to growth failure and pubertal delay or cessation of pubertal development.[46] Nutritional deficits related to inadequate food supply or bowel malabsorption and psychologic disorders, such as anorexia nervosa and depression, must also be considered.[46] Psychosocial deprivation is also known to contribute to delay in growth and maturation.

Clinical Manifestations. In some children, the first signs of puberty fail to appear at the appropriate time.

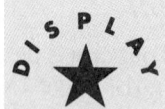

Causes of Delayed Sexual Development

HYPOTHALAMIC DISORDERS

Congenital deficiency of GnRH
  Familial or sporadic
  Kallman's syndrome
  Lawrence-Moon-Biedl syndrome
  Prader-Willi syndrome

Acquired deficiency of GnRH
  Infections
  Neoplasms
  Trauma

PITUITARY DISORDERS

Congenital gonadotropin deficiency
  Idiopathic hypopituitarism
  Isolated LH or FSH deficiency
  Midline brain defects

Acquired gonadotropin deficiency
  Neoplasms
    Craniopharyngioma, histiocytosis
    Pituitary adenomas
  Infections (meningitis, etc.)
  Trauma
  Radiation damage

GONADAL DISORDERS

Congenital gonadal deficiency
  Turner syndrome (45,XO + mosaics)
  Klinefelter's syndrome
  Gonadal agenesis or dysgenesis

  Familial testicular deficiency syndromes
  Myotonia dystrophica

Acquired gonadal defects
  Infections (gonorrhea, orchitis, etc.)
  Mechanical, postoperative, irradiation
    Torsion of ovary or testes
    Oophorectomy or orchiectomy
    Postorchiopexy atrophy
    Postirradiation necrosis
  Post-traumatic
    Spinal cord damage
    Testicular injury or atrophy

ENDOCRINE DISORDERS

Hypothyroidism or hyperthyroidism
Cushing's syndrome or congenital adrenal hyperplasia
Diabetes mellitus
Androgen insensitivity

SYSTEMIC (MAJOR ORGAN) DISEASE

Socioeconomic malnutrition
Regional enteritis or ulcerative colitis
Renal failure or renal tubular acidosis
Cyanotic heart disease
Asthma
Anemia or leukemia
Juvenile rheumatoid arthritis or systemic lupus erythematosus
Anorexia nervosa

Source: Adapted from Rallison, M. L. (1986). Growth disorders in infants, children, and adolescents (pp. 356–357); and Shenker, I. R. (1978). Pediatric Annals, 7(9), 605; and Barnes, V. D. (1975). Medical Clinics of North America, 59, 1337.

For other children, sexual maturation may begin but fail to progress. Other signs in the physical examination may alert the examiner to the presence of systemic illness or a congenital condition.

Diagnostic Studies. A comprehensive physical examination and history are required for an evaluation of adolescents who present with delayed puberty. Symptoms of systemic illness or congenital conditions indicate the need for further evaluation in a specific area.

A bone age x-ray is obtained to determine the degree of delay in skeletal maturation. A bone age of 10 years in a girl or 12 years and 6 months in a boy should correspond with the earliest signs of puberty. Children with a bone age less than this would not be expected to exhibit pubertal signs.

The measurement of sex steroids (estrogen and testosterone) and gonadotropins (LH and FSH) assists in establishing a diagnosis. The GnRH test differentiates constitutional delay from other causes of pubertal failure. In the case of primary hypogonadism, the gonadotropin levels generally increase as they attempt to stimulate un-

responsive gonads. Girls with Turner syndrome and boys with Klinefelter syndrome would have elevated gonadotropins and absent sex steroids. Low serum concentration of LH and FSH indicates lack of stimulation from the hypothalamus-pituitary axis.

★ ASSESSMENT

The child's height, weight, and growth velocity should be measured and plotted on a growth chart. A complete family and medical history should be taken, with particular emphasis on nutrition, family pubertal patterns, and history of systemic illness in childhood. The physical examination includes assessment of the Tanner stage (see Tables 66-3 and 66-4 and Figs. 66-6 to 66-9).

The adolescent's knowledge about physical maturation and feelings about delayed sexual development should be explored. It is important to determine whether relationships with peers are affected and whether the delay is causing a disturbance in self-concept and body image. Any signs of serious psychological problems, such as withdrawal, depression, poor school performance, or feelings of inferiority, should be noted and considered when treatment decisions are made.

★ NURSING DIAGNOSES AND PLANNING

Based on assessment data discussed in the previous section and the preceding chapter, the following nursing diagnoses may apply to the family and child with delayed puberty:

- Body Image Disturbance related to delayed sexual maturation.
- Impaired Social Interactions related to self-concept disturbance.
- Social Isolation related to inability to engage in satisfying personal relationships.
- Ineffective Individual Coping related to maturational crises.
- Hopelessness related to delayed sexual and physical maturation.

The nurse and child (or parents) together plan effective care based on the established nursing diagnoses. Several examples of expected outcomes are as follows:

- The child verbalizes concerns about delayed body changes and unsatisfying peer relationships.
- The child discusses strategies to enhance appearance of maturity and opportunities for socialization.
- The parents and child discuss the regimen for hormone replacement therapy.
- The child discusses potential for additional growth, sexual maturation, and reproductive capacity.

The nurse plans for the daily care of the child based on both the physician's orders and nursing diagnoses. Some general nursing care goals may include the following:

- The child and parents understand treatment options and potential outcomes.
- The child develops satisfying peer relationships.

★ INTERVENTIONS: COLLABORATIVE AND INDEPENDENT

HORMONE REPLACEMENT

The adolescent with constitutional delay who shows great concern about the lack of sexual development might benefit from a short course of hormone therapy. Boys may be given a brief series of testosterone injections to stimulate the appearance of secondary sexual characteristics. Girls may be given estrogen to stimulate pubertal development. Therapy is short term (3–12 months) for these children with normal but delayed development. The short course of therapy matures the pituitary-gonadal axis, and initiates the first signs of maturation.

Long-term replacement therapy is required for adolescents with hypothalamic-pituitary disorders (gonadotropin deficiency) and hypogonadism. Rather than attempting to mimic the pulsatile patterns of GnRH secretion, treatment consists of replacement of the end products, that is, estrogen or testosterone. Replacement therapy is started around the usual age of puberty at low dosage and is gradually increased to an adult dosage. Boys require a monthly injection of testosterone.

Girls are treated initially with a low dose of estrogen that is taken daily for about 1 year to promote breast development and statural growth. The dose is increased as needed, to promote full maturity of the breast tissue and the endometrium over 1 to 3 years. Estrogen then is given in a monthly pattern to mimic the normal menstrual cycle. Typically, girls take estrogen for the first 3 weeks of the calendar month and add progesterone during week three. Anovulatory menstruation occurs during the fourth week after the hormones are withdrawn.

Families need to be aware of the difference between using these hormones to replace what is missing and their use for other reasons. Replacement use is safe and without the side-effects seen when the hormones are used for other indications. Irregular or absent menses or heavy menstrual flow should prompt young girls to contact the health care provider. Excessive sex drive or lack of sexual ability (inability to sustain an erection or low libido) are reasons for young men to call for dosage adjustment.

PSYCHOSOCIAL SUPPORT

Any normal findings of the diagnostic evaluation such as breast budding or testicular enlargement should be pointed out to the child and parents, who may not have noticed subtle changes. Adolescents may be unaware that they are in early puberty and developing normally. Providing information about the process of sexual development and patterns of the emergence of secondary sex characteristics can be reassuring.

In children with hypopituitarism, sex steroid replacement may be delayed to allow the child more time to attain maximum height. This delay may have long-lasting negative psychological consequences that are much greater than are the centimeters in height that might be gained. The child's feelings should always be explored in order to make the decision that is best for that individual. The goals of treatment should focus on achieving a normal puberty as well as a maximal height gain.

Children with a delayed puberty have concerns, often unspoken, that must be taken into consideration. These children appear young for their age and may be considered immature by others. Discussions with parents about providing these adolescents with age-appropriate responsibilities are helpful in promoting psychological development. The nurse may suggest alterations in the adolescent's clothing, hairstyle, or other aspects of appearance that would suggest maturity. If gym classes are extremely stressful, the nurse can discuss the possibility of writing a letter to the school principal to have the classes deferred until the adolescent has achieved the physical changes already evident in classmates.

Realistic expectations about possible benefits and side-effects must be explained when pharmacologic treatment is considered as a "boost" for adolescents with delayed puberty. Children who have nonfunctional gonads (primary hypogonadism) will not be able to produce natural children; an egg or sperm donor is needed. Those children with decreased LH and FSH function (gonadotropin deficient) may be able to ovulate or produce sperm with the help of intensive hormonal intervention. These are sensitive issues that need to be broached carefully with adolescents and their family.

★ EVALUATION

The nurse and family periodically evaluate the outcomes of care given. Examples of outcomes for the child and family with delayed puberty were given under planning in this section. Have the short-term goals been met? Are the long-term goals still realistic? Planning for further nursing care takes complications into consideration.

COMPLICATIONS

Treatment with sex steroids has the potential side-effect of accelerating skeletal maturation, which eventually results in fusion of the growth plates and compromised final height. Overtreatment with testosterone may lead to priapism, aggression, and behavioral problems. Girls nonadherant to the treatment regimen may have irregular, absent, or prolonged menses and increased risk of osteoporosis in later life.

Adolescents with constitutionally delayed puberty should be followed at regular intervals to evaluate the progress of pubertal development and provide reassurance that development is progressing normally. For adolescents with GnRH deficiency and gonadal failure replacement of the sex hormones is accomplished over several years; they have a lifetime need for replacement medication.

Turner Syndrome

Definition and Incidence. Turner syndrome is a genetic disorder in girls that occurs around the time of conception when a defect occurs in the formation of the sex chromosomes. The normal female has 22 pairs of autosomes and 1 pair of sex chromosomes. The child with Turner syndrome has a karyotype without the normal female pattern (46,XX). All karotypes involve X-chromosome(s)—one is missing or abnormal. The classic form of the disorder is 45,X; only one X chromosome is present. In mosaic forms, both X chromosomes are present, but one has not been formed correctly. The defect often results in spontaneous abortion. The incidence of Turner syndrome in live births is about 1 in 2000 to 9000.[44]

Etiology and Pathophysiology. There is no known cause for the chromosome error found in Turner syndrome. Amniocentesis may reveal the distinctive chromosome pattern prior to birth. Turner syndrome may be diagnosed during childhood, adolescence, or adulthood. There is a wide variation in the expression of this disorder during childhood, ranging from short stature to life-threatening cardiac and renal anomalies.

The absence or malformation of an X chromosome leads to the inadequate development of ovarian tissue prior to birth, the hallmark of this disorder. It is unclear how this genetic anomaly can also lead to the variety of findings and health problems encountered in this population.

Some affected infants are diagnosed at birth due to severe lymphedema, the result of an inadequately developed lymphatic system. The accumulation of lymphatic fluids in the fetus causes a physical resistance to the de-velopment of various structures. When lymph accumulates in the neck, it stretches the skin, leading to the classic webbed appearance noted at birth. Accumulation of lymph also may interfere with the development of the inner structures of the head, causing the eustachian tubes to be poorly developed. Many girls do not experience lymph problems later in life, but the effects of poor drainage in utero are permanent. Other girls have poor peripheral circulation, evidenced by puffy feet and ankles, throughout their lives.

Clinical Manifestations. A list of possible clinical manifestations are presented in the accompanying display about Turner syndrome. Although these characteristics may raise suspicions, some infants have minimal physical findings. Associated defects, such as coarctation of the aorta, horseshoe kidney, and duplicated renal collecting systems, are common and may be important clues to diagnosis. However, some girls are not diagnosed until midchildhood when they seek evaluation for their significant short stature, often below the third percentile for their chronologic age. Turner syndrome may be diagnosed in adolescents when they are evaluated for delayed puberty or in adults when they are evaluated in an infertility clinic for failure to conceive a child. Undiagnosed adults typically have spontaneous puberty, but then experience irregular menstrual cycles.

With the exception of the findings of short stature and infertility, the group of girls who have Turner syn-

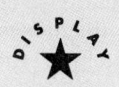

Nursing Assessment: Possible Physical Findings in Turner Syndrome

Characteristics at Birth

Small for gestational age
Edema of the feet and hands
Loose skin folds at the nape of the neck

Characteristics in Childhood

Height below the third percentile
Webbing of the neck
Low posterior hairline
Small mandible
Prominent ears
Epicanthal folds
High-arched palate
Broad chest; nipples appear widely spaced
Hyperconvex fingernails
Increased carrying angle of elbows (cubitus valgus)

Characteristics With Increasing Age

Estrogen deficiency—lack of spontaneous puberty
Pigmented nevi (may be evident in childhood)

Data from Berghman, R., & Vaughan, V. (1987). Nelson's textbook of pediatrics. (13th ed.). (p. 1236). Philadelphia: W. B. Saunders.

drome are not homogeneous in their physical characteristics. Many cases are missed because clinicians seek the classic features of Turner syndrome prior to obtaining a chromosome analysis.

Girls with Turner syndrome are smaller than their peers but grow at near-normal velocity until about the age of 6 years. Their growth rate then declines dramati-

cally, resulting in an eventual adult height range of 4 ft 4 in. to 5 ft 1 in (Fig. 56-5).[6] Affected girls may have cardiac and renal defects that further impair growth.

Children with Turner syndrome may have learning difficulties that are masked by their verbal skills. The range of intelligence in girls with Turner syndrome is the same as in the population at large, but specific learn-

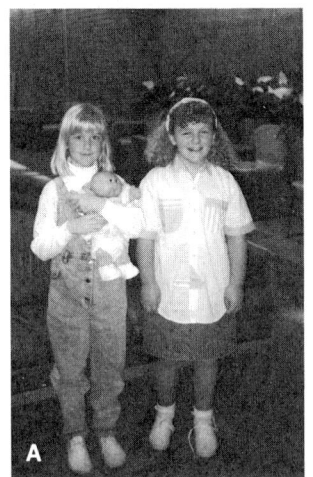

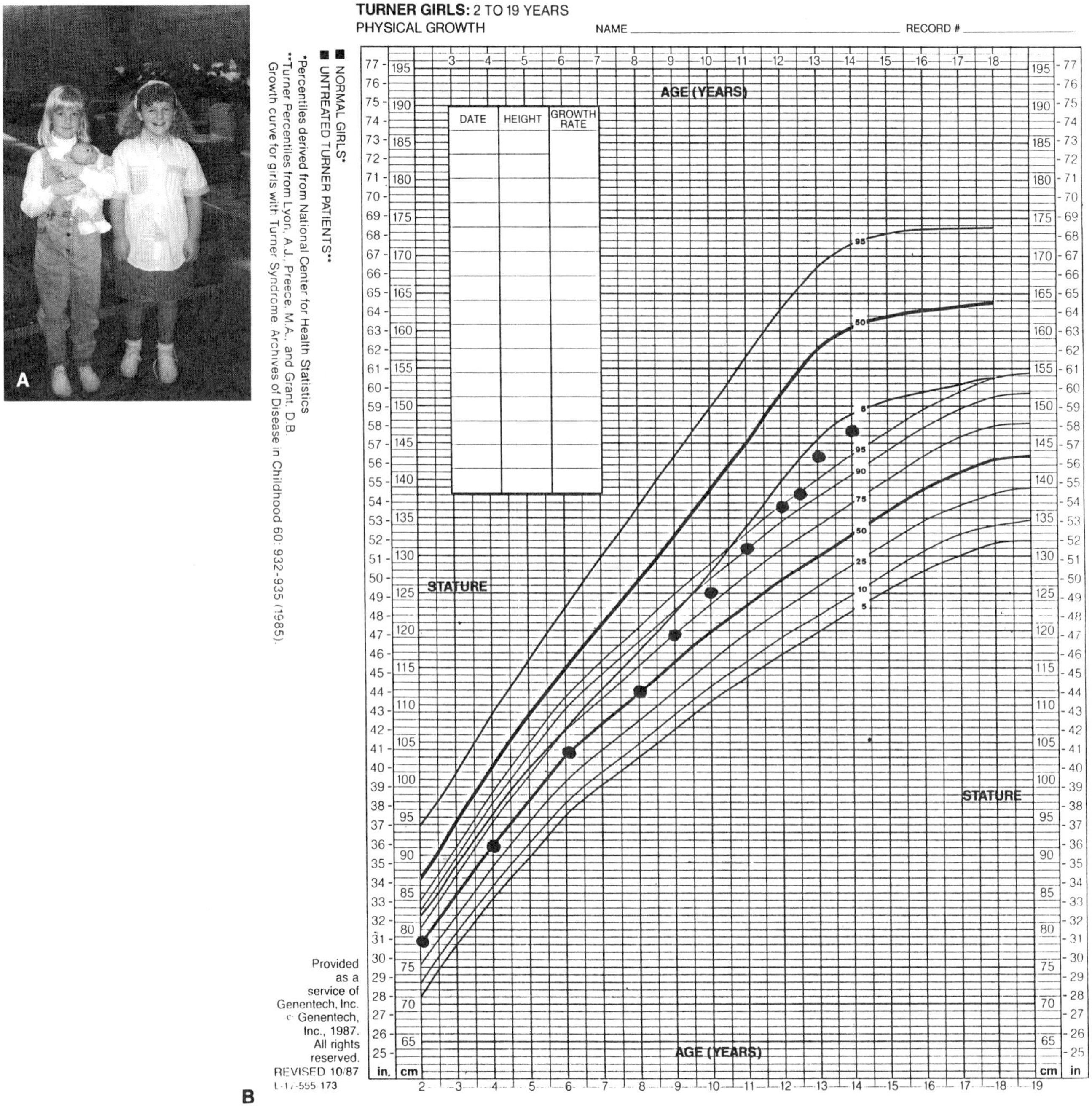

FIGURE 56-5

Turner syndrome. (**A**) A 12-year-old girl with Turner syndrome (**right**) is no taller than her 7-year-old sister. Other signs of the disorder are apparent only on closer inspection. (**B**) The growth pattern of another girl who was diagnosed with Turner syndrome at age 8. She was growing along the 50th percentile for girls with Turner syndrome at age 6, below the 5th percentile for all girls. By age 8, this speed was slower than normal and represented a further deviation for normal. Growth hormone injections increased her growth rate and allowed her to cross percentiles on the Turner syndrome chart. At age 12, her growth began to slow. By adding estrogen tablets, she again grew at a faster rate and surpassed the 95th percentile for Turner syndrome girls. Her final height of 4'10" is taller than her expected height of 4'8", given her early growth pattern along the Turner syndrome 50th percentile.

ing disabilities are common. Some girls with Turner syndrome are dysmorphic enough to be shunned by their schoolmates.

Sex organ development is normal, with the exception of the absent or underdeveloped ovaries. Chronic ear infections throughout childhood and adolescence, resulting from eustachian tube malfunction secondary to lymphedema in utero, may lead to a hearing impairment, which further impedes learning. Some girls and women with Turner syndrome have essential hypertension (high blood pressure that is unrelated to cardiac or renal findings, but the cause is unknown). Rapid and excessive weight gain is often a problem in later childhood. This finding may be related to an imbalance in hypothalamic control, but it is not well understood. Also unknown is the reason that women with Turner syndrome are likely to develop autoimmune endocrine disorders, such Hashimoto thyroiditis and diabetes mellitus.

Diagnostic Studies. Chromosome studies determine the karyotype and confirm the diagnosis. Thyroid studies (T_4 and TSH) are performed to rule out subtle deficiencies that would further hinder growth. Growth hormone studies are performed when the child and family wish to consider treatment with growth hormone. The results of growth hormone testing, however, do not always correlate with response to treatment.

A renal ultrasound is needed to look for the renal malformations commonly found in this population. Girls with renal problems, such as duplicated collecting systems and horseshoe kidney, should be referred to a nephrologist to determine whether surgical correction is indicated. These girls require an annual urinalysis to monitor the status of their kidneys, because poor renal function can further inhibit statural growth.

Cardiac echograms are needed to determine whether cardiac problems exist. Infant girls with serious cardiac problems usually present in cardiac distress at birth. However, a coarctation of the aorta may be discovered in an older child.

Psychometric testing may be performed to diagnose hidden learning problems. Testing, ideally is done prior to entering school, but it can be helpful at any time. Girls with Turner syndrome often have visual and spatial deficits.

★ ASSESSMENT

The history includes specific notations of birth size, lymphedema at birth, heart murmurs, urinary tract infections, ear infections, and school problems. A growth history is valuable and should be plotted on the specially designed Turner syndrome growth chart.

A family assessment assists in determining the meaning of this diagnosis to the family. Blame and guilt are common feelings that need to be explored privately with the parents. Possible learning, school, and social problems should be investigated.

Physical examination includes assessment of Tanner stage and accurate height and weight determinations. Blood pressure measurements in both arms and evaluation of peripheral pulses screen for undiagnosed coarctation of the aorta. The nurse assesses the child for any

of the clinical findings associated with Turner syndrome with a thorough examination that includes the skin (looking for pigmented nevi) and the nails (may be dysplastic). The mouth is examined for a high arched palate and dental crowding. Low hairline and webbing of the neck are noted if present. Arms are inspected for cubitus valgus, the distinct angulation of the elbows.

★ NURSING DIAGNOSES AND PLANNING

Nursing diagnoses listed in the previous section may be applicable. Based on assessment data discussed previously and in the preceding chapter, the following nursing diagnoses may also apply to the family and child with Turner syndrome:

- Body Image Disturbance related to distinctive physical characteristics.
- Anxiety related to need for medications to initiate growth and sexual maturity.
- Impaired Social Interaction related to short stature, delayed puberty, and distinctive physical appearance.

The nurse and child (or parents) together plan effective care based on the established nursing diagnoses. Several examples of expected outcomes are as follows:

- The child describes regimen for hormone replacement therapy.
- The child discusses how she views herself.
- The child expresses confidence in her ability to accomplish realistic goals.
- The child reports more satisfying relationships with peers.

The nurse plans for the daily care of the child based on both the physician's orders and nursing diagnoses. Some general nursing care goals may include the following:

- The child and parents understand the effects of hormone therapy.
- The parents and child have realistic expectations for future growth and development.

★ INTERVENTIONS: COLLABORATIVE AND INDEPENDENT

Girls with Turner syndrome and their families confront issues of short stature, sexuality, infertility, chronic illness, learning problems, and poor social interactions. Long-term relationships with the health care team can provide these families with the support required as the child develops. The nurse's sensitivity to these issues is important. If the primary focus is the child's short stature, the family may not feel free to initiate a discussion about other matters of concern. Support groups exist for these children and their families, and national meetings may be informative and supportive.

For parents, there may be significant and prolonged grief over their daughter's infertility and the loss of their potential natural grandchildren. They may cope with this emotion by overprotecting her. The grief of the parents may never resolve; however, the issue of infertility may be less important to the young woman.

The care of children with Turner syndrome is age-related and tailored to the needs of the child and family.

After any renal and cardiac pathologic conditions have been diagnosed and treated, the concern about short stature is usually foremost on the minds of these children. When girls are not diagnosed until mid to late adolescence, feminization may be of greatest importance.

HORMONE THERAPY

In the past, girls with Turner syndrome were believed to be short due to intrauterine growth retardation (IUGR), and the administration of growth hormone was believed to be ineffective. However, daily injections of growth hormone can increase growth velocity and lead to increased adult height in many affected girls. Estrogen replacement may be needed to promote breast development and menarche in adolescents. Weak androgens also have proven effective in augmenting growth.

Although growth hormone and anabolic steroids have proven effective in increasing growth rate in most girls with Turner syndrome, not all families choose to use these treatments. Current studies indicate an improvement in adult height in many girls when growth hormone is used, but there are many unanswered questions about the long-term effects of this treatment.

Low-dose estrogen replacement augments linear growth for a brief time while it stimulates early sexual development. Initiating estrogen replacement is individually timed because the psychosocial preparedness of the girl to accept therapy must be considered. Small doses of estrogens may be given at 9 to 10 years of age, and the dose is gradually increased over several years. Regular anovulatory menstrual cycles are induced when the girl has achieved adult breast development and has developed a sufficient endometrium. Estrogen is prescribed for 3 weeks each month; addition of progesterone tablets in the third week of the cycle is needed to mimic the normal biologic cycle. The menstrual period occurs during the fourth week, after the estrogen dose has been withdrawn.

TEACHING

Education about expected sexual development is important. Some girls may fear that they will begin to menstruate immediately when the estrogen tablets are begun; others are worried that they will never appear normal because the treatment takes too long. These girls need to be reassured that treatment for 2 to 3 years is required to complete their development. Childbearing options should be discussed early in the plan of care.

It is important for the nurse to determine the meaning that menstruation has in this family and for this girl. Mothers sometimes verbalize a negative attitude about menstruation, but the nurse can provide a different perspective. The family is encouraged to think of menarche as the "coming of age," an event to be celebrated. The nurse could suggest a small remembrance gift or special meal to mark the occasion.

SURGICAL MANAGEMENT

Some girls have an unusual physical appearance, with down-turning mouth, webbed neck, or redundant skin around the neck. They may consider plastic surgery to normalize their appearance. The procedure to remove extra neck skin can be done in childhood. In addition to cosmetic surgery, girls who have a karyotype pattern that includes a Y chromosome need surgery to remove the gonadol tissue.

PSYCHOSOCIAL SUPPORT

School and social issues are of great importance for children with Turner syndrome, who often have excellent verbal skills, but who may not do well in school without significant effort. School problems related to visual and spatial deficits can be diagnosed and addressed. Rejection from peers because of their different appearance can be a painful experience. The consultation of a health care provider with the teacher and school counselor may be beneficial in finding ways to improve social interactions.

Because these girls are small for their age and are sexually immature, they often evoke diminished expectations in adults and peers. Parents need to be interviewed to determine the family's expectations for this child. Lower expectations corresponding with the short stature and delay of sexual development tend to juvenilize the child and undermine self-esteem.

★ EVALUATION

The nurse and family periodically evaluate the outcomes of care given. Examples of outcomes for the child and family with Turner syndrome were given under planning in this section. Have the short-term goals been met? Are the long-term goals still realistic?

LONG-TERM CARE

Ongoing contact with girls who have Turner syndrome permits nurses to evaluate how well the child and family have adapted to the knowledge of the child's condition. Questioning the child about peer relationships and social activities can reveal difficulties and the need for other strategies aimed at providing psychosocial support. Referral for professional counseling or to a community support group for parents and children with congenital disorders may be indicated.

The timing of discussion about fertility is a delicate issue that must be approached on an individual basis. With ovum donor technology, it now is possible for a woman with Turner syndrome to experience pregnancy.

Premature Sexual Development

Definition and Incidence.   There are two common benign conditions often mistaken for true puberty in young children: premature thelarche and premature adrenarche. These conditions can be distinguished from true sexual precocity. The incidence is not documented, primarily owing to under-reporting by families who have not expressed concern and have not had their child evaluated.

The appearance of breast tissue or breast budding in one or both breasts is referred to as *premature thelarche*. It occurs most frequently in girls between the ages of 1 and 4 years.[60] This condition should not be confused with the breast engorgement seen in some newborns as a result of elevated maternal hormones.

Premature adrenarche is the onset of pubertal adrenal androgen activity. The normal process of adrenarche, or maturation of the adrenal gland, usually begins at 6 to 7 years of age in both boys and girls.[62] Premature adrenarche is the onset of adrenal androgen activity prior to these ages. Premature adrenarche is marked by the appearance of pubic hair.

Etiology and Phatophysiology. Premature thelarche is a benign condition. It is thought that an increase in sensitivity to estrogen or a decrease in resistance to the effects of estrogen may be responsible for the premature development.[40] Oral ingestion or absorption of estrogen through the skin also causes breast development.[48] Estrogen is obtained through creams used for labial adhesions or through the accidental ingestion of one or more birth control pills. Cases of siblings with premature thelarche have been reported, suggesting the presence of an inherited trait.

The cause of benign premature adrenarche is not well understood, but the premature appearance of pubic hair may be a family or ethnic group pattern. Late onset congenital adrenal hyperplasia (CAH) and tumors of the adrenal glands or gonads are other possible causes of precocious pubic hair development. However, these disorders have additional symptoms and serious consesquences.

Clinical Manifestations. Girls with premature thelarche have breast development that may be unilateral or bilateral. Only a small budding under the areolae may be visible, or development may be more advanced with significant amounts of breast tissue (Tanner stage 2–3). In many instances, thelarche resolves spontaneously.[40] These girls do not have progressive breast enlargement or additional signs of sexual development, such as pubic hair, axillary hair, accelerated linear growth, or advanced skeletal maturation.

The premature development of pubic hair may be accompanied by the growth of axillary hair, facial hair, increased oiliness of the hair and skin, acne, perspiration, and adult body odor.[62] These children grow at a normal velocity and do not have an advanced bone age. There is no clitoromegaly or other sign of virilization in girls with premature adrenarche.

Diagnostic Studies. A bone age determination may be the only test necessary to confirm the diagnosis of benign premature thelarche. Bone age usually is not advanced beyond the child's chronologic age and height. For most children, the diagnosis can be made with this simple test and a thorough history with physical examination. If the bone age is advanced and the child is growing at an accelerated velocity, a gonadotropin (GnRH) stimulation test may be necessary to differentiate premature thelarche from central precocious puberty. Assessment of LH and FSH in girls with premature thelarche do not demonstrate the nighttime pulses of LH apparent in either normal or precocious puberty. The LH and FSH serum concentrations are low or show pulses of FSH alone. Estradiol concentration is prepubertal.

A blood sample for measurement of dehydroepiandrosterone sulfate (DHEAS) and testosterone serum concentrations are obtained to confirm the diagnosis of premature adrenarche. An elevation in the serum concentration of DHEAS results from increased adrenal androgen production. Testosterone concentration may be slightly elevated in both boys and girls as normal variations. In some instances, adrenal and gonadal ultrasounds may be necessary to rule out the possibility of a tumor. When the bone age is advanced or there is any sign of virilization in a female, an ACTH stimulation test may be ordered to rule out the possibility of late-onset CAH.

★ **ASSESSMENT**

The child's height, weight, and growth velocity should be measured and plotted on a growth chart using standard measurement techniques. The physical examination should include an assessment of the Tanner stage and a measurement of breast tissue (see Chap. 66). The documentation of progression of sexual development is important. A careful history should be obtained to rule out the possibility of exogenous estrogen exposure or ingestion.

Parental knowledge and feelings about the child's premature development should be explored. Ideas of causality should be elicited in both parents and child to correct any misconceptions. Often, fears of breast cancer or other malignancies have prompted the referral. The effect of early development on the child's self-concept and body image should be evaluated. Observation of a child's play and artwork are valuable techniques for determining anxieties and issues.

★ **NURSING DIAGNOSES AND PLANNING**

Based on assessment data discussed in the previous section and the preceding chapter, the following nursing diagnoses may apply to the family and child with premature sexual development:

- Disturbance in Body Image related to premature development of breast tissue or pubic hair.
- Fear related to inadequate knowledge about premature development of secondary sex characteristics.

The nurse and child (or parents) together plan effective care based on the established nursing diagnoses. Several examples of expected outcomes are as follows:

- The parents discuss their fears related to the child's development.
- The child identifies positive characteristics about self.
- The parents discuss plans related to helping the child adapt to physical changes.

The nurse plans for the daily care of the child based on both the physician's orders and nursing diagnoses. A general nursing care goal may include the following:

- The parents understand that the condition is benign.
- The parents respond favorably to anticipatory guidance.

★ **INTERVENTIONS: COLLABORATIVE AND INDEPENDENT**

Premature thelarche and premature adrenarche are benign conditions that do not require medical intervention, and there are no long-term physical consequences.[62] Families require reassurance that the child's development is not the result of a life-threatening disorder and that it does not indicate the onset of true puberty. Parents need guidance to accept these changes and to continue to treat the child in an age-appropriate fashion.

The nurse should plan for private discussion of parental fears and concerns. Affected children are young and have no reason to be concerned about body changes that have developed slowly. Parents should be encouraged to avoid unintentionally generating feelings of shame in their child about these physical changes.

Breast tissue spontaneously recedes in most young girls with premature thelarche. Guidance can be given about how to minimize the appearance of breast development by dressing the child in loose-fitting clothing. Overalls are a popular choice.

A matter-of-fact approach on the part of the nurse can do a great deal to reassure the child that nothing is wrong with her. Unlike their parents, most children express little concern about these changes. Information about the physical examination and diagnostic procedures should be given in age-appropriate terms.

Many parents have difficulty discussing issues of sexuality with children of any age. Anticipatory guidance is important. Parents need to understand that *all* children have sexual feelings and that their child's questions are probably unrelated to early development. The toddler or preschool child is learning about body parts and showing sexual curiosity with games that involve exploration. School age children have a larger vocabulary and understanding of anatomy and physical development; they make comparisons with same-sex parents, siblings, and friends. By modeling open communication, the nurse can help parents understand their child's normal developmental needs.

Parents and children may need additional education about hygiene. The child with adult body odor needs more frequent bathing and may use a gentle deodorant (not an antiperspirant) to decrease odor. Oily skin and hair require more frequent washing.

Pubic hair should not be shaved because of possible injury and infection. Shaving also makes an assessment of progression in the child's development more difficult. Because axillary hair is more noticeable, shaving this area can be discussed. The child who develops acne at a young age may need referral to a dermatologist. Many over-the-counter preparations are harsh on a young child's skin. A child who develops dark facial hair may use a gentle depilatory or mild hair-bleaching agent. The pharmacist may provide assistance in identifying appropriate products.

★ **EVALUATION**

The nurse and family periodically evaluate the outcomes of care given. Examples of outcomes for the child and family with premature sexual development were given under planning in this section.

A follow-up evaluation by an endocrinologist is advised to confirm the diagnosis of premature thelarche or adrenarche. Growth parameters such as height, weight, growth velocity, bone age advancement, and progression

of pubertal development are monitored. Lack of progression of pubertal signs and of a growth spurt substantiates the diagnosis.

Precocious Puberty

Precocious puberty is characterized by sexual development outside the norms of timing for a child's maturation. Although some children who are close to expected pubertal age are able to manage the physical and emotional changes, younger children lack the necessary coping skills.

Definition and Incidence. Precocious puberty is progressive sexual development before the age of 8 years in girls and of 9 years in boys. The incidence is reported as 1 in 5,000 to 10,000 children in the United States, depending on the source providing the data.[51,58] Girls are more likely to experience precocious puberty than are boys.[58]

Precocious puberty can be classified into three groups, depending on the source of pubertal stimulation. The accompanying display lists the causes of precocious puberty. *Central precocious puberty* results from early activation of the hypothalamic-pituitary-gonadal axis in the same manner as normal puberty. This category of precocious puberty is also called *gonadotropin dependent,* because stimulation of the gonad by the gonadotropins (LH and FSH) causes the development of secondary sexual characteristics. This condition is true puberty occurring early.

The second category is *peripheral precocious puberty,* which is the result of the production of sex hormones by the adrenal gland, the gonads, or from exogenous exposure to steroids.[62] This form of puberty is also termed *gonadotropin independent,* because the gonadotropins do not stimulate the development of secondary sexual characteristics.

The third category of precocious puberty is a *combination* of central (gonadotropin-dependent) and peripheral (gonadotropin-independent) puberty. This rare combined form of precocity is related to secondary activation of the hypothalamic-pituitary-gonadal axis by elevated sex steroid levels from a peripheral source.

Etiology and Pathophysiology. The etiology of central precocious puberty is often unknown and is called *idiopathic precocious puberty.* This type of precocity occurs more frequently in girls than in boys, and it generally occurs in children older than 4 years of age.[63] A familial tendency for slightly early development may be recognized.[62] It is not known why premature activation of the hypothalamic-pituitary-gonadal axis occurs. Sometimes central nervous system disorders (a tumor, for example) are associated with central precocious puberty, particularly in boys and in children under 4 years of age.

Peripheral precocious puberty is caused by sex steroid production that has not been stimulated by the pituitary gland. These hormones may be produced by the adrenal glands or gonads or from the ingestion or absorption of steroids from food, birth control pills, makeup, creams, or lotions. Ovarian cysts or tumors that produce

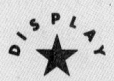

Causes of Precocious Puberty

Central Precocious Puberty

Idiopathic
Hypothalamic hamartoma
Other central nervous system lesions
    Astrocytoma, optic glioma, hydrocephalus, head
    trauma

Peripheral Precocious Puberty

Exogenous ingestion or absorption of steroids from
    birth
    Birth control pills, make-up, creams or lotions
Adrenal gland
    Enzymatic defects (congenital adrenal
    hyperplasia)
    Tumors
Ovary
    McCune-Albright syndrome
    Cysts
    Tumors
Testis
    Tumors
    Familial male precocious puberty (testotoxicosis)

*Combined Peripheral and Central
Precocious Puberty*

Congenital adrenal hyperplasia and central preco-
    cious puberty
Adrenal tumor and central precocious puberty
Ovarian tumor and central precocious puberty
McCune-Albright syndrome and central precocious
    puberty

*Source: Adapted from Pescovitz, O. H. (1990). Precocious pu-
berty. Pediatrics in Review, 11(8), 231.*

estrogen may result in premature sexual development in girls.

McCune-Albright syndrome is a cause of peripheral precocity, in which a triad of symptoms appears: precocious puberty, irregularly shaped café-au-lait spots, and polyostotic fibrous dysplasia. Precocious puberty in this syndrome is thought to be related to heightened estrogen levels associated with the development of ovarian cysts. McCune-Albright syndrome may be associated with other endocrine abnormalities, such as hyperthyroidism, Cushing syndrome, and acromegaly.[32,63] Girls with this disorder may have early menses in the absence of breast development. McCune-Albright syndrome also may appear in boys, although more unusual than in girls.

Tumors of the testes, discussed in Chapter 68, can also cause peripheral precocious puberty in boys as a result of the production of increased testosterone or androstenedione. Another cause of peripheral precocious puberty in boys is testitoxicosis, also known as familial male precocious puberty; etiology of this condition is poorly understood, but it is associated with Leydig cell hyperplasia.

Precocious puberty may be related to either hypothyroidism or Addison disease in rare instances.[62] In conditions related to hypothyroidism, growth is usually decreased and bone age delayed rather than accelerated.[64] Adrenal tumors can produce either increased androgens or estrogens and result in precocious puberty in either sex.[62]

Combined forms of sexual precocity may be seen in children who have poorly controlled CAH, adrenal or ovarian tumors, or McCune-Albright syndrome. Central or true puberty can be triggered by the high concentration of circulating hormones from any of the sources mentioned above.

Clinical Manifestations. The development of precocious secondary sexual characteristics follows the same pattern as normal puberty. In girls, breast development is the earliest change (Fig. 56-6A). Breast enlargement is followed by the pubertal growth spurt; appearance of pubic and axillary hair; increased oiliness of hair and skin; acne; adult body odor; and, finally, menarche. The ovaries and uterus enlarge. In boys, testicular enlargement is followed by the development of body hair, including pubic hair; increased oiliness of hair and skin; acne; pubertal growth spurt; and adult body odor. The voice deepens, and penile erections and emissions occur. Some boys develop an increased interest in girls and in sexual play; others exhibit an increase in aggressive behaviors. Children of both genders have increased masturbation activity.

Sex steroids are responsible for the rapidly increasing rate of skeletal maturation and premature epiphyseal fusion. Children with precocious puberty begin their growth spurt early and may be unusually tall. The growth chart in Figure 56-6B shows the dramatic changes in stature and weight associated with precocious puberty. Rapid skeletal maturation ultimately causes an early cessation of growth and loss of adult height potential.

Diagnostic Studies. Radiologic evaluation of bone age is an important part of the diagnostic process, because advanced skeletal maturation and compromised adult height are significant long-term consequences of precocious development. A cranial CT scan or MRI also may be necessary to rule out the possibility of a hypothalamic or pituitary lesion.

Blood tests are necessary to differentiate the etiology of precocious puberty, and thyroid function studies are needed to rule out hypothyroidism. Adrenal metabolites are measured to exclude possible adrenal causes for precocious development. The GnRH stimulation test is used to determine the maturity of the hypothalamic-pituitary-gonadal axis. An LH predominant response is seen after GnRH stimulation testing in children with central precocious puberty.

In peripheral precocious puberty, either little response to GnRH stimulation testing is seen or FSH is predominant, despite the commonly elevated sex steroid or adrenal metabolite levels. In the case of combined

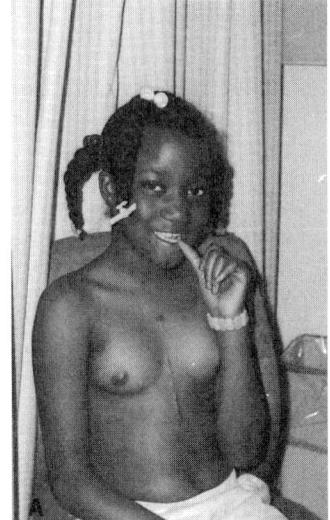

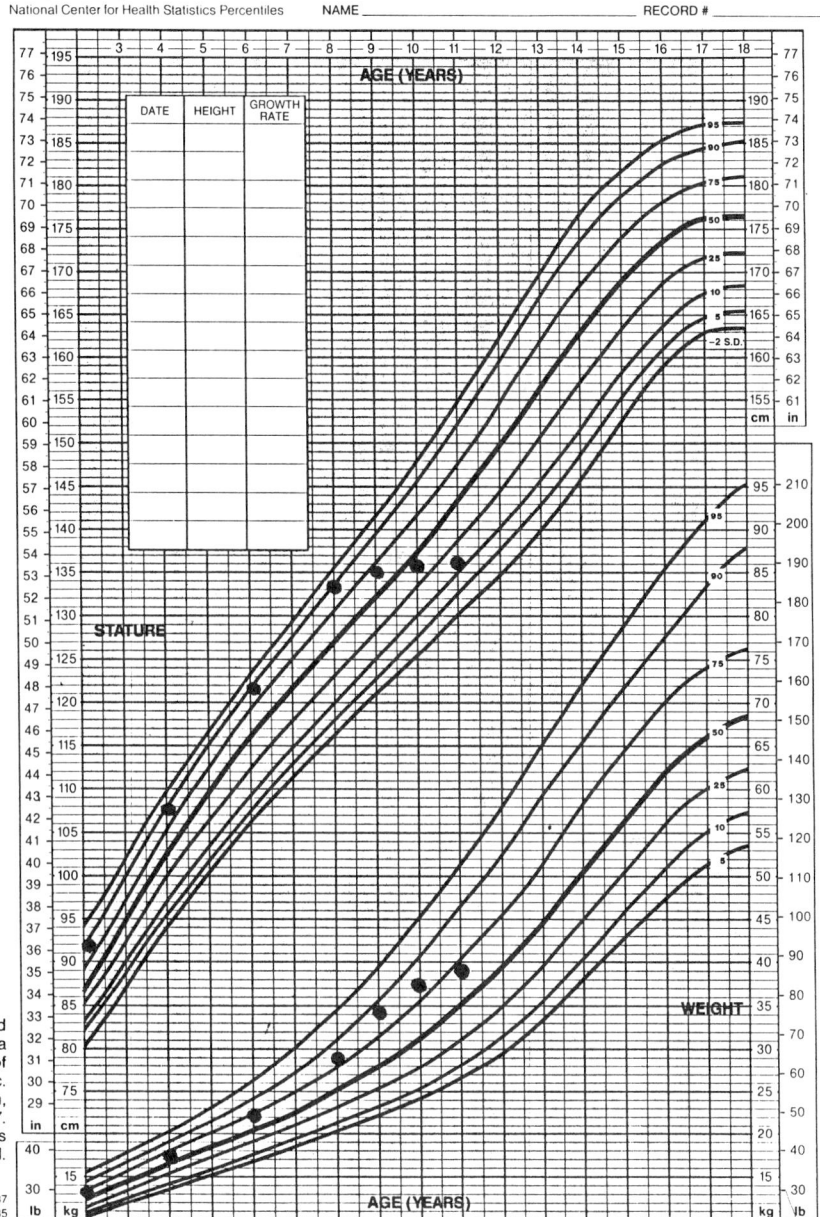

FIGURE 56-6
Precocious puberty. (**A**) A 6 year-old girl with precocious puberty. (**B**) A typical growth chart for another child with precocious puberty. At age 5, the early weight gain associated with the adrenarche that often precedes the growth spurt is seen. By age six, she has begun to cross height percentiles. Breast development at this time might not be noticed by the parents. When she is 6½, she has Tanner stage 3 breast development, downy pubic hair, and is growing at a peak growth rate. Her bone age at this time is 10–11 years.

central and peripheral precocious puberty, increased gonadotropin levels are associated with other hormonal abnormalities.

Pelvic testicular, and adrenal ultrasounds may be necessary to evaluate the size of the gonads and to rule out the presence of cysts or tumors. If McCune-Albright syndrome is suspected, a bone scan is needed to detect polyostotic fibrous dysplasia.

★ **ASSESSMENT**

The history should include any changes in behavior, emotional lability, and moodiness. The parents' and the child's knowledge about precocious puberty and their related fears also need to be assessed.

The physical examination of the child should include an assessment of the Tanner stage and measurement of breasts, testes, and penis. Growth parameters are measured and plotted on the child's growth chart to detect acceleration of growth rate. In girls a rectal exam may be used to palpate the uterus, and the vaginal mucosa may be inspected for the effects of estrogen. The examiner should be alert for evidence of sexual abuse. These children are sometimes easy targets for the adult molester because they exhibit outward signs of physical maturity and sexuality, but their innocent trust reveals their chronologic age.

Psychosocial implications vary depending on the rate of change and whether the child's environment is supportive. Based on knowledge of preadolescents' need to blend in with their peers, the nurse should examine the child's peer relationships through interviews and, when possible, direct observation. Because of their rapid growth, these children probably seek relationships with older children; however, because they develop cognitively and socially in accordance with their chronologic age, conflict and confusion with the older group will likely occur.

The parents' knowledge and feelings about their child's level of sexual development should be explored privately. The health care team should also assess whether parents relate to their child in an age- or size-appropriate manner to determine whether expectations are realistic for the child's chronologic age. Ideas of causality should be explored so that any misconceptions can be clarified.

Emotional lability, moodiness, aggressive behavior, and other changes may be noted along with the physical and hormonal changes described. These changes can be difficult for young children and their family.

★ NURSING DIAGNOSES AND PLANNING

Based on assessment data discussed in the previous section and the preceding chapter, the following nursing diagnoses may apply to the family and child with precocious puberty:

- Body Image Disturbance related to rapidly maturing body and secondary sex characteristics.
- Social Isolation related to age-appropriate interests.
- Fear related to knowledge deficit regarding maturing body and sexuality.

The nurse and child (or parents) together plan effective care based on the established nursing diagnoses. Several examples of expected outcomes are as follows:

- The child verbalizes concerns about bodily changes.
- The child participates in hygiene requirements.
- The child discusses issues related to sexuality.
- The child expresses acceptance of changes in body image.
- The child reports satisfactory peer relationships.

The nurse plans for the daily care of the child based on both the physician's orders and nursing diagnoses. Some general nursing care goals may include the following:

- The parents and child understand the physical, emotional, and social changes that will likely occur.
- The parents and child understand their options for treatment.

★ NURSING INTERVENTIONS: COLLABORATIVE AND INDEPENDENT

Treatment of precocious puberty is determined by the cause. When a cranial tumor is at fault, it will be removed or irradiated. Chemotherapy is sometimes indicated.

THERAPY FOR CENTRAL PRECOCIOUS PUBERTY

If central precocious puberty is due to a cranial tumor, surgery and possibly chemotherapy are typically required. In the absence of recognized pathology, three treatment options may be considered. The first approach is to do nothing but support and reassure the family. For the family with a healthy, well-adjusted girl 7 to 8 years old, this is the most common approach. The second approach is to administer medroxyprogesterone (Provera) to halt menses in girls and decrease symptoms of aggression in boys. This approach does not entirely shut down gonadotropin release nor does it slow the rapid skeletal maturation that leads to compromised adult height.[32] The third option is to stop the production of gonadotropins thereby stopping production of sex steroids. Several long-acting synthetic analogues of GnRH are being used experimentally to stop the production of gonadotropins. These medications inhibit the progression of secondary sexual characteristics as well as the rapid growth and skeletal maturation associated with central precocious puberty (Fig. 56-7).[62]

GnRH analogues require a daily subcutaneous injection or a nasal dosage twice daily, given at home or a monthly intramuscular injection. No serious side-effects of these medications have been reported, but the long-term effects on reproductive function are not known.[62] The analogues are costly medications.

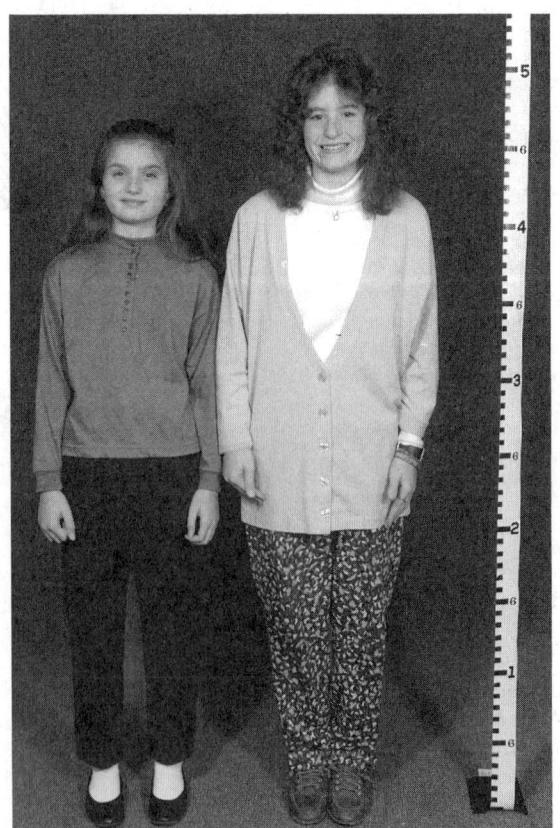

FIGURE 56-7

Therapy with GnRh has effectively inhibited the rapid growth and skeletal maturation of this 10-year-old girl (**left**), pictured here with her 13-year-old sister, who is of normal stature for her age.

Once the bone age of the child is pubertal (10 years for girls, 13 years for boys), children have already lost potential growth because of accelerated skeletal maturation. At this time, there is little reason to use GnRH analogues to enhance height. The child's predicted adult height should be considered when the decision is being made to treat an individual child. Parents need to understand the potential height range their child is expected to achieve, with or without treatment.

Given the questions about long-term effects, the expense of therapy, the need for injections, and the necessity for frequent physician visits once treatment is initiated, some families choose not to pursue GnRH analogue therapy. Children and families should be supported in whatever informed decision they make and offered continued care by a pediatric endocrinologist.

THERAPY FOR PERIPHERAL PRECOCIOUS PUBERTY

The treatment for peripheral precocious puberty depends on the specific disorder responsible for sexual development. McCune-Albright syndrome and testitoxicosis do not respond to therapy with GnRH analogues because they are gonadotropin-independent. The treatment of gonadal tumors is described in Chapter 68.

Testolactone is an investigational therapy that has been used with some success to prevent estrogen synthesis in children with McCune-Albright syndrome and, in combination with spironolactone, to inhibit testosterone synthesis and action in testitoxicosis.[49] Ketoconazole has been used to interfere with both adrenal and gonadal testosterone production in the treatment of testitoxicosis.[32,36,62]

THERAPY FOR COMBINATION PRECOCIOUS PUBERTY

Therapy for the combination of central and peripheral precocious puberty involves a combination of the treatments that have been described. The peripheral component is treated according to the specific abnormality, and the central component is treated with a GnRH analogue.

PSYCHOSOCIAL SUPPORT

Parents often have difficulty discussing their child's premature sexual development. An open, honest relationship with the professional team is essential if parents and children are to identify their concerns and fears. Time to speak privately without the child present can make this easier for the parents.

Parents need verbal and written information about precocious puberty presented in simple, direct terminology. In the case of central precocious puberty, it should be stressed that the child's development is normal but that it has occurred earlier than is usual. The long-term physical consequences of accelerated skeletal maturation should be explained. Treatment options should be discussed with the entire family.

Many parents are most concerned about their child's behavioral and psychological changes. They are often uncertain about how to respond to these changes. The issue is complicated further by the knowledge that some of the "teenage behavior" is related to hormonal changes

as well as to the child's difficulty adapting to the physical changes and to feeling different from peers.

Parents should be encouraged to treat their child age-appropriately. Fathers often feel uncomfortable continuing to hold and caress their daughters when the children have breast tissue. Little girls will not understand withdrawal of physical affection and may interpret the action as rejection. Early sexual development does not mean that the child is ready for adolescent activities.

Children's clothing should be appropriate for chronologic age rather than adolescent in appearance. Parents may need guidance about how to minimize the appearance of breast development with loose-fitting clothing or a training bra. Boys may prefer boxer short underwear and bathing suits.

Girls and their parents should be prepared for the possibility of menarche if this has not yet occurred. Menstrual hygiene becomes a significant issue for girls still in elementary school. Children with serious central nervous system disorders might be more affected by aggressive impulses than would a healthy child. One bright 8-year-old girl may not require any treatment, whereas another child the same age would need some type of management.

Parents, teachers, and health professionals all must be encouraged to treat affected children in an age-appropriate manner. Support groups may be beneficial, because parents will have the opportunity to discuss their concerns and fears with others who have similar concerns. Children may benefit from knowing that they are not alone with this problem.

Treatment may stop the progression of pubertal development, but the physical maturation that has been attained usually does not regress completely. The mature physical characteristics may be a source of discomfort for the child until the peer group catches up, or it may be viewed as a positive attribute.

The issue of sexual abuse should be discussed with the parents so that they are able to protect their child. Age-appropriate sex education is extremely important for this group of children. They need to acquire the skills of reporting to their parents or teacher any inappropriate touching or situations that occur.

A few children may experience significant problems adapting to precocious development. Any child who shows signs of serious psychological effects, such as depression, withdrawal, and aggressive behavior, should receive counseling.

★ EVALUATION

The nurse and family periodically evaluate the outcomes of care given. Examples of outcomes for the child and family with precocious puberty are given under planning in this section. Have the short-term goals been met? Are the long-term goals still realistic? Planning for further nursing care takes complications and long-term care into consideration.

COMPLICATIONS

The most serious physical consequence of untreated precocious puberty is compromised adult height. Without therapy, boys may not exceed an adult height of 5 ft 2 in., and approximately half of the girls will not exceed a height of 5 ft.[58]

The emotional impact of these disorders has not been studied. Early development may have serious emotional effects on some children.[42] Other children experience no difficulties and may not even seek evaluation.

LONG-TERM CARE

The child with precocious puberty requires an ongoing care by a pediatric endocrinologist. The response to therapy is evaluated through careful monitoring of the progression of pubertal development, growth parameters, skeletal maturation, and repeated blood tests.

The treatment of central precocious puberty with medications continues until a child reaches the normal age for puberty. When therapy is discontinued, the child is unlikely to experience resumption of the pubertal growth spurt, but otherwise, is expected to resume normally.[51] Long-term effects on fertility have not yet been documented in children treated with GnRH analogues. However, there have been anecdotal reports of pregnancies in four to six girls previously treated with these preparations.

Altered Pituitary Function

Chapter 54 reviews the structure and functions of the pituitary gland. Disorders at either the hypothalamic or pituitary level result in pituitary dysfunction. Most problems are those of hypofunction. This section includes information about several alterations in pituitary function. Isolated growth hormone deficiency (GHD), also called *hypopituitarism,* the most common pituitary problem, is distinguished from panhypopituitarism, in which all anterior pituitary hormones are absent. Decreased function of the posterior pituitary gland can occur in isolation from anterior gland function, or it may be part of panhypopituitarism. Alterations associated with hypofunction of the target glands have been discussed in the preceding sections.

Growth Hormone Deficiency: Hypopituitarism

Definition and Incidence. Growth hormone deficiency (GHD) is a rare condition affecting 1 in 10,000 children in the United States.[50] GHD exists in a classic as well as a nonclassic form. In the classic form, GHD is the failure of the pituitary to produce enough growth hormone to sustain a normal growth rate in childhood, resulting in an adult stature that is below normal. People affected with the severe form of this deficiency are commonly referred to as midgets, and medical literature may call them pituitary dwarfs. Both terms are outdated and should be avoided when discussing the condition with children and their parents.

In contrast to classic hypopituitarism, there is much controversy about the definition and treatment of children with a nonclassical form of growth hormone insufficiency.

These children are shorter than expected, given their genetic heritage, and do not have evidence of other medical conditions that affect growth. Most endocrinologists believe that short stature alone does not constitute an endocrine problem and that treatment with growth hormone is inappropriate.

Etiology and Pathophysiology. Growth hormone stimulates the growth of every tissue and organ in the body, but it has an especially powerful effect on the long bones. Growth hormone also stimulates the synthesis of insulin-like growth factor 1 (IGF-1), or somatomedin C, in most tissues but primarily in the liver. IGF-1 stimulates somatic growth, and its absence (such as in liver failure) results in poor growth.

Growth hormone is secreted in a pulsatile fashion during the day and night. During the waking hours, growth hormone production is less active. Adequate nutrition and healthy hepatic and renal systems are needed for GH or IGF-1 production. GHD may be attributed to several causes, which are outlined in the accompanying display on contributing factors. Because the course of illness varies with different causal factors, several conditions are discussed separately in this section.

Idiopathic GHD. Approximately 80% of the children with GHD have no known cause for the disorder.[6] In about two-thirds of these children, there is no other pituitary malfunction. The condition generally occurs sporadically, but familial patterns sometimes are recognized.

The incidence of idiopathic GHD is highly associated with perinatal insult, including prolonged or precipitous labor or births, breech presentation, and cesarean birth. Children with GHD typically are of normal size at birth, because fetal growth is governed by maternal factors.

Tumor. The most common tumor causing GHD is craniopharyngioma. This cystic tumor impinges on the hypothalamic-pituitary area. Although it is not a malignant tumor, the recurrence rate is high, and it may grow quickly and compress vital centers in the brain. Without surgical intervention, children may live 3 to 4 years following the onset of symptoms. Successful diagnosis and surgery increase the survival rate to 40% after 8 years.[44]

Other tumors associated with GHD include optic gliomas, adenomas, astrocytomas, and germinomas. Children with neurofibromatosis are at risk for several of these tumors, but they may cause few symptoms in a young child.

Septo-Optic Dysplasia. Developmental anomalies of the pituitary gland are associated with several congenital defects, one of which is septo-optic dysplasia, also known as *de Morsier syndrome.* This condition appears as a group of conditions, including optic nerve hypoplasia, which may cause blindness, absence of the septum pellucidum, and pituitary hormone deficiencies.[6] The child with this disorder has disabilities ranging from minor visual impairments to blindness and panhypopituitarism.

Empty Sella. Radiographic imaging of the pituitary area can reveal an absent or small pituitary gland that does not fill the sella foramen. The small gland may have been caused by pressure of cerebrospinal fluid impinging

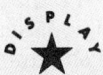

Factors Associated With Growth Hormone Deficiency

Congenital
- Septo-optic dysplasia
- Midline facial or skull defects
- Congenital absence of the pituitary gland

Trauma
- Accidental, including birth injuries
- Surgical damage to pituitary gland
- Child abuse

Infections and Other Inflammatory Diseases
- Viral encephalitides
- Bacterial infections
- Fungal infections
- Nonspecific hypophysitis (? autoimmune disorder)

Vascular
- Aneurysmal malformations of the pituitary vessels
- Pituitary infarction

Irradiation

Toxic sequelae of chemotherapy for malignancies

Tumors of the Hypothalamus and Pituitary

Histiocytosis

Sarcoidosis

Unknown Cause (idiopathic)

Hereditary (including growth hormone gene deletions)

Growth Hormone Insensitivity syndrome (Laron type)

Source: Kaplan, S. (ed.). (1990). Clinical pediatric endocrinology. Philadelphia: W. B. Saunders.

on it, possibly as a result of an incompetent sellar diaphragm, a defect of embryonic development.[44]

Radiation Treatment. The treatment for brain tumors or leukemia may include radiation to the head. Not all cranial tumors impinge on the pituitary gland, but radiation treatment in sufficient dosage causes damage to the hypothalamic-releasing hormones and pituitary function. Growth hormone is the most radiation-sensitive hormone. Children who receive a total of 2500 rads or more are particularly at risk for GHD.

Trauma. Severe head trauma from abuse or accidents can damage the pituitary gland or sever its stalk. The loss of venous supply and hypothalamic stimulation to the gland results in varying degrees of hypofunction.

Clinical Manifestations. GHD results in statural growth that is slower than is the normal velocity for the age of the child. Short stature is not the hallmark; it is the *rate of growth* that is the essential component, although slow growth over time eventually leads to short stature. Unlike people with achondroplasia, a genetic bone disorder, children with GHD have normal body proportions.

Infants with GHD may have significant hypoglycemia and be cortisol-deficient as well; both hormones are required to maintain euglycemia. Growth hormone plays a counter-regulatory role in glucose regulation. Hypoglycemia, micropenis, small testes, and prolonged hyperbilirubinemia may be present in the neonate with GHD. Poor growth may be apparent by 6 months, but may not be obvious until 2 to 4 years. Glucose regulation is rarely a problem for the older child after the first year or two of life. However, undetected long-term hypoglycemia causes permanent intellectual impairment that becomes more obvious during the school years. Chronic hypoglycemia is discussed later in this chapter.

Infants with GHD have facial features that may be described as "cherubic" in appearance. The forehead is prominent (bossing), and the eyes appear large. The nasal bridge is underdeveloped, and the nose is infantile. The cheeks are full and the chin petite. The abdomen is rounded from deposits of ripply fat (truncal adiposity). The hands and feet are small, and the skin is soft. Dental eruption often is delayed. Male infants may have small genitals, a characteristic related to additional pituitary hypofunction (GnRH deficiency).

Older children with GHD have qualities similar to affected infants; these children appear much younger than their chronologic age. Because cognitive development is not affected, children with normal developmental skills may appear precocious. Dental eruption continues to be delayed, and many children have high-pitched voices, even after puberty.

Adolescents with GHD also may have a significant delay in the onset of puberty. A bone age of 10 years for girls and 12 to 13 years for boys coincides with the beginning of puberty in the normal child. A child with untreated GHD may have a bone age many years behind the chronologic age.

Growth failure may be the presenting complaint in GHD, although headaches and visual impairments may occur. Severe manifestations of pituitary insufficiency do not occur until the pituitary gland is almost completely destroyed.

Diagnostic Studies. Many children are small for their age; by definition, 5% of children in the United States are at or below the 5th percentile on the growth curve but most of these children are normal and healthy. These children rarely require a diagnostic evaluation. However, the diagnosis of idiopathic GHD is controversial, and some endocrinologists may treat children who do not fit classic diagnostic criteria.

Children of any size who fail to grow at a normal rate, and children who are below the 5th percentile on growth charts for height, require an evaluation. Growth velocity over time is the most important diagnostic measure. Classic criteria for diagnosing GHD include short stature (height below the third percentile), failure to produce growth hormone in response to two provocative tests, delayed bone age, and slow growth velocity.

Screening Tests.   Screening tests are used to distinguish GHD from other causes of growth failure and include thyroid studies, complete blood count with sedimentation rate, and electrolytes. Urinalysis is done, along with renal and liver function studies. Serum for analysis of IGF-1 concentration is obtained as an indication of growth hormone activity; the level is below normal in children with GHD. Growth hormone secretion often can be stimulated by exercise, such as running up stairs or riding an exercise bicycle. After 15 minutes of vigorous exercise, blood is drawn for GH analysis. Growth hormone is expected to rise above 7 ng/dl. This type of testing is a basic screening tool and has a high rate of false-negative results.

A bone age study is used to determine the degree of skeletal delay. A lateral skull x-ray with sellar views is obtained to view the pituitary sella for emptiness, calcification of the pituitary gland, or tumor-related abnormalities.

Diagnostic Tests for Growth Hormone Secretion.   Children who have a low IGF-1 concentration, or who fail to produce adequate growth hormone on screening, require more extensive diagnostic testing when GHD is suspected. Laboratory studies for growth hormone assessment are complicated by the pulsatile release of this hormone. Growth hormone release can be pharmacologically stimulated; however, not all pharmacologic agents are successful even in normal subjects. Therefore, children are assessed with two stimulation tests, performed sequentially or simultaneously.

Arginine, insulin, L-dopa, glucagon, and clonidine are medications that may be used to stimulate the release of growth hormone. An intravenous heparin lock is placed, and a baseline blood concentration of growth hormone is obtained. The stimulators may be administered together, and blood is withdrawn at 30-minute intervals for 1 to 2 hours. The classic combined test (the arginine tolerance test–insulin tolerance test) requires a total of 3 hours. There is danger of profound hypoglycemia during this procedure, and constant monitoring of the child is required. Children without GHD normally produce a GH peak of at least 10 ng/dl of growth hormone in response to at least one of two provocative stimuli.

Growth hormone secretion also can be measured with an overnight study. A heparin lock is inserted, and blood is withdrawn every 10 to 20 minutes either by syringe or pump. Analysis of the samples in the normal child provides a pattern that should include several large pulses of growth hormone and an overall secretion rate that is in the normal range. Because deep sleep initiates growth hormone release, a sound sleep is essential to the quality of the results. These tests are described as overnight, physiologic, or integrated growth hormone tests. Because they require significantly more blood volume and a hospital stay, this type of test is not appropriate for all children.

Head Scans.   Children who have GHD of no known cause will have radiologic or nuclear medicine studies to rule out lesions such as tumors or empty sella. CT scans do not readily detect small tumors in the pituitary-hypothalamic region, and an MRI may be necessary.

Children with congenital GHD may have the diagnosis of septo-optic dysplasia or optic nerve hypoplasia. A head scan can determine the extent of brain structure anomalies, such as absence of the corpus callosum or septum pellucidum.

★ ASSESSMENT

INFANTS

Birth history, including such information as breech presentation, duration of labor and complications during birth, is obtained to identify perinatal insult or hypoxia. Parental heights and weights are noted, as are family members who are significantly short. Feeding difficulties and patterns of fussiness are discussed with the parents, assessing the possibility of hypoglycemia, a primary concern in infants with suspected GHD. Evidence of cortisol deficiency also is assessed.

The physical examination includes an emphasis on the possible findings listed earlier. Supine length is obtained with the use of two adults to position the infant and to ensure accuracy. Head circumference is charted. Hospitalized children should be weighed daily.

OLDER CHILDREN

Analysis of the child's growth patterns over time is the essential component of the diagnosis of GHD. If no previous height or weight measurements are available, the child may be followed for 3 to 6 months to be certain of the child's growth velocity before embarking on a complete diagnostic evaluation. Careful measurements of all children with growth concerns are obtained, using a stadiometer. The measurements should be obtained twice at each observation for reliability.

Because growth failure can occur as a result of any disease, such as renal failure and inflammatory bowel disorders, the history and physical examination are thorough. Family history of parental and sibling heights is obtained, as is the age when parental adult heights were achieved. Family interactions are noted, to identify evidence of secondary gain related to short stature. School issues and friendship patterns are analyzed to identify adaptation or learning problems.

★ NURSING DIAGNOSES AND PLANNING

Many nursing diagnoses may be needed to plan accurately for individual care, based on assessment data discussed in the previous section and the preceding chapter. The following nursing diagnoses may apply to the family and child with hypopituitarism:

- Impaired Social Interaction related to size disparity.
- Self-Esteem Disturbance related to discordant expectations by peers and adults.
- Altered Parenting related to child who is small for age.
- Fear due to knowledge deficit regarding the cause of GHD, its expected course, treatment, and outcome.

The nurse and child (or parents) together plan effective care based on the established nursing diagnoses. Several examples of expected outcomes are as follows:

- The parents demonstrate skill in administering GH by injection.
- The child identifies problematic behaviors that deter socialization.
- The child verbalizes feelings about the view of self.
- The parents verbalize beginnings of positive feelings about the child's growth and development.
- The child demonstrates an increase in behaviors appropriate to age group.
- The parents discuss future appointment dates.

The nurse plans for the daily care of the child based on both the physician's orders and nursing diagnoses. General nursing care goals may include the following:

- The parents understand the costs and benefits of GH replacement therapy.
- The parents understand the need for long-term evaluation by health care providers.
- The parents and child have realistic expectations for the child's growth gains.

★ INTERVENTIONS: COLLABORATIVE AND INDEPENDENT

GHD is usually treated by replacing the missing growth hormone with a synthetic preparation given as a daily subcutaneous injection. However, GHD that is the result of a brain tumor leads to a different set of priorities for the family. Growth hormone cannot be replaced until the activity of the tumor is ended either by surgery or radiation. Once the child has had no active disease (unchanged scans) for 6 to 12 months, the missing hormone can be cautiously replaced.

GROWTH HORMONE REPLACEMENT

Growth hormone is a complex molecule that is available only as an injectable medication, but it has been in use for more than 30 years. Initial limited supplies were obtained from human pituitary tissue, but biosynthetic growth hormone is now available in unlimited supply due to recombinant DNA technology. Growth hormone is an expensive drug, with an average wholesale cost of about $20,000 per year for a school-age child. Insurance companies and state medicaid or other payment programs recognize the diagnosis of GHD when the evaluation has been thorough and the child fulfills the classic criteria.

Growth hormone injections are given subcutaneously and are not painful. The growth hormone powder is packaged with diluent and administered with an insulin syringe. Parents or children need instruction in diluting the hormone, preparing the dose, and injecting the medication. Written instructions as well as practice in mixing and administering the injections are required.

Infants with hypoglycemia require oral cortisol and injections of growth hormone. Daily injections are associated with the best growth response, but some children may be placed on a schedule requiring injections every other day or three times a week. Current replacement is up to 0.3 mg/kg/week, and the dose is adjusted over

time as the child grows. Administration of growth hormone can be individualized for each family. The nurse works closely with the family to determine a realistic routine that can be followed faithfully.

Growth hormone replacement promotes growth at an accelerated velocity within 6 months of beginning treatment. Children who had been growing at 4 cm per year may grow 8 to 12 cm during the first year of treatment. Even with accelerated growth, it may be several years before the child catches up to the peer group. This pace can be a disappointment if the family and child are not prepared for the lengthy course of treatment. Treatment goals and expectations must be clearly communicated before beginning growth hormone replacement.

Growth hormone injections continue until the child ceases to respond to treatment, the family and adolescent indicate that an acceptable height has been achieved, or maximum growth potential is attained (epiphyseal fusion). Even with optimal response to treatment, it is unusual for children with idiopathic GHD to achieve a normal height early in their treatment course and few of these children reach their genetic potential for height.

Side effects of growth hormone replacement therapy include diabetes mellitus, the development of antibodies for synthetic growth hormone, and the risk of growth hormone excess problems. In 1985, human-derived growth hormone was associated with several cases of a fatal viral condition known as *Creutzfeldt-Jakob disease,* and it subsequently was withdrawn from the world market.[21] Additionally, an association with increased risk of leukemia has been reported in Japan, but studies of the U.S. population of children receiving growth hormone do not substantiate this observation. Some conditions that lead to GHD, such as tumors, are associated with an increased risk of secondary tumors or leukemia, but treatment with growth hormone does not appear to increase these risks. In addition to the physical side effects, psychological side effects should be considered. The child and parents may have unrealistic growth expectations and face disappointment or depression when treatment ends.

PSYCHOSOCIAL SUPPORT

Children receiving growth hormone are followed closely in the ambulatory setting, and visits are scheduled every 3 to 4 months. This routine provides the opportunity for monitoring growth velocity and dosage needs and permits emotional support during the long treatment course. Even successful treatment may not fulfill the wishes and fantasies of the child and family. Compared with normal peers, children may perceive only small gains in height. The nurse helps interpret changes on the growth chart and identifies the gains made. Each contact with the family is used to enhance the nurse's understanding of the child's expectations and perceptions.

Resistance to the injections is generally short lived, and age-appropriate defenses are seen in toddlers and preschoolers. Older children who resist the injections may be afraid to grow or afraid to lose the special status of being small. If children do not wish to grow, counseling may be appropriate. The nurse can help children express the positive and negative aspects of treatment. Working closely with the parents may empower them to continue therapeutic communications with their children.

Short children are treated differently in school by their peers; teachers and peers often cannot overlook the discordant size of the child. Adult expectations for the small child may be lower than for same-age peers, and learning may be suboptimal. Some children with GHD may accentuate their small size by wearing childish clothing and by behavior that is manipulative or helpless. Parents may benefit from counseling and support about treating the child according to chronologic age rather than appearance. Age-appropriate clothing, activities, and responsibilities may be recommended.

ANTICIPATORY GUIDANCE

Children with GHD often appear to be cognitively precocious. Relatives and strangers reinforce this impression by their comments—"My, she talks so well for being so small! She must be very bright." In fact, the 6-year-old child (who appears to be only 3 years old) may have developmental delays.

Some investigators have found that children with GHD have a high incidence of academic underachievement, learning disabilities, or slightly depressed IQ scores.[38,70] Therefore, all children with this diagnosis benefit from comprehensive psychometric testing before entering kindergarten or as soon as possible after diagnosis. Older children with GHD who are having any school problems also should have psychometric testing. Some children with GHD do well in school, but their performance should continue to be assessed over time by the nurse.

Parents may consider delaying kindergarten for a year. Small size can interfere with large muscle activities, and tiny hands have difficulty mastering writing skills. Small children sometimes are selected as school pets and often are carried about by larger children. Because children with GHD can expect a significant delay in the onset of their puberty, waiting 1 year to begin school may facilitate their adjustment in middle school as well.

Children with cranial radiation may lose significant learning potential from this treatment. These learning problems are not related to GHD or its treatment.

★ EVALUATION

The nurse and family periodically evaluate the outcomes of care given. Examples of outcomes for the child and family with hypopituitarism were given under planning in this section. Have the short-term goals been met? Are the long-term goals still realistic? Planning for further nursing care takes into consideration complications and long-term care.

COMPLICATIONS

Children who are treated with growth hormone should grow at faster than normal speed for 2 to 4 years. If growth is not improved, the cause must be discovered. Possible problems include compliance with the prescribed routine of injections, adequacy of the growth hormone dose, or medication mixing technique. Other reasons for inade-

quate growth, such as other hormone deficiencies, poor nutrition, and emotional distress, may be identified.

LONG-TERM CARE

Children with hypopituitarism who have been diagnosed and treated early have an excellent prognosis for achieving height within the normal range. Clinical research trials have begun to assess the need for growth hormone replacement into adulthood. Although growth hormone normally is produced throughout life, no current evidence supports the need to continue treatment when growth has ended.

People who have received any type of growth hormone cannot donate blood or organs, because of concerns about transmission of Creutzfeldt-Jakob disease. Children who have received only synthetic growth hormone and have not had treatment with human pituitary growth hormone extracts are not at risk.

Because idiopathic GHD may be an inherited condition, people with this diagnosis are advised to bring their children for early evaluation if they fail to grow at a normal rate.

Panhypopituitarism

Definition and Incidence. Panhypopituitarism is the loss of all anterior pituitary function resulting in deficiency of growth hormone (GH), TSH, ACTH, and gonadotropins (LH and FSH). Panhypopituitarism may also include deficiency of the posterior pituitary hormone, antidiuretic hormone (ADH).

Panhypopituitarism is a rare disorder and is estimated to occur in approximately 1 in 100,000 live births.[17] Deficiencies in GH, TSH, ACTH, or LH and FSH can occur in combination, but isolated deficiency of any hormone is possible.

Etiology, Pathophysiology, and Clinical Manifestations. Panhypopituitarism is the most complex of the pituitary disorders and usually is caused by a tumor in the pituitary region. The disorder may also occur iatrogenically as an outcome of treatment for brain tumors,[68] or as a result of encephalitis or head trauma. GH, TSH, ACTH, and gonadotropin deficiencies can occur at the same time, or their production may wane slowly as pituitary gland function is exhausted.

Growth Hormone Deficiency. GHD is the most common pituitary deficiency (isolated or combined) and may be the first hormone lost in panhypopituitarism. The previous section describes the disorder. Figure 56-8 illustrates the growth pattern associated with panhypopituitarism.

TSH Deficiency. TSH stimulates the thyroid gland to produce thyroxine; the absence of TSH results in hypothyroidism. (See section on congenital hypothyroidism for a description of clinical manifestations.) Secondary hypothyroidism due to TSH deficiency usually is not as severe as primary hypothyroidism.

ACTH Deficiency. ACTH promotes the production of cortisol. With inadequate ACTH, the adrenal cortex continues to produce aldosterone, but there is a deficiency of cortisol. Sufficient cortisol may be produced for daily function but insufficient to produce the levels of cortisol

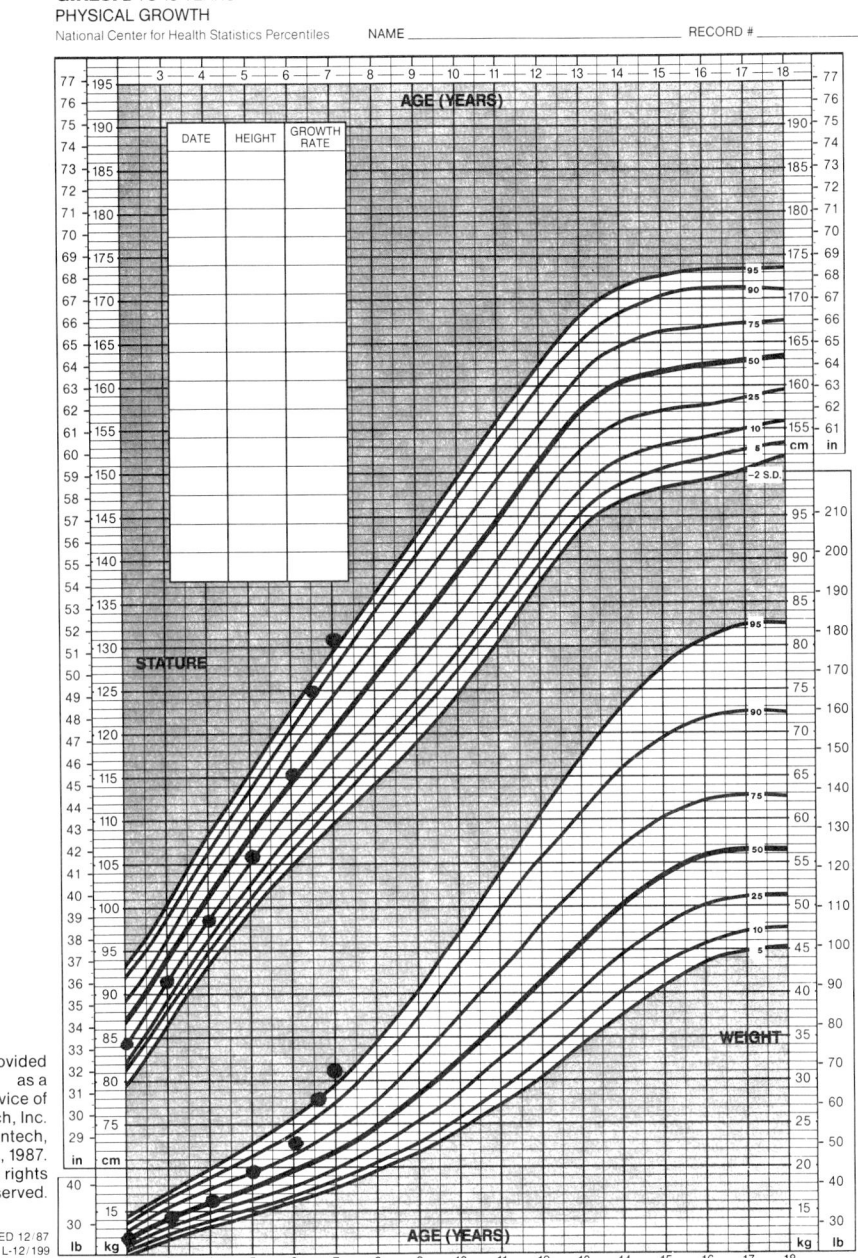

GIRLS: 2 TO 18 YEARS
PHYSICAL GROWTH
National Center for Health Statistics Percentiles   NAME _____   RECORD # _____

FIGURE 56-8

Growth pattern of a boy with panhypopituitarism. He grew normally along the 90% percentile until age 9. At that time, his growth slowed significantly, although he continued to gain weight. Three years later, he has had no change in his height, but he is still not "short." At this time, he was diagnosed with a craniopharyngioma that resulted in growth hormone deficiency.

needed during illness. The child with ACTH deficiency has the symptoms of low cortisol described in the section on alterations in adrenal function.

Gonadotropin Deficiency. Children with panhypopituitarism have intact gonads (ovaries or testes) that are inactive due to the lack of pituitary stimulation. Male infants with gonadotropin deficiency fail to produce the testosterone surge in utero that stimulates normal penile growth, resulting in a small penis at birth. Girls with congenital gonadotropin deficiency may have smaller than average labia, but this finding is difficult to assess.

Diagnostic Studies

Growth Hormone Deficiency. Provocative testing for GHD (discussed in the earlier section) is initiated in conjunction with evaluation of all pituitary hormones.

TSH Deficiency. TSH deficiency can occur alone, but it generally develops in conjunction with other pituitary losses. T_4 must be normalized before the child can be tested for GHD, because a child with hypothyroidism does not produce growth hormone in response to provocative testing. With deficient TSH, the concentration of T_4 obtained by RIA is low for age, but TSH concentration may be normal or low. Bone age is delayed if hypothyroidism is longstanding.

ACTH Deficiency. In panhypopituitarism, the morning serum cortisol level is low, and a 24-hour urine collection for urinary free cortisol yields a concentration that is below normal. Provocative growth hormone testing with insulin, glucagon, or L-dopa also can be used to test the ability of the body to mount a stress response of cortisol. A rise in cortisol to 20 μg/dl, or double the baseline value, is considered a normal response.

ACTH deficiency is the most difficult pituitary deficiency to determine. It is convenient to test for cortisol production during testing for growth hormone, but growth hormone testing cannot be done if the child is in a hypothyroid state; a child cannot be started on thyroxine if the serum cortisol level is low. The return to a normal thyroid level and metabolic rate in a child who was deficient in cortisol function could precipitate an adrenal crisis. In children with suspected multiple pituitary losses, testing must be individualized by the endocrinologist to maintain safety.

Gonadotropin Deficiency. Children with a bone age indicating the expected onset of puberty are tested with the GnRH stimulation test outlined in the section on puberty. Because the children do not produce adequate amounts of LH or FSH, they have low serum levels of sex hormones (estrogen or testosterone).

★ NURSING IMPLICATIONS

The child with multiple hormone deficiencies requires careful attention to growth parameters, such as height, weight, and pubertal status (see Tanner stage in Chap. 66). Previous sections provide guidance for specific assessment related to growth hormone, cortisol, and thyroid deficiencies.

The age at which panhypopituitarism occurs greatly influences the problems that nurses identify as needing their attention. All of the nursing diagnoses mentioned in other sections related to insufficient hormones from the pituitary's target glands may be applicable to the affected child and family.

Caring for children with panhypopituitarism is a complex nursing challenge. All of the hormones interact, and can either promote or inhibit growth. Affected children require highly specialized care by a pediatric endocrinologist. Although they are not more apt to be ill, their health is a delicate balance that requires frequent evaluation and adjustments in the replacement hormone dosages.

These children are growth hormone-deficient and height issues may be of great importance. The child with multiple hormone deficiencies faces even more significant adjustments and a more complex lifetime plan of care than children with isolated GHD.

TSH, ACTH, and gonadotropins are pulsatile hormones that have no current pharmacologic replacements. The goal of these hormones is to promote the production of other hormones. Treatment, therefore, consists of replacing the hormone produced by the target gland, as in primary gland hypofunction.

Thyroid deficiency is replaced with one daily dose of thyroxine. Hydrocortisone (Cortef) or cortisone acetate, in a dosage range of 9 to 12 mg/m²/day, is given to replace the adrenocortical hormone in three doses daily.[6] Girls are given oral estrogen supplements at a low dose to initiate early puberty, and the dose is increased progressively to levels that promote adult breast development and menstruation. Progesterone (Provera) is added to regulate the menstrual cycle. Boys are given testosterone injections monthly, beginning in the adolescent years.

Male infants who have significantly small genitals are given a short course of testosterone or HCG to stimulate enlargement of the penis and descent of the testes.

Children with well-balanced pituitary replacement should grow at a normal or catch-up rate at the beginning of treatment. Decreased growth velocity or increased weight gain may indicate a need to adjust the medications. At each visit, the medications should be re-evaluated and adjustments made before the child outgrows the dosage. Gonadotropin pulses are needed for ovulation and spermatogenesis. Children with GnRH deficiency require significant technologic assistance to reproduce.

Children with panhypopituitarism need lifelong health supervision and regulation of their replacement therapy. With adequate care, these children can expect a normal life span.

Hyperpituitarism

Disorders of overfunction of the pituitary are rare in children and generally are caused by a malignant neoplasm. Gigantism, excessive growth caused by high levels of growth hormone, usually is associated with a pituitary adenoma.[6] Tumors of the hypothalamus have also been implicated in children with excessive growth rates. Hyperpituitarism that occurs after closure of the epiphyses causes acromegaly, in which the circumference of the skull increases, the nose becomes broad, the mandible grows, and the facial features coarsen.

Fast growth and tall stature are often familial traits or normal changes associated with puberty. However, undiagnosed congenital adrenal hyperplasia also produces rapid growth. Exceptionally rapid growth is indicated on growth charts when percentiles are crossed. This change always requires careful evaluation by a pediatric endocrinologist.

Treatment options include surgery to remove tumors when possible. Radiation or radioactive implants may be used to destroy abnormal pituitary tissue. Hormone replacement therapy is indicated after destruction or removal of the existing pituitary tissue. Nursing care related to a surgical procedure is expected.

Children who are exceptionally tall, especially girls, may require intensive psychosocial support to manage feelings associated with being unlike their peers. Medical treatment (high doses of estrogen or bromocriptine) is rarely recommended but sometimes requested.

Altered Antidiuretic Hormone Function: Posterior Pituitary Dysfunction

Diabetes Insipidus

Definition and Incidence. Diabetes insipidus (DI) is the result of the deficiency in hormone antidiuretic (ADH), sometimes called vasopressin. Because the kidneys depend on ADH to concentrate urine appropriately, the lack of ADH leads to massive renal loss of fluids.

DI is also called neurogenic DI and must be differentiated from psychogenic water drinking. This condition mimics DI in the excessive amount of urine the child produces, but these children do not have an abnormality of ADH production. Children with psychogenic water drinking produce copious amounts of urine in response to the excessive quantity of fluids ingested. In DI, the child drinks copious amounts of fluid to replace the excessive loss of fluid through urine. Neither neurogenic DI nor psechogenic water drinking should be confused with nephrogenic DI, a rare, inherited disorder in which the renal tubuses are unresponsive to ADH.

Etiology and Pathophysiology. ADH works directly on the renal collecting ducts and distal tubules, to increase membrane permeability for water and urea. A deficiency in ADH allows water to diffuse into the urine. Decreased ADH secretion promotes massive water loss and retention of sodium in the serum.

Damage to the posterior pituitary gland may injure the cells responsible for the production of ADH. DI is most commonly seen in the intensive care unit as a temporary condition following cranial surgery or head trauma. In previously healthy children, ADH deficiency may be the first sign of histiocytosis X or a pituitary tumor, such as a craniopharyngioma and hamartoma. DI can be seen in conjunction with other hypothalamic-pituitary hormone deficiencies. It also can occur as an autosomal recessive deficiency, or the cause may be unknown.[7] This condition can occur at any age.

Some children with DI have damage to the thirst center in the hypothalamus. These children rapidly become gravely ill, because their diuresis is not balanced by the drive to drink fluids to replace the loss. This rare situation is the severest form of the disorder and is characterized by a fragile balance in life.

Clinical Manifestations. In psychogenic water drinking, excessive drinking habits are established over a long period. In contrast, the sudden onset of excessive thirst and polyuria are classic manifestations of DI. Frequent, abrupt trips to the bathroom are typical, with nocturia and enuresis suddenly occurring in the child who previously had gained night-time bladder control. The child awakens because of thirst at night.

Parents often state that their child will suddenly run to the bathroom to urinate, then stop to drink two or three glasses of water. Children prefer water to all other beverages; infants reject formula or breast milk in their desire for water. The thirst drive may be so intense that the child cannot eat sufficient calories to gain weight and grow.

The child's urine is extremely dilute and often colorless. The child may show signs of mild dehydration, such as a sunken fontanel in the infant, poor skin turgor, and dry mucous membranes, despite an enormous fluid intake. If the cycle of urine loss and abnormal drinking continues unchecked, the kidneys and bladder may begin to dilate to accommodate the large quantities of fluids that are ingested.

Diagnostic Studies. DI can be the presenting complaint for brain tumors or other life-threatening disorders. These children are given treatment for the ADH deficiency while being treated for their primary disease.

In the otherwise healthy child, the evaluation for DI has two steps: (1) to discover whether the excessive urination and drinking are due to ADH deficiency, and if so, (2) to determine the cause of this problem. If the child has a known organic illness that is associated with pituitary malfunction, the diagnosis of DI is made more easily. This is the case when a child has a history of brain tumor.

Initial screening tests include urine and serum specimens. Electrolytes, blood urea nitrogen, and creatinine levels are evaluated to screen for kidney disease. The sodium and osmolality of both urine and serum are analyzed and compared, and the specific gravity of the urine is analyzed. In DI, dilute urine is present although the serum is very concentrated and sodium is elevated. Children with psychogenic water drinking may have dilute urine, but the serum also is dilute and sodium is low. In nephrogenic DI, this screening test mimics true DI. Serum measurement for ADH is recommended as the most reliable diagnostic tool in conjunction with plasma osmolality.[66]

When DI is suspected, the child is hospitalized for a water deprivation test, which is potentially dangerous and requires close monitoring. Fluids are withheld and the urine volume and concentration are monitored. This test differentiates psychogenic water drinking and neurogenic or nephrogenic DI.

The water deprivation test is generally followed by a test dose of ADH, usually administered as a nasal spray of short-acting DDAVP (1-deamino-8-D-arginine vasopressin). A dose of this medication stops the abnormal diuresis that occurs in DI and results in cessation of the symptoms. DDAVP does not stop the diuresis associated with nephrogenic DI.

An MRI or CT scan of the hypothalamic-pituitary region is done in children when the cause of the DI is not known. A renal ultrasound is recommended when the condition has been long-standing to determine the extent of dilation of the renal system due to excessive urine volume.

★ **ASSESSMENT**

Children with the complaints of polyuria and polydipsia need a comprehensive physical assessment, because of the association of DI with malignant and pathologic processes. They are examined for signs of dehydration, which would prompt immediate attention. The behavior of the child during the assessment, such as requests to drink fluids and use the bathroom, should be observed. The mental status of the child generally is normal; if the child appears confused or frantic, dehydration is severe, and immediate medical attention should be sought.

History taking focuses on probable causes of the disorder. Children with no previous history to indicate an organic cause need an in-depth behavioral history. This review includes all aspects of the child's behavior, such as sleep patterns and night-time wandering; unusual foods ingested, such as dog food; the extent to which drinking and urination interrupt the child's life; choices of fluids, such as carbonated beverages or juices rather than water; drinking from unusual sources, such as toilet bowls and dog dishes; the parent-child interaction; and peer and school problems. Such questioning helps determine whether psychogenic water drinking or other emotionally based problems have led to increased urination. The assessment also aids in describing the extent to which the child seeks fluids.

The child's height and weight are obtained and plotted on a growth chart. A history of weight loss is important, because it may indicate the child's inability to consume enough calories. Height and weight gain patterns indicate the probable onset of the disorder.

★ NURSING DIAGNOSES AND PLANNING

Based on assessment data discussed in the previous section and the preceding chapter, the following nursing diagnoses may apply to the family and child with DI:

- Anxiety related to the cause of the disease and its lifetime impact.
- Fluid Volume Deficit related to excessive loss of water from the kidneys.
- Altered Comfort related to dehydration, excessive thirst, and frequent need to urinate.
- Altered Family Processes related to chronic illness and possible acute problem.

The nurse and child (or parents) together plan effective care based on the established nursing diagnoses. Several examples of expected outcomes are as follows:

- The parents and child administer the hormone therapy as prescribed.
- The child reports the cessation of abnormal urination and thirst.
- The parents or child report a period of breakthrough that is predictable (see following section).
- The child reports a return to a normal lifestyle.

The nurse plans for the daily care of the child based on both the physician's orders and nursing diagnoses. Some general nursing care goals may include the following:

- The parents and child understand the need for replacement hormone therapy and long term follow-up.
- The parents and child recognize abnormal symptoms that should be reported.

★ INTERVENTIONS: COLLABORATIVE AND INDEPENDENT

HORMONE REPLACEMENT

Most children with DI need daily replacement of vasopressin (ADH) using desmopressin (DDAVP), a synthetic analogue of ADH. Affected children usually have an intact thirst mechanism and need free access to water. DDAVP works through absorption in the highly vascularized nasal mucosa. It is available as a metered nasal spray (used largely in adults), a measured insufflation (nasal) tube, or an intramuscular injection. DDAVP has immediate action and lasts between 8 and 24 hours. DDAVP prevents diuresis only when the kidney is healthy. Nasal DDAVP

has widely replaced the use of vasopressin (Pitressin) in oil. The newer medication works more slowly and over a longer period (24–72 hours).[66]

Initial dose adjustment and education occur during the hospital stay. Careful monitoring of the child's response to treatment is necessary; evidence of adequate treatment includes daily weight gain, electrolyte balance, return to normal voiding and drinking patterns, and the ability to concentrate urine. During this adjustment period, the nurse focuses on the education of the child and family.

Administration of DDAVP is a skill that requires practice and a cooperative child or an extra adult. The accompanying display lists patient teaching guidelines for DDAVP administration The insufflation tubing generally is used for children, because the metered spray delivers a large dose (0.1 mg per spray). Most children require one or two doses daily, at bedtime and in the morning. The dose is response-based and ranges from 0.05 to 0.2 ml per day.[66]

In infants and younger children, the volume required may be so small that it cannot be properly measured in the insufflation tubing. An accurate measuring device can be constructed by cutting off the needle of a butterfly infusion set and attaching the thin tubing to a tuberculin syringe. Administration of the dose while the infant is asleep is advised to avoid the conflict that results when the nares are entered.

Children may swallow the dose instead of inhaling it when the volume is too great or their nasal surface area is too small. However, DDAVP is not absorbed in the oral cavity, the esophagus, or the stomach. When swallowing is detected, the caregiver should split the dose and give half in each naris. Liquid DDAVP also may be given successfully sublingually, but the required dosage is much higher.[66]

DDAVP is a costly medication; nevertheless, an extra bottle should be kept at home in reserve. Care must be taken to protect it from heat; refrigeration is recommended.

All children on DDAVP should have their dose adjusted to allow a daily period of "breakthrough" when symptoms are permitted to develop. Breakthrough is evidenced by a sudden desire to use the bathroom, followed by a trip to the kitchen sink for a few glasses of water. Most children experience breakthrough after school or in the evening when they are at home and can freely drink and urinate. When the child returns home after the initial hospitalization, the parents are instructed to call the health care provider if this breakthrough fails to occur.

FLUID ADJUSTMENT AT HOME

Parents are educated to note drinking patterns at home and to report any changes. For example, the child may prefer to drink rather than to eat. One or two days of increased drinking and urination are seldom cause for concern, but a pattern of changed behavior needs to be evaluated.

Free access to fluids is essential for children with deficient ADH. The preferred and recommended fluid is water. For children who are underweight, caloric beverages, such as milk and juices, should be encouraged.

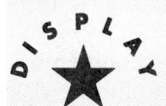

Patient Teaching: Guidelines for DDAVP Administration

Insufflation tubing is marked in various doses from 0.05 to 0.2 ml. It functions like a measuring straw, with one end used to pull up a dose and blow the medication.

General Guidelines

- Refrigerate the medication, and keep out of heat.
- Keep medication cool in an insulated thermos when traveling.
- Have an extra bottle of DDAVP at home in case of breakage, spillage, or overheating.
- Discard the medication if the medication is overheated (when several doses do not provide adequate coverage).
- Establish a single pharmacy for obtaining the medication.
- Do not repeat doses that might have been swallowed or poorly absorbed. (Overdosing is a serious medical emergency.)

Infants and Younger Children

- Construct a measuring device from a butterfly infusion set (as directed by the nurse or physician).
- Administer medication while the child is asleep to avoid conflict.
- Split the dose, and give one in each nares if the child is swallowing the medication.
- Clear the nostrils of a child with respiratory infections before giving this medication.

Self-Administration

- Insert the tube into the bottle.
- Fill up the tube to the proper dosage line.
- Hold the top of the tube closed.
- Insert the medication-filled end into the nares.
- Blow the liquid out of the tubing and into the nares.

During increased physical activity or in hot weather, adequate replacement fluid must be provided for insensible water loss.

Determination of urine specific gravity at home rarely is needed for children. However, it can be done through the use of a refractometer or urine dipsticks. These techniques can be taught to families during the initial hospitalization.

Infants with DI are weighed daily at home, and specific gravity is checked when they are ill or when weight gain is poor. They are fed every 2 hours and are offered water in addition to breast milk or formula. Parents are encouraged to keep a diary that documents the number of wet diapers and feedings during the adjustment period.

TEACHING AND COUNSELING

Children and parents should be provided education concerning the lifestyle needs and changes that take place after diagnosis. Children may desire that their teacher be given an explanation about the child's possible need to use the drinking fountain and bathroom more frequently than other children. Gym teachers and coaches must be told of the need for extra fluids and access to the bathroom. Some children increase their dose of DDAVP on the day that they plan to have a field trip or sports event. This is a safe practice if the child has an intact thirst center and has the physician's approval. All children should be encouraged to wear medical alert tags stating that they have DI.

COMPENSATED DI

In milder cases of DI, children with intact thirst centers can manage to maintain water balance without medication, by drinking enough fluids to offset fluid loss in ur-

ination. These children need to be monitored carefully to prevent kidney and bladder dilation. They may choose to use DDAVP when traveling or at night. This approach to treatment is generally chosen by the family with familial DI, when significant drinking and urinating are accepted as a family norm.

CARE OF CHILDREN LACKING A THIRST CENTER

Children who lack a thirst center require much more careful monitoring at home. They must be encouraged to drink at each meal and between meals. Children who resist drinking are tube fed to provide the water needed.[7] Their fluid replacement needs are individually calculated during the hospitalization. Daily weights, urine specific gravity measurement, and intake and output at home may be required.

★ EVALUATION

The nurse and family periodically evaluate the outcomes of care given. Examples of outcomes for the child and family with DI were given under planning in this section. Have the short-term goals been met? Are the long-term goals still realistic? Planning for further nursing care takes into consideration complications and long-term care.

COMPLICATIONS

Some children adapt to polyuria and polydipsia and do not seek adjustment of their medication as they grow. Long-term mismanagement of DI, however, can result in bladder, kidney, and pelvic damage, and central nervous system damage, vascular changes, and dehydration can occur. These complications are most likely when the cause of DI is familial, there is family acceptance, and a lack of anxiety about the condition.

LONG-TERM CARE

Many children with DI have multiple hormone deficiencies and complex health care needs. They are followed by a pediatric endocrinologist.

Syndrome of Inappropriate Antidiuretic Hormone

Syndrome of inappropriate antidiuretic hormone (SIADH), a rare disorder in children, is associated with a variety of conditions but is most often encountered as a temporary condition following brain surgery.[6] Tumors may be in the head, or there may be other tumors that have aberrant ADH production. SIADH is recognized in preterm infants with bronchopulmonary dysplasia or head trauma.[59] Drugs such as chlorpropamide, carbamazepine, analgesics, phenothiazines, nicotine, barbiturates, vincristine, and cytoxan are also recognized as causative agents.[7] SIADH can occur as a result of an overly vigorous administration of intravenous solutions.

In the normally functioning body, ADH is not be secreted when too much water is in circulation, because the excess fluid needs to be excreted. When ADH is produced in excess by tumors or by the posterior pituitary, it shuts down the normal kidney function of water filtration and loss. By keeping water in circulation, all blood components are diluted. Metabolic toxins accumulate in the blood rather than being excreted. Pressure within the central nervous system is increased by the fluid volume overload.

Weight gain occurs as fluids are retained, and the child becomes weak and lethargic. Anorexia, nausea, and vomiting develop as fluid and electrolyte balance deteriorates. The child eventually has confusion, convulsions, and coma. SIADH, therefore, is considered a life-threatening disorder.

In the presence of SIADH, laboratory studies show concentrated urine with dilute serum. Oliguria may be present. A low serum sodium level is found with a high sodium concentration in the urine. Serum studies show decreased urea, creatinine, uric acid, and albumin levels.

Children with SIADH are diagnosed within the acute care setting. The child's intake, output, and weight records are analyzed and indicate steady weight gain but deficient urine output. The child may appear bloated. The level of consciousness is assessed for changes related to fluid and electrolyte imbalance. Exposure to precipitating factors, such as possible ingestion of drugs, disease process, medications, and cranial surgery, is noted in the history.

The goals of treatment are to reduce the fluid overload and raise serum sodium level and osmolality. Fluids are immediately restricted, with intravenous infusions reduced to keep-open rates. The child may be treated with 3% normal saline intravenously and given furosemide.[7] The child may be treated with demeclocycline to induce a temporary nephrogenic DI, the condition in which the kidneys do not recognize ADH and allow maximal water excretion.[66]

Meticulous hourly intake and output records are maintained. If the child has not been catheterized, an indwelling catheter is placed to monitor hourly urine volume and specific gravity.

SIADH is a temporary crisis usually encountered in the intensive care unit. There should be no further risks to the child once the problem is corrected. In the absence of prompt and effective interventions, central nervous system damage from this incident may impair the child permanently.

Altered Pancreatic Endocrine Function

The healthy pancreas is continually active as it responds to digestive needs and blood sugar regulatory demands. Loss of the pancreas through surgery or trauma affects both digestive and glucose control functions—this is a rare event. Far more common is the failure of the cells of the endocrine system to produce adequate insulin, resulting from the autoimmune disorder, diabetes mellitus. Conversely, the islet cells may overproduce glucagon, which leads to excessively high blood sugar concentration. Most children with an endocrinopathy of the pancreas must learn to replace the missing hormones and adapt to the lifestyle changes that the disorder imposes.

Hypoglycemia

Children with a blood sugar level of less than 40 mg/dl are considered hypoglycemic and should be treated. Except for insulin reactions seen in association with diabetes mellitus, hypoglycemia is a rare condition in children. However, it is discussed briefly here and in the section on diabetes mellitus.

Premature and infants who are small-for-gestational-age are at risk for low serum glucose concentration because of their small muscle mass and glycogen stores. Infants of diabetic mothers may be hypoglycemic as a result of maternal hyperglycemia. (The infant's pancreas responds to the high levels of blood glucose that cross the placenta by pouring out insulin in large amounts. After birth, the pancreas continues to secrete insulin, but the infant's blood sugar is quickly utilized, and symptoms of hypoglycemia develop.) In other situations, liver disease or catastrophic illness may interfere with gluconeogenesis and lead to decreased circulating glucose. When low blood sugar levels persist, endocrine causes are considered.

When children present after the neonatal period with hypoglycemia, there is rarely an endocrine cause. Malnutrition, liver disease, and malabsorption must be considered. Alcohol, salicylates, insulin, and other drugs also can result in hypoglycemia.

Occasionally, a child might have pancreatic dysfunction resulting in inappropriate production of insulin, or hyperinsulinism. Other rare enzyme deficiencies, such as leucine, carnitine, or alanine deficiencies, galactosemia, and glycogen storage disease, can result in low serum blood glucose concentrations.

In the acute care setting, the nurse obtains a focused history to help validate the cause of hypoglycemia and to determine the parents' ability to care for the child at home. Linear growth and weight gain patterns are analyzed to rule out hormone deficiencies. Diagnostic studies for serum glucose may be supplemented with other evaluations of endocrine function.

Early, profound hypoglycemia may impair brain development in young children. Prevention of repeated episodes is a priority. Children with hyperinsulinism are treated with oral diazoxide and frequent feedings; surgical removal of the pancreas may be necessary. Pancreactomy, however, causes diabetes mellitus and pancreatic deficiencies for life. Children with glycogen storage disease grow poorly, and often face a childhood of feeling "different" due to their appearance and need for frequent meals throughout the day.

Diabetes Mellitus

It is estimated that 11 million people in the United States have diabetes mellitus, with approximately 500,000 new cases detected each year.[3] Children and adolescents with diabetes mellitus constitute about 10% of all cases and about 3% of all new cases detected annually.[3] Diabetes is one of the leading causes of morbidity and mortality in this country, and is a leading cause of acquired blindness, end-stage renal disease, and premature cardiovascular death.[3] In chronic illnesses among school-age children, diabetes ranks third and may contribute to increased hospitalization and school absence.

Although a cure has not been found, better understanding of the etiology and advances in treatment of diabetes have made possible the achievement of significantly better health outcomes than in the past. Whereas treatment once was directed at eliminating the overt signs and symptoms of diabetes, it is now focused on improving glycemic control in an attempt to approach euglycemia. Consequently, treatment has become increasingly complex.

Successful management of diabetes is largely dependent on the family's commitment and involvement in a regimen that includes monitoring blood glucose levels with day-to-day adjustment of insulin, diet, and exercise. Although young people need to be engaged in their own care, they should not be held responsible for their health before they are ready. The chronicity of diabetes, like many other chronic illnesses, puts a tremendous strain on the family as well as the child.

Definition and Incidence. Diabetes is a heterogeneous group of disorders that is characterized by glucose intolerance resulting from insulin deficiency or inadequate utilization of insulin. The primary features of diabetes are (1) hyperglycemia; (2) abnormalities in carbohydrate, protein, and fat metabolism; and (3) an increased incidence of eye, renal, neurologic, and premature cardiovascular diseases.[15] The metabolic alterations in diabetes occur in response either to destruction of pancreatic beta cells with absolute insulin deficiency or

as a result of peripheral insulin resistance with more normal beta-cell function (ineffective insulin action). Differences in pathogenesis reflect the heterogeneity of this group of disorders. Clinical expression of the disease and the risk of associated complications vary considerably among people and on classification of the disorder.

Three major types of diabetes mellitus have been described: type I, type II, and other types. Table 56-2 compares the three types according to etiology, clinical characteristics, and diagnostic criteria. The following discussion is limited to insulin-dependent diabetes mellitus (IDDM), the type that appears in childhood. The reader is referred to a general endocrine text for more information regarding the other categories.

The annual incidence of IDDM is about 15 new cases per 100,000 among people younger than 20 years of age. After age 20, the incidence declines to 5 new cases per 100,000. The prevalence rate (the number of cases in a defined population during a specified period) currently is about 1 in 600. The peak incidence of IDDM is between 10 and 14 years of age. Rates of expression are comparable for males and females by age 13; it is slightly more frequent among males younger than 5 years of age and slightly higher for females than males 10 to 12 years of age.[15] IDDM is about 1.5 times more common among whites than blacks and markedly less common in Hispanics, Native Americans, and Asian Americans.

Rates of expression of diabetes in children according to their country correlate with latitude, with countries furthest from the equator having the highest incidence and those closest to the equator, the lowest. Moreover, the incidence is higher during the fall and winter months than during spring and summer. Variation in incidence rates by season and geography suggests a link with infectious and environmental factors.[15]

Etiology. The etiology of IDDM is believed to be multifactorial. Genetics, autoimmunity, and environmental factors are all linked to the destruction of beta cells located within the pancreatic islets of Langerhans. Overt expression of diabetes generally does not occur until about 90% of beta-cell function is lost.[15] Although symptoms usually appear suddenly, the destruction of the beta cells is believed to be the result of a chronic, progressive autoimmune process that occurs over a period of months and years.

Genetic Factors. Genetic factors are known to play an important role in the pathogenesis of IDDM; however, the exact nature of that role is not completely understood. Genes within the human leukocyte antigen (HLA) region known as the major histocompatibility complex, located on chromosome 6, are related to the development of IDDM. This complex contains the loci (location) of several classes of genes that direct self-recognition and host-defense mechanisms. The frequency of certain HLA alleles (antigen DR3, DR4, or both) is about fivefold greater among people with IDDM.[15] Family studies also support a linkage of the HLA region with disease susceptibility. When one child within a family has IDDM, the risk of diabetes in siblings correlates with the number of HLA combinations (haplotypes) that are shared.

TABLE 56-2
Classification of Diabetes Mellitus

Class	Etiology	Clinical Characteristics	Diagnostic Criteria
Type I Insulin-Dependent Diabetes Mellitus (IDDM)	Evidence of genetic, environmental, and acquired factors associated with certain HLA types, and abnormal immune responses	1. Body build usually lean, with abrupt onset of symptoms before 20 years of age. However, onset may occur at any age 2. Insulinopenia (insulin deficient); dependent on injected insulin to prevent ketoacidosis and to sustain life	1. Classic signs and symptoms: Polyuria Polydipsia Ketonuria (may or may not be present) Weight loss 2. Fasting glucose >140 mg/dl on more than one occasion
Type II Noninsulin dependent diabetes mellitus (NIDDM) Obese and nonobese	Environmental factors superimposed on genetic susceptibility are probably involved in the onset of NIDDM types. Obesity is suspected as an etiologic factor. A subclass of type II, nonobese diabetes, has its onset in youth. Maturity onset in youth (MODY) is inherited autosomal dominant disorder	1. Usually obese, with onset >40 years of age with a strong family history. However, it may occur at any age 2. Insulin resistant, i.e., ineffective insulin response at cellular level. Insulin production may be increased, decreased, or normal 3. Not ketosis prone, although ketones may occur under unusual circumstances such as illness and surgery 4. Does not require injected insulin to sustain life	1. Unequivocal elevation of plasma glucose in addition to classic symptoms 2. Elevated fasting glucose >140 mg/dl on more than one occasion 3. Elevated plasma glucose after oral glucose challenge on more than one occasion
Other types, including diabetes associated with certain conditions and syndromes: • Pancreatic disease, e.g., cystic fibrosis, pancreatectomy • Endocrinopathies: e.g., pheochromocytoma, Cushing's syndrome • Drugs and chemicals, e.g., certain antihypertensives • Genetic syndromes e.g., hyperlipidemia	Factors are known, e.g., diabetes secondary to pancreatic disease, endocrine disease, or certain drugs In other types, there is a higher frequency of association with a syndrome or condition, as in certain genetic syndromes	1. Presence of pre-existing condition or syndrome	1. Presence of diabetes, as established by elevated plasma glucose concentration on more than one occasion or as described previously and the presence of the associated condition or syndrome.

Source: Adapted from the National Diabetes Data Group (1979). Classification and diagnosis of diabetes mellitus and other categories of glucose intolerance. *Diabetes, 28,* 1039–1057.

HLA status may determine the pathogenic mechanism of beta-cell destruction.[15] Undoubtedly, more than one gene predisposes people to IDDM. The gene may determine different pathogenic mechanisms. Distinction should be made here between an inherited disease and a predisposition to development of a disorder. A genetic disease is one in which concordance is usually 100% in identical twins; IDDM concordance rates for identical twins is less than 50%. This finding suggests that genetic susceptibility increases the risk of developing diabetes but does not ensure that it will be clinically manifested. Thus, other factors are likely to be involved in the etiology.

Environmental Factors. Evidence that implicates environmental factors in the development of IDDM exists. Drugs and infectious agents are known to induce autoimmune diseases; for example, procainimide can produce a lupuslike condition, and streptococci antigens are involved in the damage caused by rheumatic fever. However, interest has focused primarily on a viral etiology. A number of viruses are known to cause direct damage to

beta cells in animals. Viruses may act as a triggering event that initiates beta-cell destruction in a genetically susceptible person.

Although the pathogenic mechanism is not well defined, viruses are believed to cause damage by directly infecting beta cells or by disrupting normal lymphocyte function, thereby heightening autoimmune response.[16] Further evidence to support a viral origin for diabetes relates to the increased seasonal onset during the cooler months. Viral factors as initiators of autoimmune processes continue to be suspected.

Autoimmunity. The interplay of genetics and environmental factors in the etiology of IDDM remains to be determined. However, IDDM is recognized as an autoimmune disorder. A number of immunologic abnormalities have been described. Both anti-islet cell antibodies (ICAs) and insulin autoantibodies (IAA) have been found in a large number of people with new-onset diabetes. Furthermore, ICAs and IAAs have been found to precede the onset of disease by as much as a decade.[16] This latter finding may become useful in identifying people at high risk for developing IDDM. Although islet cell antibodies may react with the islet cell surface to inhibit insulin secretion, the reaction is not believed to be a primary factor in the destruction of beta cells. Rather, ICAs are believed to represent a secondary response to progressive beta-cell damage. Increasing evidence suggests that T lymphocytes mediate beta-cell destruction, probably in response to aberrant expression of HLA antigens on the surface of beta cells.[52]

Pathophysiology. Glucose is the principal fuel used by the body for energy. It is derived from dietary sources and is produced and stored in the liver and muscle as glycogen. Glucose homeostasis is regulated through a complex interaction of several hormones, including insulin and glucagon, which are produced in the endocrine pancreas in specialized cells of the islets of Langerhans. Insulin is produced by the beta cells, and glucagon is produced by the alpha cells. Both hormones are secreted directly into the bloodstream in response to changes in the plasma glucose concentration.

Insulin Deficiency. In the presence of insulin deficiency (i.e., IDDM), extracellular glucose concentration increases as a result of decreased uptake by peripheral tissues. Insulin deficiency causes an increased production of amino acids and a breakdown of fat. With excessive glucagon, a marked increase in hepatic gluconeogenesis, glycogenolysis, and ketogenesis occur.[72] An increased concentration of plasma glucose (hyperglycemia) is the hallmark of diabetes. Continued insulinopenia results in

an ongoing catabolic state with loss of weight; because glucose cannot be used for energy, the body must use alternate fuels. Therefore, glycogen, protein, and fat are mobilized from stores to meet the body's energy needs. However, in the absence of insulin, glycogen, protein, and fat cells cannot be replenished and readily become depleted. The end result is a severe state of starvation or catabolism.

Ketoacidosis. Three factors contribute to the development of hyperglycemia in the absence of insulin. First, there is a decreased rate of transfer of glucose, amino acids, and free fatty acids to the liver, muscle, and adipose tissue. Second, in the presence of glucagon, there is unrestrained glucose production by the liver through glycogenolysis (conversion of glucose from glycogen) and gluconeogenesis (formation of new glucose from amino acids and fatty acids). Finally, there is unrestrained lipolysis (fat breakdown), which further stimulates gluconeogenesis and produces excess ketone bodies. The sequence of events in the development of ketoacidosis is summarized in Figure 56-9. Failure of glucose to be taken up by peripheral tissues, combined with unrestrained glucose production by the liver, results in progressive hyperglycemia.

The increased plasma glucose concentration causes an osmotic shift in fluid from the intracellular to the extracellular compartment. In addition, more glucose must be filtered by the kidney. The renal tubules, which nor-

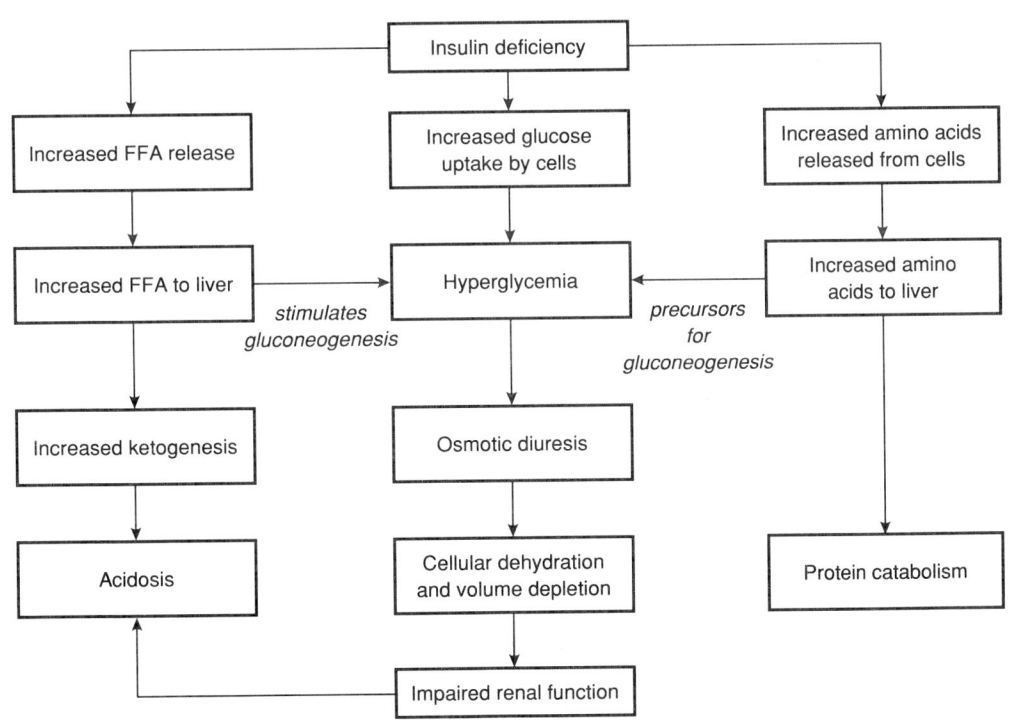

FIGURE 56-9
Metabolic consequences of insulin deficiency. Insulin deficiency generates hyperglycemia in three ways: (1) There is a decreased rate of transfer of glucose to insulin-dependent tissues; (2) there is an increase in lipolysis and free fatty acids (FFA) release, which stimulates gluconeogenesis; and (3) there is mobilization of amino acids to promote gluconeogenesis and lipolysis. Acidosis results from production of acetoacetic acid and beta-hydroxybutyric acid at a rate that exceeds the liver's ability to resynthesize triglycerides or fully oxidize these acids. (Source: Skillman, T. & Tzagournis, M. Diabetic mellitus. Upjohn Company, 1983.)

mally reabsorbs all glucose, is unable to handle the increased load. Once the renal threshold is reached (180 mg/dl), glucose spills over into the urine (glycosuria), resulting in osmotic diuresis and frequent urination (polyuria). Polydipsia (increased thirst) initially is able to compensate for the increased urine output and prevent dehydration.

In the absence of insulin, fat stores are mobilized and used as an alternate energy source. Through lipolysis, triglycerides are converted to free fatty acids and then converted to ketone bodies (acetoacetic acid and β-hydroxybutyric acid) in the liver. Ketone bodies can be used for energy by peripheral tissues at a limited rate but are not well utilized in a state of insulin deficiency. Ketone bodies are organic acids that readily disassociate to hydrogen and keto acids. An excess of ketone bodies leads to the accumulation of hydrogen ions, lowering the body pH. The concentration of hydrogen ions is regulated generally by a complex buffering system involving extracellular buffers (including bicarbonate) and the renal and respiratory systems.[72]

The initial accumulation of organic acids (ketone bodies) can be buffered through the bicarbonate system ($H^+ + HCO_3^- \rightarrow H_2O + CO_2$), the respiratory system (ventilation is increased to excrete the extra CO_2), and renal and cellular absorption of H^+ production in exchange for potassium. The serum bicarbonate level is mildly depressed, but the pH remains within the normal range. However, with increasing H^+ production, particularly when aggravated by dehydration from vomiting, the capacity of the buffering system is exceeded. As H^+ concentration increases (pH decreases), the respiratory center is further stimulated resulting in increased depth and rate of respiration (Kussmaul respirations).[72] The large loss of water from osmotic diuresis, continued vomiting, and tachypnea results in dehydration. Unless treatment is initiated promptly, dehydration progresses with increasing electrolyte imbalance, resulting in coma and death.

Clinical Manifestations.   Wide recognition of the clinical presentation of diabetes in children and adolescents contributes to early diagnosis and treatment. Consequently, diabetic ketoacidosis (DKA) is seen less frequently than in the past. Early detection has led to a marked reduction in morbidity and mortality associated with DKA. However, DKA still accounts for most diabetes-related hospitalizations, a group composed of children with new-onset and recurrent episodes associated with poor metabolic control.[25] Because DKA is life-threatening, prompt diagnosis and treatment are essential. The classic presentation of IDDM includes polyuria, polydipsia, polyphagia, and fatigue, with varying degrees of weight loss.

Both polyuria and polydipsia are directly related to osmotic diuresis secondary to hyperglycemia. However, nocturnal enuresis (bed wetting at night) is often the reason parents seek medical help. Polyphagia (increased hunger) may be present early in the course of diabetes due to the inability of the body to synthesize carbohydrate, protein, and fat. Later, however, anorexia is more likely to be present. Weight loss is variable and relates to the degree of catabolism. Loss of lean body mass from breakdown of protein, mobilization of fat, and dehydration all contribute to weight loss. Parents may be unaware of weight loss unless it is significant.

Children may complain of fatigue, headache, and general malaise, all symptoms attributed to dehydration. Visual disturbances are common but transitory and generally relate to changes in the lens secondary to hyperglycemia. As the course of the disease progresses, weight loss becomes more pronounced. Nausea, vomiting, abdominal pain, and dyspnea develop in response to increasing metabolic acidosis. Because these symptoms mimic influenza and gastroenteritis, diagnosis and treatment may be delayed. Abdominal pain can be quite severe and may be mistaken for an acute surgical condition.[15] This symptom is particularly problematic in very young children in whom the diagnosis of diabetes may not be suspected.

Dyspnea is a common complaint with DKA, and some children may have a fruity odor to their breath, which results from the excretion of keto-acids through the lungs. Unless treatment is initiated at this stage, symptoms progress to Kussmaul respirations, somnolence, and death. At this stage the child is considered dehydrated by at least 10% (see Chap. 26).

Diagnostic Studies.   Although not all diabetic children present in a state of DKA, most are symptomatic. Symptoms may range from mild to severe. Glycosuria occasionally is detected during a routine physical examination. The diagnosis of IDDM more often is made on the basis of presenting symptoms and blood glucose higher than 200 mg/dl. The classic symptoms of polyuria, polydipsia, weight loss, and fatigue (with or without ketonuria) make the diagnosis likely.[15] Although an oral glucose tolerance test is useful in the diagnosis of type II diabetes, it rarely is needed to diagnose IDDM in children. However, oral glucose tolerance tests may be used to confirm IDDM in children who have glycosuria, but are as yet asymptomatic.

★ **ASSESSMENT**

Assessment determines changes in the child's health status, the child and family's response to treatment, and their ability to adapt to changes imposed by illness. The initial assessment should include a complete history and physical examination to estimate the severity of metabolic alteration and to begin formulation of a plan of care.

The history includes a chronology of events leading to the diagnosis; whether the onset of symptoms was preceded by an infectious illness; whether there is a family history of type I diabetes; concurrent illnesses and medications; and what the family knows about the disease. Determining the families' understanding of diabetes is essential, because misinformation is common. Moreover, this line of investigation gives the family an opportunity to express their immediate concerns and fears.

The physical assessment should begin with a general observation of the child's appearance. Because varying degrees of dehydration, starvation, and metabolic acidosis may be present, attention should be given to the following areas of the examination.

GENERAL APPEARANCE AND CONDITION

What is the apparent state of health? How ill does the child appear to be? Is the child experiencing obvious difficulty such as labored breathing? What is the condition of the skin? Is it moist or dry? Are the lips cracked or sore? Are the mucous membranes dry? Is the skin mottled or are nail beds dusky? Are there sores that are not healing? Is there evidence of altered nutritional status? Has there been a recent history of increased appetite with weight loss or decreased appetite with or without vomiting? Is there a fruity or medicinal odor to the breath?

NEUROLOGIC FUNCTION

A baseline neurologic assessment is essential, particularly in children who present with DKA. Younger children may be at greater risk for neurological sequele. Cerebral edema, a rare and potentially fatal complication of DKA, usually presents within the first 12 hours of treatment and at a time when the child is actually showing signs of improvement. The neurologic status suddenly deteriorates. Changes in the following aspects of neurologic function should be reported immediately:

- Diminished level of consciousness
- Diminished pupillary response to light (a late sign of cerebral edema that may signal a sudden shift in the brain with herniation)
- Absent deep tendon reflexes, if the potassium level is low
- Diminished response to painful stimuli
- Increased dyspneic respirations, indicating acidosis

CARDIOVASCULAR FUNCTION

The functions of the cardiovascular system are preserved unless dehydration, electrolyte imbalance, and metabolic acidosis are severe. Tachycardia is a frequent finding. Cardiac arrhythmias can develop in the presence of hyperkalemia or hypokalemia. However, the decrease in potassium concentration that occurs with the initiation of fluid replacement and insulin therapy may precipitate arrhythmias. Assessment of the cardiovascular system should include the following:

- Blood pressure (hypotension is not uncommon)
- Heart rate and rhythm (rate may be increased with dehydration)
- Peripheral circulation, including peripheral pulses, skin turgor, and the presence of mottling. The nail beds are inspected for slow capillary refilling and cyanosis

RESPIRATORY FUNCTION

The metabolic disturbances of uncontrolled diabetes have direct effects on the respiratory system, resulting in increased ventilatory efforts. The respiratory assessment should include the character of respirations (rate, depth, and pattern), and signs of air hunger (restlessness and changes in skin color or mucous membranes).

RENAL FUNCTION

The kidneys play an important role in glucose homeostasis by reabsorbing glucose into the circulation from the renal tubules. When the renal threshold for glucose is exceeded (plasma glucose concentration of about 180 mg/dl), the excess is excreted in the urine. The osmotic effect of the glucose causes increased urinary output, called *polyuria*. The child with DKA may have impaired renal function in spite of excessive urine output. Because dehydration decreases the glomerular filtration rate, the rate at which ketones are excreted also decreases, resulting in progressive metabolic acidosis. The renal assessment should include history of recent urinating patterns, measurement of intake and output, current weight and history of past weight (helps estimate the amount of dehydration), and measurement of urinary ketones.

★ NURSING DIAGNOSES AND PLANNING

Based on assessment data discussed in the previous section and the preceding chapter, the following nursing diagnoses may apply to the family and child with IDDM:

- Fluid Volume Deficit related to osmotic diuresis and vomiting.
- Altered Nutrition: Less Than Body Requirements related to unrestrained catabolic activity as a result of insulin deficiency.
- Anxiety and Fear (Child) related to invasive procedures, unfamiliar environment, and knowledge deficit about diagnosis.
- Situational Low Self-Esteem related to lifestyle changes required in treatment plan.
- Altered Family Processes related to presence of child with a chronic illness.
- Altered growth and development related to effects of illness.

The nurse and child (or parents) together plan effective care based on the established nursing diagnoses. Several examples of expected outcomes are as follows:

- The child identifies preferred fluids and foods.
- The child performs aspects of self-care appropriate for age.
- The child uses effective coping mechanisms to manage anxiety.
- The child expresses a positive outlook for the future.
- The family identifies acute complications and proper responses.
- The family consults with the health care team for management advice.

The nurse plans for the daily care of the child based on both the physician's orders and nursing diagnoses. Some general nursing care goals may include the following:

- Adequate fluid and nutritional intake is maintained.
- The child and family understand all aspects of the illness and its treatment.
- The child and family integrate diabetes care into patterns of daily living.
- The child's normal growth and development patterns are restored.

★ INTERVENTIONS: COLLABORATIVE AND INDEPENDENT

The chronicity of diabetes and the complexity of treatment require a multidisciplinary approach to care. Successful management depends on the collaborative efforts of the family, the child, and the health care team. The ideal team is composed of a consulting diabetologist, primary physician, diabetes nurse educator, primary nurse, dietician, and social worker or psychologist. The nurse plays a central role in coordinating care, educating, and assisting families to master the skills necessary to manage daily requirements of diabetes.

Therapeutic management of diabetes includes insulin therapy, a structured dietary regimen, exercise, blood glucose monitoring, and a strong system of social support. Through the educational process, families learn to integrate the multiple facets of treatment into their daily lives.

Research has shown that some of the most important factors influencing metabolic and psychosocial outcomes of treatment include the philosophy of the health care provider, the family's attitude and beliefs about health or diabetes care and their ability to manage a complex disease, and the extent to which the family and health care provider agree on the goals of therapy.[1]

Increasing evidence indicates that blood glucose control over time is related to the development of long-term complications.[1] Consequently, there has been a movement toward achieving tighter metabolic control, that is, near-normal blood glucose (<80–140 mg/dl). To date, a consensus has not been reached as to what level of blood glucose control is most desirable. Until current multicenter studies provide definitive data, a reasonable goal is to strive for near normalization of the blood glucose level.

Not everyone can achieve the same level of metabolic control. Although the risk of long-term complications must be reduced, normal psychosocial development should be promoted and excessive hypoglycemia avoided. Because hypoglycemia is a serious problem for children younger than 5 years of age, most health care providers recommend stabilizing a higher blood glucose concentration (100–200 mg/dl).

DISCHARGE PLANNING

Diabetes requires an unusually high level of commitment and involvement in self-care. Consequently, parents and children must become self-managers. Successful education gives families learning experiences that enable them to provide safe and competent care. Actual experience under the guidance of a nurse helps them gain a sense of mastery.

Families are anxious at the time of diagnosis and learning cannot proceed until some of the family's anxiety lessens. Therefore, the first day of hospitalization is devoted to answering the family's questions and to discussing their immediate concerns. This approach helps to reduce anxiety and to establish a therapeutic relationship.

Learning experiences are organized sequentially, from the simple to the more complex. The child and family play an active role in the learning process, and ample opportunity for questions and answers are provided. Instructions for parents need to be written at the appropriate reading level and used to reinforce important care aspects.

Active participation is essential, for acquiring new motor skills such as injection administration and blood glucose monitoring. Opportunities must be provided for children and families to demonstrate the skills needed to ensure mastery. Knowledge is evaluated at each session to determine what has been learned, to correct errors, and to reinforce teaching. Education of the family focuses initially on the skills necessary for survival outside the hospital. The accompanying display lists basic educational needs for the diabetic child and family.

Children's participation in diabetes care is a commonly shared goal. The age at which children assume specific health care tasks requires careful, individualized assessment planning. Although many parents and some health care providers believe that children should assume responsibility for diabetes care as early as possible, recent findings suggest otherwise. In fact, there is increasing evidence that when children are given too much responsibility too soon, metabolic outcomes tend to be poor.[43]

Many children are given significant responsibility for diabetes care by age 12 years, including record keeping, monitoring their blood glucose control, weighing and measuring their food, and injecting their insulin. By age 15, many adolescents have full responsibility for diabetes care, including the more complex task of insulin dose adjustment.[41] Although responsibility for care theoretically is in the process of being transferred to children, many parents disengage from participation. Paradoxically, the transfer of responsibility occurs at a time when rates of adherence and metabolic outcomes are typically poorest.[19]

Increasing evidence indicates that the determination of readiness to assume self-care is multifactorial and includes knowledge of disease management, ability to perform self-care skills, level of cognitive development, family environment, and self-perception regarding readiness. Knowledge is a necessary prerequisite for disease management; however, it does not guarantee successful self-management behaviors. Although children

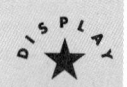

Basic Educational Needs for the Diabetic Child and Family

Insulin injections
Insulin preparations and dosages
Blood glucose and urinary ketone monitoring
Dietary management
Hypoglycemia and hyperglycemia detection
Pathophysiology
Management during illness
Exercise
Emergency phone number
Consumer information: supplies and medical
    identification
Support groups

may understand what they are supposed to do, they may not know how to do it. Thus, children must be evaluated not only for what they know, or say they know, but also by what they do.[19]

Cognitive development is an important determinant of a child's ability to assume responsibility for care. Most children are not able to comprehend the complex relationships among insulin, diet, and exercise; to anticipate probable outcomes; or to alter their behavior. Until children reach more advanced levels of cognition in the middle-to-late adolescence, they cannot conceptualize the complexities of disease management. Consequently, parents must be cautioned about transferring responsibility for care before the child or adolescent is developmentally ready.

Readiness coincides with increasing interest in learning a particular skill and with demonstration of cognitive abilities consistent with the skill. For example, in drawing up two kinds of insulin, children must have some reasoning ability as well as computational and motor skills. Readiness can be assessed in relation to the child's behavior in other areas of life. For example, the child who needs constant reminding to do homework or other tasks may not be ready to assume greater responsibility. In addition, the child's demonstration of a specific skill does not reflect readiness to assume full-time responsibility for performing that skill. Rather, care should be transferred gradually as a child demonstrates increasing competency.

Family environment is highly predictive of the child's metabolic outcomes. Families that are highly organized, flexible, and share in the responsibilities of care are more likely to have a child whose diabetes is well-regulated.[43] Conversely, families that are rigid, overprotective, and perfectionistic or indifferent and lacking cohesiveness are more likely to have a child with poor metabolic control.

Finally, children's perception about their ability to assume care is often correct. If children feel unready to assume responsibility for aspects of their care, then they probably are not. There is no particular age at which a person should be performing a certain task. General guidelines for participation in the aspects of care are given in the accompanying display.

INSULIN THERAPY

Initial management of a child with new-onset diabetes includes determination of the degree of metabolic alteration resulting from insulinopenia and initiation of insulin replacement. This initial management is outlined in the Nursing Care Plan. When the child or adolescent is not in DKA, treatment is relatively straightforward.

Because the goal of insulin therapy is to approximate normal physiologic patterns of insulin secretion, a short-acting insulin is combined with an intermediate-acting insulin and administered twice daily. This plan is commonly known as conventional insulin therapy, or the "split-mixed two shot per day" regimen. With conventional insulin therapy, normal insulin levels are sustained over 24 hours. This approach suppresses excessive glucose output from the liver and helps to maximize uptake of glucose by insulin-dependent tissues. Optimal insulin therapy is based on knowledge of insulin preparations and their pharmacologic properties, selection of an appropriate insulin regimen, and consideration of other factors that may affect insulin response and dosage requirements.

Insulin preparations are classified according to species (animal or human), purity, strength, and duration of action. Table 56-3 lists insulins available in the United States.[3] Animals species include pork, beef, or pork-beef formulations. Human insulin, which was first marketed in the early 1980s, is manufactured as either biosynthetic or semisynthetic insulin. Both biosynthetic and semisynthetic insulin are biologically equivalent and produce the desired effect of lowering blood glucose concentration.[23] Studies have demonstrated that synthetic human insulin has a more rapid onset of action.

Purity of insulin refers to the extent to which impurities are removed during the manufacturing process. Insulins in the United States are highly purified and contain fewer than 10 parts per million of other molecular proteins.[23] This standard of purity has significantly reduced the incidence of local and systemic allergic reactions and lipoatrophy (loss of subcutaneous fat at the injection site). All insulins are potentially immunogenic, although human and pork formulations are less so than are beef formulations.

U-100 insulin strength, meaning that 1 ml contains 100 U of insulin, is used in treating children with IDDM, although other concentrations are available. For very young children, insulin is sometimes diluted to U-10 or U-25 to permit smaller incremental changes in dosage. This approach substantially reduces the risk of hypoglycemia by increasing the accuracy of delivering small doses of insulin.

Insulin also is classified according to duration of action. Table 56-4 gives the approximate action time of short-, intermediate-, and long-acting insulin. Insulin pharmacokinetics vary considerably among people and in the same person from day to day.

Insulin regimens in the treatment of children with diabetes mellitus are fairly standard. With conventional insulin therapy, a short-acting insulin is combined with an intermediate-acting insulin and administered before breakfast and before the evening meal. This routine is preferred to regimens of one injection per day because it provides more adequate insulin coverage throughout the entire day. The morning injection provides insulin for breakfast (regular) and lunch (intermediate). The second injection covers the evening meal (regular) and

(text continued on page 1513)

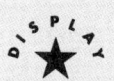

Guidelines for Ages at Which Children Are Able to Participate in Their Own Diabetic Care

- Record test results by 7–8 years
- Perform blood testing by 8–10 years
- Administer insulin by 12–14 years
- Participate in insulin adjustment by 15–17 years

Each child must be evaluated individually, according to his or her ability and not solely by age.

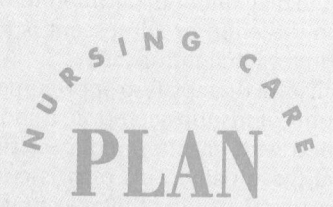

A Child With New-Onset IDDM

Assessment

Case Study Description

Lois is a 10-year-old girl with a 2-week history of polyuria, polydipsia, weight loss, and fatigue. She now presents with vomiting. Symptoms were preceded by "flu-like" illness. No first-degree relative with IDDM. Paternal grandmother is reported to have NIDDM that is treated with diet.

Assessment Data

Physical examination:

General appearance: 10-year-old girl who appears thin for height; slight fruity odor noted on breath.

Skin: Dry; mucous membranes dry; cheeks hyperemic (flushed); turgor decreased.

Cardiac: Heart rate 100 beats per min, regular rate and rhythm.

Chest: Respirations 22 breaths per min, regular rate and rhythm.

Neurologic: Alert; oriented to time and place; pupils equal and reactive to light; ankle and knee jerk within normal limits.

Blood pressure 90/50 mmHg	Serum bicarbonate (mEq/L) 16
Current weight 25 kg	Serum sodium (mEq/L) 133
Recent past weight 29 kg	Serum potassium (mEq/L) 3.5
Initial laboratory data:	Serum chloride (mEq/L) 92
Blood glucose (mg/dl) 495	Serum osmoles (mOsm/L) 302
Blood pH 7.32	Urinary ketones large
Blood urea nitrogen 17	

Nursing Diagnosis	Intervention	Rationale
1. Fluid volume deficit related to Supporting Data: • Polyuria • Polydipsia • Weight loss • Vomiting • Electrolyte imbalance: decreased NA⁺, Cl⁻, HCO₃, pH, urinary ketones positive • Dry mucous membranes • Decreased skin turgor	Assess state of hydration.	Dehydration is present in varying degrees in uncontrolled diabetes, and is more severe with vomiting.
	Record daily weights.	Weight reflects state of hydration.
	Record intake and output (output may be greater than intake owing to osmotic diuresis secondary to hyperglycemia).	Fluid intake and output reflect hydration and the need for replacement of excess urinary losses.
	Closely monitor blood pressure, vital signs, and neurologic status.	Vital signs, blood pressure, and neurologic status reflect patient response to correction of dehydration, electrolyte imbalance, and metabolic acidosis.
	Maintain fluid and electrolyte replacement.	Correct replacement therapy is essential to achieving metabolic stability.
	Observe for hyperkalemia (manifest by high-peaked T waves, wide QRS complex, and absence of P wave on electrocardiogram).	Hyperkalemia may be present at diagnosis owing to volume depletion and a shift in potassium from the intracellular to extracellular compartment.

(Continued)

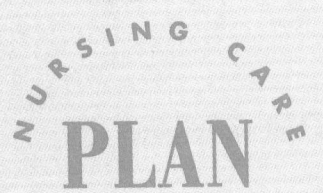

A Child With New-Onset IDDM (continued)

Nursing Diagnosis	*Intervention*	*Rationale*
	Observe for hypokalemia (manifest by low T wave, wide QT interval, and characteristic U wave on electrocardiogram).	Hypokalemia usually develops shortly after initiation of fluid and insulin replacement. A shift in potassium to the intracellular space decreases serum levels. (Both hypokalemia and hyperkalemia may result in life-threatening arrhythmias.)
	Observe for cerebral edema (manifest by decreased sensorium and changes in pupillary response to light).	Cerebral edema may occur in the first 12 hours of therapy when the patient has shown signs of improvement.
	Carefully monitor corrected serum NA^+ and serum osmoles.	Rapid decline in corrected NA^+ and serum osmoles has been implicated in the development of cerebral edema.
	Record and report changes in glucose, electrolytes, and urinary ketones.	Fluid and electrolyte replacement may change rapidly with changes in laboratory data.
2. Altered nutrition, less than body requirements related to Supporting Data: • Weight loss • Vomiting • Increased serum glucose • Urinary ketones • Fruity breath odor	Monitor insulin replacement therapy. Prime tubing with insulin solution (40 ml) before start of infusion. Piggyback insulin through a separate line. Control the rate of insulin administration with infusion pump. Administer insulin subcutaneously when metabolic acidosis resolves and intravenous infusion is discontinued. Assess knowledge of nutrition and dietary practices.	Insulin is essential to synthesis of carbohydrates, protein, and fat. Insulin may adhere to plastic. Prime intravenous tubing with insulin solution to saturate binding sites. A separate line for insulin is necessary to control the rate of administration. Rate of insulin infusion must be controlled to prevent a rapid decline in glucose, which may contribute to cerebral edema. Tissue perfusion and, consequently, subcutaneous absorption of insulin are decreased in metabolic acidosis secondary to dehydration. Dietary practices are influenced by knowledge of nutrition, eating habits, food preferences, cultural practices and financial resources.
3. Anxiety or fear related to unfamiliar environment and invasive procedures Supporting Data: • Child is fearful, cries, or verbalizes fear • Increased motor activity	Establish empathetic relationship. Assess level of anxiety. Prepare child for procedures and treatments. Provide reassurance and comfort.	Child will be more receptive to help if an empathetic relationship is established. Anxiety may interfere with mastery of self-care. Preparation for unfamiliar or painful procedures will help lessen fear. Children feel vulnerable in unfamiliar surroundings and during invasive procedures.

(Continued)

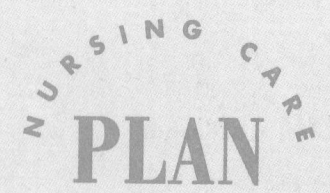

A Child With New-Onset IDDM (continued)

Nursing Diagnosis	Intervention	Rationale
	Provide opportunities for child to express feelings and concerns about injections and blood testing.	Children need acceptable ways to express their feelings, such as anger, sadness, and helplessness.
	Encourage participation in age-appropriate activities.	Play therapy provides an outlet for emotions and enhances a sense of mastery.
4. Knowledge deficit related to new diagnosis Supporting Data: • Family asks for repeated explanations • Verbalizes lack of knowledge of disease management • Questions ability to manage therapeutic regimen	Assess family's knowledge of diabetes and their learning ability. Encourage the family to verbalize their concerns and fears, and assess the family's level of anxiety. Develop teaching plan (see Teaching Plan later in Chap.).	Readiness to learn is based on knowledge of the child and family's learning needs, abilities, and learning style. Discussion of the family's immediate concerns will lessen anxiety, which may interfere with learning.
5. Self-esteem disturbance related to loss of normal pancreatic function Supporting Data: • Signs of grieving • Sadness • Loneliness • Feelings of friendlessness • Social withdrawal • Regressive behavior	Encourage the child to express feelings related to self-concept and diabetes. Help the child prepare for peer response to diagnosis. Help the child identify ways he or she is like peers. Encourage active participation in self-care appropriate to cognitive and emotional development. Provide positive feedback. Encourage peer interaction.	Children's concept of self is related to perceptions of body image and physiologic functioning. Self-esteem is based in part on peer response. Disturbance in self-esteem may be heightened by children's perception of being different from peers. Active participation enhances a sense of mastery over experiences and increases feelings of competency. Positive feedback reinforces attitudes and beliefs necessary for self-care. Peer interaction is an important developmental task that impacts self-esteem.
6. Altered family process related to situational crisis of new diagnosis Supporting Data: • Denial • Family does not communicate openly about feelings • Support is lacking	Assess family's strengths and weaknesses. Establish empathetic relationship with family. Assess family supports. Encourage participation of both parents in the care of the child. Help family problem solve regarding integration of diabetes care into daily life.	Family strengths provide the basis for successful adaptation to lifestyle change. Empathy enhances the family's receptiveness to advice. Families require support during stressful periods to adapt successfully. Shared responsibility in families correlates with more positive health outcomes. Opening up possibilities enables families to be more flexible, with greater likelihood of adaptation.

(Continued)

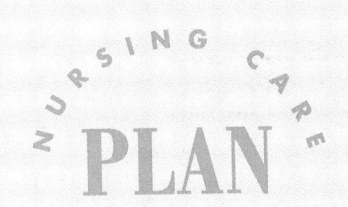

A Child With New-Onset IDDM (continued)

Nursing Diagnosis	Intervention	Rationale
	Provide anticipatory guidance regarding child's participation in care appropriate to developmental level.	Cognitive and emotional development are predictive of readiness to assume responsibility for care.
	Refer family for counseling if there is evidence of ineffective coping.	Ineffective coping may interfere with family's ability to carry out the therapeutic regimen.
	Help family identify resources in the community, such as the American Diabetes Association, Juvenile Diabetes Foundation, Diabetes Camp, and parent support groups.	Community resources extend existing supports.

Evaluation

- Vital signs are stabilized.
- Metabolic stability is achieved.
- Child is adequately hydrated and is gaining weight.

Expected Outcomes

- Family demonstrates confidence in performing blood testing.
- Family describes balanced meals and snacks eaten on time and with insulin action.
- Parents state family is sharing responsibility for diabetes care.
- Child demonstrates a positive self-esteem.

---

meets basal insulin requirements through the night (intermediate). This regimen is not without its disadvantages. Meals must be timed to coincide with the onset and peak of insulin action. Activities must be organized in relation to insulin injections and meal times. Although most families adapt to the rigid structure imposed by this regimen, it requires significant lifestyle change.

As the interest in finding regimens to achieve tighter metabolic control has grown, so have alternative insulin regimens. *Multidose insulin regimens* of three, four, or more injections per day have evolved as a means of achieving better control and providing a solution to specific problems.[3] The *three-injection-per-day regimen* is a variation of conventional insulin therapy. Combined short- and intermediate-acting insulins are given in the morning, with a short-acting insulin before the evening meal. The intermediate-acting insulin is delayed until bedtime snack. This regimen is frequently used in children who have early-morning hyperglycemia that does not respond to conventional insulin therapy.

The *four-or-more-injections-per-day regimens* use short-acting insulin just prior to meals and long-acting insulin either before breakfast or at bedtime. This regimen closely mimics normal insulin secretion, which provides continuous basal insulin secretion (long-acting insulin) with bursts of insulin in response to meals (short-acting insulin). When combined with frequent blood glucose

monitoring and adjustment of insulin dosage based on test results, this regimen can optimize control. Greater flexibility with regard to mealtimes is possible because a short-acting insulin is given when the person chooses to eat rather than at prescribed times. This regimen works particularly well for older adolescents, who may benefit from greater flexibility. However, this regimen requires greater commitment and attention to all aspects of the treatment program, including frequent self-blood glucose monitoring.

Continuous subcutaneous insulin infusion (CSII), or *insulin pump therapy*, gained popularity in the early 1980s. This system uses a small, portable infusion pump that can be programmed to deliver continuous basal insulin subcutaneously and bursts of insulin called *boluses*. This regimen requires meticulous attention to blood glucose levels. Mechanical failure and individual inability to respond to changes in control have been responsible for increased episodes of DKA with pump use.[54] Insulin pump therapy has limited clinical usefulness in the pediatric population. Implantable insulin delivery devices for children remain experimental.

Insulin requirements are affected by a multitude of factors, such as growth, puberty, activity level, diet, and intercurrent illness. Requirements are calculated based on weight and are adjusted in response to diet, exercise, and blood glucose levels. Insulin requirements remain

TABLE 56-3
Insulins Sold in the United States

Product	Manufacturer	Strength
Short-acting (usual onset 0.5–2.0 h; usual duration 3–6 h)		
Human		
Humulin regular	Lilly	U-100
Humulin BR (only external insulin pumps)	Lilly	U-100
Novolin R (regular, formerly Actrapid human)	Squibb-Novo	U-100
Velosulin human (regular)	Nordisk-USA	U-100
Novolin R Penfill (regular)	Squibb-Novo	U-100
Beef		
Iletin II regular	Lilly	U-100
Semilente	Squibb-Novo	U-100
Pork		
Iletin II regular	Lilly	U-100, U-500
Purified pork R (regular, formerly Actrapid)	Squibb-Novo	U-100
Velosulin (regular)	Nordisk-USA	U-100
Purified pork S (semilente, formerly Semitard)	Squibb-Novo	U-100
Regular	Squibb-Novo	U-100
Beef/pork		
Iletin I (regular)	Lilly	U-40, U-100
Iletin I (Semilente)	Lilly	U-40, U-100
Intermediate acting (usual onset 3–6 h; usual duration 12–20 h)		
Human		
Humulin L	Lilly	U-100
Humulin NPH	Lilly	U-100
Insulatard human NPH	Nordisk-USA	U-100
Novolin L (lente, formerly Monotard human)	Squibb-Novo	U-100
Novolin N (NPH)	Squibb-Novo	U-100
Beef		
Illetin II Lente	Lilly	U-100
Iletin II NPH	Lilly	U-100
NPH	Squibb-Novo	U-100
Pork		
Iletin II Lente	Lilly	U-100
Iletin II NPH	Lilly	U-100
Insulatard NPH	Nordisk-USA	U-100
Purified pork lente (formerly Monotard)	Squibb-Novo	U-100
Purified pork N (NPH, formerly Protaphane)	Squibb-Novo	U-100
Beef/pork		
Iletin I Lente	Lilly	U-40, U-100
Iletin I NPH	Lilly	U-40, U-100
Long acting (usual onset 6–12 h; usual duration 18–36 h)		
Human		
Humulin U (Ultralente)	Lilly	U-100
Beef		
Iletin II PZI	Lilly	U-100
Beef U (ultralente, formerly Ultratard)	Squibb-Novo	U-100
Ultralente	Squibb-Novo	U-100
Beef/pork		
Iletin I PZI	Lilly	U-40, U-100
Iletin I Ultralente	Lilly	U-40, U-100

(Continued)

TABLE 56-3
(Continued)

Product	Manufacturer	Strength
Premixed combinations		
Human		
Novolin 70/30	Squibb-Novo	U-100
Pork		
Mixtard (30% regular, 70% NPH)	Nordisk-USA	U-100

Reprinted with permission from *Physician's guide to insulin-dependent (type I) diabetes: Diagnosis and treatment.* Copyright © 1988 by the American Diabetes Association, Inc.

constant at 0.6 to 1 U/kg/day from about 2 years after diagnosis until puberty.[3]

Shortly after diagnosis, usually within weeks, children may recover some residual beta-cell function with partial return of endogenous insulin secretion. This period is known as the *honeymoon phase or remission,* and it may be marked by frequent episodes of hypoglycemia that require a reduction in exogenous insulin. The honeymoon phase is often a period of unusual stability and low insulin requirements (less than 0.5/kg/day). It may last weeks or months but rarely continues longer than 2 years.

In contrast, the pubertal years are characterized by a marked increase in insulin requirements. The increased insulin requirements during puberty are believed to be related to hormone-mediated insulin resistance; that is, decreased insulin responsiveness. Although pubertal-related insulin resistance is not completely understood, adolescents with a sexual maturity rating of Tanner stage 2 to 4 require dosages in the range of 1 to 1.5 U/kg/day.[4] Once puberty is complete, requirements usually return to 1 U/kg/day or less.

TEACHING REGARDING INSULIN THERAPY

Because "giving shots" is often a great source of anxiety, insulin injections should be the focus of the first or second educational session. Teaching should take place in a re-laxed and calm environment in which the family does not feel hurried to perform the task.

The nurse first demonstrates the correct technique for subcutaneous injections. Parents may want to practice with an orange before giving their first injection. Thereafter, parents may give their first injection to each other so that they may experience the injection as their child would. This approach also helps decrease parental fear that they will hurt their child. The child or parent also may be allowed to give an injection to the nurse. Alternate practice should not replace the parents' actually giving several injections before the child or adolescent returns home.

Children may or may not choose to learn the procedure for insulin injection at the time of diagnosis; they should never be forced to give an injection as a condition for discharge. By age 12 years, however, most children are interested in learning self-injection techniques.

Whether or not the child gives self-injections, active participation in the procedure is encouraged. For very young children, toddlers, and preschoolers, participation can take the form of choosing between different sites, wiping the site with alcohol, or pinching up the skin. Injecting children in this age group is stressful; toddlers, in particular, may exhibit periods of protest and uncooperativeness. Parents are advised to be matter of fact in

TABLE 56-4
Insulins by Relative Comparative Action Curves

Insulin	Onset (h)	Peak (h)	Usual Effective Duration (h)	Usual Maximum Duration (h)
Animal				
Regular	0.5–2.0	3–4	4–6	6–8
NPH	4–6	8–14	16–20	20–24
Lente	4–6	8–14	16–20	20–24
Ultralente	8–14	Minimal	24–36	24–36
Human				
Regular	0.5–1.0	2–3	3–6	4–6
NPH	2–4	4–10	10–16	14–18
Lente	3–4	4–12	12–18	16–20
Ultralente	6–10	?	18–20	20–30

Reprinted with permission from *Physician's guide to insulin-dependent (type I) diabetes: Diagnosis and treatment.* Copyright © 1988 by the American Diabetes Association, Inc.

their approach to minimize these occurrences. Moreover, they are encouraged to engage the child in activities that are enjoyable afterward. Play therapy with simulated syringes and dolls, for example, is helpful with this age group, because it allows children to gain a sense of mastery.

Once parents have mastered the injection technique, they can administer insulin to their child. If both parents share in this responsibility, each is relieved of carrying the total burden of care once they return home.

Families must understand insulin preparations and the techniques for mixing, aspirating, and storing the products. Families and children should be instructed to inject the insulin immediately after filling the syringes to minimize any alteration of insulin time action.

Insulin syringes for U-100 insulin are available in three sizes: 1 ml, 0.5 ml, and 0.3 ml. The introduction of the U-100 low-dose syringe (0.3 ml) has made aspirating the insulin easier because dosages for children tend to be small. The standard 1-ml syringe is calibrated in 2-U increments, whereas the low-dose syringe is calibrated in 1-U increments.

Mixing insulins of different formulations can alter insulin time action. Mixing regular (short-acting) insulin with the long-acting Lente type causes a mild delay in the onset of action of the regular type and diminishes peak insulin action. Consequently, the duration of action is prolonged.[5] This interaction does not occur when NPH and regular insulin are mixed.

Almost all children require a combination of short- and intermediate-acting insulin. Aspirating insulin from the vial for the first time requires patience and practice. Families need to be reassured that they soon will master the technique and become proficient. Practice with saline or a comparable solution can help boost confidence.

Manufacturers recommend disposing of syringes after one use; however, research has demonstrated that syringes can be safely reused without risk of infection.[35] If a needle becomes dull after two or three uses, it should be discarded. Needles can be discarded by placing them in an old coffee can or similar receptacle state and local laws may regulate disposal of biological waste. The ac-

companying display on patient teaching presents the standard procedure for mixing and administering insulin.

Insulin should be stored in the refrigerator when not in use. However, the vials in current use may be stored at room temperature for as long as 1 month without contamination or a significant loss of potency. Extremes in temperature should be avoided, because freezing and temperatures higher than 86° F reduce its potency.[5] Insulin should be transported in a separate container that is kept cool if the family travels during warm months. Extra insulin should always be kept on hand. Extra vials can be stored in the refrigerator for at least 1 year without loss of potency.

The child can participate by making the *site selection*. There are a number of anatomic sites that can be used for insulin administration. The most common are the lateral surfaces of the upper arm, the anterior and lateral surfaces of the thigh, the abdomen (avoiding the periumbilical area), and the upper outer quadrant of the buttocks (Fig. 56-10). Children need to rotate injection sites to prevent the development of hypertrophy at the injection site.

Hypertrophy is a result of growth of subcutaneous tissue at the injection site in response to repeated injection of insulin. It appears as an abnormal contour or bulge of the anatomic site. Absorption of insulin from hypertrophied tissue is erratic, making its action less predictable and control more difficult. Children should select at least two or three sites and rotate among them.

Site selection is a highly individual practice. Younger children tend to avoid the abdomen, whereas adolescents prefer it. Regardless of site selection, a consistent rotational pattern should be followed to improve the predictability of absorption and minimize fluctuations in the blood glucose. The same type of site is used at a given time of day. For example, the child could use arms for morning injections and legs for the evening. Exercise may enhance insulin absorption; therefore, a daytime site should be selected that will not be affected by exercise.

Consistent injection technique is as important as site rotation to enhance absorption. Children can place the needle into the subcutaneous tissue at either a 45- or 90-

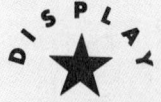

Patient Teaching: Standard Procedure for Mixing and Administering Insulin

- Insulin should be removed from the refrigerator and allowed to warm to room temperature.
- The person administering the insulin should wash their hands thoroughly.
- The tops of the insulin bottles should be wiped with alcohol.
- Intermediate- or long-acting insulin is rolled gently to ensure uniform mixture of insulin and to avoid introducing air bubbles.
- Air is placed in the intermediate-acting insulin and then in the short-acting insulin. Air should be equivalent to the amount of each insulin to be withdrawn. This equalizes care pressure in each bottle.

- Short-acting insulin is drawn up first, being careful to remove all air bubbles from the syringe.
- Intermediate-acting insulin is then drawn up. Insulin that clumps, adheres to the sides of the insulin bottle, or does not readily mix into solution should be discarded.
- The injection is given immediately upon being drawn up.

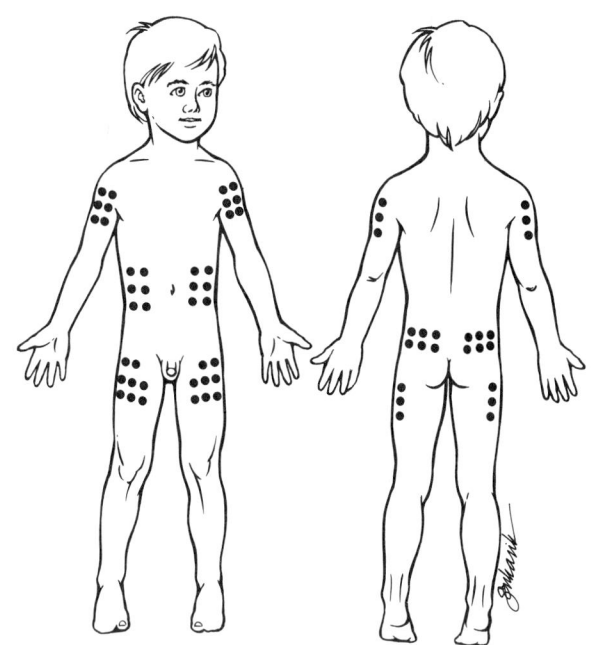

FIGURE 56-10
Insulin injection sites.

degree angle. Placing the needle in subcutaneous tissue is easier when the skin is pinched up, because most children are relatively lean. Pinching the skin separates subcutaneous tissue from underlying muscle. Although insulin can be injected into muscle, it is usually more painful, and absorption may be more rapid than desired. After inserting the needle, aspiration is not considered necessary before injecting insulin. The accompanying display on strategies provides suggestions for minimizing painful injections.

Timing of injections is important. One recommendation is that insulin be given 15 to 30 minutes prior to meals, so that the onset of regular insulin action will coincide with the postprandial increase in the level of blood glucose. This timing works best when the level of blood glucose is in the normal or above-normal range. If the blood glucose level is below normal, the hypoglycemia must be treated first.

Insulin injections are given about the same time each day for children on conventional insulin therapy. The time of insulin administration should not vary more than an hour each day. If children want to sleep late on the weekends, they are advised to get up, take the insulin, eat at the usual time, and then return to bed.

MONITORING METABOLIC CONTROL

A primary goal of therapy is for each child to achieve an optimal level of metabolic control. A reasonable goal is to strive for a preprandial glucose level between 80 and 140 mg/dl most of the time. This level is ideal, but children may not be able to achieve this degree of control all the time. Blood glucose levels may vary from day to day and throughout each day, but this variation does not always reflect poor control or poor adherence; rather, it may reflect the difficulty of precisely regulating a complex disease. Children and care providers are advised to iden-

tify probable causes of fluctuating and erratic glucose levels so that appropriate interventions can be taken.

Three aspects of metabolic control that may be assessed are blood glucose, urine glucose, and glycosylated hemoglobin. In recent years, *blood glucose monitoring* has become an integral component of diabetes care, replacing urinary glucose monitoring as the preferred method of evaluating day-to-day control. Although self blood glucose monitoring (SBGM) has many advantages, the most important is the ability to obtain an immediate and direct test result.

The disadvantages of SBGM are its cost and the invasive nature of the procedure. Start-up costs vary, but testing is usually $1 or $2 a day, depending on the number of tests performed. Although SBGM is invasive, it is nearly painless, and most children accept it. Because a variety of systems are available for purchase, the nurse needs to be familiar with all aspects of the system the family will use. Most systems employ quality assurance controls which are helpful in evaluating the precision and accuracy of the system and of the operator. Results that are questionable should be compared with those of a reference laboratory.

Until the late 1970s, *urinary glucose monitoring* was the sole method of evaluating control at home, but its use has diminished significantly because it is considered semiquantitative. Urine glucose is an indirect measure of blood glucose; therefore, results can be difficult to analyze. Glycosuria does not occur until the renal threshold is reached. Moreover, urinary glucose does not always correlate with ambient glucose concentration because of a lag time in renal excretion. A low plasma glucose concentration may be present while urinary glucose concentration is high.

Measurement of *glycosylated hemoglobin* provides a valuable method for evaluating long-term metabolic control. This test is a measure of integrated blood glucose control over a period of 1 to 3 months. *Glycosylation* refers to a chemical reaction in which glucose attaches to hemoglobin nonenzymatically, by a slow, mostly ir-

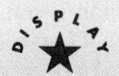

Patient Teaching: Strategies to Minimize Painful Injections

- Inject insulin at room or body temperature.
- Make sure no air bubbles remain in syringe before injecting.
- Wait until topical alcohol has evaporated completely before injecting.
- Keep injection-area muscles limber, not tense, when injecting.
- Penetrate skin quickly.
- Withdraw needle quickly.
- Do not change direction of needle while inserting or withdrawing.
- Do not reuse needles if they are becoming dull.

Reprinted with permission from Physician's guide to insulin-dependent (type I) diabetes: Diagnosis and treatment. *Copyright © 1988 by the American Diabetes Association, Inc.*

reversible, process. This process depends on the glucose concentration at the time red blood cells are exposed to glucose.[72] Thus, the higher the glucose concentration, the greater percentage of hemoglobin that is glycosylated. Because the life span of the red blood cell is 90 to 120 days, the percentage of glycosylated hemoglobin reflects the mean glucose concentration during the preceding 6 to 8 weeks.

TEACHING REGARDING MONITORING

SBGM test results help the child and family to make decisions regarding insulin, diet, and exercise and to identify both hypoglycemia and hyperglycemia. In addition, SBGM is useful for identifying glucose patterns over time if accurate records are maintained.

A wide array of blood glucose monitoring systems are available. All systems require a drop of capillary blood that can be obtained using a spring-triggered puncture device. The drop of blood is placed on a reagent strip that is chemically treated with glucose oxidase for a specific period of time. The resulting color change then can be quantified in one of two ways: the reagent strip can be read visually by comparison with a color reference chart, or it can be read with a reflectance meter that displays the result digitally. Both methods are highly reliable and accurate.[1] Accuracy, however, depends on the technical skill of the operator. Although children and adolescents have reliable technical skill, given appropriate education, most require periodic reassessment and re-education.[14]

Once a monitoring system has been chosen, education should focus on learning the correct technical skills. Practice increases proficiency but requires supervision until the desired skills are learned.

Families and children using electronic meters should be advised to follow the manufacturer's recommendations regarding general maintenance. Recently, there have been a number of reports of the transmission of hepatitis A when people share blood-letting devices. All children should have their own devices and to avoid sharing them with other children or family members. Lancets should be disposed of in the same manner as insulin syringes.

The frequency of blood glucose monitoring is individualized, taking into account the child's level of control, financial resources, and lifestyle. Children may be recommended to test three to four times a day, just prior to meals and before bedtime snack. Children are encouraged to test any time there is a change in usual routine that may alter their control. Periods of unusually strenuous activity must be followed with testing after the exercise and before bedtime to determine the need for further intervention and to avoid postexercise hypoglycemia. Although blood glucose monitoring is often the subject of negotiation among adolescents, frequent monitoring in children younger than 5 years of age is crucial to preventing significant hypoglycemic events.

Urinary ketone body measurement is another method of assessing control, because ketones are produced in response to starvation and insulin deficiency. Ketonuria is associated with poor diabetes control and impending ketoacidosis. Children generally do not need to measure urinary ketones every day. However, children and families should be advised to test for ketones when blood glucose exceeds 250 mg/dl or during periods of illness. Children are cautioned to test when vomiting is present.

The child with ketonuria requires careful monitoring. Fluid intake should be increased to help clear ketones from the urine. Vomiting associated with ketonuria must be evaluated promptly by a physician to rule out ketoacidosis. Occasionally, mild ketosis is found with a normal or below-normal blood glucose level; this state is of no significance unless it is accompanied by vomiting.

TEACHING THE CHILD TO KEEP RECORDS

Accurate record keeping is essential in establishing an individualized therapeutic regimen. Children are asked to keep records of blood glucose levels, insulin dosages, ketone measurement, their feelings, and any event that may affect metabolic control.

Although children are usually conscientious about record keeping in the beginning, accuracy often diminishes over time. Children are more likely to comply if there is some known benefit; therefore, children and families should be taught the significance of records by discussing blood glucose levels in relation to therapy and the child's notes. This effort enhances the child's understandings of the findings in relation to the behavior and expected outcomes.

Record keeping also provides a method for identifying patterns or trends in the blood glucose level. By reporting test results by time of day, patterns may emerge that suggest a need for a change in insulin, diet, or exercise. However, for record keeping to be of value, tests must be performed frequently to provide enough information for analysis.

Unfortunately, children may sometimes falsify records. Although undoubtedly misleading, the falsification is often done with the intent of meeting parental or health care team expectations. Parents should be informed that deception may be attempted. Parents and the health team are discouraged from placing blame or reinforcing guilt. Reasons should be sought for the reading but not by way of admonishment. A discussion that is age appropriate is usually all that is necessary to prevent recurrences. Repeated episodes of falsification indicates the need for close parental supervision or parental performance of the task.

DIETARY MANAGEMENT

Dietary management is one of the cornerstones of treatment, and its importance in management cannot be overemphasized. Diet is the most difficult component of treatment to manage day to day. The goals of dietary management include the following:

- Assuring consistency in the amount of calories and relative distribution of calories for carbohydrate, protein, and fat.
- Maintaining adequate nutrient intake to promote normal growth and development.
- Promoting healthy eating habits (i.e., decreased dietary fat and sodium).
- Minimizing the risk of acute and chronic complications.

The dietary intake of diabetic children or adolescents must be sufficient to sustain health and promote growth and development. Meals must be consistent from day to day, both in timing and nutrient content. Consistency is essential to minimize fluctuations in the blood glucose level and avoid hypoglycemia. Consequently, food in the recommended diet is distributed throughout the day to coincide with the onset, peak, and duration of insulin action.

Although alternative systems are available, the exchange system recommended by the American Diabetes Association (ADA) is the diet of choice. Table 56-5 shows the distribution of nutrients based on current recommendations.

Use of refined carbohydrates (sucrose) remains controversial, but recent research has shown that equivalent amounts of sucrose, as compared with carbohydrates derived from starches produce a similar glucose response.[9] This finding suggests that sucrose-containing foods probably can be used in limited quantities as part of a balanced meal plan without risk of hyperglycemia. Many sucrose-containing foods are also high in fat and may be problematic for children who are overweight or have elevated lipid profiles. Whatever the limitations, the allowance of refined carbohydrates is a boost to children who often feel deprived or compelled to engage in dietary indiscretions to minimize feeling different from their peers.

Dietary recommendations should be individualized and take into account cultural practices, food habits and preferences, and nutritional requirements. Nutritional requirements vary during childhood and adolescence. Revisions should be made periodically to reflect growth, activity, and food habits. Once growth is complete, requirements may be adjusted to maintain desirable body weight. Once requirements are established, nutrients are distributed over three meals and two or three snacks to moderate blood glucose levels and prevent hypoglycemia.

TABLE 56-5
Summary of Nutrient Recommendations and Distribution for Diabetic Children

Nutrient	Distribution of Calories (%)	Recommended Daily Intake
Carbohydrate	55–60	
Fiber		35–40 g/day
Protein	15–20	0.8 g/kg body wt
Fat (total)	<30	
Saturated fat	<10	
Polyunsaturated	≤10	
Monounsaturated	10–15	
Cholesterol		<300 mg/day
Sodium		<3000 mg/day

Reprinted with permission from *Physician's guide to insulin-dependent (type I) diabetes: Diagnosis and treatment.* Copyright © 1988 by the American Diabetes Association, Inc. Data are based on American Diabetes Association. (1987). Nutritional recommendations and principles for individuals with diabetes mellitus: 1986 (Position Statement). *Diabetes Care 10*, 126–132.

TEACHING REGARDING DIETARY MANAGEMENT

The nutritional requirements of children with diabetes should be established by a registered dietician who is familiar with the management of type I diabetes. The role of the nurse is to reinforce and support dietary education and to promote healthy dietary practices. The first step in dietary education is to provide basic information about nutrition and to provide diabetes nutritional guidelines. Basic information about the nutrient value of different food groups is provided as well as planning meals that incorporate these food groups. Table 56-6 gives the exchange list for the six different food groups used in the exchange system. Nutritional guidelines also include information about increasing complex carbohydrates, decreasing fat intake, using artificial sweeteners, limiting refined sugar, and increasing high-fiber foods.[37]

Although many of the published food exchange lists provide extensive choices, families must learn to weigh and measure food accurately to provide consistency in caloric and nutrient intake. Measuring intake helps moderate fluctuations in the blood glucose level. Periodic reassessment of this skill is helpful, because families tend to underestimate the quantity of food over time.

As families become more knowledgeable about dietary management, education can include more complex information, such as reading food labels; eating out, especially fast foods; and incorporating favorite recipes into the dietary plan. These topics expand the family's choices and introduce possibilities that may readily lend themselves to their lifestyle.

Meals and snacks must be consistently timed to coincide with insulin activity. Because fast foods are a favorite among children and adolescents, lists that provide exchanges for many fast food chains are available from the ADA. Because fast foods are generally high in fat, families are advised to limit fat intake at another meal. Because fat exchanges only minimally affect blood glucose concentration, they can be increased or decreased at a meal without affecting control. Table 56-7 gives examples of exchange equivalents that can be used at fast food restaurants. This information is not true for carbohydrates and proteins, and meal plans must be followed consistently in these regards.

School lunch programs are readily adaptable to the exchange system. Schools generally provide menus a week at a time, permitting families to assist children to select foods that are appropriate and substituting foods from home for items that are not appropriate. School parties are a special concern to parents, children, and teachers, but special treats can usually be incorporated into the diet in a limited quantity. Families must be informed of these special events far enough in advance to be able to determine exchanges and amounts.

Knowledge of dietary management for sick days is another important aspect of education. Families should be given guidelines for adapting their usual meal plan to include foods that are tolerated more readily during illness. Softer foods, such as puddings, jellos, and liquids, are recommended. For children or adolescents who are unable to eat, liquids containing sucrose can be offered in place of meals. A general rule of thumb is to

TABLE 56-6
Patient Teaching: Exchange Lists for Diabetic Diets

Exchange List	Carbohydrate (grams)	Protein (grams)	Fat (grams)	Calories
Starch/Bread	15	3	trace	80
Meat				
Lean	—	7	3	55
Medium-Fat	—	7	5	75
High-Fat	—	7	8	100
Vegetable	5	2	—	25
Fruit	15	—	—	60
Milk				
Skin	12	8	trace	90
Lowfat	12	8	5	120
Whole	12	8	8	150
Fat	—	—	5	45

Source: American Diabetes Association. (1989). *The American Diabetic Association Exchange Lists for Meal Planning*. Alexandria, VA: ADA. The Exchange Lists are the basis of a meal planning system designed by a committee of the American Diabetes Association and The American Dietetic Association. While designed primarily for people with diabetes and others who must follow special diets, the Exchange Lists are based on principles of good nutrition that apply to everyone. Copyright © 1989 by American Diabetes Association, Inc., and The American Dietetic Association.

offer the equivalent of 15 to 20 g of carbohydrate-containing liquid such as juice or carbonated beverage every hour until the child's appetite returns.

EXERCISE MANAGEMENT

Children and adolescents with diabetes can benefit from exercise with increased cardiovascular fitness, an improved sense of well-being, and weight control. In fact, exercise may improve overall metabolic control. Glucose is taken up and utilized by exercising muscle at a sub-

stantially increased rate. The blood glucose concentration is not only lower, but glucose tolerance may be improved for several days, due to increased insulin sensitivity and increased uptake by muscle to rebuild glycogen stores.[73]

However, the same benefits that improve metabolic control can also increase the risk of hypoglycemia. In people with diabetes, the rate at which glucose is made available and taken up by exercising muscle depends on circulating insulin levels. With too much insulin, the blood glucose level decreases to well below normal, as

TABLE 56-7
Patient Teaching: Exchange Equivalents for Popular Fast Food Restaurants

| Restaurant Menu Items | No. of Exchanges | | |
	Bread (Milk)	Meat	Fat
McDonald's			
Cheeseburger	2	1½	1
Big Mac	2½	3	3½
Regular french fries	1½		2
Chocolate shake	3½ (1 [2%])		½
Dairy Queen			
Brazier Chili Dog	1½	1	3½
DQ cone, small	1		1
Pizza Hut			
Thin 'N Crispy Pepperoni*	3½	2	2½
Taco Bell			
Burrito Supreme	3	2	2½
Taco	2	1½	

* Based on serving size of three slices.

a result, in part, to inhibition of glucose output by the liver. If too little insulin is available, the blood glucose level may increase during exercise as a result of increased glucose production by the liver.

Furthermore, exercise may affect insulin absorption rates from subcutaneous tissue, particularly if the exercising body part is also the site of the last injection. The increased regional blood flow increases the rate of insulin absorption. This effect is more pronounced when insulin is given less than an hour before the onset of exercise.[39] Aspects to be considered before advising about exercise are listed in the accompanying display. For children being treated with insulin, exercise must always be balanced with corresponding changes in insulin or food intake, or both.

TEACHING REGARDING EXERCISE

Exercise and physical activity are recommended for the person with diabetes. There are few contraindications to exercise; however, children should be aware that exercise may exacerbate hyperglycemia when the blood glucose

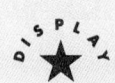

Patient Teaching: Factors to Consider Before Exercising

Type of Exercise

- Estimated intensity and duration of exercise
- Estimated caloric expenditure
- Is the exercise habitual or unusual?
- How does the exercise relate to the level of physical conditioning?

Blood Glucose

- If <100 mg/dl, take pre-exercise snack
- If 100–250 mg/dl, all right to exercise
- If >250 mg/dl, delay exercise and check urine ketones

Urine Ketones

- If negative, all right to exercise
- If positive, take insulin; don't exercise until ketones are negative

Insulin

- Type and dose
- Time of injection
- Site of injection

Food

- Time of last meal
- Preexercise snack
- Carbohydrate feedings during exercise
- Extra food after exercise

Source: Horton, E. (1988). Role in management of exercise in diabetes mellitus. Diabetes Care, 11, 206.

level is higher than 250 mg/dl and ketones are present in the urine. Once ketones have cleared, exercise may be resumed.

Exercise generally requires a corresponding adjustment in food intake or insulin dosage. The child's own response to exercise should guide intervention. Although response varies depending on intensity and duration, children should be encouraged to monitor blood glucose before, during, and after exercise. Moderate exercise of less than 45 minutes' duration requires a small snack equivalent to 50 to 100 cal. A snack composed of a complex carbohydrate or protein, or both, just prior to exercise is usually sufficient.[2] The blood glucose level ultimately determines the course of action. Blood glucose readings within the normal range require a snack, whereas a blood glucose level higher than 200 mg/dl generally does not require additional food. More intense exercise or exercise of longer duration requires snacks every 30 to 60 minutes. Simple carbohydrates may be tolerated better during exercise but should be preceded by a snack consisting of a complex carbohydrate and protein. Exercise of 2 hours' duration or longer always requires an adjustment in insulin. Although individual response should guide treatment, a downward adjustment is usually required.[2] The accompanying display lists strategies to avoid hypoglycemia or hyperglycemia with exercise.[39]

Children's exercise usually occurs as spontaneous bursts of activity. Consequently, families must be alert to changes in the intensity or duration of exercise and make appropriate adjustments in diet or insulin. Because children's activities are generally unplanned, dietary compensation is usually best. For older school-age children and adolescents who are more likely participate in organized sports, a combination of insulin reduction and dietary adjustment works well.

Prolonged periods of exercise pose the greatest risk for hypoglycemia, both during and after exercise. Postexercise hypoglycemia is common and is related to the repletion of glycogen stores. Moreover, hypoglycemic episodes may occur during the night, resulting in a more serious situation. Thus, it is important for families to check the child's blood glucose level before and after vigorous or unusual exercise and before bedtime to assure that the child has eaten sufficiently.

MANAGEMENT DURING ILLNESS AND SURGERY

Periods of illness require careful attention to blood glucose control. Metabolic needs increase during periods of illness, resulting in a corresponding increase in counterregulatory hormone action. For people with diabetes, insulin may be less effective, and requirements may increase.

Surgery also requires the adjustment of the usual insulin dosage. Because most children are NPO for varying periods, reduction in insulin is required, depending on the length and time of the surgery. Day surgery requires some alteration of both short- and intermediate-acting insulin doses. More extensive surgery may require intravenous administration of insulin with continuous monitoring of blood glucose. Families should inquire about the type of anesthesia to be used. General anesthesia requires the care of a person skilled in blood glucose mon-

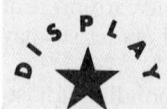

Patient Teaching: Strategies to Avoid Hypoglycemia or Hyperglycemia With Exercise

Food

- Eat a meal 1–3 h before exercise
- Take supplemental carbohydrate feedings during exercise, at least every 30 min if exercise is vigorous and of long duration
- Increase food intake ≤24 h after exercise, depending on intensity and duration of exercise

Insulin

- Take insulin >1 h before exercise
- Decrease insulin dose before exercise
- Alter daily insulin schedule

Blood Glucose Monitoring

- Monitor blood glucose before, during, and after exercise
- Delay exercise if blood glucose is >250 mg/dl and ketones are present
- Learn individual glucose responses to different types of exercise

Source: Horton, E. (1988). Role and management of exercise in diabetes mellitus. Diabetes Care, 11, 206.

itoring to provide periodic measurement of the blood glucose and, if necessary, administration of insulin or glucose, or both. With local anesthetic, children often are alert enough to perceive and symptoms of hypoglycemia.

TEACHING REGARDING ILLNESS MANAGEMENT

Monitoring blood glucose levels and urinary ketones every 4 to 6 hours is necessary during periods of illness. This routine helps identify deterioration in metabolic control and the need for additional insulin.

Families must know how to respond to changes in metabolic control. Families should receive written instructions regarding appropriate responses to changes in control. Table 56-8 provides guidelines for sick day management. The child requires insulin even if eating is impossible. Omission of insulin can lead to a rapid metabolic deterioration and, possibly, diabetic ketoacidosis. Blood glucose levels higher than 400 mg/dl generally require treatment with a supplemental dose of short-acting insulin. The presence of ketones and persistent hyperglycemia should be brought to the attention of the health care provider.

MANAGEMENT OF HYPOGLYCEMIA

Although mild hypoglycemia is a nuisance, severe hypoglycemia can result in loss of consciousness, seizures, permanent neurologic sequelae, and, in rare instances, death. A number of factors contribute to hypoglycemia. The most common are too much insulin relative to the amount of food eaten, increased physical activity without a corresponding change in insulin or food, and delayed or missed meals or snacks. Less common factors in children include gastroenteritis, surreptitious insulin administration, pregnancy, and alcohol ingestion.

Gastroenteritis may contribute to hypoglycemia as a result of slow absorption from the gastrointestinal tract or secondary to vomiting. Surreptitious insulin administration also has been documented as an uncommon but potentially serious problem in the pediatric population.[57] These children generally have significant psychopathology. Alcohol ingestion also may precipitate hypoglycemia because it augments insulin action and can inhibit gluconeogenesis.

The signs and symptoms of hypoglycemia occur in response to sympathetic nervous system stimulation and

TABLE 56-8
Sick Day Guidelines

Blood glucose level	>80 mg/dl <250 mg/dl	>250 mg/dl <400 mg/dl	>400 mg/dl	>250 mg/dl
Urinary ketones	Negative	Negative	Negative	Positive
Intervention	• Follow usual routine • Continue to monitor carefully every 4–6 hours	• Follow usual routine • Monitor carefully • Increase noncaloric fluid intake • Call physician if hyperglycemia persists	• Use additional short-acting insulin • Increase noncaloric fluid intake • Call physician if hyperglycemia persists • Monitor carefully	• Use additional short-acting insulin • Increase noncaloric fluid intake • Call physician • Monitor very carefully • Go to emergency department if vomiting occurs

central nervous system depression. The release of adrenalin and catecholamine is responsible for many of the initial symptoms of hypoglycemia. The sudden appearance of symptoms coincides with a rapid decline in blood glucose concentration. Adrenergic symptoms, such as pallor, sweating, shakiness, and tachycardia, are frequently referred to as the *early warning signs*. Late signs or symptoms of hypoglycemia develop as glucose deprivation of the central nervous system becomes more severe,[34] resulting in disruption of normal brain functions.

The behavioral changes observed in children are directly related to central nervous system dysfunction. Because some children have difficulty distinguishing hypoglycemia from hyperglycemia, blood glucose monitoring is necessary to determine the presence of hypoglycemia. An unequivocally low blood glucose level (lower than 60 mg/dl) confirms hypoglycemia. However, some children who are in poor control may experience hypoglycemic signs and symptoms at higher blood glucose levels. Children who are symptomatic should always be treated.

Children younger than 5 years of age have a significantly greater risk of severe hypoglycemia than do other age groups. They are less likely to recognize the symptoms of hypoglycemia or be able to intervene on their own behalf. Studies link even moderate levels of hypoglycemia with increased learning disabilities in children with IDDM onset before 5 years of age. Consequently, parents and other caregivers are advised to test young children more frequently and to strive for less tight metabolic control.[26]

Hypoglycemic unawareness also has been documented in older children with IDDM. The children at risk include those on intensified insulin regimens and those who do not counter-regulate well. (*Counter-regulation* refers to the hormonal response to a falling blood glucose level.[34]) Some children lack this response to a decrease in blood glucose level. Without the early warning signs associated with adrenalin release, some children develop profound, sudden hypoglycemia. These children must be advised to take extra precautions to avoid hypoglycemia.

Identifying possible factors precipitating hypoglycemia is important to prevent future recurrences. Frequent hypoglycemia may suggest the need for reduction in insulin dosage, especially if it occurs during the night. Overinsulinization can lead to hypoglycemia followed by rebound hyperglycemia. Children receiving more than 1 U/kg/day and adolescents more than 1.4 U/kg/day are at risk of being over-insulinized.[3] Blood glucose testing between 2:00 and 4:00 AM helps identify children at risk.

The treatment of hypoglycemia consists of documenting the blood glucose level if possible, treating symptoms based on their severity, preventing immediate recurrences, identifying possible causes, and modifying the regimen, if necessary (Table 56-9). For mild to moderate hypoglycemia, the oral route of treatment is indicated; simple carbohydrates work best, because they are rapidly absorbed. A general rule of thumb is to give the equivalent of 10 to 20 g of simple carbohydrates. Symptoms should resolve in 10 to 15 minutes; if not, the initial treatment should be repeated.

TABLE 56-9
Treatment Based on Degree of Hypoglycemia

Mild	Moderate	Severe
Adrenergic response to decrease in blood glucose: Hunger Shakiness Weakness Pallor Nervousness Dizziness Sweating	Mild central nervous system depression: Headache Irritability Poor coordination Combativeness Double vision Confusion	Severe central nervous system depression: Unconsciousness or inability to swallow Seizure
Can Self-Treat One fruit exchange (15 g of carbohydrate) Examples: ½ c orange juice 6 oz Coke or 7-up 7–10 Lifesavers 2 or 3 glucose tablets Repeat in 10–15 min if symptoms persist or blood glucose is <80 mg/dl. Follow with complex carbohydrate and protein if meal or snack is an hour or more away.	**May Need Assistance** If alert: One fruit exchange initially; follow with complex carbohydrate and protein snack. If symptoms do not improve in 10–15 minutes, repeat initial treatment. Follow with a snack.	**Needs Assistance** Give glucagon intramuscularly or subcutaneously (must be mixed prior to administration): Powdered tablet must be mixed with diluting solution and drawn into a syringe Dosage ½ ml—child <50 lb 1 ml—child >50 lb Repeat dosage in 15 min if there is no response, and go to the nearest emergency department. Vomiting is a common side effect; therefore, blood glucose must be monitored carefully for several hours. Follow with sugar-containing liquids. Inform physician.

Blood glucose monitoring should be performed to determine the child's response to treatment. A blood glucose level higher than 80 mg/dl does not require further treatment, unless the next meal or snack is more than an hour later. Then, the child is given a snack consisting of a complex carbohydrate and protein to help sustain the blood glucose concentration until the next meal.

Severe hypoglycemia almost always requires more intensive treatment. If the child is unconscious or unable to swallow, then 10 to 25 g of 50% dextrose should be given intravenously to restore the plasma glucose concentration. Glucagon kits are available for home use.

TEACHING REGARDING HYPOGLYCEMIA AND HYPERGLYCEMIA

Hypoglycemia occurs intermittently in almost all people treated with insulin. Children who are well controlled may experience two to three mild hypoglycemic episodes (i.e., shakiness and weakness) per week. Most health care providers believe that occasional mild hypoglycemia is an unavoidable consequence of optimal control. Early recognition of signs and symptoms is important to prevent severe hypoglycemia.

Although hypoglycemia is disconcerting to families and children, it is easily treated when recognized early. Families and children must have a clear understanding of the causes, symptoms, and treatment of hypoglycemia. Children may have difficulty discerning hypoglycemia from hyperglycemia, and for this reason, the blood glucose levels should be checked. Table 56-10 compares the differences between hypoglycemia and hyperglycemia.

If circumstances do not permit a blood glucose check, the child should treat the symptoms anyway. However, children should limit treatment to 15 g of carbohydrate (equivalent to one fruit exchange) and wait at least 10 minutes, unless symptoms become more severe. Every effort should be made to avoid severe hypoglycemia. A single severe episode is frightening for all concerned and may precipitate a change in attitude that favors less optimal control. Probable causes of the episode should always be sought to prevent recurrences.

A pattern of frequent episodes of hypoglycemia should be brought to the attention of the health care team promptly. Because hypoglycemia can occur at any time of the day, children are advised to wear some form of identification, particularly when away from home. Medical alert bracelets or necklaces are recommended because they are readily recognizable. Babysitters, teachers, bus drivers, or any responsible person entrusted with the care of a child with diabetes should have appropriate information regarding the child's condition and know how to treat hypoglycemia.

Sustained hyperglycemia indicates a deterioration in metabolic control due to insulin deficiency, but it is usually less alarming to children and families than is hypoglycemia. Symptoms of hyperglycemia develop gradually, and families need to be just as knowledgeable about the causes, symptoms, and treatment as they are for hypoglycemia. Persistent hyperglycemia may contribute to the development of long-term complications, and may lead to delayed growth and sexual maturation in children and adolescents.

TABLE 56-10
Patient Teaching: Comparison of Hypoglycemia and Hyperglycemia

Hypoglycemia	Hyperglycemia
Onset	
Rapid (usually minutes)	Gradual (hours or days)
Causes	
Too much insulin	Too little insulin
Too little food	Illness, trauma
Delayed meal or snack	Omission of insulin
Vigorous exercise without additional food	Too much food
Signs and Symptoms	
Weakness	Frequent urination (polyuria)
Fatigue	Excessive thirst (polydipsia)
Shakiness, nervousness	Excessive hunger (polyphagia)
Sweating	Dry, flushed skin
Pallor	Headache
Dizziness	Blurred vision
Hunger	Abdominal pain
Headache	Dyspnea
Visual disturbances	Vomiting
Irritability	Deep, rapid breathing (Kussmaul respirations)
Confusion	Stupor
Combativeness	Coma
Tremor	
Coma	
Seizure	

Factors that contribute to hyperglycemia include insufficient insulin, overeating, illness, and puberty-related insulin resistance. Average blood glucose levels higher than 250 mg/dl should not be ignored. Rather, these levels signal the need to continue close monitoring and to test for urinary ketones. Persistent hyperglycemia should be reported and adjustments made in insulin dosage.

MANAGEMENT OF KETOACIDOSIS

DKA is seen infrequently after the initial diagnosis, but it still accounts for a significant percentage of diabetes-related hospitalizations (many of which are recurrences in the same person). Excluding patients with new-onset IDDM, DKA is seen in fewer than 7% of the children with IDDM.[25] Its appearance after diagnosis is disturbing because it is largely preventable.

DKA constitutes a medical emergency requiring intensive medical and nursing care. Therapy is directed toward correcting the associated life-threatening metabolic abnormalities, such as dehydration, insulin deficiency, and electrolyte imbalances. Initial laboratory values associated with DKA are listed in Table 56-11.

During DKA episodes, laboratory values are measured hourly for at least the first 4 hours and every 2 to 4 hours thereafter. Bedside blood glucose and urinary ketone measurements are also performed hourly to help determine the initial metabolic status and the subsequent response of the child to therapy. The present weight should be compared with the most recent past weight to estimate the degree of dehydration. The child is placed on a cardiac monitor and the vital signs and the neurologic status are evaluated.

Correct fluid and electrolyte therapy is crucial. Initial rehydration helps to restore normal tissue perfusion and enhances the renal excretion of ketone bodies. Dehydration is usually estimated to be 10% of total body weight in children with moderate to severe DKA. However, the magnitude of acute weight loss provides the best index of degree of dehydration.[3] Electrolyte losses of sodium, potassium, chloride, phosphate, and magnesium are also substantial. Isotonic saline is almost always used initially. If the child is hyponatremic, then 0.45% saline may be used. Correction of dehydration and hyperglycemia generally proceeds slowly and with careful assessment of levels of corrected serum sodium and glucose. Rapid decline in serum osmolarity has been implicated in cerebral edema.[33] Potassium is added to intravenous fluids only after the child's renal function is established and the child has voided.

In some instances, urinary catheterization may be necessary. Despite depletion of potassium, some children may have elevated serum levels initially. However, once replacement of fluid and insulin has begun, potassium levels may decrease sharply. Consequently, children must be monitored carefully for cardiac arrhythmias associated with both hyperkalemia and hypokalemia.

In treating DKA, continuous intravenous administration of regular insulin is preferred, unless intensive care monitoring is not available. If the child has not had intermediate-acting insulin within 6 to 8 hours, an initial bolus of 0.05 to 0.1 U/kg regular insulin is administered. Thereafter, insulin is infused in normal saline at a rate of 0.05 to 0.1 U/kg/hr to decrease hepatic production of organic acids and glucose and increase glucose uptake by insulin-sensitive tissues.[25] Once the tubing is primed with 40 ml of the insulin-containing solution, the infusion is titrated to decrease the blood glucose concentration gradually at a rate of 50 to 80 mg/dl/hr.

Because metabolic acidosis resolves more slowly than does hyperglycemia, insulin infusion must be continued at an increased rate long after the blood glucose approaches normal levels. Therefore, 5% to 10% dextrose is usually added to rehydration fluids when the blood glucose level drops to 300 mg/dl. This dosage maintains glucose levels while allowing for correction of metabolic acidosis. Most children are able to resume eating as soon as peristalsis returns. This timing generally coincides with the resolution of metabolic acidosis. Children are then begun on subcutaneous insulin, and their insulin drip is discontinued.

During treatment, factors that may have precipitated DKA must be identified to prevent recurrences, and any underlying infection must be treated. For children with recent onset of IDDM, educating the family in all aspects of daily management is needed. For other families, more information regarding sick day management may be all that is necessary. In other instances, in which deliberate omission of insulin is known or suspected, a responsible

TABLE 56-11
Initial Laboratory Values for Patients Experiencing DKA

Test	Result	Remarks
Glucose	300–800 mg/100 ml	Concentration not related to severity of DKA
Ketone bodies	Strong at least in undiluted plasma	Measures only acetoacetate, not β-hydroxybutyrate
[HCO₃]	0–15 mEq/L	
pH	6.8–7.3	
[Na]	Low, normal, or high	Total body depletion; concentration dependent on relative H₂O loss
[K]	Low, normal, or high	Total body depletion; heart responsive to extra-cellular concentrations
Phosphate	Usually normal or slightly elevated; occasionally slightly low	Associated with phosphaturia; marked decrease with treatment in levels of both serum and urine phosphates
Creatinine, BUN	Usually mildly increased	May be prerenal
WBC count	Usually increased	Possibility of leukemoid reaction (even in absence of infection)
Amylase	Often increased	Predominant form of salivary gland origin
Hemoglobin, hematocrit, total protein	Often increased	Secondary to contracted plasma volume
SGOT, SGPT, LDH	Can be elevated	Spurious increases due to acetoacetate interference in older colorimetric methods

Abbreviations: [HCO₃], concentration of bicarbonate; [Na], concentration of sodium; [K], concentration of potassium; BUN, blood urea nitrogen; WBC, white blood cell; SGOT, serum glutamic oxaloacetic transaminase; SGPT, serum glutamic pyruvic transaminase; LDH, lactic dehydrogenase.

Source: Davidson M. (1981). *Diabetes mellitus: Diagnosis and treatment,* (p. 203). New York: John Wiley and Sons.

family member may need to assume responsibility for insulin administration.[27]

PSYCHOSOCIAL SUPPORT

Families usually respond to the diagnosis of diabetes with a high level of distress. Frequently, there is an initial period of shock, disbelief, and sometimes despair. This reaction is followed by an overwhelming sense of loss, confusion, and feelings of helplessness. Family distress and anxiety are often so acute initially that learning may be impaired. Thus, the amount of information must be limited, providing simple but brief explanations.

Involving both parents from the outset is useful in helping families bring their level of distress under control. Parents are able to hear the same information and to reassure and support one another. Moreover, family functioning is improved when there is a sense of equity with regard to sharing responsibilities and this is associated with better metabolic outcomes.[31] These reactions and appropriate nursing care are discussed in the nursing care plan displayed earlier in the chapter.

The Teaching Plan continues the discussion of the nurse's education of the child and parents. The nurse should provide information in a realistic but positive manner. Complications are particularly frightening to parents, and they should be given honest but fairly brief explanations that provide a hopeful outlook. Mastery of new skills usually is the best way to overcome feelings of helplessness and incompetence. Families should be given ample opportunity to practice skills and should be praised when procedures are performed correctly. Most families cope by seeking information, and the nurse should provide information by dividing it into manageable segments.

Questions regarding genetic transmission usually arise and should be discussed openly. Parents may be especially concerned about the risk to other siblings, and siblings may be concerned about "catching" diabetes. Families should be given the opportunity to express concerns regarding precipitating factors. Changes in lifestyle may be significant for families, and efforts should be made to integrate diabetes care into the family's existing lifestyle as much as possible.

Once families master the basics, they are usually ready for information that provides them with a greater range of choices. The loss of spontaneity in family activities may be acutely felt, but this feeling usually subsides in time.

The demands of diabetes superimposed on the developmental tasks of normal childhood create challenges that healthy children do not have to experience. The nurse can provide anticipatory guidance regarding developmental issues as they relate to diabetes at different ages. Such issues are discussed in Table 56-12.

Support groups are a means to help families cope with the added stress imposed by diabetes. Many are self-help groups; others may have a more psychotherapeutic format. Children, adolescents, and parents may benefit from participation. Another resource available to parents and children is a diabetes camp, which provides children an opportunity to share like experiences and learn new skills; parents are given respite from care of the child.

Although most parents are able to integrate the child's diabetes care into their daily lives successfully, there are periods when families may benefit from counseling. The onset of diabetes is a time of crisis for most families. Effective coping during the months following diagnosis sets the stage for future successes. Diabetes takes on a new meaning as children make a transition from one developmental stage to the next, and may reawaken old feelings. Families may revisit the crisis of diabetes when it is superimposed on the need to adapt to new developmental tasks. Moreover, significant life events, such as parental divorce, transition from middle school to high school, and the development of diabetes-related complications, cause disruptions and upheaval in the family's routine. Short periods of counseling may be necessary for families to move to the next life stage.

★   **EVALUATION**

The nurse and family periodically evaluate the outcomes of care given. Examples of outcomes for the child and family with IDDM were given under planning in this section. Have the short-term goals been met? Are the long-term goals still realistic? Planning for further nursing care takes into consideration complications and long-term care.

COMPLICATIONS

Diabetic children are at risk for long-term complications, including retinopathy, nephropathy, and cardiovascular disease. The duration of diabetes, level of metabolic control, and poorly understood genetic factors all play a role in the development of complications. The onset of complications rarely occurs before puberty or the fifth year of disease. Microvascular disease (functional and structural changes in small blood vessels) develops within 10 to 15 years of disease onset and leads to both retinopathy and nephropathy. However, macrovascular disease typically does not occur until after 25 years.[3]

Prevalence rates for *retinopathy* are about 50% by 10 years from disease onset and 70% to 80% by 15 years.[3] Retinopathy is categorized according to clinical findings and includes background retinopathy, preproliferative stages, proliferative stages, and macular edema. *Background retinopathy* is the development of early retinal changes that result from increased vascular permeability and occlusion of small vessels.[3] This damage results in the development of microaneurysms that can be visualized with an ophthalmoscope. No immediate intervention is required at this stage, but careful monitoring and efforts to improve diabetes control are essential.

Preproliferative retinopathy is seen as increased clustering of blot hemorrhages that suggest progression of the disease. This change also indicates that there are increased areas of nonperfused capillaries that can result in the stimulation of new growth and abnormal new blood vessels. *Proliferative retinopathy* results in the formation of new blood vessels extending from within the retina. New vessel formation is quite serious and requires laser photocoagulation therapy to prevent significant rupture and hemorrhage and subsequent retinal detachment. Macular edema also can be threatening to visual acuity with loss of retinal central vision.[3]

(text continued on page 1530)

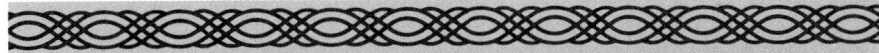

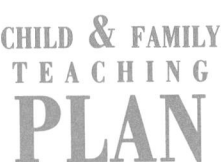

CHILD & FAMILY TEACHING PLAN

Care of a Child With IDDM

Assessment

Lois is a 10-year-old girl admitted to the hospital with new-onset IDDM in moderate ketoacidosis. Lois lives at home with both parents and her younger brother. Lois attends elementary school at the fourth grade level. Mother is employed outside the home as a school teacher and father is self-employed in the construction business. Both parents will be able to attend educational sessions. Mother has completed 4 years of college, and father has completed 1 year of college.

Parents acknowledge very little understanding of diabetes and its management. Parents state that they learn best by reading and through demonstration and practice.

Child and Family Objectives	*Specific Content*	*Teaching Strategies*
1. Describe the pathophysiology of diabetes.	1. Effects of insulin on carbohydrate, protein, and fat metabolism	1. Use videotape and drawings for discussion.
2. Identify insulin preparations and procedures and appropriate sites for injection.	2. Description of insulin preparations according to strength, species, and duration of action	2. Show parents insulin preparations and point out identifying features.
	Procedures for mixing, drawing up, and administering insulin	Demonstrate procedure, and have family return demonstration.
	Onset, peak, and duration of insulin action	Use graphs, charts, or drawings. Encourage questions.
	Appropriate sites for injection and description of rotation	Show family appropriate anatomic sites
		Have child develop chart rotation. Plan rewards for efforts.
3. Demonstrate proper knowledge and skills in blood glucose monitoring and recording.	3. Description of procedure for blood glucose monitoring	3. Demonstrate procedure and have family return demonstration.
	Common mechanical (meter) and patient errors	Provide written instructions for trouble shooting. Demonstrate common errors and problem solving.
	Explanation of when, why, what, and how to keep records	Demonstrate; have child keep records with reward for efforts.
4. Describe food groups and nutrient contents with application to meal planning.	4. Six food groups based on ADA exchange	4. Use food models, food lists, and food exchange book.
	Description of nutrient content of food and the need for consistency and timing on diabetic diet	Discuss; use food exchange lists and sample menus. Have family complete menus.
	Alternate menus for sick days	Discuss; use sample menus. Have family complete menus.
	Food substitution among different food groups	Discuss food substitution. Provide lists of alternate choices. Have family plan food substitutions.

(Continued)

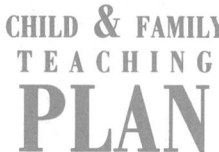

Child and Family Objectives	*Specific Content*	*Teaching Strategies*
5. Describe signs and symptoms, precipitating factors, and treatment of hypoglycemia.	5. Signs and symptoms of hypoglycemia	5. Discuss; use videotapes if available; provide written instructions.
	Treatment of hypoglycemia and contributing factors; e.g., exercise, too little food	Discuss; provide food models. Demonstrate use of glucagon, provide written instructions. Use drawings and videotape.
6. Describe signs and symptoms, monitoring procedures, contributing factors, long-term effects, and treatment of hyperglycemia.	6. Signs and symptoms and treatment.	6. Discuss; provide written instructions; use videotape.
	Procedure for urinary ketone monitoring	Demonstrate and have family give return demonstration.
	Description of factors that contribute to hyperglycemia, e.g., illness, puberty, excess food	Discuss; provide written material.
	Relationship of metabolic control and long-term complications	Discuss.
7. Describe benefits of exercise and compensatory management for exercise.	7. Physiologic effects of exercise on the cardiovascular system and glucose homeostasis	7. Demonstrate through exercise and by testing of blood glucose before and after exercise. Use written instructions
	Adjustment of food and/or insulin when exercising	Written instructions; discuss
8. Identify community resources and support.	8. Local and national resources	8. Provide written material and publications.
	Sources for medical identification bracelet	
	Describe resources for diabetes supplies	Discuss; provide written material.
	When and how to seek medical help, e.g., sick days, eye care, dental care	Discuss; provide written information.

Evaluation

- Family applies principles of disease management as evidenced by daily management.
- Family correctly identifies insulin preparations prescribed for child by strength, species, and duration of action.
- Family correctly mixes, draws, and administers insulin.
- Family correctly performs blood glucose monitoring at prescribed times.
- Family plans meals and snacks based on ADA exchange system.
- Family states how to recognize and treat hypoglycemia and hyperglycemia.
- Child engages in exercise.
- Family identifies resources and obtains supplies.

TABLE 56-12
Nursing Interventions: Anticipatory Guidance for Parents of Diabetic Children

Developmental Age	Concerns	Interventions
Infancy: Trust and object permanence	Injections, blood testing; recognition of hypoglycemia	Parents should not convey their anxieties but take a matter-of-fact approach. Once painful procedures are completed, parents may comfort and reassure their infants. Blood testing provides the most reliable method for distinguishing behaviors related to hypoglycemia.
Toddlerhood: Exploration and separate identity	Injections and hypoglycemia, food, limit setting	Consistent routines are important. Parents need to continue injection procedures begun in infancy. Toddlers can participate by wiping a finger with alcohol or choosing finger to be pricked. Limited choices are best and should be offered whenever possible. Use small portions of food, and offer carbohydrates first. Rather than force children to eat, parents set a time limit. If children do not complete all of the meal, watch for signs of hypoglycemia. Allow children limited choices regarding food preferences.
Preschoolers: Cooperation; magical thinking	Children have an intense fear of injections and blood testing. Children associate painful procedures with transgression.	Children should be assured that diabetes is not a punishment. Parents can help children recognize symptoms by matching symptoms with words. Children can be given more choices and participate in more aspects of care (e.g., pinching skin for injections or pressing button on blood testing meters). Parents may need help in "letting go" if children attend day care or preschool.
School agers: Industry, increased learning abilities, increased motor skills and social skills	Children may not understand permanence of their condition. Children are concerned about telling their friends; they may withdraw socially.	Children are interested in learning about the body. Children understand simple concepts of illness with concrete examples. The need for insulin at home should be emphasized. Children benefit from role playing answers to peers' questions. Children can be helped to identify ways they are like other children (not different). Although children take on more responsibility, parents should remain active in their care.
Adolescence: Adopting realistic body image, experimentation	Children may find it difficult to adopt a realistic body image. Adolescents may regress and seek security by becoming more dependent or disregard advice as a form of rebellion.	Children may test limits, including diabetes management (e.g., occasional omission of insulin, refusal to monitor blood glucose, dietary indiscretions). Adolescent girls may decrease their insulin dosage as an inappropriate means of losing weight. Parental supervision is still required. Nagging and threats of complications have no effect; they should be avoided.

Nephropathy develops in about 30% to 40% of children with IDDM. Both structural and functional changes occur in the kidneys and result in increased glomerular filtration, increased renal blood flow, and, eventually, proteinuria. The mechanisms that contribute to nephropathy are not completely understood, but there is increasing evidence that it is related to metabolic alterations of diabetes.[3]

Hypertension generally appears shortly after the development of incipient nephropathy and must be treated promptly and aggressively to prevent the advancement of kidney disease. The development of frank nephropathy generally progresses to end-stage renal disease within about 5 years. Life expectancy is significantly decreased a kidney transplant is performed.

Diabetic neuropathies can be divided into several discrete categories and rarely appear before adulthood. This discussion is limited to peripheral and autonomic neuropathy. *Peripheral neuropathy* is one of the most common chronic complications of diabetes. Most regions of the body can be affected, but foot damage occurs most often. The loss of sensation and decreased peripheral circulation increase the risk of infection and the need for lower limb amputation.

Autonomic neuropathy can affect autonomic function in any number of organs but is usually limited to one or two. The gastrointestinal system may be impaired, with delayed gastric emptying and delayed absorption of nutrients. This effect can result in wide swings in the blood glucose level, causing both hypoglycemia and hyperglycemia. Treatment consists of small, frequent feedings with avoidance of high-fiber foods. Cardiovascular autonomic neuropathy may also occur. Diminished pulse rate variation with inspiration and expiration is one of the earliest clinical findings. The signs include decreased exercise tolerance and tachyrhythmia. Sudden death may occur. Autonomic neuropathy is also associated with hypoglycemia unawareness.[2]

Cardiovascular disease generally tends to occur at an earlier age in diabetics than it does in the general population, and it is usually more severe. Associated risk factors include hyperlipidemia, which may occur as a result of poor control or as a genetic predisposition. Aggressive treatment of hyperlipidemia with limitation of dietary fats, improved metabolic control, and, in some instances, medication may reduce occurrence of cardiovascular disease. Hypertension, as well as cigarette smoking, compounds risk and should be aggressively treated.

Children with diabetes also can have associated *autoimmune diseases* and develop thyroiditis or adrenal failure. Annual periodic screening for thyroiditis is usually indicated, and any evidence of adrenal dysfunction should be evaluated.

LONG-TERM CARE

Diabetes requires lifelong consultation with a health care team. During childhood and adolescence, health care visits are made every 3 months, with contact by phone between visits. In the beginning, families need more frequent access to the health care team for reassurance and support. Phone calls are usually sufficient to handle most situations before the child's first return visit. During each health care visit, blood glucose records are examined in addition to insulin dose requirements, dietary needs, and other life events that may influence diabetes care.

Children require good dental care and should be examined every 6 months to a year. Ophthalmologic examinations should be performed yearly after 5 years' duration of diabetes or after the onset of puberty.

Altered Parathyroid Gland Function

The parathyroid glands produce the hormone parathormone (PTH). The action of PTH is the regulation of calcium balance through its effect on the bone, the renal tubules and the intestinal mucosa. Calcium is essential to many biologic processes, including nerve conduction, cardiac function, mitosis, muscle contraction, blood composition, and hormone synthesis.[6] Although PTH plays an important role in the calcium balance of the body, regulation is also affected by vitamin D, calcitonin (from the thyroid gland), the bones, and the serum protein.

The target organs for PTH are the bones and kidneys. A decrease in serum calcium results in the increase of PTH production. PTH causes the bones to release the needed calcium and the kidneys to spare calcium from being excreted. Conversely, a high serum calcium level suppresses PTH secretion.[44]

PTH cannot work in the absence of vitamin D.[6] Vitamin D, which is converted in the skin to its active form, is technically a hormone and not a vitamin. Its major action is to stimulate the intestinal reabsorption of calcium and mobilize the calcium from bones.

Calcitonin, a thyroid-based hormone, remains a mystery. Strangely, the loss of the thyroid gland, and therefore loss of calcitonin, does not affect calcium metabolism. Calcitonin plays a role in phosphorus and calcium balance, but there are no known disorders related to its function.[6]

The parathyroid glands do not function under the hypothalamic-pituitary feedback system. Disorders of calcium and phosphorus metabolism are rare in childhood.

Hyperparathyroidism

Hyperparathyroidism is a rare disorder seldom seen in childhood and its cause is often unknown. Hyperplasia, or a tumor in the parathyroid gland, such as an adenoma have been suggested as causal conditions.[6] Hyperparathyroidism is also associated with chronic renal disease. Excessive PTH produced in hyperfunction of the parathyroid glands causes hypercalcemia. The clinical manifestations of hypercalcemia are presented in Table 26-8. Hyperparathyroidism necessitates surgical exploration. If an adenoma is found, it is removed. If hyperplasia is discovered, a total parathyroidectomy is indicated to avoid recurrence of the problem. Postoperative observation for hypocalcemia and tetany is essential; administration of calcium gluconate may be required for a few days. If the disorder is recognized and treated early, the prognosis for complete recovery is good.

Hypoparathyroidism

Hypoparathyroidism is the decrease or absence of parathormone (PTH), which leads to hypocalcemia and hyperphosphatemia. This condition is rare in childhood but may be caused by inadvertent removal of the parathyroid glands during thyroid surgery. Absence of the glands causes acute hypoparathyroidism and calcium imbalance.

Idiopathic hypoparathyroidism sometimes occurs between the ages of 5 and 15 years, and it may be a familial condition. The parathyroid glands may be the target of autoimmune disease, because hypoparathyroidism occurs in association with other endocrine autoimmnue disorders, such as Addison disease.

A deficiency of PTH results in hypocalcemia and hyperphosphatemia. Hypocalcemia leads to increased irritability of the central and peripheral nervous systems, a precipitous decline in calcium initiates striking clinical manifestations visual and auditory problems, and diarrhea. The elevated serum phosphorus concentration is not known to cause major symptoms, but it is extremely useful in the diagnostic work-up.

The symptoms of this disorder are directly related to the level of serum calcium. Children with adequate, but low, serum calcium levels may be relatively symptom-free. Symptoms of hypocalcemia include complaints of numbness and tingling of the extremities; muscle cramps; tetany; and difficulties in vocalization. Chronic low levels of calcium result in thin, brittle nails; dry, coarse hair or alopecia; delayed dentition; and dental enamel defects. Cataracts are common in children with long-standing, untreated hypoparathyroidism, and other eye disorders, such as keratoconjunctivitis, also may occur.

Serum and urinary concentrations of calcium, phosphorus, alkaline phosphatase, and serum PTH are used to establish a diagnosis of hypoparathyroidism. These measures show low serum calcium, increased phosphorus, normal alkaline phosphatase, and low PTH levels. Levels of antibodies to the parathyroid gland are high when autoimmune disease is the cause of the disorder.

Bone x-rays that show bony changes specific to these defects may prove useful.[61] Imaging techniques, renal function studies, and ophthalmologic examination may be necessary.

★ NURSING IMPLICATIONS

Physical examination includes inspection of the skin for the ectodermal findings mentioned earlier. The reflexes may be hyperactive.

The goal of treatment is the return of normal calcium status (eucalcemia), but this goal is difficult to achieve in a growing child.[6] There is no PTH preparation currently available for therapeutic use, so therapy is aimed at mim-

icking the action of PTH. In mild hypoparathyroidism, the child is given calcium supplements—4 to 5 g of calcium carbonate daily. This dosage initially results in a mild alkalosis and an increase in symptoms. Calcium supplements may be disliked by many children, who may require encouragement from parents and the nurse. Incentives such as sticker charts may be helpful for younger children, or a small tasty reward such as a jelly bean may be given after the supplement.

Children with more severe disease require treatment with a replacement calciferol sterol, such as vitamin D_2 or dihydrotachysterol. Vitamin D increases the availability of bone calcium but has no negative feedback mechanisms that might help avoid overtreatment. These oral medications are begun at small doses to avoid dangerous hypercalcemia. The goal is to obtain calcium blood concentrations that are in the low-normal range. Some children may require oral calcium supplementation, which is given in three to four divided doses daily. If tetany, seizures, or laryngeal stridor is present, an IV infusion of 10% calcium gluconate is administered.

When adequate sterol replacement has been achieved, children can be followed with blood and urine levels of calcium and phosphorus every 2 to 4 months. Vitamin D preparations vary greatly in their onset and duration of action; therefore, they cannot be substituted for one another.[6]

Parents need to learn the signs of hypocalcemia and hypercalcemia. Hypocalcemia presents with the symptoms seen at the onset of illness. Hypercalcemia results in headache, nocturia, polydipsia, polyuria, anorexia, nausea and vomiting, lethargy, weakness, and constipation.[6] Children with this disorder need to wear a medical alert tag.

With adequate replacement, children should grow and develop normally. Children who are also receiving vitamin D and calcium therapy are monitored frequently to avoid hypercalcemia. Calcium serum concentrations are kept at the lower level of normal to avoid renal damage. Increased amounts of fluids should be taken to avoid low urine output and the formation of calcium kidney stones. Severe calcium deficiency results in respiratory stridor, convulsions, electroencephalograph changes, and mental status changes.[56]

Nonendocrine Patterns of Short Stature

The hallmark of decreased pituitary function in childhood is slow growth and eventual short stature. Although short stature is rarely the result of pituitary hypofunction, many children are evaluated for GHD due to concern about their short stature. These commonly seen patterns of growth must be understood to contrast them with the patterns seen in pituitary hypofunction. Of 270 million U.S. citizens, 8.1 million people are below the third percentile in height. Most of these people are healthy and normal.

There are several common and uncommon growth patterns that may be mistaken for GHD. It is far more likely that a short child has one of these patterns rather than GHD. Understanding these common causes of relative shortness is essential to the diagnosis of the child with suspected GHD. Constitutional delay of growth, genetic short stature, IUGR, and Prader-Willi syndrome are four nonendocrine patterns of short stature briefly presented in this section.

Constitutional Delay of Growth

Children with constitutional delay of growth exhibit a normal growth pattern that is marked by short stature in childhood but a longer prepubertal growth time and subsequent normal adult height. Growth speed decelerates in these children between 12 and 36 months of age, followed by growth at a normal speed. They may be very short during the growing years or closely follow the fifth percentile line on a growth chart. The pattern is more commonly seen in boys than in girls.

Bone age is somewhat less than chronologic age in constitutional delay and is associated with a later onset of puberty. Affected children often grow for many years longer than does their peer group. Treatment with growth hormone is a highly controversial practice, and no research has shown the long-term value for hormonally normal children.

Besides reassurance, adolescent boys with this growth pattern may benefit from several months of treatment with a low dose of an androgen to stimulate early pubertal changes. Estrogen can be used for several months in girls who have significant problems with the long wait for natural puberty. Such treatments do not alter final height.

Genetic Short Stature

Short parents can expect to produce children who are significantly short. If both parents are very short, their offspring may be even shorter and may not achieve the stature of their parents. Children who are genetically short begin life at the lower end of the growth chart and grow steadily at a normal speed. Their growth speed, which is normal, does not cause their height to catch up with their peer group.

The bone age of a child with genetic short stature is the same as their chronologic age, and they can expect to have puberty at the average age. These children are also hormonally normal and produce adequate growth hormone.

Some short parents may have undiagnosed or untreated hormone deficiency. Short children born to these parents who do not grow at a normal speed should be evaluated for this possible diagnosis.

Intrauterine Growth Retardation

When a newborn is smaller than would be expected for its gestational maturity, the baby is referred to as *small for gestational age*. Some of these infants grow quickly and catch up to normal standards of weight and length.

Those who do not grow well after birth are described as having IUGR.

The small size of affected infants may be due to intrauterine infection, placental insufficiency, chromosomal disorders, congenital anomalies, or maternal malnutrition, ingestion of drugs, tobacco, or alcohol.[6] Often, no cause can be determined. Although these children do not have altered endocrine function, they frequently are evaluated in growth clinics. Children with IUGR may have physical findings that are consistent with a defined syndrome.

One of the most common IUGR syndromes is Russell-Silver syndrome.[6] During early childhood, affected children often exhibit poor weight gain and very small appetites. They have attractive, triangular faces and may have asymmetry of their extremities, with one arm or leg longer than the other, or both. Although they are small (height below the third percentile), they have a normal head circumference, giving them an appearance of having a large head. Their intelligence is normal, but they may have a lag in developmental milestones in early childhood.

Many forms of IUGR do not fit into a classification. Of importance is the prenatal history and growth pattern after birth. Fetal alcohol syndrome (FAS) is a preventable form of IUGR. These small children have the added burden of mental deficiencies and social skill difficulties.

Psychosocial support for parents of children with IUGR is an important nursing intervention. Parents may feel guilty about having produced this very small child or may harbor fears of hidden illness. Mothers often feel that they are being blamed or are responsible for this condition. Another nursing intervention focuses on parent teaching. Some children with IUGR are extremely poor eaters and may benefit from a special diet.

Parents of children with Russell-Silver syndrome might wish to contact the Russell-Silver parents group or the Human Growth Foundation for support and education. Children with fetal alcohol syndrome require early intervention from their local school system, because they are at risk for learning difficulties. Often these children are in adoptive or foster care homes. When cared for by their biologic mother, there is no point in promoting feelings of guilt for the tragic mistakes of the past.

Children with various types of IUGR may be treated with growth hormone in an attempt to stimulate their growth. There are research opportunities for this type of treatment, but no information is available about the benefits of GH treatment in this diverse group of children.

Prader-Willi Syndrome

Prader-Willi syndrome is a chromosomal disorder with an incidence of 1 in 10,000 to 25,000 births.[29] The diagnosis is based on clinical findings that include hypotonia and poor feeding in infancy, hypogonadism with small genitals, low intellectual functioning, and a profound drive to eat that usually leads to morbid obesity in childhood. Despite their excellent nutrition, children with Prader-Willi syndrome are very short, generally below the third percentile in height. These children may seek food so persistently that their families must lock up the kitchen.[28] The cause of the disorder is unknown.

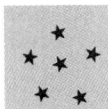

Ideas for Nursing Research

Nursing research in children with endocrine disorders needs to begin with studies of the population of normal children. Feelings and attitudes about growth and sexuality in all children will help focus care for children who experience aberrations of these life events.

Children with hypothalamic-pituitary disorders may have behaviors that arise from sources other than their hormone imbalances. Often their behaviors are attributed to "hormones," when they could result from another source. The following areas need to be explored:

- Psychological outcomes of treated versus untreated precocious puberty
- Results of self-care in medication administration of hormone replacements
- Type of peer relationships in short stature
- Teacher perceptions of children with early and late maturation
- Parental expectations of the short child
- Characteristics more likely to predict good metabolic control versus characteristics more likely to increase the risk of poor control

Analysis of the 15th chromosome of children with Prader-Willi syndrome may reveal a deletion, although this finding is not diagnostic.[29] The food-seeking behavior and hypogonadal state are seen with severe hypothalamic malfunction, and these children are often treated by endocrinologists. There is no cure for the disorder, but programs have been designed to meet the needs of these families.

Summary

The endocrine system mediates growth, metabolism, sexual development and function, and homeokinesis. Endocrine problems in children are almost exclusively those of hypofunction. Treatment is directed at replacing the missing hormones in a pattern that mimics nature, whether the deficiency is a primary problem within the endocrine gland or a secondary deficiency, such as the lack of pituitary stimulation to the endocrine gland. In children with hyperfunction, treatment is aimed at suppression of the overactive hormone.

Some conditions, such as the absence of insulin or cortisol, are lethal if not corrected. Treatment for other conditions, such as isolated GHD, may not be essential. These treatments may be viewed as unneeded or simply cosmetic by the family and child. Conversely, many families whose children do not have endocrine disorders seek treatment for perceived problems because of their mis-

understanding of normal variations in growth and sexual development.

Most endocrine disorders can be managed in the ambulatory care setting. Nurses supply ongoing interim education and follow-up by continued telephone contact. Hospitalizations are rare in this population, with the exception of children who have acute DKA.

Endocrine disorders in children are rare. Other illnesses, such as malabsorption or inflammatory bowel disease, may cause acute symptoms such as growth arrest and fatigue. Many chronic conditions or their treatments may result in endocrine abnormalities, sometimes many years later. Leukemia, brain tumors, and renal failure are examples of these problems. The nurse caring for these children must be attuned to possible future endocrine dysfunction.

Acknowledgment

The author wishes to acknowledge support for the section on diabetes in part by Grant #PHS P60 DK 20542-10 from the Diabetes Research and Training Center, Indiana University, and would also like to acknowledge the editorial advice and support of Dr. Donald Orr, Director of Adolescent Medicine.

References

1. American Association of Diabetes Educators. (1988). Prevention of transmission of blood-borne infection agents during blood glucose monitoring. *Diabetes Educator, 14,* 422–426.
2. American Diabetes Association. (1987). Nutritional recommendations and principles for individuals with diabetes mellitus (position statement). *Diabetes Care, 10,* 126–132.
3. American Diabetes Association. (1988). *Physician's guide to insulin-dependent (type I) diabetes: Diagnosis and treatment.* Alexandria, VA: ADA.
4. Amiel, S., et al. (1986). Impaired insulin action in puberty: A contributing factor to poor glycemic control in adolescents with diabetes. *New England Journal of Medicine, 315,* 215–219.
5. Anderson, J. (1990). Mixing insulins in 1990. *Diabetes Educator, 16,* 380–387.
6. Bacon, G. E., Spencer, M. L., Hopwood, N. J., & Kelch, R. P. (1990). *A practical approach to pediatric endocrinology* (3rd ed.). Chicago, Year Book Medical Publishers.
7. Bode, H. H. (1990). Disorders of the posterior pituitary. In S. L. Kaplan (Ed.), *Clinical pediatric endocrinology.* (pp. 63–86). Philadelphia: W. B. Saunders.
8. Chase, P., Jackson, W., et al. (1989). Glucose control and the renal and retinal complications of insulin-dependent diabetes. *Journal of the American Medical Association, 261,* 1155–1160.
9. Cooper, N. (1988). Nutrition and diabetes: A review of current recommendations. *Diabetes Educator, 14,* 428–432.
10. Dallas, J. S., & Foley, T. P., Jr. (1990). Hyperthyroidism. In F. Lifshitz (Ed.), *Pediatric endocrinology: A clinical guide* (2nd ed.). (pp. 483–497). New York: Marcel Dekker.
11. Dallas, J. S., & Foley, T. P., Jr. (1990). Hypothyroidism. In F. Lifshitz (Ed.), *Pediatric endocrinology: A clinical guide* (2nd ed.). (pp. 469–482). New York: Marcel Dekker.
12. Dallas, J. S., & Foley, T. P., Jr. (1990). Thyromegaly. In F. Lifshitz (Ed.), *Pediatric endocrinology: A clinical guide* (2nd ed.). (pp. 457–468). New York: Marcel Dekker.

13. Darland, N. W. (1986). Congenital adrenocortical hyperplasia: Supportive nursing interventions. *Journal of Pediatric Nursing, 1*(2), 117–123.

14. Delamator, A., Davis, S., et al. (1989). Self-monitoring of blood glucose by adolescents with diabetes: Technical skills and utilization of data. *Diabetes Educator, 15,* 56–61.

15. Drash, A. (1986). Diabetes mellitus in the child and adolescent: Part I. In J. Lockhart (Ed.), *Current problems in pediatrics.* Chicago: Year Book Medical Publishers.

16. Eisenbarth, B. (1986). Type I diabetes mellitus: A chronic autoimmune disease. *New England Journal of Medicine, 314,* 1360–1368.

17. Fisher, D. A. (1987). Effectiveness of newborn screening programs for congenital hypothyroidism: Prevalence of missed cases. *Pediatric Clinics of North America, 34,* 881–890.

18. Fisher, D. A. (1991). Management of congenital hypothyroidism. *Journal of Clinical Endocrinology and Metabolism, 72*(3), 523–529.

19. Follansbee, D. (1989). Assuming responsibility for diabetes management: What age? What price? *Diabetes Care, 15,* 347–353.

20. Fort, P. (1990). Thyroid disorders in infancy. In F. Lifshitz (Ed.), *Pediatric endocrinology: A clinical guide* (2nd ed.). (pp. 432–453). New York: Marcel Dekker.

21. Fradkin, J. E., Schonberger, L. B., Mills, J. L., Gunn, W. J., Piper, J. M., Wysowski, D. K., Thomson, R., Durako, S., & Brown, P. (1991). Creutzfeldt-Jakob disease in pituitary growth hormone recipients in the United States. *Journal of the American Medical Association, 265*(7).

22. Frasier, S. D., & Lippe, B. M. (1990). Clinical review 11: The rational use of growth hormone during childhood. *Pediatrics, 71*(2), 269–273.

23. Gallaway, J. (1980). Insulin treatment for the 80's: Facts and questions about old and new insulins and their usage. *Diabetes Care, 3,* 615–622.

24. Golden, M., & Gray, D. (1991). Diabetes mellitus in children and adolescents. In R. Rakel (Ed.), *Conn's current therapy* (pp. 502–511). Philadelphia: W. B. Saunders.

25. Golden, M., Orr, D., & Herrold, A. (1985). An approach to prevention of recurrent diabetic ketoacidosis in the pediatric population. *Journal of Pediatrics, 107,* 195–200.

26. Golden, M., Russell, B., Ingersoll, G., & Gray, D. (1985). Management of diabetes mellitus in children younger than 5 years of age. *American Journal of Diseases of Children 139,* 448–452.

27. Gray, D., Marrero, D., Godfrey, C., Orr, D., & Golden, M. (1988). Chronic poor metabolic control in the pediatric population: A stepwise intervention program. *Diabetes Care 14,* 516–520.

28. Greensway, L. R. (1990). A community outreach program for individuals with Prader-Willi syndrome. *Journal of Pediatric Health Care, 4*(1), 32–38.

29. Greensway, L. R., & Alexander, R. C. (1988). *Management of Prader-Willi syndrome.* New York: Springer-Verlag.

30. Hall, J. G., & Gilchrist, D. M. (1990). Turner syndrome and its variants. *Pediatric Clinics of North America, 37*(6), 1421–1440.

31. Hamburg, B., & Inoff, G. (1983). Coping with the predictable crisis of diabetes. *Diabetes Care, 6,* 409–416.

32. Hardin, D. S., & Pescovitz, O. H. (1991). Central precocious puberty and its treatment with long-acting GnRH analogs. *The Endocrinologist,* in press.

33. Harris, G., Fiordolisi, I., Harris, W., et al. (1990). Minimizing the risk of brain herniation during treatment of diabetic ketoacidemia: A retrospective and prospective study. *Journal of Pediatrics, 117,* 22–31.

34. Havlin, C., & Cryer, P. (1988). Hypoglycemia: The limiting factor in the management of insulin-dependent diabetes mellitus. *Diabetes Educator, 14,* 407–411.

35. Hodge, R. H., Krongaard, L., Sande, M. A., & Kaiser, D. L. (1980). Multiple use of disposable insulin syringe and needle units. *Journal of the American Medical Association, 244*(3), 266–267.

36. Holland, F. J., et al. (1985). Ketoconazole in the management of precocious puberty not responsive to LHRH-analogue therapy. *New England Journal of Medicine, 312,* 1023–1028.

37. Holler, H., & Pastors, J. (1991). Nutrition guidelines and meal planning: A step-by-step teaching process. *Diabetes Spectrum, 4,* 58–61.

38. Holmes, C. S. (1990). *Psychoneuroendocrinology: Brain, behavior, and hormonal interactions.* New York: Springer-Verlag.

39. Horton, E. (1988). Role and management of exercise in diabetes mellitus. *Diabetes Care, 11,* 201–211.

40. Ilicki, A., et al. (1984). Premature thelarche: Natural history and sex hormone secretion in 68 girls. *Acta Paediatrica Scandinavica, 73,* 756–762.

41. Ingersoll, G., Orr, D., Herrald, A., & Golden, M. (1986). Cognitive maturity and self-management among adolescents with insulin-dependent diabetes mellitus. *Behavioral Pediatrics, 108,* 620–623.

42. Jackson, P. L., & Ott, M. J. (1990). Perceived self-esteem among children diagnosed with precocious puberty. *Journal of Pediatric Nursing, 5,* 190–192.

43. Jacobson, A. M., et al. (1987). Psychologic predictors of compliance in children with recent onset of diabetes mellitus. *Journal of Pediatrics, 110,* 805–811.

44. Kaplan, S. L. (1990). Growth and growth hormone. In S. L. Kaplan (Ed.), *Clinical pediatric endocrinology* (pp. 1–62). Philadelphia: W. B. Saunders.

45. Kaplowitz, P. B. (1989). Diagnostic value of testosterone therapy in boys with delayed puberty. *American Journal of Diseases of Children, 143,*

46. Kohler, P. U. (1986). *Clinical endocrinology.* New York: John Wiley & Sons.

47. LaFranchi, A., Hanna, C. E., & Mandel, S. H. (1991). Constitutional delay of growth: Expected versus final adult height. *Pediatrics, 87,* 1.

48. Lambertina, W. F., et al. (1986). Premature thelarche in Puerto Rico. *American Journal of Diseases of Children, 140,* 1263–126.

49. Laue, L., et al. (1989). Treatment of familial male precocious puberty with spironolactone and testolactone. *New England Journal of Medicine, 320,* 496–502.

50. Lifshitz, F. (Ed.). (1990). *Pediatric endocrinology: A clinical guide* (2nd ed.). New York: Marcel Dekker.

51. Manasco, P. K., et al. (1988). Resumption of puberty after long-term luteinizing hormone–releasing hormone agonist treatment of central precocious puberty. *Journal of Clinical Endocrinology and Metabolism, 67,* 368–372.

52. Marks, J., & Skyler, J. (1991). Immunotherapy of type I diabetes mellitus. *Journal of Clinical Endocrinology and Metabolism, 72,* 3–9.

53. Martinelli, A. M., & Fontana, J. L. (1990). Thyroid storm: Potential perioperative crisis. *AORN Journal, 52*(2), 305–309.

54. Mecklenburg, R. (1989). Acute complications associated with the use of insulin infusion pumps. *Diabetes Educator, 15,* 50–55.

55. Migeon, C. J., & Lanes, R. L. (1990). Adrenal cortex: Hypo- and hyperfunction. In F. Lifshitz (Ed.), *Pediatric endocrinology: A clinical guide* (2nd ed.). New York: Marcel Dekker.

56. Mimouni, F., & Tsang, R. C. (1990). Parathyroid and vitamin D-related disorders. In S. L. Kaplan (Ed.), *Clinical pediatric endocrinology* (p. 433). Philadelphia: W. B. Saunders.

57. Orr, D., Eccles, T., Lawler, D., & Golden, M. (1986). Surreptitious insulin administration in adolescents with insulin-dependent diabetes mellitus. *Journal of the American Medical Association, 256,* 3227–3230.

58. National Institutes of Health. *Facts about precocious puberty* (DHHS Publication). Washington, D.C.: U.S. Government Printing Office.

59. Padilla, G., Leake, J. A., Castro, R., Ervin, M. G., & Leake, R. D. (1989). Vasopressin levels and pediatric head trauma. *Pediatrics, 83*(5), 700–705.

60. Pasquino, A. M., et al. (1980). Hypothalamic-pituitary-gonadotropin function in girls with premature thelarche. *Archives of Disease in Childhood, 55,* 941–944.

61. Perheentupa, J. (1990). Calcium/phosphate homeostasis disorders. In F. Lifshitz (Ed.), *Pediatric endocrinology: A clinical guide* (2nd ed.). (pp. 538). New York: Marcel Dekker.

62. Pescovitz, O. H. (1985). Precocious puberty. *Pediatrics in Review, 11,* 229–237.

63. Pescovitz, O. H., et al. (1985). Management of precocious puberty. *Journal of Pediatric Endocrinology, 1,* 85–94.

64. Pescovitz, O. H., et al. (1988). Premature thelarche and central precocious puberty: The relationship between clinical presentation and the gonadotropin response to luteinizing hormone–releasing hormone. *Journal of Clinical Endocrinology and Metabolism, 67,* 474–479.

65. Precocious puberty from ointment used for diaper rash. (1990). *Nurses Drug Alert, 9*(4).

66. Raiti, S. (1990). Diabetes insipidus. In F. Lifshitz (Ed.), *Pediatric endocrinology: A clinical guide* (2nd ed.). (pp. 863–876). New York: Marcel Dekker.

67. Schira, M. G. (1987). Steroid-dependent states and adrenal insufficiency. *Nursing Clinics of North America, 22*(4), 837–841.

68. Schultz, P. N. (1989). Hypopituitarism in patients with a history of irradiation to the head and neck area: Diagnoses and implications for nursing. *Oncology Nursing Forum, 16*(6), 823–826.

69. Speiser, P. W., & New, M. I. (1990). An update of congenital adrenal hyperplasia. In F. Lifshitz (Ed.), *Pediatric endocrinology: A clinical guide* (2nd ed.). (pp. 307–332). New York: Marcel Dekker.

70. Stabler, B., & Underwood, L. (Eds.). (1986). *Slow grows the child: Psychosocial aspects of growth delay.* Hillsdale, NJ: Lawrence Erlbaum Associates.

71. Stanhope, R., & Brook, C. G. D. (1989). Disorders of puberty. In C. G. D. Brook (Ed.), *Clinical paediatric endocrinology.* Oxford, Blackwell Scientific Publications.

72. Unger, R., & Foster, D. (1981). Diabetes mellitus. In J. Wilson & D. Foster (Eds.), *Williams textbook of endocrinology.* Philadelphia: W. B. Saunders.

73. Wasserman, D., & Abumrad, N. (1989). Physiological basis for the treatment of the physically active individual with diabetes. *Sports Medicine, 7,* 376–392.

15

UNIT

Nursing Care of Children With Altered Gastrointestinal Function

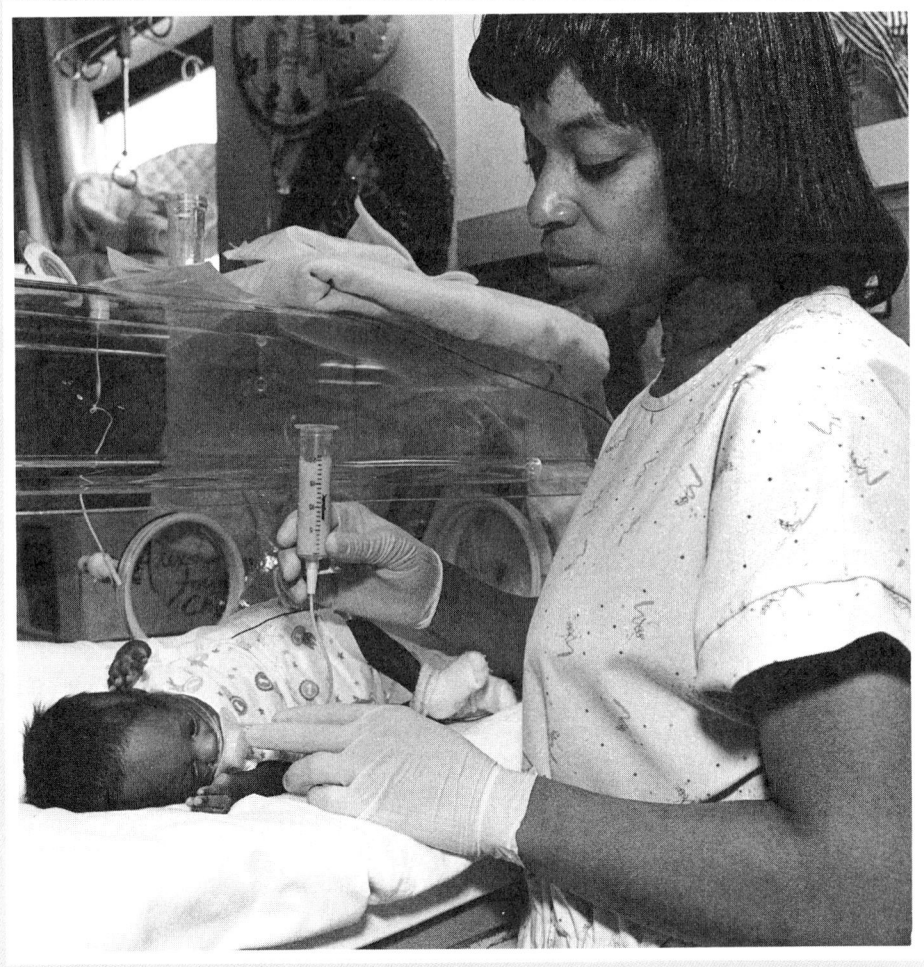

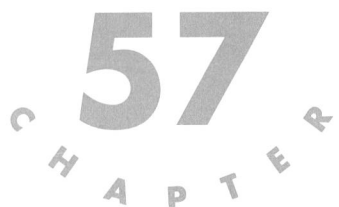

57

CHAPTER

Anatomy and Physiology of the Gastrointestinal System

FEATURE OF THIS CHAPTER

Consequences of Abnormal Embryonic Development, Table 57-1

BEHAVIORAL OBJECTIVES

Discuss embryonic development of the gastrointestinal tract.

Identify the major anatomic structures of the gastrointestinal system.

Describe the basic processes of digestion, absorption, metabolism, and elimination.

The gastrointestinal system serves as an important interface between the ingested elements from the environment and the internal milieu of the child in two ways: (1) as a major barrier to the entrance of substances such as bacteria, viruses, and potentially noxious substances, for example, undigested food proteins; and (2) as a selective inlet for other beneficial substances, such as nutrients.[5] Some of the gastrointestinal system's most important roles are in the provision of nutrients that enable the child to grow through the processes of ingestion, digestion, absorption, and elimination.

Embryonic Development

The branchial arches, foregut, midgut, and hindgut (Fig. 57-1) give rise to the gastrointestinal tract. During the fourth week of gestation, the primitive gut (foregut, midgut, and hindgut) is formed as the dorsal portion of the yolk sac is incorporated into the embryo.

Oral Cavity

Development of the oral cavity is primarily through the branchial arches, which begin to develop early in the fourth week. The first branchial arch gives rise to the development of the face. These structures are discussed in Chapter 33.

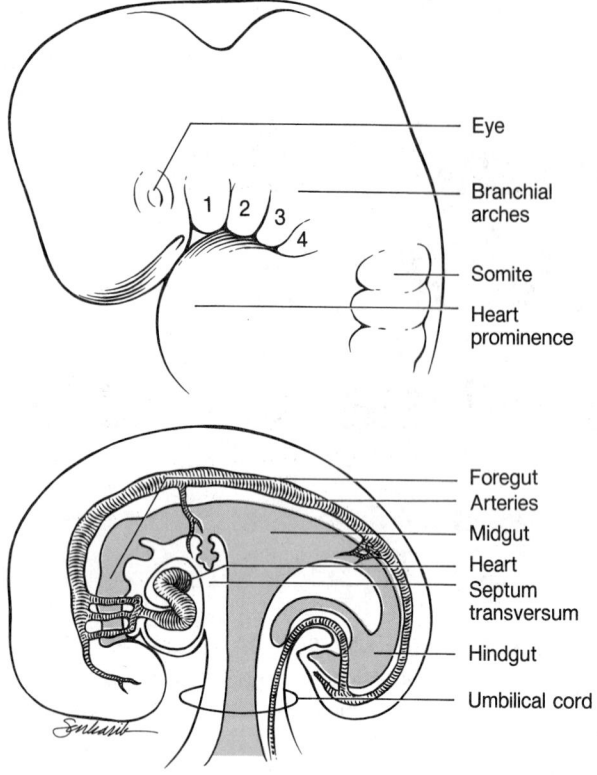

FIGURE 57-1

The human embryo. (**A**) Branchial arches. (**B**) The foregut, midgut, and hindgut. (Adapted from Moore, K. L. [1988]. *The developing human* [4th ed., p. 160]. Philadelphia: W.B. Saunders. Used with permission.)

Esophagus

The laryngotracheal groove becomes evident around 26 days' gestation. This groove divides to form the trachea and the esophagus. The laryngotracheal groove begins as a very short tube but grows rapidly. At the same time, an increase in the thickness of the epithelial lining almost obliterates the lumen, until around 8 to 10 weeks when the lumen is restored.[6]

Stomach

The stomach first appears as a fusiform dilation of the caudal portion of the foregut (around 28 days), which then enlarges and broadens. The dorsal border grows faster than the ventral border during the next few weeks, creating the greater curvature of the stomach. As the stomach becomes more like the adult-shaped stomach, it slowly rotates 90 degrees on its longitudinal axis.[8]

Duodenum

The duodenum develops from the foregut and the midgut. The junction where the foregut and the midgut fuse is just beyond the bile duct. This part of the duodenum grows rapidly and becomes a C-shaped loop. As the stomach rotates, the duodenum rotates to the right. During the fifth and sixth weeks, the lumen of the duodenum becomes temporarily obliterated due to the pro-

liferation of epithelial cells. By the end of the embryonic period, the duodenum becomes recanalized.

Jejunum Through the Midtransverse Colon

This portion of the intestines is formed from the midgut. During the sixth week of gestation the U-shaped intestinal loop herniates into the umbilical cord because of inadequate room in the abdomen. While this intestinal loop is out of the abdomen, it rotates 90 degrees. During the 10th week, the intestinal loop returns to the abdomen, rotating another 180 degrees.[8]

Like the duodenum, the rest of the gut is normally obstructed due to the epithelial cells during the fifth and sixth week, then recanalizes.

Large Intestine

The hindgut gives rise to the midtransverse colon through the superior portion of the anal canal. The inferior portion of the anal canal develops from the proctodeum. The cloaca (the caudal portion of the hindgut) is divided into the urogenital sinus and rectum by the urorectal septum. The inferior portion of the anal canal is initially separated from the superior portion by the anal membrane, but this membrane usually breaks down by the end of the eighth gestational week.

Biliary Tract

The liver bud is formed from an outgrowth of the foregut early in the fourth week. The liver bud extends into the septum transversum. The liver diverticulum rapidly enlarges and divides into two parts. Initially, both the left and right lobes of the liver are about the same size, but the right side soon becomes much larger. Hematopoiesis begins during the sixth week and is the main cause for the large size of the liver. Bile formation begins during the 12th week. The bile acid pool size of the premature infant of 32 weeks' gestation has been estimated at about 50% of that in the full-term infant.

The caudal portion of the hepatic diverticulum expands to become the gallbladder, and its stalk becomes the cystic duct. The stalk connecting the duodenum to the cystic duct and the hepatic duct becomes the bile duct. Initially, the extrahepatic biliary apparatus is occluded with endodermal cells, but it is later recanalized, similar to the duodenum.[8]

Pancreas

The pancreas develops from the dorsal and ventral pancreatic buds that arise from the caudal portion of the foregut as it is developing into the duodenum. As the pancreatic buds fuse, their ducts anastomose. The main pancreatic duct forms from the ventral bud duct and the distal part of the dorsal bud duct. The proximal portion of the dorsal bud duct often persists as an accessory pancreatic duct. There is frequently a communication between the two ducts.[8]

Consequences of Abnormal Development

As each section of the gastrointestinal system develops, disturbances in the normal pattern of events may lead to congenital birth defects. Table 57-1 lists the consequences of abnormal embryonic development.

Esophageal atresia with tracheoesophageal fistula may occur when the tracheoesophageal septum deviates posteriorly or if the lumen is not recanalized by the end of the embryonic period.[8] Malformations of the stomach are uncommon, except for pyloric stenosis, where there is a marked thickening of the pylorus. If reformation of the duodenal lumen after 6 weeks does not occur, duodenal atresia results.[8] Failure of the gut to recanalize after the sixth week causes stenosis, atresia, or duplications. Omphalocele, malrotations, or abnormalities of fixation result if the intestinal loop fails to return to the abdomen or rotates abnormally.[8] Most anorectal abnormalities (rectal atresia, fistulas) are caused by arrested growth and/or deviation of the urorectal septum.[8]

Structure and Function

The gastrointestinal system includes the mouth, pharynx, esophagus, stomach, small intestine, and large intestine and the accessory organs of the liver, gallbladder, and pancreas[13] (Fig. 57-2). Food is ingested, digested, and absorbed. Toxic material is broken down and excreted.

TABLE 57-1
Consequences of Abnormal Embryonic Development

Fetal Age (Weeks)	Structure Formed	Anomalies at Birth
4	Branchial arches	Treacher-Collins syndrome Pierre-Robin syndrome
	Incomplete closure of lateral folds	Gastroschisis
	Division of foregut into respiratory and digestive portions	Tracheoesophageal fistula
5–7	Two horizontal projections beside tongue fuse to form palate	Cleft palate
	Neural crest cells migrate into the wall of the colon	Hirschsprung's disease
	Urorectal septum fuses with cloacal membrane	Anal stenosis
8	GI tract becomes epithelialized	Esophageal atresia
		Duodenal atresia
	Anal membrane ruptures	Imperforate anus
10	Intestines return into the abdomen	Omphalocele
		Umbilical hernia
	Intestines rotate as they re-enter abdomen and become fixed	Malrotation of midgut volvulus
		Pyloric stenosis*
		Meckel's diverticulum*

* Abnormalities not identified by fetal developmental periods.

The gastrointestinal system serves as a selective, protective barrier between the outer and inner worlds of the body.

The general structure of the wall of the gastrointestinal system is similar throughout. There are four general layers: the mucosa, the submucosa, the muscularis, and the adventitia or serosa (Fig. 57-3). The mucosa is the innermost layer and includes epithelial cells that serve protective or secretory functions in varying segments of the gastrointestinal tract. The epithelial layer invaginates into the underlying tissue to form tubular exocrine glands, which secrete mucus, acid, enzymes, water, and ions into the lumen of differing portions of the gastrointestinal tract. The epithelial cells also release hormones into the blood stream. Included in the mucosa is a layer of connective tissue, lymphatic and blood capillaries, and two thin layers of muscle. The next layer is the submucosa, which consists of connective tissue with both lymphatic and blood vessels as well as a nerve fiber complex. The third layer, the muscularis, consists of two smooth muscle layers with a nerve fiber complex between the two. The muscularis layer is mainly responsible for the contractility in the gastrointestinal system. The outermost layer is the adventitia, which is connective tissue and which, when covered by a single layer of mesothelial cells, is called the *serosa*.[10] The cells of the gastrointestinal system are discussed later within each subsection in a more detailed manner. The anatomic development of the fetal gastrointestinal system by 20-week-gestation is similar to that of neonates.

The gastrointestinal tract has its own nervous system with two major nerve plexuses: the myenteric plexus and the submucous nerve plexus. The two nerve plexuses are interwoven so that neural activity in one plexus influences the activity in the other. Both the sympathetic and parasympathetic branches of the autonomic nervous system enter the tract and synapse with the neurons in the plexuses to influence the motor and secretory activity of the gastrointestinal tract. Reflexes controlling the gastrointestinal system are initiated both within and without the gastrointestinal system. Also, the neural connections permit reflexes that are independent of the central nervous system. However, the central nervous system also exerts control over the gastrointestinal tract.

In the stomach and small intestine, several different gastrointestinal hormones help regulate the volume and character of the gastrointestinal secretions. These hormones are released from the mucosa in response to the presence of food in the gastrointestinal tract; they are then absorbed into the blood and carried to glands and thereby stimulate secretions. Hormonal stimulation of the gallbladder causes the gallbladder to empty its stored bile into the duodenum.[4] Parasympathetic nerve stimulation to the gastrointestinal tract almost always increases the rates of glandular secretion. Sympathetic stimulation can have a dual effect on the gastrointestinal tract: (1) it can slightly increase secretion, but (2) if parasympathetic or hormonal stimulation is causing copious secretions, superimposed sympathetic stimulation usually reduces the secretion mainly due to decreased blood supply.[4]

The host-defense mechanisms in the gastrointestinal tract can be classified into either nonspecific, nonimmune-mediated, or specific immunologic defenses (the gut-as-

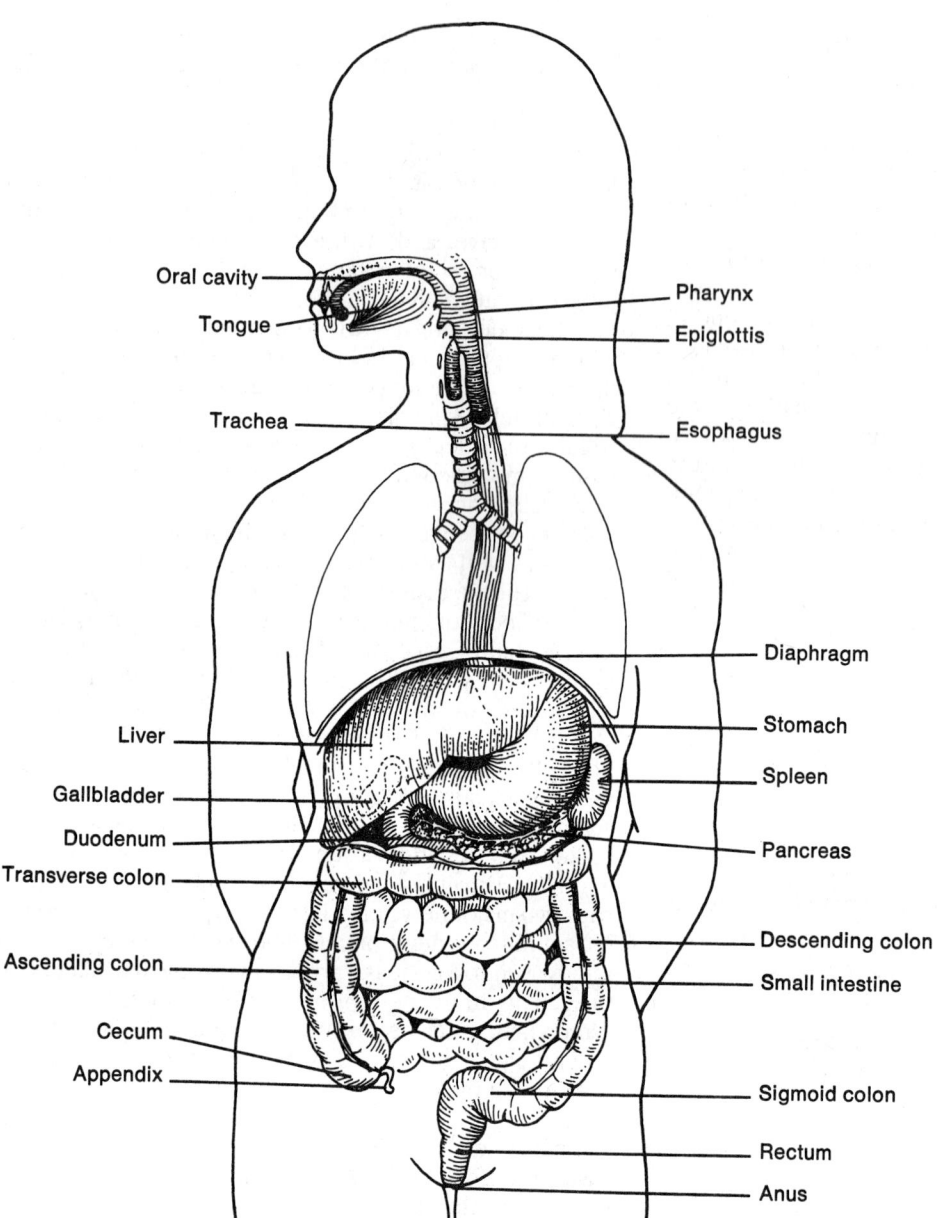

FIGURE 57-2

The gastrointestinal system. (From Broadwell, D.C., & Jackson, B.S. [1982]. Principles of ostomy care. St. Louis: Mosby.)

sociated lymphoid tissues). These defenses appear to mature along with the normal development of other organ systems. The nonspecific, nonimmune-mediated system represents the first line of defense and is composed of gastric acid, intestinal proteases, lysozymes, and bile salts, all of which contribute to the intraluminal degradation of antigens. The epithelial cell membrane and the motility of the gastrointestinal tract then serve as mechanical barriers to the influx of antigens, organisms, and their products.[5] The immunologically mediated system is composed of the secretory immunoglobulin A (IgA) antibody system and local cell-mediated immunity. The premature infant is transiently more vulnerable to antigens penetrating the intestines. The newborn still has an underdeveloped secretory immunoglobulin system. Food and microorganisms stimulate antigen production, and usually by 1 month of age almost all infants have some IgA.[11]

Oral Cavity

The oral cavity includes the lips, palate (soft and hard), tongue, teeth, gums, salivary glands, and mucous membranes. The oral cavity provides a place for food to enter the inner body and begins to convert that food to usable particles. The 1700-g premature infant mouths without effective sucking. This ineffective sucking may remain for several weeks. Premature infants weighing less than 2000 g have an immature suck-swallow pattern that may persist for weeks. Usually 34-week-gestation premature infants will be able to suck and swallow. The mature suck-swallow pattern is characterized by prolonged bursts of sucking then swallowing. Most term newborn infants acquire a mature suck-swallow pattern within a few days.

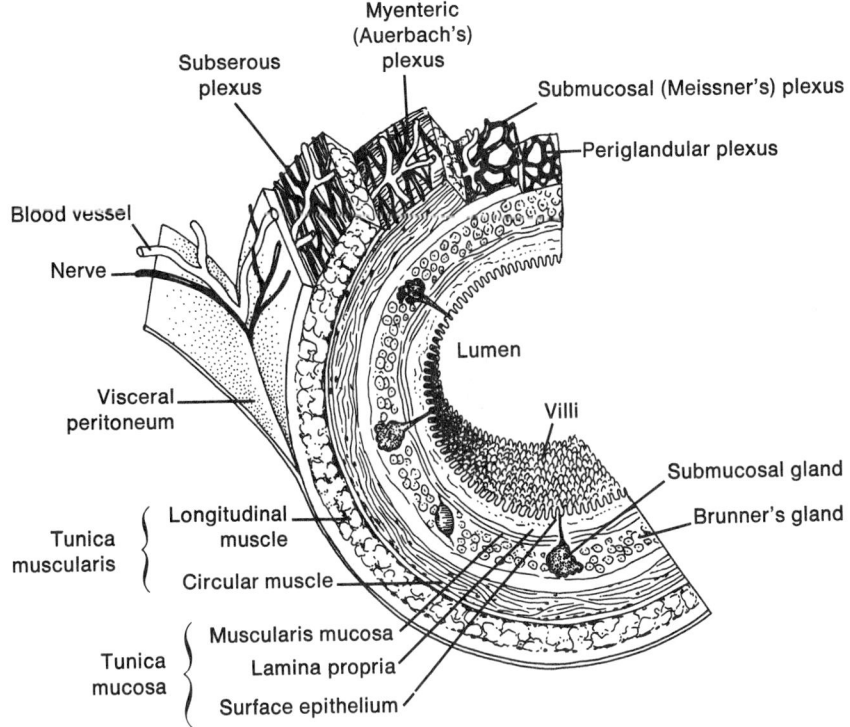

FIGURE 57-3
Layers of the gastrointestinal system. (From Broadwell, D.C., & Jackson, B.S. [1982]. Principles of ostomy care. St. Louis: Mosby.)

Sucking and swallowing are partially conscious, or voluntary, and partially unconscious, or involuntary. The infant who is unable to suck will choke and aspirate. Swallowing requires coordination with respiration because the two processes share the nasopharynx and laryngopharynx. During the voluntary stage of swallowing, the food is squeezed or rolled posteriorly in the mouth by upward and backward pressure of the tongue, forcing the food bolus into the pharynx where swallowing becomes involuntary. The food bolus in the pharynx stimulates swallowing receptor areas and impulses that then travel to the brain stem to initiate a series of automatic pharyngeal muscular contractions. The soft palate is pulled upward to close the posterior nares. The palatopharyngeal folds come together to form a slit that allows small particles to pass through to the esophagus while the vocal cords of the larynx are closely approximated to prevent passage of food into the trachea. The epiglottis also helps prevent food from entering the trachea. The upward movement of the larynx stretches the opening of the esophagus while the upper esophageal sphincter relaxes, allowing the food to move into the upper esophagus. The superior constrictor muscle of the pharynx contracts and causes a rapid peristaltic wave passing downward into the esophagus.[4]

The anterior teeth cut the food and the posterior teeth (molars) provide a grinding chewing action. Most of the muscles used in chewing are innervated by the fifth cranial nerve, and the chewing process is controlled by the hindbrain. Most of the chewing process is caused by the chewing reflex, where a bolus of food in the mouth causes reflex inhibition of the muscles of mastication, allowing the lower jaw to drop. The jaw dropping, in turn, initiates a stretch reflex of the jaw muscles, which leads to rebound contraction that raises the jaw to cause teeth closure and also compresses the bolus against the linings of the mouth, initiating another cycle of chewing.[4]

Chewing is important because the digestive enzymes only work on the surfaces of food particles. Therefore, the rate of digestion is highly dependent on the total surface area. Chewing food such as most fruits and raw vegetables is especially important because there is an undigestible cellulose membrane around their nutrient portions that must first be broken before digestion can occur.[4]

Esophagus

The esophagus is located between the oral cavity and the stomach. It is a hollow tube extending from the oropharynx through the diaphragm into the abdominal cavity and attaching to the stomach. The esophagus can be divided into three functional areas: the upper esophageal sphincter, the body, and the lower esophageal sphincter. The upper esophageal sphincter is located at the pharyngoesophageal junction, and the lower esophageal sphincter is located at the gastroesophageal junction. The esophagus has two types of glands, the esophageal and cardiac glands, both of which secrete mucus.[11]

The esophageal wall has the four general layers mentioned earlier: the mucosa, submucosa, muscularis, and adventitia. In the muscularis layer, the muscle types include striated muscle in the upper one third, a mix of striated and smooth in the middle, and smooth muscle in the lower one third of the esophagus. The adventitia layer has nerves that control the coordination of swallowing and motor functions.[11]

The esophageal arterial blood supply arises from branches of the thoracic aorta. Venous drainage occurs through three pathways: the superior vena cava, the azygous system, and the portal system.[3]

The primary function of the esophagus is to move the food to the stomach. Movement through the esophagus is involuntary. When the upper esophageal sphincter receives food, it relaxes briefly and allows passage of the food, then the food bolus is propelled down the esophageal body by a peristaltic wave. As the food bolus moves forward, the lower esophageal sphincter relaxes to allow passage of the food bolus into the stomach. With newborns the lower esophageal sphincter is immature and may stay relaxed (decreased pressure), allowing gastroesophageal reflux. In the child and adult the lower esophageal sphincter usually is closed (increased pressure) except when swallowing. The lower esophageal sphincter is affected (pressure either increases or decreases) by some drugs and hormones. The vagal nerve helps innervate the lower esophageal sphincter.

Stomach

The stomach has four segments: the fundus, body, antrum, and pyloric canal. The body of the stomach accounts for the proximal two thirds, with the antrum occupying the distal third.

The stomach's major functions include motor, endocrine, and secretory actions.[11] The motor function of the stomach includes temporary storage of the ingested food and secreted substances, a mixing of the food bolus with the gastric juices that dissolve and dilute the food, a further "kneading" of the solid material that breaks down into small particles, and then emptying the food bolus into the duodenum.[11]

The endocrine and secretory functions are performed by three types of glandular cells that produce secretions that make up gastric juice. The oxyntic cells secrete intrinsic factor (necessary for the absorption of vitamin B_{12}) and hydrochloric acid. Hydrochloric acid denatures protein, kills microbes, and changes pepsinogen to pepsin, which helps break down protein. The peptic cells secrete pepsinogen, lipase, and renin.[11] Mucous cells secrete mucus and bicarbonate, which provide a coating for the stomach mucosa. Mucus also lubricates the solid food. Water is secreted in the stomach to dissolve and dilute the food. Hydrochloric acid secretion is influenced by pH, the buffering of food, and by gastric emptying.[11] There are three mechanisms that inhibit acid secretion: receptor blockade, inhibition of cell activation by prostaglandins, and inhibition of the H^+/K^+ ATPase, which pumps acid across the parietal cell.[11]

Further regulation of gastric function is provided by the gastric mucosa, which produces gastrin and somatostatin. Gastrin stimulates pepsinogen secretion and acid secretion and also promotes mucosal growth. Somatostatin inhibits the release of gastrin. Additionally, the gastric mucosal has nerves containing peptides that also influence gastric function.[11]

The stomach is innervated by the vagus nerve. The antrum and pylorus regulate the emptying of solid food. Liquids clear the stomach faster than solids, which need to be broken down further into more liquid form for digestion.[7] Gastric emptying is prolonged by increased osmolarity, solid food, decreased pH, and increased fat content. More than 40% of term infants have a gastric emptying time of greater than 8 hours. Normal 3- to 6-month-old infants empty around 35% to 56% of formula from their stomach by 1 hour. Most infants, compared with adults, have rapid gastric emptying for the first 20 minutes, then have a curve of liquid gastric emptying similar to that of adults. Delayed gastric emptying is seen more often in infants drinking cow's milk formula than breast milk or glucose.[3]

Gallbladder

The gallbladder is located on the underside of the liver and is a pear-shaped bag that is used as a storage area for bile. The gallbladder's capacity is increased rapidly during the first 2 years of life and then grows proportionately to the other organs, including the liver. The hepatic duct joins with the cystic duct from the gallbladder to form the common bile duct, which empties into the duodenum. There are two sphincters at the end of the common bile duct.

There is a physiologic immaturity of the enterohepatic circulation of bile acids that is demonstrated by inefficient lipid digestion, delayed hepatic clearance, and metabolism of exogenous (drugs) and endogenous compounds (bile acids and bilirubin) and a cholestatic phase of liver development, with the net outcome that the newborn is prone to develop cholestasis. Other factors such as sepsis, parenteral nutrition, hormonal imbalance, or viral infection can result in hepatobiliary disease, especially in premature infants. Fat absorption also is inefficient until approximately 3 to 5 months of age, when it reaches adult functioning.[11]

The gallbladder functions as a reservoir for bile formed by the liver and concentrates the bile by actively reabsorbing sodium bicarbonate and water. This causes a tenfold increase in the concentration of nonabsorbable organic compounds stored in the gallbladder. Bile is composed of bile salts (the most abundant substance), bilirubin, cholesterol, fatty acids, and electrolytes. Bile salts have an emulsifying action on fat molecules by decreasing surface tension, which causes the fat to become solubilized. After eating, the intestinal hormone cholecystokinin causes the gallbladder to contract and the sphincter of Oddi to open, allowing bile to be released into the duodenum. Consequently, if the gallbladder is nonfunctioning or has been removed, there may be fat malabsorption.[9]

Pancreas

The pancreas is a gland that lies in the right upper abdominal quadrant, back of the peritoneum and behind the stomach. The pancreas consists of four sections: head, neck, body, and tail. The pancreatic duct (the duct of Wirsung) runs the entire length of the pancreas, with small branches draining all the lobules. The pancreatic duct connects with the common bile duct and then empties into the duodenum at the papilla.

The pancreas has dual functions: the exocrine portion aids in the digestion of food, and the endocrine portion produces insulin to regulate carbohydrate metabolism and blood glucose levels. The pancreatic acinar cells are serous cells and produce the exocrine pancreatic secretions that are emptied into the duodenum. Exocrine pancreatic secretions aid in digestion of proteins, fats, and carbohydrates and buffer the chyme from the stomach to promote an optimal milieu for enzyme activity. Each digestive enzyme's activity level develops along individual developmental rates. The activity level of all enzymes sharply increases around 26 weeks gestation. Enterokinase and trypsin activity are first noted during this period. However, enterokinase activity is extremely low compared with that of the term infant. Pancreatic enzyme activity again sharply increases between 36 to 40 weeks gestation. Infants are able to digest starches from birth.[3] However, amylase remains low until the infant is 6 months of age. Complete digestive activity is most likely not present until approximately 1½ to 2 years of age.[11]

Part of the digestive process is mediated by the vagus nerve, in which pancreatic enzymes are mobilized from the acinar cells into the ducts. When the acidic chyme enters the duodenum, the duodenal mucosa releases secretin, which in turn secretes sodium bicarbonate and electrolytes. The chyme is neutralized to a pH of 8. When protein and fat enter the duodenum, pancreatic enzyme secretion (mostly amylase, lipase, and proteolytic enzymes in their inactive forms) is stimulated by cholecystokinin-pancreozymin. The digestion and absorption of the food then proceeds.[3]

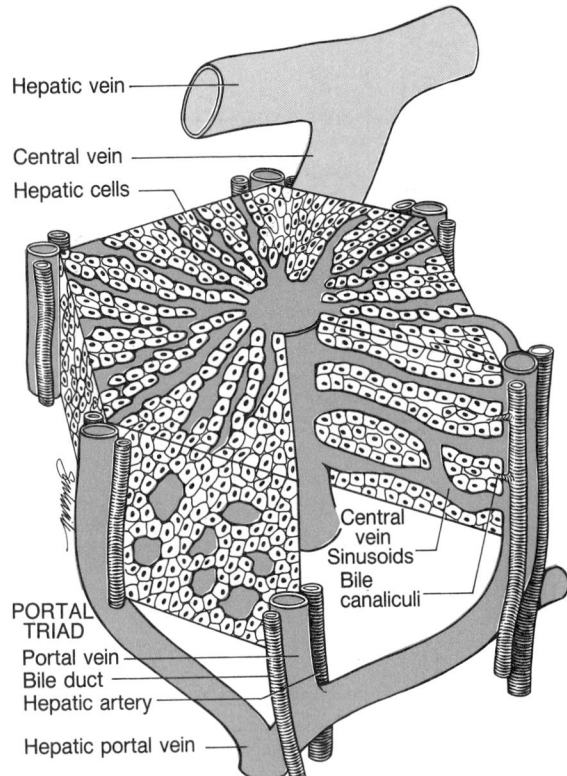

FIGURE 57-4

The liver lobule. (Adapted from Colon, A.R. [1990]. *Textbook of pediatric hepatology* [2nd ed., p. 11]. Chicago: Year Book Medical Publishers. Used with permission.)

Liver

The liver is the largest organ in the body. It is located in the right upper quadrant of the abdomen, below the diaphragm, protected in part by the rib cage. The average weight of the liver in infancy is 5% of body weight, decreasing gradually over the years up to the age of 8 years, when it remains at around 2% of the body weight. In infancy, the liver may be normally palpable up to 2 cm below the right costal margin. It may be palpated in the older child normally up to 1 cm.[1] Highly vascularized, the liver receives approximately 25% of the total cardiac output. The liver is divided into two main regions, the left and right lobes, by the falciform ligament, the ligament teres, and the ligament venosum. The functional unit of the liver is the lobule, which consists of hepatocytes (hepatic cells) around a central vein and portal triads (consisting of portal vein, the hepatic artery, and the bile duct) bounding the portal tract (Fig. 57-4). From these portal triads, hepatic artery branches and portal venous blood flow into the sinusoids, allowing slow and prolonged contact between the blood and the hepatocytes. The hepatocytes are usually two cells thick during infancy, then increase to a five- to six-cell thickness in late adolescence. The sinusoids are lined with endothelial cells; Kupffer cells, which are specialized endothelial cells and part of the reticuloendothelial system involved with

phagocytosis; and "fat cells," which are thought to play a role in fibrogenesis. The endothelial cells overlap each other loosely, leaving channels or pores through which relatively large macromolecules can move.

The liver is an extremely complex organ that has a major role in protein, carbohydrate, and lipid metabolism; detoxification of many chemicals; bile acid metabolism; hormonal regulation; vitamin absorption; and bilirubin excretion (Fig. 57-5). The major functions of the liver will be discussed later in this chapter.

The hepatocyte (liver cell) has many organelles within its structure (Fig. 57-6). The plasma membrane is an active tissue that possibly assists with the selective uptake of chemicals and their excretion into the biliary tract. Some proteins, such as albumin, cholesterol, and fibrinogen pass into the circulation through the plasma membrane. The nucleus carries genetic information. The mitochondria play a role in oxidative phosphorylation, in the production and storage of ATP for energy, in oxygen utilization, and in carbon dioxide formation. The Golgi apparatus concentrates proteins synthesized by the ribosomes and then moves them to the plasma membrane, where they are secreted. The endoplasmic reticulum is the most extensive organelle of the hepatocyte; its functions include the synthesis and transportation of proteins, lipids, and mucopolysaccharides. Lysosomes break down bacteria and other cellular debris. Ribosomes produce proteins.

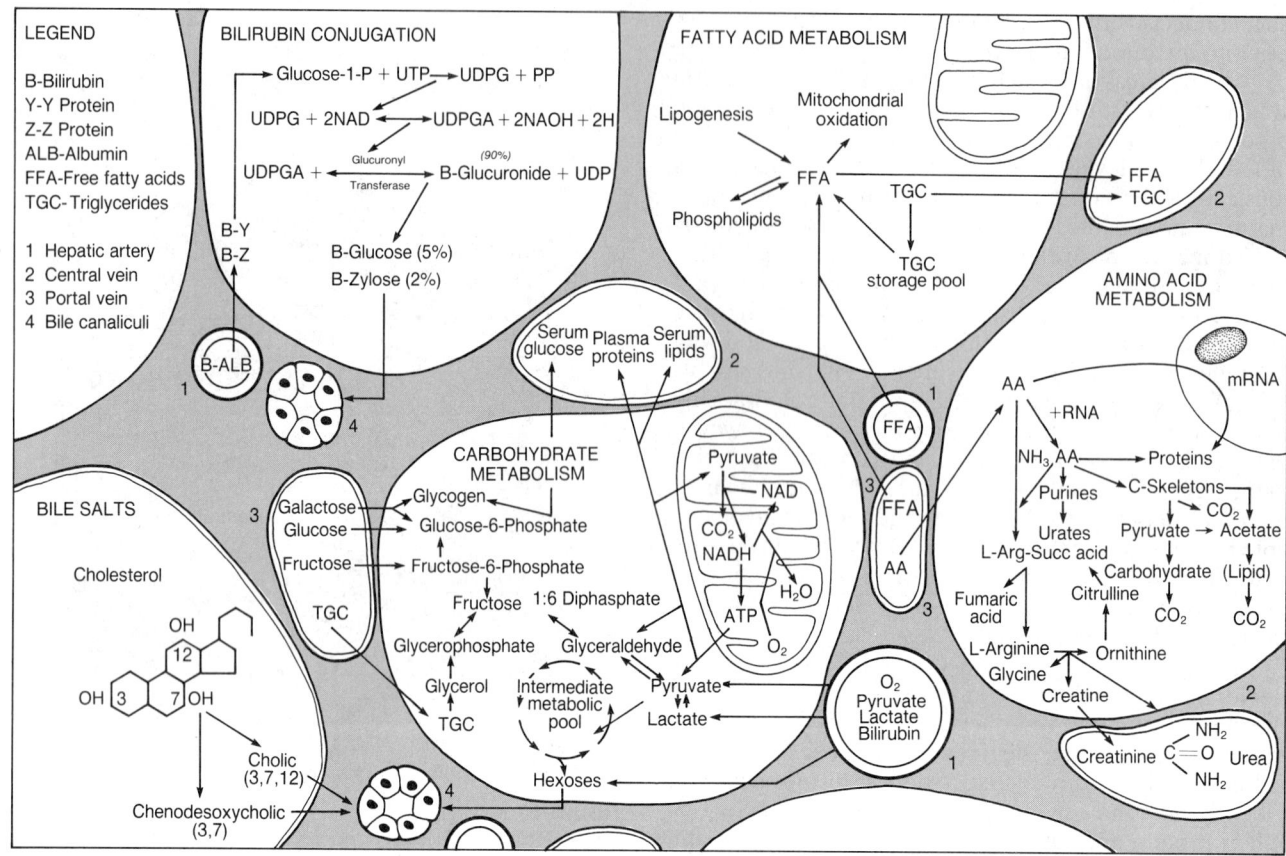

FIGURE 57-5

Metabolic overview of the liver. (Adapted from Colon, A.R. [1990]. *Textbook of pediatric hepatology* [2nd ed., p. 13]. Chicago: Year Book Medical Publishers. Used with permission.)

Small Intestine

The small intestine is attached to the stomach on one end and the large intestine on the other. There are three functional and anatomic areas in the small intestine: (1) the duodenum, followed by (2) the jejunum, and (3) the ileum. Normally, most of digestion and absorption have occurred before food reaches the middle of the jejunum.[14]

The mucous membrane of the small intestine is characterized by mucosal folds, further convoluted into villi. The mucus folds can be seen without magnification. They include mucosa and a portion of the submucosa that forms the central core. The mucous folds are more developed in the jejunum and are absent in the lower ileum. In the duodenum, finger-like villi fuse together and appear leaf shaped. In the jejunum, they appear tongue like, and in the ileum they are finger-like projections. Each villus consists of smooth muscle, an artery, a capillary meshwork, nerve fibers, and a central lymphatic or lacteal, with the basic characteristic of the lamina propria (a layer of connective tissue). The villi are covered by epithelial cells[11] (Fig. 57-7). The epithelial cell layer is the barrier that separates the fluid within the intestinal lumen from the interstitial fluid of the villi. Movement across this layer occurs several ways, including diffusion and also specific carrier-mediated transport systems.[14] DNA synthesis is performed in the Lieberkühn crypts (tubular glands that dip from the surface to the muscularis mucosa between the villi). Protein synthesis continues as the cells migrate

up the villus. The Lieberkühn crypt has all four types of epithelial cells found in the small intestine: absorptive (or columnar) cells, goblet cells, Paneth's cells, and enteroendocrine cells. The great majority of epithelial cells of the villi are absorptive cells (90%), mingled together with some goblet cells and a few enteroendocrine cells. The absorptive cells are the "brush border" of the villi. Between the epithelial cells are some lymphocytes and other white blood cells.

The small intestine is the primary site for nutrient absorption. The surface area is estimated to be 200 times the adult body surface area. The enterocyte, or intestinal cell, has all the organelles necessary for energy synthesis, catabolism, and transport. Nutrients that are transported must enter the capillary system in the lamina propria. For digestion and absorption to occur, the food must be in a suspension or a solution. The fluids involved in making solids into a solution include water, bile, gastric juice, pancreatic secretions, and salivary secretions. This solution can then contact an increased amount of microvilli, allowing greater absorption. There is a bidirectional flux of water, salts, and other small molecules. Further discussion of digestion and absorption of specific nutrients will be presented elsewhere in this chapter.

The gastrointestinal tract serves as an endocrine organ by secreting hormones. Gastrin is released from the pylorus and the duodenal mucosa at the presence of food (especially protein) or by distention of the stomach. Other peptides, such as secretin, gastric inhibitory poly-

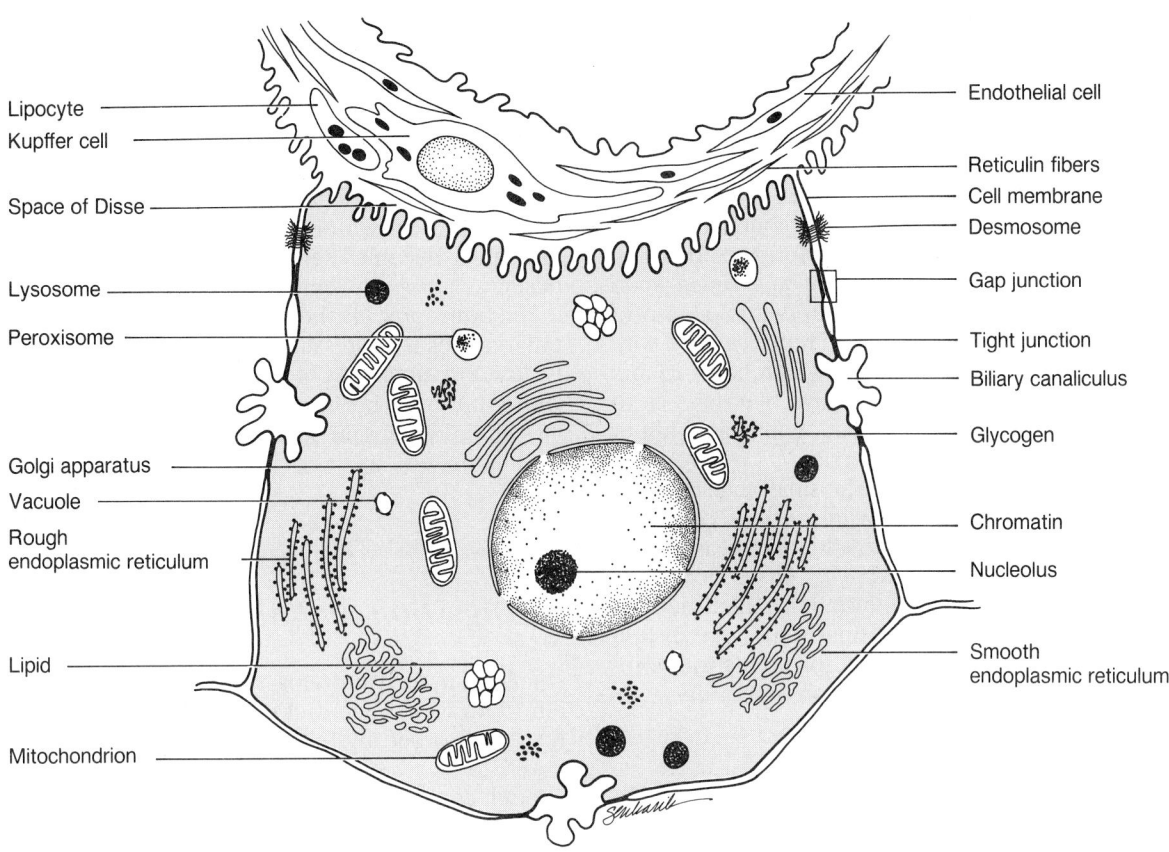

FIGURE 57-6

Organelles of liver cell. (Adapted from Sherlock, S. [1989]. *Diseases of the liver and biliary system* [8th ed., p. 12]. Oxford: Blackwell Scientific Publications. Used with permission.)

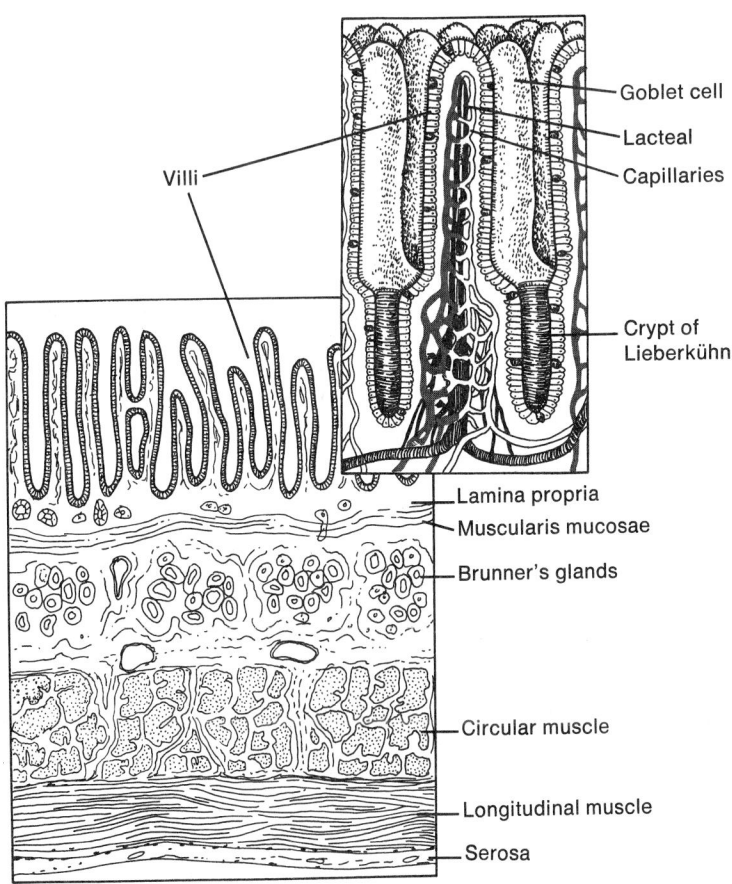

FIGURE 57-7

Structure of the small intestine villa. (From Broadwell, D.C. & Jackson, B.S. [1982]. Principles of ostomy care. St. Louis: Mosby.)

peptide, vasoactive intestinal peptide, glucagon, and calcitonin, (as well as the acidification of intestinal luminal contents), inhibit further release of gastrin. Cholecystokinin stimulates gallbladder contraction and pancreatic enzyme secretion.[11]

The motility of the small intestine has two main activities. During the fasting state, migrating myoelectric complexes, or brief periods of rhythmic contractions, occur approximately every 100 minutes, followed by irregular contractions and then by a period of quiescence. Food in the stomach or duodenum interrupts this pattern of migrating myoelectric complexes and replaces them with persistent segmenting contractions, which helps to mix the nutrients. Lipids in the ileum have been shown to slow down transit time in the duodenum and upper jejunum.[7]

There are several reflexes in the small intestine that are important for digestion. During periods of gastric emptying, contractile activity in the ileum increases. This reflex is known as the *gastroileal reflex*. Distention of the ileum causes decreased gastric motility, called the *ileogastric reflex*. Injury to the intestinal wall, large distentions of the intestine, and bacterial infections in the intestinal can cause a complete cessation of motility.[14]

Large Intestine

The large intestine (colon) has two portions, each with its own derivation and function. The proximal portion includes the cecum (and the finger-like projection of the appendix), the ascending colon, and a portion of the transverse colon. Vascular supply is from the superior mesenteric artery. The ileum connects to the colon at the ileocecal valve, which prevents retrograde reflux of fecal material into the small intestine. The distal portion of the colon includes the remainder of the transverse colon, the descending colon, the sigmoid, the rectum, and the superior portion of the anal canal. The vascular supply is from the inferior mesenteric artery.

The large intestine has a greater diameter and is about half as long as the small intestine. However, the epithelial surface area is only about $1/30$ that of the small intestine because the mucosa does not have villi like the small intestine and is not convoluted.[14] The neonatal colon measures approximately 45 cm, whereas the adult colon length is 4 to 5 ft. The mucous membrane has Lieberkühn crypts, which are associated with goblet cells intermixed with a few cylindric and enteroendocrine cells. The lamina propria contains solitary lymphoid follicles extending into the submucosa. IgA-producing plasma cells are seen in the deeper portions. The longitudinal layer of the muscularis mucosa condenses from the cecum to rectum in longitudinal bands (the teniae coli) with haustra (sacculations) between them, which gives the large intestine its characteristic look. The muscularis mucosa disappears into the anorectal canal, and the inner muscularis mucosa thickens, forming the internal anal sphincter. The external anal sphincter is formed by the sphincter ani externus muscle.[11]

The proximal colon absorbs more than 90% of sodium and chloride and a varying amount of bicarbonate. It also absorbs at least 80% of the water entering the cecum. Some glucose, amino acids, short-chain fatty acids, and vitamins are absorbed in small quantities. The distal colon functions mainly as a reservoir.[3]

The motor functions of the large intestine are mixing and propulsion. Mixing is accomplished by segmentation and circular constriction forming haustral pockets. Material enters the colon in a liquid state, and as it progresses, it becomes semisolid. Propulsion of the bolus occurs as a mass movement, when a contraction proximal to the bolus propels the material caudally in a sequence of large, positive-pressure waves. Colonic motor activity is slow and variable.[3] Colonic motility control is complex, with input from intrinsic and extrinsic innervation, hormonal and paracrine stimulation, and factors based on the amount and nature of the fecal material.[11]

System Physiology

Digestion and Absorption

Food in its natural form (carbohydrate, fat, and protein, with small quantities of vitamins and minerals) cannot be absorbed by the gastrointestinal tract. It is necessary for the food first to be broken down into small enough compounds for absorption, then to be absorbed into the gastrointestinal tract. The basic chemical process of digestion for all three major food types is hydrolysis,[4] the breakdown of a chemical bond with the addition of the elements of water (H^+ and OH^-) to the products formed.[14] The unique difference lies in the enzymes required for the food types to promote the chemical reaction (Table 57-2).[15]

Digestion and Absorption of Proteins

Intake of the essential amino acids is the cornerstone for growth and the maintenance of positive nitrogen balance. Dietary proteins are derived almost completely from meats and vegetables and consist of long chains of amino acids bound together by peptide links.

Digestion of Protein in the Stomach. The oxyntic (parietal) cells of the stomach secrete hydrochloric acid, which is mixed with the stomach contents and stomach secretions. The pH of the mixture ranges around 2 to 3. This is important to activate pepsin to begin digesting the protein. Pepsin is most active at a pH of 2 to 3 and is completely inactive at a pH greater than 5. Pepsin splits the proteins at the peptide links between the amino acids by hydrolysis.[4] Approximately 10% to 30% of total protein digestion is completed in the stomach. In the newborn, gastric pH only briefly drops to 1 to 3 after a meal, so pepsin digestion of protein is minimal.[11]

Digestion of Protein in the Small Intestine. Most protein digestion occurs at the small intestine with the assistance of the proteolytic enzymes from the pancreas (trypsin, chymotrypsin, and carboxypolypeptidase). Each of the proteolytic enzymes are specific for hydrolyzing

TABLE 57-2
Digestion and Absorption

Site	Digestion	Enzyme/Function/Secretion	Absorption
Mouth	Starch, glycogen	Salivary amylase	
	Fat	Lingual lipase	
Stomach	Protein	Gastric pepsin, gastric HCl, regulated release of peptides to upper bowel, intrinsic factor	
Duodenum	Starch, glycogen	Pancreatic amylase	Hexoses, pentoses
	Fat	Pancreatic lipase	Glycerol
	Protein	Pancreatic trypsin	Fatty acids
		Polypeptidases	Iron
		Carboxypeptidase A and B	Minerals
Jejunum	Oligopeptides	Brush border hydrolysis	Dipeptides, amino acids
	Disaccharides	Disaccharidases	Glucose, fructose, galactose
	Sucrose	Sucrase	Vitamins
	Maltose	Maltase	
	Lactose	Lactase	
	1:6 glucosides	Isomaltase or 1:6 glucosidase	Fatty acids, glycerol
Ileum	Starch	Amylase	Sugars, fatty acids
	Fat	Bile salts	Glycerol
		Cholecystokinin	Cholesterol
		Cholesterol esterase	Bile salts
	Dipeptides	Enterokinase	Amino acids, vitamin B_{12}, phosphate
Colon			Water, electrolytes

From Walker, W. A., & Hendricks, K. M.: (1985). *Manual of pediatric nutrition* (p. 102). Philadelphia; W. B. Saunders.

individual types of peptide linkages. The brush border of the small intestine contains several enzymes for hydrolyzing the remaining dipeptides and polypeptides as they come into contact with the villi epithelium. Amino acids are absorbed through the mucosa much more rapidly than intact proteins. Most of the digestion and absorption of protein occurs in the duodenum and jejunum.[4]

Digestion and Absorption of Carbohydrates

Three major sources of dietary carbohydrate exist in the usual human diet: sucrose (disaccharide known as cane sugar), lactose (disaccharide in milk), and starches (large polysaccharides that are present in almost all nonanimal food, especially in grains).

Digestion of Carbohydrates in the Mouth. When food is chewed in the mouth, it is mixed with the enzyme ptyalin (salivary amylase), which begins to break down starch into maltose and some small glucose polymers. Only 3% to 5% of all starches eaten become hydrolyzed by the time the food is swallowed.

Digestion of Carbohydrates in the Stomach. The action of ptyalin can last as long as 1 hour in the stomach, until the contents of the fundus are mixed with the gastric acid secretions, because the amylase is inactive in a *p*H below 4. Usually 30% to 40% of the starches are hydro-

lyzed by this time.[4] The salivary amylase may not be inactivated in infants because gastric secretions may not yet become acidic enough to stop its action. Salivary amylase may, therefore, play a key role for young infants in digesting starches.[2]

Digestion of Carbohydrates in the Small Intestine. Chyme (the partially digested food) mixes immediately with the pancreatic enzymes, including the pancreatic amylase, which splits starches similar to the action of salivary amylase. The epithelial cells of the brush border of the small intestine villi secrete the enzymes lactase, sucrase, maltase, and α-dextrinase. These enzymes split the disaccharides lactose, sucrose, maltose, and other small glucose polymers into their monosaccharides. The monosaccharides are then absorbed into the portal blood stream. This process is usually complete before the chyme reaches the ileum. Pancreatic amylase does not reach adult levels for several months after birth.

Digestion and Absorption of Fat

The fats in the usual diet include triglycerides (most common), phospholipids, cholesterol, and cholesterol esters. Fats are found in both animal and plant food sources.

Pancreatic lipase activity is low in young infants; therefore, nonpancreatic lipases may play a key role in the digestion and absorption of fat. Lingual lipase (derived from the base of the tongue) remains active in the low *p*H of the stomach but is inactivated by bile salts in the duodenum. Gastric lipase is produced in the stomach, with similar activity. Human milk contains several lipases, with the bile salt–stimulated lipase being the most important, because it carries on digestion in the duodenum.

Digestion of Fat in the Small Intestine. Essentially all fat digestion occurs in the small intestine, except in the young infant. First, the fat is emulsified (broken down into small globules so that water-soluble enzymes can act on the globule surfaces) with the assistance of bile salts. The major function of bile salts is to make the fat globules readily fragmentable by agitation in the small intestine. The lipases (enzymes to break down the fat molecules) are water soluble and only work on the surface of the fat globules, so it is important that the fat globules be emulsified and broken down into small particles.

The main pancreatic enzyme for the digestion of fat is pancreatic lipase. The epithelial cells of the brush border also secrete enteric lipase. Fat is digested by both enzymes through the process of hydrolysis to form monoglycerides and free fatty acids, which become dissolved in the lipid portion of the bile acid micelles. The monoglycerides and free fatty acids are "ferried" to the brush border of the villi, where they immediately diffuse through the epithelial membrane, leaving the micelle still in the chyme to ferry yet more monoglycerides and free fatty acids. With the presence of adequate amount of bile acids, approximately 97% of the fat is absorbed, whereas only 50% to 60% is absorbed if bile acids are absent. Cholesterol is absorbed through the same "ferrying" process.[4] In the young infant, the normal amount of triglyceride absorbed is 80% to 95%, varying with age and gestational maturity. Normal cholesterol absorption does not exceed 50% in young infants.[10] Medium-chain triglycerides are absorbed directly into the portal system without the assistance of lipase or bile salts, whereas all other fats require a critical micellar concentration (a certain concentration) before they are able to be absorbed.

Once the monoglycerides and free fatty acids are in the epithelial cell, most are taken up by the smooth endoplasmic reticulum where they are reformed into new triglycerides. Some of the monoglycerides are further digested into glycerol and fatty acids. The triglycerides, along with the other absorbed cholesterol and phospholipids, form a globule that is then excreted into the lymph system.[4]

Metabolism

Carbohydrate Metabolism

During the latter part of gestation, large amounts of glycogen are deposited in the liver. Glycogen is quickly mobilized after birth. Hypoglycemia may occur, especially in infants who are preterm or small for gestational age. Hypoglycemia is also common in infants born to mothers who have had gestational diabetes with continuing hyperglycemia.

Carbohydrates that have been absorbed from the intestinal tract are taken up by the liver to be utilized immediately for energy or stored as glycogen for use later by being converted to glucose during fasting.

Protein and Amino Acid Metabolism

Synthesis of proteins occurs actively in both the fetus and the newborn. Alpha-fetoprotein is the main protein seen in the fetus. Albumin serum concentration is low in preterm infants but reaches adult value by term birth. Amino acids, except cystine, have a higher concentration in the fetus than in the adult. However, the enzymes required to utilize the amino acids are not too active around birth. Thus, infants given increased protein intakes may have difficulty in assimilating and metabolizing the protein, resulting in an elevated serum amino acid concentration.

Most of the proteins in plasma are synthesized by the endoplasmic reticulum of the hepatocytes, including albumin, transferrin, ferritin, and C-reactive protein. Proteins such as fibrinogen and factors V, VII, IX, and X, necessary for the blood-clotting mechanism, are also synthesized by the liver. Vitamin K is essential for the formation of some of these clotting factors. Vitamin K–dependent factors (II, VII, IX, X) are low at birth and may drop even lower during the first week unless vitamin K is given soon after birth.

The liver quickly takes up the amino acids absorbed in the intestine and deaminates, transaminates, or utilizes them. Ammonia, a by-product of the deamination, is then converted to urea through the Krebs' cycle (the urea cycle).

Fat Metabolism

Cholesterol is synthesized in the liver, intestinal mucosa, adrenal cortex, and arterial walls and is excreted into the bile as the beginning of bile salts. Cholesterol is also the basic structure for steroid hormones. The liver metabolizes the mineralocorticoids and glucocorticoids by producing an inactive metabolite and conjugating it, which can then be excreted in the urine.

Neutral fats are oxidized within the liver to glycerol and free fatty acids. There is a constant cycle of fatty acids between the liver and the adipose tissue. The liver can only oxidize fatty acids in a limited manner; therefore, an increase in lipolysis in adipose tissue or liver problems may cause an accumulation of fat in the liver.

Medium-chain triglycerides are absorbed directly into the portal system without having to be broken down further.

Bile Metabolism

Bile is an aqueous solution, with the main contents being conjugated bile acids, bile pigments, phospholipids, cholesterol, and albumin. Bile is synthesized from cholesterol in the liver and secreted by the hepatocyte into the bile canaliculi. Bile then goes to the gallbladder for storage (Fig. 57-8). During a meal, when the gallbladder is stimulated, bile is excreted into the upper small intestines, where it is crucial in the digestion and absorption of lipids. Bile aids in the formation of micelles

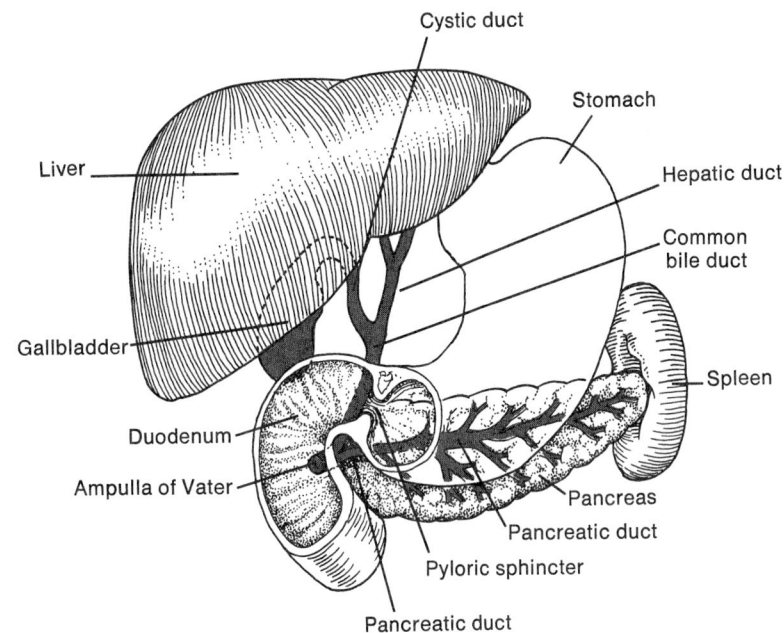

FIGURE 57-8
Biliary system. Normal anatomy of the biliary system (bile flow depicted by arrows). (From Broadwell, D.C. & Jackson, B.S. [1982]. Principles of ostomy care. St. Louis: Mosby.)

(small globules of bile salt) and increases fatty acid and monoglyceride uptake in the liver. It also activates pancreatic lipase. The absorption of fat-soluble vitamins A, D, E, and K, as well as calcium, is dependent on the bile salts. The formation of cholesterol in the liver and small intestine is controlled by bile salts.

Bile is recirculated through a system known as the *enterohepatic circulation,* which includes the liver, the biliary tract, intestine, and the portal-venous system. As much as 95% of bile is reabsorbed, by either active transport in the terminal ileum (main pathway) or passive diffusion. The neonate's liver functions are immature, and the transition to more mature functioning is gradual. Bile acid synthesis is normal in newborns, but ileal reabsorption is insufficient, leading to a reduction in the bile acid pool size and reduction in the intraluminal concentration of bile acids. If the concentration of bile acids in the intestinal lumen is below the critical micellar concentration, malabsorption of fat may occur.

Hormones

The liver is a major target organ for many hormones and frequently produces secondary messengers to further utilize particular hormones. Some hormones such as insulin, glucagon, growth hormone, corticosteroids, estrogens, and parathyroid hormone are mainly catabolized by the liver.

Drug Metabolism

Drug metabolism occurs in two steps in the liver. The first step transforms the drugs by demethylation, oxidation, or reduction. Second, the drugs are conjugated to make them more water soluble so that they can be excreted in the urine or bile. Drug metabolism in the first few months of life may be very different from the adult due to inefficient renal function, differences in the bindings of drug by serum proteins, and differences in hepatic

metabolism. Drug-metabolizing enzyme activity does not reach adult levels until approximately 3 months of age. It may be necessary to give low doses of drugs less frequently in the newborn period. In childhood, hepatic metabolism of some drugs, such as theophylline, may be increased twofold compared with adulthood.

Bilirubin Metabolism

Bilirubin is derived from hemoglobin after senescent red blood cells are taken up by the reticuloendothelial system and heme is converted to biliverdin, which is then converted to bilirubin. Serum albumin carries the bilirubin from the reticuloendothelial system to the liver, where the bilirubin passes into the hepatocyte (Fig. 57-9). Bilirubin is then transported into the endoplasmic reticulum, where an enzyme process converts bilirubin to a water-soluble form, which then is excreted into the biliary system. The bilirubin becomes part of bile that is excreted into the intestine, where it is converted to stercobilin and excreted in the stool. There is little or no enteric reabsorption of bilirubin.[1,9,11]

The fetus clears unconjugated bilirubin across the placenta in the mother's liver. After birth, the concentration of unconjugated bilirubin rises, usually peaking during the first week, then declining as the liver is increasingly able to conjugate and excrete bilirubin. Unconjugated bilirubin is cytotoxic if it enters cells, especially in the brain, and may produce an encephalopathy (kernicterus).

Elimination

Fecal continence is maintained by involuntary and voluntary control. The involuntary control includes the internal anal sphincter, which maintains a high pressure. This involuntary control is assisted by the involuntary and voluntary contraction of the external anal sphincter. Dis-

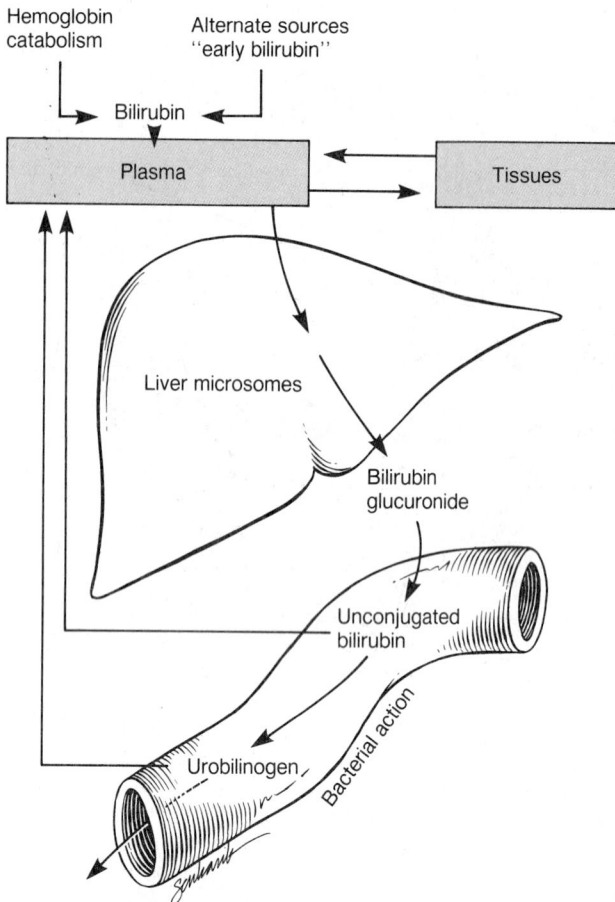

FIGURE 57-9
Bilirubin metabolism.

tention of the rectum initiates afferent signals that spread through the myenteric plexus to initiate peristaltic waves in the descending colon and sigmoid, which propels the fecal material toward the anus. When the child perceives an urge to defecate, the internal anal sphincter reflexively relaxes, and if the external anal sphincter is relaxed, defecation will occur.[4] Recognition of rectal or pelvic sensation initiates the dynamic responses to threats of continence and brings to awareness the need to defecate. Therefore, until the child can differentiate rectal sensation, incontinence will occur.

Summary

The complex multistructured gastrointestinal system plays a significant role in the overall functioning of the body. Its interaction with the external environment is complex. The ingestion, digestion, and absorption of nutrients are critical for life. The liver creates new proteins, detoxifies many harmful substances, and metabolizes other substances. Knowledge of the gastrointestinal system will provide the foundation for many aspects of nursing interventions.

References

1. Colon, A. R. (1990). *Textbook of pediatric hepatology* (2nd ed.). Chicago: Year Book Medical Publishers.
2. Greene, H. L. (1978). Gastrointestinal Development. In T. R. Johnson, W. M. Moore, J. E. Jeffries (Eds.), *Children are different: Developmental physiology*. Columbus, OH: Ross Laboratories, 150–154.
3. Gryboski, J., & Walker, W. A. (1983). *Gastrointestinal problems in the infant* (2nd ed.). Philadelphia: W.B. Saunders.
4. Guyton, A. C. (1986). *Textbook of medical physiology* (7th ed.). Philadelphia: W.B. Saunders.
5. Israel, E. J., & Walker, W. A. (1988). Host defense development in gut and related disorders. *Pediatric Clinics of North America, 35*(1), 1–15.
6. Loper, D. L. (1983). Gastrointestinal development: Embryology, congenital anomalies, and impact on feedings. *Neonatal Network 2*, 27–36.
7. Milla, P. J. (1988). Gastrointestinal motility disorders in children. *Pediatric Clinics of North America, 35*(2), 311–330.
8. Moore, K. L. (1988). *The developing human* (4th ed.). Philadelphia: W.B. Saunders.
9. Mowat, A. P. (1987). *Liver disorders in childhood* (2nd ed.). London: Butterworths.
10. Sherlock, S. (1989). *Diseases of the liver and biliary system* (8th ed.). Oxford: Blackwell Scientific Publications.
11. Silverberg, M., & Daum, F. (1988). *Textbook of pediatric gastroenterology* (2nd ed.). Chicago: Year Book Medical Publishers.
12. Sleisenger, M. H., & Fordtran, J. S. (1989). *Gastrointestinal disease: Pathophysiology, diagnosis, and treatment* (4th ed.). Philadelphia: W.B. Saunders.
13. Sordelett, S. S. (1982). Anatomy and physiology. In D. C. Broadwell & B. S. Jackson (Eds.). *Principles of ostomy care*. St. Louis: C.V. Mosby.
14. Vander, A. J., Sherman, J. H., & Luciano, D. S. (1980). *Human physiology* (3rd ed.). New York: McGraw-Hill.
15. Walker, W. A., & Hendricks, K. M. (1985). *Manual of pediatric nutrition*. Philadelphia: W.B. Saunders.

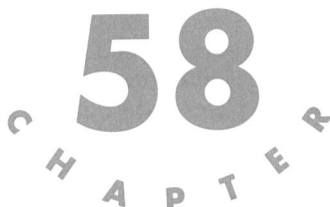

Nursing Assessment and Diagnosis of Gastrointestinal Function

CHAPTER 58

BEHAVIORAL OBJECTIVES

Use functional health patterns as a guideline for assessment of a child's gastrointestinal function.

Describe the components of a complete physical examination of a child's gastrointestinal function.

List the common diagnostic tests used to evaluate gastrointestinal function.

Interpret laboratory tests used to evaluate gastrointestinal function.

Identify nursing diagnoses that are commonly used in the care of children with gastrointestinal dysfunction.

The child health nurse plays a vital role in the assessment and diagnosis of a child's gastrointestinal (GI) function. GI function is vital to the child's nutritional status and dictates progress in growth and development. This system also plays a vital role in the integration of an infant into the family system from the first feeding of breast milk or formula and introduction of solid foods to the progression to table foods. A perception of the GI system is closely knit into every family's psychosocial (value and belief) system, and any suggested changes and interventions must be offered by the health care professional only with careful consideration of its impact on the family system. As a part of the GI system, the mouth's role in exploratory behavior and its relationship to development in the first year of life cannot be underestimated.

The purpose of this chapter is to outline the history, physical assessment, diagnostic tests, and nursing diagnoses that are commonly used to assess the child's GI system. The nurse as a child and family advocate can make this process a positive learning situation for all involved.

1553

Nursing Assessment

Child and Family History

It is important that the person providing information be a reliable historian.[3] Too often the assumption is made that the child's parents should know everything about that child. With today's population of employed mothers and various day care arrangements, the parents may not be as well informed or may not be implementing daily general health maintenance needs. Our society has many single-parent families and foster parents; thus GI function should be assessed early in the interview because further information from the grandmother, nanny, or day care provider may be required.

Health Perception and Health Management

Note the general appearance of the child and caregiver. Assess standard biographical data, including other family members, and description of living environment (home, school, sitter). Assess the general definition of health and its value to this family, including their pattern of seeking health care and any obstacles in that process. Elicit the reason for the visit from the caregiver as well as the child. When did the problem or illness begin? What has been the general health status of the child and family members in the past year? What are the child and caregivers' beliefs regarding the possible precipitating factors? Finally, what have they been doing to treat the symptoms? If the child is on medications, realize that often parents or caregivers are excellent informants of how drugs affect their child. It is also important to elicit information about any drug-nutrient interactions that may be contributing to the symptoms being described. Examples include sleepiness after hyoscyamine sulfate (Levsin) or irritability after bethanecol chloride (Urecholine) administration. Remember that symptoms may also be related to drug overdosage or toxicity. For example, liver failure may be related to acetaminophen (Tylenol) ingestion and constipation to excessive antiemetic use. Inquire into general health stress factors and illnesses of family members (blood relatives).

Nutrition and Metabolism

The nutrition of an infant and young child is often influenced by many GI illnesses. Assess the child's growth, and plot on a growth chart to delineate acute or chronic changes. What does a normal day's intake consist of? Does the child eat with the rest of the family? Is there a normal eating pattern (three meals, two snacks)? Have there been any changes in appetite? What is the child's eating behavior, and are there any conflicts over food? Is there any history of nausea or vomiting? If so, does there appear to be a causal factor? Are there any food allergies? If so, what happens when the child eats those foods? Are there any concerns regarding skin problems? Has the child seen a dentist? Is there any history of dental caries?

Elimination

Elimination is another important focus for identifying GI illness or problems. For infants, elicit from the caregiver the number of stools and frequency in a 24-hour period. What was the consistency, color, odor? Was the infant straining? Does the child have excessive flatus?

For the older child, when was the child toilet trained? What terms are used by the family for elimination, that is, "bowel movements," "BM," "number 2," and so forth? Does the caregiver report any difficulties with this process? Are there any complaints of diarrhea or constipation? If so, what was the frequency, color, odor, and/or discomfort? Is there any history of infections? If there have been problems with soiling or bedwetting, to what does the child or caregiver attribute this? Is there a history of elimination problems in other family members?

Activity and Exercise

Describe the normal family activities. What is the bathing routine (when, how, where, type of soap), and what is the child's dressing routine? What can the child do alone, and with what does the child require help (shoes, zippers)? What type of play activities are enjoyed most and least? Does the child play alone or interact with others? What are both the caregiver and child's perception of strength, stamina, coordination, and energy level? Has there been a change in the child's activity recently?

Sleep and Rest

Describe the child's sleep. How many hours of sleep does the child get in a 24-hour period? Does the child take morning and/or afternoon naps? What is the normal bedtime routine? Where does the child sleep? Does the child awaken during the night? If so, how often, and what is done to get the child back to sleep? Does the child awaken for food during the night? Is the child restless? If so, what is the caregiver and the child's perception of the reason (nightmares)? What is the family's sleeping patterns?

Cognition and Perception

What is the general affect of the child and caregiver? How do they respond to one another and to noise, objects, touch? Note speech patterns, visualization, and auditory responses. What is the family's educational level? Can the child respond to age-appropriate questions, such as name, telephone number? How does the family perceive and respond to pain? Have the caregiver and child describe what is causing pain and what seems to relieve the pain.

Self-Perception and Self-Concept

Assess the general mood of the family, caregiver, and child. How do they define their sense of worth? Does the child change moods frequently? If so, what seems to precipitate this? How does a crisis affect the child's self-perception? What is the caregiver or child concerned about relating to self-perception and self-concept? Has toilet training been a "difficult" experience?

Role Relationships

Assess roles within the family and their relationships to one another. What is the child's interaction with other family members? How does the child respond to separation? Does the child have temper tantrums or discipline problems? Has the child adjusted to the school routine? Do the caregivers voice any concerns regarding role satisfaction? Does the child volunteer any concerns regarding relationships with significant others?

Sexuality and Reproduction

Assess the child's feelings of maleness or femaleness. If the child is asking questions regarding sexuality, how is the caregiver responding? Is the family comfortable discussing issues related to sexuality and reproduction? Are topics of elimination or sexuality considered "off limits?" Are there any parental concerns?

Coping and Stress Tolerance

How does the family respond to stress? Are GI symptoms (nausea, vomiting, diarrhea) associated with stressful situations? Are support systems available and used? What coping mechanisms are used (ignoring, discussion, anger, frustration)? Does the child or caregiver volunteer any concerns?

Values and Beliefs

What does the family view as important in life? What does the child desire in the future? Are these values and desires being affected by the current problem or illness? What role does religion play in this family's lifestyle? Are there any other "rules" that influence the child and caregiver's values and beliefs?

Physical Assessment

Physical assessment of the GI tract of an infant or child begins with general observation and inspection and proceeds to the more invasive techniques of auscultation, percussion, and palpation. A parent may hold the infant or young child on their lap for most of the assessment. This helps allay the child's fear of the stranger (examiner) so that the examination may be completed in a timely fashion and allows the parent to provide a "second pair of hands" that may be needed during certain parts of the examination. Remember to focus on the infant or child, and use the verbal information given by either the child or parent in the history. Be as objective as possible.

General Approach

As a part of the general survey of any child, growth must be assessed using standard measures of weight, height, and frontal-occipital circumference (FOC) for infants younger than 36 months of age. Parameters are plotted on a growth chart, which will indicate the child's percentile for age (see Appendix). Measurements of height and weight above the 97th percentile or below the 3rd

percentile indicate a disturbance that requires further investigation. Anthropometric measures such as triceps skinfold and midupper arm circumference are indicators of fat and muscle (protein stores). Nutrition plays a vital role in brain growth in the first year of life. For this reason, the FOC is a vital measure to monitor. The GI tract function is directly related to growth. Thorough history and physical data will allow the nurse to put the pieces of data together when approaching the child holistically.[17]

Examination of Oral Cavity

Positioning of the child to allow the mouth to be visualized may be difficult but never impossible. Infants and toddlers sitting in their parent's lap can be held with the infant's back firmly against the parent's chest. Parents should place the palm of their hand on the child's forehead and tilt the head back slightly. A good way to visualize the inside of a preschooler's mouth is to teach him or her to growl like a lion. School-age children are usually willing to open their mouths to "show off their teeth." If a child clenches the teeth, a tongue blade may be advanced slowly along the lips to the posterior teeth. The blade is then eased between the teeth toward the pharynx. Press down on the tongue at the base to keep the tongue forward. This will elicit the gag reflex—the mouth will open and allow a quick moment of visibility (Fig. 58-1). The temporomandibular joint should be fully mobile, without tenderness or crepitus. If teeth are present, observe for occlusion where the top back teeth rest directly atop the lower teeth; the upper incisors slightly override the lower incisors. The lips should appear pink, moist, and without lesions.

Breast-fed babies may develop a sucking tubercle (small protrusion) in the middle of the upper lip. Buccal mucosa should appear pink, feel soft, and be without lesions, inflammation, patches, or swelling. The gums should appear coral pink. Patchy brown pigmentation may be present in dark-skinned people. Hypertrophy may appear at puberty. Pearly white cysts (Epstein's pearls) may be visualized along the gums of infants. These pinhead-

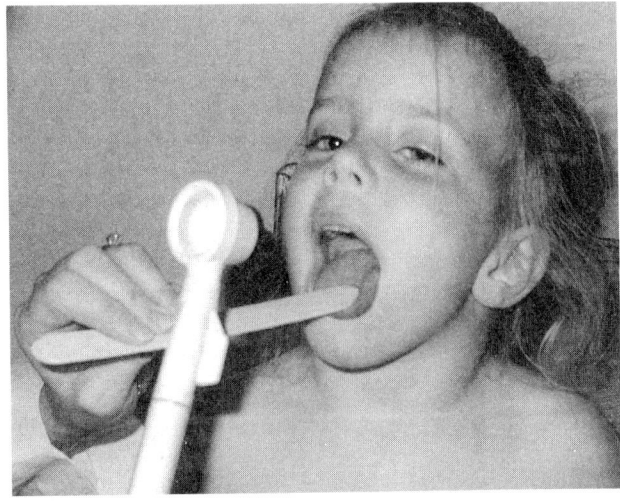

FIGURE 58-1
Eliciting the gag reflex during the oral examination.

sized, rounded elevations are due to retained secretions and disappear by 2 to 3 months of age.[2] If the infant is teething, a white line may be visualized along with gum swelling before the tooth erupts. As a general rule, primary teeth erupt in a more predictable pattern to when they are shed and secondary teeth replace them. Most infants by 7 months of age have two upper teeth and two lower central incisors. This is followed by approximately four teeth every 4 months, with a full set of 20 primary teeth usually present by 20 to 24 months. Shedding of primary teeth begins in early childhood at about age 7. This shedding coincides with the eruption of secondary teeth, which ends in early adulthood between the ages of 17 to 22 years. The tongue should be in the midline, symmetric, and pink in color without lesions or fasciculations. The frenulum may vary in thickness from a thin membrane to a thick cord. The tongue should be able to extend as far as the alveolar ridge to allow for normal speech. Dorsal and lateral portions of the tongue will contain fissures and papillae, whereas the ventral portion will be smooth, transparent pink with large veins. The floor of the mouth should appear pink and the frenulum centered without lesions.

The hard palate is pink with irregular, immovable, transverse rugae. The arch should have a gentle slope. The soft palate is pink, movable, elevated symmetrically, and smooth. Mouth odor should not be present. During inspection of the oropharynx, observe for symmetry of anterior and posterior pillars, uvula in midline, and the absence or slight visibility of tonsils. Salivary gland openings may be slightly elevated and appear like a pinpoint red marking.

Examination of Abdomen

The infant and younger child can be laid in the parents lap for examination of the abdomen. School-age children should be able to cooperate and lay on an examination table. The abdomen should be inspected first, auscultated second, and palpated third. Percussing may scare the younger child, and this may need to be done last. Nurses explain to the preschooler that they are pretending they are playing a drum on the child's abdomen prior to percussing. On *inspection,* the infant's abdomen should be the same skin tone as the rest of the body, whereas an older child's abdomen may appear lighter related to sun exposure. The skin should be smooth and soft; any scars or striae should be noted. A venous network will be more noticeable during infancy. The umbilicus should be centrally located. The umbilical stump will dry in 5 days and drop off by 2 weeks of age. Small umbilical hernias (3 cm) are considered normal and should not increase in size after 1 month of age. The normal contour the abdomen of an infant or small child is a protuberant "pot belly"; this usually disappears at or near adolescence (Fig. 58-2). The abdomen should appear symmetric without visible masses or bulges. Observe for any surface motion, such as peristalsis or pulsations (may be visible in thin children). Up to age 7, children are mainly abdominal breathers. After this age, the nurse may observe boys as chiefly abdominal breathers and girls chiefly using costal muscles. The two recti muscles of the abdominal musculature may not approximate each other. This finding is common in black children, and it should disappear during preschool years.

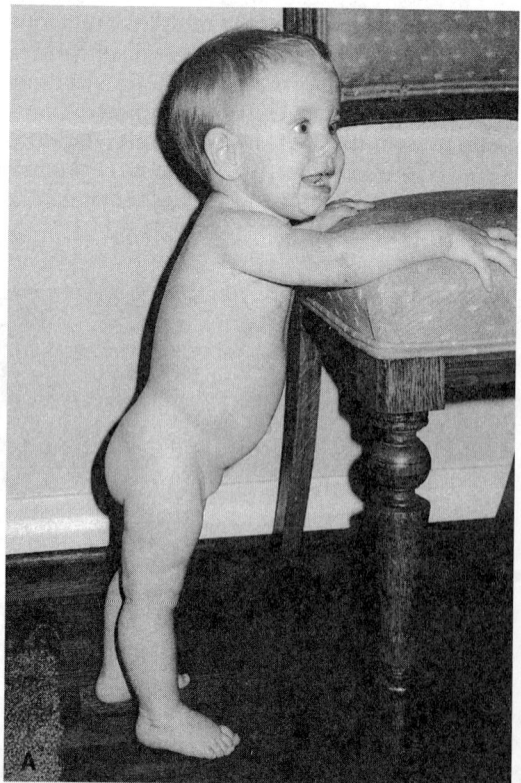 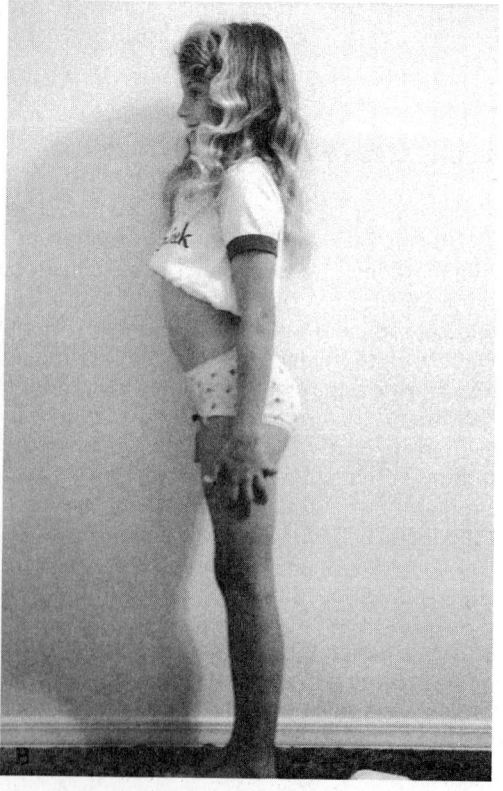

FIGURE 58-2
Contour of the abdomen. **(A)** protruding abdomen of an 8-month-old infant. **(B)** Flat abdomen of a 9-year-old child.

Auscultation should be done before palpation or percussing. Bowel sounds, dull gurgles and clicks, are heard 5 to 34 per minute. Vascular sounds and friction rubs are absent during a normal examination. *Percussion* of the infant usually reveals more air in the stomach and intestinal lumen related to swallowed air during feeding. There should be a general distribution of tympany with dullness percussed over a full bladder. The liver is percussed from approximately the sixth rib (upper border) to the costal margin (lower border). The lower border of the liver may extend 2 to 3 cm below the costal margin. Spleen percussion is done at the ninth interspace, left of the midaxillary line, at which dullness may be percussed. In infants, this may extend to 1 cm below the costal margin. *Palpation* is best achieved in a relaxed child. In an infant, relaxation may be achieved by holding the legs flexed at the knees and hips with one hand and palpate with the other. It may help an older child if nurses place the child's hand under theirs as they palpate to decrease ticklishness as well as apprehension. Light palpation should precede deep palpation. Palpate muscle tone, which should be relaxed in a nonanxious child with smooth surface characteristics. Palpate umbilical hernia if present and note size. Deep palpation should be done with one hand. The last area to be examined should be the area the child complains of as painful. Tenderness may be ascertained in midline or xiphoid process near the cecum or over the sigmoid colon. This is considered normal. The aorta, borders of rectus abdominus muscles, and feces may be palpated. The umbilical ring may be inverted or slightly everted; there should not be any bulges. The following organs may be palpated at these locations: border of liver in a 0- to 6-month-old child is 0 to 3 cm below the costal margin; 6 months to 4 years, 1 to 2 cm below the costal margin; and a child over 6 years, 1 to 2 cm or not palpable below the right costal margin. The spleen may be felt at the costal margin or under the ribs in small children. Only the spleen's tip should be palpable. The kidney lies adjacent to the vertebral column and is palpated by elevating the child's left flank with the right hand and deeply palpating at the child's left anterior costal margin. Older children can be instructed to hold their breath during this sequence (Fig. 58-3). The kidney may descend with inspiration and should have a smooth contour. Palpating an infant's bladder may result in urination, so it is advisable to lay a diaper under the infant's hips and over the boy's penis for this portion of the examination. The bladder should be a smooth midline mass between the pubis and umbilical area. If urination has just occurred, palpation may not be possible. If inguinal nodes are palpable, they are small, mobile, and nontender.

Examination of the Rectum and Anus

The rectal and anal region is usually inspected. An internal rectal examination is usually not done in a well child because of the invasiveness of the procedure. If constipation or rectal bleeding is a symptom, a rectal examination is indicated. Inspect the anal surface area; the skin may be coarse. It should be free of inflammation, lesions, scars, skin tags, fissures, lumps, swelling, or ex-

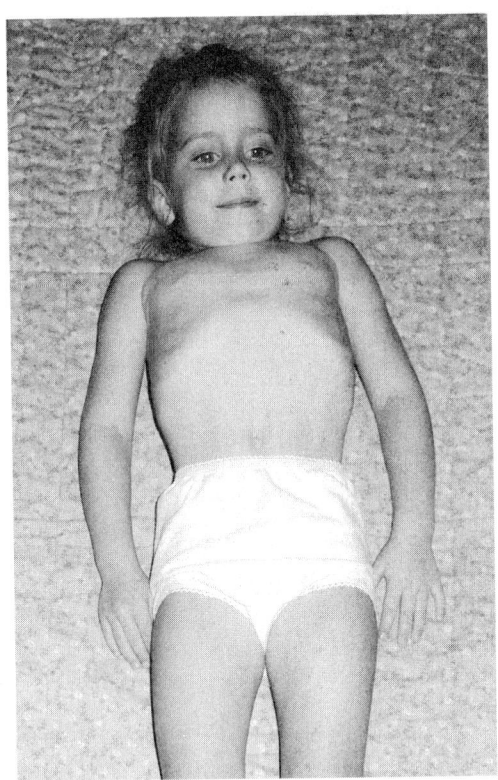

FIGURE 58-3
Child holding breath during physical examination for deep palpation.

coriation. Palpation of the coccygeal area should not elicit tenderness.

Developmental Considerations

Table 58-1 summarizes the developmental considerations when performing a physical examination on infants, children, and adolescents. Table 58-2 provides a summary of possible abnormal findings of the physical examination of which the nurse should be cognizant.

Nutritional Assessment

The importance of a nutritional assessment in childhood cannot be overstated. Researchers in the 1950s assessed physical growth and development as well as intelligence and behavioral function to determine the long-term sequelae of early nutritional deficits. Significant delays in both motor and cognitive development were exhibited by these children.[8] More recent studies have found behavioral impairment as the most permanent outcome of infant malnutrition.[12] Despite catch-up in physical growth at school age, these children exhibited an attention deficit disorder, impaired attention, poor school performance, poor memory, and easy distractibility. Extensive review of socioeconomic background in these children led Galler and Ramsey[13] to conclude that environmental factors played only a small role in the delayed mental and physical development. A prior history of malnutrition was of greater consequence in determining cognitive performance.[13]

TABLE 58-1
Developmental Considerations in Physical Examination of Gastrointestinal Function

Organ	Infant	Child	Adolescent
Mouth inspection	Age 7 months: 2 upper teeth; 2 lower teeth Age 20–24 months: full set of 20 primary teeth	Age 7: shedding of primary teeth begins	Age 17–22: full set of secondary teeth
Abdomen inspection	Protuberant contour (upright and supine position) Umbilicus deep and drops off within 2 weeks of birth Faint venous network visible	Protuberant (upright position) Concave (supine position) Cutaneous umbilical remnant may protrude or be inverted Faint venous network visible	Concave (upright and supine position) Cutaneous umbilical remnant may protrude or remain flush with skin Venous network not visible
Percussion of liver (lower border)	0–3 cm below costal margin	1–2 cm below costal margin	Costal margin, or not palpable below costal margin
Liver span	4 cm	7 cm	10 cm
Spleen	2 cm below costal margin, left midaxillary line	1 cm below costal margin, left midaxillary line	Above ninth interspace along left midaxillary line

From Bates, B. (1991). *A Guide to physical examination and history taking* (5th ed.). Philadelphia: Lippincott.

It is important for nurses to understand the components of a nutritional assessment to use these data in planning each child's care. A nutritional assessment should meet the following goals:

- Detection of malnutrition.
- Assessment of specific nutritional deficits.
- Provision of guidelines for short-term and long-term therapy and intervention.[27]

Components of a Nutritional Assessment

The tools that are used to complete a nutritional assessment may be divided into five categories of data: historical, dietary, physical findings, anthropometric, and laboratory.[23] A portion of the needed information may have been gathered with the original history and physical examination. The areas of anthropometric data and laboratory values may be gathered through the help of other health team members, such as the dietitian for collection of anthropometry and the physician for ordering laboratory specimens. A feeding assessment may be instrumental in sorting out any variables that may be contributing to malnutrition (see the accompanying display for an example of a screening tool).

Additional *historical data* must include (1) previous measurements of growth to provide a comparison to current data; (2) social and cultural history that may impact the child's eating habits; (3) previous illnesses or surgical interventions that may limit food intake while increasing metabolic needs; and (4) current medications that may compromise nutrient absorption and utilization.

Dietary data should include a nutritional history that describes (1) quantity, quality, and frequency of formula or food; (2) family eating patterns; (3) cooking and storage facilities; (4) socioeconomic status; (5) cultural habits; (6) feeding history; (7) dentition; and (8) food allergies. Dietary intakes can be determined using 24-hour recall or 3- to 7-day food record determinations. For children under the age of 5, it is important to elicit information specific to the feeding process, such as feeding milestones, oral-muscular development, feeding environment, and parental attitudes. With the help of a dietitian, this information can be compared to recommended daily allowance standards, which will point out deficiencies in the child's current diet.

Anthropometric data refers to *physical growth measurements*. Recumbent length or height, weight, and head circumference are routine measurements plotted serially on growth charts. In-depth assessments for children who do not fall within the normal growth range should include triceps skinfold thickness, which measures fat stores, and mid-arm circumference, which measures muscle stores. The mid-arm muscle circumference and area are calculated after the above measures are taken. It is important to note that infants must have their length measured in a recumbent position. Accuracy is maintained by using a calibrated measuring board, which requires two people to employ. The procedure should be repeated until two readings are within 0.5 cm of each other. Infant weights should be done in the nude, preferably on an electronic digital scale. Head circumference measurements should be done using a nonstretchable tape measure. Measurement of premature infants should be plotted on National

TABLE 58-2
Abnormal Findings on the Physical Examination of the Gastrointestinal System

	Abnormal Findings
Mouth	
Temporomandibular joint	Limited excursion, tenderness, crepitis, referred pain; movement affected by mandibular overgrowth may occur in children with rheumatoid arthritis.
Occlusion	Malocclusion (often due to hereditary predisposition), displacement, or protrusion of teeth.
Jaw size	Very small or very large; may signal congenital disease, for example, small jaw is part of Pierre Robin syndrome.
Lips	Pale, cyanotic, cherry pink, swelling, twisting, drooping cleft, dry, cracking, fissures in corners (zinc deficiency), lesions, plaques, vesicles, nodules, ulcerations; a "sucking blister" may develop on the lip of a breastfed infant due to improper positioning during feeding
Inner lips and buccal mucosa	Pale, blue, puffy, red, white patches on mucosa (oral moniliasis or thrush) that will not wipe away; excessive dry mouth may indicate dehydration or mouth breathing; excessive salivation may be seen with dental caries.
Gums	Red, pale, swelling, bleeding with slight pressure, packets of debris between teeth, tenderness, marked hypertrophy (seen in patients taking steroids, phenytoin), ulcers.
Teeth	Dark-colored teeth; decayed teeth (caries); pitted or discolored teeth (fluoride or tetracycline ingestion); green or black teeth (iron ingestion); excessive smoothness (grinding); no teeth by 1 year of age; incorrect number of teeth for age.
Tongue	Fissures, tongue too large, glossoptosis (tongue attached farther forward than usual); tongue tied (frenulum interfering with protrusion of tongue); red tongue (scarlet fever).
Floor of mouth	Red, pallor, lesions, bumps.
Hard palate	Reddened, bruising (force feeding), petechiae, clefts or absence of palate; high arch may be linked to multiple syndromes.
Soft palate	Any of the findings listed for hard palate, or discharge.
Mouth odor	Foreign body in nose; acetone or sweet smell (metabolic disease).
Oropharynx	Lateral deviation, bifid uvula; uvula with lateral deviation; pus on tonsils, swelling of tonsils; redness or exudate may be sign of sinus drainage.
Abdomen	
Inspection	
Skin color	Jaundice, redness, bruising petechiae, rashes, lesions.
Surface characteristics	Scars, taut appearance (ascites); pink, red, or purplish striae.
Venous network	Prominent or engorged veins (may indicate portal vein obstruction).
Umbilicus	Failure of the umbilical cord to heal, with granulomatous tissue or drainage from site; umbilical hernia.
Contour	Concave abdomen in a newborn may be a sign of diaphragmatic hernia; excessive distension; umbilical hernia beyond the age of 2 years for white children, 7 years for black children; hernia over 2″ long, continually growing hernia.
Symmetry	Asymmetry in the form of masses, bulges.
Surface motion	Excessive peristalsis and pulsations.
Movement with respiration	Labored, grunting, restricted movement.
Tenseness of abdominal musculature	Recti muscle misapproximate past age 6.
Auscultation	
Bowel sounds	Absence of bowel sounds; high-pitched sounds; bruit (swishing sounds); friction rub over spleen or liver.
Percussion	
	Tone—dullness; *liver*—lower border exceeds 2–3 cm below costal margin; *spleen*—spleen extends below costal margin.
Palpation	
	Cutaneous tenderness; *light*—involuntary resistance (unable to relax, masses, tenderness, congenital megacolon (Hirchsprung's disease); *deep*—local or generalized areas of tenderness; pulsating, mobile, or fixed masses; *umbilical ring*—incomplete or soft in center.

(Continued)

TABLE 58-2
(Continued)

Abnormal Findings	
Abdominal Organs	
Liver	>2 cm below costal margin, tenderness.
Spleen	Palpate more than tip.
Kidney	Nodular contour, masses.
Bladder	Distension after voiding.
Inguinal nodes	Enlarged, tender.

Center for Health Statistics (NCHS) growth charts after being corrected for gestational age. An example of this would be a 4-month-old infant who was born at 32 weeks' gestation. The corrected age is 2 months, which is the age used when plotting the growth measurements.

Laboratory data include a serum albumin, hemoglobin, hematocrit, and total lymphocyte count. Serum albumin is a long-term indicator of visceral protein status. Thus, it would take 21 days for a child on a low- or no-protein diet to show a decrease in the serum albumin level unless there is another source of protein loss (for example, chest tube, wound drain). With a level of less than 2.5 g/dl, the physical finding of pitting edema is apparent. Hemoglobin and hematocrit are useful in screening for iron deficiency, and a total lymphocyte count helps assess immunocompetency. The laboratory studies mentioned here are not by any means an all-inclusive list. Levels of serum protein and prealbumin may be needed, based of the history and appearance of the child. Electrolyte abnormalities must be corrected. Serum zinc, copper, and magnesium levels should be monitored in children with a history of short bowel and/or chronic diarrhea.

Physical findings will be related to nutritional deficiencies. Table 58-3 outlines specific nutrients, dietary sources, clinical and laboratory signs of deficiency, and conditions that place children at risk for deficiency.[16]

Undernourished children can be either acutely or chronically malnourished. Using a standard growth chart, deficiency in height for age is usually a reflection of chronic malnutrition. A weight-for-height deficit usually indicates evidence of acute malnutrition. Children who are greater than 80% of the standard are considered obese.

Children at Nutritional Risk

Practitioners advocate the use of nutritional indices as a predicting factor of prognostic outcome.[9] Certain measures of nutritional assessment can be graphed in such a way to identify those patients who are malnourished and at higher risk for complications, suboptimal treatment in response to a nutritional or metabolic derangement, or even death.[21] Preoperative assessment of nutritional risk is important because it may influence nutrient requirements, length of hospital stay, and curability of the basic disease.[4] Specific indicators, such as weight loss and albumin, may be used to assess whether the child requires nutritional repletion prior to surgery to ensure proper healing.

It has been recognized that hospitalized patients are at greater risk for developing malnutrition.[19] Almost 50% of the children surveyed at an urban hospital were noted to be less than the 10th percentile for various anthropometric measures, with a high frequency of children less than 1 year of age at nutritional risk. The finding of increasing consecutive days in-hospital was also related to nutritional status depletion. Finally, Mize and colleagues[19] recognized from their data that pediatric intensive care patients were at greater nutritional risk than other pediatric inpatients.

Nutritional assessment and support are key factors in caring for pediatric patients. Chronic underlying diseases and hospitalization place children at risk for malnutrition.[24] It is crucial to anticipate the possibility of inadequate protein and calorie intake based on the child's condition and to take these factors into consideration when planning a child's care. Criteria that can be used to identify children at high nutritional risk include the following:

Growth

- Greater than 5% body weight loss in past month.
- Length and height for age less than 5th percentile.
- Weight for height less than 5th percentile, less than 80% of standard condition or disease process.
- Any diagnosis associated with inherent protein energy malnutrition.

Laboratory

- Serum albumin less than 3 g/dl.
- Lymphocyte count less than 1000 mm³.

Infant Feeding

Infant feeding, including breast- and bottle-feeding, is discussed in Chapters 11 and 12.

Recommended Dietary Allowance

The recommended dietary allowances of the major food groups are found in Table 8-2 in Chapter 8.

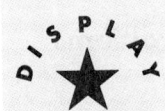

Nursing Assessment: Screening Tool for Possible Feeding Problems

I. Medical History and Clinical Exam
    A. Diagnosis _____ Age _____ Admitted _____
    B. History (check if applicable)
        aspiration _____ choking _____ gagging _____ vomiting _____
        weight loss _____ long-term NPO _____ inability to gain weight _____
    C. Physical findings
        _____ apathy   Hair: texture _____ color _____ distribution _____
        _____ irritability
        _____ pallor   Skin: color _____ dryness _____ rash _____
        _____ edema   Mouth: gum _____ dentition _____ mucous membranes _____
        _____ cachexia   GI tract: intact bowel (cm) _____ malabsorption _____
    D. Current medications _____
    E. Diet order _____
II. Feeding History
    A. Present parental concerns and view of problems.
    B. Present interviewer's concerns and view of problem.
    C. Feeding time   30 minutes _____ 45 minutes _____ 60 minutes or more _____
    D. Food preferences: likes _____ dislikes _____
        behavior displayed _____
    E. Loss of liquid/foods from mouth: more than 1/4 of feed _____
        more than 1/2 of feed _____
    F. Fatigues easily during feeds _____
    G. Poor appetite/anorexia _____
    H. Types of foods consumed: strained _____ pureed _____ table food _____
    I. Feeding skills: bottle _____ breast _____ cup _____ does the child hold _____
        feed self _____ utensils _____ finger foods _____
    J. Diet restrictions/food allergies _____
    K. Feeding environment: _____ lap _____ infant seat _____ high chair or
        feeding table _____ booster seat _____ table or chair
        _____ crib _____ other
    L. Describe child's behavior during feeding. _____
    M. Nutrient intake: daily caloric intake* _____

*Consult dietitian for diet history/calorie count.

III. Anthropometric Measurements
    A. Weight _____ 25%–50% (growth percentiles for age) _____ 5%–25%
    B. Height _____ 25%–50% _____ 5%–25% _____ less than 5% _____
        greater than 95%
    C. Weight for height _____ %
    D. FOC _____ 25%–50% _____ 5%–25% _____ less than 5%
    E. Abnormal patterns/exchanges: weight _____ height _____ FOC _____
    F. Are changes in growth Acute _____ or Chronic _____ ?

*Consult dietician for complete nutritional assessment.

IV. Laboratory Data
    A. <u>Blood Count</u>   <u>Date</u>
        WBC _____ (4.5–10.5)*
        RBC _____ (4.4–5.3)*
        HgB _____ (11–14)*
        Hct _____ (38–44)*
        MCV _____ (79–89)*
    B. Serum protein _____ (abnormal if less than 3.5–4)
    C. Serum albumin _____ (abnormal if less than 2.5–3.0) Date _____
    D. ferritin _____ Date _____ (23–350 mg/ml)*
    E. zinc _____ Date _____ (0.6–1.3 mcg/ml)*
    F. copper _____ Date _____ (70–140 mcg/ml)*
    G. other _____ Date _____

*Normal range for values.

(Continued)

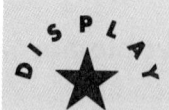

Nursing Assessment: Screening Tool for Possible Feeding Problems
(continued)

V. Oral Motor Skill Assessment
  A. Observations during feeding: _____ 1. gagging, _____ 2. inappropriate tongue thrust, _____ 3. absent suck, _____ 4. weak suck, _____ 5. uncoordinated suck/swallow, _____ 6. fatigue with eating, _____ 7. clamping on utensils, _____ 8. aversion to age-appropriate eating utensils (see overview of normal development), _____ 9. pockets of food in cheeks (Chipmunk syndrome), _____ 10. loses excessive liquids and solids with feeding, _____ weigh diaper after feeding session, _____ excessive drooling with eating.
  B. General observations: _____ 1. abnormal muscle tone, _____ arches back and hyperextends neck with increased tone, _____ curls up into fetal position with increased tone, _____ floppy with low or absent tone, _____ 2. gross motor delays* (see overview of normal development), _____ 3. fine motor delays (see overview of normal development), _____ 4. Delayed vocalization/speech* (see overview of normal development)

* For additional development/motor assessment contact Child Life or Physical Therapy.
* For additional oral assessment and evaluation contact Speech Therapy.

Interviewer _____
Date _____

Adapted from: Quay, N. (1986). *Pediatric feeding assessment and nursing interventions.* Dallas: Children's Medical Center.

Diagnostic Tests

Laboratory Tests

Urine and stool tests are the least invasive tests that require a sample of fluid or excrement to be analyzed by laboratory personnel. The specimen should be collected and handled with the appropriate infection control precautions to protect the health care provider, family, and other patients from infection. As with any body fluid, the nurse must take precaution in the collection process to send enough of the specimen required for the specific test. Most laboratories have a manual that lists the test and volume of specimen required. It is important to note whether a fresh specimen is required, and if so, how "old" the sample can be. Attention paid to these factors will prevent repeating tests unnecessarily and having to charge the patient for replicated studies. Blood and stool indices used in evaluating GI function may be found in Tables 58-4 and 58-5, respectively.

Procedures

Table 58-6 outlines various radiographic studies. Other diagnostic procedures are found in the following sections.

Colonoscopy[6,10,25]

Description

The physician gently inserts the colonoscope into the anal sphincter. Insufflation of air into the bowel lumen as the colonoscope is advanced should help with visualization and prevent perforation. This air is removed after the visualization is complete and biopsies have been taken. The scope is slowly withdrawn from the colon.

Purpose

The purpose is to visualize the intestinal mucosa of the child.

Indications

- Abnormal barium enema.
- Lower GI bleeding.
- Unexplained colonic symptoms.
- Suspected cecal or ascending colonic disease.

Contraindications

- Fulminant ulcerative colitis.
- Severe ischemic bowel disease.
- Acute radiation colitis.
- Pregnancy.

Preparation

Colonoscopy may be performed intraoperatively when a polypectomy or removal of foreign body is performed or as a single procedure in a GI laboratory (Fig. 58-4). Biopsies, cytology, and cultures are also obtained. The child and parents should have the test explained to them by the physician, and the nurse should reinforce or clarify the explanation in behavioral terms. The child should be prepped with Quick-Prep or Golytely the evening before the test. Intravenous access is established, and the child is sedated using either diazepam (Valium) or meperidine (Demerol). The child is placed in a left lateral position with knees flexed. After the child is draped, the physician lubricates the colonoscope tip with lubricant.

Developmental Considerations

Parents of an infant or toddler should be told that this test will cause a change in stooling pattern (increased gas, increased stool). Older children should be instructed that they will feel an urgency to have a bowel movement during and following the procedure. Instruct them to remain within walking distance of the bathroom until this subsides.

TABLE 58-3
Signs of Nutritional Deficiency

Nutrient	Diet Sources	Clinical Signs of Deficiency	Laboratory Signs of Deficiency	Conditions that Place Children at Risk
Protein	Meat, fish, poultry, eggs, milk, milk products (including yogurt and cheese), vegetable protein: dried peas, beans, lentils, oil seeds (e.g., sunflower), nut butters, meat analogues, tofu	Hair: dull, dry, sparse, dyspigmented, pluckable, loss of curl flag sign; moon facies; emaciation; edema; decreased muscle strength and wasting; enlarged fatty liver; flaky skin rash; poor growth	Decreased serum protein, serum albumin, prealbumin, transferrin, hemoglobin, creatinine height index; delayed hypersensitivity on skin tests	Protein-restricted diet; amino acid disorders; vegan diet; malabsorption; increased needs with surgery, burns, stress; low income
Fat	Oils, mayonnaise, margarine, butter, shortening, salad dressing, bacon, animal protein (e.g., whole milk, eggs, cheese)	Sparse hair growth; skin dry, flaky (like sandpaper); poor wound healing; loss of subcutaneous fat; poor growth	Decreased serum carotene, platelet count (linoleic acid), plasma lipids. Increased 72-hour fecal fat excretion	Malabsorption; malignancies involving GI lymphatic drainage; gluten-sensitive enteropathy; cystic fibrosis, biliary atresia, biliary obstruction; short bowel syndrome; long-term hyperalimentation; intestinal lymphangiectasia; vegan diets
Vitamin A Provitamin A (carotene)	Liver, fish oil, whole milk, egg yolk, fortified margarine and cereal, butter	Eyes: Bitot's spots, soft cornea, dry eye. Follicular hyperkeratosis	Decreased plasma, vitamin A, carotene, retinol	Gluten-sensitive enteropathy; chronic liver disease: biliary atresia, cirrhosis; cystic fibrosis
Vitamin D	Fortified milk and milk products (including yogurt and cheese), sunlight exposure	Head: frontal and parietal bossing, thin skull bones, craniotabes, open anterior fontanel; beading of ribs (rachitic rosary); legs: bow-legs, knock-knees; flared wrists	Decreased serum calcium (early and late), phosphorus, vitamin D, bone age increased alkaline phosphatase, urinary amino acids	Gluten-sensitive enteropathy; chronic liver disease; biliary atresia; cirrhosis; chronic renal disease; cystic fibrosis; antiseizure medications
Vitamin E	Vegetable oils, wheat germ, cereals, legumes, green leafy vegetables	Deficiency symptoms rare; in premature infants: irritability, edema, hemolytic anemia; ataxia; peripheral neuropathy	Decreased plasma tocopherol, increased peroxide hemolysis	Prematurity; cystic fibrosis; steatorrhea; abetalipoproteinemia
Vitamin C (ascorbic acid)	Citrus fruits, juice, other fruits (strawberries, melon, cantaloupe, acerola, papaya, guava, black currents), rose hips, vegetables (tomatoes, cabbage, potatoes)	Infantile scurvy: frog's leg position, dry, rough skin, irritability, lip tenderness, extreme sensitivity in arms and legs; bleeding, spongy gums; loose teeth; skin: petechia, dry; delayed wound healing; swollen joints; aching bones; normochromic anemia	Decreased serum ascorbic acid, alkaline phosphatase, urine ascorbic acid	Unsupplemented cow's milk formula; Feingold diet
Thiamine (Vitamin B_1)	Legumes, nuts, whole or enriched grains, pork, beef	Beriberi; infants: congestive heart failure; cyanosis; tachycardia; vomiting; sensory loss; motor weakness; calf tenderness; cardiac enlargement; anorexia, weakness	Decreased urine thiamine, erythrocyte transketolase. Increased blood pyruvate and lactate	Beriberi (rare) found in developing countries where populations subsist on polished rice
Riboflavin (Vitamin B_2)	Milk, milk products (including yogurt and cheese), green leafy vegetables, organ meats, enriched grain products	Scaling around nostrils; glossitis; photophobia; cheilosis; scrotal and vulval dermatosis; redness and fissuring of eyelid corners	Decreased urine riboflavin, plasma riboflavin, RBC count, glutathione reductase	Deficiency (rare) found in conjunction with other B vitamin deficiencies; vegan diets; unsupplemented milk-free diets
Niacin	Meat, fish, poultry, whole grain and enriched grain products, peanut butter	Pellagra; glossitis; redness and fissuring of eyelid corners; dermatitis (Casal's necklace, rash around neck); diarrhea; dementia; change in nerve cell function	Decreased urine N-methyl, nicotinamide, plasma nicotinamide. Increased RBC count.	Pellagra (rare)
Pyridoxine (Vitamin B_6)	Meat (especially liver, beef, pork), bananas, whole grain products, wheat germ	Glossitis; stomatitis; cheilosis; microcytic anemia; muscle weakness; mental depression	Decreased red blood cell count, SGPT, SGOT, decreased urine B_6 and/or pyridoxic acid. Increased urine excretion of xanthurenic acid in response to tryptophan load test	Toddler diets deficient in B_6, unsupplemented formulas
Vitamin B_{12}	Meat, fish, poultry, eggs, milk, cheese, fortified cereal, fortified soy milk, brewer's yeast	Neurologic symptoms; hyperpigmentation; glossitis; filiform papillary atrophy; pernicious anemia; macrocytic anemia	Decreased hemoglobin, reticulocyte count, serum B. Increased MCH, MCV	Vegan diets; breastfed children of vegan mothers; regional enteritis, short bowel syndrome, gastritis

(Continued)

TABLE 58-3
(Continued)

Nutrient	Diet Sources	Clinical Signs of Deficiency	Laboratory Signs of Deficiency	Conditions that Place Children at Risk
Folic acid	Green leafy vegetables, whole grain products, wheat germ, organ meats, legumes, milk (except goat's milk), brewer's yeast	Glossitis; filiform papillary atrophy; hyperpigmentation; GI disturbances; macrocytic anemia	Decreased hemoglobin, serum folate	Chronic infections, enteritis; idiopathic steatorrhea; gluten-sensitive enteropathy; hemolytic anemia; liver disease; malignancy; myeloproliferative disease; drugs: methotrexate, pentamidine, phenytoin, aminopterin, sulfasalazine
Calcium	Milk, milk products, green leafy vegetables (collard greens, mustard, turnip greens, kale, spinach), shellfish, salmon, sardines, tofu (processed with calcium), bone meal, black strap molasses	Same as symptoms of rickets	Decreased calcium (may be normal), serum phosphorus (may be normal), urine calcium, urine phosphorus, bone age; increased serum alkaline phosphatase	Gluten-sensitive enteropathy; acute pancreatitis; malabsorption; cystic fibrosis; milk-free diets; vegan diets; toddler diets; diets lacking calcium sources; chronic diarrhea
Iron	Heme sources: beef, chicken, fish, lamb, liver, pork; non-heme sources: whole or enriched grains, dairy products, eggs, soluble iron supplements	Pale skin and eye membranes; smooth tongue; spoon nails (brittle, ridged); behavioral changes: short attention span, lassitude, fatigue, weakness, irritability; microcytic hypochromic anemia	Decreased hemoglobin, MCH, MCHC, MCV, serum transferrin saturation, serum iron. Increased total iron-binding capacity	Chronic blood loss (i.e., parasites intestine); decreased food intake (poverty, esophagitis); malabsorption; toddler diets; unsupplemented infant diets
Zinc	Legumes, wheat, eggs, seafood (especially oysters), meat, poultry	Intractable diaper rash; anorexia; growth retardation; short stature; delayed wound healing; dermatitis; hypogeusia; hypogonadism; lethargy; depression	Decreased serum zinc, RBC zinc, hair zinc, urine zinc, serum alkaline phosphatase, glucose tolerance	Chronic diarrhea; sickle cell anemia; malabsorption; chronic renal disease; upper respiratory infections; malignant neoplasms; toddler diets; parenteral nutrition

SGOT = serum glutamic-oxaloacetic transaminase; SGPT = serum glutamic-pyruvate transaminase; RBC = red blood cell; MCH = mean corpuscular hemoglobin; MCHC = mean corpuscular hemoglobin concentration; MCV = mean corpuscular volume.
Adapted from Howard, R., & Winter, H. (1984). *Nutrition and feeding of infants and toddlers.* Boston: Little, Brown.

Nursing Care

The nurse should have the child breathe slowly and deeply to help relax the anal sphincter while maintaining the child in a left lateral position with knees flexed during the procedure. The patient's vital signs should be monitored every 15 minutes for the hour following the test. The nurse should instruct the child to remain in bed for 1 to 2 hours and observe for increasing abdominal pain and/or distention.

Complications

Complications include perforation of the bowel, excessive bleeding from biopsy sites, serosal tears, and retroperitoneal emphysema.

Percutaneous Liver Biopsy

Description

The physician numbs the biopsy site using subcutaneous lidocaine (Xylocaine). The needle is inserted, the biopsy material is aspirated into the needle, and the needle is removed. The biopsy site must have pressure held on it for 5 to 10 minutes while the child lies on the right side. A sterile dressing is placed over the biopsy site, and the child remains on the right side for 4 hours.

Purpose

The purpose is to obtain liver tissue for microscopic examination and/or confirmation of liver disease. The tissue may also be used for enzyme analysis, bacterial or viral culture, histochemical study, and electron microscopy.

Indications

- Cholestatic syndromes of the neonate.
- Prolonged jaundice.
- Hepatomegaly.
- Lipid and glycogen storage disease.
- Wilson's disease.
- Reye's syndrome.
- Unusual course of hepatitis.

Contraindications

- Prothrombin time greater than 2 seconds.
- Platelet count less than 50,000/mm³.
- Bleeding time prolonged more than 7 minutes.
- Significant ascites.
- Extrahepatic cholestasis (bilirubin greater than 25 mg/dl).
- Biliary obstruction with dilated ducts.
- Expected hematoma.
- Infections of peritoneum.

Preparation

Laboratory results should be current, including hemoglobin, hematocrit, prothrombin and partial thromboplastin times, platelet count, and type and crossmatch. Equipment should be assembled (liver biopsy tray) and consent signed; patient should be NPO 4 hours prior to procedure. Sedation medications, based on physician preferences, are given 30 minutes to 1 hour prior to procedure.

- For patients less than 10 years of age:
  - Demerol 2 mg/kg IM.
  - Phenergan 1 mg/kg IM.
  - Thorazine 1 mg/kg.

TABLE 58-4
Blood Indices of Gastrointestinal Function

Test	Normal Ranges	Deviations	Clinical Implications
Leukocyte	Infant: 5,000–19,000 mm^3	High	Acute infection
	Child: 5,000–14,500 mm^3		
	Adolescent: 4,500–13,000 mm^3	Low	Certain medications or treatments
Culture	No growth	Bacterial and fungal growth	Bacterial and fungal infection
Hemoglobin	Infant: 9.8–11.8 g/dl	High	People living at high altitudes
	Child: 12.3–14.7 g/dl		
	Adolescent: (male) 12.8–15.6 g/dl (female) 12.6–14.8 g/dl	Low	Anemia; prolonged hemorrhage; excessive fluid intake
Hematocrit	Infant: 29–35%	High	Erythrocytes; dehydration
	Child: 34–44%		
	Adolescent: (male) 38–46% (female) 37–44%	Low	Anemia, acute blood loss, shock
Bilirubin	Direct: 0–0.3 mg/dl	High >3 g/dl	Biliary atresia, liver disease
	Total: <1.5 mg/dl		
Alanine aminotransferase	8–36 IU/l	High	Acute liver failure, rejection with transplant, hepatitis
Transaminase	6–44 IU/l	High	Liver disease
Sodium	135–144 mEq/l	High	Dehydration, pyloric obstruction, malabsorption
		Low	Excessive losses
Potassium	3.5–5 mEq/l	High	Tissue breakdown
		Low	Vomiting, diarrhea
Chloride	98–106 mEq/l	High	Anemia
		Low	Vomiting, diarrhea
Amylase	60–160 Somogyi U/dl	High	Acute pancreatitis, pseudocyst of pancreas
		Low	Duodenal ulcer, chronic pancreatitis
Calcium	Infant: 10–12 mg/dl	High	Hypervitaminosis D
	Child: 9–11.5 mg/dl		
	Adolescent: 9–11 mg/dl	Low	Diarrhea, rickets
Phosphorus	Infant: 5–7.8 mg/dl	Low	Predisposed to rickets
	Child: 4–5.7 mg/dl		
	Adolescent: 4–5.7 mg/dl		
Triglyceride	30–200 mg/dl	High	Inadequate clearing of lipids, sepsis
Cholesterol	Infant: 70–170 mg/dl	High	Familial hypercholesterolemia
	Child: 125–170 mg/dl		
	Adolescent: 125–170 mg/dl	Low	Fat malabsorption
Protein-total	Infant: 3.6–7.4 mg/dl	Low	Shock, chronic infection, malnutrition, loss of plasma
	Child: 3.2–5 g/dl		
	Adolescent: 3.2–5 g/dl		
Albumin	Infant: 2.1–4.5 g/dl	Low	Malnutrition long-term indicator; loss of plasma
	Child: 3.2–5 g/dl		
Pre-albumin	10–40 mg/dl	Low	Malnutrition short-term indicator
Ammonia	40–80 µg/dl	High	Liver disease, metabolic disease
Alkaline phosphatase	110–220 IU/l	High	GI disease, malnutrition, gastric resection

From the Children's Medical Center of Dallas, Laboratory Department, 1990.

TABLE 58-5
Stool Indices of Gastrointestinal Function

Test	Normal Ranges	Deviations	Clinical Implications
pH	7.5	Low <7.5	Acidic diarrhea
Glucose	—	Present +1 – +4	Malabsorption due to villus damage or shortened intestinal length
Occult blood	—	Present	Infection, inflammation, diverticulitis, carcinoma, ulcerative colitis
Lipids	4.5 g/24 hr	High >4.5 g/24 hr	Malabsorption
Bacteria	Normal flora	High	Overgrowth
Ova and parasites	—	Present	Parasitic disease
Transit time	Newborn: 4 hr	Low <2 hr	Bowel resection, intestinal lumen injury

From Children's Medical Center of Dallas, Laboratory Department, 1990.

- For patients 10 years of age and older:
  - Chloral hydrate 50 mg/kg (maximum 2 g).
  - Nembutal (2 to 3 mg/kg) IM.
  - Valium (0.1 to 0.2 mg/kg) IV.

The child and family are given an explanation of the procedure before the consent is signed. The abdomen is prepared using a povidone-iodine scrub.

Developmental Considerations

Immobilization is imperative for the child's safety during this procedure. An infant may be restrained using a papoose board. Older children are placed in a supine position with arms held over their head and knees held down firmly. Children should be asked to hold their breath during needle insertion and told they will feel a sensation of pressure.

Nursing Care

The nurse should take vital signs every 15 minutes for 1 hour, then every 30 minutes for 2 hours, every 1 hour for 2 hours, every 2 hours for 4 hours, and every 4 hours overnight. Ensure that the child remains on the right side for 4 hours after the procedure. Observe for hemorrhage (tachycardia, hypotension, abdominal distension, abdominal pain, shoulder pain) or respiratory distress. The hematocrit is generally checked 4 to 6 hours after the procedure.

Complications

Complications include local pain and infection, breakage of needle, intrahepatic hematoma, bile peritonitis, pleural pain, and pneumothorax penetration of other organs, tumor seeding.

Endoscopy Procedure

Description

The endoscope consists of a lens connected by thousands of Fiberglas threads to a distal lens at the tip of the endoscope (Fig. 58-5), which allows for the passage of images to the viewer. Other channels allow for air injection, suction, passage of biopsy instruments, and removal of foreign objects and injection of varices. Photographs can be taken through the endoscope. This instrument comes in different sizes, but endoscopy is infrequently performed in small children and infants. With the child's mouth open, the endoscope is guided into the esophagus,

with further advancement under direct vision. A bite block may be needed as well as suction of the oral cavity. Once visualization of structures is complete, photographs taken, and biopsies done if indicated, the physician suctions the trapped air from the GI tract and gently withdraws the endoscope.

Purpose

An endoscopic procedure using a fiberoptic endoscope allows for visualization of mucosal lining of the esophagus, stomach, and duodenum.

Indications

- Vomiting of blood.
- Rectal bleeding.
- Inflammatory disorders.
- Biopsy.
- Excision of polyps.
- Removal of foreign bodies.

Contraindications

Low hematocrit.

Preparation

Endoscopy is usually performed under general anesthesia. Older children may be given intramuscular or oral premedication as a "pedi cocktail":

- Demerol 2 mg/kg.
- Phenergan 1 mg/kg.
- Thorazine 1 mg/kg.

The child is NPO 4 to 8 hours prior to the procedure. The child and family are given an explanation of the procedure before the consent is signed. This explanation should include a description of the drowsy feeling following preoperative medications and waking up in the recovery room if general anesthesia is used. An authorized consent is signed by parents or guardian prior to the procedure. The procedure should be completed in 20 to 30 minutes.

Developmental Considerations

The infant or toddler is restrained during this procedure. If the child is to be awake during the procedure, he or she should be told that the throat will be numbed and a bite block will be used to help hold the mouth still. The child may feel unable to swallow, so the nurse will suction the mouth, and this may cause a sore throat after the procedure. The equipment is assembled (either in a surgery suite or GI laboratory) and the child is placed on the left side. If the child is awake, the throat is anesthetized with viscous lidocaine, tetracaine (Pontocaine), or benzocaine (Cetacaine) spray or gargle.

Nursing Care

Vital signs should be monitored frequently until the child is fully awake. The child should remain in a side-lying position to prevent aspiration if nauseated or vomiting. Observe for signs and symptoms of postbiopsy bleeding. On returning to normal activities, high-risk activities such as bicycling or skateboarding are restricted for 24 hours.

Complications

Complications include bleeding, perforation, aspiration, and sore throat.

Suction Biopsy for Esophageal, Gastric, Ileal, and Jejunal Specimens

Description

The Carey Capsule consists of two metal shells with sharp-edged holes in each of the halves. The capsule is kept open by a small spring; with suction, the capsule closes instantly, thus obtaining the biopsy. Under fluoroscopy, the progress of the instrument is

TABLE 58-6
Radiographic Studies

Radiographic Study[25]	Purpose: To Rule Out	Prerequisite	Preparation	Time
Abdominal sonogram	Mass	Specify organs to be studied	<2 yr—NPO 3 hr prior to study >2 yr—NPO at midnight before study	30–60 min
Barium enema	Fistula, atresia, stricture	Specify regular or with air contrast; not if bleeding is a current problem	Enema	30–60 min
Barium swallow esophagogram	Malrotation, stricture, foreign body, varices, fistulas, atresias, gastroesophageal reflux	Clinical information; reason for test	<2 yr—NPO at 5:00 AM or 3 hr prior to study >2 yr—NPO at midnight before study	15–30 min
Biliary scan	Atresia or blockage of bile duct		<2 yr—NPO 4 hr prior to study >2 yr—NPO at midnight before study	1 hr, 24 hr with delayed films at 2, 4, 6 hr as needed
Duodenal intubation	To determine if tube is in correct position for feedings, biopsy, or aspiration of fluid	Correct tube placement	Child on right side for 30 min before exam; NPO not necessary	30 min
Operative cholangiogram		Arrange with surgery	Prep per anesthesia	2 hr
Oral cholecystogram (gall bladder series)	Cholecystitis, gall stone cholelithiasis		0–1 yr—NPO 3 hr before each >1 in Day before, give high-fat diet for breakfast and lunch; at supper, give a light fat-free diet; water only after supper (day before exam); NPO after midnight before study Telepaque, contrast used for exam, supplied as 0.5-g tablets and ordered by physician; given by mouth with juice, crush if needed, at 8:00–11:00 PM Dosage of Telepaque <30 lb: 0.07 g/lb; 30–50 lb: 4 tablets; >50 lb: 6 tablets	30–40 min 20% of tests are repeated because of poor visualization
T—Tube cholangiogram		Requires fluoroscopy and indwelling T tube	None	30 min
Meckel scan	Meckel's diverticulitis	Nuclear medicine	<2 yr—NPO 4 hr prior to study >2 yr—NPO midnight before study	1 hr
Pelvic sonogram	Mass, abscess, fluid	Echo; specify organs to be studied	Unless contraindicated, instruct toilet-trained children to drink 2–3 glasses of water 1 hr before start of test and not to empty bladder	T-tube cholangiogram
Upper GI	Study of stomach and duodenum for pyloric stenosis, ulcers, abdominal pain, diarrhea, malrotation		Specify esophagram regular upper GI or SBFT (small bowel follow-through) <2 yr—NPO at 5:00 AM or 3 hr prior to exam >2 yr—NPO at midnight before Laxatives and/or enemas are recommended, except for patients with inflammatory bowel, ulcerative colitis, Crohn's disease All computed tomography, ultrasound, nuclear medicine studies, and x-rays need to be performed before upper GI	30 min to 2 hr

From Children's Medical Center of Dallas, Department of Radiology, 1988.[7]
Adapted from Silverman, A., & Roy, C. (1983). *Pediatric Clinical Gastroenterology.* St. Louis: Mosby.

monitored. The tubing is flushed with 5 ml of air before the biopsy is taken to ensure juices, mucous, and debris are cleared out and that the capsule is fully open. A bite block may be necessary to prevent the child from biting on the tubing. The capsule is gently withdrawn, and the biopsy specimen is placed in the appropriate media (formalin for morphology; quick frozen on foil for intestinal enzymology;

glutaraldehyde for electron microscopy; and/or isopentane for immunofluorescent studies).

Purpose

The purpose of the study is to obtain full-thickness biopsy of the mucosal wall, which should aid in establishing a definitive diagnosis.

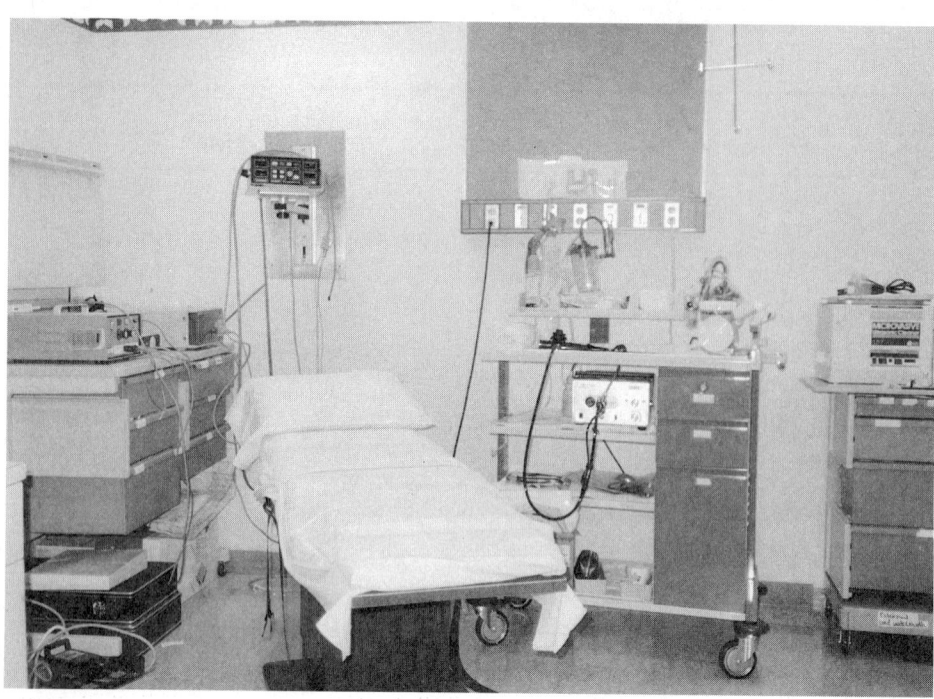

FIGURE 58-4
Gastrointestinal procedure room.

Indications

- Malabsorption syndromes.
- Iliac disease.
- Intestinal lymphangiectasis.
- Whipple's disease.

Contraindications

- Postoperative bowel resection.
- Intestinal bleeding.
- Varices.

Preparation

Patient must be NPO for 4 to 8 hours, depending on age. Prothrombin time, partial thromboplastin time, and platelet count should be checked. Consent must be signed. Explain to the child that the procedure takes 45 minutes to 1 hour. The child should be in a sitting position for the capsule and attached tube to be placed in the mouth and advanced through the throat. It usually takes 30 to 40 minutes for peristalsis to carry the capsule. Premedication is usually avoided, although metoclopramide syrup (0.1 mg/kg) orally may be given to shorten the time it takes the capsule to migrate from the stomach to the duodenum. The capsule is attached to polyethylene tubing and then to a 50- to 100-ml tight-fitting syringe.

Developmental Considerations

Small infants will swallow the capsule if it is placed at the base of their tongue; older children may need sips of water to enable swallowing. Children may need to be turned on their right side after swallowing the capsule to facilitate placement. The child should be told that the physician will have to take pictures (x-rays) during the procedure; the capsule will remove a tiny piece of lining of the intestine, which will not be felt by the child. The capsule is then removed.

Nursing Care

The child may be reunited with his or her family and resume normal activity except high-risk activities (bicycling and skateboarding) for 24

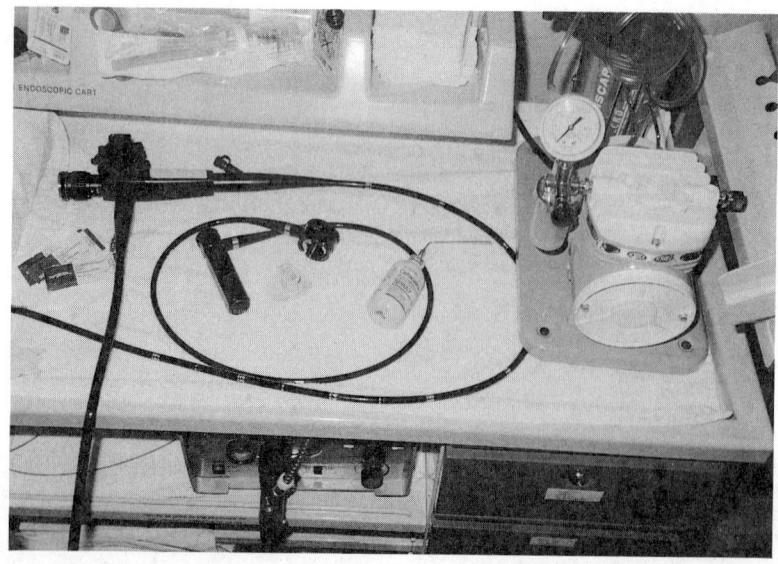

FIGURE 58-5
Endoscope.

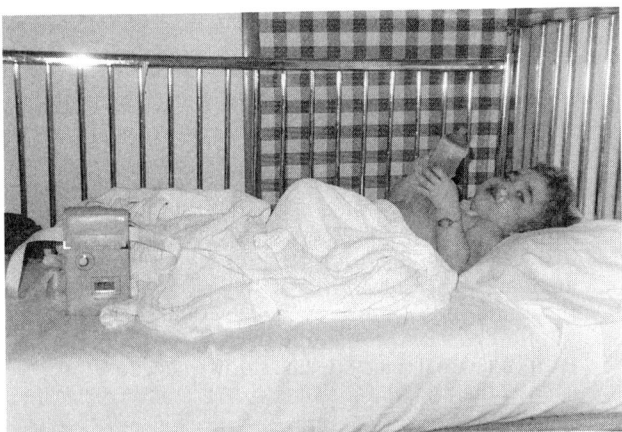

FIGURE 58-6
Portable pH probe monitoring.

hours. The child's vital signs must be monitored every 15 minutes for 1 hour. Observe for abdominal pain or distension and guaiac all emesis and stools during this time.

Complications

- Bleeding.
- Perforation.
- Aspiration.

pH Probe Monitoring

Description

The probe length is marked with adhesive tape; the end of the probe is lubricated and carefully inserted through the patient's nostril. It is taped to the infant's cheek, and placement is confirmed by chest x-ray. The proper probe placement is at the seventh vertebra, approximately 3 cm above the cardioesophageal junction. The probe is attached to the recorder, and the child is monitored, noting any changes on the graph paper such as awake time, sleep time, upright position, and supine position. The following observations are also noted: emesis, apnea, cyanosis, respiratory distress, bradycardia, or behavior changes. The child resumes regular diet and activity until termination of the test. (Some physicians prefer to limit the child's diet to apple juice and to restrict activity during the test.)

Purpose

The purpose of the test is to monitor the frequency and duration of stomach acid reflux into the esophagus.

Indications

- Unexplained irritability.
- Apnea.
- Pneumonia.
- Epigastric pain.

Contraindications

- Less than 2 weeks postoperative GI procedure
- GI bleeding.

Preparation

The infant must be NPO 2 to 4 hours prior to testing. This test can be done on either an outpatient or inpatient basis. A portable unit is also available if the child's condition warrants (Fig. 50-0). A consent is signed and the procedure is explained to the parents. The test may be run for 4, 6, or 24 hours as determined by the physician. The pH meter is calibrated by the GI nurse. If bethanechol is administered, this should also be noted on the graph paper. At the conclusion of the test, the probe is removed and the patient may be fed a normal diet.

It is important that no antacids or H_2 receptor antagonists (for example, cimetidine [Tagamet]) be given during this test.

Developmental Considerations

The parent or caregiver may remain with the infant during the entire procedure. If the infant is stable, the probe can be placed and the child may return home until the 24-hour monitoring process is complete.

Nursing Care

The nurse is responsible for placing the pH probe through the nares of the child and securing it with tape. Once the x-ray is done and correct placement is confirmed, the recorder is connected to the probe and the test initiated. At the conclusion of the test, the probe is removed and a normal diet may be resumed. Nurses notes should reflect the child's position (supine, upright, prone) and activity (chest physiotherapy [CPT], asleep or awake, vomiting, apnea or bradycardia, gagging, changes in vital signs) during the testing period.

Complications

Complications include esophageal perforation and placement of probe in tracheobronchial tree.

Pancreatic Exocrine Function

Adequate amounts of pancreatic enzymes are essential for the digestion and absorption of dietary fat and protein. Testing patients with various malabsorption syndromes (cystic fibrosis, enterokinase deficiency, pancreatic insufficiency with neutropenia [Shwachman syndrome], and chronic pancreatitis) usually help make the definitive diagnosis. Clinical symptoms such as steatorrhea and creatorrhea are present if 85% to 90% of the gland's function has been destroyed. To perform the test, a triple-lumen pediatric duodenal tube is placed for collection of duodenal juice after a 4-hour fast. Intravenous doses of the enzymes CCK-Pz and secretin 2 IU/kg body weight are given, and collections of duodenal juice are taken every 10 minutes for 50 minutes. Patients with cystic fibrosis have a reduction or absence of the enzymes lipase, trypsin, and chymotrypsin.

Motility Studies

It may be necessary to test for hypermotility in children with "short gut" or excessive stool output. A charcoal marker is placed in the infant's formula and given enterally. The time of this feeding is recorded. All stool output is inspected after this point. The time lapse between the charcoal marker intake and the time it is first observed in the stool is the transit time.

Anorectal Manometry[6,10,25]

Description

The pressure-recording device consists of a double balloon fixed to a hollow cylinder. This device is positioned at the initial anal sphincter. The test consists of recording the reflux response of the two anorectal sphincters to transient rectal balloon distension. The normal reaction is relaxation of the intestinal sphincter followed by contraction of the external sphincter. In patients with Hirschsprung's disease, the external sphincter contracts normally but the internal sphincter either fails to relax or may contract with this stimulus.

Purpose

Anorectal manometry uses a pressure-recording device to monitor anorectal mobility.

Indications

- Severe constipation.
- Suspicion of chronic fecal soiling (Hirschsprung's disease).

Contraindications

There are no contraindications.

Preparation

No analgesia is necessary. The infant or child is positioned on the side with knees flexed.

Developmental Considerations

Parents of infants and toddlers should be allowed to remain with the child to provide comfort and support. Older children should be told they may feel some pressure around the anus momentarily.

Nursing Care

The nurse inspects the anal area for any abnormalities following test.

Complications

There are no complications.

Nursing Diagnoses

After obtaining the history, performing the physical examination, reviewing results from the diagnostic tests, and tapping additional resources for information, the nurse carefully analyzes the data obtained. Nursing diagnoses appropriate for the child with GI dysfunction become apparent and are used to develop a plan of care. Selected nursing diagnoses that may be appropriate for

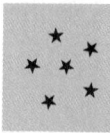

Ideas for Nursing Research

Nurses have the opportunity to observe infants and children from their first moment of life. Opportunities for nursing research exist in many areas, such as the early identification of a child with a congenital anomaly, the child's response to various foods and therapies on the gastrointestinal system,[11] and the development of the immune system relating to the gastrointestinal tract. Specific studies may develop, such as the following:

- Correlate maternal prenatal care and activities with the development of congenital anomalies of the gastrointestinal tract.
- Examine the relationship between family eating patterns, "problem eaters," and nutritional status.

the child with GI dysfunction are presented by function in Table 58-7.

Summary

The nursing assessment of the child with a known GI problem involves a number of nursing and medical pro-

TABLE 58-7
Selected Nursing Diagnoses Associated With Altered Gastrointestinal Function

Data Analysis and Conclusions	Nursing Diagnoses
Nutrition and Metabolism	
Prolonged NPO status, inadequate food intake (less than recommended daily allowance), weight loss, abnormal laboratory studies, weight and height below normal on growth chart	Altered Nutrition: Less Than Body Requirements related to inability to digest food Altered Growth and Development related to effects of physical disability
Difficulty breastfeeding	Altered Nutrition: Less Than Body Requirements related to inadequate or weak sucking and swallowing
Difficulty swallowing, coughing, choking, presence of cleft lip and/or palate, tracheoesophageal fistula	Impaired Swallowing, related to physical impairment
Elimination	
Change in bowel function, hard formed stool, painful defecation, abdominal discomfort, rectal fullness, decreased bowel sounds, history of Hirschsprung's disease	Constipation related to physical impairment
Change in bowel function, increased frequency, loose or watery stools, abdominal cramping, increased odor, increased bowel sounds, dehydration	Diarrhea related to physical impairment
Inability to control defecation, surgical intervention, trauma or injury to bowel or spinal column	Bowel Incontinence related to physical trauma High Risk for Impaired Skin Integrity related to loss of sensation due to neuromuscular impairment
Self-Perception and Self-Concept	
Change in the body secondary to surgery (ostomy) or congenital birth defect; not looking at body, does not participate in care, not involved in any social or school activities	Body Image Disturbance related to physiological impairment

cedures. The nurse's role is often much more important when the child and parents identify vague symptoms that are GI in nature but not specific. The nurse has an opportunity through a nursing history and physical, including a nutritional assessment, to identify potential and actual problems. In addition, the nurse has an opportunity to explore methods of facilitating the active participation of children and their families in their care.

References

1. Allen, S., & Harper, K. (1983). Developmental delays in infants on long term TPN. *Nutritional Support Services 3,* 43.

2. Bates, B. (1991). *A guide to physical examination* (5th ed.). Philadelphia: J.B. Lippincott.

3. Bowers, A., & Thompson, J. (1984). *Clinical manual of health assessment* (2nd ed.). St. Louis: C.V. Mosby.

4. Bozzetti, F. (1987). Nutritional assessment from the perspective of a clinician. *Journal of Enteral and Parenteral Nutrition, 11*(5), 1155–1215.

5. Byrne, W. (1988). Advances in pediatric clinical nutrition. *Nutritional Support Services, 8*(5), 10–11.

6. Children's Medical Center of Dallas, Department of Gastroenterology, 1988.

7. Children's Medical Center of Dallas, Department of Radiology, 1988.

8. Cravioto, J., & Robles, B. (1965). Evolution of adaptive and motor behavior during rehabilitation from kwashiorkor. *American Journal of Orthopsychiatry, 35,* 449–464.

9. Dempsey, D., & Mullen, J. (1987). Prognostic value of nutritional indicies. *Journal of Enteral and Parenteral Nutrition, 11*(5), 1095–1145.

10. Droske, S., & Francis, S. (1981). *Pediatric diagnostic procedures.* New York: John Wiley and Sons.

11. Frappier, P., Marino, B., & Shishmanian, E. (1987). Nursing assessment of infant feeding problems. *Journal of Pediatric Nursing, 2*(1), 37–44.

12. Galler, J. (1984). The behavioral consequences of malnutrition in early life. In J. Galler (Ed.). *Nutrition and behavior.* New York: Plenum Press.

13. Galler, J., & Ramsey, F. (1985). The influence of early malnutrition on subsequent behavioral development: VI. The role of the microenvironment of the household. *Nutrition Behavior, 2,* 161–173.

14. Gordon, M. (1987). *Nursing diagnosis: Process and application* (2nd ed.). New York: McGraw-Hill.

15. Hamosh, M. (1988). Does infant nutrition affect adiposity and cholesterol levels in the adult? *Journal of Pediatric Gastro- enterology and Nutrition, 7*(1), 10–16.

16. Howard, R., & Winter, H. (1984). *Nutrition and feeding of infants and toddlers.* Boston: Little, Brown.

17. Kennedy-Caldwell, C., & Caldwell, M. (1986). Pediatric enteral nutrition. In J. Rombeau & M. Caldwell (Eds.), *Parenteral nutrition: Clinical nutrition* (Vol. 2, pp. 434–479). Philadelphia: W.B. Saunders.

18. Mathew, O. (1988). Nipple units for newborn infants: A functional comparison. *Pediatrics, 81*(5), 688–691.

19. Mize, C., Cunningham, C., Teitell, B., Strickland, A., Dickey, E., McCarty, C., & Parker, J. (1984). Undernutrition of pediatric inpatients: Repeated nutrition status evaluation. *Nutritional Support Services, 4*(4), 27–39.

20. Nutrition Graphics. (1981). *Guide to breastfeeding; feeding your baby; feeding your preschooler.* Cowallis, OR: Nutrition Graphics.

21. Orr, M., & Allen, S. (1986). Optimal oral experiences for infants on long-term total parenteral nutrition. *Nutrition in Clinical Practice, 1*(6), 288–295.

22. Quay, N. (Ed.). (1986). *Pediatric feeding assessment and nursing interventions.* Dallas: Children's Medical Center.

23. Queen, P. (1983). Nutritional assessment of pediatric patients. *Nutrition Support Services, 3*(5), 23–31.

24. Rajah, R., Pettifor, J., Noormohamed, M., Venter, A., Rosen, E., Rabinowitz, L., & Stein, H. (1988). The effect of feeding four different formulae on stool weights in prolonged dehydration infantile gastroenteritis. *Journal of Pediatric Gastroenterology and Nutrition, 7*(2), 203–207.

25. Silverman, A., & Roy, C. (1983). *Pediatric clinical gastroenterology.* St. Louis: C.V. Mosby.

26. Smith, W., Erenberg, A., & Nowak, A. (1988). Imaging evaluation of the human nipple during breastfeeding. *American Journal of Diseases of Children, 142,* 76–78.

27. Suskind, R., & Varma, R. (1984). Assessment of nutritional status of children. *Pediatrics in Review, 5*(7), 195–202.

28. Wood, C., Isaacs, P., Jensen, M., & Hilton, H. (1988). Exclusively breast-fed infants: growth and caloric intake. *Pediatric Nursing, 14*(2), 117–124.

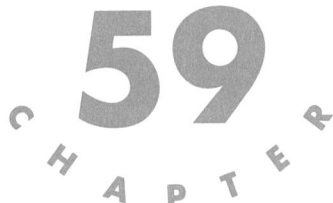

Nursing Planning, Intervention, and Evaluation for Altered Gastrointestinal Function

BEHAVIORAL OBJECTIVES

Describe the pathophysiology and clinical manifestations of common congenital and pediatric gastrointestinal abnormalities.

Discuss nursing assessment, nursing diagnoses, and nursing and collaborative interventions for the child with altered gastrointestinal function.

Describe nursing care for the child receiving enteral tube feedings, ostomy care, and total parenteral nutrition.

Identify important psychosocial needs and appropriate nursing interventions for the child with a gastrointestinal disorder.

Identify educational needs of the family and of the child with a gastrointestinal illness and discuss teaching strategies that can be used.

Gastrointestinal (GI) disorders affect children of all ages. The severity of the disease processes range from asymptomatic and unrecognized disorders to severe, overwhelming, and even fatal illness. Fortunately, most GI problems in children can be effectively treated if the symptoms are recognized early and therapeutic management is initiated promptly. Diligent nursing care of the child with a GI illness is critical to ensure early recognition of the disease and prompt implementation of appropriate therapeutic and monitoring measures. Important nursing interventions used in the care of children with GI disease include careful monitoring after abdominal surgery, close observation of feeding tolerance, implementation of specialized feeding regimens such as enteral tube feeding or total parenteral nutrition, and education of the family about home care measures. The nurse is a vital member of the health care team managing the child with a GI disorder.

measures. The nurse is a vital member of the health care team managing the child with a GI disorder.

Congenital Anomalies

Tracheoesophageal Abnormalities

Definition and Incidence. Esophageal atresia and tracheoesophageal fistulas are rare congenital malformations of the esophagus. The incidence has been variably reported as between 1 per 3000 and 1 per 4500 births.[16,62] A high percentage of infants born with tracheoesophageal abnormalities are premature or of low birthweight, and more than 40% of the infants have associated anomalies. Cardiovascular abnormalities are the most common, but pulmonary and renal anomalies, vertebral defects, anorectal malformations, and radial limb dysplasias may also occur.

Etiology and Pathophysiology. The esophagus develops during the fourth to fifth week of gestation as the foregut lengthens and forms two parallel tubes (the esophagus dorsally and the trachea ventrally) connected only at the larynx. An alteration in this process leads to esophageal or tracheal anomalies.[35] The causes of esophageal defects are not known, but there is little evidence to implicate heredity as a factor.

The various types of esophageal atresia and tracheoesophageal fistula are pictured in Figure 59-1. The most common form of these defects (85% to 90%) is characterized by a blind pouch of the upper esophageal segment and a fistula between the lower esophageal segment and the trachea. Ordinarily, the gap between the upper and lower segments is small (1 to 2 cm), and primary surgical repair is usually successful. A less common type (6% to 8%) is characterized by blind pouches of both upper and lower esophageal segments. If there is a large gap between the segments, surgical repair is more difficult.[61] Other forms of the defect may include an intact esophagus with a tracheoesophageal fistula, or esophageal atresia with fistulas between the upper or lower esophageal segments and the trachea.

Clinical Manifestations. Maternal hydramnios (an excessive amount of amniotic fluid in the amniotic sac) is commonly observed during the third trimester and at delivery of the infant with tracheoesophageal abnormality. In utero, esophageal atresia interferes with the reabsorption of amniotic fluid. Ordinarily, the amniotic fluid is swallowed by the fetus and reabsorbed by the GI tract. The esophageal obstruction blocks this process and may lead to maternal hydramnios. Immediately after birth, the infant's first cry may cause air to be forced through the fistula and into the stomach, leading to reflux and aspiration of gastric juices. If feedings are attempted, aspiration of formula can lead to severe pneumonitis. Additionally, air forced through a distal fistula into the stomach contributes to gastric distention, which further impairs ventilatory capacity.[16]

After birth, the infant with the tracheoesophageal anomaly often demonstrates excessive salivation and drooling because saliva collects in the esophageal pouch and the infant froths around the nose and mouth. With the first feeding, the infant may or may not have difficulty swallowing but will suddenly cough, choke, and often become cyanotic. Fluid may be regurgitated through the nose and mouth.

Severe pneumonia and atelectasis can result from aspiration. In the case of esophageal atresia without a tra-

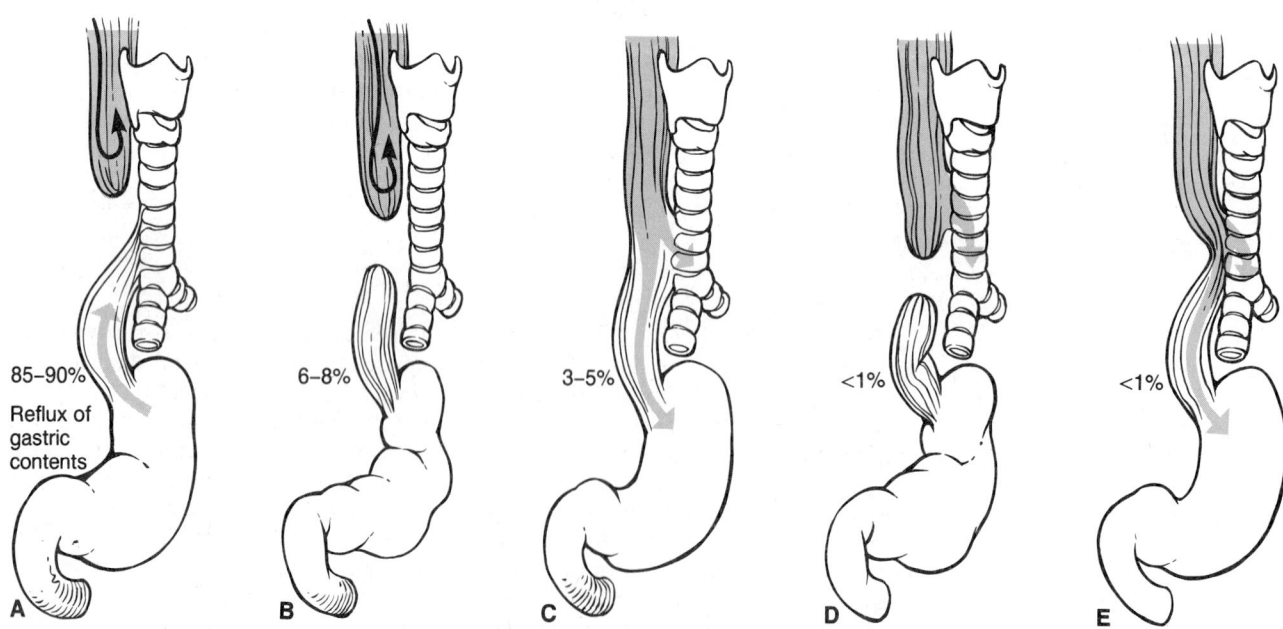

85–90%
Reflux of gastric contents

6–8%

3–5%

<1%

<1%

FIGURE 59-1

Tracheoesophageal abnormalities. Colored areas and arrows indicate path of feedings or oral secretions. (**A**) Blind pouch of upper esophageal segment with a fistula between lower segment and trachea. (**B**) Blind pouches of both upper and lower segments. (**C**) Intact esophagus with tracheoesophageal fistula. (**D**) Blind pouches of both esophageal segments with fistula between upper segment and trachea. (**E**) Esophageal atresia with fistulas between both segments.

cheoesophageal fistula, the infant may demonstrate an inability to swallow, a scaphoid abdomen, and the absence of air in the GI tract in abdominal x-rays. An infant with a tracheoesophageal fistula without esophageal atresia may not demonstrate symptoms for several months, and then repeated bouts of coughing and aspiration may be the only symptoms.[16,62]

Diagnostic Studies.   Diagnosis of esophageal atresia before the infant is fed for the first time decreases the risk of aspiration and significantly improves the prognosis. To rule out esophageal anomalies, it is recommended that every newborn be screened by passage of a semirigid rubber catheter (8 Fr) into the esophagus.[62] If the catheter passes readily, gastric secretions should be aspirated and a low pH (2 to 4) should be verified to ensure the catheter has not become coiled in the esophagus.

The type of esophageal abnormality is determined by radiographic studies. A plain lateral radiograph may be used, or a small amount of dilute radiopaque fluid may be carefully instilled into the esophagus. The introduction of radiopaque fluid into the upper esophageal pouch significantly increases the risk of pneumonia, and this approach is used only when absolutely necessary. A tracheoesophageal fistula without esophageal atresia may be difficult to demonstrate because the fistula may only be intermittently patent and symptoms may be subtle.

★ ASSESSMENT

Ideally, esophageal anomalies are diagnosed before the first feeding by passage of a catheter and careful observation of the infant for evidence of excessive amounts of mucus or drooling, difficulty with secretions, or episodes of cyanosis. A thorough assessment of an infant's response to the first feeding is a vital step in early diagnosis of esophageal abnormalities. The nurse must carefully observe the infant for coughing, choking, cyanosis, or regurgitation of fluid through the nares and mouth during the feeding. These symptoms result from an overflow of saliva or fluid from the esophageal pouch into the larynx and may lead to laryngospasm. Any of these symptoms should be well documented and reported to the physician immediately.

★ NURSING DIAGNOSES AND PLANNING

Based on the assessment data from above and from Chapter 58, the following nursing diagnoses may apply to the child with a tracheoesophageal anomaly:

- Ineffective Airway Clearance related to excessive thick secretions.
- Ineffective Breathing Pattern related to a neuromuscular impairment.
- High Risk for Infection related to regurgitation of fluid.
- Altered Nutrition: Less Than Body Requirements related to inability to procure food.
- Impaired Skin Integrity related to drooling.
- Altered Growth and Development related to physical disability effects.
- Altered Parenting related to skills deficiency concerning feeding.

The nurse and parents together plan effective care based on the established nursing diagnoses. Several examples of expected outcomes follow:

- The infant develops sucking and swallowing skills.
- The parents exhibit knowledge and skills on return demonstration of gastrostomy feedings.
- The parents describe signs of complications.

The nurse plans for the daily care of the child based on both physician's orders and nursing diagnoses. Some general nursing care goals may be the following:

- Aspiration of secretions is prevented.
- Infection is prevented.
- Regular feeding pattern is established.

★ INTERVENTIONS: COLLABORATIVE AND INDEPENDENT

PREOPERATIVE CARE

Once the diagnosis is made, preoperative care is focused on preventing aspiration of secretions and providing supportive care until surgical correction can be done. Frequent vital signs are taken, and the infant's respiratory status and amount of abdominal distention are monitored closely. To prevent further aspiration, the infant is kept NPO, and gentle intermittent or continuous suction is done through a catheter placed through the nasal passages into the proximal esophageal pouch. The infant's head and thorax are elevated 20 to 30 degrees to facilitate downward drainage of secretions. The infant is usually placed in an Isolette to minimize caloric expenditure. Oxygen is provided if the infant's respiratory status is compromised. Hydration and nutrition are maintained intravenously, and antibiotics are often prescribed to prevent or treat pneumonia. A gastrostomy tube may be inserted and placed to gravity drainage to facilitate drainage of the gastric contents and to minimize potential regurgitation of gastric contents into the trachea. The gastrostomy tube and nasal suction tube should be irrigated with air only. The nurse should maintain strict intake and output records for the infant. Surgical correction may be deferred temporarily if the infant has serious pulmonary complications or other associated anomalies, which must be corrected first. If so, a central venous catheter may be inserted, and parenteral nutrition may be used until the appropriate time for surgery.[16,62]

SURGICAL MANAGEMENT

The type of surgical correction depends on the type of esophageal abnormality. A primary repair to connect both segments of the esophagus and close the fistula is preferred in all infants when feasible. In some cases, the upper and lower esophageal segments are widely separated and a staged repair is necessary. In a staged repair, the initial surgical procedure generally includes a gastrostomy tube placement and the creation of an esophagostomy. The esophagostomy surgically diverts the upper esophageal segment externally and allows fluids to be consumed orally and drain out onto the skin just below the neck. This procedure prevents aspiration of saliva and allows the child to take feedings orally. The second stage includes closure of the esophagostomy and of the gap between esophageal segments. Occasionally, a segment of colon or gastric tissue is used to form a bridge between widely separated segments. This surgical procedure is often complicated by leaks or strictures at the anastomotic site.[16,61,62]

POSTOPERATIVE CARE

Postoperatively, the child is kept NPO and the gastrostomy tube is maintained on gravity drainage. A nasal catheter may be inserted during surgery to help drain the upper esophagus. The catheter is carefully placed to prevent pressure on the anastomotic site and should not be moved. Caution must be used when suctioning the airway to avoid injury to the anastomotic site. If tracheal suctioning is necessary, the length of suction catheter to be inserted should be measured and marked in consultation with the surgeon. The catheter length to be inserted should be communicated to all caretakers. Important nursing interventions include keeping the infant NPO until feedings are started and careful monitoring of gastric drainage. The infant's respiratory status is assessed frequently, and careful suctioning of the airway is done as needed.

Gastrostomy feedings are usually started when gastric drainage is minimal and secretions pass easily into the duodenum, usually about the second or third day postoperatively. If a primary repair has been done, oral feedings are usually started about the 10th to 14th day postoperatively. If a staged procedure is being used, the infant is fed through a gastrostomy tube until definitive repair is done.[16] If so, the esophagostomy allows external drainage of saliva and oral feedings from the upper segment.[54] Although the child does not receive nutritive benefit from oral feedings that drain out an esophagostomy, the importance of allowing the infant to develop normal oral–motor skills by practicing sucking and swallowing cannot be overemphasized.[15,50] Constant drainage of irritation can cause excoriation of the neck tissue, so the skin must be cared for meticulously. A gauze pad can be used to absorb secretions, but the pad should be changed frequently to prevent maceration of underlying tissue. A protective, occlusive ointment should be applied to the site.[55]

DISCHARGE PLANNING

Before discharge, the educational needs of the parents must be assessed. Often the parents need to learn to care for the esophagostomy and gastrostomy and how to administer gastrostomy feedings. The parents should also be instructed to observe for signs of complications such as difficulty breathing, fever, redness, or drainage at the esophagostomy or gastrostomy site or a refusal to eat. The importance of providing oral feedings must be emphasized. Gastrostomy feedings are discussed further at the end of this chapter.

★ EVALUATION

Periodically, the nurse and family evaluate the outcomes of care given. Examples of outcomes for the child with a tracheoesophageal anomaly were given under Planning in this section. Have short-term goals been met? Are long-term goals still realistic?

Care of the child with esophageal atresia is a challenge to medical, surgical, and nursing personnel, as well as to the parents. Survival and morbidity are related to birthweight, the presence of other congenital anomalies, and the development of complications that result from a delayed diagnosis. Survival for full-term infants without other congenital anomalies is close to 100%.[24,61,62]

COMPLICATIONS

Common complications of esophageal atresia include leakage or stricture at the anastomotic site or the recurrence of the fistula. Strictures may require serial dilations of the esophagus. Leaks at the anastomotic site may be treated by drainage through a chest tube or may lead to further corrective surgery. Leaks frequently lead to pneumonia, which can compromise the child's respiratory status. Recurrent fistulas and leaks must be repaired surgically. Some children develop gastroesophageal reflux, which may be treated with medications or surgical correction.[61]

Gastroschisis and Omphalocele

Definition and Incidence.   Gastroschisis and omphalocele are serious congenital malformations in which portions of the abdominal contents protrude beyond the abdominal wall. The embryologic development of these defects is not clearly understood, but they are recognized as two distinctly different abnormalities.[11,62] The incidence of gastroschisis is not well-documented, but omphalocele occurs in approximately 1 per 6000 births.[43]

Etiology and Pathophysiology.   A gastroschisis is a herniation, without a covering sac, of variable lengths of the small intestine and occasionally portions of the liver through a defect in the abdominal wall. About 60% of infants with gastroschisis are premature but rarely have associated malformations. The cause of gastroschisis is not known, and there is little evidence that it is transmitted genetically. The eviscerated intestines are usually damaged from prolonged exposure to the amniotic fluid. Peristalsis is absent at birth, and normal motility is often not present for weeks to months after surgical repair. All patients have some degree of intestinal malrotation and shortened bowel, which may cause disruption of intestinal motility and absorption of nutrients even after corrective surgery.[62]

An omphalocele is a protrusion of abdominal contents into the base of the umbilical cord. During the 6th to 10th week of gestation, the midgut grows and projects out of the abdomen into the umbilical cord because the abdomen is too small to contain it. Around the 10th to 11th week, the intestines normally migrate back into the abdomen. A failure of the intestines to migrate normally produces an omphalocele. The omphalocele is usually covered by a membranous sac, which protects the viscera. If the sac ruptures in utero, the exposed intestines may be damaged just as in gastroschisis. Infants with omphaloceles also have a high incidence of other associated abnormalities such as imperforate anus, colon agenesis, and diaphragmatic or cardiac defects.[43]

Clinical Manifestations. Most gastroschisis occur on the right side of the umbilical cord and vary in size from 2 to 15 cm. The eviscerated mass of bowel is covered by thick, gelatinous, greenish material and appears edematous and leathery. Peristalsis is absent. The peritoneal cavity is often relatively small.[62]

An omphalocele may appear as a slight enlargement at the base of the umbilical cord or as a membranous sac protruding at the umbilicus. The sac may range in size from small to gigantic and may contain liver, spleen, and a large portion of the bowel. The umbilical cord is usually inserted into the sac. If the sac has ruptured in utero, the intestines appear dark, thickened, and edematous as in gastroschisis. If the sac is not ruptured or has ruptured during delivery, the intestine appears essentially normal. Approximately one third of infants with omphalocele have associated congenital anomalies.[43,62]

Diagnostic Studies. Gastroschisis and omphalocele are diagnosed by observation at birth. The defect is occasionally noted on a prenatal sonogram. The infant is carefully assessed for the presence of associated anomalies and to determine the extent of bowel involvement.

★ ASSESSMENT

Nursing assessment includes careful observation of the newborn for abnormalities of the abdominal wall and careful pre- and postoperative assessments. An assessment of the family's understanding of the disease and coping abilities must be made.

★ NURSING DIAGNOSES AND PLANNING

Based on the assessment data from above and from Chapter 58, the following nursing diagnoses may apply to the child with gastroschisis and omphalocele:

• Impaired Skin Integrity related to altered nutritional state.
• Altered Gastrointestinal Tissue Perfusion related to altered arterial flow.
• Altered Nutrition: Less Than Body Requirements related to poor absorption.
• High Risk for Infection related to inadequate primary defenses.
• Ineffective Breathing Pattern related to musculoskeletal impairment.
• Altered Parenting related to interrupted parent–infant bonding.

Other functionally related nursing diagnoses are discussed in the Nursing Care Plan in the section on Necrotizing Enterocolitis and small bowel syndrome.

The nurse and parents together plan effective care based on the established nursing diagnoses. Several examples of expected outcomes follow:

• The infant maintains normal breathing patterns.
• The parents cuddle infant with assurance.
• The parents demonstrate understanding of care of their infant.
• The parents demonstrate ability to administer TPN.

The nurse plans for the daily care of the child based on both physician's orders and nursing diagnoses. Some general nursing care goals may be the following:

• Infection is prevented.
• Further tissue damage is alleviated.

★ INTERVENTIONS: COLLABORATIVE AND INDEPENDENT

PREOPERATIVE CARE

An infant with gastroschisis or omphalocele usually undergoes immediate surgical repair of the defect to prevent further tissue damage and infection. The nurse ensures that the defect is covered with sterile moist gauze and kept moist until surgery. Any pressure on the defect is avoided. Nasogastric suction is used to prevent further distention of the bowel, and the nurse carefully monitors the suction for amount and color of drainage. Intravenous fluids and antibiotics are initiated. Intake and output records are kept.

SURGICAL MANAGEMENT

If the defect is small enough, a primary repair is done, and the entire protrusion is placed back into the abdominal cavity. If the defect is too large, a staged repair must be performed. In this case, a protective pouch of Silastic or other synthetic material is used to encase the defect. The pouch is suspended over the infant to allow gradual return of the viscera to the abdominal cavity. The pouch is gently compressed and gradually introduced into the abdominal cavity as the abdominal musculature expands and edema of the bowel wall decreases. After the abdominal contents have completely returned to the abdomen, complete repair of the defect with closure of the skin and muscle layers is usually possible at about 2 to 3 weeks.[43,62]

POSTOPERATIVE CARE

The length of the postoperative recovery period varies considerably and depends on the size of the defect and the extent of intestinal dysfunction after surgery. Many infants experience prolonged ileus, disrupted motility, and poor absorption. Complications such as wound infection, volvulus, bowel necrosis, or intestinal fistulas may occur. Respiratory distress or diminished circulation to the lower extremities may develop due to compression of the lungs or the inferior vena cava by the replaced bowel. These infants frequently require prolonged parenteral nutrition until adequate oral feedings can be established. Although full recovery may take weeks to months, the long-term prognosis for infants with gastroschisis and omphalocele is good. Mortality is usually attributed to other congenital problems.[62]

Postoperatively, the nurse assesses the infant for evidence of potential complications including respiratory distress or sign of venous compression such as discoloration, delayed capillary refill, or edema in the lower extremities. The return of bowel function is assessed by auscultation for bowel sounds and observation of the passage of meconium or flatus.

The nurse must carefully monitor nasogastric suction for the amount and color of drainage and must administer

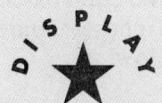

Family Teaching: Written Instructions for Total Parenteral Nutrition Home Care

When Your Child Needs TPN: Answers to the Most Common Questions

Your child may need Total Parenteral Nutrition (also known as TPN) if she or he is unable to tolerate all the calories and nutrients (food) needed through his or her gastrointestinal tract. TPN is a method of giving nutrition into a vein rather than into the mouth, stomach, and intestines. Your physician believes that TPN is the best method to supply your child with the nutrition he needs to get well. Your child may need TPN because of any or all of the following reasons:

1. Your child may have a disease that affects the absorption of food.
2. Your child may have had major surgery and may need extra nutrition to help his wounds heal and to help him grow stronger.
3. Your child may be unable to tolerate oral feedings (possibly due to nausea, emesis, or diarrhea).
4. Your child may have been born with a condition that affects his ability to swallow or digest food.
5. Your child may have a disease or treatment that has decreased his appetite.

TPN is a liquid (usually yellow in color because of the vitamins that have been added) that is infused into your child's vein. TPN contains the food your child needs for survival and healing. The TPN solution contains protein, carbohydrates, vitamins, electrolytes, and trace elements. A lipid solution is often used with the TPN solution. This solution is thick and white (it looks like milk) and contains fat, which helps supply calories and the essential fats your child needs to build stronger tissue.

The TPN solution and lipids are very concentrated and are usually infused through a special catheter in a large vein near the heart. This catheter is known as a central line or a central venous catheter. Your child may need to go to the operating room where the surgeon will carefully insert the central line catheter under general anesthesia.

Since the central line is foreign to the body, the catheter and the place where it exits your child's body (called the exit site) must be kept very clean to prevent infection and to prevent other catheter complications. If your child needs TPN at home, you will be learning how to take care of the catheter and how to administer the TPN safely.

While your child is receiving TPN, your doctor will monitor his nutritional needs closely by looking at the amount of food and TPN required, your child's physical appearance, and daily weights, and by monitoring laboratory results from samples of your child's blood. Your child may be allowed to drink some formula or eat some foods while receiving TPN. As the amount of food or formula your child can tolerate increases, the amount of TPN he receives will be decreased. When your child is doing better and can tolerate enough food through his gastrointestinal tract, the TPN will be stopped. *Usually* the central line is removed after the TPN is stopped. The surgeon may use a local anesthetic when he removes the catheter, but your child will not need to return to the operating room or be readmitted to the hospital for removal of the catheter.

DISCHARGE INSTRUCTIONS FOR TPN HOME CARE

I. TPN
    A. Run TPN at _____ cc per hour for _____ hours per day.
    B. Run lipids at _____ cc per hour for _____ hours per day.
    C. Schedule for Weaning onto TPN
        Hook up at _____ at _____ cc per hour.
      Increase rate at _____ to _____ cc per hour.
                 _____ to _____ cc per hour.
                 _____ to _____ cc per hour.
    D. Schedule for Weaning off TPN
      Decrease rate at _____ to _____ cc per hour.
                 _____ to _____ cc per hour.
                 _____ to _____ cc per hour.
      Then do Heparin flush at _____ .
    E. Change Click Lock Needle and Housing Every Day.

II. HEPARIN LOCK
    A. Flush with _____ cc of Heparin (100 units/cc) each day.
    B. Change click lock cap every week on _____ .
    C. Change extension tube every week on _____ .

(Continued)

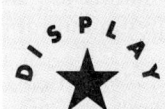

Family Teaching: Written Instructions for Total Parenteral Nutrition Home Care (continued)

III. CENTRAL LINE DRESSING
 A. Change every Monday, Wednesday, and Friday.
 B. Also change if dressing is wet, dirty, or loose.

IV. MONITORING
 A. Check temperature every day and anytime your child feels warm, is sweating, or is flushed.
 B. Check urine testape. If 1+ or more, check a chemstrip and call your doctor.

V. DIET _____

VI. TROUBLE-SHOOTING
 Call Doctor _____ at _____ for any of the following:
 A. Catheter Problems
   Fever
   Redness, drainage, or tenderness at central line exit site
   Difficulty in flushing catheter
   Occlusion alarms on pump without an obvious cause
   Broken catheter
   Difficulty breathing
   Any unusual problems with catheter
 B. Nutrition Problems
   Dry mouth or sunken eyes
   Vomiting or increased number of stools
   Sugar in urine (1+ or more on testape)
   Any unusual problems

VII. NUTRITION NURSE
 Call Nutrition Nurse _____ at _____ for any questions about procedures learned in hospital.

VIII. HOME CARE COMPANY
 Call Home Care Company at _____ for any problems with equipment or supplies.

COMPLICATIONS OF
HOME TPN THERAPY

Please read each statement then write a brief description of what you would do to remedy the situation. The nutrition nurse will go over the answers with you.

1. Your child runs out of TPN fluid.

2. Central line dressing is loose or wet.

3. The central line exit site is red and draining.

4. The TPN tubing has air in it.

5. You are unable to separate the IV tubing from the extension tubing.

6. The pump beeps "flow."

7. The pump beeps "occlusion."

8. The pump beeps "malfunction."

9. Your child has a fever and is spilling glucose in his or her urine.

10. Blood backs up the line while it is heparin locked.

11. The central line breaks.

12. The catheter is more difficult to flush than usual.

13. Your child needs to take a bath.

(With permission of Children's Medical Center of Dallas, Department of Nursing Education, August 1988.)

intravenous fluids and antibiotics. Strict intake and output records are kept. Once initiated, the tolerance of feedings is closely monitored by observing and recording stool patterns, gastric residuals, or the presence of abdominal distention.

PARENTAL SUPPORT

The birth of a child with gastroschisis or omphalocele may be a frightening experience for parents. The defect is obvious at birth, and the infant is typically whisked away to surgery immediately. The parents usually have no forewarning of the problem and need reassurance and careful explanations. Postoperatively, the parents need instruction about appropriate care for their child and appropriate feeding methods.

DISCHARGE PLANNING

If the child requires prolonged parenteral nutrition, careful instruction and discharge planning should be initiated if home parenteral nutrition is feasible.[1] The accompanying display and Figure 59-2 illustrate the nurse's discharge plans related to home TPN and materials needed for teaching handouts. An actual teaching plan for home TPN appears in the section on short bowel syndrome later in this chapter.

★ EVALUATION

Periodically, the nurse and family evaluate the outcomes of care given. Examples of outcomes for the child with gastroschisis or omphalocele were given under Planning in this section.

Necrotizing Enterocolitis

Definition and Incidence.   Necrotizing enterocolitis (NEC) is a serious disease characterized by ischemic necrosis of the small bowel or colon. NEC is seen most commonly in low birthweight infants. NEC is estimated to develop in 5% to 15% of premature, low birthweight infants. Rarely, NEC may develop in full-term infants.

Etiology and Pathophysiology.   The exact etiology of NEC is unclear and is likely multifactorial. NEC is thought to result from a shunting of blood away from the bowel, leading to hypoxia and ischemia of the bowel wall. The shunting of blood may be due to a hypoxic or stressful event that interrupts blood flow to the intestine. Several risk factors commonly associated with the development of NEC include exchange transfusions, umbilical arterial or venous catheters, perinatal asphyxia, respiratory distress syndrome, polycythemia, and congenital heart disease. The exact mechanism by which these risk factors lead to NEC is unclear. The insult to the bowel injures the mucosa, which may set the stage for colonization by gas-forming bacteria, which has been cited as a contributory cause of NEC. The gas produced by the bacteria accumulates within the bowel wall and produces a common diagnostic finding in NEC known as pneumatosis. Pneumatosis is seen radiographically as bubbly gas within the bowel wall or as free air within the peritoneal cavity.

Colonization of the mucosa can lead to extensive gangrene of the bowel and eventually bowel perforation and peritonitis.[34,62]

Most infants who develop NEC have been fed clear fluids or formula before developing symptoms. In many cases, the symptoms develop within 24 to 72 hours after the initiation of feedings. Feeding premature infants within the first 48 hours after birth or the use of hypertonic formulas may predispose the infant to NEC. However, NEC may develop in infants who have never been fed.[34,62]

Clinical Manifestations.   The classic symptoms of NEC are generally noted within the first 5 to 10 days of life. The infant usually feeds poorly and develops vomiting, abdominal distention, and bloody stools.[11] If perforation occurs, symptoms of lethargy, severe acidosis, sepsis, disseminated intravascular coagulation, and shock rapidly develop.[62]

Diagnostic Studies.   If NEC is suspected, abdominal x-rays are performed to determine the presence and extent of complications. Radiographic findings associated with NEC include ileus with moderate abdominal distention, irregular and scattered bowel loops, edema of the bowel wall, presence of fluid-filled loops and peritoneal fluid, and the presence of pneumatosis or free air in the peritoneal cavity on x-ray.[34,62]

★ ASSESSMENT

Recognition of early, and often subtle signs and symptoms of NEC is essential to decrease the risk of further progression of bowel damage. The nurse carefully assesses the newborn infant's tolerance of feedings and stool pattern. On physical examination of the abdomen, the nurse should assess bowel sounds and the tone and shape of the abdomen. Potential symptoms of NEC, such as disinterest in feedings, vomiting, absence or decrease in bowel sounds, abdominal distention, or bloody stools, must be promptly reported to the physician.

★ NURSING DIAGNOSES AND PLANNING

Based on the assessment data from above and from Chapter 58, the following nursing diagnoses may apply to the child with NEC.

- Altered Gastrointestinal Tissue Perfusion related to interrupted arterial and venous flow.
- Altered Nutrition: Less Than Body Requirements related to malabsorption.
- High Risk for Infection (peritonitis) related to potential for perforation.
- High Risk for Fluid Volume Deficit related to necrosis of intestinal mucosa.
- High Risk for Impaired Skin Integrity related to diarrhea.
- Altered Growth and Development related to nutritional deficits.
- Altered Parenting related to interrupted parent–infant bonding.
- Anticipatory Grieving related to fear of loss of newborn.
- Fear related to perceived inability to control events.

Checklist for Monitoring Home Total Parenteral Nutrition

OBJECTIVES TO BE MET BY DISCHARGE FOR MONITORING HOME TPN	Discussed Objectives With Parent/ Patient	Demonstration to Parent/ Patient	Return Demonstration by Parent/ Patient	Parent/ Patient Ready for Discharge	Comments
1. Verbalize steps of performing CVC dressing change including equipment required.					
2. Demonstrate knowledge and technical skills when performing the TPN dressing change (3 times).					
3. Describe what a healthy CVC site looks like.					
4. Describe when a CVC site looks infected.					
5. Verbalize signs and symptoms of skin sensitivity to tape and relate alternatives of care if tape sensitivity persists.					
6. Verbalize why their child is receiving TPN therapy.					
7. Verbalize the major components in the TPN solution.					
8. Demonstrate the skills to monitor the IV infusion pump.					
9. Demonstrate priming TPN tubing (3 times).					
10. Demonstrate starting the TPN infusion (3 times).					
11. Verbalize and demonstrate measuring and recording accurate intake and output on their child.					
12. Demonstrate urine glucose testing.					
13. Demonstrate use of chemstrip.					
14. Verbalize the principles of the heparin lock procedure and equipment required.					
15. Demonstrate the skills required to perform the heparin lock procedure (3 times).					
16. Demonstrate the heparin irrigation procedure (3 times).					
17. Demonstrate and relate how to perform cyclic TPN therapy.					
18. Demonstrate and relate the steps required if the line should become severed; blunt needle (2 times).					
19. Verbalize three potential complications that occur while their child is receiving TPN.					
20. Verbalize appropriate staff referrals and resources if complications occur.					

PARENT'S ACKNOWLEDGEMENT

I have received instructions from the nurse regarding the health care I should give my child after discharge from Children's Medical Center of Dallas. The nurse has explained the importance of following the appropriate instructions indicating whom I should contact regarding a question or problem.

Nurse's Name & Initials	

Parent/Guardian Signature   Date

_____

R.N.'s Signature   Date

FIGURE 59-2

Discharge planning: home total parenteral nutrition. (With permission of Children's Medical Center of Dallas, Department of Nursing Education, August 1988.)

Other functionally related nursing diagnoses are discussed in the Nursing Care Plan and in the section on Short Bowel Syndrome later in this chapter.

The nurse and parents together plan effective care based on the established nursing diagnoses. Several examples of expected outcomes follow:

- The infant passes normal stools.
- The infant tolerates initial oral feedings.
- The parents demonstrate understanding of TPN feedings.
- The parents discuss their concerns about the infant.

The nurse plans for the daily care of the child based on both physician's orders and nursing diagnoses. Some general nursing care goals may be the following:

- Infection is prevented.
- Further tissue damage is alleviated.

★ INTERVENTIONS: COLLABORATIVE AND INDEPENDENT

As soon as NEC is suspected, oral feedings are withheld, and nasogastric suction, intravenous fluids, and antibiotics are initiated.[11] Abdominal x-rays are followed frequently (every 8 to 12 hours initially) to allow early detection of perforation. If no evidence of perforation develops, the disease is managed through conservative medical treatment including nasogastric suction and the administration of intravenous antibiotics and nutrition. This treatment is continued for about 10 days until there is no radiographic evidence of pneumatosis and only a small amount of clear gastric secretions are obtained. Many cases of suspected NEC resolve spontaneously, without surgical intervention.

NEC WATCH

The infant is carefully observed for worsening symptoms, thus this conservative approach is often referred to as an "NEC watch."

During the "NEC watch" phase, an important nursing intervention is maintenance of strict NPO status for the neonate. A nasogastric tube is generally inserted and placed to intermittent suction. The nurse should observe the color and volume of nasogastric drainage and promptly report the presence of blood or a sudden increase or decrease in output. The nurse also administers intravenous antibiotics and parenteral nutrition as ordered and assists with obtaining frequent abdominal x-rays. The child must be closely monitored for any change in condition. Symptoms such as bloody stools or nasogastric drainage; abdominal distention; a taut, shiny or discolored abdomen; lethargy; fever; or hypothermia may indicate impending or actual perforation and must be reported immediately.

SURGICAL MANAGEMENT

Rapid clinical deterioration or signs of perforation or peritonitis are indications for immediate surgery. The actual operative procedure depends on the extent of necrosis. Any unquestionably necrotic or perforated bowel is resected. In some cases, a temporary ileostomy or colostomy may be placed.

POSTOPERATIVE CARE

An example of nursing care of a child with NEC is given in the accompanying Nursing Care Plan.

After surgery, the child is managed with intravenous antibiotics and parenteral nutrition. Small volumes of dilute feedings are introduced around the 10th postoperative day, and the feedings are gradually advanced. Diarrhea is common, and feeding tolerance must be monitored carefully by the nurse. Neonates with NEC often require feedings to be administered by a slow, continuous drip through a nasogastric tube. The slow perfusion of feedings through the intestine improves tolerance of the formula. Chronic complications of NEC may include long-term feeding intolerance, intestinal adhesions or obstructions, or a dependency on long-term parenteral nutrition if extensive amounts of bowel were resected.[34,62] (See section on Short Bowel Syndrome later in this chapter for teaching plan regarding home TPN teaching.)

Postoperative nursing care also includes maintaining nasogastric suction, parenteral nutrition, and intravenous antibiotics. The surgical wound is observed closely for signs of infection. Feedings are introduced slowly, and tolerance of feedings is closely monitored. A stool record should be kept detailing the frequency, color, consistency, glucose content, and pH of stool. The presence of bloody stool, abdominal distention, or vomiting is reported promptly to the physician.

PARENTAL SUPPORT

The development of NEC is often devastating for parents. The child has survived the first critical days and appears to be improving daily. Feedings are started, and parents often experience renewed hope and optimism. Suddenly, feedings must be stopped, a nasogastric tube is inserted, and the child is often rushed to surgery. The nurse can help the parents by carefully explaining what is happening to their baby and by encouraging the parents to express their feelings. After surgery or during the NEC watch, parents should be encouraged to touch and talk to their baby. If the infant is stable, holding and cuddling encourage parent–infant bonding.

DISCHARGE PLANNING

As discharge approaches, the parents are taught the signs of feeding intolerance and the importance of maintaining the diet recommended by the health care team. Many parents and grandparents are eager to introduce foods or formulas they believe will help the child. The family should be cautioned that the infant's GI system is still sensitive and the introduction of other foods could be detrimental. Some parents need to learn to administer parenteral nutrition at home or how to perform ostomy care before discharge. The family must be given adequate time to learn all the procedures and to be comfortable caring for their child well in advance of going home.

★ EVALUATION

Periodically, the nurse and family evaluate the outcomes of care given. Examples of outcomes for the child with

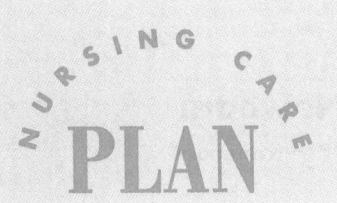

Postoperative Care of the Newborn Requiring Abdominal Surgery

Assessment

Case Study Description

Baby Boy Kyle is born prematurely. He is a 36-week AGA infant born to an 18-year-old single mother, Ms. Stuart. At 24 hours of age, he develops bloody diarrhea and a distended abdomen. An x-ray confirms the diagnosis of necrotizing enterocolitis, and he is taken to surgery for an exploratory laparotomy. The surgeon removed 20 cm of small bowel including the ileocecal valve and places a Broviac central venous catheter for postoperative total parenteral nutrition (TPN). The infant remains in stable condition and is transferred from the ICU to the general pediatric floor on postoperative day number two. The young mother appears very loving toward Kyle but is afraid to hold him because of all "the tubes." She asks when she can take him home.

Assessment Data

Alert male infant weighing 2.5 kg (down 500 g from birth weight). He is agitated. Abdominal incision is dressed, NG to low suction intact. He currently has bowel sounds and remains NPO.

Nursing Diagnosis	Intervention	Rationale
1. Anxiety related to knowledge deficit regarding postoperative care	Explain purpose of surgery.	Reinforcement of why the surgery was necessary may help Ms. Stuart understand that a recovery phase must take place.
Supporting Data: • Mother is afraid to hold infant after surgery.	Explain purpose of tubes.	Mother will take care in handling Kyle and know when to notify the nurse if something is wrong with one of "the tubes."
• Mother asks when she can take Kyle home.	Explain sequence of postoperative care without giving timeframes.	Important not to promise discharge on a certain day to prevent disappointment. Better to enforce that Kyle's progress will dictate when he may be discharged.
2. Impaired skin integrity Supporting Data: • Exploratory laparotomy, 20 cm small bowel resected. • Broviac central venous catheter placed.	Assess surgical sites as indicated for tissue granulation. Change dressing as indicated using sterile technique.	Infant's surgical site will heal without complications. Central venous access will be maintained until infant can absorb nutrition by way of gastrointestinal tract.
3. High risk for altered body temperature Supporting Data: • Premature infant. • Post surgery.	Take frequent vital signs: q4h to monitor temperature. Clothe infant and use overhead cap to prevent loss of heat. Maintain constant temperature of environment—may need Isolette.	Premature infants have less insulation (fat tissue) and may have trouble maintaining body temperature at optimal level. It is best to maintain the temperature and conserve their energy to be used toward healing. Increase in temperature may signal infection.
4. Fluid volume excess Supporting Data: • Post surgical laparotomy.	Monitor daily weight. Maintain strict intake and output. Infuse IV fluids through central venous catheter by way of infusion pump.	Prevent fluid overload. Prevent increased cardiac output in premature infant.

(Continued)

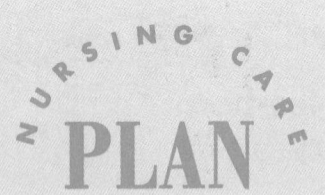

Postoperative Care of the Newborn Requiring Abdominal Surgery (continued)

Nursing Diagnosis	*Intervention*	*Rationale*
	Record frequency and consistency of output.	
	Monitor for physical signs of fluid overload (dependent edema tachypnea).	
5. High risk for fluid volume deficit Supporting Data: • Post surgical laparotomy.	Monitor daily weight. Maintain strict intake and output record. Infuse IV fluids through central venous catheter by way of infusion pump. Record frequency and consistency of output. Monitor for physical signs of dehydration (skin turgor, sunken eyes, dry mouth).	Prevent dehydration. The infant is predisposed to fluid losses related to nasogastric suction and possible electrolyte imbalance.
6. Pain Supporting Data: • Infant is agitated.	Coordinate care and procedures. Position infant to reduce tension on abdominal incision. Enlist mother in comfort measures (rocking, pacifier). Administer pain medication as ordered.	Allow infant as much uninterrupted rest time as possible.
7. Altered gastrointestinal tissue perfusion Supporting Data: • 20 cm bowel resected.	Monitor abdomen for distention. Monitor stools for blood.	Further injury to bowel will result in these symptoms.
8. High risk for infection Supporting Data: • Laparotomy incision. • Bowel surgery. • Indwelling central venous catheter.	Demonstrate good handwashing techniques. Perform sterile dressing changes to both surgical sites per protocol. Observe the appearance of the site for signs and symptoms of local infection: exudate, edema, tenderness, or erythema. Monitor infant for early signs and symptoms of sepsis: hyperthermia, hyperglycemia, glucosuria. Monitor infant for late signs and symptoms of sepsis: lethargy, hypothermia, hypoglycemia. Nurse will change IV tubing with sterile technique.	Handwashing is a priority in infection control. Prevent infection. Promote early detection of infection.
9. Altered bowel elimination Supporting Data: • NPO status. • Bowel resection, loss of ileocecal valve.	Maintain NPO status with NG tube to low suction. Check NG tube for patency, irrigate with saline to prevent blockage.	Bowel will have limited or absent motility. Gastric secretions must be removed to prevent distention or vomiting.

(Continued)

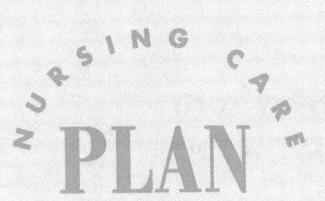

Postoperative Care of the Newborn Requiring Abdominal Surgery (continued)

Nursing Diagnosis	Intervention	Rationale
	Listen for bowel sounds when doing vital signs.	
	Tape tube securely to prevent dislodgement.	
	Measure and describe stool output.	
	Ensure frequent diaper changes to prevent skin breakdown on buttocks.	
10. Altered nutrition: less than body requirements Supporting Data: • NPO status. • Prematurity. • Post bowel resection.	Administer total parenteral nutrition by way of central venous catheter per protocol. Record accurate intake and output. Document daily weight. Plot serial anthropometrics. Obtain lab test reflecting nutritional status (serum Na, K, Cl, Ca, PO$_4$, Mg, BUN, Creatinine, Albumin, Prealbumin, Total Protein). Monitor tolerance of enteral feedings when introduced—document: vomiting, stool pH, presence of sugar in stools, consistency, frequency. Monitor diaper area for skin breakdown.	Adequate caloric intake is required during immediate postoperative phase for healing and growth. Normal weight gain for this infant would be 30 g/d. Estimated caloric intake required: 140 kcal/kg/d. After feedings are initiated, intolerance may lead to diarrhea. Bile acid content of stool can cause skin excoriation.
11. Sleep pattern disturbance Supporting Data: • Agitated infant transferred from ICU.	Dim lights during night or nap hours. Schedule procedures to decrease stress.	Infant develops sleep cycle in privacy of pediatric floor room.
12. Altered growth and development Supporting Data: • Premature infant. • Recovery phase of postoperative surgery	Post infant's care schedule on door or bed. Enlist ancillary services to evaluate child during prolonged hospitalization—Child Life (developmental testing/intervention), Physical Therapy (gross motor/fine motor), Speech Therapy (language delays), Foster Grandparents (if mother unable to stay at hospital).	Infant is maintained in the least stressful, consistent, environment possible until discharge to home. Overstimulation will be prevented.
13. Sensory/perceptual alteration: gustatory Supporting Data: • NPO. • Total Parenteral Nutrition (feeding the infant by bypassing the mouth).	Provide optimal oral experiences: encourage use of pacifier, promote hand–mouth activity, rub infant's gums with textured objects. Initiate nippled feedings (using consistent feeder) ASAP; may even begin with small amounts of sterile water. Cycle TPN–12-h infusion during night hours to promote oral intake (appetite) during day hours.	Prevent development of oral sensitivity from occurring to ensure adequate oral intake when initiated.

(Continued)

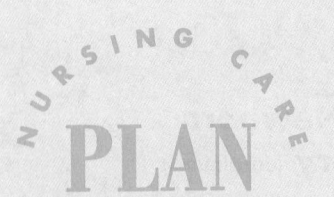

Postoperative Care of the Newborn Requiring Abdominal Surgery (continued)

Nursing Diagnosis	Intervention	Rationale
14. Altered parenting Supporting Data: • Mother separated from infant at birth. • Hospitalized infant.	Enlist mother in as much normal infant care as possible: bathing, rocking. Allow mother to have input in plan for Kyle's care. Allow mother to bring in clothes, toys from home. Explain all procedures before doing them. Allow mother time to verbalize feelings and needs. Enlist help of social worker for financial support.	The mother feels helpless during her newborn infant's hospitalization. Allow and encourage her to participate as a parent in his care.

Evaluation
- Skin integrity maintained and healing visualized.
- Body temperature maintained at 37° F axillary.
- Fluid volume overload and deficit prevented.
- Normal bowel function returns.
- Growth and development normalized as much as possible in the hospital environment.
- Oral sensitivity does not occur.
- Mother demonstrates positive parenting behaviors.

Expected Outcomes
- Mother verbalizes knowledge regarding purpose of surgery.
- Infant develops sleep/rest pattern.
- Kyle exhibits gain of average of 30 g/d through nutrition support.
- Mother demonstrates positive parenting behaviors.

A teaching plan related to home TPN appears later in this chapter.

NEC were given under Planning in this section. Revisions of short- and long-term goals may be necessary.

Anorectal Malformations: Imperforate Anus

Definition and Incidence. A variety of congenital malformations of the anorectal area have been identified. Typically, all of these anomalies are classified as imperforate anus. The various manifestations of anorectal malformations include anal stenosis, imperforate anal membrane, anal or rectal agenesis, and rectal atresia and are depicted in Figure 59-3.

Birthweight and the association of other congenital anomalies are the most important prognostic factors with anorectal abnormalities. Mortality is about 4% in infants whose birthweight is greater than 4 lb and who have no associated congenital defects. Anorectal malformations are commonly associated with other serious congenital abnormalities including genitourinary, esophageal, and cardiac anomalies.

Etiology and Clinical Manifestations. Most anorectal anomalies result from an abnormal embryologic division of the cloaca. During the fifth week of gestation, the cloaca is a common channel for the urinary, genital, and rectal areas. The urorectal septum divides the cloaca into the urogenital sinus (which becomes the bladder and urethra) and the hindgut (which becomes the rectum). A disruption in this embryologic process may lead to an anorectal malformation.

Anal stenosis accounts for about 10% of anorectal abnormalities and is characterized by a small anal aperture (opening). The severity of symptoms depends on the degree of stenosis and may not be recognized until the child is 1 year of age or older and presents with a history of difficult defecation, abdominal distention, and ribbonlike stools.[62] Ordinarily, anal stenosis can be treated with serial dilations of the anus, which may need to be continued

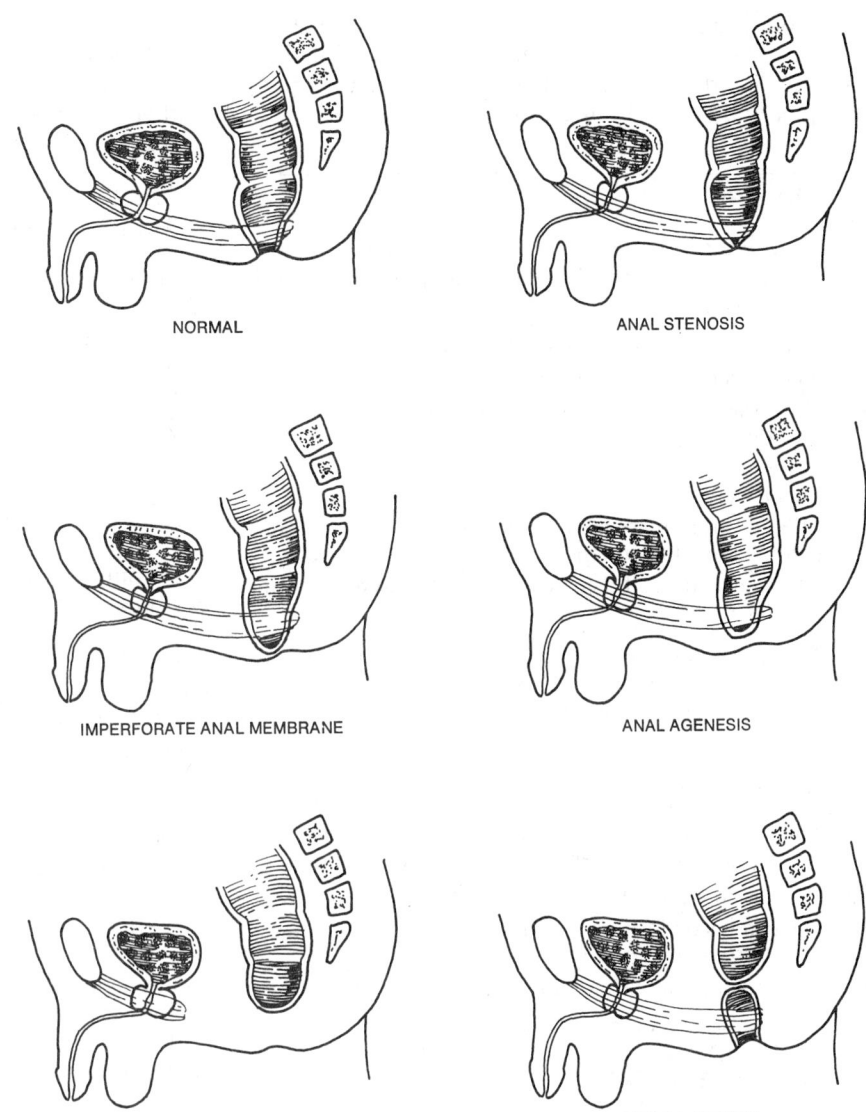

FIGURE 59-3
Various classifications of anorectal malformations.

for several months. Often parents are carefully instructed how to perform these dilatations at home.

An *imperforate anal membrane* is noted shortly after birth when the infant fails to pass meconium. A greenish, bulging membrane may be noted, or the nurse may be unable to insert a rectal thermometer. The imperforate anal membrane is treated by excision of the membrane and anal dilatations.[62]

Anal and *rectal agenesis* account for 75% to 80% of anorectal abnormalities and are typified by a rectum that ends in a blind pouch. Both of these anomalies may be associated with vaginal or uretheral fistulas.[11,62] *Rectal atresia* is characterized by a blind rectal pouch with a normal anus. The treatment of anal or rectal agenesis or atresia is through surgical reconstruction. The type of surgery is determined by the level at which the rectum terminates. If the rectum passes through the puborectalis sling of the levator ani muscle, the defect is considered a "low" defect and surgical correction usually can be done in the neonatal period by using an abdominal-perineal pull-through procedure. If the defect is high, such as in rectal agenesis where the defect is above the puborectalis

sling, it is usually necessary to perform a temporary colostomy and to do the final corrective procedure when the infant weighs 20 to 25 lb or is about 1 year of age.

Diagnostic Studies. Anorectal abnormalities are often diagnosed during a routine newborn assessment by the observation of the absence of an anal opening or the presence of a thin translucent membrane or anal dimple. Other diagnostic studies may include a urinalysis to investigate the possibility of a rectourinary fistula and radiographic studies to determine the level of the rectal pouch. During the x-ray, the infant is held in an inverted position and a radiopaque marker is placed at the usual location of the anal opening. This position allows air to ascend in the rectum and outline the level of the rectal pouch.

★ ASSESSMENT

The nurse may be the first to suspect an anorectal malformation, often when attempting to take the initial rectal temperature. Important nursing observations that should be reported include the inability to pass a rectal thermometer, the failure of the infant to pass a stool within 24 hours of birth, or meconium that appears in the urine or vagina and may indicate a fistula.

★ NURSING DIAGNOSES AND PLANNING

Based on the assessment data from above and Chapter 58, the following nursing diagnoses may apply to the child with imperforate anus:

- Constipation related to avoidance of painful defecation.
- High Risk for Wound Infection related to bowel surgery.
- High Risk for Impaired Skin Integrity related to altered nutritional state.
- Toileting Self-Care Deficit related to neuromuscular impairments.
- Altered Parenting related to unrealistic expectations regarding bowel continence.
- Situational Low Self-Esteem related to ability to perform anal dilatation.

The nurse plans for the daily care of the child based on both doctor's orders and nursing diagnoses. Some general goals may be the following:

- Wound is kept dry.
- Infection is prevented.

The nurse and child (or parents) together plan effective care based on the established nursing diagnoses. Several examples of expected outcomes follow:

- The parents perform anal dilatation procedure on return demonstration before discharge.
- The parents demonstrate ability to perform ostomy care.

★ INTERVENTIONS: COLLABORATIVE AND INDEPENDENT

The treatment of anorectal anomalies varies according to the extent of the defect. The treatment regimen ranges from excision of the anal membrane, to serial dilatations of the anus, to surgical reconstruction of the anus and rectum.

The nursing care depends on the corrective procedure. Surgical wounds must be kept clean and observed closely for evidence of infection. Due to the frequent contamination with urine and stool, the wounds are at high risk for infection. Exposing the wound to open air or a heat lamp several times each day helps keep the wound dry. If parents will be performing anal dilatations at home, ample opportunities for supervised practice of the dilatation procedure must be provided. If a temporary colostomy is created, parents are instructed about ostomy care and allowed to practice until they are comfortable with the procedure.

Many children with anorectal abnormalities have difficulty with bowel control. It is important for parents to understand that toilet training is usually affected. Most children have normal development of adequate urinary control but have a decreased awareness of rectal fullness and a short warning period of impending defecation. Children with low level defects (anal stenosis, imperforate membrane) more easily achieve continence than

children with high level defects (rectal agenesis and atresia). Most children show a gradual improvement in sensory perception and continence with age. In some cases, further corrective surgery or biofeedback training may be necessary to improve bowel control.[11,62]

★ EVALUATION

Periodically, the nurse and family evaluate the outcomes of care given. Examples of outcomes for the child with imperforate anus were given under Planning in this section. The nurse and family should determine if short-term goals have been met. A revision of long-term goals may be necessary.

Bowel Obstruction

A number of congenital abnormalities may cause an obstruction of the bowel. A bowel obstruction develops when the passage of intestinal contents is blocked by a mechanical constriction of the lumen or by abnormal muscular contraction or innervation. The symptoms and rapidity of onset vary according to the level of the obstruction. Green bile-stained emesis is the most frequent sign of a bowel obstruction.

Small bowel obstructions are characterized by a rapid onset of severe cramping and intermittent pain. Proximal to the obstruction, peristalsis increases as the bowel tries to push intestinal contents past the obstruction. High-pitched hyperactive bowel sounds may be present, and peristaltic waves may be visible on the abdomen. A rapid accumulation of fluid develops within the intestinal lumen as normal reabsorption is impaired, and large volumes of fluid may shift from the venous circulation into the bowel. Profuse, frequent vomiting is generally present, and dehydration often occurs rapidly. Some stool and flatus may be passed initially as the bowel distal to the obstruction empties. If the obstructive process continues, bacterial activity within the lumen produces toxins, which may be absorbed into the general circulation causing septic shock. Edema of the bowel wall and diminished blood supply to the bowel may cause necrosis and perforation.

Obstruction of the large bowel is characterized by a more gradual onset. Typically there are no stools and vomiting develops late. Vomitus is usually bile stained. Large bowel obstruction usually causes mild, steady pain but is often characterized by early and massive abdominal distention. Large amounts of intestinal fluids can accumulate, and the increased intraluminal pressure may lead to rupture. Pressure on the diaphragm from the abdominal distention may lead to respiratory compromise. The pathophysiologic processes involved with bowel obstruction are pictured in Figure 59-4.

Treatment of bowel obstruction usually includes intravenous fluids and electrolytes and nasogastric suction to decompress the bowel. Vital signs and all intake and output are carefully monitored. The patient is placed NPO. Abdominal x-rays are taken and reveal dilated bowel loops. The patient is usually taken to surgery to correct the obstruction as soon as fluid and electrolyte abnor-

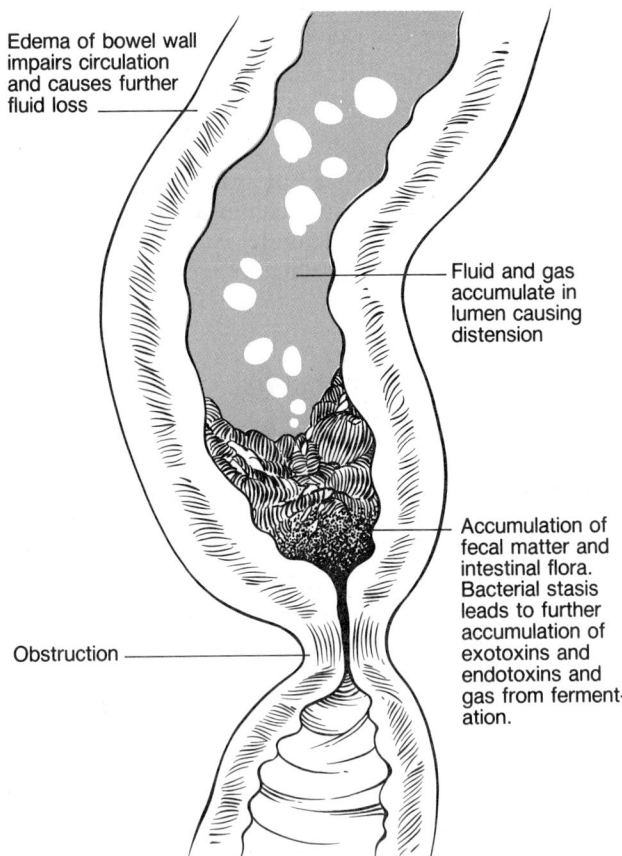

Edema of bowel wall impairs circulation and causes further fluid loss

Fluid and gas accumulate in lumen causing distension

Accumulation of fecal matter and intestinal flora. Bacterial stasis leads to further accumulation of exotoxins and endotoxins and gas from fermentation.

Obstruction

FIGURE 59-4
Pathophysiology of intestinal obstruction.

malities are corrected, and after the bowel is adequately decompressed with nasogastric suction.

Atresia or Stenosis

An *intestinal atresia* is the absence, or complete closure, of one or more portions of the GI tract. A *stenosis* is a narrowing of a portion of the GI tract. The atresia or stenosis causes a functional obstruction to the passage of nutrients and secretions. An atresia can form at any point along the GI tract but most commonly occurs in the esophagus, intestine, or anus.[11,75] Some of the common types of atresia are described here.

Esophageal Atresia. Esophageal atresia is often accompanied by tracheal malformations and other congenital abnormalities and is discussed at the beginning of this chapter.

Duodenal Atresia or Stenosis. The duodenum may be completely or partially obstructed. In cases of complete obstruction, bilious vomiting usually begins within a few hours after birth and the child often appears jaundiced. Frequently, a history of maternal hydramnios is obtained. Duodenal atresia is often associated with prematurity, trisomy 21, and other severe congenital anomalies.[62] In partial duodenal obstruction, the primary symptoms of vomiting and obstruction may occur intermittently, and diagnosis may be delayed for weeks, months, or years.[36]

Jejunal or Ileal Atresia or Stenosis. Jejunal and ileal atresias are more common than duodenal atresias and may occur together and at multiple sites within the intestine. Vascular insufficiency and viral insults in utero have been suggested as causes of jejunal atresia. Jejunal and ileal atresias are associated occasionally with cystic fibrosis or intestinal malrotations. Infants with jejunal or ileal atresia often develop vomiting of bile-stained fluid within the first 24 hours of life and may have abdominal distention. Approximately 20% to 30% of patients develop jaundice and may have minimal or no passage of meconium. A history of maternal hydramnios is evident in about 25% of cases.[62]

Colonic Atresia or Stenosis. Only about 10% of intestinal atresias or stenosis occur in the colon and are often associated with small bowel atresias or other GI abnormalities. The cause of colonic atresia is speculated to be some type of vascular insult to the fetal intestine. Signs of colonic atresia include failure to pass meconium, obstipation (severe constipation), abdominal distention, and vomiting. With colonic stenosis, the child may demonstrate failure to thrive and diarrhea.[62]

Diagnostic Studies. The diagnosis of intestinal atresia or stenosis is based on clinical and radiologic findings. Contrast studies are often used to portray the defect clearly. In some cases, definitive diagnosis cannot be made until an exploratory laparotomy is performed to allow visualization of the bowel.

★ ASSESSMENT

A careful nursing assessment of the infant's response to feedings, the presence of abdominal distention or vomiting, and passage of meconium are important factors in an early diagnosis of intestinal obstruction. The color of vomitus is particularly important. Green bile-stained emesis is often indicative of obstruction and must be reported immediately.[11]

★ NURSING DIAGNOSES AND PLANNING

Based on the assessment data from above and Chapter 58, the following nursing diagnoses may apply to the child with intestinal atresia or stenosis:

- Altered Bowel Elimination related to physical abnormality.
- High Risk for Infection (peritonitis) related to possible intestinal rupture.
- Altered Gastrointestinal Tissue Perfusion related to interrupted arterial and venous flow.
- Altered Nutrition: Less Than Body Requirements related to vomiting.
- High Risk for Impaired Skin Integrity related to vomitus.
- Altered Parenting related to fear regarding outcome.
- High Risk for Altered Growth and Development related to nutritional deficits.

Other functionally related nursing diagnoses are discussed in this chapter's Nursing Care Plan.

The nurse and parents together plan effective care based on the established nursing diagnoses. Several examples of expected outcomes follow:

- The infant tolerates initial postsurgical feedings.
- The infant passes normal stools.
- The parents demonstrate ability to perform ostomy care.

The nurse plans for the daily care of the child based on both physician's orders and nursing diagnoses. Some general nursing care goals may be the following:

- Bowel obstruction is corrected.
- Fluid and electrolyte balance is established.

★ INTERVENTIONS: COLLABORATIVE AND INDEPENDENT

When the diagnosis of atresia is suspected, the infant is made NPO and nasogastric suction is used to decompress the bowel. Intravenous fluids and electrolytes are started to correct dehydration or electrolyte abnormalities related to excessive vomiting. After diagnosis, surgical intervention is mandatory to relieve the obstruction. In most cases, the atretic or stenosed segment is resected and the remaining segments of intestine are reanastomosed. In a few cases, it may be necessary to perform an ileal, jejunal, or colonic ostomy or to do multiple bowel resections.[11,62]

Postoperatively, the child if maintained on parenteral nutrition until the anastomotic sites are healed, usually 10 to 14 days. Feedings are gradually introduced as tolerated. Complications of resections of atresias include further bowel obstructions caused by adhesions or inadequate absorption of feedings due to the shortened bowel length.[36] Severe atresias or stenoses may require extensive bowel resections leading to short bowel syndrome. These children may require prolonged parenteral nutrition. The prognosis is typically good in most cases, however, the mortality increases significantly when the defect is associated with prematurity, trisomy 21, or other congenital abnormalities.[62]

Important nursing interventions include careful monitoring of intravenous intake and nasogastric output. Strict intake and output records, including documentation of any stool or emesis, are maintained. Postoperatively, the child is assessed for evidence of wound infection and for signs of the return of bowel function including the presence of bowel sounds and the passage of stool or flatus. If an intestinal ostomy was created during surgery, the nurse must initiate a plan for ostomy care.

DISCHARGE PLANNING

In preparation for discharge, the parents need to spend time learning about the special needs of their child. The family should be warned of the possibility of formula intolerance or further bowel obstruction and should be taught to report symptoms such as an increased frequency or watery content of stool, green emesis, firm or distended abdomen, and signs of dehydration such as decreased urine output, dry mouth, or sunken eyes. If the child requires ostomy care or home parenteral nutrition, the parents need to learn these procedures.

The parents need support and encouragement from the health care team. All procedures and equipment, such as nasogastric tubes and infusion pumps, should be explained to the parents. It is often frightening for the family to perform ostomy care or home parenteral nutrition, and they should be given ample opportunities to express their fears and concerns and be allowed to practice all procedures until they feel comfortable providing care for their child.

★ EVALUATION

Periodically, the nurse and family evaluate the outcomes of care given. Examples of outcomes for the child with atresia or stenosis were given under Planning in this section. Have short-term goals been met? Are long-term goals still realistic?

Hirschsprung's Disease

Embryologically, Hirschsprung's disease is believed to result from the defective migration of ganglion cell precursors of the neural crest into the hindgut. This migration normally occurs between the 6th and 12th weeks of gestation. In Hirschsprung's disease, the ganglion cell migration is interrupted, leading to aganglionosis of the bowel. A current etiologic theory is that inhibitory nerves important for the relaxation phase of peristalsis and for relaxation of the internal sphincter synapse in the ganglion cells. Due to the absence of ganglion cells, these nerves do not function correctly and normal relaxation of the bowel cannot occur. As a result, the affected bowel remains in a constant state of contraction. A functional obstruction develops, and the normal proximal bowel becomes dilated and hypertrophied.[11,42]

Definition and Incidence. Hirschsprung's disease is a congenital disease in which the intestine lacks normal parasympathetic ganglion cells leading to inadequate or absent peristalsis. This condition leads to a functional obstruction of the intestine accompanied by marked dilatation of the segment of colon proximal to the aganglionic segment (Fig. 59-5). Variable lengths of bowel

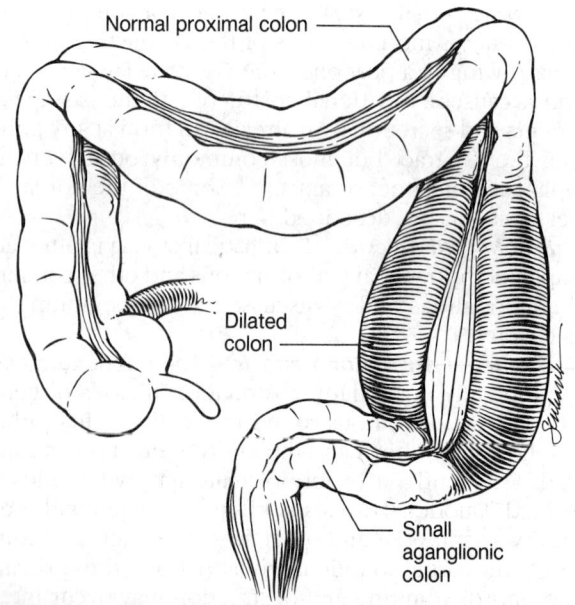

FIGURE 59-5
Hirschsprung's disease.

may be affected. Aganglionosis may involve only the area close to the internal sphincter or may affect the entire colon and parts of the small bowel. The incidence is estimated as 1 per 5000 live births and is predominantly seen in males.

Etiology and Pathophysiology. The cause of Hirschsprung's disease is unknown, but a familial history is noted in 7% to 30% of cases. A significant number of patients (5% to 10%) have Down's syndrome.[42,62]

Clinical Manifestations. Hirschsprung's disease is most commonly observed in young children; however, occasional rare cases are observed in older children, adolescents, and adults. The signs and symptoms vary with the age of the child. The newborn infant fails to pass meconium in the first 24 to 48 hours, then develops a disinterest in feeding, bilious vomiting, and abdominal distention.[42] If untreated, the condition may result in ileal, appendiceal, or colonic perforation. Hirschsprung's disease in the older infant is often associated with persistent constipation, poor feeding, and failure to thrive. The infant may have a worried or frowning appearance and may be irritable. Diarrhea is an ominous sign because it may indicate enterocolitis, which is associated with a high mortality (50%) in the first months of life.[11] Symptoms of this complication may include an unexplained fever, severe prostration, and poor tolerance of feedings followed by explosive, liquid stools, which may be bloody. Enterocolitis is seen most frequently in infants diagnosed with Hirschsprung's disease within the first 3 months of life.[62]

If the disease is not diagnosed in early infancy, the older child will demonstrate constipation with malodorous and ribbonlike stools. As the colon continues to dilate, abdominal distention increases and respiratory volume decreases. The child is often anorectic and suffers from malabsorption.[11]

Diagnostic Studies. The diagnosis is based on the history, a physical and rectal examination, radiologic studies, anorectal manometry, and an intestinal biopsy. The rectal examination typically reveals an empty rectum and snug internal sphincter. As the finger is withdrawn, flatus and malodorous, pale, liquid stools may gush out forcibly.[11,27,62] A plain abdominal film often reveals severe intestinal distention and obstruction. A barium contrast enema often demonstrates a narrowed distal segment and a dilated proximal segment of colon. The definitive diagnostic study is a rectal biopsy that reveals an absence of ganglion cells and an increase in nerve fibers.[42,62]

Other diagnostic studies may include a chemical examination of cells obtained during the biopsy. An increased activity level of the enzyme acetylcholine esterase is indicative of Hirschsprung's disease.[42] Anorectal manometry is used to evaluate the tone of the internal sphincter muscle. If this test shows a failure of the internal sphincter muscle to relax in response to distention of the rectum, it is highly suggestive of Hirschsprung's disease.[27]

★ ASSESSMENT

Preoperative nursing assessment includes careful attention to parental reports of constipation, abdominal dis-

tention, or feeding intolerance in the young infant or persistent constipation with ribbonlike stools in the older child. The presence of any of these symptoms requires further inquiry into the child's bowel function. After the diagnosis of Hirschsprung's disease is made, nursing care focuses on preparing the child and family for surgery.[11,55]

★ NURSING DIAGNOSES AND PLANNING

Based on the assessment data from above and Chapter 58, the following nursing diagnoses may apply to the child with Hirschsprung's disease:

- Constipation related to poor muscle tone.
- Ineffective Family Coping: Comprised related to situational crises.
- Knowledge Deficit regarding perianal care, ostomy care, signs of recurrent obstruction.

Other nursing diagnoses are similar to those discussed previously in the obstruction sections. Other functionally related nursing diagnoses are discussed in this chapter's Nursing Care Plan.

The nurse and child (or parents) together plan effective care based on the established nursing diagnoses. Several examples of expected outcomes follow:

- The parents discuss their concerns and coping problems.
- The parents demonstrate ability to provide ostomy care.

The nurse plans for the daily care of the child based on both physician's orders and nursing diagnoses. Some general nursing care goals may be the following:

- Continence is established.
- Normal sexual function is preserved.
- Dehydration is prevented.

★ INTERVENTIONS: COLLABORATIVE AND INDEPENDENT

Surgical intervention is the primary mode of treatment for Hirschsprung's disease. The major goals of surgery are to remove the aganglionic segment of bowel, to ensure continence, and to preserve normal sexual function (the delicate nerves of the bladder and ejaculatory mechanisms are in close proximity to the area).[42]

PREOPERATIVE CARE

Before surgery, bowel preparation is often carried out over several days to clear fecal contents from the bowel. Isotonic saline enemas are used for rectal irrigations. Tap water enemas and hypertonic phosphate enemas are contraindicated because they may lead to fluid and electrolyte disturbance.[62] Oral and systemic antibiotics may be ordered to reduce intestinal flora. The child is often kept NPO or maintained on a liquid or low-residue diet. The parents should be carefully instructed about any dietary restrictions. Infants who are NPO receive intravenous fluids to prevent dehydration. Close monitoring of the child's fluid status is essential because repeated enemas can result in dehydration or electrolyte imbalance.

SURGICAL MANAGEMENT

Surgical correction generally consists of a series of three operations. Initially, a temporary diverting colostomy is performed in a segment of bowel with normal innervation, often the sigmoid or right transverse colon. The purpose of the colostomy is to provide a period of bowel rest and to provide adequate time for the child to gain weight and achieve an improved nutritional status before the major corrective procedure. Definitive surgical correction is usually performed when the child is from 8 months to 1 year of age or has reached a weight of approximately 20 lb.[53] Common surgical procedures used for the definitive repair include Swenson's procedure, the Duhamel operation, and the Soave approach (also known as an endorectal pull-through). The Soave approach has been reported to be associated with the lowest complication rate, however, the exact surgical approach varies depending on the child's condition and the surgeon's preference. The third and final operation is closure of the colostomy, which is usually performed about 3 months after the definitive repair.[30,53]

Close follow-up between surgical procedures and the definitive correction is essential. Nutritional status must be monitored closely to ensure the child is in a good nutritional state to tolerate surgery. If necessary, the caloric density of formulas should be increased to ensure the child receives adequate calories and protein. The child's height and weight must be measured at each visit. A pediatric dietitian should be consulted if the child fails to gain weight or to maintain growth along a growth percentile.

POSTOPERATIVE CARE

After surgery, nursing care includes routine post-abdominal surgery interventions, such as maintaining nasogastric suction and monitoring for abdominal distention and return of bowel function. Additional nursing interventions include developing a routine for ostomy care and allowing parents sufficient time to become comfortable with care of the ostomy. The parents should observe the nurse performing ostomy care and should be given ample opportunities to demonstrate proficiency and to ask questions. Signs and symptoms of problems associated with the ostomy, such as skin breakdown, difficulty in keeping the appliance securely attached, and increased ostomy output indicating diarrhea, must be discussed with the parents. Additional information about ostomy care is described in Table 59-9.

After the definitive surgical correction and closure of the ostomy, perianal skin denudation can be a frustrating problem. Frequent diaper changes, careful cleansing after each stool, and application of protective ointments help alleviate the skin breakdown. Parents should be instructed about the importance of good skin care.

TEACHING

The nurse should explore the parent's perception of the ostomy and surgery. Often, the parents have many misconceptions, which can be clarified by an explanation of how the ostomy will look and a brief explanation of the care. It is important to stress that the ostomy is temporary and that they will be given adequate time and practice in learning care of the ostomy. Although the idea of a temporary colostomy may help the family adjust to the ostomy, it also necessitates further surgery, which is an added stressor for the child and family.[76]

★ **EVALUATION**

Periodically, the nurse and family evaluate the outcomes of care given. Examples of outcomes for the child with Hirchsprung's disease were given under Planning in this section. Planning for further nursing care also takes into consideration complications and long-term care.

COMPLICATIONS

After surgical correction, the prognosis for a child with Hirschsprung's disease is good. Reported mortality with the Soave procedure ranges from 0 to 1.6.[30,53] Complications that may occur include anastomotic leak, stricture, abscess, diarrhea, persistent constipation, or bowel incontinence (5% to 15% occurrence rate).

LONG-TERM CARE

Unfortunately, readmission to the hospital for surgical correction often occurs at a developmental stage when separation of the child from the parent is most difficult. Allowing the child to keep a familiar toy and providing a tape of the parents' voices helps increase the child's comfort level. Parental visitation is encouraged as much as possible. It is important to explain to the parents that regressive behavior and difficulty in separating are normal.

Malrotation and Volvulus

Etiology and Pathophysiology. Malrotation results from an abnormal rotation of the intestine during embryonic life. Normally, the intestine rotates around the superior mesenteric artery and returns to an intraabdominal position during the 10th week in utero. If the intestine moves abnormally around the superior mesenteric artery, it can cause twisting of the bowel, leading to a duodenal obstruction or may cause an infarction (volvulus) of the bowel if the blood supply is impaired. Volvulus and subsequent bowel ischemia are catastrophic events to the newborn. The area of bowel affected can be extensive and can lead to necrosis of large sections of the small bowel and colon. Malrotation can cause the formation of peritoneal bands or folds that obstruct the bowel.

Clinical Manifestations. Many people may have malrotation and remain asymptomatic throughout their lifetime. Of symptomatic cases, approximately 80% have signs of intestinal obstruction within the first 3 weeks of life.[62] Typically, infants initially feed normally, then develop bilious vomiting, abdominal distention, and the presence of visible peristaltic waves on the abdomen. If volvulus occurs, the infant may rapidly develop bloody or melenic (black, tarry) stools and evidence of sepsis, perforation, and peritonitis. About 20% of symptomatic people develop signs of malrotation during childhood or adulthood.[62] The presenting symptoms may include chronic, intermittent, and cramping abdominal pain associated with vomiting or chronic constipation.

Diagnostic Studies. Diagnosis of malrotation and volvulus is based on the clinical findings and radiographic studies including abdominal x-rays and an upper GI series. If perforation is suspected, barium contrast studies are not performed to avoid barium contamination of the peritoneal cavity.

★ ASSESSMENT

The assessment of the child with malrotation or volvulus includes careful observation for evidence of bowel obstruction, such as bilious vomiting or abdominal distention. Signs of peritonitis, bowel necrosis, or perforation, such as fever, lethargy, severe distention, abdominal firmness, or bloody stools, indicate an urgent situation and are reported immediately to the physician. The onset of symptoms may occur rapidly in a previously healthy appearing child.

★ NURSING DIAGNOSES AND PLANNING

Nursing diagnoses have been discussed under bowel obstructions. Also see this chapter's Nursing Care Plan.

★ INTERVENTIONS: COLLABORATIVE AND INDEPENDENT

Symptomatic malrotation and volvulus are treated surgically. Parents are often frightened at the need for urgent surgery and need thorough explanations of the diagnosis and treatment plan. In cases of volvulus, emergency surgery is performed to reduce the volvulus and assess the viability of the bowel. Perforated or necrotic areas of bowel are resected, but questionably compromised sections of bowel may be left alone. Commonly, a "second-look" operation is performed 36 to 48 hours later to evaluate the bowel further and resect any of the compromised bowel that has continued to deteriorate. If the obstruction is caused by peritoneal bands, the bowel is rotated correctly and the bands and adhesions are divided.

The prognosis for obstruction caused by malrotation and peritoneal bands is good, although there is about a 10% recurrence rate of intestinal obstruction. Gangrene and peritonitis are frequent complications of volvulus, and the mortality rate is about 15%.[62]

Postoperatively, the child requires routine post-abdominal surgery care, with careful observation for development of symptoms of a recurrent bowel obstruction or peritonitis. If an extensive bowel resection is necessary, the absorptive capacity of the bowel is seriously impaired and the child often requires long-term parenteral nutrition.

★ EVALUATION

Periodically, the nurse and family evaluate the outcomes of care given. Examples of outcomes were given under the evaluation section on bowel obstruction.

Meconium Ileus

Meconium ileus is an intestinal obstruction of the newborn in which the intestinal lumen is blocked by thick, tenacious meconium. Meconium ileus most commonly occurs in children with cystic fibrosis. About 10% to 15% of infants with cystic fibrosis develop this ileal obstruction.[11] Approximately 10% of cases of meconium ileus occur in patients without cystic fibrosis.[62] About one third of cases are associated with other GI complications such as volvulus, atresia, pseudocyst formation, or antenatal perforation with peritonitis.

Etiology and Pathophysiology. The thick tenacious consistency of the meconium is speculated to result from a high albumin and macromolecule content. This is probably due to the pancreatic enzyme insufficiency and from the hyposecretion of water and electrolytes from the small intestine, pancreas, and biliary system that is associated with cystic fibrosis. The thickened meconium packs the ileum, causing hypertrophy and dilatation of the bowel wall, which, in turn, leads to distention of the ileum and obstruction. Pelletlike meconium plugs are often found in the distal ileum and colon. Both the distal ileum and colon appear small and unused.[11,62]

Clinical Manifestations. The neonate with meconium ileus generally develops symptoms within the first 24 to 48 hours of life. The predominant symptoms include abdominal distention, disinterest in eating, and bile-stained vomiting. No meconium is passed. Visible peristaltic waves may be evident. Loops or masses may be palpable on the abdomen. Digital rectal examination reveals a small anal canal without the presence of meconium.

Diagnostic Studies. A family history of cystic fibrosis accompanied by evidence of intestinal obstruction is highly suggestive of meconium ileus. Abdominal x-rays are obtained, and findings usually include uneven dilatation of bowel loops, no air–fluid levels, and a bubbly granular appearance in the lower abdomen. If complications are present, interpretation may be difficult and findings may vary. A sweat chloride test must be performed. In a setting with other symptoms consistent with cystic fibrosis, three sequential tests demonstrating chloride concentrations above 60 mEq/L are considered diagnostic of this disease. Because neonates produce insufficient sweat during the first weeks of life, the testing is deferred until 4 to 6 weeks of age.[11,62]

★ ASSESSMENT

The nursing assessment of the infant with meconium ileus is similar to the care with any intestinal obstruction. The infant is observed closely for signs of obstruction, including bilious vomiting and abdominal distention. The parents should be specifically asked about a family history of cystic fibrosis.

★ NURSING DIAGNOSES AND PLANNING

Nursing diagnoses and planning have been discussed in other sections on bowel obstruction. An additional diagnosis may be Knowledge Deficit regarding disease process and implications of cystic fibrosis; ostomy care. For additional nursing diagnoses, refer to this chapter's Nursing Care Plan.

★ INTERVENTIONS: COLLABORATIVE AND INDEPENDENT

Gastrografin enemas successfully relieve the meconium obstruction in approximately over 60% of uncomplicated cases.[8] Gastrografin is highly osmotic and pulls water into the intestine to soften and release the obstruction. The Gastrografin is administered by a radiologist through a rectal catheter under fluoroscopic control and is allowed to slowly fill the distal ileum. A successful enema returns within 4 hours, and the obstruction is cleared. Occasionally, the enema may need to be repeated one or more times, 24 to 48 hours later. The high osmolality of the Gastrografin can lead to a rapid decrease of plasma volume. The child must be well-hydrated before, during, and after the procedure because the osmotic nature of enema solution can cause rapid fluid shifts. Fluid balances must be carefully monitored, including measurements of intake and output, serum electrolytes and osmolality, and hematocrit.[8,62]

Complicated cases of meconium ileus and those cases that are unresponsive to Gastrografin treatment require surgical intervention. During surgery, the obstructed loop is resected and an ileostomy is created. After surgery, the ileostomy is irrigated with Mucomyst (acetylcysteine) to allow liquefaction and evacuation of any remaining meconium. The ileostomy is closed before discharge or several months later.

Postoperatively, the infant requires routine post-abdominal procedure care including NPO status, nasogastric suction, intravenous fluids, and antibiotics. Parenteral nutrition is often started. Feedings are started with small volumes of dilute formula and advanced gradually. If the child is to be discharged before the ileostomy is closed, the parents should observe and practice ostomy care.

Nonoperative management of uncomplicated cases with Gastrografin enemas has few complications when the child is monitored closely. The mortality of surgical repair of a simple meconium ileus is about 20%, whereas the mortality rate associated with complicated cases rises to 40%.[62] Because most cases of meconium ileus are associated with cystic fibrosis, the long-term prognosis depends on the severity of pulmonary disease and other manifestations of cystic fibrosis. If the child with meconium ileus does not have cystic fibrosis, the prognosis is excellent.

If the parents are aware of the implications of a diagnosis of cystic fibrosis, the waiting period until the sweat chloride test is done is often difficult. The nurse can help the parents by encouraging ventilation of feelings and by offering to answer any questions the parents may have. If the diagnosis of cystic fibrosis is confirmed, the child should be referred to an appropriate specialist and the parents should be encouraged to seek genetic counseling.

★ EVALUATION

Periodically, the nurse and family evaluate the outcomes of care given. Examples of outcomes were given in other parts of the evaluation section on bowel obstruction.

Genetic Disorders of the Gastrointestinal Tract

Several diseases that are genetic in origin affect the GI tract. In this section, familial polyposis, Gardner's syndrome, Turcot syndrome, Peutz-Jeghers syndrome, and juvenile polyps are described. The treatment and interventions are discussed together.

Definition

Familial Polyposis. Familial polyposis, an inherited autosomal dominant trait, is characterized by progressive development of hundreds of polyps (adenomas) throughout the colon. The polyps begin to develop after puberty, and the adolescent may remain asymptomatic for several years. The concern for the adolescent with familial polyposis is the incidence of cancer related to the polyposis. Family assessments and genetic counseling play an important role in early diagnosis and treatment of familial polyposis.[11]

Gardner's Syndrome. Gardner's syndrome, a variant of familial polyposis, is also inherited as an autosomal dominant trait. GI polyps, osteomas of the skull, mandible, and long bones, and soft tissue tumors are found in Gardner's syndrome. The intestinal polyps appear in both the large and small bowel and are precancerous lesions. Manifestations of soft tissue tumors of Gardner's syndrome can include cancer of the thyroid, ampulla of Vater, and small intestine. The polyps in the intestines seem to be more scattered than what is seen in familial polyposis.[10,11]

Turcot Syndrome. Turcot syndrome describes a combination of familial polyposis and malignant central nervous system (CNS) tumors. The CNS tumors consist of glioblastomas and medulloblastomas.[10]

Peutz-Jeghers Syndrome. Peutz-Jeghers syndrome includes mucocutaneous pigmentation of the mouth, lips, hands, and feet in addition to multiple polyps in the small and large bowel. The pigmentation usually fades after puberty, with the exception of the discoloration found in the mouth. The polyps are hamartomas (i.e., they develop from glandular epitheliums supported by smooth muscles).

Juvenile Polyps. Juvenile polyps are distinctive hamartomas found in the rectum of children. The polyps do not tend to be precancerous, but may be removed if bleeding, obstruction, or intussusception occurs.[10]

Etiology and Pathophysiology. The term *polyp* refers to a discrete tissue mass that is elevated above the mucosa surface. An adenoma develops from epithelium, myoma from smooth muscle, and hemangioma from blood vessels. The most common type of colon polyp is the adenoma. Adenomas are composed of immature epithelium cells that continue to proliferate. The surface epithelium of undifferentiated cells accumulates and leads to the formation of the polyp. The relationship between polyps and cancer has been developed through longitudinal studies involving subjects with familial polyposis. The development of carcinomas in patients with colonic polyps is usually 10 to 15 years after the appearance of the benign adenomas. In familial polyposis, young people develop hundreds to thousands of colonic polyps. Cancer, in one or more polyps, generally develops before 40 years of age. The non-neoplastic polyps include mucosal polyps, hyperplastic polyps, pseudopolyps of inflammatory bowel disease, and juvenile polyps.

Clinical Manifestations. The most common presenting symptoms of the polyposis include blood in the stool, diarrhea, and cramping abdominal pain. The major concern is diagnosis of asymptomatic adolescents with familial polyposis and Gardner's syndrome because both of these disorders may lead to cancer. A careful family history and assessment of asymptomatic family members are instrumental in identifying children at risk of developing the syndromes. Clinical manifestations in Gardner's syndrome include epidermoid cysts, fibromas, lipomas, desmoid tumors, impacted teeth, mandibular cysts, sebaceous cysts, and bony tumors.

Diagnostic Studies. Diagnosis is established by digital rectal examination, colonoscopy or proctosigmoidoscopy, and air contrast barium enema. Radiography studies are used to identify osteomas found in Gardner's syndrome.

★ INTERVENTIONS: COLLABORATIVE AND INDEPENDENT

When a child is identified as a carrier of the familial trait for one of these disorders, the family is informed of the importance of regular health follow-ups to identify the presence of polyps through diagnostic studies. Colonoscopy with polypectomy may be performed for juvenile polyps or as a regular assessment and management of children with Gardner's syndrome and familial polyposis. If additional symptoms develop, the treatment necessary to manage the rectal bleeding, obstruction, or intussusception should be instituted.

Familial polyposis and Gardner's syndrome may require major abdominal surgery with total colectomy and ileostomy or total colectomy and ileoanal/sphincter saving procedures. A discussion of the care and management of children and adolescents undergoing these procedures is found later in this chapter with the discussion of inflammatory bowel disease.

The nurse must provide adequate education for children and families regarding these disorders, provide genetic counseling, and identify asymptomatic family members who may be at risk for developing problems.

★ EVALUATION

The child and family return for scheduled visits to assess the development or progression of the polyposis. An asymptomatic adolescent should be seen every 6 months for evaluation by colonoscopy for familial polyposis and Gardner's syndrome. The concern for these children is the incidence of colon cancer identified in asymptomatic young adults.

Gastrointestinal Structural Diseases

Pyloric Stenosis

Definition and Incidence. Pyloric stenosis results from a progressive hypertrophy of the circular muscle of the pylorus. This narrowing of the pyloric muscle leads to an obstruction of the gastric outlet causing gastric distention and vomiting. Pyloric stenosis is depicted in Figure 59-6. The incidence of pyloric stenosis has been estimated as 2 to 3 per 1000 births.[62,70] This disorder is one of the most common conditions requiring surgery within the first few months of life. Approximately 80% of cases of pyloric stenosis are found in males.[38]

Etiology and Pathophysiology. The causative mechanisms leading to the increase in size of the pyloric muscle are unclear; however, genetic factors appear to play a role. A familial tendency toward pyloric stenosis has been recognized. In about 5% of cases, there is a positive family history of pyloric stenosis in the father or the siblings.[62] There is a high incidence of pyloric stenosis in infants of mothers with a history of the disease. Development of pyloric stenosis in monozygotic twins and triplets has been reported numerous times. To the hypertrophy of the pyloric muscle causes a progressive obstruction of the stomach and leads to severe vomiting with consequent complications of dehydration, weight loss, and electrolyte disturbances.

Clinical Manifestations. The age of onset and patterns of symptoms are variable, but, in general, vomiting begins between 2 and 4 weeks of age in a healthy infant who eats eagerly. Initially, the vomiting may be intermittent, but it gradually increases in severity and frequency and becomes projectile. Other symptoms may include constipation and jaundice. As the vomiting persists, the infant develops dehydration, electrolyte imbalances, and weight loss. In early stages of the disease, the typical infant is alert and ravenously hungry but appears mildly

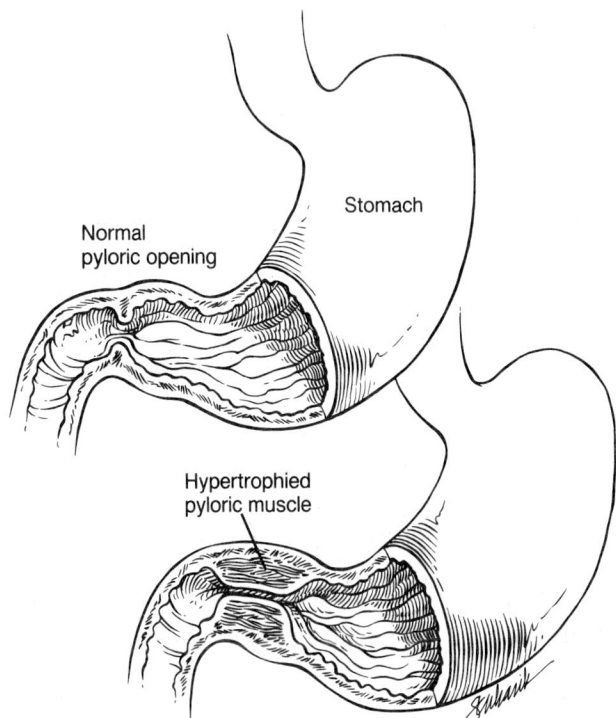

FIGURE 59-6

Normal pyloric opening compared to pyloric stenosis.

dehydrated and malnourished. As the disease progresses, the infant becomes fretful, apathetic, and appears severely dehydrated with loss of skin turgor and dry mucous membranes.[39,62,70]

Diagnostic Studies. The diagnosis of pyloric stenosis is based primarily on the history and physical examination. The characteristic physical findings are a palpable pyloric mass and visible peristaltic waves. The hypertrophied pyloric muscle is best palpated just after the infant vomits and is felt as a mobile, nontender, firm, olive-shaped mass just to the right of the umbilicus. The pyloric "olive" is a classic indicator of pyloric stenosis. Palpation of this mass is considered diagnostic of pyloric stenosis, and further diagnostic procedures are usually not indicated. Peristaltic waves are observed proceeding from the left to the right toward the pylorus and are most noticeable just after a feeding but before vomiting. If the olive-shaped mass is not easily palpated, an upper GI series with barium contrast may be done and generally reveals vigorous peristalsis, delayed gastric emptying, and the characteristic "string sign."[39] The string sign is seen as an elongation and narrowing of the pyloric channel. The degree of narrowing depends on the severity of the pyloric muscle hypertrophy. Ultrasound may also be useful to identify an increased density in the pyloric region.

★ ASSESSMENT

The nursing assessment of the child with pyloric stenosis should include particular attention to the character of vomiting and the infant's fluid status. The character, volume, and color of emesis and the timing in relationship to feedings are noted. Strict intake and output records are kept, and the infant's level of hydration is carefully assessed. The specific gravity of urine is often measured to assess the hydration state.

★ NURSING DIAGNOSES AND PLANNING

Based on the assessment data from above and Chapter 58, the following nursing diagnoses may apply to the child with pyloric stenosis:

- Fluid Volume Deficit related to structural abnormality.
- Altered Nutrition: Less Than Body Requirements related to vomiting.
- High Risk for Wound Infection related to surgery.
- Altered Parenting related to knowledge deficit about disease condition.
- Anxiety related to role functioning.
- Anxiety related to knowledge deficit regarding care of incision; feeding techniques.

The nurse and parents together plan effective care based on the established nursing diagnoses. Several examples of expected outcomes follow:

- The infant tolerates initial postsurgical feeding.
- The parents verbalize their anxiety regarding adequate role functioning.
- The parents resume skills in feeding the infant.

The nurse plans for the daily care of the child based

on both physician's orders and nursing diagnoses. Some general nursing care goals may be the following:

- Fluid and electrolyte balance is stabilized.
- Infection is prevented.

★ INTERVENTIONS: COLLABORATIVE AND INDEPENDENT

The treatment of choice for pyloric stenosis is the surgical procedure of pyloromyotomy to relieve the obstruction caused by the hypertrophied muscle. Before surgery, fluid and electrolyte abnormalities are corrected. The child is placed NPO, intravenous fluids are started, and often a nasogastric tube is inserted to decompress the stomach. The nurse carefully maintains the intravenous infusion of fluids, electrolytes, and glucose. If the child is severely dehydrated, correction of fluid and electrolyte abnormalities may take 24 to 48 hours. Surgery is performed as soon as possible after fluid and electrolyte abnormalities are corrected.

The surgical procedure is done through a small incision just below the right costal margin.[70] Postoperatively, the incision is covered with collodion or a small dressing. The wound must be kept clean and dry and monitored for signs of infection.[55]

The average postoperative stay is 2 to 3 days. Morbidity and mortality are low. Rare complications may include a perforated duodenum with peritonitis or an inadequate correction of the pyloric stenosis requiring further surgical correction.[39,62,70]

Oral feedings are generally resumed within 4 to 6 hours after surgery and gradually progressed over 1 to 2 days. Typically, feedings are started with small volumes (15 ml) of Pedialyte, and the volume is gradually increased. If volumes of 60 to 90 ml are tolerated without vomiting, formula or breast milk feedings are introduced. Most infants experience some postoperative vomiting in the first 24 to 48 hours.[39,62] The nurse carefully monitors the feeding tolerance and reports frequent or continued vomiting. The intravenous infusion is continued until full feedings are well tolerated. Positioning the child in a right side-lying position facilitates gastric emptying.

The sudden onset of pyloric stenosis in a healthy infant and the prompt surgical intervention are often upsetting to parents. The parents may feel they neglected to report vomiting early enough or that their feeding practices may have contributed to the problem. The nurse can help reassure the parents by explaining the physical cause of pyloric stenosis and the typical sudden presentation. After surgery, the nurse should explain to the parents that occasional vomiting is common and encourage the parents to participate in feedings. Often the parents are anxious about feeding the child due to the preoperative experiences. The nurse can alleviate some of the anxiety by staying with the parent during the feeding and offering positive encouragement.

★ EVALUATION

Periodically, the nurse and family evaluate the outcomes of care given. Examples of outcomes for the child with pyloric stenosis were given under Planning in this section.

Have short-term goals been met? Are long-term goals still realistic?

Intussusception

Definition and Incidence.   Intussusception occurs when one portion of the intestine invaginates or telescopes into another portion (Fig. 59-7). Most commonly, the intussusception begins at the ileocecal valve as the ileum invaginates into the cecum and colon. This form of intussusception is known as ileocolic. Other less common forms of this disorder include ileoileal, in which one portion of the ileum telescopes into another portion of the ileum, and colocolic, in which one section of colon invaginates into another portion of the colon. Intussusception is one of the most common forms of intestinal obstruction during infancy and generally affects children between the ages of 3 months and 2 years. Occasional cases are seen in the neonatal period or in older children. The disorder is three times more common in males than in females.[62,67]

Etiology and Pathophysiology.   A specific cause of the intussusception cannot be identified in the majority

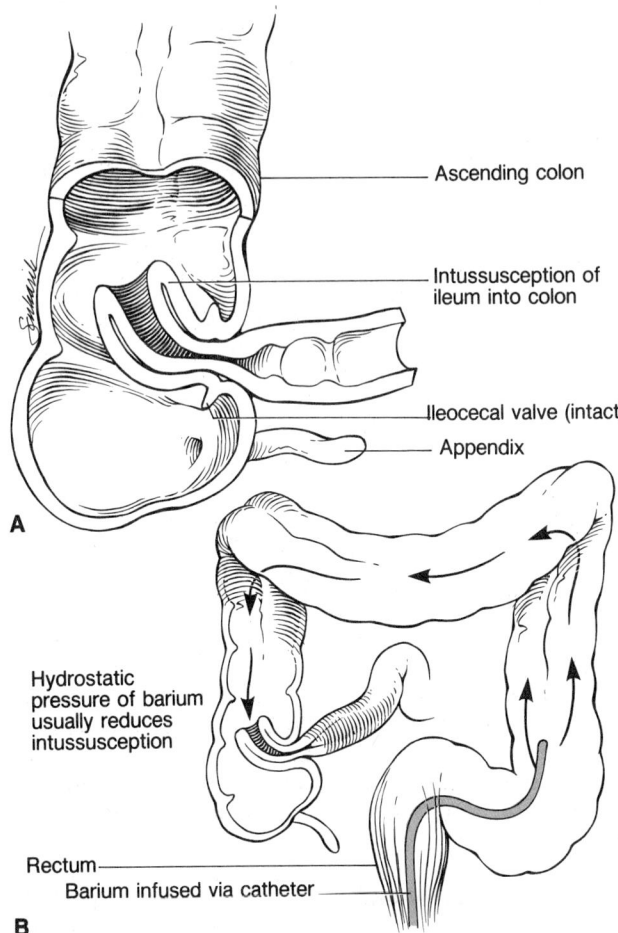

FIGURE 59-7

(A) Intussusception. (B) Schematic of colon showing how barium reduces the intussusception.

of cases. In about 5% to 6% of cases, a specific lesion such as Meckel's diverticulum, polyps, lymphosarcoma, or a foreign body can be identified as a probable trigger of the invagination.[62,70] Intussusception occurs fairly commonly among children with cystic fibrosis and has been linked to inspissated (thickened) fecal material in the ileum, appendix, or colon.[62] Many cases of intussusception occur in association with infections such as otitis media, upper respiratory infections, and rotoviral infections, which suggests a possible viral etiology.

As one portion of the intestine invaginates into another, the intestinal walls press against each other and compress the blood vessels, causing an impairment of the blood supply. The compression leads to inflammation and edema of the intestinal mucosa. If this process continues, hemorrhage and necrosis develop and perforation and peritonitis occur.[62]

Clinical Manifestations.   Intussusception classically presents as an acute and sudden onset of abdominal pain in a normal thriving infant. Characteristically, the infant suddenly screams and draws his knees up toward his chest. The episodes of pain often occur at intervals interspersed with periods when the child appears relatively normal and comfortable. Vomiting usually occurs, and the child often passes a normal stool, evacuating the colon distal to the obstruction. As the disease progresses, the infant becomes more irritable, lethargic, apathetic, and may pass currant-jelly stools (loose, red stools mixed with blood and mucus). The abdomen becomes tender and distended. Palpation of the abdomen may reveal a sausage-shaped mass in the upper abdomen and an unusual emptiness in the right lower quadrant. As the child's condition worsens, vomiting continues, becoming profuse and stained with bile or fecal material. The infant is typically febrile and develops signs of shock, dehydration, and peritonitis if perforation occurs.

As mentioned, the characteristic signs of intussusception are bilious vomiting and sudden abdominal pain, which typically appears as waves of severe pain. Bloody stools are an ominous sign that appears late in the progression of the disease. However, the diagnosis may be difficult or delayed if the disease presents with unusual or confusing symptoms such as diarrhea, constipation, or recurrent attacks of colicky abdominal pain with occasional vomiting. The latter symptom may indicate a chronic recurrent intussusception that spontaneously reduces itself. Failure to recognize and treat intussusception early is associated with serious consequences, so it is important to be alert to typical and unusual signs of this disorder and ensure the child with potential intussusception is referred for further medical intervention.[62,67,70]

Diagnostic Studies.   The clinical presentation often provides convincing evidence for the diagnosis of intussusception, but the definitive diagnosis is based on a barium enema. The barium enema usually clearly outlines the intussusception within the bowel lumen and often successfully reduces the invagination. Before performing the barium enema, the child is prepared for surgery, because immediate surgery is indicated if the intussusception is not reduced by the barium enema.

★ **ASSESSMENT**

The nursing assessment includes careful attention to the parent's report of the child's behavior. The parents often can provide an excellent description of the onset of symptoms. Ongoing assessment is essential. The nurse frequently monitors vital signs and assesses the child for evidence of worsening abdominal pain or perforation, and monitors the number and appearance of stools. Passage of more than one normal stool may indicate spontaneous resolution of the intussusception, whereas passage of increasingly bloody stools is an ominous sign indicating possible perforation.

★ **NURSING DIAGNOSES AND PLANNING**

Based on the assessment data from above and Chapter 58, the following nursing diagnoses may apply to the child with intussusception:

- Altered Gastrointestinal Tissue Perfusion related to physical abnormality.
- Acute Abdominal Pain related to disease process.
- High Risk for Infection (peritonitis) related to high risk for perforation.
- Anxiety related to knowledge deficit regarding intussusception disease process; mechanism of barium enema reduction; signs of further obstruction.

The nurse and child (or parents) together plan effective care based on the established nursing diagnoses. Several examples of expected outcomes follow:

- The infant passes normal stools.
- The parents state they understand the description of intussusception and its reduction.

The nurse plans the care for the child based on both physician's orders and nursing diagnoses. Some general nursing care goals are:

- Fluid and electrolyte balance is stabilized.
- Deterioration in infant's condition is prevented.

★ **INTERVENTIONS: COLLABORATIVE AND INDEPENDENT**

As soon as the diagnosis is suspected, the child is placed NPO and nasogastric suction and intravenous hydration are started. Intravenous antibiotics, blood, and albumin may be required if signs of shock or peritonitis are present. The majority of cases of intussusception can be treated successfully by hydrostatic reduction of the invagination by the barium enema. The diagnostic enema is continued and, as the barium flows into the bowel, it exerts sufficient pressure to push the invaginated portion of the bowel back to the original position. Reduction of the intussusception by barium enema is contraindicated if perforation or peritonitis is suspected. Surgical treatment is indicated if signs of peritonitis or shock are present, if hydrostatic reduction is unsuccessful (about 25% of cases), or if the child's condition fails to improve despite apparently successful reduction. Surgical manage-

ment includes manual reduction of the intussusception and, if indicated, resection of any necrotic bowel. The overall mortality associated with intussusception is low, 1% to 2%. Untreated cases are fatal.[62,70]

The parents may have difficulty picturing the intussusception. Using a visual aid such as a surgical glove with an invaginated finger may help the parents visualize the telescoping process. Filling the glove with water helps to depict the hydrostatic reduction of the intussusception.

After hydrostatic reduction, the nurse observes the child closely for the passage of stool or barium and for evidence of a recurrent intussusception. Recurrence develops in less than 10% of children and is usually seen within 36 to 48 hours of hydrostatic reduction.[62]

If the child requires surgery, routine post-abdominal surgery care is indicated. The nurse observes closely for evidence of further bowel obstruction.

★ **EVALUATION**

Periodically, the nurse and family evaluate the outcomes of care given. Examples of outcomes for the child with intussusception were given under Planning in this section.

Gastroesophageal Reflux

Definition and Incidence. Gastroesophageal reflux (GER) results from incompetence or immaturity of the lower esophageal sphincter, which allows return of stomach contents into the esophagus. Many infants experience some degree of regurgitation and reflux due to immature neuromuscular function of the lower esophageal sphincter. This reflux is considered normal and typically disappears without any active therapy. Studies of the natural course of the disorder have shown that, without any specific therapy, the majority of infants with GER were symptom-free by 18 months of age. Unfortunately, approximately 5% to 30% continued to manifest troublesome symptoms. GER is more common among premature infants, children with neurologic problems, cystic fibrosis, or esophageal atresia and tracheoesophageal fistula.[59,62]

Etiology and Pathophysiology. The causative mechanism of GER is not understood, but immaturity of neuromuscular function and impaired neurohormonal control of the lower esophagus and esophageal sphincter have been suggested as causative factors. Reflux of the acidic gastric contents into the esophagus may irritate the esophageal mucosa causing esophagitis. If gastric contents are aspirated into the lungs, chronic respiratory symptoms such as recurrent aspiration pneumonia, chronic coughing and wheezing, and asthmalike attacks may be seen.[62,66] Delayed gastric emptying has been increasingly recognized in association with GER and may aggravate the symptoms and complicate medical and surgical treatment.[20]

Clinical Manifestations. The pattern of emesis in GER is characterized by an initial effortless regurgitation of formula followed by more forceful vomiting. Older children may complain of chest pain or heartburn, whereas infants may become extremely irritable and fussy after vomiting. In a small number of cases, the volume and frequency of emesis are large enough to result in weight loss and failure to thrive. The acidity of the re-fluxed material can lead to esophagitis associated with occult blood loss, hematemesis, iron-deficiency anemia, and esophageal strictures. GER with chronic aspiration is associated with respiratory symptoms such as chronic cough, pneumonia, wheezing, and asthma-like attacks. Respiratory complications are most common in infants under 1 year of age and in children with diseases of the CNS or with mental retardation.[59,62]

Diagnostic Studies. Parents are frequently con-cerned if their infant spits up or vomits. A careful history and observation of the child's feeding habits are important parts of the diagnostic evaluation. Infants who demon-strate normal growth and show no signs of respiratory illness or other complications should merely be observed over time, and the parents should be reassured that some regurgitation is normal and that the child will outgrow the vomiting. Children who demonstrate delayed growth, chronic respiratory illness, or occult blood in the stools or emesis deserve further investigation for GER.[62] Com-mon diagnostic tests used to evaluate GER include a bar-ium swallow, *p*H monitoring of the esophagus, and gas-troesophageal scintigraphy.[66]

★ ASSESSMENT

The nursing assessment includes a thorough history of the infant's feeding behavior and the parents' feeding practices. Specifically, the nurse should inquire about the position the child is held in during feeding, how often he burps, or if choking, coughing, or color changes occur during the feeding. The parents are asked to describe any methods they use to help alleviate the vomiting. Often the parents have tried a number of approaches to no avail and are frustrated and may doubt their parenting skills. Explaining the physical cause of the disease and the di-agnostic tests helps reassure the parents and increase their understanding and cooperation with the treatment plan.

★ NURSING DIAGNOSES AND PLANNING

Based on the assessment data from above and Chapter 58, the following nursing diagnoses may apply to the child with GER:

- Altered Nutrition: Less Than Body Requirements related to vomiting.
- Ineffective Airway Clearance related to obstruction.
- Impaired Gas Exchange related to gastric contents in lungs.
- Altered Growth and Development related to nutritional deficiency.
- Altered Parenting related to knowledge deficit of proper feeding and burping.
- Anxiety related to perceived inadequate role func-tioning.
- Anxiety related to knowledge deficit regarding feeding and positioning techniques; medication regimen; gas-trostomy care.

The nurse and child (or parents) together plan ef-fective care based on the established nursing diagnoses. Several examples of expected outcomes follow:

- The infant retains formula.
- The infant maintains normal growth and development measured by height and weight.
- The parents verbalize their feelings of inadequacy.
- The parents state proper techniques for gastrostomy care.

The nurse plans for the daily care of the child based on both physician's orders and nursing diagnoses. Some general nursing care goals may be the following:

- The infant tolerates adequate feeding.
- The parents demonstrate comfort in feeding and burping.

★ INTERVENTIONS: COLLABORATIVE AND INDEPENDENT

The goal of treatment is to protect the esophagus and the lungs from gastric contents and to promote adequate in-take and retention of formula.[62] Conservative medical management using diet modifications, medications, and positioning maneuvers is successful in most cases and is almost always attempted before surgical treatment is con-sidered. Diet therapy includes thickening of the formula and offering small volumes of formula more frequently.

MEDICATION THERAPY

Drug therapy may include the use of antacids and ci-metidine (Tagamet) to neutralize the gastric acid and de-crease the hydrochloric acid secretion. Another medi-cation, bethanechol, may be used to increase the muscle tone of the lower esophageal sphincter. The increased tone of the sphincter muscle helps to prevent regurgi-tation of formula and gastric acids into the esophagus. For best results, bethanechol should be given 30 minutes before a feeding. Metoclopramide (Reglan) is another medication used to treat GER. Metoclopramide stimulates the smooth muscle of the stomach and relaxes the pyloric valve, improving gastric emptying. This medication is most effective if given 30 minutes before a feeding.[1] Re-glan may have undesirable extrapyramidal side-effects such as facial twitches, eye rolling, and unusual hand movements. Parents should be warned to report these symptoms promptly.

The nurse monitors the infant's response to the treat-ment plan. If vomiting occurs, the character, frequency, color, and volume are recorded. The parents are in-structed about the importance of giving the medications as scheduled. If the formula is thickened, the parents are taught how to prepare the formula. It may be necessary to enlarge the hole in the nipple slightly. The hole should be just large enough to allow the formula to flow readily as the infant sucks but not so large that the formula flows out rapidly.

SURGICAL MANAGEMENT

The majority of infants respond well to medical treatment only and are symptom-free and off treatment by 18 months of age. Surgical intervention is indicated when the symp-toms are not relieved by medical therapy. The most common surgical technique is the Nissen fundoplication. This procedure involves displacement of the distal segment of the esophagus below the diaphragm and wrapping of a portion of the stomach around the segment to improve the function of the lower esophageal sphincter. A gastrostomy tube is placed for venting of the stomach and is used for initial feedings. Children who have delayed gastric emptying in addition to GER may also require a pyloroplasty (revision of pylorus at gastric outlet) to improve gastric emptying. These procedures are associated with low morbidity and mortality and have proven successful in the relief of recurrent vomiting. A marked improvement in pulmonary symptoms and growth rates also has been noted. Complications of the Nissen fundoplication may include gastric bloating, dumping syndrome, or accidental damage to the vagus nerve.[20,56,62]

If surgical intervention in necessary, the infant requires routine post-abdominal surgery care. Feedings are gradually reintroduced through the gastrostomy tube. The nurse carefully monitors feeding tolerance and reports any emesis. Often, the parents are anxious or fearful of feeding their infant due to previous experiences with vomiting or choking. The nurse can help alleviate the anxiety by demonstrating the feeding process and offering positive reinforcement to the parents. The parents are encouraged to participate in feedings to ensure they are comfortable feeding their child before discharge.

POSITIONING

Recent research has shown that positioning the child prone with the body inclined 30 degrees may decrease reflux. Commercially produced harnesses are available to facilitate this positioning.[1] The infant is placed gently in the harness for 1 to 2 hours after feedings. Allowing the child to fall asleep on the parent's shoulder before placing him in the harness may be helpful. Patting the infant gently on the back and talking softly often soothes the infant if he is fussy or irritable. If the child is awake, visual, auditory, and tactile stimulation should be provided because the child is less mobile and less able to seek the stimulation on his own. Appropriate stimulation includes brightly colored toys within the infant's reach, a hanging mobile or mirror within the child's field of vision, or soft music on a radio or music box. The child usually outgrows the harness by the age of 4 to 5 months. Positioning the infant in a high chair provides similar upright positioning once the child has the muscular strength to sit alone. Infant seats are not used for positioning. When placed in infant seats after feeding, infants have been shown to have significantly more episodes of reflux than infants placed in a prone position.[41] The increased reflux may be due to the position of the esophagus when the infant slouches down in the seat. If a positioning harness is not used, the infant is placed in a prone position with the head turned to the side to prevent aspiration.

★ EVALUATION

Periodically, the nurse and family evaluate the outcomes of care given. Examples of outcomes for the child with GER were given under Planning in this section. The child's height and weight are monitored during follow-up visits to ensure adequate calories and protein are being consumed.

Hernias

A hernia occurs when an organ or portion of an organ protrudes through the wall of a cavity that ordinarily contains it. In children, most hernias occur due to the failure of a normal opening to close during development, either in utero or in the first months of life. Inguinal hernias are by far the most common congenital hernia. Other hernias observed in children include diaphragmatic hernias and umbilical hernias.

Diaphragmatic Hernias

Definition and Incidence.   A diaphragmatic hernia is characterized by the presence of abdominal organs in the thoracic cavity above the diaphragm. The herniated organs may include the stomach, the small or large intestine, and occasionally the liver or spleen. The most common type of diaphragmatic hernia occurs through a defect in the posterolateral portion of the diaphragm (foramen of Bochdalek). A much less common type (less than 2%) occurs through a retrosternal defect (foramen of Morgagni). The incidence of diaphragmatic hernia is estimated as 1 per 4000 live births.[62]

Etiology and Pathophysiology.   The cause of diaphragmatic hernia is unknown. Between the 8th and 10th weeks of fetal life, the diaphragm is formed and divides the coelomic cavity into the abdominal and thoracic components. At this same time, the GI tract elongates and protrudes into the umbilical pouch, then rotates and gradually returns to the abdominal cavity. A disruption of either of these two closely related processes may lead to a diaphragmatic hernia.

The herniated abdominal contents cause pulmonary compression and inhibit differentiation of the lung buds, impairing development of the lungs, resulting in pulmonary hypoplasia. The first breath of a normal infant expands the lungs, leading to a lower pulmonary vascular resistance, increased blood flow to the lungs, and closure of the foramen ovale and ductus arteriosus. In diaphragmatic hernia, the pulmonary hypoplasia and compression of lung tissue by the abdominal contents increase pulmonary vascular pressure, resulting in a right-to-left shunt. The blood that should flow through the right atrium and ventricle to the lungs for oxygenation encounters resistance due to the pulmonary hypertension. This resistance causes the blood to shunt through the patent foramen ovale to the left atrium and ventricle and out to the general circulation. This path of blood flow bypasses the lungs, resulting in severe cyanosis.[22]

Clinical Manifestations.   Most cases of diaphragmatic hernia present within the first 24 hours of life; however, the signs and symptoms vary depending on the size and location of the defect. Often, the infant appears normal at birth but rapidly develops dyspnea and cyanosis as gas fills the herniated bowel. The child may require resuscitation immediately after birth. If spontaneous respirations are established, the breathing pattern is characterized by deep and labored respirations, which are often gasping and irregular and associated with deep sternal and costal retractions. The abdomen may appear flat or scaphoid, and tinkling bowel sounds may be heard over the thorax. Percussion of the thorax often reveals dullness over the portion where lung tissue is located and tympany over the other portions where bowel tissue has migrated. A mediastinal shift occurs, and the heart and the point of maximal cardiac impulse are displaced to the side opposite the lesion. Although the predominant sign is respiratory distress, signs of intestinal obstruction may also occur. Alterations in cardiac output may lead to cool extremities and diminished peripheral pulses. If the defect is small, clinical signs may not be present for hours or days after birth and may be less severe.[46,57,60,62]

Diagnostic Studies. The diagnosis of diaphragmatic hernia is based primarily on clinical symptoms and the physical examination. A chest x-ray is performed to confirm the diagnosis.

★ ASSESSMENT

Early recognition and treatment of diaphragmatic hernia reduce morbidity and mortality. A thorough nursing assessment often allows early detection of this disorder. Progressive respiratory distress, cyanosis, and unusual findings on the abdominal and chest examination such as a scaphoid abdomen, bowel sounds over the thorax, and shifted heart sounds are strongly suggestive of diaphragmatic hernia and must be reported immediately.[46]

★ NURSING DIAGNOSES AND PLANNING

Based on the assessment data from above and Chapter 58, the following nursing diagnoses may apply to the child with diaphragmatic hernia:

- Impaired Gas Exchange related to ventilation/perfusion imbalance.
- Altered Cardiopulmonary Tissue Perfusion related to exchange problems.
- High Risk for Impaired Skin Integrity related to altered circulation.
- Sensory/Perception Alterations related to reduction of all stimuli.
- High Risk for Infection related to treatment.
- Impaired Physical Mobility related to restrictions on breathing.
- Ineffective Family Coping: Compromised related to emotional conflicts regarding illness.
- Altered Parenting related to unmet bonding and attachment needs.
- Anxiety related to fear of impending death.

Other functionally related nursing diagnoses are discussed in this chapter's Nursing Care Plan.

The nurse and parents together plan effective care based on the established nursing diagnoses. Several examples of expected outcomes follow:

- The parents verbalize their anxiety.

- The parents demonstrate techniques for bonding and attachment during this stressful period.

The nurse plans for the daily care of the child based on both physician's orders and nursing diagnoses. Some general nursing care goals may be the following:

- Skin is kept clean and dry.
- Passive range of motion (ROM) exercise is provided.
- Physical contact is limited to reduce stress.

★ INTERVENTIONS: COLLABORATIVE AND INDEPENDENT

Immediately after diagnosis, the infant is treated symptomatically. The child is endotracheally intubated, and oxygen is administered to relieve the respiratory distress. A nasogastric tube is placed to continuous suction to decompress the bowel. Surgical correction of the defect is performed as soon as possible. An abdominal approach is generally used to allow for exploration for volvulus, malrotation, or peritoneal bands and for stretching of the abdominal musculature if necessary.

After surgery, a chest tube is used to decompress the pleural space and to allow for expansion of the lung, which is often atelectatic or hypoplastic.[57,62] Blood gases are monitored frequently. Approximately half of the infants born with diaphragmatic hernia respond well to corrective surgery and to additional treatments including hyperventilation, paralysis with neuromuscular blocking agents, sedation with narcotics, and the use of pulmonary vasodilators, which help to expand the lung tissue and decrease stress on the patient. Other infants do not respond well to these treatment measures and may be candidates for extracorporeal membrane oxygenation (ECMO). ECMO is generally considered a last resort measure and is used in critically ill infants. Essentially, ECMO works as an artificial lung by diverting the pulmonary blood flow out of the body by way of a catheter inserted into the right atrium through a oxygenator and returning the oxygenated blood to the vascular system. The ECMO system is pictured in Figure 59-8. ECMO is a high-risk therapy associated with serious potential dangers including systemic emboli, intercranial hemorrhage, injury to the carotid artery, and infection.[22,46]

The prognosis depends on the promptness and excellence of diagnosis and intervention, the extent of hypoplasia of the lung, and the presence of associated anomalies. Mortality has been reported to be as high as 30% to 60%.[62] Nursing care of all infants with diaphragmatic hernia includes close observation of respiratory and circulatory status. Some centers advocate dramatically limiting the stress to which the infant is subjected. Stress reduction measures include sedation with fentanyl, ventilator support, and limiting physical contact and treatment measures to essential procedures only.[46] If a child receives ECMO therapy, nursing management includes close observation of respiratory and neurologic status, and maintenance of strict aseptic technique with the vascular catheters used with the ECMO circuit. To prevent complications from the immobilization and severe edema associated with ECMO therapy, careful attention should be paid to all pressure points to prevent skin breakdown.

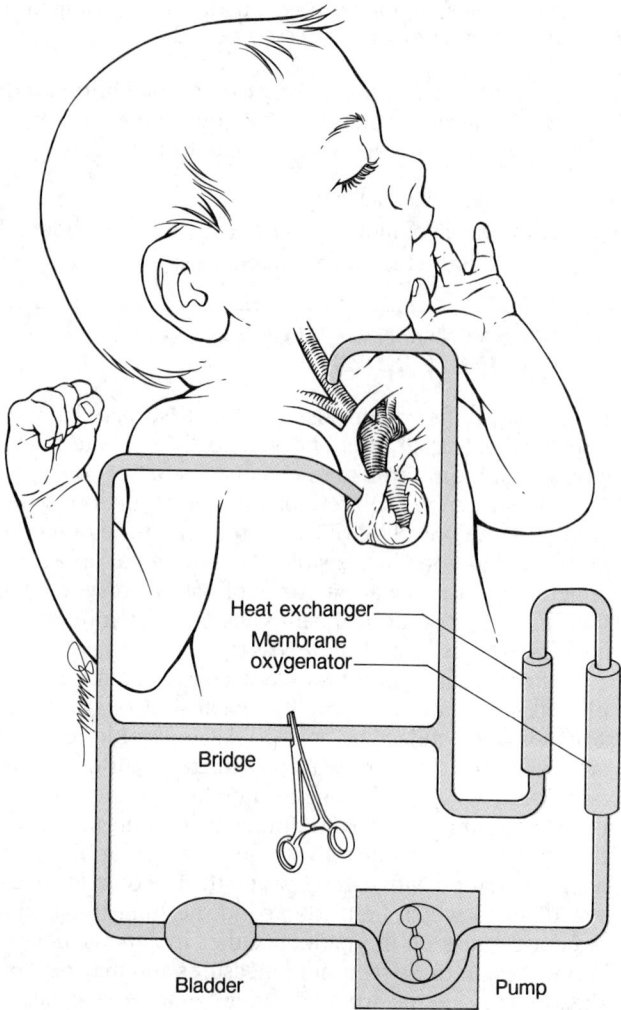

FIGURE 59-8

Extracorporeal membrane oxygenation (ECMO). Unoxygenated blood drains out of the right atrium (**A**). Blood passes through a bladder (**B**) that monitors volume. A pump (**C**) pushes the blood up toward the oxygenator. Blood passes through the oxygenator and warmer (**D**). Blood then flows into the right carotid artery (**E**).

The infant's skin should be kept clean and dry, and passive ROM exercise should be provided if tolerated.[22]

The unexpected birth of a child with diaphragmatic hernia and the subsequent emergency surgery and intensive care measures are extremely stressful for the family. Honest explanations of the child's condition and treatment measures with the encouragement of attachment behaviors (such as bringing a stuffed toy for the child) may help the family to cope with this difficult experience.

★ **EVALUATION**

Periodically, the nurse and family evaluate the outcomes of care given. Examples of outcomes for the child with diaphragmatic hernia were given under Planning in this section.

Prenatal surgeries on fetuses identified with diaphragmatic hernias have been reported with mixed success. The defect was corrected in utero, and the infants were carried to term. The impact of this experimental surgery on the early diagnosis of this disorder and the effects of treatment on the family need to be evaluated in the near future.

Inguinal Hernia

Definition and Incidence. Inguinal hernia repair is the most common operative procedure performed by pediatric surgeons. The exact incidence of inguinal hernia is unknown, due to the difficulties in tracing large populations of infants. The condition occurs more frequently in premature infants, especially low birthweight infants weighing less than 1000 g. Boys are affected much more frequently than girls, with ratios reported to be 8:1. Inguinal hernias appear as a mass in the inguinal area caused by a protrusion of a portion of the abdominal contents into an open sac, which normally closes after birth. Most cases present within the first year of life. In premature infants, the peak incidence occurs at the expected full term of gestation.[54] Inguinal hernias are the most common cause of intestinal obstruction in infants from 1 week of life to 4 months of age.[62]

Etiology and Pathophysiology. An inguinal hernia can occur when there is a persistent opening (processus vaginalis) into the inguinal canal. The processus vaginalis is a fold of peritoneum that precedes the testicle as it descends through the inguinal canal into the scrotum. Ordinarily, the proximal portion of the processus vaginalis atrophies and closes the opening, whereas the distal portion envelopes the testicle and forms the tunica vaginalis.[76] If the opening fails to close, abdominal fluid or contents can be forced into it, creating a palpable mass. The opening is present at birth; however, the hernia is symptomless until sufficient intraabdominal pressure forces abdominal contents into the sac. Most often, the small intestine herniates into the sac, but the appendix, a Meckel's diverticulum, a fallopian tube, or ovary may also be found in the hernial sac.[62] The formation of an inguinal hernia is pictured in Figure 59-9. Inguinal hernias most commonly occur on the right side, but left-sided and bilateral hernias also occur.[60] Bilateral hernias are more common in low birthweight or premature infants.[54]

Clinical Manifestations. Typically, the hernia is first noted by the parent as a painless swelling in the inguinal area. The swelling increases when the child coughs, cries, or stands and often disappears at rest. Usually, the herniated portion returns into the abdominal cavity if mild external pressure is exerted on the mass.

If the hernia cannot be manually reduced, it is considered incarcerated. Incarceration is usually associated with diminished blood supply to the herniated bowel and partial or complete intestinal obstruction. The mass is tender and painful, and the child may cry intermittently or continuously. Nausea, vomiting, and abdominal distention are commonly associated with incarceration.

Diagnostic Studies. The diagnosis of inguinal hernia is based on the physical examination and the parents' report. The scrotum is palpated gently during the examination to assess for the presence of fluid (hydrocele),

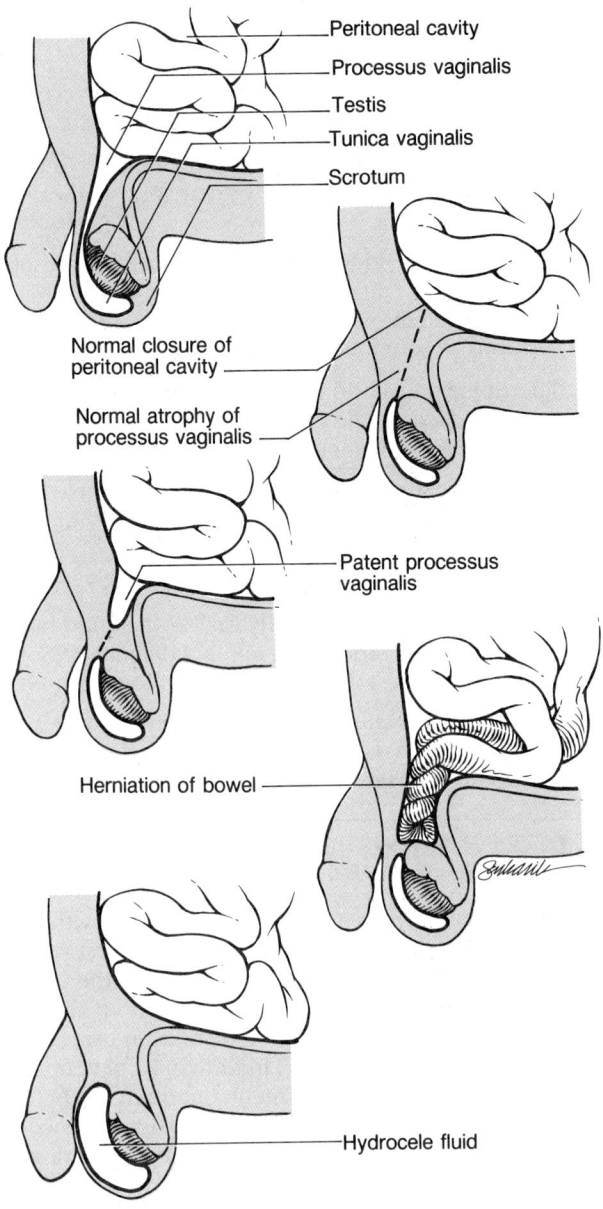

Peritoneal cavity
Processus vaginalis
Testis
Tunica vaginalis
Scrotum

Normal closure of peritoneal cavity

Normal atrophy of processus vaginalis

Patent processus vaginalis

Herniation of bowel

Hydrocele fluid

FIGURE 59-9
Inguinal hernia.

the presence of descended testes, for tenderness, and to determine the reducibility of the lesion.

★ ASSESSMENT

Parents often notice swelling in the inguinal area and mention it to the nurse during a routine examination. If the mass appears to come and go and does not appear to be painful, the parents are often uncertain of the significance of the swelling. A history of how often the mass is noted and the ease of reducibility should be elicited. An explanation of how the hernia can appear and disappear helps to assure the parents that their observations are accurate.

★ NURSING DIAGNOSES AND PLANNING

Based on the assessment data from above and Chapter 58, the following nursing diagnoses may apply to the child with inguinal hernia:

- Altered Gastrointestinal Tissue Perfusion related to interruption of arterial and venous flow.
- High Risk for Wound Infection related to surgery.
- Anxiety related to feelings of inadequacy regarding role functioning.
- Anxiety related to knowledge deficit regarding disease process; incisional care.

Other functionally related nursing diagnoses are discussed in this chapter's Nursing Care Plan.

The nurse and parents together plan effective care based on the established nursing diagnoses. Several examples of expected outcomes follow:

- The parents state they understand procedures for repair.
- The child resumes normal activities postoperatively.

The nurse plans for the daily care of the child based on both physician's orders and nursing diagnoses. Some general nursing care goals may be the following:

- Bowel obstruction is prevented.

★ INTERVENTIONS: COLLABORATIVE AND INDEPENDENT

The primary treatment for inguinal hernia is prompt surgical repair (herniorrhaphy), unless severe prematurity or another condition precludes surgery. In premature infants and in the case of left-sided hernias, the opposite side is generally explored to evaluate for a persistently open processus vaginalis. Some controversy exists as to the advisability of exploration of the opposite side in the case of right-sided hernias.[54,62]

If the hernia is suspected to be incarcerated, the infant is sedated and manual reduction is attempted. The child is placed in Trendelenburg's position with an icebag on the affected side, and gentle manual pressure is applied to the hernial sac. Surgical repair is performed after 48 hours. This waiting period allows edema to subside before repair. Immediate surgical repair is indicated if the incarceration cannot be manually reduced or if evidence of gangrenous or perforated bowel exists. Warning signs of perforation include continuous crying, vomiting, abdominal distention, bloody stools, or local redness and edema.[62]

Surgical repair of uncomplicated hernias is often done on an outpatient basis in a day surgery setting. The prognosis after repair is excellent; serious sequelae develop only rarely. The most common complications are respiratory distress and apnea (possibly related to the anesthesia and intubation during surgery) and are seen most commonly in premature infants. Wound infection or hematoma, testicular infarction or atrophy, and recurrent hernia may also occur.[60,62]

Although surgical repair of an uncomplicated hernia is considered a minor procedure by health professionals, parents are often frightened to consider that their healthy appearing child has a condition that requires surgery. The parents' concerns should be acknowledged, and the rationale for performing the procedure as a preventive measure (to prevent incarceration) should be explained.

After surgery, recovery is usually uneventful. Activity is not restricted. The wound is often covered with collodion and must be kept as clean and dry as possible to prevent infection. Frequent diaper changes or leaving the infant undiapered helps to keep the incision dry. The parents are instructed to observe for redness or drainage as warning signs of infection.[55,76] Premature infants may be admitted to the hospital overnight and placed on an apnea monitor as a precautionary measure.

After surgical reduction of an incarcerated hernia, the child is observed closely for evidence of peritonitis or bowel obstruction. Routine postoperative care generally includes intravenous fluids, antibiotics, and nasogastric suction, which is continued until bowel function returns.

★ EVALUATION

Periodically, the nurse and family evaluate the outcomes of care given. Examples of outcomes for the child with inguinal hernia were given under Planning in this section.

Umbilical Hernia

Definition and Incidence. A hernial protrusion near the umbilicus is a common defect. Approximately 40% of African-American children under 1 year of age have a detectable umbilical hernia.[62] There is an increased incidence in premature infants. Umbilical hernia is commonly seen in association with congenital diseases such as hypothyroidism, trisomy 18, and Beckwith's syndrome.

Etiology and Pathophysiology. An umbilical hernia results from an incomplete fascial closure of the umbilical ring. The umbilical ring is an embryonic structure through which the umbilical blood vessels pass in utero. Ordinarily, this ring closes spontaneously and gradually after birth. Incomplete closure of the ring allows protrusion of the omentum and intestine through the opening.[76]

Fortunately, umbilical hernias seldom cause physiologic problems. Incarceration is rare (1 in 1500 umbilical hernias). Excessive thinning of the skin with progressive enlargement of the fascial defect is uncommon but may be seen if there is increased intraabdominal pressure such as with ascites.

Clinical Manifestations. The hernia appears as a soft swelling or protrusion covered by skin and subcutaneous tissue. The size of the underlying fascial defect varies from 0.5 to 4 cm, whereas the actual protrusion may vary in size from that of a fingertip to that of an orange. The hernia often increases in size with crying or straining. Ordinarily, the hernia is easily reduced, often with a gurgling sound.[62,67]

Diagnostic Studies. The medical diagnosis is based primarily on the history and physical examination. If the defect is large, a plain abdominal x-ray may be ordered.

★ ASSESSMENT

Nursing assessment should include an evaluation of the size and softness of the defect. Symptoms to be reported promptly include a hard, tender hernia; excessively thin skin covering the defect; or symptoms of a bowel obstruction such as bilious vomiting or abdominal distention.

★ NURSING DIAGNOSES AND PLANNING

Based on the assessment data from above and Chapter 58, the following nursing diagnoses may apply to the child with umbilical hernia:

- Disturbance in Body Image related to presence of a hernia.
- Anxiety related to knowledge deficit regarding nature of normal resolution of umbilical hernia.

The nurse and child (or parents) together plan effective care based on the established nursing diagnoses. Several examples of expected outcomes follow:

- Parents verbalize their concerns regarding the hernia.
- The parents exhibit reassurance of the benign condition.
- The parents state the techniques of their care of the child.

The nurse plans for the daily care of the child based on both physician's orders and nursing diagnoses. Some general nursing care goals may be the following:

- The hernia ring closes spontaneously and unnecessary surgery is avoided.
- Child's body image is intact.

★ INTERVENTIONS: COLLABORATIVE AND INDEPENDENT

Most umbilical hernias resolve spontaneously with progressive closure of the fascial ring within the first year of life. If the fascial defect is less than 0.5 cm, the hernia almost always resolves before 2 years of age. If the ring defect is between 0.5 and 1.5 cm, resolution usually occurs by 4 years of age. Defects larger than 2 cm generally disappear slowly without treatment, but often not before the child reaches school age. Corrective surgery is commonly advised if the fascial defect exceeds 1.5 cm at 2 years of age.[67] Some evidence indicates that many of the hernias that are still present at 4 to 5 years of age will still resolve spontaneously by the time the child is 11 years old. Therefore, surgery is not always advocated unless the hernia is psychologically upsetting to the child or parents.[62] Hernias that become incarcerated or are associated with abdominal pain require surgical repair. An uncomplicated repair may be done on an outpatient basis and is seldom associated with complications or recurrences.[7]

Because the sight of the umbilical hernia may be upsetting to the parents or child, they should be reassured of the benign nature of the defect and of the normal gradual closure. Taping or strapping of the defect is not recommended because it does not expedite closure and may cause irritation or breakdown of the skin.

★ EVALUATION

Periodically, the nurse and family evaluate the outcomes of care given. Examples of outcomes for the child with umbilical hernia were given under Planning in this section. Planning for further nursing care also takes into consideration long-term care and complications.

Inflammatory Diseases

Appendicitis

Definition and Incidence. Appendicitis is an inflammation of the veriform appendix, the blind sac at the end of the cecum. Appendicitis can occur at any age. The highest incidence is among 10- to 15-year-old children. Although the disease is rare in children under 2 years of age, the highest morbidity and mortality from appendicitis are found in this group. Factors contributing to the high mortality among young children include the difficulty in establishing an early diagnosis, a thin-walled appendix, and immature physiologic defense mechanisms. Appendicitis is the most common reason for abdominal surgery during childhood.

Etiology and Pathophysiology. The exact mechanism of appendicitis is not understood, but it is generally associated with an obstruction of the appendiceal lumen. The obstruction may be caused by a fecalith (a hard stonelike fecal mass), parasites, or lymphoid tissue. The obstruction blocks the outflow of mucous secretions, causing pressure to build within the blood vessels, and leads to inflammation and ulceration of the appendiceal mucosa. The ulceration is followed by bacterial invasion and, if the process continues, necrosis and rupture of the appendix. The rupture causes fecal and bacterial contamination of the peritoneal cavity, resulting in peritonitis (an inflammation of the lining of the peritoneal cavity).[62,76]

Clinical Manifestations. Loss of appetite, abdominal pain, localized abdominal tenderness, and fever are the most common symptoms of appendicitis. Typically, loss of appetite occurs first, followed by abdominal pain. Initially, the pain is generalized throughout the abdomen or periumbilically and then localizes to the lower right quadrant. A low-grade fever (38° C) is usually present, but a high-grade fever occurs if rupture and peritonitis develop. Anorexia and vomiting are common, and frequently diarrhea or constipation are noted. An important symptom is a significant change in the child's behavior and a marked decrease in activity level. Typically, the child avoids all active movement and lies still in a side-lying posture with the knees flexed. Movement, such as riding over bumps in an automobile or climbing onto an examination table, aggravates the pain. If perforation occurs, there is a sudden, but short-lived, relief from pain, which is followed by increased abdominal pain; rapidly rising fever; rapid, shallow respirations; and restlessness. In most cases, the time course from onset of symptoms (marked by loss of appetite) to perforation is 36 to 48 hours.[62,67]

The diagnosis of appendicitis is primarily based on the clinical history and physical examination, which includes a thorough abdominal and rectal exam. A strong indication of appendicitis is a history of abdominal discomfort and tenderness that has progressed from diffuse pain to localized pain in the right lower quadrant. Other common symptoms include guarding or pain during the abdominal and rectal exam, diminished bowel sounds, fever, and a significant decrease in the child's normal level of activity.

Diagnostic Studies. The white blood cell count is mildly elevated but is rarely higher than 15,000 to 20,000/ mm^3 unless perforation has occurred.[62,67] Radiologic studies may demonstrate a fecalith or other foreign body obstructing the appendiceal lumen. Other disorders such as pneumonia, urinary tract infection, acute gastroenteritis, menstrual pain, and pelvic inflammatory disease may present with symptoms that mimic appendicitis and therefore must be ruled out.

★ **ASSESSMENT**

The nurse is often in an ideal position to recognize early signs of appendicitis. Nurses who work in private physicians' offices, ambulatory care clinics, emergency rooms, and school settings are often the first health professional to whom the symptoms are reported. The role of the nurse in these settings is to establish an early diagnosis, to refer the child for further evaluation, and to counsel the parents and child. It is essential that any child who presents with progressive abdominal pain, marked change in appetite and activity level, fever, increased vomiting, and abdominal tenderness is referred for further evaluation because optimal treatment of appendicitis depends on prompt diagnosis and intervention. Parents are counseled to avoid the use of laxatives, enemas, antiemetics, or suppositories and the application of heat to the abdomen, because these treatments stimulate bowel motility and increase the danger of perforation.[76]

★ **NURSING DIAGNOSES AND PLANNING**

Based on the assessment data from above and Chapter 58, the following nursing diagnoses may apply to the child with appendicitis:

- Altered Gastrointestinal Tissue Perfusion related to interrupted arterial and venous flow.
- High Risk for Infection (Peritonitis) related to perforation.
- High Risk for Altered Body Temperature related to disease condition.
- Altered Nutrition: Less Than Body Requirements related to infection.
- Pain related to abdominal obstruction.
- Anxiety related to threat of changes in health status.
- Ineffective Family Coping: Compromised related to temporary disorganization.
- Anxiety related to knowledge deficit regarding necessity of delaying surgery until fluid and electrolyte imbalances are corrected; postoperative signs of infection.

Other functionally related nursing diagnoses are discussed in this chapter's Nursing Care Plan.

The nurse and child (or parents) together plan effective care based on the established nursing diagnoses. Several examples of expected outcomes follow:

- The child expresses understanding of preoperative procedures.
- The parents identify reasons for delaying surgery.
- The child acts out his anxiety through therapeutic play.

The nurse plans for the daily care of the child based on both physician's orders and nursing diagnoses. Some general nursing care goals may be the following:

- Perforation is prevented.
- Infection is prevented.
- Fluid and electrolyte balance is maintained.

★ INTERVENTIONS: COLLABORATIVE AND INDEPENDENT

When appendicitis is suspected, the child must receive nothing by mouth. In preparation for probable surgery, the child is admitted to the hospital, intravenous fluids and antibiotics are started, and nasogastric suction is often initiated. Vital signs are monitored frequently, and the child is observed closely for progression of symptoms.[67]

The child and parents are usually anxious. The parents may experience guilt feelings for not having sought treatment earlier or may act angry and hostile if surgery is delayed while the child is prepared for surgery. Providing the family with calm explanations of any tests that are performed and assuring the parents that surgery is safer if the child is well-hydrated and metabolically stable before surgery are important.[19,55]

The child is often frightened by the severity of his pain and by the rapidity of the diagnosis and admission to the hospital. Frequently, this is the child's first experience in a hospital, and the unfamiliar people and machinery, coupled with the anxiety the child recognizes in the parents, can be overwhelming. Concise, age-appropriate explanations of preoperative procedures should be provided. Usually, the preoperative period is brief, and the child benefits from an opportunity to express his feelings postoperatively through therapeutic play and talking about his surgery.[19,55]

If perforation has not occurred, the treatment of appendicitis is straightforward and is associated with negligible morbidity. The treatment is the surgical removal of the appendix (appendectomy), and recovery is typically rapid and uneventful. The child is usually discharged within 2 to 5 days and may resume normal activities quickly. Contact sports and heavy lifting should be avoided in the immediate postoperative period. The incision is usually covered with collodion or a small gauze dressing. The parents are instructed to observe for evidence of redness or drainage, which indicates infection.

If rupture and peritonitis occur, surgery is delayed temporarily to allow adequate preparation of the child for surgery with intravenous fluids and electrolytes, systemic antibiotics, and nasogastric suction. Postoperatively, the treatment includes the continuation of intravenous fluids and electrolytes, intravenous antibiotics, nasogastric suction, and positioning of the child in the high or semi-Fowler's position to reduce the spread of infection to other parts of the peritoneum.[74]

In some cases, a prolonged period of ileus may occur if peritonitis is severe. The child is kept NPO until bowel function returns. If this period is prolonged, parenteral nutrition may be necessary. If a localized abscess or generalized peritonitis is present, wound irrigation and drainage are necessary. A Penrose drain or other type of wound drain is used to provide external drainage of the abscess. Thick, bulky dressings are placed over the wound to absorb the large amounts of drainage. The secretions are often thick and foul smelling and irritating to the skin. The dressings are changed frequently to prevent skin excoriation.[55] Intravenous antibiotics are administered for 7 to 10 days, and oral antibiotics are often continued after discharge. Hospitalization usually lasts for 1 to 3 weeks. The child is discharged when wound drainage is minimal and oral intake is satisfactory.

★ EVALUATION

Periodically, the nurse and family evaluate the outcomes of care given. Examples of outcomes for the child with appendicitis were given under Planning in this section. Have short-term goals been met? Are long-term goals still realistic?

Meckel's Diverticulum

Definition and Incidence. Meckel's diverticulum is a common malformation of the GI tract that results when a remnant of the omphalomesenteric duct persists as an outpouching of the ileum. The remnant may appear as a blind sac or be attached to the umbilicus by a fibrous cord or fistulous tract. This defect is found twice as often in males as in females, and complications occur three to five times more frequently in men than in women.[67]

Etiology and Pathophysiology. The omphalomesenteric duct normally leads from the midpoint of the developing gut through the umbilicus to the yolk sac during early intrauterine life. Usually, this duct atrophies and disappears, but remnants persist as a Meckel's diverticulum in 1% to 2% of the population.[27] A Meckel's diverticulum is pictured in Figure 59-10.

The majority of people with a Meckel's diverticulum are asymptomatic. The malformation creates symptoms by a variety of mechanisms. In diverticulitis, the sac becomes inflamed as in appendicitis and may perforate, leading to peritonitis. If the sac is lined with gastric mucosa, peptic ulceration, perforation, and hemorrhage may occur. Meckel's diverticulum can also act as the lead point of invagination in cases of intussusception or may cause an intestinal obstruction.

Clinical Manifestations. The majority of symptomatic cases present within the first 2 years of life. Painless rectal bleeding, which is often profuse, is the primary symptom of a Meckel's diverticulum. The hemorrhage may be massive, causing severe anemia or shock. The bleeding is commonly dark or bright red in color, and stools are seldom tarry.

Diagnostic Studies. The diagnosis of Meckel's diverticulum is strongly suspected in any young infant or child who suddenly develops massive but painless bright

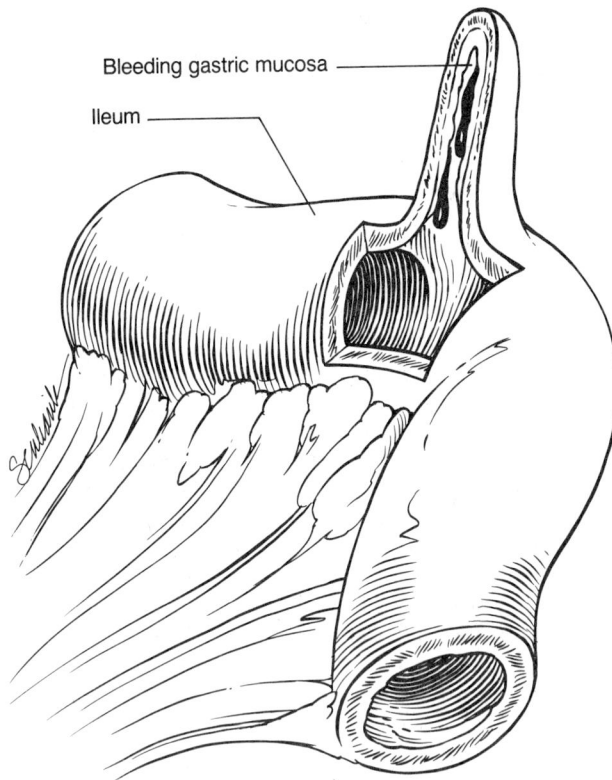

Bleeding gastric mucosa

Ileum

FIGURE 59-10
Example of Meckel's diverticulum, in which the outpouching is lined with
ectopic gastric mucosa and may ulcerate and bleed.

or dark red rectal bleeding. Rectosigmoidoscopy, upper
endoscopy, and nasogastric suction may be used to rule
out other sources of GI bleeding. Blood samples are obtained to evaluate the severity of anemia and to rule out
any bleeding disorders. Radiologic studies with contrast
are generally not helpful because the diverticulum may
not fill with barium or may be too small to be visualized.
Radionuclide imaging with a pertechnetate scan often is
useful in delineating the Meckel's diverticulum. The diagnosis is based primarily on the history and the clinical
presentation.[27,67]

★ **ASSESSMENT**

Important preoperative nursing assessments include frequent monitoring of vital signs and blood pressure to
assess for hypovolemic shock and careful recording of
the amount of blood lost in the stool. If frank bleeding
is not present, the stool is tested for occult blood.[62,67]

★ **NURSING DIAGNOSES AND PLANNING**

Based on the assessment data from above and Chapter
58, the following nursing diagnoses may apply to the child
with Meckel's diverticulum:

- Altered Gastrointestinal Tissue Perfusion related to
  hypovolemia.
- High Risk for Infection (Peritonitis) related to per-
  foration.
- Fluid Volume Loss related to active blood loss.
- Fear related to blood loss.

- Altered Health Maintenance related to ineffective individual coping.
- Anxiety related to knowledge deficit regarding disease
  process and treatment plan.

The nurse and child (or parents) together plan effective care based on the established nursing diagnoses.
Several examples of expected outcomes follow:

- The child and family verbalize fear of blood loss.
- The child and family identify reasons for blood loss.
- The parents participate in postoperative care.
- The child expresses his feelings in therapeutic play.

The nurse plans for the daily care of the child based
on both physician's orders and nursing diagnoses. Some
general nursing care goals may be the following:

- Fluid and electrolyte balance is restored.
- Surgical procedure is without complications.

★ **INTERVENTIONS: COLLABORATIVE
AND INDEPENDENT**

The treatment of this disorder is surgical removal of the
diverticulum. Preoperatively, the child may require the
administration of blood, intravenous fluids, or oxygen to
correct hypovolemic shock. If diverticulitis is suspected,
intravenous antibiotics are started. Cimetidine may be
given to decrease hydrochloric acid secretion if the diverticulum is believed to contain gastric mucosa with a
peptic ulceration.

The rapid onset of massive bleeding can be a terrifying experience for the child and family. While quickly
initiating medical interventions, the nurse must also offer
psychologic support. Age-appropriate explanations and a
calm, reassuring manner help soothe the child's anxiety.
A brief but clear explanation of the disorder and the treatment plan helps to alleviate the parents' anxiety and allows them to be supportive of their child.

★ **EVALUATION**

Periodically, the nurse and family evaluate the outcomes
of care given. Examples of outcomes for the child with
Meckel's diverticulum were given under Planning in this
section.

The postoperative prognosis is excellent, and the
child usually recovers rapidly. Recovery may be prolonged if peritonitis has developed or if portions of the
ileum were resected due to ulcerations. Postoperative
nursing measures are similar to other abdominal surgeries. The child should be given the opportunity for therapeutic play to allow him to work through his feelings.

Inflammatory Bowel Disease

Definition and Incidence.   Two chronic intestinal
disorders, ulcerative colitis and Crohn's disease, are classified under the general term of *inflammatory bowel disease* (IBD). Inflammation and ulceration of the intestinal
mucosa and symptoms of abdominal pain, weight loss,
diarrhea, protein-losing enteropathy (loss of protein by
way of the GI tract), fever, and anemia may occur with

both conditions. Despite similar epidemiologic, immunologic, and clinical features of Crohn's disease and ulcerative colitis, there are significant differences between the two disorders. Ulcerative colitis is characterized by ulcerations confined to the rectum and colon and is less severe and debilitating and more amenable to medical and surgical treatment than Crohn's disease. Ulcerative colitis can be cured by surgical removal of the colon. Crohn's disease is characterized by ulcerations that may occur anywhere in the GI tract from the mouth to the anus. There is no known cure for Crohn's disease.[47]

Over the last several decades, the incidence of ulcerative colitis has remained relatively stable, whereas the incidence of Crohn's disease appears to be increasing, although the reason for this is not known. The incidence of ulcerative colitis is about 70 to 100 patients per 100,000 population.[11] The prevalence rate of Crohn's disease is slightly lower at 30 to 40 patients per 100,000 population. IBD is more common among people at higher socioeconomic levels and among Caucasians. The disease occurs less frequently among African Americans, Orientals, and Israeli Jews, yet Jewish people living in North America and Europe appear to be at higher risk. IBD is more common in urban populations than in rural areas.[62]

Etiology and Pathophysiology. The cause of IBD is not understood, although many etiologies have been speculated. Considerable numbers of research studies have investigated possible causes, including infectious agents, allergic reactions, immunologic disorders, psychosomatic disorders, and genetic factors; however, the cause of IBD remains obscure.[45,47] Evidence indicates that some genetic factor may predispose a person to the disease. An apparent familial tendency is present in about 5% to 15% of cases.[11] Current theory holds that an environmental influence acts on this genetic predisposition and creates the characteristic symptoms of Crohn's disease or ulcerative colitis. A comparison of these disorders is presented in Table 59-1.

Clinical Manifestations. The symptoms associated with ulcerative colitis and Crohn's disease vary due to the location of the lesions and the length of time before diagnosis occurs. Children with ulcerative colitis often appear reasonably well-nourished and healthy. Common presenting symptoms include mild rectal bleeding and the frequent passage of small volume, loose, watery stools. The child often reports nocturnal diarrhea, fecal incontinence, tenesmus (painful spasms of the anal sphincter

TABLE 59-1
Comparison of Ulcerative Colitis and Crohn's Disease

	Ulcerative Colitis	Crohn's Disease
Pathology		
Bowel wall involvement	Superficial layers only (mucosa and submucosa)	Affects all layers (transmural)
Pattern of lesions	Symmetric, continuous	Asymmetric, patchy (segmental)
Primary intestinal areas affected	Colon, rectum	Entire gastrointestinal system from mouth to rectum
Clinical Manifestations		
Predominant initial symptoms	Rectal bleeding, diarrhea with pus, mucus, blood	Vague abdominal pain, fever, anorexia, weight loss
Gross rectal bleeding	Common	Infrequent
Diarrhea	Common, small volume watery stools	Mild to moderate
Abdominal pain	Mild, lower abdominal area, relieved by stool	Common, severe, exacerbated by eating
Fever	Rare	Common
Weight loss	None to moderate	Often severe
Growth retardation	Mild	Often severe
Anorexia	Mild	Often severe
Fistulas	Rare	Common
Anal lesions	Rare	Common
Response to Treatment		
Drug therapy	Good response	Fair response
Parenteral nutrition	Will not induce remission	Often induces remission
Surgery	Excellent response	Fair to poor
Prognosis		
Remissions	Common	Rare
Surgical removal of affected bowel	Curative, eliminates risk of carcinoma	Recurrence rate high
Risk of carcinoma	High if bowel not resected	Slight

with urgency to defecate), and crampy, lower abdominal pain, which is relieved by stooling. Extraintestinal or extracolonic symptoms may proceed the actual diagnosis by months and may include low-grade fever, skin lesions, and joint pain.[62] Arthritis-like symptoms in children require ruling out IBD.

The onset of Crohn's disease is often insidious; more than a year may elapse between the onset of symptoms and diagnosis. A typical presentation of the disease may include a history of recurrent, vague abdominal pain, late afternoon or evening fever, anorexia, and chronic weight loss. The abdominal pain is often triggered by eating, is much more severe than with ulcerative colitis, and is not relieved by stooling. Anorexia may ensue as the child decreases food intake in an effort to avoid abdominal pain. Diarrhea and anal lesions such as fissures or perirectal abscesses are common. Severe weight loss or growth retardation may be present at diagnosis or may occur during the course of the disease.

Both diseases are characterized by acute exacerbations interspersed with periods of remission. During remissions, the child may feel relatively well and exhibit few or no symptoms of the disease. Exacerbations often occur abruptly and are usually severe.

Diagnostic Studies. The diagnostic evaluation of a child with suspected bowel disease primarily centers on ruling out other potential causes of the symptoms and determining the extent of bowel involvement. Stool cultures are done to rule out potential infectious causes such as *Salmonella, Shigella, Campylobacter,* and amebiasis. A tuberculosis skin test is done to rule out this disease as a possible causative factor. A colonoscopy, upper endoscopy, and upper GI series with small bowel follow-through examination are done to evaluate the character and location of lesions. In ulcerative colitis, the colon may appear red and friable, but the lesions are confined to the colon only. In Crohn's disease, the lesions are characteristically patchy and may appear anywhere from the mouth to the anus. Additional diagnostic studies include plotting of the child's height and weight on standardized growth charts so that growth over time can be evaluated. Blood samples are frequently analyzed to detect evidence of anemia, hypoalbuminemia, and other nutrient deficiencies. Stool samples are analyzed to detect the presence of blood or pus.

★ **ASSESSMENT**

The nurse in a clinic or school setting may be the first to suspect that a child's subtle GI complaints may be indicative of IBD. Children with chronic abdominal pain, unusual or painful stool patterns, and weight loss or growth retardation should be referred to a physician for diagnosis.

After medical diagnosis, the nurse must carefully assess the family's understanding of the disease process and management and family dynamics, which may affect the treatment plan. The nurse works with the health care team to assess the child's response to treatment and ability to cope with this chronic illness.

★ **NURSING DIAGNOSES AND PLANNING**

Based on the assessment data from above and Chapter 58, the following nursing diagnoses may apply to the child with IBD:

- Diarrhea related to disease condition.
- High Risk for Fluid Volume Deficit related to diarrhea.
- Altered Nutrition: Less Than Body Requirements related to inability to absorb nutrients.
- Chronic Pain related to physical illness.
- Altered Health Maintenance related to ineffective individual coping.
- Powerlessness related to illness.
- Body Image Disturbance related to biophysical condition.
- Impaired Social Interaction related to self-concept disturbance.
- High Risk for Impaired Skin Integrity related to diarrhea.
- Anxiety related to knowledge deficit regarding disease process, signs of relapse, medication regimen, dietary management, ostomy care, stress reduction measures.

The nurse and child (or parents) together plan effective care based on the established nursing diagnoses. Several examples of expected outcomes follow:

- The child resumes school and other activities.
- The child eats a normal diet.
- The family demonstrates understanding of the disease process and treatment.

The nurse plans for the daily care of the child based on both physician's orders and nursing diagnoses. Some general nursing care goals may be the following:

- Nutrients are replaced.
- Fluid status is maintained.
- Normal bowel movements are resumed.

★ **INTERVENTIONS: COLLABORATIVE AND INDEPENDENT**

The therapeutic management of ulcerative colitis includes treatment of the symptoms of acute exacerbations and long-term management of the chronic symptoms. During severe, acute attacks, hospitalization is required for replacement and monitoring of fluid and electrolytes, administration of intravenous corticosteroids and antibiotics, and, in some cases, nasogastric suction and parenteral nutrition. Emergency surgery may be required for severe complications such as bowel perforation, massive GI bleeding, or with a rare but extremely serious complication known as toxic megacolon. Toxic megacolon results from a progressive dilation and inflammation of the colon leading to severe ileus and is often accompanied by shock and gram-negative sepsis. Management of ulcerative colitis requires a combination of therapies, including dietary management, drug therapy, and, in some cases, surgery.

NUTRITIONAL MANAGEMENT

The goal in nutritional management of IBD is to replace any nutrient losses associated with the inflammatory process and malabsorption, to correct any nutrient deficiencies, and to provide adequate substrates to promote a positive energy and nitrogen balance. Appropriate dietary management and regular nutrition assessment are integral factors in the care of the child with IBD to decrease the risk of depressed growth rates, retarded bone development, and delayed onset of sexual maturation. These complications have been observed in 10% to 40% of patients under 21 years of age with IBD.[45]

A high-protein, high-carbohydrate, normal- to low-fat, and high-vitamin/mineral diet is recommended. This diet helps to replace protein and nutrients such as zinc, calcium, magnesium, folate, and vitamins D and K, which may be lost from the ulcerated bowel, and to supplement inadequate intake, which may result from anorexia. Careful dietary management is most important in Crohn's disease due to the anorexia commonly associated with the disease and because of the malabsorption that often occurs secondarily due to the small bowel involvement. Encouraging the anorectic child to eat adequate amounts is often challenging. Involving the child in meal planning; offering small, frequent meals; serving meals at times when symptoms of diarrhea, mouth pain, and intestinal cramping are controlled by medication; and the use of high-protein, high-calorie foods, such as milk shakes, cream soups, and puddings, may help to increase intake. Foods that increase abdominal pain, cramping, or diarrhea are avoided. In some cases, diminished lactase activity may necessitate the use of a milk-free diet. Some children are unable to consume adequate nutrients orally and may require supplemental nasogastric drip feedings or parenteral nutrition. Supplemental feedings are often given at night so as not to interfere with the child's usual activities.

MEDICATION THERAPY

Some children develop aphthous stomatitis (most commonly with Crohn's disease, occasionally with ulcerative colitis), which further inhibits good oral intake. The appearance of the mouth ulcers may be related to emotional distress, immunologic reactions, or as a response to medications. Local applications of medications such as magnesium and aluminum hydroxide (Maalox) or lidocaine (Xylocaine Viscous) may provide temporary relief and facilitate eating and drinking.[55,61]

Drug therapy with IBD may include the use of sulfasalazine, steroids, and other immunosuppressive drugs, and antibiotics (during acute phases). These medications are used to decrease the inflammation of the bowel mucosa.

Corticosteroids are a traditional treatment method used during acute episodes and as long-term therapy in severe cases of IBD. Steroids have been shown to reduce inflammation of the bowel; however, the use of long-term steroids is associated with severe morbidity. Common complications of prolonged steroid use include weight gain, immunosuppression, acne, osteoporosis, myopathy, growth failure, aseptic necrosis of the hip, and psychosis. The large majority of children on long-term steroids eventually develop one or more of these complications; prolonged steroid use is considered highly undesirable.

Azulfidine (sulfasalazine) acts directly on the bowel mucosa to reduce inflammation and to provide protection from relapse of bowel lesions. Sulfasalazine decreases the number of exacerbations in ulcerative colitis but *not* in Crohn's disease. Unfortunately, no medication has been shown to reduce the frequency of exacerbations of Crohn's disease. The side-effects of sulfasalazine are relatively minor in comparison to steroids. Side-effects may include headache, anorexia, nausea, vomiting, allergic reaction, and bone marrow suppression. Fortunately, the bone marrow effects are usually dosage-related, and reduction of the dosage decreases the risk significantly. Children receiving sulfasalazine need periodic monitoring of blood counts to ensure early recognition of suppression. Malabsorption of folic acid often occurs with long-term sulfasalazine use, and folic acid supplementation is necessary.

The immunosuppressive drug, 6-MP (mercaptopurine), may offer new hope for children with ulcerative colitis. In low doses, this drug has an antiinflammatory effect and helps to reduce exacerbations of ulcerative colitis. Unfortunately, the response of Crohn's disease to 6-MP has been less encouraging. A potential side-effect may be bone marrow suppression. If this complication occurs, the medication should be discontinued or the dosage should be reduced accordingly.

SURGICAL MANAGEMENT

Surgical management of ulcerative colitis is undertaken when the disease is unresponsive to medical therapy or in the event of life-threatening complications such as GI hemorrhage, perforation, toxic megacolon, or carcinoma of the colon.[11,26] Additionally, the colon is usually surgically removed after 10 years have elapsed from the time of diagnosis to prevent carcinoma of the colon. Removal is usually done even before any signs of carcinoma are evident due to the extremely high risk for cancer and the difficulty of detecting the cancer at an early stage. The surgical procedure(s) generally consist of a subtotal colectomy and ileostomy and an endorectal pull-through. The surgery may be done as one operation or as a two-stage procedure. The entire colon, including the rectal mucosa, is removed, and the small bowel is brought out through the abdominal wall, forming an ileostomy. In a second procedure, the ileostomy is closed and the small bowel is "pulled through" the rectum and anastomosed to the rectal tissue. In some cases, the ileostomy stage of the procedure is skipped and the small bowel is pulled through and anastomosed to the rectum during the initial surgery. The end result of the pull-through procedure allows the child to eliminate stool out the rectum and is generally much more socially acceptable to the child and family than a permanent ileostomy. Disadvantages of this procedure include difficulty controlling the anal sphincter muscles, and frequent stooling. Removal of the diseased large bowel cures ulcerative colitis and prevents carcinoma of the colon.

A newer surgical procedure offered to children and adolescents with ulcerative colitis is the ileoanal reservoir. This procedure provides the most normal mechanism for maintaining continence and normal evacuation. The surgery requires two or three surgical procedures to complete and includes a temporary ileostomy. In the first stage, the diseased colon is removed and the mucosa lining layer of the rectal segment is stripped, leaving a muscular cuff. The rectal mucosectomy removes the mucosa and submucosa 4 to 6 cm above the dentate line. The rectal muscles and anal sphincter are left intact. A reservoir is created from a segment of terminal ileum and connected to the remaining rectal segment. The reservoir ultimately serves as a storage area for stool. A temporary ileostomy is performed to divert the stool away from the reservoir as healing of the suture lines takes place. In the second stage, the ileostomy is closed and the ileoanal reservoir begins to function. Initially, the stool is liquid and irritating to the perianal area. The frequency of the stool decreases to 6 to 12 semisolid bowel movements as the child returns to a normal diet. After a year, most children have four to six bowel movements a day.[10] Nursing inventions for children undergoing ileoanal reservoir are described in Table 59-2.

MANAGEMENT OF CROHN'S DISEASE

In Crohn's disease, surgery is not curative but may be undertaken when acute or chronic exacerbations occur that are uncontrolled by medical treatment. Surgical removal of the affected bowel may diminish symptoms, at least temporarily.

Partial bowel resection often has a favorable impact on growth, especially in prepubertal children. Unfortunately, there is a high rate of recurrence of disease in the remaining bowel. The prognosis for children with Crohn's disease is variable. A few patients may experience almost complete remission, but most continue to exhibit some symptoms that affect their quality of life throughout their lifetime. Most people with Crohn's disease are troubled with acute exacerbations, which cannot be predicted or prevented.

Enterocutaneous fistulas and anal fissures are much more common in Crohn's disease than in ulcerative colitis and can create difficult management problems. These lesions are painful and may bleed or become infected. Perirectal fistulas are most common and may cause perirectal abscesses requiring intravenous antibiotics. Metronidazole (Flagyl) has been used successfully with perianal disease. Side-effects of metronidazole includes a peripheral neuropathy, which should be observed for over time.

Many children require supplemental nutrition either by way of nasogastric drip feedings with an elemental (simple) formula or by way of parenteral nutrition at some time during the course of the disease to promote satisfactory growth, to allow the bowel to rest, or to optimize

---

TABLE 59-2
Nursing Interventions for Ileoanal Reservoirs

Nursing Action: Stage 1. Ileostomy; Ileoanal Reservoir Constructed	Rationale
1. Assess child for signs and symptoms of dehydration: dry mucous membranes, poor skin tugor, dry skin, decreased urinary output. Monitor daily weights, intake and output (urine and fecal).	1. Output from the ileostomy can be 800 to 1200 ml/24 h in adolescents because of the amount of small bowel used in the construction of the reservoir; thus, the ileostomy functions as a ''short gut.'' Weights are an excellent measure of overall fluid shifts.
2. Assess perianal skin several times a day. Use skin ointments and creams to protect the perianal skin and collect the mucus drainage with absorptive pads at night. Irrigate the reservoir daily to remove mucus drainage.	2. The mucus that collects in the reservoir contains residual digestive enzymes (this is small bowel) and can be extremely irritating to the skin.
3. Manage the ileostomy with a drainage pouch and solid wafer skin barrier. Initiate ileostomy patient teaching program, which includes: skin care, pouch management, diet, odor, and activities of daily living.	3. The adolescent needs to learn ostomy care, skin protection, and overall ileostomy management to live successfully with the temporary ileostomy.
4. Patient education and discharge planning should include: ileostomy management; Kegel exercises; intubation and irrigation of the reservoir; perianal skin care; and planned follow-up.	4. Kegel exercises are used to strengthen the sphincter muscles before the ileoanal reservoir is functional. A serious problem would be incontinence after this procedure.

Nursing Action: Stage 2. Ileostomy Closure; Ileoanal Reservoir Functioning	Rationale
1. Assess the perianal skin after each bowel movement. Avoid irritants such as nylon underwear, harsh or deodorant soaps, and fragrant toilet paper.	1. The bowel movements will be loose and frequent during this early stage.
2. Cleanse the skin with water or Domeboro (aluminum sulfate and calcium acetate) solution and cotton balls; dry with hair dryer.	2. The frequent cleansing required of the perianal area can result in irritation and denudation.
3. Apply vanishing cream and cover with a liquid skin sealant. Provide sitz baths, Balneol cleansing agents, or Tucks pads.	3. Protection of the skin is of paramount importance; it is important to be gentle in cleansing the skin.
4. Assess the frequency and consistency of the bowel movements. Encourage a regular diet. Provide psyllium (Metamucil) or loperamide (Imodium) as ordered for diarrhea.	4. Expect 10 to 20 bowel movements a day in the early postoperative period. The frequency will decrease with time and with a regular diet. If diarrhea is significant or incontinence is a problem, antidiarrheal agents may be helpful.
5. Include the following areas in discharge planning and patient teaching: perianal skin care, management of diarrhea associated with flu/viral infections; irrigation of reservoir; complications that should be reported to the physician (difficulty emptying the reservoir or irrigating, incontinence, continued diarrhea).	5. The purpose of this procedure is to provide the most ''normal'' method of elimination possible after total colectomy. The adolescent and family need to know how to manage the day-to-day activities of living with an ileoanal reservoir.

nutritional status before surgery. Parenteral nutrition can dramatically reverse growth retardation, promote closure of fistulas, and induce remission of the disease.[44,62]

MANAGEMENT OF ACUTE PHASE

During acute phases of the disease, the nurse carefully monitors the child's symptoms and responses to treatment measures. Close attention to the child's fluid status is important because severe diarrhea can lead to dehydration. Daily weights and strict intake and output are recorded. The frequency, consistency, color, and amount of stool are assessed and documented during the acute phase. Physical activity is often minimized to reduce intestinal motility. If the child is receiving parenteral nutrition, the nurse carefully monitors the infusion and the central venous catheter.

TEACHING

Comprehensive education of the child and family is essential for optimal management. The nurse must work with the health care team to ensure the family understands the disease, the medication regimen, potential side-effects of the medicines, the dietary plan, and potential complications that must be promptly reported to the physician. If indicated, the family should learn ostomy care and proper care of intracutaneous or perirectal fistulas. Perirectal ulceration and excoriation may be severe and exceedingly painful. Frequent sitz baths and meticulous skin care may alleviate some of this discomfort.

Children who undergo colectomy with the placement of an ileostomy require specific preoperative preparation. The child needs time to prepare and adjust to the impending change in body appearance. Ileostomy teaching should begin before surgery and is done by the nurse or enterostomal therapy (ET) nurse. Written and oral explanations and pictures should be provided to the child and family. Dolls with almost lifelike ostomies are available for teaching purposes. After surgery, the parents and child should be given ample opportunity to observe and practice ostomy care. Adolescents and young adults rarely accept the ostomy willingly even though it markedly reduces the pain and diarrhea and eliminates the risk of cancer of the colon. The ostomy significantly changes the child's body image and the child is encouraged to verbalize his or her feelings and to identify ways to cope with events that may be stressful such as relationships with the opposite sex.

STRESS REDUCTION

The nurse can be instrumental in helping the family identify stress reduction measures and ways to adjust to chronic illness. Stress can exacerbate the symptoms of chronic illness. During hospitalization, the nurse can reduce stress by explaining all invasive procedures and providing opportunities for therapeutic play. The child and family should be helped to recognize stressors in day-to-day life and to identify methods of reducing the stress. Common stress factors associated with the chronic illness include peer reactions to growth retardation or delayed sexual maturation, dietary restrictions, feelings of isolation from peers, altered body image from side-effects of medications such as steroids, and necessary absences from school due to acute exacerbations of the disease. Family counseling is often helpful to assist parents in dealing with chronic illness and establishing appropriate structure and discipline as well as dealing with disruptions in family function.[26,55,63]

★ EVALUATION

Periodically, the nurse and family evaluate the outcomes of care given. Examples of outcomes for the child with IBD were given under Planning in this section. Have short-term goals been met? Are long-term goals still realistic?

LONG-TERM CARE

IBD is a chronic life-disrupting illness that requires long-term medical and nursing follow-up. A collaborative team approach to these children is most effective in providing comprehensive care. The nurse's responsibilities include supportive care during acute exacerbations of the disease, education of the child and family about the disease and treatment measures, and helping the child and family identify ways to reduce stress and cope with a chronic illness.[61]

Regular follow-up visits to a clinic are required by these children and their families regardless of whether or not they "feel well." The importance of health maintenance should be stressed when teaching these children and their families about the disease, the medical treatment, and the possible surgical interventions and outcomes. Self-help groups are available in most communities. The National Foundation of Colitis and Ileitis and the United Ostomy Association are two major resource groups.

Disorders of Motility

Constipation

Definition. Patterns of bowel movements vary considerably among children. Factors accounting for this variability may include fluid and fiber content of diet, activity level, regularity of routine visits to the bathroom, and toilet training patterns. The perception of an abnormal frequency of stooling is often defined by parents as constipation. A "normal" stooling pattern may range from three stools per day to three stools per week. The actual medical diagnosis of constipation refers to the character of the stool rather than the frequency of defecation and to the association of defecation with symptoms such as difficulty in expulsion of stools, blood-streaked bowel movements, and abdominal discomfort.[62] Constipation is characterized by the passage of firm or hard stools or of small hard masses at extremely long intervals. In severe cases, constipation may be accompanied by fecal soiling (encopresis). Difficulty with defecation occurs in all age groups from infancy through adulthood. It is estimated that complaints of constipation and soiling account for up to 3% of visits to pediatric outpatient clinics.[28]

Etiology and Pathophysiology. Normal defecation and continence are characterized by several mechanisms that facilitate passage of the intestinal contents. The gastrocolic reflux is initiated by passage of food from the stomach into the small bowel, leading to rapid transit of ileal contents into the cecum and a marked increase in segmental contractions of the right colon. The segmental activity produces slow to-and-fro internal circulation of the feces but no propulsion. The segmental contractions stop, and a mass movement propels the stool to a more distal part of the colon. This process repeats itself three to four times over one to several days before delivering stool to the rectum causing relaxation of the internal sphincter and the perception of rectal distention caused by the descending fecal bolus. The conscious awareness of rectal distention results in a transient contraction of the voluntary muscles of the external anal sphincter and puborectalis sling. Voluntary relaxation of the external sphincter and puborectalis muscles and an increased intraabdominal pressure result in defecation. A squatting position raises intraabdominal pressure and facilitates sphincter relaxation and expulsion of stool.[74]

The pathophysiology of constipation is not understood. Chronic constipation has been noted to be associated with delayed intestinal transit time, decreased conscious awareness of rectal distention, formation of hard or small stools, and paradoxical contraction of the external sphincter in which there is an unconscious contraction of the sphincter during the attempted defecation. Retention of stool can be initiated by relatively innocent events, such as an anal fissure that causes pain on defecation, voluntary retention because of classroom rules, a reluctance to use an unfamiliar bathroom, or a protest against toilet training. As the feces accumulate, a vicious cycle ensues. The stool becomes larger and harder, making defecation even more difficult. As the stool becomes impacted, the rectum dilates and the awareness of a need to defecate is blunted. The internal sphincter relaxes, and liquid stool can flow around the impacted stool, causing soiling (encopresis).

Constipation may occur in association with low-fiber diets, overly aggressive approaches to toilet training, stressful events, and a variety of conditions that influence fluid content of stool, innervation of bowel or sphincter muscles, or motility of the gut. Conditions associated with constipation are listed in the accompanying display.

Clinical Manifestations. Chronic constipation is seen most often in males. The highest incidence occurs between ages 1 and 5 years; however, a significant number of cases (25%) are diagnosed under 1 year of age.[74] Parents often report the passage of large stools and involuntary soiling. The abdomen may be moderately distended, and the child may complain of abdominal pain. Large masses of stool are often palpable. Rectal examination reveals an enlarged rectal ampulla filled with a mass of stool. Stressful events such as moving or changing schools, the birth of a sibling, family problems, or intercurrent illness occur at the onset in some cases. Approximately 30% of children also suffer from enuresis or urinary tract infections.[38] In the majority of cases, some form of therapy (either a home remedy or medical treatment) has already been attempted, usually without success.

Diagnostic Studies. A careful history and physical examination are imperative. Conditions that cause or contribute to constipation, such as Hirschsprung's disease, hypothyroidism, or urinary tract disease, must be ruled out. Particular attention should be paid to a thorough diet history, age at onset of symptoms, relationship to changes in the child's environment, history of toilet training, and characteristic behaviors during defecation. A description of the frequency, consistency, and size of stools is elicited. Any medications the child receives are identified because many drugs including iron preparations, anticonvulsants, diuretics, antacids, and anticholinergics are associated

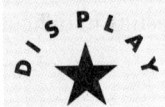

Conditions Associated With Constipation

Dietary causes
 Undernutrition
 Underhydration
 Excessive intake of cow's milk
 Low-fiber diets
Diseases of anus, rectum, colon
 Anal fissure
 Anorectal malformation or stricture
 Hemorrhoids
 Hirschsprung's disease
Spinal cord disorders
 Spina bifida
 Myelomeningocele, meningocele
 Paraplegia

Metabolic and endocrine causes
 Hypothyroidism
 Diabetes insipidus
 Pregnancy
 Hypokalemia
 Renal tubular acidosis
Psychogenic disorders
 Voluntary withholding
 Depression
 Anorexia nervosa
 Abuse of cathartics and laxatives
Drug side-effect
 Iron preparations
 Anticonvulsants
 Diuretics
 Anticholinergics
 Bismuth
 Antacids

with constipation. An abdominal x-ray typically shows a colon dilated with large amounts of stool.

★ ASSESSMENT

The nursing assessment should include a thorough history of dietary and fluid intake, stooling patterns, efforts at toilet training, and presence of any stressors that may affect bowel elimination. The physical examination should include particular attention to the presence of abdominal distention and fluid status. The primary role of the nurse is to assist in obtaining a thorough history and to educate the family about normal stooling patterns and medication and treatment regimens for chronic constipation.

★ NURSING DIAGNOSES AND PLANNING

Based on the assessment data from above and Chapter 58, the following nursing diagnoses may apply to the child with constipation:

- Constipation related to inadequate intake of low-residue foods.
- Fluid Volume Deficit related to inadequate fluid intake.
- Anxiety related to knowledge deficit regarding high-fiber diet; adequate fluid intake; toileting patterns; medication regimens.

The nurse and child (or parents) together plan effective care based on the established nursing diagnoses. Several examples of expected outcomes follow:

- The parents discuss normal stool patterns.
- The parents relate increased use of fluids and high-fiber residues in family diet.
- The child exhibits clean underwear without signs of soiling.

The nurse plans for the daily care of the child based on both physician's orders and nursing diagnoses. A general nursing care goal may be the following:

- Fluid and electrolyte balance is maintained.

★ INTERVENTIONS: COLLABORATIVE AND INDEPENDENT

Simple constipation without impaction is treated with conservative measures. Occasional episodes of infrequent or difficult stooling are normal at any age. In many cases, the parents benefit from reassurance and education concerning normal bowel habits. The intake of fluids and high-residue foods such as bran, whole grain products, fruits, vegetables, prune juice, and prunes should be increased. Stool softeners such as Colace (docusate sodium sulfosuccinate) may be prescribed. Laxatives and cathartics are generally not recommended.

Chronic constipation often requires more intensive and long-term management. The first step is to remove the fecal impaction.[32] The bowel cleansing can usually be performed at home by the use of enemas (normal saline or hypertonic phosphate) or by cathartics such as a polyethylene glycol-electrolyte solution (Golytely). Enemas may result in dramatic fluid or electrolyte shifts, and the parents must be cautioned not to exceed the number or frequency of enemas prescribed (see section

on Enema Administration). A clean bowel can be confirmed by an abdominal x-ray and physical examination.

Once the impaction has been evacuated, a regular pattern of defecation must be established. This phase of therapy includes administration of a stool-softening agent such as milk of magnesia, mineral oil, lactulose, or Colace (usually twice each day), a high-fiber diet, and placing the child on the toilet for short periods twice each day. It is best to schedule "potty" time after meals to take advantage of the gastrocolic reflex. The nurse should discuss implementation of these treatment measures into the family's routines because consistency in implementation helps to ensure success. Due to the taste and texture of the medications, getting the child to take the medicine is often challenging for the parent. In some cases, experimenting with several medicines may be necessary before a satisfactory product is identified. Medications can be mixed with juice or other fluids to increase palatability. Multivitamins may be recommended to compensate for malabsorption, which may occur secondarily to the use of medications.

★ EVALUATION

Periodically, the nurse and family evaluate the outcomes of care given. Examples of outcomes for the child with constipation were given under Planning in this section. Planning for further nursing care also takes into consideration long-term care.

LONG-TERM CARE

Establishment of normal bowel patterns may take several months, and the child is evaluated periodically to assess for compliance and the recurrence of symptoms. Signs of relapse may include excessive oil leakage, large-caliber stools, abdominal pain, decreased frequency of defecation, and soiling. Once a regular stooling pattern has been established, long-term management may require a stool softener. Behavioral modification training and biofeedback techniques have shown promising results in difficult cases.

Diarrhea and Gastroenteritis

Etiology and Pathophysiology. Diarrhea is a common problem encountered in pediatric patients. A variety of pathophysiologic mechanisms can result in diarrhea including viral and bacterial infections, malnutrition, lactase deficiency, and anatomic problems such as short bowel syndrome. A comparison of viral and bacterial infections is presented in Table 59-3. The frequency and consistency of stooling patterns among children vary considerably. A sudden *increase* in the frequency or fluid content of stool is a characteristic feature of diarrhea. The consequences of diarrheal episodes depend on the causative factor, the age and nutritional status of the patient, and the severity and duration of symptoms. In acute diarrhea, losses of fluids and electrolytes can lead to dehydration and electrolyte and acid–base imbalances. In the event of chronic diarrhea, malnutrition may develop.

Acute Viral Gastroenteritis. Most cases of diarrhea in North America have been shown to have a viral etiology.

TABLE 59-3
Characteristics of Common Causes of Pediatric Gastroenteritis

Disease Factor/ Clinical Signs	Rotovirus	Norwalk Virus	Escherichia Coli	Vibrio Cholera	Salmonella	Shigella	Staphylococcal Food Poisoning
Age group most commonly affected	6–24 mo	All age groups	0–18 mo	All ages	0–2 y	0–10 y	All ages
Incubation period	2–3 d	24–48 h	Variable	8–72 h, variable—depends on strain	12–72 h	Variable	1–6 h
Characteristic symptoms	Vomiting, fever, diarrhea, upper respiratory illness	Fever, anorexia, vomiting, diarrhea, abdominal and muscle pain	Frequent green liquid stools, fever, vomiting	Profuse, painless watery diarrhea (rice water stools), fever, vomiting, hypothermia	Diarrhea, vomiting, fever, watery stools that contain blood, pus, or mucus	Fever; abdominal pain; diarrhea; crampy abdominal pain; tenesmus; bloody, pus-containing stools	Nausea, vomiting, abdominal cramps
Duration of symptoms	48 h to 1 wk	3 d	3 d to weeks if untreated	Variable—usually about 1 wk	Several days—mild cases; several weeks—typhoid fever	Acute symptoms—1 wk; complete recovery—several weeks	24 h
Treatment	Symptomatic	Symptomatic	Symptomatic, antibiotics in severe cases	Rapid fluid and electrolyte replacement (usually orally), antibiotics	Symptomatic, antibiotics (usually ampicillin) in severe cases	Symptomatic, antibiotics	Symptomatic
Pathogenic mechanism	Mucosal inflammation, villous damage	Mucosal inflammation, villous damage	Invasion of gastrointestinal epithelium, enterotoxin production	Enterotoxin production	Invasion of gastrointestinal mucosa	Enterotoxin production	Enterotoxin production
Transmission	Person-to-person from affected individual or asymptomatic carriers	Person-to-person from affected individual or asymptomatic carriers	Person-to-person or ingestion of contaminated food, water, or equipment	Ingestion of contaminated water or seafood	Contaminated food products, particularly eggs, poultry, or milk	Fecal–oral, contaminated food, flies	Unrefrigerated, contaminated food
Season/prevalence	Winter	Winter	Year round	Developing countries, eastern coast of U.S.	Year round	Warmer months, tropical/subtropical regions	Year round

Typically, acute viral gastroenteritis is a self-limited disease that runs its course within 5 to 7 days. Viral gastroenteritis is considered highly contagious and often is the suspected cause of family and community epidemics of "intestinal flu." Most episodes of viral gastroenteritis are characterized by various combinations of diarrhea, nausea, vomiting, abdominal cramps, headache, myalgia, and low-grade fever. A number of viral agents have been speculated to be probable causative organisms of diarrhea including rotovirus, parvovirus, adenovirus, and coronavirus.

Rotovirus is the most common cause of acute nonbacterial gastroenteritis in infants and children. Rotovirus causes diarrhea worldwide and has been associated with severe outbreaks in developing countries. Nosocomial transmission of rotovirus is an important cause of diarrhea among hospitalized children. Various studies have shown that 7% to 59% of children admitted to the hospital with other diagnoses acquire rotovirus in the hospital. Children between the ages of 6 and 24 months are the most susceptible to rotoviral disease, whereas older children and adults most often have a mild or asymptomatic infection but may still transmit the disease. This illness is commonly

(20% to 40%) associated with upper respiratory symptoms. Although most cases of rotovirus are short-lived, severe illness may develop, especially in immunocompromised patients or children with other diseases.[17]

Bacterial Gastroenteritis. Diarrhea can be caused by a variety of bacterial organisms including *Escherichia coli, Vibrio cholerae, Campylobacter, Salmonella,* or *Shigella.* Bacteria are generally believed to cause diarrhea by two pathologic mechanisms.

• Rapid multiplication of bacteria after invasion of GI epithelium leading to cell destruction and ulceration of the intestinal tract wall, or
• Bacterial production of an enterotoxin that causes local tissue damage and destruction of intestinal cells.

Escherichia coli can lead to diarrhea by either invasion or enterotoxin production. Although the *E. coli* organism is normally part of the intestinal flora, specific pathogenic strains have been implicated as the causative organisms in a variety of diarrheal illnesses. *E. coli* is the organism commonly implicated in "traveler's diarrhea." The onset of *E. coli* diarrhea can be abrupt or gradual, and symptoms may range from mild to severe. The primary treatment of *E. coli* diarrhea is replacement of lost fluid and electrolytes either orally or, in severe cases, intravenously.[37]

Vibrio organisms cause diarrhea by production of a potent enterotoxin that stimulates profuse secretion of intestinal fluid. *V. cholerae* has been a major cause of epidemics of diarrhea in developing countries. Cholera is characterized by profuse, painless, watery diarrhea. The stools are initially brown in color and then become clear and contain small flakes of mucus. The stools are classically described as "rice water" stools. The fluid losses can lead to severe dehydration and death if treatment is not initiated promptly.

Another important cause of bacterial gastroenteritis is the *Salmonella* organism. *Salmonella* organisms are transmitted by contaminated food products. The most severe infection caused by *Salmonella* is typhoid fever and is caused by *Salmonella typhi*.

Milder cases of *Salmonella* gastroenteritis are characterized by a rapid onset of diarrhea, vomiting and fever, usually within 12 to 72 hours after ingestion of the contaminated foodstuff. A small number of severe cases may present with *Salmonella* bacteremia and high, spiking fevers, with or without vomiting and diarrhea. Severe *Salmonella* infections are treated with fluid and electrolyte replacement and antibiotic therapy, typically with ampicillin. Antibiotic therapy is usually contraindicated in milder cases of *Salmonella* gastroenteritis.[73]

Several species of *Shigella* can cause bacterial gastroenteritis commonly known as bacillary dysentery. *Shigella* is commonly transmitted by food handlers and flies. There is an increased risk for shigellosis with institutionalized children who are unable to learn adequate sanitary precautions and with the presence of outdoor portable toilets that lack adequate handwashing facilities. The typical case presents with fever, abdominal pain, anorexia, and vomiting. These symptoms are followed by the rapid onset of diarrhea, crampy abdominal pain, and tenesmus (spasms of the anal sphincter with urgency to defecate). Young infants and children may develop severe dehy-

dration, fever, convulsions. The acute symptoms usually persist for about 1 week, but complete recovery may take several weeks. Treatment includes fluid and electrolyte replacement as indicated and isolation of the affected person to prevent further transmission of the disease. Antibiotics are commonly used to treat severe cases and for newborn infants, young children, and people with other diseases. Although antibiotic therapy does not usually alter the course of disease for most patients, it has been shown to decrease the amount of fecal excretion of *Shigella* and decrease the risk of transmission of the disease.

Staphylococcal gastroenteritis is the most common type of food poisoning; it develops when food, particularly cream-filled pastries, milk products, cold meats, and products made with mayonnaise, become contaminated with an enterotoxin-producing strain of staphylococcus. If the food is left unrefrigerated for several hours, the organism multiplies rapidly and produces the toxin. Fluid and electrolyte replacement may be necessary in severe cases.

Diagnostic Studies. The diagnosis of diarrheal illnesses and gastroenteritis is primarily based on the history of exposure and clinical manifestations. Stool cultures and blood cultures are often used to identify the causative organism. In many cases, particularly in viral gastroenteritis, the pathogenic agent cannot be identified by readily available means.

★ **ASSESSMENT**

The nursing assessment includes a careful assessment of the child's fluid status with particular attention to mucous membranes, skin turgor, presence of sunken eyes or fontanel, and the quantity of urine output. Although it is difficult to quantify the volume of urine, parents often report that only stool and no urine has been noted in soiled diapers. The severity of dehydration must be assessed because it influences treatment measures and whether the child requires admission to the hospital.[12] Symptoms commonly associated with different degrees of dehydration are presented in Table 59-4. The nurse should inquire about any history of exposure to other children with diarrhea or foods that may have been contaminated.

★ **NURSING DIAGNOSES AND PLANNING**

Based on the assessment data from above and Chapter 58, the following nursing diagnoses may apply to the child with diarrhea:

- Diarrhea related to ingestion of contaminated food.
- Fluid Volume Deficit related to active fluid volume loss.
- High Risk for Infection transmission related to exposing other children.
- High Risk for Impaired Skin Integrity related to loose bowels.
- Anxiety related to knowledge deficit regarding oral rehydration treatment; infection control measures.

The nurse and child (or parents) together plan effective care based on the established nursing diagnoses. Several examples of expected outcomes follow:

TABLE 59-4
Assessment of Dehydration in Children

Severity	Percentage of Body Weight Lost as Water	Clinical Manifestations
Mild	Less than 5%	Decreased urine output Mild thirst
Moderate	5% to 10%	Marked thirst, little or no urine output, decreased tear formation, sunken eyes or fontanel, diminished skin turgor, dry mucous membranes, rapid breathing (due to acidosis)
Severe	More than 10%	All the symptoms of moderate dehydration plus lethargy, cool extremities, diminished peripheral pulses, tachycardia, low blood pressure

Adapted from Candy, C. (1987). Recent advances in the care of children with acute diarrhea: Giving the responsibility to the nurse and parents. *Journal of Advanced Nursing, 12,* 95–99.

- The parents relate frequent change of diapers and cleansing of skin.
- The parents describe proper handwashing after diaper changes.
- The child exhibits reestablishment of normal stools.

The nurse plans for the daily care of the child based on both physician's orders and nursing diagnoses. Some general nursing care goals may be the following:

- Fluid and electrolyte balance is reestablished.
- Diarrhea is relieved.

★ INTERVENTIONS: COLLABORATIVE AND INDEPENDENT

The treatment of diarrhea and gastroenteritis depends on the probable cause of the disease and the severity of the symptoms. The key issues in treatment include assessment of the hydration state of the child, institution of prompt rehydration, and determination of the probable causative agent to evaluate the need for antibiotic therapy. Mild cases of dehydration are often managed by substituting oral fluid and electrolyte solutions (such as Pedialyte or Pedialyte RS) for regular feedings for short periods of time. Vomiting is not a contraindication to attempting oral rehydration, however, the hydration state of the child must be assessed frequently. If the child is not progressing with oral rehydration, intravenous fluids may be indicated. Hypertonic solutions such as fruit juices and soup broth are not used for fluid replacement because the osmolality of the solution may exacerbate the diarrhea, and the concentration of sodium and potassium is inappropriate for replacement therapy. Once vomiting and diarrhea have abated, regular feedings are gradually reintroduced. More severe cases that result in greater than 5% dehydration may require hospitalization and intravenous replacement of fluids and electrolytes. A temporary lactase deficiency may develop after a severe bout of diarrhea, so it may be necessary to use lactase-free formulas when oral feedings resume. If oral feedings cannot be promptly reintroduced or if the child is already malnourished, parenteral nutrition may be necessary.

The frequent, loose stools may cause excoriation of the perineal area and diaper rash. Frequent diaper changes, thorough cleansing of the diaper area, and application of protective creams such as zinc oxide help to prevent and treat diaper rash.

Antibiotic therapy is beneficial in some episodes of bacterial gastroenteritis.[37] Antidiarrheal preparations that decrease GI motility generally are not helpful and are contraindicated in certain bacterial diarrhea. Enteric infection control measures must be instituted to prevent transmission of the disease to other family members or other hospitalized children. Careful handwashing and disposal of contaminated diapers are the most important measures to prevent transmission of the organism. Other infection control measures are described in the display on enteric precautions.

★ EVALUATION

Periodically, the nurse and family evaluate the outcomes of care given. Examples of outcomes for the child with diarrhea or gastroenteritis were given under Planning in this section.

Malabsorption

Definition. A large variety of pediatric diseases are associated with malabsorption. Malabsorption occurs when there is a disturbance in the digestion or absorption of any dietary component. Two basic processes are required for normal digestion and absorption. The first process is the chemical modification of dietary substrates within the intestinal lumen or along the mucosal surface. Secondly, the substrates must be transported across the intestinal mucosa into the bloodstream or lymphatic system. Any condition that disrupts either of these processes can lead to a malabsorptive disorder.[39,62] Many rare and common disorders affect the function of the small intestine and are associated with impaired absorption. Pediatric conditions associated with malabsorption are listed in the accompanying display.

Etiology and Pathophysiology. The etiology of malabsorptive conditions varies with the specific disorder. Many conditions are congenital, such as inborn errors of metabolism, intestinal atresias, or cystic fibrosis. Frequently, malabsorption is an acquired disease occurring secondarily to another condition such as NEC (leading to short bowel syndrome), cancer (requiring radiation therapy leading to enteritis), or gastroenteritis (causing damaged intestinal mucosa or lactose intolerance).

Depending on the particular condition, malabsorption may lead to the impaired absorption of many nutrients or, in some cases, only selected nutrients. The most common dietary substrates that are malabsorbed include carbohydrates (especially lactose), proteins, fats, fat-soluble vitamins (A, D, E, K), vitamin B_{12}, calcium,

---

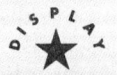

Enteric Precautions for Prevention of Transmission of Pathogens in the Feces or Oral Secretions

- Wash hands after touching patient or potentially contaminated articles such as diapers or ostomy output.
- Gloves and gowns must be worn if contact with patient or articles contaminated with fecal material is anticipated.
- Wash clothing or linen contaminated with feces in hot, soapy water and bleach if possible.
- Place hospitalized child in a private room if he or she is fecally incontinent or does not have reliable hygiene practices.
- Disinfect soiled surfaces with a 1:10 dilution of bleach or appropriate antiseptic solution.
- Dispose of contaminated articles in specially designated location.

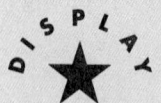

Pediatric Conditions Associated With Malabsorption

Anatomic or Structural Disorders: Lead to shortened bowel length, impaired circulation to intestine, or bacterial overgrowth and stasis, which impair acid deconjugation.

- Structural disorders requiring bowel resection as intestinal atresia, volvulus, or necrotizing enterocolitis
- Strictures or adhesions secondary previous bowel surgery
- Lymphatic drainage abnormalities (lymphangiectasis)

Functional Disorders: Interfere with the breakdown or uptake of substrates by intestinal epithelium (damaged intestinal mucosa is often present).

- Infection, viral or bacterial
- Malnutrition

- Intolerance to dietary protein, carbohydrates, or fats
- Pancreatic insufficiency (cystic fibrosis)
- Inflammatory bowel disease
- Radiation enteritis
- Inborn errors of metabolism (usually affect function of a specific enzyme system)
- Celiac disease

Miscellaneous Disorders: Impair intestinal function by a variety of mechanisms

- Immunologic disorders
- Collagen diseases
- Renal insufficiency
- Drug therapy
- Maternal deprivation (possibly due to pancreatic insufficiency)

iron, magnesium, and zinc. Inadequate amounts of these nutrients can significantly impair tissue growth and retard growth and development. In children, inadequate growth is of particular concern because of potential negative effects on critical phases of brain and bone development and because of the possibility of irreversible delays in growth.

Clinical Manifestations. Malabsorption is suspected when any of the following symptoms are noted: failure to thrive, abdominal distention, abnormal stools (diarrhea, steatorrhea), bone abnormalities (rickets, osteoporosis, fractures), skin manifestations of nutritional deficiencies (flaky dermatitis, easy bruising), stunted growth, muscle wasting, peripheral edema, apathy, irritability.

If any of these symptoms are present and are accompanied by a history consistent with a malabsorptive disorder or by a physical examination that reveals signs of malnutrition, the possibility of a malabsorptive disorder must be considered.[39]

A careful history and physical examination are a crucial step in the diagnosis of malnutrition. The examiner should obtain a careful dietary history and try to determine the relationship of the onset of symptoms and the introduction of various foods such as gluten-containing foods (cereals) or cow's milk. (Gluten is a protein factor present in wheat, rye, barley, and oats.) The physical examination should include plotting of the child's height, weight, and head circumference (for children under 2 years of age) on standardized growth charts. If feasible, previous measurements should be obtained to evaluate long-term changes (Figs. 59-11 and 59-12). Muscle tone and strength, thickness of subcutaneous fat stores, and general skin condition are also evaluated. Further diagnostic studies greatly depend on the initial clinical presentation.

A variety of studies are often obtained during the evaluation of malabsorption.

Diagnostic Studies. Stool samples may be evaluated for fecal fat content, the presence of bacteria, viruses, ova, cysts and parasites, and for occult blood. The pH of stool samples is often tested; a low pH (4.0 to 5.0) is associated with acids released during the fermentation of unabsorbed carbohydrates. The presence of reducing substances or a low pH in the stool may also indicate malabsorption of carbohydrate. Blood samples are obtained to measure a complete blood count and other hematologic studies, serum iron levels, sodium, potassium, chloride, calcium, phosphorus, magnesium, zinc, and vitamin levels (particularly fat-soluble vitamins). Abdominal x-rays and barium contrast studies may be used to identify structural intestinal problems. Bone x-rays are sometimes used to evaluate osteoporosis, rickets, and bone age. A small intestinal biopsy may be done to evaluate the intestinal mucosa. Damaged mucosa is associated with many malabsorptive conditions. A variety of enzymatic, metabolic, and immunologic studies are used if rare, malabsorptive conditions are suspected.

Intervention. The treatment of malabsorptive disorders is based on the specific condition. In cases of malabsorption of a particular nutrient (e.g., lactose intolerance or celiac disease), the offending substrate is withheld and appropriate substitutions are made. If malabsorption is caused by an anatomic defect (unrelenting ulcerative colitis), surgery may be indicated. If the intestinal mucosa has been damaged, it is often necessary to withhold or reduce feedings temporarily until the bowel recovers. Parenteral nutrition may be required during the healing phase and to correct severe malnutrition.

Several specific diseases associated with malabsorp-

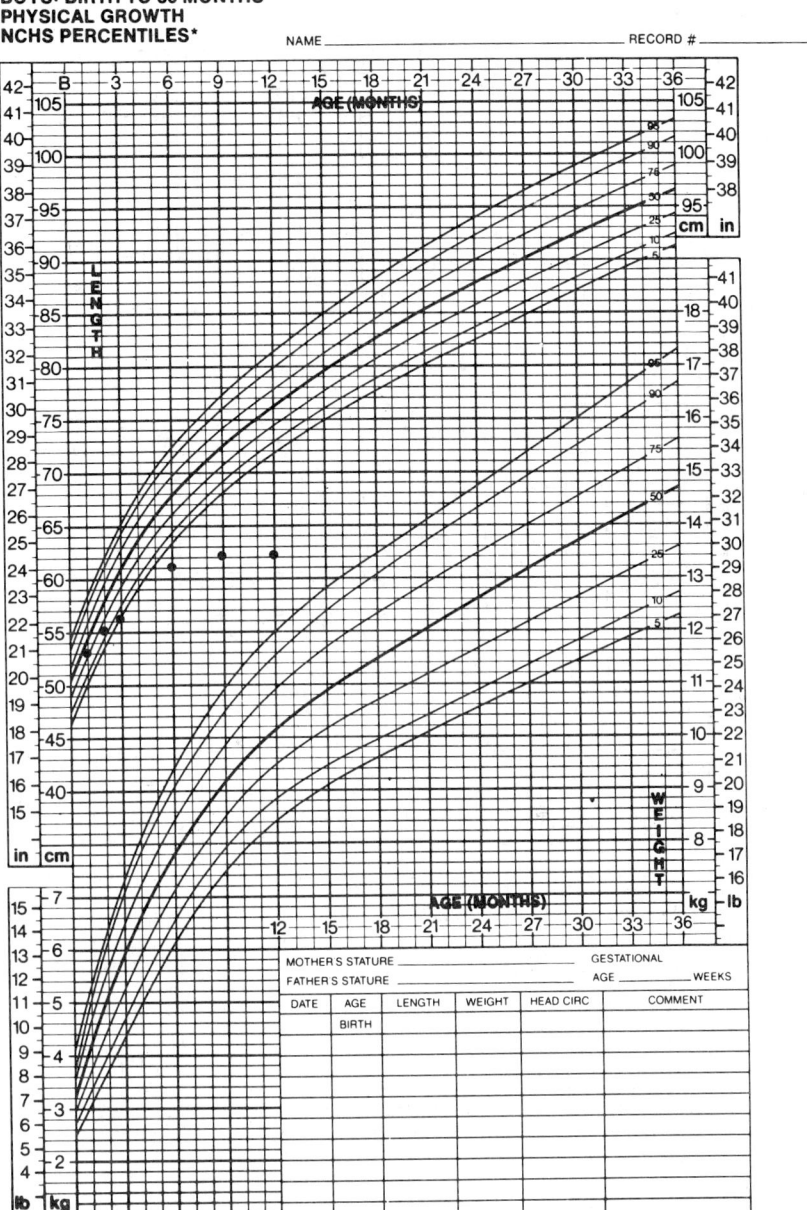

BOYS: BIRTH TO 36 MONTHS
PHYSICAL GROWTH
NCHS PERCENTILES*

NAME _____ RECORD # _____

FIGURE 59-11

Following the infant's length and weight on standardized growth charts, as shown in this example, will indicate early problems in growth. (Source: Adapted from: Hamill, P. V. V., et al. [1979]. Physical growth: National Center for Health Statistics percentiles. *American Journal of Clinical Nutrition, 32,* 607. Data from the Fels Research Institute, Wright State University School of Medicine, Yellow Springs, OH. Courtesy of Ross Laboratories.)

tion are described further in the following section with more detail provided on the interventions required based on the etiology of the malabsorption.

Lactose Intolerance

Lactose is a sugar (disaccharide) found in many common dairy products, most notably milk. The list includes breast milk; mammalian milk (whole, skim, low fat); yogurt; cheese; ice cream, cream, milkshakes; pudding; creamed soups or vegetables; mashed potatoes; many processed foods; and cookies, cakes, breads. The inability to digest lactose is marked by GI symptoms of cramps, bloating, gas, or diarrhea. The intestinal enzyme, lactase,

is required for adequate absorption. Lactase activity is decreased after infectious gastroenteritis or injury to the intestinal mucosa caused by gluten or other proteins. Therefore, it is a common practice to use infant formulas containing sucrose or glucose polymers rather than lactose for children recovering from gastroenteritis.

Etiology and Pathophysiology. Another important cause of lactose intolerance is an ethnically related lactase deficiency. The exact cause of the gradual loss of enzyme activity is unclear; however, the mutation of a regulatory gene has been theorized as a possible explanation. The age of onset of lactase deficiency varies from early childhood to late teenage years. The prevalence of lactose intolerance is highest (about 100%) among American In-

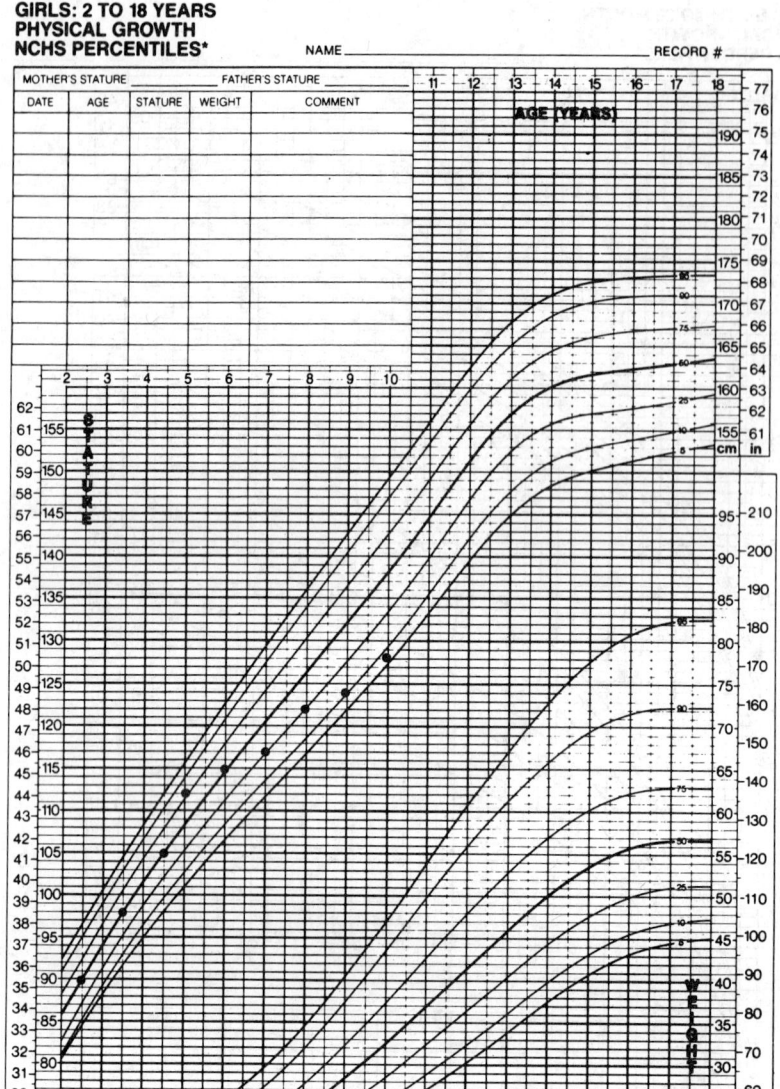

GIRLS: 2 TO 18 YEARS
PHYSICAL GROWTH
NCHS PERCENTILES*

FIGURE 59-12

Long-term follow-up of a child on a standardized growth chart shows idiosyncracies in growth, as in this example. (Source: Adapted from: Hamill, P. V. V., et al. [1979]. Physical growth: National Center for Health Statistics percentiles. *American Journal of Clinical Nutrition, 32,* 607. Data from the Fels Research Institute, Wright State University School of Medicine, Yellow Springs, OH. Courtesy of Ross Laboratories.)

dians, Eskimos, Japanese, and Chinese, whereas the prevalence among Caucasian Americans is about 20%. In African Americans, the incidence of lactose intolerance increases after 10 years of age.[39]

Diagnostic Studies. Lactose intolerance is usually diagnosed through a breath hydrogen test or by jejunal biopsy.

Intervention. Once diagnosed, the treatment of lactose intolerance involves the elimination of all or some lactose-containing products from the diet. In severe cases, lactose must be strictly restricted from the diet. In other cases, the person may be able to tolerate some lactose-containing foods such as yogurt and cheeses. In addition, many supermarkets in the United States carry special milk and milk products that contain prehydrolyzed lactose

(LactAid). Dietary counseling is often indicated for people with severe disease to ensure adequate intake of calcium and protein. Calcium supplementation is often necessary.

Celiac Disease

Definition and Incidence. Celiac disease is a disorder in which the intestinal mucosa of susceptible patients is damaged by gluten-containing foods. The exact mechanism responsible for mucosal damage is unknown, but both biochemical defects and immunologic mechanisms have been implicated. The prevalence of celiac disease is highest in western Ireland and is uncommon among blacks and Oriental populations. Celiac disease is not as commonly diagnosed in the United States as in many European countries, but it is unclear if this represents a decreased prevalence or failure to diagnose the disease.[9] Recent studies have demonstrated a decreasing incidence of celiac disease. The reasons for the lower rate of occurrence have been speculated to be related to an increase in the number of infants who are breast-fed, decreases in the antigenicity and osmolarity of infant formulas, and the trend toward the later introduction of solid, gluten-containing foods.[69]

Clinical Manifestations. The malabsorption associated with celiac disease is related to the damaged epithelium of the duodenum and jejunum caused by the gluten.[9,69] The onset of symptoms is usually related to the introduction of gluten-containing cereals, but symptoms may be subtle or may be delayed by months. The onset typically occurs between 8 and 24 months of age. The most common symptom is diarrhea, often with pale, foul, greasy, bulky stools. Other common presenting symptoms may include failure to thrive, abdominal pain or distention, vomiting, anorexia or voracious appetite, and striking personality characteristics including irritability, apathy, and extremely clingy behavior. Approximately 10% of children present with constipation and often severe fecal impaction rather than diarrhea. If malnutrition is severe, muscle wasting, stunted growth, severe abdominal distention, peripheral edema, anemia, and vitamin deficiency may be noted.

Diagnostic Studies. The diagnosis of celiac disease is based on a jejunal biopsy that shows typical mucosal lesions. If the biopsy results are consistent with celiac disease, a gluten-free diet is introduced for 18 to 24 months. A second biopsy is obtained to verify the return of normal jejunal architecture. A gluten challenge may be performed at this time to distinguish between transient gluten intolerance and celiac disease. In many cases, the gluten challenge is deferred until after puberty so as not to set back growth inadvertently by the introduction of gluten. Another biopsy is performed after the gluten challenge. If celiac disease is confirmed, permanent gluten restriction from the diet is necessary.[39,62] The introduction of this diet requires the restriction of many common foods and is considered as a severe hardship by many families.

★ ASSESSMENT

An assessment of the child's nutritional status including an accurate height, weight, and head circumference is an essential component of a thorough database. The nurse also has an important role in assessing the family's understanding of the diagnosis and compliance with dietary management.

★ NURSING DIAGNOSES AND PLANNING

Based on the assessment data from above and Chapter 58, the following nursing diagnosis may apply to the child with celiac disease:

- Altered Nutrition: Less Than Body Requirements related to inability to absorb nutrients.

- High Risk for Fluid Volume Deficit related to diarrhea.
- Altered Growth and Development related to effects of disease state.
- Diarrhea related to disease state.
- Impaired Social Interaction related to personality characteristics.
- Noncompliance (dietary restrictions) related to boredom with diet choices.
- Ineffective Family Coping: Disabling related to prolonged disease.
- Anxiety related to knowledge deficit regarding dietary management; potential consequences of dietary indiscretions.

The nurse and child (or parents) together plan effective care based on the established nursing diagnoses. Several examples of expected outcomes follow:

- The family describe celiac disease and its consequences.
- The family identify foods to be avoided in diet.
- The child exhibits use of diet.

The nurse plans for the daily care of the child based on both physician's orders and nursing diagnoses. Some general nursing care goals may be the following:

- The child maintains an asymptomatic status.
- The child's growth and development are adequate.

★ INTERVENTIONS: COLLABORATIVE AND INDEPENDENT

A primary goal of nursing intervention is education of the family about celiac disease and dietary management. Most children respond extremely well to a gluten-restricted diet and may be asymptomatic for long periods. It is often tempting for the child and parents to liberalize the diet. Occasional dietary transgressions may not cause notable symptoms and reinforces the false idea that the disease is cured and that the restricted diet is no longer necessary. Research studies have demonstrated that relapses occur in most people if dietary restrictions are not maintained.[62] Chronic illness, fatigue, and growth retardation are subtle indicators of dietary transgressions.

Many common foods such as spaghetti, hamburgers, pizza, and most cereals are restricted from the diet. Creative approaches to dietary management are important to prevent boredom with a repetitive diet. The child often feels different or isolated from peers because he or she is unable to eat the same foods. A pediatric dietitian is an excellent resource for nutrition education and can offer innovative ideas and recipes for gluten-free foods. Adolescents should be encouraged to experiment with acceptable recipes and to take responsibility for their dietary management. A number of national organizations provide lists of commercially available gluten-free foods and gluten-free recipes.[39,55]

★ EVALUATION

Periodically, the nurse and family evaluate the outcomes of care given. Examples of outcomes for the child with celiac disease were given under Planning in this section. Have short-term goals been met? Are long-term goals still realistic? Planning for further nursing care also takes into consideration complications.

COMPLICATIONS

Celiac disease is associated with rare but serious complications. A celiac crisis may be precipitated by a intercurrent infection, a prolonged fast, or anticholinergic medications. This complication is characterized by severe diarrhea and vomiting, leading to dehydration, acidosis, intestinal obstruction, and shock. Parents are instructed about the need for the child to avoid exposure to infection as much as possible and to observe their child closely if vomiting or diarrhea develops. Anticholinergic medications are often prescribed as antihistamines, mild sedatives, and for preoperative medication. The parent is taught always to report the child's celiac disease to the physician or dentist when a history is taken and to remind them of the disorder if any of these drugs are prescribed.[62]

Short Bowel Syndrome

Short bowel syndrome most commonly results from clinical conditions that require an extensive resection of the small bowel, such as NEC, intestinal atresia, or volvulus. Children who have undergone massive resections are a challenge to the health care team. This condition is usually associated with severe malabsorption due to the large loss of bowel. The outcome after bowel resection depends on a number of factors including:[13,62]

- Extent of resection—The small intestine of a normal neonate is approximately 250 cm in length. A high mortality rate is seen in children with less than 40 cm of bowel remaining, especially if the ileocecal valve is removed. A high survival rate (95%) has been reported in children with more than 60 to 75 cm of bowel remaining.
- Preservation of ileocecal valve—An intact ileocecal valve significantly improves survival because it reduces the risk of bacterial contamination from the colon into the small bowel.
- The ability of the shortened intestine to adapt—Fortunately, in many cases of bowel resection, the remaining bowel is able to adapt and compensate for the lost bowel. The mechanisms of adaptation include dilatation and elongation of the remaining small bowel, an increase in villous size, and decreased motility. These adaptive processes increase the surface area available for absorption.
- Area of small bowel resected—The ileum more readily adapts and compensates for the resected jejunum than the reverse.
- Success at reducing complications of parenteral nutrition—Many children who have undergone bowel resection require long-term parental nutrition and central venous catheterization. A number of complications of this therapy can be life-threatening including liver damage, metabolic derangements, sepsis, and thrombosis of the major veins.[1,4]

★ ASSESSMENT

Many children with short bowel syndrome are hospitalized for extended periods. A thorough initial and ongoing assessment of family dynamics, acceptance of diagnosis, and understanding and compliance with the treatment regimen is an essential component of the nursing care plan. Families often have difficulty understanding that their child who appears healthy and robust (due to parenteral nutrition) is actually in a precarious nutritional state. The family may have trouble conceptualizing the difference between oral nutrition (which enters the GI system) and parenteral nutrition (which enters the venous system).

★ NURSING DIAGNOSES AND PLANNING

Based on the assessment data from above and Chapter 58, the following nursing diagnoses may apply to the child with short bowel syndrome:

- Altered Nutrition: Less Than Body Requirements related to inability to absorb nutrients due to biologic factors.
- High Risk for Impaired Skin Integrity (perineal skin rashes) related to volume of loose bowels.
- Gustatory Sensory/Perceptual Alteration related to altered stimuli.
- High Risk for Infection (Candidal) related to inadequate primary defenses.
- High Risk for Fluid Volume Deficit related to volume of loose bowels.
- High Risk for Altered Growth and Development related to environmental deficiencies.
- Altered Parenting related to unrealistic expectations of self and child.
- Altered Health Maintenance related to ineffective individual coping.
- Knowledge Deficit regarding disease process; signs of feeding intolerance and infection; home TPN; promoting developmental activities.

The nurse and child (or parents) together plan effective care based on the established nursing diagnoses. Several examples of expected outcomes follow:

- The parents participate in daily routine of care.
- The parents exhibit understanding of TPN by return demonstration.
- The child follows structured daily schedule.
- The child participates in specially planned motor play.

The nurse plans for the daily care of the child based on both physician's orders and nursing diagnoses. Some general nursing care goals may be the following:

- The child tolerates enteral feedings.
- Infection is prevented.
- The child maintains normal growth and development on sustained feeding levels.

★ INTERVENTIONS: COLLABORATIVE AND INDEPENDENT

The management of the patient with short bowel syndrome includes a gradual introduction of enteral feedings and the provision of parenteral nutrition. Feedings are started with small volumes of a dilute formula administered as a bolus every 2 to 3 hours or administered by way of a continuous nasogastric drip. Feedings are advanced slowly according to the infant's tolerance. A large increase in stool volume, low stool pH, or the presence of reducing substances in the stool indicate the tolerance level has been reached.

Advancement of the feedings to a level where the infant can maintain normal growth and development on enteral calories only may take months to years. Parenteral nutrition by way of a central venous catheter is usually required throughout this period to provide adequate nutrition. Some oral intake should be maintained because experimental studies have suggested that oral feedings promote intestinal adaptation and reduce the incidence of feeding difficulties.[50] Close monitoring of growth parameters and developmental status is important.[13,62]

Consistent and diligent nursing care is essential to ensure optimum recovery for infants with short bowel syndrome. The severe malabsorption, lengthy hospitalization, preparation for discharge, long-term parenteral nutrition, and alterations in family dynamics all present a challenge to the nurse.

The infant's tolerance of enteral feedings is constantly monitored. Strict intake and output records and daily weights are recorded. All stools are tested for pH and glucose, and the volume, color, and consistency are documented. The presence of glucose or a low pH may indicate intolerance. Sudden changes in stool frequency or glucose content, vomiting, or gastric retention of formula also indicate formula intolerance.

Perineal skin rashes and excoriation are common due to the large volume of liquid stool output and the presence of bile acids, bile acid binding resins, and enzymes in the stool. In addition, trace element or vitamin deficiencies or a superimposed candidal infection can cause further skin breakdown. Frequent diaper changes and a thorough cleansing of the perineal region after each stool are vital in preventing skin breakdown. Protective creams such as zinc oxide should be applied liberally after the skin is cleansed. Antifungal creams are used to treat candidal infections, and cholestyramine may be used if bile acid malabsorption is suspected. Leaving the buttocks open to air or gentle drying with a heat lamp is often helpful in treating excoriated areas. The nurse and parents should avoid using commercial wipes on irritated skin.

An important nursing goal for children with short bowel syndrome is to encourage healthy family dynamics and to promote normal development of the child. The parenting relationship and family support system are often strained by the severity of the initial disease and the long-term implications of short bowel syndrome. Nurses can help parents cope with the lengthy hospitalization and complex medical care by thorough explanations of the infant's care and by encouraging parental involvement in their child's daily routine. Many children with short bowel syndrome are discharged on home parenteral nutrition. Education of the family about catheter care and TPN therapy should be started as early as possible.[1] The teaching plan for home TPN and the Nursing Care Plan for abdominal surgery outline many important details in the care of the child with short bowel syndrome. The reader is also referred to the display entitled Family Teaching: Written Instructions for TPN Home Care.

An important nursing task is to promote an atmosphere that is conducive to optimal development of the child. Some practitioners have noted an increased incidence of gross motor and language delays in children receiving long-term TPN. These developmental delays were diminished with interventions specifically designed to encourage the acquisition of developmental milestones. The use of schedules to provide structure for the child's day, the provision of opportunities for motor play, and the use of a developmental stimulation program designed specifically for the child may promote optimal development.[50]

★ **EVALUATION**

Periodically, the nurse and family evaluate the outcomes of care given. Examples of outcomes for the child with short bowel syndrome were given under Planning in this section. Have short-term goals been met? Are long-term goals still realistic?

In the future, small bowel transplantation may offer some hope for children who have had extensive bowel resections, and whose remaining bowels are unable to adapt sufficiently. A small number of human small-intestinal transplantations have been performed; however, long-term survival with this procedure has not been reported.[58]

Disorders of the Pancreas

Acute Pancreatitis

Definition and Incidence.   The diagnosis of acute pancreatitis, once considered unusual in children, is being recognized with increasing frequency. Although the actual incidence of pancreatitis is unknown, it is estimated that major pediatric centers see at least 10 new cases per year. Many mild cases may be undiagnosed or misdiagnosed. The increased frequency is attributed to improved recognition of the disorder, a rise in the number of children subjected to blunt abdominal trauma, and the increased use of therapeutic agents that can cause pancreatitis.[29]

Pancreatitis is an inflammation of the pancreas caused by a large variety of insults. Once the inflammatory process begins, pancreatic enzymes can be activated, causing autodigestion of the pancreas and surrounding tissue as well as other systemic effects. The severity of this disorder ranges from mild and often unrecognized disease to extremely serious and even fatal disease.[29,62] The child may experience complete recovery or may go on to develop chronic pancreatitis.[74]

Etiology and Pathophysiology.   A large variety of causes of pancreatitis have been identified. Blunt abdominal trauma is associated with 30% to 40% of cases. Injury may be due to child abuse but is often associated with bicycle or sledding injuries. The pancreas has a soft consistency and a plentiful vascular supply, and is not well protected by the abdominal musculature, especially in children. Thus, the pancreas is susceptible to sharp or blunt injury to the upper abdomen such as that caused by falling on bicycle handlebars. Injury to the pancreas can occur with seemingly mild trauma. Symptoms of pancreatitis may develop immediately after the injury or may

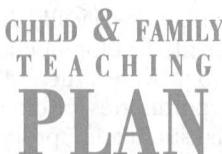

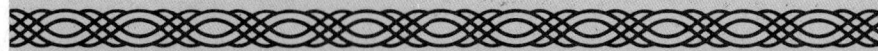

CHILD & FAMILY TEACHING PLAN

Home Total Parenteral Nutrition for an Infant

Assessment

Baby Boy Kyle diagnosed with necrotizing enterocolitis requiring subsequent small bowel resection. (Nursing Care Plan for Kyle appears earlier in Chapter.) Kyle is ready for discharge on home parenteral nutrition. The mother, Ms. Stuart, is single and resides with her mother within the city limits. Both are high school graduates. The mother and grandmother have some experience with the central line care and infusion pumps acquired during the infant's lengthy hospitalization. They identify a need to practice the procedures before discharge.

It is important to progress from simple procedures to the more complicated ones. Allow them to master one before progressing to the next. Allay fears. Build confidence.

Child and Family Objectives	Specific Content	Teaching Strategies
1. Verbalize steps in performing central venous catheter (CVC) dressing change.	1. Steps of CVC dressing change, including equipment required.	1. Use written material and pictures. Show dressing change kit and contents. Demonstrate procedure on teaching board or doll. Answer questions.
2. Demonstrate knowledge and skills when performing TPN dressing change (three times).	2. Key steps and rationale for TPN dressing change.	2. Allow them to practice on teaching board before done on infant. Discuss steps not done correctly. Allow them to be nonsterile helper first before progressing to sterile dressing change.
3. Describe a healthy CVC site.	3. Healthy CVC site description.	3. Discuss site with mother during dressing change. Use written material. Encourage questions.
4. Recognize when a CVC site looks infected.	4. Signs and symptoms (redness, drainage, tenderness, temperature 38.5° C) and location. Identify whom to contact regarding signs and symptoms.	4. Use written material regarding signs and symptoms. List of names and phone numbers to notify for infection.
5. Verbalize signs of sensitivity to tape and relate care alternatives if sensitivity persists.	5. Skin appearance if tape is irritating (excessive redness, skin breakdown). Demonstrate taping alternatives: use different tape, shift dressing to side, use Telfa over areas of breakdown.	5. Use written instructions. Describe skin appearance. Demonstrate taping alternatives.
6. State reason for Kyle's receiving TPN therapy.	6. Need for proper nutrition in infancy and method of providing it.	6. Discussion. Written instructions. Answer questions.
7. List major components in TPN solution.	7. Major components listed on bag of TPN fluid.	7. Use written material. Discuss the need and function of each.
8. Demonstrate skills to monitor IV infusion pump.	8. Display modes and alarms on infusion pump. Setting and function of each.	8. Use written material, pictures, and flow chart. Set up mock situations to troubleshoot.
9. Demonstrate the skills of priming the TPN tubing (three times).	9. Priming of tubing.	9. Use written material with pictures. Allow practice until parent can proceed without prompting.

(Continued)

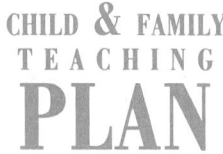

CHILD & FAMILY
T E A C H I N G
PLAN

Home Total Parenteral Nutrition for an Infant (continued)

Child and Family Objectives	Specific Content	Teaching Strategies
10. Demonstrate skill for starting TPN infusion (three times).	10. Role of sterile and nonsterile persons.	10. Use written materials; practice sessions. Discussion and demonstration. Talk through steps initially. Allow mother and grandmother to complete steps without prompting.
11. Verbalize and demonstrate measuring and recording accurate intake and output.	11. Set up recording system (dependent on physician preference). Provide notebook with columns for recording of daily intake/urine output/stool output. If stools need to be tested, demonstrate use of *p*H tape and Testape.	11. Use written material. Demonstrate and practice.
12. Demonstrate urine glucose testing.	12. Demonstrate collection method and Testape procedure. Instruction on whom to contact if glucose is greater than 180.	12. Use written material. Return demonstration.
13. Demonstrate the use of chemstrip.	13. Chemstrips are used to measure the sugar content of blood. Instruction on whom to contact if glucose is greater than 180.	13. Use written material. Demonstration and return demonstration.
14. State principles of and demonstrate skills for performing heparin lock procedure.	14. Heparin prevents a blood clot from forming in the catheter when the infusion is stopped. Use of syringe and principle of drawing medication into syringe. Stress importance of expelling all air bubbles. Demonstrate steps of placing infusion cap, heparin, irrigation, and securing line.	14. Use written material. Simulated practice. Supervise mother and grandmother performing steps until they are proficient.
15. Describe and demonstrate performance of cyclic TPN therapy.	15. Importance of weaning rate up over 1 h and back down over 1 h (prevention of hypoglycemia). Write out actual rates based on discharge description. Potential benefits of cycling TPN: increased mobility; improved appetite when off TPN; allows for a "more normal" family lifestyle.	15. Explain rationale. Written instructions and return demonstration. Review signs and symptoms of hypoglycemia. Have mother and grandmother demonstrate procedure.
16. Relate and demonstrate steps required for blunt needle repair.	16. Blunt needle repair is done when catheter breaks. Who to contact when repair is complete. Prompt repair of the catheter decreases risk of infection or occlusion. This prevents air embolism or blood loss from line.	16. Written instructions. Demonstration and return demonstration. Troubleshooting session.

(Continued)

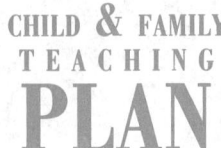

Home Total Parenteral Nutrition for an Infant (continued)

Child and Family Objectives	*Specific Content*	*Teaching Strategies*
17. List three complications that may occur.	17. "Complications of Home TPN Therapy Worksheet" serves as a tool for evaluation.	17. Worksheet. Have mother and grandmother complete. Discuss correct answers and rationale. Answer questions.
18. Describes how to elicit appropriate staff referrals and resources if complications occur.	18. List of who to call when there are problems. Discuss before discharge.	18. Written list with names and phone numbers of resources when problems arise.

Evaluation

- Mother and grandmother read written material provided.
- Mother and grandmother perform the following procedures without intervention from medical staff: central venous catheter dressing change; operate the infusion pump; prime the TPN tubing; start the TPN infusion; heparin lock; heparin irrigation; blunt needle repair.
- Mother and grandmother verbalize and display skills necessary to monitor Kyle's tolerance of the TPN infusion: urine Testape; chemstrip; cycling TPN; signs and symptoms of infection.
- Mother and grandmother recognize complications.
- Mother and grandmother describe what to do and who to call for complications and emergencies.

be delayed until hours to weeks later. When the nurse is taking a history of a patient with abdominal pain, the parent should be asked specifically about possible abdominal trauma because the episode may have been forgotten by the time the symptoms appear.[29,39]

Drug-related pancreatitis has been increasingly recognized and is estimated to cause approximately 30% of cases. L-asparaginase, used primarily in the treatment of leukemia, has been associated with fulminant pancreatitis. Valproic acid, thiazides, and steroids have all been identified as causative agents in pancreatitis. The onset of symptoms may occur days to weeks after the medication is discontinued.[29] Ethanol abuse is the most commonly recognized cause of pancreatitis in adults, and, although it is an unusual causative factor in children, the increased use of alcohol by adolescents may lead to an increased frequency of pediatric cases of alcohol-induced pancreatitis.

A number of less common causes of pancreatitis have been identified, including infection of the bile duct with the Ascaris worm, viral diseases such as mumps, measles, or hepatitis, cystic fibrosis, and congenital or metabolic diseases.[68] No specific cause can be found in about 30% of cases.

The pathophysiology of pancreatitis is due to the disruption of the pancreatic glandular tissue and of the pancreatic duct and subsequent leakage and activation of pancreatic enzymes. These enzymes have proteolytic and lipolytic activity, which can result in autodigestion of the pancreas as well as digestion of the protein and fat components of the peritoneal cavity, causing peritonitis. Spread of the enzymes by way of the bloodstream and lymphatic system accounts for many of the systemic complications. One of the most severe systemic effects and a primary cause of early death is severe hypotension leading to shock and organ failure. The decreased blood pressure is due to massive losses of blood and plasma caused by the autodigestion of blood vessels and subsequent hemorrhage.[29,39,62]

Clinical Manifestations.   Pancreatitis may present suddenly with severe symptoms that include shock and peritonitis, but, in most cases, the onset is more insidious. Abdominal pain is the most predominant symptom and occurs in at least 90% of patients. The pain is often intense and is usually localized in the epigastrium, and may radiate to the back or upper abdominal quadrants. The character of pain varies from mild to severe and is typically constant; however, intermittent pain may be observed in some patients. Pain is worsened by eating or movement. Children with pancreatitis often lie quietly on their side with the knees flexed. Nausea and vomiting occur in over 75% of cases.[39] Fever, tachycardia, abdominal fullness and distention are often present.[29]

An important complication of acute pancreatitis is the development of a pancreatic pseudocyst. This condition results from the accumulation of pancreatic products, inflammatory exudate, and plasma in a non-epithelial lined cavity near the pancreas. The pseudocyst often may be noted as a tender, palpable epigastric mass and can usually be seen with ultrasonography. The pseudocyst frequently resolves spontaneously within 4 to 12 weeks but may rupture. Rupture of the cyst is associated with a high mortality, so patients require close observation. Pseudocysts that fail to resolve spontaneously require surgical drainage.[44,74]

Diagnostic Studies. Measurement of serum amylase is the most readily available laboratory test for the assessment of pancreatitis. Levels exceeding three times the normal amount generally indicate active pancreatic inflammation.[62] Serum amylase rises within several hours after onset of symptoms but is readily cleared by the kidneys, so that elevation may be brief (hours to days) and can be missed completely. Serum lipase levels also rise shortly after the onset of symptoms and remain elevated for up to 10 days.

Pancreatic ultrasound is the most reliable, noninvasive test available to measure and monitor pancreatic inflammation and the formation of pancreatic pseudocyst or abscess. Serial ultrasounds are often obtained to facilitate early recognition of an evolving pseudocyst and to allow ongoing monitoring of its resolution. Other tests may be collected to aid in the identification of the causative agent and to monitor for possible complications. These tests include complete blood count, viral cultures, and calcium, phosphorus, and glucose levels.

★ ASSESSMENT

The nursing assessment of the child with pancreatitis includes early recognition of the potential for the disease in a child complaining of abdominal pain, especially if there is a history of trauma. After diagnosis, the nurse must assess the family's understanding of the disease and treatment.

★ NURSING DIAGNOSES AND PLANNING

Based on the assessment data from above and Chapter 58, the following nursing diagnoses may apply to the child with acute pancreatitis:

- Altered Nutrition: Less Than Body Requirements related to inability to ingest certain foods due to prescribed rest of pancreas.
- Pain related to trauma.
- High Risk for Fluid Volume Deficit related to trauma to, or hemorrhage of, pancreas.
- Impaired Physical Mobility related to therapy.
- Altered Health Maintenance related to ineffective individual coping.
- Diversional Activity Deficit related to restricted activity.
- Knowledge Deficit regarding activity restrictions; home TPN.

The nurse and child (or parents) together plan effective care based on the established nursing diagnoses. Several examples of expected outcomes follow:

- The parents discuss their guilt feelings regarding delay in seeking care.
- The parents practice home TPN.

- The child participates in self-care.
- The child expresses his or her feelings concerning therapy.

The nurse plans for the daily care of the child based on both physician's orders and nursing diagnoses. Some general nursing care goals may be the following:

- Fluid and electrolyte balance are maintained.
- Pain is controlled.
- Oral feedings are resumed.

★ INTERVENTIONS: COLLABORATIVE AND INDEPENDENT

Nursing care of the child with pancreatitis primarily involves supportive measures and ongoing maintenance of required medical therapy. The parents often feel guilty for not seeking immediate medical treatment after an apparently mild trauma. In most cases, the nurse should acknowledge the parents' guilt feelings, assure them that their reactions were appropriate, and praise them for seeking medical attention when they did. If child abuse or neglect is suspected, it must be reported to the appropriate authorities.

The primary therapies for pancreatitis include aggressive fluid and electrolyte replacement (including blood and plasma if indicated), control of pain, and complete reduction of stimulation of the pancreas. The child is placed NPO, and nasogastric suction is initiated. These measures decompress the stomach, reduce stimulation of the pancreatic enzymes, and usually diminish the pain. Meperidine (Demerol) may be required for pain relief. Morphine is not used because it has a spasmodic effect on the biliary tree. Histamine antagonists (cimetidine, ranitidine), anticholinergic drugs, and prophylactic antibiotics may be used, but their effectiveness is controversial.

In severe, fulminant cases associated with pancreatic hemorrhage or necrosis, peritoneal lavage or surgical debridement of the pancreas may be necessary. The patient may be critically ill and require intensive support. Nasogastric suction is discontinued after the initial attack subsides, generally within 4 to 10 days. Oral feedings are held until after nausea and vomiting, abdominal pain and tenderness, fever, and leukocytosis have resolved, after serum amylase and lipase levels have returned to normal, and when there is no evidence of pseudocyst formation.[29] Oral feeds are resumed cautiously, initially with clear fluids containing carbohydrates only. Oral intake of fats and proteins stimulates pancreatic secretions, and these are introduced slowly in small amounts. If symptoms recur or if serum amylase levels rise, oral feedings are withheld and parenteral nutrition is used.[29,39,62]

Surgical intervention to drain a pseudocyst is only attempted after the cyst matures (forms a fibrous capsule). This process may take 6 to 8 weeks, and the child must remain NPO throughout this time. A central venous catheter is inserted, and the child is maintained on parenteral nutrition during this period.[44]

Some children may be discharged on home TPN while awaiting maturation of the pseudocyst. Frequent follow-up of serum amylase levels and pancreatic ultrasound examinations are necessary to monitor the pseudocyst. The nurse provides opportunities for the family to observe and practice home TPN therapy before discharge[1] (see the Teaching Plan in this chapter). To diminish feelings of dependence and restriction, the child is encouraged to participate in his or her care if feasible. For example, child can assist with clamping of the catheter and handing supplies to the parent.

Pancreatitis and pseudocyst formation often occur in healthy, active school-age children. Contact sports and active play must be avoided during the recovery period. The restriction of oral intake and of normal play activities can be stressful for the child. The nurse assists the parents and child to identify alternative activities and encourages the child to express his or her feelings about the medical therapy. Therapeutic medical play is often beneficial for these children.

★ EVALUATION

Periodically, the nurse and family evaluate the outcomes of care given. Examples of outcomes for the child with abdominal trauma were given under Planning in this section. Have short-term goals been met? Are long-term goals still realistic?

Chronic Recurrent Pancreatitis

Several rare conditions result in chronic pancreatitis, including familial autosomal dominant disorders, severe metabolic abnormalities such as hyperlipidemia, or repeated bouts of pancreatitis. These conditions are associated with recurrent episodes of abdominal pain and intermittent attacks of acute pancreatitis. Ultimately, chronic pancreatitis can lead to pancreatic insufficiency requiring insulin and pancreatic enzyme replacement, narcotic dependency (for pain control), and possibly the need for total or subtotal pancreatectomy. These patients have an increased risk of pancreatic carcinoma.[39,72]

Pancreatic Insufficiency in Cystic Fibrosis

The most common cause of pancreatic insufficiency in North American and European children is cystic fibrosis. This is a genetically transmitted disease involving the exocrine glands and is characterized by chronic pulmonary disease, pancreatic insufficiency, and abnormally high sweat electrolyte levels. The pancreatic component of this disease is often associated with severe malabsorption and maldigestion of dietary proteins and fats. The clinical signs of maldigestion include chronic diarrhea with steatorrhea (bulky, foul smelling, greasy stools), abdominal distention, and malnutrition. The poor absorption of nutrients contributes to slow weight gain or growth failure, wasting of skeletal musculature, and poor nutritional reserves. Many of these children have fat-soluble vitamin deficiencies (A, D, E, K) due to fat malabsorption.[62] See Chapter 38 for further information about cystic fibrosis.

Hepatic Disorders

Liver Disease

A large variety of rare and common diseases results in liver dysfunction. Causes of liver disease include infections, congenital structural defects, metabolic disorders, tumors, and toxin-induced damage.[39] Causes of liver dysfunction are listed in the accompanying display.

A number of tests are used to assess liver dysfunction. These tests may include laboratory studies such as ALT (Alanine Aminotransferase), AST (Aspartate Aminotransferase), LDH (Lactate Dehydrogenase), and GGT (Gamma-Glutamyltransferase), which reflect leakage of enzymes from the liver and biliary tissue. However, these tests must be interpreted cautiously because elevations in levels of these enzymes may be caused by many illnesses, not just liver diseases. Serum albumin, glucose, and various clotting factors are often measured to assess the ability of the liver to synthesize these substances. Ultrasound, computed tomography (CT), and isotope scanning are used to visualize anatomic causes of liver dysfunction. Liver biopsy may be indicated for particular cases in which liver tissue is required for definitive diagnosis of the disorder.

Some liver disorders are characterized by mild or even asymptomatic presentation, whereas many other cases of liver disease are associated with severe, chronic, and life-threatening symptoms. Common signs and symptoms associated with liver disease are the following: abdominal distention; ascites; jaundice; dark urine; yellow sclera; light colored stools (gray to white); steatorrhea; prominent venous pattern on abdomen; localized ten-

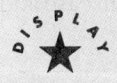

Causes of Liver Dysfunction

Infectious
  Hepatitis
  Cytomegalovirus
  Rubella
  Toxoplasmosis
Congenital structural deficits
  Biliary atresia
  Choledochal cyst
  Alagille's syndrome
Metabolic diseases
  Wilson's disease
  α_1-antitrypsin deficiency
  Glycogen storage diseases
  Tyrosinemia
  Galactosemia fructosemia
Tumors
  Hepatoblastoma
Toxin-induced damage
  Acetaminophen overdose
  Alcohol

derness in right upper quadrant or shoulder; fatigue or malaise; fever; nausea and vomiting; anorexia, weight loss, stunted growth; pruritus (itching); mental changes, irritability, lethargy (hepatic encephalopathy); upper GI hemorrhage (portal hypertension with esophageal varices); and cirrhosis.

Liver dysfunction can develop acutely and resolve spontaneously or be characterized by chronic progressive degeneration of liver function.

Hepatitis

Etiology and Incidence. Primary viral infection of the liver has traditionally been thought to be caused by either hepatitis A virus (HAV) or hepatitis B virus (HBV). Research has identified several other viruses associated with acute or chronic hepatitis including non-A, non-B hepatitis virus (hepatitis C), cytomegalovirus, herpes virus, varicella zoster, Epstein-Barr virus (EBV), rubella, and coxsackie B. These viruses can lead to inflammation of the liver as part of a generalized illness.[5]

Although a variety of organisms have been identified as causative agents, there is little difference in the clinical presentation of hepatitis caused by the various viruses. Hepatitis is often asymptomatic, especially in children. The spectrum of symptomatic disease ranges from mild flulike symptoms with low-grade fever, malaise, anorexia, and mild jaundice to fulminant disease leading to liver failure.

It is difficult to estimate the actual incidence of hepatitis. Although hepatitis is a reportable communicable disease, probably only about 25% of occurrences of the disease are reported. Many cases are asymptomatic or unrecognized, and many are simply not reported to public health agencies. In 1980, almost 60,000 cases were reported. Of these, just over 14,000 episodes occurred in children under 18 years of age. The majority of this discussion focuses on hepatitis A and hepatitis B; however, much of the information also pertains to hepatitis caused by other viruses.

Viral hepatitis has been classically divided into two distinct categories, infectious hepatitis (type A) and serum hepatitis (type B). It is apparent that the two illnesses are not as clearly delineated as previously thought. Careful serologic and clinical investigations must be undertaken to identify the causative agent and to predict the course of the disease. The traditional characteristics of Type A and Type B hepatitis are described in Table 59-5. Although

TABLE 59-5
Comparison of Type A and Type B Hepatitis

	Hepatitis A	Hepatitis B
Causative agent	Hepatitis A virus, RNA virus	Hepatitis B virus, DNA virus
Route of transmission	Primary route—fecal–oral	Primary route—parenteral
	Less frequent route—parenteral	Less frequent route—maternal–fetal, secretions (genital, oral)
Incubation period	15–30 d	3–10 wk
Clinical manifestations		
• Fever	Common	Common
• Anorexia	Severe	Mild to moderate
• Nausea & vomiting	Common	Less common
• Serum-sickness like symptoms	Very rare	Occasional
• Jaundice	Common	Common
• Hepatosplenomegaly	Common	Common
• Urticara, arthralgia	Rare	Occasional
Serologic testing	Anti-HAV-IgM	$HB_s Ag$
	Anti-HAV-IgG	Anti HB_c IgM
		Anti HB_s
		$HB_e Ag$
Complications	Very rare	10% develop chronic hepatitis, carrier state, cirrhosis
Immunization and prophylaxis		
• Immune serum globulin	Effective passive immunization if given within 2 wk of exposure, good pre-exposure prophylaxis	Provides some passive immunity
• Hepatitis B immune globulin (HBIG)	Not useful	Effective postexposure prophylaxis
• Heptavax-B	Not useful	Provides active immunity, excellent prophylaxis for high-risk groups
High-risk groups	Children in day care, institutionalized patients	Illicit drug users, infants of chronic HBV carriers, children requiring frequent blood/blood product transfusions, health professionals

there is more crossover between hepatitis A and B than previously thought, many distinctions between the two illnesses are commonly observed.

Hepatitis A is most commonly transmitted through the fecal–oral route. The feces are the predominant reservoir for HAV. The virus is transmitted during the incubation and prodromal phases of the disease when fecal excretion of the virus is present yet the person is often symptom-free. By the time jaundice appears and the diagnosis of hepatitis is suspected, susceptible contacts have already been exposed to the disease. Infants and children often have mild illness or are asymptomatic, whereas adults often have more severe symptoms. The ability of children to have undetected hepatitis and shed the virus heavily, and the difficulty in recognizing infected people in the most contagious state account for the high rates of hepatitis A seen in day care centers and crowded institutions such as for the mentally retarded.[5,14,64] Food handlers with poor hygiene practices are often implicated in epidemics of hepatitis A due to their ability to expose a large population to the virus. Some outbreaks of hepatitis A have been traced to the ingestion of water contaminated with the hepatitis virus or shellfish, such as clams and oysters, harvested from contaminated water.[39] Hepatitis A has a short incubation period (15 to 30 days) and generally has an acute, self-limited course.

In contrast to hepatitis A, HBV is most commonly spread through the parenteral route. Transmission is generally through the exchange of blood or any bodily secretion or fluid such as saliva or genital secretions. The major sources of hepatitis B are patients with acute hepatitis B or healthy, chronic carriers of the virus.[5] Transmission of the virus by way of transfused blood or blood products still occurs, although it is unusual due to careful screening for the hepatitis antigen. HBV can be spread through transfusions, through the use of contaminated needles such as with illicit drug use, from mother to infant during childbirth, and through intimate physical contact. Children at highest risk for hepatitis B infection include (1) infants of mothers who are chronic carriers, (2) hemophiliacs and others who require frequent blood or blood product transfusions, (3) children who are involved in parenteral drug abuse, (4) institutionalized children and their caretakers, and (5) children who receive organ transplants.[62,78]

The incubation period for hepatitis B is usually 3 to 10 weeks. The course of the disease may be more severe and persistent than with hepatitis A, and at least 10% of patients develop chronic hepatitis.[39] Chronic hepatitis is characterized by the continued presence of clinical or biochemical evidence of hepatitis for more than 6 months.[5] A number of patients develop a carrier state of hepatitis in which there is no obvious clinical evidence of the disease yet serologic testing is positive for the hepatitis antigen. Most chronic carriers of hepatitis B have no known history of the disease and are detected during routine screening such as before blood donation. Chronic carriers are at risk for transmission of the disease.

The transmission of hepatitis C (non-A non-B virus) is predominantly through blood transfusions. In recent years, the risk of transmission has been as high as 5% to

15%. Fortunately, the technology for screening of blood products for the hepatitis C virus has been developed and is being implemented at blood banks across the nation, and the rate of transmission should drop dramatically. The development of hepatitis C is a serious complication; up to 40% of infected people develop chronic hepatitis, and many of these progress to cirrhosis.

Pathophysiology. The hepatitis virus invades the liver cells, causing inflammation and infiltration of hepatocytes by mononuclear cells. This process may lead to degeneration and necrosis of the cell. The extent of damage is related to the severity of the insult and the ability of the host to mount an immune response. In most cases, the disease is self-limiting, and, depending on the causative agent, complete regeneration of liver tissue without permanent damage occurs.[5,62,76] Unfortunately, some forms of hepatitis are associated with continued degeneration of liver tissue. Fulminant hepatitis is characterized by rapid (1 to 8 weeks) onset of liver failure and often a fatal outcome. Liver transplant has been used successfully to treat fulminant disease. Chronic active hepatitis may develop and lead to progressive liver failure and cirrhosis.[62]

Clinical Manifestations. The clinical presentation is similar in all types of hepatitis. Many cases, particularly in children, may be asymptomatic or produce only minor symptoms. The majority of children with hepatitis are anicteric (not associated with jaundice). After the incubation period, the prodromal phase ensues and is characterized by mild flulike symptoms. Usually, this phase lasts for 5 to 7 days. Common symptoms include slight to moderate fever, anorexia, nausea and vomiting, abdominal pain, fatigue, and malaise. Occasionally, a serum-sicknesslike syndrome develops, particularly with hepatitis B, and includes a macular rash, urticaria (skin rash with wheals and severe itching), and arthralgia. Typically, at the end of the prodromal phase, the parent notes jaundice, usually as scleral icterus. On questioning, a recent history of dark urine and light colored stools can be elicited. A tender, enlarged liver is commonly palpated during the physical examination. Splenomegaly is found in 10% to 15% of cases. Over the next several days, the jaundice usually worsens but the patient clinically improves. Generally, the appetite returns; fever, vomiting, and nausea disappear; and the patient's energy level and affect improve. Meanwhile, laboratory studies often suggest worsening of the condition (rising levels of bilirubin and transaminases).

The disparity between the improvement of the patient's clinical condition and the worsening of the laboratory studies is a good prognostic factor. Deepening of jaundice with persistence or worsening of fever, anorexia, nausea, or vomiting is worrisome. These persistent symptoms are commonly seen in children who go on to develop fulminant hepatitis or chronic active hepatitis. Ordinarily, jaundice completely resolves within 4 weeks and the patient gradually regains strength. The recovery phase of acute hepatitis varies considerably. Usually, at least 1 to 3 months elapse before clinical and laboratory findings normalize and the patient feels completely well and does not experience fatigue and malaise. Children frequently recover more rapidly than adults.[5,62]

Diagnostic Studies. A diagnosis of hepatitis is often suspected on the basis of the clinical presentation of a flulike syndrome, jaundice, and a tender, enlarged liver. It is extremely important to inquire about a possible history of exposure to the disease. Laboratory studies are indicated to identify the causative agent and to assist in ruling out other liver diseases. Liver function studies including ALT, AST, bilirubin levels, and alkaline phosphatase are frequently obtained to evaluate the extent of liver injury. Blood samples are also evaluated to detect various types of antigens and antibodies present after exposure to the virus. These serologic tests are outlined in Table 59-6.

★ **ASSESSMENT**

The nurse in an outpatient setting may be the first to recognize flulike symptoms and jaundice as possible indicators of hepatitis. The child should be referred for further evaluation, and the family must be cautioned to use extremely careful handwashing techniques and to dispose diapers or other contaminated items appropriately until the diagnosis of hepatitis is ruled out. The risk of further transmission of the disease cannot be underestimated to the family. Once the diagnosis is made, the nurse helps the family identify other people who may have become infected and who may need evaluation or prophylactic treatment.

★ **NURSING DIAGNOSES AND PLANNING**

Based on the assessment data from above and Chapter 58, the following nursing diagnoses may apply to the child with hepatitis:

- Altered Nutrition: Less Than Body Requirements related to anorexia.
- Activity Intolerance related to fatigue.
- High Risk for Infection transmission related to improper health habits.
- High Risk for Fluid Volume Deficit related to vomiting.
- Altered Health Maintenance related to ineffective family coping.
- Social Isolation related to possible transfer of infection.
- Anxiety related to knowledge deficit regarding home infection control measures; avoiding use of illicit drugs.

The nurse and child (or parents) together plan effective care based on the established nursing diagnoses. Several examples of expected outcomes follow:

- The family identifies an appropriate rest and activity schedule.
- The child increases length of school day.
- The child tolerates a well-balanced diet.
- The family and child practice good hygiene measures.

The nurse plans for the daily care of the child based on both physician's orders and nursing diagnoses. Some general nursing care goals may be the following:

- The child is monitored for chronic liver disease.
- Spread of infection is prevented.

★ **INTERVENTIONS: COLLABORATIVE AND INDEPENDENT**

The primary goals in the therapeutic management of all types of hepatitis include:

- Early detection and identification of the specific causative agent
- Symptomatic support during the acute phase

TABLE 59-6
Serologic Testing for Hepatitis

Serologic Test	Time Frame	Comments
Anti-HAV IgM (antibodies of IgM class to hepatitis A virus)	Peaks 1 wk after onset of jaundice; undetectable 4–8 wk later	Presence suggests recent HAV infection
Anti-HAV IgG (antibodies of IgG class to hepatitis A virus)	Highest titers at 1–2 mo; persists for years	Confers long-term immunity and indicates previous infection
HB$_s$Ag (hepatitis B surface antigen)	Usually found 1–3 mo after exposure. Often nondetectable after onset of jaundice	If HB$_s$Ag persists longer than 6 mo, patient is considered to be a chronic carrier
Anti HB$_c$ IgM (antibodies of IgM class to hepatitis B core antigen)	Rises just after onset of jaundice, peaks at 5 mo, then declines	May be only marker of disease with appearance of anti HB$_s$Ag
Anti HB$_s$ (antibodies to hepatitis B surface antigen)	Rarely detected until 3–4 mo after onset of acute disease. Persists indefinitely (lifelong in many cases)	Presence confers long-time immunity and indicates previous infection
HB$_e$Ag hepatitis B antigen	Indicates chronic hepatitis	High titer implies a high risk for transmissibility of virus

- Monitoring for the development of chronic liver disease
- Prevention of further spread of the illness.

There is no specific treatment available for hepatitis. Nursing measures are directed at supportive care and education of the family about preventing transmission of the hepatitis virus.

TEACHING

The majority of children with mild or uncomplicated hepatitis are cared for at home. The nurse should help the family determine an appropriate rest and activity schedule. Bedrest is indicated if severe fatigue and malaise are present in the initial stages. The child is allowed gradually to resume normal activities as tolerated. There is no evidence to suggest that enforced bedrest or severe restriction of activity influences the rate of recovery or the eventual outcome. The child often limits his activities initially but soon begins to feel stronger and more energetic and wants to return to school. Although jaundice may persist, the child with hepatitis A is not considered infectious 7 to 10 days after the onset of jaundice, and the child may return to school. The child's tolerance of activity should be monitored, and extra rest periods should be encouraged. Due to easy fatigability, the child should initially be encouraged to attend a half day of school and gradually increase to a full day.

No specific dietary restrictions are indicated, however, high-fat diets may cause gastric distention and discomfort. During the initial stages of the disease when anorexia is present, the child should be allowed to select foods he or she prefers and tolerates. Thereafter, as much as possible, a well-balanced diet should be chosen. Some children have a good appetite in the morning and may tolerate breakfast better than other meals. The nurse should explain to the parents that anorexia is normal with hepatitis and that the child's appetite will gradually improve. The child should not be forced to eat. Drug therapy is seldom needed, but antiemetics may be useful if vomiting is severe. Parents are cautioned to avoid giving any medication to the child without consulting the physician. Normal doses of many common drugs are contraindicated in the child with hepatitis due to a decreased ability of the liver to detoxify and excrete the medication. Common drugs that should be avoided with liver disease include acetaminophen (Tylenol) and ferrous sulfate (iron).[5,55,76]

INFECTION CONTROL

Preventing further spread of hepatitis is vitally important and often can be achieved by the use of appropriate hygiene and isolation measures and through the use of active or passive immunization. The nurse should explain to the parent and child the usual way the hepatitis virus is spread and help the family to identify appropriate infection control measures. These measures should include:

- Careful handwashing after changing diapers or using the toilet and before eating or drinking.
- Avoiding the sharing of drinking glasses, toothbrushes, or toys that are mouthed.

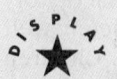

Infection Control

Caution must be exercised in the handling of all excretions. Enteric precautions should be used for HAV patients. Blood and body fluid precautions (see back cover of book) are used for HBV and non-A non-B patients. Careful handwashing after all patient contact is the most effective method of reducing transmission of the disease.

- Washing linen or clothing that is contaminated with stool or blood in hot, soapy water.
- Washing the child's eating utensils in hot, soapy water or in a dishwasher.
- Disposal of diapers, used tampons, or bandages in plastic bags.
- Avoiding intimate contact, such as kissing, with the affected person during the infectious period.[55]

If it is suspected that the child has acquired hepatitis during illicit drug use, the nurse has an important responsibility to explain the dangers of drug use and the mode of transmission of hepatitis and other bloodborne viruses. The nurse must encourage the child and family to seek counseling.

The administration of standard pooled immune globulin is effective in conferring passive immunity for people exposed to HAV. To be effective, immune globulin must be given within 2 weeks of exposure. The disease may be prevented or modified significantly in approximately 80% to 90% of cases. The immunoglobulin is given intramuscularly and is indicated for people with significant exposure to acute hepatitis A (contact with feces, household contacts, sexual contact, and workers or residents in crowded institutions such as day care centers or group homes for the mentally retarded). Immunoglobulin is also effective in providing immunity for people at high risk for exposure to the disease such as travelers to tropical and developing countries.[5]

Passive immunity to HBV can be achieved through the administration of high titer hepatitis B immune globulin (HBIG). This product is prepared from plasma preselected for a high titer of antibody against hepatitis B surface antigen (HB_sAg). This preparation is effective for one-time exposures such as accidental needlesticks or contact of contaminated material with mucous membranes. An important use of HBIG is for infants born of mothers who have acute HBV during the last trimester of pregnancy or who are chronic carriers of HB_sAg to protect the infant and prevent neonatal spread of the disease. HBIG is expensive and should be used judiciously.[5]

Heptavax-B vaccine is a major advance in providing active immunity to HBV. The vaccine is derived from the pooled plasma of chronic HB_sAg carriers or through recombinant DNA technology. The vaccine is used for preexposure prophylaxis for people at high or moderate risk for exposure to HBV. Candidates for hepatitis B vaccine include: (1) health care workers with potential blood or needlestick exposure, (2) hemodialysis patients, (3) patients receiving certain blood products, (4) clients and staff of institutions for developmentally disabled patients, (5) household contacts and sexual contacts of HBV carriers.[62] All health care workers with potential exposure to hepatitis B and all family members of HBV carriers should be immunized with the Heptavax-B vaccine. The vaccine is also used after exposure in combination with HBIG. The vaccine is given intramuscularly in three doses. The first two doses are given 1 month apart, and a booster dose is given 6 months after the first dose. No vaccine is available for hepatitis A or non-A or non-B hepatitis.

★ **EVALUATION**

Periodically, the nurse and family evaluate the outcomes of care given. Examples of outcomes for the child with hepatitis were given under Planning in this section. Have short-term goals been met? Are long-term goals still realistic?

Hospitalization of a child with hepatitis may be necessary if protracted vomiting, coagulopathy, or hepatic failure develop. Follow-up of all patients with hepatitis should include clinical examination and laboratory studies to confirm resolution of the disease and to allow early recognition of the carrier state or the development of chronic hepatitis.

Biliary Atresia

Definition and Incidence. Biliary atresia is characterized by the partial or complete absence or obliteration of the extrahepatic ducts. This malformation results in an interruption of bile drainage from the liver into the duodenum. Normal bile drainage is depicted in Figure 57-8. The altered bile flow results in liver fibrosis and severe fat malabsorption. Historically, the prognosis for children with biliary atresia has been grim, because less than 5% of affected children survived beyond 2 years of age. The prognosis improved markedly with the introduction of the Kasai procedure (hepatic portoenterostomy) in 1959. Three-year survival rates of 35% to 65% have since been reported. In most infants, the bile flow is reestablished, but the majority of children continue to suffer some morbidity ranging from mild alterations of liver enzymes to liver failure requiring transplantation.[40,52] In many cases, the Kasai procedure buys time by providing sufficient bile drainage until the child is an adequate size for transplantation and until an appropriate donor organ can be found.[71]

Etiology and Pathophysiology. The etiology of biliary atresia is unknown and under intensive investigation.[39] Researchers have observed some clusterings of cases and have noted that biliary atresia is not detected in premature and stillborn infants. These findings suggest that exposure to an infectious or toxic agent or some acquired lesion is responsible for the postnatal development of obliteration of the bile ducts.[62,79]

The obliteration disrupts bile flow and results in inflammation and progressive fibrosis of the liver. Unless the fibrotic process is interrupted by a successful Kasai procedure or by liver transplantation, the eventual outcome is cirrhosis and death. All of infants with biliary atresia not corrected by surgery die (only 1% survive until 4 years of age).[62] Inadequate bile drainage into the intestinal lumen also compromises growth and nutrition. Bile acids are required for the absorption of dietary fats; hence, the altered bile flow causes fat malabsorption and inhibits the absorption of fat-soluble vitamins.

Clinical Manifestations. In classic biliary atresia, a full-term infant presents at 2 to 3 weeks of age with jaundice. The jaundice may be noted during a well-child visit or may be observed by the parents. In some cases, jaundice can appear within the first few days of life (and be mistakenly dismissed as physiologic jaundice) or, in rare cases, the appearance of jaundice can be delayed for 2 to 3 months. The parents often have noted dark urine staining the diaper and white, gray, or light yellow stools. The skin color may appear more green than yellow. Other than jaundice, the infant seldom appears ill unless diagnosis is delayed. Mild failure to thrive may be evident when the infant's height, weight, and frontal-occipital circumference are charted on standardized growth charts. On palpation, the liver is usually enlarged and often firm or hard. The infant may scratch or dig at his skin indicating pruritis. The itching sensation is believed to be the result of increased serum bile acids. Usually, severe itching is not seen before 6 months of age. Commonly, the mother reports that the child is irritable and difficult to console.[39,62]

Diagnostic Studies. A variety of tests are performed to evaluate the possibility of biliary atresia. Blood samples usually demonstrate a steadily rising bilirubin and elevated levels of total cholesterol, alkaline phosphatase, and GGT, with mild elevations of AST and ALT levels. The absence of bile or urobilinogen in stool samples is highly suggestive of biliary atresia. Liver biopsy is used to obtain tissue for histologic exam. Fibrosis, bile duct proliferation, and bile lakes are often noted in biliary atresia. An important diagnostic study is the Tc-IDA scan. This nuclear scanning test uses an isotope that is incorporated into the hepatocyte and excreted in the bile in a manner similar to bilirubin. The accuracy of this examination is enhanced if the infant is treated with phenobarbital for 5 days before the scan, because phenobarbital stimulates bile flow. Appearance of the isotope in the intestine indicates patency of the bile ducts and excludes the diagnosis of biliary atresia.[2,39] If no isotope is visualized, an exploratory laparotomy is indicated. The combination of isotope scanning and liver biopsy is extremely reliable in identifying almost all cases of biliary atresia. Once the disorder is strongly suspected, a laparotomy is performed to confirm the diagnosis and to do the initial corrective surgery (Kasai procedure).

★ ASSESSMENT

Signs and symptoms of biliary atresia are often first recognized during a well-child exam. The nurse should be alert to evidence of jaundice in an infant and to reports of dark urine or light-colored stool. In the early stages of the disease, the infant appears relatively well except for the presence of jaundice and possibly a slight delay in growth. Once the diagnosis of biliary atresia is made, an assessment must be made of the family dynamics and support system because of the chronic nature of the disease, which will put severe stress on the family.

★ NURSING DIAGNOSES AND PLANNING

Based on the assessment data from above and Chapter 58, the following nursing diagnoses may apply to the child with biliary atresia:

- Altered Nutrition: Less Than Body Requirements related to inability to digest food.
- High Risk for Skin Integrity related to itching.
- High Risk for Fluid Volume Deficit related to active fluid loss.
- Altered Health Maintenance related to ineffective family coping.
- Altered Growth and Development related to effects of physical disease.
- Altered Parenting related to effects of stress.
- Altered Family Process related to situational crisis.
- Hopelessness related to deteriorating physical condition.
- Knowledge Deficit regarding disease process; dietary management; medication regimen; pretransplant evaluation process; signs of infection and rejection.

The nurse and child (or parents) together plan effective care based on the established nursing diagnoses. Several examples of expected outcomes follow:

- The family exhibits understanding of treatment regimen.
- The family identifies coping strengths.

The nurse plans for the daily care of the child based on both physician's orders and nursing diagnoses. Some general nursing care goals may be the following:

- The parents recognize and report signs of cholangitis.
- Growth and development are promoted.

★ INTERVENTIONS: COLLABORATIVE AND INDEPENDENT

The uncertain prognosis, the repeated and often lengthy hospitalizations, the complex medical care, and the frequent disruptions of family and work life create many difficulties for the child and family. The nurse and other medical personnel are instrumental in assuring the family is well-educated about the disease process and the treatment regimen and in assisting the family to identify coping strengths. Additionally, health care professionals must perform ongoing assessments of the child and ensure that complications are recognized promptly and that the child is referred expediently and appropriately for trans-

plantation.[79] Transplantation is discussed later in this chapter.

SURGICAL MANAGEMENT

The Kasai procedure (hepatoportoenterostomy) involves anastomosis of a segment of jejunum to the porta hepatis (area on the liver where the portal vein and hepatic artery enter and the hepatic duct leaves). This procedure allows bile to be diverted into the intestine and to bypass the obliterated bile ducts. As mentioned earlier, the procedure is successful at reestablishing bile flow in some patients. Success rates are considerably higher if the procedure is performed before the infant is 2 months of age.[2,40,71]

Frequent complications of this surgery include cholangitis, persistence of nutritional deficits, and continued progression of the disease process. Cholangitis, an inflammation of the remaining bile ducts, is a worrisome complication that occurs in over 50% of patients.[62] The mechanism responsible for cholangitis is poorly understood, but an ascending infection caused by enteric organisms migrating through the intestinal conduit to the porta hepatis is postulated as a likely explanation. Cholangitis may stimulate further liver fibrosis and hasten cirrhosis or may cause intrahepatic abscesses. This complication is suspected if symptoms of high spiking fever, chills, increased jaundice, anorexia, irritability, or light-colored stools appear. The nurse should discuss the signs and symptoms of cholangitis with the parents. Often the parents are the first to notice the early evidence of cholangitis. The parents are instructed to call the physician immediately if these symptoms are noted.[79] Early intervention may prevent additional damage to the liver. Fortunately, immediate treatment with intravenous aminoglycoside antibiotics generally leads to prompt resolution of symptoms. The incidence of cholangitis usually decreases after 1 to 2 years of age. Oral antibiotics are often used as prophylaxis against cholangitis. Phenobarbital may be used to increase bile flow.

DIET THERAPY

Persistence of growth delay and nutritional deficits are common even after "successful" establishment of bile flow. The volume of bile produced and excreted may not reach normal levels until 6 to 12 months postoperatively, if at all. Fat malabsorption usually persists, so high-carbohydrate, low-fat diets are often used. Formulas and foods containing medium chain triglycerides (which are absorbed more readily than long chain fats) as the fat source may be used to enhance absorption. Supplementation of fat-soluble vitamins is necessary in most cases.[62] Due to significant malabsorption, many children with biliary atresia require 1 1/2 to 2 times the usual amount of calories and other nutrients. Pressure on the stomach from ascites and metabolic imbalances may cause anorexia and difficulty eating. Offering small, frequent meals helps to improve intake in some children. Supplemental enteral feedings or parenteral nutrition may be necessary to provide adequate nutrients.

★ EVALUATION

Periodically, the nurse and family evaluate the outcomes of care given. Examples of outcomes for the child with biliary atresia were given under Planning in this section. Have short-term goals been met? Are long-term goals still realistic? Planning for further nursing care also takes into consideration complications.

COMPLICATIONS

As the disease progresses, or if surgical correction has been unsuccessful, chronic liver degeneration develops. Particular signs and symptoms are commonly observed with severe, chronic liver disease and are hallmarks of end-stage liver disease. These signs include portal hypertension, ascites, hepatic encephalopathy, and cirrhosis.

Cirrhosis is a disruption of the normal hepatic cellular architecture and is frequently seen in end-stage liver disease. Any severe injury or insult to the liver is capable of causing cirrhosis. The actual development of cirrhosis depends on the severity of the initial insult, the duration of exposure to the causative agent, and the delicate balance between regeneration of liver cells and the fibrotic processes that occur after the insult. A liver biopsy is the best method to diagnose cirrhosis definitively. The development of cirrhosis is an ominous sign in liver disease; however, if the offending agent can be identified and removed, the prognosis is more favorable.

The obstruction to bile flow may cause jaundice, fat-soluble vitamin deficiencies (A, D, E, K), steatorrhea, dark urine, and pale stools. Coagulation disorders may result from a diminished ability of the liver to synthesize clotting factors. Hypoalbuminemia and hypoproteinemia may result from inability of the liver to synthesize albumin and protein. Cirrhosis often leads to portal hypertension.[39,62]

Portal hypertension results from increased pressure within the portal vein caused by conditions that impede the flow of blood through the hepatic venous system. The impaired blood flow can result from an obstruction of the flow into the liver (such as with portal vein thrombosis), an increased vascular resistance within the liver (such as with cirrhosis), or an obstruction to the hepatic venous outflow. The altered hemodynamics create the characteristic clinical manifestations of portal hypertension, which are splenomegaly, ascites, a prominent abdominal venous pattern, and esophageal varices.

Esophageal varices are a worrisome complication of portal hypertension because sudden GI hemorrhage can occur when varices are present. The exact mechanism responsible for the onset of bleeding is unclear. The outcome of hemorrhage from the varices depends on the volume of blood lost and the rapidity with which it is replaced, the ability to control ongoing bleeding, and the severity of underlying disease. The bleeding often resolves spontaneously, but recurrent, and increasingly severe bleeding episodes are likely. If the bleeding does not resolve, treatment may include blood replacement, iced water gastric lavage, endoscopic evaluation, administration of vasopressin, placement of a Sengstaken-Blakemore tube with gastric and esophageal balloons for pressure on the varices, and sclerosing of varices through an esophagoscope. Melena (black, tarry stools) may develop if only a small amount of bleeding occurs from the varices. Melena may also occur simultaneously with upper GI bleeding.

Ascites is a late complication of liver disease and is characterized by the accumulation of fluid in the peritoneal cavity. The development of ascites often signifies a poor prognosis. The cause of ascites is multifactorial. Ascites is characterized by abdominal distention (which can be massive), shifting dullness during abdominal palpation, and abdominal ultrasound that reveals abdominal fluid. Ascites may be treated with dietary restrictions of fluid, sodium, and protein, and with diuretic therapy. Surgical procedures such as paracentesis or shunting of ascitic fluid may be used to drain the ascitic fluid. The treatment for ascites must be individualized for each child because the response to therapeutic measures varies significantly depending on the type and severity of the particular disease process.[62]

Hepatic encephalopathy is an alarming development characterized by neuropsychiatric symptoms in severe liver disease. Typical symptoms may include peculiar behavior, loss of memory, abnormal sleep patterns, babbling speech, incoordination of fine motor movements, and coma. Treatment of encephalopathy is directed at finding and correcting the precipitating cause if possible. Additional treatment may include the administration of lactulose to increase excretion of ammonia and a reduction in dietary protein to decrease ammonia production. An elevated blood ammonia has been implicated as one of the primary agents responsible for hepatic encephalopathy.[62]

Ulcers

Definition and Incidence. Ulcers are erosions of the mucosal tissue of the GI tract and develop most often in the stomach or duodenum. In children, ulcers are classified as primary or secondary. Primary ulcers occur in the absence of another underlying disease and occur predominantly in children 10 years of age and older. The presenting symptoms and medical treatment are often similar to that of adult ulcer patients.

Secondary ulcers, or stress ulcers, usually occur in association with a severe disease process or with the use of ulcerogenic medications. The majority of secondary ulcers occur during infancy or early childhood in association with serious conditions such as shock, sepsis, severe burns (Curling's ulcer), or intercranial lesions (Cushing's ulcer). Medications such as aspirin, indomethacin, corticosteroids, and tolazoline are often implicated in cases of secondary ulcers. In infants, about 80% of ulcers are secondary, but in older children about 70% are primary.[49] The true incidence of childhood ulcers is not known.

Etiology and Pathophysiology. Ulcers are believed to result from an inbalance of the natural mucosal defense mechanisms of the stomach and duodenum and the aggressive action of acid and pepsin secreted into the gastric or intestinal lumen.[49] A weakening of the defense mechanisms allows the acid and pepsin to erode the gastric or intestinal mucosa. Ulcers are believed to result from a complex interplay of genetic and environmental factors. Some children and adults who develop ulcers have been demonstrated to have higher amounts of gastric acid secretion than people without ulcers or with less serious ulcer disease. Ulcerogenic medications impair the mucosal defense mechanisms by inhibiting mucus secretion or by inhibiting the secretion of alkali that neutralizes the acid secretion.

Other factors have also been identified as possible contributors to the development of ulcers. Recent studies have demonstrated the presence of a bacteria (*Campylobacter pylori*) in the gastric mucosa of adults and children with peptic ulcer disease. Eradication of the organism has been associated with improved healing rates and a reduced recurrence rate.[49] Certain personality characteristics have been noted by some researchers to occur more commonly in children with ulcers than in controls. Common characteristics include difficulty handling feelings of anger and frustration, internalization of aggressive feelings, overachievement tendencies, and social withdrawal due to feelings of inadequacy. Genetic influences are recognized as playing an important role in the development of duodenal ulcer. Children with primary duodenal ulcer frequently have a family history positive for ulcer disease, but genetic factors in the development of gastric or stress ulcers have not been established.[49,62]

Clinical Manifestations. The clinical symptoms of ulcer disease in children vary considerably depending of the age of onset, location of ulcer, and the type of ulcer. Children with secondary peptic ulcers and infants with ulcers often have acute and dramatic initial symptoms, including lower GI bleeding or hematemesis. One study reported 24% of patients with secondary ulcers presenting with an intestinal perforation.[18]

In contrast, older children (over 10 years in age) and children with primary ulcer disease have milder symptoms. Abdominal pain is a common initial symptom, but the subsequent pattern of pain is variable. The pain may be either poorly localized or may be localized in the epigastrium, occurring intermittently or continuously. In older children, pain associated with duodenal ulcer resembles the pattern seen in adults. Typically, epigastric pain begins 2 to 3 hours after a meal (although a report of timing in relation to meals may be difficult to elicit in children). Pain is usually relieved by food. Pain episodes are often most severe at night and may cluster in periods of days or weeks. Vomiting or melena may occur.[73] Children with primary ulcer disease frequently have recurrence of symptoms after the original course of treatment.

Diagnostic Studies. New diagnostic methods have greatly improved the accuracy of diagnosis of ulcer disease. Fiberoptic endoscopy allows direct visualization of the esophagus, stomach, and duodenum. The diagnostic accuracy of endoscopy is high. Air contrast radiologic examinations may also be used to detect ulcers. Endoscopy and barium contrast studies are contraindicated if perforation is suspected. Gastric acid studies are generally not useful for the diagnosis of ulcers except in the case of Zollinger-Ellison syndrome, a rare disorder in which a gastrin-secreting tumor is associated with a high incidence of ulcers.[49] However, patients with recurrent ulcers need to have a gastrin level measured.

★ **ASSESSMENT**

A detailed description of the type, timing, and location of the abdominal pain is important to elicit. Any report of bloody emesis or rectal bleeding is worrisome and must be reported promptly. In addition, the nurse should inquire about any family history of ulcers and about any treatment measures that have already been tried. Potential stressors for the child and family should be assessed.

★ **NURSING DIAGNOSES AND PLANNING**

Based on the assessment data from above and Chapter 58, the following nursing diagnoses may apply to the child with ulcers:

- High Risk for Fluid Volume Deficit related to active fluid loss.
- Altered Health Maintenance related to ineffective family coping.
- Pain related to disease condition.
- Fear related to risk of bleeding.
- Ineffective Family Coping: Compromised related to situational crisis.
- Knowledge Deficit regarding disease process; medication regimen; dietary management; stress reduction.

The nurse and child (or parents) together plan effective care based on the established nursing diagnoses. Several examples of expected outcomes follow:

- The family constructs a balanced diet plan in a regular meal pattern.
- The family identifies methods of reducing stress.

The nurse plans for the daily care of the child based on both physician's orders and nursing diagnoses. Some general nursing care goals may be the following:

- Pain is reduced.
- Ulcer heals.
- Complications are prevented.

★ **INTERVENTIONS: COLLABORATIVE AND INDEPENDENT**

The primary aims of nursing therapy for children with ulcers is early recognition of symptoms and education of the family about the disease process and the treatment plan. Early recognition of symptoms such as abdominal pain or bleeding and an awareness of susceptible patients allow prompt intervention and may prevent serious complications such as perforation or hemorrhage. Frequent and consistent administration of medications is a major part of therapeutic management. It is essential that the parents and older children understand the necessity for taking the medication to prevent exacerbation or recurrence of the ulcer.

Ulcers are treated primarily by medical therapy. The goals of therapy include reduction of pain, healing of the ulcer, and the prevention of complications such as perforation or recurrent ulcer. A regular meal pattern with a balanced and nutritious diet should be established. A rigid and restricted diet is usually not necessary. Smoking and ulcerogenic medications such as aspirin must be avoided. Adolescents are cautioned to avoid alcohol.

MEDICATION THERAPY

Pharmacologic therapy is frequently used to control gastric acid secretion either by buffering the acid within the gastric lumen (with antacids) or by inhibiting acid secretion (with histamine-blocking agents). Antacids are administered frequently and often in large amounts (up to 30 ml given 1 and 3 hours after meals and at bedtime). Antacid therapy is usually continued for 6 to 8 weeks. Magnesium-containing antacids typically are alternated with aluminum hydroxide preparations to overcome the side-effects of diarrhea and constipation.[49] Liquid antacid preparations are often used, but antacid tablets may be more convenient for school-age children. Taking the antacids up to seven or eight times each day requires a great deal of motivation. The nurse can help to ensure compliance with the medication regimen by explaining that the effectiveness of the antacid to neutralize the gastric acids, reduce pain, and allow healing of the ulcer depends on frequent and consistent administration. Acknowledging the child's or parents' concerns over the difficulty in adhering to the medication schedule and a reminder that the antacids will usually be discontinued after several weeks may improve compliance. The child and parents should be given verbal instructions and a written schedule for all medications.[55]

Histamine-blocking agents, such as cimetidine, ranitidine, and famotidine, have been used in adults and children. The major therapeutic action is the reduction of acid and pepsinogen secretion. Healing of duodenal and gastric ulcers has been demonstrated after 3 to 8 weeks of therapy. Abdominal pain has been reported to be markedly reduced after several days of cimetidine therapy.[49] Cimetidine is most effective if taken before meals and at bedtime. Only rare adverse effects, including hepatic and cerebral toxicity, have been reported with cimetidine usage in children; however, long-term usage has not been extensively studied. Therefore, histamine blockers must be used cautiously in pediatric patients; however, ulcers frequently recur if long-term treatment is not used.

An anticholinergic medication (Pro-Banthine) is sometimes used in combination with antacids or histamine-blocking agents to decrease gastric motility and acid secretion. Side-effects may include drowsiness, dry mouth, constipation, and blurred vision. Children taking these medications may require more sleep and may have difficulty concentrating on school work. Adolescents should be cautioned against driving while drowsy and warned of the dangers of drinking alcohol when taking this medication.[55]

Sucralfate, a basic aluminum salt of sucrose octasulfate, has been used for many years in adult ulcer therapy. This medication has a high affinity for ulcerated gastric and duodenal mucosa and forms a protective barrier against acid, pepsin, and bile salts. Constipation is the major side-effect. Sucralfate has proven effective in the treatment of adult ulcer disease.[49] Unfortunately, it is not available in a convenient liquid form for pediatric patients. The efficacy of this medication in children has not been reported; however, it may be used in selected cases.

STRESS REDUCTION

The exact role of stress in the pathogenesis of ulcers is unclear, but stress has been implicated as possibly contributing to hyperacidity. The nurse should help the family to identify environmental or family situations that are stressful and that may have precipitated or aggravated the ulcer. The nurse should assist the parents and child to outline coping strategies to alleviate stress. Counseling may be indicated if disturbed family relationships are present or if the child needs further help in learning to cope constructively with difficult situations.[55,76]

SURGICAL MANAGEMENT

Surgical intervention may be indicated if perforation occurs or if gastric outlet obstruction persists. Perforation that occurs in association with a stress ulcer often can be treated with simple closure, but perforation as a result of a primary ulcer often requires a surgical procedure aimed at reducing gastric acidity. Highly selective vagotomy (ligation of portions of the vagus nerve) is considered the surgical treatment of choice. Recurrent ulcers or pain, vomiting, and severe hemorrhage have been reported as complications of these procedures. Experience with surgical treatment in children is limited but is indicated for children who fail to respond to medical management.[49,62]

★ EVALUATION

Periodically, the nurse and family evaluate the outcomes of care given. Examples of outcomes for the child with ulcers were given under Planning in this section. Have short-term goals been met? Are long-term goals still realistic?

Gastrointestinal Emergencies

Abdominal trauma and ingestion of foreign objects are common pediatric GI emergencies and are a significant cause of morbidity and mortality in children. Admission to the emergency room for an acute GI condition is a frightening experience for the child and for the parent. Precise nursing assessment and interventions that include clear explanations of diagnostic studies and the plan of care help to decrease the anxiety of the child and family and the morbidity of the emergency situation.

Abdominal Trauma

Definition and Incidence.   Trauma to the abdomen may present as an isolated injury to the abdomen or appear in conjunction with multisystem trauma. Multisystem trauma is responsible for more than 50% of all deaths in children from 1 to 14 years of age.[56] Abdominal injuries account for about 10% of the trauma-related deaths.[31] The spleen, liver, and kidney are the organs most commonly injured, although the pancreas, small bowel, stomach, colon, and rectum may also sustain injury. Traumas are discussed further in Chapter 30.

Etiology and Pathophysiology.   Abdominal injury may result from motor vehicle accidents, falls, blows to the abdomen, and child abuse. More than 90% of the injuries are caused by blunt trauma, whereas the remainder result from penetrating injury such as with gunshot or knife wounds.[67] The extent of injury may range from mild contusions to lacerations or rupture of the major organs. Injury to abdominal organs or laceration of major blood vessels may result in massive blood loss and shock.

Clinical Manifestations. The signs and symptoms are clearly dependent on the type and extent of injury. Abdominal injury may or may not be apparent on visual observation of the child. Ecchymosis, abrasions, or tire track marks may be noted on inspection of the abdomen.[48] Abdominal tenderness is an extremely important sign but may be difficult to assess if the child has suffered a neurologic injury. Important indicators of serious injury include shock, pain, and abdominal distention or rigidity. Signs of splenic injury may include left upper quadrant pain, tachycardia, pallor, and other evidence of blood loss.[56] Shoulder pain is an important sign of splenic damage and occurs due to referred pain from irritation of the diaphragm.

Diagnostic Studies. After a careful history and physical examination, CT is the definitive diagnostic tool for evaluation of abdominal injury.[31,48] Injuries to the spleen, liver, kidney, pancreas, and other intraabdominal organs are usually readily visualized by the CT scan. Use of the CT scan has dramatically reduced the need for surgical exploration of the abdomen to assess the degree of injury. Peritoneal lavage may be performed to assess the degree of intraperitoneal hemorrhage, especially for unstable patients with significant head injuries. A negative lavage rules out the need for emergency laparotomy.[48]

Laboratory studies generally include a complete blood count and urinalysis to assess the degree of blood loss and the possibility of renal injury. Serial hematocrits may be measured to evaluate the extent of ongoing blood loss. A serum amylase is often obtained to assess for pancreatic injury.[48,56]

★ ASSESSMENT

The nursing assessment is focused on identifying the severity of the child's injury. Of particular importance are vital signs and any symptoms of shock such as pallor, tachycardia, cold, clammy skin, and altered level of consciousness. Additional information that should be elicited includes the time of the accident, whether the child was restrained in an infant seat or seat belt, and any reports of pain or discomfort. The child's entire body must be assessed for any external evidence of injury.

★ NURSING DIAGNOSES AND PLANNING

Based on the assessment data from above and Chapter 58, the following nursing diagnoses may apply to the child with abdominal trauma:

- High Risk for Fluid Volume Deficit related to active fluid loss.
- Impaired Tissue Integrity related to pressure or tearing.
- Pain related to injury.
- High Risk for Infection related to open wound.
- Ineffective Breathing Pattern related to neuromuscular impairment.
- Activity Intolerance related to generalized weakness.

- Fear related to absence of parents.
- Anxiety related to knowledge deficit regarding activity restrictions; safety measures.

The nurse and child (or parents) together plan effective care based on the established nursing diagnoses. Several examples of expected outcomes follow:

- The family verbalize their confidence in the staff.
- The child participates in quiet play activities.
- The child exhibits correct coughing and deep breathing.

The nurse plans for the daily care of the child based on both physician's orders and nursing diagnoses. Some general nursing care goals may be the following:

- Child is stabilized.
- Complications are prevented.

★ INTERVENTIONS: COLLABORATIVE AND INDEPENDENT

The nursing care of a child with abdominal trauma centers around emergency measures aimed at stabilizing the child, offering psychologic support and clear explanations to the family, and educating the child and family about activity restrictions and other care during the recuperative period.

Therapeutic management is based on the extent of injury. If the child has sustained severe multisystem trauma, immediate resuscitation and stabilization of cardiopulmonary and circulatory function are of primary importance. The current trend in management of organ injuries is to avoid surgery if possible.[56] Many injuries heal well with conservative treatment, and nonoperative treatment protects the child from risks of emergency surgery. Conservative nonsurgical treatment is used if the child maintains stable vital signs, requires replacement of less than half of his or her blood volume, and is free of other intraabdominal injuries that require surgery.[48] The child is observed closely in the intensive care unit. A nasogastric tube is inserted to decompress the stomach, and the child is placed NPO. Vital signs and urine output are measured hourly. Electrocardiogram and blood pressure are monitored. If the child's condition deteriorates, emergency laparotomy is necessary. If surgery is not required, the child remains on bedrest for 7 days and is usually discharged from the hospital after 10 days.[56] The nurse can help the child identify play activities that do not require a lot of active movement such as reading, watching TV, or playing with dolls or other toys. Coughing and deep breathing are encouraged to prevent atelectasis. Ambulation is initiated gradually, depending on the stability of the child's condition and tolerance of activity. The patient is allowed to resume normal activity levels gradually but is often restricted from contact sports for 3 months.

Indications for surgical intervention include multisystem injuries that require exploration, an unstable hemodynamic condition, persistent hemorrhage, or a CT scan that shows multiple tissue fragments of an organ.[56] Surgical treatment may include topical application of hemostatic agents to the injured organ, suturing of the lacerated area, or partial or total resection of the damaged organ. Removal of the spleen is associated with a high risk for overwhelming infection and is avoided if at all possible. Children with abdominal injury who receive rapid and appropriate evaluation and treatment generally have an excellent prognosis. After surgery, nursing care includes routine post-abdominal surgery measures with close observation for signs of hemorrhage or infection. The nurse should keep the parents informed about their child's condition and the treatment plan. The child is often reassured if he senses that his parents understand what is happening and trust the staff.

★ EVALUATION

Periodically, the nurse and family evaluate the outcomes of care given. Examples of outcomes for the child with abdominal trauma were given under Planning in this section. Have short-term goals been met? Are long-term goals still realistic?

Foreign Body Ingestion

Definition and Incidence.   The natural tendency of young children to put objects in their mouths out of curiosity places them at high risk for ingestion of objects that will not pass through the GI tract. Ingestion or aspiration of foreign objects is the fourth most common cause of accidental death in children from 1 to 4 years of age.[33]

Etiology and Pathophysiology.   Infants and toddlers innocently place many objects in their mouths that may become lodged within the GI system. Young children do not have molars and cannot adequately chew many foods such as uncooked vegetables, large pieces of meat, and hard candies. These foods are not adequately broken down before swallowing and may become stuck in the esophagus. Additionally, children often eat while playing or laughing vigorously and may not concentrate on chewing and swallowing. Toys or objects with small, detachable parts are tempting for children to dismantle, and often these parts end up in the mouth and may be swallowed or aspirated. Older children may place inappropriate objects in their mouth and then inadvertently swallow them.

Several areas of normal physiologic narrowing are present within the esophagus. Once ingested, foreign bodies or food items may become lodged, causing erosion, edema, and the formation of granulation tissue.[33,67] Complete obstruction can result from the foreign object or from the secondary reactions. Sharp or pointed objects may cause perforation of the esophagus and lead to pneumomediastinum and mediastinitis. Ordinarily, if the foreign object passes through the gastroesophageal junction, it will safely pass through the remainder of the GI tract and be eliminated in the stool.

Clinical Manifestations.   Common signs of an esophageal foreign body include refusal to take oral feedings, increased salivation, vomiting, gagging, or pain and discomfort with swallowing. Fever accompanied by pain radiating to the sternal or back area may indicate perforation or mediastinitis. Large foreign bodies may compress the trachea and cause respiratory symptoms of stridor, coughing, or wheezing. Often, a history of foreign body ingestion can be elicited, but, in as many as 25% of cases, the parents are unaware of the ingestion.[33,67]

Diagnostic Studies.   The history and physical examination are important in forming the initial suspicion of ingestion. A history of ingestion accompanied by signs of esophageal obstruction are highly suggestive of a large foreign body. A chest x-ray, including anteroposterior and lateral views, often reveals the foreign body. CT scans are sometimes useful at outlining the object.[33]

★ ASSESSMENT

The ingestion of a foreign body must be suspected in a child who presents symptoms such as refusal to take feedings, increased salivation, vomiting, gagging, or respiratory distress but who otherwise appears healthy. The parents should be asked specifically if the child had access to any small objects such as coins, pieces of toys, buttons, or other swallowable objects. Preschool and school-age children may admit to swallowing a foreign object if questioned.

★ NURSING DIAGNOSES AND PLANNING

Based on the assessment data from above and Chapter 58, the following nursing diagnoses may apply to the child with foreign body ingestion:

- Pain related to obstruction.
- Impaired Tissue Integrity related to irritant.
- Anxiety related to stress of situation.
- Knowledge Deficit regarding follow-up observation after ingestion; general safety principles.

The nurse and child (or parents) together plan effective care based on the established nursing diagnoses. Several examples of expected outcomes follow:

- The parents identify means of collecting stools for observation for passing of object.
- The family discusses general home safety measures.

The nurse plans for the daily care of the child based on both physician's orders and nursing diagnoses. Some general nursing care goals may be the following:

- Foreign body is identified.
- Foreign body is removed or passed.

★ INTERVENTIONS: COLLABORATIVE AND INDEPENDENT

The nursing care of the child after an ingestion includes assessing the severity of the child's symptoms to assist in determining the urgency of removal and education of the family about follow-up care and general safety principles. Most small, smooth foreign bodies such as marbles or coins pass readily through the GI tract. Prompt removal of any object suspected to be lodged in the esophagus is necessary.

Once the foreign body is identified within the esophagus, it is removed by the use of esophagoscopy. During this procedure, the patient is placed under general anesthesia and is intubated. A fiberoptic telescope is inserted, and the foreign object is visualized and removed. Foreign bodies that require urgent removal include sharp or pointed objects (such as open safety pins or pull tabs from soft drink cans) or disk batteries. Disk batteries (such as in hearing aids or cameras) leak sodium or potassium hydroxide in a fluid environment and can cause rapid erosion of the esophageal mucosa if not removed. If the battery has passed into the stomach or further along in the bowel, removal may not be necessary. Usually the battery passes through the GI tract uneventfully. As with batteries, other foreign objects that reach the stomach are not surgically removed. Serial x-rays are obtained to monitor progression of the object.[33]

The parents are instructed to examine all of the child's stools to determine if the object has been expelled. If the child is toilet trained, the stool can be collected by using a stool collection device, which fits under the toilet seat, or by placing a clear piece of plastic wrap under the seat.[55] The child may eat a normal diet with some additional roughage (foods containing fiber). If severe abdominal pain, fever, or vomiting develops, the child must be examined immediately. If the object does not pass within several weeks, surgical removal is considered.

PREVENTION

The best cure for ingestion of foreign bodies is prevention. The Consumer Products Safety Act of 1979 outlined regulations for toys designated for children 0 to 3 years of age. Toys and toy pieces must be at least 1 1/4 inch in diameter and 2 1/4 inches in depth. These regulations have contributed to a decline in the number of ingestions.[33] However, these regulations do not apply to toys manufactured outside of the United States nor to the many other small objects within the home that can be ingested. The nurse should discuss general safety principles with the parents of any child who has ingested a foreign object and with any parent who is observed during routine visits to be allowing the child to play with or eat potentially dangerous objects. Parents must be cautioned to avoid giving foods that are difficult to chew to young children until their molars erupt. Additionally, children should not engage in active play while eating. Foods and objects most commonly implicated in foreign body ingestion and aspirations are listed in the accompanying display.

★ **EVALUATION**

The nurse and family evaluate the outcomes of care given. Examples of outcomes for the child with foreign body ingestion were given under Planning in this section.

Transplantation

Biliary atresia is the most common indication for pediatric liver transplantation. As many as 40% to 62% of transplanted patients are affected by biliary atresia.[3,52] Other disorders treated by liver transplantation include α_1-antitrypsin deficiency, tyrosinemia, Wilson's disease, chronic active hepatitis, hepatocellular carcinoma, and cirrhosis from a variety of causes. Dramatic improvements in post-transplantation survival were noted after the in-

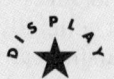

DISPLAY

Common Foreign Bodies in the Gastrointestinal Tract

*Foods**	*Objects*
Carrots	Small toy pieces
Peanuts	Coins
Apple chunks	Marbles
Hard candies	Buttons
Hot dogs	Thumbtacks
Grapes	Batteries
Chicken or fish bones	Balloon pieces
	Paperclips

Generally only problematic in children with esophageal strictures, such as with a history of tracheoesophageal fistula

---

troduction of cyclosporine A (CsA) in 1980. The average 1-year survival more than doubled from 33% to 68% immediately after the inclusion of CsA in post-transplantation regimens. Rates of survival have continued to improve with the combined use of CsA, steroids, and other immunosuppressive agents, refinements of surgical techniques, increased recognition of potential donors and recipients, and increased experience with more effective treatments for complications of the procedure.

★ **ASSESSMENT**

A potential transplantation candidate is subjected to a comprehensive evaluation, which is outlined in the accompanying display.[3] If the child is deemed to be an appropriate candidate for surgery, his name is placed on a waiting list for a donor liver. Most transplantation centers have a specialized multidisciplinary team composed of physicians, nurses, psychiatrists, social workers, and other health care personnel who evaluate the patient and assign a priority rating. The nurse assesses the family's understanding of the disease process and liver transplantation, coping mechanisms, and motivation and goals. These factors are extremely important in determining the best approaches for teaching the family and for identifying potential areas of difficulty. The priority rating is based on the child's suitability for a transplantation and the degree of urgency. These ratings are adjusted frequently as the child's clinical condition changes. Once an organ becomes available, the team must make difficult decisions regarding which child on the list would benefit the most from a transplantation at that time. The priority system helps make these decisions more objective.

Based on the assessment date from above and Chapter 58, the following nursing diagnoses may apply to the child and family before and after liver transplantation:

- Anxiety related to stress of awaiting transplant.
- Altered Growth and Development related to effects of underlying disease.
- Potential for Infection due to disease state and immunosuppressive medications.

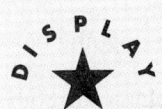

Pre-Liver Transplantation Evaluation

Laboratory studies
  Liver function studies
  Serum albumin
  Prothrombin time/partial thromboplastin time
  Trace element/vitamin level determination
  Coagulation parameters
Histocompatibility studies
  ABO blood type
  Rh factor
  HLA typing
Radiologic examination
  Abdominal ultrasound (to assess portal vein patency)
  Chest x-ray
  Extremity films (to evaluate for rickets)
Cardiopulmonary status
  Echocardiogram (to rule out congenital defects and assess myocardial function)
  ECG
  Pulmonary function test

Renal studies
  BUN, creatinine
  24-hour creatinine clearance
  Urinalysis
Immunology/virology status
  Immunization status (live vaccines are contraindicated after transplantation)
  Viral titers (hepatitis, CMV, EBV, herpes, varicella, HIV)
Growth and nutritional status
  Anthropometric studies
  Dietary history
Developmental status
  Cognitive skill testing
  Motor skill testing
Psychosocial status
  Family resources (coping patterns)
  Funding sources

The nurse and family plan effective care based on the established nursing diagnoses. Examples of expected outcomes include:

- The family identifies coping strengths.
- The family demonstrates an understanding of the treatment regimen.
- The family intervenes appropriately for complications during home care.

The nurse plans for the daily care of the child based on both physician's orders and nursing diagnoses. Some general nursing care goals are:

- The child maintains adequate growth and development.
- Infection is prevented.
- Transplant is successful.

★ INTERVENTIONS: COLLABORATIVE AND INDEPENDENT

PREOPERATIVE CARE

Waiting periods for an organ vary considerably and have been reported to range from 1 week to 18 months, depending on the child's size, condition, and blood type. The waiting period is often torturous for the family and is filled with hope and fear: hope that their child will soon receive a transplantation and fear that the child's condition will deteriorate and prevent surgery.[23] The nurse can help the family through this difficult period by allowing them to verbalize their feelings and encouraging them to maintain their hope. The nurse must be open and honest with the family and avoid giving false reassurances. The nurse should ascertain that the family understands the child will not be totally normal after transplantation. The child essentially will acquire a *new disease,* which requires daily medication and frequent

follow-up. Unfortunately, 14% to 25% of patients who need a liver transplantation die before a suitable organ is located.[3,52] The shortage of organs is related to the need for small, compatible organs and the hesitancy to ask the parents of a dying child if they are interested in organ donation. Many states have passed legislation requiring that parents be given the opportunity to consider donation if their child is a potential donor.

Promoting growth and development is essential for a child awaiting a transplantation, because an improved nutritional status increases the likelihood of a successful transplantation. The child's height and weight should be measured routinely. If growth is not progressing, more aggressive nutritional supplementation should be instituted. Tube feedings or parenteral nutrition can be administered at night to increase the child's mobility and freedom during the day. The nurse should discuss the importance of good nutrition with the child and family and help them to identify convenient and medically sound ways to improve intake.[79] The pediatric dietitian is an excellent resource to assist with nutritional assessment and counseling for the family.

INTRAOPERATIVE CARE

The transplantation procedure is often lengthy, generally lasting over 10 hours. During the transplantation surgery, the diseased organ is removed and hemostasis of the liver bed is established. The vascular anastomoses of the major hepatic vessels are performed. Once the integrity of the vascular supply is ensured, the anastomosis of the bile ducts is done. Intraoperative complications may include leakage at the vascular or biliary anastomosis, massive hemorrhage, or primary organ nonfunction in which the transplanted liver does not perfuse well when the vessels are unclamped and fails to function well postoperatively.

Most cases of primary organ dysfunction require emergency retransplantation.[52]

POSTOPERATIVE CARE

Postoperatively, the major complications include technical difficulties related to the surgical procedure (leaking or obstruction at anastomotic sites or occlusion of the hepatic artery or vein), infection, and rejection. Metabolic, graft, and pulmonary function must be monitored closely because the patient is at risk for deterioration of liver function, hypertension, metabolic alkalosis, and pulmonary compromise. The child is at high risk for bacterial or viral infections due to immunosuppressive therapy, use of many indwelling arterial and venous catheters, and the typical severe debilitation before surgery. Infection rates of 44% to 56% have been reported.[3,52] Postoperatively, the nurse closely observes for signs of infection, fluid and electrolyte abnormalities, pulmonary compromise, alternations in vital signs, and signs of rejection.[65,77]

REJECTION MANAGEMENT

Rejection can occur acutely or chronically and often can be reversed by the use of bursts of steroids or other immunosuppressive medications such as antilymphocyte globulin (ALG) or a monoclonal antibody (OKT3). Chronic rejection that fails to respond to aggressive immunosuppression may require retransplantation. Signs and symptoms of rejection may include fever, malaise, headache, abdominal pain or distention, and increased jaundice. Rejection episodes are evaluated and monitored through the use of laboratory blood studies and liver biopsies.[52]

Glucocorticoids, CsA, and azathioprine are the major immunosuppressive medications used for routine therapy. Combinations of these drugs appear to be synergistic and are effective in most cases of liver transplantations. Unfortunately, all of these medications have undesirable side-effects, which must be watched for.

DISCHARGE PLANNING

The nurse carefully instructs the family about medication administration, dosages, and side-effects in understandable terms. The parents should demonstrate measuring and administering the medications several times. Written medication schedules should be provided.

★ EVALUATION

LONG-TERM CARE

The majority of children are discharged home within 2 months of the transplantation. The child is followed primarily by the family physician who remains in close communication with the transplantation center. Long-term follow-up includes close surveillance for rejection and infection. The risk of rejection decreases over time; however, the child is at continued risk for infection, especially viral infections such as varicella, Epstein-Barr virus, or cytomegalovirus. Exposure to any of these viruses may result in life-threatening illness. The immunosuppressive process must be carefully explained to the parents. Appropriate precautions to protect their child, such as good handwashing and screening of visitors and infectious

contacts, must be discussed with the family. The child is monitored carefully by the parents on an ongoing basis for rejection or infection. Any evidence of these complications must be reported promptly to the physician. Some children are discharged with a central venous catheter after transplantation for the administration of medication and for blood sampling. Others may be discharged with supplemental nasogastric feedings or special drainage tubes. The nurse ensures that the parents are comfortable with and competent at any procedures they must perform at home.

Long-term follow-up of growth, nutritional status, and mental and motor development is essential. Some centers have demonstrated an increase in the growth chart percentiles for height and weight, which indicates catch-up growth.[3] Other studies have not clearly found improvement in linear growth. Mental and motor development has been noted to improve in many individual cases, but no significant differences in developmental scores before and after transplantation have been found.[72] Longitudinal studies are needed to determine the degree to which liver transplantation improves the quality of life and the extent of improvements in development.

Major Nursing Interventions

Feeding by Enteral Tube

Many children with NEC or other GI disorders require tube feedings into the stomach or intestine. Tube feedings are used when it is necessary to bypass the oral cavity, such as with the child who is unable to suck and swallow adequately, or a child who aspirates or has severe respiratory distress with feedings, or with a child who is unconscious. Tube feedings are also used in children with conditions such as short bowel syndrome if it is desirable to infuse small volumes of formula continuously rather than using bolus feedings of larger volumes. The feedings can be administered as a bolus infusion of formula every several hours or as a continuous drip in which a predetermined volume of formula is infused every hour. An infusion pump is used to ensure accurate delivery.

The types of tube placement are compared in Table 59-7. The most common types of tube feedings used in children are nasogastric feedings and gastrostomy feedings.

Nasogastric Feeding

To ensure optimal comfort for the child and to prevent complications of nasogastric feedings, diligent nursing care is essential. Nursing responsibilities include careful tube insertion and monitoring of feeding tolerance.[75] Additionally, the nurse often must teach the family how to insert the nasogastric tube and administer feedings at home. A variety of tubes are available for nasogastric feedings.

Moderately stiff tubes made of polyvinyl chloride are commonly used for feedings in which the tube is removed after each feeding. If these tubes are left in place, they must be replaced every 2 to 3 days. Small, soft tubes made of silicone are commonly used for feedings in which the

TABLE 59-7
Types of Tube Feedings

Type	Anatomy	Comments
Nasogastric	Tube placed through nares into stomach	Most common type. Tube can be left in place between feedings or removed after each feeding.
Orogastric	Tube placed through mouth into stomach	Commonly used in premature infants to avoid obstruction of nares because infants are obligate nose breathers.
Nasoduodenal	Tube placed through nares then into stomach and through pyloric sphincter into duodenum	Placement of tube into duodenum is difficult in some cases. Placement should be confirmed by x-ray. Insertion may need to be done under fluoroscopy.
Gastrostomy	Surgical insertion of a tube or other device (such as a gastrostomy button) through the abdominal wall and into stomach	Used for children who require long-term feedings to prevent chronic irritation of the nares and repeated tube insertions that would be necessary if a nasogastric tube was used.
Jejunostomy	Surgical insertion of a tube into jejunum	Rarely used in children.

tube remains in place indefinitely. Silicone tubes remain soft over extended periods as compared with tubes made of stiffer material such as polyvinyl chloride, which tends to become even stiffer and is therefore less comfortable and more likely to irritate the stomach. These tubes are available with and without a weight at the end. The weight may help to prevent accidental displacement of the tube, however, further research is necessary to confirm this. These tubes commonly are supplied with a stylet, which stiffens the tube and facilitates insertion. The stylet must be removed after insertion. If the stylet is required for manipulation of the tube, the entire tube must be removed from the child before the stylet is reinserted into the tube. The stylet must never be reinserted into the nasogastric tube while the tube is in place because it may lead to perforation of the esophagus.

The smallest bore feeding tube that allows infusion of the ordered formula should be selected.[51] Larger bore tubes increase patient discomfort and may obstruct the airway, particularly in neonates and infants. A larger bore tube may also compromise the function of the gastroesophageal sphincter and increase the risk of aspiration. Nursing care for the child receiving nasogastric feedings is outlined in Table 59-8.

Gastrostomy Feedings

Gastrostomy feedings are commonly used when long-term enteral tube feedings are required or when esophageal patency is impaired. Common conditions in which gastrostomy feedings are indicated include neurologic impairment that prohibits oral feedings, tracheoesophageal fistula, and severe caustic burns of the esophagus.[6] A soft tube, such as a Foley catheter or mushroom catheter, is often used for gastrostomy feedings. After insertion of the tube, the balloon is inflated to help securely hold the tube in place. Different types of gastrostomy devices are depicted in Figure 59-13.

A gastrostomy button is a new device used in lieu of the classic "tube." The button is a short device made of silicone rubber in which the tip is designed to hold the catheter in place and the outer portion has two flat wings that allow the device to lay flush against the abdominal wall. A valve at the gastric opening prevents reflux of in-

tragastric contents.[21] For feeding, a cap at the skin level is opened and an adapter is inserted. The gastrostomy button has been associated with a lower incidence of common complications seen with standard gastrostomy tubes, such as migration and accidental dislodgement.

The skin around the gastrostomy tube or button is carefully monitored for evidence of irritation or infection. The skin is routinely cleansed with dilute hydrogen peroxide or other cleansing agents to remove dried crusts and prevent infection. If a Foley catheter is used, the placement of the tube should be checked by gently pulling on the tube. Resistance to the pull is felt if the tube is in position against the abdominal wall. The tube should be taped carefully to avoid dislodgement or migration. The child should be appropriately clothed to prevent pulling on the tube. Any evidence of erythema, drainage, denudation, or leaking formula should be promptly reported.

Age Considerations

Enteral tube feedings are used in children of all ages, from newborns to adolescents. The substitution of tube feedings for normal oral feedings creates particular growth and development concerns for each age group. For the infant, if normal sucking and swallowing patterns are not stimulated, the patterns may be diminished or lost. A normal feeding situation should be simulated as closely as possible during tube feedings. If possible, the infant should be given small volumes of formula or sterile water to nipple during the feeding. If this is not feasible, the infant should be given a pacifier to encourage nonnutritive sucking. Although the pattern of sucking on a pacifier is different than that of sucking and swallowing formula, providing the pacifier at feeding times allows the infant to form an association between sucking and satiation (fullness). The infant should be cuddled, rocked, and talked to during the feeding. If the child cannot be picked up, the nurse should make eye contact with the infant and use physical contact such as stroking or gentle rubbing.

Toddlers receiving enteral feeds can be a challenge to the nurse. If the child is actively crawling, rolling, or walking, he or she must be observed closely to prevent

TABLE 59-8
Nursing Interventions: Nasogastric Feeding

Nursing Action: Tube Insertion	Rationale
1. Select appropriate tube.	1. Small soft tube increases patient comfort and decreases obstruction of nares.
2. Determine the length of tube to insert. Measure from the tip of infant's nose to the earlobe and then from the earlobe to a point midway between the xiphoid process and the umbilicus. Mark the appropriate length with tape.	2. The length to be inserted must be estimated to facilitate placement of tube in stomach. Improper placement may cause aspiration.
3. Position the child on back with the head held midline. If necessary, restrain the child's hands.	3. Proper positioning facilitates placement.
4. Gently insert tube through nares. If resistance is met or child coughs or has difficulty breathing, remove tube. Re-attempt placement in opposite nares.	4. Accidental intubation of trachea can cause coughing or choking. Excessive force may damage nasal or esophageal mucosa.
5. Verify tube placement by aspirating for gastric contents or auscultating for a gurgling sound over stomach while air is infused through tube.	5. Improper placement may cause aspiration.
6. Tape tube in place. Hypoallergenic or a transparent dressing (such as Tegaderm) may be used. Do not obstruct nares.	6. Avoid tape, which is irritating to the child's skin.

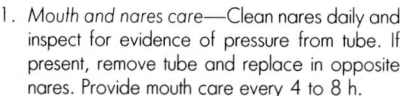

Step 2: Determining the tube length

Nursing Action: Care and Monitoring of Feedings	Rationale
1. *Mouth and nares care*—Clean nares daily and inspect for evidence of pressure from tube. If present, remove tube and replace in opposite nares. Provide mouth care every 4 to 8 h.	1. Tube may cause increased nasal secretions and mouth breathing.
2. *Feedings*—Verify correct formula and volume to infuse. For bolus feeds—allow to drip by gravity over 15–20 min.	2. Incorrect formula or volume may cause diarrhea or vomiting.
3. Aspirate gastric residual before feeding. Measure and reinstill.	3. Gastric contents are reinstilled to prevent loss of electrolytes from discarded gastric fluids.
4. Notify physician if residual is more than half of previous feeding volume. Measure residual every 2–4 h during continuous feedings.	4. High residual may indicate gastric retention.
5. Flush tube with water after bolus feedings or any medications given through tube.	5. Failure to flush tube may cause obstruction of the tube.
6. If feasible, cuddle and talk to infant during feeding. Provide pacifier.	6. Provides developmental stimulation for infant.
7. Position child on right side with head of bed elevated for 30 min after feeding (for 30–60 min after bolus feeds).	7. Promotes gravity drainage.
8. Monitor tolerance of feedings—Strict intake and output (record all oral, tube, and IV intake and all urine, stool, ostomy output). Stool record (weigh diapers to determine accurate output). Test stools for glucose. Daily weights.	8. Immature gastrointestinal function or effects of the disease process may cause feeding intolerance. Close monitoring is needed to allow early recognition of intolerance.
9. Notify physician of vomiting, increased stool output, high gastric residuals, or glucose in stools.	9. Early recognition and reporting of signs of feeding intolerance allows feeding plan to be altered before more serious complications ensue, such as dehydration or aspiration.

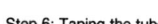

Step 6: Taping the tube

accidental dislodgement of the feeding tube. The toddler may also find the lights and sounds of the infusion pump fascinating. The pump must be placed at a safe distance from the patient. If necessary, extra extension tubes can be used to allow the pump to be placed out of the child's reach.

The school-age or adolescent child who requires tube feedings is often self-conscious about the tube. If a nasogastric tube is used, securing the tube with clear or transparent tape helps to minimize the visibility of the tube. Loose clothing usually easily conceals a gastrostomy tube. The gastrostomy button, when not attached to a formula infusion, does not require a dressing and is barely visible. In many cases, the feedings can be given at night while the child sleeps to allow increased mobility and a more normal lifestyle during the day.

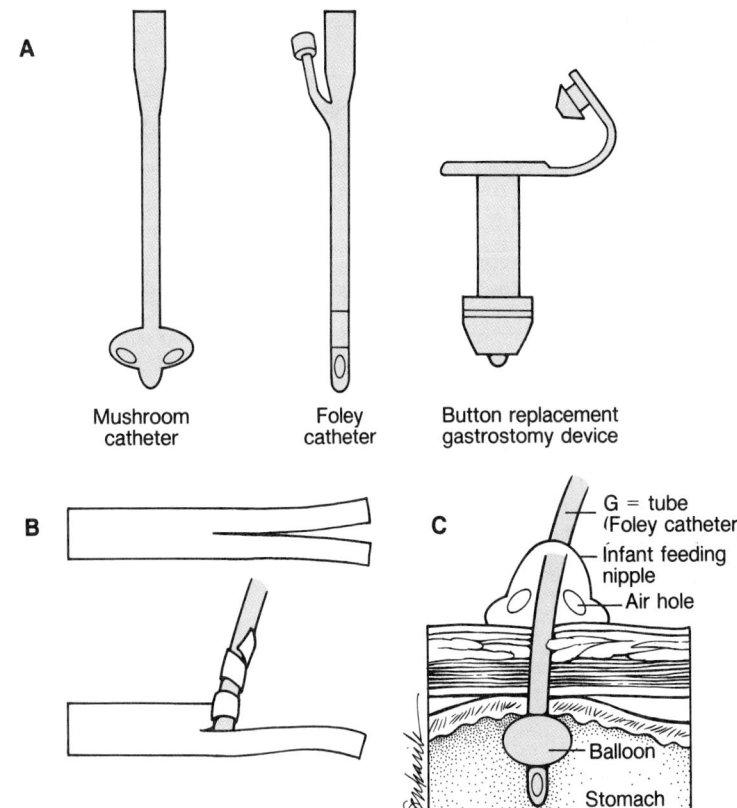

FIGURE 59-13
Different types of gastrostomy feeding devices and procedures for taping in place. (**A**) Devices. (**B**) Usual method for taping the tube. (**C**) Taping the tube by using an infant feeding nipple to secure the tube in position. (Source: **C** modified from Paarlberg, J., & Balint, J.P. [1985]. Gastrostomy tubes: Practical guidelines for home care. *Pediatric Nurs* 11(2), 99–102, 1985.)

Ostomy Care

An intestinal ostomy is a surgically created opening between the intestine and the abdominal wall. An ostomy is created either to bypass temporarily or to divert permanently stool from a segment of the intestine. An *ileostomy* is formed when the ileum is brought to the outside and a stoma (opening) is created on the right side of the abdomen. An ileostomy is performed when the entire colon is resected (such as in ulcerative colitis) or when the colon must be bypassed temporarily such as with anorectal malformations. A *colostomy* is formed by bringing the colon to the outside of the body. Colostomies are commonly created for patients with Hirschsprung's disease.

The stomal opening of an ileostomy and colostomy is usually pink or red. Due to a large number of small blood vessels in the intestinal mucosa, the stoma bleeds easily if brushed by a towel or scratched with a fingertip. Although the stoma may look raw or sore, there are no sensory nerve endings, so it is not tender or uncomfortable. However, the skin surrounding the stoma is vulnerable to breakdown (denudation) because of the presence of digestive enzymes and bile acids in the stool. The ostomy requires meticulous nursing care to protect the skin. An ostomy pouch and skin barrier are fitted around the stoma to collect stool and prevent leakage of stool contents onto the skin. The pouching system is changed as soon as any leaks develop. Nursing care of the child with an ostomy is described in Table 59-9.

Discharge Planning

Many children are discharged with an ostomy. The parents and child (if old enough) need to learn appropriate care of the ostomy and have adequate time to practice ostomy care before discharge. The nurse must assess and evaluate the parents' acceptance of the ostomy and their ability to care for it.

Body image and integrity are often concerns for the parents and child. School-age children and adolescents are often particularly anxious about the alteration in their body image and how the stoma will be viewed by peers. The nurse needs to provide accurate and detailed information to the child and family and encourage verbalization of their questions and fears.

Ideally, preparation of the family for ostomy care begins before surgery. The child should receive age-appropriate explanations. Anatomically correct dolls with stomas are available to use for teaching preoperative preparation. The family is reassured that a normal lifestyle can be expected with the ostomy. Minimal or no dietary and activity restrictions are required, and the child usually adapts readily to the ostomy.

Enema Administration

The major reason for giving an infant or child an enema is to relieve constipation. Constipation in the hospital setting may be related to inactivity; to symptoms of illness (e.g., nausea, lack of desire to drink fluids, or

TABLE 59-9
Nursing Interventions: Ostomy Care

Nursing Action: Application of the Ostomy Pouch	Rationale
1. Gather all equipment (ostomy appliance, water, towel, washcloth, measurement guide, scissors, skin barrier).	1. Having all equipment handy expedites the procedure.
2. Empty ostomy pouch before removal. Measure contents if indicated.	2. Prevents spilling of contents. Output is usually measured and tested for glucose and pH during hospitalization.
3. Position child on towel.	3. Protects underlying surface from spillage.
4. Gently remove pouch. Use a very wet gauge or, if necessary, a mild adhesive remover.	4. Gentle removal helps to avoid trauma to the skin. Press the skin away from the pouch with your fingers rather than pulling the pouch.
5. Cleanse skin around stoma gently with warm water. Remove all stool or fecal drainage. Mild cleansers specifically designed to emolify stool are available. Rinse well. Wipe the stoma gently. Pat skin dry.	5. Gentle cleaning removes irritating drainage. Stoma has no nerve endings, wiping is not painful but may cause slight bleeding. Rinse the skin well to remove residue of cleanser and soaps.
6. Use measurement guide to determine size and shape of stoma. Trim opening of skin barrier and pouch adhesive to fit stoma.	6. Individualizing size of opening improves fit of pouch and decreases chance of leakage and protects the skin from the stool.
7. Apply skin barrier to skin.*	7. Protects the skin from the adhesive of the pouch.
8. Apply skin paste to any exposed skin around the stoma.	8. Protects the skin at the base of the stoma. Smoothing out skin surface helps ensure a better seal and decreases leakage.
9. Apply pouch and smooth out any wrinkles or gaps. Direct pouch so it drains to the side or down toward the legs to facilitate the emptying.	9. Removing wrinkles and drainage in direction of a gravity flow help ensure a better seal and decreases leakage.
10. Apply skin gel to area around pouch if tape is added to protect the pouch site.	10. Gel helps protect the skin but will irritate raw or denuded skin.

Nursing Action: General Ostomy Care	Rationale
1. *Bathing*—The child can be bathed with or without pouch in place.	1. Allowing the stoma and skin to air is beneficial. Bath water will not hurt the stoma. After bathing with the pouch in place, check to ensure the pouch is well adhered.
2. Empty the pouch when it is ⅓ to ½ full.	2. The weight of stool contents of pouch can pull the adhesive loose from the skin.
3. Change the ostomy pouch only when it leaks, as long as there is a good seal.	3. The pouch can often stay on for several days; unnecessary changes irritate the skin. The usual wearing time for infants is 1–2 d, for toddlers 3–4 d, and for older children 4–7 d.
4. To minimize odor, the pouch may be rinsed between changes with cool water. Use an odorproof pouch. Use a breath mint or liquid over-the-counter breath mint in pouch.	4. Bacterial action on stored waste material (especially in colostomies) may cause odor. Over-rinsing can weaken the pouch seal resulting in leakage.

Nursing Action: Potential Complications of Ostomies	Rationale
1. Skin irritation around stoma—Ensure good fit of pouching system. Apply small amount of Karaya or stomahesive paste or other protective ostomy products, such as solid skin barrier, with the ostomy pouch. Apply a light sprinkle of stomahesive power if skin is weeping and denuded. Solid skin barrier should be applied on top of this base coat. If too much powder is used, the barrier will not adhere.	1. Residual digestive enzymes can cause skin breakdown if in contact with skin. Powder helps to form a barrier to protect skin. Certain powders, such as Karaya, sting when applied to raw skin. Many pastes contain alcohol and burn when applied.
2. White raised lesions on skin without redness—no specific treatment.	2. Lesions are probably due to sweat; will generally go away without treatment.
3. Papules with generalized redness which spread to groin area—Apply a thin coat of Nystatin powder before application of the skin barrier.	3. Papules may be indicative of a fungal (monilial) infection and require medical treatment of Nystatin powder.
4. Diarrhea (increased volume or fluid)—Monitor volume, color, consistency, and testape of stool. Notify physician of increased volume or glucose-positive stools. Administer only ordered diet. Administer any oral supplements ordered.	4. Dehydration can develop rapidly after a viral or bacterial diarrhea (especially with an ileostomy). Children (especially infants) with ostomies are quite sensitive to changes in the diet. Changes should be made under the watchful eye of physician or pediatric dietician. Children with ostomies may require sodium supplementation to replace stool losses of sodium.
5. Obstruction—Observe for warning signs of obstruction such as little or no stool output, associated nausea, vomiting, cramping, or abdominal distention. Notify the physician if these symptoms occur.	5. Obstruction can lead to necrosis and perforation of bowel.
6. Prolapse (protrusion of bowel out of abdomen—Observe closely for evidence of impaired circulation to stoma or bowel (blue or gray color). Notify physician immediately if color change is noted.	6. As long as bowel remains pink or red, the prolapse is more of a nuisance than a dangerous complication. Impaired circulation of bowel can lead to necrosis. Crying often puts pressure on blood flow to stoma resulting in a darker color of stoma, which readily changes to red.

(Continued)

TABLE 59-9
(Continued)

Nursing Action: Parent Education	Rationale
1. Start ostomy teaching as soon as possible. Ideally, begin initial explanations preoperatively.	1. Family and child need time to adjust to idea of ostomy and to have adequate practice to become competent with ostomy care.
2. Allow family to observe ostomy care and then perform skills at their own pace.	2. Pushing parents to learn before they are ready may increase anxiety and delay the learning process.
3. Discuss potential complications and interventions with family. Provide written and oral instructions. Provide the name and phone number of resource person if problems develop.	3. Family must be prepared for potential problems and must know appropriate actions to take. Knowing that a resource person is available is reassuring for the family.

*Note: Pouching systems are available that already have solid skin barriers attached. These may be easier for parents and children to apply.

medications); or to treatment measures. Because enemas are an intrusive procedure, care must be taken to try all nonintrusive methods of relieving constipation first. Nonintrusive measures include: increased fluid intake, increased bulk and roughage in diet, increased exercise and mobility, added defecation-inducing foods (e.g., prunes) to the diet. Enemas may also be given for preparation for surgery, diagnostic testing, or therapeutic interventions for children with GI disorders.

As with suppositories, enemas involve intrusion into an orifice in the perineal area. Toddlers and preschoolers may be distressed by the procedure. Older children and adolescents may understand the necessity of the procedure but are concerned about privacy and may be embarrassed about exposing an intimate body area. Sphincter control, and thus retention of an enema, is impossible for infants and young toddlers; difficult and limited for older toddlers and preschoolers; and possible for school-age children and adolescents. Infants and young toddlers can be positioned on their backs with the head and back raised and a small bedpan used under the buttocks, whereas older children may be placed in a knee–chest position (Fig. 59-14). Adolescents are positioned on the left side with the right knee drawn up toward the chest.

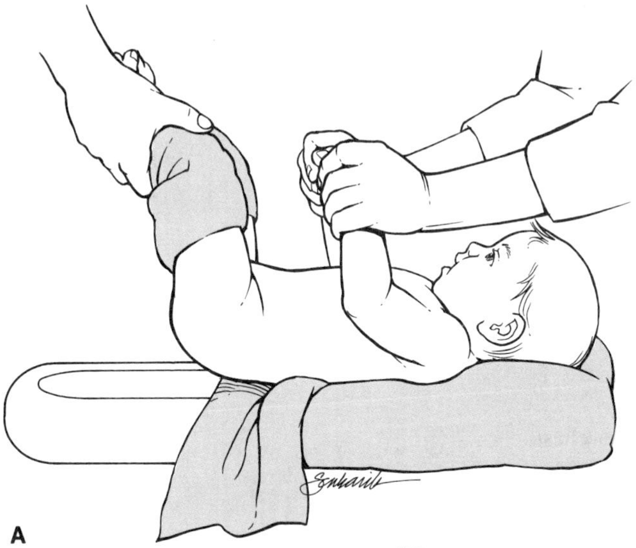

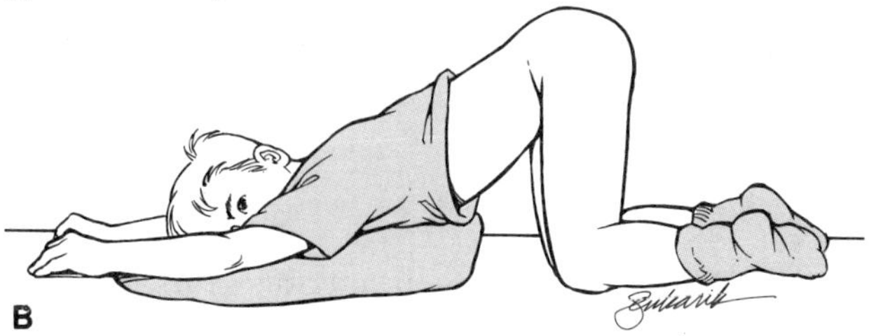

Isotonic solutions should be used for infants and young children to prevent the risk of water intoxication and fluid and electrolyte imbalance, which may occur if nonisotonic solutions are used. An isotonic saline solution can be prepared by mixing 5 ml of salt with 500 ml of water. To prevent cramping and to increase the retention time of the enema, the water should be warmed to 37 to 39° C. Commercially prepared pediatric enemas may occasionally be used.

When preparing the equipment, all air should be eliminated from the tubing. The tube is lubricated. The height of the enema bag is slowly elevated to ensure a slow rate of flow of the solution into the rectum. For infants, this may be 7.5 to 10 cm (3 to 4 inches) up to a maximum of 30 cm for older children. Adolescents may need adult elevations. The tube is inserted gently into the rectum. The distance will vary with age, and special considerations are noted in the accompanying display. Once the enema is expelled, the nurse needs to observe the results and chart the success of the procedure. The accompanying display summarizes special considerations for giving enemas to children.

Provision for Total Parenteral Nutrition

Total parenteral nutrition (TPN) is used if a child is unable to assimilate adequate calories and nutrients through the GI tract. The TPN solution usually contains glucose (10% to 35% concentration), amino acids, vitamins, minerals, and trace elements. A fat emulsion solution may also be given to provide essential fatty acids and extra calories.[25] Many GI disorders (other than short bowel syndrome) impair the absorptive capacity of the bowel or require a time period during which the child must remain NPO. GI conditions in which TPN is used commonly include:

- Postoperative management of congenital GI disorders (such as volvulus, gastroschisis, intestinal atresia, tracheoesophageal abnormalities)

FIGURE 59-14
Positions for enema administration in children. (A) Position of infant or small toddler. (B) Knee–chest position.

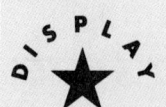

Special Considerations for Giving Enemas to Children

Infancy

Positioning:	Head and back raised, hips over a padded bedpan.
Size of catheter:	10–12 Fr
Amount of solution:	50–150 ml
Distance of insertion into rectum:	2.5 cm (1 inch)
Special considerations:	If retention is required, nurse must manually hold buttocks together. Because the amount given may be quite small, the barrel of a 50-ml syringe may be more appropriate than an enema can or bag. Two people will likely be required to perform the procedure.

Toddler

Positioning:	As per infant or left lateral Sims' or knee–chest.
Size of catheter:	10–12 Fr
Amount of solution:	100–200 ml
Distance of insertion into rectum:	5 cm (2 inches)
Special considerations:	As per infant. Also, may prefer to expel contents in potty if toilet-trained. Two people will likely be required to perform the procedure.

Preschooler

Positioning:	Left lateral Sims' or knee–chest
Size of catheter:	12–14 Fr
Amount of solution:	200–300 ml
Distance of insertion into rectum:	6–7.5 cm (2½–3 inches)
Special considerations:	A preschooler will have difficulty holding a retention enema for longer than 1–2 min. Threat to genital region most intense at this age. May wish to expel contents in potty or toilet.

School-Age Child

Positioning:	Left lateral Sims' or knee–chest
Size of catheter:	14–16 Fr
Amount of solution:	300–500 ml
Distance of insertion into rectum:	7–8 cm (2½–3½ inches)
Special considerations:	Should be able to hold enema contents for 5 min, if requested. Privacy is important. Will probably wish to expel contents in the toilet.

Adolescents

Positioning:	Left lateral Sims' or knee–chest
Size of catheter:	14–16 Fr
Amount of solution:	500–800 ml
Distance of insertion into rectum:	7.5–10 cm (3–4 inches)
Special considerations:	Should be able to hold the enema contents for 5 to 10 min. Privacy is very important. Will wish to expel contents in the toilet.

- Inflammatory bowel disease
- Intractable diarrhea
- Pancreatitis with pseudocyst formation
- Pre- and postoperative management of liver transplantation patients

TPN may be used for short intervals (1 to 2 weeks) or for extended periods (months to years). An unfortunate few short bowel patients with ultrashort bowel will probably require TPN throughout their lifetime. TPN may be administered through a peripheral vein or into a central vein (such as the jugular or superior vena cava). The glucose concentration of a peripheral TPN solution should not exceed 12.5%. Solutions with higher glucose concentrations are too hypertonic and may damage the vein, causing rapid infiltration. Due to the limitation on the glucose concentration, it is difficult to provide adequate calories by way of a peripheral vein without giving large volumes of fluid, which can lead to fluid overload. If the child is fluid restricted, has poor venous access, or requires long-term TPN (more than 2 weeks), TPN is administered through a central vein. The rapid flow of blood through these large veins quickly dilutes the concentrated TPN solution, preventing hypertonic damage to the vein.

Central TPN

Central TPN is commonly administered through a tunneled central venous catheter (Fig. 59-15). These catheters are most often inserted in the operating room with the child under general anesthesia. To insert the catheter, the surgeon first makes a small incision and locates the vein to be used and creates a subcutaneous tunnel along the chest wall. The catheter is threaded through the tunnel and into the vein and advanced so that the catheter tip lies at the junction of the right atrium and superior vena cava. The tissue in the tunnel gradually adheres to a small Dacron cuff on the subcutaneous portion of the catheter. This cuff helps to secure the catheter. The catheter can remain in place indefinitely. It is not removed unless it is no longer required or if complications such as infection or occlusion develop and do not respond to treatment.

Occasionally, central venous catheters are inserted into the saphenous or femoral vein and threaded into the inferior vena cava. These catheters are usually tunneled along the abdominal wall. Extra care must be taken to prevent soiling of the dressing by urine, stool, or ostomy drainage. Covering the site with a water-repellant dressing such as Tegaderm helps to keep the site clean.

Nursing Implications

Meticulous nursing care is required to diminish the risk of catheter complications. All catheter procedures should be done according to a standardized protocol. If the child is active or uncooperative, two people should perform the procedure. One person should perform all sterile steps of the procedure while the other acts as a nonsterile assistant and helps to restrain the child. Nursing care measures that reduce the incidence of complications include aseptic technique for all catheter manipulations, a secure dressing to protect the catheter from trauma, the use of only smooth edge clamps to clamp catheter, the use of luer lock connectors to prevent accidental disconnection of tubing, and the use of an infusion pump to regulate closely the rate of infusion and to provide an early warning of air in the tubing system or the presence of an occlusion. The child should be dressed appropriately to prevent pulling on or playing with the catheter.

Infants receiving parenteral nutrition (TPN) require close observation for catheter complications and metabolic complications of TPN.[1,4] The most common central venous catheter complications include sepsis and occlusion. The child is observed closely for evidence of a

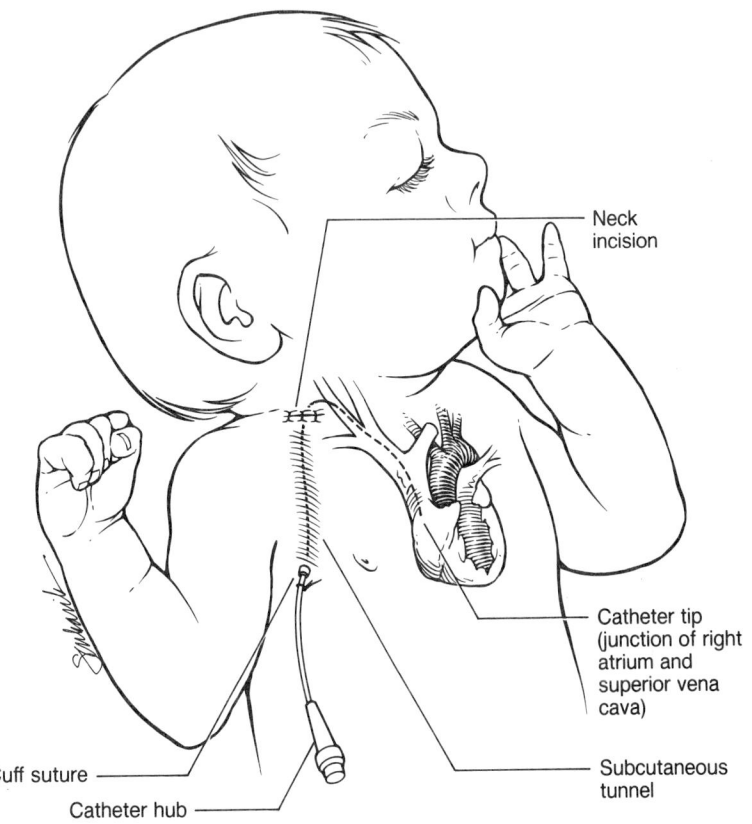

FIGURE 59-15
Placement of a tunneled central venous catheter.

Neck incision

Catheter tip (junction of right atrium and superior vena cava)

Subcutaneous tunnel

Cuff suture

Catheter hub

catheter-associated infection including redness or drainage at the catheter insertion site, fever, glucosuria, or a change in behavior such as irritability, lethargy, or poor feeding. Late signs of sepsis may include hypothermia, mottling, or apnea. As soon as infection is suspected, blood cultures are drawn and intravenous antibiotics are started. If the cultures remain negative, the antibiotics are usually discontinued after 72 hours. If the cultures are positive, antibiotics are continued for 10 to 14 days. Many catheter infections can be treated successfully without removal of the catheter. If the child's condition deteriorates, the catheter is removed. Catheter-related sepsis can cause fatal, overwhelming sepsis; therefore, prompt recognition and treatment of infection are crucial. Meticulous nursing care of the catheter is the most effective method of preventing catheter infection. Aseptic technique must be used for all catheter manipulations to avoid accidental contamination of the catheter. Local infections at the catheter exit site must be recognized and treated promptly to prevent spread of the organism into the bloodstream.

Catheter occlusions may be caused by precipitant or fibrin blockage of the catheter lumen. Warning signs of a catheter occlusion include difficulty flushing or withdrawing blood from the catheter or an "occlusion" warning alarm from the infusion pump. Precipitant formation commonly results from interactions among components of the TPN solution (usually calcium and phosphorus), the administration of incompatible medications through the catheter, or with the use of medications with a high probability of precipitation, such as Dilantin. Many precipitant occlusions can be prevented by close observation of the TPN bag and tubing for precipitant formation and by the avoidance of the administration of incompatible medications. Precipitant occlusions are difficult to treat. Measures that have been used with some success include a slow normal saline infusion through the catheter or the installation of a low pH solution (such as 0.1 normal hydrochloric acid) into the catheter to increase the solubility of the precipitated substances.

Occlusions may also be caused by fibrin formation at the catheter tip or within the catheter lumen. Frequently drawing blood through the catheter or inadvertently leaving the infusion pump turned off increases the risk of catheter occlusion. Fibrin-related occlusions are often treated successfully with urokinase, which is administered through the catheter. Urokinase is an enzyme used to induce the degradation of fibrin.

Many other rare and common catheter complications may occur, including breakage or dislodgement of the catheter, air embolism, pleural effusion, or cardiac tamponade. These complications are characterized by a usually rapid onset of respiratory distress, tachycardia, and chest pain.

A number of metabolic complications of TPN may develop. Abnormalities of any electrolyte, vitamin, or mineral levels and other blood studies may occur. Routine monitoring of blood samples is important to allow for early recognition of these problems. Altered liver functions and bile stasis develop in some children receiving TPN. Fortunately, these abnormalities are almost always reversible when the TPN is discontinued. It is worrisome

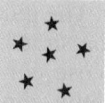

Ideas for Nursing Research

The child health nurse who works with children with gastrointestinal diseases faces a variety of clinical situations because of the number and interrelationships of the organs of digestion and absorption. The following areas need to be explored:

- Determine which feeding tubes are least likely to become dislodged or to be associated with other complications.
- Identify the safest and most expedient methods of central venous catheter care.
- Identify the most effective ways to treat central venous catheter complications.
- Evaluate the effectiveness of teaching methods used for education of the child and family (e.g., one-to-one teaching, video tape, group sessions).
- Identify more effective methods to prevent and treat the diaper rash associated with large volumes of stool output.
- Evaluate the effectiveness of interventions used to prevent feeding difficulties.

if altered liver functions develop in children who require long-term TPN. The cause of the liver damage is unclear. Children at the highest risk for liver damage include premature infants, infants with surgery of the ileum, and infants who require high doses of intravenous amino acids.

Summary

The nurse has a critical role in the care of the child with a GI illness. A thorough understanding of the etiology, pathophysiology, clinical manifestations, and course of the disease is essential so that the nurse can offer accurate information to the family and can develop an appropriate and comprehensive care plan. A detailed nursing assessment of the child's symptoms and response to treatment, and of the family dynamics and understanding of the child's illness is a vital component of the nursing care plan. Many nursing interventions focus on education of the child and family about the disease process and any home care that is required. Due to the long-term consequences and the acute and severe nature of many GI diseases, the nurse is an integral part of the psychosocial support for the family. An example of the implementation of nursing care of the child after abdominal surgery may be found in the nursing care plan and in the child and family teaching plan.

References

1. Allen, S. (1989). *Home care instructions* (2nd ed). Dallas: Children's Medical Center.

2. Altman, R. P., & Stolar, C. J. (1985). Pediatric hepatobiliary disease. *Surgical Clinics of North America, 65*(5), 1245–1265.

3. Andrews, W., Fyock, B., Gray, S., Cohn, D., Hendrickse, W., Siegel, J., Belknap, B., Hogge, A., Benser, M., Kennard, B., Stewart, S., & Albertson, N. (1987). Pediatric liver transplantation: The Dallas experience. *Transplantation Proceedings, 19*(4), 3267–3276.

4. Baker, S. S., Dwyer, E., & Queen, P. (1986). Metabolic derangements in children requiring parenteral nutrition. *JPEN. Journal of Parenteral and Enteral Nutrition, 10*(3), 279–281.

5. Balistreri, W. F. (1988). Viral hepatitis. *Pediatric Clinics of North America, 35*(2), 375–402.

6. Beckom, L., Perez, R., Beckom, L., Jebara, L., Lewis, M. & Patenaude, V. (1984). Care of the child with a gastrostomy tube: Common and practical concerns. *Issues in Comprehensive Pediatric Nursing, 7,* 107–119.

7. Benjamin, B., Vinocur, C., Wagner, C., & Weintraub, W. (1987). A closed technique for umbilical hernia repair. *Surgery, Gynecology and Obstetrics, 164*(5), 473–474.

8. Boyd, A., Carachi, A., Azmy, A., Raine, P., & Young, D. (1988). Gastrografin enema in meconium ileus: A persistent approach. *Ped Surg International, 3,* 139–140.

9. Branski, D., & Lebenthal, E. (1981). Celiac disease. In E. Lebenthal (Ed.), *Textbook of gastroenterology and nutrition in infancy,* vol. 2. New York: Raven Press.

10. Broadwell, D. C. (1989). Gastrointestinal system. In J. M. Thompson, G. K. McFarland, J. E. Hirsh, S. M. Tucker, & A. C. Bowers (Eds.). *Clinical nursing,* pp. 731–875. St. Louis: Mosby.

11. Broadwell, D. C., & Jackson, B. S. (1982). *Principles of ostomy care.* St. Louis: Mosby.

12. Candy, C. (1987). Recent advances in the care of children with acute diarrhea: Giving responsibility to the nurse and parents. *Journal of Advanced Nursing, 12,* 95–99.

13. Clark, J. H. (1984). Management of short bowel syndrome in the high-risk infant. *Clinics in Perinatology, 11*(1), 189–197.

14. Crawford, F., & Vermund, S. H. (1985). Hepatitis A in day care centers. *Journal of School Health, 55*(9), 378–381.

15. De Bear, K. (1986). Sham feeding: Another kind of nourishment. *American Journal of Nursing, 86*(10), 1142–1143.

16. Dienno, M. (1987). Esophageal atresia: Corrective procedures and nursing care. *AORN Journal, 45*(6), 1356–1367.

17. Donowitz, L. G. (1988). *Hospital-acquired infection in the pediatric patient.* Baltimore: Williams & Wilkins.

18. Drumm, B., Rhoads, J. M., Stringer, D., Sherman, P., Ellis, L., & Durie, P. (1988). Peptic ulcer disease in children: Etiology, clinical findings, and clinical course. *Pediatrics, 82*(3), 410–444.

19. Edwinson, M., Arnbjornsson, E., & Ekman, R. (1988). Psychologic preparation program for children undergoing acute appendectomy. *Pediatrics, 82*(1);30–35.

20. Fonkalsrud, E. W., Berquist, W., Vargas, J., Ament, M. E., & Foglia, R. P. (1987). Surgical treatment of the gastroesophageal reflux syndrome in infants and children. *American Journal of Surgery, 154*(1), 11–17.

21. Gauderer, M. W., Olsen, M., Stellato, T., & Dokier, M. (1988). Feeding gastrostomy button: Experience and recommendations. *Journal of Pediatric Surgery, 23*(1), 24–28.

22. Gerraughty, A. B., & Younie, L. J. (1985). ECMO: The artificial lung for gravely ill newborns. *American Journal of Nursing, 85*(5), 655–688.

23. Gold, L. M., Kirkpatrick, B., Fricker, F. J., & Zitelli, B. (1986). Psychosocial issues in pediatric organ transplantation: The parent's perspective. *Pediatrics, 77*(5), 738–743.

24. Gutierrez-Sanroman, C., Villa-Carbo, J., Segarra-Llido, V., Garcia-Sala, C., & Ruiz-Compary, S. (1988). Long-term nutritional evaluation of 70 patients operated on for esophageal atresia. *Pediatric Surgery International, 3,* 123–127.

25. Haas-Beckert, B. (1987). Removing the mysteries of parenteral nutrition. *Pediatric Nursing, 13*(1), 37–41.

26. Hagenah, G. C., Harrigan, J., & Campbell, M. A. (1984). Inflammatory bowel disease in children. *Nursing Clinics of North America, 19*(1), 27–39.

27. Harries J. T. (1977). *Essentials of paediatric gastroenterology.* Edinburgh: Churchill Livingston.

28. Hatch, T. (1988). Encopresis and constipation in children. *Pediatric Clinics of North America, 35*(2), 257–280.

29. Hillemeier, C., & Gryboski, J. (1984). Acute pancreatitis in infants and children. *Yale Journal of Biology and Medicine, 57,* 149–159.

30. Joseph, V. T., & Sim, C. (1988). Problems and pitfalls in the management of Hirschsprung's disease. *Journal of Pediatric Surgery, 23*(5), 398–402.

31. Kane, N. M., Cronan, J., Dorfman, G. S., & DeLuca, F. (1988). Pediatric abdominal trauma: Evaluation by computed tomography. *Pediatrics, 82*(1), 11–15.

32. Katz, C., Drongowski, R. A., & Coran, A. G. (1987). Long-term management of chronic constipation in children. *Journal of Pediatric Surgery, 22*(10), 976–978.

33. Kenna, M. A., & Bluestone, C. D. (1988). Foreign bodies in the air and food passages. *Pediatric Review, 10*(1), 25–30.

34. Kliegman, R. M., & Walsh, M.C. (1987). Neonatal necrotizing enterocolitis: Pathogenesis, classification, and spectrum of illness. *Current Problems in Pediatrics, 17*(4), 219–288.

35. Kluth, D., Steding, G., & Seidl, W. (1987). The embryology of foregut malformations. *Journal of Pediatric Surgery, 22*(5), 389–393.

36. Kokkonen, M. L., Kalima, T., Jaaskelainen, J., & Louhimo, I. (1988). Duodenal atresia: Late follow-up. *Journal of Pediatric Surgery, 23*(3), 216–220.

37. Krugman, S., Katz, S. L., Gershon, A. A., & Wilfert, C. (1985). Infectious diseases of children (8th ed.). St. Louis: Mosby.

38. Levine, M. D. (1975). Children with encopresis: A descriptive analysis. *Pediatrics, 56,* 412–416.

39. Levy, J. (1988). *Practical approaches to pediatric gastroenterology.* Chicago: Year Book Medical.

40. Lilly, J., Hall, R., Vasquez-Estevez, J., Karrer, F., & Shikes, R. (1987). The surgery of "correctable" biliary atresia. *Journal of Pediatric Surgery, 22*(6), 522–528.

41. Lynn, M. R. (1986). Use of infant seats for gastroesophageal reflux. *Journal of Pediatric Nursing, 1*(2), 127–129.

42. Martin, L. W., & Torres, A. M. (1985). Hirschsprung's disease. *Surgical Clinics of North America, 65*(5), 1171–1180.

43. Martin, L. W., & Torres, A. M. (1985). Omphalocele and gastroschisis. *Surgical Clinics of North America, 65*(5), 1235–1243.

44. Millar, A. J., Rode, H., Stunden, R. J., & Cywes, S. (1988). Management of pancreatic pseudocysts in children. *Journal of Pediatric Surgery, 23*(2), 122–127.

45. Motil, K., & Grand, R. (1985). Nutritional management of inflammatory bowel disease. *Pediatric Clinics of North America, 32*(2), 447–469.

46. Moynihan, P., & Gerraughty, A. (1985). Diaphragmatic hernia: Low stress—higher survival. *American Journal of Nursing, 85*(6), 662–665.

47. Myer, S. A. (1984). Overview of inflammatory bowel disease. *Nursing Clinics of North America, 19*(1), 3–9.

48. Newman, K. D., Eichelberger, M., & Randolph, J. (1988). Abdominal injury. In M. Eichelberger & G. Pratsch (Eds.). *Pediatric trauma care,* pp. 101–105. Rockville, MD: Aspen.

49. Nord, K. (1988). Peptic ulcer disease in the pediatric population. *Pediatric Clinics of North America, 35*(1), 117–137.

50. Orr, M., & Allen, S. (1986). Optimal oral experiences for infants on long term parenteral nutrition. *Nutrition in Clinical Practice, 1*(6), 288–295.

51. Paine, J. S. (1986). Practical aspects of nasogastric feeding in pediatric patients from a ward nursing perspective. *Nutritional Support Services, 6*(2), 11–14.

52. Paradis, K. J., Freese, D., & Sharp, H. (1988). A pediatric perspective on liver transplantation. *Pediatric Clinics of North America, 35*(2), 409–433.

53. Polley, T. Z., Coran, A. G., & Wesley, J. (1985). A ten-year experience with ninety-two cases of Hirschsprung's disease. *Annals of Surgery, 302*(3), 349–354.

54. Powell, T. G., Hallows, J. A., Cooke, R. W., & Pharoah, P. O. (1986). Why do so many small infants develop an inguinal hernia? *Archives of Disease in Childhood, 61,* 991–995.

55. Rockenhaus, J. M. (1988). Ingestion, digestion, and elimination. In S. James and S. Mott (Eds.), *Nursing care of children and families.* Menlo Park, CA: Addison-Wesley.

56. Ryckman, F. C., & Noseworthy, J. (1985). Multisystem trauma. *Surgical Clinics of North America, 65*(5), 1287–1301.

57. Schaffer, A. J., & Avery, M. E. (1977). *Diseases of the newborn.* Philadelphia: Saunders.

58. Schwartz, M. Z. (1988). Small-bowel transplantation. *Pediatric Surgery International, 3,* 318–325.

59. Shepard, R. W., Wren, J., Evans, S., Lander, M., & Ong, T. H. (1987). Gastroesophageal reflux in children. *Clinical Pediatrics, 26*(2), 55–60.

60. Shun, A., & Puri, D. (1988). Inguinal hernia in the newborn. *Pediatric Surgery International, 3,* 156–157.

61. Sillen, U., et al. (1988). Management of esophageal atresia: Review of 16 years' experience. *Journal of Pediatric Surgery, 23*(9), 805–809.

62. Silverman, A., & Roy, C. C. (1983). *Pediatric clinical gastroenterology* (3rd ed.). St. Louis: Mosby.

63. Simmons, M. A. (1984). Using the nursing process in treating inflammatory bowel disease. *Nursing Clinics of North America, 19*(1), 11–25.

64. Smith, D. P. (1986). Common day-care diseases: Patterns and prevention. *Pediatric Nursing, 12*(3), 175–179.

65. Smith, S. (1985). Liver transplantation: Implications for critical care nursing. *Heart & Lung, 14*(6), 617–618.

66. Sondheimer, J. M. (1988). Gastroesophageal reflux: Update on pathogenesis and diagnosis. *Pediatric Clinics of North America, 35*(1), 103–115.

67. Sperhac, A. M. (1988). Gastrointestinal emergencies. In S. Kelley (Ed.). *Pediatric emergency nursing.* Norwalk, CT: Appleton & Lange.

68. Spicer, R. D., & Cyrves, S. (1988). Pancreatitis in childhood. *Pediatric Surgery International, 3,* 33–36.

69. Stevens, F. M., Egan-Mitchell, B., Cryan, E., McCarthy, C. F., McNicholl, B. (1987). Decreasing incidence of coeliac disease. *Archives of Disease in Childhood, 62*(1), 465–468.

70. Stevenson, R. J. (1985). Non-neonatal intestinal obstruction in children. *Surgical Clinics of North America, 65*(5), 1217–1235.

71. Stewart, B. A., Stewart, B., Hall, R., & Lily, J. (1988). Liver transplantation and the Kasai operation in biliary atresia. *Journal of Pediatric Surgery, 23*(7), 623–626.

72. Stewart, S., Uauy, R., Belknap, W., Kennard, B., Waller, D., & Andrews, W. (1987). One year follow-up of mental/motor development and growth in children after successful liver transplantation. *Pediatric Research, 21*(4), 278.

73. St. Geme, J. W., Flodes, H., Marcy, S. M., Pickering, L. K., Rodriguez, W. J., McCracken, G. H., & Nelson, J. D. (1988). Consensus: Management of *Salmonella* infection in the first year of life. *Pediatric Infectious Disease Journal, 7,* 615–621.

74. Walker-Smith, J. A., Hamilton, J. P., & Walker, W. A. (1983). *Practical pediatric gastroenterology.* London: Butterworth.

75. Weibley, T., Adamson, M., Clinkscales, N., Curran, J., & Bramson, R. (1987). Tube insertion in the premature infant. *MCN: American Journal of Maternal Child Nursing, 12*(1), 24–27.

76. Whaley, L. F., & Wong, D. L. (1987). *Nursing care of infants and children* (3rd ed.). St. Louis: Mosby.

77. Williams, L., & Rzucidlo, S. E. (1985). Care of the pediatric liver transplant patient in the ICU. *Critical Quality Care, 8*(1), 13–25.

78. Withers, J., & Bradshaw, E. (1986). Preventing neonatal hepatitis B infection. *MCN: American Journal of Maternal Child Nursing, 11*(4), 270–272.

79. Zink, M. (1985). Biliary atresia: Nursing diagnosis and management. *Journal of Enterostomal Therapy, 12,* 128–139.

16 UNIT

Nursing Care of Children With Altered Musculoskeletal Function

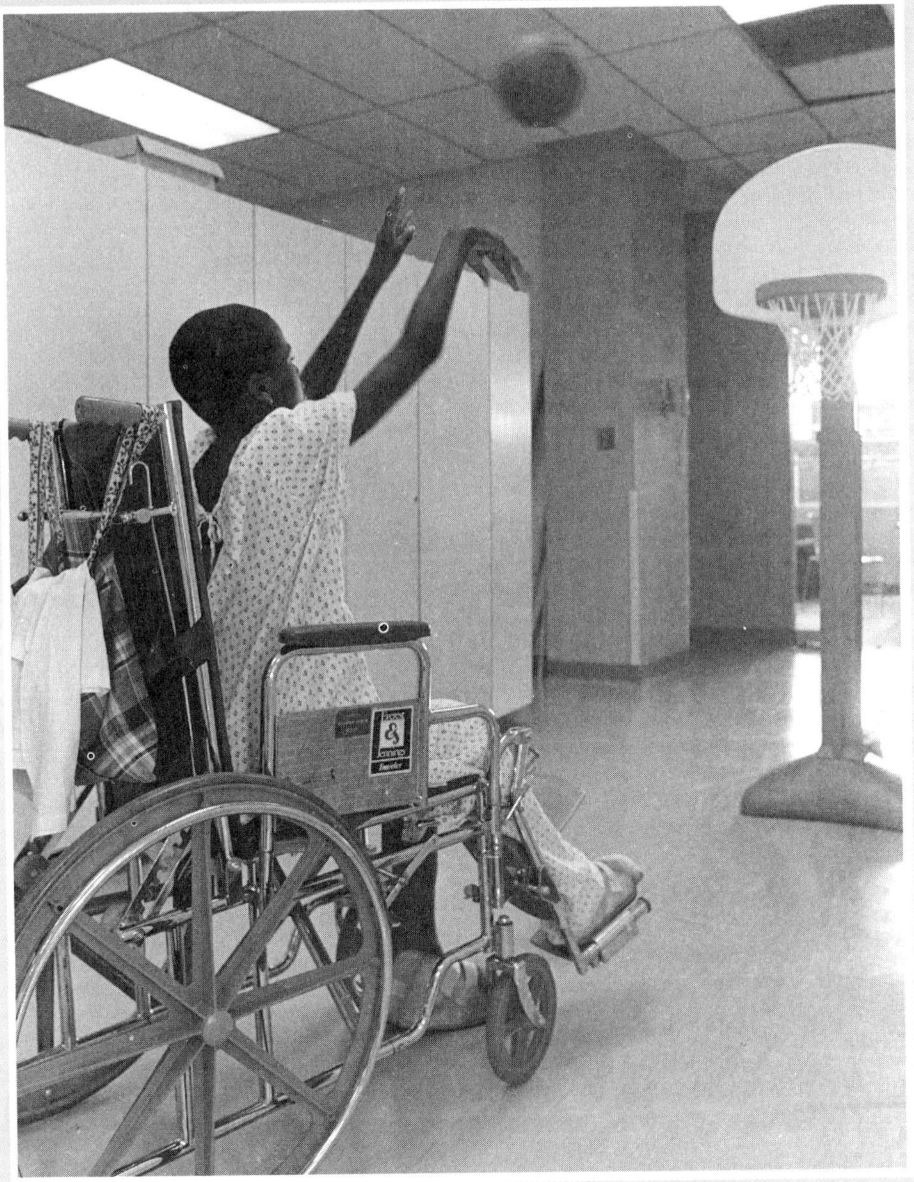

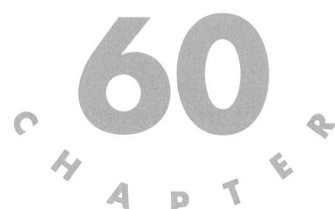

60
CHAPTER

Anatomy and Physiology of the Musculoskeletal System

BEHAVIORAL OBJECTIVES

Describe the embryonic development of the musculoskeletal system.

Discuss the consequences of abnormal fetal development.

List the functions of the musculoskeletal system.

Identify the different types of joints and their actions.

Differentiate among smooth, skeletal, and cardiac muscle functions.

Define the most common types of movements produced by skeletal muscles.

Summarize the ossification process of bone formation.

Discuss muscle stimulation, contraction, and relaxation.

Describe milestones in the development of mobility.

The musculoskeletal system includes the bones, joints, muscles, and connective tissue. These components work in harmony to produce the actions that allow a child independence in exploration and discovery. The skeleton is the framework of the human body, but the muscles produce movement by exerting a force on the bones to which they are attached. This chapter reviews the anatomy and physiology of the musculoskeletal system and the consequences for the child and family when there is an abnormal development of this system.

Embryonic Development

Development of the musculoskeletal system is controlled by genetic makeup. However, environmental factors *in utero* also can affect the developing fetus. During the third week after conception three germ layers (ectoderm, mesoderm, and endoderm) are formed from the inner cell mass of the embryo and give rise to all of the tissues and organs of the developing fetus.[7] The musculoskeletal system is derived from the mesoderm layer.

1655

Skeleton

Bone formation begins about the eighth week of gestation and involves the delivery of bone cell precursors to the sites of bone formation and the aggregation of these cells at the primary center of ossification.[5] During early fetal life the fetal skeleton is composed mostly of hyaline cartilage, which eventually undergoes ossification and bone formation. Intramembranous ossification occurs when osteoblasts in the flat bones form and secrete a matrix that calcifies and acts as a precursor to osteocytes. This network of matrix and osteocytes forms the basis of spongy bone. Endochondral ossification is the means by which cartilage develops into bone in the long bones. This ossification begins in the shaft (*diaphysis*) and the ends (*epiphyses*) of the bones. The formation of bone from cartilage continues until two thin strips remain at the ends of the bones (*epiphyseal plates*). Any teratogenic insult to these plates may result in abnormal growth patterns for the child during prenatal and postnatal growth and development. During the fourth week of gestation the upper limb buds appear and are followed by the lower limbs around the seventh week. This cephalocaudal growth pattern is retained throughout embryonic development.

Joints

Joints begin to develop during the sixth week, and by the end of the eighth week they closely resemble adult joints.[7] Synovial joints (e.g., knee and elbow) are formed when the mesoderm between the bones forms a capsule and differentiates into articular cartilage and synovial membranes. The resulting space forms the joint cavity. Fibrocartilaginous joints are formed when mesoderm between the developing bones differentiates between hyaline cartilage (e.g., *costochondral joints*) and fibrocartilage (e.g., *symphysis pubis*). Fibrous joints are formed when the mesoderm in the joint differentiates into dense, fibrous connective tissue (e.g., sutures of the skull).

Vertebral Column and Ribs

During the fourth week mesodermal cells from the somites migrate and form the vertebral column dorsally and the ribs ventrally. Ossification becomes evident in the vertebral column around the eighth week. By 40 weeks' gestation the vertebral column consists of three bony parts, the centrum and two halves of the vertebral arch, which are all connected by cartilage.

The ribs form from the mesodermal costal processes of the thoracic vertebrae. Initially the ribs are cartilaginous, but by the 13th to 14th week they begin to ossify.

Skull

The fetal skull develops from the mesoderm surrounding the developing brain. The fetal skull separates into the parietal, frontal, temporal, and occipital bones by weeks 20 to 24. These bones are separated by dense connective tissue membranes that form fibrous joints called *sutures*. The fibrous areas where the sutures meet are called *fontanels*. These sutures and fontanels enable the fetal skull to accommodate brain growth and to change shape during the birth process. This accommodation of the fetal cranial vault is called *molding*.

Muscles

All muscles except those of the iris form from myoblasts that are derived from the mesoderm (Fig. 60-1). Skeletal muscles show their classic cross-striations and multinucleations by the 12th week. Smooth muscles evolve from myoblasts that elongate and develop contractile characteristics. Cardiac muscle forms from the splanchnic mesoderm that surrounds the heart tubes during the third week. The first heartbeat occurs around the fourth week of gestation.

Ultrasound can detect fetal muscle movement in the neck, trunk, and limbs by the seventh week. By the 11th week the fetus demonstrates sucking and swallowing reflexes. The 12th week brings about fetal responses to skin stimulation. By the end of the 12th week the fetus can bend, flex, and turn its body all around the uterus. However, these movements are so minute and weak that they cannot be felt by the mother. As the fetal skeleton and musculature continue to develop, fetal movements usually can be felt by the 20th week. This sensation is called quickening.

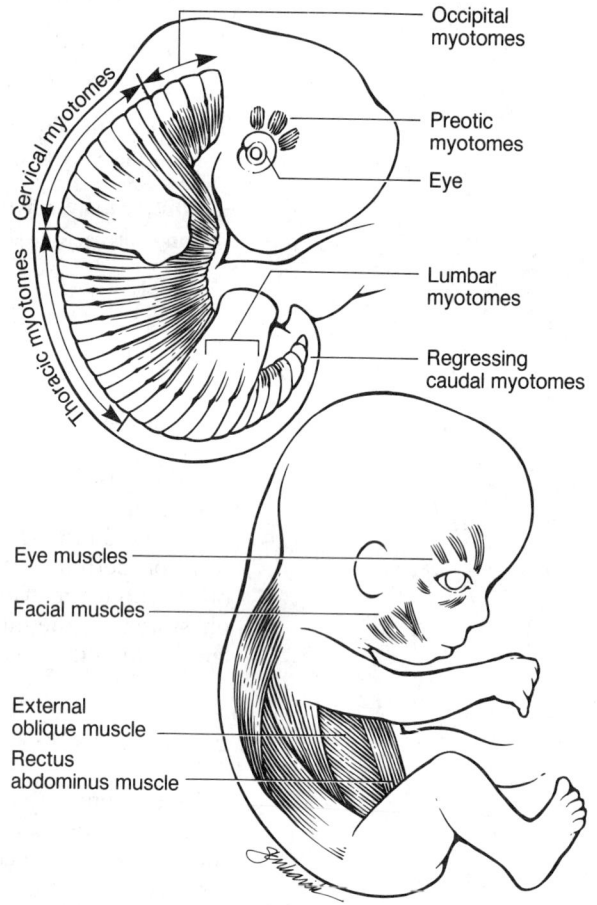

FIGURE 60-1

The developing muscular system. (**A**) A 6-week embryo, showing the myotome regions of the somites that give rise to most skeletal muscles. (**B**) An 8-week embryo, showing the developing superficial trunk musculature. (Redrawn from Moore, K. L. [1989]. *Before we are born: Basic embryology and birth defects.* Philadelphia: W.B. Saunders.)

Consequences of Abnormal Development

The period during which limb development is critical is from 24 to 42 days after fertilization.[7] Consequently, any environmental or teratogenic agent to which a pregnant woman is exposed or ingests during this crucial time may result in congenital anomalies or musculoskeletal deformities. Genetic factors over which the parents have no control also may cause these abnormalities. Interruption in the normal development of the musculoskeletal system during the prenatal period can have deleterious effects on the spinal column, hips, and limbs, creating serious problems with ambulation and activities of daily living.[9] Prenatal detection of fetal abnormalities can be accomplished through the maternal history and physical examination, ultrasonography, radiology, fetoscopy, and blood tests. Table 60-1 provides information on abnormal embryonic development.

Structure and Function

Components of the musculoskeletal system include bones, muscles, tendons, joints, bursae, ligaments, and cartilage. Although each structure is described separately, it is the interdependence of these structures that allows a pattern of normal growth and development for the child. The musculoskeletal system provides the framework and voluntary movements that assist the child in maintaining activities of daily living and exploring the environment. The skeletal and muscular systems are discussed independently to enhance clarity.

Skeletal System

Structure

The skeleton is composed of 206 bones that determine the size of the body and the framework. The main functions of the skeletal system follow:

- Support
- Protection

TABLE 60-1
Consequences of Abnormal Embryonic Development

Fetal Age	Structure	Anomalies at Birth
4 weeks	Neural tube, spinal column	Spina bifida
4 weeks	Limbs	Amelia (absence of limbs)
5–6 weeks	Limbs	Meromelia (partial absence of limbs)
5–6 weeks	Maxilla, palate	Cleft palate
6 weeks	Upper lip	Cleft lip
6–7 weeks	Ankles, feet	Talipes equinovarus (congenital club foot)
Throughout	Limbs	Amniotic band deformities (constriction bands, amputation)
Throughout	Acetabulum	Congenital hip dysplasia

- Movement
- Storage
- Hematopoiesis

The skeleton is buried deep within the muscles and other soft tissues, providing a support structure for the entire body.[11] The skeleton is like the stationary steel girders in a building except the bones can move toward, around, and away from each other. Various internal organs are protected by different parts of the skeleton. For example, the skull protects the brain; the rib cage protects the heart and lungs; and the spinal column protects the spinal cord.

Movement is accomplished through a direct relationship between the bones and the muscles that are attached to them. This relationship enables a child to proceed from reflexive movements in infancy to purposeful, graceful locomotion and ambulation as a young child.

Bones serve as storage for important minerals, such as phosphorus and calcium. During periods of hypocalcemia, the bones can release calcium into the bloodstream to enable the body to maintain homeostasis.

Hematapoiesis (blood cell formation) occurs in the red bone marrow of the long bones. There is a reserve supply of blood cells in the marrow available during physiologic stress. The increased amount of red bone marrow found in an infant's and child's body decreases as the body ages.

Divisions of the Skeleton

The skeleton is divided into two parts: the axial skeleton and the appendicular skeleton[4] (Fig. 60-2). The axial division is composed of bones that establish the longitudinal axis of the body and include the skull, rib cage, vertebral column, sacrum, and coccyx. These 80 bones form the body cavities and protect the internal organs.

The appendicular skeleton includes the bones of the upper and lower extremities and the shoulder and pelvic girdles. These 126 bones attach to the axial skeleton and form the free-moving appendages of the body.

Shapes of Bones

Bones are most often classified according to their shape (i.e., short, long, flat, or irregular). Short bones are irregularly or cube-shaped and consist of a core of cancellous or spongy bone enclosed in a thin sheath of compact bone. These bones include those of the wrist, ankles, and toes.

Long bones, found in the arms and legs, have an elongated shape and provide support and strength to the body[1] (Fig. 60-3). Each bone consists of a proximal and distal epiphysis, which are knobby in shape. This area provides space for muscle and ligament attachments near the joint. The diaphysis is made of hard, compact bone, which contributes to the bone's rigidity and strength. The metaphyses lie between the diaphysis and epiphysis, which are at both ends of the long bone and contain the epiphyseal plate and newly formed bone. This area is not fused during childhood to allow for optimal growth. The articular cartilage is a thin layer of cartilage that covers each epiphysis and acts as a cushion against trauma. The

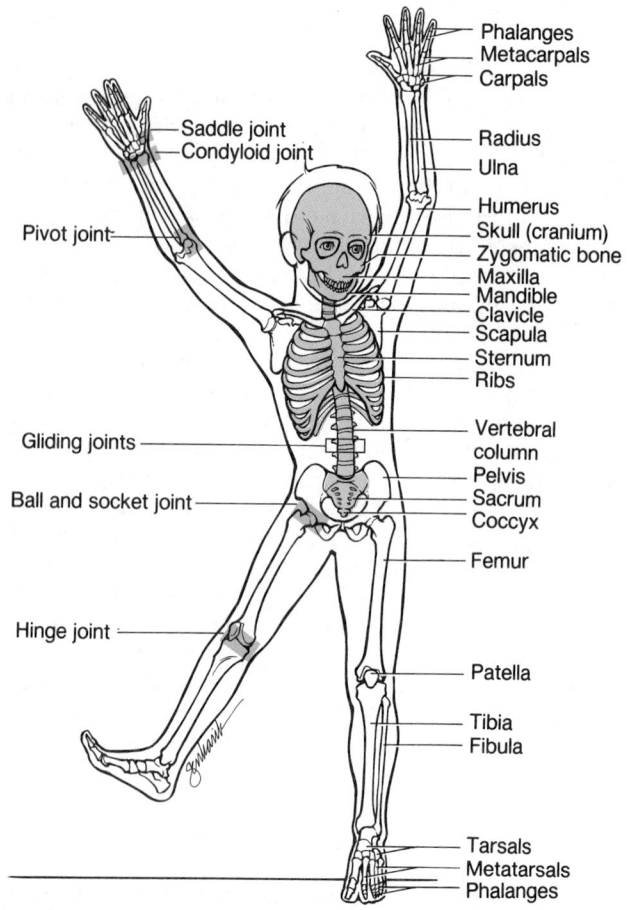

FIGURE 60-2

The axial (grey) and appendicular (blue) skeleton. Diarthrotic joints are indicated by arrows.

grow between the two articulating bones and join them together. The joints of the skull are an example. During fetal and infant development, these joints or sutures remain open to allow for normal brain growth. The skull usually becomes ossified by 18 months.

Amphiarthroses (cartilaginous joints) are slightly movable joints. The articulating bones are connected by cartilage. Examples of amphiarthrodial joints include the symphysis pubis, intervertebral disks, and joints between the ribs and the sternum.

Diarthroses (synovial joints) are freely movable joints that allow movement in various directions. A thin, smooth, white layer of cartilage (articular cartilage) covers and pads the articulating surfaces. The ends of the bones are enclosed by a joint capsule. This capsule is filled with a lubricating fluid (synovial fluid) that helps to reduce friction and allows easier movement in the joint cavity. Synovial joints are classified according to their structure and range of movement they produce.[6]

Ball and socket joints contain the spherical end of one bone fitting into the cup-shaped end of another bone. This type of joint permits the maximum freedom of movement and includes the hip and shoulder joint. *Gliding joints* allow flat bone surfaces to slide over each other in all directions. The carpals, tarsals, and intervertebral joints are examples of gliding joints. *Pivot joints* contain a small projection on one bone rotating in an arch of another. Examples include the joint between the first and second cervical vertebrae, allowing head rotation, and the joint between the distal end of the humerus and the proximal end of the radius, allowing the hand to pronate and supinate.

Hinge joints allow movement in opposite directions by changing the angle between the articulating bones. Joints in the fingers, elbows, and knees are hinge joints.

periosteum is a thick, white, fibrous membrane that covers the rest of the long bone. Because of the periosteum's rich blood supply, and nerves, bone growth, bone repair, and bone nutrition take place here. The periosteum also serves as a point of attachment for tendons, muscles, and ligaments.

Flat bones are composed of cancellous and compact bony material and are shaped exactly as their name suggests. They provide broad surfaces for muscle attachments and are important sites for hematopoiesis. The bones of the skull, ribs, scapulae, and sternum are examples of flat bones.

Irregular bones are similar in makeup to short bones but are irregular in shape. Examples of irregular bones are the vertebrae, ossicles of the ear, and patella.

Joints

The site where two or more bones are attached is called a joint or articulation.[5] The primary function of joints is to provide mobility and stability to the skeleton. The joint's location and structure determine the resulting movement or stability. Joints are classified according to the degree of movement they permit.

Synarthroses (fibrous joints) are immovable joints. Interlocking projections and fibrous connective tissues

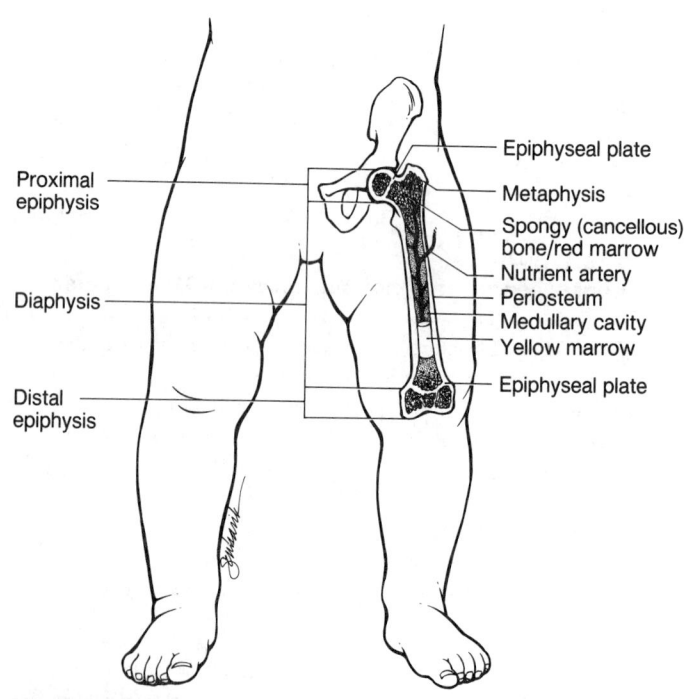

FIGURE 60-3

Portions of the long bone.

Condyloid joints allow movement when oval-shaped articular surfaces fit into elliptical cavities. An example is the wrist between the bones of the forearm. *Saddle joints* have deep articulating surfaces and allow for the human thumb's versatile movement. Without this joint the pincher grasp for picking up or grasping an object would be impossible.

Ligaments

Ligaments are short, flat bands of distinct fibrous connective tissue that connect bones to each other and provide support to the joints between them. Ligaments help to prevent instability and uncoordinated muscular actions. The two types of ligaments are those that connect viscera to each other and those that connect one bone to another.[1] Ligaments may be collagenous or elastic. Collagenous (white) ligaments as those in the knees do not move or stretch yet provide stability and resiliency to the joint. Elastic (yellow) ligaments as those located in the vertebral column allow for great flexibility, movement, and stretching to the involved joint.

Bursae

Bursae are small, flat sacs lined with synovial membrane and filled with synovial fluid. The main function of bursae is to help ease movement and reduce friction around areas subject to stress. Bursae are located around the joints that are susceptible to pressure and trauma, such as the knee, shoulder, elbow, and hip.

Cartilage

Cartilage is a type of connective tissue made up of collagenous fibers that give strength, form, support, and flexibility to surrounding structures. These musculoskeletal structures include the joints, vertebral disks, ribs, and embryonic skeleton. Cartilage is composed of chondrocytes, collagen, and matrix, which form a dense, firm, gelatinous material that is organized into a system of fibers. Articular cartilage covers the ends of the long bones and helps to reduce friction in the joints and to distribute the force of weight bearing.[5] Because cartilage does not contain blood vessels, nutrients must diffuse through the matrix to reach the chondrocytes.

Muscular System

The skeletal system provides the framework for the body, yet it is incapable of movement by itself. Movement of body parts is achieved through the contraction and relaxation of muscles that are attached to bones. Muscle mass comprises 25% of an infant's and 50% of a child's total body weight. An infant's upper body muscles develop before the lower muscles, thereby illustrating cephalocaudal development.

Classification of Muscles

Muscles are classified as involuntary or voluntary. Involuntary muscles are those over which the child has no control. They contract independent of conscious effort. The two types of involuntary muscles are cardiac muscle and smooth muscle.

Cardiac muscle, which forms the majority of the heart wall, is called the myocardium. The size and thickness of the myocardium depend on the work load of the different heart chambers. Smooth or visceral muscle is found along the walls of the hollow structures of the body, such as the digestive tract, ureters, and blood vessels. Contractions of smooth muscle aid in peristalsis, vasodilation, and vasoconstriction.

Voluntary muscles contract in a controlled, willful manner. It is this type of muscle, skeletal muscle, that is the basis of the musculoskeletal system and is discussed in depth.

Structure of Skeletal Muscle

Skeletal muscles are considered organs because they possess multinucleated, contractile cells (myocytes) and a connective tissue framework. This framework supplies the muscle with a network of nerve fibers, blood vessels, and lymphatic channels. Muscle cells are long and slender with numerous contractile fibers (myofibrils) running lengthwise. As these threads contract the entire cell shortens; when they relax the entire cell lengthens.

Each skeletal muscle is encased in a three-layered connective tissue framework called *fascia*.[4] The outer layer, the epimysium, is located on the surface of the muscle. The second layer, the perimysium, surrounds small bundles of fibers. The third layer, the endomysium, binds the individual muscle fibers found in the bundles of fibers. Each muscle cell is surrounded by a cell membrane called a sarcolemma.

Each muscle fiber is further divided into sarcomeres, which are the contractile units of the myofibril. Sarcomeres contain thick and thin myofilaments. The thick myofilament contains the contractile protein myosin, while the thin myofilaments are twisted double strands containing actin, troponin, and tropomyosin. Actin and myosin lie beside each other and partially overlap, causing the myofibril to have alternating light and dark bands.[1] The light bands containing actin filaments are called I bands. The dark bands containing myosin filaments and part of the actin filaments are called A bands. In the middle of the light band is the dark line called the Z line.

The muscle cells also contain sarcoplasm, which is the cytoplasm of the muscle cells that supplies the cell with proteins and enzymes. The numerous mitochondria provide the energy source for the cell. The sarcoplasmic reticulum helps to transport calcium into the sarcomere to initiate muscle contractions.

Tendons

Muscles connect to bones through a network of fibrous connective tissue called *tendons* that form a cord between the body of the muscle and the bones to which it is attached (Fig. 60-4). When these connective tissues connect over a large expanse of bone, such as the skull or vertebrae, the attachment is called an aponeurosis. Tendons possess great tensile strength and are difficult to injure.

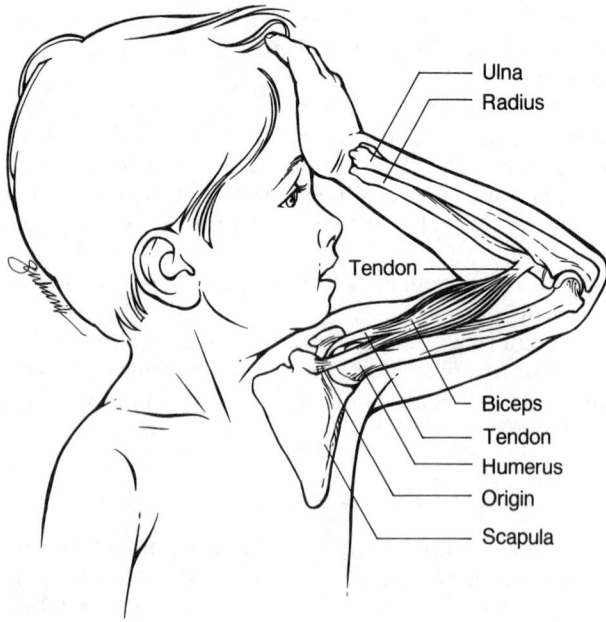

FIGURE 60-4
The biceps muscle attached to the bones of origin and insertion by its tendons.

Functions

In addition to movement the muscular system is responsible for posture or muscle tone and heat production. Muscles produce movement by pulling the bones they connect toward or away from each other. During muscle contractions the involved bones remain slightly fixed or stationary (origin) or mobile (insertion).

Certain movements can involve the interaction and coordination of various muscles. The main muscle involved is called the prime mover or agonist. The muscles that indirectly contribute to that movement are called synergists. The muscles that oppose the agonist are called the antagonist. Muscle fibers contract in only one direction. Other muscle fibers must reverse or relax the contraction.

Muscle tone refers to a partially contracted state of the muscle that is normal when the muscles are not in use.[6] These muscle contractions are called tonic contractions and they help maintain body posture. Skeletal muscles facilitate posture by counteracting the forces of gravity.

Skeletal muscles also produce heat and maintain body temperature through two methods. First, energy and heat are released from the breakdown of adenosine triphosphate (ATP) during a muscle contraction. This heat helps maintain homeostatic body temperature. Second, shivering or uncontrolled, rapid muscle activity produces energy that is retained in its entirety as heat.

Types of Muscle Contractions

The body depends on other types of muscular contractions in addition to tonic contractions. These contractions include isometric, isotonic, twitch, and tetanic.

Isometric contractions do not change the muscle length but increase the muscle tension. Consequently,

the muscle increases in size and strength. An example of isometric contractions occurs when a child pushes against an immovable object. *Isotonic contractions* maintain a constant muscle tension but change the muscle's shape and length, thus producing movement. Walking, running, and playing sports are examples of isotonic contractions. A *twitch* is a spasmodic contraction of a portion of a muscle in response to a single stimulus. It usually lasts less than $\frac{1}{10}$ of a second. *Tetanic contractions* (tetany) last longer than a twitch and are produced by a series of stimuli rapidly attacking the muscle. These muscle spasms can be very frightening and painful for a child but usually can be reversed once the etiology is identified.

Types of Movements

The interdependence between the skeletal and muscular systems is best illustrated when body movements are discussed. The shape of the bones, the type of movable joint, and the structure of the muscles and tendons enable the child to move through the environment. Opposing muscles work in contrast to each other to help the body maintain proper alignment, anatomic position, and movement. Range of motion is illustrated in Figures 61-2 and 61-6.

Flexion is defined as movement that decreases the angle between two bones at the joint. Another term for flexion is bending. *Extension* counteracts flexion by increasing the angle between two bones at the joint, as in straightening or stretching movements. *Adduction* means movement toward the center or midline of the body. *Abduction* means moving away from the center or midline of the body. *Rotation* is the process of turning around a longitudinal axis. *Supination* occurs when the palm of the hand is turned upward. *Pronation* is when the palm of the hand is turned downward. *Dorsiflexion* is movement that elevates the top of the foot and tips it up, such as when a child walks on the heels. *Plantarflexion* occurs when the foot is pointed downward, such as seen in toe-walking. *Inversion* is turning inward toward the body, while *eversion* is turning outward away from the midline.

System Physiology

Children are able to define and explore their world through the intricate functions of their musculoskeletal system. Whether threading beads on a string or running for the winning touchdown, fine and gross motor coordination allows the child to succeed at such activities. The health and integrity of the musculoskeletal system facilitates the child's passage from a dependent infant to an independent adolescent.

Bone Formation

Bones are living organs that require their own network of nerves, lymph, and blood. Bone evolves from cartilage present during embryonic life, as noted previously in this chapter. The elements of bone tissue include specific bone cells and bone matrix. Each type of bone cell has a unique function.

Osteoblasts are specialized bone-forming cells and lay the foundation for the transformation of embryonic cartilage into bone. Osteocytes are formed when bone matrix surrounds the osteoblast and calcifies it. Osteocytes function by maintaining and modifying bone matrix and maintaining mineral (calcium and phosphorus) balance.[5] Osteoclasts are directly responsible for resorption or breakdown of bone. The direct relationship between the osteoblasts and osteoclasts model growing bone into its ultimate shape. Bone matrix is composed of collagen fibers, proteins, glycoproteins, and bone minerals. Bone matrix is what gives bones their tensile strength (resistance to being pulled apart) and their compressive strength (resistance to being crushed).

There are two types of bone tissue: dense (compact) and spongy (cancellous). Although both types of tissue contain the same elements, the organization and distribution of these elements differentiate them. Compact bone is highly organized, dense, and very strong. It is found in the diaphysis of the long bones and outer layer of other bones. The structural unit of compact bone is the haversian system. Each system is a cylindrical, tube-like structure that maintains the viability of the bone. In the center of the haversian system is the haversian canal, which contains the blood vessels and nerve fibers. The blood vessels pass through transverse tubes called Volkmann's canals and form a network between the periosteum and the medullary cavity. This network helps to deliver nutrients to the osteocytes and waste products away from them. The concentric rings of calcified matrix surrounding the haversian canal are called *lamellae*.

The tiny spaces found between the lamellae are called *lacunae* and contain the osteocyte. Minute, finger-like projections called *canaliculi* connect the lacunae to each other and to the haversian canal, and they supply oxygen and nutrients to the osteocyte.

Cancellous bone is less intricate and does not contain a haversian system. Instead the lamellae form a meshwork of bony plates called *trabeculae*. The structure and design of the trabeculae are determined by the amount and direction of stress that is placed on the bone. These trabeculae are surrounded by red bone marrow, which is responsible for hematopoiesis. As the child matures the red marrow partially converts to yellow marrow, which

contains fat. Cancellous bone is found at the ends of the long bones and at the center of other bones.

Bone Growth

Bones grow in length from the epiphyseal plates (endochondral ossification) and in thickness from the periosteum (intramembranous ossification).[2] Two areas of the bone are responsible for growth (Fig. 60-5). The primary center of ossification is located in the shaft (diaphysis) of fetal cartilage. Growth and ossification extend toward either end of the developing bone. The secondary centers of ossification are located at the epiphyses of the bones and extend from the epiphyseal cartilage to the articular cartilage. While the secondary centers of ossification do not contribute to bone length, they do contribute to formation of the epiphyses and joints.

Bones continue to grow from these centers throughout infancy and childhood. New cells are constantly being formed on the distal side of the cartilaginous epiphyseal plates, causing ossification and increased bone length. Remodeling takes place in the shaft of the long bones, causing the center of the diaphysis to become strong and compact enough to withstand pressure and stress.

As bones grow in length, they also grow in circumference. Osteoblasts on the periosteal surface secrete bone matrix, which calcifies and adds to the diameter of the bone. At the same time osteoclasts on the medullary surface resorb bone, causing the medullary cavity to increase in size for red and yellow marrow production.

A child usually reaches adult height by late adolescence when the epiphyseal plates close and all the cartilage is replaced with bone. Any injury to these plates during a child's growth spurt could cause abnormal bone growth patterns. Examiners are able to detect a child's growth potential and physical maturity by studying the epiphyseal areas of the wrists and hand through radiography.

Rate of bone growth varies with each age level.[10] Growth spurts occur during infancy and adolescence. During the early years of life growth patterns for both sexes are similar, but as children approach adolescence these patterns change. Girls usually experience their growth spurt between 10 and 12 years of age, while boys

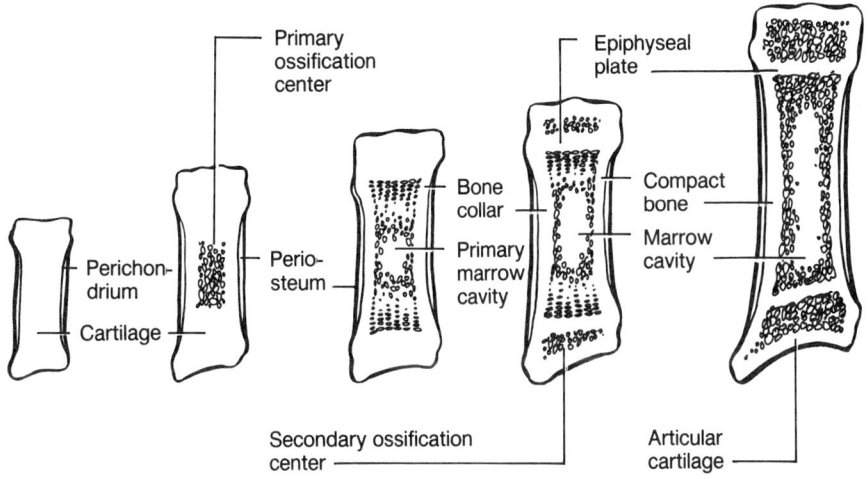

FIGURE 60-5

Stages of bone formation and centers of ossification.

Primary ossification center

Epiphyseal plate

Perichondrium

Periosteum

Bone collar

Compact bone

Marrow cavity

Primary marrow cavity

Cartilage

Secondary ossification center

Articular cartilage

experience it between 12 and 14 years. Prior to adolescence the lower limbs grow more rapidly than the trunk. During adolescence, a child's height increases as a result of growth in the trunk rather than in the lower limbs.

Factors Affecting Bone Growth

Remodeling is the process by which bone forms and resorbs during a person's lifetime. Under normal conditions a child should be able to attain normal adult stature. Several factors can affect the growth pattern.

Calcium and phosphorus are the extracellular minerals that help to support and strengthen bone formation and growth.[4] These minerals combine with the collagen fibers of bone to give bone its great tensile and compressional strength. Normal serum calcium and phosphorus levels are maintained through adequate dietary intake. Parathyroid hormone is responsible for maintaining serum calcium levels when dietary intake is deficient. When calcium levels are low, parathyroid hormone secretion increases, helping the body to absorb more calcium from the intestinal tract and to promote the formation of osteoclasts. Osteoclasts break down bone tissue, which releases calcium into the body. Conversely, when serum calcium levels are elevated, parathyroid hormone production decreases drastically. Exactly how calcium affects the formation of new bone is unknown.

Vitamin D promotes bone calcification by enhancing calcium and phosphorus absorption from the intestines. Vitamin D is believed to encourage calcium migration across cell walls.

Calcitonin is a hormone that helps to reduce serum calcium levels, especially in children in whom bone remodeling occurs at a rapid rate. Calcitonin encourages the growth and activity of osteoblasts and discourages the growth of osteoclasts. The result is decreased serum calcium levels. The opposing effects of calcitonin versus parathyroid hormone should be noted.

The sex hormones, estrogen and testosterone, affect bone growth primarily during puberty. Estrogen stimulates osteoblast activity and enables girls to reach their adult height before the epiphyseal plates close. Testosterone has the same effect on bone growth for boys.

Growth hormone causes linear bone growth by increasing cartilage formation. It also helps to widen the epiphyseal plates and increase the amount of bone matrix in the ends of the long bones. Other factors that affect bone formation and growth include weight bearing, gluticosteroids, malnutrition, vitamin deficiencies, and mechanical trauma.

Muscle Contractions

Properties of muscle tissue include excitability, contractility, extensibility, and elasticity. *Excitability* is the ability of the muscle to respond to a stimulus, while the actual shortening and thickening of the muscle is known as *contractility*. *Extensibility* permits the muscle cells to stretch, and *elasticity* ensures that the muscle will return to its original length once it has relaxed.

A stimulus is necessary to induce a myofilament in the skeletal muscle to contract.[1] This stimulus usually is a nerve impulse that originates in the spinal cord and travels down the nerve axon to the junction where it contacts the muscle (neuromuscular junction). Acetylcholine is released, causing the action potential of the muscle cell membrane to alter its permeability to sodium. The action potential transmits a message to the sarcoplasmic reticulum to release calcium. The calcium binds with the proteins troponin and tropomyosin and releases their cohesion with actin. The exposed actin slides over the myosin and causes a shortening or contraction of the sarcomere and eventually the entire muscle. This sliding over or attraction between the actin and myosin is called the sliding filament theory.

Muscle relaxation occurs when the calcium pump in the sarcoplasmic reticulum breaks the link between calcium and troponin and tropomyosin. This breakage allows troponin and tropomyosin to recover the actin filaments and inhibits the attraction to myosin. Without the configuration between the actin and myosin, the sarcomere units extend, causing muscle relaxation.

An energy source must be available for muscle contractions to occur.[3] The first source of energy is adenosine triphosphate (ATP), an enzyme that is readily available in resting muscle cells. Once that energy source has been depleted, phosphocreatine supplies the cell with a phosphate ion to maintain ATP production and function. Another source of energy is that released by the process of digestion and glycolysis. The last source of energy is from aerobic and anaerobic metabolism.

Muscle Growth

The makeup and size of muscles vary with chronologic age. Between birth and adolescence the number of muscle nuclei increases in the body 14 times in boys and 10 times in girls. The growth of fibers is directly related to the range of movement the muscle performs. The development of a muscle results from the tension level exerted against it by the antagonist.

During infancy the muscles of the head, trunk, and upper extremities are heavier than the poorly developed muscles of the lower extremities. An infant's muscles required for breathing and sucking are well developed to prevent respiratory compromise and poor feeding. Pelvic muscles develop during childhood, as illustrated by the graceful movements demonstrated by children as they approach adolescence. During adolescence muscle growth is a major contributing factor to weight gain.

Development of Mobility

Children are born with crawling and stepping reflexes. These reflexes disappear during early infancy, and the actual motions of crawling and walking need to be perfected and developed in later infancy and toddlerhood. The development of ambulation depends on maturation of the central nervous system, which also develops in a cephalocaudal direction.

During the first 3 months of life infants progress from raising the chin while lying on the abdomen to lifting the head erect when in a prone position.[8] From 3 to 6 months infants progress from sitting with support to pulling

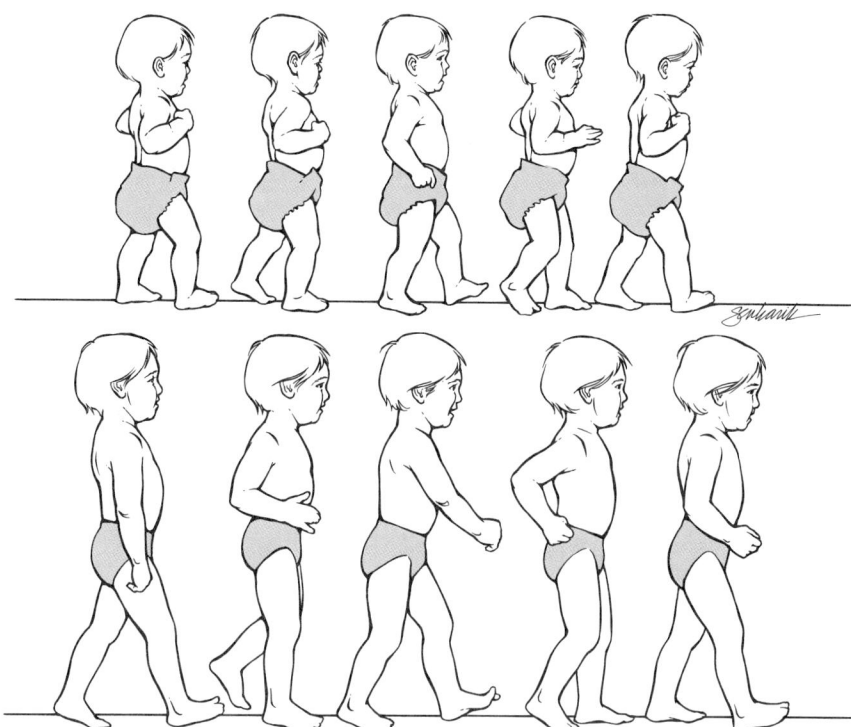

FIGURE 60-6

Comparison of posture and gait between a 1-year-old child and a 3-year-old child.

themselves to a sitting position unsupported for a short period of time. Between 6 and 9 months infants master creeping or crawling and can pull themselves to their feet by holding onto support. They also can bear weight on their feet and take steps with help. Between 9 and 12 months they can sit from a standing position without help, may stand unsupported for a few seconds, walk around furniture, and walk with help for longer distances. The lumbar and dorsal curves also develop while learning to walk. By 15 months a child becomes more independent with walking and can creep up stairs. Increased ambulation with running occurs at 18 months, and by 24 months the child is able to walk, balance, and bend over without falling. An adult pattern of gait develops between 3 and 5 years of age.[10]

While observing the stages of mobility, one is able to distinguish the difference in gross motor development of ambulation between infants and toddlers (Fig. 60-6). Infants have a wide base, hyperflexed hips and knees, extended and abducted arms, and jerky and abrupt movements. As children mature mobility and coordination increase. The base narrows, reciprocal arm swing is present, stride and walking speed increase, and movements become more smooth and graceful.

Summary

The ability of children to investigate and explore their environment is partially due to the intricate relationships within the musculoskeletal system. Many prenatal and postnatal factors can affect the integrity of this system.

The ability to recognize normal growth and development patterns of bones and muscles assists nurses and parents to have realistic expectations about a child's attainment of gross motor and fine motor mobility.

References

1. Bullock, B. L., & Rosendahl, P. P. (1992). *Pathophysiology: Adaptations and alerations in function.* (3rd ed.). Philadelphia: J.B. Lippincott.
2. England, M. A. (1990). *A color atlas of life before birth: Normal development.* London: Wolfe Medical Productions.
3. Guyton, A. C. (1991). *Textbook of medical physiology.* Philadelphia: W.B. Saunders.
4. Gylys, B. A., & Wedding, M. E. (1988). *Medical terminology: A systems approach.* Philadelphia: F.A. Davis.
5. McCance, K. L., & Huether, S. E. (1990). *Pathophysiology: The biologic basis for disease in adults and children.* St. Louis: C.V. Mosby.
6. Memmler, R. L., & Wood, D. L. (1987). *Structure and function of the human body* (4th ed.). Philadelphia: J.B. Lippincott.
7. Moore, K. L. (1989). *Before we are born: Basic embryology and birth defects.* Philadelphia: W.B. Saunders.
8. Murray, R. B., & Zentner, J. P. (1989). *Nursing assessment and health promotion strategies through the life span* (4th ed.). Norwalk, CT: Appleton and Lange.
9. Purtilo, D. T., & Purtilo, R. B. (1989). *A survey of human diseases* (2nd ed.). Boston: Little, Brown.
10. Tachdjian, M. O. (1990). *Pediatric orthopedics* (2nd ed.) (vols. 1 & 4). Philadelphia: W.B. Saunders.
11. Thibodeau, G. A., & Anthony, C. P. (1988). *Structure and function of the body.* (8th ed.). St. Louis: Times Mirror/ Mosby College.

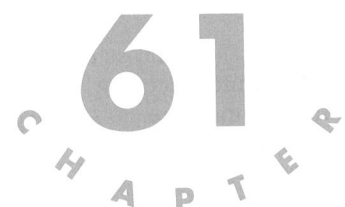

61 CHAPTER

Nursing Assessment and Diagnosis of Musculoskeletal Function

BEHAVIORAL OBJECTIVES

Use functional health as a guideline for assessment of the child's musculoskeletal function.

Describe the components of a complete physical examination of the child's musculoskeletal function.

Differentiate among various studies and diagnostic tests used in determining musculoskeletal function.

Identify nursing diagnoses that are used often in the care of children with musculoskeletal dysfunction.

Many factors affect musculoskeletal function, including normal developmental changes, the environment, and the onset and duration of a musculoskeletal disorder. Musculoskeletal disorders comprise a significant proportion of children's health problems, and these disorders may cause alterations or disturbances in a child's function.[4] Accurate assessments can lead to early detection of musculoskeletal dysfunction and may help diminish their severity and disabling effects.

The most accurate musculoskeletal diagnoses are based on a detailed family history and a comprehensive physical examination.[3] Gaining the trust and cooperation of the child and family is crucial to effective assessment and interpretation of the findings. Being acutely attuned to voiced complaints, parent-child interactions, and visible musculoskeletal deficits can help guide the nurse in providing expert care and coordination of resources for the child and family.

Nursing Assessment

Child and Family History

The health history of the child and family serves as a foundation for the physical and diagnostic assessment. Content of the health history varies depending on the reason for the visit and the severity of the problem. Using functional health patterns to organize the history of a child who has a musculoskeletal disorder results in a comprehensive data base that will guide the physical examination and the formation of nursing diagnoses.

Health Perception and Health Management

To determine factors that affect the musculoskeletal system, the health history should include the child's physical health since birth, genetic and inherited familial diseases, and the mother's prenatal history. Intrauterine conditions affecting the musculoskeletal system's growth and development may have slight or marked influences on growth, development, and movement as the child progresses through life. Medication such as tranquilizers and broad-spectrum antibiotics taken during pregnancy have been related to musculoskeletal anomalies. Maternal viral infections, such as rubella, varicella, and mumps, also have a high coincidence with the development of congenital anomalies affecting orthopedic structures.[6]

The family's general perceptions, health management, and preventive practices in regard to health and illness are explored. Age is of particular importance in comparing the child's developmental motor skill level with the norms for that age group. Do the parents view the child as developing normally for age? Delays in developmental milestones may indicate pathologic conditions such as cerebral palsy or congenital hip dysplasia.

Accurate documentation of the child's immunization record is necessary. Do the parents understand the detrimental results of delinquent immunizations for their child? Polio and tetanus can have devastating effects on the musculoskeletal system.

Information about the family's financial status may be appropriate because health maintenance may not be a priority for families with limited incomes. Some musculoskeletal disorders require multiple health services, and the expenses incurred can be staggering if affected children are to reach their maximum level of functioning.

Nutrition and Metabolism

Assessing the nutritional–metabolic health pattern includes describing the patterns of food and fluid consumption relative to the indicators of local nutrient supply and metabolic demand. Evidence of adequate nutrition may include firm, well-developed muscles; straight spine; symmetric extremities; and flexible joints with full range of motion. Knowledge of a child's diet will help the nurse determine if the child is receiving enough calories, fats, carbohydrates, proteins, vitamins, and minerals. Indicators of unmet metabolic needs include altered growth and development patterns and malnutrition.

The family should be questioned about the child's typical daily food intake, vitamin supplements, dietary restrictions, or dental problems. Some children who have musculoskeletal disorders also have neurologic involvement such as seizures or increased intracranial pressure, and they may require daily doses of phenobarbital and

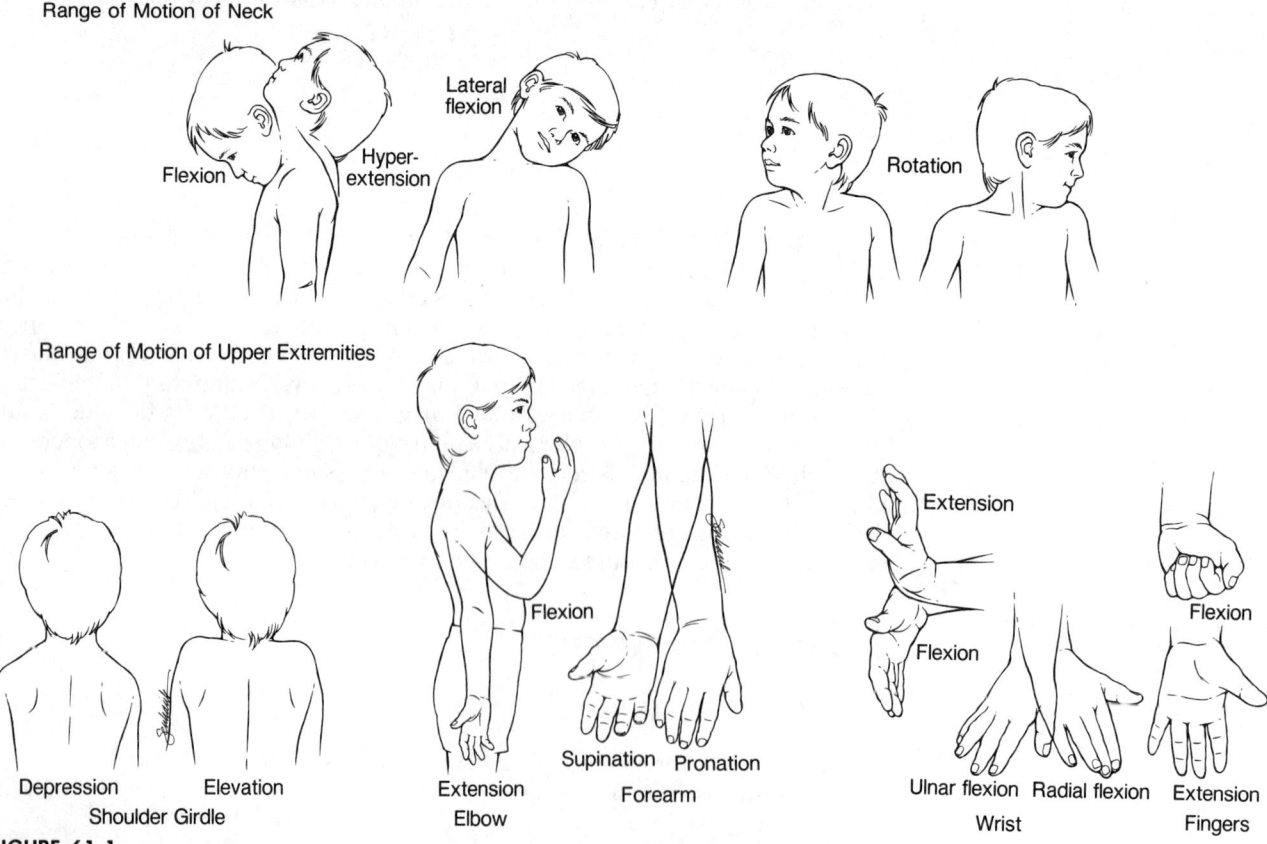

FIGURE 61-1

Normal range of motion.

phenytoin. These drugs can cause gingival hyperplasia, which may lead to mechanical difficulties with chewing, swallowing, oral hygiene, and dental caries.

Elimination

Bowel and urinary elimination patterns may vary in the presence of different musculoskeletal disorders. Is the child continent of urine and stool and able to take care of personal elimination needs? What is the child's normal pattern of elimination? Children who have limited mobility may suffer from chronic constipation. They may be dependent on laxatives or enemas related to decreased peristalsis secondary to immobility.

Meticulous skin care is important to prevent skin breakdown and body odor caused by casts, braces, and dressings. Body cast care can be a challenge to the family, especially if the child is not toilet trained. What measures is the family using to promote elimination patterns and protect the integrity of the cast and skin?

Activity and Exercise

The nurse should assess the child's level of independence in meeting self-care health needs. Many musculoskeletal disorders can render a child incapable of activities of daily living and general mobility. Contractures and loss of muscle tone force children to be dependent on their caregivers for hygiene, feeding, and safety. Range

of motion, discussed under the Physical Examination and summarized in Figure 61-1, is necessary to perform accurate and pain-free activities of daily living.

Leisure activities should be identified because these patterns describe the recreational activities necessary for a productive life. Developmentally, children need opportunities to express themselves through play. Because play is the child's natural medium of expression, precise coordination of the musculoskeletal system is needed to enable the child to run, jump, and interact with the environment. What types of games does the child like to play? Are they appropriate for the child's developmental and chronologic age? What factors contribute to the child's increased mobility and independence, involvement in play activities, and maintenance of sufficient energy to participate in diversional activities?

Sleep and Rest

How much time is allotted for rest and relaxation? Is the bed specially designed to accommodate conditions of immobility? What is the child's perception of the quality and quantity of sleep and rest? Many musculoskeletal disorders require children to wear splints and braces intermittently throughout their sleep cycles. Removal and application of these devices may interrupt the child's sleep, causing stress and fatigue. Other equipment, such as casts and traction, diminish the possibility of changing positions, causing pressure areas and discomfort. What measures has the family discovered that facilitate the child's sleep and rest?

Range of Motion of Lower Extremities

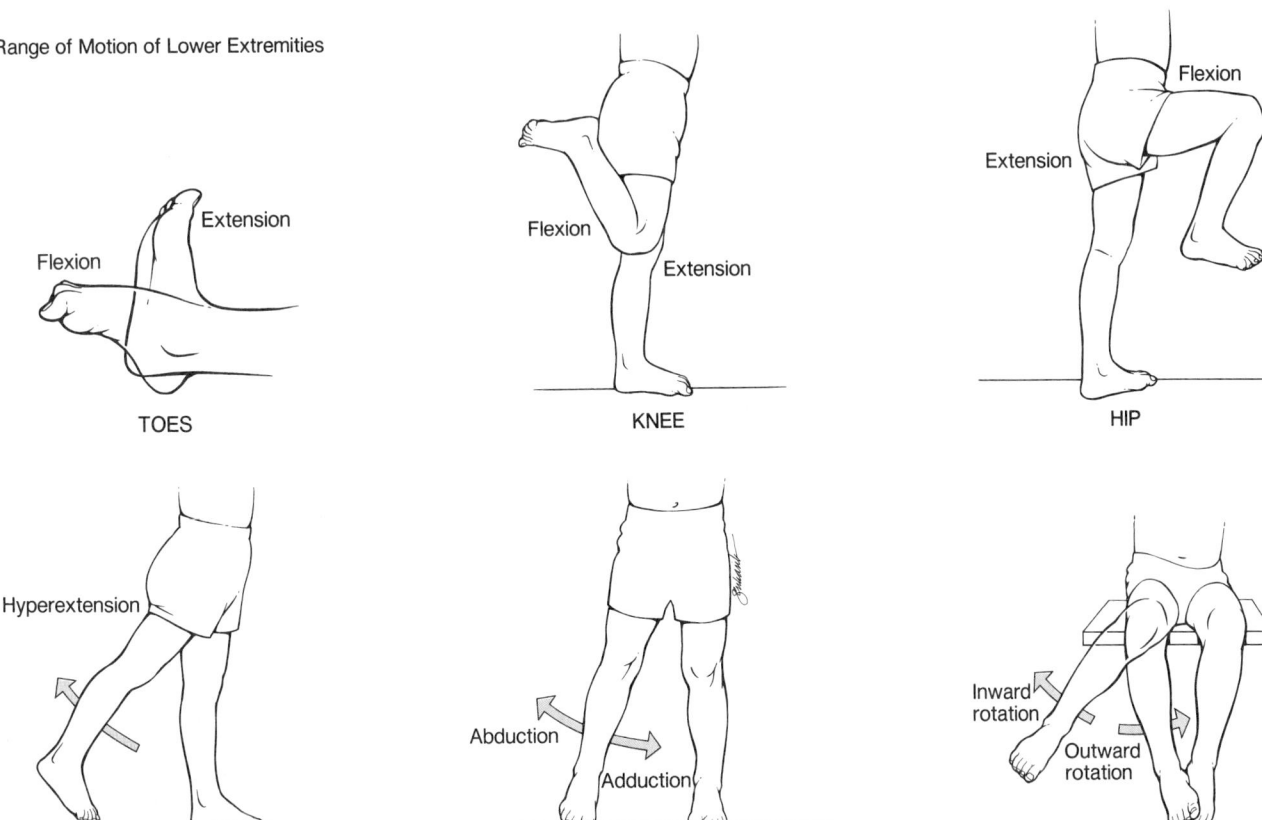

FIGURE 61-1 (Continued)

Cognition and Perception

Because of the complexity of many musculoskeletal disorders, the child may not have the cognitive functions of language capacity, memory, problem solving, and decision making. How does the family interpret the needs of the child? Who is ultimately responsible for decision making on behalf of the child?

Multiple surgical procedures may be needed to correct congenital musculoskeletal disorders. Likewise, some musculoskeletal problems, such as juvenile arthritis, cause chronic pain. Altered comfort levels and pain may interfere with a child's daily functioning. Does the child have a high or low threshold of pain? Postoperative analgesics can cause basic sensory alterations, such as confusion, impaired sensorium, slurred speech, and drowsiness. How is the family helping the child to manage chronic pain?

Self-Perception and Self-Concept

Feelings of powerlessness and lack of control experienced by children and their families during a crisis greatly affect their self-perception and self-concept. High levels of anxiety in the child and caregiver can inhibit the development of a positive self-image. Families have perceptions and concepts about their image in the community and their competencies to deal with life. Any threat to these perceptions can result in depression, isolation, aggression, or passivity.

What is the posture and movement of the child during the assessment? Does the child make eye contact? Children who have a negative self-concept may withdraw and avoid direct eye contact with the interviewer. How do the parents interact with the child? When questioning a child, do the parents always respond? Does the child feel that people are listening to him or her? Children treated with respect feel valued and are likely to develop positive self-perceptions.

Role Relationships

Disruption in the child's social roles can negatively influence overall adjustments and role relationships. Chronic musculoskeletal disorders may require frequent hospitalizations, surgeries, and separation from families and significant others. Does the child have many friends? Have they been nonjudgmental toward the child's disability? Is the child included in his or her peers' social events? Peer acceptance is important for children of all ages.

Sexuality and Reproduction

A child's care providers usually control how the child learns about sexuality, reproduction, and contraception. Is the subject of sexuality freely discussed in the family? Does the caregiver believe that the physically disadvantaged child needs information, recognition, and acceptance of feelings regarding sexuality? Parents of children with musculoskeletal problems may ignore this aspect of the child's growth and development. Adolescents who are wheelchair bound have special challenges to confront with respect to dating, sexuality, and intimacy. Careful consideration also must be given to the fact that physically disabled children are vulnerable to manipulative adults and are at high risk for sexual abuse and sexual exploitation.

Coping and Stress Tolerance

Acquired musculoskeletal disorders, such as traumatic fractures and amputations, can threaten or challenge a family's coping abilities. Is the threat perceived to be beyond their control? What resources do they have? How fragile or strong are the family dynamics to withstand the stressful conditions? While some families are able to work through the stressors in life, other families may decompensate or disintegrate from the stress that accompanies illness and chronic musculoskeletal disorders.

Values and Beliefs

If the child has a permanent musculoskeletal disability, what impact does it have on the child's life goals or desires for the future? Does the child or family value mobility and independence to such an extent that life without these characteristics has diminished meaning? Do the child and family have spiritual beliefs that help them cope with the child's illness? Do they have religious practices that they wish to revive or maintain during the illness?

Physical Examination

Assessment of the musculoskeletal system is directed toward structure and function primarily by inspection, palpation, assessment of muscle strength against resistance, and determination of range of motion.[3] Developmental norms listed in Table 61-1 must be considered when examining the musculoskeletal system in children.

The physical examination should begin with observation of normal movement. Functional mobility includes walking, sitting, running, playing, controlling the head, and displaying primitive reflexes in infants and children who are neurologically impaired. These actions may be nonthreatening for the child, and they facilitate the assessment process by promoting a trusting relationship between the child and the nurse. To continue in a therapeutic manner the examination should advance from general to specific observation, inspection, and palpation.[5]

Inspection of the musculoskeletal system includes visual scanning of the two sides of the body for symmetry, contour, and size.[8] Posture and body alignment should be viewed from the front and the back.

Active and passive range of motion is tested on all joints. Any abnormalities, such as pain, crepitation, or limited range of motion should be noted. Findings are described as normal range of motion, restricted motion, severe weakness, or paralysis. A *goniometer* (Fig. 61-2) is used to measure range of motion and aids in determining the degree of flexion and extension of specific joints.

TABLE 61-1
Developmental Considerations in the Physical Examination of Musculoskeletal Function

Area or Action	Infant	Child	Adolescent
Legs	Bowlegged	Knock-knees	Straight
		Shin pain common, especially at night ("growing pains")	
Range of motion to all joints	Hypermobility	Full range of motion and mobility	Full range of motion and mobility
Gait	Walking reflex disappears around 4 months	Feet far apart, a wide base for stability; external rotation of femurs	Feet point straight ahead; 0° angle of gait; no external rotation
Neck	Short with skin fold; full range of motion	Lengthens; full range of motion	Lengthens: full range of motion
Spine	Rounded or C-shaped	Lumbar lordosis	Straight; symmetrical hips and shoulders
Feet	Flat, broad, arch covered by fat pad	Flatfoot	High arch, flatfoot

Evaluation of Muscle Function

Muscles are inspected and palpated for tone, strength, symmetry, mass, and paralysis. Muscle tone is described as normal, rigid, weak, or spastic. During passive range-of-motion exercises the child's muscle tone may be evaluated by feeling the movement of the muscles on the relaxed limb held in the examiner's hand. A slight resistance normally is felt.

Assessment of muscle strength is important to help diagnose musculoskeletal conditions and supply information about the child's need for assistance with activities of daily living. Muscle strength is tested by asking the child to resist movement or to move against restrictions applied by the nurse. A simple procedure for testing muscle strength is to ask the child to pull a toy from the examiner's hand. While strength is expected to be greater on the dominant side, the nurse should be alert for any unilateral weakness, often indicative of hemiparesis or pain.

Evaluation of Stance and Gait

Stance and gait stability can be observed simply by watching the child run and walk the length of the hallway.[7] Depending on the age the child should wear only a diaper, underwear, or shorts. Inspection of the stance includes base of support, weight-bearing stability, and posture. The angle that the long axis of the foot makes with the direction the child is walking is noted. Observation of whether the posture is erect or stooped is included. Stride length should be equal on both sides. Deviated strides such as wide-based, propulsive, shuffling, or limping may indicate conditions such as hamstring or heel cord tightness, deformity, or pain in the lower back, hip, or leg.

Evaluation of Upper Torso and Upper Extremities

Evaluation of the upper torso begins with assessment of the head and neck. Observation of the head includes facial structures, muscle development, and temporomandibular joint function. The neck is observed for range of motion (see Fig. 61-1). Nuchal (neck) rigidity may indicate meningeal irritation. Tightness of the sternocleidomastoid muscle may indicate torticollis or "wry neck." The clavicles and scapulae are palpated for size and symmetry; limited range of motion and a painful lump may indicate a fractured clavicle, especially in the neonate as a result of birth trauma.

The hands and wrists are assessed for size, color, temperature, mobility of the joints, crepitation, and bony enlargements. The size and number of the fingers and palmar creases are included in the examination. Short, broad extremities, hyperextensive joints, and simian creases in the palms may indicate Down syndrome.

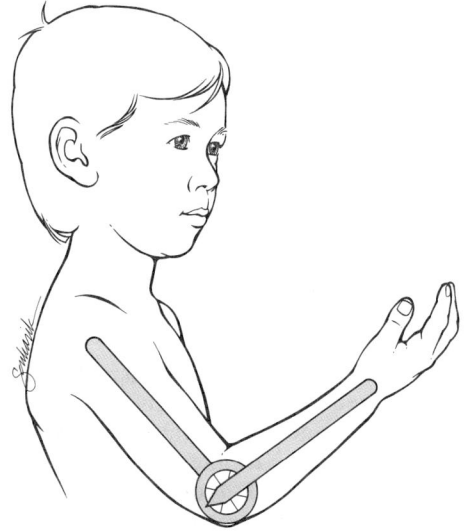

FIGURE 61-2
Goniometer used to measure the range of joint motion.

The arms normally form a smooth, continuous line of approximately 180 degrees. Muscle strength and tone of the arm are assessed by palpation of the biceps and triceps. Any muscle atrophy, weakness, tenderness, or swelling should be documented. Range of motion of the fingers, wrists, elbows, and shoulders also is included during examination of the upper extremities (see Fig. 61-1).

Evaluation of Spine

The spine is evaluated for posture, curvature, and range of motion. While the child is bending at the waist with the arms dangling, the spine is assessed from the front, back, and sides. The nurse should be able to identify the cervical, thoracic, and lumbar curves. Any signs of lordosis (anterior convexity of the spine), kyphosis (angulation of the posterior spinal curve), or scoliosis (lateral curvature of the spine) should be further evaluated (Fig. 61-3). Spinal curves that are evident while the child is standing but disappear when the child bends forward may indicate poor posture. Palpation of the paravertebral bodies should reveal equally strong muscle strength and tone.

Evaluation of Hip Function

Hip evaluation begins with assessment of gait and pelvic obliquity or angulation. Obliquity is best detected by placing the examiner's hands on the child's iliac crests and noting the level and symmetry. All neonates and children should have thorough hip evaluations to rule out congenital hip dysplasia (Fig. 61-4). Some of the signs of congenital hip dysplasia include unequal thigh folds, apparent short femur (Galeazzi's sign), and limited abduction of the thigh. A positive Trendelenburg sign is manifested by a downward tilt of the pelvis toward the unaffected side when the child stands on the affected leg and raises the normal leg. Ortolani's sign or hip click is readily detectable in a relaxed, quiet neonate.

Hip flexion contractures can be detected by the Thomas test (Fig. 61-5). This test requires the examiner to assist the child to maximally flex both hips as the child lies on his or her back. While holding one hip in position, the examiner slowly brings the other hip into maximum extension. The presence of any contractures, decreased range of motion, or abnormalities is noted.

Evaluation of Lower Extremities

Lower-extremity evaluation includes observing the child's gait; measuring limb length; and assessing muscle bulk or atrophy, patellar stability, muscle strength, and range of motion. Range of motion of the lower extremities is shown in Figure 61-1. Manual compression of the patella against the front of the femur (Fairbank's test) may reveal lateral displacement or subluxation of the patella. Many pathologic conditions affecting the knee joint are accompanied by thigh or calf atrophy.

Both legs are assessed for symmetry, length, shape, and strength. Genu varum (bowlegs) is a lateral curvature of the tibia (Fig. 61-6). Genu valgum (knock-knees) is identified when the knees touch and the medial malleoli are more than 3 inches apart (see Fig. 61-6). Tibial torsion is the abnormal rotation or bowing of the tibia. The ex-

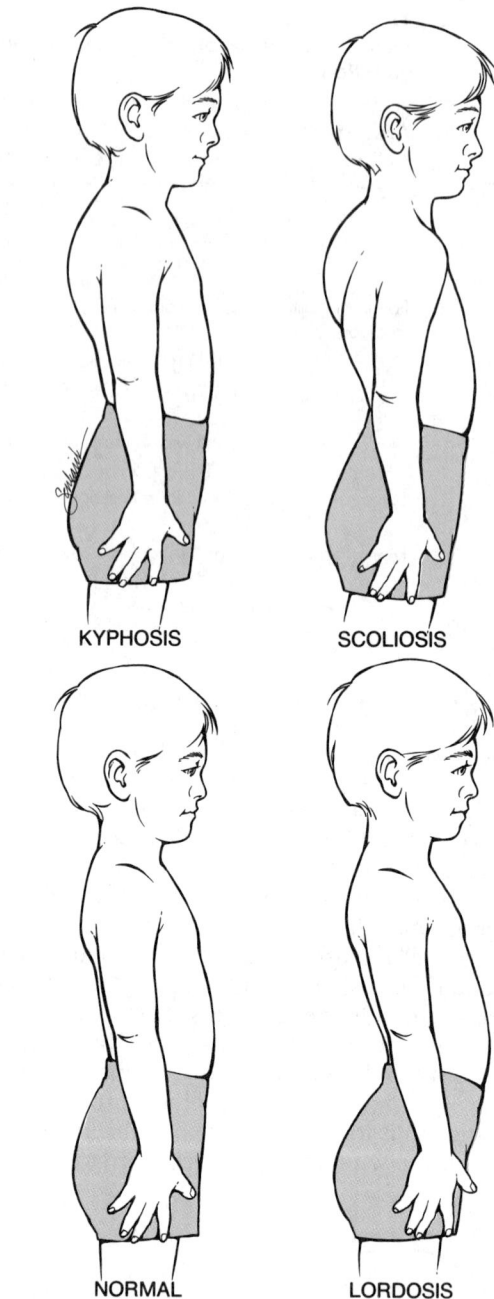

FIGURE 61-3
Profiles of children with normal and abnormal spinal curves.

aminer notes any inward rotation of the tibia as the child sits on the edge of the examination table with the legs dangling.

The best method of evaluation of the feet is to observe the child's barefoot gait for the angle of the foot to the floor and stability during standing. Evidence of high arches, flat feet, or toe walking is noted. Toe walking is common during the first several months after a child starts to walk. Continued toe walking may be a sign of mild cerebral palsy or congenitally tight heel cords (see Fig. 61-6). Talipes (clubfoot) is noted when the child's foot twists inward, the forefoot is adducted, and the foot is in plantar flexion (talipes equinovarus) or when the foot twists outward, with the forefoot adducted (talipes equinovalgus).

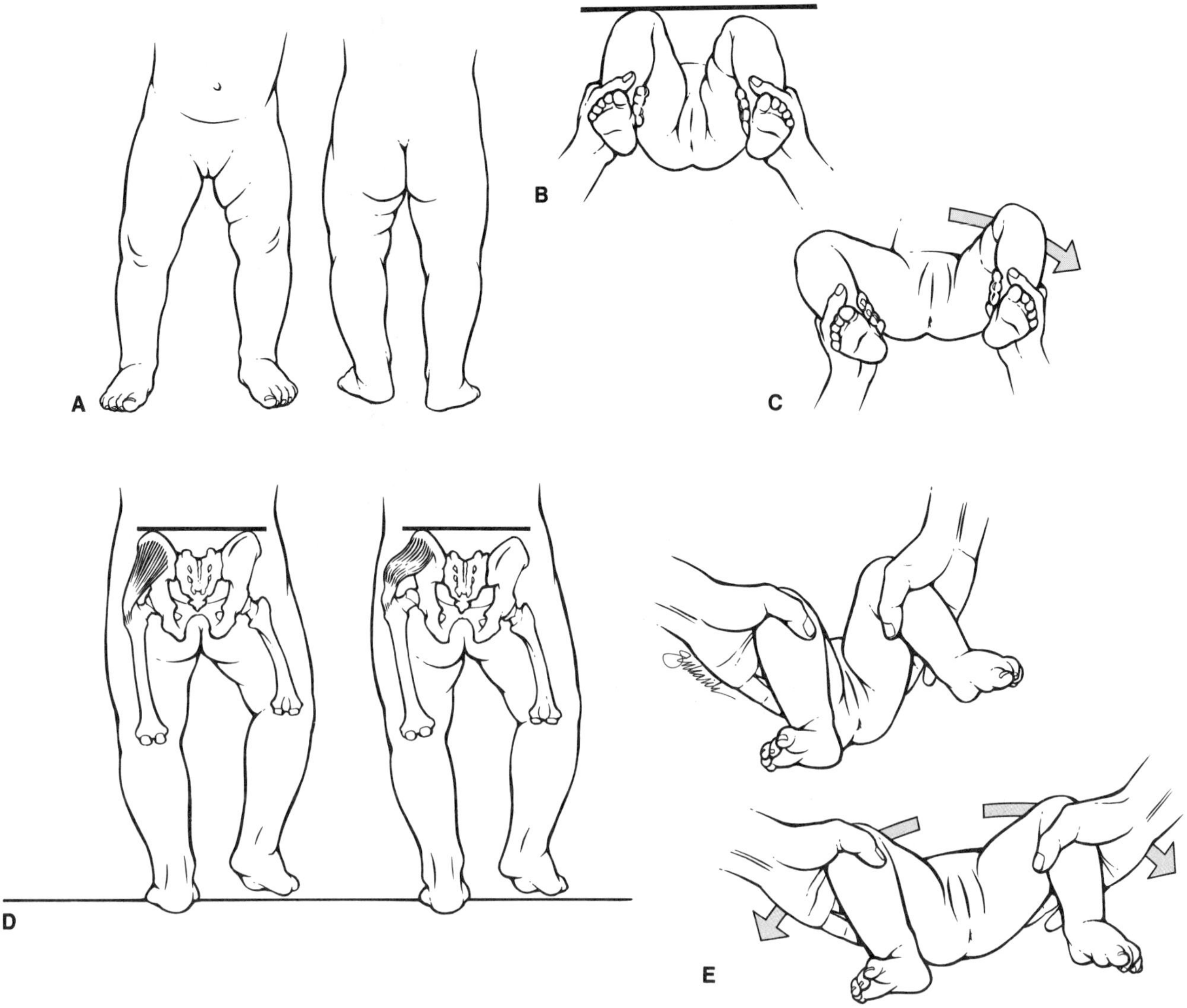

FIGURE 61-4

Common clinical findings depicting congenital hip dysplasia. (**A**) Unequal thigh folds, (**B**) apparent short femur (Galeazzi's sign), (**C**) limited abduction of affected hip, (**D**) downward tilt of pelvis on affected side (Trendelenberg's sign), and (**E**) a "click" felt when dislocated hip is abducted (Ortolani's sign).

Diagnostic Studies

Many studies are used to diagnose, validate, and evaluate musculoskeletal disorders. While many of these tests are noninvasive and painless, some are invasive, painful, and produce anxiety for the child and family.[1] Nurses must prepare children for the sensations and feelings they may experience to help allay their anxiety and facilitate the performance of the tests. Individual institutional policies dictate when consent forms are needed, usually for invasive procedures.

Laboratory Tests

Laboratory studies used to diagnose or evaluate musculoskeletal problems are limited. Blood indices, however, are commonly used in diagnostic workups. Normal

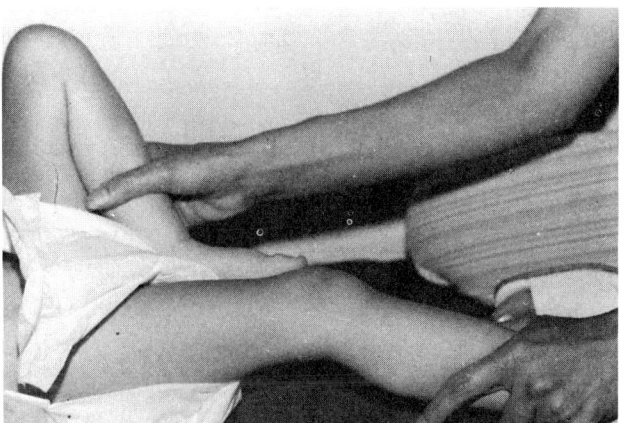

FIGURE 61-5

The Thomas test: The nurse attempts to fully extend one hip while maintaining full flexion in the other.

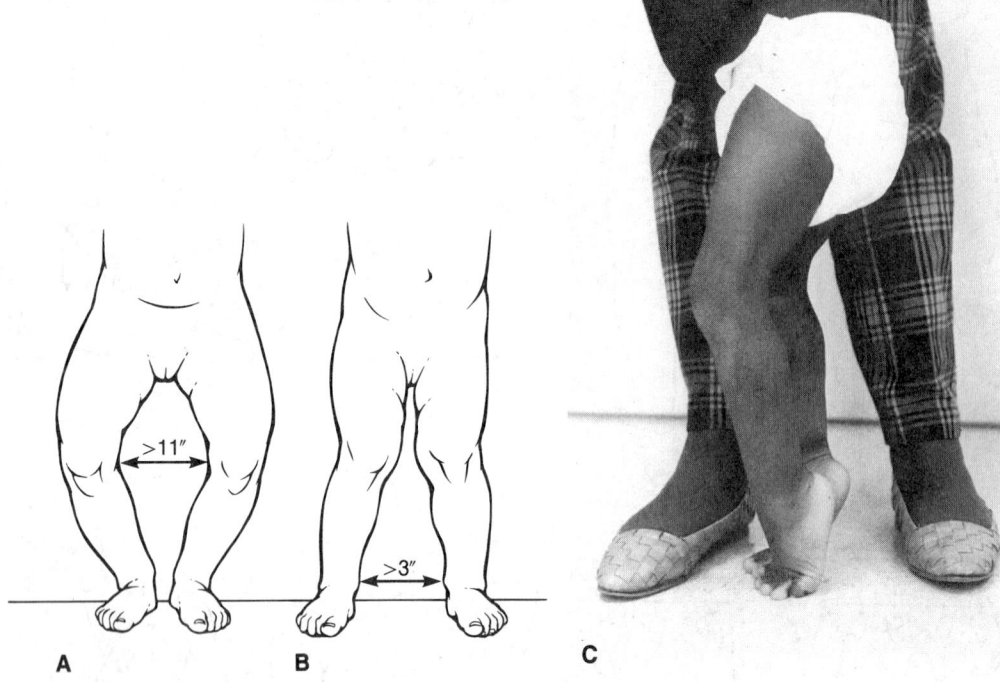

FIGURE 61-6
Variations of the lower extremities in children. (**A**) Bowleg (genu varum). (**B**) Knock-knees (genu valgum). (**C**) Toe walking caused by congenital heel cord tightening.

values for blood studies that may indicate musculoskeletal problems are presented in Table 61-2.

Procedures

Preparation of children for diagnostic procedures depends on their cognitive and developmental levels. Parents also need preparation with thorough explanations of the procedures so they will be able to comfort and assist children effectively. Older children need time to prepare themselves for the testing to help decrease their anxiety. No matter what age the child is, the nurse must be honest with the explanations and descriptions of the sensations that the child will experience.

Roentgenography (X-Ray)

Description/Definition
Obtaining images on film using roentgen rays.

Purpose
Initial diagnosis can be made by providing identification and observation of numerous pathologic conditions.

Indications
- Suspected bone fractures.
- Suspected child abuse.
- Suspected pathologic changes.

Contraindications
Pregnancy—unknown effects on fetus.

Preparation
Nurses should reinforce instructions and explanations from the primary care provider to the child and family. Infants and young children may require heavy sedation or restraints to ensure immobility. Older children may be able to practice being absolutely still for short periods of time to familiarize themselves with the feeling of immobility.

Nursing Implications
Because the child is left alone in the x-ray room, verbal contact by the nurse from the control room helps to soothe and comfort the child. The child's safety needs to be ensured during the tests through the use of safety belts or side rails. Breast shields are used on adolescent females, and gonad shields are used on children of all ages.

Complications
Overexposure to radiation from multiple x-rays could adversely affect the reproductive organs.

Magnetic Resonance Imaging

Definition/Description
Magnetic resonance imaging (MRI) uses a magnetic field and radio waves to image body tissue; it depicts hydrogen density of body tissues.[9]

Purpose
MRI provides excellent anatomic delineation of joint structures; it is able to distinguish among muscles, tendons, and ligaments.

Indications
- Defects in bone, spinal, or joint structure.
- Suspected pathologic changes in bones and muscles.

Contraindications
- Pregnancy—unknown effects on fetus.
- Sickle cell anemia—use of contrast dye interferes with oxygen-carrying capacity of red blood cells.

TABLE 61-2
Blood Indices of Musculoskeletal Function

Test	Appropriate Ranges	Deviations	Clinical Implications
Erythrocyte sedimentation rate	Infant: 0 to 2 mm/h	Increased	Polymyositis
			Osteomyelitis
	Child: 0 to 10 mm/h		Juvenile rheumatoid arthritis
	Adolescent: Males: 0 to 15 mm/h	Decreased	Degenerative joint disease
	Females: 0 to 20 mm/h		
Creatine phosphokinase	Infant: 68 to 580 U/L	Increased	Polymyositis
			Muscular dystrophy
	Child: 15 to 50 U/L		Response to electro-myelography or vigorous exercise
	Adolescent: Males: 25 to 90 U/L		Birth trauma in neonates
	Females: 10 to 70 U/L		
Aldolase	Infant: 12 to 24 U/dl	Increased	Polymyositis
			Muscular dystrophy
	Child: 6 to 16 U/dl	Decreased	End-stage muscular dystrophy
	Adolescent: 3 to 8 U/dl		
Rheumatoid factor	Infant, child, and adolescent: Negative (<1:20)	Increased	Polymyositis
			Juvenile rheumatoid arthritis
White blood cells	Infant: 5.0 to 19.5 $\times$ 1000 mm^3	Increased (leukocytosis)	Osteomyelitis (acute phase)
	Child: 4 to 7 y: 5.5 to 15.5 $\times$ 1000 mm^3		Juvenile rheumatoid arthritis
	8 to 13 y: 4.5 to 13.5 $\times$ 1000 mm^3		
	Adolescent: 4.5 to 11.0 $\times$ 1000 mm^3		
Blood culture	Infant, child, and adolescent: Negative; no pathogens	Positive	Osteomyelitis
Alkaline phosphatase	Infant: 40 to 300 U/L	Increased	Rickets
	Child: 60 to 270 U/L		Osteomalacia
	Adolescent: 20 to 90 U/L		Osteogenic sarcoma
			Bone tumors
Calcium	Infant: 10 to 12 mg/dl	Increased (hypercalcemia)	Immobilization
	Child: 8 to 11.5 mg/dl		Multiple fractures
	Adolescent: 8.5 to 11 mg/dl		Metastatic cancer in bones
		Decreased (hypocalcemia)	Rickets
			Osteomalacia
Phosphorus	Infant: 4.5 to 6.7 mg/dl	Decreased (hypophosphatemia)	Rickets
	Child: 4.5 to 6.5 mg/dl		Osteomalacia
	Adolescent: 2.5 to 4.5 mg/dl		
Iron	Infant: 40 to 100 μg/dl	Decreased	Juvenile rheumatoid arthritis
	Child: 50 to 200 μg/dl		
	Adolescent: Male: 60 to 170 μg/dl		
	Female: 50 to 130 μg/dl		

- Claustrophobia—the child lies in the middle of the MRI machine, which resembles a long, narrow tube; it is noisy, and the child is unable to see anyone during imaging procedure.
- Presence of objects, such as cardiac pacemakers, metal vascular clips, metal prostheses, and replacement heart valves—these objects contain ferrous material and may interfere with magnetic field.
- Implanted insulin pump—interferes with mechanism of pump.

Preparation

The child and family are given complete explanations about the procedure and instructions on the necessity to remain immobile. Some children may require sedation. General anesthesia is contraindicated because of the inaccessibility of the child once inside the machine. Removal of all external metal objects is crucial because they can interfere with the magnetic field. The child is warned that the MRI machine is noisy and makes loud knocking, hammering sounds.

Nursing Implications

Some children may experience claustrophobia; the nurse remains with the child, talking and encouraging throughout the procedure. Some children may find it helpful to think of the MRI machine as a spaceship and helmet.

Complications

Fever—radio waves may slightly increase body temperature.

Computerized Axial Tomography Scan

Definition/Description

A combination of x-rays and computer technology is used to show cross-sectional images of various layers or slices of body tissue and tissue density.

Purpose

A computerized axial tomography (CAT) scan determines the size and position of bony tumors or lesions. A CAT scan is helpful in diagnosing a disease early in the disease process.

Indications

- Suspected bone tumors.
- Soft tissue masses.

Contraindications

- Pregnancy.
- Allergy to iodine used in contrast dye.

Preparation

Explanations should be given, including the possibility that the physician may decide to use intravenous contrast dye to enhance the pictures. A picture of a CAT scanner may be helpful to familiarize the child with the size and shape of the machine. Infants and young children may need to be sedated to ensure immobility throughout the procedure. Nurses should reiterate that the procedure will not hurt.

Nursing Implications

The child will be strapped to the scanner table during the procedure to ensure immobility and safety. A humming noise emanates from the scanner and may frighten the child as the surface on which the child is lying automatically moves slowly through a large donut-shaped machine. Some institutions may allow the parent in the room with the child. If this is not allowed, the nurse will be in the control room and can talk to the child during the procedure. Emergency drugs should be available to counteract possible allergic reactions to the contrast material.

Complications

- Overexposure to radiation with multiple procedures.
- Allergic reaction to contrast dye.

Tomography

Definition/Description

This special technique used with x-rays shows detailed images of structures in a selected plane of tissue by blurring images or structures in all surrounding planes.

Purpose

Tomography is used in addition to x-ray for further detail of the tissue or bone being studied.

Indications

- Bone fracture.
- Pathology of bones.

Contraindications

Pregnancy.

Preparation

See x-ray.

Nursing Implications

See x-ray.

Complications

See x-ray.

Electromyelography

Definition/Description

Electromyelography (EMG) measures electrical activity of muscles by means of needle electrodes inserted into the muscles to be tested. Electrical activity is measured at rest and during movement. EMG elicits information on the quality of the nerve impulses to the muscles as well as the response of those muscles to the nerve impulses.

Purpose

EMG differentiates between muscle and nerve disorders.

Indications

- Low back pain.
- Myasthenia gravis.

Contraindications

None.

Preparation

Thorough explanation to the child and parents is essential. Children will experience some discomfort; the sensation may be compared to mosquito bites or described as tingling. Infants and young children may need sedation.

Nursing Implications

Before the test the physician should be asked about withholding medications, such as muscle relaxants, anticholinergics, and cholinergics that could interfere with the test results. Nursing responsibilities during the procedure are mainly supportive. The importance of immobility is stressed. The child's pain should be acknowledged, and praise should be given for cooperation.

Complications

None.

Muscle and Bone Biopsy

Definition/Description

Biopsy is the removal of a sample of muscle tissue, bone, or skin. The sample is stained with a histologic agent for laboratory analysis.

Purpose

Biopsy helps to diagnose lower motor neuron disease, degeneration, inflammatory reactions, bone disease, bone lesion, and connective tissue disorders.

Indications

- Suspected neoplasms.
- Lower motor neuron disease.
- Muscle degeneration.
- Differentiation of benign from malignant bone lesions.

Contraindications

Thrombocytopenia.

Preparation

The nurse explains the procedure to the child and includes the fact that there will be some discomfort at the biopsy site. A shave or skin scrub may be required prior to the procedure.

Nursing Implications

After the procedure, the nurse should be alert for signs and symptoms of hemorrhage. Dressings to the biopsy site should be changed as needed. Activity is limited during the first 24 hours depending on the biopsy site, but after 24 hours activity is allowed as tolerated to help prevent stiffness at the biopsy site. The child's need for analgesics should be assessed and treated appropriately.

Complications

Infection of the biopsy site.

Myelography

Definition/Description

A study conducted by injecting radiopaque dye into the subarachnoid space of the lumbar spine.

Purpose

Myelography detects deformities or abnormalities of the spinal cord using fluoroscopy.

Indications

- Trauma.
- Spinal mass.
- Lesions.
- Herniated intervertebral discs.
- Metastatic tumors.
- Congenital malformations.
- Low back pain.

Contraindications

Allergy to iodine used in contrast dyes.

Preparation

Only clear liquids are permitted after midnight, depending on institutional policies. The nurse explains the procedure and describes the equipment for the child. Practice of the side-lying, knee-chest position helps the child to become familiar with it. A cleansing enema may be ordered to remove feces and gas for improving visualization. Adequate time should be allowed for the child to ask questions and to express fears and concerns.

Nursing Implications

The child is restrained with the use of several straps in a side-lying, knee-chest position. Comforting is needed during the administration of the local anesthetic at the puncture site. The child will be tilted in various directions to help distribute the dye and visualize the spinal cord. After the films are obtained, another lumbar puncture will be performed to remove the contrast dye. The child should be praised for cooperation and self-control during the procedure. A bandage is applied to the puncture site. The head of the bed is elevated 30 to 45 degrees or perfectly flat depending on the type of contrast dye used in the study. Fluids are encouraged to replace cerebrospinal fluid loss. Vital signs are monitored every 30 minutes for the first 2 hours and then every hour for the next 4 hours until stable. Neurovascular checks are needed to determine the presence of dorsiplantar flexion in the lower extremities. The child should void within 8 hours postmyelogram; therefore, intake and output should be monitored.

Complications

Adverse reaction to contrast material, which may cause meningeal irritation.

Arthrography

Definition/Description

Arthrography requires injection of a radiopaque substance or air into a joint, usually the knee or shoulder.

Purpose

The purpose of arthrography is to detect abnormalities of the cartilage or ligaments and to outline soft-tissue structures and joint contours.

Indications

- Meniscal and ligamental tears.
- Synovial abnormalities.
- Internal derangement of joints.

Contraindications

Allergy to iodine used in contrast dye.

Preparation

Children are restricted from fluids (NPO) after midnight, but infants are kept NPO only 4 hours prior to the procedure. Infants and young children need sedation. An explanation should be given that there will be some pain at the injection site. The knee or shoulder site is prepared with a surgical scrub using aseptic technique.

Nursing Implications

Comfort and emotional support should be given to the child. The physician may need assistance in rotating the joint to distribute the contrast material evenly. After the procedure an ice bag is applied to the affected joint to decrease swelling and bleeding. The child is instructed to rest the affected joint for 12 hours after the procedure and then to resume activity as tolerated. Analgesics are offered as needed.

Complications

Infection at the injection site or in the joint.

Arthroscopy

Definition/Description

This endoscopic procedure allows direct visualization of a joint, especially the knee, shoulder, and ankle.

Purpose

Direct visualization of the specific joint for diagnostic data.

Indications

- Meniscal, patellar, and synovial disease.
- Ligament damage.
- Chondromalacia.

Contraindications

Infection in the affected joint.

Preparation

The affected joint is prepared with an aseptic scrub. The child is kept NPO after midnight for general or spinal anesthesia. Ventilation of feelings and anxiety should be permitted, and explanations about the procedure should be provided.

Nursing Implications

The surgical site is assessed for signs and symptoms of bleeding, swelling, or redness. The pressure dressing applied after the procedure is assessed for tightness; circulation to the extremity should be ensured. Analgesics are provided as needed. Orders regarding immobilization of the joint depend on the extent of the procedure, but the child usually is instructed to avoid extensive use of the joint for 2 to 3 days.

Complications

Infection; effusion.

Arthrocentesis

Definition/Description

Insertion of a needle into a joint for aspiration of synovial fluid. The procedure may be performed at the bedside or in the treatment room.

Purpose

Examination of synovial fluid to determine the causative microorganism for the probable infection.

Indications

- Knee injury.
- Aseptic inflammatory process.

Contraindications

Use of anticoagulant medication or other drugs containing aspirin.

Preparation

The procedure is explained to the child and family. The joint is scrubbed with an antiseptic soap prior to the procedure.

Nursing Implications

Strict asepsis during the procedure needs to be assured. All collection tubes are accurately labeled and sent to the laboratory. A pressure dressing and ice pack are applied after the procedure, and the joint is assessed frequently for signs and symptoms of hemorrhage, bruising, or inflammation. The child is encouraged to rest the joint for 12 to 24 hours postprocedure. Discomfort after the procedure is assessed frequently and analgesics are given as ordered.

Complications

Infection of the involved joint.

Bone Scan

Definition/Description

Parenteral injection of bone-seeking radioactive isotopes and use of x-ray to evaluate bones.

Purpose

Increased concentration of isotope uptake in certain areas indicates skeletal disease sites. Bone scans detect abnormal pathology much earlier than x-rays.

Indications

- Detect early bone disease.
- Inflammatory skeletal disease (osteomyelitis).
- Suspected metastatic bone disease.
- Suspected osteoporosis.
- Suspected Paget's disease.
- Healing activity of fractured bones.
- Unexplained bone pain.

Contraindications

None.

Preparation

The nurse should explain to the child and family the purpose of the scan and the technique used. There is a waiting period between injection of the radionuclides and the actual scanning, usually about 2 to 3 hours. The injection may be given at the bedside or in the treatment room. Fluid intake is then encouraged to facilitate circulatory distribution of the radioisotope. Although activity is permitted prior to the scan, the child may need to be immobilized for up to 1 hour during the scan. Sedation may be required for infants and young children. The child should be reminded to void before the scan to diminish bladder activity and to increase visibility in the pelvic bones.

Nursing Implications

Support and comfort during venipuncture for injection of the radioactive isotopes is an important nursing intervention. The child and family may be reassured that the bone scan itself is painless. They also should be informed that the radioactive substance is not harmful to anyone, and it is excreted from the body in 6 to 24 hours. The child must be transported to radiology at the specified time after injection of radioactive isotopes.

Complications

- Two radionuclides administered in 1 day may interfere with each other and therefore should be avoided.
- Dehydration prior to imaging could affect the results.

Selected Nursing Diagnoses

After obtaining the history, performing the physical examination, reviewing results from the diagnostic tests, and tapping additional resources for information, the nurse carefully analyzes data obtained. Nursing diagnoses appropriate for the child with musculoskeletal dysfunction become apparent and are used to develop a plan of care.[2] Selected nursing diagnoses that may be appropriate for the child with musculoskeletal dysfunction are presented by function in Table 61-3.

Summary

Musculoskeletal disorders comprise a significant proportion of children's health problems. Accurate assessment leads to early detection of musculoskeletal dysfunction and may help lessen severity and disabling effects. Assessment of musculoskeletal function is directed toward structure and function primarily by inspection, palpation, assessment of muscle strength against resistance, and observation range of motion. The physical examination begins with observation of normal movement. The functional mobility evaluation includes walking, sitting, running, playing, controlling the head, and displaying primitive reflexes in neonates and infants. Posture and body alignment should be viewed from the front and back.

TABLE 61-3
Selected Nursing Diagnoses Associated With Altered Musculoskeletal Function

Data Analysis and Conclusion	Nursing Diagnosis
Self-Perception and Self-Control	
Verbalization of fear of strangers or loss of independence; muscle tightness; fatigue; irritability; crying, screaming; nightmares; tachycardia, tachypnea	Fear related to actual or anticipated loss of a body part, hospitalization, invasive procedure, surgery, disease, or disability
Sensory—Perceptual	
Ability to localize source of pain	Pain related to fractures, casts, traction, braces, surgery, ambulation, position
Crying, moaning	
Limited range of motion to affected part	
Muscle spasms; tenderness	
Irritability; withdrawal	
Admission of pain when oral analgesic offered; denial of pain when parenteral analgesic offered	
Activity Exercise	
Inability to move in bed, ambulate, or transfer	Impaired Physical Mobility related to limited use of lower or upper extremities, amputation, external corrective devices
Limited range of motion	
Limited muscle strength	
Altered coordination	
Unstable gait	
Non–weight-bearing to lower limbs	
Weak, absent, spastic motor function	
Elimination	
Hard, formed stools	Constipation related to lack of privacy, immobility, analgesics
Painful defecation	
Defecation less than three times per week	
Decreased bowel sounds	
Moderate abdominal distention	
Minimal flatulence	
Activity, Exercise	
Inability to dress, feed, bathe, or use toilet independently	Self-care Deficit related to pain, nonfunctioning or missing limb, immobility, external corrective device
Health Perception—Health Management	
Parent states, "I don't know how to take care of my child with all this equipment"	Altered Health Maintenance related to lack of knowledge of external corrective devices
Parent refuses to participate in child's care	
Parent states, "All this equipment scares me"	
Child exhibits anxious behavior, such as increased verbalization, inappropriate laughing, restlessness, inability to concentrate or retain information	
Role Relationship	
Parent expresses concern about change in parental role	Parental Role Conflict related to illness, hospitalization
Parent states, "The doctors and nurses are making all of the decisions for my child; I don't know what I'm supposed to do"	
Parent states, "I feel so guilty and angry"	
Parent unable to stay with sick child because of siblings at home	
Parent states, "How will I ever be able to care for my child at home when he can't walk?"	
Nutrition, Metabolic	
Skin under cast becomes wet	Impaired Skin Integrity related to immobility, maceration, external corrective devices
Inability to turn in bed	
Imposed bedrest	

(Continued)

TABLE 61-3
(Continued)

Data Analysis and Conclusion	Nursing Diagnosis
Disruption of skin layers	
Skin erythematous, chaffed, excoriated, pruritic	
Activity—Exercise	
Muscle atrophy	High Risk for Disuse Syndrome related to pain, fracture, amputation, immoblity, external corrective devices
Contracture	
Decreased muscle tone, muscle strength	
Joint degeneration	
Paralysis	
Coping, Stress Tolerance	
Child states, "I'm bored"	Diversional Activity Deficit related to monotony of confinement
Restless, fidgeting in bed	
Frequent use of call bell	
Long-term hospitalization	
Loss of ability to perform favorite activities	
Hostility	
Lack of appropriate toys	

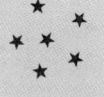

Ideas for Nursing Research

The unique nature of many pediatric musculoskeletal disorders makes them especially amenable to nursing research. Issues of family involvement, pain control, and family adjustment to the chronicity of some of these disorders are areas of research that need to be explored. The following areas are possible topics for nursing research:

- Cooperation of children during diagnostic studies with or without parents present.
- Possible standardization of defining charcteristics of the nursing diagnosis, "Impaired Physical Mobility" as it pertains to musculoskeletal function.
- Correlation between a child's perceived pain while immobilized and peer–sibling visitation.
- Parents' perceptions of altered health maintenance when caring for a child in a body cast.
- Correlation between adolescents' increased knowledge of sports injuries and long-term negative effects and decrease in incidence of injuries.

Right and left sides of the body should be examined for symmetry, contour, and size. Any abnormalities, such as pain, crepitation, or limited range of motion, should be noted. Findings are described as normal range of motion, restricted motion, severe weakness, or paralysis.

References

1. Smeltzer, S. C., & Bare, B. G. (1992). *Brunner and Suddarth's textbook of medical surgical nursing* (7th ed.). Philadelphia: J.B. Lippincott.
2. Carpenito, L. (1992). *Nursing diagnosis. Application to clinical practice* (4th ed.). Philadelphia: J.B. Lippincott.
3. Farrell, J. (1986). *Illustrated guide to orthopedic nursing* (3rd ed.). Philadelphia: J.B. Lippincott.
4. Gordon, M. (1987). *Nursing diagnosis, process and application* (2nd ed.). New York: McGraw-Hill.
5. Linley, J. (1987). Screening children for common orthopedic problems. *American Journal of Nursing, 87,* 1312–1316.
6. Mourad, L. (1988). *Nursing care of adults with orthopedic problems* (2nd ed.). New York: John Wiley and Sons.
7. Renshaw, T. (1986). *Pediatric orthopedics.* Philadelphia: W.B. Saunders.
8. Schoen, P. (1986). *The nursing process in orthopaedics.* Norwalk, CT: Appleton-Century-Crofts.
9. Zubay, R. (1988). *Understanding magnetic resonance imaging from a nursing perspective. Orthopaedic Nursing, 6,* 17–23.

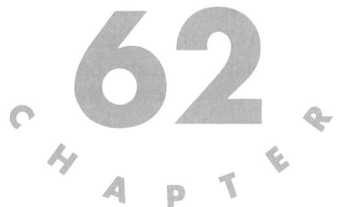

62

C H A P T E R

Nursing Planning, Intervention, and Evaluation for Altered Musculoskeletal Function

BEHAVIORAL OBJECTIVES

Identify critical assessment variables and nursing diagnoses for a child with altered musculoskeletal function.

Discuss nursing interventions to maintain skin integrity, prevent and control infection, avoid neurovascular compromise, and alleviate pain.

Examine the effects of various musculoskeletal disorders on the growth and development of a child.

Review the unique characteristics of fractures and healing in children.

Explain the principles of caring for a child in an immobilizing device.

Analyze the psychosocial impact of impaired mobility on the child and family.

Examine the nurse's role in the multidisciplinary management of a child with altered musculoskeletal function.

A normal functioning musculoskeletal system is critical to the growth and development of children. When the system is impaired, children must learn new ways to explore their environment. Parents are often so overwhelmed with the diagnosis and potential physical limitations of their child that they are unable to identify ways to normalize the child's environment. Therefore, the nurse is challenged to work closely with the child and family to mobilize their strengths and maximize the child's physical potential.

Musculoskeletal disorders may be present at birth or may be acquired during

1679

some stage of the child's development. The birth of a less-than-perfect child or the development of a musculoskeletal disorder during childhood can be traumatic. Often the physical development and abilities of a healthy child are a source of pride to the child and family.

Children may develop musculoskeletal disorders as a result of injury, infection, or inflammation. Sometimes these problems may affect the child's growth plate, resulting in altered skeletal growth and deformity. These children often require frequent surgeries, hospitalizations, and extensive follow-up care. The nurse has the opportunity to develop long-term relationships with the child and family and positively influence the outcomes of care.

Knowledge of growth and development and keen observational abilities are essential when caring for children with musculoskeletal disorders. Any delay in the child's physical development should alert the nurse to the possibility of a musculoskeletal disorder. Furthermore, the nurse is in an excellent position to prevent musculoskeletal injuries by providing anticipatory guidance about age-appropriate safety issues.

Musculoskeletal disorders can occur for a variety of reasons. This chapter begins with disorders that appear at birth and continues with disorders that affect the growth plate. Other acquired disorders, including those associated with infection and inflammation, are addressed. Finally, injuries common to the musculoskeletal system are reviewed, followed by a section on special interventions for treatment of musculoskeletal disorders. The final section includes information about care of children in casts, traction, and special beds.

The accompanying display lists resources for the nurse to give families of children with altered musculoskeletal function.

Congenital Disorders

Although the etiology differs for each congenital musculoskeletal disorder, the common thread for health care providers is the parents' reaction, adaptation, and bonding with a less-than-perfect baby. The nurse is ideally positioned to initiate early intervention and decrease the disabling potential of these disorders.

Brachial Plexus Palsy

Definition and Incidence.   Brachial plexus palsy results when the natural position and relationship of the neck, shoulder, and arm is interrupted. Sometimes referred to as obstetric paralysis, brachial plexus palsy is caused when excessive traction has been applied to the brachial plexus during the birth process. Reported incidence ranges from 0.4 to 2.5 per 1000 live births.[19]

Etiology and Pathophysiology.   Obstetric risk factors are usually present when a brachial plexus injury has occurred in the newborn. These factors include high birthweight, prolonged maternal labor, shoulder dystocia, breech presentation, and forceps delivery.[19] Injuries to the brachial plexus can range from mild stretching to complete disruption of the continuity of the nerve trunk, cords, or nerve root.[41] A classification of the three types of brachial plexus palsy is given in Table 62-1. Damage to the brachial plexus includes rupture or avulsion of the nerve roots ranging from C5 to T1.[37]

Clinical Manifestations.   Brachial plexus palsy is usually obvious at birth. The clinical manifestations include loss of abduction and external rotation of the

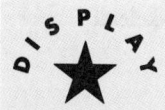

Resources for Families of Children With Altered Musculoskeletal Function

Muscular Dystrophy Association of America, Inc.
810 7th Avenue
New York, NY 10019

March of Dimes Birth Defects Foundation
1275 Mamaroneck Avenue
White Plains, NY 10605

National Scoliosis Foundation, Inc.
Post Office Box 547
Belmont, MA 02178

Scoliosis Research Society
2225 Prospect
Suite 127
Park Ridge, IL 60068

Clubfoot
Medic Publishing Co.
P.O. Box 89
Redmond, WA 98073-0089

Osteogenesis Imperfecta Foundation, Inc.
P.O. Box 14807
Tampa, FL 34629-4807

Arthritis Foundation (AF)
1314 Spring Street, NW
Atlanta, GA 30309

American Juvenile Arthritis Organization (AJAO)
(Same address as AF)

National Arthritis and Musculoskeletal and Skin Disease Information Clearinghouse
Box AMS
Bethesda, MD 20892

TABLE 62-1
Classification of Brachial Plexus Palsy

Type	Cause	Manifestations
Erb's palsy (Erb-Duchenne paralysis)	Injury to the upper trunk at Erb's point or the junction of C5 and C6	Paralysis of the deltoid, elbow flexors, and brachioradialis
Erb-Duchenne-Klumpke palsy	Injury to the entire brachial plexus from C5 to T1	Complete paralysis of affected limb
Klumpke's palsy	Injury from the C8 to T1 nerve roots	Shoulder girdle and elbow flexors functional; intrinsic muscles to the hand and wrist affected; lower arm nonfunctional

shoulder, loss of flexion at the elbow, loss of supination of the forearm, and compromised hand function.[2] Three types of brachial plexus injuries have been identified according to the degree of paralysis and the level of the lesion (see Table 62-1).

Diagnostic Studies. Many studies can assist the health care provider in diagnosing brachial plexus palsy. A complete roentgenographic study of the cervical spine, shoulder girdle, and clavicle should be performed. Cervical myelography with contrast medium helps to depict root avulsion injuries. Computed tomography (CT) helps to define better the degree and extent of brachial plexus injury. A combination of myelography and CT scan helps to reduce the margin for error and the misdiagnosis of the disorder.

Electromyelography (EMG) studies reveal the degree of muscle and nerve involvement in the affected limb. Magnetic resonance imaging (MRI) provides clear images of nerve grafts and determines nerve viability[43] (see Chap. 61).

★ ASSESSMENT

Newborns who are at risk for brachial plexus injuries should be carefully examined in the delivery room and the newborn nursery. It is necessary to determine whether the injury is related to brachial plexus involvement or a fractured clavicle, humerus, or cervical spine. Documenting the degree and extent of palsy helps to determine the type of injury that has occurred.

Assessment includes careful inspection of the head, neck, and cervical spine. The clavicles and shoulder are palpated to determine skeletal integrity. The nurse performs passive range of motion to all joints of the affected limb and observes for any spontaneous movements. If there is damage to the fifth and sixth cervical nerve, the infant appears hypotonic with flaccid arm muscles. Assessment of newborn reflexes reveals abnormal moro and tonic neck responses. Palpation of the radial pulse on the affected side determines if there is any vascular involvement. Dusky, cool skin and edema may indicate arterial and venous disruption.

★ NURSING DIAGNOSES AND PLANNING

Based on assessment data discussed previously and in the preceding chapter, the following nursing diagnoses may apply to the family and child with brachial plexus palsy:

- Impaired Physical Mobility related to paralysis.
- High Risk for Altered Parenting related to parental concerns about increased injury to the child.
- High Risk for Disuse Syndrome related to paralysis.

The nurse and parents together plan effective care based on the established nursing diagnoses. Several examples of expected outcomes follow:

- The family demonstrate bonding with their newborn by touching, talking to, and maintaining eye contact with their infant.
- The family demonstrates how to perform passive range of motion exercises.

The nurse plans for the daily care of the child based on physician's orders and nursing diagnoses. Some general nursing care goals may include the following:

- Atrophy and contracture of the muscles of the affected arm are prevented.
- Range of motion of the shoulder, elbow, wrist, and finger joints is maintained.

★ INTERVENTIONS: COLLABORATIVE AND INDEPENDENT

Even with advances in obstetric techniques and prenatal monitoring, brachial plexus injuries still occur. Careful documentation of pelvimetry, fetal monitoring during labor, and excellent communication between the nurse and obstetrician can help to reduce the incidence of brachial plexus palsy.

Early recognition and treatment of brachial plexus palsy facilitates full recovery. Consulting with an orthopedic surgeon helps the nurse and family to establish a plan of care that ensures maximum use of the dysfunctional arm. Informing parents of the prognosis for recovery helps them to set realistic goals for their child.

Daily passive range of motion exercises may be helpful in maintaining joint mobility and muscle integrity. Teaching the caregiver to perform these exercises at home is an important nursing intervention. Sometimes orthoses may be needed to maintain joint position and motion. The nurse needs to teach the caregiver how to apply these devices and to prevent skin irritation.

Surgical intervention, including nerve grafts and neurolysis, may be indicated in some cases. Nursing interventions include preoperative and postoperative teaching, pain management, and teaching the caregivers about home care.

★ EVALUATION

The recovery time is usually within the first 12 months with additional improvements noted in the second 12 months. The degree of injury and site of lesion determine the functional ability of the affected extremity. Some palsies may be mild and require minimal intervention be-

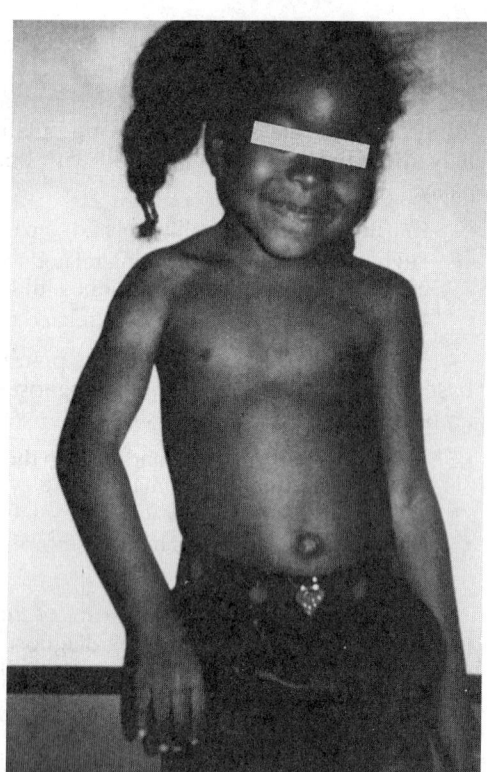
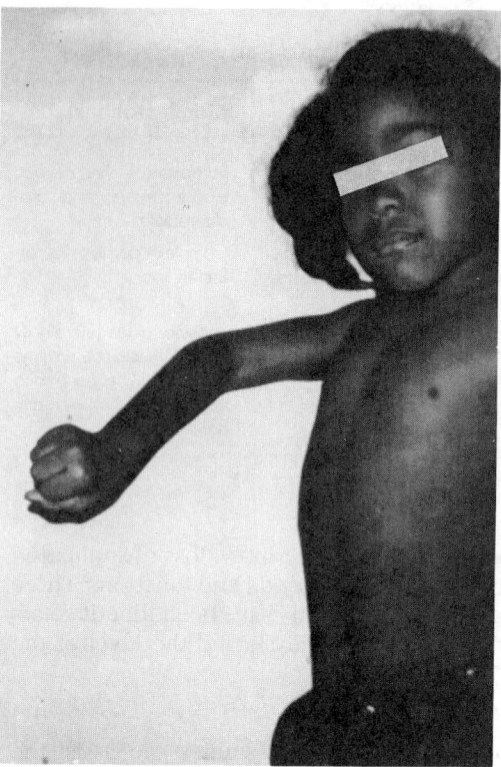

FIGURE 62-1
Child with Erb's palsy shows resting and active motion. Note residual loss of proximal muscle mass and abduction-external rotation. (Morrissy, R. T. [1990]. Lovell and Winter's pediatric orthopaedics [3rd ed.]. [Vol. II]. Philadelphia: J. B. Lippincott.)

yond exercises. If avulsion or complete disruption of the nerve roots has occurred, the prognosis for return of normal function is poor (Fig. 62-1).

Congenital Muscular Torticollis

Congenital muscular torticollis, referred to as *wry neck*, is a muscular condition resulting from abnormal contraction or injury of the sternocleidomastoid muscle. The condition may be the result of intrauterine positioning or local trauma to the soft tissues during delivery. Often the problem is associated with breech or difficult forceps deliveries. Some theories suggest that the condition may be caused by the occlusion of venous outflow from the sternocleidomastoid muscle resulting in edema, degeneration of muscle fibers, and subsequent fibrosis of the muscle. When fibrosis occurs the normal muscular stretching associated with growth is impeded.

An astute neonatal nurse will discover the condition during an initial neonatal assessment. For the first 4 to 6 weeks following birth, a firm, movable, and nontender mass is palpable in the midsternocleidomastoid muscle. Later the mass is replaced by fibrous tissue that lacks the normal stretching properties of muscle. The infant may display a contracture and abnormal positioning of the neck. The head tends to tilt toward the affected side with the chin rotating toward the opposite shoulder. Head rotation and tilting usually are limited.

Head and facial asymmetry may develop if the con-

dition is not diagnosed in early infancy. Infants with torticollis tend to position their head on the affected side. The infant may develop a flat face appearance on the affected side due to molding. In addition, the position of the eyes and ears may be distorted. Therefore, the importance of early diagnosis and treatment cannot be overemphasized.

Treatment usually consists of gentle stretching exercises. The nurse often is responsible for teaching parents. Parents are taught to turn the infant's face toward the affected muscle and tilt the head in the opposite direction with the neck extended. The exercises are repeated 10 times twice a day. The exercises usually are easier to perform if one person is available to hold the infant's torso while another person manipulates the head. The nurse should assess the parents' understanding of these exercises and reinforce the importance of performing the procedure as instructed. The nurse needs to plan creative ways to ensure that the infant will turn its head actively. For example, toys should be arranged so that the infant is encouraged to turn toward the affected side. Positioning the infant to ensure movement of the neck in the appropriate direction during feedings and play should be part of the instruction.

If torticollis is not recognized during early infancy, the treatment plan may be more extensive. Some children require surgical release of the sternocleidomastoid muscle. In addition head traction or special bracing may be needed. Early diagnosis and treatment decreases the possibility of facial and skull deformities that may result from a fixed torticollic posture. Once the deforming pull of the sternocleidomastoid muscle is released, the asymmetry of the skull and face should improve with growth.

Syndactyly

Syndactyly or "webbed fingers" is one of the most common hand anomalies seen in children. The defect is found most frequently between the ring and middle finger and the ring and little finger. Severity of the anomaly can range from fingers being joined by a skin bridge with each finger having its own tendons, nerves, and bone structures to complete webbing of the entire hand.

Assessment data include limited flexion and extension of the digits due to the different lengths of the metacarpals and phalanges. Treatment options include surgical separation and reconstruction of the involved fingers. One of the main complications of surgical correction is vascular compromise to the fingers. While nerves can be split and directed to separate fingers, blood vessels cannot.

Polydactyly

Polydactyly is the presence of supernumerary digits on the thumb or fifth finger of the hand. It is an autosomal dominant condition that can express itself in a variety of forms. Polydactyly is found more frequently in African Americans than in white children.

Careful assessment is needed to determine if the extra digit is simply a skin tag or actually contains bony elements. Skin tags can be surgically incised during the neonatal period under local anesthesia. If the digit contains osseous material, removal is usually delayed until a more thorough evaluation of motor function is obtained. For cosmetic reasons, the extra digit should be removed prior to school age.

Congenital Limb Deficiency

Definition and Incidence. Limb deficient children (also called juvenile amputees) encompass a group of children who are either born with limbs that are partially deformed or absent (congenital) or who lose a limb through trauma or disease (acquired). Increased attention and research has been given to congenital limb deficiencies since the thalidomide calamity during the 1950s. Thalidomide was a widely prescribed drug for pregnant women to combat nausea and vomiting during the first trimester of pregnancy. These women produced a high number of children with multiple congenital limb deformities.

Congenital limb deficiencies are more prevalent than acquired limb deficiencies; incidence is evenly distributed between the sexes. Upper limbs are involved twice as often as lower limbs and include multiple limbs in approximately 30% of the children.[33]

Etiology and Pathophysiology. Malformations are caused by chromosomal aberrations, genetic disorders, or environmental factors.[31] Genetic factors are present at conception, while most environmental limb deficiencies occur during the embryonic phase of gestation.

Environmental factors include hormones, drugs, viruses, and irradiation. During the third to eighth week of gestation, teratogenic factors may inhibit the orderly differentiation of the highly sensitive cellular components that are rapidly changing.[48A] The limb deficiency is either the result of arrested development in the embryonic limb or some form of destructive process to the limb already formed.

Several systems have been devised for classification of this disorder. The most widely used system, devised by Frantz and O'Rahilly,[11] groups congenital limb deficiencies according to the absence of limb parts. Despite the fact that it was developed more than 30 years ago, this system, as shown in the accompanying display, is still widely accepted in the United States as the basis for limb deficiency identification.

Clinical Manifestations. Defining characteristics of congenital limb deformities depend on the specific category and limb that is affected. The terminology described in the display can be used to identify the type of deficiency. In addition specific names identify certain disorders.

For example, *congenital absence of the radius* (radial club hand) is one of the most common deficiencies of the long bones. It is a longitudinal upper intercalary deficiency known as a longitudinal radial hemimelia according to the Frantz and O'Rahilly classification. Con-

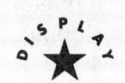 **Frantz and O'Rahilly System for Classifying Limb Deficiencies**

TERMINOLOGY IDENTIFYING ABSENT SKELETAL PARTS

Amelia:	Complete absence of a limb
Hemimelia:	Absence of a major portion of a limb
Phocomelia:	Central portion of a limb missing; hand or foot attached to the trunk

TWO TYPES OF LIMB DEFICIENCIES

Terminal:	No unaffected parts distal to the named deformity
Intercalary:	The middle part of the limb deficient but the areas proximal and distal to it intact

SUBDIVISIONS OF TERMINAL AND INTERCALARY TYPE

Longitudinal (paraxial):	Defect extends the length of the limb; preaxial and postaxial parts of limb absent
Transverse:	Defect extends transversely across entire width of the limb

Frantz, C. H., & O'Rahilly, R. (1961). Congenital skeletal limb deformities. Journal of Bone and Joint Surgery. 43, 1202.

genital absence of the radius is characterized by radial hand deviation of 90 degrees, shortening of the forearm, and underdevelopment or absence of the thumb.[33] The ulna is usually short and bowed, while the muscles, tendons, nerves, and blood vessels are absent or abnormal. Most cases are bilateral.

Another example of a limb deficiency is phocomelia or "seal limbs." This deficiency includes all proximal portions of the lower limb. With this deficiency the feet attach directly to the trunk. Digits may be absent or present with partial mobility, function, and range of motion. The joints (if present) are unstable and hyperextensible.

With each type of limb deficiency, there is a group of specific characteristics. Nurses need to understand the nature of these deficiencies in terms of the individual's functional abilities.

Diagnostic Studies.   Roentgenogram (x-ray) is the best method of detecting the extent of congenital upper limb deficiencies. EMG may be used to evaluate muscle function relative to the involved limb (see Chap. 61).

★ ASSESSMENT

Because limb deficiencies are present at birth, a thorough assessment should be completed in the delivery room or the newborn nursery. An in-depth maternal health history may reveal hereditary or environmental factors that may be the cause of the limb deficiency. Because some of the limb deficiencies can be grotesque, careful attention must be given to family and infant attachment.

As the child develops, the assessment parameters change. The nurse should assess the child's development and ability to perform self-care activities. Assessing the child's ability to function provides valuable data about the child's needs.

★ NURSING DIAGNOSES AND PLANNING

Based on the assessment data and the specific clinical manifestations for the affected child, the following nursing diagnosis may be considered:

- Self-Care Deficit related to dysfunctional limbs.
- High Risk for Impaired Skin Integrity related to malfitting prostheses.
- Altered Parenting related to impaired bonding.
- Impaired Social Interaction related to unacceptability of appearance to peers or family.
- Self-Esteem Disturbance related to congenital anomaly.
- Dysfunctional Grieving related to loss of "normal" baby.

The nurse and child (or parents) together plan effective care based on the established nursing diagnoses. Several examples of expected outcomes follow:

- The parents express normal reactions to the birth of a child with physical anomalies.
- The parents discuss their reactions openly.
- The parents hold and talk to the infant.
- The parents demonstrate techniques for maintaining skin integrity around the prosthesis.
- The child participates in school activities.

The nurse plans for the daily care of the child based on both physician's orders and nursing diagnoses. A general nursing care goal may include the following:

- The child obtains optimal development.

★ INTERVENTIONS: COLLABORATIVE AND INDEPENDENT

One of the primary roles of the nurse is to prevent the deficiency. During the critical period for limb formation (3 to 8 weeks' gestation), many women do not know they are pregnant. Nurses may have opportunities during family planning sessions or general health programs to stress the importance of lifestyle changes prior to conception.

The nurse is often the coordinator of the multidisciplinary team with the family. Team members should include physicians, surgeons, nurses, geneticists, social workers, a discharge planning coordinator, physical therapists, occupational therapists, clergy, and school teachers. By including the different disciplines in the care of the child, a holistic, comprehensive approach to the care of the child is supported.

PSYCHOSOCIAL SUPPORT

The identification of prenatal and postnatal physical anomalies is a devastating family crisis that shatters the usual excitement of the birth of a new baby. Parents may react with disbelief, shock, anger, and denial. Nurses are often the first individuals whom the parents encounter when they receive the devastating news. Support, empathy, and a strong commitment to facilitating parent-infant attachment are essential nursing interventions.

Prostheses have revolutionized the self-care abilities of children afflicted with limb deficiencies (Fig. 62-2). Fenestrated, artificial limbs are available for children with complete phocomelia. Clothing designers and occupational therapists can help to design clothing and adaptive devices to make a child's life easier and provide more control over the environment.

The nurse should stress the importance of maintaining skin integrity while the child wears the prosthesis. Excessive perspiration, irritating prosthetic material, ill-fitting devises, and physical abuse of the prosthesis can result in skin excoriation, blisters, and abrasions.

Anticipatory guidance is invaluable for parents in terms of their child's developmental level. Most children with congenital limb deformities are not developmentally delayed. Therefore, the nurse should help parents design ways for the child to meet developmental milestones despite some of the motor skill deficits.

Encouraging active participation in school activities is helpful to parents and children.[16] The nurse may offer to meet with teachers, to emphasize the need for normalcy and social interactions for the child. If realistic expectations are identified for the child, success should be rewarding and self-esteem increased.

Adolescence has its own inherent problems because of issues of body image, dating, sexuality, and independence. The nurse should provide ongoing counseling for the child with a limb deficiency during this critical stage of development. Psychosocial support may be provided through regular meetings with a group of similarly af-

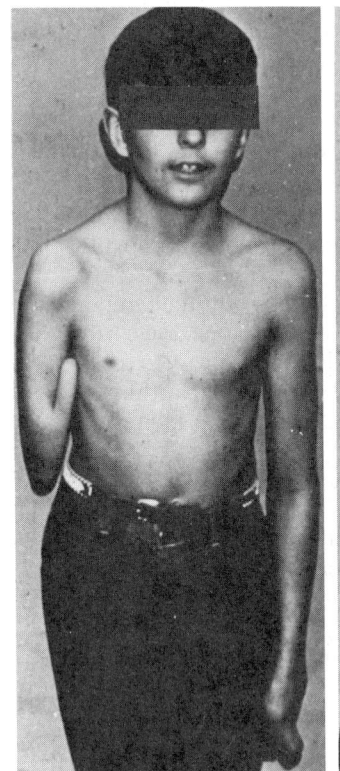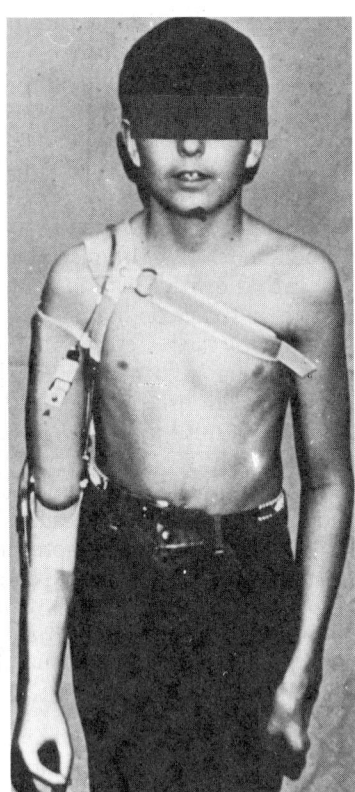

FIGURE 62-2
Ulnar hemimelia with a nonfunctional monodigital hand and severe flexion contracture at the elbow treated by surgical conversion to an elbow disarticulation, followed by appropriate prosthetic fitting. (Morrissy, R. T. [1990]. Lovell and Winter's pediatric orthopaedics [3rd ed.]. [Vol. II]. Philadelphia: J. B. Lippincott.)

fected teens under the leadership of a clinical nurse specialist or other professional.

SURGICAL MANAGEMENT

Surgical intervention may be necessary for some children to correct or reconstruct their limb deficiency. Preoperative teaching should be provided at the child's developmental level. Stressing the positive outcome of surgery will help the child and family through the trauma of hospitalization.

Nurses who care for children in all health care settings can help to ease the transition of the limb-deficient child into the mainstream of life. Continuous monitoring of the child's progress, health status, school life, prosthesis fittings, and family relationships is necessary. The child's independence is facilitated, and the family's acceptance of the defect is promoted.

Congenital Dislocation of the Hip

Definition and Incidence. Congenital dislocation of the hip (CDH), also called congenital hip dysplasia, is a condition in which the femoral head does not sit properly in the acetabulum. The term refers to a range of hip joint problems that have been classified into the subgroups in the accompanying display.[26]

The incidence of CDH varies according to the degree of instability. Approximately 11.7 of every 1000 infants has some degree of hip instability, with subluxable hips occurring in 9.2 of every 1000 infants, dislocatable hips in 1.2 of every 1000 infants, and dislocated hips in 1.3 of every 1000 infants.[25]

Seventy percent of dislocated hips occur in girls and they occur more often in firstborn children. In addition, CDH is more prevalent in children carried or delivered in breech position. Congenital dislocation of the hip is seen 60% of the time in the left hip, 20% in the right hip, 20% in both hips, and 75% unilaterally.[28]

Etiology and Pathophysiology. While the etiology of CDH remains unknown, some risk factors or predisposing factors have been identified. There is a family history of the defect in about 33% of the cases, and there is a 10-fold increase of risk in a second child if the first child has CDH.[26] Maternal estrogens and hormones affecting maternal pelvic laxity prior to birth may temporarily cause

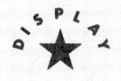

Classification of Unstable Hip Joints in Children

Dislocated hip—The femoral head has completely displaced from the acetabulum and requires reduction.
Dislocatable hip—The femoral head is in the acetabulum but can be completely displaced by adducting the thigh and applying slight force.
Subluxable hip—The femoral head can be moved significantly but does not completely leave contact with the acetabulum.

laxity of the pelvic joint and hip capsule in a newborn and lead to joint instability.

At birth the ball-and-joint socket structures of the hip are largely cartilaginous. As ossification of the hip proceeds, the head of the femur must be contained within the acetabulum for normal hip configuration to develop. If the head of the femur is not positioned well within the joint, adaptive changes cause varying degrees of deformity in the femur, acetabulum, soft tissues, and joint capsule.

In the newborn with CDH, the hip structures are close to normal. If the condition is diagnosed early, the femoral head usually can be returned to the normal position easily. After the femoral head is reduced, it is necessary to maintain this relationship of the head of the femur within the acetabulum until the joint capsule returns to its normal configuration.

If left undiagnosed or untreated, normal use, activity, and stress on the hip joint causes adaptive changes in the hip, and CDH becomes more difficult to reduce. Treatment becomes more complex and the possibility of success is greatly reduced as the child becomes older. The muscles around the hip become contracted, and the acetabulum and femoral head become dysplastic.

Clinical Manifestations. All newborns should be checked for signs of hip instability or dislocation. In the newborn period the hip is examined for excessive looseness that causes the head of the femur to slide in and out of the acetabulum. After the newborn period, the adaptive changes occurring in the hip make other signs and symptoms more apparent. The following are commonly recognized: asymmetry of gluteal or thigh folds, an apparent shortening of the femur, limitation in abduction of the hip, a telescoping or pistoning action of the thigh, and a positive Trendelenburg's sign (see Fig. 61-4).

Diagnostic Studies. In the newborn, the diagnosis of CDH is based on clinical examination in which an attempt is made to either dislocate or reduce the dislocated hip. Routine radiologic evaluations of infants are not always reliable because the structures of the hip are primarily cartilaginous and therefore radiolucent. As the child grows and ossification occurs, the radiologic evaluation is more diagnostic. Ultrasound is sensitive to the cartilaginous structures of the hip and may be beneficial in the newborn. The hip arthrogram can be used to determine whether concentric reduction has occurred.

⋆ ASSESSMENT

The nurse plays a significant role in the diagnosis of the child with CDH. Signs of the condition should be identified during physical examination or routine baby care. Two tests to determine if the hips can be easily dislocated and reduced are performed routinely in the newborn: Ortolani's reduction test and the Barlow dislocation test. These tests should be performed only by an experienced examiner.

For the Ortolani test the baby is placed on the back with hips and knees flexed to 90 degrees. The examiner grasps the thigh and places the middle finger over the greater trochanter. The thigh is lifted to bring the femoral

head from its dislocated position to opposite the acetabulum and is abducted to reduce the head into the acetabulum. The test is positive if the examiner hears or feels a "clunk" on reduction. The Ortolani test is illustrated in Figure 61-4.

In the Barlow test the examiner attempts to dislocate the hip, as shown in Figure 62-3. The baby's hips and knees are flexed to 90 degrees. The thigh is adducted and pressure is exerted downward. The hip may be felt to dislocate. If either test is positive, the physician should be notified immediately for prompt treatment.

As the infant matures and adaptive changes occur in the hip, other signs and symptoms of CDH become more evident. The lower extremities are examined for asymmetric gluteal or thigh folds. The infant is held upright and the legs are inspected anteriorly and posteriorly (see Fig. 61-4). Asymmetric skin folds are sometimes seen in infants without CDH. A positive finding along with other signs and symptoms alerts the nurse to the possibility of dislocation and the need to refer the child for definitive diagnosis.

Further testing may be performed with the infant in a supine position with hips and knees flexed and abducted. Limitation in abduction is caused by contracted and shortened hip adductor muscles. An apparent shortening of the femur is seen by placing the child supine with hips and knees flexed and with feet placed on the examining surface. If one knee is lower than the other, a positive Allis's or Galeazzi's sign is present (see Fig. 61-4). In the same position with hips and knees flexed, if the femur can be moved freely up and down, this action is called pistoning or telescoping. With the child standing on the leg of the dislocated side, the unaffected side droops. Due to tightness of the hip abductors in the affected side. The child may walk with a limp or a waddling gait.

⋆ NURSING DIAGNOSES AND PLANNING

Based on assessment data discussed previously and in the preceding chapter, the following nursing diagnoses may apply to the family and child with CDH:

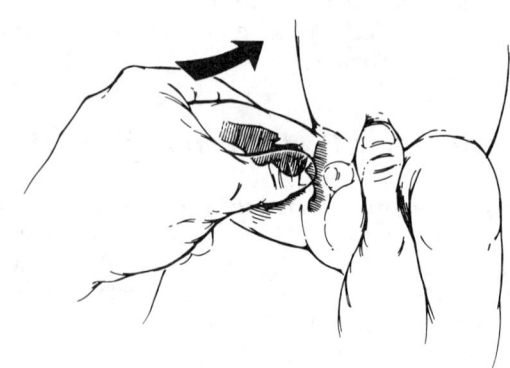

FIGURE 62-3

Barlow test. The thumb is placed on the inner aspect of the thigh. Adduction and posterior pressure toward the examining table may produce a "clunk" of subluxation or dislocation. (Oski, F. A., DeAngelis, C. D., Feigin, R. D., & Warshaw, J. B. [Eds.]. [1990]. *Principles and practice of pediatrics.* Philadelphia: J. B. Lippincott.)

- Anxiety related to knowledge deficit regarding genetic potential for future pregnancies, plan of treatment, development aspects of immobility, support groups, and home care needs.
- Impaired Physical Mobility related to the condition and treatment.
- High Risk for Injury (Neurovascular Impairment) related to improper application of treatment device.

The nurse and parents together plan effective care based on the established nursing diagnoses. Several examples of expected outcomes follow:

- The parents verbally explain techniques for neurovascular assessment.
- The parents demonstrate correct neurovascular assessment.
- The parents provide developmentally sound activities for the child.
- The parents return demonstration of basic care for the child in cast or traction.
- The parents state they have contacted a support group.

The nurse plans for the daily care of the child based on physician's orders and nursing diagnoses. Some general nursing care goals may include the following:

- The correct position of femur and acetabulum is maintained.
- Injury is avoided.

⭐ **NURSING INTERVENTIONS: COLLABORATIVE AND INDEPENDENT**

Treatment is usually initiated in the physician's office or in an ambulatory care setting. The treatment plan focuses on reduction of the head of the femur into the acetabulum. The earlier the reduction, the fewer adaptive changes required. Treatment involves many months of care. The nurse is able to monitor family needs related to continuous medical management and care of the child.

All activities should be clarified at the beginning of the treatment plan and shared with the family throughout the course of care. The family may need assistance in focusing on the child's strengths and in helping the child continue to develop normally.

During the hospital stay, each nurse must be a skilled care provider in all the techniques of proper hip management for CDH.

MEDICAL MANAGEMENT

Various types of positioning devices are used in the child from birth to 6 months. Triple diapers were used in the past but now are considered ineffective. The diapers do not produce flexion, and the amount of abduction achieved is unpredictable.[17] The head of the femur, which is largely a cartilaginous structure in the infant, is vulnerable to vascular insufficiency. For this reason rigid braces and forced abduction should be avoided.[17] The Pavlik harness, a cloth positioning device that provides abduction and hip flexion, is a popular form of treatment (see Figure 62-4). The harness is worn for many weeks until the hip is stable. Parent teaching is discussed in the Teaching Plan for a child with a Pavlik harness.

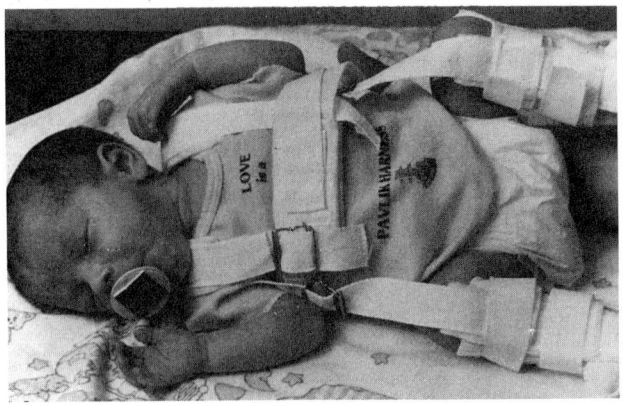

FIGURE 62-4
Proper positioning of an infant in a Pavlik harness. The harness is composed of shoulder straps, stirrups, and a chest strap. It is placed on both legs, even if only one hip is dislocated. (Morrissy, R. T. [Ed.]. [1990]. Lovell and Winter's pediatric orthopaedics [3rd ed.]. [Vol. II]. Philadelphia: J. B. Lippincott.)

Children older than 6 months who have been diagnosed late or in whom early treatment has been unsuccessful may need a period of traction to stretch the soft-tissue structures of the hip prior to reduction. The traction reduces the risk of developing avascular necrosis to the head of the femur. (See section on Care of a Child in Traction later in this chapter.) Traction is carried out at home or in the hospital. The goal of treatment is to bring the head of the femur below the level of the acetabulum to achieve a safe reduction. Once the hip is safely reduced, a spica cast is applied until satisfactory development of the hip is achieved. (See section on Care of a Child in a Cast later in this chapter.) Casts are changed every 6 to 8 weeks. If the head of the femur cannot be safely reduced, a surgical procedure is necessary. Postoperatively, a spica cast is used for 4 to 6 months (see Table 62-16).

CONTINUOUS MONITORING

The nurse continues to monitor neurovascular status of the child in traction, cast, or following surgery. Assessment should include motion, color, temperature, pain, capillary refill, edema, sensation, tingling, and numbness. The importance of neurovascular assessment cannot be overemphasized. Problems related to neurovascular compromise must be considered an emergency and treated immediately.

GROWTH AND DEVELOPMENT PROMOTION

The child being treated for CDH is forced into some form of immobility at a time when growth and development demands activity. The nurse's knowledge of normal aspects of development is used to offer the family advice and direction on how to foster development in a child who is confined. The nurse can help the family focus on the activities the child is able to do. For example, the child in a cast or traction has upper body mobility. Play activities should be designed to encourage movement of the upper body—balls, large bright toys, overhead mobiles, music and sound-producing activities, and visual activities. Additionally, the child can almost always be placed in a stroller or some kind of mobile device to

(text continued on page 1690)

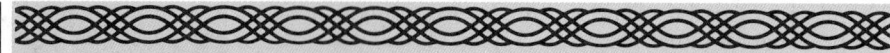

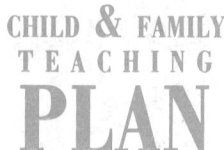

CHILD & FAMILY
T E A C H I N G
PLAN

Care of a Child With a Pavlik Harness for Congenital Dislocation of the Hip

Assessment

A routine physical examination was performed on Charisse Henderson at 2 days old. Her birth was by cesarean delivery because of a breech presentation. While performing the Ortolani test on Charisse's hips, the pediatric nurse practitioner (PNP) was able to palpate a "clunk" as the right femoral head was reduced into the acetabulum. The Barlow test enabled the PNP to dislocate gently the right femoral head out of the acetabulum. A positive Galleazzi's sign was noted when Charisse was placed supine in her bassinet, and the right knee appeared lower than the left knee. Asymmetric gluteal skin folds also were noted, along with limited abduction of the right thigh. None of these maneuvers caused any discomfort to Charisse. After conferring with the pediatrician, a diagnosis of right congenital dislocation of the hip was identified.

A Pavlik harness was chosen as the form of treatment because of its mobility, effectiveness, and simplicity. Charisse was fitted for a Pavlik harness and discharged home to her parents with instructions to bring her to the orthopedic clinic weekly for adjustments to the harness.

Child and Family Objectives	*Specific Content*	*Teaching Strategies*
1. Strengthen parent-infant bonding.	1. Feelings surrounding birth and concerning Charisse's dysfunction	1. Explore parental feelings of guilt, self-blame for child's disorder
	Recognition of infant stressors: hunger, wet diaper, fatigue, limited range of motion	Validate feelings of grief, frustration, inadequacy, fears
	Importance of holding, touching, fondling infant	Point out positive features Charisse's
	Share child care, household responsibilities between parents	Provide positive reinforcement
		Use audiovisuals
	Positive feedback for compliance with proper use of Pavlik harness	Identify parent support groups
	Adequate stimulation and interaction between parents and infant	
2. Perform activities of daily living with minimal interference from the Pavlik harness.	2. Bathing: • Remove harness for short periods of time if allowed. • Keep infant's legs apart with 2 to 3 cloth diapers or receiving blanket while not in harness. Clothing: • Wear undershirts under the harness. • High socks under leg pieces. • One piece stretch suits with snaps or Velcro under harness. • Buntings in cold weather. • Baggy clothes to accommodate harness and position of legs.	2. Provide instruction packets. Use audiovisuals. Suggest support groups. Demonstrate and use return demonstration for various aspects of care.

(Continued)

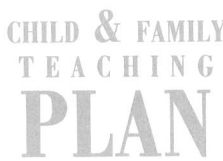

CHILD & FAMILY
T E A C H I N G
PLAN

Care of a Child With a Pavlik Harness for Congenital Dislocation of the Hip (continued)

Child and Family Objectives	*Specific Content*	*Teaching Strategies*
	Feeding: • Assure adequate leg abduction while nursing baby. • Feed in upright position if possible. • Avoid soiling harness with food. Toileting: • Keep harness clean and dry. • Avoid soiling of appliance. • Keep child in harness during diaper change. • Pay special attention to skin care in inguinal skin folds. Safety: • Unable to use conventional car seats • Infant carriers • Back packs • Grocery carts	
3. State complications related to improper application and nonuse of the Pavlik harness.	3. Skin integrity: redness, chafing, irritation Turning schedule every 2 hours to reduce pressure areas and decrease respiratory compromise Circulatory status: • Neurovascular checks to toes • Mottling of skin Follow-up appointments: • Weekly for Pavlik harness adjustments • As needed for other problems. • Phone availability of health care providers. Potential complications: redislocation, casting, traction, surgery, impaired ambulation, avascular necrosis of the femoral head	3. Demonstrate and have return demonstration. Use written instructions for reinforcement.
4. Demonstrate correct application and removal of Pavlik harness	4. Parts of Pavlik harness: stirrups, buckles, chest straps, shoulder straps, crossbands Application of Pavlik harness: • Hips in proper flexion position • Straps secure but not too tight • Keep straps off abdominal area	4. Discuss diagrams. Provide written instructions. Have parents discuss use of harness parts. Use role playing. Provide question-and-answer time. Give individualized instructions. Use short teaching sessions.

(Continued)

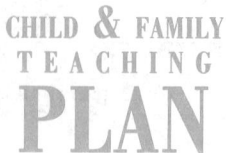

CHILD & FAMILY TEACHING PLAN

Care of a Child With a Pavlik Harness for Congenital Dislocation of the Hip (continued)

Child and Family Objectives	*Specific Content*	*Teaching Strategies*
	Time frame for wearing Pavlik harness Care of harness: • Clean with mild soap • Air dry, machine dry on low temperature setting Removal of harness: • Locate strap marks for identification for easier reapplication • Inspect skin for signs/symptoms of skin excoriation	• Demonstrate and have parents return demonstration.
5. Verbalize an understanding of the need for the Pavlik harness.	5. Normal versus abnormal pathophysiology of the newborn's hips: • Relationship between head of femur and acetabulum • Position and function of hip ligaments Risk factors for CHD: breech delivery, genetics, fetal position *in utero* Ortolani's maneuvers • Palpate "clunk" on right hip Purpose of Pavlik harness: • Stabilize hip joint • Prevent further dislocation and complications	5. Use colorful diagrams, charts, audiovisuals of normal and abnormal hip positions. Explain x-ray pictures of their child's hip joints. Provide individualized instructions. Provide written handouts. Demonstrate Ortolani's maneuvers.
Evaluation	• Both parents demonstrate commitment to treatment process. • Both parents demonstrate parent-infant bonding. • Charisse's weight and height remain at 75th percentile. • Parents gradually wean Charisse from harness as instructed at 6 months. • Parents state they are pleased with success of Pavlik harness therapy. • Charisse shows signs of sitting unsupported.	

provide a change of scenery. Even the traction equipment can be made mobile by fitting it with wheels or adapting it to fit into a wagon. A reclining wheelchair can be used for an older child in a hip spica. The nurse also demonstrates basic care, such as bathing, diapering, and changing position. A bean bag chair is an excellent positioning device for the child in a cast.

DISCHARGE PLANNING

The care of the child with CDH occurs primarily in the home. Parents should receive an overview of the plan of care at the onset. The family must be familiar with all

phases of the home care treatment plan. They must be able to verbally explain and then demonstrate, correctly and without assistance, the techniques of neurovascular assessment and the method of treatment being used, whether it is cast care, harness care, traction application, or brace care.

The nurse demonstrates the correct methods of application and use of all devices required by the child. The nurse includes proper home management of all aspects of the care in the teaching plan. The nurse should reinforce the teaching and training program with written materials. The teaching plan outlines the discharge preparation given to parents of a child in a Pavlik harness for treatment of CDH.

The family also should receive information related to support groups involved in the care of the child with CDH. A consistent support person who also understands the plan of care is a great asset to the family. Treatment of hip dislocation can take many months, and parents need continuous support.

⋆ EVALUATION

During follow-up visits, the nurse assesses the proper use of the therapeutic device. The nurse also evaluates the coping mechanisms of the family as they continue through the planned treatment program. The nurse may find it necessary to contact a home care nursing agency to assist with care of the child.

The nurse also discusses with the family the activities they are using for developmental stimulation. Parental responses provide cues for altering the existing plan.

COMPLICATIONS

The earlier CDH is diagnosed and the earlier the treatment is initiated, the better the outcome. Children treated before walking age generally have a better prognosis than those treated after walking age. The adaptive changes that occur as the child matures make remodeling of the hip more difficult in the older child. Most children with CDH are successfully treated in the newborn period; few untreated cases persist to develop a more difficult treatment plan. Radiographs are taken periodically to determine hip development.

Congenital Dislocation of the Knee

Congenital dislocation of the knee is a disorder characterized by anterior displacement of the tibia. Displacement ranges from mild hyperextension of the knee to severe hyperextension with complete anterior dislocation of the tibia from the femur.[41] The disorder is usually bilateral and affects girls more than boys.

Congenital dislocations of the knee may be hereditary or may be the result of positioning *in utero* with the feet hooked underneath the mandible. Some conditions associated with this disorder include fibrosis of the vastus lateralis and quadriceps, oligohydramnios, arthrogryposis multiplex congenita, and CDH.

The knee becomes dislocated when the posterior capsule is very loose, the anterior capsule is contracted, and the cruciate ligaments are either stretched, hypoplastic, or absent.[33,46] The tibia may be bowed anteriorly, and the hamstrings function as extensors of the knee.

Congenital dislocation of the knee is immediately apparent at birth. The knee is in hyperextension and the hip in hyperflexion with the toes touching the anterior chest wall or chin.[49] Knee flexion is limited, yet the knee can be further extended from its hyperextended state. Transverse skin folds are noted on the ventral side of the knee.

Prenatal ultrasonography may reveal congenital dislocation of the knee. Following the birth of the child, roentgenographic studies reveal the true nature of the

deformity. The proximal end of the tibia may be partially or completely displaced anteriorly over the distal end of the femur. CT and MRI studies are useful in depicting pathologic changes.

NURSING IMPLICATIONS

A newborn assessment should include documentation of range of motion for all the extremities. The degree of hyperextension of the infant's knees can be validated using a goniometer. Palpation of the popliteal area reveals the presence of the femoral condyles. Because of the high incidence of other associated congenital anomalies, the nurse should screen for other musculoskeletal disorders.

Goals are directed toward preventing permanent loss of function and physical deformity. The nurse works closely with the family to ensure that the infant is encouraged to reach developmental milestones. This goal as well as those related to the teaching and support of the family is of paramount importance to the nurse.

Early recognition and treatment during the neonatal period is essential to prevent permanent loss of function and physical deformity. Skeletal traction is usually the treatment of choice for gentle repositioning of the dislocated knees. The traction forces initially pull the proximal end of the tibia around the distal end of the femur. Then traction forces are manipulated to encourage gradual knee flexion. Pin site care is usually prescribed by the physician or the standards of the agency. Regardless of the type of skin care prescribed, the nurse must observe for drainage, swelling, erythema, pain, and tenting around the site. (See section on Care of a Child in Traction later in this chapter.)

Once the infant is out of traction, serial casting is performed every 2 weeks to ensure gradual, progressive knee flexion. Cast care instructions are reviewed with the parents special emphasis is placed on safety, hygiene, and neurovascular status. (See section on Care of a Child in a Cast later in this chapter.) This mode of treatment lasts for 6 to 8 weeks.

Once knee flexion is achieved, passive range-of-motion exercises are performed several times a day to promote further knee flexion. Careful attention is given to avoid forcing the knees through flexion exercises. Teaching the parents how to perform these exercises helps them participate in the rehabilitation process for their child. Parents can then begin to feel a sense of control over what has happened.

Once the child is able to maintain knee flexion and the casts are removed, a Pavlik harness is used intermittently throughout the day and night to maintain the attained degree of flexion (see Fig. 62-4). Parents are instructed to exercise the knees to increase the range of motion and enhance muscle tone without forcing the knees beyond the point of resistance.

If closed reduction is not successful in infancy, open reduction is indicated. Timing for surgery is crucial because it should be performed before the child starts bearing weight on the affected leg. Preoperative and postoperative instructions are reviewed with the parents.

Special attention must be given to the parent-infant attachment process. Because of the imposed immobility and hospitalization required during the newborn period, the infant is at risk for diminished social interaction. Parents are encouraged to touch their baby and participate in as many of the activities of daily living with which they feel comfortable. If possible, the parents should be provided with the opportunity to "room in" with their infant. It is also important to recognize that the parents need time to be alone as a couple or with the rest of their family. The nurse should act as an advocate in making arrangements to suit the needs of the family and the infant.

Complications such as pin site infection and neurovascular compromise can adversely affect the outcomes of treatment. Children are considered fortunate if they are able to attain 90-degree flexion of the affected extremity. Continued follow-up and evaluation are needed to ensure that the child reaches the developmental potential.

Congenital Disorders of the Foot and Ankle

Definition and Incidence.   Foot and ankle disorders are among the most common congenital anomalies. Approximately 1 in every 700 infants is born with some form of foot or ankle deformity. Disorders vary in severity depending on the areas affected and the degree of rigidity and flexibility. When the ankle and foot are involved, the term *talipes* is used. Forefoot involvement includes the metatarsal area of the foot. Definitions and illustrations of various types of foot and ankle disorders are included in Table 62-2.

The term *clubfoot* is often used broadly to define any of the various combinations of ankle equinous or calcaneus, hindfoot, and forefoot varus or valgus. However, there are only two types of true clubfeet. Talipes equinovarus is the most common type, accounting for 95% of all cases. The calcaneovalgus variety is seen in approximately 5% of the reported cases. The disorder occurs in 1 of every 1000 newborns and is twice as common in boys as in girls.[18] Because of its multifactorial inheritance pattern, a familial tendency has been noted with this disorder.

Metatarsus Varus or Valgus.   Disorders that only affect the forefoot or metatarsus are often mistaken for clubfoot. Metatarsus varus (adductus) is the most common congenital foot deformity. This mild varus deformity is characterized by a unilateral or bilateral "toeing in" of the affected feet. Mild valgus deformities that result in a child's feet "toeing out" are termed metatarsus valgus.

TABLE 62-2
Common Foot and Ankle Disorders

Type	Description	Type	Description
Metatarsus varus (adductus)	"Toeing in." The forefoot turns toward the midline of the body, and the heel remains straight.	Talipes calcaneovalgus	The foot is dorsiflexed at the ankle. Toes point upward and outward—type of "clubfoot."
Metatarsus valgus	"Toeing out." The forefoot turns away from the midline of the body, and the heel remains straight.	Talipes varus	Foot and ankle bend toward the midline of the body.
Talipes equinovarus	The foot and ankle deviate toward the midline of the body and plantar flexion of the forefoot, most severe type of "clubfoot" deformity.	Talipes valgus	Foot and ankle bend away from the midline of the body.

Etiology and Pathophysiology. Even though the cause of many of these ankle and foot disorders remains unknown, several theories about the etiology have been proposed. The disorders are generally believed to be associated with either intrauterine positioning or arrested or anomalous fetal development.

Deformities associated with intrauterine positioning tend to be more flexible than those associated with fetal development. The metatarsal disorders generally fit into this category. Intrauterine molding may occur as a result of mechanical forces exerted by firm uterine and abdominal muscles, oligohydramnios, or a breech position.

Often clubfoot is associated with other congenital disorders as myelodysplasia or arthrogryposis. Some theorists believe that a primary germ plasm defect results in dysplasia of the talus and other associated changes. Others suggest that the normal inversion and eversion of the foot that occurs *in utero* is somehow arrested in the early trimesters. If the foot fails to go through this normal process, a rigid deformity may result. Finally, some consideration has been given to the possible influences of environmental factors, drugs, or diseases on the interuterine development of the foot and ankle.

Clubfoot is a three-dimensional deformity that includes a combination of forefoot and hindfoot varus or valgus and equinous or calcaneus of the ankle. The disorder varies in severity from a foot that is very flexible and easily corrected to a foot that has a very rigid bony structure. Even without a bony deformity, the soft tissues still may be tight and short. In the more severe forms of clubfoot, the bone, soft tissue, and muscles are involved. Shortening of the soft tissues along with the nerves, blood vessels, and skin tends to occur on the medial and posterior aspect of the foot. On the lateral aspect of the foot, laxity of these tissues and nerves is often observed.

Metatarsal Disorders. Metatarsus varus (adductus) and metatarsus valgus originate at the tarsometatarsal joint. Movement of the joint influences the adduction and inversion of all five metatarsals. Varying degrees of flexibility and rigidity depend on the amount of bone and soft-tissue involvement. However, the majority of these children have only a soft-tissue deformity. Involvement is usually bilateral and associated with tibial torsion. The condition differs from true clubfoot because there is no deformity of the heel or ankle.

Clinical Manifestations. Depending on the degree of involvement, clinical manifestations of foot and ankle disorders are usually obvious at birth. The infant's feet usually assume one of the positions described in the preceding sections. Generally the foot can be passively overcorrected and returned to the original position. If bony involvement is extensive, however, manipulation of the foot may be impossible.

Clubfoot. With true clubfoot, full range of motion is limited. The affected foot presents with forefoot adduction and supination through the midtarsal joint. There is heel varus or valgus through the subtalar joint and ankle equinus or calcaneus. The entire foot deviates medially relative to the knee.

Metatarsal Disorders. Children with metatarsal disorders present with adduction or abduction and inversion or eversion of the forefoot. There is no heel or ankle deformity. With these disorders, especially in bilateral cases, a lateral or twisting rotation of the tibia may be present. The space between the great and second toe may be wider than normal with varus deformities.

Generally the foot is pliable and easily rotated through the normal range of motion. If these deformities are not identified before the child begins to walk, a characteristic gait will be evident. Children with metatarsus varus tend to "toe in," giving a pigeon-toed appearance. A duck walk appearance related to toeing out is seen in children with metatarsus valgus.

Diagnostic Studies. Diagnosis is usually readily made at birth. However, radiographic studies are needed to differentiate positional deformities from those that involve the bony structures. Anteroposterior, lateral, and oblique views of the foot and ankle will reveal any displacements relative to the talus in the affected foot and ankle.

★ ASSESSMENT

Assessment of the child with a congenital foot disorder usually begins shortly after birth. At this time the parents are overwhelmed with the whole experience of the birth. Even though this disorder is not life-threatening, the misshapen foot of their newborn can be quite distressing to new parents. Despite the fact that the condition may appear minor to the nurse, the nurse should be sensitive to the emotional needs of the family during the assessment process.

Data about the family's genetic history and the birth history of the child must be carefully collected. Often such information gathering causes the parents to feel guilty and responsible for their child's deformity. Therefore, the nurse also assesses the family's coping patterns.

Physical assessment includes a description of the position and appearance of the affected foot. Gentle, passive range of motion should be performed to determine the degree of mobility. If the child is ambulating, the gait and the position of the feet in relation to the tibia should be noted. In addition, a developmental history should be obtained. The child's psychosocial and motor development should be considered.

★ NURSING DIAGNOSES AND PLANNING

Based on assessment data discussed previously and in the preceding chapter, the following nursing diagnoses may apply to the family and child with a congenital disorder of the foot or ankle.

- Grieving related to perceived loss of a normal child.
- High Risk for Altered Parenting related to inability to attach to newborn.
- Anxiety related to knowledge deficit regarding the disorder and treatment plan.
- Impaired Physical Mobility related to position of feet.
- High Risk for Injury (Neurovascular) related to compromise associated with casting.
- Altered Growth and Development related to inability to meet developmental milestones of ambulation.

- Pain related to manipulation, casting, and operative procedures.
- High Risk for Impaired Skin Integrity related to frequent casting and taping procedures.
- Body Image Disturbance related to inability to participate in age-related activities.

The nurse and parents together plan effective care based on the established nursing diagnoses. Several examples of expected outcomes follow:

- The family discusses their feelings about the birth of an "imperfect" child.
- The parents demonstrate correct care required for their child.
- The child's skin remains intact without any signs of neurovascular impairment.
- The child demonstrates relief from pain and discomfort.
- The child continues to develop normally.

The nurse plans for the daily care of the child based on physician's orders and nursing diagnoses. Some general nursing care goals may include the following:

- The child attains maximum function of the feet and ankles.
- The child accepts any limitations imposed by the deformity.

★ INTERVENTIONS: COLLABORATIVE AND INDEPENDENT

The three levels of medical treatment options are based on the severity of the disorder and the associated rigidity of the soft tissues and bony structures. Mild deformities may respond to gentle manipulation and splinting. As the deformity becomes more rigid, serial casting followed by splinting may be indicated. Very rigid and nonresponsive deformities usually require surgical intervention.

Generally, following the diagnosis of a foot and ankle disorder, a treatment plan is initiated. The nurse can support parents by helping them express their concerns, answering questions about the rationale for the treatment plan, and providing them with helpful resources. A booklet or information about the defect is an excellent resource for parents.

EXERCISING

If the disorder is diagnosed at birth and the infant's foot is very pliable, gentle but firm manipulation of the foot can be effective. The nurse can help the family plan a schedule that coincides with the infant's care routines and ensures that the exercises will be performed at least five to six times daily. Nurses can teach the parents to hold the infant's heel firmly while gently stretching the forefoot. By positively reinforcing the parents' performance, the nurse can help to ensure that parents will comply with the treatment plan.

CASTING

If the exercise program is not effective, the physician will initiate serial castings of the infant's affected extremity. Taping of the extremity is sometimes used as an alternate treatment. The purpose of these procedures is to stretch the tight structures gradually and constrict the lax structures of the foot. Weekly manipulation and casting is usually needed to accomplish this goal.

In preparation for weekly casting, parents are asked to remove the old cast by soaking it in a vinegar and water solution. This procedure is often very tedious and time-consuming for parents. The nurse can suggest that the parents position themselves comfortably on the floor with a basin of the solution between their legs. The infant can be held against the parent's abdomen and be comforted and talked to as the baby's legs dangle in the basin of solution.

The serial casting treatment is continued until correction is achieved. Observing and participating in these procedures can be upsetting to the parents. The nurse can offer support and reassurance to the parents.

In addition, nurses need to teach parents about caring for their infant in a cast. (See section on Care of a Child in a Cast later in this chapter.) Because of the infant's rapid growth rate, special attention must be focused on the infant's neurovascular status and skin integrity. Any signs of cast pressure must be reported to the physician, and the cast must be removed immediately.

SURGICAL MANAGEMENT

Rigid deformities that do not respond to exercising or casting require surgical intervention. To realign the bones, a posteromedial release is usually performed. The bones are internally positioned with pins, and a long-leg cast that is flexed at the knee is applied. This position helps to prevent cast slippage as well as to discourage weight bearing. After 6 weeks this cast is usually changed, and the pins are removed. The length of time the child is in the cast varies but is typically about 4 months.

Nursing interventions should focus on preparing the parents and child for the procedure. The parents' anxiety about the procedure will readily be communicated to their infant. By letting the parents discuss their feelings and providing information about what to expect, the parents' anxiety should be reduced. A young child can be prepared for the procedure by playing with some of the casting materials and storytelling. Rather than give extensive information about the procedure, nurses should focus on describing sensations the child will feel.

The nurse is responsible for providing postoperative care to the child. A review of the nursing interventions needed following orthopedic surgery is included in Table 62-3.

ORTHOTIC DEVICES

Following correction of the deformity, some type of splint with corrective shoes is required. Outflare or reverse-last prewalker shoes attached to a Denis Browne splint generally are used for infants. The Denis Browne splint is shown in Figure 62-5. Older children wear a reverse-last shoe with special heel and sole wedges.

During this stage of treatment, the parents find it difficult to make their infants wear these orthotic devices for 16 to 23 hours per day. Nurses need to be sensitive to the parents' feelings as they reinforce the need to continue with the schedule. When shoes do not fit well, blistering and chafing may occur. The nurse needs to emphasize that the parents must replace these shoes with

TABLE 62-3
Nursing Interventions: Care Following Orthopedic Surgery

Intervention	Action
Assessment of neurovascular status	Assess color, sensation, capillary refill, movement, pain, and pulses at least every 1 hour for the first 4 hours and then every 2 to 4 hours.
	Encourage frequent movement of toes or fingers to improve circulation.
Assessment of blood loss	Review any decreases in hemoglobin and hematocrit levels.
	Take vital signs at least every 2 to 4 hours, and note any decrease in blood pressure or elevation in pulse rate from the preoperative assessment.
	Circle the amount of serosanguinous drainage on the cast with the date and time.
	Report significant increases of drainage to the surgeon.
	Describe any behavioral changes, such as restlessness, thirst, or increased pallor.
Assessment of complications	Assess for compartment syndrome and fat emboli (described in Table 62-14).
Maintain comfort	Assess pain level, and administer analgesics regularly for at least the first 24 to 48 hours.
	Support extremity with pillows and bolsters.
	Provide diversional activities.
Decrease edema	Elevate the extremity above the level of the heart (unless otherwise contraindicated).
	Place ice packs over the surgical site (cast) for the first 24 hours.
Maintain body alignment	Turn and reposition child every 2 hours.
Preserve pulmonary function	Provide deep breathing exercises every 4 hours (blow bottles; incentive spirometry; inflate gloves with faces).
Force fluids	Encourage clear, noncarbonated beverages, but limit milk and milk product intake to two to three glasses per day.
	Infants and Toddlers: 1500 ml/d
	Preschoolers: 2000 ml/d
	School-agers: 3000 ml/d
	Adolescents: 3500 ml/d

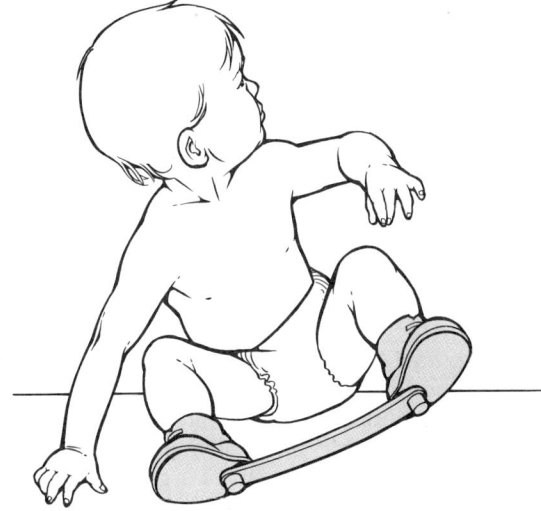

FIGURE 62-5
A Denis Browne splint with shoes attached is used in congenital disorders of the foot.

ones that fit properly. Because replacements may be expensive for the family, the nurse may need to direct the family to resources to help them with payment.

TEACHING

The challenges of caring for an infant are intensified when the infant is in a cast or orthotic device. Initially, their restricted movement may interfere with normal sleep patterns. However, extreme fussiness may be a sign of cast pressure.

Positioning an active infant with a cast or splint for feeding and dressing can be difficult. The nurse can suggest that the parent place a small pillow under the infant's legs for self-protection. Because infant clothing is not designed to fit over a cast or orthotic device, parents need suggestions for adapting clothing. The parents may be disappointed that the infant is unable to wear some of the gifts they have received.

Infant equipment should be carefully examined for safety. Some car seats and infant seats will not secure the infant with a cast or orthotic device. The nurse needs to provide anticipatory guidance for parents about the purchase and use of special infant equipment.

Nurses also provide anticipatory guidance for the parents about the developmental needs of their infant. Parents need to be assured that their infant should develop normally despite some of the limits imposed by the treatment plan. Nurses should emphasize the importance of holding and cuddling their infant. In addition parents need information about activities that will facilitate development.

⭐ **EVALUATION**

The outcomes of treatment are usually best when treatment is initiated soon after the birth of the child. The nurse plays an important role in reinforcing the treatment plan and ensuring by the parents' cooperation. By helping the parents through each stage of the treatment plan, the nurse will facilitate their coping.

If correction has been achieved, the child is able to participate in play and sports activities without difficulty. However, the affected extremities may appear slightly atrophied.

During each stage of treatment, the goals and objectives should be evaluated. Ensuring that the child is able to meet developmental milestones and the family is able to emotionally bond with their child are as important as goals related to the physical outcomes.

LONG-TERM CARE

Even after correction has been achieved, the child requires follow-up care. Often the deformity will recur and require additional surgical intervention. With each surgical procedure, the foot becomes less functional. Careful observation of changes in the extremity is an important aspect of the long-term plan of care.

Osteogenesis Imperfecta

Definition and Incidence. Osteogenesis Imperfecta (OI), the most common genetic disorder of the bone, occurs in 1 of every 20,000 live births. This inherited disorder is equally prevalent in all races and in both sexes. OI is a disorder of the connective tissue that affects the bone, soft tissues, and ligaments. The disorder is characterized by brittle bones and associated deformities, shortness of stature, scoliosis, and various metabolic problems.

Etiology and Pathophysiology. OI is a genetically heterogeneous disorder classified by four types of inherited patterns with variations in manifestations, as shown in Table 62-4. There may be an obvious genetic link, or the disorder could be the result of a genetic mutation. The degree of severity of these manifestations varies with each type and tends to decrease as the child reaches puberty.

OI is characterized by ligamentous laxity, structural abnormalities of the bones, and multiple fractures. The abnormal development of the collagen fibers in the connective tissue of these individuals may be responsible for the variety of manifestations.

The bones are generally slender and short with thin cortices and trabeculae. The narrow diaphysis of the long bones contributes to the fractures and bowing deformities. Instead of the normal smooth lamellae, a woven pattern of bone is evident. The haversian system is usually poorly developed. Often the bones lack the minerals needed to form bone matrix, and result some degree of osteopenia is usually present. In the more severe types of OI the design of the bone is greatly disrupted. Despite these major defects in the bone, the child's calcium, phosphorus, magnesium, vitamin D, and parathyroid hormone concentrations are normal.[54]

Even though fractures heal easily, the callus tends to have a plastic appearance. The bones are easily deformed by normal forces associated with movement. The laxity of the ligaments results in joints that are hypermobile and increase the potential for dislocations. These deformities are uncontrollable and may limit the child's physical capabilities.

Clinical Manifestations. The nature of the clinical manifestations depends on the type and severity of the disorder. The primary manifestation is soft, fragile bones that fracture easily. Children with OI tend to have bowing of the long bones and to develop spinal deformities from frequent vertebral fractures; therefore, children with OI tend to be short in stature. The laxity of the ligaments results in joints that are hypermobile and easily dislocated. In the pelvic area the acetabula may protrude.

The facial features of children with OI are typically distinct. The distance between the temporal areas of their skull is wide. However, the rest of the face narrows into a small triangular shape. The base of the skull is soft, broad, and flat, and the anterior fontanel is enlarged, delaying closure. These characteristics of the skull may predispose the child to neurologic problems.

The loose arrangement of the collagen fibers and the subsequent connective tissue disorder affect other body systems. The skin is characterized by a very thin and translucent appearance with signs of vascular fragility and bruising. In fact bruising and edema generally do not occur at fracture sites.

Affected teeth are soft, translucent, and bluish gray to brown. Children with OI also tend to have involvement of the cornea and the bony labyrinth of the middle ear. Some children may present with blue sclerae and tympanic membranes, as well as middle ear deafness.

Systemic manifestations, such as epistaxis and diaphoresis, may also be present. Affected children have difficulty tolerating high temperatures and sometimes have mild hyperpyrexia. Furthermore, tachycardia and tachypnea may be present at rest.

The severity of the clinical manifestations varies. Some newborns have multiple fractures and crushing injuries; other children have a history of occasional fractures. A careful evaluation of the total clinical picture is essential so that these children are not mislabeled as battered.

Diagnostic Studies. Radiologic studies are performed to examine the structure and density of the bones. The findings vary with the type of disorder and the time of the study. X-rays taken in the newborn may not reveal any deformity. Slender, long bones with thin cortices and deformities from multiple fractures may indicate OI.

Recently, Ultrasound studies have revealed some significant abnormalities in children with OI.[54] The collagen fibers of the bone and other tissue are thinner and arranged in a more variable pattern than in healthy children. Excessive levels of glycogen also have been found in the osteoblasts.

★ **ASSESSMENT**

Whenever a child presents with a history of frequent fractures, a complete nursing history is needed. Data should be collected about the family's genetic history and about the birth history of the child. A complete developmental assessment is also important. Even though delays in motor development may be evident, the child's psychosocial

TABLE 62-4
Classification of Osteogenesis Imperfecta

Type and Inheritance	Clinical Manifestations
I Autosomal dominant	Mild bone fragility; fractures usually appear during the preschool years; blue sclerae; deafness by age 20–30; teeth affected in some children
II Autosomal recessive	Fatal during perinatal period; dark blue sclerae; very brittle bones with multiple fractures at birth
III Autosomal recessive	Fractures occur at birth; progressive deformities; normal sclerae and hearing; severe growth failure
IV Autosomal dominant	Mild to moderate bone fragility; variable deformities; normal sclerae; normal hearing; teeth affected in some children

Adapted from Lovell, W. W., & Winter, R. B. (Eds.). (1986). *Pediatric orthopaedics.* Philadelphia: J. B. Lippincott.

development should not be limited. Questioning older children with OI about perceptions of their bodies may reveal important data about their body image and self-esteem.

The parents also may feel threatened and sensitive because of questions about the reasons for their child's frequent fractures. Therefore, it is important that the nurse be sensitive to these feelings when incidents associated with the child's fractures are examined.

The physical assessment should begin with a record of the child's vital signs. Any patterns indicating periods of increased heart and respiratory rate as well as elevated temperature are noteworthy. The skin should be carefully examined for color, elasticity, translucency, and any signs of edema or bruising.

A physical description of the position and appearance of the child's trunk and extremities as well as the facial characteristics is also important. The height of the child in terms of expected growth for chronologic age should be considered. Any signs of scoliosis or laxity of the ligaments are noted. Assessment of range of motion, both actively and passively, may indicate such problems.

A complete assessment of the child's sight and hearing may alert the nurse to sensory problems associated with OI. The appearance of the sclerae and the tympanic membranes should be described. Any defect of the primary and permanent teeth and gums should be noted.

OI is a disorder that involves many body systems. Even though the assessment parameters described are specific for this disorder, the nurse needs to perform a complete psychosocial and physical assessment.

★ NURSING DIAGNOSES AND PLANNING

Children with OI and their families have very specialized needs. Based on assessment data discussed previously and in the preceding chapter, the following nursing diagnoses may apply to the family and child with OI:

- High Risk for Injury (Fractures) related to fragility of bones.
- Pain related to frequent bone fractures and dislocations.
- Impaired Physical Mobility related to frequent fractures and deformities.
- High Risk for Altered Growth and Development related to physical and psychosocial limitations associated with treatment and protection from fractures.
- Fear (Child) related to frequent fractures, pain, and casting procedures.
- Anxiety (Parental) related to safe care of their child.
- Diversional Activity Deficit related to frequent immobilization.
- Altered Family Processes related to the chronic nature of their child's disorder.
- Grieving (Parental) related to preceived loss of their "normal" child.
- Powerlessness (Parental) related to inability to prevent injury to their child.
- Self-Care Deficit related to limited mobility and limb deformity.
- Body Image Disturbance related to feelings about limb deformities.

The nurse and child (or parents) together plan effective care based on the established nursing diagnoses. Several examples of expected outcomes follow:

- The family plans activities to optimize the child's developmental potential.
- The child participates in safe, age-appropriate activities.
- The child performs activities of daily living at the preinjury level.
- The child discusses fears and concerns about injuries and treatment procedures.
- The child and family express feelings about the impact of the disorder on their lives.
- The caretaker returns a demonstration of the care required for the child at home.
- The parents seek genetic counseling.

The nurse plans for the daily care of the child based on physician's orders and nursing diagnoses. Some general nursing care goals may include the following:

- Further injury is prevented.
- The child undergoes a rehabilitation plan to maintain mobility.
- The child returns to preinjury level of mobility following fracture healing.
- The child is free from pain.

★ INTERVENTIONS: COLLABORATIVE AND INDEPENDENT

Because there is no known cure for the disorder, interventions are primarily supportive. To address the variety of needs exhibited by these children, an interdisciplinary approach is essential. The focus of the team is on prevention of further injury and deformity while supporting the child and family through the treatment process. Consequently, many of the interventions are directed toward the education of the family.

MEDICAL MANAGEMENT

The treatment of fractures is often a challenge because of the child's abnormal bone structure and the laxity of the ligaments. Generally, fractures are treated using the closed reduction method and stabilized using a cast or splinting device.

When fractures occur repeatedly in the same area, an intramedullary rod has been effective. With this procedure a telescoping rod that elongates with growth is used to stabilize the fracture. This approach has enabled nonambulatory children to walk by stabilizing the fracture area. However, the possibility that the rod may penetrate the cortex or fail to expand causes further problems. Also, these rods may bend with the impact of falls.

Postoperative care requirements are more extensive for children with OI. These children tend to lose large amounts of fluid through their skin, blood loss often is extensive. In addition any thoracic deformities may impair chest expansion and the ability of the child to effectively cough and deep breathe. Although the standard requirements for a child following orthopedic surgery are followed (see Table 62-3), intensive monitoring of all body systems is needed for at least 24 to 36 hours. These children are discharged from the hospital with some type of cast or splinting device. The nurse must ensure that the parents know how to care for their child in a cast or splint. (See section on Care of a Child in a Cast later in this chapter.)

Splinting devices are generally used to stabilize the bones and protect against additional fractures. They also facilitate ambulation and decrease problems of osteoporosis associated with disuse.[12]

For infants devices such as custom molded contour seating provide support and the beginnings of an upright posture. Standing frames are used to further support an upright position. Special long-leg lightweight braces are available for children who are able to ambulate. Various types of lightweight polypropylene splints also are used for support.

Nurses have a responsibility to help the parents learn how to apply these devices and to watch for any signs of pressure. The principles of skin care discussed in the section on Care of a Child in a Cast later in this chapter also are followed.

SAFETY PROMOTION

Children with OI are always at risk for injury. The challenge for the nurse and the family is to find ways to protect the child without inhibiting physical and psychosocial needs. At the same time the family needs to understand that injuries can occur even without trauma.

Children with OI must be handled very gently. The trunk and extremities need to be supported whenever they are moved. Parents need to be shown how to change a diaper, bathe, dress, and even hold their baby. The nurse can guide the parents to use pillows and blankets for support when holding and cuddling their baby. As parents learn how to safely manage their child's care, their abilities need to be reinforced. Nurses need to allow parents to suggest ways that they can safely care for their child when hospitalized.

If the child is very fragile, the mattress should be firm and the sides of the bed padded. In addition to the usual child-proofing measures, parents need to assess the home environment to ensure that areas are appropriately cushioned and that obstacles are eliminated.

EXERCISING

Physical therapy is advocated for muscle strengthening and prevention of disuse fractures. Exercises that offer light resistance may be part of the plan. Swimming is an excellent sport for children with OI. However, a qualified physical therapist needs to be involved when planning the exercise and ambulation programs.

If complete immobilization is required for healing, gentle physical therapy should be initiated to the unaffected extremities. Efforts to keep the unaffected areas mobile may prevent further fractures.

GROWTH AND DEVELOPMENT PROMOTION

Opportunities for normal exploration of the environment are often limited for the child with OI. Some children may have sensory perceptual deficits related to hearing or vision. Often parents of infants with OI are afraid to provide the tactile stimulation so necessary for development. Therefore, it is essential that the nurse guide the parents to create opportunities to stimulate devel-

opment and reinforce those areas where the parents are already providing stimulation.

Stimulation is important not only for the physical development of the child, but also to build confidence and a sense of well-being. The child with OI suffers many disruptions in life. Besides frequent hospitalizations, the child misses the opportunity to attend school on a regular basis and may be restricted from participating in sports activities. In addition changes in body structure, especially with the approach of adolescence, can be very distressing. Children need to talk about these issues to someone who will let them express their feelings.

The nurse is often the best person to help a child ventilate concerns and fears. Sometimes young children express themselves through artwork. Older children may feel comfortable writing about their experiences. In either instance the nurse needs to be attuned to cues that the child is giving. Thus, activities such as picture drawing and writing may be suggested as positive outlets for expression.

Once the child's feelings are expressed, the nurse can provide anticipatory guidance for the child and family. If the child really wants to participate in a particular sport, the nurse can suggest appropriate alternatives. Children who have milder types of the disorder may participate in an alternate noncontact sport like swimming. The nurse can assist the child and family to find a sports and exercise activity that is satisfying and safe.

PSYCHOSOCIAL SUPPORT

Regardless of the age of the child at the time of diagnosis, the news is always devastating to the family. If the diagnosis occurs soon after the birth of the child, the family is overwhelmed with feelings of grief and despair. If the child is older, the family has probably had to deal with accusations of child abuse each time the child was taken for treatment of a fracture. A nonjudgmental, supportive approach may help the family to express some of their feelings.

A diagnosis of OI brings with it the knowledge that there is a long road ahead for treatment. All members of the family, including the siblings, need to be involved in the care. Despite the extensive care needs of their sibling, other children in the family need to be treated as individuals with their own needs. Some families separate with the burden of such knowledge, but others seem to build stronger bonds. The nurse can direct families to organizations such as the Osteogenesis Imperfecta Foundation, Inc., where they may have contact with families with similar problems. By helping the family to build a stronger support system, the nurse provides a strong foundation for the long-term care of their child.

TEACHING

One of the major responsibilities of the nurse is teaching the family about the disease and the child's abilities. Safety and care of the child following treatment for a fracture were addressed earlier. The family needs to learn that general signs such as fever, irritability, and refusal to eat may be signs of a fracture. The family needs a review of first aid principles for fractures and cast care. (See section on Care of a Child in a Cast later in this chapter.)

In addition the family needs to be taught how to observe for manifestations of the disorder on other body systems. Some of these children may develop cataracts, which limits their vision; others may develop middle ear deafness. Any signs of sensory impairment should be brought to the attention of a physician who is familiar with OI. Parents need to be taught to provide good dental care. These children often have dental involvement, which leads to frequent caries and fillings that will not adhere.

Every time the child comes in contact with a nurse, information about home care should be reinforced. The nurse also can provide anticipatory guidance about age-appropriate safety issues. Each visit with the nurse should be an opportunity to reassess and re-educate the family about needs that may have changed because of the child's age or other situations.

★ EVALUATION

Periodically the nurse and family evaluate the outcomes of care given. The progressive nature of OI requires continuous follow-up care and teaching. The long-term goals for care of the child should be reexamined with the family frequently. If the child's condition has changed significantly, these goals may not be reasonable. The nurse should ensure that follow-up and long-term care is being provided to meet the many needs of these children and their families.

The nurse will probably coordinate the care with other members of the interdisciplinary team. In addition to the follow-up care provided by the orthopedist, children with OI require monitoring by a qualified ophthalmologist and audiologist. Regular visits to these specialists may make detection of vision and hearing problems possible in the early stages. Because of the risk of dental involvement, regular visits to a dentist who is familiar with this disorder are warranted.

Follow-up regarding the families' learning needs should continue with each health care visit. Genetic counseling should be encouraged for the family. Guidance about realistic activity and career planning for the child should be part of the long-term plan. All of these plans, however, must be individualized according to the severity of the child's disorder.

Muscular Dystrophy

Definition and Incidence. The term *muscular dystrophy* refers to a group of congenital disorders characterized by progressive degeneration of muscle fibers without neural or sensory defects. There are approximately 13 pure muscular dystrophies, which are classified by mode of inheritance, age of onset, muscle involvement, and severity of degeneration. The seven most common types affecting the pediatric population are compared in Table 62-5. The most common muscular dystrophy of childhood is Duchenne's muscular dystrophy, also known as pseudohypertrophic muscular dystrophy. It primarily affects boys with an incidence of 1 per 3500. This section focuses on Duchenne's muscular dystrophy.

Etiology and Pathophysiology. More than half of the identified cases of muscular dystrophy are inherited

as a sex-linked recessive trait. The remaining cases appear as spontaneous or fresh mutations. Symptoms usually appear before age 5, after the child has started to ambulate independently. No current mode of therapy has been influential in arresting or reversing the disease process.

Initial muscle weakness and degeneration are noted in the hips, shoulders, and spine. Fat and fibrous tissue replace the normal muscle fibers. Progressive weakness and wasting of symmetric muscle groups occur with increasing deformity. The muscle wasting and weakness eventually involve all the muscle groups, including the respiratory and cardiovascular systems.[13] Death usually occurs during young adulthood as a complication of respiratory infections or cardiac failure.

Clinical Manifestations. Children present to the health care provider with the classic symptoms of Duchenne's muscular dystrophy. The parents state that their child is having difficulty running, riding a bicycle, walking up the stairs, and maintaining the activity level of his or her friends. The child walks with a wide base and waddling gait from affected muscles in the hip girdle; frequent falls are typical. A positive Gowers' sign reveals the necessity for the child to use the upper extremity muscles to compensate for weak hip extensors by "climbing up" his or her legs with the hands until in an upright position (Fig. 62-6).

Shoulder girdle weakness and wasting also are apparent. The child presents with a characteristic "slipping through" of the arms when the examiner attempts to lift the child from under the axilla.[41]

The classic sign of Duchenne's muscular dystrophy is the pseudohypertrophy of the calf muscles. Although these muscles appear healthy and large, in actuality muscle fibers have been replaced with fibrous tissue and fat deposits. Consequently, these muscles have a firm, rubbery consistency.

Children with muscular dystrophy lose the ability to ambulate between the ages of 9 and 12 and, over time, become confined to a wheelchair. The hyperlordosis that is seen initially gradually progresses to include scoliosis and kyphoscoliosis. Mental ability and intelligence testing reveal that children with muscular dystrophy function slightly lower than normal.

Diagnostic Studies. A definitive diagnosis of Duchenne's muscular dystrophy can be made through a combination of clinical manifestations, muscle biopsy, EMG, electrocardiogram, and serum enzyme levels. Muscle biopsy reveals that normal muscle has been replaced by fibrous tissue and fat. Seventy-five percent of these children have abnormal electrocardiograms.

EMG studies denote changes in skeletal musculature and motor neuron deficits. One of the most significant findings in this condition is the extreme increase in serum creatine phosphokinase (CPK), an enzyme normally found in muscle tissue. Because the CPK levels are elevated at birth, Duchenne's muscular dystrophy can be detected in the high-risk male neonatal population. Although CPK levels are grossly elevated at birth, they gradually decline to normal levels as the child approaches young adulthood and death.

TABLE 62-5
Comparison of Major Muscular Dystrophies in Children

Type	Mode of Inheritance	Age of Onset	Muscle Involvement	Severity of Degeneration
Duchenne muscular dystrophy	Sex-linked recessive	3–5 years	Progressive involvement of voluntary and involuntary muscles	Rapid progression with no remission Wheelchair bound by 10 years Death in early 20s
Becker's muscular dystrophy	Sex-linked recessive	Second decade—may occur between 5 and 15 years	Milder variant of Duchenne	Slower progression Prolonged survival Inability to walk by 27 years Death at 42 years but may live to sixth decade
Congenital muscular dystrophy	Autosomal recessive	In utero	Muscle atrophy, hypotonia, muscles of respiration, including diaphragm	Death usually by 1 year
Facioscapulohumeral muscular dystrophy (Landouzy-Dejerine)	Autosomal dominant	Second decade	Weakness and atrophy of facial and shoulder girdle muscles	Slow progression compatible with normal life span Most benign form
Limb-girdle muscular dystrophy (also juvenile dystrophy of Erb)	Autosomal recessive	Late childhood, adolescence, or adulthood	Proximal muscles of pelvic and shoulder girdle	Variable progression but usually slow Disability may be minimal or may be incapacitating May reach advanced age
Ocular myopathy	Not clear	Childhood or adolescence	Extraocular muscles	Progressive ophthalmoplegia Pigmentary degeneration of retina Heart block Progressive ataxia Nerve deafness Growth retardation Sudden death possible due to cardiac conduction defect
Myotonic dystrophy (Steinert's disease)	Autosomal dominant	Commonly in young adulthood Can begin in infancy, childhood, or adolescence	Distal extremities Weakness and atrophy Poor suck and hypotonia in infants In children facial, jaw, and temporalis muscle weakness Bilateral ptosis	Guarded prognosis in children Disability usually severe in 15–20 yrs. after onset Rarely obtain normal life span

★ ASSESSMENT

Assessment begins by identifying families that are at risk for Duchenne's muscular dystrophy. A thorough nursing history is needed to determine when the child started to manifest the symptoms of muscular dystrophy. Ongoing assessment is necessary to help the family work through their anger and anticipatory grief. It is especially important to determine how long the child has remained ambulatory, the degree of muscle weakness and hip contracture, and quality of respiratory function. Questioning the child about the presence of headaches, nightmares, difficulty sleeping, fatigue or daytime somnolence, difficulty chewing or swallowing, and weight loss may alert the nurse to the insidious beginning of respiratory failure.[18]

★ NURSING DIAGNOSES AND PLANNING

Based on assessment data discussed previously and in the preceding chapter, the following nursing diagnoses

may apply to the family and child with Duchenne's muscular dystrophy:

- Constipation related to immobility.
- Impaired Gas Exchange related to weak respiratory musculature.
- Spiritual Distress related to a fatal disease.
- Impaired Physical Mobility related to altered musculature.
- Altered Growth and Development related to musculoskeletal impairment.
- Self-Care Deficit related to progression of disease.
- Powerlessness related to lack of control over the outcome of the disease.
- Anticipatory Grieving related to terminal illness.
- Altered Nutrition: More Than Body Requirements related to sedentary lifestyle.

The nurse and child (or parents) together plan effective care based on the established nursing diagnoses. Several examples of expected outcomes follow:

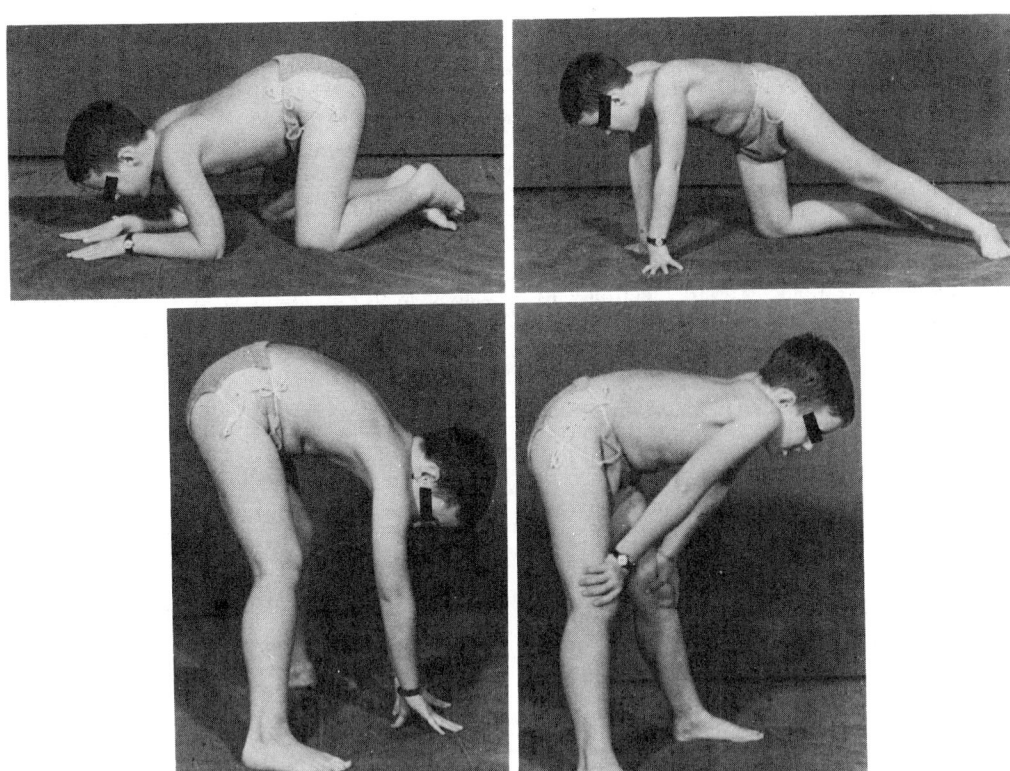

FIGURE 62-6
Gowers' sign. A series of maneuvers is necessary to achieve an upright posture in all types of pelvic and trunk weakness. The child climbs up his or her legs when rising from the floor. (Morrissy, R. T. [Ed.]. [1990]. Lovell and Winter's pediatric orthopaedics [3rd ed.]. [Vol. I]. Philadelphia: J. B. Lippincott.)

- The parents participate in the child's exercise program.
- The parents obtain assistive devices as suggested.
- The parents construct a nutritional daily dietary program for the child.
- The parents state they have scheduled genetic counseling.
- The parents discuss their feelings of guilt, frustration, anxiety, fear, and hopelessness.

The nurse plans for the daily care of the child based on physician's orders and nursing diagnoses. A general nursing care goal may include the following:

- The child remains ambulatory as long as possible.

The primary goal of treatment is to help the child and family accept the limitations on their lifestyle that the disease will impose, while encouraging independence, ambulation, and socialization for as long as possible. Attention is focused on keeping the child ambulatory as long as possible.

★ INTERVENTIONS: COLLABORATIVE
AND INDEPENDENT

Because there is no effective treatment for Duchenne's muscular dystrophy, only palliative interventions can help prolong function and longevity. An interdisciplinary approach to helping the child and family accept this incapacitating, progressive, fatal disease is recommended. The nurse often acts as a coordinator for the various aspects of care.

OCCUPATIONAL AND PHYSICAL THERAPY

Exercise is very important to maintain muscle strength and prevent contractures. Teaching the family passive range-of-motion exercises and active resistance exercises can help to prevent joint contractures that are common to children with muscular dystrophy. Occupational therapists can suggest assistive devices, such as Velcro closures on clothes and shoes, elevated commode seats, and bathtub rails.

NUTRITIONAL MANAGEMENT

Dietary consultations are recommended because children who are wheelchair bound are at risk for obesity secondary to immobility. Increased fluid intake is encouraged to prevent urinary stasis and bladder infections.

RESPIRATORY THERAPY

Respiratory therapists can teach diaphragmatic breathing techniques and postural drainage to help compensate for respiratory muscle weakness. Effective airway clearance will help to minimize the risk of pneumonia.

SURGICAL INTERVENTION

Surgical interventions are indicated when the child loses the ability to ambulate. Heel cord lengthening, release of hip flexor muscles, and spinal instrumentation are indicated to maintain posture in children with Duchenne's muscular dystrophy. In addition to the standard nursing interventions following orthopedic surgery, these children need aggressive mobilization, range-of-motion exercises, and pulmonary exercises to prevent muscle weakness, atrophy, and respiratory failure. Approximately 3% of the child's muscle strength will be lost per day if he or she is kept on bedrest.[41]

COUNSELING

If there is a family history of Duchenne's muscular dystrophy, parents are encouraged to seek genetic counseling. Elevated CPK levels in female carriers can be detected with 70% to 80% accuracy. Greater accuracy in detecting the female carrier status can be accomplished with phosphorylation of erythrocyte protein and genetic markers.

Grief counseling may be indicated because muscular dystrophy is a fatal disease. Feelings of guilt, frustration, anxiety, fear, and hopelessness should be addressed during clinic visits.

★ EVALUATION

Periodically, the nurse and family evaluate the outcomes of care given. Examples of outcomes for the child and family with Duchenne's muscular dystrophy were given under Nursing Diagnoses and Planning in this section. Have short-term goals been met? Are long-term goals still realistic?

LONG-TERM CARE

Ongoing evaluation of the child and family is necessary to ensure that the goals are met. Maintaining adequate respiratory function and social interactions and normalizing the child's life as much as possible will assist the family during the course of the disease. Emotional support, grief counseling, and parent support groups can assist families in accepting the outcome of this fatal disorder.

Disorders Related to Musculoskeletal Growth

This group of disorders includes a variety of conditions that occur during periods of rapid growth. These disorders directly affect the musculoskeletal system by causing changes to the epiphysis, the structure of the musculoskeletal system, or the composition of the bones. Generally these disorders occur during childhood before skeletal maturity is reached. With all of these disorders there is a possibility of skeletal deformity even with the initiation of prompt treatment. The associated sequelae can be present throughout the remainder of the child's life.

Legg-Calvé-Perthes Disease*

Definition and Incidence. Legg-Calvé-Perthes disease (LCPD) is referred to as Perthes disease, Legg-Perthes disease, osteochondritis deformans juvenilis, and coxa plana. In this disease the proximal femoral epiphysis

* This section was written by Marilyn L. Boos, MS, RN.

of the femur becomes avascular, dies, and is then gradually replaced by living bone.

LCPD is relatively common, appearing between the ages of 3 and 10 years. Peak incidence is around 6 years. Boys are affected about four times as often as girls. It occurs with equal frequency in the left or right hip, and bilateral involvement occurs in 15% of those affected.[3]

Etiology and Pathophysiology. While the exact cause is unknown, it is generally agreed that LCPD is caused by an interruption of the blood supply to the growing proximal femoral epiphysis. Hormonal, genetic, infectious, and traumatic factors may play a role also. Perhaps the most plausible theory is that synovitis of the hip joint causes increased pressure within the hip capsule. Repeated episodes of synovitis or increased pressure cause tamponade of retinacular vessels and decreased blood supply to the epiphysis.[53]

LCPD, a self-limited condition, proceeds through the cycle of avascular necrosis, revascularization, resorption of necrotic bone, and replacement of living bone. The process is predictable and takes 3 to 4 years. Table 62-6 describes the stages of LCPD referred to by Bowen and Miller.[3]

Clinical Manifestations. One of the earliest symptoms of LCPD is a limp that may or may not be painful. Symptoms are insidous, but a history of trauma can be obtained in approximately one third of patients. Pain of long-standing (several months') duration can be elicited on questioning. Pain may be exacerbated by running, walking, or engaging in increased activities or movement. The pain may radiate to the groin, anterior thigh, or knee. Rest provides relief from pain.

Observation of gait demonstrates a limp with less time spent in weight bearing on the affected side. Motion is limited, particularly abduction and internal rotation. Symptoms usually are mild. Parents may note a child who is typically active seeking out rest periods. Parents frequently do not seek immediate treatment of attention for many weeks after the clinical onset.

Diagnostic Studies. The diagnosis and follow-up is made by radiographic evaluation. Because the condition follows the stages in Table 62-6, it is important that the radiographs be reviewed sequentially to evaluate the stage and degree of femoral head involvement. Arthrography is used mainly to determine the shape of the femoral head and the degree of flattening that has occurred. The relationship of the femoral head to the acetabulum is also studied. Bone scans are helpful in determining the extent of epiphyseal involvement. CT scans and MRI may be used to evaluate the involvement of the femoral head.

★ ASSESSMENT

The nurse plays a significant role in the assessment of the child who presents with a typical history of LCPD. The school nurse in particular can easily observe children who display persistent symptoms. Discomfort in the hip is increased by activity, running, or walking. Pain, when it is present or acknowledged, occurs in the knee, groin, or thigh, but it is usually relieved by rest. A typically active

TABLE 62-6
Stages of Cycle of Legg-Calvé-Perthes Disease

Stage	Action	Description	Duration
1	Necrotic stage	Joint capsule bulges secondary to synovitis. Infarctions appear in bony epiphysis. Articular cartilage continues to grow, but growth is asymmetric. Avascular femoral epiphysis cannot support the usual mechanical stress and vertical compression, and the epiphysis is reduced in height.	5.7 months
2	Fragmentation stage	Necrotic tissue is resorbed, and fibrocartilage fills in resorbed areas. Femoral epiphysis may deform with resulting femoral neck widening.	7 months
3	Reossification stage	Reossification occurs, and normal bony density returns. Alterations in femoral neck shape become apparent.	20–38 months
4	Remodeling	Head continues to remodel until child reaches skeletal maturity.	

child who frequently seeks out rest periods during physical activity suggests that something may not be right. In addition a persistent limp with or without pain may be observed. Trauma may be part of the history. Of particular concern is the child with persistent symptoms.

Range of motion can be assessed by the nurse. Typically, the child with LCPD has limitation in abduction and external rotation. Abduction is assessed by placing the child on the back with hips flexed. A limitation in abduction is present in the affected hip. Internal rotation is assessed by placing the child on the abdomen, with the knees flexed. The hip can be internally rotated by moving the lower leg away from the midline. The nurse who observes any of these signs and symptoms should discuss concerns with the parents.

The nurse must assess the family's understanding of the long-term nature of the treatment plan for LCPD and the importance of completing the prescribed therapy.

★ NURSING DIAGNOSES AND PLANNING

Based on assessment data discussed previously and in the preceding chapter, the following nursing diagnoses may apply to the family and child with LCPD.

- High Risk for Injury (Neurovascular Compromise) related to improper application of traction, cast or brace, and pressure over peripheral nerves.
- Impaired Physical Mobility related to condition and treatment.
- High Risk for Impaired Skin Integrity related to treatment.
- Anxiety related to knowledge deficit about disease process, treatment protocol, and developmental issues related to treatment.

The nurse and child (or parents) together plan effective care based on the established nursing diagnoses. Several examples of expected outcomes follow:

- The child returns to school.
- The family states friends come to visit the child at home.
- The parents state the signs and symptoms of potential problems.
- The parents demonstrate proper application of mechanical devices.

- The parents exhibit acceptable techniques of neurovascular assessment.

The nurse plans for the daily care of the child based on physician's orders and nursing diagnoses. Some general nursing care goals may include the following:

- Deformity of the femoral head and acetabulum is minimized.
- Full range of motion of the hip is attained and maintained.
- The head of the femur is contained within the acetabulum.

★ INTERVENTIONS: COLLABORATIVE AND INDEPENDENT

MEDICAL MANAGEMENT

Treatment in the past emphasized prolonged non–weight bearing. The hope was that the hip would reform in a round configuration, corresponding to the contours of the uninvolved acetabulum. The process of reformation of the femoral head with new bone takes 18 to 36 months, which is a long time to keep the child on bedrest.

The principal treatment has changed from non–weight bearing to containment. In this plan of management the avascular segments of the femoral head must remain beneath the coverage of the acetabulum during the period of reformation. The idea is that containment will cause the new femoral head to be congruent with the femoral head, making a joint that glides smoothly through a range of motion. At present the principle of containment seems to be valid with improved long-term results.

Containment and the method by which it is achieved are controversial. When only small portions of the femoral head, such as the anteromedial portion, are affected by avascular necrosis, no treatment is required. The femoral head will reform in a contained and congruent fashion.

When the lateral portion of the femoral head or the whole head is involved in the avascular process, approaches vary. Prolonged bracing in devices that hold the avascular parts of the head beneath the bony acetabulum seems to be effective in producing a congruent joint.

Compliance with a bracing program by parents and patients is essential to achieve a good result.

Osteotomies of the pelvis or the proximal femur to give better lateral coverage of the reforming femoral head offer an advantage of shorter overall immobilization time compared to bracing. There is considerable controversy about the long-term results of operative containment compared to bracing.

RANGE-OF-MOTION PROMOTION

Painless range of motion is accomplished by physical therapy and generally by administering nonsteroidal anti-inflammatory drugs, such as aspirin. A non–weight bearing position using skin traction with the hips in progressive abduction aids in range of motion. The child may or may not be hospitalized at this time. Serial casts, such as the Petrie or broomstick casts, may be used to achieve abduction. Containment methods of treatment include abduction orthosis (Fig. 62-7), casts, braces, or surgery. (See traction, section on Care of a Child in a Cast later in this chapter, and Table 62-3 earlier in this chapter for nursing care requirements following orthopedic surgery.)

GROWTH AND DEVELOPMENT PROMOTION

Because school is a significant focus in the child's life and peer and social activities occur daily in the school environment, it is important that the child return to school as soon as possible. With planning the child may return to school in most cases. The school nurse is the contact person to assist in ensuring that the environment is safe and accessible. Students with LCPD may return to school in a brace or cast, ambulatory with or without crutches, or in a wheelchair. The child may need an elevator, or someone may be needed to assist with toileting. Special transportation may be necessary to accommodate the

child in a Petrie cast or brace. The nurse works closely with the school nurse to make an easy transition.

The child who cannot return to school needs encouragement in maintaining peer contacts, and the family is encouraged to arrange contacts with friends. The developmental level of the child provides guidance in the type of activities that will be enjoyed if physical limitations become a short-term problem.

Family coping may be a problem if the child is unable to attend school. Parents who work outside the home may find it necessary to make arrangements for someone to stay in the home with the child.

TEACHING

The location of the treatment site determines the teaching to be carried out. If in the hospital, the family can easily be instructed in skin care, safety in the use of the various treatment modalities, neurovascular assessment, and the importance of fostering normal growth and development. The family should be taught room exercises and the signs and symptoms of potential problems, such as decreasing abduction and internal rotation. Correct application of all devices is stressed. The family is given reference materials with detailed information so that the treatment plan can be followed at home.

The importance of neurovascular assessment for anyone in a brace, cast, or traction cannot be overemphasized. A feared complication known as compartment syndrome is described in Table 62-7 and considered an emergency. Application of corrective devices and therapeutic skin care should be taught well. Making the home environment safe and accessible also is a major nursing concern.

Because most of the care of the child with LCPD occurs in the home, the nurse who initially teaches the family must determine if a home care nursing referral is nec-

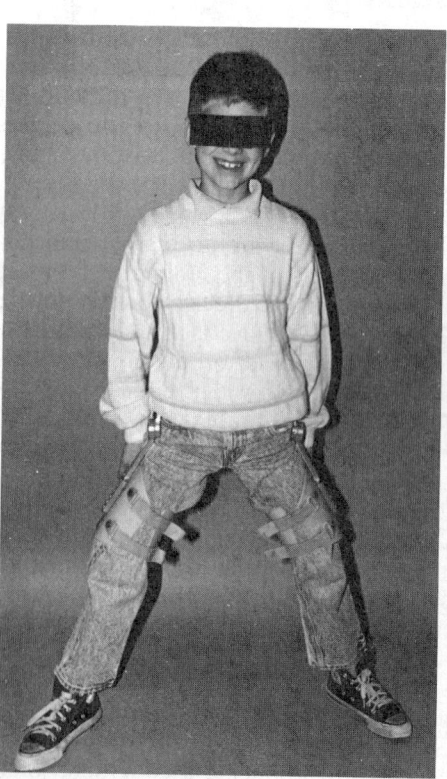
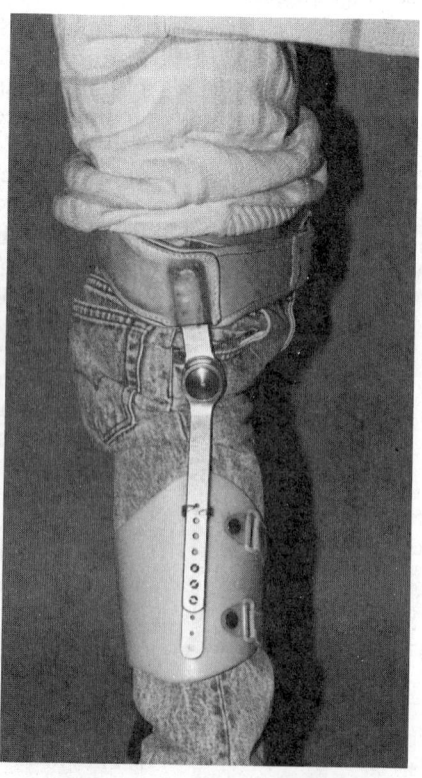

FIGURE 62-7

An abduction orthosis provides for containment by abduction but allows free motion of the knee and ankle. (Morrissy, R. T. [Ed.]. [1990]. Lovell and Winter's pediatric orthopaedics [3rd ed.]. [Vol. II]. Philadelphia: J. B. Lippincott.)

TABLE 62-7
Major Complications of Fractures

Complication	Etiology	Clinical Manifestations	Interventions
Neurovascular impairment	Restriction of circulation and nerve function resulting from injury or the immobilizing device	Absence of pulse distal to the injury, discoloration, edema, pain, decreased sensory and motor function	Release of pressure by bivalving or windowing cast (if physician is not available, the nurse MUST perform this procedure)
Compartment syndrome	Excessive swelling around injury site, causing increased pressure in a closed compartment; fascia (covers and separates muscles) unable to compensate for increased edema	Severe pain (unrelieved by medication) and with passive motion; paresthesia, diminished reflexes, loss of motor function; peripheral pulses distal to injury may remain normal (different from neurovascular compromise)	Elevation of extremity and release of constricting devices; monitoring of pressures with a small catheter; fasciotomy if pressure is not relieved
Volkmann contracture	Massive infarction of muscle resulting from arterial occlusion to the area	Pallor or cyanosis; absence of pulses; edema, loss of sensation, sometimes severe pain	Removal of constricting devices and extension of joint; surgery may be needed to increase blood supply to area
Fat emboli	Fat globules from the fracture site (major long bones) released into systemic circulation and sometimes lodge in lung capillaries	Rapid onset; occurs within first 24–72 hours postinjury; restlessness, dyspnea, substernal chest pain, tachycardia, low-grade fever, diaphoresis, pallor, cyanosis	Child placed in semi-Fowler's position; oxygen administered; and respiratory support provided

essary. The referring nurse must also ensure that the home care agency understands the treatment protocol.

⭐ **EVALUATION**

The various stages in the treatment of LCPD can take as long as 3 to 4 years. The outcome is determined by the final shape of the head of the femur. Prognosis depends on the extent of the femoral head involvement, the age of the child at onset, and compliance and follow through with the treatment plan. The best results generally occur when less than 50% of the femoral head is affected and when the result is a more spheric femoral head. The younger the child, the better the results. Despite treatment, however, this condition can become progressively worse.

At each office or ambulatory care visit, the nurse should ensure that the family is correctly performing neurovascular assessment and cast or brace care. The parents should be asked to demonstrate all activities, and teaching needs are reviewed.

Osgood-Schlatter Disease

Although Osgood-Schlatter disease is classified with other juvenile osteochondroses, it is not considered a true osteochondrosis. The disorder has been referred to as a tendonitis of the distal portion of the patellar tendon. The disease is characterized by a partial separation of the tibial tuberosity. The separation may be caused by sudden or continuous stress on the patellar tendon during periods of rapid growth. Some theories suggest that flexion of the knee against a tight quadriceps may precipitate the problem.

The condition usually presents itself in boys between the ages of 10 and 16 who are active in sports. Manifes-

tations of the disorder include pain in the anterior portion of the knee with inflammation and thickening of the patellar tendon. The pain is exacerbated by activities that promote exertion of the anterior knee or tibial tubercle and subsides with cessation of the activity. Generally, no fluid in the knee is palpable. The patella may be displaced anteriorly and there may be prominence of the involved tubercle. The disorder is self-limiting and resolves with closure of the growth plate.

Adolescents with Osgood-Schlatter disease are usually treated in an ambulatory care setting. The goal of treatment is to prevent further irritation during the healing process. Conservative treatment includes rest and discontinuation of the activity that causes pain. Although this disorder can be considered mild, it is often very distressing to the adolescent who is actively involved in sports programs. The nurse assists the adolescent in making decisions about lifestyle alterations until healing has occurred. Aspirin or ibuprofen therapy is often helpful to relieve the discomfort. The adolescent will probably respond to some type of physical therapy program during this period of immobilization. Maintaining muscle tone in the athletic adolescent enhances body image and feelings of self-esteem.

More intensive treatment may be needed if rest and analgesics do not resolve the discomfort. Sometimes casts or braces are applied to ensure immobilization of the extremity. If bony fragments are present in the patellar tendon, surgery may be necessary.

Following treatment, the adolescent may begin to return to usual activities. Sometimes the affected knee needs to be strapped to prevent discomfort. By the time the adolescent reaches 18 years of age, the problem should resolve. However, the patella on the affected side may remain elevated, and lateral dislocation of the knee may occur. If complete healing has not occurred before the adolescent returns to normal activities, degenerative arthritis may occur.

Slipped Capital Femoral Epiphysis

Definition and Incidence. Slipped capital femoral epiphysis (SCFE) is the displacement of the femoral head from the femoral neck at the epiphyseal plate. The femoral neck rotates externally and slides upward, while the femoral head remains in the acetabulum (Fig. 62-8). Slippage is classified according to the amount of displacement and can be acute or chronic.

The incidence of SCFE is closely linked to puberty and the rapid growth that occurs in early adolescence. The disorder is seen two to three times more often in boys. The incidence also is higher in African Americans.[34] A significant number of adolescents will have bilateral SCFE.

Etiology and Pathophysiology. The exact cause of the slippage of the upper epiphysis is unknown. Children who are overweight and large or tall and thin are at risk for this disorder. Other identified factors include trauma, inflammation or autoimmune response, and intrinsic malformation of the epiphyseal plate. Adolescent endocrine factors, such as an imbalance between excessive growth hormone and insufficient estrogen or testosterone, have been cited as predisposing factors. Weakening of the epiphyseal plate also occurs during the adolescent growth spurt, thus rendering the epiphyseal line weak and vulnerable to slippage. Because a family history has been associated with the disorder, genetic factors may also contribute to the problem.

When this disorder occurs the femoral shaft externally rotates away from the epiphysis or the femoral head. As this process continues, the epiphyseal plate appears to slip posteriorly and the femoral neck changes shape and contour. In severe situations the femoral shaft may completely separate from the epiphyseal plate and press against the acetabulum.

Blood supply to the femoral neck remains intact as long as the slippage is chronic. During an acute slippage the blood supply to the femoral neck is interrupted and may result in avascular necrosis of the femoral head and neck. Chondrolysis also may occur as a complication of this disorder. With chondrolysis the cartilage of both the femoral head and acetabulum is destroyed. Regardless of the position of the femoral head, remodeling of the femoral head will occur spontaneously, and if untreated, deformity may result.

Clinical Manifestations. Any child who presents with complaints of pain, limping without any significant injury, and loss of hip motion especially with internal rotation should be suspect for SCFE. Referred pain may include the knee, thigh, and hip. If the etiology is traumatic and acute, the presenting symptoms may be severe pain and inability to bear weight on the affected side.

With SCFE the hip externally rotates with flexion. Abduction and internal rotation also is limited. Any attempts to position the hip will cause severe pain in the groin area. This pain is associated with the synovitis that accompanies the disorder.

Diagnostic Studies. Roentgenographic studies confirm the diagnosis of SCFE. Anteroposterior views of the hip may reveal a widening of the epiphyseal line and changes in the contour of the femoral head and neck. A biplanar or frog leg view should always be included in the diagnostic studies because anteroposterior views may miss the initial posterior slippage.

★ **ASSESSMENT**

Any pubescent child who complains of hip or leg pain and walks with a limp should be carefully screened for SCFE. Questions about trauma or sports injuries should be included in the assessment process. The nurse should assess the onset and severity of pain and the child's ability to bear weight.

Physical assessment includes an examination of the range of motion of the affected extremity. Assisting the child to move the leg through range of motion can help determine the degree of limitation. When the thigh is flexed, limitations in internal rotation and abduction are noted. When chronic slippage occurs, thigh atrophy and shortening of the affected leg also can be observed.

★ **NURSING DIAGNOSES AND PLANNING**

Based on assessment data discussed previously and in the preceding chapter, the following nursing diagnoses may apply to the family and adolescent with SCFE:

FIGURE 62-8

In slipped capital femoral epiphysis, the hip rotates externally as it is flexed by the examiner. (Oski, F. A., DeAngelis, C. D., Feigin, R. D., & Warshaw, J. B. [Eds.]. [1990]. *Principles and practice of pediatrics*. Philadelphia: J. B. Lippincott.)

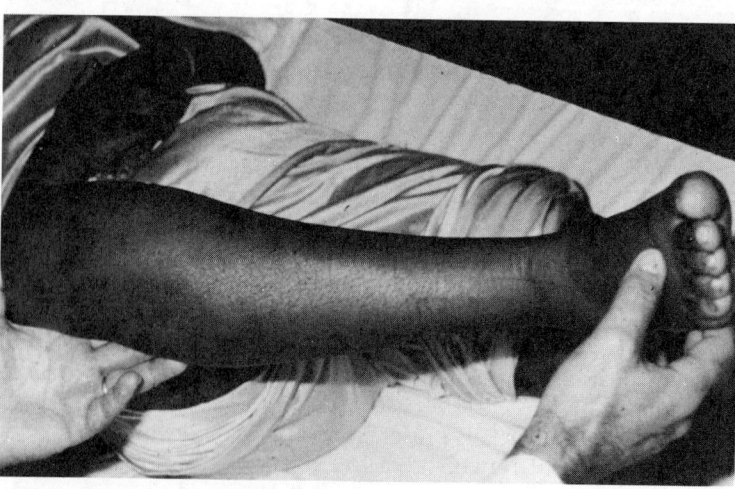

- Pain related to slippage of the femoral epiphyses.
- Impaired Physical Mobility related to imposed bedrest and treatment restrictions.
- Body Image Disturbance related to changes in body structure and function during a critical period of psychosocial development.
- Altered Growth and Development related to altered bone structure and disturbance to the epiphysis.

The nurse and adolescent (or parents) together plan effective care based on the established nursing diagnoses. Several examples of expected outcomes follow:

- The adolescent expresses feelings about body image.
- The family demonstrates care of the adolescent in hip spica cast.
- The adolescent participates in age-appropriate developmental activities.
- The adolescent participates in nutritional meal planning.

The nurse plans for the daily care of the child based on physician's orders and nursing diagnoses. A general nursing care goal may include the following:

- Further slippage is prevented.

★ INTERVENTIONS: COLLABORATIVE AND INDEPENDENT

Early detection and treatment is essential to prevent hip abnormalities and degenerative bone changes.

The parents and the child should be aware that the overall goal for treatment is to prevent further slippage and avoid avascular necrosis and chondrolysis. The nurse works closely with the child and family to ensure that all aspects of the treatment plan are understood and followed. At the same time it is important that the child be encouraged to express feelings about body image.

As soon as SCFE is detected, the child is told not to bear weight on the affected side. The overall treatment plan is dependent on the severity of the slippage. Sometimes the child may be placed in traction to gently return the epiphysis to the normal position and decrease muscle contractions. Various types of surgical stabilization and correction of the deformity are possible. Internal fixation by pinning is used to stabilize the femoral head and neck. Using a percutaneous technique, the fixation device can be accurately placed without requiring a long hospitalization.[34] When this procedure is used, individuals with chronic slips can be stabilized and begin to bear weight within 1 to 2 weeks. The nurse should reinforce any instruction that is given to the child about crutch walking and teach the family about safety issues.

Individuals with more severe acute slips usually require at least 6 weeks of immobilization. A severely displaced epiphysis may require osteotomies to correct the deformity or, in rare cases, a total joint replacement. Regardless of the type of surgical procedure, the nurse is involved in providing preoperative instruction and postoperative care. The principles of postoperative nursing care are outlined in Table 62-3. If extended immobilization is required following surgery, a hip spica cast is applied. The nurse must teach the family how to care for the adolescent in a hip spica cast. (See section on Care of a Child in a Cast later in this chapter.) This responsibility may be very challenging for the family because of the size of the child and the weight of the cast.

Because of impaired mobility and treatment options, such as pin fixation, bedrest, and spica casting, psychosocial issues such as embarrassment, change in body image, and social isolation need to be addressed. The child is placed in a dependent position at a time when independence is so important, and any opportunity for independence must be supported. Ventilation of feelings about these imposed restrictions on lifestyle and changing body image should be encouraged. The nurse also should encourage continued involvement with school work so that the child does not fall behind in his or her studies. Follow-up with school counselors can help the child to maintain his or her grade status.

Dietary and nutritional counseling is indicated for children who are overweight. The nurse needs to stress the relationship between obesity and stress on the joints and muscles. Encouraging the child's input with meal planning may help to encourage compliance and weight loss.

★ EVALUATION

Because slippage may occur in the opposite hip, the child and family should be taught how to recognize the signs and symptoms of a SCFE. Any pain or symptoms of decreased range of motion should be reported to the orthopedist.

Follow-up is continued until the growth plate closes. If there is premature closure of the growth plate, growth retardation and deformity may occur. During this period the child is monitored for any signs of avascular necrosis or chondrolysis. Even with prompt treatment, these children may develop osteoarthritis or degenerative hip problems as they age.

Limb-Length Discrepancy

Definition and Incidence. Many people have minor variations in the length of the lower limbs. Discrepancies up to 2 cm usually can be treated with shoe orthotics or can be ignored. When the discrepancy is greater than 2 cm, surgical intervention is indicated regardless of the cause. Limb length discrepancy (LLD) is not selective according to race or gender.

Etiology and Pathophysiology. LLD can be categorized three ways: those that cause a difference in length but not growth rate, those that cause a difference in growth rate but not initially in length, or a combination of both.[33] There are six main etiologies associated with limb length discrepancies, as listed in Table 62-8. Poliomyelitis used to be a major cause of LLD, but this viral disease has been virtually eradicated from the United States since the discovery of the polio vaccine.

The area of bone most sensitive to alteration is the physeal plate or growth center.[24] Depending on the cause and extent of injury to this area, irreparable damage may result in complete growth arrest. Conversely, any condition that causes hyperemia to the limb or excessive

TABLE 62-8
Causes of Limb-Length Discrepancy

Cause	Shortening	Lengthening
Congenital	Hemiatrophy	Vascular malformations
	Skeletal dysplasias	
Infection	Growth plate damage from osteomyelitis	Metaphyseal osteomyelitis
		Septic arthritis
Paralysis	Poliomyelitis	
Tumors	Echondromatosis	Hemangioma
	Osteochondromatosis	Neurofibromatosis
Trauma	Growth plate damage	Healing fractures
	Overriding fractures	Diaphyseal operations
Other	Legg-Perthes disease	
	Slipped capital femoral epiphysis	
	Radiation therapy	

proliferation of physeal growth cartilage can cause overgrowth of that limb.

Clinical Manifestations. The degree of limping is related to the difference in the length of the lower limbs. The typical gait of the child with LLD is characterized by a stepping down onto the short leg and vaulting over the long limb.[36] This atypical gait leads a child to flex the knee of the long limb or walk on the toes of the short limb. This pattern of walking causes fatigue and increased energy expenditure during ambulation.

Scoliosis may result from the pelvic obliquity, which tilts the lumbosacral junction. This postural scoliosis disappears when the child is seated or blocks are placed under the short leg to compensate for the difference. There also is a correlation between uncorrected LLD and low back pain later in life.

Diagnostic Studies. Diagnostic studies are initiated to distinguish between an apparent and an absolute (true) LLD. To determine the mode of treatment for the child, accurate measurements of the limbs are essential. Serial x-rays predict future growth patterns based on the child's skeletal age.

Limb length can be measured by various types of roentgenograms. Results show the amount of discrepancy between the legs and the location of the discrepancy. Single exposures of both legs produce a long film that is beneficial for children who cannot be still for multiple exposures. Multiple-exposure films can be more accurate, but most children have difficulty remaining quiet for long periods of time.

Deformities also can be measured by placing premeasured blocks under the short leg until the pelvis is level. Photographs are taken showing the level pelvis and the amount of blocks necessary to achieve this. CT scans are an effective method of measuring LLD. A combination of these four methods of evaluating LLD can facilitate identification of correction goals.

★ ASSESSMENT

When assessing a child with LLD it is important to view the child holistically instead of strictly from a structural perspective. While the physician evaluates multiple factors to determine the appropriate treatment option, the nurse assesses the functional health patterns of the child and family. The nurse is particularly concerned with the child's ability to handle the treatment requirements and restrictions.

Attention is given to the child's psychologic makeup. Many of the treatment regimens require the child's complete cooperation. Assessment of the child's level of independence and ability to follow instructions is essential. The nurse also needs to examine the impact of the deformity on the child's lifestyle and self-esteem. Many children with deformities look for a guarantee that surgical correction will cure them of their disfigurement. Nurses must point out that outcomes of surgical intervention are never entirely certain. While girls may be content being shorter than their peers, boys may prefer a limb-lengthening procedure rather than a shortening one.

Physical assessment includes a description of the child's limb as well as gait. Measurement of the discrepancy from the anterosuperior iliac spine to the medial malleolus reveals the absolute discrepancy. The apparent discrepancy is measured from the umbilicus to the medial malleolus. Any limitations in motion should be noted. Observation of the child standing with both feet flat on the ground reveals any associated postural deviations between the iliac crests, knees, and ankles. Any deviations in the skeletal structure resulting from compensatory mechanisms also should be described.

A baseline assessment of vital signs and neurovascular status is important for comparison following surgery. Hypertension has been associated with some of the limb-lengthening procedures.

★ NURSING DIAGNOSES AND PLANNING

Many of the nursing diagnoses will be determined by the mode of treatment selected. Based on assessment data discussed previously and in the preceding chapter, the following nursing diagnoses may apply to the family and child with an LLD:

* Activity Intolerance related to energy expenditure during ambulation.
* Altered Growth and Development related to discrepancy in limb length.
* Body Image Disturbance related to feelings about discrepancy in limb length.
* Anxiety related to lack of knowledge of treatment parameters and surgical intervention.
* High Risk for Infection related to limb-lengthening devices.
* Impaired Physical Mobility related to alteration in lower limb and treatment limitations.
* Impaired Tissue Integrity related to insertion site of external fixator.
* High Risk for Injury related to position of the limb lengthening and the need to ambulate.

The nurse and child (or parents) together plan effective care based on the established nursing diagnoses. Several examples of expected outcomes follow:

- The child uses a shoe prosthesis.
- The child states he or she is resuming activities of daily living.
- The child states he or she is using leg exercises.
- The child demonstrates an understanding of proper patient-controlled analgesia (PCA) following surgery.
- The child performs range-of-motion exercises.
- The parents demonstrate knowledge of care of pin site.
- The parents and child discuss safety in the home and school.

The nurse plans for the daily care of the child based on physician's orders and nursing diagnoses. Some general nursing care goals may include the following:

- The discrepancy in limb length is decreased.
- The child's mobility is improved.
- Structural and postural deformities are prevented.

★ INTERVENTIONS: COLLABORATIVE AND INDEPENDENT

Many methods are available for correction of an LLD. The projected discrepancy at skeletal maturity is the major premise for determining which method will be used. Treatment options are either nonsurgical or surgical. If the LLD is less than 2 cm, intervention is not advocated. The discrepancy should not cause any deleterious effects on the child's growth or ability to ambulate.

Nonsurgical interventions are used when the discrepancy is between 2 and 5 cm. These interventions include heel or shoe lifts and extension prostheses that add stability to the ankle and are more acceptable for cosmetic reasons. Nurses should encourage the child to wear the prosthesis to facilitate normal activity levels and growth and development. Unsightly prostheses and shoe orthoses make noncompliance a problem with adolescents.

SURGICAL MANAGEMENT

Surgical interventions include shortening the long leg, lengthening the short leg, or a combination of both. During the growth period, limb shortening can be accomplished through epiphysiodesis or surgical destruction of the growth plate of the longer leg. Correction of the LLD is achieved by normal growth of the short leg with interruption of growth in the longer leg. Nursing care requirements are the same as those for any child undergoing an orthopedic procedure followed by immobilization in a cast.

EXTERNAL FIXATION DEVICES

Mechanical devices have been shown to be very effective in limb length equalization. The Wagner lengthening apparatus is used for children with LLD greater than 6 cm.[48] Other criteria include a stable hip joint, range of motion of the knee, intact musculature and soft tissue to the thigh, and no vascular compromise to the short leg. The surgery is performed in three steps and requires long periods of hospitalization, several months of rehabilitation, and years of avoiding contact sports and activities.

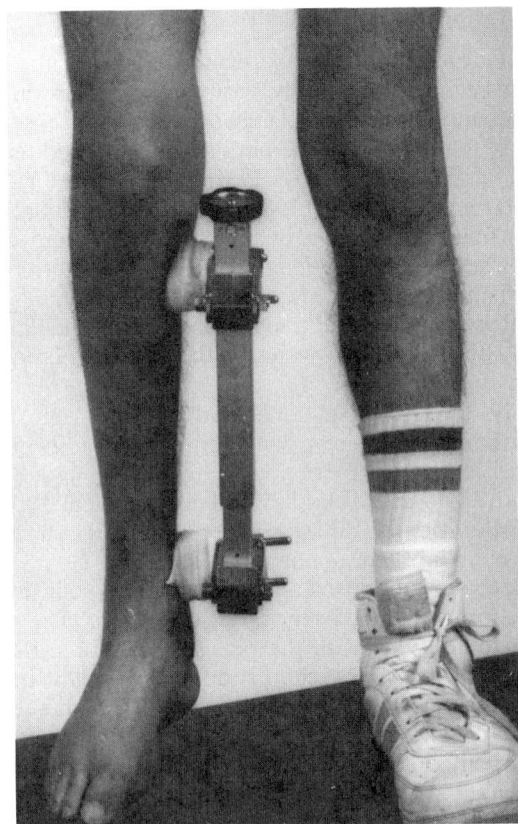

FIGURE 62-9
Wagner lengthening device. Patients with the Wagner device can be up and about and apply partial weight bearing. (Morrissy, R. T. [Ed.]. [1990]. Lovell and Winter's pediatric orthopaedics [3rd ed.]. [Vol. II]. Philadelphia: J. B. Lippincott.)

The Wagner apparatus, illustrated in Figure 62-9, includes an external telescoping device that is attached parallel and lateral to the femoral shaft by a series of screws. A knob that is attached to the device is turned once a day to achieve distraction (separation) at the site of the osteotomy. The amount of distraction determines how long the device remains in place. Once the device is removed, the child gradually resumes activities of daily living and progressive weight bearing.

The Ilizarov external fixator is another device that can lengthen and widen bones or immobilize fractures.[38] A corticotomy (osteotomy through only the cortex of the bone) is performed, and the fixator is applied. Distraction usually takes place at 1 mm/day. Once the prescribed limb length is achieved, treatment is stopped. The apparatus remains in place until the limb strength is sufficient to bear weight without pain, limp, or edema.

TEACHING

Preoperative teaching and preparation for the distraction device are essential for these children and their families to assure their commitment to the treatment program. The physical therapist will instruct the child in leg exercises that will help to stretch and tone the muscles as the limb is being lengthened. Instructions also include crutch walking and operation of the specific device that will be applied.

POSTOPERATIVE CARE

Following the application of a distraction device, the child should be assessed carefully for any signs of neurovascular compromise. Neurovascular compromise is caused by damage to the femoral and popliteal arteries and lengthening of the femoral, popliteal, and peroneal nerves. Regular monitoring of blood pressure is essential. Hypertension may be caused by stretching of the sympathetic nerves adjacent to the femoral and popliteal arteries.[48] Observation of the pin sites for any purulent drainage or sensitivity is part of the postoperative assessment. Pin care should be instituted according to the protocol of the physician or agency.

The use of patient-controlled analgesia (PCA) enables the child to receive pain medication readily during the early postoperative period. Following the initial postoperative period the child should not experience any severe pain from the device. Severe pain may indicate an underlying problem or complication.

Range-of-motion exercises are started as soon as possible and are directed by the physical therapist. The nurse needs to continue with the plan and reinforce the instructions given to the child and family. Administration of analgesics prior to the exercises decreases the child's discomfort and improves participation. As soon as the child's condition is stable, crutch walking is taught. Small, frequent elongation steps cause the child less pain, tingling, numbness, and circulatory problems than single step increments.[15]

DISCHARGE PLANNING

Discharge instructions should reinforce all the care requirements that were taught in the hospital. The parents need to learn about pin care, signs of pin site infection, and evidence of neurovascular compromise. Maintenance of the limb-lengthening device includes daily turning of the screws to ensure distraction.

The safety of the home environment should be discussed. Adaptations may need to be made to ensure the child's safety. Damage to the device can cause pain and severe compromise to the limb.

PSYCHOSOCIAL SUPPORT

The nurse needs to assess the child's adjustment to the device and the imposed restrictions. The child should be given an opportunity to express feelings and concerns either verbally or through play. The nurse can then suggest approaches to deal with some of the perceived problems. Adaptable clothing enhances the child's appearance and self-esteem. Fostering independence and social interactions enables the child to adapt to the activity restrictions yet remain involved in activities of daily living, school projects, and play.

★ **EVALUATION**

Children who have undergone leg-lengthening procedures receive long-term follow-up in an ambulatory care setting. The amount of distraction achieved and the condition of the muscles around the device are evaluated with each visit.

Follow-up care is essential to promote a positive outcome for the child. Continuous evaluation of home care may determine the need for home health nursing care.

COMPLICATIONS

Soft-tissue contractures may result from extensive time in the device. During office visits for follow up, the child's adherence to the exercise program should be evaluated. Range-of-motion exercises and physical therapy can prevent the development of knee flexion contracture. The child's crutch walking ability also should be assessed. Nonunion of the lengthened bone may be the result of inadequate mobilization or an appliance malfunction.

The pin sites should be carefully examined for any signs of infection. Signs of systemic infection also should be considered. Osteomyelitis can occur because of the break in the integrity of the skin and bone. The neurovascular status as well as the child's blood pressure should be checked with each visit.

Acquired Disorders

These disorders are categorized together because they are acquired during the child's development. The characteristics of these disorders are mixed. Some have congenital etiologies as well as etiologies associated with growth.

Curvature of the Spine

Curvatures of the spine usually occur as a result of persistent poor posture (functional) or structural changes in the vertebrae. Structural changes may be caused by congenital abnormalities, neuromuscular disorders, disease, or trauma, or they may be idiopathic. Regardless of the cause, most of the deviations become evident during periods of rapid skeletal growth.

The various types of curves are defined according to their vertebral location and the convexity or concavity of the curve. Treatment is determined by the type and degree of the curve and by the underlying vertebral abnormalities.

Definition and Incidence. There are three types of spinal curvatures: kyphosis, lordosis, and scoliosis (see Fig. 61-3). The definitions and incidence of these curves vary. Some common elements exist in the classification of these curves; they are listed in the accompanying display.

Kyphosis. Kyphosis (hunchback) is a mild to severe convex angulation in the thoracic area of the spine. The incidence of kyphosis in school-age and adolescent children is approximately 4% and is equally distributed between boys and girls.[41] Postural forms usually develop insidiously in children around puberty. Pain is not associated with the problem. Structural kyphosis, also called Scheuermann's disease, is more prevalent in boys.

Lordosis. Lordosis (swayback) is an exaggerated concave curvature of the lumbar spine. Children may have a genetic predisposition to lordosis, but most are idiopathic in nature. Postural lordosis is normally present in toddlers and should disappear by age 8. This type of curve is usually compensatory for other types of curvatures. Obese children, especially pubescent girls, may develop

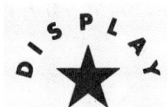

Causes of Spinal Curvatures

FUNCTIONAL (POSTURAL) CHANGES

- No vertebral changes
- Flexible curve
- Associated with chronic slouching
- Sometimes compensatory for other musculoskeletal deviations
- Insidious during puberty
- Usually no pain
- Easily corrected with bending or exercise

STRUCTURAL CHANGES

- Changes in spine and supporting structures
- Decreased flexibility
- Rotation of affected vertebrae causes physiologic alterations in spine, chest, and pelvis

Congenital
- Malformation of vertebrae during third to fifth week of fetal development

Neuromuscular (Paralytic)
- Muscular imbalance produces the curvature
- Upper and lower motor neurons may be involved as a result of underlying pathology

- Associated with neuromuscular or myopathic diseases, such as cerebral palsy, muscular dystrophy, neurofibromatosis, myelomeningocele

Idiopathic
- May be infantile, juvenile, or adolescent
- Type varies with age of onset
- Cause is unknown although familial tendency

Traumatic
- Associated with spinal fractures, tumors, or irradiation

Diseases
- Associated with nutritional disorders, such as rickets
- Associated with metabolic and inflammatory disorders, such as renal osteodystrophy and rheumatoid arthritis
- Associated with dwarfism
- Associated with connective tissue disorders, such as osteogenesis imperfecta, arachnodactyly, arthrogryposis multiplex congenita

---

a compensatory lordosis. Hamstring tightness also may be associated with lordosis. The muscles are unable to support the erect position.[50] Consequently, the spine begins to sag, and strain is placed on the ligaments, causing pain and fatigue. Lordosis may appear secondary to such disorders as CDH or SCFE. Unresolved lordosis also may be associated with degenerative changes of the vertebrae later in life.

Scoliosis. Scoliosis is a lateral curvature of the spine associated with rotation of the vertebral bodies around their vertical axes. The curve may be C-shaped or S-shaped and may be related to functional or structural changes in the vertebrae.

Scoliosis affects approximately 100 out of every 1000 individuals. However, only about 2 of every 1000 individuals with scoliosis require treatment to arrest the curve.[5] Idiopathic scoliosis is the most common type and accounts for about 70% of all cases. The other 30% are functional and usually can be corrected through noninvasive treatment. It occurs about seven to eight times more frequently in adolescent girls than boys.

Etiology and Pathophysiology. Etiologies of the various types of spinal curvatures are outlined in the display. The pathophysiologic processes that occur with curvature of the spine depend on the flexibility of the vertebral column.

Functional or postural types are caused by chronic slouching or poor posture, which may be compensatory mechanisms associated with musculoskeletal deviations in other areas. A compensatory curvature often develops

secondary to a leg length discrepancy, which tilts the pelvis down on the short side. With functional curvatures, marked spinal curvature is noted, but there are no changes in the spine or supporting structures. The spine is very flexible and returns to its normal shape with bending.

Structural curvatures are characterized by changes in the spine or supporting structures with decreases in flexibility. With congenital types of curvature, one side of the vertebrae either incompletely develops or fails to grow, causing wedging. There may be anterior narrowing of the vertebrae. Narrowing of the intervertebral disk spaces also occurs. Rotation of the affected vertebrae causes physiologic alterations in the spine, chest, and pelvis. These changes can be congenital or result from structural damage to the spine.

Curvatures that have neuromuscular origins result from an uneven pull on the spine by the muscles and ligaments. Upper and lower motor neurons may be involved as a result of the underlying pathology.

The physiologic changes that occur with development of spinal curvatures can best be understood by reviewing the process of spinal growth. The spine grows to maintain the body's balance. The musculature on either side of the spine supports this process. When curvatures develop, the spine and ribs rotate toward the convex portion of the curve. The forces exerted by this rotation may cause the vertebrae to change shape. On the concave side of the curve, the muscles and ligaments become contracted and thickened. Conversely, they become atrophied on the convex side. A compensatory curve usually develops to maintain the posture and balance of the body.

Curves rapidly progress during growth spurts and continue until skeletal maturity is reached.

Clinical Manifestations. The appearance of the child's spinal curve and the associated manifestations vary with the type of defect, the degree of curvature, and the location. Children with kyphotic curvatures may have a hunchback or rounded appearance to their dorsal spine. They may have difficulty being fitted for sweaters and shirts. Lumbar lordosis often develops in these children to compensate for the kyphotic changes.

The child who presents with poor posture and swayback should be evaluated for lordosis. There may be vague complaints of lower back pain, hip pain, and fatigue. The chest and abdomen may protrude depending on the degree of the curvature. The pelvis inclines forward to accommodate the rearrangement of the spinal column.

The classic appearance of a child with scoliosis is that of uneven shoulders and hips and a rib hump or paraspinal muscle prominence with bending. A prominent scapula is seen on the convex side of the curve. The thoracic cage is asymmetric with displacement of the sternum from the midline as the ribs rotate. If the curve is greater than 50 degrees, respiratory function can be adversely affected.

Unless the curve is severe, these changes can only be seen if the child is undressed. Pain is not common except in cases of severe deformity in which degenerative changes have occurred. Most of the time the parent brings the child for a routine health visit and may comment that clothing does not seem to fit right.

Diagnostic Studies. Accurate measurement of a spinal curvature is essential for determining the degree of curvature and any progression in the pathology. Standing anteroposterior and lateral radiographs assist the health care team in measuring and documenting spinal curvature. Radiographs enable the health care provider to classify the curvature according to extent, degree, mobility, and location. Skeletal maturation, an important variable in determining the treatment plan, also can be identified on radiographs.

Special imaging techniques are now used to monitor a child's curve. This approach decreases the need for frequent radiographs. Laminography (tomography) is used when congenital anomalies are suspected. Images of spinal structures in a selected plane are detailed by blurring images of proximate structures in all other planes. Myelography is used for evaluating any neurologic impairment secondary to the curvature.

The angle of trunk rotation can be measured with a scoliometer. This is a helpful tool for nurses during school screening. Any angle less than or equal to 5 degrees requires follow-up consultation.

Pulmonary function tests may be performed to determine if respiratory compromise has occurred. Decreased lung expansion and tidal volume may result from the thoracic curvature.

The age of onset, pattern of the curve, and progression of the curve are all diagnostic indicators for future treatment. Kyphosis, lordosis, and scoliosis are diagnosed from the clinical and radiologic findings. Progressive

curves or curvatures greater than 25 degrees need referral to an orthopedic surgeon.

★ ASSESSMENT

A health history should be obtained for every adolescent who is suspect for scoliosis. Because most of these clients are adolescents, their privacy needs to be respected. They may be more comfortable discussing their concerns without their parents present. The nurse may need to ask the parents to wait while some of the initial history information is collected. The nurse needs to ask the youth about the possibility of injury. Also the nurse should determine through discussion the nature of any discomforts experienced. The adolescent may complain of fatigue, dyspnea, and backache.

Adolescents tend to be very modest. A complete physical assessment of scoliosis, however, must include observations of the youth's bare back. When assessing a child for scoliosis, the nurse looks for any signs of asymmetry through the shoulders, back, and waist. A curvature of the spine may be palpated by locating the spinous processes. As the child bends forward, the angular deformity of the spine becomes apparent. Assessment includes noting any protrusion of the chest or abdomen and the alignment of the trunk.

Assessment also includes a review of other body systems. The asymmetry of the trunk can cause major compromises to other systems of the body.

★ NURSING DIAGNOSES AND PLANNING

Because idiopathic scoliosis is the most common type of spinal curvature, the focus of this section is on this disorder. The nursing diagnoses and interventions, however, are relevant to the other types of spinal curvatures. Treatment plans and consequently the nursing interventions can be selected based on the individual needs of the adolescent with any type of spinal curvature.

Based on assessment data, the following nursing diagnoses may apply to the family and adolescent with scoliosis.

- Ineffective Breathing Pattern related to impact of curvature on ventilation and immobility.
- Impaired Skin Integrity related to bracing device and surgical incision.
- Impaired Physical Mobility related to restrictions associated with spinal curvature and treatment modalities.
- Constipation related to decreased bowel motility secondary to spinal surgery and immobility.
- Acute Pain related to spinal surgery.
- High Risk for Infection related to break in skin integrity secondary to surgical incision.
- Self-Esteem Disturbance related to altered body structure.
- Ineffective Management of Therapeutic Regimen related to incompatibility between treatment plan and developmental needs.
- Anxiety related to lack of knowledge about expectations regarding the treatment regimen.

The nurse and adolescent (or parents) together plan effective care based on the established nursing diagnoses. Several examples of expected outcomes follow:

- The adolescent discusses the importance of correct posture.
- The adolescent uses postural exercises.
- The adolescent describes the correct use of the brace and hygiene related to its use.
- The adolescent identifies the importance of compliance with brace use and exercises.
- The adolescent contacts another adolescent who has had corrective surgery.
- The adolescent coughs every 2 hours following surgery.
- The adolescent moves the extremities regularly while on bedrest.

The overall goal of treatment is to arrest the spinal curvature. The nurse needs to work closely with the child and family to define objectives that relate specifically to the individualized treatment plan. Outcomes should include return to activities of daily living within activity limitations, maintenance of a positive body image, and a smooth transition to home.

★ NURSING INTERVENTIONS: COLLABORATIVE AND INDEPENDENT

Many options are available for the treatment of scoliosis. These options range from simple observation, exercise, bracing, and electric stimulation to surgery with internal fixation. The orthopedic surgeon recommends the mode of treatment based on the degree and progression of the curvature. Variables such as skeletal maturity also are included in the decision. Regardless of the treatment method, the nurse plays an integral role in supporting and educating the adolescent and family.

NONOPERATIVE TREATMENT

Nonoperative treatment includes observation, exercise, and bracing. This treatment method is usually selected for individuals with curvature less than 40 degrees. The type of brace selected depends on the location of the curvature. Two types of braces are shown in Figure 62-10. Generally, Milwaukee braces are used to control high

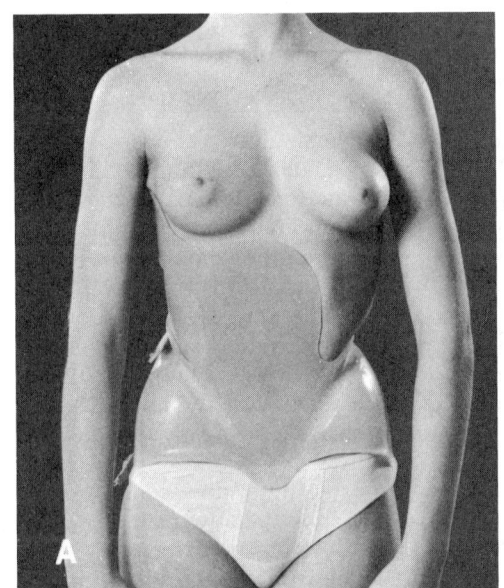
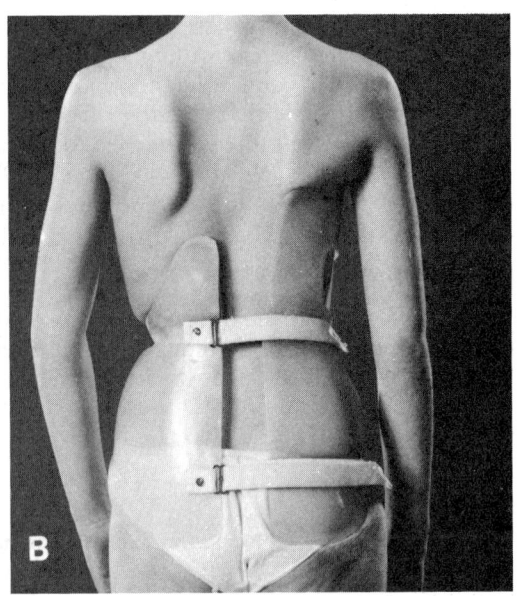
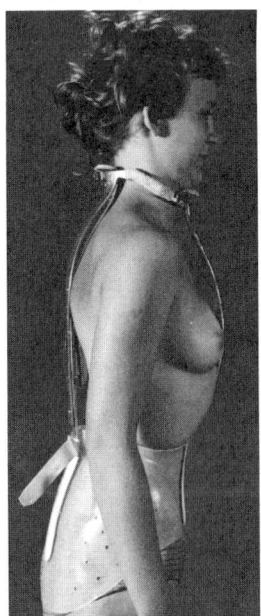
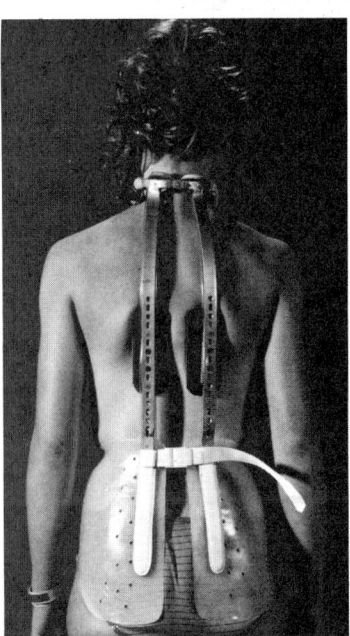

FIGURE 62-10
Above, a thoracolumbar sacral orthosis for the treatment of a lumbar idiopathic curvature. Below, A Milwaukee brace for kyphosis. (Morrissy, R. T. [Ed.]. [1990]. Lovell and Winter's pediatric orthopaedics [3rd ed.]. [Vol. II]. Philadelphia: J. B. Lippincott.)

thoracic curvatures. The Lyon brace and the Boston brace are underarm braces that are used to treat thoracic and thoracolumbar curvatures.[4] The latter braces are often more acceptable because they can be concealed under loose clothing.

The orthopedist recommends the number of hours that the adolescent is required to wear the brace. Some physicians require that the brace be removed only 1 hour a day for hygiene and exercise. When these restrictions are made, however, compliance is usually a problem. The current trend is to allow time out of the brace for participation in gym and other desired physical sports.

Another nonoperative approach to prevent progression of the curvature is the lateral electric surface stimulator (LESS).[10] The electrodes are strategically placed on the thoracic curvature and stimulate underlying muscles to contract. The ribs move toward each other causing the spine to straighten. The therapy may be uncomfortable at first, but the child is usually acclimated to it within 7 days. The child is required to use the LESS 8 hours a night until skeletal maturity is attained.

The success of any of these nonoperative approaches depends on the individual's willingness to cooperate. The nurse is involved in counseling the adolescent about the program and assessing the degree of compliance expected. Ongoing counseling is needed to determine adherence to the treatment regimen. Table 62-9 outlines nursing strategies for individuals who require nonoperative treatment.

SURGICAL MANAGEMENT

Despite attempts at the more conservative treatment methods, some adolescents require surgical intervention. Surgery is usually indicated for skeletally immature individuals whose curvature has progressed beyond 40 degrees. Depending on the type of curvature and the surgeon's preference, various types of instrumentation are used. The Harrington rod, Luque wire, or Cotrel-Dubousset instrumentation is used for posterior spinal fusion. Adolescents with a flexible thoracolumbar or lumbar curvature usually require an anterior spinal fusion with Zielke instrumentation. Regardless of the type of surgery, nursing care is focused on the preparation and care of a child undergoing spinal surgery.

PREOPERATIVE CARE

The nurse has a primary role in preparing the adolescent for surgery. The adolescent and family need specific information about what to expect with the surgical procedure. It is sometimes helpful to give the adolescent the name of another person who has undergone the procedure.

These adolescents usually require 4 to 6 units of blood for surgery. The autologous method of transfusion is recommended. The units of blood are drawn during a series of scheduled preoperative visits. Supplements of ferrous sulfate are prescribed to ensure an adequate hemoglobin. If possible, the nurse should use these opportunities to further discuss the upcoming surgery.

POSTOPERATIVE CARE

Nursing care following a spinal fusion can be extensive. Besides assessing the usual postoperative variables, the nurse needs to pay particular attention to the adolescent's neurologic and respiratory function. The upper and lower extremities should be assessed for motion, strength, and sensation at least every 4 hours for the first 72 hours following surgery. Because of the large incision, adolescents are often reluctant to cough and deep breath. To mobilize secretions, coughing and deep breathing should be encouraged every 2 hours. During this time the nurse should auscultate breath sounds, and abnormalities should be reported.

These adolescents experience a considerable amount of postoperative pain. The procedures used to manipulate the spine are extensive. Often a bone graft is taken from the iliac crest, resulting in pain in the donor area. PCA helps these children better manage their pain. If this therapy is not available, intramuscular or intravenous (IV) analgesics are given regularly for the first 48 hours. Once the child is able to tolerate a regular diet, oral analgesics can be administered as needed.

The operative incision is usually covered for the first 2 days. The nurse needs to assess the area for bleeding and any unusual drainage. Some patients have drains inserted into the graft site. Assessment of the amount of drainage in this device is also important. The nurse should assess for any local or systemic signs of infection. Many times these children receive prophylactic antibiotics for the first 72 hours after surgery.

When assessing other body systems, the nurse needs to listen to the patient's bowel sounds and assess bowel motility. Because of the stretching associated with spinal correction, these patients may develop an ileus. Therefore, it is important to progress fluids and diet gradually until bowel motility is fully restored.

Early mobilization of individuals undergoing spinal fusion decreases the risk of pulmonary emboli and phlebitis. Patients need to be encouraged to move their ex-

TABLE 62-9
Nursing Intervention: Nonoperative Management of Scoliosis

Nursing Action	Rationale
Encourage correct posture.	Functional spinal malformations can be corrected through good posture.
Review physical exercises that will help decrease the severity of spinal malformations.	Postural exercises and sports can strengthen the back muscles and may help decrease the severity of the curvature.
Instruct the child in correct use of the brace. Include application, time worn, and potential problems encountered, such as chafed skin, and pressure areas.	The brace is a noninvasive treatment option for spinal malformations. It is worn under clothes and should be worn at all times except during showering and personal hygiene. The physician needs to be aware of any problems that are encountered.
Stress the importance of compliance in wearing the brace to help decrease spinal curvature and disfigurement.	Teenagers' acute awareness of body image and body changes may lead to noncompliance with the orthotic device and therapy.
Conduct school screening clinics to detect spinal malformations early.	School screening clinics have proved to be effective in early detection of spinal malformations.

tremities while on bedrest. The nurse should ensure that the child is pain free before attempting mobilization. Usually by the fourth to fifth postoperative day, these individuals are ambulating. Sometimes a molded orthosis is needed for added support.

DISCHARGE PLANNING

Children may be discharged within 1 week of the spinal fusion. At that time they are usually independent in self-care. Parents need to be taught about any activity restrictions and medications. Patients are usually given a prescription for an oral analgesic, an iron supplement, and a stool softener.

Initially, children who have had spinal fusion are advised to avoid twisting and bending activities or lifting heavy objects. Contact or high-impact sports are discouraged for up to 2 years. Swimming and cycling, however, can usually be resumed in 3 to 4 months. They should be encouraged to plan rest periods during the day. Usually these children return to school in 4 to 6 weeks. A homebound tutor needs to be arranged for the time they are absent from school.

The care of the adolescent with scoliosis presents many challenges to the nurse. Children requiring a spinal fusion have problems with increased blood loss, immobility, pain control, and imposed dependence. Because many patients with scoliosis are adolescents, body image and growing independence are major factors that need to be addressed. Adolescents should be encouraged to make as many decisions about their treatment and care as possible. Negotiating with adolescents gives them a sense of control over appearance, self-esteem, and interpersonal relationships.

★ EVALUATION

Periodically, the nurse and family evaluate the outcomes of care given. Examples of outcomes for the child and family with curvature of the spine were given under Nursing Diagnoses and Planning in this section. Have short-term goals been met? Are long-term goals still realistic?

LONG-TERM CARE

Children who require nonsurgical management of their spinal curvature are followed in an ambulatory care setting until skeletal maturity is reached. The nurse is in an excellent position to evaluate compliance with the plan and to offer suggestions for making the treatment more acceptable to the adolescent.

When operative treatment is required, the nurse should evaluate the outcomes of the plan of care while the child is hospitalized. These children are carefully monitored in an ambulatory care center following discharge from the hospital. The nurse can reinforce the need to restrict activities until stabilization of the fusion occurs. Sometimes high-impact activities may be restricted for up to 2 years. Internal fixation devices may be removed if they start to protrude or if the physician feels that fixation has been achieved.

If treatment is successful, balance will be restored, and the muscles will be strengthened. The adolescent will have very erect posture, and the goals for treatment will be achieved. Recognizing the adolescent's improved posture will help the individual to reestablish a positive body image.

Additional follow-up may be needed in adulthood. Changes such as pregnancy may place added stress on the vertebrae, and treatment or modification of activities may be suggested.

Benign Neoplasms of the Skeletal System

Malignant or benign neoplasms of the skeletal system are common in children. Osteosarcoma and Ewing's sarcoma, common malignant bone tumors, are addressed in Chapter 31. The following benign tumors are addressed in this section: osteochondromas, osteoblastomas, unicameral bone cysts, and aneurysmal bone cysts.

Definition and Incidence. The most common type of benign bone tumor in children is osteochondroma. The tumor, which is primarily composed of bone and cartilage, may occur as multiple or single tumors. Multiple osteochondromas are referred to as exostoses. Because of the nature of the tumor and its prevalence during periods of rapid skeletal growth, it is sometimes considered a developmental malformation instead of a true tumor.

Osteoblastomas (osteoid osteomas) are small benign vascular tumors. Generally these tumors occur more frequently in males younger than age 20 but are not usually not seen in individuals older than age 40.

Unicameral bone cysts are tumor-like solitary fluid-filled bone cysts that affect children between the ages of 5 and 15 years. These tumors commonly occur in the proximal humerus, femur, and tibia. Aneurysmal bone cysts are more common in children than adults. This lesion can be differentiated from a unicameral bone cyst by the greater number of thin-walled vessels involved. Although the lesion can affect any bone, the predominant location is the metaphysis of the long bones. There is no variation in incidence between boys and girls.

Etiology and Pathophysiology. Benign bone tumors originate in the bone tissue or cartilage, grow slowly, and do not destroy supporting or surrounding tissues. There are, however, variations in the etiology and pathology of each type of bone tumor.

Osteochondromas are generally developmental. Multiple osteochondromas usually follow an autosomal dominant inheritance pattern. The tumor is primarily cartilaginous with increasing ossification as skeletal maturity is reached. A small cartilaginous nodule often originates in the periosteum and begins to form a stalk or mushroom as endochondral ossification progresses. The muscles, tendons, joints, blood vessels, and nerves may be affected. When skeletal maturity is reached, growth of the tumor is usually arrested.

Osteoblastomas usually occur in poorly formed bone and fibrous tissue of the vertebrae, femur, tibia, or upper extremities. Bone erosion and resorption is associated with the tumor.

The pathophysiology and etiology of unicameral bone cysts and aneurysmal bone cysts are similar. They may be caused by a developmental defect resulting in a vascular anomaly. The defect causes a transitory disturbance in the circulation of the affected bone with dysplasia of the tissue of the metaphysis. These tumors usually contain large cavities and are capable of expanding the cortex of the bone. With aneurysmal bone cysts, however, the capacity to expand the bone is greater, and the tumor site is more variable.

Clinical Manifestations.   The presence of a bone tumor may not be revealed until children are evaluated for injuries associated with sports and play activities. Pain is not a primary indicator of a benign bone lesion except with osteoblastomas. Even when pain is present, children often have difficulty describing and localizing the pain.

Depending on the location of the tumor, a mass may be palpable. Because of the thin muscle covering, lesions located in the ankle and hand are easier to palpate. If the arteries are affected, pulsations of the mass may be visible near the epiphyseal plate of the long bones. In these situations a bruit can be auscultated, and arterial insufficiency is evident distally.

With most benign bone tumors function is limited to a varying degree. If significant bone erosion has occurred, pathologic fractures may develop. When lesions are close to a joint, synovial effusion may be responsible for decreases in motion. Pressure on peripheral nerves also causes limitation of movement as well as decreased sensation and numbness. Because most benign neoplasms affect the extremities, a limp may be evident.

Diagnostic Studies.   Sometimes bone neoplasms are difficult to visualize using roentgenography because the cartilaginous part of the lesion is radiolucent. Also, localization of the lesion based on historical data from the child is often a challenge. A tomogram may be needed to identify the exact geometry of the lesion. Depending on the extent of the lesion, an arteriogram and myelogram may be indicated.

Biopsies are often performed to confirm the histologic nature of the lesion. If a malignancy is suspected, other laboratory tests may be prescribed.

★ ASSESSMENT

The nurse usually begins the assessment by collecting data about the child's usual activities. Any limitations in these activities related to pain or function should be noted. If a limp is present, the child and family should be asked when it was first noticed and what activities precipitate it. The nurse should note if the child has just entered a period of rapid growth.

Children often have difficulty describing the nature and location of their pain. The nurse may have to use pain tools to obtain these data. Any pain that is described as burning or stinging should alert the nurse to further assess this area. Pain that is prevalent at night and is dramatically relieved with mild analgesics may suggest the presence of an osteoblastoma. Sometimes the pain may be referred to nearby joints.

The position and appearance of the affected extremity should be assessed. If a mass is palpable, the size and

any changes in the lesion should be described. Localized edema and muscular atrophy also may be visible. To provide comparative data, measurements of these findings may be indicated. The range of motion of the extremities and the extension and flexion of the joints also should be assessed.

Finally, the neurovascular status of the affected extremity should be evaluated. Changes in sensation and tenderness over the lesion may be important variables in identifying the extent of the lesion.

★ NURSING DIAGNOSES AND PLANNING

Based on assessment data discussed previously and in the preceding chapter, the following nursing diagnoses may apply to the family and child with benign neoplasms of the skeletal system. Variations may exist based on the type of lesions identified and the clinical manifestations.

- Pain related to limitations in movement and pressure from the tumor on underlying structures.
- Altered Tissue Perfusion related to possible hemorrhage associated with excision of vascular lesions.
- Sleep Pattern Disturbance related to nocturnal pain.
- Impaired Physical Mobility related to pressure from the bone tumor on the peripheral nerves.
- Anxiety related to the child's diagnosis.
- Fear related to lack of knowledge about treatment and home care following excision of the tumor.

Because many bone tumors grow slowly and do not impair function, the plan may be to continue to observe the child for any changes in tumor size, function, or pain. If the tumor interferes with function, the lesion is usually excised. Expected outcomes for a child after excision of a bone tumor may include the following:

- The child sleeps throughout the night.
- The child demonstrates correct non–weight-bearing or partial weight-bearing crutch walking.
- The family reviews questions and concerns about their child's diagnosis with the nurse.
- The family demonstrates how to care for their child.

The nurse plans for the daily care of the child based on physician's orders and nursing diagnoses. Some general nursing care goals may include the following:

- The child maintains maximum function of the affected extremity without any adverse effects from the tumor or associated treatment.
- The child remains pain free.
- The child does not hemorrhage following excision of a vascular tumor.

★ INTERVENTIONS: COLLABORATIVE OR INDEPENDENT

When parents first discover that their child may have a bone tumor, they are often unprepared for the diagnosis. The word tumor may have many negative connotations and generate much anxiety in the parents. At the time of the initial diagnosis, the surgeon may be unsure of the type of tumor. Therefore, the parents will need a considerable amount of emotional support from the nurse in the form of listening, presence, and empathy. Once a definitive diagnosis is made, the nurse should be available to clarify any misconceptions about the nature of the tumor.

If the decision is to excise the tumor, the nurse is usually responsible for explaining the surgical experience to the child and family. It is important to emphasize how the child will look and feel following the surgery. Younger children should be given the opportunity to play with some of the equipment that will be used. Realistic explanations about what to expect will be helpful to both the child and family.

The nurse provides postoperative care for the child. The standard of care for a child undergoing an orthopedic procedure should be followed. (See Table 62-3) Because of the vascular nature of many bone tumors, the vital signs and blood pressure should be assessed frequently. The extremity, which is usually covered with a supportive wrap or cast, should be elevated above the level of the heart. If a dressing covers the incision, specific instructions for wound care are usually prescribed.

Prior to discharge from the hospital, the child will be taught how to use crutches. The physician usually prescribes the type of weight bearing, and the physical therapist initiates the instruction. The nurse is usually responsible for following through with the teaching initiated by the physical therapist. In addition the nurse teaches the family how to care for their child in a cast. (See section on Care of a Child in a Cast later in this chapter.)

★ EVALUATION

Periodically, the nurse and family evaluate the outcomes of care given. Examples of outcomes for the child and family with benign neoplasms of the skeletal system were given under Nursing Diagnoses and Planning in this section. Follow-up care is continued on an outpatient basis. During each visit the functional capacity of the extremity is evaluated. Once the tumor has been removed, the child should not have complaints of pain.

Some bone tumors may recur. If sections of an osteochondroma are not removed, there will be recurrences. Although these recurrences may be distressing to the family, they are rarely malignant. Repeated excisions are not recommended unless the tumor limits function. Aneurysmal bone cysts are large, progressive tumors that are difficult to excise. Radiation therapy is sometimes prescribed when the surgeon is unable to excise the entire lesion. With each follow-up visit it is important that the nurse emphasize the benign nature of these tumors. Families will need continuous assurance, especially when tumors recur.

Rickets

Rickets is a disturbance of normal bone ossification and weakening of the skeletal structures resulting from a deficiency in any combination of calcium, phosphorus, or vitamin D. The development of the disorder is usually related to poor nutritional intake, absorption problems, or inadequate exposure to sunlight.

The prevalence of fad diets or pica could contribute to the development of rickets in this country. If breast-feeding mothers do not consume an adequate intake of vitamin D, the deficiency could be transmitted to their infants. Infants born prematurely may not have the advantage of the large amounts of phosphorus and calcium that are usually transferred from the mother to the fetus during the last trimester of pregnancy.

Other causes of rickets are related to various problems with absorption in the gastrointestinal, hepatic, or renal system. Various diseases or the associated treatments for these diseases may contribute to the development of rickets. Absorption problems also may be directly related to genetic factors. Vitamin D-resistant rickets is inherited through an X-linked dominant trait and is characterized by a decrease in the ability to absorb calcium.

Regardless of the cause of rickets, the pathologic and clinical pictures are similar. Before any deformities are noticed in the bony structure, decreases in serum calcium and phosphorus and elevations in parathyroid levels are present. Radiologic views of the bones reveal thin cortices with signs of resorption. The growth plate is usually enlarged, and the blood supply to this area is altered. The presence of a layer of unmineralized bone surrounding a mineralized segment is a significant finding with all types of rickets.

The manifestations of the disorder vary with the severity of the deficiency; generally the manifestations are vague. Children with rickets may appear apathetic and irritable with a short attention span. They may complain of pain in their muscles.

A head-to-toe assessment of the skeletal system may reveal a softening of the cranial bones with a prominence of frontal bones. The skull may appear flat and depressed with delayed closure of the fontanel. There is usually an enlargement of the costal cartilages of the chest with indentation of the lower ribs and sometimes a sharp protrusion of the sternum. The spine may be curved, producing scoliosis, kyphosis, or lordosis. The long bones of the lower extremities are usually shortened with bowing and varus deformities present in the upper extremities. Not only is bending and distortion of the bones present, but the ligamentous structures do not offer the needed support. Therefore, the risk for fractures is increased. Other systems are also affected by the deficiency.

★ NURSING IMPLICATIONS

The nurse has a primary role in prevention and detection of this disorder. Early intervention can prevent some of the deformities associated with untreated rickets. The nurse needs to be alert to children who are at risk for developing rickets. A history of the dietary habits of infants and young children may alert the nurse. Detailed nutritional assessments are especially important when caring for preterm infants, infants who are breast-fed, African American and Asian children, and any children who have limited exposure to sunlight. The nurse should recommend vitamin D supplements for preterm infants and infants who do not receive vitamin D in their diets.

If the child does not have an adequate intake of calcium, vitamin D supplements are of little value. Therefore, the nurse must help the family plan meals that will provide the needed calcium. The importance of these nutrients to the development of the child also should be explained. With each follow-up visit, the nurse should review records of the child's growth and development. Any decline in skeletal growth should alert the nurse to the possibility of rickets.

If the child has rickets, the nurse needs to provide ongoing teaching to the family about diet and dietary supplements. Regardless of the cause of rickets, treatment always includes replacement therapy with some form of vitamin D. Replacement therapy is carefully monitored through frequent evaluation of blood levels of calcium. An explanation of the reason for these frequent blood tests may alleviate the parents' anxiety. Reviewing some of the signs and symptoms of overdose from supplements may help to reinforce the reasons for the precautions.

Parents should be advised against using any over-the-counter drugs or supplements that are not prescribed by the physician. Sometimes parents may feel that more vitamins may speed up their child's recovery. Generally, healing begins in 2 to 4 weeks. If rapid healing does not occur, then vitamin D-resistant rickets may be suspected.

In severely affected children the treatment plans are more extensive. The nurse must plan care based on the effect of the disorder on the skeletal system as well as on other body systems. Because of the fragile bony deformities, gentle body positioning to maintain alignment is needed. The parents need to be taught how to apply and care for any supportive splints or braces. Frequent turning and positioning are important to prevent further deformities and respiratory infections.

Because children with rickets may have degeneration of the spleen and liver, care should always be focused on the prevention of infection. Also, these children are at risk for developing tetany from extremely low calcium levels. A solution of 10% calcium gluconate should be available in case rachitic tetany develops. During hospitalizations, seizure precautions should be instituted, and parents should be taught safety measures related to seizure management at home.

Infection and Inflammation

Juvenile Rheumatoid Arthritis*

Several terms associated with arthritis are defined in the accompanying display. Arthralgias are painful joints without restricted movement, swelling, or inflammation. Arthritis is a painful joint with swelling, heat, or tenderness. The difference between juvenile rheumatoid arthritis (JRA) and rheumatoid arthritis is outlined in Table 62-10.

Definition and Incidence. A subcommittee of the American Rheumatology Association (ARA) has adopted the term *juvenile rheumatoid arthritis* as the commonly accepted diagnostic term for children with chronic, inflammatory, idiopathic arthritis in which other forms of

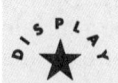

Terms Associated With Arthritis

Arthralgia: Pain in joint without swelling, warmth, or restricted range of motion noted on physical examination
Arthritis: Inflammation of a joint, usually accompanied by pain, swelling, and restricted range of motion in structure (Pain itself is not sufficient for a diagnosis of arthritis.)
Rheumatoid arthritis: Chronic systemic disease with inflammatory changes in joints and related structures that result in deformities
Juvenile rheumatoid arthritis: Chronic, inflammatory, systemic disease that may cause joint or connective tissue damage and visceral lesions in the body (Other possible diagnoses, such as rheumatic disease, infectious arthritis, nonrheumatic bone and joint conditions, and occasionally systemic disease are eliminated.)

arthritis have been excluded.[7] Children with JRA are younger than 16 and have arthritis continuously in one or more joints for a minimum of 6 weeks.

The ARA subcommittee also recommends that JRA be classified into three onset subtypes after 3 months' disease duration. These subtypes are systemic, pauciarticular, and polyarticular. Table 62-11 summarizes these subtypes. Pauciarticular JRA involves four or fewer joints with no systemic features. Polyarticular JRA involves five or more joints with few systemic features. These children tend to have more stiffness and pain than those who have the pauciarticular form. Systemic JRA is characterized by high fevers, a distinctive rash, and arthritis of one or more joints.

TABLE 62-10
Differentiation Between Rheumatoid Arthritis and Juvenile Rheumatoid Arthritis

Rheumatoid Arthritis	Juvenile Rheumatoid Arthritis
Small joint	Large joint
Chronic inflammation and joint changes	Remission in two thirds
Rheumatoid factor positive in 80%	Rheumatoid factor positive in 20%
Adults develop ulnar drift	Pericarditis
	Uveitis
	Hepatitis
	Rash
	Fever
	Radial drift at metacarpophalangeal joints

Data from Kovalesky A., Boutaugh, M., Erlandsen, D., Fubro, J., Jacobowitz, S., Mahy, M., Shields, C., & Tehan, M. (1987). *Understanding Juvenile Arthritis—A Health Professional's Guide to Teaching Children and Parents.* Atlanta: Arthritis Foundation.

TABLE 62-11
Subtypes of Juvenile Rheumatoid Arthritis

Mode of Onset and Frequency (% of Patients)	Incidence	Laboratory Findings	Clinical Manifestations	Course of Joint Disease	Prognosis
Systemic 20%	Age: no peak age/variable Sex: F = M	Anemia, leukocytosis, elevated sedimentation rate, ANA positive in 15%, RF negative, HLA-B27 negative	Spiking fever (>104°F), rash (90%) consisting of discrete confluent salmon-colored macules, hepatosplenomegaly, pleuritis, pericarditis, leukocytosis, anemia, lymphadenopathy, myalgia, fatigue, muscle atrophy, weight loss	25% have severe chronic arthritis after systemic manifestations have subsided	25% to 40% have permanent disability
Polyarticular (five or more joints)/seronegative 30%	Age: 1–3 years/9 years Sex: F > M (2:1)	Elevated sedimentation rate, ANA positive in 25% to 40%, RF negative	Multiple symmetric joint involvement pattern (small and large joints/usually not spine), cervical spine involvement, modest systemic symptoms such as low-grade fever, anemia, malaise, weight loss, adenopathy		10% to 15% have permanent disability
Polyarticular (five or more joints)/seropositive 10%	Age: late childhood (older than 8 years) Sex: F > M	Elevated sedimentation rate, RF positive in 100%, ANA positive in 25% to 40%	Symmetric small-joint involvement, rheumatoid nodules, vasculitis, mild systemic symptoms such as low-grade fever, anemia, and malaise	Destructive and disabling arthritis in 50%	Worse in all the subtypes/poor
Pauciarticular or oligoarticular (four or fewer joints) 20%	Age: early childhood 1–4 years Sex: F > M	ANA positive in 60%, elevated sedimentation rate, RF negative	No systemic symptoms, chronic iridocyclitis (10% to 50%), asymmetric joint involvement, large-joint involvement (knees, ankles, wrist, or elbows/not hips or sacroiliac joint)	60% go into remission	Excellent except for the complication of uveitis (can yield blindness in 10% of patients)
Pauciarticular (four or fewer joints) 20%	Age: late childhood (10 years) Sex: F < M	Elevated sedimentation rate, RF negative, ANA negative, HLA-B27 positive in 60% to 75% (juvenile ankylosing spondylitis)	Asymmetric joint involvement (hip and back involvement such as sacroiliitis)	Increased risk for developing ankylosing spondylitis or Reiter's disease	Good

Key: ANA, antinuclear antibody; RF, rheumatoid factor; HLA-B27, human leukocyte antigen B27; F, female; M, male.

JRA is the most common rheumatic disease of childhood. Its peak incidence is in the second year of life.[45] More girls than boys have this disease with sex and age ratios differing in the various subtypes.

Etiology and Pathophysiology. The cause of JRA is unknown. Multiple factors such as autoimmunity, trauma, stress, infection, and immunogenetic predisposition are thought to contribute. JRA may result from multiple etiologic events or a single pathologic event with multiple clinical factors. It rarely occurs in more than one child in a family.

The basic pathology underlying JRA is a joint's inflammation of synovial membrane. Ongoing inflammation of the synovium yields increased production of synovial fluid, increased pressure within the joint, and thickening of the synovial membrane. Increased blood flow stimulates bony overgrowth at the area of the inflamed joint. Chronic synovitis can yield deformity, subluxation, and fibrous or bony ankylosis of a joint (Fig. 62-11).

Continued inflammation can ultimately lead to progressive erosion and destruction of articular cartilage and bone. Extra-articular manifestations of JRA include growth retardation, chronic iridocyclitis, pericarditis, lymphadenopathy, tenosynovitis, myositis, rheumatoid nodules, and hepatosplenomegaly. The disease course varies considerably with exacerbations and remissions; however, the majority of children do not suffer permanent joint damage and disability.

Clinical Manifestations. Signs and symptoms of arthritis may be insidious. Some general clinical manifestations include morning stiffness, objective arthritis, increased irritability, anorexia, guarding of the joints, a limp or refusal to walk, increased fatigue, weight loss, and failure to grow. The child frequently will *not* complain of pain. Studies of children with JRA have shown that complaints of pain have been found to correlate poorly with other measures of activity or severity of the disease.[7]

Diagnostic Studies. JRA is a "diagnosis by exclusion." Other causes for the arthritis must be eliminated. Conditions that cause similar symptoms and are ruled out including other rheumatic diseases, infectious arthritis, inflammatory bowel disease, neoplastic conditions, nonrheumatic conditions of bones and joints, and hematologic and psychogenic conditions. JRA is a clinical diagnosis and therefore depends on details from a thorough history and physical.

No specific laboratory or radiologic test is diagnostic for JRA. Laboratory tests (such as an erythrocyte sedi-

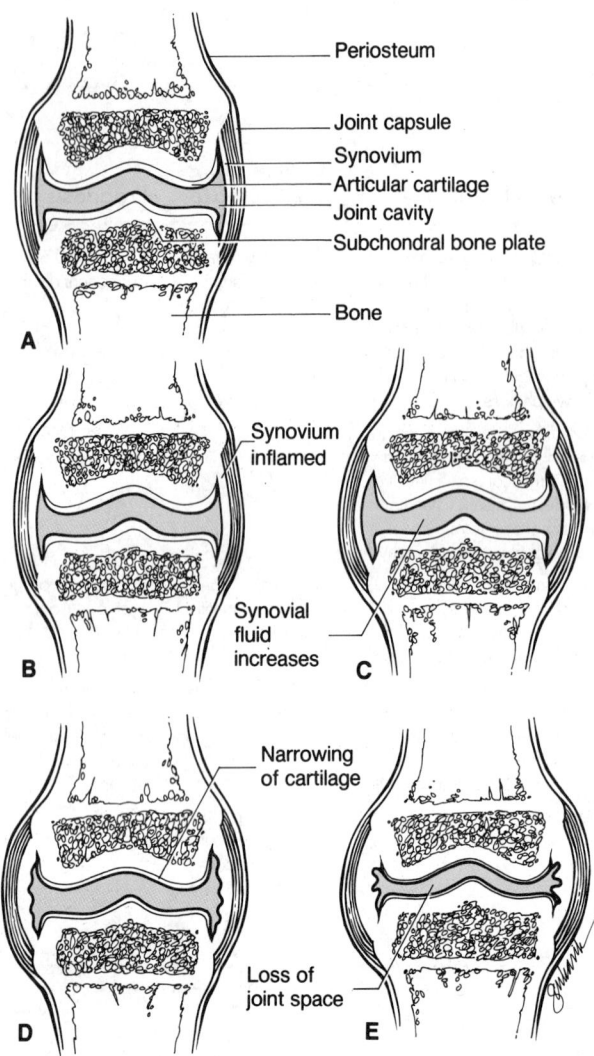

FIGURE 62-11

Joint changes due to rheumatoid arthritis. Ongoing inflammation of the synovium (**A**) causes increased production of synovial fluid and the appearance of an enlarged joint (**B**). Progressive destruction of the inflamed joint may occur (**C**). The synovial membrane thickens and the cartilage is compressed (**D**). Chronic synovitis eventually erodes and destroys cartilage and bone (**E**).

mentation rate, antinuclear antibody, rheumatoid factor, and human leukocyte antigen), while not diagnostic, are often helpful in classifying symptoms and may assist in the exclusion of other disorders. The ESR may or may not be elevated. ANA is positive in low to moderate titers in approximately 40% of the children with JRA, and rheumatoid factors are negative in 85% of cases. Laboratory findings in the specific subtypes are outlined in Table 62-11.

Radiographs of the joints are helpful as a baseline to assess articular growth or possible damage later and to rule out infection, fracture, or tumor. Radiographs are not diagnostic except when revealing late characteristic signs of articular damage.

★ ASSESSMENT

The effects of JRA can have a physical and psychological impact on the child's activities of daily living, school per-

formance, sports participation, and social interactions. The impact of chronic disease on family functioning and dynamics also should be considered. To determine the extent of its impact the nurse needs to ask specific questions, such as the following: What is the duration, time, and pattern of the child's stiffness and pain? Is the child able to perform the activities of daily living, and if so which ones? Have the roles of the family members changed since the child was diagnosed with a chronic illness, and if so, to what extent? In the course of the day what activities does he or she find difficult to perform? Has the child's personality and outlook on life changed? How does the child feel about having a chronic illness? What observations does the child make about limitations or appearance? These are only a few of the questions that may be posed to a child with JRA or to his or her family.

★ NURSING DIAGNOSES AND PLANNING

Based on assessment data discussed previously and in the preceding chapter, the following nursing diagnoses may apply to the family and child with JRA:

- Pain related to stiffness.
- Impaired Physical Mobility related to joint stiffness and contractures.
- Activity Intolerance related to decreased mobility.
- Fatigue related to decreased mobility and stiffness.
- Self-Care Deficit related to joint stiffness and contractures.
- Self-Esteem Disturbance related to decreased mobility.
- Altered Growth and Development related to decreased mobility.
- Anxiety related to lack of knowledge about disease and its unpredictable nature.
- Altered Family Processes related to stresses imposed by chronic illness.
- Family Coping: Potential for Growth related to stress imposed by chronic illness.

The nurse and child (or parents) together plan effective care based on the established nursing diagnoses. Several examples of expected outcomes follow:

- The child and family discuss the diagnosis and therapy program.
- The family identifies lifestyle changes needed to adapt to the child's chronic illness.
- The family establishes priorities for daily and weekly activities to conserve the child's energy.
- The child participates in age-appropriate activities that stimulate and balance physical, cognitive, affective, and social domains.
- The parents state they are giving support to each other.
- The child states that he or she has taken responsibility for activities of daily living, medications, and therapies according to age level.

The nurse plans for the daily care of the child based on physician's orders and nursing diagnoses. Some general nursing care goals may include the following:

- Joint inflammation is relieved.
- Joint range of motion, muscle strength, and tone are increased and maintained.
- Pain is relieved.

• The child's activities are kept as normal as possible to promote physical and psychosocial development.

★ INTERVENTIONS: COLLABORATIVE AND INDEPENDENT

JRA is best managed by a coordinated, multidisciplinary approach that involves a number of professionals, including a pediatrician, pediatric rheumatologist, nurse specialist, physical therapist, occupational therapist, social worker, dietician, ophthalmologist, psychologist, orthopedist, and possibly a psychiatrist. Including the child and family as a part of this team is extremely important. Their cooperation is key to the success of any interventions.

There is no cure for JRA; therefore, most of the treatment is supportive, not curative.[27] Treatment is done at home or as an outpatient, with the child being hospitalized only during periods of disease exacerbation.

MEDICATION THERAPY

The natural history of JRA without pharmacologic intervention is unknown. Several groups of medications are used in the treatment of JRA. To achieve the desired effect these medications may be used alone or in combination. Traditionally, the philosophy of management is to begin with the safest, simplest, and most conservative measures. The progression from one group of medications to another depends on a number of factors, such as the extent of the disease, age, previous medication (successes and failures), functional capacity, anticipated follow-up and compliance, medication toxicity, and the physician's philosophy of management. No matter what medication is prescribed, parents need information about the medication, why it has been prescribed, common side-effects and interactions, the dosage schedule, and what to expect as a result of its administration. Children on any of these medications need to be monitored for their response and any indications of side-effects. For more information on these medications, see Table 62-12.

Nonsteroidal anti-inflammatory drugs (NSAIDs) are traditionally the first level of medication used. They are used primarily for their anti-inflammatory properties, and it usually takes 2 to 4 weeks for a therapeutic threshold of these medication to be reached. Because of some concern with the safety and efficacy of these first-line agents, some rheumatology centers recently have begun to inject triamcinolone hexacetonide into the most commonly affected joint (usually the knee) of children with pauciarticular JRA. This treatment has effectively suppressed synovitis of the involved joint and has maintained resolution of inflammation for up to 6 months after an injection.[27]

Second-line medications, referred to as disease-modifying antirheumatic drugs, are thought to retard or change the course of the disease and may even induce a remission. These medications are frequently taken in conjunction with NSAIDs. Medications within this group may take several weeks to several months to effect a response.

Although oral steroids have a number of side-effects, such as growth suppression, osteoporosis, and muscle wasting, potent anti-inflammatory agents are very beneficial in some situations. The usual indication that the drugs are needed is serious extra-articular manifestations of the disease. During a period of an acute exacerbation, a large dose of methylprednisolone (30 mg/kg intravenously) is used to decrease inflammation quickly or to act as a temporary "bridge" medication until a newly initiated medication begins to work.

Other immunosuppressive agents, such as chlorambucil, cyclophosphamide, and cyclosporin A, are considered experimental and are reserved for serious disease courses that have been unresponsive to more conventional forms of therapy.[44] Another relative newcomer to the medication regimen has been IV gamma globulin; studies of its efficacy are in progress.

THERAPEUTIC EXERCISE

Therapy programs are crucial to the successful management of a child with JRA. Individualized exercise pro-

TABLE 62-12
Medications for Juvenile Rheumatoid Arthritis

Group	Medications	Indications	Common Side-Effects
Nonsteroidal anti-inflammatory drug (NSAID)	Aspirin (acetylsalicylic acid), Tolectin (tolmetin sodium)	Anti-inflammatory	Gastrointestinal irritation (give with food)
Disease-modifying anti-inflammatory drug (DMARD)	Injectable gold (Myochrysine), Ridaura (Auranofin), Azulfidine, methotrexate, Plaquenil (hydroxychloroquine sulfate), Cuprimine (D-penicillamine)	Retards or modifies disease course	Skin rash Oral ulcerations
	Prednisone (corticosteroids)	Potent anti-inflammatory	Growth failure, weight gain, hypertension, immune suppression, fractures
Cytotoxic	Chlorambucil, Cytoxan (cyclophosphamide), cyclosporin A	Serious disease courses Unresponsive to conventional forms of therapy	Infertility, oncogenicity, infection

grams to maintain or increase joint range of motion are essential to preventing deformity and dysfunction of the joints. Simple and practical exercise programs that the child and family can learn to do at home seem to accomplish these goals most effectively. Focusing on the joints that are most affected and suggesting a limited number of exercises is a useful approach.[39] A child's activities of daily living, play routines, and gym classes offer many opportunities for incorporating therapeutic exercises into existing routines. If possible, children should be allowed to help choose the activities. Activities should be gradually increased and performed during the child's peak performance time. Scheduling regular periods for rest is very helpful.

Children with arthritis tend to flex their joints while at rest. Splinting the affected joints in a functional position with maximum strength or motion enables children to remain active and to prevent future complications from flexion contractures. Children with arthritis in a number of joints may benefit from assistive devices for use at home or in school. For example a raised toilet seat and a large pen or pencil allow the child increased independence.

SURGICAL MANAGEMENT

Very few surgical interventions are beneficial to children with JRA. A synovectomy may be helpful to relieve the mechanical impairment of joint motion related to joint pain or synovial hypertrophy. Other surgical interventions that may be useful in a child with a severe contracture of the knee or hips are soft-tissue releases, tendon lengthening, posterior capsulotomy, or tenosynovectomy. Children with marked disability and pain may need reconstructive surgery, such as a total hip replacement.

PAIN RELIEF

Stiffness is a major source of discomfort, as is decreased mobility, particularly in the morning or during periods of inactivity. Smaller children may manifest stiffness by unusual gaits or irritability and crankiness. Heat is widely used and has been shown to be beneficial in decreasing the joint stiffness associated with arthritis. Warm tub baths, showers, heating pads, or electric blankets with a timer set to come on 1 hour before the child awakens in the morning are commonly used to combat stiffness and discomfort.

TEACHING

Helping the child and family to learn about the chronic disease and teaching a management style for the therapeutic regimen that fits their personality and lifestyle helps them adapt to the chronicity and uncertainty of JRA. To help increase compliance to the therapy regimen, it is crucial to reinforce teaching about the disease, therapies being used, and the rationale for these therapies. Parents frequently need additional parenting skills on how to foster the child's growth, development, and independence, and how to set limits on behavior. Teaching parents advocacy skills also assists them in dealing with systems, such as the school, insurance companies, and hospitals.

PSYCHOSOCIAL SUPPORT

The disease course of JRA is variable and very frustrating to children and families who are used to dealing with concrete or predictable issues. Some helpful interventions include the following: Provide a system in which caregivers or children with a chronic illness can verbalize feelings; offer constructive suggestions for how they might cope in certain situations; discuss fears related to exacerbations of the disease; and explore the child's feelings about having a chronic illness. The nurse needs to be alert for cues that signal undue anxiety or guilt within the family. Referring the family to agencies that provide special services demonstrates the nurse's advocacy role.

★ EVALUATION

Periodically, the nurse and family evaluate the outcomes of care given. Examples of outcomes for the child and family with JRA were given under Nursing Diagnoses and Planning in this section.

The most important goal to keep in mind when treating a child with JRA is to keep his or her life as normal as possible. The overall prognosis is good. Seventy to ninety percent of children with JRA have satisfactory outcomes without serious disability.[7] Less than 5% have recurrences as adults. Ten percent of those with JRA enter adulthood with severe functional disability. Because each child's course may vary greatly, treatment should be aimed at decreasing residual deformity or impaired function.

Osteomyelitis

Definition and Incidence. Osteomyelitis is an infection of the bone that usually involves the cortex or the marrow cavity. The rapid growing ends of the bones and the long bones of the lower extremity are the most susceptible. Acute osteomyelitis has an abrupt onset, usually within 7 days of the beginning symptoms. Chronic osteomyelitis is a bone infection that persists longer than 4 weeks or an infection that has failed the initial course of antibiotic therapy for acute osteomyelitis.[30] Osteomyelitis is four times more prevalent in boys. Eighty-five percent of known cases have been reported in children younger than 16 years of age.[41]

Etiology and Pathophysiology. *Staphylococcus aureus* is the most common pathogen, causing more than 90% of the cases of osteomyelitis. Other organisms that have been implicated include *Haemophilus influenzae, Pneumococcus, Streptococcus, Escherichia coli,* and *Pseudomonas.*[35] The source of infection can be either hematogenous—the bacteria are carried by the bloodstream—or exogenous from a penetrating injury to the bone or by indirect extension from nearby infected tissue.

The organisms gain entry into the bone through the metaphysis, which is porous and vascular. The inflammatory response is characterized by leukocytoses and increased vascularization of the subperiosteal space. Pus and an abscess are formed. As the pus escapes through the metaphyseal cortex, pressure increases, causing the periosteum to pull away from the bone and its vascular supply. The elevated periosteum remains viable because its blood supply comes from the overlying muscles. The avascular area of bone becomes necrotic and is called a sequestrum. Because of inhibited blood supply to the sequestrum, bacteria may remain viable, causing chronic osteomyelitis. If the infection remains untreated, the periosteum ruptures, releasing purulent drainage into the nearest joints.

The same infection can manifest itself differently in children of different ages.[14] Infants younger than 18 months are at risk for infiltration into the epiphyseal plate. After 18 months the growth plate acts as a barrier against pathogens to the epiphysis.

Clinical Manifestations.   Signs and symptoms of osteomyelitis vary depending on the extent and location of the infected bone. Any child complaining of localized bone pain that is rapid in onset and severe enough to cause limited movement of the extremity should be suspicious for acute hematogenous osteomyelitis. Some children with osteomyelitis present with the signs and symptoms of sepsis, which include malaise, irritability, restlessness, elevated temperature, tachycardia, and tachypnea. Localized swelling, tenderness, and warmth over the metaphysis are present in the majority of cases.

Diagnostic Studies.   Osteomyelitis is diagnosed by clinical symptomatology. Laboratory studies are used only to confirm the diagnosis. Blood studies may show leukocytosis, an elevated erythrocyte sedimentation rate, and anemia. Blood, urine, sputum, and pharyngeal cultures should be obtained before antibiotics are initiated to determine the source of the infection.

Bone scintigraphy may be used to help confirm the diagnosis of osteomyelitis.[32] If the bone fails to attract the circulating radioisotope, it may indicate diminished blood supply to the sequestrum and require aggressive therapy.

Radiographic findings reveal soft-tissue swelling during the early stages of osteomyelitis. Actual bone changes will not be detected for at least 10 to 14 days after the onset of the infection.

Bone aspiration is the most useful test in diagnosing osteomyelitis.[35] The aspiration of pus confirms the presence of infection in that specific area. Tentative identification can be made on the aspirate through Gram's stain. Bone aspiration can also determine the need for surgical intervention.

★ ASSESSMENT

Children with acute hematogenous osteomyelitis present with a complaint of bone pain for several days. Infants may be irritable and cry when the affected limb is manipulated. The pain may be severe enough to cause limping or restricted use. Swelling and erythema of the infected limb may be localized unless the infection has spread to the surrounding tissue. The nurse should collect data about the onset of symptoms, including a history of recent systemic infection or a recent puncture injury.

When performing the physical assessment, the nurse should examine the affected area last. Children who frightened and in pain will be uncooperative if the nurse causes them further discomfort early in the physical examination. At the completion of the physical assessment,

the inflamed area should be inspected for erythema and palpated for temperature and swelling.

Assessing vital signs determines the presence of systemic infection. Not all children who have osteomyelitis, however, will have an alteration in vital signs. Laboratory studies are performed to identify the responsible pathogen. Information about drug allergies, especially to antibiotics, should be included in the assessment process.

★ NURSING DIAGNOSES AND PLANNING

Based on assessment data discussed previously and in the preceding chapter, the following nursing diagnoses may apply to the family and child with osteomyelitis:

- Pain related to bone infection.
- Hyperthermia related to the infectious process.
- Impaired Tissue Integrity related to bacterial infiltration.
- Impaired Physical Mobility related to imposed bedrest.
- Altered Growth and Development related to involvement of the growth plates.
- Diversional Activity Deficit related to boredom, bedrest.

The nurse and child (or parents) together plan effective care based on the established nursing diagnoses. Several examples of expected outcomes follow:

- Parents demonstrate commitment to treatment plan.
- Parents demonstrate parent-infant attachment.
- Parents demonstrate correct use of IV drugs.
- Child maintains correct body alignment in bed.
- Child uses trapeze bar regularly to assist in movement.
- Child participates in self-care activities.
- Child participates in quiet play in bed.
- Friends visit the child.

The nurse plans for the daily care of the child based on physician's orders and nursing diagnoses. Some general nursing care goals may include the following:

- Infectious organism is eliminated.
- Intact bone structure and pain control are maintained.
- Normal growth and development are supported.

A successful outcome depends on a commitment by the parents and child to follow the rigorous medication and treatment plan.

★ INTERVENTIONS: COLLABORATIVE AND INDEPENDENT

Nursing care for a child with osteomyelitis involves careful assessment for local and systemic signs and symptoms of acute infection. Lengthy hospitalizations may be required for antibiotic therapy and surgery, thereby causing increased anxiety for the child and family. The accompanying Nursing Care Plan gives an example of nursing care of a child with osteomyelitis.

Bedrest and immobilization are indicated during the acute phase of the illness. Weight bearing on the affected extremity is not permitted. Appropriate diversional activity helps the child overcome boredom and fear.

The nurse is responsible for monitoring the child's vital signs and identifying when the child is in pain. An-
(text continued on page 1726)

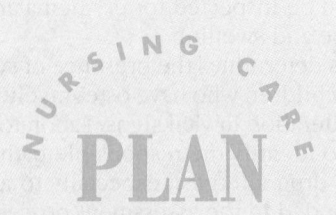

A Child With Osteomyelitis

Assessment

Case Study Description

Jerry, a 9-year-old boy, contracted impetigo on his face and neck at summer day camp. Three days later he started to complain of acute pain and decreased mobility to his left leg. His mother was concerned because Jerry rarely complained of minor illnesses. At the pediatrician's office a pediatric nurse practitioner obtained a thorough nursing history and carefully examined Jerry's leg. After extensive tests and conferring with the pediatrician, a diagnosis of acute hematogenous osteomyelitis was made.

Assessment Data

Vital Signs: Temperature, 37.6°C; pulse, 112; respirations, 28; blood pressure, 110/62.

Musculoskeletal Assessment: Decreased range of motion to left hip and left knee. Acute pain to lower left femur; pain radiates above and below the area. Ambulates with a limp to the left leg. Guarding of left leg on examination.

Skin: Swelling, erythema, warmth over lower left femur.

Behavior: Irritable, weak, malaise, frightened

Diagnostic Studies: Red blood cells: 4.7 m/mm^3; hemoglobin, 14.2 g/dl. White blood cells: 32,000/mm^3; hematocrit, 43.1 g/dl. Platelets: 350,000 mm^3; erythrocyte sedimentation rate, 26 mL/hour.

X-ray: Marked soft-tissue swelling noted around left distal femur.

Bone Scan: Increased uptake of radionuclide isotopes at left distal femur.

Nursing Diagnosis	Intervention	Rationale
1. Acute pain Supporting Data: • Guarding behavior • Statements of pain • Crying • Facial mask of pain	Assess pain characteristics on standardized pediatric pain level scale.	Children relate better to visual pain assessment scales than numbers.
	Administer analgesics and monitor effectiveness.	Timely administration and evaluation of effective analgesics help to control pain.
	Maintain correct body alignment.	Correct alignment helps to reduce stress and tension on the limb.
	Support and elevate limb.	Dependent edema and further trauma to the affected limb are reduced.
	Inspect immobilizing agent for fit and application.	Proper application of device decreases chance of vascular compromise, further tissue destruction and contracture.
	Avoid unnecessary handling of infected extremity.	Manipulation of limb causes increased pain and possible spread of infection.

(Continued)

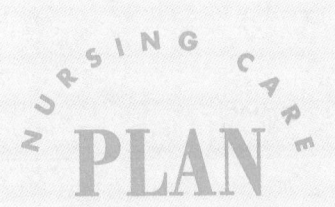

A Child With Osteomyelitis (continued)

Nursing Diagnosis	*Intervention*	*Rationale*
2. Impaired physical mobility related to musculoskeletal impairment	Encourage activities that exercise muscles other than in affected leg.	Other muscles need to be exercised to prevent atrophy.
Supporting Data: • Pain to left leg • Limited range of motion • Hesitant to move leg • Mechanical device restricting movement	Apply trapeze bar to head of bed.	Trapeze bar increases independence and exercises upper extremities.
	Involve physical therapy in exercise program.	Physical therapy specializes in correct muscle movement and exercise.
	Observe for complications of immobility.	Phlebitis, pressure ulcers, neurovascular compromise, and decreased respiratory function are all examples of complications of immobility.
	Teach child methods of self-care activity while restricted to bedrest.	Self-care activities increase independence and sense of control.
3. High risk for infection transmission	Initiate wound and skin isolation precautions.	Isolation protects the health care workers and others from pathogens.
Supporting Data: • Possible draining wound • Gram-positive or -negative infected wound	Institute health teaching about mode of pathogen transmission.	Direct and indirect contact with the pathogens can cause its spread.
	Assign child to private room.	Private room helps to decrease the spread of infection to a susceptible host.
	Administer antibiotics as ordered.	Strict adherence to medication schedule maintains constant serum levels to ensure bactericidal action of antibiotic.
	Monitor for evidence of drug reactions.	Multiple antibiotics may cause adverse drug interactions and side-effects.
4. High risk for altered body temperature related to bone infection	Monitor vital signs every 4 hours and as needed, and record pattern.	Alteration in vital signs are early indicators of progression of infection.
Supporting Data: • Elevated temperature • Flushed, pale appearance • Tenderness over affected area • Leukocytosis	Assess for pain, swelling, and erythema over affected area.	Any change in status of affected area may indicate further bacterial infiltration.
	Maintain adequate nutrition and hydration.	Increase in basal metabolic rate due to infection increases need for calories and fluid.
	Maintain comfortable temperature control: — Bathe with cool water. — Use cotton sheets. — Use fan in room to circulate air. — Change damp clothing as needed.	Stable external environmental factors can help to control a person's homeostasis.
	Administer antipyretics as needed.	Antipyretics help to decrease temperature by acting on the hypothalamus. High fevers in children predispose them to seizures.

(Continued)

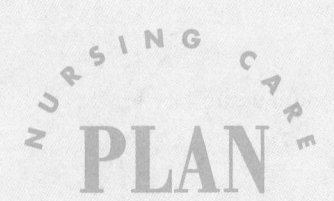

A Child With Osteomyelitis (continued)

Nursing Diagnosis	*Intervention*	*Rationale*
5. Diversional Activity deficit related to immobility Supporting Data: • Confinement to room • Flat affect ("I have no one to play with.") • Restlessness • Bedrest • Constant use of call bell system	Provide diversional activity appropriate to the child's condition and developmental level.	Play is the child's natural medium of expression.
	Allow the child to participate in planning his or her care and making choices when applicable.	A sense of control helps a child to feel independent and involved with his or her surroundings.
	Encourage play therapist to visit child while socially isolated.	Recreational therapists have access to many toys and games that will encourage the child to participate in social activities.
	Solicit parental involvement in child's care and treatments.	Parents will have a sense of control and maintain their parental role for the child while in the hospital.
	Encourage sibling, playmate, teacher visitation, if allowed.	Helps to maintain contact with the outside world.
	Be creative and spontaneous when engaging the child in diversional activities.	Stimulating the child's senses through sight, smell, touch, hearing, and tasting dispels boredom.

Evaluation
• Effective pain control is maintained.
• No complications of immobility are observed while Jerry remains on bedrest.

Expected Outcomes
• Jerry states three ways to decrease the spread of infection to other people.
• Jerry's vital signs return to normal parameters.
• Jerry participates in playing with model cars, puzzles, and board games.
• Jerry maintains school work as recognized by his being named "Student of the Month."

algesics should be provided on a regular basis to decrease some of the discomfort.

Careful monitoring of fluid and electrolytes, intake and output, and therapeutic serum antibiotic levels is ongoing. Parenteral antibiotic therapy continues for 7 to 10 days.

A diet high in calories, protein, vitamin C, and calcium helps to promote bone healing. Small, frequent meals may help decrease anorexia and increase caloric intake.

If the treatment includes surgical intervention, such as wound drainage and débridement or muscle flaps, monitoring for postoperative complications is indicated. Continuous irrigation and suction of the infected bone aids in the débridement and drainage of the pus and the offending pathogens.

Because many children are discharged on IV antibiotics, special parental instruction is needed. Monitoring IV sites, mixing antibiotics, and flushing heparin locks

are all part of the discharge instruction. The child is eventually switched to oral antibiotics for the remainder of the drug therapy. Cast care instruction may be needed for children who require immobilization with a cast. Referrals to home health nurses may help ease the transition from the hospital to home care.

★ EVALUATION

The importance of early recognition and treatment of osteomyelitis cannot be overemphasized. Delayed or inaccurate diagnosis can result in permanent damage and growth retardation to the affected limb. Ongoing education is necessary for the child who is on home parenteral antibiotic therapy. Patient compliance, adequate response to IV therapy, and availability of laboratory facilities to determine serum antibiotic levels are the keys to successful oral antibiotic treatment.

Follow-up is needed to ensure that the antibiotics

have been effective. Long-term care is needed to ensure that there is not a recurrence. Bones that are weakened by osteomyelitis are more susceptible to repeated invasion by organisms.

Skeletal Tuberculosis

Because of the recent increased incidence of tuberculosis, the effect of this disease on the skeletal system warrants some discussion. If the disease is left untreated, the bones may become infected through hematogenous dissemination from the primary tubercular lesion.

In young children the bones of the feet and hands may be affected. Manifestations usually include painless spindle-shaped swelling and tenderness of the surrounding soft tissues with periods of remission. If the disease is untreated, permanent deformities may result.

The vertebrae of older children are usually affected, producing a kyphotic curve. The affected thoracic spine is usually painful, but symptoms may be intermittent. Children tend to guard the painful area by assuming postures to ease the discomfort. Once the disease is diagnosed, antibiotic therapy and drainage of the tubercular abscess is initiated. A spinal fusion may be needed to correct the spinal deformity. Nursing care requirements are similar to those for a child with scoliosis.

The epiphyses of the femoral head and the hip joint are another focal areas for tuberculosis. The primary manifestation is a limp prevalent on arising and after exercise. The lesion is painful and progressive. Muscle spasms may develop. Also, the femur may become fixed in the acetabulum in an adducted and internally rotated position. Antimicrobial therapy with bedrest and traction are the treatments of choice. If the deformity is severe, a hip fusion may be needed.

The primary role of the nurse in the care of children with tuberculosis is early recognition and prevention. If lesions are recognized early, progression and damage to the skeletal system should not occur. Therefore, the nurse needs to provide anticipatory guidance to families about the need for periodic screening.

Traumatic Injuries

With society's current emphasis on participation in sports at an early age, the potential for musculoskeletal injury is increased. Each year, the incidence of sports-related injuries is as high as 1 out of every 100 children.[51] This rate does not take into account other accidental injuries. The mechanisms of injury as well as the anatomic characteristics of the immature skeleton contribute to the occurrence of strains, sprains, and fractures in children.

Fractures

Definition and Incidence. A fracture is any complete or incomplete break in the continuity of the bone that occurs when more stress is placed on the bone than the bone is able to absorb. Fractures are usually classified as open or closed depending on how they communicate with the external environment. The pattern or the direction of the fracture line and the location of the fracture also distinguish fractures.

The direction of the fracture line usually occurs in a recognizable pattern. The various configurations are described in the accompanying display and Figure 62-12. Another way to describe fractures is by location. In reference to the long bones, fractures can be described as proximal, distal, or midshaft. Further description should indicate if the fracture is located in the epiphyseal, metaphyseal, or diaphyseal area.

The incidence of fractures in children varies with the type of fracture and location. Clavicle fractures, which usually result from birth trauma or falls on an outstretched arm or shoulder, are the most common fracture in child-

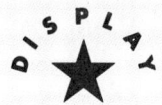

Classification of Fracture Patterns

Buckle (torus): Impaction injury characterized by a raised or bulging projection near the metaphysis (Incidence decreases with skeletal maturity.)

Closed (simple): Fracture with no open wound

Comminuted: Bone splintered or crushed (Related to high impact forces; occurs more frequently in children and older adolescents.)

Complete: Fracture involves entire cross-section of bone.

Compression: Two bones crushed or squeezed together (Usually occurs in vertebral area.)

Depressed: Bone dented inward (Fracture of skull sometimes called "ping-pong" fracture.)

Double: Bone fractured in two places

Greenstick: Bone bends and splits but does not break completely. (Common in children because their bones are still soft and pliable. Incidence decreases with skeletal maturity.)

Impacted: One fragment of bone driven into another

Incomplete: Fracture does not involve complete cross-section of bone

Longitudinal (fissure): Crack runs length of bone

Oblique: Fracture slants across bone shaft

Open (compound): Bone breaks through skin, causing an open wound.

Pathologic (spontaneous): Fracture occurring without force or injury sufficient to break a normal bone (May occur in such conditions as certain types of malnutrition, porous bones, cancer, and as a complication of cortisone and adrenocorticotropic hormone therapy.)

Spiral: Fracture twists around bone (Associated with a twisting force.)

Transverse: Fracture at right angles to bone shaft (Occurs in infants and small children.)

Closed fracture—No open wound

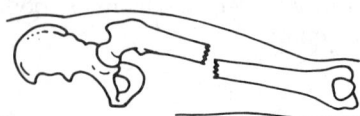

Longitudinal fracture—Break runs parallel with bone

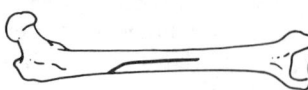

Greenstick fracture—Bone broken, bent but still securely hinged at one side

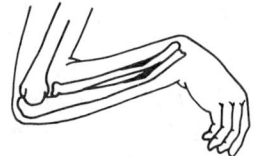

Open fracture—Wound in skin communicates with fracture

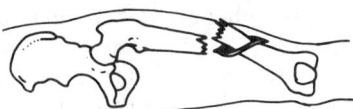

Transverse fracture—Break runs across bone

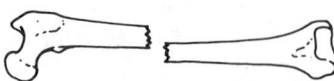

Impacted fracture—Bone broken and wedged into other break

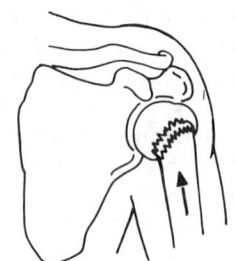

Extracapsular fracture—Bone broken outside joint

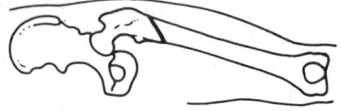

Oblique fracture—Break runs in slanting direction on bone

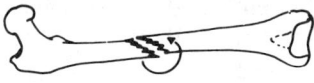

Intracapsular fracture—Bone broken inside joint

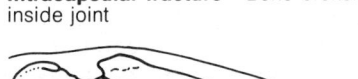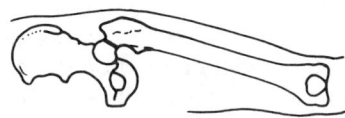

Spiral fracture—Break coils around bone

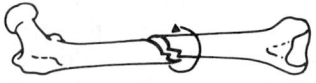

Fracture dislocation—Break complicated by bone out of joint

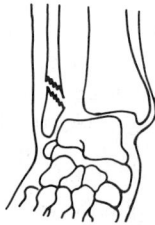

Comminuted fracture—Bone splintered into fragments

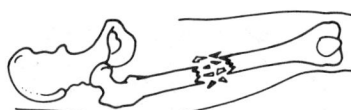

Pathologic fracture—Break is at site of bone disease

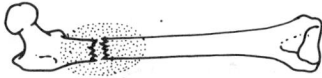

Depressed fracture—Broken skull bone driven inward

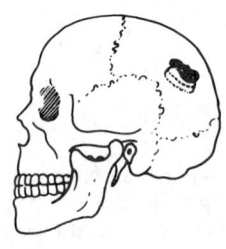

FIGURE 62-12
Types of fractures.

hood. Greenstick fractures are common in young children, but spiral fractures sometimes indicate child abuse. Skeletal injuries must be carefully evaluated in young children because of their effect on bone growth. Epiphyseal injuries account for approximately one third of all skeletal injuries in children.

Etiology and Pathophysiology. The active nature of children despite their limited motor ability predisposes them to injuries to the musculoskeletal system. Fractures may be caused by direct and indirect trauma, repeated stress on the bony structures or pathologic conditions. Trauma results from motor vehicle and pedestrian accidents, falls during play or sports, or child abuse. Motor vehicle accidents are a common cause of injury in children between the ages of 4 and 7. Injuries sustained in this manner usually affect the child's femur, trunk, and head. The type of activities in which a child engages and the use of equipment such as rollerskates, skateboards, bicycles, and trampolines may be responsible for the high incidence of skeletal injury in children.

Other injuries may be unrelated to trauma. Pathologic

conditions, including neoplasms, osteogenesis imperfecta (OI), osteopetrosis, metabolic disorders, and nutritional deficiencies, may increase the child's tendency for fractures.

A stress fracture results from repeated wear and tear on a bone. Children who are involved in sports activities are especially prone to this type of injury. Forces transmitted to the musculoskeletal system affect children differently because of their size and strength. Their ligamentous structures are very flexible and the epiphyses are open, further predisposing them to injuries.[47] Stress fractures are related to the effect of repeated muscle contractions on an athlete's bony structures. This problem is usually associated with sports such as running, gymnastics, and basketball, all of which require repetitive weight bearing.

The training of young athletes is intensive. Often they do not condition their bodies to increase their strength and endurance. Instead they try to challenge themselves beyond their limits. Sometimes they fail to use the necessary protective equipment.

There are several anatomic, biomechanical, and physiologic elements that differentiate a child's bone structure from that of an adult. These factors relate to the mechanisms of injury as well as the healing process.

The child's periosteum is thicker, stronger, and contains a more profuse blood supply than that of the adult. This leads to more rapid healing of the fracture in young children. Nonunion of bones rarely occurs in children. The increased blood supply, however, tends to stimulate growth for 6 to 12 months following the injury, and an overgrowth in the long bones may result.

Children's bones tend to be very porous and lack the density of adult bones. This characteristic allows bones to bend, buckle, and break in unusual ways. Consequently, bone deformity may be present before an actual fracture occurs. Bowing, referred to as a plastic deformation, may occur on the compression side adjacent to another bone. Bowing of these adjacent bones may interfere with reduction of the fracture. Buckle and greenstick fractures, which are unique to young children, are related to the increased porosity and flexibility of their bones.

Often the ligamentous structures are stronger than the bones and growth cartilage. Therefore, the joint capsule and ligaments are often more resistant to stress than the bones and growth cartilage. As a result, joint injuries, dislocations, sprains, and strains are less common in young children.

Epiphyseal Injuries. Injury to the epiphysis is a much more serious condition. The epiphysis, referred to as the growth plate, is a thick, elastic portion of the bone where growth occurs. Sometimes injury to this area is not evident until new bone begins to form. The epiphysis serves to absorb shock and protect the joint from injury. Despite this property the epiphysis is weaker than the surrounding bone and cartilage and therefore is more subject to injury that may result in asymmetric growth. Injury to the epiphysis can cause a progressive angular deformity, a line length discrepancy (LLD), and joint inequality. The relationship of the fracture to the growth plate is usually defined according to the Salter-Harris system, outlined in Table 62-13. This classification system

TABLE 62-13
Salter-Harris Classification System of Growth Plate Injuries

Type	Description
I	Epiphysis is completely separated from the metaphysis, without fracture.
II	Transverse fracture line extends through the separated epiphyseal plate through the metaphysis, producing a triangular fragment.
III	Fracture plane extends through part of the epiphyseal plate into the joint.
IV	Fracture extends through the epiphyseal plate and through part of the metaphysis.
V	An area of the epiphyseal plate is crushed but not displaced.

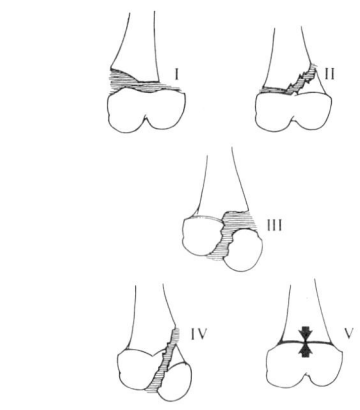

Adapted from Joy, C. (1989). *Pediatric trauma nursing.* Gaithersburg, MD: Aspen Publishers.

lists epiphyseal injuries in order of increasing risk of permanent epiphyseal damage and potential growth disturbance. When used with data about the mechanism of injury, the system provides a guide for treatment.

Type I injuries are usually seen in young children with thick epiphyseal plates. Often these injuries are associated with birth trauma. Frequently, there is no displacement, and the periosteum remains intact. Consequently, radiologic findings are inconclusive, and the injury may be confused with a type V injury. Before an accurate diagnosis can be made, the mechanism of injury must be considered. If the blood supply to the epiphysis remains intact, the outcome for this type of injury is excellent. Healing generally occurs in 3 weeks or less.

Type II epiphyseal injury occurs most often in children older than 10 years. Type II is the most common type of epiphyseal injury. Because the periosteum is torn on only one side, the fracture is easily reduced. Again, the prognosis is excellent when the blood supply to the epiphysis is not compromised.

Type III injuries are usually seen in children who are approaching skeletal maturity. Despite the fact that the growth plate is partially closed, growth disturbances are not significant. Because this fracture involves the joint space, accurate reduction is essential. If the joint surface and vascularity are restored, the outcome will be positive.

With type IV injuries there is vertical splitting of the epiphysis. Often the fracture fragment migrates toward the diaphysis. Unless there is perfect anatomic alignment, growth will be affected. Joint stiffness and deformity also are associated with this type of injury.

The most severe type of epiphyseal injury is classified as type V, which usually occurs following a crush injury to the epiphyseal plate. Because there is not a clear fracture line or displacement, radiologic findings are often inconclusive. An understanding of the mechanisms of injury is essential. Type V injuries may occur with other types of epiphyseal injuries, and this type of injury affects bone growth.

Healing. Healing of fractures occurs much more rapidly in the immature skeleton. In general the younger the child, the more rapid the healing process. This property is related to the osteogenic nature of the periosteum and its characteristic thickness. The rapid formation of subperiosteal bone that bridges the fracture site is assisted by parts of the periosteum that remain intact.

The bone healing process follows a sequence of five stages, as summarized in the accompanying display. In children, however, the process is accelerated, and the remodeling capacity is unique. Children's bones remodel regardless of the anatomic position of the bone fragments. Remodeling serves to restore a portion of the normal bone structure despite significant malalignment. The capacity for remodeling is related to the type and location of the fracture, the age of the child, the amount of angulation that exists at the fracture site, and the position of the bone fragments. The younger the child, the greater the potential for remodeling. Remodeling is also accentuated when the injury is close to the epiphysis and takes place in the plane of motion of the adjacent joint. Therefore,

the chance of deformity is enhanced in children because of the possibility of undetected fractures or incorrect alignment of the fracture fragments.

When an injury occurs the muscles and soft tissues also respond. The muscles contract and physiologically splint the area. The force of the muscle contraction may pull the fracture fragments out of alignment. Contusions accompanied by bleeding into the surrounding tissues may occur in the soft tissues. These tissues become edematous, and a hematoma usually forms. Shock may occur in response to the bleeding and pain of the injury. The severity of the physiologic response to a musculoskeletal injury varies according to the degree of damage to underlying structures and area of injury.

Clinical Manifestations. When children experience a fracture to some area of the musculoskeletal system, they display the usual signs and symptoms, including pain with movement, edema, ecchymosis, crepitus, and guarding. The pain may be localized or in the form of muscle spasm, or there may be obvious deformity at the fracture site. In addition there may be loss of motor function and impaired sensation.

Children, however, may not be able to verbalize what they are experiencing. If a child refuses to walk or use an extremity following an injury, a fracture should be suspected. Children tend to guard the injured area, and the range of motion to that area is decreased. However, the fracture may remain stable if the periosteum is intact. In these situations children may continue to use the affected extremity.

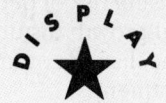 ## Stages of Bone Healing

I. HEMATOMA FORMATION (PROCALLUS)

- Occurs 24 to 48 hours postinjury.
- Blood from the torn vessels in the bone fragments and soft-tissue leak between and around fracture fragments.
- Hematoma serves as a fibrin meshwork for subsequent cellular invasion.
- Granulation tissue begins to invade area.
- Osteoblastic (bone forming) activity is stimulated.

II. CELLULAR PROLIFERATION (FIBROCARTILAGINOUS CALLUS)

- Occurs within 2 weeks of injury.
- Blood supply increases and brings fibroblasts, endothelial cells, and nutrients to the area.
- Hematoma changes to granulation tissue to form a framework for bone-forming cells (osteoblasts).
- Ends of fracture fragments become necrotic and die.
- Osteoblasts multiply and differentiate into fibrocartilaginous callus.
- Callus forms a soft collar around the fracture site to bridge and connect bone fragments.

III. CALLUS FORMATION (BONY CALLUS)

- Occurs 3 to 4 weeks postinjury.
- Osteoblasts enter the area and produce a "sticky" osteoid matrix causing the fibrin bridge to become firm.

IV. OSSIFICATION

- Occurs 3 to 10 weeks postinjury.
- Union occurs—the final laying down of bone.
- Mature bone replaces callus.
- Callus is reabsorbed by osteoclasts.

V. REMODELING

- Occurs after 9 months.
- Resorption of excess bony callus that develops within marrow space and encircles external aspect of fracture site.
- Bone responds to mechanical stress by becoming thicker and stronger.

The clinical manifestation may vary with the type and location of the fracture. When injury occurs to the supracondylar structures of the humerus and femur, nerve and vascular damage may occur. Evidence of neurovascular compromise includes the five "Ps" of ischemia: pain, pallor, pulselessness, paresthesia, and paralysis. Usually these signs are present in the extremity distal to the injury. The best discriminators of upper-extremity injury are gross deformity and point tenderness.[42] Lower-extremity injuries are distinguishable by the presence of gross deformity and pain with movement.

Diagnostic Studies. Following an initial evaluation of the clinical manifestations and a review of the mechanisms of injury, radiologic studies are performed. Because the ossification process in children often is not complete until the child reaches 18 to 21 years of age, the appearance of the bone is altered. Much of the skeleton of infants and young children is composed of radiolucent growth cartilage that is not visible on radiograms. Therefore, alterations in the epiphysis often are difficult to detect. Comparisons of the unaffected extremity generally are needed to evaluate the injury. Sometimes arthrography, ultrasonography, or computer-assisted tomography is needed for a reliable diagnosis. Radiographic studies are performed following reduction of the fracture and at various stages in the healing process.

When severe soft-tissue, muscle, and bone injury occur, laboratory studies may be warranted. When red blood cells are damaged, there may be a rise in bilirubin and a decrease in the hemoglobin and hematocrit level. The inflammatory response to the injury may produce a slight elevation in the neutrophils of the white blood cells. If an infection occurs, these findings are elevated significantly. Muscle damage may stimulate an increase in serum enzymes that are usually contained within the muscle cells. Serum levels of creatinine, alkaline phosphatase, serum glutamic-oxaloacetic transaminase, and lactate dehydrogenase may increase relative to the degree of muscle involvement.

★ ASSESSMENT

Assessment begins with data collection about the mechanism and cause of the injury. Data about the mechanism reveal whether the injury occurred by such activities as flexion, extension, torsion, or direct assault. The cause of injury refers to the vehicle of injury, such as an automobile, a bicycle, or another person. The child may not be a reliable source of data because of limited vocabulary or the circumstances surrounding the injury. If the child was engaged in a forbidden activity, the child may be afraid to give accurate information for fear of punishment; the parents may be unaware of the true cause of the injury. In cases of child abuse, the parent usually does not give accurate information. The nurse may need to talk with the child alone using various play and story-telling techniques.

Because data related to the mechanism and cause of injury may be limited, the physical assessment is even more important. To ensure cooperation of the child, the nurse must be careful not to inflict any pain during this part of the assessment. Initially, the nurse should observe for the presence of any spontaneous movement in the affected extremity.

Assessment of an injury to the musculoskeletal system always includes evaluation of the extremities for the presence of the five Ps mentioned in the section on Clinical Manifestations above. Children often have difficulty identifying and locating the source of their pain. The nurse must be alert to signs such as unreasonable crying, restlessness, guarding of an area, and other nonverbal indicators of pain. If the child is cooperative, age-appropriate pain assessment scales and pictures can be used. Children who are hospitalized for musculoskeletal injuries usually experience a greater number of painful events and bodily symptoms than children hospitalized for other reasons.[53A] Parents often are a valuable resource in helping their child to identify the source of their pain.

A baseline assessment of vital signs and respiratory status also should be included as part of the initial assessment. The possibility of developing a fat embolism is greatest in the first 24 to 72 hours following an injury. Any signs of respiratory difficulty or elevated blood pressure may indicate an embolism.

The child and family may be very anxious about the experience, and their anxiety may intensify the child's pain. Therefore, the assessment always should include data about the child and the family's level of anxiety and any coping strengths that are noted.

★ NURSING DIAGNOSES AND PLANNING

Based on assessment data discussed previously and in the preceding chapter, the following nursing diagnoses may apply to the family and child with a fracture during the acute phase of the injury. Nursing diagnoses for the child in traction or in a cast can be found in the appropriate sections.

- Pain related to extremity manipulation, muscle damage, and ischemia.
- Altered Peripheral Tissue Perfusion related to edema and pressure.
- Impaired Gas Exchange related to release of fat globules in the systemic circulation.
- High Risk for Infection related to immobility, skin disruption from open fractures, pin insertion, or external fixation device.
- Impaired Physical Mobility related to limits imposed by the injury.
- Anxiety related to knowledge deficit about treatment and care procedures.
- Fear related to feelings about the cause of the injury and unfamiliarity with treatment procedures.

The nurse and child (or parents) together plan effective care based on the established nursing diagnoses. Several examples of expected outcomes follow:

- The child demonstrates decreased pain.
- The child does not develop osteomyelitis.
- The child moves all unaffected extremities through full range of motion.
- The child expresses fears through discussion or play acting.
- The family discusses the rationale for the treatment plans and the expected outcomes.

- The family demonstrates how to care for their child in a cast.

The nurse plans for the daily care of the child based on physician's orders and nursing diagnoses. Some general nursing care goals may include the following:

- The child's fracture is reduced with a minimum of deformity and without complications.
- Optimum function is restored to the affected extremity.
- The family and child understand the treatment plan.

★ INTERVENTIONS: COLLABORATIVE AND INDEPENDENT

Nursing interventions are initiated based on the physician's treatment plan and the needs of the child. Medical treatment approaches vary according to the type of injury. Table 62-14 indicates some options. The decision to hospitalize a child or to treat the child on an outpatient basis is based on several criteria. Hospitalization is required when surgical intervention and reduction by internal or external fixation is warranted. Common orthopedic procedures are explained in the accompanying display. When traction is needed, the child also requires hospitalization.

In most situations immobilization by closed reduction is effective treatment for the fractures in young children. This method is generally successful because of the young child's bone remodeling capability. The open reduction method with internal fixation is usually reserved

TABLE 62-14
Common Childhood Fractures

Management of Anatomic Site	Assessment, Treatment, and Other Implications
Clavicle	Shoulder on affected side droops forward and inward; lower than unaffected shoulder. Treated with a figure-8 splint.
Humerus	Inability to move arm, pain with passive movement, ecchymosis and edema at site. Treated with a sugartong splint from the wrist to the axilla with 90-degree elbow flexion; supported with a sling and bound by a soft wrap around the arm and chest.
Supracondylar area	Complete fracture reveals an s-shaped configuration of the arm, marked ecchymosis and swelling at site, pain on movement; potential for vascular and nerve damage and muscle ischemia. Treatment involves splinting with 20 to 30 degrees of elbow flexion and closed or open reduction.
Radius, ulna, wrist, and hand	Often overlooked when treating more serious problems.
Femur	Potential for significant vascular and nerve compromise, including large blood loss. Treatment may include traction or external fixation, open reduction, and internal fixation.
Below knee	Potential for development of compartment syndrome; ankle fractures may affect the epiphysis; treatment may be closed reduction and casting or open reduction and fixation.

Adapted from Campbell, L. S., & Campbell, G. D. (1991). Musculoskeletal trauma in children. *Critical Care Nursing Clinics of North America, 3*(3), 445–446.

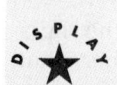

Terms for Common Procedures Used in Orthopedics

Arthroplasty: Reconstruction or replacement of a joint to correct a congenital deformity or repair a damaged joint

Closed reduction: External manipulation of bone to force into alignment

External fixation: Device that provides rigid immobilization of bony fragments on the exterior of the extremity; includes casts, splints, traction, single bar appliances, and frame appliances (Hoffmann and Wagner devices)

Fusion: Merging together of two or more bones as seen when vertebrae are fused in a spinal fusion

Internal fixation: Devices applied to the bone fragments through an open incision; hardware used to stabilize the fragments may include wires, screws, pins, plates, staples, rods, and prosthesis

Open reduction: Internal manipulation of bony fragments through an open incision

Osteotomy: Sawing or cutting of the bone to enable stabilization and realignment

for situations in which there is tissue damage or injury to the nerves or arteries. Fractures of the femur or supracondylar fractures of the distal humerus are examples of fractures that usually require open reduction and internal fixation.

Occasionally external fixation devices are used in the treatment of fractures. The use of these devices is generally reserved for open injuries and fractures in the multiply injured child. Distraction bars are attached proximally and distally to the bone fragments with pins. These devices allow for treatment of the open wound while maintaining the alignment of the bone fragments. In addition the child is able to ambulate earlier and thus decrease some of the negative effects of immobilization on other body systems.

Traction may be part of the treatment plan. The type of traction depends on the age and size of the child as well as the nature of the injury. The purpose of traction is to hold the bone fragments in place while gently decreasing the negative forces from muscle contractions and spasms.

Regardless of the overall treatment plan, casting is usually required at some stage. Because the interventions associated with casting and traction are addressed in another section, only the interventions related to the immediate care of the child with a fracture are discussed here.

PAIN RELIEF

Pain relief is a necessary intervention for a child with a fracture. The key component in achieving pain relief is the ability of the nurse to assess the child's pain level accurately (see Chap. 28). A pain flow sheet and appropriate pediatric pain scales can aid in determining the intensity of the child's pain, the child's response to pain, and the effect of pain-relieving interventions.

Nonpharmacologic and pharmacologic approaches to pain relief should be used. Some nonpharmacologic approaches include repositioning and the application of ice as prescribed. Providing the child with age-appropriate activities while immobilized provides some distraction. Allowing the child to vent frustrations by using hammer toys and punching bags is also helpful.

Positioning of the extremity above the level of the heart promotes venous return and decreases edema. These effects serve to decrease the pressure on the nerve endings that may be responsible for the pain. Support should always be applied above and below the fracture site because any movement may potentiate pain. If ice is prescribed, the nurse must make sure that the ice packs are changed. Ice promotes vasoconstriction, thereby regularly decreasing edema and pain.

Analgesics should be prescribed and given regularly to ensure adequate blood levels of the medication. Whenever possible, children should be given oral or IV analgesics. Older children may be taught to provide their own relief by using a PCA pump. Sometimes children develop muscle spasms around the fracture area. It is important for the nurse to determine the type of pain so that appropriate medications are prescribed. If the child is experiencing periodic spasms, muscle relaxants may be needed. Whenever medications are prescribed for the management of pain, the nurse must assess the effectiveness. If pain relief is not achieved, the nurse must further evaluate the source of the pain. Severe pain may indicate neurovascular compromise, which necessitates immediate medical intervention.

NEUROVASCULAR STATUS ASSESSMENT

The nurse must assess the five Ps of ischemia at least every hour for the first 24 hours of treatment. Depending on the type of injury and treatment, the frequency of assessment can be progressed to every 2 to 4 hours for the remainder of the treatment. Any signs that indicate neurovascular compromise must be reported immediately to the physician. Early detection ensures prompt treatment and the prevention of permanent injury from tissue necrosis and nerve damage.

INFECTION PREVENTION

If the treatment plan involves open reduction or external fixation, the nurse must be alert for any signs of infection. Local manifestations include erythema, edema, and purulent drainage at the site. Fever, restlessness, tachycardia, and tachypnea are signs that may indicate a systemic infection. Assessment of vital signs should be continued at least every 4 hours throughout the initial treatment phase. Protocol for care of the pin site usually varies with physician. Therefore, the nurse needs to follow the prescribed protocol and report any abnormalities to the physician.

ACTIVITY PROMOTION

Because of the naturally active nature of children, problems of disuse syndrome are not present in children. However, the usual activity of children must be curtailed to ensure adequate immobilization and healing of the fracture. The nurse should collaborate with the phy-

sician and the physical or occupational therapist to design activities that enhance muscular movement and maintenance.

The nurse needs to be creative when designing an activity program that maintains the child's physical and psychosocial development and ensures healing of the affected extremity. Allowing the child to perform self-care activities helps to maintain muscle strength as well as the child's self-esteem. Diversional activities that are developmentally appropriate and encourage movement of the unaffected extremities should be planned.

PSYCHOSOCIAL SUPPORT

The child who is undergoing treatment for a fracture must manage fears related to the cause of the injury as well as those associated with unfamiliar surroundings and procedures. Because children often will not discuss their fears, opportunities for allowing the child to vent some of these feelings must be provided. Some children express their feelings through play or through artwork. Sometimes the use of hammer toys or punching bags is helpful. Older children may prefer to write about their feelings. The nurse needs to select interventions that will allow the child to express fears and frustrations in a positive manner. Once the fears are identified, the nurse can intervene to dispel unrealistic fears and anxieties.

Socialization with other children also should be encouraged. If the child is confined to a bed, the bed with the immobilizing equipment can be moved to the playroom. If the child attends school, parents should be encouraged to bring in assignments so that the child will not fall behind with school work. Visiting by siblings and school mates should be encouraged. If visiting is not permitted, pictures and cards by friends and siblings can be recommended. If the nurse is able to maintain some degree of normalcy in the child's routine, the child's fears related to loss of control may be decreased.

TEACHING

The child and family must be involved in the treatment plan. The nurse is often the intermediary in explaining the treatment plan to the child and the family. Frequent reassurance is often needed. Once the child and family feel comfortable with the explanations about the injury and treatment, they should be more open to the extensive instructions that are needed for cast care and home care. These instructions are discussed in the section on Care of a Child in a Cast later in this chapter.

★ EVALUATION

Follow-up as an outpatient is required to ensure that healing has occurred with a minimum of deformity. Generally, healing is rapid, and problems of nonunion are not seen in children. However, if damage to the epiphysis or bone overgrowth have occurred, asymmetry of the extremities may be apparent. In situations in which the fracture site was exposed, the possibility of osteomyelitis must be considered.

Follow-up involves ensuring that optimal function of the extremities is achieved. Physical therapy may be needed to improve the function of the affected extremity. Depending on the nature of the injury and the type of complications encountered, follow-up may be continued until skeletal maturity is reached. During this time the nurse should provide anticipatory guidance to the child and family about prevention of injuries. Each developmental age offers new challenges to families regarding the safety of their children.

COMPLICATIONS

If the nurse carefully assesses the child and evaluates outcomes, any complications should be easily detected. Major complications that can result from a fracture include neurovascular impairment, compartment syndrome, Volkmann's contracture, and fat emboli. A description of these complications and the treatment parameters are included in Table 62-7. All of these complications demand immediate intervention.

Sprains and Strains

Definition and Incidence.   Sprains and strains, referred to as acute overload injuries, result from sudden stress to soft-tissue structures. Damage to these structures accounts for most sports-related injuries in older children. In younger children the effects of abnormal forces are usually transmitted to the weakest area of the musculoskeletal system, the epiphysis. As skeletal maturity is reached, the muscles, tendons, and ligamentous structures respond to the stress.

A sprain is a complete or incomplete tear to the tendons, muscles, or ligaments in contact with a joint. Muscular damage that occurs as a result of overuse or overstretching is referred to as a strain. Both sprains and strains are graded according to the degree of severity. Although sprains may occur in any joint, they are most common in the ankle joint. Strains commonly occur in the lumbar and cervical spine area. However, strains also may appear around the elbows and shoulders.

Etiology and Pathophysiology.   A twisting or rotational stress to a joint usually results in a sprain. This motion may result in a complete ligamentous tear or rupture or an incomplete tear. Sometimes a chip of bone is attached to the torn ligament. Often damage to the blood vessel, nerves, tendons, and muscles accompanies a sprain.

A strain is generally caused by some type of physical effort associated with stretching of the musculotendinous unit. The effects from overstretching may occur immediately or over a period of time.

Healing of soft-tissue injuries generally occurs without sequelae. If muscle contractions exert pressure on the injured tissues before healing has occurred, however, tendons may heal in a lengthened position. The healing process is initiated by fibroblasts from the tendon sheath or connective tissue. Capillary beds in the area provide the fibroblasts with the necessary nutrients for the production of large amounts of collagen. Healing occurs over 4 to 5 weeks. During that time the collagen bundles strengthen the ligamentous structures.

Clinical Manifestations.   The clinical manifestations of sprains and strains are sometimes difficult to dif-

ferentiate. The variations in symptoms are related to the degree of injury. Discomfort associated with strains may be acute or chronic with minor complaints of stiffness. Generally, acute pain is identified with more severe damage around the area of muscle origin or tendon insertion. Often there is no visible evidence of injury. Bleeding, however, may occur within the affected muscle prior to the development of edema.

Minor sprains may be difficult to distinguish from strains. Symptoms vary from minor sprains with normal or limited joint movements to severe sprains with considerable joint laxity. Pain and edema associated with moderate to severe sprains usually take longer to resolve than with strains. The external joint surface is usually discolored and warm to the touch. Ecchymosis usually indicates local hemorrhage and joint effusion. Whenever abnormal joint movements are associated with other complaints, a sprain should be suspected. Children with severe sprains may state that they heard a snapping or popping sound. Although pain may not be a primary manifestation of a severe sprain, children will usually be reluctant to bear weight on the affected joint.

Diagnostic Studies.   Diagnosis is primarily based on the clinical findings. Radiologic studies may be performed to validate the nature of the injury. Unless there is bone avulsion (a forceable tearing away) with the sprain, the soft-tissue edema damage that occurs with a sprain or strain will not be visible on x-ray.

⭐ **ASSESSMENT**

The initial assessment usually begins with collection of data about the mechanism of injury. It is important to note whether the injury has occurred before. The nurse needs to determine if the injury followed any twisting or rotation of the joint or if a direct blow to the area preceded the injury. In addition questions about the type of sports activities engaged in should be asked.

An assessment of the pain also should be included. If the child is able to indicate when the pain started, the nurse needs to direct the assessment to identify variations in the level of pain. Pain assessment tools may be necessary to help the child describe the intensity of pain.

The nurse should begin the physical assessment by observing the child for any limitation of function or guarding of the injured area. Often children will not bear weight or use the injured extremity. Additionally, the nurse should note any abnormal movements of affected joints. Without touching the joint, the nurse can assess the appearance and position of the extremity. A neurovascular assessment should be performed to determine the possibility of damage to nerves and blood vessels. The extent of edema to the area needs to be described. By carefully touching the area, any point tenderness can be noted.

⭐ **NURSING DIAGNOSES AND PLANNING**

Based on assessment data discussed previously and in the preceding chapter, the following nursing diagnoses may apply to the family and children with a sprain or strain:

- Pain related to increased edema and stretching or tearing of the ligamentous structures.
- Impaired Physical Mobility related to limited or abnormal movement of the injured part.
- Fear related to pain and unfamiliar surroundings.
- Anxiety related to knowledge deficit about treatment procedures.

The nurse and child (or parents) together plan effective care based on the established nursing diagnoses. Several examples of expected outcomes follow:

- The child and family identify sports and recreational activities appropriate for the child's size and strength.
- The child participates in the rehabilitation plan.
- The child discusses fears and concerns related to the injury and treatment modalities.

The nurse plans for the daily care of the child based on physician's orders and nursing diagnoses. Some general nursing care goals may be the following:

- The child is free from pain.
- The child regains maximum function of the injured structure.

★ INTERVENTIONS: COLLABORATIVE AND INDEPENDENT

Similar principles are followed in the treatment of strains and sprains. Rest and immobilization of the injured area is paramount in the management of both injuries. Within the first 12 hours after the injury, ice should be applied for 20 to 30 minutes. Other components of the treatment plan are dictated by the extent of the injury.

Muscle strains are usually immobilized until the pain and edema have subsided. When the cervical or lumbar area of the spine is affected, more extensive treatment is required. Sometimes, bedrest with traction is prescribed. The application of heat and massage to the area decreases muscle spasms and increases comfort. The child needs to be taught exercises and proper body mechanics to reduce the possibility of reinjury. Teaching adolescents to maintain good body posture can be a real challenge for the nurse; creative teaching methods are needed.

Management of minor sprains includes rest, ice, and support of the injured part. Usually the area is covered with a wet compression bandage to support and transfer cold to the injury. The wrap should provide support without affecting the neurovascular status, which should be assessed frequently (Table 62-16). The skin under the ice pack should be protected with a single layer of the wrap.

The affected extremity should be supported and elevated above the level of the heart. This procedure promotes venous return and decreases edema formation in the injured area. In addition the child will be more comfortable in this position. Mild analgesics should be given as prescribed to further alleviate the discomfort.

When ligaments are torn in joints such as the knee or ankle, casts or elastic splints may be required (Fig. 62-13). With severe sprains, open reduction may be needed to repair the torn ligamentous structures. Immobilization for 3 to 4 weeks with gentle passive exercises typically is needed. Children should be taught how to perform

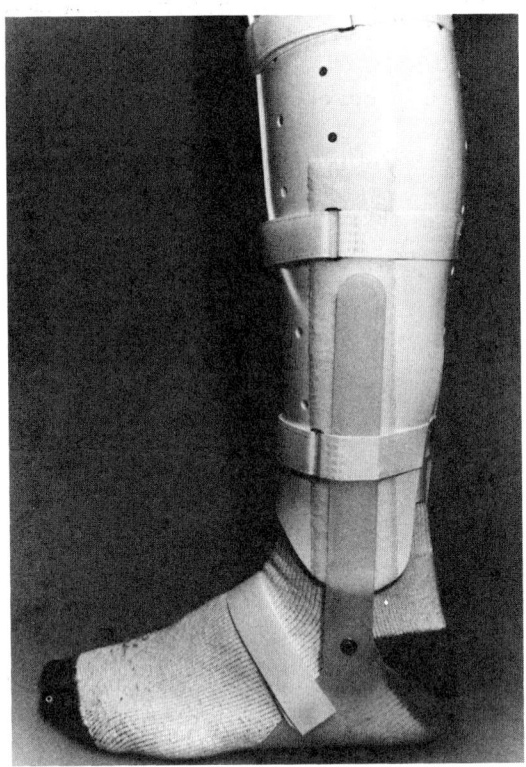

FIGURE 62-13
The articulate ankle–foot orthosis, readily available and easily adjusted, is useful for severe-grade ankle sprains. (Morrissy, R. T. [Ed.]. [1990]. Lovell and Winter's pediatric orthopaedics [3rd ed.]. [Vol. II]. Philadelphia: J. B. Lippincott.)

muscle-setting exercises. These exercises help to maintain the child's muscle tone and facilitate return to normal activities. Once sufficient healing has occurred, active exercises of the joint can be initiated.

★ EVALUATION

Healing usually occurs within 6 weeks of the injury. Treatment and follow-up are managed on an outpatient basis. During each visit the nurse and the physician evaluate the function of the affected area and determine if the expected outcomes have been met. Guidance regarding safety and the child's participation in sports activities should be provided. The importance of body conditioning for endurance and strength should be emphasized. In addition, discussion about the use of protective equipment in sports activities should be addressed. If the child is actively involved in a sports program, the nurse should discuss the outcomes of treatment and follow-up plans with the child's athletic trainer.

Special Interventions in Musculoskeletal Dysfunction

Care of a Child in a Cast

Definition. Casts are used to immobilize fractured bones and for orthopedic correction of skeletal deformities. Types of casts and their functions are summarized

TABLE 62-15
Types and Functions of Casts

Types of Casts	Functions
Short arm	Stabilizes fractures of the metacarpals, carpals, or distal radius
Long arm	Immobilizes unstable fractures of the carpals, stable fractures of the distal humerus, and fractures of the radius, ulna, or both
Hanging arm	Exerts traction on the humerus
Thumb spica (gauntlet)	Immobilizes fractures of the carpal navicular, thumb metacarpal, and phalanges
Shoulder spica	Immobilizes unstable fractures of the shoulder girdle and humerus
Short leg (bootcasts)	Immobilizes stable fractures of the ankle, metatarsals, and fractures of the talus, calcaneus, navicular, cuboid, and cuneiform bones
Long leg	Immobilizes fractures of the tibia, fibula, and ankle joint
Hip spica	Immobilizes fractures of the femur and associated joints; maintains surgical correction (e.g., congenital dislocated hips)
Petrie	Immobilizes hips in abduction and internal rotation for treatment of Legg-Calvé-Perthes disease
Risser (body cast)	Stretches the ligamentous structures and muscles on each side of the spine to allow more surgical correction for scoliosis
Queen Anne body cast	Immobilizes cervical and thoracic spine after posterior spinal fusion
Minerva	Immobilizes the head and spine

Long arm cast

Gauntlet or Thumb spica cast

Short leg cast   Long leg cast with walker

Body cast   Short leg hip spica cast

Bilateral long-leg hip spica cast

in Table 62-15. When a cast is applied to immobilize a fractured bone, the amount of surface area covered depends on the completeness of the fracture, bone involvement, and the amount of weight bearing that will be permitted during bone healing. The joints above and below the fracture site also may be immobilized to eliminate the possibility of movement of a fractured bone in the extremity.

Casting Materials. Cast materials have become more lightweight and water resistant due to the use of fiberglass and polyurethane resin. Such casts are often used for immobilizing arms and for infant hip spica casts. The synthetic cast materials are more expensive than plaster, but are easy to clean, resist soiling, and are stronger than plaster. They dry and harden minutes after application and are less susceptible to denting. These characteristics make synthetic casts preferable for infants and children. The synthetic casts are available in fashion colors, including neon and camouflage. The child is provided with the opportunity to select a favorite color for the cast before application. The traditional plaster of Paris casting material is used for larger casts, especially for body, leg, and larger hip spica casts. Even the traditionally white plaster cast may be covered by a layer of the colored synthetic material at the time the cast is trimmed and finished.

★ NURSING DIAGNOSES

The child who is immobilized in a cast has many needs. Some nursing diagnoses, derived from the needs assessment, may include the following:

* Impaired Physical Mobility related to restrictions of cast.
* Self-Care Deficit related to restricted movement.
* Body Image Disturbance related to immobilization.

- Diversional Activity Deficit related to long-term confinement.
- Constipation related to lack of exercise.
- High Risk for Impaired Skin Integrity related to immobility.
- Impaired Tissue Integrity related to constriction.
- Altered Growth and Development related to restricted movement.

★ INTERVENTIONS: COLLABORATIVE AND INDEPENDENT

PREPARATION FOR CASTING

Before the cast is applied, the nurse assesses what the child knows about the casting procedure and wearing a cast. Explaining the procedure based on the child's developmental level with the use of dolls with casts reduces anxiety and increases cooperation. In addition, the nurse may suggest how the child can help during cast application.

The area of the body to be casted is cleaned, dried, and thoroughly inspected for the presence of cuts, abrasions, skin lesions, bruises, or other alterations in skin integrity. These baseline data assist the nurse in evaluating the child's complaints of pain or tenderness under the cast. A baseline neurovascular assessment also is performed and documented before casting. Jewelry or other items that may cause constriction secondary to edema are removed. It may be desirable to administer analgesia to reduce discomfort during manipulation and cast application.

ASSISTING WITH CAST APPLICATION

The nurse may be asked to assist with the cast application. Assistance may require holding the body part to be casted or handing the casting materials to the physician as the procedure is performed. Rubber gloves and a plastic apron are worn during the procedure. Nursing responsibilities during the cast application include the following:

- Gather materials needed, preparing materials according to manufacturer's instructions.
- Make baseline data assessments.
- Prepare the injured area (may need to be washed and dried or shaved).
- Position or restrain the child as directed.
- Wrap the area to be casted with stockinette or other wadding material.
- Explain the procedure to the child. (The child should have been prepared beforehand with a casted doll.)
- Reassure and comfort the child during the procedure.

The casting materials are wrapped around the area while a smooth surface is maintained. A follow-up x-ray is usually taken after the casting to make sure the bone is aligned. The area is cleaned immediately following the procedure before the material hardens. Cast material is never placed in a regular sink.

CARE FOLLOWING CASTING

A plaster cast may take 24 to 72 hours to dry completely. Therefore, special attention must be given to correct handling of the damp cast to prevent dents and flat spots.

The palmar surface of the hand with fingers extended is used when supporting the cast so that fingertips do not touch the plaster. The skin around the cast is washed with warm water to remove any splashes of the casting material.

The cast is elevated on pillows slightly above the level of the heart to reduce swelling and promote venous return (Fig. 62-14). Ice bags are sometimes ordered to minimize excessive swelling. To prevent dents in the cast, the ice bags are placed along the sides of the cast. They are checked frequently for positioning and may be removed in 48 hours.

The child is repositioned every 2 to 3 hours to prevent skin breakdown. A neurovascular assessment is performed every hour for the first 4 hours (Table 62-16). Subsequent assessments are performed every 4 hours or as ordered by the physician. Nursing judgment should be used to determine the need for more frequent neurovascular assessments. A serious complication related to neurovascular compromise in a casted extremity is compartment syndrome (see Table 62-7). Compartment syndrome is an orthopedic emergency in which excessive swelling around the injury site, results in increased pressure in the fascia. The increased edema cannot be accommodated by the fascia.

When the cast has fully dried and swelling has subsided, the nurse inspects the cast edges for roughness. Adhesive cast petals, 3 × 1½ inch pieces of waterproof tape or moleskin, are overlapped around the raw edges of the cast to provide a smooth, finished surface (Fig. 62-15).

DAILY CAST CARE

Cast care is performed at least twice a day and involves visual inspection of the skin at the cast edges and under the cast. The nurse may use a flashlight to inspect the skin under the cast, observing for drainage, foreign objects, and odors. Alcohol is applied to the skin surrounding the cast edges with alcohol wipes, and a stockinette soaked with alcohol may be threaded under the cast to clean and toughen the skin and assess for breakdown.

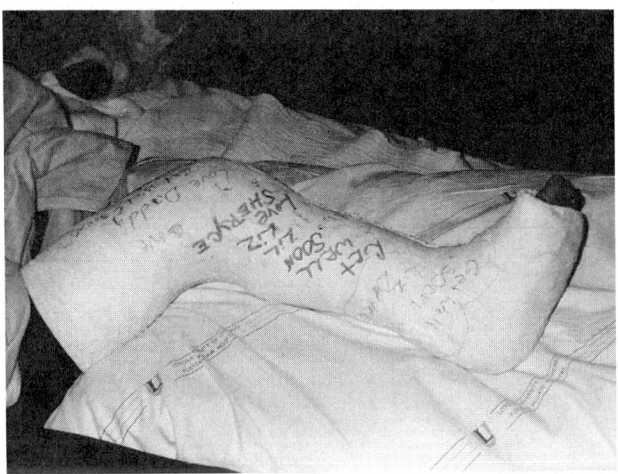

FIGURE 62-14
The cast is elevated on pillows above the level of the heart. (Skale, N. [1992]. *Manual of pediatric nursing procedures*. Philadelphia: J. B. Lippincott.)

TABLE 62-16
Nursing Assessment: Neurovascular Assessment

Parameter	Finding
Color	Pink, pale, bluish
Edema	Absent, mild, moderate, severe
Temperature	Warm, cool, cold, hot
Pulse (distal)	Strong, weak, absent
Pain	Present, absent
Capillary refill	Rapid (<2 seconds), sluggish, absent
Sensory nerve function (ulnar, median, radial nerves or peroneal, tibial nerves)	Present, tingling, numbness
Motor nerve function (ulnar, median, radial nerves or peroneal, tibial nerves	Present, decreased, absent

Pressure sores may develop under the cast as a result of foreign objects inside the cast or areas of decreased blood supply to the skin. As the sore develops, the cast above the area may feel warm (a "hot spot"). The child may complain of a burning sensation followed by numbness and tingling, foul odor, and bloody drainage or secretions. Management involves cutting out a window in the cast to inspect the skin and to treat the pressure sore. The nurse must then observe the area for window edema and the development of a secondary pressure area.

DISCHARGE PLANNING

Prior to discharge, home care instructions for the child in a cast should include information about general cast care, neurovascular assessment, turning, toileting and diapering, safety, nutrition and hydration, and activities to promote growth and development.

Children and families should be instructed never to stick anything down inside of the cast. If the skin under the cast itches, a hair dryer used on the cool setting may provide some relief. Lotions and powders should not be used on the skin under or surrounding the cast. A sticky buildup of lotion and powder may predispose the child to skin irritation and breakdown.

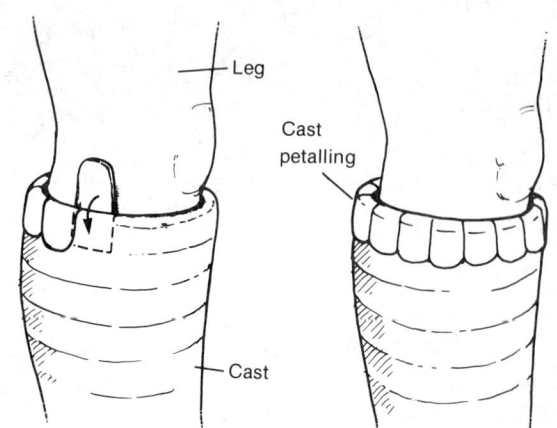

FIGURE 62-15
Adhesive cast petals are overlapped around the edge of the cast for protection against tough edges. (Skale, N. [1992]. Manual of pediatric nursing procedures. Philadelphia: J. B. Lippincott.)

Parents may ask about how to keep the cast clean. A soiled synthetic cast may be washed with a mild abrasive detergent and dried with a hair dryer used on the low, cool setting. A severely soiled plaster cast may have to be changed because, unlike the synthetic cast, plaster casts are not water resistant. When wet, they soften and crumble and therefore cannot be washed.

The child in a hip spica cast may use a urinal or fracture pan to void. Parents are instructed in methods to keep the cast free of urine and feces. One method is to make a funnel around the perineal area of the cast with six 10×5 inch plastic strips. These strips are tucked inside the cast, and the ends are placed inside the fracture pan creating the funnel. The child should be elevated so that urine and feces will pass through the funnel into the fracture pan without soiling the cast.

Parents caring for an infant in a hip spica cast should be instructed to diaper the infant in layers. The first layer may be a sanitary napkin followed by a disposable diaper and a layer of plastic. The infant should be checked frequently and the diaper changed immediately to prevent cast soiling.

Another method of keeping the cast from becoming soiled with feces or urine is to use a split Bradford frame for the incontinent child. The frame helps keep the cast dry by the use of gravity produced when the head of the frame is elevated. Urine and feces naturally flow through a plastic funnel into a bedpan positioned under an opening in the frame. (See section on Care of a Child in Special Beds and Frames later in this chapter.)

To prevent constipation related to decreased mobility, parents are encouraged to provide a diet high in bulk and fiber. Adequate fluid intake also reduces the likelihood of constipation and renal calculi. Increased protein in the child's diet aids in bone healing.

CAST REMOVAL

The cast is removed with a special saw. The saw oscillates back and forth, although it appears to be rotating. The blade will not cut the patient. The process needs to be described to the child beforehand, because the noise and dust may frighten the child. The nurse wears gloves and sometimes protective eyewear for the procedure. Other actions taken by the nurse include the following:

- Assemble the equipment.
- Explain the procedure, and demonstrate the saw's noise and oscillation.
- Cut vertically the lateral and medial sides of the cast, using the cast cutter.
- Use the cast spreader to separate the sides of the cast.
- Cut sheet wadding under the cast with a large bandage scissors.
- Remove the cast.
- Inspect the skin under the cast.
- Remove dead skin gently with warm soapy water.
- Apply lotion or mineral oil.

Care of a Child in Traction

Definition and Principles. Methods of applying traction may differ from physician to physician and institution to institution. Therefore, nurses need to understand the basic principles of traction.

Traction is the application of a pulling force along the long axis of a body part. It is provided by attaching weights, such as sand, water, or steel, to ropes and pulleys connected to orthopedic devices placed on the body part. Traction is used for the following reasons:

- To correct and maintain skeletal alignment
- To reduce fractures or dislocations and maintain alignment
- To decrease muscle spasms and pain
- To immobilize a body part to promote rest
- To prevent or correct contracture deformities

Three types of traction are used in the care of children with musculoskeletal dysfunction: manual, skin, and skeletal. In manual traction the hands provide a steady pulling force to reduce fractures during cast application. Frequently, it is the nurse who applies this force during casting. Manual traction is also used in halo application (discussed later in this section).

With skin traction, a light pull is applied to the skin or soft tissue. Traction may be applied and removed intermittently. Noninvasive orthopedic devices, such as elastic bandages, skin adherents, or foam boots, may be used for the traction.

In skeletal traction a strong pull is applied to the bone. A 15- to 40-pound weight may be applied to the extremities. Skeletal traction should not be removed without a physician's order.

Specific types and uses of traction are illustrated and described in Figure 62-16.

Bed equipment for traction therapy for a child or adolescent may include an overhead frame to which a trapeze is attached. The overhead frame and trapeze help to increase the child's mobility and independence while in bed. A firm mattress is also necessary to assure traction efficiency and to avoid possible contracture deformities.

Countertraction. For traction to be effective there must be countertraction, which is achieved by applying a pulling force to the body in the opposite direction from the traction. Countertraction may include one of the following:

- Another traction set-up (weights, pulleys, ropes, and orthopedic devices)
- The child's own body weight
- Jacket restraints to maintain the child's position.

A jacket restraint is illustrated in Figure 25-1C. An increase in countertraction may be applied by elevating the head or foot of the bed or traction frame.

★ ASSESSMENT

Before a child is placed in traction, the nurse assesses the child's and family's knowledge of traction therapy. Explaining the procedure based on the child's developmental level is necessary if treatment is to be successful. Sample traction set-ups using teaching dolls are important visual instructional tools. School-age children and adolescents may respond well to discussing traction therapy with a peer who is in traction.

Data collected prior to application of traction should include any history of allergy to tape or foam rubber and problems with circulation and sensation. The nurse inspects the skin to be covered by traction prior to application for any alterations in skin integrity (e.g., rashes, abrasions, or bruises). Skin lesions are documented in the chart before they are covered, and the physician is notified of their presence. A baseline neurovascular assessment is completed before traction is applied (see Table 62-16). The presence of any pain, including the location, degree, and description is also identified.

★ NURSING DIAGNOSES

Needs based on assessments will determine nursing diagnoses for the child in traction. The following are often seen in children in traction:

- Diversional Activity Deficit related to immobility.
- Altered Growth and Development related to restricted movement.
- High Risk for Impaired Skin Integrity related to immobility and effects of friction.
- Impaired Tissue Integrity related to constriction.
- Impaired Physical Mobility related to traction therapy.
- Constipation related to immobility.

★ INTERVENTIONS: COLLABORATIVE AND INDEPENDENT

MAINTAINING TRACTION

Several factors underlying effective traction must be maintained. They include countertraction, friction, line of pull, continuity, positioning, and safety. The nurse assesses these factors and intervenes when there is a problem.

The nurse must assess *countertraction* every 3 hours to determine if the child's body is being gradually pulled to the foot of the bed. The nurse supports the involved body part and assists the child to move to the head of the bed. Restraints also should be inspected and reapplied if they become too tight or are improperly positioned secondary to the child's sliding.

Friction disrupts the pull of traction and may be caused by bed linens, the traction set-up, or the child's body. Points along the traction from the child to the weights should be inspected for impingements. Some common causes of friction include knots pressing against pulleys; weights caught on the bed; footplates, spreaders, or splints touching the foot of the bed; and bed linens covering the ropes or straps.[9]

The *line of pull* is inspected regularly to ascertain that the child's body is resting in line with the pull of the traction. Positioning is particularly important with skeletal traction and fracture reduction when the traction is maintaining bone alignment.

For traction to be effective it must be *continuous*; children in skeletal traction remain in traction 24 hours a day. Children in skin traction may come out of traction for a set amount of time each day, usually 2 to 4 hours, depending on the treatment protocol. Compliance may be a problem for all children who developmentally learn about their world through movement and exploration. A mutually agreed on schedule between the child or family and nurse may increase compliance. Adolescents may respond well to a contract outlining their responsibility for

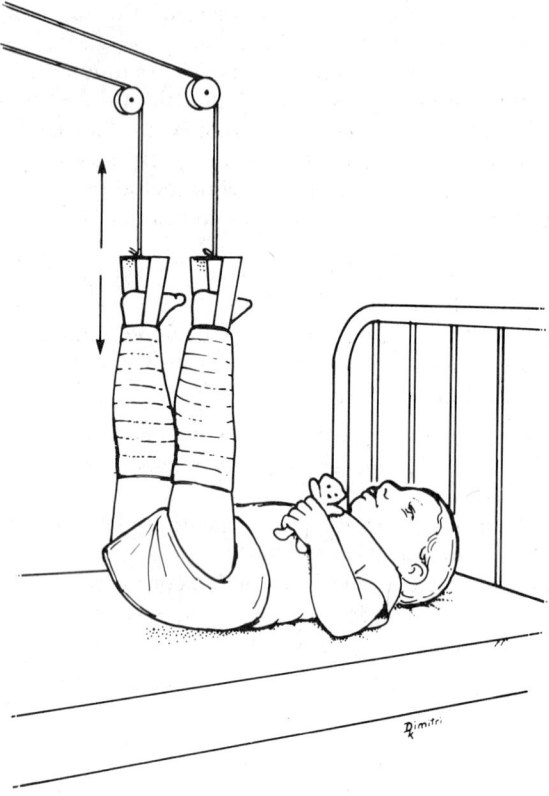

Bryant's Traction
- Skin traction
- Vertical suspension
- Always applied bilaterally
- Used in children older than 2 years or less than 31 pounds
- Used to treat fractures of the femur and in congenitally dislocated hip
- Countertraction supplied by weight of child

Buck Extension Traction
- Skin traction
- Used to correct bone deformities or contracture and for short-term immobilization
- Countertraction supplied by weight of child

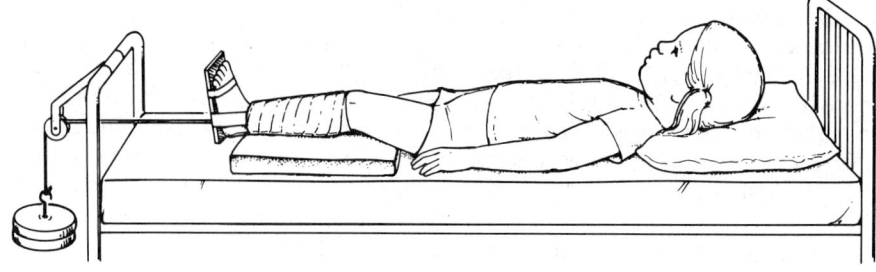

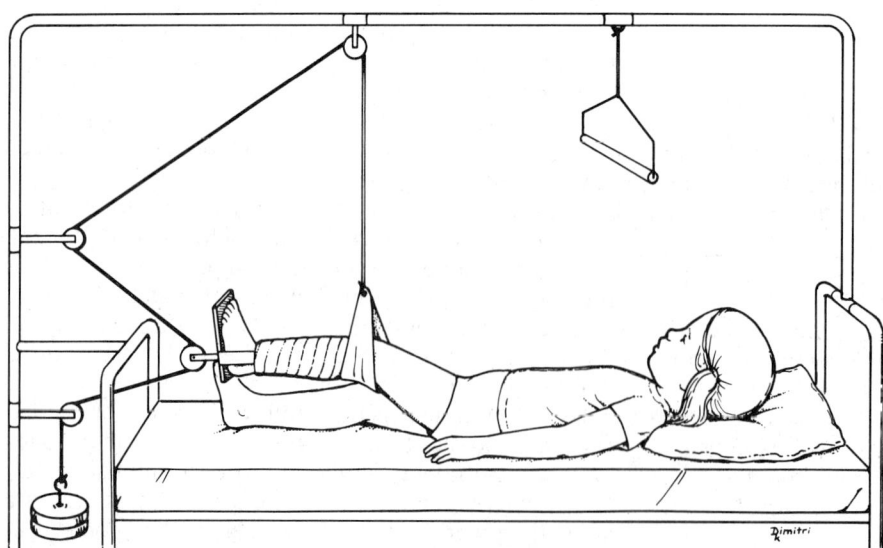

Russell Traction
- Used to treat knee injuries and fractures of the hip and femur
- Similar to Buck extension with the addition of a padded suspension sling under the knee
- Used most frequently for treatment of femoral shaft fractures

FIGURE 62-16
Types, uses, and considerations in traction. (Adapted from Skale, N. [1992]. Manual of pediatric nursing procedures. Philadelphia: J. B. Lippincott.)

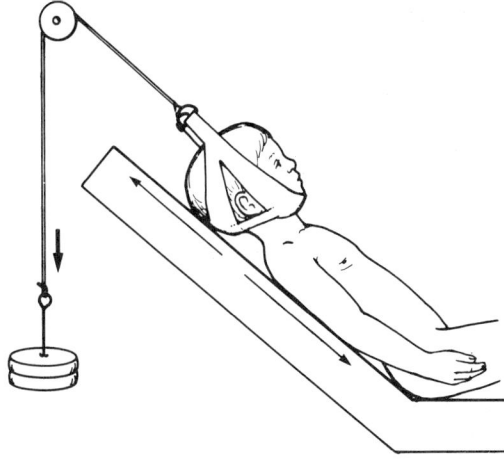

Cervical Head Halter
- Provides immobilization in a neutral position
- Used in spinal fractures, muscle spasms, or spinal injuries

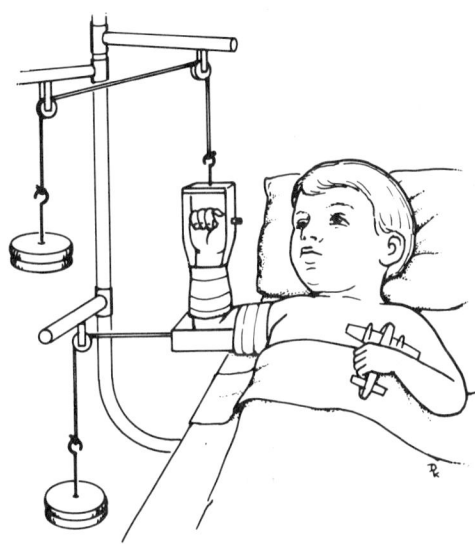

Dunlop Traction
- Used to treat fractures of the humerus
- Similar use as sidearm traction but vertical force of child's body eliminates need for countertraction

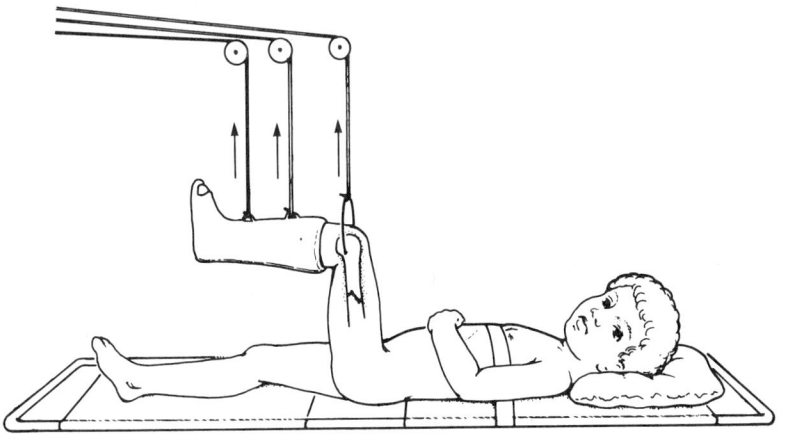

Ninety-Ninety Skeletal Traction
- Used to treat fractures of the femoral shaft in children > 2 years
- A boot cast is applied to the lower leg, and skeletal pins or wires are placed through the distal femur
- Maintains 90-degree flexion of knee and hip

FIGURE 62-16 (Continued)

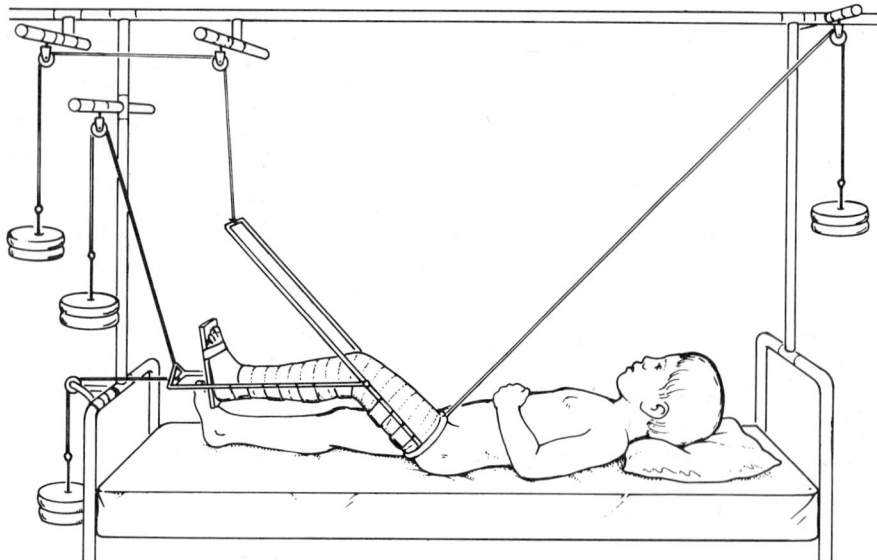

Crutchfield Tongs
- Used to reduce fractures and dislocations of the cervical spine
- Head of bed may be elevated for mild countertraction by physician's order
- Regular or special bed may be used
- Illustrated in Figure 53-11

Balanced Suspension With Thomas Splint and Pearson Attachment
- Used to suspend the leg in flexion to relax the hip and hamstring muscles
- May be used with skin or skeletal traction

Halo Device
- Allows greater mobility with minimal risk to spinal alignment
- Steel bars anchor device to body cast or vest
- Used to immobilize the child with cervical injuries
- Illustrated in Figure 53-11

FIGURE 62-16 (Continued)

maintaining the traction schedule. Age-appropriate diversional activities and school work should be incorporated in the child's plan of care.

The child should be *positioned* in correct body alignment on a firm mattress or frame (e.g., Bradford frame; see section on Care of a Child in Special Beds and Frames later in this chapter). When needed, support is provided to shoulders, head, or legs to alleviate muscle strain. The child's position is checked frequently. Repositioning may be necessary to realign the child's head and pelvis perpendicular to the bed and to maintain a supine position.

The nurse is responsible for assuring the *safety* of the child in traction. The nurse should inspect the traction set-up at least every 8 hours for frayed ropes, loosened clamps, or knots.

WIRE AND PIN-SITE CARE

The wires or pins of skeletal traction should be observed for movement that may indicate migration in the bone. This condition is confirmed by x-ray and may be a risk to normal bone growth in children if the pin migrates into the epiphyseal plate (growth plate).

Care of skeletal pins and wires is established by individual institutions or physicians. There is diversity of opinion concerning how skeletal traction pin sites should be treated, if at all. Despite some inconsistency, there are common core clinical behaviors that are used across institutions.[21] Generally, either hydrogen peroxide, betadine, normal saline, sterile water, or soap and tap water are used to clean the pin insertion sites. Hydrogen peroxide is the most popular cleansing agent. Cleansing is followed by the application of betadine, polysporin oint-

ments, or alcohol. The majority of institutions use clean rather than sterile technique.[21]

Skeletal traction pin site care is performed by the nurse according to institutional policy, usually two to three times a day. The nurse observes the pin site for signs of infection, including redness, odor, and exudate. The child with a skeletal pin tract infection may be febrile, have an elevated white blood cell count, and exhibit general malaise and poor feeding. Treatment may include more frequent pin site care and antimicrobial therapy after culturing the pin site.

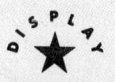

Complications of Traction Therapy

- Circulatory impairment
- Volkmann ischemic contracture
- Neurologic impairment
- Nonunion of bone fragments
- Malunion of bone fragments
- Epiphyseal plate damage
- Osteomyelitis
- Emboli
- Hypercalciuria
- Pressure sores
- Achilles tendon contracture

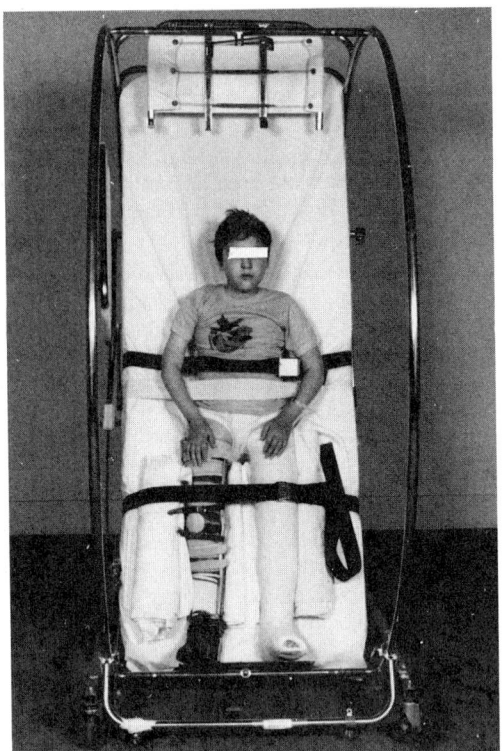

FIGURE 62-17
The electronically powered circle bed is effective in removing pressure, stabilizing the body, and useful in nursing care. (Morrissy, R. T. [Ed.]. [1990]. Lovell and Winter's pediatric orthopaedics [3rd ed.]. [Vol. II]. Philadelphia: J. B. Lippincott.)

ASSESSMENTS

Nursing care of a child in traction requires frequent skin assessments because of immobility and friction created by the pull of the traction. The child's head, heels, and major bony prominences should be assessed carefully for signs of redness or skin breakdown. Even the child's ears are potential pressure points.

PREVENTION OF SKIN BREAKDOWN

Massaging the high-risk areas increases circulation and prevents cell anoxia. The child's position should be changed every 2 to 3 hours. Lamb's wool may be placed on areas of potential skin breakdown. Other potential complications of traction are summarized in the accompanying display.

ACTIVITY PROMOTION

Exercise maintains muscle tone and normal elimination and increases circulation; it should be a part of the child's care. Movement of all unaffected extremities is encouraged. Children may accomplish exercise through play. The foot of the affected leg in traction also should be exercised with either passive or active range of motion to prevent contracture of the Achilles tendon.

FLUID AND NUTRITIONAL MANAGEMENT

The child should be encouraged to maintain adequate fluid intake. Favorite beverages are offered in small amounts at frequent intervals because the child's thirst and appetite may be poor. A diet high in bulk, fiber, and

TABLE 62-17
Special Beds and Frames

Types	Purpose	Advantages	Disadvantages
Kinetic therapy bed (KTB) or oscillating bed	Patients with unstable cervical or thoracic spines who need frequent turning; multiple trauma patients	Fewer pulmonary complications; rotates pressure points; easily adapted to all types of traction; good for children who cannot tolerate the prone position.	Not tolerated well by children who have increased intercranial pressure; only available in adult size, but can be used by children.
Wedge turning frame	Spinal cord injury clients; patients requiring strict immobilization after spinal surgery	Can be turned by one person; no weight bearing with turning; spinal alignment maintained with turning.	Frames are narrow and cannot be used with obese clients; chin support may cause neck extension; impaired pulmonary expansion; pressure on occipital area; turning may be uncomfortable for client
Foster frame	For spinal stabilization or alignment; stretching prior to spinal fusion	Can be used with halofemoral or halopelvic traction; maintain spinal alignment while turning	Frames are heavy and difficult to handle; two people are needed for turning; others as stated with wedge turning device
CircO-electric bed	Used for vertical turning of highly immobilized clients	Electronically operated—only requires one person to operate; anterior frame can be adjusted to the size of the child; cervical traction can be attached; can be positioned in upright, reclining, or trendelenburg position	Weight bearing occurs with turning—cannot be used with clients who have unstable spines; head and chin straps on anterior frame may cause neck extension
Solid Bradford frame	To assist with immobilization and alignment for young children in lower extremity traction	Small area makes immobilization of small children easier; countertraction can be easily applied by lowering the head of the frame	Children may resist confinement; canvas covers may be uncomfortable unless they are covered with foam mattress
Split Bradford frame	Used with incontinent children in hip spica cast to keep the cast clean and dry	Position of frame with head elevated keeps urine from flowing up into the cast; elevated position allows child to see surroundings	Elevated position may contribute to perineal edema following hip surgery; restraining the small child may limit normal exploratory behavior; parents need to find new ways of providing stimulation

Data from a variety of sources, including Ceccio, C. M. (1990). Understanding therapeutic beds. *Orthopedic nursing, 9*(3), 57–70.

protein helps promote normal elimination and bone healing.

Care of a Child in Special Beds and Frames

Special beds and frames are sometimes used as an adjunct to the care of children with musculoskeletal alterations. These devices provide a healing environment to relieve pressure, stabilize the spine, or prevent some of the complications of immobility (Fig. 62-17). The use of these devices often facilitates nursing care. The nurse can easily position the patient and provide comfort measures.

Preparation of the child is essential before placement in special beds and frames. If possible, every opportunity should be given to the child to try out the device before it is used. The child should experience some of the sensations and feelings associated with turning. Many of the frames are very narrow. Children need to feel safe and comfortable with the turning procedures. Therefore, the nurse and the child should decide on a signal that will indicate when the turn will be started. Sometimes children enjoy practicing by turning their favorite nurse. (The nursing staff should review the use of frames by practicing turning each other. By experiencing some of the sensations, they may be better able to prepare children for the event.)

Many of the frames are designed for easy turning by one person. The variety of beds and frames is discussed in Table 62-17. As an added safety measure, however, two people should be in attendance while the child is being turned. Straps are placed around the frames to provide a feeling of security to the child. The child's arms and legs should be aligned within the bed before beginning the turn. Children usually need to be turned every 2 to 4 hours. The nurse should always check the child's skin with each turn. When the oscillating bed is used, skin checks can be planned with scheduled treatments.

Whenever a special bed or frame is used, the child's mobility is restricted. Plans should include opportunities for the child to participate in as much self-care as possible. When children are in the prone position, for example, they can feed themselves if the small tray is attached to the bed frame. In this position the child can do school work or other activities. When children are in the supine position, a special bookboard can be placed over them. Prism glasses assist a supine person to better visualize their environment. The nurse needs to be creative in planning diversional activities that are age appropriate and stimulating for the immobilized child.

Summary

A multidisciplinary approach to children with musculoskeletal disorders promotes holistic care for the child and family. The nurse is in a key position to coordinate the care. Many organizations are available to families to assist with the emotional, physical, and financial aspects of the child's dysfunction.

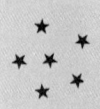

Ideas for Nursing Research

The diversity of musculoskeletal disorders in children suggests that the area has great potential for generating nursing research. The following areas need to be explored:

- Relationship between intrapartal nurse's attitude about congenital musculoskeletal deformities and the parents' ability to bond with their infant
- Relationship between a modified ambulation program and a decrease in fractures in children with osteogenesis imperfecta
- Relationship, if any, between peer support groups for adolescents with scoliosis and their compliance with bracing and exercise restrictions
- Effectiveness of support groups for parents with children with disfiguring congenital musculoskeletal disorders and an increase in parents' abilities to be advocates for their child
- Comparison of various types of pin care and the development of a pin tract infection in children with skeletal traction
- Display of overt signs of anxiety by children prepared for casting procedures using sensory descriptions compared to signs of anxiety in children given only descriptions of the procedure itself
- Effectiveness of alcohol for prevention of skin irritation and breakdown in children with casts

Children with chronic musculoskeletal disorders require multiple hospital admissions and extensive rehabilitation. Frequent contact gives the nurse an opportunity to intervene with these children and their families on numerous occasions. The nurse is rewarded when children are able to reach their maximum potential within the family unit and society. The effectiveness of nursing care is thereby validated.

References

1. Barrett, J. B., & Bryant, B. H. (1990). Fractures: Types, treatment, perioperative implications. *AORN Journal, 52*(4), 755–771.
2. Boome, R. S., & Kaye, J. C. (1988). Obstetric traction injuries of the brachial plexus. *Journal of Bone and Joint Surgery, 70B*, 571–576.
3. Bowen, J. R., & Miller, G. (1992). Legg-Calve-Perthes disease. In R. A. Balderston, R. H. Rothman, R. E. Booth, & W. J. Hozack (Eds.). *The hip.* (pp. 134–151). Philadelphia: Lea & Febiger.
4. Brosnan, H. (1991). Nursing management of the adolescent with idiopathic scoliosis. *Nursing Clinics of North America, 26*(1), 17–31.
5. Bunnell, W. P. (1988). The natural history of idiopathic scoliosis. *Clinical Orthopaedics and Related Research, 229*, 20–25.
6. Campbell, L. S., & Campbell, J. D. (1991). Musculoskeletal trauma in children. *Critical Care Nursing Clinics of North America, 3*(3), 445–456.
7. Cassidy, J. T., & Petty, R. E. (1990). *Textbook of pediatric rheumatology* (2nd ed.). New York: Churchill Livingstone.

8. Ceccio, C. M. (1990). Understanding therapeutic beds. *Orthopedic Nursing, 9*(3), 57–70.

9. Farrell, J. (1986). Illustrated guide to orthopedic nursing (3rd ed.). Philadelphia: J.B. Lippincott.

10. Francis, E. (1987). Lateral electrical surface stimulation: A treatment for scoliosis. *Pediatric Nursing, 3*, 157–160.

11. Frantz, C. H., & O'Rahilly, R. (1961). Congenital skeletal limb deficiencies. *Journal of Bone and Joint Surgery, 43A*, 1202–1224.

12. Gerber, L. H., Binder, H., Weintrob, J., Grange, D. K., Shapiro, J., Fromherz, W., Berry, R., Conway, A., Nason, S., & Marini, J. (1990). Rehabilitation of children and infants with osteogenesis imperfecta: A program for ambulation. *Clinical Orthopaedics and Related Research, 251*, 254–262.

13. Gilgoff, I., et al. (1989). Patient and family participation in the management of respiratory failure in Duchenne's muscular dystrophy. *Chest, 95*, 519–524.

14. Green, N. E., & Edwards, K. (1987). Bone and joint infections in children. *Orthopedic Clinics of North America, 18*, 555–576.

15. Green, S. A. (1989). Ilizarov orthopedic methods. *AORN Journal, 49*, 215–230.

16. Hart, M. D. (1987). Classroom aids for a child with severe upper limb deficiencies. *American Journal of Occupational Therapy, 41*, 467–469.

17. Herring, J. A. (1990). Congenital dislocation of the hip. In R. T. Morrissey (Ed.), *Lovell and Winter's pediatric orthopaedics* (p. 815–850). Philadelphia: J.B. Lippincott.

18. Hooker, C. W., & Greene, W. B. (1983). Congenital malformations. In F. C. Wilson (Ed.), *The musculoskeletal system* (2nd ed.). Philadelphia: J.B. Lippincott.

19. Jackson, S. T., et al. (1988). Brachial-plexus palsy in the newborn. *Journal of Bone and Joint Surgery, 70A*, 1217–1220.

20. Jacobs-Zacney, J., & Horn, M. (1988). Nursing care of adolescents having posterior spinal fusion with Cotrel-Dubousset instrumentation. *Orthopedic Nursing, 7*, 17–21.

21. Jones-Walton, P. (1991). Clinical standards in skeletal traction pin site care. *Orthopedic Nursing, 10*(2), 12–16.

22. Joy, C. (1989). *Pediatric trauma nursing.* Gaithersburg, MD: Aspen Publishers.

23. Kyzer, S. P. (1991). Congenital idiopathic clubfoot. *Orthopaedic Nursing, 10*(4), 11–18.

24. Lovell, W. W., & Winters, R. B. (1986). Pediatric orthopedics (2nd ed.). Vols. 1 & 2. Philadelphia: J.B. Lippincott.

25. MacEwen, G. D., & Bassett, G. S. (1984). Current trends in the management of congenital dislocation of the hip. *International Orthopaedics, 8*, 103–111.

26. MacEwen, G. D., & Millet, C. (1990). Congenital dislocation of the hip. *Pediatrics in Review, 11*, 249–252.

27. Malleson, P. N., & Petty R. E. (1990). Remodelling the pyramid—A pediatric perspective. *Journal of Rheumatology, 17*(7), 867–868.

28. McCluskey, W., & Bunnell, W. P. (1992). Congenital dislocation of the hip. In R. A. Balderston, R. H. Rothman, R. E. Booth, & W. J. Hozack (Eds.). *The hip.* (pp. 95–133). Philadelphia: Lea & Febiger.

29. McCullough, F. L. (1989). Skeletal trauma in children. *Orthopaedic Nursing, 8*(2), 41–46.

30. Martin, M. E. (1989). Oral antibiotic treatment of patients with chronic osteomyelitis. *Orthopedic Nursing, 8*, 35–38.

31. Mason, K. J. (1991). Congenital orthopedic anomalies and their impact on the family. *Nursing Clinics of North America, 26*(1), 1–16.

32. Merkel, K. D., et al. (1984). Scintigraphic evaluation in musculoskeletal sepsis. *Orthopedic Clinics of North America, 15*, 401–416.

33. Morrissey, R. T. (1990). Lovell and Winter's pediatric orthopedics (3rd ed.). Vols. 1 & 2. Philadelphia: J.B. Lippincott.

34. Morrissey, R. T., & Selman, S. (1991). Slipped capital femoral epiphysis. *Orthopaedic Nursing, 10*(1), 11–20.

35. Morrissey, R. T., & Shore, S. L. (1986). Bone and joint sepsis. *Pediatric Clinics of North America, 33*, 1551–1564.

36. Moseley, C. F. (1987). Leg lengthening discrepancy. *Orthopedic Clinics of North America, 18*, 529–535.

37. Narakas, A. O., & Hentz, V. R. Neurotization in brachial plexus injuries. *Clinics in Orthopedics, 237*, 43–56.

38. Newschwander, G. E., & Dunst, R. M. (1989). Limb lengthening with the Ilizarov external fixator. *Orthopedic Nursing, 8*, 15–21.

39. Page-Goertz, S. S. (1989). Even children have arthritis. *Pediatric Nursing, 15*(1), 11–16.

40. Reilly, P. (1992). Juvenile rheumatoid arthritis. In P. L. Jackson & J. Vessey (Eds.), *Primary care of the child with chronic condition* (pp. 336–354). St. Louis: C.V. Mosby.

41. Renshaw, T. (1986). Pediatric orthopedics. Philadelphia: W.B. Saunders.

42. Rivara, F., Parish, R., & Mueller, B. (1986). Extremity injuries in children: Predictive value of clinical findings. *Pediatrics, 78*, 803–807.

43. Roger, B., et al. (1988). Imaging of posttraumatic brachial plexus injury. *Clinics in Orthopedics, 237*, 57–61.

44. Rosenberg, A. M. (1989). Advanced drug therapy for juvenile rheumatoid arthritis. *Journal of Pediatrics, 114*(2), 171–178.

45. Schumacher, H. R. (Ed.) (1988). *Primer on the rheumatic diseases* (9th ed.). Atlanta: Arthritis Foundation.

46. Skale, N. (1992). Manual of pediatric nursing procedures. Philadelphia: J.B. Lippincott.

47. Smrcina, C. M. (1991). Stress fractures in athletes. *Nursing Clinics of North America, 26*(1), 159–166.

48. Stout, J. A., & Gibbs, K. R. (1981). The child undergoing a leg-lengthening procedure. *American Journal of Nursing, 81*, 1152–1155.

48A. Swagman, A. (1986). Caring for limb-deficient children and their families. *Maternal and Child Nursing, 11,* 46–52.

49. Tachjian, M. O. (1990). Pediatric orthopedics (2nd ed.). Vol. 4. Philadelphia: W.B. Saunders.

50. Turek, S. (1984). Orthopedics: Principles and their application. Philadelphia: J.B. Lippincott.

51. Tursc, A., & Crost, M. (1986). Sports related injuries in children. *American Journal of Sports Medicine, 14*(4), 294–299.

52. Wallace C. A., & Levinson, J. (1991). Juvenile rheumatoid arthritis: Outcome & treatment for the 1990's. In B. H. Athreva (Ed.), *Rheumatic Disease Clinics of North America* (pp. 891–905). Philadelphia: W.B. Saunders.

53. Weinstein, S. (1990). Legg-Calve-Perthes disease. In R. T. Morrissy (Ed.), *Lovell and Winter's pediatric orthopaedics.* (pp. 851–883). Philadelphia: J.B. Lippincott.

53A. Wong, D., & Baker, C. (1988). Pain in children: Comparison of assessment scales. *Pediatric Nursing, 14,* 9–17.

54. Zaleske, D. J., Doppelt, S. H., & Mankin, H. J. (1986). Metabolic and endocrine abnormalities of the immature skeleton. In W. W. Lovell & R. B. Winter (Eds.), *Pediatric orthopaedics* (2nd Ed.). (pp. 92–101, 111–116). Philadelphia: J.B. Lippincott.

UNIT 17

Nursing Care of Children With Altered Integumentary Function

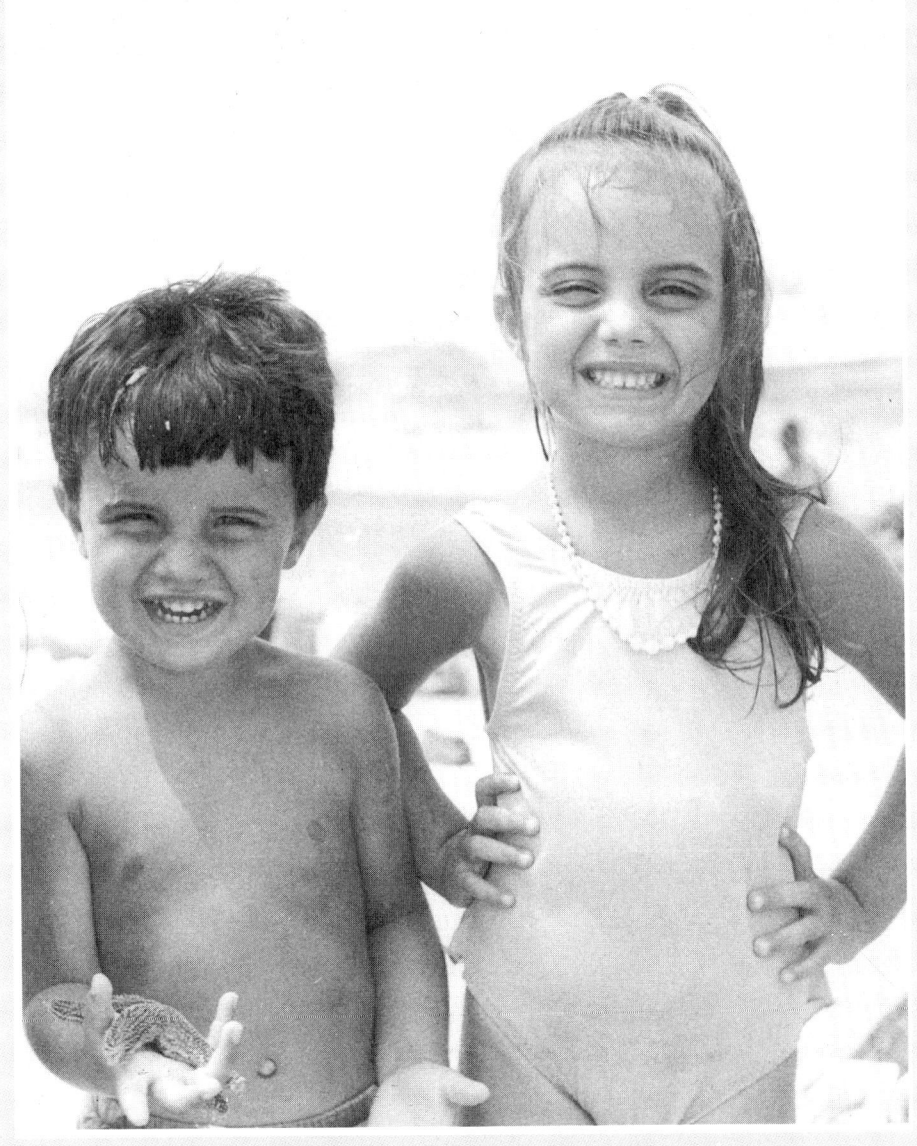

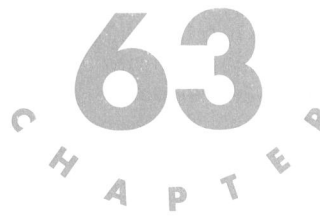

Anatomy and Physiology of the Integumentary System

BEHAVIORAL OBJECTIVES

Explain the embryogenesis of the skin.

Identify the major anatomic structures of the skin and their functions.

Describe epidermal appendages and their functions.

Explain the functions of the skin as an organ.

Delineate differences among preterm, newborn, childhood, and adult skin.

FEATURES OF THIS CHAPTER

Consequences of Abnormal Embryonic Development of the Skin, Table 63-1

Functions of the Skin

Structural Differences in Premature and Newborn Infant Skin, Table 63-2

The skin is the largest organ of the body. Functionally, it provides the link between the person and the surrounding environment and affords protection from external elements. Apart from being a protective organ, the skin is also an interactive organ. The skin is a powerful and complex communication channel that feeds a person information about the environment and provides the environment feedback about the person.

For the nurse, understanding the development, structure, and function of the skin offers important insights into the impact of disease on the skin and serves as the basis for skin assessment. This valuable information is necessary for planning care. An important note, however, is that the skin is not static but is ever changing, adapting to the environment and responding to internal conditions of the body. The skin reflects emotions and overall well-being of a person. Because the skin is the interface with the environment, it may provide evidence of internal disease as well as cause substantial human suffering as a result of disability, discomfort, and disfigurement.

Beginning with the development of skin in utero, the skin progresses through the stages of newborn skin, childhood skin, adult skin, and finally enters the stage of elderly skin. Differences in structure and function, which are evidence of the ongoing development and aging of the integument, can be identified at each stage.

The primary focus of this chapter is to acquaint the nurse with the perspective of the skin as a vast and complex organ. Special emphasis is given to the embryology of the skin, the structure and function of normal skin, and the differences between skin of infants and children and that of mature adults.

Embryonic Development

The skin of the embryo begins to form during the first 20 to 50 days of embryonic life. The earliest skin is organized into layers consisting of an epidermis, dermis, and subcutaneous tissue. Embryonic ectoderm and mesenchyme serve as origins of human skin, which develops in a fluid environment vastly different from the environment it experiences at birth. The role amniotic fluid plays in skin development is unknown; however, it is hypothesized that considerable interaction does occur. Two major stages of development of the skin are the embryonic and fetal periods.

Embryonic Period

The first 2 months of gestation mark the embryonic period. During this period, the epidermis is formed from the ectoderm and consists of the basal and periderm layers. The embryonic basal layer is equivalent to the adult basal layer. The periderm is the outermost layer of the skin. It is unclear to investigators whether the periderm is the true first layer of skin or if it is formed by the single layer of basal cells of the epidermis. Skin development in humans has been studied only in embryos older than 30 days' estimated gestational age (EGA), because tissue before this time has not been available.[15] The periderm remains on the surface of developing skin until keratinization of the cells of the epidermis is complete. The function of the periderm is unknown, but it probably plays a role in the interaction between the fetus and the amniotic fluid, such as secretion of material into the amniotic fluid, transportation of substances from amniotic fluid to developing skin, and protection of the developing skin.[14]

Other components of the skin are present at this stage, but in an immature form. Recognition of certain cell-specific markers indicates that Langerhans cells and melanocytes have already migrated to the epidermis as early as 43 days EGA.[15] No epidermal appendages are present at this stage of epidermal development. The embryonic dermis, formed from the mesoderm, is a thin but loosely woven network of mostly mesenchymal cells and a small amount of collagen. Fluid present in intercellular spaces composes as much as 90% of the dermal bulk. The embryonic subcutaneous tissue is difficult to distinguish from the dermis because it also contains mesenchymal cells and has no fat cells at this stage.

Fetal Period

The third month of prenatal life marks the transition from embryo to fetus. This is an important stage in the establishment of a pattern of skin development because during this time the epidermis becomes stratified with initial keratinization of cells. The basal cell layer gives rise to the intermediate layer and also begins to form certain epidermal appendages. From approximately 80 days' gestation, the pilosebaceous structures, apocrine glands, eccrine glands, and nails begin to form.[15] Langerhans cells and melanocytes are easily identifiable, but Merkel cells are not yet present.

During this period, dermal development is more gradual. The dermis becomes less cellular and fluid with the increase of fibrous connective tissue composed of collagen types I, III, and V. Fibroblasts, macrophages, and mast cells are present. From approximately 12 weeks' EGA, papillary and reticular zones may be identified. The dermis is still relatively thin and poorly demarcated from subcutaneous tissue; however, vascular plexus help to differentiate between the two dermal layers.

Approximately the fourth month EGA, keratinization of the hair cone begins. Melanocytes begin to synthesize melanin, and the last of the immigrant cells, Merkel cells, appear. Also at this time the sebaceous gland shows evidence of lipogenesis, nails are keratinized, the epidermal ridges of the plantar and palmar surfaces are well defined, and fat is first seen in adipocytes of the subcutaneous tissue. The dermis still contains approximately 80% water despite an increase in fibrous connective tissue.[15]

At the end of the second trimester of pregnancy, the rest of the epidermis begins to keratinize, and the last two layers of the epidermis are formed. After keratinization, the periderm is sloughed, revealing an epidermis consisting of a few layers of cornified cells, a single layer of granular cells, two to three layers of spinous cells, and a single basal layer. Vernix caseosa, the cheesy white coating often still present on the skin at birth, is seen first at this stage due to the secretion of sebum by the sebaceous glands and sloughing of the periderm. Hair is also visible on the skin surface at this time. Elastin fibers are first seen in the dermis at the end of the second trimester.

At the beginning of the third trimester all skin structures are present. From this point on, the skin matures and adds connective tissue to the dermis. The fat cells of the subcutaneous tissue gradually enlarge, adding bulk to the skin. A sudden increase in thickness of the stratum corneum occurs just before birth. The dermis increases in bulk, and maturation of connective tissue components continues after birth.

Consequences of Abnormal Development

Numerous primary developmental anomalies of the integument are known. In addition, the skin is often secondarily involved in aberrations of underlying tissues. Some skin anomalies are local and benign, others may be severe and life-threatening, and still others may provide valuable clues to the identity of dysmorphic syndromes. Anomalies of the skin may be placed into three categories.[1] First are deformities that occur because of the skin's inherent elasticity and growth potential. Unusual enlargement or stretching of the underlying structures from such conditions as prenatal edema, massive abdominal distension, or congenital hip dislocation can result in redundant skin or aberrant skin creases. Second are disruptions associated with severe, prolonged pressure on the skin, injury from procedures such as amniocentesis, or from amniotic bands. Ulcers, skin dimpling, or cicatricial constriction rings may result. The final group are dysplasias, or more generalized abnormalities that cause structural changes in the epidermis, dermis, melanocyte distribution or function, and capillaries. Conditions in this category are listed in Table 63-1.

TABLE 63-1
Consequences of Abnormal Embryonic Development of the Skin

Fetal Age (wk)	Structure	Anomalies at Birth
6–7	Melanocyte migration and function	Congenital nevi Mongolian spots Café-au-lait spots
	Collagen fiber bundle formation	Ehlers-Danlos syndrome
9–10	Epidermal stratification	Ichthyosis
	Development of anchoring and attachment structures	Epidermolysis bullosa
14–15	Formation of epidermal appendages	Ectodermal dysplasias
16–17	Synthesis of melanin by melanocytes	Albinism
23–24	Elastin fiber formation	Cutis laxa
unknown	Vasculature	Salmon patch Port wine stain Hemangioma

Structure

The skin is divided into three basic structural layers (Fig. 63-1). The outermost layer is the epidermis, the middle layer is the dermis, and the innermost layer is the subcutaneous tissue. Although each layer has distinct differences, they do not function independently. Rather, each layer relies on the other for regulation, modulation, and support. The three layers of the skin are composed of a variety of cells and fibers that are essential to the structure and function of the skin. In addition, several appendages are also present: the pilosebaceous units, nails, eccrine glands, and apocrine glands. The skin is also well supplied with blood vessels, lymphatics, and nerves (see Fig. 63-1).

Epidermis

The epidermis is the outermost portion of the skin and varies in thickness from approximately 0.04 to 1.5 mm.[16] This portion is arranged in four layers, with specialized cells called keratinocytes gradually moving from the inner layer to the outer layer over a period of 3 to 4 weeks. This process is referred to as *differentiation*. As the keratinocytes migrate through the epidermal layers, they transpose from fragile, round, fluid-filled cells to tough, flat, dehydrated cells. Differentiation enables the epidermis to regenerate constantly while at the same time to provide a tough protective barrier. Figure 63-2 is a detailed illustration of the components of the epidermis.

Layers of the Epidermis

Epidermal layers are differentiated by the certain characteristics of the keratinocytes within each layer. Differentiation, also referred to as keratinization, is a progressive, genetically programmed series of events that includes: (1) development and alteration of the intracellular protein keratin, (2) loss of cell nucleus and other cytoplasmic organelles, (3) increase in cell size and flattening of the shape, (4) dehydration, and (5) changes in cell metabolism.[16] The end point of keratinization is a dead keratinocyte, which is eventually desquamated. A keratinocyte takes 14 days to move from the basal layer to the stratum corneum, and another 14 days to move through the stratum corneum. The number of layers remains constant among different body regions. An addi-

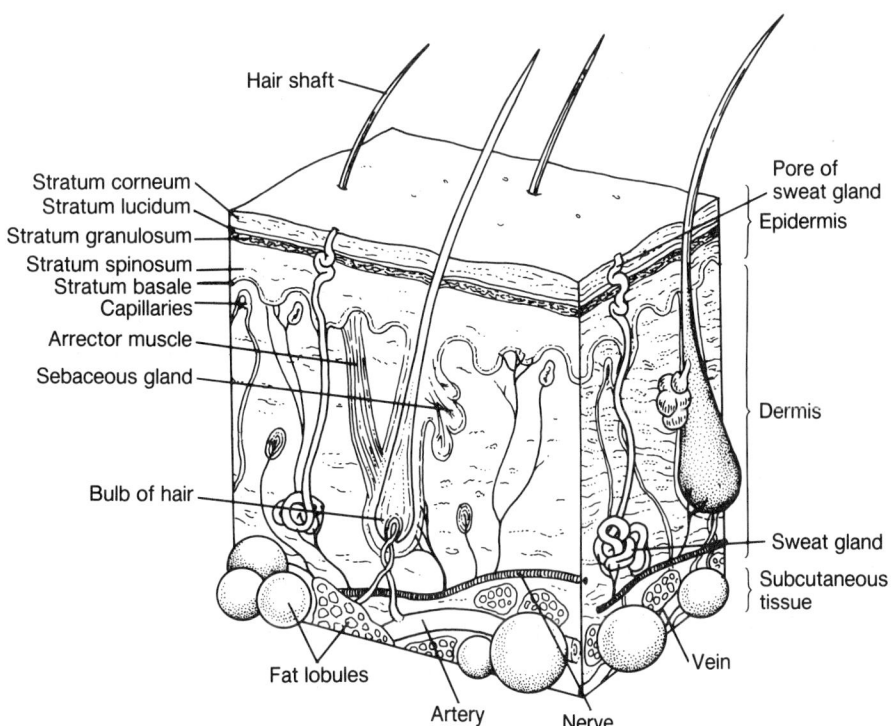

FIGURE 63-1
Structure of the skin.

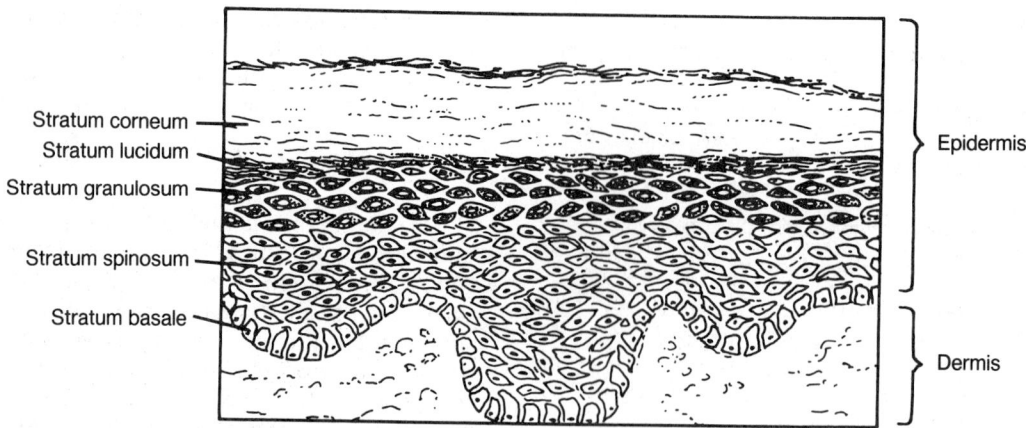

FIGURE 63-2

Epidermal layers and the epidermal melanin unit.

tional layer, the stratum lucidum, is present on the palms and soles, where the epidermis is the thickest. This layer is only several cell layers thick and lies between the stratum spinosum and the stratum corneum.

Basal Cell Layer (Stratum Basale). The stratum basale is the innermost layer of the epidermis and rests on the basement membrane zone (BMZ). This layer contains a single layer of mitotically active keratinocytes called basal cells that give rise to the keratinocytes, which move through the more superficial layers of the epidermis. The main function of the stratum basale is to maintain the epidermis by continually renewing the population of keratinocytes. However, not all basal cells are mitotically active at the same time. Certain conditions such as injury or carcinogens can stimulate nonactive cells to provide additionally needed keratinocytes. Also, by its firm attachment to the BMZ, the stratum basale plays an important role in preserving epidermal architecture.

Spinous Cell Layer (Stratum Spinosum). This layer, sometimes referred to as the prickle cell layer, is so named for the spines or desmosomes on the cell margins. Desmosomes extend from the keratinocyte and anchor the cells of the epidermis together. As the keratinocytes move through this layer, they continue to differentiate by enlarging and flattening. Keratohyaline granules, which help to form the barrier proteins of the outermost layers of the epidermis, first appear in the keratinocytes of the stratum spinosum.

Granular Cell Layer (Stratum Granulosum). The stratum granulosum is so named because of the high concentration of keratohyaline granules present in the keratinocytes. The granules synthesize the barrier proteins. As the keratinocyte moves through this layer, it loses its nucleus, continues to flatten, and dehydrates; the intracellular contents consist of barrier proteins (keratins) and dense matrix material.

Horny Cell Layer (Stratum Corneum). The stratum corneum layer provides the major barrier for the skin. This is the layer that is in direct contact with the envi-

ronment. Without this layer of the epidermis, the skin would be similar to mucous membrane. The overall thickness of this zone depends on the region of the body it covers. For example, the face has a thinner stratum corneum than the posterior trunk.

In this layer, the keratinocyte, which has become a cornified cell, is fully differentiated and at its largest size. This cell is flattened and has no nucleus or cytoplasmic structures. Keratin accounts for as much as 80% of the cornified cell contents with the remaining contents being comprised of water, water-soluble proteins, amino acids, sugars, urea, minerals, and some lipids.[16] These substances help maintain skin integrity, act as buffers and lubricants, and enable the skin to bind water. The flattened cells are arranged in well-organized layers and aligned in columns with overlapping cell edges. The outer portion of the horny cell layer is gradually sloughed and replaced with other fully keratinized cells that have migrated through the epidermis.

Cells of the Epidermis

Approximately 80% of the cells composing the epidermis are keratinocytes. However, three other types of cells are present in much smaller numbers and have distinctly different functions. These cells are often called immigrant cells because they arrive in the epidermis during embryonic development and are of different origins than keratinocytes. Approximately 5% to 10% of the epidermal cells are melanocytes, 5% are Langerhans cells, and less than 1% are Merkel cells.[9]

Melanocytes. Melanocytes are derived from the neural crest and arrive early in the epidermis during embryonic development. Their main function is the production of skin pigment, which serves to protect the skin and underlying structures from ultraviolet radiation. These cells are confined to the basal cell layer; however, their extending cell processes, referred to as *dendrites,* associate them with a specific number of keratinocytes. This association is called the epidermal melanin unit and extends into the more superficial layers of the epidermis.

Melanosomes are the specialized cellular parts of the

melanocyte in which melanin is synthesized. Melanosomes are transported along dendrites and transferred to keratinocytes, giving the skin its characteristic pigment. The skin color is determined by the size and organization of the melanosomes, not the amount present. Melanosome size and organization are genetically determined, with black skin having large, grouped melanosomes and skin that is lighter in color having small, single melanosomes. This genetically determined skin color is called *constitutional skin color*. *Facultative skin color* is the additional pigmentation of skin that has been stimulated by ultraviolet light, hormones, or low-grade cutaneous inflammation. The intensity of facultative skin color depends on the number of melanosomes, their dispersion, and how fast they produce melanin.[21]

Langerhans' Cells. Langerhans cells can be found in all layers of the epidermis with the exception of the stratum corneum and are distributed fairly evenly over various regions of the body. Like melanocytes, they arrive early during embryonic development; however, they are derived from precursor cells in the bone marrow and migrate into the epidermis from systemic circulation. The main function of Langerhans cells is to protect against environmental antigens. They stimulate T-cell activity and are involved in cell-mediated hypersensitivity reactions and in sensitization associated with donor graft rejection. The activity of Langerhans cells is impaired by skin exposure to ultraviolet light. Additionally, they have been found to be reduced in number in people with certain skin diseases such as psoriasis, sarcoidosis, and contact dermatitis.[16]

Merkel's Cells. Merkel cells were originally thought to be derived from the neural crest like melanocytes. More recently, however, evidence suggests that they originate from the ectoderm like keratinocytes.[15] These cells are confined to the basal layer and can be found in specific regions of the body such as glabrous skin of digits, lips, oral cavity, hair follicle, and collected in specialized structures called tactile disks or touch domes. Merkel cells are considered part of the sensory receptor system of the skin, and they frequently are associated with nerve fibers. The exact role of Merkel cells, however, is unclear. They are thought to be receptors that transmit a stimulus to the neurite by way of a chemical synapse or serve as a neuromodulator by influencing the threshold of the sensory nerve ending by way of the release of a neuropeptide.[16]

Basement Membrane Zone

The basement membrane zone (BMZ) is the interface between the epidermis and the dermis. This zone acts as a semipermeable membrane and regulates epidermal differentiation and repair. The primary function of the BMZ is to maintain epidermal and dermal adhesion. In several genetic blistering disorders, such as epidermolysis bullosa, this region is altered, resulting in separation of the epidermis and dermis and the subsequent formation of a blister.

Dermis

The dermis is the second layer of the skin and makes up the greatest proportion of skin mass. From region to region, it varies in thickness from 1 to 4 mm (see Fig. 63-1). The dermis is largely acellular, with the exception of fibroblasts, macrophages, and mast cells being scattered throughout. Connective tissue fibers, such as collagen and elastin, compose most of the dermis. Various other structures, including blood vessels, lymphatic vessels, nerves, and the deeper portions of epidermal appendages, complete the components of the dermis.

Layers of the Dermis

The dermis is organized into two layers: the papillary dermis and the reticular dermis. The papillary dermis is next to the epidermis, molds to its contours, and is approximately the same thickness. The bulk of the dermis is the reticular dermis, which extends to the subcutaneous tissue. The two regions are distinguished by the size of collagen bundles and their respective cell and blood vessel populations. Strictly cutaneous disorders characterized by edema and erythema tend to involve the papillary dermis and its abundant capillary supply. Systemic diseases with skin manifestations primarily tend to involve the reticular dermis.[9]

Connective Tissue of the Dermis

The dermis is made up of two main types of connective tissue—collagen and elastin. These tissues provide the dermis with its dense, interwoven, and fibrous characteristics. Collagen fibers account for the largest portion of dermal connective tissue. These fibers provide the tensile strength and some elasticity by interweaving fiber bundles to form a basketweave structure. Several types of collagen are present in the dermis and scattered in various locations. Elastin fibers are present in all regions of the dermis along with collagen. These fibers line the basketweave structure of the collagen bundles and enable the skin to recoil to its original shape after being stretched.

Cells of the Dermis

Although the dermis essentially is acellular, a few cells can be identified. They are highest in concentration in the papillary dermis, particularly around blood vessels. Cells indigenous to the dermis include the fibroblast, macrophage, and mast cells. Lymphocytes, plasma cells, and other blood-derived leukocytes enter the dermis from the blood vessels in response to various stimuli (e.g., inflammation).

The dermal cell most significant in number is the fibroblast, which synthesizes and degrades collagen and elastin. A second dermal cell is the macrophage. This cell synthesizes and secretes enzymes necessary for the body's defense against microorganisms, components of the complement system, and other soluble factors such as interleukin, prostaglandins, and interferon. Another important dermal cell is the mast cell, which is a specialized secretory cell that releases histamine, causing vasodilation and dermal edema. The mast cell is also responsible for immediate type hypersensitivity reactions. The macrophage and masts cell along with the Langerhans cells of the epidermis play a significant role in the body's immune response (Chap. 27).

Subcutaneous Tissue

The subcutaneous tissue functions primarily as a cushion and temperature regulator for the body. This layer also allows the skin to move easily over underlying structures and molds body contours. The subcutaneous tissue lies beneath the dermis and is composed primarily of adipose or fat (see Fig. 63-1). The transition from the fibrous dermis to the fatty subcutaneous, also referred to as hypodermis, is often abrupt. The two regions are closely related, however, by way of nerves, blood vessels, and appendages that course through both areas. Fibrous connective tissue is present in the subcutaneous region to provide a framework for fat deposition. Thickness of the subcutaneous tissue varies from region to region. For instance, the skin thickness of the pretibial area on the lower leg is much thinner than that on the abdomen. The amount of subcutaneous tissue in each of these regions accounts for its thickness. Along with site variation, the amount of subcutaneous tissue in a person is controlled by circulating hormones, heredity, age, and eating habits.

Epidermal Appendages

Pilosebaceous Unit

Pilosebaceous units (see Fig. 63-1) are integrated structures consisting of the hair follicle and the sebaceous gland, and they are found on all areas of the skin except the palms and soles. The size and number vary across regions of the body.

Sebaceous Gland. The sebaceous gland is a lobulated structure connected to the hair follicle wall by the sebaceous duct at the level of the infundibulum. This gland produces and secretes sebum, an oily substance that passes through the sebaceous duct into the hair canal and onto the skin surface. Sebum secretion is a continual process under the control of hormones such as estrogens and androgens. Elevations of temperature, however, increase sebum flow to the skin surface. The actual function of sebum has not been fully explored. One hypothesis suggests that sebum enhances barrier properties, moisturizes the skin, and serves as an antibacterial or antifungal agent, but this remains a speculation.

The largest sebaceous glands can be found on the face and scalp. In general, they are smaller on the trunk, and sebaceous glands along the midline of the body are larger than on the lateral surface. The smallest sebaceous glands are found on the extremities.[16]

Hair Follicle. The hair follicle can be divided into sections defined by specific landmarks. The three major landmarks are the sebaceous gland duct opening, the at-

tachment site bulge of the arrector pili muscle, and the bulb (see Fig. 63-1). The infudibulum is the uppermost portion of the follicle that lies between the skin surface and the sebaceous gland duct opening. The arrector pili muscle consists of smooth muscle cells that contract under sympathetic nerve stimulation, pulling the follicle into a vertical position and elevating the hair. This muscle attaches to the hair follicle wall producing a bulge. The area lying between the duct opening and the bulge is called the isthmus.

The portion of the follicle between the bulge and the bulb is the lower follicle. This area is transient and grows or atrophies, depending on the phase of the hair growth cycle. The bulb is the lowest portion of the hair follicle. Contained within the bulb are germinal cells that produce the hair and melanocytes that give the hair its color. The hair follicle is positioned in the skin at an angle, and the hair emerges from the follicle on a slant. On the arms and legs, the hair projects downward away from the midline of the body. On the trunk, the hair grows downward. On areas such as the sacrum and the scalp, the hair is whorled.[3]

The hair has two distinct regions, the outer cuticle and the inner cortex. The cortex is the pigmented part of the hair and varies in thickness depending on hair type. Some hairs have a third region called the medulla located at the center of the hair shaft.

An important feature of the hair follicle is the hair growth cycle (Fig. 63-3). The hair growth activity of the follicle is intermittent. During the active growth cycle of the hair, or *anagen,* the hair follicle is at its largest size, often extending deep into the dermis. Toward the end of anagen, the follicle bulb constricts and the distal end of the hair shaft becomes keratinized forming the "club" hair. This transition phase is called *catagen.* As the club hair moves toward the skin surface and the lower follicle

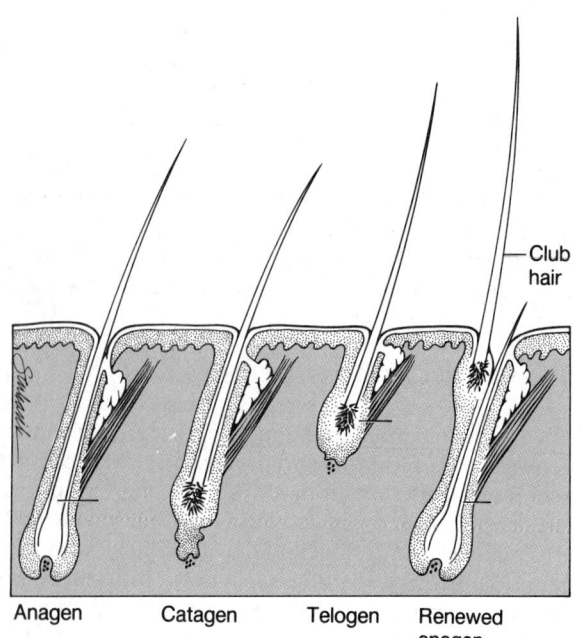

FIGURE 63-3
Hair growth cycle.

shrinks, the hair follicle enters the resting phase, or *telogen*. Several weeks after the hair is shed, the next cycle starts. In the human scalp at any one time, the majority of scalp hairs are in anagen, with less than 1% of the follicles in catagen and about 13% in telogen.[4]

Several types of hair are found on the body at various ages and sites. Lanugo hairs are the first hairs formed by fetal follicles. These hairs are fine, soft, and lightly pigmented. The first growth is shed in utero at the seventh or eighth month of gestation. A second growth, usually shorter, grows and is shed, often unnoticed, soon after birth. Vellous hairs are fine, soft, short, and lightly pigmented and grow after the loss of lanugo. Scalp hair follicles quickly convert from vellous hair to terminal hair growth. Others, such as axilla, pubic, and beard hair in males, are converted later in life as the result of hormonal stimulation. This same hormonal stimulation can revert terminal hairs to vellous hair in areas like the scalp, most frequently seen in adult males. Terminal hair is long, coarse, and pigmented. The color and length are genetically determined. Terminal hair is found on regions of the body such as the scalp, eyebrows, beard, axilla, and pubis. This is the only type of hair that may have a central medulla.

Eccrine Sweat Glands

Eccrine sweat glands (see Fig. 63-1) are distributed over nearly the entire body surface and excrete sweat as a normal response to exercise and increased body temperature. This function helps the body to maintain thermal control through heat loss by way of water evaporation. Eccrine sweat glands also perform an excretory role by removing various end products of metabolism or drugs from the body. They help to maintain body homeostasis by reabsorption of electrolytes and fluid.

An eccrine sweat gland consists of a coiled secreting segment located in the deep dermis or subcutaneous tissue, and the duct, which ascends vertically to the skin surface. The duct serves as a pathway where sweat composition is changed by reabsorption processes on its way to the skin surface. Sweat glands respond to sympathetic stimulation from the temperature regulatory center in the hypothalamus when it senses an increase in core temperature. Emotional stress can also stimulate eccrine sweat gland function. This response is usually confined to the palms, soles, axilla, and forehead; however, it can occur over the entire body surface.

Apocrine Sweat Glands

Apocrine development and function depend on sex hormone stimulation. Apocrine glands do not become functional in humans until just before puberty. Structurally, these glands are similar to eccrine glands; however, they are usually larger, the coil is located deeper in the skin, and they are restricted to the face, scalp, axilla, and anogenital regions. They produce a clear, oily substance that is odorless when first secreted. Subsequent bacterial action is necessary for odor production. The duct opens into the infundibulum of the hair follicle where apocrine secretion and sebum merge. Specialized apocrine glands are located in the auditory meatus and secrete cerumen. Montgomery tubercles are specialized apocrine glands on the breast areolae. The role apocrine glands play in humans is unclear. In many animal species, they are important for territorial marking, thermal regulation, and increasing friction resistance of foot pads on paws. Because they do not begin to function until puberty and are odor producing, apocrine glands are thought to have some type of function as a sexual attractant in humans.[16] The apocrine glands may have played an important role earlier in the evolution of humans; however, they are now considered to be of minor importance physiologically. On the other hand, they do play a significant economic role in the cosmetic and fragrance industry.

Nails

The nail is a hard keratinized plate at the tips of digits and is the end product of terminally differentiated epidermal cells originating in the nail matrix. The main function of the nail is to provide a splint for the soft tip of the finger and aid in fine grasp. Nail growth is slow and continuous. Growth of the nail depends on the particular digit and its innervation as well as the age, nutritional state, and general health of the person.

The nail is divided into four distinct zones (Fig. 63-4). The first zone is the epidermal tissue, which lies above and covers the deepest portion and sides of the nail plate. This area is called the *nail fold*. The cuticle is a thin ridge of stratum corneum that adheres to the nail plate at the proximal portion of the nail fold and forms a loose seal protecting the deep nail matrix. The *nail matrix* is the second zone and is composed of a thick epithelium where the nail plate is formed. The nail matrix is continuous with the *nail bed*, the third zone, which is well supplied with capillary networks and nerves. The nail bed adheres to the under surface of the nail plate. The point of separation of the nail bed and the nail plate creates the fourth zone, referred to as the *hyponychium*. Cells shed from the stratum corneum collect beneath the nail, forming a seal that protects the nail bed.[2]

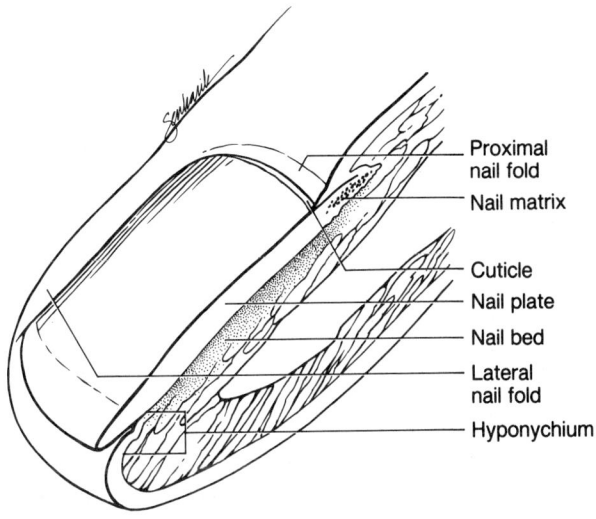

FIGURE 63-4
Nail unit.

Blood Supply

Blood vessels that supply the skin penetrate the subcutaneous tissue, enter the reticular dermis, and ascend, forming capillary loops that extend into the papillary dermis. At many points in the reticular dermis, vessel branches provide circulation to coils of sweat glands and bulbs of hair follicles. The epidermis is avascular and depends on the dermis for its vascular support.

The abundance of vessels in the skin is more than is needed to meet its metabolic requirements. The vascularity of the skin allows the body to shunt blood in varying amounts to assist with temperature and blood pressure regulation. In comparison to the vasculature of other organs, vessels of the skin have thicker walls as well as extra support from connective tissue and smooth muscles, which allows them to withstand greater forces.

Lymphatics

The lymphatic channels present in the skin are most prominent at the junction between the papillary and reticular dermis. The lymphatic system is important in regulating the interstitial fluid and in clearing tissue of cells, proteins, fluid, and degraded substances from sites of inflammation.

Nerves

The skin is supplied with somatic sensory and sympathetic autonomic nerve fibers, which conduct stimuli from Merkel cells in the epidermis and specialized receptors found in regions of thick skin and hair follicles. Sensory fibers are the most widespread and function as receptors of touch, pain, temperature, itch, and mechanical stimuli. The density and type of fibers are regionally variable, which accounts for the variation in acuity at different sites of the body. Sympathetic fibers are codistributed with sensory fibers except for branches that innervate sweat glands, blood vessel walls, and arrector pili muscles.

Function

The role that the skin plays in maintaining the health of a person becomes more evident after reviewing the anatomy of the skin. Skin functions can be described as protective, metabolic, and interactive as listed in the accompanying display.

Protection

As long as the stratum corneum is intact, it is the major protective structure in the skin.[3] The stratum corneum allows humans to live in a dry environment and avoid dehydration. Its thickness and overlapping structure retard the entrance of toxic agents from the environment. In addition, the Langerhans cells within the epidermis play an immune surveillance role by stimulating activation

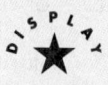

Functions of the Skin

Protective

Fluid and electrolyte regulation
Entrance of toxic environmental agents retarded
Colonization and invasion of microorganisms inhibited
Immune surveillance
Ultraviolet light damage inhibited
Low-voltage current damage resisted
Mechanical trauma cushioned
Temperature regulation

Metabolic

Vitamin D synthesis
Drug absorption
Excretion of metabolic end products
Fat storage

Interactive

Sensory perception
Physical intimacy
Social and sexual communication

of T-cell-dependent immune responses against infectious or noninfectious agents to which the skin is continuously exposed.[16] The dryness and multilayered structure of the skin inhibit the colonization and invasion of microorganisms. The protein and melanin it contains absorb ultraviolet radiation; skin provides electrical resistance by maintaining a low water content. The stratum corneum, dermis, and hypodermis maintain the structural strength of the skin and provide cushioning to protect the underlying structures from mechanical trauma.

The skin is also an important organ in maintaining a constant core temperature when the environmental temperature fluctuates. The vascular, eccrine gland, and neurologic responses, as well as the relatively poor thermal conductivity of dry skin, protect the body from extreme heat or cold.[3]

Metabolism

The metabolic functions of the skin include synthesis of vitamin D from a form of cholesterol in the skin when exposed to sunlight. The skin also degrades and metabolizes topically applied medications by skin enzyme systems. The eccrine glands excrete electrolytes and nonelectrolytes such as urea and lactate, and the subcutaneous tissue serves as a storage depot for fat.

Sensation

As a tactile organ the skin plays a vital role in the physical, emotional, and behavioral development of the person. The skin is abundantly supplied with sensory nerves, which are capable of receiving stimuli of heat, cold, touch, and pain. Neurologic stimulation is necessary for the continued neurologic development in the child.

Touch is the language of physical intimacy to which emotional meanings become attached. Research with animals has demonstrated the importance of touch on the survival of the newborn. Maternal behaviors such as licking and grooming of the young appear necessary for survival in many animal species.[17] Human survival is also thought to rely heavily on sensory stimulation. In human newborns, the tactile rooting reflex assists the child to find nourishment, and a mother's caressing and communication of affection through touch have a dramatic effect on comforting a distressed infant.

Several investigators have observed positive physiologic and developmental responses in low birth weight infants who were given body massage and kinesthetic stimulation daily when compared to a control group.[8,29] Other investigations have suggested that healthy human infants deprived of touch and handling for long periods develop a kind of infant depression that leads to withdrawal and apathy.[27]

In a child with skin disease, the normal parental contact is altered. Parents may be afraid to touch the child's skin, or the normal spontaneous touching and stroking become a task restricted by necessity and time constraints.[22] Instead of being a pleasurable interaction, skin care can actually lead to discomfort. To a certain extent, touch is controlled by cultural norms; however, the basic need for human contact is universal.

The skin also functions as a major organ of social and sexual communication, playing a vital role in first impressions and attraction, both of which are based on superficial appearance. It has been suggested that early experiences of closeness and skin contact with parental figures have an impact on the development of adult sexuality.[19] Dysfunction of this organ has an enormous impact on the development of self-image. A visit to the local drug store with a stroll from the magazine counter to the cosmetic counter gives insight into the importance placed on appearance in our society. Feeling accepted and appearing "normal" are major issues for children and adolescents.[25] Parental expectations and dreams regarding their unborn child may be dashed when faced at birth with a child who has disfiguring skin lesions.[22] Skin disorders have significant impact on the development of self-esteem and long-lasting social implications.

Developmental Differences

Preterm Infant Skin

The skin of a preterm infant corresponds with the gestational age and nutritional status of the child. Basically, it is the skin of a third-trimester fetus with a thin epidermis, less fibrous connective tissue, partial or nonfunctional sweat glands, and immature vascular and neurologic networks (Table 63-2). The subcutaneous tissue is well developed; however, the fat cells are small. This along with the underdeveloped dermis accounts for the scrawny appearance of the preterm infant. Because of im-

TABLE 63-2
Structural Differences in Preterm and Newborn Infant Skin

Skin Structure	Preterm	Newborn
Epidermal layers	Thinner	Same
Melanocytes	Little melanin production	Low melanin production
Hair follicles	Thick lanugo growth, scalp hair in telogen	Thin lanugo growth, scalp hair in telogen
Sebaceous glands	Actively secreting	Actively secreting
Eccrine glands	Present but nonfunctioning	Present but poor sweating response
Apocrine glands	Nonfunctioning	Nonfunctioning
Dermal layers	Edematous, thin, regions indistinct	Thin, edematous, regions less distinct
Dermal collagen	Small bundles widely spaced	Intermediate size bundles
Dermal elastin	Immature, sparse, tiny	Small, immature, same distribution
Dermal cells	Abundant	Moderately abundant
Blood vessels	Structurally and functionally immature	Structurally and functionally immature
Nerves	Structurally and functionally immature	Structurally close to maturity; functionally immature
Subcutaneous	Well developed, but thin	Well developed

maturity, a preterm infant is more susceptible to enhanced permeability of the skin, fluid imbalance, skin injury, and impaired temperature control.

The barrier properties of preterm infants' skin have been shown to be decreased in several instances, allowing for increased percutaneous absorption of toxic compounds.[11,20,28] The outer layer of the epidermis, the stratum corneum, gives the skin its barrier properties. In the preterm infant, the stratum corneum has only a few cell layers and is markedly thinner than that of the newborn or the adult[14] and therefore functions as a relatively permeable membrane.[18] Additional factors in the neonate such as decreased plasma protein binding and immature kidney functioning lead to drug toxicity at lower doses, placing the child at even greater risk for toxicity from topically applied products.[28] The thin stratum corneum and the underdeveloped connective tissue in the dermis make the skin particularly vulnerable to trauma. The already imperfect barrier is further weakened when it is traumatized by the use of adhesive tape, caustic substances,[24] or the placement and removal of monitoring probes and electrodes.[10,13]

The preterm infant is also predisposed to insensible skin fluid loss due to the imperfect cutaneous barrier and high fluid content of the dermis. Excessive fluid losses have been observed during the early neonatal period in infants of 30 weeks' gestation or less.[7,13] Insensible water loss in the skin is also a major source of heat loss and can be a contributing factor to hypothermia in small infants.[23,26] The delayed functioning of eccrine glands and the subsequent anhidrosis in the preterm infant inhibits temperature control by sweating when the rectal temperature is elevated even to 37.8°C.[12] Although this phenomenon can protect the infant from additional insensible fluid loss, it also can put the infant at risk for hyperthermia. The fragility of preterm infants' thermoregulation mechanisms highlights the enormous importance of environmental control.

Once exposed to the dry outside environment, the skin of the preterm infant quickly adapts. Infants less than 31 weeks' EGA demonstrate striking epidermal maturation with increased thickness of the epidermis and a fully developed stratum corneum that may be nearly as effective as that of an adult within the first 2 weeks after birth.[5]

Newborn Infant Skin

In many aspects the skin of a full-term newborn infant is similar in structure and function to that of an adult. Several features, however, are still immature (see Table 63-2). In the newborn, the epidermis is nearly identical to the adult epidermal structure, with excellent barrier capabilities as well as functional hair follicles and sebaceous glands.[6] On the other hand, melanin production by melanosomes is decreased, and eccrine gland function is reduced. The dermis exhibits even greater difference between the two age groups, with newborn dermis being thinner, and having incompletely developed connective tissue. Vascular and neurologic networks also are functionally and structurally immature.[15] These features of newborn skin account for the development of certain transient cutaneous conditions such as milia, acne neonatorum, and cutis marmorata (see Chap. 65).

With mature barrier function of full-term newborn skin, the risk for dehydration and hypothermia related to insensible fluid loss is greatly diminished. Excessive skin permeability is also reduced; however, newborns are still susceptible to toxicity from percutaneous absorption of topical compounds due to their increased volume-to-skin-surface ratio as well as metabolic differences.

Healthy infants born at term have not yet attained full development of eccrine sweating function. The onset of sweating ranges from the 2nd to the 18th day of life.[12] Therefore, until that time, their ability to dissipate heat from the body by sweating is impaired.

The melanocyte population in the basal layer of the epidermis is believed to be the same as in the adult. However, melanin production by melanosomes at this age is low.[15] In addition, the skin pigment of a newborn is influenced only by constitutional skin color. The skin has not been exposed to factors, such as ultraviolet light, that are responsible for facultative skin color. As a result, the skin pigment of a newborn of any race is lighter at birth. This feature is more pronounced in darker pigmented races, such as an African-American infant who may be fair at birth. Skin pigment darkens with age as melanin production increases, and the skin pigment is influenced by facultative factors. It is unclear when melanin production in the newborn reaches adult levels; however, it is thought to be nearly the same by 1 year of age.

Childhood Skin

Childhood skin differs only slightly from adult skin. The epidermis is equivalent to that of an adult. However, there is some functional variation. The amount of hair in anagen, or the active growth cycle, is highest in children. Hair in sexual sites, such as the groin and axilla, remain vellous until puberty when, under hormonal influence, they become terminal hair. Sebaceous gland activity becomes quiescent between 6 and 12 months of age. Sebum production begins to increase as early as age 6 in girls and age 7 in boys, probably stimulated by androgens from adrenal glands. More marked increase of sebum production occurs at puberty and in later teens. As a result, at puberty or slightly before, disorders of sebaceous glands, such as acne, are seen (see Chap. 65). Complete neurologic control of eccrine sweating may not be in place until 2 or 3 years of age. At that time, the sweating mechanism is similar to that of an adult except for a lower concentration of sodium chloride.[12] The apocrine glands remain nonfunctional until stimulated by hormones at puberty.

The dermis continues its development during the childhood years. After an initial growth spurt during the first 2 weeks of life, the dermis remains fairly constant in thickness during the first year. At this age, it begins to increase in thickness and to develop more connective tissue. By the age of 7, it is double the thickness of newborn dermis. After puberty, the skin again gains in thickness until, in a young adult, the dermis is approximately 3.5 times the thickness of newborn dermis. The vascular system pattern within the dermis and hypodermis is well developed by the end of the second year of life. By comparison, many investigators believe that cutaneous nerves continue to develop until puberty or even later.[15]

Summary

The skin is a complex organ acting as an interface between the environment and the person. The epidermis, dermis, and hypodermis, along with the other structures of the skin, work together to form the integument. All skin structures are present at birth. From this point on, they continue to mature as well as to undergo modification and resynthesis throughout life. The skin tends to stay healthy as long as it remains intact. However, preterm or diseased skin interferes with its barrier functions, leaving the person susceptible to a number of environmental factors. The interactive functions are also altered by disease, influencing the child's psychological and social development. The nurse's knowledge of cutaneous structure and function is necessary to provide comprehensive health care for the child and family.

References

1. Aase, J. M. (1990). *Diagnostic dysmorphology*. New York: Plenum.
2. Baden, H. P., & Zaias, N. (1987). Biology of nails. In T. B. Fitzpatrick (Ed.), *Dermatology in general medicine* (3rd ed.), p. 219. New York: McGraw-Hill.
3. Blank, I. H. (1987). The skin as an organ of protection. In T. B. Fitzpatrick (Ed.), *Dermatology in general medicine* (3rd ed.), p. 337. New York: McGraw-Hill.
4. Ebling, J. J. (1987). Biology of hair follicles. In T. B. Fitzpatrick

(Ed.), *Dermatology in general medicine* (3rd ed.), p. 213. New York: McGraw-Hill.

5. Evans, N. J., & Rutter, N. (1986). Development of the epidermis in the newborn. *Biology of the Neonate, 49,* 74.

6. Fairley, J. A., & Rasmussen, J. E. (1983). Comparison of stratum corneum thickness in children and adults. *Journal of the American Academy of Dermatology, 8,* 652.

7. Fanaroff, A. A., et al. (1972). Insensible water loss in low birth weight infants. *Pediatrics, 50,* 236.

8. Field, T., et al. (1987). Massage of preterm newborns to improve growth and development. *Pediatric Nursing, 13,* 385.

9. Fitzpatrick, T. B., et al. (1987). Correlation of pathophysiology of skin. In T. B. Fitzpatrick (Ed.), *Dermatology in general medicine* (3rd ed.), p. 69. New York: McGraw-Hill.

10. Golden, S. M. (1981). Skin craters: A complication of transcutaneous oxygen monitoring. *Pediatrics, 67,* 514.

11. Goutieres, F., & Aicardi, J. (1977). Accidental percutaneous hexachlorophene intoxication in children. *British Medical Journal, 2,* 663.

12. Green, M. (1982). Comparison of adult and neonatal skin eccrine sweating. In H. I. Maibach & E. K. Boisits (Eds.), *Neonatal Skin: Structure and Function,* p. 35. New York: Marcel Dekker.

13. Harpin, V. A., & Rutter, N. (1983). Barrier properties of newborn infant's skin. *Journal of Pediatrics, 102,* 419.

14. Holbrook, K. A. (1982). A histological comparison of infant and adult skin. In H. I. Maibach & E. K. Boisits (Eds.), *Neonatal Skin: Structure and Function,* p. 3. New York: Marcel Dekker.

15. Holbrook, K. A., & Sybert, V. (1988). Basic science. In L. A. Schachner & R. C. Hansen (Eds.), *Pediatric dermatology,* p. 3. New York: Churchill Livingstone.

16. Holbrook, K. A., & Wolff, K. (1987). The structure and development of skin. In T. B. Fitzpatrick (Ed.), *Dermatology in general medicine* (3rd ed.), p. 93. New York: McGraw-Hill.

17. Montagu, A. (1971). *Touching: The human significance of the skin.* New York: Columbia University Press.

18. Nachman, R. L., & Esterly, N. B. (1971). Increased skin permeability in preterm infants. *Journal of Pediatrics, 79,* 628.

19. Nadelson, T. (1978). A person's boundaries: A meaning of skin disease. *Cutis, 21,* 90.

20. Pyati, S., et al. (1977). Absorption of iodine in the neonate following topical use of povidone-iodine. *Journal of Pediatrics, 91,* 825.

21. Quevedo, W. C., et al. (1987). Biology of melanocytes. In T. B. Fitzpatrick (Ed.), *Dermatology in general medicine* (3rd ed.), p. 225. New York: McGraw-Hill.

22. Rauch, P., & Jellinek, M. S. (1988). Psychosocial development in children with cutaneous disease. In L. A. Schacner & R. C. Hansen (Eds.), *Pediatric dermatology,* p. 139. New York: Churchill Livingstone.

23. Rutter, N., & Hull, D. (1979). Water loss from the skin of term and preterm babies. *Archives of Disease in Childhood, 54,* 858.

24. Schick, J. B., & Milstein, J. M. (1981). Burn hazard of isopropyl alcohol in the neonate. *Pediatrics, 68,* 587.

25. Selekman J. (1983, April). The development of body image in the child: A learned response. *Topics in Clinical Nursing,* 12.

26. Sinclair, J. C. (1972). Thermal control in premature infants. *Annual Review of Medicine, 23,* 129.

27. Thayer, S. (1988). Close encounters. *Psychology Today, 22,* 31.

28. West, D. P., et al. (1981). Pharmacology and toxicology of infant skin. *Journal of Investigative Dermatology, 76,* 147.

29. White-Traut, R. C., & Goldman, M. B. C. (1988). Premature infant massage: Is it safe? *Pediatric Nursing, 14,* 285.

64 CHAPTER

Nursing Assessment and Diagnosis of Integumentary Function

BEHAVIORAL OBJECTIVES

Use functional health as a guideline for assessment of the child's integumentary function.

Define skin lesions according to type, pattern of distribution, and arrangement.

Describe various diagnostic tests used in skin disorders.

Identify nursing diagnoses that may be used in the care of children with cutaneous disorders.

Describe the components of a complete physical examination of the child's integumentary function.

The visibility and accessibility of the skin make its assessment and examination distinctly different from other organ systems. However, because of the prevalence of various skin disorders, it is always important to have the child or parent identify the problem with which they are concerned.[13] The nurse must not assume that the most visible lesion is the one that prompted their seeking medical consultation. For example, an adolescent with facial acne may be more concerned about a wart on the bottom of his or her foot. This situation allows the health care team to provide additional health care and teaching, but identifying the primary problem from the view of the child or parent fosters their trust and respect.

Nursing Assessment

Nursing assessment of the skin begins with assessment of the child's functional health to provide an overall view of the health patterns of the child and family.[8] When caring for children, the nurse not only deals with the child but also must rely on an accompanying parent or adult for the historic or current information regarding health patterns and the presenting health problem.

The examination of the skin is the second step in assessment. This information is combined with other health data to establish the nursing diagnoses. The baseline information is used for comparison in all future evaluations.

1761

Child and Family History

The focus of functional health assessment is to identify current and past health behaviors of the child and family that affect the integument. Functional and dysfunctional health patterns are used to direct nursing care and teaching.

Health Perception and Health Management

Assessment of health perception and health management provides a basis for understanding the overall health status, past and current skin health status, skin care practices, frequency of skin problems, and previous experiences in obtaining care for skin ailments. It is also important to establish if the child or parent perceives previous treatment to be successful and what their expectations are in relation to treatment of the skin. Sample questions used in this assessment follow: What is the child's current skin problem? When and where did the skin problem start? Has it spread? Are there accompanying symptoms such as pain or itching? How long has the skin problem been present, and are there factors that make it better or worse? Has the child had this problem before? What other skin problems has the child had in the past?

How is the overall health of the child and the family? Does the child have any other medical problems? Does the child have any allergies? Is the child using any medication? Does the child administer his or her own medications and treatments? If not, who does?

What are the child's normal skin and hair care routines? How are bug bites, scrapes, and cuts routinely cared for? Who are the family members that help the child care for his or her skin?

What do you think caused this problem? What have you done in the past to treat this problem? Was the action helpful? Have you sought help for this or any other skin problem in the past? Was the past treatment successful? Were you able to follow the treatment directions you were given? If not, how did you change them? How can we be most helpful to you?

Nutrition and Metabolism

Nutritional and metabolic assessment in relationship to the skin includes patterns of food and fluid consumption and indicators of metabolic need. Sample questions include: How is the child's appetite? Does ingestion of any foods cause the child's skin to break out in a rash? Has the child ever had difficulty healing an area of the skin that has been injured?

Elimination

Assessment of elimination patterns in relationship to the skin focuses on skin integrity and functioning of eccrine and apocrine sweat glands. Is the child wearing diapers or toilet trained? Has the child had problems with diaper rash or any skin problems associated with bowel or urinary elimination? Does the child have an ostomy? If so, are there any associated skin problems? Does the child have any problems with sweating or excessive odor?

Activity and Exercise

Assessment of the activity and exercise pattern emphasizes the level of the child's self-care abilities and the ability and availability of the caregiver. Information regarding work, play, and exercise activities may give clues to actual or potential skin problems as well as how skin treatments can be incorporated into daily life. What work, play, and exercise activities does the child participate in? What is the child's daily routine? What is the caregiver's daily routine?

Sleep and Rest

Assessment of quality and quantity of sleep and rest along with energy level provides information regarding interference by skin-related symptoms such as pruritis or pain. Does the child complain of skin symptoms, such as pain or itching, during the night? Does the child have difficulty going to sleep or wake often because of these symptoms?

Cognition and Perception

Language, memory, decision making, and sensory capabilities of the child and parent are assessed to evaluate the ability of the child or parent to understand the disease process and treatment recommendations and to communicate with the nurse. Obtaining information regarding how the child or parent best learns new skills is important for planning health teaching. What does the child or parent understand about the disease and how to carry out the treatments? Does the child have any symptoms, such as pain or itching, associated with his or her skin problem? If so, what have you done to relieve these symptoms in the past? Was it helpful?

Self-Perception and Self-Concept

Disorders of the skin often have an effect on a child's body image and self-concept. The nurse should assess how the child or parent thinks the skin problem has affected the child's body image, feelings of self worth, and perception of abilities. Has there been any changes in what the child does or how he or she feels about herself since the start of the skin problem?

Role Relationship

How satisfied is the child with family and social roles? Information regarding past or present skin conditions of family members and social contacts may also be obtained. Skin disease often interrupts the child's ability to participate in social activities and can disrupt the entire family functioning. Sample questions include the following: What is the family structure? (Draw a family diagram, include extended family members.) Does any immediate or extended family member have a similar skin problem? What skin problems have family members had in the past? How do other family members feel about the illness?

Does the child belong to any social groups or have close friends? Does the child spend a lot of time alone? Does anyone in these social groups have a similar skin problem as the child? What is the effect of the skin problem on the child's willingness to participate in school or peer group social activities? Does the presence of the skin problem affect peer relationships at school or in the community?

Sexuality and Reproduction

The skin plays a major role in sexual communication and physical intimacy. Disturbances of the integument may influence the development of the child's sexuality. Sexually active adolescents may be at risk for contracting a sexually transmitted skin infection. Age-appropriate sample questions should be asked. Does the skin disease interfere with the child's relationships with peers of the opposite sex? Does the skin disease interfere with the child's ability to dress in the fashions of his or her peers? Has the child ever had a sexually transmitted disease, such as genital warts?

Coping and Stress Tolerance

The nurse must assess the ability of the family to adapt to the demands of the child's skin ailment and treatment. The nurse should look for changes in family routines as well as additional demands placed on family members and the impact that change has had on the family. Child and family support systems must be assessed. What family activities have changed because of the child's skin problem? How has this change affected the family? Who does the child or family look to for support and help (i.e., extended family, school friends, neighbors, and so forth?) Does the child or family member use medicine, illicit drugs, or alcohol?

Values and Beliefs

The nurse should assess the impact of the child's skin problem on future goals of the child or family. The nurse notes what is important to the child and family in their lives and how these beliefs influence health-related decisions and actions. Will the skin problem affect future goals or aspirations held by the parents for the child? Has this skin disease caused the child or parents to reevaluate their goals, beliefs, or priorities?

At the completion of the assessment, the nurse should inquire if there is anything else the child or parent would like to mention or if they have any questions.

Physical Examination

Developmental differences expected in the physical examination of the skin, hair, and nails of children are described in Table 64-1.

Physical examination of the child requires careful inspection and palpation of the entire skin surface. The examination should take place in a well-lit room, preferably with natural lighting or a good untinted light source. Elaborate tools are not needed. Instead, the nurse must rely on his or her own visual and tactile senses. A magnifying lens is helpful for examining the fine features of the skin, and a metric measuring tape or ruler is needed to document the exact size of various skin lesions. Ideally, the child is completely disrobed and covered with a loose gown or sheet to provide privacy. The room should be a comfortable temperature to prevent chilling. Handwashing is vital to prevent transmission of infection, and gloves are needed to palpate mucous membranes and open areas of the skin.

While obtaining the history and physical examination, the nurse also has the opportunity to observe some general characteristics of the child and parent and their interactions. The child's and parent's body posture, eye contact, and voice inflections are observed. Likewise, nonverbal interaction patterns between family members and how supportive a parent is to the child are assessed. The child's and parent's attention span and vocabulary level are also evaluated.

A total skin examination is a necessary part of the first evaluation of any well or ill child. This opportunity can be used to establish a baseline against which future

TABLE 64-1
Developmental Considerations in the Physical Examination of Integumentary Function

Organ/System	Infant	Child	Adolescent
Skin	Dry, soft texture	Dry, soft texture	Oily texture in sebaceous areas
	Many skin folds	Normal skin folds	Normal skin folds
	Lighter pigment	True genetic pigment	True genetic pigment
Hair	Eyebrow and scalp hair terminal	Eyebrow and scalp hair terminal	Eyebrow, scalp, and hair in sexual sites terminal
	Vellus hair in remaining sites	Vellus hair in remaining sites	Vellus hair in remaining sites
	Lanugo hair at birth		
	Scalp hair may be scant		
Nails	Soft and thin	Firmer and thicker	Firmer and thicker

findings can be compared and also to identify potentially malignant lesions or lesions that are markers for systemic disease. For instance, the presence of the characteristic hypopigmented macule commonly called an ash leaf macule is a sensitive and early sign of tuberous sclerosis. The extent of future examinations must be individualized for each child depending on the skin disease and the time interval between examinations.

The nurse initially stands back and notes the child's general health appearance. This survey should include an assessment of the general skin color. Normal skin color varies greatly from one child to the next, depending on the particular mix of the four biochromes in the skin. The two biochromes in the epidermis are melanin, which is brown, and carotenoids, which are yellow. The other biochromes are found in the dermis. Oxyhemoglobin, which is red, is found in arterioles and capillaries of the papillary layer. Reduced hemoglobin, which is bluish-red, is found in the subpapillary layer. The whiteness of the skin in lightly pigmented children can be attributed to dermal connective tissue.[7] Cyanosis, flushing, and yellowing of the skin can all be signs of systemic health problems.

In addition to skin color, the overall examination of the skin focuses on assessment of moistness, turgor, texture, and temperature. Moisture is assessed by observing the characteristics of the skin surface for dryness, sweating, or oiliness. Turgor, on the other hand, refers to tissue hydration and can be best assessed by grasping the skin on the forehead or chest between the forefinger and the thumb and pulling upward. In a child who is dehydrated, the skin remains in the pinched position for a while before resuming the normal contour. Tactile assessment of the skin reveals its texture and whether the skin is soft, smooth, rough, hard, or tense. Olfactory assessment for abnormal body odors should be done, along with examination of the skin for presence or lack of sweat.

Assessment of Lesions

Pattern of Distribution. While standing back several feet from the child, the nurse views the skin surface as a whole. This perspective enables the nurse to assess the general skin features and the pattern of distribution over the skin surface of any lesions present. Their location and the extent of involvement of the skin surface are noted. Skin disorders such as impetigo may be localized periorally and found only on that area of the skin surface. In diseases like herpes zoster, the skin lesions are regional, involving a dermatome. Not uncommonly, skin problems are generalized and involve a large portion or all of the skin surface, possibly including mucous membranes.

The examiner should determine whether there is a specific pattern to the location of the skin lesions. Figure 64-1 shows patterns of distribution. Is the pattern symmetric and found on both sides of the body, or is it unilateral, involving only one side? Skin lesions produced or exacerbated by exposure to the sun are found on regions of the skin such as the outer aspects of the arms, backs of the hands, face (sparing the upper eyelids), back of neck, and the "V" of the chest. Certain skin eruptions may occur predominantly on the trunk or the extremities.

Intertriginous distribution involves areas of folded skin such as the axillae, groin, or inframammary regions. In infants, the neck region is a common intertriginous area for skin rashes. Flexural or extensor surface involvement may be seen on the extremities. The pattern of distribution often is important information for the complete nursing assessment.

Primary and Secondary Lesions. After an overall inspection of the skin, the nurse looks closely at the skin lesions. According to the pathologic process and the location in the skin, cutaneous lesions assume distinct characteristics. The nurse must be able to distinguish the primary skin lesions, those that present initially and make up the disease process, and secondary lesions, those that result from an alteration (e.g., scratching of the primary lesion). Often it is possible to observe the evolution of the skin eruption on one child by identifying new primary lesions and older secondary lesions. Table 64-2 describes primary and secondary lesions, provides visual descriptions of the lesions, and gives examples. Tactile assessment is helpful in determining the characteristics of the eruption and identifying the type of lesion. Observation of the color of individual lesions can also provide clues to the skin disorder. Skin lesions can be found in hues of red, purple, white, brown, and black.

Vascular Lesions. Vascular lesions are a result of an alteration of the cutaneous vessels. *Telangiectasias* are dilated capillaries. The color of telangiectasias disappears with the application of pressure on the overlying skin. *Purpura* is caused by extravasation of red blood cells into surrounding tissue. This color does not disappear with pressure. *Petechiae* are small pinpoint purpuric spots, and *ecchymoses* are larger areas of purpura.

Shape of Individual Lesions. After identification of the primary and secondary lesions, the shape of the individual lesions should be noted. *Annular* lesions are ring shaped. Other rounded lesions include *arcuate* (arclike), *iris* (bull's eye or targetlike), *nummular* (coin-shaped), *ovoid* (oval), and *discoid* (disclike). Individual lesions can also be *linear* (in a line), *gyrate* (coiled or spiral-like), *pedunculated* (on a stalk), *verrucous* (wartlike), and *umbilicated* (with a central depression).[10]

Arrangement of Multiple Lesions. The arrangement of lesions in relationship to each other is another important observation in assessment of the skin (Fig. 64-2). Like individual lesions, multiple lesions may take on an *annular* or *linear* configuration. Cutaneous lesions may also be isolated from each other and are therefore referred to as *solitary* or *discrete*. *Satellite* lesions are individual lesions in close proximity to a larger group. *Grouped* lesions are clusters of primary or secondary lesions, which may or may not be *confluent* or merging together. *Zosteriform* describes grouped lesions that occur in a bandlike arrangement following a dermatome. Additional terms used to describe multiple lesions include *reticulated* (netlike), *guttate* (droplike), *serpiginous* (snakelike), *punctate* (pointlike), *polycyclic* (oval lesions containing more than one ring), and *polymorphous* (occurring in several forms).[10]

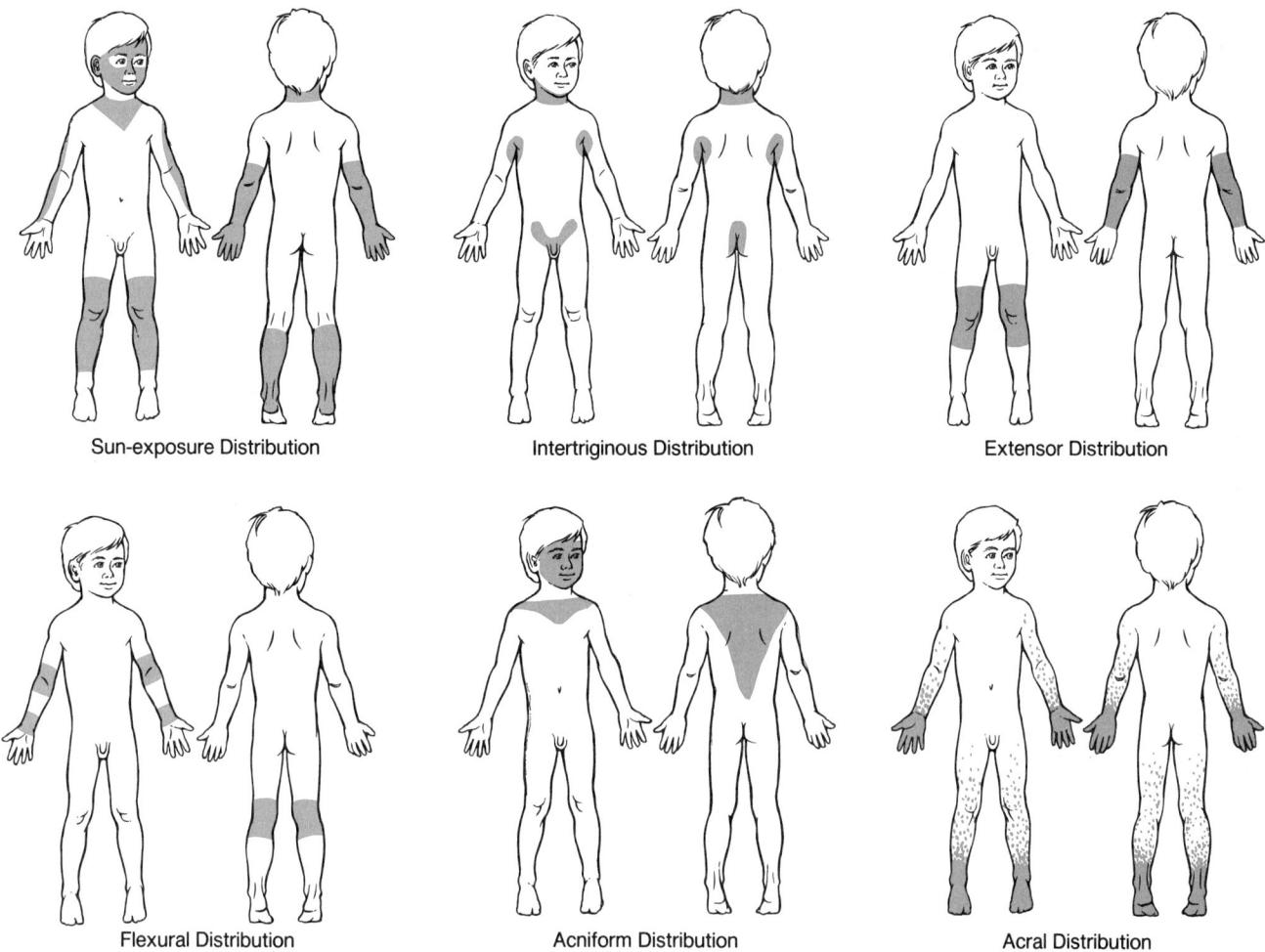

Sun-exposure Distribution

Intertriginous Distribution

Extensor Distribution

Flexural Distribution

Acniform Distribution

Acral Distribution

FIGURE 64-1

Patterns of distribution of skin lesions.

Assessment of Hair

In assessment of the hair, several features are important to observe, including the type, amount, and distribution of body hair. In preterm and full-term infants, the presence or absence of lanugo should be noted, and, in infants, normal patterns of hair loss should be noted. A common observation in a child of 3 months is an area of alopecia over the occipital region. The hairs in this area do not enter telogen until after birth. At that time, they all convert about the same time, remain on the scalp for 8 to 12 weeks, and then fall. The parietal region also has a considerable portion of hair in telogen immediately after birth, resulting in sparse hair in this region at 3 months. After this initial shedding of hair, a random pattern of anagen to telogen hair more characteristic of the adult pattern is developed. However, it is not uncommon for infants to have little scalp hair for several months after the initial telogen fall.[1] Developmental differences in hair are described in Table 64-1.

During puberty, areas of skin normally bearing only vellus begin to bear terminal hair under the influence of androgen production. The process begins in the pubic region followed by the axillae. Tanner staging is a standardized assessment tool for grading sexual hair devel-

opment.[11,12] (See Chapter 56 for a detailed discussion of Tanner Developmental Staging.) Looking for excessive hair development (hirsutism) in females can provide information regarding endocrine function.[5]

Color and texture of the hair should also be assessed. Normal hair color has a broad spectrum. Early graying or patchy loss of hair pigment are sometimes seen with conditions such as vitiligo. There are a wide variety of abnormalities that affect the shape or composition of the hair shaft. These abnormalities can result in increased hair fragility or uncontrollable hair. Nutritional deficiencies and certain metabolic disorders can interfere with the production of hair pigment and also can cause the hair shaft to be abnormally dry, coarse, or brittle.

Assessment of Nails

All nails should be assessed for presence, color, change in appearance, thickness, and shape. The surrounding nail fold should also be assessed for erythema, inflammation, drainage, or the presence of telangiectasia.[2] The nails can provide evidence of systemic disease with an alteration such as discoloration, pitting, ridging, or clubbing. An important diagnostic finding in children with

TABLE 64-2
Primary and Secondary Skin Lesions

Primary Skin Lesions: Original lesions arising from previously normal skin

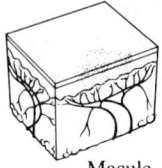
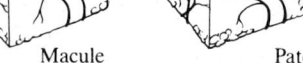
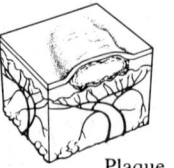
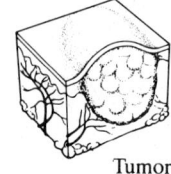

Macule   Patch   Papule   Plaque   Tumor

Macule, Patch

- *Macule:* <1 cm, circumscribed border
- *Patch:* >1 cm, may have irregular border
- Flat, nonpalpable skin color change (color may be brown, white, tan, purple, red)

Examples:

Freckles, flat moles, petechia, rubella, vitiligo, port wine stains, ecchymosis

Papule, Plaque

- *Papule:* <0.5 cm
- *Plaque:* >0.5 cm
- Elevated, palpable, solid mass
- Circumscribed border
- Plaque may be coalesced papules with flat top

Examples:

Papules: Elevated nevi, warts, lichen planus
Plaques: Psoriasis, actinic keratosis

Nodule, Tumor

- *Nodule:* 0.5–2 cm
- *Tumor:* >1–2 cm
- Elevated, palpable, solid mass
- Extends deeper into the dermis than a papule
- Nodules circumscribed
- Tumors do not always have sharp borders

Examples:

Nodules: Lipoma, squamous cell carcinoma, poorly absorbed injection, dermatofibroma

Tumors: Larger lipoma, carcinoma

Secondary Skin Lesions: Lesions resulting from changes in primary lesions

Erosion

- Loss of superficial epidermis
- Does not extend to dermis
- Depressed, moist area

Examples:

Ruptured vesicles, scratch marks

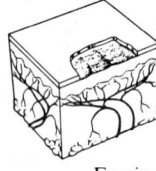

Erosion

Pustule

- Pus-filled vesicle or bulla

Examples:

Acne, impetigo, furuncles, carbuncles

Cyst

- Encapsulated fluid-filled or semisolid mass
- In the subcutaneous tissue or dermis

Examples:

Sebaceous cyst, epidermoid cyst

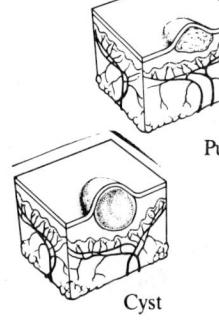

Pustule

Cyst

Vesicle, Bulla

- *Vesicle:* <0.5 cm
- *Bulla:* >0.5 cm
- Circumscribed, elevated, palpable mass containing serous fluid

Examples:

Vesicles: Herpes simplex/zoster, chickenpox, poison ivy, second-degree burn (blister)
Bulla: Pemphigus, contact dermatitis, large burn blisters, poison ivy, bullous impetigo

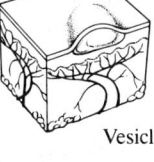

Vesicle

Bulla

Scar (Cicatrix)

- Skin mark left after healing of a wound or lesion
- Represents replacement by connective tissue of the injured tissue
- Young scars: red or purple
- Mature scars: white or glistening

Example:

Healed wound or surgical incision

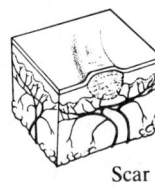

Scar

Wheal

- Elevated mass with transient borders
- Often irregular
- Size, color varies
- Caused by movement of serous fluid into the dermis
- Does not contain free fluid in a cavity as, for example, a vesicle

Examples:

Urticaria (hives), insect bites

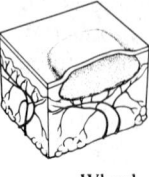

Wheal

Ulcer

- Skin loss extending past epidermis
- Necrotic tissue loss
- Bleeding and scarring possible

Examples:

Stasis ulcer of venous insufficiency, decubitus ulcer

Fissure

- Linear crack in the skin
- May extend to dermis

Examples:

Chapped lips or hands, athlete's foot

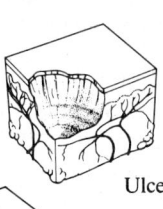

Ulcer

Fissure

(Continued)

TABLE 64-2
(Continued)

Secondary Skin Lesions: Lesions resulting from changes in primary lesions (*Continued*)

Scales
- Flakes secondary to desquamated, dead epithelium
- Flakes may adhere to skin surface
- Color varies (silvery, white)
- Texture varies (thick, fine)

Examples:

Dandruff, psoriasis, dry skin, pityriasis rosea

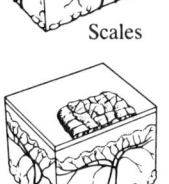

Scales

Crust
- Dried residue of serum, blood, or pus on skin surface
- Large adherent crust is a scab

Examples:

Residue left after vesicle rupture: impetigo, herpes, eczema

Crust

Keloid
- Hypertrophied scar tissue
- Secondary to excessive collagen formation during healing
- Elevated, irregular, red
- Greater incidence in blacks

Example:

Keloid of ear piercing or surgical incision

Keloid

Atrophy
- Thin, dry, transparent appearance of epidermis
- Loss of surface markings
- Secondary to loss of collagen and elastin
- Underlying vessels may be visible

Examples:

Aged skin, arterial insufficiency

Atrophy

Lichenification
- Thickening and roughening of the skin
- Accentuated skin markings
- May be secondary to repeated rubbing, irritation, scratching

Lichenification

Example:

Contact dermatitis

From Fuller, J., & Schaller-Ayers, J. (1990). Health assessment: A nursing approach. Philadelphia: Lippincott.

systemic lupus erythematosus and dermatomyocytis is telangiectasia in the proximal nail fold. Not uncommonly in children, the nail fold becomes infected by *Candida* or papilloma virus, resulting in inflammation or distortion of the nail and surrounding skin. Developmental differences in the nails are described in Table 64-1.

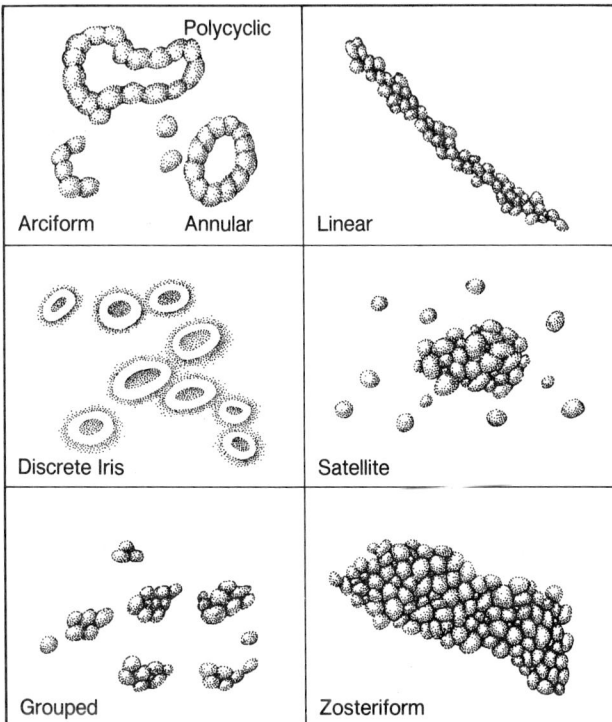

FIGURE 64-2
Arrangement of multiple lesions.

Assessment of Mucous Membranes and Anogenital Skin

The mucous membranes and anogenital skin should be visualized and assessed. These areas are often involved in systemic disease as well as localized disease. Color, skin integrity, and alterations in appearance should be noted. The mucous membranes indicate the child's state of hydration. The tongue may show color changes such as the strawberry tongue associated with Kawasaki's disease. Heat, moisture, and occlusion in the anogenital region as well as irritation in a child wearing diapers provide an ideal setting for infection or irritant dermatitis. If the child has an ostomy, the area should also be observed for integrity of the mucous membrane and the surrounding skin.

Diagnostic Tests

In skin examination, the initial inspection is often not enough and various diagnostic techniques are necessary to augment the existing database or to confirm the initial impression.[14-16] How to inspect, rub, press, or scrape a cutaneous lesion is a skill that takes practice to learn. For a child, these procedures may be frightening; the nurse can make these experiences less traumatic for the child and parent. Many of these procedures seem threatening to the child. However, because the skin is so easily accessible, the majority of the diagnostic techniques are not painful. Careful explanation, demonstration, and acquaintance with the tools can ensure the retrieval of useful information with minimal trauma for the child.

Laboratory Tests

The following laboratory tests are used in assessing integumentary function: potassium hydroxide preparation, Gram's stain, Tzanck smear, visualization of ectoparasites, darkfield examination, skin cultures, patch testing, photo or photo-patch testing, skin biopsy, and fetal amniocentesis and biopsy.

Potassium Hydroxide (KOH) Preparation

Description/Definition

A specimen is collected by scraping the skin with a round-bellied blade (#15 blade). The scale, hair fragments, or vesicle contents are placed on a microscope slide. After one drop of 20% potassium hydroxide is added to the collected specimen, it is covered with a cover slip. At this point, the slide is heated slightly or allowed to sit for 5 to 10 minutes to allow the keratinized cells to dissolve. Before viewing under low power magnification, it is often helpful to gently press on the cover slip to flatten the specimen and allow for better visualization.

Purpose

This technique allows for microscopic examination of samples from the stratum corneum. It is most useful in diagnosis of superficial fungal infections of the skin, hair, and nails. Recognition of spores, hyphae, or infected hair fragments takes practice under the guidance of an experienced practitioner.

Indications

- Superficial dermatophyte infections.
- Candidiasis.
- Tinea versicolor.

Contraindications

None.

Preparation

- Gather the necessary equipment: glass slide, cover slip, #15 scalpel blade, potassium hydroxide solution, heat source, microscope.
- Explain the procedure to the child and parent. Assure both that the procedure will not cause discomfort.

Developmental Considerations

In extremely fearful young children who may make abrupt movements, a blunt instrument such as a tongue depressor may be used to collect the specimen. This technique, however, is less successful in obtaining an adequate specimen.

Nursing Care

Assist the child to remain still during specimen collection.

Complications

Injury to the child during specimen collection.

Gram's Stain

Description/Definition

Gram's stain is a common microscopic technique in which the collected specimens are stained and visualized under the microscope. Gram-positive organisms stain a deep blue; gram-negative organisms stain a pale pink to red. The collected specimen is placed on a glass slide, heat-fixed, and the following steps are performed: (1) stain with gentian violet or crystal violet, (2) rinse with water and stain with iodine solution, (3) rinse with water and then rinse with 95% alcohol, (4) counter stain with safranin, a red dye, (5) rinse with water, air dry, and visualize.

Purpose

Gram's stain is used to identify various bacteria and yeasts that infect the skin. Most cutaneous bacterial infections are gram-positive organisms such as staphylococci and streptococci.

Indications

Suspected bacterial or candidial skin infections.

Contraindications

None.

Preparation

- Gather the necessary equipment: glass slide, #15 scalpel blade, stains, microscope.
- Explain the procedure to the child and parent. Assure both that the procedure will not cause discomfort.

Developmental Considerations

None.

Nursing Care

Assist the child to remain still during specimen collection.

Complications

Injury to the child during specimen collection.

Tzanck Smear

Description/Definition

The Tzanck smear is a microscopic staining technique used to identify multinucleated giant cells in vesicular herpetic conditions. The best results are obtained by selecting an intact vesicle and applying its contents along with the scrapings of the vesicle base on a slide. The material is stained with Wright's or Giemsa stain and visualized under low power on the microscope.

Purpose

This technique is used to examine contents of vesicles and is most commonly used in cutaneous lesions of herpes simplex, varicella, and herpes zoster.

Indications

- Blistering disorders.
- Areas of the skin with superficial erosions.

Contraindications

None.

Preparation

- Gather the necessary equipment: glass slide, #15 scalpel blade, stain, cover slip, microscope.
- Explain the procedure to the child and parent. Assure both that only minimal discomfort will be experienced during specimen collection.

Developmental Considerations

None.

Nursing Care

- Assist the child to remain still during specimen collection.
- Appropriate wound care is given after collection of the specimen.

Complications

Injury to the child during specimen collection.

Visualization of Ectoparasites

Description/Definition

This technique allows visualization and identification of ectoparasites that may infest the skin or hair. The techniques vary according to the ectoparasite sought. The suspected material is removed from the skin or hair and placed on a microscope slide. KOH preparation or immersion oil may be used to keep the specimen in place.

Purpose

To provide a definite diagnosis when skin infestation by lice, scabies, or ticks is suspected.

Indications

*   Pruritis and excoriated papules especially in intertriginous areas, between fingers, or on the inner wrists.
*   Pruritis of the scalp with presence of nits.
*   Pruritis of the trunk with excoriated papules and wheals.

Contraindications

None.

Preparation

*   Gather the necessary equipment: glass slide, cover slip, tweezers or #15 blade, immersion oil, microscope.
*   Explain the test to the child and parent. Assure both that only minimal discomfort will be experienced during specimen collection.
*   In suspected scabies infestation, the lesion to be scraped is painted with oil before scraping to aid transfer of the specimen from the skin to the slide.

Developmental Considerations

None.

Nursing Care

*   Assist the child to remain still during specimen collection.
*   Cleanse the site after specimen collection and administer proper wound care.

Complications

*   Mild bleeding may occur.
*   Injury to the child during specimen collection.

Darkfield Examination

Description/Definition

The darkfield examination uses a special microscope to visualize organisms difficult to see with a regular microscope.

Purpose

This examination is used to identify spirochetes in cutaneous lesions of syphilis.

Indications

*   Suspected primary syphilis lesions.
*   Secondary syphilis lesions that are ulcerative or exudative.

Contraindications

None.

Preparation

*   Gather the necessary equipment: darkfield microscope, microscope slides and cover slips, gloves, and gauze pads.
*   Explain the procedure to the child and parent. Assure both that only minimal discomfort will be experienced during specimen collection.

Developmental Considerations

None.

Nursing Care

Cleanse the collection site and administer appropriate wound care.

Complications

None.

Skin Cultures

Description/Definition

Cultures isolate and enable identification of the etiologic agent of various cutaneous infections. It is important that adequate specimens are obtained and that they are placed in the appropriate medium for growth.

Purpose

To identify the variety of fungal, yeast, bacterial, or viral microorganism causing the skin infection for confirmation of diagnosis or determination of appropriate treatment.

Indications

*   Dermatophyte infection.
*   Candidiasis.
*   Bacterial infection.
*   Viral infection.

Contraindications

None.

Preparation

*   Gather the necessary equipment: instrument to collect the specimen (this could include a scalpel blade, tooth brush, or cotton-tipped applicator) and culture media (Fig. 64-3).
*   Explain the procedure for collection of the culture specimen to the child and parent. Assure them the procedure will not cause discomfort.

Developmental Considerations

None.

Nursing Care

*   Specimen collection: Collecting specimens for fungal and yeast cultures is similar to collecting specimens for a KOH preparation.

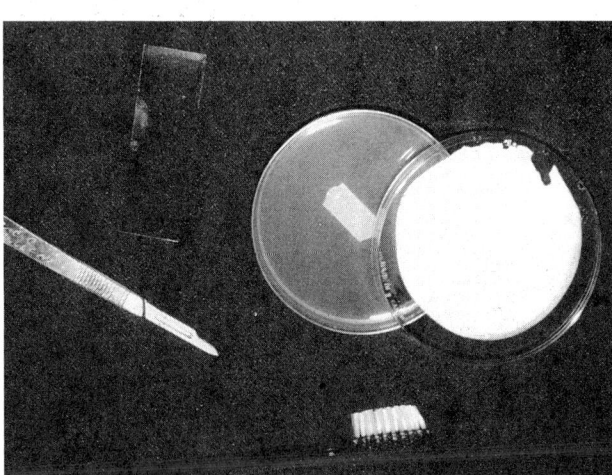

FIGURE 64-3

Fungal culture equipment. A scalpel blade or tooth brush may be used to collect scale or broken hair and apply it to the fungal culture medium.

The use of a toothbrush to obtain specimens from suspected scalp areas has been found to provide excellent specimens as well as being nonthreatening for the child. Material collected is placed on dermatophyte test media (DTM) and loosely covered, labeled, and incubated at room temperature. Dermatophytes grow within 2 weeks and turn the media red. Collecting specimens of bacterial cultures of the skin is best done by rubbing the site with a moistened cotton-tipped applicator. The applicator is placed in a transport container, labeled, and sent to the laboratory for culture and sensitivity. Viral culture specimens are obtained by selecting an intact blister and using a scalpel blade to unroof the blister. The base of the blister is scraped, and the collected material is placed in viral transport media, labeled, and immediately sent to the laboratory.

- Appropriate wound care is given to any specimen collection sites.

Complications

Potential injury to the child if a scalpel blade is used for specimen collection.

Patch Testing

Description/Definition

Patch testing is a procedure in which suspected allergens are placed on the skin in a manner that allows the identification of an irritant or allergic sensitivity. Usually the most appropriate test is the closed patch test, in which a small amount of suspected allergen is placed on normal skin by means of a specially designed patch called a Finn chamber (Fig. 64-4). In an open patch test, the substance is applied directly to normal skin and left uncovered. Application is repeated twice a day for 2 or more days.

Purpose

The patch test is performed to identify or confirm a suspected allergy to a substance that is contacted by the skin. It is also used to differentiate irritant reactions from allergic reactions.

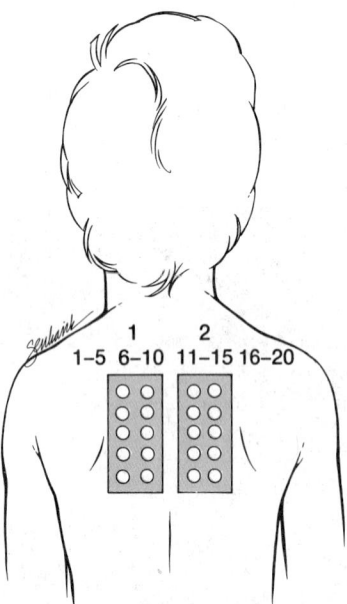

FIGURE 64-4
Patch test application. A small amount of testing material is placed in each disk of the Finn Chamber and applied to the upper back. Each disk is identified by a number that corresponds with the testing material for later reference when reading the patch test.

Indications

- In suspected contact allergic dermatitis based on history and distribution pattern of eruption.
- In chronic dermatitis that is unresponsive to treatment, especially when involving the hands or feet.

Contraindications

Patch testing should not be performed in children with extremely active dermatitis or if the test area is inflamed.

Preparation

- Gather the necessary equipment: Finn chambers, hypoallergic paper tape, allergen samples, skin marking pen.
- Determine if the patient has used corticosteroids within the past week or antihistamines in the past 3 days.
- Hairy test areas must be shaved, preferably with electric clippers.
- Explain the procedure to the child and parent and that moderate pruritis may be experienced while the patches are in place.

Developmental Considerations

None.

Nursing Care

- Select normal appearing, nonhairy, flat surfaces for patch testing. The back, except over the spine, is the preferred site for patch testing. An alternative site may be the inner aspect of the forearm.
- Carefully number each site to allow for allergen identification after removal of the Finn chambers. Apply the allergens to the patches and apply the patches to the test area. Reinforce the patches with hypoallergic paper tape.
- Instruct the child (1) to avoid strenuous exercise, especially activity that involves stretching movements or induces perspiration; (2) to avoid rubbing or scratching the test area; (3) to keep the test area completely dry; (4) not to take antihistamines or use corticosteroids during the test period; and (5) to return for removal of the patches.
- The patches are removed in 48 hours and read after waiting for 30 minutes to allow the skin reaction from the tape removal to subside. Irritant, allergic, or nonreactions are noted in the patient's chart. The numbering of the patches may need to be replaced on the skin for easy identification at the second reading.
- The child is instructed to return in 24 hours for the second reading and to continue to follow the same guidelines as the previous 2 days. Later readings may also be requested by the physician because delayed reactions of 3 days or more may occur.
- The following interpretation codes are used to record findings:[6,14]
  - + = weak nonvesicular reaction with erythema and mild induration.
  - ++ = strong microvesicular reaction with erythema and induration.
  - +++ = extreme vesicular or bullous reaction with spreading erythema. May be ulcerative.
  - ? = doubtful reaction with macular erythema only.
  - IR = irritant reaction.
  - − = negative reaction.
- Caution the child that reactions may take several weeks to subside. Cool compresses may help to relieve pruritis, or the physician may prescribe topical steroids to be applied to the test areas.

Complications

- Dermatitis may worsen or recur.
- Patch testing may elicit an "angry back" reaction where every test site reacts and determination of allergy is impossible. This reaction requires retesting at a later date when the dermatitis has subsided.
- Anaphylactic allergic reactions are extremely rare.

Photo Testing/Photo-Patch Testing

Description/Definition

Photo testing involves the exposure of small areas of skin to well-controlled doses of ultraviolet A (UVA) and/or ultraviolet B (UVB) light from a specially designed light unit. This test is performed on normally unexposed skin, usually the buttock. A grid is used to allow increased exposure doses to each section of the grid by covering a section at set dose increments. The test site is observed in 24 hours for UVB or 48 hours for UVA, to determine the child's minimal erythema dose (MED). During photo testing, the child's eyes and skin surface, excluding the test area, are protected from light exposure. When photo testing is performed on an area of the skin to which an allergen has been applied, the procedure is called photo-patch testing.[3,16]

Purpose

Photo testing is performed to discover or confirm the skin's response to ultraviolet light, especially in children presenting with a history of abnormal sensitivity to sunlight. It may also be used to determine the initial treatment dose in children who are beginning phototherapy for a photoresponsive skin disease. Phototherapy is initiated at 80% of the MED. Photo-patch testing is performed to discover or confirm a photo-contact allergy and to identify a causative agent in children who develop a dermatitis on areas of the skin that contact the allergen and are exposed to ultraviolet light (usually UVA wavelengths).

Indications

- Psoriasis.
- Atopic dermatitis.
- Solar urticaria.
- Polymorphous light eruption.
- Photo-allergic contact dermatitis.

Contraindications

Photo testing should not be performed in children unable to follow instructions to stand or lie still and to keep their eyes and protected skin covered during the test procedure.

Preparation

- Gather the necessary equipment: ultraviolet light source, adhesive tape, drapes to cover unexposed skin, skin marking pen, goggles for eye protection.
- Explain the procedure to the child and parent noting that the child may feel warm during the test period, but otherwise no discomfort will be experienced.
- Prepare the test grid on the skin test site, and mark the test areas to enable accurate reading at a future time. Place the protective goggles over the child's eyes, and drape all skin, excluding the test site area.

Developmental Considerations

None.

Nursing Care

- Determine skin type (see section in Chap. 65 on photosensitivity).
- Select normal appearing, easily exposed skin sites. Apply the grid, and drape all remaining skin. Apply protective goggles to the eyes. Mark the test site with a skin marking pen.
- Perform the test according to the ultraviolet light doses prescribed by the physician or protocol dose according to skin type.
- Inform the child and parent that no special care needs to be given to the test site after the procedure.
- Instruct the child and parent to return in 24 or 48 hours for reading of the test site.

Complications

Sunburn.

Skin Biopsy

Description/Definition

A skin biopsy is the removal of a small portion of skin tissue for microscopic study or culture. A shave, punch, incisional, or excisional biopsy may be performed. The choice of biopsy technique is based on the type of skin lesion and which method will provide tissue representative of the pathologic alteration and result in the smallest, if any, cosmetic defect. A *shave biopsy* provides a thin disc of tissue that protrudes above the skin surface and is shaved off at or slightly below skin surface. A *punch biopsy* provides a plug of tissue by means of a specially designed instrument varying in size from 2 to 6 mm. An *incisional biopsy* is used when a slightly larger of tissue is needed than can be provided with a punch biopsy. An *excisional biopsy* is the largest and deepest biopsy performed. It may or may not remove the entire lesion and is used when a large piece of tissue is needed.

Purpose

Usually the tissue obtained with the biopsy is taken for histopathologic study. However, biopsies are also used for other purposes, such as immunofluorescent testing to detect connective tissue or bullous diseases, electron microscopy for distinguishing various types of epidermolysis bullosa, or to set up a tissue culture for deep skin infections.

Indications

- Inflammatory conditions, tumors, or growths, especially those for which diagnosis cannot be easily determined by inspection.
- Potentially malignant lesions.

Contraindications

Children who have bleeding disorders.

Preparation

- Gather the necessary equipment: biopsy punch or scalpel with blade, local anesthesia, needle and syringe, forceps, scissors, suture and needle holder, labeled specimen bottle, appropriate wound care and dressing materials.
- Explain the procedure to the child and parent explaining that some discomfort will be experienced only when the local anesthetic is injected. Ensure that written consent is obtained from the parent.
- Position the child, and cleanse the biopsy site.

Developmental Considerations

None.

Nursing Care

- Provide support during the biopsy procedure. Assist to stabilize the biopsy area.
- Administer appropriate wound care and apply wound dressing.
- Instruct the child and parent how to care for the wound at home.

Complications

- Bleeding.
- Infection.

Fetal Amniocentesis and Biopsy

Description/Definition

Fetal diagnostic procedures include amniocentesis and fetal biopsy by fetoscopy. In amniocentesis, a sample of the amniotic fluid is withdrawn for genetic testing. Fetoscopy is used to visualize the fetus in utero. A biopsy forceps is inserted into the cannula of the fetoscope, and samples of skin are obtained. Fetal biopsy is performed in relatively few centers and may not be available.[9]

Purpose

Amniocentesis is helpful in diagnosis of sex-linked disorders of the skin or skin disorders with specific gene abnormalities. Diseases involving the epidermis or the basement membrane zone are most amenable to prenatal diagnosis by fetal biopsy. Disorders that affect primarily the dermis are poor candidates for intrauterine diagnosis because of the immaturity of the fetal dermis.

Indications

- Diseases of keratinization, such as ichthyosis.
- Bullous disorders, such as epidermolysis bullosa.
- Pigment cell defects, such as albinism.
- Disorders that affect epidermal appendages, such as x-linked hypohydrotic ectodermal dysplasia.

Contraindications

- Women with a history of premature labor or incompetent cervix.
- In the presence of placenta previa and abrupto placentae.

Preparation

- Gather the necessary equipment: anesthetic, spinal needle, fetoscope, specimen container.
- Explain the procedure to the parents.
- Have the mother void just before the test.
- Position the mother and cleanse the skin at the test site with an antiseptic solution.
- Obtain and record fetal heart tones.
- Inform the mother that she may experience short-lived feelings of nausea, vertigo, or mild cramping during the procedure.

Developmental Considerations

Amniocentesis is performed at 14 to 18 weeks estimated gestational age (EGA), and fetal biopsy is performed at 19 to 21 weeks EGA.

Nursing Care

- Provide support to the mother during the procedure, and assist her to relax.
- Administer appropriate wound care, and apply a dressing.
- Check blood pressure, pulse, respirations, and fetal heart tones every 15 minutes for the first half hour after test completion.
- Instruct the mother to notify the physician if she experiences amniotic fluid loss, signs of labor onset, abdominal pain, bleeding, elevated temperature, chills, unusual fetal activity, or lack of movement.

Complications

- Fetal loss in 5% of all cases.
- Premature birth in 10% of all cases.
- Hemorrhage in mother or fetus.
- Infection in mother or fetus.
- Persistent amniotic leak.
- Placenta injury.
- Rh sensitization.
- Scarring of the fetus.

Procedures

The following physical diagnostic techniques and procedures are performed on the child with possible skin problems: Darier's sign, Nikolsky's sign; Auspitz sign; diascopy; hair pull test; dermatographism; and Wood's lamp examination.

Darier's Sign

Description/Definition

The development of a hivelike swelling with surrounding erythema 1 to 10 minutes after rubbing or firmly stroking a lesion with the finger or a blunt instrument.

Purpose

To aid in the diagnosis of conditions resulting from dense collections of mast cells, which release histamine when rubbed. These conditions include urticaria pigmentosa and cutaneous mastocytosis.

Indications

Children presenting with:

- A single or multiple yellow-brown or reddish-brown flat or slightly elevated lesion.
- A history of swelling lesions with or without accompanying pruritis.

Contraindications

None.

Preparation

- Explain test procedure and purpose.
- Reassure the child and parent that the test does not cause pain but may be accompanied by pruritis of the lesion.

Developmental Considerations

In children under the age of 3 years, a blister may form at the test site.

Nursing Care

- Reassure the child and parent that the eruption will subside in a short time.
- If a blister is formed, instruction is given on care of the blister.

Complications

None.

Nikolsky's Sign

Description/Definition

The development of a sheetlike loss of the epidermis or blister formation when normal appearing skin is pushed, rubbed, or rotated with the finger.

Purpose

This test is performed on uninvolved skin to detect disadherence of the epidermis in blistering disorders such as epidermolysis bullosa, staphylococcal scalded skin, or toxic epidermal necrosis. A positive Nikolsky's sign is only suggestive and must be accompanied by a skin biopsy to determine the level of separation in the skin.

Indications

Children presenting with one or more of the following:

- Large blisters.
- Large areas of intensely erythematous skin.
- Large areas of superficial erosions with crusting.

Contraindications

None.

Preparation

- Explain the test to the child and parent.

Developmental Considerations

None.

Nursing Care

- Appropriate wound care is given to blisters or erosions.
- Parents are instructed on wound care and ways to avoid friction to the skin.

Complications

Wound infection.

Auspitz Sign

Description/Definition

The development of tiny pinpoint areas of bleeding in red, elevated, scaling lesions when the overlying scale is gently scraped off with a blunt instrument or finger.

Purpose

The Auspitz is a characteristic sign in psoriasis and is a clinical manifestation of the exaggerated and highly vascularized dermal papillae covered by a thin epidermis. A positive Auspitz sign is not diagnostic of psoriasis but must be accompanied by a positive history, physical examination, and possibly a skin biopsy.

Indications

Children presenting with discrete, elevated, scaly, erythematous lesions.

Contraindications

None.

Preparation

Explain the test to the child and parent. Assure both that the test will not cause discomfort.

Developmental Considerations

None.

Nursing Care

Appropriate wound care is given to any areas of bleeding.

Complications

Infection.

Diascopy

Description/Definition

Inspection of a lesion while pressure is applied over the area with a glass slide or a piece of clear plastic.

Purpose

This procedure empties blood from the superficial vessels and differentiates areas of vascular dilation from areas of blood extravasation. In purpuric areas, the color remains unchanged under pressure, whereas in areas of vascular dilation, the erythema blanches and disappears.

Indications

- In petechial, purpuric, and telangiectatic eruptions.
- In granulomatous conditions such as sarcoid or granuloma annulare.

Contraindications

None.

Preparations

- Gather the necessary equipment: piece of hard clear plastic or a glass slide.
- Explain the test to the child and parent. Assure both that the test will not cause discomfort.

Developmental Considerations

None.

Nursing Care

The child is encouraged to hold still to permit good visualization of the lesion.

Complications

If a glass slide is used for visualization, careful pressure should be applied to prevent breakage and possible injury to the skin.

Hair Pull Test

Description/Definition

This technique involves grasping close to the scalp, 60 adjacent hairs with the thumb and index finger. A slow constant pressure is applied to the hair as the thumb and index finger are slowly moved along the length of the hair. The intent is only to epilate loose hair, therefore a jerking motion is not used. Count the number of hairs epilated. This test should be conducted at several sites on the scalp.

Purpose

The hair pull test is used to evaluate the amount of hair loss and can be useful in children with suspected rapid hair loss. A normal count would be up to four hairs. More than six hairs is suggestive of excessive hair loss.[13]

Indications

- Active alopecia areata.
- Telogen effluvium.
- Drug-induced hair loss.
- Any child complaining of excessive hair loss.

Contraindications

None.

Preparation

Explain the test to the child and parent. Assure both that the test will not cause discomfort.

Developmental Considerations

None.

Nursing Care

The child is encouraged to hold still to prevent jerking and ensure epilation of only loose hair.

Complications

The results of this test are somewhat dependent on the hair combing and shampooing habits of the child. When hair loss is expected, it is common to keep combing and shampooing to a minimum. This practice can result in a false-positive test.

Dermatographism

Description/Definition

The development of hives or urticaria at sites of normal appearing skin where it is stroked or scratched with a blunt instrument.

Purpose

To detect an exaggerated response by the mast cells with release of histamine when stroked or rubbed. Writing on the skin normally results in mild erythema where the skin is touched. However, in children with urticaria, vivid red hives develop; in children with atopic dermatitis, it may result in blanching or "white dermatographism."

Indications

- Children complaining of swelling, redness, and pruritis after scratching or rubbing.
- Atopic dermatitis.

Contraindications

None.

Preparation

Explain the test to the child and parent. Assure both that the test will not be painful; however, it may cause mild pruritis.

Developmental Considerations

None.

Nursing Care

Assure the parent and child that the reaction will subside over the next 30 to 60 minutes.

Complications

None.

Wood's Lamp Examination

Description/Definition

The Wood's lamp (Fig. 64-5) emits a low-intensity, long-wave ultraviolet light, more commonly known as a "black light." This examination should be conducted in a windowless room with all lights turned off except for the Wood's lamp. The lamp is held 4 to 5 inches from the skin and moved along until the entire skin surface is visualized.

Purpose

To induce a visible fluorescence in pigmentary or infectious conditions, which can help to make a diagnosis. Areas of hypopigmentation appear blue-white, whereas areas of depigmentation appear bright white. Additionally, certain bacterial or fungal organisms can be identified by their reaction to the Wood's lamp.

Indications

- Pigmentary disorders.
- Dermatophyte infections.
- *Pseudomonas* infections.

Contraindications

None.

Preparation

- Gather the necessary equipment: Wood's lamp.
- Explain the procedure to the child and parent. Assure both that the light is not harmful to the skin or eyes.

Developmental Considerations

None.

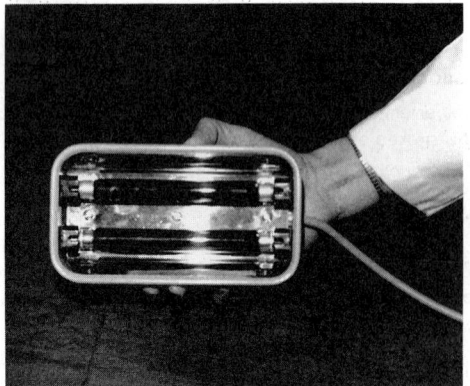

FIGURE 64-5
A small, hand-held Wood's lamp is used for examination of skin lesions under long-wave ultraviolet lighting.

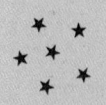

Ideas for Nursing Research

The multiple purposes served by the skin reflect its vital role in the well-being of infants and children. Because nurses have to spend extended periods of time with children under their care, scholarship related to the integumentary system is possible. The following areas need to be explored:

- Identification of sensitive screening questions to obtain accurate cutaneous historic data.
- Evaluation of skin care techniques used in intensive care nurseries and normal newborn nurseries.
- Identification of nursing care measures directed at maintaining skin integrity in high-risk infants and children.
- Development of methods to provide tactile sensory stimulation to ill infants and children in acute care settings.
- Examination of the impact of skin disease on the interactive functions of the skin.

Nursing Care

Have the patient undress and wear a drape or gown.

Complications

None.

Selected Nursing Diagnoses

After obtaining the history, performing the physical examination, reviewing results from the diagnostic tests, and tapping additional resources for information, the nurse carefully analyzes the data obtained. Nursing diagnoses appropriate for the child with integumentary dysfunction become apparent and are used to develop a plan of care.[4] Selected nursing diagnoses that may be appropriate for the child with integumentary dysfunction are presented by function in Table 64-3.

Summary

Nursing assessment and diagnosis of the skin are based on careful collection of information regarding functional health patterns and close examination of the skin by visual inspection and tactile palpation supplemented by information obtained from various diagnostic tests. Cutaneous disorders affect all areas of human functioning: physical, psychological, and social. Identifying the impact of the disorder on the individual child and family depends on skilled information gathering, diagnostic reasoning, and verification of conclusions.

TABLE 64-3
Selected Nursing Diagnoses Associated With Altered Integumentary Function

Data Analysis and Conclusions	Nursing Diagnosis
Health Perception and Health Management	
Disruption of mucous membrane or integumentary tissue. Presence of primary or secondary lesions, edema, erythema, exudate.	Impaired Skin Integrity related to skin lesions and inflammatory response.
Verbalization of noncompliance or nonparticipation or confusion about therapy. Direct observation of behavior indicating noncompliance.	Noncompliance related to financial cost of therapy; complex, unsupervised, or prolonged therapy; knowledge deficit; poor self-esteem.
Examples: Missed appointments, partially used or unused medication, persistence of symptoms, progression of disease, occurrence of undesired outcomes (skin infections).	
Verbalizes a deficiency in knowledge for health promotion or health maintenance.	Altered Health Maintenance related to lack of knowledge of need for preventive behavior.
Reports or demonstrates an unhealthy practice or lifestyle.	
Examples: Malodorous and unclean skin, nails, or hair; skin lesions (pustules, rashes, dry or scaly skin); sunburn, unusual skin color; pallor; unexplained scars.	
Nutrition and Metabolism	
Output is greater than intake. Increased serum sodium. Dry skin/mucous membranes.	Fluid Volume Deficit related to lack of skin integrity or skin structure immaturity.
Examples: Premature birth, increased body temperature associated with widespread erythema, decreased skin turgor.	
Temperature fluctuations related to limited metabolic compensatory regulation in response to environmental factors.	Ineffective Thermoregulation related to large surface area relative to body mass, prematurity.
Evidence of risk factors such as altered production of leukocytes, altered immune response, altered circulation, presence of favorable conditions for infection. History of frequent skin infections.	High Risk for Infection related to altered integumentary system.
Activity and Exercise	
Inability to move purposefully within the environment, ambulation.	Impaired Physical Mobility related to pain and inflammation in the skin.
Sleep and Rest	
Difficulty falling or remaining asleep.	Sleep Pattern Disturbance related to pain or pruritis.
Example: Skin symptoms causing interrupted sleep patterns.	
Cognition and Perception	
The child reports or demonstrates discomfort.	Altered Comfort related to pain or pruritis.
Examples: Contagious disease (chickenpox), inflammatory skin disease (atopic dermatitis, psoriasis).	
Verbalizes a deficiency in knowledge or skill/request for information.	Anxiety related to lack of information about new medical condition, complex regimen, lack of education or readiness.
Expresses ''inaccurate'' perception health status. Does not correctly perform a desired or prescribed health behavior.	
Self Perception	
A change in body image, self-esteem, role performance, or personal identity.	Disturbance in Self-Concept related to chronic illness, severe trauma (burns), appearance, and response of others.
Examples: Refusal to touch or look at body part, refusal to look in a mirror, unwillingness to discuss disfigurement, withdrawal from social contacts.	
Role Relationships	
Family system cannot or does not adapt constructively to crisis, communicate openly and effectively among family members.	Altered Family Processes related to disruption of family routines, emotional changes, and financial burden of treatments.
Reports inability to establish or maintain stable, supportive relationships.	Impaired Social Interaction related to chronic disease or physical disfigurement.
Examples: Altered appearance, lack of self-esteem.	

References

1. Barth, J. H. (1987). Normal hair growth in children. *Pediatric Dermatology, 4,* 173.
2. Barth, J. H., & Dawber, R. P. R. (1987). Diseases of the nails in children. *Pediatric Dermatology, 4,* 275.
3. Bernhard, J. D., et al. (1987). Abnormal reactions to ultraviolet radiation. In T. B. Fitzpatrick, et al. (Eds.), *Dermatology in general medicine,* p. 1481. New York: McGraw-Hill.
4. Carpenito, L. J. (1992). *Nursing diagnosis: Application to clinical practice* (4th ed.). Philadelphia: Lippincott.
5. Ferriman, D., & Gallwey, J. D. (1961). Clinical assessment of body hair growth in women. *Journal of Clinical Endocrinology, 21,* 556.
6. Fisher, A. A. (1986). *Contact dermatitis* (3rd ed.). Philadelphia: Lea & Febiger.
7. Fitzpatrick, T. B., & Bernhard, J. D. (1987). The structure of skin lesions and fundamentals of diagnosis. In T. B. Fitzpatrick, et al. (Eds.), *Dermatology in general medicine* (3rd ed.), p. 20. New York: McGraw-Hill.

8. Gordon, M. (1987). *Nursing diagnosis: Process and application* (2nd ed.). New York: McGraw-Hill.

9. Holbrook, K. A., & Sybert, V. (1988). Basic science. In L. A. Schachner & R. C. Hansen (Eds.), *Pediatric dermatology*, p. 3. New York: Churchill Livingstone.

10. Leider, M., & Rosenblum, M. (1976). *A dictionary of dermatological words, terms and phrases.* New Haven, CT: Dome Laboratories.

11. Marshall, W. A., & Tanner, J. M. (1969). Variations in pattern of pubertal changes in girls. *Archives of Disease in Childhood, 44,* 291.

12. Marshall, W. A., & Tanner, J. M. (1970). Variations in pattern of pubertal changes in boys. *Archives of Disease in Childhood, 45,* 13.

13. Molde, S. (1986). Understanding patients' agendas. *Image, 18,* 145.

14. Pariser, D. M., et al. (1986). *Techniques for diagnosing skin and hair disease.* New York: Thieme.

15. Rasmussen, J. E. (1988). Principles of diagnosis. In L. A. Schachner & R. C. Hansen (Eds.), *Pediatric dermatology*, p. 159. New York: Churchill Livingstone.

16. Rosen, T., et al. (1983). *The nurse's atlas of dermatology.* Boston: Little Brown.

65

C H A P T E R

Nursing Planning, Intervention, and Evaluation for Altered Integumentary Function

BEHAVIORAL OBJECTIVES

Describe the basic principles of care in healthy skin.

Describe care in wound healing.

Identify the more common disorders of the skin in children.

Describe the clinical manifestations in various skin diseases in children.

Discuss the psychosocial impact of skin diseases in children.

Apply the nursing process in the care of children with skin disease.

There are more than 2000 recognized skin disorders, some of which are more common than others. Skin disorders may be seen at any age. These disorders can be the result of a wide variety of etiologic factors, including genetic factors, external factors that produce a reaction in the skin, or systemic factors of which the lesions are a cutaneous manifestation. Disease of the skin is often symptomatic with people experiencing discomfort from pain, pruritus, or alteration in local feeling or sensation. Moreover, because the skin is so visible and its disorders are often cosmetically disfiguring, dermatologic conditions can cause considerable psychological and social stress.

Nurses caring for children are in the unique position to have a major impact on the protection, observation, and care of the skin. Working in both inpatient and outpatient settings, nurses have the opportunity for close inspection and early detection of cutaneous changes. This proximity helps the nurse to determine the psychosocial impact of the skin disorder and to take measures that enable children to cope with these problems. Another major role of the nurse is education of the child and family in strategies that enhance the skin's protective function. Instruction on care of the skin can maintain the health of skin and prevent future skin problems. The accompanying display lists various organizations as resources for educational materials on skin care and skin conditions.

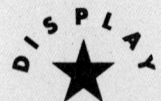

Resources for Families With Skin Disorders

Foundation for Ichthyosis and Related Skin Types
(F.I.R.S.T.)
P.O. Box 20921
Raleigh, NC 27619–0921

Dystrophic Epidermolysis Bullosa Research Association
(DEBRA)
141 Fifth Avenue
New York, NY 10010

Eczema Association for Science and Education
1221 SW Yamhill, Suite 303
Portland, OR 97205

Canadian Psoriasis Foundation
1565 Carling Ave., Suite 400
Ottawa, Ontario, Canada K1Z8R1

National Psoriasis Foundation
6443 SW Beaverton Highway, Suite 210
Portland, OR 97221

Herpes Resource Center
c/o American Social Health Association
P.O. Box 13827
Research Triangle Park, NC 27704

National Pediculosis Association
P.O. Box 149
Newton, MA 02161

Melanoma Foundation
750 Menlo Ave #250
Menlo Park, CA 94205

National Cancer Institute
National Institutes of Health
NIH 31, 9000 Rockville Pike
Bethesda, MD 20892

Skin Cancer Foundation
245 Fifth Avenue, #2402
New York, NY 10016

Large Congenital Nevocytic Nevi Registry
Oncology Section, Skin and Cancer Unit
New York University Medical Center
562 First Avenue
New York, NY 10016

National Vitiligo Foundation
Box 6337
Tyler, TX 75711

National Alopecia Areata Foundation
714 "C" Street, Suite 216
San Rafael, CA 94901

National Congenital Port Wine Stain Foundation
125 East 63rd Street
New York, NY 10021

This chapter describes some of the most common skin disorders seen in children. The skin diseases are categorized in groups and, in many instances, the nursing process is applied to a whole disease category rather than to individual conditions.

General Skin Care

Before discussion of specific dermatologic disorders, it is important to review general skin care measures for normal healthy children, ill children, and preterm infants. Basic skin care principles that apply to skin care in any setting are included in the following section.

Skin Care in Healthy Children

Promotion of the "tenderness of baby skin" is more of an advertising gimmick than fact. Unlike what many advertisers of skin care products would like us to believe, routine skin care requires little more than water, mild soap, and possibly an emollient. This is true throughout childhood.

A change in the skin care regimen may be required at adolescence with the onset of increased sebaceous gland activity. Additional skin oil production at this age may require more frequent cleansing of the skin and hair and may decrease the need for lubrication. Ethnic background also has an impact on care of the skin. Cutaneous characteristics are different in white, African-American, and Asian-American children. Skin care practices also vary among ethnic groups.

★ ASSESSMENT

Assessment of the skin includes a history of previous skin problems and a thorough examination for skin integrity, turgor, temperature, and moisture. The parents' knowledge of skin care for their child and current beliefs and practices related to skin care are also assessed.

★ NURSING DIAGNOSES

Based on assessment data from above and Chapter 64, the following nursing diagnoses may apply to general skin care of the family and child:

- High Risk for Impaired Skin Integrity related to developmental factors.
- Anxiety related to knowledge deficit regarding skin care.

★ INTERVENTIONS: COLLABORATIVE AND INDEPENDENT

The goal of hygiene and care of healthy skin is to maintain clean, well-hydrated skin with avoidance of irritation, drying, or the development of sensitivity. Education of the child and family on appropriate skin care measures can help prevent skin problems.

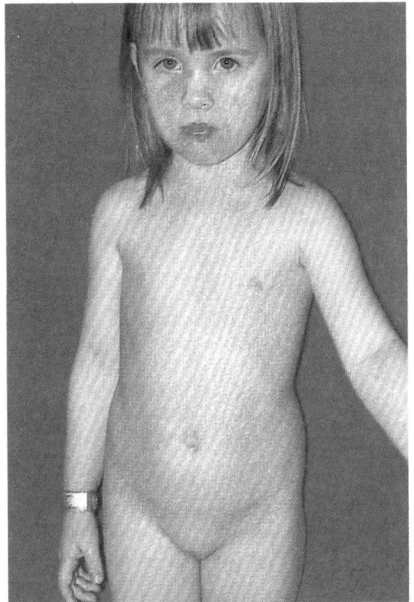

Punctate erythema rash of scarlet fever

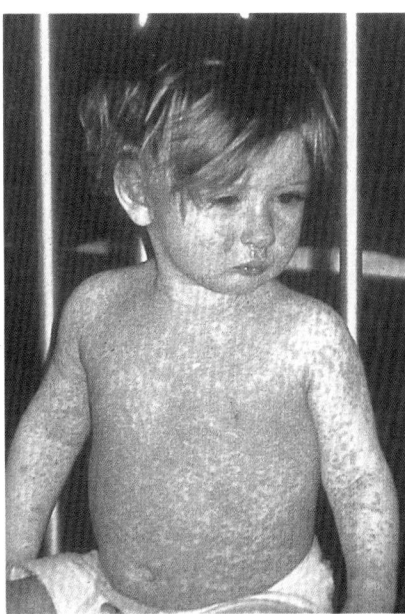

Purpuric rash of measles

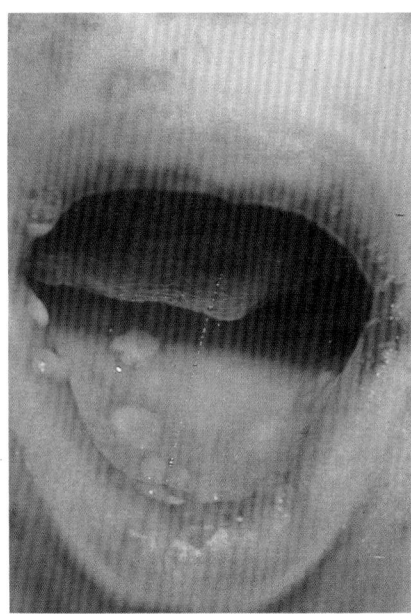

Oral lesions of chickenpox

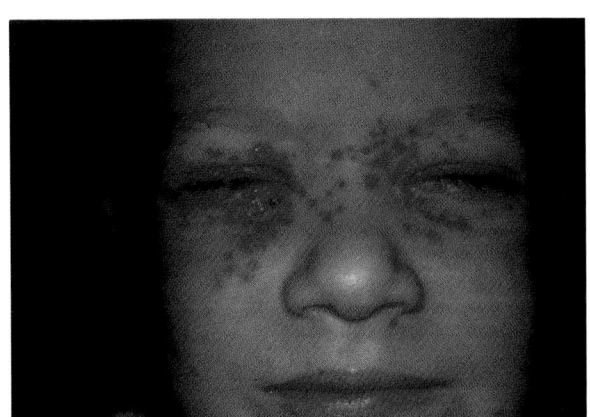

Primary herpes simplex around the eyes

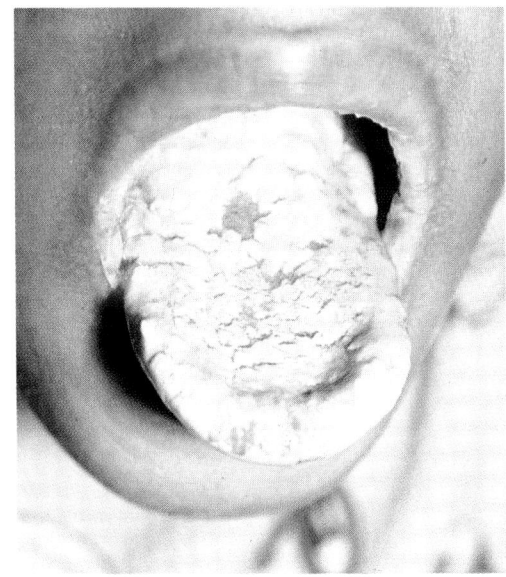

Oral candidiasis in AIDS

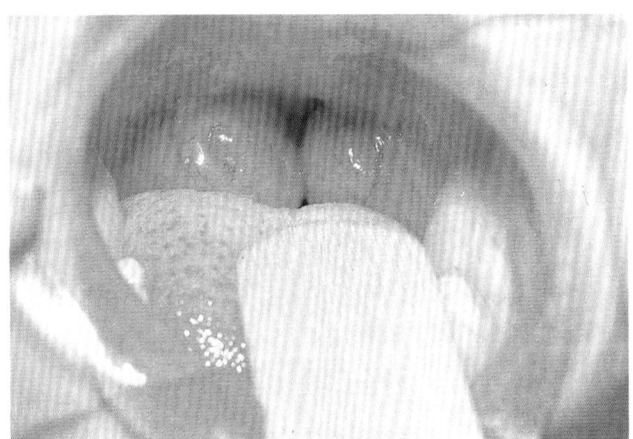

Tonsillitis

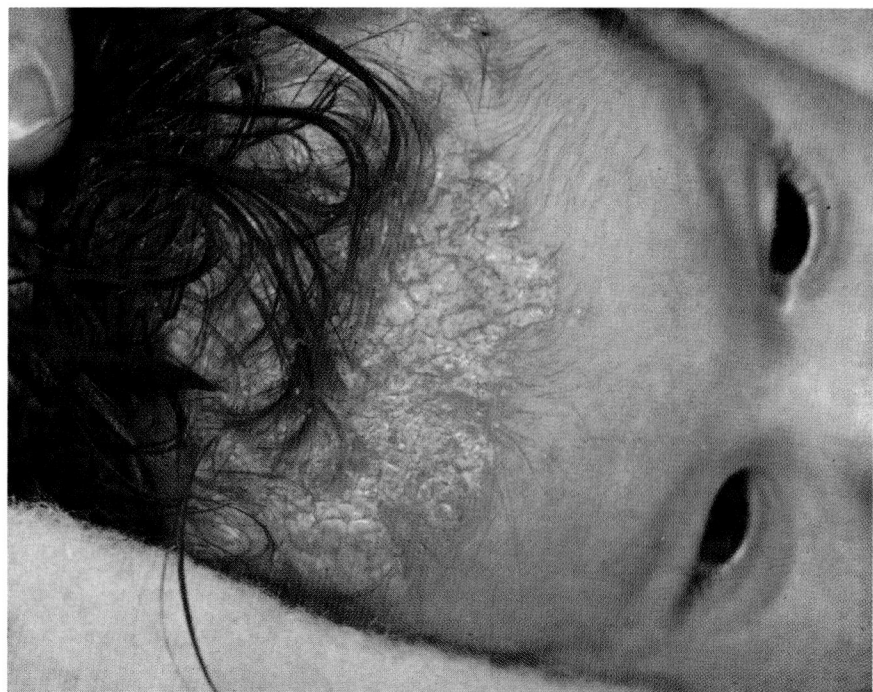

Seborrheic dermatitis of infancy

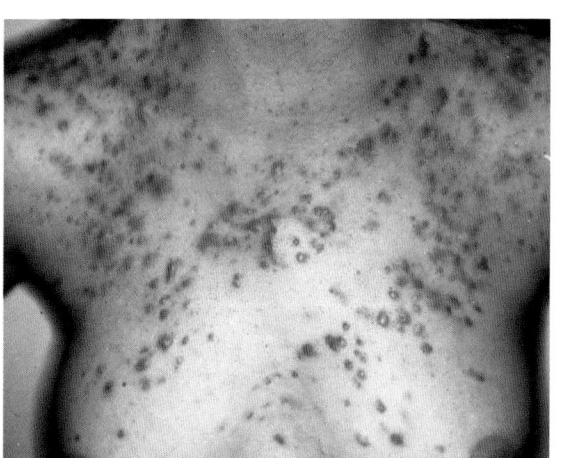

Severe acne of the chest

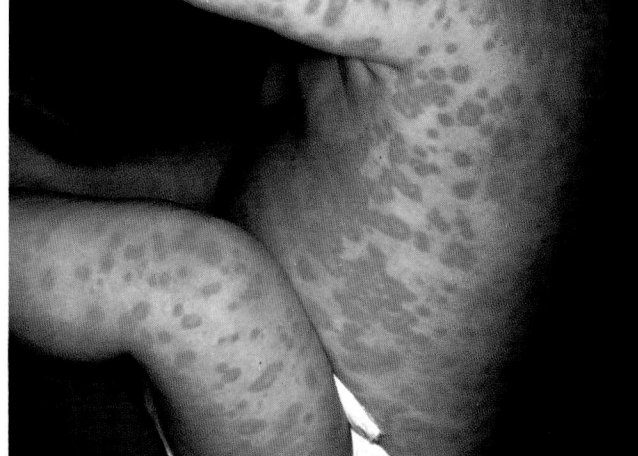

Acute urticaria from penicillin

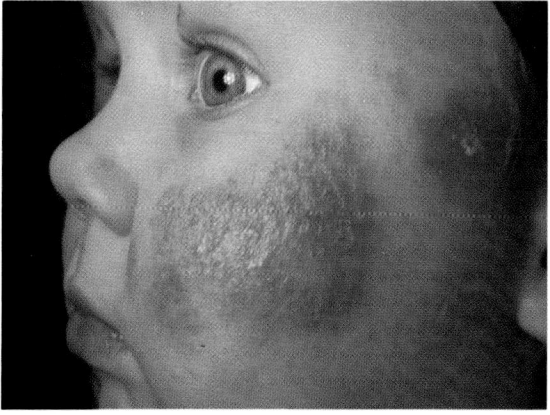

Atopic eczema in an infant

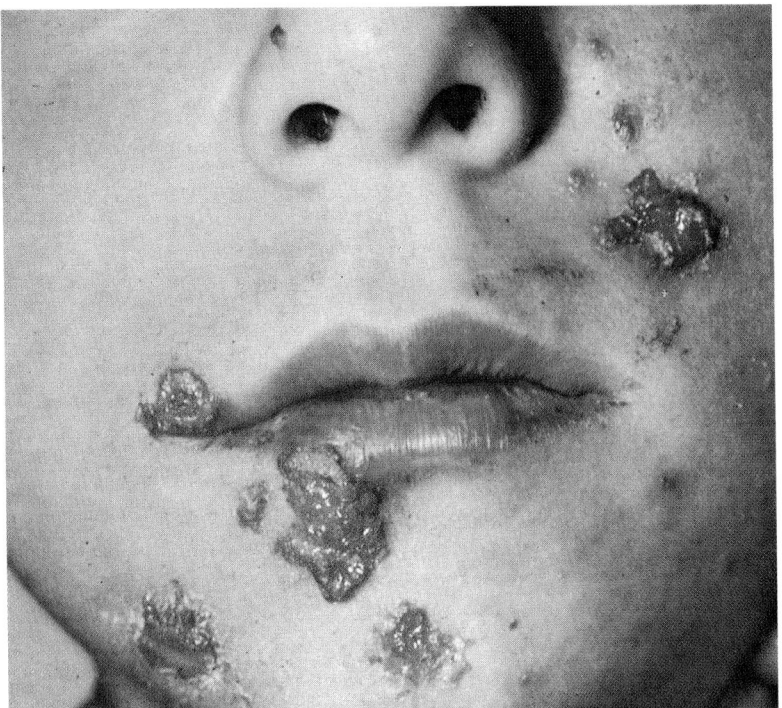

Impetigo of the face

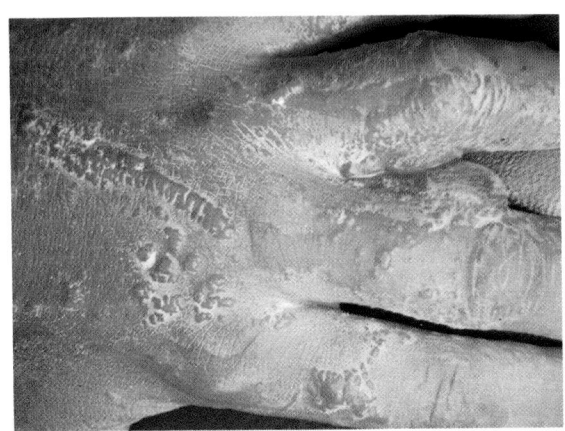

Contact dermatitis from poison ivy

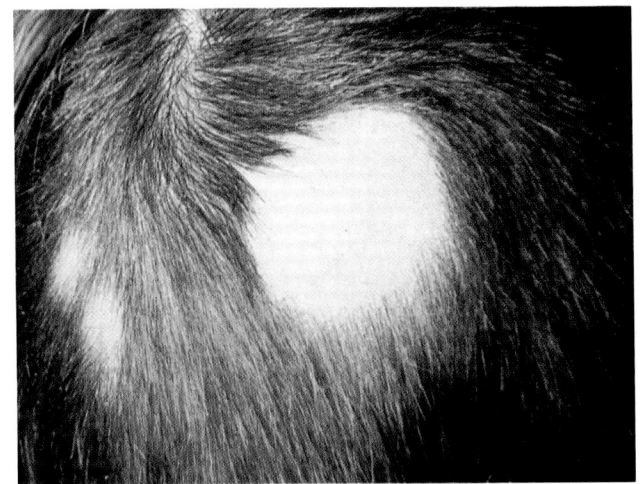

Tinea of the scalp

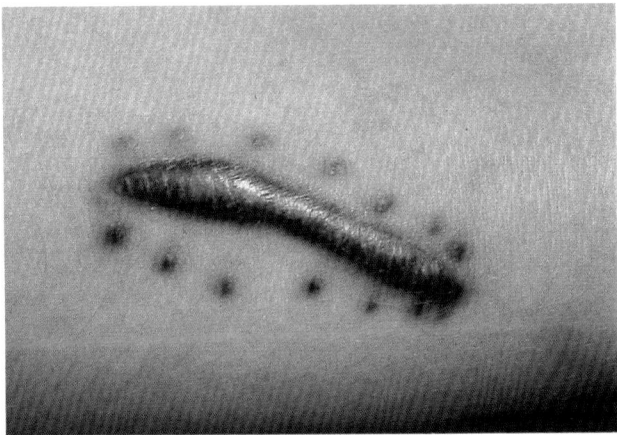

Keloid formed on surgical repair site

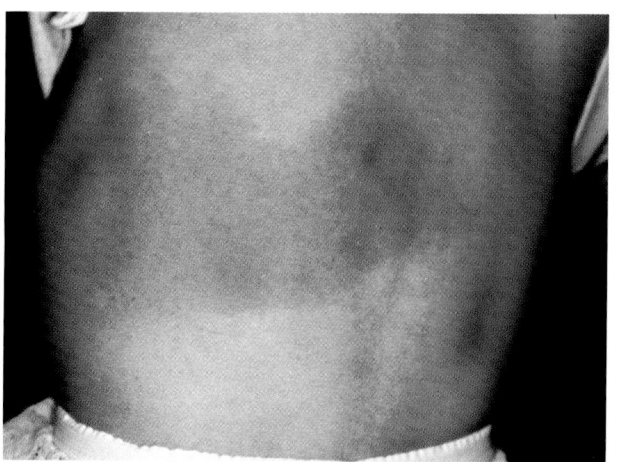

Mongolian spot on back

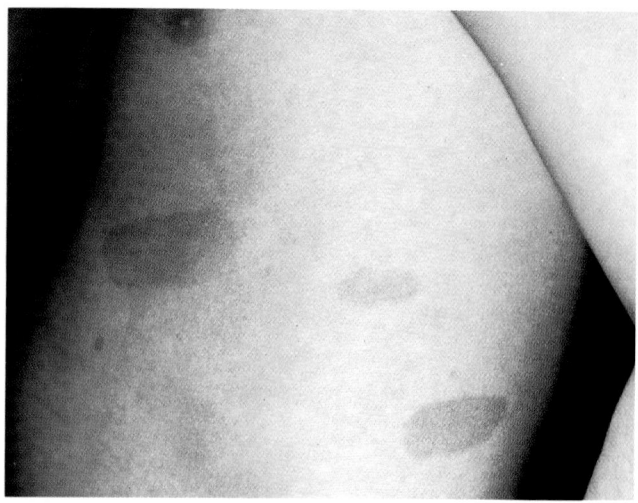

Cafe-au-lait lesions

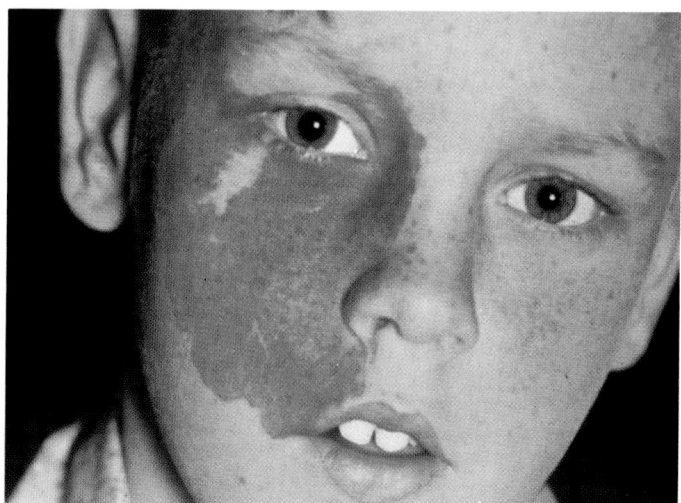

Port-wine stain

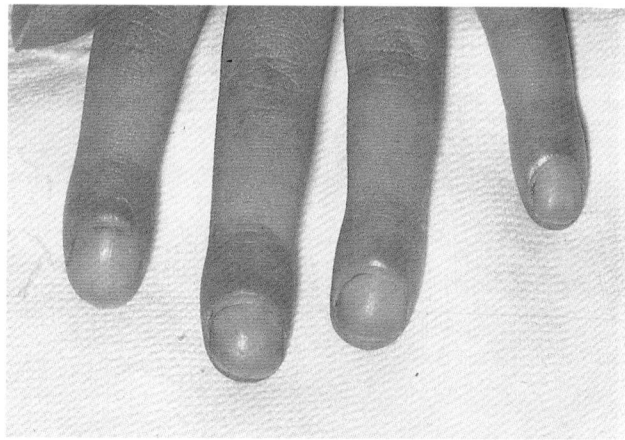

Clubbing of the nails

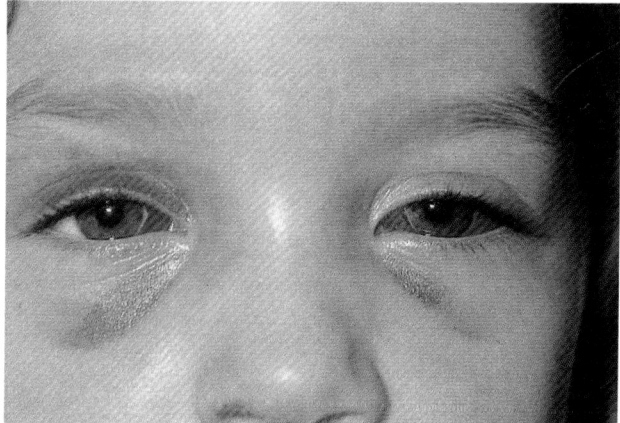

Periorbital bruising and subconjunctival hemorrhage in acute leukemia

A simple skin care regimen is encouraged. Bathing in plain warm water (body temperature or slightly warmer) with a mild soap and gentle nonfrictional cleansing is best. Daily bathing may or may not be necessary, and soap should be used only in areas not well-cleansed with plain water, such as the groin, hands, feet, nails, and face if drooling or nasal discharge is present.

CARE OF NEWBORNS AND INFANTS

In neonates, cleansing and drying one anatomic part before proceeding to the next area prevents excessive chilling. Tub bathing should be postponed until after detachment of the umbilical cord, generally around 7 to 14 days of age. To facilitate detachment and decrease bacterial colonization, alcohol is applied to the base of the umbilical cord several times daily. The diaper is placed below the cord to avoid irritation against the material. Any signs of infection, such as presence of erythema and malodorous, purulent discharge, are reported. Parents are instructed on signs of infection and that a small amount of bleeding when the cord does separate is normal. Gentle pressure should stop the bleeding. If not, the physician should be notified.

Skin care after circumcision depends on the type of procedure used. The care is directed at promotion of wound healing while taking measures to decrease pain and prevent infection. If a Gomco clamp is used, a petrolatum gauze dressing is applied loosely to keep the area moist and prevent adherence to the diaper. The petrolatum gauze also protects the wound from urine and stool. If the Hollister Plastibell is used, no special dressing is required. The diaper is changed frequently and is applied loosely to prevent rubbing and pressure on the penis. Any evidence of bleeding or unusual swelling is reported to the physician. Parents are instructed on wound care and to watch for signs of infection.

BATHING AND HYDRATION

As the child gets older, bath time often becomes an enjoyable and playful time for both the child and the parent. The ability of the stratum corneum to bind water makes spending extended periods of time soaking in water a healthy activity for the skin. However, the benefits of this time are reversed by the use of bubble baths, soaps, and other water additives that are often heavily scented and contain many irritating and sensitizing substances. Delaying the use of soap until the end of the bath not only decreases the amount that is needed, but also prevents prolonged contact with the skin while the child is playing in the water.

Bathing not only removes soil from the skin, but also removes the natural lubricant barrier that prevents water evaporation from the skin. If this lubricant barrier is not replaced, the water absorbed during bathing quickly evaporates and can produce dry skin. A tendency for dry skin can be a familial pattern but dry skin may develop because of a particular lifestyle or environmental conditions. Low humidity, for example, can rapidly draw the water from the skin. This is why dry skin often worsens during the winter months when exposed to cold, wind, and the low humidity of heated rooms. Summer conditions, such as air-conditioned rooms and overexposure to the sun, can also dry skin.

Hydration of the skin is accomplished by drinking plenty of fluids and soaking the skin in water. The use of emollients immediately after bathing decreases the tendency to develop dry skin. Emollients replace the oil barrier on the skin and prevent water evaporation; they do not add moisture to the skin. Emollients work best when applied while the skin is still moist. In choosing an emollient, simplicity is the key (Table 65-1). Lotions that contain higher quantities of water may be used for mildly dry skin. Creams and ointments, which are more occlusive, may be necessary for severely dry skin.

Emollients containing urea or lactic acid improve the binding of water in the skin and prevent evaporation by way of occlusion. If the skin is irritated, mild stinging may be experienced for a few minutes immediately after application. This stinging should quickly resolve with improvement of the skin's integrity.

Heavily scented preparations and those containing other topical sensitizers should be avoided. Petrolatum, or a similar product, continues to be the most effective emollient. Applying a thin layer while the skin is still moist and toweling off the excess provides an excellent barrier and decreases the oily feel. Unfortunately, many find this product cosmetically undesirable.

Various environmental conditions, including sun or wind exposure, temperature, and humidity, can make the skin susceptible to breakdown or cause injury. (See "Photosensitivity" in this chapter for a detailed discussion on the use of sunscreens in children.) Windy and cold conditions increase the water evaporation from the skin. Skin hydration and the use of emollients protect the skin under these conditions. Heat and humidity can cause the skin to become macerated, particularly in intertriginous sites. Frequent cleansing and drying of the skin decrease the incidence of skin breakdown from overhydration. Drying compounds, such as powder, may be helpful in decreasing maceration. However, these products must be used cautiously. A small amount of powder should be applied to the hand and then directly to the skin, removing any excess. This procedure prevents inhalation of the

TABLE 65-1
Emollients That Protect the Skin From Drying

Most Protective		Least Protective
Ointments/Oils	Creams	Lotions
White petrolatum	Eucerin	Eucerin
Aquaphor	Moisturel	Moisturel
Mineral oil	Lubriderm	Lubriderm
	Curel	Curel
	Purpose	Neutraderm
	Complex 15*	Complex 15*
	Aquaderm*	Aquaderm*
	Neutraplus*	Carmol*
		Aquacare*
		Lacticare†

* Contains urea.
† Contains lactic acid.

powder, which can occur with vigorous shaking, and avoids application of excessive amounts. Old powder left on the skin for prolonged periods can serve as an excellent medium for bacterial growth. All powder should be removed carefully when cleansing the skin and before additional applications.

★ **EVALUATION**

With appropriate skin care practices, the skin is protected and its integrity is maintained. The nurse should have the child or parent describe the prescribed skin care routine. The nurse should determine the ability of the child and family to incorporate the skin care principles into daily life. The skin should be monitored for signs of breakdown or injury.

Skin Care in Ill Children

Illness can be demanding on the skin. Numerous systemic diseases affect the skin because they interfere with circulation and oxygenation of tissue, nutrition, and mobility, as well as the breakdown and elimination of metabolic end products. Surgery, intravenous or intraarterial access, ostomies, or cutaneous monitoring devices interrupt the continuous cutaneous barrier. Table 65-2 lists systemic conditions frequently associated with skin manifestations. Types of skin lesions and distribution patterns are discussed and illustrated in Table 64-2 and Figures 64-1 and 64-2. Wound healing is a natural process of the skin in which the structure and function of cells are restored. The healing process is accomplished one of three ways:

- *Resolution*—recovery of damaged cells
- *Regeneration*—replacement of damaged cells with new cells

TABLE 65-2
Systemic Disorders Affecting the Skin

Disorder	Skin Effect
Nutritional disorders	Skin breakdown
	Delayed wound healing
	Xerosis
	Pallor
Cardiovascular disorders	Impaired circulation
	Purpura, ecchymosis
	Cyanosis
Hepatic disorders	Jaundice
	Xerosis
	Pruritus
Renal disorders	Edema
	Pruritus
	Xerosis
Endocrine disorders	Hirsutism
	Acne
	Xerosis
Neurologic disorders	Impaired tactile sensation

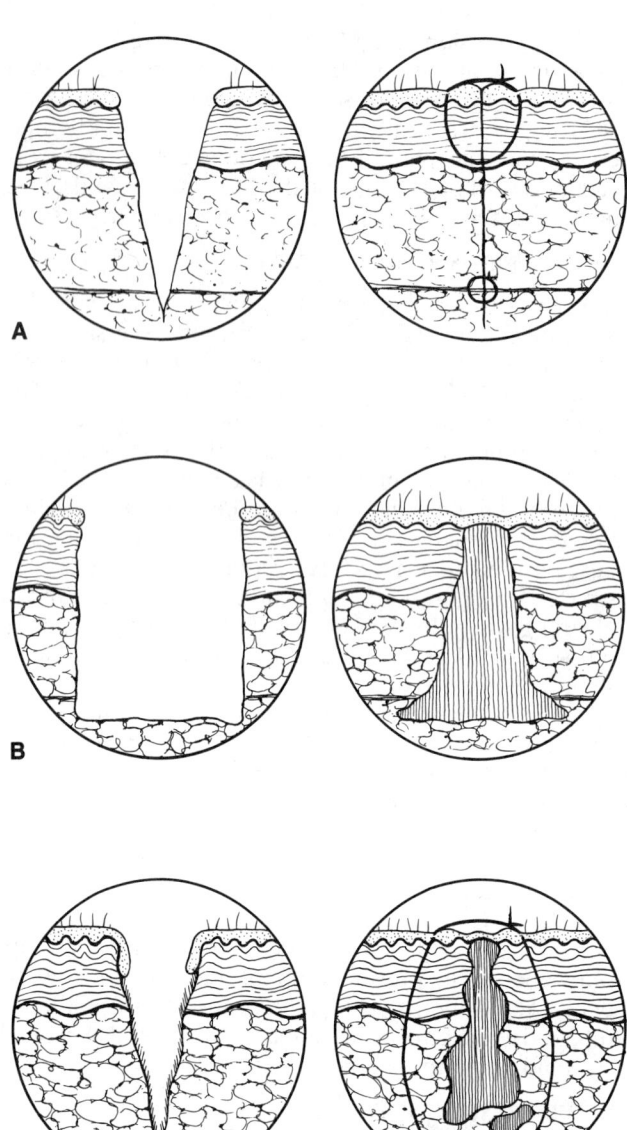

FIGURE 65-1
Mechanics of wound healing. (**A**) Smoothly separated wound edges are held together with suture facilitating first intention healing. This is the optimum method of healing because it ensures minimal scar formation. (**B**) Second intention healing requires that the body produce material to fill the area between separated wound edges. Healing takes place slowly from the wound margin toward the center. (**C**) Third intention healing shows delayed closure, early formation of granulation tissue around the margin of the edges, and then the use of suture to join the wound edges together. (Source: Timby BK, Lewis LW. [1992]. *Fundamental skills and concepts in patient care* [5th ed.]. Philadelphia: J.B. Lippincott.)

- *Scar formation*—substitution of destroyed cells with connective tissue

Factors that influence the outcome of wound healing include the following[67]:

- Extent of injury
- Blood supply to the injury
- Type of injured tissue
- Presence of debris
- Presence of infection
- General health of child

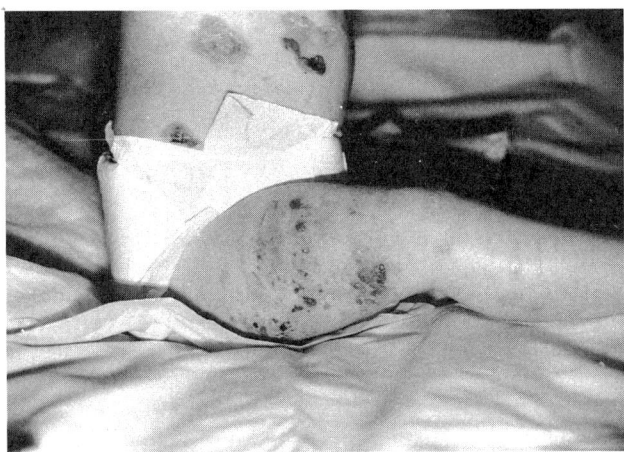

FIGURE 65-2
Epidermolysis bullosa. Hemorrhagic blisters and erosions of recessive dystrophic epidermolysis bullosa involving the trunk and proximal lower extremity. (Courtesy of the National Epidermolysis Bullosa Registry.)

Three mechanisms are used in wound healing: first, second, and third intention (Fig. 65-1). In *first intention healing,* the wound edges are close to each other. Only a narrow space needs to be filled in, and a small scar results. In *second intention healing,* the wound edges are relatively far apart and they cannot be stretched to meet for closure. Granulated tissue fills in the space. The nurse must be careful not to dislodge the tissue and reinjure the wound. In *third intention healing,* wound edges are widely separated, and the wound usually is deep and may contain fluid. The amount of scar tissue formed with third intention healing is similar to that of second intention healing.

★ ASSESSMENT

Assessment of the skin in ill children focuses on examination for skin integrity, temperature, moisture, turgor, and color. Valuable information can be obtained from a history of any previous skin problems and an assessment of current nutritional state. The nurse should carefully observe skin sites that are more prone to skin breakdown, such as bony prominences and intertriginous areas. The nurse should also look for cutaneous reactions to substances applied to the skin, such as lotions or tape, or to systemic medications. The skin should be assessed for signs of xerosis, infection, pruritus, maceration, or decreased circulation. A bony prominence with redness lasting more than 15 minutes is an early sign of reduced circulation and imminent skin breakdown.

In children with wounds and skin breakdown, the RYB color code[18] can be used as an assessment tool to document wound progress and guide wound care. This tool is based on determination of the color of an open wound: red, yellow, or black. It may be applied to any wound allowed to heal by secondary intention. A black (brown to gray to black) wound signals the presence of thick eschar. In a yellow wound, the tissue is not damaged enough to form eschar and, instead, is covered with a yellow fibrous or viscous exudate. A red wound signals the presence of granulation tissue and a wound that is

"ready to heal." The nutritional status and blood supply to the area of injury influence the shade of red observed.

★ NURSING DIAGNOSES AND PLANNING

Based on assessment data from above and Chapter 64, the following nursing diagnoses may apply to the family and child with skin dysfunction related to illness:

• Impaired Skin Integrity related to altered metabolic state.
• Pain related to physical injury.
• Altered Comfort (Pruritus) related to metabolic factors.
• High Risk for Infection related to traumatized tissue.
• Altered Nutrition: Less Than Body Requirements related to inability to digest food.

The nurse and child (or parents) together plan effective care based on the established nursing diagnoses. Several examples of expected outcomes follow:

• The child verbalizes relief from pruritus.
• The parents verbalize their understanding of cleaning the wound and when to call the physician.
• The child verbalizes feelings of improved comfort.

The nurse plans for the daily care of the child based on both physician's orders and nursing diagnoses. Some general nursing care goals include the following:

• Infection is prevented.
• Comfort is achieved and maintained.

★ INTERVENTIONS: COLLABORATIVE AND INDEPENDENT

Nursing care of the skin in ill children focuses on promotion of healing and comfort along with maintenance of skin integrity. Nursing measures that maintain skin hydration and replace the lubricant skin barrier are carried out. The skin should be kept clean with the use of mild cleansers or plain water, especially in intertriginous areas.

Careful attention is given to the child's diet to ensure adequate nutrition, which plays an important role in prevention of skin breakdown and promotion of wound healing. Additionally, children with limited mobility associated with paralysis, sedation, traction, or weakness require frequent turning and careful positioning to enable adequate blood circulation at skin pressure points. Special mattresses and mattress overlays may also be used to reduce pressure and prevent skin breakdown. Choosing the appropriate mattress surface can be a difficult task. Willey[71] has developed a tool to use in the clinical setting to aid in choosing the most clinically appropriate and cost-effective equipment based on assessment of the child's condition. Willey's detailed decision tree can aid in making a determination in light of the child's individual needs.[72]

WOUND CARE

Appropriate skin prepping and wound care are necessary to prevent infection when invasive procedures are required. The incidence of infection is low in wounds that are kept clean. Emphasis is placed on cleansing and not disinfecting, because most disinfecting agents are toxic to healing tissue and may impair the healing process.[5] In general, the use of tap water or normal saline is all that is required to cleanse a red wound. Gentle cleansing with a bulb syringe helps to remove exudate. Occasionally, a dilute solution of an antiseptic, such as hydrogen peroxide, is used in wounds with heavy drainage.

Yellow and black wounds signal the presence of necrotic tissue requiring debridement.[19] Wound irrigation, wet to dry gauze dressings, chemical debridement with Dakin's solution or topical enzymes, and surgical debridement are methods used to remove necrotic tissue. Once the wound bed is red, gentler wound care is instituted to promote tissue granulation and wound healing.

After cleansing, the wound bed may be covered with a thin layer of antibiotic ointment (polysporin, bacitracin, or mupirocin). This ointment not only is helpful in preventing infection but also keeps the wound bed moist. Neosporin should not be used because of the high incidence of allergic reaction to neomycin. Petrolatum-impregnated gauze also is effective in maintaining a moist wound. It is well-recognized that wounds kept moist and covered heal faster than air-exposed, dry wounds.

Wound dressing is an area of increasing technological advancement. Choosing the type of dressing can be difficult and requires consideration of the child's condition and cost effectiveness. Although occlusion influences both epidermal resurfacing and dermal repair, risks are associated with the use of occlusive dressings. There is some concern that semipermeable wound dressings are associated with increased frequency of bacterial growth underneath the dressing and potentially contribute to the development of sepsis.[42] Interestingly, in a study looking at the effect of semiocclusive dressings on the microbial population in superficial wounds, Mertz and Eaglstein found that the number of bacteria in wounds under an occlusive dressing was substantially greater than in wounds open to the air. Despite this finding, the occluded wounds healed 21% faster and the incidence of infection was not increased.[48] These same investigators demonstrated that dressings such as Op-site or Vigilon protected 50% of wounds challenged with *Staphylococcus aureus* and under Duoderm neither *Staphylococcus aureus* or *Pseudomonas aeruginosa* were recovered when challenged. Op-site and Vigilon did not protect against *P. aeruginosa*.[49] Assuming that the organisms responsible for many wound infections are delivered to the wound from an exogenous source or distant site on the child and that most wound infections in the nursery are caused by *Staphylococcus aureus,* occlusive dressings can play a role in preventing wound infection and promoting wound healing. The wound, however, must be closely observed for signs of infection.

Frequent dressing changes, careful wound cleansing, and the appropriate use of topical antibiotics (Polysporin, bacitracin, or mupirocin) prevent infection and provide the optimal environment for wound healing.[5] The child and family need to be instructed on appropriate wound care and the early signs of infection.

★ EVALUATION

When evaluating skin care in ill children, the nurse should determine if skin integrity has been maintained, if the healing has occurred, and if infection or skin breakdown has been prevented. The nurse should assess whether discomfort from pain or pruritus is relieved and if adequate nutrition has been maintained.

Skin Care in Preterm Infants

Preterm infant skin is incompletely developed with a thin epidermis and, therefore, is susceptible to enhanced permeability and injury. The extent of immaturity depends on both the gestational age and the nutritional status of the infant. The first few weeks of life appear to be the most critical time for the skin of the preterm infant. Once exposed to the outside environment the skin is adaptable and the stratum corneum is nearly as effective as that of an adult by 2 weeks of age.

Simplicity is the key in caring for the preterm infant's skin. However, due to its immaturity, precautions must be taken to prevent disruption of this delicate barrier. During the short period of time until an effective epidermal barrier is developed, gentleness is important.

★ ASSESSMENT

Assessment of preterm skin should include careful monitoring of intake and output, weight, and temperature. Frequent total skin examinations should be conducted for early identification of edema, xerosis, maceration, fissuring, irritation, erosion, or infection. The nurse should pay particular attention to skin sites where monitoring equipment, infusions, or other apparatus come in contact with the skin.

★ NURSING DIAGNOSES AND PLANNING

Based on assessment data from above and Chapter 64, the following nursing diagnoses may be used concerning the skin of a preterm infant:

- Impaired Skin Integrity related to immaturity.
- High Risk for Infection related to traumatized tissue.
- Fluid Volume Deficit related to faulty thermoregulatory mechanisms.
- Sensory/Perceptual Alterations (Tactile) related to noxious environmental stimuli.
- Parental Anxiety related to lack of knowledge about skin care.
- Ineffective Management of Therapeutic Regimen related to knowledge deficit regarding skin care.

The nurse and parents together plan effective care based on the established nursing diagnoses. Several examples of expected outcomes follow:

- The parents touch and cuddle the newborn.
- The parents discuss skin care needs of the infant.
- Weight loss due to chilling is minimal.
- Skin integrity is maintained.

The nurse plans for the daily care of the child based on both physician's orders and nursing diagnoses. Some general nursing care goals may be the following:

- Infection is prevented.
- Injury of the skin is prevented.

- Thermoregulation is maintained with minimum disturbance of fluid-electrolyte balance.

★ INTERVENTIONS: COLLABORATIVE AND INDEPENDENT

Highly skilled nursing care is required to accomplish the goals of caring for preterm skin. Many advances have been made, resulting in significant improvement in the survival of children previously thought unable to live. Many of these advances require continual, careful monitoring of oxygen and carbon dioxide levels, cardiac function, temperature, as well as providing ventilation, fluids, and nutrition. These measures often place great demands on immature skin.

CLEANSING AND SKIN PROTECTION

Warm water baths are preferred for preterm infants, and warm sterile water should be used on irritated or denuded skin. Soaps and cleansing agents, which may dry and irritate the skin, should be avoided. The use of emollients should be restricted to petrolatum to avoid percutaneous absorption of ingredients contained in other products. Applying a thin coat of petrolatum is thought to decrease skin fragility, improve wound care, and help to protect these infants.[41]

Cleansing of the skin before an invasive procedure is important and may necessitate the use of harsh agents. Isopropyl alcohol and povidone-iodine are commonly used germicides. Because of the potential for isopropyl alcohol to be extremely drying to the skin and of povidone-iodine being absorbed percutaneously causing elevated levels of iodine in the plasma, it is imperative that these products be used in a limited area and be removed with water after the procedure is completed.

Prevention of physical injury to the skin is of primary concern. Adhesive tape should be used sparingly. The use of tincture of benzoin before tape application should be avoided, because tight adherence of the tape to the skin increases skin damage when the tape is removed. The lowest effective heat on transcutaneous oxygen monitors should be used to prevent burns. It is also recommended that the site of the temperature probe be changed every 2 hours to prevent the development of erythema and skin craters at the probe site. When ventilators or intravenous catheters need to be secured, the use of Hollihesive, Op-site, or a similar dressing over the skin and securing the equipment with tape applied to the dressing prevents the need to apply the tape directly to the skin. Removal of adhesives can be accomplished with water-soaked gauze, patience, and care. Use of solvents or other chemicals is not recommended because of the risk of chemical injury to the skin and the potential for absorption.

Despite following the above recommendations, skin breakdown may occur and application of the principles of moist wound healing are required. In preterm infants, areas of skin breakdown should be cleansed with sterile water. Application of a thin layer of antibiotic ointment may be recommended. For sites that require a dressing, the use of a transparent semipermeable dressing is recommended. The skin is cleansed with plain sterile water and allowed to dry completely. A dressing is cut to size allowing for adherence to intact skin and placed on the site. The dressing is held firmly for 1 to 2 minutes to permit molding and adhesion.

The most important nursing measure in the prevention of infection in the preterm infant is conscientious handwashing by staff and other contacts before and after handling the infants. Person-to-person contact is the major route for transmission of *Staphylococcus aureus* in neonatal nurseries. (See "Bacterial Skin Infections" in this chapter for further discussion.)

THERMOREGULATION

Thermal regulation of preterm infants is generally maintained by overhead infrared warmers and monitored by a control probe on the abdomen. Although successful in maintaining body temperature, these radiant warmers cause increased insensible water loss and possibly increased oxygen consumption. Infants of 32 weeks gestational age or less are at high risk for fluid loss through the skin. This transepidermal water loss is increased with the infant's activity as well as its being placed under a radiant warmer. By increasing the ambient humidity from 20% to 60%, an early gestational age infant shows a 100% decrease in transepidermal water loss.[7] As soon as possible, the infant should be moved from the radiant warmer to an Isolette for better control of the humidity. Infants should be weighed as frequently as necessary to evaluate their state of hydration.

TOPICAL APPLICATIONS

Percutaneous absorption is also a major concern in infants because of the immature skin barrier and the greater ratio of surface area to body weight than adults. Topically applied drugs and other substances must be carefully considered for their potential toxic effects. In general, topical applications should be limited to water and petrolatum, or a similar product. If skin prepping with an antiinfective or other agent is required, its use should be limited only to the area needed and removed with water as soon as possible.

ENVIRONMENTAL INTERVENTION

Because of the need for monitoring, regulating, and assisting the preterm infant to function, the postnatal environment may seem hostile and abusive in comparison to the serene intrauterine environment. A study conducted by Medoff-Cooper[46] suggests that preterm infants are sensitive to routine handling and experience tachycardia, tachypnea, and bradycardia, physiologic responses attributed to an immature neurologic system. Infants thus reacted with signals of distress to stimuli from their environment.

On the other hand, preterm infants sometimes experience relatively little touching for comfort. Little is known about the effect of diminished physical contact with other humans. Field and associates[24] found that tactile/kinesthetic stimulation of preterm infants enhanced weight gain and responsiveness. Developmental readiness seems to be a primary consideration in determining how much stimulation a preterm infant needs.

"Skin-to-skin" care, also referred to as "kangaroo care" has been practiced in various European hospitals for up to 3 years.[2] This practice allows parents, usually mothers, to hold their diaper-clad infants upright and prone between their breasts, skin to skin, with a blanket covering. The infant must be physiologically stable and developmentally ready before instituting kangaroo care.

★ EVALUATION

Evaluation of nursing intervention in skin care for preterm infants includes observation for maintenance of skin integrity, moisture, and temperature. If invasive procedures are required or skin breakdown has occurred, the nurse should evaluate the areas for absence of infection and progress of wound healing. The nurse should observe the infant's reaction to tactile stimulation and parents' participation in the infant's care. The nurse should evaluate the parents' understanding and independence in the care of their infant.

Transient Cutaneous Conditions in the Newborn

Definition and Incidence. The first anxious questions of many new parents relate to the appearance of their newborn's skin. Infant skin differs from adult in that it seems to reflect bodily changes more easily. During the first few days to weeks of life, many transient skin conditions appear and disappear. Few infants escape this stage without exhibiting one or more of these conditions.

Etiology and Pathophysiology. The transient cutaneous conditions seen in newborns are related to events occurring during birth, immaturity of various physiologic systems, or to influence of maternal hormones. In general, affected infants appear healthy and in no apparent distress.

Clinical Manifestations. At birth, a normal infant's skin is purplish-red in color and brightens quickly to a reddish-pink hue. It is soft, smooth, and covered with a grayish-white greasy material called *vernix caseosa*. Familial and racial factors contribute to establishing the range of an infant's skin color. The child's skin color also varies from one moment to the next depending on the state of activity. Not uncommonly, the hands and feet develop a bluish hue, especially when they have been exposed or chilled. This condition is termed *acrocyanosis* and is more commonly seen in full-term than preterm infants.

Another physiologic response to chilling is *cutis marmorata*. This is a transient bluish, reticulated, mottling of the skin on the trunk and extremities. It occurs in both full-term and preterm infants, and is thought to be the result of poor autonomic nervous system control of blood vessels.

A color change observed most frequently in premature infants, but which can be seen in full-term infants, is *harlequin color* change. This phenomenon occurs when the infant is lying on its side. The lower half of the body reddens, with a simultaneous blanching of the upper half. The head and genitalia may be spared. A distinct line of demarcation runs along the midline of the body. The color change may occur quickly and may last for

several minutes to a half hour. It appears to be related to the immaturity of the hypothalamic centers which control the tone of peripheral blood vessels. Harlequin color change is most frequently seen at 3 to 4 days of age, but may be seen up to 3 weeks of age.

Physiologic jaundice, also known as *icterus neonatorum*, occurs in one-third to one-half of all normal newborns and is thought to be caused by the increased destruction of red blood cells no longer needed after birth. The immature newborn liver is unable to excrete bilirubin in sufficient quantities. Although almost all newborns experience elevated bilirubin levels, only about half demonstrate observable signs of jaundice. Physiologic jaundice first appears after 24 hours in full-term infants or by 48 hours in preterm infants. Postterm infants have little or no physiologic jaundice. Extent of involvement varies widely and may be noted only as slight yellowing of the sclerae or the entire skin surface may be discolored. This condition rarely causes ill effects, unlike hyperbilirubinemia that begins in the first 24 hours of life, which should always be considered pathologic.

Trauma during labor and birth also may cause transient skin conditions in the newborn. Prolonged labor may result in *edema* or *hematomas* of the scalp or buttocks, depending on the infant's presentation. *Forceps marks* located on the cheek and jaw area are often alarming for parents but rarely cause problems and resolve in several days. Erosions on the scalp from fetal monitor probes may also be seen in newborns. In most instances, these erosions heal without complications. However, cutaneous complications associated with fetal scalp electrode-induced erosions include herpes simplex infection and scalp abscesses that are contracted when the infant passes through the birth canal or with prolonged ruptured membranes and amnionitis.[34]

Various lumps and bumps may be present during the newborn period. *Erythema toxicum*, also called *urticaria neonatorum*, is characterized by transient blotchy, red macules with or without a papule or yellowish-white pustule centrally. Erythema toxicum occurs in 30% to 70% of full-term infants and may be present at birth. The skin lesions are asymptomatic and may be found on any body surface except the palms or soles. They usually disappear by 7 to 10 days of life. The etiology is unknown.

A condition closely related to erythema toxicum, but seen less frequently, is *transient neonatal pustular melanosis*. This is a vesiculopustular and pigmented disorder seen predominantly in African-American infants, but may also be seen in white infants. After rupture of the vesiculopustular lesions, postinflammatory hyperpigmented macules remain and usually resolve in one to several months. Again, the etiology is unknown.

A skin lesion that often raises much concern when initially seen, but resolves on its own without treatment, is a solitary bulla or erosion on the dorsum of the fingers, thumb, or the lower arm. It results from vigorous sucking in the prenatal period. The infant may continue sucking in the same area after birth, giving a clue to the diagnosis. The presence of a *sucking blister* initially raises the suspicion of some form of epidermolysis bullosa (EB). However, the characteristic location and failure of additional blisters to develop can rule out EB.

Several cutaneous lesions in the newborn result from

underdeveloped skin appendages. *Miliaria* results from keratin plugging of immature sweat ducts and sweat leaking into the skin below the obstruction. Nearly every newborn develops some form of miliaria. *Miliaria rubra* (prickly heat) are discrete erythematous papules or pustules. *Miliaria crystallina* are clear, superficial, pinpoint vesicles without accompanying erythema. Miliaria often occurs in crops with predilection for intertriginous areas, but it also is seen on the face and scalp.

Milia occur as a result of keratin and sebaceous retention in the pilosebaceous apparatus of vellus hair. They most commonly occur on the face and appear as pearly white papules. Milia usually disappear spontaneously during the first 3 to 4 weeks of life. *Bohn's nodules and Epstein's pearls* are similar to milia except they occur in the oral mucosa, especially at the gum margins or midline of the hard palate. They are small cysts containing keratinous debris that rupture spontaneously and heal without treatment during the first few months of life.

A common neonatal skin condition resulting from maternal androgen stimulation is *acne neonatorum*. This condition usually is noted at 2 to 4 weeks of age with the appearance of papules, pustules, and comedones over the face, chest, back, and groin. The extent of involvement varies and may be present for several months. Usually this condition resolves spontaneously.

Diagnostic Studies. Diagnosis of these skin lesions is made by their clinical features. Due to the benign nature of these conditions, additional laboratory studies usually are not required. An exception is a child with physiologic jaundice in whom a serum bilirubin level is obtained.

★ ASSESSMENT

Initially, a description of the onset, duration, and treatment attempts for the skin manifestation is obtained. Because many of these conditions have a transient nature, the nurse should attempt to determine situations that may be associated with their appearance.

Physical assessment includes observing the skin for color changes at regular intervals. Jaundice is assessed most reliably by observing the color of the sclera, nails, and skin. Applying direct pressure to the skin causing blanching may make the yellow color more apparent. Careful observation should be made of the skin with documentation of the onset and resolution of the skin condition as well as the types of skin lesions present, their distribution, and pattern.

★ NURSING DIAGNOSES AND PLANNING

Based on assessment data from above and Chapter 64, the following nursing diagnoses may apply to the family and newborn with transient cutaneous conditions:

- Impaired Skin Integrity related to common physiologic changes.
- High Risk for Infection related to broken skin.
- Ineffective Family Coping: Compromised related to temporary preoccupation with the skin condition.
- Anxiety related to knowledge deficit about skin disorder.

The nurse and parents together plan effective care based on the established nursing diagnoses. Several examples of expected outcomes follow:

- The infant's skin condition improves.
- The parents discuss their concern about the infant's skin condition.
- The parents touch and cuddle the infant.
- The parents demonstrate good infant skin care.

The nurse plans for the care of the child based on both physician's orders and nursing diagnoses. Some general nursing care goals include the following:

- Infant is protected from complications during phototherapy.
- Adequate fluid balance is maintained.
- Infection is prevented.
- Parental anxiety is diminished.

★ INTERVENTIONS: COLLABORATIVE AND INDEPENDENT

In conditions such as acrocyanosis or cutis marmorata, rewarming of the skin with clothing or blankets results in quick resolution. In harlequin color change, no therapy is required. Increased activity such as crying usually abates the color change. Because recurrent episodes are common with all of these skin color changes, parents should be prepared for possible recurrences.

As long as physiologic jaundice is minimal, no treatment is necessary. However, with an elevated serum bilirubin level and pronounced jaundice, phototherapy with full-spectrum, 20-W fluorescent bulbs with a 400- to 500-nm wavelength spectrum may be prescribed by the physician. Several precautions are taken for infant protection during phototherapy. The infant's closed eyes are covered by opaque eye shields to provide secure and complete coverage of the eyes. The shields protect the eyes from possible burns and increased risk of cataract formation as a result of prolonged exposure to ultraviolet lights. Complications that may arise if correct placement or fitting is not obtained include occlusion of the nares, excoriation of the corneas, and excessive pressure on the lids.

The infant is placed nude at a distance of 42 to 45 cm between the upper surface of the child and the lights. Skin surfaces not exposed to the light retain their jaundiced appearance, so the infant must be repositioned every 2 to 4 hours to allow for maximal light exposure. The environmental temperature is maintained by a radiant heat warmer or a servocontrolled incubator and monitored by a thermistor attached to the infant to prevent hypothermia or hyperthermia. Increased insensible fluid loss occurs during light exposure; therefore fluid intake should be increased an additional 25% over normal intake. A Plexiglas shield between the infant and the light bulbs filters out some of the ultraviolet rays that could cause burning of the infant's skin. This shield also protects the infant from injury due to accidental breakage of the light bulbs.

Documentation of phototherapy should include the number, type, and photometer measurement of light intensity in milliwatts as well as the exposure interval lengths, safety precautions instituted, infant's distance from the light bulbs, repositioning, temperature, fluid intake, the infant's response to the therapy, and any complications. Phototherapy is generally discontinued when the indirect bilirubin level falls below 10 mg/dL.

Edema and hematomas resulting from trauma during labor and delivery require only observation and verification of resolution. The edema most commonly is noted around the eyes and on the face, legs, dorsum of hands and feet, scrotum, or labia. Any open lesions should be cleansed with sterile water, covered with petrolatum, Polysporin, or bacitracin ointment and observed for any signs of cutaneous infection.

Dressing infants appropriately for the weather with loose clothing and reducing the environmental temperature decrease sweating in conditions such as miliaria. Mild keratolytics, such as emollients containing urea (see Table 65-1), may be prescribed for milia and neonatal acne. However, no treatment is necessary, because these conditions are self-limited.

Much parental anxiety can be relieved with explanations about these common conditions, how newborn skin differs from adult skin, the transient, self-healing nature of these conditions, and instruction on newborn skin care. Regardless of how benign the condition is, parents require explanation and reassurance. During pregnancy, parents develop expectations about their infant's appearance and imperfections are a disappointment. Parents may even secretly blame themselves by attributing the skin condition to unrelated events during pregnancy, such as not eating the right foods. Reviewing these private theories and providing factual reassurances and care instructions are therapeutic. Guilt is eased and parents are provided with measures they can take to help their infant.

★ EVALUATION

Periodically, the nurse and family evaluate the outcomes of care given. Examples of outcomes for the child and family with transient neonatal cutaneous conditions were given under planning in this section. Because minimal treatment or intervention is required in these conditions, the infants are followed to confirm resolution of the skin lesions. The nurse should review the infant skin care practices with the parents and determine if they have any additional questions or concerns regarding their child's skin condition.

Genodermatoses

Genodermatoses is a group of hereditary cutaneous disorders. Many of these disorders are accompanied by manifestations in other structures and organs. As many as 200 separate entities are described in the dermatology literature. Many of these conditions are rare. This section focuses only on ichthyosis and epidermolysis bullosa.

Ichthyosis

Definition. Ichthyosis is a family of genetically determined disorders in which the orderly process of epidermal desquamation is the most obvious functional impairment. The term *ichthyosis* is derived from the Greek root for fish, *ichthy.* The term is applied to these disorders because of the resemblance of the skin to fish scales.

Clinical Manifestations. These disorders are characterized by the presence of dryness and scaling of the skin. The severity of these disorders spans from mild scaling often described as "dry skin" (ichthyosis vulgaris) to an ichthyosis that is incompatible with life (harlequin fetus).

Ichthyosis vulgaris is the most common and mildest form of ichthyosis.[1] The scaling is usually noted after the third month of life. Often, the milder forms of this disorder are undiagnosed, and the symptoms are instead attributed to "dry skin." Ichthyosis vulgaris often improves with age, high humidity, and warm temperatures. It involves predominantly the extensor surfaces of the extremities with sparing of the flexural areas. The scales on the pretibial aspects of the lower legs are usually large and platelike. With involvement of the trunk and the upper extremities, a fine, white scale is seen. Increased palmar and plantar creases, atopic background, and keratosis pilaris are frequently associated with ichthyosis vulgaris.

Thick, adherent scaling with deep grooves and intertriginous involvement often occurs in the more severe forms of ichthyosis. Maceration and bacterial colonization of the scale can result in a foul odor of the skin. This odor can be distressing to the child and family.

Diagnostic Studies. The different sizes and shapes of the scale as well as the sites of involvement, history, genetic transmission, and microscopic appearance are the basis for the distinction among the types of ichthyosis. Skin biopsy of a well-developed area of ichthyosis is used for microscopic examination, but, unfortunately, is not always diagnostic.[73]

Prenatal diagnosis requires amniocentesis and fetoscopy for fetal skin biopsy. Urinary estrogen levels are measured in the third trimester of pregnancy for prenatal diagnosis of X-linked ichthyosis.[73] Postnatal serum lipoprotein electrophoresis identifies elevations of cholesterol sulfate in the child with X-linked ichthyosis.

★ ASSESSMENT

Historical information regarding the presentation of skin manifestations and history of other family members with similar symptoms is obtained. The characteristics of the scale are assessed as well as sites of involvement, and whether odor is present. Presence of erythema or blisters is noted, and palmar and plantar surfaces are examined for increased skin markings and hyperkeratosis. Skin examination includes observation for ectropion, eclabium, alopecia, and nail dystrophy. It is also important to determine the family's understanding of the disease process and treatment recommendations, as well as the family coping abilities and the effect of the disorder on the child's self-image. Because ichthyosis is a chronic condition, the family's resources and support systems also should be assessed.

★ NURSING DIAGNOSES AND PLANNING

Based on assessment data from above and Chapter 64, the following nursing diagnoses may apply to the family and child with ichthyosis:

- Ineffective Thermoregulation related to obstructed sweat glands.
- Impaired Skin Integrity related to altered state of skin.
- High Risk for Infection related to broken skin.
- Body Image Disturbance related to body odor and knowledge deficit regarding disease process and treatment.
- Ineffective Management of Therapeutic Regimen related to knowledge deficit regarding disease process and treatment.

The nurse and child (or parents) together plan effective care based on the established nursing diagnoses. Several examples of expected outcomes follow:

- The child verbalizes psychosocial impact of the condition.
- The child performs good skin care.
- The family participates in education regarding the disease and its treatment.

The nurse plans for the daily care of the child based on both doctor's orders and nursing diagnoses. Some general nursing care goals include the following:

- Skin hydration is maintained.
- Scaling is decreased.
- Infection is prevented.
- Healthy body image is achieved.

★ INTERVENTIONS: COLLABORATIVE AND INDEPENDENT

Collaborative measures involve the use of various topical and oral medications, skin therapies, and genetic counseling. Soaking in a tub of plain water once or twice a day is the best way to hydrate the hyperkeratotic areas of skin. Emollients in an ointment or cream form, with or without keratolytics, are the mainstay of treatment. Keratolytics aid in softening the stratum corneum, and they promote desquamation. Occlusion with plastic wrap or a sauna suit increases the action of these medications. Salicylic acid is used cautiously in young children because of absorption and the potential for metabolic acidosis.[73]

Oral retinoids, such as isotretinoin, are especially useful in relieving the hyperkeratosis associated with ichthyosis. Unfortunately, because of the toxicity potential, retinoids are reserved for use only in severe ichthyosis.[60] Methotrexate has been reported to be helpful but is rarely used.

As the child grows, issues such as nutrition, thermoregulation, body image, and family education must be addressed. Any of the hyperproliferative states places a strain on the body's iron stores. Iron supplements along with regular testing for anemia are therefore important in severe cases.

Heat prostration due to obstruction of eccrine glands by hyperkeratosis is a potential problem especially with strenuous physical activity. External cooling measures such as dousing with cool water help prevent hyperthermia. Topical measures to reduce the thickness of scale are most effective in preventing this complication.

Families need extensive teaching regarding the pathogenesis of the disease, how the medications work, and how to apply the topical treatments. In children with bullous ichthyosis, measures are taken to avoid blistering similar to those used in children with EB. (See "Epidermolysis Bullosa, Interventions: Collaborative and Independent" in this chapter.)

Depending on the extent of involvement, ichthyosis can have an enormous impact on the development of body image. In children for whom body odor is a problem and hyperkeratosis affects their appearance, understanding and patience are necessary. The child and family need to understand that this is a lifelong disorder and that continuous treatment is necessary. Families need a great deal of support in dealing with the psychosocial issues of this disease. The National Ichthyosis Foundation and the Ichthyosis Foundation of America provide support and information.

★ EVALUATION

Periodically, the nurse and family evaluate the outcomes of care given. Examples of outcomes for the child with ichthyosis were given under planning in this section. Planning for further nursing care takes into consideration complications.

COMPLICATIONS

Depending on the extent of involvement, children with ichthyosis may be at risk for developing a variety of complications. With the presence of thick scale, particularly when present in intertriginous areas, maceration, bacterial colonization, and odor may result. Ectropion and eclabium may occur with facial tautness. Involvement of the scalp may lead to alopecia, and nail dystrophy may be present when there is marked inflammation of the nail folds. As the child grows, eccrine obstruction may lead to hypohidrosis and heat intolerance.

Epidermolysis Bullosa

Definition and Incidence. Epidermolysis bullosa (EB) is a group of inherited disorders characterized by the spontaneous development of bullous lesions as a result of varying degrees of friction or mechanical trauma. Disorders range in severity from mild forms, in which the lesions are subtle and trivial, to more severe forms that are mutilating with multiorgan involvement that threatens both the length and quality of life. Estimates by the U.S. Department of Health and Human Services in 1984 state there are between 25,000 and 50,000 Americans with some form of EB. This estimate is thought to be low because many milder forms go unreported or undiagnosed. EB affects all races and both sexes.[60]

Etiology and Pathophysiology. The disorders of EB are divided into three classes based on the level in the skin where separation occurs to form the blister. This location usually correlates with the clinical findings. In the *epidermolytic* form, the blistering occurs in the lower layers of the epidermis but above the basement membrane zone (BMZ). This pathology explains the lack of scar formation in this group. In *junctional* EB, the skin separation takes place within the BMZ. In this group, skin atrophy may be seen in areas of healed lesions. In *dermolytic, dystrophic* EB, the blisters develop below the BMZ in the papillary dermis; scarring is prevalent and often debilitating.[16]

The EB disorders are further distinguished by the mode of inheritance, onset, distribution of lesions, degree of trauma required, and the intensity of the bullous reaction. Children with EB who present with lesions of the oral mucosa are most likely to have junctional or dystrophic forms of the disease.

Clinical Manifestations. Vesicles, bullae, and erosions are the primary clinical manifestations of EB (see Table 65-2). The sites of involvement, extent of blistering, and presence of atrophy or scarring vary with the different types of EB. Epidermolytic EB variants may have mild to severe involvement but do not tend to be scarring. Sites affected may include extremities (particularly hands and feet), nails, and oral mucosa. In junctional EB variants, extremities, nails, hair, teeth, mucosa, and systemic organs may be affected. Depending on the number of skin sites and organs involved, prognosis varies, but dermolytic EB variants have the poorest prognosis, with the possibility of scarring and contractures. These forms of EB may be widespread and debilitating, drastically affecting the child's expected life span.

Diagnostic Studies. The presence of EB is diagnosed based on the clinical features exhibited by the child. However, to determine the particular variant of EB, a skin biopsy with electron microscopy and immunofluorescence mapping to the dermal–epidermal junction is necessary.[60] Microscopic or macroscopic vesicles may be induced by using the Nikolsky technique (see Chap. 64). This procedure may be done in the biopsy area just before obtaining the biopsy.

Prenatal diagnosis has been successful in some cases. Fetal biopsy by fetoscopy at 17 to 20 weeks' gestation is beginning to play a significant role in the diagnosis of EB.[60]

A hoarse cry is a reliable feature to distinguish between the junctional form of EB and the less severe dystrophic forms in the first weeks of life. The hoarse cry signals laryngeal involvement. The major cause of death occurs from tracheal strictures in junctional EB during the first 2 years of life.[16]

★ ASSESSMENT

Information is obtained regarding the presence of EB in other family members. The entire skin surface and mucous membranes should be examined for the presence of blisters and scarring. Evidence of corneal clouding, fusions of the fingers and toes, delayed tooth eruption, malformed teeth, alopecia, and abnormal nails are noted during the skin exam. Weight and height are measured and documented. Families are assessed for understanding of the disease process and treatment, as well as their coping skills and support systems.

★ NURSING DIAGNOSES AND PLANNING

Based on assessment data from above and Chapter 64, the following nursing diagnoses may apply to the family and child with EB:

- High Risk for Injury (Trauma) related to skin disorder.
- Interrupted Breastfeeding related to oral trauma.
- Altered Nutrition: Less than Body Requirements related to inability to ingest food.
- Sensory/Perceptual Alterations (Tactile, Gustatory) related to altered environmental stimuli.
- Body Image Disturbance related to recurrent blisters.
- Altered Family Processes related to protection and care of child.

The nurse, child, and parents together plan effective care based on the established nursing diagnoses. Several examples of expected outcomes follow:

- The family touches and cuddles the infant.
- The family performs daily care of the newborn in the hospital.
- The family demonstrates understanding of the principles of skin and wound care.
- The family participates in planning a safe home environment for the growing child.

The nurse plans for the daily care of the child based on both physician's orders and nursing diagnoses. Some general nursing care goals include the following:

- Trauma is avoided.
- Complications are avoided.
- Child's nutritional needs are met.
- Family is informed about the disease, treatments, and available resources.

★ INTERVENTIONS: COLLABORATIVE AND INDEPENDENT

The types of EB that exhibit multiorgan system problems require a multidisciplinary approach. The profound effect of the birth of a child with EB on the family must not be overlooked. Psychosocial, educational, rehabilitative, and genetic counseling must be provided. The amounts and types of therapies given to a child with EB and the family depend on the child's particular variant of EB.

CARE OF NEONATES AND INFANTS

For neonates, trauma avoidance begins immediately by removing any source of mechanical trauma, such as identification bands. The infants are handled carefully, lifting them by supporting the back of their heads and buttocks, not under their arms. Rubbing is avoided. Instead, cleansing of the skin is accomplished by soaking and compressing. Dressings are secured with soft fleece or gauze bandages. Flotation mattresses and sheepskin, soft blankets, and loose, nonrestrictive clothing are used. Axillary temperatures are taken.

Wound care is directed at promotion of healing and prevention of infection. Bullae are punctured carefully with a sterile scalpel or iris scissors using a crescent incision. This procedure allows release of the fluid but keeps the blister roof intact. The areas are covered with petrolatum gauze or mupirocin and telfa. Dry, adherent dressings are avoided. If necessary, dressings are removed by soaking in warm water.

Because of the increased protein loss with large denuded areas and wound healing demands, these infants require twice the basal requirements of caloric intake as compared to the normal neonate. For formula feeding, a cool formula with a small nipple or rubber-tipped syringe is used. Breast-feeding is encouraged unless the baby's mouth is severely affected. Formula may be added for supplement of protein, carbohydrates, vitamins, and iron. Nasogastric feedings are avoided due to the risk of injury to the mucous membrane with insertion of the nasogastric tube.

Antibiotics are used for control of infection. Analgesics for pain, and antihistamines for suppression of pruritus are also used periodically when needed. Topical medications such as mupirocin, parfenac, glutaraldehyde, and aluminum chloride are used as adjunctive treatments. Mupirocin has replaced other topical antibiotics, proving to be a more effective and safe topical therapy for patients with long-standing EB erosions and ulcers.[60] Glutaraldehyde and aluminum chloride are used to decrease friction and, therefore, blister formation on the hands and feet. Parfenac is a nonsteroidal antiinflammatory topical treatment.

DISCHARGE PLANNING

The family of an infant with EB should be involved in the baby's care from the first day to prepare them for the enormous task of caring for the child at home. They must understand the pathologic process of EB, the principles of skin and wound care, the nutritional requirements, and how to meet the emotional needs of both the infant and themselves. The family may be afraid to handle the infant for fear they will induce blister formation, thereby depriving the infant of much-needed tactile stimulation.

The burden of providing time-consuming care, fear of leaving the child in someone else's care, and anxiety associated with public ridicule due to the child's appearance places considerable stress on the family. Support and counseling are vital for maintaining the family integrity and promoting the growth and development of the child. The Dystrophic Epidermolysis Bullosa Research Association (DEBRA) of America, Inc., provides emotional support and guidance to families. The National Epidermolysis Bullosa Registry is a data collecting and coordinating center that also can be a resource for families. Genetic counseling should begin when a definitive diagnosis is made, to assist the family in future family planning.

TRAUMA PREVENTION

When the child goes home from the hospital and as he or she grows, measures must be taken to maintain skin integrity and prevent injury. Loose, soft clothing in a jumper style and soft canvas shoes with double socks are the most comfortable and easy on the skin. Overheating is avoided, and, if sweaty feet are a problem, holes may be cut in the canvas to provide ventilation. When the child

begins to crawl, foam pads sewn into the clothing at the knees and elbows help to protect the skin. Hands may be covered with socks to prevent sucking on the fingers.

Environmental control is necessary to avoid slipping and rough, sharp surfaces. Pads may be placed on beds, high chairs, walkers, and swings. Soft rubber or foam toys, mobiles, music, and conversation provide stimulation while minimizing injury. As children grow older and their range of activities widens, contact sports and activities that involve running should be avoided. Stretching and swimming activities provide exercise with a minimum of trauma. A cool environment is important because most forms of EB are exacerbated by increased ambient temperature.

NUTRITIONAL MANAGEMENT

Providing adequate nutrition poses a challenge both to the health care team and the family. Oral, dental, and esophageal sequelae can include oral strictures and scarring with microstomia, tooth enamel loss, esophageal strictures, and obstruction. Nutritional assessment and interventions may be one method for improving morbidity and mortality associated with this disease.

The pain and discomfort associated with mucosal lesions make it difficult to consume a solid diet. Meals that begin and end with cool, soft, palatable food, such as Jello, pudding, ice cream, or sherbet, ease this discomfort. Soft purees minimize mucosal trauma. Meals of this sort may need to be supplemented with high protein mixtures.

Oral hygiene measures are encouraged to decrease destruction of the teeth, a feature of severe junctional and dystrophic EB in children. After meals, care of the mouth and teeth includes the use of a moist cotton-tipped applicator and, at 1 to 2 years, a short-handled, multitufted, soft toothbrush or a pulsating water device designed for teeth cleaning. Comprehensive periodontal care is mandatory. Parents should be warned about the dental hazards of prolonged bottle feeding with sugary solutions and the dangers of sugary snacks and drinks between meals.

★ EVALUATION

Periodically, the nurse and family evaluate the outcomes of care given. Examples of outcomes for the child and family with epidermolysis bullosa were given under planning in this section. Have short-term goals been met? Are long-term goals still realistic? Planning for further nursing care takes into consideration complications and long-term care.

COMPLICATIONS

Prognosis in EB depends on the variety and severity of the disease. In nonscarring forms of EB, blisters become less severe with age. However, in the severe scarring forms, disability and disfigurement can be extensive and may cause death during infancy or childhood. The complications associated with EB are many and are listed in the accompanying display.

LONG-TERM CARE

The effectiveness of the therapeutic measures to prevent blistering, infection, and scarring, and to promote wound healing and comfort is evaluated. The family is reassessed

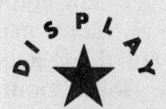

Complications of Epidermolysis Bullosa

Nonhealing erosions resulting in:
  Loss of blood and protein
  Malabsorption and difficulty eating
  Malnourishment
  Anemia
  Growth retardation
Infection
Scarring resulting in:
  Joint contractures
  Oral strictures
  Esophageal webbing, obstruction, perforation
  Airway obstruction
  Auditory canal stenosis
  Genitourinary obstruction

Squamous cell carcinoma
Otitis externa
Tooth enamel loss
Corneal, globe, and conjunctival ulceration resulting in:
  Symblepharon
  Ectropion
  Duct obstruction

for understanding necessary skin care measures and incorporating these measures into their daily routines. The nurse should determine if the family has developed effective coping strategies and support systems. Referral for rehabilitative and psychosocial services may be needed by the child and family. It is the responsibility of the nurse to ensure that communication channels are established and maintained among the various disciplines caring for a child with EB.

Papulosquamous Disorders

The term *papulosquamous disorder* refers to a group of inflammatory conditions of the skin characterized by a papular or raised quality with a squamous or scaling component. The most common disorders of this group include atopic dermatitis (AD), seborrheic dermatitis, contact dermatitis, psoriasis, and pityriasis rosea. Dermatitis represents the majority of papulosquamous diseases seen in infants and children.

Dermatitis simply means inflammation of the skin. A modifying adjective is added to specify the particular type based on the pattern of distribution or etiologic factor, such as AD, contact dermatitis, or diaper dermatitis.

Atopic Dermatitis

Definition and Incidence.   Atopic dermatitis is a genetically determined disorder of unknown etiology. (The term *eczema* is used by much of the general public to describe this disorder.) AD is defined as a chronic skin disorder characterized by red itchy skin and frequent exacerbations associated with elevated IgE levels and a personal or family history of AD, allergic rhinitis, and/or asthma.

AD is seen most frequently in infancy and childhood with decreasing incidence in adolescence and adulthood. The exact incidence is difficult to estimate. AD affects males and females equally and is particularly common in white and Asian children. It is also more common in highly industrialized countries.[41]

Etiology and Pathophysiology.   The cause of AD is unknown, but it is thought to have a strong genetic component. A child has a 60% chance of developing AD if one parent exhibits atopy and an 80% chance if both parents are affected. In comparison, the incidence of AD in nonatopic families is only 19%.[41] The immunologic component is not clear and continues to be debated. AD has both humoral and cell-mediated immunity aspects. Children with AD have elevated serum IgE levels, and these elevated levels may be directed to a wide variety of antigens including common pollens, molds, foods, and insects.

Histamine is thought to be the main chemical released in the various reactions in AD. The release of histamine causes pruritus, inhibits chemotaxis, and depresses T cell production.[41] By producing pruritus and erythema, histamine is the initiator of the itch–scratch cycle that produces the eczematous lesions.

Children with AD have a higher staphylococcal colony count on both involved and uninvolved skin when compared to children with psoriasis or the normal population.[41] The higher colony counts increase their risk for developing cutaneous infections.

Clinical Manifestations.   AD is a disease of continually changing cutaneous manifestations with periods of exacerbations and remissions. The most important symptom and the major cause of morbidity is pruritus. Many of the child's activities, as well as sleep, are interrupted by itching. The constant rubbing and scratching to relieve the itch are responsible for many clinical changes seen in the skin.

The clinical signs most characteristics of AD include extremely dry and sensitive skin, erythema, lichenification, excoriations, hyperpigmentation or hypopigmentation, vesicles, pustules, and crusting. There are three distinct clinical phases of AD based on the age of the patient and the distribution of the skin lesions. These phases may overlap or they may be separated by a period of remission. The *infantile phase*, which extends from birth to 2 years of age, is characterized by the skin eruption appearing on the cheeks and lateral aspects of the lower arms and legs. The diaper area is usually clear. The lesions are symmetric, erythematous papules or patches and may be accompanied by exudate and crusting. The hair is often dry with scaling in the scalp. In the *childhood phase*, the skin lesions are most often found in the antecubital and popliteal areas with the neck and flexures of the wrists and ankles frequently involved. In this phase, the more chronic features of AD are seen, such as excoriations and lichenification. The fingernails may become shiny and buffed from constant rubbing. Finally, in the *adult phase*, which starts at puberty, the clinical signs become redistributed involving the body more diffusely with more scaling and less exudate.

Seasonal variation is often observed. The low humidity and cold temperatures of winter most often cause flare-ups. However, summer heat and sweating cause exacerbations in some children, and others have more trouble when pollen counts are high in the spring or fall.

Various skin lesions are also typically seen in association, although not exclusively, with AD. Hyperkeratotic follicular papules called *keratosis pilaris* are seen on the extensor aspect of the upper arm or thighs as well as the cheeks. The lesions are asymptomatic but produce a rough texture to the skin when rubbed. *Pityriasis alba*, or hypopigmented, dry patches with fine scale, are seen on the face, arms, legs, and occasionally on the trunk. Pityriasis alba tends to be more prominent in darker pigmented children. Hyperlinear palms and soles frequently occur in children with AD. Atopic pleats under the eyes of children with AD, caused by inflammation, are called *Dennie-Morgan folds*. *Lichen spinulosus* are round pruritic patches of grouped hyperkeratotic papules found scattered on the trunk of children with AD. *White dermatographism* (see Chap. 64) is thought to be a diagnostic feature of AD and appears to be due to vasoconstriction of the skin vessels.

Seborrheic Dermatitis

Definition and Incidence. Seborrheic dermatitis occurs in young infants and adolescents. It is an erythematous eruption with a greasy scale that occurs predominantly in areas of greatest sebaceous activity, such as the scalp, face, postauricular, presternal, and intertriginous areas. It is usually a benign, trivial disease; yet, in rare cases, its presence can signal histiocytosis-X, Leiner's disease, or acquired immunodeficiency syndrome (AIDS).[41] Seborrheic dermatitis is often confused with AD but has a much better prognosis. Distinguishing between the two conditions is important.

Etiology and Pathophysiology. The cause and pathogenesis of seborrheic dermatitis are unknown. The name implies a role of sebum. However, no increase of sebum production is associated with the eruption. The age of occurrence suggests a role for maternal or pubes-

cent hormones, but there is no evidence to support this theory.[41]

Clinical Manifestations. In infants, the eruption begins during the first month of life. The first manifestation is often "cradle cap," a diffuse, tenacious, yellowish scale on the vertex of the scalp. The eruption is asymptomatic and often spreads to involve areas behind the ears, neck, and axillae. Commonly, well-demarcated, scaly, erythematous patches coexist in the inguinoanal region. The intertriginous areas may become macerated and superinfected with *Candida.* In severe cases, the face and trunk also may become involved.

In adolescence, seborrheic dermatitis usually begins on the scalp and is commonly referred to as "dandruff." In more severe cases, the condition is accompanied by erythema, pruritus, and greasy hair. Sites of further involvement may include the eyebrows and paranasal, auricular, presternal, infrascapular, and pubic regions.

Seborrheic dermatitis is differentiated from AD by its early onset, lack of pruritus and stigma of atopy, the greasy yellowish scale, well-circumscribed nature of the lesions, and its predisposition for the scalp and intertriginous areas.

Contact Dermatitis

Definition and Incidence. Contact dermatitis is an inflammation of the skin that results from contact with any of a variety of natural or manufactured substances. When these substances contact the skin, they may provoke a primary irritation reaction (irritant contact dermatitis) or an allergic delayed-type hypersensitivity reaction (allergic contact dermatitis). **Diaper dermatitis** is the most common type of irritant contact dermatitis in childhood.

Allergic contact dermatitis is not diagnosed as frequently as irritant contact dermatitis in children. Contact responsiveness seems to mature somewhat slowly with age. Children younger than 5 years of age generally are less contact-sensitive. Even preteens are not as likely as teenagers or adults to develop allergic contact dermatitis. Dermatitic skin, in general, is more permeable to allergens, and, thus, children with conditions such as AD are more susceptible to developing allergic contact dermatitis.

Irritant Contact Dermatitis

Etiology and Pathophysiology. Irritant contact dermatitis results from disruption of the physiologic barrier properties of the stratum corneum and the development of an inflammatory reaction in the skin. The resulting reaction depends on the constitutional composition of the person and the strength of the offending substance. It may develop after the initial exposure to primary irritants, such as lye, gasoline, turpentine, or paint remover, that are strong enough to cause a demonstrable reaction and actual physical damage to the skin. These strong primary irritants tend to affect almost everyone. Mild irritants, such as soaps, bleaches, and other cleansers, affect fewer people. Often, repeated exposure to these substances is required before an inflammatory response develops. Any substance can act as an irritant provided the concentration and the length of exposure are sufficient.

Practically no infant escapes the diaper years without an occasional bout of diaper dermatitis. Several factors have been associated with the development of diaper dermatitis. The frequency of diaper rash relates to the age of the infant, with the rash occurring more frequently in the latter part of the first year of life. Diet also may be an important factor in the etiology of diaper dermatitis. It is believed that breast-fed babies experience less diaper rash than formula-fed infants, although the clinical data supporting this conclusion are limited. A higher frequency of intestinal carriage of *Candida albicans* is seen in infants with active diaper rash and has been strongly associated with the more severe forms of diaper dermatitis. Finally, the frequency and duration of contact of the infant's skin to excreta have an impact on the incidence and severity of diaper dermatitis. Children with diarrhea are especially at risk for developing diaper dermatitis.

Clinical Manifestations. The typical skin lesion produced by an irritant reaction includes erythema, edema, vesiculation, erosions, and crusting. These lesions may be accompanied by pruritus, pain, or burning.

Diaper dermatitis results from irritation by urine, stool, and topical preparations as well as occlusion and friction. The reaction of erythema, edema, vesicles, and weeping involves the genitalia, perineum, buttocks, and may extend onto the thighs. Skin creases are usually spared. If the eruption is present long enough, the involved skin becomes secondarily infected. *Candida albicans* is the organism recovered most frequently in cultures of diaper dermatitis.

Allergic Contact Dermatitis

Etiology and Pathophysiology. Allergic contact dermatitis is a form of delayed hypersensitivity or cell-mediated immunity. Poison ivy is probably the most common offending agent in children. Other common sensitizers include paraphenlyenediamines (shoe dyes), nickel, cosmetics, and topical medications containing sulfonamides, antihistamines, or neomycin.

Clinical Manifestations. Development of the allergic reaction occurs in two phases. The *sensitization phase* occurs with exposure to the chemical or antigen, which must remain in contact with the skin for at least 18 to 24 hours. The antigen combines with a protein carrier on the membrane of a Langerhans cell and is presented to the T lymphocytes in the regional lymph nodes. The T lymphocytes become sensitized cells that react to that specific antigen. The *elicitation phase* occurs after reexposure of the skin to the allergen. The antigen again combines with the Langerhans cell, however, this time it is recognized by the sensitized T cells that are circulating through the body. A delayed hypersensitivity reaction is set in motion with the development of erythema, edema, and vesiculation. The reaction may be elicited as quickly as 6 to 24 hours or it may take up to 2 to 4 days to appear.[41] The skin involvement may be confined to the site of contact with the allergen, or a more generalized response

may be seen. The allergic reaction may first appear the second time the skin is exposed to the antigen or may not be seen until after numerous exposures.

Psoriasis

Definition and Incidence. Psoriasis is a chronic proliferative disease of the epidermis characterized by erythematous scaling papules and plaques frequently localized to areas such as the scalp, elbows, and knees. It may, however, generalize to involve any area of the skin surface including the nails. Although psoriasis is considered to be fairly uncommon in childhood, it is said to account for 4% of all dermatoses seen in pediatric patients under the age of 16 years.[10] Psoriasis is more common in whites and is much less common in African Americans, Asian-Americans, and North and South American Indians.

Etiology and Pathophysiology. The etiology and pathogenesis of psoriasis remain unclear. Genetic factors are thought to be involved in the development of psoriasis. This belief is supported by the tendency for psoriasis to run in families.[10] However, genetics appears to be only one factor of many.

The skin lesions of psoriasis result from hyperproliferation of keratinocytes. In psoriasis, the keratinocyte reaches the outer layer of the epidermis as quickly as 3 days after it is initially formed in the stratum basale. Hyperproliferation and short transit time accounts for the large amount of scales and poor barrier qualities of the affected skin.

Clinical Manifestations. Several forms of psoriasis exist. The classic is *psoriasis vulgaris* or plaque-type psoriasis. The skin lesion is an asymptomatic or pruritic erythematous plaque with silvery-white scales. It is well-demarcated from surrounding normal-appearing skin. When the scale is removed, pinpoint areas of bleeding are seen (Auspitz sign). This type of psoriasis is commonly seen on the elbows, knees, and scalp. However, it may be widely distributed on the skin surface. Involvement of the intertriginous areas, palms, and soles is common. In infants, the diaper area is generally involved.

Guttate (droplike) psoriasis is a form seen most often in children and young adults. Skin spots may be the first manifestation of psoriasis in a child and characteristically occurs a few weeks after a streptococcal upper respiratory infection. The eruption appears abruptly with multiple small, erythematous scaling papules and plaques that are often pruritic and spread to a generalized distribution.

Pustular psoriasis is seen less frequently in children. This form of psoriasis tends to have an abrupt onset and is associated with systemic symptoms, such as elevated temperature, chills, and generalized malaise. Initially, children complain of tender, burning skin. Crops of multiple sterile pustules appear along with intense pruritus. Considerable mortality is associated with widespread pustular psoriasis.

Erythrodermic psoriasis is also associated with considerable mortality. It is seen more often in adults than in children.

Psoriatic arthritis is an inflammatory erosive joint disorder seen in a few children with psoriasis. Joint involvement is often asymmetric. Patients usually complain of pain, stiffness, and swelling in the distal interphalangeal joints of the hands and feet. Tendon sheath involvement and sausage digits are common. Many children are initially misdiagnosed as having juvenile rheumatoid arthritis; however, in psoriatic arthritis the rheumatoid factor is absent in the serum. Disease activity in children is intermittent and appears to regress with time. Long-term prognosis is usually good, with minimal or no permanent joint derangement.

Nail involvement occurs in 25% to 50% of children with psoriasis.[41] The most common manifestation is pitting of the nail plate. Other changes include yellowish-brown spots (also called oil-spots) beneath the nail plate, onycholysis, and subungual hyperkeratosis. Complete loss of the nail may occur during times of acute flaring of the psoriasis.

The *koebner response* is a reaction to various traumatic insults to the skin resulting in the eruption of psoriatic lesions at the site of injury. Injuries such as sunburn, abrasions, removal of adhesive tape, excoriations, lacerations, and venipuncture have all been cited as causes of the Koebner reaction in psoriasis. Other papulosquamous disorders may exhibit this same reaction.

Pityriasis Rosea

Definition and Incidence.   Pityriasis rosea (PR) is a benign, acute, inflammatory skin disorder. The pediatric age group makes up approximately 45% of all cases, with most cases occurring in the winter months.[10]

Etiology and Pathophysiology.   PR lacks a definite, identified etiology. Because it is acute, self-limited, and frequently associated with prodromal symptoms such as headache, malaise, and pharyngitis, most clinicians attribute it to a viral infection. The low rate of recurrence also seems to favor an infectious etiology.

Clinical Manifestations.   The initial presentation of PR is generally with the development of a solitary, annular, erythematous scaly lesion called a *herald patch*. Within 1 week, many smaller, scaly lesions develop on the trunk, extremities, and neck. The distribution of the skin lesions is symmetric, often following the lines of skin cleavage exhibiting the characteristic "Christmas tree" appearance on the posterior trunk. Pruritus is associated in varying degrees, or the lesions may be asymptomatic. In general, children feel well and go about their normal life routines, bothered mostly by the cosmetic appearance of their skin. Treatment is generally limited to symptomatic treatment for the pruritus.

Care in Papulosquamous Disorders

Diagnostic Studies.   Diagnosis of papulosquamous diseases is generally made by obtaining the history and observing the characteristic skin eruption. Laboratory testing is seldom required unless complications or other systemic disorders are suspected. Bacterial, viral, or fungal cultures may be obtained if infection is suspected. A skin biopsy may be needed if the eruption does not respond to usual therapeutic intervention. Allergy testing in AD has been shown to be of little benefit. Patch testing in contact dermatitis can be helpful in identification of the offending allergen (see Chap. 64).

★ ASSESSMENT

Nursing assessment in papulosquamous conditions includes obtaining a history of the skin eruption and associated symptoms. The presence of a positive family history of similar conditions, asthma, allergies, and arthritis is also noted. It is common for the parents to have previously treated the skin before seeking medical attention. The nurse should question parents regarding previous remedies used and their effect on the skin.

Physical examination focuses on the types of cutaneous lesions, their distribution, and pattern. The distribution and lesion pattern are important keys in differentiating among the various papulosquamous disorders. In AD, the areas most easily reached by the child to scratch have the most involvement, and areas covered by clothing are less involved. Contact dermatitis and irritant dermatitis usually begin at the point of contact with the antigen or irritant substance. For instance, the initial lesion of poison ivy is often a linear streak where the leaf brushed against the skin. In AD, the diaper area is often spared, unlike seborrheic, irritant dermatitis, or psoriasis. Scalp involvement is seen in seborrheic dermatitis and psoriasis with thick scaling and erythema. AD in the scalp is less common and tends to have fine scaling. Facial involvement differs in that the cheeks are usually involved in AD compared to forehead and eyebrow involvement in seborrheic dermatitis.

In addition to the history and physical examination, it is important to assess the impact of the disorder, especially if it is chronic, on the child's sleep, play, and social interactions. Parents are also questioned on their ability to cope and the impact the disorder is having on family life.

★ NURSING DIAGNOSES AND PLANNING

Based on assessment data from above and Chapter 64, the following nursing diagnoses may apply to the family and child with papulosquamous disorders:

- Impaired Skin Integrity related to scratching.
- High Risk for Infection related to traumatized tissue.
- Sleep Pattern Disturbance related to nocturnal pruritus.
- Self-Esteem Disturbance related to appearance of skin.
- Impaired Social Interaction related to self-concept.
- Ineffective Family Coping: Compromised related to chronic skin condition.
- Anxiety related to knowledge deficit regarding disease process and treatment plan.

The nurse and child (or parents) together plan effective care based on the established nursing diagnoses. Several examples of expected outcomes follow:

- The parents demonstrate their understanding of recommended bathing and skin care.

- The parents state child is finding relief from itching.
- The child discusses embarrassing situations and possible solutions.
- The child states he or she has found a developmental area in which to excel.

The nurse plans for the care of the child based on both physician's orders and nursing diagnoses. Some general nursing care goals may be the following:

- Skin heals.
- Medications are used safely.
- Inflammation and pruritus are controlled.
- Infection is prevented.

★ INTERVENTIONS: COLLABORATIVE AND INDEPENDENT

Good patient/parent education coupled with a carefully designed treatment plan is fundamental to effective management of a child with a papulosquamous disorder. Most children with these disorders are treated on an outpatient basis, which requires active involvement of the parent. However, because these disorders are relatively common, they are often seen in children hospitalized for other reasons. Although the intervention techniques outlined below focus on outpatient care, they are also applicable to the hospitalized child. The accompanying display outlines the interventions in papulosqamous disorders.

HYDRATION

Hydration of the skin is thought to be the key to treatment of papulosquamous disorders.[51] Children with AD lack water in their skin, not oil. One way to hydrate the skin is to soak in plain lukewarm bath water for 15 to 20 minutes. Another way is to apply a wet wrap of tap water–soaked soft cloths or clothing to the skin followed by dry clothing or a plastic sweat suit to slow evaporation.[51] The room temperature is kept warm to prevent chilling. Socks and tubular dressings can be used to secure the wet wrap

to the head, hands, and feet. After the bath or wet wrap, an occlusive emollient is applied while the skin is still damp.

RELIEF OF PRURITUS

Pruritus is a common and often intense symptom associated with papulosquamous disorders. In chronic conditions such as AD and psoriasis, itching can be particularly detrimental because it interferes with the child's ability to concentrate and sleep. Frequently, this symptom is the most frustrating part of the illness for the child and parent. An itchy child is often impossible to satisfy, fussy, and irritable. Antihistamines may be prescribed and are particularly useful at night when the pruritus tends to be the most intense and the usual daily distractions are not present. Unfortunately, antihistamines are not a good option for school-age children because of their sedative effects. Keeping the child cool while sleeping helps to reduce the itching. Because of the damage to the skin caused by scratching, the child's nails are kept short and may be covered with socks or gloves at night. In severe cases, where antihistamines are not effective, a short-acting sedative may be temporarily prescribed.

PREVENTION OF INFECTION

Infection is the most common complication of papulosquamous skin disease. Prevention is accomplished by keeping the skin clean and intact. The vast majority of infections are caused by *Staphylococcus aureus*. In mild cases, the topical antibiotic mupirocin may be prescribed; however, systemic antibiotic therapy is most effective with a quicker response.

MEDICATION THERAPY

Topical corticosteroids are frequently prescribed for their ability to reduce inflammation and pruritus. These medications are available in a wide range of strengths and vehicles (Table 65-3). Topical corticosteroids are used on an as-needed basis. They are applied in a thin layer once or twice daily to the involved areas and discontinued once the eruption subsides. Due to the side effects of skin thinning with the development of skin fragility and striae, topical corticosteroids are used cautiously and restricted to low to midpotency prescriptions in children. These side effects occur more frequently in areas where the skin is the thinnest, such as the face, axillae, and groin. Only low-potency corticosteroids are used in these sites. In most children, an ointment preparation is preferred because of its occlusive qualities. Occasionally, another vehicle is chosen for sites such as the scalp or intertriginous areas or when a more drying quality is desired.

Systemic steroids are generally not used in the treatment of chronic conditions such as AD or psoriasis. In these conditions, their use is restricted to severe, incapacitating exacerbations. In severe contact dermatitis with widespread involvement, a tapering course of prednisone over 14 to 21 days is prescribed. If a shorter course is prescribed, the lesions tend to rebound.

Scaling in the scalp occurs frequently in papulosquamous disorders, especially in seborrheic dermatitis and psoriasis. Antiseborrheic shampoos containing pyrithione zinc, selenium, salicylic acid, or tar may be used to facilitate removal of the scale. Presoftening of the scale

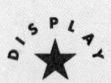

Nursing Interventions in Papulosquamous Disorders

- Hydrate and protect skin
  - Plain lukewarm water bathing
  - Oral fluid hydration
  - Occlusive emollients
- Control pruritus
  - Antihistamines
  - Topical steroids
  - Hydration
- Control infection
  - Lukewarm water soaks
  - Topical or systemic antibiotics
  - Topical antifungals
- Reduce inflammation
  - Topical glucocorticosteroids
  - Avoidance of irritating substances

TABLE 65-3
Topical Glucocorticosteroids

Potency	Name	Vehicle	Strength
Super Potent I	Temovate (clobetasol propionate)	Ointment/cream	0.05%
	Diprolene (betamethasone dipropionate)	Ointment/cream	0.05%
	Psorcon (diflorasone diacetate)	Ointment	0.05%
Potent II	Cyclocort (amcinonide)	Ointment	0.1%
	Diprosone (betamethasone dipropionate)	Ointment	0.05%
	Florone (diflorasone diacetate)	Ointment	0.05%
	Maxiflor (diflorasone diacetate)	Ointment	0.05%
	Lidex (fluocinonide)	Ointment/cream/gel	0.05%
	Topicort (desoximetasone)	Ointment/cream/gel	0.25%
	Maxivate (betamethasone dipropionate)	Ointment	0.05%
	Halog (halcinonide)	Cream	0.1%
III	Aristocort A (triamcinolone acetonide)	Ointment	0.1%
	Valisone (betamethasone valerate)	Ointment	0.1%
	Diprosone (betamethasone dipropionate)	Cream	0.05%
	Florone (diflorasone diacetate)	Cream	0.05%
	Maxiflor (diflorasone diacetate)	Cream	0.05%
	Maxivate (betamethasone dipropionate)	Cream	0.05%
Midpotent IV	Synalar (fluocinolone acetonide)	Ointment	0.025%
	Cordran (flurandrenolide)	Ointment	0.05%
	Westcort (hydrocortisone valerate)	Ointment	0.2%
	Aristocort (triamcinolone acetonide)	Ointment	0.1%
	Kenalog (triamcinolone acetonide)	Ointment	0.1%
	Topicort LP (desoximetasone)	Cream	0.05%
V	Elocon (mometasone furoate)	Ointment/cream	0.1%
	Cordran (flurandrenolide)	Cream	0.05%
	Synalar (fluocinolone acetonide)	Cream	0.025%
	Valisone (betamethasone valerate)	Cream	0.1%
	Westcort (hydrocortisone valerate)	Cream	0.2%
	Aristocort (triamcinilone acetonide)	Cream/lotion	0.1%
	Kenalog (triamcinolone acetonide)	Cream	0.1%
	Diprosone (betamethasone dipropionate)	Lotion	0.2%
Low Potent VI	Aclovate (alclometasone dipropionate)	Ointment/cream	0.05%
	DesOwen (desonide)	Cream	0.05%
	Tridesilon (desonide)	Ointment/cream	0.05%
	Valsone (betamethasone valerate)	Lotion	0.05%
	Synalar (fluocinolone acetonide)	Solution	0.01%
Very Low Potent VII	Hytone (hydrocortisone)	Ointment/cream/lotion	1% 2.5%
	Nutracort (hydrocortisone)	Cream/lotion	1% 2.5%
	Hexadrol (dexamethasone)	Cream	0.04%
	Medrol (methylprednisolone acetate)	Ointment	0.25%
	Metiderm (prednisone)	Cream	0.5%
VIII	Cortaid (hydrocortisone)	Cream	0.5%

with oil and salicylic acid or salicylic acid gel followed by shampooing may be necessary in more severe cases.

Tar preparations, particularly in an oil or ointment vehicle, frequently are used to treat psoriasis and also may be helpful in AD. Tar in combination with ultraviolet B (UVB) radiation has been helpful in treating childhood psoriasis. This treatment method is referred to as the Goeckerman regimen. The tar preparation is applied to the skin for 6 to 8 hours and then washed off. This process is followed by exposure to ultraviolet light (UVL) outdoors or in a specially designed light unit that emits UVB light, 290 to 320 nm. The use of a light unit is generally preferred because it permits careful control of the UVL dose and provides total body exposure. Side effects include cataracts with increased risk for skin cancer and wrinkling. Patients are advised to protect their eyes during UVL exposure with specially designed glasses and to protect their skin from UVL except during treatment.

The use of anthralin, a potent keratolytic and irritant, in the treatment of skin disease is limited to psoriasis. Short-contact therapy with application of 0.1% to 1% concentrations for 15 to 30 minutes and then washed off has been an effective therapeutic alternative. Careful application instructions are necessary because of the risk of skin irritation and staining.

Systemic therapies in psoriasis are reserved for the most severe cases. Psoralen plus ultraviolet A (PUVA) light therapy is not recommended for children under the age of 12 years. Methotrexate is used only under extreme conditions due to its hepatic and hematopoietic toxicity. Etretinate (Tegison), a retinoid, is also reserved for severe psoriasis due to its liver and bone effects.[58]

CARE DURING DIAPER USE

In diaper dermatitis, keeping the diaper area clean, dry, and protected is most important to promote healing and prevent the development of a diaper rash. Frequent diaper changes, as soon after soiling as possible, are followed by washing the diaper area with water and a mild soap. The area is allowed to dry before application of a zinc-oxide based ointment. Commercially premoistened towelettes should be avoided with inflamed skin. These preparations contain many preservatives and are heavily scented. Nonintact skin is at high risk for developing contact sensitivity to these common sensitizers. Mild topical steroids may be prescribed for 7 to 10 days in cases of severe dermatitis. If *Candida* infection is suspected, an antifungal agent also may be prescribed. Avoidance of talcum powder is generally recommended due to the risk of aspiration and powder's tendency to cake.

Controversy continues regarding the type of diaper and its effect on diaper dermatitis. A study conducted by Procter and Gamble showed that both the frequency and severity of diaper dermatitis were significantly lowered with the exclusive use of disposable diapers than with the use of only cloth diapers or a combination.[38] However, other studies have shown the opposite or that there is no difference between cloth or disposable diapers on diaper rash.[39] In another series of clinical studies also conducted by Procter and Gamble, increased bathing frequency and the use of zinc-oxide based ointments had a greater impact on reducing the incidence and severity of diaper rash than did diaper change frequency or type of diaper used.[39]

NUTRITIONAL MANAGEMENT

The role that diet plays in the treatment of papulosquamous disorders such as psoriasis and AD continues to be controversial. The significance of food allergens in AD is not known. Because of this controversy, the current recommendation is to avoid foods that appear to cause problems. If new foods are introduced, they should be introduced one at a time with sufficient time between to determine if there is any effect on the skin.

PSYCHOSOCIAL SUPPORT

The psychological and social impact of diseases such as AD and psoriasis can be significant. The discomfort and embarrassment caused by these diseases may have an impact on the personal development of the child and family relationships. The presence of disfiguring disease may interfere with the development of body image and self-esteem. By looking at and touching the child's skin without hesitation or awkwardness, the nurse can present a comforting and nonjudgmental attitude. Reviewing situations that caused embarrassment and suggesting behavioral alternatives for similar future situations increase the child's feelings of control over their lives. Helping and encouraging children to develop an area of expertise in which they can excel is a strategy for increasing self-esteem.

Parents are also in need of reassurance, support, understanding, and praise. It is important for them to realize that the feelings of anger, hopelessness, frustration, guilt, and incompetence are normal. It is also normal for parents to try to identify a cause for their child's problem and to feel an urgency for their child to be well.

The regimens outlined for treatment of these chronic skin conditions are complicated and time consuming. Reassurance and praise for both the child and the parent are necessary. The nurse should review with the family how the treatments can be incorporated into their daily routines causing minimal disruption. It is also important for the child and the parent to understand that even when they have put forth their best efforts in skin care, flares may still happen.

Individual and family counseling may be helpful for discovering how the illness is adversely affecting family life. It is also helpful in preadolescent and adolescent years when appearance and identity are so important. The Eczema Association and the National Psoriasis Foundation are resources to children and their families.

★ EVALUATION

Periodically, the nurse and family evaluate the outcomes of care given. Examples of outcomes for the child and family with papulosquamous dermatitis were given under planning in this section. Have short-term goals been met? Are long-term goals still realistic? Planning for further nursing care takes into consideration complications and long-term care.

COMPLICATIONS

Viral and bacterial skin infections are the most frequent complications associated with AD. The excoriations often produced by scratching to relieve pruritus interrupt the normal protective skin barrier allowing secondary infections to develop. *Staphylococci aureus* and group A beta-hemolytic streptococci are also a frequent culprit. The onset of infection is signaled by the development of serous exudate, crusting, and pustules. Secondary bacterial infection should be considered whenever a flare of AD develops or fails to respond to conservative therapy. The infection responds quickly to water soaks and systemic antibiotics.

An explosive vesicular eruption in a child with AD

may signal the development of **eczema herpeticum**. This condition occurs when a child with AD contracts herpes simplex from close contact with a playmate or family member who has a cold sore on the lips or any other herpetic lesion. The eruption usually begins with the development of vesicles in the areas of eczema and quickly spreads to normal skin. Depending on the extent of involvement, compresses, systemic antibiotics, fluid and electrolyte management, and use of IV acyclovir may be necessary.

In addition to secondary infection by bacteria and herpes simplex virus (HSV), children with AD appear to have a tendency to develop verrucae, molluscum, and tinea infections.

Complications in the remaining papulosquamous diseases are mainly attributed to secondary infection due to the lack of skin integrity. However, because most of these conditions are chronic, exacerbations are common. In infants, if seborrheic dermatitis is not treated, it tends to resolve spontaneously by the age of 8 to 12 months. However, it has a tendency for chronicity and recurrence in adolescents.

LONG-TERM CARE

Because recurrence is common, the nurse should determine if the child and family are aware that the problem may return, of possible exacerbating factors, and what measures to take for early treatment. The nurse should take note of how the child feels about him or herself and how the child interacts socially.

Fortunately, most children with AD tend to experience improvement of their condition with age. Over 50% of infants and toddlers with AD clear by the age of 2, and the skin eruptions usually do not recur. Of the remaining 50%, one half of the children clear by adolescence; in the rest, AD usually persists into adulthood.[41]

Skin Infections

Skin infections are common reasons for parents to seek medical care for their children. In addition to serving as a primary site for infection, the skin often exhibits early warning signs for life-threatening systemic infection.

The microflora of the skin can be divided into three groups (see the accompanying display). The *resident* skin flora includes a fairly small number of organisms that are found regularly on the skin and are not easily removed. These organisms can take up residence, multiply, and survive on the skin. The *transient* flora is a much larger group of organisms that are deposited on the skin from the environment. These microorganisms do not proliferate and are easily removed by washing the area. In the normal host, neither resident nor transient flora cause skin infections. However, these organisms have been blamed for "opportunistic" infections in debilitated or immunocompromised patients. *Pathogenic* flora are found on the skin when placed there by some external or internal source. A disruption of the normal skin defense mechanisms allows these organisms to take up residence and establish an infection. Although the distinction among the kinds of microbes in each of these categories is somewhat arbitrary, and clinically significant infections may be

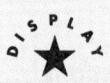

Microflora of the Skin

RESIDENT MICROFLORA

Staphylococcus epidermidis
Propionibacterium acnes
A diverse group of aerobic diphtheroids
Malassezia ovalis (Pityrosporon ovale)

TRANSIENT MICROFLORA

Gram-negative microorganisms derived from fecal microflora
Sarcina species

PATHOGENIC MICROFLORA

Staphylococcus aureus
Streptococcus pyogenes

caused by organisms considered nonpathogens, the distinction is useful as a general guide.

Bacterial Skin Infections

Bacterial infections, common during childhood, can be divided into five categories:

- Gram-positive bacterial infections
- Gram-negative bacterial infections
- Rickettsial infections
- Cutaneous tuberculosis
- Hansen's disease (leprosy)

Gram-positive bacteria are the most frequent pathogens in children's skin infections, followed by gram-negative bacterial infections and rickettsial infections. Cutaneous tuberculosis and Hansen's disease are rare and are not included in this discussion.

Etiology and Pathophysiology. Infection of the skin by bacteria depends on several factors affecting both the host and the bacterial organism. These factors are listed in the accompanying display. By maintaining a dry, intact epidermal barrier, normal competitive microflora, and regular epidermal shedding, the skin contributes to the host's defenses.

Several pathogenic properties of the microorganism influence the development of skin infections. Certain virulent organisms, such as pneumococcus, are able to multiply rapidly and resist phagocytosis. The ability of the bacteria to produce toxins also assists in their ability to grow in and invade tissue. The skin environment and nutritional requirements also influence the development of a skin infection. Skin microorganisms need warm temperatures, high humidity, and abundant nutrients to grow. Thus, the microbial counts are highest in body folds such as the gluteal cleft, axillae, nail folds, and toe webs.

How the organism reaches the involved area influ-

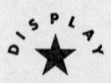

Factors Influencing the Development of Skin Infections

Virulence of the bacteria
Portal of inoculation
Presence or absence of competitive local microflora
Nutritional requirements for bacterial growth
Ability of the bacteria to produce toxins
Dry, intact epidermal barrier
Normal process of skin desquamation
Presence of sebum
Nutritional status of the host
Immunocompetence of the host

ences the clinical signs of infection. Local inflammation and pus formation are the initial signs of a direct bacterial invasion of the skin. When the bacteria is carried to the skin by way of the vascular system, inflammatory changes in and around blood vessels produce petechiae, purpura, and vasculitis.

Newborn skin is essentially sterile at birth and develops a flora population comparable to that of an adult by the age of 6 weeks. Cutaneous infection in the neonate is due to *Staphylococcus aureus* in the vast majority of cases. The circumcision site in males and the umbilical stump in both sexes provide fertile environments for colonization of *Staphylococcus aureus*.

As a child grows older, other predisposing factors increase the risk of developing skin infections. Insect bites, burns, wounds, cuts, and maceration damage the skin or render it less capable of coping with microbial invasion. Illness producing edematous limbs and immunosuppression or requiring insertion of various indwelling catheters and the use of drugs such as systemic and topical steroids, place a child at increased risk for skin infection.

The gram-positive organisms, *Streptococcus pyogenes* and *Staphylococcus aureus,* are the two most important pathogenic skin microorganisms causing skin infections in children (Table 65-4). They account for many primary pyodermas and are frequent secondary invaders of injured skin in conditions such as AD, psoriasis, and contact dermatitis. The basic pattern of staphylococcal infection is localized and circumscribed individual lesions, whereas skin invasion by streptococci produces a spreading cellulitis and early lymphatic involvement.[30]

The primary streptococcal pyodermas are due almost exclusively to group A beta-hemolytic streptococci (GABHS). These bacteria are unable to survive on intact skin and require at least superficial damage to the stratum corneum to take hold and proliferate. The hallmarks of GABHS infection are profuse edema, rapid spread in the tissue, and the relatively thin exudative response.[30]

Streptococcal infection is spread by close person-to-person contact. People with GABHS skin infections may harbor the same organism in their pharynx, which is often the source for spread of the infection. Infection may also

spread to the skin by way of the lymphatic or hematogenous routes and result in a fulminant clinical course.

Staphylococcus aureus can colonize intact skin and frequently is found distributed over the skin, particularly in nasal carriers. Epidemiologic studies suggest that transmission of *Staphylococcus aureus* occurs predominantly by way of direct personal contact rather than through the air.[71] Infection is specifically associated with *Staphylococcus aureus* of phage group II. The hallmarks of infection by this organism are fragile bullae, varnish-like crust, and desquamation. The cutaneous response is caused by an extracellular exfoliative toxin (exfoliatin) produced by *Staphylococcus aureus.*

The gram-negative organisms, *Pasteurella multocida, Neisseria meningitidis, Hemophilus influenzae, Pseudomonas aeruginosa,* and *Borrelia burgdorferi* (Table 65-5), are responsible for the majority of gram-negative infections. These infections are spread by close contact with an infected person or by an animal vector. The cutaneous lesions are varied.

Rickettsial infections are caused by bacteria, which are obligate intracellular parasites, transmitted by blood-sucking arthropods, such as the body louse, flea, tick, and mite. These arthropods serve both as the vector and the reservoir.

Clinical Manifestations

Gram-Positive Infections.   Impetigo (see Table 65-4) is by far the most common bacterial skin infection in children. Prevalence varies with the season of the year. Impetigo occurs more often in hot, humid environments at lower altitudes. Sparse clothing, poor hygiene, skin trauma, and crowded conditions also contribute to the spread of impetigo.

A variety of lesions are seen in impetigo. Nonbullous impetigo (Fig. 65-3*A*) starts as a tiny vesicle or pustule that soon ruptures and is replaced by expanding crusts. Bullous impetigo (Fig. 65-3*B*) begins with a large superficial bullae that quickly ruptures, revealing moist, denuded skin. As the lesion ages it develops thin collarettes of serosanguineous scale. In general, impetigo is asymptomatic, although pruritus may be present.

Ecthyma (see Table 65-4) is a deep ulcerative type of pyoderma commonly seen on the lower extremity and buttocks of children. It is caused by GABHS[68] and often follows skin trauma from an insect bite, a cut, or varicella.

Folliculitis (see Table 65-4) or superficial infection of the hair follicles, frequently occurs on the scalp, face, buttocks, and extremities. Nasal and perianal carriage has been associated with frequent recurrences. A less common cause of folliculitis is *Pseudomonas aeruginosa* more recently reported in association with the use of hot tubs. It is important to remember that folliculitis may also result from contact with irritating substances such as tar or occlusive dressings. These lesions may be sterile or culture out *Staphylococcus epidermidis.*

Furunculosis (see Table 65-4) usually develops from a preceding folliculitis as a painful deep follicular infection, whereas *carbunculosis* (see Table 65-4) occurs slower than furunculosis.

Cellulitis (see Table 65-4) is a full-thickness infection of the skin involving dermal and subcutaneous tissue. In

TABLE 65-4
Gram-Positive Bacterial Skin Infections

Organism and Infection	Cutaneous Lesions	Systemic Symptoms	Complications	Treatment
Staphylococcus aureus				
Bullous impetigo	Large superficial bullae that rupture easily leaving denuded skin and serosanguineous crusts; each lesion resolves in 12–14 days	None	Local or systemic spread	Mupirocin, penicillinase-resistant penicillin, erythromycin, soaks
Folliculitis	Painless superficial follicular pustule with narrow red areola, and a hair shaft in center	None	Furunculosis	Warm compresses, mupirocin
Furunculosis	Deeper inflammation with central pustulation and necrosis, tender, 1–5 cm diameter	Pain	Lymphangitis, carbunculosis, cellulitis, sepsis, scarring	Warm compresses, incision and drainage, penicillinase-resistant penicillin, erythromycin
Carbunculosis	Extremely painful, deep abscess with pustulation and necrosis, 3–10 cm diameter	Fever, malaise	Cellulitis, sepsis	Same as above
Staphylococcal scalded skin syndrome	Generalized erythema, thin walled flaccid bullae and exfoliation, crusting, Nikolsky's sign +	Fever, malaise, irritability, skin tenderness	Sepsis, endocarditis, mortality 4%	Fluid hydration, analgesics, penicillinase-resistant antibiotics
Toxic shock syndrome	Scarlatiniform sunburn, edema, mucous membrane hyperemia, fine desquamation, Nikolsky's sign −	High fever, myalgia, hypotension, vomiting, diarrhea	Cardiac, respiratory, or renal failure, mortality 3%	Fluid hydration, cloxacillin or cephalexin, antihypotensives, oxygen
Streptococcus pyogenes				
Nonbullous impetigo	Superficial papule that erodes with crusts and local adenopathy. Little surrounding erythema	None	AGN, lymphangitis, scarlet fever, ecthyma, cellulitis	Soaks, mupirocin, penicillin, erythromycin
Ecthyma	Painful lesion with intense erythema, craterlike ulcer, thick crust that may scar	Pain	Scar, cellulitis, scarlet fever, lymphangitis	Penicillin, erythromycin, mupirocin, soaks
Erysipelas	Demarcated erythematous patch that spreads peripherally, skin is warm, border palpable	Pain, headache, fever, myalgia, malaise	Lymphangitis, sepsis, AGN, endocarditis	Penicillin, cephalosporin, erythromycin, bedrest, warm compresses
Cellulitis	Patch of erythema, edema, and tenderness with vague border	Pain, fever, malaise	Meningitis, septic arthritis, sepsis	Penicillin, erythromycin, warm compresses, bedrest
Lymphangitis	Tender, red streak extending from site of injury or infection	Pain, fever	Lymphadenitis, scarlet fever	Penicillin, erythromycin
Scarlet fever	Diffuse erythema, sandpaper-textured skin followed by fine desquamtion	Fever, pharyngitis, nausea and vomiting, malaise, headache, chills	Tonsillar abscess, otitis media, cervical adenitis, AGN, rheumatic fever	Penicillin, erythromycin, bedrest, fluids, soft diet

AGN = acute glomerulonephritis

a series of children with cellulitis, 84% of the cases involved the limbs, especially the legs.[30] Most cases occur after trauma or interruption of the cutaneous barrier.

A distinctive type of cellulitis caused by GABHS is called *erysipelas* (see Table 65-4). The infection is frequently heralded by a severe systemic reaction. Erysipelas is seen most commonly in infants, young children, and older adults. Children with nephrotic syndrome appear particularly susceptible to erysipelas. The most frequently involved sites are the face, scalp, and lower extremities. In neonates, it may be seen at the umbilical stump.

Acute lymphangitis (see Table 65-4), more commonly known as "blood poisoning," is an inflammatory process involving lymphatic channels of the skin and subcutaneous tissue. Lymphangitis usually follows a cutaneous injury or infection and presents with a tender red streak ascending the arm or leg. The red streak varies in length and width and originates from the site of injury or infection.

Scarlet fever (see Table 65-4) is one of the toxic syndromes caused by bacterial infection of the skin or mucous membranes. It is seen almost exclusively between

TABLE 65-5
Gram-Negative Bacterial Skin Infections

Organism and Infection	Cutaneous Lesion	Systemic Symptoms	Complications	Treatment
Pasteurella multocida				
Focal abscess	Focal soft tissue swelling after animal exposure	Pain	Lymphangitis, chronic skin ulcer, infection of tendon, bone, joint	Penicillin, chloramphenicol, incision and drainage
Neisseria meningitidis				
Meningococcemia meningitis	Tender erythematous macules, papules, petechiae, purpura acrocyanosis, skin necrosis	High fever, headache nausea and vomiting, diarrhea, hypotension, stupor, seizures	Ischemic necrosis, purpura fulminans, renal impairment, gangrene	Ampicillin, aminoglycoside, intensive care, central venous pressure, blood pressure, renal output
Hemophilus influenzae Type B				
Cellulitis	Raised, warm, tender, erythematous area on face	Pain, fever, irritability	Meningitis, sepsis	Ampicillin, chloramphenicol
Bacteremia	Exanthematous rash over trunk and extremities			
Pseudomonas aeroginosa				
Folliculitis	Pruritic papules, deep violaceous nodules; lesions resolve in 1–2 wk	Fever, malaise, lymphadenopathy	Ecthyma gangrenosum, septicemia	Aminoglycosides, penicillin, acetic acid soaks
Septicemia	Ecthyma gangrenosum, purpura			
Borrelia burgdorferi				
Lyme disease	Erythema chronicum migrans (a red, expanding, doughnut-shaped lesion)	Headache, stiff neck, fatigue, memory loss, paresthesia	Chronic arthritis, cardiac and neurologic abnormalities	Tetracycline, penicillin, erythromycin

the ages of 2 and 10 years. Females are more frequently affected than males. Infants and children under the age of 2 do not develop scarlet fever, due, in part, to transplacental transference of antibodies and poorly developed ability to localize an infection. Most children have only one episode of scarlet fever because of the development of specific antitoxin antibodies.[30]

The onset of scarlet fever is acute with the development of fever, chills, pharyngitis, nausea, vomiting, malaise, headache, generalized lymphadenopathy, and diffuse abdominal pain. The rash, which consists of both an exanthem and an enanthema, develops 24 to 48 hours after the onset of pharyngitis. Up to 2 months after the onset, nails may be marked with transverse lines (Beau's lines).

Another of the toxic syndromes caused by bacteria is *staphylococcal scalded skin syndrome* (SSSS; see Table 65-4). This syndrome is primarily seen in children under

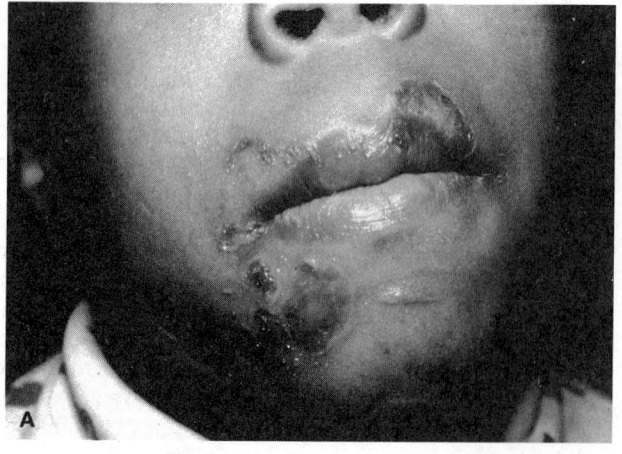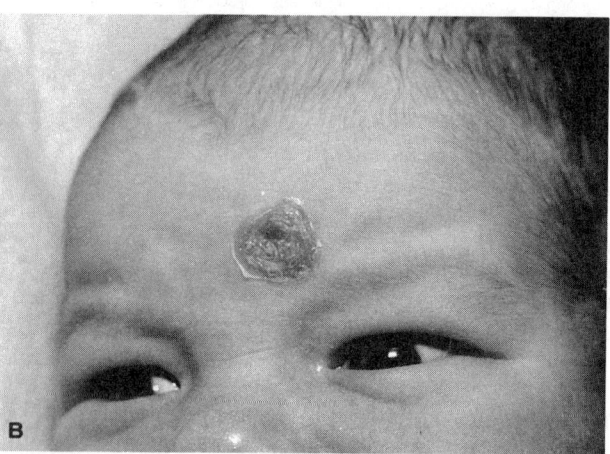

FIGURE 65-3
Impetigo. (**A**) Nonbullous impetigo. Moist expanding perioral crusts with minimal surrounding erythema characteristic of streptococcal infection of the skin. (Courtesy of Bernard A. Cohen, M.D.) (**B**) Bullous impetigo. Erythematous lesion with varnished appearance and collarette of scale characteristic of staphylococcal infection on the forehead of an infant.

the age of 5 years, but has been reported in adults. Older children and adults, unless they are immunocompromised, develop a specific antistaphylococcal antibody, are better able to metabolize and excrete the toxin, and generally do not develop SSSS.[30]

Another toxic syndromes is *toxic shock syndrome* (TSS; see Table 65-4), discussed in Chapter 68.

Gram-Negative Infections. *Pasteurella multocida* (see Table 65-5) is primarily an animal pathogen found in the mouths of cats and dogs. The distribution of this organism is worldwide. Most human infections are related to animal bites. However, a bite is not always necessary for contraction of the infection. Although the youngest children (0 to 4 years) are at greatest risk, *Pasteurella multocida* infection may occur at any age. The disease caused in humans may range from a focal abscess to septicemia and endocarditis.

Infection caused by *Neisseria meningitidis* (see Table 65-5) is found worldwide, with children under the age of 5 years accounting for 50% of all infections. The disease has a rapid onset and fulminant course. The fatality rate varies from 8% in major medical centers to 70% in Third World countries. Most cases occur in the late winter to early spring.[30] Transmission is by respiratory droplet and inhalation of secretions of an infected person or carrier.

Meningococcal bacteremia without sepsis is seen in older children and adults. It has not been reported in infants. Clinically, only a fever is observed without cutaneous manifestations.

Meningococcemia varies from more benign forms to a severe life-threatening form. The benign form is preceded by a prodrome similar to a mild upper respiratory tract infection. This stage is followed within 24 to 48 hours by high fever, headache, nausea, and diarrhea. A petechial rash occurs on the skin and mucous membranes consisting of bright red or pink tender macules and papules. The macules and papules may have hemorrhagic centers and be arranged in a reticulated pattern. This form carries with it a 50% fatality rate.[30] Survivors often have renal impairment and extensive skin necrosis.

Meningitis may follow bacteremia and seeding of the meninges with severe headache, stiff neck, nausea and vomiting, stupor, seizures, and coma. *Chronic meningococcemia* is characterized by periodic episodes of fever, arthralgia, and petechial skin lesions. The child is relatively free of symptoms between episodes. Cutaneous manifestations are some of the most important clues in the diagnosis of this life-threatening infection.

Although infection with *H. influenzae* type B (HIB; see Table 65-5) results in bacteremia, cutaneous manifestations are frequently seen with this strain. Infection with this organism is primarily a disease of young children under the age of 5 years who lack immunity to the organism. HIB is the major cause of meningitis in most regions of the United States.[30]

Transmission occurs mainly by direct contact with secretions or fomites, but may be a result of airborne droplet transmission. The bacteremia associated with infection spreads the organism throughout the child's body, resulting in meningitis, pneumonia, empyema, septic arthritis, cellulitis, osteomyelitis, pericarditis, endocarditis, peritonitis, glossitis, and epiglottitis.

The most common skin infection caused by *Pseu-* *domonas aeruginosa* (see Table 65-5) is hot tub folliculitis. The cutaneous signs of this infection occur 8 to 48 hours after bathing in a hot tub or whirlpool that has not been adequately disinfected. Superficial pruritic papules, pustules, and/or deep violaceous nodules are most dense in areas covered by a bathing suit. If not reexposed, the lesions resolve in 1 to 2 weeks.

Pseudomonas septicemia is accompanied by several types of skin lesions. Ecthyma gangrenosum is considered pathognomonic for this infection and begins as a solitary erythematous macule. The lesion quickly becomes indurated, then bullous or pustular and evolves into a thick, black-crusted erosion surrounded by a ring of tender inflammation. Other skin manifestations reported in *Pseudomonas* septicemia include widespread purpura, maculopapular rash, and nodules or bullae that do not ulcerate or become necrotic.[25] The organism may be cultured from the blood or skin lesions.

First described in 1975, *Lyme disease* (see Table 65-5) is named for Lyme, Connecticut, where the first cases were recognized. It is the most prevalent vectorborne illness in the United States. The organism is transmitted by a deer tick. Outbreaks of Lyme disease are seen in people who live in wooded areas that are heavily populated with deer or the common field mouse, both reservoir hosts to the tick. The major predisposing factors include summer activity and travel to endemic areas such as the northeastern and upper midwestern United States. However, Lyme disease has occurred in 43 states and cases have also been reported in Europe, China, the former Soviet Union, Canada, and Australia. A recent survey indicated that May and June are the months of greatest risk, with a secondary peak in October and November.[43]

Often, Lyme disease is difficult to diagnose because the infection does not follow a consistent pattern. There are many possible symptoms that resemble other diseases. In addition, the symptoms tend to be intermittent and to change. Recognition of the characteristic skin lesion plays a major role in early diagnosis of this infection.

Rickettsial Infections. The illnesses caused by rickettsial bacteria include endemic typhus, Rocky Mountain spotted fever (RMSF), rickettsial-pox, Q fever, scrub typhus, epidemic typhus, trench fever, Queensland tick typhus, North Asian tickborne rickettsiosis, and boutonneuse fever. Of these infections, only the first four listed are seen in the United States. Rickettsial infections are seen more commonly in temperate and tropical climates. It has been estimated that more human lives worldwide have been lost from rickettsial disease than from any other infection except malaria.[30] Early diagnosis and the proper use of antimicrobial agents are the most important factors in decreasing the risk of mortality in rickettsial infections.

Because rickettsiae invade the endothelial cells of small blood vessels, virtually all rickettsial diseases of humans produce a rash except for Q fever. RMSF, the most common rickettsial infection seen in the United States, is discussed here.

Despite its name, *Rocky Mountain spotted fever* (RMSF) is found primarily in the southeastern and south central United States. However, it has been reported in every state except Vermont, in Canada, and in several Central and South American countries.[30]

RMSF is caused by *Rickettsia rickettsii,* which is transmitted to humans by a bite of an infected tick. The illness is seen in all ages from spring to fall, with the highest incidence in July. Occupational and recreational activities in areas where there is contact with ticks increase the risk of contracting RMSF.

Manifestations of RMSF can range from mild to fulminant and fatal. Onset is with fever, malaise, muscle and joint aches, photophobia, anorexia, nausea, and vomiting. One to 4 days later, a macular erythematous rash develops, more marked on extremities including the palms and soles. The rash gradually becomes generalized, developing a more papular nature with a darker hue. In 2 to 3 days, petechiae and purpura may be seen. In severe cases, gangrene may develop on terminal parts of the body such as the fingers, toes, earlobes, and scrotum. Accompanying nonpitting, nondependent edema frequently occurs, especially periorbital edema in children. Diseases with which it may be confused include meningococcemia, measles, juvenile rheumatoid arthritis, and systemic lupus erythematosus.

Diagnostic Studies. Diagnosis of bacterial skin infection is made by the characteristic clinical findings along with several laboratory tests that confirm or rule out certain diagnoses. An aerobic bacterial skin culture is the most common diagnostic test along with a Gram's stain. The accuracy is improved for both of these tests if the specimen is obtained from a recently unroofed vesicle or under a crust. A moistened cotton-tipped applicator helps in applying the specimen onto the culture medium. Cultures may also be taken from sites distant from the skin lesions such as the throat, nasal mucosa, blood, or cerebrospinal fluid (CSF).

SSSS must be differentiated from toxic epidermal necrolysis (TEN), a drug, or viral-induced process with similar clinical features (see Table 65-16 on drug reactions). Although SSSS and TEN are similar in appearance, they require drastically different treatments. They can be distinguished easily by determining the point of cleavage in the skin with a skin biopsy.[30] In SSSS, superficial necrosis of the epidermis is seen. In TEN, a full-thickness necrosis of the epidermis is present.

Specific tests are available for Lyme disease that detect antibodies present in the child's blood. Unfortunately, the antibodies are hard to detect in the earliest stages of the disease or if the patient has taken antibiotics. Several new tests have been approved.[43] One measures the T-cell response and may detect Lyme disease in patients who have already taken antibiotics. Another is a quick test that produces results in 7 minutes and can be done in the physician's office. In some instances, a culture of the spirochete can help to establish a definitive diagnosis. A skin biopsy of erythema chronicum migrans (ECM) shows features of an arthropod bite reaction.

Diagnosis of rickettsial infection is made by clinical examination, which may be supported by a serologic test for rickettsial antibody titers. In RMSF, no rise in antibody titers is detected until late in the second week of the illness. A more rapid diagnosis is possible by culture and identification of rickettsiae by monocyte culture or in tissue by direct immunofluorescence.

★ ASSESSMENT

Assessment of children presenting with bacterial infections of the skin include obtaining a complete history of the eruption and any treatment measures taken. Recent exposure to someone with the same infection, the presence of infection in other family members, recent hiking or playing in wooded areas, or travel to endemic areas should be noted.

A total skin examination is done with a description of the lesion morphology and distribution. Temperature is taken to assess systemic involvement.

★ NURSING DIAGNOSES AND PLANNING

Based on assessment data from above and Chapter 64, the following nursing diagnoses may apply to the family and child with a bacterial skin infection:

- Impaired Skin Integrity related to bacterial invasion.
- Altered Comfort (Pain) related to skin disorder.
- Anxiety related to knowledge deficit regarding illness, treatment, and prevention.
- Ineffective Management of Therapeutic Regimen related to knowledge deficit regarding treatment and prevention.

The nurse and child (or parents) together plan effective care based on the established nursing diagnoses. Several examples of expected outcomes follow:

- The parents and child demonstrate their understanding of skin care needs.
- The parents state steps to avoid spreading of infection in home.
- The child exhibits signs of comfort.

The nurse plans for the care of the child based on both physician's orders and nursing diagnoses. Some general nursing care goals include the following:

- Skin heals.
- Spread of infection and other complications are prevented.

★ INTERVENTIONS: COLLABORATIVE AND INDEPENDENT

Bacterial infections of the skin are common afflictions during the childhood years. A major nursing concern in the care of children is prevention of skin infections. Certain measures are taken while caring for children and parents are educated on measures to prevent infection in the child. The Nursing Care Plan and Teaching Plan, for example, discuss care of a preschooler with impetigo.

Most bacterial infections are managed on an outpatient basis. However, due to systemic effects, certain types of cellulitis, SSSS, TSS, meningococcemia, and infections with complications require hospitalization. (Refer to Tables 65-4 and 65-5 for medical management of bacterial infections.)

Nursing responsibilities in the care of a hospitalized child with a bacterial skin infection include maintenance of isolation, administration of medication, employment of measures that ensure comfort and safety of the child, and maintenance of optimum hydration and nourishment.

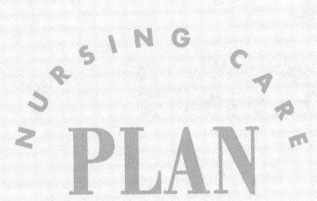

A Preschooler With Impetigo

Assessment

Case Study Description

Jason is a 4-year-old white male seen in an outpatient pediatric office. Jason is the oldest of two children. Both of his parents work outside of their home. His mother is a dental hygienist, and his father is a math teacher at the local middle school. Both parents are involved in the personal care of Jason, including bathing and dressing. Jason attends day care 5 days a week. At day care, one teacher and two assistants are responsible for Jason's care. Jason is accompanied to the office by his mother.

Assessment Data

Subjective:

Mother reports that Jason first developed a red spot on his chin 5 days ago. Since that time, the area has enlarged, started to ooze clear fluid, and become crusted. Two days ago, new red areas began to appear around Jason's mouth and right nostril. The spots do not seem to bother Jason. However, his mother has seen Jason pick the areas occasionally. Jason's mother initially thought the spots were bug bites and applied calamine lotion, but now she is concerned because new areas are appearing. Jason's teacher at day care told her that several other children have similar lesions and she has advised all parents to take the child to their doctor. Mother states Jason has no allergies to medications and has had no recent or chronic skin problems.

Objective:

Jason is a happy, somewhat shy child. He is cooperative with physical exam and procedures while sitting on his mother's lap. He is afebrile, and other vital signs are within normal limits.

There are 3 irregularly shaped erythematous, moist erosions with honey-colored crust at the perimeter of each lesion. Surrounding erythema is very minimal, and there is no regional lymphadenopathy. The sites of involvement are limited to the chin, right nostril, and upper lip. Jason does not complain of discomfort when the areas are touched.

The remaining physical exam is within normal limits. Growth and development are normal for his age.

Bacterial culture is positive for *Staphylococcus aureus*.

Nursing Diagnosis	Intervention	Rationale
1. Impaired skin integrity Supporting Data: • Presence of erosions • Presence of exudate	Apply warm tap water compresses three to four times daily.	Moisture aids removal of crusts and exudate.
	Gently cleanse lesions with a diluted antibacterial soap.	Keeping the lesions clean prevents secondary infection.
	Administer topical or oral antibiotics as ordered.	Antibiotic ensures elimination of the causative organism and reduces the risk of complications.
2. High risk for infection related to impaired skin integrity, presence of pathogen, and frequent close contact with family members and playmates.	Monitor for signs of new areas of infection.	Impetigo is a highly contagious disease, and appropriate care techniques at the pediatrician's office, home, and day care are vital to prevention of transmission.

(Continued)

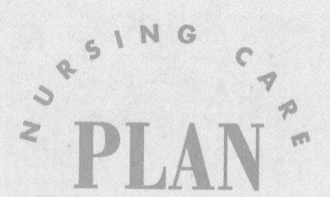

A Preschooler With Impetigo (continued)

Nursing Diagnosis	*Intervention*	*Rationale*
Supporting Data: • Jason has a younger sibling. • Jason attends day care 5 days a week. • Ability of *Staphylococcus aureus* to colonize on intact skin. • Transmission occurs by direct contact.	Use strict handwashing techniques before and after caring for infected areas. Develop a teaching plan for transmission prevention. (See "Child and Family Teaching Plan: Care of a Preschooler With Impetigo." in this chapter.)	
3. Parental anxiety related to lack of information regarding the disease process, treatment plan, and home care regimen. Supporting Data: • Newly diagnosed • Parents asking multiple questions	Explain disease process and treatment in terms the parents can understand. Provide verbal and written information on the infection, treatment, and home care regimen. Review signs of healing, such as decreased erythema and exudate with return of skin integrity. Review side-effects of prescribed medication: • Allergic reactions • GI disturbances • Resistance of organism Demonstrate the appropriate method for application of prescribed topical medications and wet compresses.	Successful treatment of impetigo depends on parental understanding and adherence to the treatment regimen. Fears can be relieved with adequate information.

Evaluation

• Skin lesions are resolved.
• Entire course of antibiotic has been completed as prescribed.
• No new impetigo lesions are present.

Expected Outcomes

• Family members and playmates maintain skin free of impetigo.
• Family expresses understanding of disease, transmission, treatment, and prevention.

INFECTION PREVENTION

Infection prevention begins in the nursery with careful cleansing of the umbilical stump and circumcision site coupled with strict adherence to policies of handwashing before and after handling infants. These measures are vital in the prevention of nosocomial infection in the neonatal nursery. The period of time before discharge is a prime opportunity to teach parents about general skin and wound care. This instruction is followed-up and reinforced at subsequent well-child care visits to the pediatrician. The nurse may also provide written material and reading suggestions for parents on this subject.

When impetigo occurs in an infant during the first 2

weeks of life, the newborn nursery that cared for the child is notified so that follow up regarding infection control in the nursery can be initiated. In school-age children, the school is notified by the parent when impetigo occurs.

Preventing infection is paramount to minimizing the risk of contracting various vector-borne infections such as Lyme disease and RMSF or *Pasteurella multocida* infections as a result of contact with animals. Children are taught to avoid areas of tall grass and low brush and contact with wild or domestic animals. Parents should examine children closely after they have been in infested areas and should remove ticks only with a tweezers. Light-colored, tightly woven clothing enhances the recognition of ticks. Long pant-legs and long sleeves with the bottom

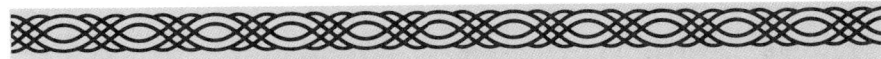

CHILD & FAMILY
T E A C H I N G
PLAN

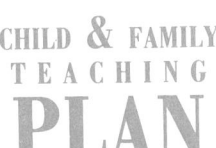

Care of a Preschooler With Impetigo

Assessment

Jason is a 4-year-old, white male seen in an outpatient pediatric office for rapidly spreading skin lesions on his face. The diagnosis was confirmed as bullous impetigo with a positive bacterial culture for *Staphylococcus aureus.*

Jason is the oldest of two children and lives with his parents and sibling. Both parents have attended school past high school, and both are employed outside of the home. Jason's parents share the responsibility for the personal care of Jason and his sibling. Jason attends day care 5 days a week where one teacher and two assistants are responsible for Jason's care.

Mother states she has heard of impetigo but does not know what causes it or how it is spread from one person to another. Because impetigo is an acute disease, the teaching is done at the office visit with follow-up by phone with the parents and day care facility or office visit in 10 days.

Child and Family Objectives	*Specific Content*	*Teaching Strategies*
1. Administer medication correctly by return demonstration.	1. Topical or oral antibiotic administration by medication cup or other liquid measurement device.	1. Demonstrate application of topical medication to skin lesions. Demonstrate accurate measurement and administration of liquid oral medication
2. State signs and symptoms of recurrence or spread.	2. Review signs of recurrence (erythema, vesicles, erosions, exudate)	2. Discuss recurrence and spread with mother. Provide written material for her to review at home and give to father and day care teacher.
3. Identify measures to decrease risk of infection transmission. Mother will communicate information to father and day care teachers.	3. Instruct mother on infection control measures: • Good handwashing • Administer full course of medication • Clip Jason's fingernails short and keep them clean. • Wash Jason's personal items (clothing and linens) separately in hot water. • Bathe Jason daily alone, not with sibling, until all lesions have resolved. • Jason should not return to day care until treated for 24 hours with oral antibiotic or 48 hours with topical antibiotic. • Do not share Jason's personal items with family members or contacts at day care. • Change pillowcase, washcloth, and towel daily, including similar items used at day care until all lesions are resolved.	3. Assess hygiene practices and health habits at home and at day care. Demonstrate good handwashing techniques. Provide written materials outlining teaching content for mother to refer to at home and review with father and day care teachers.

(Continued)

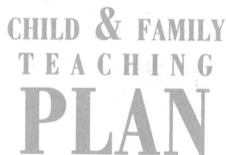

Child and Family Objectives   *Specific Content*   *Teaching Strategies*

- No swimming until skin integrity has returned.
- Attempt to determine possible source.
- Provide balanced diet.

Evaluation
- Mother demonstrates accurate medication administration.
- Mother verbalizes signs of recurrence and spread.
- Mother demonstrates good handwashing
- Mother describes good health and hygiene practices to follow at home and day care.
- Mother communicates information to father and day care teachers.

---

of the pant-legs tucked into socks and the shirt tucked into pants make it difficult for the ticks to reach open skin. Repellents containing the ingredient diethyltolvamide (DEET) may be applied to the skin or clothing to repel the ticks. Pets that spend time outdoors should wear tick collars and be inspected often for attached ticks. These animals should be kept off furniture, especially beds. Wound care after an animal bite includes thorough cleansing and debriding of the wound. Surgical closure is avoided because of the high incidence of wound infection with wound closure.[30]

TEACHING

Education is important to the recovery of the child. The expected course of the infection is discussed with the family. The nurse should review with the family the importance of handwashing and not touching the infected area unless applying compresses or medication. Squeezing of furuncles or carbuncles is avoided. Measures to prevent spread should be taken, such as keeping all of the child's linen and clothing separate and washing them in hot water. Parents are also taught how to administer the medication, including the importance of continuing therapy for the prescribed period of time.

MEDICATION THERAPY

The primary tool for treatment of skin infections is systemic antibiotics. A general rule for the use of antibiotics in skin infection is that *Staphylococcus aureus* should be considered penicillin-resistant until proven otherwise, and all GABHS may be considered penicillin-sensitive.[30]

Until recently, topical antibiotics have played a minor role in the treatment of skin infection. However, with the development of mupirocin (Bactroban), a much more effective topical antibiotic is available. Mupirocin is active against some gram-positive pathogens, most notably

Staphylococcus aureus and GABHS. Due to its unique chemical structure, novel mode of action, and its use restricted to topical application, the associated development of cross-resistance with other clinically important antibiotics is nonexistent. In addition, the potential for development of contact sensitization and phototoxicity is low.

The nurse is responsible for administration of medication ordered or making sure parents understand administration procedures. Frequently, treatment of skin infections involves topical measures such as soaks, compresses, or wet wraps to cleanse the skin and remove crusts. (See ''Papulosquamous Disorders'' in this chapter for guidelines for administering these topical treatments.)

★ **EVALUATION**

Evaluation of nursing intervention in bacterial skin infections involves examination for resolution of all skin lesions. In uncomplicated cases, symptoms should resolve in 7 to 14 days with appropriate treatment. Additional nursing care may be required if complications develop.

COMPLICATIONS

Refer to Tables 65-4 and 65-5 for a listing of the complications in gram-positive and gram-negative skin infections. Local complications of impetigo are rare. The lesions are shallow and usually heal without scarring. However, scarring is common in ecthyma. Transient hyper- or hypopigmentation may be seen after healing. Occasionally, the infection may invade deeper tissue, developing furuncles, carbuncles, ecthyma, lymphangitis, or cellulitis. Acute glomerulonephritis (AGN) after impetigo has been well-documented, and scarlet fever may be associated with nonbullous impetigo.[30]

Complications of RMSF are a result of extensive bleeding into the skin and include cardiac failure, shock, and disseminated intravascular coagulation.[30]

Viral Skin Infections

Viruses are ultramicroscopic organisms that grow only within living cells. They are capable of producing several different types of skin lesions ranging from a rash with erythema, macules, papules, and vesicles to localized growths such as warts and molluscum contagiosum (MC). Viral infection of the skin is common.

The following discussion reviews cutaneous viral infections seen in children and includes common viral exanthems, the herpesvirus family (herpes simplex, varicella, herpes zoster, cytomegalovirus infection, Epstein-Barr infection). Cutaneous manifestations of human immunodeficiency virus (HIV) infection are included. In addition, cutaneous viral lesions such as warts and MC are reviewed.

Three mechanisms are responsible for producing the skin lesion in viral infections. The first mechanism is direct invasion of the skin by way of the bloodstream or by direct contact. Typically, such invasion produces vesicular, ulcerative, or tumor-like lesions. Varicella, herpes simplex, certain enteroviral infections, and warts are examples of conditions resulting from direct invasion. The second mechanism probably accounts for the presence of most viral rashes is viruses in the skin reacting with circulating cell-mediated immune factors. In such instances, the virus can be recovered from areas of involved skin as in rubeola and rubella. Circulating immune factors may also cause cutaneous abnormalities even without the presence of the virus or viral antigen in the skin. This process is thought to be the third mechanism, which results in acute urticaria, erythema multiforme, and purpura fulminans seen in some viral illnesses.[28]

The mode of transmission also varies depending on the organism. In the case of warts and herpes simplex, infection occurs as a result of direct inoculation of the skin. In these conditions, shedding of the virus from human skin to human skin occurs. The skin also can become infected during viremia in which the virus is transferred to the skin by way of the bloodstream as is the case in varicella and most viral exanthems. The viremia is a result of transmission by respiratory droplet, fecal–oral, or direct contact routes. Local spread of the virus to the skin after reactivation of a latent viral infection occurs in cases of herpes simplex and herpes zoster.

Viral Exanthems

Definition and Incidence. Exanthem is a general term used to describe an eruption of the skin that is accompanied by inflammation. Over 50 specific viral agents, including 30 enteroviruses, are known to cause viral exanthems.[23] Enanthems, which are eruptions of the mucous membranes, may also accompany an exanthem. The viral exanthems discussed in this section include rubella (German measles), rubeola (measles), roseola infantum, erythema infectiosum, enterovirus infection, and papular acrodermatitis of childhood (PAC; Table 65-6).

Viral exanthems are common communicable infections in children.

Rubella (German measles; see Table 65-6) is rarely seen in young infants but is common in children and young adults.

Rubeola (measles) is a highly contagious, acute viral infection (see Table 65-6) of childhood that is seen more frequently in infants and young children in urban areas, whereas infection is more common in school-age children in rural areas.[28]

Roseola infantum (exanthema subitum) is a disease of infants and young children (see Table 65-6) seen primarily in children under 4 years of age.

Erythema infectiosum (fifth disease; see Table 65-6) is characterized by a "slapped cheek" appearance of the face and a lacy erythematous eruption on the extremities. It is seen most in children ages 5 to 14 and in females more than males. A human parvovirus has been identified as the etiologic agent.

TABLE 65-6
Viral Exanthems

Infection and Organism	Transmission	Incubation	Communicability Period	Immunity
Rubella (rubella virus)	Respiratory droplet / Direct contact / Transplacentally	14–21 days	5–7 days before to 3–5 days after onset of rash	Transplacental transfer / Postinfection vaccination
Rubeola (rubeola virus)	Respiratory droplet / Direct contact	1–11 days	From beginning of prodromal period to 4 days after onset of rash	Transplacental transfer / Postinfection vaccination
Roseola infantum (unknown)	Unknown, thought to be relatively noncontagious	5–15 days	Unknown	Unknown
Erythema infectiosum (human parvovirus)	Unknown probably respiratory droplet	1–14 days	Unknown	Unknown
Enterovirus infection (enteroviruses)	Fecal–oral / Respiratory droplet	Varied	Unknown	Unknown
Papular acrodermatitis of childhood (Several associated viruses, hepatitis virus?)	Not considered contagious	Unknown	Not applicable	Unknown

Enteroviruses (see Table 65-6) are thought to be the leading cause of childhood exanthems in the summer and fall. Children are more susceptible than adults because the development of specific antibodies increases with age. Enteroviruses cause a wide array of clinical symptoms with associated exanthems. Historically, enteroviruses were subdivided based on the antigenic properties: (1) polioviruses, (2) coxsackie groups A and B, and (3) echoviruses. Due to similarities, they are labeled in one group as enteroviruses. More than 30 types of enteroviruses have been associated with exanthems.[28]

Papular acrodermatitis of childhood (Gianotti-Crosti; PAC) is an erythematous papular rash (see Table 65-6) that affects primarily the face and extremities with relative sparing of the trunk. It is associated with mild constitutional symptoms and anicteric hepatitis. A similar disorder exhibits the rash without hepatitis.

Etiology and Pathophysiology. Table 65-6 outlines the etiology, transmission, incubation period, period of communicability, and immunity for the six viral exanthems discussed here.

Clinical Manifestations. In *rubella*, a prodrome of low-grade fever, headache, malaise, conjunctivitis, sore throat, rhinitis, cough, and lymphadenopathy precedes the rash by 1 to 4 days and resolves rapidly with appearance of the rash. Cutaneous lesions appear first on the face and spread rapidly to the neck, arms, trunk, and legs. The rash consists of reddish-pink macules and papules that are discrete and remain so on the extremities but coalesce on the trunk. After 2 to 3 days, the rash disappears and may be followed by a fine desquamation. An enanthem is seen at the end of the prodromal period or the beginning of the rash and consists of pinhead-size red spots scattered over the soft palate. These are referred to as *Forschheimer spots.*

The clinical course of *rubeola* consists of three phases: (1) an asymptomatic incubation period of 10 to 11 days after exposure; (2) a prodromal period with fever, malaise, cough, coryza, and conjunctivitis with development of *Koplik's spots* in the mouth; and (3) a macular and papular rash. The rash first appears behind ears and over the forehead, spreads down the neck and trunk, and then appears distally over the upper and lower extremities. Hands and feet are often involved. A fine desquamation may occur as the rash heals.

In *roseola infantum*, the child initially has a fever ranging from 38.8° to 40.5° C, which lasts 3 to 5 days. Exanthema subitum is first seen with disappearance of the fever. Discrete 3- to 5-mm macules or papules with a halo are most pronounced on the trunk and, to a lesser extent, on the proximal extremities, neck, and face. The rash is present for approximately 24 hours but may last up to 2 days.

After the incubation period of *erythema infectiosum*, a low-grade fever, malaise, and headache may be present for a day or two. The exanthem consists of three stages: (1) a fiery red, macular erythema on the cheeks with circumoral pallor; (2) discrete erythematous macules and papules appear on the proximal extremities and may spread to the trunk; and (3) the eruption waxes and wanes in intensity. Changes in the environmental temperature,

exposure to sunlight, exercise, crying, and emotional factors may contribute to the variability of the eruption. In general, the children appear well except for the skin rash. No isolation is necessary due to the mild nature of the disease.[28]

The clinical manifestations of *enterovirus infection* depend on the age at the time of the infection. Exanthems are more common in young children and central nervous system (CNS) symptoms are more common in older children. Cutaneous manifestations are highly variable. Systemic manifestations may include fever, upper respiratory symptoms, malaise, sore throat, cervical adenopathy, aseptic meningitis, encephalitis, and pneumonia.

Hand, foot, and mouth (HFM) syndrome is probably the most distinctive enteroviral exanthem. The presence of vesicles on the buccal mucosa, tongue, hands, and feet is the most common manifestation. These vesicles may be found on the buttocks in young infants. The exanthem is usually preceded 1 to 2 days by a brief prodrome of low-grade fever, anorexia, malaise, and sore throat.

The cutaneous manifestations of *PAC* are characterized by multiple, discrete, erythematous papules varying in size from 2 to 5 mm. These lesions may be hemorrhagic, and some may have a lichenoid quality. Pruritus may or may not be present. They are distributed on the face, neck, buttocks, and extremities. The trunk, antecubital, and popliteal fossae are generally spared. An upper respiratory infection may precede an abrupt appearance of the rash. Mild constitutional symptoms of malaise, low fever, and diarrhea often accompany the cutaneous eruption. When it is associated with hepatitis, hepatomegaly and lymphadenopathy are also seen. However, the incidence of its association with hepatitis is rare in the United States.[28]

Diagnostic Studies. It is not unusual that a child presents with a rash and the specific etiologic diagnosis never is made. Most viral illnesses are benign and self-limited, making specific diagnosis unnecessary in the normal healthy child. However, there are several cases in which specific diagnosis is vitally important. Because of the risk to the fetus with infections such as rubella, diagnosis during pregnancy is important. In an immunocompromised person, specific diagnosis is important. Viral infections also need to be distinguished from treatable bacterial and rickettsial diseases and from a rash caused by sensitivity to a particular drug. Diagnosis is also important in settings where isolation of patients or immunization of exposed people might be necessary to prevent epidemic outbreaks.

Few laboratory studies provide firm supportive evidence for diagnosis of a viral infection, short of culturing the responsible viral agent. Diagnosis of a viral exanthem is usually made by observation of the rash characteristics. This is especially true for roseola, where no etiologic agent is known. Bacterial cultures, complete blood count with differential, or liver function studies may be done to rule out certain diagnoses such as bacterial infection and hepatitis. If a drug eruption is suspected, the detection of eosinophilia may signal a hypersensitivity reaction. Patients with hemorrhagic eruptions should have a platelet count and possibly coagulation studies.

Viral cultures are helpful in enteroviral exanthems

when taken from several sites such as stool, urine, throat, nose, CSF, or a vesicular skin lesion. The rubella, rubeola, and parvovirus organisms are difficult to culture. In most instances, cultures are best obtained as early in the disease as possible.

Acute and convalescent serum antibody titers, usually drawn 10 to 21 days apart, are helpful in diagnosis confirmation. These tests do not give rapid results because it is necessary to have both titers for comparison.

★ ASSESSMENT

Nurses in ambulatory care settings, emergency rooms, and schools are often the first health professionals to see the signs of a viral exanthem. A thorough assessment with proper referral for treatment is essential in the prevention of complications and spread of the illness. A history of the onset, progression of the exanthem, associated symptoms, and medications is obtained as well as a history of upper respiratory infection, exposure to hepatitis, or other infections. Both the skin and mucous membranes should be examined closely, noting the distribution and morphology of cutaneous lesions. The eyes, ears, nose, and pharynx are also assessed for changes. Temperature is recorded as well as presence of lymphadenopathy, hepatomegaly, or splenomegaly.

★ NURSING DIAGNOSES AND PLANNING

Based on assessment data from above and Chapter 64, the following nursing diagnoses may apply to the family and child with viral skin infection:

- Impaired Skin Integrity related to scratching.
- Hyperthermia related to infection.
- High Risk for Infection (Secondary) related to scratching.
- Anxiety (Parental) related to knowledge deficit regarding disease and treatment.
- Ineffective Management of Therapeutic Regimen related to knowledge deficit regarding treatment.

The nurse and child (or parents) together plan effective care based on the established nursing diagnoses. Several examples of expected outcomes follow:

- The parents demonstrate effective care of their child during fever.
- The parents discuss the care they will provide for the child at home.
- The parents state steps to avoid spreading of infection at home.
- The parents state that their children have received all required vaccinations.
- The child expresses relief from itching.

The nurse plans for the care of the child based on both physician's orders and nursing diagnoses. Some general nursing care goals include the following:

- Spread of infection is prevented.
- Complications are prevented.
- Comfort is promoted.

★ INTERVENTIONS: COLLABORATIVE AND INDEPENDENT

Medical management of the child with a viral exanthem is usually symptomatic with the use of antipyretics for fever and antibiotics for secondary infection. If pruritus is a problem, oral antihistamines or a mild topical corticosteroid may be prescribed.

The amount of itching experienced varies. Lukewarm baths followed by a cream or ointment emollient, possibly containing menthol or phenol, provide relief in mild to moderate pruritus. Antihistamines are most effective if administered on a regular basis and before the pruritus becomes severe. Avoiding overheating also decreases itching. Scratching, with disruption of the skin barrier, is a major cause of secondary infection by bacteria. Keeping the child's fingernails short and taking measures to control itching, as well as keeping the skin clean are important to preventing impetiginization.

Temperature-lowering measures are most important with roseola due to its association with high fever. Parents are instructed regarding tepid baths, and any child with a history of febrile seizures should have seizure precautions instituted. In certain cases, anticonvulsants may be prescribed.

Several of the exanthems require isolation. Children with rubella or rubeola should be isolated for 5 days after the rash appears. Hospitalized children are kept in respiratory isolation. It is especially important for pregnant females to avoid contact with children suffering from rubella infection. No isolation is necessary for erythema infectiosum due to the mild nature of the disease, and children with enteroviral infection are placed in enteric isolation if hospitalized; otherwise, no specific isolation is needed. No special precautions are recommended in PAC or roseola.

Bedrest is recommended if the child is feverish or experiencing other systemic symptoms. Bedrest with quiet activity is especially recommended during phase two of rubeola. Otherwise, most children with viral exanthems may be as active as is tolerated.

Several additional measures may be taken, depending on the child's symptoms. Photophobia may be experienced by some children with rubeola. In these cases, dim lighting increases comfort. A cool mist vaporizer may be used if the child has a cough or coryza. Fluids and soft bland foods are recommended if the child has mucous membrane involvement.

The majority of children with viral exanthems convalesce at home. Time spent teaching parents about the disease course and measures to be taken while caring for their child goes a long way toward decreasing parental anxiety. Written guidelines provide parents something to which they may refer at home.

Prophylaxis of viral infection has been far more successful than specific treatment of an established infection. Vaccines have been extremely useful in prevention of a variety of illnesses. Effective vaccines for rubella and rubeola are available and administered at the age of 15 months. All prepubertal children, susceptible adolescents, and adult females of childbearing potential should be vaccinated against rubella. Pregnancy is avoided for 3 months after vaccination. There is no reported risk of administering rubella vaccine to a child if the mother is pregnant.[28]

★ EVALUATION

Periodically, the nurse and family evaluate the outcomes of care given. Examples of outcomes for the child and family with viral skin infection were given under planning in this section. Planning for further nursing care takes into consideration complications.

COMPLICATIONS

Rubella is essentially a benign disease with complications occurring rarely. Arthritis and arthralgia are complications that occur more with increased age. A mild encephalitis, which resolves completely without effect on intellectual function, has been reported. Thrombocytopenic purpura and peripheral neuritis also occur rarely.[28] The most serious complications occur with exposure of the fetus to rubella.

The devastating effects of rubella infection in the fetus were first described in 1941. Infants who are exposed to rubella in the first trimester of pregnancy experience multiple congenital defects of the heart, eyes, CNS, skin, ears, and the bone marrow. The earlier the infection occurs in gestation, the more severe the fetal damage. The accompanying display provides a list of potential congenital defects occurring as a result of prenatal infection.

Cutaneous manifestations during the immediate neonatal period include petechiae, purpura, and "blueberry muffin" spots (BMS). BMS are areas of extramedullary hematopoiesis and are the most common skin manifestation. Initially, the lesions are macular with a dark blue, dark red, or blue-gray color. They may become papular and measure up to 7 to 8 mm in diameter and persist for as long as 8 weeks before fading. BMS are usually seen on the trunk, scalp, or neck but may be seen on the extremities and face also. The characteristic macular rash of rubella seen in older children is not found in neonates.

Uncomplicated rubeola usually runs a self-limited course, lasting about 10 days with no sequelae; however, the prognosis in rubeola worsens in the presence of malnutrition or immunodeficiency.[28] Complications that have been associated with rubeola include encephalitis in approximately 1 of 800 cases, purpura secondary to thrombocytopenia, otitis media, and pneumonia.[28]

Roseola and erythema infectiosum generally run a benign course without sequelae. Rare febrile seizures have been reported in roseola, and neurologic sequelae, arthritis, encephalitis, and pneumonia are rarely associated with erythema infectiosum. Children with PAC are observed for signs of hepatitis.

Herpesvirus Infection

Definition and Incidence. *Herpes simplex virus* (HSV) is caused by two closely related herpes simplex viruses, type 1 and type 2. These are similar but distinct viruses that eventually infect most humans. They rarely cause life-threatening disease, but, in immunocompromised hosts, severe lesions can occur. Children with defects in cell-mediated immunity have more severe and persistent herpetic infections.

Oral-facial herpes simplex infection (gingivostomatitis) afflicts between 25% and 40% of people in the United States.[8] This is the most common manifestation of infection with HSV. Genital infection with HSV has been increasing in the past two decades, especially in the young adult population.

Varicella-zoster virus (VZV) infection, caused by the herpesvirus varicella-zoster virus, results in *varicella* or *herpes zoster*. Humans are the only known hosts for this virus.

Varicella (chickenpox) is a common, acute, and highly contagious infection. Around 96% of susceptible children develop the infection within 1 month of exposure. Varicella can occur at any age. However, 90% of the cases occur in children 1 to 14 years of age.[54]

Herpes zoster (shingles) is a sporadic disease. The majority of affected people are over the age of 60. The incidence increases with age and is low in children. Infection with herpes zoster is most common in children with depressed immunity. The illness does not develop as a result of exposure to someone with varicella. On the other hand, exposure to herpes zoster can lead to development of varicella in a nonimmune person. Second episodes occur in only 40% of people.[11]

Cytomegalovirus (CMV) infection may occur congenitally, or it may be acquired postnatally. CMV is an opportunistic pathogen in immunocompromised hosts. In neonates infected in utero and children with leukemia, or organ transplant recipients, this infection can be serious. However, infection postnatally or later yields a fairly benign course in the immunocompetent host. In the United States, 20% to 80% of adults have antibodies to CMV.[28]

The most common syndrome associated with *Epstein-Barr virus* (EBV) is *infectious mononucleosis.*

★ DISPLAY
Congenital Defects Associated With Prenatal Rubella Infection

Intrauterine growth retardation
Central nervous system effects
  Microcephaly
  Hydrocephaly
  Seizures
  Severe mental retardation
Visceral abnormalities
  Eyes: Microphthalmos
    Cataracts
    Retinopathy with black pigment deposits
  Heart: Patent ductus arteriosus
    Ventricular septal defect
  Ears: Delayed hearing loss
Bone marrow effects resulting in skin lesions
  Thrombocytopenia
  Blueberry muffin spots
  Petechiae
  Purpura

Infectious mononucleosis is considered endemic in adolescents and young adults in the United States. However, it is seen worldwide, and the incidence in young children appears to occur more frequently than originally believed.[28]

Etiology and Pathophysiology. Table 65-7 describes the etiology, transmission, incubation period, and the period of communicability for herpesvirus infections.

Intrauterine or neonatal infection by any of the herpes-viruses is much more likely to cause a life-threatening infection than in older children and adults. *Herpes simplex neonatorum* is estimated to occur in 1 out of every 3500 deliveries.[65] It is further estimated that there are about 20,000 pregnancies each year in the United States that potentially could be complicated by HSV infection.[36] Preterm birth increases the risk of disseminated infection, possibly related to the decreased opportunity for the transplacental transmission of antibodies. Infants exposed to HSV because of primary infection in the mother have a 50% risk of acquiring HSV in comparison to a 4% risk in infants whose mothers have recurrent infection. Approximately 70% of infants presenting with cutaneous manifestations progress to develop systemic infection.[36] The first month of life appears to be crucial because infection acquired during the first 28 days of life is more likely to disseminate and produce visceral complications than is disease acquired in older infants. Dissemination in otherwise healthy infants and children beyond this period usually does not occur.

Most neonatal HSV infection is with type 2 virus, although HSV type 1 infection is increasing in incidence.[32] The major mode of viral transmission is believed to be exposure to maternal genital infection at the time of delivery.[4] Intrauterine infection by way of transplacental transmission has been considered but not yet substantiated in several cases.[32] Intrauterine infection by the ascending route from an infected cervix occurs with prolonged rupture of membranes.

Maternal varicella infection is estimated to occur in 1 to 2.3 per 10,000 pregnancies, but *congenital varicella* occurs less often.[65] Most infants born to mothers with varicella in the first trimester appear to be normal. However, maternal infection early in pregnancy may cause the congenital varicella syndrome. The risk of *neonatal varicella* is approximately 24% when maternal chickenpox occurs in the 21 days preceding delivery.[65] Varicella infections after 10 days of age are acquired as a result of postnatal exposure.

Clinical Manifestations. *Primary herpetic infection* follows initial inoculation of a previously seronegative person. Clinical manifestations of primary infection may range from no apparent disease to a severe reaction with florid lesions, lymphadenopathy, fever, and systemic illness. The characteristic herpetic lesion is grouped vesicles on an erythematous base (Fig. 65-4). Mucosal lesions tend to ulcerate quickly. Pain or pruritus may accompany the eruption.

Reactivation of herpetic infection resulting in *secondary herpetic infection* may occur at all sites of primary infection. Recurrent episodes of facial–oral infection are most common on the vermilion border of the lip and is known as herpes labialis or a "cold sore."

Neonatal herpetic infection may be categorized as disseminated, local, or asymptomatic. Disseminated infection usually is rapidly progressive, with hepatic and adrenal necrosis, encephalitis, and pneumonia. The relative frequency of the various forms is unknown. Skin or mucous membrane lesions, consisting of the typical grouped vesicles on an erythematous base that quickly ulcerate, are present in 50% to 75% of infected neonates.[32,65] The initial site of involvement is frequently the area that first comes into contact with maternal HSV le-

TABLE 65-7
Herpesvirus Infection

Name	Etiology	Transmission	Communicability Period	Incubation
Herpes simplex virus (HSV) infection		Direct mucocutaneous contact	From prodromal period to healing of lesion	1–26 days Persistent viral shedding?
Oral, facial	Predominantly HSV type 1			
Genital	Predominantly HSV type 2			
Varicella	Varicella zoster virus	Respiratory droplet Direct contact Transplacentally	2 days before to the 8th day after onset of the rash	14–16 days
Herpes zoster	Varicella zoster virus	Direct contact can result in varicella in susceptible individuals	Until healing of skin lesions	Acute reactivation of an endogenous infection
Cytomegalovirus infection	Cytomegalovirus	Respiratory droplet Transplacentally	Opportunistic infection	Unknown Persistent viral shedding?
Epstein-Barr virus infection				
Mononucleosis	Epstein-Barr virus	Direct contact	Unknown	10–16 days

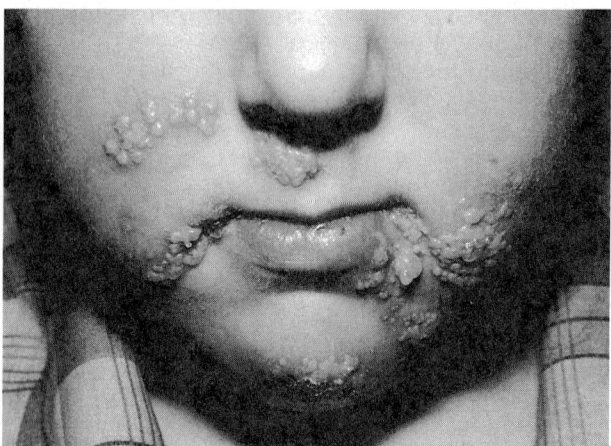

FIGURE 65-4
Herpes simplex. A florid eruption of grouped vesicles on an erythematous base characteristic of primary herpes simplex on the face of a child.

sions. Along with the typical appearance of the cutaneous lesions, infants with HSV infection have presented with a variety of other lesions.

Clinical manifestations of *varicella* include a variety of cutaneous and systemic signs and symptoms. Most recognizable is the vesicular exanthem that usually begins on the scalp or trunk and spreads to the face and extremities. The eruptions occur in crops and may first appear as erythematous macules that rapidly develop into vesicles with an erythematous base. A "dew drop on a rose petal" appearance is characteristic (Fig. 65-5). Crusts are formed on the lesions within a few hours to 1 or 2 days and gradually heal. Mucous membranes frequently are affected with lesions seen on the hard palate, uvula, tonsillar pillars, conjunctiva, and vulva. The number of cutaneous lesions varies from a few to several hundred. Children under 1 year of age, adolescents, and adults are at greater risk for a more severe course. A higher concentration of lesions may be found in areas of skin injury or irritation, thereby accounting for the higher incidence of a severe course seen in children with chronic skin disorders. In rare instances, other skin lesions may accompany infec-

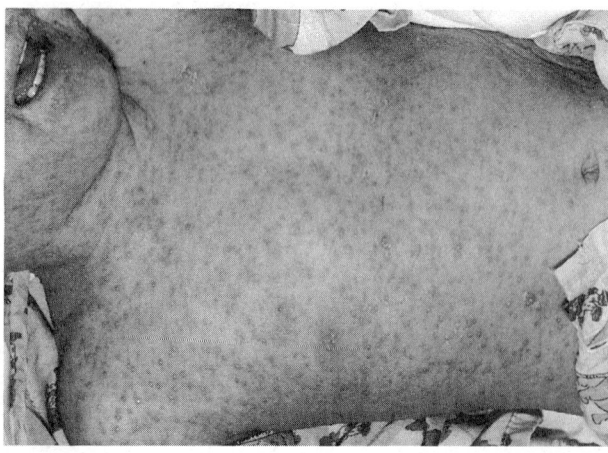

FIGURE 65-5
Varicella. Discrete vesicles on an erythematous base ("dew drop on a rose petal") characteristic of widespread varicella eruption.

tions, but this problem generally is seen in people more severely affected or immunocompromised.

Congenital varicella syndrome produces multiple congenital defects of the extremities, eyes, skin, and CNS. Late gestational infection causes neonatal varicella within the first 10 days after delivery. *Neonatal varicella* may be severe, with mortality ranging between 5% and 31%.[65] Characteristic cutaneous lesions are often accompanied by lesions in the lungs, liver, brain, kidneys, adrenals, and myocardium.

Herpes zoster represents an acute reactivation of an endogenous infection at the root ganglia by VZV that has persisted in latent form after a preceding varicella infection. If the person's immune response decreases below a certain level, the infection is reactivated, causing neuralgia and spread of the virus to appropriate sensory nerve endings in the skin and development of the dermatomal rash.[11] Development of the skin lesions is unilateral and generally involves from one to three dermatomes. The dermatomes most commonly involved are the ophthalmic branch of the trigeminal nerve and the thoracic dermatomes.

The cutaneous eruptions associated with *acquired CMV infection* are cutaneous ulcers and generalized exanthematous eruptions. Systemic symptoms include fever, lymphadenopathy, malaise, or mild hepatitis. In bone marrow transplant recipients and cardiac patients, a fatal interstitial pneumonia may develop. *Congenital and neonatal CMV infection* is rare.

The onset of the clinical manifestations of *infectious mononucleosis* may be acute or insidious, and the severity of symptoms varies greatly. These characteristics are believed responsible for the under-reporting that is thought to occur in this infection. Characteristic systemic manifestations include malaise, fatigue, fever, upper respiratory infection symptoms, and pharyngitis. Often, the pharyngitis is accompanied by cervical adenopathy and a membrane-like exudate. Hepatosplenomegaly may also occur and accounts for the abdominal pain experienced more commonly in older children. The clinical manifestations are usually less severe in younger children.

Younger children typically develop a rash along with the systemic symptoms. The rash is predominantly maculopapular but may take on a variety of forms including petechial, scarlatiniform, papulovesicular, or urticarial. An exanthem of petechiae or macules may also be seen on the palate.

Diagnostic Studies. Diagnosis of HSV infection is aided by the Tzanck test, viral culture, or skin biopsy. In addition, immunologic assays for the detection of HSV antigens in lesions are used. Viral culture of intact vesicular or pustular lesions yields a positive result in close to 100% of cases but only 34% to 72% in crusted lesions. A viral culture enables differentiation between HSV types 1 and 2. The Tzanck test of the base of an intact vesicle is a quick and simple diagnostic method that has a high correlation of 94% with viral cultures.[36] A skin biopsy is generally not necessary.

Laboratory tests in uncomplicated varicella are rarely necessary. Diagnosis is made by observing the characteristic cutaneous findings. A viral culture of vesicular fluid during the first 3 days of illness frequently is positive.

Acute and convalescent serum may be tested for complement fixing antibodies to confirm infection. A Tzanck smear and skin biopsy showing multinucleated giant cells demonstrates a herpesvirus infection but is not specific for varicella.

Diagnosis of herpes zoster is made by the characteristic appearance of the eruption along with the presence of pain. A Tzanck preparation and viral culture early in the course of the disease help to confirm the diagnosis.

Urine culture for CMV is the most specific test for this infection. The urine should be cultured immediately after collection or stored at 4°C. For general screening of neonates suspected of congenital CMV infection, the rheumatoid factor is most convenient. However, the rheumatoid factor is also positive in toxoplasmosis, syphilis, and rubella. Anticomplement immunofluorescence for CMV-specific nuclear antigens and monoclonal antibodies are new diagnostic tests that are diagnostic in 91% of infected neonates. These tests use urine samples and provide results within 16 to 24 hours.[65] A skin biopsy of the exanthematous eruption may demonstrate cytomegalic nuclear inclusions in the endothelial cells of cutaneous blood vessels.[28]

Diagnosis of EBV infection is made by obtaining a complete blood count with differential and monospot. Lymphocytosis is seen in approximately 70% of cases with white counts reaching 30,000 to 50,000. Atypical lymphocyte counts vary widely and may reach 90%. Mild thrombocytopenia may also be seen.

The most sensitive test for EBV infection is the monospot, which is a heterophile antibody test. The monospot quickly confirms the diagnosis in most cases; however, the incidence of false-negatives increases in children under the age of 4 years. The older heterophile antibody test using sheep red blood cells or EBV-specific antibody tests are available when the monospot is negative and EBV infection is still suspected.[66]

★ ASSESSMENT

Assessment in herpesvirus infections includes obtaining a history of the eruption and possible exposure. Notation is made of infection in family members and other close contacts (e.g., babysitters). In HSV, determination of whether the infection is primary or recurrent is an important consideration in planning care. The immunocompetence of the child is also established.

A total skin and mucous membrane examination is done, making note of the distribution of the skin lesions along with the morphology. The stage of evolution of the eruption, such as vesicular or crusting, provides clues as to how long the lesion has been present and whether the patient is still contagious. Temperature is also recorded.

★ NURSING DIAGNOSES AND PLANNING

Based on assessment data from above and Chapter 64, the following nursing diagnoses may apply to the family and child with herpesvirus infection:

- Impaired Skin Integrity related to open lesions.
- High Risk for Infection related to scratching.
- Hyperthermia related to infection.

- Pain related to skin lesions.
- Altered Oral Mucous Membranes related to spread of lesions.
- Altered Nutrition: Less Than Body Requirements related to oral lesions.
- Anxiety related to knowledge deficit regarding illness, treatment, and prevention.
- Ineffective Management of Therapeutic Regimen related to knowledge deficit regarding treatment and prevention.

The nurse and child (or parents) together plan effective care based on the established nursing diagnoses. Several examples of expected outcomes follow:

- The parents demonstrate they understand effective oral care of their child.
- The parents describe the care they will provide for the child during the infection.
- The pregnant woman maintains a regular prenatal schedule of visits with her health care provider.
- The family exhibits an understanding of the course of the disease and its prognosis.
- The child exhibits signs of comfort.

The nurse plans for the care of the child based on both physician's orders and nursing diagnoses. Some general nursing care goals include the following:

- Spread of infection is prevented.
- Secondary infection is prevented.
- Strategies are successful in promoting comfort.
- Anxiety about the child's illness, treatment, and prognosis is diminished.

★ INTERVENTIONS: COLLABORATIVE AND INDEPENDENT

Treatment often is limited to symptomatic care. Topical measures play a big role in accomplishing many of the goals of treatment, especially in HSV and VZV infections in which vesiculation and crusting are present. Cool wet compresses assist in cleansing moist open lesions and relieving pruritus. Soaks with Burow's solution may help promote drying during the weeping stage. The compresses are followed by application of drying agents, such as calamine lotion. It is recommended that topical benadryl be avoided due to the high incidence of hypersensitivity. A hair dryer set to low heat setting may also help in drying the lesions.

Gingivostomatitis often interferes with the child's ability to eat food and take fluids. Anesthetic mouthwashes, such as viscous lidocaine, may reduce the pain and are helpful when administered before eating. A diet of soft, cool food and cleansing the mouth with cool water rinses and a soft toothbrush increase the child's comfort.

MEDICATION THERAPY

A variety of systemic medications may be prescribed in the treatment of herpesvirus infections. Analgesics, antipyretics, antihistamines, and antibiotics are prescribed on an as-needed basis, depending on the symptoms the child experiences. Aspirin is avoided in children with varicella due to the increased risk of Reye's syndrome.

Systemic corticosteroids may be prescribed in herpetic eye lesions.

Acyclovir and vidarabine are two antiviral medications shown to be helpful in severe HSV and VZV infections in which dissemination or other complications are likely. These medications are not useful in the treatment of CMV or EBV infection. Acyclovir is the drug of choice in most instances and may be administered orally, parenterally, and topically. The topical form has been shown to be effective only in shortening the course of primary HSV infection and has not proven beneficial in recurrent HSV infection. Intravenous acyclovir is used in the treatment of immunocompromised hosts with mucocutaneous HSV or VZV infection and in neonatal infection. Oral acyclovir may be used to treat widespread infection in immunocompromised patients or those with eczema herpeticum. Acyclovir is also used in low doses over prolonged periods to decrease reactivation rates in genital herpetic infection and for prophylaxis of HSV or VZV infection in high-risk patients such as bone marrow transplant recipients who have especially high rates of HSV infection. However, the risks of long-term suppressive therapy are unknown.

Therapy in CMV and EBV infection is limited to supportive measures. Antiviral therapies are not beneficial. Oral corticosteroid administration in EBV is recommended if there are complications such as airway obstruction, severe thrombocytopenia, or hemolytic anemia.

PREVENTION OF INFECTION

Successful prophylaxis against most herpesvirus infections has not been developed. However, passive immunization with VZV hyperimmune globulin has helped to modify or prevent illness in high-risk people. The vaccine is administered within 72 hours after exposure to patients with leukemia or lymphoma, to patients receiving chemotherapy or other immunosuppressive drugs, and to newborns whose mothers have developed primary varicella within 5 days of delivery. A safe, live attenuated vaccine has been developed in Japan that appears to provide adequate immunity. Once available in the United States, this vaccine will probably be given to immunocompromised children but its use in well children is still debated.[54]

Because HSV infection is so common, infants are at risk of infection during the postpartum period. Transmission may occur if newborns come into contact with people (health professionals or family members) with HSV infection from direct contact (i.e., kissing or with inadequate handwashing techniques). An infant is particularly at risk for serious HSV infection during the newborn period if the mother has never had HSV and no antibody has been transmitted.[4] A confounding factor in identifying infants at risk is that 50% of mothers who have neonates with HSV have no history, signs, or symptoms suggestive of current or previous herpesvirus infection.[65] Furthermore, 70% of affected infants are born to mothers who have no signs or symptoms of genital herpesvirus infection at the time of delivery.[36]

In the nursery, any infant suspected of having a congenital or neonatal infectious disease is placed in strict isolation, and any pregnant personnel are cautioned to avoid contact. Any hospitalized child with herpesvirus infection should be placed in isolation to prevent spread

to other susceptible patients. There is no evidence that HSV is contracted by way of respiratory droplets or contact with inanimate surfaces. Also, the presence of any halogenated compound, such as chlorine, bromine, or iodine in water, immediately inactivates HSV.[18] Therefore, respiratory isolation is not required in herpes simplex infection. On the other hand, varicella infections in hospitalized patients can create monumental problems because it is so highly contagious and transmitted by way of respiratory droplets. Strict respiratory isolation is needed for both infected and susceptible children. At home, children with varicella should be kept isolated until the vesicles have dried, approximately 1 week after onset. Children with herpes zoster should be isolated from children with no history of varicella. No isolation recommendations are given for CMV or EBV infection except avoidance of direct contact.

TEACHING

Education plays a major role in the management of herpesvirus infections. The child and parents are taught about the course and prognosis of the infection, including a discussion regarding recurrent lesions in HSV infection, modes of transmission, and possible complications. The treatment plan is reviewed, and written instructions are given. Families with infants suffering from congenital infection are taught any special handling techniques required. If sequelae are present, the family is referred to appropriate agencies for assistance in dealing with the various problems that may arise. The Herpes Resource Center is a good resource for educational materials.

Activity restrictions generally depend on the degree of symptomatology and what the child can tolerate. It is recommended that children with EBV infection refrain from contact sports or heavy lifting for 2 to 3 weeks or longer if infection is accompanied by splenomegaly.

★ EVALUATION

Periodically, the nurse and family evaluate the outcomes of care given. Examples of outcomes for the child and family with herpesvirus infection were given under planning in this section. Have short-term goals been met? Are long-term goals still realistic? Planning for further nursing care takes into consideration complications.

COMPLICATIONS

Herpetic infection of the eyes with ulceration of the cornea and damage to deeper structures is a leading cause of blindness. Children with preexisting skin disorders, such as AD or blistering disorders, are at increased risk for widespread cutaneous and systemic infection. Development of HSV infection in this setting is referred to as eczema herpeticum. Herpetic infection of a digit may result in herpetic whitlow, which is often painful. Prepubertal children who present with genital herpes should be assessed for the possibility of sexual abuse. Devastating effects are seen in neonatal herpes simplex infection. Outside of these settings, HSV has coexisted with humans for centuries, causing fairly benign disease in the majority of cases.

The complications associated with varicella are many and serious. Virtually all cases with CNS involvement occur in normal children, whereas cases of pneumonia are seen in both normal and immunocompromised children.[28] The most common complication is bacterial infection of the skin by *Staphylococcus aureus* or GABHS. Cutaneous scarring is common and may be distressing, especially with keloidal scarring. Pneumonia, encephalitis, Reye's syndrome, hepatitis, arthritis, nephritis, meningoencephalitis, and aseptic meningitis are a few of the possible complications.

Complications associated with herpes zoster occur in both normal and immunosuppressed patients. Generalization of the herpes zoster eruption may occur within 1 week of onset of the eruption. Generalization is usually associated with internal involvement including pulmonary, hepatic, and CNS lesions. Postherpetic pain is rare in younger children. Scarring and anesthesia of the involved skin may occur with severe eruptions. Involvement of the eyes may lead to blindness.

CMV rarely causes complications in an immunocompetent child. However, when infection occurs in an immunosuppressed child, neurologic sequelae, pneumonia, and death may occur.

Prognosis in infectious mononucleosis is excellent, with approximately 95% of patients recovering completely.[2] However, convalescence of adolescents and young adults has been reported to take several months in some instances. Complications are varied and rare.

Tumor-Forming Viral Infections

Definition and Incidence. Several viruses have the ability to infect epidermal cells and produce tumor-like lesions known as molluscum contagiosum and warts. These lesions are commonly seen in children. Incidence of molluscum contagiosum ranges from 2% to 8%,[31] with the highest rates of incidence seen in children under the age of 5 years. The incubation period is from 2 to 8 weeks.[28]

Human papillomavirus (HPV) is a group of viruses that infect a wide variety of mammalian species. Cutaneous and mucous membrane infection with HPV produces a skin lesion commonly known as a wart. The incidence of warts is difficult to determine because many go unreported. From 0.8% to 10% of the population in the United States is estimated to experience warts,[31] but this figure is believed to be fairly low. Warts may be seen at any age but are more frequently seen in children and young adults.

Etiology and Pathophysiology. *Molluscum contagiosum* (MC) is a common viral infection in children that is restricted to the skin. It is caused by a pox virus that is the largest virus known to infect humans. MC is a contagious illness and is transmitted by person-to-person direct contact with the infective material, by fomites, or by autoinoculation.

Over 50 different human *papillomavirus* types have been identified. Some HPV types have been detected in cutaneous and genital cancer. It is believed that these types are oncogenic and probably play a role in malignancy.

The role that host immune factors play in the acquisition of warts is not understood. Certain apparently healthy people appear to be susceptible to HPV infection, whereas other family members never develop warts despite close contact. Cellular immunity rather than humoral immunity appears to play the important role in the control and spontaneous regression of warts.[31] Immunocompromised people are at risk for widespread infection, and future discoveries in this area may eventually lead to the development of a vaccine against HPV infection.

Transmission of HPV occurs by contact with infected stratum corneum either by direct contact with a wart on another person or indirectly by contact with infected scale on inanimate surfaces, such as locker room floors. Autoinoculation occurs frequently. Understanding the transmission of condyloma is of particular importance because of the association of possible sexual abuse in infected children. In sexually active adolescents and adults, they are transmitted by sexual contact. Acquisition in children may occur by autoinoculation, by contact with a caretaker who has warts, by contact with a sibling with whom they may have been bathing, or by exposure at delivery if the mother had genital lesions. All of these modes of transmission must be investigated thoroughly when a child presents with condyloma acuminata.

Clinical Manifestations. The typical MC lesion is a discrete, dome-shaped, waxy papule, which may or may not be umbilicated. The center of the papule contains a cheesy, keratotic core in which the virus lives and multiplies. The lesions vary in size from 1 to 5 mm, although larger lesions have been reported. Most MC lesions are white, pink, or skin-colored. Signs of inflammation may be seen in those that are irritated frequently. In general, the lesions are asymptomatic, although pruritus and pain may accompany the larger irritated papules.

The face, neck, axilla, abdomen, and thighs are the most common sites of involvement in children. Genital lesions are usually found in adults due to sexual transmission. Genital lesions in children are thought to more likely be caused by autoinoculation. However, the possibility of sexual abuse must be considered, especially in the absence of other cutaneous lesions.

Infection of the skin with HPV causes cell hyperplasia with eventual development of intraepidermal tumors or warts. These tumors vary in size and shape and are clas-

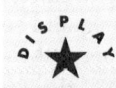

Clinical Classification of Warts

Verruca vulgaris	Common wart
Verruca plana	Slightly elevated flat-topped wart
Condylomata acuminatum	Anogenital wart
Mosaic verrucae	Extensive plantar warts
Verruca plantaris	Plantar warts
Filiform verruca	Stalk-like wart
Periungual verruca	Wart located in nail fold areas

sified according to their morphology and clinical location, as shown in the accompanying display. Warts are generally flesh-colored or tan, firm papules or plaques with a rough or smooth surface. Common warts occur most frequently on the hand, especially fingers, and are generally asymptomatic, unless they occur around or under the fingernail. Plantar warts are found on the plantar surface of the foot and can be painful when they are present at pressure points. Filiform warts are stalk-like lesions commonly seen on the face or hairy areas of the skin. Flat warts are skin-colored, slightly elevated, flat-topped papules that are often difficult to visualize. Condyloma acuminata are pink to white papules, found on and around the mucosal surface of the vagina, rectum, and urethra.

Diagnostic Studies. The majority of MC cases are diagnosed by the clinical findings. A crush preparation of the cheesy, keratotic core enables visualization of molluscum inclusion bodies after staining with Gram's, Giemsa, or Wright's stain. This study helps to confirm the diagnosis. Skin biopsy is rarely necessary.

Usually the diagnosis of warts is straightforward and made by clinical appearance. If the diagnosis is uncertain, paring off some of the hyperkeratotic material may reveal small, pinpoint, black dots or areas of bleeding characteristic of warts. Identification of the wart viral types is specialized and is generally not available unless the tissue is sent to a specialized laboratory.

Hard to visualize warts, especially those located in the anogenital region, may be more easily identified by applying 5% acetic acid. After soaking for 10 to 15 minutes, the warts turn white and become more visible.

★ ASSESSMENT

Nursing assessment of a child presenting with MC or warts includes obtaining a history of the lesion and possible exposure. Also, immunocompetence should be established, along with the presence of any chronic skin disorder.

At the initial visit, a total skin examination is done to determine the number and sites of lesions. If multiple lesions are present, it is often helpful to map sites to enable determination of resolution or new eruptions at future visits. The presence of MC or warts in other family members is also noted.

If genital or rectal lesions are present and sexual abuse is suspected, a thorough examination is conducted for other signs of abuse. Cultures for gonorrhea and serology for syphilis may also be obtained to rule out the presence of other sexually transmitted diseases. If there is reason to believe sexual abuse has occurred, the case is reported to the proper authorities for follow-up.

★ NURSING DIAGNOSES AND PLANNING

Based on assessment data from above and Chapter 64, the following nursing diagnoses may apply to the family and child with any of a variety of warts:

- Impaired Skin Integrity related to the tumor-like lesions.
- High Risk for Infection related to spread of virus.
- Anxiety related to knowledge deficit regarding illness, treatment, and prevention.

The nurse and child (or parents) together plan effective care based on the established nursing diagnoses. Several examples of expected outcomes follow:

- The parents describe the care they are to provide at home after treatment of the warts.
- The parents and child exhibit an understanding of the course of the treatment.
- The parents and child return for scheduled follow-up visits.

The nurse plans for the care of the child based on both physician's orders and nursing diagnoses. Some general nursing care goals include the following:

- Infection is eradicated.
- Further infection is prevented.
- Scarring is prevented.

★ INTERVENTIONS: COLLABORATIVE AND INDEPENDENT

Spontaneous regression is common with MC and warts. In the case of MC, nearly all lesions spontaneously resolve, although it may take several months to several years to occur.

Due to the high probability of spontaneous regression, the decision whether to treat depends on several factors. The duration, location, and number of lesions, especially if they are causing discomfort or are a cosmetic problem, are considered. Because younger children generally have a low tolerance for medical procedures, the age of the child and the amount of discomfort determine the type of treatment chosen. Cost, immunocompetence of the child, risk of scarring, risk of spread, and parental desires are also important factors. For instance, a healthy 5-year-old child with one plantar wart may not be treated. However, a child of the same age on immunosuppressive medication for asthma or renal disease would be aggressively treated. If no treatment is administered, parents are reassured about the benign nature of the condition and instructed on measures to prevent spread and infection. Treatment always remains an option for the future.

In many instances, treatment is undertaken because of the risk of transmission. In MC, several topical preparations may be used to induce blistering or irritation producing evacuation of the lesion. Most effective and least painful is the use of cantharidin 0.9% in flexible collodion. This preparation is carefully applied in the physician's office with a toothpick to induce a blister and enough inflammation to evacuate the lesion.

Additional treatment modalities include application of 25% podophyllin, retinoic acid, or benzoyl peroxide, as well as surgical curettage. Podophyllin may cause pain 24 hours after application, and the effectiveness of retinoic acid and benzoyl peroxide is questionable.

The only effective way to treat warts is to destroy the epidermal tissue in which the virus lives. Destruction can be accomplished with the use of several chemical agents or surgically. No one treatment modality is 100% effective, accounting for the frustration frequently experienced in the treatment of warts.

Salicylic acid in a combination with lactic acid is a useful and effective treatment. Other medications that may be used in the treatment of warts include application of trichloroacetic acid or cantharidin once a week after paring of the wart. These medications are applied in the physician's office and require repeated visits for treatment. Podophyllin also is used in the treatment of condyloma acuminata. A combination of salicylic acid, podophyllin, and cantharidin has been reported to be effective in 80 out of 100 children in the treatment of plantar warts.[17] However, this treatment can be used on only one or two warts at a time. Interlesional injections of bleomycin have also been successful but tends to be a more painful procedure. Extensive, widespread warts are extremely difficult to treat and can be disfiguring.

More aggressive surgical techniques for treatment of both MC and warts include curettage and cryotherapy. Carbon dioxide laser has also been used successfully. Care is taken when treating with surgical techniques to avoid scarring. All of these procedures involve a certain amount of discomfort and are poorly tolerated by younger children. Postoperative wound care instructions are reviewed and given to the child and parent to promote healing and prevent infection.

The possibility of autosuggestion in stimulating spontaneous regression cannot be overlooked. Every person involved in the treatment of warts for very long can relate a story about seemingly mysterious spontaneous regression.

Often the success in the treatment of MC or warts depends on the extent of teaching that is given to the patient and family. It is important that the nurse help the family to understand the importance of becoming a participant in the treatment plan. The biologic behavior of warts and MC should be discussed in understandable terms along with the importance of persistent treatment. Complete candor along with an optimistic outlook is vital in the face of often frustrating treatment. Follow-up visits for treatment are often necessary. The family needs to understand the importance of these visits to the success of treatment.

★ EVALUATION

Periodically, the nurse and family evaluate the outcomes of care given. Examples of outcomes for the child and family with warts were given under planning in this section. Planning for further nursing care takes into consideration complications.

COMPLICATIONS

Complications that may be associated with MC and warts include inflammation and secondary bacterial infection if lesions are excoriated. Fortunately, this response may result in resolution of the lesion. On the other hand, the inflammation may also lead to autoinoculation by spreading of the viral organisms. In addition, children with AD or other generalized skin eruptions and immunosuppressed patients may experience widespread cutaneous infection. Extensive inflammation and infections may result in scar formation. Periocular MC may be associated with conjunctival molluscum and conjunctivitis. However, ocular infection rarely results in permanent structural damage. Warts located on laryngeal structures have been reported to obstruct the airway and cause breathing difficulties.

Cutaneous Manifestations of Acquired Immunodeficiency Syndrome

The first pediatric cases of AIDS caused by HIV were reported in 1982. Since that time, the incidence of AIDS in children has reflected the increased frequency of HIV infection in women of childbearing age. As of June 30, 1992, 3898 children with AIDS have been reported.[13] Transmission of HIV to children occurs in utero or perinatally, or by receiving contaminated blood products. AIDS is discussed in Chapter 27.

The presence of opportunistic infections or neoplasms in addition to positive HIV serology is necessary to make the diagnosis of AIDS in children. The primary cutaneous manifestations are also listed in the accompanying display.

The most frequent cutaneous manifestation of pediatric AIDS is persistent oral and diaper candidiasis.[56] Oral thrush in children over the age of 1 year and younger children with oral or diaper candidiasis that does not respond to conventional therapy may suggest the possibility of underlying HIV infection in the absence of other factors causing immune suppression.

Other skin infections that have been reported to occur more frequently in HIV-positive children than in healthy children include herpes simplex, herpes zoster, and widespread MC.[56] It is also believed that children with AIDS are more susceptible to bacterial infections such as impetigo, ecthyma, and cellulitis than adults with AIDS.[34] Staphylococcal skin infections are especially prevalent.

The most common noninfectious skin manifestation of AIDS is a generalized eruption with features of seborrheic dermatitis such as erythema and scaling.[59] Intertriginous sites, the scalp, and forehead are most commonly

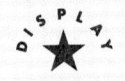

Cutaneous Manifestations of AIDS in Childhood

INFECTIOUS

Candidiasis
Herpes simplex
Herpes zoster
Molluscum contagiosum
Impetigo
Ecthyma
Cellulitis
Pseudomonas otitis externa
Tinea corporis
Onychomycosis
Cryptococcosis

NONINFECTIOUS

Seborrheic dermatitis
Thrombocytopenic purpura
Vasculitis
Cutaneous changes associated with
   nutritional deficiencies
Kaposi's sarcoma

involved. In addition, psoriasis may be exacerbated and purpuric or ecchymotic lesions associated with thrombocytopenia or vasculitis may also be seen.[59] Skin changes suggestive of nutritional deficiencies, such as pellagra, acrodermatitis enteropathica, and scurvy, are seen in children with AIDS due to the anorexia, malabsorption, and weight loss that often accompany this infection.[34,69] Kaposi's sarcoma is rare in AIDS during childhood.[9]

A propensity to develop pruritic skin lesions has been observed in adults with AIDS. In one series of patients studied, the pruritic skin lesions were the presenting manifestation in 79% of patients. The lesions included erythematous macules, papules, or nodules on the trunk, face, and extremities. These lesions tend to persist and do not respond well to any therapeutic regimen. Similar types of skin eruptions have not been reported in children. However, because of the high incidence in adults with AIDS, it is important to determine the prevalence in children. This is also true for other cutaneous manifestations that have been observed in adults but have not yet been reported in children.

The ability of the nurse to recognize the cutaneous manifestations of AIDS in children assists in early recognition of an opportunistic infection and permits prompt treatment as well as enables early detection of HIV infection.

Fungal Skin Infections

Definition and Incidence. Fungal infections are extremely common among children and widespread around the world. The skin is, by far, the organ most often affected by fungi. These organisms do not depend on humans for their existence; instead, they are able to thrive on inanimate surfaces in the environment as well as on the skin. Three types of fungal organisms infect the skin: the dermatophytes, *Pityrosporon* organisms, and the yeastlike fungi, *Candida.*

Fungal infection of keratinized tissues of the epidermis, nails, and hair by a dermatophyte fungus is called dermatophytosis. Dermatophyte infections of the skin are commonly referred to as ringworm or tinea. Table 65-8 lists terms used to indicate fungal infections at various

TABLE 65-8
Classification of Dermatophyte Infections

Name	Infection Site
Tinea corporis	Smooth skin not otherwise designated
Tinea faciei	Face
Tinea capitis	Scalp and hair
Tinea barbae	Bearded areas of the face and neck
Tinea manum	Hands
Tinea unguium	Nailbed and nail folds
Tinea pedis	Feet
Tinea cruris	Groin, perineum, and perianal areas
Otomycosis	Ear
Onychomycosis	Nails

cutaneous sites. Tinea capitis and tinea corporis are the most common forms of dermatophytosis found in children.

Pityriasis versicolor, also known as tinea versicolor, is a superficial fungal infection of the stratum corneum. Although this is a common skin infection in susceptible people, it often goes undiagnosed because of its benign nature. It most often develops after puberty but may be present at any age.

Candida infections are largely opportunistic infections contingent on diminished defense mechanisms in the host. People at greatest risk for developing candidiasis include the very young, very old, and immunocompromised. Candidiasis of the integument can be classified as mucous membrane involvement, cutaneous involvement, a combination of the two as in chronic mucocutaneous candidiasis, or systemic involvement.

Oral candidiasis, also known as thrush, is infection of the oral cavity including the tongue, soft and hard palate, and buccal and gingival mucosae. It is found most often in infants. Cutaneous candidiasis in children may occur on any surface of the skin where the appropriate growing conditions exist. Dark, warm, moist areas, such as the axillae, skin folds, and diaper area are most frequently involved. Candidiasis is the most frequent cause of infectious vulvovaginitis before puberty, although it occurs more often in adolescents.[62]

Etiology and Pathophysiology. Skin, hair, and nails become infected in dermatophytosis. This infection is caused by the colonization with one or more of the dermatophytes belonging to the genera *Trichophyton, Microsporum,* and *Epidermophyton.* Of the 39 species of dermatophyte recognized, most human infections in the United States are caused by only five species. These are *T. rubrum, T. tonsurans, T. mentagrophytes, E. floccosum* and *Microsporum canis.*[62]

During the past 25 years, *T. tonsurans* has become responsible for the majority of tinea capitis infections in the United States.[55] Boys and girls are affected equally; however, African-American children account for 90% of patients with tinea capitis.[27] The reason for this racial predilection is not known.

In childhood, the disease types (see Table 65-8) follow fairly regular patterns. Young children exposed to cats, dogs, or other animals often contract tinea capitis and corporis caused by *M. canis* or *T. mentagrophytes.* School-age children frequently become involved with institution-centered epidemics and are infected with tinea capitis caused by *T. tonsurans.* These infections are often brought home and shared with family members. By adolescence, tinea pedis and cruris become more common. Tinea pedis is generally caused by *T. rubrum, T. mentagrophytes,* or *E. floccosum.* The predominant causative organism for tinea cruris in the United States is *T. rubrum.* However, *T. tonsurans* infections seem to be on the increase. Infections of the hands, feet, and nails are less common before puberty. Dermatophytes do not depend on humans for their growth. Transmission occurs from inanimate objects such as combs, towels, brushes, hats, and pillows as well as person-to-person contact.

Pityriasis versicolor is caused by an organism called *Pityrosporon orbiculare* or *Malassezia furfur.* This organism is not a dermatophyte and, therefore, the name pityriasis versicolor is preferred over the more common name of tinea versicolor. *Malassezia furfur* is part of the normal flora of human skin; however, it proliferates in certain people, producing the characteristic rash. It is not understood what pathologic factors predispose a person to develop pityriasis versicolor, but it appears that warm temperatures, high humidity, and occlusion of the skin, along with certain genetic factors, play a role. Cushing's disease, immunosuppression, and malnutrition also predispose a person to develop pityriasis versicolor.[63]

Candidiasis is an infection caused by a yeast, *Candida albicans* or, on occasion, by other yeasts of the genus *Candida.* It is usually confined to the skin, nails, mucous membranes, and gastrointestinal tract but can be systemic and infect internal organs. The normal flora population on mucous membranes generally prevents overgrowth of *C. albicans.* Certain predisposing factors, listed in the accompanying display, may alter this ecologic balance, allowing overgrowth and infection by these yeasts. The most critical variable in predisposing children to *Candida* infection is their immune function.[63] Environmental factors, prematurity, endocrine function, intestinal flora, and medications also play important roles. Infants born of mothers with vaginal candidiasis have at least a 50% chance of developing thrush. But if the mother is not infected, the risk is as low as 1%. Prolonged hospitalization and care in a specialized unit also increase the risk of oral candidiasis in neonates.

Clinical Manifestations. *Tinea capitis* infection is characterized by hair loss, dandruff, and inflammation. The earliest sign is usually the appearance of dandruff followed by hair loss and inflammation after long-standing infection. Hair loss is usually the reason for seeking medical care. Close examination of the scalp reveals a fine, white, adherent scale. Tiny perifollicular pustules and hair stubs that have broken off at the surface of the scalp (so-called black dots) may also be present. The hair loss frequently appears in a "moth eaten" pattern.

The *tinea corporis* lesion starts as red scaly papules that multiply and spread peripherally, eventually forming scale-covered plaques. The typical lesion is annular and may have central clearing. It is usually accompanied by varying degrees of pruritus. As in tinea capitis, dramatic inflammatory reactions develop in those with hypersensitivity to the fungal antigen.

Tinea pedis, or athlete's foot, and *tinea manum,* a dermatophyte infection of the hands, are similar in their clinical presentation. Tinea pedis ordinarily starts in the toe web spaces with erythema, scaling, and maceration. The infection quickly spreads to involve adjacent areas of the foot. The overlying stratum corneum becomes thickened and white. Tinea manum is usually accompanied by tinea pedis. It appears as dry, scaly hyperkeratosis and commonly affects only one hand. It is thought to occur from contact of the hand with the infected foot.[63] Both forms can be pruritic and often occur in the same patient simultaneously.

Tinea cruris usually begins on the upper medial portion of the thighs and is similar in appearance to tinea corporis with erythema, scaling, and inflammation. Pustules and vesicles may be present on the advancing bor-

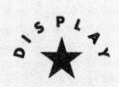

Predisposing Factors in *Candida* Infections

CONGENITAL

Maternal intrauterine device
Maternal cervical suture
Amniocentesis

NEONATAL

Maternal *Candida* infection
Invasive procedures
Hyperalimentation

INFANCY AND OLDER

Local occlusion with maceration
Skin trauma
Malnutrition
Extremes of age
Intestinal flora
Menstruation
Immunodeficiency
Diabetes mellitus
Cushing's syndrome
Uremia
Malignancy
Down's syndrome
Radiation therapy
Medications

ders of the plaque, and maceration frequently occurs. Tinea cruris is extremely pruritic, and persistent scratching may result in thickening of the skin or lichenification. It may be accompanied by tinea pedis.

The most common presentation of *pityriasis versicolor* is bilateral and symmetric scaly hypopigmented or hyperpigmented macules or patches on the chest, back, and neck. As the infection progresses, it may also involve the face, abdomen, groin, and proximal extremities. Slight erythema may be present. The scale is fine and superficial, and, if not immediately evident, light stroking of the involved areas with a dull blade or a fingernail causes it to become visible.

Candida infection causes the skin to develop a deep red color, often described as "beefy red." The raw skin area usually is edematous and oozing with pustules and crusting at the periphery. Small vesicopustule satellites on a red base occur away from the main area of involvement.

Cutaneous candidiasis usually presents in intertriginous sites because of the predilection of *C. albicans* for colonizing in warm, moist, macerated folds of skin. In infants, the most common presentation is in the diaper area (Fig. 65-6A), but frequently the neck area also is involved. In candidiasis of the diaper area, the recessed areas of the inguinal folds are usually involved as compared to primary irritant diaper dermatitis in which the inguinal folds are spared. In boys, the scrotum and the penile shaft are often inflamed, and, in girls, the vulva may be involved.

Clinically, *thrush* appears as white to gray, often "cheesy" looking patches on the oral mucosa. These patches are easily scraped off, revealing a raw, brightly erythematous surface. Other sites of involvement include the web spaces between the fingers and toes, the intergluteal fold, axillae, or on the backs of bedridden patients and around wounds being dressed with occlusive dressings. In obese children, the folds of the skin may become

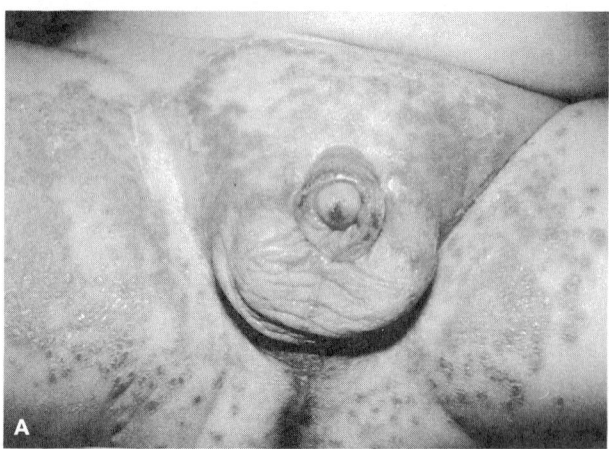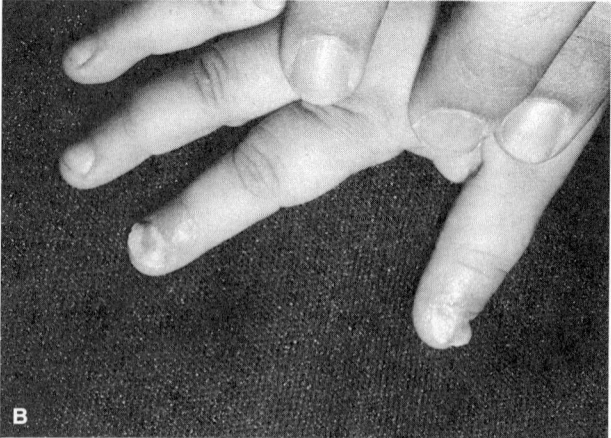

FIGURE 65-6
Candidiasis. (**A**) Cutaneous candidiasis. Erythematous papules and plaques with satellite lesions and involvement of the skin folds characteristic of cutaneous candidiasis in the diaper area. (Courtesy of Bernard A. Cohen, M.D.) (**B**) Candidal onychomycosis demonstrating erythema, inflammation, and nail distortion associated with *Candida* infection of the paronychia.

infected with *Candida,* especially in warm humid weather. *Paronychia,* inflammation of the periungual area, is often due to *Candida* in children who suck their fingers or toes (see Fig. 65-6B). *Congenital candidiasis* with systemic or cutaneous lesions is fairly uncommon.

Neonatal candidiasis develops after the first week of life and is usually limited to mucocutaneous lesions. Thrush is present in most cases of neonatal candidiasis, with diaper or intertriginous areas frequently involved. Systemic infection may be acquired as a result of invasive procedures.

In vulvovaginal candidiasis, the vulva exhibits varying degrees of erythema and edema along with pustules, maceration, and a whitish discharge. It is generally accompanied by intense pruritus. Its presentation in prepubertal children could signal the possibility of diabetes mellitus.

Diagnostic Studies. Diagnosis of fungal infections of the skin is made by the clinical appearance along with microscopic examination of a potassium hydroxide (KOH) preparation of the hair or scale and culture of the fungus on selective media. Treatment frequently is instituted before culture confirmation, which requires 2 weeks. Clinical appearance and a positive KOH warrant starting treatment because of the risk of contagion and potential complications that may result from failure to treat the fungal infection.

Diagnosis of pityriasis versicolor is by demonstration of short nonbranching hyphae and numerous spores in a KOH preparation. Culture is not useful in diagnosis because *Malassezia furfur* can be cultured from normal skin.

Diagnosis of cutaneous candidiasis is best done by visualization of the pseudohyphae and spores in a KOH preparation. Occasionally, a culture is helpful; however, findings may be misleading because it is possible to culture *Candida* from normal skin especially in the diaper area and oral mucosa. For infants suspected of having systemic involvement, cultures are made of their urine, CSF, and blood.

★ **ASSESSMENT**

Nursing assessment in fungal infections includes obtaining a history of the skin lesions, possible contacts, and accompanying symptoms. Physical examination is made of the scalp and skin, especially intertriginous areas, for the characteristic cutaneous manifestations of fungal infection. This information provides the basic subjective and objective data. Further inquiry is made into the presence of similar signs and symptoms in other family members or playmates.

Examination with a Wood's lamp may provide additional information. Tinea capitis caused by *Microsporum canis* fluoresces green. The pigmentary changes in pityriasis versicolor intensify under the Wood's lamp, and margins of involvement may be more readily seen. Infected areas may show a gold-to-orange fluorescence.

★ **NURSING DIAGNOSES AND PLANNING**

Based on assessment data from above and Chapter 64, the following nursing diagnoses may apply to the family and child with fungal skin infection:

- Impaired Skin Integrity related to oozing of lesions.
- High Risk for Infection related to spread of fungus.
- Altered Comfort (Pruritus) related to lesions.
- Ineffective Management of Therapeutic Regimen related to knowledge deficit regarding the spread of fungus, treatment, and prevention.

The nurse and child (or parents) together plan effective care based on the established nursing diagnoses. Several examples of expected outcomes follow:

- The parents and child demonstrate an understanding of how to prevent spread of the fungus to other family members and classmates.
- The parents state how the treatment is to proceed.

- The parents and child return for scheduled follow-up visits.

The nurse plans for the care of the child based on both physician's orders and nursing diagnoses. Some general nursing care goals include the following:

- Healing is promoted.
- Further infection is prevented.

★ INTERVENTIONS: COLLABORATIVE AND INDEPENDENT

Prompt identification with appropriate treatment of fungal infections is important to prevent their spread and potential complications. At one time, massive epidemics of tinea infections, especially tinea capitis, occurred regularly and were difficult to treat. Today, treatment with oral griseofulvin 10 to 20 mg/kg daily is effective for tinea capitis and resistant cases of other dermatophyte infections.

Adequate child/parent teaching is vital for successful treatment of tinea capitis. It is important for the parent to understand that the drug must be administered systemically so that it becomes incorporated into the growing hairs. Treatment should be continued for 2 weeks beyond the time of apparent resolution of infection, possibly as long as 6 to 8 weeks. If the medication is stopped too quickly, the infection will recur. Absorption of griseofulvin is enhanced by taking it with food, especially food with high fat content. Ketoconazole may be prescribed when griseofulvin is not tolerated or is ineffective. The use of selenium sulfide 2.5% as a shampoo three times a week is suggested to decrease shedding of the fungus and transmission of the infection. Failure to treat appropriately may lead to scarring and permanent alopecia.

Topical antifungal treatment, although not effective in treating tinea capitis, may be used alone for treating the remaining dermatophyte infections as well as pityriasis versicolor and candidiasis (Table 65-9). The antifungal preparation is applied one or more times a day, rubbed into an area larger than what is clinically infected, and continued for 1 week after apparent eradication. The skin surface should be kept cool and dry, avoiding occlusion. Warm, humid climates encourage growth of the fungus. Frequent diaper changes and allowing the skin to dry before rediapering decrease moisture.

Along with topical therapy, resistant cases of candidiasis may be treated with oral nystatin. In the case of disseminated candidiasis, amphotericin B, flucytosine, or ketoconazole is administered. In thrush, nystatin suspension applied four times a day is effective.

Multiple dermatophyte infections are common, with spread to family members and schoolmates. Early detection and treatment are vital to preventing continued transmission. Parents are instructed to wash all barrettes, ribbons, combs, brushes, headgear, pillows, coats, and linen frequently during treatment. These items should not be shared among family members. The school is informed of infection; however, children under treatment may return to school. A protective hat may be worn to contain broken hairs and scales. Follow-up examinations in 1 to 2 months after discontinuation of treatment help to identify reinfection.

★ EVALUATION

Evaluation of a child with a fungal infection includes inspection of the skin for resolution of the lesions. If any scale persists, a repeat KOH examination or culture may

TABLE 65-9
Topical Antifungal Medications

Name	Vehicle	Activity
Lotrimin (clotrimazole)	Cream, lotion, solution	Broad-spectrum
Mycelex (clotrimazole)	Cream, solution, troche, vaginal cream or tablets	Broad-spectrum
Monistat-Derm (miconazole)	Cream, lotion	*Trichophyton mentagrophytes, Trichophyton rubrum, Epidermophyton floccosum, Candida albicans, Malassezia furfur*
Mycostatin (nystatin)	Cream, ointment, powder, troche, oral suspension, vaginal tablet	*Candida albicans*
Nilstat (nystatin)	Cream	*Candida albicans*
Fungizone (amphotericin B)	Cream, lotion, ointment	*Candida albicans*
Halotex (haloprogin)	Cream, solution	Dermatophytes *Malassezia furfur*
Nizoral (ketoconazole)	Cream	Broad-spectrum
Spectazole (econazole nitrate)	Cream	Broad-spectrum
Loprox (ciclopirox olamine)	Cream	Broad-spectrum except *Trichophyton tonsurans*
Terazol (terconazole)	Vaginal cream and suppositories	*Candida albicans*
Exelderm (sulconazole nitrate)	Cream	Dermatophyte
Oxistat (oxiconazole nitrate)	Cream	Dermatophyte

be performed. The child or parent may be asked to describe the procedure followed in administration of the medication. The nurse also should question the family regarding symptoms of fungal infection in people who have close contact with the child. The nurse should determine if complications such as secondary infection and resistance to treatment are present.

COMPLICATIONS

Fungal infections in humans usually are not life-threatening. However, they can be fatal in children compromised by immune dysfunction or inadequate nutrition. Fungal infections become life-threatening when they no longer are confined to the skin surface, but infect deep into the skin and other organs of the body.

Candidiasis limited to the skin has a favorable prognosis. On the other hand, mortality in congenital systemic candidiasis is 50%.[65] The prognosis in neonatal candidiasis is excellent and is generally not responsible for infant deaths.[65]

Infestations of Lice and Scabies

Definition and Incidence. Infestation by lice (pediculosis) and scabies has plagued humans for centuries. The incidence is worldwide and affects all races, ages, and both sexes. Despite many years of awareness, infestations by lice and scabies may be on the increase.

Lice may be found on the head, body, or pubic regions. Head lice preferentially infests whites, Asians, Hispanics, North American Indians, and females. Head lice infest people at all levels of society and is a common problem in elementary school. The prevalence of body lice is unknown, but infestation is almost always confined to people of deprived social status because of poor personal and clothing hygiene. The ability to bathe and wash clothing regularly makes a person an unlikely host for continuing infestation.

Traditionally, pubic lice ("crabs") is considered a sexually transmitted disease. However, transmission also may occur by sharing of linen or beds. The presence of pubic infestation in children requires consideration of the possibility of sexual abuse.

Scabies is an infestation of the epidermis by the mite, *Sarcoptes scabiei.* The incidence of human infestation with scabies is believed to be increasing, although no accurate epidemiologic data are available. Scabies indiscriminately affects people worldwide, of all ages, either sex, and across all social classes.

Etiology and Pathophysiology. Only three species of lice infest humans: *Phthirus pubis,* the crab louse, *Pediculus humanus capitis,* the head louse, and *Pediculus humanus corporis,* the body or clothing louse. These insects are known to transmit vectorborne diseases such as endemic typhus, murine typhus, trench fever, and louse-borne relapsing fever. More deaths have occurred due to this louse than from any other insect except for the malaria mosquito.[67] Much concern exists about the potential for head lice to transmit diseases among children in the school or day care environment.

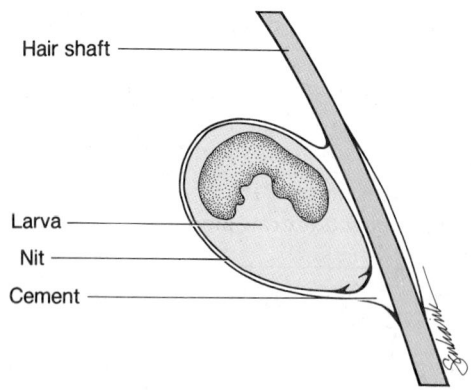

FIGURE 65-7

Head louse. The microscopic appearance of the head louse larva encased in a nit that has been attached to the shaft of a hair with an adherent cement.

Pediculus humanus capitis, the head louse (Fig. 65-7), ranges in size from 2 to 3 mm with a life span of approximately 40 to 50 days. The adult female deposits an egg, which is encased in an egg case or nit. The nit is attached to human hair 1 to 2 cm from the scalp with a cement-like substance (see Fig. 65-9). Over the next 7 to 10 days, the egg matures and hatches. *Pediculus humanus capitis* is able to survive away from the host for only 6 to 20 hours.

Pediculus humanus corporis, the body louse, ranges in size from 2 to 4 mm with a life span of 30 to 40 days. The louse normally lives in the bedding and clothing of the affected person, emerging only to feed on the host. Eggs are laid by the female in or near the seams of clothing, bedding, and mattresses.[67]

Phthirus pubis, the crab louse, generally infests the pubic hair but may be found in any hairy area of the body such as the moustache, beard, axillae, eyelashes, or scalp. Crab lice are the smallest of human lice, ranging in size from 0.8 to 1.2 mm. They attach nits to the hair shaft with an adherent cement similar to *Pediculus humanus capitis.* Empty egg cases resemble dandruff. However, the cases are not easily removed from the hair.

Like pediculosis, the scabies mite, *Sarcoptes scabiei* (Fig. 65-8), has infested humans for centuries. Transmission occurs through close personal contact with an infested person. Human scabies mites remain alive and well enough to infest a host for at least 36 hours after they are dislodged from the host.

Clinical Manifestations. Lice live by feeding on human blood. The individual feeding sites are difficult to see on the scalp. Usually, cases of head lice and pubic lice are first detected because of the pruritus that develops several weeks after infestation. On close examination, erythema, scaling, and excoriations may be seen on the scalp or skin with nits adherent to the hairs. Pyoderma, secondary to excoriations of the scalp, is a common complication of pediculosis capitis.

The bite of *Pediculus humanus* is relatively painless. The clinical manifestations are a result of the host reaction to the saliva injected by the louse into the dermis at the time of feeding. This reaction varies according to the degree of host sensitivity. The eruption consists of 2- to 3-

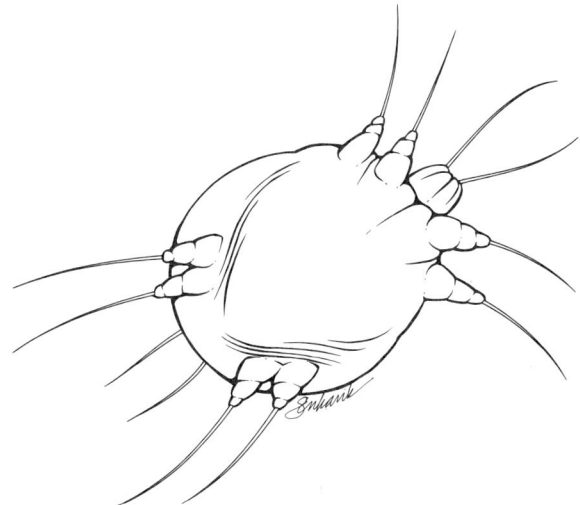

FIGURE 65-8
Female scabies mite. The microscopic appearance of the female scabies mite that is responsible for the cutaneous eruption associated with infestation of scabies. It is pinpoint in size and barely visible to the unaided eye.

mm erythematous macules or papules and *maculae cerulae*, blue-green macules indicating areas of old hemorrhage. In highly sensitive people, hivelike reactions may occur. Intense itching, especially at night, generally accompanies infestation.

The condition produced by infestation of *Sarcoptes scabiei* is a papular-pustular-vesicular eruption with crusting and intense pruritus. The characteristic lesion of scabies is a burrow, 5 to 15 mm in length, which is produced by the female scabies mite as it works its way into the epidermis and lays eggs. Many of the skin lesions are reactive inflammatory papules caused by the release of toxic or antigenic secretions and excretions of the female mite. The eruption is more pronounced in intertriginous sites, although it may be generalized.

In children and infants, the palms, finger webs, wrists, buttocks, intergluteal cleft, soles and medial aspect of the feet, periauricular area, umbilicus, and skin folds of the neck are the most common sites of infestation. These sites are where evidence of burrowing will be found. Children often present with complaints of severe itching that becomes particularly intense at night. Several other members of the household may also be experiencing itching. The pruritus generally does not begin until 2 to 6 weeks after exposure and infestation.

Diagnostic Studies. Diagnosis of pediculosis is made by identification of the oval nits firmly attached to the hair or actually seeing the louse on the skin or in clothing. Confirmation of the diagnosis is accomplished by removing the hair or the louse and inspecting it under the microscope (see Chap. 64).

Accurate diagnosis of scabies infestation can be difficult but is the key to eradication of this extremely disconcerting disorder. Diagnosis is made by microscopic identification of the mite, eggs, or feces on a skin scraping (see Chap. 64). Successful scrapings are most often taken from a new, nonexcoriated burrow on the hands, wrists, or feet. Multiple scrapings may be necessary to identify

the mite; however, failure to find the mite does not rule out scabies.

★ **ASSESSMENT**

Children who present with complaints of pruritus on the scalp should be closely examined for the possibility of head lice. The nits closely resemble dandruff but cannot be easily removed from the hair shaft. Regular screenings are conducted in many schools to identify infestations early. Once head lice is identified in the school setting, a notice encouraging frequent examinations is sent home to parents.

Children with scabies also tend to present with complaints of pruritus. Physical examination reveals the typical skin lesions and excoriations from scratching.

In all cases of infestation, an attempt to identify a history of exposure is important to prevent reinfestation. Family members, schoolmates, and playmates should be examined. When infestation occurs in young children and infants, intimate contact is much more common than with older children. In these cases, the school or day care center should be notified by the parents that their child has been diagnosed with pediculosis or scabies.

★ **NURSING DIAGNOSES AND PLANNING**

Based on assessment data from above and Chapter 64, the following nursing diagnoses may apply to the family and child with lice or scabies infestation:

- Impaired Skin Integrity related to itching.
- High Risk for Infection (Secondary) related to scratching.
- Altered Comfort (Pruritus) related to allergic reactions.
- Social Isolation related to fear of spread.
- Anxiety related to knowledge deficit regarding disease, treatment, and prevention.
- Ineffective Management of Therapeutic Regimen related to knowledge deficit regarding disease, treatment, and prevention.

The nurse and child (or parents) together plan effective care based on the established nursing diagnoses. Several examples of expected outcomes follow:

- The parents and child demonstrate an understanding of how treatment is applied.
- Parents state they have followed through on treatment and washing/cleaning household items.
- Treatment is effective in eradicating infestation.

The nurse plans for the care of the child based on both physician's orders and nursing diagnoses. Some general nursing care goals include the following:

- Infestation is eradicated.
- Transmission and reinfestation are prevented.
- Itching is relieved.

★ **INTERVENTIONS: COLLABORATIVE AND INDEPENDENT**

Lindane 1% (Kwell, Scabene) is the treatment of choice in most cases of head and body lice. Lindane is available as a cream, lotion, or shampoo. Clear administration instructions are necessary to ensure adequate treatment. In the case of head lice, the shampoo is rubbed into the hair and on the scalp for 10 minutes and then rinsed out. After treatment, the nits are removed with a fine-toothed comb because lindane may not kill the nits. A 50% vinegar and 50% water solution applied to the hair for 1 hour may help to dissolve the cement and facilitate nit removal. A system for nit removal has been developed called Step 2. This system includes a comb and creme rinse containing a chemical that appears to loosen the powerful natural adhesive that bonds the nits to the hair shaft. Reapplication of lindane in 7 to 9 days kills any lice that were not removed and that hatched since the first treatment. Over-the-counter products such as RID, Nix, and A-200 Pyrinate are also available. Despite the therapy used, the child is examined frequently over the subsequent 2 weeks to ensure a cure.

RID is the preferred treatment for pediculosis pubis because of its effectiveness in a shorter period of time and with less toxicity potential than lindane.[67] The shampoo is applied for 5 minutes. Repeated application in 7 to 9 days is recommended to ensure eradication of the infestation. When eyelashes are infested, RID is not used; instead, petrolatum is applied two to five times daily for 8 days. This treatment causes the lice to suffocate and die.

In all cases of lice infestation, decontamination of inanimate objects is recommended. Linens, clothing, and headgear are washed in hot water (above 125°C) and dried in a hot dryer or dry cleaned. Items that cannot be cleaned are sealed in a plastic bag for 10 days. Floors and furniture should be thoroughly vacuumed. This removes all loose hairs with attached eggs. Hair combs and brushes may be coated with the pediculicide for 15 minutes and then washed in hot soapy water. In the case of body and pubic lice, furniture and carpeting may be treated with an insecticide spray. However, only products approved for such uses should be used. Household or agricultural sprays or powders should not be used.

Therapy for scabies requires treatment of the infested child and all close personal contacts simultaneously. Transmission at school is thought to be unlikely, but anyone sharing beds, linen, or other types of close contact over the past 4 to 6 weeks should be treated. All symptomatic or asymptomatic contacts are treated at the same time.

The drug of choice for scabies is 1% lindane (Kwell, Scabene) lotion or cream. One to 2 oz is required to treat each adult, and less is required for children and infants. The cream or lotion is applied from the neck down over the entire body in a single application before bed. A bath or shower before application is not recommended because hydration of the skin increases the systemic absorption of lindane. Infants and children with scalp or facial involvement should have the lindane carefully applied to those areas avoiding the eyes, mouth, and nose. Special attention is also paid to intertriginous area such as the neck, postauricular folds, axillae, umbilicus, gluteal cleft, wrist, finger or toe webs, and subungual regions. It may be necessary to cover the child with clothing as much as possible, including socks over the hands, to avoid oral contact with the medication. The lindane should remain on the skin 6 to 8 hours and is washed off completely in the morning.

One treatment is generally sufficient to treat scabies infestation unless the child is exposed. Frequently, pruritus continues after treatment for several days to 2 weeks. Retreatment is not recommended unless reinfestation is documented with a positive scraping, but no sooner than 7 days after the last treatment. Antihistamines may be prescribed for the pruritus along with regular use of a cream or ointment emollient.

Because of the social stigma associated with infestation, it is important to reassure parents the condition is common and does not automatically mean the child has received inadequate care. Teaching the parents methods of eradication helps to dispel anxiety. The National Pediculosis Foundation, a parent-sponsored consumer advocacy group that encourages research and public education, is available as a resource for health care professionals and parents.

★ EVALUATION

Evaluation of the child with an infestation includes examination for resolution of the skin lesions and pruritus. The skin is inspected for signs of reinfestation or complications such as secondary infection and xerosis. The nurse should determine whether close contacts of the child were treated and if any are experiencing symptoms of infestation. In schools where students with infestations have been identified, regular examinations of all students are required for early diagnosis and treatment.

Disorders of Appendageal Structures

Hair, nails, sebaceous glands, eccrine glands, and apocrine glands are appendageal structures of the skin. Disorders of these specialized structures may occur independently or in association with systemic or cutaneous disorders. Acne and several disorders affecting the hair are described in this section. In addition, nail alterations are briefly reviewed.

Acne Vulgaris

Definition and Incidence.   Acne vulgaris is a common disorder of the pilosebaceous unit that involves intrafollicular hyperkeratosis and increased sebum production, with or without inflammation. The disorder is almost universal in adolescents. Acne also is seen frequently in children as early as 9 or 10 years of age; it is also seen occasionally in infants as a result of maternal hormone stimulation.

Etiology and Pathophysiology.   The pathophysiology of acne has become clearer in the past few decades. One of the basic underlying abnormalities is an alteration of keratinization in the upper third of the hair follicle that

Factors in the Pathogenesis of Acne

ENDOGENOUS FACTORS

Sex steroid hormones
Bacterial colonization
Individual host immune responses
Defect of keratinization

EXOGENOUS FACTORS

Cosmetics
Season
Medications

renders it more sticky. The accumulated material, keratin and sebum plus bacteria, within the dilated follicle makes up the acne lesion.[45]

Several underlying factors are important in the pathogenesis of acne vulgaris as listed in the accompanying display. The first is hormonal, namely androgenic hormones. This process is evident with acne occurring under maternal hormone influence in the neonate, at puberty in the adolescent, premenstrually in the menstruating female, and in association with polycystic ovarian disease or adrenal disorders. People with acne complain of flare-ups during times of stress, such as before final exams at school, giving further credence to the hormonal basis of acne.

The second factor contributing to the development of acne is bacterial colonization. *Propionibacterium acnes* and *Micrococcus* are part of the skin's normal flora. However, people with severe acne have higher colony counts of these organisms, particularly *Propionibacterium acnes,* than do people without acne or those mildly affected.

A third factor is the individual host immune response, which determines the degree of inflammation and differentiates mild from moderate or severe acne. This is the newest causal factor of acne to be studied and has provided evidence that the effectiveness of antibiotics in acne may be related to their antiinflammatory action over their antibacterial action.

The final factor considered as an etiological factor is a defect in keratinization that causes plugging of the follicular orifice.

All of these endogenous factors act together to determine the type and severity of acne. In addition, various exogenous factors may be added to the etiology formula. Cosmetics, oily hair pomades, hair spray, yearly seasons, and drugs are examples of exogenous factors in acne. Fortunately, many cosmetic products specifically designed for acne-prone skin are available. Some people note improvement of their acne in the summer. In other individuals, however, acne is aggravated by sweating. Many note improvement with UVL exposure. Drugs that are known to cause acneiform eruptions include corticosteroids and lithium. Diet is not considered a major factor in the acne process.

Clinical Manifestations. The cutaneous sites most often affected by acne vulgaris are the face, upper chest, and upper back. In severe cases, acne lesions may also be seen on the scalp, neck, buttocks, and proximal extremities.

The primary acne lesion is the microcomedo (Fig. 65-9). These lesions are difficult to see and are easier to feel by lightly rubbing a fingertip over the skin. As more keratin accumulates, the microcomedo develops into a

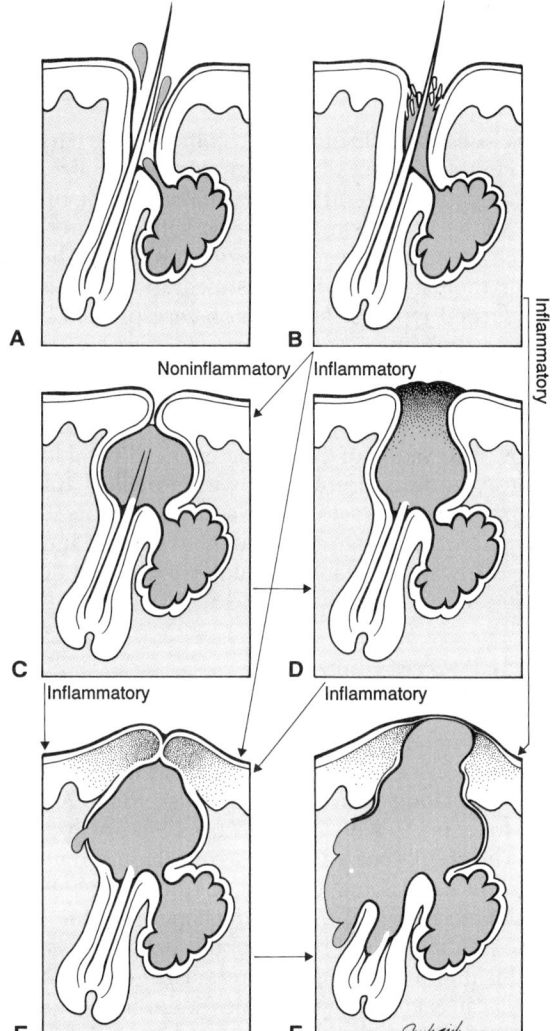

FIGURE 65-9

Pathogenesis of acne. (**A**) The normal pilosebaceous unit as compared to changes of the pilosebaceous units in acne. (**B**) The microcomedo is the primary acne lesion demonstrating early retention of epithelial cells. (**C**) The closed comedo (whitehead) is an enlargement of the microcomedo that results from obstruction of the pilosebaceous unit opening and further retention of the epithelial cells. (**D**) The open comedo (blackhead) is a mature comedo in which the opening has dilated and is obstructed with a dark plug of epithelial cells and sebum. A closed or open comedo may develop into (**E**) an inflammatory papule if the follicular wall ruptures, expelling the pilosebaceous unit contents into the dermis resulting in an ensuing inflammatory reaction. As the lesion enlarges the lesion may become (**F**) pustular or cystic. (Redrawn with permission from Dermatological Division, OrthoPharmaceutical Corporation, Raritan, NJ.)

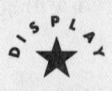

Classification of Acne Lesions

NONINFLAMMATORY ACNE

Microcomedones
Closed comedones
Open comedones

INFLAMMATORY ACNE

Papules
Pustules
Nodules

visible closed comedo or an open comedo. The dark color of the central portion of an open comedo is a result of oxidization of the central material, turning it black in color. As the condition progresses with rupture of the follicular wall, inflammatory lesions are seen. These include erythematous papules, pustules, and nodules. Typically, several types of acne lesions are present on the skin at any one time. The accompanying display provides the classification of acne lesions.

Diagnostic Studies. Diagnosis of acne vulgaris is made by observation of the characteristic clinical lesions. Laboratory findings are usually within normal limits in acne patients. Occasionally, serum androgens are screened in women with acne and other signs of androgen excess, such as hirsutism, irregular menses, or delayed menarche.

★ ASSESSMENT

The initial evaluation of children with acne requires assessment of general medical history, historic data regarding disease onset and progression, previous treatment, and results, along with associated symptoms. A family history for acne, as well as a menstrual history in girls, is noted. The child's current skin care regimen is reviewed, and current topical and systemic medications are documented. The family's current understanding of the pathogenesis, treatment, and beliefs about how acne is exacerbated is important for a comprehensive database.

Physical examination includes identification of the skin lesions, noting their pattern and distribution. An assessment of sexual development and growth is also made, especially noting hirsutism in females.

★ NURSING DIAGNOSES AND PLANNING

Based on assessment data from above and Chapter 64, the following nursing diagnoses may apply to the family and child with acne:

- Impaired Skin Integrity related to hormonal influence.
- High Risk for Infection (Secondary) related to picking and squeezing the lesions.
- Self-Concept Disturbance related to altered physical appearance.

- Anxiety related to knowledge deficit regarding the cause of acne and effective treatment.
- Ineffective Management of Therapeutic Regimen related to knowledge deficit regarding illness and treatment.

The nurse and child (or parents) together plan effective care based on the established nursing diagnoses. Several examples of expected outcomes follow:

- The parents and adolescent demonstrate an understanding of treatment and prognosis.
- The adolescent discusses healthy cleansing of the face.
- The adolescent discusses importance of compliance with treatment regimen.
- The adolescent states he or she feels less self-conscious about appearance.

The nurse plans for the care of the child based on both physician's orders and nursing diagnoses. Some general nursing care goals may be the following:

- Infection and scarring are prevented.
- Appearance is improved.

★ INTERVENTIONS: COLLABORATIVE AND INDEPENDENT

Successful treatment of adolescent acne depends on developing an individualized treatment plan along with patient/parent education. The primary components of treatment for acne are medications, education, and psychosocial support of the adolescent.

MEDICATION THERAPY

Table 65-10 outlines current topical and systemic medications prescribed for the treatment of acne. These medications may be used individually or in combination. All

TABLE 65-10
Topical and Systemic Acne Medications

Name	Vehicle	Action
Topical Medication		
Benzoyl peroxide (2.5%, 5%, 10%)	Gel, lotion, wash, soap	Comedolytic, bacteriostatic
Tretinoin (0.025%, 0.01%, 0.05%, 0.1%)	Cream, gel	Increase cell turnover in follicular wall
		Decrease stickiness of follicular contents
		Prevent microcomedo formation
Topical antibiotics (erythromycin, clindamycin, tetracycline)	Gel, lotion, solution, cream	Decrease colonization of *P. acnes*
Systemic Medication		
Systemic antibiotics (tetracycline, minocycline, erythromycin)		Decrease colonization of *P. acnes*
		Antiinflammatory
Hormonal therapy		Decrease sebum production
Accutane (isotretinoin)		Decrease sebum production
		Decrease sebaceous gland size
		Increase cell turnover in the follicular wall

topical medications may cause skin drying and sun sensitivity. To avoid these effects, treatment is started slowly and increased in dose and frequency as tolerance develops. For truly effective treatment, the medications must be applied regularly in a thin film to all acne-prone areas. If medications are used only on active lesions, the preventive quality of the medication is lost. Children and parents are warned about sun sensitivity and advised to use noncomedogenic sunscreens or to avoid sun exposure during treatment. Patients are also warned that benzoyl peroxide may cause bleaching of colored clothing and linen.

The preferred topical regimen for mild to moderate acne is benzoyl peroxide or tretinoin alone once or twice daily or in combination. When combination therapy is prescribed, the benzoyl peroxide and tretinoin are never applied at the same time because of the ability of benzoyl peroxide to oxidize tretinoin and render it useless.[70] If benzoyl peroxide is not tolerated, a topical antibiotic may be used.

Systemic treatment is reserved for inflammatory acne. Tetracycline and erythromycin are the mainstays in systemic antibiotic treatment of acne. At the outset, antibiotic therapy in acne needs to be continued for at least 6 to 12 months and then tapered to be successful. Minocycline is a second-generation tetracycline that also is clinically effective in the treatment of acne.

Severe nodular acne has been an extremely difficult disease to control. In 1955, isotretinoin (Accutane), a vitamin A derivative, was synthesized. Subsequently, this drug has produced dramatic results in people with this severe inflammatory form of acne. However, because of the potential for acute and chronic toxicity and extreme teratogenicity, isotretinoin is approved for use only in severe, recalcitrant, nodular acne that is unresponsive to conventional treatment.

Despite strong evidence of the impact isotretinoin has on severe acne, its availability is threatened by continued accidental fetal exposure and subsequent development of severe congenital malformations or fetal death. Extensive educational efforts have been directed at preventing fetal exposure. The nurse plays an important role in educating and monitoring females of childbearing potential on isotretinoin. Effective contraceptive measures do exist and if used appropriately, the fetus should not be exposed to isotretinoin.

Nonsteroidal antiinflammatory drugs (NSAIDs) and hormonal therapy are other options for the treatment of acne. As a result of recent investigations into the role of inflammation in acne, clinical trials are in progress to evaluate the effectiveness of NSAIDs alone or in combination with tetracycline in the treatment of acne. Although not a standard part of acne therapy, NSAIDs may become a relatively safe addition to the therapeutic options in the treatment of acne.[45]

Hormonal therapy is reserved for women in whom an endocrine abnormality has been documented. Estrogen, low-dose glucocorticosteroids, or antiandrogens such as spironolactone may be prescribed in these cases.

SUPPORT OF ADOLESCENT

A myth that is commonly associated with acne is that it comes from dirty skin. This belief often results in the use of harsh and abrasive skin cleansing techniques. Many medications used to treat acne also have a drying and irritating effect on the skin. Therefore, a gentle cleansing regimen is recommended. The affected area is washed with a gentle cleanser or soap no more than twice daily. Rough scrubbing, picking, and squeezing of the lesions are avoided. Only noncomedogenic cosmetics and sunscreens should be used on affected areas.

Adolescents are particularly sensitive about their appearance and obtain much of their self-confidence and self-esteem from their own sense of attractiveness. Self-consciousness about their appearance may contribute to adolescents' withdrawal and social isolation. Adolescents also tend to have an "act now" approach to life and desire a "quick fix" for their acne, making waiting for the medication to be effective difficult. Nonadherence is the major cause for treatment failure in acne.[57]

The nurse needs to be aware of these characteristics in adolescents in order to establish an alliance with the teenager for development of a shared treatment plan. Time is spent helping the adolescent understand his or her acne problem and discussing how treatment can fit into his or her lifestyle. Acne is a chronic problem during the teenage years, and nurses should also foster realistic expectations regarding treatment and the effort required on the part of the teenager to obtain the optimum effect.

Adolescents are also strongly influenced by peers and media advertisement. They often switch from product to product. The nurse can discuss various myths about acne to help increase adherence to treatment and to prevent disappointment with therapy.

★ **EVALUATION**

The nurse evaluates the skin to determine the effectiveness of the prescribed treatment and the presence of complications, such as dryness, irritation, sun sensitivity, and infection. The child is asked to describe the procedure followed in cleansing the skin and application of medications. The nurse should determine the use of effective birth control measures in females using tetracycline or isotretinoin. The nurse also should assess the impact of the condition on the development of self-esteem and social relationships.

Prognosis in acne is generally good, especially with compliance to recommended treatment. Adolescent acne usually abates by late teens to early twenties. However, in some instances, acne continues into adulthood. Permanent scarring may occur and is especially prevalent in the more inflammatory types of acne. With increased understanding of the pathophysiology, some researchers believe that early treatment of comedonal acne may prevent the development of scarring inflammatory acne.[40,45]

Disorders of the Hair

Definition and Incidence. During the period of hair growth, the normal cyclic pattern may be interrupted by a variety of factors. (See Chap. 63 for review of the hair growth cycle.) The disorders of hair discussed in this section relate only to hair loss and include telogen effluvium, anagen effluvium, alopecia areata (AA), and traumatic hair loss. (See *Dermatology in General Medicine*[8] for additional information on other types of hair disorders, which include hair shaft abnormalities, pigment abnormalities, and hypertrichosis or hirsutism [excessive hair growth].)

Conditions that cause hair loss are a common problem in children. Because of the effect of hair loss on appearance, children, adolescents, and their parents often become concerned. The exact incidences of telogen effluvium (trauma- or stress-related hair loss), anagen effluvium (hair loss related to environmental chemical exposure), and traumatic hair loss are unknown.

Alopecia areata is defined as the sudden appearance of well-circumscribed patchy hair loss. This condition is fairly common in both children and adults. Ten to 20% of affected people have a positive family history for AA.[8]

Etiology and Pathophysiology. *Telogen effluvium* is fairly common and represents hair loss after some type of stressful event. In this condition, the normal anagen phase of hair growth is shortened with early conversion to telogen phase and subsequent hair loss. This condition may occur after a febrile illness, surgical shock, crash diet, injury, emotional stress, pregnancy, or the use of certain drugs such as anticoagulants, beta-blocking agents, or estrogen-dominated oral contraceptives.[36]

Anagen effluvium occurs as a result of the use of antimitotic chemotherapy agents, such as those used in the treatment of cancer. It is a much less common disorder than telogen effluvium. Excessive irradiation of the scalp can also cause anagen effluvium as well as ingestion of chemicals such as lead, thallium, arsenic, bismuth, or Coumadin.[8]

The cause of alopecia areata (AA) is unknown; however, recent evidence points to an autoimmunologic process.[8] The hair loss is a result of follicular damage with interruption of the growth cycle. The hair follicle shrinks and remains small, not progressing past early anagen, as long as the disease is active. Disorders in which an increased incidence of AA is seen include Hashimoto's thyroiditis, pernicious anemia, adrenal disease, vitiligo, diabetes, AD, and Down's syndrome.

Traumatic alopecia results from forceful removal of the hair causing hair shaft breakage or extraction of the entire hair. Traumatic alopecia may result from hair styles that include the use of tight braids, ponytails, or curlers. The use of a hot comb for hair straightening or curling can result in traumatic hair loss. Hair loss of this type is referred to as *traction alopecia*.

Traumatic hair loss may also occur with prolonged bedrest in one position. The most common situations in which this type of hair loss is seen are with the chronically ill or after a prolonged surgical procedure in which the head is kept in one position for extended periods of time. It also may be seen in neglected infants who are left in a crib or playpen for extended periods of time.

Trichotillomania is a self-induced, traumatic hair loss caused by pulling, twisting, or rubbing the hair. The most common area of involvement is the scalp, but eyebrows and eyelashes may also be involved. This disorder may signal an unconscious habit, emotional stress, or a deep-rooted psychological problem.[37]

Clinical Manifestations. The amount of hair loss experienced by the child in *telogen effluvium* is variable and depends on the proportion of follicles affected. The hair loss is generalized and noted by overall hair thinning and increased hair loss during grooming. In *anagen effluvium*, the hair follicle converts to a modified growth phase producing fine velluslike hair. The amount of hair loss depends on the degree of toxicity of the offending agent. Frequently, profound hair loss results.

Typically, *AA* presents suddenly with one or more, round or oval patches of total hair loss (Fig. 65-10). Occasionally, the patch is irregularly outlined. This hair loss may occur on any hair-bearing surface of the skin. Characteristically, the skin of the involved scalp area is smooth, soft, and ivory-white in color. Loose "exclamation mark" hairs with large bulbs and short stumps may be detected, especially at the perimeter of the hair loss patch. "Exclamation mark" hairs are considered pathognomonic for AA.

Trichotillomania appears as irregularly shaped patches of hair loss, which are never completely bald. The hairs within these areas are often short, broken off, and of varying lengths. Other types of *traumatic hair loss* are noted at the site of the trauma. Areas where the hair is parted and the occipital region are most frequently involved.

Diagnostic Studies. Diagnosis of hair disorders is made by observation of the typical clinical appearance along with several office and laboratory tests that aid in further delineating the problem. The hair pull test (see Chap. 64) is useful to determine how active the hair loss is at the time of examination. The hair bulbs of epilated hairs may be examined under the microscope to determine the growth cycle stage. A KOH may be done of scale or broken hair to rule out tinea capitis. A skin biopsy of an affected site is often helpful, especially in AA or trichotillomania.

★ **ASSESSMENT**

Nursing assessment of hair disorders includes obtaining a history regarding the onset and progression of the dis-

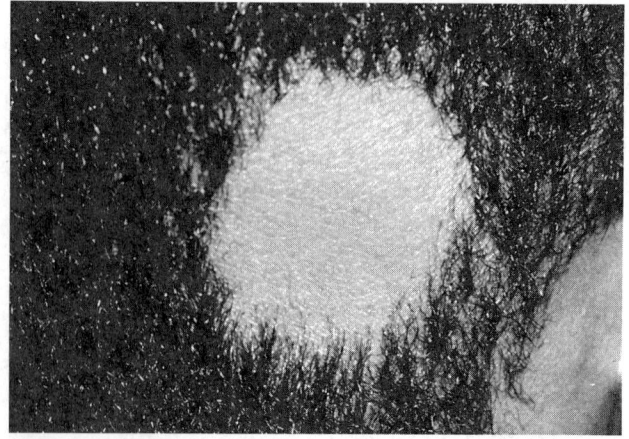

FIGURE 65-10
Alopecia areata. An annular patch of complete hair loss on the scalp of a child. The scalp surface is normal.

order as well as a family history of hair problems. The child's past medical history is reviewed to identify an immunologic disease, stressor, or medication that may be related to the hair loss.

On physical examination, the distribution and pattern of hair loss are observed. The total cutaneous surface is examined for hair loss of vellus and terminal hair. The appearance of the skin in the area of hair loss is also observed, noting erythema, scaling, excoriations, or other abnormalities in appearance.

★ NURSING DIAGNOSES AND PLANNING

Based on assessment data from above and Chapter 64, the following nursing diagnoses may apply to the family and child with hair loss:

- Self-Esteem Disturbance related to hair loss.
- Anxiety related to knowledge deficit regarding illness and treatment.
- Ineffective Management of Therapeutic Regimen related to knowledge deficit regarding illness and treatment.

The nurse and child (or parents) together plan effective care based on the established nursing diagnoses. Several examples of expected outcomes follow:

- The parents and child demonstrate an understanding of recommended hair care.
- The parents and child discuss the illness and treatment options.
- The child demonstrates a more positive image of self.

The nurse plans for the care of the child based on both physician's orders and nursing diagnoses. Some general nursing care goals include the following:

- Hair regrowth is promoted.
- Parents and child discuss aspects of the condition and its treatment.

★ INTERVENTIONS: COLLABORATIVE AND INDEPENDENT

No effective treatment is available for telogen or anagen effluvium. Careful explanation of the cause and its favorable prognosis helps to dispel anxiety. No special hair care is required; however, parents often feel better following guidelines for general hair maintenance as outlined in the accompanying display. A cooling hat or occlusive scalp tourniquet applied immediately before drug administration may be helpful in anagen effluvium. This practice is thought to decrease blood flow to the hair follicles and, therefore, decrease the amount of drug to which the hair unit is exposed.

A variety of medications or treatments may be prescribed for treatment of AA. The effectiveness of these treatment measures is variable. Topical midpotent corticosteroids, applied alone or under occlusion, have been helpful in some cases. Intradermal corticosteroid injections at the site of hair loss are effective at inducing hair regrowth; however, the hair may quickly fall out again once the corticosteroid effect is ended. Topical treatments such as anthralin, PUVA, or DNCB, which induce irritation, are believed to increase blood flow to the hair unit and stimulate hair growth. Minoxidil (Rogaine), the an-

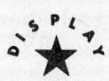

Patient Teaching: General Guidelines for Maintaining Good Scalp and Hair Hygiene

- Keep the hair clean with gentle products and shampoo regularly (every 2 to 4 days).
- Avoid high heat from dryers and combs when drying and styling the hair.
- Comb or brush gently to minimize undue strain on the hair.
- Avoid braids, pony tails, tight barrettes, or bands.
- Do not sleep with rollers in the hair.
- Use a satin pillowcase to decrease friction between the hair and pillowcase.
- Avoid harsh chemical hair treatments, such as coloring or permanent waving.

tihypertensive drug that causes hirsutism, has been approved for topical use in hair loss. This drug has shown variable results in adults, and the data on its effects in children are not available.[8]

Discussion of practices causing hair loss in traction alopecia often increases awareness on the part of the parent or child, leading to behavior change and hair regrowth. In cases of persistent trichotillomania, the child is referred for psychological evaluation and treatment.

PSYCHOSOCIAL SUPPORT

Losing hair can be emotionally challenging, especially for those children with extensive hair loss. Because of the visibility of hair loss, the child or parent may decide to cover the head or replace the hair. Several alternatives, including caps, scarves, or turbans, are available for covering the head and may be a good option for children with more temporary hair loss. In other cases, a fashionable wig or hair prosthesis can be a good option and can enhance self-image. A variety of wigs are available. Human hair wigs tend to be more expensive and need more servicing. Synthetic wigs are less expensive, easier to style, wash easily, dry quickly, and need less care. Both can look natural.

A hair prosthesis is the latest technological advance in replacing lost hair. They are made to adapt to all lifestyles. The prosthesis is form-fitted and individually designed. Prosthetic hair washes easily, dries quickly, and needs minimal care. It is the most natural in appearance, the most flexible in application, and the most expensive.

Creative use of eye makeup and artificial lashes may be helpful in disguising loss of eyelashes and eyebrows.

A careful hair care regimen is suggested to prevent further hair loss from trauma as well as to provide optimal conditions for regrowth. Children with hair loss are often hesitant to comb or brush the hair for fear it will cause additional hair loss. Parents appreciate being taught general guidelines for hair care, which were given in the Patient Teaching display.

Emotional support is vital for the child with hair loss because of the impact on the development of self-confidence and self-image. It is important for the child and family to know that others are afflicted with these conditions and to share their reactions and feelings. This support may be provided by a nurse, physician, psychologist, or a self-help group such as the National Alopecia Areata Foundation.

⭐ EVALUATION

Evaluation in the child with hair loss includes assessment of the response to treatment. Serial photographs of the affected area can be helpful in identifying subtle changes. The nurse should ask the child or parent to describe their normal hair care routine to determine understanding and adherence to recommendations. The nurse should assess the effectiveness of coping strategies, such as wigs, and support systems.

LONG-TERM CARE

The prognosis in telogen effluvium is excellent, with spontaneous regrowth unless the stressful event recurs. It may, however, take up to 6 months for complete regrowth. Regrowth occurs in anagen effluvium with elimination of the offending agent.

Spontaneous regrowth may occur in AA; however, alopecia lasting more than 1 year is considered to have a poor prognosis for regrowth.[37]

The prognosis in traumatic alopecia is totally reliant on discontinuation of the causative practices. On occasion, if the trauma is repeated over a prolonged period of time to the same site, permanent hair loss will result.

Disorders of the Nail

The human nail can be affected by a wide variety of acquired or congenital disorders. Various anatomic parts of the nail may be damaged by external agents, may be involved in localized or generalized cutaneous disease, or may reflect an underlying systemic disorder. Table 65-11 summarizes alterations in the nail plate, nailbed, and nail folds and lists disorders in which they are seen.

Disorders of Pigmentation

Skin pigmentation is produced by melanocytes and serves to protect the skin and underlying structures from UVL (see Chap. 63). The amount and distribution of melanin account for the color of one's skin. In normal skin, essentially all melanin is in the epidermis. If too little melanin is produced or the melanocytes are absent, hypopigmentation or depigmentation results. If too much melanin is produced or if the pigment is distributed in a different fashion, hyperpigmentation results. Disturbances of melanization may be generalized or localized, and they may occur congenitally or be acquired. Skin pigmentation is an important cosmetic and cultural characteristic. Disorders of pigmentation may range from relatively minor pathologic consequences to potentially life-threatening conditions. As with many disorders of the skin, the effect of altered pigment on the child's appearance can have an enormous impact on the development of body image and self-esteem.

TABLE 65-11
Disorders of the Nails

Disorder	Definition	Association
Onycholysis	Separation of nail plate from the nailbed	Congenital, dermatoses, drugs, systemic disease, trauma
Beau's lines	Transverse depressions on nail plate caused by periods of reduced growth	Times of physical stress
Clubbing	Increased downward curvature of the nail plate	Congenital, cardiovascular, pulmonary, gastrointestinal disease, malnutrition, AIDS
Koilonychia	Upward curvature of the nail plate	Congenital, dermatoses, iron deficiency
Leukonychia	White nail plate	Trauma, systemic disorders, poisons, drug toxicity
Anonychia	Absence of nail plate	Congenital, traumatic, severe paronychia
Micronychia	Smaller nail plate	
Onychomadesis	Complete separation with loss of nail plate	Severe paronychia, trauma, severe illness, drug toxicity
Nail pits	Punctate depressions in the nail plate	Dermatoses (psoriasis, alopecia)
Nail dystrophy	Thickening of the nail plate	Congenital, infection, dermatoses
Nail dyschromia	Alteration in color of the nail plate or bed	External agents, drugs, infections, dermatoses, systemic disease, trauma, nevi, tumors
Ingrown toenail	Entrapment of portions of the nail plate in lateral nail folds	Congenital, ill-fitting shoes, trauma
Paronychia	Painful, red, swelling of nail folds	Trauma, infections, drugs
Prominent nail fold capillaries	Enlargement of nail fold capillaries	Scleroderma, dermatomyositis

Pigment Loss

Definition and Incidence.   Three disorders of pigment loss are discussed. These include a genetic disorder, albinism; a disorder believed to have autoimmune etiology, vitiligo; and a common phenomenon, postinflammatory hypopigmentation.

Albinism is a group of 14 clinical syndromes with congenital lack of skin, hair, and eye pigment. Oculocutaneous albinism, with skin, hair, and eye involvement, accounts for the majority of cases. The general incidence of albinism is 1 per 20,000 births. All varieties have an autosomal-recessive inheritance pattern, with the exception of X-linked ocular albinism. Both sexes are affected equally, with a higher prevalence in African Americans over whites.[44,50]

Vitiligo is a relatively common acquired disorder of hypomelanosis. Approximately 1% to 4% of people in the United States develop this disorder.[22] Fifty percent of these people are affected before the age of 18 years. Both sexes are affected equally, and the incidence is fairly constant among various racial groups.

Postinflammatory hypopigmentation is the decreased skin pigment that remains apparent on the skin after resolution of skin inflammation. This is a common occurrence, but is more noticeable in those with darker skin pigment.

Etiology and Pathophysiology.   The disorders of pigment loss are all a result of several factors that affect the production of melanin by melanocytes. Melanocytes are present in the epidermis of people with albinism. The absence of skin pigment is due to a defect of the tyrosinase enzyme, resulting in insufficient production of melanin.

On the other hand, the exact pathogenesis of vitiligo is unknown. Genetic factors are believed to be involved in vitiligo, but their precise role is still unclear. The pigment loss occurs as a result of degeneration with eventual disappearance of melanocytes in the areas of involvement. Histologically, all the other skin structures are normal. Several hypotheses have been proposed to account for this selective melanocyte destruction. The strongest one suggests that immunologic abnormalities are responsible.

Postinflammatory hypopigmentation is a result of temporary interruption of normal melanin production.

Clinical Manifestations.   Children with albinism present with a variety of manifestations, depending on their particular variant of albinism. Those with oculocutaneous albinism present with snow-white hair, pinkish-white skin, and blue-gray irises. Visual acuity is poor, with moderate to severe strabismus. Freckles and pigmented nevi are not acquired with age, and the skin and the eyes are exquisitely sensitive to sunlight.

Vitiligo is characterized by the development of patchy pigment loss, which enlarges peripherally. Children present with macules and patches of depigmentation that vary greatly in size. The distribution is generally symmetric with a predilection for periorificial sites, particularly around the eyes, mouth, and genitalia. Areas of trauma are also more frequently involved, such as the elbows, knees, and hands. The extent of involvement varies from one or two macules to widespread depigmentation. Scalp involvement leads to loss of pigment in the hair follicle with development of white hair in those areas.

Vitiligo has been described as medically benign but psychologically malignant.[22] The effect this disorder has on appearance can be dramatic. In general, children with vitiligo are healthy, but they have an increased frequency of autoimmune diseases when compared to a healthy control group.[22] Vitiligo has been associated with disorders such as Addison's disease, Hashimoto's thyroiditis, pernicious anemia, diabetes mellitus, hypoparathyroidism, and autoimmune hemolytic anemia as well as AA and scleroderma.

Postinflammatory hypopigmentation appears as areas of decreased pigment at sites of previous inflammation. It is differentiated from vitiligo by the characteristic poor margination and absence of milk-white color under Wood's lamp examination. Pityriasis alba, AD, psoriasis, and pityriasis versicolor are examples of inflammatory conditions that produce hypopigmentation.

Excessive Pigment

Benign Pigmented Lesions

Definition and Incidence.   *Café au lait spots* are congenital pigmented lesions that are seen in 25% of children.[44] They are differentiated from congenital melanocytic nevi by their even pigment and normal skin surface texture and appearance. The border is distinct but may have a variable contour. They enlarge in proportion to body growth and, once stabilized, remain for the entire life span. By far, the majority of children with these lesions have no other associated abnormalities. However, multiple large café au lait spots may be a sign of one of three multiorgan syndromes: neurofibromatosis, Albright's syndrome, or Watson's syndrome.[44]

Freckles, also referred to as *ephelides*, are the common, small pigmented macules seen in predisposed children, especially in those with fair skin and red hair. They tend to become less noticeable in adult life and with decreased sun exposure.

The term *lentigo* refers to a small brown spot that results from an increased number of epidermal melanocytes. There are several different types of lentigines: lentigo simplex, solar lentigo, and lentigo maligna. Despite the presence of melanocytic hyperproliferation, the majority of these lesions are considered benign, without malignant potential.[44] Multiple *lentigo simplex* lesions are associated with several multisystem diseases including the leopard syndrome and Peutz-Jeghers syndrome. The presence of *solar lentigines* signals considerable sun exposure.

A *Becker's nevus* is a large, unilateral patch with hyperpigmentation and dark hair growth. These lesions are most often found on the upper trunk of males. The Becker's nevus represents a benign process without malignant potential.[44]

The *mongolian spot* is a hyperpigmented macule or patch most commonly seen in children of African-American, Asian, or Hispanic races. It is much less common in whites. The blue-gray color of the spot is due to the position of the melanocytes in the deeper dermis. These lesions usually regress by the age of 4 to 6 years.[44] These areas sometimes are mistaken for ecchymosis in cases of suspected child abuse; therefore, it is important to document the presence of a mongolian spot in the child's medical record.

Postinflammatory hyperpigmentation occurs after an inflammatory dermatosis. It is seen in all people capable of producing melanin but is more pronounced in people with darker skin color. Dermatoses that affect the BMZ of the epidermis produce the most postinflammatory pigmentation. Generally, the lesions fade within 6 months, although they can be permanent in darkly pigmented people, when the pigment moves into the dermis and acts as a tattoo.

Etiology and Pathophysiology. Benign pigmented lesions are a result of either excessive production of melanin by epidermal melanocytes or hyperproliferation of melanocytes in the epidermis or dermis. Refer to Table 65-12 for the etiology of each individual lesion. All these pigmentary alterations are considered to be totally benign and have no potential for malignant degeneration.

Clinical Manifestations. Table 65-12 describes the clinical manifestation of the various benign pigmented lesions.

Melanocytic Nevi

Melanocytic nevi are collections of melanocytes in the epidermis or the dermis. These lesions may be acquired or congenital. They are important because of their relationship to cutaneous melanoma and the disfigurement that occurs when they are present on prominent areas of the skin. The pigmented lesions described in this section include congenital melanocytic nevi, common acquired melanocytic nevi, dysplastic melanocytic nevi, halo nevi, and blue nevi. Table 65-13 compares the various melanocytic nevi and melanoma.

Congenital Melanocytic Nevi

Congenital melanocytic nevi (CMN) are pigmented areas apparent at birth.

Etiology and Pathophysiology. CMN consist of melanocytes in the epidermis or dermis. They are classified into categories of small, medium, and large or giant. There is no other satisfactory way to place nevi into these categories. However, classification based on actual size and ease of removal is most popular. CMN are classified as small if they measure less than 1.5 cm. These lesions can be excised easily and the wound defect can be closed primarily without causing significant deformity. CMN are classified as medium if they measure between 1.5 and 19.9 cm and as large or giant if they measure more than 20 cm. Excision of medium and large CMN is difficult and may require staged excisions, tissue-expanding techniques, skin flaps, or grafts, all of which can result in significant deformity.[61]

Clinical Manifestations. CMN present in a wide variety of sizes, shapes, and forms (Fig. 65-11 and Table 65-13). Fortunately, the majority of CMN are of the small variety and occur singularly. CMN generally have well-circumscribed borders. However, the surface may be smooth or irregular with an even color or variations in shades of brown or blue throughout the lesion. The lesion may also be asymmetric with irregular borders. The surface may be verrucous or contain papules or nodules as well as hair. Giant or "garment" CMN may cover a large section of skin such as the bathing trunk area, an extremity, or larger area.

TABLE 65-12
Benign Pigmented Lesions

Name	Etiology	Onset	Clinical Manifestations
Café au lait	↑ Epidermal melanin without melanocytic proliferation	Congenital Seen in 25% of children[44]	Uniform tan-brown, round or oval macule/patch Enlarge in proportion to growth of child
Freckles	↑ Epidermal melanin without melanocytic proliferation	Acquired Seen first at 2–4 years of age	Small red-brown macules that enlarge and darken with sun exposure
Lentigo simplex	↑ Epidermal melanocytes	Congenital or acquired	Small, discrete tan or brown macules, <5 mm in diameter. Do not darken with sun exposure.
Solar lentigo	↑ Epidermal melanocytes	Acquired with excessive sun exposure, especially in fair-skinned people	Circumscribed pigmented macules present on sun-exposed skin surfaces
Becker's nevus	↑ Epidermal melanin and melanocytic hyperproliferation	Acquired in males during or after puberty	Large, slightly thickened, irregular, unilateral, hairy, pigmented patch often found on the trunk
Mongolian spot	Deep dermal melanocytic hyperproliferation	Congenital More common in darker pigmented races	Blue-gray pigmented patch >75% present in the sacrogluteal region[44]
Postinflammatory hyperpigmentation	↑ Epidermal melanin stimulated by inflammation	Acquired Seen in all persons capable of producing melanin	Macular or patchy areas of ↑ pigment at sites of previous inflammation

TABLE 65-13
Comparison of Melanocytic Lesions

	Congenital melanocytic nevi	Acquired melanocytic nevi	Dysplastic melanocytic nevi	Malignant melanoma
Definition	Lesion composed of nevus cells apparent at birth	Lesion composed of nevus cells	Lesion composed of nevus cells with melanocyte dysplasia	Cancer of melanocytes
First seen	Birth	After 6 months of age	Puberty or later	Rare in children Peak incidence 45–55 y
Size	Small <1.5 cm Medium 1.5–19.9 cm Large/giant >20 cm	<5 mm	>5 mm	>5 mm

Shape	Widely varied	Round or oval
		  Junctional—flat
		  Compound—raised
		  Interdermal—dome-shaped
			Irregular	Irregular, indentations or notches

Border	Regular or irregular, well-demarcated	Regular Well-demarcated	Irregular, fades into surrounding skin	Irregular, fades into surrounding skin
Color	Variations of brown or blue	Uniformly light to dark brown	Widely varied, brown, pink, blue, flesh-colored	Haphazard shades of blue, black, brown, red, white, or flesh-tone
Surface	Smooth or uneven, may contain hair	Smooth, may contain hair	Uneven topography	Uneven topography, ulcer, crust, scale, bleeding
Number	Usually one, may be multiple	15–20 Whites 2 African Americans	Tend to be multiple	Primary—one Metastatic—may be multiple

The major concern with CMN is the potential for regression into malignant melanoma. The relationship of giant congenital nevi and melanoma has been well-documented. However, confusion still exists as to the malignant potential of the various classifications of CMN. The literature concerning the cumulative lifetime risk for developing melanoma is unclear.

Acquired Melanocytic Nevi

Definition and Incidence. Acquired melanocytic nevi (AMN; see Table 65-13) are collections of melanocytes present in the epidermis (junctional nevi), the der-

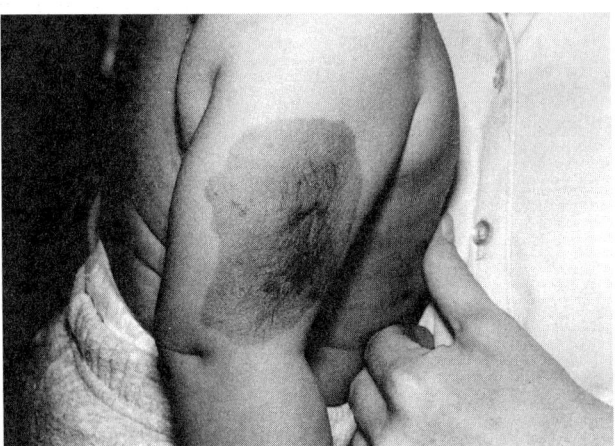

FIGURE 65-11
Congenital melanocytic nevus. A well circumscribed medium-sized congenital melanocytic nevus with some variability of surface pigmentation and dark terminal hair on the arm.

mis (intradermal nevi), or in both (compound nevi). Most people develop at least one AMN over their lifetime. However, they occur in larger numbers in whites. The average number commonly seen in whites ranges from 15 to 40, whereas African Americans average 2.[44]

Etiology and Pathophysiology. AMN are acquired pigmented areas that may present on any cutaneous area. They first appear after the first 6 to 12 months of life, and, if the child lives a normal life span, they disappear by the later stages of life. In most cases, acquired nevi are considered benign lesions. It is generally believed that AMN evolve through a life cycle, first becoming apparent in childhood, peaking in number during the second and third decades of life, and disappearing during the seventh to ninth decades.

Clinical Manifestations. The clinical characteristics of AMN vary according to the type. The junctional nevus is the most common type seen in the early years of life. These lesions are small and tend to be macular and light to dark brown. Over time, the nevus cells migrate into the epidermis while continuing to proliferate in the epidermis. This causes the nevus to become more papular and forms the compound nevus. Finally, the nevus cells completely migrate into the dermis, forming the intradermal nevus. These nevi become smooth, dome-shaped papules and may lose their pigment and become flesh-colored. Typically, AMN have a round or oval shape and even coloring with well-demarcated smooth borders. The surface of the nevus may have hair growth that is more apparent than the hair of the surrounding normal skin.

A *halo nevus* is a pigmented melanocytic nevus sur-

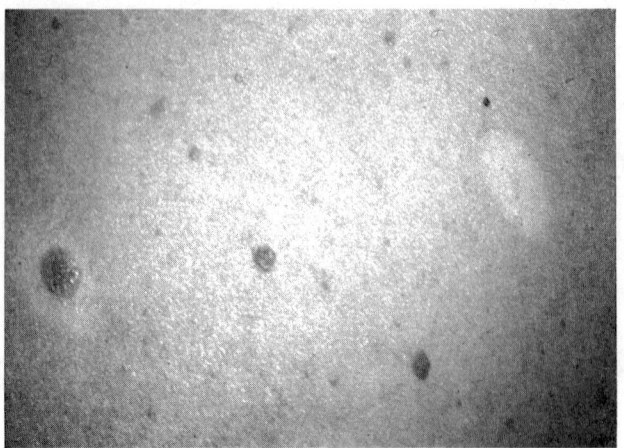

FIGURE 65-12

Halo nevi. Left lesion is an interdermal nevus surrounded by a depigmented halo. In the right lesion, the central melanocytic nevus portion has totally disappeared, leaving only an area of depigmentation.

rounded by a depigmented halo (Fig. 65-12). This phenomenon can be found at any age and is thought to represent an immunologic response that destroys the nevus cells and some of the normal epidermal melanocytes at the periphery of the lesion.

Blue nevi are collections of deep dermal melanocytes accounting for the blue color. They are uncommon in children under the age of 10 years but can be seen in later childhood.[44] These lesions are discrete papules and tend to measure less than 0.75 cm in diameter. The natural history is unknown, but it is believed that the majority of these lesions are benign.

Dysplastic Melanocytic Nevi

Definition and Incidence. Dysplastic melanocytic nevi (DMN; see Table 65-13) are collections of melanocytes that are characterized by melanocytic dysplasia on histologic examination. These lesions are atypical appearing when compared to the normal AMN. DMN are important because of their strong association to malignant melanoma. DMN are much less common than AMN. These lesions are usually not seen in children until puberty or later.

Etiology and Pathophysiology. Familial dysplastic nevus syndrome (FDNS), also known as the familial, atypical, multiple-mole melanoma (FAMMM) syndrome, is autosomal dominantly inherited and greatly increases the lifetime risk of family members for developing melanoma to 18%. This risk becomes even more significant with the lifetime risk of melanoma approaching 100% in children with two or more extended first-degree family members who have atypical moles and melanoma.[33]

How early a FDNS mole can clinically be distinguished from an ordinary nevus is still unknown. One case study reported identification as early as age 2 years. Obtaining this information requires lifelong, intensive surveillance and management programs.

Clinical Manifestations. The determination that a nevus is dysplastic can only be done on histologic ex-

amination. However, several clinical characteristics have been associated with these lesions, and their presence may lead one to suspect dysplasia. These characteristics include asymmetry, border, color, and diameter, which are easily remembered with the acronym of ABCD.[29] DMN tend to be irregularly shaped with an uneven topography. When the lesions are divided in half, the halves are not equal. The borders are not smooth and well-demarcated but rather have an irregular contour or fade into the surrounding skin. DMN tend to have dark pigmentation or a haphazard deposition of multiple hues of brown, pink, blue, or flesh tone. The last characteristic is diameter; DMN tend to be 5 mm or larger in size.

DMN also tend to be multiple, ranging from 1 to 200, often exceeding the total average number for ACN in one small area of the person's back. However, only one DMN is necessary to give rise to melanoma. DMN may be found anywhere on the skin surface, but do tend to be more prevalent on the posterior trunk (Fig. 65-13).

Melanoma

Definition and Incidence. Malignant melanoma (MM; see Table 54-13) is a cancer of the melanocytes and represents the leading fatal illness arising in the skin. MM in children is fairly rare. The incidence of MM is least common in the first decade of life and increases during the teenage years. Understanding MM and associated risk factors are important to the childhood years because of the impact of lifestyle on the development of MM. Also, identification of children at risk may enable early diagnosis of melanoma with an improved prognosis.

Etiology and Pathophysiology. The precise predisposing factors of childhood melanoma are unclear and are thought to be an interaction of genetic factors with environmental and lifestyle factors. MM in childhood is usually associated with CMN, but additional factors influence the development of MM in adolescence. The incidence of childhood melanoma is somewhat higher in girls as well as children with skin type I or II (see Table

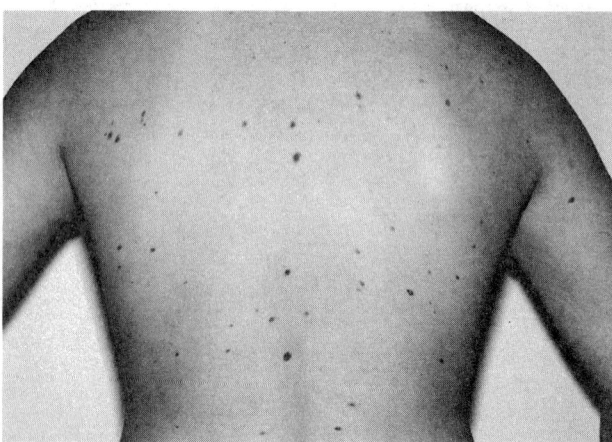

FIGURE 65-13

Dysplastic melanocytic nevi. The back of an adolescent with many irregularly shaped, large melanocytic nevi. This child has more nevi on his back than the average number of the normal adult over the entire cutaneous surface.

TABLE 65-14
Skin Types and Skin Reactivity

Skin Type	Reaction to Sun	Examples
I	Always burns easily and severely (painful burn); tans little or none and peels.	People with fair skin. Blue or even brown eyes, freckles; unexposed skin is white.
II	Usually burns easily and severely (painful burn); tans minimally or lightly, also peels.	People with fair skin, red, blond or brown hair, blue, hazel, or brown eyes; unexposed skin is white.
III	Burns moderately; tans about average.	Average Caucasian; unexposed skin is white.
IV	Burns minimally; tans easily and above average with each exposure; exhibits IPD (immediate pigment darkening) reaction.	People with white or light brown skin, dark brown hair, dark eyes; unexposed skin is white or light brown.
V	Rarely burns, tans easily and substantially; always exhibits IPD reaction.	Brown-skinned persons; unexposed skin is brown.
VI	Never burns and tans profusely; exhibits IPD reaction.	Blacks; unexposed skin is black.

Developed by Pathak, A., Fitzpatrick, T. B., Parrish, J. A., & Mosher, D. B., Harvard Medical School, Massachusetts General Hospital, Boston, MA; and Greiter, F. J., Vienna, Austria.

65-14). A family history of melanoma and the presence of palpable benign nevi are the strongest risk factors in childhood MM.[47] The relationship of sun exposure to melanoma is unclear. The incidence of MM does increase in solar-intense areas close to the equator. However, MM is more often associated with short but intense sun exposure as well as accumulative exposure, especially those that result in severe burns.[3]

Clinical Manifestations. MM usually presents as an asymptomatic, pigmented lesion that has recently changed. The development of asymmetry, irregular borders with indentations or notches, a haphazard pigment pattern, and an increase in size are all early signs of malignant degeneration. Ulceration, bleeding, and pruritus are all found in advanced tumors. Frequently, MM is associated with a dark blue or black color. However, it may also appear in all shades of brown, red, pink, or even without obvious pigment (amelanotic melanoma). The melanoma subtypes include superficial spreading melanoma, nodular melanoma, lentigo maligna melanoma, acral-lentiginous melanoma, and amelanotic melanoma. Of these types, only lentigo maligna does not occur in children.

Diagnostic Studies in Pigmentation Disorders.
For the majority of disorders of pigmentation, diagnosis is made by identification of the clinical features. A Wood's lamp is useful for differentiating hypopigmentation from depigmentation. It is also useful to differentiate epidermal and dermal melanin pigment in people with skin types I to IV but is not helpful in skin types V and VI (Table 65-14). Epidermal melanin increases in intensity under Wood's lamp exposure, but dermal melanin does not.

At the initial evaluation for vitiligo, several laboratory studies are obtained to rule out any asymptomatic internal disease. These studies include a complete blood count and differential, thyroid function tests, fasting blood sugar level, and an antinuclear antibody test (ANA). A skin biopsy is invaluable for diagnosis of dysplasia or malignancy

in melanocytes and also enables determination of prognosis by identifying the depth of MM.

⭐ **ASSESSMENT**

Nursing assessment in children with disorders of pigmentation include obtaining an in-depth family history of these disorders. It is also necessary to assess the child's sun exposure habits and measures for sun protection that are routinely practiced by the family. Assessment also includes obtaining an accurate description of the evolution of the skin lesion. The total cutaneous surface is examined to determine the child's skin type and the pattern, distribution, and type of skin lesion.

⭐ **NURSING DIAGNOSES AND PLANNING**

Based on assessment data from above and Chapter 64, the following nursing diagnoses may apply to the family and child with a disorder of pigmentation:

- High Risk for Injury related to sunburn.
- Chronic Low Self-Esteem related to pigmentation disorder.
- Social Isolation related to altered physical appearance.
- Anxiety related to knowledge deficit regarding illness, treatment, prognosis, and prevention.
- Ineffective Management of Therapeutic Regimen related to knowledge deficit regarding illness, treatment, prognosis, and prevention.

The nurse and child (or parents) together plan effective care based on the established nursing diagnoses. Several examples of expected outcomes follow:

- The parents and child state the importance of limiting sun exposure.
- The parents and child discuss importance of early identification of melanoma.
- The child demonstrates knowledge of self-examination of skin.
- The child demonstrates a more positive image of self.

The nurse plans for the care of the child based on both physician's orders and nursing diagnoses. Some general nursing care goals may be the following:

- Injury from sun exposure is prevented.
- Suspicious lesions are identified through regular self-examination.
- Child will identify positive characteristics about self.

★ INTERVENTIONS: COLLABORATIVE AND INDEPENDENT

Nursing interventions for children with disorders of pigmentation include prevention of injury from sun exposure, early identification of melanoma, and education of the child and family regarding prevention and early identification.

CARE OF CHILDREN WITH ALBINISM AND VITILIGO

There is no cure or specific treatment for albinism. Children with this disorder cannot lead the same type of lives as do their normal counterparts because of the extreme sensitivity of their skin and eyes to sunlight. The nurse's responsibility is to educate both the child and parent on protection of the skin and eyes from UVL. Sun exposure should be avoided with encouragement of indoor activities during the daylight hours. When sun exposure is unavoidable, protection is achieved with dark-colored, tightly woven clothing and broad-spectrum sunscreens (Table 65-15). Ultraviolet filtering sunglasses are used for photophobia.

There also is no cure for vitiligo, nor is there an entirely effective treatment. Oral or topically applied psoralen and UVA exposure (PUVA) can increase skin pigmentation and provides the most efficacious results. However, the use in children, especially under the age of 2, is controversial due to potential for burning and long-term effects of premature skin aging and skin cancer. There is general agreement that due to the psychological and social impact of vitiligo on the child that it should be treated. For children and adolescents with less than 20% to 25% involvement, with ocular abnormalities or other conditions that contraindicate oral PUVA, topical PUVA is used. Oral PUVA is reserved for children with

TABLE 65-15
Sunscreen Agents

Preparation	Ultraviolet Spectrum
Physical blocking agents	
Titanium dioxide	UVA + UVB
Zinc oxide	UVA + UVB
Chemical sunscreen agents	
PABA	UVB
PABA esters	UVB
Salicylates	UVB
Cinnamates	UVB
Anthranilates	UVB, weakly UVA
Benzophenones	UVB, weakly UVA
Butyl methoxydibenzoylmethane (parsol 1789)	UVA

greater than 25% involvement, those recalcitrant to other therapeutic modalities, and those older than 9 years of age.[22] PUVA treatments require a commitment to long-term therapy.

On rare occasions, depigmentation with monobenzylether or hydroquinone has been used as an alternative in children with rapidly progressing vitiligo that is recalcitrant to other treatments. Midpotent topical corticosteroids (see Table 65-3) may also be used, although their effectiveness is variable.

Corrective cosmetics are specifically designed to camouflage alterations in skin color and are effective in hiding the depigmented areas of vitiligo. When applied correctly, they provide a waterproof, smudge-resistant, therapeutic option for a frustrating and cosmetically disfiguring disorder. Several skin stains are also available, but their use is limited due to the inability to obtain an acceptable skin color match for a great number of children.

It is important to stress the daily use of broad-spectrum sunscreens on all depigmented patches to prevent sunburn and chronic actinic damage. The nurse should review with the child and parent methods of sun protection (see "Photosensitivity" in this chapter). Because the natural protective skin pigment is absent in children with albinism and vitiligo, regular follow-up skin exams for premalignant and malignant skin tumors are necessary.

The psychosocial problems experienced by children with albinism and vitiligo are often of major proportion. Children with albinism often experience social isolation because of their inability to participate in outdoor activities during the day. Also, children with albinism or vitiligo are subject to a great deal of ridicule from playmates because of their appearance, causing psychological trauma.

Parents of children with vitiligo are often anxious, dissatisfied, and frustrated because the etiology of vitiligo cannot be satisfactorily explained, no clear prediction of the course of the disease can be offered, there is little chance of spontaneous recovery, treatment options are limited, and no cure is available. Nurses have the opportunity to discuss with the family what is understood about vitiligo. Patients of any age and their families often benefit from talking with others who have a similar condition. The National Vitiligo Foundation can serve as a resource for information and support.

CARE OF CHILDREN WITH BENIGN PIGMENTED LESIONS

Benign pigmented lesions that carry no malignant potential do not require treatment unless desired by the patient or parent because of its cosmetic significance. On the other hand, pigmented lesions with malignant potential such as CMN and DMN do require close follow-up, total body photographs, periodic excision, and extensive education on sun protection measures, self-skin examination, and the necessity of regular pediatric follow-up visits.

CARE OF CHILDREN WITH MELANOMA

Melanoma is treated by excisional surgery. The extent of surgery and whether associated lymph nodes are also removed depend on the depth of the tumor. Metastatic melanoma has no curative treatment. However, radiation or chemotherapy is used to extend life expectancy, and immunotherapy has been used experimentally. Children with melanoma that is successfully excised require long-term follow-up because they are at increased risk for developing a second melanoma. Observation for up to 15 years may be necessary to be certain of a cure.[61]

Nursing intervention in children at increased risk for melanoma is directed at early detection and prevention. The nurse can help to identify those people with suspicious lesions. Nurses in all types of medical settings have the opportunity to examine a child's skin during routine system assessment, bathing, and otherwise caring for the child.

Children and their parents need to be taught about the warning signs of melanoma. Providing clear, accurate information is a vital part of the nurse's role. The ABCD system is easy to understand and remember.[29] The nurse should instruct the parent and child on how to use this system in self-skin examination. If any suspicious lesion is noted, they are instructed to seek prompt medical attention. These skin examinations are conducted once a month in good lighting and are aided by photographs of existing lesions that are being followed.

Although the exact role sun exposure plays in the development of melanoma is not clearly understood, much evidence suggests a correlation between sun exposure and the incidence of MM. Children at risk for the development of melanoma and their parents should be instructed on measures of sun protection (see "Photosensitivity" in this chapter).

The Skin Cancer Foundation, American Cancer Society, the National Cancer Institute, and the American Academy of Dermatology have excellent patient education materials, which can be provided for children and families to assist them in self-skin examinations, recognition of the warning signs of melanoma, and understanding methods of sun protection.

★ EVALUATION

Because many nursing interventions are directed at prevention and early detection, evaluation includes the determination of the success of prevention strategies and if complications, such as skin injury from sunburn or malignant regression, have occurred. The nurse should note if the child and family can identify the warning signs of melanoma and their ability to incorporate skin protection measures into their daily life. Also, the nurse should evaluate the effectiveness of strategies to alleviate parental anxiety and promote good self-esteem in the child.

COMPLICATIONS

Prognosis in disorders of pigment loss varies with the type of disorder. The prognosis in albinism is for a normal life span as long as precautions are taken early in the child's life. Without adequate medical follow-up, cutaneous malignancies from ultraviolet radiation damage can be the direct cause of death relatively early in life. In vitiligo, only about 10% of lesions repigment spontaneously, and this disorder does tend to progress with age. Postinflammatory hypopigmentation eventually resolves, taking as long as 6 to 12 months for the original skin color to return in some people.

In determining the prognosis in MM, several prognostic indicators must be considered. These indicators include the depth of invasion, the MM subtype, and the cutaneous site. Several methods associating prognosis and tumor depth have been developed. Thin MM, less than 0.76 mm, have a high cure rate, with the rate of metastasis increasing along with the tumor thickness.[20]

Children with superficial spreading melanomas have a better prognosis than do those with nodular melanomas. Also, the biologic behavior of melanoma of the extremities is believed to be fairly aggressive with a worse prognosis. Locations with higher risk of mortality include the palms, soles, scalp, midback, anterior chest, and genital region. Low-risk areas include the thighs and forearms.

Photosensitivity

Photosensitivity occurs as a result of exposure of the skin to UVL alone or simultaneous exposure to UVL and a chemical. Several systemic disorders noted for photosensitivity are listed in the accompanying display. The most common harmful effect from sunlight exposure in children is a phototoxic reaction, namely sunburn. Photoallergy may also occur but is seen much less frequently. Both phototoxic and photoallergic reactions are described in this section.

Phototoxic Reactions

Sunburn

Definition and Incidence. People vary a great deal in the type of response their skin produces when exposed to sunlight. This variability is attributed to the melanin

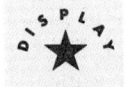

Systemic Disorders With Photosensitivity

Genodermatoses
    Xeroderma pigmentosum
    Bloom's syndrome
    Cockayne's syndrome
    Hartnup disease
    Rothmund-Thomson syndrome
Porphyria
    Congenital erythropoietic protoporphyria
    Porphyria cutanea tarda
    Variegate porphyria
    Hepatoerythropoietic porphyria
Pellagra
Connective tissue disease
    Lupus erythematosus
    Dermatomyositis
Pigmentary disorders
    Albinism
    Vitiligo
    Phenylketonuria

content in unexposed skin (constitutive skin color) and the ability of the skin to tan (facultative skin color).[53] Constitutive skin color and facultative skin color, both of which are genetically determined, together define a person's skin type (see Table 65-14). Natural hair and eye color, how easily children sunburn, and how well they are able to suntan are factors in the determination of skin type.

Sunburn is most often seen in children with skin types I to III. The sunburn reaction is seen quickly in children with skin type I and takes longer exposure times with each successive skin type. Sunburn does occur in skin types V and VI; however, prolonged, intense UVL exposure is required to produce the reaction.

In addition to skin type increasing the risk of a child obtaining a sunburn, various environmental factors also play a role. These factors include the time of day, season, altitude, and latitude, as well as the presence of reflective surfaces. The UVL rays are most intense at the equator and least intense at the poles. UVL is also more intense in higher altitudes and during the summer. Water, sand, snow, and Astroturf are extremely reflective of UVL and increase exposure intensity.

Etiology and Pathophysiology. Concern about excessive sun exposure and sunburn has increased because of the link of sun exposure to skin cancer. Several observations are the basis for this association[25]:

• The higher incidence of skin cancer in lighter pigmented people when compared to those with darker skin pigment.
• The prevalence of skin cancer on sun-exposed surfaces of the skin.
• The increased incidence of skin cancer in regions of the world that have warm climates and are more solar-intense.
• The greater incidence of skin cancer in older people who have accumulated substantial sun exposure.
• The increased incidence of skin cancer in people with outdoor versus indoor occupations.
• The excessively high incidence of skin cancer in people with genetic diseases characterized by intolerance to sunlight.

Because skin cancer is rare in children, it may be unclear why sun exposure during childhood is important. Several facts must be realized. First, nonmelanoma skin cancer is related to cumulative sun exposure.[25] The more sun exposure a person gets, the greater the risk of skin cancer. Second, MM is related to both cumulative sun exposure and short, high dose, traumatic sun exposure resulting in severe, blistering sunburns, particularly if they occur before the age of 20 years.[3] Finally, it is estimated that by the time a child reaches 18 years of age, he or she has already received the majority of their lifetime dose of ultraviolet radiation.[64] Therefore, sun protection in the first and second decades of life can have a substantial impact on the development of skin cancer as an adult.

Clinical Manifestations. Sunburn is characterized by erythema, pain, and edema. If the sunburn is severe enough, vesiculation may also occur. This reaction manifests itself several hours after exposure, reaches a peak in 14 to 20 hours, and resolves in 24 to 48 hours. The reaction is usually followed by desquamation and hyperpigmentation.

Ultraviolet light has rays of different length. Ultraviolet A (UVA) rays are the longest (between 320–400 nanometers) and can penetrate into the dermis; Ultraviolet B (UVB) rays are between 200–290 nanometers and penetrate only as far as the epidermis. A sunburn reaction is generally a result of UVB wavelength exposure. Erythema is produced by UVA, but much longer exposure times are required. UVA is thought to have a greater effect on the connective tissue of the dermis.

Phototoxic Contact Dermatitis

Definition and Incidence. Phototoxic reactions occur when the skin is simultaneously exposed to a chemical and UVL. This condition is fairly common in children and adults.

Etiology and Pathophysiology. Several systemically or topically administered substances can serve as a photosensitizer, producing the phototoxic reaction. This reaction does not require previous exposure but may be seen for the first time when these conditions occur. Examples of such substances include psoralen, tetracycline, sulfonamides, thiazides, retinoids, coal tar and its derivatives, and various oils such as lime, cedar, vanilla, lavender, and sandalwood. *Berloque dermatitis* is a specific photosensitivity reaction resulting from the use of oil of bergamot, a common component of perfumes and colognes.[21]

Clinical Manifestations. Phototoxic contact dermatitis is manifested clinically as an exaggerated sunburn reaction followed by pigmentation on sun-exposed surfaces of the skin. The severity of such a reaction depends on the amount of photosensitizing substance administered and the dose of UVL. The skin eruption spontaneously resolves and only recurs under similar exposure conditions.

Photoallergic Reactions

Definition and Incidence. Photoallergy is an allergic reaction that is produced when the skin is exposed to the sun with an ensuing cutaneous reaction. Unlike phototoxicity, photoallergy is not dose-related, but rather is immunologically controlled. For some people, even slight exposure to sunlight can cause a severe reaction. Photoallergic reactions occur much less frequently in children than do phototoxic reactions.

Three types of photoallergic disorders are seen in susceptible people.[21] *Solar urticaria* is an example of an immediate photoallergic response that may follow even short periods of sun exposure. It is fairly rare in young children but may be seen in later childhood or adolescence. The solar urticarial reaction is also seen in erythropoietic protoporphyria.

Polymorphic light eruption (PMLE) is an example of a delayed photoallergic response elicited with sun exposure. PMLE is seen at any age, in either sex, and tends to flare-up every spring and improve over the summer.

Photoallergic contact dermatitis is a form of delayed allergic hypersensitivity that is elicited when the skin is simultaneously exposed to a chemical and UVL. This condition is also seen at any age and in either sex.

Etiology and Pathophysiology. Solar urticaria occurs within minutes after exposure to UVL and may last up to several hours. Most children with this disorder react to UVL rays shorter than 370 nm. In contrast, PMLE becomes evident several hours or days after UVL exposure. In most cases, PMLE results from exposure to UVL in the 290- to 320-nm range, although reactions to longer wavelengths have occurred. As the summer progresses, PMLE eruption decreases and may disappear with repeated sun exposure, which is thought to be the result of desensitization.[21]

Unlike phototoxic contact dermatitis, photoallergic contact dermatitis requires previous exposure and much lower concentrations of the chemical to produce a photoallergic eruption. Examples of substances that are frequently associated with photoallergic contact dermatitis include fragrances (musk ambrette, methylcoumarin), hexachlorophene and closely related substances (widely used as antiseptics), and sunscreens (para-aminobenzoic acid [PABA], cinnamate, and benzophenone). Several agents that produce phototoxic reactions are also capable of producing photoallergic reactions. These include phenothiazines, promethazine hydrochloride and sulfonamides.[21]

Clinical Manifestations. The solar urticaria eruption consists of urticarial wheal formation ("hives") with pruritus and a burning sensation. Previous areas of involvement may develop a reaction if a distant site is challenged with UVL. This commonly occurs during phototesting, in which only a small area of the buttock may be exposed but the eruption is also seen on the face or V of the upper chest.

PMLE is a chronic disorder of photosensitivity. It is characterized by the development of erythema, papules, vesicles, and urticaria on sun-exposed sites. Affected children experience remission and flaring depending on the amount and intensity of UVL exposure.

The clinical manifestations of photoallergic contact dermatitis include a sunburn-like reaction with erythema, papules, and possibly bullae or fissuring. The eruption is seen on sun-exposed surfaces of the skin and disappears when the photocontactant is avoided.

Diagnostic Studies in Photosensitivity. In addition to obtaining the clinical history and observation of the cutaneous lesions, several diagnostic tests may be ordered to assist in making a definitive diagnosis. A complete blood count with differential, antinuclear antibody, Ro and La antibody, RBC protoporphyrin, and urinary porphyrins may be obtained to rule out systemic disorders that exhibit photosensitivity such as systemic lupus erythematosus or porphyria.

Phototesting includes a determination of the minimal erythema dose (MED) to both UVA and UVB. Photopatch testing may also be completed if a chemical is thought to be associated with the eruption. (See Chap. 64 for descriptions of phototesting and photopatch testing.) A skin biopsy of a representative lesion also may be helpful in confirming or rejecting certain diagnoses.

★ ASSESSMENT

Nursing assessment in photosensitivity includes obtaining historic elements as well as conducting a physical examination. The following guide is used in conducting the assessment:

• Determination of the child's skin type.
• Assessment of the child's sun exposure habits and sun protection practices.
• Assessment of the child's and parent's knowledge and attitudes regarding effects of sun exposure on the skin.
• Review of recent medications both systemic and topical.
• Determination of family history of sun reactions or skin cancer.
• Review historic aspects of the skin eruption: When did it first appear, how long did it last, and how was it related to sun exposure?
• Review of unusual recent trips, exposures to plants, fruit or vegetable juices.
• Determination of other medical problems.
• Examination of the skin, noting lesion type, pattern, and distribution.

★ NURSING DIAGNOSES AND PLANNING

Based on assessment data from above and Chapter 64, the following nursing diagnoses may apply to the family and child with photosensitivity:

• Impaired Skin Integrity related to knowledge deficit about the sun's effect and skin protection
• Pain or pruritis related to phototoxic or photoallergic reactions
• Ineffective Management of Therapeutic Regimen related to knowledge deficit regarding disease, treatment, and prevention

The nurse and child (or parents) together plan effective care based on the established nursing diagnoses. Several examples of expected outcomes follow:

• The parents and child state the importance of limiting sun exposure.
• The parents and child make a selection of the proper sunscreen to be used.
• The child demonstrates knowledge of effective application of the sunscreen and the dangers of using indoor tanning beds.

The nurse plans for the care of the child based on both physician's orders and nursing diagnoses. Some general nursing care goals include the following:

• Healing is promoted.
• Causative agent is identified.
• Complications are prevented.

★ INTERVENTIONS: COLLABORATIVE AND INDEPENDENT

Treatment of acute photosensitive reactions includes the use of oral analgesics, cool compresses, and bland emollients. The use of topical anesthetics such as benzocaine is avoided because of the potential for sensitization, causing allergic contact dermatitis. Oral antihistamines may be prescribed for pruritus.

Photoallergy may be treated by several medications including topical or systemic corticosteroids, antimalarial medications, and beta-carotene.[21] Children with PMLE may be desensitized by administering small amounts of UVL with incremental increases over a period of several months. UVB or PUVA phototherapy may be used to increase the child's tolerance to the sunlight.

Exposure to the photosensitizing agent must be eliminated to treat photocontact dermatitis effectively. The child is also advised to minimize sun exposure for at least 2 weeks after an acute reaction.

Current sun exposure habits appear to be difficult to change. A strong misconception exists that a glowing tan is desirable and healthy. Nurses are in the unique position to provide much needed education on sun effects and sun protection. In addition, nurses frequently have the opportunity to reinforce and review this information during subsequent check-ups and visits.[15,35]

TEACHING REGARDING SUN PROTECTION

Education on sun protective measures is important for both prevention of skin damage from chronic UVL exposure and treatment of various photosensitivities.[15,25] The focus of education regarding sun protection should begin as a newborn and include information regarding general skin care. This information should be reinforced at subsequent well-child visits to the pediatrician.

The following information is reviewed in education regarding sun protection:

- How UVL affects the skin.
- Skin type and various risk factors that may increase sun sensitivity.
- The type of environment the family lives in and the impact that altitude, latitude, and seasons have on skin reaction to the sun.
- The variability of UVL intensity over the course of a day.
- The role of reflective surfaces in increasing sun exposure.
- The use of tanning parlors.
- The use of clothing and sunscreens or sunblocks for skin protection.

Sun protection begins with sun avoidance, especially during the hours of 10 AM to 2 PM (11 AM to 3 PM daylight savings time) when UVL is most intense. Outdoor activities can be planned during the early morning or late afternoon hours. These precautions also apply to cloudy days, when 80% of the sun's rays pass through clouds and can cause sunburn. Shade provides protection unless reflective surfaces are near.

Sun protection also may be obtained by the use of adequate clothing as well as the use of sunscreening agents. Closely woven brown, orange, and red fabrics are the best for protecting against UVL. White cotton material provides minimal protection, especially once it is wet with water or perspiration.[53] Clothing manufacturers have begun attaching sun protection factors, similar to sunscreens, to clothing, thereby providing valuable information to the public when choosing clothing for outdoor activity.

The sunscreen market has changed drastically over the last decade. Originally, these topical preparations were regarded as cosmetics. They are now classified by the Federal Drug Administration (FDA) as drugs intended to protect the structure and function of the skin against sun damage.

Sunscreens are classified as physical blocks or chemical screens (see Table 65-15). Sunblocks screen all UVL and some visible light and are available in the form of opaque pastes or creams. Because these products are visible on the skin, they are often undesirable. They are, however, available in a variety of bright colors making them more appealing to children.

Chemical sunscreens filter UVL but allow for passage of visible light. Their potency is measured by a sun protection factor (SPF). The SPF relates only to UVB and is a ratio of the least amount of UVB energy required to produce skin erythema through a sunscreen film to the amount of energy required to produce the same reaction on skin without sunscreen protection:

$$SPF = \frac{\text{Minimal erythema dose of sun-protected skin}}{\text{Minimal erythema dose of unprotected skin}}$$

A person who experiences initial reddening of the skin in 10 minutes without sunscreen will experience the same reddening of the skin in 150 minutes when the skin is protected with a sunscreen with an SPF of 15.

A variety of chemicals have been approved by the FDA as safe, effective sunscreens (see Table 65-15). These chemicals vary in their effectiveness in screening UVB and UVA rays. The performance of a sunscreen depends on its concentration and its ability to remain on the skin. To obtain the higher SPF, these chemicals are increased in concentration or combined in a single preparation. Swimming, heat, high humidity, and sweating reduce the effectiveness of a sunscreen.

Although sunscreens have many qualities that make them effective, they become useless if they are not applied correctly to the skin. Sunscreens are available as creams, lotions, and gels. They should be applied liberally and evenly to all sun-exposed surfaces 1 to 2 hours before sun exposure to allow adequate penetration of the chemical into the horny layer of the skin. They also should be reapplied after swimming or excessive sweating.

A new UVA-absorbing agent, butyl methoxydibenzolmethane (parsol 1789), appears to have much better UVA absorption than previous sunscreens. Photoplex is the only sunscreen available in the United States containing this chemical and has provided substantial relief for people with photosensitivity to UVL in the UVA wavelength range.

The use of sunscreens on children under 6 months of age is not recommended. These children should not be in the sun for extended periods of time. From 6 months on, the regular use of a sunscreen with an SPF of 15 or higher is recommended.

TEACHING REGARDING TANNING BEDS

Nurses have the opportunity to take a leading role in educating the public about the use of indoor tanning beds. One must receive 30 to 45 minutes of repeated exposure to this intense light to develop a tan. This exposure drastically increases the total accumulated dose of UVL. Increased photosensitivity, premature skin aging, cataracts, and skin cancer are associated with UVA exposure in a tanning bed. Cases of temporary blindness have been reported because of UVA-induced corneal damage received from inadequate eye protection in a tanning bed.[12] Tanning salons are not federally regulated and represent a significant threat to the health of the children and adults who use them.

★ EVALUATION

The response of the skin reaction to treatment and any residual skin manifestations are evaluated. The skin is assessed for any signs of complications of photosensitive reactions, such as infection and scarring. The nurse should determine the child and family's understanding of the cause of the reaction and their ability to incorporate appropriate measures for sun protection into their daily activities.

Hemangiomas

The term *hemangioma* refers to a number of vascular nevi with varying clinical features. These lesions are among the most common cutaneous birthmarks that occur in children. Hemangiomas are classified according to their tendency to resolve spontaneously over time and whether they are palpable. Macular hemangiomas (nevus flammeus), which are variably persistent, include salmon patches and port wine stains. Involuting palpable hemangiomas include strawberry (superficial capillary) hemangiomas, deep cavernous hemangiomas, and mixed strawberry/cavernous hemangiomas. Some hemangiomas also have a lymphangioma component and are referred to as hemangiolymphangiomas.

Macular Hemangiomas

Definition and Incidence. There are two distinct types of macular hemangiomas. The *salmon patch*, also referred to as an angel's kiss or stork bite, is a benign lesion that occurs in over half of all newborns. These well-demarcated macules are evident at birth and are pink or dull red in color. The *port wine stain* is a congenital vascular formation involving mature capillaries. They are seen much less frequently than salmon patches.

Etiology and Pathophysiology. Salmon patches result from distended dermal capillaries and are believed to represent persistent fetal circulatory patterns in the skin.[14] Crying and physical activity make these lesions more apparent. A port wine stain is also the result of distended dermal capillaries in which dilatation increases gradually, not explosively as in palpable hemangiomas.

Clinical Manifestations. Salmon patches at the nape of the neck account for 80% of the macular hemangiomas. Less common sites include the forehead, eyelid, glabella, and nasolabial regions of the face. These macules are always situated on the midline or bilaterally symmetric. Frequently, children have more than one.

The face and neck are the most common sites for a port wine stain, but they may be seen anywhere on the body. Clinically they appear as light to dark red macules or patches that can vary a great deal in size from one child to another. The distribution is usually unilateral and may follow a dermatomal distribution. They differ from palpable hemangiomas in that they persist and tend to darken with age, developing a purple hue.

Palpable Hemangiomas

Definition and Incidence. Palpable hemangiomas occur in 10% of all infants. They may be found on any cutaneous surface, but, like most vascular nevi, they have a predilection for the head and neck.

Strawberry (superficial capillary) hemangiomas account for about 60% of all palpable vascular nevi and are more common in females.[14] *Cavernous hemangiomas* are palpable vascular nevi that involve deep cutaneous capillaries. *Mixed hemangiomas* have features of both a strawberry and a cavernous hemangioma.

Palpable hemangiomas are often inapparent at birth and manifest in the first few months of life. Occasionally, however, a newborn exhibits a telltale red macule, papule, or telangiectasia surrounded by a pale halo at birth.

Etiology and Pathophysiology. Palpable hemangiomas seem to progress through three phases from onset to complete involution. The first phase is the growth phase in which the hemangioma enlarges rapidly. This growth phase ends between 6 to 12 months of age, and the hemangioma enters a stationary phase for several months when it grows only in proportion to the child's growth. Approximately 1 year after the initial appearance of the hemangioma, involution begins. In general, by 5 years of age, half the lesions involute with little or no residual effect. By 7 years of age, most are clear, and any residual hemangiomas continue to improve through later childhood and adolescence.

Clinical Manifestations. Clinically, strawberry hemangiomas are bright red, slightly elevated with well-defined borders. They grow quickly into solid, rubbery masses that partially blanch on palpation. The size ranges from a few millimeters to more than 20 cm in diameter.

Clinically, cavernous hemangiomas may present as poorly demarcated subcutaneous masses with absent overlying cutaneous changes or as a well-circumscribed intradermal nodule that produces a bluish discoloration of the overlying skin. They protrude above the skin surface and, on palpation, have the consistency of a "bag of worms."

A mixed hemangioma has features of both a strawberry and a cavernous hemangioma with a red surface and a deep rubbery subcutaneous mass (Fig. 65-14).

Several rare congenital syndromes are associated with vascular nevi. Sturge-Weber syndrome (SWS) is a leptomeningeal vascular formation in which the port wine stain involves the ophthalmic distribution of the trigeminal nerve. Seizures occur in 55% to 97% of children with this

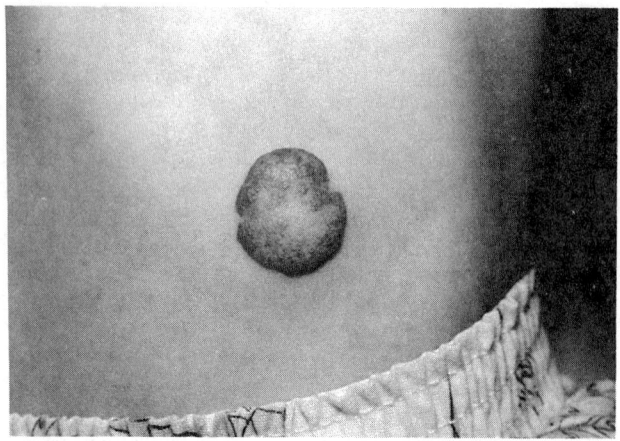

FIGURE 65-14
Hemangioma. A well defined, bright red rubbery mass on the flank of a child characteristic of a strawberry hemangioma. This lesion shows evidence of early involution with spotty loss of the red color.

syndrome.[52] Klippel-Trenaunay-Weber syndrome (KTWS) has both a nevus flammeus component and a cavernous hemangiolymphangioma component. These lesions cause hypertrophy of the bone and soft tissue. Cutis marmorata telangiectatica congenita (CMTC) presents with persistent, patchy, bluish mottling of the skin. This condition differs from physiologic cutis marmorata (see "Transient Cutaneous Conditions in the Newborn" in this chapter) in that it is not influenced by ambient temperature.

Diagnostic Studies in Hemangiomas. By far, the majority of hemangiomas are diagnosed on the basis of their clinical appearance. Laboratory studies are normal in most of these children. Additional studies are required only with the more serious forms of presentation. Platelet counts may be done in children with rapidly enlarging lesions. Children with port wine stains involving the orbit area should have an ophthalmologic examination to screen for eye involvement.

★ ASSESSMENT

Nursing assessment of a child presenting with a hemangioma includes a total cutaneous examination to identify and document the number and sites of lesions. The surface of the hemangioma is also examined closely to note signs of involution and the presence of any areas of skin breakdown. All lesions are carefully measured and photographed at the initial visit and each follow-up visit. This procedure enables careful documentation of the progression of the hemangioma through the various growth and involution stages.

Because of the profound psychological impact the presence of a hemangioma can have on both the child and parent, it is important for the nurse to assess the psychosocial impact this lesion is having on the child and parent as well as its effect on the family process. Parents are interviewed about their beliefs and concerns regarding the hemangioma and public reaction to their child's appearance.

★ NURSING DIAGNOSES AND PLANNING

Based on assessment data from above and Chapter 64, the following nursing diagnoses may apply to the family and child with hemangioma:

- Anxiety related to knowledge deficit regarding the disorder and treatment
- Self-Esteem Disturbance related to appearance.
- Ineffective Family Coping: Compromised related to progress of lesions.

The nurse and child (or parents) together plan effective care based on the established nursing diagnoses. Several examples of expected outcomes follow:

- The parents demonstrate an understanding of signs of complications.
- The parents contact a support group.
- The parents and child state the measures they are using to combat social reactions to the hemangioma.
- The parents and child make recommended follow-up visits.

★ INTERVENTIONS: COLLABORATIVE AND INDEPENDENT

The majority of hemangiomas require no treatment. In port wine stains, the treatment is limited and generally unsatisfactory. Excision, radiation, cryotherapy, and dermabrasion all have been unsuccessful, resulting in considerable scarring. The use of lasers has shown the most promise for treatment.

The current recommendations in the treatment of involuting palpable hemangiomas is the avoidance of aggressive therapy and the use of compression and massage in selected lesions, along with carefully planned parent counseling.

An option in conservative management of hemangiomas is the application of compression bandages to selected lesions and the use of gentle massage. Neither of these treatment modalities has undergone systematic clinical evaluation; however, they are harmless and provide the parents with an active therapeutic option for their child.

In some instances, restorative plastic procedures may be necessary if the lesion resolves with loose atrophic skin or scarring after ulceration or infection. This surgery is not done, however, until complete involution has occurred.

COUNSELING AND TEACHING

Much time is spent with parents at the initial evaluation visit discussing the natural evolution of hemangiomas and helping them to understand that in most cases no treatment is the best option. This approach is often difficult for parents to accept while they watch the appearance of their perfect child become distorted. Parents often experience feelings of shock, grief, fear, and guilt. The extent of parental reaction is not always related to the seriousness of the defect. It is important, therefore, that the nurse remain unbiased in dealing with parents of children with birthmarks and instead provide acceptance and support based on the parents' actual need. The nurse may also want to involve extended family members, who are part of the immediate family's support system, in the educational process. Having family members present helps the parents to feel that they do not have to bear the burden of this experience alone.

In addition to information regarding the natural course of hemangiomas, it is important that parents are instructed on the signs of complications and how to care for the cutaneous surface of a hemangioma if it should be abraded or ulcerated. Meticulous skin care is required to reduce the risk of secondary bacterial infection. Parents are instructed to notify their physician at the first sign of infection.

In addition to watching the growth of the hemangioma during the first stage, frequent follow-up visits provide an opportunity to reinforce the information initially discussed and to observe how the parents and family are coping. Provision of written literature is important. The National Congenital Port Wine Stain Foundation is an excellent resource for information and support. Parents may also find it reassuring to be able to talk with another family that has had a child with a hemangioma.

★ EVALUATION

Involution of the hemangioma is determined by clinical observation of a decrease in the size of the hemangioma, as well as a surface color change and softening of the lesion. Serial photographs are extremely helpful in accurately monitoring the progression of a hemangioma. The nurse should also note whether the family understands the conservative treatment plan and review their coping strategies.

COMPLICATIONS

Complications such as ulceration, secondary bacterial infection, and septicemia are rare. Sometimes the hemangioma becomes so large it causes considerable deformity of adjacent structures. Deformities involving the nose, mouth, ear, eye, urethra, and anus are most worrisome, and obstruction of these structures requires prompt treatment.

Even rarer are more serious life-threatening complications. The Kasabach-Merritt syndrome may be seen in children with rapidly enlarging hemangiomas. In these children, the syndrome is signaled by the development of ecchymosis and other signs of bleeding as a result of thrombocytopenia secondary to platelet sequestration within the hemangioma. Hemangiolymphangiomas have a poor prognosis because of their tendency to involute; this characteristic is not shared by lymphangiomas.

Cutaneous Drug Eruptions

Definition and Incidence. Medication use is common in the United States with approximately 55,000 drug products available on the market. The actual incidence of drug reactions in children is not known; however, drug eruptions are seen frequently. The incidence in children is believed to be lower than in adults because fewer drugs are administered to children, thereby limiting their ex-

posure to these chemicals. Factors that influence the development of a drug reaction are the following:

- Age: Children develop drug reactions less frequently than do adults
- Presence of serious disease
- The number of drugs administered
- Disease that affects the liver or kidneys
- Gender: Drug reactions occur more frequently in females

Etiology and Pathophysiology. Adverse reactions to drugs are seen more often in the skin than in any other organ. Cutaneous reactions to drugs are classified in two ways:

- Drug allergies resulting from immunologic mechanisms
- Drug hypersensitivity resulting from nonimmunologic mechanisms

Drug hypersensitivity is activated in a variety of ways, including overdosage, UVL exposure, drug interactions, metabolic alterations, or exacerbation of preexisting dermatoses. Most cutaneous reactions occur within 1 week of exposure to the drug.

Clinical Manifestations. Table 65-16 outlines the most common drug eruptions in the order of frequency along with the drugs that are the leading causes of these various eruptions.

Diagnostic Studies. Identifying the etiology of a skin eruption can be difficult, particularly in seriously ill children. Determining whether the reaction is a result of a drug or viral infection in immunocompromised children is especially difficult. In these more complicated cases, the identification of the etiologic culprit requires meticulous investigation guided by several key elements. The key elements include the type of eruption elicited, the drugs that are the most common offenders, other agents that are capable of producing similar reactions, and the timing of events. All of these variables must be considered when attempting to implicate the causative agent.

Routine laboratory data are usually not helpful and show no specific changes. The presence of peripheral eosinophilia in drug eruptions is not a consistent finding, and controversy exists as to its value in diagnosis. Certain laboratory tests may be done to rule out other etiologies for the rash. A skin biopsy may be helpful to identify the type of eruption to rule out certain diagnoses; however, it is impossible to differentiate the particular causative agent in reactions, such as exanthematous eruptions, that can be caused by several agents. Skin testing is only reliable in penicillin allergy.

★ ASSESSMENT

The history provides the primary clues for determining the offending drug. A detailed history of all prescription and nonprescription medications taken over the past 2 to 3 weeks is obtained. Previous exposure of the child to any current medication is also noted, in addition to a family and personal history of previous drug reactions.

TABLE 65-16
Drug Eruptions With Associated Drugs

Eruption	Associated Drug	Eruption	Associated Drug
Morbilliform (exanthematous)	Penicillin and related antibiotics	Exfoliative eruption	Carbamazepine
	Carbamazepine		Cimetidine
	Allopurinol		Gold salts
	Gold salts		Isoniazid
	Phenytoin		Lithium salts
	Sulfonamides		Nitrofurantoin
	Trimethoprim		Hydantoin derivatives
	Nitrofurantoin		Pyrazolone derivatives
	Chloramphenicol		Streptomycin
	Erythromycin	Photosensitivity	Amiodarone
	Blood products		Thiazide diuretics
Urticaria	Penicillin and related antibiotics		Phenothiazines
	Radiographic contrast media		Psoralens
	Enzymes		Nonsteroidal antiinflammatory drugs
	Sulfonamides		Sulfonamides
	Glafenine		Tetracyclines
Erythema multiforme	Sulfonamides		Protriptyline
	Phenytoin		Nalidixic acid
	Pyrazolone derivatives	Purpura	Sulfonamides
	Barbiturates		Thiazides
	Penicillins		Quinidine
	Carbamazepine		Phenytoin
Toxic epidermal necrosis	Sulfonamides		Nonsteroidal antiinflammatory drugs
	Barbiturates		Radiographic contrast media
	Oxyphenbutazone	Acneiform eruptions	Androgenic hormones
	Nonsteroidal antiinflammatory drugs		Corticosteroids
	Allopurinol		Oral contraceptives
Fixed drug eruption	Barbiturates		Phenytoin
	Phenacetin		Phenobarbital
	Sulfonamides		Lithium salts
	Tetracyclines		Halogens
	Phenolphthalein		

The nurse should also inquire as to any possible infectious exposures. An accurate account of the eruption course is vital to determining the timing of events.

A complete physical examination provides information regarding the morphology of the eruption and enables classification of the type of reaction.

★ NURSING DIAGNOSES AND PLANNING

Based on assessment data from above and Chapter 64, the following nursing diagnoses may apply to the family and child with a drug eruption:

- Impaired Skin Integrity related to medication allergy.
- Anxiety related to knowledge deficit regarding the skin eruption, its treatment, and prognosis.

The nurse and child (or parents) together plan effective care based on the established nursing diagnoses. Several examples of expected outcomes follow:

- No long-term adverse effects are present.
- The parents and child state they understand the danger in the particular family of drugs being used.

The nurse plans for the care of the child based on both physician's orders and nursing diagnoses. Some general nursing care goals may be the following:

- Causative agent is identified.
- Treatment plan is followed as recommended.
- Skin exhibits signs of healing.

★ INTERVENTIONS: COLLABORATIVE AND INDEPENDENT

The treatment of a drug eruption includes the discontinuation of the drug, administration of epinephrine or corticosteroids in widespread severe reactions, or administration of antihistamines in less serious urticarial reactions. When the drug is needed and equally effective drugs are not available, it may be necessary to complete the course of therapy despite the presence of a cutaneous reaction. These children must be carefully monitored, and the drug should be discontinued quickly if more serious systemic reactions develop.

When the nurse suspects a drug reaction, all further doses of the medication should be held and the physician should be notified of the eruption. Careful documentation of the course of events and the appearance of the eruption are extremely helpful in determining the causative agent.

The child and parent are instructed on what drug or group of drugs caused the reaction and the risk if the drug is taken again. They are also advised to obtain identification jewelry or a card that is carried at all times listing the child's drug sensitivities.

★ EVALUATION

Following discontinuation of the offending drug and interventions with therapeutic measures, the nurse and family evaluate the outcomes of care given. Examples of outcomes for the child and family with a drug eruption were given under planning in this section. Have the goals been met? The nurse also should confirm that the drug reaction is well-validated in the child's records so that future allergic reactions can be avoided.

Summary

The skin is more than a simple, flexible, passive covering for the body's internal organs. Instead, it is a dynamic, complex organ with many protective, metabolic, immunologic, and interactive tasks of its own. The skin is the outer self we present to the world. When it is healthy and attractive, it boosts morale and self-confidence. However, when it is marred by lesions or trauma, it can become a physical, social, and emotional handicap.

Disorders of the skin are numerous and occur frequently in children. They may be conditions that are localized to the skin, or they may be manifestations of systemic conditions. Skin problems affect children, not only physically, but psychologically and socially as well. Knowledge of the skin, its disorders, and the principles of skin care enable the nurse to provide the essential care to children with skin problems and to children with other conditions that may affect the skin. This knowledge also serves as the basis for education of children and their parents about skin care and protection techniques so vital to preserving the interface between a person and the environment.

Acknowledgments

I wish to acknowledge and express my gratitude to several people who have made substantial contributions to the development of this manuscript. Bernard A. Cohen, M.D., Director of Pediatric Dermatology at John's Hopkins Hospital has shared with me a great deal of knowledge and insight in the care of children with skin disease. A very special thanks to him for the many hours he spent reviewing the material presented in this Unit, as well as for contributing ideas and clinical photographs. I would also like to thank my husband, Thomas Rudy, Ph.D., and my son, Ian Rudy, for their patience, assistance, and support during the development of this manuscript.

Sherrill Rudy

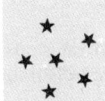

Ideas for Nursing Research

Research in skin structure, skin function, and skin disorders is progressing at a phenomenal rate. This research is yielding greater understanding of the role skin plays in the overall body functions. These advances will influence on the treatment and care of children with conditions such as severe burns, immunodeficiency, genetic disorders, and many other conditions. In addition, skin research is increasing our understanding of the role of skin in emotional and cognitive development. The following areas need to be explored:

- Psychological distress associated with persistent pruritus.
- Success of pruritus control methods in children.
- Effects of knowledge and teaching method on family skin health protective practices.
- Impact of social supports and social networks on family coping in families of children with chronic skin disorders.
- Coping abilities in parents of children with disfiguring disorders.
- Value of therapeutic and physical touch on self-image in children with skin disorders.
- Impact of chronic skin disease on the quality of life.

References

1. Alper, J. C. (1988). Ichthyosis. In K. E. Greer (Ed.), *Common problems in dermatology* (p. 185). Chicago: Year Book Medical.
2. Anderson, G. C. (1989). Skin-to-skin: Kangaroo care in western Europe. *American Journal of Nursing, 89,* 662.
3. Armstrong, B. K. (1988). Epidemiology of malignant melanoma: Intermittent or total accumulated exposure to the sun? *Dermatologic Surgery and Oncology, 14,* 8.
4. Arvin, A. M. (1984). Herpes simplex infections during pregnancy and in infants. *Seminars in Dermatology 3,* 102.
5. Atwater, E. A. (1989). Care of the surgically created granulating wound. *Dermatology Nursing, 1,* 43.
6. Barton, L. L., & Friedman, A. D. (1987). Impetigo: A reassessment o etiology and therapy. *Pediatric Dermatology, 4,* 185.
7. Baumgart, S. (1982). Radiant energy and insensible water loss in the premature infant nursed under a radient warmer. *Clinical Perinatology, 9,* 483.
8. Bertolino, A. P., & Freedburg, I. M. (1987). Hair. In T. B. Fitzpatrick et al. (Eds.), *Dermatology in general medicine* (p. 627). New York: McGraw-Hill.
9. Buck, B. E., et al. (1983). Kaposi sarcoma in two infants with acquired immune deficiency syndrome. *Journal of Pediatrics, 103,* 911.
10. Caputo, R. V. (1988). Papular squamous disease. In L. A. Schachner & R. C. Hansen (Eds.), *Pediatric dermatology* (p. 725). New York: Churchill Livingston.
11. Caro, I. (1988). Herpes zoster. In K. Greer (Ed.), *Common problems in dermatology* (p. 169). Chicago: Year Book Medical.

12. Centers for Disease Control. (1989, May 19). Injuries associated with ultraviolet tanning devices—Wisconsin. *MMWR, 38*(1).

13. Centers for Disease Control (June 30, 1992). Update: Acquired immunodeficiency syndrome–United States. *MMWR, 41*(24).

14. Cohen, B. A. (1987). Hemangiomas in infancy and childhood. *Pediatric Annals, 16,* 17.

15. Coody, D. (1987). Pediatric nurses—sun protection advocates and educators. *Skin Cancer Foundation Journal, 5,* 16.

16. Cooper, T. W., & Bauer, E. A. (1984). Epidermolysis bullosa: A review. *Pediatric Dermatology, 1,* 181.

17. Coskey, R. J. (1984). Treatment of plantar warts in children with a salicylic acid-podophyllin-cantharidian product. *Pediatric Dermatology, 2,* 71.

18. Crumpacker, C. S. (1987). Herpes simplex. In T. B. Fitzpatrick et al. (Eds.), *Dermatology in general medicine* (p. 2301). New York: McGraw-Hill.

19. Cuzzell, J. Z. (1988). The new RYB color code. *American Journal of Nursing, 88,* 1342.

20. Day, C. L., Jr., et al. (1982). The natural break points for primary-tumor thickness in clinical stage I melanoma. *New England Journal of Medicine, 305,* 115.

21. Deleo, V. A., & Harber, L. C. (1986). Contact photodermatitis. In A. A. Fisher (Ed.), *Contact dermatitis* (3rd ed.), p. 454. Philadelphia: Lea & Febiger.

22. Esterly, N. B., et al. (1986). Management of vitiligo in children. *Pediatric Dermatology, 3,* 498.

23. Esterly, N. B. (1984). Viral exanthems: diagnoses and management. *Seminars in Dermatology, 3,* 140.

24. Field, T., et al. (1987). Massage of preterm newborns to improve growth and development. *Pediatric Nursing, 13,* 385.

25. Fitzpatrick, T. B., & Sober, A. J. (1985). Editorial: Sunlight and skin cancer. *New England Journal of Medicine, 313,* 818.

26. Flemming, G., et al. (1987). *Pseudomonas* septicemia with nodules and bullae. *Pediatric Dermatology, 4,* 18.

27. Frieden, I. F. (1987). Diagnosis and management of tinea capitis. *Pediatric Annals, 16,* 39.

28. Frieden, I. J., & Penneys, N. S. (1988). Viral infections. In L. A. Schachner & R. C. Hansen (Eds.), *Pediatric dermatology* (p. 1371). New York: Churchill Livingston.

29. Friedman, R. J., et al. (1985). *The ABCD's of moles and melanoma*. New York: The Skin Cancer Foundation.

30. Galen, W., et al. (1988). Bacterial infections. In L. A. Schachner & R. C. Hansen (Eds.), *Pediatric dermatology* (p. 1261). New York: Churchill Livingston.

31. Gellis, S. E. (1987). Warts and molluscum contagiosum in children. *Pediatric Annals, 16,* 69.

32. Glover, M. T., & Alterton, D. J. (1987). Congenital infection with herpes simplex virus type I. *Pediatric Dermatology, 4,* 336.

33. Greene, M. H., et al. (1986). Acquired precursors of cutaneous malignant melanoma. *New England Journal of Medicine, 312,* 91.

34. Gupta, A. K., & Rasmussen, J. E. (1988). What's new in pediatric dermatology. *Journal of the American Academy of Dermatology, 18,* 239.

35. Hill, M. (1988). Dermatology nurses: Proponents of skin cancer awareness. *Skin Cancer Foundation Journal, 6,* 41.

36. Hurwitz, S. (1988). Herpes simplex neonatorum. In K. Greer (Ed.), *Common problems in dermatology* (p. 169). Chicago: Year Book Medical.

37. Hurwitz, S. (1988). Hair disorders. In L. A. Schachner & R. C. Hansen (Eds.), *Pediatric dermatology* (p. 575). New York: Churchill Livingston.

38. Jordon, W. E., et al. (1986). Diaper dermatitis: Frequency and severity among a general infant population. *Pediatric Dermatology 3,* 198.

39. Jordon, W. E., & Blaney, T. L. (1982). Factors influencing infant diaper dermatitis. In H. I. Maibach & E. K. Boisits (Eds.), *Neonatal skin: Structure and function* (p. 205). New York: Marcel Dekker.

40. Kligman, A. M. (1989, April). An update on topical retinoids. Presentation at Pittsburgh Academy of Dermatology Meeting, Pittsburgh, PA.

41. Krafchik, B. R. (1988). Eczematous dermatitis. In L. A. Schachner & R. C. Hansen (Eds.), *Pediatric dermatology* (p. 695). New York: Churchill Livingston.

42. Lane, A. T. (1987). Development and care of the premature infant's skin. *Pediatric Dermatology, 4,* 1.

43. Lastavica, C. C., et al.(1989). Rapid emergence of a focal epidemic of Lyme disease in coastal Massachusetts. *New England Journal of Medicine, 320,* 133.

44. Levine, N. (1988). Pigmentary abnormalities. In L. A. Schachner & R. C. Hansen (Eds.), *Pediatric dermatology* (p. 529). New York: Churchill Livingston.

45. Lucky, A. W. (1987). Update on acne vulgaris. *Pediatric Annals, 16,* 29.

46. Medoff-Cooper, B. (1988). The effects of handling on preterm infants with bronchopulmonary dysplasia. *Image, 20,* 132.

47. Melnik, M. K., et al. (1986). Malignant melanoma in childhood and adolescence. *American Surgeon, 52,* 142.

48. Mertz, P. M., & Eaglstein, W. H. (1984). The effect of semi-occlusive dressing on the microbial population in superficial wounds. *Archives of Surgery, 119,* 287.

49. Mertz, P. M., et al. (1985). Occlusive wound dressings to prevent bacterial invasion and wound infection. *Journal of the American Academy of Dermatology, 12,* 662.

50. Mosher, D. B., et al. (1987). Disorders of pigmentation. In T. B. Fitzpatrick et al. (Eds.), *Dermatology in general medicine* (p. 794). New York: McGraw-Hill.

51. Nicol, N. H. (1987). Atopic dermatitis: The wet wrap. *American Journal of Nursing, 87,* 1560.

52. Paller, A. S. (1987). The Sturge-Weber syndrome. *Pediatric Dermatology, 4,* 300.

53. Pathak, M. A., et al. (1987). Preventive treatment of sunburn dermatoheliosis, and skin cancer with sunprotective agents. In T. B. Fitzpatrick et al. (Eds.), *Dermatology in general medicine* (p. 1507). New York: McGraw-Hill.

54. Preblud, S. T., et al. (1984). Varicella: Clinical manifestations, epidemiology and health impact in children. *Pediatric Infectious Disease Journal, 3,* 505.

55. Prevost, E. (1983). The rise and fall of fluorescent tinea capitis. *Pediatric Dermatology, 1,* 127.

56. Prose, N. S., et al. (1987). Pediatric human immunodeficiency virus infection and its cutaneous manifestations. *Pediatric Dermatology, 4,* 67.

57. Rauch, P., & Jellinek, M. S. (1988). Psychosocial development in children with cutaneous disease. In L. A. Schachner & R. C. Hansen (Eds.), *Pediatric dermatology* (p. 139). New York: Churchill Livingston.

58. Rosinka, D., et al. (1988). Etretinate in severe psoriasis of children. *Pediatric Dermatology, 5,* 266.

59. Rubenstein, A. (1986). Pediatric AIDS. *Current Problems in Pediatrics, 16,* 363.

60. Schachner, L. A., & Press, S. (1988). Vesicular, bullous and pustular disorders. In L. A. Schachner & R. C. Hansen (Eds.), *Pediatric dermatology* (p. 775). New York: Churchill Livingston.

61. Sober, A. J. (1987). Screening patients at risk for melanoma. Risk profiles. *Skin Cancer Foundation Journal, 5,* 21, 1987.

62. Solomon, L. M. (1980). The management of congenital nevi. *Archives of Dermatology, 116,* 1017.

63. Stein, D. H. (1988). Fungal, protozoa and helminth infections. In L. A. Schachner & R. C. Hansen (Eds.), *Pediatric dermatology* (p. 1415). New York: Churchill Livingston.

64. Stern, R. S., et al. (1986). Risk reduction for nonmelanoma skin cancer with childhood sunscreen use. *Archives of Dermatology, 122,* 537.

65. Storer, J. S., & Hawk, R. J. (1988). Neonatal skin and skin disorders. In L. A. Schachner & R. C. Hansen (Eds.), *Pediatric dermatology* (p. 267). New York: Churchill Livingston.

66. Sumaya, C. V., & Ench, Y. (1985). Epstein-Barr virus, infectious mononucleosis in children. II. Heterophile antibody and viral-specific responses. *Pediatrics, 75,* 1011.

67. Taplin, D., & Menking, T. (1988). Infestations. In L. A. Schachner & R. C. Hansen (Eds.), *Pediatric dermatology* (p. 1465). New York: Churchill Livingston.

68. Timby, B. K., & Lewis, L. W. (1992). *Fundamental skills and concepts in patient care* (5th ed.). Philadelphia: Lippincott.

69. Tong, T. K., et al. (1986). Childhood-acquired immunodeficiency syndrome manifesting as acrodermatitis enteropathica. *Journal of Pediatrics, 108,* 426.

70. Tunnessen, W. W. (1984). Acne: An approach to therapy for the pediatrician. *Current Problems in Pediatrics, 14,* 1.

71. Tunnessen, W. W. (1985). Practical aspects of bacterial skin infections in children. *Pediatric Dermatology, 2,* 255.

72. Willey, T. (1989). High-tech beds and mattress overlays: A decision guide. *American Journal of Nursing, 89,* 1142.

73. Williams, M. L. (1988). Ichthyosis and disorders of cornification. In L. A. Schachner & R. C. Hansen (Eds.), *Pediatric dermatology* (p. 389). New York: Churchill Livingston.

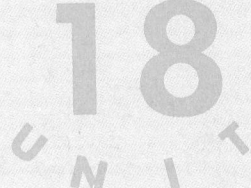

Nursing Care of Children With Altered Reproductive Function

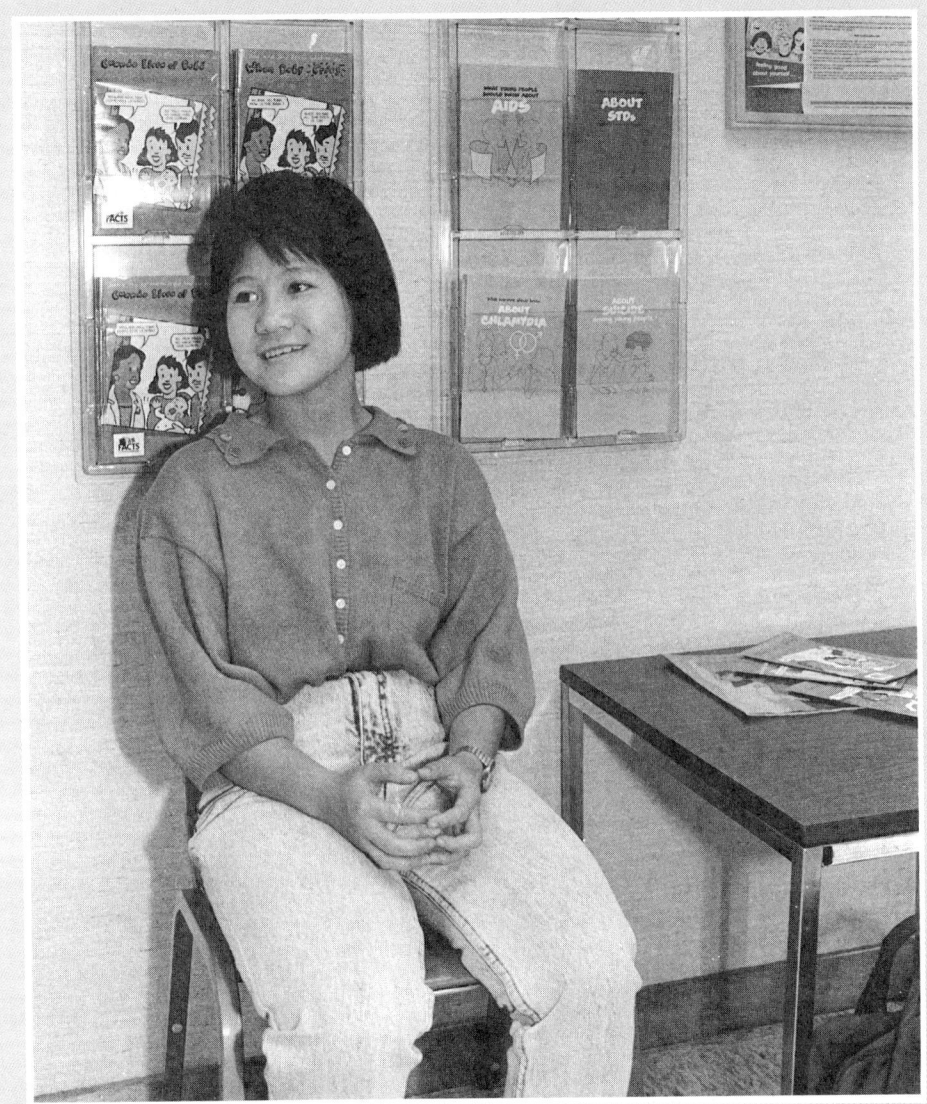

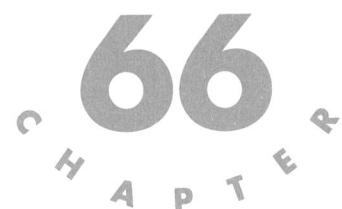

Anatomy and Physiology of the Reproductive System

BEHAVIORAL OBJECTIVES

Describe the process of differentiation of the sexes during embryonic development.

Identify the internal and external structures and function of the male and female reproductive systems.

Describe the events at puberty and the development of female and male secondary sexual characteristics.

Summarize the physiologic events that occur during a female's monthly menstrual cycle.

Describe male sperm production and the process of ejaculation.

Development of the male and female reproductive systems *in utero* and at puberty is the result of a series of complex physiologic events that require and are controlled by male and female hormones. Understanding these physiologic events as well as the consequences of abnormal embryonic development is an integral part of a thorough comprehension of the male and female reproductive systems.

Embryonic Development

The importance of knowing the embryologic development of the fetal reproductive system lies in the ability to identify influences during the prenatal period that can contribute to congenital malformations or other reproductive system deviations that appear later in life.

The human reproductive system for both sexes is embryologically derived from the same primitive gonad (Fig. 66-1). The chromosomal sex of the fetus determines the differentiation of the indifferent gonad into that of a male or female.[1,2,4,7]

Each mature ova contains 22 autosomes and one X sex chromosome. Each spermatozoon contains 22 autosomes and either one X or one Y sex chromosome. At conception, the spermatozoon's X or Y sex chromosome is added to the ovum's X sex chromosome, thus determining the genetic sex of the fetus. The male's chromosomal pattern is 46 XY, and the female's is 46 XX.[1,2,4]

1851

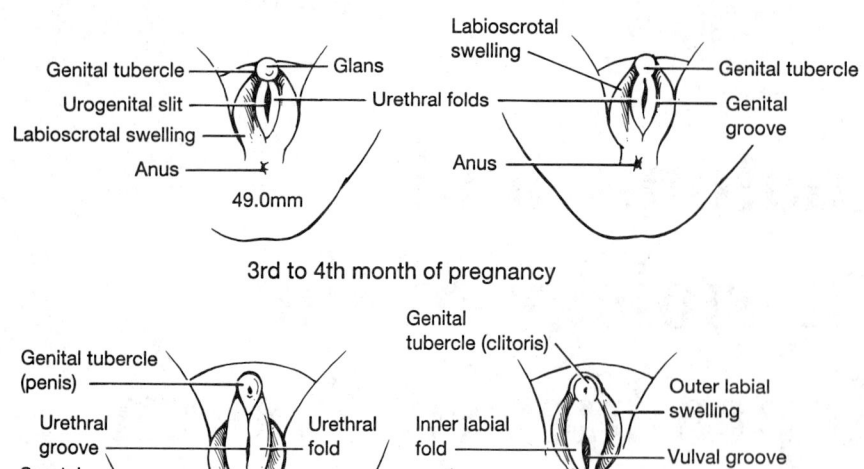

3rd to 4th month of pregnancy

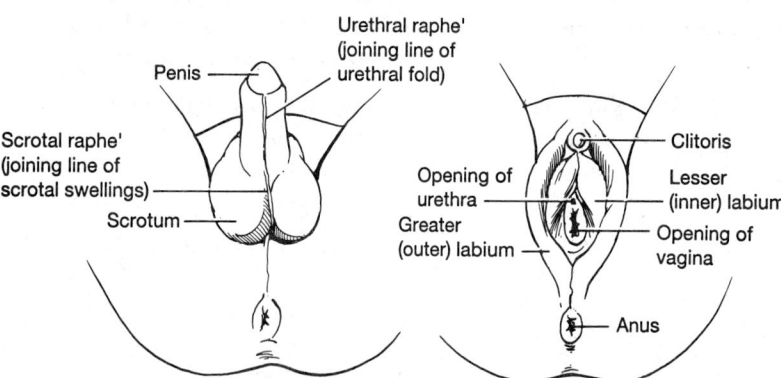

Time of birth

FIGURE 66-1

(A) Male and female external genitalia are identical at 7 weeks, but changes occur after the third month, and genital differentiation continues until birth. (B) Differentiation of internal sex organs of the male and female.

The process of male gonadal differentiation requires functional testes, the secretion of testosterone, müllerian inhibiting factor (MIF) and the presence of the histocompatibility-Y (H-Y) antigen. The H-Y antigen is commonly found in males of the mammalian species. H-Y antigen is a male determinant and is necessary for testicular differentiation during fetal development.[1] During the fifth or sixth week of gestation, the H-Y antigen's presence will stimulate the indifferent gonad to develop into a testis and produce the androgens, testosterone, and the testosterone metabolite, dihydrotestosterone. Additional testosterone production by the Leydig's cells, located in the testes, is stimulated by the placental secretion of large amounts of chorionic gonadotropin.[1] Between the eighth and twelfth week of fetal gestation, the complete process of masculinization of the external and internal genitalia occurs as a result of the androgen hormones. Testosterone stimulates the wolffian ducts to differentiate into the epididymis, vas deferens, and seminal vesicles. Dihydrotestosterone influences the urogenital sinus to form the urethra and scrotum and the penis to be formed from the urogenital tubercle.[1,2,4] MIF is a hormone produced by the Sertoli's cells of the fetal testes during the gestational period. MIF represses the differentiation of the müllerian ducts into female sex organs.[1,7]

Differentiation of the gonad into a female is not as complex as that of the male. The process of differentiation does not require the existence of functional ovaries secreting estrogen. Sexual differentiation of the female takes place due to the lack of the four male determinants and begins to occur prior to the appearance of ovaries during the 12th week.[1,7] The first steps in female differentiation take place when the wolffian duct regresses and the uterus and fallopian tubes develop from the müllerian ducts[1,2,7] (see Fig. 66-1). The vagina is formed from the urogenital sinus. The clitoris begins its development like the penis, but the urogenital folds do not fuse as they do with the penis. Instead, the urogenital folds remain open and become the labia minora. The labia majora are the unfused labioscrotal folds.[7] Figure 66-1 illustrates the progression of external and internal genital sexual differentiation.

Consequences of Abnormal Development

Examples of alterations in the reproductive system that originate in the prenatal period are gonadal dysgenesis, cryptorchidism, alterations in reproductive organ development, and imperforate hymen. These embryo-

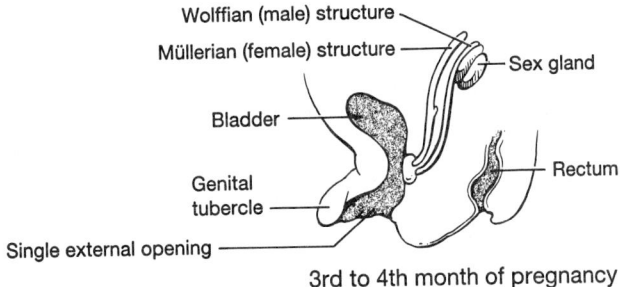

3rd to 4th month of pregnancy

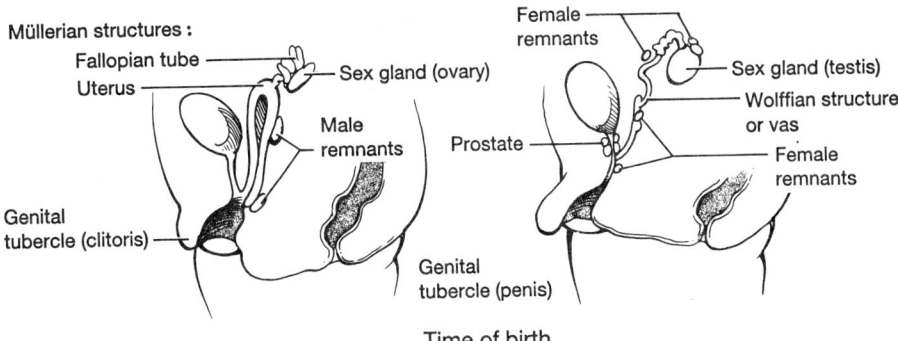

Time of birth

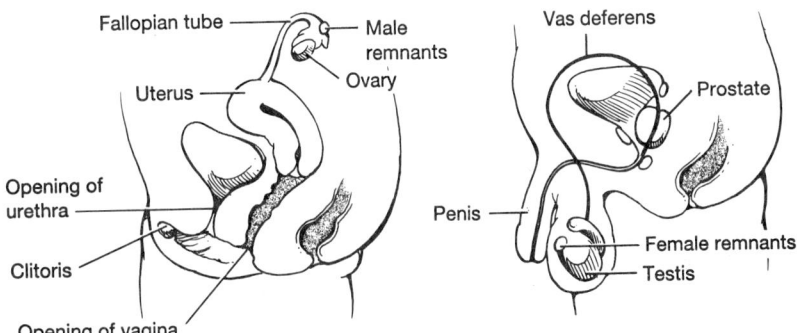

FIGURE 66-1 (Continued)

logic alterations and their origins are highlighted in Table 66-1.

Structure and Function

Female Organs

Internal Organs

The main internal structures of the female reproductive system—the ovaries, fallopian tubes, uterus, cervix, and vagina—are illustrated in Figure 66-2. Together the internal structures produce and transport the ova, accept and transport the sperm, and provide an acceptable environment in which conception and fetal growth can occur.

Ovaries. At birth, the elongated ovaries lie above and behind the fallopian tubes suspended by two sets of ligaments, the suspensory and ovarian ligaments. Each ovary contains the precursors of the ova or primordial follicles. The primordial follicle contains an oocyte. Each female is born with approximately 140,000 to 2 million follicles. This number gradually declines through child-

hood, and the number at puberty has been estimated to be anywhere from 18,000 to 48,000.[2,5,7] The ovaries, fallopian tubes, and uterus are located high in the abdomen during childhood. By 10 years of age, the ovaries have grown and changed to an oval shape and have begun their descent into the pelvis along with the fallopian tubes and uterus.[9]

The blood supply to the ovaries comes from the ovarian arteries that branch from the aorta. The nerve supply

TABLE 66-1
Consequences of Abnormal Embryonic Development

Fetal Age	Structure	Anomalies at Birth
Conception	Chromosomal structure Gonads	Gonadal dysgenesis
7–10 weeks	Forming of urogenital folds and closure of urethral groove	Hypospadias Epispadias
	Failure of fusion of caudal parts of müllerian duct and uterine development	Double uterus Bicornuate uterus Unicornuate uterus
	Failure of canalization or development of vaginal plate	Absence of vagina Double vagina

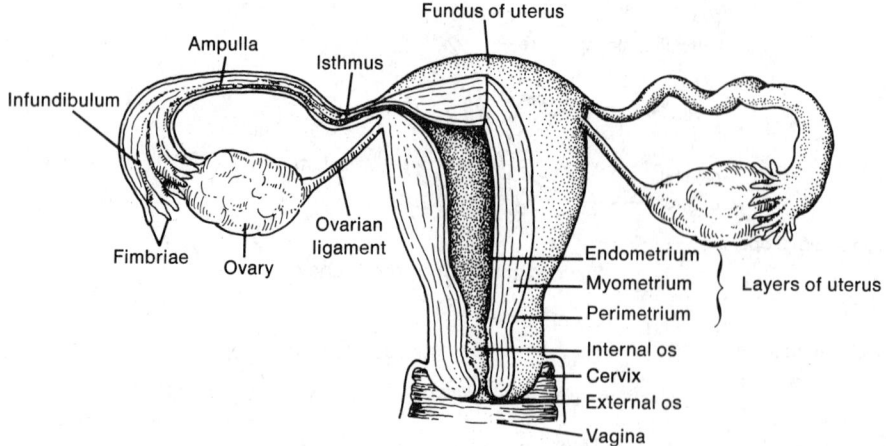

FIGURE 66-2

Anterior view of the internal female reproductive organs. The ovum is released into the abdominal cavity while the fimbriae of the fallopian tubes reach out for it.

is from the renal and aortic plexuses. Lymphatic pathways lead to nodes in the lateral periaortic area, near the renal veins and the hypogastrium.[5,9]

Fallopian Tubes. Fallopian tubes are small, convoluted tubules located along the upper border of the broad ligament. At birth, the tubes have a muscle layer, mucosal villi, and fimbriae. By the age of 10 years, the tubes have grown in size, are straighter in shape, and have descended into the pelvis. Internally, the mucosa has begun to create complex folds, and the cilia that sweep its surfaces and aid in the transport of the ova begin to appear. At menarche, the fallopian tubes are approximately 12 cm long, spread out from the uterus, and curve downward and medially toward the ovaries. The section of the fallopian tubes closest to the ovary is called the *ampullary segment.* The fimbriae flare out from the wide opening of the ampullary segment and act to guide the ovum to the tube, as shown in Figure 66-2. The isthmus is the narrower midsection of the fallopian tube. The intramural section enters the uterus. The blood supply to the tubes is from both the ovarian and uterine arteries. The broad ligament provides the greatest support for the fallopian tubes. The infundibulopelvic ligament, which is derived from the broad ligament, secures the tubes against the pelvic wall.[9]

Uterus and Cervix. At birth, the uterus is about 3 cm long and weighs 3 g. It becomes smaller as maternal hormone stimulation decreases after birth. From infancy onward, the uterus grows very slowly. At about 10 years of age, the uterus and cervix are equal in length, but at menarche the uterus doubles in size owing to the proliferation of the myometrium and assumes its characteristic anteflexion shape.[5,9]

At menarche, the uterus is located between the bladder and rectum. The uterus is a thick, muscular organ composed of three layers: the endometrium (innermost to the uterine cavity), the myometrium, and the peritoneum (outermost to the uterine cavity). The mucosal changes in the endometrium at puberty and during menarche will be discussed in a later section.[5,7]

The cervix is the portion of the uterus that extends into the vagina. At menarche, the cervix resembles a knob and is cylindric in shape, with the cervical canal traversing

its length. The canal is lined by mucosa and ends in the cervical os. The canal enlarges at menarche and continues to enlarge for a time afterward.[5,7]

The uterus is held in place chiefly by the broad ligament. The cervix is held in place by the cardinal ligaments and the sacrouterine ligaments. The round ligaments are musculofibrous bands that attach at the uterus and terminate at the labia majora. The uterine artery is the blood supply to the uterus, cervix, and vagina.[9]

Vagina. The vagina measures about 4 cm at birth. Vaginal length is doubled between the ages of 2 and 8 years and triples by adolescence. The child's vagina is not as elastic or distensible as that of the postmenarchial adolescent; thus, examination in the preadolescent age group is much more difficult. The vagina's surface is not smooth but is composed of ridges or rugae that allow the walls to expand during sexual intercourse and the birth process. The vagina's development is said to be a sensitive indicator of approaching puberty. The lengthening and thickening of the mucosa as well as other changes are early signs of increased estrogen levels. The blood supply to the vagina is from the vaginal artery.[5,7]

External Organs

The external genital structures of the female reproductive system, collectively known as the *vulva,* are the labia minora, labia majora, clitoris, and hymen (Fig. 66-3). The urinary meatus and vaginal orifice are also located within the vulva.

At birth, the precursors of the labia majora resemble two round fat pads on either side of the vulvar vestibule. The labia minora at birth are larger and thicker and function to provide a protective covering over the opening of the vulvar vestibule. As the child develops, the protective function is taken over by the enlarged labia majora. At birth, the clitoris is also quite large owing to hormonal stimulation but decreases in size as the flow of hormones ceases. The urethral meatus in the infant can be located just above the point where the labia minora converge anteriorly.[5,9]

As the child grows, the labia minora and majora become thinner and flatten. The clitoris enlarges and the hymen, which is found at the vaginal introitus, becomes

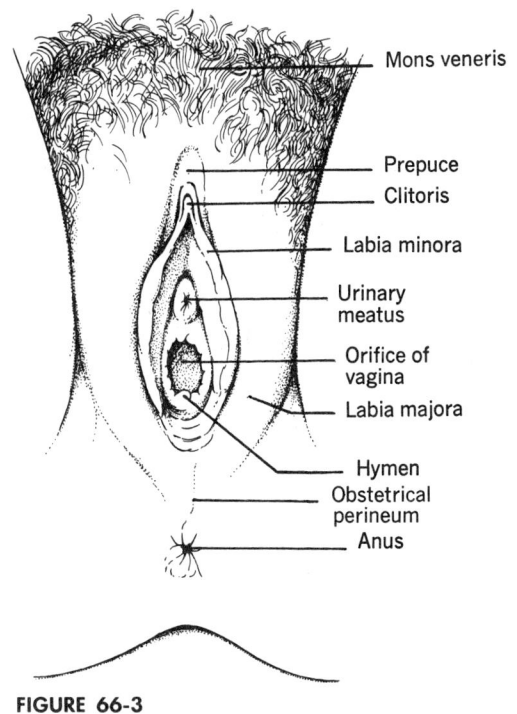

FIGURE 66-3
External genitalia of the female.

Mons veneris

Prepuce

Clitoris

Labia minora

Urinary meatus

Orifice of vagina

Labia majora

Hymen

Obstetrical perineum

Anus

thinner and more membranous. Early signs of the commencement of the maturation process are the increase in pubic hair growth and increase in size of the mons pubis and labia majora. The vaginal mucosa becomes thickened and pink as menarche approaches.[5,9] At maturation, the mons pubis is round and covered by curly pubic hair. The vaginal introitus is enclosed on either side by the labia majora. The labia minora are pigmented, firm, and hairless.[5,9]

The blood supply to the area is provided by the internal pudendal artery and its branches. The sacral nerves and the pudendal nerve supply the region.[9]

Male Organs

Internal Organs

The internal structures of the male are the testes and the structures that compose the ejaculatory system. The ejaculatory system includes the seminiferous tubules, epididymis, vas deferens and ampulla of the vas deferens, prostate gland, seminal vesicle, ejaculatory duct, internal urethra, and the urethral and bulbourethral (Cowper's) glands.

Testes. In infancy, the testes are formed by layers of cells known as the *testis cords*. Interstitial cells fill the space between the testis cords. As the child matures, these interstitial cells degenerate and leave space. The seminiferous tubules are derived from this open space. Inside the tubules are spermatogonia. Mitotic activity of the spermatogonia increases at puberty, and spermatids appear shortly thereafter. As these events unfold during childhood, the testes gradually increase in size. Major

testicular growth occurs at puberty. Normal adult testicular size will be reached during mid to late adolescence.[9]

The testes begins to descend through the inguinal canal into the scrotum during the latter part of intrauterine life. They reach their final destination at the end of the normal 40 weeks of gestation or by the first month of life.[7,9] Three arteries supply blood to the testes: the internal spermatic, the deferential artery, and the external spermatic artery.[9]

Ejaculatory System. Each testicle contains approximately 900 coiled, seminiferous tubules. These tubules may be as much as 2 ft in length. The sperm formed in the seminiferous tubules empty into the epididymis, another coiled tube. The epididymis becomes the vas deferens, which enlarges into the ampulla of the vas deferens and terminates at the prostate.[4,9] Figure 66-4 depicts the duct system of the testes.

The three accessory glands in the male reproductive system are the seminal vesicles, the prostate, and the bulbourethral (Cowper's) glands. Figure 66-5 depicts the relationship of these glands to the rest of the male reproductive system. Semen, which nourishes and transports sperm during ejaculation, is formed from the fluids of these glands. Approximately 1 to 2 ml per day of prostatic fluid is secreted after puberty. The fluid has a pH of 6.5 and is a mixture of citric acid, calcium, acid phosphate, a clotting enzyme, and a profibrinolysin. Its function is to add to the bulk of semen as well as to neutralize the acidity of the fluid secreted by the vas deferens, thereby enhancing the motility and viability of sperm. Seminal vesicle fluid is high in fructose and is thought to nourish sperm. The bulbourethral (Cowper's) gland secretes mucus. The prostate gland is located underneath the bladder and is formed from several lobes. The posterior lobe is prone to malignancy in adult men, and the other lobes frequently undergo benign hypertrophy in old age.[4,9]

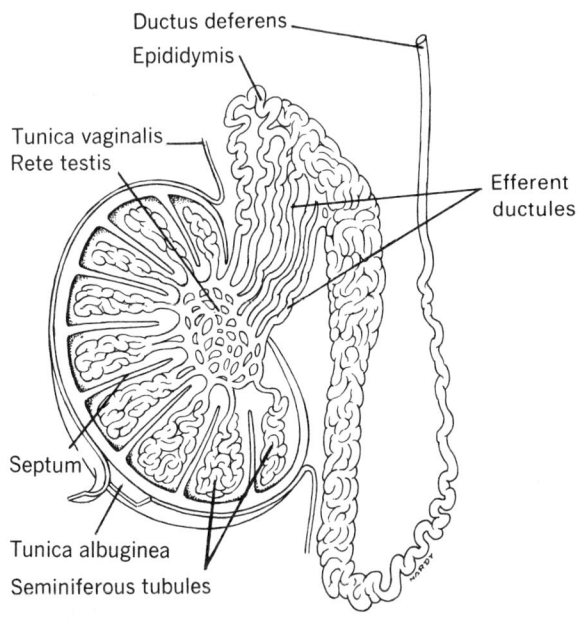

Ductus deferens

Epididymis

Tunica vaginalis

Rete testis

Efferent ductules

Septum

Tunica albuginea

Seminiferous tubules

FIGURE 66-4
Diagram of structural features of the testis and epididymis.

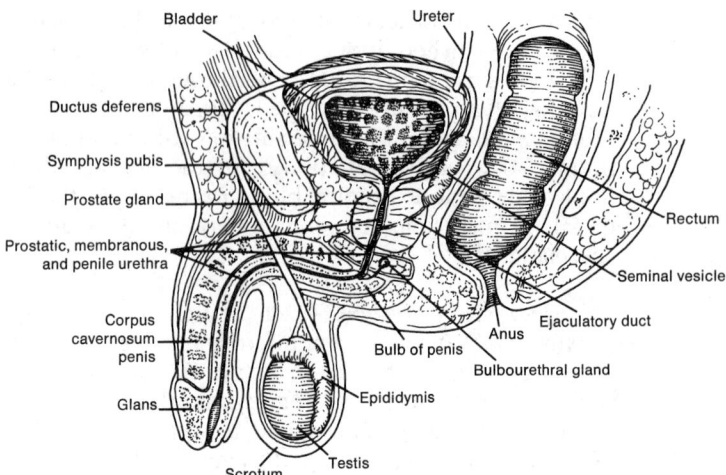

FIGURE 66-5
Male reproductive system.

External Organs

Penis. The penis is fully developed at birth except for its size. At birth, the prepuce covers and adheres to the glans penis. Normal separation of the prepuce from the glans to visualize the urethral meatus cannot be accomplished in approximately half of newborn males. In uncircumcised boys, the percentage of a fully retractable prepuce drops to 10% by the age of 3 years, which is considered normal. Later in childhood, most boys have a fully retractable foreskin.[3,6]

Smegma is part of natural foreskin separation and consists of shed epithelial cells between the glans penis and inner prepuce. In the adolescent, smegma is a combination of sebaceous material and shed epithelium.[3,6]

The penis grows slowly during childhood until adolescence when its length doubles or triples in size. The testes begin their rapid growth and pubic hair appears prior to significant penile growth (see the section on male secondary sexual characteristic development). The urethra runs through the penis (see Fig. 66-5). Erectile tissue is contained in the corpus spongiosum and corpus cavernosum. The corpus spongiosum contains the urethra. During sexual excitement, the erectile tissue fills with blood that is supplied to the penis via the internal pudendal artery.[9]

Scrotum. The scrotum contains the testes, which are suspended in the scrotal sack by the spermatic cord. The scrotum is composed of six layers of tissue. The outermost skin layer overlies the scrotal epithelium, the external spermatic fascia, and the tunica vaginalis. The tunica vaginalis attaches to the testes.[9]

System Physiology

Puberty

Pubertal events are influenced by significant changes in the hypothalamic-pituitary-adrenal system. As these changes take place, the hormones secreted initiate the internal maturation of the reproductive system, development of secondary sexual characteristics, and accelerated physical growth that characterize puberty.[8,9] The three significant changes in the hypothalamic-pituitary system are (1) the increased release of luteinizing hormone (LH) during sleep; (2) an increase in gonadotropins, LH, and follicle-stimulating hormone (FSH) secreted by the pituitary; and (3) the development of a positive feedback system in the female whereby large amounts of estrogen produced by the ovaries stimulate an increase in gonadotropin-releasing hormone (GRH), a subsequent increase in LH, and initiation of ovulation. At the same time, the adrenals are independently beginning their secretion of androgens.[1,8,9]

In prepubertal boys, the rise in sleep-related LH causes an increase in testicular secretion of testosterone. As LH and FSH levels rise, further release of testosterone by the maturing testes occurs. Testosterone then stimulates those pubertal events that outwardly signal that puberty is occurring. These events are development of the penis, scrotum, prostate, and seminal vesicles; growth of pubic, facial, and axillary hair; accelerated linear growth; increase in muscle mass; and a deepening of the voice.

Male pubertal development ordinarily begins at approximately 11.6 years, with a range between 9.5 and 13.5 years. The average number of years over which pubertal change takes place is 3 years, but the process can take from 2 to 5 years.[1,8]

Puberty in females occurs at an average of 11.2 years of age. There is a wide variation. Girls enter puberty anytime from 8 years to 13.5 years or even later.[5,9] Changes occur throughout the body but most noticeably are breast development, broadening of the hips, accelerated linear growth, appearance of pubic and axillary hair, and the maturation of the internal reproductive system. Normally, pubertal changes occur over a 4-year period; however, the range can be from 1.5 to 8 years.[8]

Prepubertal girls' hormonal changes are similar to that of boys. They, too, have changes in the hypothalamic-pituitary system that lead to an increase in the release of FSH and LH. A more detailed discussion can be found in the section on menarche. FSH stimulates the development of ovarian follicles as well as influences the ovary to increase its production of estrogen. LH influences androgen secretion from the ovaries and progesterone synthesis from the corpus luteum. Estrogen stimulates development of the reproductive organs and breasts and increases the body's fat mass. Linear growth in girls is influenced by low levels of estrogen and testosterone. If high levels of estrogen are produced, the rate of epiphyseal closure will increase. Testosterone and adrenal androgens also influence the development of pubic and axillary hair in girls. Estrogen influences the uterine endometrium to proliferate while progesterone converts it to a secreting endometrium. Table 66-2 describes the major action of pubertal hormones in males and females.[8]

Normal adolescent physical development follows a typical pattern. An English physician, J. M. Tanner, studied adolescent development and published a classification system that he had devised based on the typical patterns he had observed. The classification system is called *Tanner staging*, or the *sexual maturity rating scale* (SMR; see Tables 66-3 and 66-4 and Figs. 66-6 through 66-9). The scale is used to assess where the adolescent falls in the secondary sexual characteristic development continuum and to identify more accurately adolescents who do not fit the norms. The scale rates the development of pubic hair and breasts in girls and pubic hair and genitals in boys on a scale from 1 to 5. A stage of 1 is the least developed, and 5 is the most developed.[9,10] Adolescents

TABLE 66-2
Primary Action of Major Hormones of Puberty

Hormone	Action	
	Male	Female
Follicle-stimulating hormone (FSH)	Stimulates gametogenesis	Stimulates development of primary ovarian follicles
		Stimulates activation of enzymes in ovarian granulosa cells to increase estrogen production
Luteinizing hormone (LH)	Stimulates testicular Leydig cells to produce testosterone	Stimulates ovarian theca cells to produce androgens and the corpus luteum to synthesize progesterone
		Midcycle surge induces ovulation
Estradiol (E$_2$)	Increases rate of epiphyseal fusion	Stimulates breast development
		Low level enhances linear growth while a high level increases the rate of epiphyseal fusion
		Triggers midcycle surge of LH
		Stimulates development of labia, vagina, uterus, and ducts of the breasts
		Stimulates development of a proliferative endometrium in the uterus
		Increases fat mass of the body
Testosterone	Accelerates linear growth	Accelerates linear growth
	Increases rate of epiphyseal fusion	Stimulates growth of pubic and axillary hair
	Stimulates development of the penis, scrotum, prostate, and the seminal vesicles	
	Stimulates growth of pubic, facial, and axillary hair	
	Increases larynx size and thus deepens the voice	
	Stimulates sebaceous gland secretion of oil	
	Increases libido	
	Increases muscle mass	
	Increases red blood cell mass	
Progesterone		Converts a proliferative uterine endometrium to a secretory endometrium
		Stimulates lobuloalveolar breast development
Adrenal androgens	Stimulates pubic hair and linear	Stimulates pubic hair and linear growth

Source: adapted from Neinstein, L. S. (1984). *Adolescent health care: A practical guide.* Baltimore: Urban & Schwarzenberg; reproduced with permission from Adolescent Health Care by Lawrence S. Neinstein, M.D., copyright 1984, Urban & Schwarzenberg, Baltimore-Munich.

TABLE 66-3
Tanner Staging in Females

Stage	Breasts	Pubic Hair	Other*
I	None	None	
II	Breast budding (thelarche): areolar hyperplasia with small amount of breast tissue, erect papillae	Long, downy pubic hair over mons veneris or labia majora; may occur with breast budding or several weeks or months later (pubarche)	Thickening of vaginal epithelium tissue, lowering of vaginal pH
III	Further enlargement of breast tissue and widening of areola with no separation of their contours	Increase in amount of hair (dark, coarse and curly) spread sparsely over junction of pubes	Peak height spurt begins; enlargement of uterus; axillary hair begins to appear
IV	Double contour form: areola and papillae form secondary mound on top of breast tissue	Adult appearance but less area covered, no spread to medial aspects of thighs	Axillary hair present, uterus enlarges, vaginal discharge
V	Larger, mature breast with single contour form	Adult distribution and quantity with spread to medial aspects of thighs	Adult characteristics present

* Criteria not included in original Tanner stages.
Source: Adapted from Tanner, J. M.: (1969). *Growth at adolescence,* 2nd ed. Oxford, Blackwell Scientific Publications; and Marshall, W. A., & Tanner, J. M. (1969). Variations in pattern of pubertal changes in girls. *Archives of Disease in Childhood, 44,* 291–303.

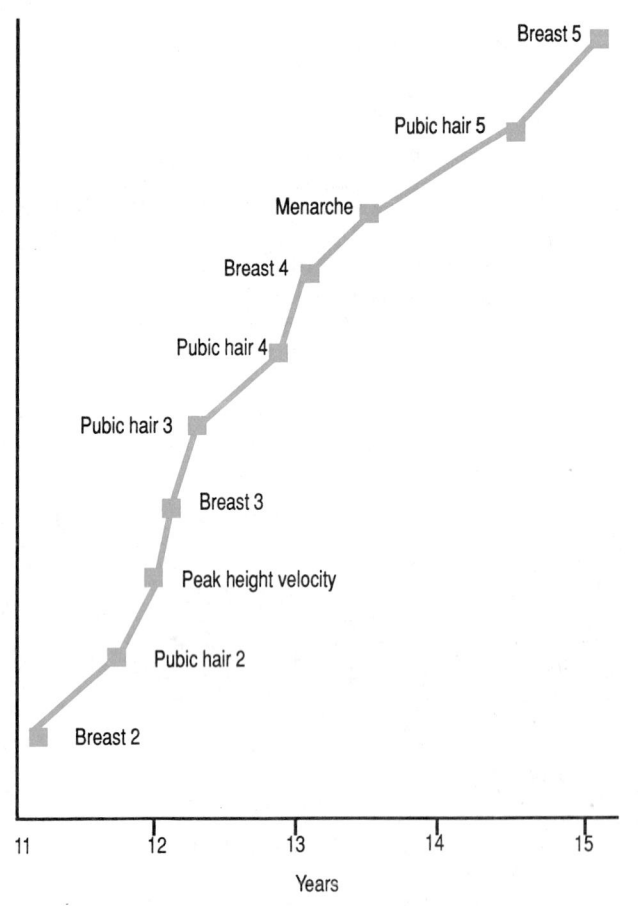

FIGURE 66-6
Sequence and mean age of pubertal events in girls, based on Tanner staging. (Source: Root, A. W. [1973]. Endocrinology of puberty. *Journal of Pediatrics, 83,* 187–200.)

may be at differing stages of genital, breast, or pubic hair maturation at any one time. For example, a boy may be at stage 3 genital growth and stage 4 for pubic hair. A girl may be at stage 4 breast development and stage 5 for pubic hair. The interrelationship of the SMR and pubertal events is illustrated in Figures 66-6 and 66-8.

Development of Female Secondary Sexual Characteristics

The first sign of the female's transition into puberty is the appearance of the breast bud. Estrogen is the primary hormone that influences breast development.[8] A mound is formed by the developing breast tissue and papilla and the areola increases in size. No protrusion of the nipple or papilla is evident as the breast continues to enlarge. The next stage is characterized by continued growth of the breast, with the areola and papilla forming a distinctive second mound on the breast. Contour and separation of the breasts are apparent. The mature breast has a flattened areola, and only the nipple projects. Figure 66-7 depicts these changes in the breast.

The appearance of the pubic hair in the adolescent girl precedes axillary hair and has a significant pattern of development. When pubic hair first appears, it is scant, straight, and distributed along the labia. Later, the hair is dark, thicker, and covers the mons pubis in a triangular shape. Pubic hair then becomes curled, more dense, and spread out. At maturity, pubic hair has spread onto the medial aspect of the thighs and is quite thick.[8] Sexual maturity ratings of the pubic hair are pictured in Figure 66-7.

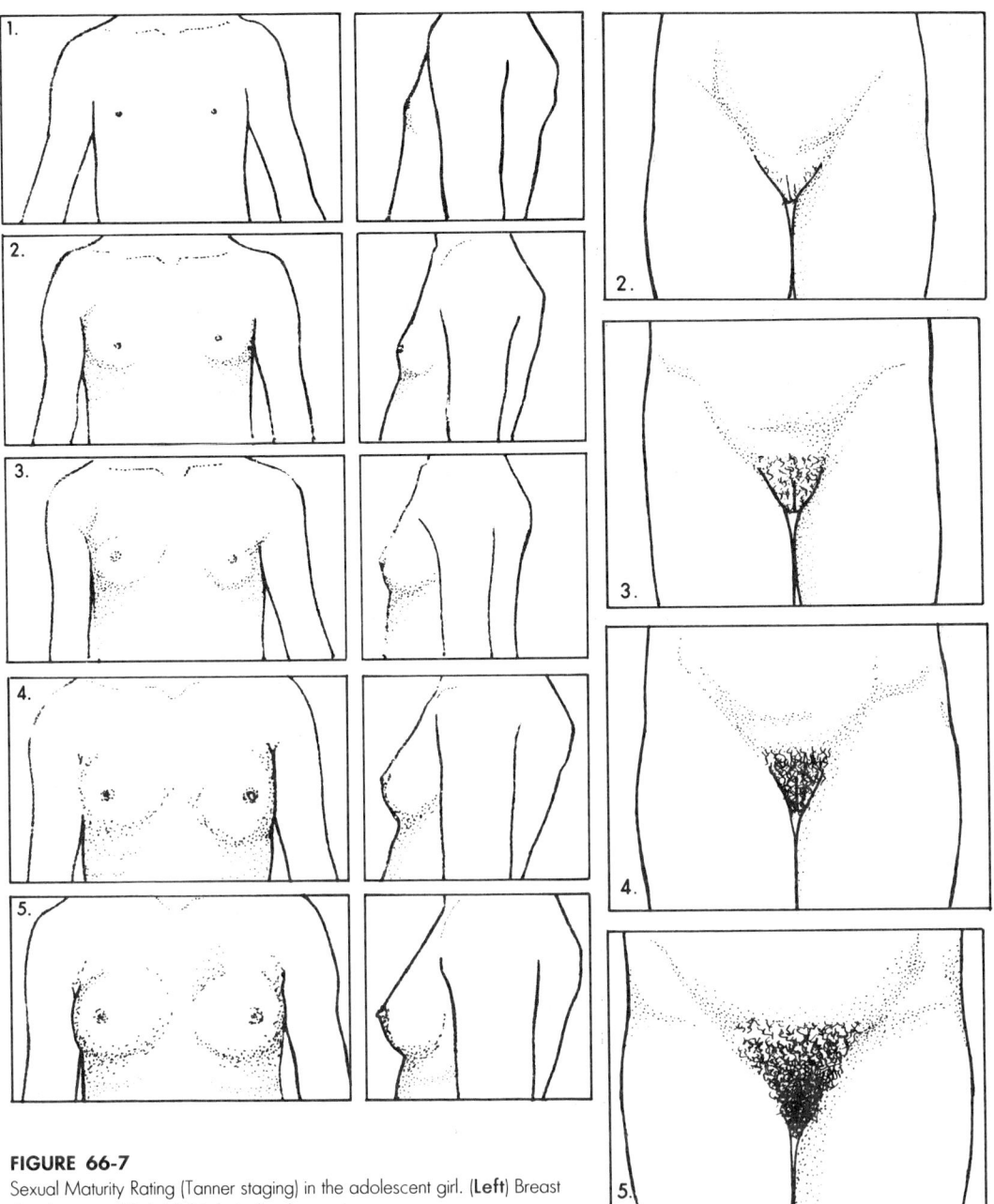

FIGURE 66-7
Sexual Maturity Rating (Tanner staging) in the adolescent girl. (**Left**) Breast development. (**Right**) Pubic hair development.

Menarche and the Menstrual Cycle

The physical and hormonal events leading to the initiation of menarche in the female are complex. The gonadotropins, FSH, and LH are part of a complex hormonal axis called the *hypothalamic-pituitary-adrenal-gonadal axis*. During development, the fetus secretes FSH and LH. The level gradually increases and reaches its peak at about 150 days of gestation. At birth, the hormonal levels have dropped considerably as a result of negative feedback systems. During infancy and childhood, this hormonal feedback system suppresses the gonadotropins.

As puberty approaches, the secretion of GRH increases from the hypothalamus, which, in turn, increasingly sensitizes the pituitary and causes it to be more responsive to the GRH. The pituitary response is to release FSH and LH.[9]

Menarche commences at the average age of 12 years. The normal range is from 8 to 17 years.[5,8,9] Since the beginning of this century the mean age of menarche has been decreasing. Most recent international statistics reveal that the downward trend is slowly diminishing and in many Western countries is remaining more constant.[8] Improved nutrition, socioeconomic status, heredity, and

TABLE 66-4
Tanner Staging in Males

Stage	Pubic Hair	Penis	Testes and Scrotum
I	None	Childhood size and proportion	Childhood size and proportion
II	Sparse growth of long, slightly pigmented, downy hair, straight or only slightly curled, chiefly at the base of the penis	Slight or no enlargement	Testes larger; scrotum larger, somewhat reddened, and altered in texture
III	Darker, coarser, curlier hair spreading sparsely over the pubic symphysis	Larger, especially in length	Further enlarged
IV	Coarse and curly hair, as in the adult; area covered greater than in stage 3 but not as great as in the adult and not yet including the thighs	Further enlarged in length and breadth, with development of the glans	Further enlarged; scrotal skin darkened
V	Hair adult in quantity and quality, spread to the medial surfaces of the thighs but not up over the abdomen	Adult in size and shape	Adult in size and shape

Source: Tanner, J. M. (1969). *Growth at adolescence* (2nd ed.). Oxford, Blackwell Scientific Publications.

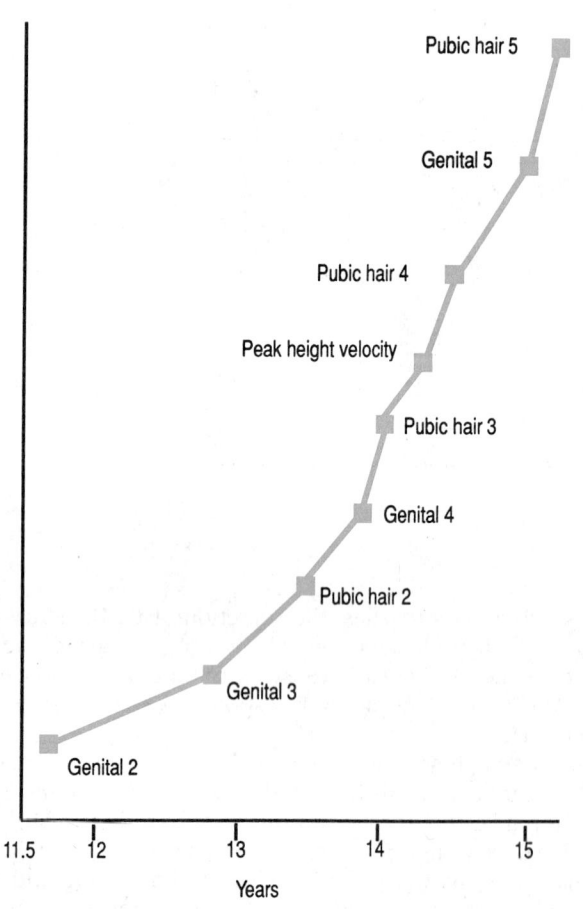

FIGURE 66-8
Sequence and mean age of pubertal events in boys, based on Tanner staging. (From Root A. W. [1973]. Endocrinology of puberty. *Journal of Pediatrics, 83,* 187–200.)

cultural and racial differences contribute to a female's age of menarche. Nutrition status and maintenance of body fat at 24% of total body mass are major determinants in achieving and maintaining regular menstrual cycles. Research that has been conducted using female athletes and dancers supports this theory. Menarche may also be delayed in girls who live in higher altitudes, in rural areas, and in large families.[5,8] Refer to Chapter 68 for further discussion on delayed and precocious puberty.

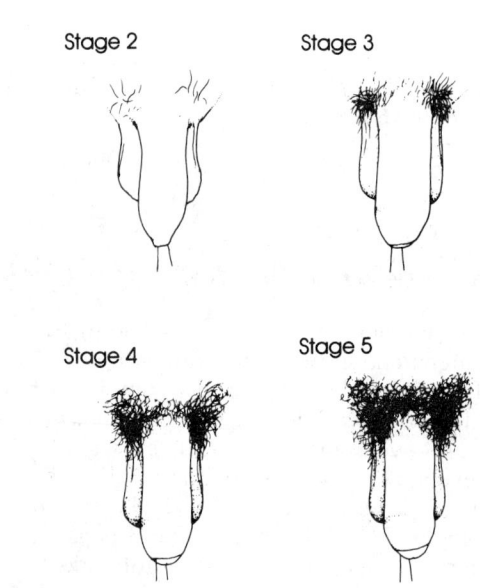

FIGURE 66-9
Sexual maturity rating (Tanner staging) in the adolescent boy based on development of penis, scrotum and testes, and pubic hair.

The Menstrual Cycle

The major milestone of an adolescent girl's pubertal development is the commencement of the menstrual cycle. The menstrual cycle averages 28 days in length, but there is an individual variation of from 23 to 35 days. An alteration in the number of days in a cycle will result in variations of the proliferative phase of the sequence.[5] The events of the menstrual cycle can be divided into two parts: the endometrial cycle and the ovarian cycle, as shown in Figure 66-10. There are three phases in the endometrial cycle: the proliferative, the secretory, and the menstrual.[4] Each phase moves smoothly into the next so that the entire cycle is continuous. The *proliferative or estrogen phase* begins after menstruation. Estrogen influences the regeneration of the epithelium, which rebuilds the endometrium within 3 to 7 days after the beginning of menstruation. This phase continues for approximately 2 weeks whereby the endometrium becomes about 3- to 4-mm thick. A thin, stringy mucous that guides the sperm into the uterus is secreted by the endometrial glands and lines the cervical canal.[4]

The corpus luteum is a glandular structure that develops from the ovarian follicle under the influence of LH. The corpus luteum secretes primarily progesterone and some estrogen. Progesterone stimulates the endometrial lining of the uterus to prepare for implantation. This portion of the endometrial cycle is the *secretory or progestational phase*. As a result of the swelling and the secretory development of the lining, the endometrium becomes about 5- to 6-mm thick. The secretory endometrium contains stored nutrients that provide the hospitable environment for implantation. If the ovum is fertilized, the corpus luteum enlarges and becomes the corpus luteum of pregnancy. If the ovum is not fertilized, the corpus luteum degenerates 10 to 12 days following ovulation.[4]

The *menstrual cycle* begins as a result of a sharp drop in estrogen and progesterone approximately 2 days prior to the end of the monthly cycle. The endometrium rapidly reduces to about 65% of its previous thickness. The layers are shed during menstruation for an average blood loss of 35 ml. Approximately 35 ml of serous fluid is also lost at this time. Uterine contractions expel the blood and fluid. Normally, clotting of menstrual fluid does not occur because of the release of fibrinolysin. Clotting will occur if there is excessive bleeding due to insufficient amounts of fibrinolysin being released. The endometrium is usually completely re-epithelialized within 3 to 7 days after the commencement of menstruation.[4]

The *ovarian cycle* begins with oogenesis (see Fig. 66-10). Oogenesis is the process by which the primitive ova, the oogonia, develops into a mature ova. These transformations are initiated during fetal life and remain dormant during childhood owing to normal negative feedback of the hypothalamic-pituitary-gonadal system. Oogenesis remains an ongoing process during each ovarian cycle.[4,7]

In utero the oogonia undergo mitotic division and develop into primary oocytes. The primary oocytes remain

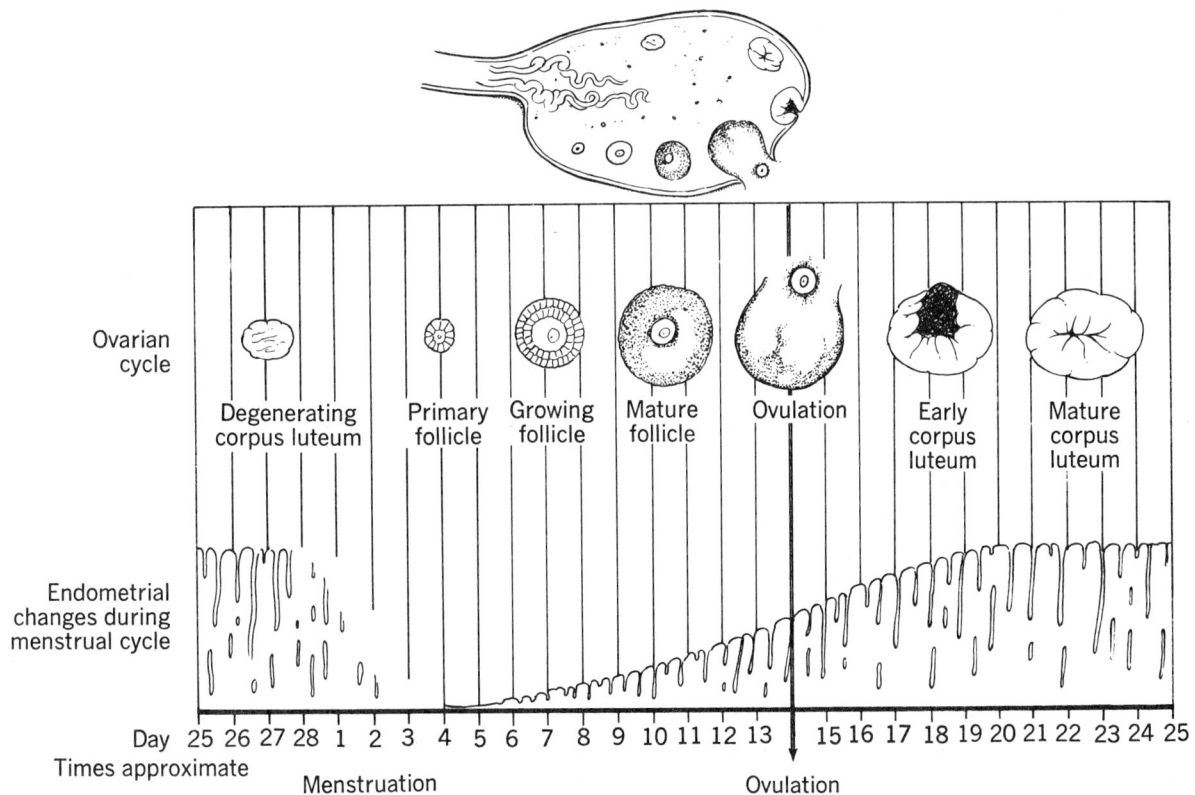

FIGURE 66-10

Schematic representation of one ovarian cycle and the corresponding changes in thickness of the endometrium. The endometrium is thickest just before the onset of menstruation and thinnest just as menstruation ceases.

dormant until puberty, at which time they then enlarge. At puberty, FSH stimulates the growth of from 5 to 12 primary follicles. Usually only one follicle matures and ruptures through the ovary to release its ovum. A surge of LH is required for ovulation to occur. If there are inadequate levels of LH, anovulation will result. Ovulation takes place approximately 14 days after the last menstrual period in an average 28-day cycle. At ovulation the ovum is surrounded by the zona pellucida and the corona radiata, which the sperm must penetrate to fertilize the ovum.[4,7]

Development of Male Secondary Sexual Characteristics

Testicular enlargement is the first physical sign of puberty in males. As puberty begins, the pubic hair is scant and usually light. The penis and testes have enlarged somewhat, and the scrotum is no longer smooth. As the adolescent male matures, the penis, testes, and scrotum have increased their size. The pubic hair is more apparent and darker and extends across the pubis. Later, the pubic hair is darker, curly, and very abundant. The genitals are much larger, with dark pigmentation of the scrotum. At maturity, the pubic hair extends onto the inner aspect of the thighs. Figure 66-9 depicts the male development[8] (also see Table 66-4 and Fig. 66-8).

Axillary and facial hair appear sometime after the commencement of pubertal events. Normally, the sequence of appearance is pubic hair, axillary hair, and about 6 months later, the facial hair. Hair growth is stimulated by the hormone testosterone.[9]

Sperm and Sperm Production

Sperm production begins at puberty, or approximately 13 years of age, owing to secretion of LH-releasing hormone by the hypothalamus. Spermatogenesis will continue throughout a man's life. Sperm are produced in the seminiferous tubules. The sperm remain in the epididymis while they undergo a maturational process from a nonmotile to a motile, fertile state.[4] Most sperm are stored in the ampulla of the vas deferens and the vas deferens itself. Sperm can remain fertile for several months if no sexual activity occurs.[4]

A mature sperm consists of a head and tail. The head contain enzymes that are thought to facilitate penetration of the ovum during fertilization. The tail is composed of three pieces that provide motility to the sperm.[4]

Process of Ejaculation

The process of ejaculation results from a complex series of interactions in the neuromuscular system. During sexual stimulation, signals are sent along the parasympathetic nervous system to the penis, which elongates and becomes engorged with blood. As the penis becomes engorged it becomes firm and erect. Ejaculation occurs with the continued, intense stimulation of the penile muscles until they suddenly and forcefully expel the semen.[4]

Newborn baby boys often have erections due to hormonal stimulation. The adolescent male will probably begin having nocturnal emissions due to hormonal stimulation at about an SMR rating of 3. Some sperm is present in semen if ejaculation occurs at this time, but the male is relatively infertile. When the adolescent reaches SMR 4, enough sperm are present for fertility.[8,9]

Summary

The differentiation of the sexes begins shortly after conception. A complex neuroendocrine feedback system inhibits the infant's and child's reproductive development until puberty. At puberty, complex hormonal events trigger the physical and emotional changes that govern the adolescent years.

References

1. Behrman, R. E., Vaughn, V. C., & Nelson, W. E. (1987). *Nelson textbook of pediatrics* (13th ed.). Philadelphia: W. B. Saunder
2. Freis, P. C. (1983). The physiological basis of sexuality. In R. M. Russo (Ed.), *Sexual development and disorders in childhood and adolescence* (2nd ed.). New Hyde Park, NY: Medical Examination Publishing. pp. 19–27.
3. Gibbons, M. B. (1984). Circumcision: The controversy continues. *Pediatric Nursing 10*(2), 103–109.
4. Guyton, A. C. (1986). *Textbook of medical physiology* (7th ed.). Philadelphia: W. B. Saunders.
5. Huffman, J. W., Dewhurst, C. J., & Capraro, V. (1981). *The gynecology of childhood and adolescence* (2nd ed.). Philadelphia: W. B. Saunders.
6. Klauber, G. T., & Sant, G. R. (1985). Disorders of the male external genitalia. In P. P. Kekalis, L. R. King, & A. B. Belman (Eds.). *Clinical pediatric urology* Vol. 2 (2nd ed.). Philadelphia: W. B. Saunders. pp. 825–863.
7. Moore, K. L. (1989). *Before we are born* (3rd ed.). Philadelphia: W. B. Saunders.
8. Neinstein, L. S. (1984). *Adolescent health care: A practical guide.* Baltimore: Urban and Schwarzenberg.
9. Russo, R. M. (1983). *Sexual development and disorders in childhood and adolescence.* New Hyde Park, NY: Medical Examination Publishing.
10. Tanner, J. M. (1962). *Growth at adolescence* (2nd ed.). Oxford: Blackwell Scientific.

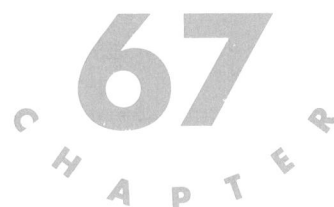

Nursing Assessment and Diagnosis of the Reproductive System

BEHAVIORAL OBJECTIVES

Use functional health as a guideline for assessment of the child's reproductive function.

Describe the components of a complete physical examination of the child's reproductive function.

Describe tests used to diagnose reproductive dysfunction.

Identify nursing diagnoses that are commonly used in the care of children with reproductive dysfunction.

A thorough assessment of the reproductive system includes a broad range of information gathered by the nurse using a skillful interviewing technique. This chapter begins by discussing components of a successful interview as well as pertinent topics and questions for a reproductive health assessment using functional health. Additional data for assessment of a child's reproductive health system are gathered by physical examination, diagnostic tests, and procedures, which include special techniques and observations specifically but not limited to the reproductive system. Finally, appropriate, selected nursing diagnoses with sample client statements and data analysis are described.

Nursing Assessment

Child and Family History

A primary concern of the nurse when interviewing a client about the reproductive system, regardless of age, is to assure privacy and confidentiality. Many of the questions about the reproductive system require the child or adolescent to reveal private thoughts, feelings, and activities. There are three keys to a successful interview on reproductive health or sexuality, including (1) setting the stage; (2) unbiased or nonjudgmental approach and attitude; and (3) constructive approach to the subject.

Setting the stage includes choosing the time and place to pose sexual or reproductive health questions. Both are important elements to consider before the interview begins. Another consideration is providing an environment in which privacy and confidentiality can be achieved. Readiness for interviewing in a hospital room or in a clinic can be determined by observing whether family or friends are visiting or present; whether the noise level is high in the interviewing area; and whether the client is ready emotionally and psychologically to listen and respond.

The nurse should choose a setting that will provide the most privacy. If there are visitors in the hospital room or in the clinic examining room, they must be asked to leave. The adolescent has a right to privacy and confidentiality. If the parent accompanies the adolescent, it should be explained at the beginning of the interview that the nurse will speak to both together but at some point the parent will leave so that the adolescent can answer questions alone. If the parent refuses to leave, the nurse would conclude the interview and indicate that additional questions will be asked at some future time. Confrontation is rarely appropriate or necessary.

The nurse's attitude should be nonjudgmental and reflect honesty and sensitivity to the child's or adolescent's responses; and the nurse should be aware of underlying or hidden meaning in responses. When the nurse asks sensitive questions in an open, nonjudgmental manner it signals the client that it is permissible to talk about private topics and that the nurse will assist by providing information.

Beginning with the least sensitive issues and progressing toward the most sensitive is usually a successful interviewing technique. Another approach that works well with the adolescent client is to ask questions that are global in scope and, based on their responses, continues along a continuum to more specific topics. This concept is illustrated in Figure 67-1.

When assessing the child, adolescent, and family, it is helpful to use the functional health patterns as a guide to systematically gather data concerning the reproductive health system. At times these categories overlap as the data gathering progresses. Appropriate questions to ask concerning the client and family's history, recent changes or problems, and general symptoms are discussed under each functional health pattern.

Health Perception and Health Management

The age of the client will determine to whom the interview will be addressed and which direction the interview will follow. For example, if the client is an infant, toddler, or preschooler, questions are appropriately directed toward the parent or other caregiver. The school-age and adolescent client should always be included in the interview and allowed the opportunity to give responses to all questions. The parent may clarify if necessary.

Certain topics are appropriately addressed in private when interviewing the adolescent client. Examples of these include questions concerning their sexuality. Re-

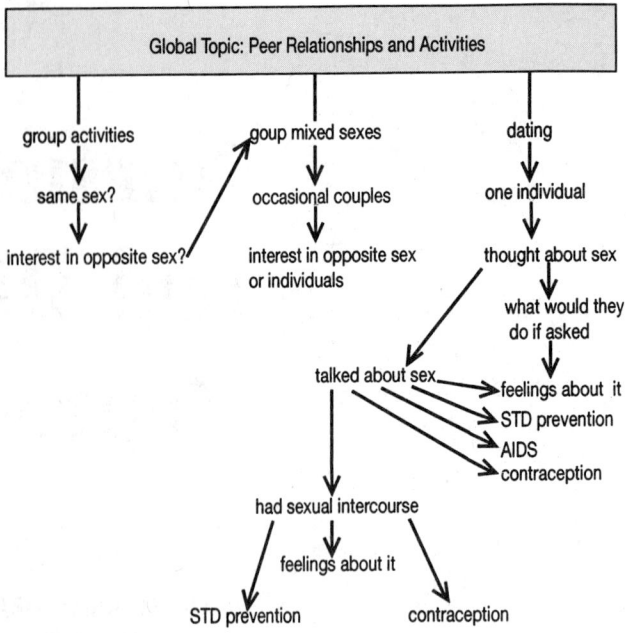

FIGURE 67-1

Flow chart for approaching the adolescent regarding peer relationships, activities, and sexuality.

lated to this topic are peer relationships; menstruation; breast, penile, or other physical changes; sexual activity; access to and use of birth control methods; and knowledge concerning prevention of sexually transmitted diseases. An assessment of the adolescent's knowledge related to self-examination of breasts or testicles is also pertinent. Other topics to address in private are the adolescent's use or abuse of alcohol or drugs, or both, that affect reproductive function and frequently contribute to reproductive health problems, such as pregnancy and sexually transmitted diseases. Problems such as identity confusion, low self-esteem, or poor self-concept related to sexuality or another reproductive health problem may lead to suicidal thoughts or attempts. It is also appropriate to inquire about instances of violence or abuse in the adolescent's life because precocious or aberrant sexual behavior may subsequently occur. The answers to all of these topics may reveal further assessment data that might not otherwise have become known in the normal interviewing process of the adolescent.

Additional appropriate assessment questions would be information regarding general preventive health care routines, such as immunization status and childhood diseases. Financial and transportation resources should also be addressed with the adolescent or parent, or both. The relevancy of these topics can be shown with an example. In the instance of the pregnant adolescent, the nurse needs to know if the girl has had rubella or whether she has had rubella immunization. If the adolescent is still in school, she may have been immunized recently, perhaps during the first months of her pregnancy. This information must be relayed to other members of the health care team. Exposure to any of the common communicable diseases during pregnancy may be life threatening or have long-term consequences for the adolescent as well as for the fetus she is carrying. In addition, if the adolescent has financial or transportation problems, these may affect her obtaining appropriate prenatal care and postdelivery access to birth control methods.

Another example related to the health management topic concerns the parent who has given birth to an infant with gonadal dysgenesis or has a child with cancer of the reproductive system. There is a strong relationship between women who take drugs, especially hormones, during pregnancy and the development of either problem in their offspring. An example is the hormone, diethylstilbestrol, which was prescribed to pregnant women for management of threatened abortion. Studies in the 1970s indicated a strong correlation between women prenatally exposed to diethylstilbestrol and subsequent development of vaginal adenocarcinoma, structural defects of the genital tract, and genitourinary anomalies.[1,4]

Nutrition and Metabolism

The interaction between the reproductive system and the client's nutritional assessment may be less obvious; therefore, an assessment of the nutritional status and dietary practices appropriate for age and physical status is necessary. In the child and adolescent age groups the nurse should also pay particular attention during the interview to weight fluctuations. A loss may indicate anorexia, bulimia, or other eating disorders in the adolescent. A weight gain may indicate a tendency toward obesity in any age group. A female adolescent with sudden weight gain should be questioned about her last menstrual period and approached about the possibility of pregnancy. Denial of pregnancy is frequently encountered, especially in young adolescent girls. Either a weight gain or loss may be an emotional response to sexual abuse. Further investigation is always appropriate. Other possible causes that need further confirmation might be an endocrine or other biologic disorder or other emotional problem.

There are other problems or natural milestones in a child's development that should be considered during the nutritional assessment. These may have an impact on the reproductive system or may be a consequence of an alteration of the system. For instance, menstruation may cease with excessive weight loss or gain. Anemia is a possibility if the menstrual periods are frequent and heavy. The possibility of pregnancy would have an effect on the nutritional plan of care. The adolescent growth spurt increases nutritional requirements.

Elimination

Certain topics are appropriately assessed in this category as they relate to the reproductive system. An assessment of the client's normal baseline urinary and bowel function is necessary. A history of urinary tract or vaginal infections would correctly lead the nurse into a discussion of hygiene practices associated with toileting. This is relevant for the client of any age.

Questions regarding pain associated with urination or defecation should be included. Examples of what the nurse might assess for are the presence of urinary tract infections, hemorrhoids, or anal fissures. A history of or current problem with constipation should be investigated. Further questioning might reveal sexual abuse or, in the sexually active adolescent, sexual practices that may contribute to the alterations in function described.

The female adolescent who has reached menarche should be queried regarding her menstrual hygiene practices. These questions should include the use and frequency of changing pads or tampons. This is often a good opportunity to assess for practices that might put the adolescent at risk for toxic shock syndrome, such as the frequency of changing tampons.

The use of personal hygiene products such as deodorants, douches, powders, and perfumes in the perineal area should always be discussed with the mother and with the adolescent. It is important to include the adolescent's mother because the daughter's hygiene practices are frequently initiated or encouraged by the mother, and the adolescent can become confused with the conflicting advice given by the nurse and her mother. If the client is an infant, the use of powders and other perfumed products on the perineum should be reviewed with the caregiver. Aspiration of talcum powder by infants has caused some deaths in this age group; therefore, prevention of complications by increasing the parent's knowledge is essential.[8] Related points to emphasize, as appropriate, during the assessment phase are the following:

- The skin's sensitivity to the perfumes in most personal hygiene products.
- Douching upsets the normal vaginal flora and may contribute to infections, especially yeast.
- The vagina produces a small amount of normal mucus discharge that serves to cleanse the vagina; if there is an odorous discharge or an irritating, large amount of discharge, it should be assessed and treated because it is never normal.

Activity and Exercise

Total body grooming and hygiene practices as they relate to potential detection and transmission of sexually transmitted diseases is germane. The parent of a child with ambiguous genitalia might be hesitant about being in public or interacting with family members. The adolescent with delayed or precocious puberty may be acting out their feelings with inappropriate social activities and behavior. The sexually molested child or victim of rape may be withdrawn from normal childhood activities with family or peers, or both. A school phobia or unusual fear of adults may be described. These are but a few examples where activities that are reported by the client or caregiver could lead to additional in-depth questioning by the interviewer.

Sleep and Rest

An assessment of adequate sleep time is part of the normal head-to-toe assessment for all age groups. Additional questions might be posed pertaining to nightmares if the interviewer believes this may be helpful, especially if there is a question about depression, sexual abuse, or rape.

Cognition and Perception

When interviewing the child, adolescent, or adult, information concerning the client's ability to think in the abstract is necessary. The relationship between a client's ability to think in the abstract and the reproductive system is subtle. So much of what relates to the reproductive system requires the child or adolescent to be able to act on something that is not tangible and that requires an ability to think in abstract terms. Examples are using birth control to prevent pregnancy or prevention measures for sexually transmitted diseases. Another dimension of the adolescent's cognitive ability is to assess the compliance with taking or using routine medications, including birth control pills or other contraceptive methods or keeping appointments.

The capability of the adolescent to think beyond the present or that which they have experienced is an important concept to understand and apply during an interviewing situation. If the nurse is interviewing a concrete thinker, that fact will dictate how questions are phrased. Most children and young adolescents think in concrete terms. As the person grows into adulthood, the ability to think in the abstract develops. However, there are many adults who have never mastered the ability to think abstractly so age cannot dictate how one formulates questions during the interview. As the nurse conducts the assessment, it will become apparent how the client thinks. All clients, especially children and adolescents, benefit by the addition of visual images for teaching but a concrete thinker may also require detailed, step-by-step instructions during patient teaching.

Self-Perception and Self-Concept

This functional area can be assessed with questions to the client related to his or her feelings about sexuality and reproductive function. Parental attitudes toward sex and reproductive function greatly influence the child and adolescent's attitudes. If the parent is embarrassed and considers sex to be dirty or the child's normal stages of sexual development to be unnatural and needing to be inhibited or punished, the child possibly will develop dangerous behavioral responses. For example, the adolescent may become rebellious or act out in an extreme way. The parent with a child who is a hermaphrodite or has Turner's or Klinefelter's syndrome might have a diminished self-concept related to his or her ability to have a normal child. They may be concerned about how friends and family may think of them as reproductive beings.

A child's or adolescent's self-concept or self-perception is frequently influenced by an alteration in reproductive function. Knowing that identification and acceptance by one's peers are an important part of an adolescent's identity, the nurse should assess the adolescent with precocious or delayed puberty for an altered or confused self-concept.

Role Relationship

This topic may have been partially covered under the categories of activity and self-perception depending on the client's age and situation. To assess role relationship adequately, sufficient information should be gathered concerning the client's relationship with peers, family members, teachers, or other significant persons. The nurse should be alert for any signs of an unusual relationship with a family member. Does the child react in a negative, fearful, or embarrassed way when describing who lives in the home?

Sexuality and Reproduction

The adequate assessment of this functional area necessarily overlaps with all previously described sections. It is necessary to keep in mind that questions related to sexuality are emotionally charged and require a great deal of sensitivity and openness on the part of the interviewer. A further discussion of how to conduct this type of interview is contained in the section on child and family history.

In general the nurse should examine all aspects of sexuality and the reproductive system as it relates to the client's age, physical situation, and psychological state. The complexity of these subjects and how they interrelate with all the functional areas can be illustrated by these examples. The sexually active teenager with frequent urinary tract infections and pain on defecation may lead the nurse to investigate that person's sexual practices and partners. The teenager's responses may steer the interview toward further discussion by both the teenager and the nurse related to role relationships, values, and self-concept. Another example of the interrelatedness of the functional areas in reproductive health is asking the parent questions related to the young child's developing sex role. For example, do children ask questions related to the parent's body?; do they play house or nurse or doctor with playmates?; do they show an interest in their own genitals and the differences between males and females?

If the child or adolescent has an acute or chronic disease, any medications taken in association with the disease process as well as the disease's potential or actual impact on sexual development, reproductive capability, or sexual satisfaction should be explored. Any functional disturbance that might alter the child's sexual satisfaction or reproductive capability should be discussed as well.

In general, the adolescent's knowledge related to sexual functioning, self-care, hygiene practices, contraception, sexually transmitted diseases, and pregnancy should always be assessed. The adolescent girl who is postmenarche should be questioned regarding the impact of dysmenorrhea on activities, such as school attendance, and methods used to relieve the problem. When a disabling condition complicates the adolescent's health, it is also important to include questions related to these areas. If a child needs the help of a caregiver owing to mental or physical impairment, these same questions should be addressed, as much as possible, both to the client and to the caregiver. The adolescent who has a significant, intimate relationship with another person should be asked questions that assess the emotional satisfaction and, if appropriate, the physical satisfaction of the relationship, including any pain associated with intercourse.

By matching for tone and body language, the nurse will provide an interviewing situation that is nonjudgmental and leads to open communication. Only when this atmosphere is created can such questions provide an opportunity for the client and nurse to explore further these emotionally charged topics.

Coping and Stress Tolerance

The broad topic to be explored in this functional area relates to the client and family's ability to respond and adapt to the client's maturing body. A narrower focus might be if the child has been sexually abused or raped. Questions then need to be addressed about their coping mechanism and support systems available to them and those used by the child and family.

Values and Beliefs

Any questions related to the religious or cultural acceptability of the child's or adolescent's sexual behavior or practices should be included in the interview. Again, this is a point for which the nurse must not be judgmental.

Physical Examination

Assessment of the reproductive system should be approached systematically. Certain information should be collected regardless of the child's age. Vital signs, height, and weight should be taken at each visit. For accuracy, these last two measurements must be done in the same manner at every visit. For example, the height is always taken with shoes off, and weight is taken with a minimum of clothing. The results of the height and weight measurements should be recorded on a growth chart and trends noted. This information can frequently aid the nurse in identifying children with some types of gonadal dysgenesis, such as Turner's and Klinefelter's syndrome.

The skin should be inspected in all age groups for the presence of a rash or lesion, scarring, or growths. Skin abnormalities may indicate the presence of a sexually transmitted disease, sexual abuse, rape, or trauma. Examples are a painless, indurated ulcer with a small amount of yellow serous discharge on the penis or the vulva, which is an indication of primary syphilis; multiple scars around the vagina or anus of a toddler may indicate sexual manipulation, trauma, or abuse.

Equipment

A comfortable examining table, height and weight scales, and a sphygmomanometer are the only equipment necessary to carry out a physical assessment of the reproductive system for most children. The nurse can use inspection for most of the examination. Additional equipment is needed for the reproductive examination of a female who requires a pelvic examination. A table with stirrups (not always necessary, especially with children; see Chap. 68 for additional information on examining children), vaginal specula, and lubricant are needed.

Specula come in various sizes for children and adolescents or adults who have never had intercourse, as well as larger sizes for sexually active adolescents.

Positioning

Positioning depends on the age or developmental stage of the child. Young children are examined supine (Fig. 67-2*A* and *B*). The head may be raised 30 degrees so the child is comfortable. A frog-leg position may be used for females. Boys older than 3 years of age may sit in the tailor position with knees bent and feet either flat or ankles crossed (see Fig. 67-2*C*). This is the best position for examining the placement of the testicles in the scrotum.

The nurse may part the young girl's labia with her thumb and forefinger for examination (see Figs. 67-2*A* and *B*). To help distract the child during the examination, the nurse may use the young female's fingers and hands to part the labia (see Fig. 67-2*D*).

Inspection and Palpation

The genitals of all age groups should be inspected for the presence of discharge, rash, lesions, scarring, and growths. The presence of any of these is more than likely abnormal and may indicate a history of trauma, sexual abuse, rape, or sexually transmitted disease. Documentation of circumcision or the ability to retract the foreskin in uncircumcised males should be noted in male infants and children. The testes of the infant or child should be palpated for descent into the scrotum. The presence of a hydrocele should also be noted. This is most likely found in the neonatal period.

The female infant, child, and adolescent should be examined for a normal introitus and vulva. An imperforate hymen may be noted, but more than likely this will not be noted on examination until adolescence and the beginning of menstruation. Different types of hymens are illustrated in Chapter 68. A pelvic examination should be routinely done if the adolescent is sexually active, is beginning a birth control method, or has a family history of early genital tumors.

An overall sexual maturity rating should be done using Tanner's staging scale on both adolescent boys and girls. Pubic hair and genitalia are scored separately. A total score is the average of both. All scores (not just the total) should be noted in the examination documentation. A detailed discussion of Tanner staging (sexual maturity rating) is found in Chapter 66.

Children and adolescents should be examined for the presence of and distribution of axillary, facial, or pubic hair. The common order of appearance is pubic, axillary (shortly thereafter), and facial (approximately 6 months later). Pubic hair distribution is noted according to Tanner's sexual maturity rating. The abnormal presence of or lack of body hair may indicate a genital tumor or gonadal dysgenesis.

In all age groups, breasts should be inspected for symmetry of nipple placement and, in boys, the presence of gynecomastia. Breasts should be palpated for the presence of nodules or masses and discharge from nipples.

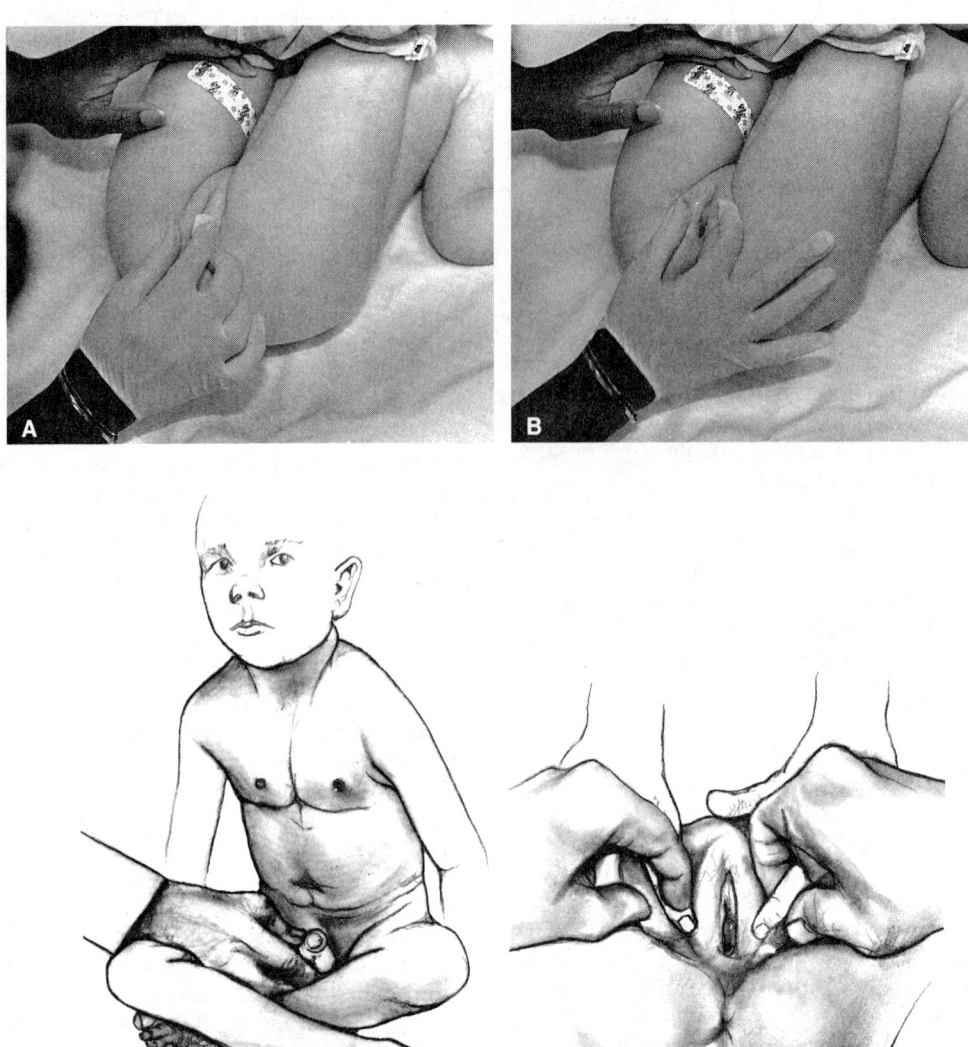

FIGURE 67-2

Positioning for genital examination. (**A** and **B**) In young girls, the nurse parts the labia with her thumb and forefinger for examination. (**C**) Boys older than 3 years of age may sit in the tailor position. This is the best position for examining the placement of the testicle in the scrotum. (**D**) Young girls may be distracted from the examination by having the nurse use the child's fingers to spread the labia for observation. (Source of **C** and **D**: Bates, B. [1991]. *A guide to physical examination and history taking.* [5th ed.]. Philadelphia: J. B. Lippincott.)

The examination can be used as a teaching opportunity to teach the adolescent breast self-examination (see Chap. 68 for a description of the female breast self-examination.) Children and adolescents who show some breast development should be evaluated according to the Tanner sexual maturity ratings. Early or late breast development may indicate precocious or delayed puberty or gonadal dysgenesis.

The child or adolescent undergoing a maturation of the penis and scrotum should be evaluated according to Tanner's sexual maturity rating. In addition, testes should be palpated for nodules and the examination can be used as an opportunity to teach the adolescent testicular self-examination (see Chap. 68 for a description of the testic-

ular self-examination). The presence of a nodule may indicate a testicular tumor. Always note whether the adolescent male is circumcised when documenting the examination.

Diagnostic Tests

Laboratory Tests

Many of the tests done as part of the assessment data collection process for alterations in the reproductive system are collected from blood, urine, genital secretions, or tissue samples. These indices are discussed in Tables 67-1 and 67-2.

TABLE 67-1
Blood Indices of Reproductive Function

Test	Normal Ranges		Deviations	Clinical Implications
Rubella Titer	Negative or positive		Negative in childbearing years	If negative, requires vaccination
VDRL/RPR	Negative		Positive with increasing titers	History of or presently infected with syphilis
Pregnancy Test	Negative		Positive	Pregnancy
Serum Testosterone (ng/dl)	<8 yr 8–10 yr 10–13 yr >13 yr >18 yr	<10 <15 5–55 15–55 10–55	< normal levels	Alteration or lack of normal pubertal events
Serum Luteinizing Hormone (mIU/ml)	*Female* 4–10 yr 10–13 yr >13 yr *Male* Prepubertal Pubertal	<9 2–15 3–20 <8 2–17	< normal levels	Alteration or lack of normal pubertal events
Serum Follicle-Stimulating Hormone (mIU/ml)	*Female* 4–10 yr 10–13 yr >13 yr *Male* Prepubertal Pubertal	<5 1–12 3–12 <5 2–17	< normal levels	Alteration or lack of normal pubertal events
Serum Estradiol (E$_2$) (ng/dl)	<8 yr 8–10 yr 10–13 yr >13 yr	<2 <2 1–12 2.5–25	< normal levels	Alteration or lack of normal pubertal events
Serum Progesterone (ng/dl)	*Female* <8 yr 8–10 yr 10–13 yr >13 yr *Male* Prepubertal Pubertal	 <40 10–50 <10–100 10–150 <10–30 <10–80	< normal levels	Alteration or lack of normal pubertal events
Complement Fixation	Negative		Rise in titer	Cytomegalovirus

(Data source for hormone levels: Greydanus, D. E., & Shearin, R. B. [1990]. *Adolescent sexuality and gynecology*. Philadelphia: Lea & Febiger.)

TABLE 67-2
Urine Indices of Reproductive Function

Test	Normal Range	Deviation	Clinical Implications
Bacteria	Negative	*Escherichia coli, Klebsiella,* or *Proteus*	Urinary tract infection
Human chorionic gonadotropin	Negative	Positive	Pregnancy

Procedures

The following procedures are performed on males or females. The indices for these procedures are given in Table 67-3.

Buccal Smear
Description and Definition
Scraping of cells from inside the mouth.

Purpose
Provide tissue for sex chromatin typing (see Table 67-3).

TABLE 67-3
Tissue and Genital Secretion Indices of Reproductive Function

Test	Normal Ranges	Deviations	Clinical Implications
Buccal Mucosa (Genetic Screening)	Normal complement of sex chromosomes (46,X female or 46,Y male)	45,X 47,XXY	Turner's syndrome Klinefelter's syndrome Ambiguous genitalia
Vaginal or Penile Smear	Negative	Sperm	Recent sexual intercourse
		Trichomonads	*Trichomonas* infection
		Yeast buds or hyphae	Yeast infection
		Chlamydia (cultured on special medium)	Pelvic inflammatory disease
		Gonorrhea (typical colony and Gram's stain morphology, positive oxidase reaction)	Pelvic inflammatory disease
Tissue Biopsy	Negative	Presence of virus	Condylomata acuminata Cytomegalovirus Herpes

Indications

Ambiguous genitalia.

Contraindication

None.

Preparation

Provide information to the parents about the test.

Developmental Considerations

Infants only: no preparation necessary.

Nursing Implications

Teaching and emotional support is given the parents.

Complications

None.

Pelvic Examination and Pap Smear

Description and Definition

Insertion of vaginal speculum; examination and manipulation of internal and external female reproductive organs. Obtaining tissue and secretion samples from vaginal wall and cervix.

Purpose

Examination of the female reproductive system to determine the presence of masses or cancer cells, or both, and rule out sexual abuse (see Table 67-3).

Indications

- Sexual molestation
- Rape
- Trauma to the genitalia
- Vaginal discharge
- Sexually active
- Using birth control
- Family history of early reproductive organ cancer

Contraindication

None.

Preparation

Decrease anxiety.

Developmental Considerations

- Infant: Allow mother to hold infant; use digital examination only.
- Child: Position for comfort and privacy in nonthreatening environment; proceed slowly with examination, being sensitive to anxiety and fear; use digital examination or smallest vaginal speculum, or both.
- Adolescent: Same as above. Use family language for body parts, and include proper terminology as well. Refer to Chapter 68 for further information.

Nursing Implications

Teaching and emotional support appropriate to the development level is given.

Complications

None.

Penile Smear and Testicular Examination

Description and Definition

Penile smear is obtaining a specimen with a sterile cotton-tipped applicator and saline.

Testicular examination is manually palpating the testes.

Purpose

Penile smear is examining any discharge from the penis for infectious organisms or for the presence of sperm (see Table 67-3).

Testicular examination is to examine the testes for nodules and masses.

Indications

- Undescended testes
- Tumors
- Penile discharge

TABLE 67-4
**Selected Nursing Diagnoses Associated With Altered Reproductive
and Sexual Function**

Data Analysis and Conclusions (Defining Characteristics)	Nursing Diagnosis
Health Perception and Health Management	
Verbalization of noncompliance or nonparticipation or confusion about therapy	Noncompliance related to side effects of prescribed treatment (for contraception or for sexually transmitted disease)
Direct observation of behavior indicating noncompliance	
Examples: Missed appointments, partially or unused medications, persistence of symptoms, progression of disease process, occurrence of undesired outcomes (pregnancy)	Knowledge deficit regarding importance of therapy
Sample client statements: "I stopped taking my pills because they made me sick/gain weight/afraid I would get cancer." "I keep forgetting to take my pills"	
Nutrition and Metabolism	
Presence of favorable conditions for infection.	High risk for infection related to hygiene or sexual practices
Examples: lack of hygiene, intercourse without use of condoms.	
Loss of weight with adequate or inadequate food intake according to metabolic requirements	Altered nutrition: less than body requirements related to growth spurt, anorexia, bulimia, excessive menstrual blood loss
20% or more under ideal body weight	
Lack of interest in food	
Aversion to eating	
Menstrual periods > 7 days a month or more frequent than every 3 weeks with or without heavy flow.	
Elimination	
Reported history of urinary tract infection	Altered urinary elimination related to hygiene or sexual practices
Pain with urination	
Urgency and frequency	
Report wiping perineum from back to front	
Nocturia	
Enuresis	
Anal intercourse	
Hard, formed stool	Constipation related to sexual practices or sexual molestation
Defecation less than 3 times a week	
Pain or difficulty with defecation	
Reported history of anal intercourse	
Sexual molestation	
Disruption of mucous membrane tissue of vagina, perineum	Impaired tissue integrity related to mechanical friction of tampon use
Expresses inadequate knowledge of appropriate use of tampons	Knowledge deficit regarding tampon use
Activity and Exercise	
Parent refuses to touch or change infant. Parent may be unwilling to discuss the sex of the child and denies that there is a problem. Parent exhibits signs of grieving.[3]	Situational low self-esteem related to child with ambiguous genitalia
Sleep and Rest Pattern	
Reports having nightmares, insomnia, difficulty staying awake during school	Sleep pattern disturbance related to being awakened during the night from nightmares or trouble initially falling asleep
Reports of past or present sexual abuse or rape	Fear related to past experience of rape or sexual abuse, present or past
Cognition and Perception	
Reports of discomfort during menstrual cycle	Pain related to menstruation
Expresses lack of knowledge regarding any of these topics	Knowledge deficit regarding body development, reproduction, pregnancy prevention, prevention or treatment of sexually transmitted disease

(Continued)

TABLE 67-4
(Continued)

Data Analysis and Conclusions (Defining Characteristics)	Nursing Diagnosis
Self-Perception and Self-Concept	
Expresses hostility or anger toward those who are healthy	Self-esteem disturbance related to unhealthy sexual development or alteration in reproductive functioning
Withdrawal from social contacts, peers, family, friends	
Unwillingness to discuss a limitation, deformity or disfigurement, or denial of same	
Reports nonacceptance of fact that client cannot reproduce normally or at all	Impaired adjustment related to lack of acceptance of inability to reproduce normally, physical status, or infertility
Nonacceptance that chronic disease impacts the client's sexuality or reproductive capability	
Role Relationship	
Child reacts negatively, fearfully, or with embarrassment when describing with whom he or she lives	Fear related to past or current sexual abuse
Sexuality and Reproduction	
Identification of sexual difficulties, limitations, or changes[3]	Sexual dysfunction related to physiologic limitations
Sexual performance limitation due to disease or therapy impairment	
Reports of problems with sexual function	Altered sexuality patterns related to change or loss of body part
Altered relationships with significant others	
Dissatisfaction with sexual role	
Misinformation or lack of knowledge regarding sexuality or function	Knowledge deficit regarding sexuality or reproductive function
Coping and Stress Tolerance	
Inability to meet role expectations	Ineffective individual coping related to feelings of inadequacy, confused role perception, inability to adapt to maturing reproductive function
Change in usual communication patterns	
Alterations in social participation[3]	
Reports sexual assault	Rape-trauma syndrome
Values and Beliefs	
Feelings of cultural or religious conflict/guilt/ambivalence regarding sexual expression or activity	Spiritual distress related to conflict between religious and cultural beliefs and sexual expression or activity
Reports of sexual experimentation with same sex, feelings of attraction to same sex, confusion related to these feelings of attraction	Anxiety related to identity and role confusion
	Ineffective individual coping related to inability to meet role expectations
Feeling different from peers/family/role expectations	Situational low self-esteem related to peer/family/role pressures

Contraindications

None.

Preparation

Decrease anxiety.

Developmental Considerations

- Infant: Be gentle (see the section in Chapter 68 on cryptorchidism).
- Child: Be gentle; provide privacy; be sensitive to anxiety and fear.
- Adolescent: Same as above.

Nursing Implications

Teaching and emotional support appropriate to development level is provided.

Complications

None.

Selected Nursing Diagnoses

After obtaining the history, performing the physical examination, reviewing results from the diagnostic tests, and tapping additional resources for information, the nurse carefully analyzes data obtained. Nursing diagnoses appropriate for the child with reproductive dysfunction become apparent and are used to develop a plan of care. Selected nursing diagnoses that may be appropriate for the child with reproductive dysfunction are presented by function in Table 67-4.

Summary

Assessment of the child's and adolescent's reproductive health and sexuality is complex. The interviewing process

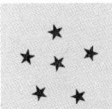

Ideas for Nursing Research

The reproductive system will always be important to children and adolescents as they learn about where they came from and how their bodies work. There are many opportunities for nursing research in the care of children and adolescents with altered reproductive health or in the normal course of development of the reproductive health system. Nurses have an opportunity to be innovative. The following areas need to be explored:

- Identification of the nurse's role in managing sexual abuse in children and adolescents.
- Evaluation of the success of nurses in educating and changing patterns of teenage pregnancy and sexually transmitted diseases.
- Effectiveness of nurses in parental education in contraception use by adolescents and parental communication with their adolescents regarding its use.
- Role of substance abuse in early sexual experimentation.
- Development of special approaches or methods of meeting the distinctive reproductive needs of mentally or physically disabled adolescents.

takes great sensitivity and understanding on the part of the nurse. Nurses frequently interview and conduct assessments of adolescents in hospital and clinic settings and because of the adolescent's changing reproductive system and sexuality, the nurse is able to assess the adolescent using functional health and gathering information on many dimensions of the adolescent's life and health.

References

1. Behrman, R. E., Vaughn, V. C., & Nelson, W. E. (1987). *Nelson textbook of pediatrics.* (13th ed.). Philadelphia: W. B. Saunders.
2. Bellack, J. P. (1984). *Nursing assessment.* Monterey, CA: Wadsworth Health Sciences.
3. Carpenito, L. J. (1989). *Nursing diagnosis: application to clinical practice.* (3rd ed.). Philadelphia: J. B. Lippincott.
4. Creasy, R. K., & Resnik, R. (1989). *Maternal-fetal medicine: principles and practice.* (2nd ed.). Philadelphia: W. B. Saunders.
5. Greydanus, D. E., & Shearin, R. B. (1990). *Adolescent sexuality and gynecology.* Philadelphia: Lea & Febiger.
6. Moore, J. B. (1984). *The pocket guide to clinical nursing process for the pediatric client.* New York: Miller Press.
7. Muscari, M. E. (1987). Obtaining the adolescent sexual history. *Pediatric Nursing, 13*(5), 307–310.
8. Wagner, T. J., & Hindi-Alexander, M. (1984). Hazards of baby powder? *Pediatric Nursing, 10*(2), 124–125.

68

CHAPTER

Nursing Planning, Intervention, and Evaluation for Altered Reproductive Function

BEHAVIORAL OBJECTIVES

Discuss *congenital anomalies*
of reproductive function.

Describe nursing care for children
with injuries or trauma
to the genitalia.

Differentiate assessment of disorders
related to puberty and menstruation.

Perform testicular or breast
self-examination as preparation
for teaching it to others.

Plan teaching regarding prevention
of sexually transmitted diseases
and pregnancy.

Discuss physical and psychological
complications in the homosexual
adolescent.

The possible alterations in reproduction are diverse and complex in their causes and interventions. The alterations discussed in this chapter range from those manifested in easily resolved physical changes, such as selected congenital anomalies and physiologic bleeding, to alterations that have strong, lasting psychosocial sequelae and physical impact. Examples of the latter are sexual molestation or rape, teenage pregnancy, and homosexuality. The impact of many alterations straddle the physical and psychosocial arenas. Examples are childhood injuries or trauma, tumors (benign and malignant), precocious or delayed puberty, menstrual disorders, and sexually transmitted diseases (STDs). Each area includes a general background discussion followed by the implications for the child health nurse. Resources that can be useful to children and families with altered reproduction function and to the nurse caring for them are listed in the accompanying display.

Contraception is an integral part of the reproductive system, although it cannot be considered a reproductive alternation. However, contraception is discussed in this chapter under Problems for the Sexually Active Adolescent.

Congenital Anomalies

Congenital anomalies of the reproductive system are relatively rare. Generally they occur in less than 1% of all live births. The congenital anomalies discussed in

1875

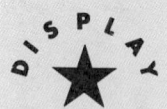

Resources for Children and Families With Altered Reproductive Function

Crisis Intervention Agencies

Hotlines for child abuse prevention, rape crisis, runaways, missing children, suicide, and mental health crisis can be accessed by contacting local mental health organizations, public health departments, and in some phone books under Crisis Intervention Agencies.

Tumors of the Reproductive System

American Cancer Society for community-based support groups such as:
    Support groups for adolescents
    Make A Wish Foundation
    Candlelighters
    Prosthesis advisors and those who can give one-on-one support based on personal experience

Congenital Anomalies; Precocious and Delayed Puberty

Support groups for children, adolescents, and their families coping with systemic diseases, such as kidney failure

and arthritis. Examples are Kidney Foundation, Arthritis Foundation, and American Cancer Society.

Toxic Shock Syndrome

Teaching unit on toxic shock syndrome in Cestaro-Seifer, D. J. (1983). Developing an instructional unit on toxic shock syndrome for adolescent girls. *Issues in Comprehensive Pediatric Nursing, 6*(2).

Sexually Transmitted Diseases

Centers for Disease Control STD Treatment Guidelines, Technical Information Services, Center for Prevention Services, Centers for Disease Control, Atlanta, Georgia 30333.
American Social Health Association Hotline for STD Information 1-800-227-8922
Local AIDS support groups

---

this chapter are related to gonadal dysgenesis (ambiguous genitalia, Turner's and Klinefelter's syndromes), cryptorchidism, and imperforate hymen. Some of these may be readily apparent on observation at birth, but others may be discovered much later in a child's life.

Gonadal Dysgenesis

Forms of gonadal dysgenesis that the nurse is most likely to encounter in caring for infants and children are ambiguous genitalia, Turner's syndrome, and Klinefelter's syndrome.

Definition, Incidence, Etiology, and Clinical Manifestations. The normal sex chromosomes XX (female) and XY (male) determine gonadal differentiation. The gonads develop into ovaries in the XX fetus. In the XY fetus the testes begin to develop and produce androgens and the müllerian inhibitor. Both of these substances continue to differentiate and develop the external male genitalia and internal reproductive system. The müllerian inhibitor acts to prevent further development of the female uterus, vagina, and fallopian tubes.[1,8]

An aberration of the X or Y chromosome or an additional chromosome affects normal sexual differentiation and development. Turner's syndrome, Klinefelter's syndrome, or some forms of ambiguous genitalia generally result. The lack of adequate production of androgens or müllerian inhibitor or the inability of the end organs to respond to either substance also can cause various forms

of gonadal dysgenesis, with ambiguous genitalia being the most prominent feature.[1,8]

Ambiguous Genitalia. Genitalia that are not clearly male or female are described as ambiguous (Fig. 68-1). This is considered a rare occurrence.[1,8,17] The karyotype can be XX or XY. The cause for the ambiguous genitalia is sometimes clear after chromosomal testing, or it may never be clearly understood.

The *in vitro* virilization of a female fetus results in ambiguous genitalia. The most common cause is congenital adrenal hyperplasia. The effect on the fetal reproductive system's development is an enlarged clitoris and fused labia. Frequently the vagina and urethra share a common opening. Internally the female reproductive organs are normal. In addition to the external abnormalities there is a 50% possibility of the existence of salt wasting, which is life-threatening.[1]

Ambiguous genitalia also may be caused by chromosomal aberrations or hormone defects. The external genitalia are ambiguous, but internally ovarian and testicular tissue exist. The presence of both types of tissue defines a true hermaphrodite. Approximately 50% to 80% of true hermaphrodites have a 46,XX karyotype. The rest are divided between the karyotype 46,XY and mosaics (46,XX/46,XY).[1,8,10,15] Ambiguous genitalia in infants with an XY karyotype may be due to an inadequate production of testicular androgens as a result of deficiencies in necessary enzyme production. The failure of end organs to respond to normal amounts of androgens or müllerian inhibitor also may result in ambiguous genitalia.

Turner's Syndrome. Turner's syndrome is a dis-

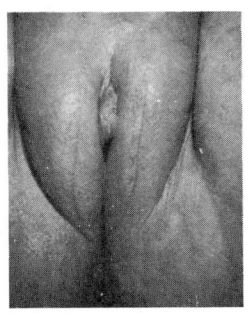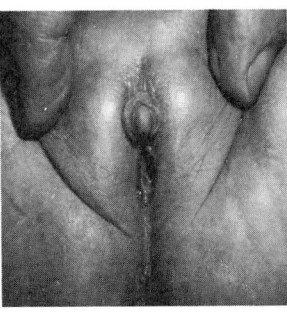

FIGURE 68-1

Ambiguous genitalia. This newborn was considered a normal girl at birth. At 6 months a nurse practitioner questioned the nature of the symmetrical masses in the labia majora (**left**). Spreading the labia (**right**) discloses the obvious enlargement of the phallus and foreshortened introitus. Throughout the diagnostic procedures and following surgical procedures, every effort was made to support the parents by assuring them that the gender role assigned at birth remained correct. This case serves to underscore the importance of careful examination of neonatal genitalia. (Source: Oski, F. A., DeAngelis, C. D., Feigin, R. D., & Warshaw, J. B. [1990]. *Principles and practice of pediatrics.* Philadelphia: J.B. Lippincott.)

order of the X chromosome. It is discussed in Chapter 56 under Altered Gonadal Function.

Klinefelter's Syndrome. Klinefelter's syndrome occurs in 1 in 400 to 1000 live born boys. It is more common than Down's syndrome. Maternal age has a minor influence on the chromosomal aberration that is typical of this syndrome. In some cases, however, maternal age does seem to be a factor. The typical karyotype is 47,XXY. The mosaic karyotype is XY/XXY.[1] The syndrome is rarely discovered in boys until puberty when they fail to develop sexually. Although they appear normal externally, the testes of boys with Klinefelter's syndrome remain small, and there is an absence of spermatogenesis due to hyalinization of the seminiferous tubules and Leydig's cell hyperplasia. The phallus may be smaller than normal with cryptorchidism or hypospadias. Despite the lack of genital development at puberty, some androgen activity may occur, which leads to the appearance of facial hair and a growth spurt. In approximately 40% gynecomastia develops due to the decreased ratio of testosterone to estrogen.[17]

Diagnostic Studies. Cells scraped from the buccal mucosa (buccal smear) can be used to screen for sex chromatin. In addition cells from the vagina, hair root, or amniotic fluid can be used. A full chromosomal analysis of the structural arrangements of sex chromosomes and genes is necessary.[1,8]

The infant with ambiguous genitalia should be screened for congenital adrenal hyperplasia. Electrolytes should be drawn and examined for low sodium and chloride levels with high potassium levels. Definitive tests for congenital adrenal hyperplasia in infants younger than 1 month are urine or blood pregnanetriol or testing blood levels for 17-hydroxyprogesterone. A 24-hour urine collection is performed, and a 17-ketosteroid assay is performed on older children. An elevated 17-ketosteroid titer in children between 1 month and 1 year is significant.[8]

The child with XX chromosomes should receive radiologic examinations, which include urethrovaginog-

raphy or endoscopy, to identify a vagina or cervix. Ultrasound can identify internal organs, such as the ovaries and uterus. The XY child should be studied for normal testicular androgen production. In the prepubertal child this is accomplished by measuring human chorionic gonadotropin (hCG) levels.[1]

The child with suspected Turner's syndrome must have a chromosomal analysis. In addition, blood is tested for elevated follicle-stimulating hormone (FSH), especially if the child is an infant or is older than 10 years.

Boys with suspected Klinefelter's syndrome require chromosomal analysis. Baseline plasma levels of FSH, luteinizing hormone (LH), response to gonadotropin-stimulating hormone, and hCG are normal in boys younger than 10 years. During the midstage of puberty the gonadotropins become elevated, and testosterone is lower than normal. In boys with gynecomastia a high estradiol to testosterone ratio is found. Testicular biopsy may be performed to determine functional abnormalities.[1]

★ **ASSESSMENT**

A nurse's knowledge and observational skills in identifying the physical characteristics of infants with gonadal dysgenesis are crucial for early diagnosis and treatment. Identifying early signs of congenital adrenal hyperplasia in association with ambiguous genitalia will improve the infant's ability to survive. These early signs are failure to gain weight, progressive weight loss, and dehydration. Vomiting and lack of appetite also occur. Progressive dehydration will lead to cardiac abnormalities of rate and rhythm, cyanosis, and breathing difficulties. Without medical intervention these infants will die.[1] Equally important to caring for the physical needs of infants with ambiguous genitalia or Turner's syndrome is the nurse's assessment of the parents' knowledge base, anxiety level, and coping skills during the uncertain time before definitive diagnosis and gender identification.

Children with Turner's and Klinefelter's syndromes are not always easily identified by physical signs. Therefore, nurses can contribute to their identification by carefully listening to parental concerns regarding the child's lack of growth or sexual development. Documentation on growth charts and monitoring the child's development will aid in early identification. Initially adolescents with Turner's or Klinefelter's syndromes and their parents should be assessed for their knowledge base regarding sexual functioning and fertility associated with these syndromes. Concurrently signs of disturbance in self-esteem, such as verbal expression of shame or guilt, must be assessed.

★ **NURSING DIAGNOSES AND PLANNING**

Based on assessment data discussed previously and in the preceding chapter, the following nursing diagnoses may apply to the family and child with a form of gonadal dysgenesis:

- Fluid Volume Deficit related to salt wasting.
- Anxiety related to threat to self-concept.
- Sexual Dysfunction related to altered body structure.
- Self-Esteem Disturbance related to sexual functioning.

- Anxiety related to knowledge deficit regarding condition, genetic involvement, treatment, and prognosis.
- Ineffective Management of Therapeutic Regimen related to knowledge deficit regarding treatment and prognosis.

The nurse and child (or parents) together plan effective care based on the established nursing diagnoses. Several examples of expected outcomes follow:

- The parents demonstrate an understanding of genetic counseling.
- The family participates in planning for the future.
- The adolescent client discusses concerns about sexual functioning.

The nurse plans for the daily care of the child based on physician's orders and nursing diagnoses. Some general nursing care goals may be the following:

- Gender is determined through chromosomal analysis.
- Reconstructive surgery is accomplished successfully.

★ INTERVENTIONS: COLLABORATIVE
AND INDEPENDENT

The approach for treatment of ambiguous genitalia is to first determine gender through chromosomal analysis. Once this is established, discussion with parents regarding the external organ configuration and the genetic identification of the infant as female or male takes place. The gender by which the child will be identified and raised is considered and mutually agreed upon by the parents. The need for reconstructive surgery to assist in the external physical appearance is addressed. In most cases the infant is genetically female, and surgery is required to reconstruct the external genitalia to emulate a female. In cases in which the chromosomes are XY the infant's genitals may be constructed as a female with external genitalia and vagina due to the difficulty of constructing a functioning penis. Additionally, the gonads of an XY infant should be removed due to the 15% to 30% incidence of gonadal malignancy.[1,8,15,17]

Estrogen replacement with a progression toward estrogen–progesterone cyclic therapy is the usual treatment for girls with Turner's syndrome. The age when this therapy should begin is debatable because of the concern of estrogen's effects on growth and closure of epiphyseal plates. However, the benefits of treatment seem to outweigh the actual effect of the hormones on growth.

Boys with Klinefelter's syndrome also are treated with replacement hormones beginning at 11 or 12 years of age. Long-acting testosterone is used.[1]

Independent nursing interventions consist of teaching and emotional support for these children or adolescents and their families. The nurse bases the teaching content on areas of knowledge that were initially assessed to be lacking. Parents almost always need to know why they have a child with gonadal dysgenesis. The complexity and uncertainty of genetically related problems present a challenge to the nurse. Nurses must be knowl edgeable and must present the information related to the diagnosis, its possible causes, and the plan of care in simple terms. Pictures and diagrams frequently are useful in clarifying explanations. The future of these children regarding sexual development, sexual performance, and

fertility should be discussed with the parents. Emotional support to decrease anxiety and any disturbance in self-esteem should be provided to the child and family.

★ EVALUATION

Periodically, the nurse and family evaluate the outcomes of care given. Examples of outcomes for the child and family with gonadal dysgenesis were given under Nursing Diagnoses and Planning in this section.

LONG-TERM CARE

Ongoing evaluation and management of medical and psychosocial needs are required for these families. Difficulties with gender identity have caused emotional problems and even suicide in children and young adults. Genetic counseling and follow-up for families who desire more children also are imperative.[1,8]

Cryptorchidism

Definition and Incidence. *Cryptorchidism* means that one or both testes are undescended into the scrotum. Either undescended testis may be located in the inguinal canal or intra-abdominal cavity. The testes normally descend down the inguinal canal into the scrotum during the seventh month of gestation. Infants born before this gestational stage have a 100% incidence of undescended testes. The incidence of undescended testes in full-term infants is 3.4%. The occurrence of undescended testes drops to .7% to 1% by 1 year of age, and the majority of testes descend by the age of 3 months. After 1 year the testes do not drop spontaneously. In 30% of cases cryptorchidism is bilateral.[1,17]

Etiology and Pathophysiology. The cause of cryptorchidism is unclear except when birth occurs before the seventh month of gestation. Possible causes of undescended testes in a full-term infant are genetic reasons, testicular dysgenesis, anatomic obstruction, or gonadal hormone deficiencies.[17]

There are five possible sequelae of undescended testes: infertility, tumors, hernias, torsion, and psychological effects. Infertility varies depending on whether the cryptorchidism is bilateral or unilateral. In adults who had unilateral cryptorchidism at birth, there is a 50% chance of infertility, which supports the theory that the descended testis may be congenitally abnormal or functionally damaged. If bilateral undescended testes are untreated, there is a 100% chance of infertility. Those who are treated decrease the risk of infertility to less than 30%. Overall, the rate of fertility can be increased if surgical intervention and correction takes place at an early age.[1]

Malignant tumors occur in 20% to 44% of men who had cryptorchidism at birth. Men at greatest risk for developing malignant tumors are those with a history of untreated intra-abdominal cryptorchidism or who had surgical correction for the problem at puberty or later. Sixty percent of malignant tumors in men with cryptorchidism are seminomas; this is twice the rate seen in men who had normally descended testes at birth.[1]

Inguinal hernias are always present with true undescended testes. The excessive mobility of the undescended testis frequently leads to testicular torsion. Finally, the psychological effects of having only one normally descended testis may be considerable.[1]

Clinical Manifestations. Upon careful examination of the testis in the scrotum, the clinician should feel a small nodular area in each testis. An undescended testis will not be felt in the scrotum. When handling the scrotum the examiner must take care not to allow the retraction of either testicle into the inguinal canal by the cremasteric reflex, giving the false impression that either testis is undescended.

Diagnostic Studies. Occasionally, ultrasonography is used to locate the testis in the inguinal canal or intraabdominal cavity. If there is no palpable testicle, a baseline level of serum testosterone is measured, and a second measurement is taken after the infant is given hCG. If a positive response is achieved with a rising level of testosterone, an abdominal exploration may be elected.[1,17]

★ ASSESSMENT

The nurse is able to evaluate for the presence of both testes at birth and during the first well-child visit. While the infant is in a supine position, a small nodule should be felt on both sides as the nurse gently compresses both inguinal canals. When examining an older child a sitting or squatting position helps eliminate the cremasteric reflex so that the testes can be felt (see Fig. 67-2*C*). It is essential that an assessment for the condition and any necessary intervention take place before 2 years of age because of malignant changes and infertility associated with cryptorchidism.[1]

★ NURSING DIAGNOSES AND PLANNING

Based on assessment data discussed previously and in the preceding chapter, the following nursing diagnoses may apply to the family and child with cryptorchidism:

- Anxiety related to the procedure.
- Body Image Disturbance related to the boy's physical appearance.
- Anxiety related to knowledge deficit regarding condition, treatment, and prognosis.

The nurse and child (or parents) together plan effective care based on the established nursing diagnoses. Several examples of expected outcomes follow:

- The parents demonstrate that they are prepared to be with the infant in the recovery room.
- The parents discuss the potential complications of infertility or cancer.
- The adolescent client performs testicular self-examination.

The nurse plans for the daily care of the child based on physician's orders and nursing diagnoses. A general nursing care goal may be the following:

- Testes are successfully brought into the scrotum.

★ NURSING INTERVENTIONS: COLLABORATIVE AND INDEPENDENT

Orchiopexy is the preferred surgical intervention and treatment for cryptorchidism. With this procedure the testes are located and brought down into the scrotum, and the associated inguinal hernia is repaired. Occasionally a controversial medical treatment is attempted prior to orchiopexy. The infant is given hCG or an LH-releasing hormone. In some cases the hCG is believed to facilitate surgery. The hormones aid in the descent of retractile testes, which remain in the inguinal canal due to an exaggerated cremasteric reflex. The hCG treatment should never be used in place of surgical repair for true undescended testes.[1]

Most surgery is performed during the child's first year of life in outpatient or same-day surgery facilities. Teaching usually is parent focused and is concerned with preoperative preparation and postoperative care. The effects of anesthesia and the postsurgical recovery phases should be discussed. For example if parents are allowed in the recovery room, they should be introduced to the room and its equipment. Generally they should be told what to expect preoperatively and postoperatively. It is always wise to assess and validate how much a parent wants to know and how they are assimilating what the nurse, anesthesiologist, or surgeon has told them.

Immediate postoperative evaluation includes care of the incision site until healed and any lingering concerns expressed by parents. Depending on the patient's age when corrective surgery is performed, a schedule should be developed that allows for the resumption of the child's normal activities. How quickly a child is allowed to or is willing to participate in normal activities is a good indicator of a child's return to normalcy following surgery.

Important cultural considerations include the role of the man as heir in each culture and the man's ability to procreate. This is especially true in Asian and Hispanic cultures. The family's concerns may be focused in these areas. If the patient is an adolescent, teaching should address the possibility of infertility and of the development of testicular cancer. At the postsurgery checkup the steps of a testicular self-examination should be demonstrated and time should be allowed for questions.

★ EVALUATION

Periodically the nurse and family evaluate the outcomes of care given. Examples of outcomes for the child and family with cryptorchidism were given under Nursing Diagnoses and Planning in this section.

LONG-TERM CARE

In the rare instances when this type of condition is corrected in adolescence, additional counseling should be considered because of the very low fertility rate that occurs and the possibility of developing testicular cancer.[1]

Imperforate Hymen

Definition, Incidence and Etiology. The opening to the vagina is covered by the hymen, a thick, fibrous, nonelastic band of tissue. An imperforate hymen has a nonexistent or very small opening. The incidence is thought to be 0.1% of all girls.[17] The hymen is thought to be the remains of the urogenital membrane,[8] and the imperforate hymen is considered to be derived from an aberration during gestational development.[8]

Clinical Manifestations and Diagnostic Studies. During a vaginal examination the hymen may be seen in a variety of configurations, as illustrated in Figure 68-2. The cribriform hymen is punctured by many small holes and looks almost web-like. There may be one or more openings in a very underdeveloped-looking hymen as in the septate hymen, or it may be completely imperforate.[1,8,17] The diagnosis is made by clinical evaluation.

★ ASSESSMENT

Occasionally the imperforate hymen is noticed on examination of an infant or little girl. More frequently it is visualized during an examination of the pubertal adolescent female.[1] The earlier the discovery, the better. If discovered after menstruation begins, retention of vaginal secretions occurs with associated amenorrhea and lower abdominal pain and swelling or bulging at the introitus. The hymen will appear yellowish, bluish, or gray-white depending on the secretions behind it.[1,8,17]

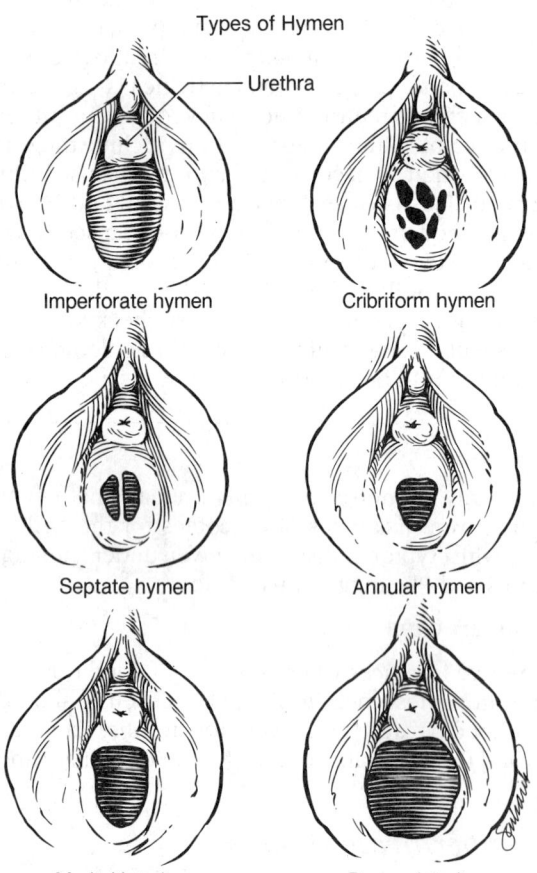

Types of Hymen

Urethra

Imperforate hymen

Cribriform hymen

Septate hymen

Annular hymen

Marital introitus

Parous introitus

FIGURE 68-2
Types of hymen seen on speculum examination.

★ NURSING DIAGNOSES AND PLANNING

Based on assessment data discussed previously and in the preceding chapter, the following nursing diagnoses may apply to the family and child with an imperforate hymen:

*   Anxiety related to threat to change in health status.
*   Pain related to swelling.
*   Self-Care Deficit: Hygiene or Toileting related to discomfort.
*   Altered Urinary Elimination related to urinary tract infection.
*   Knowledge Deficit regarding condition, treatment, and prognosis.

The nurse and child (or parents) together plan effective care based on the established nursing diagnoses. Several examples of expected outcomes follow:

*   The parents demonstrate an understanding of the condition and its treatment.
*   The parents verbalize their understanding that normal sexual development will occur.
*   The adolescent client discusses concerns related to normal sexual activities.
*   The adolescent verbalizes an understanding of sexual development.

The nurse plans for the daily care of the child based on physician's orders and nursing diagnoses. Some general nursing care goals may be the following:

*   Surgical management is successful.

★ NURSING INTERVENTIONS: COLLABORATIVE AND INDEPENDENT

Surgical intervention is always needed to open the hymen. The nurse should be alert for any surgical or anesthesia-related complications. Examples are infection, either systemic or at the surgical site, or reactions to the anesthesia. Child and family teaching is related to the condition, surgical procedure, and follow-up care. Psychosocial support provided by the nurse helps allay the anxiety of the child and her parents.

The postoperative management of the child or adolescent with imperforate hymen greatly depends on the age of the client and the type of defect that was surgically corrected. Most often there is very little need for any type of follow-up. Reassurance that normal sexual development will occur, if it has not already, and that the child will be able to have normal vaginal intercourse when the time comes is necessary.[1,8,17]

★ EVALUATION

Periodically the nurse and family evaluate the outcomes of care given. Examples of outcomes for the child and family with an imperforate hymen were given under Nursing Diagnoses and Planning in this section. Planning for further nursing care takes into consideration complications.

Physiologic Bleeding in Infants and Children

Physiologic bleeding from the vagina in infants and children occurs for a variety of reasons. When physiologic bleeding occurs in newborn girls it is due to maternally influenced estrogens. The withdrawal of these maternal hormones after birth causes a small amount of vaginal bleeding in approximately 25% of newborn girls. In children the cause of physiologic bleeding is almost invariably from an exogenous or organic source. Examples of these causes are trauma to internal organs or genitalia; foreign bodies that have been introduced into the vagina or rectum; vaginitis caused by bacteria, viruses, or yeasts; and precocious puberty.[5]

If the cause is pathologic, a vaginal examination, occasionally using a speculum, may be required. Refer to the section on childhood injuries of the reproductive system for an explanation of how to assess a female child.

The assessment is conducted to rule out childhood injuries, sexual molestation, STDs, and precocious puberty. The nursing diagnoses are similar to those related to any of these etiologies and can be found elsewhere in this chapter. No intervention is required if the cause is withdrawal of maternal hormones. Other primary etiologies of the bleeding are treated.

Childhood Injuries and Trauma

The most common types of childhood injury or trauma to the genitalia are due to accidents or sexual molestation. Injuries to the genitourinary tract are third in frequency behind skeletal and central nervous system injuries. Boys are unlikely to have testicular injury before puberty because of the small size of the testes.[1,8]

Accidents

Etiology. There are many causes of external or internal genital injury. These could be accidentally or intentionally perpetrated. Likely reasons for injury include falls on sharp or penetrating objects that tear or maim; trauma caused by crushing, kicking, whipping, or beating during physical abuse, athletic activities, motor vehicle accidents, or other accidents; or trauma caused during sexual molestation.[1,8,17]

Clinical Manifestations. During a careful and gentle inspection of the male external genitalia, the examiner might find signs of bruising or signs of some other disfigurement. A girl may have perineal, vulvar, or vaginal hematomas or lacerations.[8] The extent of the injuries may appear to be minimal during an external physical examination. Any external injuries should be investigated because of their frequent association with urinary tract or intra-abdominal organ damage.[17]

Diagnostic Studies. Ultrasound or laparoscopy may be used for internal examination of the reproductive organs, especially in girls. A urinalysis may detect urinary tract involvement.

★ ASSESSMENT

The key to a thorough nursing assessment in many of these cases is the interview with the child or parent using the techniques discussed in Chapter 67. Collecting data that might aid in determining whether the circumstances were accidental or intentional will make it easier to formulate medical and nursing diagnoses.

Preparing the child or adolescent for the physical examination also is essential. Positioning should promote comfort and decrease anxiety. A very young child can be examined in the parent's lap or on a table in a knee-chest position. The key to facilitating the examination is gaining the child's cooperation, which will decrease discomfort and reduce fear. In young girls the rectal examination is the best method to examine the uterus or palpate for internal masses or foreign bodies. A finger is placed in the rectum while the other hand palpates the abdomen. Prepubertal children can be examined while their feet are on a table, grasping their ankles and allowing their legs to fall open. In most cases visual inspection of the external genitalia and vaginal opening using an otoscope for illumination is adequate. For more detailed examinations or to view the cervix of the prepubertal child or virginal adolescent, specially sized vaginal specula are available. The smallest size that allows for good visualization should always be selected.[1]

★ NURSING DIAGNOSES AND PLANNING

Based on assessment data discussed previously and in the preceding chapter, the following nursing diagnoses may apply to the family and child with a genital injury:

- Anxiety related to situational crises.
- Pain related to procedure.
- Powerlessness related to health care environment.
- Ineffective Individual Coping related to personal vulnerability.
- Self-Care Deficit: Hygiene or Toileting related to discomfort.
- Altered Urinary Elimination related to urinary tract infection.
- Impaired Tissue Integrity related to mechanical irritants.

The nurse and child (or parents) together plan effective care based on the established nursing diagnoses. Several examples of expected outcomes follow:

- The child expresses degree of pain.
- The child expresses normal emotional range related to hospitalization.
- The adolescent client discusses concerns related to normal sexual activities.

The nurse plans for the daily care of the child based on physician's orders and nursing diagnoses. Some general nursing care goals may be the following:

- Hemorrhaging is successfully controlled.
- Lacerations are repaired.

- Antibiotic therapy is used to prevent infection.
- Possible abuse is reported to the hospital's abuse team.

⭐ **NURSING INTERVENTIONS:**
  COLLABORATIVE AND INDEPENDENT

In many cases initial intervention will consist of assisting with the surgical control of hemorrhaging and repair of lacerations. Once the child is out of danger, collaborative interventions involve antibiotic therapy to prevent or treat infections. The child should be monitored for any signs of additional internal injuries that were missed on initial assessment. All complaints of pain should be evaluated and symptoms of shock reported immediately to the physician.[1] The nurse is an integral part of the health care team's coordinated effort to manage the pain and anxiety associated with all collaborative interventions.

During the assessment phase, if the injury was determined not to be accidental, the hospital's child abuse team should be consulted. Law enforcement authorities also will need to be involved. However, if the injury was accidental, preventive measures should be discussed with the child and parents. The child with major injuries to the genital area will need additional psychosocial support and teaching to allay anxiety and uncertainty about the ability to have sexual intercourse and about future reproductive capabilities.

⭐ **EVALUATION**

Periodically the nurse and family evaluate the outcomes of care given. Examples of outcomes for the child and family with genital injury were given under Nursing Diagnoses and Planning in this section.

LONG-TERM CARE

Children whose injuries are the result of child abuse need long-term follow-up. The child and parents should be monitored by authorities and participate in family and individual therapy. Nurses are involved in the referral process and occasionally in the monitoring of these children, especially when the child makes periodic visits for health examination.

Sexual Molestation and Abuse

Definition and Incidence. Sexual molestation or abuse is difficult to define in specific terms that apply to all cases. The definition usually is determined by state or federal statute. These laws range from vague to very specific in relation to the victim's age, the act, the age of the perpetrator, and the intent. Value judgments and community standards frequently enter into the definition. According to the National Legal Resource Center for Child Advocacy and Protection, the term *sexual abuse* could be used to define a sexual act committed by an adult that the child knows. The center suggests that *sexual exploitation* be used when a commercial component is involved, such as children prostituting themselves or being sold as models for pornography or prostitution.[7] Everstein and Everstein propose one definition of sexual molesta-

tion as an "adult's caressing, fondling, kissing, or masturbating a child without making bodily penetration."[4]

The incidence of sexual abuse or molestation is difficult to determine because of the nature of the act and the age of the victims. It has been estimated 2.5% to 8.7% of the male population has committed sexual molestation and that 9% to 10% of the male population has been sexually molested.[4] Girls are thought to be molested more frequently than boys, at a ratio of 2:1. Therefore, the incidence in the female population could be estimated to be twice that of males or approximately 18% to 20%. Girls are molested more frequently by family members, whereas boys usually are molested or abused by nonfamily members. In almost every instance the boy is molested by a man.[4]

A second difficulty in evaluating the true incidence of sexual abuse of children is the type of research and methodology used in this area. Comparison of groups and generalization to the population are difficult because of the variation in samples of victims, operational definitions, and methods used to gather data, such as surveys and interviews.[7]

Clinical Manifestations. If the molestation has been done clandestinely (as opposed to prostitution), the child may exhibit somatic complaints, such as gastrointestinal disturbances, general or specific aches and pains, sudden changes in toilet habits, or enuresis. Phobias may develop, such as a school phobia or a refusal to play outside the home. Nightmares and withdrawal from normal activities may occur. Some of these symptoms may mask depression or internalization of the anxiety related to the abuse. Behaviors such as running away from home, substance abuse, or other self-destructive acts; inappropriate sexual behavior; or inappropriate anger and hostility actually may be an "acting out" of emotions related to the abuse.[4]

Diagnostic Studies. Studies to rule out organic causes of molestation complaints may be indicated. An upper or lower gastrointestinal radiography study may be indicated for symptoms of gastrointestinal disturbance. Play therapy or psychological testing may be used to solicit additional data for school or emotional problems.

⭐ **ASSESSMENT**

Frequently the child is brought into the clinic or emergency room with a somatic complaint as described previously. The nurse should be aware that unless he or she has already had a trusting relationship with the child or adolescent, the child will seldom disclose the incidence of sexual abuse at an initial interview. Therefore, during the course of the interview the nurse should be aware of any body language or inappropriate verbal response that could lead to further questions and the suspicion of sexual abuse. Examples of body language that would lead to further questioning may be little or no eye contact or nervous acts. Inappropriate responses might be anger or hostile behavior displayed by the child toward those trying to help; evasiveness or vagueness in answering questions about adults with whom the child lives or sees frequently; fear of the perpetrator being nearby; or asking the nurse not to tell a specific individual that the incident was disclosed, for fear of reprisal.

★ NURSING DIAGNOSES AND PLANNING

Based on assessment data discussed previously and in the preceding chapter, the following nursing diagnoses may apply to the family and child experiencing sexual molestation and abuse:

- Anxiety related to situational crises.
- Fear related to further abuse.
- Powerlessness related to interpersonal interactions.
- Ineffective Individual Coping related to personal vulnerability.
- Self-Esteem Disturbance related to unjustified feelings of guilt.
- Altered Family Processes related to situational crises.
- Altered Parenting related to unrealistic expectations of the child.
- Altered Sexuality Patterns related to impaired relationships.
- Hopelessness related to long-term stress.

The nurse and child (or parents) together plan effective care based on the established nursing diagnoses. Several examples of expected outcomes follow:

- The child verbally expresses anxiety and fear.
- The child expresses desire to change the situation.
- The adolescent discusses concerns about sexual relationships.

The nurse plans for the daily care of the child based on physician's orders and nursing diagnoses. Some general nursing care goals may be the following:

- Professional psychological support is obtained.

- A safe and supportive environment is found for the child.
- Abuse is reported to hospital's abuse team.

★ NURSING INTERVENTIONS: COLLABORATIVE AND INDEPENDENT

An important nursing intervention for this group of children or adolescents is to identify information gathered during the assessment (see Chap. 67) and help them obtain the professional psychological support that they need to get well. Helping them become established in a safe and supportive environment also may be included in the nurse's role.

★ EVALUATION

Periodically the nurse and family evaluate the outcomes of care given. Examples of outcomes for the child and family with sexual molestation and abuse were given under Nursing Diagnoses and Planning in this section.

LONG-TERM CARE

For long-term management of children or adolescents who have been sexually molested or abused, see the nine variables in the accompanying display.

Rape

Definition and Incidence. *Rape* is defined by law, and like sexual abuse, its meaning can be all-encompassing or very specific. However, generally rape is considered penetration of a child's anus or vagina by an adult's finger, penis, or other object. In some states forced oral copulation also is considered rape.[4,7] *Date rape* is a phenomenon that was defined in the 1980s as

---

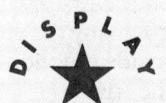

Variables in Long-Term Management of Sexually Abused Children

- *Age of the victim.* The youngest are considered the most vulnerable. Older children seem to be hurt most by the social stigma associated with sexual abuse.
- *Psychological condition of the child.* If there are prior emotional problems to which sexual abuse is added, the child usually will have more difficulty in resolving the psychological trauma.
- *Sexual knowledge or experience.* Children with no prior sexual experience seem to be most vulnerable.
- *Type of assault.* It has been shown that the greatest extent of psychological trauma is correlated with a higher degree of violence or bodily penetration. There is also the extent to which the child considers his or her body disfigured or injured.

- *Repeated assaults* are considered more traumatic than a single episode.
- *Molestation by a stranger* is considered less damaging than victimization by a known or trusted person.
- *Reactions of others*, especially negative reactions by the victim's family or peers, contribute to a poor outcome.
- *Not being believed or supported* contributes to a poor outcome.
- *Those who receive therapy* are more likely to recover.

Everstine, D. S., & Everstine, L. (1989). Sexual trauma in children and adolescents. (p. 68). New York: Brunner/Mazel.

forced sexual intercourse during a date with someone the victim is acquainted with. This phenomenon also has been termed acquaintance rape. Date rape appears to be more commonly reported on college campuses and may be related to an increased use of alcohol and drugs. Changes in social morals, attitudes, and acceptable dating behaviors, as well as peer education, have helped young women to identify that they are not "at fault" and that they can report the rape and receive compassionate help.[14]

As in sexual abuse the incidence of rape is usually underreported. In greater than 30% of all cases of reported rape, the victim is an adolescent.[1] Date rape has been occurring for many years, but it has only recently been identified and its reporting encouraged; therefore, date rape may be significantly underreported.

Clinical Manifestations. There are two types of rape: (1) the child or adolescent reports the rape and seeks evaluation and treatment and (2) the victim does not seek help. The latter is called *silent rape*. With silent rape the victim comes in or is brought in to the clinic or emergency room with other complaints that are similar to those discussed in the section on sexual molestation and abuse. Frequently, date rape is not reported and is a form of silent rape.[4]

Diagnostic Studies. In a reported rape the evidence is very important and must be collected to exacting specifications. Only nursing and medical personnel who have been trained in evidence collection should participate in this part of the examination. Usually evidence is collected from clothing, hair, and nail scrapings. Photographs are taken. Cultures for gonorrhea and blood for syphilis testing are taken. Pap smears and wet mounts should be performed to validate the presence of sperm.[16]

★ **ASSESSMENT**

The child is brought in or walks in to the clinic or emergency room with vague somatic complaints, such as aches and pains, sudden changes in toilet habits, or gastrointestinal disturbances. Associated complaints might be behavioral changes, such as a withdrawal from normal activities, nightmares, or school phobias. The nurse should be aware of the possibility that the child might be a victim of sexual abuse or rape. A private and trusting environment should be provided in which questions can be asked that would elicit vital information. Such questions might concern what is frightening the child or where the pain is and what precipitated its onset.

The very young child will most likely respond to rape trauma by being fearful, but his or her greatest concern is the pain they are experiencing. Once the pain has subsided the child needs to be assessed for a fear of strangers or fear of a known person if the perpetrator was an acquaintance. The older child and adolescent will typically respond in a sequence of steps similar to the grieving process.

Everstine and Everstine have described a response to rape that is typical of the older child and adolescent. They call this the *rape trauma response*. After the attack begins there is a disbelief that it is happening to them. The instinctive decision to fight back follows. After the

child is released or escapes, the post-trauma recovery cycle begins. This cycle is described as a series of emotional responses. These are shock, denial, depression, mood swings, anger, philosophic reflection, and laying to rest.[4] Using Everstine and Everstine's stages, the nurse observes the child's or adolescent's behavior and verbal responses to determine the appropriate intervention.

★ **NURSING DIAGNOSES AND PLANNING**

Based on assessment data from above and the preceding chapter, the following nursing diagnoses may apply to the family and child who has been raped:

• Pain related to abusive physical trauma.
• Rape-Trauma Syndrome related to chronic abuse.
• Self-Esteem Disturbance related to chronic abuse.
• Fear related to threats made by abusive person.
• Altered Family Processes related to stresses imposed by chronic abuse.

The nurse and child (or parents) together plan effective care based upon the established nursing diagnoses.

★ **INTERVENTIONS: COLLABORATIVE AND INDEPENDENT**

Collaborative interventions initially center on the presence of traumatic injury, injury repair, and the collection of evidence for prosecution. Once that is accomplished the treatment focuses on the prevention of STDs and pregnancy. If there is a lapse of time between the rape trauma and the child seeking assistance, treatment of an existing sexually transmitted disease or pregnancy may need to take place. In either case psychological reactions need to be addressed and therapy provided if necessary.

★ **EVALUATION**

As in the case of sexual abuse, individual and family therapy are vital in achieving a positive outcome. Nurses who work in rape crisis centers frequently accompany the victim through the perpetrator's trial and provide emotional support for the victim during and after the trial.

Tumors of the Reproductive System

Tumors of the reproductive system can be benign or malignant. In the female pediatric population the benign variety of tumor, polycystic ovaries or polycystic breasts (fibroadenoma), is more common than malignant tumors of either organ. However, in the adolescent and young adult male population, the incidence of testicular malignancy is at its highest incidence.

Testicular Tumors

Definition and Incidence. Teratoma-type tumors are found most often in prepubertal boys. In infants younger than 2 months of age, 10% of these tumors are malignant. The rate of malignancy increases to 50% to

70% of all teratomas diagnosed in prepubertal boys.[15] The incidence for prepubertal boys peaks before the age of 2. Other germ cell tumors are diagnosed most often in postpubertal and young adult men. The incidence peaks after the age of 14.[1,15,19]

Testicular tumors are a significant cause of death in male adolescence through early adulthood. Testicular tumors are estimated to cause 14% of all cancer deaths in this age group. The incidence is 2.3 in 100,000 males, which makes the testicular tumor the most common solid tumor in males 15 to 34 years of age. Other less common solid tumors are embryonal cell carcinomas, choriocarcinomas, Sertoli's cell tumors, and Leydig's cell tumors.[1,15] For unknown reasons testicular cancer is seen more commonly in white males in higher social classes than in other groups of males.[19] The risk of testicular malignancy is 48 to 50 times greater in male adolescents with a history of cryptorchidism.[1,15]

Etiology and Pathophysiology and Clinical Manifestations. The origins of most malignant, testicular tumors can be traced to the germ cell.[1,17] Germ cell tumors typically occur in the gonads but occasionally are found in extragonadal sites due to an error in the migration of germ cells during fetal development. The most common solid tumor seen in newborns is the sacrococcygeal teratoma (1 in 40,000 live births).[1] This teratoma usually is felt in the area of the sacrum and buttocks. If it is not detected at birth, its growth will eventually obstruct the urinary tract or rectum.[1]

The most common testicular tumor found in prepubertal boys, especially those younger than 2 years of age, is the teratoma. Its presence at birth can go undetected because of the presence of a hydrocele. Occasionally the tumor is mistaken for a hydrocele. The tumor is usually felt while palpating the testicle in the scrotum.[1]

Sexual precocity is rare in boys 4 to 6 years of age. Gynecomastia is a typical example of its manifestation. Leydig's cell tumors of the testes are the most common cause.[1]

In postpubertal men other types of testicular tumors, the seminoma or the choriocarcinoma, occur. The seminoma occurs mostly in very late adolescence or early adulthood. In approximately half of these boys there are no symptoms other than a small, firm, painless mass or nodule felt on testicular examination. The other half experience a gradual swelling of the testicle with pain and tenderness over the span of several weeks. Occasionally the first clinical manifestations are due to complications of malignant cell metastasis to the retroperitoneal lymph nodes or the lungs.[1]

Diagnostic Studies The best tool the health care provider has for diagnosing the presence of a testicular tumor is careful examination of the scrotum and observation of any unusual clinical signs such as gynecomastia. After discovery the tumor can be visualized by ultrasound or computed tomography (CT) scan. Excision and biopsy of the tumor are important to establish its histologic origins. Retroperitoneal lymph node metastasis can be detected by CT scan of the abdomen. Other metastasis can be detected by bone scan and CT scan or roentgenogram of the chest.[1]

★ **ASSESSMENT**

The nurse can be a key player in early detection of testicular tumors because of his or her ability to assess the knowledge base of the at-risk male population. According to one large study in which the average age was about 15 years, 28% had heard of the cancer, none knew how to perform a self-examination, and less than 2% were taught how to perform the self-examination even though they had recently received a physical examination.[19] If the nurse is performing the examination, he or she can demonstrate to the adolescent the correct method with an emphasis on performing this routinely for early detection.

★ **NURSING DIAGNOSES AND PLANNING**

Based on assessment data discussed previously and in the preceding chapter, the following nursing diagnoses may apply to the family and child with testicular cancer:

- Anxiety related to threat to health status.
- Body Image Disturbance related to biophysical changes.
- Sexual Dysfunction related to altered body structure.
- Anxiety related to knowledge deficit regarding self-examination.

The nurse and child (or parents) together plan effective care based on the established nursing diagnoses. Several examples of expected outcomes follow:

- The adolescent client performs self-examination as a return demonstration.
- The male client discusses his concerns related to future sexual activity.

The nurse plans for the daily care of the child based on physician's orders and nursing diagnoses. Some general nursing care goals may be the following:

- The tumor is surgically removed.
- Chemotherapy or radiation therapy is begun.

★ **NURSING INTERVENTIONS:**
   COLLABORATIVE AND INDEPENDENT

Surgical removal of the tumor and chemotherapy or radiation therapy are necessary treatments for testicular tumors. Radiation is most effective with seminoma tumors. If a tumor has been detected and excised, teaching is focused on postsurgical recovery and long-term follow-up for detection of metastasis of the cancer to the chest, abdomen, or bone. Additional teaching and emotional support are directed toward helping the adolescent develop a healthy self-concept concerning his sexuality and altered body image. This is especially important if a testicle has been removed.

The primary independent nursing intervention is teaching related to early detection. The nurse can use the examination time for teaching. The accompanying display on testicular self-examination prepares the male for self-examination.

The American Cancer Society recommends that the following points be emphasized when teaching a male to do testicular self-examination.

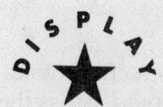

Patient Teaching: Testicular Self-Examination

Your best hope for early detection of testicular cancer is a simple 3-minute monthly self-examination. The best time is after a warm bath or shower, when the scrotal skin is most relaxed.

Roll each testicle gently between the thumb and fingers of both hands. If you find any hard lumps or nodules, you should see your doctor promptly. They may not be malignant, but only your doctor can make the diagnosis.

Following a thorough physical examination, your doctor may perform certain x-ray studies to make the most accurate diagnosis possible.

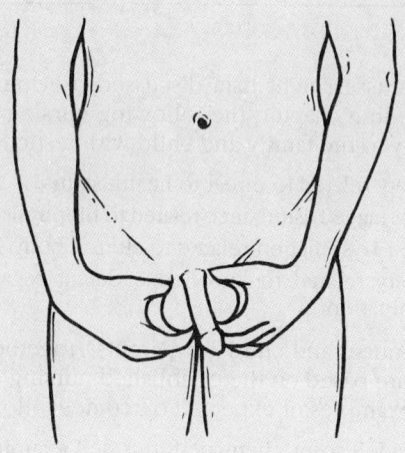

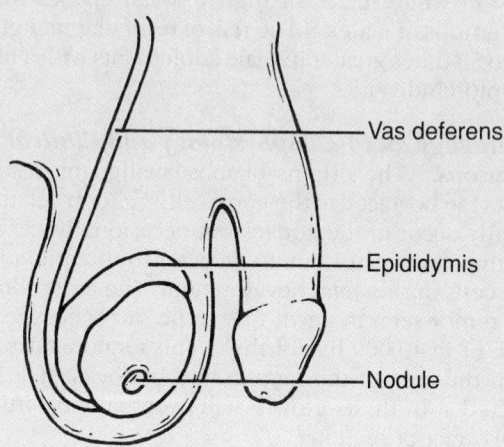

Vas deferens

Epididymis

Nodule

- Examine testes during or after a hot bath or shower.
- Examine testes with the index and middle fingers on the underside of the testicle and the thumb on top of the testicle.
- Gently roll the testicle between the thumb and fingers.
- Do not mistake the epididymis for an abnormality.
- If an abnormality, such as a lump, is found, report it immediately.
- Examine each testicle once a month.[15]

★ EVALUATION

Periodically the nurse and family evaluate the outcomes of care given. Examples of outcomes for the child and family with a testicular tumor were given under Nursing Diagnoses and Planning in this section.

LONG-TERM CARE

Long-term management using radiation therapy and chemotherapy has greatly improved the long-term survival of boys with testicular tumors. During clinic visits the nurse should constantly assess the learning needs and emotional support requirements of the adolescent and his parents.

Breast Tumors

Definition and Incidence. Malignant breast tumors in children and adolescents are extremely rare.[1,8,10] Fi-

broadenoma is the most common type of benign breast tumor, occurring in 76% to 90% of all benign breast lesions in female adolescents.[15] The malignant tumors found in children and adolescents are very slow growing, and most are localized in the breast. Occasionally they metastasize to the axilla.[1,8,10]

Clinical Manifestations and Diagnostic Studies. The examiner might find unilateral or bilateral breast enlargement. The malignant nodule usually is circumscribed, firm, and painless, although some tenderness has been reported. Because malignant tumors are so rare in children and adolescents, the mass usually is observed through at least one complete menstrual cycle. An increase in size and tenderness close to menstruation is more consistent with fibroadenomas.[1,8,10] Fibroadenomas frequently are described as unilateral, "rubbery," and mobile. Occasionally they are bilateral and multiple. They usually grow slowly.[1,8,10]

Mammography is an important noninvasive tool used in early detection of tumors. Ultrasound also can be used to visualize tumors. If malignancy is suspected, the most important procedure for confirmation is biopsy, usually performed by needle aspiration under local anesthesia.

★ ASSESSMENT

As with testicular tumors the nurse can be a key person in the early detection of breast tumors. During preparation for physical examinations or at family planning visits, the nurse can assess the adolescent's family history of breast cancer and knowledge of breast self-examination. It has been reported that girls with a family history tend to develop breast cancer 10 to 12 years earlier than those who have no family history.[10]

★ NURSING DIAGNOSES AND PLANNING

Based on assessment data discussed previously and in the preceding chapter, the following nursing diagnoses may apply to the family and child with a breast tumor:

- Anxiety related to surgical procedure.
- Body Image Disturbance related to mastectomy.
- Sexual Dysfunction related to altered body structure.
- Anxiety related to knowledge deficit regarding self-examination.

The nurse and adolescent (or parents) together plan effective care based on the established nursing diagnoses. Several examples of expected outcomes follow:

- The adolescent performs self-examination as a return demonstration.
- The adolescent discusses her concerns related to future sexual activity.
- The adolescent contacts a support group.

The nurse plans for the daily care of the child based on physician's orders and nursing diagnoses. Some general nursing care goals may be the following:

- The tumor is surgically removed successfully.
- The adolescent discusses the long term implications of fibroadenoma and the role of self-examination.

★ NURSING INTERVENTIONS: COLLABORATIVE AND INDEPENDENT

Nurses can assist adolescent girls in the early detection of breast tumors by teaching them how to do breast self-examination and constantly reinforcing the need to perform the procedure. The accompanying display on breast self-examination describes the proper steps of a breast self-examination. If a tumor is found, surgical intervention usually is required, especially if the tumor is malignant or if the benign fibroadenoma is large and growing.[1,8]

Preoperatively, nursing interventions to prepare the adolescent include increasing her knowledge, which in turn assists in decreasing anxiety. If the breast appearance has been altered during the surgical removal of the tumor, postoperative nursing support is directed toward assisting the adolescent to accept her altered body image. Information on available options concerning prostheses and reconstructive surgery should be made available as soon as the adolescent is ready. Referrals to support individuals or groups available through the American Cancer Society branches also should be made.

★ EVALUATION

Periodically the nurse and family evaluate the outcomes of care given. Examples of outcomes for the adolescent and family with a breast tumor were given under Nursing Diagnoses and Planning in this section.

LONG-TERM CARE

Malignant changes have been reported in mammary fibroadenomas; therefore, careful, ongoing evaluation is necessary for girls with such a history. Because tumors in adolescent girls are mostly localized, additional chemotherapy or radiation therapy is rarely required. However, breast self-examinations and yearly mammograms are indicated to detect a recurrence.[1,8,15]

Ovarian Tumors

Definition, Incidence, and Etiology. Ovarian tumors are masses found on the ovary during pelvic examination. They are not common in children and adolescents but have two peaks of incidence similar to testicular tumors. The first peak is before age 2, and the second greatest incidence occurs after age 6. Eighty-four percent of germ cell tumors seen in girls younger than 10 years of age are malignant.[1]

There are two major types of ovarian tumors seen in children and adolescent girls; both arise from germ cells. Cystic teratoma tumors develop from ovarian mesenchymal tissue and are mostly benign; however, malignancy must always be ruled out. They produce estrogen and progesterone and cause bone maturation and development of secondary sexual characteristics. Usually they are too small to be palpated. An extremely malignant, solid tumor is the teratomatous choriocarcinoma, which is easily palpated, grows extremely fast, and metastasizes quickly to the lungs, lymph nodes, and bone.[1,17]

Clinical Manifestations and Diagnostic Studies. The tumor might be discovered during an examination to establish the cause of precocious pubertal development. Complaints of nausea, vomiting, and pain also may be early clinical signs. The adolescent may have menstrual irregularities and other symptoms that simulate pregnancy. An abdominal mass may be palpated during a routine examination during which no specific complaints were made. Occasionally ovarian torsion causes appendicitis-like symptoms.[1]

Ultrasound, laparotomy, and biopsy are used to confirm the diagnosis. Metastasis can be detected by ultrasound and CT scan.

★ ASSESSMENT

Listening to concerns or complaints of the child or adolescent is necessary to help identify ovarian tumors. Because ovarian tumors can be missed in this age group, it is important to be aware that they can cause precocious sexual development or produce symptoms similar to appendicitis.

★ NURSING DIAGNOSES AND PLANNING

Based on assessment data discussed previously and in the preceding chapter, the following nursing diagnoses may apply to the family and child with an ovarian tumor:

- Fear related to surgical procedure.
- Anxiety related to chemotherapy.

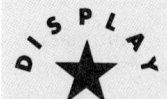

Patient Teaching: Breast Self-Examination

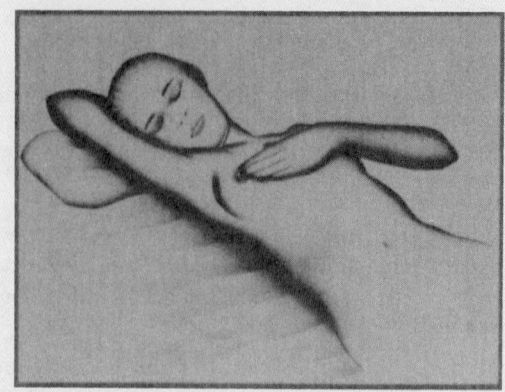

Why Do the Breast Self-Examination?

There are many good reasons for doing the breast self-examination (BSE) each month. One reason is that breast cancer is most easily treated and cured when it is found early. Another is that if you do BSE every month, it will increase your skill and confidence when doing the examination. When you get to know how your breasts normally feel, you will quickly be able to feel any change. Another reason is that it is easy to do.

When to Do BSE

The best time to do BSE is about 1 week after your period, when breasts are not tender or swollen. If you do not have regular periods or sometimes skip a month, do BSE on the same day every month.

How to Do BSE

1. Lie down, and put a pillow under your right shoulder. Place your right arm behind your head.
2. Use the finger pads of your three middle fingers on your left hand to feel for lumps or thickening. Your finger pads are the top third of each finger.
3. Press firmly enough to know how your breast feels. If you're not sure how hard to press, ask your health care provider, or try to copy the way your health care provider uses the finger pads during a breast examination. Learn what your breast feels like most of the time. A firm ridge in the lower curve of each breast is normal.
4. Move around the breast in a set way. You can choose either the circle (**A**), the up and down line (**B**), or the wedge (**C**). Do it the same way every time. It will help you to make sure that you've gone over the entire breast area and to remember how your breast feels each month.
5. Now examine your left breast using right hand finger pads.
6. If you find any changes, see your doctor right away.

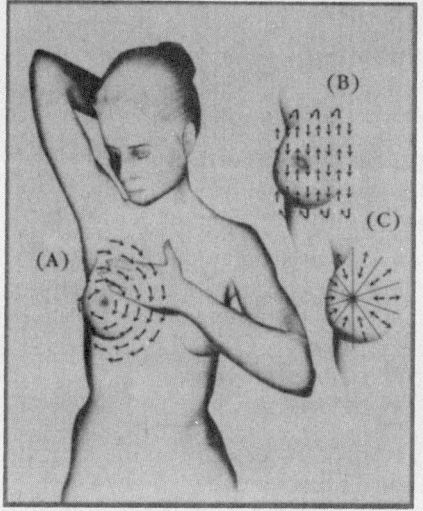

For Added Safety

You might want to check your breasts while standing in front of a mirror right after you do your BSE each month. See if there are any changes in the way your breasts look: dimpling of the skin, changes in the nipple, or redness or swelling. You might also want to do an extra BSE while you're in the shower. Your soapy hands will glide over the wet skin, making it easy to check how your breasts feel.

Remember: BSE could save your breast—and save your life. Most breast lumps are found by women themselves, but, in fact, most lumps in the breast are not cancer. Be safe, be sure.

Reprinted by permission of the American Cancer Society, Inc.

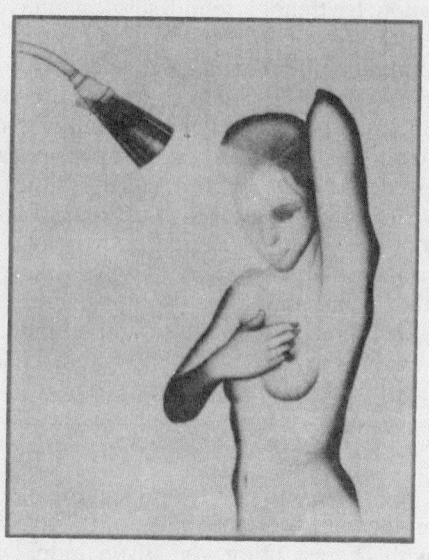

- Body Image Disturbance related to surgical procedure.
- Hopelessness related to deteriorating physical condition.

The nurse and adolescent (or parents) together plan effective care based on the established nursing diagnoses. Several examples of expected outcomes follow:

- The adolescent verbalizes concerns about surgery and chemotherapy.
- The adolescent states actions that will be taken to address side-effects of chemotherapy.
- The adolescent discusses her concerns related to future sexual activity.

The nurse plans for the daily care of the child based on physician's orders and nursing diagnoses. Some general nursing care goals may be the following:

- The tumor is surgically removed successfully.
- Side-effects of chemotherapy are managed.

★ NURSING INTERVENTIONS: COLLABORATIVE AND INDEPENDENT

Treatment for ovarian tumors is similar to that described for testicular tumors of germ cell origin. Surgical removal and histologic examination of the tumor are done. A combination of chemotherapy and radiation therapy follows.

Emotional support and teaching by nurses focuses on preoperative preparation to decrease fear and anxiety and to increase the adolescent girl's knowledge base related to surgery and postoperative care. Postoperatively, nursing care involves administering chemotherapy and teaching related to its side-effects. Chemotherapy usually is begun in an outpatient setting soon after discharge. Psychosocial support may deal with any feelings of hopelessness or anxiety regarding the future, especially if metastasis has occurred. If the tumor is benign, the adolescent girl may require assistance in incorporating a different body image into her self-identity.

★ EVALUATION

Periodically the nurse and family evaluate the outcomes of care given. Examples of outcomes for the child and family with an ovarian tumor were given under Nursing Diagnoses and Planning in this section.

LONG-TERM CARE

Long-term management is done on an outpatient basis with periodic visits to detect a recurrence or metastasis. At all visits the nurse should repeatedly assess the girl and her family for needed psychosocial support and additional knowledge.

Polycystic Ovarian Disease

Definition, Incidence, and Etiology. Polycystic ovarian disease is a disorder of the hypothalamic-pituitary-ovarian system. The exact starting point or triggering mechanism is not known. In general the dysfunction is related to inappropriate secretion of gonadotropins,

which causes LH levels to remain high instead of fluctuating. FSH levels remain at low or low normal levels. The abnormal circulating hormones create a lack of maturing follicles, anovulation, less than normal secretion of estrogen and progesterone, and an abnormally high level of androgens. The high androgen level is converted to additional estrogens, which further increase LH levels. A vicious cycle is created.[15]

Clinical Manifestations and Diagnostic Studies. Adolescents with polycystic ovarian disease can be divided into three groups based on symptoms. The smallest group consists of girls with greatly enlarged ovaries, secondary amenorrhea or oligomenorrhea, hirsutism, and obesity (Stein-Leventhal syndrome). The second largest group are girls with normal or slightly enlarged polycystic ovaries and signs of hyperandrogenism such as hirsutism. The third group have polycystic ovaries without signs of hyperandrogenism. The latter two groups are considered atypical and other causes, such as adrenal hyperplasia or enzyme deficiencies, should be investigated and ruled out.[15]

The diagnosis can be made based on clinical findings and hormone assays of serum LH, FSH, and testosterone. Normal levels of FSH are seen, and the LH level is two to three times higher. Testosterone is frequently high normal or in the normal male range. Laparoscopy with biopsy of the ovarian tissue should be performed if malignancy is suspected.[8,15]

★ ASSESSMENT

The adolescent may seek advice because she never started menstruating or has had a few cycles and is now menstruating infrequently or not at all. She may have excessive facial hair and may be obese. A complete initial assessment involves gathering data that facilitate eliminating familial or exogenous causes of the menstrual problem. Examples are familial hirsutism, pregnancy, or taking hormones.[1,8,15]

★ NURSING DIAGNOSES AND PLANNING

Based on assessment data discussed previously and in the preceding chapter, the following nursing diagnoses may apply to the family and child with polycystic ovarian disease:

- Body Image Disturbance related to biophysical changes.
- Anxiety related to knowledge deficit regarding causes and management of symptoms.

The nurse and child (or parents) together plan effective care based on the established nursing diagnoses. Several examples of expected outcomes follow:

- The adolescent verbalizes concerns about bodily changes.
- The adolescent states actions that treatment will correct.

The nurse plans for the daily care of the adolescent based on physician's orders and nursing diagnoses. Some general nursing care goals may be the following:

- Successful hormonal treatment is begun.
- The adolescent identifies the lifelong nature of the treatment protocol.

★ NURSING INTERVENTIONS:
COLLABORATIVE AND INDEPENDENT

The hypothalamic-pituitary-ovarian cycle will not correct itself; therefore, provision of the missing hormones will aid its return to normal functioning and the disappearance of external symptoms. If the adolescent has developed hirsutism or other symptoms of excessive androgen production, oral contraceptives or corticosteroids are used. Amenorrhea associated with polycystic ovarian disease can be corrected with oral contraceptives as well. The long-term use of estrogen without progesterone can lead to endometrial cancer, so its use should be very limited.[15]

Nurses can increase the adolescent's knowledge regarding the origin of the problem and the treatment plan. Emotional support may be related to the adolescent's body image.

★ EVALUATION

Periodically the nurse and family evaluate the outcomes of care given. Examples of outcomes for the adolescent and family with polycystic ovarian disease were given under Nursing Diagnoses and Planning in this section.

LONG-TERM CARE

The treatment plan for polycystic ovarian disease using hormone therapy is lifelong. Follow-up is similar to that of girls on oral contraceptives. Regular visits for Pap smears and pelvic examinations are made to determine the progress of cyst growth.

Precocious and Delayed Puberty

The origins of precocious and delayed puberty are varied. The most serious consequences of either seem to be emotional, psychological, and social. Each is discussed in Chapter 56.

Precocious Puberty

Precocious puberty can be defined broadly as a child, more commonly female than male, who develops one or more sexual characteristics before the normal age of puberty. Associated with external signs is gonadal development with ovulation and spermatogenesis.[15,17] Because of the variable age of onset of puberty, there is no well-defined age at which a child is considered to be developing precociously. However, in general a girl may be considered to be precocious if she develops breasts or pubic hair before age 8. Boys are precocious if genital development occurs before age 9.[15,17] Precocious puberty is discussed in Chapter 56 as altered gonadal function.

Delayed Puberty

Delayed puberty can be defined generally as sexual maturity ratings that fail to progress beyond certain guidelines or a time lapse of 5 years between the initiation of genital growth and its completion.[15] Delayed sexual development is discussed in Chapter 56 as altered gonadal function.

Disorders Associated With the Menstrual Cycle

The physiology of the menstrual cycle was discussed in Chapter 66. This section describes disorders that are associated with the menstrual cycle: dysfunctional uterine bleeding, amenorrhea, dysmenorrhea, endometriosis, premenstrual syndrome (PMS), and toxic shock syndrome (TSS).

Dysfunctional Uterine Bleeding

Definition and Incidence. *Dysfunctional uterine bleeding* is another term for abnormal menstrual bleeding. Irregular menstrual bleeding is very common in adolescents, especially in the first year after menarche; however, in 90% of cases of adolescent abnormal bleeding, the cause is thought to be dysfunctional uterine bleeding, and an etiology must be sought.[8,15]

Etiology. Irregular or excessive bleeding can be a symptom of an immature hypothalamic-pituitary-ovarian axis, anovulatory menstrual cycles, or an organic disease such as thyroid problems.[8] For the most part the cause of the abnormal bleeding is unknown. Other possibilities are an ectopic pregnancy, threatened abortion, endometritis, intrauterine device (IUD), or oral contraceptives.[15]

Clinical Manifestations. In general normal menstruation does not occur more often than every 21 days from the beginning of one cycle to the beginning of the next. Flow should not last more than 6 to 7 days, and the heaviest flow should use no more than 6 well-soaked perineal pads or 10 tampons in 24 hours.[8] Anything outside of these parameters should be considered abnormal. In general it is difficult to judge what the adolescent's normal cycle is, especially if no cycles have occurred in any rhythm. To accurately define what is abnormal the clinician should evaluate the adolescent through several menstrual cycles.

Diagnostic Studies. A pelvic examination should be performed and should include a Pap smear and culture for gonorrhea. If indicated, testing for pregnancy and liver and thyroid function should be done to determine any possible demonstrable etiology. In addition, a complete blood and platelet count and clotting time should be performed to determine if the heavy flow may be associated with abnormal bleeding or if the bleeding has caused an anemia.[8,15]

★ ASSESSMENT

A complete nursing assessment for dysfunctional uterine bleeding includes a comprehensive evaluation of the adolescent's menstrual cycle. The adolescent may be asked to keep records during her next menstruation to more accurately define the amount of flow by her use of pads or tampons. The accompanying display on dysfunctional uterine bleeding contains information that should be assessed. Complete information pertaining to the interviewing process of an adolescent can be found in Chapter 67.

★ NURSING DIAGNOSES AND PLANNING

Based on assessment data discussed previously and in the preceding chapter, the following nursing diagnoses may apply to the family and adolescent with dysfunctional uterine bleeding:

- Altered Health Maintenance related to ineffective individual coping.
- Altered Nutrition: Less Than Body Requirements related to iron deficiency.
- Anxiety related to changes in health status.

The nurse and adolescent (or parents) together plan effective care based on the established nursing diagnoses. Several examples of expected outcomes follow:

- The young person describes the need for iron and vitamin C in the diet.
- The person responsible for planning meals and cooking in the family plans iron-rich meals.
- The child states facts regarding puberty and the menstrual cycle.

The nurse plans for the daily care of the adolescent based on physician's orders and nursing diagnoses. Some general nursing care goals may be the following:

- A cause of dysfunctional bleeding is established.
- The cause is successfully treated.

★ NURSING INTERVENTIONS: COLLABORATIVE AND INDEPENDENT

Initially, interventions involve the control of excessive bleeding and correcting any systemic problem that is causing or contributing to dysfunctional uterine bleeding. Contraceptives or other hormonal therapy are used to correct problems in the hypothalamic-pituitary-ovarian axis and anovulatory menstrual cycles.[15] If the cause is from an IUD, the device is removed and another form of contraception selected. Occasionally, when the cause is the use of one of the oral contraceptives, the adolescent is switched to another brand based on the estrogen–progesterone content necessary to correct the dysfunctional bleeding.

Nutrition-related teaching should take place if the adolescent's hemoglobin or hematocrit levels are less than normal. An acceptable hemoglobin level is greater than 11, and the hematocrit should be greater than 34% to 35%.[1] The adolescent should be taught which foods are rich in iron. If iron therapy is prescribed as well, the adolescent should be informed about possible side-effects, such as constipation, and encouraged to take the iron with a source of vitamin C, which improves the iron's absorption.

Frequently, the adolescent lacks a knowledge of her body and how her reproductive system functions. In addition, the parent, most often the adolescent's mother, may have her own questions regarding the normal reproductive system and the deviations occurring in her child.

★ EVALUATION

Periodically the nurse and family evaluate the outcomes of care given. Examples of outcomes for the adolescent

---

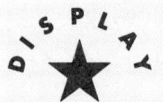

Nursing Assessment: Dysfunctional Uterine Bleeding

AGE OF MENARCHE

- If less than 1 year since menarche, irregular periods are common.
- If greater than 1 year since menarche, pregnancy, endocrine, or other organic problems may be the etiology.

SEXUAL ACTIVITY

- If positive response, pregnancy should be first concern.

CONTRACEPTIVE USE

- If using pills, problem may be related to them.
- If using an IUD, bleeding will be increased.

HISTORY OF PREGNANCY/RECENT ABORTION (SPONTANEOUS OR THERAPEUTIC)

- Retained remnants of placenta

SYSTEMIC DISEASE AND MEDICATION USE

- Endocrine disorder
- Hematologic abnormality
- Use of tranquilizers

TRAUMA

- Recent trauma to the genitals, including rape or sexual molestation

MENSTRUAL CYCLE INFORMATION

- Timing between one cycle and the next (in days)— 3 to 6 weeks between cycles is normal.
- Number of days period lasts—1 to 7 days is normal.
- Amount of flow—estimate number of pads and saturation in 24 hours and type used (e.g., regular, super).
- Pain associated with cycle—when it occurs, what is taken or done to relieve pain.

and family with dysfunctional uterine bleeding were given under Nursing Diagnoses and Planning in this section.

LONG-TERM CARE

Any long-term management depends on the etiology of the problem. Most of the demonstrable causes of dysfunctional uterine bleeding can be corrected with no long-term follow-up needed. If hormonal therapy is required, appropriate visits must be scheduled for a pelvic examination with Pap smears and any other associated tests. These are usually scheduled every 6 months to 1 year depending on how closely the adolescent must be followed. Girls in their early to midteens and those just beginning hormone use should be followed at least every 3 to 6 months. However, any teen whose ability to comply is in doubt should be seen more frequently. Each visit will ensure appropriateness of pill selection as evidenced by a normal menstrual cycle with pill use, determine compliance, and evaluate for blood pressure elevation or other side-effects.

The pelvic examination with Pap smear usually is done once a year. A history of certain STDs (herpes simplex, venereal warts) or a previously abnormal Pap smear will dictate more frequent Pap smears.

Amenorrhea

Definition. There are two types of amenorrhea, primary and secondary. *Primary amenorrhea* occurs when there is no spontaneous bleeding by age 16, and the development of breasts or pubic hair is absent. The term also is used for an 18-year-old who has not had a menstrual period despite the development of breasts and pubic hair. An adolescent with diagnosed Turner's syndrome and no menstrual periods would be defined as having primary amenorrhea. *Secondary amenorrhea* is the commencement of uterine bleeding and then an absence of menstrual flow for the equivalent of 3 consecutive cycles or 6 months.[8,15]

Incidence and Etiology. The incidence of amenorrhea is generally unknown and depends on the etiology. Most primary causes are relatively rare. Amenorrhea secondary to another problem is more common.[8,15]

Primary amenorrhea generally is due to one of three possibilities: (1) gonadal failure secondary to a genetic problem, such as Turner's syndrome or testicular feminization; (2) hypothalamic-pituitary-ovarian axis problem; or (3) a genital tract problem, such as a congenital absence of the uterus. Secondary amenorrhea may be due to stress, excessive weight loss, or excessive exercise. A pituitary tumor or ovarian failure may be alternate etiologies of secondary amenorrhea.[8,15]

Clinical Manifestations and Diagnostic Studies. The reported absence of menstruation and the presence or absence of secondary sexual characteristics are the common reasons an adolescent or her parent seeks help. Other signs are associated with the primary or secondary etiology. An example of associated clinical signs are the classic manifestations of Turner's syndrome, such as webbed neck and short stature.

Diagnostic studies are related to the suspected primary or secondary etiology (Fig. 68-3). Most are hormonal studies, such as measuring sex hormone levels in suspected hypothalamic-pituitary-ovarian axis problems. Genetic studies might be conducted to rule out Turner's syndrome.[8,15]

★ ASSESSMENT

The most important part of the assessment for amenorrhea is a thorough history. Because amenorrhea is a symptom of another problem, information must be systematically gathered, which aids the nurse to determine the direction of further questioning.

★ NURSING DIAGNOSES AND PLANNING

Based on assessment data discussed previously and in the preceding chapter, the following nursing diagnoses may apply to the family and adolescent with amenorrhea:

- Altered Health Maintenance related to ineffective individual coping.
- Anxiety related to self-concept.
- Knowledge Deficit regarding the cause of the problem and how to solve it.

The nurse and adolescent (or parents) together plan effective care based on the established nursing diagnoses. Several examples of expected outcomes follow:

- The young person verbalizes an understanding of the underlying problem.
- The young person states why the problem may recur if causative habits are not changed.

The nurse plans for the daily care of the adolescent based on physician's orders and nursing diagnoses. Some general nursing care goals may be the following:

- The cause of amenorrhea is established.
- The adolescent is successfully treated.

★ NURSING INTERVENTIONS: COLLABORATIVE AND INDEPENDENT

The interventions depend on the final diagnosis. Interventions for gonadal dysgenesis or a hypothalamic-pituitary-ovarian axis problem, tumor, or ovarian failure are described elsewhere in this chapter. If the cause is stress or excessive weight loss or excessive exercise, the source of these problems must be determined and eliminated. In many cases psychological intervention might be indicated. Education is helpful in preventing a recurrence of a preventable etiology.

★ EVALUATION

Periodically the nurse and family evaluate the outcomes of care given. Examples of outcomes for the child and family with amenorrhea were given under Nursing Diagnoses and Planning in this section.

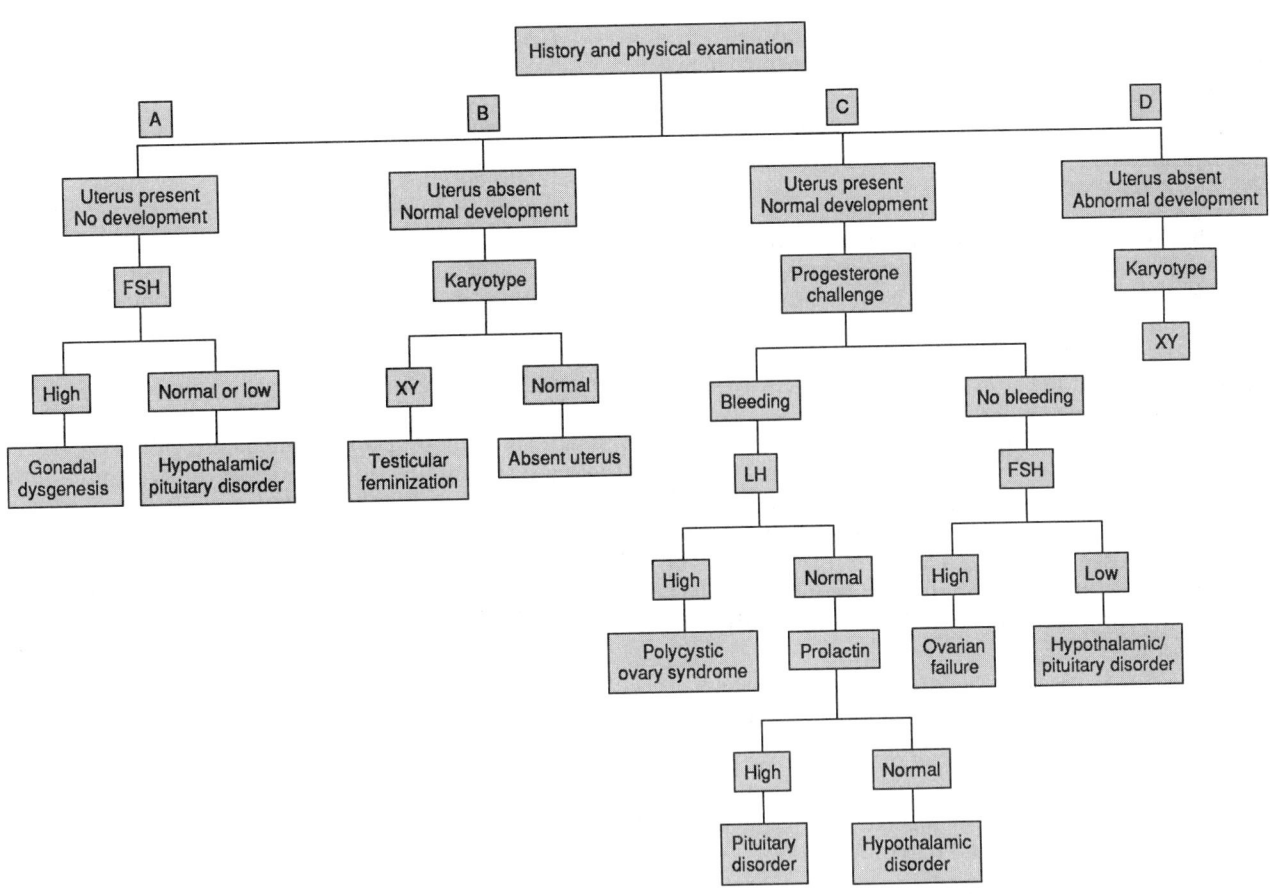

FIGURE 68-3

Flowchart for evaluation of primary amenorrhea. Evaluation is indicated if menses are absent by age 16 with normal development, by age 14 without development, or by 4 years after onset of puberty. Section A diagrams the most common situation. Section B diagrams a congenital anomaly. Section C presents an evaluation similar to that for secondary amenorrhea (after a negative pregnancy test). Section D shows an unusual circumstance in which the patient has either an enzyme defect or absent gonads that prevented normal male development. *Abbreviations:* FSH, follicle-stimulating hormone; LH, luteinizing hormone. (Source: Oski, F. A., DeAngelis, C. D., Feigin, R. D., & Warshaw, J. B. [1990]. *Principles and practice of pediatrics.* Philadelphia: J.B. Lippincott.)

Dysmenorrhea

Definition and Incidence.   Primary dysmenorrhea is described as the onset of pain just before or at the commencement of menstruation.[6,9] An associated problem is called *mittelschmerz* or the pain of ovulation.[10] The incidence of both is common, and they are referred to as "cramps." It is estimated that as many as 45% to 60% of all postpubescent girls experience dysmenorrhea.[15] Some girls describe the pain as sharp, low pelvic pain. Others may describe a dull, aching sensation in the lower back or pelvic region. *Secondary dysmenorrhea* can be differentiated from primary because it may occur during any phase of the menstrual cycle.

Etiology.   Primary dysmenorrhea usually is attributed to a high level of prostaglandins, which cause uterine spasms. Prostaglandins are fatty acids that are manufactured in endometrial tissue under the influence of progesterone. The associated gastrointestinal and vascular smooth muscle symptoms are caused by the prostaglandin's effect on smooth muscle.[10] The pain of mittel-

schmerz is a result of peritoneal irritation from the leakage of fluid around the ovary at ovulation.[10]

Secondary dysmenorrhea has several possible origins. Examples are pelvic inflammatory disease (PID), fibroids, endometriosis, endometrial cancer, problems associated with early pregnancy, or IUD-related problems.[6,9]

Clinical Manifestations and Diagnostic Studies.   Primary or normal menstrual cramping usually occurs after a pattern of ovulation is established. Typically cramping first occurs about 6 to 12 months after menarche. It may occur intermittently or consistently during a woman's entire reproductive years. Approximately half of those who have dysmenorrhea experience associated symptoms, such as fatigue, nausea and vomiting, dizziness, nervousness, diarrhea, backache, and headache.[15] In some adolescents dysmenorrhea is so severe that it can be incapacitating, and they may miss significant amounts of school.

Secondary dysmenorrhea can occur during any phase of the menstrual cycle. Usually secondary dysmenorrhea increases with time unless its primary problem is resolved.

Dysmenorrhea should not be considered "normal," and a cause should be sought.[6,9,10] Diagnostic studies, such as a pelvic examination and related tests, are used to rule out any of the possible demonstrable etiologies.

★ ASSESSMENT

As with all the alterations in reproductive health, the most important element in the assessment process is a thorough health, sexual, and reproductive history. This information will aid the health care team in diagnosing the problem by excluding many other possibilities. A physical examination, including pelvic examination, will assist the clinician in finding evidence of endometriosis, polyps, fibroids, or uterine or cervical anomalies.[15]

★ NURSING DIAGNOSES AND PLANNING

Based on assessment data discussed previously and in the preceding chapter, the following nursing diagnoses may apply to the adolescent and family with dysmenorrhea:

- Pain related to menstrual cycle.
- Anxiety related to knowledge deficit regarding the origin and appropriate interventions for dysmenorrhea.

The nurse and adolescent (or parents) together plan effective care based on the established nursing diagnoses. Several examples of expected outcomes follow:

- The young person states that she has found comfort measures to alleviate pain.
- The young person verbalizes an understanding of the use of medications for relief of pain.

The nurse plans for the daily care of the adolescent based on physician's orders and nursing diagnoses. A general nursing care goal may be the following:

- Pain is controlled by pharmacologic or nonpharmacologic measures.

★ NURSING INTERVENTIONS: COLLABORATIVE AND INDEPENDENT

Primary dysmenorrhea or mittelschmerz is treated by either aspirin or ibuprofen (prostaglandin inhibitors). For long-term treatment aspirin usually is tried first because ibuprofen is more expensive. Some adolescents report that sleeping with a heating pad helps.[6,9] Intervention for secondary dysmenorrhea depends on the cause. For example if the cause is PID, it is treated with antibiotics. If the cause is an IUD, it is usually removed.

Independent nursing interventions include helping the adolescent determine the best method to relieve the pain and monitoring the pain's effect on the adolescent's lifestyle, especially as it relates to school attendance and other routine activities.

★ EVALUATION

Periodically the nurse and family evaluate the outcomes of care given. Examples of outcomes for the child and family with dysmenorrhea were given under Nursing Diagnoses and Planning in this section.

Endometriosis

Endometriosis occurs when endometrial-type tissue is found exterior to the uterus. Usually it is seen in the pelvis, or outside of the pelvic cavity. In some studies in which adolescents were evaluated for cyclic or chronic pelvic pain, endometriosis was diagnosed in 47% to 65% of the cases.[10]

The cause of endometriosis is still not certain, but several theories have been proposed. A controversial and partly refuted theory is that endometriosis is caused by the endometrium's ability to proliferate if it "escapes" during menstruation due to reflux of menstrual flow through the fallopian tubes. Another theory is that transplanted endometrial cells stimulate metaplasia in tissues with a resulting functional endometrium forming in the pelvic cavity or elsewhere.[10]

The symptoms mimic many other menstrual-related problems, such as irregular menses, sudden onset of dysmenorrhea after years of being pain-free, increased vaginal discharge, and pain on intercourse or when defecating due to implants in the vagina, cervix, or bowel. The most common diagnostic tool is the use of a laparoscope with tissue examination. The laparoscope is used to visualize the extent of tissue implantation in various abdominal sites without extensive abdominal exploratory surgery.[10]

Nursing assessment includes a thorough history, including an evaluation of the adolescent's menstrual cycle. Because endometriosis mimics many other problems, the history and physical examination must be used to exclude other possible etiologies.

Adolescents usually are treated with oral contraceptives. In older women pregnancy seems to improve symptoms of endometriosis; therefore, the pseudopregnancy that is created with the use of oral contraceptives is recommended for adolescents for which pregnancy is never appropriate as a remedy. As a last resort surgery may be used to remove endometrial tissue from affected organs.[10]

The adolescent should be taught relaxation techniques and other pain relief skills. Education should be offered regarding the use of oral contraceptives to suppress endometriosis, the progress of endometriosis, and the effect it has on fertility. The need for long-term follow-up due to hormone therapy should be discussed with the adolescent.

Premenstrual Syndrome

PMS covers many different symptoms that occur during the luteal phase of the menstrual cycle. Due to the great diversity of possible symptoms, this is considered a fairly common syndrome. However, the intensity of the symptoms' effects on each female's ability to function varies. Its causes are unknown.[6]

The most common symptoms of PMS can be divided into two broad categories: behavioral and physiologic as shown in the accompanying display on most common PMS symptoms. An individual's symptoms can be a combination of any of these. Behavioral symptoms can become acute and debilitating.

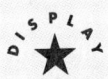

Most Common Premenstrual Syndrome Symptoms

BEHAVIORAL

Depression
Anxiety
Irritability
Tension
Inability to concentrate

PHYSIOLOGIC

Breast tenderness
Fluid retention (average 2 to 5 lb a month, some as much as 10 lb)
Fatigue
Headache
Food cravings (especially salt, sugar, and chocolate)

Data from Hatcher, R. A., Guest, F., Stewart, G. K., Trussell, J., Bowen, S., & Cates, W. (1988). Contraceptive technology, 1988–1989. (14th Ed.). New York: Printed Matter/Irvington Publishers.

Nursing assessment is similar to that in the previous sections. Perhaps the most important tool to help assess for PMS is the cyclic charting of symptoms by the adolescent.[6] The nurse can give the girl a calendar and ask her to write down any behavioral or physiologic symptoms she is feeling each day and what she does to relieve them. This gives the nurse a baseline of information on which to plan interventions.

Because the etiology of PMS is unknown, interventions are tried on an experimental basis. What works for some will not always work for others. Some successful measures are oral contraceptives or manipulating the diet by eliminating possible sources of sensitivity, such as caffeine and alcohol. Eliminating smoking and increasing exercise also have been successful for some adolescents.[6]

The nurse can support the adolescent by helping her to integrate the prescribed treatments into her lifestyle. Nurses can aid in decreasing the fear and anxiety related to PMS with emotional support and education regarding the syndrome. Pain-alleviation measures can be discussed and tried in relation to the headaches and breast tenderness. Diet measures to prevent or alleviate fluid retention, such as a reduction of salt at certain times, also might be appropriate.

Toxic Shock Syndrome

Definition and Incidence. TSS was first described in children in 1978. It is a generalized infection of the bloodstream (sepsis) caused by toxins from bacteria that migrate from the site of invasion into the circulation. It is a relatively rare combination of symptoms that may occur in close proximity to the menstrual period, usually during or immediately after. If the syndrome is not recognized and treated immediately, shock, coma, and death can quickly ensue. Although toxic shock is generally as-

sociated with women who are menstruating and using tampons, TSS is also found in males.

Mortality due to TSS in 1980 was 10%. By 1983 it had dropped to 2.6%. This drop is believed to be related to rapid recognition and treatment of TSS. Another possible contributing factor is the addition of inserts in tampon packages that describe the symptoms and warn the user of the risks. An additional factor was the removal of certain brands of tampons that were correlated with a great many of the cases. The risk is believed highest in the 15- to 24-year-old age group.[6]

Etiology. The cause of TSS is believed to be a form of toxin produced by the bacteria *Staphylococcus aureus*. Tampon use is implicated in 99% of the menstrual cases of TSS. Other episodes of TSS have been associated with the postpartum period, after an initial episode of the syndrome, and with the use of certain contraceptives, such as the diaphragm. TSS may develop from an *S. aureus* infection elsewhere in the body, which may explain its occurrence in men.[6]

Clinical Manifestations. The danger signals appear during or immediately after the girl has finished menstruating. These signs are high fever (101° F or higher), diarrhea, vomiting, muscle aches, and a sunburn-like rash. There may be other flu-type symptoms associated with the danger signs. The most significant combination is fever and rash or desquamation (peeling) of skin.[6]

Desquamation appears about 1 week to 10 days after the onset of the symptoms. Children with TSS are generally much sicker than adults and frequently require hospitalization.

Diagnostic Studies. There is no definitive diagnostic test for TSS. The diagnosis is based on the history along with nonspecific hematologic findings. Laboratory studies will reveal proteinuria; hematuria; elevated blood urea nitrogen; decreased albumin and total protein; and prolonged prothrombin time and partial thromboplastin time. Hypocalcemia and hyponatremia also may be found. One definitive diagnostic tool is a positive vaginal culture of the bacteria.

★ ASSESSMENT

The most important part of the assessment is to link all of the symptoms together. The symptoms that were previously described, such as a high fever with rash and desquamation of the skin, are hallmarks of the syndrome. The timing of the symptoms during or at the end of menstruation is the final link in the early identification of TSS.

★ NURSING DIAGNOSES AND PLANNING

Based on assessment data discussed previously and in the preceding chapter, the following nursing diagnoses may apply to the family and adolescent with TSS:

• Hyperthermia related to infectious process (fever).
• Fluid Volume Deficit related to hypotension (secondary to inflammatory process).

- High Risk for Infection related to invasion of body by microorganisms.
- Disabling Ineffective Family Coping related to life-threatening illness.
- Knowledge Deficit regarding menstrual hygiene and tampon use.

The nurse and adolescent (or parents) together plan effective care based on the established nursing diagnoses. Several examples of expected outcomes follow:

- The young person states that she is comfortable following fever reduction.
- The adolescent female describes proper use of tampons.
- The adolescent female describes proper hygiene during the menstrual period.
- The family verbalizes a feeling of confidence regarding the child's recovery from the illness.

The nurse plans for the daily care of the adolescent based on physician's orders and nursing diagnoses. Some general nursing care goals may be the following:

- Fever is reduced.
- Fluids and electrolytes are balanced.

★ NURSING INTERVENTIONS: COLLABORATIVE AND INDEPENDENT

Early intervention is most successful before septic shock occurs. Treatment is supportive and includes the administration of fluids, steroids, and medications to combat hypotension. Antibiotics specific for staphylococcus also are given, although they do not change the immediate course of the disease.

Nursing management of the child or adolescent with TSS is directed toward supportive care. Large amounts of intravenous fluids are given to combat the hypovolemia. These need to be carefully monitored to prevent fluid overload. The child is at risk of respiratory complications from fluid overload. Vital signs also must be monitored

for continuing signs of deterioration. Antipyretics given as ordered will assist in maintaining comfort.

The child with TSS may be critically ill. Skilled nursing care is essential; in addition the parents and child need a calm, reassuring atmosphere. Information should be given as indicated; however, anxiety and fear will interfere with parental understanding in many instances.

TEACHING

Teaching relating to appropriate use of tampons and prevention of TSS is an effective nursing action. The cause and those at highest risk have been identified; therefore, each time the nurse identifies an at-risk adolescent girl, she must be instructed how to minimize the risk factors and identify the early warning signs of TSS. Steps in reducing risk are given in the accompanying display on minimizing TSS risk.

The Federal Drug Administration (FDA) is developing standardized absorbency testing for tampons. The object is to label tampon boxes with instructions on how to interpret and select the lowest absorbency needed.[18] If the adolescent has had an episode of TSS, she should be instructed never to use tampons at least until the *S. aureus* is eliminated from the vagina. The adolescent who has never had TSS should be instructed to use a combination of pads and tampons during each menstrual period rather than tampons exclusively. Tampons during the day and pads at night might be an option. The adolescent also should be instructed not to change the tampons too frequently. Tampons should be changed when they are saturated and slip out easily. If they are removed too soon and are not saturated, the tampons might create microscopic abrasions that allow the bacteria to enter the bloodstream and cause the infection. The adolescent should be instructed to use a combination of tampon absorbencies or tampons and pads to guard against this problem. They should be taught to notify a physician immediately if any signs of TSS are noted during the menstrual period, including fever, rash, vomiting, or diarrhea.

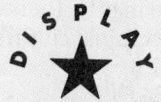

Patient Teaching: Minimizing Toxic Shock Syndrome (TSS) Risk

TAMPON USE

- If you have had TSS, do not use tampons again until *Staphylococcus aureus* is completely eliminated from the vagina.
- Use sanitary pads to eliminate risk.
- Wash hands before inserting anything into the vagina.
- Handle tampons carefully so they are not exposed to infectious surfaces.
- Change your tampon every 8 hours.
- Allow a tampon-free interval every day (e.g., tampons during the day and pad at night).

CONTRACEPTIVE PRODUCT USE

- Do not leave any contraceptive product (e.g., diaphragm, sponge) in place longer than recommended.
- Do not use contraceptives during a menstrual period.
- If there is a history of TSS, do not use a barrier method of contraception.

FOLLOWING PREGNANCY

- After any type of abortion or pregnancy, wait 6 to 12 weeks before using any barrier method. Use condoms or oral contraceptives instead.

Know the danger signs, and seek immediate care if you have fever, rash, vomiting, or diarrhea.

Periodically the nurse and family evaluate the outcomes of care given. Examples of outcomes for the child and family with TSS were given under Nursing Diagnoses and Planning in this section.

Problems for the Sexually Active Adolescent

In the last few decades the age at which sexual activity is begun has decreased, and sexual activity has increased. Increased sexual activity causes increased complications for which the adolescent usually is not prepared. Complications discussed in this chapter are STDs, genital infections, and adolescent pregnancy. Contraceptive methods are discussed here also. Although they are not a problem (and in fact are an answer to infections and pregnancy), the adolescent has to choose the method carefully.

Finally, the complications of a homosexual lifestyle are considered. Homosexuality is an alternative to heterosexual activity; it is not considered abnormal. However, homosexual activity does present some psychological and physical complications, some of them life-threatening.

The nurse needs to have knowledge of STDs, adolescent pregnancy and its alternatives, contraceptive methods, adolescent fatherhood, and homosexuality to meet educational and counseling needs of the adolescent.

Sexually Transmitted Diseases and Genital Infections

The 1970s and 1980s saw a runaway infection rate of known STDs and the emergence of new varieties, such as human immunodeficiency virus (HIV), herpes simplex virus (HSV), and human papillomavirus (HPV). Resistant strains of gonorrhea have appeared. The long-term physical and societal consequences of STDs are manifested in a high rate of infertility, ectopic pregnancy, and rapidly changing social values regarding sexual promiscuity and its consequences.[6]

Prevention is the key issue in any discussion of STDs and genital infections in general. Barrier methods, such as condoms with spermicide, are considered to be somewhat effective in protecting against bacterial infections and HIV. However, barrier methods do not protect the individual from other viruses such as HPV or HSV, which may pass from infected vaginal secretions or from scrotal lesions. Additional preventive methods for transmitting STDs are celibacy, monogamy or a significantly reduced number of sexual partners, avoidance of sexual partners who have had many sexual contacts, discussion of sexual history with a new partner, and examination of a new partner for lesions. Little else has been shown to be effective in prevention of STDs.[6]

The following discussion examines the more common STDs or related diseases. These are various types of vaginitis, gonorrhea, chlamydia, genital warts, genital herpes, cytomegalovirus, PID, syphilis, and pediculosis pubis. Acquired immunodeficiency syndrome (AIDS) is discussed in Chapter 27 as an immunodeficiency disorder. Table 68-1 also summarizes the major types of STDs.

Sexually Transmitted Diseases in Infants and Children

STDs are much more prevalent in adolescents and adults. However, there has been a sufficient increase in the incidence of some STDs in infants and children to warrant an examination into these two groups. For example, the reporting of gonorrhea in the 0- to 9-year-old age group increased by 90% between 1960 and 1979. The numbers are small (3100) and may be due to more case finding and better reporting.[20]

When investigating the etiology of STDs in infants or children, it is helpful to divide them into three age groups: infancy, childhood, and adolescence. The majority of infants are infected with STDs by *in utero* exposure or during the birth process. Examples of these diseases are congenital syphilis, perinatal gonococcal ophthalmia, chlamydia, hepatitis B, and group B streptococci. All cases of STDs in children beyond the immediate neonatal period should be presumed a result of sexual abuse until proven otherwise. Rarely these children are infected from fomites, such as bedding, or by infected peers during normal experimentation.[20]

Vaginitis

Vaginitis is an infection or inflammation of the vaginal tissue from a variety of causes. Bacteria or other STDs account for most of its diagnosis. Other less frequent causes are the estrogenic effect of birth control pills, stress, chemical irritants, tampons left in place, trauma, or allergies. It is thought that almost one third of all women will have had at least one episode of vaginitis during their lifetime. First episodes usually occur during adolescence, especially if the girl is sexually active.[15]

Normally the vagina has defenses that inhibit vaginitis from developing. The defenses are an acid *p*H; a protective, thick epithelium; normal bacterial flora that help combat *Candida albicans*; and physiologic mucous secretion that aids in cleansing the vagina. If any of these factors are altered, a woman's chances of developing vaginitis are increased.[15]

Candida Albicans. *Candida* is normally present in 25% to 50% of the healthy female population. Certain medications or physical conditions allow an overgrowth to occur. Antibiotic therapy, use of oral contraceptives, immune suppression therapy, diabetes mellitus, and steroid therapy increase the possibility of candidal infections. The greatest incidence of candidal infection occurs in the 16- to 30-year-old age group.[6]

On physical examination the patient will describe having (or the nurse will see) a milky-white cottage cheese-like discharge. Usually this does not have any odor but will cause itching, burning, and other signs of irritation. The nurse will see on a wet mount slide, prepared with saline or potassium hydroxide, budding yeast with

TABLE 68-1
Major Sexually Transmitted Diseases

Infection and Agent	Transmission	Symptoms	Possible Complications	Prevention
Gonorrhea Gonococcus Neisseria gonorrhoeae	Sexual contact; mother to fetus during delivery	Yellow mucopurulent discharge of the genital area, painful or frequent urination, pain in the genital area; may be asymptomatic	Sterility, cystitis, arthritis, endocarditis	Public should be educated on safe sex practices. Mother should be tested before delivery. Newborn's eyes should be treated with silver nitrate. All contacts should be treated with antibiotics.
Chlamydia Bacteria Chlamydia trachomatis	Sexual contact; mother to fetus during vaginal delivery	Mucopurulent genital discharge, genital pain, dysuria	Sterility	Public should be educated about safe sex practices. Sexual contact should be avoided when lesions are present. Infected mothers should have a cesarean delivery.
Genital herpes Virus Herpes simplex type 2	Sexual contact; mother to fetus during vaginal delivery	Genital soreness, pruritus, and erythema; vesicles appear that usually last for about 10 days, during which time transmission of virus is likely		Public should be educated about safe sex practices. Sexual contact should be avoided when lesions are present. Infected mothers should have a cesarean delivery.
Syphilis Spirochete Treponema pallidum	Sexual contact; mother to fetus via placenta; blood transfusion if donor is in early stage of disease and undiagnosed	Primary stage: genital lesion, enlarged lymph nodes. Secondary stage (6 weeks later): lesions of skin and mucous membrane, with generalized symptoms of headache and fever	Tertiary stage: central nervous system and cardiovascular damage, paralysis, psychosis	Public should be educated about safe sex practices. Screen blood donors. Do serologic testing before and during pregnancy. Avoid contact with body secretions from infected patients.
Acquired immunodeficiency syndrome (AIDS) Human immunodeficiency virus (HIV)	Sexual contact; exposure to blood or blood products; mother to fetus	Active phase: rash, cough, malaise, night sweats, lymphadenopathy. Asymptomatic phase: no symptoms, but test is positive for HIV antigens. AIDS-related complex (ARC): lymphadenopathy, diarrhea, oral candidiasis, weight loss, fatigue, skin rash, recurrent infections, fever. AIDS: rare infections such as Pneumocystis carinii pneumonia or rare cancers such as Kaposi's sarcoma or B-cell lymphomas	Neurologic impairment	Public should be educated about safe sex practices, especially high-risk groups. Blood or blood products used for transfusion should be carefully screened. Intravenous drug abusers should not share needles. Universal precautions should be used consistently in all health-care settings. Institute measures to avoid needlesticks among health-care workers.

Source: Craven, R. F., & Hirnle, C. J. (1992). *Fundamentals of nursing: Human health and function.* Philadelphia: J. B. Lippincott.

pseudohyphae. Potassium hydroxide is the preferred fixative because it is able to destroy epithelial cells and allow the examiner to see the yeast more clearly. A Gram's stain has a greater sensitivity in visualizing yeast. Yeast appear as gram-positive oval masses with tube-like structures.[6,15]

Treatment varies by physician and sometimes by patient preference. Topical agents such as nystatin suppositories, clotrimazole vaginal tablets and cream, or miconazole cream or suppositories are the most commonly used medications. Additionally, sources of reinfections or other factors that put the patient at risk should be eliminated. Some sources of reinfection might be a diaphragm, underwear, and oral–genital sexual contact.[6,15]

Trichomonas Vaginalis. *Trichomonas* is caused by a flagellated protozoon. It is the most frequently diagnosed sexually transmitted disease. It is most often transmitted sexually, but the protozoon has been found to survive for 1½ hours on a wet sponge, so transmission by fomites might occur. Its peak incidence occurs in adolescence and early adulthood. The most common sites are the vagina, urethra, and periurethral glands.[15]

Symptoms do not always occur in women. The most common symptoms are itching and a discharge. The discharge is frequently described as malodorous, frothy, and greenish or yellow. In some cases dysuria is reported. All of these may be seen during a pelvic examination. In addition some edema and erythema of the external genitals or vagina may be seen.[6,15]

Diagnosis can be made easily by examining a wet mount microscopically for the presence of trichomonads, which usually are motile. The most effective treatment is metronidazole (Flagyl) for the patient and his or her partner(s).[6,15]

Gardnerella Vaginitis. This particular vaginitis also is very common among sexually active adolescents. It is also known as *Hemophilus vaginalis* or *Corynebacterium* vaginitis. If seen in a patient, it is almost certain to be found in his or her partner.[15]

Less than half of the patients with this STD exhibit symptoms. Those who do complain of a grayish-white discharge, which the examiner can see adheres to the vaginal wall. There may be no odor, or there may be a fishy type of odor.[6,15] The diagnosis is made by visualizing under a microscope the "clue cells," which are epithelial cells covered by small gram-negative rods.[15]

Treatment is either with metronidazole (Flagyl) or ampicillin. Partners also should be treated with either medication.[6,15]

Gonorrhea

Gonorrhea is the most commonly reported communicable disease in the United States. It is caused by the bacteria *Neisseria gonorrhoeae*, which is seen under the microscope as a gram-positive diplococcus.[6]

Dysuria is a commonly reported symptom. Men also report urinary frequency and a urethral discharge. Women report an abnormal vaginal discharge. Many times the person is asymptomatic. If the person has developed pharyngeal gonorrhea, he or she might have pharyngitis.[6] A definitive diagnosis is made with a positive culture that is oxidase reactive. Treatment is usually with a single dose of penicillin and 1 week of tetracycline to treat the commonly concurrent chlamydia infection.[6]

The most common complication of gonorrhea in the infant is gonococcal conjunctivitis, which, if untreated, will lead to blindness. In female adolescents the most common complication is PID with resultant pelvic abscess and frequently sterility. Occasionally arthritis may occur. In male adolescents epididymitis, sterility, and urethral stricture may occur.[6]

Chlamydia

Chlamydia is the primary cause of nongonococcal urethritis. It has a greater incidence of occurrence than gonorrhea. An inexpensive, reliable, and fast diagnostic test is not available to most clinicians; therefore, its diagnosis is made primarily by exclusion. Many men complain of dysuria, urinary frequency, and urethral discharge. Many men and women are asymptomatic.[6,15]

A diagnosis of chlamydia is made if tests for gonorrhea are negative, and symptoms are present with white blood cells seen on a Gram's stain of the urethral or vaginal discharge. Some studies have shown that there is a high incidence of concurrent chlamydial infection with a positive test for gonorrhea.[6,15]

Medical treatment is tetracycline or if contraindicated, erythromycin. If untreated, the complications are similar to those seen with gonorrhea.[6,15]

Genital Warts (Condyloma Acuminatum)

Genital warts are caused by HPV. HPV is considered to be the most common viral STD in the United States. As many as 3 million cases per year are seen. There is a high incidence in men and women who began sexual activity early, who have had multiple partners, and who have not regularly used contraception, especially the barrier methods.[6]

Genital warts may occur on the penis, urethra, and perineum; around the anus; or in the vulvovaginal area. They are usually painless and may be found as a single or multiple soft, fleshy growth. Occasionally they are diagnosed by Pap smear and clinically.[6]

Treatment is most often with 10% to 25% podophyllin. This treatment should not be used during pregnancy or with cervical, oral, urethral, or anorectal warts. Sometimes cryotherapy, CO_2 laser surgery, or surgical removal is used. The most common problem associated with genital warts is that they may be a precursor to tissue dysplasia and malignancy. During pregnancy the warts sometimes enlarge and obstruct the birth canal if present in the vagina or on the cervix.[6]

Genital Herpes

HSV types 1 and 2 cause this sexually transmitted disease. It is estimated that 200,000 primary infections occur per year.[6]

The most visible symptom is single or multiple vesicles that spontaneously rupture to form a shallow, painful ulcer. The ulcers usually resolve spontaneously with minimal scarring. The initial infection usually lasts a mean of 12 days. Recurrent infections last 4 to 5 days and are usually milder. The virus is shed intermittently without symptoms during the latency period. Type 2 genital infections are five times more likely to recur than type 1 infections. Either type can be found as an oral or genital infection. HSV is definitively diagnosed by Pap smear and culture. On examination of the Pap smear multinucleated giant cells with intranuclear inclusions are seen.[6]

There is still no cure for herpes. The drug acyclovir has been successful at reducing or suppressing symptoms. Sometimes the use of condoms will help protect partners from infection. Annual Pap smears for women are recommended due to the risk of dysplasia and malignancy.[6]

The most devastating complication is from an active maternal herpes infection during a vaginal delivery. The infant will develop neonatal herpes, which causes a wide range of infectious processes to multiple organ systems. There is a high fatality rate, especially if the central nervous system is involved. This complication is best prevented by detection and delivery by cesarean section.[6]

Cytomegalovirus

Cytomegalovirus is a member of the herpesvirus family. The most disastrous sequelae occur with infection during pregnancy. CMV infections occur in approximately 1.5% of all pregnancies in the United States. Approximately 50,000 infants are affected in 1 year. If a pregnant adolescent becomes infected from a sibling who contracted the virus in day care or from another source, her infant may experience multiple-organ system disease, with the most common problems being microcephaly and hearing loss.[6]

CMV symptoms are usually nonspecific. The adolescent may present with a febrile illness, mononucleosis, pneumonitis, hepatitis, or a combination of these. A diagnosis is made with a rise in titer of complement fixation, immunofluorescent testing of the serum, or identification of the virus in tissue.[6] Caution must be taken when caring for infected individuals because the virus is shed in all body fluids, including breast milk.

Treatment is primarily supportive, due to the self-limiting nature of the disease; however, if the individual is immunosuppressed, complications or death may occur.[6]

Pelvic Inflammatory Disease

PID is the most common, serious complication of certain STDs, such as gonorrhea and chlamydia. The highest rates of acute salpingitis are seen in teenage and young adult women, especially when multiple partners are involved. Frequently the girl reports she is monogamous and only becomes aware of her partner's infidelity when she is infected and develops PID. The use of an IUD places the adolescent girl at greater risk, and the IUD is generally contraindicated in this age group. Organisms cultured from intra-abdominal sites can be divided into three groups: (1) one third of cases are caused by gonorrhea, (2) one third by chlamydia and gonorrhea, and (3) one third by nongonoccocal aerobic and anaerobic bacteria.[15]

Typically the adolescent girl reports severe, continuous abdominal pain in the bilateral lower quadrants. The pain usually increases with movement or sexual intercourse. Other symptoms may be vaginal discharge, fever, chills, nausea, and vomiting.[15]

Treatment usually can be accomplished with antibiotics on an outpatient basis. However, there are times when the adolescent may be hospitalized for treatment with intravenous antibiotics. The physician may choose to hospitalize a girl with PID if she is severely ill, pregnant, noncompliant with oral therapy, or has failed to respond to treatment.[15]

Recurrence takes place in about one third of cases and is much higher if the partner is not sufficiently treated. Infertility is highest when multiple episodes of PID occur with time.[15]

Syphilis

The spirochete *Treponema pallidum* causes this STD. It is not as common as in the past, but its incidence is rising, especially in populations such as drug abusers and lower socioeconomic groups. This increase may be attributed to a variety of factors, the most important being a scarcity of resources for case finding and treatment of those who cannot afford to pay for it. Syphilis in the adolescent population is relatively uncommon. Congenital syphilis is seen in about 1 in 10,000 pregnancies per year.[6]

Syphilis develops in three phases. A chancre is seen during the primary phase. This is a painless indurated ulcer at the exposure site. Secondary syphilis is characterized by a skin rash, lymphadenopathy, and other variable signs. There are no clinical symptoms during the latent or third phase.[6]

Diagnosis during the primary phase is by clinical symptoms and a positive serologic test. Titers usually rise in active cases. The spirochetes can be visualized by darkfield microscopy from chancre or lymph node material. Secondary phase diagnosis also is by clinical signs and with a strongly reactive serologic test. During the latent phase a serologic test is the only tool with which a diagnosis can be made.[6]

Treatment is most successful with benzathine penicillin. Nontreatment can result in congenital syphilis or central nervous system or cardiovascular system involvement, leading to death.[6]

Pediculosis Pubis

This infection is caused by the pubic louse. It is 1 to 4 mm long and has claws with which it clings to pubic hairs. Transmission occurs by close physical contact but not necessarily sexual contact. It is included in discussions of STDs because it is most often transmitted during sexual contact. It is relatively common, and women report slightly more episodes than men.[6]

Symptoms can range from slight discomfort to severe itching. The examiner will see erythematous papules with lint-like nits clinging to hairs.[6]

Diagnosis and treatment is by history and clinical symptoms. Treatment is with Kwell (lindane 1%) or other similar insecticide. Additional teaching includes information about disinfecting clothing and linen by washing in hot water or by dry cleaning so transmission does not occur.[6]

Nursing Implications

When counseling adolescents with STDs it is most important that they have a clear understanding of the disease process and the reasons for compliance with the treatment protocol. After this is well understood the next topic to emphasize is prevention.

Abstinence from sexual activity during which bodily fluids such as semen or blood are transmitted or skin-to-skin contact is made should be stressed. An emphasis on risk-free options is important. These include monogamous relationships between uninfected partners or complete abstinence from all sexual activity.[6] The nurse should bear in mind that most adolescents believe that they are indestructible and that infections will not happen to them. Most adolescents do not recognize that what they do now may have future consequences. They are probably the least compliant with the use of preventive methods unless they feel that they have a vested interest in using that method. Emphasizing how prevention of STDs can help them usually is the most successful argument to use with an adolescent.

The accompanying Teaching Plan gives an example of a nurse teaching an adolescent about prevention of STDs and the use of birth control methods.

Choice of Contraceptive Methods

Contraceptive methods are grouped for discussion into barrier methods, oral contraceptive methods, IUDs, over-the-counter methods, natural family planning, coitus interruptus, abstinence, and postcoital contraception. Each group is examined for its general mechanism of action, benefits, contraindications, or special information of which the nurse should be aware for counseling. The relative effectiveness of each group of contraceptive method is described in the accompanying display. Finally, some principles of patient education and counseling are addressed as they relate to contraception. A more detailed discussion of these methods is beyond the scope of this chapter, and the reader is encouraged to seek additional information in the resources used for this chapter as well as others.

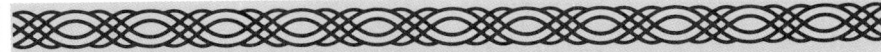

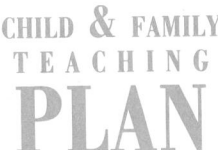

CHILD & FAMILY
T E A C H I N G
PLAN

Prevention of Sexually Transmitted Disease and Introduction to Birth Control Methods

Assessment

Tanya, a 16-year-old African American adolescent girl, has been hospitalized on the adolescent unit for treatment of pelvic inflammatory disease (PID). During the initial assessment the nurse discovers that Tanya has been having unprotected intercourse with her 19-year-old boyfriend, Anton, for the past 3 months. Tanya did not know how she became infected with gonorrhea. She has never been pregnant, and this is her first experience with sexual intercourse.

During the nurse's conversation with Tanya she realizes that she must speak in very simple terms and have Tanya repeat the questions she is asking to make sure Tanya understands what the nurse is asking. Occasionally the nurse uses street slang as the correct terminology to get across the meaning.

Tanya will be discharged with 1 month's supply of birth control pills, foam, and condoms.

Child and Family Objectives	Specific Content	Teaching Strategies
1. Identify the reason for developing PID and how gonorrhea is transferred from one person to another.	1. Discuss confidentiality of interview. Explain what organisms (gonorrhea, chlamydia) cause PID. Discuss which pelvic structures and other systems the disease affects and other sequelae. Discuss how the bacteria are transferred from one individual to another (e.g., vaginal or anal intercourse, orally). Reinforce the necessity for a follow-up culture for test of cure and treatment of any contacts. Answer questions and dispel any myths.	1. Provide a teaching place that is quiet and private. Allow enough time for the teaching so that there is good comprehension. If necessary, the nurse may need to break up the content into smaller segments. The nurse may need to repeat the information several times before there is adequate comprehension. Ask for adolescent's definition first. This will give the nurse a baseline to assess how much information needs to be given and how much needs to be corrected. Use a diagram of internal female reproductive system to trace path of bacteria and the infection's progress.

2. State how birth control pills work, when to start the first pack of pills, what to do if pills are missed, and what precautions to take during the first month on the pill.	2. Discuss the following:
	• How the pills work: Combination pills contain two hormones, estrogen and progestin. These hormones work by stopping ovulation.
	• When to start taking pills. Choose one of three ways:
	  1. Start pack on first day of period.
	  2. Start pack on first Sunday after period begins.
	  3. Start pack on fifth day after period begins.
		2. Use a sample pack of prescribed pills, calendar, and package insert. Give written instruction sheet if available. Always test the adolescent's reading ability. For example, have them read the instructions out loud and repeat their understanding of the instructions to you.

(Continued)

CHILD & FAMILY
T E A C H I N G
PLAN

Prevention of Sexually Transmitted Disease and Introduction to Birth Control Methods
(continued)

Child and Family Objectives	*Specific Content*	*Teaching Strategies*

	• Read the package insert.
	• Taking the pill: pills work best when taken once a day at the same time. This will keep hormone levels steady.
	• When pills are missed during a cycle:
	
	1. If one pill is missed, take it as soon as you remember it. Take the current day's pill at the regular time.
	
	2. If two pills in a row are missed, take two pills as soon as you remember and two the next day. Some spotting may occur. Use backup method until you get your next period (foam and condoms).
	
	3. If more than two pills in a row are missed, your ovaries will probably produce an egg, and you could become pregnant. This also may happen if you miss taking pills during the month. If either of these situations occur, start using your backup birth control method (foam and condoms). You might start your period. Do one of two things:
	
	    Option 1: Take two pills a day for 3 days, and use a backup method of birth control.
	
	    Option 2: Throw away the old pack of pills and start a new pack on the next Sunday or on the fifth day of your period. Use a backup method of birth control.
	
	4. If you become sick with *severe* diarrhea or vomiting for several days, use a backup method of birth control until your next period.	

(*Continued*)

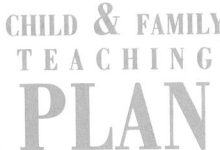

CHILD & FAMILY TEACHING PLAN

Prevention of Sexually Transmitted Disease and Introduction to Birth Control Methods
(continued)

Child and Family Objectives	*Specific Content*	*Teaching Strategies*
3. Demonstrate an understanding of how to use foam and condoms.	3. Explain how during the first month, a backup method of birth control (such as foam and condoms) should be used.	3. Use one or two different kinds of contraceptive foam and condoms for demonstration. It is important to demonstrate every phase. For example, demonstrate the difference in foam before and after the required shaking; how the foam spreads, so it blocks the cervix; and how to take apart and clean the insertion device. Have the adolescent repeat all the instructions in the proper order and do a return demonstration. Follow the same method with the condom. Let the adolescent feel it and demonstrate with two fingers how the condom fits over the fingers, how to hold on while removing it. Be visual and graphic in detail.
4. State what steps to take if a period is missed or spotting occurs.	4. Explain what to do for missed periods: If a period is missed after completing a cycle of pills, start taking the next pack of pills. If a second cycle is missed, call the clinic, nurse practitioner, or physician. If one or more pills are missed and you miss a period, use your backup method of birth control, and call the clinic to schedule a pregnancy test. If spotting occurs, continue taking the pill as usual. This is common and will usually stop after 1 or 2 months.	4. Use written instructions to reinforce what you are saying.
5. State the possible side-effects of birth control pills and what to do if they occur.	5. Emphasize that any time you see a nurse or doctor for any reason, mention that you are taking birth control pills, particularly if you are admitted to a hospital. Discuss side-effects. *Serious*: Hypertension (high blood pressure), blood clotting disorders, peripheral venous thrombosis or cerebral thrombosis (stroke), myocardial infarction (heart attack), biliary disease (jaundice).	5. Use written instructions to reemphasize the information.

(Continued)

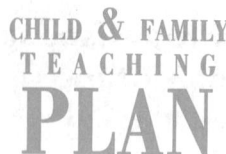

Child and Family Objectives	*Specific Content*	*Teaching Strategies*
	If any of these occur call your health care provider right away.	
	Nonserious: Breast tenderness or enlargement, weight gain, nausea, vomiting, abdominal bloating or cramps, breakthrough bleeding, change in menstrual flow, skin changes, loss of hair, change in sex drive.	
	Explain that any of these will usually resolve in 3 months. Do not stop taking the pills. Consult with your health care provider if they do not resolve.	
6. State when and where to go for her follow-up appointment.	6. Discuss date, time, and place of follow-up appointment. Reinforce reasons for appointment: • Checking on pill tolerance • Satisfaction with selection of birth control method • Refill	6. Use written instruction with the information inserted into an appropriate blank space with the appointment time, date, place, and who to see as well as who to call if questions or problems arise.

Evaluation

• Tanya verbalizes her understanding of how one contracts PID and gonorrhea.
• Tanya states when she will start pills and how and when to take them.
• Tanya demonstrates how to use foam and condoms.
• Tanya discusses steps to take if she misses a period.
• Tanya lists possible side-effects of pills.
• Tanya repeats instructions for her follow-up appointment.

Barrier Methods

The use of a barrier is one of the oldest contraceptive measures. Current barrier methods include the diaphragm, condom, cervical cap, and contraceptive sponge. They create a barrier that prevents sperm from entering the cervical canal and uterus. The condom fits over the penis preventing sperm from entering the vagina. The diaphragm, cervical cap, and contraceptive sponge fit over the cervical os, thus preventing the sperm from entering. A special spermicidal gel or cream is used with these mechanical products to improve their effectiveness. An added benefit with any of these methods is that all provide some protection against STDs. In addition the diaphragm protects against cervical neoplasia.[6]

Any of these barrier methods might be contraindicated in adolescents who are allergic to the latex rubber or spermicidal gel or cream; who have vaginal anatomic abnormalities that make a good fit impossible; who might not use the method every time sexual intercourse takes place due to age or motivation; and who have a history of TSS.[6]

Oral Contraceptives

Oral contraceptives contain estrogen or progestin, both of which act on the reproductive cycle to prevent ovulation. The progestin-only (mini) pills work slightly differently. The progestin-only pill alters the cervical mucus, which disrupts sperm transport up the cervical canal and alters the luteal phase of the reproductive cycle.[6] Research has demonstrated that ovulation is prevented in only 15% to 40% of cases in which progestin-only pills are used. There are three types of oral contraceptives on the market today: (1) the combination pill with a constant amount of estrogen and progesterone; (2) the triphasic

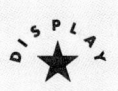

Effectiveness of Various Contraceptive Methods

MOST EFFECTIVE

Abstinence
Combination birth control pills
Progestin-only pills
Intrauterine devices

EFFECTIVE IF COMPLIANCE IS GOOD

Barrier methods used alone or with over-the-counter
    spermicidal products
Natural family planning methods
Postcoital contraceptive methods

LEAST EFFECTIVE

Coitus interruptus or the withdrawal method
Over-the-counter spermicidals used alone

pill, which varies the amount of progesterone; and (3) the progestin-only pill. The newer triphasic pills have been in use in the United States since 1984. They are being prescribed more frequently because they use less progestin and there are fewer metabolic effects on lipids, carbohydrate metabolism, and blood pressure because of the lower dose of progestin.[6]

Contraindications to the adolescent taking the combined birth control pill or progestin-only pill are a history of one or more of the following: cardiovascular disease, thrombophlebitis, coronary artery disease, breast cancer or other estrogen-dependent neoplasia, pregnancy, liver tumor, and undiagnosed abnormal genital bleeding. The pill should never be prescribed in any of these cases. Other contraindications are hypertension, diabetes, gall bladder disease, sickle cell disease, major surgery planned within 1 month, injury to the lower leg, or a long leg cast.[6]

Intrauterine Devices

The IUD is theorized to work in any or all of the following ways: (1) a hostile environment for sperm implantation may be created by the presence of the IUD; (2) the motility of the ovum through the fallopian tube may be increased, which then decreases the chance for fertilization; (3) sperm may be immobilized; or (4) the viscosity of cervical mucus may be increased.[6]

Major contraindications to the use of the device is an active pelvic infection and pregnancy. Among the many additional risk factors are multiple sexual partners, history of recurrent pelvic infection, undiagnosed bleeding disorders, and blood coagulation disorders. The IUD is widely used outside of the United States, but it has decreased in popularity due to the high incidence of pelvic infection and infertility associated with its use.[6] In general the IUD is not recommended for use as a birth control method in adolescents.

Over-the-Counter Methods and Vaginal Spermicides

Over-the-counter methods of contraception include condoms, which were discussed previously, and the vaginal spermicides, such as foam; contraceptive cream, gel, or jelly; and suppositories. All are relatively easy and safe to use. The spermicidal preparations are composed of an inert base, such as foam or cream. This base acts by forming a barrier at the cervical os. The chemical used as a spermicide usually is nonoxynol-9 or octoxynol-9. For greatest efficacy all of these methods should be used in combination with condoms or another method of birth control.[6]

The contraindications include an allergy to the spermicidal preparation, noncompliance or lack of motivation to use the method every time sexual intercourse takes place, or any physical disability that interferes with the preparation being used effectively. A major benefit with the use of the spermicidal preparations is their ability to kill a number of organisms that cause STDs, especially gonorrhea.[6]

Natural Family Planning

Natural family planning has been used for many years. The menstrual cycle is charted by the woman. She and her partner avoid having sexual intercourse during the days she is most likely to be fertile. This method is used by members of religious groups for which all other methods of contraception are forbidden. Natural family planning in all its forms requires great compliance and an awareness of bodily changes. For these reasons it is probably the least desirable method of birth control for the adolescent.[6]

Coitus Interruptus

This method is also known as withdrawal. The penis is removed from the vagina before ejaculation, which should take place completely away from the vagina and external genitalia of the woman. It is one of the least effective methods because frequently the pre-ejaculatory fluid contains sperm, especially if there has been a recent ejaculation. The self-control needed by the couple and the effect on their pleasure make it an unreliable method of birth control.[6]

Abstinence

In this age of increasing incidence of teenage pregnancy, AIDS, herpes, and other STDs, abstinence is becoming more acceptable and common. Alternative methods of sexual gratification can be encouraged that do not include penis-in-vagina intercourse. Certain medical situations necessitate the use of an alternative to intercourse. Examples are an acute episode of a sexually transmitted disease; pelvic, genital, or urinary tract infection; late third-trimester pregnancy; or postabortion.[6]

Several programs for teenagers have been developed that use peer pressure and other methods to encourage abstinence from sexual intercourse, thereby lowering the teen pregnancy rate.[6] One of these programs should be implemented especially if the nurse is providing family planning counseling to many adolescents.

Postcoital Contraception

Another common term used for this method is the "morning-after" pill. Its use is most common after a woman is raped. These pills are a combination of estrogen and progestin. The hormones act to disturb the luteal phase, the development of the endometrium, and the transport of the fertilized ovum.[6]

RU 486 is a new, politically controversial, postcoital product currently available only outside of the United States. It is a progesterone antagonist and is an early abortifacient and midcycle contraceptive. Complete abortion occurs in 85% of cases when it is orally administered within 10 days of a missed period.[6]

Nursing Implications

Some principles to use when counseling or educating clients about contraceptive methods have been stated in other parts of this unit. The following teaching principles should be used.

Always have the actual method available for demonstration as well as written material in simple language for the client to take home. Make each session short, but provide enough time for the client to repeat and demonstrate what has been taught. Be consistent among caregivers so confusion is minimized. Encourage questions and be nonjudgmental. Finally, the environment in which the counseling is provided should be confidential.[6] The teaching plan gives an example of teaching regarding birth control and prevention of sexually transmitted disease.

Nurses should be aware of their state's law regarding the age of legal consent for seeking contraception and the legal necessity for parental involvement. In cases in which the parents do not have to be told, the nurse must use good judgment in encouraging the adolescent to tell his or her parents. The nurse should never become an obstacle between the adolescent and parents' communication. In most cases in which an adolescent becomes pregnant, communication barriers already exist between the girl and her parents. The nurse can facilitate communication with encouragement and support.

Adolescent Pregnancy

To effectively intervene in the prevention of teenage pregnancy, the nurse must have some idea of the scope of the problem. According to data published in 1985 by the Centers for Disease Control, the number of female 15 to 19 year olds declined between 1970 and 1980; however, the number of pregnancies increased, while the number of births decreased because of an increased abortion rate.[11]

There are many possible reasons for the rising teenage pregnancy rate. One reason is that the age of menarche has declined in the last 100 years. In the late 19th century it occurred in the midteens; now it occurs at approximately 12 to 13 years. Another possibility is the increased use of contraceptives in the general population and the greater acceptability or tolerance of early sexual activity or experimentation, including greater peer pressure to begin sexual activity.[15]

The Problem

Despite the widespread availability of contraceptives, their accessibility is still an issue. Two thirds of sexually active adolescents never or occasionally use contraception.[15] The reasons for this are varied, but the most successful outreach to teenagers regarding contraception is school-based clinics that provide a variety of health related care, contraception being only a small portion.

Research has suggested that certain common threads run through groups of pregnant adolescents. These are poor academic achievement, poor family relationships, lower self-esteem than those who postpone pregnancy, a perceived lack of options, and a feeling that pregnancy is the only way out.[12]

The generally poor outcome of teenage pregnancy is related to many factors. One is inadequate prenatal care, lack of postnatal care for mother and infant, and inadequate parenting knowledge and skills.[15] In prenatal clinics that have specialized programs for teenagers, the maternal and fetal outcomes are greatly improved. In these clinics additional education is provided regarding nutrition, social and parenting skills, contraception, and methods the teenager can use to increase self-esteem. Without this comprehensive and aggressive support, the outcomes are not substantially improved. The accompanying Nursing Care Plan for a pregnant 14-year-old addresses some of these issues.

Why is the teen and her fetus at such risk? There is an increased risk of mortality to the mother during the pregnancy and delivery due to complications such as pre-eclampsia; poor nutrition, which can lead to anemia and contributes to an increased risk of preeclampsia; and the social problems that may impact the adolescent girl for the rest of her life. Among these are a lack of education, unemployment, and the likelihood of her being on welfare. The greatest fetal risk is the increased incidence of low birth weight in this group, which contributes to the high mortality rate in the first year of life.[15]

Alternatives to Pregnancy

The alternatives for pregnant teens are keeping the baby, abortion, and adoption. For 96% of unmarried teens keeping the baby is the most acceptable choice. Even though at the time of this writing abortion is legal, many barriers have been erected that do not allow easy access for a teenager to obtain an abortion. In addition to the legal reasons, in many socioeconomic groups abortion is not acceptable. Adoption is probably the least commonly used alternative in this age group.[15]

Programs for the Future

There is a movement toward aggressively preventing subsequent pregnancies by a variety of methods. The most successful programs seem to be those that help direct the adolescent back into school soon after delivery, pro-

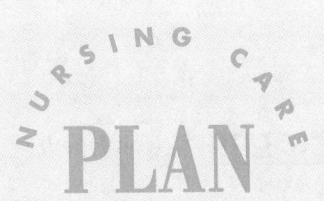

A 14-Year-Old Girl Who Is Pregnant

Assessment

Case Study Description

Stella is a 14-year-old girl who comes to the clinic for a pregnancy test. She has been complaining of nausea and vomiting, especially in the morning, for the past 2 months. She has missed school at least 2 to 3 days a week because of it. She is also experiencing some pelvic pain this week. She is single, and her mother is with her at the clinic visit. During the interview while the mother is present, Stella is quiet with a flat affect.

When interviewed alone the adolescent is tearful and states that the 16-year-old father of the child denies paternity, and she has not seen him for the past 2 weeks. Her last intercourse was 2 weeks ago. They never used birth control because he said he would pull out in time and that if they used anything, it would ruin the moment.

Assessment Data

Menstrual history—Stella started her periods at 13, and she has irregular cycles. Her last menstrual period (LMP) was 5 months ago, she thinks. Her pregnancy test (urine) was positive. Her pelvic examination showed positive signs for pregnancy. The fundal height is 17 weeks. There is a yellowish discharge with numerous white blood cells on wet mount. Gonorrhea culture is positive. Her blood tests showed the following: syphilis, negative; rubella titer, positive; hematocrit, 32%.

Nursing Diagnosis	Intervention	Rationale
1. Knowledge deficit regarding positive gonorrhea (GC) culture, pregnancy, birth control Supporting Data: • Stella has not been able to state how she contracted GC or how to prevent it. • Stella is unable to state how to care for herself during the pregnancy. • Stella is not able to state how to prevent further pregnancies or what types of contraception are available.	Determine Stella's reading ability. Use written instructions and ask Stella to read and interpret. Develop teaching plan for treatment and prevention of gonorrhea and birth control methods (see Teaching Plan presented in this chapter).	Reading ability varies from person to person. Assess each person's ability to determine what written instructions, if any, should be provided. All clinic health care providers should follow the same plan and give similar information. This avoids confusing the adolescent, reinforces her trust and confidence in what clinic personnel say, and supports compliance with treatment plan and visits. Introducing a discussion of birth control methods at this time helps to dispel myths and lays a foundation for prevention of further STD episodes during pregnancy. This information should be repeated during the third trimester and postpartum.
	At each clinic visit, using fundal height progress, pictures, diagrams, and other audiovisual aids, show pregnancy progress.	Most adolescents think in concrete terms and are visually oriented. Using meaningful audiovisual aids helps the adolescent interpret what is happening inside their bodies. This also involves the adolescent in her pregnancy and aids in the identification and attachment process with the fetus.

(Continued)

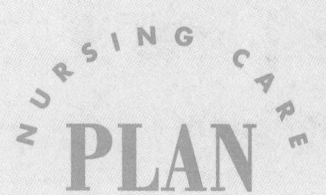

A 14-Year-Old Girl Who Is Pregnant (continued)

Nursing Diagnosis	Intervention	Rationale
2. Noncompliance related to meeting clinic appointments and taking iron pills Supporting Data: • Mother works during clinic hours so Stella must take the bus • Stella is young and mother states that she hates taking pills	Provide written schedule of appointments, instructions on what will take place at each visit, and what to do if she can't make an appointment (call and reschedule).	Set behavior expectations, limitations, and consequences if these expectations are not met.
3. Altered nutrition less than body requirements Supporting Data: • Adolescent pregnancy • Hematocrit (Hct) 32%	Provide verbal and written instructions for taking iron pills. State what will happen if Hct drops (iron injections). Have Stella follow Hct levels with you at each visit.	More opportunities for questions and answers lead to a greater understanding by Stella of why you are asking her to take iron Involving Stella in the positive and negative consequences of her behavior (Hct going up or down) will help compliance and bring about a better outcome.
	Refer Stella to nutritionist.	Using an expert consultant to assess and follow Stella's dietary habit is part of the team approach to following pregnant adolescents.
4. Self-esteem disturbance related to pregnancy Supporting Data: • Denial of pregnancy • Anger at father of child • Tearful and depressed about pregnancy • Doesn't want to return to school • Has stopped seeing her friends	Provide nonjudgmental clinic atmosphere, emotional support, and understanding for both Stella and her mother. Encourage school attendance or attendance at a school for pregnant girls. Provide encouragement and opportunities for success. Expectations should be reasonable and slowly increase as Stella demonstrates achievement.	Provide a safe, trusting, supportive environment in which compliance is expected. Success and positive achievements help build self-esteem. This will minimize the tendency to quit school and have more babies. Staying in school helps to increase self-esteem.
	Refer Stella to social worker.	Using the skills of the social worker to provide additional emotional and social support is an important component of the team approach for pregnant adolescents.

Evaluation

• Gonorrhea infection is resolved with the repeat GC negative culture.

Expected Outcomes

• Stella takes iron pills three times a day as indicated by increased serial Hcts.
• Stella uses prescribed diet and gains weight appropriately.
• Stella states she is getting sufficient rest.
• Stella verbally demonstrates signs of her accepting the pregnancy.
• Stella maintains regular appointment schedule.

vide child care options, and provide guidance with alternatives and options in their lives and increasing their self-esteem.[12]

Adolescent Fatherhood

Only recently has a focus encompassed the adolescent father. The most successful programs involve the father early in the pregnancy and provide education regarding the pregnancy, parenthood, and subsequent pregnancy prevention not only to the expectant mother, but to the father as well.[15] In studies with adolescent parents the recurring themes are those of powerlessness and a struggle to provide psychological and financial support to the mother. Frequently, unrealistic expectations are expressed.[3] It is clear that intervention and support for adolescent fathers are as important to the success of raising a healthy baby as they are for the adolescent mother.

The Homosexual Adolescent

Homosexuality is defined as seeking sexual gratification or participating in sexual activity with a person of the same sex. Homosexuality also can be an orientation to the same sex; that is, the person is attracted to that sex but does not necessarily act on that attraction. During adolescence homosexual behavior is frequent and most often experimental in nature and does not necessarily mean that the teenager is homosexual. It is considered a normal part of seeking one's own sexual identity. When adolescents continue to have a preference for their own sex into adulthood, they then can define themselves as homosexual.[15,21]

Historically, depending on how safe it was to reveal a homosexual orientation, it has been difficult to estimate the prevalence of homosexuality and lesbianism.[21] It is thought that 35% to 50% of teenage boys have had some homosexual contact. It is thought that approximately 10% of all male adults are exclusively homosexual for at least 3 years of their lives and 5% for all of their lives.[15] Women are more difficult to estimate because society does not question women living together as adults as often as it does men. When men live together as adults, it is often thought that they are homosexual. Rarely is it thought women living together are lesbian. The incidence of lesbianism is approximately 50% of the incidence in men.[15]

Why does one become homosexual? There is no one accepted reason. Many theories exist with little substantiated research to support any of them to the exclusion of another. Some of the suggested hypotheses are prenatal hormonal effects, genetics, or environmental factors.[15] However, the reader must be cautious because most studies dealing with the gay and lesbian population have been poorly constructed, and there has been little clear evidence of pathology in the family backgrounds of this group.[13]

During adolescent development, the task of achieving a sexual identity is accomplished (psychosexual development was discussed in Chap. 16). There are three components to this identity: inner sense of being a man or woman, behaving in accordance with one's gender role

as culturally defined, and determining one's sexual partner orientation. The gay or lesbian youth differs from his or her heterosexual peers only in the last component.[2]

★　ASSESSMENT

The need for a sexuality assessment is emphasized. In addition a discussion of the adolescent's sexual identity should be offered. Bidwell states that "for most gay teens there is no trusted friend in whom to confide."[2] This is not surprising because most nurses and physicians are not comfortable discussing this side of the adolescent's lifestyle. Because of the negative reaction from many health care workers and society in general, gay men and lesbian women are likely to be extremely sensitive to subtle changes in the interviewer's voice or manner, which might signal discomfort or disapproval.[21] Therefore, it is crucial that an adolescent's sexual orientation or confusion relating to this identity be explored due to the estimated high incidence (one third) of gay or bisexual adolescents who have attempted suicide.[2]

After the nurse has established a rapport with the adolescent during the interviewing process, an appropriate question might be posed in this way: "Many teens are worried about feeling attracted to others of their own sex. Have you ever had these feelings or worried about them?"[2] If they express a positive response, a further exploration of any source of concern should take place (Fig. 68-4).

It may be too soon to ask the teen to disclose any other information. As a trusting relationship evolves, the nurse should gently explore additional information concerning the relationship. Perhaps the issue may be that the teen is experimenting and is experiencing considerable confusion about sexual identity. Questions to ask should relate to the nature of the sexual expression, types and frequency of sexual practices, number of partners, and any concurrent use of alcohol or drugs. Each issue should then be addressed individually with appropriate teaching and counseling.

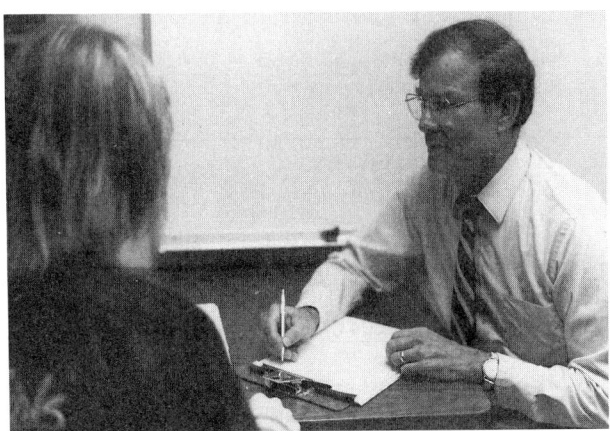

FIGURE 68-4
School and clinic nurses, who have developed rapport with their clients, can be very effective in helping adolescents understand the consequences of their sexual activity. (Courtesy of Overlake Hospital Medical Center, Bellevue, WA.)

During interviews with older adolescents many nurses tend to ask questions that have heterosexual values tied to them. The nurse may compare the following examples put forth by Williamson: "Are you married?" versus "Whom shall I contact if you become seriously ill?" Another example is "How often do you have intercourse?" versus "Are you sexually active?" A third example is "Is there any need for birth control" versus "What birth control method do you use?"[21] The second selection in the examples modify the interview questions to minimize heterosexual values.

★ NURSING DIAGNOSES AND PLANNING

Based on assessment data discussed previously and in the preceding chapter, the following nursing diagnoses may apply to the family and adolescent with homosexual orientation:

- Anxiety related to unconscious conflict about essential values.
- Body Image Disturbance related to psychosocial factors.
- Altered Family Processes related to situational crises.
- Altered Sexuality Patterns related to conflict with sexual orientation.
- High Risk for Infection related to sexual partners.
- Ineffective Individual Coping related to personal vulnerability.
- Hopelessness related to long-term stress.
- Ineffective Management of Therapeutic Regimen related to knowledge deficit regarding "safe sex" practices.

The nurse and adolescent together plan effective care based on the established nursing diagnoses. Several examples of expected outcomes follow:

- The young person verbalizes his or her conflicts regarding sexual orientation.
- The adolescent states that a "safe sex" method is being used during sexual activity.
- The family verbalizes a better understanding of the stresses the adolescent is undergoing.

The nurse plans for the daily care of the adolescent based on physician's orders and nursing diagnoses. Some general nursing care goals may be the following:

- Rapport for further counseling is established.
- Infection is treated.

★ NURSING INTERVENTIONS: COLLABORATIVE AND INDEPENDENT

Most interventions relate to the possible complications of male homosexual practices both physically and psychologically. The accompanying display lists complications of sexual practices of homosexual men.

Gonorrhea is most typically cultured from the pharynx or the anorectal area. Syphilis and hepatitis B are on the rise in this high-risk population. Gay bowel syndrome is a combination of amebiasis, giardiasis, shigellosis, gonorrhea, syphilis, chlamydia, rectal warts, trauma, polyps, abscesses, and fistulas. Most commonly this syndrome is seen in male homosexuals; however, any of these

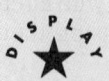

Complications of Sexual Practices of Homosexual Men

Gonorrhea (anorectal or pharyngeal)
Syphilis
Hepatitis type B
Gay bowel syndrome
Venereal warts (penis and rectal area)
Herpes simplex virus
Acquired immunodeficiency syndrome

Data from Neinstein, L. S., & Lawrence, S. (1984). Adolescent health care: A practical guide. *Baltimore: Urban & Schwarzenberg.*

problems can occur in females with a history of anal intercourse. Venereal warts are usually on the penis and rectal area. HSV has become commonplace among homosexuals as well as heterosexuals. Finally the most lethal of the complications is AIDS.[15]

Women are most at risk later in life for breast or endometrial cancer if they are childless. They have a very low risk of sexually transmitted disease except for the transmission of HSV. Gay men and lesbian woman do seem to exhibit a very high rate of alcohol and drug abuse, which should be addressed in the health care plan.

Nursing interventions should be closely aligned with the medical treatment plan. There is a considerable need for ongoing teaching and counseling, particularly in the adolescent population in which this lifestyle may be only transitory, but its effects may be life-threatening. A total team approach with medicine, nursing, and often psychological or social work involvement is necessary because of the impact on the adolescents and their relationships with family and peers.

The 1980s saw the creation of many support groups for gays and lesbians. One group is Parents and Friends of Lesbians and Gays, P.O. Box 24565, Los Angeles, CA 90024. However, there are still relatively few support groups for adolescents and their families; often these people are forced to struggle alone.

★ EVALUATION

Periodically the nurse and family evaluate the outcomes of care given. Examples of outcomes for the child and family with complications related to homosexual orientation were given under Nursing Diagnoses and Planning in this section.

Summary

Children from infancy through adolescence may experience alterations in their reproductive function. The nurse must be knowledgeable about these alterations so that he or she may intervene early, make appropriate referrals, and provide counseling, education, and emotional

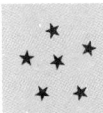

Ideas for Nursing Research

Nurses have traditionally been important in preventing or minimizing the reoccurrence of altered reproductive function. Health promotion to families and their children in this sensitive area continues to be a nursing responsibility. The following areas for research may determine ways to improve care of children and adolescents with a reproductive health problem:

- Methods that effectively aid the nurse in providing effective counseling and teaching.
- Methods that motivate the child or adolescent to participate in prevention programs.
- Development of strategies for effectively identifying victims of date rape.
- Effectiveness of educational programs designed to reduce date rape on college campuses.
- Development of approaches to teaching adolescents from different cultures regarding topics in reproduction.
- Assessment of reproductive informational needs for physically or mentally disabled adolescents and their parents.

support when necessary. Resources are available for children and their families to assist in the education, prevention, and treatment of problems related to the reproductive system. Nurses are also in a key position to provide valuable new knowledge through research.

The explosion of sexual activity among today's adolescents has created new problems for young people who are already confused about other factors of adolescent growth and development. STDs and genital infections are on the rise. Pregnancy and single parenthood among adolescents has become a major socioeconomic issue. Nurses actively become involved in prevention and counseling of these young people. Adolescents may experiment with others of the same sex, or older adolescents may feel strongly about their homosexual orientation. The nurse, after establishing rapport, can give such young people counseling regarding the physical and psychological issues that may result.

References

1. Behrman, R. E., Vaughn, V. C., & Nelson, W. E. (1987). *Nelson textbook of pediatrics.* (13th ed.). Philadelphia: W.B. Saunders.
2. Bidwell, R. J. (1988). The gay and lesbian teen: A case of denied adolescence. *Journal Pediatric Health Care, 2*(1), 3–8.
3. Caparulo, F., & London, K. (1981). Adolescent fathers: Adolescents first, fathers second. *Issues in Health Care of Women, 3*(1), 23–33.
4. Everstine, D. S., & Everstine, L. (1989). *Sexual trauma in children and adolescents.* New York: Brunner/Mazel.
5. Fischl, F., & Vytiska-Binstorfer, E. (1984). Diagnosis and therapy of genital bleeding in infancy and childhood. *Pediatric and Adolescent Gynecology, 2*(2), 201–211.
6. Hatcher, R. A., Guest, F., Stewart, F., Stewart, G. K., Trussell, J., Bowen, S., & Cates, W. (1988). *Contraceptive Technology 1988–89.* (14th ed.). New York: Printed Matter/Irvington.
7. Haugaard, J. J., & Repipucci, N. D. (1988). *The sexual abuse of children.* San Francisco: Jossey-Bass.
8. Huffman, J. W., Dewhurst, C. J., & Capraro, V. J. (1981). *The gynecology of childhood and adolescence.* Philadelphia: W.B. Saunders.
9. Khoiney, F. (1988). Adolescent dysmenorrhea. *Journal of Pediatric Health Care, 2*(1), 29–37.
10. Lavery, J. P., & Sanfilippo, J. S. (1985). *Pediatric and adolescent obstetrics and gynecology.* New York: Springer-Verlag.
11. Miller, K. A. (1986). Epidemiologic concepts of adolescent pregnancy. *Seminars in Adolescent Medicine, 2*(3), 175–179.
12. Moore, M. L. (1989). Recurrent teen pregnancy: Making it less desirable. *MCN American Journal of Maternal Child Nursing, 14*(2), 104–108.
13. Moses, A. E., & Hawkins, R. O. (1982). *Counseling lesbian women and gay men, a life issues approach.* St. Louis: C.V. Mosby.
14. Muehlenhard, C. L. (1988). Misinterpreted dating behaviors and the risk of date rape. *Journal of Social and Clinical Psychology, 6*(1), 20–37.
15. Neinstein, L. S. (1984). *Adolescent health care, a practical guide.* Baltimore: Urban & Schwarzenberg.
16. Niehaus, M. A. (1986). Rape. In J. Griffith-Kenney (Ed.), *Contemporary women's health.* (pp. 221–235). Menlo Park, CA: Addison-Wesley.
17. Russo, R. M. (1983). *Sexual development and disorders in childhood and adolescence.* New Hyde Park, NY: Medical Examination Publishing.
18. Scherer, P. (1989). Clinical news: Rating tampons to reduce toxic shock. *American Journal of Nursing, 89*(1), 14.
19. Vaz, R. M., Best, D., & Davis, S. (1988). Testicular cancer, adolescent knowledge and attitudes. *Journal of Adolescent Health Care, 9*(6), 474–479.
20. Whitner, M. S., & Anderson, M. V. (1987). Sexually transmitted diseases in children. *Health Care for Women International, 8*(1), 9–18.
21. Williamson, M. (1986). Lesbianism. In J. Griffith-Kenney (Ed.), *Contemporary women's health.* (pp. 278–296). Menlo Park, CA: Addison Wesley.

Appendices

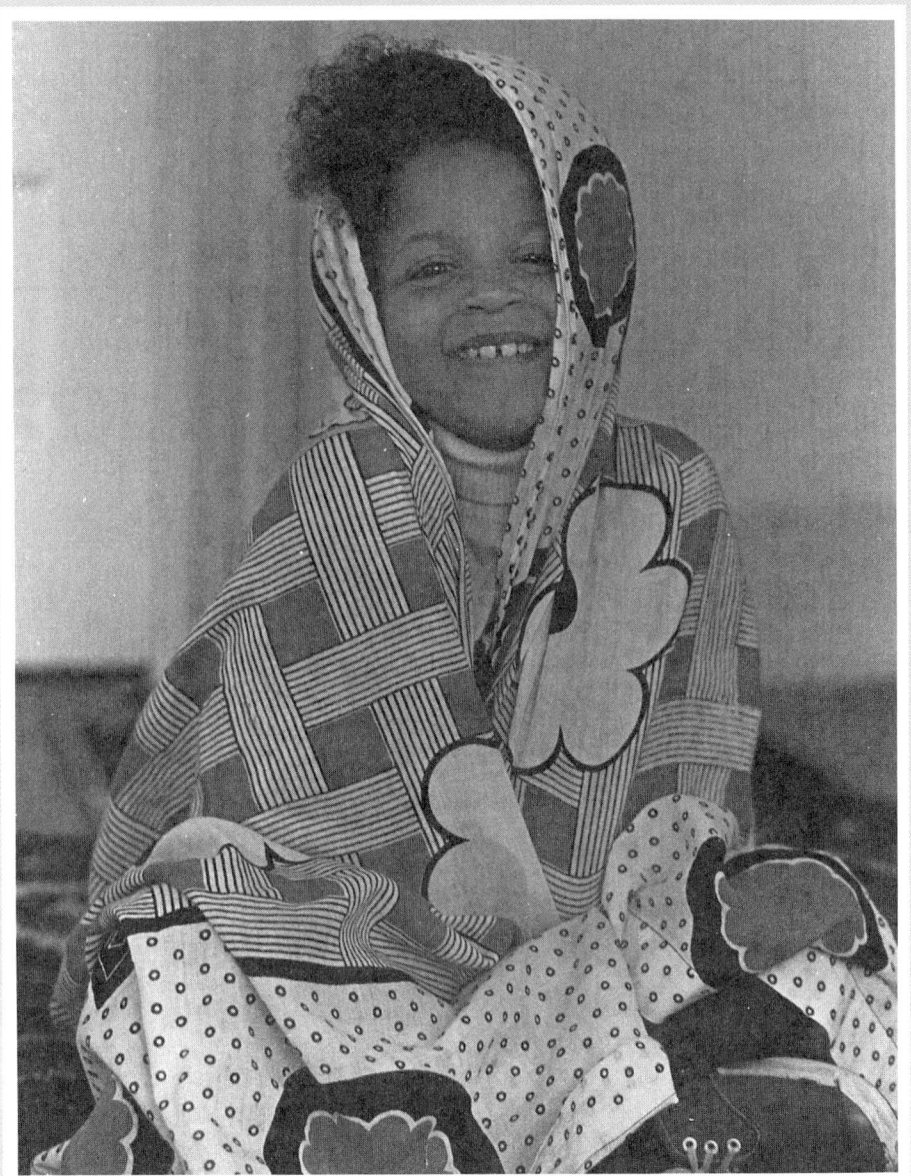

APPENDIX A Normal Range of Laboratory Values

Norms for laboratory studies are seldom precise. This listing of norm ranges provides a guide, but variations among reporting institutions should be expected. In most cases, where an adult laboratory value is given in this table, it is also applicable to an adolescent. More details on aspects of these tests are discussed in the Assessment sections of chapters in the text.

To simplify the interpretation of laboratory results reported in International System (SI) units, conversion factors (from SI to conventional units) are provided. SI base units are the gram (g), the liter (L), and the mole (mol). Other abbreviations used throughout this chapter are listed below.

SI Prefixes

Factor	Prefix	Symbol
10^3	kilo	k
10^{-1}	deci	d
10^{-2}	centi	c
10^{-3}	milli	m
10^{-6}	micro	μ
10^{-9}	nano	n
10^{-12}	pico	p
10^{-15}	femto	f

Abbreviations

CI	confidence interval
d	day
F	female
h	hour
Hb	hemoglobin
M	male
MCHC	mean corpuscular hemoglobin concentration
MCV	mean corpuscular volume
mEq	milliequivalent
min	minute
RBC	red blood cell
s	second
SD	standard deviation
U	unit
WBC	white blood cell
yr	year

Blood

Test	SI Reference Range	Conversion Factor	Conventional Units Reference Range
Adrenocorticotropic hormone (ACTH)	Cord: 130–160 ng/L 1st week: 100–140 Adult 0800 h: 25–100 1800 h: <50		Cord: 130–160 pg/mL 1st week: 100–140 Adult 0800 h: 25–100 1800 h: <50
Alanine aminotransferase (ALT)	<1 yr: 5–28 U/L >1 yr: 8–20		Same as SI
Albumin	35–50 g/L		3.5–5.0 g/dL
Aldolase	Newborn: <32 U/L Child: <16 Adult: <8		Same as SI

(Continued)

Blood
(Continued)

Test	SI Reference Range	Conversion Factor	Conventional Units Reference Range
Aldosterone	Newborn: 0.14–1.66 nmol/L 1 wk–1 yr: 0.03–4.43 1–3 yr: 0.14–1.66 3–5 yr: <0.14–2.22 5–7 yr: <0.14–1.39 7–11 yr: 0.14–1.94 11–15 yr: <0.14–1.39	nmol/L × 36.1 = ng/dL	Newborn: 5–60 ng/dL 1 wk–1 yr: 1–160 ng/dL 1–3 yr: 5–60 ng/dL 3–5 yr: <5–80 5–7 yr: <5–50 7–11 yr: 5–70 11–15 yr: <5–50
Alkaline phosphatase	Infant: 150–400 U/L 2–10 yr: 100–300 11–18 yr (M): 50–375 11–18 yr (F): 30–300 Adult: 30–100		Same as SI
α_1-antitrypsin	2–4 g/L		200–400 mg/dL
α-fetoprotein	Fetal: peak of 2–4 g/L Cord: <0.05 g/L >1 yr: <30 μg/L		Fetal: 200–400 mg/dL Cord: <5 >1 yr: <30
Ammonia nitrogen	9–34 μmol/L	μmol/L × 1.4 = μg/dL	13–48 μg/dL
Amylase	Newborn: 5–65 U/L >1 yr: 25–125		Same as SI
Androstenedione	Child: 0.17–1.7 nmol/L Adult (M): 2.4–5.2 Adult (F): 2.7–8.0	nmol/L × 28.7 = ng/dL	Child: 5–50 ng/dL Adult (M): 70–150 Adult (F): 76–228
Angiotensin-converting enzyme	<670 nmol·L^{-1}·S^{-1}	nmol·L^{-1}·S^{-1} × 0.06 = nmol/mL/min	<40 nmol/mL/min
Anion gap [Na − (Cl + HCO$_3$)]	7–14 mmol/L		7–14 mEq/L
Aspartate amino-transferase (AST)	<1 yr: 15–60 U/L >1 yr: ≤20 U/L		Same as SI
Bicarbonate	<2 yrs: 20–25 mmol/L >2 yrs: 22–26 mmol/L		<2 yrs: 20–25 mEq/L >2 yrs: 22–26
Bilirubin (total)	_Preterm_ _Full term_ Cord: <34 <34 μmol/L 0–1 d: <137 <103 1–2 d: <205 <137 3–5 d: <274 <205 Thereafter: <34 <17	μmol/L × 0.05848 = mg/dL	_Preterm_ _Full term_ Cord: <2 <2 mg/dL 0–1 d: <8 <6 1–2 d: <12 <8 3–5 d: <16 <12 Thereafter: <2 <1
Bilirubin (conjugated)	0–3.4 μmol/L	μmol/L × 0.05848 = mg/dL	0–0.2 mg/dL
Calcium (ionized)	1.12–1.23 mmol/L	mmol/L × 4 = mg/dL	4.48–4.92 mg/dL
Calcium (total)	Preterm <1 wk: 1.5–2.5 mmol/L Term: <1 wk: 1.75–3 Child: 2–2.6 Adult: 2.1–2.6	mmol/L × 4 = mg/dL	6–10 mg/dL 7–12 8–10.5 8.5–10.5
Carbon dioxide (CO$_2$ content)	22–26 mmol/L		22–26 mEq/L
Carbon monoxide (carboxyhemoglobin)	_% total HB_ Nonsmokers: <0.02 Smokers: <0.01 Toxic: >0.20		_Fraction of HB sat_ Nonsmokers: <2 Smokers: <10 Toxic: >20
Carotene	Infant: 0.37–1.30 μmol/L Child: 0.74–2.42 Adult: 1.12–3.72	μmol/L × 53.7 = μg/dL	Infant: 20–70 μg/dL Child: 40–130 Adult: 60–200
Ceruloplasmin	1–12 yr: 300–650 mg/L >12 yr: 150–600 mg/L		1–12 yr: 30–65 mg/dL >12 yr: 15–60

(Continued)

Blood
(Continued)

Test	SI Reference Range	Conversion Factor	Conventional Units Reference Range
Chloride	94–106 mmol/L		94–106 mEq/L
Cholesterol	Infant: 1.81–4.53 mmol/L	mmol/L × 38.61 = mg/dL	Infant: 53–135 mg/dL
	Child: 3.11–5.18		Child: 70–175
	Adolescent: 3.11–5.44		Adolescent: 120–200
	Adult: 3.63–6.48		Adult: 140–250
Complement, C_3	1 mo: 0.61–1.30 g/L		1 mo: 61–130 mg/dL
	6 mo: 0.87–1.36		6 mo: 87–136
	Adult: 1.11–1.71		Adult: 111–171
Complement, C_4	Newborn: 0.16–0.39 g/L		Newborn: 16–39 mg/dL
	Adult: 0.15–0.45 g/L		Adult: 15–45
Complement, total hemolytic (CH 50)	75–160 U/mL		75–160 U/mL
Copper	0–6 mo: 3.1–11 µmol/L	µmol/L × 6.353 = µg/dL	0–6 mo: 20–70 µg/dL
	6 yr: 14–30		6 yr: 90–190
	12 yr: 12.6–25		12 yr: 80–160
	Adult (M): 11–22		Adult (M): 70–140
	Adult (F): 12.6–24		Adult (F): 80–155
Cortisol	0800 h (or pre-ACTH): 225–505 nmol/L	nmol/L × 0.0362 = µg/dL	0800 h (or pre-ACTH): 8–18 µg/dL
	Post-ACTH: twice pre-ACTH value		Post-ACTH: twice pre-ACTH value
Creatine kinase	Newborn: 76–600 U/L		Same as SI
	Adult (M): 38–174		
	Adult (F): 96–140		
Creatine kinase isoenzymes	_Fraction of total activity_		_% Activity_
	CK-BB (CK-1): absent or trace		CK-BB (CK-1): absent or trace
	CK-MB (CK-2): 0.04–0.06		CK-MB (CK-2): 4%–6%
	CK-MM (CK-3): 0.94–0.96		CK-MM (CK-3): 94%–96%
Creatinine	Newborn: 27–88 µmol/L	µmol/L × 0.0113 = mg/dL	Newborn: 0.3–1.0 mg/dL
	Infant: 18–35		Infant: 0.2–0.4
	Child: 27–62		Child: 0.3–0.7
	Adolescent: 44–88		Adolescent: 0.5–1.0
	Adult (M): 53–106		Adult (M): 0.6–1.2
	Adult (F): 44–97		Adult (F): 0.5–1.1
Dehydroepiandrosterone (DHEA)	Child: 3–10 nmol/L	nmol/L × 0.2884 = µg/L	Child: 1–3 µg/L
	Adult (M): 6–15		Adult (M): 1.7–4.2
	Adult (F): 7–18		Adult (F): 2–5.2
Dehydroepiandrosterone sulfate (DHEA-S)	1–4 days: <52 µmol/L	µmol/L × 0.37 = µg/mL	1–4 days: <20 µg/mL
	Child: 1.6–6.6		Child: 0.6–2.54
Estradiol	_Males_	pmol/L × 0.2723 = pg/mL	
	Pubertal stage: I: 7–29 pmol/L		2–8 pg/mL
	II: 40		11
	III: >73		>20
	Adult: 29–132		8–36
	Females		
	Pubertal stage: I: 0–84 pmol/L		0–23 pg/mL
	II: 0–242		0–66
	III: 0–385		0–105
	IV: 73–1101		20–300
	Follicular: 37–330		10–90
	Midcycle: 367–1835		100–500
	Luteal: 184–881		50–240
Free fatty acids	Child: <1.10 mmol/L	mmol/L × 28.25 = mg/dL	Child: <31 mg/dL
	Adult: 0.3–0.9		Adult: 8–25

(Continued)

Blood
(Continued)

Test	SI Reference Range	Conversion Factor	Conventional Units Reference Range
Ferritin	Child: 7–144 μg/L		Child: 7–144 ng/mL
	Adult (M): 30–265		Adult (M): 30–265
	Adult (F): 10–110		Adult (F): 10–110
Fibrinogen	2–4 g/L		200–400 mg/dL
Folate	4–20 nmol/L	nmol/L × 0.4413 = ng/mL	1.8–9.0 ng/mL
Folate (RBCs)	340–1020 nmol/L packed cells	nmol/L × 0.4413 = ng/mL	150–450 ng/mL
Follicle-stimulating hormone (FSH)	Prepubertal: <5 IU/L		Prepubertal: <5 mIU/mL
	Adult (M): 1.5–16		Adult (M): 1.5–16
	Adult (F): 2–17.2		Adult (F): 2–17.2
Fructose	55–330 μmol/L	μmol/L × 0.018 = mg/dL	1–6 mg/dL
Galactose	Newborn: 0–1.11 mmol/L	mmol/L × 18.02 = mg/dL	Newborn: 0–20 mg/dL
	Thereafter: <0.28		Thereafter: <5
Gamma glutamyl transferase (GGT)	0–3 wk: 0–130 U/L		Same as SI
	3 wk–3 mo: 4–120		
	3 mo–1 yr (M): 5–65		
	3 mo–1 yr (F): 5–35		
	1–15 yr: 0–23		
	Adult: 0–35		
Gastrin	<100 ng/L		<100 pg/mL
Glucagon	50–100 ng/L		50–100 pg/mL
Glucose	Preterm: 1.1–3.6 mmol/L	mmol/L × 18.02 = mg/dL	Preterm: 20–65 mg/dL
	Full term: 1.1–6.1		Full term: 20–110
	1 wk–16 yr: 3.3–5.8		1 wk–16 yr: 60–105
	>16 yr: 3.9–6.4		>16 yr: 70–115
Haptoglobin	0.4–1.8 g/L		40–180 mg/dL
Hemoglobin A$_{1c}$	0.039–0.077 fraction of total Hb		3.9%–7.7% of total Hb
β-Hydroxybutyrate	<100 μmol/L	μmol/L × 0.01041 = mg/dL	<1 mg/dL
17-Hydroxyprogesterone	Prepubertal (M): 0.3–0.91 nmol/L	nmol/L × 0.33 = ng/mL	Prepubertal (M): 0.1–0.3 ng/mL
	Prepubertal (F): 0.61–1.52		Prepubertal (F): 0.2–0.5
	Adult (M): 0.61–5.45		Adult (M): 0.2–1.8
	Adult (F):		Adult (F):
	Follicular: 0.61–2.42		Follicular: 0.2–0.8
	Luteal: 2.42–9.10		Luteal: 0.8–3.0
Immunoglobulins A, G, M	*IgA*	*IgG*	*IgM*
	Newborn: 0–0.05 g/L	6.4–16 g/L	0.06–0.24 g/L
	1–3 mo: 0.03–0.66	3.0–10.0	0.15–1.50
	3–6 mo: 0.04–0.90	1.4–10.0	0.15–1.10
	6–12 mo: 0.45–2.25	4.0–11.5	0.43–2.25
	1–2 yr: 0.35–2.40	3.5–12.0	0.36–2.40
	2–6 yr: 0.40–1.90	5.0–13.0	0.50–1.99
	6–12 yr: 0.40–2.70	7.0–16.5	0.50–2.60
	12–16 yr: 0.50–2.32	7.0–15.5	0.45–2.40
	Adult: 0.70–3.90	6.5–15.0	0.40–3.4
Immunoglobulin E	Newborn: 0–24 μg/L		Newborn: 0–10 U/mL
	6–12 yr: 0–480		6–12 yr: 0–200
	Adult: 0–960		Adult: 0–400
Insulin, fasting	3–23 mU/L		3–23 μU/mL
Iron	Newborn: 20–48 μmol/L	μmol/L × 5.587 = μg/dL	Newborn: 110–270 μg/dL
	4–10 mo: 5.4–12.5		4–10 mo: 30–70
	3–10 yr: 9.5–27.0		3–10 yr: 53–119
	Adult: 13.0–33.0		Adult: 72–186

Blood
(Continued)

Test	SI Reference Range	Conversion Factor	Conventional Units Reference Range
Iron-binding capacity	Newborn: 10.6–31.3 μmol/L Thereafter: 45–72	μmol/L × 5.587 = μg/dL	Newborn: 59–175 μg/dL Thereafter: 250–400
Lactate	Venous: 0.5–2.0 mmol/L Arterial: 0.3–0.8	mmol/L × 9.01 = mg/dL	Venous: 5–18 mg/dL Arterial: 3–7
Lactate dehydrogenase	Newborn: 160–1500 U/L Infant: 150–360 Child: 150–300 Adult: 100–250		Same as SI units
Lactate dehydrogenase isoenzymes		*Fraction of total* LD 1 (heart): 0.24–0.34 LD 2 (heart, RBCs): 0.35–0.45 LD 3 (muscle): 0.15–0.25 LD 4 (liver, muscle): 0.04–0.10 LD 5 (liver, muscle): 0.01–0.09	
Lead	<1.16 μmol/L	μmol/L × 20.7 = μg/dL	<24 μg/dL

Lipids	95th %ile values—mmol/L (mg/dL)		5th %ile values—mmol/L (mg/dL)

	VLDL (Cholesterol)	*LDL (Cholesterol)*	*HDL (Cholesterol)*
	M — F	M — F	M — F
5–9 yr:	0.47 (18) 0.62 (24)	3.34 (129) 3.62 (140)	0.98 (38) 0.93 (36)
10–14 yr:	0.57 (22) 0.59 (23)	3.41 (132) 3.52 (136)	0.96 (37) 0.91 (35)
15–19 yr:	0.67 (26) 0.62 (24)	3.36 (130) 3.49 (135)	0.80 (31) 0.91 (35)
		mmol/L × 38.61 = mg/dL	

Test	SI Reference Range	Conversion Factor	Conventional Units Reference Range
Luteinizing hormone	Prepubertal: <5 IU/L Adult (M): 3.9–18 Adult (F): 2.0–22.6		Prepubertal: <5 mIU/mL Adult (M): 3.9–18 Adult (F): 2.0–22.6
Magnesium	0.75–1.0 mmol/L	mmol/L × 2 = mEq/L	1.5–2.0 mEq/L
Methemoglobin	<46 μmol/L	μmol/L × 0.0065 = g/dL	<0.3 g/dL
Osmolality	285–295 mmol/kg		285–295 mOsm/kg
Phosphorus	Newborn: 1.36–2.91 mmol/L 1 yr: 1.23–2.00 2–5 yr: 1.13–2.20 Adult: 0.97–1.45	mmol/L × 3.097 = mg/dL	Newborn: 4.2–9.0 mg/dL 1 yr: 3.8–6.2 2–5 yr: 3.5–6.8 Adult: 3.0–4.5
Phytanic acid	<0.003 fraction of total serum fatty acids		<0.3% of total serum fatty acids
Potassium	<10 days: 3.5–6.0 mmol/L >10 days: 3.5–5.0		<10 days: 3.5–6.0 mEq/L >10 days: 3.5–5.0
Progesterone	*Males* Prepubertal: 0.35–0.83 nmol/L Adult: 0.38–0.95	nmol/L × 0.314 = ng/mL	0.11–0.26 ng/mL 0.12–0.30
	Females Prepubertal: ≤0.95 Pubertal stage II: ≤1.46 III: ≤1.91 IV: 0.16–41.34 Follicular: 0.06–2.86 Luteal: 19.08–95.40		≤0.30 ≤0.46 ≤0.60 0.05–13.0 0.02–0.9 6.0–30.0
Prolactin	Newborn: <200 μg/L Adult: <20 μg/L		Newborn: <200 ng/mL Adult: <20 ng/mL
Protein, total	Preterm: 40–70 g/L Term newborn: 50–71 1–3 mo: 47–74		Preterm: 4.0–7.0 g/dL Term newborn: 5.0–7.1 1–3 mo: 4.7–7.4

(Continued)

Blood
(Continued)

Test	SI Reference Range	Conversion Factor	Conventional Units Reference Range
	3–12 mo: 50–75		3–12 mo: 5.0–7.5
	1–15 yr: 65–86		1–15 yr: 6.5–8.6
Pyruvate	0.03–0.10 mmol/L	mmol/L × 8.81 = mg/dL	0.3–0.9 mg/dL
Renin	Adults: 0.30–1.14 ng·L⁻¹·S⁻¹	ng·L⁻¹·S⁻¹ × 3.6 = ng/mL/h	Adults: 1.1–4.1 ng/mL/h
Sodium	135–145 mmol/L		135–145 mEq/L
Somatomedin C	0–2 yr: 220–1000 IU/L		0–2 yr: 0.22–1.00 U/mL
	3–5 yr: 270–1600		3–5 yr: 0.27–1.60
	6–10 yr: 370–2100		6–10 yr: 0.37–2.10
	11–12 yr: 450–2800		11–12 yr: 0.45–2.80
	13–14 yr: 1100–4000		13–14 yr: 1.10–4.00
	15–17 yr: 1000–2900		15–17 yr: 1.00–2.90
	Thereafter: 460–1500		Thereafter: 0.46–1.50
Testosterone, free	Prepubertal: 2.08–13.19 pmol/L		Prepubertal: 0.06–0.38 ng/dL
	Adult (M): 48.6–201		Adult (M): 1.40–5.79
	Adult (F): 6.94–25		Adult (F): 0.20–0.73
Testosterone, total	Prepubertal: 0.35–0.70 nmol/L		Prepubertal: 10–20 ng/dL
	Adult (F): 0.8–2.6		Adult (F): 23–75
	Adult (M): 9.5–30		Adult (M): 275–875
Thyroid-stimulating hormone (TSH)	Cord: 0–17.4 μU/L		Cord: 0–17.4 mIU/mL
	1–3 days: 0–13.3		1–3 days: 0–13.3
	Thereafter: 0–5.5		Thereafter: 0–5.5
Thyroxine (T₄), total	Cord: 95–168 nmol/L	nmol/L × 0.0775 = μg/dL	Cord: 7.4–13.0 μg/dL
	<1 mo: 90–292		<1 mo: 7.0–22.6
	1 mo–1 yr: 93–213		1 mo–1 yr: 7.2–16.5
	1–5 yr: 94–194		1–5 yr: 7.3–15.0
	5–10 yr: 83–172		5–10 yr: 6.4–13.3
	10–15 yr: 72–151		10–15 yr: 5.6–11.7
	Adult: 55–161		Adult: 4.3–12.5
Thyroxine (T₄), free	9–22 pmol/L	pmol/L × 0.0777 = ng/dL	0.7–1.7 ng/dL
Transferrin	Newborn: 1.30–2.75 g/L		Newborn: 130–275 mg/dL
	Adult: 2.20–4.00		Adult: 220–400

Triglycerides	Normal upper limits—mmol/L (mg/dL)		
	Male	*Female*	
	0–4 yr: 1.12 (99)	1.26 (112)	
	5–9 yr: 1.14 (101)	1.19 (105)	
	10–14 yr: 1.41 (125)	1.48 (131)	
	15–19 yr: 1.67 (148)	1.40 (124)	
		mmol/L × 88.55 = mg/dL	

Test	SI Reference Range	Conversion Factor	Conventional Units Reference Range
Triiodothyronine (T₃)	Cord: 0.23–1.16 nmol/L	nmol/L × 65.1 = ng/dL	Cord: 15–75 ng/dL
	<1 mo: 0.49–3.70		<1 mo: 32–240
	1 mo–1 yr: 1.70–4.31		1 mo–1 yr: 110–280
	1–5 yr: 1.62–4.14		1–5 yr: 105–269
	5–10 yr: 1.45–3.71		5–10 yr: 94–241
	10–15 yr: 1.28–3.31		10–15 yr: 83–215
	Adult: 1.08–3.14		Adult: 70–204
Triiodothyronine-resin uptake	0.25–0.35		25%–35%
Urea nitrogen	2–7 mmol/L	mmol/L × 2.8 = mg/dL	5–20 mg/dL
Uric acid	120–420 μmol/L	μmol/L × 0.0169 = mg/dL	2–7 mg/dL
Vitamin A	Newborn: 1.22–2.62 μmol/L	μmol/L × 28.65 = μg/dL	Newborn: 35–75 μg/dL
	Child: 1.05–2.79		Child: 30–80
	Adult: 1.05–2.27		Adult: 30–65

(Continued)

Blood
(Continued)

Test	SI Reference Range	Conversion Factor	Conventional Units Reference Range
Vitamin B_6	14.6–72.8 nmol/L	nmol/L × 0.247 = ng/mL	3.6–18 ng/mL
Vitamin B_{12}	96–579 pmol/L	pmol/L × 1.355 = pg/mL	130–785 pg/mL
Vitamin C	11.4–113.6 μmol/L	μmol/L × 0.176 = mg/dL	0.2–2.0 mg/dL
Vitamin D_3 (1,25 dihydroxy)	60–108 pmol/L	pmol/L × 0.417 = pg/mL	25–45 pg/mL
Vitamin E	11.6–46.4 μmol/L	μmol/L × 0.043 = mg/dL	0.5–2.0 mg/dL
Zinc	10.7–22.9 μmol/L	μmol/L × 6.54 = μg/dL	70–150 μg/dL

Hematology

Age	HB (g/dL) Mean	HB (g/dL) −2 SD	Hematocrit (%) Mean	Hematocrit (%) −2 SD	MCV (fL) Mean	MCV (fL) −2 SD	MCHC (g/dL RBC) Mean	MCHC (g/dL RBC) −2 SD	Reticulocyte (%)	WBC (1,000/mm³) Mean	WBC (1,000/mm³) 95% CI	Platelets (1,000/mm³) Mean (Range)
Term (cord blood)	16.5	13.5	51	42	108	98	33.0	30.0	3.0–7.0	18.1	9.0–30.0	290
1–3 days	18.5	14.5	56	45	108	95	33.0	29.0	1.8–4.6	18.9	9.4–34.0	192
2 weeks	16.6	13.4	53	41	105	88	31.4	28.1		11.4	5.0–20.0	252
1 month	13.9	10.7	44	33	101	91	31.8	28.1	0.1–1.7	10.8	5.0–19.5	
2 months	11.2	9.4	35	28	95	84	31.8	28.3				
6 months	12.6	11.1	36	31	76	68	35.0	32.7	0.7–2.3	11.9	6.0–17.5	
6–24 months	12.0	10.5	36	33	78	70	33.0	30.0		10.6	6.0–17.0	(150–300)
2–6 years	12.5	11.5	37	34	81	75	34.0	31.0	0.5–1.0	8.5	5.0–15.5	(150–300)
6–12 years	13.5	11.5	40	35	86	77	34.0	31.0	0.5–1.0	8.1	4.5–13.5	(150–300)
12–18 years (M)	14.5	13.0	43	36	88	78	34.0	31.0	0.5–1.0	7.8	4.5–13.5	(150–300)
12–18 years (F)	14.0	12.0	41	37	90	78	34.0	31.0	0.5–1.0	7.8	4.5–13.5	(150–300)

Urine

Test	SI Reference Range	Conversion Factor	Conventional Units Reference Range
Aminolevulinic acid	8–53 μmol/d	μmol/d × 0.131 = mg/d	1–7 mg/d
Calcium	<0.1 mmol/kg/d	mmol/d × 40 = mg/d	<4 mg/kg/d
Copper	<0.6 μmol/d	μmol/d × 63.7 = μg/d	<40 μg/d
Coproporphyrin	<300 nmol/d	nmol/d × 1.527 = μg/d	<200 μg/d
Cortisol, free	70–340 nmol/d	nmol/d × 0.362 = μg/d	25–125 μg/d
Creatinine	Infant: 71–177 μmol/kg/d	μmol/kg/d × 0.113 = mg/kg/d	Infant: 8–20 mg/kg/d
	Child: 71–194		Child: 8–22
	Adolescent: 71–265		Adolescent: 8–30
Cystine	40–260 μmol/d	μmol/d × 0.12 = mg/d	5–31 mg/d
Dehydroepiandrosterone (DHEA)	<5 yr: <0.3 μmol/d	μmol/d × 0.288 = mg/d	<5 yr: <0.1 mg/d
	6–9 yr: <0.7		6–9 yr: <0.2
	10–15 yr: <1.4		10–15 yr: <0.4
	Adult (M): <8.0		Adult (M): <2.3
	Adult (F): <4.2		Adult (F): <1.2
Epinephrine	<55 nmol/d	nmol/d × 0.183 = μg/d	<10 μg/d

Urine
(Continued)

Test	SI Reference Range	Conversion Factor	Conventional Units Reference Range
Fluoride	<50 μmol/d	μmol/d × 0.019 = mg/d	<1 mg/d
Homovanillic acid (HVA)	*mmol/mol creatinine*	mmol/mol creatinine × 1.61 = μg/mg creatinine	*μg/mg creatinine*
	1–12 mo: 0.75–21.7		1–12 mo: 1.2–35.0
	1–2 yr: 2.5–14.3		1–2 yr: 4.0–23.0
	2–5 yr: 0.43–8.4		2–5 yr: 0.7–13.5
	5–10 yr: 0.31–5.6		5–10 yr: 0.5–9.0
	10–15 yr: 0.15–7.4		10–15 yr: 0.25–12.0
	15–18 yr: 0.31–1.24		15–18 yr: 0.5–2.0
Metanephrines	*mmol/mol creatinine*	mmol/mol creatinine × 1.74 = μg/mg creatinine	*μg/mg creatinine*
	<1 yr: 0.001–2.64		<1 yr: 0.001–4.6
	1–2 yr: 0.15–3.09		1–2 yr: 0.27–5.38
	2–5 yr: 0.20–1.72		2–5 yr: 0.35–2.99
	5–10 yr: 0.25–1.55		5–10 yr: 0.43–2.70
	10–15 yr: 0.001–0.38		10–15 yr: 0.001–1.87
	15–18 yr: 0.03–0.69		15–18 yr: 0.001–0.67
Norepinephrine	<590 nmol/d	nmol/d × 0.169 = μg/d	<100 μg/d
Osmolality	50–1200 μmol/kg		50–1200 mOsm/kg
Oxalate	110–440 μmol/d	μmol/d × 0.088 = mg/d	10–40 mg/d
Porphobilinogen	0–8.8 μmol/d	μmol/d × 0.226 × mg/d	0–2 mg/d
Potassium	25–125 mmol/d (varies with diet)		25–125 mEq/d
Pregnanetriol	<7.4 μmol/d	μmol/d × 0.3365 = mg/d	<2.5 mg/d
Protein	10–140 mg/L		1–14 mg/dL
Steroids: 17-hydroxycortico-steroid	Prepubertal: 2.76–15.5 μmol/d	μmol/d × 0.3625 = mg/d	Prepubertal: 1–5.6 mg/d
	Adult (M): 11–33		Adult (M): 4–12
	Adult (F): 11–22		Adult (F): 4–8
Steroids: 17-ketosteroids	<1 mo: ≤6.9 μmol/d	μmol/d × 0.2884 = mg/d	<1 mo: ≤2 mg/d
	1 mo–5 yr: <1.73		1 mo–5 yr: <0.5
	6–8 yr: 3.47–6.9		6–8 yr: 1–2
	Adult (M): 21–62		Adult (M): 6–18
	Adult (F): 14–45		Adult (F): 4–13
Uric acid	1.48–4.43 mmol/d	mmol/d × 169 = mg/d	250–750 mg/d
Vanilylmandelic acid (VMA)	*mmol/mol creatinine*	mmol/mol creatinine × 1.75 = μg/mg	*μg/mg creatinine*
	1–6 mo: 1.71–9.71		1–6 mo: 3–7
	6–12 mo: 1.14–8.57		6–12 mo: 2–15
	1–5 yr: 1.14–5.71		1–5 yr: 2–10
	5–10 yr: 0.86–4.00		5–10 yr: 1.5–7
	10–15 yr: 0.57–3.43		10–15 yr: 1–6
	>15 yr: 0.57–3.43		>15 yr: 1–6

Cerebrospinal Fluid

Cell Count Range

Preterm: 0–25 WBC $\times$ 10^6 cells/L (57% polymorphonuclears)

Term: 0–22 WBC $\times$ 10^6 cells/L (61% polymorphonuclears)

Child: 0–7 WBC $\times$ 10^6 cells/L (0% polymorphonuclears)

Cell Count Percentiles

	Total WBC			Polymorphonuclears			Monocytes		
	25%	50%	75%	25%	50%	75%	25%	50%	75%
<6 wk	0.50	2.57	5.16	0	0	2.42	0	0.83	2.71
6 wk–3 mo	0.34	1.86	3.75	0	0	0.66	0	0.96	2.78
3–6 mo	0.00	1.11	2.31	0	0	0.40	0	0.43	1.64
6–12 mo	0.41	1.47	3.25	0	0	0.52	0.03	0.93	2.32
>12 mo	0.00	0.68	1.82	0	0	0	0	0.25	1.45

Test	SI Reference Range	Conventional Units Reference Range
Glucose	Preterm: 1.3–3.5 mmol/L	Preterm: 24–63 mg/dL
	Term: 1.9–6.6	Term: 34–119
	Child: 2.2–4.4	Child: 40–80
Protein	Preterm: 0.65–1.50 g/L	Preterm: 65–150 mg/dL
	Term: 0.20–1.70	Term: 20–170
	Child: 0.05–0.40	Child: 5–40
Pressure	<200 mm H_2O	<200 mm H_2O

This table was prepared by Peter C. Rowe, Assistant Professor of Pediatrics, University of Ottawa School of Medicine, Children's Hospital of Eastern Ontario, Ottawa, Ontario, Canada, and is borrowed from Oski FA, DeAngelis CD, Feigin RD, and Warshaw JB (eds.) (1990). *Principles and practice of pediatrics.* Philadelphia: J.B. Lippincott Co., with permission.

APPENDIX B Physical Growth Charts
(NCHS Percentiles)

BOYS: BIRTH TO 36 MONTHS
PHYSICAL GROWTH
NCHS PERCENTILES*

NAME _____   RECORD # _____

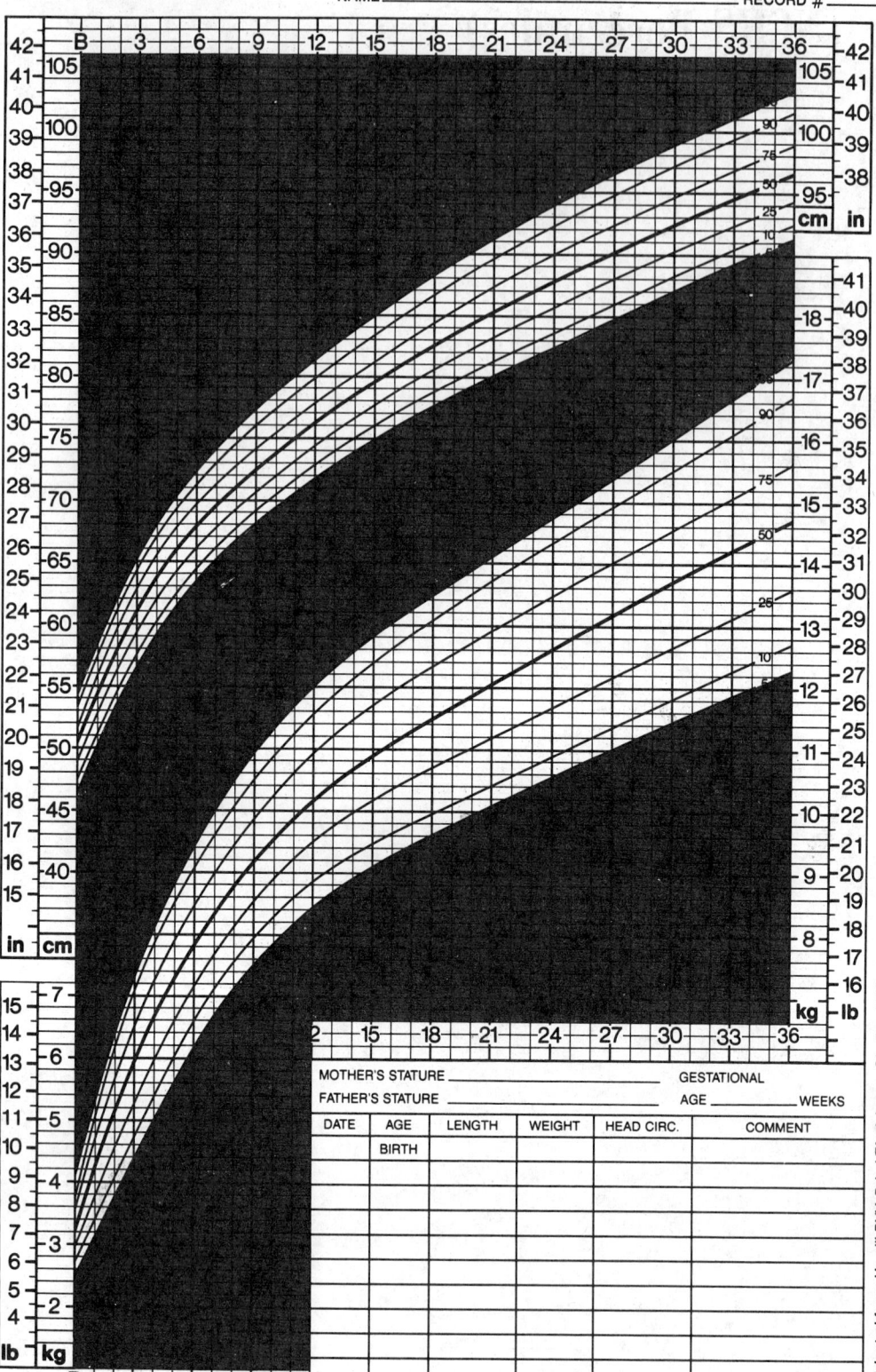

MOTHER'S STATURE _____   GESTATIONAL

FATHER'S STATURE _____   AGE _____ WEEKS

DATE	AGE	LENGTH	WEIGHT	HEAD CIRC.	COMMENT
	BIRTH				

Ross
Growth &
Development
Program

*Adapted from: Hamill PVV, Drizd TA, Johnson CL, Reed RB, Roche AF, Moore WM: Physical growth: National Center for Health Statistics percentiles. AM J CLIN NUTR 32:607-629, 1979. Data from the Fels Longitudinal Study, Wright State University School of Medicine, Yellow Springs, Ohio.

© 1982 Ross Laboratories

BOYS: BIRTH TO 36 MONTHS
PHYSICAL GROWTH
NCHS PERCENTILES*

NAME _____   RECORD # _____

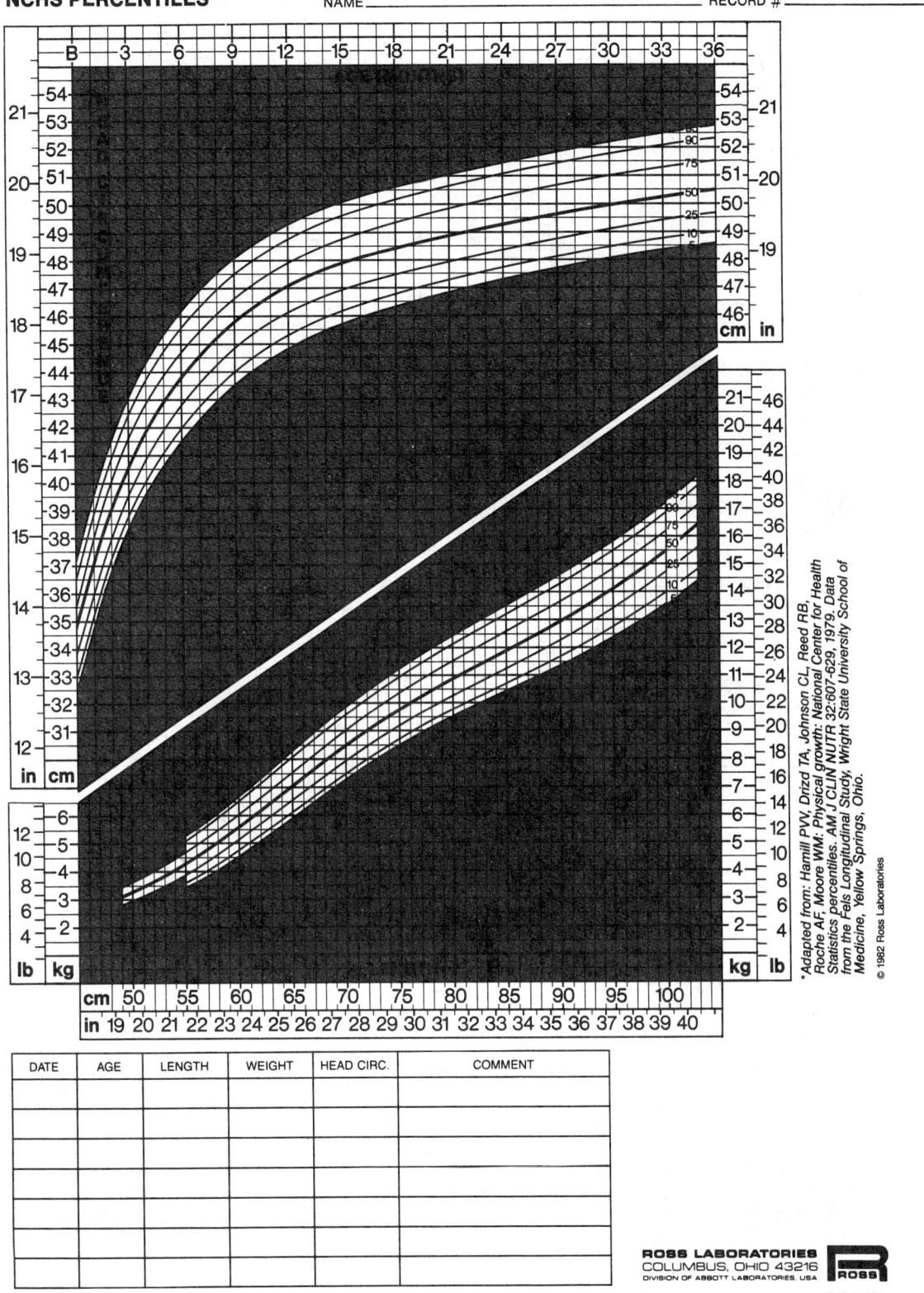

*Adapted from: Hamill PVV, Drizd TA, Johnson CL, Reed RB, Roche AF, Moore WM: Physical growth: National Center for Health Statistics percentiles. AM J CLIN NUTR 32:607-629, 1979. Data from the Fels Longitudinal Study, Wright State University School of Medicine, Yellow Springs, Ohio.

© 1982 Ross Laboratories

DATE	AGE	LENGTH	WEIGHT	HEAD CIRC.	COMMENT

ROSS LABORATORIES
COLUMBUS, OHIO 43216
DIVISION OF ABBOTT LABORATORIES, USA

G105(0.05)/JANUARY 1986   LITHO IN USA

GIRLS: BIRTH TO 36 MONTHS
PHYSICAL GROWTH
NCHS PERCENTILES*

NAME _____ RECORD # _____

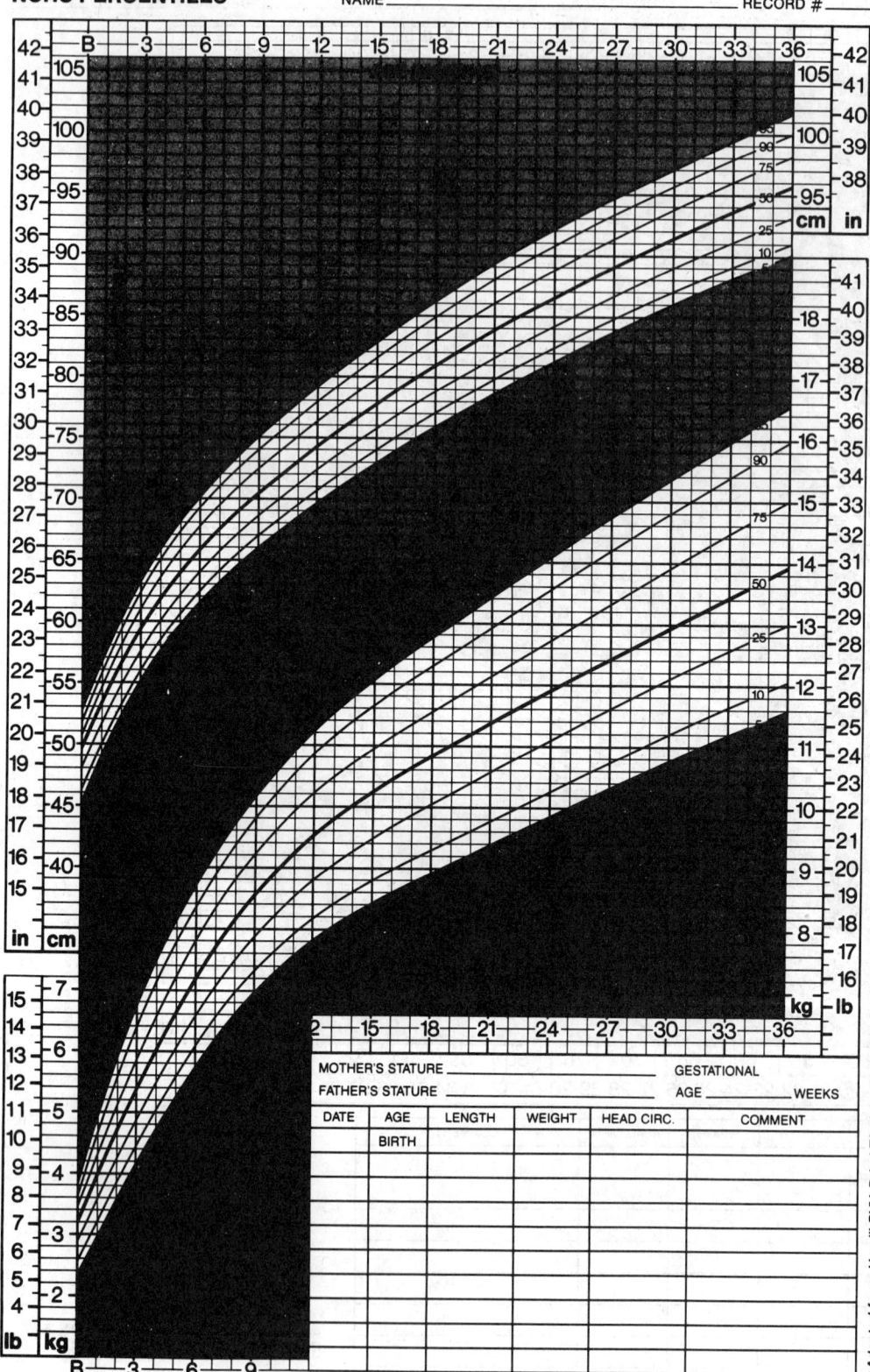

* Adapted from: Hamill PVV, Drizd TA, Johnson CL, Reed RB, Roche AF, Moore WM: Physical growth: National Center for Health Statistics percentiles. AM J CLIN NUTR 32:607-629, 1979. Data from the Fels Longitudinal Study, Wright State University School of Medicine, Yellow Springs, Ohio.

© 1982 Ross Laboratories

Ross Growth & Development Program

DATE	AGE	LENGTH	WEIGHT	HEAD CIRC.	COMMENT
	BIRTH				

MOTHER'S STATURE _____ GESTATIONAL
FATHER'S STATURE _____ AGE ___ WEEKS

GIRLS: BIRTH TO 36 MONTHS
PHYSICAL GROWTH
NCHS PERCENTILES*

NAME _____   RECORD # _____

* Adapted from: Hamill PVV, Drizd TA, Johnson CL, Reed RB, Roche AF, Moore WM: Physical growth: National Center for Health Statistics percentiles. AM J CLIN NUTR 32:607-629, 1979. Data from the Fels Longitudinal Study, Wright State University School of Medicine, Yellow Springs, Ohio.

© 1982 Ross Laboratories

DATE	AGE	LENGTH	WEIGHT	HEAD CIRC.	COMMENT

BOYS: 2 TO 18 YEARS
PHYSICAL GROWTH
National Center for Health Statistics Percentiles   NAME_____ RECORD #_____

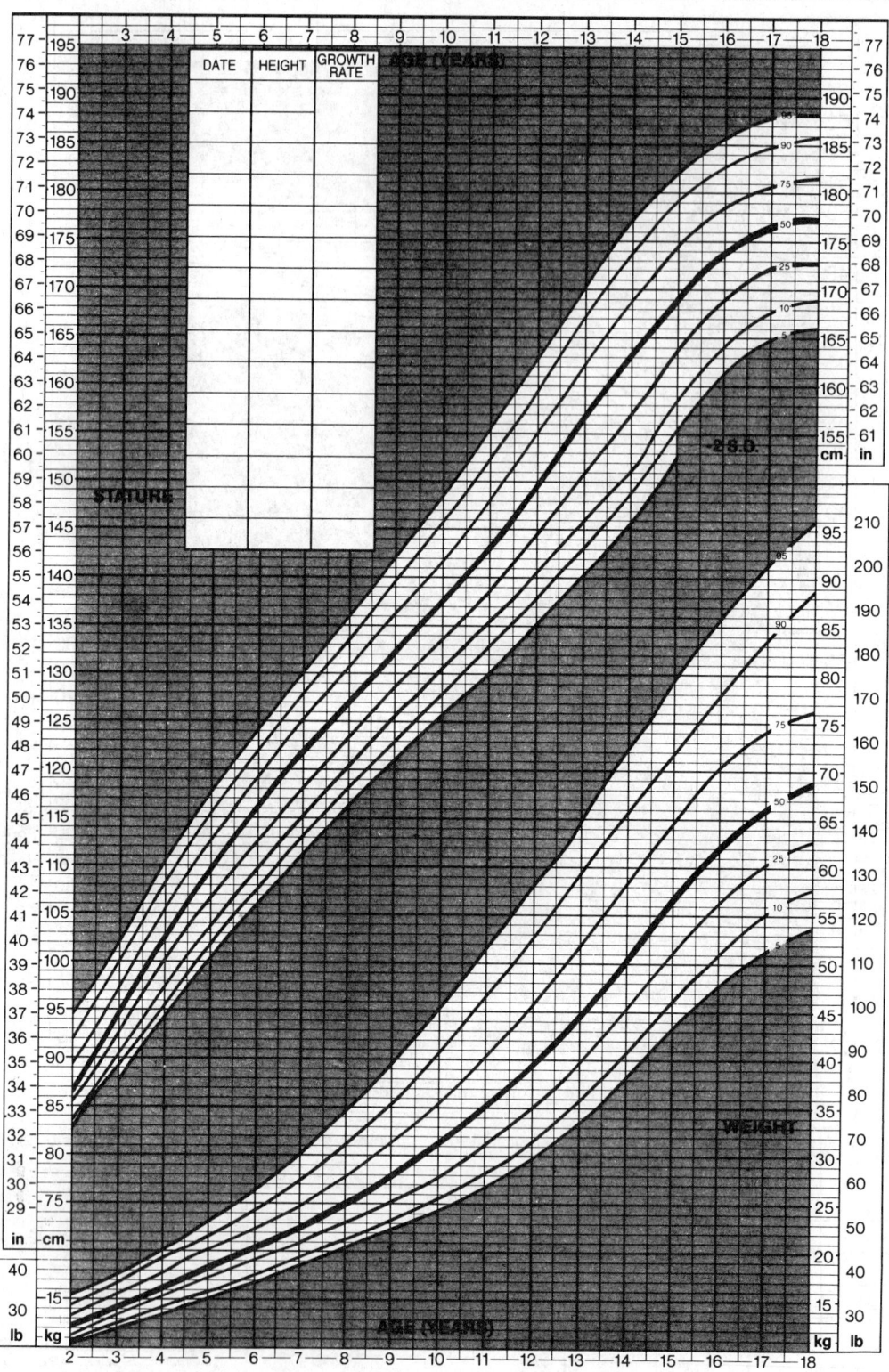

Provided as
a service of
Genentech, Inc

G70048-RO

GIRLS: 2 TO 18 YEARS
PHYSICAL GROWTH
National Center for Health Statistics Percentiles   NAME _____ RECORD # _____

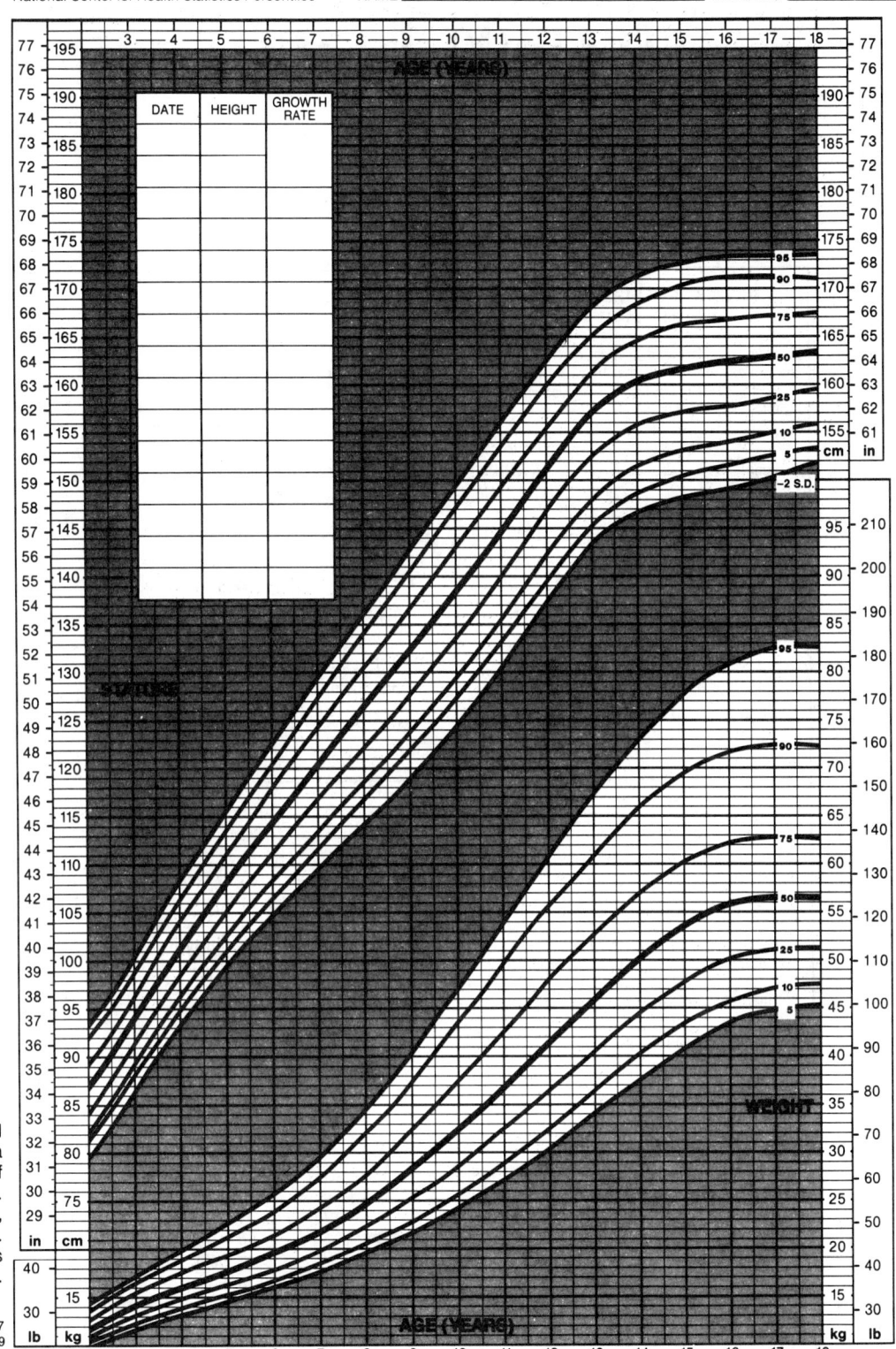

Denver Articulation Screening Exam

DENVER ARTICULATION SCREENING EXAM
for children 2½ to 6 years of age

Instructions: Have child repeat each word after you. Circle the underlined sounds that he pronounces correctly. Total correct sounds is the Raw Score. Use charts on reverse side to score results.

Name:

Hosp. No.:

Address: _____

_____

Date: _____ Child's age: _____ Examiner: _____ Raw score: __
Percentile: _____ Intelligibility: _____ Result: _____

1. table	6. zipper	11. sock	16. wagon	21. leaf
2. shirt	7. grapes	12. vacuum	17. gum	22. carrot
3. door	8. flag	13. yarn	18. house	
4. trunk	9. thumb	14. mother	19. pencil	
5. jumping	10. toothbrush	15. twinkle	20. fish	

Intelligibility: (circle one)
1. Easy to understand
2. Understandable ½ the time
3. Not understandable
4. Can't evaluate

Comments:

Date: _____ Child's age: _____ Examiner: _____ Raw score: __
Percentile: _____ Intelligibility: _____ Result: _____

1. table	6. zipper	11. sock	16. wagon	21. leaf
2. shirt	7. grapes	12. vacuum	17. gum	22. carrot
3. door	8. flag	13. yarn	18. house	
4. trunk	9. thumb	14. mother	19. pencil	
5. jumping	10. toothbrush	15. twinkle	20. fish	

Intelligibility: (circle one)
1. Easy to understand
2. Understandable ½ the time
3. Not understandable
4. Can't evaluate

Comments:

Date: _____ Child's age: _____ Examiner: _____ Raw score: __
Percentile: _____ Intelligibility: _____ Result: _____

1. table	6. zipper	11. sock	16. wagon	21. leaf
2. shirt	7. grapes	12. vacuum	17. gum	22. carrot
3. door	8. flag	13. yarn	18. house	
4. trunk	9. thumb	14. mother	19. pencil	
5. jumping	10. toothbrush	15. twinkle	20. fish	

Intelligibility: (circle one)
1. Easy to understand
2. Understandable ½ the time
3. Not understandable
4. Can't evaluate

Comments:

A

(A) *Denver Articulation Screening Examination (DASE) for children 2½ to 6 years of age.* (B) *Percentile rank. (From A.F. Drumwright, University of Colorado Medical Center, 1971)*

To score DASE words: Note raw score for child's performance. Match raw score line (extreme left of chart) with column representing child's age (to the closest previous age group). Where raw score line and age column meet number in that square denotes percentile rank of child's performance when compared to other children that age. Percentiles above heavy line are ABNORMAL percentiles, below heavy line are NORMAL.

PERCENTILE RANK

Raw Score	2.5 yr.	3.0	3.5	4.0	4.5	5.0	5.5	6 years
2	1							
3	2							
4	5							
5	9							
6	16							
7	23							
8	31	2						
9	37	4	1					
10	42	6	2					
11	48	7	4					
12	54	9	6	1	1			
13	58	12	9	2	3	1	1	
14	62	17	11	5	4	2	2	
15	68	23	15	9	5	3	2	
16	75	31	19	12	5	4	3	
17	79	38	25	15	6	6	4	
18	83	46	31	19	8	7	4	
19	86	51	38	24	10	9	5	1
20	89	58	45	30	12	11	7	3
21	92	65	52	36	15	15	9	4
22	94	72	58	43	18	19	12	5
23	96	77	63	50	22	24	15	7
24	97	82	70	58	29	29	20	15
25	99	87	78	66	36	34	26	17
26	99	91	84	75	46	43	34	24
27		94	89	82	57	54	44	34
28		96	94	88	70	68	59	47
29		98	98	94	84	84	77	68
30		100	100	100	100	100	100	100

To score intelligibility:		**NORMAL**	**ABNORMAL**
	2 ½ years	Understandable ½ the time, or, "easy"	Not understandable
	3 years and older	Easy to understand	Understandable ½ time Not understandable

Test result: 1. NORMAL on Dase and Intelligibility = NORMAL
2. ABNORMAL on Dase and/or Intelligibility = ABNORMAL

*If abnormal on initial screening rescreen within 2 weeks.
If abnormal again child should be referred for complete speech evaluation.

B

APPENDIX D Denver II

(Developmental Screening Test)

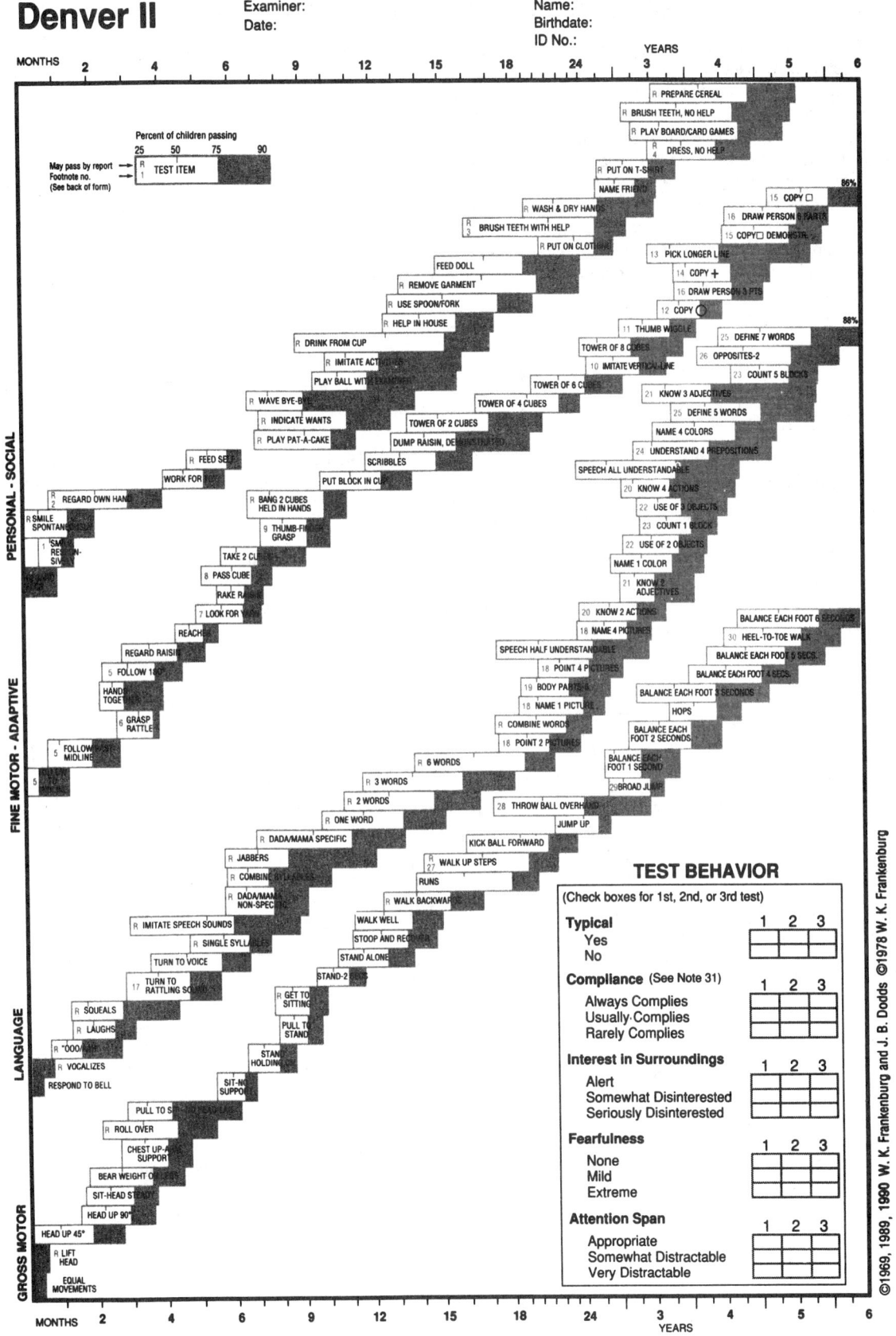

Denver II

Examiner:
Date:

Name:
Birthdate:
ID No.:

©1969, 1989, 1990 W. K. Frankenburg and J. B. Dodds ©1978 W. K. Frankenburg

DIRECTIONS FOR ADMINISTRATION

1. Try to get child to smile by smiling, talking or waving. Do not touch him/her.
2. Child must stare at hand several seconds.
3. Parent may help guide toothbrush and put toothpaste on brush.
4. Child does not have to be able to tie shoes or button/zip in the back.
5. Move yarn slowly in an arc from one side to the other, about 8" above child's face.
6. Pass if child grasps rattle when it is touched to the backs or tips of fingers.
7. Pass if child tries to see where yarn went. Yarn should be dropped quickly from sight from tester's hand without arm movement.
8. Child must transfer cube from hand to hand without help of body, mouth, or table.
9. Pass if child picks up raisin with any part of thumb and finger.
10. Line can vary only 30 degrees or less from tester's line. $\sqrt{}$
11. Make a fist with thumb pointing upward and wiggle only the thumb. Pass if child imitates and does not move any fingers other than the thumb.

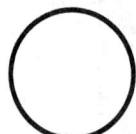   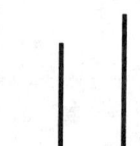   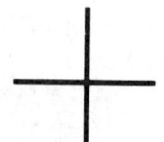   

12. Pass any enclosed form. Fail continuous round motions.
13. Which line is longer? (Not bigger.) Turn paper upside down and repeat. (pass 3 of 3 or 5 of 6)
14. Pass any lines crossing near midpoint.
15. Have child copy first. If failed, demonstrate.

When giving items 12, 14, and 15, do not name the forms. Do not demonstrate 12 and 14.

16. When scoring, each pair (2 arms, 2 legs, etc.) counts as one part.
17. Place one cube in cup and shake gently near child's ear, but out of sight. Repeat for other ear.
18. Point to picture and have child name it. (No credit is given for sounds only.)
   If less than 4 pictures are named correctly, have child point to picture as each is named by tester.

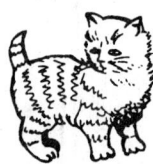   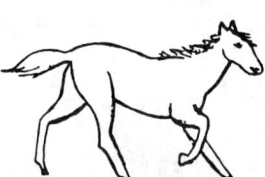   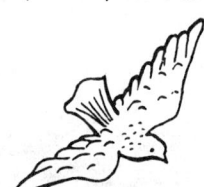   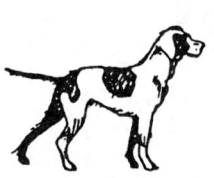   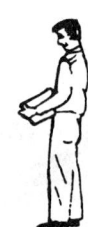

19. Using doll, tell child: Show me the nose, eyes, ears, mouth, hands, feet, tummy, hair. Pass 6 of 8.
20. Using pictures, ask child: Which one flies?... says meow?... talks?... barks?... gallops? Pass 2 of 5, 4 of 5.
21. Ask child: What do you do when you are cold?... tired?... hungry?   Pass 2 of 3, 3 of 3.
22. Ask child: What do you do with a cup? What is a chair used for? What is a pencil used for?
   Action words must be included in answers.
23. Pass if child correctly places <u>and</u> says how many blocks are on paper. (1, 5).
24. Tell child: Put block **on** table; **under** table; **in front of** me, **behind** me. Pass 4 of 4.
   (Do not help child by pointing, moving head or eyes.)
25. Ask child: What is a ball?... lake?... desk?... house?... banana?... curtain?... fence?... ceiling? Pass if defined in terms of use, shape, what it is made of, or general category (such as banana is fruit, not just yellow). Pass 5 of 8, 7 of 8.
26. Ask child: If a horse is big, a mouse is __? If fire is hot, ice is __? If the sun shines during the day, the moon shines during the __? Pass 2 of 3.
27. Child may use wall or rail only, not person. May not crawl.
28. Child must throw ball overhand 3 feet to within arm's reach of tester.
29. Child must perform standing broad jump over width of test sheet (8 1/2 inches).
30. Tell child to walk forward, ∞∞∞∞➔ heel within 1 inch of toe. Tester may demonstrate.
   Child must walk 4 consecutive steps.
31. In the second year, half of normal children are non-compliant.

OBSERVATIONS:

APPENDIX E # Family Profile
Based on the
Circumplex Model

Clinical Rating Scale (CRS)
for the
Circumplex Model of
Marital and Family Systems

Family Social Science
University of Minnesota
290 McNeal Hall
St. Paul, Minnesota 55108

Instructions for Use of the Clinical Rating Scale

There are three primary dimensions in the Circumplex Model: **family cohesion, family (change)**; and a facilitating dimension of **family communication**. Each dimension has several concepts which help define and describe the global dimension. Before doing a clinical assessment of a couple or family, the therapist or interviewer should review all the concepts and descriptions on the rating scale for cohesion, adaptability (change) and communication.

In doing a clinical assessment, the therapist should evaluate a couple or family in terms of each of the concepts for each dimension. The clinical interview can be semi-structured in an attempt to elicit this information. Although no specific clinical techniques or format is recommended for the interview, we have found it useful to encourage the couple or family to dialogue with each other regarding how they handle these general issues, i.e., time, space, discipline, etc. Asking the family to describe what a typical week is like and how they handle their daily routines, decision-making and conflict is often illuminating.

After the interview has been completed, the therapist should **carefully read the descriptions** for each concept and **select the scale value** that is **most relevant** for that couple or family as a unit. Although some individuals or dyadic units might be classified in different ways, it is important to remember that the final classification should be based on how the **couple or family functions as a group.**

If one or more persons functions differently from the rest of the family, a separate description of that person can be made using the **Coalitions and Disengaged Individuals: Cohesion Subscale.** For example, it is possible to have a "Rigidly Enmeshed" family with a "Chaotically Disengaged" husband.

A **global** rating should be made for each dimension (cohesion, adaptability and communication). **The global rating should be based on an overall evaluation or gestalt rather than a sum of the sub-scale ratings.** Then it becomes possible to classify the couple or family into one of the four levels of **cohesion** (disengaged, separated, connected or enmeshed) and one of the four levels of family **adaptability** (rigid, structured, flexible and chaotic).

This clinical assessment is designed so that a therapist can describe the type of marital and family system and also identify what characteristics might be most useful to focus on in terms of **intervention.**

In closing, we hope you find these rating scales of value in your clinical and research work. We would appreciate any feedback you have regarding their usefulness and are open to suggestions for change and additions.

Coalitions & Disengaged Individuals: Cohesion Subscale

Instructions:

The functioning of some families can be adequately described through a **global assessment** on the cohesion dimension of the Circumplex Model. However, many families include individuals or dyadic units whose functioning may be somewhat different from that of the family as a whole. A subsystem or individual's functioning may be markedly different from the family as a group.

This rating scale provides a way of noting coalitions and disengaged individuals patterns in family systems. After observing the family's interactions, the coalitions or disengaged individuals should be noted by checking the relevant categories below.

Coalition: An enmeshed subsystem is typified by extreme emotional closeness and over involvement with each other. During family interaction, the dyad is very connected to each other, often to the exclusion of other family members.

Disengaged Individual(s): These individuals are emotionally separated from the rest of the family. There is low involvement and interaction.

Coalitions

_____Mother-Son
_____Mother-Daughter
_____Father-Son
_____Father-Daughter
_____Son-Daughter
_____Same Sex Siblings

Disengaged Individuals

_____Disengaged Mother
_____Disengaged Father
_____Disengaged Child(ren)

Figure 1: Circumplex Model: Sixteen Types of Marital and Family Systems

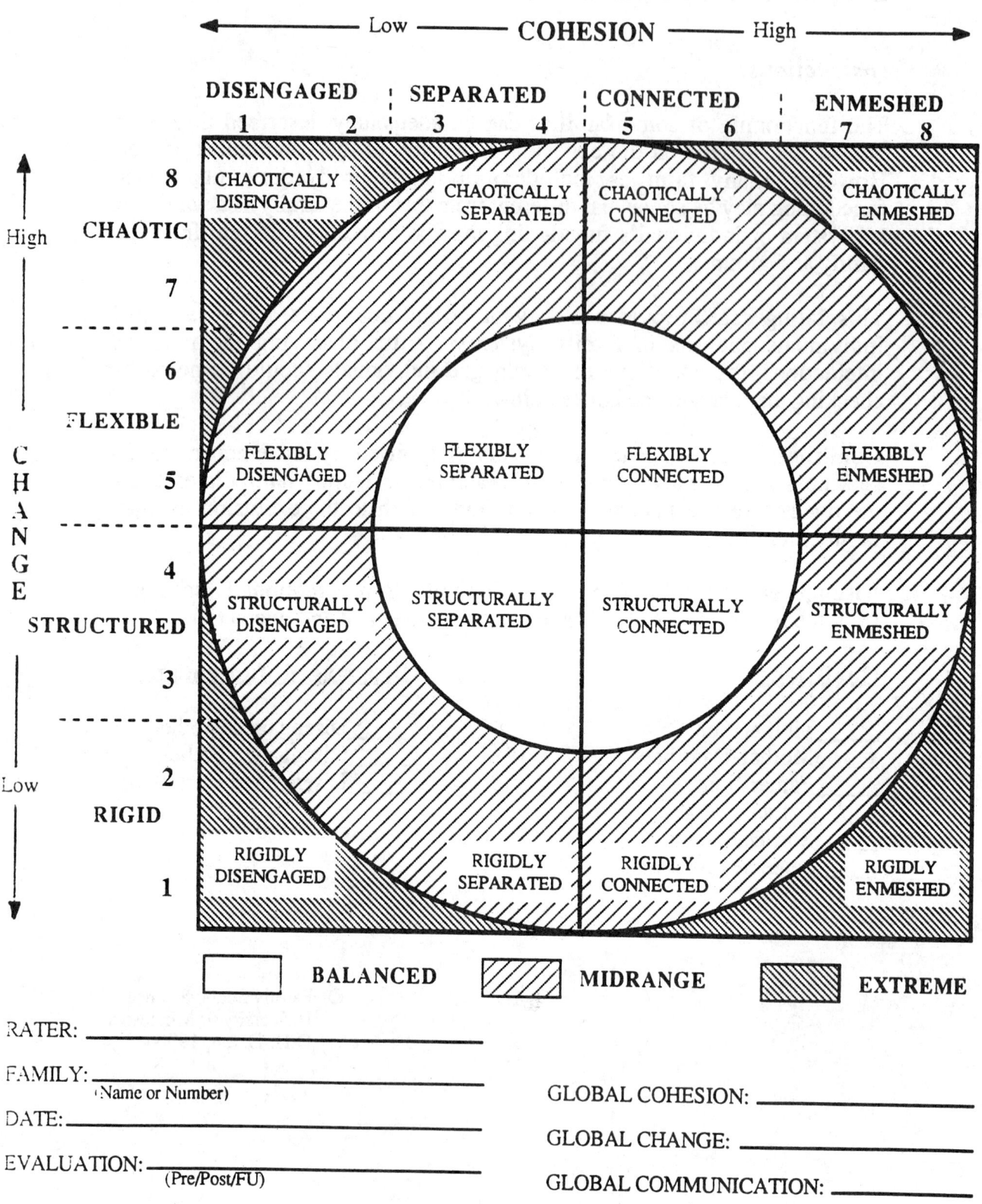

FAMILY PROFILE
Based on the Circumplex Model

	DISENGAGED		SEPARATED		CONNECTED		ENMESHED	
COHESION	1	2	3	4	5	6	7	8
Emotional Bonding	•	•	•	•	•	•	•	•
Family Involvement	•	•	•	•	•	•	•	•
Marital Relationship	•	•	•	•	•	•	•	•
Parent-Child Relationship	•	•	•	•	•	•	•	•
Internal Boundaries	•	•	•	•	•	•	•	•
External Boundaries	•	•	•	•	•	•	•	•
GLOBAL RATING	•	•	•	•	•	•	•	•

	RIGID		STRUCTURED		FLEXIBLE		CHAOTIC	
CHANGE	1	2	3	4	5	6	7	8
Leadership	•	•	•	•	•	•	•	•
Discipline	•	•	•	•	•	•	•	•
Negotiaton	•	•	•	•	•	•	•	•
Roles	•	•	•	•	•	•	•	•
Rules	•	•	•	•	•	•	•	•
GLOBAL RATING	•	•	•	•	•	•	•	•

	LOW ←		Facilitation		→ HIGH	
COMMUNICATION	1	2	3	4	5	6
Listener's Skills	•	•	•	•	•	•
Empathy						
Attentive Listening						
Speaker's Skills	•	•	•	•	•	•
Speaking for Self						
Speaking for Others						
(*Reversed Scoring)						
Self-Disclosure	•	•	•	•	•	•
Clarity	•	•	•	•	•	•
Continuity/Tracking	•	•	•	•	•	•
Respect and Regard	•	•	•	•	•	•
GLOBAL RATING	•	•	•	•	•	•

TABLE 1: COUPLE & FAMILY COHESION

COUPLE/FAMILY SCORE	DISENGAGED		SEPARATED		CONNECTED		ENMESHED	
	1	2	3	4	5	6	7	8
EMOTIONAL BONDING	Extreme emotional separateness. Lack of family loyalty.		Emotional separateness; limited closeness. Occasional family loyalty.		Emotional closeness, some separateness. Loyalty to family expected.		Extreme emotional closeness, little separateness. Loyalty to family demanded.	
FAMILY INVOLVEMENT	Very low involvement or interaction. Infrequent affective responsiveness.		Involvement acceptable; personal distance preferred. Some affective responsiveness.		Involvement emphasized personal distance allowed. Affective interactions encouraged and preferred.		Very high involvement. Fusion; over-dependency; High affective responsiveness and control.	
MARITAL RELATIONSHIP	High emotional separateness; limited closeness.		Emotional separateness; some closeness.		Emotional closeness, some separateness.		Extreme closeness, fusion; limited separateness.	
PARENT-CHILD RELATIONSHIP	Rigid generational boundaries; Low p/c closeness.		Clear generational boundaries; Some p/c closeness.		Clear generational boundaries; High p/c closeness.		Lack of generational boundaries; Excessive p/c closeness.	
INTERNAL BOUNDARIES	*Separateness dominates*		*More separateness than togetherness*		*More togetherness than separateness*		*Togetherness dominates*	
TIME (physical & emotional)	Time apart maximized Rarely time together.		Time alone important Some time together.		Time together important. Time alone permitted.		Time together maximized. Little time alone permitted.	
SPACE (physical & emotional)	Separate space needed and preferred.		Separate space preferred; sharing of family space.		Sharing family space. Private space respected.		Little private space permitted.	
DECISION MAKING	Individual decision making. (Oppositional)		Individual decision making but joint possible.		Joint decisions preferred.		Decisions subject to wishes of entire group.	
EXTERNAL BOUNDARIES	*Mainly focused outside the family.*		*More focused outside than inside family.*		*More focused inside than outside family.*		*Mainly focused inside the family.*	
FRIENDS	Individual friends seen alone.		Individual friendships seldom shared with family.		Individual friendships shared with family.		Family friends preferred limited individual friends.	
INTERESTS	Disparate interests.		Separate interests.		Some joint interests.		Joint interests mandated.	
ACTIVITIES	Mainly separate activities.		More separate than shared activities.		More shared than individual activities.		Separate activities seen as disloyal.	
GLOBAL COHESION RATING (1-8)	Very Low		Low to Moderate		Moderate to High		Very High	

TABLE 2: COUPLE & FAMILY CHANGE (ADAPTABILITY)

COUPLE/FAMILY SCORE	RIGID		STRUCTURED		FLEXIBLE		CHAOTIC	
	1	2	3	4	5	6	7	8
LEADERSHIP (control)	Authoritarian leadership. Parent(s) highly controlling.		Primarily authoritarian but some equalitarian leadership.		Equalitarian leadership with fluid changes.		Limited and/or erratic leadership. Parental control unsuccessful; Rebuffed.	
DISCIPLINE (for families only)	Autocratic "law & order." Strict, rigid consequences. Not lenient.		Somewhat democratic. Predictable consequences. Seldom lenient.		Usually democratic. Negotiated consequences. Somewhat lenient.		Laissez-faire and ineffective. Inconsistent consequences. Very lenient.	
NEGOTIATION	Limited negotiations. Decisions imposed by parents.		Structured negotiations. Decisions made by parents.		Flexible negotiations. Agreed upon decisions.		Endless negotiations. Impulsive decisions.	
ROLES	Limited repertoire, strictly defined roles; Unchanging routines.		Roles stable, but may be shared.		Role sharing and making. Fluid changes of roles.		Lack of role clarity, role shifts and role reversals; Few routines.	
RULES	Unchanging rules. Rules strictly enforced.		Few rule changes. Rules firmly enforced.		Some rule changes. Rules flexibly enforced.		Frequent rule changes. Rules inconsistently enforced.	
GLOBAL COHESION RATING (1-8)	Very Low		Low to Moderate		Moderate to High		Very High	

The global rating is based on your overall evaluation, not a sum score of the sub-scale.

1940

TABLE 3: FAMILY COMMUNICATION

LOW ◄──────── **Facilitating** ────────► HIGH

COUPLE/ FAMILY SCORE	1	2	3	4	5	6
LISTENER'S SKILLS Empathy Attentive Listening		Seldom evident Seldom evident		Sometimes evident Sometimes evident		Often evident Often evident
SPEAKER'S SKILLS Speaking for Self Speaking for Others* (*Note reverse scoring)		Seldom evident *Often evident*		Sometimes evident *Sometimes evident*		Often evident *Seldom evident*
SELF-DISCLOSURE		Infrequent discussion of self, feelings and relationships.		Some discussion of self, feelings and relationships.		Open discussion of self, feelings and relationships.
CLARITY		Inconsistent and/or unclear verbal messages. Frequent incongruencies between verbal and non-verbal messages.		Some degree of clarity; but not consistent across time or across all members. Some incongruent messages.		Verbal messages very clear. Generally congruent messages.
CONTINUITY/TRACKING		Little continuity of content. Irrelevant/distracting non-verbals and asides frequently occur. Frequent/inappropriate topic changes.		Some continuity but not consistent across time or across all members. Some irrelevant/distracting non-verbals and asides. Topic changes not consistently appropriate.		Members consistently tracking. Few irrelevant/distracting non-verbals and asides; facilitative non-verbals. Appropriate topic changes.
RESPECT and REGARD		Lack of respect for feelings or message of other(s); possibly overtly disrespectful or belittling attitude.		Somewhat respectful of others but not consistent across time or across all members. Some incongruent messages.		Consistently appears respectful of other's feelings and message.
GLOBAL FAMILY COMMUNICATION RATING (1-6)		**The global rating is based on your overall evaluation, not a sum score of the sub-scale.**				

APPENDIX F Family Apgar With Supplement

The following questions have been designed to help us better understand you and your family. You should feel free to ask questions about any item in the questionnaire.

Comment space should be used if you wish to give additional information or if you wish to discuss the way the question applies to your family. Please try to answer all questions.

"Family" is the individual(s) with whom you usually live. If you live alone, consider family as those with whom you now have the strongest emotional ties.

	For each question, check only one box		
	Almost always	Some of the time	Hardly ever
I am satisfied that I can turn to my family for help when something is troubling me. Comments:	☐	☐	☐
I am satisfied with the way my family talks over things with me and shares problems with me. Comments:	☐	☐	☐
I am satisfied that my family accepts and supports my wishes to take on new activities or directions. Comments:	☐	☐	☐
I am satisfied with the way my family expresses affection, and responds to my emotions, such as anger, sorrow, or love. Comments:	☐	☐	☐
I am satisfied with the way my family and I share time together. Comments:	☐	☐	☐

Who lives in your home?* List by relationship (eg, spouse, significant other,** child, or friend).

Please check below the column that best describes how you now get along with each member of the family listed.

Relationship	Age	Sex	Well	Fairly	Poorly
_____	___	___	☐	☐	☐
_____	___	___	☐	☐	☐
_____	___	___	☐	☐	☐
_____	___	___	☐	☐	☐
_____	___	___	☐	☐	☐
_____	___	___	☐	☐	☐

If you don't live with your own family, please list below the individuals to whom you turn for help most frequently. List by relationship, (eg, family member, friend, associate at work, or neighbor).

Please check below the column that best describes how you now get along with each person listed.

Relationship	Age	Sex	Well	Fairly	Poorly
_____	___	___	☐	☐	☐
_____	___	___	☐	☐	☐
_____	___	___	☐	☐	☐
_____	___	___	☐	☐	☐
_____	___	___	☐	☐	☐
_____	___	___	☐	☐	☐

* If you have established your own family, consider home to be the place where you live with your spouse, children, or significant other; otherwise, consider home as your place of origin, eg, the place where your parents or those who raised you live.
** "Significant other" is the partner you live with in a physically and emotionally nurturing relationship, but to whom you are not married.

Smilkstein G, Ashworth C, Montano D: Validity and reliability of the family APGAR as a test of family function. *The Journal of Family Practice* 15:2, 303–311, 1982. Reprinted by permission of Appleton & Lange, Inc.

APPENDIX G West Nomogram for Calculation of Body Surface Area

A straight line is drawn from the child's height (in the left column) to the child's weight (in the right column). Body surface area is determined by the intersection of this straight line with the column labeled SA (surface area), which is calculated in square meters (m²).

$$\text{Estimated child's dose} = \frac{\text{BSA of child (in m}^2)}{1.7\ \text{m}^2\ (\text{BSA of adult})} \times \text{Adult dose}$$

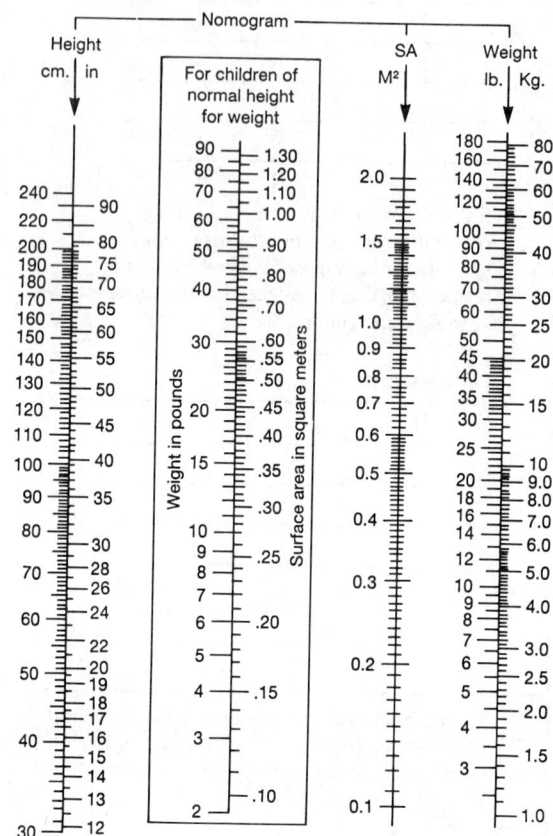

The Food Guide Pyramid (USDA)

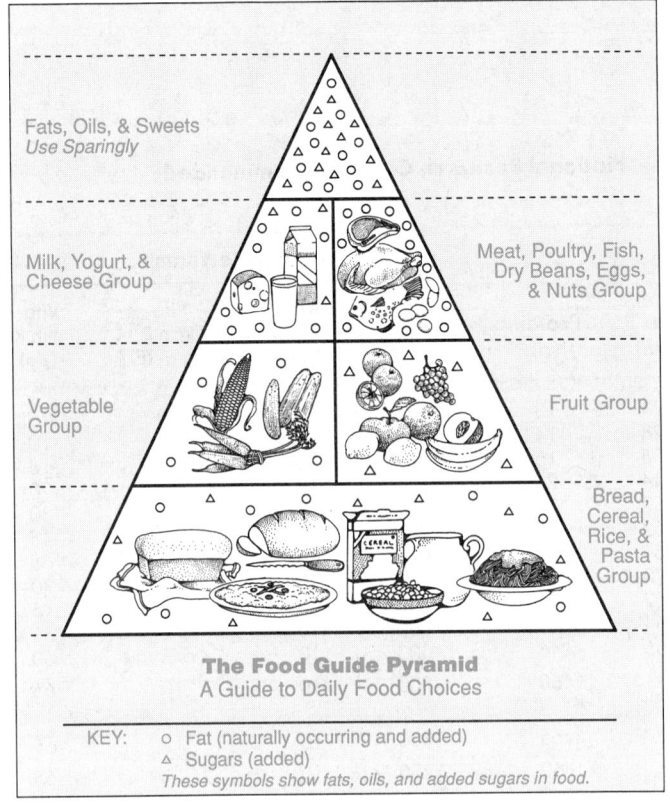

The Food Guide Pyramid
A Guide to Daily Food Choices

KEY: o Fat (naturally occurring and added)
△ Sugars (added)
These symbols show fats, oils, and added sugars in food.

USDA's Food Guide Pyramid. Published by Human Nutrition Information Service. U.S. Department of Agriculture, Hyattsville MD, 1992. Home and Garden Bulletin #249. (The Food Guide pyramid in relationship to the well child is discussed in Chapter 8, Growth and Development of Children.)

APPENDIX I Recommended Dietary Allowances (RDAs)

Food and Nutrition Board, National Academy of Sciences—National Research Council Recommended Dietary Allowances, Revised 1989*

Category	Age (yr) or Condition	Weight† (kg)	(lb)	Height† (cm)	(in)	Protein (g)	Fat-Soluble Vitamins Vita-min A (µg RE)‡	Vita-min D (µg)§	Vita-min E (mg α-TE)‖	Vita-min K (µg)
Infants	0.0–0.5	6	13	60	24	13	375	7.5	3	5
	0.5–1.0	9	20	71	28	14	375	10	4	10
Children	1–3	13	29	90	35	16	400	10	6	15
	4–6	20	44	112	44	24	500	10	7	20
	7–10	28	62	132	52	28	700	10	7	30
Male	11–14	45	99	157	62	45	1000	10	10	45
	15–18	66	145	176	69	59	1000	10	10	65
	19–24	72	160	177	70	58	1000	10	10	70
Females	11–14	46	101	157	62	46	800	10	8	45
	15–18	55	120	163	64	44	800	10	8	55
	19–24	58	128	164	65	46	800	10	8	60
Pregnant						60	800	10	10	65
Lactating 1st 6 months						65	1300	10	12	65
2nd 6 months						62	1200	10	11	65

* The allowances, expressed as average daily intakes over time, are intended to provide for individual variations among most normal persons as they live in the United States under usual environmental stresses. Diets should be based on a variety of common foods to provide other nutrients for which human requirements have been less well defined.

† The use of these figures does not imply that the height-to-weight ratios are ideal.

‡ Retinol equivalents. 1 retinol equivalent = 1 µg retinol or 6 µg β-carotene.

§ As cholecalciferol. 10 µg cholecalciferol = 400 IU of vitamin D.

‖ α-Tocopherol equivalents. 1 mg d-α tocopherol = 1 α-TE.

¶ NE (niacin equivalent) is equal to 1 mg of niacin or 60 mg of dietary tryptophan.

Adapted from Recommended Dietary Allowances, 10th edition, © 1989 by the National Academy of Sciences. Published by National Academy Press, Washington, DC.

Water-Soluble Vitamins							Minerals						
Vita-min C (mg)	Thia-min (mg)	Ribo-flavin (mg)	Niacin (mg NE)¶	Vita-min B₆ (mg)	Fo-late (µg)	Vita-min B₁₂ (µg)	Cal-cium (mg)	Phos-phorus (mg)	Mag-nesium (mg)	Iron (mg)	Zinc (mg)	Iodine (µg)	Sele-nium (µg)
30	0.3	0.4	5	0.3	25	0.3	400	300	40	6	5	40	10
35	0.4	0.5	6	0.6	35	0.5	600	500	60	10	5	50	15
40	0.7	0.8	9	1.0	50	0.7	800	800	80	10	10	70	20
45	0.9	1.1	12	1.1	75	1.0	800	800	120	10	10	90	20
45	1.0	1.2	13	1.4	100	1.4	800	800	170	10	10	120	30
50	1.3	1.5	17	1.7	150	2.0	1200	1200	270	12	15	150	40
60	1.5	1.8	20	2.0	200	2.0	1200	1200	400	12	15	150	50
60	1.5	1.7	19	2.0	200	2.0	1200	1200	350	10	15	150	70
50	1.1	1.3	15	1.4	150	2.0	1200	1200	280	15	12	150	45
60	1.1	1.3	15	1.5	180	2.0	1200	1200	300	15	12	150	50
60	1.1	1.3	15	1.6	180	2.0	1200	1200	280	15	12	150	55
70	1.5	1.6	17	2.2	400	2.2	1200	1200	300	30	15	175	65
95	1.6	1.8	20	2.1	280	2.6	1200	1200	355	15	19	200	75
90	1.6	1.7	20	2.1	260	2.6	1200	1200	340	15	16	200	75

APPENDIX J Conversion Charts

Conversion of Pounds to Kilograms

Pounds	0	1	2	3	4	5	6	7	8	9
0	—	0.45	0.90	1.36	1.81	2.26	2.72	3.17	3.62	4.08
10	4.53	4.98	5.44	5.89	6.35	6.80	7.25	7.71	8.16	8.61
20	9.07	9.52	9.97	10.43	10.88	11.34	11.79	12.24	12.70	13.15
30	13.60	14.06	14.51	14.96	15.42	15.87	16.32	16.78	17.23	17.69
40	18.14	18.59	19.05	19.50	19.95	20.41	20.86	21.31	21.77	22.22
50	22.68	23.13	23.58	24.04	24.49	24.94	25.40	25.85	26.30	26.76
60	27.21	27.66	28.12	28.57	29.03	29.48	29.93	30.39	30.84	31.29
70	31.75	32.20	32.65	33.11	33.56	34.02	34.47	34.92	35.38	35.83
80	36.28	36.74	37.19	37.64	38.10	38.55	39.00	39.46	39.91	40.37
90	40.82	41.27	41.73	42.18	42.63	43.09	43.54	43.99	44.45	44.90
100	45.36	45.81	46.26	46.72	47.17	47.62	48.08	48.53	48.98	49.44
110	49.89	50.34	50.80	51.25	51.71	52.16	52.61	53.07	53.52	53.97
120	54.43	54.88	55.33	55.79	56.24	56.70	57.15	57.60	58.06	58.51
130	58.96	59.42	59.87	60.32	60.78	61.23	61.68	62.14	62.59	63.05
140	63.50	63.95	64.41	64.86	65.31	65.77	66.22	66.67	67.13	67.58
150	68.04	68.49	68.94	69.40	69.85	70.30	70.76	71.21	71.66	72.12
160	72.57	73.02	73.48	73.93	74.39	74.84	75.29	75.75	76.20	76.65
170	77.11	77.56	78.01	78.47	78.92	79.38	79.83	80.28	80.74	81.19
180	81.64	82.10	82.55	83.00	83.46	83.91	84.36	84.82	85.27	85.73
190	86.18	86.68	87.09	87.54	87.99	88.45	88.90	89.35	89.81	90.26
200	90.72	91.17	91.62	92.08	92.53	92.98	93.44	93.89	94.34	94.80

Conversion of Pounds and Ounces to Grams for Newborn Weights

Pounds	0	1	2	3	4	5	6	7	8	9	10	11	12	13	14	15	Pounds
												Ounces					
0	—	28	57	85	113	142	170	198	227	255	283	312	430	369	397	425	0
1	454	482	510	539	567	595	624	652	680	709	737	765	794	822	850	879	1
2	907	936	964	992	1021	1049	1077	1106	1134	1162	1191	1219	1247	1276	1304	1332	2
3	1361	1389	1417	1446	1474	1503	1531	1559	1588	1616	1644	1673	1701	1729	1758	1786	3
4	1814	1843	1871	1899	1928	1956	1984	2013	2041	2070	2098	2126	2155	2183	2211	2240	4
5	2268	2296	2325	2353	2381	2410	2438	2466	2495	2523	2551	2580	2608	2637	2665	2693	5
6	2722	2750	2778	2807	2835	2863	2892	2920	2948	2977	3005	3033	3062	3090	3118	3147	6
7	3175	3203	3232	3260	3289	3317	3345	3374	3402	3430	3459	3487	3515	3544	3572	3600	7
8	3629	3657	3685	3714	3742	3770	3799	3827	3856	3884	3912	3941	3969	3997	4026	4054	8
9	4082	4111	4139	4167	4196	4224	4252	4281	4309	4337	4366	4394	4423	4451	4479	4508	9
10	4536	4564	4593	4621	4649	4678	4706	4734	4763	4791	4819	4848	4876	4904	4933	4961	10
11	4990	5018	5046	5075	5103	5131	5160	5188	5216	5245	5273	5301	5330	5358	5386	5415	11
12	5443	5471	5500	5528	5557	5585	5613	5642	5670	5698	5727	5755	5783	5812	5840	5868	12
13	5897	5925	5953	5982	6010	6038	6067	6095	6123	6152	6180	6209	6237	6265	6294	6322	13
14	6350	6379	6407	6435	6464	6492	6520	6549	6577	6605	6634	6662	6690	6719	6747	6776	14
15	6804	6832	6860	6889	6917	6945	6973	7002	7030	7059	7087	7115	7144	7172	7201	7228	15

Conversion of Fahrenheit to Celsius

Celsius	Fahrenheit	Celsius	Fahrenheit	Celsius	Fahrenheit
34.0	93.2	37.0	98.6	40.0	104.0
34.2	93.6	37.2	99.0	40.2	104.4
34.4	93.9	37.4	99.3	40.4	104.7
34.6	94.3	37.6	99.7	40.6	105.2
34.8	94.6	37.8	100.0	40.8	105.4
35.0	95.0	38.0	100.4	41.0	105.9
35.2	95.4	38.2	100.8	41.2	106.1
35.4	95.7	38.4	101.1	41.4	106.5
35.6	96.1	38.6	101.5	41.6	106.8
35.8	96.4	38.8	101.8	41.8	107.2
36.0	96.8	39.0	102.2	42.0	107.6
36.2	97.2	39.2	102.6	42.2	108.0
36.4	97.5	39.4	102.9	42.4	108.3
36.6	97.9	39.6	103.3	42.6	108.7
36.8	98.2	39.8	103.6	42.8	109.0
				43.0	109.4

$(°C) \times (9/5) + 32 = °F.$

$(°F - 32) \times (5/9) = °C.$

Index

Note: Page numbers in *italics* indicate illustrations; page numbers followed by t indicate tables; page numbers followed by d indicate display material.

A

AB blood group, 1072, 1072t
ABC analysis, for behavioral/emotional
    problems, *411*, 411–412
ABCD system, in skin self-examination,
    1834, 1837
ABCs, of emergency care, 674, 689d, 690d,
    690–691, *691*, 692d, 706–708
Abdomen
    in endocrine disorders, 1450t, 1452
    examination of, 167, *168*, *1556*, 1556–
        1557, *1557*, 1558t–1560t
        in neonate, 208t, 213
        in renal disorders, 1151–1153, *1152*
        in urinary assessment, 1233
    ultrasonography of, 1567t
Abdominal breathing, in infant, 876
Abdominal contour, assessment of, *1556*,
    1556, 1559t
Abdominal mass
    in infant and child, 1234
    malignant, 733
    in neonate, 1234
    neuroblastoma presenting as, 741–742
    Wilms' tumor presenting as, 742
Abdominal muscles, examination of, 1556,
    1557, 1559t
Abdominal pain
    in acute pancreatitis, 1626
    in appendicitis, 1605
    in bowel obstruction, 1588
    in diabetes, 1506
    in inflammatory bowel disease, 1609
    in intussusception, 1597
    stress-related, 425, 426
    in ulcers, 1636
Abdominal restraint, 553, *555*
Abdominal surgery. *See also* Surgery
    in neonate, nursing care plan for, 1583–
        1586
Abdominal trauma, 719–720, 1637–1639
    pancreatitis and, 1623–1626
Abdominal wall defect, in prune belly
    syndrome, 1260, 1264
Abdominopelvic computed tomography,
    1236
Abducens nerve, 1325t
    assessment of, 1337t, 1341–1342
Abduction, 1660, *1667*
Abduction orthosis, in Legg-Calvé-Perthes
    disease, 1703, *1703*
ABGs. *See* Arterial blood gases
A blood group, 1072, 1072t
Abortion, induced, 1906
Abrasion, corneal, 834–836
Abruptio placentae, 195

Abscess, brain, 1392–1393
Absence (petit mal) seizures, 1401, 1401t
Absolute neutrophil count, 1085t, 1086,
    1119, 1120
Absorption, nutrient
    deficient. *See* Malabsorption
    physiology of, 1548–1550
Abstinence, sexual, 1905–1906
Abuse
    child. *See* Child abuse
    sexual. *See* Sexual abuse
    substance. *See* Substance abuse
Acceleration head injury, 1365
Acceptance, of death and dying, 768, 769
Accessory nerve, 1325t
    assessment of, 1337t, 1342
Accidental injuries. *See* Trauma
Accidental loss, 394
Accident prevention. *See* Safety
    precautions
Accommodation
    in Piaget's cognitive theory, 127
    visual, 794–795
Accommodative strabismus, 829d
Acculturation, 54
Accutane (isotretinoin), for acne, 1826t,
    1827
Acetaminophen, 649t
    for otitis media, 843
    poisoning by, 697, 698t
Acetylcholine, in bladder control, 1222
N-Acetylcysteine (NAC; Mucomyst), for
    acetaminophen poisoning, 697,
    698t
Acid
    definition of, 603–604
    volatile, 604
Acid-base balance, 603–605
    disturbances of, 612–613
    renal regulation of, 1145
    respiratory system in, 878
Acidosis
    metabolic, 613
        after cardiac surgery, 1059
        in diabetes, *1505*, 1505–1507, 1524–
            1526, 1525t
    renal tubular, 1194–1195, 1195t
    respiratory, 612–613, 878
        after cardiac surgery, 1059
Acinar cells, 1545
Acne neonatorum, 803t, 1784
Acne vulgaris, 383, 803t, 1824–1827, *1825*
    premature, 1486, 1487
Acoustic nerve, assessment of, 1337t, 1342
Acoustic otoscopy, in otitis media, 841–
    842

Acoustic reflex testing, 848
Acquaintance rape, 1883–1884
Acquired immunity, 621
Acquired immunodeficiency syndrome,
    633d, 633t, 633–635, 634d, 1397–
    1399, 1898t. *See also* Human
    immunodeficiency virus infection
    in adolescents, 371
    as chronic illness, 486
    cutaneous manifestations of, 1817d,
        1817–1818
    in hemophiliacs, 1130, 1131
    neurologic complications in, 1397–1399
    in pregnancy, 199
Acrocephalopolysyndactyly, 818
Acrocyanosis, 137, 212, 1784, 1785
Acroencephalosyndactyly, 818–819, *819*
Acromegaly, 1498
ACTH, 1438, 1439t
    in congenital adrenal hyperplasia, 1473,
        1474
    deficiency of, in panhypopituitarism,
        1496–1498
    excess of, 1476–1479
    normal values for, 1914t
ACTH stimulation test, 1454t
    in iatrogenic adrenal insufficiency, 1476
Actinomycin-D (Cosmegan), 736t
Activated charcoal, 696–697, 698t
Active alert state, in neonate, 223
Active immunity, 621, 623
Active ion pump mechanism, 600
Active sleep state, in neonate, 223
Activity and exercise
    in acute poststreptococcal
        glomerulonephritis, 1192
    for adolescents, 381
    after cardiac surgery, 1060
    assessment of, 21t, 23d
    in asthma, 941
    in bronchopulmonary dysplasia, 950,
        952
    cardiovascular function and, 994, 997,
        1004t
    in chronic renal failure, 1172
    in cystic fibrosis, 946
    in diabetes, 1520–1521, 1521t
    in edema, 1183
    endocrine function and, 1449, 1455t
    in epidermolysis bullosa, 1789
    in fracture immobilization, 1733
    gastrointestinal function and, 1554
    head and neck function and, 800
    hematologic function and, 1080, 1089t
    in hemolytic uremic syndrome, 1189
    in hypospadias repair, 1258–1259

Amylase
  pancreatic, 1545, 1549
    in acute pancreatitis, 1627
    normal values for, 1565t, 1915t
  salivary, 1549
ANA. *See* American Nurses' Association
    (ANA)
Anaclitic depression, in infants, 440
Anagen effluvium, 1828–1830
Anagen hair growth, 1754, *1754*
Anal. *See also under* Anorectal; Anus
Anal agenesis, 1586–1588, *1587*
Anal canal, embryonic development of,
    1540
Analgesia, 700t
  for circumcision, 661
  for dysmenorrhea, 1894
  for fractures, 1732–1733
  gate control theory and, 647
  goals of, 645–646
  in home care, 654
  inadequate, 641–643, 651–652
  for injections, 661
  for juvenile rheumatoid arthritis, 1722
  in mechanical ventilation, 965
  nonpharmacologic, 662–666
    acupuncture in, 666
    distraction in, 664
    heat and cold in, 665–666
    hypnosis in, 665
    nursing care plan for, 662–663
    parental role in, 661–663
    play and activity in, 663
    relaxation techniques in, 664–665
    teaching in, 661
    TENS in, 666
    touch in, 664
  nursing care plan for, 662–663
  nursing research in, 666
  orders for, requesting change in, 646,
    646d
  for otitis media, 843
  patient-controlled, 660–661, 661d
  pharmacologic, 648–662. *See also*
    Analgesics
  for sickle cell crisis, 1116
  for suturing, 661
Analgesics
  adjuvant drugs for, 654
  narcotic, 650–654
    action and effects of, 650–652, 651t
    addiction to, 642
    advantages and disadvantages of, 650
    continuous spinal infusion of, *659,*
      659–660
    continuous subcutaneous infusion of,
      660, *660*
    delivery options for, 658–661
    dependence on, 652–654
    dosage of, 649t, 651t, 655, 656t
    frequency of, 655
    home administration of, 654
    intravenous, 657–659, 658d, 659d
    intraventricular infusion of, 660
    PRN vs. around-the-clock, 655, *657*
    respiratory depression and, 642
    route of administration of, 655–658
    side effects of, 649t, 650, 651t
    teaching plan for, 653
    tolerance to, 652
    withdrawal from, 652–654
  non-narcotic, 648–650, 649t
  selection of, 648
  topical, for teething, 271

Anal membrane, imperforate, 1585–1588,
    1587
Anal sphincters, 1548, 1551–1552
Anal stage, 124t
Anal stenosis, 1586–1588, *1587*
Anaphylactoid purpura, 1127
  nephritis in, 1193
Anaphylaxis, 625, 685
  immunization-induced, 172t, 173, 173t,
    175, 176, 177
Anasarca, 610
Anastomosis, Glenn, 1056d
Androgen(s)
  for aplastic anemia, 1097
  excess of, in congenital adrenal
    hyperplasia, 1473
  in polycystic ovarian disease, 1889–1890
  prenatal sexual differentiation and, 1435
  production and effects of, 1439t, 1441
  in puberty, 1857, 1857t
Androstenedione, normal values for, 1915t
Anemia
  aplastic. *See* Aplastic anemia
  assessment in, *1078*, 1078–1079, *1079*
  Blackfan-Diamond, 1101–1103
  cancer-related, 1103–1104
  cardiomegaly in, 1094
  in chronic renal failure, 1170
    Epoetin alfa in, 1172
  classification of, 1083–1085
  client teaching in, 1094, 1095t
  Cooley's, 1111–1112
  diagnostic tests for, 1084t
  dysfunctional uterine bleeding and,
    1891
  Fanconi's, 1096
  in G6PD deficiency, 1117–1118
  hemolytic, 1112–1118
    in hemolytic uremic syndrome, 1188
  in hereditary spherocytosis, 1118
  iron-deficiency. *See* Iron-deficiency
    anemia
  nutrition and metabolism in, 1080
  physiologic, 1072
  prevention and early detection of, 1108d
  psychosocial support in, 1095t, 1096
  in pyruvate kinase deficiency, 1118
  restoration of erythrocyte production in,
    1094–1096, 1095t
  sickle cell. *See* Sickle cell anemia
  in thalassemia, 1111, *1111*
  tissue oxygenation in, 1094, 1095t
  in transient erythroblastosis of
    childhood, 1103
Anencephaly, 1323, 1354–1355, 1436t
Anesthesia, 537
  in diabetes, 1521–1522
  inhalation, in pregnancy, 185t
Aneurysmal bone cysts, 1715–1717
Angel's kiss, 137, 207t, 212, 1841, 1842–
    1843
Anger
  aggression and, 395–396
  in death and dying, 767, 768, 773
  temper tantrums and, 286–288, 287t, 395
Angiocardiography, 1003–1004
Angiography, cerebral, 1348
Angioplasty
  balloon. *See* Balloon angioplasty
  cardiac catheter, 1052–1053, *1053*
Angiotensin, 1146
Angiotensin-converting enzyme, normal
    values for, 1915t

Angiotensin-converting enzyme inhibitor,
    for hypertension, 1052t
Animism, in preschooler, 314
Anion gap, normal values for, 1915t
Anions, 602
Anisocoria, 1368
Anisometropia, 831–832
Ankle
  congenital disorders of, *1692,* 1692–
    1695
  edema of, in pregnancy, 193t
  fractures of, 1732t
  sprains and strains of, 1732–1735, *1735*
Ankle-foot orthosis, *1735*
Ankyloglossia, 791
Annular lesions, 1764, *1767*
Anogenital skin, examination of, 1767
Anogenital warts, 1815–1817, 1898t, 1899
Anomalous pulmonary venous return,
    1035, 1035–1036
  balloon septoplasty for, 1052, *1052*
Anonychia, 1830t
Anorectal injuries, 720
Anorectal manometry, 1569–1570
  in Hirschsprung's disease, 1591
Anorexia
  in cancer, 745
  diet in, 1610
  in hepatitis, 1632
Anorexia nervosa, 119, *447,* 447t–449t,
    447–451
Antacids
  for chronic renal failure, 1172t
  for gastroesophageal reflux, 1599
  for ulcers, 1636–1637
Antecubital fossa, blood sampling from,
    564t, 565
Antenatal care, 179–200. *See also*
    Pregnancy
Anterior fontanel, 791, *792,* 803t, 1324
  bulging, in hydrocephalus, 1356, 1358
  examination of, 816, 1340
Anterograde amnesia, 1376
Anthrin, for psoriasis, 1796
Anthropometric measurements, 1150–
    1151, 1555
  in nutritional assessment, 1558–1559,
    1561d
Antianxiety drugs, with analgesics, 654
Antibiotics
  for acne, 1826t, 1827
  for bacterial meningitis, 1390
  for bacterial tracheitis, 913
  for chronic renal failure, 1172t
  for cutaneous bacterial infections, 1806
  for cystic fibrosis, 946
  for endocarditis, 1043, 1044d
  for epiglottitis, 909
  for leukocyte disorders, 1120
  for neutropenia, 1121
  for otitis externa, 847
  for otitis media, 843, 843t
  for pneumonia, 923–924
  prophylactic
    client teaching for, 1312, 1312t
    for endocarditis, 1043, 1044d
    in leukocyte disorders, 1120
    for meningitis, 1390
    in rheumatic fever, 1041
    in ventricular septal defect, 1025
    in vesicoureteral reflux, 1311–1312,
      1312t
  for sinusitis, 852
  for tonsillitis, 860

female virilization and, 1473, 1474–
1475, 1876, *1877*
Hypercyanosis, in tetralogy of Fallot, 1032
Hyperemia, 833
Hyperextension, *1666, 1667*
Hyperglycemia, in diabetes, *1505,* 1505–
1506, 1524
vs. hypoglycemia, 1524t
Hyperinsulinism, 1502, 1503
Hyperkalemia, 603, 610t, 611
in acute renal failure, 1165–1166
in adrenal insufficiency, 1469
in chronic renal failure, 1170
in diabetic ketoacidosis, 1525
management of, 1166
Hyperkeratosis, in ichthyosis, 1787
Hyperlipidemia, in nephrotic syndrome,
1176
Hypermagnesemia, 603
Hypernatremia, 602–603
in chronic renal failure, 1170
dehydration in, 607–608, 608t
Hyperopia, *820,* 820–822
Hyperparathyroidism, 1530–1531
Hyperphosphatemia
in chronic renal failure, 1170, 1171
hypoparathyroidism and, 1531
Hyperpigmentation, 1831–1832
in Addison disease, 1469, 1472
Hyperpituitarism, 1498
Hyper-resonance, on percussion, 889t
Hypersensitivity, 624t, 624–625, 1792. *See
also* Allergies
anaphylaxis in, 625, 685
leukocytes in, 1073–1074
to vaccines, 172t, 173, 173t, 175, 176,
177
Hypertelorism, ocular, 818d
Hypertension, 1049–1052
in acute poststreptococcal
glomerulonephritis, 1192
in acute renal failure, 1166
after cardiac surgery, 1059
in chronic renal failure, 1170, 1172t
clinical manifestations of, 1050
definition of, 1049–1050
diabetic, 1530
diagnostic studies in, 1050
drug therapy for, 1050–1052, 1051t–
1052t
etiology and pathogenesis of, 1050
incidence of, 1050
in increased intracranial pressure. *See*
Increased intracranial pressure
interventions for, 1050–1052, 1051t–
1052t
pheochromocytoma and, 1478
portal, in biliary cirrhosis, 1635
in pregnancy, 198–199
primary (essential), 1050
secondary, 1050
vesicoureteral reflux and, 1315
Hyperthermia, analgesic, 665–666
Hyperthyroidism, 465–1468, 1465–1468
goiter in, 1465, 1468, *1468*
Hypertonic dehydration, 607–608, 608t
Hypertonic solutions, 615, 615t, 616t
Hypertrophic cardiomyopathy, *1041,*
1041–1042
Hyperuricemia, chemotherapy-related, 751
Hyperventilation, 888t
central neurogenic, in increased
intracranial pressure, 1368
for increased intracranial pressure, 1370

presuctioning, 965
respiratory alkalosis and, 613
stress-related, 425, 426
Hypervolemia, 609–610. *See also* Edema
Hyphema, 715, 835
Hypnosis, for pain relief, 665
Hypoalbuminemia, in nephrotic syndrome,
1176
Hypocalcemia, 603, 611–612, 612t, 1564t
in chronic renal failure, 1170
hypoparathyroidism and, 1531
in renal tubular acidosis, 1194
Hypodermis, 1754
Hypogammaglobulinemia, 632–633
Hypoglossal nerve, 1325t
assessment of, 1337t, 1342
Hypoglycemia, 1502–1503
in adrenal insufficiency, 1469
in diabetes, vs. hyperglycemia, 1524t
in growth hormone deficiency, 1493,
1495
neonatal, 1502, 1550
in Reye's syndrome, 1394
Hypogonadism, delayed puberty and,
1479–1482
Hypokalemia, 603, 610t, 610–611
in Bartter's syndrome, 1194
in diabetic ketoacidosis, 1525
in renal tubular acidosis, 1194
Hypomagnesemia, 603
hypokalemia and, 610, 611
Hyponatremia, 602–603
in adrenal insufficiency, 1469, 1474
in chronic renal failure, 1170
dehydration in, 608, 608t
hypokalemia and, 611
Hyponychium, 1755, *1755*
Hypoparathyroidism, 1531
Hypophysis. *See* Pituitary
Hypopigmentation, 1831
Hypopituitarism, 1492–1496. *See also*
Growth hormone deficiency
delayed puberty and, 1479, 1480d, 1481
Hypoplastic left heart syndrome, *1038,*
1038–1039
Hypospadias, 209t, 213, 1215, 1215t, *1256,*
1256–1259
Hypotension
in increased intracranial pressure, 1368,
1370
in shock, 686t
Hypothalamic-pituitary-adrenal-gonadal
axis, 1859
Hypothalamic-pituitary system, pubertal
changes in, 1856
Hypothalamic-pituitary-target cell
feedback, *1437*
Hypothalamus
disorders of, delayed sexual
development and, 1479, 1480d
embryonic development of, 1434
structure and function of, 1326, 1435–
1437, *1437,* 1437t
Hypothermia
induced, in open heart surgery, 1055–
1057
in near drowning, 699
Hypothyroidism, 1461–1465, 1465t
acquired (juvenile), 1461, *1462*
congenital, 1461
neonatal, test for, 215
in panhypopituitarism, 1496–1498
precocious puberty and, 1488
Hypotonic dehydration, 608

Hypotonic solutions, 614, 615t, 616t
Hypoventilation
atelectasis and, 930
respiratory acidosis and, 612–613
Hypovolemia, 606
management of, 613–616, 615t, 616t, 687
prerenal failure and, 1162, 1164
Hypovolemic shock, 684t, 685, 686t, 707.
See also Shock
in adrenal insufficiency, 1469, 1470
fluid therapy for, 614–616, 615t, 616t,
687
Hypoxemia
in congenital heart disease, 1031–1032
oxygen therapy for, 584–586
in pulmonary stenosis, 1019
Hypoxia
after cardiac surgery, 1058
in bronchopulmonary dysplasia, 949–
950
cardiopulmonary arrest and, 689–692
finger clubbing and, 885, *887*
oxygen therapy for, 584–586
perinatal, cerebral palsy and, 1416–1417,
1417t
treatment of. *See* Oxygen therapy

I

Iatrogenic conditions, 1460
Ibuprofen (Motrin), 649t
Ichthyosis vulgaris, 1786
resources for, 1778, 1787d
Icterus neonatorum. *See* Jaundice,
neonatal
ICU. *See* Intensive care unit
Id, 123
Identification procedures, for neonate, 217
Identity
development of, 132, 365–369, 366t,
368t–369t
vs. role confusion, in adolescence, 124t,
125, 365–369
Idiopathic nephrotic syndrome, 1174
Idiopathic thrombocytopenic purpura,
1122–1124, 1123t
assessment in, 1123
clinical manifestations of, 1123
definition of, 1122
diagnosis of, 1086, 1086t, 1123, 1123t
etiology and pathophysiology of, 1123
evaluation in, 1124
incidence of, 1123
interventions in, 1124
nursing care plan for, 1124–1125
nursing diagnoses and planning in,
1123–1124
IgA, 621, 622t, 623
normal values for, 1917t
secretory, in breast milk, 236
IgD, 621, 622t
IgE, 621, 622t
normal values for, 1917t
IgE-mediated hypersensitivity, 624t, 624–
625
IGF-1. *See* Insulin-like growth factor
IgG, 621–622, 622t, 623
for idiopathic thrombocytopenic
purpura, 1124
normal values for, 1917t
platelet-associated, in idiopathic
thrombocytopenic purpura, 1123
IgM, 621–622, 622t
normal values for, 1917t

Approved Nursing Diagnoses, North American Nursing Diagnosis Association, 1992

Activity Intolerance
Activity Intolerance, High Risk for
Adjustment, Impaired
Airway Clearance, Ineffective
Anxiety
Aspiration, High Risk for
Body Image Disturbance
Body Temperature, High Risk for Altered
Breastfeeding, Effective
Breastfeeding, Ineffective
· Breastfeeding, Interrupted
Breathing Pattern, Ineffective
· Caregiver Role Strain
· Caregiver Role Strain, High Risk for
Communication, Impaired Verbal
Constipation
Constipation, Colonic
Constipation, Perceived
Decisional Conflict (Specify)
Decreased Cardiac Output
Defensive Coping
Denial, Ineffective
Diarrhea
Disuse Syndrome, High Risk for
Diversional Activity Deficit
Dysreflexia
Family Coping: Compromised, Ineffective
Family Coping: Disabling, Ineffective
Family Coping: Potential for Growth
Family Processes, Altered
Fatigue
Fear
Fluid Volume Deficit
Fluid Volume Deficit, Potential
Fluid Volume Excess
Gas Exchange, Impaired
Grieving, Anticipatory
Grieving, Dysfunctional
Growth and Development, Altered
Health Maintenance, Altered
Health-Seeking Behaviors (Specify)
Home Maintenance Management, Impaired
Hopelessness
Hyperthermia
Hypothermia
Incontinence, Bowel
Incontinence, Functional
Incontinence, Reflex
Incontinence, Stress
Incontinence, Total
Incontinence, Urge
Individual Coping, Ineffective
· Infant Feeding Pattern, Ineffective
Infection, High Risk for
Injury, High Risk for
Knowledge Deficit (Specify)
Noncompliance (Specify)
Nutrition, Altered: Less Than Body Requirements
Nutrition, Altered: More Than Body Requirements

Nutrition, Altered: Potential for More Than Body Requirements
Oral Mucous Membrane, Altered
Pain
Pain, Chronic
Parental Role Conflict
Parenting, Altered
Parenting, High Risk for Altered
· Peripheral Neurovascular Dysfunction, High Risk for
Personal Identity Disturbance
Physical Mobility, Impaired
Poisoning, High Risk for
Post-Trauma Response
Powerlessness
Protection, Altered
Rape Trauma Syndrome
Rape Trauma Syndrome: Compound Reaction
Rape Trauma Syndrome: Silent Reaction
· Relocation Stress Syndrome
Role Performance, Altered
Self-Care Deficit
   Bathing/Hygiene
   Feeding
   Dressing/Grooming
   Toileting
Self-Esteem, Chronic Low
Self-Esteem, Situational Low
Self-Esteem Disturbance
· Self-Mutilation, High Risk for
Sensory-Perceptual Alterations (Specify)
   (visual, auditory, kinesthetic, gustatory, tactile, olfactory)
Sexual Dysfunction
Sexuality Patterns, Altered
Skin Integrity, High Risk for Impaired
Skin Integrity, Impaired
Sleep Pattern Disturbance
Social Interaction, Impaired
Social Isolation
Spiritual Distress
Suffocation, High Risk for
Swallowing, Impaired
· Therapeutic Regimen, Ineffective Management of
Thermoregulation, Ineffective
Thought Processes, Altered
Tissue Integrity, Impaired
Tissue Perfusion, Altered (Specify Type)
   (renal, cerebral, cardiopulmonary, gastrointestinal, peripheral)
Trauma, High Risk for
Unilateral Neglect
Urinary Elimination, Altered
Urinary Retention
· Ventilation, Inability to Sustain Spontaneous
· Ventilatory Weaning Response, Dysfunctional
Violence, High Risk for: Self-directed or directed at others

· *New diagnoses from 1992 conference*

(From North American Nursing Diagnosis Association Classification of Nursing Diagnosis: Proceedings of the Tenth Conference, Philadelphia, J.B. Lippincott Company, 1993)